CBSPD Dedicated to Education

Introducing

TARGET HIGH™ Digital Pro

Now Target High Book is at your fingertips

Be smart, Go PHYGITAL...

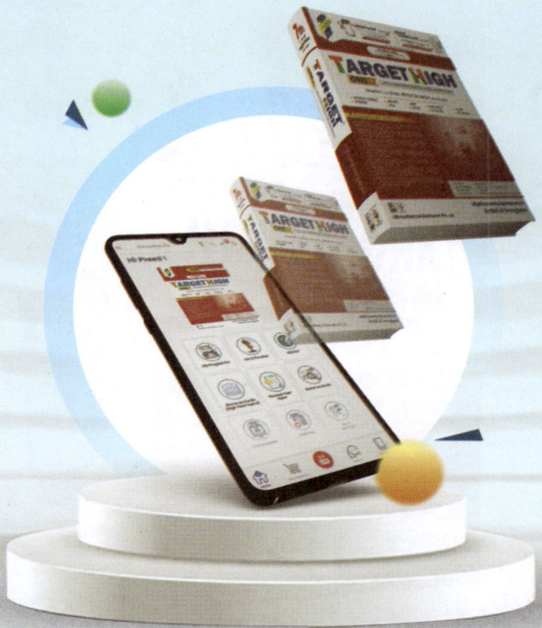

My Phygital Pro
Synopsis, MCQs, Golden Points, Key Points, IBQs, VBQs, CBQs & Recent Qs of all 13 Subjects/All Topics in Read & Practice form.

See & Perceive
Subject wise Golden points in Podcast form, 500+ Conceptual videos with voice over and animated video

My Test
Subject & topic wise tests, Mini tests with subject combinations, IBQ Tests and Grand tests based on Important National & State level Exams incl. NORCET

Revise on the Go
Important Appendices, Tables & Images for quick reveiw

Previous Year Papers
150+ Exam papers in Practice and Review mode (with Rationales of Selective papers)

Search on the Go
Mapping of 1000+ Important Topics of All subjects in searchable format

TH Olympiads
12 Olympiads with National Level Rankings and Rewards

ADD ONs
Recent Updates, Current Affairs, Nursing Skill Procedures, Study Tips and E-book (optional)

Be in Spotlight
Special section for TH Contributors, Reviewers, Rank holders, Happy Users

Any Doubt Ask Amli
Get your TH Queries resolved by Ms Amli, Your TH Educator (24*7 Query assistance)

Why to Choose Target High Digital PRO?

Real-time updates	Accessibility	Interactivity & Engagement	Multimedia Integrartion	Progress tracking
No need to wait for any latest updates and revision	Anytime and Anywhere access to the content	Read and practice approach on a single platform	Next level study preparation with videos, animations podcasts and infographic	Assess your preparation for the targeted exams

About the Authors

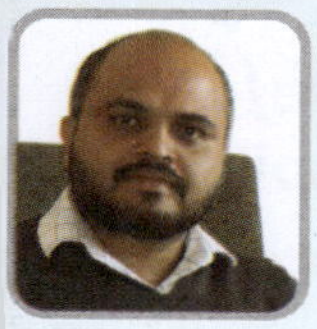

Muthuvenkatachalam Srinivasan PhD (INC Consortium), MSc (AIIMS), D Pharma, RN (NMBA Australia) is currently working as an Assistant Professor at Institute of Human Behaviour and Allied Sciences (IHBAS), New Delhi. He is former Associate Professor in College of Nursing, All India Institute of Medical Sciences (AIIMS), New Delhi. He obtained Doctorate in Psychiatric Nursing from INC Consortium (in collaboration with RGUHS, Karnataka) in 2017. He is a Postgraduate in Psychiatric Nursing from AIIMS, New Delhi and has also completed a Diploma in Pharmacy. He is also a Registered Nurse with the Nurses and Midwifery Board of Australia. He has published numerous research papers in national and international journals of repute. He is Deputy Editor of Indian Journal of Psychiatric Nursing. He has contributed chapters in textbooks and training manuals of Govt. of India. He is an executive body member of Indian Society of Psychiatric Nurses (ISPN). He received 'Best Researcher Award' from ISPN in the year 2016. Last but not least, the author attended IRON programme for Registered Nurses in Australia, International conferences in USA and Canada with travel grant from ICMR and conference organization.

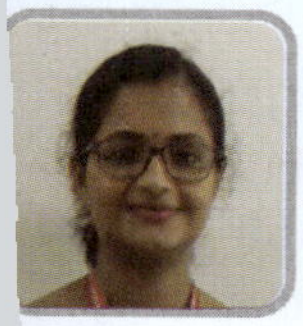

Ambili M Venugopal MSc Pediatric Nursing (AIIMS), BSc (Hons) Nursing (AIIMS) is pursuing PhD in Pediatric Nursing from National Consortium for PhD in Nursing. She is currently working as a Tutor, College of Nursing, at All India Institute of Medical Sciences, Mangalagiri, Andhra Pradesh. She is a Postgraduate in Pediatric Nursing from AIIMS, New Delhi and former Nursing Officer in AIIMS, New Delhi. She has published several research papers in reputed journals. She has secured top ranks in several competitive exams including NO, AIIMS, Delhi, SNO, AIIMS Bhubaneswar (AIR-1), Nursing Tutor, AIIMS Kalyani (AIR-1), AIIMS Deoghar (AIR-1), AIIMS Nagpur and AIIMS Manglagiri

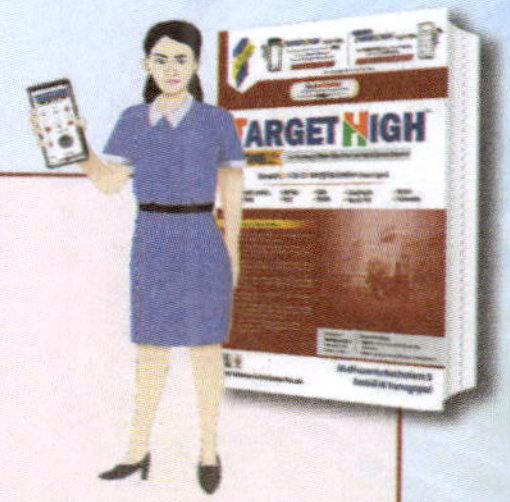

Golden Points
Podcast
Listen & Recall

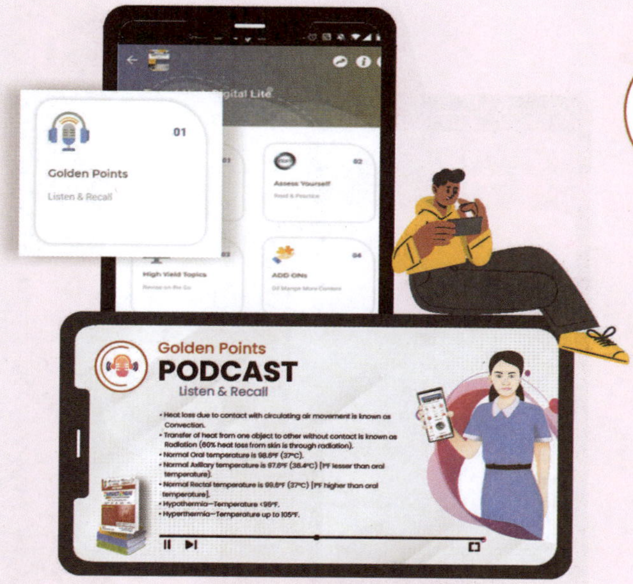

Get
3000+
Golden Points in Podcast Form
(Covering important one-liners from all the subjects)

Elevate Your Learning Skills Through Active Listening

With **AMLI** (*The* **TH** *Educator*)

DON'T FORGET TO
Assess Yourself
Read & Practice

Success Rises With Every Question: Practice for Achievement

Get Yourself Assessed with
AMLI

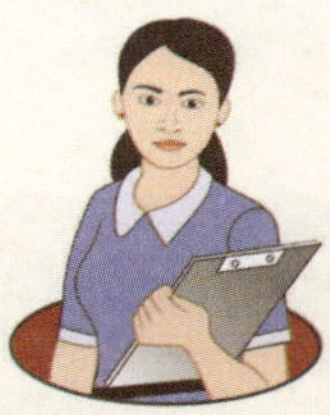

80+ Tests
(Subject-wise Tests & IBQ tests)
covering **8000+ Questions**

48 Grand Tests
based on **new exam pattern of NORCET (Pre/Mains)**
covering **4800 questions**

Real-time Approach and National Level Ranking

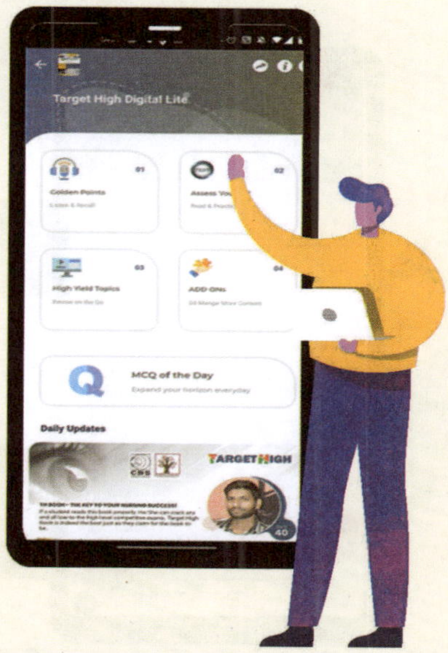

Make your prep easy with Target High Hybrid Digital Edition
The content in this book is excellent, comprehensive and informative . It contains quality MCQs with rationales that will push the registered nurses toward their Targets. Now it is in Hybrid form - Target High Digital Lite which makes your nursing competitive exams prep easy.
Sunil Kumar Choudhary *(Nagaur, Rajasthan)*

A concoction of Nursing excellence!
The Target High Hybrid book is a unique compendium covering all the important subjects needed to excel in your staff nurse entrance exams. The content is well explained. There are ample IBQs and previous year papers in the application and book that will make your learning journey highly efficient.
Rakesh Kumar Yadav *(Behror, Rajasthan)*

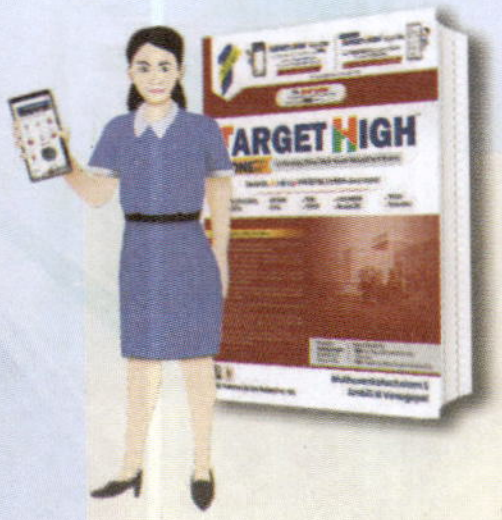

High Yield Topics

Revise on the Go...

Get Important

300+

High-Yield Topics

(Subject-wise important Tables and Images) with their descriptions for quick access at your Fingertips

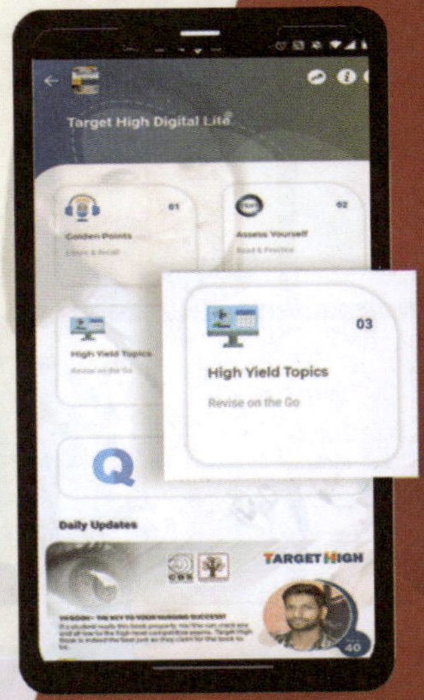

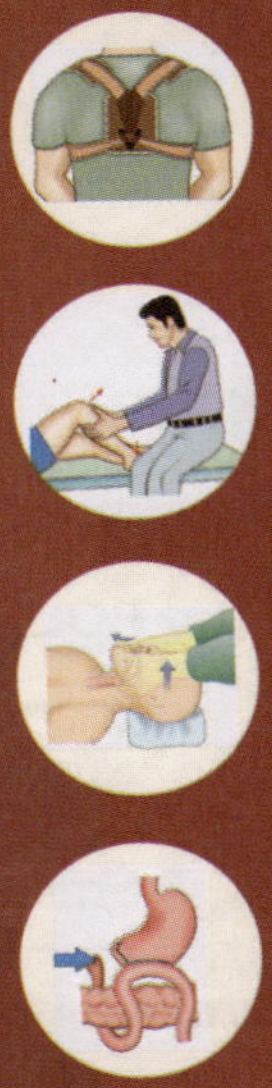

Get

Add ONs

Dil Mange More Content

Unleash Your Potential For Free: Dive Into Extra Learning Content

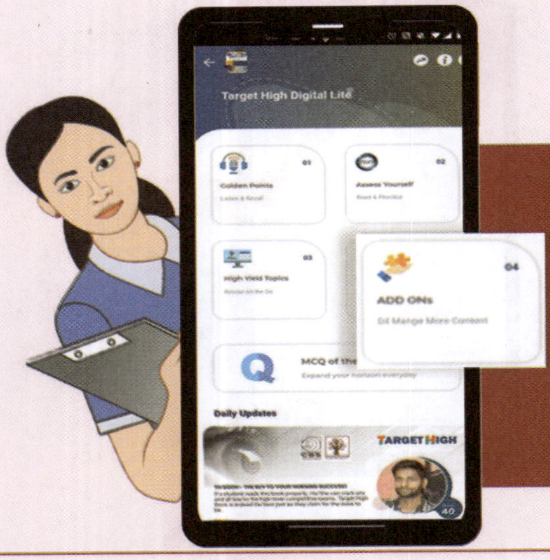

- **115+** Previous Year Papers (from 2023-2004) of all State/ National Level Exam) including NORCET. Selective Papers are given with Rationale.
- **75+** Appendices
- **Study Plan** – Decoding the case scenario-based questions?
- How to prepare for NORCET – Pre & Mains (an overview)
- Monthly Current Affairs
- Nursing Skill Procedures
- How to Crack Nursing Competitive Exams & Interview Section

THE BEST IS HERE!

The Hybrid feature of Target High is more than enough: It has any doubt, ask AMLI feature, ""be in Spotlight"" that highlights the rank holders, current affairs in dil mange more, and many more to make your learning journey highly effective.

Shankar Raj *(Nalanda, Bihar)*

Target High Hybrid book is a broad spectrum of literary work!

Hybrid features of this book are all the important points, high yield topics, previous year papers and much more for you to level up for your exams. It has explained everything in a broad manner to remove complexity for you. Amazing book overall!"

Kana Ram Maurya (Nawa, Rajasthan)

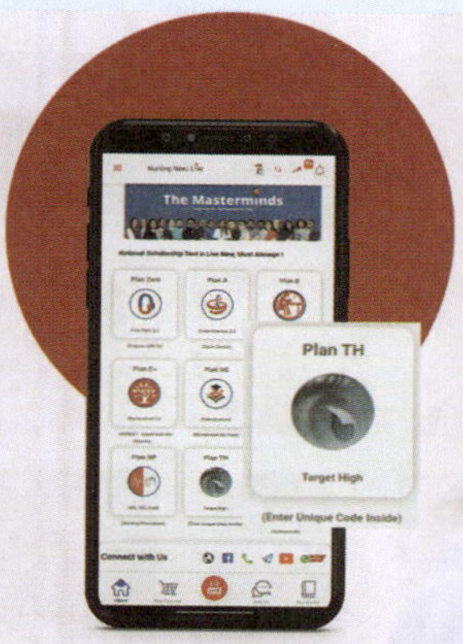

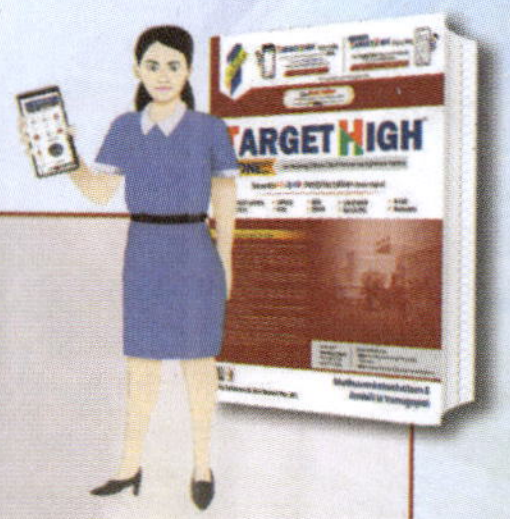

Bridging the Gap Between Theory & Practice through

Conceptual & Animated Videos

200+

Conceptual Videos on Important Topics
in Infographic Form with voice-over
for easy learning

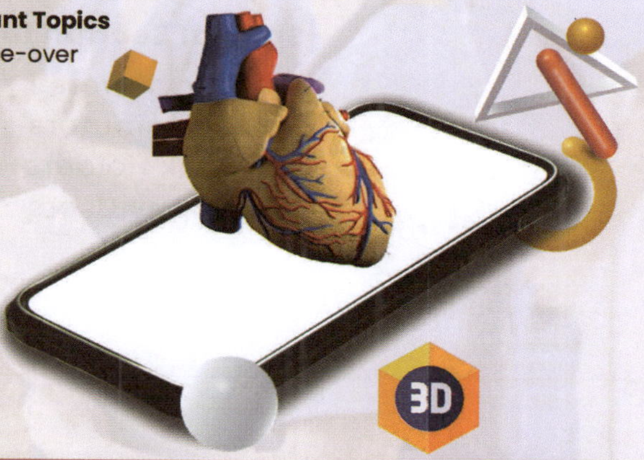

5

3D Animated videos with their descriptions

1. *Positions & Presentations of fetus during labor*
2. *Parts and Diameter of fetal skull*
3. *Body planes & movement*
4. *Respiration: Exchange of gases*
5. *Anatomy of Heart & Cardiac Cycle*

Clinical Learning

It's time to explore the advanced level learning!!

400+	50+	1000+
Image-Based Questions	Video-Based Questions	Clinical Case-based Questions

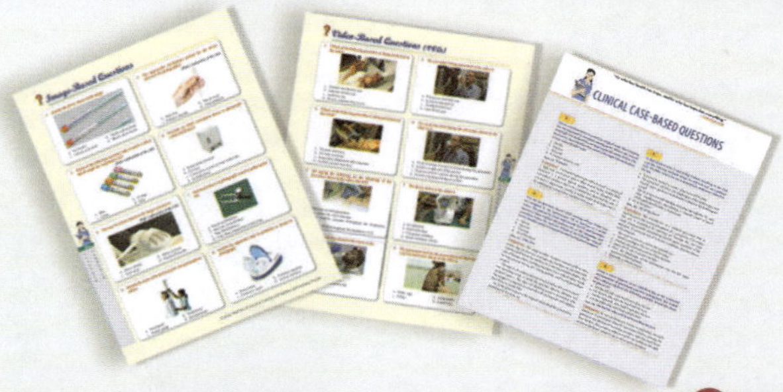

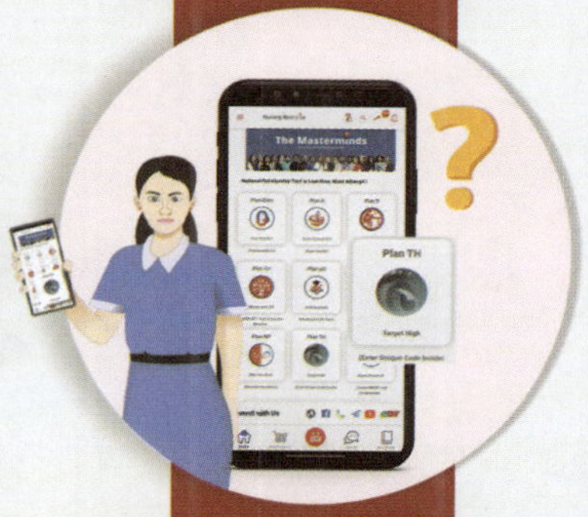

Target High Digital Lite - Best companion for Nursing Aspirants!
This book has proved to be the best preparation companion for any and all nursing exams. Target High Digital Lite has updated new features like chapter-wise and subject-wise clinical based MCQs and the clinical highlights between the synopses, which make reading & practicing MCQs more interesting. This book will always keep you updated.
Zahoor Ahmad Shaikh (Kulgam, J & K)

Target High Hybrid Digital edition: Dil Maange More!
I am much of a book reader but once I started studying the Hybrid features of Target High, I could feel the difference. It has described every single topic and subject in a very precise and intricate manner that made my study quite comprehensive for me. Highly recommended for all.
Shafat Ahmad Naikoo (Pulwama, J & K)

Download the App
Nursing Next Live

Access
TARGET HIGH Digital Lite

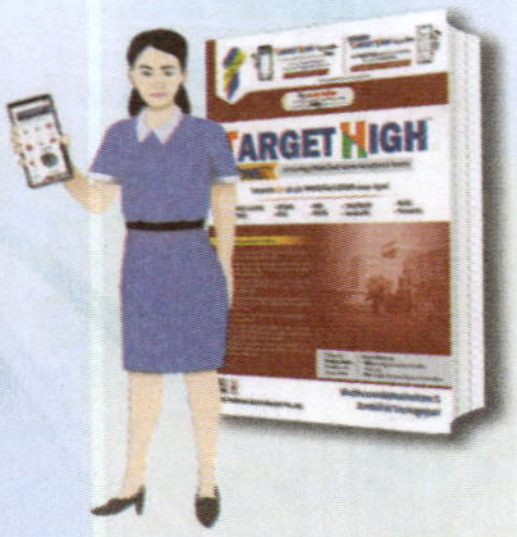

Be in Spotlight

Claim Your Moment: Flourish in the Spotlight by Sharing your success story and feedback

Special Section for

Reviewers
Contributors
Rank Holders
Happy Users

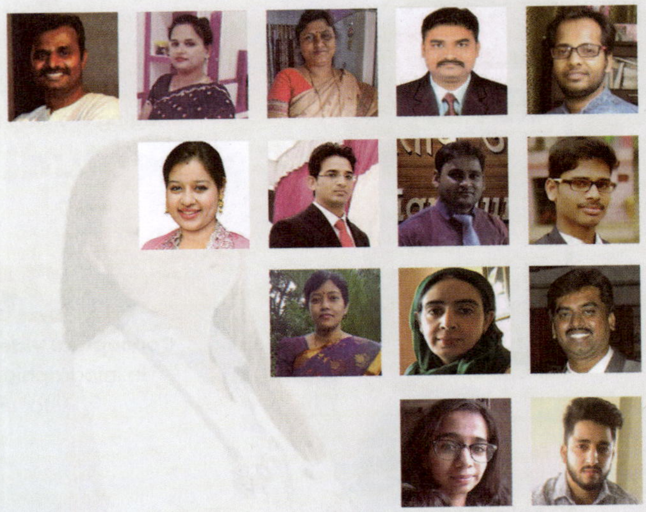

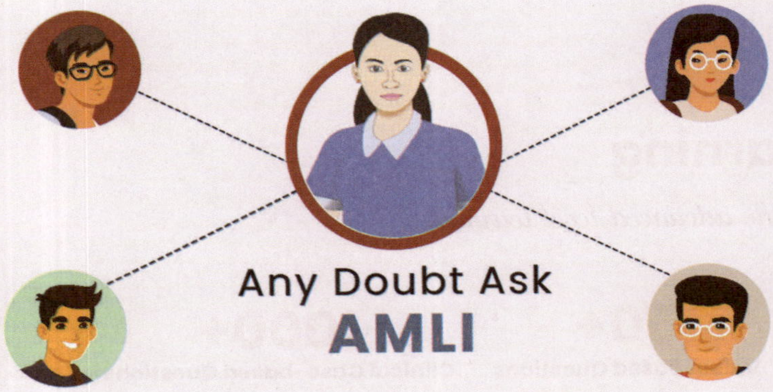

Any Doubt Ask
AMLI

Get your
TARGET HIGH
Queries Resolved from
AMLI (The **TH** Educator)

FROM DOUBTS TO CONFIDENCE
Expert Counseling & Guidance for NORCET Exam

Target High played a vital role in my preparations especially Golden Points
"This book has played an important role in my preparations. I could prepare with all the given features that are listen and recall, assess yourself by tests, etc. You should definitely go for it."
Kana Ram Chotiya *(Jayal, Rajasthan)*

Target High with Updated Features – HIGHLY RECOMMENDED FOR ALL
The content of the Target High Book is excellent and adequate. The target high digital lite has new updated features like "Assess Yourself" in which chapter-wise and subject-wise MCQs are available which will help you to gain confidence in single subject and help you to achieve your ultimate goal.
Shobha Kumari *(Ranchi, Jharkhand)*

Download the App
Nursing Next Live

Access
TARGET HIGH Digital Lite

TARGET HIGH™

ONE NATION NORCET BOOK on Nursing Officer/Staff Nurse Recruitment Exams

Seventh COLORED PHYGITAL Edition *(Book+Digital)*

- NORCET (AIIMS)
- PGIMER
- JIPMER
- ESIC
- RRB
- DSSSB
- CHO/MLHP
- Kerala PSC
- HAAD
- Prometric

FREE *Add On* BOOKLET

Get Free *Add On* BOOKLET with Target High 7/e
containing Target High Digital Lite Table of Content and General Knowledge & Aptitude

Authors

Muthuvenkatachalam Srinivasan
PhD (INC Consortium), MSc Nursing (AIIMS Delhi), D Pharm
RN (NMBA Australia)
Assistant Professor
Institute of Human Behaviour and Allied Sciences (IHBAS)
Govt. of NCT
New Delhi

Ambili M Venugopal
MSc Pediatric Nursing (AIIMS), BSc (Hons) Nursing (AIIMS)
Tutor/Clinical Instructor
College of Nursing
All India Institute of Medical Sciences
Mangalagiri, Andhra Pradesh

Foreword

Roy K George
Sandhya Gupta
Reddemma K
Indarjit Walia

Recommended By

- Usha Ukande
- Ratna Prakash
- Sandhya Ghai
- B V Kathyayni
- Indarjit Walia
- Sabina Ali
- Harinder Jeet Goyal
- B Valli
- Jeyaseelan M Devadason
- Prema P
- Rashmi E John
- T Samuel Ravi
- Shyamala D Manivannan
- Sr Rojamma
- Jacintha D'Souza
- HC Rawat
- Jyoti Sarin
- Sunita Lawrence
- Deepika C Khakha
- Sr Mary Lucita
- L Gopichandran
- Radha Saini
- Saumya Srivastava

CBSPD Dedicated to Education
Nursing Knowledge Tree

CBS

CBS Publishers & Distributors Pvt Ltd
• New Delhi • Bengaluru • Chennai • Kochi • Kolkata • Lucknow
• Mumbai • Hyderabad • Nagpur • Patna • Pune • Vijayawada

TRADEMARK

Target High is now a registered trademark title of CBS Publishers and Distributors Pvt Ltd and all rights are reserved with the publisher. You are prohibited to use Target High name in any form (book, Facebook page, coaching institute, etc.). Kindly note, the affiliations of the authors are mentioned at the back cover and they don't run any coaching institute with the name Target High. Also, there is only one registered Facebook page of Target High by CBS Publishers and Distributors Pvt Ltd. Any other Facebook page, book or coaching institute are not connected with us.

DISCLAIMER

Target High is a reference title and not a standard resource of information. Careful efforts have been invested in compiling/editing of the concerned data/information given in this book in various sections. However, it is likely that some errors might have crept in despite being vigilant. In such a case, please refer to standard publications for verification, and authors and publishers would not be held responsible in case any of the readers attempts a wrong answer in any of his/her examinations. We are grateful to the authors of the standard textbooks that have been referred to while compiling the text of the book. Questions given in the book are memory based and we do not claim that they are the originally asked questions in examinations. Any such similarity would be purely coincidental.

SET ISBN: 978-93-94525-20-7

Seventh Edition: 2024

Sixth Edition (Revised Reprint): 2022

Published by **Satish Kumar Jain** and produced by **Varun Jain** for

CBS Publishers & Distributors Pvt Ltd

4819/XI Prahlad Street, 24 Ansari Road, Daryaganj, New Delhi 110 002, India.
Ph: +91-11-23289259, 23266861, 23266867 Website: www.cbspd.com
Fax: 011-23243014
e-mail: delhi@cbspd.com; cbspubs@airtelmail.in.

Corporate Office: 204 FIE, Industrial Area, Patparganj, Delhi 110 092
Ph: +91-11-4934 4934 Fax: 4934 4935
e-mail: feedback@cbspd.com; bhupesharora@cbspd.com

Branches

- **Bengaluru:** Seema House 2975, 17th Cross, K.R. Road, Banasankari 2nd Stage, Bengaluru-560 070, Karnataka
  Ph: +91-80-26771678/79 Fax: +91-80-26771680 e-mail: bangalore@cbspd.com
- **Chennai:** 7, Subbaraya Street, Shenoy Nagar, Chennai-600 030, Tamil Nadu
  Ph: +91-44-26680620, 26681266 Fax: +91-44-42032115 e-mail: chennai@cbspd.com
- **Kochi:** 68/1534, 35, 36-Power House Road, Opp. KSEB, Cochin-682018, Kochi, Kerala
  Ph: +91-484-4059061-65 Fax: +91-484-4059065 e-mail: kochi@cbspd.com
- **Kolkata:** Hind Ceramics Compound, 1st Floor, 147, Nilganj Road, Belghoria, Kolkata-700056, West Bengal
  Ph: +033-2563-3055/56 e-mail: kolkata@cbspd.com
- **Lucknow:** Basement, Khushnuma Complex, 7-Meerabai Marg (Behind Jawahar Bhawan), Lucknow-226001, Uttar Pradesh
  Ph: +0522-4000032 e-mail: tiwari.lucknow@cbspd.com
- **Mumbai:** PWD Shed, Gala No. 25/26, Ramchandra Bhatt Marg, Next to J.J. Hospital Gate No. 2, Opp. Union Bank of India, Noor Baug, Mumbai-400009, Maharashtra
  Ph: +91-22-66661880/89 Fax: +91-22-24902342 e-mail: mumbai@cbspd.com

Representatives

- **Hyderabad** +91-9885175004
- **Pune** +91-9623451994
- **Patna** +91-9334159340
- **Vijayawada** +91-9000660880

Printed at : Goyal Offset Works Pvt. Ltd. Haryana (INDIA)

Foreword to 7th Edition

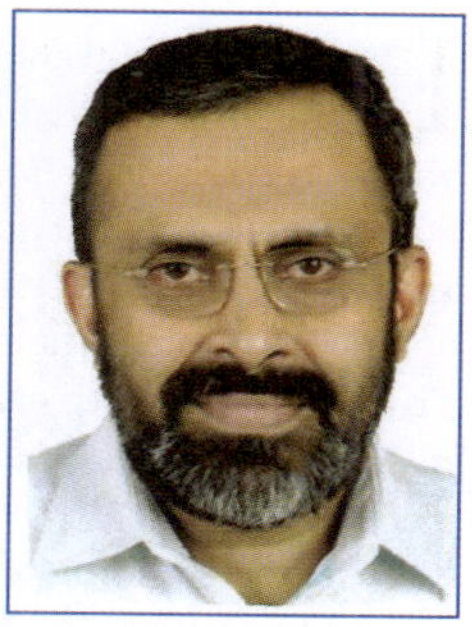

It gives me immense pleasure to introduce this thoroughly Revised and Updated 7th Edition of "Target High: Nursing Entrance Exam Guide." In this edition, authors have meticulously curated a comprehensive and all-encompassing resource to empower aspiring nursing professionals with the knowledge and skills needed to excel in their journey toward success. With a keen focus on latest developments, all the most recent information, current affairs, programs, policies, and the latest exam patterns up to July 2023 have also been incorporated in this edition.

This book continues to be testament to authors' commitment of providing the most relevant and up-to-date content for nursing aspirants. With a keen eye toward enhancing your preparation strategy, a separate section has been dedicated to decoding case-scenario based questions, along with insightful guidance on navigating NORCET 5.0 Stage I-Prelims and NORCET Stage II-Mains.

In alignment with the evolving landscape of nursing education, this edition organizes all subjects according to the New Revised INC Curriculum. Furthermore, the authors have expanded the scope of this book by including two new subjects, *Applied Psychology and Sociology*, along with *Forensic Nursing*, ensuring that students are well-prepared for the diverse challenges of the nursing profession.

To facilitate effective learning, an attractive layout that combines theory with previously-asked questions from important exams, including NORCET 2023, 2022, and the latest state-level exams has been followed. Within these pages, you will find more than 1000 important key points, meticulously crafted synopses for Fundamentals of Nursing, Obstetrics and Gynecology, Pediatric Nursing, and Community Health Nursing, and over 1000 illustrative tables, images, flowcharts, and illustrations which will help you in clarifying the concepts.

The digital age demands a strong digital support system so, Target High has been supported with a digital boost having a variety of features. With over 25,000 MCQs, including 500+ new questions, 5,000 MCQs with rationale, 15,000 practice questions, and an array of integrated clinical-based and case-based questions, this edition is a treasure trove of learning and practice opportunities.

As you embark on this transformative journey, authors have rest assured that you have in your hands a comprehensive and powerful tool that has been honed and perfected over time. The inclusion of 116+ previous year papers, 3000+ golden points for last-minute revisions, and a wide array of appendices further solidify the status of edition as a beacon of knowledge and guidance.

I extend my heartfelt gratitude to the authors of this book who have tirelessly worked to bring this edition to fruition, and I wish all nursing aspirants the very best in their pursuit of excellence. May "Target High: Nursing Entrance Exam Guide" be your steadfast companion, guiding you toward success and accomplishment in the dynamic and rewarding field of nursing.

Prof. (Dr) Roy K George
National President TNAI
Member Indian Nursing Council
Director Academics, Baby Memorial Hospital
Kozhikode, Kerala

Foreword to 6th Edition

I know Dr Muthuvenkatachalam when he joined as student for postgraduate studies at AIIMS, New Delhi followed by PhD which also he did under my guidance from PhD consortium of Indian Nursing Council and Rajiv Gandhi University of Health Sciences. And thereafter, we have done some research projects together. I would like to emphasize here that he is a highly motivated to improve the standard of nursing education. His dedication is visible from the way he has been putting efforts to update this 6th edition of book *Target High* which is already on runaway success and enjoys greater acceptance and appreciation by all readers.

In my opinion, the book has the original contents, which are well thought out, keeping in mind ever changing health science, treatment protocols and health care delivery system. The work in this book requires praise for the author in doing evidence-based updating of content of *Target High 6th Edition* from each reader who will get oneself ready for all competitive exams in Nursing Science.

The *Target High 6th Edition* is prepared with interactive approach and the content is supported with several examples and illustrations for better understanding of complex content. This book is one single platform for students who are looking forward to crack any of the entrance exams, particularly for the nursing officer's and staff nurse positions in the country.

I congratulate Dr Muthuvenkatachalam Srinivasan for bringing out *Target High 6th Edition at the right time when the competition is all time high.* Dear readers, this book is well referenced from standard books and will work as guide for you for all areas in nursing science and will motivate you to excel in your professional practice in addition to success in entrance exams.

Dr Sandhya Gupta

Formerly-Principal (Actg.) & Associate Professor
College of Nursing, AIIMS, New Delhi

15.9.2021

Foreword to 4th & 5th Edition

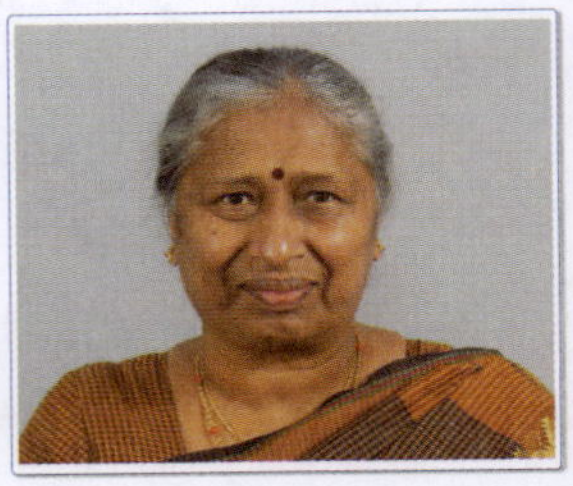

In this fast-paced world, the healthcare industry has become an area of utmost importance. People have become more aware about their bodily needs and they are ready to spare their valuable time for keeping themselves hale and hearty. In such circumstances, the personnel working in the field of nursing have to perform a crucial role. To perform their roles with dexterity and sheer determination, the nursing professionals have to keep themselves updated with the modern techniques of healthcare and for this, they have to explore the nursing examination system.

It is my privilege to write the foreword of a book which is a gem of a book available for the staff nurses and nursing officers' exam. There is no dearth of books for the nursing recruitment examination but it is a fact that the aspirants need something which could prove a panacea for such examinations, and the book, *Target High* for Nursing Officer/Staff Nurse Recruitment Exam is one such effort of the authors. Dr Muthuvenkatachalam Srinivasan and Mrs Ambili M Venugopal have produced a wonderful book which will undoubtedly help the aspirants in hitting the bull's eye. The authors are masters of their fields and so they have included everything which is needed by the aspirants of this exam.

In addition to this, renowned reviewers have reviewed the important topics of this book and these topics enhance the accuracy and authenticity of this book. After going through I can say with authority that this book has certainly an edge over the other books available for *Nursing Officer/Staff Nurse Recruitment Exam.*

I wish the authors all the luck and success, and really appreciate their commendable efforts which is a boon in true sense for the nursing officers/staff nurses' aspirants.

Reddemma K

Nodal Officer, National Consortium for PhD in Nursing
Formerly, Senior Professor and HOD
Department of Nursing
NIMHANS
Bengaluru, India

From Authors' Desk

We extend our heartfelt wishes to you and your loved ones, hoping that you are in good health and navigating the challenges posed by the lingering pandemic with resilience and safety. These past three years have brought about unprecedented trials the global community has borne witness to, a series of unfortunate events. The unwavering dedication of health care professionals has provided us with a beacon of hope and care.

Among these health care heroes, nurses have stood at the forefront, selflessly tending to our well-being, playing a pivotal role in saving lives. Today, we stand united in expressing our deepest gratitude to all nurses and health care workers. As we look forward to the future, it is heartening to envision a collaborative journey ahead, where you will join hands with fellow health care champions.

As we present the 7th Edition of Target High, we extend our profound gratitude to all health care workers and nurses, and readers who have propelled this journey of knowledge and excellence. May this edition serve as a guiding light for all Nursing Officer Aspirants, equipping them with the knowledge and insights needed to excel in their career.

Serving its purpose profitably with 6 successful editions, Target High has now come out with more valuable and informative content. Change is the law of nature and the need of the hour, and with this vision, Target High 7th Edition has been thoroughly revised, updated and upgraded in all aspects.

With the motive of **Aim High, Achieve High,** we have changed the motto of Target High from **One Nation, One Book** to **One Nation, One NORCET, One Book,** keeping in mind the changing trends in the examination pattern, giving due importance to the top-level examinations. All the reviewers, contributors and readers have played a pivotal role in making this compendium reach the next level by covering all the required study material that targets Nursing Recruitment Examination held in India and in foreign countries.

In this edition, we have covered synopsis of each and every subject that has been updated and wrapped in an integrated manner by emphasizing the clinical importance and focusing on the futuristic approach of the Nursing Officer Examination. This time two new subjects have been added as per the revised INC Syllabus, i.e., Applied Psychology and Sociology. The whole edition has been thoroughly revised and updated as per the changing examination trends. The text of Target High has been supplemented with a number of **Key Point boxes** that cover important facts, **Points to Remember** boxes that cover Must-Know-Information, **Clinical Corner** that covers all the relevant scenario-based questions, **Practice Questions section** that covers important questions, **Recent Questions** section that covers recently held examinations' questions, like NORCET 2023, NORCET 2022, CNCI 2020 and many more.

Special emphasis has been given to Subject-wise cum Topic-wise Clinical Case-based questions of the core nursing subjects, like Fundamentals of Nursing, Medical Surgical Nursing, Psychiatric Nursing, Obstetrics and Gynecological Nursing and Pediatric Nursing as per the NCLEX examination pattern and recently changed NORCET Exam pattern. Multiple Choice Questions of each subject have also been arranged under various topics in Subject-wise cum Topic-wise manner.

The answers to all the questions have been authenticated from various reference resources and controversial questions have been supplemented with their explanations for doubt clarification. Question banks have been enhanced by adding more exam-oriented questions to give an extensive coverage of questions from all the topics along with Important one-liners at the end of every subject, in a Podcast Format.

New Important and Quick Glance topics have been covered under Appendices. All latest Previous Year Papers up to July 2023 have been added to provide glimpses on the recently held examination in one go. General Knowledge, English, Numerical Ability and Reasoning section have been covered in detail in a separate booklet.

Last but not the least, Target High has come up with the Hybrid Edition this time. The Hybrid Edition is an amalgamation of 'the book and the digital platform'. Readers, can now read theory from the book and practice from the Nursing Next Live App. This integrated approach will help students enhance their comprehension, knowledge and level of practice.

With its meticulously curated content and innovative approach, the Hybrid Edition of Target High serves as a panacea, addressing every facet of your Nursing Exam preparation. It is our fervent hope that you embrace this edition with the same enthusiasm and affection that you have shown for the previous editions.

As you embark on this journey, we encourage you to prepare with utmost diligence and dedication, leaving no stone unturned in your pursuit of excellence. May this edition serve as the catalyst that propels you toward your long-cherished dream job, a culmination of your relentless efforts and aspirations.

Muthuvenkatachalam Srinivasan

Ambili M Venugopal

Acknowledgements

Thanking the Almighty for His Immense Blessings!!!

With humility, we acknowledge our indebtedness to all. The task of writing a book and updating the matter in accordance with the changing scenario is harder than we thought and more rewarding than we could have ever imagined. None of this would have been possible without your all-incredible support. We are eternally grateful to all of you for playing a vital role during our struggle and success for the *Target High Sixth Edition*. Now, with the blessing and support from all of you, we are presenting **Target High Seventh Premium Colored Hybrid Edition** with a new look, updated and upgraded content, additional features and digital support as per the need and demand of the time.

From the inception, with profound love, we owe sincere gratitude to our parents, siblings and daughters for their unconditional love, support, understanding and forbearance throughout the ups and downs in the journey of this book.

It is very well said that *a teacher is a great source of knowledge, prosperity and enlightenment by which anybody can be benefited.* Our teachers deserve the credit for the gift of their guidance, invaluable suggestions, constructive criticism and perpetual inspiration, which inspired us in our difficult time, kept us motivated and enabled us to complete this book.

We are forever grateful to our teacher, mentor and a great motivator **Dr Sandhya Gupta**, Formerly-Principal (Actg.) and Associate Professor, College of Nursing, AIIMS, New Delhi, for inspiring us and inculcating confidence into us to write a book. We are indebted to her for the constant support and encouragement in this endeavor. We also want to thank **Dr Latha Venkatesan**, Professor cum Principal, College of Nursing, AIIMS, New Delhi for being a constant support and a mentor.

Words fail to express our gratitude to **Dr Ratna Prakash**, Professor and Academic Director (Former Principal), Pal College of Nursing and Medical Sciences, Haldwani, Uttarakhand for her unconditional support and encouragement on initiating this book. We are fortunate to have her in our path.

We wish to express our heartfelt thanks and regards to all those, who have contributed appropriate and relevant information to this book. Without their cooperation, this endeavor might not have been possible.

These acknowledgments will be incomplete without mentioning the role of our beloved students, who have always been our well-wishers, constant supporters and source of learning and encouragement.

We appreciate the support of **Mr Satish Kumar Jain** (Chairman) and **Mr Varun Jain** (Managing Director), M/s CBS Publishers and Distributors Pvt Ltd for their wholehearted cooperation in publication of this book. We have no words to describe the role, efforts, inputs and initiatives undertaken by **Mr Bhupesh Arora** (Sr. Vice President – Health Sciences Division, Publishing & Marketing), for his endeavor toward the development of the book.

We sincerely thank the entire CBS team for bringing this colorful edition with utmost care and amazing presentation. We would like to thank Ms Nitasha Arora (Publishing Head & Content Strategist – PGMEE & Nursing Division), Ms Daljeet Kaur (Assistant Publishing Manager), Dr Anju Dhir (Product Manager cum Commissioning Editor – Medical), Mr Shivendu Bhushan Pandey (Senior Manager and Team Leader), Mr Ashutosh Pathak (Senior Proofreader cum Team Coordinator) for putting their hard work and efforts to bring out this book on time and all the production team members for devoting laborious hours in designing and typesetting of the book.

Our special thanks are due to entire Sales, Marketing and Tech team—Mr Chiradeep Bose (General Manager–Central Marketing and Sales Offline Unit), Ms Neetu Jindal (Senior Digital Marketing Manager) and Ms Preeti Arora (Tech and Operation Head) for their special contributions in offline & online marketing and strong tech support.

We owe special thanks to all Branch Heads for their contributions toward making the book available throughout India and turning our idea of "**ONE NATION, ONE NORCET, ONE BOOK**" into a reality.

We are also thankful to our colleagues who helped us to formulate ideas when they did not even know that they were helping. Their involvement has triggered and nourished our intellectual maturity. Once again, we express our heartfelt gratitude to the unstinting support given by our friends and everyone in our team.

Finally, we would like to thank everybody who is important to the successful realization of this book and express our apology if we missed anyone's name, which we assure is completely inadvertent.

From Publisher's Desk

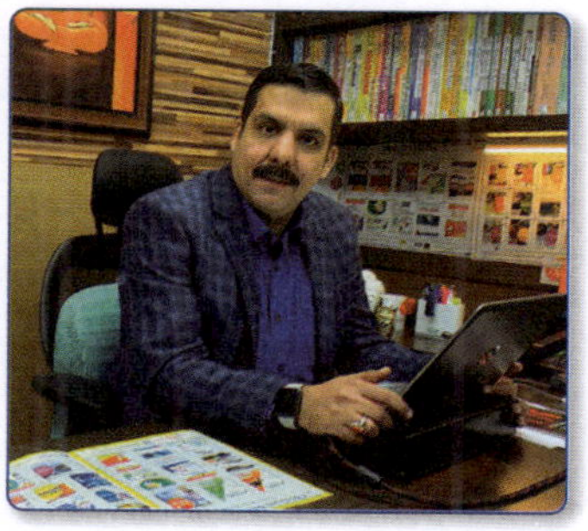

Education is the most powerful weapon which you can use to change the world. - Nelson Mandela

With a firm belief that quality education can change the world, I on behalf of CBS Publishers & Distributors would like to show my gratitude to all the readers of Target High across India. With the huge success of previous editions of Target High, making it the 'Best-Seller', we have come up with the new updated 7th edition to provide "Nothing but the Best" for nursing aspirants.

We are delighted to announce that CBS Publishers & Distributors have completed 50 glorious years of publishing. The journey of these 50 years hasn't been easy but phenomenon. Your love and support have helped us to come up with various quality health science books and educational platforms.

Over the past fifty years, the publishing industry has undergone significant changes. Publishers used to be just intermediaries between authors and readers. They didn't actively participate in quality checks or stay up to date with examination trends, which led to users receiving content without proper vetting.

CBS and the Nursing Knowledge Tree division have adapted to the changing scenario and are dedicated to delivering top-notch education. As with huge success comes huge responsibility, we believe Improving the quality of books is imperative to enhance the standard of nursing education and students. And to do so, the approach has always been a thorough quality check at various levels and inputs to/from authors as per the current examination trends.

Target High embarked on its journey in 2016 with the aim of creating a book that is complete in itself aiding the needs of nursing aspirants. I am pleased to share that we have undoubtedly accomplished our vision over the past six years. More than 3,00,000 Students nursing aspirants have read and referred to Target High with a belief that it has played a significant role in their success.

Every single word of this edition has been meticulously analyzed by experts to meet the highest standards of authenticity and credibility. The goal has always been to create an unparalleled source of information for nursing aspirants, one that is flawless and complete. The journey which started with just one book has come a long way with a series of Target High books

1. Target High NEXT - Nursing Decode for Nursing Undergraduate 1st, 2nd, 3rd and 4th year
2. Target High CHO Entrance
3. Target High MSc Entrance
4. Target High Kerala PSC Entrance
5. Target High Digital Lite (App)
6. Target High Digital Pro (Forthcoming)
7. Target High NEXT NCLEX (Forthcoming)

The trust and faith students have shown in Target High Brand has given us confidence and boast to cover complete exam prep segment from UG to NORCET, Indian State & National Level exams to NCLEX and from Book to Digital App.

Our previous editions have proven to be valuable assets and so we present you with our latest edition to exceed your expectations. We believe, no matter how good a book is, there is always a scope for improvement. We request you to keep sharing your constant feedback so that we could provide you with the best.

I would be happy to get your valuable feedback or if you have any new ideas which can be implemented in target high series kindly do share it with me at **bhupeshaarora@cbspd.com** and you can also connect with me at 9555590180

Bhupesh Aarora
Sr. Vice President – Health Sciences Division (Publishing & Marketing)
CBS Publishers and Distributors Pvt Ltd

ATTENTION TO THE READERS!

STOP PIRACY! PROMOTE ORIGINALITY!

Dear All

Target High Staff Nurse Recruitment Examinations has been conceptualized and developed with a sole purpose of benefitting the thousands of staff nurse aspirants across the country by providing them a one-stop solution to everything they need to excel. Authors, publisher and everyone associated with this project aimed to channelize your efforts with this book so as to save your time and money you invest in referring various different resources for the same information.

However, it has come to our notice that widespread illegal distribution of photocopies and PDFs is already taking place in the market. We would like to acquaint you with the fact that Indian Reprographic Rights Organization (IRRO), a copyright society registered under the Copyright Act, permits only up to 15% of a copyrighted work to be reproduced. Also, the usage should be non-commercial and non-profitable. Photocopying the whole book/uploading PDFs or images of the book without the due permission of author or publisher is punishable under the copyright act as it weighs against the fair use policy because completely copying and distributing the work for free online and physically would hinder the economic viability of creating and maintaining the source.

We are aware of the resources from where these practices are emerging and coming into existence. In case, anyone of you come across such practice going around you, please reach us at +91 9555353330 or bhupeshaarora@cbspd.com We would take strict legal actions against the alleged without any prior notice. If your information is found genuine, we will also reward you. Please note that in this whole process, we assure that your identity would be kept confidential.

Piracy and infringement lead to demotivation of the complete author and publishing fraternity. If the same content would be circulated all the time, there would be no new original work and hence, the growth in knowledge propagation would be hampered considerably. Therefore, in interest of everyone, let's stop this illegal practice of piracy and give due respect to the intellectual creation of everyone.

Today it's someone else's work! Tomorrow it could be Yours!

Publisher

Luminaries in Nursing

We overcome with felicity in showcasing our gratitude toward the Luminaries in Nursing for they have recommended Target High Series wholeheartedly. A book becomes great because of two important reasons, firstly, the efforts put in by the authors and secondly, when the book is recommended by the elite faculty members. Here, as far as Target High is concerned, the topnotch Luminaries, by their recommendations, have made its success twofold. We express our heartfelt thanks to the Luminaries who always support quality education in Nursing and they believe that quality education should, in every form, be provided to the Nursing Students and Nursing Fraternity.

We, the Target High team, have maintained the high standards of quality education. And the outcome is that the splendid luminaries combinedly proclaim that they recommend Target High as "One Nation, One NORCET, One Book" for Nursing competitive exams.

CBS Team Extends its Whole-Hearted Thanks *to All The Luminaries*

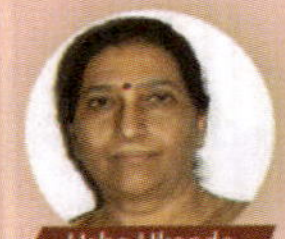
Usha Ukande
PhD, MSc OBG (N)
Former Principal
Choithram CON
Indore, Madhya Pradesh

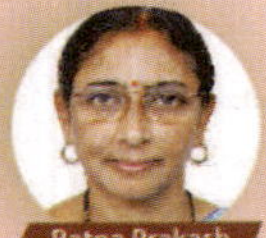
Ratna Prakash
PhD, MSc (MSN)
Prof. & Academic Director (Former Principal)
Pal College of Nursing
Haldwani, Uttarakhand

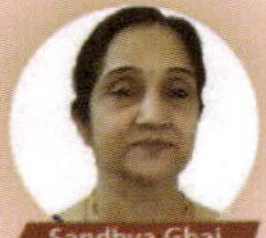
Sandhya Ghai
PhD, MSc (N)
Former Principal
NINE, PGIMER
Chandigarh, Punjab

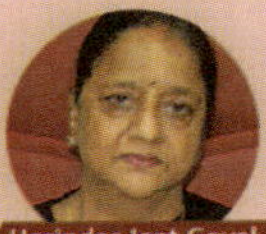
Harinder Jeet Goyal
PhD, MSc (MSN)
Former Principal
RAKCON
New Delhi

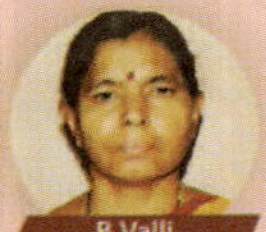
B Valli
MSc (MSN)
Principal
Govt. CON, Guntur
President, TNAI
AP State Branch

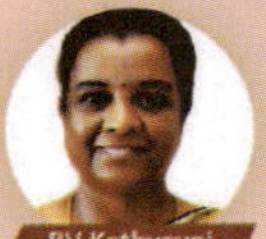
BV Kathyayni
MSc (Pediatric Nursing)
Principal
College of Nursing, NIMHANS
Bangalore

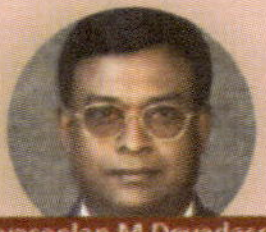
Jeyaseelan M Devadason
PhD, MSc (N)
President TNAI
Tamil Nadu, Branch Dean
Annai JKK Sampoorani Ammal CON
Komarapalayam

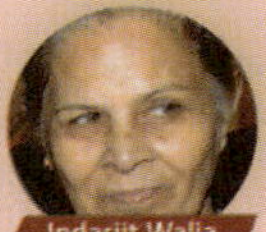
Indarjit Walia
PhD (Community Medicine)
MSc (CHN)
Formver Principal
PGI NINE
Chandigarh, Punjab

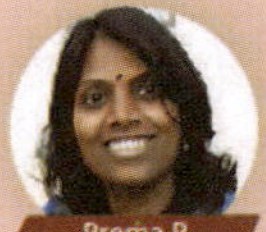
Prema P
PhD (N), MSc (CHN)
Principal
Muzaffarnagar Nursing Institute
Muzaffarnagar
Uttar Pradesh

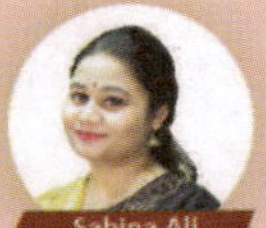
Sabina Ali
RN, RM, MSc (MSN)
(Critical Care Nursing)
Senior Content Strategist
Nursing Next Live - CBS Publishers & Distributors Pvt Ltd.
New Delhi

"Target High is a Book Worth Reading and hence, Worth Buying"

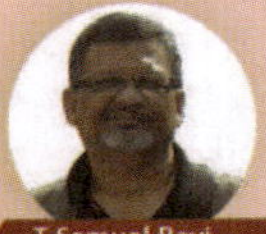
T Samuel Ravi
Retired Head Emergency Nursing
Trauma Center Coordinator
Christian Medical College
Vellore, Tamil Nadu

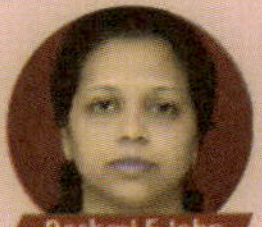
Rashmi E John
MSc (N)
Principal
KGMU
Lucknow, Uttar Pradesh

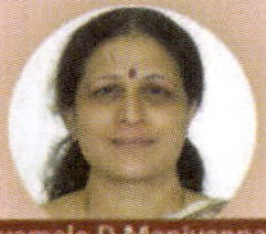
Shyamala D Manivannan
RN, RM, MSc, PhD (CHN)
Professor and Director
Dr MGR Educational & Research Inst. University
Chennai, Tamil Nadu

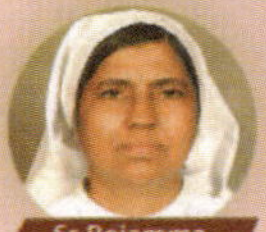
Sr Rojamma
MSc (Psychiatric Nursing)
Professor
JMJ CON, Hyderabad
President, TNAI
Telangana State Branch

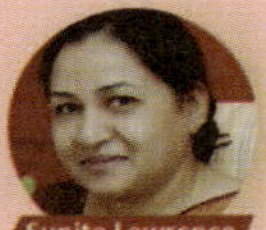
Sunita Lawrence
MSc OBG (N)
PhD (Nursing Education)
Principal
Pragyan Nursing College
Bhopal, Madhya Pradesh

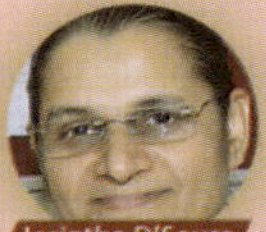
Jacintha D'Souza
MPhil (N)
Principal and Professor
Father Muller CON
Mangalore, Karnataka

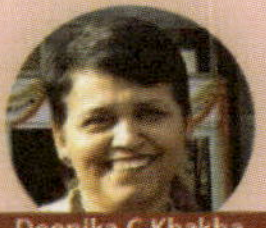
Deepika C Khakha
PhD, MSc (N), MA (Psychology)
Nursing Advisor, DGHS
Ministry of Health & Family Welfare
Government of India
New Delhi

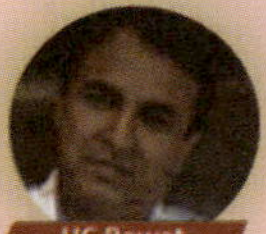
HC Rawat
MSc (Pediatric Nursing)
Principal
University CON, BFUHS
Faridkot, Punjab

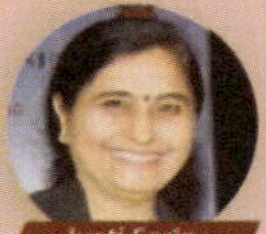
Jyoti Sarin
Director Principal
M.M. College of Nursing
Ambala, Haryana

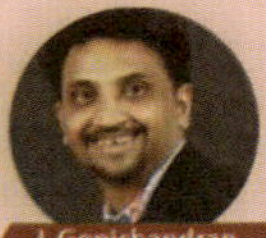
L Gopichandran
Associate Professor
College of Nursing, AIIMS, New Delhi
President, TNAI
Delhi Branch

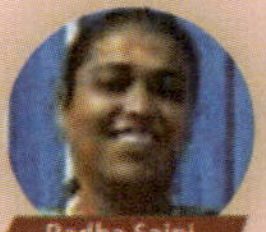
Radha Saini
MSc (CHN)
Fellow
UICC
Geneva

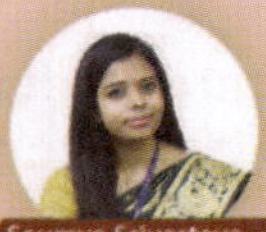
Saumya Srivastava
MSN (Oncology Nursing), RN, RM
Nursing Tutor
Vivekananda College of Nursing
Lucknow, Uttar Pradesh

Our luminaries believe
TARGET HIGH™
Series comes with **Unique Features**

#QualityNursingEducation #TargetingNORCET #UGCentricApproach #UpdatedEdition

#OneNationOneNORCETOneBook #UGSeNORCETvTak #NursingCompendiumWithDigitalSupport RecommendedForAllNursingExams

"The more that you read, the more things you will know. The more that you learn, the more places you will go." —Dr Seuss

Our Valuable Reviewers & Contributors

Approximately 500+ Reviewers & Contributors from 22 States & 2 Union Territories & 120 Cities from India

We, the authors and the publisher, are grateful to all the reviewers who spent some time from their busy schedules and invested it in reviewing the book, making it most authentic and unique quality compendium.

A

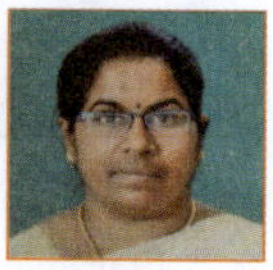

A Helen Mary Perdita
Madurai, Tamil Nadu

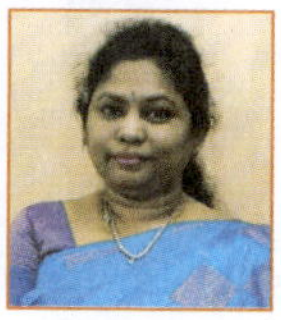

A Jayasudha
Coimbatore, Tamil Nadu

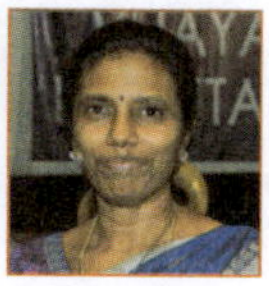

A Vimala
Chennai, Tamil Nadu

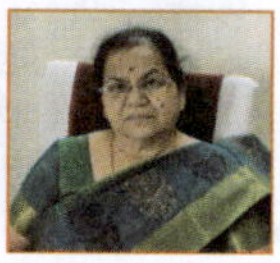

Asha Ramesh Shimgekar
Nagpur, Maharashtra

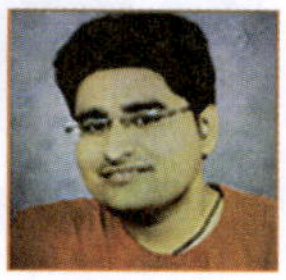

Atul Sharma
Patna, Bihar

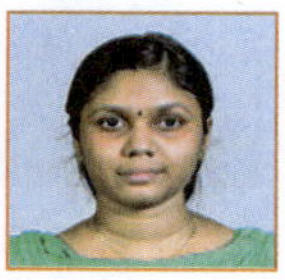

Ambily V Vijayakumar
Kottayam, Kerala

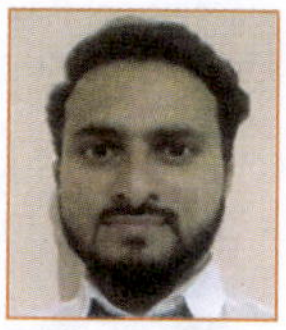

Arshid Nazir Shah
Baramulla, J&K

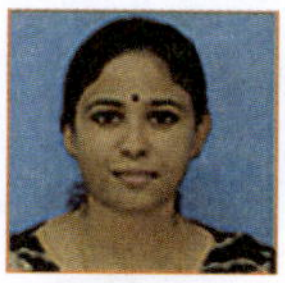

Ajitha Paul Sebastian
Thiruvananthapuram
Kerala

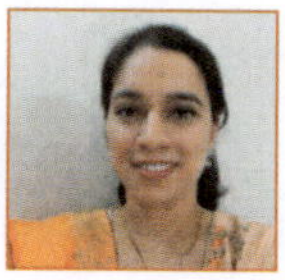

Amandeep Kaur
Gurgaon, Haryana

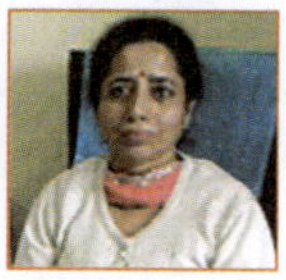

Amita Sareen Puri
Shimla
Himachal Pradesh

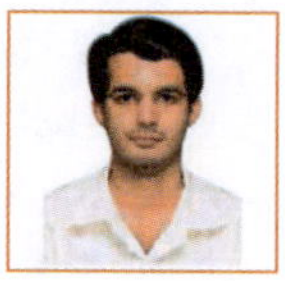

Athar Javeth
Patna, Bihar

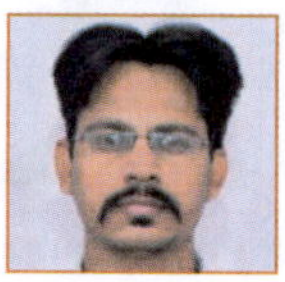

Abhishek Sharma
Alwar, Rajasthan

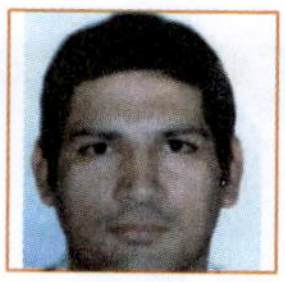

Akash Gaur
Jaipur, Rajasthan

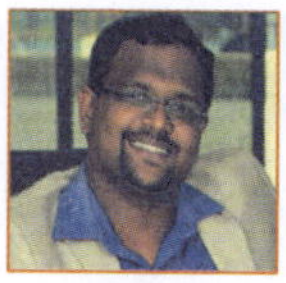

Albert Blesson V
Patna, Bihar

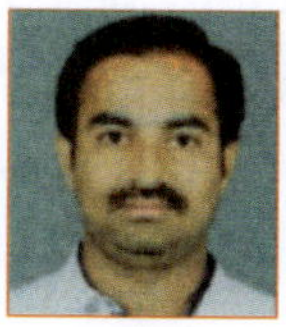

Anand GH
Gokak, Karnataka

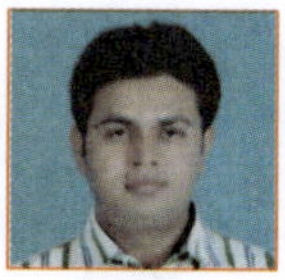

Anish Pathan
Bikaner, Rajasthan

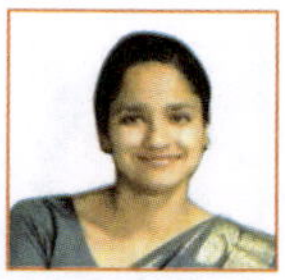

Ankita Sharma
Rishikesh, Uttarakhand

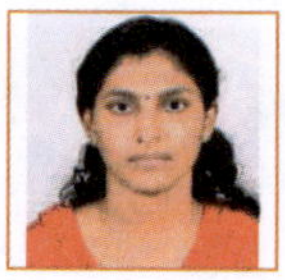

Anu C Vijay
Mangalagiri
Andhra Pradesh

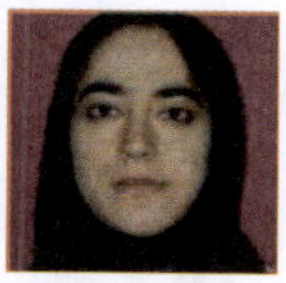

Asifah
Charar-i-Sharief
Srinagar, J&K

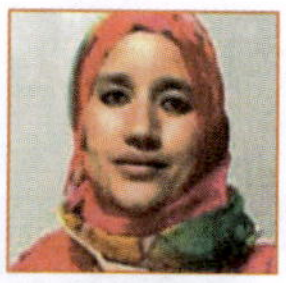

Ather U Nisa
Srinagar, J&K

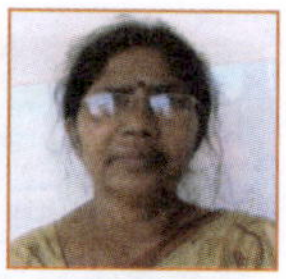

Amrita Lenka
Bhubaneswar, Odisha

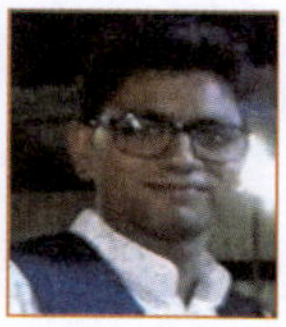

Amar Kumar
Rajasthan

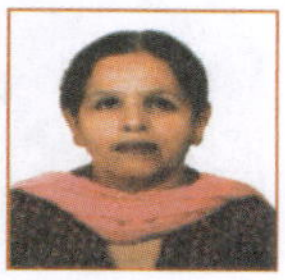

Avinash Kaur Rana
Chandigarh, Punjab

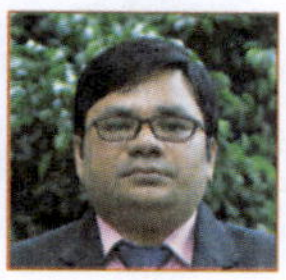

Anil Sharma
Anand, Gujarat

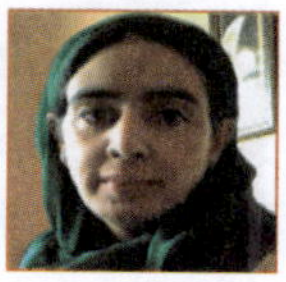

Anjum Khurshid
J&K

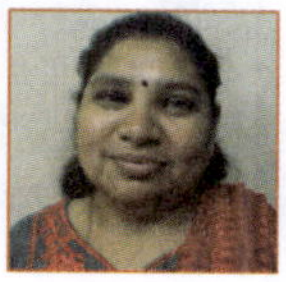

Amudha K
Bengaluru, Karnataka

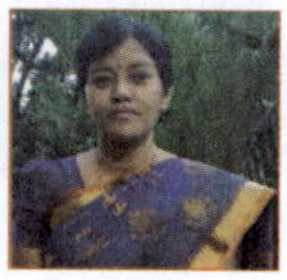

Anita Yuvraj Nawale
Pune, Maharashtra

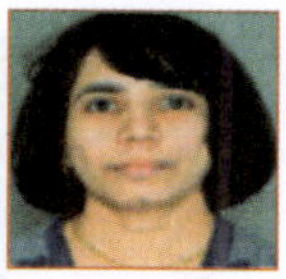

Avani Oke
Mumbai, Maharashtra

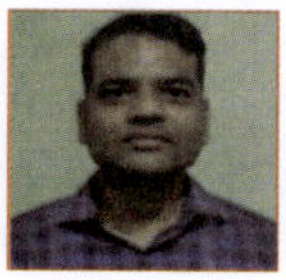

Ankush Jain
New Delhi

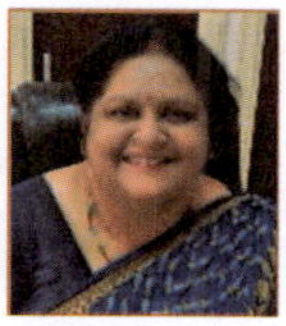

Alka Saxena
Gwalior, Madhya Pradesh

For details of all reviewers & contributors refer TH Lite

New reviewers of TH 7/e covered in TH Lite (App)

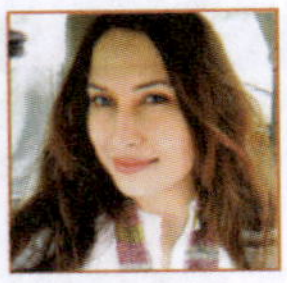

Anupinder Dhaliwal
Patiala, Punjab

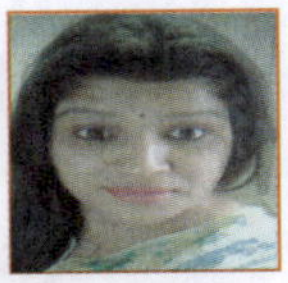

Alka Chauhan
Lucknow, Uttar Pradesh

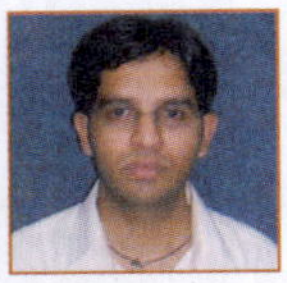

Anil Parashar
Haldwani, Uttarakhand

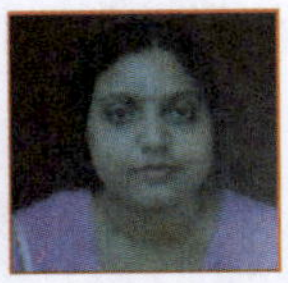

Antara Roy
Kolkata, West Bengal

B

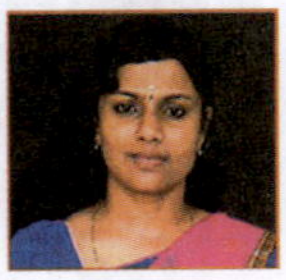

B Gomathi
Bhubaneswar, Odisha

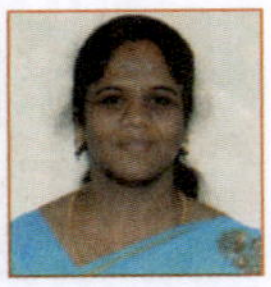

B Menaga Gandhi
Thiruvannamalai
Tamil Nadu

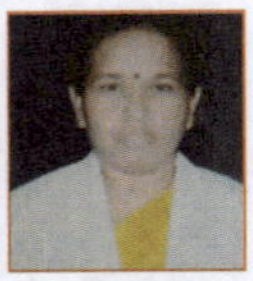

Bharati S Mokhasi
Vijayapur, Karnataka

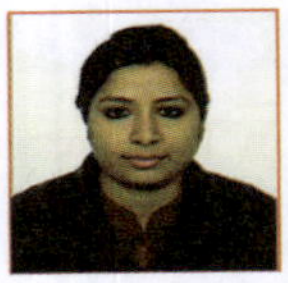

Betsy Chakraborty
Greater Noida
Uttar Pradesh

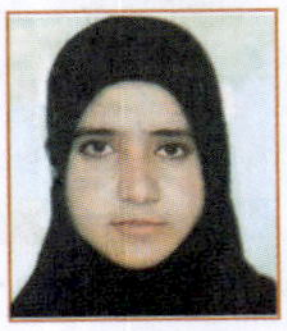

Bilqees Ara
Srinagar, J&K

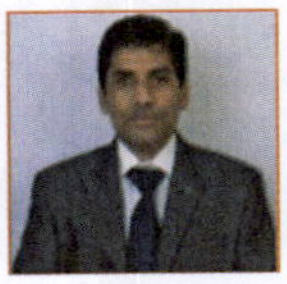

Binu Joe
Gujarat

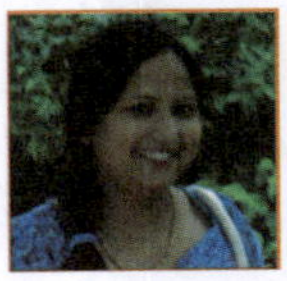

Bandana Bisht
Rajpura, Punjab

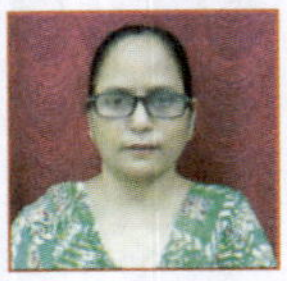

Bhupinder Kaur
Faridkot, Punjab

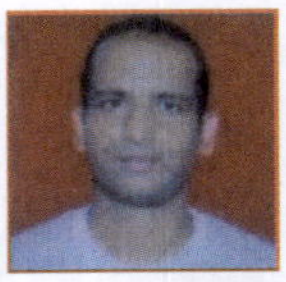

Bheru Singh Jodha
Bikaner, Rajasthan

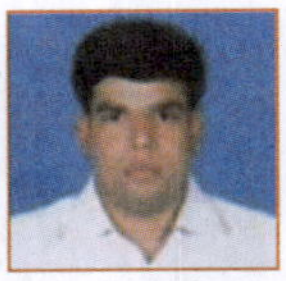

Bhupendra Jain
Jaipur, Rajasthan

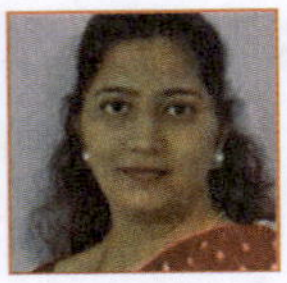

Beulah Philips Kothapally
Hyderabad, Telangana

C

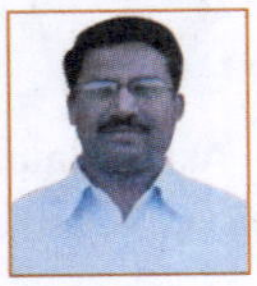

Chandrashekhar H
Hassan, Karnataka

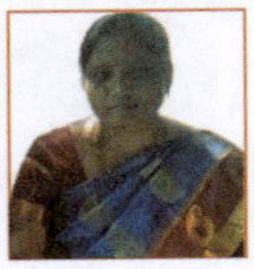

Christy Mekala V
Dharapuram, Tamil Nadu

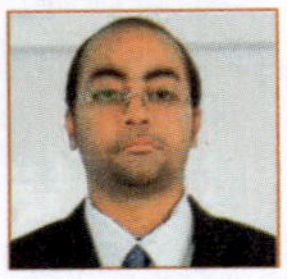

Chandan Pradhan
Bhubaneswar, Odisha

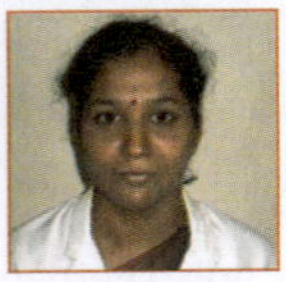

C Kulanthaiammal
Sangrur, Punjab

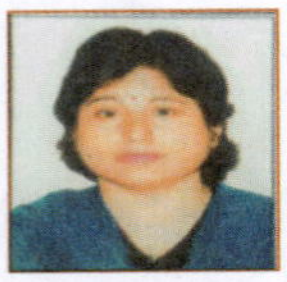

Chander K Sarin
Chandigarh

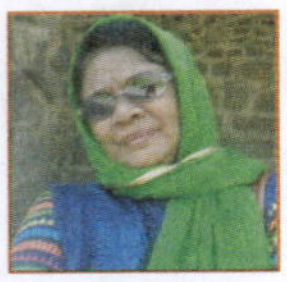

Christin Anil Kumari D
Hoskote, Karnataka

D

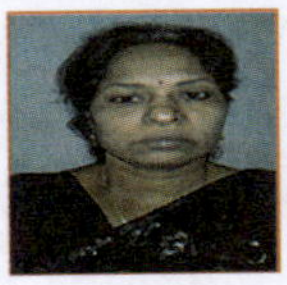

Dr P Shanthi Ida Sophia
Greater Noida
Uttar Pradesh

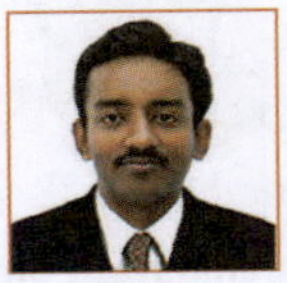

Dr P Prakash
Puducherry, Tamil Nadu

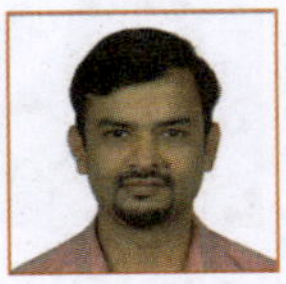

Dr Aldrin Vas
Moodabidri, Karnataka

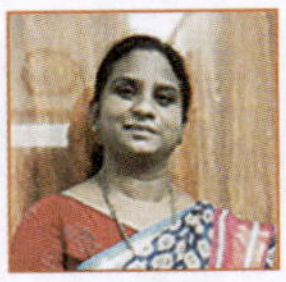

Dr J Anitha
Chennai, Tamil Nadu

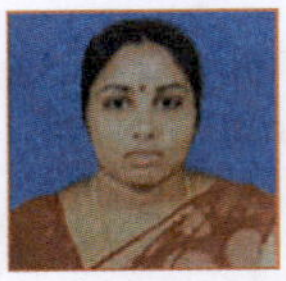

Dr G Dhanalakshmi
Chennai, Tamil Nadu

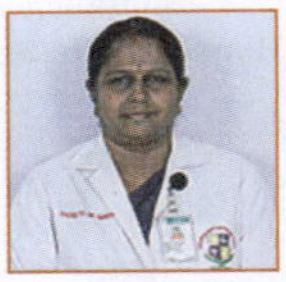

Dr Prof Hema VH Sushresh
Chennai, Tamil Nadu

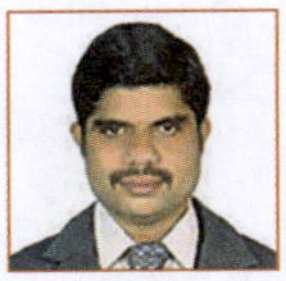

Dr Padmakumar S
Thiruvananthapuram
Kerala

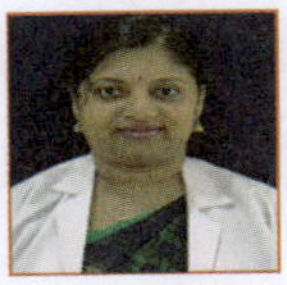

Dr Shwetha Rani CM
Lakhimpur
Uttar Pradesh

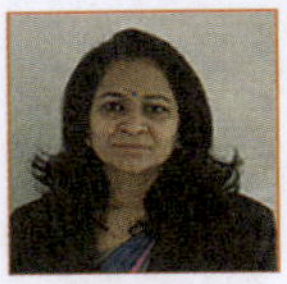

Dr Manju Rajput
Noida, Uttar Pradesh

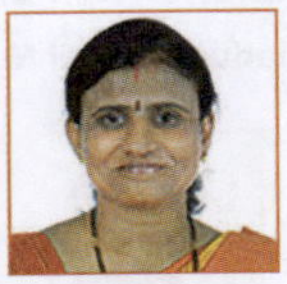

Dr Sheela Shenai NA
Alappuzha, Kerala

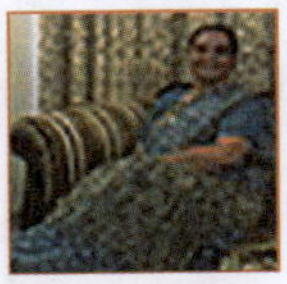

Dr Kirandeep Kaur Dhaliwal
Mullana, Punjab

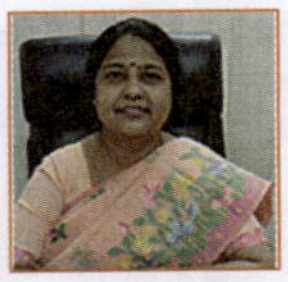

Dr Prachi H Dharap
Thane, Maharashtra

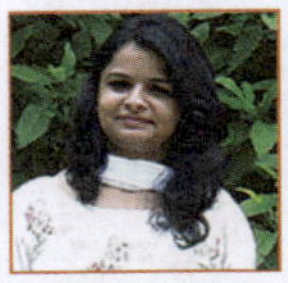

Deepika Bajwan
Greater Noida
Uttar Pradesh

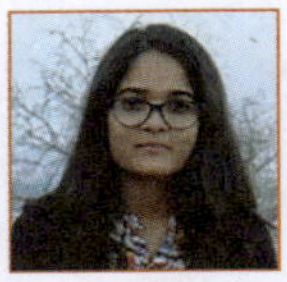

Deeksha Patel
Bhopal
Madhya Pradesh

For details of all reviewers & contributors refer TH Lite

New reviewers of TH 7/e covered in TH Lite (App)

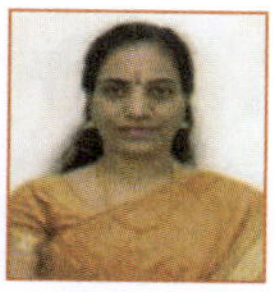
Dr Danasu
Mangalagiri
Andhra Pradesh

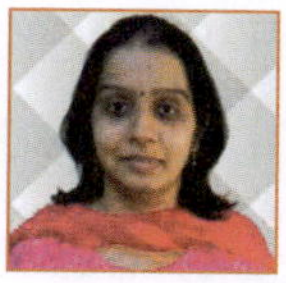
Dr Swati Mehra
New Delhi

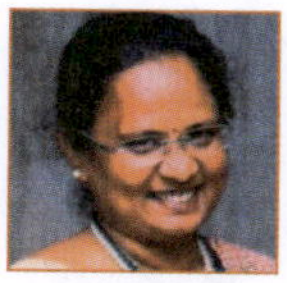
Dr A Maria Therese
Puducherry, Tamil Nadu

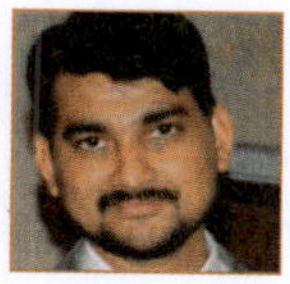
Dr Neeraj Kumar Bansal
Gwalior, Madhya Pradesh

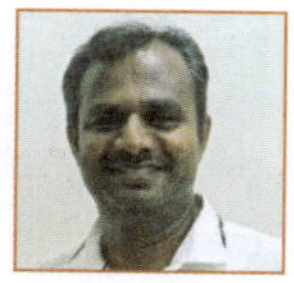
Dhanasekar V M
AIIMS, Mangalagiri

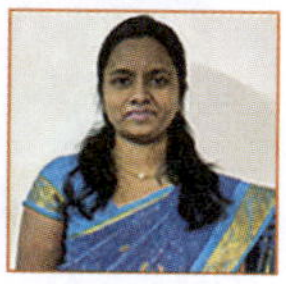
Deva Pon Pushpam I
Tirunelveli, Tamil Nadu

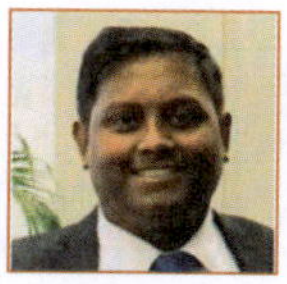
Dr Siraj Ahmad
New Delhi

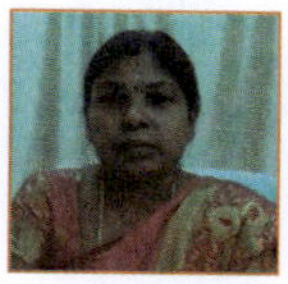
Dr C Susila
Chennai, Tamil Nadu

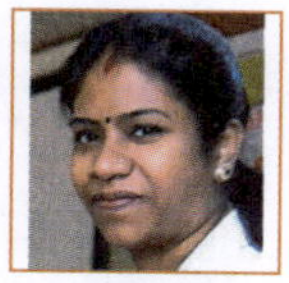
Dr Renuka K
Puducherry, Tamil Nadu

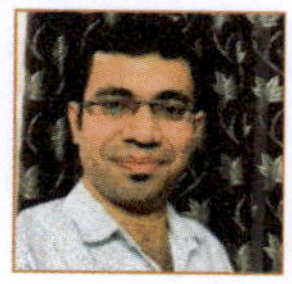
Dinesh Sharma
Kota, Rajasthan

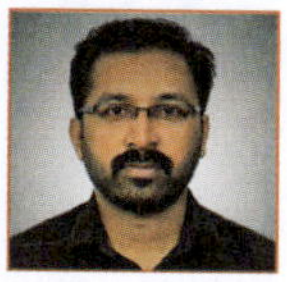
Don Jose K
Ernakulam, Kerala

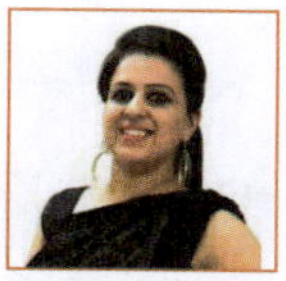
Dr Mrinalini Bakshi
New Delhi

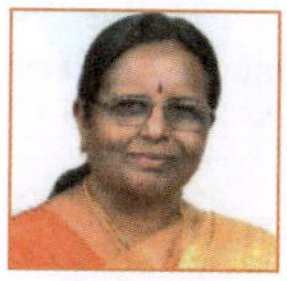
Dr C Kanniammal
Kancheepuram, Tamil Nadu

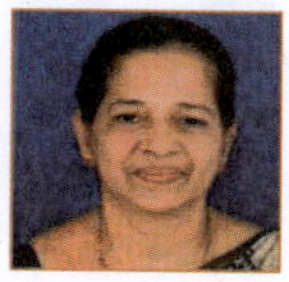
Dr Selliyamma Kuruvila
Kothamangalam, Kerala

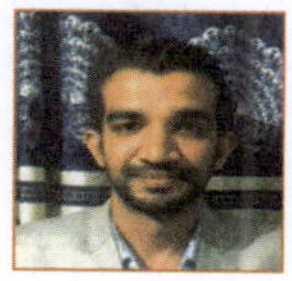
Dipak Patidar
Mehsana, Gujarat

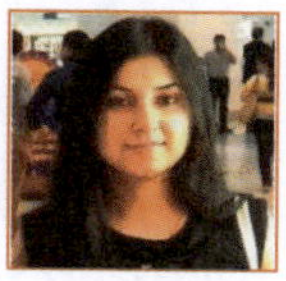
Dr Puja Singh
New Delhi

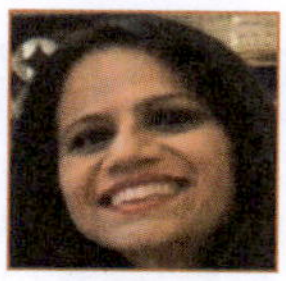
Dr Mansi Midha
New Delhi

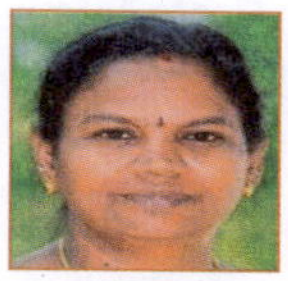
Dr G Muthamilselvi
Kirumampakkam
Puducherry, Tamil Nadu

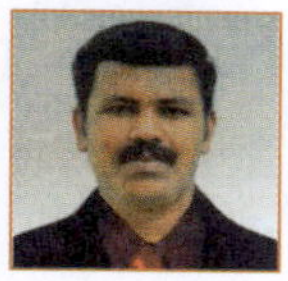
Dr Siva Jeya Anand T
Pandalam, Kerala

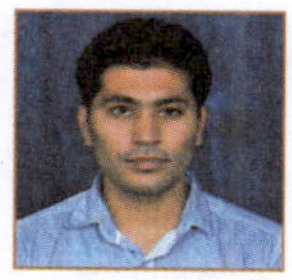
Deepesh Swami
Bikaner, Rajasthan

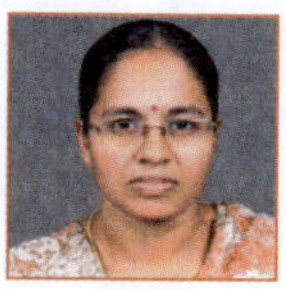
Dr G Vimala
Maharashtra

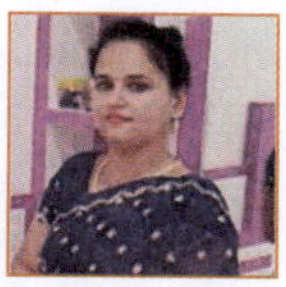
Dr Sandeep Kaur
Amritsar, Punjab

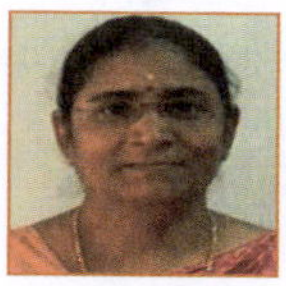
Dr K Kamala
Karaikal, Tamil Nadu

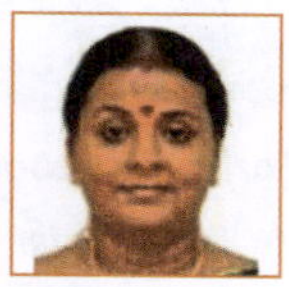
Dr Sindhu Devi
Ambalamugal, Kerala

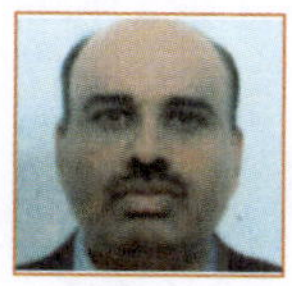
Dayal D Patidar
Gujarat

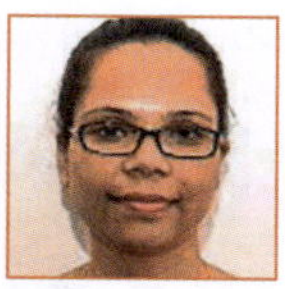
Dr Nurnahar Ahmed
Tezpur, Assam

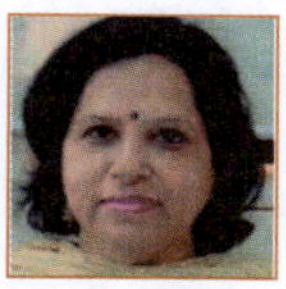
Dr Anju Dhir
New Delhi

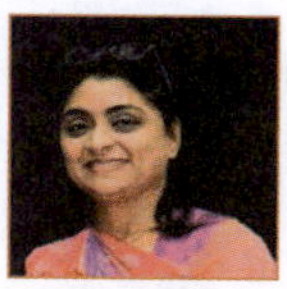
Dr Mallika Vhora
Vadodara, Gujarat

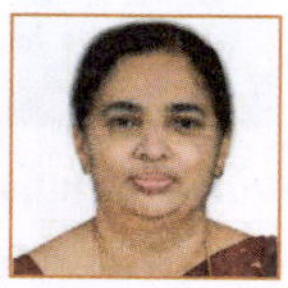
Dr Theyamma Joseph
Kottayam, Kerala

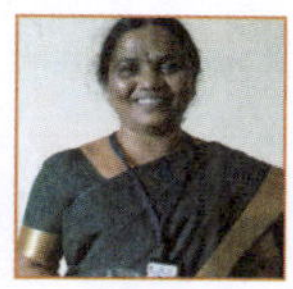
Dakshayini K P
Mysore, Karnataka

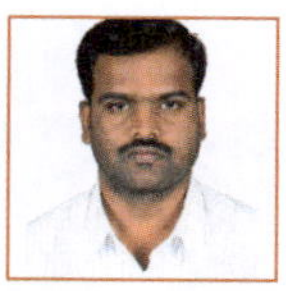
Dr T Sivabalan
Maharashtra

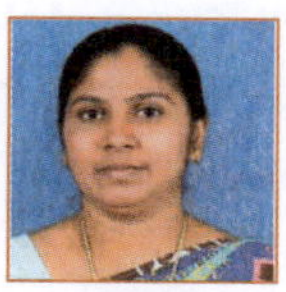
Dr A Jebarna Kiruba Mary
Kambipura, Karnataka

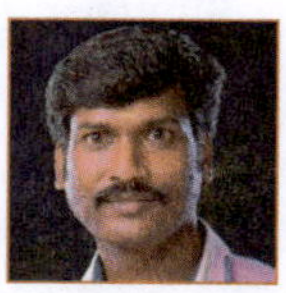
Dr Manikandan T
Kirumampakkam
Puducherry, Tamil Nadu

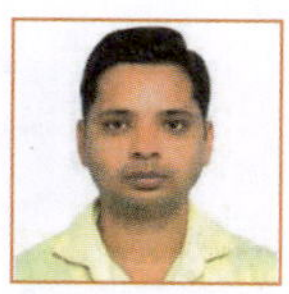
Deepak
Meerut, Uttar Pradesh

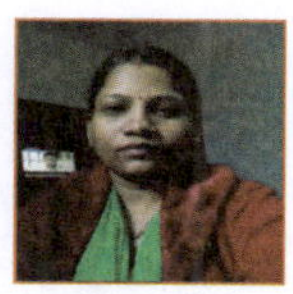
Dharitri Swain
Bhubaneswar, Odisha

For details of all reviewers & contributors refer TH Lite

New reviewers of TH 7/e covered in TH Lite (App)

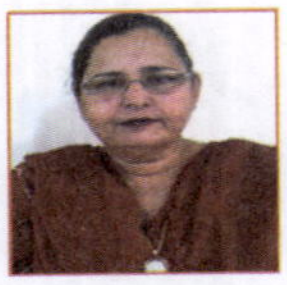

Darshan Kaur Sohi
Amritsar, Punjab

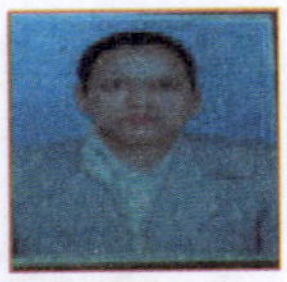

Davinder Kaur
Punjab

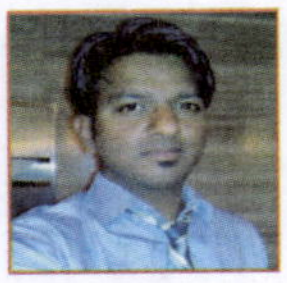

Deepak Shandilya
Mandi Gobindgarh
Punjab

E

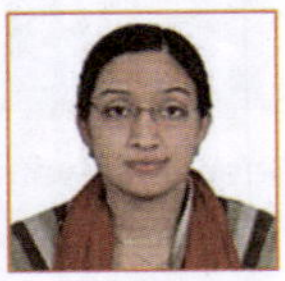

Emin Elsa Thomas
New Delhi

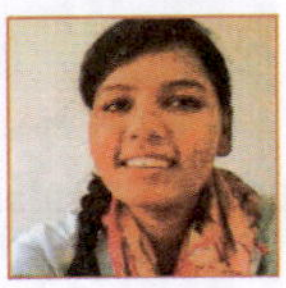

Eleena Kumari
Amritsar, Punjab

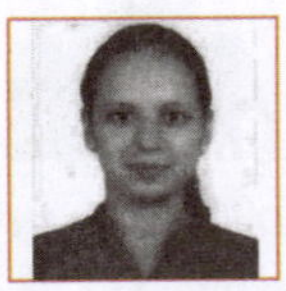

Eenu
Haryana

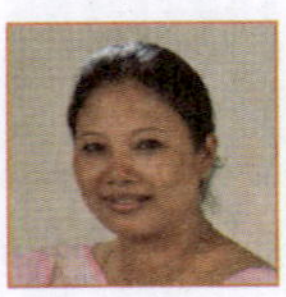

Elsa Sanatombi
Karnataka

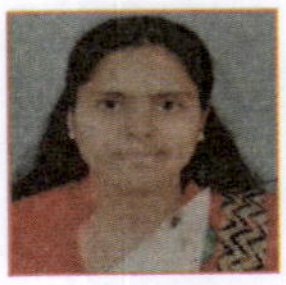

Elizabeth Chinadore
Bengaluru, Karnataka

F

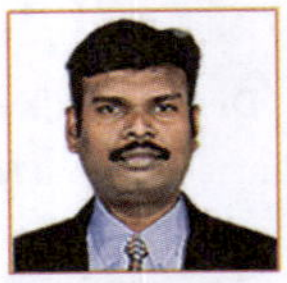

Frank J C
Tirunelveli
Tamil Nadu

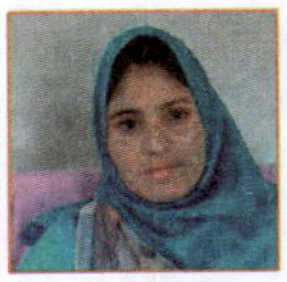

Fancy Rasool
Srinagar, J&K

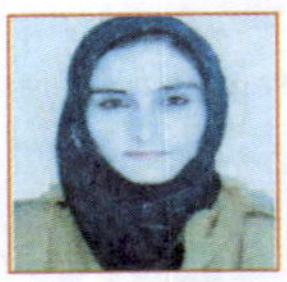

Foziya Manzoor
Awantipora, J&K

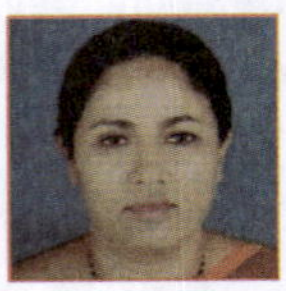

Firdose Fathima
Mysore, Karnataka

G

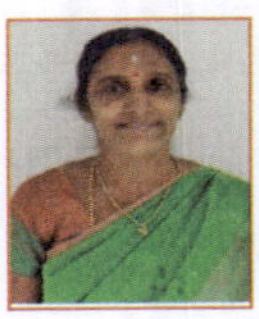

G Karpagam
Chennai, Tamil Nadu

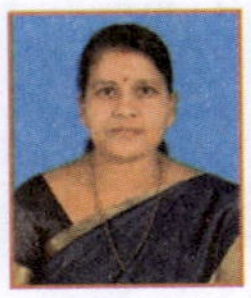

G Maheswari
Namakkal
Tamil Nadu

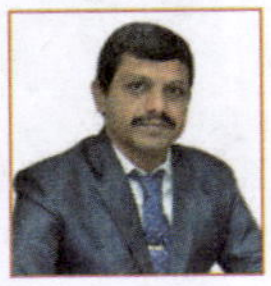

Gangadhar S Isarannavar
Ankola, Karnataka

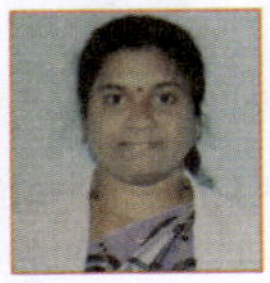

Geeta Toravi
Vijayapur, Karnataka

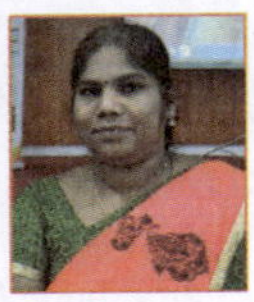

Geetha B
Bangalore, Karnataka

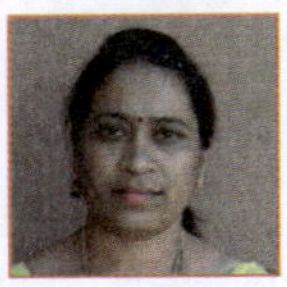

Geetha
Bengaluru, Karnataka

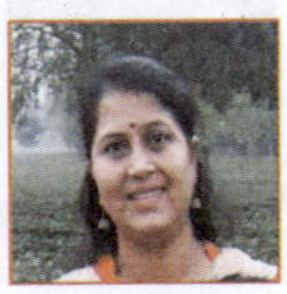

Gitumoni
Guwahati, Assam

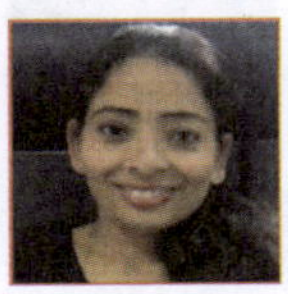

Ghodasara Jalpaben C
Rajkot, Gujarat

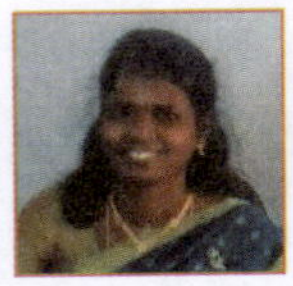

Gowri
Bengaluru, Karnataka

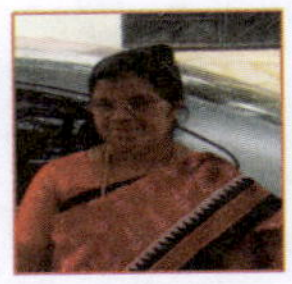

Gracy V C
Mysore, Karnataka

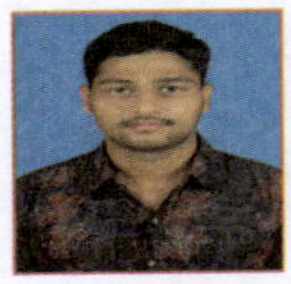

G Srinivasan
Lucknow, Uttar Pradesh

H

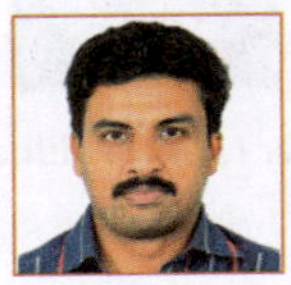

Harikrishna Beena
Kerala

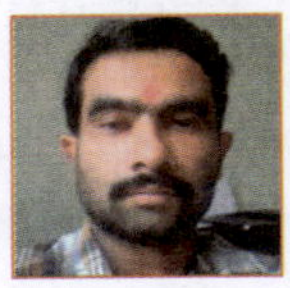

Hardik Kumar A Sharma
Ahmedabad, Gujarat

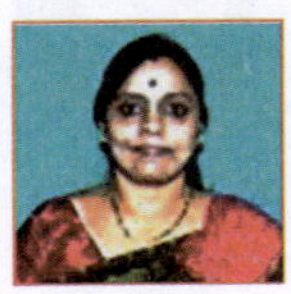

HN Chandrakala
Tumkur, Karnataka

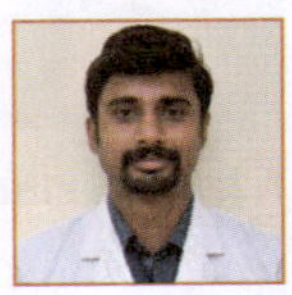

Harish Kumar Nair
Abu Road, Rajasthan

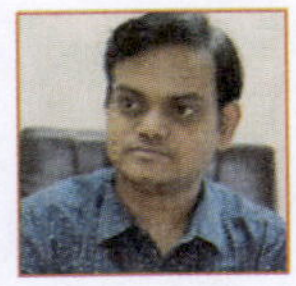

Hansmukh Jain
Patna, Bihar

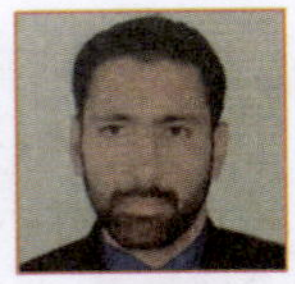

Haseeb Ali
Srinagar, J&K

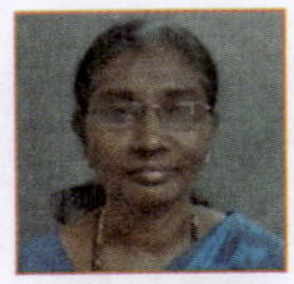

Helena D'silva
Mysore, Karnataka

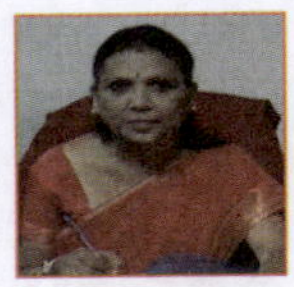

Hemavathy S
Bengaluru, Karnataka

I

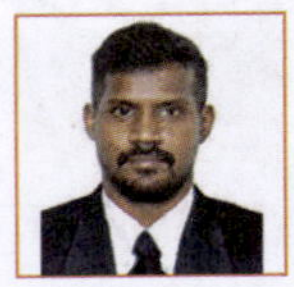

Israel Jeba Prabu
Madurai, Tamil Nadu

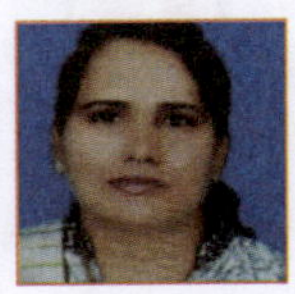

Indravati
Gujarat

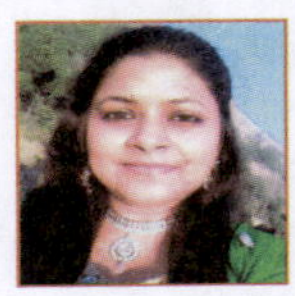

Indu Rathor
Solan, Himachal Pradesh

For details of all reviewers & contributors refer TH Lite

New reviewers of TH 7/e covered in TH Lite (App)

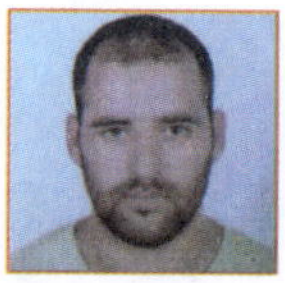

Iqbal Majid Dar
M A Road, Srinagar
J&K

J

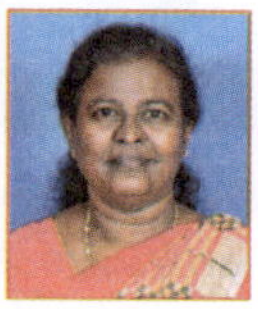

J Jasmine
Puducherry, Tamil Nadu

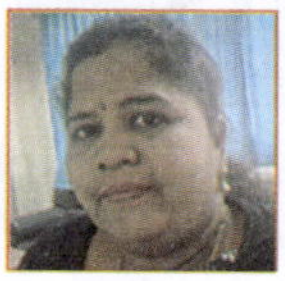

J Jeayareka
Raipur, Chattisgarh

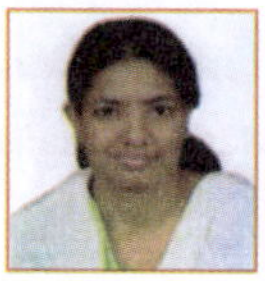

Jaya Shanthi Mani
Madurai, Tamil Nadu

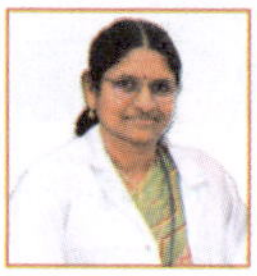

JC Helen Shaji
Chengalpattu, Tamil Nadu

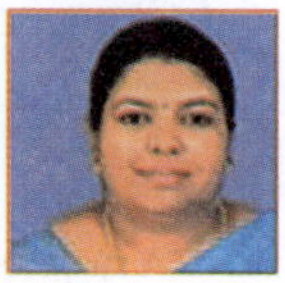

Jishi S Das
Thiruvananthapuram
Kerala

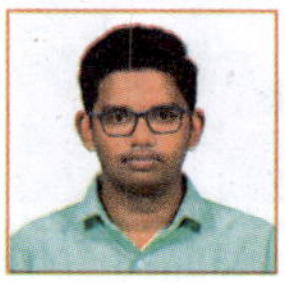

Joshwa
Saket, New Delhi

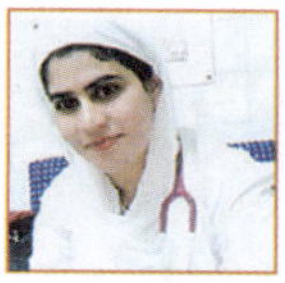

Joziea Farooq
Anantnag, J&K

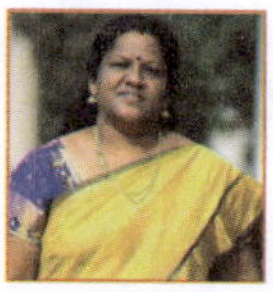

Julie Jestin A
Eluru, Andhra Pradesh
Vijayawada, Andhra Pradesh

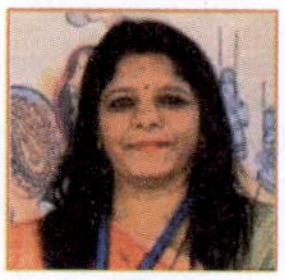

Jyoti Nirapure
Betul, Madhya Pradesh

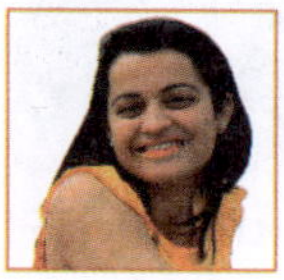

Jyoti Ruhil
New Delhi

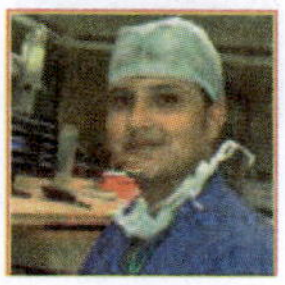

Jakir Husain Mansuri
New Delhi

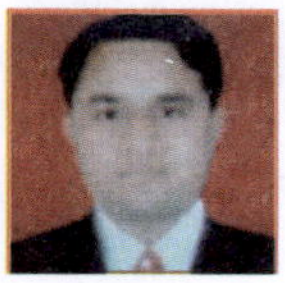

Jagdish Kumar
Jodhpur, Rajasthan

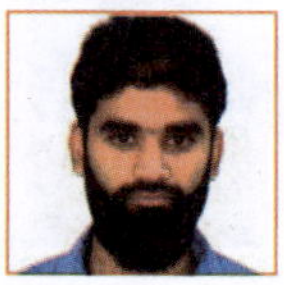

Javaid Ahmad Mir
Srinagar, J&K

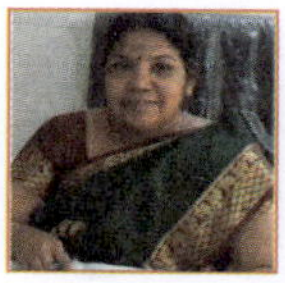

Jayalakshmi
Tumkur, Karnataka

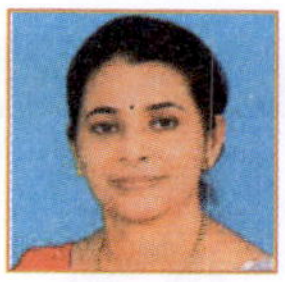

Jincy John
Kochi, Kerala

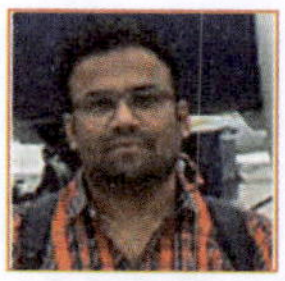

Jitendra Kumar
Jodhpur, Rajasthan

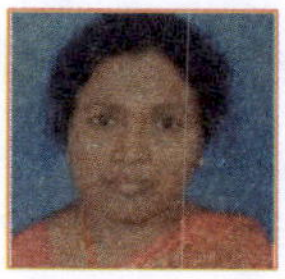

Joice Kalavathi
Bengaluru, Karnataka

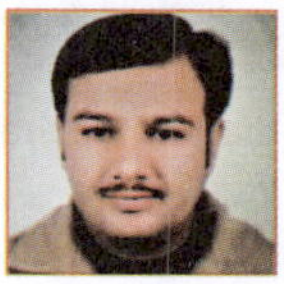

Jitendra Singh
Kishtwar, J&K

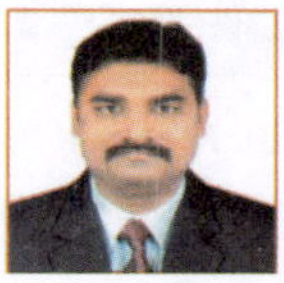

Jeenath Justin Doss K
Rajkot, Gujarat

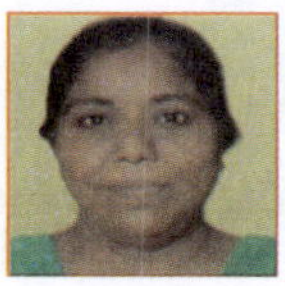

Judith Margret Morris
Ahmedabad, Gujarat

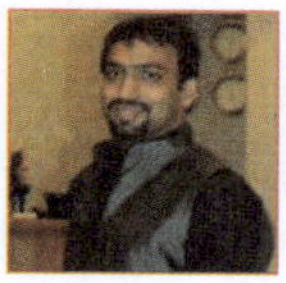

Jaideep Herbert
Haryana

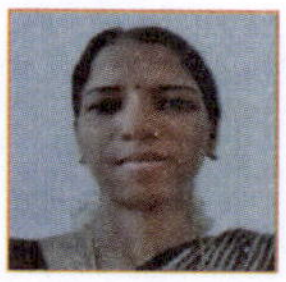

Jeeva Subramaniam
Karnataka

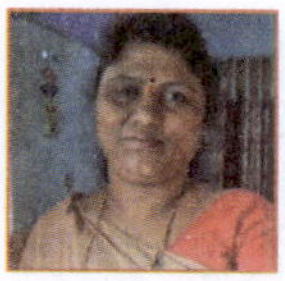

Jyothi
Bengaluru, Karnataka

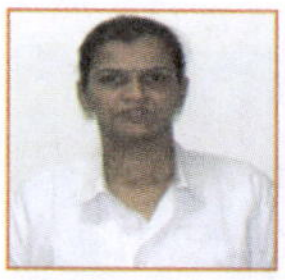

Jyotsna R Deshpande
Pune, Maharashtra

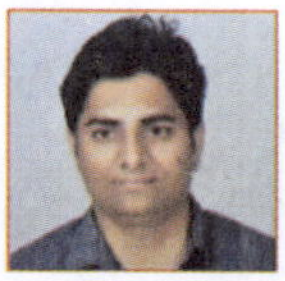

Jitendra Kumar Nagar
Rajasthan

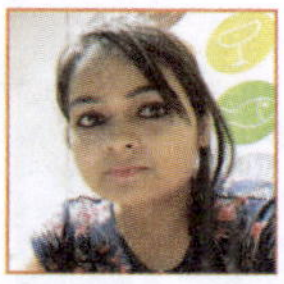

Jyoti Godhiyal
Lucknow, Uttar Pradesh

K

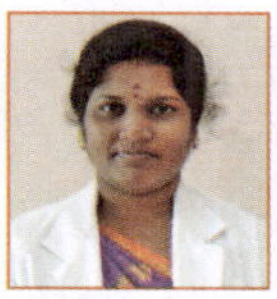

K Geetha
Karaikal, Puducherry
Tamil Nadu

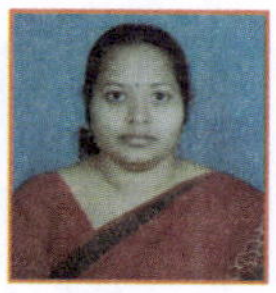

K Lakshmipriya
Tamil Nadu

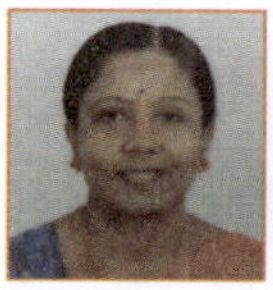

K N Jayanthi
Bangalore, Karnataka

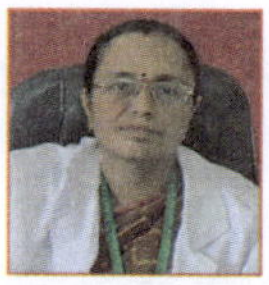

K P Abarnadevi
Chengalpet, Tamil Nadu

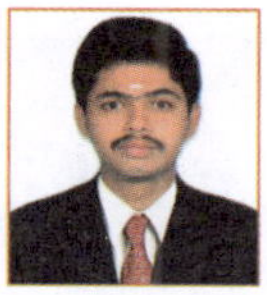

K Sesha Kumar
Valligatla Chittoor
Andhra Pradesh

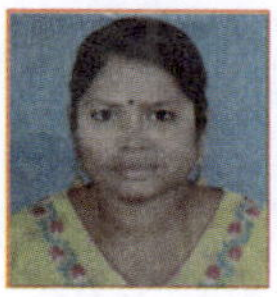

Kanitha D
Bangalore, Karnataka

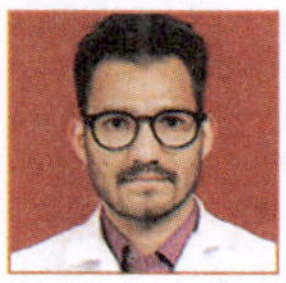

Kondal Naik. Megavath
Nalgonda, Maharashtra

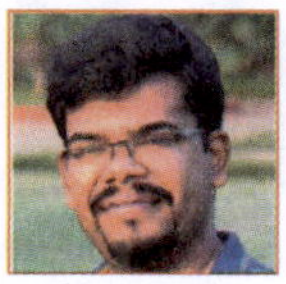

K Jayakrishnan
Kalyani, West Bengal

Our Valuable Reviewers & Contributors

For details of all reviewers & contributors refer TH Lite

New reviewers of TH 7/e covered in TH Lite (App)

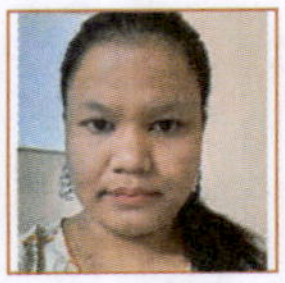

Khumukcham Anupama D
Patna, Bihar

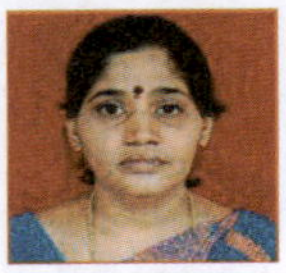

KS Mamatha
Tumkur, Karnataka

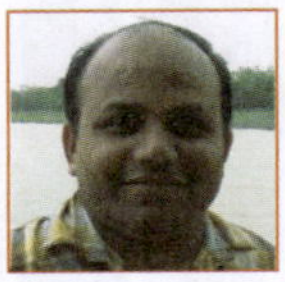

Khemchand
Himachal Pradesh

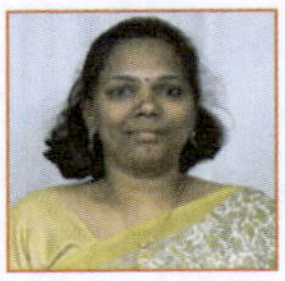

Krishnaveni Murugesh
Patna, Bihar

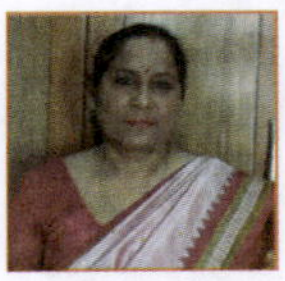

Krishna Das
Guwahati, Assam

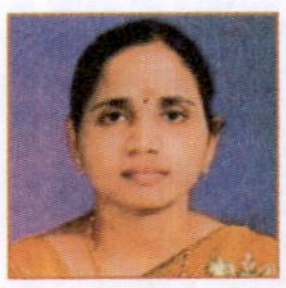

K Lakshmi Prasanna
Patna, Bihar

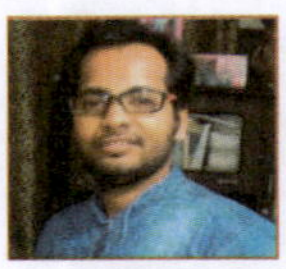

Kaushal Kishore
Chandigarh

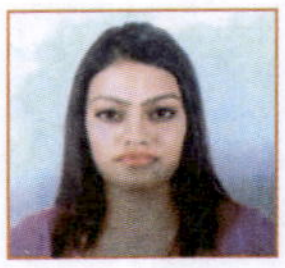

Kirandeep Kaur Parmar
Chandigarh

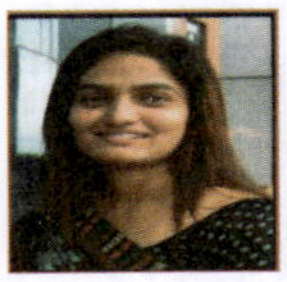

Kanika Rai
Ambala, Haryana

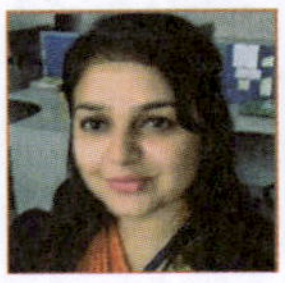

Kamini Chauhan
Gurgoan, Haryana

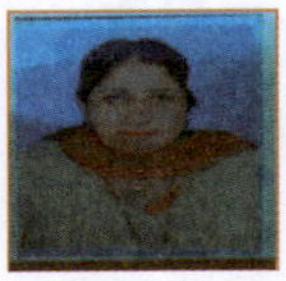

Krishna Dhawan
Himachal Pradesh

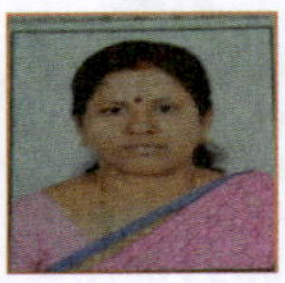

Kodimalar P
Bengaluru, Karnataka

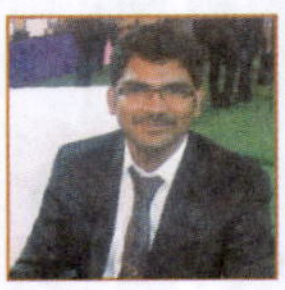

Karthikeyan Pethuswamy
New Delhi

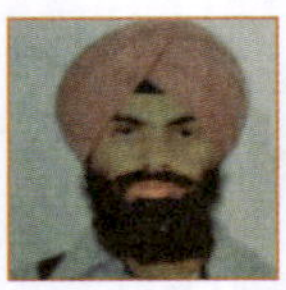

Kartar Singh
Gurdaspur, Punjab

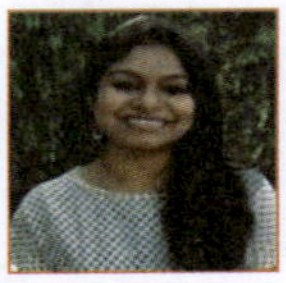

Keerthi Mohannan
Patna, Bihar

L

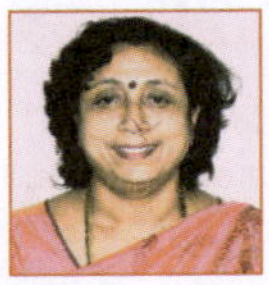

L Lakshmi
Chennai, Tamil Nadu

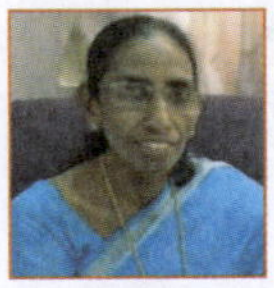

Lizzie Raveendran
Coimbatore
Tamil Nadu

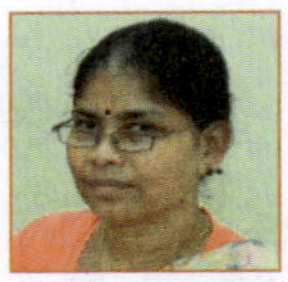

Latha Damodaran
Kollam, Kerala

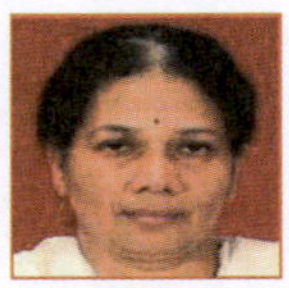

Lt Col. Meera K Pillai
Thiruvananthapuram
Kerala

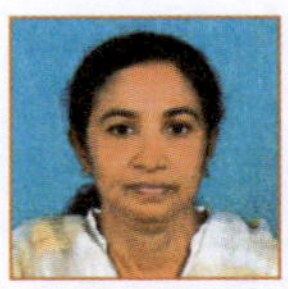

Lt Col. Sheela Paul (Retd)
Ernakulam, Kerala

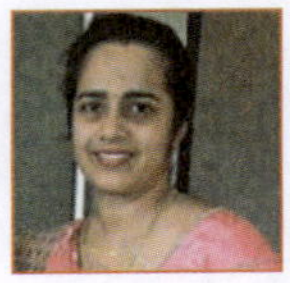

Lolita Dsouza
Mangalore
Karnataka

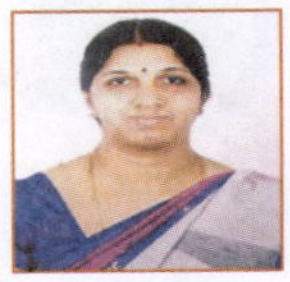

Lakshmi A
Bengaluru, Karnataka

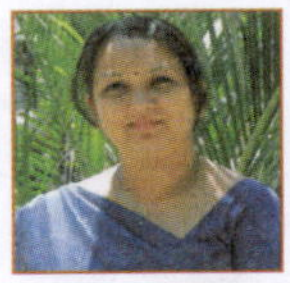

Lily Podder
Pune
Maharashtra

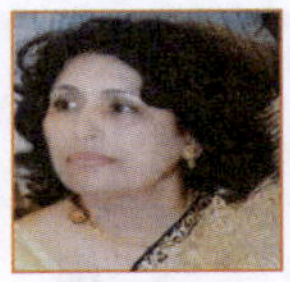

Liza Sharma
Punjab

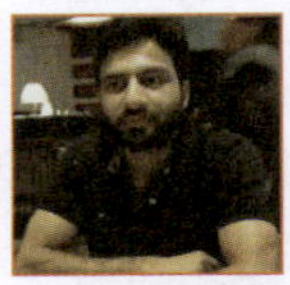

Laxhman Yadav
Rajasthan

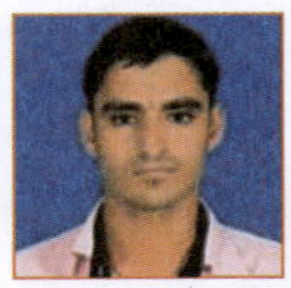

Lakshman Chaudhary
Rajasthan

M

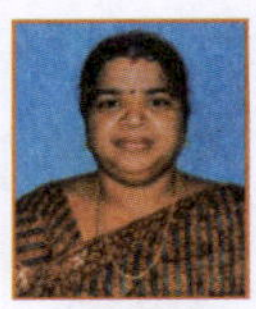

M Hemamalini
Chennai, Tamil Nadu

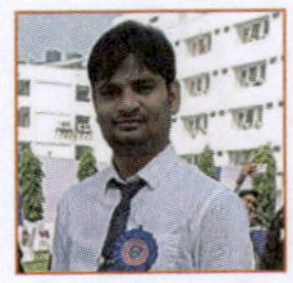

Madan Mohan Gupta
Lucknow
Uttar Pradesh

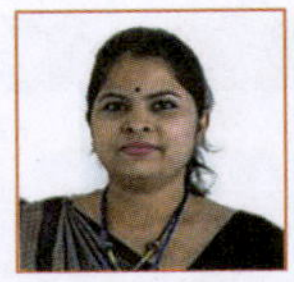

Madhusmita Nayak
Bhubaneswar, Odisha

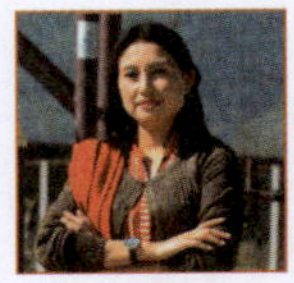

Maibam Ranita Devi
Imphal, Manipur

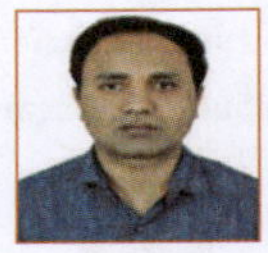

Manjunatha H
Bangalore
Karnataka

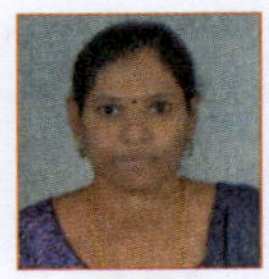

Menaga P
Bangalore,
Karnataka

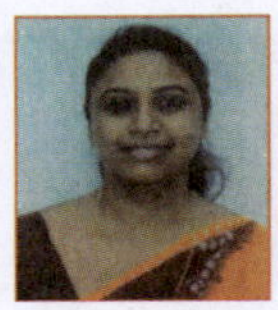

Mercy A Anjore
Nagpur
Maharashtra

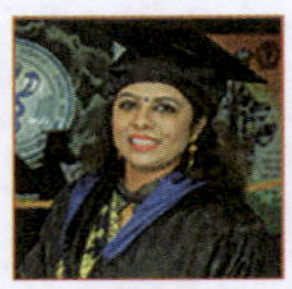

Monika Kankarwal
New Delhi

For details of all reviewers & contributors refer TH Lite

New reviewers of TH 7/e covered in TH Lite (App)

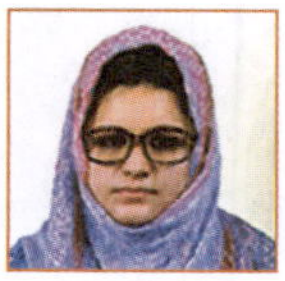
Mujasam Rasool
Khanabal Handwara
J&K

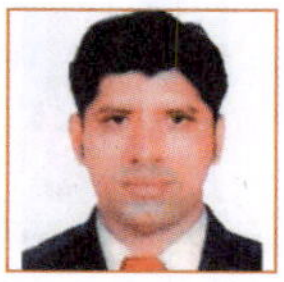
Mohd. Atif Muzammil
Mumbai
Maharashtra

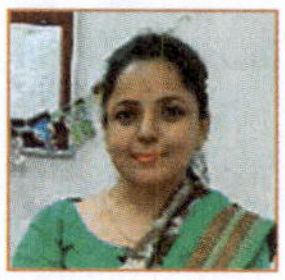
Manvirpal Kaur
Ludhiana, Punjab

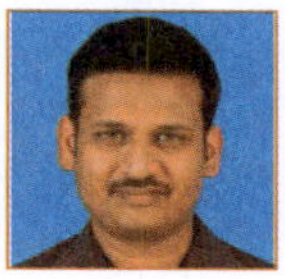
M Jawahar Babu
New Delhi

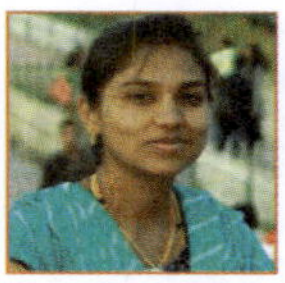
Manjula S
Ramanagara, Karnataka

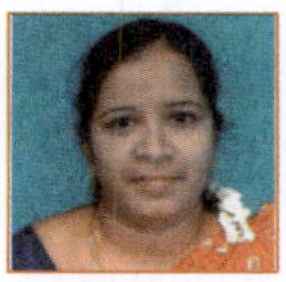
M Angelin Dhanalakshmi
Kancheepuram
Tamil Nadu

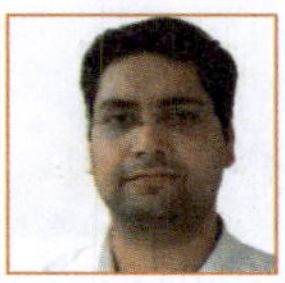
Manish Kumar Tripathi
Bhilwara, Rajasthan

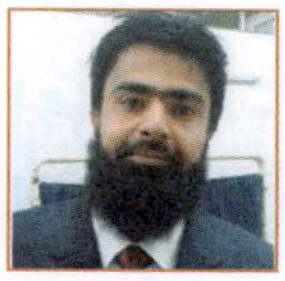
Mohd Suhail Jogi
Srinagar, J&K

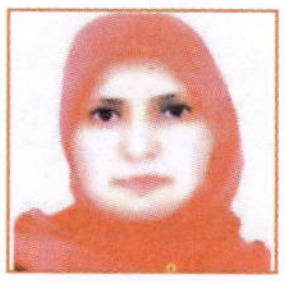
Mubashir Bashir
Awantipora, J&K

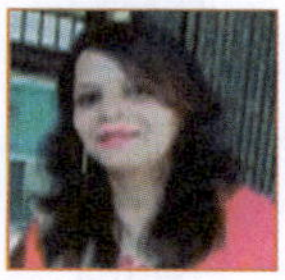
Mubina Akhtar
Srinagar, J&K

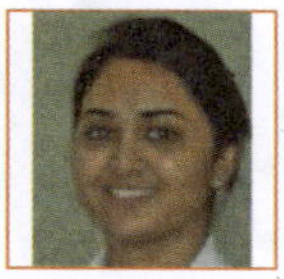
Monika Thakur
New Delhi

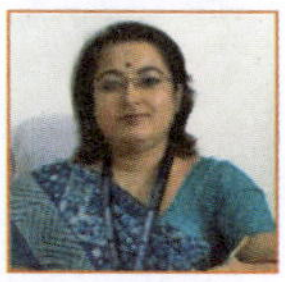
Manashi Sengupta
Assam

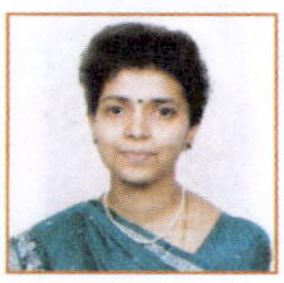
Manju Dhandapani
Chandigarh, Punjab

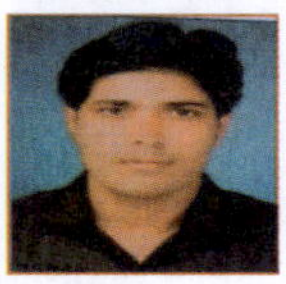
Mukesh Malav
Chandigarh

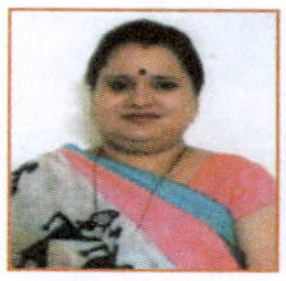
Monika Sharma
Himachal Pradesh

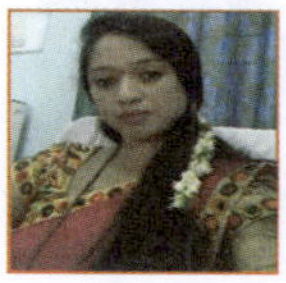
Mangala V
Bengaluru, Karnataka

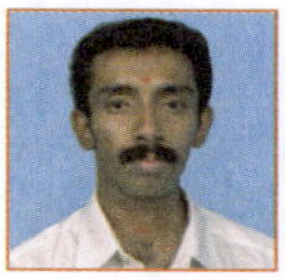
Manikuttan N
Kerala

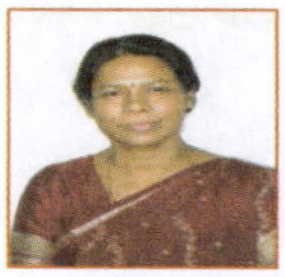
Manju Joshi
Indore, Madhya Pradesh

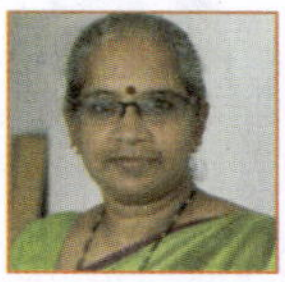
Mangalam Sriram
Thane, Maharashtra

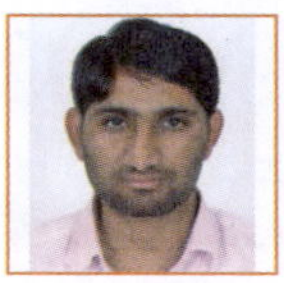
Mahaveer Singh
New Delhi

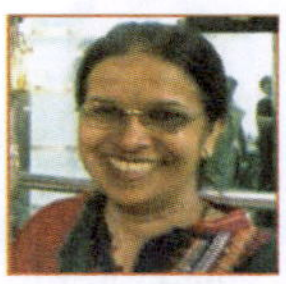
Molly Babu
New Delhi

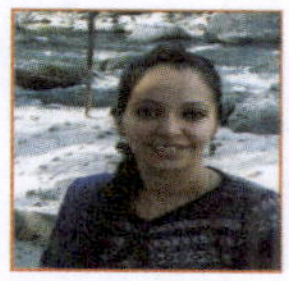
Madhuri Kashyap
Punjab

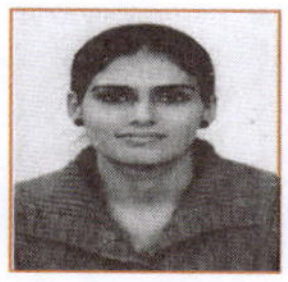
Maninder Kaur
Punjab

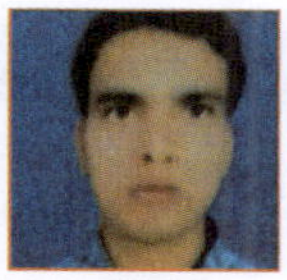
Manish Saraswat
Jodhpur, Rajasthan

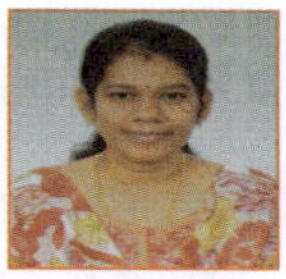
M P Saraswathy
Chennai, Tamil Nadu

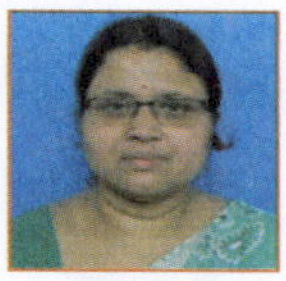
Mamita Dey
Kolkata, West Bengal

N

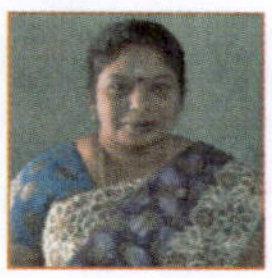
N Kalaikuruselvi
Tamil Nadu

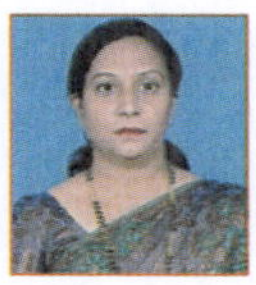
Namratha N
Chamarajanagar
Karnataka

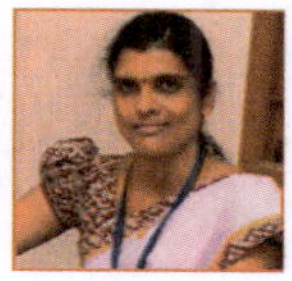
N Gowri
Thanjavur, Tamil Nadu

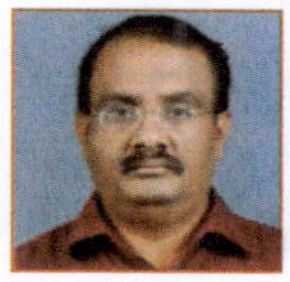
N Thanga Durai
Chennai, Tamil Nadu

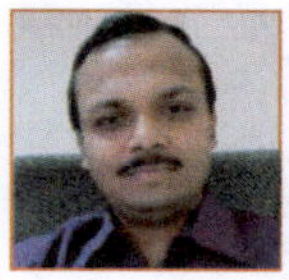
Naveen Kumar Sharma
Patna, Bihar

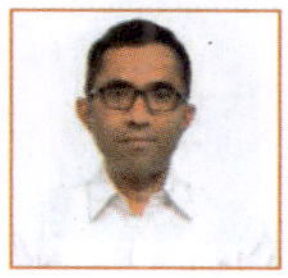
Nitish Dubey
New Delhi

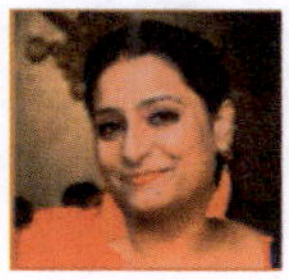
Nitasha Arora
New Delhi

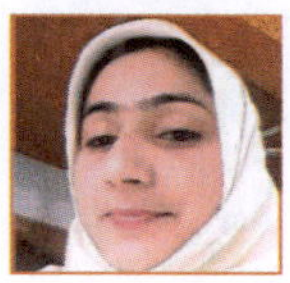
Nahida Shafi
Srinagar, J&K

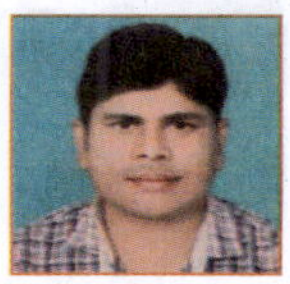
Nanak Chand Sumar
Alwar, Rajasthan

Our Valuable Reviewers & Contributors

For details of all reviewers & contributors refer TH Lite

New reviewers of TH 7/e covered in TH Lite (App)

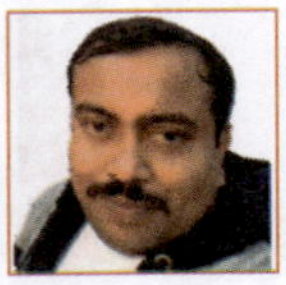

Naveena JH
Gurugram, Haryana

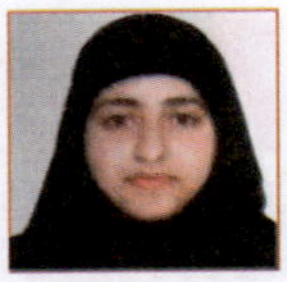

Nazimah Parvaiz Khan
Srinagar, J&K

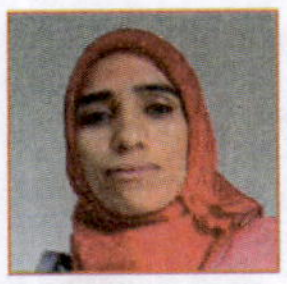

Nazneena Akhter
Srinagar, J&K

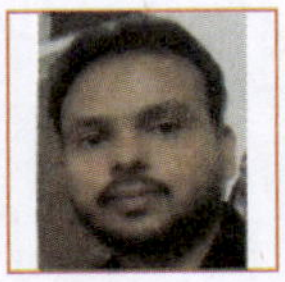

Navneet Mudgal
Rajasthan

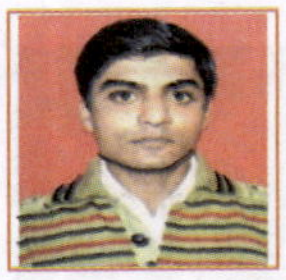

Narendra Kumar Sharma
Gujarat

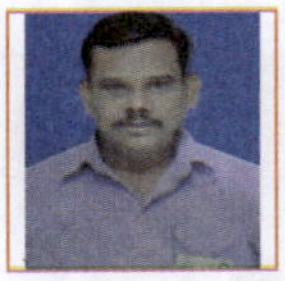

Navin Kumar
Rajkot, Gujarat

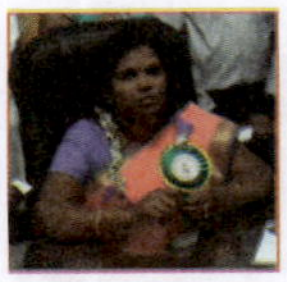

N T Aruna Devi
Mysore, Karnataka

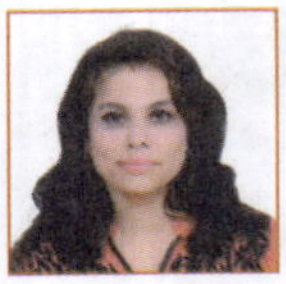

Nisha S Naik
Pune, Maharashtra

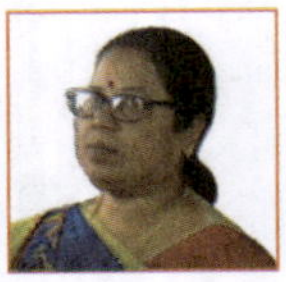

Niyati Das
Bhubaneswar, Odisha

P

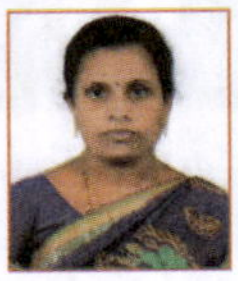

P Sathiavathy
Puducherry, Tamil Nadu

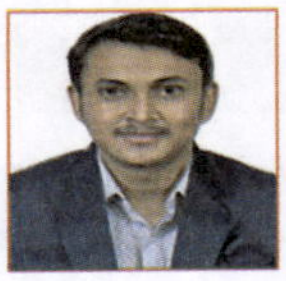

Praful Damor
Vadodara, Gujarat

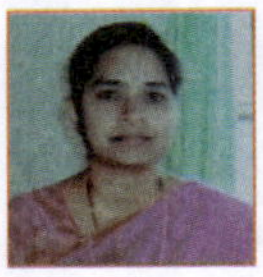

Pratibha Swami
Bangalore, Karnataka

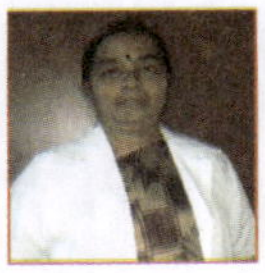

Prema Anbalagan
Chennai, Tamil Nadu

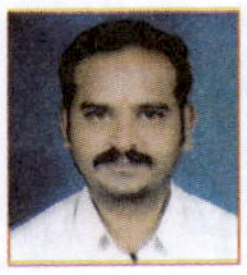

Punithamani G
Chitradurga, Karnataka

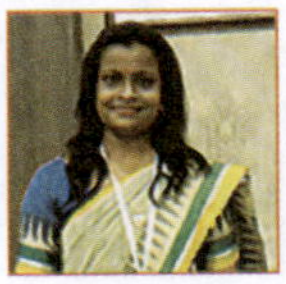

Purnima Sahoo
Bhubaneswar, Odisha

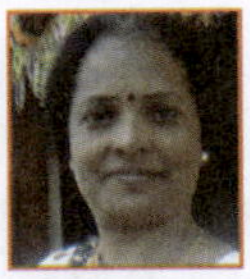

Pushpalata G Sandimani
Karnataka

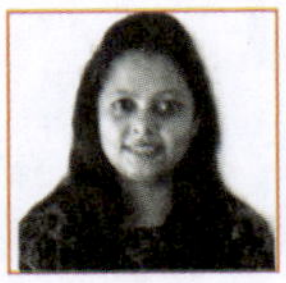

Priyanka
Amritsar, Punjab

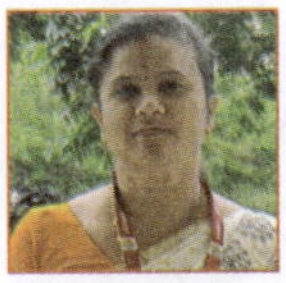

Priya M
AIIMS, Mangalagiri

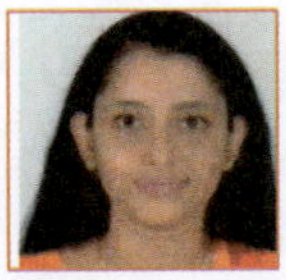

Priyanka Elizabeth Thomas
Patna, Bihar

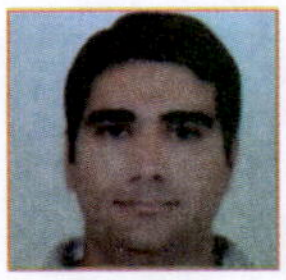

Prakash Mahala
Rishikesh, Uttrakhand

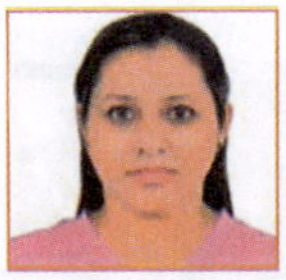

Payal Kahol
New Delhi

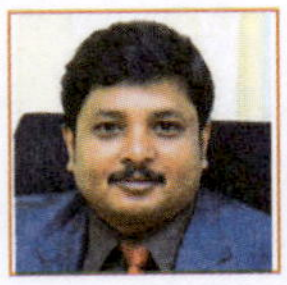

P Karthikeyaprasath
Bengaluru, Karnataka

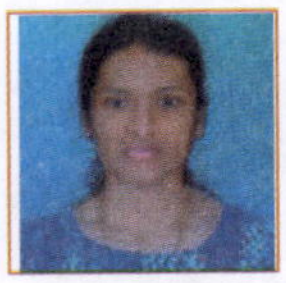

Prabhavati Savant
Dandeli, Karnataka

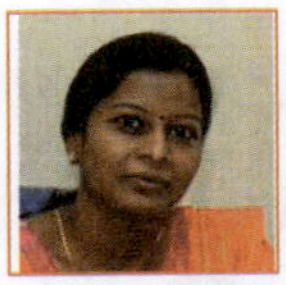

Preetha
Chikmagalur, Karnataka

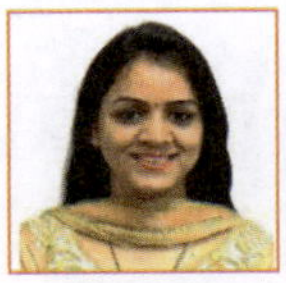

Priya Sharma
Vishakhapatanam
Andhra Pradesh

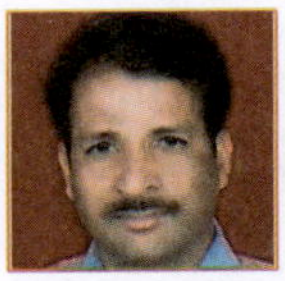

Prof Vir Vikram Sahdev Singh
Meerut, Uttar Pradesh

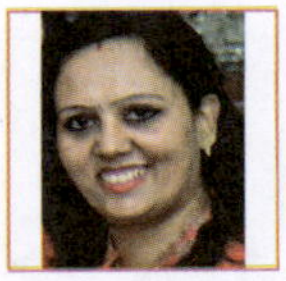

Poonam Sharma
Una, Himachal Pradesh

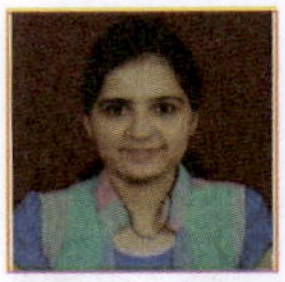

Priyanka Malhotra
Rishikesh, Uttarakhand

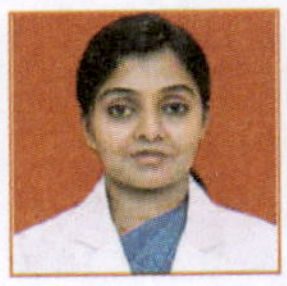

Pratiti Haldar
Haldwani, Uttarakhand

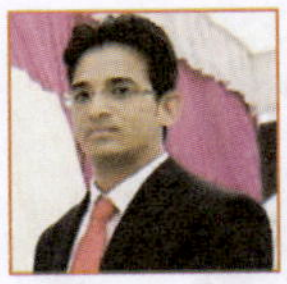

Prahlad Devenda
Jodhpur, Rajasthan

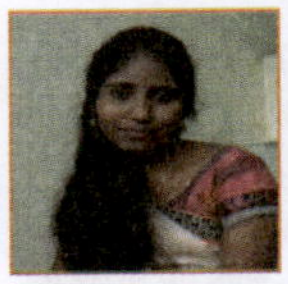

P Thulasiammal
Chandigarh

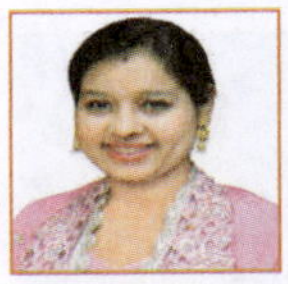

Parmees Kaur
Chandigarh

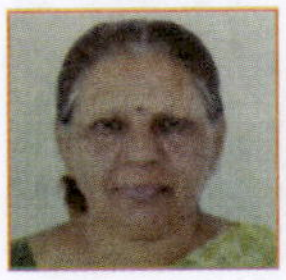

Pratima Mali
Ahmedabad, Gujarat

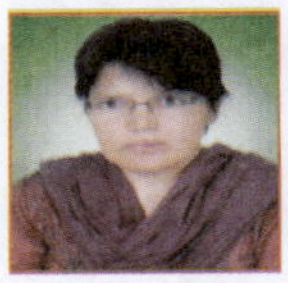

Prabha Kashyap
Shimla, Himachal Pradesh

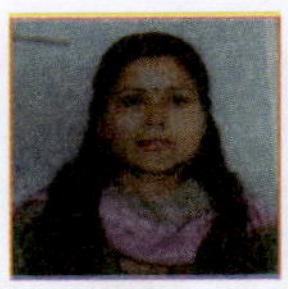

Pushpa Panwar
Shimla, Himachal Pradesh

For details of all reviewers & contributors refer TH Lite

New reviewers of TH 7/e covered in TH Lite (App)

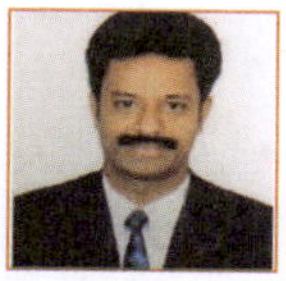

P Muniyasamy
Chitradurga, Karnataka

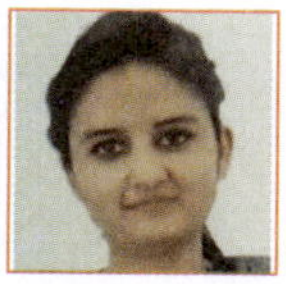

Prabhjot Kaur
Amritsar, Punjab

R

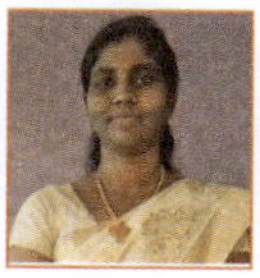

R Arul Malar
Coimbatore, Tamil Nadu

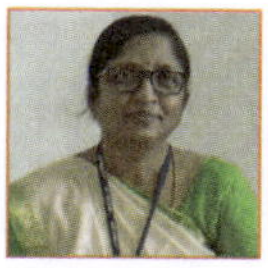

R Revathi
Madurai, Tamil Nadu

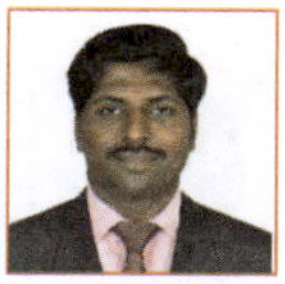

R Velmurugan
Bhopal, Madhya Pradesh

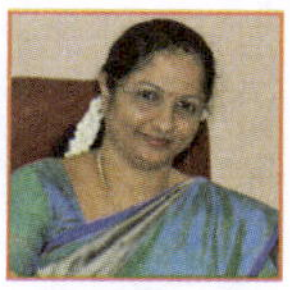

R Vijayalakshmi
Chennai, Tamil Nadu

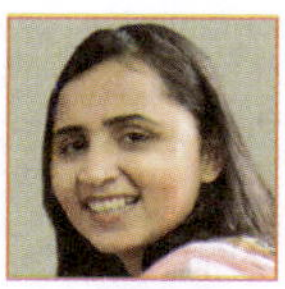

Ramandeep Kaur
Chandigarh

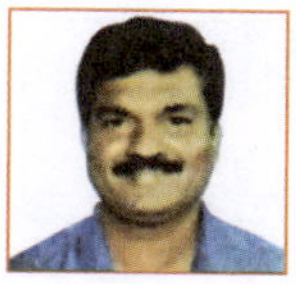

Raveesh Kumar
Vidyanagar, Hubli
Andhra Pradesh

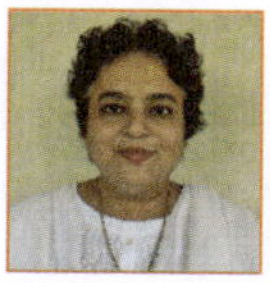

Rebecca Jadhav
Jabalpur, Madhya Pradesh

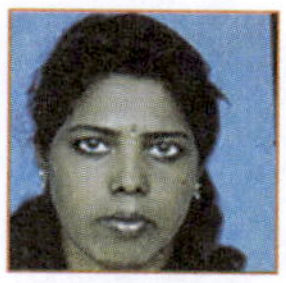

Renu B
Thiruvananthapuram
Kerala

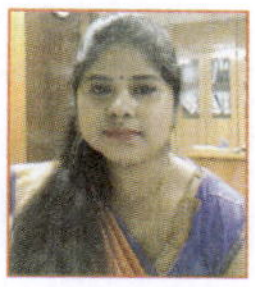

Renuka Malladad
Bangalore, Karnataka

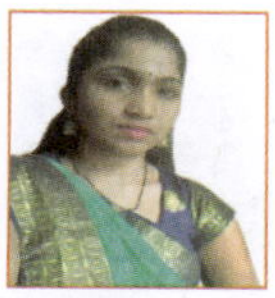

Reshma Kharvi
Bangalore, Karnataka

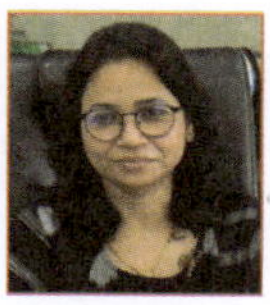

Rupa Ashok Verma
Nagpur, Maharashtra

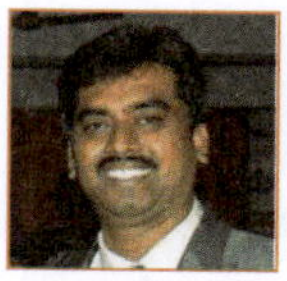

Redeppa Sree Raja Kumar
Greater Noida
Uttar Pradesh

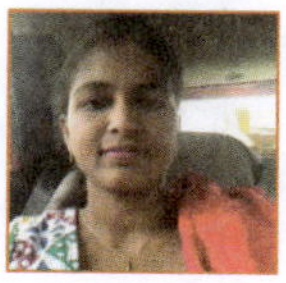

Rajeshwari G
New Delhi

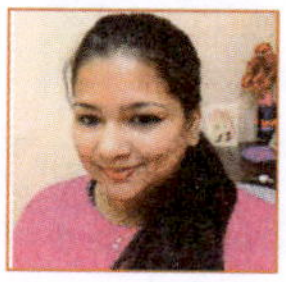

Rebecka Thananki
Patna, Bihar

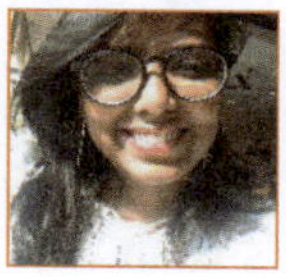

Rachel Dutt
New Delhi

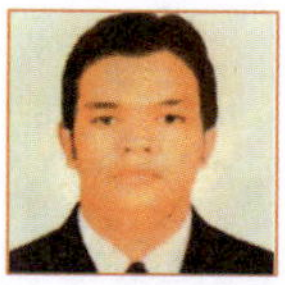

Rajesh Joshi
Mehsana, Gujarat

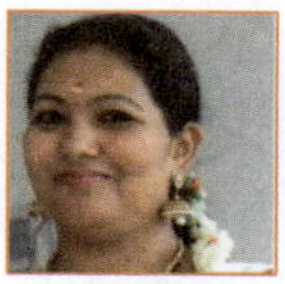

Rakhi Nath
Bengaluru, Karnataka

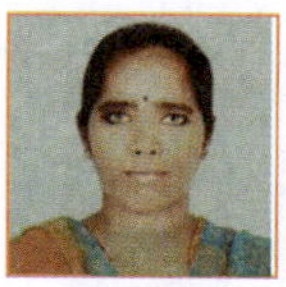

Ranganayaki L
Amritsar, Punjab

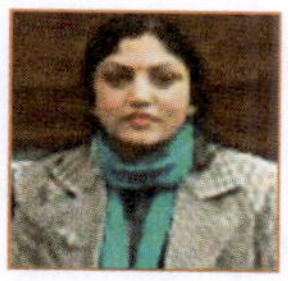

Reena Dogra
Shimla, Himachal Pradesh

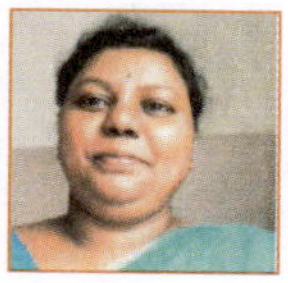

Regina Shoba Dass
Bengaluru, Karnataka

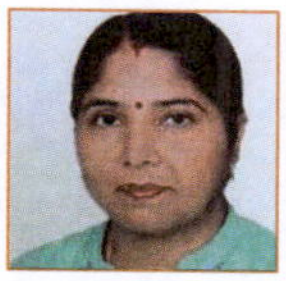

Rekha Anil Kumar
New Delhi

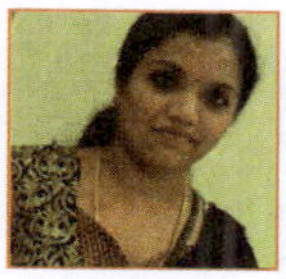

Revathy Duraiswami
Kelambakkam
Tamil Nadu

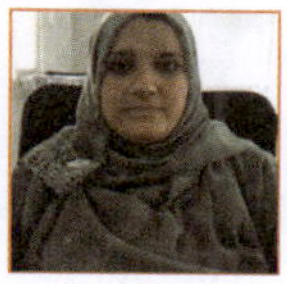

Rohi Jan
Awantipora, J&K

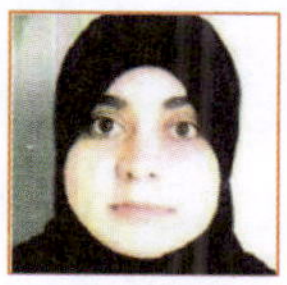

Rohi Jan
Srinagar, J&K

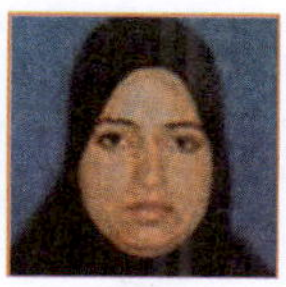

Roohi Jan
Awantipora, J&K

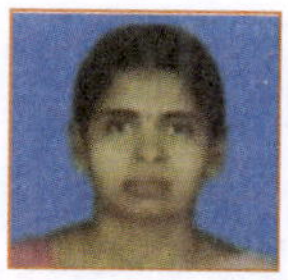

Reena Govindraja
Andhra Pradesh

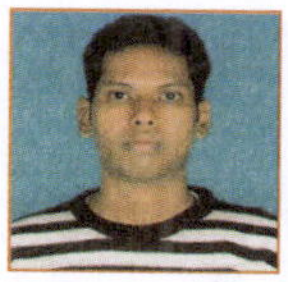

Rohit Yadav
Udaipur, Rajasthan

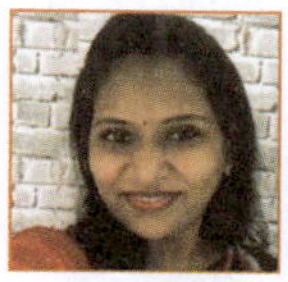

Renu Nagar
Navi Mumbai
Maharashtra

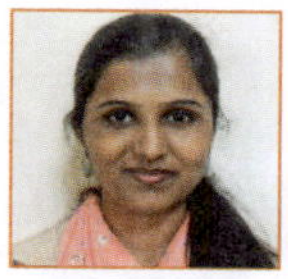

Ramya Vasanth
Patna, Bihar

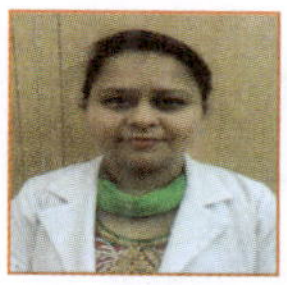

Rajbeer Kaur
Chandigarh

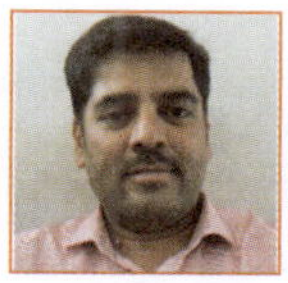

Ravindra JH
Gujarat

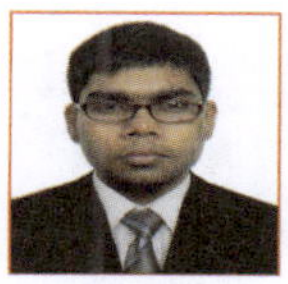

Rupindra A Bharathi
Shimla,
Himachal Pradesh

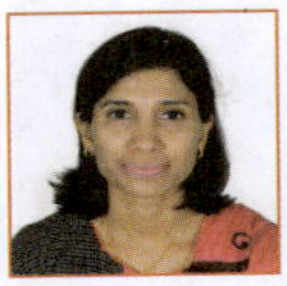
Reena George
Bengaluru, Karnataka

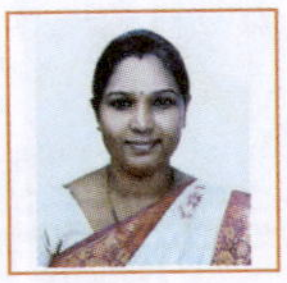
Rakhi Phandse
Indore
Madhya Pradesh

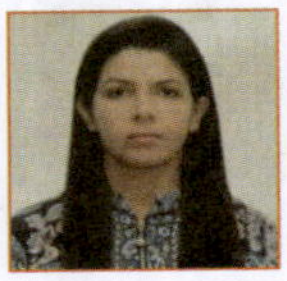
Rachna Sharma
New Delhi

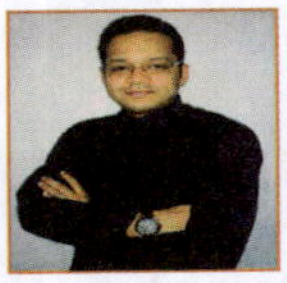
Ranjan Patel
New Delhi

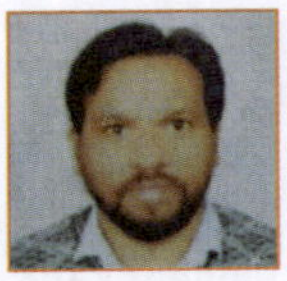
Rizwan Khan
Jalalabad, Punjab

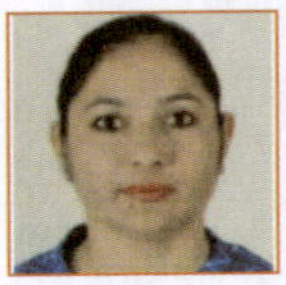
Rupinder Kaur
Amritsar, Punjab

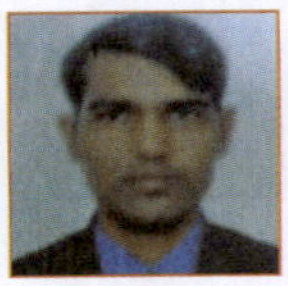
Ram Lakhan Mali
Dera Bassi,
Punjab

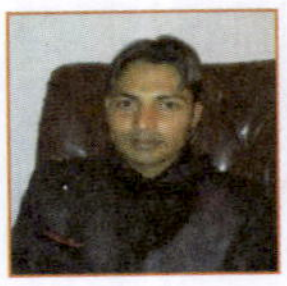
Raghunandan Singh
Punjab

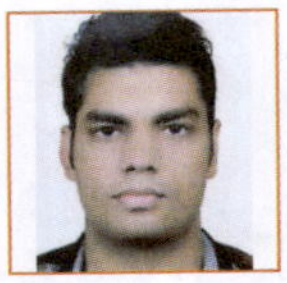
Ravi Prakash Jangid
Deoli (Tonk)
Rajasthan

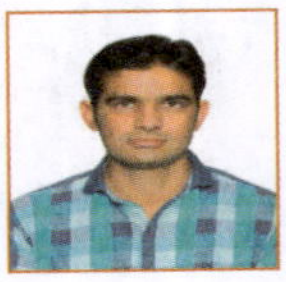
Rajesh K Bhaira
Sikar, Rajasthan

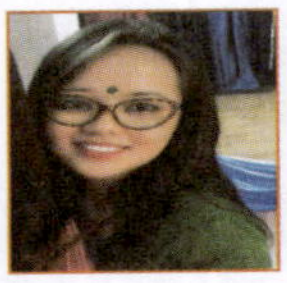
Reshma Tamang
Sikkim

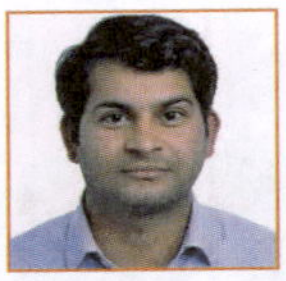
Rajesh Kumar Kataria
Rishikesh, Uttarakhand

S

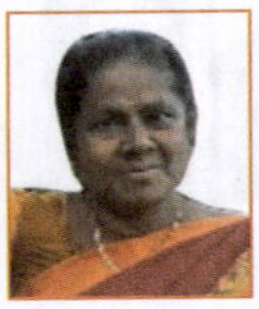
S Kamalam
Puducherry, Tamil Nadu

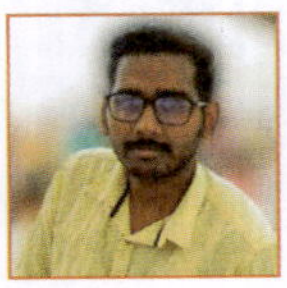
S Karthi
AIIMS Delhi

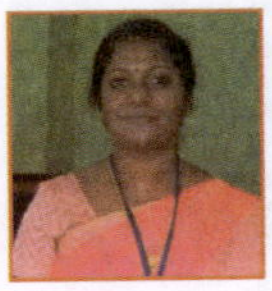
S Punitha Josephine
Tamil Nadu

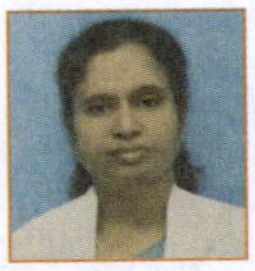
S Rajamani
Madurai, Tamil Nadu

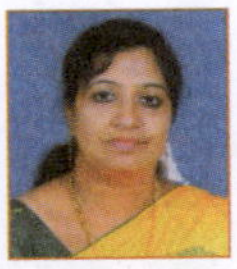
S S Sharmila Jansi Rani
Neyyoor, Tamil Nadu

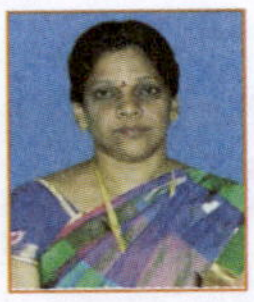
S Tamilselvi
Tiruvannamalai
Tamil Nadu

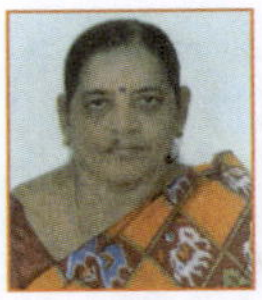
S Thaiyalnayaki
Chennai, Tamil Nadu

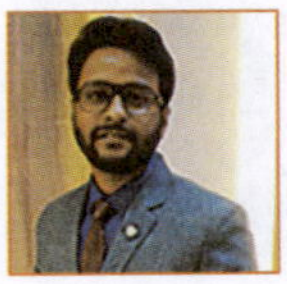
Sahil George
Varanasi
Uttar Pradesh

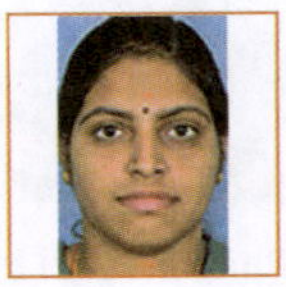
Sandhya Ramachandran
Chennai, Tamil Nadu

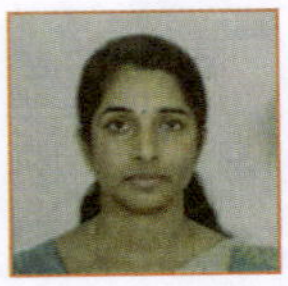
Sangeetha Freddy
Thiruvananthapuram,
Kerala

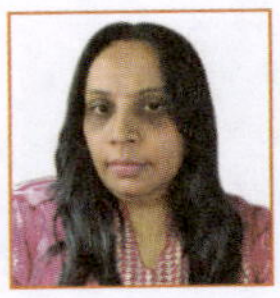
Sangeetha K
Bangalore
Karnataka

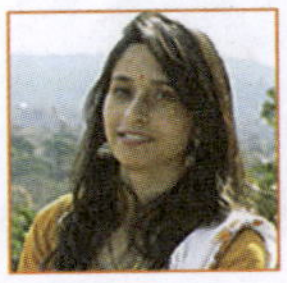
Sanjana Kumari
Greater Noida
Uttar Pradesh

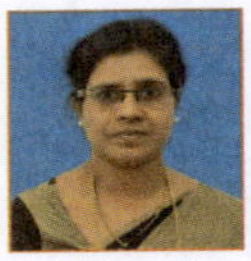
Santhi Appavu
Neyyoor
Tamil Nadu

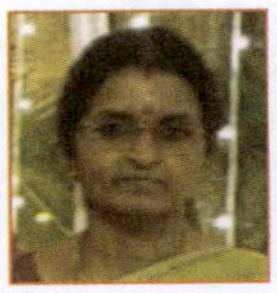
Santhi N
Coimbatore
Tamil Nadu

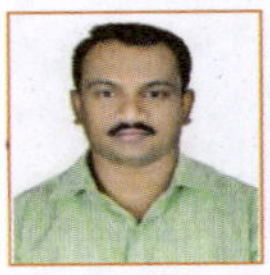
Santosh Shindhe
Bhandara
Maharashtra

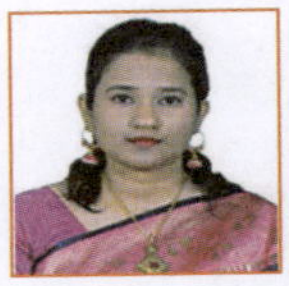
Sarbattama Nayak
Bhubaneswar, Odisha

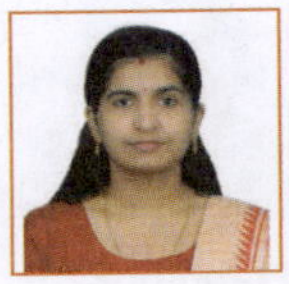
Sarika M L
Bhubaneswar
Odisha

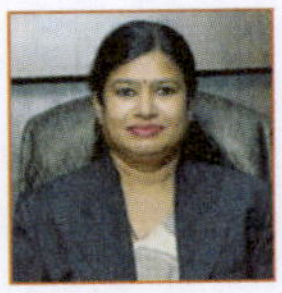
Seema Singh
Nagpur
Maharashtra

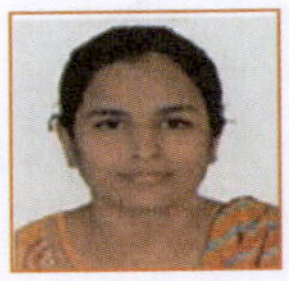
Shailaja M J Mathews
Pune, Maharashtra

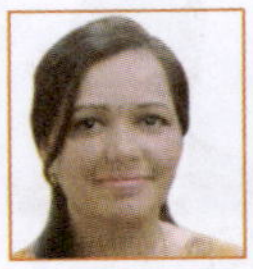
Shankarevva
Bangalore, Karnataka

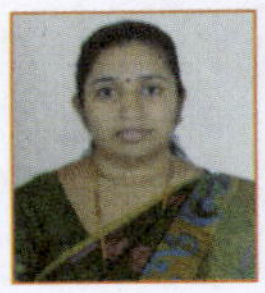
Shini Raju Gouli
Davangere, Karnataka

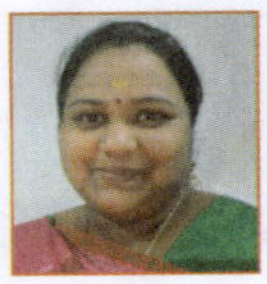
Shiny Mol K
Tamil Nadu

For details of all reviewers & contributors refer TH Lite

New reviewers of TH 7/e covered in TH Lite (App)

Our Valuable Reviewers & Contributors

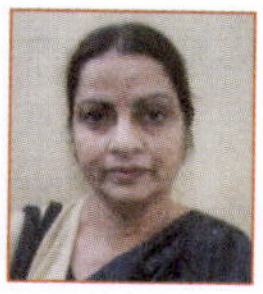

Shobha Dahiya
Bangalore, Karnataka

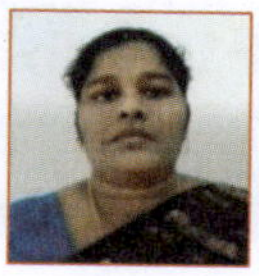

Suja Venisha
Tirunelveli, Tamil Nadu

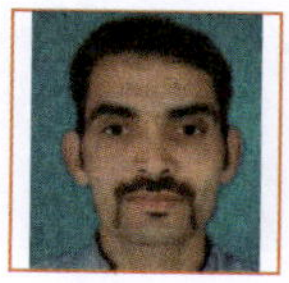

Shravan Kumar
Patna, Bihar

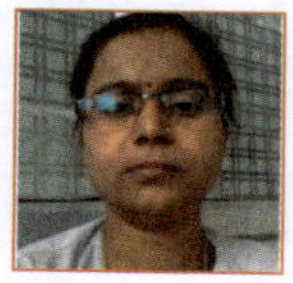

Sarita K Gaurav
Lucknow, Uttar Pradesh

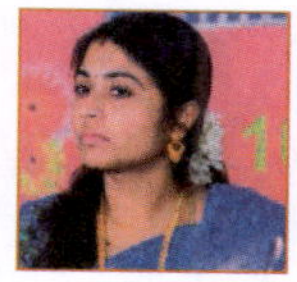

Shruthi N
Shivamogga, Karnataka

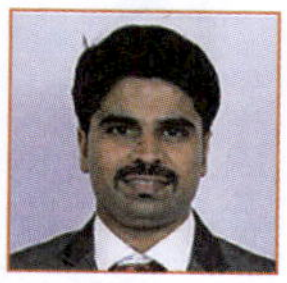

Shrikant Desai
Rishikesh, Uttrakhand

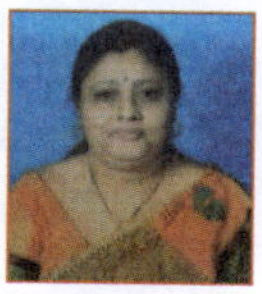

Suneeta Davey
Akola, Maharashtra

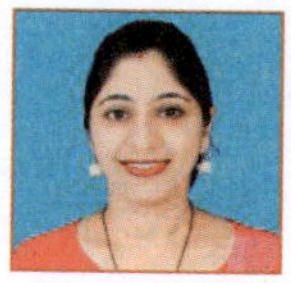

Sushma Pandey
Mumbai, Maharashtra

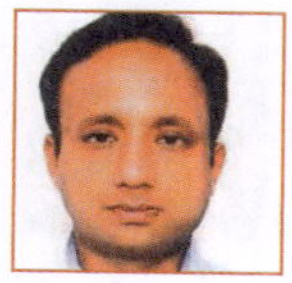

Salish Chand Bansal
Badal, Punjab

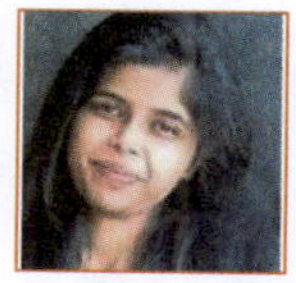

Shweta
Jamia Hamdard
New Delhi

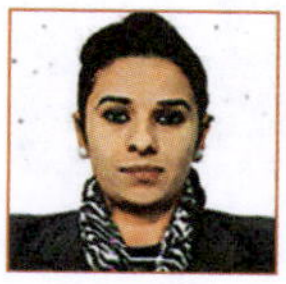

Sonia Singh
Greater Noida
Uttar Pradesh

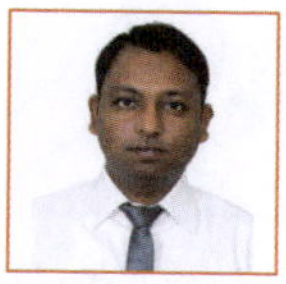

Sunil Singh
Ludhiana, Punjab

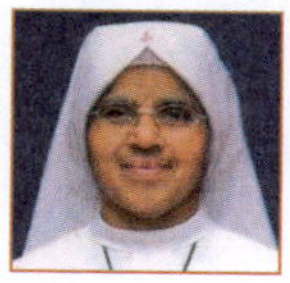

Sr Rubeena
Ernakulam, Kerala

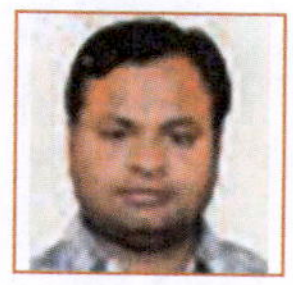

Shakil Ahmad
Alwar, Rajasthan

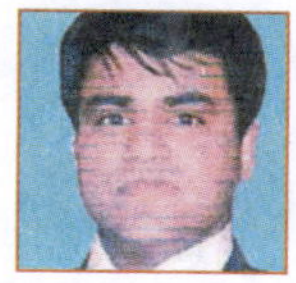

Sumit Kumar Sharma
Jaipur, Rajasthan

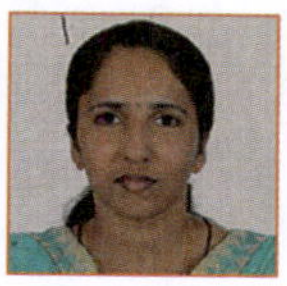

Sony Thomas
Kottayam, Kerala

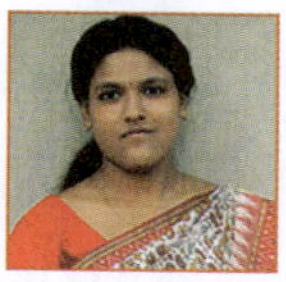

Suvashri Sasmal
Kolkata, West Bengal

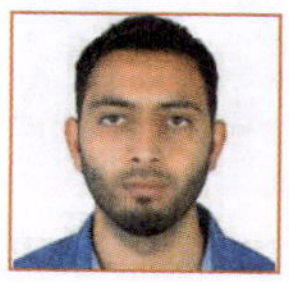

Sameer Ahmad Dar
Srinagar, J&K

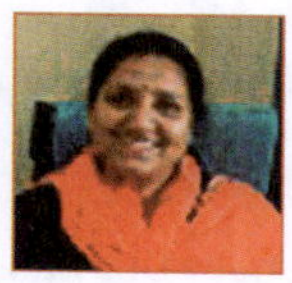

Shashi Sharma
Shimla, Himachal Pradesh

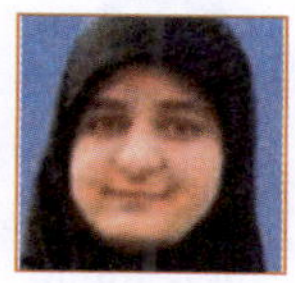

Sumyra Nazir
Gurugram, Haryana

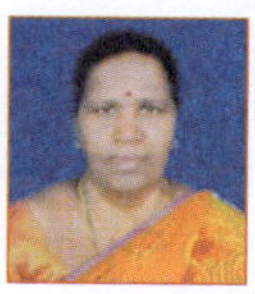

Subhadramma M Rajolli
Kalaburgai, Karnataka

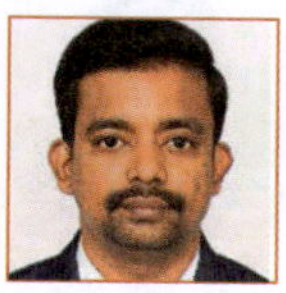

Srinivasan P
Mangalagiri
Andhra Pradesh

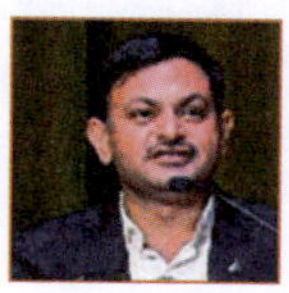

Sandeep Kumar
Rohtak, Haryana

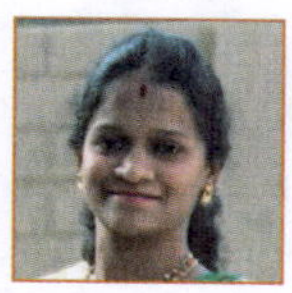

Shashirekha M
Davangere, Karnataka

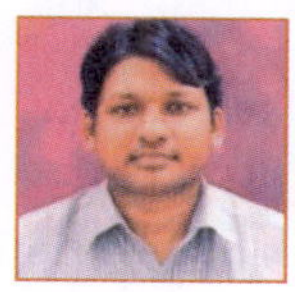

Sunil Kumar Garg
Badal, Punjab

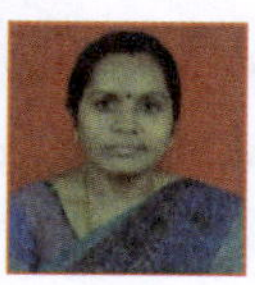

Sudha Maheswari R
Theni, Tamil Nadu

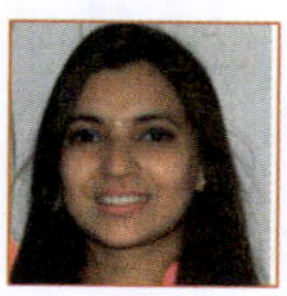

Saloni Sharma
New Delhi

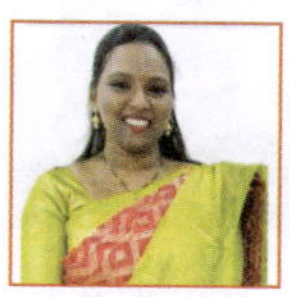

Sandhya C
AIIMS, Mangalagiri

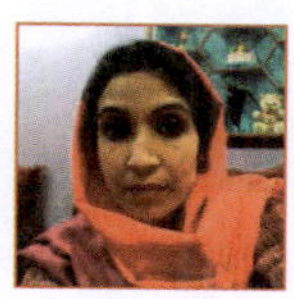

Shazia
Srinagar, J&K

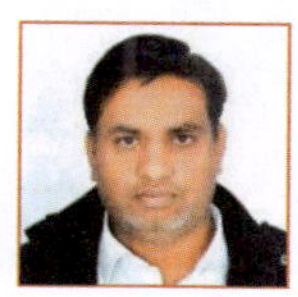

Sunil Kumar Joshi
Udaipur, Rajasthan

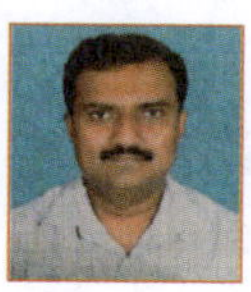

Sudhakar H H
Bangalore, Karnataka

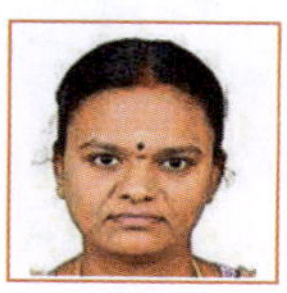

Sathiyakala K
Patna, Bihar

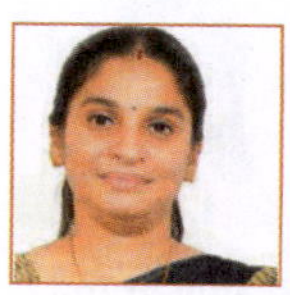

Sarika Sukesh Nair
Navi Mumbai
Maharashtra

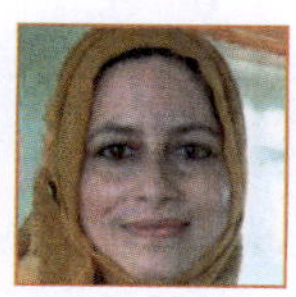

Sheema Bashir
Srinagar, J&K

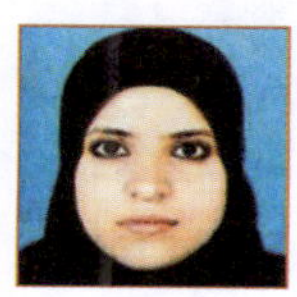

Syed Arifa
Srinagar, J&K

For details of all reviewers & contributors refer TH Lite

New reviewers of TH 7/e covered in TH Lite (App)

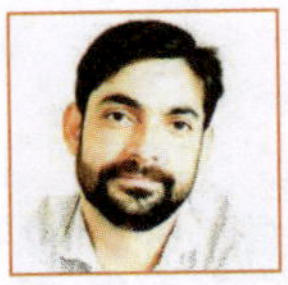

Syed Shahid Siraj
Charar-i-Sharief
Srinagar, J&K

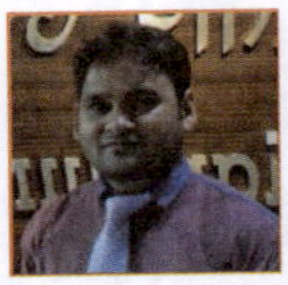

Semant Prashar
Bhopal, Madhya Pradesh

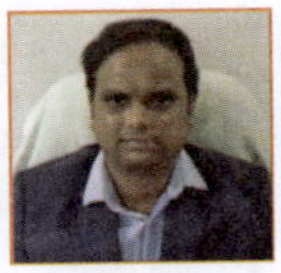

Sanjay Dixit
Gujarat

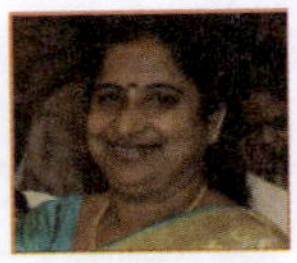

Sujatha
Tumkur, Karnataka

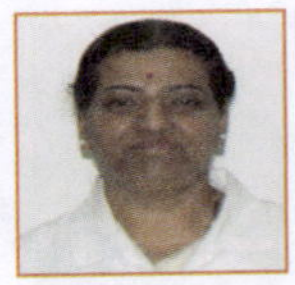

Sneha A Pitre
Pune, Maharashtra

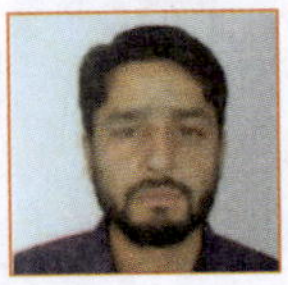

Syed Tajamul Islam
Srinagar, J&K

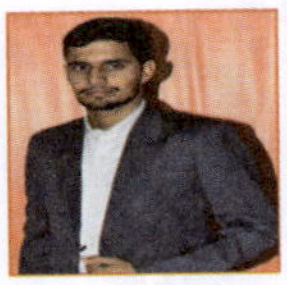

Suresh Krishniya
Sikar, Rajasthan

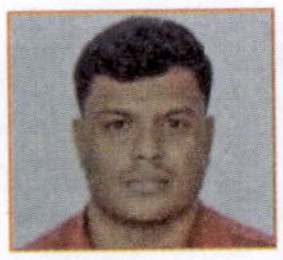

Siyad Farook
Kangra, Himachal Pradesh

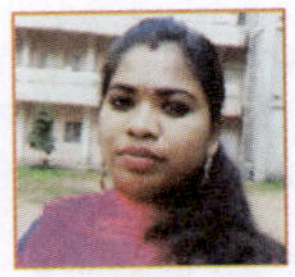

Sofiarani
Bengaluru, Karnataka

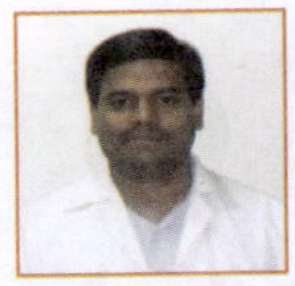

Suresh Ray
Pune, Maharashtra

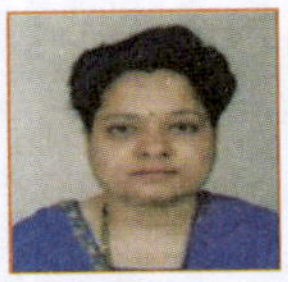

Shubhangi Dumbray
Pune, Maharashtra

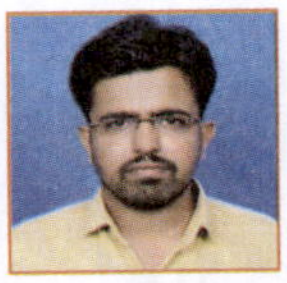

Shakti Soni
Rajasthan

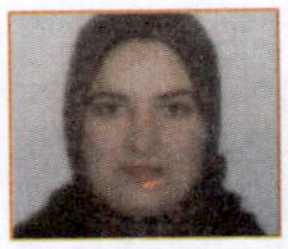

Shazia Afroze
Srinagar, J&K

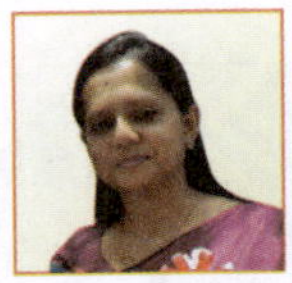

Shweta Pattnaik
Indore, Madhya Pradesh

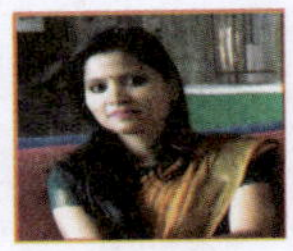

Sarita Nadiya Ahwal
New Delhi

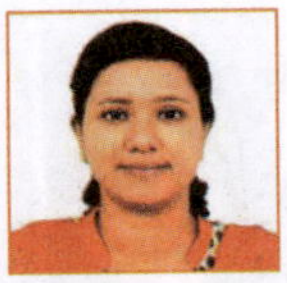

Soney Toppo
Bhopal, Madhya Pradesh

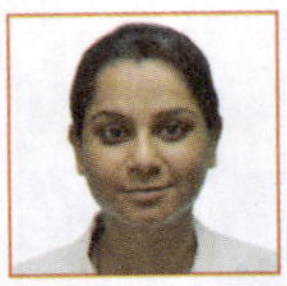

Shelly Dhawan
Patna, Bihar

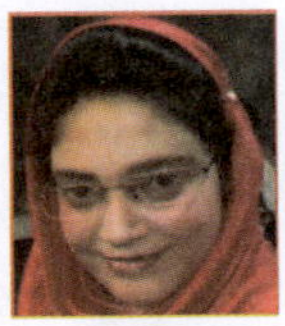

Shazia Nabi
Srinagar, J&K

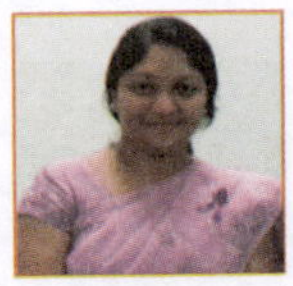

Shreeja Vijayan
Indore, Madhya Pradesh

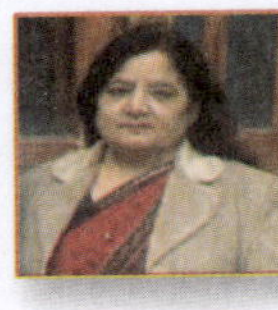

Sarita Mehta
New Delhi

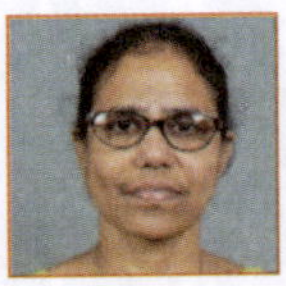

S Rajeswari
Goa

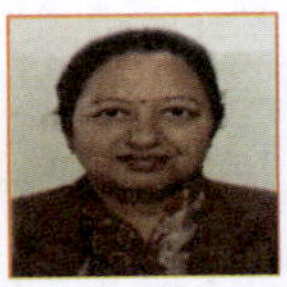

Sushma Kumari Saini
Chandigarh, Punjab

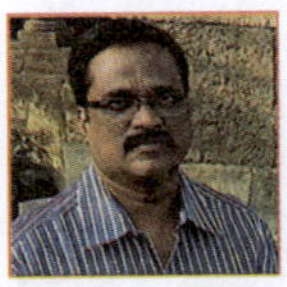

S F Bilali
Devangere, Karnataka

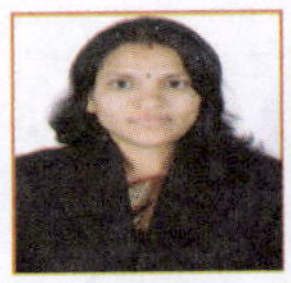

Sunita Choubey
Bhopal, Madhya Pradesh

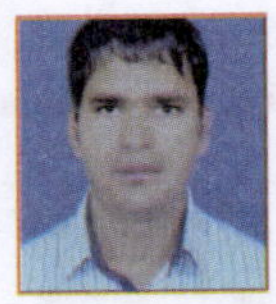

Shivraj Singh Meena
New Delhi

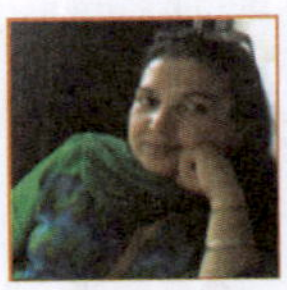

Sukhwinder Kaur
Patiala, Punjab

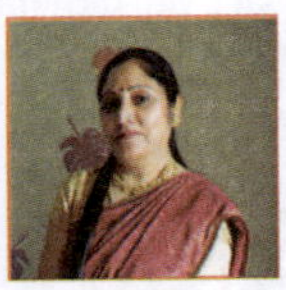

Sukhpal Kaur
Chandigarh, Punjab

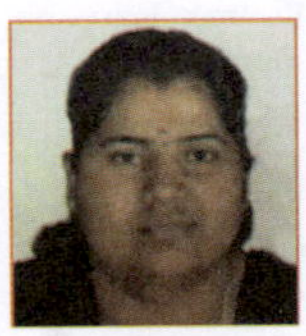

Sumathy S
Bengaluru, Karnataka

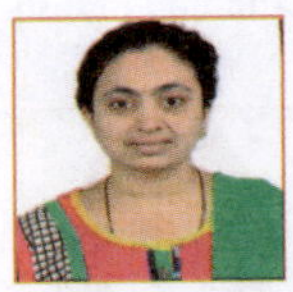

Sadhna U Adhyapak
Pune, Maharashtra

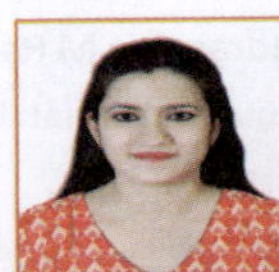

Swati Tiwari Bakshi
New Delhi

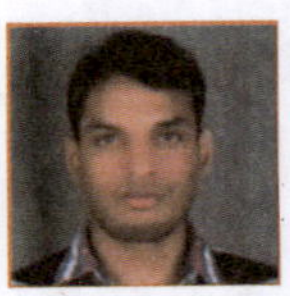

Sanjay Mittal
Rajasthan

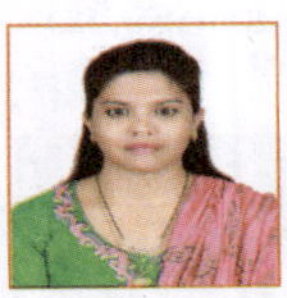

Shweta Patras
Raipur, Chhattisgarh

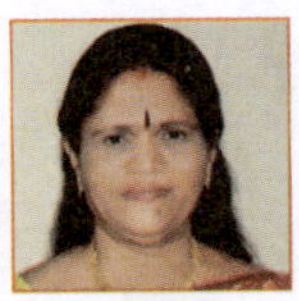

Shivamma
Bengaluru, Karnataka

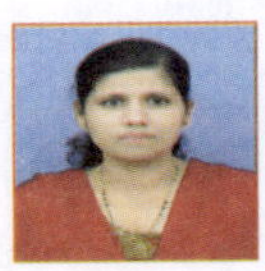

Shweta Joshi
Pune, Maharashtra

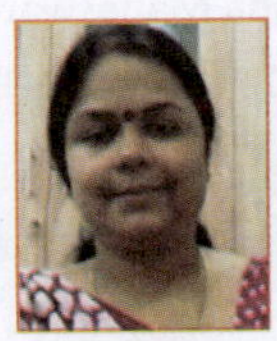

Sasmita Das
Bhubaneswar, Odisha

For details of all reviewers & contributors refer TH Lite

New reviewers of TH 7/e covered in TH Lite (App)

Our Valuable Reviewers & Contributors

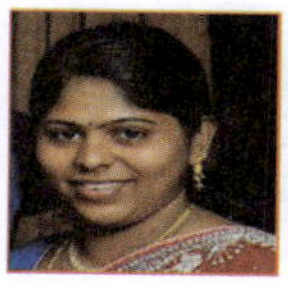

Subhatra
Bhubaneswar, Odisha

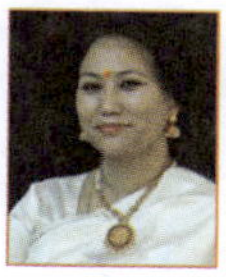

Suman Bodh
Kangra, Himachal Pradesh

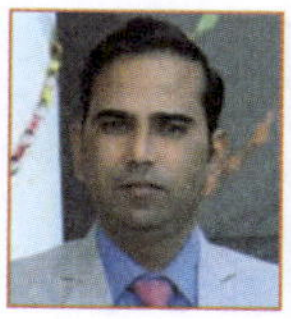

Santosh Kumar
Sangrur, Punjab

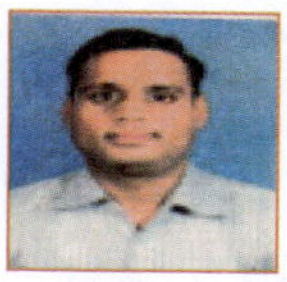

S K Maheshwari
Faridkot, Punjab

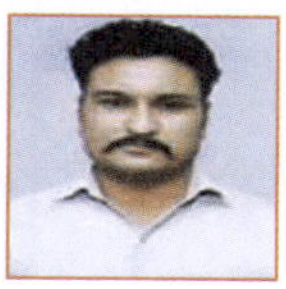

Surender Moond
Sikar, Rajasthan

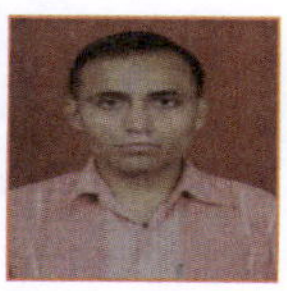

Suresh Kumar
Jaipur, Rajasthan

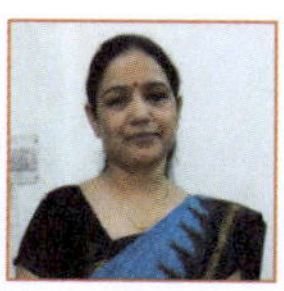

Samta Soni
Jaipur, Rajasthan

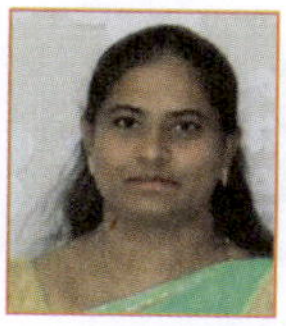

S Queen Mary
Hyderabad, Telangana

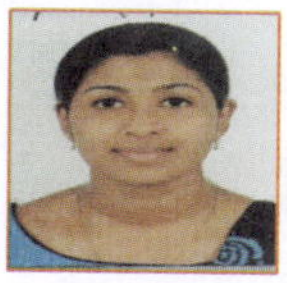

Sunu Anna Punnoose
Lucknow, Uttar Pradesh

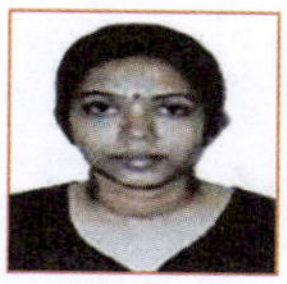

Soumyasree Sarkar
Kolkata, West Bengal

T

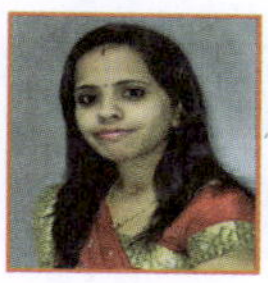

Tejeshwari B V
Bangalore, Karnataka

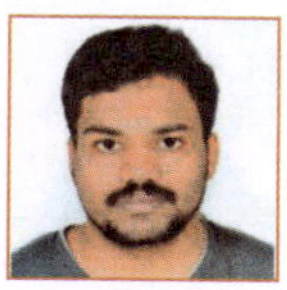

Thivakar J
Bhubaneswar, Odisha

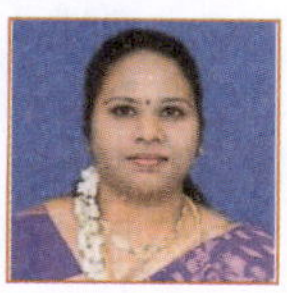

Thenaruvi R
Vellore, Tamil Nadu

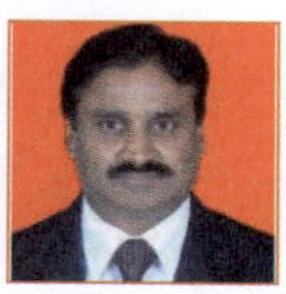

T E Setyanarayana
Bengaluru, Karnataka

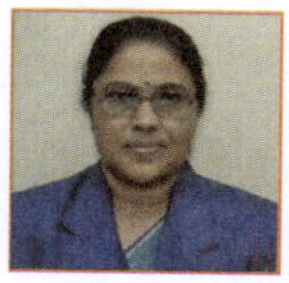

Thressiamma PM
Bengaluru, Karnataka

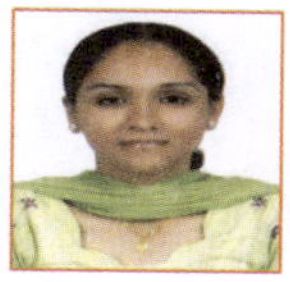

Talwinder Kaur
Punjab

U

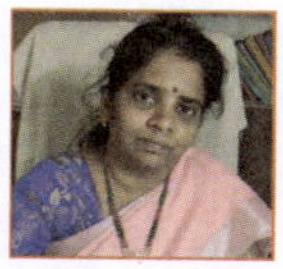

U Jhansi Rani
Andhra Pradesh

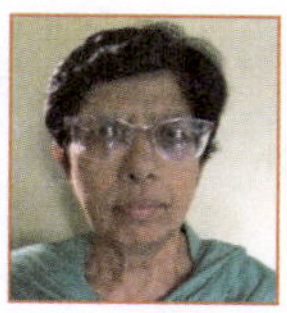

Usha Behl
Hoshiarpur, Punjab

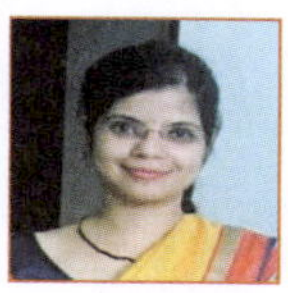

Urvashi
Lucknow, Uttar Pradesh

V

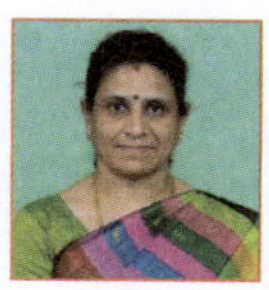

V Selvanayaki
Salem, Tamil Nadu

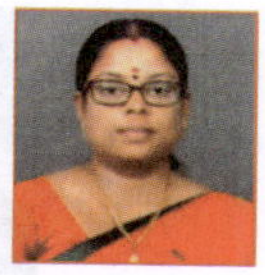

Visala Pandian V
Nagapattinam
Tamil Nadu

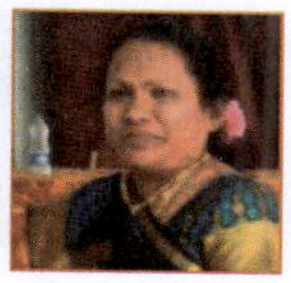

Vasanthamma A
Gulbarga, Karnataka

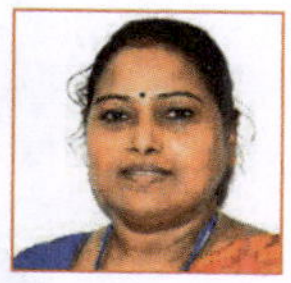

Veena M Joseph
Kanchipuram, Tamil Nadu

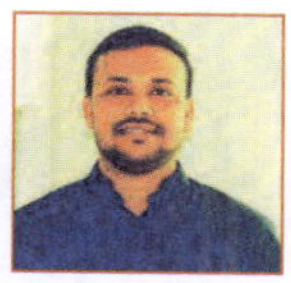

Vikrant Nesari
Belagavi, Karnataka

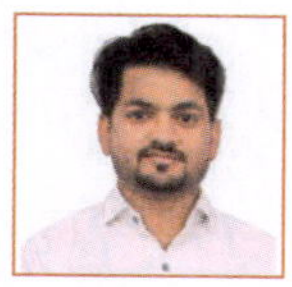

Vikram Singh
Rank 1, 2015

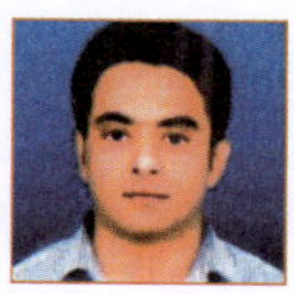

Vipin Kumar Pillai
Udaipur, Rajasthan

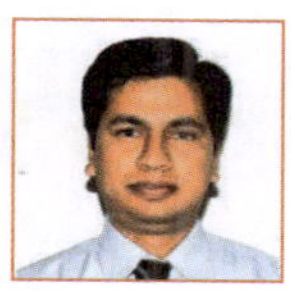

Vishal Tak
Jaipur, Rajasthan

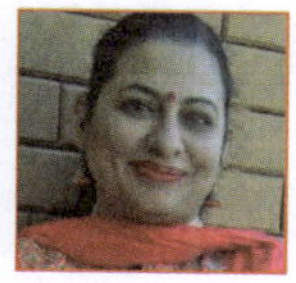

Varinder Kaur
Himachal Pradesh

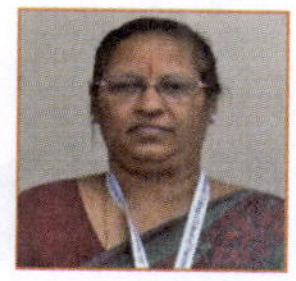

V Sujatha
Tamil Nadu

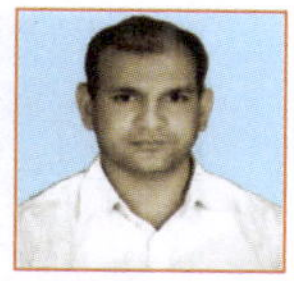

Virendra Chaudhary
Faridkot, Punjab

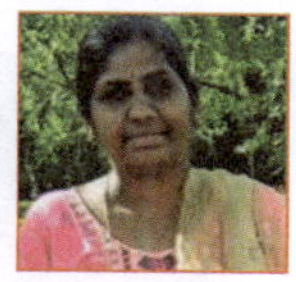

Vijayasanthi
Dehradun, Uttarakhand
Jaipur, Rajasthan

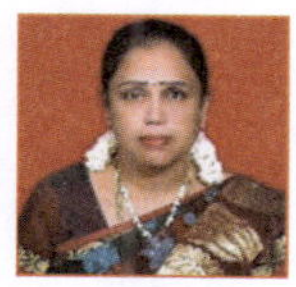

Vasantha Chitre
New Delhi

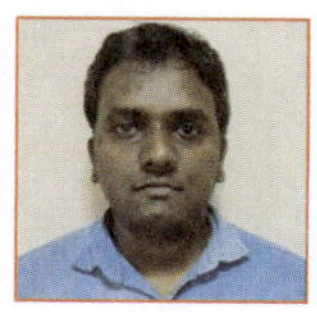

Visanth VS
Patna, Bihar

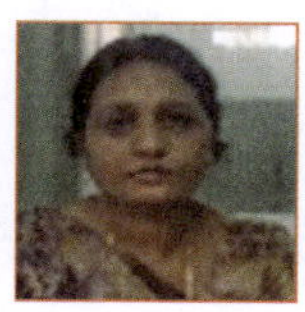

Vandna Chansoriya
Raipur, Chattisgarh

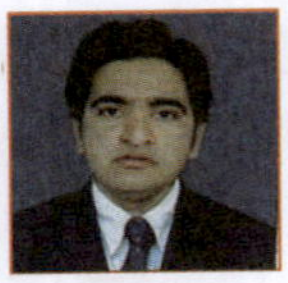

Vipin Vageriya
Anand, Gujarat

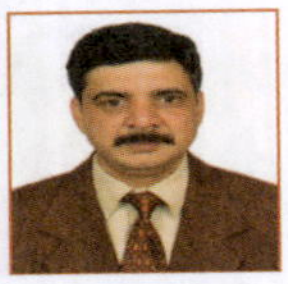

Vikas Sood
Shimla, Himachal Pradesh

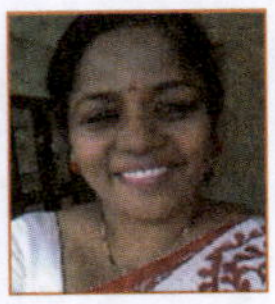

Vidya Raju Saliyan
Bengaluru, Karnataka

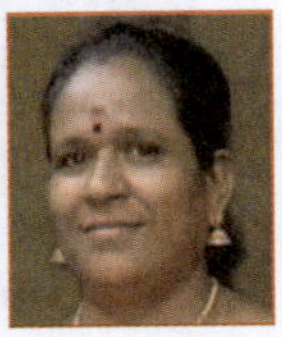

Vanmathisaravanan
Bengaluru, Karnataka

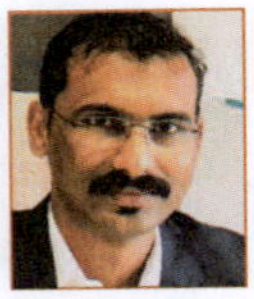

Vinayak I Patil
Karnataka

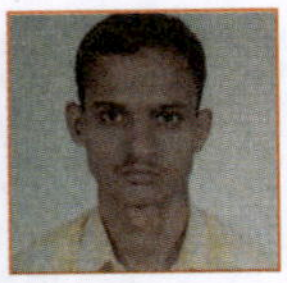

Veerendra Patel
Davangere, Karnataka

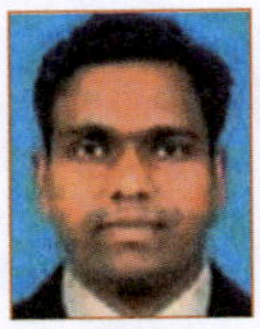

Vijayreddy Vandali
Nashik, Maharashtra

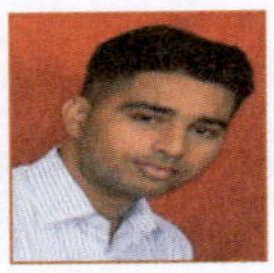

Vishaldeep Singh Batth
Gharuan, Punjab

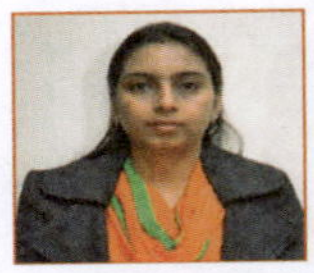

Vandana
Faridkot, Punjab

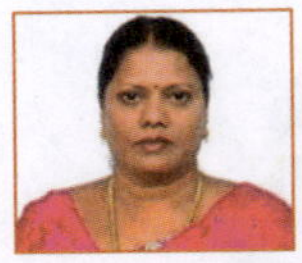

V Hemavathy
Chennai, Tamil Nadu

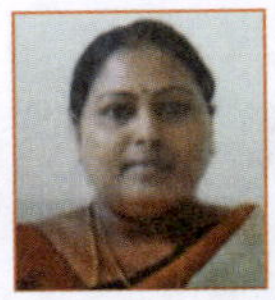

Veena M Joseph
Kelambakkam
Tamil Nadu

Y

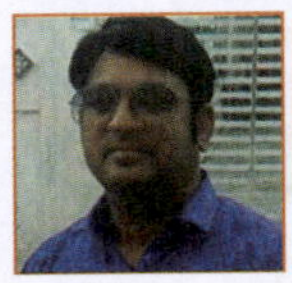

Yugal Swarnkar
Udaipur, Rajasthan

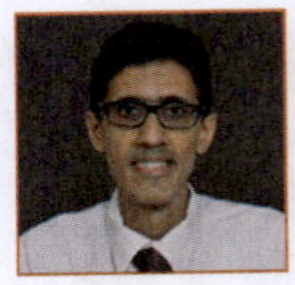

Yogesh Gulati
Lucknow, Uttar Pradesh

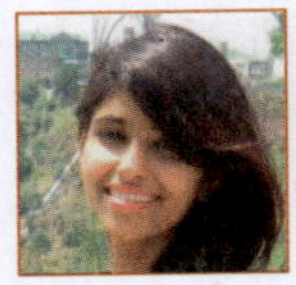

Yogita Kumari Shringi
Chandigarh

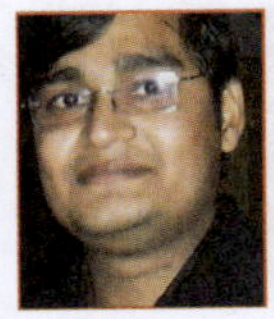

Yogendra Garg
Karnataka

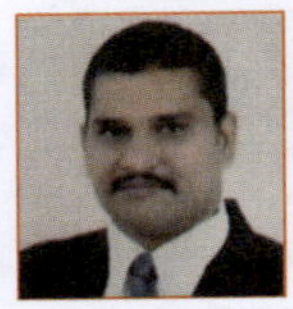

Yogeshwar Puri
Udaipur, Rajasthan

And many more... (Page 4)

6 Reasons to Choose Nursing Next Live as Your Study Partner for Guaranteed Success

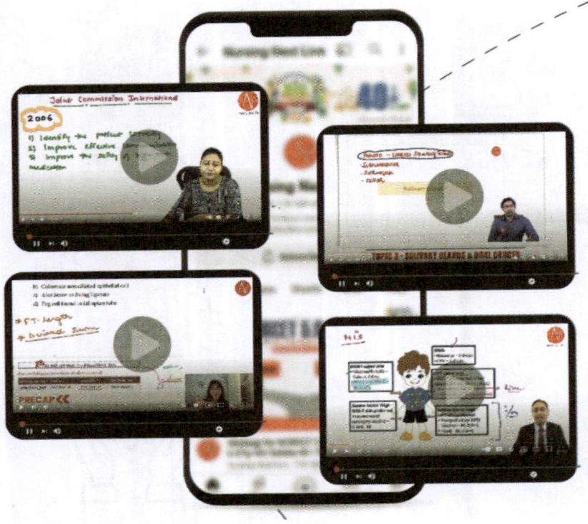

1 Advance Video Lectures by the Masterminds (Top Educators)

- Master the NORCET exam with our updated video lectures by the top-tier Medical and Nursing Educators.
- With **over 1700+ Hours of conceptual lectures (in Hinglish And English)**, we comprehensively cover all subjects and topics according to NORCET's latest exam pattern.
- Learn and retain the high-yield topics using our **1000+ conceptual videos** encompassing theoretical concepts, skill procedures and clinical case scenarios.
- All the lectures are given in the guided-study form of **Foundation, Intermediate & FastTrack Revision**

2 Interactive Live Classes and Doubt Sessions

- Experience our innovative blend of **recorded lectures and live teaching.**
- Engage in **High Yield Topics discussion, Fast Track Classes, Probable Questions Discussion, Golden Points Chanting Sessions, and Clinical Case-Based Scenario Questions** through live sessions conducted by the Mastermind Faculty.
- **Monthly Doubt Sessions** with the faculty to ensure uninterrupted learning.

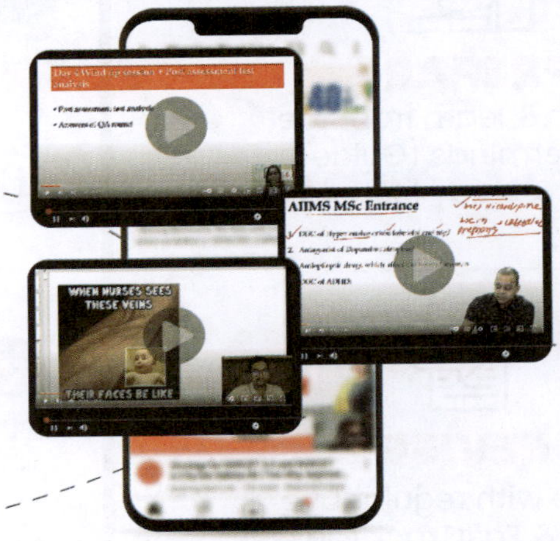

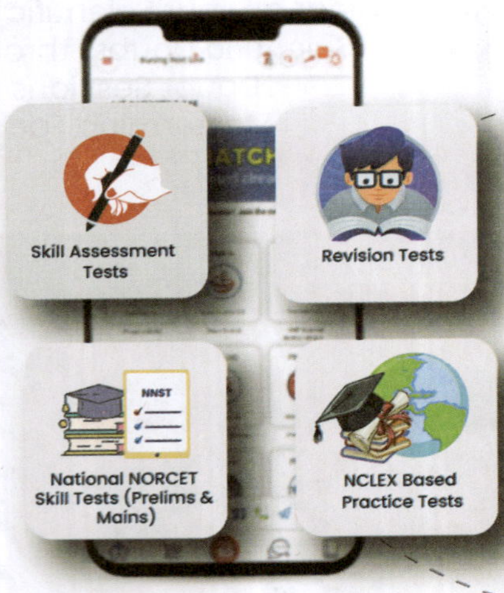

3 Practice Practice Practice

- Learning through practice; knowledge through practice. Our exclusive **Real-Time Exam-Based Approach** offers a 360-degree Test Series, encompassing **50,000+ questions** with varying complexities: **MCQs, CBQS, IBQS, VBQS, Priority Interventions, all with rationale explanations.**
- Assess your progress at every step with **Monthly Tests, National NORCET Skill Tests (Prelims & Mains)**, providing negative marking and national rankings among 5000-7000 students.

4 Comprehensive Study Material

- Quality study material is the cornerstone of preparation. NNL adopts a 4-way learning approach for providing you with the **extra-mile study material:**
  1. **Lecture Notes** (PDFs) from Mastermind Lectures
  2. Comprehensive **Revision Notes (3 Vol)** covering **High-Yield Topics, Last-Minute Pointers, and Most Probable Questions**
  3. Innovative **Nursing E-Flash Cards** (150-300), with a one card one concept approach.
  4. **E-Workbooks** for self assessment in Fast Track Classes and making last-minute revision notes

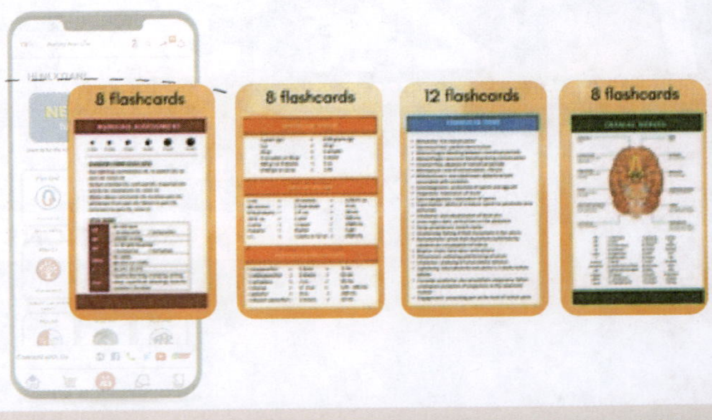

Nursing Next Live Exam Prep Pvt Ltd | Patparganj Industrial Area, New Delhi | Vol 3 | 18th July, 2023 | No Monetary Investment Gold Value

Nursing Next Live
The Next Level of NURSING EDUCATION

THE NURSING NEXT LIVE BULLETIN

ONE NATION e-RESOURCE

18th July, 2023

The Next Level of Nursing Education

Tuesday

AIIMS NORCET TOPPERS (2020 - JUNE 2023)

NEXTIANS TAKE THE LEAD YET AGAIN

All India Ranks In Open Category

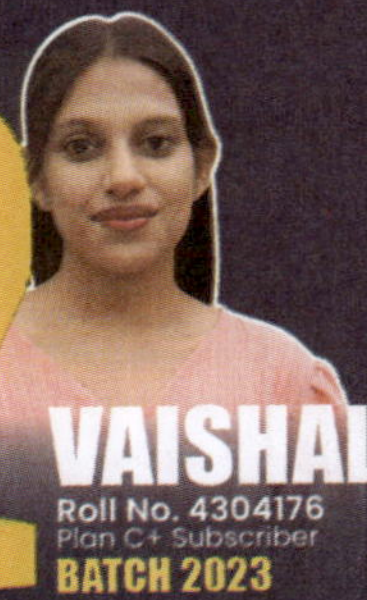

2 VAISHALI
Roll No. 4304176
Plan C+ Subscriber
BATCH 2023

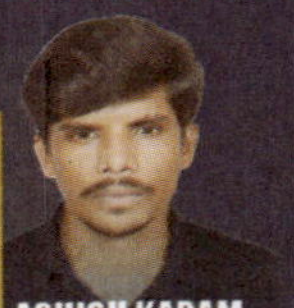

AIR 1 ASHISH KADAM
Roll No. 4112461
Plan C+ Subscriber
BATCH 2022

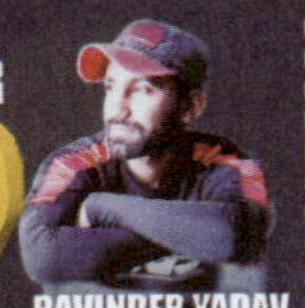

AIR 2 RAVINDER YADAV
Roll No. 9783050
Plan C+ Subscriber
BATCH 2021

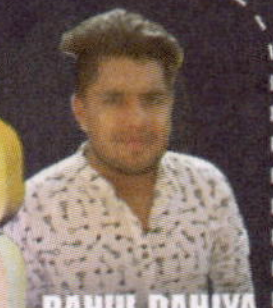

AIR 3 RAHUL DAHIYA
Roll No. 9016060
Plan C+ Subscriber
BATCH 2020

AIR 3 Amit Sehrawat
Roll No. 4301742
Plan C+ Subscriber
BATCH 2023

AIR 4 Subhadip Tripathi
Roll No. 4202513
Plan C+ Subscriber
BATCH 2023

AIR 6 Riya Ghosh
Roll No. 4258133
Plan C+ Subscriber
BATCH 2023

AIR 7 Uma
Roll No. 4244885
Plan C+ Subscriber
BATCH 2023

AIR 8 Shubham Kavhad
Roll No. 4255490
Plan C+ Subscriber
BATCH 2023

ALL INDIA OPEN CATEGORY RANKS IN TOP 100 (NORCET-JUNE 2023)

- AIR 11 Sunidhi Patial, Roll No. 4255490, Plan C+
- AIR 14 Diksha Minocha, Roll No. 4273517, Plan C+
- AIR 15 Muskaan Sharma, Roll No. 4225951, Plan C+
- AIR 18 Geeta Borkhatariya, Roll No. 4259925, Plan C+
- AIR 19 Rakesh Panwar, Roll No. 4261606, Plan C+
- AIR 20 Dinesh Gehlot, Roll No. 4239629, Plan C+
- AIR 26 Muthamil Selvam, Roll No. 4301892, Plan C+
- AIR 34 Pooja, Roll No. 4273919, Plan C+
- AIR 36 Heena, Roll No. 4252484, Plan C+
- AIR 37 Atika Aktara, Roll No. 4291601, Plan C+
- AIR 38 Sumit Rathod, Roll No. 4204636, Plan C+
- 39 Tamanna, Roll No. 4269899, Plan C+
- AIR 42 Bheemanagouda, Roll No. 4280212, Plan C+
- AIR 44 Imran, Roll No. 4219450, Plan C+
- AIR 45 Abhishek, Roll No. 4200108, Plan C+
- AIR 46 Sushma kumari, Roll No. 4270265, Plan C+
- AIR 50 Sudipa, Roll No. 4275835, Plan C+
- AIR 51 Vandana Kushwaha, Roll No. 4258307, Plan C+
- AIR 52 Pankaj, Roll No. 4221309, Plan C+
- AIR 55 Khodbhaya, Roll No. 4219606, Plan C+
- AIR 61 Priyanka, Roll No. 4284124, Plan C+
- AIR 69 Renu Bisht, Roll No. 4254957, Plan C+
- AIR 79 Devendra, Roll No. 4278881, Plan C+
- AIR 80 Nancy, Roll No. 4265449, Plan C+
- AIR 84 Abhilasha, Roll No. 4249584, Plan C+
- AIR 90 Kakoli Khatun, Roll No. 4256474, Plan C+
- AIR 92 Rajni Pal, Roll No. 4215405, Plan C+
- AIR 96 Shameema, Roll No. 4235551, Plan C+

and many more

TOP 100 RANKS IN NORCET FOR 3 CONSECUTIVE YEARS

BATCH 2022

AIR 1 ASHISH KADAM
Roll No. 4112461
Plan C+ Subscriber

- AIR 10 Pushpa, Roll No. 4130466, Plan A
- AIR 12 Azra Fatima, Roll No. 4103618, Plan C+
- AIR 13 Suresh, Roll No. 4170313, Plan C+
- AIR 17 Anjali Saini, Roll No. 4177368, SUPER 40
- AIR 22 Sutapa Gantait, Roll No. 4115442, Plan C+
- AIR 27 Satwinder Kaur, Roll No. 4161718, Plan C+
- AIR 36 Radheshyam, Roll No. 4128407, Plan RRR
- AIR 41 Vaishali Solanki, Roll No. 4103724, Plan C+
- AIR 45 Melari Maring, Roll No. 4147098, Plan A
- AIR 55 Komal, Roll No. 4188608, Plan MSc
- AIR 59 Vishaakha, Roll No. 4123040, Plan B
- AIR 60 Shoaiab, Roll No. 4153003, Free User
- AIR 62 Monika, Roll No. 4165818, SUPER 40
- AIR 72 Chetna, Roll No. 4105029, Plan C+
- AIR 74 Akshay, Roll No. 4182798, Plan A
- AIR 82 Shrinath, Roll No. 4182798, Plan C+
- AIR 83 Deveshri, Roll No. 4151828, Plan C+
- AIR 87 Sneha, Roll No. 4122964, Plan C+

BATCH 2021

AIR 2 RAVINDER YADAV
Roll No. 9783050
Plan C+ Subscriber

- AIR 9 BHAVNESH, Roll No. 9757509, Plan C+
- AIR 10 Nishant Kumar, Roll No. 9710853, Plan C+
- AIR 19 Satyam, Roll No. 9711718, Plan RRR
- AIR 20 Chanchal, Roll No. 9794394, Plan C+
- AIR 21 Sunil Chahar, Roll No. 9757345, Plan C+
- AIR 22 Aditya Whaval, Roll No. 9778071, Plan B
- AIR 41 Yogita, Roll No. 9778071, Plan C+
- AIR 42 Monika, Roll No. 9774436, Plan C+
- AIR 48 Vinod
- AIR 53 Vikas, Roll No. 9701891, Plan C+
- AIR 56 Manisha, Roll No. 9797937, Plan RRR
- AIR 59 Priya Gupta, Roll No. 4239629, Plan C+
- AIR 75 Priti Prajapati, Roll No. 9722223, Plan C+
- AIR 76 Shweta, Roll No. 9792030, Plan A
- AIR 92 Amit
- AIR 93 Jyoti, Roll No. 9725260, Plan C+
- AIR 94 Adrija, Roll No. 9741131, Plan C+
- AIR 97 Anita, Roll No. 9781151, Plan C+
- AIR 99 Yogesh, Roll No. 9726062, Plan C+
- AIR 100 Arif, Free User

BATCH 2020

AIR 3 RAHUL DAHIYA
Roll No. 9016060

- AIR 12 Nisha Singla, Roll No. 9101820
- AIR 14 Arushi Mittal, Roll No. 9079646
- AIR 51 Komal Dhull, Roll No. 9024458
- AIR 72 Shivani Bourai, Roll No. 9092877
- AIR 79 Nivedita Saini, Roll No. 9004587
- AIR 89 Rupali Garg, Roll No. 9054544

LET THE NUMBERS DO THE TALKING

- 1.80L+ Downloads
- 40k+ Active Users
- 5000+ Selections in 2019-2023
- UP TO 90% Strike Rate in Exams
- 3000+ Cities
- 4.8 Stars Rating on Google Play Store

Contents

Preliminary Pages

Foreword to 7th Edition IX
Foreword to 6th Edition X
Foreword to 4th & 5th Edition X
From Authors' Desk XI
Acknowledgements XII
From Publisher's Desk XIII
Luminaries in Nursing XVI
Our Valuable Reviewers & Contributors XVII
Contents XXXV
How to Prepare for NORCET (Prelims and Mains): An Overview XLII
Decoding the Case Scenario-based Questions XLIII
Video-Based Questions (VBQs) LI
Appendices A-3 to A-42

SECTION A

Subject-wise Synopsis, CBQs, IBQs & MCQ's

Fundamentals of Nursing

Synopsis

Florence Nightingale's Contribution to Nursing 3
Milestones of Nursing in India 3
Basic Characteristics of a Profession 4
Different Roles of Nurses 4
Trends in Nursing 4
Nursing Programs in India 4
Ethics in Nursing 5
Sources of Law 5
Legislation and Nursing Practice 6
Legislation Issues in Nursing Practice 6
Professional Values 7
Nursing Process 7
Documentation and Reporting 10
Admission and Discharge 11
Vital Signs 12
Techniques of Physical Examination 20
Types of Nursing Modalities 24
Medical and Surgical Asepsis-Terminologies 25
Basic Principles of Surgical Asepsis 26
Stages of Infection 27
Methods of Sterilization and Disinfection 30
Biomedical Waste Management 32
Specimen Collection 32
Bed Making 36
Personal Hygiene 36
Back Massage Techniques 38
Pressure Ulcers 38
Medication Administration 41
Nursing Theories 45
Basic and Advanced Life Support 46
Complementary Therapies 47
Loss and Grief 48
Activity and Exercise 49
Oxygenation 49
Incentive Spirometer 53
Suction 53
Oral Airway 54
Chest Tube/Intercostal Drainage 55
Fluids 56
Electrolyte Abnormalities 56
Acid-Base Balance 59
Hot and Cold Applications 60
Sleep 61
Positions 61
Pain and its Management 64
Nutrition 66
Enteral Tube Feeding 67
Parenteral Nutrition 68
Bladder Elimination 68
Bowel Elimination 70
Colostomy 72
Body Mechanics and Mobility 73
Venous Thromboembolism (VTE) 74
Wound Drains 74
Suture 75
Needle 76
Key Nursing Roles in Important Procedures 76
Triage 77
Intravenous Fluid Administration Drop Rate Calculation 77
Insulin Syringe Preparation (Mixing Regular with NPH) 78
Hemoglobin 79
Renal Function 79
Liver Function Test (Normal Values) 79
Pulmonary Function Test 80
Endocrine Function 80
Blood Sugar Profile 80
Cardiac Markers 80
Urine Routine and Microscopy 81
Cerebrospinal Fluid (CSF) 81
Neurological Values 81
Arterial Blood Gas (ABG) Values 81
First Aid 82
Color Coding of Medical Gas Cylinder 84
Comfort Devices 84

Clinical Case-Based Questions 88

Image-Based Questions 106

Multiple Choice Questions 112

Medical Surgical Nursing/ Adult Health Nursing

Synopsis

Inflammation and Wound Healing 168
- Inflammation 168
- Wound Healing 168
- Gangrene 170

Multiple Choice Questions 172

Immune System 175
- Overview of Immune System 175
- Immunoglobulins 176
- Blood Products, Storage Temperature, Shelf Life and Compatibility 176
- Types of Transfusion Reactions 176
- Immunological Disorder 177

Multiple Choice Questions 180

Musculoskeletal System 184
- Anatomy and Physiology of Musculoskeletal System 184
- Classification of Bones 185
- Review Points 186
- Anatomy of Bone 188
- Types of Joints in Human Body 189
- Vertebral Column 190
- Diagnostic Evaluation 190
- Disorders of Musculoskeletal System 191
- Orthopedic Surgeries 195
- Crutches 196
- Gout 197

Tendinitis 197
Bursitis 197
Osteoarthritis 198
Rheumatoid Arthritis 198
Osteomyelitis 198
Osteoporosis 198
Osteomalacia 199
Paget's Disease 199
Rhabdomyolysis 199
Spinal Column Deformities 199
Prolapsed Intervertebral Disk 200
Amputation of the Lower Extremity 200
Pott's Disease 200
Carpel Tunnel Syndrome 200
Disorders of Lower Limb 201

Multiple Choice Questions 202

Gastrointestinal and Hepatobiliary System 218

Gastrointestinal System 218
Hepatic Biliary System 236

Multiple Choice Questions 246

ENT System 271

Anatomy of Ear 271
Physiology of Hearing 272
Disorders of Ear 274
Disorders of Nose 275
Disorders of Throat 276

Multiple Choice Questions 278

Ophthalmology 284

Anatomy and Physiology of Eye 284
Assessment and Diagnostic Tests 286
Disorders of Eye 289

Multiple Choice Questions 296

Integumentary System and Burns 302

Integumentary System 302
Burns 308
Zones of Burn Wound 310

Multiple Choice Questions 312

Respiratory System 321

Anatomy and Physiology 321
Classification of Respiratory System 322
Assessment and Diagnostic Tests 325
Disorders of Respiratory System 327

Multiple Choice Questions 335

Cardiovascular System 349

Anatomic and Physiologic Overview of Heart 349
Diagnostic Tests 357
Hemodynamic Monitoring 357
Disorders of Cardiovascular System 361
Coronary Artery Diseases 365
Nursing Care of Patient Undergoing CABG (Coronary Artery Bypass Graft) 366
Other Diseases of Heart 367
Arterial Diseases 368

Multiple Choice Questions 374

Hematology 397

Anatomy and Physiology of Hematologic System 397
Blood Groups and Blood Typing 400
Blood Coagulation 400
Diagnostic Tests 401
Hematological Diseases and Disorders 401
Blood Transfusion 406

Multiple Choice Questions 408

Renal System 422

Anatomy and Physiology of Renal System 422
Functions of Kidney 425
Investigations 427
Disorders of Renal System 429
Renal Transplant 434
Miscellaneous Urinary Diseases 434

Multiple Choice Questions 436

Endocrine System 447

Anatomy and Physiology of Endocrine System 447
Diagnostic Tests in Endocrinology 450
Disorders of Endocrine System 450
Thyroid Gland 452
Parathyroid Gland 453
Endocrine-Pancreas 454
Adrenal Cortex 456
Adrenal Medulla 457
Gonads 458

Multiple Choice Questions 459

Nervous System 471

Anatomy and Physiology of Nervous System 471
Classification of Nervous System 472
Assessment and Diagnostic Tests 477
Seizure Disorders 481
Stroke 481
Head Trauma/Head Injury 482
Intracranial/Brain Herniation 483
Spinal Cord Injuries 483
Meningitis 484
Encephalitis 485
Brain Abscess 485
Multiple Sclerosis 485
Myasthenia Gravis 485
Guillain-Barre Syndrome 486
Trigiminal Neuralgia 486
Bell's Palsy 486
Parkinson's Disease 486
Alzheimer's Disease 487
Huntington's Disease 487
Amyotrophic Lateral Sclerosis (ALS) 487
Brain Tumor 487
Neurocysticercosis 488

Multiple Choice Questions 489

Oncology 511

Cancer 511
Few Common Cancers 512
Bone Marrow Transplantation (BMT) 520

Multiple Choice Questions 522

Male Reproductive System 536

Anatomy and Physiology of Male Reproductive System 536
Accessory Sex Glands 537
Male Sexual Development and Function 537
Diagnostic Tests 538
Disorders of Male Reproductive System 539
Prostate Cancer 539

Multiple Choice Questions 542

Perioperative Nursing Care 547

Introduction 547
Types of Surgeries 547
Surgical Approaches 547
Preoperative Nursing Care 547
Preoperative Period: Nursing Responsibility 548
Intraoperative Period: Nursing Responsibility 548
Pain 548
Types of Anesthesia 550
Common Positions Used During Surgeries 550
Sutures 552
Surgical Needles 554

Multiple Choice Questions 555

Homeostasis, Emergency and Critical Care Nursing 561

Stress 561
Shock 561
Anaphylaxis 563
Fluid Imbalances 563
Edema 563
Understanding Acid-Base Imbalance 564

Causes of Other Acid-Base Disorders 564
Electrolytes 565
Hemorrhage 566
Emergency Nursing - Prioritization of Care 566
Priorities of Care and Triage Categories 566
Common Equipment in Critical Care Area 567
Defibrillator 568
Stages of Death and Dying (Kubbler Ross Stages of Dying) 569
Multiple Choice Questions 571
Clinical Case-Based Questions 584
Image-Based Questions 616

Pharmacology

Synopsis

Key Terminologies 655
Prodrugs 656
Therapeutic Index (TI) 656
Different Routes of Administration, its Advantages and Disadvantages 657
Special Drug Delivery System 657
Conversion Equivalence of Weight 658
Conversion Equivalence of Volume 658
Drug Calculation 658
Antimicrobial Agents 659
Cardiac Drugs 660
Drugs Acting on Central Nervous System 662
Sedative and Hypnotics 662
Antipsychotic Drugs 663
Antidepressants 664
Mood Stabilizers 664
Deaddiction Drugs 665
Anticonvulsants 666
Analgesics 666
Anti-Gout Agents 666
Sympathomimetic (Adrenergic) Drugs 667
Cholinergic Drugs 667
Drugs Affecting the Respiratory System 667
Drugs Acting on Gastrointestinal Tract 668
Insulin 669
Oral Hypoglycemic (Antidiabetic) Agents 669
Adrenocorticosteroids and Analogues 669
Posterior Pituitary Hormones 670
Calcitonin and Calcium Salts 670
Thyroid Drugs 670
Antithyroid Drugs 671
Diuretics 671
Antitubercular Drugs 671
Anticancer Drugs 672
Anticoagulants 672
Thrombolytic Medications 672
Antiplatelet Drug 672
Specific Antidotes Against Poisoning 673
Disease and Drug of Choices 673
Adverse Effects of Some Common Drugs 676
Drug Safety During Pregnancy 677
Drug Safety During Breastfeeding 677
Image-Based Questions 680
Multiple Choice Questions 681

Community Health Nursing

Synopsis

Concepts and Determinants of Health and Well-Being 708
Indicators of Health 709
Levels of Healthcare and Health for All 710
Millennium Development Goal and Sustainable Development Goal 711
Levels of Prevention 711
Introduction to Epidemiology 713
Mortality Rate and Ratios 714
Incidence and Prevalence of Disease 715
Epidemiological Method 716
Epidemiological Triad 717
Surveillance and Monitoring for Disease 718
Iceberg Phenomenon 718
Immunity 719
Cold Chain 721
Adverse Events Following Immunization 722
National Immunization Schedule/Universal Immunization Program 724
Communicable Diseases 724
Ebola Virus 726
COVID-19 (Refer to Annexure for Detailed Note of COVID-19) 727
Nipah Virus Infection 727
Gastrointestinal Disorders 727
Food Poisoning 728
Parasitic Infections 729
Arthropod-Borne Infections 730
Zoonoses 731
Leprosy (Hansen's Disease) 732
Tetanus 733
Sexually Transmitted Diseases (STDs) 733
Purification of Water 734
Noncommunicable Disease 736
Health Programs in India 739
Demographic Trends in India 739
National Population Policy 2000 741
Contraceptive Methods/Family Planning Methods (Fertility Regulation Method) 741
Barrier Methods 742
Hormonal Methods 744
Depot Formulations 746
Subdermal Implants 747
Vaginal Rings 747
Post-Conceptional Methods 747
Prenatal Advice 749
Intranatal Care 749
Mother and Child Health (MCH) 749
Reproductive Child Health Program (RCH) 750
Under 5 Clinic 751
School Health Services 752
Nutrition And Health 752
Disaster Management 754
Occupational Hazards 754
Health Policy and Planning 757
Healthcare of the Community 758
Primary Healthcare 758
Healthcare Delivery System 758
National Health Mission (NHM) 762
Differences Between NRHM and NUHM 763
Programs Under NRHM 764
Urban Poverty Alleviation 765
National Health Programs 765
International Health Agencies 766
Image-Based Questions 770
Multiple Choice Questions 778

Psychiatric Nursing

Synopsis

Introduction 830
Mental Health 830
Mental Illness 830
Development of Personality 831
Theories of Personality Development 831
Defense Mechanism 833

Therapeutic Communication 834
Neurotransmitters 835
Psychosocial Therapies 836
ICD 10 Classification of Psychiatric Disorders 837
General Psychopathology 838
Organic Mental Disorders 841
Substance Use Disorders 842
Schizophrenia 844
Personality Disorders 846
Mood Disorders 848
Somatoform Disorders 850
Stress and Adaptation 850
Phobia 850
Obsessive Compulsive Disorder (OCD) 852
Adjustment Disorder 852
Eating Disorders 853
Sleep Disorders 853
Seasonal Affective Disorder 854
Sexual Disorders 855
Electroconvulsive Therapy (ECT) 855
Childhood Psychiatric Disorders 855
Attention Deficit Hyperactive Disorder (ADHD) 856
Mental Retardation (Intellectual Disability) 856
Management 857
Learning Disabilities and Disorders (Specific Learning Disorder) 857
Psychopharmacology 857
National Mental Health Program (NMHP) 860
Objectives of District Mental Health Program (DMHP) 860
Deaddiction Drugs/Antabuse Drugs 860
Crisis and Crisis Intervention 861
Psychiatric Emergencies 862
Glossary of Common Terminologies 863

Clinical Case-Based Questions 869

Image-Based Questions 882

Multiple Choice Questions 886

Pediatric Nursing

Synopsis

Growth and Development 940
Growth Chart 943
Milestones 943
Theories of Growth and Development 944
Essential Newborn Care 945
Thermoregulation in Newborn 947
Kangaroo Mother Care (KMC) 948
High Risk Newborn 949
Newborn Resuscitation 950
Common Respiratory Conditions in Newborns 950
Feeding in Children 951
Immunization 952
Under-Five Clinics 957
Jaundice 957
Neonatal Care 958
Birth Injuries 959
Integrated Management of Neonatal and Childhood Illness (1995) 961
Baby Friendly Hospital Initiative 961
Child Welfare Programs 961
Child Welfare Milestones 962
Types of Play Among Children 962
Protein Energy Undernutrition 963
Disorders of Respiratory System 964
Disorders of Gastrointestinal System 967
Cleft Lip and Cleft Palate 970
Tracheoesophageal Fistula and Esophageal Atresia 971
Hypertrophic Pyloric Stenosis 972
Congenital Diaphragmatic Hernia (CDH) 972
Umbilical Cord Anomalies 974
Disorders of Hepatic System 975
Disorders of Cardiovascular System 976
Disorders of Genitourinary System 982
Disorders of Central Nervous System 984
Orthopedic Problems in Children 986
Disorders of Skin 991
Disorders of ENT 991
Disorders of Eye 992
Pediatric Emergency 992
National Immunization Schedule 992
Genetic Disorders 995
Behavioral Disorders in Children 997
Challenged Children 997
Drugs in Pediatrics 997
Common Pediatric Nursing Procedures 998
Fetal Circulation 1001

Clinical Case-Based Questions 1004

Image-Based Questions 1020

Multiple Choice Questions 1031

Obstetric and Gynecological Nursing

Synopsis

Anatomy of Female Reproductive System-Overview 1091
Menstrual Cycle 1095
Fundamentals of Reproduction 1097
Development of the Inner Mass Cells 1098
Human Chorionic Gonadotropin 1099
Principal Events of Embryonic and Fetal Development 1099
The Placenta and Fetal Membranes 1099
Placental Abnormalities 1100
Amniotic Fluid 1103
Amniotic Fluid Disorders 1103
Umbilical Cord 1104
Umbilical Cord Abnormalities 1104
Fetal Circulation 1106
Physiological and Emotional Changes During Prenatal Period 1106
Diagnosis of Pregnancy 1107
Estimation of EDD and Gestational Age 1108
Screening Tests During Pregnancy 1109
Antenatal Assessment of Fetal Well-Being 1113
Anatomy and Types of Female Pelvis 1118
Pelvic Diameter 1120
Fetal Skull 1121
Fetus in Utero (Lie, Presentation and Position) 1123
Positions and Presentations of Fetus During Labor 1124
Different Positions and Presentations During Labor 1126
Labor and Delivery 1127
Difference Between True and False Labor 1128
Assisted Deliveries/Operative Vaginal Deliveries 1136
Forceps Deliveries 1136
Postpartum Nursing Care 1138
Puerperium 1138
Induction of Labor 1139
Contraceptive Method (Fertility Regulation Method) 1140
Abortion 1141
Medical Termination of Pregnancy 1142
Intra-Uterine Fetal Death (IUFD) 1143
Gestational Trophoblastic Disorders 1143
Multiple Pregnancy 1143
Antepartum Hemorrhage 1143
Hyperemesis Gravidarum 1148
Anemia in Pregnancy 1148
HIV in Pregnancy 1149
Rh Incompatibility 1149
Gestational Diabetes Mellitus (GDM) 1150
Heart Disease in Pregnancy 1150
Hypertension in Pregnancy 1150
Postpartum Hemorrhage (PPH) 1151

Injuries to Birth Canal 1152
Prolonged Labor and Obstructed Labor 1153
Preterm Labor and Post-Term Pregnancy 1154
Premature Rupture of Membranes 1155
Pharmacology in OBG 1155
Operative OBG 1156
Common Gynecological Disorders 1156
Fibroid Uterus 1157
Gonorrhea, Syphilis and Pelvic Inflammatory Disease 1157
Cervical Cancer Screening 1157
Lactation and Feeding 1157
GTPAL 1159
Clinical Case-Based Questions 1165
Image-Based Questions 1172
Multiple Choice Questions 1179

Applied Microbiology

Synopsis

Historical Perspectives of Microbiology 1242
The Normal Bacterial Flora of Human Body 1242
Staining Techniques 1243
Types of Microscope 1243
Culture Media 1243
Biochemical Reactions 1244
General Guidelines for Collecting Culture Specimen 1244
Classification of Bacteria 1245
Virus 1247
Fungus 1248
Parasites 1248
Image-Based Questions 1250
Multiple Choice Questions 1252

Applied Biochemistry and Nutrition

Synopsis

Applied Biochemistry 1265
- Introduction 1265
- The Cell 1265
- Transport Mechanisms 1266
- pH, Buffers and Acid-Base Balance 1267
- Enzymes and Coenzymes 1267
- Carbohydrates 1269
- Lipids 1270
- Proteins 1271
- Amino acids 1271
- Vitamins, Minerals and Electrolytes 1273

Applied Nutrition 1276
- Calorie 1276
- Metabolism 1276
- Classification of Foods 1276
- Food Preservation Methods 1277
- Common Adulterants Used in Food Materials 1278
- Tests to Detect Common Adulteration 1278

Multiple Choice Questions 1281

Applied Sociology and Psychology

Synopsis

Applied Sociology 1297
- Introduction 1297
- Socialization 1297
- Family 1298
- Marriage 1299
- Society 1300
- Crowd 1301
- Community 1301
- Culture 1302
- Social Change 1302
- Social Control 1302
- Norms 1303
- Social Stratification 1303
- Social Mobility 1303
- Social Problems 1304
- Population Explosion 1306
- Urbanization 1306

Applied Psychology 1307
- Introduction 1307
- Pure Psychology versus Applied Psychology 1307
- Branches of Pure Psychology 1307
- Branches of Applied Psychology 1307
- Importance of Psychology for Nurses 1308
- Mind 1308
- Behavior 1309
- Attention 1309
- Perception 1309
- Learning 1309
- Memory 1311
- Forgetting 1311
- Thinking 1312
- Reasoning 1312
- Problem-Solving 1312
- Intelligence 1312
- Stress 1312
- Conflict 1313
- Attitude 1314
- Personality 1314

Multiple Choice Questions 1317

Nursing Research and Statistics

Synopsis

Introduction 1327
Definition 1327
Steps in the Quantitative Research Process 1327
Steps in the Qualitative Research Process 1327
Research Process 1327
Research Designs 1329
Mixed Method Research 1333
Major Types of Data Collection Methods 1334
Sample and Sampling Technique 1336
Ethics in Research 1338
Data Analysis and Interpretation 1338
Numerical Data Properties and Measures 1340
Application of Inferential Statistics 1343
Image-Based Questions 1347
Multiple Choice Questions 1352

Nursing Education

Synopsis

Education 1373
Indian Nursing Council (INC) 1374
Nursing Programs in India 1375
Nursing Education in India 1375
International Council of Nurses (ICN) 1375
State Nursing Councils in India 1375
Trained Nurses Association of India (TNAI) 1375
Curriculum 1375
Educational Objectives 1376
Audio-Visual Aid 1377
Maxims of Teaching 1378
Pedagogy vs Andragogy 1378
Principles of Teaching 1378
Evaluation 1380
Continuing Nursing Education 1381
In-Service Education 1381

Johari Window 1381
Accreditation in Higher Edcuation 1382
Educational Learning Theories 1382
Innovative Methods of Teaching 1382
Multiple Choice Questions 1384

Nursing Administration and Management

Synopsis

Organization 1391
Administration 1391
Management 1391
Leadership 1394
Budgeting 1394
Material management 1395
Inventory Control 1395
Staff Development 1396
Quality Management 1396
Nursing Audit 1397
Norms of Staffing (SIU—Staff Inspection Unit) 1397
Norms of (as per INC and TNAI) 1397
Teacher-Student Ratio for Nursing Programs as per Indian Nursing Council (INC) 1398
Multiple Choice Questions 1399

Computer/Health and Nursing Informatics

Synopsis

Basic Key Terms 1410
History of Computers 1410
Generations of Computers 1410
Classification of Computers 1411
Hardware and Software 1411
Computer Networking 1416
Multiple Choice Questions 1418

Forensic Nursing and Indian Laws

Synopsis

Introduction 1427
Importance 1427
Areas of Forensic Nursing Practice 1427
Scope and Practice of Forensic Nursing 1427
Milestones in Forensic Nursing 1427
Subspecialties in Forensic Nursing 1428
Ethical Issues in Forensic Nursing 1428
Forensic Team 1429
Evidence and Sample Collection in Forensic Nursing 1429
Comprehensive Forensic Nursing Care 1430
Violence 1430
Sexual Abuse 1431
Death 1431
Fundamental Rights 1431
Rights of Victim 1431
Rights of Accused 1432
Human Rights Commission 1432
Indian Nursing Council Act 1432
State Nursing Registration Council 1433
Overview of the Indian Judicial System and Laws 1433
Civil Case Procedure 1434
Criminal Case Procedure 1434
Indian Penal Code (IPC) 1434
Criminal Procedure Code (CrPC) 1434
Indian Evidence Act 1434
Multiple Choice Questions 1436

Section B

Previous Year Papers

1. NORCET (June) 2023 (Memory Based) (NEW) 1443
2. AIIMS Jodhpur (SNO) 2023 (NEW) 1451
3. AllMS Bibinagar (Tutor) 2023 (NEW) 1459
4. AllMS Bibinagar Associate Professor 2023 (NEW) 1463
5. Sree Chitra Tirunal Institute for Medical Science and Technology (NO) 2023 (NEW) 1468
6. Uttar Pradesh University of Medical Sciences (NO) 2023 (NEW) 1473
7. NORCET (NO) 2022 (Memory Based) (NEW) 1483
8. Staff Nurse Examination Himachal Pradesh 2022 (NEW) 1491
9. Western Coalfields Limited 2022 (NEW) 1497
10. Odisha Subordinate Staff Selection Commission (NO) 2022 (NEW) 1501
11. Gujarat Nursing Service (Nursing Officer/Principal) 2022 (NEW) 1506
12. NORCET (NO) 2021 (Memory Based) (NEW) 1514
13. CNCI (NO) 2021 1520
14. NORCET (NO) 2020 1525
15. Combined AIIMS (NO) (Bhopal, Jodhpur, Patna & Raipur) 2020 1533
16. AIIMS Nagpur (NO) 2020 1542
17. AIIMS Patna (NO) 2020 1547
18. Nursing Officer Exam, JIPMER 2020 1555

Papers in Nursing Next Live

(Under Target High Digital Lite Package)

1. NORCET (June) 2023 (Memory Based) (NEW)
2. AIIMS Jodhpur (SNO) 2023 (NEW)
3. AllMS Bibinagar (Tutor) 2023 (NEW)
4. AllMS Bibinagar Associate Professor 2023 (NEW)
5. Sree Chitra Tirunal Institute for Medical Science and Technology (NO) 2023 (NEW)
6. Uttar Pradesh University of Medical Sciences (NO) 2023 (NEW)
7. NORCET (NO) 2022 (Memory Based) (NEW)
8. Staff Nurse Examination Himachal Pradesh 2022 (NEW)
9. Western Coalfields Limited 2022 (NEW)
10. Odisha Subordinate Staff Selection Commission (NO) 2022 (NEW)
11. Gujarat Nursing Service 2022 (Nursing Officer/Principal) (NEW)
12. NORCET (NO) 2021 (Memory Based) (NEW)
13. Combined AIIMS (NO) (Bhopal, Jodhpur, Patna & Raipur) 2020
14. AIIMS Raipur (Lecturer) 2021
15. AIIMS NORCET 2020
16. AIIMS Nagpur (Nursing Officer) 2020
17. AIIMS Patna (Nursing Officer) 2020
18. AIIMS Raipur (Nursing Officer) 2019
19. AIIMS Bhatinda (Nursing Officer) 2019
20. AIIMS Raipur (Nursing Officer) 2019; Shift 1
21. AIIMS Raipur (Nursing Officer) 2019; Shift 2
22. AIIMS Raipur (Nursing Officer) 2019; Shift 3
23. AIIMS Bhubaneshwar (Senior Nursing Officer) 2019
24. AIIMS New Delhi (Nursing Officer) 2019
25. AIIMS New Delhi (Nursing Officer) 2018

26. AIIMS Nagpur (Nursing Officer) 2018
27. AIIMS Jodhpur (Senior Nursing Officer) Grade 1: 2018
28. AIIMS Bhopal (Senior Nursing Officer) 2018
29. AIIMS Bhopal (Nursing Officer) 2018; Shift 1
30. AIIMS Bhopal (Nursing Officer) 2018; Shift 2
31. AIIMS Mangalagiri (Nursing Officer) Grade-II; 2018; Shift 2
32. AIIMS Bhubaneswar (Nursing Officer) 2018
33. AIIMS Raipur (Nursing Officer) 2017; Shift 1
34. AIIMS Raipur (Nursing Officer) 2017; Shift 2
35. AIIMS Raipur (Nursing Officer) 2017; Shift 3
36. AIIMS Raipur (Nursing Tutor) 2017
37. AIIMS Jodhpur & Rishikesh (Nursing Officer) 2017
38. AIIMS Raipur (Senior Nursing Officer) 2017
39. AIIMS Bhopal (Nursing Officer) 2016
40. AIIMS New Delhi (Nursing Officer) 2016
41. AIIMS Bhopal (Senior Nursing Officer) 2016
42. CNCI (Nursing Officer) 2021
43. BFUHS 2021
44. ESIC Paramedical 2019; Shift 1
45. ESIC Paramedical 2019; Shift 2
46. ESIC (Nursing Officer) 2016; Shift 1
47. ESIC (Nursing Officer) 2016; Shift 2
48. ESIC (Nursing Officer) Banglore Shift 1: 2016
49. ESIC (Nursing Officer) Banglore Shift 2: 2016
50. ESIC (Nursing Officer) Delhi 2016
51. ESIC (Nursing Officer) Banglore 2013
52. ESIC (Nursing Officer) Chennai 2012
53. ESIC (Nursing Officer) Grade II: 2011
54. ESIC (Nursing Officer) Ahmedabad 2011
55. Kerala PSC 2021
56. Kerala PSC (Nursing Officer) 2017
57. Kerala PSC (Nursing Officer) 2016
58. Kerala PSC (Nursing Officer) 2014
59. Kerala PSC (Nursing Officer) Grade II: 2011
60. Kerala PSC (Nursing Officer) Set C: 2011
61. Kerala PSC (Nursing Officer) 2010
62. BHU (Nursing Officer) 2019
63. BHU (Nursing Officer) 2018
64. BHU (Nursing Officer) 2016
65. BHU (Nursing Officer) 2015
66. Safdarjung (Nursing Officer) 2019
67. Safdarjung (Nursing Officer) 2018
68. JIPMER (Nursing Officer) 2020
69. JIPMER (Nursing Officer) 2013
70. JIPMER (Nursing Officer) 2012
71. UK State MSc (Nursing Officer) 2016
72. UK Nursing Tutor (Paper 1- Set B)
73. RRB (Nursing Officer) 2019; Shift 1
74. RRB (Nursing Officer) 2019; Shift 2
75. RRB (Nursing Officer) 2019; Shift 3
76. RRB (Nursing Officer) 2019; Shift 4
77. RRB (Nursing Officer) 2019; Shift 5
78. RRB Paramedical PHN 2015
79. RRB (Nursing Officer) 2015; Set A
80. RRB (Nursing Officer) 2015; Set B
81. RRB (Nursing Officer) 2015; Set C
82. RRB Secunderabad (Senior Nursing Officer) 2015
83. RRB (Nursing Officer) 2012
84. HPSSC (Nursing Officer) 2016
85. HP (Nursing Officer) 2016
86. RAK MSc Entrance Exam 2018
87. RAK New Delhi Entrance Exam 2017
88. GMCH (Nursing Officer) 2019
89. GMCH (Nursing Officer) 2016
91. Northern Coal Field Limited, Singrauli (Nursing Officer) 2019
92. PGIMER Chandigarh (Nursing Officer) 2016
93. CHO Haryana 2021
94. CHO Rajasthan 2020
95. CHO Madhya Pradesh 2020
96. CHO Madhya Pradesh 2019 Shift-1
97. CHO Uttar Pradesh 2018
98. RUHS MSc Nursing Entrance Exam 2018
99. RUHS MSc Nursing Entrance Exam 2016
100. RUHS Post Basic Basic Nursing Entrance Exam 2016
101. LNJP Hospital Delhi (Nursing Officer) 2012
102. DSSSB Shift I (NO) 2019
103. DSSSB Shift II (NO) 2019
104. DSSSB PHN 2015
105. DSSSB ANM 2015
106. Jhalawar Hospital and Medical College Society 2012
107. TNPSC Maternal and Child Health Officer 2015
108. RML Hospital (Nursing Officer) 2011
109. Insurance Medical Services (Nursing Officer) 2004
110. RRC (Nursing Officer) 2012
111. SCTIMST (Nursing Officer) 2015
112. Rohtak (Nursing Officer) 2020
113. NIMHANS (Nursing Officer) 2019 (Memory Based)
114. SKIM (Nursing Officer) 2020 Paper
115. Gujarat Staff (Nursing Officer) 2021
116. Jr. Grade Nurse/Jr. Staff Nurse/Jr. Nurse 2020
117. UPPSC Staff Nurse 2021
118. Uttarakhand Assistant Professor 2021
119. Daman & Diu (NO) 2018

How to Prepare for NORCET (Prelims and Mains): An Overview

The recent changes in NORCET exam pattern have brought two stages of exams: Stage I – NORCET Preliminary and Stage II- NORCET Mains.

NORCET examination will be conducted in two successive stages as described below:

Stage I: NORCET Preliminary

Stage II: NORCET Mains

The overview of NORCET new pattern and how TARGET HIGH can be effectively used for preparation is illustrated below.

	Stage I- NORCET Prelims	Stage II- NORCET Mains
Exam pattern	• 100 MCQs – 100 marks • 80 Questions from nursing subjects at BSc nursing level • 20 Questions from GK & Aptitude. • Computer-based test	• 100 MCQs – 100 marks • Case scenario-based questions • Nursing skill related questions • Computer-based test
Time duration	**90 mins**	**90 mins**
Negative marking	1/3 per wrong answer. (-0.33 per wrong answer)	1/3 per wrong answer. (-0.33 per wrong answer)
Scheme of exam	**Qualifying in nature** • 50% for UR/EWS • 45% for OBC • 40% for SC & ST • Additional 5% relaxation for PWBD However, NOT all eligible candidates will be called (shortlisted) for Stage-II exam. Only 5 times the total seats in each category (UR, OBC, SC, ST, EWS) will be shortlisted to write Stage-II-Mains exam. For example, if the vacancy position is UR-100, OBC-25, SC-15, ST-7, & EWS-10), then the number of candidates shortlisted will be UR-500, OBC-125, SC-75, ST-35 & EWS-50. The qualified candidates who are in tie with the last shortlisted candidates also will be called for Stage-II exam. All qualified PWBD candidates will be called for Stage-II exam.	The qualifying marks in the Stage-II, NORCET Mains Examination will be: • 50% for UR/EWS • 45% for OBC • 40% for SC & ST. • Additional 5% relaxation for PWBD Merit rank list shall be prepared based on performance in CBT as per qualifying criteria in Stage-II NORCET Mains.
Difficulty level	**Easy to moderate**	**Moderate to difficult**
How to prepare using TARGET HIGH	**Theory:** • Synopses in the 7th edition is thoroughly revised, particularly the FON to enhance knowledge in basic nursing procedures and concepts. • All the subjects as per the new INC syllabus have been included. • Focus on reading the synopses of all subjects. • Give attention to Key points, Practice questions and Questions from recent NORCET exams provided side-by-side in the synopsis for better understanding. • Read, revise and reinforce the Golden Points given at the end of each synopsis. Those golden points are high yield points which are more likely to be asked in the Stage-I Prelims. • **GK & Aptitude:** Keeping in mind the 20% weightage, the GK & Aptitude content is improved and enriched with all recent updates, verbal and numerical reasonings, quantitative aptitude, etc. Most importantly, the GK & Aptitude section is provided as a separate booklet.	**Theory:** • Case scenario-based questions (CBQs) and Nursing Skill based questions are the only focus in the Stage II-Mains exam. • They provide a strong foundation in disease conditions, signs and symptoms, physiological parameters, pharmacology, drug effects, and pathophysiology which are crucial for solving these questions effectively. • Target High 7th Edition contains comprehensive information on these concepts, particularly in the synopsis part. The synopsis part also includes Case scenario-based questions side-by-side. • The inclusion of 1000+ Case scenario-based questions with rationales in the book's various sections is seen as a valuable tool for test-takers to practice and enhance their understanding. • Practicing these Case scenario-based questions can indeed be a beneficial strategy to refine and improve one's knowledge and problem-solving skills for the exam.
How to boost preparation using TARGET HIGH Digital Lite	• You can prepare on the go with the Target High Digital Lite App. • All the Target High readers are free to use this feature. • Subject wise tests and Grand tests as per the recent pattern are provided from time to time. • Voice over of Golden points can heard on the move. This will reinforce your memory of important key points.	• Review and Practice additional Case scenario-based questions provided in the App to boost your preparation. • Take Grand tests on the NORCET Mains pattern in the App.

Decoding the Case Scenario-based Questions

INTRODUCTION

Decoding the scenario-based clinical multiple-choice questions (MCQs) in nursing requires a systematic and strategic approach. Such questions assess a nurse's ability to apply clinical knowledge, critical thinking, and clinical judgment in various patient situations. To navigate these questions effectively, a step-by-step strategy can be employed.

This strategy involves a detailed 5-Points approach which is as follows:

1. Analyzing the question stem and options
2. Prioritizing nursing actions or interventions
3. Categories of case scenario-based questions
4. Normal vs abnormal and nursing action vs physician action
5. Answering complex case scenario-based questions using clinical judgment

Each of these approaches has been discussed in detail with suitable examples:

ANALYSING THE QUESTION STEM AND OPTIONS

- The Scenario-based MCQs will have two parts. The stem and the four options, out of which one option would be correct. Options other than the correct answer are known as distractors.
- The goal of these scenario-based MCQs is to assess the nurse's ability to apply knowledge, clinical reasoning, and critical thinking skills to make the best decision in a given patient situation.
- As a test-taker, it is crucial to carefully read and analyze both the stem and the options before selecting the most appropriate response based on your nursing knowledge and judgment.

The Stem

- **Stem provides the context** and information about the patient or clinical situation.
- **Understanding the stem** and identifying the key terms or strategic terms is very important to answer the question.
- **Read the stem carefully:** Start by reading the stem carefully and pay close attention to the patient's condition, symptoms, vital signs, and any other relevant information.
- **Stem usually has two parts:** 1. *Scenario/Event:* The case scenario for which a nurse in caring for. 2. *Query:* What the nurse is expected to do (nursing action).
- **Identify the main issue:** Determine the main problem or issue that the question is addressing. It could be:
  - a specific symptom
  - a change in vital signs
  - a complication, or
  - a potential risk to the patient.

Note: Considering the time limit (one minute per question), it is very important to read quickly and carefully to understand the key term or strategic term.

- **Look for quantitative information:** Keep an eye out for specific numerical data, such as vital signs, laboratory values, or medication doses. These values can be essential in identifying abnormal findings or trends.
- **Note qualitative descriptions:** Look for descriptive terms or adjectives that provide clues about the severity or character of the patient's condition. For example, words like "severe," "acute," "mild," "chronic," "sudden," or "gradual" can impact the urgency of the response.
- **Recognize key terms or strategic terms:** Recognize key terms or phrases which guide you to choose the correct answer. The key terms include: **first, initial, best, essential, priority, immediately, early, late, most appropriate, inappropriate, EXCLUDE, INCLUDE, increased, decreased.**
- **Positive vs negative stem:** Look for key word to determine whether the stem is positive or negative.
  - **Positive terms:** Positive terms in the stem include **Appropriate, True, Indicated** and **Understand.** For example, which statement **best** represents how the nurse should document these findings? In this case, you should be looking for a positive response (appropriate or right method) from the options.
  - **Negative terms:** Negative terms in the stem include **Not, Never, further (....further education or intervention required), Least, Avoid, Contraindicated.**

  For example, which intervention should be given the **least** priority in this case? In this case, you should be looking for least important intervention (or inappropriate or unsuitable intervention) form the options.

Example Question

Positive Stem

During the discharge process of a 12-year-old child with hemophilia, the nurse advises the parents regarding the **most appropriate** sport activity for the child. What sport activity does the nurse recommend?

a. Swimming b. Football c. Field hockey d. Basketball

Ans. (a) Swimming

Explanation: Hemophilia is a bleeding disorder characterized by a deficiency or dysfunction of clotting factors in the blood. Therefore, high-impact or contact sports should generally be avoided to minimize the risk of bleeding and injury. With that in mind, the nurse should recommend low-impact and non-contact sports. So, among the given options most appropriate sport activity for the child is swimming.

STRATEGY: The key word **Most appropriate** leads to a positive or suitable or appropriate sports activity for the child with hemophilia.

Example Question

Negative Stem

Nurse Ramya, a palliative care nurse, is providing nursing care to a terminally ill patient during the dying and grieving process. She is aware that the **least important** goal of nursing intervention in this client is:

a. Providing comfort measures
b. Promotion of rest and sleep
c. Increase self-esteem through cosmetic improvement
d. Pain management

Ans. (c) Increase self-esteem through cosmetic improvement

Explanation: The nursing interventions should target pain management through pain-reduction techniques and analgesia, providing comfort measures, promotion of sleep and rest, and energy conservation for this patient. Though dying with dignity and self-esteem is important, increase of self-esteem through cosmetic improvement is not important for this client.

STRATEGY: The negative key term "least important" leads to choose the unimportant interventions among given options.

ALERT

Double negatives in the stem: While using the key word strategy, please be cautious about double negatives in the stem. If the stem has two negative terms, then you should be looking for positive response. For example, Stem: all of the following interventions are **contraindicated** in a patient with diabetes mellitus, **except.** In this stem, there are two negative key words; 'contraindicated' and 'except' which guide you to choose the positive or suitable intervention.

Example Question

Double Negatives

A 45-year-old patient has recently undergone a colostomy surgery. The nurse is providing dietary education to the patient. The nurse advises the patient **to avoid** the following foods to ensure optimal recovery, **except:**

a. Consume high-fiber diet
b. Encourage raw vegetables
c. Encourage intake of legumes
d. Encourage cereals made from refined flour

Ans. (d) Encourage cereals made from refined flour

Explanation: The question is asking for the food that the nurse should not advise the patient to avoid. Cereals made from refined flour are low in fiber and easy to digest, so they are not a concern after a colostomy surgery. The other answer choices are all foods that are high in fiber and should be avoided after a colostomy surgery.

STRATEGY: Identify the double negative terms in the stem; **'to avoid'** and **'except'.** This leads you to choose the appropriate or suitable diet for the patient with colostomy.

- **Pay Attention to time frames:** If time-related information is provided in the stem, consider how it might influence your response. For instance, the urgency of the intervention might differ between immediate actions and actions that can be taken later. On the other hand, time frame is important in deciding what is the appropriate action/intervention to be taken.

Example Question

Time Frame

A 2-year-old child weighing about 35 kg was brought to the emergency department **30 minutes** after accidental ingestion of 12 tablets of Paracetamol 650 mg. Which of the following intervention is the priority for this child?

a. Administer N-Acetylcysteine
b. Administer activated charcoal
c. Perform gastric lavage
d. Administer 5% dextrose in half normal saline

Ans. (b) Administer activated charcoal

Explanation: Treatment guidelines for oral Paracetamol (acetaminophen) ingestion in children:

- Less than 4 hours after ingestion – Consider activated charcoal if dose is >150 mg/kg (activated charcoal is not advised if the ingested dose is unknown)
- 4–24 hours – Obtain plasma acetaminophen level as soon as possible. Start with N-Acetylcysteine (NAC) administration.
- Longer than 24 hours – NAC administration

STRATEGY: Time-related information is key to solve this question. Time frame 30 minutes (<4 hours) is the key factor for the treatment option. If time frame exceeded 4 hours, the answer would be a. Administer N-Acetylcysteine.

Options

By following the previous steps, you have read the stem carefully and understood the client conditions, and parameters, and identified the key terms. Now, you read the options carefully and try to match:

- Positive key terms with positive options (appropriate or suitable interventions)
- Negative key terms with negative options (inappropriate or non-suitable interventions)
- Double negative key terms with a positive options (appropriate or suitable interventions)

Note: The examples for these 3 scenarios were given earlier in this chapter.

Identify words or phrases in the options that have strong connection or similarity to words in the stem. Sometimes, the words in the options may be closely linked but not identical.

Example Question

Connection Words

A patient develops anaphylactic reaction to an IV medication, which of the following should be the **immediate** response of a nurse?

a. Call for emergency help
b. Stop the medication administration immediately
c. Administer IM Epinephrine
d. Start CPR

Ans. (b) Stop the medication administration immediately

Explanation: The immediate response of the nurse should be removing the allergen (stopping IV medication in this case). The next step is to call rapid response and start basic life support (BLS/CPR) until the help arrives.

STRATEGY: Look for connection word 'immediately' in the stem and the option which guides the test-taker to option b.

Consider the following strategies while trying to choose right option:

1. **Use Elimination Process:**
   - Always apply the process of elimination.
   - Carefully read each option, and after eliminating options, re-read the question before making your final choice.
2. **Compare and Eliminate:**
   - Identify comparable or similar options and eliminate them from consideration.
   - It is one of the key strategies in elimination process. If two options are similar or alike or comparable, then both are not the correct answer, so it can be eliminated.

Example Question

Eliminate Similar or Alike Options

All of the following statements are true about SIADH lab values, EXCEPT (AIIMS Bibinagar, Faculty 2023)

a. SIADH causes increased urine osmolarity
b. SIADH causes elevated urine sodium concentration
c. SIADH causes decreased plasma osmolarity
d. SIADH causes increased plasma osmolarity

Ans. (d) SIADH causes increased plasma osmolarity

STRATEGY: Eliminate a and b because both are similar statements [elevated urine sodium concentration (b) = increased urine osmolarity (a)].

Explanation: Syndrome of Inappropriate Antidiuretic Hormone (SIADH) results in Increased. Antidiuretic Hormone (ADH) secretion, leading to increased water retention and dilution of the blood's solutes. The excess water retention causes the blood to become more diluted, resulting in a lower concentration of solutes in the blood and decreased plasma osmolarity. The other statements (a, b, and c) are true about SIADH lab values.

3. Consider encompassing or **umbrella options:** Check if any option covers a broader concept or scenario; it might be the correct choice. An example of umbrella options is **Administer fluids.** This option encompasses all of the different types of fluids that can be administered to patients, such as IV fluids, oral fluids. Another example of umbrella option is **Provide emotional support** which encompasses options such as listening to the patient's concerns, offering words of encouragement, and providing touch therapy.
4. Watch for close-ended words: If you find close-ended words in options, the option is likely incorrect. Examples of close-ended words include '**Always**', '**Never**', '**Must**'.
   The words 'Always' and 'Never' imply that there is no exception to the rule. In reality, there is often exception to the rule.

Example Question

Close-Ended words

During the discharge instructions, the nurse explains the concept of feedback in communication to the patient's family. In the context of healthcare communication, which understanding of feedback aligns with the principle that "communication is interaction perspective"?

a. Feedback is **never** intentional
b. Feedback is sometimes unintentional
c. Feedback is **always** intentional
d. Feedback is seldom useful

Ans. (b) Feedback is sometimes unintentional

STRATEGY: Option a, c has close-ended words **'never'** and **'always'** respectively. Hence, they are unlikely the correct answer. Option (d) feedback is seldom useful is factually incorrect so it is easy to eliminate.

5. **Utilize therapeutic communication:** For communication questions, use therapeutic communication techniques. Focus on the client's emotions, concerns, fears, and thoughts.
6. **Delegate with guidelines:** Use delegation and job description of Nursing personnel (Staff Nurse/Incharge-Nurse/Supervisor/Nurse Manager, and others) to align the client's needs with the health care provider's scope of practice.
7. **Pharmacology considerations:** If a question involves medication, apply pharmacology guidelines to choose the correct option.
8. Whenever the listed options include "notify the physician" or "document the findings," apply the strategy discussed later in this section to select or eliminate them.

Prioritizing Nursing Actions or Interventions

- Prioritization is a crucial skill in nursing, and it involves determining the order of actions when faced with multiple tasks or patient needs.
- **Apply ABCs, Maslow's Hierarchy, and Nursing Process:** For prioritization questions, apply the ABCs (airway, breathing, circulation), Maslow's Hierarchy of Needs, and the nursing process steps to choose the right answer.

ABCs (Airway-Breathing-Circulation)

Recognize the critical importance of maintaining and prioritizing the client's airway, breathing, and circulation (in its order) in emergency situations.

The order of priority is Airway – Breathing – Circulation. To understand this better, let's expand on each element with reference to a nursing care scenario involving a patient who is brought to the Emergency Department after a Road Traffic Accident:

- **Airway:**
  - The first priority for the nurse is to assess the patient's airway to ensure it is clear and unobstructed. Noe that the airway is always the priority nursing action.

    Note: During Cardiopulmonary Resuscitation (CPR), the order is CAB (Compression/Circulation, airway and breathing)

  - The patient is unconscious and may have suffered injuries to the head and neck due to the accident, increasing the risk of airway obstruction.
  - The nurse quickly opens the patient's airway using the jaw-thrust maneuver or head-tilt chin-lift technique, while maintaining spinal precautions if there is suspicion of cervical spine injury.
- **Breathing:**
  - After securing the airway, the nurse assesses the patient's breathing to ensure it is adequate.
  - The patient may have compromised breathing due to chest trauma or internal injuries, and respiratory distress is a common concern in trauma cases.
  - The nurse assesses the rate, depth, and quality of the patient's breaths and provides supplemental oxygen if needed.

- **Circulation:**
  - Once the airway and breathing are stabilized, the nurse assesses the patient's circulation to check for signs of shock or hemorrhage.
  - The patient may have sustained internal bleeding or other injuries resulting in hypovolemic shock.
  - The nurse checks the patient's pulse, blood pressure, and skin perfusion to evaluate circulation and starts appropriate interventions, such as intravenous (IV) access and fluid resuscitation, if indicated.
  - Other interventions: (This step usually follows after ABC is addressed)
  - The nurse performs a thorough head-to-toe assessment to identify all injuries and prioritize care accordingly.
  - Collaborating with the healthcare team, the nurse may request imaging studies, such as X-rays or CT scans, to further evaluate and diagnose any internal injuries or fractures.
  - Pain management is initiated using appropriate medications to alleviate the patient's discomfort and reduce stress response.

Example Question

A-B-C

An unconscious patient is brought to the emergency room after a road traffic accident. Which of the following is the priority intervention in this patient?

a. Assess for level of consciousness
b. Assess vital signs
c. Airway management
d. Management of bleeding

Ans. (c) Airway management

STRATEGY: Apply A-B-C to prioritize nursing action in the given scenario which leads to airway management option.

Maslow's Hierarchy of Needs

Understand the priority of addressing physiological needs before addressing higher-level needs. The hierarchy of Maslow's theory is as follows:

- **Physiological needs:** Air (oxygen), water (fluid), food, rest, and hygiene
- **Safety and Security needs:** Protection from injury or physical harm, Safe environment.
- **Love and Belonging needs:** Social relationship, trusting interpersonal relationship, love and affection, sense of belonging.
- **Self-esteem needs:** Self-confidence, achievement, status and sense of accomplishment
- **Self-Actualization needs:** Realizing personal goals, pursuing creative activities, state of fulfilment.

Example Question

Maslow's Hierarchy of Needs

A nurse is assigned to four patients in the surgical ward. Which patient's needs should the nurse address first according to Maslow's hierarchy of needs?

a. A patient who is requesting assistance to reposition in bed due to discomfort.
b. A patient who is feeling lonely and asks to talk to a friend on the phone.
c. A patient who is postoperative and requires pain medication for incisional pain.
d. A patient who wants to participate in an art therapy session in the recreation room.

Ans. (c) A Patient who is postoperative and requires pain meds……

STRATEGY: Apply Maslow's hierarchy of needs. Physiological needs, such as pain relief, take precedence over higher-level needs (comfort, need for relationship and recreation) in the hierarchy.

Nursing Process

Utilize the steps of the nursing process (assessment, diagnosis (analysis of problem), planning, implementation, and evaluation) to prioritize the nursing action.

Let's explore how each step of the nursing process can guide the test taker in answering Case Scenario-based questions:

Assessment: If the question stem lacks specific details about the client's condition or assessment outcomes, the test taker should prioritize selecting the assessment option that will provide crucial data to guide further action.

For example, if the question involves a client with a suspected infection but lacks specific vital signs or laboratory results, choosing the assessment option related to collecting vital signs or obtaining a culture sample would be the appropriate first step.

The following key words in the 'option' indicate that it is related to assessment:

- Determine
- Find out
- Assess
- Ascertain
- Collect
- Check
- Identify
- Gather
- Monitor
- Obtain information
- Recognize
- Observe

Example Question

Nursing Process - Assessment

Two days after the coronary angiography, the client reports increased pain and discomfort at the catheter site, what should the nurse do?

a. Explain the client that it is normal after coronary angiography
b. Assess the signs for infection
c. Elevate the affected extremity
d. Give massage to the pain site

Ans. (b) Assess the signs for infection

STRETEGY: The client's report of pain and discomfort at catheter site indicates the possibility of infection. So, the nurse should assess for signs of infection to decide further action.

Diagnosis (Analysis of problem): If the question stem provides assessment data or specific client information, the test taker should proceed to analyze the data and identify the most relevant patient problem (nursing diagnosis) which needs to be addressed. For instance, if the question describes a client with shortness of breath, wheezing, and a history of asthma, the test taker would recognize that the nursing diagnosis "Impaired Gas Exchange related to bronchoconstriction" is appropriate based on the presented data.

Planning: If the problem is clearly stated in the question stem, the test taker should focus on selecting appropriate nursing interventions or actions to address the client's needs. For example, if the problem stated is "patient with acute pain related to surgical incision," the test taker would indeed choose interventions such as administering pain medication, using comfort measures, and repositioning the client for pain relief.

However, if any of the options present an assessment action, such as "assess the level of pain," the test taker should prioritize selecting the assessment option. Assessing the level of pain is critical to understanding the intensity and nature of the client's pain, which is essential for choosing the most effective pain management intervention. By assessing the pain level, the nurse can determine the appropriate type and dosage of pain medication or other comfort measures needed to provide optimal pain relief.

Implementation: In this step, the test taker should consider the selected nursing interventions and determine which action to implement first based on the client's immediate needs and safety.

For instance, if the nursing interventions include wound dressing, administration of insulin, and patient education, the test taker would prioritize administration of insulin to address the client's immediate physiological needs.

Apply ABC, Maslow's hierarchy of needs and nursing process steps to prioritize the nursing interventions (as discussed above).

Evaluation: This is the final step of nursing process. In evaluation, the nurse assesses the client's response to the nursing interventions and compares it to the expected outcomes set during the planning phase. If the question stem explicitly asks the test taker to identify the effectiveness of the implemented nursing interventions or determine whether the client's desired outcomes have been achieved, then the appropriate response would be options related to evaluation.

If the question stem states that the client's desired outcomes have been met, the test taker would choose options related to reinforcing the successful interventions or documenting the positive outcomes.

Example Question

Concept: Evaluation (NORCET 2021)

A 17-year-old student has a long history of bronchial asthma and has experienced several severe asthmatic attacks during the school year. The school nurse is required to administer 0.2 mL of 1/1000 solution of epinephrine SC during an asthma attack. How does the school nurse evaluate the effectiveness of this intervention?

a. Increased pulse rate
b. Increased expectorate of secretions
c. Decreased inspiratory difficulty
d. Increased respiratory rate

Ans. (c) Decreased inspiratory difficulty

STRATEGY: The stem has key word **"nurse evaluate"**. The expected outcome after administration of Epinephrine SC during asthma attack should be evaluated. Think of a positive outcome among given options.

Categories of Case Scenario-based Questions

Case scenario-based questions are designed to assess the nurse's ability to:

- Provide safe and Effective care environment
- Provide care to maintain physiological integrity of patients
- Provide care to maintain psychosocial integrity of patients
- Promote health maintenance in patients.

Provide Safe and Effective Care Environment

Questions in this category assess the nurse's ability to:

- Provide safe nursing care to clients.
- Collaborate effectively with other healthcare team members to ensure optimal client care
- Protect clients, their significant others, and healthcare personnel from environmental hazards.

Key Focus Areas for Safety-related Questions:

- **Hand washing:** Give stress on the importance of proper hand hygiene to prevent the transmission of infections.
- **Asepsis:** Emphasize the importance of maintaining a sterile environment during procedures to minimize the risk of infections.
- **Call lights or bells:** Address the significance of promptly responding to clients' calls for assistance to ensure their safety and comfort.
- **Bed positioning:** Explain the appropriate positioning of clients to prevent complications such as pressure ulcers and respiratory issues.
- **Appropriate use of side rails:** Discuss the safe use of side rails to prevent falls while considering individual client needs.
- **Use of standard and other precautions:** Review the implementation of infection control practices to safeguard against the spread of communicable diseases.
- **Triage:** Describe the process of prioritizing patients based on the severity of their conditions in emergency situations.
- **Emergency response planning:** Highlight the importance of having well-defined protocols to manage emergencies effectively and efficiently.

Physiological Integrity of Patients

These questions in the Physiological Integrity category assess the nurse's ability to:

- Provide care related to comfort and assistance with activities of daily living for clients.
- Administer medications and parenteral therapies safely and accurately.

These Questions also Evaluate the Nurse's Capability to:

- Minimize the client's risk of developing complications or health problems related to treatments, procedures, or existing medical conditions.
- Deliver care to clients with acute, chronic, or life-threatening physical health conditions.

Key Focus Areas for Physiological Integrity Questions:

- Care related to comfort and activities of daily living
- Medication administration
- Parenteral therapy safety
- Minimizing the risk of complications
- Understanding procedures and treatments
- Assessing and monitoring clients
- Client education

Psychosocial Integrity of Patients

These questions focus on providing nursing care that helps clients and family members cope, adapt, and solve the problems in challenging situations, such as illnesses, disabilities, or stressful events, like abuse, neglect, or violence.

Within this category, test takers may encounter communication-type questions that assess how the nurse responds to clients, their family members, significant others, or other members of the health care team.

When approaching psychosocial integrity questions, it is essential to use therapeutic communication techniques. These techniques are effective in promoting a supportive and healing communication process between the nurse and the client or significant others. The nurse should choose options that address the thoughts, feelings, concerns, anxieties, or fears of the client, their family members, or significant others.

In answering psychosocial integrity questions, the nurse should consider the client's emotional and mental well-being as well as his social context. This may involve demonstrating sensitivity to cultural differences, respecting client's autonomy and decision-making, and collaborating with other health care team members to provide comprehensive and patient-centered care.

Example Question

Psychosocial Integrity

A nurse is caring for a client who has recently been diagnosed with a chronic illness. The client appears anxious and expresses concerns about managing the condition and its impact on daily life. Which therapeutic communication response by the nurse is most appropriate?

a. "I understand how difficult this must be for you. You'll get through this."
b. "Don't worry; the treatment for this illness is very effective."
c. "You should focus on the positive aspects of your life and not dwell on the illness."
d. "Tell me more about your concerns and how this diagnosis is affecting you."

Ans. (d) "Tell me more about your concerns and how this diagnosis is affecting you."

Explanation: Option d demonstrates therapeutic communication by actively listening to the client's concerns and inviting them to share his thoughts and feelings openly. It acknowledges the client's emotional state and allows him to express his fears and anxieties related to the chronic illness. This response promotes trust and rapport between the nurse and the client, which is essential in supporting the client's psychosocial well-being.

Options a and b may be dismissive and closing the conversation. It does not encourage the client to express his feelings. Option c may come across as minimizing the client's emotions and may not effectively address his concerns.

Example Question

A nurse is caring for a client who has been diagnosed with a terminal illness. The client appears distressed and says, "I'm scared of what the future holds." Which response by the nurse is most appropriate?

a. "You have nothing to be scared of. Everything will be okay."
b. "Why are you feeling scared about the future?"
c. "Don't worry about the future. Focus on the present."
d. "Can you tell me more about your concerns?"

Ans. (d) Can you tell me more about your concerns?"

Explanation: Option d is the most appropriate response as it asks the client to share more about his concerns, the nurse encourages open communication and creates a supportive environment for the client to express his emotions. This therapeutic communication approach allows the nurse to understand the client's fears and provide appropriate emotional support.

Options a, and c do not address the client's feelings effectively and may not provide the opportunity to client to express further concern. While Option b is attempting to understand the client's feelings, it uses a non-therapeutic communication technique by asking "why."

Promote Health Maintenance in Patients

This category of questions assess the nurse's ability to provide and direct nursing care to promote and maintain the client's health.

These questions focus on assisting client and significant others during the normal expected stages of growth and development, as well as providing care related to the prevention and early detection of health problems.

When approaching health promotion and maintenance questions, it is essential to keep the following points in mind:

- **Focus on client teaching:** If the question involves client teaching, use the Teaching and Learning theory to guide your response. Remember that the client's willingness, desire, and readiness to learn should be the first priority.

  Consider the client's individual learning needs and preferences when providing education and ensure that the information is delivered in a way that is easily understandable and applicable to the client's situation.

Example Question

Assess Readiness to learn Before Teaching Client

A nurse is providing education to a client diagnosed with diabetes mellitus. The client seems disinterested and unmotivated to learn about blood glucose monitoring and insulin administration. What is the nurse's best approach?

a. Continue providing the education despite the client's lack of interest.
b. Suggest involving the client's family in the teaching session.
c. Assess the client's readiness to learn and address any barriers to learning.
d. Offer to reschedule the teaching session to a later time.

Ans. (c) Assess the client's readiness to learn and address any barriers to learning

Explanation: The nurse's first priority should be to assess the client's readiness and willingness to learn. If the client seems disinterested, it is essential to identify any barriers to learning and address them before proceeding with the education. This approach ensures that the information is delivered effectively and is applicable to the client's situation.

Example Question

A nurse is providing education to a client with diabetes about self-monitoring blood glucose. The client states, "I'm terrible at remembering things. I don't think I can do this." What is the nurse's best response?

a. "Diabetes management is crucial. You need to find a way to remember."
b. "Don't worry; I'll remind you every day to check your blood glucose."
c. "It's normal to feel overwhelmed. Let's discuss strategies to help you remember."
d. "If you can't remember, we might need to admit you to the hospital."

Ans. (c) It's normal to feel overwhelmed. Let's discuss strategies to help you remember."

Explanation: The nurse should acknowledge the client's concerns and offer to discuss strategies to help him remember to self-monitor his blood glucose. Option *a* may sound demanding and not empathetic, and Option *b* may foster dependency. Option *d* is an extreme response that is not warranted in this situation. Option *c* shows understanding and promotes problem-solving to address the client's concern effectively.

- **Address normal growth and development:** For questions related to normal expected stages of growth and development, **consider the age and developmental milestones of the client**.

  Nurses should be familiar with typical growth and developmental patterns to identify any deviations or concerns that may require intervention.

Example Question

A nurse in the well-baby clinic assessing a 12-month-old infant. The infant's parent expresses concern about the child not walking yet. What is the nurse's best response?

a. "Don't worry; all children develop at their own pace."
b. "Your child should be walking by now. Let's discuss possible causes for the delay."
c. "Walking typically starts between 10 and 15 months. Your child is still within the normal range."
d. "It's concerning that your child is not walking yet. I will refer you to a pediatric specialist."

Ans. (c) "Walking typically starts between 10 and 15 months. Your child is still within the normal range."

Explanation: The nurse should provide reassurance by explaining that walking typically starts between 10 and 15 months, and the child is still within the normal range of development.

Option a is supportive, but option c provides more specific information about the typical age range for walking and addresses the parent's concern appropriately.

- **Focus on preventive care:** Health Promotion and Maintenance questions may involve preventive care measures to avoid the development of health problems. Consider how the nurse can proactively support a client in adopting healthy behaviors, such as promoting regular exercise, healthy eating habits, and adherence to recommended screenings and vaccinations.
- **Be mindful of negative event queries:** Negative event queries are frequently used in Health Promotion and Maintenance questions related to client education. These queries may present scenarios where a client lacks knowledge or understanding about a specific health-related topic. The nurse's role is to identify gaps in knowledge and provide appropriate education to improve the client's understanding and self-care abilities.

Normal Vs Abnormal & Nursing Action Vs Physician Action

- Often, the scenario-based questions have options such as "**notify the physician**" or "**Document the findings**". Understanding this strategy will help you to choose between these options.
- Understanding normal and abnormal physiological parameters and laboratory values will help solve many questions. As a Nurse, you are expected to differentiate normal from abnormal.

The following steps will help you to choose the appropriate correct options in such a scenario-based Question.

Step 1: Read the Scenario Carefully. Take your time to read the scenario thoroughly and understand the patient's condition, symptoms, and any other relevant information provided. Pay attention to vital signs, laboratory values, and the patient's chief complaints.

Step 2: Identify Normal vs. Abnormal Parameters Once you have a clear understanding of the scenario, identify the physiological parameters or laboratory values mentioned. Determine whether they fall within the normal range or if they are abnormal. You should have a good understanding of the typical reference ranges for various vital signs and lab values. (Refer to the Synopsis for the Normal values)

Step 3: Analyze the Severity of Abnormality if you come across abnormal parameters. Some abnormal values may be only slightly out of range and might not require immediate intervention. Others may indicate a more serious condition that needs prompt attention.

Step 4: Consider the Nurse's Scope of Practice. If the scenario presents abnormal parameters that can be managed within the nurse's scope of practice, you can **consider implementing nursing interventions before notifying the physician**. Nursing interventions may include providing comfort measures, repositioning the patient, administering prescribed medications, or addressing other immediate needs based on your training and facility's policies.

Step 5: Determine if Immediate Physician Notification is Required. If the abnormality is severe and beyond the nurse's scope of practice, immediate notification of the physician or other relevant health care provider may be necessary.

Step 6: Consider the Overall Clinical Condition. Assess the patient's overall clinical condition and any other pertinent factors that could influence your decision. These factors might include the patient's medical history, comorbidities, recent interventions, and responses to previous treatments.

Step 7: Choose the Appropriate Response. Based on your analysis of the scenario, select the most appropriate response from the available options.

If the parameters are within the normal range, you might choose to **Document the findings.** If the abnormality can be managed within the Nurse's scope of practice, you could choose to "Any of the nursing interventions given as options". If immediate physician intervention is necessary, you may choose to "Notify the physician."

Example Question

Normal Findings

Nurse Ramya is assessing a male newborn following circumcision and observes that the circumcised area appears red with a slight amount of bloody drainage. What would be the most appropriate nursing action in this situation?

a. Apply gentle pressure to the area
b. Reinforce the dressing
c. Document the findings
d. Notify the physician

Ans. (c) Document the findings

Explanation: After circumcision, it is normal for the circumcised area to appear red and have a small amount of bloody drainage. This is a common and expected finding in the immediate postcircumcision period. By documenting these findings, the nurse is maintaining an accurate record of the newborn's condition, which is important for ongoing assessment and communication among healthcare providers.

STRATEGY: Understand the normal Physiological and clinical Parameters. Understanding of the nurse that the redness and small amount of bloody drainage is normal findings after a circumcision procedure. This leads to the option "Document the Findings".

When the respiratory rate of a 12-month-old child is 35 breaths/min, the most appropriate nursing action is:

a. Notify the physician
b. Administer oxygen
c. Reassess respiratory rate in 15 minutes
d. Document the findings

Ans. (c) Document the findings

Explanation: The respiratory rate of a 12-month-old child is typically 30–60 breaths/min. So, a respiratory rate of 35 breaths/min is within the normal range. Therefore, the most appropriate nursing action in this situation is to document the findings.

STRATEGY: Understand the normal physiological and clinical parameters.

Example Question

Abnormal Findings

A client is in active labor with twins and the cervix is 5 cm dilated. The nurse observes that contractions are occurring every 7 to 8 minutes in a 30-min period. The most appropriate action by the nurse would be to:

a. Administer oxygen at 4 liters by mask
b. Note the fetal heart rate patterns
c. Notify the physician immediately
d. Instruct the client to relax during the contractions

Ans. (c) Notify the physician immediately

Explanation: Given the scenario of a client in active labor with twins, a 5 cm dilated cervix, and contractions occurring every 7 to 8 minutes in a 30-min period, it is important to consider the possibility of hypotonic uterine contractions, which are characterized by weak and infrequent contractions that can slow down labor progress. The most appropriate nursing action would be to "Notify the physician immediately" (option c). Hypotonic uterine contractions can lead to labor complications, and the physician needs to be informed promptly so that appropriate interventions, such as administering oxytocin to augment contractions can be considered.

Example Question

Infective endocarditis client developed sudden left leg pain with pallor, paresthesia, and a loss of peripheral pulses. Priority nursing action is:

a. Elevate the leg to promote venous return.
b. Apply constrictive elastic bandage
c. Notify the physician
d. Use blood blocks to elevate foot end

Ans. (c) Notify the physician

Explanation: The sudden onset of pain, pallor, paresthesia, and loss of peripheral pulses in a client with infective endocarditis are signs of a possible embolic event, such as a clot or vegetation breaking off from the heart and traveling to the leg. This is a serious medical emergency that requires immediate medical attention.

STRATEGY: Determine that "Immediate Physician Notification" is required if the abnormality is severe and beyond the nurse's scope of practice, immediate notification of the physician.

Answering Complex Case Scenario-based Questions Using Clinical Judgment

All the strategies discussed above may help you solve a case scenario-based question, however, there is no alternative to sound subject knowledge and clinical judgement of the situation.

The following points need to be carefully considered while solving complex case scenario-based questions.

- Read the question stem carefully and identify the key information, the client scenario and vital details.
- Identify the main issue in the question. The question stem may have too many details out of which the main issue needs to be identified. This will direct the test-taker to choose correct answer.
- Consider safety and prioritization: Read the options carefully and assess the urgency and potential risks associated with each option.
- Apply clinical knowledge: Use your knowledge of anatomy, physiology, pathophysiology, and pharmacology to make the best decision.
- Use your clinical judgment to weigh the risks and benefits of each option and make the best decision for the patient.
- Consider the patient's age, gender, and cultural background while making clinical judgement.
- Think about the setting in which the question is taking place (Emergency room, General ward, ICU, OT or Community setting). The response may vary depending on the setting.
- Use the process of elimination (as discussed above)

Negative Marking:

- Negative marking of 1/3 for each wrong answer makes it the guess work a big challenge. If you don't know the exact answer and would like to guess the answer, be extra cautious due to this 1/3 negative marking.
- If you guess randomly on a 4-option MCQ, you have a 1/4 chance of getting the answer right and a 3/4 chance of getting it wrong. This means there is a probability to get 1/12 mark for each MCQ that you guess.
- However, if you can eliminate (confidently) two of the wrong answers, then you have a 1/2 chance of guessing the correct answer and a 1/2 chance of getting it wrong. On average, there is a probability to get 1/6 mark for each MCQ that you guess.

Video-Based Questions (VBQs)

Video Based Questions — Watch these VIDEOS in TARGET HIGH Digital Lite

1. Which of the following procedure is being performed in the video?

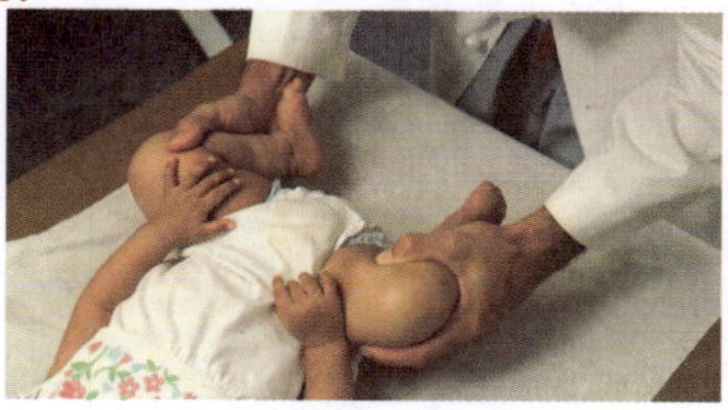

a. Ortolani and Barlow test
b. Anterior drawer test
c. Lachman test
d. Flexion rotation drawer test

2. Which of the following procedure is being performed in the video?

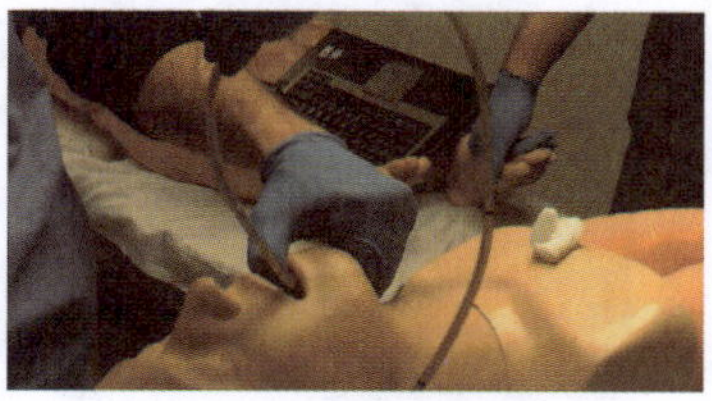

a. NG tube insertion
b. OG tube insertion
c. Sengstaken-Blakemore tube insertion
d. Guedel's airway insertion

3. All among the following are the advantage of the procedure shown in the video; EXCEPT:

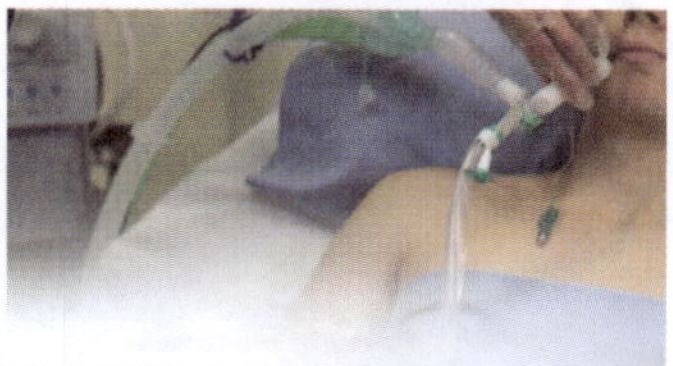

a. Minimize aerosol generation
b. Less chance for cross infection
c. Apply negative pressure throughout the respiratory cycle
d. Maintain PEEP throughout the respiratory cycle

4. The specimen collection shown in the videos is for:

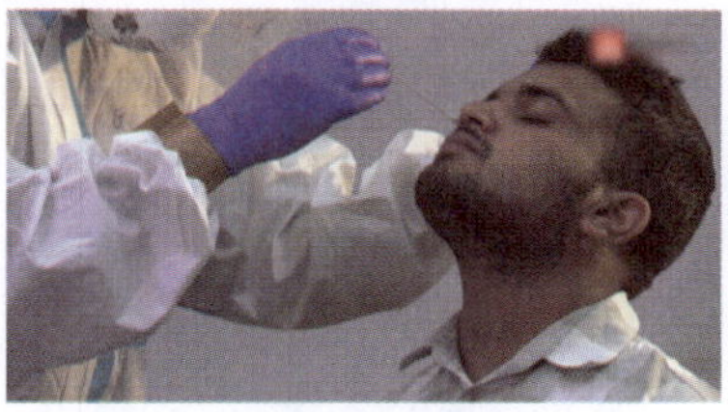

a. RT-PCR
b. Rapid antigen test for COVID
c. Sputum culture and sensitivity test
d. Both a & b

5. The procedure being performed in the video is:

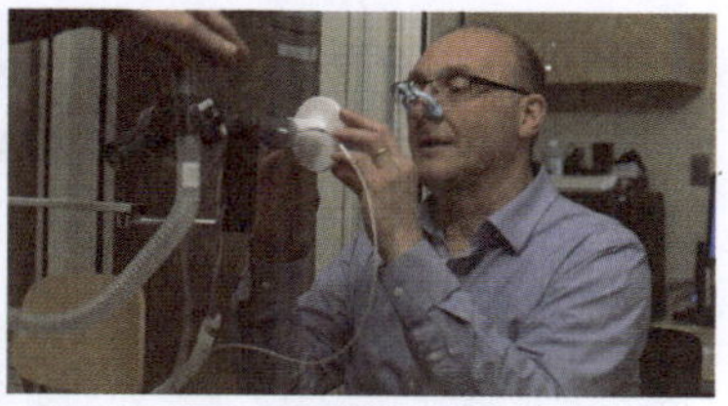

a. Pulmonary function test
b. Incentive spirometry
c. Alcohol breath test
d. Urea breath test

6. The nasal clip used during the procedure shown in the video is to:

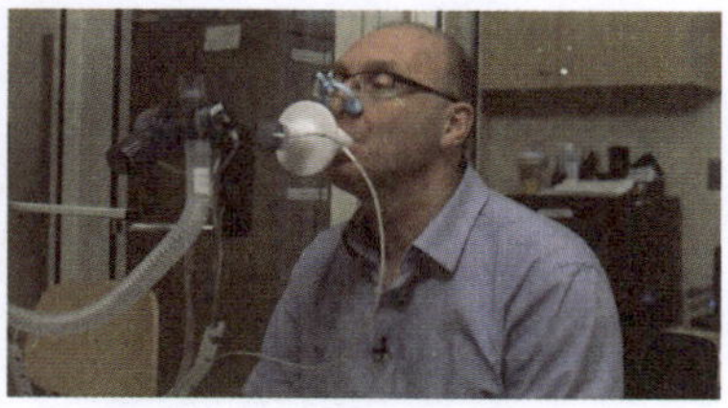

a. Avoid drainage of nasal secretion during the procedure
b. Achieve a tight seal of the airway
c. Improve patient comfort during the procedure
d. Prevent sneezing during procedure

7. The device shown in the video is:

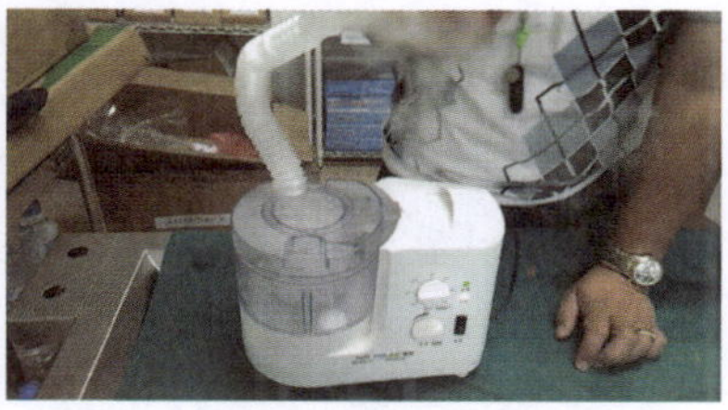

a. Jet nebulizer
b. Mask nebulizer
c. Ultrasonic nebulizer
d. Steam inhalation device

8. The instrument used for the measurement of Mid-Upper Arm Circumference shown in the video is:

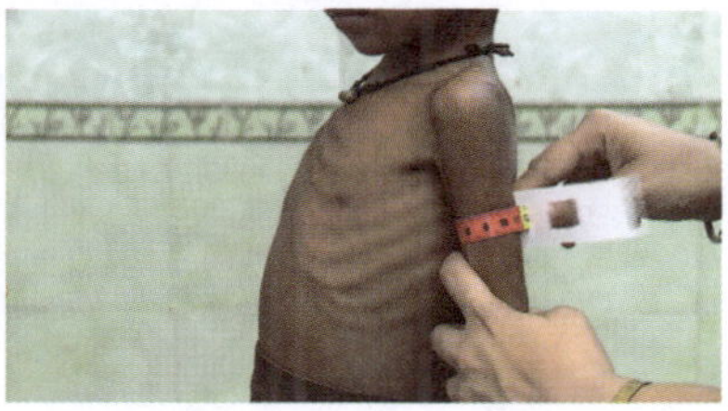

a. Shakir tape
b. Stadiometer
c. Edtape
d. Gulick tape

Ans.

1. a
2. b
3. c
4. d
5. a
6. b
7. c
8. a

9. The test shown in the video is usually performed before:

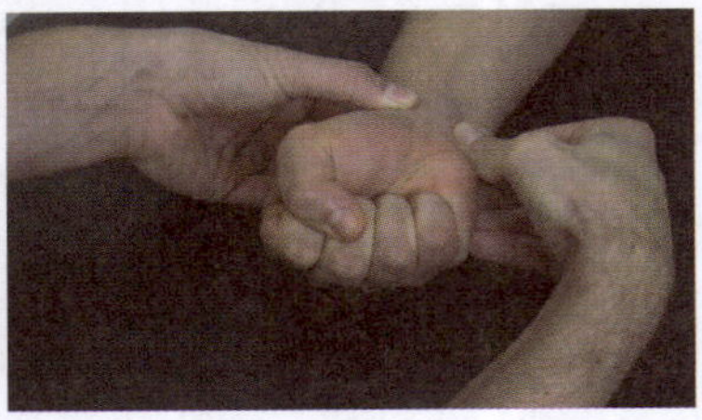

a. Intravascular cannulation
b. Taking an arterial sample
c. Blood pressure assessment
d. All of the above

10. The response of the patient to the test shown in the video is:

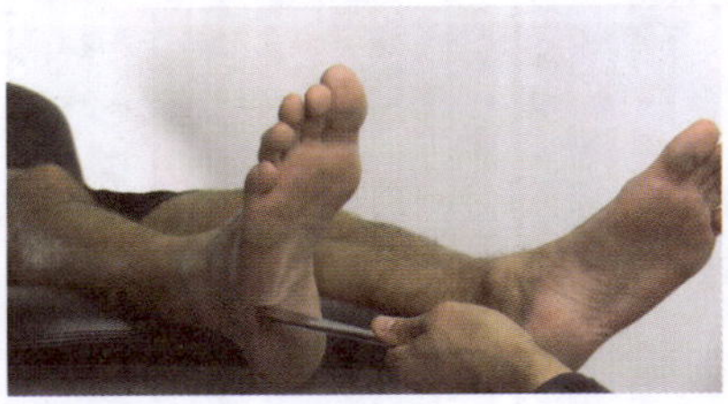

a. Negative Babinski reflex
b. Positive Babinski reflex
c. Normal plantar response
d. All of the above

11. The response of the patient to the test shown in the video is:

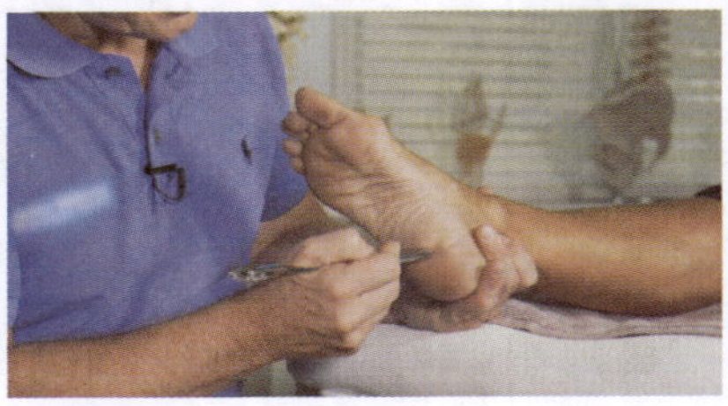

a. Negative Babinski reflex
b. Positive Babinski reflex
c. Extensor plantar response
d. All of the above

12. Bubbling shown in the chest tube drainage system indicates:

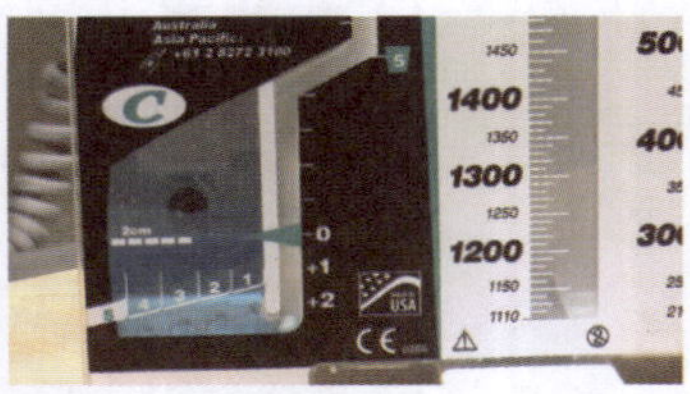

a. Normal functioning of the system
b. Leakage somewhere in the system
c. Kinking of the chest tube
d. None of the above

13. Oscillation shown in the chest tube drainage system is an indicates:

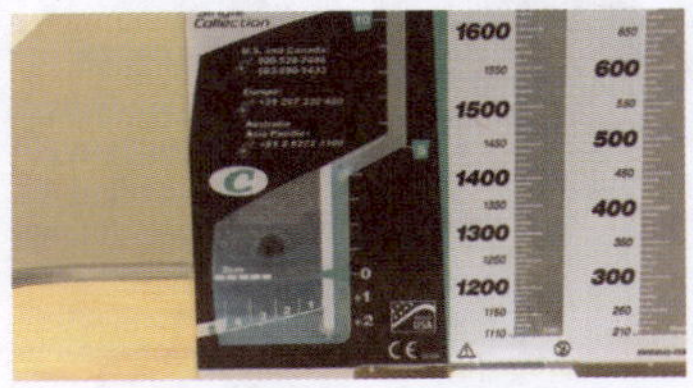

a. Normal functioning of the system
b. Leakage somewhere in the system
c. Kinking of the chest tube
d. None of the above

14. Name of the procedure being performed in video is:

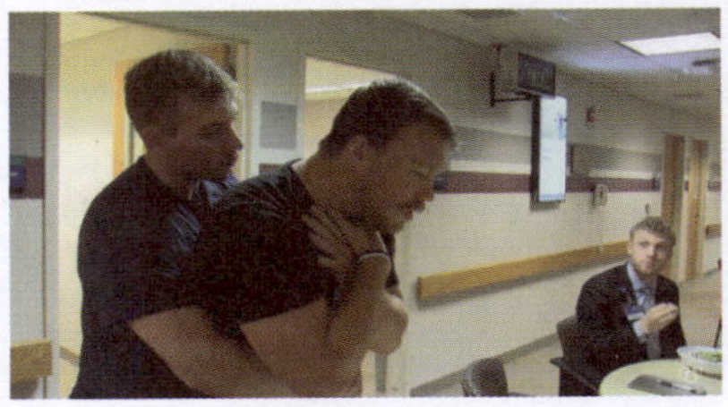

a. Abdominal thrust maneuver
b. Heimlich maneuver
c. Chest compression
d. Both a & b

15. The instrument used during the CPR procedure shown in the video is known as:

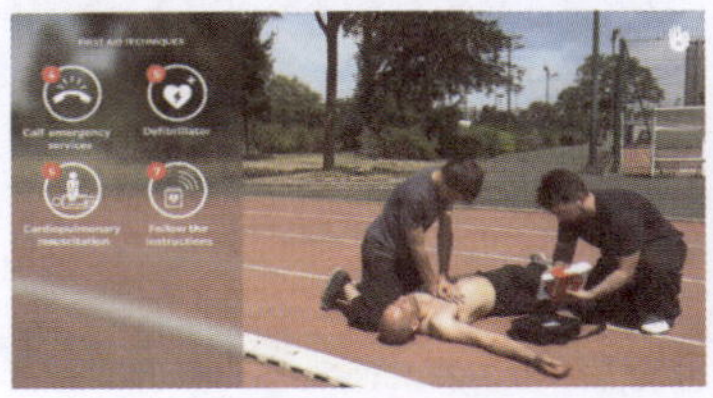

a. Automated external defibrillator
b. Manual external defibrillator
c. Manual internal defibrillator
d. Portable cardiac defibrillator

16. In the video, the nurse is preparing for which of the following procedure?

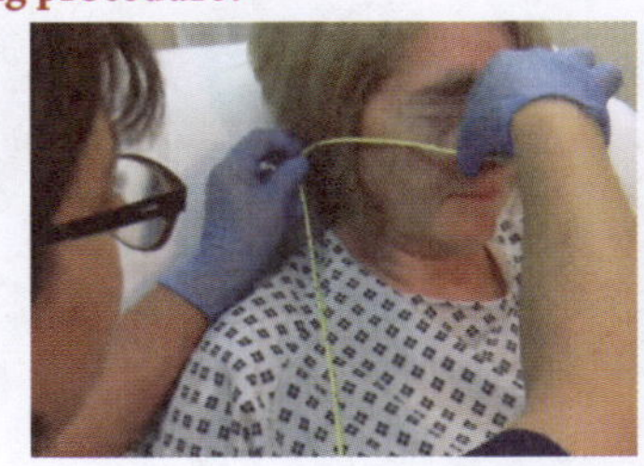

a. OG tube insertion
b. NG tube insertion
c. Sengstaken Blakemore tube insertion
d. PEG tube insertion

Ans.

9. b
10. b
11. a
12. b
13. a
14. d
15. a
16. b

17. In the video, the nurse is confirming the placement of:

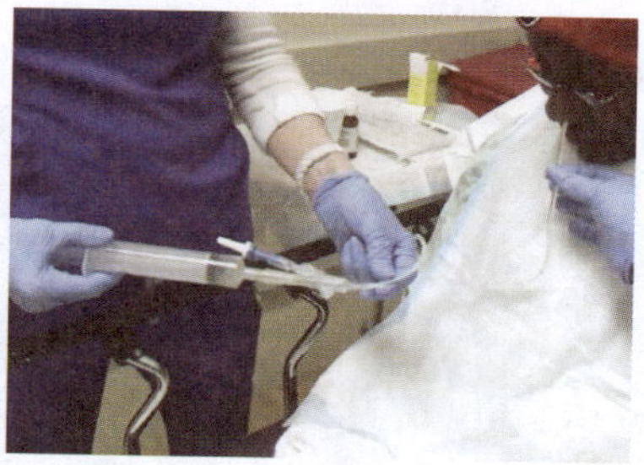

a. Orogastric tube
b. Nasogastric tube
c. Sengstaken-Blakemore
d. PEG tube

18. The procedure demonstrated in the video is related to:

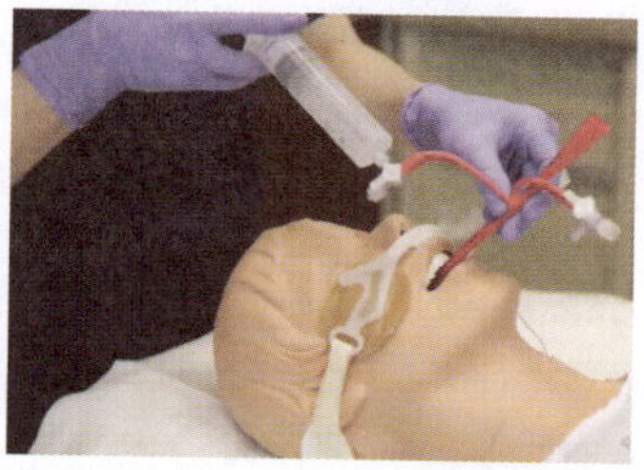

a. NG tube insertion
b. OG tube insertion
c. Sengstaken-Blakemore tube insertion
d. PEG tube placement

19. The procedure demonstrated in the video is:

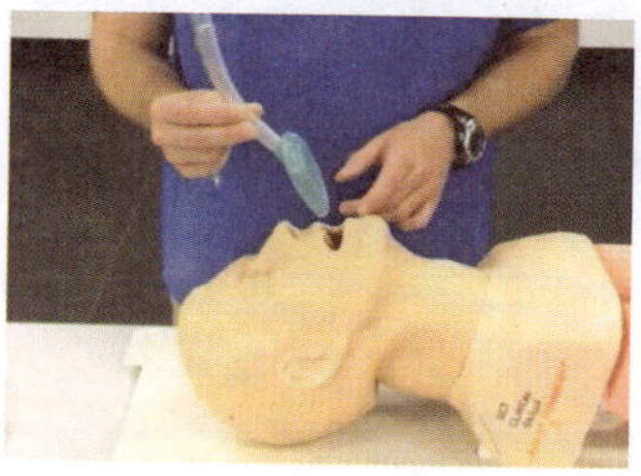

a. Endotracheal tube insertion
b. Guedel's airway insertion
c. Laryngeal mask airway insertion
d. Oropharyngeal airway

20. The procedure demonstrated in the video is:

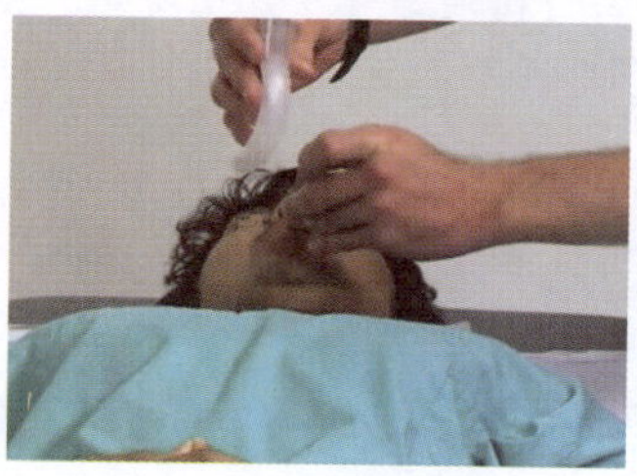

a. Endotracheal tube insertion
b. Guedel's airway insertion
c. Laryngeal mask airway insertion
d. Oropharyngeal airway

21. The procedure shown in the video is:

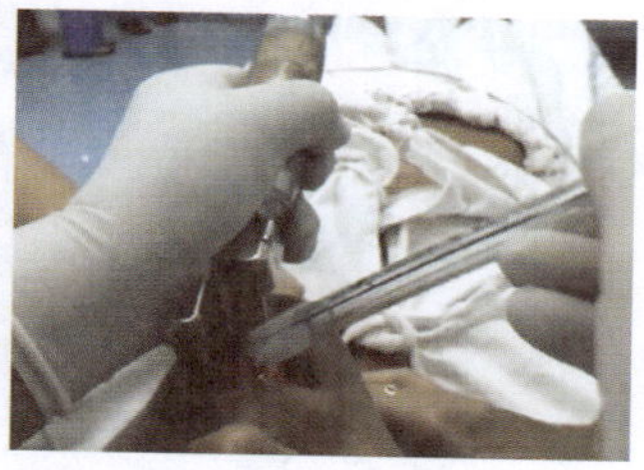

a. Oropharyngeal intubation
b. LMA intubation
c. Endotracheal intubation
d. Ryle's tube insertion

22. The purpose of the procedure demonstrated in the video is to:

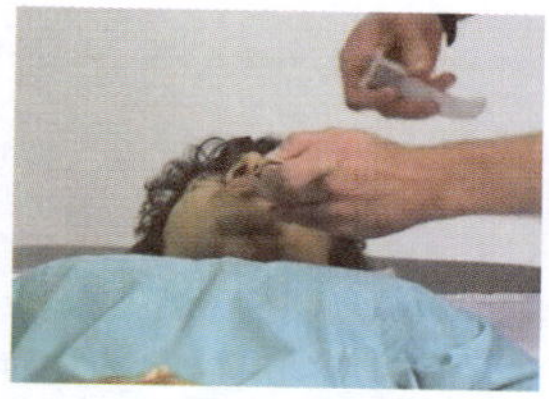

a. Open and maintain patient's airway
b. Prevent the tongue from covering the epiglottis
c. Prevent obstruction of airway from relaxed upper airway muscle
d. All of the above

23. The equipment shown in the video is used to:

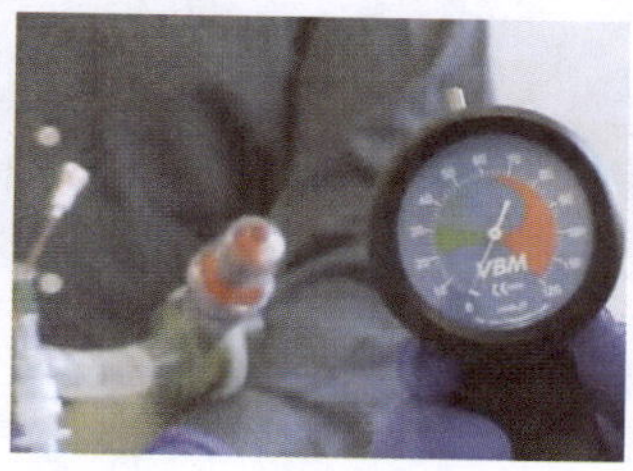

a. Assess cuff pressure in endotracheal tube
b. Adjust cuff pressure in endotracheal tube
c. Both a and b
d. To confirm the placement of ET tube

24. The name of the handheld instrument used in he procedure is:

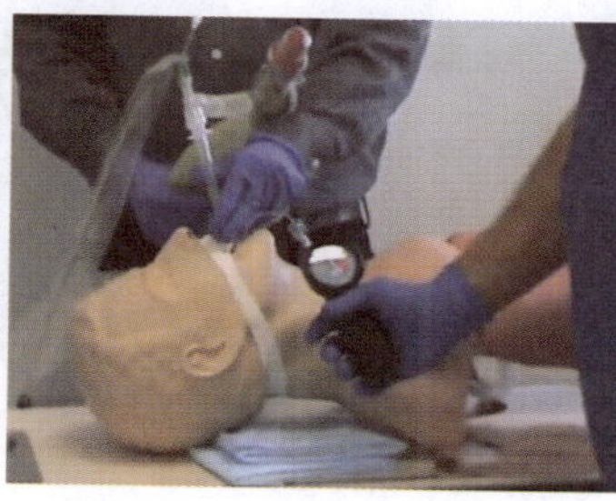

a. Cuff Sphygmomanometer
b. Cuff monitor
c. Cuff manometer
d. Cuff barometer

Video-Based Questions (VBQs)

Ans.

17.	b
18.	c
19.	c
20.	b
21.	c
22.	d
23.	c
24.	c

25. Name the step of the procedure shown in the video during assessment using transcutaneous bilirubin meter?

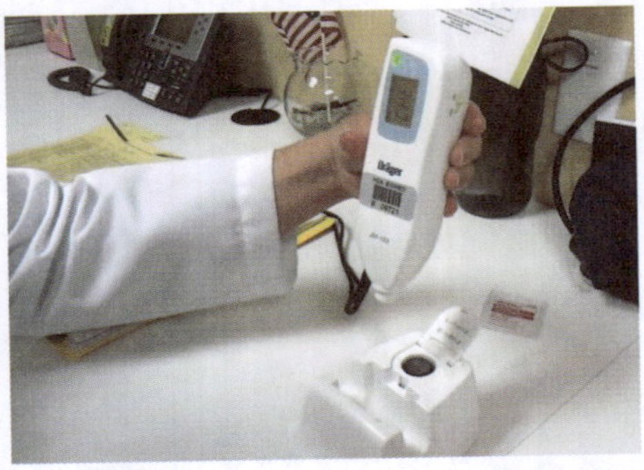

a. Assessing calibration
b. Reading the result
c. Checking battery
d. All of these

28. A patient with ataxia is undergoing the test shown in the video. What is the possible interpretation if the patient tests positive for the test?

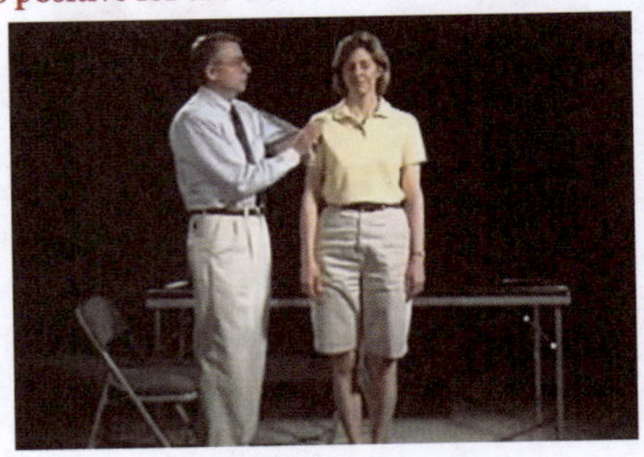

a. Ataxia is cerebellar in nature
b. Ataxia is sensory in nature
c. Ataxia is due to toxic reaction
d. Ataxia is due to cerebral palsy

26. In the video, the healthcare worker is assessing the bilirubin level of the newborn using transcutaneous bilirubin meter. Apart from the site used for assessment in the video, which other site is also preferred for the assessment?

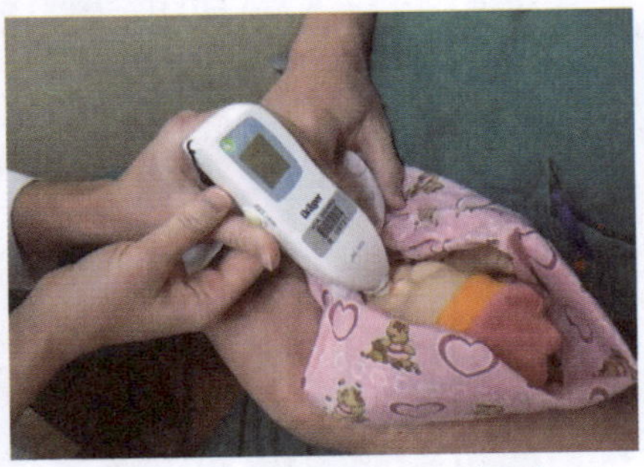

a. Ear pinna
b. Forehead
c. Anterior thigh
d. Abdomen

29. The assessment procedure shown in the video is:

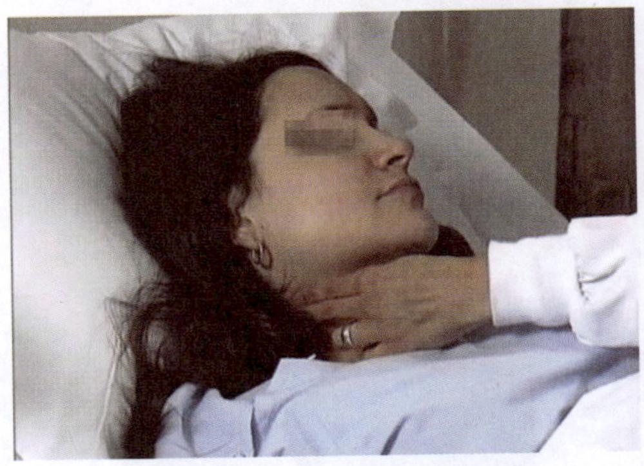

a. Bruits
b. Nuchal rigidity
c. Carotid pulse
d. Apical pulse

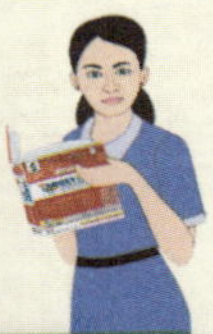

Ans.

25. a
26. b
27. b
28. b
29. c
30. a

27. The procedure shown in the video is:

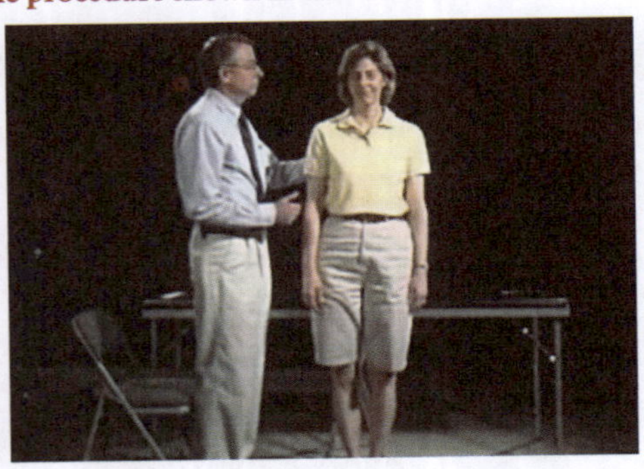

a. Rinne's test
b. Romberg's test
c. Assessment of 7th cranial nerve
d. Tandem gait test

30. Which of the following is being assessed in the video:

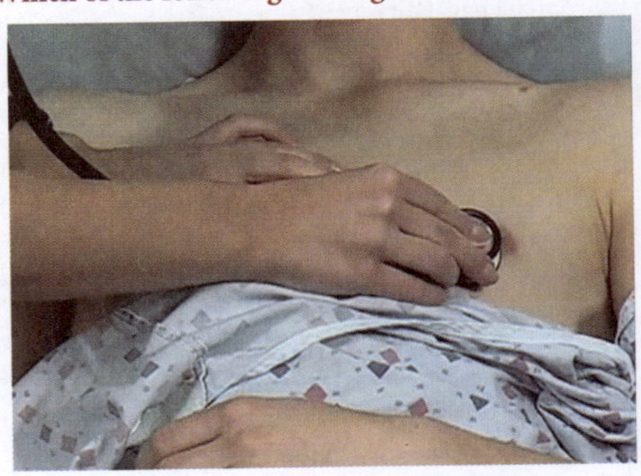

a. Apical pulse
b. Lung sound
c. Aortic regurgitation
d. None of these

Appendices

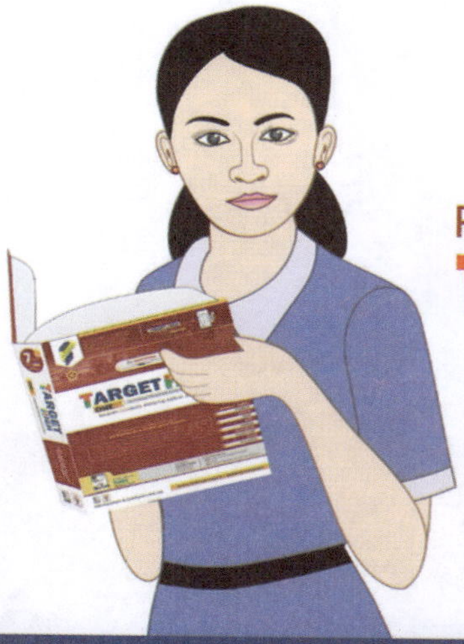

Read from **TARGET HIGH** *Book*

APPENDICES COVERED *(in Book)*

1. Updates on Tuberculosis
2. Decontamination of Equipment and Unit
3. Some Disease Conditions and their Primary Signs/Symptoms
4. Instruments
5. Equipment/Instruments
6. Obstetrics and Gynecological Instruments
7. Tubes and Catheters
8. Recent Updates on Community Health Nursing
9. Demography of India
10. Review of Health Programs in India, Launch Year and Objectives
11. Vitamins: Functions, Sources and Deficiency Diseases
12. Health Planning in India
13. Frye's ABCDE Cascade for Prioritizing Care
14. Triage Categories
15. Arterial Blood Gas
16. Shocks: Types, Management and Solutions
17. ECG Waveforms and Pathological Findings
18. Common Scales used for Assessment/Treatment
19. Level of Spinal Cord Injury and Associated Motor Loss
20. Some Important Social Welfare/Health/Development Program Launched by Government of India from August 2014 till June 2023 (New)
21. Cold Chain Methods and Equipment

Appendices Covered in

Nursing Next Live > Target High Digital Lite

Turn overleaf

Read from
TARGET HIGH Digital Lite App

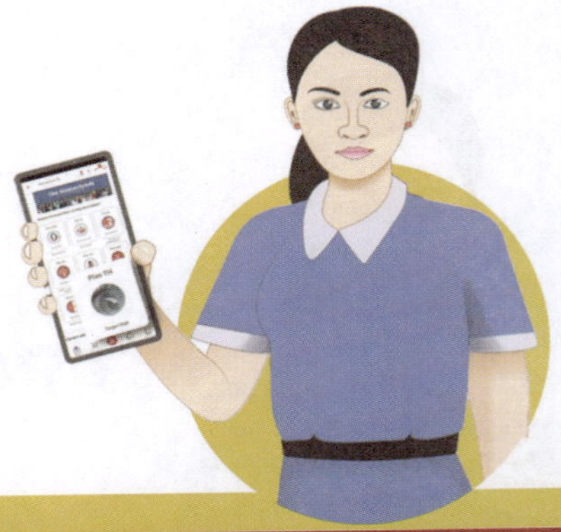

APPENDICES COVERED *(in App)*

1. Updates on COVID-19 (New)
2. Management of COVID-19 in Pregnancy (New)
3. Mucormycosis (Black Fungus) (New)
4. Updates on Tuberculosis (New)
5. Updated Questions on COVID-19
6. Slings and Splints
7. Decontamination of Equipment and Unit
8. Some Disease Conditions and their Primary Signs/Symptoms
9. Fetal Circulation and its Postnatal Changes
10. Positions
11. Instruments
12. Equipment/Instruments
13. Obstetrics and Gynecological Instruments
14. Tubes and Catheters
15. Recent Updates on Community Health Nursing
16. Norms for Health Personnel/Centers in Community
17. Cold Chain Methods and Equipment
18. Demography in India
19. Review of Health Programs in India, Launch Year and Objectives
20. Vitamins: Functions, Sources and Deficiency Diseases
21. Health Planning in India
22. Frye's ABCDE Cascade for Prioritizing Care
23. Triage Categories
24. Arterial Blood Gas
25. Shocks: Types, Management and Solutions
26. Skeletal and Skin Traction
27. ECG Waveforms and Pathological Findings
28. Biomedical Waste Management Rules 2016
29. Common Scales used for Assessment/Treatment
30. Level of Spinal Cord Injury and Associated Motor Loss
31. Neurotransmitters' Chart
32. Interpretation of BMI
33. Positions and Presentations of Fetus during Labor
34. Some Important Social Welfare/Health/Development Programs Launched by Govt. of India from August 2014 Till June 2023
35. Conversion from Celsius (°C) to Fahrenheit (°F)
36. Quadrants of Abdomen
37. Fetal Skull
38. Cranial Nerves, their Types and Functions
39. Types of Joints in Human Body
40. Functions of Sympathetic and Parasympathetic Nervous System
41. Normal Values
42. Communicable Diseases
43. Levels of Prevention
44. Vaccines used to Prevent Diseases
45. Immunization Schedule
46. Community Nutrition Program
47. Types of Insulin
48. Glasgow Coma Scale
49. Lung Volumes and Capacities
50. Immunoglobulins and their Characteristics
51. Drugs and their Actions
52. Growth and Development
53. Comparison of Components for Adults, Children, and Infants BLS/CPR
54. Stages of Personality Development
55. EGO Defense Mechanisms with Examples
56. Phases of Wound Healing Process
57. Classification of Mental Retardation
58. Phobias
59. Blood Groups
60. Specific Antidotes against Poisoning
61. Drug Storage Temperature
62. Leopold's Maneuver
63. Abbreviations
64. Sequence of Donning and Doffing of PPE while Caring for COVID-19 Patients
65. Blood Supply of Heart
66. Lobes of Brain and their Functions
67. Color Coding for Medical Gas Cylinders
68. Acts and Legislations
69. Radiating Pain/Referred Pain
70. Endocrine Glands and Hormones
71. Acute Coronary syndromes and their Treatment
72. Burns

1

"All healing is first a healing of the heart."
—Carl Townsend

UPDATES ON TUBERCULOSIS

- In 2020, the RNTCP was renamed the National Tuberculosis Elimination Program (NTEP) to emphasize the aim of the Government of India to eliminate **TB in India** by 2025.
- Prime Minister of India launched TB Free India campaign at 'Delhi End TB Summit' on 13th March, 2018
- India has committed to **End TB by 2025**, 5 years ahead of the global SDG target
- Estimated Incidence of Tuberculosis in 2019 is **26.9 lakh TB cases (199/lakh population)**
- **Updates on Lab test**
    - Nucleic acid amplification tests (NAATs) have been used as a **diagnostic tool for tuberculosis** (TB)
    - **Cartridge-based nucleic-acid amplification test (CB NAAT)** is the preferred first diagnostic test in children, extrapulmonary TB, contact of Drug resistant TB patients, Smear Negative Chest X-ray positive patients.
- **Sample collection (sputum) and transportation to be in falcon tubes in cold chain (quantity – minimum 5 mL)**

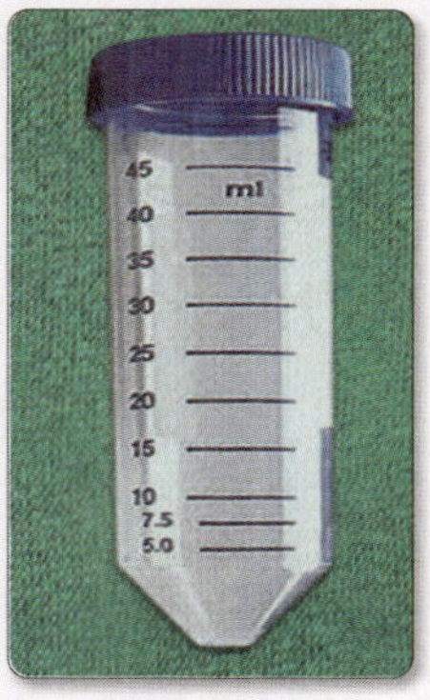

Falcon tube

Treatment of Drug Sensitive TB

Type of TB case	Treatment Regimen Intensive Phase (IP)	Treatment Regimen in Continuation Phase (CP)
New OR Previously treated	(2) HRZE	(4) HRE
• The drugs are given daily • The doses of drugs are according to body weight • Fixed Dose Combination (FDC) tablets are used • No need for extension of IP • CP may be extended by 12–24 weeks in certain forms of TB like CNS TB, Skeletal TB, Disseminated TB, etc.		

Treatment of TB-Adult

Weight category	Number of tablets (FDCs)	
	Intensive phase (2 months)	Continuation phase (4 months)
	Combined dose: [H (75 mg), R (150 mg), Z (400 mg), E (275 mg)]	Combined dose: [H (75 mg), R (150 mg), E (275 mg)]
25–34 kg	2	2
35–49 kg	3	3
50–64 kg	4	4
65–75 kg	5	5
≥75	6	6

Note: If patient gains or loses weight, the dose has to be adjusted accordingly during the course.

Nikshay Poshan Yojana

- ₹500 at the beginning of each month for every notified TB patient for the full treatment period
- Direct Benefit Transfer only

2

"Children have more need of role model than of critics."
—Joseph Jonbert

DECONTAMINATION OF EQUIPMENT AND UNIT

Strengths of Chemical and their Actions on Equipment and Supplies

Chemical	Strength	Types of instruments	Action and time
Glutaraldehyde	2%	Spirometry tubing Dialyzer Reuse of laparoscopic instrument Rubber instruments or plastic	High level disinfectant for medical equipment such as endoscope 10–20 minutes
Isopropyl alcohol	70%	All metal instruments Scope lenses Ambu bag and its face mask Thermometer probes Clinical glass thermometer Trolley tops Electric razors	Disinfection of articles in 10 minutes
Sodium hypochlorite	0.5% (Add 500 mL of 1% sodium hypochlorite in 500 mL of boiled water to make total quantity of 1 L)	All types of metal, glass, plastic and rubber items scope lenses	Decontamination, disinfection of articles in 10 minutes Fresh solution to be prepared daily
Chlorhexidine gluconate	Add 100 mL 0.5% solution in 900 mL of boiled water to make 1 L	Bedpans Furniture	Disinfection in 10 minutes
Clean solution of phenol	2%	All metal instruments Toughened plastics Glass Delicate items Tubing	Sterilization in 12 hours at room temperature of 20°C
Formalin	7 gm per cubic meter	All metal instruments Toughened plastics Glass Delicate items Tubing	Disinfection in 10 minutes
Savlon	5% pure solution	Cheatle forceps Clinical glass Thermometer Furniture instruments	Disinfection in 20 minutes

Cleaning, Disinfection of Various Items

Procedure	Rationale	Scientific principle
Glass items: Disinfect the items by immersing in 0.5% chlorine/sodium hypochlorite Chlorhexidine solution minimum for 5 minutes in plastic container covered with lids.	To decrease the number of microorganisms on the surface of the items	Chlorine kills many microorganisms by releasing free oxygen
Enamel wares: Immerse the items in a chlorine solution of 0.5%.	To disinfect	Disinfection can kill most of the bacteria and viruses like hepatitis B virus (HBV), human immunodeficiency virus (HIV), (microbiology)
Stainless steel items: Always immerse in 0.5% of chlorine solution for five minutes.	To disinfect	Disinfection destroys many of the pathogens

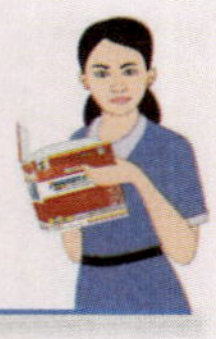

Contd...

Procedure	Rationale	Scientific principle
Needles: Decontaminatė all types of needles attached to syringe and flush with 0.5% chlorine solution/chlorhexidine/sodium hypochlorite immediately after use.	To render the article safe for use	To decontaminate and make the article availability for reuse
Proctoscope and bronchoscope: Immerse both obturator and speculum in a 0.5% chlorine solution minimum for 10 minutes, then rinse in water, boil for 10 minutes. Then send for autoclaving.	To decontaminate	To decontaminate and make the article availability for reuse
Sharp instruments: Immerse the sharp instruments in a 0.5% chlorine solution or in 2% glutaraldehyde (CIDEX) for 12 minutes at 20°C. Add antirust agents, e.g., sodium nitrate, 0.1%, if available.	To disinfect and sterilize the instruments	Disinfection destroys many of the pathogens
Laryngoscope: Detach the blade separate and immerse it in a 2% glutaraldehyde solution for 12 minutes	To decontaminate	By decontaminating we can make it ready for next use

Commonly Used Skin Disinfectants and Antiseptics

Biocides	Most commonly used dilution
Alcohols (ethanol, isopropanol, n-propanol)	60–95%
Chlorhexidine gluconate	Aqueous or detergent preparations containing 0.5% or 0.75% chlorhexidine alcohol preparations containing 4% chlorhexidine
Chloroxylenol (parachlorometaxylenol: PCMX)	0.3–3.75%
Hexachlorophene	3%
Iodophors (povidone-iodine)	7.5–10%
Quaternary ammonium compounds	0.05–0.2% quat
Triclosan	0.2–2%

3

"The human brain starts working the moment you are born and never stops until you stand up to speak in public."
—George Jessel

SOME DISEASE CONDITIONS AND THEIR PRIMARY SIGNS/SYMPTOMS

Disease/condition	Important signs/symptoms
Addison's disease	Bronze-like skin pigmentation
Angina	Crushing, stabbing pain relieved by Nitroglycerin (NTG)
Appendicitis	Rebound tenderness at McBurney's point Rovsing's sign (palpation of LLQ elicits pain in RLQ) Psoas sign (pain from flexing the thigh to the hip)
Asthma	Wheezing on expiration
Basilar skull fracture	Raccoon eyes (periorbital ecchymosis) Battle's sign (mastoid ecchymosis)
Buerger's disease (Inflammation and thrombosis in small and medium-sized blood vessels)	Intermittent claudication (pain at buttocks or legs from poor circulation resulting in impaired walking)
Bulimia	Chipmunk faces (parotid gland swelling)
Candidiasis	White cheesy odorless vaginal discharges
Cataract	Blurry vision
Chancroid	Painful chancres

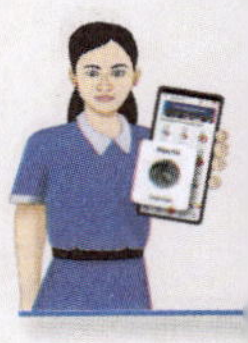

Contd...

Disease/condition	Important signs/symptoms
Chicken pox	Pleomorphism: All stages of the rash (papules, vesicles and crusts) are seen simultaneously
Chlamydia	Milky discharge and painful urination
Cholecystitis	Murphy's sign (pain in the Right Upper Quadrant)
Cholera	Rice-watery stool and washer woman's hands (wrinkled hands from dehydration)
Cirrhosis of liver	Spider angioma
COPD	Barrel-chest
Cushing's syndrome	Moon face appearance and buffalo hump
Cushing's triad	Bradypnea (irregular decreased respiration) Bradycardia Systolic hypertension
Cytomegalovirus (CMV) infection	Owl's eye appearance of cells (huge nucleus in cells)
Deep vein thrombosis (DVT)	Homan's sign
Dengue	Thrombocytopenia, fever, rash, and headache, positive Herman's sign
Dengue	Petechiae
Diabetes mellitus	Polydipsia, polyphagia, polyuria
Diabetic ketoacidosis	Acetone breathe
Diphtheria	Pseudomembrane formation
Down syndrome	Protruding tongue, single crease on palm, flat nasal bridge, epicanthal fold, flat facial profile
Emphysema	Barrel chest
Gastroesophageal reflux disease (GERD)	Heartburn
Genital Warts	Warts are 1–2 mm in diameter
Glaucoma	Tunnel vision
Gonorrhea	Green, creamy discharges and painful urination
Grave's disease (hyperthyroidism)	Exophthalmos (bulging of the eye out of the orbit)
Guillain-Barre syndrome	Ascending muscles weakness
Hepatitis	Icteric sclera (yellowish discoloration of sclera)
Herpes Simplex Type II	Painful vesicles on genitalia
Hirschsprung's disease (toxic megacolon)	Ribbon-like stool
Hyperthyroidism	Exophthalmos
Intussusception	Sausage-shaped mass, current jelly like stool
Kawasaki disease	Strawberry Tongue
Leprosy (Hanson's disease)	Leonine faces (faces that resemble that of a lion)
Malaria	Stepladder like fever with chills
Measles	Koplik's spots (clustered white lesions on buccal mucosa)
Meningitis	Brudzinski's sign (forced flexion of the neck elicits a reflex flexion of the hips) Kernig's sign (stiffness of hamstrings causing inability to straighten the leg when the hip is flexed to 90 degrees)
Multiple sclerosis	Charcot's Triad: Nystagmus, intention tremor, and dysarthria
Mumps	*Parotitis (swollen, painful salivary glands)*
Myasthenia gravis	Descending muscle weakness, ptosis (drooping of eyelids)
Myocardial infarction (MI)	Levine's sign (clutching of the chest) Crushing, stabbing pain radiating to left shoulder, neck, and arms. Not relieved by NTG
Pancreatitis	Cullen's sign (ecchymosis of the umbilicus), Grey Turner's sign (bruising of the flank)
Parkinson's disease	Pill-rolling tremors
Patent ductus arteriosus	Washing machine-like murmur
Pernicious anemia	Beefy red tongue (Schilling's Test)

Contd...

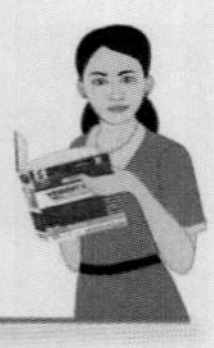

Disease/condition	Important signs/symptoms
Pneumonia	• Rust-colored sputum or • Greenish rusty sputum
Pregnancy induced hypertension (PIH)	Proteinuria, hypertension, edema
Pulmonary tuberculosis (PTB)	Low-grade afternoon fever
Pyloric stenosis	Olive-like mass, projectile vomiting
Retinal detachment	Flashes of light, shadow with curtain across vision
Syphilis	Painless chancres
Systemic lupus erythematosus	Butterfly rash
Tetanus	Risus sardonicus or rictus grin
Tetany	Hypocalcemia, [+] Trousseau's sign (jerky movements); Chvostek sign (muscle twitching face)
Tetralogy of Fallot • Pulmonary stenosis • Overriding of aorta • Ventricular septal defect • Right ventricular hypertrophy	Characterized by clubbing of fingernails
Thrombophlebitis	Homan's sign
Trichomoniasis	Yellow, itchy, frothy, and foul-smelling vaginal discharges
Typhoid	Rose spots in the abdomen

4

"A surgeon should be young a physician old."
—French Proverb

INSTRUMENTS

Name of the instruments

Adson thumb forceps
- For holding and manipulating delicate tissues.

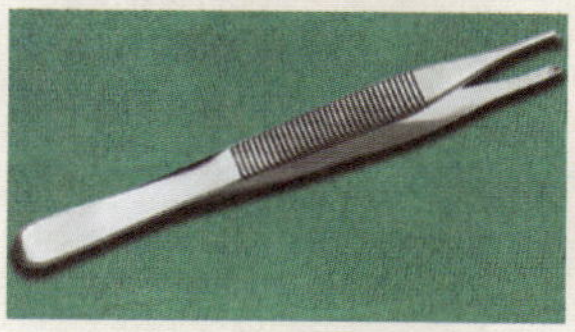

Babcock forceps
- Used to grasp delicate tissue in laser procedures. They are frequently used with intestinal and laparotomy procedures.

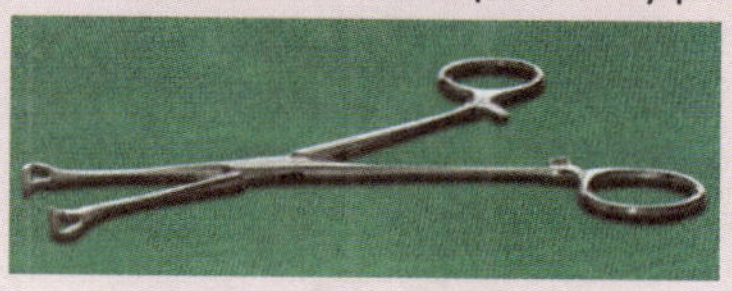

Alli's/Alli's tissue forceps
- Alli's tissue forceps are used for grasping organs and slippery or dense tissue during electrosurgery.

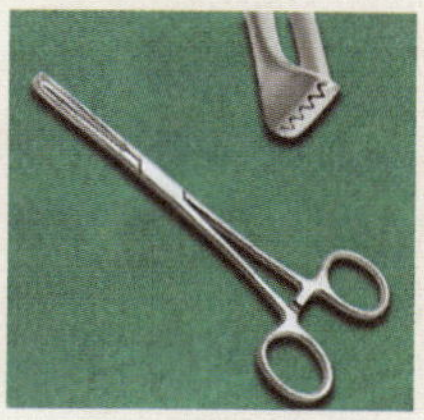

Vulsellum
- Used in gynecological operations to hold the tip of cervix.
- This structure is similar to Alli's forceps except they are very long.

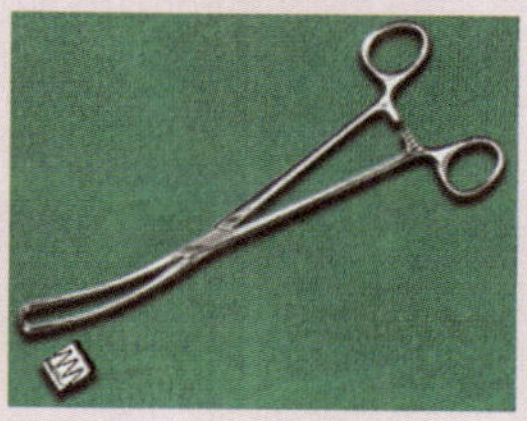

Contd...

Name of the instruments

Artery forceps
- Used for grasping, compressing, and holding the end of an artery during ligation.

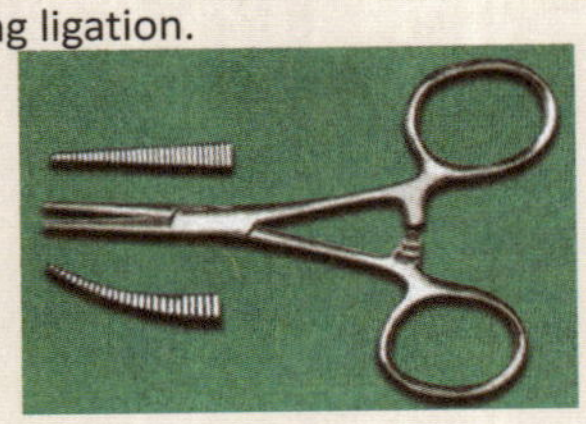

Right-angled artery forceps
- To isolate, encircle and ligate vessels or ducts, especially those present in depths.

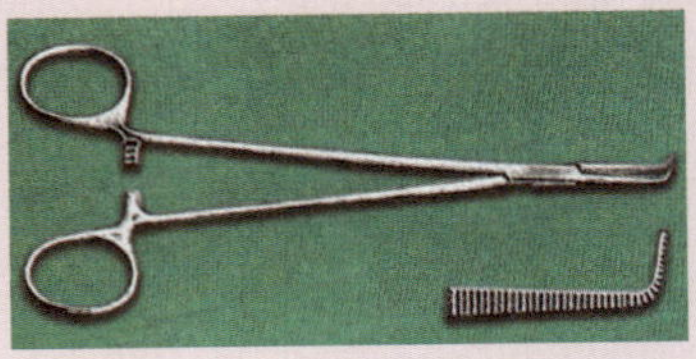

Kocher's Forceps
- To hold securely superior thyroid pedicle vessels.
- Hold retracting cut ends of vessels in tough fibrous tissue.
- Hold ribs during rib resection.
- To cause artificial rupture of gestational membrane.

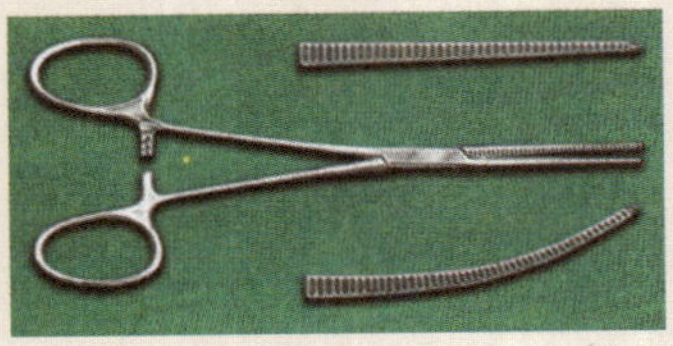

Cautery or electrocautery
- Removal of unsightly warts.
- To burn or coagulate the specific area of tissue.

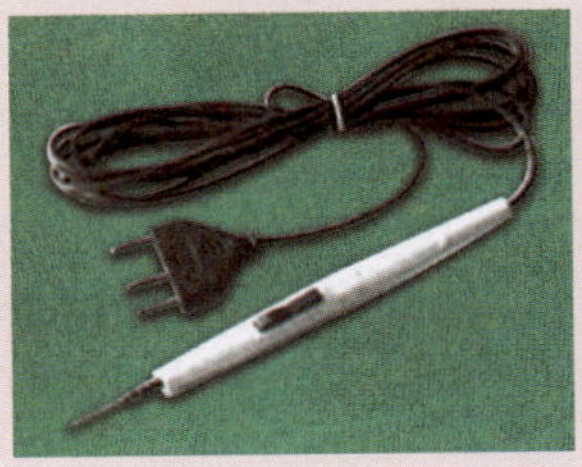

Trochar
- To create holes in body part, e.g., to create holes before laparoscopic surgery.

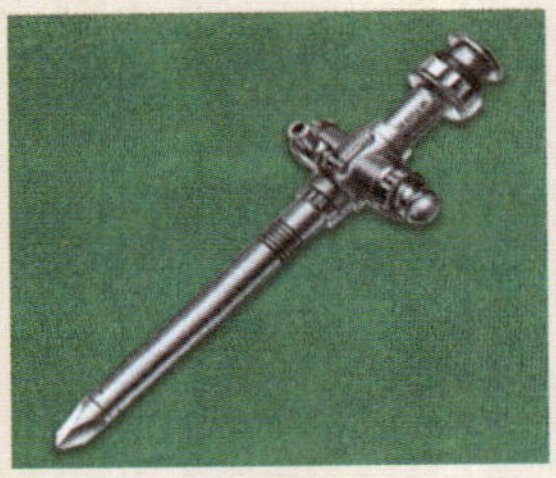

Kidney tray
- To collect waste material following surgery or any procedure.

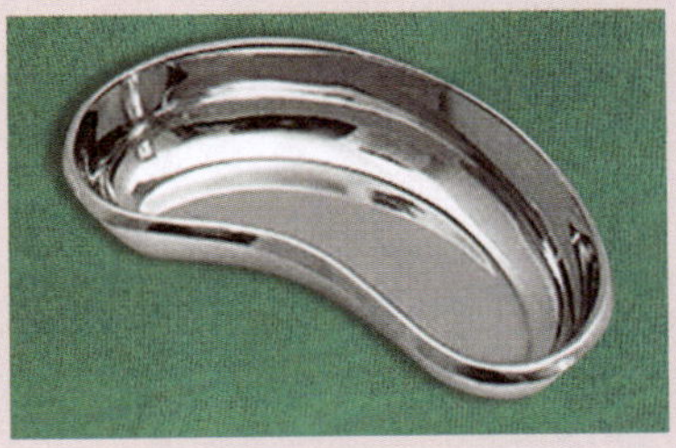

Bard parker handle or scalpel handle (Also known as BP Handle or Blade Holder)
- Intended to be used with BP Safety Blades for tissue separation, and other procedures that require a sharp surgical blade to puncture or cut.

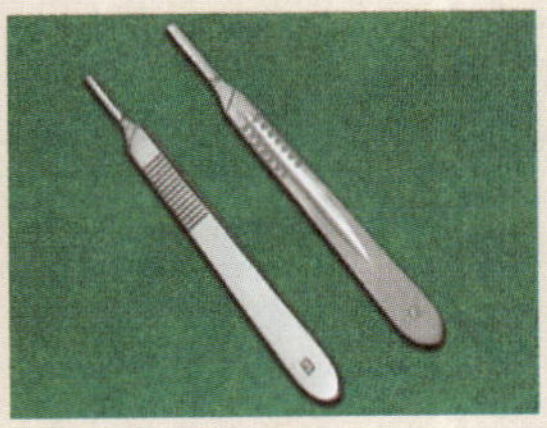

Deavers retractor
- Used to hold back the abdominal wall during abdominal or thoracic procedures.

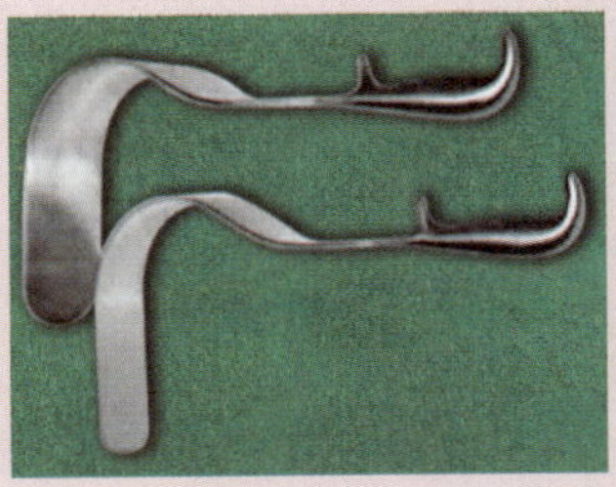

Cheatle forceps
- Used to remove sterilized instruments from boilers and formalin cabinets. The forceps are placed in a container of methylated spirits when not in use.

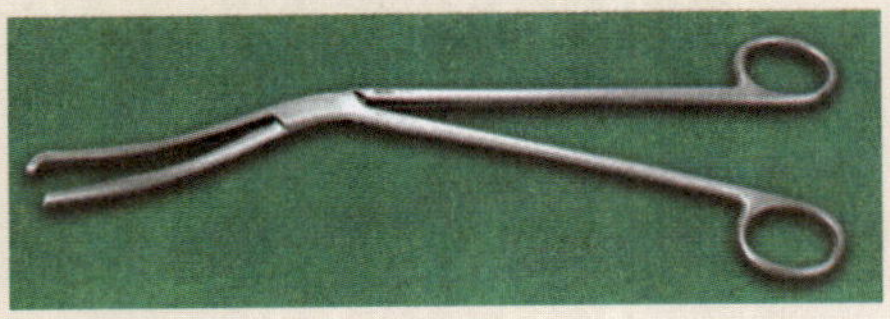

Doyen's towel clip
- Used to fix draping towels.
- Used for fixing diathermy cables, suction tubes, etc.

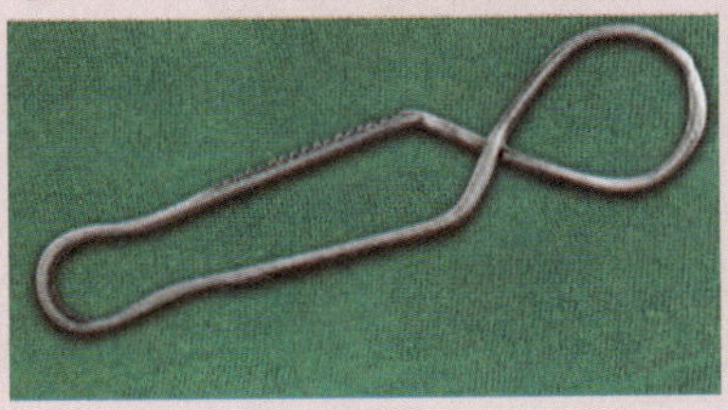

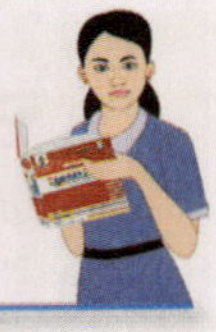

Contd...

Name of the instruments

Doyens-retractor

- Used in pelvic surgery.

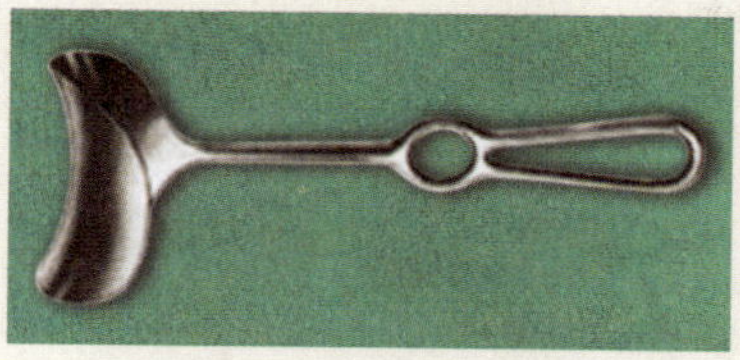

Cat's Paw/Volkman's retractor

- Retraction of skin and tough fascia.

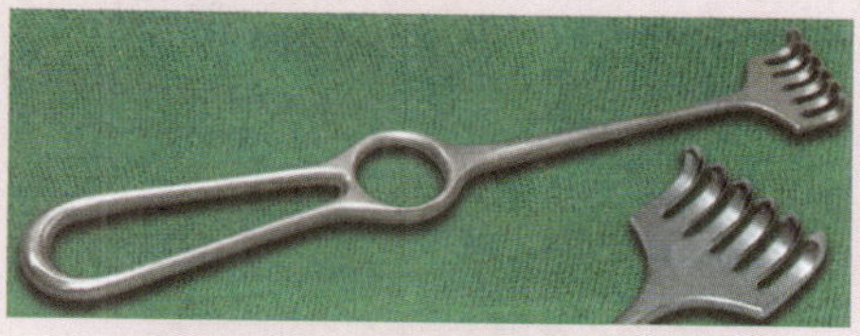

Langenbeck retractor

- In operation involving a lot of dissection in superficial muscle pain which requires retraction, e.g., Hernioplasty, Thyroidectomy.

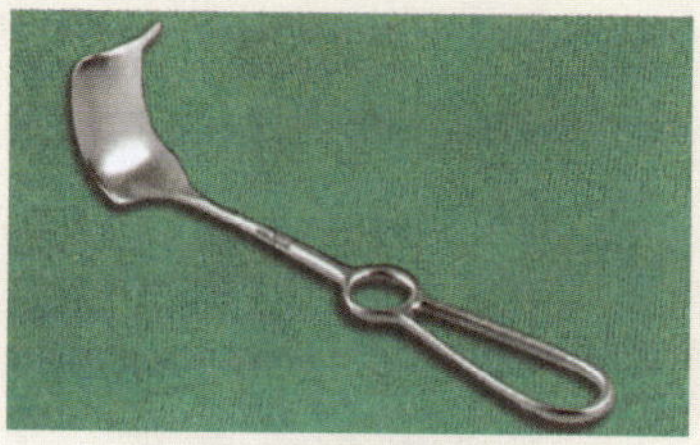

Mayo's towel clip

- Fix drapes in a manner to expose operative field only.
- Also used to fix tubing's and cautery wire to drapes in a way that they don't fall.

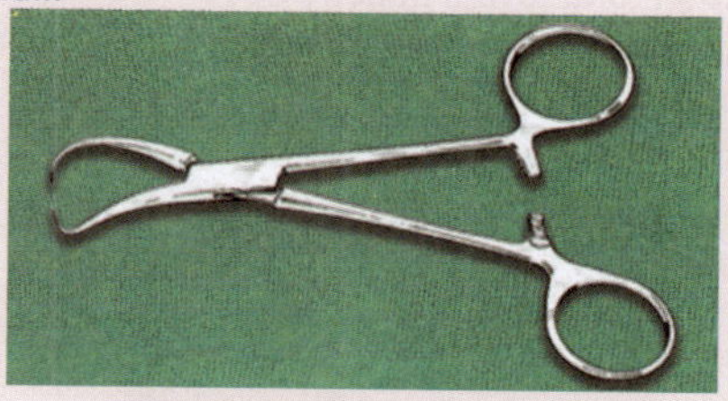

Morris double ended retractor

- To retract strong structures like abdominal wall muscles and it gives wider space to work.

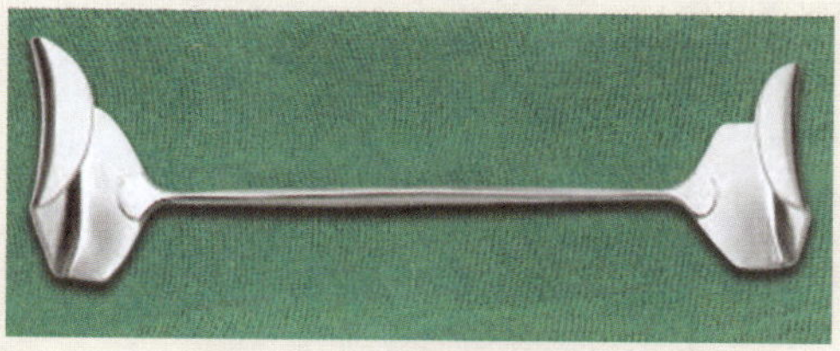

Mosquito artery forceps or small artery forceps

- As a hemostat, holding cut edges, to open up abscess, hold free ends of the suture, hold cut end of the sutures, breaking loculi, etc.

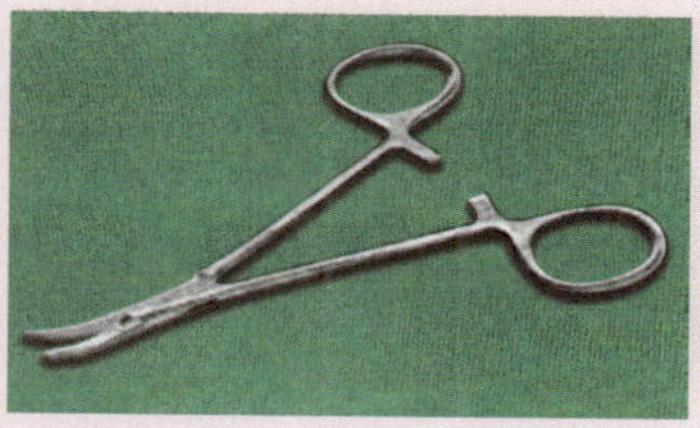

Needle-Holder
(Mayo Hager Needle Holder)

- Used to hold a suturing needle for closing wounds during suturing and surgical procedures.

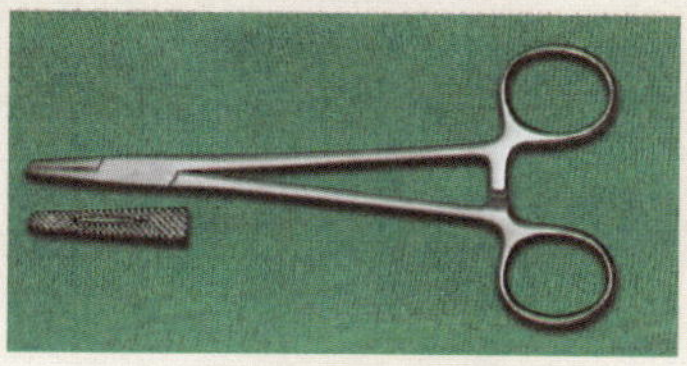

Self-retaining retractor

- Self-retaining retractors allow hands free operation during a surgery.

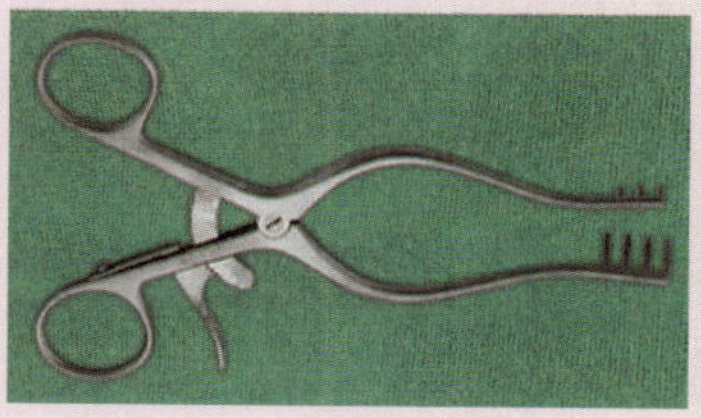

Scissors

- Are used for sharp as well as blunt dissection and also for cutting various tubing's, surgical dressings, gauze, sutures, etc.

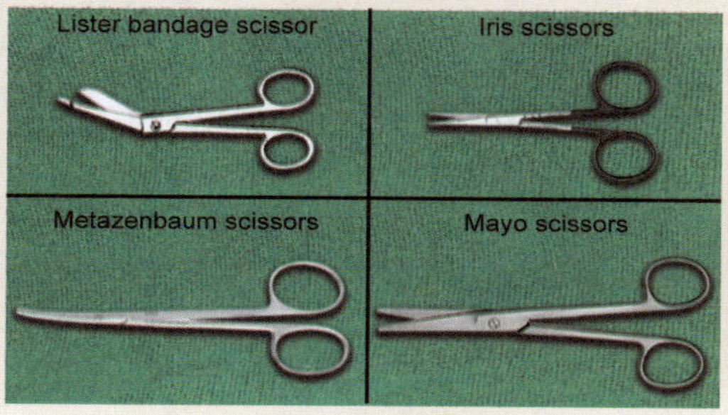

Scalpel blade

- For incisions.

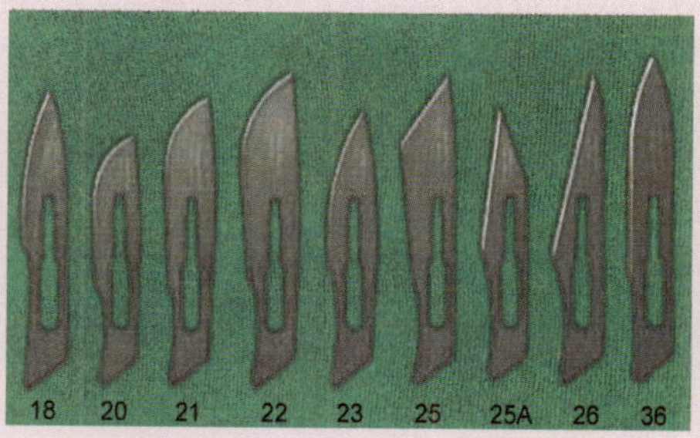

Contd...

Name of the instruments

Ear syringe
- To instil irrigating solutions into the ear.

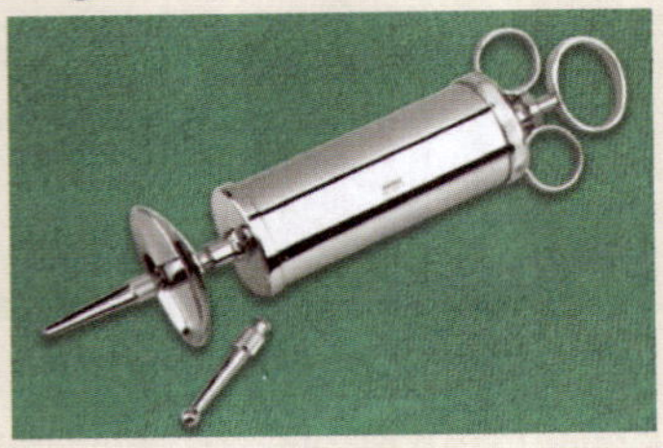

Iris scissors
- It is a scissor with sharp pointed tips used during ophthalmic surgery.

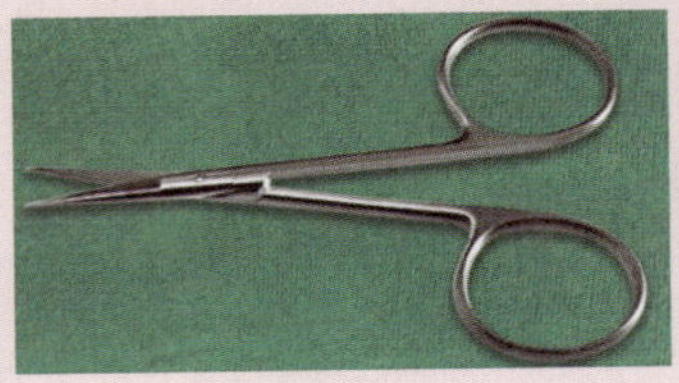

Sputum mug
- To collect expectorate from patient.
- Before collecting expectorate some disinfecting solutions should be poured into the mug.

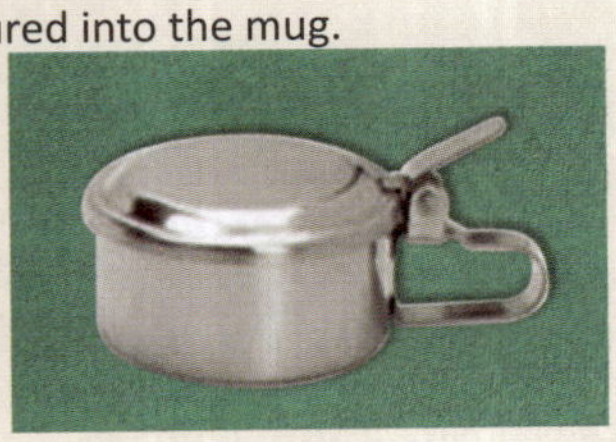

Rampleys sponge holding forceps
- To hold cotton or sterile gauze piece with or without antiseptic solution to clean body part before medical, diagnostic or surgical procedure.

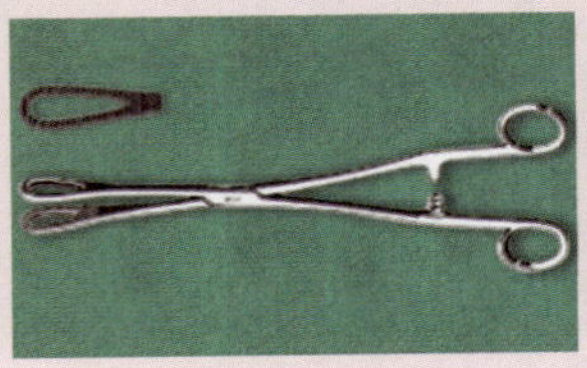

Tongue forceps
- To hold tongue during oral surgeries without causing any damage or injury to it.

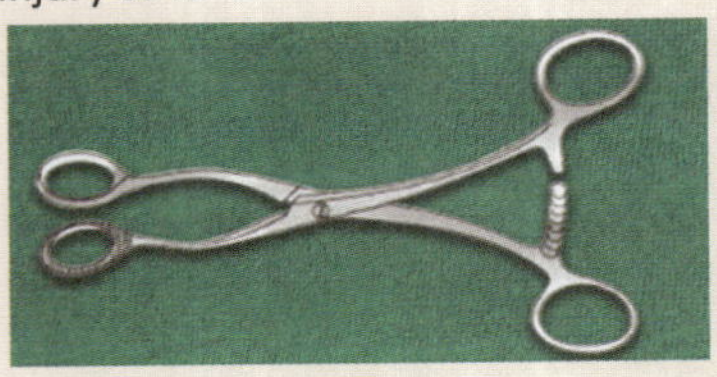

Aneurysm needle
- To hold delicate structures such as blood vessels and nerves during procedures.

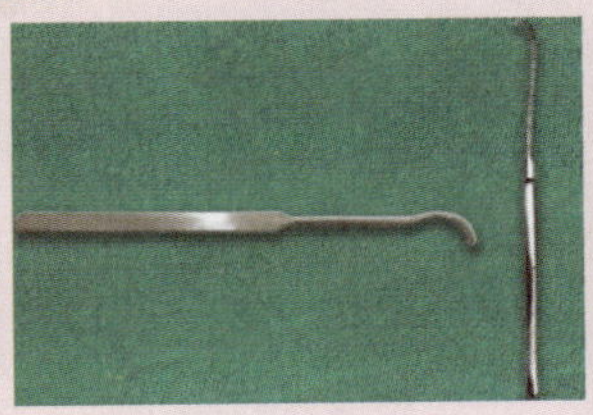

Bone chisel
- Used for cutting and shaping the bone during the procedure.

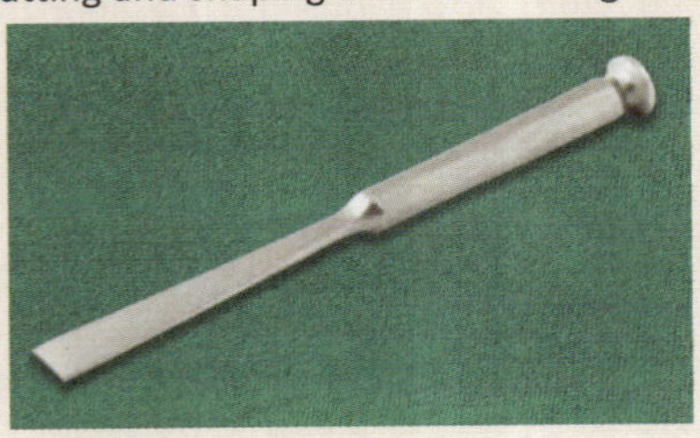

Nontoothed dissecting forceps
- Used in the reconstruction of eyelid surgery.

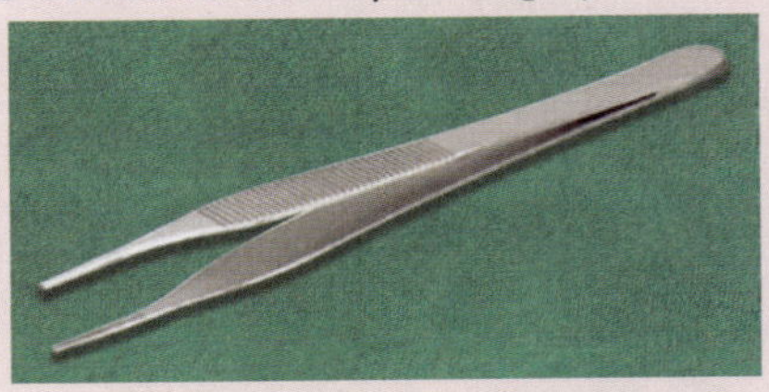

Reflex hammer
- To elicit deep tendon reflexes during neurological and physical examination to assess the functioning of central and peripheral nervous system.

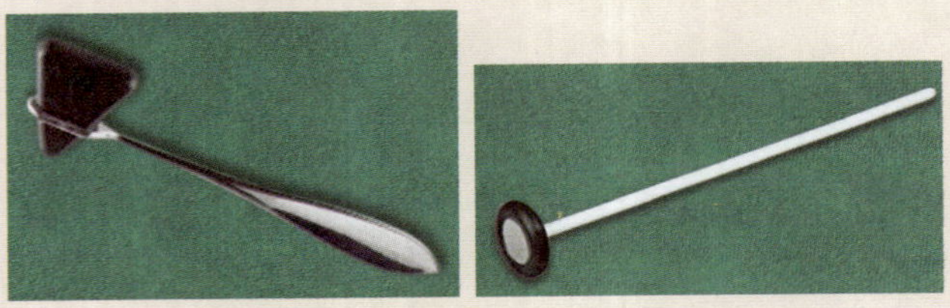

Proctoscope/rectoscope
- To examine anus, rectum and sigmoid colon.

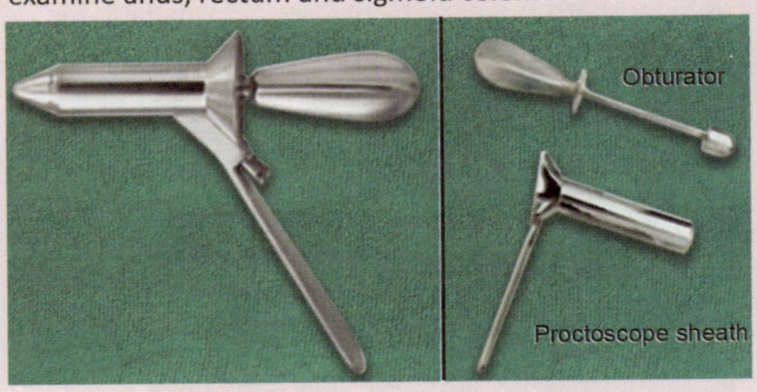

Contd...

Name of the instruments

Tracheal dilator

- Used to widen the opening made in the trachea during procedures like tracheostomy and to keep the tracheal opening patent.

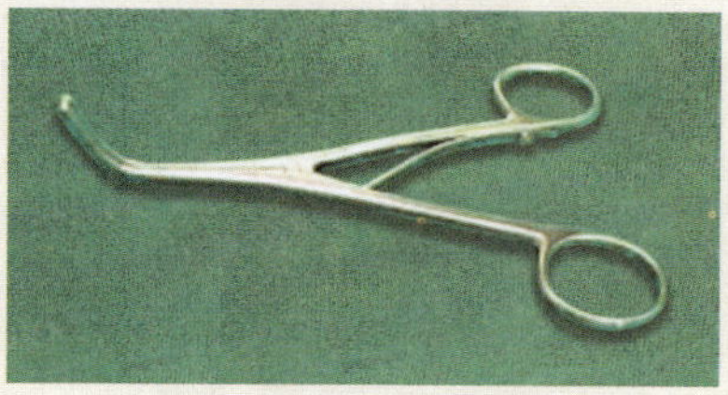

Adsons Pickup forceps (Adsons Tissue forceps)

- Adson Tissue Forceps are used for holding and manipulating delicate tissues. These **forceps** have a wide and flat thumb grasp area that is commonly serrated.

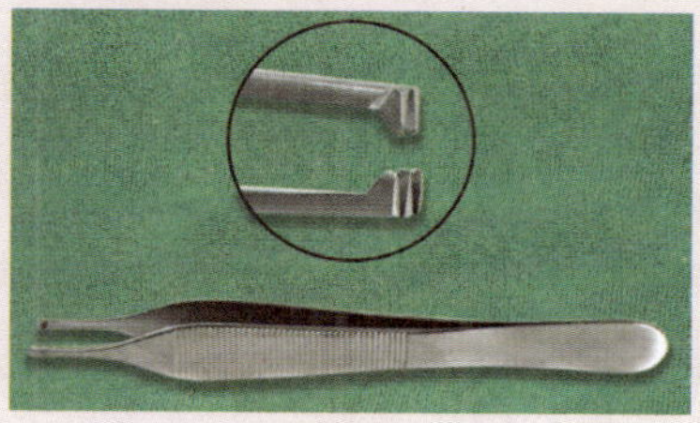

Magill forceps

- It is a right-handed instrument used to place ET tube correctly in laryngeal inlet.
- It is also used to remove foreign bodies and throat packs.

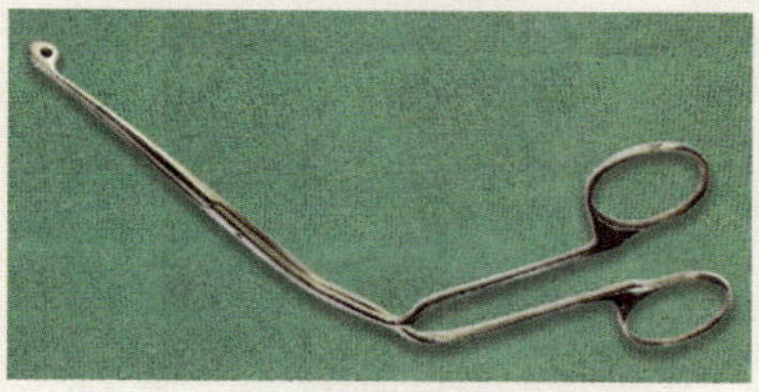

AMBU bag

- Artificial manual breathing unit or bag valve mask unit used to provide positive pressure ventilation to those patients who all are breathing inadequately.

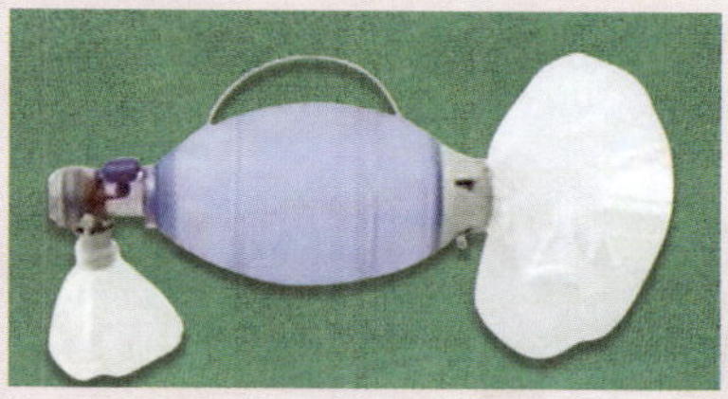

Asepto syringe

- Irrigation of wound or cavities.

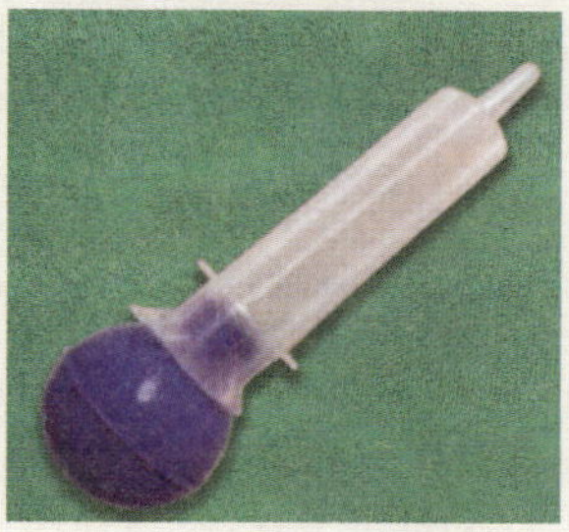

Crocodile forceps/hartmann alligator forceps

- Used to remove foreign body during ENT procedure.

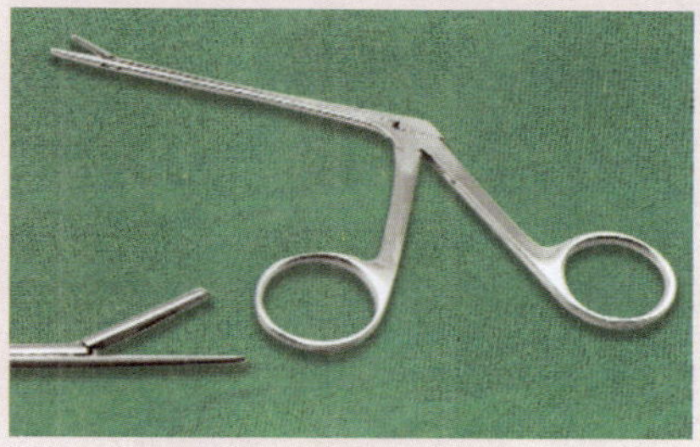

Bone cutting forceps

- Used for cutting bones during surgery or following infection in a particular part of bone.

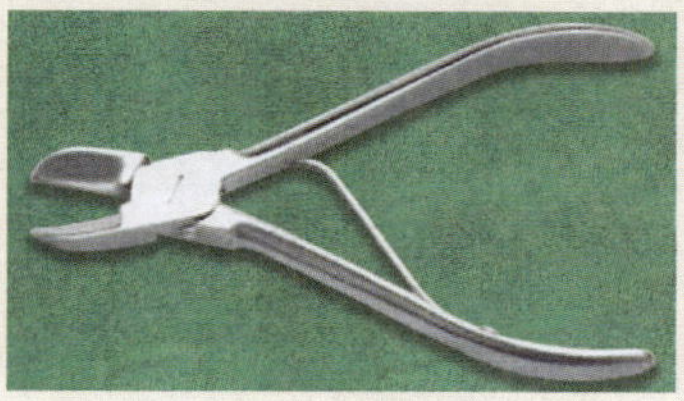

Bandage scissors

- Used for sizing dressing and removing circumferential bandages
- Also used to cut plaster, fabric occasionally.

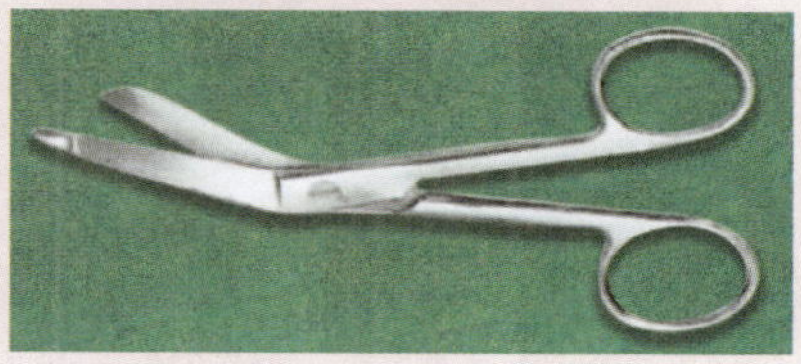

Punch biopsy forceps

- To obtain biopsy from various body organs.
- To remove embedded hair follicles, callous formations and tiny cysts or nodules.

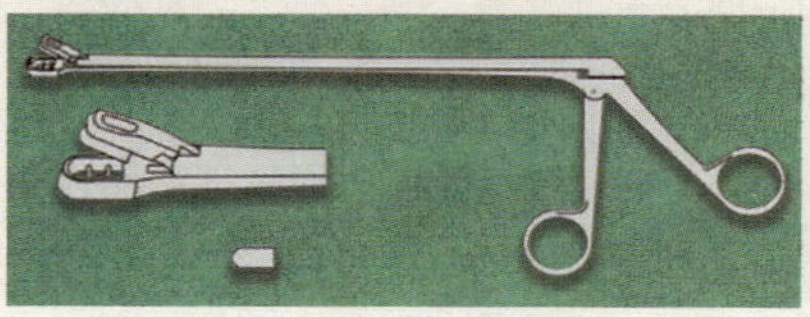

Nelson inhaler

- Used for steam inhalation purpose. Hot water mixed with medication is poured into the jar before inhalation.

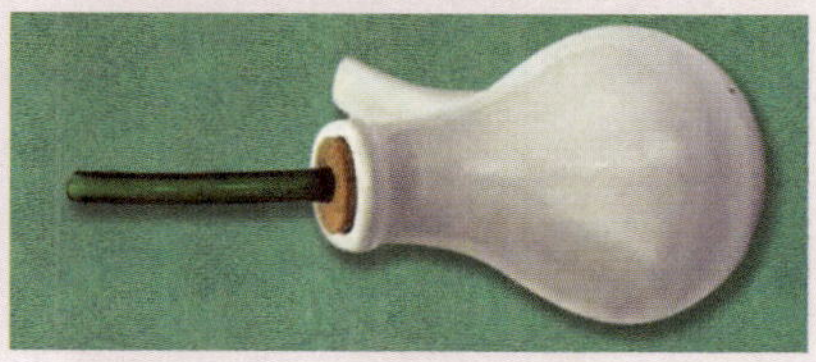

Contd...

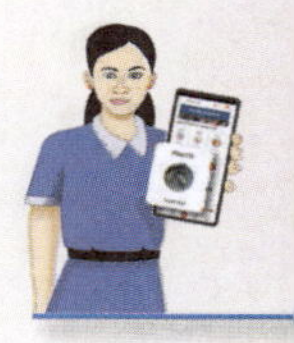

Name of the instruments

Laryngoscope

- Helps in visualization of larynx and helps in ET intubation. Curved blades are known as macintosh and straight blades are known as miller.

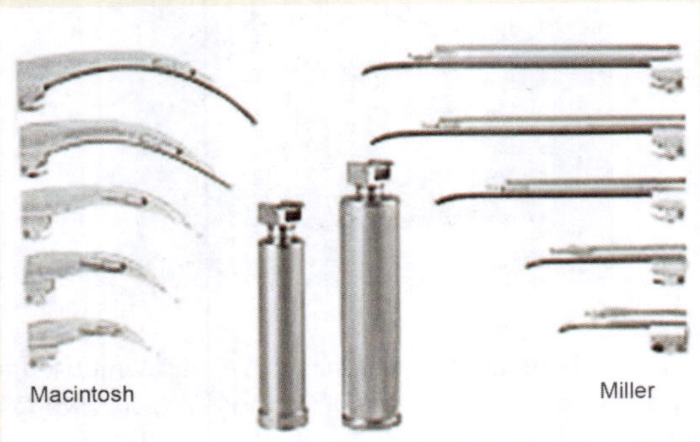

Suction cannulas aural speculum

- It is used for ear examination and ear surgeries.

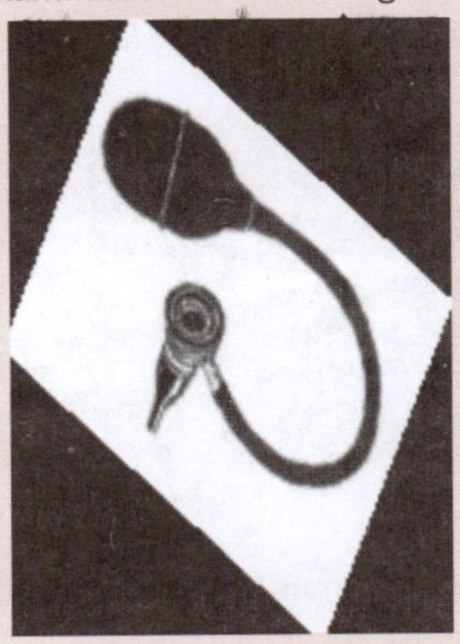

Otoscope/auriscope

- Allows the visualization of inner ear structures.

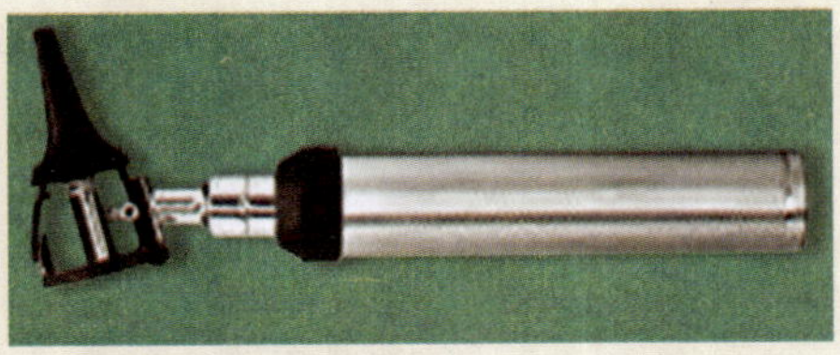

Jolles thyroid retractor

- Self-retaining thyroid retractor used in thyroid surgeries to retract skin.

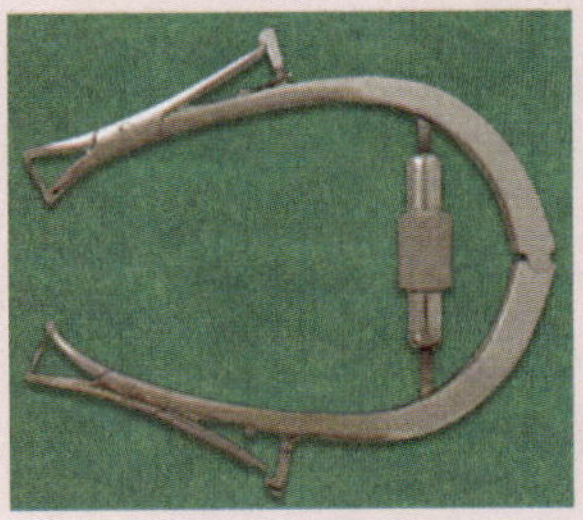

Balfour with bladder blade retractor

- Also known as balfour abdominal retractor.
- It is a self-retaining retractor.
- Used during specific abdominal procedures, cesarean sections and bowel resection.

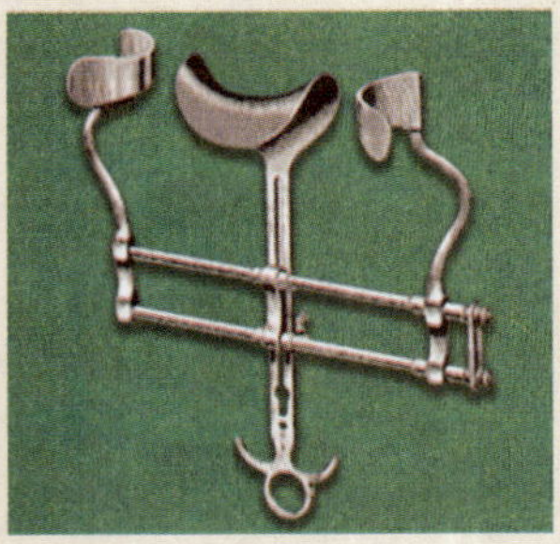

Army-navy retractor

- It is also known as right angle retractor or US army retractor.
- It is a double-ended retractor with fenestrated handle used to retract small or shallow incision.
- Mainly used during plastic surgery procedure to expose skin.
- Usually they are used in pairs to provide traction and counter traction.

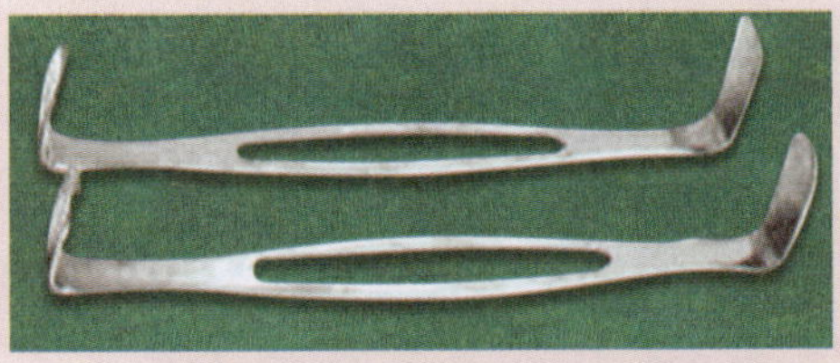

Weitlaner retractor

- Self-retaining retractor used during basic plastic surgeries, large bone and joint surgeries and mastoid surgeries.

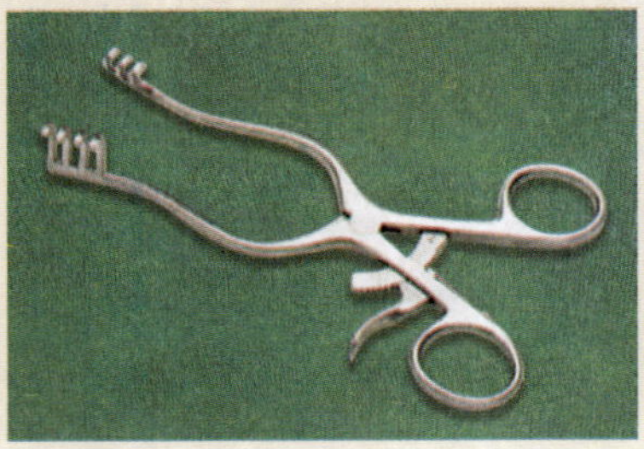

Gelpi retractor

- Used in small surgical site.
- It is self-retaining retractor.

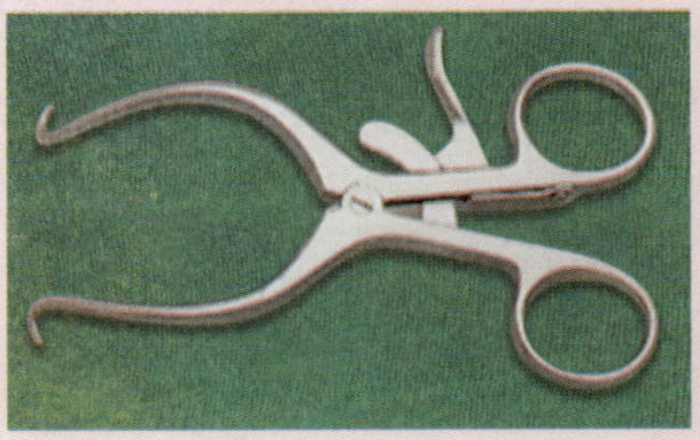

Contd...

Name of the instruments

Goulet retractor

- It is a handheld retractor used for holding back tissue from small, and superficial incisions.

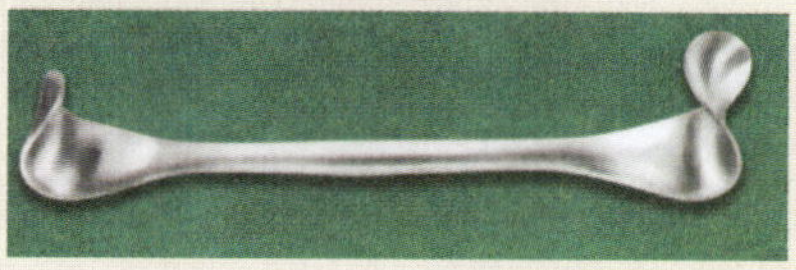

Ophthalmoscope/ funduscope

- Allows the visualization of the fundus of eye.

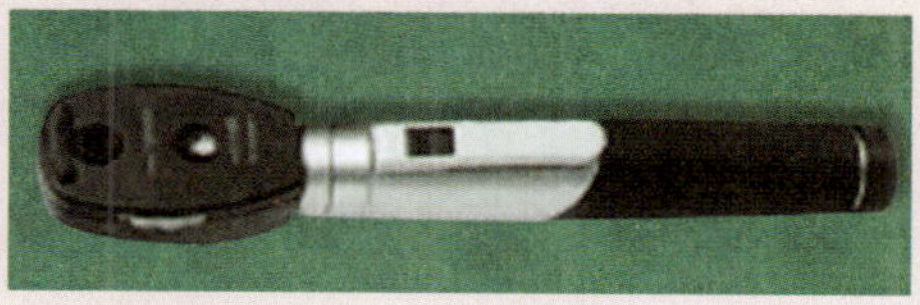

Kelly hemostat (Kelly forceps)

- This instrument is available as curved and straight forms.
- Used to clamp large blood vessels and to dissect tissues.

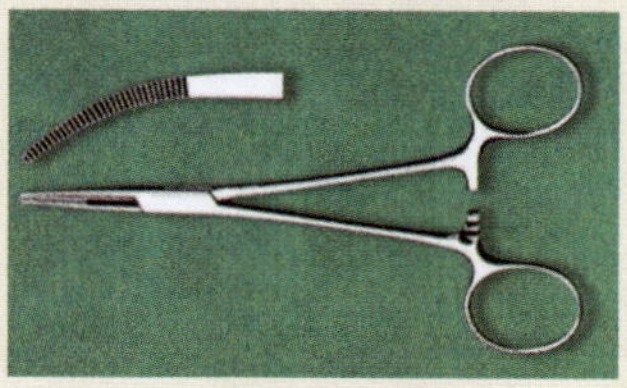

Curved artery forceps

- Used for grasping large sections of tissue or passing sutures in abdominal procedures. They have long shanks and short jaws with full and horizontal serrations.

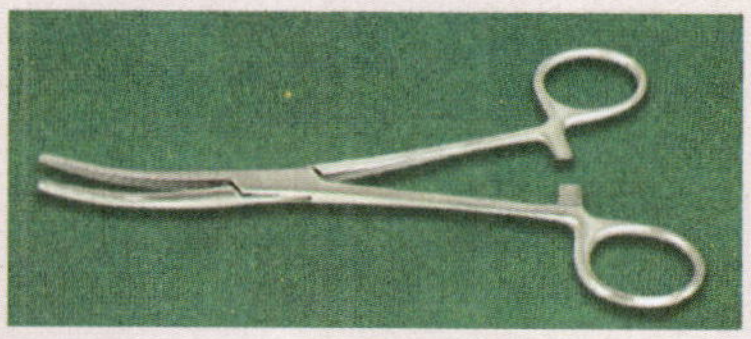

Hemoclip applier with hemoclips

- Hemoclip applicator is used to apply hemoclip and to ensure good ligation.

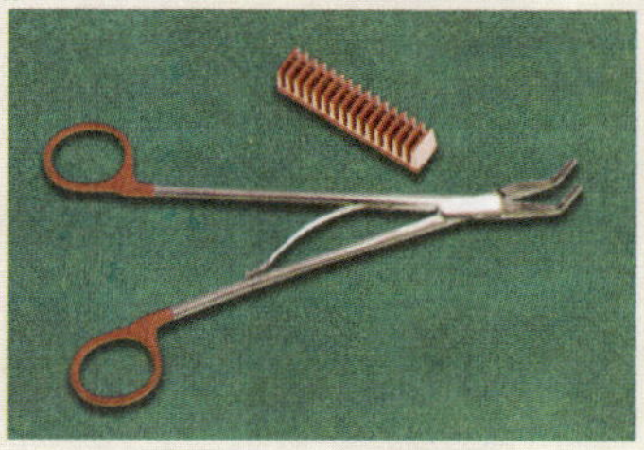

Thudichum nasal speculum

- Speculum widens the nasal cavity and allows the better visualization of nasal cavity during therapeutic and diagnostic procedures.

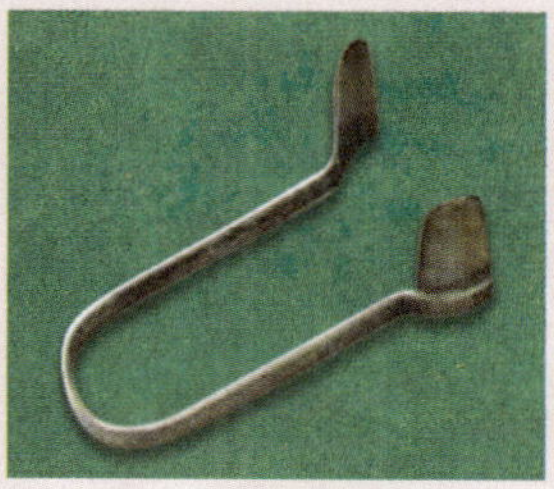

Dressing forceps

- Dressing forceps are thumb forceps used for holding dressing material during dressing or surgery procedures.

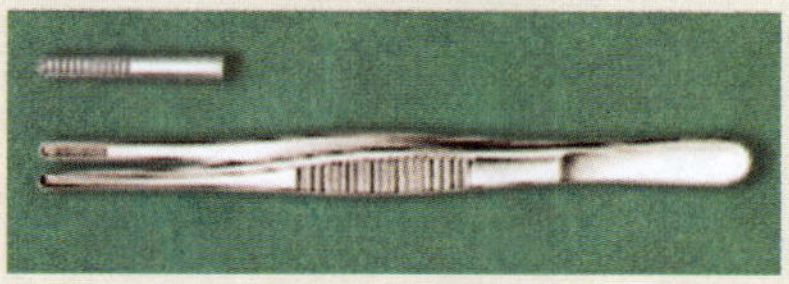

Debakey forceps

- A traumatic forceps used during vascular procedure to avoid tissue damage during manipulation.

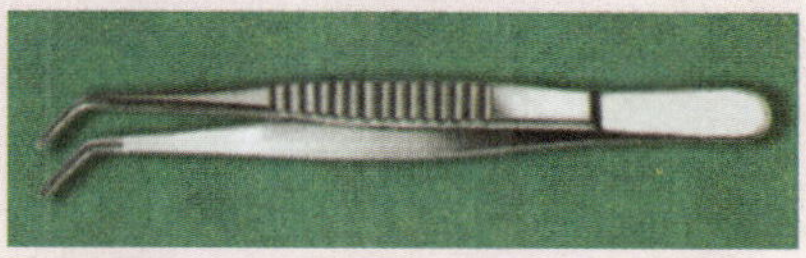

Tongue depressor

- These are the instruments which allow us to depress the tongue and allow the visualization of mouth and throat.
- Nowadays wooden type disposable tongue depressors are commonly used than stainless steel type tongue depressor.

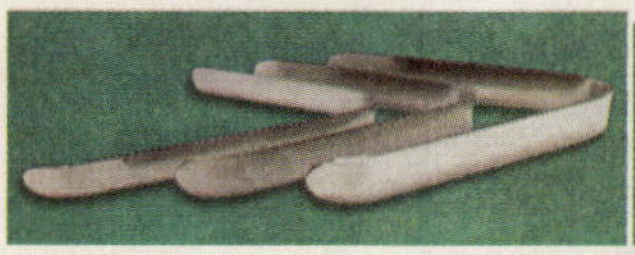

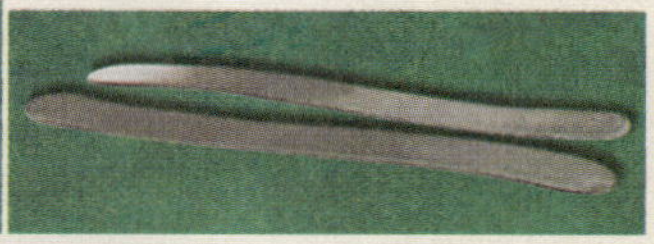

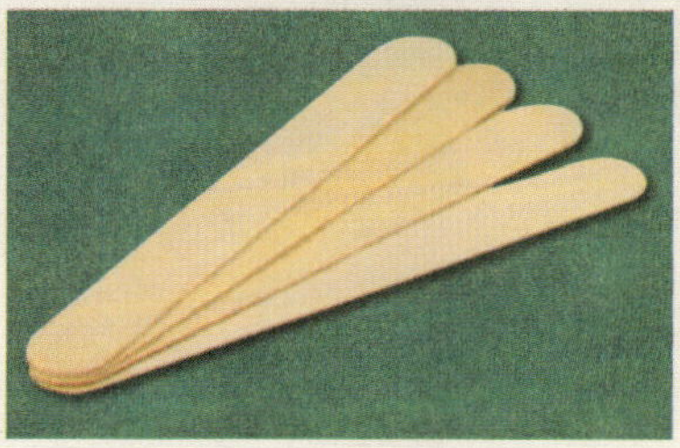

Russian tissue forceps

- Used to hold dense tissue during procedures such as wound debridement and closure.

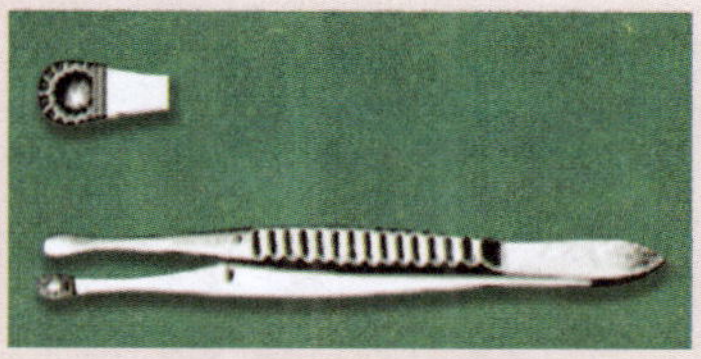

Toothed dissecting forceps

- Used to hold tissue during procedures.

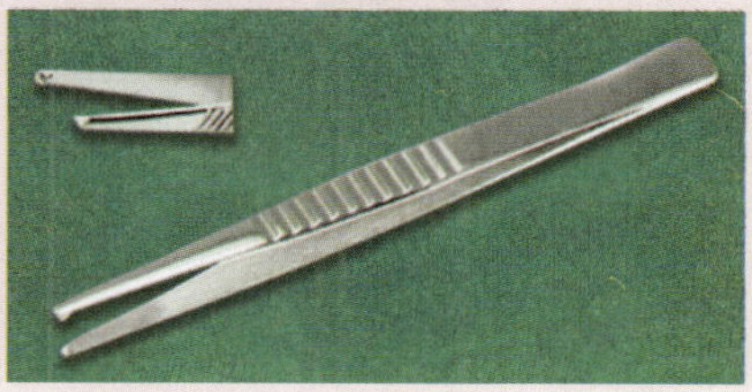

5

"Your body is a temple, but only if you treat it as one."
—Astrid Alauda

EQUIPMENT/INSTRUMENTS

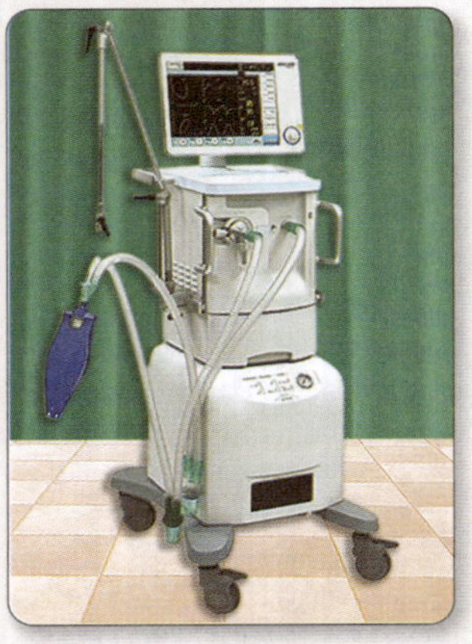

Ventilator/mechanical ventilator

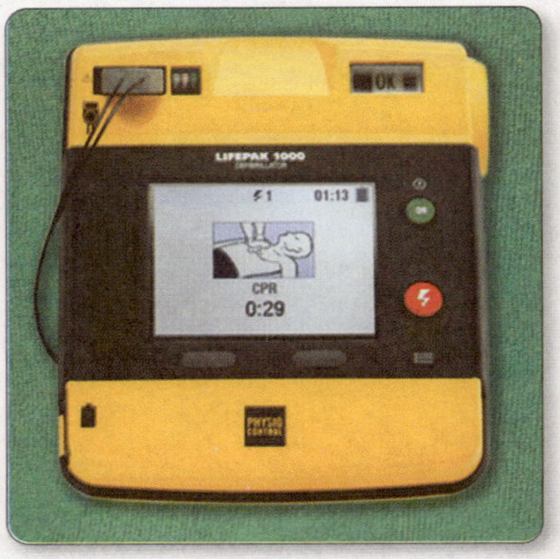

Automatic external defibrillator (AED)

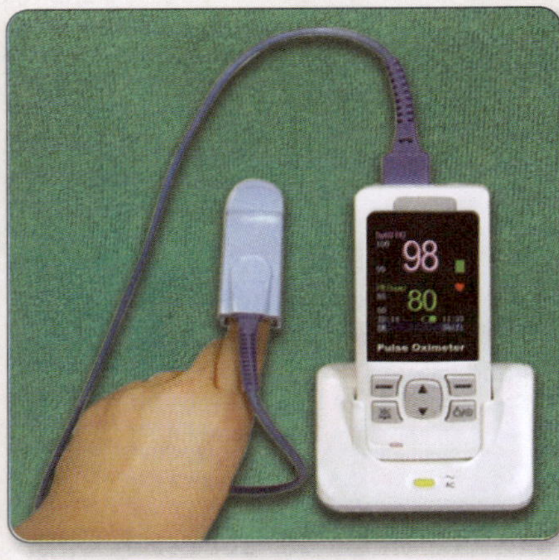

Pulse-oximeter

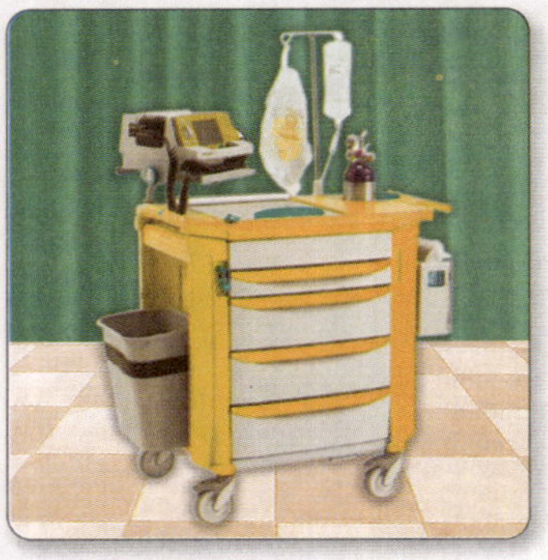

Crash cart trolley

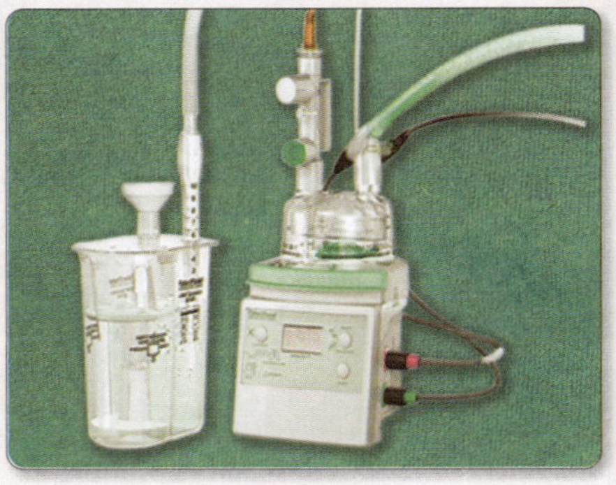

Bubble CPAP

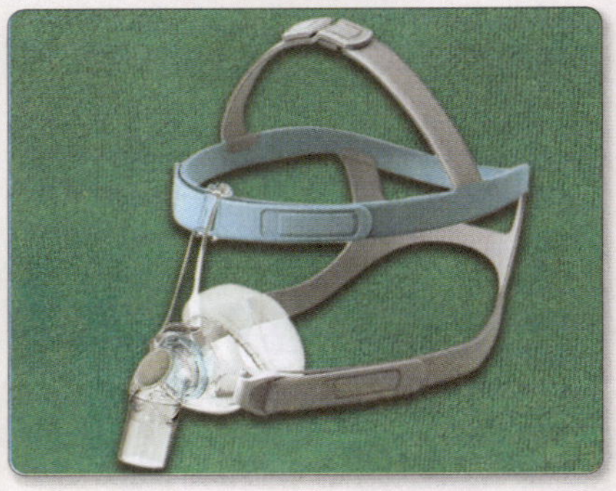

CPAP mask

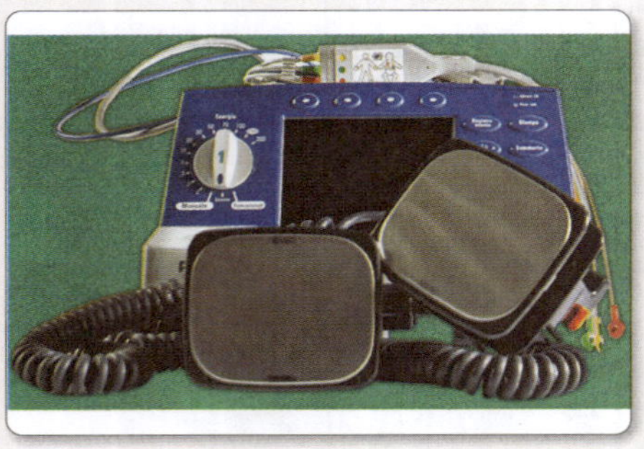

Defibrillator

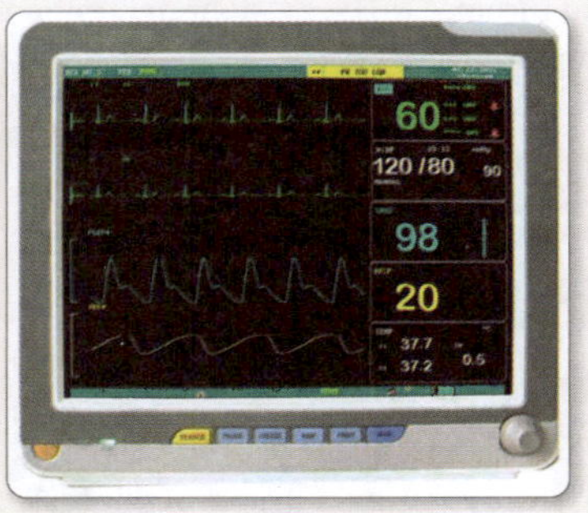

Cardiac monitor

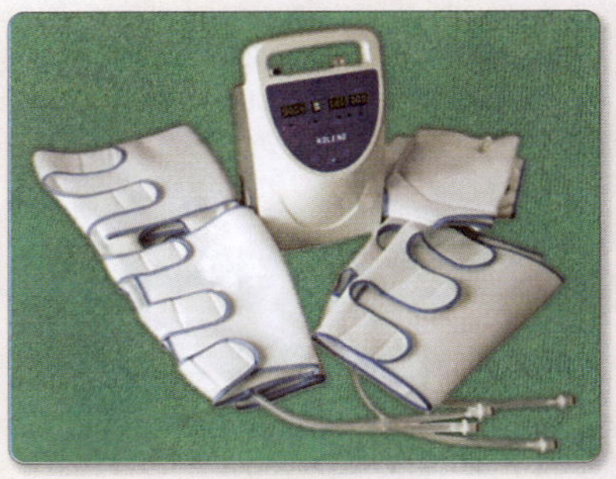

DVT pump

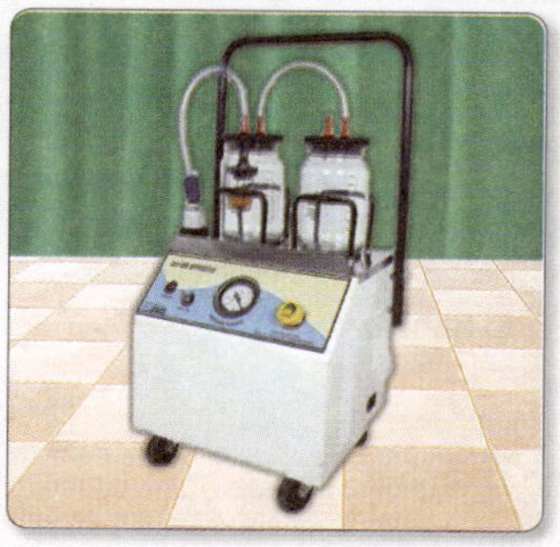

Portable suction machine

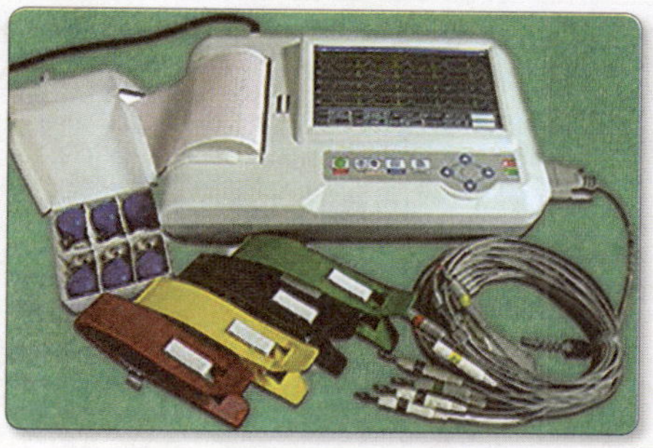

ECG machine

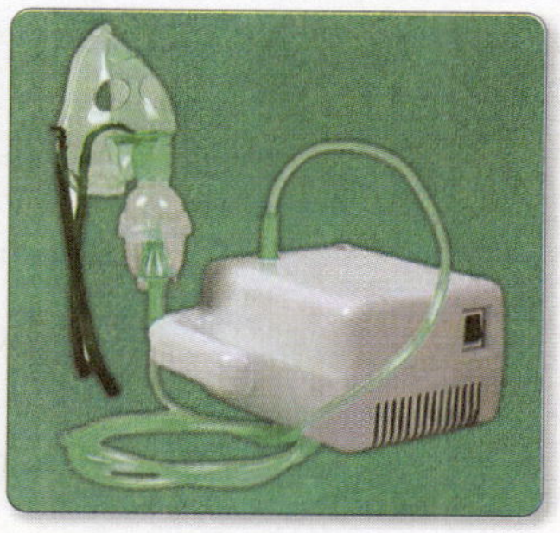

Nebulizer

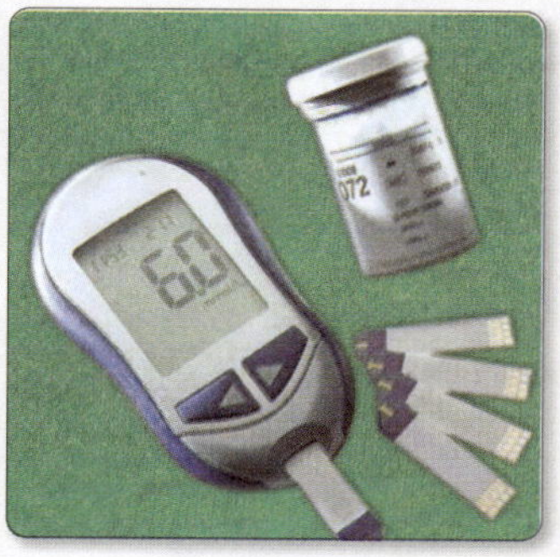

Glucometer

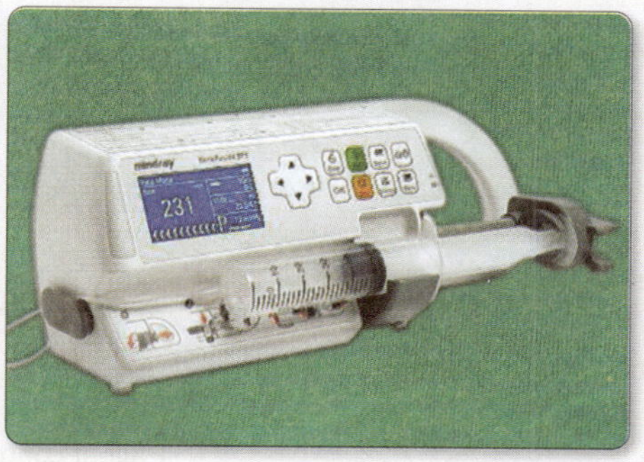

Syringe pump

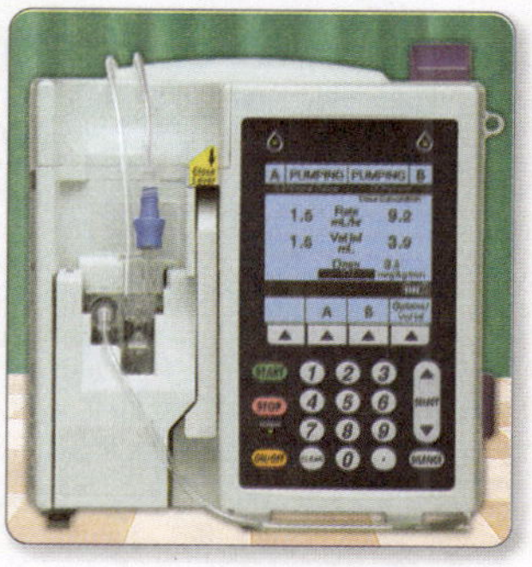

Infusion pump

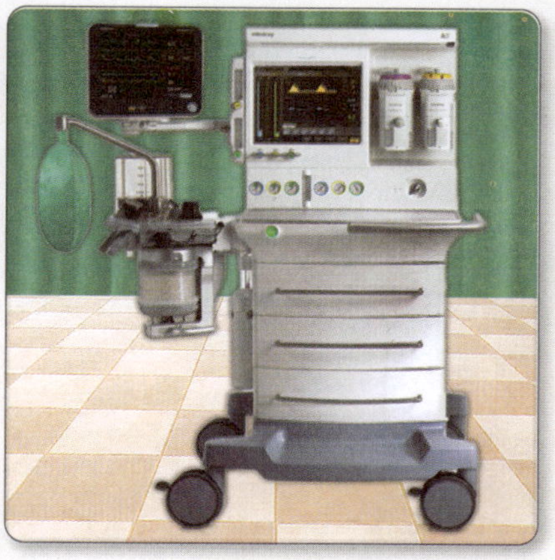

Anesthesia machine

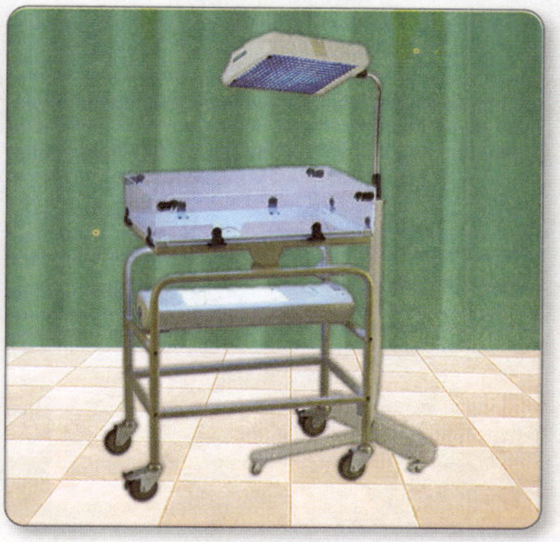

Phototherapy unit

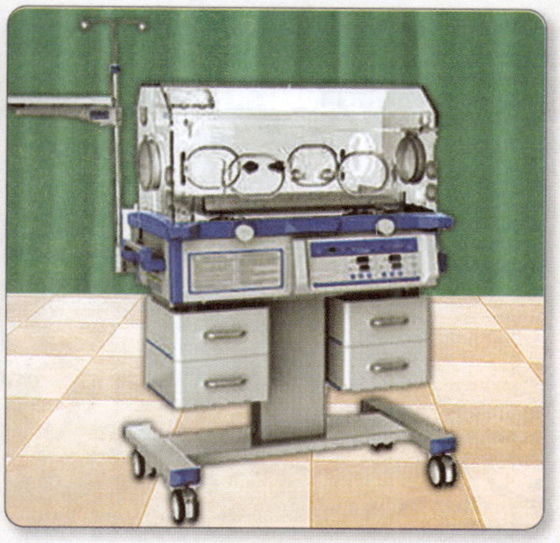

Incubator/closed care system

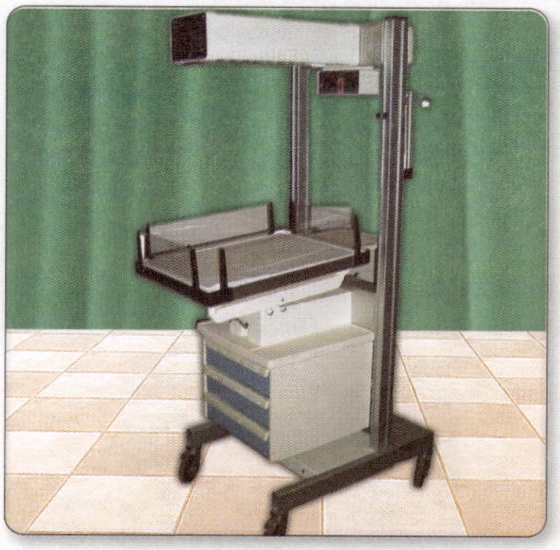

Radiant warmer/open care system

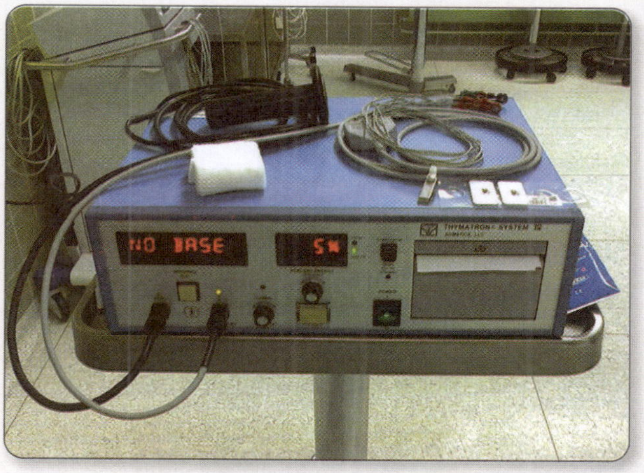

ECT machine

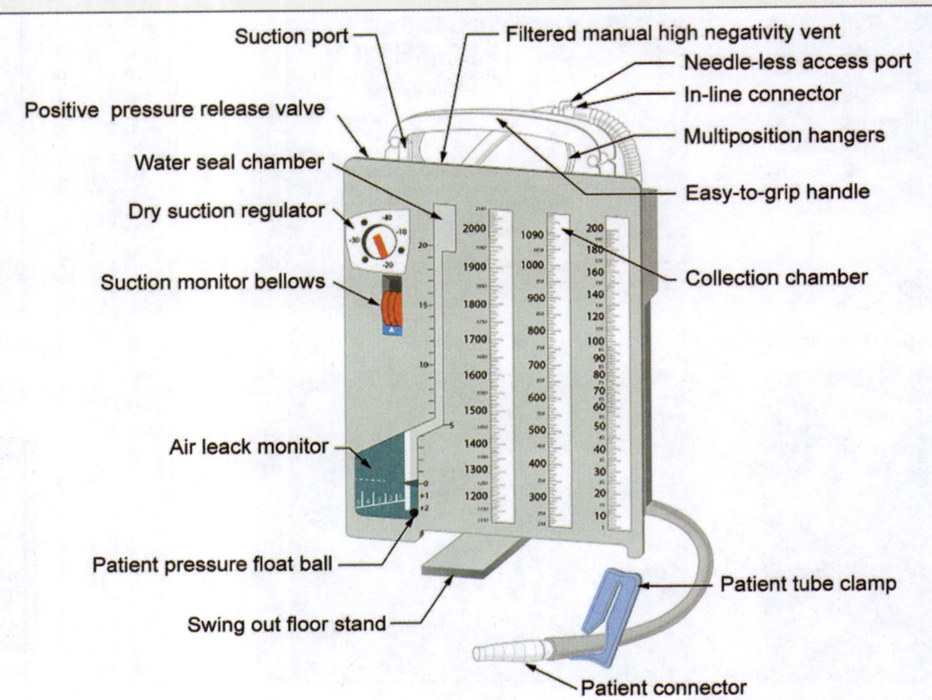

Intercostal drainage system

Name of the instruments

Guedel airway (oropharyngeal airway)

- To maintain or open a patient's airway. It does this by preventing the tongue from covering the epiglottis, which could prevent the person from breathing.

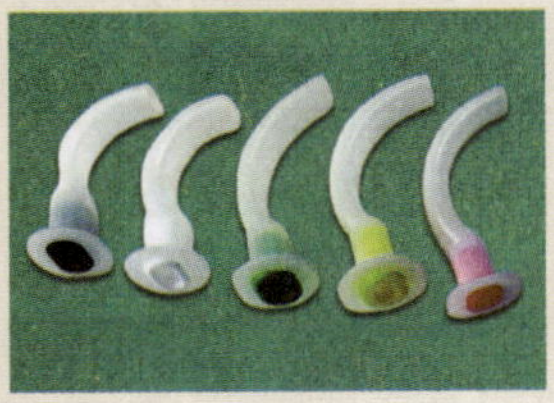

Doppler fetal monitor

- It is a hand-held ultrasound transducer used to detect the fetal heartbeat for prenatal care.

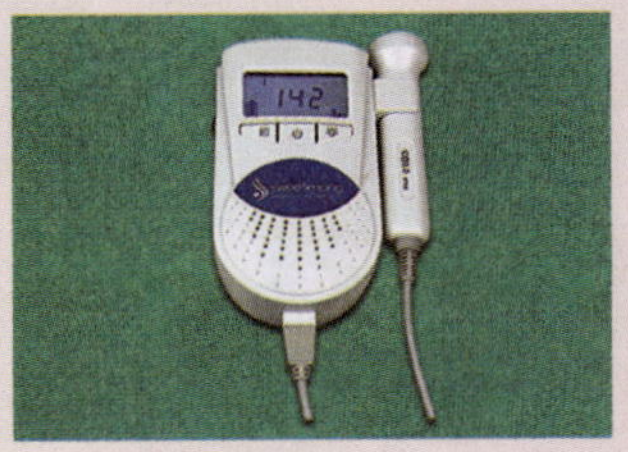

Ice lined refrigerator

- It is used for storage of vaccines.

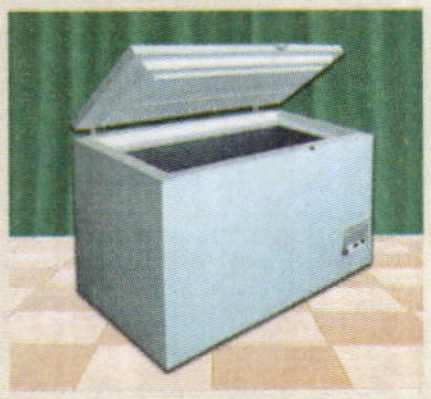

Deep freezer

- It is used for transportation of vaccines.

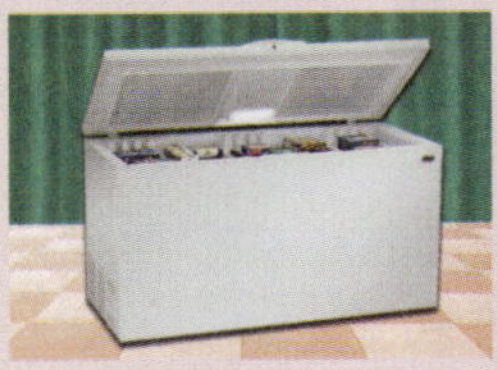

Cold box

- It is used for safe transportation of vaccines.

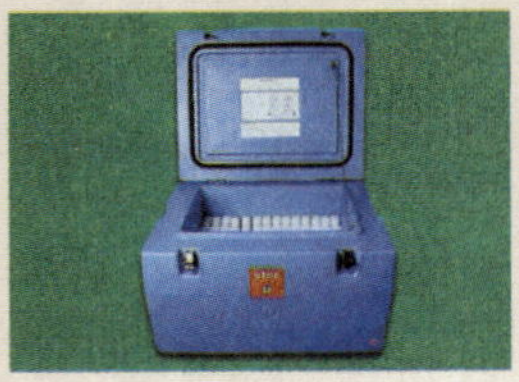

Vaccine carrier (vaccine carrier has a strap)

- It is used for transportation of vaccines.

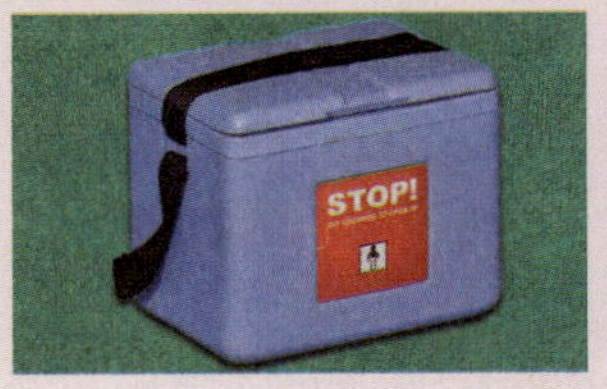

Contd...

Name of the instruments

Incentive spirometer

- It is used to facilitate a sustained slow deep breath.
- Incentive spirometer is designed to mimic natural sighing by encouraging patients to take slow, deep breaths.

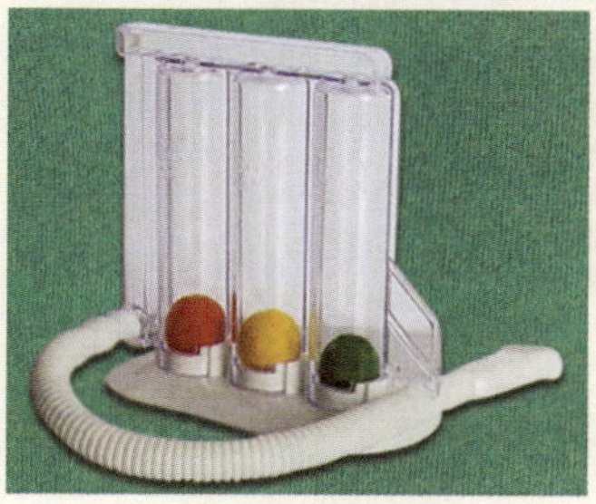

Single-use clinical thermometer (disposable thermometer)

Procedure

- Unwrap the thermometer and place in the mouth under the tongue into either heat pocket for 60 seconds.
- Remove thermometer and wait for 10 seconds.
- Read the temperature by looking at the last blue dot and discard after use.

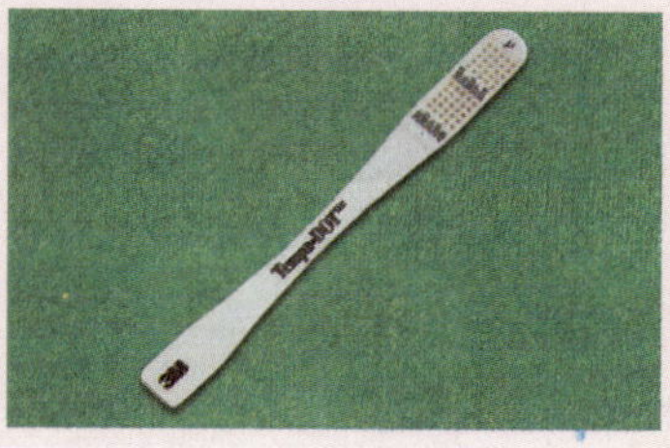

Oxygen hood

- It is used for babies who can breathe on their own but still need extra oxygen.

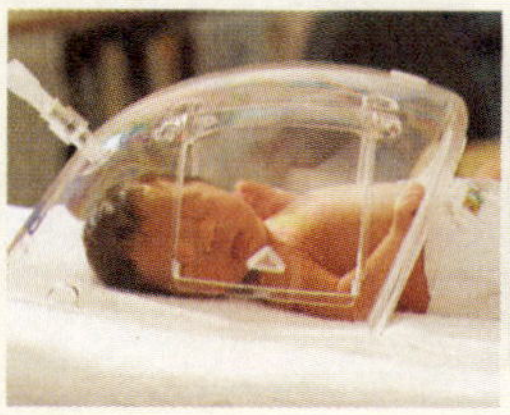

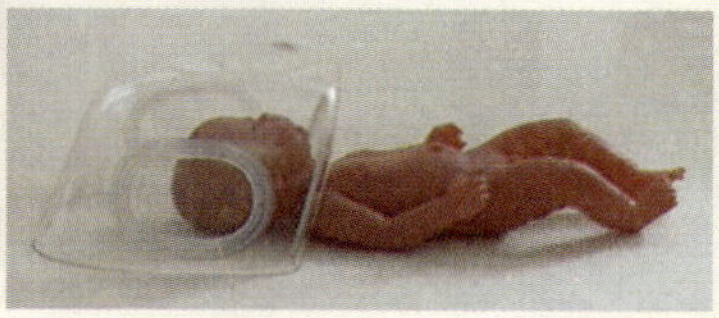

Ice pack vaccine carrier

- It is used for transportation of vaccines.
- Ice-packs are used to keep vaccines cool inside the vaccine.

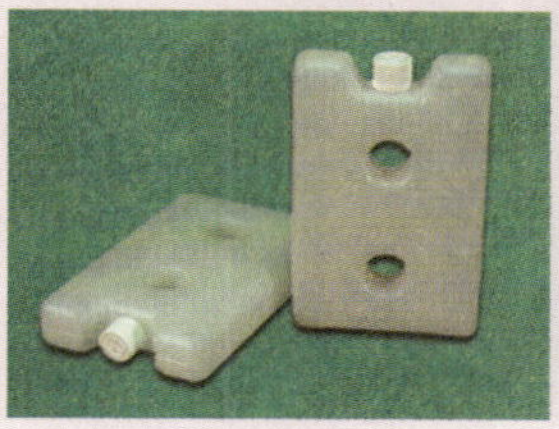

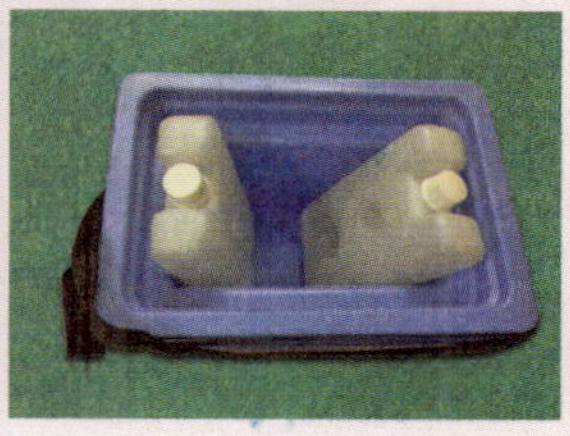

Needle destroyer

- It is used to destroy the used disposable **needles.**

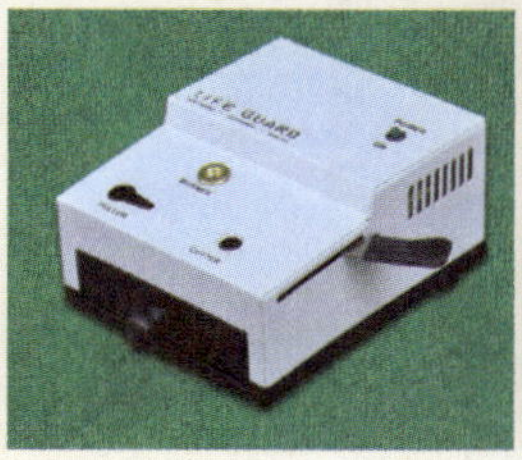

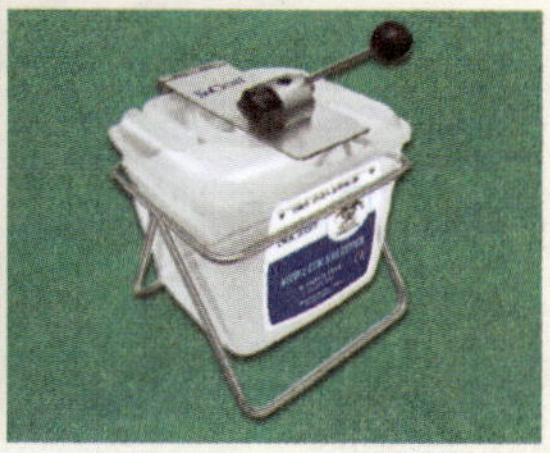

Suction machine (wall mount)

- It is used for suction in hospital settings.

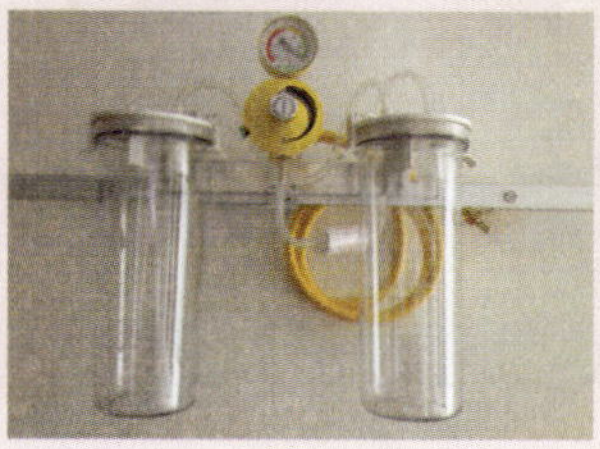

Walk-in freezer

- It is used for storage of vaccines on large scale.

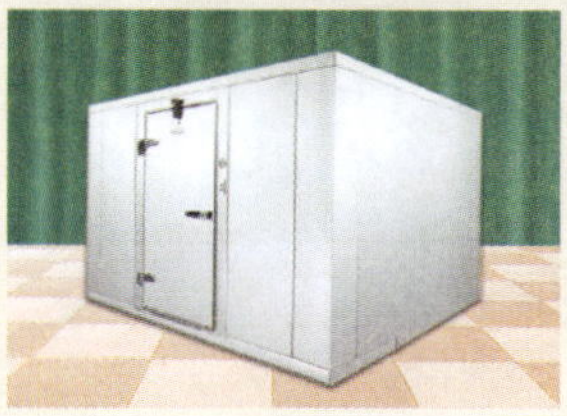

Neonatal jaundice meter

- The transcutaneous jaundice meter is a noninvasive method for screening babies for jaundice.

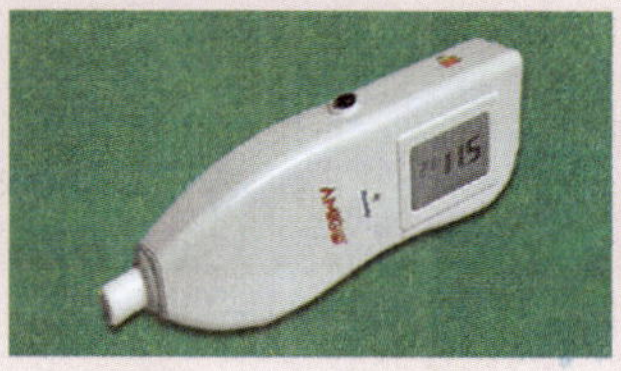

Mouth suction device/nasal aspirator

- For mouth suction and nasal aspiration of babies without backflow.

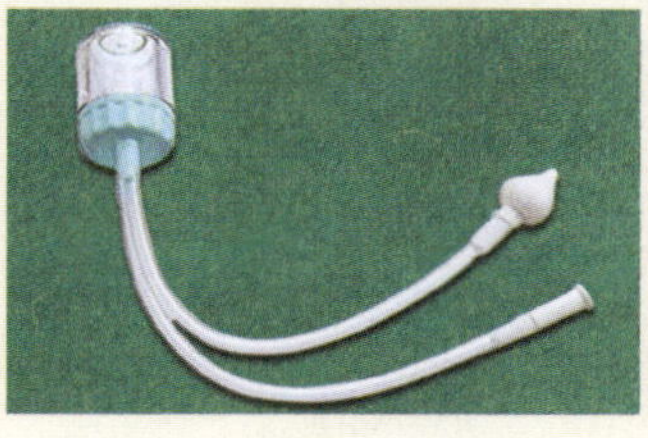

Mucous extractor

- It is used with a suction machine to maintain an airway by removing secretions from the mouth, throat or lungs.

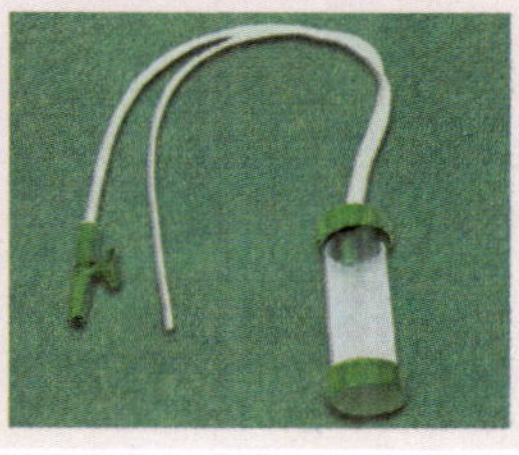

Contd...

Name of the instruments

Metallic vacuum cup (vacuum delivery)

- It is used to assist delivery of a baby using a vacuum device
- It is a mushroom-shaped metal cup varying from 40 mm to 60 mm in diameter.

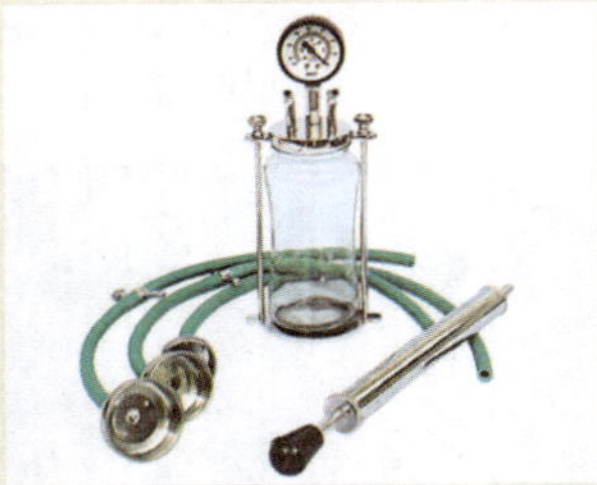

USG machine (ultrasound machine)

- It uses high-frequency sound waves to capture live images from the inside of your body. Used for diagnostic purpose.

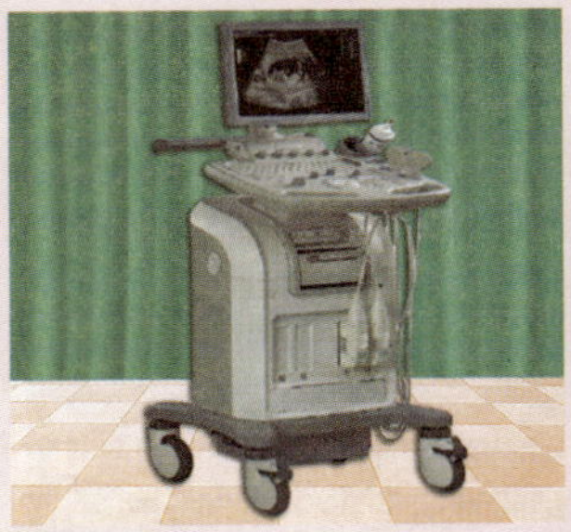

Cardiotocography machine (CTG)

- It is used to perform non-stress test during antenatal period.

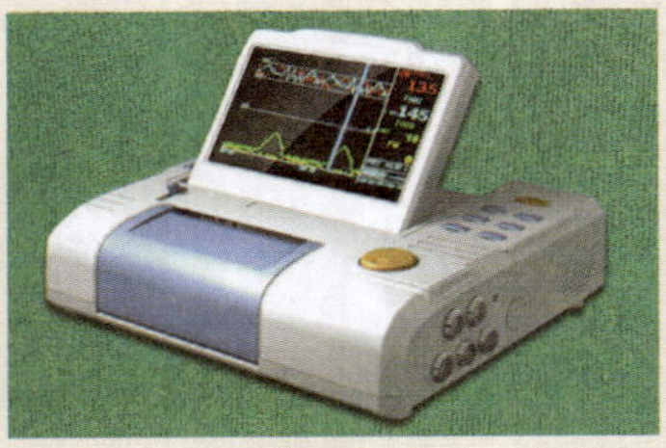

Pinard fetoscope

- It is a type of stethoscope used to listen to the heartbeat of a fetus during pregnancy.

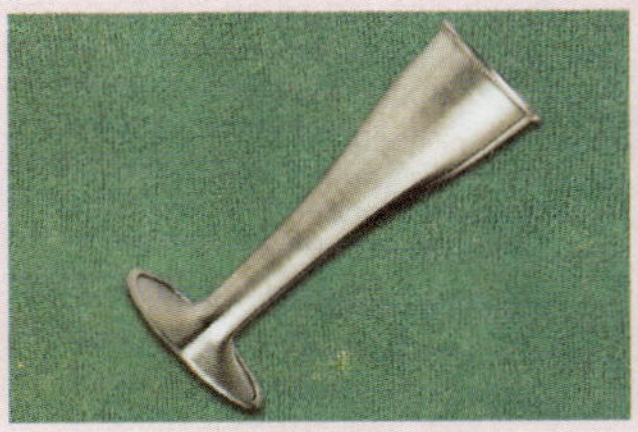

Skin stapler

- It is used to close both internal and skin wounds.

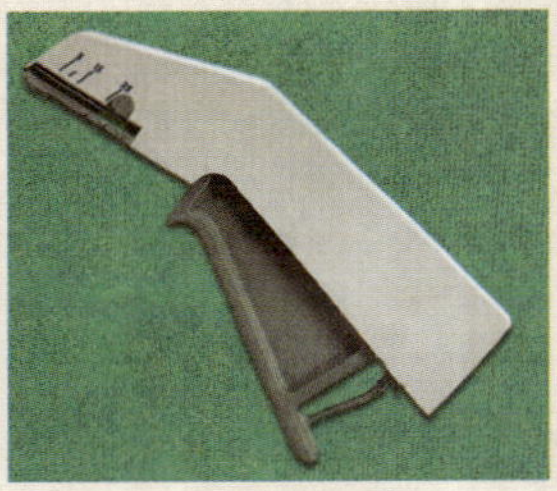

Video laryngoscope

- It helps in indirect visualization during intubation.

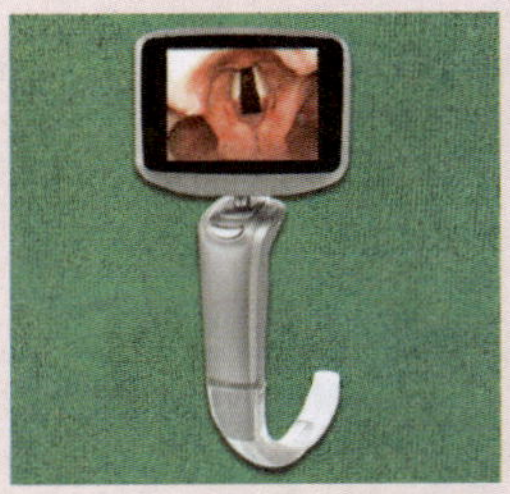

CPR machine

- It is used as an adjunct to CPR during advanced cardiac life support by professional health care providers.

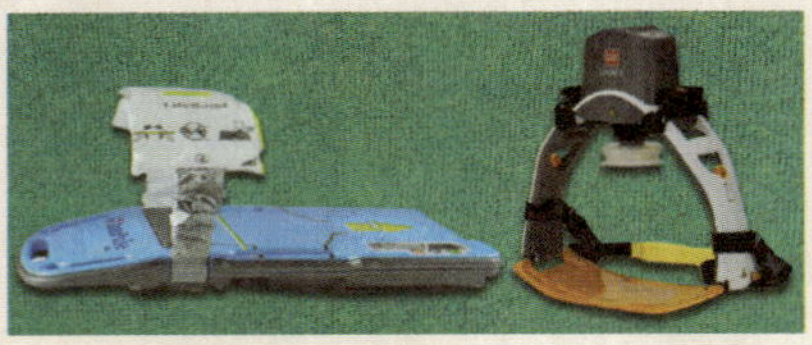

Skin stapler remover

- It is used for removal of skin staples.

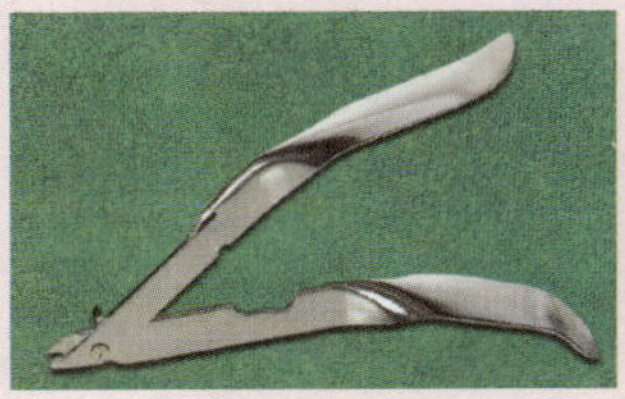

Cuff manometer

- Cuff manometer is used to check pressure in ET tube or LMA.
- Cuff pressure should be maintained at 20–30 H_2O.

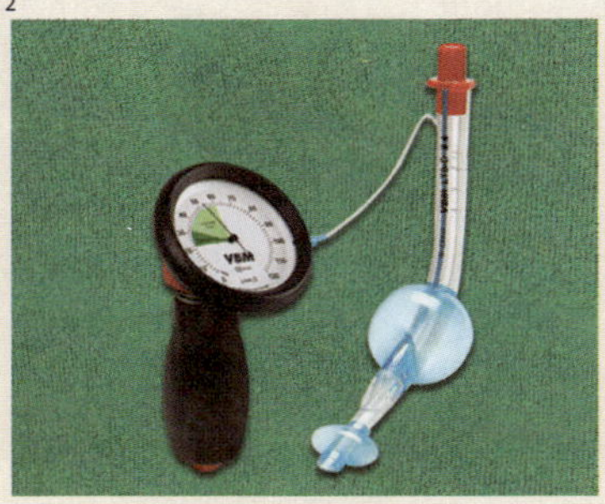

6

"A surgeon should be young a physician old."

—French Proverb

OBSTETRICS AND GYNECOLOGICAL INSTRUMENTS

Name of the instruments

Uterine sound

- It is used to measure the length and depth of the uterine cavity.

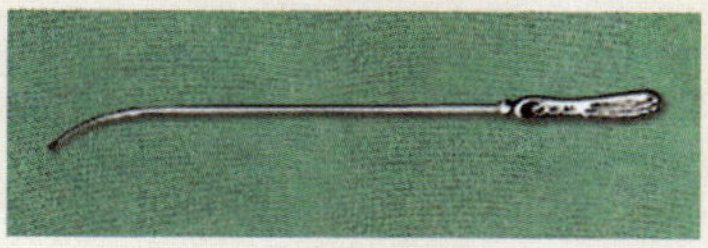

Sims' anterior vaginal wall retractor

- It helps to allow easy visualization of cervix and vagina.

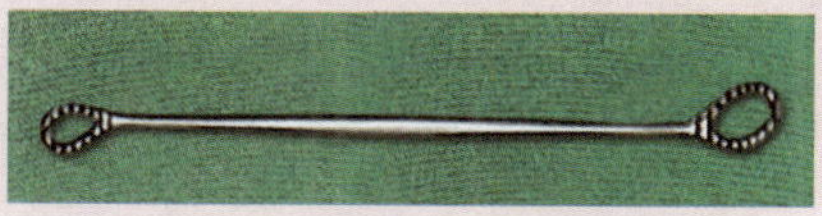

Ovum forceps

- It is used to remove placental fragments and product of conception inside the uterus.
- Also used as hemostatic clamp.

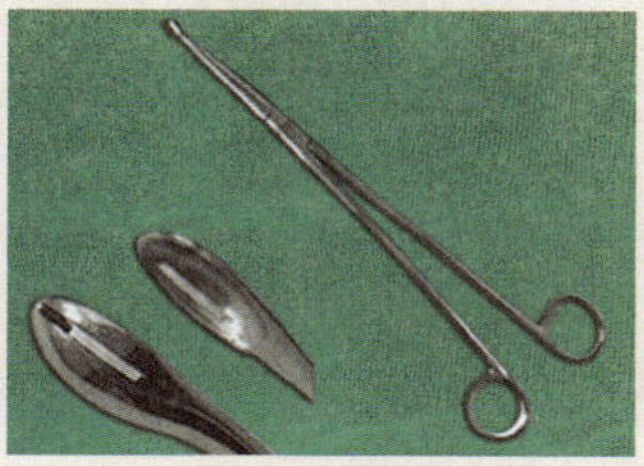

Ayre's spatula

- This instrument is used to collect PAP smear. The broad end is for vaginal sample collection and narrow end is for cervical sample collection.

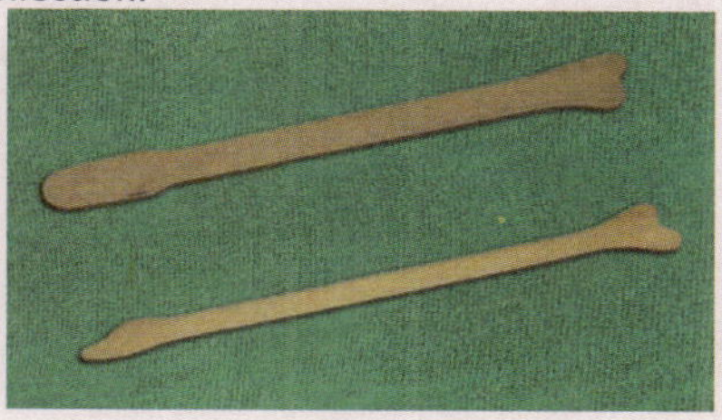

Uterine curette

- It is used to scrap endometrial cavity or uterine cavity to obtain samples.

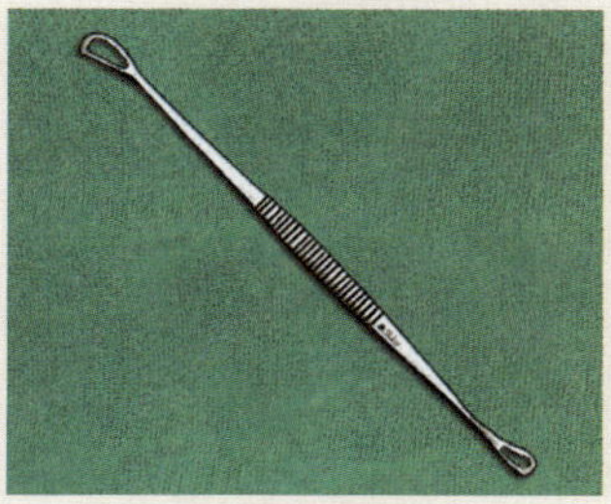

Episiotomy scissors

- It is used to provide episiotomy during second stage of labor.
- It is used to perform episiotomies during delivery and labor.

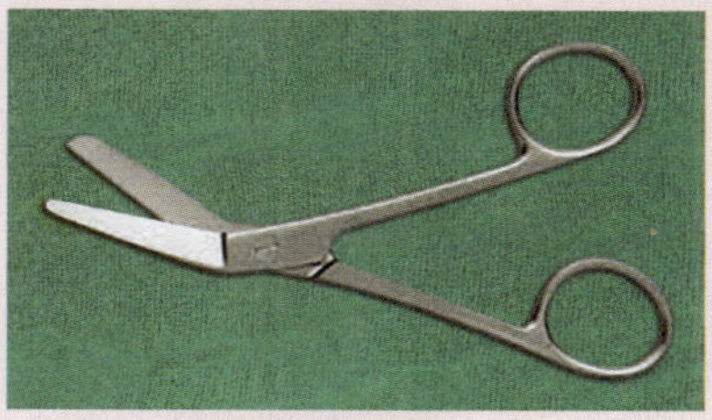

Sims' vaginal speculum

- It is a double-bladed speculum used during gynecological examination to examine vagina and cervix.

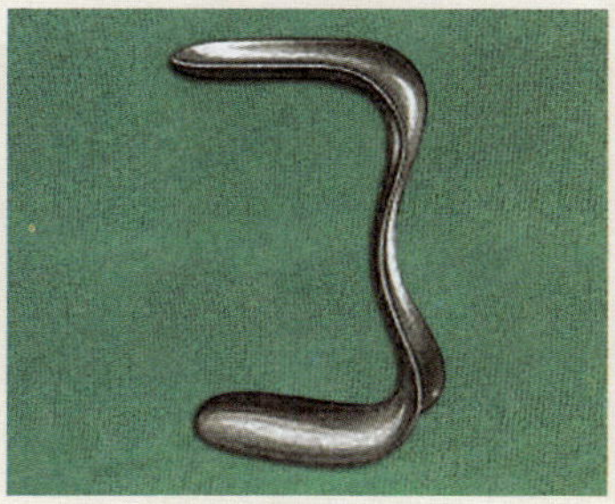

Cusco's speculum

- It is a self-retaining double-bladed vaginal speculum used to examine vagina and cervix.

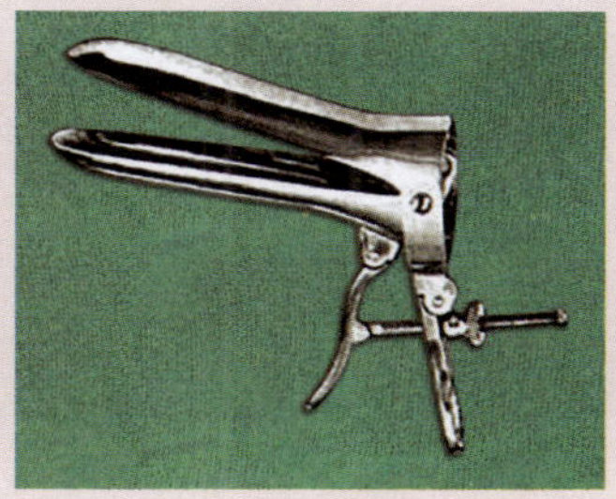

Contd...

Name of the instruments

IUCD removing hook
- It is used to remove the intrauterine contraceptive device.

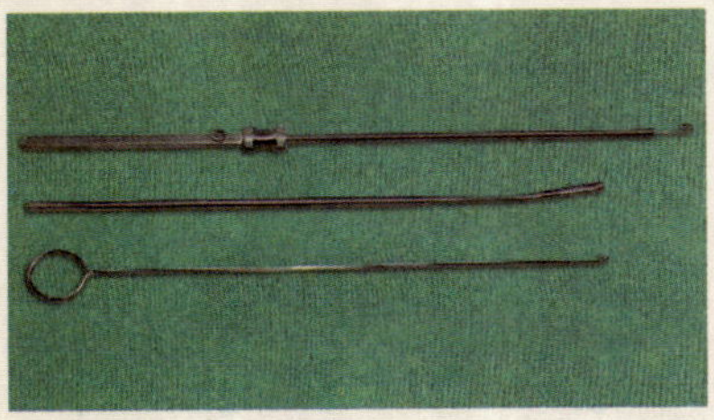

Umbilical scissors/cord cutting scissors
- It is used to cut the umbilical cord following delivery of the baby.

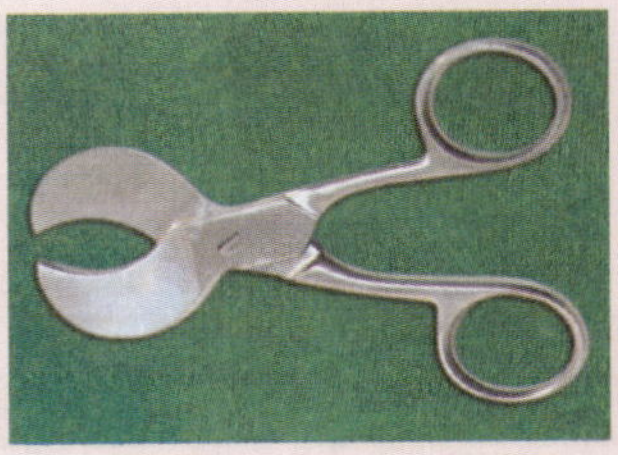

Metal ventose cup
- These are the cups used during assisted vacuum deliveries.

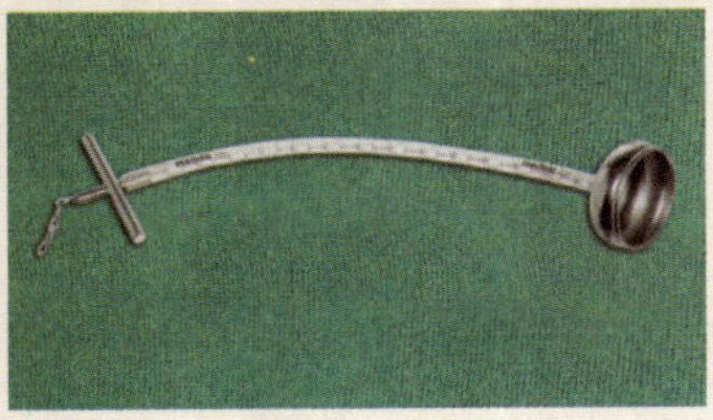

Silastic ventose cup

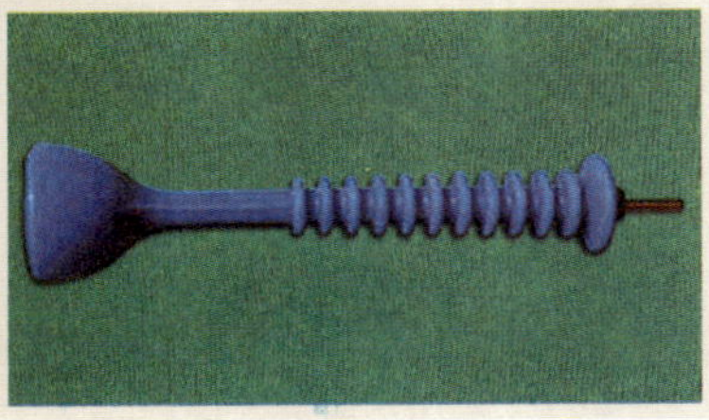

Hegar dilator
- These are the dilators of varying sizes used to increase size from few millimetres.
- These dilators are used to treat vaginismus and to increase cervical dilation.
- These dilators are also used to increase the size of stoma following colostomy.

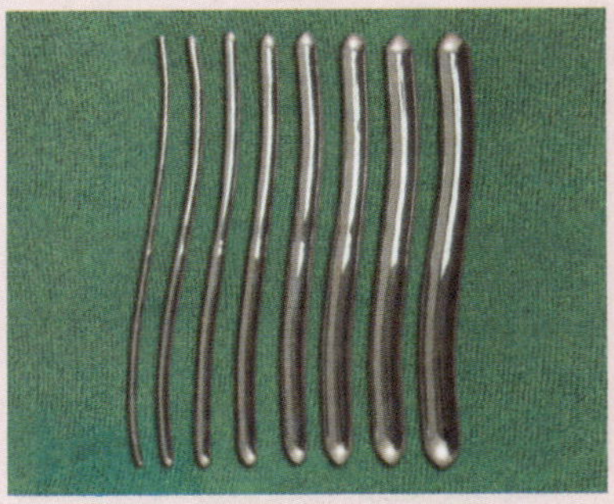

Copper T
- It is an intrauterine birth control device used for birth control and spacing.

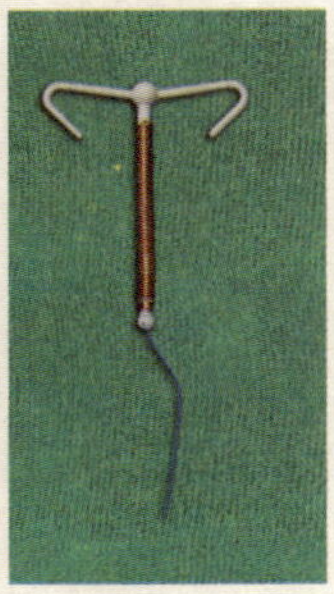

Uterine dressing forceps
- It is used for packing uterine cavity.
- It is used to remove tissue and intrauterine devices during gynecological procedures.

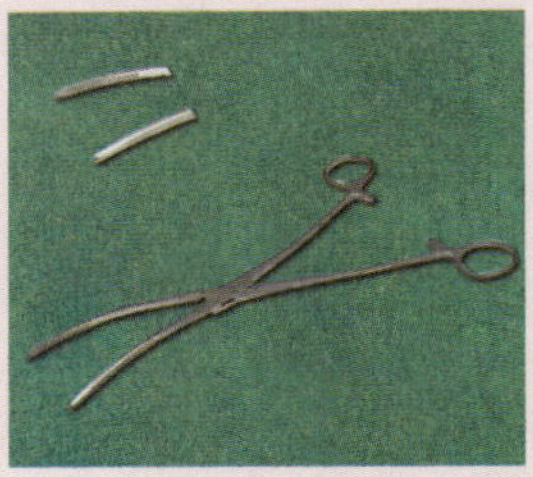

Umbilical cord clamp
- It is used to clamp the umbilical cord following delivery.

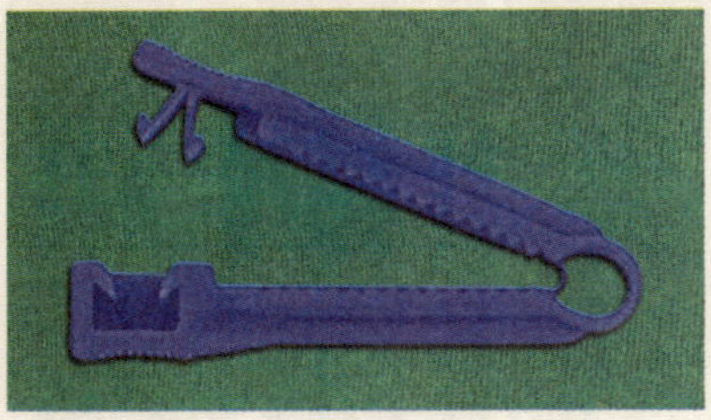

Fergussons tubular vaginal speculum
- It is a tubular speculum used to diagnose vaginal and cervical conditions.

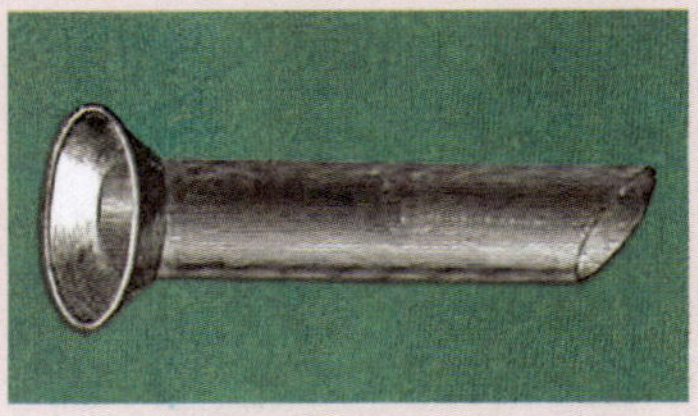

Contd...

Name of the instruments

Simpson perforator

- It is used to remove fetus or to perforate fetus skull in an arrested labor where mother's life is at risk.

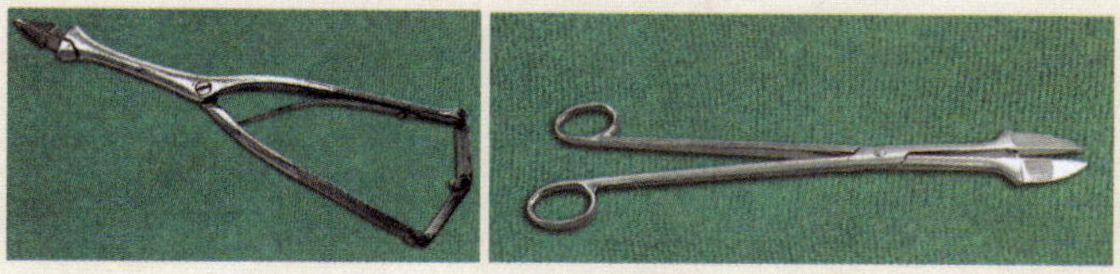

Doyen's myoma screw

- Used to remove fibroids from endometrium during myomectomy.

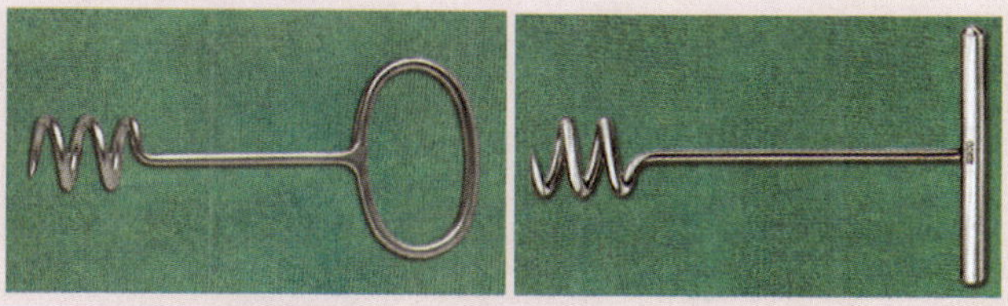

Craniotomy forceps

- Also known as cranioclast.
- They are heavy-toothed instruments used for breaking up the skull of fetus.
- They are used as last resource in difficult labor or obstruct labor when the fetus died in the womb.

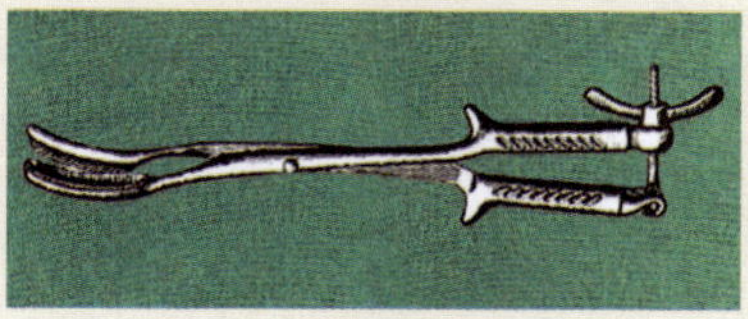

Wilet Scalp traction forceps

- Used during labor to ease the delivery of a new-born by grasping its scalp with the smooth flattened blades.

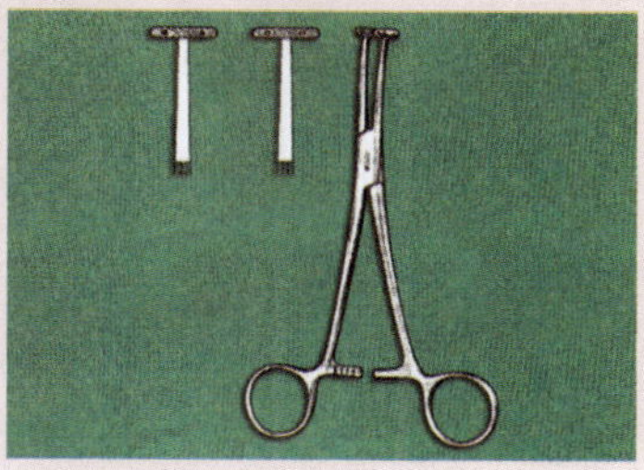

Amniotic perforator

- Instrument used to rupture amniotic membrane with minimal risk to mother and fetus.

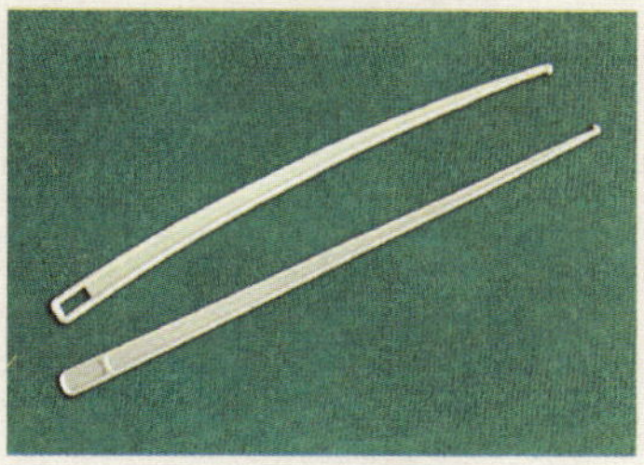

Cleidotomy scissors

- In case of dead fetus with shoulder dystocia for bulk reduction of one or both clavicles are divided using this instrument.

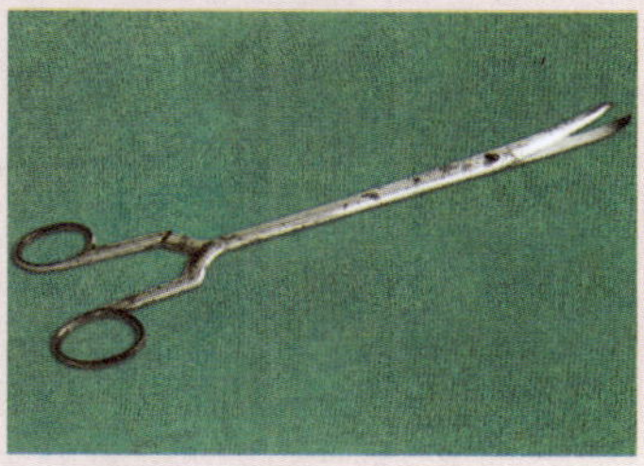

Breech hook

- In difficult breech delivery, head or trunk of the unborn fetus is extracted by inserting blunt hook around the neck or shoulder.

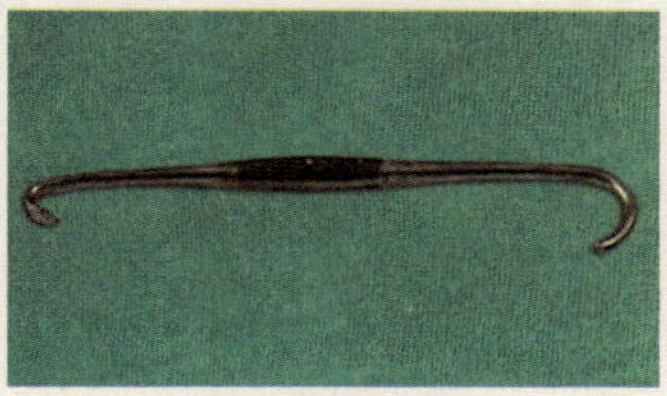

Richardson retractor

- Used during appendectomy surgery, cesarean sections and laparotomy to hold and retract back muscles.

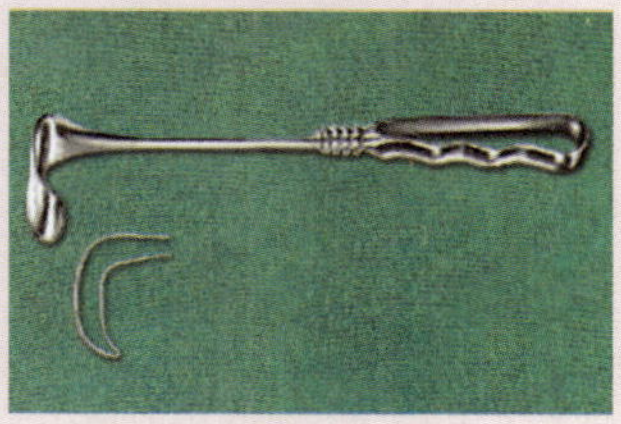

Wrigley outlet forceps

- These forceps are used to deliver head of the baby when it is at +3 station.
- These forceps are used at the end of second stage when there is urgency to deliver in terms of fetal distress or maternal issues.

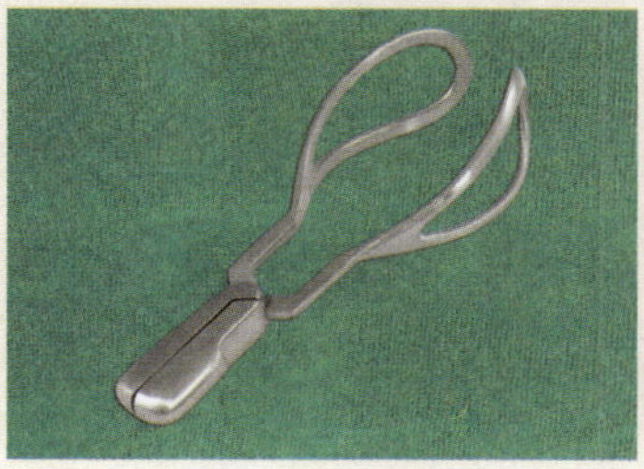

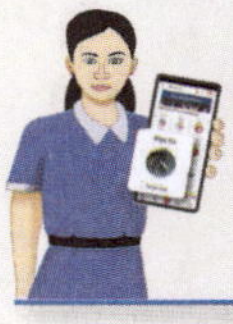

7

"An expert is one who knows more and more about less and less."
—Nicholas Murray Butler

TUBES AND CATHETERS

Name of tubes/ catheter	Images	Descriptions	Usages
Blood transfusion set	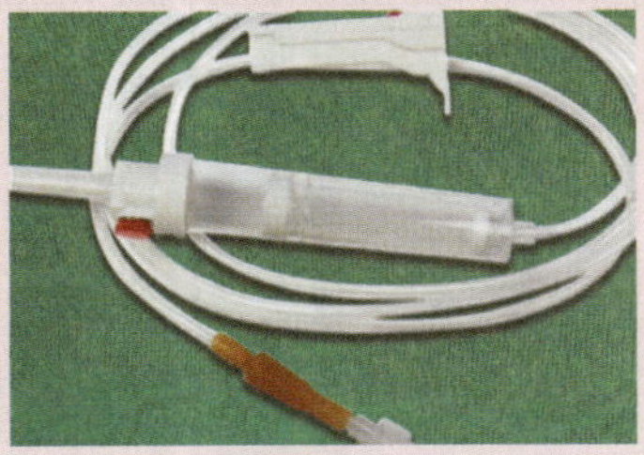	Set contains one filter inside the chamber as compared to IV set, in order to remove clots or small clumps of platelet during transfusion.	• Blood transfusion.
Endotracheal tube	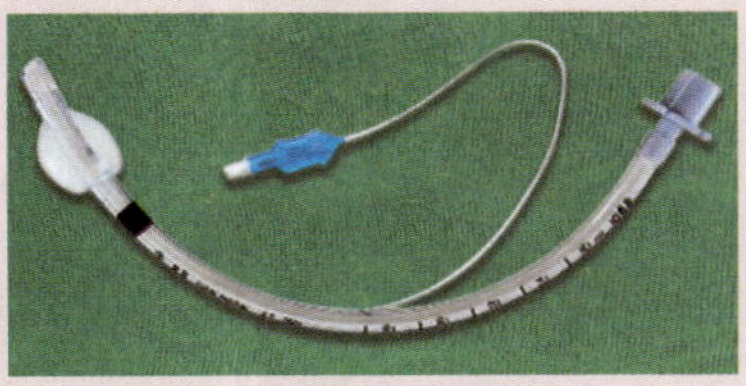	Tube is placed in the trachea through mouth in order to provide artificial ventilation.	• Establish and maintain airway patency. • To prevent aspiration.
Foley's catheter	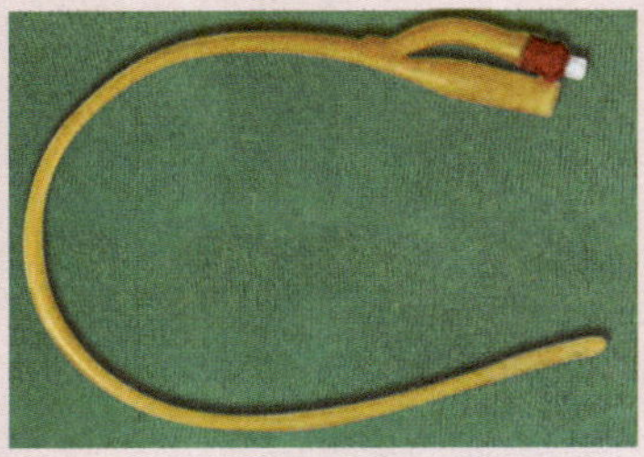	Tube passes through urethra into bladder in order to drain urine. It has got two lumens one for connecting the urinary bag and other for inflating the balloon.	• Urinary drainage.
IV set	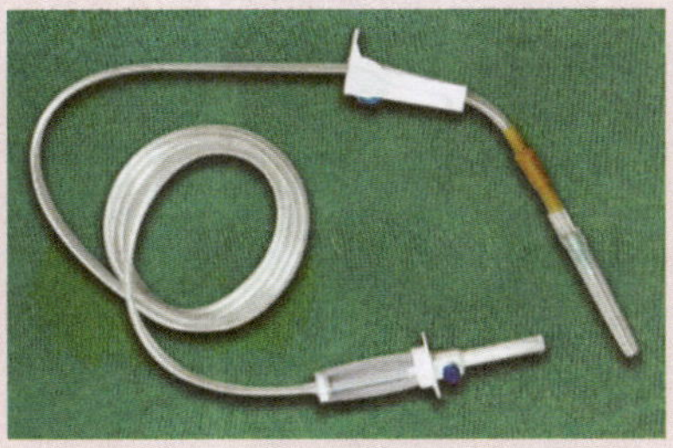	Its needle is inserted into the vein, or the tip is connected to the cannula inserted into the vein.	• IV administration of fluids. • IV administration of drugs.
IV cannula	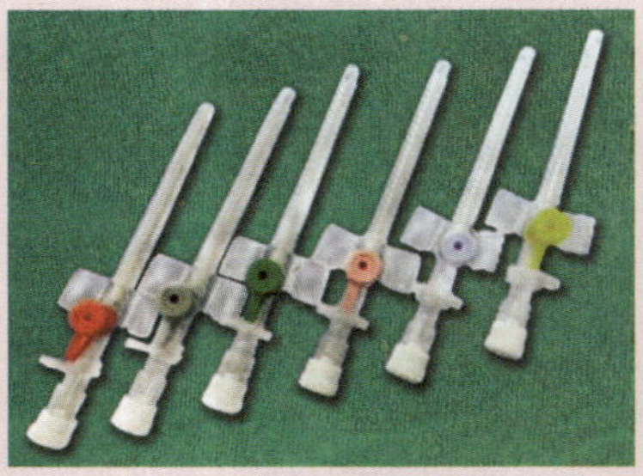	Cannula is a medical device placed inside a vein to provide venous access. It is available in various gauges (14–24 gauge, i.e., orange to yellow), lengths (19–44 mm), compositions, and designs. Orange is the biggest size cannula while the yellow is the smallest.	• To create venous access.

Contd...

Name of tubes/ catheter	Images	Descriptions	Usages
Laryngeal mask airway	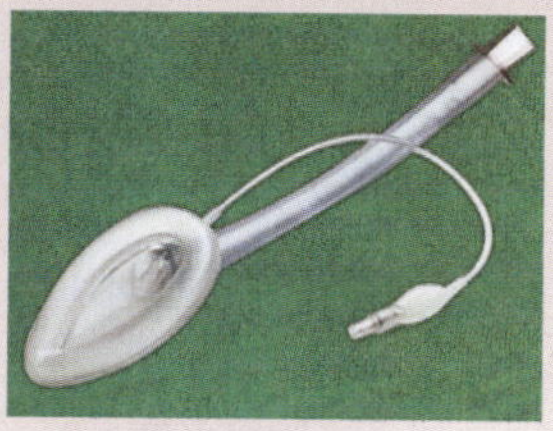	It is a device used to create airway during procedures and in emergency situations where ET intubation is difficult or failed.	• To create patent airway.
Nasogastric tube	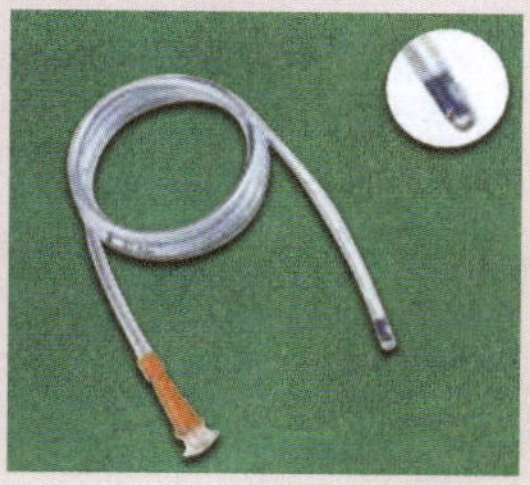	It is a tube inserted into the stomach via nostrils.	• To provide feed and medicine. • For gastric lavage.
Sengstaken-Blakemore tube	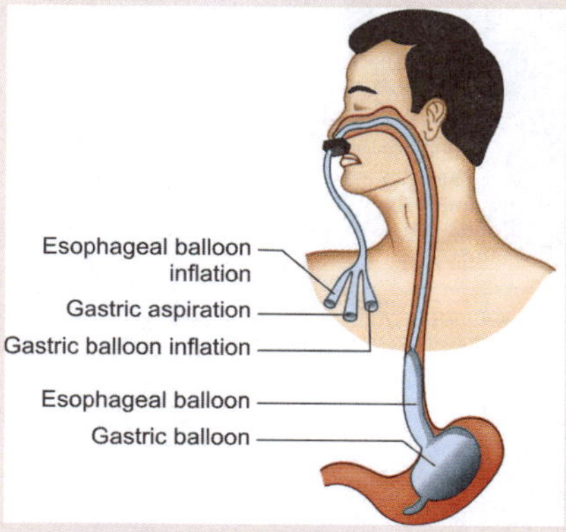	It is a three-way catheter with 2 balloons, one balloon will rest in the esophagus and other in the stomach. Inflated balloon helps to control variceal bleeding.	• Patient with massive esophageal vericeal bleeding.
Pig-tail drainage catheter	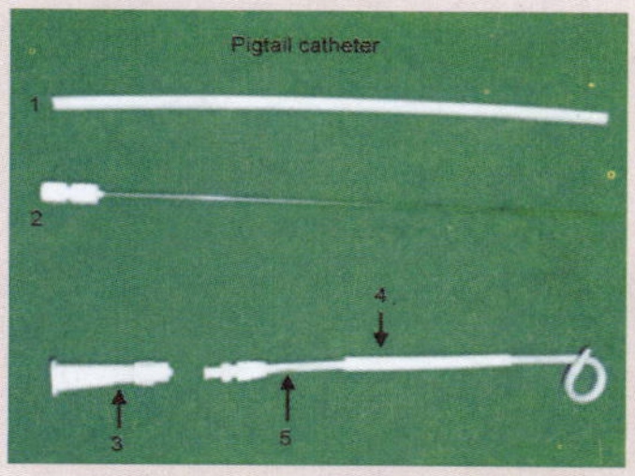	Pig tail catheters inserted into the body under strict aseptic technique with the purpose of removing unwanted body fluids from an organ, cavity or abscess. Its locking tip looks like pig tail and it has got several holes which facilitate drainage.	• To remove unwanted body fluids from an organ, cavity or abscess.
T-tube	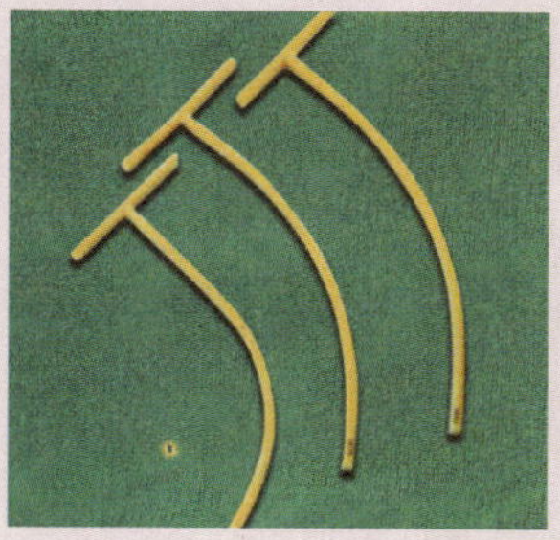	Placed in common bile duct during GB surgery or in radiology attached to a drainage bag but not sutured in. It is an external port that is placed into common bile duct and extends outside the body. The port is an easy access to allow drainage of bile and stone from the bile duct.	• To drain bile.
Tracheostomy tube	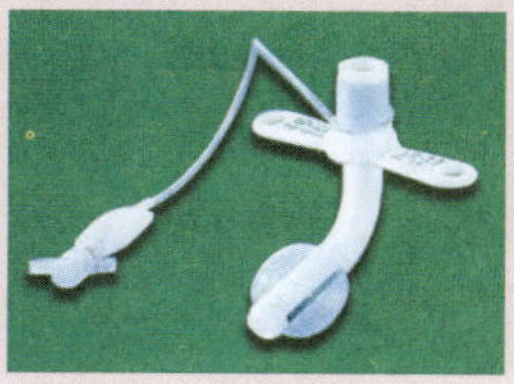	It is a tube inserted directly into the trachea via surgical incision on trachea.	• To create patent airway. • Prolonged intubation. • Upper airway obstruction. • Inability to intubate.

Contd...

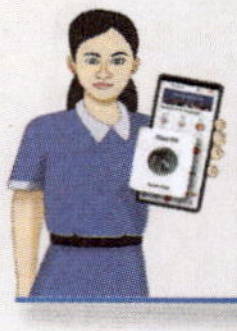

<table>
<tr><th>Name of the instruments</th><th>Picture of the instruments</th><th>Uses</th></tr>
<tr><td>Combi-tube (or) double lumen airway tube</td><td>
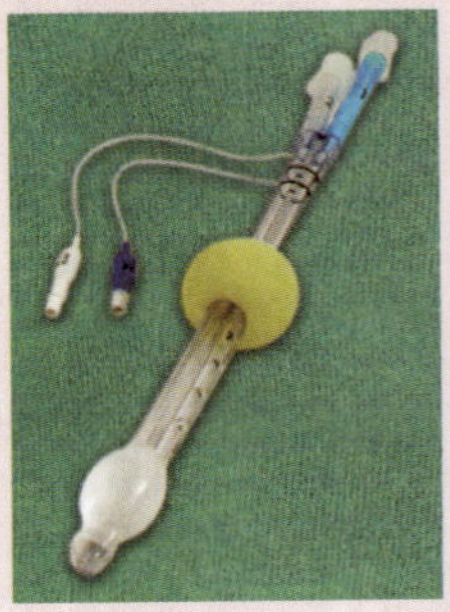
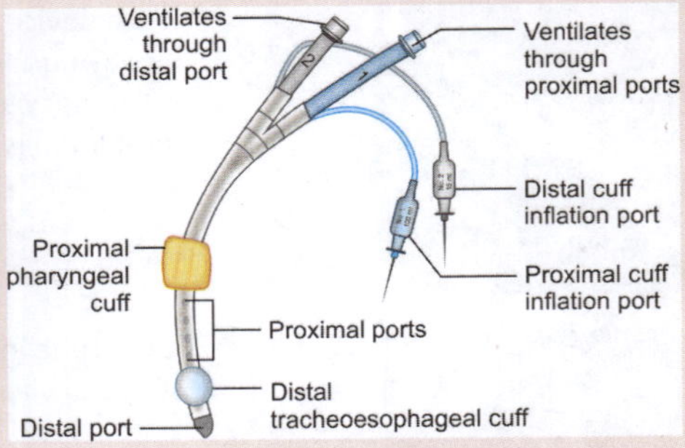

</td><td>
<ul><li>It is a type of endotracheal tube which is used in tracheal intubation during thoracic surgery and other medical conditions to achieve selective, one-sided ventilation of either the right or the left lung.</li></ul>
</td></tr>
<tr><td>Gastrostomy tube (PEG tube)</td><td>
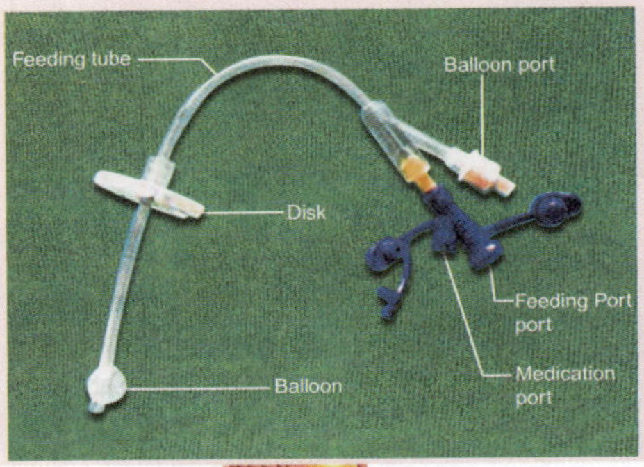

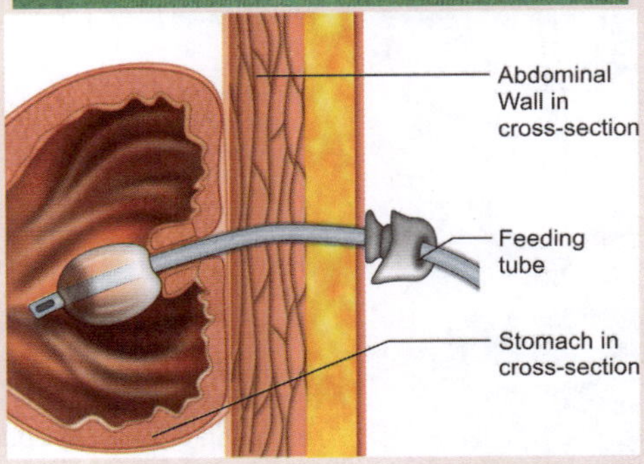

</td><td>
<ul><li>PEG—Percutaneous Endoscopic Gastrostomy.</li>
<li>It is a flexible feeding tube placed through the abdominal wall and into the stomach.</li>
<li>PEG allows nutrition, fluids and/or medications to be put directly into the stomach, bypassing the mouth and esophagus.</li></ul>
</td></tr>
<tr><td>Nasojejunal (NJ) feeding tube</td><td>
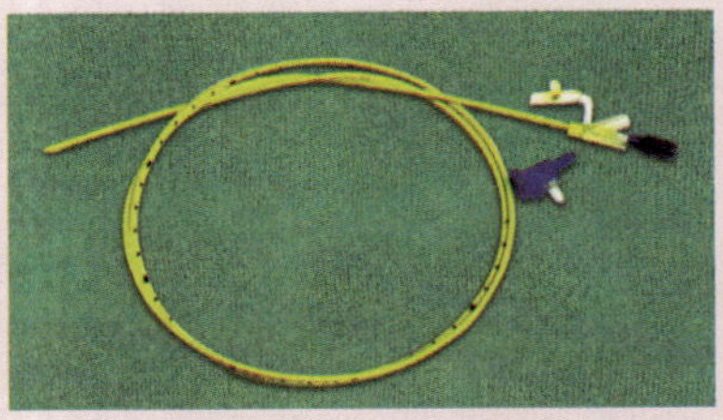
</td><td>
<ul><li>NJ feeding tubes are frequently used for long-term enteral nutrition.</li></ul>
</td></tr>
<tr><td>Butterfly scalp vein cannula (winged infusion set)</td><td>
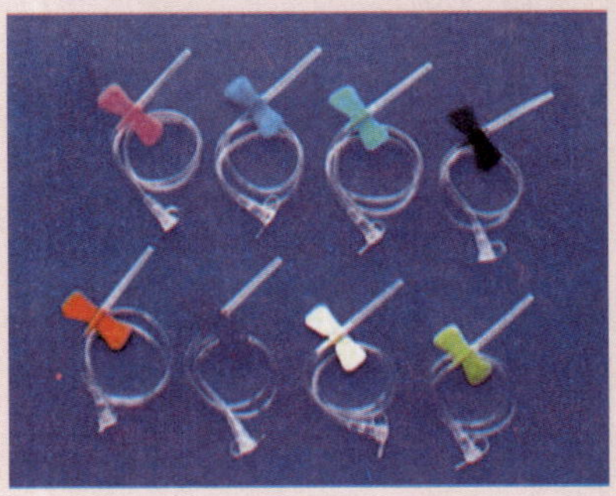
</td><td>
<ul><li>It is primarily used for venepuncture.</li>
<li>It consists of a:
<ul><li>Hypodermic needle.</li>
<li>Two bilateral flexible wings.</li>
<li>Flexible small bore transparent tubing (20–35 cm long).</li>
<li>A connector (female Leur).</li></ul></li></ul>
</td></tr>
</table>

Contd...

Name of the instruments	Picture of the instruments	Uses
Silicone catheter	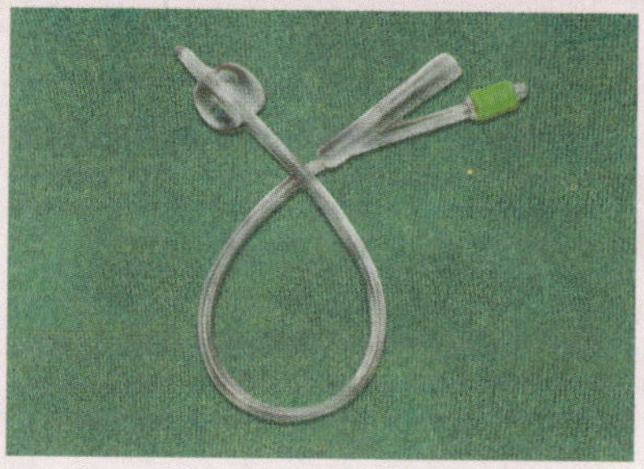	• **Compared to rubber catheters, silicone catheters** cause less injuries and reduce substantially irritation of the urinary mucosa. It is recommended for patients requiring longterm indwelling urinary catheters.
Three-way Foley catheter	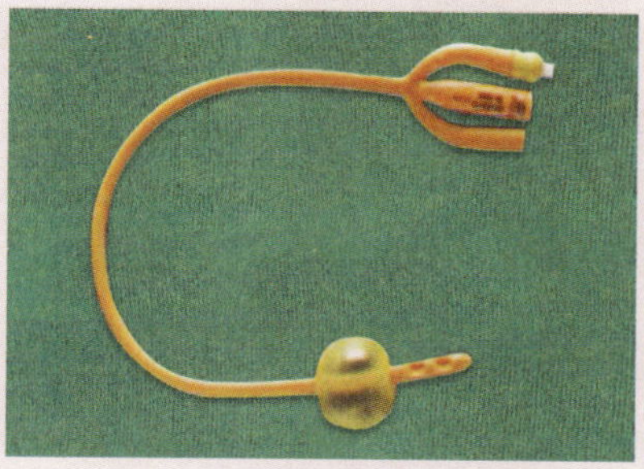	• Just like two-way Foley catheter, one connector of the three-way catheter is used to drain the urine while the other is used to inflate the balloon. • The third channel allows for continuous bladder irrigation that helps in removing debris and blood clots.
Suprapubic catheter (SPC)	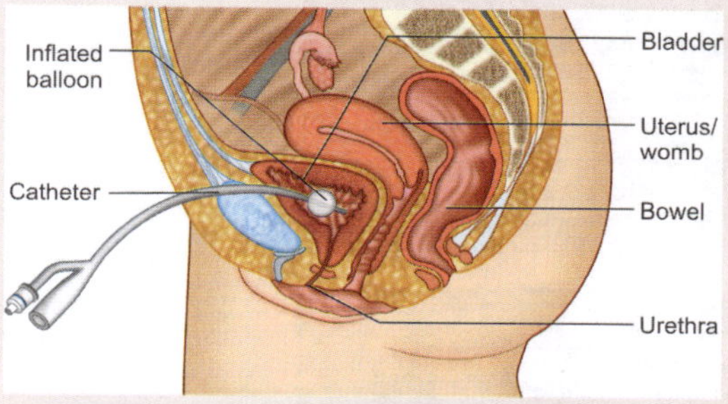 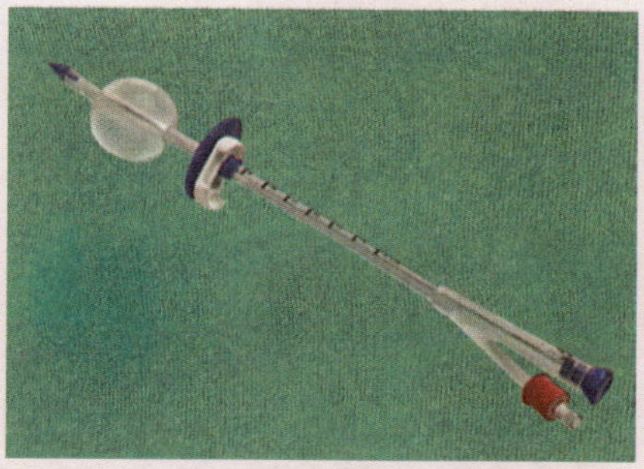	• It is inserted into the bladder through a incision in the abdomen, a few inches below the umbilicus.
Red rubber catheter	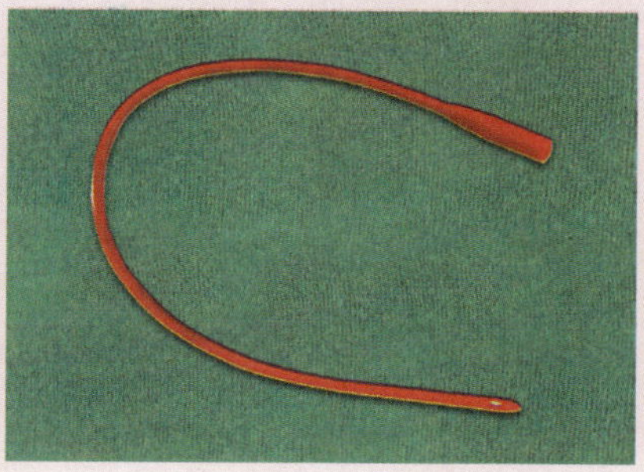	• **Red rubber catheters** are used like other straight catheters. The catheter is inserted through the urethra into the bladder. • **Red rubber catheters** are designed to be used once and then thrown away.

Contd...

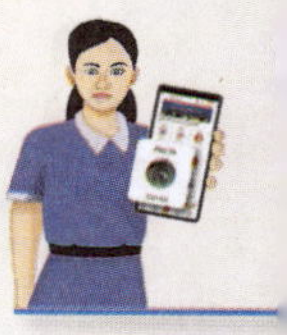

Name of the instruments	Picture of the instruments	Uses
Suction catheter	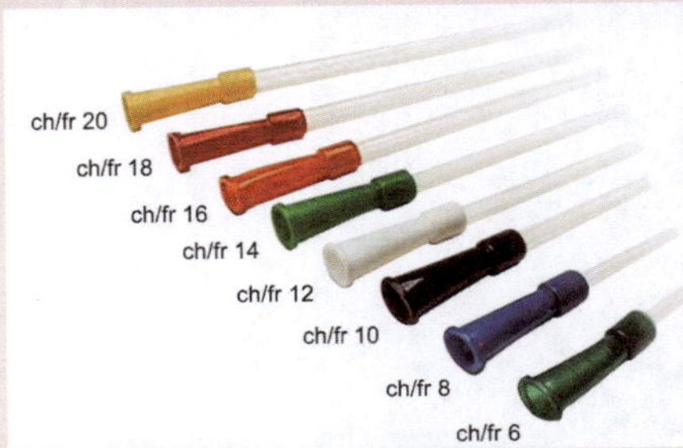 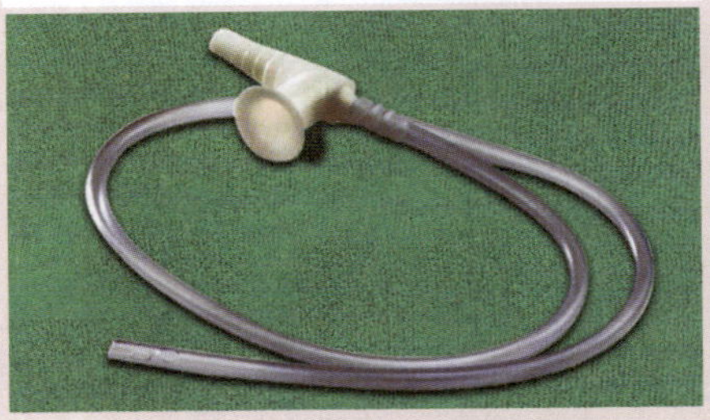	• Used to extract bodily secretions, such as mucus or saliva from the upper airway. • It has color coded connectors for fast size identification.
Metallic catheter	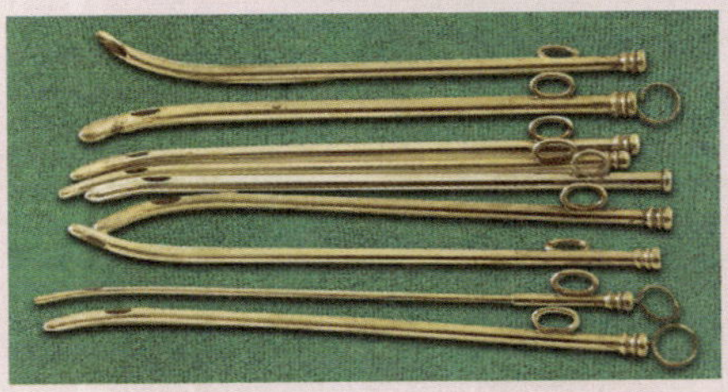	• Catheter made up of metal.
Colostomy bag (stoma bag or ostomy bag)	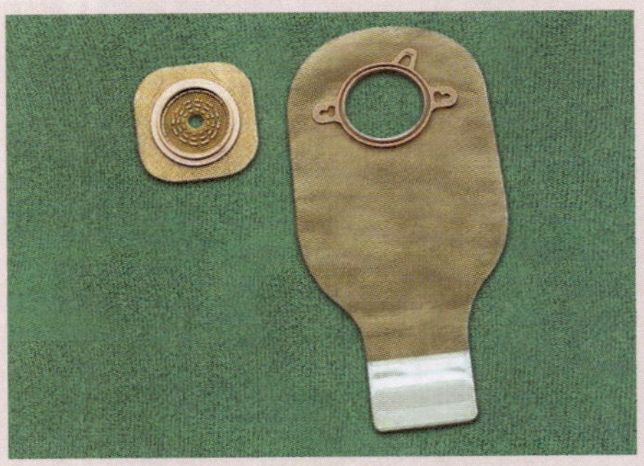	• Waterproof **pouch** used to collect waste from the bowel.
Bakri baloon	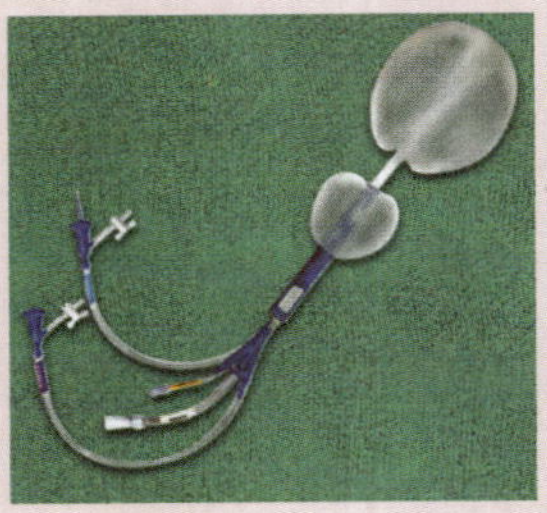 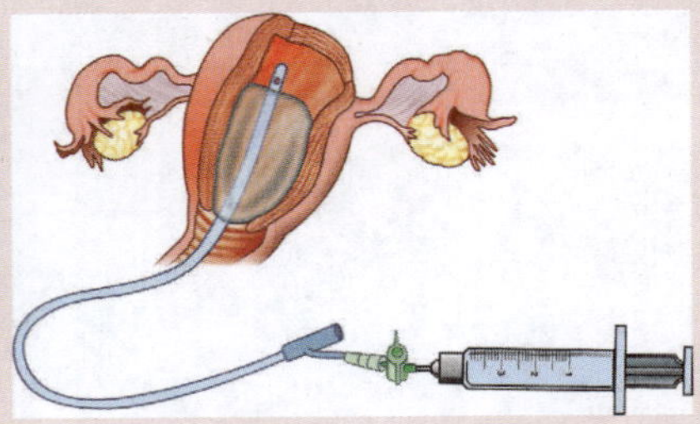	• The **Bakri Balloon** is a silicone, obstetrical balloon specifically designed to treat postpartum hemorrhage (PPH).

8

"Words are the most powerful drug used by the mankind."

—Rudyard Kipling

RECENT UPDATES ON COMMUNITY HEALTH NURSING

Update Topic	Remarks
PM Atmanirbhar Swasth Bharat Yojana	Launched on October 2021 Focus on strengthening healthcare infrastructure across the country. It will provide support to set up 17,788 rural Health and Wellness centers in 10 high focus states.
Ayushman Bharat Digital Mission (ABDM)	Launched on September 2021 Previously known as National Digital Health Mission (NDHM) ABDM aims to develop the backbone necessary to support the integrated digital health infrastructure of the country. It will bridge the existing gap amongst different stakeholders of Healthcare ecosystem through digital highways.
National Digital Health Mission (NDHM)	Launched on August 15, 2020. NDHM aims to make India Atmanirbhar or Self-reliant in providing universal health coverage to all the citizens in the country. It aligns with the goals and objectives of the National Health Policy (NHP) 2017
LaQshya Programme	It is a quality improvement initiative which aims to ensure Quality of Care during intrapartum and immediate post-partum period in Labour Room and Maternity OT. It targets all Government Medical College Hospitals, District Hospitals & equivalent health facilities, designated FRUs as well as high case load CHCs. 283 obstetric high dependency unit (HDU) /Intensive care unit (ICU) have been approved in high caseload tertiary care facilities across the country.
Ayushman Bharat Yojana (ABY)	Ayushman Bharat Yojana (ABY) launched in September 2018. It has two sub-missions: • **Establishment of Health and Wellness Centers (HWCs)** for primary care, providing Comprehensive Primary Health Care (CPHC) with free essential drugs and diagnostic services. • **Pradhan Mantri Jan Arogya Yojana (PM-JAY)** offers cashless treatment up to ₹5 lakh at secondary and tertiary levels for poor citizens, covering pre-existing diseases and post-hospitalization.
eSanjeevani OPD	In view of the COVID-19 pandemic, the Ministry of Health and Family Welfare (MoHFW) launched eSanjeevani OPD free teleconsultation system for people to get medical consultation from the safety of home.
National Nutrition Mission (NNM) or *Poshan Abhiyaan*	• *Launched on March 8, 2018 from Jhunjhunu, Rajasthan* • **Goal:** To improve nutritional outcomes for children, pregnant women, lactating mothers, and children from 0 to 6 years of age. • Cost of Food grains, its transportation and management born by Central Govt under PM POSHAN scheme. • Cooking cost and payment to cooks shared by Central and State govt on 60:40 basis.
First Dengue vaccine	Dengvaxia (CYD-TDV) is a live recombinant tetravalent dengue vaccine developed by Sanofi Pasteur. It was first approved in Mexico for marketing in December 2015. Till date (July, 2023), India has not approved Dengvaxia for marketing in the country. The ICMR has tied up with two biotech companies – Panacea and Serum Institute of India – to conduct a phase III trial of their dengue vaccines
Mission Parivar Vikas (MPV)	Launched on July 11, 2017 (World population Day) MPV is a strategic approach to substantially increase the access to contraceptives and family planning services in these 145 districts. There are 145 high fertility districts (TFR ≥3) spread over 7 states in India (UP, Bihar, Rajasthan, MP, Chhattisgarh, Jharkhand and Assam). **Goal:** To accelerate the efforts to meet the goals of achieving Total Fertility Rate of 2.1 by 2025 in the these districts.
CHHAYA (Centchroman)	Ormeloxifene (Centchroman) is a non-hormonal, non-steroidal oral contraceptive. Available in 30 mg tablet. Developed by the CSIR-Central Drug Research Institute's (CSIR-CDRI) It is the world's first non-steroidal birth control pill. A single tablet should be taken twice a week (Sunday and Wednesday) for first 3 months and then once a weekly (every Sunday). Other barrier methods (e.g., Condom) should be used for the first month.

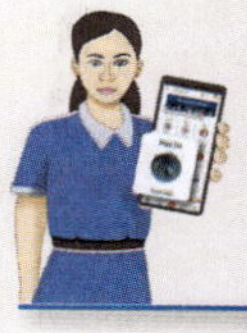

Contd...

Update Topic	Remarks
Pradhan Mantri Surakshit Matritva Abhiyan (PMSMA)	PMSMA was launched on June 9, 2016. The objective of the program is to boost the health care facilities for pregnant women, especially the poor women. Women will be provided free health check-up and treatment for free on 9th day of every month. These facilities were made available at all Government hospitals.
Mother's Absolute Affection (MAA)	MAA was launched in August 2016. Efforts on promotion, protection and support of breastfeeding practices through health services. Components of MAA include: Community level interventions: Capacity building Health facility strengthening Monitoring
Pneumonia vaccine	Single largest infectious cause of death among under-five children worldwide. *Streptococcus pneumoniae* is the most common cause of bacterial pneumonia in children. Hib is the second common cause of pneumonia. The recommended vaccine for pneumonia is **Pneumococcal Conjugate Vaccines (PCV-13).** **PCV** is frozen sensitive vaccine. Discard if frozen. New **PCV for pneumonia** was launched by Minister of Health and Family Welfare, J P Nadda at Mandi in Himachal Pradesh on May 2017.
Measles-Rubella Campaign	Intensification of 1st and 2nd dose of measles vaccination coverage was undertaken under **Mission Indradhanush** from the year 2015. Measles-Rubella vaccination campaign was launched at Bangalore, Karnataka in February 2017. Started in 5 states (Karnataka, Tamil Nadu, Puducherry, Goa and Lakshadweep).
Rotavirus vaccine	Rotavirus is the leading cause of acute severe diarrhea in under-five children worldwide. Rotavirus vaccine was launched under Universal Immunization Programme on **March 26, 2016.** Launched in four states (Odisha, Himachal Pradesh, Andhra Pradesh and Haryana) in the first phase.
HPV vaccines	Prevention of cervical cancer is best achieved through immunization of girls, prior to sexual debut. 3 types of HPV vaccine: Bivalent, Quadrivalent, Nonavalent HPV vaccine.
New TB drugs	BEDAQUILINE and DELAMANID. Drugs Controller General (India) approved Bedaquiline 10 mg tablet (14.1.2015) and Delamanid 50 mg tablet (2.8.2017) for the treatment of Tuberculosis under RNTCP program for treatment of TB patients with specific indications.

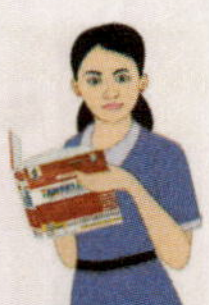

9

"I learnt a long time ago that minor surgery is when they do the operation on someone else, not you."

—Bill Walton

DEMOGRAPHY OF INDIA

Vital Statistics at a Glance (SRS 2020)

Brith Rate and Fertility Rate (per 1000 live birth)

Indicator	Total	Rural	Urban
Crude Birth Rate (CBR)	19.5	21.1	16.1
Total Fertility Rate	2.0	2.2	1.6
Gross reproduction rate	0.9	1.0	0.8

Mortality indicators

Indicator	Total	Rural	Urban
Crude Death Rate (per 1000 population)	**6.0**	**6.4**	**5.1**
Under-five Mortality Rate	32	36	21
Infant Mortality Rate	28	31	19
Neo-natal mortality rate	20	23	12
Early neo-natal mortality rate	15	17	9
Peri-natal Mortality Rate	18	21	12
Still birth rate	3	4	3

States with Highest and Lowest Indicators of Vital Statistics

Indicator	State	Max./Min. Values	Values
Birth rate	Uttar Pradesh	Maximum	28.5
	Kerala	Minimum	11.4
Death rate	Chhattisgarh	Maximum	8.5
	Jammu & Kashmir	Minimum	4.4
Infant mortality rate	Madhya Pradesh	Maximum	48
	Kerala	Minimum	6

Source: SRS Statistical Report (2020), Govt of India.

Demography in India

Variables	Value
Total Fertility Rate (India)	2.0
Highest Total Fertility Rate State	Bihar- 3.0
Lowest Total Fertility Rate State	Delhi- 1.4
Life Expectancy at birth (2016-20)	70.0 yrs
Life expectancy in male	68.6 yrs
Life expectancy in females	71.4 yrs
Lowest life expectancy STATE	Chhattisgarh – 65.1 yrs
Highest life expectancy STATE	Delhi – 75.8 yrs
Sex Ratio	907 female per 1000 male
Highest sex ratio state	Kerala – 974 female per 1000 male
Lowest sex ratio state	Uttarakhand – 844 female per 1000 male
Number of districts	766
Percentage of URBAN population	68.8% (census 2011)
Percentage of RURAL Population	31.2% (census 2011)
Population density (census 2011)	382 per sq. km
Highest population density state	Delhi (11320 per sq. km)
Lowest population density state	Arunachal Pradesh (17 per sq. km)
Elderly (60 yrs+) % (census 2011)	8.6%
Literacy rate (2021)	74.04%
Highest literacy rate state	Kerala (94%)
Lowest literacy rate state	Jammu and Kashmir (68.7%)

Most common causes of:

Maternal Mortality : Hemorrhage (38%)
Maternal Mortality : Hemorrhage (38%)
Neonatal mortality : Prematurity/preterm birth
Infant mortality : Prematurity/low birth weight (35.9%)
Death (all ages) : Most common: Cardiovascular disease (23.5%)
Second most common: Stroke

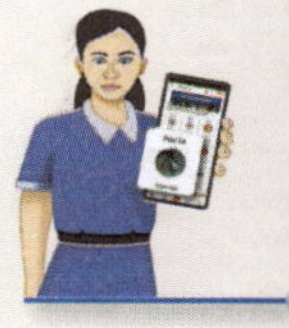

10

"A sad soul can kill you quicker than a germ."
—John Steinbeck

REVIEW OF HEALTH PROGRAMS IN INDIA, LAUNCH YEAR AND OBJECTIVES

Name of the programs	Year	Main objectives
National Anti-Malaria Program converted to National Malaria Eradication Program	1953 1958	To eradicate malaria once and for all from the country
Urban Malaria Scheme	1971	To reduce or interrupt malaria transmission in town and cities
National Filaria Control Program	1955	Filarial control strategy includes vector control through anti-larval operations, source reduction, detection and treatment of microfilaria carrier
Kala-azar Control Program	1990–1991	To bring down the incidence rate of kala-azar
National Leprosy Control Program	1955	To achieve control of leprosy through early detection of cases and dapsone monotherapy
National Leprosy Eradication Program	1983	National Leprosy Eradication Program was launched as a continuation of the National Leprosy Control Program of 1955
National Tuberculosis Control Program Revised National Tuberculosis Control Program (RNTCP)	1962 1992	To reduce the TB in the community to that level when it ceases to be a public health problem
National AIDS control Program	1987	To prevent further transmission of HIV, to decrease morbidity and mortality
National Program for Control of Blindness	1976	To reduce the prevalence of blindness from 1.4% to 0.3%
Iodine Deficiency Disorders Program	1962	To reduce the incidence of goiter through fortification of common salt
Pulse Polio Immunization Program	1995	To eradicate polio by providing additional polio drops
National Rural Health Mission	5th April 2005	To improve rural health care delivery system
National Guinea Worm Eradication Program	1984	To reduce the disease significantly in the affected area
National Cancer Control Program	1975–76	To prevention, early diagnosis and treatment of cancer
National Mental Health Program	1982	To ensure mental health care services to all, to encourage application of mental health knowledge in general health care
National Program for Control and Treatment of Occupational Diseases	1998–1999	To prevent, control and treatment of occupational health problems
Integrated Disease Surveillance Project	Nov 2004	To detect early warning signals of impending outbreaks and help initiate an effective response in a timely manner
National Water Supply and Sanitation Program	1954	To provide safe water supply and adequate drainage facilities

11

"We first make our habits and then our habits make us."
—John Dryden

VITAMINS: FUNCTIONS, SOURCES AND DEFICIENCY DISEASES

Vitamins	Functions	Sources	Deficiency diseases
Vitamin A (Retinol)	• Contributes to the production of retinal pigments • Required for the normal functioning of epithelial and glandular tissues • Supports growth especially skeletal growth • It is anti-infective	Liver, egg, butter, cheese, whole milk, fish, meat, yellow and green fruit, some roots such as carrot	• Night blindness • Conjunctival xerosis • Bitot's spot • Corneal xerosis • Keratomalacia • Xerophthalmia
Vitamin D (1,25 dihydroxy-cholecalciferol)	• Promotes intestinal absorption of calcium and phosphate • Stimulates normal mineralization • Permits normal growth	Liver, egg yolk, butter, cheese, exposure to sunlight	• Rickets • Osteomalacia
Vitamin E (Tocopherol)	Antioxidant property	Vegetable oil, cotton seed, sunflower seed, egg yolk, butter	
Vitamin K	Stimulates or helps in the production of certain anticoagulant factors	Green leafy vegetables, Cow's milk	Prolonged blood clotting time
Vitamin B1 (Thiamine)	This vitamin is essential for the oxidative pathway of glucose	Whole grain cereals, wheat, yeast, pulses, oilseed and nuts Meat, fish egg, vegetables and fruits contain only small amount	• Beriberi • Wernicke's encephalopathy
Vitamin B2 (Riboflavin)	• Fundamental role in cellular oxidation • Maintains the integrity of mucocutaneous structure.	Milk, egg, liver, green leafy vegetables	Angular stomatitis
Vitamin B3 (Niacin)	• Essential for metabolism of carbohydrate • Essential for the normal functioning of skin, intestinal and nervous tissue	Meat, poultry, fish, legumes, groundnut	Pellagra characterized by 4Ds • Diarrhea • Dermatitis • Dementia • Death
Vitamin B6 (Pyridoxine)	Important for the metabolism of carbohydrate and amino acid	Milk, liver, meat, egg yolk, fish, whole grain cereals, legumes and vegetables	Peripheral neuritis
Vitamin B5 (Pantothenic acid)	Specific role in the biosynthesis of corticosteroids		
Vitamin B12 (cyanocobala-min)	It cooperates with folate in the biosynthesis of DNA	Meat, fish, egg, milk, cheese	Megaloblastic anemia (Pernicious anemia)
Vitamin C (Ascorbic acid)	• Antioxidant and plays an important role in tissue oxidation • Synthesis of collagen	Fresh fruits and green leafy vegetable, fresh meat, fish,	Scurvy

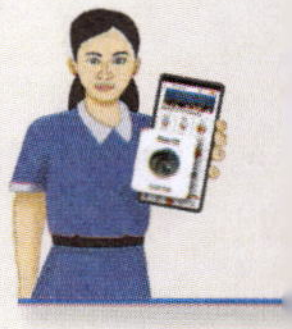

12

"Do small things with great love."
—Mother Teresa

HEALTH PLANNING IN INDIA

Year	Committee	Main features
1946	Bhore Committee	• Sir Joseph Bhore was the chairman • Also known as **Health Survey and Development Committee** • Comprehensive proposal for the development of National Program of Health Services. • Integration of preventive and curative services at all levels • Recommended Development of **Primary Health Centers (PHC)** in 2 stages.
1948	Chopra Committee	• Integrating the several systems of medicine with allopathic system and evolution of an integrated system of medical education.
1957	Balwant Rai Mehta Committee	• Recommended setting up of 3 Tier system of Panchayati Raj at village, block and district level
1962	Mudaliar Committee	• Commonly known as **health survey and planning committee** • Advice for the strengthening of existing primary health care centers before new centers were established • Strengthening of the district hospital with specialist services to serve as central base of regional services • Integration of medical and health services as recommended by Bhore committee • Constitution of All India Health Service on the pattern of Indian Administrative Services
1963	Chadha Committee	• Monthly home visit should be implemented through basic health workers • The workers were envisaged as **multipurpose workers** to look after additional duties of collection of vital statistics and family planning, in addition to malaria vigilance • The family planning health assistants were to supervise 3–4 of these basic health workers
1965	Mukherjee Committee	• Separate staff for the family planning program • The committee also recommended to delink malaria activities from family planning
1966	Jain Committee	• 1 bed per 1000 population, 50 beds hospital at taluka level • Health insurance for large population coverage
1966	Mukherjee Committee	• The committee worked out the details of the basic health services which should be provided at the block level, and some consequential strengthening required at higher levels of administration
1967	Jungalwalla Committee	• Integration of health services from top to bottom, similar seniority and unified cader to be implemented • Elimination of private practice by government doctors
1972–73	Kartar Singh Committee	• The Government of India constituted a committee in 1972 known as **the Committee of Multipurpose Workers** under health and family planning under the chairmanship of Kartar Singh
1974–75	Shrivastav Committee	• The MoHFW, GOI (1974) setup "Group on Medical Education as Support Manpower" popularly known as the Shrivastav Committee. This committe recommended **"Three tier system of health care delivery in rural area."**
1977	Rural Heath Scheme	• Following the recommendation of Shrivastav Committee Government launched Rural Health Scheme in 1977 • The main aim of program was to train community health workers
1981	Health for All by 2008	• To identify the goal for health for all by 2000 AD and to outline with that perspective the specific Programs for the sixth five-year plan
1983	Krishnan committee	• Revamping of Primary urban health services– Health posts in urban slums. • Basic health and Family welfare services to be made available within 1–3 km of dwelling, with appropriate link to secondary and tertiary care centers
1986	Bajaj Committee, 'Expert committee for Health Manpower Planning, Production and Management'.	• Formulation of a national medical and health education policy • Formulation of a national health manpower policy • Establishment of health science universities. • Vocationalization of education at 10 + 2 level with regards to health. • Carry out realistic health manpower survey.

13

"The physician heals, nature makes well."

—Aristotle

FRYE'S ABCDE CASCADE FOR PRIORITIZING CARE

Frye's ABCDE cascade provides a framework for prioritizing care by identifying the most important treatment concerns.

A **Airway: The airway is the first priority in any emergency situation.** This includes everything that affects a patent airway, e.g, a foreign object, fluid from an upper respiratory infection, and edema from trauma or an allergic reaction.

B **Breathing:** Once the airway is open, you should assess the patient's breathing. This includes everything that affects the breathing pattern, including hyperventilation or hypoventilation and abnormal breathing patterns, such as Kussmaul's breathing.

C **Circulation:** The next priority is to assess the patient's circulation. This includes everything that affects the circulation, including fluid and electrolyte disturbances and disease processes that affect cardiac output.

D **Disease processes:** Once the airway, breathing, and circulation have been assessed, you should then assess the patient for any other medical conditions that may be affecting them. Give priority to the disease process that poses the greatest immediate risk. For example, if a patient has terminal cancer and hypoglycemia, hypoglycemia is a more immediate concern.

E **Everything else:** This category includes such issues as writing an incident report and completing the patient chart. When evaluating needs, this category is never the highest priority.

14

"What mental health needs is more sunlight, more candor and more unashamed conversation."

—Glenn Close

TRIAGE CATEGORIES

Immediate/Emergent Category

These casualties require immediate life-saving treatment.

Urgent Category

These casualties require significant intervention as soon as possible.

Delayed Category

These patients will require medical intervention, but not with any urgency.

Triage Category	Priority	Color	Conditions
Immediate/Emergent	1	Red	Chest wounds, shock, open fractures, 2–3 burns
Delayed/Urgent	2	Yellow	Stable abdominal wound, eye and CNS injuries
Minimal	3	Green	Minor burns, minor fractures, minor bleeding
Expectant	4	Black	Unresponsive, high spinal cord injury

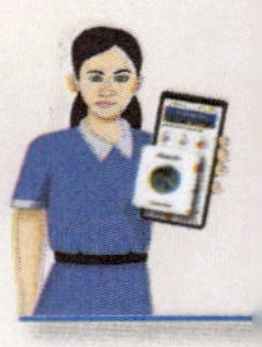

15

"Fasting is a natural method of healing."
—Paramahansa Yogananda

ARTERIAL BLOOD GAS

Normal ABG Value

pH	7.35–7.45
$PaCO_2$ (mm Hg)	35–45
HCO_3^- (mEq/L)	22–26
PaO_2 (mm Hg)	80–100

INTERPRETING ABG VALUES

Step 1: Determine whether the pH value is normal or shows acidosis or alkalosis.

- pH below 7.35 - Acidosis
- pH above 7.45 - Alkalosis

Step 2: (to find the cause is Respiratory or Metabolic)

Use ROME mnemonic to determine whether the acid base imbalance is due to Respiratory or Metabolic Cause:

- **ROME:** Respiratory Opposite, Metabolic Equal.
- **Respiratory opposite:** If the pH and PCO_2 values move on opposite direction from its normal value – It is due to respiratory cause. For example, If pH is 7.2 (below normal) and PCO_2 is 50 (above normal) it is Respiratory Acidosis. If pH is 7.5 (above normal) and PCO_2 is 30 (below normal), it is Respiratory alkalosis.
- **Metabolic equal:** If the pH and HCO_3 values move on same direction from its normal value- It is due to metabolic cause. For example, If pH is 7.2 (below normal) and HCO_3 is 20 (below normal), it is metabolic acidosis. If pH is 7.5 (above normal) and HCO_3 is 28 (above normal), it is metabolic alkalosis.

Step 3: To determine whether it is compensated, partially compensated or Uncompensated.

Once the respiratory and metabolic components of acid-base balance has been identified, then use the following method to determine whether it is compensated, uncompensated or partially compensated.

- **Fully compensated:** The pH is within normal limits but both the PCO_2 and HCO_3 are deranged.
- **Partially compensated:** pH is deranged; both PCO_2 and HCO_3 are also deranged.
- **Uncompensated:** pH is deranged; Either PCO_2 or HCO_3 only deranged.

Examples

Case 1: Measurement of arterial blood gas shows pH 7.2, $PaCO_2$ 70 mm Hg, HCO_3^- 26 mEq/L, and PaO_2 59 mm Hg. How would you interpret this?

Interpretation: This patient has **respiratory acidosis (uncompensated).**

Rationale: pH 7.2 indicates acidosis. The increased CO_2 (and reduced O_2) indicates respiratory acidosis. If the CO_2 is normal and the HCO_3^- is less than normal in this case (below 21) it could be **Metabolic acidosis**.

Case 2: Measurement of arterial blood gas shows pH 7.2, PaO_2 100 mm Hg, $PaCO_2$ 25 mm Hg, and HCO_3^- 10 mEq/L. What is your assessment?

Interpretation: These results show that he/she has metabolic acidosis (Partially compensated) with respiratory compensation (low CO_2).

Rationale: Low pH (7.2) indicates acidity & Low HCO_3^- indicates metabolic acidosis. Note that the $PaCO_2$ 25 mm Hg is also below normal. This means the respiratory compensation (hyperventilation) has happened to increase the pH. Hence it is Metabolic acidosis (partially compensated) with respiratory compensation.

Case 3: Measurement of arterial blood gas shows pH 7.42, PaO_2 115 mm Hg, $PaCO_2$ 28 mm Hg, and HCO_3^- 18 mEq/L. What does this mean?

Interpretation: Respiratory alkalosis (Fully compensated)

Rationale: Normal pH (7.42) indicates fully compensated Respiratory alkalosis. Low CO_2 indicates that the condition is Respiratory alkalosis. Low HCO_3^- indicates that there is a metabolic compensation to counter the decrease in pH. This lead to normal pH (full compensated).

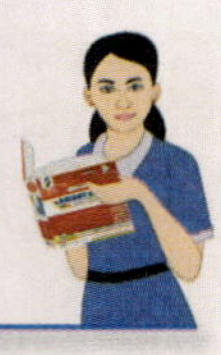

16

"Walking is man's best medicine."
—Hippocrates

SHOCKS: TYPES, MANAGEMENT AND SOLUTIONS

Types	Causes	Pathophysiology	Clinical feature	Treatment
Hypovolemic	• Hemorrhage • Dehydration	• Preload ↓ • Contractility normal or ↑ • Afterload (SVR) ↑	• HR ↑ • BP ↓ • Cardiac output ↓ • CRT Delayed • Extremities cool and pale • Weak thready pulse	• Prevent losses • Secure large bore IV access, Fluid resuscitation with crystalloids
		Distributive		
1. Septic	• Infections • Sepsis	• Preload ↓ • Contractility normal or ↓ afterload ↓	• HR ↑ • BP ↓ • Cardiac output ↓ • CRT Flash/delayed • Extremities warm and pink	• IV Antibiotics, Fluids • IV Noradrenaline →drug of choice
2. Anaphylactic	• Anaphylaxis	• Preload ↓ • Contractility variable • Afterload ↓	• HR ↑ • BP ↓ • Cardiac output ↓ • CRT Flash/delayed • Extremities warm	• IV Epinephrine, Fluids
3. Neurogenic	• Spinal cord injury • Traumatic brain injury (TBI)	• Preload ↓ • Contractility normal • Afterload (SVR) ↓ • Loss of sympathetic tone	• HR ↓ • BP ↓ • Cardiac output ↓ • CRT Flash/normal • Extremities warm	• High flow O2 • Fluid resuscitation • Vasopressors
Cardiogenic	• Myocarditis • Dysrhythmia	• Preload ↓ • Contractility ↓ • Afterload (SVR) ▪ ↑ (Rt ventricular) ▪ ↓ (Left ventricular)	• HR ↑ • BP ↓ • Cardiac output ↓ • CRT delayed	• Inotropes • Cautious use of fluids, ECMO • DOC: Noradrenaline
Obstructive	• Tamponade • Tension pneumothorax • Pulmonary embolus • Chest trauma	• Preload ↓ • Contractility normal • Afterload (SVR) ↑	• HR ↑ • BP ↓ • Cardiac output ↓ • CRT Delayed • Extremities cool	• Pericardiocentesis • Chest tube
Dissociative	• CO poisoning • Cyanide	• Variable	• HR ↑ • BP Normal or ↑ • Cardiac output ↑ • CRT normal • Extremities normal	• Antidotes • Hyperbaric oxygen therapy

Courtesy: VD Agrawal, PRIMES 2nd Edition, CBS Publishers.

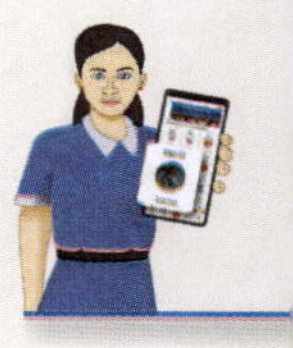

Types of Shock and its Management

Types of shock	Management
All Types of Shock	• Increase perfusion to vital organs • Increase peripheral perfusion • Decrease myocardial oxygen demand and workload • Relieve pulmonary congestion • Correct acid-base imbalances • Ensure adequate oxygenation
Cardiogenic Shock	• Administer an inotropic medication, such as dobutamine, dopamine, milrinone, or inamrinone
Hypovolemic Shock	• Increase intravascular volume with the appropriate solution, such as blood or a blood product, a colloid preparation, a plasma expander, or a crystalloid solution
Distributive Shock: Anaphylactic Shock	• Administer adrenalin and an antihistamine

Types of Solutions

Type of parenteral solution	Examples	Indications
Hypertonic Solution	• Dextrose 5% in normal saline solution • 3% NaCl • Dextrose 10% in water	• To treat severe hyponatremia • To treat hypoglycemia
Hypotonic Solution	• Half-normal saline solution	• To expand the intracellular compartment • To replace free water • To replace sodium and chloride
Isotonic Solution	• Normal saline solution	• To increase extracellular fluid volume • To treat hypovolemia • To replace sodium and chloride
	• Lactated Ringer's solution	• To treat hypovolemia and fluid lost from burns and GI tract • To provide electrolyte replacement • To maintain fluid volume;
	• Dextrose 5% in water (D5W)	• To provide free water to treat hypernatremia and hyperkalemia

Colloid Solution

- Albumin
- Fluid resuscitation
- Dextran
- Hydroxyethyl starch
- Gelofusine

17

"Constant attention by a good nurse may be just as important as a major operation by a surgeon."

—Dag Hammarskjold

ECG WAVEFORMS AND PATHOLOGICAL FINDINGS

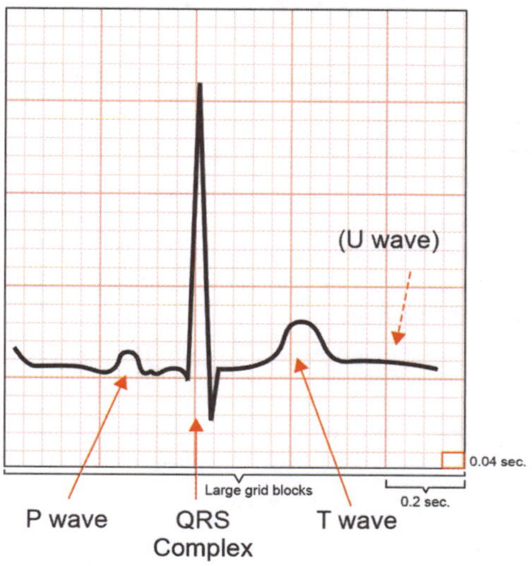

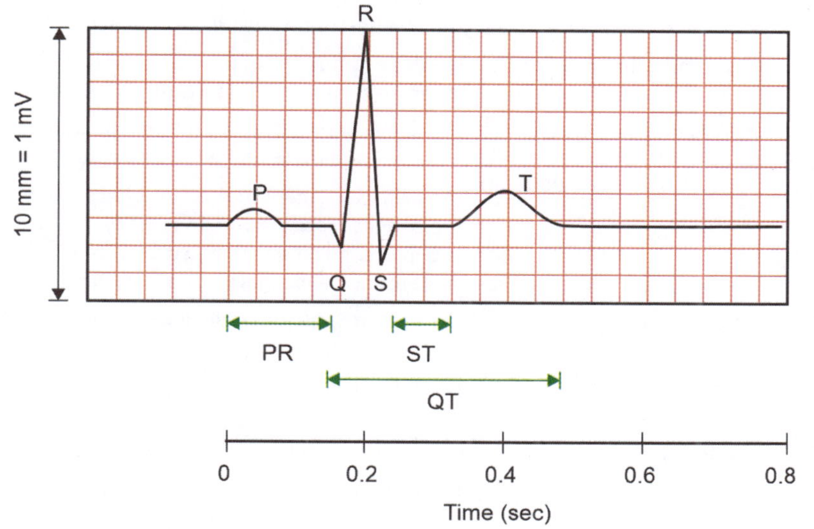

WAVEFORMS

- P wave: Atrial depolarization (contraction)
- QRS complex: Ventricular depolarization (contraction)
- T wave: Ventricular repolarization (relaxation of ventricles)
- (U wave: unknown)

P wave (0.08 - 0.10 s)
P-R interval (0.12 - 0.20 s)

QRS (0.06 - 0.10 s)
$Q\text{-}T_c$ interval ($\leq$ 0.44 s)*

$^*Q\text{-}T_c = QT/\sqrt{RR}$

- Each second = large grid blocks.
- Each large block= 0.2 sec.
- Each small block = 0.04 sec.

ECG Changes and Interpretations

ECG changes	Interpretations
Shortened QT Interval	Hypercalcemia, some drugs, certain genetic abnormalities, hyperkalemia
Prolonged QT Interval	Hypocalcemia, some drugs, certain genetic abnormalities
Flattened or Inverted T-waves	Coronary ischemia, hypokalemia, left ventricular hypertrophy, digoxin effect, some drugs
Hyperacute T-waves	Possibly the first manifestation of acute myocardial infarction, where T waves become more prominent, symmetrical, and pointed
Peaked T wave, QRS wide, prolonged PR, QT short	Hyperkalemia, treat with calcium chloride, glucose and insulin or dialysis
Prominent U-waves	Hypokalemia

Contd...

Abnormal ECG Tracing

• Peak T wave	Hyperkalemia
• T wave inversion	Myocardial infarction
• ST segment depression	Angina pectoris
• ST segment elevation	Myocardial infarction
• Widening of QRS complexes	Arrhythmia
• Positive U wave	Hypokalemia

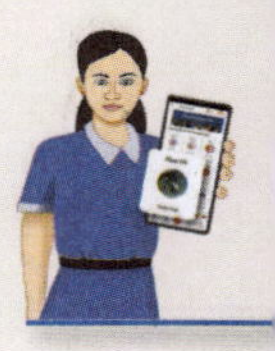

18

"Don't be afraid to fail, be afraid not to try."
—Michael Jordon

COMMON SCALES USED FOR ASSESSMENT/TREATMENT

1	GCS	The **Glasgow Coma Scale (GCS)** is the most common scoring system used to describe the level of consciousness in a person following a traumatic brain injury. Score ranges from 3 to 15. The first description was in 1975 by Jennett and Bond.
2	Asia impairement scale	The American Spinal Injury Association (ASIA) as a universal classification tool for Spinal Cord Injury based on a standardized sensory and motor assessment.
3	Behavioral pain scale	The Behavioral Pain Scale (BPS) can be used to assess pain in adults, including those in the ICU. It can be used for intubated patients and nonintubated patients.
4	CPOT	The pain assessment tool, CPOT is based on four domains: The patient's facial expressions, body movements, compliance with ventilator (or voice use for non-intubated patients), and muscle tension. The total score can vary between 0 and 8, where 0 indicates no pain behavior and 8 indicates clear signs of pain behavior.
5	Braden scale	The Braden Scale for Predicting Pressure Ulcer Risk, is a tool that was developed in 1987 by Barbara Braden and Nancy Bergstrom.
6	Norton scale	The Norton Scale was developed in the 1960s and is widely used to assess the risk for pressure ulcer in adult patients.
7	Waterlow Scale	It provides predictive information about the risk of developing a pressure sore.
8	VIP scale	The Visual Infusion Phlebitis (VIP) score tool for assessment of the early signs of phlebitis, along with prompt removal of peripheral intravenous cannulas.
9	CPIS	Clinical pulmonary infection score (CPIS) as a screening tool in ventilatory associated pneumonia (VAP).
9	BOAS scale	The Beck Oral Assessment Scale and the mucosal-plaque score were used to assess the oral cavity.
10	ROSIER	The Recognition of Stroke in the Emergency Room (ROSIER) scale as a stroke recognition tool.
11	NIHSS	The National Institutes of Health Stroke Scale, or NIH Stroke Scale (NIHSS) is a tool used by healthcare providers to objectively quantify the impairment caused by a stroke.
12	FLACC scale	The Face, Legs, Activity, Cry, Consolability scale or FLACC scale is a measurement used to assess pain for children between the ages of 2 months and 7 years or individuals that are unable to communicate their pain.
13	CRIES scale	A new neonatal postoperative pain measurement score. C--Crying; R--Requires increased oxygen administration; I--Increased vital signs; E--Expression; S--Sleeplessness.
14	FOUR score	FOUR: **F**ull **O**utline of **U**n**R**esponsiveness. The **FOUR Score** is a clinical grading scale designed for use by medical professionals in the assessment of patients with impaired level of consciousness.
15	GCS–Pupils score	GCS Pupils Score (GCS-P) was constructed to bring together information about a patient's responsiveness as reflected in the GCS Score and the pupil reaction The GCS-P is calculated by subtracting the Pupil Reactivity Score (PRS) from the Glasgow Coma Scale (GCS) total score: **GCS-P = GCS - PRS**
16	CDR Scale	The **Clinical Dementia Rating** or **CDR** is a numeric scale used to quantify the severity of symptoms of dementia.
17	RASS	The Richmond Agitation and Sedation **Scale (RASS)** is a validated and reliable method to assess patients' level of sedation in the intensive care unit.

Contd...

18	ABBEY pain scale	The Abbey Pain Scale is a standardized pain assessment tool developed for use in demented nonverbal patients.
19	MMSE **(Folstein** test)	The **Mini-Mental** State Exam **(MMSE)** is a 30-point questionnaire, widely used test of cognitive function. Any **score of** 24 or more **(out of** 30) indicates a normal cognition.
20	PANAS	Positive and Negative Affect Schedule (PANAS) is a self-report questionnaire that consists of two 10-item scales to measure both positive and negative effects.
21	SOFA Score	**Sequential organ failure assessment score (SOFA score)**, previously known as the **sepsis-related organ failure assessment score** is used to track a person's status during the stay in an intensive care unit (ICU) to determine the extent of a person's organ function or rate of failure.
22	APACHE II Score	APACHE - Acute Physiology, Age, Chronic Health Evaluation The **APACHE II** Scoring System is designed to measure the severity of disease in patients admitted to the intensive care unit.
23	**CAGE Questionnaire (CAGE)**	The CAGE questionnaire is a series of four questions that doctors can use to check for signs of possible alcohol dependency.

19

"When you are sick of your sickness, you are no longer sick."
—Chinese Proverb

LEVEL OF SPINAL CORD INJURY AND ASSOCIATED MOTOR LOSS

Levels of spinal injury	Associated motor loss
C1 – C4	• Quadriplegia and loss of respiratory function
C4 – C5	• Quadriplegia and may affect respiratory function if edema damages the phrenic nerve
C5 – C6	• Quadriplegia • Gross motor movement of the arms remains intact with use of the scapular elevators; diaphragmatic breathing remains intact but may not be able to support ventilation because of the loss of intercostal muscle innervation
C6 – C7	• Quadriplegia • Diaphragmatic breathing remains intact but may not be able to support ventilation; arm muscles remain innervated and capable of elbow flexion, wrist extension, and weak thumb grasp
C7 – C8	• Quadriplegia • Diaphragmatic breathing remains intact, but ventilation and airway secretion removal may be compromised because of loss of intercostals muscle innervations. Biceps and triceps muscles respond to voluntary control, and wrist flexion may be possible
T1 and L1 – L2	• Paraplegia • Voluntary motor function of the arms remains intact • Loss of some intercostals muscle innervations may affect ventilation and secretion removal
Cauda equina	• Mixed loss of motor, sensory, bowel, bladder, and sexual function and depends on which roots are damaged
Sacral spinal nerves	• Loss of bowel, bladder and sexual function

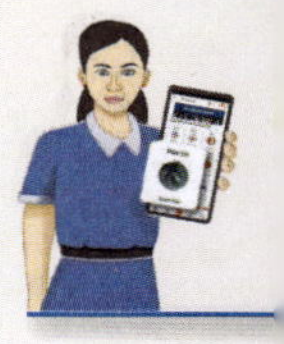

20

"Nothing is impossible. The word itself says I am possible."

—Audrey Hepburn

SOME IMPORTANT SOCIAL WELFARE/HEALTH/DEVELOPMENT PROGRAM LAUNCHED BY GOVERNMENT OF INDIA FROM AUGUST 2014 TILL JUNE 2023

Program	Launch date	Objectives and features
PM Pranam Yojana	June 28, 2023	• Aims to reduce the use of chemical fertilizers by incentivizing states to adopt alternative fertilizers.
Amrit Dharohar Yojana	June 5, 2023	• To Promote values of local communities in conserving Wetland Ecosystem
Ayushman CAPF Healthcare Scheme	November 2, 2021	• Joint initiative by the MHA and NHA to help Central Armed Police Force (CAPF) personnel access healthcare services pan India.
PM Atmanirbhar Swasth Bharat Yojana	October 25, 2021	• Focus on strengthening healthcare infrastructure across the country. • Provide support to set up 17,788 rural Health and Wellness Centers in 10 high focus states • IT-enabled disease surveillance system through the development of a network of surveillance laboratories
PM GatiShakti-National Master Plan	October 13, 2021	• This program aimed at integrating and implementing various infrastructure schemes in the next four years.
Ayushman Bharat Digital Mission	September 27, 2021	• Earlier known as National Digital Health mission • Aims to create a seamless online platform through the provision of a wide range of data, information, and infrastructure services
e-SHRAM	August 26, 2021	• Unorganized sector workers, linked with Aadhaar, will receive an e-SHRAM card through which Social security schemes can be accessed.
Swachh Bharat Mission-Urban 2.0	August 1, 2021	• Aims to to eliminate open defecation and improve solid waste management
AMRUT 2.0	August 1, 2021	• To make cities self-reliant and ensure water security
Start-up India Seed Fund Scheme (SISFS)	April 1, 2021	• Aims to provide financial assistance to start-ups for proof of concept, prototype development, product trials, market entry and commercialization.
PM Umeed Scheme	April 1, 2021	• To provide skill training to youths to help them become entrepreneurs till 2025-26.
Gram Ujala Scheme	March 24, 2021	• To raise awareness against climate change and save electricity • LED bulbs will be distributed at Rs. 10 per bulb in five states: Uttar Pradesh, Bihar, Telangana, Andhra Pradesh, and Karnataka.
Mission COVID Suraksha	November 29, 2020	• The Government of India launched the 'Mission COVID Suraksha', a development program for Indian candidates and researchers working on the COVID-19 vaccine.
SERB-POWER Scheme (Promoting Opportunities for Women in Exploratory Research)	October 29, 2020	• The main objective of this project is to mitigate gender disparity in science and engineering research funding in various S&T programs in Indian academic institutions and R&D laboratories.
Ayushman Sahakar Scheme	October 19, 2020	• Ayushman Sahakar Fund will be made available by the National Cooperative Development Corporation (NCDC). Any cooperative society with suitable provision to undertake healthcare-related activities would be able to access the NCDC fund. • Term loans to prospective cooperatives to the tune of ₹10,000 crore shall be provided.
Mission Karmayogi	September 2, 2020	• It aims to establish the new national architecture for civil services capacity building at individual, institutional and process levels. • It will cover around 46 lakh central employees between 2020–2025.

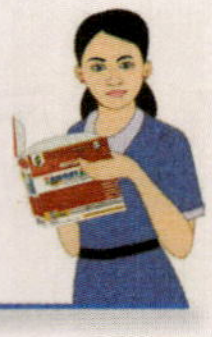

Contd...

Program	Launch date	Objectives and features
Sahakar Mitra Scheme	June 12, 2020	• The aim of the program is to provide a learning experience to young professionals about the cooperative sector and bring out innovative solutions; making them self-reliant.
Prime Minister Street Vendor's AtmaNirbhar Nidhi (PM SVANidhi)	June 1, 2020	• It will provide affordable working capital loans to street vendors who are left affected by the novel coronavirus pandemic.
Atmanirbhar Bharat Scheme	May 12, 2020	• PM Modi announced a relief package of Rs 20 lakh crore to ease the coronavirus distress.
Mission Sagar	May 2020	• Mission Sagar was a COVID-19 relief mission launched by the Government of India in May 2020 as a part of its efforts to provide essential aid to the Indian Ocean countries (Maldives, Mauritius, Madagascar, Comoros and Seychelles)
SVAMITVA Scheme	April 24, 2020	• Survey of Villages and Mapping with Improvised Technology in Village Areas • Scheme is a reformative step toward establishment of clear ownership of property in rural inhabited (Abadi) areas.
DHRUV – PM Innovative Learning Programme	October 10, 2019	• Started by Ministry of Human Resource Development, GoI to identify and encourage talented children to enrich their skills and knowledge.
Pradhan Mantri Kisan Mandhan Yojana	Effective from August 9, 2019	• Farmers between 18 and 40 years of age will get ₹3,000 monthly pension after attaining the age of 60
Pradhan Mantri Kisan Samman Nidhi	February 24, 2019	• All small and marginal farmers will get up to ₹6,000 per year as minimum income support
Ayushman Bharat Yojana or Pradhan Mantri Jan Arogya Yojana or National Health Protection Scheme	September 23, 2018	• Aims to help economically vulnerable Indians who are in need of healthcare facilities
Pradhan Mantri Ujjawala Yojana	May 1, 2016	• To provide LPG connections to 5 crore BPL families
Setu Bharatam Project	April 4, 2016	• To make national highways free of railway crossings by 2019
Shyama Prasad Mukherji Rurban Mission	February 21, 2016	• To develop smart village on the line of smart cities • 300 Rurban clusters developed in 3 years
Pradhan Mantri Fasal Bima Yojana	February 18, 2016	• Agriculture insurance scheme • Is in force since Kharif 2016
Ujwal DISCOM Assurance Yojana (UDAY)	November 5, 2015	• Energy efficiency and conservation • Reduction of cost of generation of power • Development of renewable energy
Stand Up India, Start Up India	August 15, 2015	• To promote bank financing for business start-ups • To promote entrepreneurship and job creation
Nai Manzil Scheme	August 8, 2015	• To address educational and livelihood needs of minorities • Focus on skill development for 17–35 age group
Deen Dayal Upadhyaya Gram Jyoti Yojana	July 25, 2015	• Subsumed Rajiv Gandhi Gramin Vidyutikaran Yojana • To achieve 100% rural electrification
Pradhan Mantri Krishi Sinchai Yojana	July 2, 2015	• To attain water efficiency by 2020 will be achieved through converging existing programmes
Smart Cities Mission	June 25, 2015	• Focus is on building urban infrastructure
Mission Housing for All—Urban	June 25, 2015	• To provide housing to all eligible by 2022
AMRUT Yojana	June 25, 2015	• Atal Mission for Rejuvenation and Urban Development • To develop infrastructure in 500 towns and cities
Namami Gange Yojana	May 14, 2015	• Integrated Ganga Conservation Mission • Focus is on pollution abatement and socio-economic development
Pradhan Mantri Jeevan Jyoti Bima Yojana	May 9, 2015	• To provide for life insurance cover to the needy • Offers ₹2 lakh coverage for ₹330 premium • Administered by the LIC India
Atal Pension Yojana	May 9, 2015	• To enhance old age income security of the working poor • Fixed pension between ₹1000 and 5000 per month

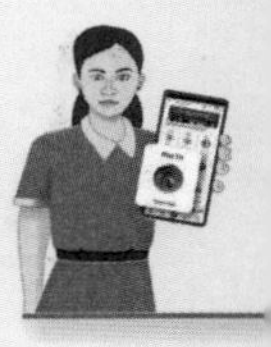

Contd...

Program	Launch date	Objectives and features
Pradhan Mantri Suraksha Bima Yojana	May 9, 2015	• Offers death and disability cover (1–2 lakh) on account of an accident • Annual premium of ₹12 only.
Pradhan Mantri MUDRA Yojana (PMMY)	April 8, 2015	• Micro Units Development and Refinance Agency Ltd. • Has three categories—Shishu, Kishor and Tarun • Provides loans between 50,000 and 10 lakh rupees
Soil Health Card Scheme	February 19, 2015	• To improve farm productivity. **Slogan:** *Swasth Dharaa Khet Haraa*
Beti Bachao, Beti Padhao	January 22, 2015	• Launched first in the state of Haryana • To address the declining Child Sex Ratio issue • To celebrate the girl child and facilitate her education
HRIDAY Yojana	January 21, 2015	• To promote inclusive and sustainable development of heritage sites
Mission Indradhanush	December 25, 2014	• To achieve full immunization coverage for all children by 2020 • Coverage against 7 life-threatening diseases, i.e. Diphtheria, Whooping Cough, Tetanus, Polio, Tuberculosis, Measles, Hepatitis B
Saansad Adarsh Gram Yojana	October 11, 2014	• Village development scheme under MPLADs
Swachh Bharat Mission	October 2, 2014	• To make India 100% open defecation free by 2019 • Focus is on attitudinal change of people toward clean India
Make in India	September 25, 2014	• To make India a global manufacturing hub, Aimed to create 1 crore jobs per year
Deen Dayal Upadhyaya Antyodaya Yojana	September 25, 2014	• To alleviate poverty in rural and urban areas • Implemented by Rural Development and Housing and Urban poverty alleviation ministries
Pradhan Mantri Jan Dhan Yojana	August 28, 2014	• To achieve 100% financial inclusion; 22 crore bank accounts opened so far. **Slogan:** *Mera Khata – Bhagya Vidhaata*
SKILL India Mission	August 28, 2014	• Skill Development in Youth • Aimed to skill 300 million people by 2022
Digital India	August 26, 2014	• To achieve digitally empowered knowledge economy • Transformed version of National e-Governance Plan • Worth 1 lakh crore rupees

21

"Nurses are the heart of healthcare."
—Donna Wilk Cardillo

COLD CHAIN METHODS AND EQUIPMENT

Equipment		Temperature	Location of use
Electrical	Walk-in-freezer (WIF)	–15 to –25°C	National, State and Regional vaccine store
	Walk-in-Coolers (WIC)	2 to 8°C	Government medical store depot, state and regional vaccine store
	Deep Freezer (DF)	–15 to –25°C	District level and above For freezing of ice packs at sub-district levels
	Ice lined refrigerator (ILR)	2 to 8°C	District and sub-district level
	Domestic refrigerator (Front load refrigerator)	2 to 8°C	Private clinic, Nursing home
Non-Electrical	Cold boxes	Fully frozen ice packs are placed at bottom and sides	Used for transportation of vaccine in all peripheral centers
	Vaccine carriers	4 fully frozen ice packs are used	Used for outreach section and can carry 16 to 20 vials at a time
	Day carrier	2 fully frozen ice packs are used	Can carry 6 to 8 vials for few hours, mainly used in a nearby session

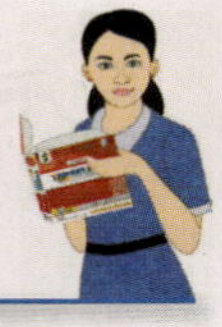

Source: Govt. of India (2016). Handbook for Vaccine and Cold Chain Handlers. 2nd Edition. MoHFW, New Delhi. India 2016

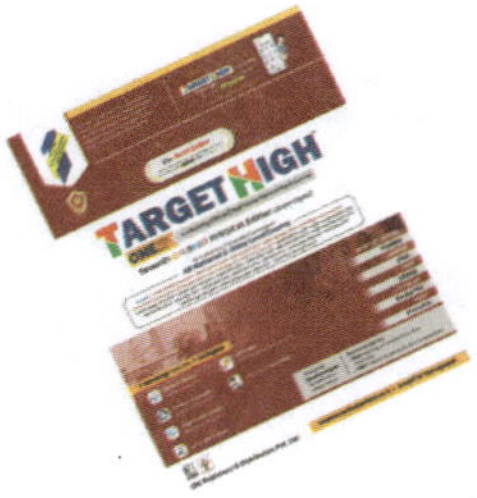

Read from TARGET HIGH Book

Section A

Subject-wise Synopsis CBQs, IBQs & MCQs

SUBJECTS COVERED

- Fundamentals of Nursing
- Medical Surgical Nursing/Adult Health Nursing
- Pharmacology
- Community Health Nursing
- Psychiatric Nursing
- Pediatric Nursing
- Obstetric and Gynecological Nursing
- Applied Microbiology
- Applied Biochemistry and Nutrition
- Applied Sociology and Psychology
- Nursing Research and Statistics
- Nursing Education
- Nursing Administration and Management
- Computer/Health and Nursing Informatics
- Forensic Nursing and Indian laws

Practice from TARGET HIGH Digital

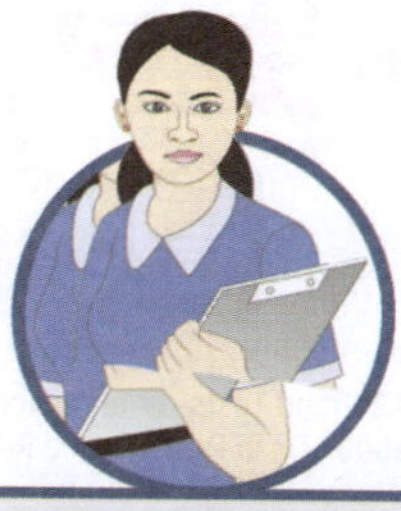

Don't Forget to **Assess** Yourself

Get Your Study Assessed with AMLI

Subjects	MCQs Tests		IBQs Tests		Total Tests
	No. of Tests	No. of Qs	No. of Tests	No. of Qs	
Fundamentals of Nursing	8	800	2	40	10
Medical Surgical Nursing/Adult Health Nursing	6	600	1	30	7
Pharmacology	6	600	2	20	8
Community Health Nursing	8	800	2	40	10
Psychiatric Nursing	4	1200	2	30	6
Pediatric Nursing	8	800	1	20	9
Obstetric and Gynecological Nursing	8	800	2	40	10
Applied Microbiology	2	150	-	-	2
Applied Biochemistry and Nutrition	4	350	-	-	4
Applied Sociology and Psychology	1	20	-	-	1
Nursing Research and Statistics	3	200	-	-	3
Nursing Education	3	150	-	-	3
Nursing Administration and Management	3	150	-	-	3
Computer/Health and Nursing Informatics	2	100	-	-	2
Forensic Nursing and Indian laws	1	20	-	-	1
GK	3	160	-	-	3
Total	70	6900	12	220	82

80+ Tests (Subject-wise Tests & IBQs Tests) Covering **7500+** Questions

"One day in perfect health is much."

—Arabic proverb

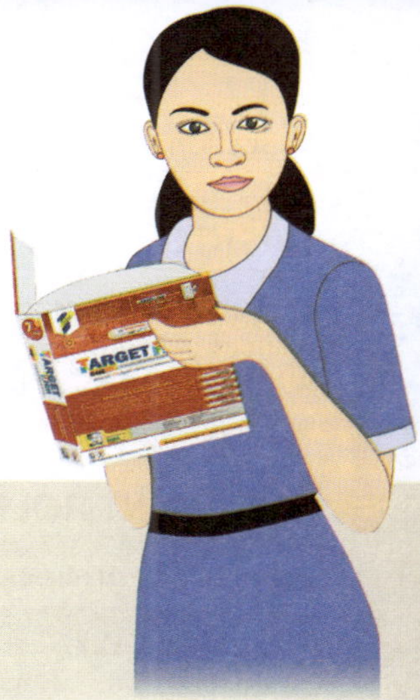

CHAPTER 1

FUNDAMENTALS OF NURSING

SYNOPSIS

- The term "nursing" has been derived from a Latin word "nurtix" which means to nourish.
- Definition of nursing by Virginia Henderson—"The unique function of the nurse is to assist the individual, sick or well, in the performance of those activities contributing to health or its recovery (or to peaceful death) that he would perform unaided if he had the necessary strength, will or knowledge."
- Definition of nursing by the American Nurses Association (ANA)—"protection, promotion, and optimization of health and abilities, prevention of illness and injury, alleviation of suffering through the diagnosis and treatment of human response, and advocacy in the care of individuals, families, communities, and populations."

FLORENCE NIGHTINGALE'S CONTRIBUTION TO NURSING

- Florence Nightingale was born in Florence, Italy on May 12, 1820 and died on August 13, 1910.
- Every year, International Nurses Day is celebrated on 12th May.
- She developed first organized nursing program for nurses in the year 1860.
- She started her program in the Nightingale Training School for Nurses at St. Thomas' Hospital in London.
- She volunteered herself during Crimean War in the year 1853.
- She is known as **"Lady with the Lamp"** for taking care of soldiers with lamp at night.

KEY POINTS

- **Florence Nightingale** defined nursing as **"the art of utilizing the environment of patients to assist them in their recovery."**
- **Environment** is the focus of nursing care in Nightingale's theory.
- A profession requires an extended education/training of its members as well as a basic foundation.

MILESTONES OF NURSING IN INDIA

1871	The first school of nursing with 4 students was started in Government General Hospital, Madras (now Chennai) with 6 months Diploma in Midwives' Program.
1908	Trained Nurses' Association of India (TNAI) was formed.
1926	Madras state (now Tamil Nadu) formed first registration council to provide basic standards in education and training.
1946	The first four years' bachelor's degree program was established at RAK College of Nursing in New Delhi and Christian Medical College, Vellore, Tamil Nadu
1947	The Indian Nursing Council Act was passed by ordinance on December 31.
1948	Nursing Council Act came into existence in 1948 to constitute a council of nurses.
1949	The Indian Nursing Council constituted under the Indian Nursing Council Act, 1947.
1959	First master's nursing course of 2 years duration started at RAK College of Nursing, New Delhi.
1986	MPhil in Nursing was started by RAK College of Nursing, Delhi.
1992	Doctoral program in nursing was started by RAK CON under Department of Nursing, University of Delhi.
2017	Indian Nursing Council launched nurse practitioner in critical care nursing program.
2023	The National Nursing and Midwifery Commission Bill 2023 (NNMC 2023) was passed in Lok Sabha on July 28. NNMC was passed in Rajya Sabha on 08 August 2023.

KEY POINTS

Principles of nursing: Safety, therapeutic effectiveness, comfort, resource utilization and good workmanship

characteristics of a profession:

- Profession has a theoretical body of knowledge leading to defined skills and abilities.
- A profession provides a specific service.

BASIC CHARACTERISTICS OF A PROFESSION

- Specialized education
- Body of knowledge
- Continuous research activity
- Service orientation
- Code of professional ethics
- Autonomy
- Professional organization

DIFFERENT ROLES OF NURSES

Table 1: Role of nurses

Role	Description
Autonomy and accountability	Nurse should be able to initiate independent nursing action without medical orders within the scope of practice. E.g., initiation of cold sponging to a client with fever. Nurse is always responsible and answerable for the quality of care provided to the client.
Caregiver	Caregiver helps the client to achieve maximum level of functioning independently by providing good care.
Advocate	Nurse acts as an advocate to client by protecting client's rights.
Educator	Nurse educates the client about the disease process and its management. Nurse demonstrates and educates clients on health-related activities and promotes healthy lifestyle.
Communicator	It's an integral part of a good relationship. Nurse communicates to the client about disease process, its management and progress.
Manager	Nurse managers are responsible for managing nurses within a healthcare environment and are responsible for creating an environment that promotes a culture aimed at enhancing the quality of life for patients.

TRENDS IN NURSING

Table 2: Trends in nursing

Trend	Description
Evidence-based practice	To provide high-quality nursing care through evidence-based practice.
Quality and safety education for nurses	Provide regular education to stay updated with health care changes.
New technologies	Emerging technologies that contribute to sophisticated diagnostic and treatment modalities, development of e-health and tele medicine, etc.
Genomics	It is the study of inheritance and nurse should use these study findings ethically and for the upliftment of the mankind.
Public perception of nursing	Nowadays, public is aware about the consumer rights and rights of a patient. Always provide high-quality competent care to the client to avoid medical errors.

NURSING PROGRAMS IN INDIA

Table 3: Nursing programs in India

Name of the program	Duration	Basic qualification
Auxiliary Nurse Midwife	18 months and 6 months internship	10+2
GNM	3 years and 6 months	10+2
BSc Nursing	4 years	10+2 Science
Post Basic Nursing	2 years	GNM
MSc Nursing & Nurse Practitioner in Critical Care (NPCC)	2 years	BSc Nursing or Post Basic Nursing with 1 year of experience (INC criteria) NOTE: AIIMS Institutes does not require 1 year experience.

Contd...

KEY POINTS

- **Nurse as a Client Advocate:** Defends the client's right to be treated equally without any harm intentionally or unintentionally.
- **Nurse Researcher:** Investigates the role of nurses which further improves the nursing practice.

Clinical Corner

CASE SCENARIO 1:

A nurse is caring for a patient who has been diagnosed with a serious medical condition that requires immediate treatment. However, the patient is refusing to undergo the recommended treatment. The patient's family insists the nurse to persuade the patient to accept the treatment. What should the nurse do?

a. The nurse should attempt to convince the patient to accept treatment.
b. The nurse should take legal action through court to force the patient to accept treatment.
c. The nurse should discuss with another registered nurse to decide further course of action.
d. The nurse should respect the patient's autonomy and allow him to refuse treatment.

Ans. (d) The nurse should respect the patient's autonomy and allow him to refuse treatment.

Name of the program	Duration	Basic qualification
MPhil Nursing	1 year course for regular candidate and 2 year course for part-time candidate	MSc in nursing (NOTE: M.Phil course is abolished as per new NEP)
PhD Nursing	3 years—full time 5 years—part time	• MSc Nursing is essential qualification. • 3 years of experience after MSc Nursing for National Consortium for PhD in Nursing. • Other Universities have their own criteria but MSc Nursing is essential.

ETHICS IN NURSING

Table 4: Ethics in nursing

Ethical principle	Definition	Example
Autonomy	Respecting and supporting others' decisions	Respecting a patient's decision to refuse treatment
Beneficence	Doing good for others	Administering pain relief to a suffering patient
Nonmaleficence	Avoiding harm to others	Avoiding unnecessary procedures that may cause harm
Justice	Equal and fair treatment	Providing equal care to all patients, regardless of background
Fidelity	Faithfulness to agreements and promises	Respecting patient's confidentiality and privacy
Veracity	Being truthful or telling truth	Informing a patient about his/her diagnosis truthfully
Accountability	Answerable to oneself and others for own action	Owning up to a medication error and reporting it
Responsibility	Liability for specific duties in a particular role	A nurse ensuring proper care of patients in his/her charge

Code of Ethics for Nurses

- Code of ethics serves as a means of self-regulation and sets the standard of individual behavior for the profession.
- Professional code of ethics is a system of rules and principles and nurses adhere to the professional practice standards by following these.
- An international code of ethics for nurses was first adopted by the **International Council of Nurses in 1953.**
- The **ICN code of ethics** for nurses, most recently, was **revised in the year 2012.**
- **Four principal elements of ICN code of ethics:**
  1. Nurses and people
  2. Nurses and practice
  3. Nurses and the profession
  4. Nurses and co-workers
- The fundamental responsibility of the nurse is in four areas, namely
  1. To promote health
  2. To prevent illness
  3. To restore health
  4. To alleviate suffering

SOURCES OF LAW

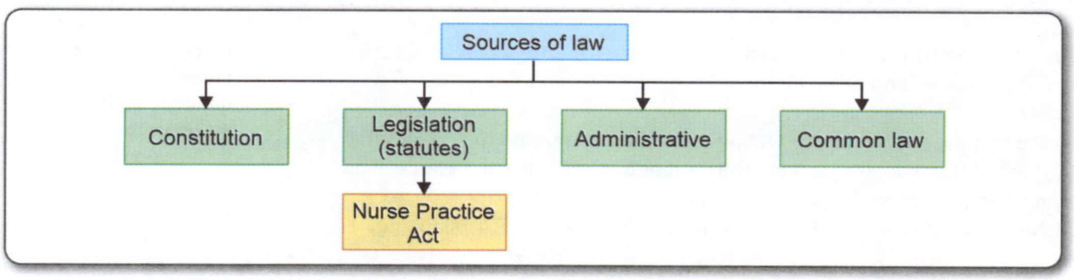

Figure 1: Sources of law

KEY POINTS

- The International Council of Nurses is founded in 1899.
- ICN is an independent, nonpartisan, non-governmental federation of national nurses' associations.

Clinical Corner

CASE SCENARIO 2:

Two patients with similar medical conditions are admitted to a hospital. Both require immediate medical attention, but there is only one available bed in the ICU. What ethical principle should guide the nurse's decision-making process in this situation?

a. Beneficence
b. Fidelity
c. Justice
d. Autonomy

Ans. (c) Justice

(Providing equal and fair treatment to all patients, regardless of background)

Recent Question
(NORCET 2022)

1. **Nurses Day theme 2021 was:**
   a. Nurses: a voice to lead - a vision for future healthcare.
   b. Nurses: A voice to lead - Nursing the World to Health.
   c. Nurses: A voice to lead - Health for All.
   d. Nurses: A voice to lead - Health is a Human Right.
   Ans: a.

Ans. (a) Nurses: a voice to lead - a vision for future healthcare.

Table 5: Types of law

Type	Description	Example
Constitutional Law	It is the body of law that outlines fundamental principles and structures by which government exercises its authority	Freedom of speech
Statutory Law	Laws created by elected bodies, at state or national level	Nurse Practitioner Act
Regulatory Law	Rules and regulations by administrative agencies	State nursing council regulations
Common Law	Laws made by judges through courts	Informed consent, patient's right to refuse treatment, negligence, malpractice
Criminal Law	Laws to protect society and punish crimes • **Misdemeanors:** Lesser offenses, fines or brief imprisonment • **Felonies:** Serious offenses, longer imprisonment or death	Violations of nurse practice act, illegal possession of controlled substances, active euthanasia
Civil Law	Laws to protect patient rights, fair treatment for violations	Malpractice, negligence

LEGISLATION AND NURSING PRACTICE

Table 6: Nursing practice and legislation

Term	Description
Licensure	Allows professionals to provide specific skills/service to the public and safeguards them from legal proceedings (e.g., state nursing councils providing valid registration for RNs).
Good Samaritan Law	Legally protects professionals providing emergency services (e.g., a nurse providing emergency care at a road traffic accident scene within his/her practice limits is protected even if the patient develops complications later).
Public Health Law	Applies to nurses working in community settings who have obligations to report vital events and major community issues (e.g., elder or child abuse, domestic violence, communicable disease outbreaks, school immunization status).
Uniform Death Determination Act	Medical death confirmation methods: • Cardiopulmonary method: Requires irreversible cessation of circulatory and respiratory functions. • Whole brain standard: Requires irreversible cessation of all brain functions. Nurses should be aware of the death declaration methods in their work area.
Autopsy	Also known as postmortem, performed when death occurs under nonnatural circumstances.
Death with Dignity/ Physician-Assisted Suicide	Carried out upon verbal or written request of a person in the terminal stage of illness when recovery is not possible. Medication is given to end life in a dignified manner. **Not practiced in India due to legal and cultural reasons.**

LEGISLATION ISSUES IN NURSING PRACTICE

Torts	Tort is a wrongful act or omission made against a person or property. It can be classified into intentional, unintentional, and quasi-intentional. **Intentional torts** **Assault**: It is threatening the patient or pretending to hit the patient and that places the patient under significant fear. E.g., threatening the patient by stating that CT scan will be done after applying restraint when the patient refuses to give consent. **Battery:** It is touching patient's body without consent from the patient. E.g., slapping, pinching, pulling.

Contd...

Clinical Corner

CASE SCENARIO 3:
A nurse is caring for a bedridden patient who is at risk of hip external rotation due to his position in bed. The nurse wants to implement a comfort device to prevent this external rotation of the hips. Which of the following comfort devices should the nurse use?

a. Trochanter rolls
b. Hand roll
c. Trapeze roll
d. Sandbags

Ans. (a) Trochanter rolls

Clinical Corner

CASE SCENARIO 4:
A first aid rescuer provides hands only CPR to a victim collapsed in front of him outside a coffee shop. Which of the legal principle supports the rescuer from being successfully sued for wrongdoing?

a. Statutory law
b. Misdemeanor
c. Good Samaritan laws
d. Administrative law

Ans. (c) Good Samaritan laws

Good Samaritan laws are laws that protect people who help others in an emergency from being sued for wrongdoing.

Practice Question

1. **Nurse Ramya posts derogatory comments about her supervisor on social media. This act refers to:**
   a. Intrusion
   b. Slander
   c. Libel
   d. Battery

   Ans. (c) Libel

	False imprisonment: When the patient is intentionally restricted from moving from one place to another or restrain the patient without any legal reason. E.g., not allowing the patient to meet the family members. **Unintentional torts** **Negligence:** When the standard of care falls below the minimum, it is known as negligence. It results in unintended harm to the patient due to the unintentional act or omission of act from nurse's side. E.g., failure to monitor patient at required time interval; not reporting changes in patients' status correctly; failure to give medications **Malpractice:** In this, nurse willingly or knowingly does something which results in harm to the patient. E.g., transfusing blood to wrong client; administering a medication with known allergy to the patient. **Quasi-intentional tort** **Invasion of privacy**: it means patient does not want anyone to enter in his or her personal matter. Releasing patient information to anyone without patient's consent is also a type of invasion of privacy. **Defamation of character:** It means release of false information about patient's character which may affect patient's reputation. It can be of two types, **Slander** and **libel.** ***Slander*** means verbal wrong information about patient. ***Libel*** means written information which causes defamation of character
Informed consent	It is patients' agreement for a medical procedure or investigation after receiving complete information about it. Patient has right to refuse the treatment or investigation. **Physician/surgeon is responsible to obtain the informed consent.** Informed consent is to be obtained when the patient is conscious, not under the influence of opioids, and explained in a language he/she can understand and witnessed by another person.

PROFESSIONAL VALUES

Professional values are the guiding beliefs and principles that influence work behavior.

- **Altruism**: Selfless concern of a nurse for the well-being of patients and others, e.g., advocating for vulnerable patients and mentoring other health care professionals.
- **Autonomy**: Right to self-determination, e.g., nurse should respect patient's rights to make decisions on their treatment, e.g., plan of care in consultation with patients.
- **Integrity**: The quality of being honest and acting in accordance with code of ethics, e.g., providing honest information to patients and family, taking responsibility for own actions and accurate documentation.
- **Human dignity:** Respect for the uniqueness of individuals/people, e.g., culturally competent care to patient, respecting patient's privacy and maintaining confidentiality of patient's information.
- **Social justice:** "Acting in accordance with fair treatment regardless of economic status, ethnicity, age, citizenship, disability, or sexual orientation" (American Association of College of Nursing, 2007), e.g., facilitate universal access to health care and nondiscrimination in delivery of nursing care.

NURSING PROCESS

- Nursing process is a continuous holistic and fundamental approach while providing care to a client.
- It is the systematic way of providing individualized care to the client.

Five steps are:

1. **Assessment:** Data collection (subjective or objective)
2. **Nursing diagnosis:** Problem of the client
3. **Planning:** How to manage the problem
4. **Implementation:** Putting plan into action
5. **Evaluation:** Check the plan whether it is working

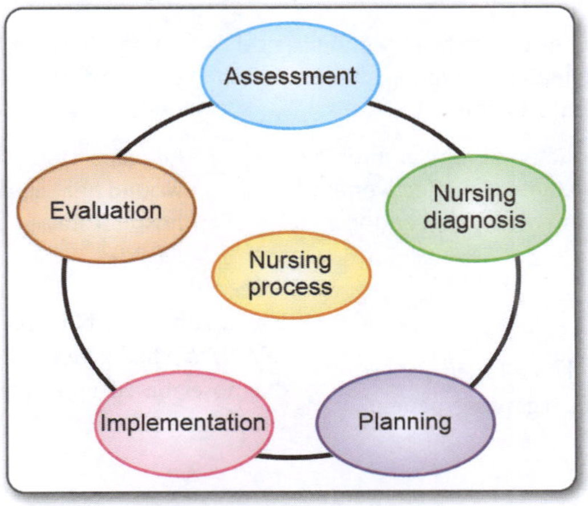

Figure 2: Nursing process

RECENT UPDATE:

National Nursing and Midwifery Commission (NNMC) Bill:

- The Govt of India passed the NNMC Bill, 2023 on 24 July 2023 in the Lok Sabha.
- The NNMC Bill aims to set up National Nursing and Midwifery Commission (NNMC), and will repeal the Indian Nursing Council Act, 1947, to streamline nursing education in India.
- The Central Government shall establish three Autonomous Boards under the overall supervision of the National Commission to carry out specific functions as per this Act. These boards are:
  - The Nursing and Midwifery Undergraduate and Postgraduate Education Board
  - The Nursing and Midwifery Assessment and Rating Board
  - The Nursing and Midwifery Ethics and Registration Board

KEY POINTS

- Colour coding for Other Medical Gas Cylinders in India:
- Air - Grey body & White and black neck.
- Cyclopropane - Orange body and neck.
- Ethylene - Violet body and neck

Characteristics of Nursing Process

- Cyclic
- Systematic
- Client-centered
- Problem focused
- Decision making
- Universally applicable
- Interpersonal and collaborative style
- Use critical thinking and logical reasoning

Nursing Assessment

- Assessment is the collection, organization, interpretation, and validation (cross-checked/double verified) of data regarding patients to understand their current and past health issues and coping strategies.
- Collection of data can be done through:
  - History collection
  - Physical examination
  - Interview
  - Medical records
  - Observation of patient and significant others.
- Sources of data can be primary, secondary and tertiary.
  - **Primary:** Information given by the client.
  - **Secondary:** Information given by significant others of client or people within the reference of client. For an unconscious client or a child, secondary data source is most important.
  - **Tertiary**: It is the data obtained regarding client's condition from medical literature and journals.
- Collected data can be either subjective or objective
  - **Subjective data**: Feelings or complaints by the patient that can't be observed directly. Examples: pain, nausea and a feeling of uneasiness.
  - **Objective data**: Measurable or observable data about a patient's health status. Examples: vomiting, high blood pressure, fever and skin discoloration.

KEY POINTS

- **Admission assessment:** Comprehensive nursing assessment completed at the time of admission, which includes patient history, general appearance, physical examination and vital signs.
- **Shift assessment:** Brief nursing assessment at the beginning of each shift OR if patient condition changes at any other time of the shift.
- **'Real time' progress notes:** Nursing documentation written in a timely manner during the shift.
- **'End of shift' progress notes:** Nursing documentation written as a summary at the end of shift.

Types of Assessment

Table 7: Types of nursing assessment

Types of assessment	Description	Example
Initial assessment	Performed after admission within a specific time to determine the nature of the problem.	Assessment conducted upon admission to the ward or emergency department.
Problem-focused assessment	Determines the status of a particular problem identified during the initial assessment.	Monitoring a patient's temperature every 2 hours when they complain of fever.
Emergency assessment	Conducted during emergency situations to identify life-threatening events.	Rapid assessment of ABCs for a client brought to the emergency room following a road traffic accident.
Time-lapsed assessment	Performed several months after the initial assessment to determine changes in the client's health status.	Assessment conducted during subsequent follow-up visits.
Comprehensive assessment	Includes health history and physical examination, covering all aspects of a patient's health.	Comprehensive assessment of a patient during his/her first visit to a primary care provider.
Ongoing assessment	Conducted at regular intervals to evaluate the effectiveness of treatment or interventions.	Regular assessment of a patient's wound healing process during his/her hospital stay.

Nursing Diagnosis

- Nurse will critically analyze the collected data in the assessment and conclude regarding patient's problem from the collected data.
- North American Nursing Diagnosis Association (**NANDA**) has given a list of possible nursing diagnoses based upon the nursing research and work.

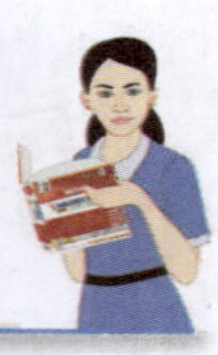

Clinical Corner

CASE SCENARIO 5:

A nurse has received 34-year-old male patient from the OPD with the chief complaints of allergic rhinitis, including episodic cough, wheeze, itchy red watery eyes and a runny, itchy nose. Patient had a history of Asthma since 2015. After performing the initial assessment which type of health assessment the nurse will perform?

a. Comprehensive Health Assessment
b. Focused Health Assessment
c. Episodic Health Assessment
d. Emergency Health Assessment

Ans. (b) Focused Health...

Types of Nursing Diagnosis

Table 8: Types of nursing diagnosis

Types	Description
Problem focused/actual	These are the diagnoses related to the problem present in the client during assessment. It has three components: 1. Nursing diagnosis 2. Related factors 3. Defining characteristics **Example**: Impaired skin integrity related to pressure over bony prominence.
Risk diagnosis	These diagnoses represent conditions not currently present in the client but may develop in the future due to vulnerability or the presence of risk factors. It has two components only (NO related factors) 1. Nursing diagnosis 2. Defining characteristics **Example:** Risk for falls *as evidenced by* muscle weakness.
Health promotion diagnosis or wellness diagnosis	It is the diagnosis related to the desire/ motivation of client to improve his/her health status. It is only one component statement. Examples: Readiness for enhanced knowledge, readiness to enhanced parenting.
Syndrome diagnosis	A syndrome diagnosis is a clinical evaluation of a set of related problems or risks, anticipated to arise from a specific situation or event. Example: Chronic pain syndrome.

Components of NANDA Nursing Diagnosis

Table 9: Components of NANDA Nursing diagnosis

Component	Description
Problem statement	Actual problem of the client E.g., ineffective breathing pattern
Etiology	Cause of the health problem in the client E.g., related to brain injury
Defining characteristics	Cluster of signs and symptoms or characteristics of the health problem E.g., as evidenced by difficulty in breathing or dyspnea.

Planning

- In planning, goal and intervention will be set to solve or reduce client's health problems.
- **Planning starts** when client has **first contact with the health care facility**.
- The planning involves **collaborating and consulting with the patient to develop a plan of care** that addresses the patient's individual needs and preferences.
- Outcomes are defined as expected changes in patient's activity, behavior or physical state and evaluate the nursing intervention.
- Outcomes should be based on **SMART**: Specific, measurable, attainable, realistic and time bound.
- While planning goals and expected outcome, it should be:
  - Patient-oriented
  - Focused on singular goal or outcome

Types of Planning

- **Initial planning:** Planning done for a client after initial assessment.
- **Ongoing planning:** Continual and ongoing planning while the client stays in the health care facility.
- **Discharge planning:** Planning done for the client after discharge to meet his/her needs.

Components of Planning

- Setting priorities: Prioritize nursing care plan as high, intermediate, and low. Prioritization is mostly based on:
  - ABC (Airway > Breathing > Circulation) or
  - Maslow's Hierarchy of needs (Physiological needs > Safety and Security > Love and belonging > Self-esteem)
- Establishing goal: For each diagnosis, a short-term or long-term goal will be set.
- Select appropriate nursing intervention: Any action/ treatment initiated by nurse to improve clint's health status.
- Writing individualized nursing interventions on care plan.

Practice Questions

2. Which of the following is the most important assessment during the acute stage of an unconscious patient?

a. Coherence and sense of hearing
b. Level of awareness and response to pain
c. Papillary reflexes and response to sensory stimuli
d. Patency of airway and adequacy of respiration

Ans. (d) Patency of airway and adequacy of respiration

If you are not able to use ABC or if it is not applicable, use actual to potential concept. The intervention which addresses the actual problem (at present) should be given priority over the interventions which are concerned about the future risk (potential risk).

3. A patient with head injury is confused, drowsy and has unequal pupils. Which of the following nursing diagnosis is a priority at this time?

a. Altered level of cognitive function
b. High risk for injury
c. Altered cerebral tissue perfusion
d. Sensory perceptual alteration

Ans. (c) Altered cerebral tissue perfusion

Tips: High risk for injury is a potential risk which comes after taking care of actual risks. Use Maslow's hierarchy of needs model to choose from remaining three options. Maintaining perfusion is a priority compared to cognitive function and perception.

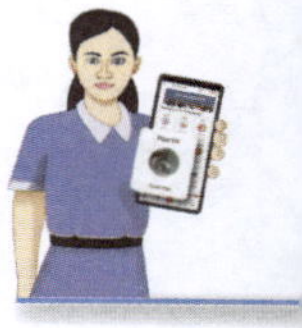

Nursing Interventions

Nursing interventions are the actions planned by a nurse for the client to improve the health status.

Types of Interventions

Table 10: Types of interventions

Type	Description
Independent	Actions a licensed nurse can carry out within the scope of practice.
Dependant	Activities carried out by a nurse under the supervision of a physician.
Collaborative	Interventions carried out by nurse along with other professionals or health care team members.

Implementation

Putting planned nursing interventions to action is known as implementation.

Evaluation

Evaluation is the monitoring of client's health status after implementation to evaluate the effectiveness of interventions.

DOCUMENTATION AND REPORTING

Documentation: It is the written information about patient and the problem, decision and interventions done by the nurse and patient's response to that.

Purposes

- Interprofessional and intraprofessional communication.
- Legal documentation.
- Medical claim/insurance reimbursement.
- Auditing and monitoring.
- Research activities.
- Education of medical and nursing students.

Guidelines for Quality Documentation

- Factual
- Accurate
- Complete
- Current and logical order
- Organized
- Use only standard abbreviations.
- Signed by the person who wrote the document with date.
- Confidentiality

POINT TO REMEMBER

Nursing assessment focuses on collecting data and information about the patient's health status, while the **Evaluation** focuses on determining the effectiveness of the nursing interventions provided to the patient.

KEY POINTS

Basic purposes of an accurate and completely written patient records:

- It is a legal record of care
- It is a permanent record for accountability
- Sometimes used by Government agencies for evaluation
- Can be used for research and teaching

Methods of Documentation

Table 11: Methods of documentation

Types	Description
Source oriented	• In this method, each department will have separate page to make their entry. • It is the traditional method • Narrative charting is a part of traditional recording. On this, story-like format will be used for documentation. E.g., admission department will make entry in admission sheet, physician will write in physician order, nurse will write in nurses order
Problem oriented medical record (POMR)	• Developed by **Lawrence Weed.** • It has **four components**: Data base, problem list, plan of care and progress note. • **Data base:** All available assessment information in relation to the patient. E.g., history, physical examination, etc. • **Problem list:** It contains different problems pertaining to physiological, psychological, social, cultural, spiritual etc. New problems can be added to the list. • **Plan of care/care plan:** Person who identifies the problem can write care plan for the patient. Doctor writes medical care plan, while nurses write nursing care plan. • **Progress note:** Health care providers note patient's condition and write the progress note as client improves. • Progress note can be written in various formats such as: ▪ SOAP—subjective-objective-assessment-plan ▪ SOAPIE—subjective-objective-assessment-plan-intervention-evaluation ▪ SOAPIER—subjective-objective-assessment-plan-intervention-evaluation, revision ▪ DAR—data-action-response ▪ PIE—problem-intervention-evaluation
Charting by exception	Any deviation from normal or any abnormality will be recorded.
Case management and critical pathway	• It is the method of providing care to a client by collaborating all inter-professional and document the care provided. • Critical pathway helps to identify client's problem, interventions and expected outcome in the patient within the specified time.

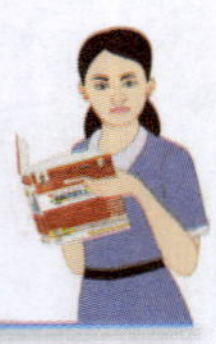

Clinical Handovers Formats for Nurses

Clinical handover refers to the transfer of professional responsibility and accountability for some or all aspects of patient care to another nurse or health care professional on a temporary or permanent basis. Two commonly used formats for handover are SBAR and ISOBAR.

- **SBAR**—Stands for Situation, Background, Assessment and Recommendation
  - **S**ituation—Briefly describe the patient's current situation
  - **B**ackground—Provide relevant background information about the patient
  - **A**ssessment: Describe the patient's current assessment findings and vital signs
  - **R**ecommendation: Provide recommendations for next steps and interventions
- **ISOBAR**—Introduction, Situation, Observation, Background, Assessment and Recommendation. In addition to SBAR, Introduction and Observation have been added in ISOBAR.
  - **I**ntroduction: Introduce yourself and your role in the patient's care.
  - **O**bservation: Describe any observations you have made about the patient, including changes in vital signs.

ADMISSION AND DISCHARGE

Admission

It is allowing the patient to stay in a health care facility for observation, diagnosis or treatment of the problem.

Types of Admission

Table 12: Types of admission

Type of admission	Description
Routine admission	Priorly planned admission for a client for diagnostic procedure or treatment
Emergency admission	Admission of client with life-threatening medical conditions.
Long-term admission	Hospital stay will be for long duration.
Short-term admission	Hospital stay will be for short duration.
Diagnostic admission	Admission is for undergoing investigation/diagnostic procedure.
Therapeutic admission	Patient who needs medical care for his/her conditions will be admitted.
Medicolegal issues related admission	**Chief Medical Officer and Police need to be informed** about such admissions and these records should be kept confidential with proper label.

Important Points to Consider in Case of Admission of Medicolegal Cases

- **Physician must be informed immediately** after the arrival of the patient.
- Patient's records are **confidential** and should be **kept under lock and key.**
- Patient's belongings should be kept under custody as per hospital policy.
- While handing over patient belongings to police or relatives, record the complete details and take signature of the receiver, and inform the treating physician.
- Female patient should be examined by a **female physician** or in the presence of a female health care worker.
- Maintain complete records of body fluid, description including color, amount, smell, and consistency, and do not discard them without physician's permission.
- No evidence related to the patient should be destroyed.
- **Informed consent** must be taken from patient or relative before doing any invasive procedures.
- If a patient needs, then allow family members to stay with the patient.
- Inform higher authority such as medical superintendent, chief nursing officer, chief medical officer, security officer and police regarding the MLC as per hospital policy.

Discharge

It is the release from health care facility. It starts when the patient is admitted to the facility.

Types of Discharge

- **Planned discharge:** Patient is relieved from the hospital once the purpose of admission is completed.
- **LAMA (Leave Against Medical Advice):** Patient leaves the health care facility against medical advice for various reasons. The recent terminology for LAMA is **Discharge Against Medical Advice (DAMA).**
- **Referral/transfer:** Patient is transferred to another health care facility for better treatment or other reasons.
- **DOPR (Discharge on patient request):** Patient requests to leave the hospital and leaves against medical advice with the consent of the treating doctor.
- **Absconding:** Patient runs away from the health care facility. If it occurs, inform immediate supervisor and the Chief Medical Officer.
- **Parole:** In mental health facility, a patient who has not been discharged from a hospital can be sent home for 2–3 days, if requested by the relatives and approved by treating psychiatrist. If patient fails to return, then discharge procedure should be carried out as per the hospital policy.

KEY POINTS

Key responsibilities of a nurse during admission of a patient:
- Orient patient to the hospital.
- Confirm that the patient understands diagnostic tests and procedures.
- Monitor patient's ability to ambulate independently.
- Monitor patient's ability to operate hospital bed, call light and emergency button.

KEY POINTS

- On admission, initial nursing assessment and health history are usually done once the patient is settled in his/her room.
- Red color wrist band indicates that the patient has allergies.
- Staff nurse or in-charge nurse is primarily responsible for discharge planning.
- Concern about actual and potential health problems and potential outcome of treatment are the usual concerns of patient upon admission.

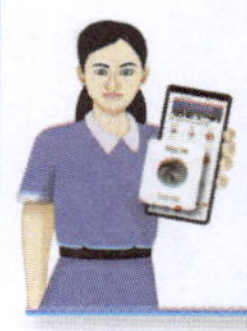

Important Points to Consider in Case of Discharge of Medicolegal Cases

- Patient's record should not be handed over to police or legal authority without written permission from the physician.
- Name and complete details of the person should be entered to whom patient's records and belongings handed over.
- If MLC patient is going on LAMA or DAMA or death occurred, Chief Medical Officer should be informed about the event.
- Discharge records should be kept under lock and key.
- Prior permission from the chief medical officer should be obtained before handing over unclaimed dead bodies to the police.

VITAL SIGNS

- Vital signs are also known as cardinal signs.
- These are the parameters that are easy to measure and give the complete picture of client's health status.
- Temperature, pulse, respiration and blood pressure are the major vital signs.
- SPO_2 and pain levels are also assessed along with other vital signs.

Normal values (adult)

Vital sign	Normal value
Temperature (oral)	37 °C (Range: 36.5°C to 37.5°C)
Pulse	72 bpm (Range: 60–100 bpm)
Respiration	12–20 bpm
BP	Systolic <120 mm Hg Diastolic <80 mm Hg
SPO_2	≥95%

Contd...

Temperature

- It is the balance between heat produced (thermogenesis) and heat lost (thermolysis) in the body.
- Two types of temperatures are surface temperature and core body temperature.
  1. **Surface temperature:** Temperature of skin, subcutaneous tissue and fat. It fluctuates in response to environmental temperature. E.g., Axillary temperature
  2. **Core body temperature:** Temperature of the deep tissues of the body such as abdominal cavity and pelvic cavity. It remains relatively constant. E.g., temporal, tympanic, oral, esophagal, urinary bladder, rectal, pulmonary.
- **Hypothalamus** is the temperature **control center** of the body.
- Anterior hypothalamus controls **heat loss;** posterior hypothalamus controls **heat production** (Tip to remember: Production can be linked to posterior).
- **Hormones that increase body temperature:** Thyroxin, testosterone and progesterone
- Body temperature is usually lowest between 1:00 am and 4:00 am (early morning) and maximum temperature is by 4:00 pm (evening).

POINT TO REMEMBER

Pain is considered as 5th Vital Sign.

Mechanism of Heat Loss from the Body

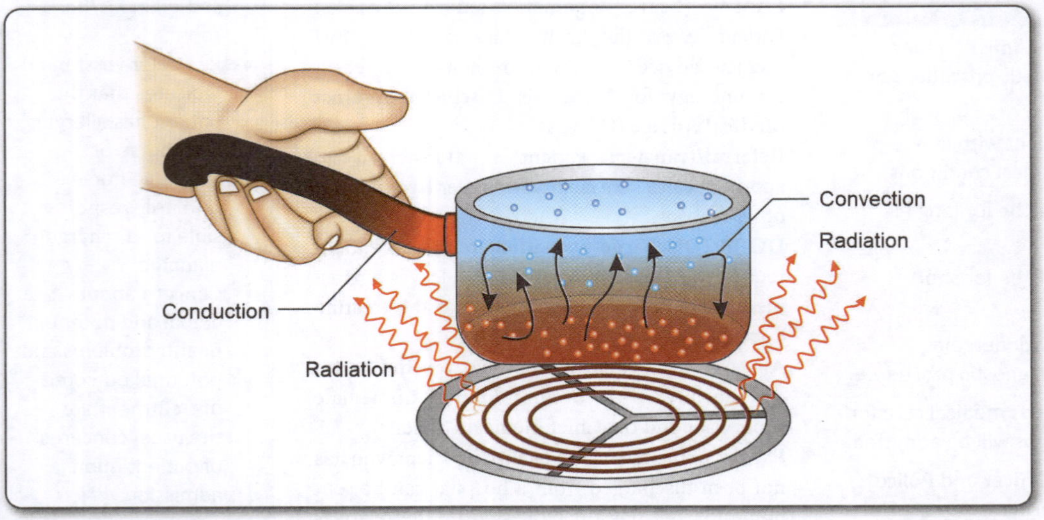

Figure 3: Conduction, convection and radiation

Practice Question

4. Discharge summary includes all of the following, except
a. Short- and long-term goals for care
b. Learning needs of patient
c. Estimated cost for follow-up care
d. Health education completed for the patient

Ans. (c) Estimated cost for follow-up care

Clinical Corner

CASE SCENARIO 6:

You have measured the body temperature of your assigned patient and found that the patient is febrile. You have instructed the patient that you may lose body heat through perspiration. The patient then asks the nurse about the mechanism of heat loss followed in this condition.
a. Conduction
b. Convection
c. Evaporation
d. Radiation

Ans. **(c) Evaporation**

It occurs when sweat is produced by the sweat glands and comes into contact with the skin's surface. As the sweat evaporates, it absorbs heat from the body, leading to cooling.

Clinical Corner

CASE SCENARIO 7:

A client brought to the emergency with the complaint of abdominal pain. Nurse Linda recorded vital signs of the client. What phase of nursing process is done by the nurse here?
a. Assessment
b. Planning
c. Implementation
d. Evaluation

Ans. **(a) Assessment**

Monitoring vital sign helps to obtain information related to client. So this is considered as assessment of the client.

Mechanism of heat loss	Description
Conduction	Heat loss from one object to another through direct contact **Application**: Applying several layers of clothes or woollen clothes (hard conductor) helps to reduce this type of heat loss. E.g., while touching a cold object, we lose heat from body to the object. Hot application, cold application.
Convection	Heat transferred from the body to the surrounding air that is in movement (circulation). E.g., fan promotes convectional heat loss
Evaporation	Heat loss occurs when liquid is converted to vapor. E.g., sweating
Radiation	Transfer of heat from object to another without any physical/direct contact between two. E.g., loss of body heat in the cold environment.

Temperature normal level:
- **Normal oral:** 37°C (98.6°F)
- **Normal rectal:** 37.5°C (99.5°F), which is 0.5°–1°F (0.3°–0.6°C) higher than the oral temperature.
- **Normal axillary:** 36.5°C (97.7°F), which is 0.5°–1°F (0.3°–0.6°C) lower than the oral temperature.

Conversion from Celsius (°C) to Fahrenheit (°F)
- **The formula is** (°C × 9/5) + 32 = °F or (°F – 32) × 5/9 = °C
- Let us convert 37°C to Fahrenheit
  37°C × 9/5 + 32 = 98.6°F
- Let us convert 98.6°F to Celsius
  (98.6°F – 32) × 5/9 = 37°C

Thermometers

Thermometers are the instruments used to measure the temperature.

Table 13: Different types of thermometer along with their pictures

Name of the thermometer	Picture
Glass thermometer Or Mercuric thermometer	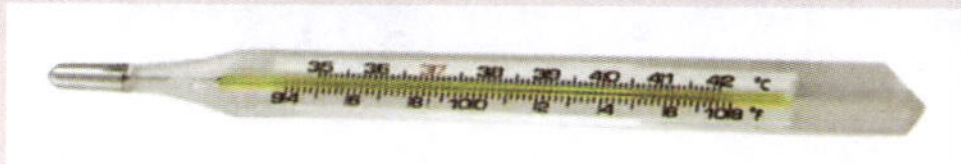
Electronic thermometer	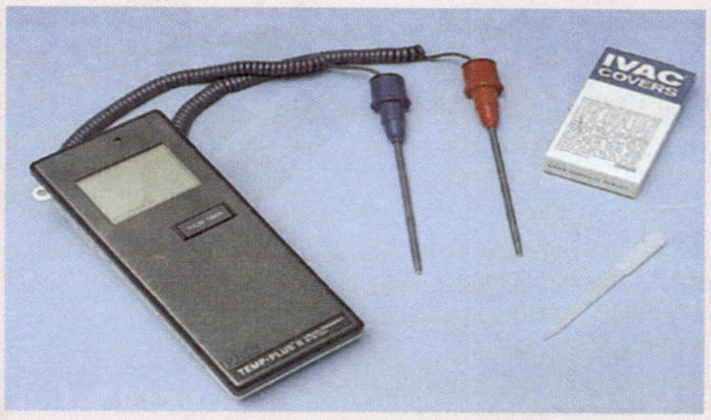
Digital thermometer	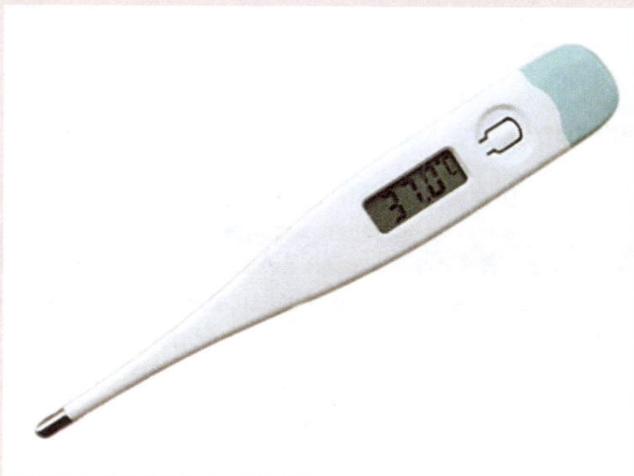

Contd...

Recent Question (NORCET 2023)

2. **Identify the steps of urinary catheterization to a female client?**
   a. Clean the site with betadine - apply lubricant on tip of catheter - Insert catheter - check for urine - inflate the balloon
   b. Apply lubricant on tip of catheter - clean the site with betadine - insert catheter - inflate the balloon - check for urine
   c. Clean the site with betadine - apply lubricant on tip of catheter - insert catheter - inflate balloon - check for urine
   d. Insert Catheter---Clean the site with betadine----Apply lubricant on the tip of catheter----Check urine---- Inflate balloon.

Ans. (a) Clean the site ...

Recent Questions (NORCET 2021)

3. **A nurse measures the temperature of the child as 38.2°C. What will be his temperature in Fahrenheit?**
   a. 101.4°F
   b. 102.6°F
   c. 100.7°F
   d. 99.8°F

Ans. (c) 100.7°F
To convert Celsius to Fahrenheit, you can use the following formula:
°F = (°C * 9/5) + 32
So, 38.2°C * 9/5 + 32 = 100.7°F.

4. **A patient complains of pain, HR 76 beats/min, RR 24/min, BP 90 mm Hg, temp. 37.6 degree. What is the 5th vital sign?**
   a. RR
   b. HR
   c. BP
   d. Pain

Ans. (d) Pain

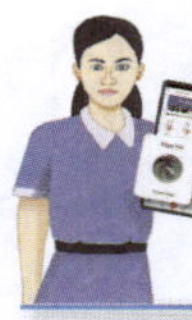

Name of the thermometer	Picture
Tympanic thermometer **Note:** Cerumen (ear wax) impaction can affect tympanic temperature values by as much as 0.3°F lower than the unobstructed ear.	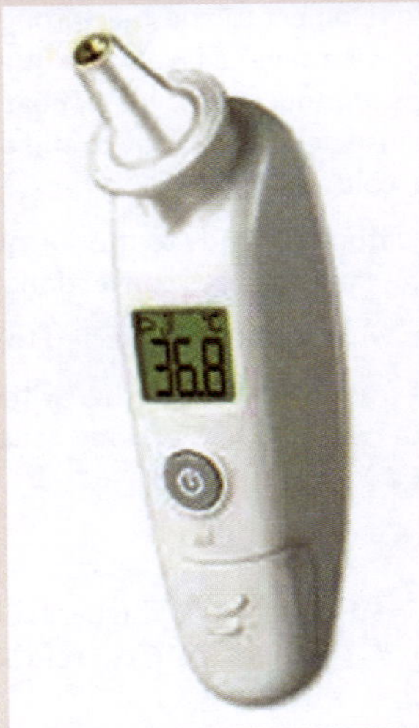
Non-contact digital infrared thermometer (Forehead thermometer) **Note:** To use forehead thermometer, the environmental temperature should be between 60.8-104°F (16-40°C) and relative humidity below 85%.	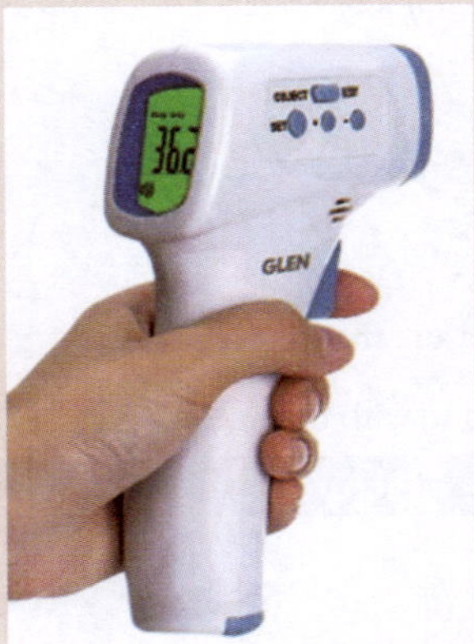
Disposable thermometer strip **Note:** • Have patient open mouth and place the grid end of the thermometer far back in mouth under tongue. • After at least 60 seconds has elapsed, remove thermometer from patient's mouth.	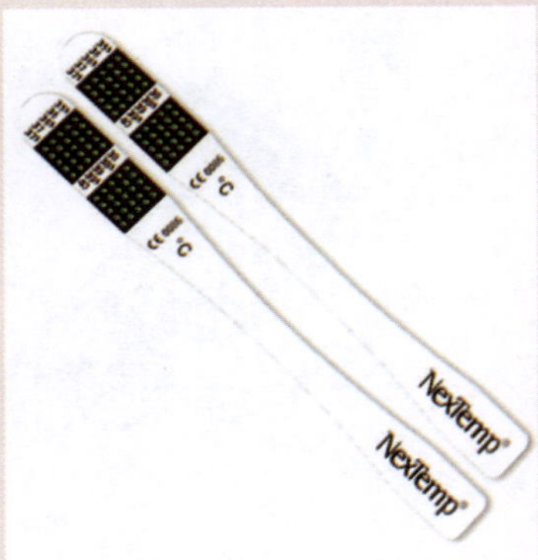

Methods for Measuring Temperature

Table 14: Methods for measuring temperature along with advantages and disadvantages

Method	Advantages	Disadvantages
Oral	Easily can be done in conscious, alert and cooperative patient.	• Not usable for child <5 years. • Recent consumption of hot and cold items alters the measurement. • Oral surgery and trauma are contraindications.
Rectal	Can be done easily in children and unconscious patient.	Hemorrhoids, rectal surgery and fistula are the contraindications.

Contd...

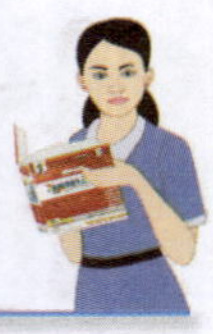

Clinical Corner

CASE SCENARIO 8:

You went into the patient's room to monitor the patient vital signs, and noticed that the patient is holding a hot cup of coffee in his hand. You informed the patient that you have to monitor his body temperature. Patient replied, "Ok! Sure, I have almost finished my coffee". Select the most appropriate response made by the nurse in this situation?

a. The nurse waits for 30 minutes then after that monitor the oral body temperature.

b. The nurse will ask the patient to gargle his mouth with water and apply the thermometer.

c. The nurse will check the other vital sign first then check the oral temperature.

d. The nurse will inform the patient that the temperature will be checked in next shift.

Ans. (a) The nurse waits for 30 minutes then after that monitor the oral body temperature.

To obtain a reliable body temperature measurement, it is necessary to wait until the patient's oral cavity has cooled down from the hot coffee. Waiting for approximately 30 minutes allows sufficient time for the mouth to return to a normal temperature before taking the oral temperature.

Method	Advantages	Disadvantages
Axillary	• Most preferable, easy and **commonly used** method. • Can be used in young children and older adult.	• Long duration of measurement. • Does not reflect core body temperature.
Tympanic membrane	• Sensitive to core body temperature • Rapid measurement	• If hearing aid is there, that needs to be removed. • Ear wax needs to be removed. • Ear surgery is the contraindication.
Noncontact digital infrared thermometer (Forehead thermometer)	• Convenient, safe and accurate. • No direct contact. • Rapid assessment.	If the person's forehead is sweaty, dirty, or covered in hair, the thermometer may not provide accurate readings.

Points to Remember While Taking Temperature

- In case of oral temperature, it can be measured 20-30 minutes after taking anything hot or cold.
- While checking oral temperature, thermometer needs to be placed in the sublingual pocket.
- While taking tympanic temperature, ear pinna needs to be held.
  - **Downward and backward** in children less than 3 years and
  - **Upward and backward** among children more than 3 years.
- Before taking temperature – Clean thermometer from bulb to stem
- After taking temperature—Clean from stem to bulb.
- Glass thermometer is indicated only in patients who are alert and cooperative and can understand instructions and can hold thermometer in the mouth.
- For taking rectal temperature, client needs to be positioned in Sim's position
- While taking rectal temperature, insert thermometer **2.5–3.5 cm (1–1.5 inch) beyond anal sphincter.**

Fever

Body temperature above normal is known as fever or hyperthermia.

Types of Fever

Table 15: Types of fever along with its description and conditions

Types of fever	Description	Conditions seen in (examples)
Low-grade fever	Temperature between 37.1°–38.2°C (98.8°–100.8°F) and lasts for more than 24 hours	Tuberculosis
High-grade fever	Temperature above 38.2°C (100.8 °F)	Influenza
Hyperpyrexia	Temperature above 40°C (above 104°F)	Heat stroke
Sustained fever	Body temperature remains constantly above 38°C (100.4°F) with minimal fluctuation	Typhoid fever
Intermittent fever	Fever is present and body temperature reaches normal at least once in 24 hours	Malaria, kala-azar, pyemia, septicemia
Remittent fever	Continuous fever and fever spikes and falls are there, but temperature never reaches to the normal level	Typhoid infection, infective endocarditis
Relapsing fever	Fever episodes are separated by intervals of normal temperature for days or weeks	Borrelia infections
Inverse fever	Characterized by temperature rise in the early morning rather than in the evening	
Crisis	Sudden return of temperature to the normal range from a very high temperature	Bacterial endocarditis

Contd...

KEY POINTS

- The rectal route is the most accurate for assessing core temperature.
- Body temperature of a healthy person is higher in the evening than in the morning.
- The range of marking in glass/clinical thermometer is **95°–110°F and 35°–43.3°C**.
- Best site for assessment of temperature in children is **Axilla.**
- Tympanic temperature = Oral temperature.

KEY POINTS

- **Wait 30 minutes** if patient ingested hot or cold food before taking an oral temperature.
- **Rectal temperature** taking is considered to be very accurate, but it is inconvenient and unpleasant for patients.
- **Rectal temperature** taking is contraindicated for patients with Myocardial Infarction.

POINT TO REMEMBER

With **intermittent fever**, the temperature is elevated but falls to normal (37.2°C or below) each day, while in a **remittent fever**, the temperature falls each day but not to normal.

POINT TO REMEMBER

Infant Radiant warmer warms by **IR energy**. The IR energy is absorbed by the infant's skin and blood flow in the skin transfers heat to rest of the body through **convection method**.

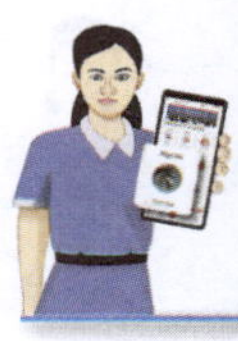

Types of fever	Description	Conditions seen in (examples)
Lysis	Temperature falls in a zigzag manner (step-ladder pattern) for days or week before reaching the normal temperature	Viral infections
Continuous fever	Also known as constant fever in which temperature variation is not more than 2°C between morning and evening and the temperature does not reach the normal	Urinary tract infections
Rigor	Sudden rise in body temperature along with shivering	Malaria

Heat Stroke

- Body temperature above 40° C along with hot dry skin, delirium, convulsion and coma.
- Signs and symptoms: giddiness, confusion, coma, muscle cramps, visual disturbance, thirst, nausea, increased body temperature, tachycardia, hypotension.
- **Management**: Rapid cooling , moving patient to a cooler environment, remove excess of clothes, use fan, irrigating stomach and lower bowel with cool solutions, hypothermic blankets.

Heat Exhaustion

- Heat exhaustion is a condition when there is profuse diaphoresis, and excessive electrolyte loss occurs.
- **Management**: Transporting victim to a colder environment and replace fluid and electrolyte.

Frostbite

- When body is exposed to subnormal temperature, ice crystals form inside the cells. Fingertip, ear lobe, nose, fingers and toes are susceptible to this condition.
- **Management**: gradual rewarming, analgesics, protection of inured body part.

Pulse

Pulse is the palpable bounding blood flow felt on blood vessels due to the contraction of left ventricle. Normal pulse rate is 60–100 beats/ min.

Sites for Monitoring Pulse

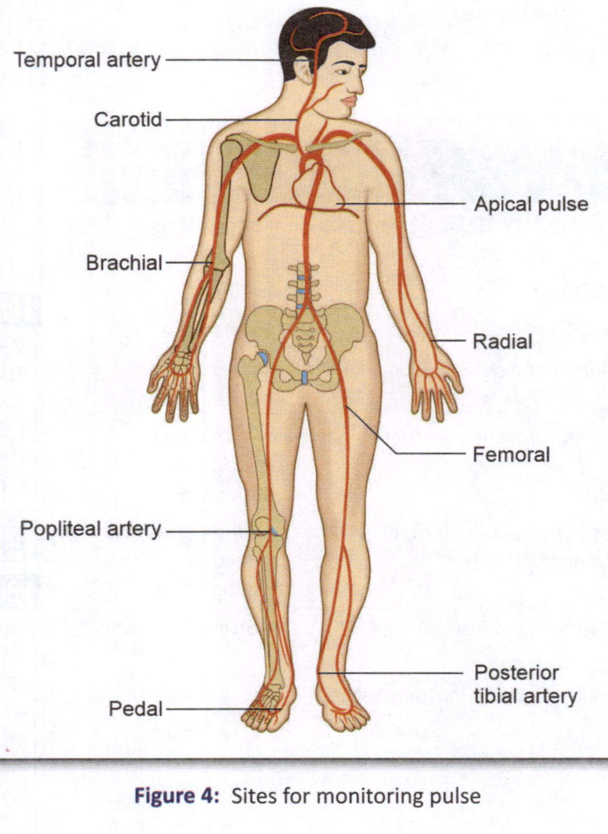

Figure 4: Sites for monitoring pulse

Clinical Corner

CASE SCENARIO 9:
You have received a patient in the ED. The assessment findings are: increased body temperature, hot, dry erythemic skin and no visible perspiration. The pulse rate is rapidly increasing and then slows down as the blood pressure falls. The patient complains of dry mouth nausea and vomiting. Identify the possible cause on the basis of assessment findings?

a. Hypothermia
b. Relapse Fever
c. Heat stroke
d. Heat exhaustion

Ans. (c) Heat stroke

Heat stroke is a life-threatening condition that occurs when the body's temperature rises to dangerously high levels. The assessment findings in the question are consistent with heat stroke.

POINTS TO REMEMBER

- While checking pulse, use fingertips of middle and index finger or middle three fingers of hands. Fingertips are most sensitive part.
- **Never use thumb** for checking pulse as it has **its own pulsation** which may interfere with the checking.
- Apical pulse is checked with the help of a **stethoscope.** It can be measured in the 5th intercostal space at the left midclavicular line.
- **Never measure simultaneously** carotid pulse on both sides as it impairs the blood flow to the brain.

Variations in Pulse

- **Tachycardia**: heart rate above 100 bpm
- **Bradycardia**: heart rate below 60 bpm.
- **Arrhythmia**: An irregular heartbeat or rhythm
- **Pulse deficit:** difference between apical pulse and radial pulse. To assess these, 2 people simultaneously assess radial pulse and apical pulse and then compare the rate. Pulse deficit is often **associated with abnormal rhythms.**
- **Water hammer pulse/ Corrigan pulse**: Condition caused by **aortic regurgitation** that results in a rapid and forceful pulse **resembling the sound of a water hammer.**
- **Paradoxical pulse:** A decrease in systolic blood pressure during inspiration greater than 10 mm Hg, often accompanied by a decrease in pulse strength or amplitude. It is seen in pericardial tamponade, constrictive pericarditis, severe obstructive lung disease.

Respirations

- Respirations is the exchange of gas between atmosphere and blood.
- Respiration mainly includes three processes: **ventilation, diffusion, and perfusion.**
- Inspiration is an active process.
- Expiration is a passive process.
- The respiratory center is located in the medulla oblongata and pons, in the brainstem.
- The most important factor in controlling the respiration is the **CO_2 in the arterial blood.** If CO_2 increases, rate and depth of respiration increase and vice versa.
- **Capnography**: It is the measurement of CO_2 in the exhaled air throughout the exhalation.
- **Eupnea**: Normal breathing pattern.
- **Normal respiratory rate:** 12–20 breaths/min.

KEY POINTS

- Apical pulse is measured with the help of stethoscope in the fifth intercostal space at left midclavicular line.
- Suitable site to check pulse in newborn is **Apical Pulse.**
- When a pulse rate is irregular, it is best to count the Apical pulse for a full minute.

Mechanism of Respiration

Table 16: Mechanism of respiration

Mechanism	Inspiration	Expiration
Diaphragm (*primary muscle responsible for inspiration*)	Contracts	Relax
External Intercostal muscles	Contracts	Relax (passive)
Abdominal organ	Moves downward and forward	Moves upward and back to position
Volume of chest cavity	Increases	Decreases
Pressure in the lung	Less as compared to atmospheric pressure	More as compared to atmospheric pressure

KEY POINTS

- The sequence of vital signs assessment in newborn is **R**espiratory Rate, **P**ulse and **T**emperature.
- Always count pulse for one full minute.
- **Normal respiratory rate adult:** 12–18 bpm.
- Paradoxical respiration is seen in flail chest due to **Blunt Chest Trauma.**

Abnormality in Respiration

- **Tachypnea:** Respiratory rate >20 breaths/min. Regular rapid breathing can be seen in this.
- **Bradypnea**: Respiratory rate <12 breaths/min. Regular slow breathing can be seen in this.
- **Dyspnea:** Difficulty in breathing or labored breathing.
- **Apnea:** Cessation of breathing for >20 seconds.
- **Hyperpnea:** It is increased depth of breathing when required to meet metabolic demand of body tissues, such as during or after exercise, or when the body lacks oxygen (hypoxia), for instance on high altitude or as a result of anemia.
- **Orthopnea:** Patient can breathe only in upright position. Shortness of breath (dyspnea) occurs while lying flat.
- **Hyperventilation:** Hyperventilation is rapid or deep breathing that can occur with anxiety or panic. It is also called overbreathing.
- **Hypoventilation:** The state in which a reduced amount of air enters the alveoli in the lungs, resulting in decreased levels of oxygen and increased levels of carbon dioxide in the blood.
- **Hypoxia:** Decreased amount of oxygen in the tissues
- **Hypoxemia:** Decreased amount of oxygen in the arterial blood.
- **Cheyne-Stokes respiration**: Respiratory cycle begins as slow shallow respiration which gradually increases to abnormal rate and depth (hyperventilation) then again becomes slow and shallow followed by apnea.
- **Kussmaul's respiration:** Respirations are abnormally deep, regular and with increased rate. It is also known as fruity acetone breath. It is often associated with severe metabolic acidosis.
- **Biot's respiration:** Respirations are abnormally shallow for two to three breaths, followed by periods of apnea. Seen in patients with increased intracranial pressure, associated with spinal meningitis and other central nervous system disorders.

Recent Questions (NORCET 2021)

5. Normal respiration in adults is:

a. 8 beats/min
b. 10 beats/min
c. 14 beats/min
d. 30 beats/min

Ans. (c) 14 beats/min

6. A patient has a respiratory rate of 36/min, this condition is known as:

a. Eupnea
b. Dyspnea
c. Bradypnea
d. Tachypnea

Ans. (d) Tachypnea

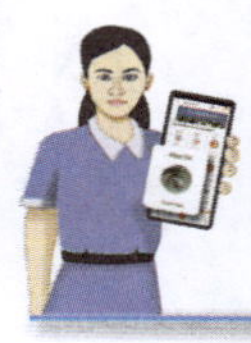

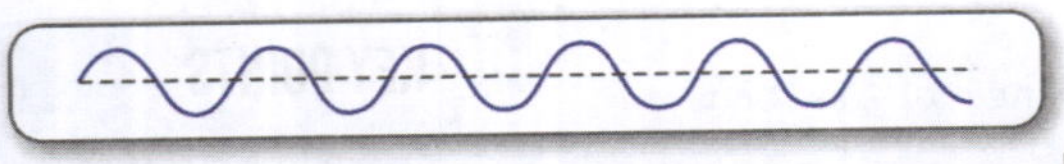

Eupnea (Normal Breathing, regular rate and Depth)

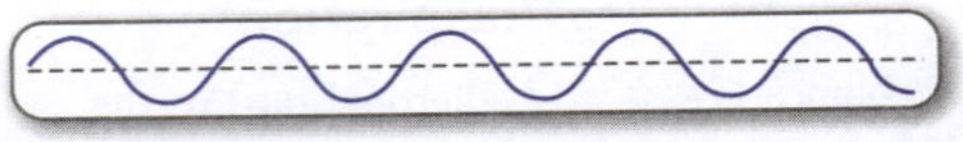

Bradypnea (Slow rate and shallow breath)
Causes: Medications, cardiovascular disorders, CNS depression)

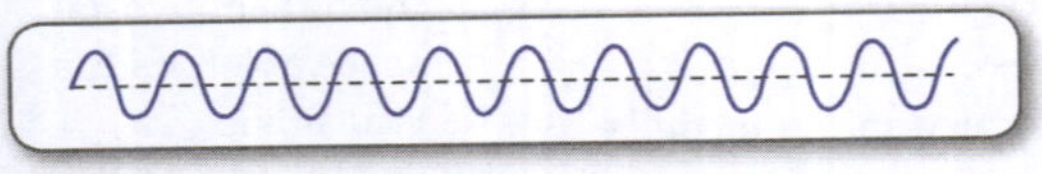

Tachypnea (Fast rate and shallow breath)
Causes: Stress, anxiety, exercise, cardiac diseases, respiratory infections)

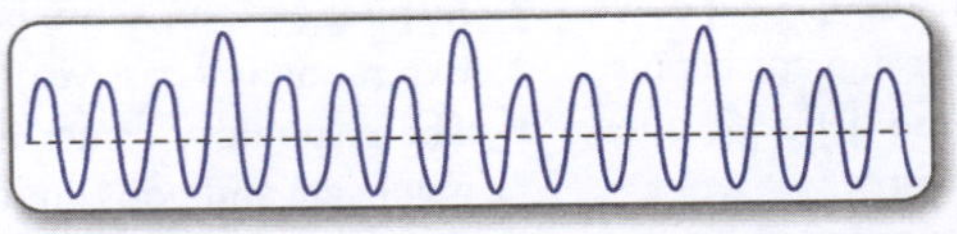

Sighing (frequent sighs interspersed with regular breathing)
Causes: Dyspnea, anxiety, respiratory disorders

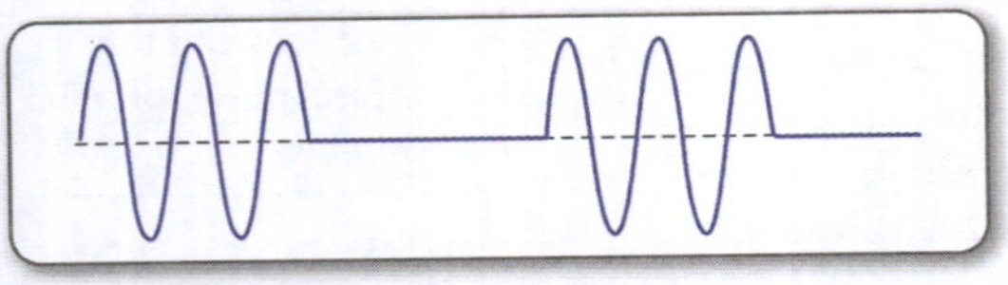

Biot's respiration [Deep breathing with periods of sudden pauses)
Causes: Meningitis, brainstem damage, head injury

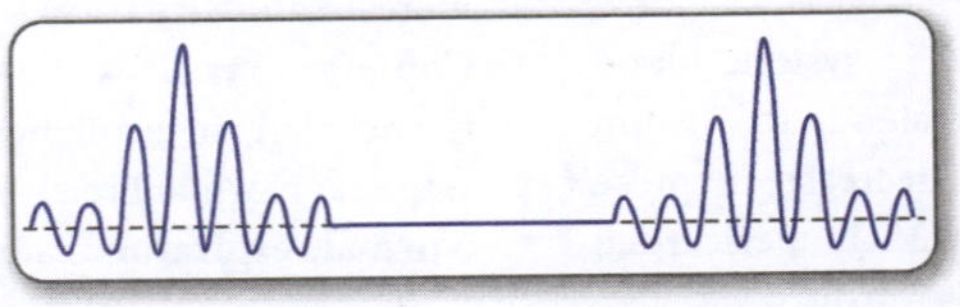

Cheyne-Stokes (cycles of varying depth and rate of breathing)
Causes: Stroke, traumatic brain injury, brain tumors, decompensated congestive heart failure

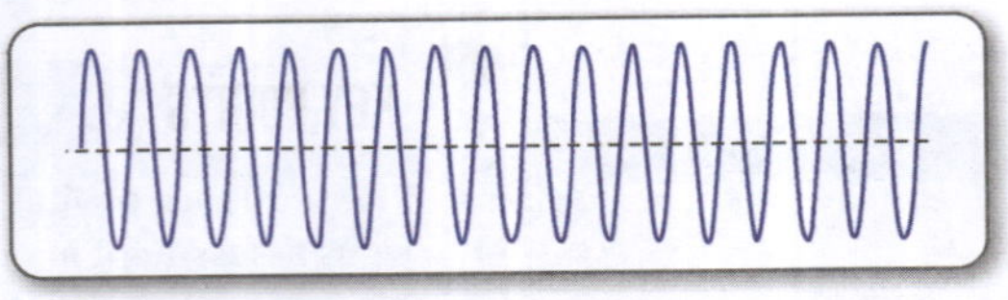

Kussmaul's respiration [Fast and deep breath]
Causes: Diabetic ketoacidosis (DKA), kidney failure

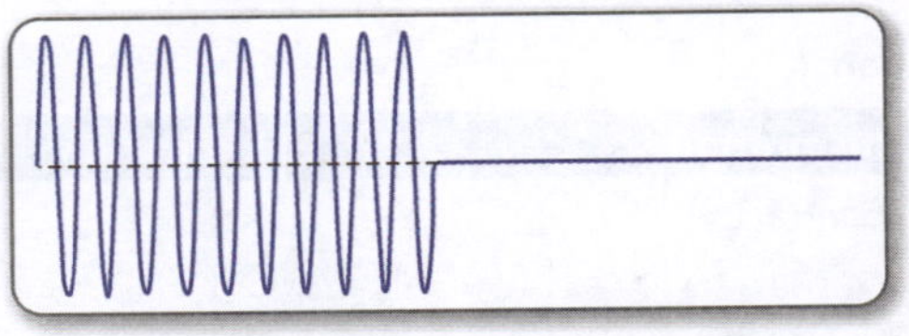

Central sleep apnea [Apnea during sleep]
Causes: Heart failure, kidney failure

Blood Pressure

- Blood pressure is the force exerted by the blood against the wall of the artery.
- **Systolic blood pressure (SBP):** Maximum pressure exerted by blood on the blood vessel during left ventricular contraction (ejection).
- **Diastolic blood pressure (DBP):** Pressure exerted by blood on the wall of the artery during diastole (resting and filling) of the heart.
- **Pulse pressure:** Difference between systolic and diastolic pressure. Normal range is 30-50 mm Hg.
- While measuring BP, the sounds heard are known as Korotkoff sounds.
- **Normal blood pressure:** 120/80 mm Hg.

Factors Affecting BP

- BP increases
  - As the cardiac output increases
  - As the peripheral vascular resistance increases
  - As the viscosity or hematocrit increases
  - As the elasticity of blood vessel **decreases**
  - When smoking
  - During stress and anxiety
  - During acute pain
- After puberty, males tend to have higher BP than females of similar age.
- After menopause, females tend to have higher BP than males of similar age.

Abnormal BP

Table 17: Abnormal BP

Blood pressure category	SBP (mm Hg)		DBP (mm Hg)
NORMAL	<120	and	<80
Elevated BP	120–129	and	<80
Hypertension Stage–I	130–139	or	80–89
Hypertension Stage–II	≥140	or	>90
Hypertensive Crisis	>180	and/or	>120

Ref: American Heart Association

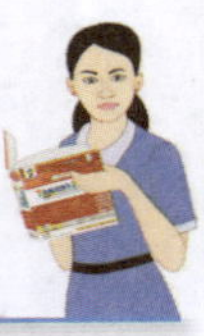

Recent Question
(NORCET 2021 & 22)

7. Difference between systolic and diastolic blood pressure is called:
a. Pulse pressure
b. Pulse deficit
c. Auscultatory gap
d. Korotkoff sounds

Ans. (a) Pulse pressure

Recent Question
(NORCET 2022)

8. A person has a central venous catheter in place. Which of the following data can be assessed with this?
a. Central venous pressure
b. Blood pressure
c. Urine output
d. Pulse pressure

Ans. (a) Central venous pressure

(NORCET 2023)

Normal Blood pressure of an adult: 120/80

Clinical Corner

CASE SCENARIO 10:
Nursing student was taking BP of a client admitted in general ward. Student selected large cuff for the client. What finding should be expected by the instructor?
a. Falsely high
b. Falsely low
c. Correct reading
d. It can be high or low

Ans. (b) Falsely low

The width of the bladder of the blood pressure cuff should be approximately 40% of the circumference of the upper arm midway between the olecranon and the acromion. The length of the bladder of the cuff should encircle 80–100% of the circumference of the upper arm at the same position. If the cough is large, it will give falsely low reading and a small cough will give falsely high BP value.

- **Orthostatic hypotension:**
  - It is also known as postural hypotension.
  - It refers to a sudden drop in blood pressure when a person changes from lying down to sitting or standing up position.
  - It is diagnosed when SBP falls 20 mm Hg or more, or DBP falls 10 mm Hg or more within 3 minutes of position change.

Blood Pressure Equipment

Table 18: Blood pressure equipment

Equipment	Picture
Sphygmomanometer	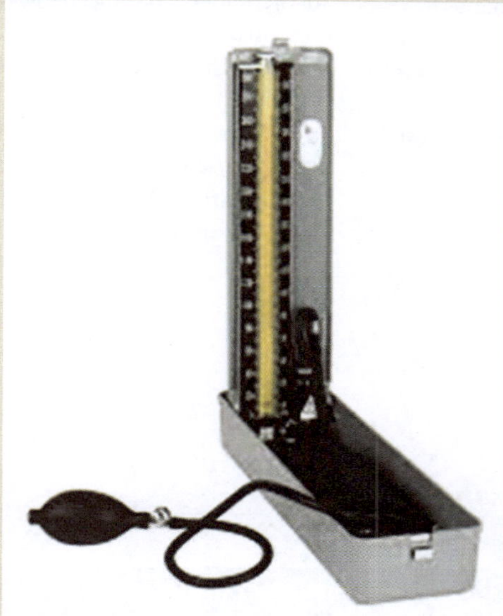
Aneroid manometer	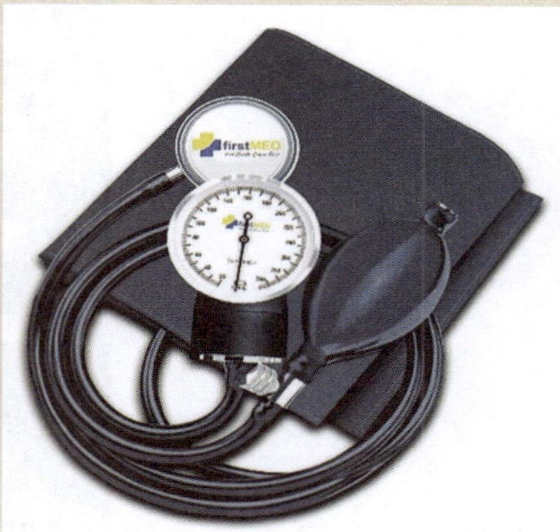
Electronic BP device	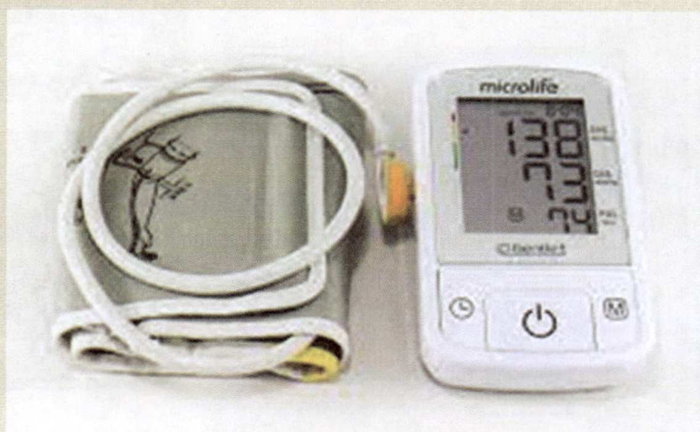

POINTS TO REMEMBER

- Width of the BP cuff is 40% of arm circumference and length of the bladder within the cuff should encircle 80–100% of the circumference of upper arm.
- While measuring BP, make sure that client has not ingested caffeine or smoked 20–30 minutes before as it increases reading.
- **Use appropriate size cuff.** *Small sized cuff* results in Falsely high BP reading and **large sized cuff** results in Falsely low BP reading.
- While measuring BP, place the arm of the patient at the level of heart. Placing arm above the level of heart causes falsely low BP reading.
- Remove constrictive clothing while checking BP as it causes elevated BP reading.

TECHNIQUES OF PHYSICAL EXAMINATION

- **Inspection**: Visual examination of the client or systematic observation of different body parts to collect data regarding health status of the client.
- **Palpation:** The act of feeling with the hand; application of the fingers with light pressure on the surface of the body for the purpose of determining the conditions of the parts beneath. Bimanual palpation refers to palpation with both hands.
- **Percussion:** It is the tapping over body parts and listening to the sound produced to assess the condition of the organs. Sounds produced during percussion include tympany, hyper-resonant, resonant, dull and flat.

Sound	Organ
Hyper-resonant	Hyper inflated lung tissue
Resonant	Normal lung tissue
Dull	Liver, Spleen
Flat	Bone
Tympany	Fluid filled organs such as bladder, stomach, intestine, etc.

- **Auscultation**: It is the technique of listening to the sounds produced by body organs using stethoscope.
  - **Bell** of the stethoscope is used to hear **low-pitched sound.**
  - **Diaphragm** of stethoscope is used to listen to **high-pitched sound.**
- **Manipulation:** It is the technique of assessing flexibility and movement of body parts.

POINTS TO REMEMBER

- The sequence/order of doing physical examination: Inspection, Palpation, Percussion and Auscultation
- In abdominal examination, the sequence is inspection, auscultation, percussion and palpation. Here, auscultation should be performed before percussion and palpation to avoid stimulating bowel activity, which could alter bowel sounds and frequency.
- While wearing gloves, first wear gloves in the **dominant hand.**

Instruments used for Physical Examination

Table 19: Instruments used for physical examination

Instruments	Purpose	Picture of the instrument
Ophthalmoscope	Examining the eyes	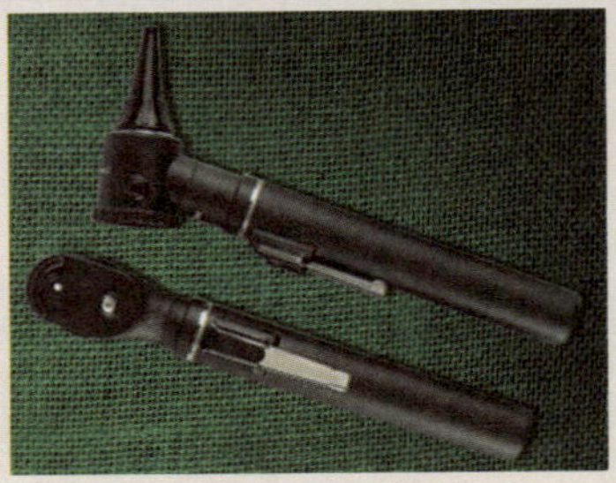
Otoscope	Examining ear	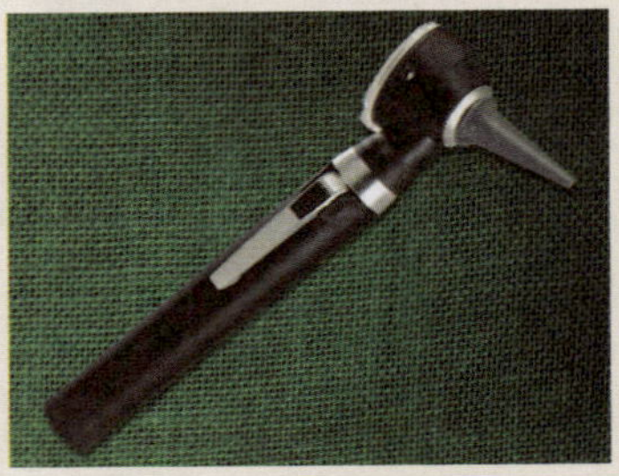
Stethoscope	Auscultation (listening to body sounds)	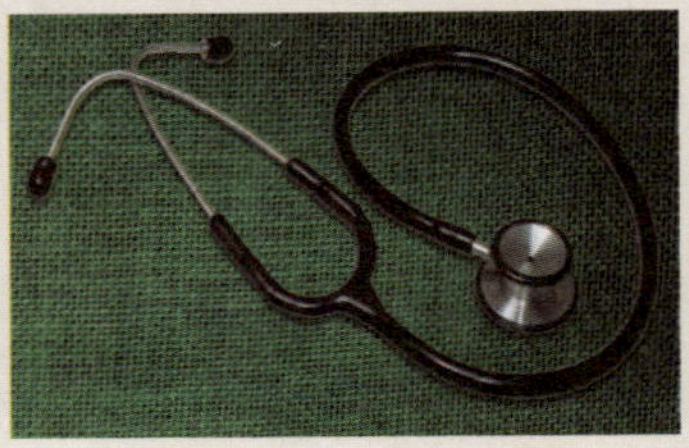

Contd...

Instruments	Purpose	Picture of the instrument
Sphygmomanometer	To measure BP	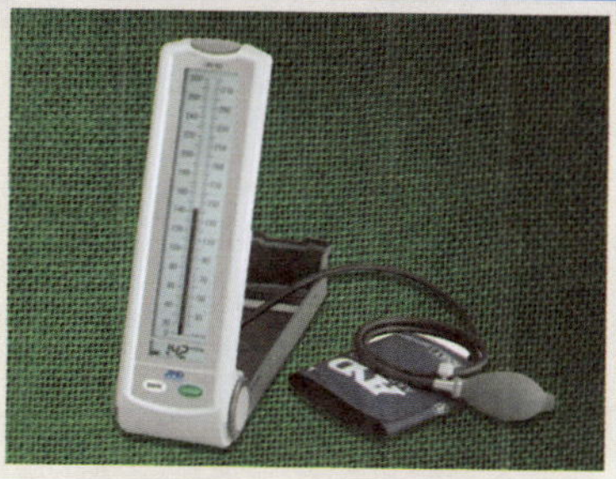
Thermometer	To measure the body temperature	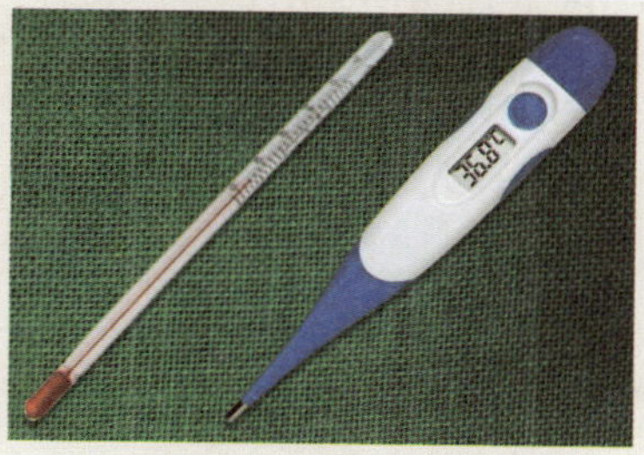
Urinometer	To measure the specific gravity of urine	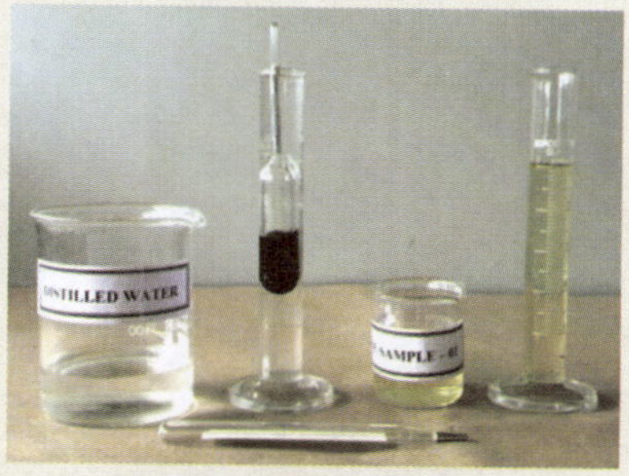
Glucometer	To measure the blood glucose level	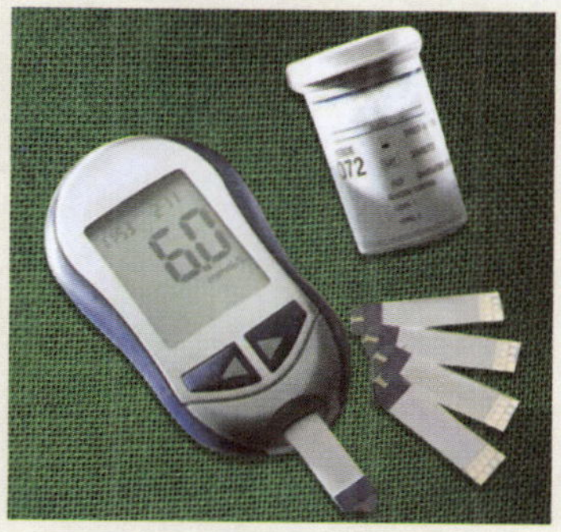
Snellen chart	To measure the visual acuity	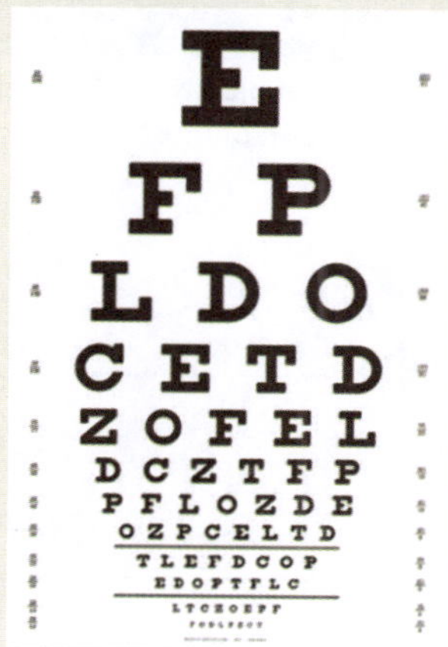

Contd...

Instruments	Purpose	Picture of the instrument
Tongue depressor	To examine the oral cavity, by suppressing the tongue	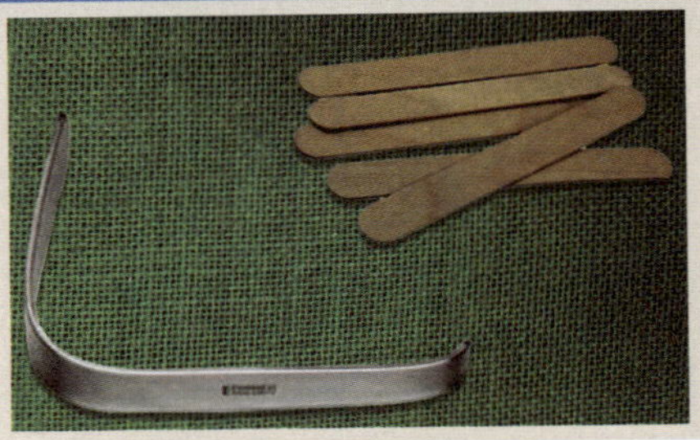
Laryngoscope	To visualize larynx	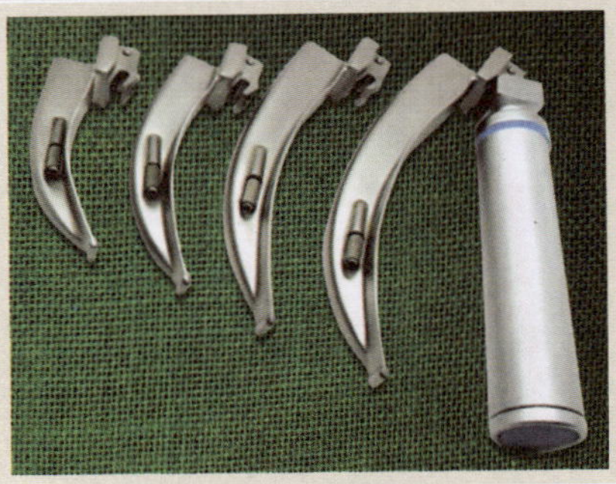
Nasal speculum	To examine the nasal cavity	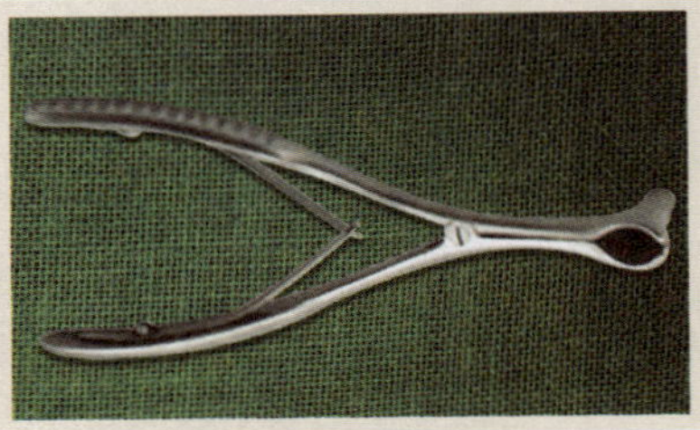
Percussion hammer	To check the reflexes	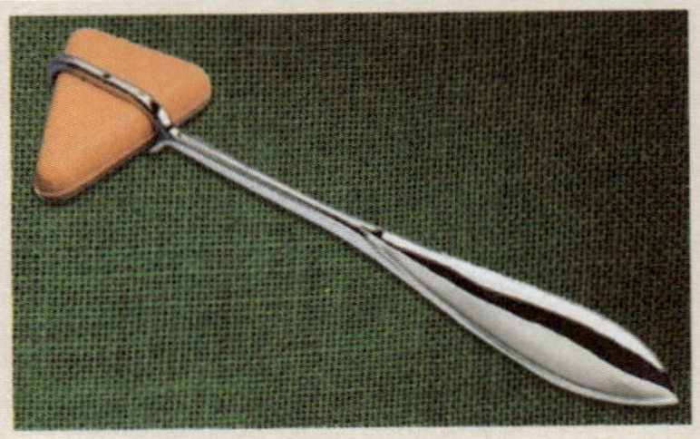

Reflexes

Table 20: Different types of reflexes

Name of the reflex	Response	Picture of procedure
Biceps reflex	Tapping of biceps tendon causes contraction of muscle.	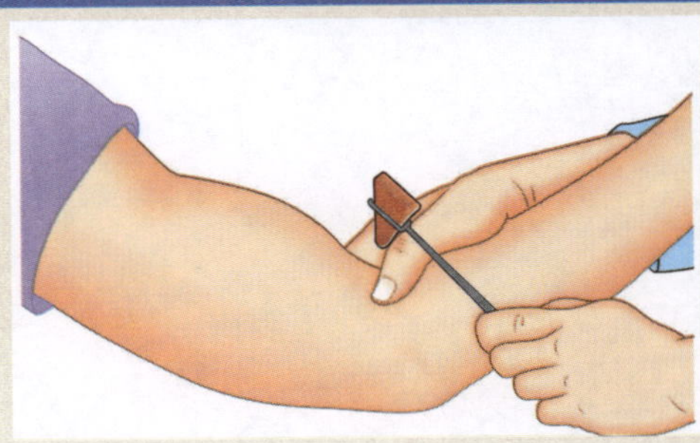

Contd...

Name of the reflex	Response	Picture of procedure
Triceps reflex	Tapping over olecranon process causes straightening of upper arm.	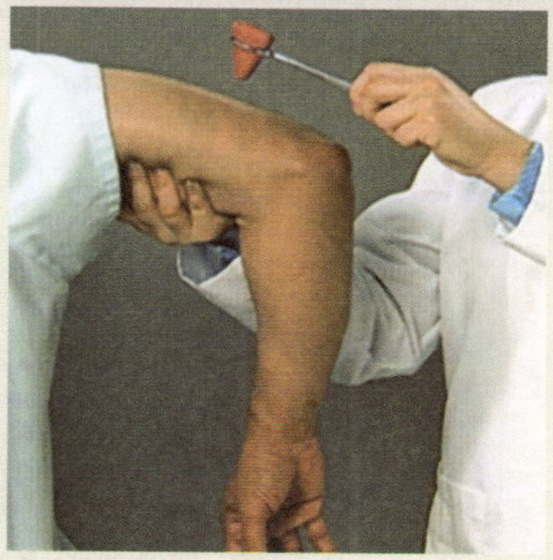
Patellar reflex	Tapping just below the knee (patella) causes forward kicking movement of leg.	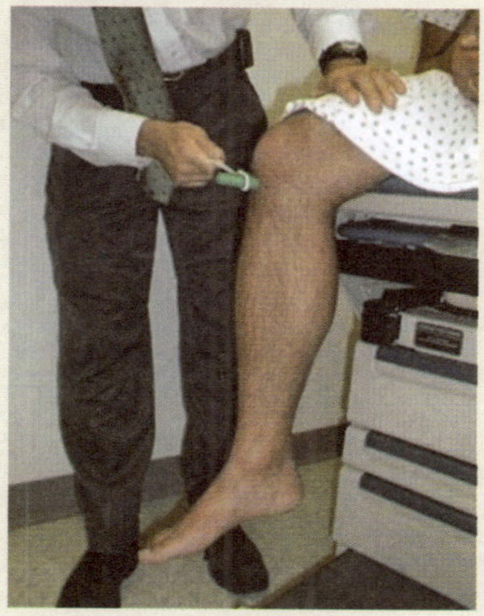
Achilles reflex	Tapping over the Achilles tendon causes downward jerky movement.	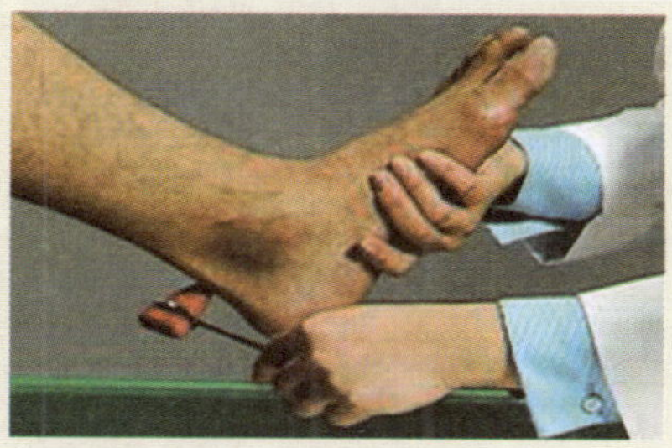
Plantar reflex (Babinski reflex)	Stroking over the sole causes toe to bend downward, it is negative Babinski and is normal for adult. But in children, stroking over the sole causes toe to move upward and outward, that is called positive Babinski and is normal for children up to 2 years of age. Positive Babinski is considered abnormal for adults.	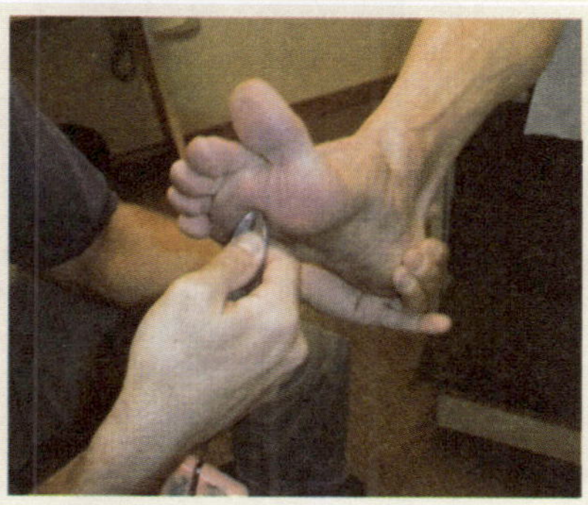

Romberg's Test/Romberg's Sign (for balance)

- In this test, ask the person to stand with feet together and eyes closed. If the patient is able to maintain the equilibrium, then test is normal. But if the person falls down, then Romberg's test is positive which means patient has balancing problem.

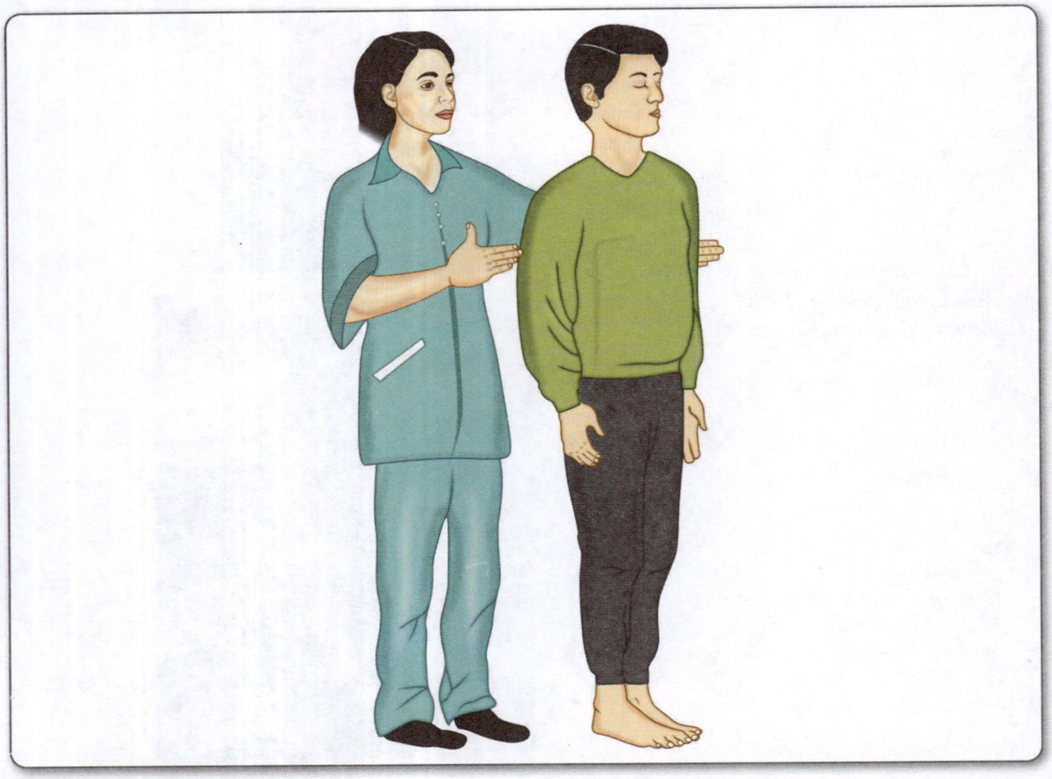

Figure 5: Romberg's test

TYPES OF NURSING MODALITIES

Primary Nursing

- Each nurse is assigned to a small group of patients.
- The nurse assumes 24-hour responsibility for each patient's total care continuously until discharge (even when the nurse is technically off duty).
- She may be assisted by an associate nurse, but the primary nurse is contacted, if needed.
- **Common use areas:** Hospice care and home health.

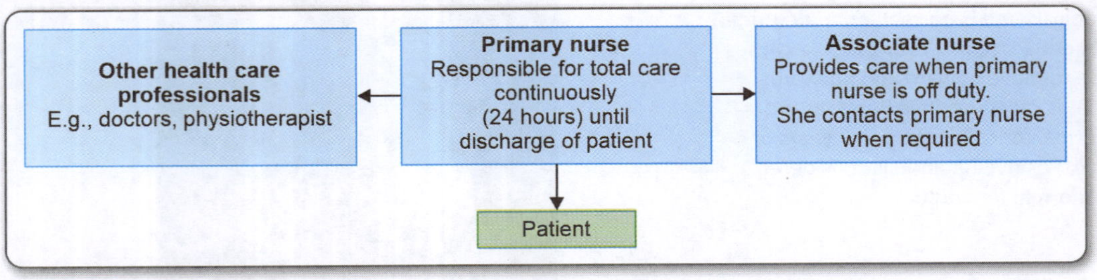

Figure 6: Primary nursing structure

POINT TO REMEMBER

Ensuring patient safety is the most important nursing intervention during Romberg's test. The nurse should stand close to the patient to prevent potential injury if the patient were to fall (as shown in Figure 2).

Clinical Corner

CASE SCENARIO 11:

Nurse Liza is performing abdominal assessment for a client with complaint of abdominal pain. Which among the following is correct?

a. Assess the quadrant of abdomen with pain first
b. Assess the quadrant of abdomen with pain at the last
c. Perform abdominal quadrant assessment from left to right
d. Any area of the abdomen can be assessed as per the convenience of nurse

Ans. (b) Assess the quadrant of abdomen with pain at the last

While performing abdominal examination, the nurse should systematically assess all areas of the abdomen. The symptomatic area of the abdomen should be examined at last. If symptomatic quadrant palpated first, it will elicit pain in the symptomatic area, causing the muscles in other areas to tighten. This would interfere with further assessment.

Team Nursing

- A head nurse or nurse manager supervises and coordinates a team of nurses.
- The nurse manager assigns a group of patients to an individual nurse [Registered Nurse (RN)].
- Each nurse is responsible for most of each patient's care. Some of the duties are assigned to other nurses or nursing assistants.
- Includes nurses at all levels of knowledge, i.e., Registered Nurses, Practical Nurses and Nursing Assistants.

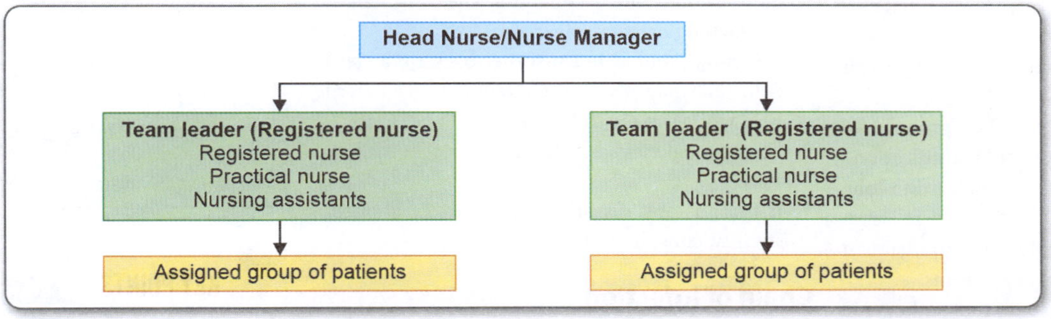

Figure 7: Structure of team nursing

Modular Nursing

- Modular nursing is a modification of team nursing.
- Patient unit is divided into modules (geographical area/unit) with an RN as team leader.
- The same team of caregivers is consistently assigned to same geographical area.

Functional Nursing

- Nurses are assigned a specific task and do only that duty.
- The nurse performs a particular task for every patient in the ward. For example, medication nurse, dressing nurse, IV nurse, etc.
- **Common use area:** Operation theater.

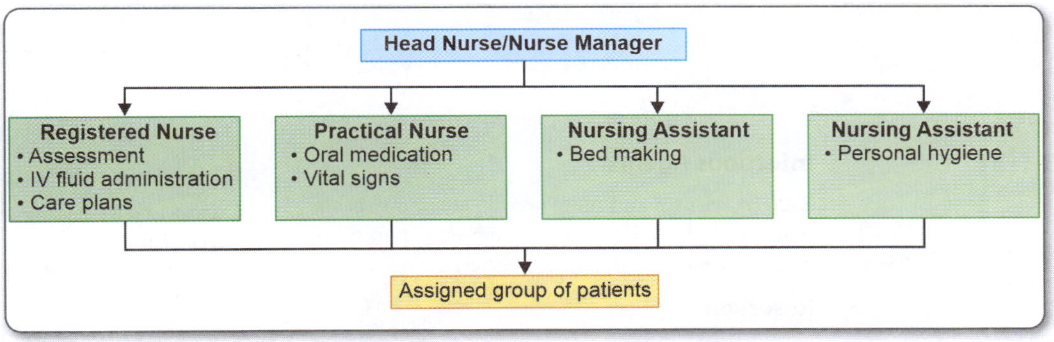

Figure 8: Structure of functional nursing

Nursing Case Management

- Role of nurse is a case manager.
- A registered nurse as case manager advocates, manages and coordinates care for patients.
- Applicable in clinics, hospitals and in community.

Private Duty Nursing

The nurse is responsible for the total care of one individual patient generally at home.

MEDICAL AND SURGICAL ASEPSIS-TERMINOLOGIES

- **Asepsis:** It refers to techniques used to prevent the growth and spread of harmful microorganisms in health care settings.
- **Medical asepsis: Reduction in the number** of disease-causing agents and their spread. Clean and dirty are the terms used to denote articles in medical asepsis. E.g., handwashing, barrier nursing, environmental cleaning, etc.

POINT TO REMEMBER

The team nursing model is similar to the functional nursing method, but provides care on a larger scale.

Clinical Corner

CASE SCENARIO 12:
Collaboration in providing care to a group of patients under the supervision of a professional nurse is referred to as:
OR
Nurse manager assigned responsibility of a group of patient to a team of nurses. This kind of patient care is known as:

a. Primary nursing
b. Functional nursing
c. Team nursing
d. Case method

Ans. (c) Team nursing

In team nursing, a group of nurses provide care to a group of fixed patients.

Primary nursing is one type of patient care delivery that requires a one-to-one relationship between an RN and the patient, with responsibility for planning and managing care clearly established.

Functional nursing is one in which the leader of the ward assigns different tasks to specific nurses based on the nursing care plans for different patients.

Case method is a useful strategy for helping the students learn how to analyse a case, identify problems and solutions, compare alternate decisions, and arrive at conclusions about different aspects of patient care.

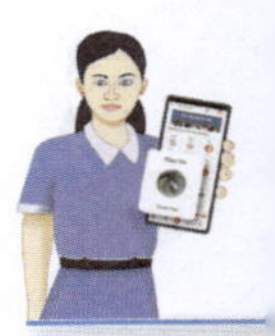

- **Surgical asepsis: Complete elimination** of disease-causing agents. Sterile is the term that denotes surgical asepsis.
- **Antiseptic:** The substance that is **applied to living tissue** or skin to reduce the possibility of infection, sepsis or putrefaction.
- **Disinfectant:** The substance that is **applied on non-living surfaces or objects** to eliminate or reduce the number of microorganisms.
- **Bacteriostat:** Substance which inhibits the growth of microorganisms.
- **Culture:** Used to promote the growth of microorganisms for the purpose of identification.
- **Cross infection:** Spread of infection from one person to another.
- **Carrier:** Person who carries microorganism without showing the signs and symptoms.
- **Disinfection:** Destroys most of the pathogenic organisms.
- **Concurrent disinfection:** All articles are disinfected immediately after use.
- **Terminal disinfection:** Articles are disinfected once the patient is discharged or death of the patient occurs.
- **Sterilization:** Killing microorganisms including spores is known as sterilization.

Isolation vs Quarantine

- **Isolation:** Refers to the separation of infected persons from a non-infected person for the period of communicability under conditions. This will prevent the transmission of infection to others.
- **Quarantine:** It is detention or isolation of a healthy person who has come in contact with an infectious disease for a period of time equal to the longest incubation period of that disease.

BASIC PRINCIPLES OF SURGICAL ASEPSIS

- Only a sterile object is used to touch another sterile object.
- While opening a sterile package, the first edge of the wrapper is to be projected away from the nurse to prevent the sterile surface touching unsterile clothing.
- The outer surface of the sterile package is considered contaminated.
- **One inch (2.5 cm)** of the outside edge of a sterile field is considered contaminated.
- A wet field is considered contaminated if the surface below (paper or cloth used as a field for sterile set up) is unsterile.
- Avoid spilling any solution/liquid on a paper or cloth used as a field for sterile set up. This will allow moisture to penetrate through the sterile cloth and carry microorganisms along.
- Sterile objects are to be held **above the level of waist.**
- To prevent contamination from droplet, the nurse should avoid coughing, sneezing, talking or reaching over a sterile field.
- The nurse should not turn her back on a sterile field that may result in contamination of sterile field while it is out of her view.
- Forceps soaked in disinfectant are not considered sterile.
- If there is any doubt about an object about its sterility, consider it unsterile.

Chain of Infection

Six components of infection cycle.

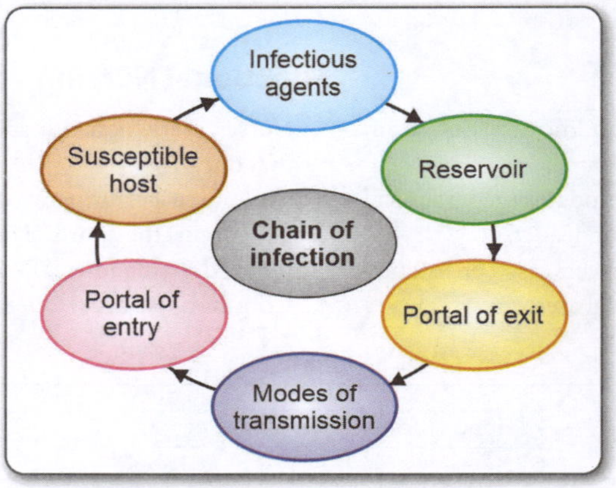

Figure 9: Chain of infection

Infectious Agents

Bacteria, viruses and fungi are the common agents that cause infections. Most common infection-causing agents in hospitals are bacteria.

Reservoir

The reservoir is a source of natural habitat of the microorganisms. Reservoirs of pathogenic organisms include humans, animals, food, water, milk and inanimate objects.

Portal of Exit

Portal of exit is the site from where the microorganisms leave the host (reservoir). Common portals of exit in humans include the respiratory (nose or mouth), gastrointestinal (feces), genitourinary tracts and breaks in the skin.

KEY POINTS

- **Quarantine duration** = upper range of the incubation period of the disease. (for individuals who have been exposed but are not yet sick)
- **Isolation duration** = Period of communicability. (for individuals who are already infected)

KEY POINTS

- **One inch (2.5 cm)** of the outside edge of a sterile field is considered contaminated.
- Sterile objects are to be held **above the level of waist.**
- The nurse **should not turn her back on a sterile field** that may result in contamination of sterile field

Practice Questions

5. Which of the following type of asepsis method eliminates all microorganisms?
a. Surgical asepsis
b. Medical asepsis
c. Both a and b
d. None of the above

Ans. (a) Surgical asepsis

6. The primary purpose of aseptic procedure is to:
a. Protect patients
b. Protect health care workers
c. Protect both patients and health care workers
d. None of the above

Ans. (c) Protect both patients and health care workers

Modes of Transmission

An organism can be transmitted from its reservoir through various modes of transmission.

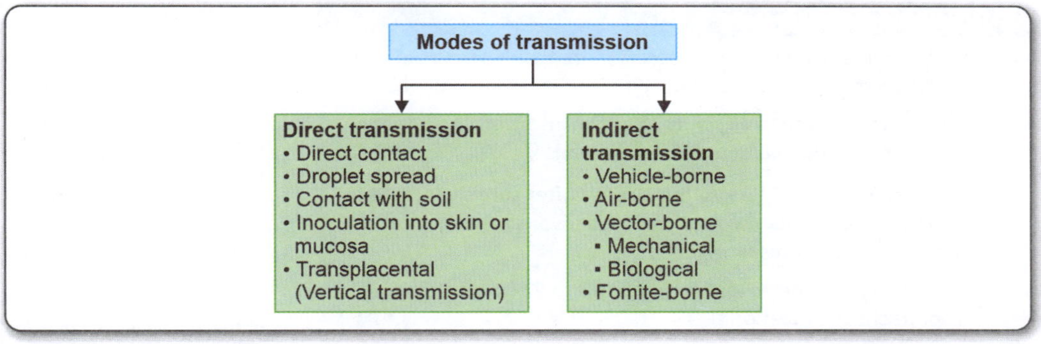

Figure 10: Modes of transmission

Portal of Entry

The portal of entry is the point from where the microorganisms enter the susceptible host. The point of entry is almost same as the point of exit. Pathogens enter the body through mucous membranes, skin, respiratory, gastrointestinal, urinary and reproductive tracts.

Susceptible Host

The person who is at risk of developing a disease from an infection is known as susceptible host. Factors that make the person more susceptible to infections include age (young and elderly), weakened immune system, malnutrition, certain medications and chronic illnesses.

STAGES OF INFECTION

Most infectious diseases have four stages:

1. **Incubation period:** Time from initial contact with infectious agent to first signs of symptoms.
2. **Prodromal stage:** Early signs and symptoms of the disease are present. Mild and generalized symptoms (fatigue, malaise, headache, and low-grade fever).
3. **Clinical stage/invasive stage/full stage of illness:** Signs and symptoms specific to the disease appear.
4. **Convalescent period:** Recovery period from the disease.

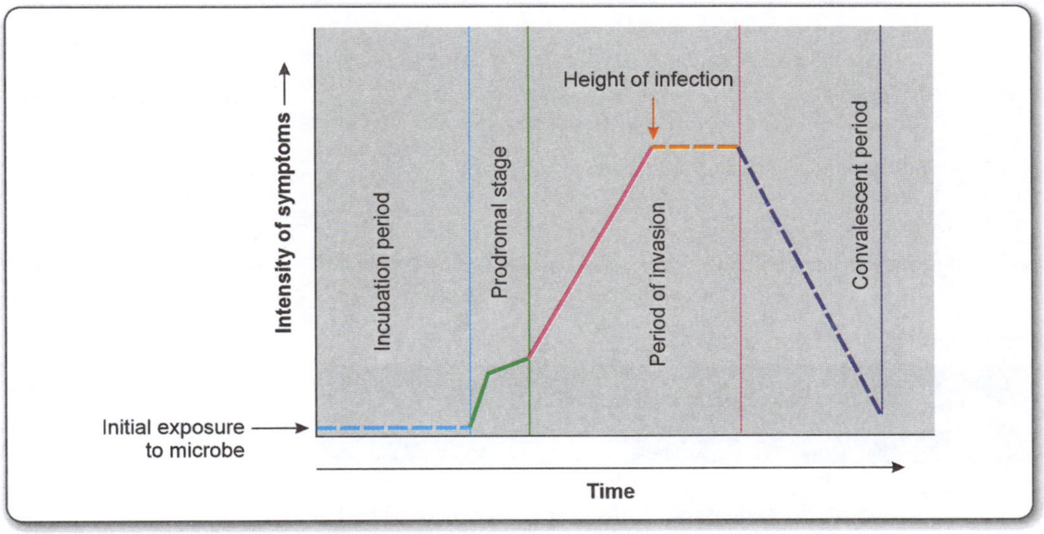

Figure 11: Stages of infection

Health Care-Associated Infections (HAIs)

- Hospital acquired infections are now commonly referred to as health care associated infections.
- HAIs are also known as health care acquired infections or nosocomial infections
- HAIs manifest **after 48 hours of hospital admission.**

KEY POINTS

- The chain of infection can be interrupted most readily at mode of transmission.
- Universal precautions are mandatory regulations enforced by Occupational Safety and Health Administration (OSHA) in all health care settings as part of its blood-borne pathogens standard.

Clinical Corner

CASE SCENARIO 13:

Nurse is caring for a client with diagnosis of MRSA. While caring for this client, nurse needs to understand that the type of isolation required for this client is:

a. Respiratory isolation
b. Contact isolation
c. No isolation needed
d. Reverse isolation

Ans. (b) Contact isolation

Use contact precautions when caring for patients with MRSA. Contact precautions mean whenever possible, patients with MRSA will have a single room or will share a room only with someone else who also has MRSA. Healthcare providers will put on gloves and wear a gown over their clothing while taking care of patients with MRSA. Visitors may also be asked to wear a gown and gloves. When leaving the room, hospital providers and visitors remove their gown and gloves and clean their hands. Patients on contact precautions are asked to stay in their hospital rooms as much as possible.

Types of HAIs

Table 21: Types of HAIs

Types of HAI	Time-related definition
Central line-associated bloodstream infection (CLABSI)	A bloodstream infection that occurs more than **48 hours after the insertion** of a central line or **within 48 hours of its removal.**
Cather-associated urinary tract infection (CAUTI)	UTI occurs more than **48 hours after the insertion** of a urinary catheter or **within 48 hours of its removal.**
Surgical site infection (SSI)	An infection that occurs **within 30 days after surgery** (or **within one year if an implant** was placed) and involves the surgical incision, deep tissues or organs.
Ventilator-associated pneumonia (VAP)	Pneumonia that develops **more than 48 to 72 hours** after endotracheal intubation
Hospital-acquired pneumonia (HAP)	Pneumonia that occurs **48 hours or more after admission** to the hospital and did not appear to be incubating at the time of admission

Iatrogenic Infection

Iatrogenic infection is the infection that occurs as a result of invasive, diagnostic or therapeutic procedure.

Prevention of Cross Infection in Hospital

- Handwashing (most important)
- Maintain good ventilation
- Maintain general cleanliness of hospital
- Safe food and water supply
- Safe disposal of excreta
- Destruction of microorganisms through disinfection and sterilization

Isolation/Barrier Nursing

Definition

- **Isolation nursing:** It is carried out by placing the patient in a single room.
- **Barrier nursing:** Nursing technique by which a patient with an infectious disease is prevented from infecting other people.

Table 22: Types of isolation and barrier techniques

Types of isolation	When it is required	Technique used
Respiratory isolation Droplet infection		Wear mask
Enteric isolation	Pathogens are transmitted via feces	Wear gloves and gown while handling soiled articles
Wound and skin isolation	Pathogens are present in wound and can be transmitted while coming in contact with the infected wound	Wear gown and gloves
Blood isolation	Pathogens are found and spread via blood	Wear gloves while coming in contact with blood

Table 23: Transmission-based precautions

Types of PPE	Modes of transmission			
	Contact	Droplet	Airborne	For Aerosol generating procedures
Mask 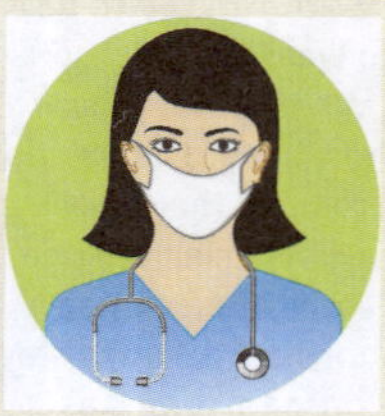	NO	YES	YES (N95 or equivalent or higher)	YES (N95 or equivalent or higher)

Contd...

Clinical Corner

CASE SCENARIO 14:

Nurse Ramya is working in the triage area of the Emergency Department. A patient reports a cough with blood-streaked sputum for almost two months with night sweats and an unintended 10 kg weight loss. Nurse suspected these as signs and symptoms of tuberculosis (TB). Which of the following type of precautions is appropriate to provide nursing care for this patient?

a. Contact
b. Droplet
c. Airborne
d. Contact and Droplet

Ans. (c) Airborne

Nurse caring for the patient must wear appropriate respiratory protection such as an N95 respirator or PAPR (powered air-purifying respirator).

CASE SCENARIO 15:

A previously healthy 40-year-old woman is admitted to the medical unit with symptoms of fever, cough and body pain for three days. She is tested positive for seasonal influenza. Which of the following precaution is appropriate for this patient?

a. Standard
b. Droplet
c. Airborne
d. Contact

Ans. (b) Droplet

The nurse should follow droplet precautions and wear a surgical face mask while coming in contact with the patient.

Types of PPE	Modes of transmission			
	Contact	Droplet	Airborne	For Aerosol generating procedures
Gown 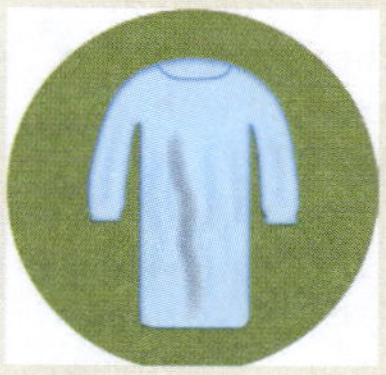	Yes	No	No	Yes
Gloves 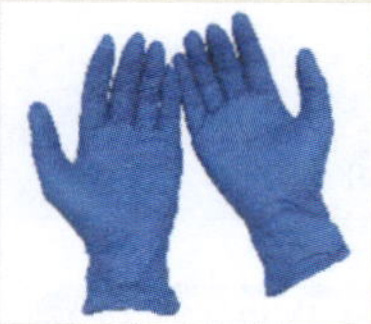	Yes	No	No	Yes
Goggles or Eyeshield 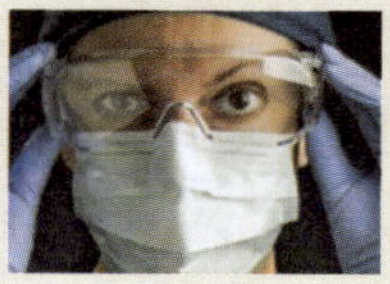	No	No	No	Yes

Ref: Infection control manual, AIIMS New Delhi & CDC

Examples of Aerosol generating procedures:

- Intubation
- Noninvasive positive pressure ventilation
- Tracheotomy
- Cardiopulmonary resuscitation
- Bronchoscopy
- Sputum induction
- **Medical aseptic practices:** These include practices that protect patient and his environment from transmission of disease. Practices include:
  - Cleaning of articles
  - Handwashing (medical handwashing)
  - Wear all personal protective equipment
- **Surgical asepsis:** This is the procedure used to keep areas and articles completely free from microorganisms. Practices include:
  - Handwashing (surgical handwashing)
  - Opening sterile packages properly
  - Use of sterile gloves and gown

Handwashing

There are five moments of hand hygiene in health care.

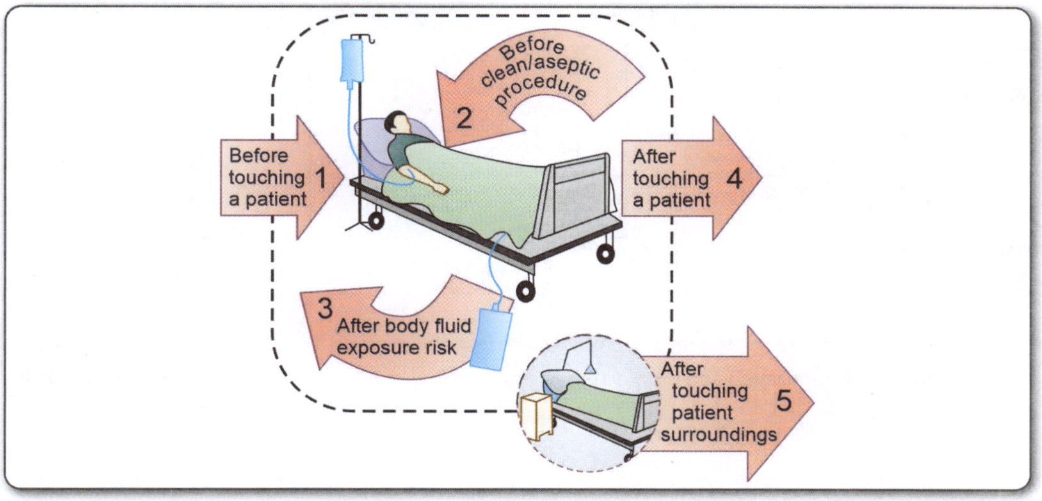

Figure 12: Five moments of hand hygiene

Source: WHO Guidelines on Hand Hygiene in Health Care: A Summary (2009).

Clinical Corner

CASE SCENARIO 16:

Nurse Ramya is caring for a 65-year-old patient with large draining wound on his hip. The wound is difficult to keep covered and draining onto his linens. Nurse is aware that this patient needs to be placed under:

a. Standard precautions
b. Contact precautions
c. Droplet precautions
d. Airborne isolation precautions

Ans. (b) Contact Precautions

Contact precautions should be considered when a patient has a wound draining. Contact precautions are also considered for patients with uncontrollable diarrhea and other scenario when the environment may become contaminated.

KEY POINTS

Types of masks:

- Surgical Masks - Protect against large droplets and splashes **(does not require fit-testing)**

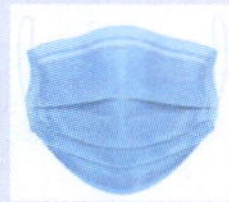

- N95 respirators - Protect against dusts, fumes, mists, microorganisms **(requires fit-testing)**

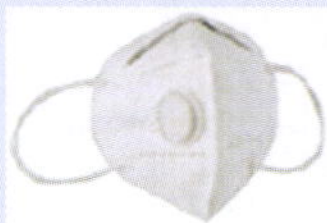

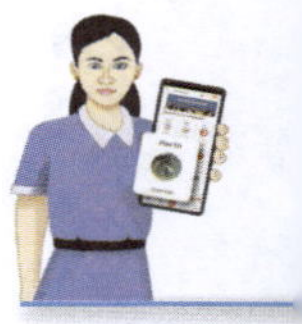

Steps of Handwashing *(Six Steps of Handwashing as per WHO are Highlighted)*

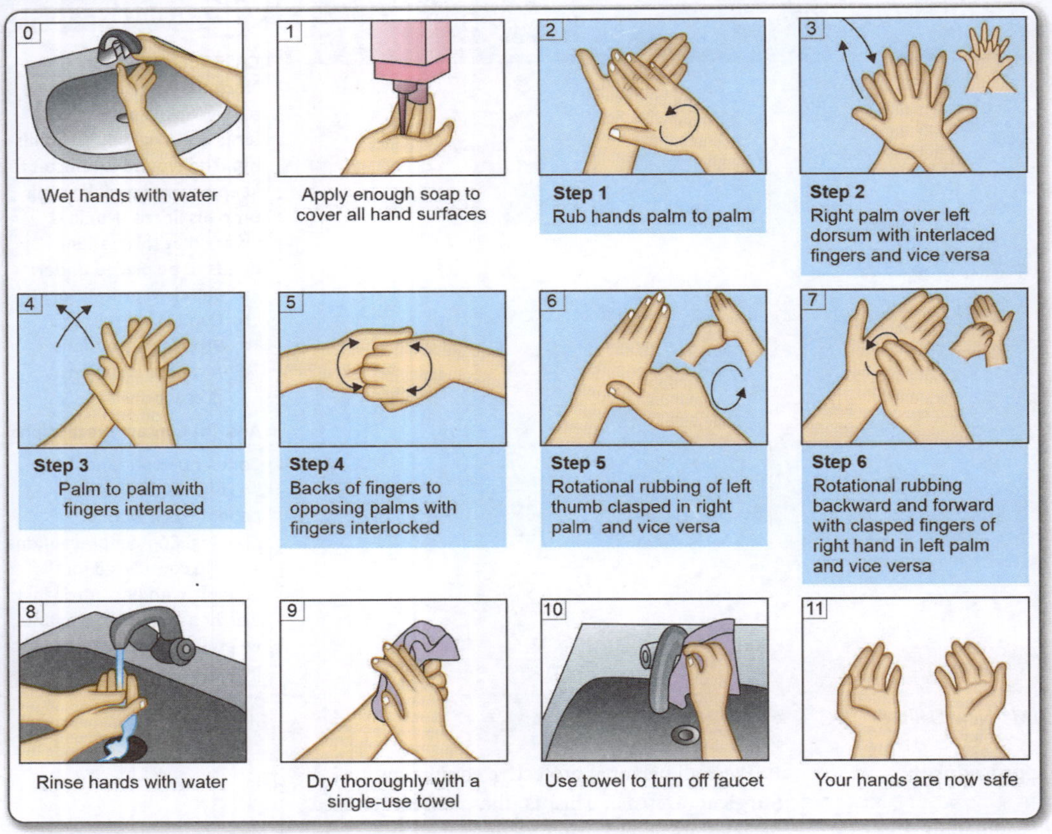

Figure 13: Hand hygiene technique with soap and water

Source: WHO Guidelines on Hand Hygiene in Health Care: A Summary (2009).

METHODS OF STERILIZATION AND DISINFECTION

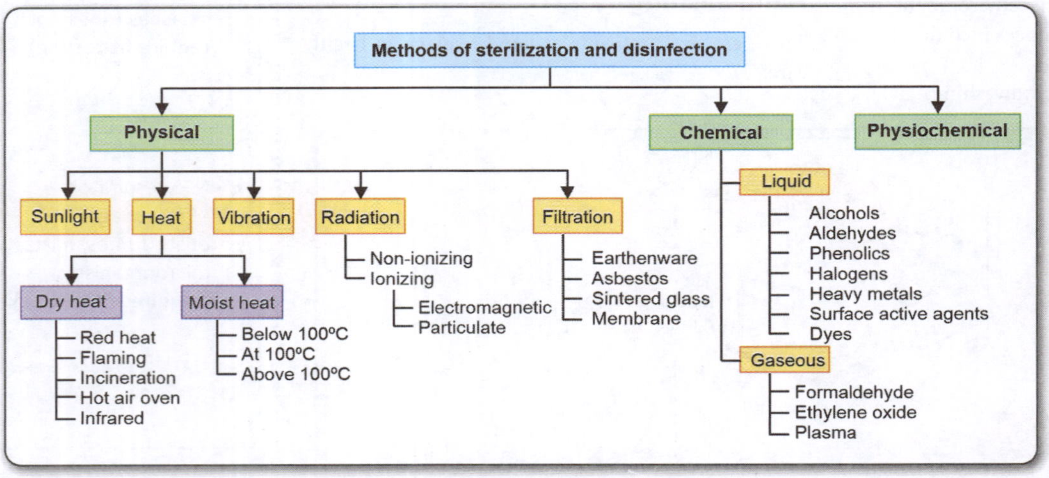

Figure 14: Methods of sterilization and disinfection

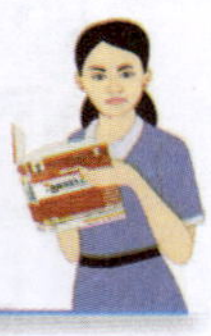

Recent Question

9. Which of the following PPE is appropriate for the nurse who is going to perform tracheostomy suction in a patient with COVID-19?

a. Surgical mask, goggles, gown
b. N95 mask, face shield, gown, gloves
c. N95 mask, gown, face shield
d. Surgical mask, face shield, gown, gloves

Ans. (b) N95 mask, face...

POINTS TO REMEMBER

Handwashing is the single most effective method of prevention of microorganism transfer from one person to another in the hospital setting.

- Handwashing is the most important step to control and prevent infection
- Duration of handwashing is 40–60 seconds
- Duration of hand rub is 20–30 seconds.

Recent Question (NORCET 2023)

10. Hand hygiene consists of all except

a. Cut short nails
b. Handwash for 40 sec
c. Don't use artificial nails
d. Use Alcohol based hand rub when hands are visibly soiled

Ans. (d) Use Alcohol...

Recent Question (NORCET 2021)

11. WHO, recommended time for hand washing by hand rub is:

a. 20–30 seconds
b. 40–60 seconds
c. 1–3 minutes
d. 3–5 minutes

Ans. (a) 20 to 30 seconds

Table 24: Sterilization methods of articles/instruments and their advantages and disadvantages

Sterilization method	Articles/instruments sterilized	Advantages	Disadvantages
Boil water for 10–15 minutes; add 2% sodium carbonate to boiling water to kill spores	Syringes, needles, bowls, trays, rubber articles, cautery wires and metallic instruments	Easy, cheap and no special gadgets required	Spores are not killed; Instruments rattle; damage to sharpness of instruments
Autoclaving	Blunt metallic instruments; rubber and glass articles; linen and bandages; non-absorbable suture materials	Kill spores; no rattling of instruments; storage possible for 5-6 days	Special gadgets required; expensive; thermolabile articles cannot be sterilized
Hot-air sterilization (dry heat)	Talcum powder; glass items; culture media	No rattling; used in microbiology	Needs special gadget; not fit for endoscope
Chemical sterilization (carbolic acid, cetrimide, lizol, formalin, iodine, 70% alcohol)	Sharp metallic instruments	Easy; no special gadget required	
Gas sterilization (Ethylene Oxide; Formaldehyde)	Respirators; endoscopes; Heart lung machines; Glass and rubber articles. Fumigation of wards, theaters, furniture and clothing	Shelf life is more	Expensive; special chambers and gases are required
Gamma radiation (Cobalt-60 is used)	Gloves, catheters, tubes, syringes, drapes	Cheap; indefinite storage	Available in selected centers only

Table 25: Indicators for sterilization methods

Sterilization method	Biological indicator	Mechanical indicator	Chemical indicator
Steam (autoclaving) (Pressure: 15 psi, temperature: 121°C, duration: 15–30 minutes)	*Bacillus stearothermophilus spore strips*	Time and temperature recorders Pressure gauges	Chemically treated strips for temperature and humidity Pellet in glass for time and temperature (Bowie Dick test for pre-vacuum)
Dry heat (Hot air oven)	*Bacillus subtilis spore type*	Time and temperature recorders	–
Ethylene oxide gas	*Bacillus subtilis spore type*	Time and temperature graphs, Humidity gauge, Gas pressure gauge	Exposure sensitive tapes, Chemically treated strips for temperature, humidity and pH
Liquid chemical glutaraldehyde	–	–	Reagent strips for appropriate chemical concentrations

Care of Linen

- Protect clean linen until it is distributed for use.
- Do not leave extra linen in patients' rooms.
- Avoid shaking clean linen. It releases dust and lint into the room.
- Clean soiled mattresses before putting clean linen on them.

Spill Management

There are two types of spills:

- **Small spills (<10 mL):** 1:100 dilution of sodium hypochlorite solution should be used to decontaminate small spills.
- **Large spills (>10 mL):** A 1:10 dilution of sodium hypochlorite solution should be used for first application (before cleaning) to reduce the risk of infection before cleaning. After first application, any visible organic matter should be removed with absorbent material (paper, towels, etc.) and then, a terminal disinfection with 1:100 dilution sodium hypochlorite solution should be done.
- After disinfection, thorough cleaning of the floor with soap and water is necessary.
- Avoid splashing or generating aerosol during the clean-up.

Spillage Kit

- The spillage kit contains:
  - PPE (mask, cap, shoe cover, heavy duty gloves, gown, plastic apron, goggles, gum boots)
  - Yellow polythene bag
  - Absorbable materials (paper/waste cloth/duster)
  - Sodium hypochlorite solution
  - Cleaning up scoop and scrapper
  - Spillage slide

KEY POINTS

- Autoclaving pressure: 15 psi
- Autoclaving temperature: 121°C
- (Duration: 15 - 30 mins)

POINTS TO REMEMBER

- Small spills - less than 10 mL
- Large spills - More than 10 mL.

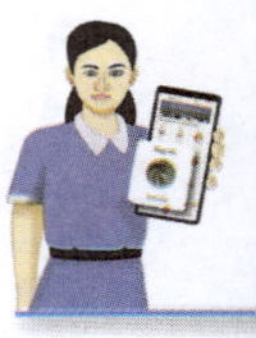

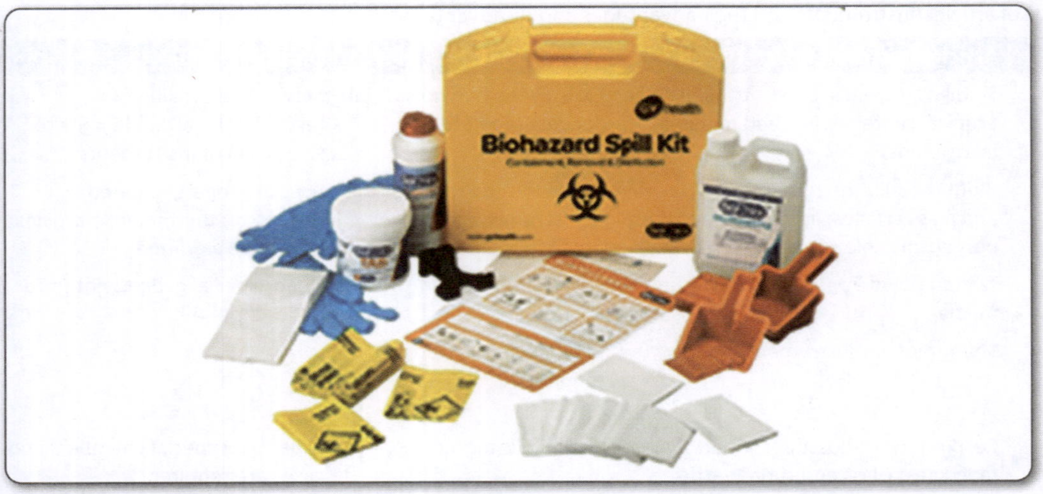

Figure 15: Biohazard spill kit

BIOMEDICAL WASTE MANAGEMENT

Biomedical waste (BMW) means any waste, which is generated during the diagnosis, treatment or immunization of human beings or animals or research activities pertaining thereto or in the production or testing of biological or in health camps.

Color Coding for Disposal of BMW

Black	Yellow	Red	Blue	White
General waste which has no contact with any infectious or hazardous material.	Item contaminated with blood and body fluids	Contaminated plastic waste	Glassware items	Contaminated sharps
Newspaper Food waste Water bottles Packing material Cardboard box	Human anatomical waste, Routine mask, cap, gown Dressing material such as cotton, gauze bandage, Expired/discarded medicine, Blood bag	All plastic tubing, plastic IV bottle, catheter, drains, urobag, syringes without needle, IV cannula, gloves, vacutainer	Broken ampules, medicine vial, metallic body implant, test tubes	Scalpel, needle, suture needle, syringe with fixed needle

SPECIMEN COLLECTION

Urine Collection

Table 26: Types of urine collection methods

Types of urine specimen	Remarks
Randomly collected specimen	• Not regarded as specimen of choice • Chance of dilution of specimen if collected after the patient has consumed large amount of fluid
First morning specimen	• Considered the specimen of choice for urinalysis and microscopic analysis • Generally more concentrated specimen

Contd...

POINT TO REMEMBER

A 1:100 dilution of 5.25–6.15% sodium hypochlorite solution provides 525–615 ppm of available chlorine.

Practice Question

7. Which of the following infection control specific form should be filled after completing the clean up procedure of a blood spill?

a. Critical incident report form
b. Postexposure evaluation form
c. Work completion report form
d. Staff illness report form

Ans. (b) Postexposure evaluation form

Recent Question (NORCET 2022)

12. Doctor orders the removal of the NG tube for a patient. The nurse follows the order and removes it. She knows that after the removal of NG tube, it has to be discarded in:

a. Yellow bin
b. Red bin
c. Blue bin
d. Black bin

Ans. (b) Red bin

Recent Question (NORCET 2023)

13. For which exposure post exposure prophylaxis is not given

a. HIV
b. Hep B
c. Hep C
d. Tetanus

Ans. (d) Tetanus

Types of urine specimen	Remarks
Mid-stream clean catch specimen	• Recommended for microbiological culture and sensitivity test • Before collecting the urine, the genitalia should be cleaned properly with soap and water
Timed collection specimen	Required for quantitative measurement of certain analytes, e.g., Creatinine, urea, sodium, potassium, uric acid, amino acids, calcium, citrate, cortisol, etc.
Collection from catheter and collection during catheterization	• Syringe is used to collect sample followed by transfer to a specimen tube or cup • Urine can also be drawn directly from the catheter to an evacuated tube using an appropriate adaptor
Suprapubic aspiration	• A needle is inserted through the abdominal wall into the bladder in order to obtain the specimen • It may be necessary for a nonambulatory patient who cannot be catheterized or if there is any problem in obtaining a sterile specimen through conventional sampling methods
24 hours collection	• A variety of preservative agents (E.g., boric acid, concentrated HCl, formalin and chloroform) need to be added to the collection bag/ bottle • The first urine in the morning is discarded
Pediatric specimens (bag collection)	A special urine specimen collection bag can be adhered to the skin surrounding genitalia

Table 27: Color of urine and interpretations

Color of Urine	Interpretation
Pale yellow to clear	Well-hydrated; **normal urine**
Transparent yellow	**Normal urine**
Dark yellow	Mildly dehydrated; **normal urine**
Amber or honey-colored	Dehydrated; **normal urine**
Light orange	Mild dehydration; possible liver or bile duct problem
Orange	Dehydration; possible liver or bile duct problem OR intake of **Rifampicin**
Pink or reddish	Presence of blood in urine; possible UTI or kidney stones
Brown or tea-colored	Presence of old blood in urine; possible liver or kidney disease
Blue or green	Rare genetic disorder (familial benign hypercalcemia) or presence of certain medications or foods
Cloudy or milky	Presence of pus or bacteria in urine; possible urinary tract infection

Table 28: Some diagnostic tests on urine to determine the presence of selected substances

Test	To determine	Color indicating presence (positive)
Cold test/hot test	Urine albumin	Cloudy
Benedict test/Fehling's test	Sugar	Green < Yellow < Orange < Red (in increasing intensity)
Sulfur powder test (Hay's test)	Bile salts	Sulfur powder sinks to bottom of the test tube
Iodine test (Smith's test)	Bile pigments	A green ring between the layers of solutions indicates positive
Rothera Nitroprusside test	Ketone bodies/acetone	Purple

Recent Question
(NORCET 2021)

14. In which color bag Placenta is discarded?
a. Red
b. Yellow
c. Blue
d. Black

Ans. (b) Yellow

KEY POINTS

- First morning urine specimen is considered the specimen of choice for urinalysis and microscopic analysis.
- In 24 hours urine specimen collection, All urine, after the first flushed specimen, must be saved, stored, and kept refrigerated.
- Preservatives such as boric acid, concentrated HCl, formalin or chloroform need to be added to the collection bag in case of 24 hours urine collection.

Practice Question

8. Which type of urine specimen collection is recommended for quantitative measurement of certain analytes, such as creatinine, urea, and sodium?
a. Mid-stream clean catch specimen
b. Timed collection specimen
c. Collection from catheter and during catheterization
d. Suprapubic aspiration

Ans. (b) Timed collection specimen

Timed collection specimen involves collecting all urine voided by the patient over a specific period, usually 24 hours, to obtain accurate measurements of these analytes.

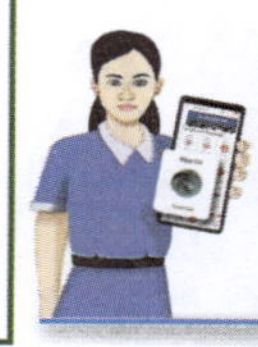

Sputum Collection

Sputum is examined for:
- Gross appearance
- Microscopic
- Gram staining
- Cytology

Procedure

- For most examinations, first **morning sample is considered the best**.
- Ask the patient to rinse the mouth with plain water to remove contaminants from mouth.
- Sputum mug or wide mouthed specimen container with cover is used to collect sputum sample.
- Instruct the patient to bring out sputum by deep cough.
- Sputum for culture should be collected in a sterile container.
- Label the specimen container before collection of sample.
- Transport to the laboratory immediately.
- For sputum AFB throat swab, patient can be told to hold the tongue out with paper.
- Swab for AFB can be kept in a test tube and sterile cotton swab should be used to cover the test tube.
- Patient should not be receiving any antibiotic before collecting sample for AFB or culture sensitivity.
- Do not send saliva. It may give false negative results.

Stool Collection

Definition

- Stool collection is the process of obtaining sample of a patient's feces for diagnostic purpose.
- It is used to identify infectious organisms, mucus, fat, parasites, or blood in the stool (melena).

Procedure

- A specimen of freshly passed feces of ½–1 ounce (15–30 g) is collected, without contamination of urine or toilet tissue, into a small container with a small spatula for easier collection of the sample.
- Adults/older children can collect the specimen by passing feces into a plastic bag stretched loosely over the toilet bowl. A portion from the sample can then be transferred into the container.
- For young children and infants wearing diapers, a plastic wrap can be lined with the diaper. A urine bag can be attached to the child to ensure that the stool specimen is not contaminated with urine.
- Specimen bottle should not be over filled. Avoid contamination of outer surface of specimen bottle.
- Label the container before collecting sample.
- The specimen should be sent for lab examination as soon as possible.
- Stool specimen for culture should be collected in a sterile container.
- For best result, stool should be examined for three consecutive days.

Preparation of Patient

- If occult blood is suspected, a mild laxative should be given to the patient and he should avoid eating foods rich in meat extracts or leafy vegetables three days prior to the test.
- In case of bleeding of gums, the mouth should be cleansed with mouthwash and wiped with a cloth to avoid blood entering the digestive system. This will prevent contamination of stool specimen.
- The patient should avoid having antacids, oily foods and drugs and antibiotics as they may interfere with stool analysis.
- Barium sulfate should be excluded two weeks prior to the test, and medical procedure dyes three weeks prior to the test.
- If fat in stool is suspected, the patient is asked to collect the samples in preweighed airtight containers.
- Feces passed in a 24-hour period is collected for 2 or 3 days consecutively and is sent daily for analysis.

Nursing Responsibilities

- Watery feces will not be suitable for a test to identify fat present in stool.
- Delay in sending the specimen for testing may give false reading because it results in either death or multiplication of organisms present in the feces.
- Patient should be educated to inform medical staff about any medication that he is taking currently, as sometimes elements of the drugs may also be present in the feces.

Blood Collection

Blood may be tested for:
- Complete blood study: Hb, TLC, DLC, ESR, CT, grouping and cross match, etc.
- Culture and sensitivity
- Urea, sugar, LFT, lipid profile and enzymes
- Electrolyte
- Antigens and antibodies

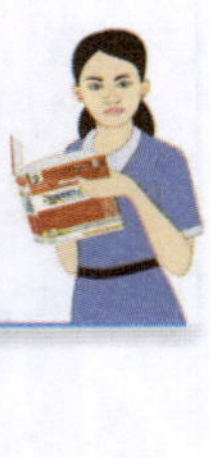

KEY POINTS

- Right specimen, Right time, Right amount and Right container are the four rules to be followed while collecting specimens.
- The best time to collect a sputum specimen is first thing in the morning.
- When collecting a 24-hour urine specimen, the urine must be stored in refrigerator or on ice.
- While collecting a 24-hour urine specimen, the first urine of first day is discarded.
- Guaiac Fecal Occult Blood Test (gFOBT) finds occult blood in the stool.

KEY POINT

While doing finger prick for sugar monitoring, use lateral side of fingers and heels as this area has less nerve supply.

Practice Question

9. Nurse Ramya instructs the patient to collect urine specimen after voiding is initiated and before it is finished. This specimen is known as:
   a. Patient collected-specimen
   b. Midstream specimen
   c. Sterile specimen
   d. Contaminated specimen

Ans. (b) Midstream specimen

Table 29: Blood collection containers guide

Cap color	Additives	Volume required	Suitable for
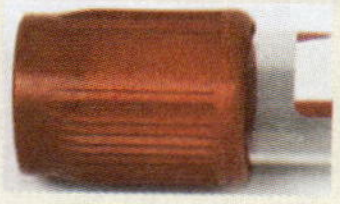	Plain, clot activator	6 mL	• Cryoproteins cold agglutinin cryoglobulin + EDTA • Immunohematological test that requires clotted blood
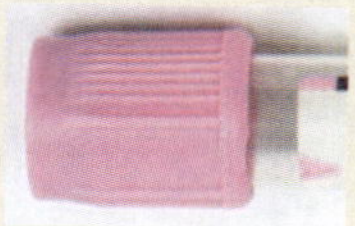	K2EDTA (Di-Potassium Ethylene Diamine-tetraacetate)	6 mL	• Group and cross match • Antibody screen • Blood group • Coombs test • Cryofibrinogen + red top • Transfusion testing
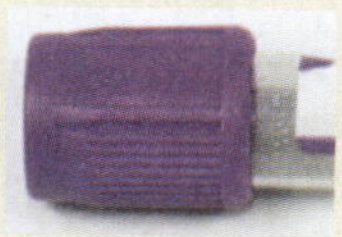	K2EDTA	3 mL	• Most hematological tests including Hgm, TLC, DLC, PS for MP, MF, electrophoresis, typhoid • HbA1c, cyclosporine, homocysteine and molecular genetics test • Malaria • Lymphocyte surface markers • HFE gene
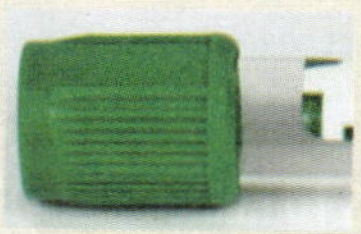	Lithium heparin	4 mL	• They are used for plasma determinations in chemistry • Chromosome studies • Lead • Lymphocyte Surface markers • Vitamin B_1 • Vitamin B_6
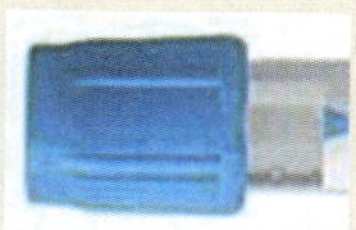	Sodium citrate	2.7 mL	• Coagulation studies • Prothrombin time (PT), activated partial thromboplastin time (APTT); International normalized ratio (INR); Bleeding Time (BT); Clotting time (CT)
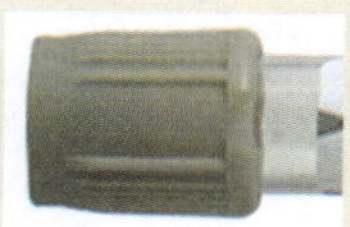	Sodium fluoride/ potassium oxalate	6 mL	• Blood sugar levels • Glucose • Glucose tolerance tests • Blood alcohol
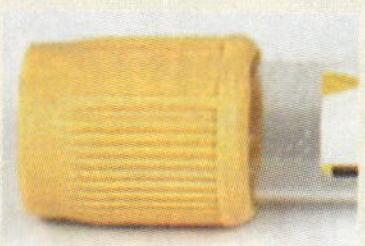	Plain, ST II, clot activator and serum gel separator	3–5 mL	• Biochemistry and serology • S. Electrolytes • Liver function test (LFT), kidney function test (KFT), serum urea, serum creatinine, serum bilirubin • Thyroid function test • Lipid profile, iron studies, immunology • HIV, hepatitis, dengue serology, virology, rheumatoid factor • Vitamin D, troponin-T, insulin, iron studies, digoxin

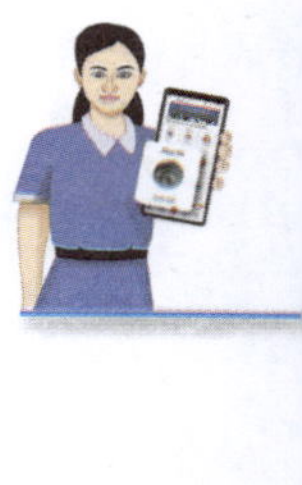

BED MAKING

Principles Involved in Bed Making

- Microorganisms are present everywhere, so nurse needs to take care for the prevention of transmission of microorganisms from source to new host.
- A safe and comfortable bed will ensure rest, sleep and prevent several complications in bedridden patient.
- Good body mechanism followed by the nurse will maintain good body alignment and prevent fatigue.
- Systematic way of functioning saves time, energy and material.

Types of Bed

Table 30: Types of bed and their descriptions

Bed	Description
Closed bed	It is an empty bed, which is not occupied by any patient. After the admission of patient, closed bed is converted to open bed.
Open bed	This bed is about to be occupied by a new patient or an ambulatory patient.
Admission bed	The bed is made as an open bed, the patient gets into the bed after thorough bath and changing into hospital dress.
Occupied bed	This bed is for those patients who cannot move out of the bed.
Operation bed/postanesthesia bed/ recovery bed	This bed is for those patients who are getting recovered from the effect of anesthesia.
Cardiac bed	This kind of bed helps the patient attain a sitting position with least strain and also helps to relieve dyspnea.
Fracture bed	The bed is prepared for patient with fracture. It provides support to the fractured part using a firm mattress, which rests on fracture board or bed board.
Amputation bed/stump bed	This bed helps to take off the weight of bed linen on the amputated part.
Burn bed	It consists of a long bed cradle which takes off bed linen weight from all over the body.

PERSONAL HYGIENE

Oral Care

Solutions used for mouth care:
- Hydrogen peroxide—1:20
- Condy's solution (potassium permanganate)—1:5000 to 1:10000 concentration
- Sodium bicarbonate

Positions while providing oral care:
- **For conscious patients:** Seated position, Semi-Fowler's position or supine position.
- **For unconscious patients:** Lateral recovery position (preferred)- the patient is placed on side, with head tilted slightly downward, and a towel or basin is used to collect excess water or saliva.

Key points to remember during oral care:
- In unconscious patient, use Yankauer suction to remove excessive secretions.
- Avoid oral care with hydrogen peroxide if oral thrush or oral lesions present.
- If dentures present, remove and gently brush and rinse. Soak dentures overnight.

Clinical Corner

CASE SCENARIO 17:

Nurse Amli in the general ward is preparing occupied bed. Identify the incorrect statement regarding occupied bed:

a. Roll the patient to far side of the bed
b. Tuck the top sheet and blanket at the bottom of the bed
c. Ask the patient to sit on a chair beside the bed
d. Place pillow at the head end of the bed

Ans. (c) Ask the patient to sit on a chair beside the bed

Occupied bed is a bed prepared with a patient in it, the one who cannot get out of the bed. Except option c, all other options are incorrect regarding occupied bed.

POINTS TO REMEMBER

- While removing linen from bed, always hold soiled linen away from uniform.
- Do not shake soiled linen in the air because shaking can disseminate dirt and microorganisms in the air.

Clinical Corner

CASE SCENARIO 18:

Rahul is working in critical care area as Registered Nurse. He was providing bed bath to his client. While cleaning the lower extremities he uses long, firm strokes from the distal to the proximal areas. This is because:

a. To increase the range of motion in the extremities and to prevent foot drop
b. Proximal area is cleaner than the distal area of the extremities
c. To increase venous return and to prevent venous stasis
d. To assess the skin integrity

Ans. (c) To increase venous...

Table 31: Oral diseases with their descriptions

Problem	Description
Halitosis	Bad odor of breath
Dental caries	Commonly known as cavities. Destructive process causing decalcification of enamel which leads to cavitation
Dental plaque	Soft thin layer of debris and epithelial cell deposited on the teeth which provides a medium for the growth of microorganisms
Calculus/tartar	Dental plaque becomes hard and forms calculus
Bottle mouth syndrome	Dental caries occur in children because of use of bottles with liquids other than water
Periodontal disease/pyorrhea	Socket of teeth filled with pus is known as pyorrhea
Periodontitis	Inflammation of gum which spreads to other parts around the teeth is called periodontium.
Sordes	Brown crust formed on teeth and lips is known as sordes
Cheilosis	Cracking and ulceration of the lips and angles of the mouth
Glossitis	Inflammation of tongue
Stomatitis	Inflammation of mucous membrane of mouth
Gingivitis	Inflammation of gum

Eye care—points to remember.

- Clean the eyes from inner canthus to outer canthus.
- Use different cotton balls for cleaning the eye.
- If one eye is infected, then clean the non-infected eye first, then the infected eye.
- Among unconscious patients defective eye closure leads to exposure keratopathy.

Ear care—points to remember.

- Never use any sharp object into the ear canal to remove the ear wax.
- Perforated tympanic membrane is a contra-indication for ear irrigation.
- To straighten the ear canal, adult and children above 3 years of age hold the pinna upward and backward. Among children less than 3 years of age, hold the pinna downward and backward.
- Use solution at body temperature to irrigate the ear to prevent dizziness and vertigo.

Care of Skin/Bathing

Types of Baths

- **Complete bed-bath:** Nurse administers complete bath to a totally dependent patient.
- **Partial bed bath:** Bathing only those body parts, which are left unbathed by patient who is unable to reach all body parts.
- **Tub bath:** Patient is immersed in a tub of water. It allows thorough cleaning and washing. Patient needs nurse assistance.
- **Shower:** Patient sits or stands under a continuous stream of water.
- **Therapeutic bath:** Bath with healing and medicinal qualities. Whirlpool bath is done in a tub which can agitate water. Starch or oatmeal bath is used in patients with dermatitis. Sitz bath is used to apply moist heat and clean the perineal or anal area.

Bath—points to remember.

- Do not soak feet and hand into the water basin of patient with diabetes or peripheral vascular disease as it may lead to maceration of the skin.
- Do not use long firm stroke while caring lower limb of patients with high risk of deep vein thrombosis.

Care of the Hair

Common hair problems

Dandruff	Scaling of the scalp accompanied by itching. Severe cases may affect ear canal and eyebrow.
Hair loss	Permanent thinning and loss of hair.
Ticks	Small gray brown parasite that bites into the tissue and sucks blood.
Pediculosis (lice)	• Lice is a parasite that infests mammals. • Infestation of lice is known as pediculosis. ▪ **Pediculosis capitis:** Lice found on the scalp ▪ **Pediculosis pubis:** Lice found in pubic hair ▪ **Pediculosis corporis:** Lice found in the body
Scabies	• Contagious skin infection by itch mite. • Characteristic lesions are burrow produced by female itch mite. • The mite causes intense itching. • Treatment includes application of scabicide lotion.
Hirsutism	Growth of excessive hair in the body.

Practice Question

10. Bacterial growth and odor of the skin are due to:

a. Fatty acid + minerals + nitrogenous waste
b. Fatty acid + proteins + nitrogenous waste
c. Amino acid + proteins + minerals
d. Amino acid + proteins + nitrogenous waste

Ans. (b) Fatty acid + proteins + nitrogenous waste

KEY POINT

Bed bath (sponge bath) is for patients who must remain in the bed and are unable to bathe themselves.

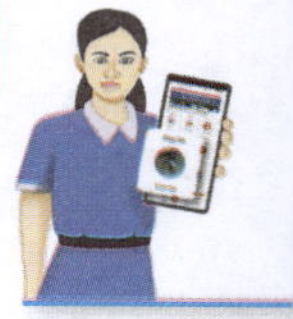

Pediculosis Treatment

Pesticides used for pediculosis treatment include:

- DDT 5% or 10%
- Carbonic lotion 1:40
- Equal part of kerosene and equal part of hair oil.

Care of Hands and Feet

Common foot and nail problems

Callus	Thickened portion of epidermis caused by local friction or pressure.
Corns	Caused by friction and pressure from shoes seen over bony prominence.
Plantar warts	Fungal lesions appearing on feet and soles caused by papilloma virus.
Athlete's foot (tinea pedis)	Fungal infection of the foot caused by wearing constricting footwear.
Ingrown nail	Toe nails or finger nails grow inward into the soft tissue.
Paronychia	Inflammation of the tissue surrounding the nail.
Foot odor	Due to excessive perspiration promoting microbial growth.

KEY POINTS

- While giving bed bath, wash patient's extremities from distal to proximal. This will promote venous return.
- Hold the brush at 45° angle while brushing the teeth of a patient.
- The hair found on Scalp, Eyebrows, Axillae, Perineum and Legs is called terminal hair.
- Vellus hair is found all over the body.
- Excess shedding of epidermal layer of scalp is dandruff.
- Hair helps to maintain temperature.
- Healthy nail beds are convex in shape.
- Podiatrist is a specialist of foot care.

BACK MASSAGE TECHNIQUES

Effleurage	A massage technique that involves using long, sweeping strokes with the hands or fingers to apply gentle pressure and create a soothing and relaxing effect on the muscles.
Petrissage	A massage technique that involves kneading and stroking the muscles using the thumb and fingers
Friction	A massage technique that involves using deep circular or back-and-forth movements with the fingers, thumbs, or palms to apply pressure and create heat in a specific area of the body.
Hand over hand	A massage technique that involves using both hands in a rhythmic and alternating motion to apply pressure to a specific area of the body.
Brush strokes	A gentle, relaxing massage technique that uses long, flowing strokes to promote relaxation
Kneading	A type of massage that involves compressing and squeezing the muscles with rhythmic, circular movements using the hands, fingers or the elbows
Tapping (tapotement)	Tapping involves rhythmic tapping, pounding or patting movements applied to the body with the fingertips, fists or the side of the hand.

PRESSURE ULCERS

- Pressure ulcers are also known as bed sores or decubitus ulcers. Pressure causes a local area of tissue necrosis. Most often pressure ulcer occurs at bony prominence.
- Another main factor along with pressure in the development of pressure ulcer is shearing force.
- Braden scale is the tool used for predicting bedsore risk.

Table 32: Components of Braden scale

Sensory perception	1 Completely limited	2 Very limited	3 Slightly limited	4 No impairment
Moisture	1 Constantly moist	2 Moist	3 Occasionally moist	4 Rarely moist
Activity	1 Bed rest	2 Chairfast	3 Walk occasionally	4 Walks frequently
Mobility	1 Completely immobile	2 Very limited	3 Slightly limited	4 No limitation
Nutrition	1 Very poor	2 Probably inadequate	3 Adequate	4 Excellent
Friction and shear	1 Problem	2 Potential problem	3 No apparent problem	------

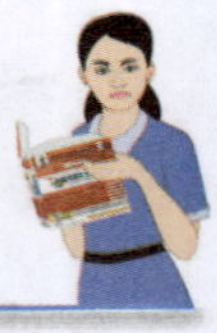

- Total score is 23.
- A lower Braden score indicates higher level of risk for pressure ulcer development.
- **Score 19–23:** Not at risk
- **Score 15–18:** Mild risk
- **Score 13–14:** Moderate risk
- **Score 10–12:** High risk
- **Score ≤9:** Very high risk

Table 33: Stages of pressure ulcer

Stages	Characteristics
Stage 1	Nonblanchable redness of a localized area.
Stage 2	Partial thickness skin loss involving epidermis or dermis. Looks like an abrasion or blister.
Stage 3	Full thickness skin loss. Extended to subcutaneous tissue which is damaged or necrotic.
Stage 4	Full thickness skin loss with damage to muscle, bone or supporting structures.

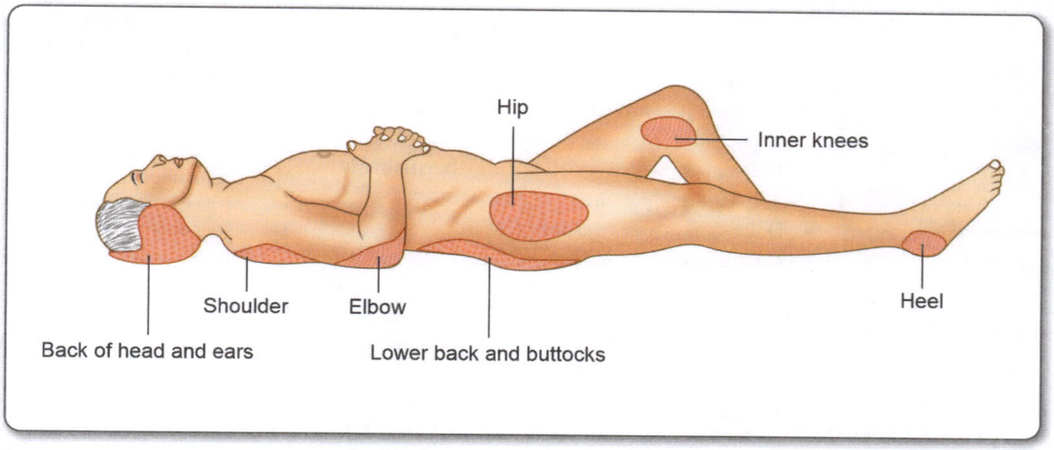

Figure 16: Pressure points

Risk Factors

Friction, shear, impaired sensory perception, impaired physical mobility, altered level of consciousness, fecal and urinary incontinence, malnutrition, dehydration, excessive body heat, advanced age, chronic medical conditions like diabetes, cardiovascular diseases.

Stages of Pressure Ulcer

Staging systems for pressure ulcers are based on the depth of tissue destroyed.

Stage I: Nonblanchable Redness of Intact Skin

- Intact skin presents with nonblanchable erythema of a localized area usually over a bony prominence.
- Discoloration of the skin, warmth, edema or pain may also be present.
- Stage I indicates "at-risk" persons.
- Involves only the epidermal layer of skin.

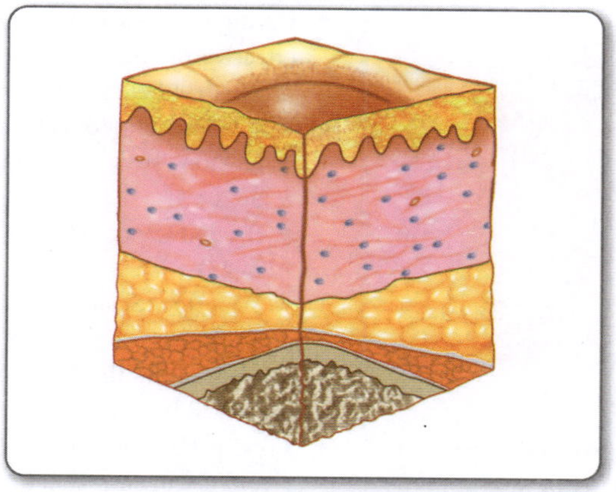

Figure 17: Stage I

KEY POINTS

Common pressure ulcer sites:

- **Sitting position:** Sacrum, Ischial Tuberosity, heels.
- **Wheelchair pressure points:** Scapula, elbow, sacrum and coccyx, ischial tuberosity, heels, plantar surface of foot.
- **Supine position:** Scapula, occipital bone, sacral region, elbow and heels.
- **Side lying position:** Malleolus of ankle joint, condyles, trochanter, scapula, ribs and ear.
- **Prone position:** Frontal and mandible bone, sternum, humerus, Tibia and Tuberosity of pelvis.

Practice Question

11. While assessing a 60-year-old bedridden patient for pressure ulcer, the nurse noted a full loss of skin tissue that is extending to the subcutaneous tissue. She documented the pressure ulcer as:

a. Stage I
b. Stage II
c. Stage III
d. Stage IV

Ans. (c) Stage III

KEY POINT

Application of **topical insulin** on wound and use of **water proof ointment** during dressing are recommended (e.g., Zinc oxide) to treat pressure ulcer.

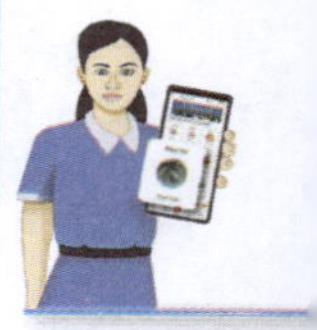

Stage II: Partial-thickness Skin Loss or Blister

- A partial thickness loss of dermis presents as a shallow open ulcer with a red-pink wound bed without slough.
- Stage II does damage to the epidermis and the dermis.
- In this stage, the ulcer may be referred to as a blister or abrasion.

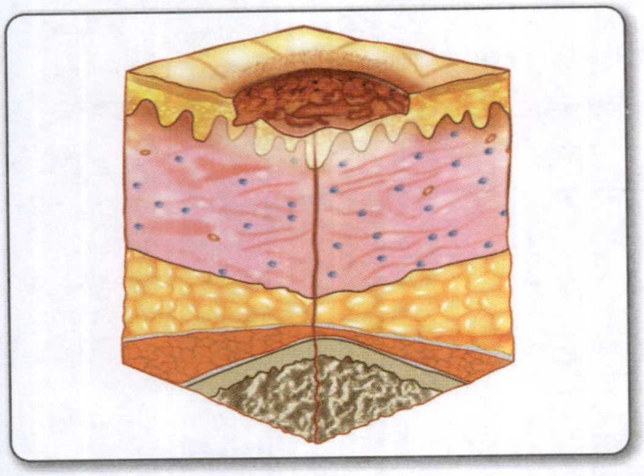

Figure 18: Stage II

Stage III: Full-thickness Skin Loss (Fat Visible)

- A stage III ulcer is a full-thickness tissue loss.
- Subcutaneous fat may be visible, but bone, tendon, or muscle are not exposed.
- Epidermis, dermis and subcutaneous tissues are involved.
- Subcutaneous layer has a relatively poor blood supply; so, it is difficult to heal.

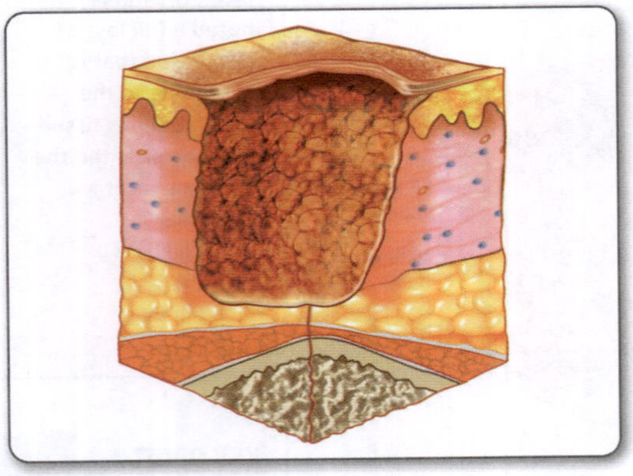

Figure 19: Stage III

Stage IV: Full-thickness Tissue Loss

A stage IV ulcer is the deepest, extending into the muscle, tendon or even bone.

Full thickness tissue loss occurs with exposed bone, tendon or muscle.

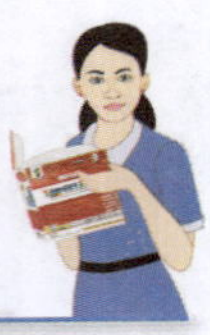

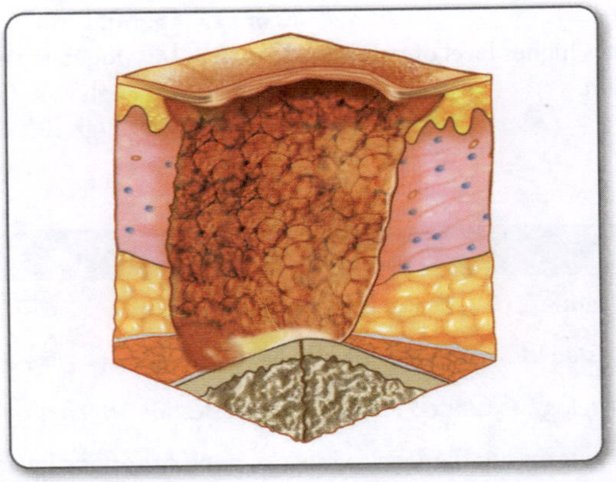

Figure 20: Stage IV

Prevention of Pressure Ulcer

- Changing position
  - **Every 15 minutes** in a wheelchair bound patient
  - **Every 2 hours**, even during the night, in a bedridden patient
- Daily skin inspections for pressure sores.
- Nutritional management.
- Adequate hydration to maintain the skin integrity.
- **Exercise**: Daily exercise improves circulation.
- **Use pressure-relieving devices** such as air mattress (alpha bed, ripple bed), water mattress.
- **Using support surfaces:** These are special cushions, pads, mattresses and beds that relieve pressure on an existing sore and help protect vulnerable areas from further breakdown.

Key Nursing Responsibilities in Prevention and Care of Pressure Ulcer

- **Change of position every two hours** is the most effective method of prevention of pressure ulcer in a bedridden patient.
- Risk assessment tools for pressure ulcer:
  - Norton scale (5 categories; scoring range: 5–20)
  - Braden Scale (6 categories; scoring range: 6–23)
  - Waterlow Scale (10 categories; scoring range: 1–64)
- Do not allow the skin to remain wet. Clean as soon as it becomes wet.
- Provide bath regularly.
- Avoid use of soap that dries the skin.
- Apply cream on dry, scaly skin.
- Prevent skin from coming in contact with feces and urine.
- Use pressure reducing devices.
- Further trauma to the wound should be avoided by reducing friction and cuts.
- Prevent further infection by covering the wound (wherever applicable).

Practice Question

12. A home care nurse is providing care to a 60-year-old male patient with a paralysis of all four extremities after a CVA. The patient's daughter provides care to the patient at home. On assessment, the nurse found that the patient has a stage I pressure ulcer on the sacral area. While teaching the patient's daughter on prevention of further breakdown of the current pressure ulcer, the nurse would include all of the following, except:

a. 2-hourly repositioning of the patient.
b. Active and passive exercise of extremities.
c. Use comfort devices on elevated bony prominences.
d. Keep the skin moist around sacral area and layer with extra sheet.

Ans. (d) Keep the skin moist around sacral area and layer with extra sheet.

Rationale: Keep the pressure ulcer dry and clean, and avoid extra sheets. Extra layer of sheet will increase the risk of moisture and chance of wrinkles and friction.

KEY POINTS

- Change of position every 2 hours is the most effective method of prevention of Pressure ulcer.
- Risk assessment tools for pressure ulcer:
  - Nortan scale
  - Braden Scale
  - Waterlow scale.

MEDICATION ADMINISTRATION

Route	Description
Oral route	Easy and the most common method to administer medication. Oral medication has slower onset of action but has prolonged effect than parenteral route.
Sublingual route	Medication is administered under the tongue. Instruct the patient to not swallow or drink anything until the medication is completely absorbed.
Buccal administration	Administering medication in the mouth against the mucous membrane of cheek until it is absorbed.
Parenteral route	It involves the injection of medication into the body tissues. The major types are: • **Intradermal** Injecting medication under the skin or below the epidermis. • **Subcutaneous:** injecting medication into the subcutaneous tissues. • **Intramuscular:** injecting medication into the muscles. • **Intravenous:** injecting medication into the vein.
Epidural	Medication is administered into the epidural space.
Intrathecal	Medication is administered into the subarachnoid space or into the ventricles of brain.
Intraosseous	Medications are administered into the bone marrow. Most used among children with poor IV access.
Intraperitoneal	Administering medications into the peritoneal cavity.
Intrapleural	Administering medications into the pleural space.
Intra-arterial	Administering medications into the arteries.
Intracardiac	Administering medications into the cardiac tissue
Intra-articular	Administering medications into the joint.
Topical administration	Medications are administered into the skin and mucous membrane for local effect. E.g., eye drops, eye ointment, suppository into the rectum or vagina, ear drop, nasal instillation, irrigation of body cavity.
Inhalation route	• Medications are administered into the pulmonary tissue either via nasal or oral inhalation or via endotracheal tube or tracheostomy tube. • Inhaled medications are readily absorbed because of the rich capillary network present in the pulmonary system.
Intraocular route	Medications are administered into the eyes in a manner that contact lenses are applied. This medication may remain in place for some duration.

Subcutaneous Injection

- Subcutaneous injections are also known as hypodermal injections.
- Subcutaneous tissues have less blood supply as compared to muscular tissues so medications absorption is slower.
- Best site for S/C injections
  - Outer posterior aspect of upper arm.
  - Abdomen below the costal margin to the iliac crest.
  - Anterior aspect of the thigh.
  - Alternative sites include scapular areas of the upper back, upper ventral and dorsal gluteal areas.
- For administering subcutaneous injection, needle is inserted at 45° angle.

KEY POINTS

- Clients with pressure ulcer lose large amount of protein in wound exudates, hence, require 4000 kcal/day or more to remain anabolic.
- Poor nutrition, poor hydration, incontinence, and immobility are the major risk factors for pressure ulcer.
- Moisture may contribute to skin maceration.
- The most widely used risk assessment scale for pressure ulcer is the Braden scale. It consists of six subscales, namely: activity, mobility, moisture, nutrition, sensory perception and friction.

Clinical Corner

CASE SCENARIO 19:

Nurse Amli is educating a client regarding sublingual medication administration. Which statement by the client indicates need for further teaching?

a. These are the medications administered on the floor of the mouth
b. These medications are absorbed directly into blood stream from the oral mucosa
c. These medications bypass the GI and hepatic system
d. These are the medications administered on top of the tongue

Ans. (d) These are the medications administered on top of the tongue

Sublingual administration means medications are administered under the tongue to dissolve and for easy and early absorption. They are not administered on the top of the tongue.

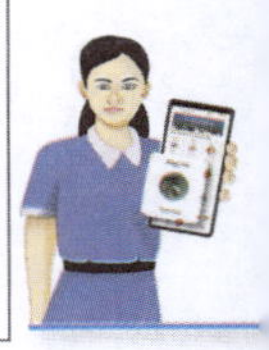

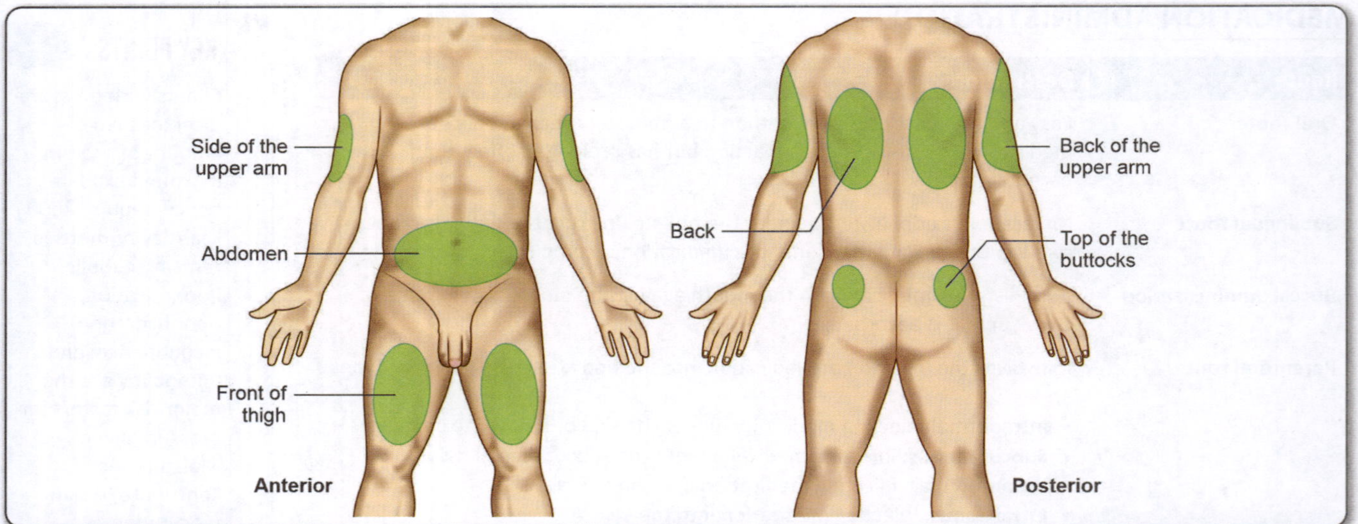

Figure 21: Sites of subcutaneous injection administration

Intramuscular Injection

- IM injection provides faster medication absorption as muscular tissues are highly vascular.
- Angle of insertion of IM injection is 90°
- Z track method is the recommended method to administer IM injection as this method helps to reduce the local skin irritation and also seal the medication within the muscle.
- Z track method: it is the displacement of skin and subcutaneous tissue by pulling them laterally or downward.

Sites of IM injection

Site	Location	Picture
Ventrogluteal	• It involves the use of gluteus medius. • Use nurse right hand for patient's left hip and vice versa and place palm of your hand on greater trochanter of the patient and forearm is perpendicular to the femur. • Thumb is pointing toward the groin • Index finger at anterior-superior iliac spine and extend middle finger to the back toward the buttocks. • Index finger and middle finger form the V-shaped triangle and the midpoint of the triangle is the injection site.	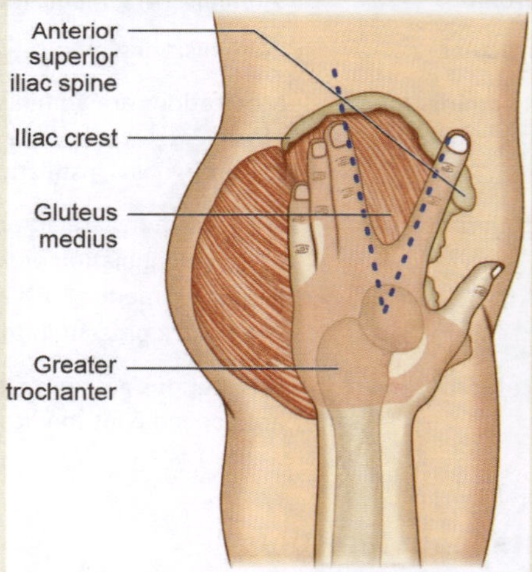
Vastus lateralis	• This muscle is in the anterior and lateral aspects of the thigh. • In adult, it extends from hand breadth above the knees to hand breadth below the greater trochanter of the femur. Injection into the outer middle third of the muscle.	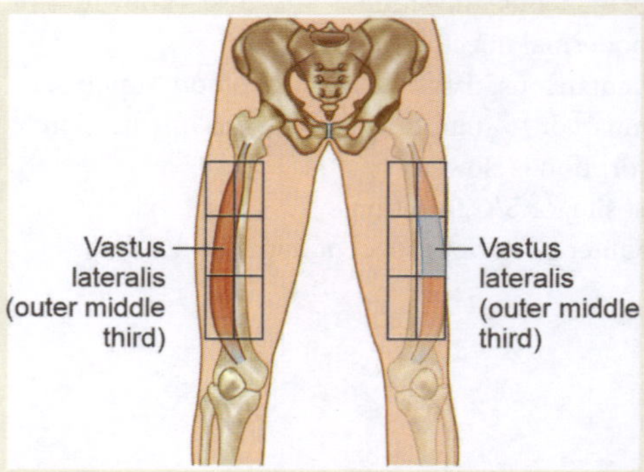 Correct place to give shot in the thigh muscle

Contd...

Site	Location	Picture
Deltoid	• Site is located one to three fingers below the acromion process. • There is a potential damage to blood vessel (brachial artery) and nerves (axillary, radial, brachial and ulnar) as they lie within the upper arm under the triceps • Site is useful for administering small volume of medications usually 2 mL or less.	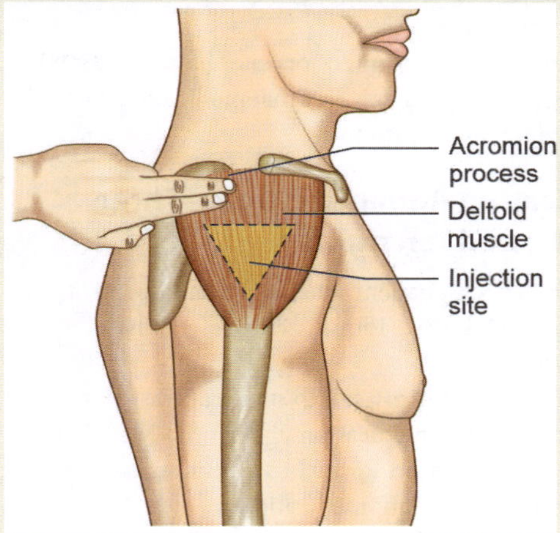
Dorsogluteal	• This is the least preferred muscle tissue because of its proximity to sciatic nerve. • Patient in prone position or standing position • Muscle located in the upper outer quadrant of the buttocks. • This muscle can be also located by drawing an imaginary line between posterior superior iliac spine and the greater trochander.	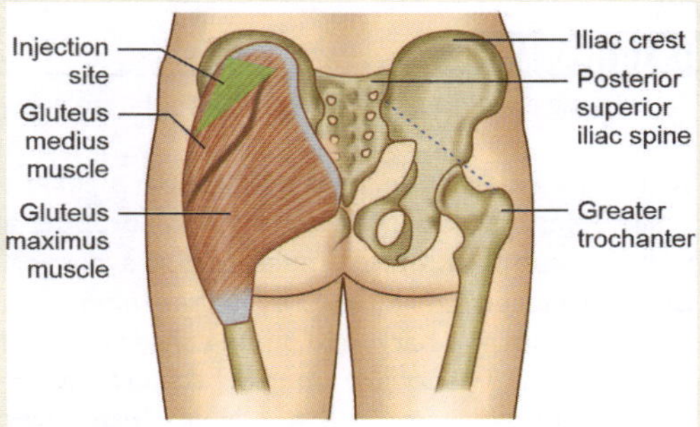
Rectus femoris	• The rectus femoris is one of the four quadriceps muscles located at the front of the thigh. It is the only one of the four quadriceps muscles that crosses both the hip and knee joints. The muscle originates from the anterior inferior iliac spine (AIIS) of the hip bone and runs down the front of the thigh to its insertion point on the patella (kneecap) via the quadriceps tendon. • The injection site is typically located at the midpoint of a line drawn between the anterior superior iliac spine (ASIS) and the superior border of the patella (kneecap).	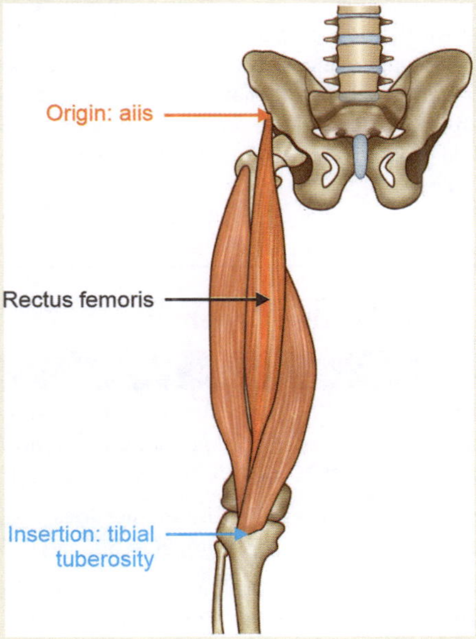

Intradermal Injection

- Intradermal injection are used for skin testing and sensitivity test.
- Here, blood supply is less, and medications are not absorbed promptly into the circulation.
- These type of injections help us to study the sensitivity to an injection and reactions.
- Sites for ID injections are lightly pigmented, free from lesion and relatively hairless.
- Inner surface of the forearm and upper back below the scapula are the locations.
- Hypodermic syringes are used for ID injections.

- Angle of injection is 5°–15°.
- After giving ID injection, bleb will be formed at the site of injection.
- If bleb is not formed or site bleeds after ID injection, there is a chance that medication entered the subcutaneous tissue.

Medication Administration—Three Checks and Ten rights

- Three checks, patient interaction and ten rights to be followed while administering medicines.
- Three checks:
  1. **Before administering medication**, compare the label of medication against the Medication Administration Record (MAR) to ensure right patient and right medication.
  2. **While preparing medication for administration**, check label against MAR to ensure right medication is being prepared for right patient.
  3. **Before administering medication to the patient**, check the medication, dose, and right route of administration again, to ensure that the right medication is being given to the right patient, in the right dose, and via the right route.
- **Patient interaction:** Inform patient what medication you are giving and ask for any known allergies
- **Ten rights** include right patient, right drug, right time, right dose, right route, right documentation, right to refusal, right education, right assessment, right evaluation.

POINTS TO REMEMBER

- Calculating drug dose for pediatric population is always based upon body weight or body surface area.
- While doing instillation, **hold the dropper 1 cm above** the body part.
- While doing instillation, **never touch the dropper at any of the body part.**
- **Instill ear drops at room temperature** to avoid vertigo, dizziness or nausea.
- Ear canal can be straightened by holding pinna:
  - Downward and backward among children less than 3 years of age
  - Upward and backward among children above 3 years of age.
- While performing eye instillation, **never instill medications directly into the cornea**.
- After the instillation of eye drop, apply gentle pressure with fingers to block the nasolacrimal duct to prevent the flow of medication into the nasal and pharyngeal passes.
- If patient has eye drop and eye ointment at a time, **apply drop first followed by ointment**.
- A patient who is on inhalation therapy with corticosteroid should be advised to rinse the mouth with water or brush the oral cavity after each dose to reduce the incidence of fungal infection.
- While preparing injection, after dilution roll the vial between palm, should not shake it as it creates bubbles.
- When there is a need to mix injection from both vial and ampule in the same syringe, withdraw medications from vial first, then use filter needle to withdraw medications from ampules.

Types of Medication Order

Types	Description
Standing order (routine medication order)	These are the orders that need to be carried out until the physician cancels the order or the time duration mentioned in the order is achieved. E.g., Inj. augmentin 625 mg IV × TDS (8 hourly), Calcitriol sachet 60,000 IU once in a week x 6 weeks.
PRN orders	These are the medications that need to be administered when the patient requires them. E.g., Inj. PCM 500 mg IV SOS
Single- or one-time order	These are the medications ordered at a specific time. E.g., Inj. atropine 1 mg IV before shifting to OT.
STAT order	These are the medications that need to be administered only once and immediately. E.g., Inj. hydrocortisone 25 mg IV STAT
Now order	These are the medications that need to be administered only once after receiving the order. Unlike STAT orders, these medications can be administered within 90 min by the nurse. E.g., Inj. Colistin 7 lakh IU per 1000 mL of PD fluid.

Clinical Corner

CASE SCENARIO 20:
Nurse Amli is preparing Inj. Augmentin to administer. While diluting this medicine, to ensure complete dilution nurse should:

a. Warm the diluents
b. Shake medicine vial vigorously
c. Roll the vial between the palm
d. After adding diluents keep the vial as it is

Ans. (c) Roll the vial between the palm

After reconstituting powdered form of medication with saline or water for reconstitution it should be rolled between palms. It should not be shaken vigorously.

Recent Question

(AIIMS Bibinagar, Tutor 2023)

15. The route of administration in which the drug is rubbed into the skin to get absorbed to produce a systemic effect is:

a. Inunction
b. Dermojet
c. Iontophoresis
d. Topical application

Ans. (a) Inunction

KEY POINTS

- **Instill ear drops at room temperature** to avoid vertigo, dizziness or nausea.
- If patient has eye drop and eye ointment at a time, **apply drop first followed by ointment**.
- STAT order need to be administered only once and immediately.

NURSING THEORIES

- "Theories are a set of interrelated concepts that give a systematic view of a phenomenon (an observable fact or event) that is explanatory and predictive in nature." —**Kerlinger**
- Nursing theories provide rationale for nursing interventions.
- Four concepts (metaparadigms of nursing) of nursing theory are:
  1. Person
  2. Environment
  3. Health
  4. Nursing

Classification of Nursing Theories

- **Metatheory:** It refers to 'theory of theories'. It focuses on philosophical issues and methodological issues of nursing theory, e.g., J. Dickoff's and P. James's Theory of Theory.
- **Grand theory:** It is the most complex and broadest in scope. Therefore, it focuses on nonspecific and abstract concepts. Concepts lack operational definition, e.g., Orem, Roy and Roger's theory.
- **Middle range theory:** It targets specific concepts or phenomena, e.g., Hildegard Peplau theory of interpersonal relations.
- **Practice theory:** It is least complex in nature. It addresses specific goals and explores specific actions needed to achieve them.

KEY POINT

The most important concept in nursing theory is the **'person'.**

Table 34: Summary of nursing theories

Nursing theorist	Year of theory	Central theme
Florence Nightingale	1860	• Environmentalist theory. • Focuses on environmental cleanliness and concerns for ventilation, temperature, light and noise.
Hildegard Peplau	1952	• Theory of interpersonal relationship. • Interventions are directed to support therapeutic interpersonal relationship.
Virginia Henderson	1955	• Nursing need theory. • Focus is on assisting the patient in performance of those activities contributing to health or its recovery. • Theory focuses on increasing the patient's independence.
Faye Abdellah	1960	• Focus is on providing nursing care to meet health-related needs of the patient and family. • 21 nursing-care problems were determined to ascertain patient needs.
Ida Jean Orlando	1961	• Theory focuses on providing solutions to problems in order to diminish the distress of the patient that will enhance well-being.
Myra E Levine	1967	• Conservation Model. • Conservation of energy, structural integrity, personal integrity and social integrity.
Martha Rogers	1970	• Science of unitary human beings. • Major concepts are energy field, open field, pattern and pan dimensionality.
Dorothea Orem	1971	• Self-care deficit theory. • Self-care deficits require nursing interventions.
Imogene King	1971	• Theory of **Goal Attainment.** • Nurses and patients communicate to manage mutually set goals.
Betty Newman	1972	• Systems model. • Based on individual's reaction to stressors in the environment. • Focuses on keeping the patient system stable and assisting patient adjustments to stressors.

Contd...

KEY POINTS

- **According to Virginia Henderson,** "Nurses help patient to perform 14 basic needs."
- **Neuman's system model:** Stress reduction is the goal of systems model of nursing practice.
- **Peplau's theory** focuses on interpersonal relationship (4 phases of interpersonal relationship).
- **Callista Roy** developed the adaptation model, known as Roy's Adaptation Model.
- **Dorothea Orem:** Self-care deficit nursing theory.
- The theory that involves care and helps the patient attain total self-care is **Orem's theory.**

Nursing theorist	Year of theory	Central theme
Sr Callista Roy	1974	• Roy Adaptation Model. • Human beings strive to maintain a balance between biological, psychological and social systems. • Nursing interventions are needed when patient demonstrates ineffective adaptive response to environment.
Madeleine Leininger	1978	• Theory of Transcultural Nursing or Culture Care Theory. • Caring is the central theme of nursing (care, knowledge and practice).
Jean Watson	1979	• Holistic health care is central to the practice of nursing care.

BASIC AND ADVANCED LIFE SUPPORT

Comparison of Components for Adults, Children and Infants BLS/CPR

Table 35: A comparison of the components for adults, children and infants BLS/CPR

Component	Adults	Children	Infants
Recognition	Unresponsive (for all ages)		
	No breathing or no normal breathing (i.e., only gasping)	No breathing or only gasping	
	No pulse palpated within 10 seconds for all age groups (HCP only)		
CPR sequence	C-A-B		
Compression rate	100 to 120/min		
Compression depth	At least 2 inches (5 cm)	At least 1/3 AP diameter about 2 inches (5 cm)	At least 1/3 AP diameter About 1.5 inches (4 cm)
Chest wall recoil	Allow complete recoil between compressions HCPs Rotate compressors every 2 minutes		
Compression interruptions	Minimize interruptions in chest compressions Attempt to limit interruptions to <10 seconds		
Airway	Head tilt-chin lift (HCP suspected trauma: jaw thrust)		
Compression-to-ventilation ratio (until advanced airway placed)	30:2 1 or 2 rescuers	30:2 Single rescuer 15:2 2 HCP rescuers	
Ventilations: when rescuer untrained or trained and not proficient	Compressions only		
Ventilations with advanced airway (HCP)	1 breath every 6–8 seconds (8–10 breaths/min) Asynchronous with chest compressions about 1 second per breath Visible chest rise		
Defibrillation	Attach an AED as soon as available. Minimize interruptions in chest compressions before and after shock; resume CPR beginning with compressions immediately after each shock		

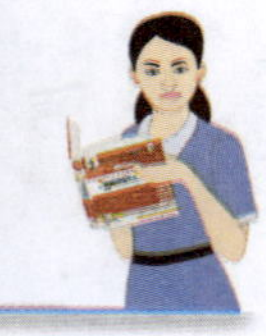

Clinical Corner

CASE SCENARIO 21:

You are working in Neurological ICU and assigned to provide care to a patient who is lightly sedated. You are doing the documentation into the electronic medical system and notice that the patient is continuously doing a non-purposeful action by tapping the side rails of the bed which is very disturbing in work. You went to the patient bed side and threaten him that you will apply the restraint if he doesn't stop. Identify the most appropriate legal term for this scenario.

a. Battery
b. Assault
c. Liability
d. Respondent superior

Ans. **(b) Assault**

Recent Question (NORCET 2021)

16. During child CPR, chest compressions should be given at:

a. Upper half of sternum
b. Xiphisternum
c. Lower half of sternum
d. Below sternum

Ans. **(c) Lower half of sternum**

KEY POINTS

Compresion to Ventilation ratio:

- For adult - 30:2 (for 1 or 2 rescuers).
- For children/infant -
  - 30:2 (single rescuer)
  - 15:2 (2 rescuers).
- For neonate- 3:1

COMPLEMENTARY THERAPIES

Complementary therapies are used along with conventional treatment. As the name indicates, these therapies complement the conventional treatment.

Classifications

Name of the therapy	Description
Acupuncture	Part of **Chinese medicine** In this, needle is inserted into specific body part.
Alexander technique	The Alexander technique helps to identify harmful habits and promotes natural balance through gentle, energy-saving movements, using only the appropriate amount of energy.
Tai chi	A slow, **graceful martial art** that combines breathing techniques and meditation in motion to promote self-healing by improving the flow of energy and calming the mind.
Qi-gong	It is the use of breathing technique and meditation to improve flow of energy around the mind.
Aromatherapy	This therapy is based on the fact that smell can influence one's mood, stress level, sexual desire, and metabolism. The smell releasing oils influence the hypothalamus which is the hormone releasing center of the body. E.g., for oil: chamomile, lavender, peppermint, rosemary, eucalyptus, sandalwood, and tea tree.
Chiropractic	It is a hands-on approach and manipulation of spinal column to aid in the healing. It includes exercises as well as nutritional counseling.
Herbal medicine	Involves the preparation of plant based medicine for specific sign or symptom.
Massage	Manipulation of soft tissue through stroking, rubbing, kneading to improve the blood flow and to relax the muscles. **Five basic strokes in Swedish massage** are effleurage, friction, petrissage, vibration, and percussion.
Reflexology	Applying different amounts of pressure to specific body parts such as hands, foot, and ear.
Cupping	Using heated cup to create vacuum at different body parts which helps to increase the blood flow and to reduce the inflammation.
Meditation	It focuses on rhythmic breathing to calm down the mind and to relax the body.
Relaxation and deep breathing	These are helpful to relieve muscle tension, relieve breathlessness, lessen the stress and anxiety.
Landscape	It is the therapy used for distraction and to manage pain and anxiety. In this, picture/ video of landscape will be show in a darkened room via slide show, video show or art books.
Music therapy	This will help to address physical, psychological, cognitive and social issues. It involves listening to or playing music.
Biofeedback	Process involves visual or auditory information to control thoughts, emotions, or behaviors.
Guided imagery	It involves a group of images to distract the mind to create positive mental images and desired outcome.
Hypnotherapy	It is done by a therapist to induce deep relaxation.
Therapeutic touch	It involves gentle touch to assess energy field changes and relieve stress, fatigue, headache and muscle pain by directing energy from practitioner to patient.
Reiki therapy	It has its roots in Buddhist rituals. Practitioner places hand on client body and energy is transferred from practitioner hand to needed body part of client.
Magnet therapy	Therapy involves placing magnet on patient body to reduce pain and to relax the body.

Non-allopathic Medicine System

A	Ayurveda	It **originated in India**. Ayurvedic treatment consists of products from plant, diet, exercises, and lifestyle modifications.
Y	Yoga and naturopathy	This is a drugless system of medicine. It **originated in India**. It is a mind-body therapy that emphasizes good body posture, breathing technique and meditation to improve overall health.
U	Unani	It is based on **Perso-Arabic system of health**. Unani theory of illness is based on the imbalance between certain fluids in the body.
S	Siddha	It is the **Indian system of medicine** which focuses on balance between human body and the physical environment, climate conditions, stress, physical activities, etc.
H	Homeopathy	It **originated in Germany**. In this system, tiny amount of natural substance is taken from plants and animals and it is believed that it stimulates healing process.

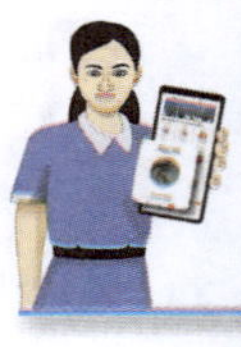

LOSS AND GRIEF

Loss: It is the process or act of losing someone or something.

Grief: It is the emotional response to the loss.

Mourning: It is the social and outward expression of grief which helps the individual to successfully adapt to the loss. E.g., cultural and religious customs surrounding death.

Bereavement: It is a period of grief and mourning after a loss. It includes both emotional response and outward social behavior of the person.

Types of Loss

Type	Description
Actual loss	It is a loss occurs following a real event and it happens when a person can no longer see, hear, or touch an object or a person. This can be recognized and verified by others. E.g., Amputation of extremity, death of a loved one
Perceived loss	It is a loss perceived by the person himself. Others can't verify this type of loss. E.g., loss of confidence
Maturational loss Or Developmental	It is a loss occurs due to normal life transitions. E.g., adolescent going to college by leaving home, loss of teeth and hair with age, menopause in women, marriage, birth of a child.
Situational loss	Loss occurs due to sudden or specific life events. E.g., death of loved one following road traffic accident, sudden loss of job.

Types of Grief

Type	Description
Anticipatory grief	This type of grief is expected, and one prepares himself for the loss. Anticipation does not necessarily ease the pain of loss. E.g., Chronic cancer patient died after years of suffering
Disenfranchised grief	Explained by **Kenneth Dokain** in the year 1989. Grief experienced following loss cannot be openly acknowledged, publicly mourned, or socially supported. E.g., Physician experiences death of patients
Normal grief or Uncomplicated grief	It is the normal universal grief reaction to the loss which is characterized by complex responses.
Complicated grief Or Prolonged grief disorder	Person experiences significant problems to move forward after the loss. Types of complicated grief are: • **Chronic grief:** a person experiences normal grief for longer duration which may be years. • **Exaggerated grief:** person may show self-destructive and maladaptive behaviors. • **Delayed grief**: emotional reaction to the loss is delayed or postponed because of many reasons. • **Masked grief**: people experiencing grief do not express their emotions and suppress them and try to behave like normal.

Takosubo cardiomyopathy (Broken heart syndrome): it is a condition which weakens the left ventricles due to severe emotional or physical stress such as illness, loss of loved one or due to natural disasters (flooding) or accidents etc. It is exclusively seen among women and it resolves within a few months.

Stages of Grief and Dying

The stages of grief were given by Kubler Ross.

The stages include **DABDA** = Denial (D), Anger (A), Bargaining (B), Depression (D), Acceptance (A)

- **Denial:** Whenever one hears about the terminal illness or death of a loved one, at first the person can't accept it. The person will simply deny the fact. It is a form of psychological protection to overcome immediate shock associated with it.

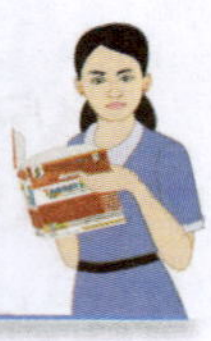

Practice Question

13. The process of preparing families for impending death and continues immediately following death and up until patient death refers to:

a. End of life care
b. Bereavement care
c. Crisis intervention
d. Both b and c

Ans. (b) Bereavement care

Rationale: Bereavement is the period of grief and mourning after a death. Bereavement care is an essential component of hospice care that includes anticipating grief reactions and providing ongoing support for the bereaved.

Recent Question (NORCET 2023)

17. Feeling of loss and sadness, Loneliness is seen in which stage of Kubler ross model?

a. Bargaining
b. Acceptance
c. Depression
d. Denial

Ans. (c) Depression

KEY POINTS

Tasks that facilitate passage from grief to closure are:

- Accepting the reality of loss
- Experiencing the pain of grief
- Adjusting to the new environment that excludes the lost person or object
- Channeling emotional energy into new relationships

- **Anger:** Once the denial is over, then the person expresses intense emotions or anger at the situation, to a person or to the God.
- **Bargaining:** It is the negotiation by the client to the supreme power or higher authority or God to delay the events. E.g., Client may ask God to let the person live till a major event like marriage, birthday etc.
- **Depression**: In this phase, the person realizes the impact of loss.
- **Acceptance**: Person accepts the truth and incorporates it into life.

ACTIVITY AND EXERCISE

- **Activity:** It is an energetic action and being in a state of movement.
- **Body alignment:** It is the geometrical relationship of one body part to another either in a horizontal or on a vertical plane.
- **Body mechanics:** It is the efficient and well-co-ordinated use of the body to produce motion, balance and activity.
- **Range of motion:** It is the maximum movement possible at a particular joint.

Types of Exercise

Type	Description
Isotonic (dynamic)	A type of physical activity in which muscles contract and relax while working against a constant resistance. E.g., walking, running, swimming
Isometric (static)	A type of strength training exercise that involves contracting a muscle without changing its length. Useful to maintain the strength of an immobilized muscle. E.g., strengthening of abdominal muscle, neck isometrics to treat spondylosis.
Isokinetic (resistive)	Isokinetic exercise involves performing movements at a constant speed against a resistance. It can be either isotonic or isometric. E.g., push-ups

Contd...

OXYGENATION

Oxygenation is a process that comprises both inspiration and expiration and the exchange of gases in the body.

- **Ventilation**: It is the process of moving gas into and out of the lung through inspiration and expiration
- **Inspiration**: Movement of oxygen into the lung
- **Expiration:** Movement of carbon dioxide out of the lung.
- **Perfusion:** It is the process of intake of oxygen by tissue and return of carbon dioxide into the lung.
- **Atelectasis**: Collapse of the alveoli which prevent air exchange.
- **Hypoxia**: Decreased oxygen level in the tissue
- **Hypoxemia**: Decreased oxygen level in the blood.
- **Peripheral chemoreceptors** of respiration are in the **carotid and aortic bodies.**
- **Peripheral chemoreceptors** are more sensitive to PaO_2.
- **Central chemoreceptors** of respiration are located in the **ventrolateral surface of medulla oblongata.**
- **Central chemoreceptors** are more sensitive to change in H^+ ion.
- **Capnography:** It is the noninvasive measurement of the carbon dioxide level in the expired gas. It is known as end tidal CO_2.
- Humidification of oxygen helps to prevent the dryness of the airway.
- In a COPD patient, decreased level of oxygen in the blood is the respiratory drive. So, do not administer oxygen at high flow rate.
- Atmospheric air contains **21% oxygen.**
- Expired air contains **16% oxygen.**
- Neonate exposed to high level of oxygen may develop **retinopathy of prematurity.**
- Oxygen is a flammable gas; so, there is a risk of fire accident.

KEY POINT

In a **COPD patient,** decreased level of oxygen in the blood is the respiratory drive. So, do not administer oxygen at high flow rate.

POINTS TO REMEMBER

- Wide base of support helps to maintain balance.
- More balance can be achieved by bringing center of gravity down and near to the wide base of support.

Clinical Corner

CASE SCENARIO 22:
Upon assessment of the client, the nurse notices bradycardia, wheezing, and a respiratory rate of 10 breaths/minute. These signs are indicative of which of the following condition?

a. Delirium
b. Hyperventilation
c. Hypoxia
d. Hyperpnea

Ans. (c) Hypoxia

The signs of wheezing, bradycardia, and a respiratory rate of 10 breaths/minute collectively suggest that the patient is experiencing hypoxia, which refers to a deficiency of oxygen in the tissues and organs of the body. Hypoxia can have various causes, such as respiratory conditions, cardiac disorders, or inadequate oxygen delivery.

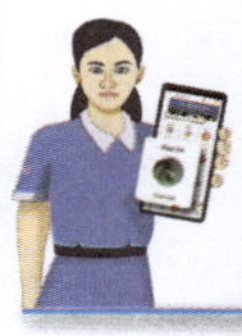

Oxygen Administration Methods

Sl. no.	Name	Points to remember	Image
Low-flow system			
1	Nasal cannula	**Flow rate:** 1-6 L/min. Flow rate higher than 4 L/min has drying effect on mucosa. Patient can talk and eat while receiving the oxygen therapy. **Limitations:** easily dislodged, not useful in mouth breathing patient, not useful in patient with polyps, deviated nasal septum and nasal block, drying of nasal mucosa.	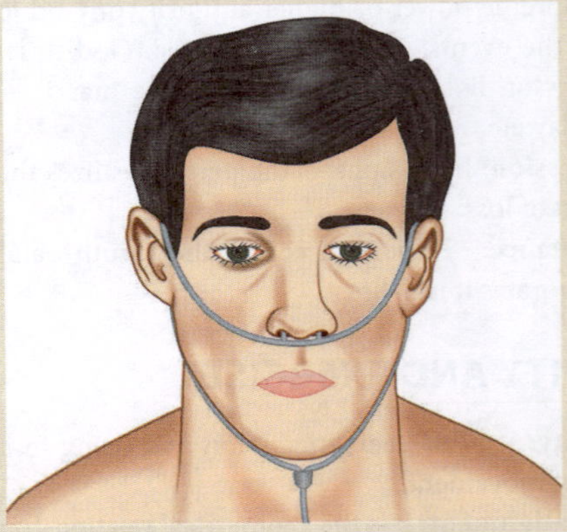
2	Nasopharyngeal catheter	• Nasopharyngeal catheters are passed into the nose and through to the posterior pharynx. • Useful when a patient's mouth is difficult to open in conditions like angioedema and trismus. • Mucosal irritation is the disadvantage of this method.	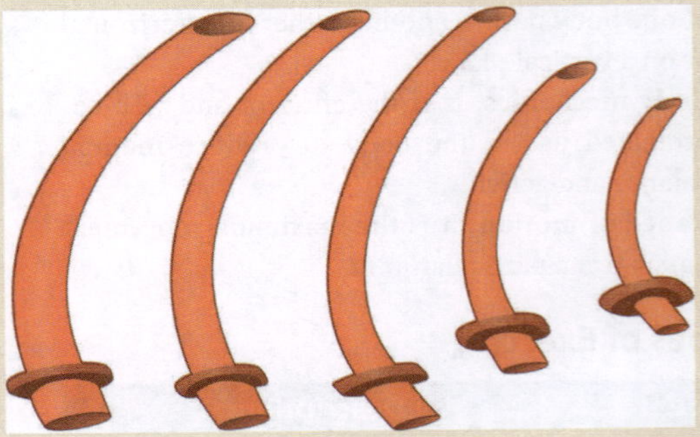
3	Face mask/ simple oxygen mask	• It fits over nose and mouth of the patient. • It has a metal clip to fit over the nose and elastic band to adjust the tightness of the mask. • It has holes on the sides (exhalation ports) which remain always open and aid in carbon dioxide exhalation. • **Flow**: 6-12 L/min • **Limitations**: difficult to talk and eat while wearing mask.	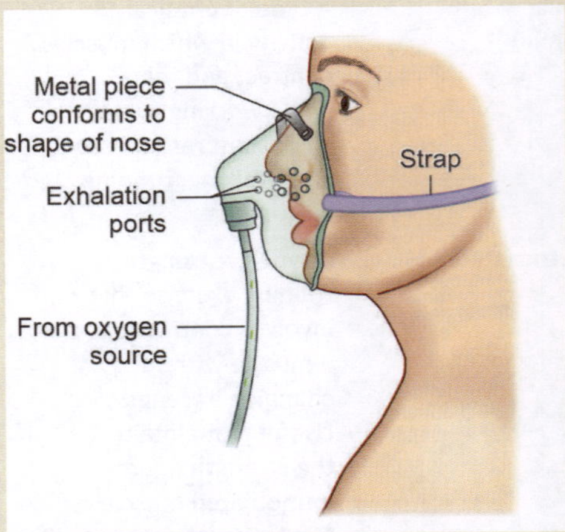
High flow system			
4	Face tent	• Mask covers face and nose but does not create a tight seal around the nose. • It helps to provide oxygen to patient with facial trauma or burn injury. • It is difficult to achieve high concentration of oxygen with this.	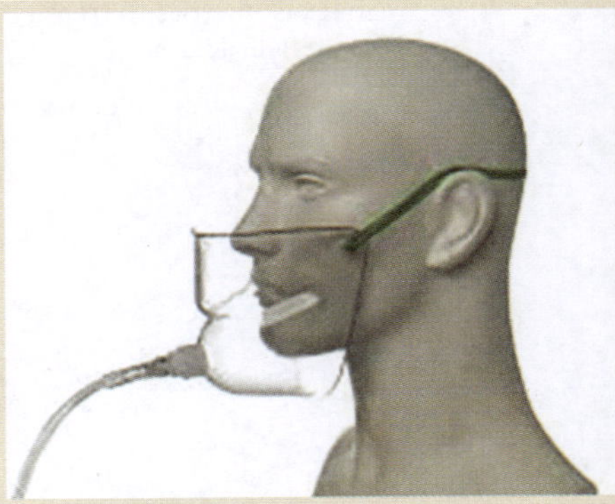

Contd...

Sl. no.	Name	Points to remember	Image
5	Transtracheal oxygenation	• In a patient with chronic use of oxygen, Teflon catheter is inserted directly into trachea between 2nd and 3rd tracheal ring. • This method helps to bypass the dead space in the upper airway and deliver oxygen directly into the trachea. • Infection and irritation are the most common risk factors associated with this.	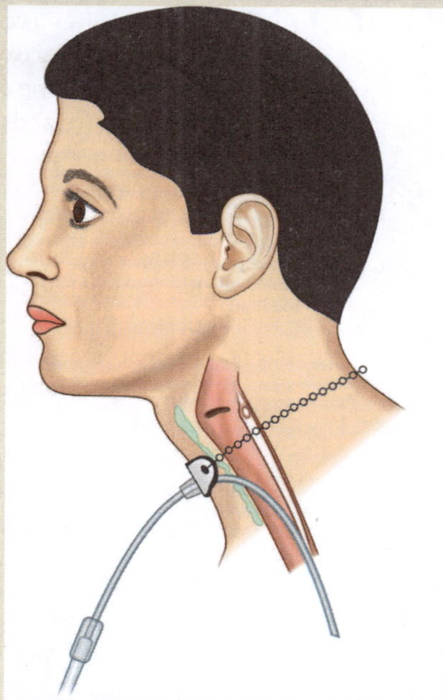
6	Nonrebreather mask *(Qs asked in NORCET 2023)*	• It has a mask with a bag and one-way valve between them. • During inspiration, one-way valve opens and patient takes air only from the bag and exhalation port remains closed. • During exhalation, one-way valve remains closed and the exhaled air is directed to the exhalation ports which remain open during exhalation. • **Limitations:** Risk of suffocation if gas flow is interrupted. Bag should not be deflated completely. It interferes with speaking and eating. • **Flow**: 10-15 L/min	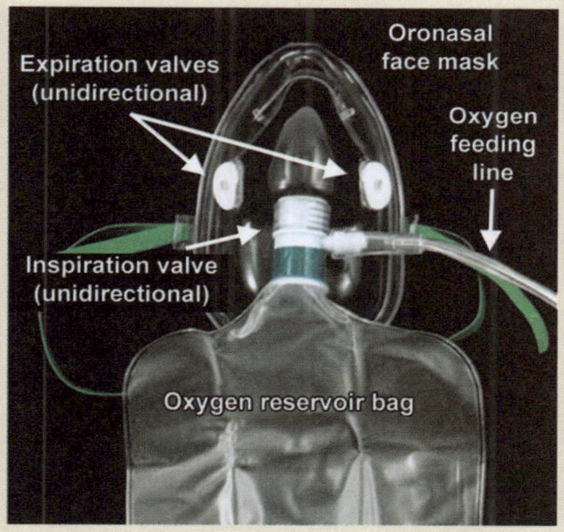
7	Partial rebreather mask	• It has a mask and the reservoir attached to it. • It has a two-way valve between mask and the reservoir. • The two-way valve allows first 150 mL of the exhaled air to go to the reservoir bag and to mix with oxygen and to use for the next respiration. Exhalation port remains closed during expiration. • The reservoir bag should remain partially inflated. • **Limitations:** interfere with eating and talking • **Flow**: 10-15 L/min	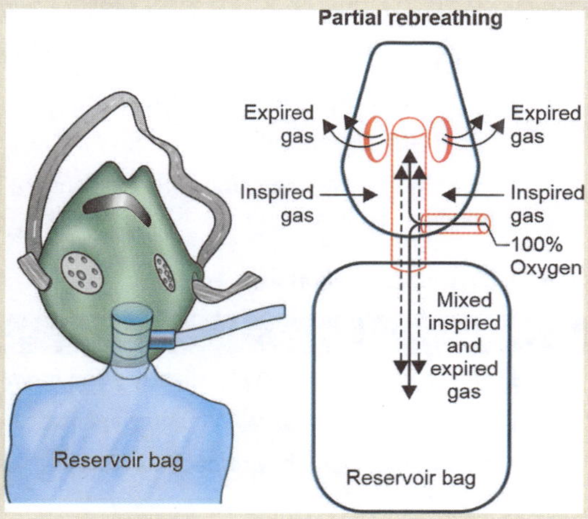

Contd...

Sl. no.	Name	Points to remember	Image
8	Venturi mask	• Used to deliver a controlled and precise concentration of oxygen to a patient. • It works by mixing air with a high-flow oxygen source and using the Venturi effect to deliver a specific oxygen concentration to the patient. • The mask consists of a mask body, a connecting tube, and a variety of interchangeable Venturi hoods with different sized air holes. • Different hoods can be easily interchanged to change the oxygen concentration as needed. • Delivers 24-60% oxygen • Flow rate: 2–15 L/min • Flow rate varies with color Blue = 2–4 L/min = 24% O_2 White = 4–6 L/min = 28% O_2 Yellow = 8–10 L/min = 35% O_2 Red = 10–12 L/min = 40% O_2 Green = 12–15 L/min = 60% O_2	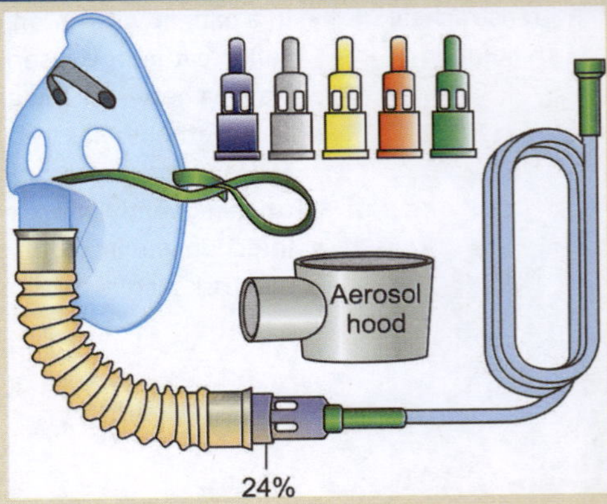

Postural Drainage Positions—Adults

Sl. no.	Position	Lobe
1	High Fowler's	Both lungs
2	Sitting on side of bed	Apical segment
3	Supine with head elevated	• Right upper lobe anterior segment • Left upper lobe anterior segment
4	Right-side lying-in Trendelenburg position	Left lower lobe lateral segment
5	Left side lying in Trendelenburg position	Right lower lobe lateral segment
6	Prone with right side of the chest elevated in Trendelenburg position	Right lower lobe posterior segment
7	Prone with thorax and abdomen elevated	Right middle lobe posterior segment
8	Side lying with right side of the chest elevated on pillows	Right upper lobe posterior segment
9	Left lateral position	Right upper lobe apical segment
10	Side lying with left side of the chest elevated on pillows	Left upper lobe posterior segment
11	Supine with Trendelenburg position	Both lower lobe anterior segment
12	Prone with Trendelenburg position	Both lower lobe posterior segment
13	Three fourth supine position with dependent lung in Trendelenburg position	Right middle lobe anterior segment

Postural Drainage—Babies

Sl. no.	Position	Segment
1	Sitting on care giver lap with slightly bend forward	B/L apical segment
2	Sitting on care giver lap with leaning against care giver	B/L middle and anterior segment
3	Lying on care giver lap with back supported	B/L lobe anterior segment

INCENTIVE SPIROMETER

- Incentive spirometer has visual feedback mechanism, that's why it is called incentive spirometry.
- Spirometer is of two types:
  - Volume based
  - Flow based (triflow exerciser)

Indications

- Postoperative patients
- Atelectasis
- Decreased ventilation

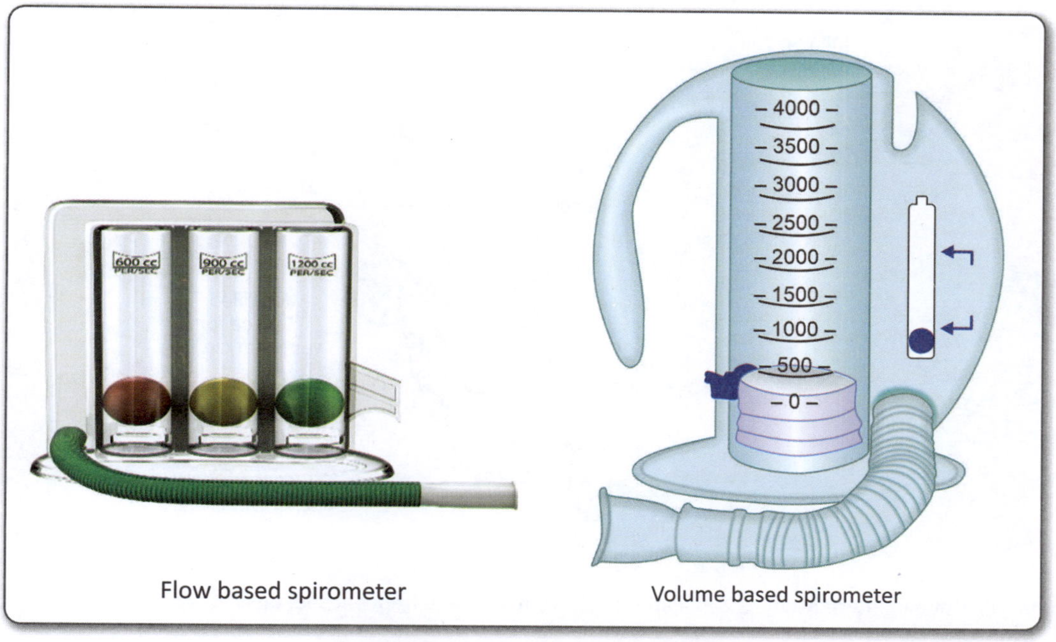

Figure 22: Incentive spirometer

Contraindications

Use of spirometer is contraindicated if patient is experiencing:

- Wheezing
- Chest tightness
- Dyspnea.
- Hemoptysis of unknown origin
- Uncontrolled hypertension
- Aneurysm

SUCTION

Suction is the application of negative pressure to remove secretions from tracheobronchial tree.

POINTS TO REMEMBER

- **Hyperoxygenation with 100% FiO_2** should be done before airway suctioning.
- **Never apply pressure while inserting** the suction catheter.
- **Apply suction while withdrawing** the suction catheter.
- While removing, **use rotatory motion to withdraw** the catheter as it aids in removing secretions adhered to the side of the airways.
- While to suctioning mouth and nose, **first do oral then nasal** otherwise risk of aspiration is there.
- Each suction session **should not be longer than 10 seconds.**

POINTS TO REMEMBER

- Use incentive spirometry in sitting or standing position.
- Keep the device straight at eye level while performing the test
- Use bronchodilators if prescribed (inhaler/nebulization) before using spirometry.
- Support suture site in case of post operative patient.
- Do not perform this immediately after meal or a strenuous activity.
- Maximum flow through the triflo incentive spirometry is 1200 cc/sec
- Maximum volume of volume-based incentive spirometry is 4000 mL.
- Work of breathing is less with volume-based incentive spirometry than flow-based incentive spirometry.
- Volume-based incentive spirometers are giving diaphragmatic exercises.
- Flow-based incentive spirometers focus on muscles of the upper chest.

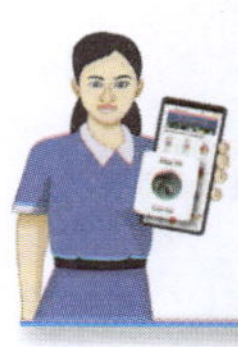

Open suction	Closed suction (in-line suction)
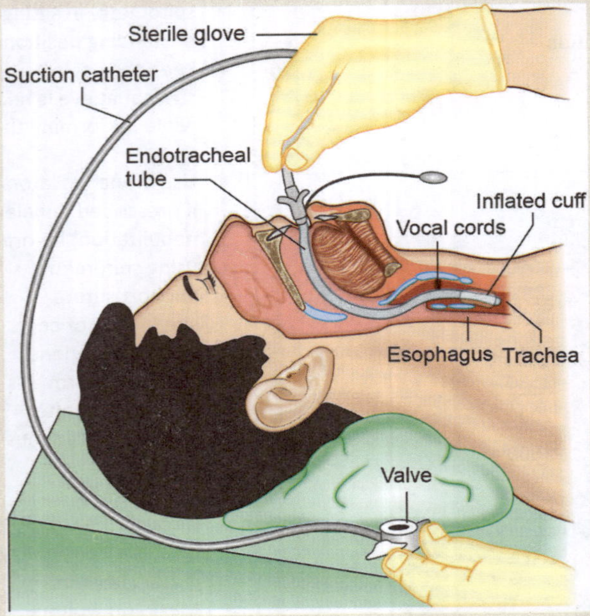	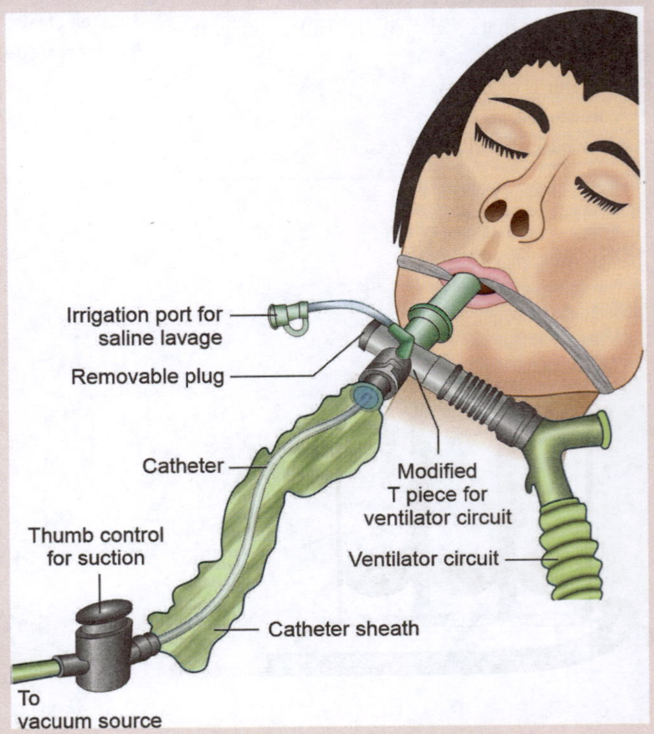
Patient recently removed from ventilator and intermittent suction is needed	Patient is on ventilator and frequent suction is needed.
Patient needs to be disconnected from ventilator and single use suction catheter is used	No need to disconnect from the ventilator. One-way valve allows suction catheter insertion without removing the ventilator.
Airway remains open to the environment, and there is a loss of PEEP, which can result in decreased alveolar pressure and reduced lung expansion and can lead to atelectasis.	Closed suction maintains PEEP and pressure levels within the airway
Open suction increases the risk of contamination and infection	Reduces the risk of infection by providing a closed system

Suction Pressure

Adult	120–150 mm Hg
Children	60–100 mm Hg
Infant	40–60 mm Hg

ORAL AIRWAY

- Oral airway is also known as **Guedel airway**.
- Guedel airway helps maintain an open airway and prevents the tongue from blocking the airway.
- Size of the airway is determined from the corner of mouth to the angle of the jaw.
- If airway used is small, then tongue does not stay in the anterior portion of mouth.
- If airway used is big, then it forces the tongue toward epiglottis and obstructs the airway.

KEY POINT

Guedel airway is an example of Oropharyngeal airway.

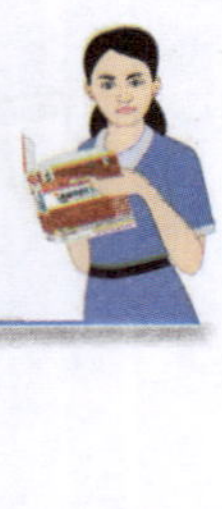

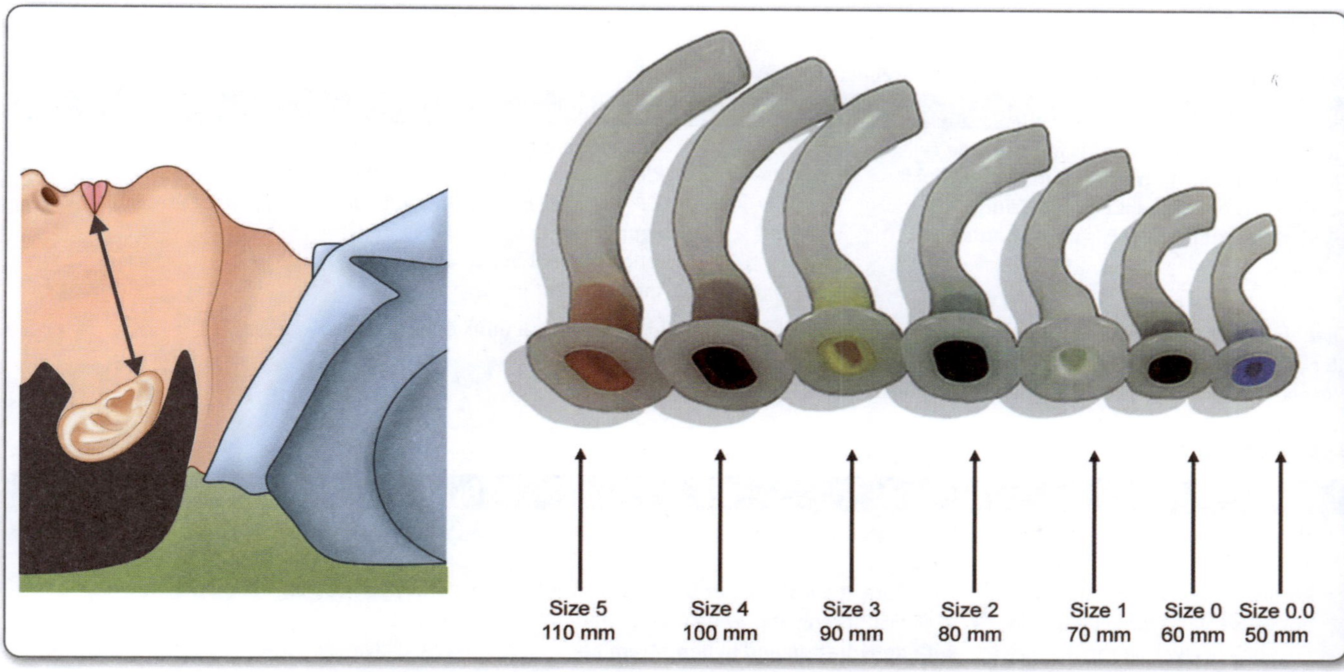

Figure 23: Guedel airway (Common adult sizes)

CHEST TUBE/INTERCOSTAL DRAINAGE

- Chest tube is also known as a **pleural catheter**.
- It is a flexible tube inserted into the pleural cavity through the chest wall to drain fluid or air that has accumulated in the pleural space.
- For **pneumothorax,** chest tube is inserted at **2nd and 3rd intercostal space at mid clavicular** line.
- For **hemothorax,** chest tube is inserted at **4th or 5th intercostal space at mid axillary line.**

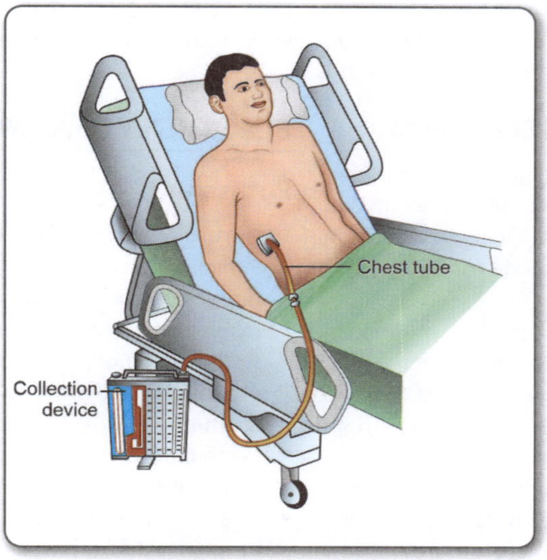

Figure 24: Chest tube drainage system

Indications

- **Pneumothorax**: Air accumulates in the pleural space.
- **Hemothorax**: Blood accumulates in the pleural space.
- **Pleural effusion**: Fluid accumulates in the pleural space.
- **Empyema**: Pus accumulates in the pleural space.

Recent Question
(NORCET 2023)

18. A nurse taking care of a patient with chest tube drainage suddenly notices that there is no fluctuation in the water seal tube. Which of the following action should the nurse take first?

a. Turn the patient to the unaffected side
b. Inform the physician
c. Check the tubing to ensure there is no kinking
d. Start milking the chest tube

Ans. (c) Check the tubing to ensure there is no kinking

POINTS TO REMEMBER

- Chest tube system should be closed and below the level of patient
- Chest tube should be secured to client's chest
- Make sure that water level is maintained in the water seal chamber.
- Check tidaling (fluctuation of water column) in chest tube to ensure the working of chest tube.
- Bubbling in the chest drainage indicates air leakage.
- Clamping of chest tube is contraindicated as it can lead to pneumothorax.
- Routine milking and stripping of chest tube are not recommended.
- If any accidental dislodge of chest tube happens, then cover the area of insertion.

FLUIDS

Body fluids are in two compartments, i.e., intracellular and extracellular

Intra cellular fluid (ICF)	Extracellular fluid (ECF)
ICF refers to the fluid that is found inside cells. ICF is about two-thirds of the total body fluid. Cation present in the ICF is **potassium.** Anion present in the ICF is **phosphorus.**	Fluid found outside the cell is known as ECF. ECF is approximately 1/3rd of the total body water. ECFs are intravascular (plasma), interstitial, and transcellular (CSF, pleural fluid etc). Cation present in ECF is **sodium.** Anion present in ECF is **chloride.**

Osmolarity: It is a measure of the total concentration of solutes in a fluid, expressed in units of osmoles per liter (Osm/L).
Normal osmolarity of plasma is **280-295 mOsm/L.**

Types of Fluids

Isotonic	Hypotonic	Hypertonic
• Solutions that have the same osmotic pressure as body fluids. • Administration of this fluid will not cause significant changes in fluid balance within the body. • It is used to treat dehydration in clinical setting.	• Lower osmotic pressure compared to body fluids. • Therefore, it causes **water to move into cells.** • In clinical setting, it may be used in **patient with dehydration and hypernatremia.** • Use cautiously in patients with heart, liver and kidney failure.	• Higher osmotic pressure compared to body fluids. So, **fluid moves out of the cells.** • It may be used for the **management of edema.** • While giving, closely monitor client for hypervolemia, hypertension and breathing difficulties.
• (0.9% NaCl), Ringer's lactate, and plasma-lyte, 5% dextrose in water	• 0.45%NS, • Saline (NaCl) solutions with <0.9% concentration • 2.5% Dextrose (<5% dextrose concentration)	• 3% NS, 5% D in NS, 5%D in RL, D10, D25, D50 • DNS (Dextrose [5%] in NS) • D5 in 0.45% NaCl

Movement of Fluid and Electrolyte

- **Active transport:** It refers to movement of solutes from an area of low concentration to an area of high concentration against their concentration gradient. This requires ATP and specific transport proteins.
- **Diffusion:** It refers to passive movement of substances or molecules from higher concentration to lower concentration due to natural concentration gradient until equilibrium is reached.
- **Osmosis:** It refers to passive movement of water molecules from an area of high water concentration (lower solute concentration) to an area of low water concentration (higher solute concentration) across a semi-permeable membrane, in response to a difference in solute concentration. The direction of osmosis is determined by the relative concentration of solutes on either side of the membrane.
- **Facilitated diffusion:** It refers to movement of water soluble solutes across the cell membrane with assistance of proteins.

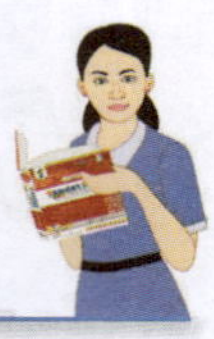

ELECTROLYTE ABNORMALITIES

Potassium

- Normal range: **3.5–5.2 mEq/L**
- Potassium is essential for regulation of fluid balance, muscle contractions, and the maintenance of a normal heart rhythm.
- Reabsorption of potassium mainly takes place at **proximal convoluted tubule** (65–85%) and **thick ascending loop of Henle (10–20%).**
- Potassium secretion mainly occurs at the **distal convoluted tubule** and **collecting duct**.
- The secretion of potassium is regulated by the hormone **Aldosterone**.
- Aldosterone promotes the **uptake of sodium** and the **excretion of potassium** by the kidneys.

Foods rich in potassium: Banana, leafy vegetables, root vegetables (potato, sweet potato), dried apricot, dark chocolate, dates, beans, tomato, raisins, yogurt, milk, orange juice.

Recent Question
(AIIMS Bibinagar, Faculty 2023)

19. Which of the following statements is FALSE regarding electrolytes?
a. Balances your body's acid/base (pH) level
b. Moves nutrients into your cells
c. Helps in blood production
d. Balances the amount of water in your body

Ans. (c) Helps in blood production

Recent Question
(NORCET 2023)

20. The type of fluid which causes water to shift from cells into blood stream?
a. Hypotonic
b. Hypertonic
c. Isotonic
d. Albumin

Ans. (b) Hypertonic

Hypokalemia

Low level of potassium in the blood.

Causes

- Decreased potassium intake
- Excessive vomiting or diarrhea
- Certain medications, such as laxatives, corticosteroids, and insulin.
- Adrenal insufficiency (Cushing syndrome)
- Excess aldosterone secretion
- Diuretic use

Signs and symptoms

- Weakness/cramps
- Paralysis
- Fatigue
- Muscle twitching
- Arrhythmias
- Metabolic acidosis
- Constipation
- Respiratory paralysis

ECG changes

- T-wave flattening initially
- ST-segment depression
- T-wave inversions
- Abnormal U wave

Hyperkalemia

High level of potassium in the blood

Causes

- Increased potassium intake
- Kidney failure
- Oliguria
- Addison's disease
- Hypoaldosteronism
- Rhabdomyolysis
- Potassium-sparing diuretics such as spironolactone
- Release of potassium from tissue following injury such as burns

Signs and symptoms

- Arrhythmias
- Muscle cramps
- Muscle weakness
- Rhabdomyolysis
- Myoglobinuria

ECG changes

- Spiky T wave
- Flat P wave
- Prolonged PR interval
- Widening of QRS complex
- Sine wave pattern

Sodium

- **Normal range: 135–145 mEq/L**
- Plays an important role in acid-base balance and the fluid balance in the body.
- Supports proper nerve and muscle function.
- Sodium regulation happens at kidney (osmotic balance maintenance).
- **Proximal tubule** is the part where majority of the **sodium is reabsorbed** into the body.
- **Foods rich in sodium:** table salt, processed food, fast food, deli meats, cheese, sauce, pickled food, smoked food, canned meat.

Hyponatremia

Serum sodium level is <135 mmol/L.

Causes

- Excessive water intake
- Diuretic use
- Kidney disease
- Addison's disease
- Heart failure
- Liver disease
- Low sodium consumption
- Increased loss of sodium
- Increased ADH hormone
- Hypoaldosteronism

Signs and symptoms

- It cause neurological manifestations
- Headaches
- Confusion and drowsiness
- Nausea
- Delirium.
- Vomiting
- Seizure
- Muscle cramps
- Irritability
- Restlessness

Hypernatremia

Serum sodium levels are >145 mmol/L.

Causes

- Increased sodium intake
- Decreased water intake
- Excessive water loss (diarrhea, fever, vomiting, sweating).
- Hormonal imbalance (Cushing syndrome)
- Decreased ADH (diabetes insipidus)
- Osmotic diuresis in diabetes mellitus
- Dehydration
- Hyperaldosteronism
- *Prolonged cortisone use*

Signs and symptoms

- Dehydration
- Lethargy
- Weakness
- Irritability
- Seizure and coma
- Fever
- Edema
- Thirst
- Dry mouth
- Nausea and vomiting
- Confusion
- Neuromuscular excitability
- Hyperreflexia, seizures

KEY POINTS

- Excessive water intake leads to **Hyponatremia.**
- Decreased water intake OR excessive water loss leads to **Hypernatremia.**

Recent Question
(AIIMS Bibinagar, Tutor 2023)

21. All of the following statements are true about SIADH lab values EXCEPT

a. SIADH cause increased urine osmolarity
b. SIADH cause elevated urine sodium concentration
c. SIADH cause decreased plasma osmolarity
d. SIADH cause increased plasma osmolarity

Ans. (d) SIADH cause increased plasma osmolarity

Syndrome of Inappropriate Antidiuretic Hormone (SIADH) results in increased antidiuretic hormone (ADH) secretion, leading to increased water retention and dilution of the blood's solutes. As a result, plasma osmolarity decreases rather than increases in SIADH. The excess water retention causes the blood to become more diluted, resulting in a lower concentration of solutes in the blood and decreased plasma osmolarity. The other statements (a, b, and c) are true about SIADH lab values.

STRATEGY: Option c and d are opposite statements. So, the either c or d must be the answer.

Eliminate a and b because both are similar statements (elevated urine sodium (b) = increased urine osmolarity(a)).

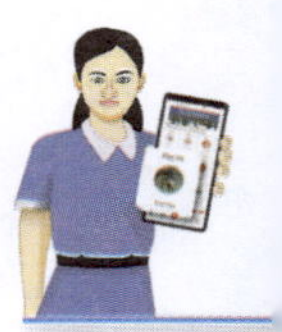

Calcium

- **Normal range: 8.5-10.5 mg/dL**
- Responsible for building and maintaining strong bones and teeth, nerve and muscle functions, blood clotting, hormone secretion and enzyme function.
- It is abundantly present in the ECF.

Dietary sources: dairy products, such as milk and cheese, leafy green vegetables, such as kale and spinach, nuts, and seeds such as almonds and sesame seeds.

Hypocalcemia

Low calcium levels in the blood, <8.5 mg/dL.

Causes

- Deficiency of parathyroid hormone (hypoparathyroidism).
- Deficiency of Vitamin D.
- High level of phosphorus
- Low level of albumin
- Malabsorption (Crohn's disease, celiac disease, pancreatitis).
- Kidney disease
- Phenytoin use
- Severe burn injury

Signs and symptoms

- **Osteoporosis**
- **Muscle weakness and cramps**
- Mood changes
- Numbness and tingling in the fingers, toes, and face.
- Confusion and disorientation
- Joint and bone pain
- Seizure
- **Slow and irregular heartbeat**
- **Tetany**
- **Trousseau's sign:** Carpopedal spasm will be present during the inflation of BP cuff.
- **Chvostek's sign:** Tapping the patient's facial nerve near the ear causes ipsilateral contraction of muscle.

Hypercalcemia

High calcium level in the blood, >10.5 mg/dL.

Causes

- Hyperparathyroidism
- Hyperthyroidism
- Multiple myeloma, breast and lung cancer
- Vitamin D toxicity
- Prolonged immobilization
- Sarcoidosis (granulomas)
- Dehydration
- Bone cancer (Paget's disease)
- Thiazide diuretics
- Long-term lithium use
- Excessive ingestion of calcium carbonate ('milk alkali syndrome')

Signs and symptoms

- Musculoskeletal pain and pathological fracture
- Renal colic (flank pain)
- Abdominal pain
- Nausea and vomiting
- Constipation
- Anorexia
- **QT shortening potentially leading to ventricular fibrillation arrest.**
- Confusion and coma (severe case)
- Lethargy
- Polyurea
- **Nephrolithiasis**
- Excess urination
- Dehydration
- Muscle cramps and weakness
- Bone pain

Magnesium

- **Normal range:** 1.46–2.86 mg/dL
- It is an intracellular cation involved with ATP metabolism, contraction and relaxation of muscles, proper neurological functioning, and neurotransmitter release.

Dietary sources: Dark chocolate, avocados, nuts, legumes, seeds (**flax, pumpkin, and chia seeds), whole grains (wheat, oats, and barley), banana, spinach**

Contd...

Recent Question
(AIIMS Bibinagar, Tutor 2023)

22. ________ is the hormone that helps in reabsorption of sodium, chloride and water in the renal tubules to maintain the water balance.
a. Thyroxin
b. Aldosterone
c. Growth hormone
d. Calcitonin

Ans. (b) Aldosterone

Recent Question
(NORCET 2022)

23. A patient who has undergone thyroidectomy shows the symptoms of carpopedal spasm. Which medication is to be administered to this patient?
a. Calcium carbonate
b. Calcium gluconate
c. Calcium lactate
d. Calcium citrate

Ans. (b) Calcium gluconate

KEY POINTS

- Positive Trousseau's sign and Chvostek's sign indicate Hypocalemia.
- QT shortening, Nephrolithiasis and renal colic are notable complications of hypercalcemia.

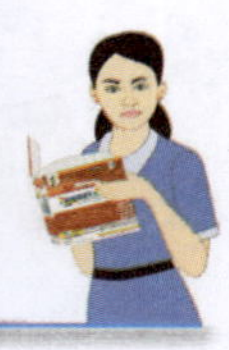

Hypomagnesemia
Low serum magnesium <1.46 mg/dL
Causes
- Decreased intake
- Malabsorption in Crohn's disease, celiac disease
- Chronic alcoholism
- Intake of certain drugs such as diuretics, proton pump inhibitors, and aminoglycoside antibiotics
- Kidney disease
- Diabetes mellitus
- Sweating

Signs and symptoms
- Muscle weakness and cramp
- Generalized weakness
- Cardiac ischemia and death
- Nervousness
- Irritability
- Nausea and vomiting
- Confusion

Hypermagnesemia
High level of magnesium >2.86 mg/dL
Causes
- Decreased renal excretion
- Increased intake
- Milk-alkali syndrome

Signs and symptoms
- Weakness
- Nausea
- Dizziness
- Confusion
- Decreased reflexes
- Bladder paralysis
- Flushing
- Headache
- Constipation
- Bradycardia
- Blurred vision

Phosphorous

- **Normal range:** 2.5–4.5 mg/dL
- Important mineral with the functions of bone and teeth health, necessary for ATP production, nerve and muscle functions, DNA and RNA synthesis.

Dietary sources: Dairy products, meats and whole grains

Hypophosphatemia
Serum phosphate level <2.5 mg/dL.
Causes
- Inadequate intake
- Intestinal malabsorption
- Chronic diarrhea
- Hyperparathyroidism
- Refeeding syndrome
- Alcoholism
- Drugs such as antacids

Signs and symptoms
- Muscle weakness
- Fatigue
- Breathing difficulty
- Numbness and tingling
- Confusion
- Osteomalacia

Hyperphosphatemia
Serum phosphate level >4.5 mg/dL.
Causes
- Renal failure
- High intake of phosphorus
- Excessive use of phosphate-containing laxatives or enema
- Vitamin D intoxication
- Hypoparathyroidism
- Acromegaly
- Thyrotoxicosis
- Tumor lysis syndrome

Signs and symptoms
- Nausea and vomiting
- Muscle weakness and cramps
- Confusion and altered mental status
- Tetany

ACID-BASE BALANCE

- Normal blood pH is 7.35–7.45
- Decrease in pH <7.35 is acidosis, and increase in pH >7.45 is known as alkalosis.
- **Acid:** Any substance that yields H^+ ion in a solution.
- **Alkali (base):** Any substance that yields OH^- in the solution.

Normal values of ABG interpretation
- pH = 7.35–7.45
- pCO_2 = 35–45 mm Hg
- pO_2 = 75–100 mm Hg
- HCO_3^- = 22–26 mEq/L
- O_2 Sat = >95%

Buffer System

- A buffer system is a mechanism in the body that helps to maintain a stable pH in the blood and other bodily fluids.
- Buffer is any solution which contains a weak acid, weak base and their salts.

Practice Question

14. A 50-year-old male patient with a history of COPD is brought to the emergency room with shortness of breath and fever. Arterial blood gas shows pH 7.3, $PaCO_2$ 65 mm Hg, HCO_3 29 mmol/L, and PaO_2 60 mm Hg. Which of the following is the correct interpretation of the ABG analysis?
a. Metabolic acidosis, partially compensated
b. Respiratory acidosis, partially compensated
c. Respiratory acidosis, fully compensated
d. Respiratory acidosis, uncompensated

Ans. (b) Respiratory...

KEY POINTS

- **Metabolic acidosis** is the most common acid-base imbalance in acute kidney injury, caused by impaired excretion of metabolic fixed acid.
- **Metabolic alkalosis** can occur in repeated episodes of vomiting due to loss of HCL from stomach.
- **Metabolic acidosis** can occur in diarrhoea due to the loss of bicarbonate (HCO3-) through GI tract.

Recent Question
(AIIMS Bibinagar, Faculty 2023)

24. Geetha, a 6-year-old girl had severe diarrhoea and her body lost too much of sodium bicarbonate. This led to:
a. Hyperchloremic acidosis
b. Calcaemic acidosis
c. Diabetic ketoacidosis
d. Lactic acidosis

Ans. (a) Hyperchloremic acidosis

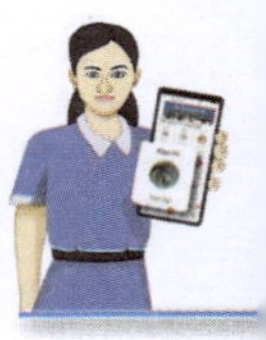

- Most important types of buffer systems include:
  - Bicarbonate buffer (HCO_3^-/CO_2): Ratio of bicarbonate buffer system is 20:1 (HCO_3^-: CO_2). It is the major buffer in the ECF (blood plasma).
  - Hemoglobin buffer (in erythrocytes)
  - Phosphate buffer system
  - Protein buffer system
  - Ammonium buffer

Mechanism of Regulation of pH

Front Line Mechanism

- Buffer in the blood
- Respiratory buffer

Second Line Buffer Mechanism

- Renal mechanism

Dilution Defense

- Acid/base entered or produced in the body will be equally distributed throughout the ECF and therefore, change in pH will be negligible.

ABG Analysis/Acid Base Balance has been discussed in detail in Appendices.

HOT AND COLD APPLICATIONS

There are two types of applications: hot application and cold application.

Hot Application

Hot application is the application of a hot agent, either in a moist or dry form on the surface of the body.

Purposes:

- To relieve pain and congestion
- To provide warmth
- To promote suppuration (pus formation) and soften the exudates
- To promote healing
- To decrease muscle tone

Contraindications of Hot Application:

- Impaired kidney, heart or lung functions
- Malignancies
- Acutely inflamed areas
- Open wounds
- Edema associated with venous or lymphatic disease
- Clients with paralysis
- Clients with metabolic disorder
- Headache
- Very young and very old clients

Clinical Corner

CASE SCENARIO 23:
Which of the following statements is CORRECT regarding the use of hot applications for patients?

a. Extended periods of hot application is recommended.
b. Hot applications should be applied directly to the skin without any protective barrier to ensure effective heat transfer.
c. Hot applications are contraindicated for patients with acute inflammation.
d. Hot applications can be applied directly to open wounds to promote healing.

Ans. (c) Hot applications are contraindicated for patients with acute inflammation.

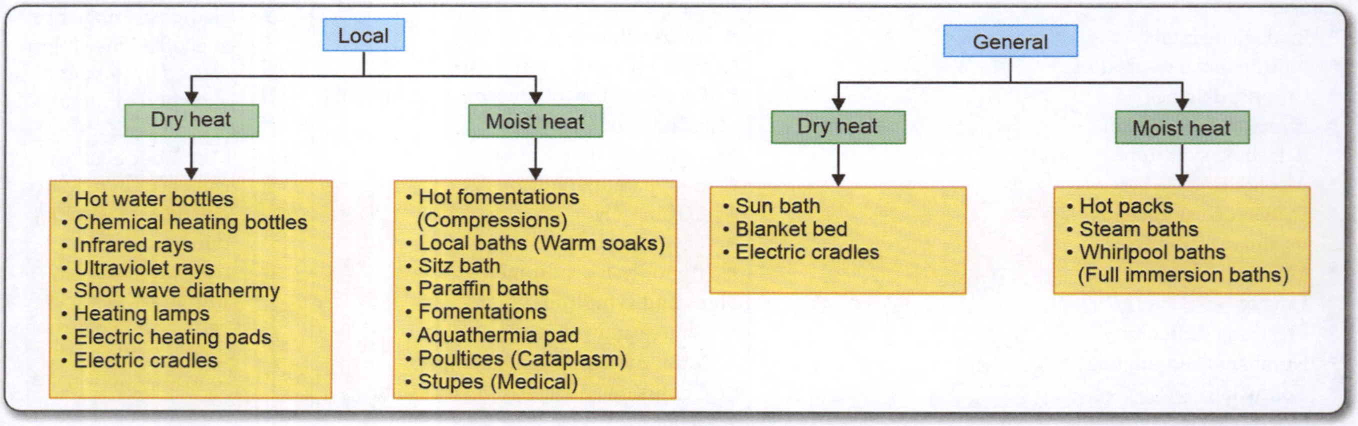

Figure 25: Classification of hot application

Cold Application

Cold application is the application of a cold agent, either in a moist or dry form on the surface of the skin.

Purposes:

- To reduce pain, inflammation and body temperature
- To anesthetize body area
- To control the growth of bacteria
- To control hemorrhage
- To prevent edema and gangrene

Contraindications of cold application:

- Client in a state of shock and collapse
- Muscle spasm
- Impaired sensation
- Diseases associated with impaired circulation/perfusion
- Edema
- Client with shivering or low temperature

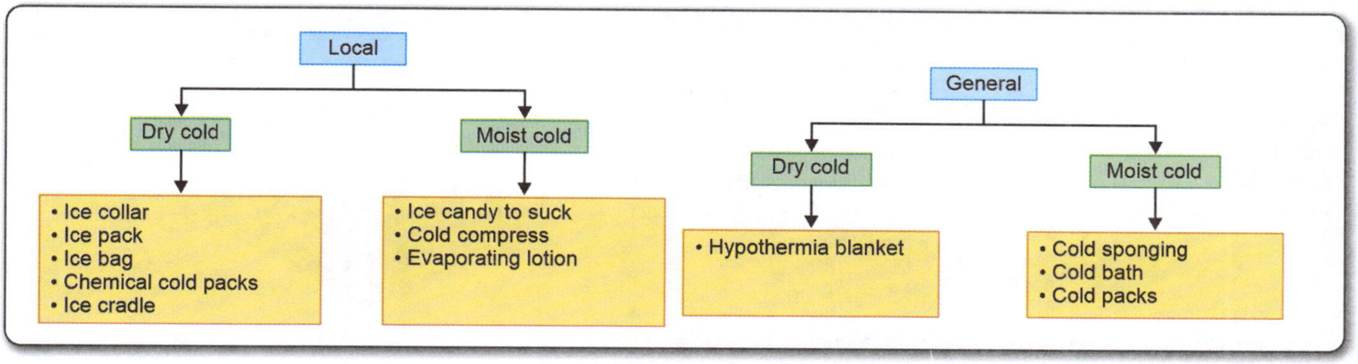

Figure 26: Classification of cold application

Table 36: Temperature for hot and cold applications

Application	Description	Temperature	
		Celsius	Fahrenheit
Ice bag	Very cold	Below 15°C	Below 59°F
Cold packs	Cold	15°–18°C	59°–65°F
Cold compresses	Cold	18°–27°C	65°–81°F
Alcohol sponge bath	Tepid	27°–37°C	81°–99°F
Warm bath	Warm	37°–40°C	99°–104°F
Hot soak, hot compresses	Hot	40°–46°C	104°–115°F
Hot water bag for adults	Very Hot	Above 46°C	Above 115°F

Table 37: Comparison between cold and hot applications

Effects	Hot application	Cold application
Effect on blood vessels	Vasodilation	Vasoconstriction
Capillary permeability	Increased	Decreased
Oxygen consumption	Increased	Decreased
Local metabolism	Increased	Decreased
Blood and lymph flow	Increased	Decreased
Motility of WBC	Increased	Decreased
Blood viscosity	Decreased	Increased
Muscle tone	Decreased	Increased

Recent Question (NORCET 2023)

25. After a liver biopsy, the best position for the client is:

A. High Fowler
B. Prone
C. Supine
D. Right lateral

Ans. (d) Right lateral

SLEEP

Detailed explanation in psychiatric nursing synopsis

POSITIONS

Position name with description	Uses	Picture
Supine position (dorsal recumbent) The supine position in nursing refers to a patient lying flat on back with face and torso facing upward. The patient lies flat on back with head, neck, and spine in a neutral position. The patient's arms may be positioned close to the body.	• Induction of anesthesia • Surgery of thorax and abdomen • Examination of anterior part of the body. • Vital sign measurement • Catheterization of male patient. • Lung biopsy	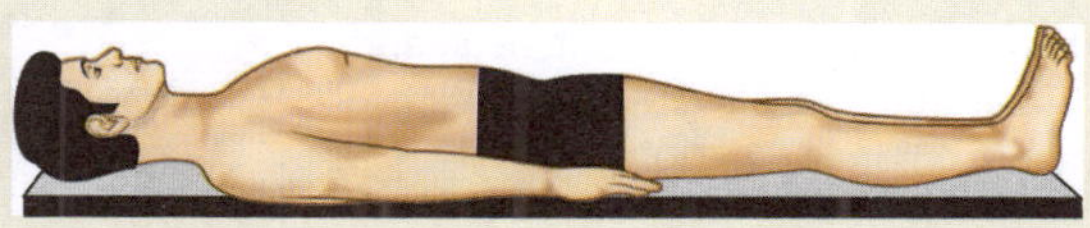

Contd...

Position name with description	Uses	Picture
Prone position The prone position is a position in which a person lies on stomach with head turned to one side and arms at sides or above head. The legs may be straight or slightly bent at the knees.	• Back surgeries • Improving oxygenation in patients with acute respiratory distress syndrome (ARDS) • To relieve pressure on coccyx • In case of neural tube defect • Renal biopsy	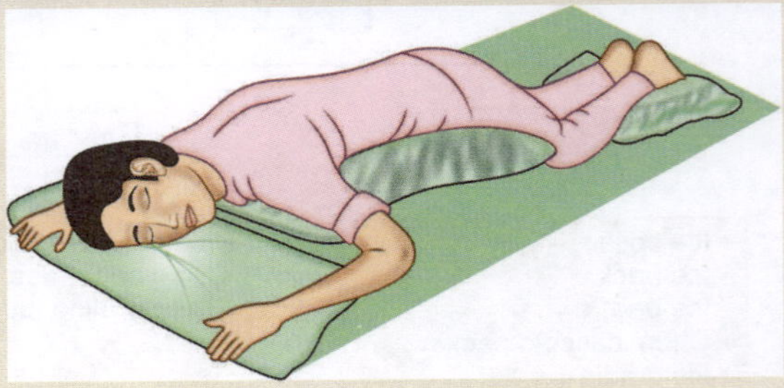
Dorsal recumbent position It is a supine position in which a person lies on back with knees bent and feet flat on the surface. The arms are typically placed at the sides or across the chest.	• Rectal pelvis and vaginal examination • Female catheterization • PV examination • Perineal care	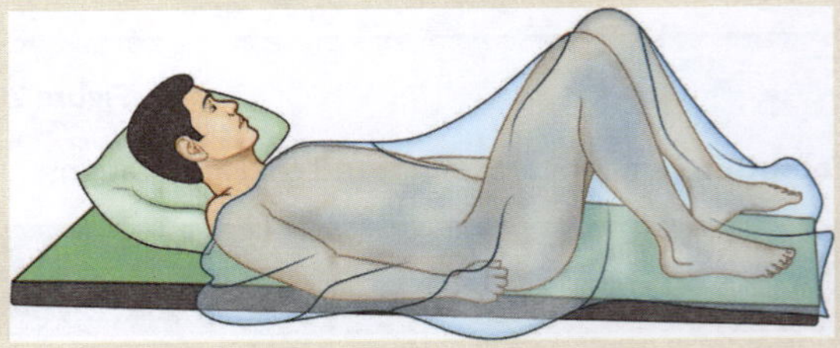
Left lateral position It is a side-lying position in which a person lies on left side, left arm behind back and right arm in front of body. The legs may be straight or slightly bent at the knees.	• Colonoscopy • Enemas • Sigmoidoscopy • Rectal temperature • Air embolism	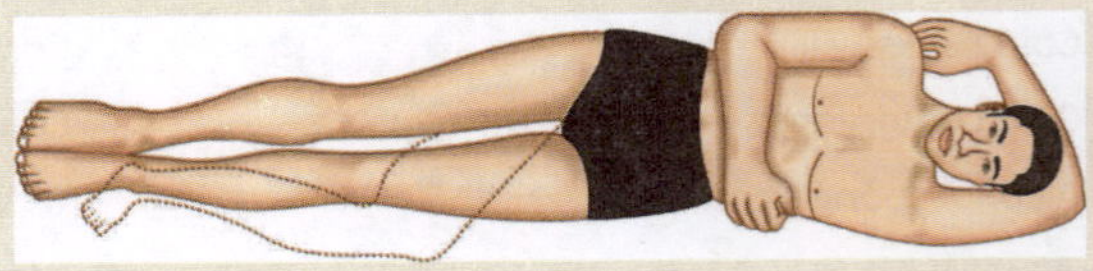
Right lateral position The right lateral position is a medical position where a patient is lying on right side.	• To relieve pressure on back and coccyx • After liver biopsy • Pyloric stenosis	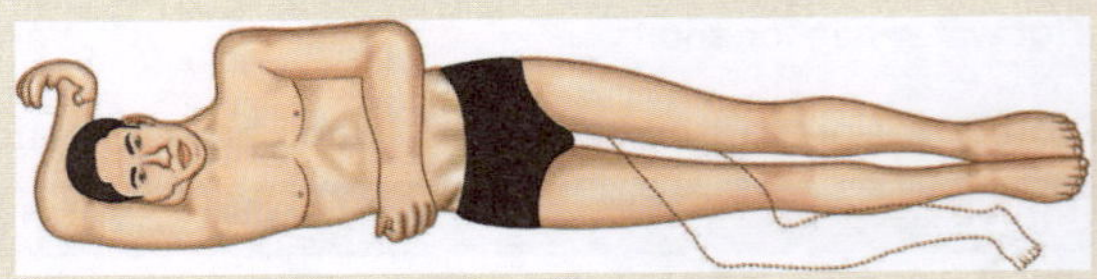
Sim's position (recovery position) The patient lies on left side at an angle of 45°. Left arm is behind back, right arm is flexed at the elbow and rests in front, and right leg is flexed at the hip and knee.	• Rectal examination • Enemas and medicine adminis-tration	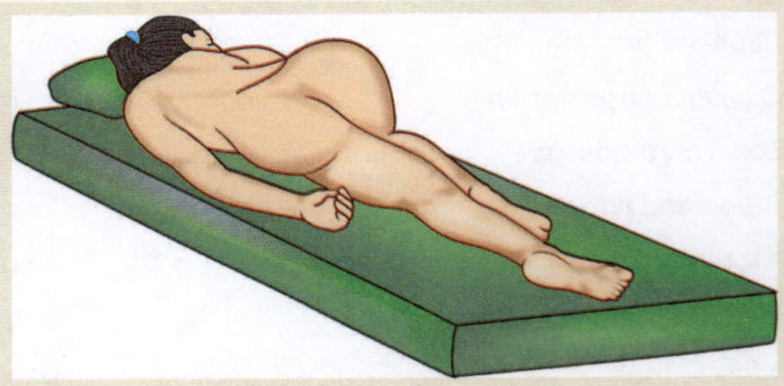
Fowler's position The Fowler's position is a semi-sitting position in which the head and upper body are elevated to varying degrees. **Low Fowler's position:** The head and upper body are elevated at an angle of approximately **15°–30°.** **Semi-Fowler's position:** The head and upper body are elevated at an angle of approximately **30°–45°.** **High Fowler's position:** The head and upper body are elevated at an angle of approximately **60°–90°.**	• Improve breathing • Reduce the risk of aspiration • Improve lung expansion • To relieve dyspnea • In case of increased ICP. • To reduce tension on abdominal suture • During gastric gavage	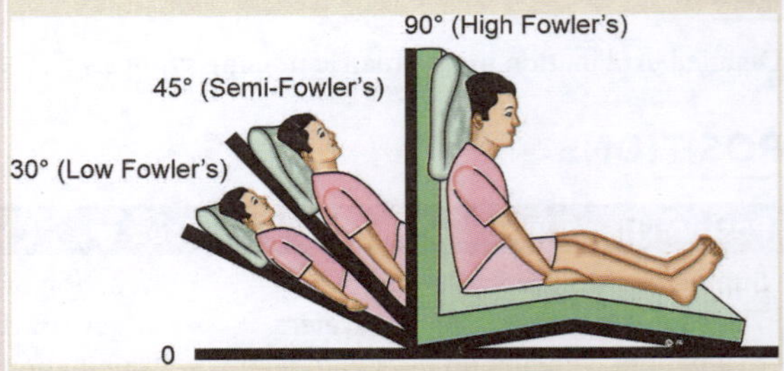

Contd...

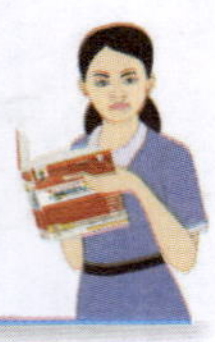

Position name with description	Uses	Picture
Orthopneic position (tripoid position) The orthopneic position is a sitting position in which a person sits upright, leaning slightly forward and getting support from a table or pillows placed on a surface.	• Patients who have difficulty breathing • COPD • Heart failure • Thoracentesis • Pericarditis	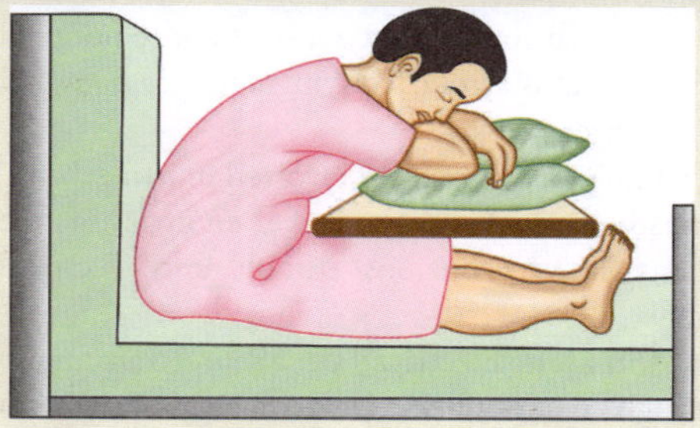
Trendelenburg position: Person lies flat on back with head lower than feet. The body is tilted at an angle of about 15°–30°, with the feet elevated above the head.	• Genitourinary surgery. • Shock • Hypotension • To promote venous return • Cord prolapse **Contraindications** Head injury and increased ICP	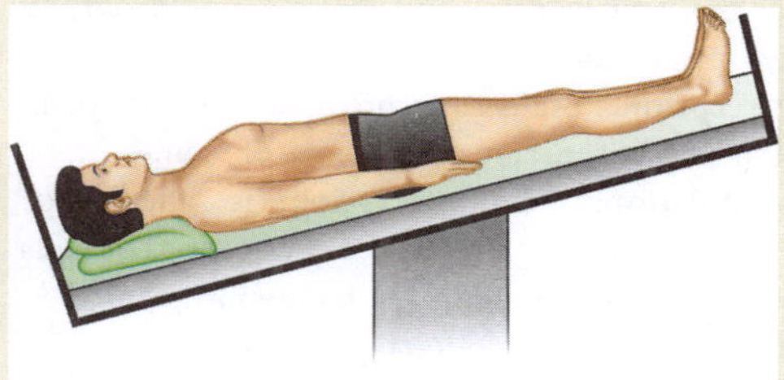
Reverse Trendelenburg Position (anti-Trendelenburg) Patient's head is elevated above the level of heart, and feet are positioned downward.	**Patient with GERD** Certain gynecological surgeries	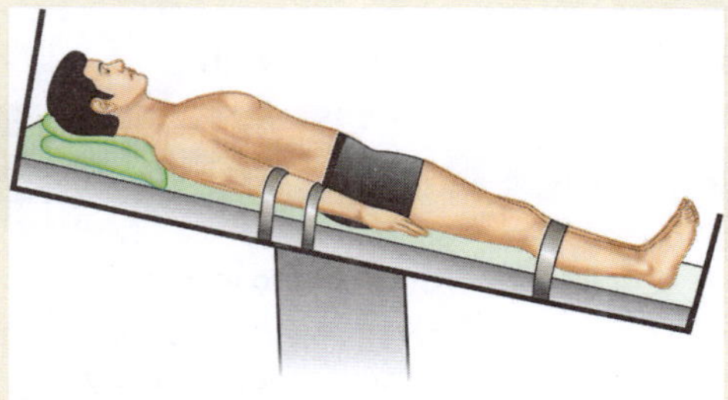
Lithotomy position Patient lies on back with legs elevated and flexed, supported by stirrups, and feet rest in the air.	• Gynecological, urological, and colorectal surgical procedures • Normal delivery	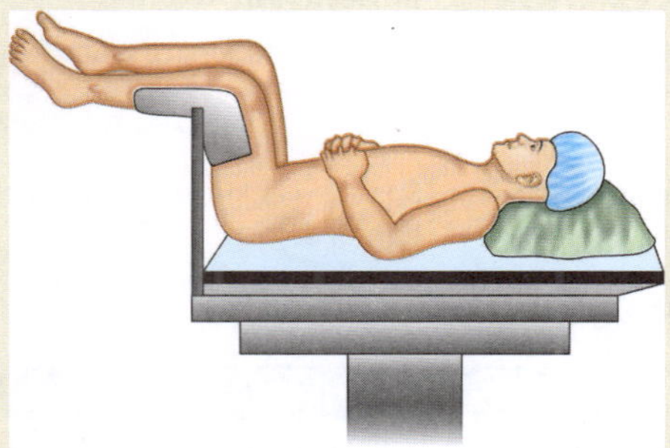
Knee chest position Patient is positioned on knees and chest with face down. It can be given as **prone knee chest position** in which buttocks are in the air or it can be given as **lateral knee chest position.**	• Vaginal examination • Rectal examination • Sigmoidoscopy • Cord prolapses • Lumbar laminectomy • Lumbar puncture (LKP)	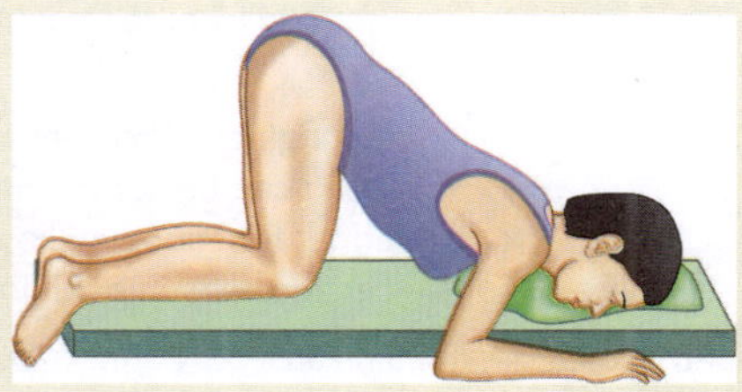 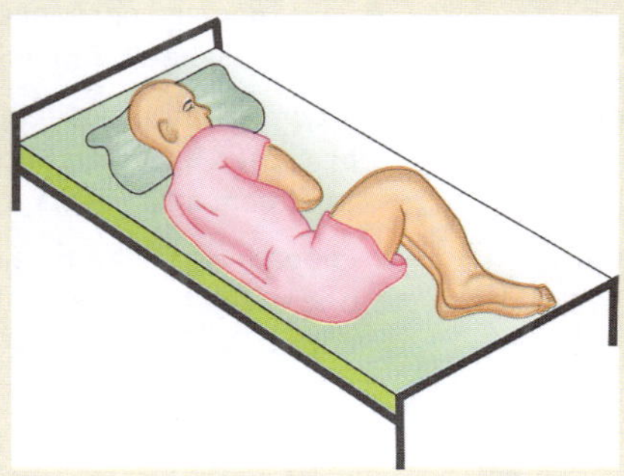

PAIN AND ITS MANAGEMENT

Pain: Pain is an unpleasant sensory and emotional experience that is associated with actual or potential tissue damage.

Four physiological processes involved in pain:

1. **Transduction**: Sensory nerve endings in the organs convert noxious stimuli into electrical signals.
2. **Transmission**: Electrical signals are transmitted through nerve fibers **(A-delta and C fibers)** to the spinal cord and brain, modulated by neurotransmitters.
3. **Perception**: Brain interprets signals as pain, resulting in conscious experience of pain.
4. **Modulation**: Pain perception is altered or suppressed through release of endogenous opioids (endorphins), serotonin, norepinephrine, GABA, or cognitive and emotional processes.

Hyperalgesia: Hyperalgesia is a condition in which an individual experiences an increased sensitivity to painful stimuli.

Allodynia: This is a type of hyperalgesia in which an individual experiences pain in response to a stimulus that is not normally painful, such as a light touch or a gentle pressure.

Gate Control Theory of Pain

- Gate control theory was first proposed by Melzack and Wall in 1965.
- Small diameter fibers open the gate for pain, while large diameter fibers close the gate for pain.
- Rubbing or massaging the injured area opens the large diameter fibers and closes the pain transmission via small diameter fibers.

Acute Pain versus Chronic Pain

Characteristic	Acute pain (transient pain)	Chronic pain (persistent noncancer pain)
Duration	Short duration Few weeks to months	Long duration Months or even years.
Underlying cause	Identifiable cause or tissue damage. It warns about the injury so **protective in nature**.	Nerve damage, underlying medical conditions or psychological factors.
Treatment	Pain medication, rest and physical therapy	Combination of medications, physical therapy, psychological therapy and lifestyle changes.
Examples	Sprained ankle, a cut or burn and dental pain.	Low back pain, fibromyalgia and neuropathic pain.

Types of Pain

Types	Description
Somatic pain	Originates from the skin, muscles, bones, or connective tissues, and is usually sharp and localized pain. Easy to locate. E.g., sprained ankle, a cut, or a broken bone
Visceral pain	Pain originates from internal organs and is described as a dull, difficult to locate ache. It can be accompanied by symptoms such as nausea or changes in bowel/bladder function, unlike somatic pain. E.g., heart attack, the pain of a stomach ulcer, or the pain of an inflamed appendix
Neuropathic pain	Pain caused by abnormal activity in the nervous system. This can occur due to nerve damage or changes in pain signal processing. It can be due to conditions such as diabetes, multiple sclerosis, stroke, spinal cord injuries and infections.
Cancer pain	A type of chronic pain that is caused by cancer or cancer treatment. It can be caused by factors such as tumor growth, nerve damage, inflammation or treatment side effects.
Idiopathic pain	Idiopathic pain is a type of chronic pain that has no clear underlying cause or origin. The term 'idiopathic' means that the cause of the pain is unknown or not easily identifiable.

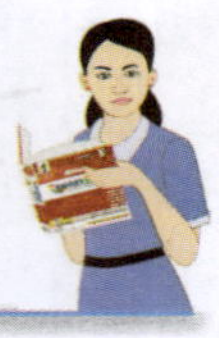

Clinical Corner

CASE SCENARIO 24:

A patient presents with chronic pain that has become hypersensitive to painful stimuli. Which of the following terms describes the condition where the individual experiences an increased sensitivity to painful stimuli?

a. Hyperesthesia
b. Hyperpathia
c. Hyperalgesia
d. Allodynia

Ans. (c) Hyperalgesia

CASE SCENARIO 25:

A patient is experiencing chronic pain, and upon examination, it is found that the pain perception is suppressed through the release of endogenous norepinephrine and GABA. Which of the following processes is responsible for this altered of pain perception?

a. Transduction
b. Transmission
c. Perception
d. Modulation

Ans. (d) Modulation

Practice Question

15. A patient presents with a chronic, dull, difficult to locate ache that is originating from internal organs. The pain is often accompanied by symptoms such as nausea or changes in bowel/bladder function. Which type of pain does this description best fit?

a. Somatic pain
b. Visceral pain
c. Neuropathic pain
d. Cancer pain

Ans. (b) Visceral pain

Pain Scales

Pain scales are tools used by health care professionals to assess and measure the intensity of pain experienced by a patient.

<table>
<tr><th>Pain scale</th><th>Description</th><th>Picture</th></tr>
<tr><td>Numerical rating scale</td><td>The numerical rating scale is an 11 point pain scale that asks patients to rate their pain from 0 (no pain) to 10 (worst pain imaginable).</td><td>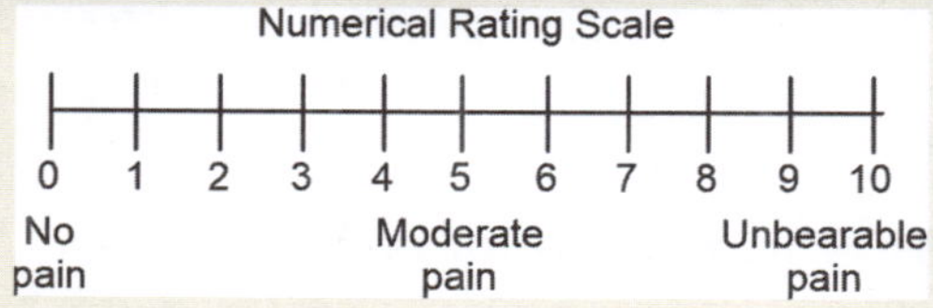
</td></tr>
<tr><td>Verbal descriptor scale</td><td>This type of pain scale uses descriptive words such as 'no pain,' 'mild,' 'moderate,' 'severe,' and 'very severe' to rate the intensity of pain.</td><td>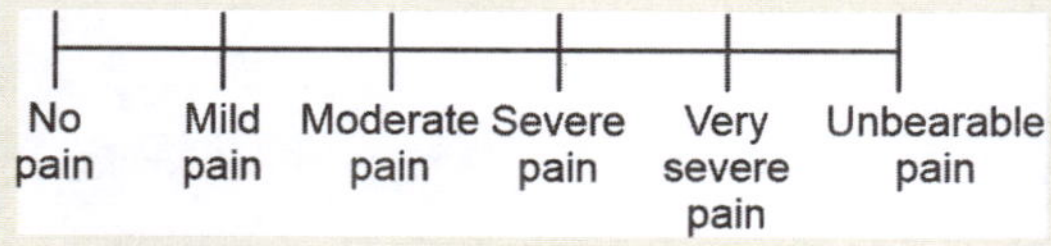
</td></tr>
<tr><td>Visual Analog Scale</td><td>This type of pain scale uses a line with end-points labeled with 'no pain' and 'worst pain imaginable,' and the patient is asked to mark the point on the line that corresponds with their level of pain.</td><td>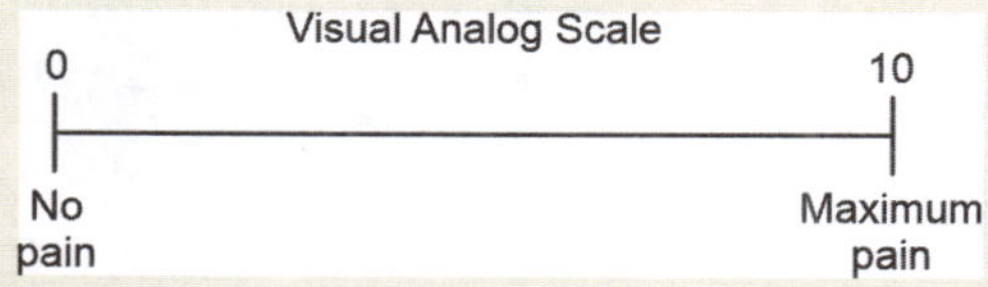
</td></tr>
<tr><td>Faces pain scale</td><td>This type of pain scale uses a series of faces with different expressions to represent different levels of pain, and the patient is asked to choose the face that best represents pain.</td><td>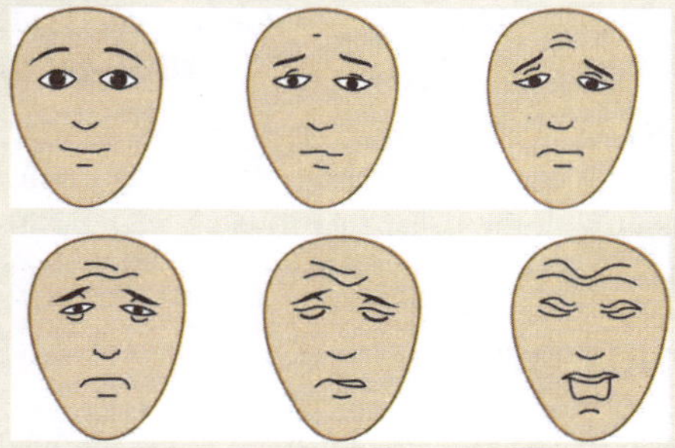</td></tr>
<tr><td>Wong-Baker FACES Pain Rating Scale</td><td>This pain scale uses faces to indicate pain severity, with each face depicting a different level of pain.</td><td>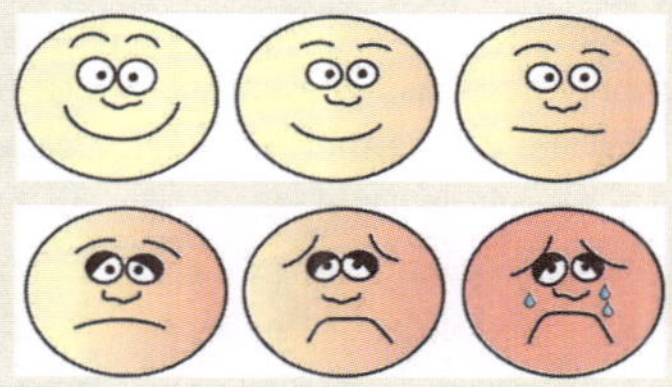</td></tr>
</table>

Nonpharmacological Pain Management

- **Biofeedback:** It involves using sensors to monitor bodily functions such as heart rate and muscle tension, and teaching patients how to control these functions to reduce pain.
- **Cognitive-behavioral therapy (CBT):** CBT is a type of talk therapy that can help patients to identify and change negative thoughts and behaviors that may be contributing to their pain.
- **Physical therapy:** Physical therapy can help to improve strength, flexibility and mobility, which can reduce pain and improve function.
- **Acupuncture:** Acupuncture involves inserting thin needles into specific points on the body to stimulate the body's natural pain-relieving mechanisms.
- **Mind-body techniques**: Mind-body techniques such as yoga, meditation and mindfulness can help to reduce stress and anxiety, which can exacerbate pain.
- **Transcutaneous electrical nerve stimulation (TENS):** TENS involves applying a mild electrical current to the affected area, which can help to reduce pain by blocking pain signals to the brain.
- **Massage therapy**: Massage therapy can help to reduce muscle tension, improve circulation, and promote relaxation, which can help to reduce pain.
- **Guided imagery:** Guided imagery is a relaxation technique that uses mental images to reduce stress, anxiety, and pain. This technique involves a trained professional or an audio recording guiding the patient through calming images and visualizations to help the patient focus his/her mind and relax. The steps involved in guided imagery include preparation, visualization, sensory experience, and positive affirmation.

Recent Question
(AIIMS Bibinagar, Asso. Prof 2023)

26. Which of the following is a multi-dimensional pain assessment tool with three main components as sensory intensity, the cognitive evaluation of pain and the emotional impact of pain?
   a. Visual Analogue Scale (VAS)
   b. McGill Pain Questionnaire (MPQ)
   c. FLACC scale
   d. Numeric Rating Scale (NRS)

Ans. (b) McGill Pain Questionnaire (MPQ)

- **Distraction:** It is a pain management technique that involves redirecting a patient's attention away from the source of pain toward a more engaging or pleasurable activity or experience. The goal of distraction is to reduce the perception of pain by shifting the patient's focus to something else.

Pharmacological Management of Pain

Analgesics: These are the medications used to relieve pain.

- Non-opioids including acetaminophen and NSAIDs
- Opioids
- Adjuvant or coanalgesics

WHO Three Steps Analgesics

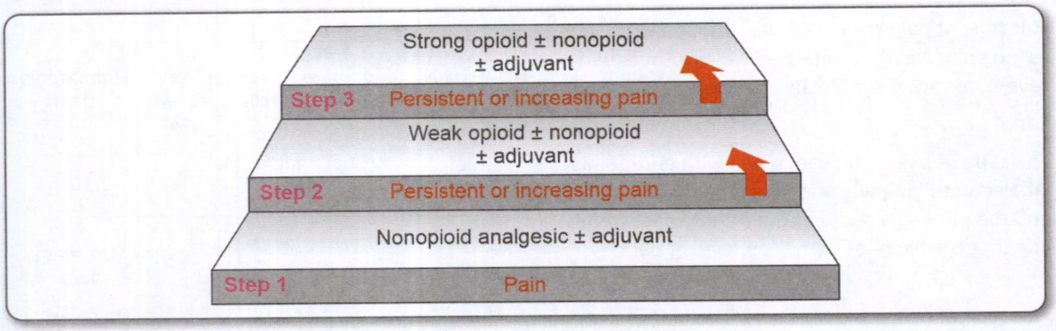

Figure 27: WHO analgesic ladder

Placebo: A placebo is a substance or treatment that has no active therapeutic effect but is given to a patient with the belief that it will have a positive effect.

NUTRITION

- **Basal metabolic rate (BMR):** It is the minimum amount of energy or calories that a person's body needs to perform basic, essential functions while at rest. This includes functions such as breathing, circulating blood, maintaining body temperature, and other metabolic activities.
- BMR is expressed in kilocalories.
- Factors affecting BMR:
  - Body size
  - Body composition
  - Age
  - Gender
  - Hormonal factors
  - Climate

Nutrients

Nutrients are substances that the body requires for growth, maintenance, and repair. (Refer to Biochemistry and Nutrition chapter for detailed information on this topic)

Nutrient	Key points
Carbohydrates	• Primary source of energy for the body • Broken down into glucose for use by cells • Energy: 4 Kcal/g • Found in grains, fruits, vegetables, and dairy products
Proteins	• Essential for building and repairing tissues • Energy: 4 Kcal/g • Made up of amino acids • Found in meat, fish, eggs, beans, and dairy products
Fats	• Provide energy and help absorb certain vitamins • Energy: 9 Kcal/g • Can be saturated or unsaturated • Found in oils, nuts, seeds, and fatty meats
Vitamins	• Essential for growth, development, and various bodily functions • There are 13 different vitamins, including B complex, A, C, D, E, and K • **A, D, E and K are fat soluble vitamins.**
Minerals	• Essential for maintaining healthy bones, teeth, and other bodily functions • There are many different minerals, including calcium, iron, and potassium
Fiber	• Helps promote regular bowel movements • Can help lower cholesterol and regulate blood sugar levels • Found in fruits, vegetables, whole grains, and legumes

Recent Questions (AIIMS Bibinagar, AP 2023)

27. Which analgesic is commonly used for cancer patients with severe pain?
a. Non-steroidal anti-inflammatory drugs (NSAID)
b. Opioid medicine
c. Acetylated salicylates
d. Non-acetylated salicylates

Ans. (b) Opioid medicine

28. Which type of analgesics are commonly used in ICU?
a. NSAID
b. Antiepileptic drugs
c. Non-opiod analgesics
d. Opiod analgesics

Ans. (d) Opiod analgesics

Practice Question

16. Which of the following nutrient provides highest amount of energy per gram?
a. Carbohydrate
b. Protein
c. Fat
d. Vitamin A

Ans. (c) Fat

Fat provides 9 Kcal per gram. Carbohydrate and Protein provides 4 Kcal per gram each.

ENTERAL TUBE FEEDING

- Enteral nutrition is a method of providing nutrients to the body through a feeding tube that is inserted into the gastrointestinal tract.
- Enteral nutrition can be administered through different types of feeding tubes, such as nasogastric tubes, gastrostomy tubes, percutaneous endoscopic gastrostomy, jejunostomy tubes or percutaneous endoscopic jejunostomy tube.
- Elevate the head end to a minimum of 30° preferably 45° if medically not contra indicated during feeding and up to 1 hour following feeding.
- Delayed gastric emptying is suspected if gastric residual volume is 250 mL or more during two consecutive measurement and 500 mL or more in a single measurement.

Confirmation of Tube Placement

- pH testing: Gastric fluid has a pH range of 1–5, while intestinal fluid has a pH range of 6–7. Using a pH strip or pH meter, you can measure the pH of the aspirated fluid from the enteral tube to determine its location.
- Auscultation: Place a stethoscope over the stomach or abdomen and inject air into the enteral tube. If you hear a gurgling sound, the tube is likely in the stomach.
- Radiography: **This is the most accurate** method to confirm the position of the enteral tube. An X-ray image can show the position of the tube relative to the anatomy of the patient.

Aspiration Precaution While Giving Oral and Enteral Feed

- Provide Fowler's position to the client as it facilitates swallowing
- Use thickened food items they are easy to control in the mouth than liquids and help to prevent aspiration.

Feeding the Client

- Provide the client with high Fowler's position
- Give feed always at room temperature. Hot formula inures the GI tract, while cold formula causes cramping and discomfort.
- If aspiration of GI content is done before the feed, push it back to the GI system to prevent electrolyte imbalance.
- Before opening the feeding tube, pinch the proximal end of the tube to prevent air entry into the GI system and also to prevent leakage of GI content.
- After feeding, give some water to prevent the clogging of the feeding tube.

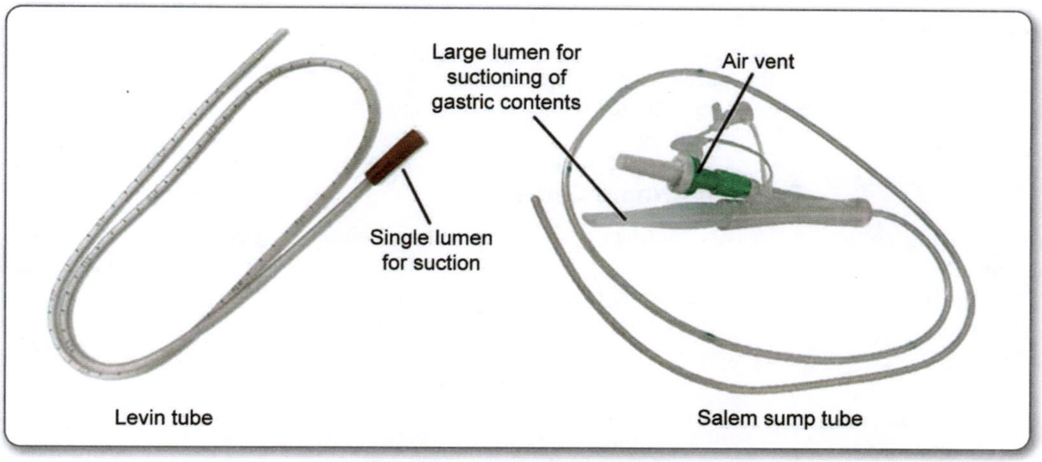

Figure 28: Feeding tubes

Removing Feeding Tube

- Provide patient with high Fowler's position unless contraindicated
- While removing the tube, ask the patient to take a deep breath and hold it to avoid the aspiration of gastric content.

Gastric Decompression

- Gastric decompression is a medical procedure that involves the removal of gas or fluid from the stomach to relieve symptoms such as bloating, nausea, vomiting, or abdominal distention.
- Small size feeding tubes are used for enteral feeding, while large size tubes are used for decompression purpose.
- Levin and salem sump are the most commonly used tubes
- Levin tube: It is a single-lumen nasogastric tube commonly used for decompression or aspiration of gastric contents.

POINTS TO REMEMBER

Inserting feeding tube

- Basilar skull fracture, nosebleeds, Oro-facial surgery, facial trauma, nasal septal deviation require careful assessment before inserting feeding tubes.
- While inserting the feeding tube, it should be inserted in the most patent nares.
- While inserting the feeding tube, give high Fowlers position unless contraindicated because it prevents aspiration as well as promotes swallowing.
- For adult patient, length of nasogastric to be inserted is calculated from tip of nose to ear lobe to xiphoid process of sternum.
- For pediatric patient, length of NG tube is calculated from tip of nose to ear lobe to mid-way between xiphoid process and umbilicus.
- While inserting the feeding tube, it should not be advanced during inspiration or cough as tube may end up in respiratory tract.

- The Salem Sump tube is a double-lumen nasogastric tube that is also used for gastric decompression. The second lumen is a vent that allows air to flow in and out of the stomach, preventing a vacuum from forming and reducing the risk of tissue damage or irritation.

PARENTERAL NUTRITION

- Parenteral nutrition (PN) is a medical treatment that involves providing nutrients directly into a patient's bloodstream via an intravenous (IV) catheter.
- PN is typically used when a patient cannot consume food orally or absorb nutrients from the digestive system due to illness, surgery, or other medical conditions.
- TPN is a complex mixture of individual components including lipids, dextrose, amino acids, vitamins, electrolytes, minerals, and trace elements.
- TPN is administered through central venous line which ends at superior vena cava or right atrium.
- Some time peripherally inserted central catheters (PICC) are also used.
- PICC lines into the basilic, cephalic, brachial, or median cubital vein.
- Basilic vein is often preferred for PICC line insertion because of its larger size and superficial location.
- Once the central line is inserted, before using it position needs to be confirmed with X-ray.
- While inserting the catheter, ask the patient to hold the breath and bear down (Valsalva maneuver). This will help to create increased venous pressure and prevent air from entering the bloodstream and this helps to prevent air embolus.
- When a patient is suspected of having an air embolism, he/she should be immediately placed in the left lateral position. This helps to prevent further air from entering the bloodstream and can improve blood flow to the vital organs.
- Total parenteral nutrition (TPN) has a high osmolarity that can cause irritation and damage to peripheral veins; so, it is not recommended for peripheral parenteral nutrition (PPN).
- PPN is typically administered with a lower osmolarity solution, usually less than 900 mOsm which requires larger volume feedings and higher fat content.
- Complications associated with TPN include electrolyte and mineral imbalance, hyperglycemia, osmotic diuresis, and dehydration etc.

BLADDER ELIMINATION

- Micturition: The act of urination, or the process of emptying the bladder.
- Hematuria: blood in the urine
- Proteinuria: protein in the urine.
- Dysuria: painful micturition
- Bacteriuria: presence of bacteria in the urine
- Urinary retention: inability to empty the bladder partly or completely.
- Post residual volume: Volume of urine left in the bladder after voiding.
- Urinary incontinence: involuntary loss of urine.

Urine Sample Collection—Points to Remember

- Midstream urine collection is recommended for sampling in a self-voiding client.
- Midstream urine collection: To collect a midstream urine sample, the individual first cleans the external genital area with an antiseptic wipe or soap and water. The individual then begins urinating into the toilet or urinal, allowing the first few seconds of urine to pass before collecting a sample of the midstream urine in a sterile container.
- Never collect urine from bag in a catheterized client.
- Clamp and clean the catheter and then using a sterile syringe, aspirate the desired amount of urine from the catheter tubing and inject it into the collection container.
- In 24-hour urine collection, discard the first voided urine at the starting time of collection and add the last voided urine at the time of finishing the collection.
- Send the collected sample as soon as possible to the laboratory.

Types of Urinary Catheter

- Urinary catheters are made up of latex, silicon, rubber, or PVC.
- Size of the urinary catheter is French in size.
- Size in French reflects the internal diameter of the catheter. 12 Fr means internal diameter is 12.

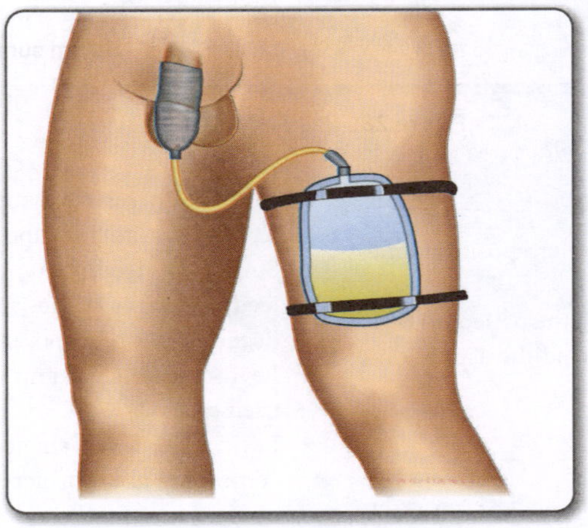

Figure 29: Condom catheter

Clinical Corner

CASE SCENARIO 26:
Nursing instructor completed a class on parenteral nutrition. Which among the following identified by student as not a route for parenteral nutrition indicates that class was effective?

a. Subclavian
b. PIC line
c. Femoral vein
d. PEG line

Ans. (d) PEG line

Parenteral nutrition means infusing specialized form of nutrition via veins. Subclavian, PIC line and femoral vein are the different routes for establishing parenteral nutrition. PEG line means percutaneous endoscopic gastrostomy tube which allow to receive nutrition directly into stomach. So, it becomes enteral route.

KEY POINT

Basilic vein is often preferred for PICC line insertion because of its larger size and superficial location.

KEY POINTS

- Never collect urine from bag in a catheterized client.
- In 24-hour urine collection, discard the first voided urine at the starting time of collection and add the last voided urine at the time of finishing the collection.

Type	Description	Picture
Single lumen	It is used for intermittent or straight catheterization	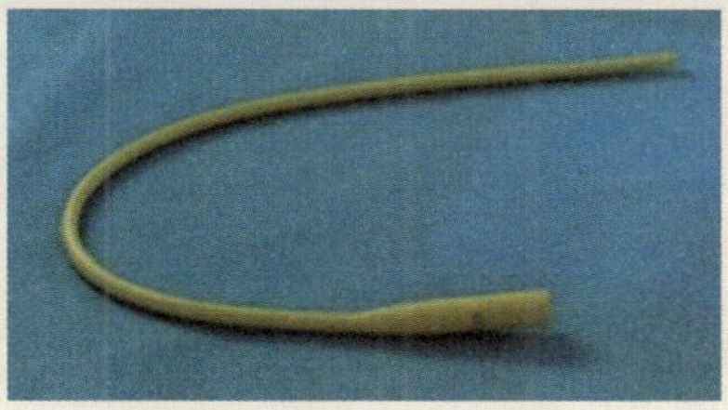
Double lumen	One lumen for inflating balloon Second lumen for urinary drainage	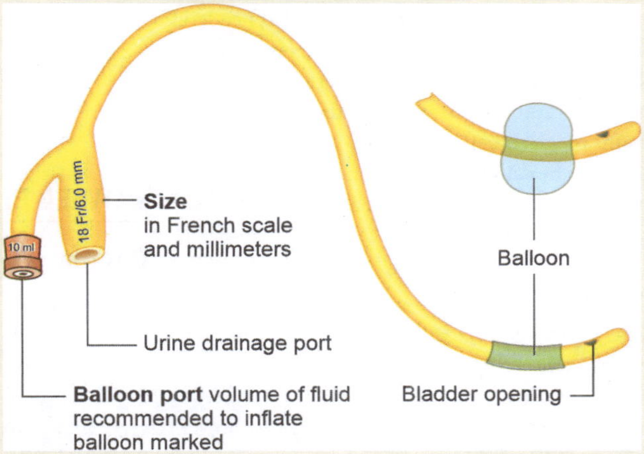
Triple lumen	One lumen for inflating balloon Second lumen for urinary drainage. Third lumen for bladder irrigation.	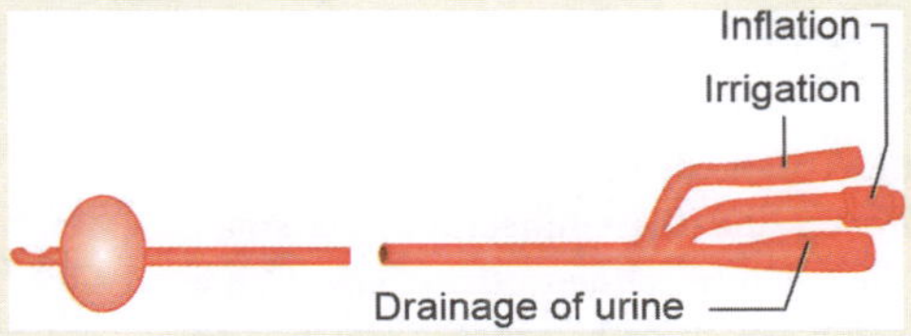

Suprapubic Catheter

- Suprapubic catheter is used to drain urine from the bladder when a person is unable to urinate normally. It involves the insertion of a catheter through the skin and into the bladder, bypassing the urethra.
- It is used when urethral catheterization is not possible in conditions like enlarged prostate, urethral stricture, etc.

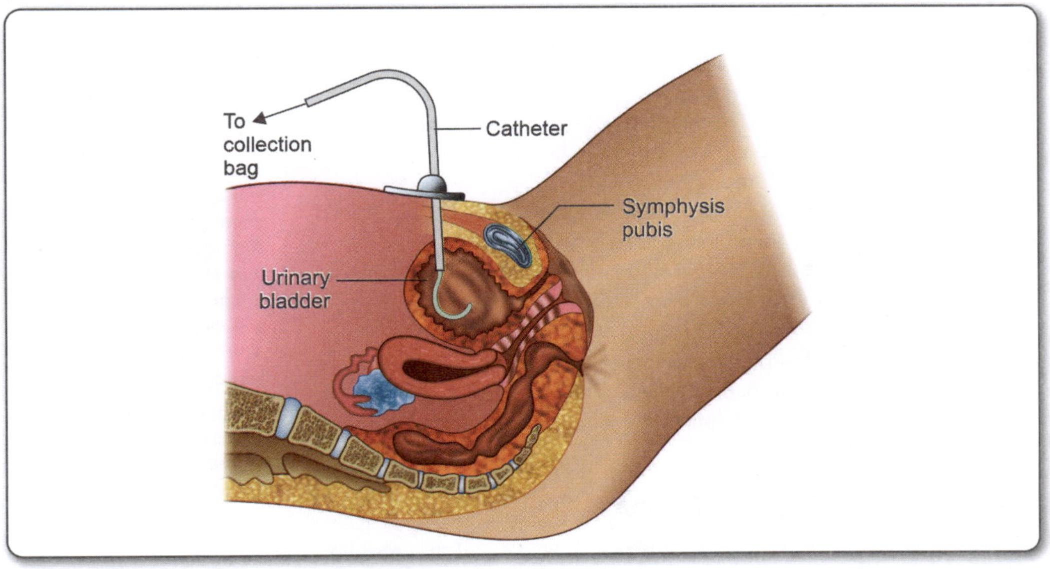

Figure 30: Suprapubic catheter

Clinical Corner

CASE SCENARIO 27:
Foley's catheter of a patient was removed 24 hours before. On assessment, the nurse found that the urine output is below the expected volume. What would be the primary nursing action among the following options?

a. Administer Inj. Lasix 20 mg IV
b. Ambulate the patient
c. Check bladder for distension
d. Notify the doctor

Ans. (c) Check bladder...

After a Foley catheter is removed, the bladder may not be able to empty completely on its own. This can lead to urinary retention, which is a condition in which urine builds up in the bladder. The priority nursing action is to check the bladder for distension.

Condom Catheter

- Condom catheter is also known as an external catheter or penile sheath.
- It is used to manage urinary incontinence in men.
- It consists of a flexible sheath made of silicone or latex that is placed over the penis and connected to a drainage bag.
- The condom catheter collects urine as it is released from the bladder and directs it into the drainage bag, which can be emptied and replaced as needed.
- Condom catheters are associated with less chances of urinary tract infection than other methods.
- It is important to ensure that there is a small amount of space between the tip of the penis and the end of the catheter because the space allows for proper urine flow and prevents any obstruction or backflow of urine.

Urinary Diversion

- Urinary diversion is a surgical procedure that involves redirecting the flow of urine from the bladder to stoma.
- Stoma is usually located in the right lower quadrant of the abdomen.

Types

- **Ileal conduit**: This involves the creation of a stoma in the abdomen and the connection of a small section of the small intestine to the stoma. Urine is collected in a pouch or bag that is attached to the stoma.
- **Continent urinary diversion**: This involves the creation of a pouch or reservoir inside the body that collects urine. The pouch is connected to a stoma in the abdomen, and the individual uses a catheter to empty the pouch periodically.
- **Orthotopic neobladder**: This involves the creation of a new bladder using a section of the intestine. The new bladder is connected to the urethra, allowing the individual to urinate normally.

Urinary Catheterization—Points to Remember

- While doing catheterization for female patients, provide dorsal recumbent position; for male patients provide supine position with leg extended and thighs slightly abducted.
- While inserting catheter to a female patient, ask her to bear down (it helps to relax the sphincter) and advance the catheter.
- In female patients, insert catheter for 5– 7.5 cm or until you get urinary back flow.
- In male patients, hold the penis at 90° angle and ask the patient to bear down.
- In male patients, insert catheter for a length of 17–22.5 cm or until you get backflow.

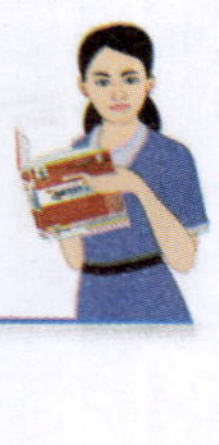

- In female patients, secure the catheter to the inner thigh and in male patients, secure the catheter to the top thigh or lower part of the abdomen.

Pelvic Floor Exercise

- Pelvic floor exercise is also known as Kegel exercise.
- It involves contracting and relaxing the muscles of the pelvic floor.
- These exercises can help strengthen the muscles that support the bladder, uterus, and rectum, and may be recommended for individuals with urinary or bowel incontinence, pelvic organ prolapse, or other pelvic floor disorders.

BOWEL ELIMINATION

Enema

- **Definition:** The administration of a substance in liquid form into the rectum for the evacuation of feces or for drug administration.
- The enema should be administered at a temperature of 40.5°–43.3°C.
- Position to administer enema is sim's position (left side lying) because natural curve of rectum and sigmoid colon holds enema as well as aids in gravitational flow of enema.
- Quantity should not be >100–250 mL while giving retained enema so that rectum is not distended to cause peristalsis.
- Expel the air from enema to prevent abdominal distention.
- The small, lubricated tube is inserted 3–4 inches (7.5–10.0 cm) into the adult's rectum, 2–3 inches in child's rectum and 1–1.5 inches in infant's rectum.
- Insert suppositories about 4 cm into the rectum, usually using the index finger.
- Normally hang the solution 30 cm (12 in) above the rectum.
- 12–18 inches or 30–45 cm height should be maintained from the bed level for giving high cleansing enema.
- 20 cm or 8 inches height should be maintained from rectum in retention enema.
- Abdominal cramps and discomfort are expected findings while administering enema. If they occur, slow down the flow rate.
- If abdomen becomes rigid and client complains of pain or bleeding occurs during enema, then discontinue the procedure and inform the doctor on duty.

Types of Enema

- **Cleansing enema**: It is a medical procedure that involves introducing liquid into the rectum and colon to help remove stool and other waste

POINTS TO REMEMBER

- Always hang the urine drainage bag below the level of bladder to promote the gravity drainage.
- Urine bag should not touch the floor to prevent the contamination.
- Empty the urine drainage bag when it is half to one third full to prevent the trauma to the urethra due to the traction (pulling) from the bag.
- Medications like rifampicin, phenazopyridine may cause urine orange red in color.

Clinical Corner

CASE SCENARIO 28:

During the history collection, a 30-year-old female complaints to the nurse that she passes small amount of urine while she coughs or sneezes. Nurse identified this as:

a. Urge incontinence
b. Stress incontinence
c. Overflow incontinence
d. Functional incontinence

Ans. (b) Stress incontinence

In stress incontinence, urine leaks out at time of increased intra-abdominal pressure such as cough or laugh.

Urge incontinence: Urine leaks as you feel a sudden, intense urge to pee, or soon afterwards. **Overflow incontinence (chronic urinary retention):** Unable to fully empty the bladder, which causes frequent leaking.

Functional incontinence is also known as disability associated urinary incontinence. It occurs when the person's bladder and/or bowel is working normally but he/she is unable to access the toilet.

material. Purpose is to help relieve constipation, empty the bowels before a medical procedure or surgery, or to prepare for a diagnostic test, such as a colonoscopy.

- **Tap water:** Type of enema where plain water is used to cleanse the rectum and colon. It is hypotonic and moves from intestine into the interstitial space. Repeated administration can cause water intoxication and circulatory overload.
- **Normal saline enema:** It is the safest enema to administer as it has same osmolarity as that of the interstitial fluids. This enema nullifies the risk of fluid imbalance. They work by softening the stool and increasing the volume of water in the colon, which helps to stimulate bowel movements.
- **Hypertonic solutions enema**: In this enema, a solution with higher osmotic pressure is used to cleanse the rectum and colon. It draws water out of the body's tissues and into the colon, which helps to stimulate bowel movements and loosen stool.
- **Soapsuds enema:** It is a type of enema where soap is added to the water to cleanse the rectum and colon. The soap helps to soften the stool and facilitate bowel movements.
- **Retention enema:** This type of enema is used to administer medication and oil into the patient's rectum. Types of oil and medications include nutritive, antibiotics, and anthelmintics.
- **Carminative enema:** It is a type of enema that is used to relieve gas and bloating in the digestive system. Example for carminative enema is magnesium, glycerin, and water (MGW) enema. The solution is designed to soften stool, relieve constipation, and promote bowel movements.
  - Magnesium sulfate, also known as Epsom salt, is a laxative which softens stool.
  - Glycerin is a lubricant that helps to soften and ease the passage of stool.
  - Water is added to dilute the solution and make it easier to administer.

Temperature of enema solution:
- For adults: 105°F
- For child: 98.6°F

- For giving cleansing enema, use 22 French (F) for adults, 14-18 F for school age child and 12 F for an infant.
- **High enema:** Enema is administered to clean the large intestine as much as possible. It is usually high volume and high-pressure enema to reach all parts of large intestine. During this enema, client may be asked to change the position (Sims' position to dorsal recumbent then to right lateral) several times to ensure that enema solution reaches all parts of the gut.
- **Low enema:** Enema is administered to the rectum and sigmoid colon. It is usually low volume and low-pressure enema.

Contraindications for Enema

- Appendicitis
- Bowel perforation
- Increased ICP
- Glaucoma
- Recent rectal/addominal/prostate surgery

Digital Removal of Stool

- Digital removal of stool is also known as manual fecal disimpaction.
- It involves the manual removal of stool from the rectum and lower colon.
- The procedure involves the use of a gloved finger or fingers to gently break up and remove the impacted stool.
- It may cause vasovagal response. (Stimulation of the vagus nerve during digital removal of stool may cause a temporary decrease in heart rate or blood pressure, which can result in light-headedness or fainting in some individuals.)

Practice Questions

18. While administering enema, the patient complains of abdominal cramps. Which of the following is the appropriate action by the nurse?

a. Continue giving enema as it is an expected reaction
b. Slow down the rate of administration
c. Stop giving enema
d. Administer analgesic

Ans. (c) Stop giving enema

19. The purpose of giving purgative enema is to:

a. Destroy intestinal worms
b. Provide anesthesia
c. Provide nutrition
d. Improve peristalsis

Ans. (d) Improve peristalsis

Practice Question

17. A Harris flush drip (Return flow enema) is ordered for an adult patient with flatulence. In comparison to cleansing enema, what should the nurse do that is unique to a return flow enema?

a. Solution container should be raised 12 inches above the anus
b. Insert the rectal tube 3–4 inches into the anus
c. Solution container is lowered after instilling about 150 mL of solution
d. Lubricate the last 5 cm of the rectal tube with water soluble lubricant

Ans. (c) Solution container is lowered after instilling about 150 mL of solution.

Rationale: Steps given in options a, b and d are common to cleansing and return flow enema. In return flow enema, the solution container is lowered to create a siphon effect that pulls the instilled fluid back out through the rectal tube into the solution container.

KEY POINTS

Temperature of enema solution:
- For adults: 105°F
- For child: 98.6°F

For giving cleansing enema, use
- 22 French (F) for adults,
- 14-18 F for school age child
- 12 F for an infant.

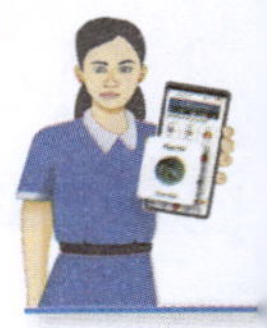

COLOSTOMY

A colostomy is a surgical procedure that creates an opening, called a stoma, in the abdomen through which a portion of the colon is brought to the surface and connected to a collection bag.

Types of Colostomies (Based on Location of Stoma)

Name	Location	Stool characteristics
Ascending colostomy	Stoma on ascending colon	Liquid stool
Transverse colostomy	Stoma on transverse colon	Semi liquid stool
Descending colostomy	Stoma on descending colon	More solid stool
Sigmoid colostomy	Stoma on sigmoid colon	Formed stool

Types of Colostomies (Based on Stoma Configuration)

Type and description	Picture
Double-barrel colostomy This type of colostomy involves dividing the colon and creating two separate stomas on the abdomen. One stoma is created to expel fecal matter, and the other stoma is created to expel mucus. The two stomas are independent and do not connect.	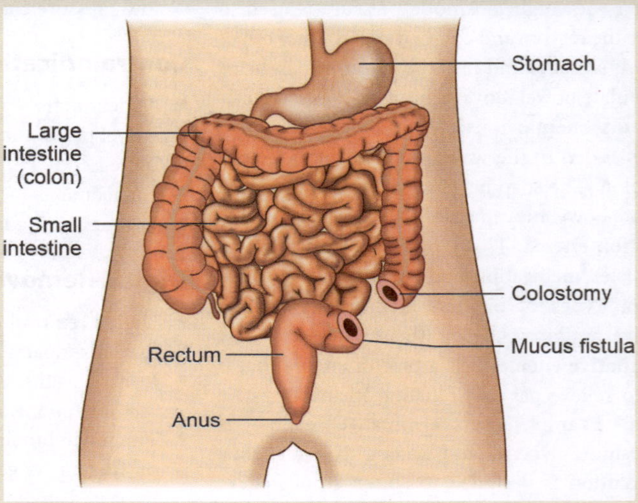
Loop colostomy This type of colostomy involves creating a loop of colon that is pulled through the abdomen to form a stoma. The loop is then divided, and one end is brought to the surface to form the stoma, while the other end is left in the abdomen and sutured & closed. This type of colostomy is often temporary and can be easily reversed.	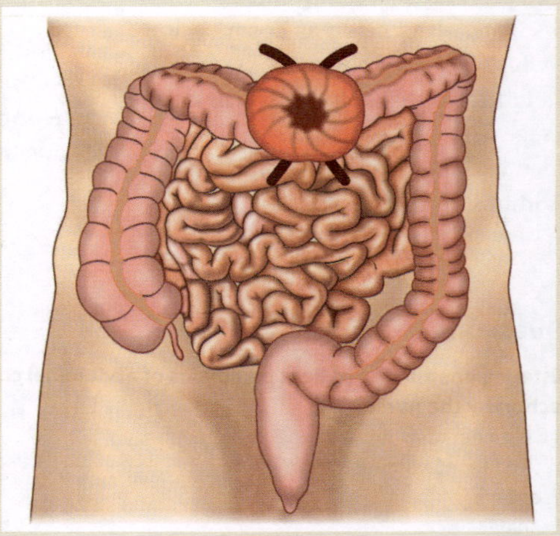 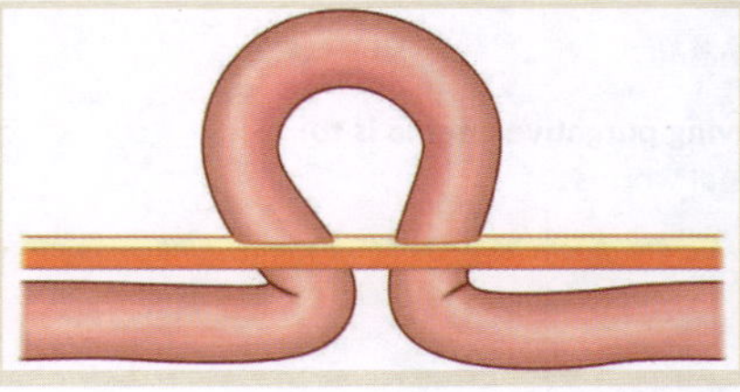

Contd...

Type and description	Picture
End colostomy This type of colostomy is created when the end of the colon is brought to the surface to form the stoma. This is the most common type of colostomy and can be temporary or permanent.	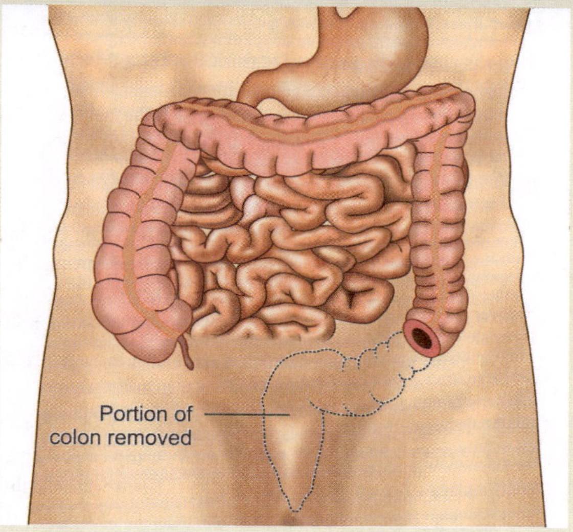

POINTS TO REMEMBER

- A healthy stoma should be pink or red in color and moist while touching.
- As such there is no diet restriction for patients with colostomies
- Food items like fish, egg and onion may produce offensive gas. Educate client regarding this.
- People with ileostomy have liquid stool and there is a chance of loss of water and salt. So, maintain water and electrolyte balance.
- Food blockage is often present in people with ileostomy due to the incomplete digestion of certain food material.
- Empty the colostomy pouch when it is half to one third full because its weight may disrupt the seal and adhesion with the skin.
- Necrotic stoma will be dry with purple or black color.
- The sigmoid colostomy is the most common type of colostomy, while the transverse colostomy is the second most common.
- Output from the colostomy is known as effluent.
- Newly created colostomy will be functional after 2–4 days.

Clinical Corner

CASE SCENARIO 29:
Nursing instructor was observing student's assistance to transfer the client from bed to chair. Which among the following body mechanism is wrong?

a. Taking wide base of support
b. Bending at the level of waist and knee
c. Bending the back and lift the client
d. Face the client before shifting from bed

Ans. (c) Bending the back and lift the client

In body mechanisms, bending at the back is not recommended. Bending at the level of waist and knee is recommended.

BODY MECHANICS AND MOBILITY

Body mechanics: It refers to the proper use and coordination of the body's muscles, joints, and bones to perform various physical activities with efficiency and safety.

Principles of Body Mechanics

- Maintain a stable base: Keep your feet shoulder-width apart, with one foot slightly in front of the other, to provide a stable base of support.
- Use your leg muscles: While lifting or carrying objects, bend your knees and use the muscles in your legs to lift the weight, rather than straining your back.
- Maintain a neutral spine: Keep your back straight, with your shoulders back and down, and your pelvis in a neutral position to reduce stress on your spine.
- Use the weight of your body: Use your body weight to help you move objects, such as by shifting your weight forward or backward, rather than relying solely on your muscles.
- Avoid twisting or bending at the waist: While lifting or carrying objects, avoid twisting or bending at the waist, which can strain your back muscles.
- Position yourself close to the object: Move the object as close to your body as possible to reduce the strain on your arms and back.
- Get help when needed: For heavy or awkward objects, ask for help from a co-worker or use equipment, such as a dolly or lift, to assist with the task.

Range of Motion Exercise

- Range of motion (ROM) refers to the amount of movement that a joint or series of joints can perform in a particular direction. It is a measure of the flexibility and mobility of the body.
- ROM can be measured actively or passively.
- Active ROM refers to the range of motion that an individual can achieve on his/her own through voluntary muscle contractions.
- Passive ROM refers to the range of motion that can be achieved with the assistance of an external force, such as a therapist or a device.

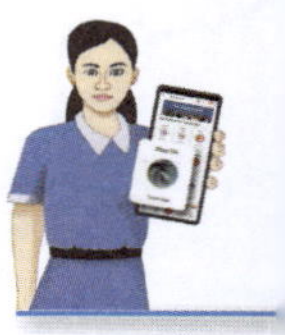

Planes of Body and Movement

Plane	Description	Movements
Sagittal	Divides the body into left and right portions	**Flexion:** Bending a joint to decrease the angle between two body parts. **Extension:** Straightening a joint to increase the angle between two body parts. **Hyperextension:** Excessive straightening of a joint beyond its normal range. **Dorsiflexion:** Bending the foot upward at the ankle. **Plantar Flexion:** Pointing the foot downward at the ankle. **Eversion/Inversion:** Turning the sole of the foot outward (eversion) or inward (inversion).
Frontal plane (coronal plane)	Divides the body into front and back portions	**Abduction:** Moving a body part away from the midline of the body. **Adduction:** Moving a body part toward the midline of the body.
Transverse plane	Divides the body into upper and lower portions	**Rotation:** Turning or twisting a body part around its axis. **Supination:** Turning the palm or foot upward. **Pronation:** Turning the palm or foot downward.

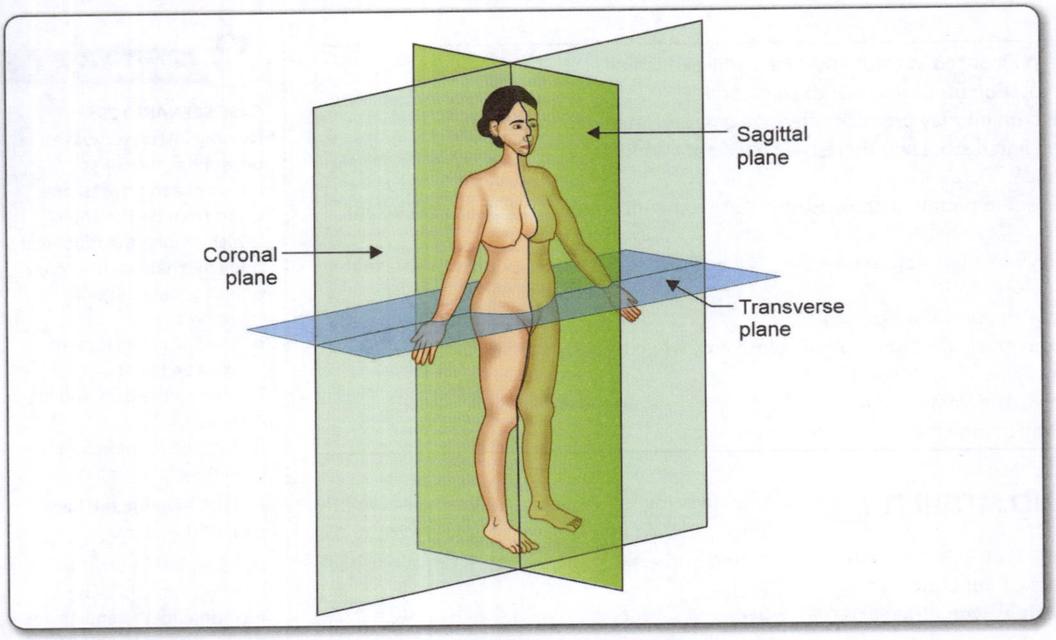

Figure 31: Planes of body

VENOUS THROMBOEMBOLISM (VTE)

- VTE is a condition in which a blood clot (thrombus) forms in a vein, which can then break loose and travel through the bloodstream to another part of the body, causing blockage of blood flow in vital organs such as the lungs, heart, or brain.

There are two main types of VTE:

- **Deep vein thrombosis (DVT):** A blood clot that forms in a deep vein, typically in the leg or pelvis. Symptoms may include pain, swelling, warmth, and redness in the affected area.
- **Pulmonary embolism (PE):** A blood clot that travels to the lungs, causing sudden chest pain, shortness of breath, rapid breathing, and sometimes coughing up blood.

WOUND DRAINS

Wound drains are devices used to remove fluid, such as blood or lymphatic fluid, from a surgical site or wound.

- **Jackson-Pratt drain:** A bulb-like device that is attached to a flexible tube which is placed in the surgical area. The bulb is compressed to create suction, which pulls fluid out of the wound and into the bulb.

Clinical Corner

CASE SCENARIO 30:

Mr. Ravi, a 65-year-old patient, has been admitted to the hospital with mobility challenges due to a recent hip surgery. The nurse is assessing the room setup and equipment needs to ensure his safety and comfort during his hospital stay. The nurse notices a trapeze bar installed in the room. What is the main function of the trapeze bar for Mr. Ravi's care?

a. Handing IV solution/drip
b. Repositioning the patient while sleeping
c. Acting as a safety rail on a hospital bed
d. Assisting Mr. Ravi in sitting up and getting into and out of bed.

Ans. (d) Assisting Mr. Ravi in sitting up and getting into and out of bed.

Clinical Corner

CASE SCENARIO 31:

The nurse puts mechanical calf pumps to a patient who is admitted after prolapsed L1-L2 disc. The rationale behind it is

a. Prevention of deep vein thrombosis
b. To help stimulate neural recovery
c. Mechanical calf pumps are not essential. Log rolling can be done
d. To prevent spontaneous flexor spasms

Ans. (a) Prevention of deep vein thrombosis

The application of mechanical pumps over the client's calf muscles will provide regular interval of compression and prevent the clot formation. This will help the client from the development of DVT and the pulmonary embolism.

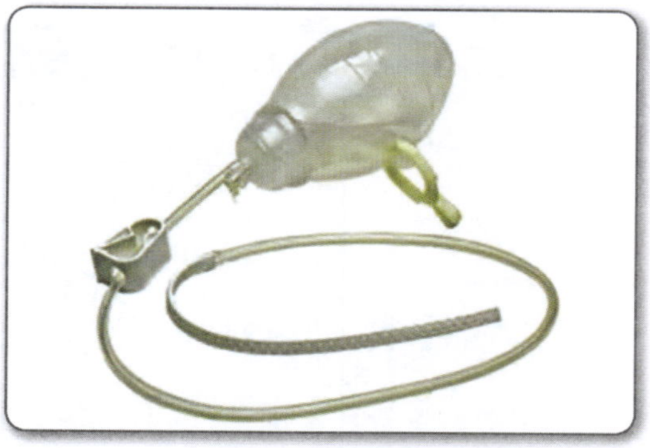

Figure 32: Jackson-Pratt drain

- **Hemovac drain:** A flat, spring-like device that is also attached to a flexible tube. The device is compressed to create suction, which pulls fluid out of the wound and into a collection chamber.

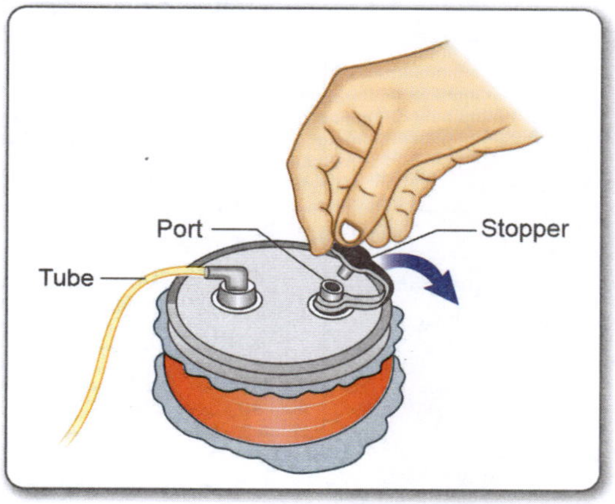

Figure 33: Hemovac drain

- **Blake drain:**. A long, thin tube is inserted into the surgical area and connected to a collection chamber. Drains have four continuous channels that provide greater tissue contact area than regular perforated drains and offer multiple drainage routes to resist clogging.

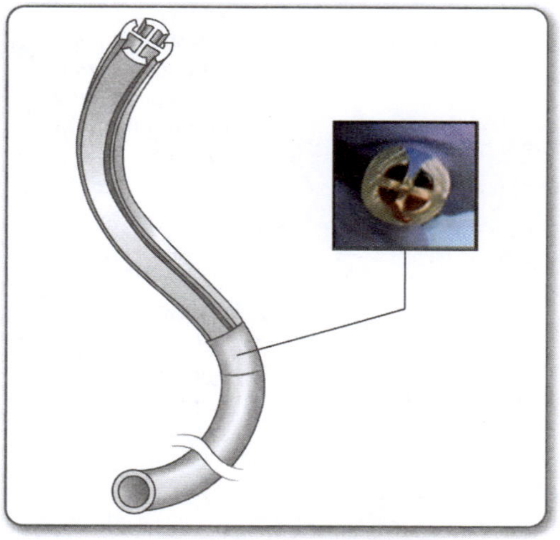

Figure 34: Blake drain

- **Penrose drain:** A Penrose drain is a flexible tube inserted into a wound to allow fluid to drain out by gravity. It is typically used after surgery to prevent fluid build-up. A Penrose drain is typically made of latex or silicone. The drain is typically secured in place with a suture or clip or pin.

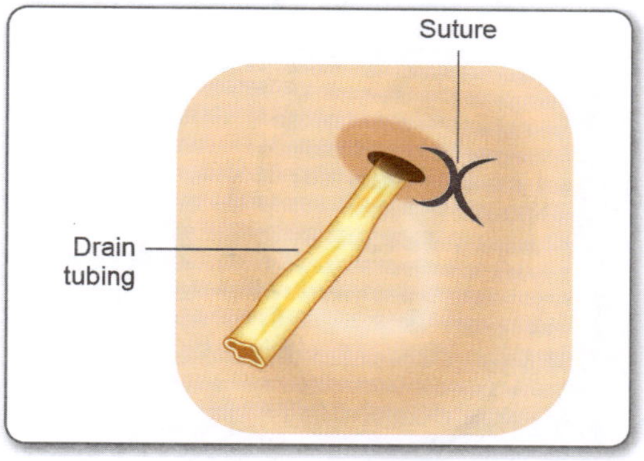

Figure 35: Penrose drain

SUTURE

- **Sutures or stitches:** As a method for closing cutaneous wounds.
- Type A: According to nature of absorption
  - **Absorbable suture:** The sutures which are absorbable and will break down harmlessly in the body within 60–90 days are known as absorbable sutures. **Absorbable sutures include** Polyglycolic acid sutures, Polyglactin 910, Catgut, Poliglecaprone 25 and Polydioxanone sutures.
  - **Nonabsorbable suture:** Manually removed if they are not left indefinitely. **Nonabsorbable sutures include** Polypropylene sutures, nylon (polyamide), polyester, PVDF, silk and stainless steel sutures.
- Type B: On the basis of material structure
  - **Monofilament** sutures and **multifilament** or **braided** sutures. Braided sutures provide better knot security, whereas monofilament sutures provide better passage through tissues.
  - **Polyglycolic** acids are known for their high quality and undoubted performance. Made-up of braided and coated 100% polyglycolic acid.
  - **Catgut** is pliable, absorbable, sterile, surgical suture composed of highly purified connective tissue. Chromic catgut lasts for 2–3 weeks and is used for ligatures and tissue suture.
  - **Braided suture** is usually made of natural products (silk, linen or cotton). It is acceptable in many situations, but is contraindicated in a wound that is, or may be, contaminated.
  - **Poliglecaprone** suture is a fast absorbing suture made of a synthetic absorbable monofilament composed of glycolide and epsilon-caprolactone copolymer (usually called PGCL suture). It comes in dyed (violet) and undyed (clear) form, and is a monofilament suture.

Clinical Corner

CASE SCENARIO 32:

A 42-year-old woman with cancer of breast underwent mastectomy. A Jackson-Pratt drain is placed to help empty excess fluid from the wound site. After emptying a Jackson-Pratt bulb, the nurse needs to reestablish the negative pressure in the system. Which of the following actions is required to reestablish negative pressure?

a. Place the bulb lower than chest level
b. Fill the bulb with normal saline
c. Compress the bulb and open the valve
d. Compress the bulb and close the valve

Ans. (d) Compress the bulb and close the valve

Jackson-Pratt drain has a soft plastic bulb with a valve (stopper) and a flexible tube attached to it. The drainage end of the tubing (flat white part) is placed into surgical site through a small opening near incision. A suture will hold it in place. The rest of the tube will extend outside the body and will be attached to the bulb.

The nurse has to squeeze the bulb when the stopper is open and then close the valve. When the bulb is compressed (squeezed) with the valve (stopper) is closed, a constant gentle suction is created. The bulb should be compressed at all times, except when the drainage being emptied.

NEEDLE

Surgical Needles

All surgical needles have three basic components:
- Eye (or Swage)
- Body
- Point

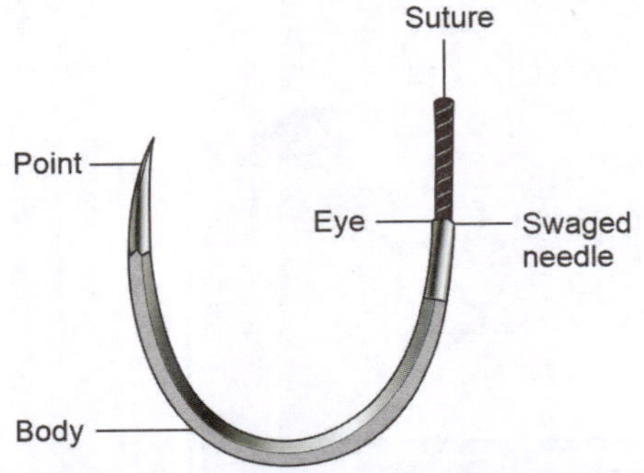

Figure 36: Basic needle design

- **Round bodied:** For soft (subcutaneous) tissues such as muscle, fascia, mucous membrane. The middle of the needle is flat for better seating in the needle holder and easy entry.
- **Cutting:** For firm tissue, sclerotic vessels and prostheses.
- **Trocar:** Trocar needles have a sharp tip but a round body. They are useful, necessary to perforate tough tissues.
- **Spatula needle:** Used in ophthalmic and microsurgery procedures. It has a flattened needle body that is hand ground laterally

KEY NURSING ROLES IN IMPORTANT PROCEDURES

Checking temperature	• Patient should not take anything hot or cold 10–20 minutes prior to the checking of oral temperature. • Insert rectal thermometer 3.5–4 cm in adults, 1.5 cm in infants and 2.5 cm in children. • Duration to be kept while taking temperature from different routes through mercuric thermometer is: ▪ Oral: 2 minutes ▪ Axillary: 3 minutes ▪ Rectal: 1 minute • Before taking temperature, thermometer needs to be cleaned from bulb to stem and after taking temperature, from stem to bulb. • Axillary temperature is one degree lower than oral temperature. • Rectal temperature is one degree higher than the oral temperature.
Assessment of pulse	• Both carotid pulses should not be palpated at same time as it can cause reflex drop in pulse or BP. • During cardiac arrest among adults, carotid pulse is assessed. • In infants during cardiac arrest, brachial or femoral pulse is assessed. • Never use thumb for pulse checking because thumb has its own pulsation and can be mistaken as patient's pulse.
BP monitoring	• BP should not be measured on patient's arm with fistula or shunt or on the same side of the radical mastectomy. • The ideal cuff bladder length is ≥80% of the patient's arm circumference. The ideal cuff bladder width is ≥40% of the patient's arm circumference. • If the cuff is small for patient's arm size—BP reading will be high. • If cuff is large for patient's arm size—BP reading will be low.

Contd...

KEY POINTS

The ideal suture material should cause minimal inflammation and tissue reaction while providing maximum strength in the lag phase of wound healing.
- **Characteristics of tissue reaction:** Fibrous cell reaction, absorption, potentiation of infection, and allergic reaction.
- **Swaged, or atraumatic** needles with sutures comprise a pre-packed eyeless needle attached to a specific length of suture thread.
- **A swaged needle** is ideal for a running suture line and thus is often selected for **obstetric applications.**

Recent Questions (NORCET 2021)

29. Rapid and weak pulse is known as:
a. Bounding pulse
b. Thready pulse
c. Strong pulse
d. None of the above

Ans. (b) Thready pulse

30. In an emergency, patient is admitted with cardiac arrest. Which pulse is used to assess PR in the patient?
a. Carotid
b. Brachial
c. Apical
d. Femoral

Ans. (a) Carotid

31. Difference between apical pulse and radial pulse is called:
a. Atrial flutter
b. Atrial fibrillation
c. Pulse deficit
d. Sinus bradycardia

Ans. (c) Pulse deficit

Eye care	• Clean the eyes from inner canthus to outer canthus. • Clean the non-infected eye first then the infected eye.
Instilling eye drops	• If more than one eye drop is ordered, instill with an interval of 10–15 minutes. • If there is order of applying eye drop and ointment, apply drop first then ointment. • OD—right eye • OS—left eye • OU—both eyes
Tracheostomy suction	• Position: Semi-Fowler's or Fowler's position. • Pressure: ▪ Adult: 100–120 mm Hg ▪ Child: 80–100 mm Hg ▪ Infant: 50–80 mm Hg • Hyperoxygenate the patient before applying suction. • Insert 10–12.5 cm or until the patient coughs. • Apply intermittent suction by occluding 'Y' port with thumb. • Do not apply suction for more than 10 seconds.
Lumbar Puncture	• Position for procedure: Fetal position (Knee chest position). • Site for lumbar puncture: Below the conus medullaris (L3/L4 or L4/L5 interspinous levels). • Provide supine position after procedure. • Measure blood glucose level immediately after or just before the procedure. • Headache and pain at puncture site are the most common side effects.

TRIAGE

At the time of disaster, **Simple Triage and Rapid Transport (START)** can be used to categorize patients.

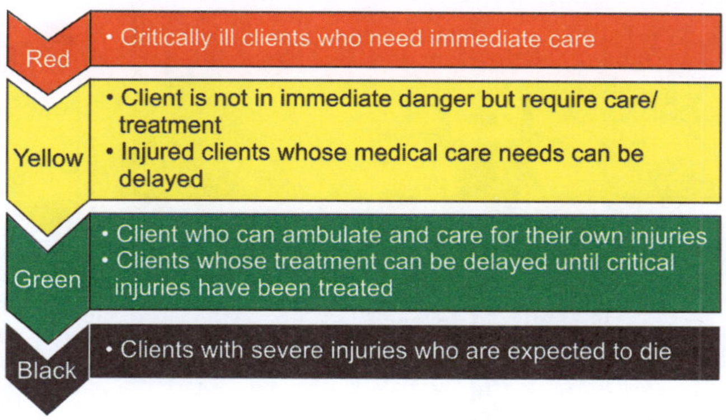

Figure 37: Categories of patients in Triage

INTRAVENOUS FLUID ADMINISTRATION DROP RATE CALCULATION

When intravenous fluid is administered to a patient and regulated manually, the nurse should be able to calculate IV flow rate (drops per minute to be administered). It can be calculated from amount of liquid, time period and a drop factor (gtts/mL).

Formula

$$\frac{\text{Volume (mL)}}{\text{Time (min)}} \times \text{Drop factor (gtts/mL)} = \text{Y (Flow rate in gtts/min)}$$

KEY POINTS

- Site for lumbar puncture: Between L3/L4 or L4/L5.
- During tracheostomy suction, DO NOT apply suction for more than 10 seconds.

Clinical Corner

CASE SCENARIO 33:

Mr. Rajesh, 40-year-old male, was brought to ER after a road traffic accident with a laceration on the forehead. Upon assessment, patient is conscious, RR- 35/min, radial pulse absent, and capillary refill time >2 seconds. Which triage category would this client be assigned to?

a. Black
b. Green
c. Red
d. Yellow

Ans. (c) Red

In the given scenario, the client had a head trauma with related signs and symptoms. Hence the patient needs an immediate intervention and resuscitation. In the triage category, red one should be applied for the emergency condition, yellow should be applicable for urgent condition and green should be indicated in the standard or minimal condition.

Questions & Answers

For Example

Q. Calculate the IV flow rate for 1000 mL of NS to be infused in 8 hours. The infusion set is calibrated for a drop factor of 20 gtts/mL.

$$\frac{\text{Volume (mL)}}{\text{Time (min)}} \times \text{Drop factor (gtts/mL)} = \text{Y (Flow rate in gtts/min)}$$

Convert 8 hours to minutes

8 hours × 60 min = 480 minutes

$$\frac{1000 \text{ mL}}{480 \text{ min}} \times 20 \text{ gtts/mL} = 41.66 = 42 \text{ gtts/min}$$

Q. Calculate the IV flow rate for 500 mL of 5% dextrose over 4 hours. Infusion set has drop factor of 15 gtts/mL.

$$\frac{\text{Volume (mL)}}{\text{Time (min)}} \times \text{Drop factor (gtts/mL)} = \text{Y (Flow rate in gtts/min)}$$

$$\frac{500 \text{ (mL)}}{4 \text{ hrs} \times 60 \text{ minutes}} \times 15 \text{ gtts/mL} = 31.25 = 31 \text{ gtts/min}$$

INSULIN SYRINGE PREPARATION (MIXING REGULAR WITH NPH)

- Wash hands
- Roll the NPH vial gently between palms for 10 minutes
- Wipe the top of vials with alcohol swab
- Draw back amount of air in the syringe that is equal to total dose
- Inject air equal to NPH dose into NPH vial (needle tip not to touch with insulin)
- Inject air equal to regular insulin dose into regular vial
- Invert regular insulin vial and withdraw regular insulin dose
- Invert NPH vial and withdraw NPH insulin dose. Do not push syringe content back into vial as this will contaminate NPH insulin with regular insulin.

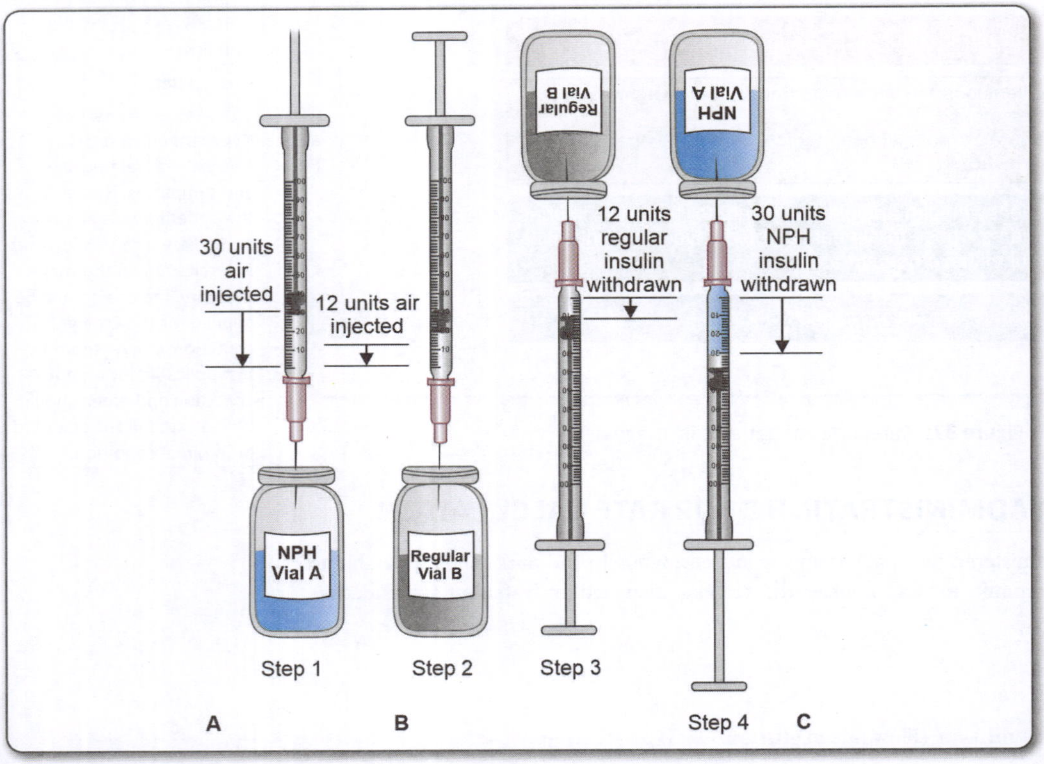

Figure 38: How to draw and mix NPH and regular insulin

Remember: RN (Regular first and NPH next while mixing)

Practice Question

20. Nurse is preparing inj. Albumin to administer. Prescription is inj. Albumin 100 mL IV over 4 hours. The drop factor is 40 drops per mL. Nurse understands that the prescribed flow rate is ....

a. 12 drops/min
b. 15 drops/min
c. 17 drops/min
d. 21 drops/min

Ans. (c) 17 drops/min

Calculation:

(100 mL/240 mins) x 40 = 16.6

Rounded off to 17 drops/min

POINT TO REMEMBER

Since it is not possible to give a patient a fraction of a drop, it is typical to round off answers for these problems (up or down) to the nearest whole number.

KEY POINTS

- Sites for insulin injection should be separated from one another by one inch (2.5 cm) and should be done every week or two.
- NPH (Neutral Protamine Hagedorn) insulin is an insoluble intermediate-acting insulin preparation.
- NPH insulin has an onset of 1–3 hours after injection, peaks 4–12 hours later, and is effective for about 12–16 hours.
- The most likely time for a hypoglycemic reaction to occur is 6 to 14 hours after NPH insulin administration.

HEMOGLOBIN

Hemoglobin Male : Female:	 13.5–17.0 g/dL 11.5–16.0 g/dL
Hematocrit Male : Female:	 0.40–0.51 or 40–51% 0.34–0.48 or 34–48%
RBCs	4.5–6 million/mm^3 or 4.5–6.0 x 10^{12}/L of blood
WBCs	4000–11000 cells/mm^3
Platelets	1,50,000–4,00,000 cells/mm^3 of blood

Interpretations of Abnormal CBC

- Decrease in hemoglobin (anemia) is due to iron or other deficiency, bleeding or marrow suppression such as chemotherapy. Hemoglobin is increased in polycythemia vera.
- WBC increases due to steroid use, infection or leukemia, decreases due to marrow suppression.
- Platelet decreases due to increased consumption of platelet in ITP or splenomegaly, or decreased production due to marrow suppression. Platelet count drops in case of dengue.

Coagulation Studies

INR (International Normalized Ratio of PT or prothrombin time) Therapeutic Coumadin (Warfarin) Mechanical heart valves	0.9–1.1 2.0–3.0 2.5–3.5	
PTT (Partial thromboplastin time) Therapeutic heparin	21–33 seconds 60–85 seconds	
PT Bleeding Time Thrombin time	10–14 seconds 3–7 minutes 11–15 seconds	

RENAL FUNCTION

Sodium	135–145 mEq/L
Potassium	3.5–5.5 mEq/L
Chloride	98–107 mEq/L
Bicarbonate	24–28 mEq/L
Blood urea nitrogen (BUN)	7–20 mg/dL or 2.5–8.0 mmol/L
Creatinine	0.6–1.2 mg/dL or 60–125 mmol/L

- Electrolyte disturbances may be due to renal failure, alterations in hydration (hypo or hyper), drug use (diuretics), alterations in pH (acidosis or alkalosis), diabetic ketoacidosis, adrenal disease, etc.
- Renal failure (and increasing BUN and creatinine) may be due to acute tubular necrosis (due to hypotension), glomerulonephritis, diabetic nephropathy, urinary tract infection, etc.

LIVER FUNCTION TEST (NORMAL VALUES)

Albumin	3.5–5.0 g/dL
Total bilirubin	0.3–1.2 mg/dL
Direct bilirubin (conjugated)	0.1–0.4 mg/dL
Indirect bilirubin (unconjugated)	0.2–0.8 mg/dL
Aspartate aminotransferase (AST)	10–42 U/L
Alanine aminotransferase (ALT)	10–40 U/L

In liver failure (due to hepatitis or cirrhosis), serum albumin will be decreased due to reduced production, serum bilirubin will be increased due to loss of liver metabolic function, serum enzymes will be increased due to 'leakage' of contents of damaged cells.

KEY POINTS

Hemoglobin criteria for anemia:

- Anemia in pregnant women: Hb <11 g/dL in venous blood.
- Anemia in nonpregnant women: Hb <12 g/dL
- Anemia in men: Hb <13 g/dL
- Anemia in under-five children: Hb <11 g/dL in venous blood.
- Anemia in children 5–11 years: Hb <11.5 g/dL
- Anemia in children 12-14 years: Hb <12 g/dL

POINT TO REMEMBER

INR and PTT may be elevated due to loss of factor production in liver disease, due to congenital deficiency such as hemophilia or suppression with drugs such as coumadin or heparin.

KEY POINTS

- **Sodium (Na^+)** is the most abundant cation in extracellular fluid.
- **Chloride (Cl^-)** is the most abundant anion in extracellular fluid.
- **Potassium (K^+)** is the most abundant cation in intracellular fluid.
- **Phosphate (HPO_4^-)** is the most abundant intracellular anion.
- **Calcium** is the most abundant mineral in the body.

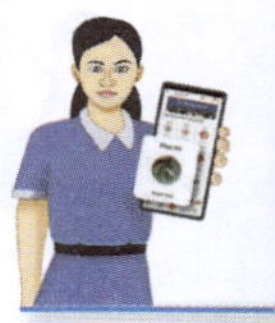

PULMONARY FUNCTION TEST

PFT (Pulmonary Function test) **FEV_1** (Forced Expiratory Volume in one second: total volume of air a patient is able to exhale in the first second during maximal effort)	
Normal	>75%
Mild disease	<60%
Moderate disease	40–60%
Severe disease	<40%

ENDOCRINE FUNCTION

- **Normal calcium level:** 9–10.5 mg/dL
- Calcium levels will be reduced with dietary vitamin D or calcium deficiency, loss of parathyroid function (for example post thyroid surgery), etc.
- TSH is depressed with excess exogenous thyroid hormone, Grave's disease or a secreting thyroid adenoma.

Thyroid Function Test

- **Normal TSH** : 0.35–5.00 mIU/L
  Suppressed : <0.10 mIU/L
  Elevated : >15.0 mIU/L
- ADF:
  T3 (triiodothyronine) - 80–180 ng/dL
  T4 (thyroxine) - 4.6–12 mcg/dL

BLOOD SUGAR PROFILE

Random Blood Glucose (Random)	70–125 mg/dL
Glucose (Fasting) 70–100 mg/dL	
Glucose (Post prandial)	<140 mg/dL
HbA1c (Glycated Hemoglobin) *(To identify the three-month average plasma glucose concentration)*	4–6%
HbA1c level 5.7–6.4: High risk for diabetes HbA1c level >6.4: Diabetes	

CARDIAC MARKERS

Table 38: Cardiac markers and their normal ranges

Cardiac markers	Normal range and onset
Troponin I	0–0.1 ng/mL (onset: 4–6 hours, peak: 12–24 hours, return to normal: 4–7 days)
Troponin T	0–0.2 ng/mL (onset: 3–4 hours, peak: 10–24 hours, return to normal: 10–14 days)
Myoglobin (Male)	10–95 ng/mL (onset: 1–3 hours, peak: 6–10 hours, return to normal: 12–24 hours)
Myoglobin (Female)	10–65 ng/mL (onset: 1–3 hours, peak: 6–10 hours, return to normal: 12–24 hours)
Troponin I	0–0.1 ng/mL (onset: 4–6 hours, peak: 12–24 hours, return to normal: 4–7 days)
Creatinine kinase Index (CK-Index)	0–3
Creatinine kinase-MB (CK-MB)	0–3 ng/mL
Total creatinine kinase	38–120 ng/mL

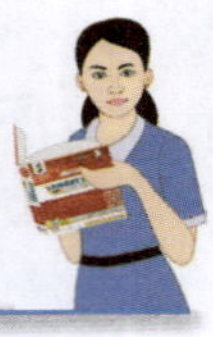

KEY POINTS

- An AST/ALT ratio equal to one (ALT is equal to the AST) is suggestive of **acute viral hepatitis or drug-related liver toxicity.**
- An AST/ALT ratio higher than one (AST is higher than ALT) is suggestive of **cirrhosis.**
- An AST/ALT ratio of less than one (ALT is significantly higher than AST) is suggestive of **non-alcoholic fatty liver disease.**

POINT TO REMEMBER

Pulmonary Function Test (PFT) is the confirmatory test for COPD.

KEY POINTS

- TSH is elevated in hypothyroidism due to primary thyroid deficiency.
- Normal TSH level during pregnancy is lower than the normal nonpregnancy level.
- Increased serum glucose may be related to undiagnosed diabetes, or poorly controlled diabetes due to noncompliance or the 'brittleness' of the underlying disease.
- Decreased serum glucose is typically due to insulin overdose or inadequate dietary intake of calories in the face of insulin or oral hypoglycemic use.

URINE ROUTINE AND MICROSCOPY

Table 39: Normal values of urine

Color	Straw
Specific gravity	1.005–1.030
pH	4.6–8.0
Na	40–220 mEq/24 hrs
K	25–125 mEq/24 hrs
Cl	80–250 mEq/day
Total nitrogen	10–20 g/24 hrs
Creatinine	1.0–2.0 g/24 hrs
Calcium	0.1–0.7 g/24 hrs
Protein	1–15 mg/dL
Osmolality	80–1300 mOsm/L
Urine bilirubin	Negative
Urine blood	Negative
Urine ketone	Negative
Urine leukocytes	Negative
RBCs	0–2/HPF
WBCs	0–2/HPF
RBC casts	0/HPF

CEREBROSPINAL FLUID (CSF)

Appearance	Clear
Glucose	40–80 mg/dL
Osmolality	290–298 mOsm/L
Pressure	70–80 mm/H_2O
Protein	15–45 mg/dL
Total cell count	0–5 cells
WBCs	0–6/μL

NEUROLOGICAL VALUES

Cerebral perfusion pressure	70–90 mm Hg
Intracranial pressure	5–15 mm Hg or 5–10 cm H_2O

ARTERIAL BLOOD GAS (ABG) VALUES

pH	7.35–7.45
$PaCO_2$	35–45 mm Hg
HCO_3	22–26 mEq/L
O_2 saturation	96–100%
PaO_2	85–100 mm Hg

KEY POINTS

- Biomarkers are used to help diagnose acute coronary syndrome (ACS) and cardiac ischemia.
- Troponin (I or T)—this is the most commonly ordered and most specific of the cardiac markers.
- Myoglobin is an early marker but has **poor clinical specificity (60–90%)** due to the presence of large quantities of myoglobin in skeletal muscle.
- Fresh urine sample collected any time of the day is suitable for routine examination.

POINTS TO REMEMBER

Urine specimen

- Random collection—for routine screening
- Fasting and postprandial—for diabetes mellitus
- 24 hours sample—for quantitative tests
- Midstream clean catch urine—for culture as well as routine
- Catheterized—for culture
- Suprapubic aspiration—for bladder culture

KEY POINTS

- Normally, CSF is clear and colorless.
- The glucose test of CSF helps in diagnosing bacterial infection or tumors.
- Increased protein level in CSF may be a sign of a tumor, bleeding, nerve inflammation, or injury.

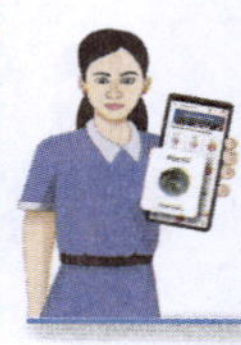

FIRST AID

- First aid provides immediate care for injuries or illness to preserve life, prevent further harm, and promote recovery.
- Fundamental rules of first aid are to ensure safety of rescuer and victim, assess the situation for safety, and call for help, if necessary.
- Red Cross offers training courses for basic and advanced first aid techniques to the public.

Asphyxia

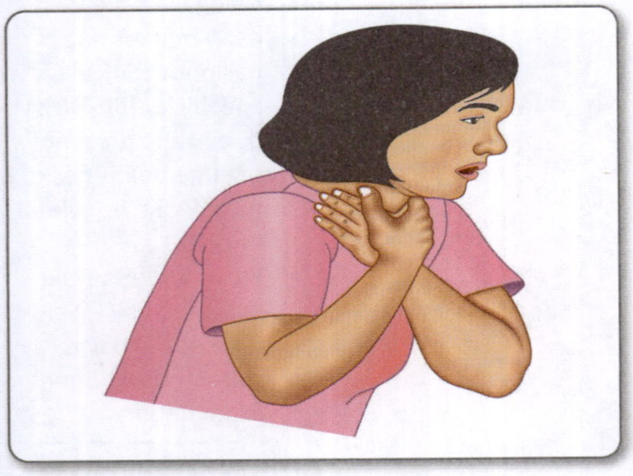

Figure 39: universal choking sign

- Choking occurs when an object blocks the airway, making it difficult or impossible to breathe.
- The universal sign of choking is hands grasping the throat.
- Never perform a blind sweep during choking.

Adult

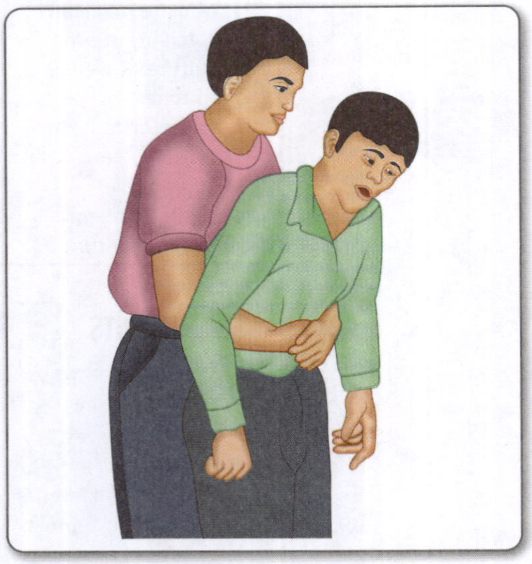

Figure 40: Heimlich maneuver

- Ask the person if he/she is choking: If the person can speak or cough, it may mean that airway is partially blocked. Encourage the person to cough forcefully to try to dislodge the object.
- Perform Heimlich maneuver by standing behind the person, making a fist above the navel, and pulling in and up sharply. Repeat this until object is dislodged.
- For pregnant or obese victims, place your fist just below the xiphisternum instead of the naval.

Infant and Younger Children

- Administer back blows and chest thrust: Hold the child face down on your forearm with its head lower than chest and give up to five sharp blows between its shoulder blades with the heel of your hand. If this does not dislodge the obstruction, perform up to five chest thrusts by placing two fingers in the center of the child's chest, just below the nipple line, and giving up to five quick thrusts.
- Repeat this blow and thrust until the object is dislodged or child becomes unconscious.

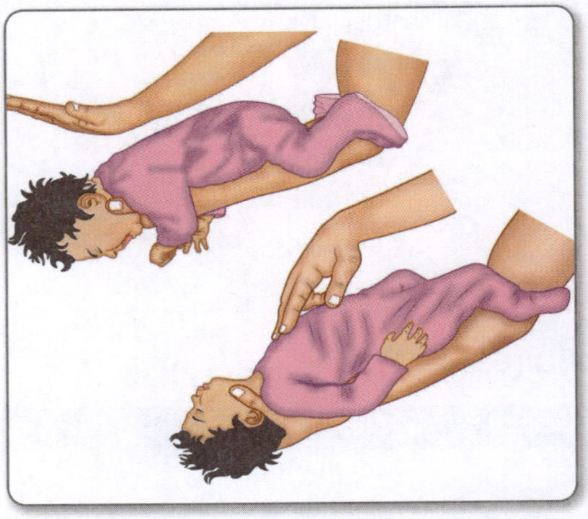

Figure 41: Back blows and chest thrust

First Aid Management for Open Wound

- Stop the bleeding.
- Clean the area under running water, if cut is small, pressure from the water is enough to stop bleeding.
- Apply pressure over the cut using a clean cloth.
- Wash out the dirt if it is present.
- Seek medical help if cut is deep and big.

First Aid Management of Dog Bite

- Wash the wound thoroughly with soap and water for at least 5 minutes. This can help reduce the risk of infection.
- Control any bleeding by applying pressure with a clean, dry cloth or bandage.
- Apply an antibiotic ointment to the wound and cover it with a sterile dressing.
- Shift the victim to the hospital.
- If dog is known, obtain the vaccination status of dog; if not known, observe the dog for 10–15 days.

Clinical Corner

CASE SCENARIO 34:

During a first aid class, the teacher quizzes the students on identifying the cardinal signs of choking in child correctly. Which of the following signs should they NOT consider as a cardinal sign of choking in a child?

a. Inability to speak
b. cyanosis
c. Collapse
d. Vomiting

Ans. (d) Vomiting

The cardinal signs of choking in child include:
1. Inability to speak
2. cyanosis (blue color)
3. Collapse
Vomiting is not a sign of chocking.

KEY POINTS

Signs of chocking in adults:

- Clutching the neck (universal sign of choking)
- Weak or no cough
- Unable to make noise or talk
- Little or no breathing
- Appears cyanotic (lips and fingertips)

Clinical Corner

CASE SCENARIO 35:

Ten-month-old infant chokes and becomes unconscious. After opening the airway, what is the first step of action by the nurse?

a. Look for foreign object in the mouth
b. Do blind sweep
c. Give back blows
d. Call emergency response number

Ans. (a) Look for foreign object in the mouth

Once the airway is open, then look for the foreign object in the mouth.
Blind sweeps are not recommended. If foreign objects are not visible, then back blow is indicated.

First Aid Management of Burn Injury

Thermal burn	Chemical burn	Electrical burn
• Remove the person from source of burn injury.		
Stop the burning process by pouring water. Application of ice is not recommended as it causes peripheral vasoconstriction.	Rinse the affected area with large amounts of running water.	Turn off the power source or remove the person from the source of electricity, if possible.
Cover the person with a thick cloth or blanket immersed in water to stop burning process.		
Ask the victim to drop and roll on the ground.		
• Move the victim to a safe place. • Remove any jewelry or clothing that may be in contact with the burned area, but do not remove any clothing that is stuck to the burn. • Place the client in a recovery position and look for breathing. • If patient is unresponsive, then start with CPR.		

First Aid Management of Poisoning

Ingested Poison

- Try to find out the type of poison ingested.
- Check for ABC of victim. If the victim is not responding, then start with CPR.
- Never induce vomiting if poison is not identified. Acid, alkali, and chemical poison may cause burning of GI tract and further injury.
- Call poison control center and follow the instructions.
- Provide symptomatic management and seek medical help.

Inhaled Poison

- Ensure scene safety and call for help.
- Stop further injury either by turning off the source or moving the person out to a safe open place. If movement is not possible, open the doors and windows of the room.
- If the person is unconscious or having difficulty breathing, start CPR or rescue breathing, as appropriate.
- If the person is conscious, make him/her sit upright and breathe slowly and deeply. This can help reduce the amount of poison in lungs.
- If the poison is a gas, remove contaminated clothing and wash any exposed skin with soap and water.
- If the poison is a particulate (such as dust or powder), help the person remove any contaminated clothing and flush the affected area with water.

First Aid Management of Snake Bite

- Call emergency services immediately.
- Keep the person calm and still. Movement causes the venom to spread more quickly through the body.
- Keep the affected limb below the level of the heart, if possible. This can help slow the spread of venom.
- Remove any tight clothing or jewelry around the bite area.
- Clean the bite wound with soap and water, but do not attempt to suck out the venom or cut the wound.
- Apply firm, but not tight, bandage or dressing over the bite; **do not apply a tourniquet**.
- Monitor the breathing and pulse; perform CPR or rescue breathing, if necessary.
- Try to identify the snake, if possible, but do not attempt to capture or kill it. The doctors will need to know the type of snake to provide the appropriate antivenom.

Recent Questions
(NORCET 2022)

32. Patient in ED is admitted with a history of chemical burns. What is the priority nursing intervention?
a. Wash with running water
b. Call doctor
c. Apply povidone cream
d. Apply antibiotic cream

Ans. (a) Wash with running water

Chemical burns can be caused by acids or bases that come into contact with tissue. Prompt wound irrigation with running water is the most critical aspect in limiting the extent of dermal burns from exposure to chemicals

33. A patient with circumferential burn comes to the emergency. The patient should be assessed for which complication?
a. Fluid status
b. Urine output
c. Engorged neck veins
d. Absent peripheral pulse

Ans. (d) Absent peripheral pulse

Recent Question
(NORCET 2023)

34. Gastric lavage Procedure should be avoided in which of the following situation?
a. Kerosene Poisoning
b. Arsenic Poisoning
c. Organophosphate Poisoning
d. Ethanol Poisoning

Ans. (a) Kerosene Poisoning

Kerosene is a petroleum-based product, and inducing vomiting or using gastric lavage can lead to aspiration of the kerosene, which can cause aspiration pneumonia.

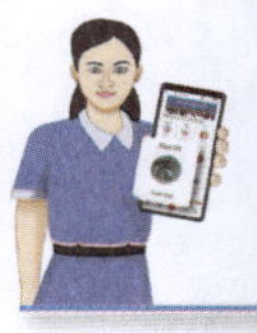

COLOR CODING OF MEDICAL GAS CYLINDER

Cylinder name	Picture
Oxygen cylinder white neck with black body	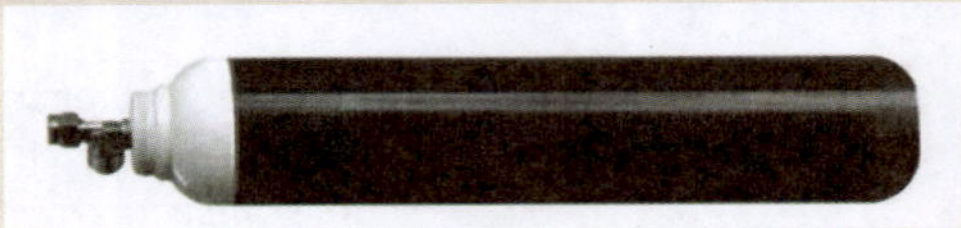
Nitrous oxide (laughter gas) blue color	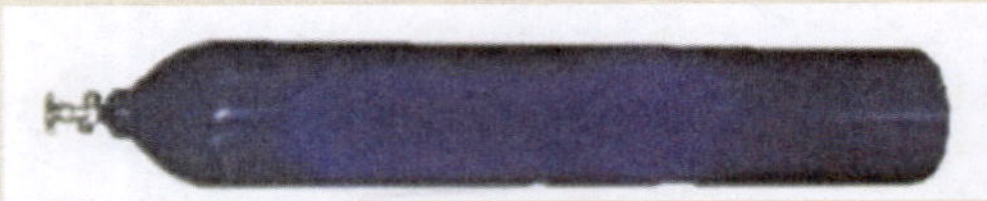
Carbon dioxide gray color	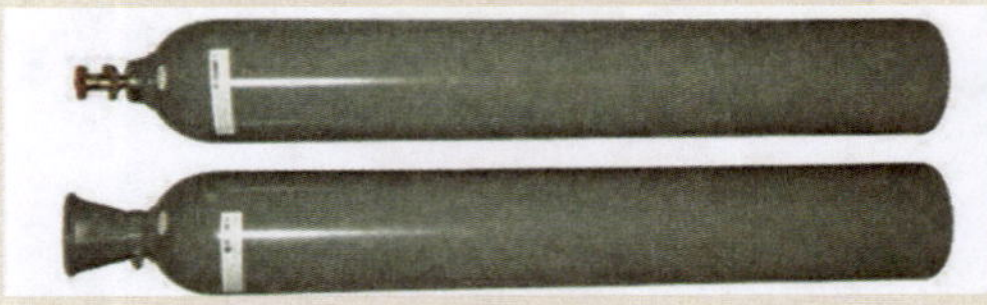
Nitrogen black color (**Note:** Aluminium Alloy cylinder - Black at the vavle end; body should not be pained)	
Helium brown color	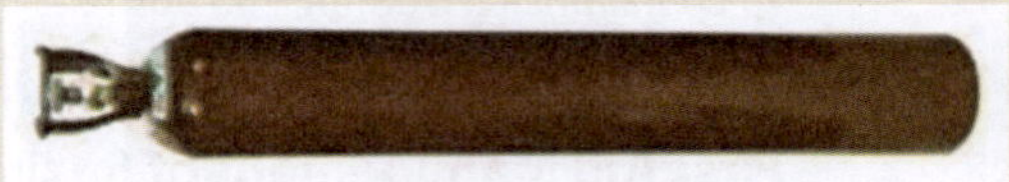

Recent Question (HPSSB 2020)

35. Colour coding for nitrous oxide cylinder is:
a. Black
b. Black with white shoulder
c. French blue
d. Grey

Ans. (c) French blue

KEY POINTS

- Color coding for Other Medical Gas Cylinders in India:
- Air - Grey body & White and black neck.
- Cyclopropane - Orange body and neck.
- Ethylene - Violet body and neck

POINTS TO REMEMBER

- In case of Aluminium Alloy Gas Cylinders, the body of the cylinder shall not be painted.
- The identification colour to be applied to the valve end of the Cylinder.

COMFORT DEVICES

Comfort devices are used to provide comfort and relief to patients who are undergoing medical treatment or are recovering from an illness or injury.

Comfort device	
Backrest • A backrest comfort device is a device used to provide support and comfort to the back while sitting or lying down. • This device helps to ease the work of breathing in a patient. 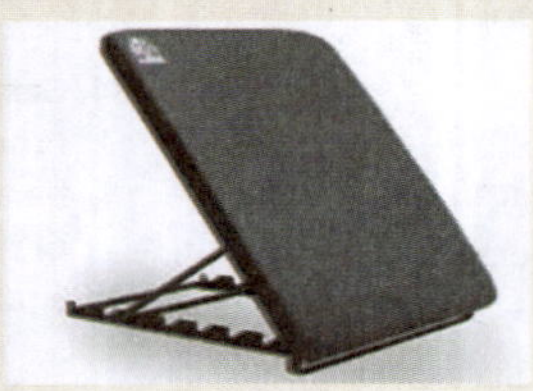	**Foot rest/Foot board** • To provide proper alignment of foot and to prevent foot drop. • It should be perpendicular to bed and parallel to the plantar surface of the foot. 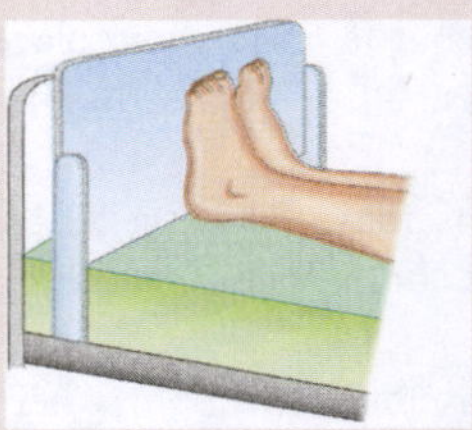
Bed cradle • This device helps to take off the weight of the top linens. • In burn patients, this device helps to prevent the linen from touching the body. 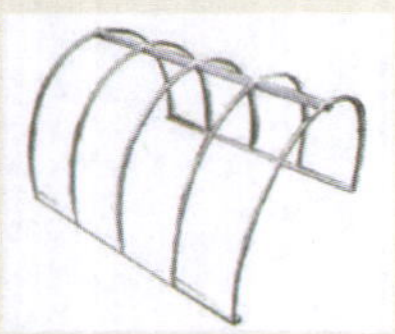	**Cardiac table** Patient can lean on the table during therapeutic and diagnostic procedures and it also helps to facilitate breathing. 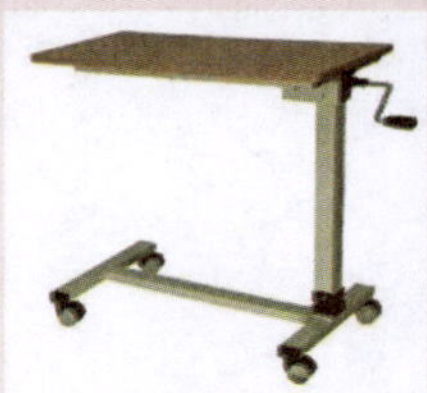

Contd...

Comfort device

Sand bag

To immobilize a particular part.

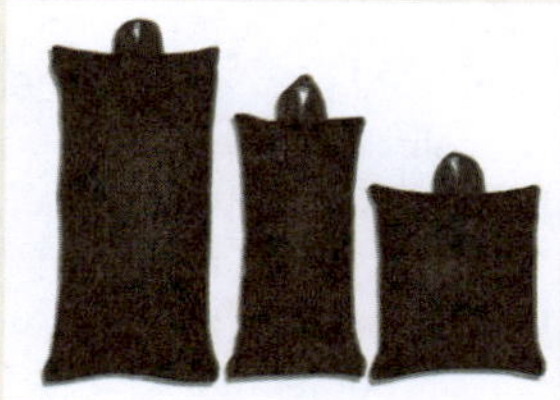

Trapeze bar

- It is positioned over the head.
- It helps the patient to mobilize/reposition self.

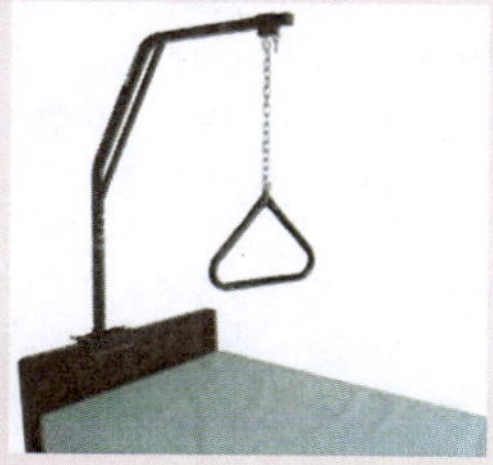

Air mattress/Water Mattress

This type of mattress is filled with water or air and it helps to equally distribute the pressure exerted on the body. It helps to prevent the development of bed sore.

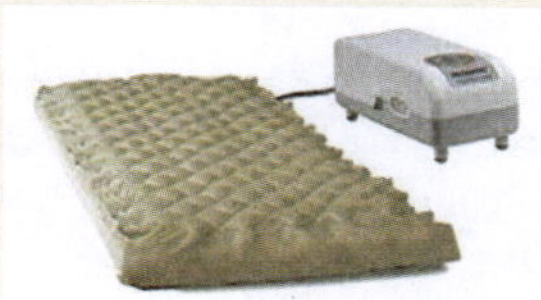

Trochanter roll

It helps to prevent the external rotation of the legs when the patient is in supine position.

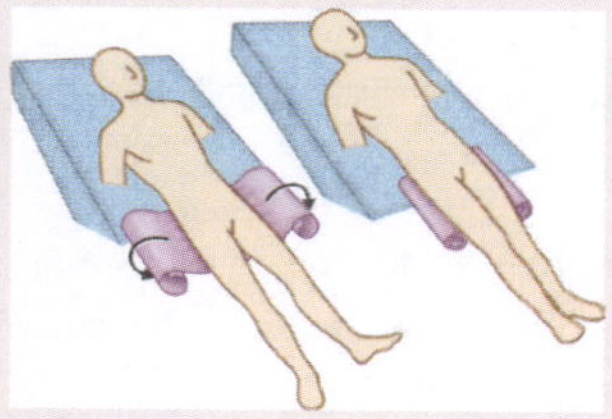

Bed blocks

- These blocks are kept at either head end or foot end according to the position given to the client.
- This block helps to provide Trendelenburg and reverse Trendelenburg positions to the client.

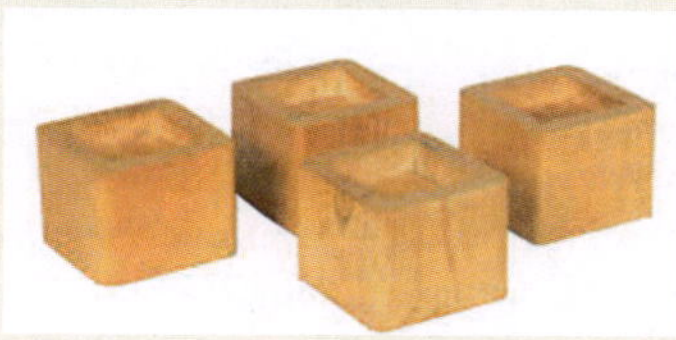

Air cushion

It is made of rubber and round in shape. It is used to relieve pressure at pressure points in the body.

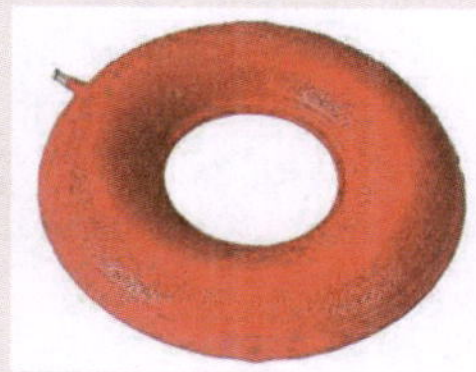

Cotton ring

- It is made of rubber and covered with cotton.
- It is used to provide support to the pressure points.

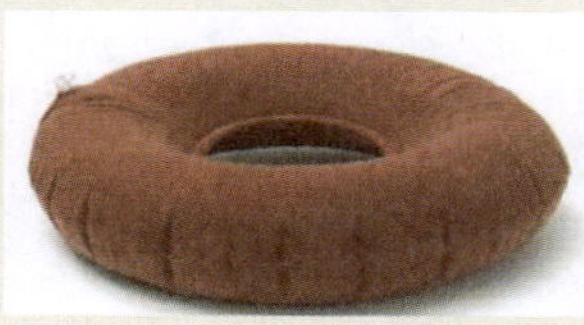

Pillows

Used to support the body parts and also to maintain proper alignment of body parts.

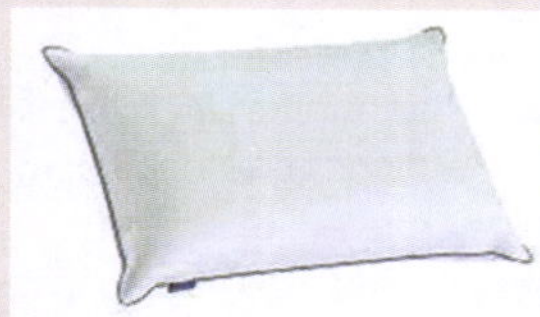

Hand roll

Used to maintain thumb in adducted position and in apposition to other fingers

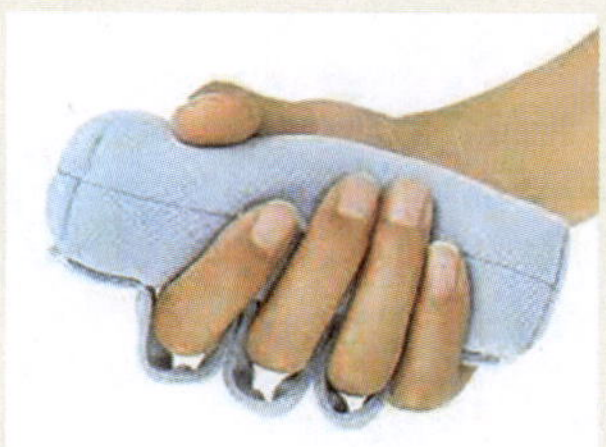

Hip abduction pillow

It is also known as wedge pillow. It is used to maintain hip in abduction position in patients after total hip replacement.

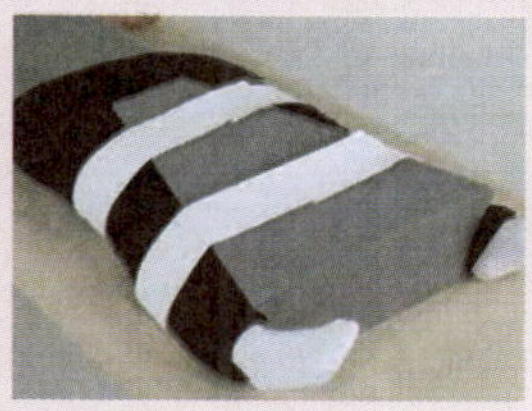

Golden Points to Remember

- Heat loss due to contact with circulating air movement is known as **convection**.
- Transfer of heat from one object to other without contact is known as **radiation** (60% heat loss from skin is through radiation).
- Normal **oral temperature is 98.6°F** (37°C).
- Normal **axillary temperature is 97.6°F** (36.4°C) [**1°F** lesser than oral temperature).
- Normal **rectal temperature is 99.6°F** (37°C) [**1°F** higher than oral temperature].
- **Hypothermia**—Temperature <95°F.
- **Hyperthermia**—Temperature up to 105°F.
- **Hyperpyrexia**—Temperature >105°F.
- Rectal temperature is the most reliable to assess core temperature.
- To assess rectal temperature, the thermometer is inserted 1.5 inch in adult and 1 inch in children. Position – Left lateral.
- Wipe the thermometer from **bulb to stem** with **moist swab before taking temperature**.
- Wipe the thermometer from **stem to bulb** with **dry swab after taking temperature.**
- **Relapsing fever:** Fever episodes are separated by intervals of normal temperature for days or weeks.
- **Lysis:** Temperature falls in a zigzag manner (step-ladder pattern).
- **Crisis:** Sudden return of temperature to the normal range from a very high temperature.
- **Rigor:** Sudden rise in body temperature with shivering as seen in malaria.
- **Inverse fever:** Temperature rises in the early morning rather than in the evening.
- Increased depth of breathing with normal respiratory rate is called **hyperpnea.**
- **Cheyne-Stokes Respiration** is characterized by altered period of tachypnea and apnea.
- **Kussmaul respiration** (air hunger) is associated with severe metabolic acidosis and diabetic ketoacidosis.
- Always count pulse for one full minute.
- **Pulse pressure** refers to the difference between systolic blood pressure and diastolic blood pressure.
- Pulse Pressure = Systolic Blood Pressure – Diastolic Blood Pressure
- Width of the cuff should be 40% of the arm circumference and length of the cuff should be 80% of the **arm circumference**.
- A **blood pressure cuff** that is too large will give falsely low reading of BP.
- A **blood pressure cuff** that is too small will give falsely high reading of BP.
- **Nonmaleficence** is an ethical principle that obliges one to not inflict intentional harm (to do no harm).
- **Intentional torts** include assault, battery, false imprisonment, intentional infliction of emotional distress, libel, slander and trespassing.
- **Beneficence:** Doing good for patients and providing benefit balanced against risk.
- **Fidelity:** Being loyal and faithful to commitments and accountable for responsibilities.
- **Veracity:** Telling the truth and not intentionally deceiving or misleading patients.
- **Slander** refers to crime of making false spoken statement damaging to a person's reputation.
- A patient whose life is threatened and who is comatose is assumed to give **implied consent.**
- Movement of an extremity away from the body midline is called **abduction.**
- **Adduction**: Moving toward midline of the body.
- **Extension**: Straightening a joint.
- **Flexion**: Bending motion that decreases the angle of joint.
- **Isotonic solutions** allow free movement of water across the membrane without changing concentration of solutes on either side, e.g., 0.9% NaCl.
- **Hypotonic solution:** Solutions in which solutes are less concentrated than in the cells, e.g., 0.45% NS.
- **Hypertonic solution:** Fluids with solutes more concentrated than in cells, e.g. 5% dextrose.
- Hospital has to keep MLC record up to **Ten Years,** because it serves to demonstrate professional integrity.
- The **order** of techniques during physical examination (except abdominal exam) is **Inspection – Palpation – Percussion – Auscultation.**
- For abdominal exam, the order of examination technique is **Inspection – Auscultation – Percussion – Palpation.** It is because percussion or palpation may alter the bowel sound.
- **Surgical asepsis** or "sterile technique" is used in surgery and invasive procedures.
- Medical asepsis or "clean technique" involves procedures to reduce the number and transmission of pathogens.
- Sterilization aims at killing all microorganisms and their spores. To be effective, the autoclave must reach 121°C and maintain temperature for at least 30 minutes.
- The most unreliable method of sterilization is **sunlight.** Microbicidal activity takes place due to the presence of UV rays. It does not kill spores.
- Gently pulling and inverting **gloves** when removing them decreases the risk of spreading the pathogens.
- Oxygen has a drying effect on mucous membrane that results in damage to the airways, secretions may become thick and difficult to clear, and it also causes airway obstructions. Oxygen has to be humidified before administration.
- Taping the Foley catheter to upper thigh helps to prevent accidental removal, decreases the trauma to urethra/bladder.
- If a patient has taken cold or hot drink, wait for 10–20 minutes in order to measure the right oral temperature.
- If a patient develops chills and headache during blood transfusion, the immediate action is to **stop the transfusion.**
- **Common indication of infiltration** of a peripheral intravenous infusion is cool skin around the insertion site. Other signs

Contd...

include swelling, burning sensation, discomfort and feeling of tightness.

- **Redness and swelling** around the insertion site (IV cannula) might indicate the signs of **infection/inflammation.**
- The nurse must stop IV infusion and remove cannula immediately if patient complains of pain and has redness with swelling at the site of IV.
- **Mask** is the only PPE needed when the nurse is assigned to a patient who has a bacterial pneumonia and is under droplet precautions (if no other indications).
- The stages of infection in sequence—**Incubation, Prodromal, Illness** and **Convalescence** stages.
- Factors that can produce falsely low reading of oxygen saturation (SpO_2) by pulse oximetry (SaO_2) include methemoglobinemia, anemia, inadequate peripheral circulation, blue or green nail polish and edema.
- Adult basal metabolic rate (BMR) decreases with an increase in body fat. Normal BMR in women is 1493 calories and normal BMR in men is 1662 calories.
- Patient's position to perform colonoscopy: **Make the patient lie on his/her left side of the body with legs bent.**
- The ideal length of insertion of rectal suppository in an adult is 4 cm beyond internal sphincter.
- **Vastus lateralis muscle** is the preferred site of intramuscular injections in infants.
- **Intramuscular injection (IM)** is given at an angle of **90°.**
- Maximum volume of medication for a single IM injection in adult is **5 mL**.
- **Subcutaneous injection** is given at an angle of **45°.**
- Maximum volume of medication for a single subcutaneous injection in adult is **1–1.5 mL**.
- **Intravenous injection** is given at an angle of **25°.**
- **Intradermal injection** is given at an angle of **10°–15°.**
- Maximum volume of medication for a single **Intradermal injection** is 0.1 mL.
- Palliative treatment is meant to **relieve symptoms and improve quality of life.**
- Cold application is also known as **Cryotherapy.**
- **Patient incident report** is also known as accidental report, which is the documentation of the incidence or any accident in detail.
- **Discharge planning** of a patient ideally begins at the time of the admission of a patient.
- Nursing informatics is a field of nursing that incorporates nursing, computer and information sciences to improve patient care outcomes.
- A **Kardex** or **Rand System** is a medical information system used by nursing staff to communicate a quick summary of individual patient needs that is updated at every shift change.
- Active, inactive, potential and resolved problems that serve as the index for charting documentation is known as **problem list**.
- Traditional **nursing chart** is divided into sections or blocks. It also uses graphics and narrative charting.
- Narrative charting is considered traditional **charting method.**
- Personal assessment and judgment of incident should not be considered while filling up an **incident report**.
- Using a score that rates each patient by severity of illness is known as **acuity charting.**
- Problem oriented charting is focused on the patient's problems.
- Components of SOAP format are **S**ubjective data, **O**bjective data, **A**ssessment and **P**lan.
- Managed care is a systematic approach to care that provides a framework for the coordination of medical and nursing interventions.
- The most important nursing interventions for dryness of the skin are:
  - Increase fluid intake
  - Use of non-irritating soap
  - Apply moisturizing lotion
- If the client reports abdominal cramping while administering enema, the instillation must be stopped immediately. An assessment must be made before continuing the administration possibly with a slower rate of administration.
- When bathing a patient's extremities, the nurse should use long, firm strokes from the distal to the proximal areas to facilitate venous blood return.
- The fecal occult blood test (FOBT) is a test to assess for occult blood in the stool. It is commonly used for screening of colorectal cancer.
- Tryptophan is a natural sedative (sleep-inducing amnio acid). Protein foods such as milk and milk products contain tryptophan.
- Legal responsibilities of nurse while restraining patient include:
  - Obtain written order from physician except in an emergency
  - Document the type of restraints used and the patient's behavior
- Tenderness, burning sensation, swelling, warm and erythematous skin around IV site are indications of phlebitis.
- The nurse should roll the vial gently between the palm to ensure homogenization when diluting powdered medication in a vial.
- While preparing insulin injection, the nurse should draw up the shorter-acting, clear insulin (regular) before the longer-acting, cloudy insulin (NPH) to ensure accurate measurements.
- While examining a patient with abdominal pain, the nurse should assess the symptomatic quadrant last.
- The nail polish of patients scheduled for surgery is removed **to detect any cyanosis caused by low oxygen level.**
- In Europe and Japan, Catgut sutures have been banned due to concerns that **they could transmit bovine spongiform encephalopathy (mad cow disease).**

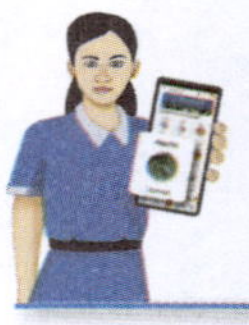

"He who has health has hope; and he who has hope has everything."

—Arabian proverb

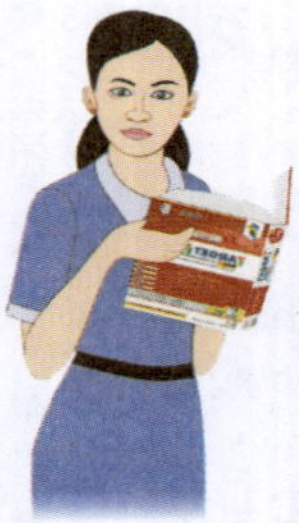

CLINICAL CASE-BASED QUESTIONS

1

Sireen, a trainee nurse, is posted in surgical ward. She is helping the nursing head in inventory management. Where she noticed that high-risk medications are kept separately under locker. The head nurse then asked her that which of the high-risk medication is kept under double lock?

a. Insulin
b. Digoxin
c. Fentanyl
d. Potassium chloride 10%

Ans. (c) Fentanyl

Explanation: Among the options provided, fentanyl is considered a high-risk medication and is often stored under double lock. Fentanyl is a potent opioid analgesic and is classified as a controlled substance due to its potential for abuse and the risk of respiratory depression. Storing it under double lock helps ensure its safekeeping and prevents unauthorized access.

2

You are an operation theater (OT) nursing officer. Today you are assigned in the laparoscopic OT to function as a scrub nurse. The patient has been taken inside the OT and the entire operative team verified the patient, site of the operation, and procedure before the incision. Which of the following surgical safety checklist point is being performed in the given scenario?

a. Sign in
b. Sign out
c. Time out
d. All of the above

Ans. (c) Time Out

Explanation: The surgical safety checklist consists of three main points: Sign in, time out, and sign out. The time out checklist point is performed before the incision to verify the patient's identity, the site of the operation, and the procedure. It is a critical safety check to help prevent wrong-site, wrong-patient, and wrong-procedure surgery.

The sign in checklist point is performed before the patient enters the operating room to verify the patient's identity, allergies, and medical history. The sign out checklist point is performed after the surgery is complete to ensure that all instruments and supplies have been accounted for.

So, in the given scenario, the surgical safety checklist point being performed is the time out.

3

A clinical instructor is providing bedside teaching to the 2nd year BSc nursing students about the whoosh test on a patient with NG tube. Select the most appropriate statement related to the test.

a. It is used to assess the correct placement of NG tube.
b. The examiner will place the diaphragm of the stethoscope over the left upper quadrant of abdomen to listen to the bubbling air sound.
c. The air is injected with the help of syringe through the NG tube while simultaneously auscultating, a whoosh sound is heard which indicates the tube is in stomach.
d. All of the above.

Ans. (d) All of the above.

Explanation: The whoosh test is a bedside procedure that is used to assess the correct placement of a nasogastric (NG) tube. The test is performed by injecting air through the NG tube while simultaneously auscultating the left upper quadrant of the abdomen. If a whoosh sound is heard, it indicates that the tube is in the stomach.

The steps on how to perform the whoosh test:

1. Attach a syringe to the end of the NG tube.
2. Aspirate any stomach contents from the tube.
3. Inject 10–20 mL of air into the tube.
4. Place the diaphragm of the stethoscope over the left upper quadrant of the abdomen.
5. Listen for a whoosh sound.

4

When a nurse suspects an air embolism due to the accidental disconnection of parenteral nutrition tubing from the central line catheter, which of the following position should the client be placed in?

a. On the left side, with head lower than the feet.
b. On the left side, with the head end elevated.
c. On the right side, with head lower than the feet.
d. On the right side, with head end elevated.

Ans. (a) On the left side, with head lower than the feet.

Explanation: In case of suspected venous air embolism, Durant's maneuver is performed. Durant's maneuver involves placing the patient in the left lateral decubitus position, with the head lower than the feet. This position helps to trap the air bubble in the right atrium of the heart, where it can be more easily absorbed.

5

You are working as a home care nurse and observed that your client has developed swelling over the left ankle. The client then reported about the left ankle sprain. Select the best possible instruction to be given by the nurse to manage the ankle sprain.

a. Apply the ice pack to the injured area for a period of 10–20 minutes
b. Apply ice pack to the injured area for a period of 1–2 hours
c. Apply the hot pack to the injured area for a period of 2 hours, followed by cold application
d. Maintain the left leg in dependent position

Ans. (a) Apply the ice pack to the injured area for a period of 10–20 minutes

Explanation: Applying an ice pack to the injured area for a short period of time is a common first aid measure for managing acute injuries like sprains. Ice helps reduce swelling and inflammation by constricting blood vessels and numbing the area.

The recommended duration for applying an ice pack is typically 10-20 minutes at a time, allowing for a break in between to prevent potential tissue damage from prolonged exposure to cold.

6

You are posted in the coronavirus screening zone. As per the Indian Government directives, the health care provider has to take nasopharyngeal /oropharyngeal (Throat) swab. It may cause discomfort to the clients during administration, but the benefits of early recognition of this coronavirus both for the individual and society, outweigh the temporary discomforts. Which principle is involved in this situation?

a. Nonmaleficence
b. Respect for autonomy
c. Beneficence
d. Principle of justice

Ans. (c) Beneficence

Explanation: Beneficence is the principle of doing good. In this situation, the healthcare provider is doing good by taking the nasopharyngeal/oropharyngeal swab, even though it may cause discomfort to the client. The benefits of early recognition of the coronavirus, both for the individual and society, outweigh the temporary discomforts.

7

A nurse cares for terminally ill cancer patients with the prognosis of 6 months by providing physical, psychological, social, and spiritual care for the patients, their families, and other loved ones. What type of care is the nurse providing?

a. Respite care
b. Palliative care
c. Hospice care
d. Extended care

Ans. (c) Hospice care

Explanation: Hospice care is a specialized form of care provided to individuals who have a terminal illness with a prognosis of approximately six months or less to live. The focus of hospice care is on providing comprehensive support to address the physical, psychological, social, and spiritual needs of the patients and their families during the end-of-life journey.

In the given situation, the nurse is providing physical, psychological, social, and spiritual care for the patients and their families. This is consistent with the goals of hospice care, which is to provide comfort and support to terminally ill patients and their families. Therefore, the answer is (c).

8

A nurse inspects a two-day-old intravenous site and identifies erythema, warmth, and mild edema. The client reports tenderness when the area is palpated. What should the nurse do first?

a. Irrigate the IV tubing
b. Discontinue the infusion
c. Slow the rate of the infusion
d. Obtain a prescription for an analgesic

Ans. (b) Discontinue the infusion

Explanation: The presence of erythema (redness), warmth, mild edema (swelling), and tenderness at the intravenous site may indicate the development of phlebitis, which is inflammation of the vein. To prevent further complications and promote the client's well-being, the nurse should first discontinue the infusion. This action stops the administration of any potentially irritating substances into the inflamed vein and reduces the risk of further inflammation or infection.

9

A 45-year-old client is admitted for an exacerbation of emphysema. On assessment, the nurse determines that the client has a fever, chills, and difficulty breathing on exertion. Considering the client's present condition, what is the priority nursing action?

a. Checking for capillary refill
b. Encouraging increased fluid intake
c. Suctioning secretions from the airway
d. Administering a high concentration of oxygen

Ans. (b) Encouraging increased fluid intake

Explanation: In a client with an exacerbation of emphysema who is experiencing fever, chills, and difficulty breathing on exertion, encouraging increased fluid intake is important for multiple reasons: replacing fluid loss from fever and decreasing viscosity of secretions.

10

A 50-year-old client is admitted with emphysema and undergoing treatment. The patient experiences a sudden episode of breathlessness and is diagnosed with a spontaneous pneumothorax. Which of the following is the most likely reason for the onset of spontaneous pneumothorax?

a. Pleural friction rub
b. Penetrating injury to chest wall
c. Tracheoesophageal fistula
d. Rupture of a subpleural bleb

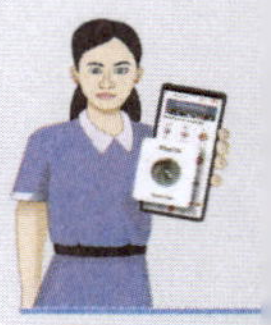

Ans. (d) Rupture of a subpleural bleb

Explanation: A spontaneous pneumothorax is a condition in which air leaks into the space between the lung and the chest wall. This can cause the lung to collapse. It typically happens due to the rupture of a subpleural bleb, which is a small, thin-walled air-filled sac located on the surface of the lung. These blebs can form due to weak spots in the lung tissue and are more commonly found in individuals with emphysema.

11

A client with esophageal varices is admitted to the hospital and requires a blood transfusion. The physician orders a blood transfusion of one unit. What nursing actions should be taken?

a. Record the vital signs in accordance with institutional policy and check the blood product against the client's ID bracelet in the presence of the nursing supervisor.
b. Obtain vital signs, confirm the blood product with another nurse using the client's ID bracelet, and monitor vital signs as per institutional policy.
c. Hang the blood and monitor the client's vital signs every 15 minutes until the transfusion is absorbed.
d. Take the vital signs after hanging the blood and return in 15 minutes to monitor the vital signs.

Ans. (b) Obtain vital signs, confirm the blood product with another nurse using the client's ID bracelet, and monitor vital signs as per institutional policy.

Explanation: When administering a blood transfusion, it is important to ensure patient safety and monitor for any adverse reactions. The nursing actions in option (b) encompass the necessary steps for proper blood transfusion administration. Obtain baseline vital signs before administering blood products. Two registered nurses should verify patient and blood product data, and monitor vital signs throughout the procedure as per institutional policy.

12

During a simulation training session, a nursing supervisor is observing a junior nurse who is practicing the open suctioning of an Endotracheal Tube (ET) on an adult medium fidelity mannequin. Which step performed by the junior nurse requires correction from the nursing supervisor?

a. She has set the pressure of the suction apparatus at 110 mmHg before suctioning.
b. She has pre-oxygenated the patient prior to suctioning and in between suctioning procedure for 5 minutes
c. She has not applied negative pressure while inserting the suction catheter inside the endotracheal tube.
d. She maintained sterility as open suctioning is a sterile procedure.

Ans. (b) She has pre-oxygenated the patient prior to suctioning and in between suctioning procedure for 5 minutes

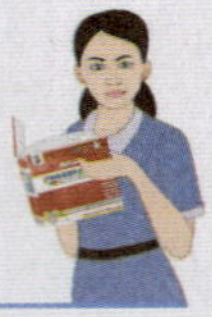

Explanation: The step that should be corrected by the nursing supervisor is option b. The nurse has pre-oxygenated the patient prior to suctioning and in between suctioning procedures for 5 minutes.

During open suctioning of an endotracheal tube, pre-oxygenation is typically performed prior to the procedure to ensure adequate oxygenation of the patient and prevent hypoxemia. However, pre-oxygenation is not required in between suctioning procedures.

13

Nurse Ramya is caring for a patient who is on mechanical ventilation. She has instruction to perform suctioning of an ET tube without disconnecting it from the mechanical ventilator. Which type of suction catheter should be used for ET tube suctioning in this case?

a. Closed suction catheter
b. Thumb pressure control suction catheter
c. Plain suction catheter
d. Fingertip pressure control suction catheter

Ans. (a) Closed suction catheter

Explanation: A closed suction catheter is a type of suction catheter that is used to suction an endotracheal tube without disconnecting the tube from the mechanical ventilator. The catheter has a Y-connector that allows the suction apparatus to be connected to the catheter without disconnecting the tube from the ventilator.

14

You are assigned to provide care to the intubated patient shifted from the emergency ward with a history of congestive heart failure. On initial assessment, you have observed that the doctor has ordered for an ETT cuff pressure monitoring in each shift. Which device you will use to check the cuff pressure and what reading will you document as normal cuff pressure reading?

a. Capnogram, 10–20 cm H_2O
b. Cuff manometer, 20–30 cm H_2O
c. CVP monitor, 20–30 mmHg
d. Sphygmomanometer, 20–30 mmHg

Ans. (b) Cuff manometer, 20–30 cm H_2O

Explanation: A cuff manometer is a device that is used to measure the pressure in the cuff of an endotracheal tube. The normal cuff pressure reading is 20–30 cm H_2O.

15

The nurse has inserted the thumb pressure control suction catheter into an ETT until she felt the resistance. After that she pulled back the suction catheter at 1–2 cm above the resistance in order to avoid which complications?

a. Bradycardia
b. Tachycardia
c. Infection
d. Hypotension

Ans. (a) Bradycardia

Explanation: When suctioning an endotracheal tube (ETT), it is important to avoid excessive suctioning that can stimulate the vagus nerve and lead to a vagal response, resulting in bradycardia (slow heart rate).

By pulling back the suction catheter at 1–2 cm above the resistance, the nurse ensures that the catheter is not suctioning too deeply into the ETT, which can stimulate the vagus nerve and potentially trigger a bradycardic response.

16

Ramya, a registered nurse, is selected as one of the members for code blue (cardiac arrest) team. In her shift duty, code blue has been announced and the victim is a 3-year-old child. Ramya is performing the chest compression, while another code blue team member is providing respiration by using bag-valve mask. What is the correct ratio of chest compressions to ventilations which Ramya and other team member will follow during resuscitation?

a. 1:5
b. 3:2
c. 15:2
d. 30:2

Ans. (c) 15 : 2

Explanation: The American Heart Association (AHA) recommends compression to ventilation ratio of 15:2 in case of two rescuers for children who are 1–8 years old.

17

You have found a 9-month-old baby lying on the bed and is unresponsive. What is the best preferred site of pulse you will select to assess for the need of resuscitation?

a. Temporal
b. Carotid
c. Femoral
d. Brachial

Ans. (d) Brachial

Explanation: If the infant or child is unresponsive and not breathing (gasps do not count as breathing), healthcare providers may take up to 10 seconds to attempt to feel for a pulse (brachial in an infant and carotid or femoral in a child). [AHA guidelines, 2010]

18

When you are eating at a restaurant, suddenly a lady shouted, "Help Please help, my baby (6-month-old) has ingested something". You reached at the incident point and noticed that the baby is choking. What will be the first action you will do to save the life of that victim?

a. 5 back slaps followed by 5 chest thrusts
b. 15 chest compression followed by 2 ventilation
c. Try to remove the obstructed object by using your finger
d. Performing abdominal thrust

Ans. (a) 5 back slaps followed by 5 chest thrusts

Explanation: For a choking infant under 1 year of age, the recommended initial action is a combination of back slaps and chest thrusts. This technique is known as the "5 and 5" method:

- 5 back slaps: The rescuer should deliver five firm back slaps between the baby's shoulder blades using the heel of their hand.
- 5 chest thrusts: After the back slaps, the rescuer should provide five chest thrusts. This is done by using two fingers in the middle of the infant's chest, just below the nipple line, and giving gentle inward and upward thrusts.

19

You are walking in a garden, suddenly you observed that a young man collapsed across the garden area. Arrange the following action in a sequence which is to be performed by a rescuer:

i. 30 chest compression
ii. Scene safety
iii. Check the carotid pulse and respiration
iv. 2 ventilation
v. Activate the emergency response system
vi. Check response of the victim

a. vi, ii, iii, v, i, iv
b. v, ii, vi, iii, iv, i
c. iii, vi, ii, v, i, iv
d. ii, vi, v, iii, i, iv

Ans. (d) ii, vi, v, iii, i, iv

20

You have received a victim with a history of fall from 3rd floor and on examination, the victim is unresponsive. Which method the nurse will use to assess the airway in this victim?

a. Jaw thrust maneuver
b. Head-tilt-chin lift maneuver
c. Heimlich maneuver
d. None of these

Ans. (a) Jaw thrust maneuver

Explanation: The jaw thrust maneuver is the appropriate method to assess the airway in a victim with suspected spinal injury. This maneuver is performed without tilting the head or neck and involves gently lifting the jaw forward while keeping the head in a neutral position. It helps to open the airway without potentially exacerbating any spinal injury.

21

Ramya, a nursing staff, has been shifted from the surgical ward to ICU. During the orientation period, Ramya is assisting other ICU nurses to get familiar with the nature of procedures being performed in ICU. While assisting in endotracheal tube suctioning, she asked the assigned nurse for the duration to perform the endotracheal tube suctioning at a time. Select the most appropriate response to be made by the assigned nurse.

a. 5 seconds
b. 10 seconds
c. 20 seconds
d. 30 seconds

Ans. (b) 10 seconds

Explanation: The American Association of Critical-Care Nurses (AACN) recommends that endotracheal tube suctioning be limited to 10 seconds at a time.

22

After the doctor has removed the patient's plaster cast and examined the extremity, the nurse will direct the housekeeping personnel to dispose of the plaster cast in which biomedical waste bin?

a. Yellow bin
b. Red bin
c. Black bin
d. Blue bin

Ans. (a) Yellow bin

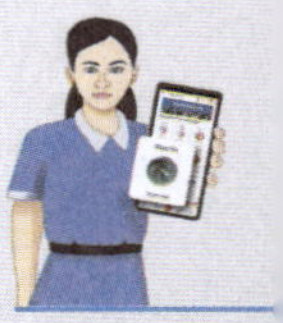

23

Kripa is assigned to provide care to a patient who is on ventilator Synchronized Intermittent Mandatory Ventilation (SIMV). She is well aware that her patient is at risk of developing which type of hospital-acquired infection?

a. Upper respiratory tract infection
b. Ventilator associated pneumonia
c. Ventilator-associated infection
d. Acute respiratory infection

Ans. (b) Ventilator-associated pneumonia

Explanation: Ventilator-associated pneumonia (VAP) is a type of hospital-acquired infection (HAI) that occurs in patients who are on mechanical ventilation. Ventilator-associated pneumonia is defined as pneumonia occurring more than 48 hours after patients have been intubated and received mechanical ventilation.

24

You are assigned to provide care to a patient admitted in the surgery ward for laparoscopic cholecystectomy. In order to prevent the risk of surgical site infection (SSI), the nurse will perform all the following actions; except:

a. Part preparation by using a surgical blade
b. Antiseptic bath before surgery
c. Maintains the vital parameter of the patient
d. Arrange appropriate antibiotic prophylaxis

Ans. (a) Part preparation by using a surgical blade

Explanation: The use of a surgical blade for part preparation is not a standard procedure to prevent surgical site infections (SSIs) in a laparoscopic cholecystectomy. The other options mentioned, such as antiseptic bath before surgery, maintaining vital parameters of the patient, and arranging appropriate antibiotic prophylaxis, are all important measures in preventing SSIs.

25

The nursing intern has provided bolus NG tube feeding with the help of 60 mL syringe to conscious bedridden patient. Which of the following action by the nurse is recommended to prevent regurgitation after NG tube feeding?

a. Place the patient in left lateral position for 1 hour after feeding
b. Place the patient in Fowler's position for 1–2 hours after feeding
c. Place the patient in Fowler's position for 30–60 minutes after feeding
d. Place the patient in supine position after NG tube feeding

Ans. (c) Place the patient in Fowler's position for 30–60 minutes after feeding

Explanation: Regurgitation is the backward flow of stomach contents into the esophagus. It can occur after NG tube feeding, especially in conscious bedridden patients. To prevent regurgitation, the nurse should place the patient in Fowler's position for 30–60 minutes after feeding. This will help to keep the stomach contents down in the stomach.

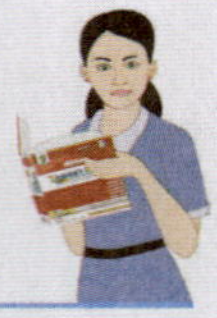

26

Nurse Ramya received a patient from outpatient department with the provisional diagnosis of stroke. Upon admission the nurse will assess the patient for the risk of fall. Identify the scale commonly used to assess the fall risk.

a. Modified Morse
b. Ramsay scale
c. Muscle power grading scale
d. Richmond Agitation sedation

Ans. (a) Modified Morse

Explanation: Modified Morse Scale is a scale commonly used to assess the risk of fall in older adults. It is a 10-item scale that assesses factors such as history of falls, balance, gait, and mobility. The scale is scored from 0 to 24, with a higher score indicating a higher risk of fall.

The other options are not correct.

- Ramsay scale is a scale used to assess the level of consciousness in critically ill patients.
- Muscle power grading scale is a scale used to assess the strength of muscle contractions.
- Richmond Agitation Sedation Scale is a scale used to assess the level of agitation and sedation in critically ill patients.

27

The nurse had received a patient from OPD who is infected with Methicillin resistant Staphylococcus aureus. The on-duty doctor orders to shift this patient into the isolated room where 2 other patients with the same infection are already present. Which type of isolation is maintained in this case?

a. Cohort isolation
b. Airborne isolation
c. Standard isolation
d. Droplet isolation

Ans. (a) Cohort isolation

Explanation: Cohort isolation is a type of isolation in which patients with the same infectious agent are grouped together in a single room. This type of isolation is used for patients who are infected with highly contagious organisms, such as Methicillin-resistant Staphylococcus aureus (MRSA).

28

A BSc nursing student posted in medicine ward is helping the morning shift nurses in their bedside work. The student is assisting the nurse who is preparing the medication of the patient with NG Tube. The student then asks the nurse about the most suitable form of medication that can be administered through NG tube. Select the best response made by the nurse.

a. Elixir
b. Enteric coated tablet
c. Sustained release tablet
d. Sublingual tablet

Ans. (a) Elixir

Explanation: Elixirs are liquid medications that are typically flavored and sweetened. They are the most suitable form of medication that can be administered through NG tube. Enteric coated tablet and sustained release tablet should not be crushed before administration, so they cannot be administered through NG tube. Sublingual tablets need to be placed under tongue, not to be administered through NG tube.

29

Nurse Ramya, assigned to a postoperative ward, encountered an incident where a 35-year-old surgical patient fell from the bed on the 3rd day after surgery, resulting in the accidental dislodgment of the nasogastric (NG) tube from the nose. Upon assessment, the patient exhibited signs of irritability and reported pain at the surgical incision site. The above-mentioned issue was to be documented as an unusual event. Which of the following report is considered by Ramya to record the above-mentioned issue?

a. Employee incident report
b. Offense incident report
c. Patient incident report
d. Shift incident report

Ans. (c) Patient incident report

Explanation: A patient incident report is a document that is used to record any unusual event that happens to a patient during their stay in a healthcare facility. This includes falls, injuries, medication errors, and other events that could potentially harm the patient.

30

You have received a patient in the emergency department with a history of overdose of aspirin. All of the following are the possible complications of aspirin poisoning; except:

a. Onset of pulmonary edema
b. Metabolic acidosis
c. Respiratory alkalosis
d. Metabolic alkalosis

Ans. (d) Metabolic alkalosis

Explanation: Aspirin overdose can lead to a number of complications, including respiratory alkalosis, metabolic acidosis, and pulmonary edema. Metabolic alkalosis is a condition in which the body has too much bicarbonate. This is not a complication of aspirin overdose.

Salicylate-induced pulmonary edema (SIPE) can occur in both acute and chronic users of aspirin or salicylate products. Salicylate poisoning causes respiratory alkalosis (due to hyperventilation) and, by an independent mechanism, metabolic acidosis.

31

During the dietary assessment of a patient who follows a vegan diet, the nurse should prepare to provide dietary education that emphasizes the consumption of food items rich in which vitamin, considering the absence of that vitamin in a vegan diet?

a. Vitamin A
b. Vitamin B_1
c. Vitamin B_{12}
d. Vitamin C

Ans. (c) Vitamin B_{12}

Explanation: Vitamin B_{12} is a nutrient that is found in animal products, such as meat, fish, and dairy products. Vegans do not consume these products, so they are at risk of being deficient in vitamin B_{12}.

32

If the patient develops tachycardia while doing suctioning, what is the priority nursing action?

a. Stop suction and oxygenate the patient
b. Continue suction
c. Inform the physician
d. Give left lateral position

Ans. (a) Stop suction and oxygenate the patient

Explanation: Suctioning can cause a number of adverse effects, including tachycardia. If a patient develops tachycardia while being suctioned, the priority nursing action is to stop suction and oxygenate the patient. This will help to reduce the patient's anxiety and improve their oxygen levels.

33

A patient with diarrhea has been diagnosed with clostridium difficile. Along with standard precautions, which kind of transmission-based precautions will be used when the nurse is caring for this patient?

a. Droplet precautions
b. Contact precautions
c. Isolation precautions
d. Airborne precautions

Ans. (b) Contact precautions

Explanation: Clostridium difficile (C. difficile) is a bacterium that can cause diarrhea. It is spread through contact with the stool of an infected person.

Contact precautions are used to prevent the spread of infection through contact with the patient's body fluids or contaminated surfaces. These precautions include:

- Wearing gloves and gown when caring for the patient.
- Washing hands thoroughly after contact with the patient or their environment.
- Declaring the patient's room as "contact isolation" and cleaning it thoroughly after the patient is discharged.

34

To provide free water and intracellular fluid hydration for a patient with acute gastroenteritis who is NPO, the nurse would expect administration of which infusion?

a. Dextrose 5% in water
b. Dextrose 10% in water
c. Lactated Ringer's solution
d. Dextrose 5% in normal saline (0.9%)

Ans. (a) Dextrose 5% in water

Explanation: Dextrose 5% in water is a type of IV fluid that is used to provide free water and intracellular fluid hydration. It is a clear, colorless solution that is isotonic to the blood.

- Dextrose 10% in water is too concentrated and can cause fluid shifts.
- Lactated Ringer's solution is a balanced electrolyte solution, but it does not provide as much free water as dextrose 5% in water.
- Dextrose 5% in normal saline (0.9%) is a hypertonic solution, which can cause fluid shifts.

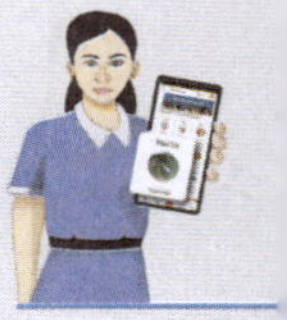

35

A patient, who is a heavy caffeine user has been NPO all day. He is scheduled for surgery in the evening. The nurse monitors the patient for effects of caffeine withdrawal that may include all, except:

a. Headache
b. Drowsiness
c. Irritability
d. Shortness of breath

Ans. (d) Shortness of breath

Explanation: The severity of symptoms of caffeine withdrawal varies from individual to individual, and the most common symptoms include headache, fatigue, decreased energy/activeness, decreased alertness, drowsiness, decreased contentedness, depressed mood, difficulty concentrating, irritability, and feeling foggy/not clearheaded. Shortness of breath is not a symptom of caffeine withdrawal.

36

A mother brings her child in emergency department and complains that her child has accidently ingested something while she was busy in cooking. What clinical manifestation would be most suggestive that the poison was a corrosive product?

a. Tinnitus
b. Disorientation and unresponsiveness.
c. Stupor, lethargy and coma
d. Edema of the lips and tongue

Ans. (d) Edema of the lips and tongue

Explanation: Corrosive products can cause damage to the mouth, throat, and stomach. This can lead to edema of the lips and tongue, as well as pain and difficulty swallowing.

37

The first aid nurse is handling a patient with an open wound on the right wrist which is bleeding profusely. As an immediate measure, the nurse has applied the direct pressure over the wound by using the sterile dressing but the bleeding still continues. Identify the next measure which the nurse will perform to control the bleeding.

a. Application of tourniquet
b. Apply indirect pressure over the pressure points
c. Elevation of the affected limb above the heart level
d. All of the above

Ans. (c) Elevation of the affected limb above the heart level

Explanation: Raising the affected limb above the heart level will reduce the bleeding due to gravity. This is because the blood will flow back to the heart more easily, which will help to reduce the pressure in the bleeding area.

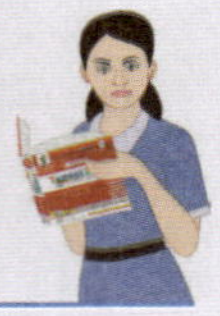

38

Ramya is a trainee nurse who works in a central sterile supply department. She developed an acute respiratory illness and is not responding to conventional therapies. Her physician suspects her illness to be linked to a workplace exposure. What is the best place from where the nurse can obtain information regarding her potential workplace exposure?

a. Health record of department
b. Material safety data sheets
c. Medical record department
d. Hospital information system

Ans. (b) Material safety data sheets

Explanation: MSDS are documents that provide information about the hazards of chemicals and other substances. They include information about the physical and chemical properties of the substance, its potential health hazards, and first aid procedures. In the case of the trainee nurse, her treating doctor suspects that her illness may be linked to a workplace exposure to a hazardous substance. The best place for the nurse to obtain information about her potential workplace exposure is from the MSDS for the substances that she works with.

39

During a routine round, a nurse enters a patient's room and observes the patient attempting to read their ultrasonography report. The patient asks the nurse to provide the report's result, to which the nurse responds, "According to this report, you have grade 2 liver enlargement and multiple calculi in the gallbladder." Which ethical principle the nurse adheres to in this scenario?

a. Principle of fidelity
b. Principle of veracity
c. Principle of nonmaleficence
d. Principle of autonomy

Ans. (b) Principle of veracity

Explanation: Veracity is the ethical principle of telling the truth. In this scenario, the nurse is telling the patient the truth about the results of his ultrasound report. This is important because the patient has a right to know about his medical information.

The other options are not as accurate. The principle of fidelity (option a) is the ethical principle of keeping promises. The principle of nonmaleficence (option c) is the ethical principle of doing no harm. The principle of autonomy (option d) is the ethical principle of respecting patient autonomy.

40

A nurse is checking the clinical progress sheet of his patient in order to identify any new treatment to be added by the attending doctor after his morning clinical rounds. The nurse noticed that the doctor has mentioned the patient's pulse as 3+ grade. Select the most appropriate statement which best describes this patient pulse.

a. Absent pulse
b. weak, barely palpable, easily obliterate
c. Strong and bounding pulse
d. Normal pulse

Ans. (d) Normal pulse

Explanation: The pulse is graded on a scale of 0 to 4+:

- 0 indicating no palpable pulse;
- 1 + indicating a faint, but detectable pulse;
- 2 + suggesting a slightly more diminished pulse than normal;
- 3 + is a normal pulse; and
- 4 + indicating a bounding pulse.

41

A nurse has received a 75-year-old female patient into the surgical ward with the diagnosis of osteoarthritis. On admission, the nurse has given a room orientation to the patient and placed her on bed with side rails up. This action of the nurse is justifying which level of Maslow Hierarchy for the patient?

a. Esteem need
b. Physiological need
c. Safety and security need
d. Self-actualization need

Ans. (c) Safety and security need

Explanation: The first level Maslow's hierarchy is physiological needs, which are the basic needs for survival, such as food, water, and shelter. The second level is safety and security needs, which are the needs for protection from harm and danger.

In this scenario, the nurse is placing the patient on bed with side rails up to protect the patient from falling out of bed. This is an example of meeting the patient's safety and security needs.

42

A nurse is assigned to care for two patients with the tracheostomy tube. As per the doctor's order, the nurse is supposed to provide tracheostomy tube dressing in her shift duty for both the patients. While preparing for the procedure, she noticed that there is only one sterile dressing set available and she was having the fear that if she hasn't done the dressing, the doctor will scold her. She used the same dressing set for both the patients due to which the second patient develops serious infection later on. Which option best describes this scenario?

a. Negligence
b. Assault
c. Fraud
d. Battery

Ans. (a) Negligence

Explanation: Negligence is a failure to act in a reasonable and prudent manner, resulting in harm to another person. In this scenario, the nurse failed to use a sterile dressing set for both patients, which resulted in the second patient developing a serious infection.

43

While working in the morning shift with another nursing staff member on the surgical floor, you overhear the nurse making negative comments about the attending doctor of your patient. The nurse claims that the doctor never participates in clinical rounds, is always occupied with private patients, and makes other false statements. Which option accurately depicts this situation?

a. Libel
b. Slander
c. Defamation
d. False imprisonment

Ans. (b) Slander

Explanation: Slander is the spoken form of defamation, while libel is the written form. In this scenario, the nurse is making false statements about the doctor, which could damage his reputation. This is an example of slander.

Tips to Remember: Libel = Literature (written material)

44

You are assigned to provide care to a patient posted for arthroplasty surgery. You have to make sure that the patient must sign the informed consent before being shifted to preoperative area. Which of the following are the nursing responsibilities in context to an informed consent?

a. Assessing the patient's level of knowledge whether the patient's knowledge level is sufficient to give consent.
b. Describe the nature of surgery, associated risk factor and expected complications, and get the consent form signed by the patient.
c. Witness the client's signature on the consent form.
d. a and c

Ans. (d) a and c

Explanation: The surgeon is responsible for obtaining the informed consent. Assessing the patient's knowledge and educating about the procedure, and being witness for consent form are the responsibilities of a nurse. So, options a and c are correct.

45

You are taking care of a patient who is on mechanical ventilator and the patient is very agitated, trying to remove all the line and tubes. The doctor orders for the application of restraint and has taken the informed consent from the patient's family member. The nurse should know that the order for restraints is valid up to:

a. 24 hours
b. 48 hours
c. 72 hours
d. Till the patient gets discharged

Ans. (a) 24 hours

Explanation: In India, the order for restraints is valid up to one calendar day, i.e., maximum of 24 hours. If restraint is initiated by registered nurse in emergency situation, the concerned physician needs to be informed within 12 hours.

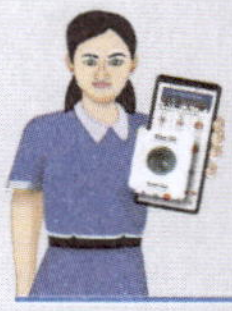

46

A nursing intern assisting the mentor nurse is identifying the patient need. The mentor nurse, after collecting the detailed history, is making the nursing care plan for her patient. The nursing intern asked the assigned nurse about the purpose of formulating the nursing diagnosis.

a. Recognize the patient's response toward an illness
b. Center on disease and pathology
c. Offer the nurse's subjective view of the patient
d. All of the above

Ans. (a) Recognize the patient's response toward an illness

Explanation: A nursing diagnosis is a clinical judgment concerning a human response to health conditions/life processes, by an individual, family, group, or community. A nursing diagnosis provides the basis for selecting nursing interventions to achieve outcomes for which the nurse has accountability.

47

A nurse is formulating a nursing care plan for a newly admitted patient with left below knee amputation. While formulating the nursing care plan, the nurse found two nursing diagnoses closely similar to each other. How will the nurse recognize which diagnosis will most accurately reflect the patient's needs?

a. Reassess the patient condition
b. Both nursing diagnoses can be utilized
c. Review the defining characteristics
d. All of the above

Ans. (c) Review the defining characteristics

Explanation: The nurse should review the defining characteristics associated with each nursing diagnosis to determine which one accurately reflects the patient's needs. By carefully examining the defining characteristics, the nurse can differentiate between the two closely similar nursing diagnoses and choose the one that aligns best with the patient's specific condition and presenting symptoms.

48

Nurse Ramya is checking the progress of doctor sheet for any new treatment after the doctor's clinical round. She noticed that the attending doctor has mentioned 'up ad lib' order for the patient. The nurse understands that this means:

a. The patient can engage in activities as directed.
b. The patient can engage in activities as desired.
c. Activity of daily living.
d. Activity intolerance.

Ans. (b) The patient can engage in activities as desired

Explanation: When the attending doctor mentions an "up ad lib" order for the patient, it means that the patient may be up and about as desired. Hence, the patient can engage in activities or actions as desired, if the patient so desires.

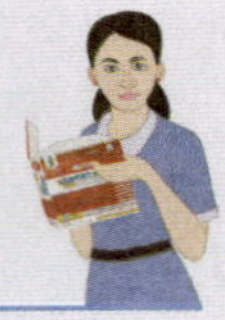

49

You are assigned to provide care to a patient admitted with malaria. On assessment, the patient face is pale, pulse is feeble and rapid, and the temperature is 40°C. You have informed the attending doctor that the patient is experiencing rigor. Identify the stage of rigor on the basis of findings.

a. Hot stage
b. Cold stage
c. Fever stage
d. Stage of sweating

Ans. (b) Cold stage

Explanation: In malaria, the disease is characterized by cyclic episodes of fever and chills, which are collectively known as rigor. The different stages of rigor include the hot stage, cold stage, and stage of sweating.

In the given scenario, the patient's symptoms of pale face, feeble and rapid pulse, and a high temperature of 40°C indicate that the patient is experiencing the cold stage of rigor. During this stage, the patient typically experiences intense shivering, feeling cold, and a rapid rise in body temperature.

50

On 25th June, you have received a patient in day care for the administration of Injection penicillin. After 10 days again the patient came for the administration of injection penicillin. But now the patient has developed an anaphylactic reaction after receiving intravenous penicillin. Which among the following statement conclude the cause of this reaction?

a. An acquired atopic sensitization occurred.
b. Antibodies to penicillin developed after previous exposure.
c. It is a passive immune response of the body.
d. Potent antibodies were produced when the infusion was administered second time.

Ans. (b) Antibodies to penicillin developed after previous exposure.

Explanation: Anaphylaxis is a severe allergic reaction that can be life-threatening. In the case of the patient who received penicillin twice, he developed an anaphylactic reaction after the second exposure. This suggests that he developed antibodies to penicillin after the first exposure. These antibodies caused him to have a more severe reaction to the second exposure.

51

You are assigned to provide care to the patient admitted into the medical floor. You have monitored the vital signs of the patient as temperature = 98.7°F, Pulse = 72 beats/min, Respiration = 20 breaths/min, BP = 135/85 mmHg. While documenting the vital sign report, a Junior Resident asked you what is the pulse pressure of this patient? Select the most appropriate response of nurse.

a. 100
b. 1.6
c. 214
d. 50

Ans. (d) 50

Explanation: The pulse pressure can be calculated as:
- Pulse Pressure = SBP - DBP
- Pulse Pressure = 135 mmHg - 85 mmHg
- Pulse Pressure = 50 mmHg

52

You are assigned to provide care to the patient admitted with the complaint of fever and diarrhea. During your morning shift, the temperature of the patient was 99.8°F orally. While the evening shift nurse recorded the temperature 103°F orally. The nurse will classify this fever as:

a. Constant fever
b. Intermittent
c. Relapsing
d. Remittent

Ans. (d) Remittent

Explanation: Remittent fever refers to a fever pattern in which the body temperature fluctuates throughout the day, but it never returns to normal (baseline). In this scenario, the patient's morning temperature was 99.8°F, and the evening temperature increased to 103°F. The fact that the temperature remains elevated and does not return to normal indicates a remittent fever.

53

Ramya, a registered nurse, is assigned to provide care to a patient with the diagnosis of right lower lobe pneumonia in the medicine ward. While monitoring the vital signs, the nurse auscultates the right lower lobe. What findings of breath sounds the nurse would expect to note?

a. Breath sound will be absent
b. Vesicular
c. Bronchial
d. Broncho-vesicular

Ans. (c) Bronchial

Explanation: Pneumonia involves inflammation and infection in the lung tissue, leading to consolidation and decreased air movement in the affected area. As a result, the breath sounds may change from the normal vesicular breath sounds to bronchial breath sounds. Bronchial breath sounds are characterized by a louder, harsher quality with a higher pitch compared to vesicular breath sounds.

54

Due to shortage of the nursing staff, the supervisor has adapted functional nursing approach and you are assigned to measure the vital signs of all the patients admitted in the unit. While documenting the blood pressure, which among the following patients BP reflect orthostatic hypotension?

a. 118/68 mmHg when standing and 110/60 mmHg when lying down.
b. 140/80 mmHg, Heart rate 82 beats/min when sitting and 130/75 mmHg, Heart rate 98 beats/min when standing.
c. 146/88 mmHg when lying down and 125/78 mmHg when standing, and reports feeling dizzy.
d. 126/72 mmHg lying down and 133/80 mmHg when sitting, and reports shortness of breath.

Ans. (c) 146/88 mmHg when lying down and 125/78 mmHg when standing, and reports feeling dizzy.

Explanation: A decline of ≥20 mm Hg in systolic or ≥10 mm Hg in diastolic blood pressure after 3 minutes of standing = orthostatic hypotension.

55

You have measured the body temperature of your assigned patient and found that the patient is febrile. You have instructed the patient that you may lose body heat through perspiration. The patient then asks the nurse about the mechanism of heat loss followed in this condition.

a. Conduction
b. Convection
c. Evaporation
d. Radiation

Ans. (c) Evaporation

Explanation: Evaporation occurs when sweat is produced by the sweat glands and comes into contact with the skin's surface. As the sweat evaporates, it absorbs heat from the body, leading to cooling. This process helps regulate body temperature by dissipating excess heat.

56

A nursing intern is measuring the cardinal sign of a patient and while recording, she asked the assigned nurse about the factors that may affect a patient's blood pressure. Which statement accurately described by the assigned nurse best supports the nursing intern question?

a. Blood pressure is usually lowest while getting up in the morning.
b. Blood pressure decreases with age.
c. Blood pressure increases after eating food.
d. Blood pressure decreases with increased cardiac output, peripheral vascular resistance.

Ans. (a) Blood pressure is usually lowest while getting up in the morning.

Explanation: Blood pressure can show diurnal variation, meaning it can fluctuate throughout the day. In many individuals, blood pressure tends to be lower in the morning upon arising and gradually increases throughout the day.

57

A nurse is assigned to provide care to a 7-year-old child during her shift duty. As per the doctor's order she has to assess the patient vital signs after every 2 hourly. To assess the fifth vital sign, the nurse has used a series of faces ranging from a happy face at 0, or "no hurt", to a crying face at 10, which represents "hurts like the worst pain imaginable". Identify the name of the scale being used by the nurse to assess the fifth vital sign.

a. Wong Baker Pain scale
b. FLACC pain scale
c. VAS
d. All of the above

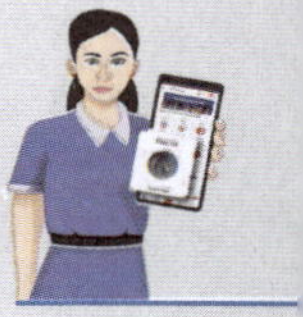

Ans. (a) **Wong Baker Pain scale**

Explanation: The Wong Baker Pain scale is a commonly used pain assessment tool for children. It consists of a series of faces depicting various levels of pain intensity, ranging from a happy face at 0 (indicating no hurt/pain) to a crying face at 10 (representing hurts worst). The child is asked to choose the face that best represents their current level of pain.

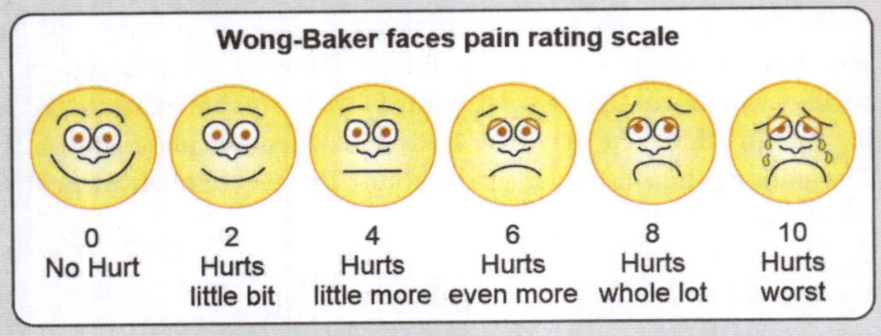

58

You are taking care of an adult patient who is on synchronized intermittent mandatory ventilation (SIMV) mode. To keep the airway patent, doctor recommended for the open suctioning procedure which is to be performed every 4-hourly. Before doing the procedure, you have checked the patient unit and the suction apparatus for proper functioning. What pressure you will set on the wall mounted suction apparatus for performing suction on this patient?

a. 50–100 mmHg
b. 100–150 mmHg
c. 150–200 mmHg
d. 250–300 mmHg

Ans. (b) **100–150 mmHg**

Explanation: The wall mounted suction apparatus is used to remove secretions from the airway. The suction pressure should be set at a level that is sufficient to remove the secretions without causing harm to the patient. In the case of an adult patient who is on SIMV mode, the suction pressure should be set at 100–150 mmHg.

59

You are providing care to an unresponsive patient whose weight is 110 kg. As per the doctors order, you need to reposition the patient every hourly in order to prevent the risk of pressure ulcer. Which of the following intervention to be applied first by the nurse while moving the patient?

a. While turning the patient, keep the patient's body as close as possible
b. Inform the team leader for assistance
c. Keep the elbow close and knees apart
d. Administer analgesics to reduce the pain level due to repositioning

Ans. (b) **Inform the team leader for assistance**

Explanation: When repositioning a patient, it is important to have assistance from another nurse or healthcare provider. This is especially important for patients who are unresponsive or who have a high body weight. Having assistance will help to prevent the nurse from straining their back or other muscles.

60

You are assigned to provide care to a patient admitted in nephrology ward. The doctor has prescribed a 24-hour-urine sample for creatinine clearance test. Select the most appropriate statement related to 24-hour-urine collection.

a. Instruct the client, the first void should be discarded
b. Keep the urine specimen on ice or refrigerated
c. A 24-hour urine collection container has a preservative that should not be refrigerated
d. All of the above

Ans. (d) **All of the above**

61

Team leader has assigned one patient Mr. Ramesh who is on airborne precaution to nurse Ruby in her evening shift. As an assigned nurse to this patient, which action done by the nurse indicates her poor understanding related to airborne precaution?

a. Use of N95 mask while providing care to patient
b. Use surgical mask in order to protect herself from the infection
c. Strict hand hygiene maintained by nurse
d. Patient should be placed in a negative pressure room

Ans. (b) **Use surgical mask in order to protect herself from the infection**

Explanation: When caring for a patient on airborne precautions, it is essential for the nurse to have a clear understanding of the appropriate personal protective equipment (PPE) required. The use of a surgical mask, in this case, is not sufficient to protect the nurse from airborne infections.

62

The patient is admitted as a case of Hemophilus influenza type b. The nurse in-charge understands that in addition to standard precautions, the nurse would initiate which type of transmission-based precaution for this patient?

a. Isolation precaution
b. Airborne precaution
c. Droplet precaution
d. Contact precaution

Ans. (c) Droplet precaution

Explanation: Haemophilus influenzae type b (Hib) is primarily transmitted through respiratory droplets. Therefore, to prevent the spread of infection, the nurse would implement droplet precautions when caring for a patient with this condition.

63

The doctor has planned the dietician referral for the assigned patient who is on NG tube feeding. The assigned nurse has informed the dietician and booked the 3:00 pm slot. The dietician came and changed the current nutritional requirement of the patient. After the dietician referral the nurse read the orders given by the dietician to increase the rate of the patient's NG feeding. Which of the following orders should the nurse question?

a. Advance tube feeding rate by 100 mL/hour every 8 to 12 hours to target rate of 250 mL/hour over 12 hours.
b. Increase by 50 mL per feeding per day until total volume is achieved to meet patient's caloric needs according to dietician's referral.
c. Strictly monitor the intake and output of the patient
d. None of the above

Ans. (a) Advance tube feeding rate by 100 mL/hour every 8 to 12 hours to target rate of 250 mL/hour over 12 hours.

Explanation: Increasing the tube feeding rate by 100 mL/hour every 8 to 12 hours to reach a target rate of 250 mL/hour over 12 hours is a significant rate of advancement. Such a rapid increase in the feeding rate may not be appropriate or safe for all patients, especially those who are at risk for complications such as refeeding syndrome or intolerance to rapid feeding increases.

64

The nurse is inserting an indwelling urinary catheter into a male patient admitted in medicine ward with the complaint of urinary incontinence. The nurse has inserted the tip of the catheter into the urethra, immediately the urine begins to flow into the tubing. At what point the nurse should inflate the balloon?

a. Soon after urine begins to flow into the catheter inflate the balloon
b. Advance the urinary catheter till the bifurcation point and then inflate the balloon
c. Insert the catheter 2.5 to 3 cm then inflate the balloon
d. Before inserting the catheter inflate the balloon

Ans. (b) Advance the urinary catheter till the bifurcation point and then inflate the balloon

Explanation: In a male patient, you should always insert an indwelling catheter up to the catheter's Y bifurcation before you inflate the balloon. This ensures that the balloon isn't inflated while in the prostatic urethra, which would cause pain and bleeding.

65

Babita, a registered nurse is working in the Surgery ward. During her morning shift she is assigned to provide care to a female patient who is posted for laparoscopic cholecystectomy. Before shifting the patient to the pre-operative area, the nurse has to insert the urinary catheter. Nurse Babita will use which size of urinary catheter for catheterization procedure?

a. 8 to 10 French
b. 12 to 16 French
c. 14 to 16 French
d. 18 to 20 French

Ans. (b) 12 to 16 French

Explanation: The size of the urinary catheter that is used for catheterization will depend on the patient's anatomy and the type of surgery that they are having. For a female patient who is having laparoscopic cholecystectomy, a 12 to 16 French catheter is typically used.

A French catheter is a unit of measurement that is used to measure the diameter of a catheter. A 12 French catheter is about 3.3 mm in diameter, and a 16 French catheter is about 4.7 mm in diameter. In this case, the nurse should use a 12 to 16 French catheter because it is a good compromise between ease of insertion and drainage capacity.

66

Nurse Deepti is working in a medical surgical department where the team lead has assigned four patients to her. While performing the risk assessment for the development of pressure ulcer among the following which patient is on highest risk for pressure ulcer?

a. Patient with the diagnosis of quadriplegia
b. Patient admitted as a case of typhoid fever
c. Patient who has hypertension with controlled diabetes and ambulating independently
d. All are at high risk for pressure ulcer

Ans. (a) Patient with the diagnosis of quadriplegia

Explanation: Patients with quadriplegia are often immobile or have limited mobility, which puts them at a significantly higher risk for pressure ulcers. The lack of movement and pressure relief can lead to prolonged pressure on certain areas of the body, increasing the likelihood of tissue damage and the development of pressure ulcers.

For other patients, the immobility factor is less likely.

67

Aditya, an evening ICU nursing officer, is taking handover of his assigned patient with central venous line. He asked the morning staff about when the transparent dressing over the CVP line needs to be changed. Select the appropriate answer given by the morning staff.

a. Every 7 days or when it gets soiled
b. Every 10 days
c. Every day
d. Every 12 days

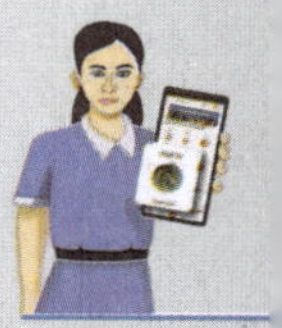

Ans. (a) Every 7 days or when it gets soiled

Explanation: Transparent dressings over CVP lines are typically changed every 7 days as a routine practice. However, if the dressing becomes soiled, wet, or compromised in any way, it should be changed immediately to maintain a clean and sterile environment around the CVP line.

68

You are assigned to provide care to a patient admitted for status epilepticus. After the doctor's round you have checked the medication administration record sheet for any new order. The attending doctor has mentioned injection Dilantin 0.3 g PO. Dilantin is available as 120 mg/2 mL in your stock. How much volume should the nurse administer to the patient?

a. 2 mL
b. 5 mL
c. 10 mL
d. 15 mL

Ans. (b) 5 mL

Explanation: The ordered dose of Dilantin is 0.3 g, which is equal to 300 mg.

- The available stock concentration is 120 mg/2 mL, which means there are 120 mg of Dilantin in 2 mL of solution.
- To find the dose per 1 mL, we divide 120 mg by 2 mL, resulting in 60 mg per 1 mL.
- Now, we can calculate the volume needed to administer 300 mg of Dilantin:
- 300 mg / 60 mg/mL = 5 mL
- Therefore, the nurse should administer 5 mL of Dilantin solution to provide a dose of 300 mg

69

At the end of your evening shift, one of the patients become hypoglycemic with the blood glucose level of 45 mg/dL. You have informed the nursing supervisor and looking for the doctor to inform him. But unfortunately, the doctor wasn't available at that time. You made a call to the doctor and informed him about the patient's condition and received the telephonic orders. Which of the following statement is related to the "joint commission read-back requirement" policies?

a. Repeat and confirm
b. Write, read back and confirm
c. Listen, repeat and confirm
d. Document and proceed with the orders

Ans. (b) Write, read back and confirm

Explanation: The Joint Commission's read-back requirement is a policy that requires healthcare providers to repeat and confirm verbal or telephone orders. This policy is designed to prevent errors in medication administration.

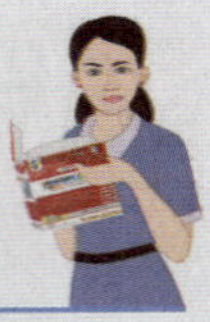

70

A registered nurse is measuring the blood pressure of 58-year-old patient admitted in orthopedic ward with the diagnosis of osteoarthritis. The nurse knows that BP is often higher in older adults. Which among the following options best support the nurse statement?

a. Decreased elasticity of arterial wall
b. Decrease in peripheral resistance
c. Decrease of muscle mass
d. All of the above

Ans. (a) Decreased elasticity of arterial wall

Explanation: As individuals age, the elasticity of the arterial walls tends to decrease. This loss of elasticity can lead to stiffening of the arteries and increased peripheral resistance to blood flow, resulting in higher blood pressure.

71

Nurse Sheela is caring a patient who has difficulty in falling asleep. She is aware that the following interventions help the patient to fall asleep; except:

a. Provide a warm glass of milk before the bedtime
b. Turn on quiet music in patient's room
c. Provide back massage to the client
d. Encourage short nap after lunch.

Ans. (d) Encourage short nap after lunch.

Explanation: It is normal to feel a little sleepy after eating lunch. However, sleeping after lunch may lead to difficulty in falling asleep in the night. Warm glass of milk before the bedtime, listening to quiet music of patient's choice and back massage promotes sleep.

72

Nurse is caring for client with a communicable disease. While providing isolation to the client, which among the following characteristic is most important for the nurse to know?

a. Causative agent and mode of transmission
b. Causative agent and treatment options
c. Immune power of the host
d. Diagnostic methods available

Ans. (a) Causative agent and mode of transmission

Explanation: Knowledge regarding causative agent and its mode of transmission is most important in deciding isolation method/technique for the infected client. The use of type of PPE (gown/glove/mask) depends on the mode of transmission. For example, wearing mask is necessary if the mode of transmission is droplet. Gown and glove are essential if the mode of transmission is direct contact. Immune power of the host and diagnostic methods are not relevant here as the patient is already infected and is diagnosed. Treatment options do not influence the decision of isolation method.

73

Nurse Shalini is educating her client regarding the collection of sputum for culture and sensitivity. Which among the following statement by the client indicates that teaching was effective?

a. Collect sputum in a wide-opened mouth sterile container
b. Collect sputum in the morning after rinsing with mouthwash
c. Collect sputum in a plastic container and cover it with plastic wrap to prevent contamination
d. Collect sputum at bed time after taking prescribed medications

Ans. (a) Collect sputum in a wide-opened mouth sterile container

Explanation: The best quality sample is usually obtained early in the morning upon rising. Mouth should be rinsed out with water or saline prior to collection (not with mouthwash). Food should not be ingested for 1–2 hours prior to collection. It is very important that the sputum is the material coughed up from the lungs, and not saliva "spit". For culture and sensitivity, the sputum must be collected in a sterile container. Collection of sputum at bedtime after taking medications is not recommended.

74

A client with IV line in situ for the last 72 hours is complaining of swelling and pallor at the site. These signs indicate:

a. Phlebitis
b. Infection
c. Infiltration
d. Dislodgement

Ans. (c) Infiltration

Explanation: Infiltration is a complication in IV line. When IV fluids or medications leak into the surrounding tissue, it is known as infiltration. It is caused by improper placement or dislodgment of the catheter. Manifestations include redness around the site, swelling, puffy or hard skin around the site, blanching (lighter skin around the IV site), pain or tenderness around the site, IV not working, cool skin temperature around the IV site or of the scalp, hand, arm, leg or foot near the site.

75

Nurse is preparing inj. Insulin for her client. Which among the following statement is correct?

a. Two types of insulin should not be mixed
b. Draw up regular insulin, then NPH insulin
c. Draw up long-acting insulin then short acting insulin
d. Use two separate syringe to administer different types of insulin

Ans. (b) Draw up regular insulin, then NPH insulin

Explanation: When you mix regular insulin with another type of insulin, always draw the regular insulin into the syringe first. NPH (neutral protamine hagedorn) is an intermediate-acting insulin. The rapid- or short-acting insulin (clear) is drawn up first to prevent the intermediate-acting insulin (cloudy) from getting into the rapid- or short-acting insulin bottle and affecting the onset, peak, and duration.

76

While collecting history from a client admitted in the emergency department, which among the following reported by the client is considered subjective data?

a. Weakness
b. Icterus
c. Hemoptysis
d. Melena

Ans. (a) Weakness

Explanation: Subjective data are the symptoms which are felt by the patient and others can't be seen such as weakness, tiredness, etc. All other options are objective data or sign which others can also observe. It includes icterus, melena, hemoptysis, etc

77

Which among the following statement is wrong regarding transferring a patient from bed to chair?

a. Place the patient flat on the bed
b. Help the patient to sit on the edge of the bed with legs dangling
c. Nurses need to stand by facing the patient
d. Place the chair by facing the head of the bed

Ans. (a) Place the patient flat on the bed

Explanation: Except option a, all others are the steps involved in transferring patient from bed to chair or wheelchair.

78

An asthmatic patient is getting discharged from the respiratory unit. Nurse has given health education to the client regarding asthma and its management. After teaching the client, nurse asks the client to repeat the instructions. Which of the following professional role is performed by the nurse?

a. Advocate
b. Educator
c. Adviser
d. Manager

Ans. (b) Educator

Explanation: While educating a client about his or her own disease and its management, nurse performs the role of an educator.

79

Which among the following is the responsibility of a scrub nurse in the operation theater?

a. Verify the informed consent
b. Assist the surgeon in gowning and gloving
c. Receiving the patient
d. Maintain the count of instruments used

Ans. (d) Maintain the count of instruments used

Explanation: In the operating room, maintaining the count of instruments is the responsibility of scrub nurse. All the other given options are the responsibilities of a circulatory nurse.

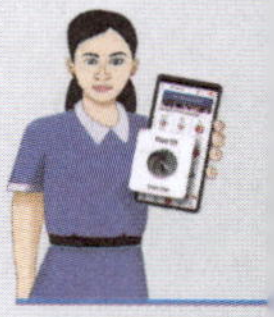

80

Nurse Ramya is advised to provide continuous enteral feed to his client. Which among the following action by nurse indicates lack of knowledge in this area?

a. Providing fowlers position to the client
b. Administering feeds at room temperature
c. Maintain prescribed flow rate
d. Hang the enteral feed for one day

Ans. (d) Hang the enteral feed for one day

Explanation: Continuous enteral nutrition: gravity administered or by feeding pump continuously for 12 hrs/day or more. Except option d, all other options are correct related to continuous enteral feed.

81

Nurse Jisha is caring for a client in postoperative unit with Jackson-Pratt wound drain in situ. Which of the following action performed by nurse Jisha is correct regarding the care of drain site?

a. Clean the drain site from inner to outer in circular motion
b. Clean the drain site from outer to inner with a linear stroke
c. Remove the drain and clean the site
d. Wear all PPE while providing drain site care

Ans. (a) Clean the drain site from inner to outer in circular motion

Explanation: Drain site is considered clean and the site has to be cleaned from inner to outer (more clean to less clean area) using circular strokes. Cleaning from outer to inner and the removal of drain and cleaning the site are also not recommended. While cleaning the drain site, one needs to wear sterile gloves rather than PPE.

82

Which among the following nursing diagnosis is most important while caring for a female client with deep vein thrombosis?

a. Risk for injury related to increased venous blood flow
b. Altered tissue perfusion related to venous congestion
c. Fluid volume overload related to edema
d. Risk for infection related to altered skin integrity

Ans. (b) Altered tissue perfusion related to venous congestion

Explanation: Deep vein thrombosis leads to decreased tissue perfusion. So most appropriate nursing diagnosis is altered tissue perfusion related to venous congestion.

83

Nurse John is reviewing his nursing care plan for the assigned client and decided to revise the nursing care plan for his client. In which step of the nursing process revision takes place?

a. Assessment b. Planning
c. Implementation d. Evaluation

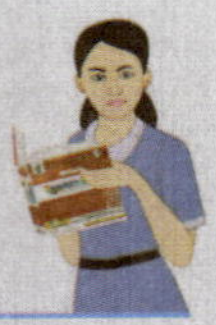

Ans. (d) Evaluation

Explanation: During the evaluation step of the nursing process the nurse determines whether the goals established have been achieved and evaluates the success of the plan. Assessment involves data collection. Planning involves setting priorities, and implementation is the actual intervention.

84

Nurse Alice working in recovery room received a client following cholecystectomy surgery. Which among the following nursing diagnosis takes highest priority in the immediate postoperative period?

a. Impaired skin integrity related to surgical incision
b. Fluid volume deficit related to blood loss during surgery
c. Risk for aspiration related to general anesthesia
d. Acute pain related to surgery

Ans. (c) Risk for aspiration related to general anesthesia

Explanation: In the recovery room nurse is receiving client immediately after surgery. In the immediate post-operative period, airway is the most important priority. So, option c is the correct answer.

85

A client is on frusemide therapy. Which among the following food items if selected by the client indicate his/her knowledge regarding frusemide therapy?

a. Banana and orange
b. Egg and dairy products
c. Sea food items
d. Cereals

Ans. (a) Banana and orange

Explanation: Frusemide is a loop acting diuretic which eliminates water and potassium via urine. By giving food items such as banana and orange, it helps to replenish the potassium storage in the body.

86

Nurse is performing physical examination of musculoskeletal system and noticed lack of voluntary coordination of muscle movements. She records this finding as:

a. Ataxia
b. Aphasia
c. Tic
d. Anisocoria

Ans. (a) Ataxia

Explanation: Given description is related to ataxia. Aphasia is a language disorder that affects a person's ability to communicate. Tic is a **sudden, repetitive, nonrhythmic motor movement or vocalization involving discrete muscle groups**. Anisocoria is the unequal pupil size.

87

Nurse Linda is collecting history and preparing care plan for her client. In which step of nursing process the nurse identifies the problem with the client?

a. Assessment
b. Diagnosis
c. Planning
d. Implementation

Ans. (b) Diagnosis

Explanation: The nursing assessment includes gathering information concerning the patient's individual physiological, psychological, sociological, and spiritual needs. Diagnosis is formulating a nursing diagnosis by using clinical judgment; what is wrong with the patient. Planning involves developing a care plan which incorporates goals, potential outcomes, interventions. Implementation is performing the task or intervention. Evaluation is to check whether intervention is successful or unsuccessful.

88

A client is brought to the emergency department with the complaint of chest pain. Health care team immediately orders for ECG and trop-t. What kind of assessment is this?

a. Emergency assessment
b. Focused assessment
c. Concurrent assessment
d. Terminal assessment

Ans. (b) Focused assessment

Explanation: Emergency assessment is done during emergency procedures. For example, ABC assessment in emergency. Focused assessment is looking closely at a particular problem or disorder. Here by ordering ECG and Trop t, nurse focuses her assessment on chest pain. Concurrent assessment means evaluation going on side by side. Terminal assessment means at the end of a program assessment is done. Concurrent and terminal assessment are the part of nursing education and evaluation.

89

Nurse is recording vital signs of a client who is admitted just now in the ward. If there is no contraindication, which is the most preferred position for vital sign assessment?

a. Sitting
b. Supine
c. Prone
d. Left lateral

Ans. (a) Sitting

90

Nurse instructor asks students regarding the importance of hand washing. Students correctly said hand washing helps to remove:

a. Transient flora
b. Visible contaminant
c. Both a and b
d. Resident flora

Ans. (c) Both a and b

Explanation: Handwashing helps to remove the visible contaminant in the hands as well as the transient flora which all temporarily colonize in the hand. Residual flora is the microorganism that usually occupy certain body parts.

91

Nurse is preparing a client for contrast MRI and asks regarding history of any allergies. Client reports that he/she doesn't have any allergies. How the nurse reports this finding in the report?

a. NKA
b. NKDA
c. NFA
d. NA

Ans. (a) NKA

Explanation: NKA means no known allergies. NKDA means no known drug allergies.

92

A client comes to the nurse with history of UTI. Nurse teaches the client regarding measures to prevent UTI. Which among the following identified by the client indicates need for further teaching?

a. Wipe the perineal area from front to back
b. Wear cotton undergarments
c. Increase the fluid intake
d. Promote tub bath rather than shower bath

Ans. (d) Promote tub bath rather than shower bath

Explanation: Tub bath increases the risk for UTI as compared to shower bath. So in a client with UTI, shower bath needs to be promoted than tub bath.

93

A client with ascending colon colostomy came for follow up with the complaint of liquid feces from the stoma. What should be the immediate nursing response?

a. Report the physician
b. Educate client that it's normal finding
c. Ask the client's dietary history
d. Prescribe antimotility drugs

Ans. (b) Educate client that it's normal finding

Explanation: Ascending colon is the initial part of large intestine. So, in this part, stool are not well formed and water is also not absorbed completely. So feces from colostomy will be in liquid form only.

94

A client admitted to the GI ward with complaint of diarrhea. Nurse Luzy listed down the following nursing diagnosis for the client. Which among the following has the most priority?

a. Disturbed body image
b. Fluid volume deficit
c. Social isolation
d. Impaired skin integrity

Ans. (b) Fluid volume deficit

Explanation: In the above given nursing diagnosis, if we prioritize them based on ABC fluid volume, deficit will come as a prior nursing responsibility for a client with diarrhea.

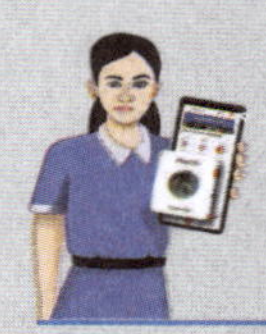

95

Nurse Linda is caring for a group of clients. She arranged fracture bedpan for her client. Which among the following clients need fracture bedpan?

a. Total knee replacement client
b. Multiple sclerosis client
c. Spinal cord injury client
d. Client with Alzheimer's

Ans. (c) Spinal cord injury client

96

Nurse is assisting a client for enema administration. Which among the following positions is needed to give this client?

a. Lithotomy
b. Left lateral
c. Semi fowler's
d. Prone

Ans. (b) Left lateral

Explanation: In left lateral position enema solution flows down by gravity along with natural curve of the sigmoid colon and rectum.

97

Nursing instructor is evaluating the student nurses ET suction procedure. Which among the following is the incorrect step of doing ET suction?

a. Preoxygenate the client with 100% oxygen
b. Apply intermittent suction while inserting the catheter
c. Withdraw suction catheter in rotation manner
d. Wear gloves and mask while performing suction

Ans. (b) Apply intermittent suction while inserting the catheter

Explanation: Apply intermittent suction while withdrawing the catheter in circular motion is indicated. Applying suction while introducing catheter is not recommended.

98

In a preoperative unit, nurse was teaching incentive spirometry exercise to a group of clients. Which among the following statements indicate that teaching was effective?

a. To perform this exercise, one has to breathe out on the mouth piece.
b. Exercise needs to be performed three times a day.
c. Mouthpiece needs to be disinfected with cidex after every use.
d. This exercise helps to prevent pulmonary complication.

Ans. (d) This exercise helps to prevent pulmonary complication.

Explanation: Correct statement related to incentive spirometry is, this exercise helps to prevent pulmonary complication and helps to increase inspiratory volume and maintains alveolar ventilation and prevents atelectasis. To perform this exercise, client needs to exhale normally then keeping mouthpiece in the mouth, should take slow deep breaths to elevate the balls. This exercise must be done 4–5 times hourly. Once done, clean the mouthpiece with water and shake it to dry.

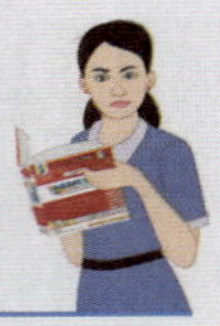

99

Client admitted in the emergency department with the history of cramping legs and lethargy. On detailed history, nurse understood that the client is suffering from diarrhea for the last one week. What should the nurse do first?

a. Administer antidiarrheal medications
b. Give IV fluid
c. Monitor serum electrolyte
d. Collect stool for C/S

Ans. (c) Monitor serum electrolyte

Explanation: Diarrhea for the last one week leads to fluid and electrolyte abnormality. This client is at risk for developing hypokalemia. So serum electrolyte monitoring is the primary responsibility.

Regarding the fluids, if the child can take fluid via mouth there is no need for IVF.

100

Nurse monitored 22-year-old client's respiration and found the RR to be 15 bpm. How the nurse will record this finding?

a. Tachypnea
b. Eupnea
c. Bradypnea
d. Slow breathing

Ans. (b) Eupnea

Explanation: In an adult patient, 12–16 breaths per minute is considered normal. Here the RR is 15 bpm, hence, the finding is documented as eupnea. Respiratory rate more than usual (fast breathing) is documented as tachypnea and respiratory rate less than normal (slow breathing) is documented as bradypnea.

101

Nurse Richa is giving discharge teaching to her client. In the discharge summery Syp. PCM 3 teaspoon PO TDS is written. While educating client she needs to tell that at a time client needs to take .... mL of syp PCM.

a. 10 mL
b. 15 mL
c. 30 mL
d. 45 mL

Ans. (b) 15 mL

Explanation: One teaspoon is 5 mL. So three teaspoon is $5 \times 3 =$ 15 mL.

102

In a prescription order for IV fluid its written as 25 gtt/min. Gtt indicates...............

a. Drop
b. Volume
c. Time
d. Speed

Ans. (a) Drop

Explanation: GTT is the abbreviation used for drops.

103

What is PRN order for medications?

a. Immediately
b. Whenever necessary
c. At bed time
d. Early morning

Ans. (b) Whenever necessary

Explanation: PRN means **Pro Re Nata**. It's a Latin word which means as the situation arises or when the need arises.

104

More nurses are assigned in emergency department on a day with shortage of nurses. Which ethical principle is followed here?

a. Autonomy
b. Beneficence
c. Nonmalficence
d. Justice

Ans. (d) Justice

Explanation: Justice is fairness. As per this principle, care must be fairly, justly, and equitably distributed among a group of patients.

105

Confused client was left alone on the bed without enough safety and had a fall injury and hip fracture. What it is called?

a. Battery
b. Assault
c. Negligence
d. Tort

Ans. (c) Negligence

Explanation: Negligence is defined as doing something or failing to do something that a prudent, careful, and reasonable nurse would do or not do in the same situation.

106

You are signing a consent form as witness. Here your sign means:

a. You have heard all the explanation given by the physician
b. You have seen the sign given by the person
c. You are aware about the outcome and complications of the procedure
d. Can withdraw from the procedure

Ans. (b) You have seen the sign given by the person

Explanation: Signing as witness means you have seen that the person or client is signing the consent by self without any force or threat from anyone else.

107

Code of ethics for nurses is given by:

a. WHO
b. ANA
c. TNAI
d. NABH

Ans. (b) ANA

Explanation: Code of Ethics for Nurses is developed by the American Nurses Association (ANA).

108

Client admitted in the ward refuses a treatment option. This will come under:

a. Nurse Practice Act
b. Common law
c. Civil law
d. Statutory law

Ans. (b) Common law

Explanation: Informed consent, the patient's right to refuse treatment, negligence, and malpractice comes under common law.

109

Transcultural nursing theory is given by:

a. Florence Nightingale
b. Betty Newman
c. Madeleine Leininger
d. Orem

Ans. (c) Madeleine Leininger

Explanation:

Florence Nightingale	Environmental theory
Betty Newman	Health care system model
Madeleine Leininger	Transcultural nursing
Orem	Theory of self-care

110

Nurse suspects a client with IV fluid therapy for the occurrence of air embolism. Position recommended in this situation is:

a. Right side head lower than feet
b. Right side head higher than feet
c. Left side head lower than feet
d. Left side head higher than feet

Ans. (c) Left side head lower than feet

Explanation: Immediately place the patient in the left lateral decubitus (Durant maneuver) and Trendelenburg position. This helps to prevent air from traveling through the right side of the heart into the pulmonary arteries which leads to right ventricular outflow obstruction (air lock).

111

After the transfusion of one unit of cryoprecipitate, nurse expects order for which of the following laboratory test?

a. Coagulation factors
b. Hemoglobin
c. Serum electrolyte
d. Platelet level

Ans. (a) Coagulation factors

Explanation: Cryoprecipitate is rich in coagulation factors. Cryoprecipitate is prepared from plasma and contains fibrinogen, von Willebrand factor, factor VIII, factor XIII and fibronectin. Cryoprecipitate is the only adequate fibrinogen concentrate available for intravenous use.

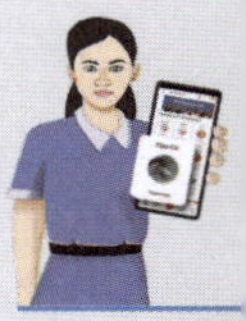

Image-Based Questions

1. **Identify the device shown in the image:**

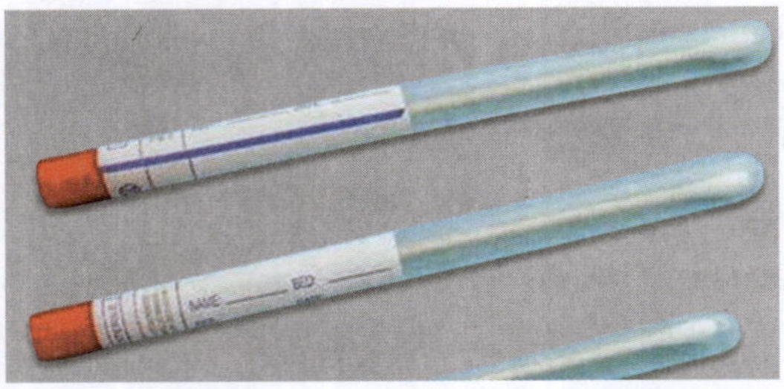

a. Vacutainer | b. Tissue culture bottle
c. Culture swab stick | d. Blood culture bottle

2. **Which of the following vacutainer tube is used to collect blood sample for coagulation test?**

(Refer explanation at the end)

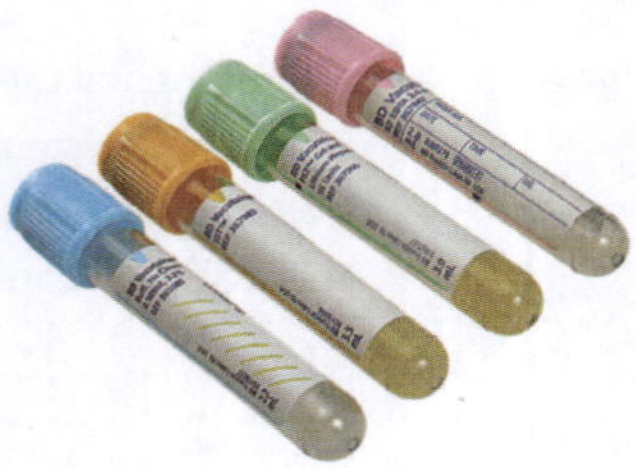

a. Blue | b. Orange
c. Green | d. Pink

3. **The type of restrain shown in the image is known as:**

(Refer explanation at the end)

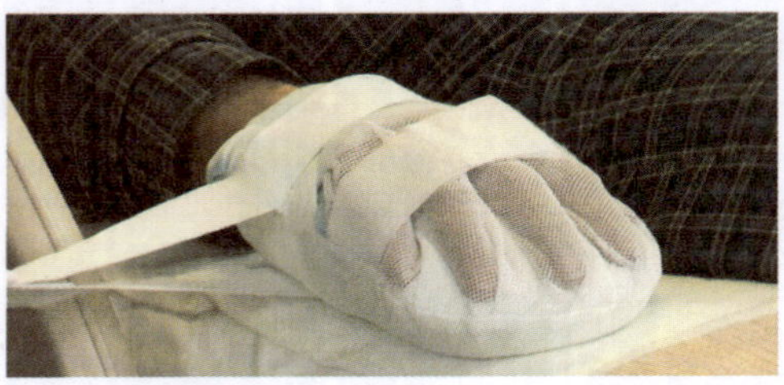

a. Allen restrain | b. Mitten restrain
c. Vests wrap | d. Handcuff bracelet

4. **Identify the name of the device used to measure height in adults:**

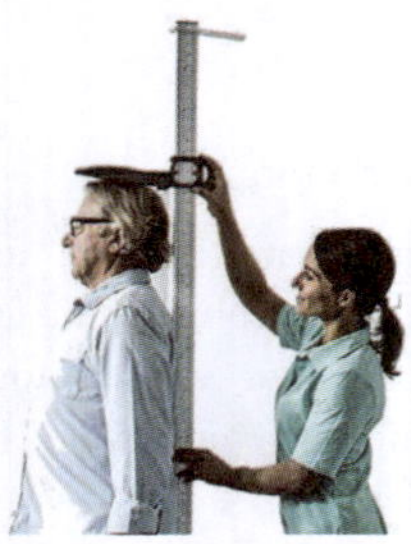

a. Nomogram | b. Stadiometer
c. Vernier gauge | d. Interferometer

5. **The appropriate sterilization method for the device shown in the photograph is:**

(Refer explanation at the end)

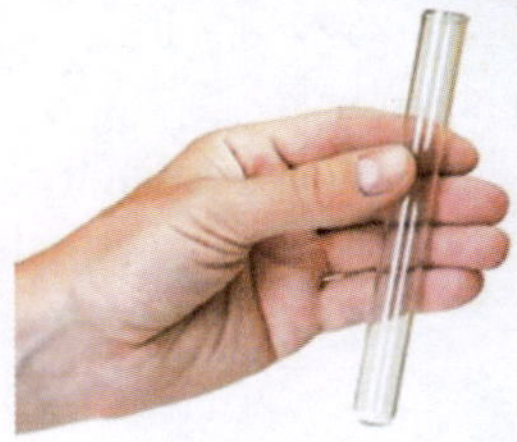

a. Autoclave | b. Hot air oven
c. Ethylene dioxide | d. Gluteraldehyde

6. **Principle on which instrument shown in photograph causes sterilization:**

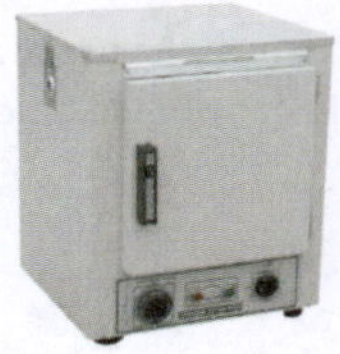

a. Steam under pressure
b. Dry heat
c. Convection current in water molecules
d. Tyndallization

7. **Instrument shown in photograph is used in public health for:**

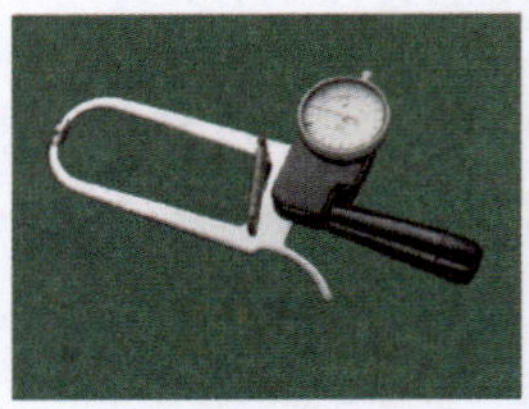

a. Head circumference
b. Mid arm circumference
c. Skin fold thickness
d. Cold chain temperature monitoring

8. **Identify the apparatus used in pediatrics as shown in photograph:**

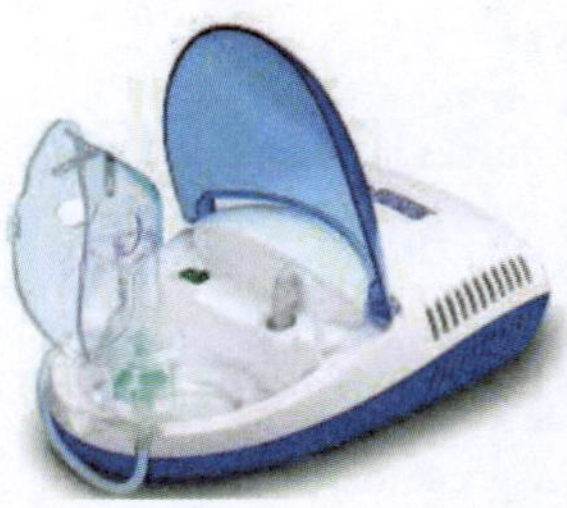

a. Resuscitator | b. Nebulizer machine
c. Irradiance meter | d. Suction machine

Ans.

1. c
2. a
3. b
4. b
5. b
6. b
7. c
8. b

[*Courtesy*: PHOTON-20® 3th ed. by Vivek Jain, CBS Publishers and Distributors Pvt Ltd]

9. The response shown by the adult in the following picture is:

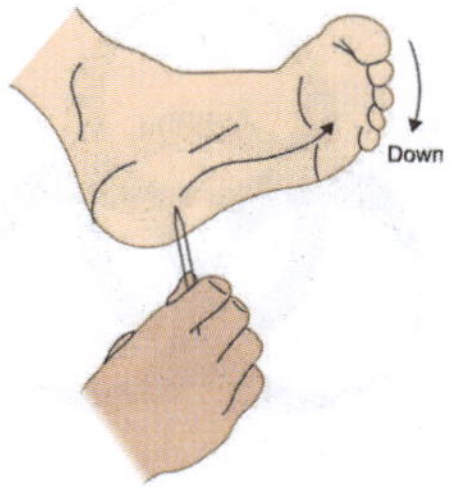

a. Flexor planter reflex b. Babinski reflex
c. Ankle reflex d. Tow reflex

10. The response shown by the adult in the following picture is:

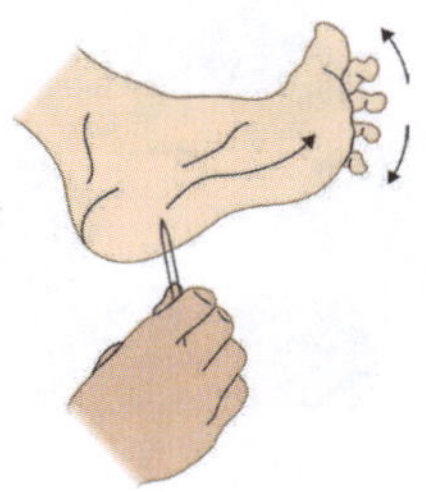

a. Extensor plantar reflex b. Babinski reflex
c. Both a and b are correct d. Flexor plantar reflex

11. The physician is examining the patient's abdomen to diagnose possible ________.

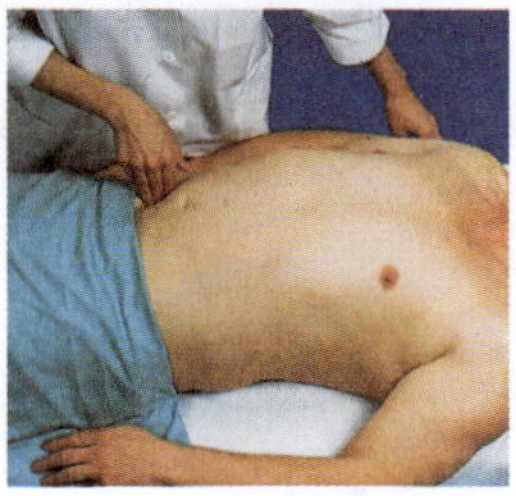

a. Cullen's sign b. Ulcerative colitis
c. Appendicitis d. Diverticulitis

12. Name the maneuver:

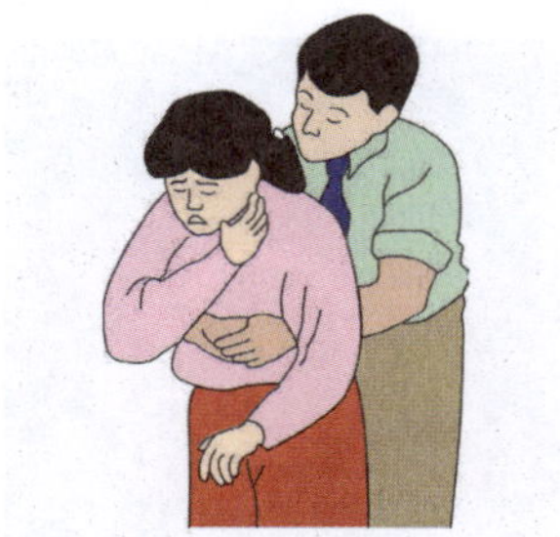

a. Semont maneuver b. Heimlich maneuver
c. Epley maneuver d. Chock maneuver

13. The patient is being assessed for:

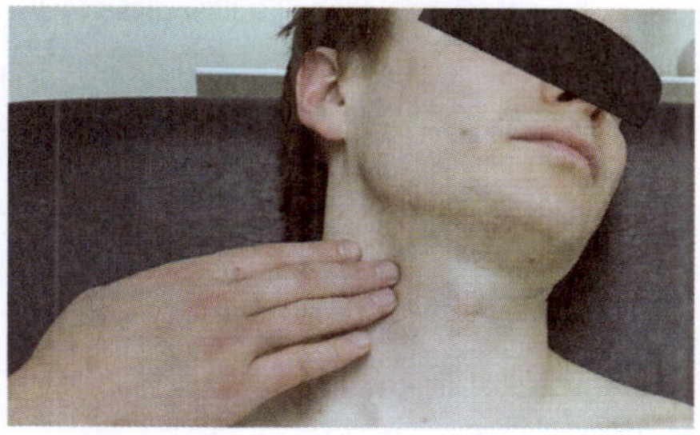

a. Radial pulse b. Femoral pulse
c. Carotid pulse d. Tibial pulse

14. Name the instrument in the following image:

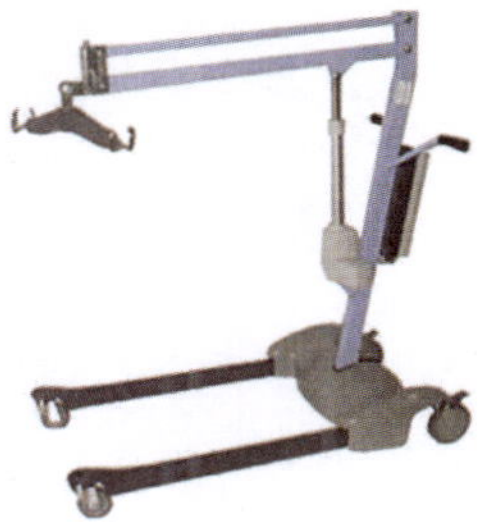

a. Patient sling b. Patient hoist
c. Recline lift d. Patient Walker

15. Name of the examination shown in image is:

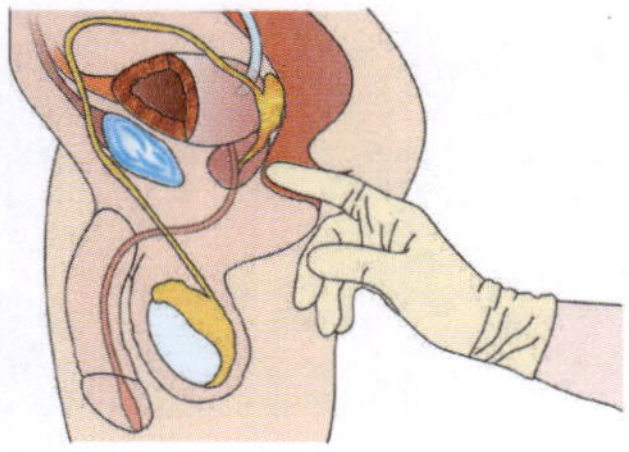

a. Digital rectal Examination
b. Manual rectal Examination
c. Proctoscope
d. Rectoscopy

16. The diameter (size) of shown image starts from:

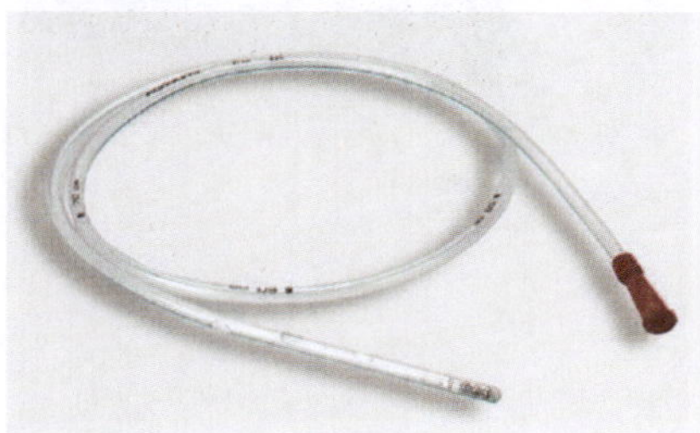

a. 4 mm b. 4.5 mm
c. 5 mm d. 5.5 mm

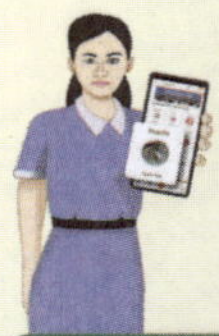

Ans.

9.	a
10.	c
11.	c
12.	b
13.	c
14.	b
15.	a
16.	c

17. A nurse is assessing the blood pressure of a hypertensive patient as given in the picture. The recorded BP would be:

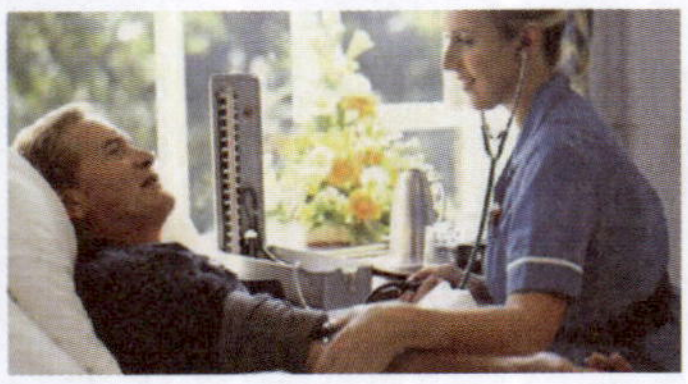

a. Same as actual BP
b. Higher systolic but lower diastolic
c. Higher systolic and diastolic
d. Lower systolic and diastolic

18. Identify the position shown in the photograph:

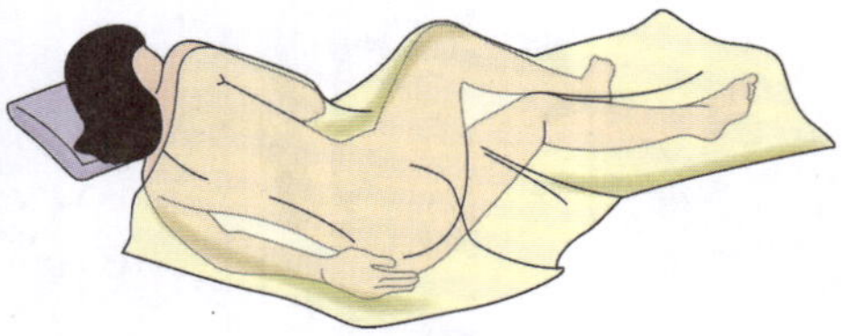

a. Trendelenburg position
b. Sim's position
c. Fowler position
d. Lloyd Davis position

19. What is this?

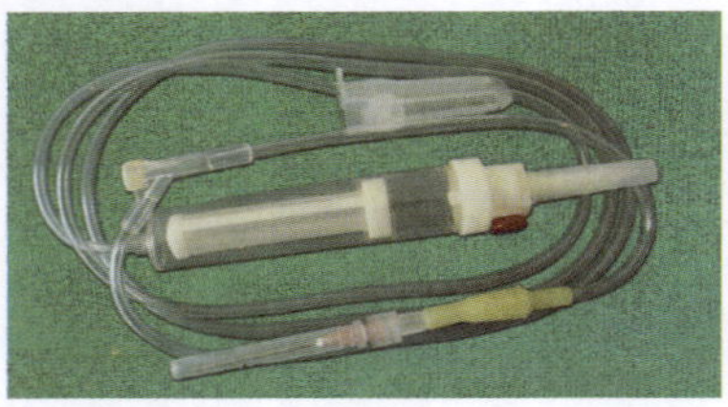

a. Intravenous fluid infusion set
b. Blood set
c. Arterial line
d. CVP line

20. Route of drug administration shown in photograph is:

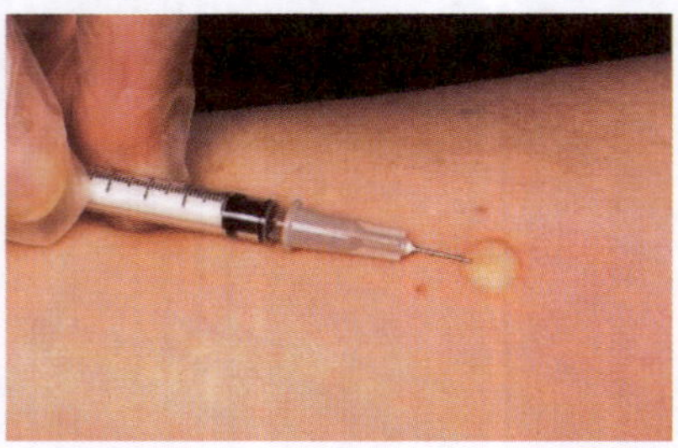

a. Subcutaneous
b. Dermojet
c. Intradermal
d. Pellet implant

21. Identify the symbol shown in photograph:

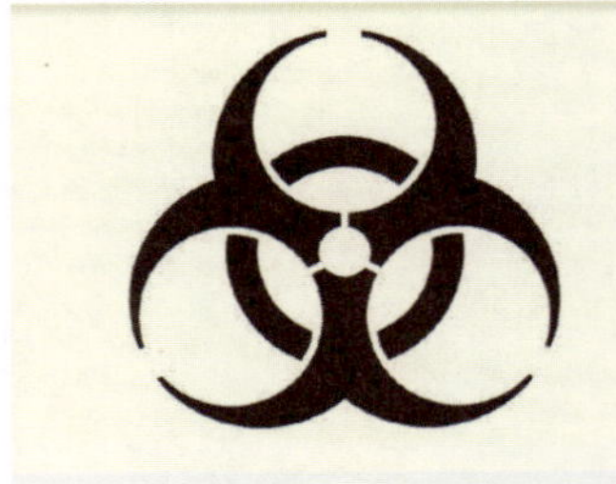

a. Radiation hazard
b. Biohazard waste
c. Cytotoxic waste
d. Biodegradable waste

22. Identify the symbol shown in photograph:

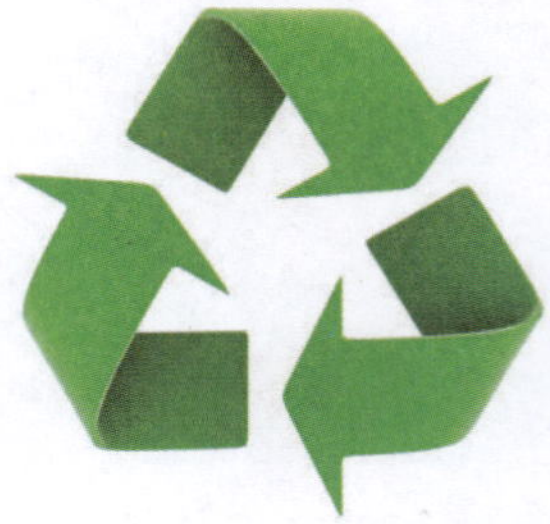

a. Recyclable waste
b. Biohazard waste
c. E-waste
d. Food waste

23. Identify the symbol shown in photograph:

a. Radiation hazard
b. Biohazard waste
c. Cytotoxic waste
d. Biodegradable waste

24. Identify the symbol shown in photograph:

a. Radiation hazard
b. Biohazard waste
c. Cytotoxic waste
d. Biodegradable waste

Ans.

17.	a
18.	b
19.	b
20.	c
21.	b
22.	a
23.	a
24.	c

25. Identify the instrument shown in photograph:

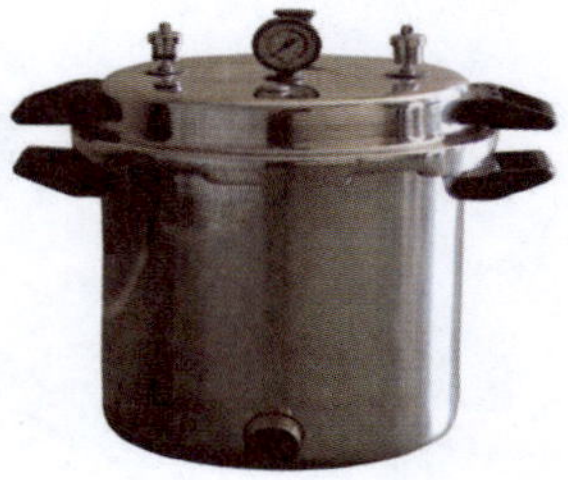

a. Hot air oven b. Autoclave
c. Hydroclave d. Microwave

26. Identify the test done by instrument shown in the photograph:

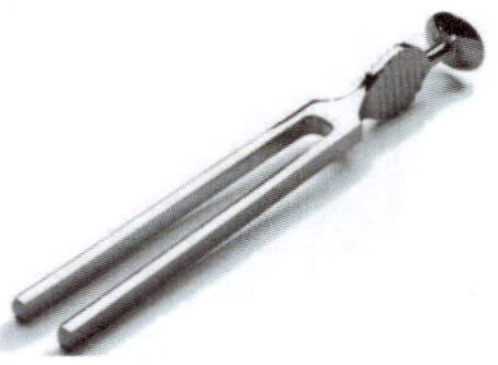

a. Rinne's test
b. Weber's test
c. Modified Schwabach's test
d. All of the above

27. Site (arrow) shown in the photograph is used for:

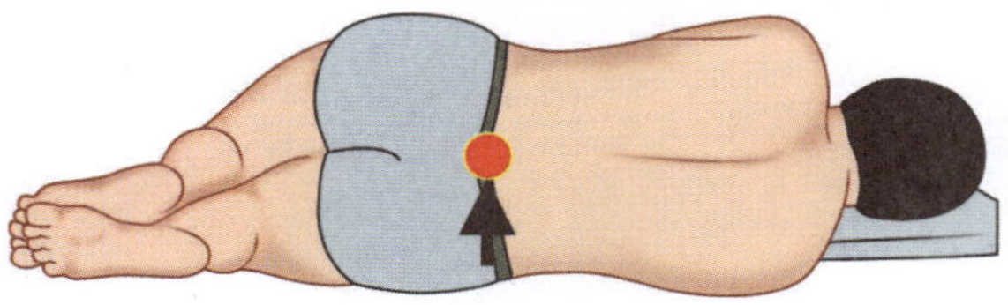

a. Pleural fluid aspiration
b. Ascitic tap
c. Lumbar puncture
d. Bone marrow aspiration

28. Identify the instrument shown in photograph, used for artificial nutrition support:

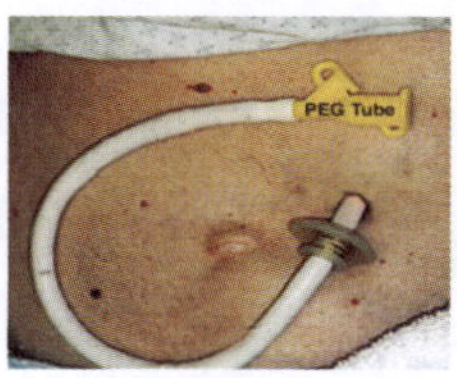

a. Gastropexy tube
b. Percutaneous endoscopic gastrostomy tube
c. Esophagogastroduodenoscope
d. Fine bore feeding tube

29. Identify the instrument shown in photograph, used during general anesthesia:

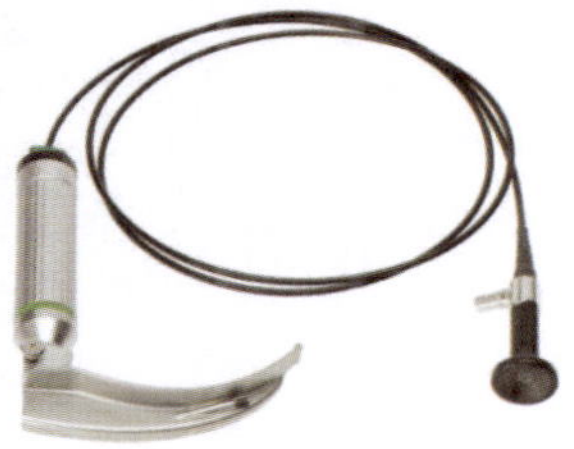

a. Laryngoscope b. Endotracheal tube
c. Laryngeal mask airway d. Fibro-optic laryngoscope

30. Unit shown in the photograph is stored in Blood bank at .... temperature.

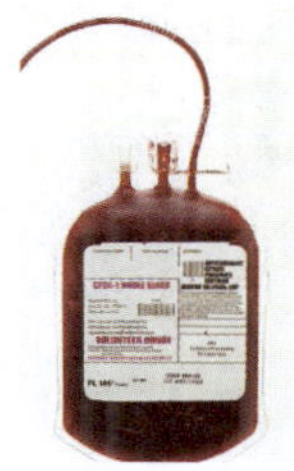

a. +4°C b. –4°C
c. +24°C d. –60°C

31. Identify the type of splint shown in photograph:

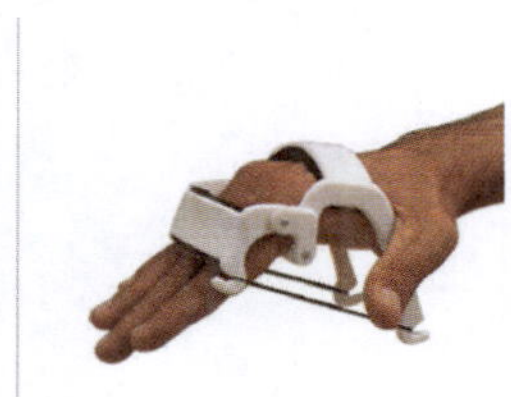

a. Aeroplane splint
b. Thomas splint
c. Knuckle bender splint
d. Cock-up splint

32. What is the use of this?

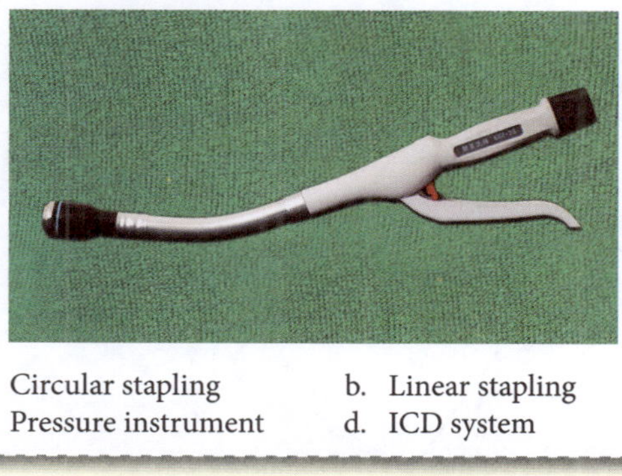

a. Circular stapling b. Linear stapling
c. Pressure instrument d. ICD system

Ans.

25.	b
26.	d
27.	c
28.	b
29.	d
30.	a
31.	c
32.	a

33. Type of CT scan technology shown in photograph is:

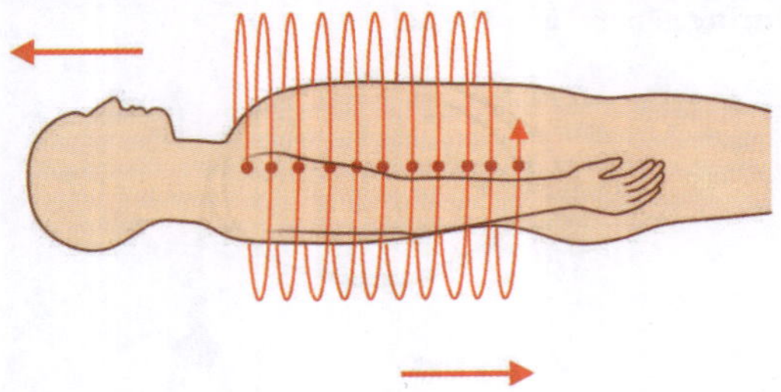

a. Multi-slice CT
b. High resolution CT
c. Electron beam CT
d. Spiral CT

34. Identify the gas cylinder shown in the photograph:

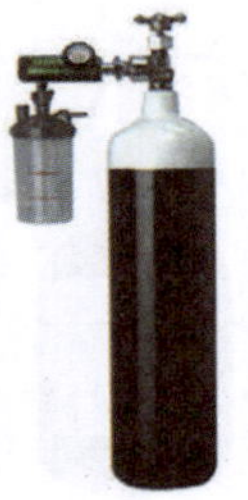

a. Oxygen
b. Cyclopropane
c. Nitrous oxide
d. Thiopentone

35. Identify this tube:

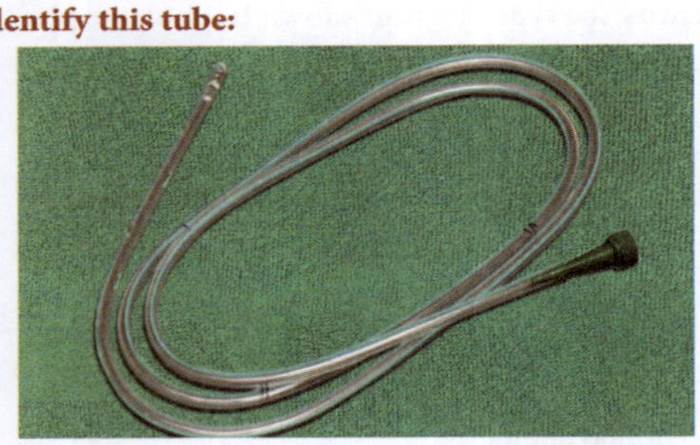

a. Ryles
b. Sengstaken Blakemore
c. Malecot's
d. Minnesota

36. What is the name of this catheter?

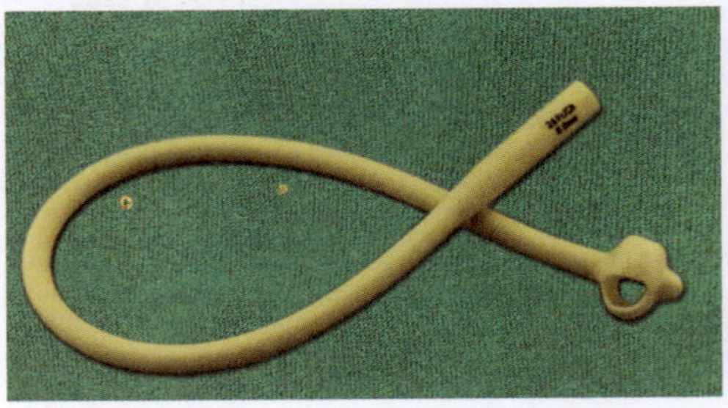

a. Mallecot' s
b. Foleys
c. Sengstaken
d. Hudd's

37. Which one of the following statements is TRUE regarding this Instrument? *[Recent Question 2016]*
(Refer explanation at the end)

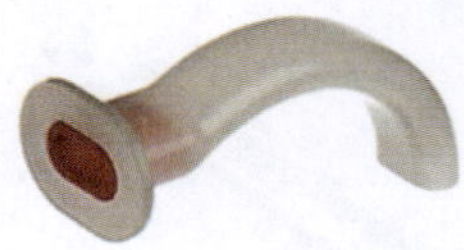

a. Prevents tongue from falling on posterior pharyngeal wall or epiglottis
b. It is called Berman oral airway
c. Best inserted during a seizure to prevent tongue bite
d. Inserted into the mouth with concavity towards tongue

Ans.

33.	d
34.	a
35.	a
36.	a
37.	a

Explanations of Image-Based Questions

2. Ans. (a) Blue

A light blue Vacutainer tube is commonly used to collect blood samples for coagulation tests. The light blue-top tube contains sodium citrate, an anticoagulant that is specifically used for coagulation studies. Sodium citrate prevents blood from clotting by binding calcium ions, which are necessary for the coagulation cascade to occur. By preserving the blood sample in an anticoagulated state, it allows accurate measurement of clotting factors and clotting times during coagulation testing.

3. Ans. (b) Mitten restrain

A soft mitt prevents the patient from being able to grasp things, but they are still able to move their arms. Soft wrist and ankle restraints may be used to prevent a patient from interfering with cares, such as pulling at an IV or other tubes or removing a dressing.

5. Ans. (b) Hot air oven

The most effective and used method of sterilization of glassware is dry heat treatment using hot air oven. On exposing the glassware to dry heat, the inhibition in growth occurs due to denaturation of proteins and oxidation of biomolecules.

37. Ans. (a) Prevents tongue from falling on posterior pharyngeal wall or epiglottis

[Ref. Ajay Yadav, 4/e p40]

- Guedel airway **(Photograph)** is the MC type of airway used while also preventing tongue falling back on posterior pharyngeal wall

"Sometimes the remedy is worse than the disease."

—Francis Bacon

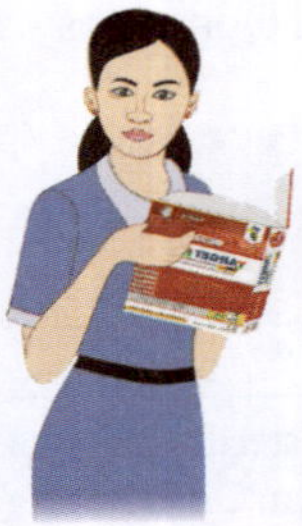

MULTIPLE CHOICE QUESTIONS

(Including Explained and Practice Questions)

DEFINITION OF NURSING

1. Which of the following phrase best describes 'the science of nursing'?

a. Application of clinical skills
b. Holistic approach in patient care
c. Body of nursing knowledge
d. Art of specialized nursing care

2. "The unique function of the nurse is to assist the individual, sick or well, in the performance of those activities contributing to health or its recover". This definition of nursing is stated by:

a. Florence Nightingale b. Dorothea Orem
c. Virginia Henderson d. Calista Roy

3. "The act of assisting others in the provision and management of self-care to maintain or improve human functioning at home level of effectiveness". The given statement regarding the Nursing professional is proposed by:

a. Florence Nightingale b. Dorothea Orem
c. Virginia Henderson d. Calista Roy

4. The definition given by the Florence Nightingale mainly focuses on:

a. Love and affection
b. Evidence based practice
c. Reliable and valid care
d. Utilizing the environment for Recovery.

5. "Nursing encompasses autonomous and collaborative care of individuals of all ages, families, groups and communities, sick or well and in all settings." Which of the following Institution has given this definition regarding Nursing Professions in the year of 2002?

a. INC b. WHO
c. TNAI d. ICN

6. Which of the following agency defines the nursing and its values as "Nursing is the protection, promotion, and optimization of health and abilities, prevention of illness and injury, alleviation of suffering through the diagnosis and treatment of human response"?

a. World Health Organization
b. Indian Nursing Council
c. American Nurse association
d. International council of Nurses

7. Adaptation Model of Nursing with Five major needs for human physiology was developed by the Sister:

a. Callsita Roy b. Betty Neumann
c. Dorothea Orem d. Henderson

8. The Word "Nurse" is rendered from the Latin word "NutriX" which refers the actual meaning of:

a. Care b. Cure
c. Nourish d. Nutritious

9. The Knowledge-based Nursing practices and core skills for this profession mainly depend on the:

a. Reporting and Documentation
b. Research and Analysis
c. Diagnosis, Intervention and Evaluation
d. History collection and Assessment

Explanation: By performing the Appropriate diagnosis for a condition and treating the condition with the actual intervention and evaluating the result will enhance the knowledge-based practice and limit the occurrence of error.

10. International council for Nurses was first established in the year of:

a. 1899 b. 1908
c. 1923 d. 1945

HISTORY OF NURSING

11. The first school of nursing was established by: *(AIIMS Raipur Grade II 2017)*

a. Virginia Henderson b. Theodor Fliedner
c. Florence Nightingale d. Isabel Hampton

Explanation: In 1836, Pastor Theodor Fliedner established the Kaiserswerth School for Nursing in his parish in Kaiserswerth, Germany. It was one of the first formally established schools of nursing in the world. Florence Nightingale established St. Thomas' Hospital and the Nightingale Training School for Nurses in 1860.

12. International day for nurses is celebrated on:

a. December 1 b. May 12
c. June 2 d. May 1

Explanation: International nurses day is celebrated on May 12, which is the birth day of Florence Nightingale

13. Florence Nightingale was born on: *(Recent Question 2012)*

a. May 12th 1820 b. May 12th 1832
c. April 7th 1820 d. June 7th 1842

14. In 1860, Nightingale set up the first nursing training school at: *(ESIC Chennai May 2012)*

a. St. Thomas' Hospital, London
b. University of Edinburgh
c. Petersburg, Virginia
d. None of the above

15. ICM theme for International Nurses Day 2023 is ... *New Q*

a. Closing the gap: Millennium Development Goals
b. Our Nurses. Our Future
c. Nurses: A voice to lead – Invest in Nursing and respect rights to secure global health
d. Nurses: A voice to lead - Health for All

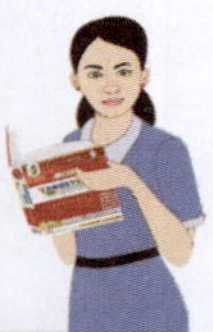

Ans.

1.	c
2.	c
3.	b
4.	d
5.	d
6.	c
7.	a
8.	c
9.	c
10.	a
11.	b
12.	b
13.	a
14.	a
15.	b

Explanation:

The themes of International Nurses Day for last 7 years are given below:

2023	Our Nurses. Our Future
2022	Nurses: A voice to lead - Invest in Nursing and respect rights to secure global health
2021	Nurses: A voice to lead - A vision for future healthcare
2020	Nurses: A voice to lead - Nursing the World to Health
2019	Nurses: A voice to lead - Health for All
2018	Nurses: A voice to lead - Health is a Human Right
2017	Nurses: A voice to lead - Achieving the Sustainable Development Goals

16. In which year, the Florence Nightingale award was instituted by Ministry of Health and Family Welfare, Govt of India? *New Q*

a. 1947 b. 1952
c. 1965 d. 1973

Explanation: The Ministry of Health and Family Welfare instituted the National Florence Nightingale Awards in 1973 to recognize the outstanding services rendered by nurses and nursing professionals to society. The award is presented annually on May 12th, which is celebrated as International Nurses Day in honor of Florence Nightingale, the founder of modern nursing.

LEGAL AND ETHICAL ASPECTS IN NURSING

17. What should be done if a female MLC patient is brought to the hospital with no female physician available for examination? *New Q*

a. The patient should be examined by a male physician due to nonavailability of female physician.
b. The patient should be examined by a male physician with a female healthcare worker present.
c. The patient should not be examined until a female physician is available.
d. The patient should be sent to a different hospital with a female physician.

Explanation: For MLC admission, a female patient should be examined by a female physician or in the presence of a female healthcare worker. If no female physician is available, a male physician may examine the patient with a female healthcare worker present to ensure adequate privacy.

18. Which of the following is not a value essential for a professional nurse? *(AIIMS-BBS SNO 2019)*

a. Human dignity
b. Dependence
c. Social Justice
d. Integrity

Explanation: Dependence is the state of relying on or being controlled by someone and it is an undesirable quality. The nurse is expected to have professional nursing values such as principles of human dignity, integrity, altruism, and justice.

19. The doctrine of informed consent deals with: *(AIIMS BPL NO 2018)*

a. Full disclosure of all relevant facts to the patient
b. Informing higher authorities about the patient's condition
c. Notification of diseases
d. Patient confidentiality

Explanation: Informed consent is taken from the patient or significant others before conducting any type of invasive procedure to communicate full disclosure of relevant facts regarding the procedure. In this the patient and/or their attendants are informed about the condition of the patient along with the possible treatment strategies and the expected prognosis.

20. Patient whose life is threatened and who is comatose is assumed to give what kind of consent for life sustaining treatment? *(AIIMS Raipur NO 2019)*

a. Informed b. Implied
c. Direct d. Expressed

Explanation: Implied consent is an assumption of permission to do something that is inferred from an individual's actions rather than explicitly provided. In case of emergency when delayed treatment would be dangerous, informed consent is not needed.

21. Which of the following is not an ethical principle? *(AIIMS-BBS SNO 2019)*

a. Autonomy b. Non-maleficence
c. Justice d. Non-beneficence

22. Principles of ethical practice includes the following; EXCEPT: *(ESIC 2019)*

a. Maleficence
b. Beneficence
c. Justice
d. Respect for autonomy

Explanation: **Maleficence** means to harm some and is opposite of non-maleficence which means "to not harm". Maleficence should not be used as principle for performing nursing action. Non-maleficence is an ethical principle that obliges one to not inflict intentional harm.

Beneficence Refers to taking positive actions to help others.

Ethical principles include principle of respect for autonomy, principle of non-maleficence, principle of beneficence, principle of justice, principle of veracity, etc.

23. All of the following are true regarding deontology; EXCEPT? *(AIIMS-BBS SNO 2019)*

a. It focuses on the consequences of actions
b. It encompasses natural law
c. It incorporates dutiful actions of an individual
d. It is also known as formalism

Explanation: Deontology is an ethical theory that says the morality of an action should be based on whether that action is right or wrong under a series of rules, rather than based on the consequences of the action.

24. When a nurse enters the patient's room for administering medications, she notices that the patient's food remained on the table. Helping the patient in providing food and then administering the medication is an act of: *(AIIMS Raipur Grade II 2017)*

a. Beneficence b. Non-maleficence
c. Maleficence d. Empathy

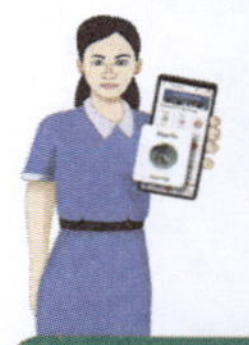

Ans.

16.	d
17.	b
18.	b
19.	a
20.	b
21.	d
22.	a
23.	a
24.	a

Explanation: Beneficence is defined as an act of charity, mercy, and kindness with a strong connotation of doing good to others including moral obligation. Non-maleficence means to do no harm. Maleficence is the act of harming or evil. Empathy is the ability to understand and share the feelings of another.

25. Which of the following ethical principles refers to doing good to the client?

a. Beneficence   b. Non-maleficence
c. Autonomy   d. Justice

Explanation:

- **Beneficence:** Doing good for the client
- **Non-maleficence:** Doing no harm
- **Autonomy:** Self-determination of client
- **Justice:** Treat equally

26. Nurse fails to administer correct medication to the patient. This action is known as:

a. Negligence   b. Crime
c. Tort   d. Battery

Explanation: Negligence is a type of malpractice. It refers to doing of something which a reasonably prudent person would not do, or the failure to do something which a reasonably prudent person would do, under circumstances similar to those shown by the evidence.

- Crime is an action or omission which constitutes an offence and is punishable by law.
- A tort, in common law jurisdictions, is a civil wrong that unfairly causes someone else to suffer loss or harm resulting in legal liability for the person who commits the tortious act, called a tortfeasor.
- Battery is the unlawful and unwanted touching or striking of one person by another, with the intention of bringing about a harmful or offensive contact.

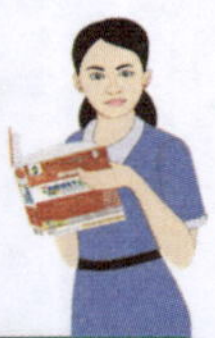

27. An intentional touching of the patient's body without consent is termed: *(DSSSB PHN, 2015)*

a. Negligence   b. Assault
c. Battery   d. Malpractice

28. Immunization causes pain in child but it will also provide protection against certain diseases. Which of the following ethical principle is applicable here?

a. Justice   b. Beneficence
c. Non-maleficence   d. Autonomy

29. Which of the following ethical principles in nursing is defined as treating all patients fairly and equally, without discrimination? *New Q*

a. Autonomy   b. Non-maleficence
c. Beneficence   d. Justice

Explanation: Justice is an ethical principle in nursing that refers to the obligation to treat all patients fairly and equally, without discrimination.

30. Physician ordered blood transfusion for a client, but her father refused blood transfusion. Which among the following is the appropriate action by healthcare workers?

a. Try to make the father willing for blood transfusion
b. Get court order for blood transfusion
c. Do blood transfusion without listening to father
d. Abide by the father's wishes and inform the healthcare provider

31. A nurse administered a wrong dose of medication to a client. Upon realizing the mistake, she immediately reported to the authority and did incidental reporting. This shows:

a. Accountability   b. Responsibility
c. Authority   d. Decision making

32. Which of the following nursing actions is an example of malpractice? *New Q*

a. Administering medication without proper training or certification.
b. Failing to document a patient's vital signs accurately.
c. Failing to follow a physician's orders without proper justification.
d. Failing to follow infection control practices.

Explanation: Malpractice is a term used to describe any professional misconduct, negligence, or breach of duty by a healthcare provider that causes harm or injury to a patient. Administering medication without proper training or certification (without having registration as Nurse) is an example of malpractice because it puts the patient's health and safety at risk.

Failing to document a patient's vital signs accurately or failing to follow a physician's orders without proper justification or failing to follow infection control practices are examples of professional negligence, but not necessarily malpractice.

33. The patient's right to refuse treatment is an example of:

a. Common law
b. Religion clause
c. Statutory law
d. Nursing Council Act

Explanation: The right to refuse medical treatment is indeed based on the common law right of self-determination of one's body and the ethical principle of respect for autonomy.

34. Code of ethics for registered nurse defines the:

a. Uniformity of care to all clients
b. Principles by which nurses' provide care to their clients
c. Protocols to be followed during nursing procedures
d. SOPs for patient safety

35. Which of the following is the nurse's best legal safeguard?

a. Collective bargaining
b. Competent practice
c. Written or implied contracts
d. Patient education

36. The intention of a nurse to do no harm to the patient while providing care is the ethical principle of:

a. Beneficence   b. Justice
c. Non-maleficence   d. Fairness

PROFESSIONAL VALUES

37. Which ethical principle promotes self-determination by the client?

a. Autonomy   b. Non-maleficence
c. Justice   d. Fidelity

Explanation: Option a, autonomy means self-determination by the client. It means let the client and significant others to determine what they wish to do. Non-maleficence means doing no harm, justice means treat everyone equally, fidelity means faithfulness.

Ans.

25. a
26. a
27. c
28. b
29. d
30. d
31. a
32. a
33. a
34. b
35. b
36. c
37. a

38. Which one of the following is not an attribute of a professional?

a. Concerned with quantity
b. Concerned with quality of outcome
c. Independent
d. Self-directed

39. Which values of Nursing practice refer to the act of selfless concern of a nurse for the wellbeing of patients?

a. Autonomy b. Empathy
c. Altruism d. Compassion

Explanation: The word altruism refers to the genuine selfless kind of concern for the other's goodness and wellbeing.

40. Registered Nurse had various rights to practice and perform their sound skills in the clinical settings. Among the rights, which of the following values refers to the Right of self-determination?

a. Integrity b. Autonomy
c. Dignity d. Justice

41. Among the following professional values, which value speaks about the Respect for uniqueness of the individual considering their personal and cultural values?

a. Validity b. Social Norms
c. Social Justice d. Human dignity

42. Defamation that comes under the Intentional tort consists of:

a. Assault and battery b. Fraud and crime
c. Malice and felony d. Libel and slander

43. Nurse should respect the patients' right to make decision on their treatment is the professional value of:

a. Human dignity b. Social justice
c. Autonomy d. Integrity

44. The Nurse Ramya is reporting the patient's false lab results during the doctors round, though she knows that values are not real, because she hadn't send the sample at the appropriate time. This act of intentional behavior comes under:

a. Slander b. Malice
c. Libel d. Malpractice

45. The act of damaging a certain person's reputation by means of publishing through the spoken or verbal word would be referred to as:

a. Felony b. Slander
c. Tort d. Libel

46. The act of damaging a certain person's reputation by means of spreading or propagating through written form or pictures or through prints refers to the:

a. Felony b. Slander
c. Tort d. Libel

47. The act of being responsible and answerable for whatever action a Nurse does in her working environment is explained in the professional values of:

a. Accountability b. Reliability
c. Validity d. Genuineness

48. Which of the following professional values defines the services that are provided by the nurse that enhances the likelihood of positive outcomes:

a. Autonomy
b. Validity
c. Quality of care
d. Dignity

49. The value that a Nurse holds in her Career for being voice for their patients and facilitates what is best for them is known as:

a. Generous b. Advocacy
c. Autonomy d. Leadership

Explanation: Advocacy is one of the major roles of nurse that enables the patients to attain their rights and benefits during the time of helplessness in their place where they got treated.

ADMISSION & DISCHARGE PROCEDURE

50. Which of the following is the purpose of a nursing discharge summary? *New Q*

a. To document the patient's medical history and treatment plan.
b. To communicate the patient's status and care needs to the healthcare team.
c. To provide instructions to the patient and family regarding post-discharge care.
d. To ensure that the patient's insurance provider is appropriately billed for services rendered.

Explanation: The nursing discharge summary is a document that outlines the patient's medical status, treatment plan, and instructions for post-discharge care. The purpose of the nursing discharge summary is to ensure that the patient and their family are fully informed about the patient's condition and care needs after leaving the healthcare facility.

51. What is the full form of LAMA?

a. Leave against medical advice
b. Leave and medication advice
c. Leave alone with medical application
d. Leave against medication apply

Explanation: LAMA is an acronym that stands for "Leave Against Medical Advice." When a patient leaves the hospital against the advice of their physician, it is called LAMA. This decision can be made for a variety of reasons, such as financial constraints, personal obligations, or dissatisfaction with the quality of care received. However, leaving the hospital against medical advice can be risky and may lead to negative health outcomes. Therefore, healthcare providers typically advise patients against LAMA and encourage them to follow the recommended treatment plan to ensure the best possible health outcomes.

52. The primary response of a nurse during admission of a client is to:

a. Orient the client to hospital routine
b. Prepare admission sheet
c. Receive the client in a courteous manner
d. Fill consent form

53. What should be done if an Medico-Legal Case (MLC) patient decides to leave the hospital against medical advice (DAMA)? *New Q*

a. The patient should be allowed to leave without any intervention.
b. The physician should inform the Chief Medical Officer and the Police.
c. The patient should be convinced to stay in the hospital.
d. The patient's records and belongings should be handed over to the police.

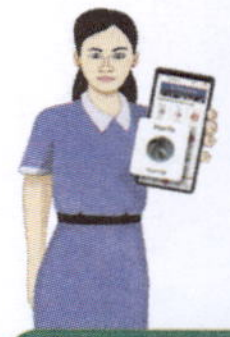

Ans.

38.	a
39.	c
40.	b
41.	d
42.	d
43.	c
44.	b
45.	b
46.	d
47.	a
48.	c
49.	b
50.	c
51.	a
52.	c
53.	b

Explanation: If an MLC patient decides to leave the hospital on DAMA (Discharge Against Medical Advice), the physician should inform the Chief Medical Officer and the police. This is to ensure that proper procedures are followed and the patient's safety is not compromised.

54. Discharge planning of the patient begins:
a. When the physician orders for discharge
b. When patient starts showing positive response to the treatment
c. At the time of initiation of treatment
d. At the time of admission

55. A patient who decides to leave the hospital against medical advice (LAMA) must sign a form. What is the purpose of this form? **New Q** *(LNJP H D 2012)*
a. To release the physician and hospital from legal responsibility for the patient's health status
b. To ethically illustrate that the patient has control of his or her own care and treatment
c. To use in the event of readmission
d. To indicate the patient's wishes

Explanation: The purpose of signing a form while leaving on LAMA is to document the patient's decision and ensure that they are making an informed choice. The form may also help protect the healthcare providers legally by demonstrating that they provided the patient with appropriate information and advice, and that the patient was aware of the risks of leaving the hospital against medical advice.

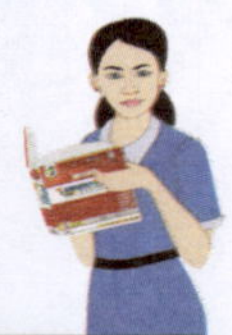

56. Disinfection of patient's unit after the death/discharge of patient is termed as:
a. Concurrent disinfection b. Terminal disinfection
c. Sterilization d. Quarantine

57. Which of the following nursing actions should be given highest priority when admitting the patient into the operating room? *(ESIC Chennai May 2012)*
a. Level of consciousness
b. Patient identification and correct operative consent
c. Positioning and skin preparation
d. Vital signs

NURSING PROCESS

58. Which type of assessment is performed after admission within a specific time to determine the nature of the problem? **New Q**
a. Initial assessment
b. Problem-focused assessment
c. Emergency assessment
d. Time-lapsed assessment

59. What is the primary purpose of an on-going assessment? **New Q**
a. Identify life-threatening events
b. Determine the status of a particular problem
c. Evaluate the effectiveness of treatment or interventions
d. Compare changes in the client's health status over time

60. Which type of assessment is conducted several months after the initial assessment to determine changes in the client's health status? **New Q**
a. Emergency assessment b. Time-lapsed assessment
c. Comprehensive assessment
d. On-going assessment

61. Which of the following is not a component of planning in the nursing process? **New Q**
a. Setting priorities
b. Establishing goals
c. Selecting nursing interventions
d. Evaluating the nursing diagnosis

Explanation: The components of planning in the nursing process include setting priorities, establishing goals, selecting nursing interventions, and writing individualized nursing interventions on the care plan. Evaluating the nursing diagnosis is a part of the evaluation phase.

62. ____ is a tool of Nursing Process: *(Safdarjung NO 2018)*
a. Personal history b. Present illness
c. Socioeconomic status d. Planning

Explanation:
- The tools of nursing process include Assessment, Nursing diagnosis, Planning, Intervention and Evaluation.
- **Planning** is establishing priorities of care and is an important tool or element of nursing process. It is a base for implementation.

63. Nursing care that is based on identifying and meeting the needs of a patient is called: *(AIIMS BPL NO 2018)*
a. Client-oriented b. Prioritization
c. Goal-oriented d. Target realization

Explanation: **Client-oriented** approach or patient-centered care means that the nursing care is based on assessing and meeting the needs of the client as per the nursing process.

64. Which of the following statements is true about nursing diagnosis? *(AIIMS BPL NO 2018)*
a. It predicts the prognosis
b. It aids in the quality of care to meet the client's needs
c. It studies the cause and effect of the illness
d. It identifies the disease

Explanation: Nursing diagnosis usually points toward the potential problems that can occur in a client. Nursing diagnosis is developed based on data obtained during the nursing assessment. This is need based and is prioritized as per the urgency to provide quality care.

65. A post-operative patient receives a stat dose of injection Pethidine intramuscularly. After one hour, the nurse checks on pain relief. Which step of the nursing process is the nurse using here? *(Daman & Diu NO 2018)*
a. Evaluation b. Assessment
c. Implementation d. Planning

Explanation: Evaluation helps the nurse to assess her own interventions and also give her opportunity to improve it. The aim of the nurse is to evaluate the action of Pethidine on post-operative pain. So, the nurse uses the last step of nursing process that is evaluation. **Assessment** refers to collection of subjective and objective data, usually before planning for intervention.

66. An example of an objective data is: *(AIIMS Bhopal Grade-I 2018)*
a. Feeling of worry b. Discoloration of the skin
c. Itching d. Nausea

Ans.

54.	d
55.	a
56.	b
57.	b
58.	a
59.	c
60.	b
61.	d
62.	d
63.	a
64.	b
65.	a
66.	b

Explanation: Objective data are measurable and overt data ("signs") obtained through observations, physical examination and diagnostic examinations. Whereas subjective data are the information from patient's point of view ("symptoms") including feelings, perceptions and concerns obtained through interview.

67. Nurse obtains vital signs and determines level of comfort for the patient. Which standard of practice is performed?

a. Assessment
b. Diagnosis
c. Planning
d. Implementation

Explanation: Obtaining vital signs is objective data and determining level of comfort by asking the patient is subjective data. Obtaining subjective and objective data from patient is known as assessment in nursing process. Nursing process includes assessment, nursing diagnosis, planning, implementation and evaluation.

68. Information verbalized or stated by the patient is known as:

a. Objective data
b. Subjective data
c. Signs
d. All of these

Explanation: Subjective data are collected or obtained via personal interactions with patient. Objective data are observable and measurable (signs) through physical examination, observation and or laboratory findings.

69. Type of assessment in which more data is collected about already identified problem is:

a. Initial assessment
b. Focus assessment
c. Emergency assessment
d. Time lapsed assessment

Explanation: Option b is the correct answer. In initial assessment, the assessment is done when the person enters the healthcare facility. Emergency assessment refers to assessment which is done in a life-threatening situation/emergency. Time lapsed assessments are carried out after initial assessment.

70. The first part of the nursing diagnosis is:

a. Problem
b. Etiology
c. Risk factor
d. Evaluation

Explanation: The first part of the nursing diagnosis is problem.

71. Which type of nursing diagnosis represents conditions not currently present in the client but may develop in the future due to vulnerability or the presence of risk factors? *New Q*

a. Problem-focused diagnosis
b. Risk diagnosis
c. Health promotion diagnosis
d. Syndrome diagnosis

Explanation: Risk diagnosis represents potential conditions or situations that may develop in the future due to client vulnerability or presence of risk factors.

72. Which type of nursing diagnosis is related to the desire/motivation of the client to improve their health status? *New Q*

a. Problem-focused diagnosis
b. Risk diagnosis
c. Health promotion diagnosis
d. Syndrome diagnosis

Explanation: Health promotion diagnosis is related to the client's motivation and desire to improve their health status by adopting healthy behaviors.

73. Which type of nursing diagnosis is a clinical evaluation of a set of related problems or risks, anticipated to arise from a specific situation or event? *New Q*

a. Problem-focused diagnosis
b. Risk diagnosis
c. Health promotion diagnosis
d. Syndrome diagnosis

Explanation: Syndrome diagnosis is a clinical evaluation of a set of related problems or risks that are expected to arise from a specific situation or event. It involves identifying the patterns of symptoms or risk factors that are commonly associated with a particular condition or situation.

74. How many components are there in a problem-focused nursing diagnosis? *New Q*

a. One
b. Two
c. Three
d. Four

Explanation: A problem-focused nursing diagnosis has three components – nursing diagnosis, related factors, and defining characteristics.

75. Planning phase of nursing process will determine:

a. Expected outcome
b. Intervention needs to be provided
c. Change in client condition
d. Actual problem of client

Explanation: In planning phase, the nurse will determine the goal or expected outcome. Each problem (nursing diagnosis) is assigned a clear, measurable goal for the expected beneficial outcome.

76. When should planning in the nursing process begin? *New Q*

a. After evaluation of the patient's health status
b. At the time of the patient's discharge
c. When the patient has the first contact with the healthcare facility
d. During ongoing care of the patient in the healthcare facility

Explanation: Planning in the nursing process should begin when the patient has the first contact with the healthcare facility to develop a plan of care that addresses the patient's individual needs and preferences.

77. The nursing process provides a:

a. Basis for nursing theories
b. Knowledge component of nursing
c. Systematic process for delivery of nursing care
d. Basis for acquiring body of knowledge

78. Which of the following is an objective data?

a. Chest pain
b. Complaint of dizziness
c. An evaluation of blood pressure
d. Complains of nausea

79. 'The patient will remain free from pain throughout hospitalization'. This statement is an example of a (an):

a. Short term goal
b. Long term goal
c. Nursing diagnosis
d. Expected outcome

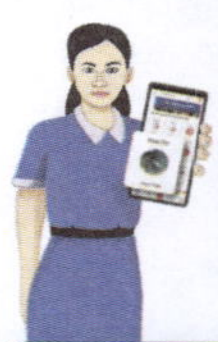

Ans.

67.	a
68.	b
69.	b
70.	a
71.	b
72.	c
73.	d
74.	c
75.	a
76.	c
77.	c
78.	c
79.	a

Explanation: In nursing process, goals and expected outcomes are both important components of the planning phase. Although these terms are often used interchangeably, there is a subtle difference between them.

Goals (long-term and short-term) are broad statements that describe what the healthcare team hopes to achieve, whereas expected outcomes are derived from goals and provide more specific, measurable indicators of progress toward achieving those goals.

For example, a goal in pain management could be "The patient will be free from pain throughout hospitalization." The expected outcomes derived from this goal could be:

The patient will rate their pain level as less than 3 out of 10 on the pain scale.

The patient will report relief from pain after receiving pain medication.

The patient will be able to participate in activities of daily living without experiencing pain.

80. First step of nursing process is:
a. Assessment b. Diagnosis
c. Planning d. Implementation

81. Collection of subjective data from patient is carried out in:
a. Assessment phase b. Nursing diagnosis phase
c. Implementation phase d. Planning phase

82. Which of the following is an example of nursing diagnosis?
a. Hypertension b. Pain
c. Shock d. Hyperglycemia

83. The interpretation of the information collected about the patient represents the:
a. Assessment of the patient
b. Plan of care
c. Health problems of the patient
d. Nursing interventions implemented for the patient

84. Action phase of nursing process includes:
a. Subjective assessment b. Planning
c. Implementation d. Evaluation

85. Priorities of planning in nursing process is done based on:
a. Information processing model
b. Maslow's hierarchy of human needs
c. Erik Erikson's theory
d. Health-Illness continuum model

86. Patient-oriented outcomes should be derived from:
a. Nursing diagnosis
b. Assessment
c. Evaluation
d. Planned interventions

87. Which of the following takes priority in planning nursing care for a client?
a. Physician order b. Nurse's condition
c. Client's condition d. Hospital policy

88. The clinical manifestation that are objective are:
a. Signs b. Symptoms
c. Disease d. Syndrome

89. The nurse compares the characteristics of acute renal failure with those of chronic renal failure and at the end selects acute renal failure. This process is called:
a. Data collection b. Data interpretation
c. Data comparing d. Data lustering

90. Total number of steps in nursing process are:
a. Three b. Four
c. Five d. Six

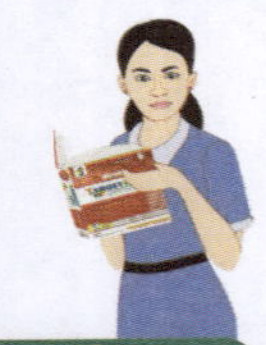

Ans.

80.	a
81.	a
82.	b
83.	c
84.	c
85.	b
86.	a
87.	c
88.	a
89.	b
90.	c
91.	c
92.	c
93.	c
94.	c
95.	b
96.	c
97.	a

91. The primary source of data for evaluation is:
a. Doctor b. Nurse
c. Client d. Family

92. Which of the following is subjective data of nursing assessment?
a. Vomiting, pulse 82/min.
b. Respirations 22/min., blood pressure 120/70 mm Hg
c. Nausea and abdominal pain
d. Pale skin and moist hands

93. Conditions that increase vulnerability to a disease are known as:
a. Etiology b. Precipitating factor
c. Risk factors d. Pathophysiology

Explanation: Correct answer is option c. A risk factor of predisposing factor is any attribute, characteristic or exposure of an individual that increases the likelihood of developing a disease or injury.

94. Data that include all the measurable and observable pieces of information are called: *(AIIMS BPL NO 2018)*
a. Subjective data b. Hearsay data
c. Objective data d. Documented data

Explanation: ***Objective*** data are observable and measurable data ("signs") obtained through observation, physical examination, and laboratory and diagnostic testing. Subjective data are gathered when the patient himself tells the nurse about it.

95. When considering a client's symptoms, how should the nurse categorize a client's complaint of tinnitus? *(RAK MSc 2018)*
a. Objective b. Subjective
c. Prodromal d. Functional

Explanation:
- Tinnitus is a ringing sensation experienced in the ears that can only be felt by the person experiencing it and cannot be observed by the health personnel. Hence it is a subjective data. Subjective data is what the patient tells as his/her their symptoms are, including feelings, perceptions and concerns.
- **Objective data** is the one which a nurse can observe in the patient.

96. A method of data interpretation among the following is: *(AIIMS BPL NO 2018)*
a. Interview b. Observation
c. Prioritization d. Listening

Explanation: Interview, observation and listening are the methods of data collection not data interpretation whereas prioritization is an action (interpretation) that can be done after collection of data.

Strategy: Find the odd one out.

97. Nurse uses the nursing process as a method of: *(ESIC 2019)*
a. Planning, organizing and delivering patient care
b. Communicating with patients and families
c. Meeting the legal requirements and standards in nursing
d. Meeting public expectations of nurse

Explanation: The purpose of nursing process is primarily to organize and deliver care to the patient. Communicating with patients, meeting legal requirements and standards, meeting public expectations are duties and responsibilities that are part of nursing process.

98. The type of assessment that includes data related to a client's biological, cultural, spiritual and social need is called: *(AIIMS-BBS SNO 2019)*
   a. Behavioral assessment
   b. Screening assessment
   c. Comprehensive assessment
   d. Focused assessment

Explanation: Comprehensive means including everything. Assessing biological, cultural, spiritual and social needs is called comprehensive assessment. Behavioral assessment is a method used to assess behavior. Screening is a process for evaluating the possible presence of a particular problem. Detailed nursing assessment of specific body system(s) relating to the presenting problem is known as screening.

99. Purpose of assessment is to:
   a. Make nursing diagnosis
   b. To collect basic data regarding client's health status
   c. To provide intervention
   d. For giving health education

Explanation: Assessment provides basic data regarding the client, which helps us to find out the actual and potential problem as well as the changes occur in client's health during the treatment course.

DOCUMENTATION & REPORTING

100. What does SOAP stand for in progress note documentation? New Q
   a. Situation, Observation, Assessment, Plan
   b. Subjective, Objective, Assessment, Plan
   c. Situation, Objective, Assessment, Plan
   d. Subjective, Observation, Assessment, Plan

Explanation: SOAP stands for Subjective, Objective, Assessment, Plan and is one of the progress note documentation methods used in problem-oriented medical records.

101. What is the purpose of charting by exception? New Q
   a. To document any deviation from normal or any abnormality
   b. To provide a detailed narrative of patient care
   c. To document all aspects of patient care in chronological order
   d. To provide a problem-oriented medical record

Explanation: Charting by exception is a documentation method that focuses on documenting any deviation from normal or any abnormality.

102. What is the purpose of clinical handover in nursing? New Q
   a. To transfer professional responsibility and accountability for patient care
   b. To document patient care for legal purposes
   c. To provide medical insurance reimbursement
   d. To educate medical and nursing students

Explanation: Clinical handover refers to the transfer of professional responsibility and accountability for some or all aspects of patient care to another nurse or healthcare professional on a temporary or permanent basis.

103. What is the purpose of a problem list in the problem-oriented medical record (POMR)? New Q
   a. To provide relevant background information about the patient
   b. To identify different problems pertaining to the patient
   c. To list the patient's current assessment findings and vital signs
   d. To provide recommendations for next steps and interventions

Explanation: The problem list in the POMR is used to identify different problems pertaining to the patient, which can be added to the list as needed.

104. Which of the following is the most important guideline for quality documentation? New Q
   a. Use only standard abbreviations
   b. Provide a detailed narrative of patient care
   c. Document all aspects of patient care in chronological order
   d. Ensure the documentation is factual, accurate, complete, current, and in logical order

105. When handing over the belongings of a medicolegal case (MLC) patient to the police or relatives, what should be done? New Q
   a. Record the details and signature of the receiver
   b. Record the details and signature of the receiver and inform the treating physician.
   c. The belongings of the patient should never be handed over to anyone.
   d. Destroy any evidence related to the patient before anyone could see it.

Explanation: When handing over the belongings of a MLC patient to the police or relatives, the complete details and signature of the receiver should be recorded, and the treating physician should be informed. This ensures proper documentation and accountability of the belongings, and maintains the confidentiality and security of the patient's records.

106. Your patient says that he "urinates at night" and it is affecting his daytime alertness. You would document this as: *(AIIMS Bhopal Grade-I 2018)*
   a. Oliguria b. Nocturia
   c. Dysuria d. Polyuria

Explanation: Nocturia or nocturnal polyuria is defined as the need to wake (one or more times) and pass urine at night. It should be distinguished from enuresis, where urine is passed unintentionally during sleep.

107. A post-operative patient is brought to the postsurgical ward. The receiving nurse assessed the patient for patent airway and stable vital signs. Which of the following should be performed next?
   a. Complete the admission file work
   b. Log roll the patient to evaluate cleanliness of bed linens
   c. Assess dressings for bleeding
   d. Pain assessment on a scale of 1 to 10

108. Time limit for registering birth is within: *(AIIMS Bhopal Grade-I 2018)*
   a. 21 days b. 10 days
   c. 14 days d. 7 days

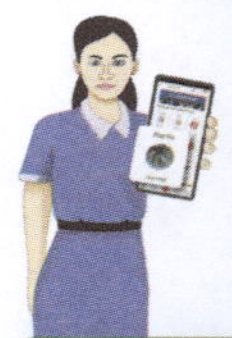

Ans.
98. c
99. b
100. b
101. a
102. a
103. b
104. d
105. b
106. b
107. c
108. a

Explanation: The registration of births and deaths act passed in 1969, for the regulation of registration of births and deaths and for matters connected therewith. The normal period of 21 days (from the date of occurrence) has been prescribed for reporting the birth, death and still birth events.

109. The disadvantages of Electronic Health Records are the following; EXCEPT: *(AIIMS Raipur Grade II 2017)*

a. Expensive
b. Lack of integration
c. Downtime processes
d. Increased medical errors

Explanation: The disadvantages of electronic health records are expensive, Lack of integration and downtime process.

110. The primary purpose of the patient record is:

a. Education
b. Communication
c. Research
d. Funding

111. Which of the following records refers to short and objective description of incidents or events that are important to the observer?

a. Admission record
b. Anecdotal record
c. Observation checklist
d. Investigation report

112. All of the following are principles of record writing; EXCEPT: New Q

a. Accurate
b. Error-free
c. Use standard abbreviation
d. Data redundancy

Explanation: Data redundancy refers to the repetition of information in a record. This can make the record longer and more difficult to read, and may lead to confusion or errors.

Avoidance of data redundancy is one of the principle of record writing.

113. What is the primary purpose of an incident report?

a. Identifying risks
b. Staff evaluation
c. Disciplinary action
d. Audiotape report

114. How would the nurse record smoking history on a patient who has smoked 2.5 packs of cigarettes per day for 10 years? *(RAK MSc 2018)*

a. Patient has smoked cigarettes for 10 years
b. Patient smokes 2.5 packs of cigarettes per day
c. Patient has a 12.5 pack-year smoking history
d. Patient has a 25 pack-year smoking history

Explanation:

- The formula for calculating "pack years" for a patient who smokes is:

Pack years = No. of packs smoked per day × No. of years person smoked

As per the above data,

Pack years = 2.5 × 10
= 25

So, the nurse records smoking history on a patient who has smoked 2.5 packs of cigarettes per day for 10 years as Patient has a 25 pack-year smoking history.

VITAL SIGNS

115. Which of the following is not a heat loss mechanism from the body?

a. Conduction
b. Convection
c. Evaporation
d. Diffusion

Explanation: All the given options except option d are heat loss mechanism from the body. Diffusion is not a heat loss mechanism. Diffusion is the movement of a substance from an area of high concentration to an area of low concentration.

- **Conduction:** Heat loss occurs when two bodies with different temperature come in direct contact with each other.
- **Convection:** Air current carries away the temperature.
- **Evaporation:** When water is converted to vapor, the body temperature will be used that induces hypothermia.

116. Before taking temperature, thermometer needs to be cleaned from:

a. Bulb to stem
b. Stem to bulb
c. Middle to stem
d. Middle to bulb

117. Cleaning of thermometer needs to be done in .... direction after taking temperature.

a. Bulb to stem
b. Stem to bulb
c. Midway between stem and bulb to stem
d. Midway between stem and bulb to bulb

Explanation: After taking temperature, cleaning has to be done from stem to bulb, i.e., more clean to less clean area. Before taking temperature, it has to be cleaned from bulb to stem.

118. The nurse in-charge measures a patient's temperature at 102°F. What is the equivalent Centigrade temperature? *(AIIMS Raipur NO 2019)*

a. 39 degree
b. 49 degree
c. 38.9 degree
d. 48.1 degree

Explanation: To convert Fahrenheit scale to Celsius scale:

C = (F – 32) × 5/9
C = (102 – 32) × 5/9
C = 70 × 5/9
C = 38.9°

119. The type of fever in which the temperature fluctuates more than 2°C, all above normal, during a 24 hour period is: *(AIIMS Raipur Grade II 2017)*

a. Intermittent fever
b. Remittent fever
c. Recurrent fever
d. Relapsing fever

Explanation: Intermittent fever is a type of fever in which there is an interval where temperature is elevated for several hours followed by an interval where temperature drops back to normal. Recurrent fever can be a symptom of various illnesses such as periodic fevers, aphthous ulcers, pharyngitis and adenopathy. Relapsing fever is a vector-borne disease caused by bacteria in the genus Borrelia, which are transmitted through the bites of lice or soft-bodied ticks.

120. What is the normal 'oral temperature' of an adult? *(AIIMS Bhopal Nursing Officer, 2018)*

a. 90.0°F
b. 98.6°F
c. 91.5°F
d. 90.6°F

Explanation: 98.6°F is the normal 'oral temperature' of an adult. Rectal temperature is 0.5°C or 1°F higher than oral temperature while axillary temperature is 1°F less than the oral temperature.

121. Which of the following method is the most appropriate to measure temperature in a patient who underwent oral surgery?

a. Rectal
b. Axilla
c. Oral
d. Central line

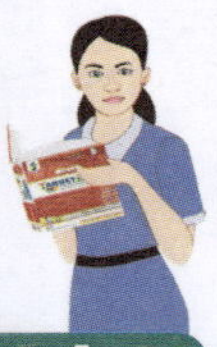

Ans.

109.	d
110.	b
111.	b
112.	d
113.	a
114.	d
115.	d
116.	a
117.	b
118.	c
119.	b
120.	b
121.	b

Explanation: Taking temperature from Axilla is the most appropriate method and easily accessible site in this client.

After oral surgery, the oral cavity may be sensitive, inflamed, or have an open wound, which can make it difficult or painful for the patient to use the oral route to measure temperature.

Using a rectal thermometer may be invasive and uncomfortable, and may increase the risk of infection. Similarly, using a central line is invasive and increase the risk of complications such as infection, bleeding, or dislodgement.

122. What is the difference in temperature between oral cavity and rectum in a patient at same time?

a. 0.5°F b. 1°F
c. 2°F d. 3°F

Explanation: Oral temperature is 1°F higher than axillary and 1°F Less than rectum.

123. If highest temperature is recorded in the morning and lowest temperature in the evening. This kind of fever is known as:

a. Inverse fever b. Lysis
c. Crisis d. Remittent fever

Explanation: In inverse fever, the temperature rises in the morning rather than in the evening. Option b means fall in temperature in a zig-zag manner. Option c means sudden return to normal temperature. Option d, Remittent fever refers to a fever pattern in which temperature varies during each 24-hour period but never reaches normal.

124. Rectal thermometer needs to be inserted up to:

a. 0. 5-1. 5 inch b. 1-2 inch
c. 1. 5-2. 5 inch d. 2-3 inch

Explanation: Rectal thermometer needs to be inserted up to 0. 5-1. 5 inch.

125. Which of the following methods is the most accurate for measuring core body temperature in critically ill patients? *New Q*

a. Oral temperature measurement
b. Axillary temperature measurement
c. Tympanic membrane temperature measurement
d. Pulmonary artery catheter temperature measurement

Explanation: Core body temperature is the temperature of the deep tissues of the body, including the brain, heart, and liver. Accurate measurement of core body temperature is important in critically ill patients, as even small deviations from normal can have significant clinical implications.

Pulmonary artery catheter temperature measurement is considered the most accurate method for measuring core body temperature in critically ill patients. This method involves inserting a catheter into the pulmonary artery, which allows for direct measurement of the blood temperature as it returns to the heart from the core tissues.

126. Which of the following is a potential challenge of using an infrared tympanic thermometer for temperature measurement? *New Q*

a. Skin irritation or trauma
b. Inaccurate temperature readings
c. Infection transmission
d. Impacted cerumen affecting temperature readings

Explanation: Cerumen (ear wax) impaction can affect tympanic temperature values by as much as 0.3°F lower than the unobstructed ear. It is important for nurses to ensure that the ear canal is clear of obstructions before taking a temperature measurement.

127. Who invented the first prototype of thermometer known as thermoscope? *(ESIC Chennai May 2012)*

a. Celsius b. Galileo Galilee
c. Lord Kelvin d. Thomas J. Manning

Explanation: The thermometer was not invented by a single person. Rather, the development of the thermometer has been a gradual process over several centuries, involving contributions from many scientists and inventors.

One of the earliest recorded temperature measurements was made by **Galileo Galilei** in the 16th century using a rudimentary thermoscope. Later, in the 17th century, scientists such as **Robert Fludd, Santorio Santorio, and Cornelis Drebbel** made further advancements in temperature measurement, including the use of mercury in thermometers.

128. A clinical thermometer indicates temperature in degree Fahrenheit from: *(ESIC Chennai May 2012)*

a. 94 to 108 b. 94 to 110
c. 96 to 108 d. 96 to 110

129. In a child with fever, oxygen demand increases because:

a. Metabolic need increases
b. Blood sugar level decreases
c. Patient is less active
d. Patient is more alert

130. Temperature regulation is under the control of:

a. Lungs
b. Pituitary gland
c. Hypothalamus
d. Pineal gland

131. Assessment of rectal temperature is recommended if patient has

a. Arm in a cast b. Nasal packing
c. External hemorrhoids d. Gastrostomy feeding tubes

132. The fall of temperature step by step in a zig-zag manner is termed:

a. Lysis b. Crisis
c. Homeostasis d. Thermostasis

133. Relapsing fever is characterized by:

a. Recurring episodes of fever
b. The fall of temperature in zig-zag manner to normal
c. In the morning, temperature is higher than the evening
d. Temperature comes to normal at least once in a day

134. Which of the following is the characteristics of inverse fever?

a. The sudden fall of temperature from high to normal
b. The fall of temperature in zig-zag manner to normal
c. In the morning, temperature is higher than in the evening
d. Temperature comes to normal at least once in a day

135. The sudden return to a normal temperature from very high fever is called:

a. Lysis b. Crisis
c. Thermostasis d. Homeostasis

136. Temperature difference between axillary and rectal route is:

a. 1°F b. 2°F
c. 3°F d. 4°F

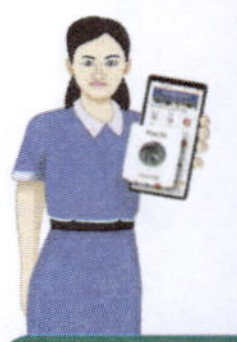

Ans.

122. b
123. a
124. a
125. d
126. d
127. b
128. a
129. a
130. c
131. a
132. a
133. a
134. c
135. b
136. b

137. Temperature difference between axillary and oral route is:

a. 0°F b. 1°F
c. 2°F d. 3°F

138. 97°F is equal to:

a. 36.1°C b. 36.8°C
c. 37.1°C d. 37.5°C

Explanation:

To convert Fahrenheit to Celsius, we use the formula:
C = (F – 32) × 5/9
Where C is the temperature in Celsius and F is the temperature in Fahrenheit.
So, to convert 97°F to Celsius:
C = (97–32) × 5/9 = 36.1 degrees Celsius
Therefore, 97°F – 36.1°C

139. 37°C is equal to:

a. 98.0°F b. 98.6°F
c. 99.6°F d. 99.8°F

Explanation:

To convert Celsius to Fahrenheit, we use the formula:
F = (C × 9/5) + 32
Where F is the temperature in Fahrenheit and C is the temperature in Celsius.
So, to convert 37°C to Fahrenheit:
F = (37 × 9/5) + 32 = 98.6 degrees Fahrenheit
Therefore, 37°C = 98.6°F

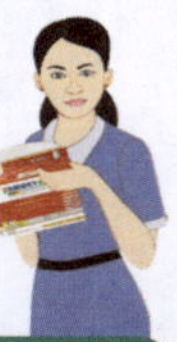

140. Body tissue works better with temperature of:

a. 32–34°C b. 34–36°C
c. 36–38°C d. 38–40°C

Explanation: Best functioning of body tissue ensured with optimal body temperature of 36-38°C.

141. The primary source of heat in the body is:

a. Sunlight
b. Metabolism
c. Heart beat
d. Circulation

142. If a patient's blood pressure is 160/96, his pulse pressure is: *(AIIMS Raipur NO 2019)*

a. 64 b. 96
c. 160 d. 256

Explanation: Pulse pressure is the difference between the systolic and diastolic blood pressure. Normal pulse pressure is 30-50 mm Hg.
Pulse pressure = Systolic BP – Diastolic BP = 160–96 = 64 mm Hg

143. Pulse deficit refers to the difference between:

a. Apical pulse and radial pulse
b. Radial pulse and femoral pulse
c. Two radial pulse obtained with 5 minutes gap
d. Two apical pulse obtained with 5 minutes gap

Explanation: The pulse deficit (difference between heartbeats and pulsations at the periphery) is determined by simultaneous palpation at the radial artery and auscultation at the apex of the heart. In other words, it is the difference between heart rate and pulse rate.

144. Location of auscultation for apical pulse is:

a. 5th intercostal space at the right mid-axillary line
b. 5th intercostal space at the left mid-clavicular line
c. 5th intercostal space at the right mid-clavicular line
d. 5th Intercostal space at the left mid-axillary line

Explanation: Location of auscultation of apical pulse is 5th intercostal space at the left mid-clavicular line, where the apex of the heart is located.

145. Apical pulse is assessed by placing the diaphragm of the stethoscope at the area of: *(DSSSB 2013)*

a. Aortic area b. Pulmonic area
c. Mitral area d. Tricuspid area

Explanation: The apical pulse is the heartbeat that can be heard at the apex of the heart, which is located at the fifth intercostal space in the mid-clavicular line.

The mitral area is also known as the apex beat or point of maximal impulse (PMI), which is the area where the apical pulse can be heard most clearly. To assess the apical pulse, the nurse should place the diaphragm of the stethoscope at the mitral area, which is located on the left side of the chest, just below the nipple line.

146. The difference between systolic and diastolic blood pressure is known as: *(Staff Nurse G II 2014)*

a. Pulse difference b. Cardiac pressure
c. Systolic pressure d. Pulse pressure

147. The difference between the apical and radial pulse rates is called the: *(LNJP H D 2012)*

a. Rhythm deficit b. Heart amplitude
c. Pulse deficit d. Pulse amplitude

148. Core body temperature is highest at:

a. Early morning b. Noon
c. Later afternoon d. Night

149. Other name for collapsing pulse is:

a. Thread pulse b. Water-hammer pulse
c. Bounding pulse d. Pulse deficit

Explanation: Collapsing pulse, also known as a water hammer or Corrigan's pulse, is a medical term used to describe a pulse that quickly rises and falls in intensity, often with a sharp or abrupt collapse.

150. Appropriate time duration to assess pulse is:

a. 15 seconds b. 30 seconds
c. 45 seconds d. 1 minute

151. The pulse assessed from the neck to the side of the wind pipe is called:

a. Brachial pulse b. Carotid pulse
c. Nuchal pulse d. Popliteal pulse

152. Appropriate site to verify radial pulse measurement is:

a. Temporal artery b. Femoral artery
c. Brachial artery d. Apex of the heart

Explanation: To verify the accuracy of the radial pulse measurement, the brachial artery is typically used. The brachial artery is located in the upper arm, and it is the major artery that supplies blood to the arm. To verify the accuracy of the radial pulse measurement, the nurse should palpate the brachial artery with their fingers while simultaneously taking the radial pulse measurement.

Ans.

137. b
138. a
139. b
140. c
141. b
142. a
143. a
144. b
145. c
146. d
147. c
148. c
149. b
150. d
151. b
152. c

153. Poor oxygenation of the blood ordinarily will affect the pulse rate and cause it to become:

a. Bounding b. Faster than normal
c. Irregular d. Slower than normal

154. The nurse is examining an 8-year-old boy with tachycardia and tachypnea. Which one of these non-invasive tests can determine the extent of hypoxia? *(AIIMS Raipur NO 2019)*

a. Pulmonary function test b. Pulse oximetry
c. Peak expiratory flow d. Chest X-ray

Explanation: Arterial oxygen can be monitored non-invasively and continuously using pulse oximeter probe on finger or toe.

155. What is the term used for normal respiratory rhythm and depth in a client? *(Safdarjung NO 2018)*

a. Eupnea b. Apnea
c. Bradypnea d. Tachypnea

Explanation: Eupnea is normal, good, unlabored ventilation, sometimes known as quiet breathing or resting respiratory rate. It is derived from the words eu-, "well" + pnoia, "breath."

156. The cardinal signs of the body includes the following; EXCEPT: *(AIIMS Raipur Grade II 2017)*

a. Temperature b. Blood pressure level
c. Blood glucose level d. Heartbeat

Explanation: Cardinal signs or Vital signs include Body temperature, Pulse (Heart rate), Respiration, and Blood Pressure. It may also include pain and oxygen saturation (pulse oximetry). Blood glucose level is not a cardinal sign of the body.

157. Increased depth of breathing with normal respiratory rate is called: *(AIIMS Bhopal Nursing Officer, 2018)*

a. Hyperpnea b. Bradypnea
c. Orthopnea d. Kussmaul's breathing

Explanation: Increased depth of breathing with normal respiratory rate is known as Hyperpnea

- **Bradypnea:** Abnormally slow breathing
- **Orthopnea:** Discomfort in breathing while lying down flat
- **Kussmaul's breathing:** Deep and labored breathing associated with severe metabolic acidosis

158. Gradual increase in rate and depth of respiration is known as:

a. Hyperventilation b. Hypoventilation
c. Kussmaul respiration d. Cheyne-Stokes

Explanation: Kussmaul breathing (respiration) is a type of hyperventilation that is the lung's emergency response to metabolic acidosis. In this condition, the hydrogen ion combine with bicarbonate and form carbonic acid, it disintegrates and forms water and carbon dioxide. The carbon dioxide needs to be eliminated from the body. So the rate and depth of respiration will increase. Kussmaul respiration is most commonly associated with conditions that cause metabolic acidosis, particularly diabetic ketoacidosis.

Cheyne-Stokes respiration is an abnormal pattern of breathing characterized by progressively deeper and sometimes faster breathing followed by a gradual decrease in breathing and apnea.

- Hyperventilation means breathing fast.
- Hypoventilation refers to reduced amount of air entering the alveoli.

159. The normal breath rate of human beings is: *(ESIC Chennai May 2012)*

a. 12–15 per minute b. 22–25 per minute
c. 15–18 per minute d. 20–24 per minute

160. Volume remaining in the lungs and airways following a maximum expiratory effort is known as: *(ESIC Chennai May 2012)*

a. Residual volume b. Total lung capacity
c. Vital capacity d. Tidal capacity

161. The most reliable way to assess the respiratory rate of a patient is:

a. Observe the chest rising and falling
b. Listen and feel the air movement
c. Count the respiration 10 sec and multiply with six
d. Use cardiac monitor

162. An abnormally slow breathing rate is called:

a. Bradypnea b. Bradycardia
c. Tachypnea d. Tachycardia

163. Kussmaul breathing is a deep and labored breathing pattern often associated with:

a. Diabetic ketoacidosis
b. Hepatitis
c. Hepatomegaly
d. Acute renal failure

164. Irregular respiration characterized by apnea and hyperventilation is known as:

a. Cheyne-Stokes respiration
b. Hyperventilation
c. Kussmaul's respiration
d. Sighing

165. Rate of ventilation exceeding normal range is known as:

a. Cheyne-Stokes respiration
b. Hyperventilation
c. Kussmaul's respiration
d. Sighing

166. Respiration is abnormally deep but regular is:

a. Cheyne-Stokes respiration
b. Hyperventilation
c. Kussmaul's respiration
d. Sighing

167. Hypoxia is:

a. Lack of oxygen in the tissues
b. Lack of oxygen in the blood
c. Bluish discoloration of mucosa
d. None of the above

168. Hypoxemia is:

a. Lack of oxygen in the tissues
b. Lack of oxygen in the blood
c. Bluish discoloration of mucosa
d. None of the above

169. While measuring blood-pressure in upper arm, Korskoff's sound is auscultated in .... blood vessel

a. Axillary artery b. Brachial artery
c. Femora. d. Ulnar artery

170. While measuring blood-pressure from leg, Korskoff's sound is auscultated in:

a. Femoral artery b. Popliteal artery
c. Ulnar artery d. Axillary artery

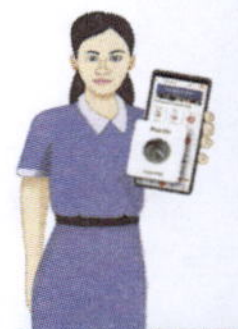

Ans.

153. b
154. b
155. a
156. c
157. a
158. c
159. c
160. a
161. a
162. a
163. a
164. a
165. b
166. c
167. a
168. b
169. b
170. b

HEALTH ASSESSMENT/PHYSICAL EXAMINATION

171. When assessing blood pressure, the sound that is heard through a stethoscope placed over the artery is termed:

a. Crackles b. Korotkoff sound
c. Brachial sounds d. Murmurs

172. The instrument used to measure blood pressure is: *(ESIC Chennai May 2012)*

a. Electrocardiograph b. Stethoscope
c. Rotameter d. Sphygmomanometer

173. Which site is used to assess the status of circulation to lower arms and auscultate blood pressure? *(AIIMS Bhopal Nursing Officer, 2018)*

a. Apical b. Temporal
c. Axillary d. Brachial

Explanation: Circulation to lower arms and BP is measured in brachial artery.

174. Low blood pressure that happens when a person stand up from sitting or lying position is known as:

a. Postural hypotension b. Orthostatic hypotension
c. Supine hypertension d. Both a and b

Explanation: Orthostatic hypotension—also called postural hypotension—is a form of low blood pressure that happens when person stands up from sitting or lying down. Orthostatic hypotension can make the person feel dizzy or lightheaded, and maybe even faint.

175. In a patient with postural hypotension, what is the minimum expected decrease in systolic BP after standing for at least one minute? *(AIIMS MSc 2012)*

a. 5 mm Hg b. 10 mm Hg
c. 15 mm Hg d. 20 mm Hg

Explanation: Systolic blood pressure decrease of at least 20 mm Hg or a diastolic blood pressure decrease of at least 10 mm Hg within three minutes of standing.

176. Which of the following blood pressure readings should be reported immediately to the physician? *(AIIMS Raipur Staff Nurse Grade I-2018)*

a. 130/98 mm Hg b. 140/88 mm Hg
c. 110/70 mm Hg d. 138/82 mm Hg

Explanation: Among the given values, option a has the highest diastolic blood pressure. Diastolic blood pressure gives best idea related to the risk for heart disease or stroke.

177. If a narrow cuff is used for measuring BP, then what will the outcome?

a. Actual reading will be obtained
b. Falsely high reading will be obtained
c. Falsely low reading will be obtained
d. BP can't measure

Explanation: Use of narrow cuff leads to falsely high reading and use of large cuff will cause falsely low reading. The width of the BP cuff should be 40% of the circumference and length of the cuff should be 80% of the circumference.

178. Movement of a body part toward the body's midline is termed as:

a. Abduction b. Adduction
c. Extension d. Pronation

179. Movement of a body part away from the body's midline is termed as:

a. Abduction b. Adduction
c. Extension d. Pronation

180. Bending of a part, or decreasing the angle between two parts is known as:

a. Abduction b. Adduction
c. Flexion d. Extension

181. Increasing the angle between two parts is known as:

a. Abduction b. Adduction
c. Flexion d. Extension

182. Inward movement of the foot is termed as: *New Q*

a. Pronation b. Supination
c. Inversion d. Eversion

Explanation: The tilting of the sole toward the midline of the body (inward movement of the foot) during movement is known as Inversion. Eversion is the movement of turning the sole of the foot outward, away from the midline.

183. Health promotion activities can include all; EXCEPT:

a. Balanced nutrition
b. Habitual drinking of alcohol
c. Exercise
d. Safe sexual practice

184. Which of the following statements accurately defines the term 'health'?

a. Health is a state of optimal functioning
b. Health is an absence of illness
c. Health is always an objective data
d. Health is not determined by the patient

185. Patient's health is determined based upon:

a. Behavior b. Family support
c. Knowledge d. Education

186. Characteristic of a chronic illness is:

a. Has reversible pathologic changes
b. Has a predictable clinical course and prognosis
c. Results in permanent deviation from normal
d. Always starts with an acute illness and then gradually deteriorates

187. Health promotion in the older adult is primarily focused on:

a. Adherence to medication
b. Avoid smoking
c. Teaching positive health behaviors
d. Talking to others

188. A sudden redness of the skin is termed as:

a. Flush b. Jaundice
c. Cyanosis d. Pallor

189. Bad breath is known as:

a. Periodontal disease b. Halitosis
c. Cheilosis d. Sordes

190. First heart sound S1 indicates closure of ....valves.

a. Mitral and tricuspid
b. Aortic and pulmonic
c. Mitral and pulmonic
d. Tricuspid and aortic

191. Second heart sound S2 indicates closure of ....valves.

a. Mitral and tricuspid
b. Aortic and pulmonic
c. Mitral and pulmonic
d. Tricuspid and aortic

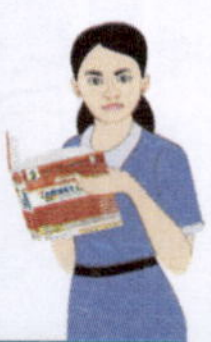

Ans.

171. b
172. d
173. d
174. d
175. d
176. a
177. b
178. b
179. a
180. c
181. d
182. c
183. b
184. a
185. a
186. c
187. c
188. a
189. b
190. a
191. b

192. The nurse is collecting data on a patient with a ruptured appendix that is painful. Where would the nurse expects the patient's pain to be located? *(RAK MSc 2018)*

a. Right upper quadrant b. Right lower quadrant
c. Left upper quadrant d. Left lower quadrant

Explanation: The nurse is collecting data from a patient with a ruptured appendix that is painful. The nurse expects the patient's pain to be located at right lower quadrant. This is known as Rovsing's sign. In ruptured appendix, the pain becomes more diffuse and abdominal distention develops as a result of paralytic ileus.

193. During physical assessment of children, asymmetry of the skull indicates: *(AIIMS Raipur Grade II 2017)*

a. Hydrocephalus b. Craniotabes
c. Craniosynostosis d. Osteogenesis imperfect

Explanation: Craniotabes are softening or thinning of skull in infants and children especially seen in newborns. Osteogenesis imperfecta are genetic disorders that affect bones. Hydrocephalus is a condition in which there is an accumulation of CSF in brain.

194. A low-pitched, continuous gurgling sounds caused by secretions in the large airways is called: ***New Q*** *(AIIMS Raipur Grade II 2017)*

a. Wheezing b. Rhonchi
c. Coughing d. Stridor

Explanation: Rhonchi is a type of adventitious breath sound that is heard during auscultation of the lungs. It is a low-pitched, continuous gurgling sound that is caused by secretions in the large airways.

Wheezing is a high-pitched, musical sound that is heard during expiration and is caused by narrowing of the airways, often due to inflammation or constriction.

Stridor is a harsh, high-pitched sound that is heard during inspiration and is caused by obstruction of the upper airway, such as in cases of croup or epiglottitis.

195. When a nurse is doing a physical examination for a patient, she notices the patient's grimace. The nursing diagnostic process the nurse used here is: *(AIIMS Raipur Grade II 2017)*

a. Data interpretation
b. Data clustering
c. Concept mapping
d. Data Collection

Explanation: Data clustering refers to collection and clubbing of data from different sources such as physical examination, observation and laboratory details. A concept map is a diagram that depicts relationship between concepts mostly used by engineers, designers as a graphical tool to organize and structure knowledge.

196. Positive Babinski is:

a. Abnormal for adults
b. Abnormal for children
c. Abnormal for all age groups
d. All of the above

Explanation: Stroking over the sole causes toe to bend downward, it is negative Babinski and is normal for adults. But in children stroking over the sole causes toe to move upward and outward, that is called positive Babinski and is normal for children up to 2 years of age. Positive Babinski is considered as abnormal for adults.

197. Instrument used for examining eye is:

a. Otoscope b. Proctoscope
c. Ophthalmoscope d. Endoscope

Explanation: Ophthalmoscope, also called funduscope, is an instrument used for inspecting the interior of the eye. Otoscope is used for examining ears and proctoscope is used to examine the anal cavity, rectum and sigmoid colon. Endoscope is used to visualize body cavity.

198. Which among the following data will give more accurate information regarding an end stage renal disease client's fluid status?

a. Daily weight of the client b. Intake and output chart
c. Electrolyte level d. Bowel movement

Explanation: Daily weight of the client gives more accurate information. 1 L = 1 kg (Approx)

199. Visual acuity can be assessed with:

a. Ophthalmoscope b. Snellen chart
c. Goniometer d. Refractometer

Explanation: Visual acuity can be assessed through Snellen's chart. Ophthalmoscope is used to see inside the fundus of the eye and other structures. Goniometer is an instrument for the precise measurement of angles, especially one used to measure the angles between the faces of crystals.

200. In Weber test and Rinne's test cranial nerve examined is:

a. Cranial nerve 1 b. Cranial nerve 2
c. Cranial nerve 7 d. Cranial nerve 8

Explanation: Cranial nerve 8, acoustic is examined through these tests. Cranial nerve 1 is olfactory which helps in smelling, cranial nerve 2 is optic which is assessed with the help of Snellen's chart. Cranial nerve 7 is facial.

201. Goniometer is used to assess: *(DSSSB 2013)*

a. Auditory faculty b. Muscle strength
c. Range of motion of joints d. Visual acuity

Explanation: An instrument for the precise measurement of angles, especially one used to measure the angles between the faces of crystals and it measures range of motion of joints angles of the body, thereby helps to track the progress of the rehabilitation program.

202. Lateral curvature of the spine is called as: *(DSSSB 2013)*

a. Kyphosis b. Lordosis
c. Scoliosis d. Pectus Excavatum

Explanation: Anterior curvature of spine = Lordosis
- **Posterior curvature of spine = Kyphosis**
- **Lateral curvature of spine = Scoliosis**

203. The equipment used in the examination of ears is: *(DSSSB 2013)*

a. Laryngoscope b. Ophthalmoscope
c. Otoscope d. Proctoscope

Explanation: An otoscope or auriscope is a medical device which is used to look into the ears. Healthcare providers use otoscopes to screen for illness during regular check-ups and also to investigate ear symptoms. An otoscope potentially gives a view of the ear canal and tympanic membrane or eardrum.

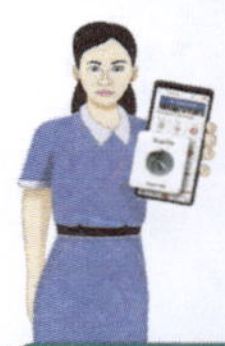

Ans.

192. b
193. c
194. b
195. b
196. a
197. c
198. a
199. b
200. d
201. c
202. c
203. c

204. The nurse is auscultating the client's lung fields. The systematic pattern used for comparison is:

a. Anterior to posterior b. Interspace to intraspace
c. Side to side d. Top to bottom

Explanation: Intensity, pitch, duration and quality of breath sounds are compared side to side on auscultation of lung fields.

205. History and physical examination of a client will help the nurse in:

a. Evaluation of the therapy
b. Health teaching
c. Assessment
d. Nursing diagnoses and collaborative problems

206. Instrument to detect the color of a solution is: *(Banaras HU 2015)*

a. Calorimeter b. Flame photometer
c. Chromatography d. Colorimeter

207. Which of the following lung sounds is predominant in a patient with asthma in exacerbation?

a. Rhonchi b. Crakes
c. Pleural rub d. Wheezes

208. Crackling sounds bilaterally at the bases of lungs is referred to as:

a. Rhonchi b. Wheezing
c. Rales d. Pleural rub

209. Redness over the bony prominence of a bed ridden patient suggests:

a. Ulceration b. Bedsore
c. Poor nutritional status d. Wound infection

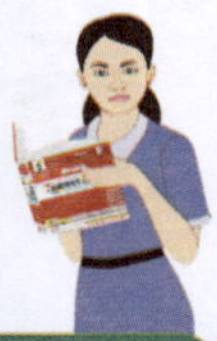

210. Which of the following strategy is not effective in enhancing a patient's impaired vision?

a. Use bright colors around patient
b. Stand in patient's field of vision
c. Use of fluorescent lighting
d. Ensure enough light inside the room

211. Which of the following causes crackles in breath sounds?

a. Pulmonary emboli b. Moisture in air passages
c. Narrowed bronchioles d. Dryness in the upper airway

212. Deep palpation is used to assess:

a. Internal Organs b. Internal masses
c. Skin turgor d. Both a and b

213. Which of the following substances is likely to increase the urine excretion?

a. Mushrooms
b. Caffeine-containing drinks, such as coffee and cola
c. Urinary analgesics
d. NSAIDs

214. Which of the following assessment data is a normal finding when performing percussion of the client's chest?

a. Resonance b. Hyperresonance
c. Tympany d. Dullness

215. Which among the following physical examination techniques requires stethoscope?

a. Observation b. Percussion
c. Palpation d. Auscultation

216. Normal biceps reflex response is:

a. Flexion of arm at elbow b. Extension of arm at elbow
c. Extension of leg at knee d. Flexion of leg at knee

217. Normal triceps reflex response is:

a. Flexion of arm at elbow b. Extension of arm at elbow
c. Extension of leg at knee d. Flexion of leg at knee

218. Normal patellar reflex response is:

a. Flexion of arm at elbow b. Extension of arm at elbow
c. Extension of leg at knee d. Flexion of leg at knee

219. Normal achilles reflex response is:

a. Flexion of arm at elbow b. Extension of arm at elbow
c. Extension of leg at knee d. Plantar flexion of foot

220. Normal plantar (Babinski) reflex response in adult is:

a. Flexion of arm at elbow b. Extension of arm at elbow
c. Extension of leg at knee d. Bending of toe downward

Explanation: In adults, **a normal plantar reflex response** (also known as Babinski reflex) is characterized by a downward curling of the toes, with no fanning or extension of the toes. When the sole of the foot is stroked with a blunt object, the big toe should move downward, while the other toes may flex slightly but should not move upward or fan out.

An abnormal response, also known as a positive Babinski sign, is characterized by the extension of the big toe and fanning out of the other toes

221. Muscle strength 5 means:

a. Normal b. Good
c. Fair d. Poor

222. While assessing cranial nerve of a patient, the nurse asks the patient to raise the eyebrow, smile and show the teeth. The nurse is examining ______ cranial nerve.

a. Vagus b. Optic
c. Olfactory d. Facial

223. Level of consciousness of a client is assessed using: *(DSSSB 2013)*

a. Lund Browder method b. Braden Scale
c. Glasgow Coma scale d. Snellen chart

Explanation: Option c is the answer. Lund Browder method is for the assessment of extent of burn injury assessment, Braden scale is used for the assessment of risk of bedsore, and Snellen chart is for assessment of visual acuity. Glasgow Coma Scale (GCS) contains three domains such as eye opening, motor response and verbal response. Maximum score is 15 and minimum is 3.

224. Which of the following is used for assessing the pain in children? *(DSSSB 2013)*

a. Verbal descriptor scale
b. Numerical rating scale
c. Visual analogue scale
d. Wong Baker Faces pain rating scale

Explanation:

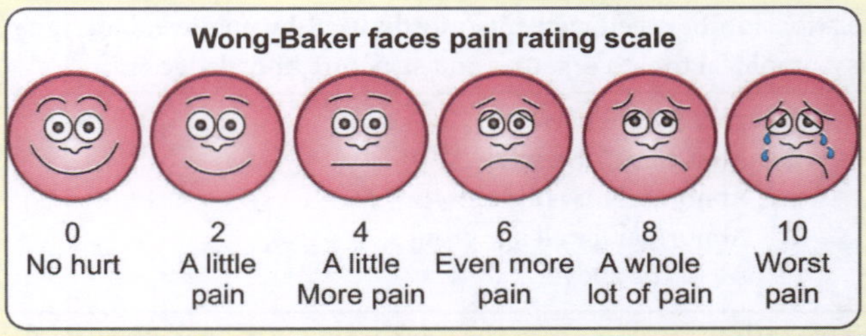

225. Use of pain scale is an example of adherence to .... intellectual standard

a. Specificity b. Accuracy
c. Consistency d. Responsibility

Ans.

204.	c
205.	d
206.	d
207.	d
208.	c
209.	b
210.	c
211.	b
212.	d
213.	b
214.	a
215.	d
216.	a
217.	b
218.	c
219.	d
220.	d
221.	a
222.	d
223.	c
224.	d
225.	c

Explanation: Different nurses use same scale to collect data thus adhere to consistency in data collection.

226. A comprehensive health assessment of an older person includes: *(LNJP H D 2012)*

a. Functional assessment
b. Clinical assessment
c. Psychosocial assessment
d. All of these

227. The first assessment performed by the nurse while initiating nurse-patient relationship is:

a. Vital signs
b. Appearance and behavior
c. Observing specific body systems
d. Collection of a detailed health history

228. Reassessment of client is:

a. Carried out when the client complains of discomfort
b. Done as per the nurse's convenience
c. Carried out during emergency situations
d. A continuous process

229. At what time nurse assess the gait of an ambulatory patient?

a. After the neurologic assessment
b. At the end of the physical examination
c. While the patient is lying supine on the examining table
d. When the patient walks into the room

230. During the examination of ear of a 2-year-old child, the pinna needs to be held in .... direction:

a. Upward and backward
b. Downward and backward
c. Straightly back
d. Pull it downward

Explanation: For examination of ear, straighten the patient's ear canal by pulling the pinna downward and backward in children <3 years. Pull upward and backward in children aged 3 years and above.

231. Adequacy of collateral circulation before radial artery cannulation is done with the help of .... test:

a. Allen's test b. Weber's test
c. Rinnie's test d. Cold's test

Explanation: Allen's test will be performed to find out the adequacy of ulnar circulation before radial artery cannulation. Option b and c belong to hearing assessment. Cold test is a urine test done to examine urine for albumin.

232. Which of the following is used to assess the function of brain stem? *(DSSSB 2013)*

a. Cold calorie test
b. Glasgow Coma scale
c. Braden scale
d. Intracranial pressure

Explanation: Cold calorie test is performed to assess the function of brain stem.

233. Air conduction and bone conduction is tested using which among the following test?

a. Weber's test
b. Rinne's test
c. Romberg's test
d. Allen's test

234. Apart from Vital signs, which of the following assessment would provide most important assessment information of a ten month old infant with diarrhea and dehydration?

a. Stool specimen analysis
b. Infant's body weight
c. Inspection of infant's posterior fontanel
d. Urine specimen analysis

235. All are the components of Braden scale; EXCEPT:

a. Sensory perception
b. Shear
c. Mobility
d. Length of hospital stay

Explanation: Length of hospital stay is not a component. Components of Braden scale include sensory perception, moisture, activity, mobility, nutrition, and friction or shear.

236. All of the following are the methods to calculate extent of burn injury; EXCEPT:

a. Rule of nine b. Waterlow method
c. Lund Browder method d. Palmar method

Explanation: Waterlow method is used to assess the risk of pressure ulcer in a bedridden client. Other methods are used in calculation of area of burn injury. Rule-of-nine estimates the body surface area on an adult that has been burned by using multiples of nine. Lund Browder is a method for estimating the extent of burns that allows for the varying proportion of body surface in persons of different ages. In Palmar method scattered burn percentage is calculated by considering patient's own palm as 1%.

237. The type of assessment that includes data related to a client's biological, cultural, spiritual and social need is called: *(AIIMS-BBS SNO 2019)*

a. Behavioral assessment
b. Screening assessment
c. Comprehensive assessment
d. Focused assessment

Explanation: Comprehensive means including everything. Assessing biological, cultural, spiritual and social needs is called comprehensive assessment. Behavioral assessment is a method used to assess behavior. Screening is a process for evaluating the possible presence of a particular problem. Detailed nursing assessment of specific body system(s) relating to the presenting problem is known as screening.

238. The nurse in charge is assessing a patient's abdomen. Which examination technique should the nurse use first? *(AIIMS Raipur NO 2019)*

a. Auscultation b. Palpation
c. Percussion d. Inspection

Explanation: While performing physical examination, the sequence of techniques: 1. Inspection, 2. Palpation, 3. Percussion, and 4. Auscultation.

While performing abdominal examination, the sequence of techiques: 1. Inspection, 2. Auscultation, 3. Percussion and 4. Palpation. Because palpation and percussion can alter bowel sounds, so auscultation should be performed before percussion and palpation.

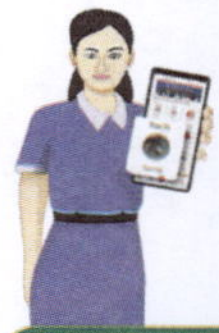

Ans.

226. d
227. b
228. d
229. d
230. b
231. a
232. a
233. b
234. b
235. d
236. b
237. c
238. d

TYPES OF NURSING MODALITIES

239. Which of the following is the responsibilities of the staff nurse? *(AIIMS Raipur Staff Nurse Grade I-2018)*

a. Quality care b. Observation & reporting
c. Record keeping d. All of these

240. The nursing care that focuses on patient care along with the family needs, in the scope of multidisciplinary healthcare team is called: *(AIIMS Bhopal Nursing Officer, 2018)*

a. Team based care b. Case management
c. Patient navigation care d. Primary care

Explanation: Above given definition indicates case management. Team based care means redistribution of work among members of a practicing team. Patient navigation care means an individual or patient navigator helps the individual to go through treatment and care. Primary care is the day to day healthcare given by healthcare provider. Typically this provider acts as first level of contacting and principal point of continuing care.

241. A single nurse is assigned for care and she is responsible for directing and coordinating other nurses and other personnel. This type of nursing is known as:

a. Functional nurse b. Primary nurse
c. Team nursing d. Total patient care

Explanation: Option b is the correct answer. Functional nursing is task oriented. Team nursing is decision-making that occurs over a single shift; largely by team leader or nurse manager. In total patient care, decision-making occurs over a single shift—either by an RN caring for the patient or by a charge nurse.

242. Which of the following is a type of nursing modality in which the principal idea is that nurses to be assigned tasks, not patients?

a. Team nursing b. Functional nursing
c. Primary nursing d. Case method nursing

Explanation: In functional nursing, Nurses are assigned to specific task and do that duty only. The nurse performs a particular task for every patient in the ward. For example, Medication Nurse, Dressing Nurse, IV Nurse, etc. In team nursing, nurse is responsible for most of the each patient's care. Some of the duties are assigned to other nurses or nursing assistants.

243. Which nursing modality involves assigning a specific task to each nurse to perform for every patient in the ward? *New Q*

a. Primary Nursing b. Team Nursing
c. Modular Nursing d. Functional Nursing

244. Which of the following patient care models is suitable when there are many patients but very few nurses:

a. Total patient care
b. Functional nursing
c. Team nursing
d. Advanced Nursing

245. Which nursing modality, The Nurse Manager assigns a group of patients to an individual Registered Nurse? *New Q*

a. Primary nursing
b. Team nursing
c. Modular nursing
d. Functional nursing

246. Which of the following nursing modality is commonly used in Hospice care and home health? *New Q*

a. Primary nursing
b. Case management
c. Modular nursing
d. Functional nursing

247. In a hospital setting, who is responsible for informing the patient about surgery along with possible outcome, risk, complications and benefits?

a. Nurse b. Nurse in-charge
c. Surgeon d. ANS

248. Clients are referred to as 'residents' in:

a. Day care centers
b. Long-term care facilities
c. Hospitals
d. Custodial care centers

249. The type of nursing care assignment best suited in an intensive care unit is: *(RAK MSc 2018)*

a. Case method b. Functional method
c. Primary care method d. Team method

Explanation: Case method is the oldest method of patient care delivery. One professional nurse assumes total responsibilities of providing complete care to one or more patients. This method is frequently used in ICU's.

250. The nursing care that focuses on patient care along with the family needs, in the scope of multidisciplinary healthcare team is called: *(AIIMS BPL NO 2018)*

a. Team based care b. Case management
c. Patient navigation d. Primary care

Explanation: Case management is a collaborative process of assessment, planning, facilitation, care coordination, evaluation and advocacy for options and services to meet an individual's and family's comprehensive health needs through communication and available resources to promote quality cost effective outcomes.

251. Collaborative intervention refers to therapies that requires:

a. Physician and nurse interventions
b. Nurse and client interventions
c. Nursing team interventions
d. Multiple healthcare professionals

MEDICAL AND SURGICAL ASEPSIS

252. Medical asepsis differs from surgical asepsis in that it is aimed at: *(ESIC 2019)*

a. Preventing transmission of microorganisms
b. Preventing entry of microorganisms into the body
c. Sterilizing all equipment
d. Killing all microorganisms

Explanation: Surgical asepsis or "sterile technique" is used in surgery and invasive procedure. It aims to prevent entry of microorganisms into the body, sterilizing all equipment and at killing all microorganisms and spores (sterilization). Whereas the medical asepsis or 'clean technique' that involves procedures to reduce the number and transmission of pathogens.

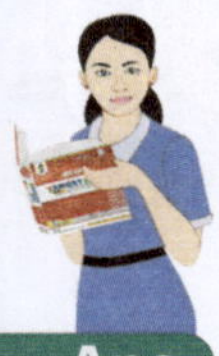

Ans.

239. d
240. b
241. b
242. b
243. d
244. b
245. b
246. a
247. c
248. b
249. a
250. b
251. d
252. a

253. Sterile technique is also called:

a. Medical asepsis
b. Surgical asepsis
c. Autoclaving
d. Disinfection

Explanation: Surgical asepsis (sterile technique); Practices that keep an area or object free from all microorganisms non-pathogenic and pathogenic including spores and viruses.

254. An agent which kills pathogenic bacteria is called: *(RRB SSNE 2015)*

a. Asepsis b. Disinfectant
c. Fomite d. Bacteriostat

255. Which of the following techniques is appropriate for wound dressing:

a. Medical asepsis
b. Surgical asepsis
c. Septic technique
d. Medical and surgical asepsis

256. An agent which has the power to kill bacteria is:

a. Antiseptic b. Bacteriostatic
c. Bactericidal d. Disinfectant

257. The amount of moisture in the air is recorded with: *(Staff Nurse G II 2014)*

a. Anemometer b. Hygrometer
c. Barometer d. Six's thermometer

258. What is the other name of thumb forceps? *(LNJP H D 2012)*

a. Needle holder b. Mosquito forceps
c. Kelly's forceps d. Mouse's teeth

259. Which of the following agents is used to eliminate disease-causing organisms by loosening and removing dirt and grime to which the organisms are attached? *New Q*

a. Antiseptic agent b. Chemical disinfectant
c. Cleansing agent d. Sterilizing agent

Explanation: A cleansing agent is a type of agent that is used to remove dirt and other materials from a surface or object. This can help to eliminate microorganisms that may be attached to the surface, thereby reducing the risk of infection.

BASIC PRINCIPLES OF SURGICAL ASEPSIS

260. Before the surgical procedure, obtaining informed consent is the responsibility of:

a. Physician b. CNO
c. Head nurse d. Nurse

Explanation: Obtaining informed consent is the responsibility of physician.

261. All of the following statements are correct regarding surgical asepsis; EXCEPT:

a. Sterile objects to be held above the level of waist
b. One inch of the outside edge of the sterile field is considered as contaminated
c. Never reach across the sterile field
d. Forceps soaked in disinfectant are considered to be sterile

Explanation: Forceps soaked in disinfectant are not considered to be sterile. Other important principles of surgical asepsis are:

- Only a sterile object to touch another sterile object
- **One inch (2.5 cm)** of the outside edge of a sterile field to be considered as contaminated.
- A wet field is considered as contaminated if the surface below (paper or cloth used as a field for sterile set up) is unsterile.
- Avoid spilling any solution/liquid on a paper or cloth used as a field for sterile set up.
- Sterile objects to be held **above the level of waist.**
- To prevent contamination from droplet, the nurse should avoid Coughing, sneezing, talking or reaching over a sterile field.
- The nurse should not turn her back on a sterile field that may prevent contamination of sterile field while it is out of her view.
- Never reach across the sterile field
- Forceps soaked in disinfectant are not to be considered as sterile.
- If there is any doubt an object of its sterility, considered it as unsterile

262. While wearing sterile gloves, first glove needs to be worn in ....hand?

a. Any hand b. Dominant hand
c. Non-dominant hand d. Always right hand

Explanation: Putting on the dominant hand glove first can minimize the risk of ripping or contamination to the hand that is likely used most.

263. You are irrigating a draining wound with sterile saline solution. Which of the following would be the most appropriate procedure to follow: *(LNJP H D 2012)*

a. Prepare sterile field, put on sterile gloves and remove soiled dressing, wash hands
b. Wash hands, wear clean gloves, remove soiled dressing, remove gloves, wash hands, wear sterile gloves, prepare sterile field
c. Remove soiled dressing, flush wound and wash hands, prepare sterile field
d. Pour solution, wash hands and remove soiled dressing, prepare sterile field

264. Which of the following term refers to the meaning of freedom or liberty from the disease causing Organism;

a. Sterility b. Sepsis
c. Asepsis d. Disinfectant

265. While rinsing the hand for the preparation of medical asepsis, the hand should be held:

a. Upward
b. Downward
c. Sideward
d. Toward the other hand.

266. The hand to be held upwards in which type of asepsis procedure?

a. Surgical asepsis
b. Medical asepsis
c. Both surgical and medical asepsis
d. None of the above

Explanation: In surgical asepsis, the hand to be held upwards in order to prevent any accidental contamination before any surgical procedure.

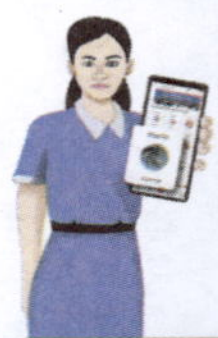

Ans.

253. b
254. b
255. b
256. c
257. b
258. d
259. c
260. a
261. d
262. b
263. b
264. c
265. b
266. a

267. The Nurse in the scrubbing area should consider what distance from the edges of the sterile field as contaminated?

a. 1 inch/2.5 cm b. 0.5 inch/1 cm
c. 3 inch/7 cm d. 3.5 inch/8.5 cm

Explanation: The distance of 2.5 cm to 3 cm (1 inch) around the outer edges of the sterile filed would be considered as contaminated and sterile materials should not be placed in this area.

268. What should a Nurse do when her sterile field made with sterile cloth or paper become wet?

a. Clean the area with dry gauze
b. Cover the area using sponge
c. Considered as a contaminated one
d. Considered as a sterile one.

269. What would be the primary objective of aseptic techniques and the procedure followed by the nurse in her working area?

a. Protect the healthcare worker
b. For the safety of the patient
c. Restrict and get rid of microorganism
d. To protect both Nurse and patient.

270. If a nurses turns back to the sterile field it would be considered as:

a. Still sterile
b. Contaminated
c. Nurse got contaminated
d. None of the above

Explanation: Although a Nurse made herself sterile by following the asepsis technique, the back of the person is considered as a nonsterile field.

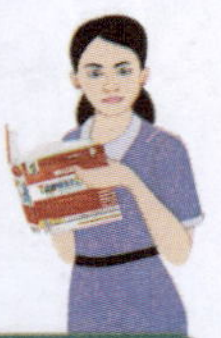

271. During a surgery, a new circulatory nurse mistakenly touches the sterile field, what is the main action the circulatory nurse needs to do?

a. To correct his mistake and not to do again
b. Immediately inform the operating surgeon
c. Not to tell anyone regarding this error
d. None of the above

CHAIN OF INFECTION

272. A toxin or other foreign substance that induces an immune response in the body is known as:

a. Complement b. Antigen
c. Antibody d. All of these

273. The most efficient way to break the chain of infection is by:

a. Hand hygiene b. PPE
c. Wearing gloves d. Isolation of patient

274. The diseases that can be transmitted directly from one person to another person is termed:

a. Contact diseases
b. Communicable diseases
c. Vector borne diseases
d. Air borne diseases

275. What is the First and Primary step in the stages of Infection:

a. Reservoir host b. Portal of exit
c. Infectious Agents d. Portal of entry

276. If a human being acts as a reservoir in the phase of chain of infection, he/she would be referred to as:

a. Host b. Carrier
c. Transporter d. Agent

277. The mode of transmission of infectious agent takes via various agents. If a disease gets contracted from the animal to the human being, it would be referred to as:

a. Zoonoses b. Xerophilous
c. Zygotic d. Fomites

278. If a person receives certain kind of vaccination for a particular infectious disease, it will break which link in the chain of infection?

a. Portal of entry
b. Portal of exist
c. Mode of transmission
d. Susceptible host

279. A male teenager fell from his cycle and injured his hand. His mother cleans the wound and bandaged the area. These interventions will break which link in the chain of infection?

a. Portal of exit
b. Portal of entry
c. Mode of transmission
d. Infectious agent

280. A Nurse washes her hand regularly after every contact with the contaminated materials, this would break which link in the chain of infection?

a. Mode of transmission
b. Infectious agent
c. Portal of exit
d. Portal of entry

281. A nurse working in the TB ward, directing the patients to wear mask regularly over their mouth and nose. These kind of actions will break which link in the chain of infection?

a. Mode of transmission b. Portal of entry
c. Portal of exit d. Reservoir

Explanation: Wearing mask on the facial region will prevent of organism exited to the outer atmosphere rapidly and reduce the transmission of disease.

282. Actions taken to destroy and eliminate the polluted standing water thereby to reduce the mosquito growth and population, will break which link in the chain of infection:

a. Susceptible Host
b. Reservoir
c. Mode of transmission
d. Portal of entry.

STAGES OF INFECTION

283. During infection, which among the following values will be elevated?

a. RBC b. WBC
c. Platelet d. ESR

Explanation: WBCs are responsible for fighting against infection, so this value will be elevated first.

284. In the stages of infection, what would referred to the period between a person get infected with a microorganism and the appearance of first signs and symptoms related to that condition?

a. Prodromal stage
b. Incubation period
c. Convalescence period
d. Decline stage

Ans.

267. a
268. c
269. c
270. b
271. b
272. b
273. a
274. b
275. c
276. b
277. a
278. d
279. b
280. a
281. c
282. b
283. b
284. b

285. Infected people don't realize their symptoms more, but the pathogen gets multiplied within their body and they spread that infection to other people. This stage of infection is referred to as:

a. Prodromal stage b. Incubation period
c. Illness stage d. Convalescence stage

286. A person feels specific signs and symptoms to the infectious agent that he/she got infected in his/her body, refers to which stage of infection?

a. Convalescence stage b. Incubation period
c. Illness stage d. Prodromal stage

287. In which stage of the disease stage, the person gets back to his/her healthy life and all the signs and symptoms get subsided and experience the recovery from the infection?

a. Incubation period b. Predromal stage
c. Convalescence stage d. Prodromal stage

288. In the infectious stage, the term describing the "Severity of a disease" following an infection is referred to as:

a. Harmfulness b. Virulence
c. Pathogenicity d. Infectivity

289. What would be the name of a microorganism that lives on another organism for its metabolic growth and development and it lives completely depending on other organism:

a. Pathogen
b. Host
c. Parasite
d. Vector

290. In this stage of infection, the immune response gets intensively triggered and manifests excessive symptoms in a person's body:

a. Incubation Period b. Illness period
c. Prodromal stage d. Convalescent period

Explanation: Immune system fights very high and stirs excessively during the illness period comparing to the other stages of infection.

291. The term that refers to the origin, which is either animate or inanimate that would be the etiology and beginning point that links the infectious cycle is:

a. Pathogens b. Vector
c. Source d. Host.

292. All of the following are vector borne diseases; EXCEPT:

a. Encephalitis b. Dengue
c. Lyme disease d. Typhoid

293. The mechanism that enables the HIV virus to bind with the White Blood Cells of human beings:

a. Tapered hooks b. Slime mechanism
c. Viral spikes d. Protein binds

PREVENTION OF CROSS INFECTION IN HOSPITAL

294. Germ theory of disease was propounded by: *(Staff Nurse G II 2014)*

a. Darwin b. Freud
c. Louis Pasteur d. Erickson

295. Which of the following concept of health is associated with germ theory of disease?

a. Biomedical concept b. Holistic concept
c. Psychosocial concept d. Ecological concept

296. Iatrogenic infections are infections developed due to:

a. Hospital admission
b. Therapeutic procedure
c. Exposure to affected person
d. Low immunity

297. The best way to decrease the risk of transferring pathogens to a patient when removing contaminated gloves is to: *(AIIMS Raipur NO 2019)*

a. Wash the gloves before removing them
b. Gently pull on the fingers of the gloves when removing them
c. Gently pull just below the cuff and invert the gloves when removing them
d. Remove the gloves and then turn the inside out

298. The nurse is assigned to a patient who has a bacterial pneumonia and is under droplet precautions, which personal protective equipment (PPE) will she wear to deliver the meal tray? *(ESIC 2019)*

a. No PPE required
b. Only mask is needed
c. Special filtration mask and gloves
d. Gown, mask, gloves, shoe covers

Explanation: Only mask is needed for protection against droplet infection. Gloves or gown are not necessary to protect from droplet infection.

299. The most common site of hospital-acquired infection is: *(AIIMS BPL NO 2018)*

a. Surgical sites b. Respiratory tract
c. Urinary tract d. Eyes

Explanation: Urinary infections are the most common nosocomial infection; 80% of infections are associated with the use of an indwelling urinary catheter.

300. What type of isolation precaution is in use when a patient is asked to wear mask? *(AIIMS Raipur Staff Nurse Grade I-2018)*

a. Blood safety b. Contact
c. Droplet d. Standard

Explanation: Droplet infections are transmitted from one individual to another by droplets of moisture expelled from the upper respiratory tract through coughing or sneezing. By wearing the mask this kind of infection can be prevented.

301. Infection occurs following treatment modality or procedures is known as:

a. Iatrogenic infection b. Nosocomial infection
c. Concurrent infection d. Fomite infection

Explanation: Iatrogenic infection occurs as a result of diagnostic and, or therapeutic procedures on a patient. Nosocomial infections are those infections that occur in patient after 48 hours of hospital stay. Concurrent infection is the term used when a patient has two or more simultaneous infections. Fomite infections refer to infections transmitted by objects.

302. Most effective way to prevent cross infection in hospital setting is:

a. Hand washing
b. Use alcohol based hand rub between patients
c. Screen the visitors
d. Ensure adequate ventilation

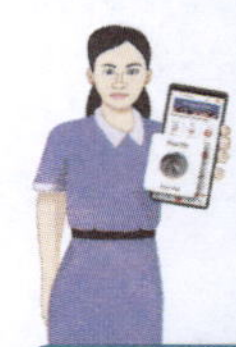

Ans.

285. a
286. c
287. c
288. b
289. c
290. b
291. c
292. d
293. c
294. c
295. a
296. b
297. c
298. b
299. c
300. c
301. a
302. a

Explanation: Hand washing is the most effective way. Alcoholic hand rubs are not a substitute for hand washing.

303. What type of isolation is most appropriate for a patient diagnosed with methicillin resistant staphylococcus aureus (MRSA) pneumonia?

a. Standard precautions b. Contact isolation
c. Respiratory isolation d. Reverse isolation

Explanation: The hands of healthcare workers are the principal mode of transmission for MRSA. In the given example, the organism is limited to sputum. As the principal mode of transmission is through hands of healthcare personnel, contact isolation is necessary with a private room, Body Substance Isolation (barrier protection using gloves, mask, gown, goggle, etc.), and good hand washing techniques.

304. Which of the following infections agent can be transmitted by blood transfusion? *(LNJP H D 2012)*

a. Hepatitis b. HIV
c. Plasmodium d. All of these

305. Which of the following procedures requires a nurse to wear gloves?

a. Back massage b. Providing passive exercise
c. Feeding d. Providing Oral hygiene

306. The mode of transmission of trachoma from one person to other person is: *(AIIMS Raipur Grade II 2017)*

a. Air borne b. Direct and indirect contact
c. Blood borne d. Iatrogenic

Explanation Trachoma spreads by direct contact with fingers or fomites (indirect, e.g., washcloths, handkerchiefs) contaminated with eye discharge from an infected person or by eye-seeking flies.

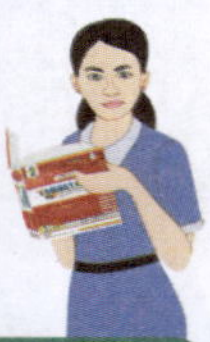

Ans.
303. b
304. d
305. d
306. b
307. c
308. d
309. b
310. a
311. a
312. b
313. d

METHODS OF STERILIZATION AND DISINFECTION

307. The process by which, medium is placed at 100°C in flowing steam for 30 minutes each on 3 successive days is: *(AIIMS Raipur Grade II 2017)*

a. Steam under pressure b. Autoclave
c. Tyndallization d. Inspissation

Explanation: Autoclaves are used to sterilize equipment and supplies at high pressure saturated steam at 121°C for around 15-20 minutes. Tyndallization is a method of heating article for three successive days, first day at 85°C for 60 minutes, second day 75 to 80°C for 20 minutes and third day 75 to 85°C for 20 minutes.

308. To sterilize disposable syringes, the method of sterilization used is: *(AIIMS Raipur Grade II 2017)*

a. Autoclaving
b. Infrared radiation
c. Ultraviolet radiation
d. Gamma radiation

Explanation: Ethylene oxide is used to sterilize devices that incorporate electronic components, plastic packaging or plastic containers. Infrared radiation is used to sterilize articles such as syringes and catheters. UV radiations are used for disinfecting enclosed areas such as operation theaters and laboratories.

309. Sharp instrument should not be sterilized by: *(AIIMS Raipur Staff Nurse Grade I-2018)*

a. Cooling b. Boiling
c. Hot air oven d. Antiseptic solution

Explanation: Boiling the sharp instruments lose their sharpness through repeated boiling. Other methods are suitable for sharp instruments as they keep the instruments functional.

310. Tubes and catheters are disinfected with:

a. 2% Glutaraldehyde b. 1% hypochlorite
c. Formalin d. Korsolex

Explanation: 2% Glutaraldehyde - To disinfect tubes and Catheters

1% hypochlorite - Surface disinfection; blood spillage, liquid waste disinfection

Formalin - Used for preservation of tissue and anatomical specimens

Korsolex - Used to disinfect heat sensitive instruments

311. Immediate disinfection of all articles and bodily discharge during the course of disease is known as:

a. Concurrent disinfection b. Recurrent disinfection
c. Terminal disinfection d. Sterilization

Explanation: Concurrent disinfection refers to application of disinfective measures as soon as possible after discharge of infectious material from the body of an infected person, or after soiling of articles with such infectious discharges. Concurrent disinfection is done for urine, feces, clothes, dressings, etc., throughout the course of illness.

Recurrent (prophylactic) disinfection refers to prevention of an infection by chlorination of water, pasteurization of milk, hand washing, etc.

Terminal disinfection refers to application of disinfective measures after the patient has been removed, e.g., by death, or has ceased to be a source of infection.

Sterilization is different from disinfection and bactericidal refers to a, b.

312. What do you mean by cold sterilization?

a. Sterilization under a temperature range of 1–80°C
b. Disinfection using disinfectant
c. Sterilization done under minus degree Celsius temperature
d. All of the above

Explanation: *Cold* (chemical) *sterilization* is the use of liquid chemical solutions (disinfectants) to *sterilize* medical instruments. In other words, disinfection done using disinfectant is known as cold sterilization.

313. Identify incorrect statement regarding care of rubber article used in hospital setting?

a. Rubber articles will be destroyed by heat
b. Do not fold rubber articles, roll them instead
c. Do not pin on rubber articles
d. Rubber articles are sterilized using dry heat method

Explanation: Rubber articles are sterilized by autoclaving or Ethylene Oxide Gas Method. In autoclaving method, Temperature must not exceed 134°C (250°F) for 15 minutes. All reusable rubber and plastic products with the exception of cushion masks may be sterilized using ETO if sufficient aeration is provided.

314. All of the following statements regarding boiling as a sterilization method is true; EXCEPT:
a. Most economical way of sterilizing articles
b. Some bacteria, viruses and spores are resistant to boiling
c. It is not a suitable method for those articles which will be destroyed by heat and moist
d. Effective boiling time for articles is 10 minutes

Explanation: Boiling works on microorganisms by changing the physical properties of proteins, causing them to coagulate and stop functioning. Boiling the object(s) for a minimum of 30 minutes is required for effective sterilization.

315. The solution used to disinfect the bed linen of HIV positive patient is: *(DSSSB 2013)*
a. Dettol b. Lysol
c. Savlon d. Sodium hypochlorite

Explanation: Sodium hypochlorite is used to disinfect the bed linen of HIV patient. Linen should be soaked for 20 minutes. Sodium Hypochlorite is also known as polar solution.

316. Inoculating loop is sterilized by: *(Banaras HU 2015)*
a. Hot air oven b. Autoclave
c. Flaming d. Radiation

317. Residual chlorine in water is determined by: **New Q**
a. Starch iodide method
b. Orthotolidine method
c. Both a and b
d. Oxidation test

318. All these are sterilized by chemicals; EXCEPT: *(ESIC Chennai May 2012)*
a. Endoscopes b. Gauze
c. Scissors d. Cables

319. Recommended disinfectant used for handling spills is: *(LNJP H D 2012)*
a. 10% sodium hypochlorite
b. 5% bleach solution
c. 1% sodium hypochlorite
d. 2% bleach solution

320. Which of the following chemicals is most powerful disinfectant? *(LNJP H D 2012)*
a. Dettol b. Lysol
c. Phenol d. $KMnO_4$.

321. Fresh bleaching powder contains: *(RRB Feb 2012)*
a. 0.033% chlorine b. 33% chlorine
c. 0.33% chlorine d. 3.3% chlorine

322. HIV contaminated waste products can be decontaminated by:
a. Formaldehyde b. Sodium hypochlorite
c. Glutaraldehyde d. All of these

323. Temperature range used in autoclaving is:
a. 121-123°F b. 150-200°F
c. 250-254°F d. 260-275°F

324. Pressure range used in autoclaving is:
a. 10-12 pounds b. 15-17 pounds
c. 18-20 pounds d. 20-22 pounds

325. Solution of choice for disinfecting enamelware item is:
a. 0.5% chlorine
b. 2% glutaraldehyde
c. 50-70% alcohol
d. Savlon

326. Fiber optic items are disinfected with:
a. 0.5% chlorine b. 2% glutaraldehyde
c. 50-70% alcohol d. Salvon

327. Solution used in suction bottle before suctioning with disinfection purpose is:
a. Sodium hypochlorite b. Savlon
c. Chlorine d. Cidex

328. Agent used to inhibit the growth of bacteria:
a. Antiseptic b. Bacteriostatic
c. Bactericidal d. Disinfectant

329. Cidex is also known as:
a. Glutaraldehyde b. Formaldehyde
c. Korsolex d. Hypochlorate

SPECIMEN COLLECTION

330. Mantoux test is to determine: *(LNJP H D 2012)*
a. Tuberculosis
b. Measles
c. Diphtheria
d. AIDS

331. Urine bile can be tested through .... test:
a. Hay's test
b. Benedict Test
c. Fehling's Test
d. Cold test

Explanation: Hay's test is used to detect urine bile presence. Benedict's and Fehling's tests are used to detect urine sugar and cold test and hot test are used to detect urine albumin.

332. The most appropriate time for the nurse to obtain a sputum specimen for culture is: *(AIIMS Raipur NO 2019)*
a. Early in the morning
b. After the patient eats a light breakfast
c. After aerosol therapy
d. After chest physiotherapy

Explanation: Fresh early morning sample is preferred because secretions accumulate overnight. Secretions must be of sputum for accurate findings.

After breakfast, sputum will be mixed with food and findings will be altered. Sample after aerosol therapy will alter findings. Chest therapy may help in excretion of secretion, but the sample should be fresh in the morning.

333. Which test is done for identifying the presence of occult blood in stool? *(AIIMS BBS NO 2018)*
a. Fouchet's test b. Benzidine test
c. Orthotolidine test d. Guaiac test

Explanation: The stool guaiac test screens for hidden (occult) blood in a stool sample. It is the most common type of fecal occult blood test (FOBT). The test involves placing a fecal sample on guaiac paper and applying hydrogen peroxide which, in the presence of blood, yields a blue reaction product within seconds.

334. Which is the preservative used in 24 hour urine collection?
a. Toluene b. Boric acid
c. 50% Acetic acid d. All of these

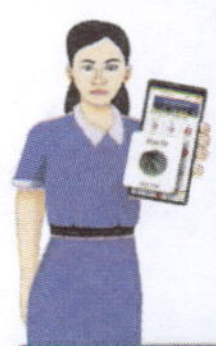

Ans.
314. d
315. d
316. c
317. c
318. b
319. c
320. c
321. b
322. d
323. c
324. b
325. a
326. b
327. a
328. b
329. a
330. a
331. a
332. a
333. d
334. d

Explanation: All of the above mentioned preservatives and concentrated HCl and chloroform are also used as a preservative agent in 24 hours urine collection.

335. All of the following are the methods used to assess urine specific gravity; EXCEPT:

a. Urinometer b. Refractometer
c. Reagent strips d. Biuret method

Explanation: Biuret method is used to determine protein in urine. All other methods are used for measurement of urine specific gravity. Most commonly used method is urinometer, which is simple and easy to carry out in the bed side of patient.

336. Elevated specific gravity can be seen in:

a. Diabetes insipidus
b. Dehydration
c. Hypervolemia
d. Polyuria

Explanation: Adults generally have a specific gravity in the range of 1.010 to 1.030. Elevated specific gravity of urine is observed in dehydration and SIADH (Syndrome of Inappropriate Anti Diuretic Hormone). Low specific gravity is seen in diabetes insipidus, hypervolemia and polyuria.

337. All of the following can be a cause of milky-white color urine; EXCEPT:

a. Urinary tract infection
b. Uric acid crystals from eating purine-rich foods
c. Strenuous exercise
d. Phosphate crystals from excess parathyroid hormone

Explanation: Strenuous exercise can sometime result in blood getting into urine, hence turns the urine color into red. Cause of milky-white colored urine include uric acid crystals from eating purine-rich foods, such as anchovies, herring, and red meat (lamb, beef, and pork), and phosphate crystals from excess parathyroid hormone.

338. EDTA-containing tubes are not suitable for sample collection meant for coagulation studies because:

a. They will lead to thrombolysis
b. They binds the calcium which is needed for coagulation
c. Calcium concentration will increase in the sample
d. They activate the fibrinogen to form fibrin.

Explanation: EDTA strongly binds to calcium in the sample which is needed for coagulation. It will affect the coagulation time. EDTA tubes are purple or lavender-colored tube which is used for complete blood counts (CBC).

339. Anticoagulant of choice for estimating blood glucose is:

a. EDTA b. Sodium Fluoride
c. Sodium Citrate d. Heparin

Explanation: Sodium fluoride inhibits the system involved in glycolysis and preserve the glucose.

340. Sputum sample for AFB should be collected:

a. Morning after wake up
b. After breakfast
c. In the evening
d. Whenever the person coughs

Explanation: Early morning sputum is ideal for mycobacteriological exam for tuberculosis. Cough reflex is usually suppressed at night. Thus, the first early morning expectoration represents overnight secretions accumulated in the chest.

341. Lipid profile does not include: *(Banaras HU 2015)*

a. HDL b. Total Cholesterol
c. SGOT d. VLDL

342. In Benedict's test which of the end color indicates absence of sugar in urine? *(Banaras HU 2015)*

a. Yellow b. Green
c. Orange d. Blue

343. What should be the sequence of events during collection of blood sample?

a. Ask the patient his name → verify from file → collect blood → Label the sample at bedside
b. Look at the file → Collect sample → Label the sample at bedside
c. Prelabel the sample vials → Check the file patient details → Collect sample
d. Collect sample → Confirm name from file → Label the sample vial

344. Clay colored stool is suggestive of: *(JIPMER 2012)*

a. Amoebic dysentery b. Typhoid
c. Ulcerative colitis d. Obstructive jaundice

345. The reagent used for testing urine sugar is: *(RRB Feb 2012)*

a. Benedict's reagents b. Sahli's reagent
c. Rothera's reagent d. None of these

346. Stool specimen for guaiac fecal occult blood testing is done to screen for:

a. Colorectal cancer b. Irritable bowel syndrome
c. Fistula d. Cancer prostate

347. Which among the following blood tests is recommended to a client on heparin therapy?

a. Bleeding time
b. Clotting time
c. Prothrombin time
d. Activated partial thromboplastin time (APTT)

348. Which among the following blood tests is recommended to a client on warfarin therapy?

a. Bleeding time
b. Clotting time
c. Prothrombin time (PT)
d. International normalized ratio (INR)

349. The correct method to collect urine sample for culture from urinary collecting system is:

a. Collect from catheter
b. With needle aspiration
c. Empty urine from bag
d. Any of the above methods

350. Glycated hemoglobin (HbA1c) is primarily measured to identify mean plasma glucose concentration of:

a. Over 7 days b. Over 30 days
c. Over 60 days d. Over 90 days

351. Which of the following is one of the component of a solution present in blood transfusion bag?

a. Sodium citrate b. Heparin
c. EDTA d. Warfarin

352. The 'Kahn Test' for syphilis is an example of: *(AIIMS Bhopal Nursing Officer, 2018)*

a. Tube flocculation test b. Slide flocculation test
c. Coombs test d. Ring precipitation test

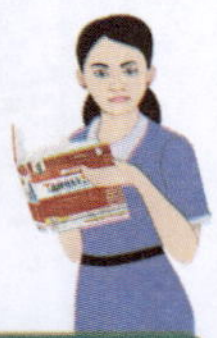

Ans.

335. d
336. b
337. c
338. b
339. b
340. a
341. c
342. d
343. a
344. d
345. a
346. a
347. d
348. d
349. b
350. d
351. a
352. a

Explanation: Kahn Test for syphilis is an example of tube flocculation test. Slide flocculation test was employed as the routine serologic test for syphilis.

COMFORT DEVICES

353. Complication that can be prevented by using foot rest: *(Safdarjung NO 2018)*

a. Bedsore b. Foot edema
c. Foot drop d. Rash

Explanation: **Foot drop** is a gait abnormality in which the dropping of the forefoot happens due to weakness, irritation or damage to the common fibular nerve including the sciatic nerve, or paralysis of the muscles in the anterior portion of the lower leg. Foot board or Foot rest is a comfort device used to prevent foot drop. The board supports legs and prevents planter flexion of legs.

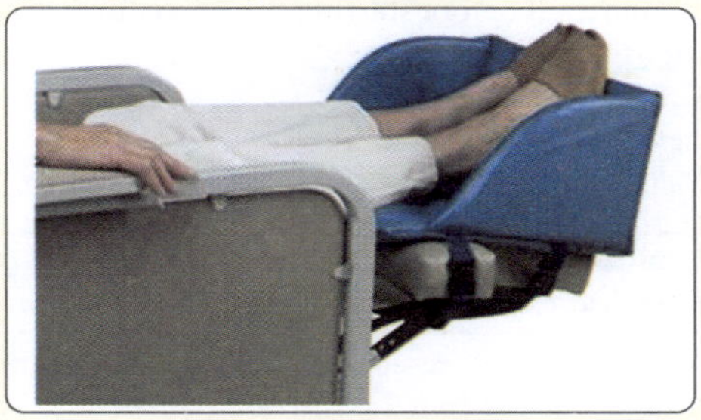

354. This comfort device is used to support hips and thighs, preventing external rotation and keeping the feet in alignment in case of paralysis, fracture of femur and hip surgery. *(Safdarjung NO 2018)*

a. Trochanter roll b. Sand bags
c. Bed boards d. Bed block

Explanation:

- **Trochanter roll** is a safety device which helps to support hips and legs so that the femur does not rotate outward.

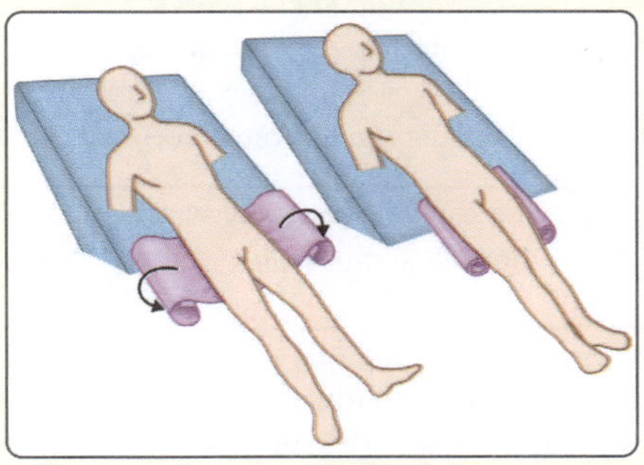

Figure: Trochanter roll

355. Comfort device used to prevent foot drop is:

a. Bed cradle b. Foot board
c. Sand bag d. Pillow

Explanation: Foot drop occurs because of injury to peroneal nerve. Foot board helps to maintain the alignment of foot and thereby helps to prevent foot drop.

356. Risk for fall injury is highest among:

a. School aged children b. Adolescents
c. Toddlers d. Older adults

BED MAKING

357. In which strength Savlon will be used to carbolize cot and mattress during bed making procedure? *(Safdarjung NO 2018)*

a. 1:40 to 1:50 b. 1:20 to 1:40
c. 1:30 to 1: 1:40 d. 1:40 to 1:60

Explanation: Strength of Savlon (Chlorhexidine Gluconate) to be used for bed cleaning is in the ratio of 1:33 aqueous solution (33 mL made up to in 1 L of water). It is also used for the treatment of wounds and burns, swabbing in obstetrics.

358. Which of the following actions has to be avoided to prevent contamination of the environment during bed making?

a. Strip all linens at the same time
b. Embrace soiled linens
c. Fanning soiled linens
d. Finishes both sides at the time

359. The bed which contains extra firm mattress with overhead frame is called?

a. Cardiac bed b. Fracture bed
c. Fowler's bed d. Operation bed

360. Which type of bed should be kept ready for receiving the new patient?

a. Open bed b. Closed bed
c. Admission bed d. Post operative bed

361. In which of the following type of beds, the top covers are pulled up to the head of the bed over the bottom covers and a pillow is placed on top of the linens or is covered with the bedspread?

a. Open bed b. Closed bed
c. Admission bed d. Post operative bed

362. A Nurse had done the one side of the bed while doing bed making. She is planning to turn the patient toward her side and move away to make other side, before moving she should:

a. Raise the head end
b. Cover the patient's side with blanket
c. Raise the foot end
d. Raise the side rails

Explanation: Before turning the patient toward her side and moving away to make the other side of the bed, the nurse should raise the side rails.

Raising the side rails helps to prevent the patient from accidentally rolling out of bed and injuring themselves while the nurse is making the other side of the bed. It also helps to provide a safe and secure environment for the patient during the bed-making process.

363. What should a Nurse do if she witnessed an unoccupied bed that soiled and looks wet:

a. Use hot water to clean the bed
b. Bed should be fumigated
c. Wipe the moisture with disinfectant and dry thoroughly
d. Change the bedsheet with waterproof mattress

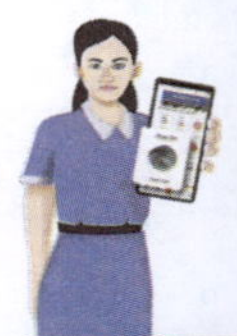

Ans.

353. c
354. a
355. b
356. d
357. b
358. c
359. b
360. b
361. b
362. d
363. c

364. Before going to make an unoccupied bed, A nurse should primarily ensure which of the following things for an ideal bed making:
a. Use sterile gloves
b. Keep Laundry Bag near the Bed
c. Call bell should kept near to the Nurse
d. Keep the Bed at comfortable working height

365. A Nurse is preparing a Bed for a post-surgical patient who had undergone surgery over abdominal region. During this scenario, the Nurse should place the waterproof pad on which part of the bed:
a. Over the Top sheet
b. Place over the bottom sheet
c. Just over the mattress
d. Avoid waterproof pad for this patient

366. The nurse who is making the bed should avoid which of the following actions to prevent environmental contamination and her uniform from contamination:
a. Using the bare hand to prepare bed
b. Having fan and AC to function
c. Shaking the linen to wipe off dust
d. Keeping the windows open

367. The Nurse should follow which of the precautions while changing soiled bed linen to prevent the risk of microorganism transmission:
a. Do hand hygiene and wear clean gloves
b. Roll all the soiled linens outside the bottom sheet
c. Fresh linen should be placed over the foot end of the bed
d. Hold the soiled linen away from uniform and place it on the floor

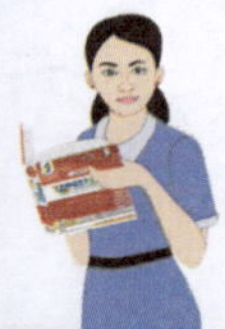

Explanation: Hand hygiene and standard precautions are the most effective and primary method to prevent the microorganism get transmitted. Roll all the soiled linens inside the bottom sheet and holds them away from uniform and place them in the linen hamper or laundry bag, not on the floor. Place the fresh linen on the client's chair or overbed table (not the foot end); do not use another client's bed.

Ans.
364. d
365. b
366. c
367. a
368. d
369. b
370. a
371. d
372. b
373. c
374. c
375. a
376. b

PERSONAL HYGIENE

368. Most important aspect of hand washing is:
a. Time
b. Type of soap
c. Surface tension
d. Friction

Explanation: Friction is the most important aspect while doing hand washing.

369. Arrange the following steps of hand washing in order:
1. Wash palm and fingers
2. Wash fingers and knuckles
3. Wash thumbs
4. Wash back of hands

Options
a. 1, 2, 3 and 4
b. 1, 4, 2 and 3
c. 4, 3, 2 and 1
d. 2, 3, 1 and 4

Explanation: Steps of hand washing are as follows. 1. Wash palm and fingers. 2. Wash back of the hands. 3. Wash fingers and knuckles. 4. Wash thumbs. 5. Wash finger tips. 6. Interlocking of hands. 7. Wash wrists

370. Which of the following is not included in the 5 moments of hand washing?
a. Before touching patient's surroundings
b. Before touching a patient
c. After touching patient's surroundings
d. After body fluid exposure risk

371. Universal precautions in hospital involve: *(LNJP H D 2012)*
a. Gloving
b. Mask, gowning
c. Hand washing
d. All of the above

372. The Nurse is planning to provide oral care to the unresponsive patient. Assessing for which of the following is most important before starting the procedure?
a. Moisture of the oral cavity
b. Gag reflex
c. Level of consciousness
d. Pain level

Explanation: Assessing gag reflex before providing oral care is very important because absence of gag reflex may lead to aspiration.

373. The Nurse should re-educate the patient with Diabetes Mellitus about the foot care, if the patient makes which of the following statements regarding the foot care:
a. I will check my foot daily with the mirrors
b. I will shorten and keep my nails neat and safe
c. I will try to walk with barefoot in my garden at least once a day
d. I will try to get microcellular rubber footwear

374. The nurse is providing a complete bed bath to a patient. The nurse should provide all of the following comforts to the patient; EXCEPT:
a. Curtain should be covered properly
b. Room temperature should be raised
c. Make sure water temperature is not warmer than 50 degree Celcius
d. Place towels under the person to keep the bed dry

Explanation: During the bed bath, the water temperature should not exceed **110°F (43°C)** to ensure the comfort and safety of the patient.

375. The Nurse is providing personal hygiene care to the ill patient. The Nurse should follow which of the following actions to reduce the risk of infection transmission and provide sterility;
a. Clean from less contaminated to highly contaminated area
b. Clean from highly contaminated to less contaminated area
c. Use circular motion to wipe the soiled area
d. Method of cleaning depends on the level of contamination

376. The Nurse is providing the oral care to an unresponsive patient; which of the following actions is appropriate for this care?
a. Keep the mouth gag while doing the care
b. Provide chlorhexidine spray to moisture the cavity
c. Wipe off the moisture content and maintain dryness
d. Both a and b

Explanation: Unresponsive client cannot able to have oral rinse with chlorhexidine, hence swabbing or spraying with this liquid will provide good care to the oral region.

377. How frequently should a nurse change the position of a bedridden patient to prevent bedsores? *New Q*

a. Every 30 mins　　b. Every 1 hour
c. Every 2 hours　　d. Every 4 hours

378. The Nurse should educate the client that hair care will promote:

a. Healing process
b. Good self-image
c. Confident and self-esteem
d. Sense of independence

379. While providing hygiene care for an elderly patient the Nurse should keep the fact in mind, that the skin of the old age person:

a. Is more moist and resilient
b. Is subjective to bruising is very less
c. Sweat and sebaceous glands are highly active
d. Requires less frequent bathing

Explanation: The old age skin has very less moisture and highly subjective to bruising, hence the frequent bathing and wiping the skin leads to unnecessary bruising and wound formation.

PRESSURE ULCER/BEDSORE

380. Identify the risk factors for bedsore:

a. Shearing force
b. Moisture
c. Impaired peripheral circulation
d. All of the above

381. Braden Scale is used for assessing the risk for: *(DSSSB 2013)*

a. Decubitus ulcer　　b. Diabetes Mellitus
c. Hypertension　　d. Urinary tract infection

Explanation: Braden scale is a tool that was developed in 1987 by Barbara Braden & Nancy Bergstrom. The purpose of this scale is to assess the patient for the risk of pressure ulcer (decubitus ulcer). Braden scale has following six criteria. 1. Sensory perception. 2. Moisture. 3. Activity. 4. Mobility. 5. Nutrition. 6. Friction and shear.

382. Which of the following interventions can best prevent bedsore? *(Kerala PSC 2016, DSSSB 2013)*

a. Massage reddened areas with lotion or oils
b. Change the position every two hourly
c. Use special water mattress
d. Keep skin clean and dry

Explanation: Changing position is the most effective way to prevent bedsore in bed-ridden patient. It is advised to change position of a bed-ridden patient at least every 2 hours and wheelchair-bound patient at least every 15 minutes. Dry skin is more easily damaged.

383. Which of the following nursing interventions is most appropriate in prevention of pressure sore?

a. Provide frequent bath to patient
b. Maintaining the patients' skin moist
c. Frequent turning and repositioning of the patient
d. Frequent feeding

384. Cleaning of bedsore has to be done from:

a. Inner to outer
b. Outer to inner
c. Wound part near to the care giver first then the further part
d. None of the above

Explanation: Bedsore is considered as a contaminated wound, in this wound periphery is considered as more clean, so cleaning of the wound has to be done from outer to inner. In surgical wound cleaning has to be done from inner to outer.

385. Which of the following is a hazard of immobility?

a. Loss of bone calcium *(Safdarjung NO 2018)*
b. Increased vital capacity
c. Venous vasoconstriction
d. A positive nitrogen balance

Explanation: The process of bone demineralization increases in immobility. Immobility causes slow bone formation while breakdown increases. That is when someone is immobile, the cells that make bone (osteoblasts) are not able to work. In addition, there is more activity of the cells that breakdown bone (osteoclasts). Moreover, during bed rest there is an increased loss of calcium and phosphorus in the urine and often higher blood calcium levels. Thus, loss of bone calcium takes place.

386. Among the following, the factor that contributes to pressure ulcer is: *(AIIMS BBS NO 2018)*

a. Edema　　b. Chronic disease
c. Shearing forces　　d. Malnutrition

Explanation: The major factors contributing to pressure ulcers are Friction and shearing forces, loss sensory perception, exposure to moisture, lack of activity, and mobility.

Edema, chronic disease and malnutrition may indirectly contribute to pressure ulcer but shearing forces are the direct cause of pressure ulcer.

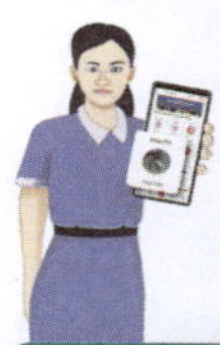

387. In which stage of pressure ulcer, hyperemia, increased temperature and redness with pressure is noticed?

a. Stage I　　b. Stage II
c. Stage III　　d. Stage IV

388. Which of the following sites is at high risk for pressure sore in side lying position?

a. Rib cage　　b. Buttocks
c. Ear　　d. Occiput

389. All of the following sites are at high risk for pressure sore in side lying position; EXCEPT:

a. Ear　　b. Hip
c. Elbow　　d. Sacral region

390. While assessing the client for pressure sore, the nurse noted skin loss and damage involving the top-most skin layers. This suggests:

a. Grade I pressure sore
b. Grade II pressure sore
c. Grade III pressure sore
d. Grade IV pressure sore

391. Which of the following guidelines has to be followed when caring for bedsore?

a. Wound must remain moist
b. Tight packing of the wound
c. Dressing to dry before removal
d. All of the above

Ans.

377.	c
378.	b
379.	d
380.	d
381.	a
382.	b
383.	c
384.	b
385.	a
386.	c
387.	a
388.	c
389.	d
390.	b
391.	c

392. Flush is defined as a:
- a. Sudden redness of the skin
- b. Bluish discoloration of the skin
- c. Pale skin
- d. None of the above

FLUID AND ELECTROLYTE BALANCE

393. Potential adverse effects of surgery and anesthesia are as follows; EXCEPT: *(ESIC 2019)*
- a. Thrombosis from compression of blood vessels or stasis
- b. Malignant hyperthermia/hypothermia
- c. Dehydration and electrolyte imbalance
- d. Myocardial depression, bradycardia, circulatory collapse

Explanation: Dehydration and electrolyte imbalance are not the side effects of anesthesia. Hydration level and electrolyte balance can be maintained by adequate administration of intravenous fluid before, during and after surgery. Conditions given in other options are potential adverse effects of surgery and anesthesia.

394. Skin turgor test is used to assess: *(AIIMS BPL NO 2018)*
- a. Hydration status
- b. Level of pain
- c. Consciousness
- d. Infection

Explanation: Skin turgor means the elasticity of skin. Elasticity is usually seen when the skin is well hydrated and nourished. Poor skin turgor is a late sign of dehydration.

395. Slow infusion of isotonic fluid into subcutaneous tissue is called: *(AIIMS BPL NO 2018)*
- a. Dialysis
- b. Hypodermoclysis
- c. Plasmapheresis
- d. Enteroclysis

Explanation: Hypodermoclysis, also called interstitial infusion or subcutaneous infusion, is the subcutaneous administration of fluids to the body.

396. The nurse is caring for a patient with acute kidney injury. Which of the following actions should the nurse take to obtain the most accurate assessment of fluid balance for the patient? *(RAK MSc 2018)*
- a. Document voiding pattern
- b. Obtain daily weight
- c. Review laboratory studies
- d. Observe skin turgor

Explanation: Daily assessment of patient's weight is a reliable indicator of fluid overload in a patient admitted with acute kidney injury or acute renal failure.

397. Which type of solution causes water to shift from the cells into plasma? *(AIIMS Raipur staff nurse grade I-2018)*
- a. Hypertonic
- b. Hypotonic
- c. Isotonic
- d. Alkaline

Explanation: Hypertonic solution shifts fluids from cells to plasma while hypotonic solution shifts fluid from plasma to cells. Isotonic solution has same osmolality as that of blood plasma. Alkaline solutions are those solutions which have pH more than 7.

398. Which among the following signs/symptoms will be present in a patient with hypovolemia?
- a. Increased heart rate
- b. Hypertension
- c. Bounding pulse
- d. Urine output 30 mL/hr

Explanation: In patients with hypovolemia, an increase in heart rate can be noted to maintain adequate tissue perfusion.

399. Calcium balance in the body is regulated with the help of:
- a. Aldosterone
- b. Calcitonin
- c. Parathormone
- d. Both b and c

Explanation: Calcitonin produced by thyroid gland helps to mobilize calcium from blood to bone and parathormone produced by parathyroid gland helps to mobilize calcium from bone to blood, both these hormones are involved in calcium metabolism.

400. Plasma protein which determines oncotic pressure is:
- a. Albumin
- b. Globulin
- c. Heme
- d. Prothrombin

Explanation: Albumin is the plasma protein responsible for determining oncotic pressure. Decrease in albumin causes edema over the body.

401. Isotonic saline contains ----------- amount of NaCl.
- a. 0.9 gm/dL
- b. 9.0 gm/dL
- c. 4.5 gm/dL
- d. 5 gm/dL

Explanation: 0.9 gm of NaCl (Sodium Chloride) is present in 100 mL of isotonic saline (normal saline).

402. Which of the following IV fluid administration is contraindicated in patients with lactic acidosis and impaired liver function?
- a. Normal Saline
- b. Ringer Lactate
- c. Mannitol
- d. Dextran

Explanation: Ringer lactate solution (RL) is also known as sodium lactate solution and Hartmann's solution. It can be used to treat metabolic acidosis, if the cause of acidosis is other than lactic acidosis. Administration of RL is contraindicated in severe metabolic acidosis (caused by lactic acidosis) or alkalosis and in severe liver disease or anoxic states which affects lactate metabolism.

403. Clinical manifestation of hypokalemia include:
- a. Spiky T wave
- b. Prolonged PR interval
- c. Positive Chvostek sign
- d. Muscle weakness

Explanation: Muscle weakness, paralytic ileus, abdominal distention. ST wave depression, abnormal U wave are the characteristic of hypokalemia. Option a and b indicate hyperkalemia, option c indicates hypocalcemia.

404. Which one is the most abundant anion in extracellular fluid?
- a. Sodium
- b. Potassium
- c. Bicarbonate
- d. Chloride

Explanation: Major anions and cations:
- Extracellular fluid:
  - Major anion: Chloride
  - Major cation: Sodium
- Intracellular fluid:
  - Major anion: Phosphate
  - Major cation: Potassium

405. Patient with liver problem develops edema because of:
- a. Fall in oncotic pressure
- b. Increase in hydrostatic pressure
- c. Fall in osmotic pressure
- d. Rise osmotic pressure

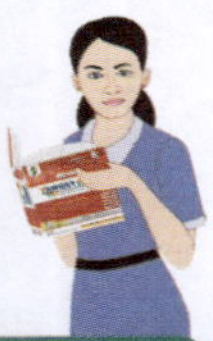

Ans.

392. a
393. c
394. a
395. b
396. b
397. a
398. a
399. d
400. a
401. a
402. b
403. d
404. d
405. a

Explanation: Albumin is produced in the liver and is responsible for oncotic pressure, due to the fall in oncotic pressure edema occurs in a patient with liver problem.

406. Solution of choice for bladder irrigation for a patient who is undergoing Transurethral Resection of Prostrate: *(AIIMS 2016)*

a. Glycine b. NS
c. RL d. Isolate P

Explanation: Glycine 1.5% and sterile water are the most widely used irrigating fluids in urological endoscopic surgeries (TURP and certain transurethral procedures).

407. All of the following are the signs and symptoms related to hypocalcemia; EXCEPT:

a. Numbness and tingling sensations
b. Shortened QT interval in ECG
c. Chvostek sign
d. Trousseau sign

Explanation: Hypocalcemia characteristically causes prolongation of the QT interval in the electrocardiogram. Prolongation of the QT interval is associated with early after-depolarizations and triggered dysrhythmias. Although electrocardiographic conduction abnormalities are common, serious hypocalcemia-induced dysrhythmias, such as heart block and ventricular dysrhythmias, are infrequent.

408. Major electrolyte imbalance that occurs in water intoxication is:

a. Hypernatremia b. Hyponatremia
c. Hypokalemia d. Hyperkalemia

Explanation: Water intoxication is a life-threatening disorder (hypo-osmolar syndrome) accompanied by brain function impairment due to severe dilutional hyponatremia. Inappropriate water retention causes the *dilutional hyponatremia.*

409. Which of the following is used in the management of Hyperkalemia? *(DSSSB 2013)*

a. Insulin with glucose b. Sodium Bicarbonate
c. Potassium Chloride d. Magnesium Sulfate

Explanation: Drugs used in the treatment of hyperkalemia include the following:

- Calcium Gluconate: It is the antidote of potassium.
- Insulin administered with glucose: Facilitates the uptake of glucose into the cell, which brings potassium with it.
- Diuretics: Causes potassium loss through the kidney.
- Nebulization with salbutamol also helps to decrease the potassium level in the blood. Because bronchodilators such as Beta 2-adrenergic agonists: Promote cellular reuptake of potassium.

410. Which of the following ECG findings indicates the presence of hypokalemia? *(DSSSB 2013)*

a. Tall, peak T wave b. ST segment depression
c. Widening of QRS complex d. Prolonged PR interval

Explanation: ST segment depression and abnormal U wave are the characteristics of hypokalemia.

411. Chvostek sign is an indication of: *(DSSSB PHN, 2015)*

a. Hypernatremia b. Hypercalcemia
c. Hyponatremia d. Hypocalcemia

412. The symptoms of severe dehydration in an adult include all of the following; EXCEPT: *(Banaras HU 2015)*

a. Decreased thirst b. Dizziness
c. Weakness d. Palpitations

413. Hypokalemia is suspected when a client has serum potassium level falling below: *(Kerala PSC, Nov 2014)*

a. 5.0 mEq/L b. 3.52 mEq/L
c. 4.5 mEq/L d. 5.5 mEq/L

414. Which of the following solutions is isotonic? *(Recent Question 2012)*

a. 0.9% saline b. Dextran
c. 0.45% saline d. Dextrose saline

415. The most important electrolyte of intracellular fluid is: *(Recent Question 2012)*

a. Potassium b. Calcium
c. Sodium d. Chloride

416. Lugol's solution contains: *(Recent Question 2012)*

a. Potassium iodide b. Sodium bromide
c. Ammonium chloride d. Calcium chloride

417. Quantity of sodium chloride required to make 1 L of normal saline is: *(LNJP H D 2012)*

a. 900 grams
b. 0.9 grams
c. 9 grams
d. 90 grams

418. A patient on Furosemide therapy complaining of muscle weakness, which among the following laboratory values the nurse needs as to assess first?

a. Serum glucose
b. Serum potassium
c. Serum Albumin
d. Serum sodium

419. Which among the following patients requires a sodium restricted diet?

a. Patient with fracture
b. Patient with heart failure
c. Patient with gastroenteritis
d. Patient with inflammatory disease

420. Which among the following electrolytes has to be replaced in a client with vomiting and diarrhea?

a. Sodium b. Potassium
c. Calcium d. Magnesium

421. Patient with which of the following condition is at greatest risk for developing hypocalcemia?

a. Hyperthyroidism b. Appendicitis
c. Acute pancreatitis d. Cardiomyopathy

422. An adult client with meningitis is receiving IV fluids and oral fluids. The fluid intake of the client should be monitored because fluid overload may cause:

a. Hypovolemic shock b. Bradycardia
c. Cerebral edema d. Dehydration

423. All of the following are clear fluids; EXCEPT:

a. Juice b. Shakes
c. Soups d. Lemon soda

424. Extracellular fluid constitutes:

a. 33% of the body fluid b. 47% of the body fluid
c. 53% of the body fluid d. 67% of the body fluid

425. Intracellular fluid constitutes:

a. 33% of the body fluid b. 47% of the body fluid
c. 53% of the body fluid d. 67% of the body fluid

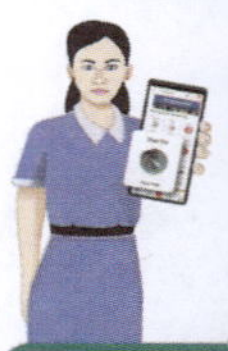

Ans.

406. a
407. b
408. b
409. a
410. b
411. d
412. a
413. b
414. a
415. a
416. a
417. c
418. b
419. b
420. b
421. c
422. c
423. b
424. a
425. d

426. The chief intracellular cation in our body is:
a. K^+ b. Na^+
c. Ca^{++} d. Mg^{++}

427. The chief extracellular cation in our body is:
a. K+ b. Na+
c. Ca^{++} d. Mg^{++}

428. Organ with major role in fluid regulation is:
a. Kidney b. Lung
c. Skin d. Intestine

429. The chief intracellular anion in our body is:
a. Potassium b. Sodium
c. Phosphate d. Chloride

430. The chief extracellular anion in our body is:
a. K^+ b. Na^+
c. Cl^- d. HCO_3^-

431. Osmolarity is defined as:
a. Moles per mL of solvent
b. Moles per deciliter of solvent
c. Moles per kg of solvent
d. Moles per liter of solvent

432. Hypoparathyroidism and vitamin D deficiency predisposes to:
a. Hpokalemia b. Hperkalemia
c. Hypercalcemia d. Hypocalcemia

433. 5% Dextrose in water is _________ solution.
a. Hypotonic b. Isotonic
c. Colloidal d. Hypertonic

434. 0.45% sodium chloride solution is:
a. Hypotonic b. Isotonic
c. Hypertonic d. Colloidal

435. Function/s of sodium is/are:
a. Maintain normal blood pressure
b. Maintain normal function of muscles and nerves
c. Both a and b
d. None of the above

436. Functions of potassium in the body is:
a. Crucial to heart function
b. Skeletal and smooth muscle contraction
c. Normal digestive and muscular function
d. All of the above

437. Causes of hypernatremia includes:
a. Nasogastric drains b. Diabetes insipidus (DI)
c. Cushing syndrome d. All of these

438. Causes of hyperkalemia includes:
a. Immediate period burn injury
b. Addison's disease
c. Renal failure
d. All of the above

439. Cause of hypercalcemia includes:
a. Hyperthyroidism b. Hyperparathyroidism
c. Malignancy d. All of these

440. Characteristic feature of hyponatremia includes:
a. Nausea and vomiting b. Confusion
c. Spasms and cramps d. All of these

441. Which of the following is the most significant symptom of hypokalemia?
a. Increased pulse rate
b. Muscle weakness
c. Muscle irritability
d. Hypertension

442. Laryngospasm with stridor is common among clients with:
a. Hypernatremia
b. Hyponatremia
c. Hypercalcemia
d. Hypocalcemia

443. Trousseau's sign is associated with:
a. Hypocalcemia b. Hyponatremia
c. Hypercalcemia d. Hypernatremia

ACID-BASE BALANCE

444. A patient who is in unresponsive situation is reported to the emergency triage with unknown history. On assessment it is found, respiration are deep and rapid. ABG values are pH, 7.20; $PaCO_2$, 21 mm Hg; PaO_2, 92 mm Hg and HCO_3, 8. You interpret these values to indicate:

(AIIMS Bhopal Grade-I 2018)

a. Respiratory alkalosis b. Metabolic acidosis
c. Respiratory acidosis d. Metabolic alkalosis

Explanation: Metabolic acidosis is a type of acid-base imbalance in which a total concentration of buffer base (HCO_3^-) is lower than the normal with relative increase in the hydrogen ion (H+) concentration which is caused due to renal insufficiency or many more other reasons can be there like severe diarrhea, malnutrition, etc. To compensate for the acidosis, deep and rapid respirations (Kussmaul's respirations) occur as the lungs attempt to exhale the maximum CO_2.

445. Which patient is at risk for metabolic acidosis?

(Kerala PSC, Nov 2014)

a. Patient with uncontrolled diabetes mellitus
b. Patient with emphysema
c. Patient with chronic bronchitis
d. Elderly patient receiving IV therapy

446. Acid base imbalance that develops in acute renal failure is:

(JIPMER 2012)

a. Metabolic acidosis b. Respiratory acidosis
c. Respiratory alkalosis d. Metabolic alkalosis

447. Interpret the following ABG results:
pH - 7.53
$PaCO_2$ - 38 mm Hg
HCO_3 – 31 mEq/L
a. Respiratory alkalosis, uncompensated
b. Metabolic alkalosis, uncompensated
c. Respiratory alkalosis, fully compensated
d. Metabolic alkalosis, partially compensated

448. Interpret the following ABG results:
pH - 7.35 $PaCO_2$ - 70 mmHg
HCO_3 – 36 mEq/L
a. Respiratory acidosis, uncompensated
b. Respiratory acidosis, fully compensated
c. Respiratory alkalosis, fully compensated
d. Metabolic acidosis, partially compensated

449. Arterial blood gas levels of patient shows: pH, 7.25; $PaCO_2$, 37 mm Hg; PaO_2, 92 mm Hg; and HCO_3^-, 18. These laboratory values indicates:
a. Metabolic acidosis b. Metabolic alkalosis
c. Respiratory acidosis d. Respiratory alkalosis

450. Burn injury, diabetic ketoacidosis, etc. will lead to:
a. Respiratory acidosis b. Respiratory alkalosis
c. Metabolic acidosis d. Metabolic alkalosis

Ans.
426. a
427. b
428. a
429. c
430. c
431. d
432. d
433. b
434. a
435. c
436. d
437. d
438. d
439. d
440. d
441. b
442. d
443. a
444. b
445. a
446. a
447. b
448. b
449. a
450. c

451. Vomiting, prolonged gastric suctioning, Cushing syndrome, hyperaldosteronism may lead to:

a. Respiratory acidosis b. Respiratory alkalosis
c. Metabolic acidosis d. Metabolic alkalosis

452. Depression of the respiratory center or severe asthma attack will lead to:

a. Respiratory acidosis b. Respiratory alkalosis
c. Metabolic acidosis d. Metabolic alkalosis

453. Excessive elimination of carbon dioxide from the body will leads to:

a. Respiratory acidosis b. Respiratory alkalosis
c. Metabolic acidosis d. Metabolic alkalosis

VARIOUS POSITIONS

454. While attaching temperature probe on the skin, most preferred site for a patient with supine position is right hypochondriac region. Why?

a. Liver is located in that region
b. Easy to attach
c. Large surface area
d. All of the above

Explanation: Liver is present in right hypochondriac region, which is the site for metabolism, so by attaching the probe there, more accurate information regarding peripheral temperature can be obtained.

455. When a client change his position from lying down to standup, his pulse rate increases from 72 to 120 beats/min and patient becomes dizzy. It is suggestive of:

a. Malignant hypertension b. Orthostatic hypotension
c. Primary hypertension d. Rebound hypertension

456. For assessing inguinal hernia what the physician will ask to do?

a. Lie down with leg flexed *(AIIMS 2016)*
b. Sit in squatting position and bear down
c. Stand erect with hands drawn behind the back
d. Sit on a chair with hands drawn behind the back

Explanation: Option b is the correct answer, in this position when the patient bears down or coughs or sneezes, hernia protrudes easily and doctor can observe it easily.

457. A 35-year-old male patient developed air embolus while receiving parenteral nutrition through central venous catheter. Which among the following is the immediate nursing action?

a. Raise head of bed to 90 degrees
b. Notify the physician immediately
c. Turn patient to left lateral decubitus position
d. Instruct the patient to perform Valsalva maneuver

458. The most accurate method to check the position of a newly placed NG tube:

a. Placing an order for X-ray to check position
b. Observing the color of gastric contents
c. Testing the pH of the gastric contents
d. Auscultating over the gastric area as air is injected into the tube

459. After nasogastric feeding head end of the patient should be raised for:

a. 30-60 degree at least for 15 minutes
b. 30-60 degree at least 30 minutes
c. 45-60 degree at least for 15 minutes
d. 45-60 degree at least for 30 minutes

460. A child is admitted to the emergency department with dyspnea related to bronchospasm. The nurse should place the client in which of the following positions? *(RAK MSc 2018)*

a. High Fowler's b. Side-lying
c. Prone d. Supine

Explanation: High Fowler's position is recommended in case of dyspnea as this position minimizes the tension of abdominal muscles which provide more space for lungs to expand, resulting in improvement in breathing. The High Fowler's position is a position in which a patient is placed when the head of the bed needs to be elevated as high as possible. The upper half of the patient's body is between 60° and 90° in relation to the lower half of their body.

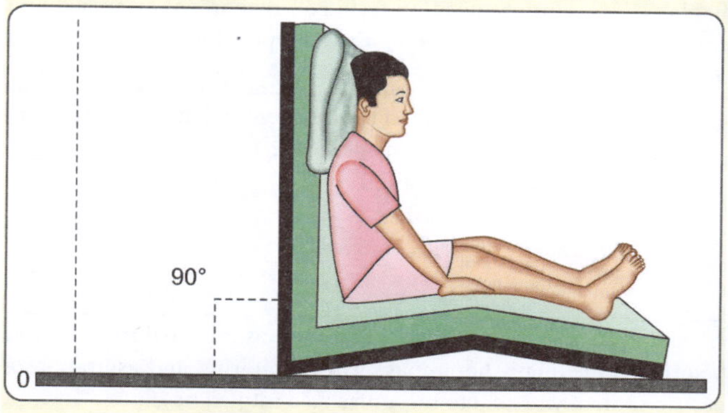

Figure: High Fowler's position

461. When a patient experiences difficulty in breathing, the most appropriate position to place him/her in is:

a. Lateral position *(AIIMS BBS NO 2018)*
b. Fowler's position
c. Dorsal recumbent position
d. Sims' position

Explanation: Fowler's position is a standard patient position in which the patient is seated in a semi-upright sitting position and may have knees either bent or straight. It is an intervention used to promote oxygenation via maximum chest expansion.

462. Position given to the client while administering enema is:

a. Sims' left lateral b. Prone
c. Knee chest d. Sitting

Explanation: Position the patient on left side, lying with the knees drawn to the abdomen. This eases the passage and flow of fluid into the rectum. Gravity and the anatomical structure of the sigmoid colon also suggest that this will aid enema distribution and retention. So option a is the correct answer.

463. Best position for a client in hypovolemic shock is:

a. Knee chest position b. Trendelenburg
c. Fowler's d. Lateral position

Explanation: Trendelenburg position promotes venous return in patient with hypovolemic shock.

464. Best position given to an unconscious client while performing oral care is:

a. Supine b. Sitting
c. Side lying d. Fowler's

Explanation: Side lying position is the best indicated position, because it reduces the risk of aspiration.

Ans.

451.	d
452.	a
453.	b
454.	a
455.	b
456.	b
457.	c
458.	a
459.	b
460.	a
461.	b
462.	a
463.	b
464.	c

465. Other name for Genupectoral position is:

a. Lithotomy b. Trendelenburg
c. Knee chest d. Sims' position

Explanation: Genupectoral position is also known as knee chest position.

466. Fowler's position given to a client with dyspnea helps to relieve dyspnea by:

a. Making patient more comfortable
b. Facilitating expansion of the thorax
c. Reducing oxygen demand
d. All of the above

Explanation: Upright position facilitates diaphragm excursion and enhances thorax expansion. So Fowler's position helps to relieve dyspnea.

467. Before providing NG feed to the client, what all are the pre-procedural care a nurse needs to do?

a. Provide Fowler's position
b. Take abdominal girth
c. Aspirate the gastric content
d. All of the above

Explanation: All of the above are the actions expected from a nurse before NG feeding. Abdominal girth monitoring and aspiration of gastric content will help to recognize feed intolerance.

468. Position used during pleural tapping is:

a. Orthopneic b. Supine
c. Prone d. Knee chest

Explanation: Patients who are alert and cooperative are most comfortable in a seated position leaning slightly forward and resting the head on the arms or hands or on a pillow, which is placed on an adjustable bedside table. This position facilitates access to the posterior axillary space, which is the most dependent part of the thorax. Orthopneic position is the one in which a person sits upright in a bed, possibly bending forward.

469. While giving NG tube feeding which of the following nursing actions prevents complications? *(DSSSB 2013)*

a. Advance tube 2 cm
b. Flush with 20 mL of air
c. Provide high Fowler's position
d. Plug the air vent during feeding

Explanation: High Fowler's position helps in easy administration and also to prevent regurgitation.

470. Which of the following positions is given to a patient with severe breathing difficultly? *(DSSSB 2013)*

a. Dorsal recumbent b. Fowler's
c. Supine d. Trendelenburg

Explanation: Fowler's position helps in proper expansion of lung by moving diaphragm downward and promoting lung expansion.

471. The position to be maintained for a patient with increased ICP is: *(DSSSB PHN, 2015)*

a. Fowler's position
b. Trendelenburg's position
c. Side lying
d. Supine position

472. Position in which the patient is to be cared after lower extremity amputation is: *(JIPMER 2012)*

a. Left lateral
b. Supine with head turned to one side
c. Side lying with amputated side up
d. Prone

473. Patient recovering from general anesthesia should be positioned in: *(Recent Question 2012)*

a. Supine position b. Fowler's position
c. Trendelenburg position d. Side lying position

474. Position for administration of enema: *(RRB Feb 2012)*

a. Left lateral b. Supine
c. Right lateral d. Prone

475. Which of the following is the best position for examining the rectum using proctoscopy? **New Q**

a. Lithotomy
b. Sims'
c. Knee-chest
d. Prone

Explanation: In knee-chest position, the patient kneels on the examination table with their buttocks elevated and their chest resting on the table. This position may be preferred for certain specialized types of rectal examinations, such as proctoscopy. In these procedures, a flexible or rigid instrument is used to visually inspect the inside of the rectum and lower colon. The knee-chest position helps to create a clear line of sight.

476. To perform catheterization, the nurse should place a woman in the:

a. Dorsal recumbent position
b. Lithotomy position
c. Supine position
d. Side lying

477. Which of the following nursing interventions decreases the risk of aspiration while feeding a patient with dysphagia?

a. Sit the patient upright in a chair
b. Provide liquid only at the end of the meal
c. Provide only soft food
d. Instruct the patient to lie down for 45 minutes after food

478. Appropriate position to provide oral care of a conscious patient is:

a. Supine position with head turned sideways
b. Left lateral position
c. Trendelenburg position
d. Fowler's position

479. Position given to patients while inserting gavage tube is:

a. Knee chest b. Supine position
c. Mid-Fowler's position d. High-Fowler's position

480. When helping a stroke patient, nurse should assist: *(Recent Question 2012)*

a. From behind b. On weak side
c. On strong side d. From back

481. Position given to patients during sigmoidoscopy is:

a. Supine b. Prone
c. Lithotomy d. Left lateral

Explanation: The left lateral (Sims') position, in which the patient lies on his or her left side with the hips and knees flexed and parallel, is probably the position most commonly used for rigid sigmoidoscopy. Knee-chest position is preferred for Proctocopy

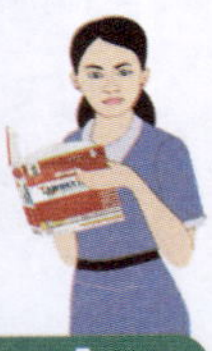

Ans.

465. c
466. b
467. d
468. a
469. c
470. b
471. a
472. c
473. d
474. a
475. c
476. a
477. a
478. d
479. d
480. b
481. d

482. To provide Fowler's position, the head end of the client should be elevated to:
a. 15° angle
b. 35° angle
c. 45° angle
d. 60° angle

483. Which of the following positions is appropriate to do percussion and promote postural drainage of lower lobe of lungs in a patient with bronchiectasis?
a. Fowler's position
b. Semi Fowler's position
c. Prone position
d. Decubitus position

484. After spinal injury, position given to the patient is:
a. Supine
b. Prone
c. Lateral
d. Lithotomy

485. Position used for visualizing internal sex organs is:
a. Knee chest
b. Trendelenburg
c. Lithotomy position
d. Prone position

486. Position used for flatus tube insertion is:
a. Left lateral
b. Right lateral
c. Knee chest
d. Prone

487. All of the following positions are used for enema administration; EXCEPT:
a. Sims' position
b. Prone position
c. Knee-chest position
d. Supine with knees flexed and legs separated

488. For assessing rectum, position given to the patient is:
a. Sims Position
b. Knee Chest
c. Both a and b
d. Lithotomy

489. In postural drainage, anterior segments of left upper lobes can be drained by providing ....position.
a. Supine with head elevated
b. Leaning forward 30 degrees
c. Left side lying with pillow under the chest
d. Right side lying with pillow under the chest

490. In postural drainage, apical segment of upper lobe can be drained by providing .... position.
a. Semi-Fowler's position
b. Leaned backwards from sitting position
c. Left side lying with pillow under the chest
d. Right side lying with pillow under the chest

491. In postural drainage, posterior segment of lower lobes can be drained by providing ....position.
a. Prone in Trendelenburg's position
b. Supine in Trendelenburg's position
c. Right side lying with pillow under the chest
c. Bed forward about 30 degrees

492. In postural drainage, anterior segments of lower lobes can be drained by providing which of the following positions?
a. Upright at 30 degree forward leaning
b. Semi-Fowler position
c. Prone in Trendelenburg's position
d. Supine in Trendelenburg's position

493. Bed used to provide various positions during postural drainage:
a. Nelson's bed
b. Cardiac bed
c. Orthopedic bed
d. Divided bed

494. Identify the components of proper body mechanics:
a. Move as close to the patient's bed as you can
b. Set your feet into a comfortable and solid wide base of support when lifting.
c. Keep the head upright and hold your shoulders up
d. All of the above

Explanation: Body mechanics is a broad term used to denote an effort coordinated by the muscles, bones and nervous system. It can either be good or bad and can be directly related to the occurrence of back pains. All of the above mentioned rules are correct regarding body mechanics.

495. When planning to move a patient, two workers lifting together:
a. Allow more time to do tasks
b. Will reduce the workload by 50%
c. Provide more comfort to the patient
d. Will make work boredom free

496. Which of the following Range of Motion (ROM) cannot be applied to a wrist?
a. Abduction and adduction
b. Flexion and extension
c. Inversion and eversion
d. Radial and ulnar flexion

497. What is the rule of thumb in lifting or transferring a patient?
a. Always ask for help even if you can do it alone
b. Do not attempt to lift more than 60% of your body weight
c. Do not attempt to lift more than 35% of your body weight
d. Always ask the patient to walk first

498. All of the following range of motion (ROM) can be applied to neck and cervical spine; EXCEPT:
a. Lateral flexion and extension
b. Flexion and extension
c. Abduction and adduction
d. Hyperextension

499. Which of the following is not a correct practice?
a. Avoid bending from the waist
b. Work at height that is comfortable for you
c. Carry objects away from the midline of your body
d. Be aware of the maximum weight that is safe to carry

500. The nurse needs to ________ while lifting or carrying heavy object.
a. Keep the knees close to each other
b. Maintain a wide base or support
c. Bend the back perpendicular to the body
d. Hold objects away from the body

HOT AND COLD APPLICATION

501. Hot application causes all of the following; EXCEPT:
a. Peripheral vasodilation
b. Increased capillary permeability
c. Increased oxygen consumption
d. Decreased motility of leucocytes

Explanation: Hot application causes peripheral vasodilation, increased capillary permeability, increased oxygen consumption, increased local metabolism, decreased blood viscosity, decreased muscle tone, increased blood flow, increased lymph flow and motility of leucocytes.

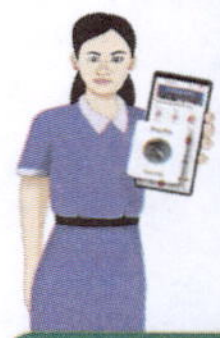

Ans.
482. c
483. c
484. a
485. c
486. a
487. b
488. c
489. a
490. b
491. a
492. d
493. a
494. d
495. b
496. c
497. c
498. c
499. c
500. b
501. d

502. What should be the temperature of water used for cold sponging? New Q *(RRB SSNE 2015)*
- a. 100°F
- b. 95°F
- c. 70°F
- d. 30°F

503. Therapeutic effect of hot application include:
- a. Vasoconstriction
- b. Increased lymph flow
- c. Decreased lymph flow
- d. None of these

504. On application of hot compress to a client, heat is transmitted through:
- a. Conduction
- b. Convection
- c. Evaporation
- d. Radiation

505. Heat application causes:
- a. Vasodilation
- b. Decreases blood viscosity
- c. Both a and b
- d. Vasoconstriction

506. Cold application causes:
- a. Vasodilation
- b. Decreases blood viscosity
- c. Both a and b
- d. Vasoconstriction

507. All of the following are types of dry cold application; EXCEPT:
- a. Ice bag
- b. Ice pack
- c. Cold compress
- d. Ice collar

508. Identify the solutions used for sitz bath:
- a. Potassium permanganate 1:5000
- b. Boric acid 1 dram to 1 pint
- c. Eusol/Dettol (1:40)
- d. All of the above

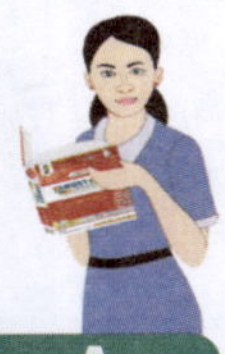

DRUG ADMINISTRATION

509. Which of the following is the highest priority nursing intervention for a newly admitted patient who is receiving blood transfusion?
- a. Instruct the patient to report any itching, shortness of breath, or chest pain
- b. Warm the blood to room temperature before transfusion
- c. Documentation of blood transfusion in the patient's chart
- d. Check the vital signs of the patient every 30 minutes from initiation of blood transfusion till completion

510. In a patient receiving IV fluids, sluggish flow, redness and tenderness at the site of cannula indicates: *(AIIMS BPL NO 2018)*
- a. Venous spasm
- b. Thrombophlebitis
- c. Infection
- d. Nerve damage

Explanation: Sluggish flow, redness or blanching and tenderness at the venipuncture site are the features of venous spasm, while thrombophlebitis has severe discomfort, redness and hard vein. Infection has an additional feature of local temperature increase at site. Nerve damage is a delayed effect associated with extreme painful numbness and muscle contraction.

511. Which of the following would be a common indication of infiltration of a peripheral intravenous infusion? *(NCFL 2019)*
- a. Redness and swelling around the insertion site
- b. Blood return in the cannula
- c. Difficulty regulating the flow with gravity
- d. Cool skin distal to the insertion site

Explanation:
- Infiltration happens when intravenous fluid or medications leak into nearby tissues due to the dislodgment or improper placement of intravenous catheter. The signs of infiltration include swelling, burning sensation, discomfort, feel of tightness, cool skin, blanching, reduced or flow rate stopped.
- Redness and swelling – signs of infection/inflammation.
- Blood return in the cannula and Difficulty regulating the flow with gravity indicates blockage of IV cannula.

512. A nurse has just administered medication via orogastric tube. What is the priority nursing action following nursing action? *(AIIMS Raipur NO 2019)*
- a. Check tube placement
- b. Re-tape the tube
- c. Flush the tube
- d. Remove the tube

Explanation:
- Failure to flush the tube before and after both drugs administration can result in tube clogging, which may necessitate removal and insertion of new tube.
- Patient must receive the prescribed dose of medication, so the tube is flushed to administer the drug completely.

513. Patient complains of pain and has redness with swelling at the site of IV. The nurse must: *(ESIC 2019)*
- a. Stop infusion and remove IV cannula
- b. Start nasal oxygen
- c. Change IV tubing and the solution
- d. Apply warm moist pack to the reddened area

Explanation: Pain, redness and swelling and IV site are the signs of thrombophlebitis and further infusion can complicate the condition. The nurse must stop infusion and remove IV cannula.

514. Which of the following is the reason for intradermal injection to be used for testing allergic reactions? *(Daman & Diu NO 2018)*
- a. It is less painful
- b. It is easy to administer
- c. It diffuses rapidly
- d. It diffuses slowly

Explanation: The test for allergy requires the medicine to get absorbed slowly else it can result into serious anaphylaxis. So it is given through intradermal route as the blood supply in this layer is less which delays absorption. Additionally, the body's reaction to substances is more easily visible since it is closer to the surface. The layer underneath the epidermis contains a large number of immune cells, mainly dermal dendritic cells.

515. The preferred site for intramuscular injection with Z-track technique in an adult is: *(RAK MSc 2018)*
- a. Deltoid
- b. Rectus femoris
- c. Ventrogluteal
- d. Vastus lateralis

Explanation: The Z-track method is a type of IM injection technique used to prevent tracking (leakage) of the medication into the subcutaneous tissue. As the gluteal muscles are the largest muscles, it is considered as the best site for administering intramuscular injection using z-track technique to prevent the passage of medicine into subcutaneous layer and minimizing the local irritation. The Ventrogluteal site provides the greatest thickness of gluteal muscle, is free of penetrating nerves and blood vessels.

Ans.

502.	c
503.	b
504.	a
505.	c
506.	d
507.	c
508.	d
509.	a
510.	a
511.	d
512.	c
513.	a
514.	d
515.	c

516. The method used for administering medication into the ear is called: *(AIIMS Bhopal Grade-I 2018)*

a. Instillation b. Injection
c. Inhalation d. Infiltration

Explanation: Instillation is the term used for administration of medication into the ear. Injection refers to parenteral administration of medication using a needle. Inhalation refers to administration of drugs that are gases or those are dispersed in an aerosol. Infiltration refers to administration of drugs that results in drugs passing into tissue spaces or into cells.

517. Which among the following is a complication of spinal anesthesia? *(AIIMS Bhopal Grade-I 2018)*

a. Tachycardia b. Hypotension
c. Hypertension d. Dyspnea

Explanation: The most common neurological complications after spinal anesthesia are postural puncture, headache and hypotension. Hypotension after spinal anesthesia is a physiological consequence of sympathetic blockade

518. An immunologic reaction to a drug to which a person has already been sensitized is known as: *(AIIMS Bhopal Grade-I 2018)*

a. Drug tolerance b. Drug allergy
c. Drug toxicity d. Drug intolerance

Explanation: A drug allergy is the abnormal reaction of the immune system to a medication.

Drug tolerance refers to patient's reduced reaction to a drug following its repeated use. Drug intolerance or drug sensitivity refers to an inability to tolerate the adverse effects of a medication.

Drug toxicity refers to gradual accumulation of too much of a drug in the blood stream.

519. Which of the following sites is recommended for adults as a safe site for the majority of intramuscular injection? *(AIIMS Bhopal Grade-I 2018)*

a. Ventrogluteal site b. Vastus lateralis site
c. Dorsal gluteal site d. Rectus femoris

Explanation: Ventrogluteal I/M injections are considered to be safest because this area is free from major blood vessels and nerves.

520. Which is the most important route of excretion of drugs? *(AIIMS Raipur Staff Nurse Grade I-2018)*

a. Kidney b. Saliva and sweat
c. Exhaled air d. Feces

Explanation: Kidney is the most common route for excretion of drugs, all others are minimally involved in excretion of drugs.

521. Which of the following drugs induces sleep?

a. Hypnotics
b. Analgesics
c. Antipyretics
d. Antihistamines

Explanation: Hypnotics are the group of drugs which induce sleep. Analgesics relieve pain. Antipyretics bring down temperature and antihistamines are used for treating allergy.

522. What is the ideal length of insertion of rectal suppository in an adult?

a. 2 inches beyond internal sphincter
b. 4 inches beyond internal sphincter
c. 9 inches beyond internal sphincter
d. 10 inches beyond internal sphincter

Explanation: Ideal length of insertion of rectal suppository in an adult is 4 inches beyond internal sphincter

523. How should a nurse administer an iron injection to an adult? *(AIIMS Bhopal Nursing Officer, 2018)*

a. Intradermal in the forearm
b. Intramuscular in the deltoid
c. Subcutaneous in the arm
d. Z track intramuscular in the gluteal

Explanation: Iron injection is irritable, so it is administered in well-developed muscles as deep I/M. To prevent leak of injection it is administered as deep I/M using Z track technique.

524. Which of the following nursing interventions is incorrect when using the Z-track method of injection? *(DSSSB 2013)*

a. Prepare the injection site with alcohol
b. Use a needle that is at least 1" long
c. Aspirate for blood before injection
d. Rub the injection site vigorously after the injection

Explanation: Z-track method is an intramuscular injection technique. In this procedure, skin and tissue are pulled and held firmly while a long needle is inserted into the muscle. After the medication is injected, the skin and tissues are released. The needle track that forms during this procedure takes the shape of the letter "Z". This zig-zag track line prevents medication from leaking from the muscle into surrounding tissue which minimizes skin staining and irritation.

Rubbing the injection site is contraindicated because it may cause the medication to leak into the surrounding tissue and skin.

525. Which of the following medication orders is immediately administered? *(DSSSB 2013)*

a. PRN order b. STAT order
c. Single order d. Standing order

Explanation: STAT order means the medication needs to be administered immediately. PRN medications are given on an "as needed" basis for specific signs & symptoms. A "standing order" is a prewritten medication order and specific instructions from the Physician to administer a medication to a person in clearly defined circumstances.

526. The most appropriate and safest way to verify the patient's identity before administration of medication is:

a. State the name of the patient aloud and ask her/him to repeat
b. Check the room number and bed number of the patient
c. Check the patient's identification band
d. Ask the patient his/her name

Explanation: Checking the identification band is the safest way to verify the identity before administration of medication irrespective of whether the patient is conscious or unconscious. The nurse should ask the name of the patient only after checking the identification band.

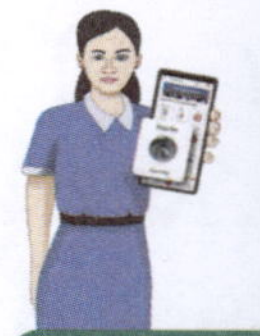

Ans.

516. a
517. b
518. b
519. a
520. a
521. a
522. b
523. d
524. d
525. b
526. c

527. Which is the most serious complication caused by bolus administration of KCl?

a. Arrhythmia and cardiac arrest
b. Respiratory depression
c. Paralytic ileus
d. All of the above

Explanation: Arrhythmia and cardiac arrest is the complication caused by bolus administration of KCl.

528. While administering albumin to a client, nurse needs to give this drug:

a. Rapidly and restrict water intake
b. Rapidly and increase the water intake
c. Slowly and increase water intake
d. Slowly and restrict the water intake

Explanation: The therapeutic effect of albumin will be achieved if it is administering slowly along with restricted water intake.

529. A client is receiving prednisolone. Which among the following is the most important nursing intervention?

a. Check the urine output hourly
b. Check hourly urine specific gravity
c. Check blood sugar hourly
d. Check the blood level of the drug

Explanation: Prednisolone causes increase in blood sugar level, so the nurse needs to check hourly blood sugar level. The abrupt withdrawal of the drug needs to be avoided because it will lead to insufficiency of adrenal cortical hormones.

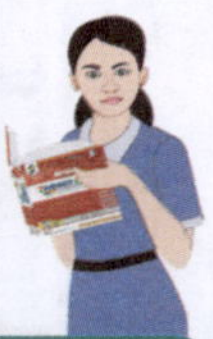

530. Intradermal injection is given at an angle of:

a. 15 degrees b. 30 degrees
c. 45 degrees d. 90 degrees

Explanation: ID at 15 degrees; Subcutaneous (SC) at 30-45 degrees; Intramuscular (IM) at 90 degrees

531. Antidote for Heparin is: *(DSSSB 2013)*

a. Vitamin K
b. Protamine sulfate
c. Aminocaproic acid
d. Amiodarone

Explanation: Protamine sulfate is an antidote for heparin. Protamine sulfate is a drug that reverses the anticoagulant effects of heparin by binding to it.

532. A patient's GRBS is 40 mg%. The immediate management is to administer: *(DSSSB 2013)*

a. 5% dextrose
b. 50% dextrose
c. 5% dextrose in normal saline
d. Normal saline

Explanation: Emergency and immediate management of low blood sugar is 50% dextrose to restore blood glucose level.

533. Sensitivity and reaction are tested by administering the drug *(DSSSB 2013)*

a. Intradermally b. Intramuscularly
c. Intravenously d. Subcutaneously

Explanation: Sensitivity and reaction are tested by administering a low dose of the drug intradermally. The allergic reaction can be easily observed on the skin if the drug or allergen is injected through intradermal route and the absorption is slower compared to other parenteral route.

534. Medications used for nausea and vomiting are known as: *(DSSSB 2013)*

a. Analgesics b. Antipyretics
c. Antiemetics d. Antibiotics

Explanation: Antiemetics are the medications used for nausea and vomiting. Analgesics for pain relief. Antipyretics to bring down temperature and antibiotics to treat infections.

535. The appropriate needle size for insulin injection is: *(DSSSB 2013)*

a. 18 G, 1 ½" long b. 22 G, 1" long
c. 22 G, 1 ½" long d. 25 G, 5/8" long

Explanation: 25G, 5/8" needle is the recommended size for insulin injection because insulin is administered by the subcutaneous route.

536. Which of the following is the preferred site for intramuscular injection in infants? *(DSSSB 2013)*

a. Deltoid b. Rectus Femoris
c. Vastus lateralis d. Ventrogluteal

Explanation: Vastus lateralis site is the preferred site for IM injections in infants.

537. Which among the following abbreviations indicates 'once a day'?

a. OD b. BD
c. TD d. HS

Explanation:

OD - Once a day
BD - Twice a day
TDS - Thrice a day
HS - At bed time
STAT - At immediately (or at once)
SOS - If necessary (in emergency)
PRN - As needed (for example, if paracetamol is prescribed on PRN basis, then it is to be taken whenever there is a pain.

538. The preferred site for giving IM injection to infants is: *(DSSSB PHN, 2015)*

a. Gluteal
b. Deltoid
c. Vastus Lateralis
d. Umbilicus

539. What is the maximum volume that can be given as IM injection in adult? *(JIPMER 2012)*

a. 0.5 mL b. 1 mL
c. 2 mL d. 5 mL

540. Which of the following is not a Parenteral route of administration of drugs? *(ISRO)*

a. Subcutaneous
b. Intramuscular
c. Rectal
d. Intravenous

Ans.

527. a
528. d
529. c
530. a
531. b
532. b
533. a
534. c
535. d
536. c
537. a
538. c
539. d
540. c

541. While administering medication, client stated that he is not remembering that he was getting this medication before. Appropriate nursing action is:
a. Administer medication
b. Record client's statement
c. Verify the medication order again
d. Inform physician

542. Long term use of sedative and hypnotics in older persons lead to:
a. Headaches and nausea
b. Altered level of consciousness
c. Depression and anxiety
d. Sleep disruption

543. A patient is on oral paracetamol 2 tablets every 3 hours. Priority nursing action for this client is:
a. The patient's level of pain
b. Temperature of the patient
c. The amount of daily dose
d. Risk for bleeding

Explanation: The maximum daily dose of paracetamol for adults is 4 grams (4000 mg) per day. Therefore, it is important to check the total amount of paracetamol the patient is taking in a day to ensure that they are not exceeding this maximum safe dose.

544. A drug that relieves flatulence is known as:
a. Carminatives b. Purgatives
c. Antacids d. Astringents

545. Which of the following is not classified under parenteral route of drug administration?
a. Intramuscular b. Intradermal
c. Sublingual d. Intravenous

546. Intradermal injection is given at an angle of:
a. 15 degrees b. 30 degrees
c. 45 degrees d. 90 degrees

547. Subcutaneous injection is given at an angle of:
a. 15 degrees b. 30 degrees
c. 45 degrees d. 90 degrees

548. Intramuscular injection is given at an angle of:
a. 15 degrees b. 30 degrees
c. 45 degrees d. 90 degrees

549. Size of the needle used for IM injection is...................
a. 16-18 gauge b. 18-20 gauge
c. 22-25 gauge d. 25-28 gauge

550. Hypodermal injection commonly known as ....
a. Intradermal
b. Subcutaneous
c. Intramuscular
d. Intravenous

551. 'After meal' is abbreviated as:
a. PRN b. PM
c. PC d. HS

552. Patient on continuous IV infusion develops edema at the IV site. It suggests:
a. Pain b. Infiltration
c. Phlebitis d. Thrombosis

553. Immediate nursing action in a client with infiltration is ......
a. Stop IV infusion
b. Hot application
c. Cold application
d. Inform the doctor

554. All of the following are sites for subcutaneous injection in adult; EXCEPT:
a. Scapula b. Upper arm
c. Lower abdomen d. Anterior upper thigh

Explanation: The scapula is not typically recommended for subcutaneous injections in adults due to the risk of injury to underlying structures such as nerves and blood vessels.

All other sites mentioned above are common sites for subcutaneous injection.

555. Which among the following sizes of IV cannula has the largest diameter?
a. 16 G b. 18 G
c. 20 G d. 22 G

556. Massaging medication over the skin is:
a. Inunction b. Inhalation
c. Instillation d. Irrigation

557. Taking medication directly into the respiratory tract is termed as:
a. Inunction b. Inhalation
c. Instillation d. Irrigation

558. Administration of medication directly into the eyes is known as:
a. Inunction b. Irrigation
c. Instillation d. Inhalation

559. Most commonly used steam inhaler is:
a. Ultrasonic b. Nelson's inhaler
c. Jet inhaler d. Marsh's inhaler

560. Current RIGHTS of medication administration are:
a. Five Rights b. Seven Rights
c. Eight Rights d. Ten Rights

561. Adjuvant drug used during anesthesia is:
a. Halogen b. Medicated air
c. Nitrous oxide d. Propofol

Explanation: Agents that are administered along with anesthetics to improve delivery, increase effectiveness, or decrease required dosage are known as adjuvants, e.g., Nitrous oxide, Sedatives, etc.

Propofol is an anesthetic agent.

562. What should be added to normal saline solution which is connected to arterial line measuring blood pressure?
a. Protamine b. Calcium
c. Potassium d. Heparin

Explanation: Heparin can be added to normal saline solution that is connected to an arterial line measuring blood pressure to prevent the formation of blood clots within the line.

563. The nurse should check the prescription ________ times before administering the medicine to a patient.
a. One b. Two
c. Three d. Four

Explanation: The label on the medication must be checked for name, dose, and route, and compared with the Medication Administration Record (Prescription) at three different times:
1. When the medication is taken out of the drawer.
2. When the medication is being poured (e.g., loaded in syringe or poured in container etc.).
3. When the medication is being put away/or at bedside.

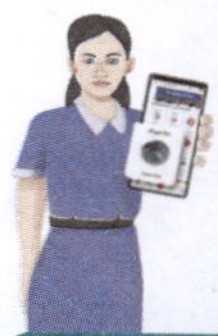

Ans.

541. c
542. d
543. c
544. a
545. c
546. a
547. c
548. d
549. c
550. b
551. c
552. b
553. a
554. a
555. a
556. a
557. b
558. c
559. b
560. d
561. c
562. d
563. c

564. Which of the following methods is used to administer BCG vaccine?

a. Subcutaneous injection
b. Intradermal scratch injection
c. Intravenous injection
d. Z-track injection

565. When administering penicillin injection, the nurse observes a fine rash on the patient's skin. The immediate nursing action would be to:

a. Administer the medication with CPM
b. Administer the medication and notify the physician
c. Withhold the medication and notify the physician
d. Apply ice packs on rashes

566. Cone shaped or oval shaped drug which is inserted into the rectum and which melt at body temperature is known as:

a. Suppository
b. Enema
c. Foley's catheter
d. Rectal tube

567. Administration of medication into the sub arachnoid space is known as:

a. Intrathecal
b. Intraosseous
c. Intradermal
d. Subcutaneous

568. Administration of medication into the bone is known as:

a. Intrathecal
b. Intraosseous
c. Intradermal
d. Subcutaneous

569. Name the nerve which is more likely to get injured in improper dorso gluteal IM injection:

a. Peroneal
b. Sciatic
c. Brachial
d. Femoral

570. Method used while administering irritating medication via IM route is:

a. Z track method
b. Deep IM method
c. Sealing method
d. All of the above

571. The following statement is true about Z track method of injection: *(ISRO)*

a. Painless
b. Prevent leakage of medication into the subcutaneous tissue
c. Easy to administer
d. A type of intradermal injection

572. In which of the following conditions blood transfusion is contraindicated? *(AIIMS Bhopal Nursing Officer, 2018)*

a. Bleeding hemorrhoids
b. Hemorrhage
c. Congestive cardiac failure
d. Hemophilia

Explanation: In congestive heart failure, already fluid overload is there. So, blood transfusion may worsen the condition. In all other conditions blood transfusion is the treatment of choice.

573. Which of the following equipment is the most essential to prevent the risk of cardiac dysrhythmias in a patient receiving multiple transfusion of blood?

a. ECG Machine
b. Cardiac monitor
c. Blood warmer
d. Syringe pump

Explanation: Rapid transfusion of cold blood places the patient at risk for cardiac dysrhythmias. ECG machine and Cardiac monitor are used to assess the cardiac function but not for prevention of dysrhythmias. Syringe pump is used for infusion of very small amount of drugs but not used for blood transfusion. Blood warmer is needed to rewarm the cold blood to body temperature before transfusion.

574. Which of the following techniques during IM injection helps to prevent the leakage of medication from the tissues? *(AIIMS 2015)*

a. Massaging the skin with antiseptic solution before injection
b. Stretching the skin
c. Administration at an angle of 90°
d. Slow push of injection

Explanation: Stretching the skin leads to Z track technique. Stretching leads to zig-zag arrangement of skin and tissues which prevents leakage of medication.

575. Commonly used solutions for mouth care include:

a. $KMnO_4$ 1: 5000
b. Hydrogen peroxide 1:8
c. Sodium chloride 1 teaspoon to 1 pint of water
d. All of the above

Explanation: All of the above solutions are used for mouth care. Other than these, commercially available solutions can also be used.

576. The appropriate needle size for blood transfusion in an adult is:

a. 12 to 16 G
b. 16 to 20 G
c. 18 to 24 G
d. 22 to 26 G

577. The nurse has to administer ear drop to a 7-year-old boy. How does the nurse pull the patient's ear?

a. Outward
b. Backward
c. Upward and outward
d. Upward and backward

578. Reason for administering Fresh Frozen Plasma (FFP) for a patient admitted after heavy bleeding related to Road Traffic accident is:

a. To increase platelet count and treat platelet dysfunction
b. To provide clotting factors
c. To increase hemoglobin
d. To increase hematocrit

579. All of the following are the components of VAP care bundle; EXCEPT:

a. Good hand hygiene practices
b. Regular oral hygiene for patient
c. Ensure limited patient movement while on ventilator
d. Elevation of the head end of the bed by 30-45 degrees

580. Digoxin 75 mcg = ? mg:

a. 0.75 mg
b. 0.075 mg
c. 7.5 mg
d. 750 mg

Explanation:
1 mg = 1000 mcg
1 mcg = 1/1000 mg
75 mcg = 75/1000
75 mcg = 0.075 mg

Ans.

564. b
565. c
566. a
567. a
568. b
569. b
570. a
571. b
572. c
573. c
574. b
575. d
576. b
577. d
578. b
579. c
580. b

581. gtt is an abbreviation of:
a. Drop b. Milliliter
c. Liter d. Gallon

582. The size of the intravenous cannula used for neonates is: *(DSSSB 2013)*
a. 18 Gauze b. 20 Gauze
c. 22 Gauze d. 24 Gauze

Explanation: Sizes of Cannula:
- 14 G- (Orange) adolescent and adult.
- 16 G- (Grey) adolescent and adult major surgery and trauma.
- 18 G- (Green) adolescent and adult major surgery and trauma.
- 20 G- (Pink) Older children, adolescent and adult.
- 22 G- (Blue) Older children, adolescent and elderly adult.
- 24 G-(Yellow) Neonate, infant and toddler.

NURSING THEORIES

583. Which of the following is a model based on an individual's relationship to stress the reaction to it and reconstitution factors that are dynamic in nature? *(AIIMS-BBS SNO 2019)*
a. Parse's Human Becoming Theory
b. Universality Theory
c. Roy's Adaptation Model
d. Neuman's System Model

584. The theory which intends to provide a unifying focus for approaching a wide range of nursing concerns and for understanding fundamental nursing phenomena: the client, the environment, health and nursing is: *(AIIMS Raipur Grade II 2017)*
a. Roy's theory of nursing
b. Neuman's theory of nursing
c. Nightingale's theory of nursing
d. Scudder theory of nursing

Explanation: The Neuman Systems Model views the client as an open system that responds to stressors in the environment. Roy's theory of nursing sees the individual as a set of interrelated systems such as biological, psychological and social. Florence Nightingale developed Environmental theory of nursing which believed "Healthy surroundings (environment) were necessary for proper nursing care." Scudder theory of nursing describes discipline of nursing should be a human science because it studies how nurses care for patients.

585. The theory that involves care and helps through which the client attains total self-care is: *(AIIMS Raipur NO 2019)*
a. Nightingale theory b. Orem's theory
c. Paplau's theory d. Roy's theory

Explanation:

Table

Theorists	Theories
Orem's theory	Self-care deficit theory which helps client to attain total self-care.
Nightingale's theory	Environment as the focus of nursing care.
Peplau's theory	Focuses on interpersonal relationship.
Roy's theory	Roy developed an adaptation model, known as RAM.

586. In Maslow's hierarchy of physiologic needs, the human need of greatest priority is: *(RAK MSc 2018)*
a. Love b. Elimination
c. Nutrition d. Oxygen

Explanation: As per Maslow's hierarchy of needs, physiological needs must be met first. These include food, water, oxygen, warmth and rest. Out of all of options, oxygen is the highest priority as it is must for survival. Without oxygen, survival is not possible even for few minutes.

587. Highest level of need According to Maslow's hierarchy is:
a. Physiologic needs b. Safety and security
c. Love and belongings d. Self-actualization

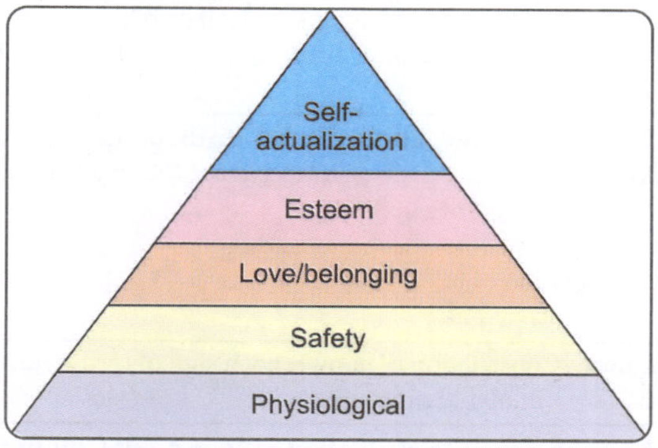

Explanation: Self-actualization is the highest need as per Maslow.

588. The four major concepts in nursing theory are:
a. Nursing, Physician, Environment, Patient
b. Nursing, Person, Environment, Cure
c. Nursing, Person, Environment, Health
d. Prevention, promotion, Treatment, Rehabilitation

589. 'Nursing is a theoretical body of knowledge that prescribes analysis and action to care for an ill person'. This is proposed by:
a. Callista Roy b. Virginia Henderson
c. Martha Rogers d. Betty Neuman

590. Who defined that 'the nurse/patient relationship evolve through *orientation, identification, exploitation and resolution*'
a. Madeleine Leininger
b. Dorothea Orem
c. Hildegard Peplau
d. Betty Neuman

591. A system model that focuses on the response of the client system to actual or potential environmental stressors was developed by:
a. Martha Rogers
b. Betty Neuman
c. Dorothea Orem
d. Virginia Henderson

592. Self-care theory was developed by:
a. Dorothea Orem b. Callista Roy
c. Martha Rogers d. Betty Neuman

593. Four conservation principles, i.e., energy, structural integrity, personal integrity and social integrity was described by:
a. Leininger b. Peplau
c. Levin d. Rogers

Ans.
581. a
582. d
583. d
584. b
585. b
586. d
587. d
588. c
589. a
590. c
591. b
592. a
593. c

BASIC AND ADVANCED LIFE SUPPORT

594. A nurse enters a room and finds a client lying on the floor. Which action should the nurse perform first? *(AIIMS BPL NO 2018)*

a. Ask the client what happened
b. Call for help to get the client back in bed
c. Establish whether the client is responsive
d. Assist the client back to bed

Explanation: The first priority is to assess the patient's condition, therefore, assessing the response of the patient should be the first thing, which is then followed by calling for help to shift the client, assist client back to bed and then ask the client to explain the incidence. If the patient is unresponsive, Call or tell someone to call 911. Check the person's airway, breathing, and pulse. If necessary, begin CPR.

595. All of the below are signs of cardiopulmonary arrest; EXCEPT: *(AIIMS Bhopal Nursing Officer, 2018)*

a. Constriction of pupil
b. Immediate loss of consciousness
c. Dilatation of pupil
d. Absence of pulse

Explanation: Constriction of pupil is not a sign of cardiopulmonary arrest. It is seen in opioid poisoning.

596. The compression to ventilation ratio in adult CPR in case of single rescuer is: *(DSSSB PHN, 2015; LNJP H D 2012)*

a. 5:2 b. 15:2
c. 30:2 d. 2:30

597. The compression to ventilation ratio in adult CPR in case of two rescuer is: *(Recent question)*

a. 5:2 b. 15:2
c. 30:2 d. 2:30

598. The compression to ventilation ratio for CPR in child/infant in case of one rescuer is: *(Recent question)*

a. 5:2 b. 15:2
c. 30:2 d. 2:30

599. While doing CPR in an infant what is the compression ventilation ratio with two rescuers: *(LNJP H D 2012)*

a. 15:1 b. 5:1
c. 15:2 d. 30:2

600. The compression to ventilation ratio for CPR in neonate is: *(Recent question)*

a. 3:1 b. 1:3
c. 30:2 d. 15:1

601. Rate of chest compression in one person CPR is: *(Recent Question 2012)*

a. 150-170/min b. 100-120/min
c. 60-70/min d. 80-100/min

602. Carotid pulse should be checked for: *(LNJP H D 2012)*

a. 15–20 seconds
b. Less than 5 seconds
c. 5–10 seconds
d. 10–15 seconds

603. Chest compression in an unresponsive victim will be started: *(LNJP H D 2012)*

a. After giving two breaths to victim
b. After making an emergency call to ambulance service
c. After checking carotid pulse of the victim and find the pulse is absent
d. As soon as you find an unresponsive victim

604. CPR stands for:

a. Cardiopulmonary revival
b. Cardiopulmonary resuscitation
c. Cardiopulmonary recycle
d. Cardiopulmonary recovery

OXYGEN THERAPY

605. Blood vessel that extends and branches out from an artery and leads to capillaries is:

a. Venule b. Arteriole
c. Capillary d. Sinus

Explanation: Arterioles are the blood vessels in the microcirculation that extend and branch out from an artery and lead to capillaries. A very small vein, especially one collecting blood from the capillaries and return to vein. Capillary beds can consist branch from arterioles and provide exchange between cells and the blood, and short vessels that directly connect the arterioles and venules at opposite ends of the beds.

606. The factors that interfere correct function of pulse oximeter include all; EXCEPT:

a. Carbon monoxide poisoning
b. Hypertension
c. Pulse volume
d. Vasoconstriction

Explanation: Several factors can interfere with the correct function of a pulse oximeter including:

- Light – bright light (such as the operating theater light or sunlight) directly on the probe may affect the reading.
- Shivering – movement may make it difficult for the probe to pick up a signal.
- Pulse volume – the oximeter only detects pulsatile flow. When the blood pressure is low due to hypovolemic shock or the cardiac output is low or the patient has an arrhythmia, the pulse may be very weak and the oximeter may not be able to detect a signal
- Vasoconstriction reduces blood flow to the peripheries. The oximeter may fail to detect a signal if the patient is very cold and peripherally vasoconstricted.
- Carbon monoxide poisoning may give a falsely high saturation reading. Carbon monoxide binds very well to haemoglobin and displaces oxygen to form a bright red compound called carboxyhemoglobin. This is only an issue in patients following smoke inhalation from a fire.

Source: WHO Pulse Oximetry Training Manual (WHO, 2011).

607. After receiving a patient from OT following cardiac surgery, most priority nursing intervention is:

a. Connect the patient to cardiac monitor
b. Ensure patent airway
c. Check vital signs of the patient
d. Start the medication and IV fluids

Explanation: ABC are the priority. So ensure that the client is having an open airway.

608. The priority nursing intervention for a patient during the immediate post-operative period is:

a. Observing for hemorrhage
b. Maintaining a patent airway
c. Recording the intake and output
d. Checking the vital signs every 15 minutes

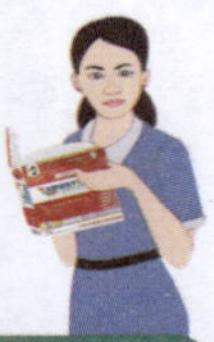

Ans.

594. c
595. a
596. c
597. c
598. c
599. c
600. a
601. b
602. c
603. c
604. b
605. b
606. b
607. b
608. b

609. The nurse is administering oxygen to a client with chest pain who is restless. What is the method of oxygen administration that is least likely to increase apprehension in the client? *(RAK MSc 2018)*

a. Nasal Cannula
b. Catheter
c. Venturi mask
d. Rebreather mask

Explanation:
- Nasal **cannula** is the best method for administering oxygen as it does not interfere with the usual activities of drinking, eating and mobility. A nasal cannula is generally used wherever small amounts of supplemental oxygen are required.

610. Equipment used to measure the oxygen saturation is:

a. Billy blanket
b. Pulse oximeter
c. Ophthalmoscope
d. Goniometer

Explanation: Pulse oximeter is the instrument used to measure the oxygen saturation. Billy blanket is used in double surface phototherapy.

611. The percentage and the flow of oxygen in a red color venturi mask is: *(DSSSB 2013)*

a. 31% and 6 L/min
b. 35% and 8 L/min
c. 40% and 10 L/min
d. 60% and 15 L/min

Explanation:

Color	% of O_2
Blue	24%
White	28%
Orange	31%
Yellow	35%
Red	40%,
Green	60%

612. Color coding for oxygen cylinder is:

a. Black
b. Black with white shoulders
c. Light blue
d. Gray

Explanation: Nitrous oxide cylinder is blue in color, oxygen cylinder is black with white cap, Chlorine: yellow and nitrogen: black

613. All of the following are complications associated with oxygenation; EXCEPT:

a. Peau d'orange
b. Paul Bert effect
c. Lorrain Smith effect
d. Retinopathy of prematurity

Explanation: Peau d'orange is not a complication associated with oxygenation. A pitted or dimpled appearance of the skin, especially as characteristic of some cases of breast cancer or due to cellulite is Peau d'orange.

All other options are complications related to oxygen administration. Oxygen toxicity in central nervous system condition is called Paul Bert effect, and the pulmonary condition is called as Lorrain Smith effect. Oxygen toxicity in premature infant is known as retinopathy of prematurity.

614. In which of the following conditions is oxygen therapy has high risk of causing hypercapnia? *New Q*

a. Chronic obstructive pulmonary disease (COPD)
b. Acute respiratory distress syndrome (ARDS)
c. Acute exacerbation of asthma
d. Carbon monoxide poisoning.

Explanation: In patients with COPD, oxygen therapy may be contraindicated or not indicated in some cases because it can cause a decrease in respiratory drive and lead to retention of carbon dioxide, which can worsen respiratory acidosis and respiratory failure. Therefore, in patients with COPD, oxygen therapy should be carefully monitored and titrated to avoid hypercapnia and respiratory acidosis.

615. Oxygen therapy is recommended in: *(ESIC Chennai May 2012)*

a. Severe respiratory distress
b. Acute myocardial infarction
c. Severe trauma
d. All of the above

616. What is the recommended flow rate of oxygen via nasal cannula?

a. 1-4 L/min
b. 3-6 L/min
c. 4-7 L/min
d. 6-8 L/min

617. The dose of oxygen to be delivered through a nasal mask to a patient with chronic respiratory failure is:

a. 1 L/min
b. 2 L/min
c. 5 L/min
d. 10 L/min

618. Concentration of oxygen present in expired air is:

a. 78. 04%
b. 13.6% - 16%
c. 4% - 5.3%
d. 1%

Explanation: 78.04% nitrogen; 13.6% - 16% oxygen: 4% - 5.3% carbon dioxide; 1% argon and other gases.

619. The purpose of humidifying oxygen during oxygen therapy is that the oxygen is:

a. A hot air and it may burn trachea
b. Easily absorbed because humidification adds H-ion to it
c. Free of pathogens by humidification
d. A dry gas may thicken the mucus

620. Which of the following symptoms would the nurse assess to determine the oxygen status of patient with iron deficiency anemia?

a. Increased breathlessness but increased activity tolerance
b. Increased breathlessness and decreased activity tolerance
c. Decreased breathlessness and increased activity tolerance
d. Decreased breathlessness and decreased activity tolerance

621. A prescribed amount of oxygen is required for a patient with Chronic Obstructive Pulmonary Disease (COPD) to prevent:

a. Increased partial pressure of carbon dioxide in arterial blood ($PaCO_2$)
b. Inhibition of the respiratory hypoxic stimulus
c. Hypervolemia
d. Respiratory stimulation

622. Objectives of the Incentive spirometry includes all; EXCEPT:

a. To reduce transpulmonary pressure
b. To increase inspiratory volumes
c. To maintain airway patency
d. To prevent atelectasis

Ref: AARC Clinical Practice Guideline.

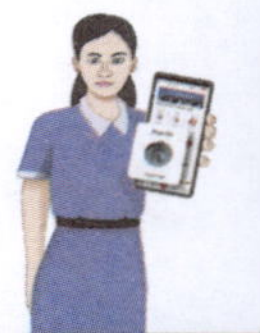

Ans.

609. a
610. b
611. c
612. b
613. a
614. a
615. d
616. a
617. b
618. b
619. d
620. b
621. b
622. a

Explanation: Incentive spirometry is designed to mimic natural sighing or yawning by encouraging the patient to take long, slow, deep breaths. The objectives of incentive spirometry procedure are to:

- Increase transpulmonary pressure and inspiratory volumes
- Improve inspiratory muscle performance
- Re-establish or simulate the normal pattern of pulmonary hyperinflation.
- When the procedure is repeated on a regular basis, airway patency may be maintained and lung atelectasis prevented and reversed.

623. While measuring central venous pressure, the zero point of the manometer is adjusted to: *(DSSSB 2013)*

a. Anterior axillary line
b. Mid axillary line
c. Posterior axillary line
d. Shoulder level

Explanation: Zero level of the manometer is adjusted to mid axillary line, at the level of patient's right atrium.

624. While performing lumbar puncture in an adult, the needle is inserted between: *(DSSSB PHN, 2015)*

a. L3-L4 or L4-L5
b. Ll-L2 or L2-L3
c. L2-L3 or L3-L4
d. L1-L2 or L3-L4

625. Which of the following is an indication for Bag-valve-mask ventilation? *(AIIMS Bhopal Nursing Officer, 2018)*

a. Meconium stained delivery
b. Diaphragmatic hernia
c. Baby is apneic with heart rate less than 100 beats
d. Good respiratory efforts at birth with heart rate of 120 beats

Explanation: As per the guidelines, bag and mask ventilations is indicated if baby is apneic and heart rate is less than 100. In Meconium stained delivery and in Diaphragmatic hernia bag and mask ventilations is contraindicated. Good respiratory efforts at birth with heart rate of 120 beats is a good sign and there is no need of bag and mask ventilation.

NURSING ROLES IN IMPORTANT NURSING PROCEDURES

626. All of the following precautions are true while recording oral temperature of a patient; EXCEPT: *(Banaras HU 2015)*

a. Measurement of temperature should be done on a fixed time of the day
b. It is measured at least 3 min after keeping the thermometer sublingually with lips closed
c. Not to record in patients who have recently smoked
d. In patients on oxygen inhalation, stop the oxygenation before recording oral temperature

627. All of the following are precautions in the care of a patient with high fever; EXCEPT: *(Banaras HU 2015)*

a. Never leave a patient with high fever alone
b. Rigors and convulsions may occur any time
c. Administer antipyretic drugs
d. Tepid cold sponging is not useful in patient not responding to antipyretics

628. Patient has intravenous fluids infusing in the right arm when taking a blood pressure on this patient, the nurse would: *(LNJP H D 2012)*

a. Take the blood pressure in the left arm
b. Take the blood pressure in the right arm
c. Use the smallest possible cuff
d. Report inability to take the blood pressure

629. Pre-procedural preparation before taking oral temperature includes:

a. Make sure that patient performed oral hygiene before the procedure
b. Make sure that patient has not taken anything cold or hot 10-20 min before the procedure
c. Make sure that patient is not wearing any denture while performing the procedure
d. All of the above

630. A patient in the unit has a 103.7°F temperature. Which intervention would be most effective in restoring normal body temperature?

a. Use a cooling blanket while the patient is febrile.
b. Administer antipyretics on an around-the-clock schedule.
c. Provide increased fluids and have the UAP give sponge baths.
d. Give prescribed antibiotics and provide warm blankets for comfort.

631. The patient has voided only 50-100 mL of urine after the removal of Foley's catheter. What is the priority nursing action?

a. Check for bladder distention
b. Encourage fluid intake
c. Re-catheterize the client
d. Monitor I/O chart

632. What is the important nursing intervention while assisting for peritoneal dialysis catheter insertion?

a. Explain the procedure and get consent from the patient
b. Check the renal function of the patient
c. Ask the patient to empty the bladder
d. Arrange emergency trolley near to bedside

Explanation: Option c is the correct answer to avoid injury to the bladder, Option a is the physician's responsibility.

633. Which of the following nursing interventions can prevent increase of intracranial pressure (ICP) in an unconscious child? *(Banaras HU 2015)*

a. Avoid activities that cause pain or crying
b. Lower the position of head (Trendelenburg position)
c. Provide environmental stimulation
d. Turn head side to side every hour

634. When the patient vomits, the most important nursing objective is to prevent: *(ESIC Chennai May 2012)*

a. Rupture of suture line
b. Metabolic Alkalosis
c. Dehydration
d. Aspiration

635. Physician ordered oral as well as nasal suction to a client. You will do suction first in:

a. Mouth
b. Nose
c. Where the secretion is more
d. Where the secretion is less

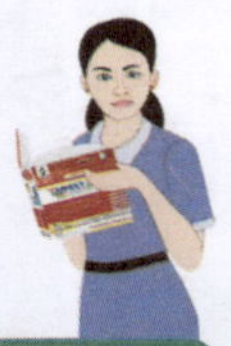

Ans.

623.	b
624.	a
625.	c
626.	d
627.	d
628.	a
629.	b
630.	b
631.	a
632.	c
633.	a
634.	d
635.	a

Explanation: Always do first suction in the mouth, then the nose because doing suction first in the nose will stimulate pharynx and cause aspiration. To avoid this, always do suction first in the mouth.

TIPS: M comes before N in the alphabet.

636. Methods used to reconfirm the position of NG tube each time before administering a feeding is/are:

a. By dipping tip of the tube in bowl of water
b. Pushing some air and auscultating
c. pH testing of the aspirated fluid
d. All of the above

Explanation: X-rays are currently the gold standard for NGT placement confirmation because they can visualize the course of the NGT tube. However, dipping tip of the tube in bowl of water to observe for air bubbles, pushing some air and auscultating, or pH testing of the aspirated fluid are the methods used to reconfirm NG tube position each time before administering feeding because the tube can become displaced later.

637. Length of insertion of NG is measured from:

a. Tip of nose to earlobe then to xiphoid process
b. Tip of nose to xiphoid process
c. Tip of nose to forehead and to xiphoid
d. Tip of nose to stomach

Explanation: NG tube insertion length is measured from tip of nose to ear lobe then to xiphoid process.

638. While cleaning eye, it has to be cleaned from:

a. Inner canthus to outer canthus *(AIIMS 2016)*
b. Outer canthus to inner canthus
c. Middle of the eye to outer canthus
d. Middle of the eye to inner canthus

Explanation: Cleaning has to be done from more clean to less clean area, so inner canthus to outer canthus.

639. Mr. Alex was receiving transfusion of packed RBC's. He suddenly developed difficulty in breathing, chills and flushing. Which of the following nursing interventions should take priority?

a. Place the client on semi-fowler position
b. Check the client's temperature
c. Stop the transfusion
d. Administer oxygen

Explanation: The patient is experiencing blood transfusion reaction. The priority action of the nurse is to stop the transfusion immediately before initiating other interventions.

640. Find out the true statement regarding eye irrigation:

a. Irrigate right eye first then left eye
b. Irrigate from outer canthus to inner canthus
c. Most commonly using solution for eye irrigation is mannitol
d. Irrigate least infected eye first then more infected eye

Explanation: Option D is the only correct statement regarding eye irrigation. While irrigating eye, least infected eye is irrigated first not the right eye. Irrigation has to be done from inner canthus to outer canthus, most commonly used solutions for eye irrigation are normal saline, 2% boric acid and 1% silver nitrate.

641. Find out the incorrect statement regarding colostomy irrigation:

a. It is a clean procedure
b. NS and water can be used to irrigate the stoma
c. As the fluid moves in cramps can happen
d. Irrigation is recommended for patient with stomal prolapse

Explanation: Colostomy irrigation of patient with stomal prolapsed can increase the risk of further prolapse. Option a, b, c are correct statement regarding colostomy irrigation.

642. Which of the following statements is not TRUE regarding paracentesis?

a. Empty the bladder to avoid injury to bladder before the procedure
b. It can be done at 2 cm below the umbilicus in the midline
c. It can be done at 5 cm superior and medial to the anterior superior iliac spines on either side
d. Paracentesis is usually performed with the patient in side lying position

Explanation: Paracentesis is a procedure in which a needle or catheter is inserted into the peritoneal cavity to obtain ascitic fluid for diagnostic or therapeutic purposes. Paracentesis is usually performed with the patient in supine position. The bed is flat or the head is slightly elevated. The face-down position with the fluid pooled in the dependent abdomen permits drainage of the last few milliliters of fluid.

643. Frequent swallowing in a patient following tonsillectomy indicate:

a. Hemorrhage b. Active gag reflex
c. Thirst in patient d. None of these

Explanation: Frequent swallowing following tonsillectomy suggestive of hemorrhage in the patient.

644. Chest drain should not be clamped. Why?

a. It leads to accumulation of more blood
b. It leads to tension pneumothorax
c. Patient will complain pain
d. None of the above

Explanation: There is a risk of the patient developing a tension pneumothorax if chest drainage is clamped.

645. Milking of drainage tube will create:

a. Negative pressure b. Positive pressure
c. Occlude the tube d. None of these

Explanation: Milking of chest drain is only to be done with written orders from medical staff. Milking drain creates a high negative pressure that can cause pain, tissue trauma and bleeding

646. For managing hemothorax, ICD is inserted in a patient. Continuous bubbling in the water seal indicates:

a. It is a normal finding
b. Air leakage
c. Time to remove the ICD
d. Fully expanded chest

Explanation: In a person with hemothorax, bubbling in the water seal indicates air leakage. In pneumothorax, it is a normal finding.

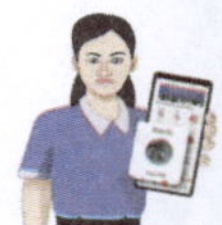

Ans.

636. d
637. a
638. a
639. c
640. d
641. d
642. d
643. a
644. b
645. a
646. b

647. Go through the following statements regarding swing of fluids in ICD and identify the correct statement:

a. The water in the water seal chamber will rise and fall with respirations
b. The swing will diminish as the pneumothorax resolves
c. Unexpected cessation of swing may indicate the tube is blocked or kinked
d. All of the above

Explanation: All of the above statements are correct in relation to swing of fluid in ICD drainage.

648. While shifting the patient from stretcher to bed, accidental dislodging of ICD occurred, which is the most appropriate nursing action?

a. Apply pressure to the exit site and seal
b. Call the doctor immediately
c. Try to reinsert the tube
d. None of the above

Explanation: Apply pressure to the exit site and seal with steri-strips. Placing an occlusive dressing over the top is the most appropriate nursing action.

649. Which of the following need to be performed before radial arterial cannulation to evaluate radial and ulnar arterial patency? *(DSSSB 2013)*

a. Allen's test b. Angiography
c. Buerger's test d. Capillary refill test

Explanation: A test for occlusion of radial or ulnar arteries: the patient makes a tight fist so as to express the blood from the skin of the palm and fingers; the examiner makes digital compression on either the radial or ulnar artery. Failure of blood to return to the palm and fingers when the hand is opened indicates obstruction of the blood flow in the artery that has not been compressed. Either this test or a doppler ultrasound examination should always be performed prior to insertion of a radial artery line.

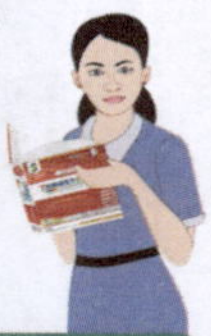

650. While instilling ear drops, the ear canal of an adult is straightened by pulling the pinna: *(DSSSB 2013)*

a. Down and back
b. Up and back
c. Straight down
d. Straight back

Explanation: For adults, gently pull the upper ear up and back. For children, gently pull the lower ear down and back.

651. All of the following instructions are given to a patient before computed tomography (CT) scan; EXCEPT: *(Banaras HU 2015)*

a. Wear comfortable, loose-fitting clothing
b. Remove all metallic objects such as hairpin, dentures, jewelry, etc.
c. It will not affect the outcome of pregnancy in case of female patient
d. Nil per oral several hours before the scan

652. Insertion of a needle into the pleural cavity is: *(Kerala PSC, Nov 2014)*

a. Endoscopy b. Paracentesis
c. Thoracentesis d. Evisceration

653. Which of the following nursing measures should be avoided in a patient with increased intracranial pressure? *(Recent Question 2012)*

a. Suctioning for prolonged time
b. NG tube feeding
c. Fowler's position
d. Catheterization

654. Choosing the appropriate catheter depends on: *(ESIC Chennai May 2012)*

a. Knowledge of any allergies to latex or plastic
b. The expected duration of catheterization
c. The size of the patient's urethral canal
d. All of the above

655. Curved or coude catheters have: *(ESIC Chennai May 2012)*

a. A rounded curved tip
b. A single lumen with a small 1 1/24 cm opening
c. A single lumen with a small 1 ¼ cm opening
d. An inflatable balloon that encircles the tip near the lumen or opening

656. Tracheostomy is usually performed between the tracheal rings of cartilage of: *(LNJP H D 2012)*

a. Fourth and fifth b. Third and fourth
c. Second and third d. First and Second

657. Most important concern while providing oral care to an unconscious client is:

a. Use ordered mouth care solution
b. Preventing aspiration
c. Look for denture
d. Provide oral care in each shift

658. After a surgical procedure, stockings are usually used to:

a. Prevent varicose veins
b. Promote venous return to the heart
c. Prevent muscular atrophy
d. All of the above

659. Post-operative period respiratory complications can be prevented by:

a. Deep breathing b. Coughing exercises
c. Incentive spirometer d. All of these

660. Which of the following teaching approach is appropriate for a client with chest pain having emergency cardiac catheterization?

a. Selling approach b. Telling approach
c. Trusting approach d. All of these

661. Chest tube drainage is useful in which of the following conditions:

a. Pneumothorax b. Pleural effusion
c. Hemothorax d. All of these

662. Slow administration of NG feed helps to reduce:

a. Flatulence b. Distension
c. Regurgitation d. Indigestion

663. Anthelmintic enema is given to:

a. Soften hard fecal matter
b. Destroy intestinal parasites
c. Remove flatus
d. Remove foreign particles from large intestines

664. Which of the following is a type of evacuant enema?

a. Nutrient enema b. Sedative enema
c. Cold enema d. Anesthetic enema

Ans.

647. d
648. a
649. a
650. b
651. c
652. c
653. a
654. d
655. a
656. c
657. b
658. b
659. d
660. b
661. d
662. c
663. b
664. c

Explanation: The cold water enema energizes the muscles and nerves of the intestine which is most effectual as a means of relieving constipation through its tonic effects upon the structures of the rectum and mucous membrane.

665. Carminative enema is given to: *New Q*
a. Remove gas accumulation
b. Destroy intestinal parasites
c. Reduce body temperature
d. Induce sleep

Explanation: Carminative enema is called anti-spasmodic enema. It is used to remove the gaseous accumulation in abdomen. This enema consisted of glycerin, magnesium sulfate (epsom salts) and water. The combination of ingredients stimulated peristalsis resulting in a bowel movement in which feces and flatus are expelled.

666. The procedure that involves insertion of a tube through nose into stomach is known as:
a. Nasogastric irrigation b. Nasogastric intubation
c. Gastric gavage d. Endotracheal intubation

667. To avoid pulling the urinary catheter, nurse should tape the catheter on patient's: *(Recent Question 2012)*
a. Lower thigh b. Upper thigh
c. Hind leg d. Foot

668. Site for bone marrow aspiration is:
a. Iliac crest b. Sternum
c. Both a and b d. None of these

669. The preferred site for bone marrow aspiration in children is:
a. Posterior superior iliac crest
b. Anterior inferior iliac crest
c. Posterior inferior iliac crest
d. Anterior inferior iliac crest

670. The preferred site for bone marrow aspiration in obese patient is:
a. Posterior superior iliac crest
b. Anterior iliac crest
c. Inferior iliac crest
d. None of the above

Explanation: In obese patients, the anterior iliac crest may be preferred due to its greater accessibility and the potential for fewer complications.

671. Complications of blood transfusion include:
a. Anaphylactic reaction
b. Fluid overload
c. Hemolytic reaction
d. All of the above

672. Bronchoscopy is performed for all of the following purposes; EXCEPT: *New Q*
a. To view abnormalities of the airway
b. To obtain tissue specimens of the lung in a variety of disorders
c. To remove secretions, blood, or foreign objects lodged in the airway
d. To obtain accurate measurement of oxygen saturation levels

673. A colostomy in the right side of the colon is known as:
a. Dry colostomy
b. Wet colostomy
c. Double barrel colostomy
d. Loop colostomy

674. A colostomy in the left side of the colon is known as:
a. Dry colostomy
b. Wet colostomy
c. Double barrel colostomy
d. Loop colostomy

Explanation: A "dry colostomy" refers to a colostomy created in the left side of the colon (descending/sigmoid colon), where the fecal content is typically more formed and solid in consistency. This is due to the fact that the left colon is responsible for absorbing water and electrolytes from the intestinal contents, resulting in a more solid stool.

Conversely, a "wet colostomy" refers to a colostomy created in the **right side of the colon** (ascending colon), where the fecal content is typically more liquid in consistency.

675. Which part of the colon is the preferred site for permanent colostomy? *New Q*
a. Ascending colon
b. Transverse colon
c. Descending colon
d. Sigmoid colon

Explanation: The preferred site for a permanent colostomy is often the sigmoid colon, which is located in the lower left side of the abdomen. This is because the sigmoid colon tends to produce formed stool that is easier to manage with an ostomy appliance or bag. In addition, the sigmoid colon is located closer to the surface of the skin, which can make it easier to create the stoma and manage the colostomy.

676. While performing colostomy irrigation, what is the maximum height at which fluid container can be kept:
a. 25 cm b. 30 cm
c. 35 cm d. 45 cm

677. Length of catheter needs to be inserted into the stoma while performing colostomy irrigation is:
a. 5 cm b. 10 cm
c. 15 cm d. 20 cm

Explanation: A depth of 10 cm (4 inches) is considered sufficient to direct the flow of solution into the bowel and facilitate effective elimination of stool.

Insertion of a catheter that is too short, such as **5 cm**, may not reach deep enough into the stoma and can lead to leakage of irrigation fluid around the catheter.

On the other hand, insertion of a catheter that is too long, such as 15 cm or 20 cm, may cause trauma to the mucosa and lead to discomfort or other complications.

678. Which of the following advices is given to a client with plaster of Paris?
a. Elevate the casted extremity
b. Cast should not to wet, cut, heat
c. Move the digits
d. All of the above

679. A procedure used to visualize and examine the female pelvic organs through the vagina is known as: *New Q*
a. Laparoscopy
b. Culdoscopy
c. Gastroscopy
d. Endoscopy

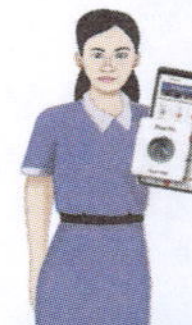

Ans.
665. a
666. b
667. b
668. c
669. a
670. b
671. d
672. d
673. b
674. a
675. d
676. d
677. b
678. d
679. b

Explanation: **Culdoscopy** is a procedure used to examine the female pelvic organs, including the uterus, fallopian tubes, and ovaries. It involves the insertion of a thin, lighted instrument called a culdoscope through the vagina and into the pelvic cavity.

Laparascopy - Visualization of abdominal organs through the opening in the abdominal wall.

Gastroscopy - a medical procedure that uses a flexible endoscope to examine the inside of the stomach and upper digestive tract.

Endoscopy - a medical procedure that uses a thin, flexible tube with a camera and light attached that is inserted through a natural opening to view the inside of the body (eg. Stomach, intestine etc)

680. Antroscopy is a visualization of the:

a. Maxillary sinus b. Bone
c. Stomach d. Hollow organ

681. In barium swallow the type of barium used is:

a. Barium sulfate b. Barium Meta bisulfate
c. Barium bromide d. Barium citrate

682. Radiographic examination of the spinal cord using contrast dye is referred as *New Q*

a. Myelography b. Electromyography
c. Myography d. Tomography

Explanation:

Myelography: Radiographic examination of the spinal cord using contrast dye.

Myography: The recording of the electrical activity produced by muscle fibers.

Electromyography: The diagnostic test that assesses the electrical activity of skeletal muscles.

Tomography: Medical imaging technique that produces detailed, cross-sectional images of the body using X-rays, magnetic fields, or other forms of radiation (not specific to spinal cord)

Salpingography: Imaging procedure that uses contrast dye to visualize the fallopian tubes and uterus.

683. During blood transfusion the most important nursing responsibility is:

a. Draw a sample from the patient before each unit is transfused
b. Maintain patency of IV catheter with dextrose solution
c. Warm the blood to body temperature to prevent chilling
d. Start the blood transfusion at a slower rate during the first few minutes

684. Tube inserted into the rectum for the expulsion of gas is called as: *New Q*

a. Flatus tube b. Enema tube
c. Foley's catheter d. Rectal tube

685. Cleaning of surgical wound is performed in .... direction.

a. Inner to outer
b. Outer to inner
c. Divide the wound into equal half and clean each half
d. All of the above

686. Solutions used for bladder irrigation is/are:

a. Distilled water/normal saline
b. Sodium nitrate 1:8000
c. 2%boric acid
d. All of the above

687. Eye irrigation is performed using:

a. Normal saline b. 2% boric acid
c. 1% silver nitrate d. All of these

688. Which of the following statements is not true regarding eye irrigation procedure?

a. Use strict aseptic technique
b. Irrigate less infected eye first then more infected eye
c. Irrigate from inner canthus to outer canthus
d. Fluid flow should be allowed to fall directly onto the cornea

Explanation: When performing an eye irrigation procedure, the fluid flow should not be allowed to fall directly onto the cornea, as this can cause additional irritation and potentially damage the cornea. Instead, the fluid should be directed toward the inner canthus of the eye and allowed to flow out of the outer canthus. This helps to flush out any debris or irritants that may be present in the eye while minimizing the risk of injury or discomfort.

689. Incorrect statement related to abdominal paracentesis is: *New Q*

a. It is performed midway between the symphysis pubis and umbilicus
b. The position given to the patient for abdominal paracentesis is Fowler's position
c. Ask the patient to urinate before the procedure
d. Paracentesis is performed using a regular IV catheter.

Explanation: A paracentesis needle is specialized needle and is different from an IV cannula needle. A paracentesis needle is a long, thin needle used to remove fluid from the abdominal cavity.

690. Which among the following things require/indicate proper function of chest tube?

a. Chest drainage should be upright and below the level of insertion
b. Water seal fluctuate with patient's inspiration and expiration
c. Bubbling in water seal
d. All of the above

691. A procedure that involves the administration of food or medications directly into the stomach via a tube passed through the nose or mouth is known as *New Q*

a. Gastric lavage b. Gastric gavage
c. Gastrostomy d. PEG

Explanation:

Gastric gavage - A procedure that involves the administration of food or medications directly into the stomach via a tube passed through the nose or mouth.

Gastric lavage - a procedure that involves the irrigation of the stomach with a saline solution to remove ingested toxins or other substances.

Gastrostomy - a surgical procedure that involves the creation of an opening in the stomach through the abdominal wall for the purpose of feeding or administering medications.

PEG (Percutaneous endoscopic gastrostomy) - A flexible tube is inserted through the abdomen directly into the stomach under endoscopic guidance.

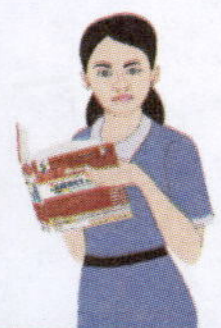

Ans.

680. a
681. a
682. a
683. d
684. a
685. a
686. d
687. d
688. d
689. d
690. d
691. b

692. Which of the following is not a skin traction?
- a. Buck's traction
- b. Bryant's traction
- c. Russell's traction
- d. Crutchfield traction

693. Plaster of Paris (POP) is chemically:
- a. Calcium carbonate
- b. Calcium sulfate
- c. Calcium phosphate
- d. Calcium magnate

694. When a patient is getting shifted from the ward for CT scan a nurse should do the following: *(ISRO)*
- a. Administer laxatives
- b. Explain the procedure
- c. Administer a radio isotope
- d. Give plenty of fluids

695. The nurse is caring for a patient who is bleeding from the punctured wound. Which of the following intervention should the nurse use to control the arterial bleeding? *(RAK MSc 2018)*
- a. Pressure at the puncture site
- b. Application of a tourniquet
- c. Pressure point massage
- d. Pressure dressing

Explanation:
- The best method to prevent bleeding from a punctured wound is to apply firm pressure at the punctured site as it slows down the blood flow to the wound site, favoring clot formation and also preventing any further blood loss.
- If severe bleeding does not stop with direct pressure and elevation, apply direct pressure to an artery. Use direct pressure on an artery along with elevation and direct pressure on the wound.

696. Which of the following actions should be taken first for a patient who is found with hyperthermia? *(RAK MSc 2018)*
- a. Undress the patient
- b. Use tepid water as a mist spray
- c. Remove patient from the hot environment
- d. Place patient in continual breeze from electric fans

Explanation:
- The priority intervention would be that which prevents further exposure to the harmful stimuli, therefore, removing patient from the hot environment is preferred over all others.

697. The nurse inserting a Ryle's tube for an adult patient is aware that the distance between incisor teeth and Gastroesophageal junction is:
- a. 20 cm
- b. 30 cm
- c. 40 cm
- d. 50 cm

698. Recommended duration for completing suctioning of the tracheostomy tube is:
- a. 5-10 seconds
- b. 10-20 seconds
- c. 20-30 seconds
- d. 30-45 Seconds

699. A lethargic patient has fever, vomiting, and headache. The nurse has to prepare him for which of the following procedure?
- a. Blood culture
- b. Lumbar puncture
- c. CAT scan
- d. Ultrasound scan

700. Patient complains of pain, muscles spasm and resistance while the nurse was doing a passive ROM exercise. Which of the following is most appropriate action in this scenario?
- a. Assess degree of pain
- b. Stop the exercise
- c. Administer pain medication
- d. Call physician

701. Regarding the request of organ and tissue donation at the time of death, the nurse needs to be aware that: *(AIIMS Bhopal Grade-I 2018)*
- a. Requests are usually made by the nurse who case for the patient at time of death
- b. Professionals need to be very selective in whom they ask for organ and tissue donation
- c. Specially educated personnel make requests
- d. Only patients who have given prior instruction regarding donation become donors

Explanation: Regarding the request of organ and tissue donation at the time of death, Individuals specially trained in requesting organ donations facilitate the process. They are skilled in talking compassionately to people who have suffered a tragic, sudden loss and have answers to many questions that people have regarding the donation process.

702. At the time of death of patient, it is appropriate to make request for organ donation by:
- a. Specially educated counsellor
- b. Nurse caring for the client
- c. Family doctor
- d. Any healthcare worker

703. All of the following are the responsibilities of a nurse while caring for a patient suffering from thrombophlebitis; EXCEPT:
- a. Educate client to avoid straining during defecation
- b. Leg should not be massaged
- c. Administer ordered anticoagulant
- d. Keep the leg in dependent position

Explanation: Option d is incorrect. While caring for a person with thrombophlebitis, educate that person to keep the leg slightly elevated on pillows, and slightly flexed at the level of knee in order to enhance venous return

704. What is the management of persistent hiccups?
- a. Ask person to drink water
- b. Administer 3-10% carbon dioxide
- c. Ask the person to walk in an open space
- d. All of the above

Explanation: Hiccups are diaphragmatic spasm which can be relieved by administering 3-10% carbon dioxide.

705. Nursing measures for a patient who is complaining of difficulty with micturition includes:
- a. Sound of running water
- b. Stroking in the inner thigh
- c. Pour lukewarm water over the perineum
- d. All of the above

Explanation: All of the above mentioned are correct nursing measures in a person who is complaining of difficulty with micturition. Other than these, slight pressure over the bladder can also be applied which is known as Credé's maneuver.

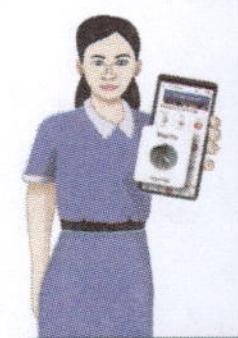

Ans.

692. d
693. b
694. b
695. a
696. c
697. c
698. a
699. b
700. b
701. c
702. a
703. d
704. b
705. d

706. Thoracentesis is the treatment of choice of:

a. Hemothorax b. Empyema
c. Hydrothorax d. All of these

Explanation: Thoracentesis is a procedure to remove fluid from the space between the lungs and the chest wall called the pleural space. It is indicated in all of the above conditions.

707. The tube introduced into the rectum of patient to relieve gas is known as:

a. Rectal tube b. PEG tube
c. Foley's catheter d. NG tube

Explanation: A rectal tube to facilitate expulsion of flatus. Foley's catheter is a type of indwelling urinary catheter. NG tube is inserted into stomach through nostrils. PEG tube stands for percutaneous endoscopic *gastrostomy.*

708. Collection of lymph fluid in the pleural space:

a. Hemothorax
b. Pneumothorax
c. Chylothorax
d. None of the above

Explanation: Collection of lymph fluid in the pleural space is known as chylothorax. Chylothorax or chyle leak is a type of pleural effusion, resulting from lymph formed in the digestive system called chyle accumulating in the pleural cavity due to either disruption or obstruction of the thoracic duct.

709. Which of the following is the appropriate measures to prevent DVT and its complication?

a. Patients should wear elastic compression stockings.
b. Patients should observe special body positioning and perform indicated exercise.
c. Patients should use intermittent pneumatic compression.
d. All of the above

Explanation: Intermittent pneumatic compression (IPC) devices increase blood flow through the veins and prevent blood clot. Elastic compression stockings help increase circulation and prevent blood clot formation. Special body positioning and specific exercises also help improving the blood circulation.

710. Which of the following intervention can prevent increased intracranial pressure in a patient with head trauma?

a. Maintain well lit room
b. Elevate the head end of the patient
c. Frequently change the position of the patient
d. Elevate the foot end of the patient

711. A nurse caring a patient who is on pancreatic enzyme replacement therapy should assess for:

a. Weight gain b. Orthostatic hypotension
c. Bradycardia d. GIT irritation

712. Best method to make sure the functionality of intercostal drainage tube is to observe for:

a. Continuous bubbling in water-sealed bottle
b. Oscillation of water column in drainage bottle
c. Continuous bubbling from suction tube
d. All of the above

713. A nurse stands to protect the needs and wishes of the patient. What role does she exhibit?

a. Caregiver b. Counselor
c. Client advocate d. Nurse manager

714. A nurse in the critical care unit explains to the client and family regarding the future treatment and surgery options. Here nurse is performing the role of:

a. Advocate
b. Caregiver
c. Researcher
d. Leader

715. Which of the following statements best describe 'knowing the patient'?

a. Anticipating the patient's personal preferences of shift nurse
b. Identify the patient's preference on physician
c. Collecting task-oriented information during assessment
d. Establishing an understanding of a specific patient

716. Holistic care refers to:

a. Disease, spirit, and environmental interactions
b. Emotions of the patient
c. Mind-body-spirit of patients and their families
d. Muscles and neurological disorders

717. All of the following are the goals of restraining the patient; EXCEPT:

a. To prevent injuries due to fall
b. To prevent self-directed violence
c. To prevent pressure ulcer
d. To impose control on behavior

718. Which of the following is the most common source of client injury?

a. Medication error and falls
b. Transfer from bed
c. Bedsore
d. Needle stick injury

719. A method used to assist individuals with disability or chronic illness to attain and maintain maximum function:

a. Restorative care b. Rehabilitation
c. Reconstruction d. All of these

BACK CARE

720. Which massage technique involves using long, sweeping strokes with the hands or fingers to create a soothing and relaxing effect on the muscles?

a. Petrissage b. Friction
c. Effleurage d. Tapotement

721. Which massage technique involves compressing and squeezing the muscles with rhythmic, circular movements using the hands, fingers, or elbows?

a. Kneading b. Tapotement
c. Hand over hand d. Petrissage

722. Which massage technique involves rhythmic tapping, pounding, or patting movements applied to the body with the fingertips, fists, or the side of the hand?

a. Brush strokes
b. Kneading
c. Friction
d. Tapotement

Explanation: Tapotement is also known as tapping, a massage technique involves rhythmic tapping, pounding, or patting movements applied to the body with the fingertips, fists, or the side of the hand.

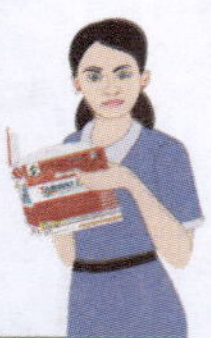

Ans.

706. d
707. a
708. c
709. d
710. b
711. a
712. b
713. c
714. a
715. d
716. c
717. c
718. a
719. b
720. c
721. a
722. d

723. Which of the following is the purpose of a nursing discharge summary?
- a. To document the patient's medical history and treatment plan.
- b. To communicate the patient's status and care needs to the healthcare team.
- c. To provide instructions to the patient and family regarding post-discharge care.
- d. To ensure that the patient's insurance provider is appropriately billed for services rendered.

Explanation: The nursing discharge summary is a document that outlines the patient's medical status, treatment plan, and instructions for post-discharge care. The purpose of the nursing discharge summary is to ensure that the patient and their family are fully informed about the patient's condition and care needs after leaving the healthcare facility.

ENEMA

724. All are retention enema; EXCEPT:
- a. Stimulant enema
- b. Nutrient enema
- c. Oil enema
- d. Emollient enema

725. The maximum height at which the enema should be held while giving it is: *(Recent Question 2012)*
- a. 66 cm
- b. 45 cm
- c. 37 cm
- d. 30 cm

726. If a client complains of severe abdominal cramps while administering enema, the nurse should: New Q
- a. Continue to administer enema
- b. Slow the rate of enema
- c. Stop giving enema
- d. Administer analgesic

Explanation: If a client experiences severe cramping and bloating during an enema administration, the appropriate nursing intervention is to stop the flow, wait for 30 seconds and restart with a slower flow rate and instruct the client to take short, panting breaths. This can help the client to relax and alleviate discomfort.
Ref: Rushing Jill. Administering an enema to an adult. Nursing 33(11):p 28, November 2003.

727. Solutions used for evacuant enema is/are:
- a. Soap and water
- b. Normal saline
- c. Tap water
- d. All of these

728. Amount of evacuant enema used in adult is:
- a. 250-500 mL
- b. 500-1000 mL
- c. 1000-1500 mL
- d. 1500-2000 mL

729. Amount of evacuant enema used in child is:
- a. 250-500 mL
- b. 500-1000 mL
- c. 1000-1500 mL
- d. 1500-2000 mL

730. Solutions used in oil enema is/are:
- a. Olive oil
- b. Sweet oil
- c. Castor oil and olive oil 1:1
- d. All of the above

731. Enema which irritates the mucosal lining and stimulate peristalsis is:
- a. Oil enema
- b. Purgative enema
- c. Carminative enema
- d. Astringent enema

732. Anti-spasmodic enema is also known as:
- a. Oil enema
- b. Purgative enema
- c. Carminative enema
- d. Astringent enema

733. Enema which contracts the tissue/blood vessels, check bleeding and inflammation is:
- a. Oil enema
- b. Purgative enema
- c. Carminative enema
- d. Astringent enema

734. Enema used to destroy and expel the worm is:
- a. Oil enema
- b. Purgative enema
- c. Carminative enema
- d. Anthelminthic enema

735. Size of rectal tube used in adults while giving enema is:
- a. 10-14 Fr
- b. 12-18Fr
- c. 18-22 Fr
- d. 22-30 Fr

736. Size of rectal tube used in children while giving enema is:
- a. 10-14 Fr
- b. 12-18 Fr
- c. 18-22 Fr
- d. 22-30 Fr

737. How long the patient should be encouraged to retain the enema solution?
- a. 10-15 min
- b. 15-20 min
- c. 20-35 cm
- d. 30-45 cm

738. Length to which rectal catheter needs to be inserted while giving enema is:
- a. 5 cm
- b. 10 cm
- c. 15 cm
- d. 20 cm

SUTURES

739. If wound eviscerations occur, the immediate nursing action is: *(ESIC Chennai May 2012)*
- a. Cover the wound with sterile dry gauze
- b. Leave the wound uncovered and pull the skin edges together
- c. Cover the wound with sterile gauze moistened with sterile NS
- d. Cover the wound with water-soaked gauze

740. Catgut suture belongs to which among the following categories?
- a. Synthetic absorbable suture
- b. Synthetic non-absorbable suture
- c. Natural non-absorbable suture
- d. Natural absorbable suture

741. Which of the following procedures is likely to be performed in a patient who manifests symptoms of meningitis?
- a. Culture and Sensitivity of blood
- b. Lumbar puncture
- c. CAT scan
- d. USG

742. Catgut is made from the intestine of:
- a. Pig
- b. Human
- c. Sheep
- d. All of the above

Explanation: Catgut is made of collagen derived from healthy sheep or cattle. It is tanned with chromium salts to improve handling and to resist degradation in tissue.

Ans.

723. c
724. c
725. b
726. c
727. d
728. b
729. a
730. d
731. b
732. c
733. d
734. d
735. d
736. b
737. b
738. b
739. c
740. d
741. b
742. c

743. The image shown below is which type of suture:

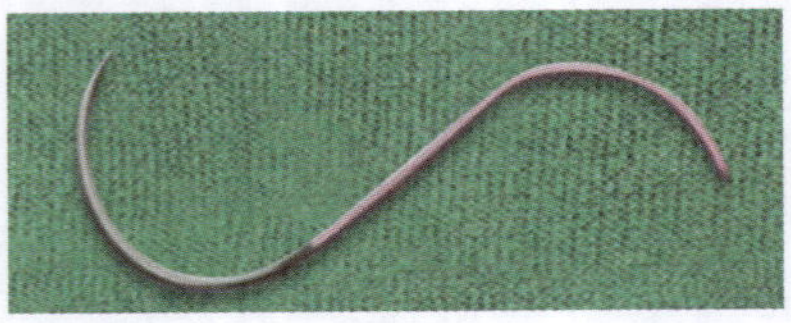

a. Ethilon b. Polydiaxanone
c. Plain catgut d. Silk

744. Polydiaxanone suture is normally absorbed in:

a. 8 weeks b. 6 weeks
c. 4 weeks d. 6 months

745. Tissue reaction is most commonly seen in which type of suture?

a. Silk b. Polydiaxanone
c. Chromic catgut d. Vicryl

746. Which surgeon introduced catgut suture in surgery?

a. Lord Lister b. Astley Cooper
c. Syme d. John Hunter

747. Name the following instrument:

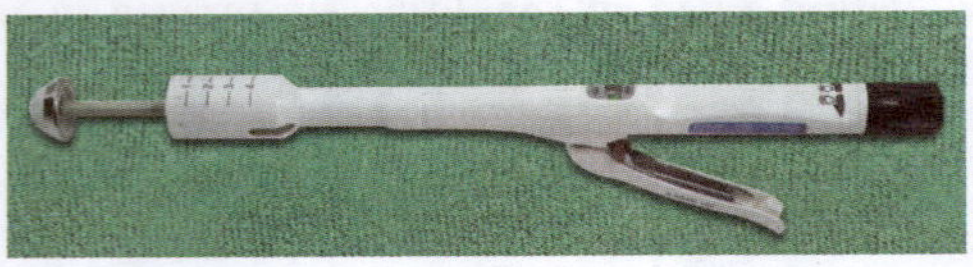

a. Circular stapler
b. Head skin stapler
c. MIRUS hemorrhoids stapler
d. Linear cutter

Explanation: MIRUS hemorrhoids stapler is a three row approach for Minimally Invasive Procedure for Prolapsed Hemorrhoids.

748. Which of the following preservatives is used for packing catgut suture?

a. Formaldehyde b. Gluteraldehyde
c. Isopropyl alcohol d. Sodium hypochlorite

GRIEF PROCESS

749. Identify the correct order of Kubler Ross grieving stages:

a. Depression – anger – bargaining – denial – acceptance
b. Denial – bargaining - anger - depression - acceptance
c. Denial – acceptance – bargaining – depression – anger
d. Denial – anger – bargaining – depression – acceptance

750. The type of loss in which the client is aware that a loss will occur is known as: *(AIIMS-BBS SNO 2019)*

a. Anticipatory loss b. Observable loss
c. Actual loss d. Perceived loss

Explanation: ***Anticipatory*** grief refers to a feeling of grief occurring before an impending ***loss***. Typically, the impending ***loss*** is the death of someone close due to illness.

751. 'Hospice' is the treatment concept for: *(AIIMS Raipur staff nurse grade I-2018)*

a. Terminally ill cancer patient
b. Psychiatric patients
c. Cardiac patients
d. All of the above

Explanation: Hospice care is the best compassionate care for those patients who all are facing life limiting chronical disease condition. It is planned according to patient's wishes and to meet medical need, pain management, emotional support and spiritual need of the patient.

752. 'No, not me' reaction of the patient is seen in which stage of death (terminal patients)?

a. Bargaining
b. Denial
c. Anger
d. Acceptance

Explanation: The "No, not me" reaction of the patient is typically seen in the denial stage of the Kübler-Ross model, which is the first stage of the grieving process. In this stage, the patient may initially deny the reality of the terminal illness or impending death, and may exhibit feelings of shock, disbelief, or numbness. This is a common coping mechanism used by individuals when faced with a traumatic or overwhelming situation.

Denial, Anger, Bargaining, Depression and Acceptance are the various stages of grief process.

753. The key aspect of palliative care is:

a. Pain relief
b. Emotional support
c. Ostomy care
d. General care

754. What is the appropriate nursing measure, when the wife of a person is just diagnosed with cancer?

a. Tell the person that it is normal for everyone
b. Provide comfort measures
c. Provide anticipatory support for grief
d. Discuss the situation of the client with other nurse

755. What is the final stage of Kubler Ross stages of grief?

a. Denial b. Acceptance
c. Anger d. Bargaining

TRIAGE

756. In triage, yellow color indicates: *(DSSSB PHN, 2015)*

a. Emergent b. Urgent
c. Non-urgent d. Dead

757. Which is considered as an internal disaster: *(Safdarjung NO 2018)*

a. Patient fall
b. The massive spread of pneumonia
c. A computer hacking episode
d. Unexpected staff absences due to illness

Explanation:

- WHO defines an internal disaster as an event that occurs within the confines of the hospital, and affects the patient. Patient fall is considered as internal disaster.
- The massive spread of pneumonia is an example of external disaster.
- A computer Hacking episode is an example of information technology disaster.
- Unexpected staff absences due to illness can be considered as staff crisis.

Ans.

743. b
744. d
745. a
746. d
747. c
748. c
749. d
750. a
751. a
752. b
753. a
754. c
755. b
756. b
757. a

758. In a hospital, there are 4 patients who require attention of the nurse. Whom of the following should the nurse attend first? *(AIIMS Bhopal Nursing Officer, 2018)*

a. 21-year-old post-op patient complaining of pain
b. 34-year-old asthma patient asking to ambulate
c. 66-year-old waiting to be discharged
d. 66-year-old with a pneumothorax complaining of shortness of breath

Explanation: As per ABC rules, patient with airway or breathing problem needs immediate attention.

759. Which of the following nursing actions takes priority for a patient who is brought to emergency room complaining of mid-sternal chest pain?

a. History collection with emphasis on preceding events
b. Chest examination with auscultation
c. Electrocardiogram
d. Assessment of vital signs

760. The process of assessing patients and determining the management priorities during emergency is known as:

a. Collage
b. Lavage
c. Labeling
d. Triage

761. A 42-year-old unconscious patient is brought to the casualty following road traffic accident. His blood pressure was 80/60 mm Hg. What you will do first?

a. Protect the airway
b. Infuse 2 L of crystalloid
c. Order for CT scan of the head
d. Start vasopressor

762. Deficiency of oxygen in the tissue is known as:

a. Hypoxia
b. Hypoxemia
c. Cyanosis
d. Apnea

Explanation: Deficiency of oxygen in the tissue is hypoxia, if it is in the blood it is known as hypoxemia. Bluish discoloration of skin and mucous membranes due to the lack of oxygen is known as cyanosis. Apnea is absence of respiration for more than 20 seconds.

763. In an adult patient, length of insertion of Guedel's airway is measured between the first incisors to the:

a. Angle of the mandible
b. Nasopharnyx
c. Oropharynx
d. Ear lobe

764. An accident victim is able to obey commands and walk, this patient comes under which color in triage?

a. Red
b. Black
c. Green
d. Yellow

765. From the following clients, which client should be treated first according to triage?

a. 86-year-old male client with head injury
b. 16-year-old female client with severe bleeding
c. 56-year-old client with severe cardiac abnormalities
d. 45-year-old female client with fracture of femur

Explanation: In a triage scenario, the 16-year-old female client with severe bleeding (option b) should be treated first becasue severe bleeding can be life-threatening and requires immediate medical attention to control the bleeding and stabilize the patient. In addition, a 16-year-old patient having highest life expectancy.

While the 86-year-old male client with a head injury (option a) and the 56-year-old client with severe cardiac abnormalities (option c) may also require urgent medical attention, they are not as immediately life-threatening as severe bleeding. The 45-year-old female client with a fracture of femur (option d) may require medical attention but is generally considered a lower priority than other cases.

766. Which of the following clients would be triaged with 'black color'?

a. Client with distended abdomen
b. Client with tingling sensation in the lower leg
c. Client with spinal cord injury
d. Client has decerebrate posturing

Explanation: Decerebrate posture is an abnormal body posture that involves the arms and legs being held straight out. This posture is associated with a stuporous or comatose mental status and increased intra cranial pressure and the prognosis is very poor.

767. While triaging, which of the following clients should be given priority treatment?

a. An unresponsive head injury client
b. Patient with burn injury of 55%
c. Patient with sucking chest wound
d. Patient with clavicle fracture

Explanation: Sucking chest wound is a life-threatening condition and is survivable emergency if it is treated first. Treatment for a client with clavicle fracture can be delayed. Unresponsive client with head injury has less prognosis.

Note: The highest priority is to be given for airway so the client with sucking chest wound is given priority over a patient with burn injury.

768. Which of the following conditions will be treated as triage color 'green'?

a. An unresponsive client with head injury
b. Client with sucking chest wound
c. Client with abdominal injury
d. Clients with bruises in their legs and sprain in ankle

Explanation: Clients with bruises in their legs and sprain in ankle can be able to move and can be able to treat their own injury. So, these clients are treated as green in triage category.

FLUID AND DRUG CALCULATION

769. A child is to receive dexamethasone (Decadron) intravenously at the ordered dosage of 7.6 mg. The drug concentration in the vial is 4 mg/mL. Which of the following amounts would the nurse administer? *(RAK MSc 2018)*

a. 0.05 mL
b. 0.72 mL
c. 1.9 mL
d. 3.8 mL

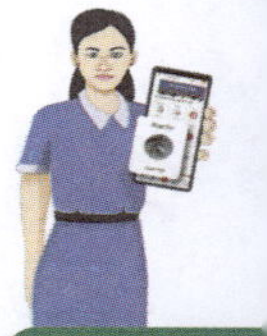

Ans.

758. d
759. d
760. d
761. a
762. a
763. a
764. c
765. b
766. d
767. c
768. d
769. c

Explanation:
Calculation of Drug dose of Liquid Drugs: $\frac{D}{H} \times Q = X$
D = Dose Desired
H = Dose on Hand
Q = Quantity
X = Dose to be administered
According to the given question: D = 7.6 mg; H = 4 mg; Q = 1 mL
$X = \frac{D}{H} \times 1 = 1.9$ Dose to be administered is 1.9 mL.

770. A child is to receive 500 mL of an IV solution over 12 hours via tubing that delivers micro drips at 60 drops/mL. The nurse would infuse solution at which of the following rates? *(RAK MSC 2018)*

a. 42 drops/minute
b. 48 drops/minute
c. 63 drops/minute
d. 84 drops/minute

Explanation:
Total volume of fluid to be infused = 500 mL
Drop factor = 60 drops/mL
Total time of infusion = 12 × 60 (To convert hours into minutes)
= 720 minutes
Therefore,
Flow rate = Volume of infusion in mL × Drop factor (in drops/mL)/ Time of infusion in minutes
Flow rate = 500 × 60/720 = 41.66 or 42 drops/min

771. 500 mL of IV fluids needs to be administered over 5 hr. Drop factor is 20. Calculate drops/minute?

a. 32 drops/min
b. 33 drops/min
c. 34 drops/min
d. 35 drops/min

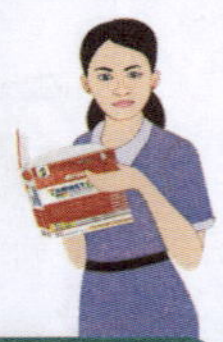

Ans.
770. a
771. b
772. d
773. b
774. b
775. c
776. a
777. b

Explanation: Formula:
Drops per minute = (volume in mL × drop factor)/(time in minutes)
Here. . . . Time in minutes = 5 × 60
So. . . = (500 × 20)/(5 × 60)
= 33. 33
33. 33 is converted to nearest whole number.
i.e., 33 drops/min

772. A physician orders 1000 mL of Normal Saline to be infused over 8 hours. What is the flow rate a nurse has to set if drop factor is 15 drop per mL? *(ISRO)*

a. 20 drops/min
b. 24 drops/min
c. 28 drops/min
d. 31 drops/min

Explanation:
Drops per minute = (volume in mL × drop factor) / (time in minutes)
First, let's find the total number of minutes in 8 hours:
Total time = 8 hours × 60 minutes/hour
Total time = 480 minutes
Now we can apply the given values into the formula:
Drops per minute = (1000 mL × 15 drops/mL)/480 minutes
Drops per minute = 15000 drops/480 minutes
Drops per minute = 31.25 drops/min
Round down to the nearest whole number:
Drops per minute = 31 drops/min

773. How much will be the drop rate/min if 500 mL of fluid is to be administered over 24 hours via ordinary drip set with drop factor 15 drops/mL. *(Recent Question 2012)*

a. 3 drops/min
b. 5 drops/min
c. 24 drops/min
d. 50 drops/min

774. A client is ordered 75 milligrams of Amoxicillin orally. 125 milligrams in 5 milliliters of Syrup is available. How many milliliters will you administer?

a. 2.5 mL
b. 3 mL
c. 3.5 mL
d. 4 mL

Explanation:
Here's the step-by-step calculation:
1. **Calculate the concentration of the syrup:**
   Concentration = Amount of medication available / Volume available
   Concentration = 125 mg / 5 mL
   Concentration = 25 mg/mL
2. **Determine how many milliliters are needed for the 75 mg dosage:**
   Volume to administer = Amount of medication ordered/ Concentration
   Volume to administer = 75mg / 25mg/ml
   The "mg" units will cancel out:
   Volume to administer = 3 mL

775. Frusemide 90 mg IV is charted. Stock dose is 20 mg/mL. How many mL would you give?

a. 0.45 mL
b. 0.9 mL
c. 4.5 mL
d. 9 mL

Explanation:
1. **Calculate the concentration of the available stock:**
   Concentration = Amount of medication available / Volume
   Concentration = 20 mg/mL (given in the problem)
2. **Determine how many milliliters are needed for the 90 mg dosage:**
   Volume to administer = Amount of medication ordered / Concentration
   Volume to administer = 90 mg / 20 mg/mL
   The "mg" units will cancel out:
   Volume to administer = 4.5 mL

776. A patient requires 8 mg of Morphine IV. Morphine is available as 20 mg/mL. How many mls will you draw up?

a. 0.4 mL
b. 0.8 mL
c. 1.2 mL
d. 1.6 mL

777. Physician's order reads: Eltroxin 60 mcg po daily. Available dose: Eltroxin 0.12 mg tab. How many tablets will you administer?

a. ¼ tab
b. ½ tab
c. 2 tabs
d. 5 tabs

Explanation:

1. Since the available dose is given in milligrams (mg), we should convert the ordered dose from micrograms (mcg) to milligrams (mg).
   1 mg = 1000 mcg
   1 mcg = 1/1000 mg
   So, 60 mcg = 60 x 1/1000mg
   ordered dose=0.06 mg
2. Next, we'll find out how many tablets are needed:
   Tablets to administer = Ordered dose / Available dose per tablet
   Tablets to administer = 0.06 mg / 0.12 mg/tab
   The "mg" units will cancel out:
   Tablets to administer = 0.5 tab
   So, you will administer half a tablet.

778. A patient must receive 30 units of Humulin regular insulin. The label reads 100 units = 1 mL. How many milliliters should the nurse administer?

a. 0.2 mL b. 0.3 mL
c. 0.5 mL d. 1.0 mL

779. The physician's order reads "Administer 1 g cefotaxime in 150 mL of normal saline solution in 60 minutes." What is the flow rate if the drop factor is 20 gtt = 1 mL?

a. 25 gtt/min b. 38 gtt/min
c. 50 gtt/min d. 72 gtt/min

780. Physician's order – Streptomycin 25 mg/kg IM q 12 hr; Available dose: Streptomycin 0.35 Gm/mL. How many mL will you administer for each dose to a 70 kg patient?

a. 2 mL b. 5 mL
c. 7 mL d. 10 mL

Explanation: First, let's calculate the total amount of Streptomycin required per dose for a 70 kg patient:
Total Streptomycin per dose = Dose per kg × Patient's weight
Total Streptomycin per dose = 25 mg/kg × 70 kg
Total Streptomycin per dose = 1750 mg
Convert the total Streptomycin per dose to grams, as the available dose is given in grams:
1 g = 1000 mg
Total Streptomycin per dose = 1750 mg × (1 g/1000 mg)
Total Streptomycin per dose = 1.75 g
Next, find out how many milliliters of the available Streptomycin solution are needed for each dose:
Available dose = 0.35 g/mL (given in the problem)
Volume to administer = Total Streptomycin per dose / Available dose
Volume to administer = 1.75 g / 0.35 g/mL
The "g" units will cancel out:
Volume to administer = 5 mL

781. Doctor's Order: Infuse 500 mL DNS over 6 hr; Drop factor: 15 gtt/mL. What flow rate will you set?

a. 21 drops/min
b. 30 drops/min
c. 42 drops/min
d. 45 drops/min

782. Doctor's Order: Infuse 1200 mL of NS at 125 mL/hr; Drop Factor: 20 gtt/min. How many drops per minute will you set in the IV set?

a. 21 drops/min b. 42 drops/min
c. 45 drops/min d. 60 drops/min

783. Doctor's Order: ½ L of RL to infuse over 4 hrs 10 mins; Drop factor: 20 gtt/mL. How many gtt/min will you regulate the IV?

a. 20 gtt/min b. 40 gtt/min
c. 50 gtt/min d. 60 gtt/min

784. Calculate the IV flow rate for 100 mL over 1 hour. Drop factor is 20 gtt/mL.

a. 22 drops/min b. 33 drops/min
c. 36 drops/min d. 40 drops/min

NORMAL LAB VALUES

785. Normal oral temperature is:

a. 97°F b. 97.6°F
c. 98.6°F d. 99.6°F

786. Urinary bag of a Foley's catheterized patient needs to be kept:

a. At the waist level of patient
b. Below the level of patient
c. On the lap of patient
d. Above the waist level of patient

Explanation: Gravity promotes the drainage of urine, so it should be kept below the waist level of patient. Above the waist level of patient can cause back flow of urine and serious complications in the patient.

787. The normal intraocular pressure is: *(DSSSB 2013)*

a. 12-22 mm Hg b. 16-25 mm Hg
c. 20-35 mm Hg d. 19-38 mm Hg

Explanation: Intraocular pressure (IOP) is the pressure within the eyes and is measured with tonometry. Normal range is 12-22 mm Hg. Increased IOP causes glaucoma.

788. Normal serum potassium Level in mEq/L is: *(DSSSB 2013)*

a. 2. 5 to 3. 5 b. 3. 5 to 5. 1
c. 5. 5 to 6. 5 d. 6. 5 to 7. 5

Explanation: The normal range is 3. 5 to 5. 1 mEq/L.

789. Normal serum level of sodium is:

a. 135-145 mEq/L b. 145-155 mEq/L
c. 3.5-5.2 mEq/L d. 9-11 mEq/L

790. Normal potassium value is:

a. 135-145 mEq/L b. 3.5-5 mEq/L
c. 8-11 mEq/L d. 98 – 107 mEq/L

791. Normal serum chloride level is:

a. 135 – 145 mEq/L b. 120 – 130 mEq/L
c. 98 – 107 mEq/L d. 50 – 70 mEq/L

792. One teaspoon = ... mL.

a. 1 mL b. 3 mL
c. 5 mL d. 7 mL

Explanation:

- One teaspoon = 5 mL
- One tablespoon = 15 mL
- One fluid ounce = 30 mL

793. The normal Cholesterol level is: *(DSSSB 2013)*

a. 100-150 mg/dL b. 150-200 mg/dL
c. 200-250 mg/dL d. 250-300 mg/dL

Explanation: As per American Heart Association, desirable level of cholesterol is less than 200 mg/dL.

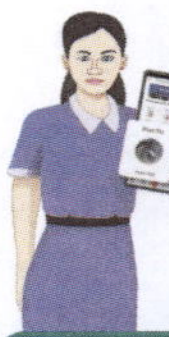

Ans.

778.	b
779.	c
780.	b
781.	a
782.	b
783.	b
784.	b
785.	c
786.	b
787.	a
788.	b
789.	a
790.	b
791.	c
792.	c
793.	b

794. One tablespoon is equal to: *(DSSSB PHN, 2015)*

a. 5 mL b. 15 mL
c. 30 mL d. 20 mL

795. What is the normal CSF pressure when the individual is lying on his side? *(Kerala PSC, Nov 2014)*

a. 15 cm H_2O b. 20 cm H_2O
c. 10 cm H_2O d. 25 cm H_2O

796. The normal adult intracranial pressure is: *(Staff Nurse G II 2014)*

a. 0–15 mm Hg b. 60–70 mm Hg
c. 80–100 mm Hg d. 20–40 mm Hg

797. 1200 mL is equal to ______ liters.

a. 1.2 b. 12
c. 120 d. 12000

798. Two teaspoon is equal to:

a. 6 mL b. 10 mL
c. 20 mL d. 30 mL

799. 1 fluid ounce is approximately equal to:

a. 15 mL b. 30 mL
c. 50 mL d. 100 mL

800. A patient with cirrhosis of the liver has a serum bilirubin level of 30 mg/dL. In order to evaluate these laboratory results, you need to know that the normal serum bilirubin level is: *(LNJP H D 2012)*

a. 0.2 to 1.0 mg/dL b. 10 to 20 mg/dL
c. 3 to 10 mg/dL d. 20 to 30 mg/dL

801. Normal fetal heart rate is: *(LNJP H D 2012)*

a. 120 to 140 regular
b. 120 to 160 regular
c. 90 to 100 irregular
d. 100 to 120 irregular

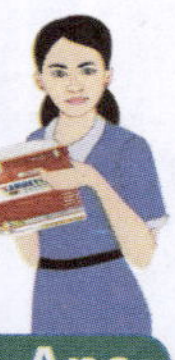

802. The fasting blood sugar value is: *(DSSSB PHN, 2015)*

a. 70-110 mg% b. 50-90 mg%
c. 120-180 mg% d. 180-200 mg%

803. Stroke volume is:

a. 50 mL b. 70 mL
c. 90 mL d. 120 mL

804. Four teaspoon is equivalent to:

a. 12 mL b. 20 mL
c. 40 mL d. 60 mL

Explanation:
1 teaspoon = 5 ml
4 teaspoon = 4 x 5 ml = 20 ml

805. Normal pH of urine is in the range of:

a. 4.5 to 8.0 b. 3.0 to 5.0
c. 7.5 to 8.5 d. 7.35 to 7.45

806. Normal RBC range in adults

a. 4.3- 5.7 trillion cells/L
b. 4.5 -5.5 million/mm³ of blood
c. 150-450 billion/L
d. 2000-3000 million/mm³ of blood

807. Normal WBC range in adults:

a. 2000-4000/mm³ of blood
b. 4000-10000/mm³ of blood
c. 7000-20000/mm³ of blood
d. 10000-25000/mm³ of blood

808. Normal platelet range in adults

a. 50000 to 150000 cells/mm³ of blood
b. 150,000 to 450,000 cells/mm³ of blood
c. 350,000 to 600,000 cells/mm³ of blood
d. 500,000 to 700,000 cells/mm³ of blood

809. 1 Ounce is equal to .... teaspoon:

a. 2 teaspoons b. 4 teaspoons
c. 5 teaspoons d. 6 teaspoons

810. 1 liter is approximately equal to:

a. 33 ounce b. 34 ounce
c. 40 ounce d. 45 ounce

Explanation:
We have the conversion factors:
1 liter = 1000 milliliters
1 fluid ounce = 29.5735 milliliters
Now, we can calculate how many ounces are in 1 liter:
No. of Ounces in 1 liter = 1000 milliliters/29.5735 milliliters/ounce
No. of Ounces in 1 liter = 33.814 ounces
Convert to the nearest whole number:
1 liter is approximately equal to 34 ounces.

811. One teaspoon is:

a. 5 mL b. 7 mL
c. 10 mL d. 15 mL

812. One fluid ounce is equal to:

a. 10 mL b. 15 mL
c. 25 mL d. 30 mL

813. Body Mass Index (BMI) Range for overweight is: *(ISRO)*

a. Above 30 b. 18.5-24.9
c. 22.9-27.9 d. 25.0-29.9

814. During the time of any infection what will happen to the WBC count? *(AIIMS Raipur staff nurse grade I-2018)*

a. Increased
b. Decreased
c. Remain unchanged
d. Fluctuating

Explanation: WBCs are the fighter cells in the blood. If a person affected with any kind of infection, WBC count will increase.

BIOMEDICAL WASTE MANAGEMENT

815. Yellow color code is used for which type of hospital waste? *(AIIMS Bhopal Grade-I 2018)*

a. Body parts b. Glassware
c. Plastic d. Sharps

Explanation: According to Indian Society of Hospital Waste Management (ISHWM- July, 2018), Yellow color coded container is used to dispose the Cat 1, 2, 3 and cat 6 waste (Human and animal waste, microbial and biological waste, and soiled waste).

816. Which of the following colored containers must be used for discarding Human anatomical waste in hospital?

a. Yellow b. Red
c. Blue d. Black

Refer Appendices for complete information on color coding used in biomedical waste management.

Ans.

794. b
795. a
796. a
797. a
798. b
799. b
800. a
801. b
802. a
803. b
804. b
805. a
806. b
807. b
808. b
809. d
810. b
811. a
812. d
813. d
814. a
815. a
816. a

Explanation: **Yellow bag:** Human Anatomical Waste, Animal tissues, organs, Body parts carcasses, bleeding parts, fluid, blood and experimental animals used in research, Microbiology and Biotechnology waste.

817. The color of bag in which the infectious solid wastes are disposed is: *(DSSSB PHN, 2015)*

a. Red b. Black
c. Blue d. Yellow

818. Infectious non-sharp waste is collected in: *(LNJP H D 2012)*

a. Black bag b. White bin
c. Yellow bag d. Red bag

819. Yellow plastic bags containing biomedical wastes are treated by: *(RRB Feb 2012)*

a. Microwaving b. Autoclaving
c. Shredding d. Incineration

820. Discarded medicines and chemical wastes are discarded in .... color bag.

a. Yellow
b. Black
c. Blue
d. Puncture proof container

821. In Hospital waste management which colored plastic bag is not used: *(ISRO)*

a. Green b. Red
c. Yellow d. Blue

822. Which color-coded disposal container should be used for general waste, such as newspapers, food waste, and water bottles, that has no contact with infectious or hazardous materials? *New Q*

a. Black b. Yellow
c. Red d. Blue

823. In which color-coded disposal container should contaminated plastic waste, such as gloves, IV cannula, and vacutainer, be placed? *New Q*

a. Black b. Yellow
c. Red d. Blue

824. Which color-coded disposal container is designated for contaminated sharps, such as scalpels, needles, and suture needles? *New Q*

a. Black b. Yellow
c. White d. Blue

825. Glassware items, such as broken ampules, medicine vials, and test tubes, should be disposed of in which color-coded container? *New Q*

a. Black b. Yellow
c. Red d. Blue

COMMUNICATION AND THERAPEUTIC RELATIONSHIP

826. Choose the most therapeutic response to Mr. Sham's question: "Am I going to die?" *(NCFL 2019)*

a. "We all are going to die one day."
b. "What has your doctor told you?"
c. "You really don't want to talk about death, do you?"
d. "Would you like to talk about your condition and prognosis?"

Explanation:
- The response, "would you like to talk about your condition and prognosis?" Makes the patient to ventilate his/her feelings thereby it leads clarification why the patient is thinking out that 'he is going to die' (Therapeutic technique used here is mental ventilation)
- Other responses are antitherapeutic communication techniques.

827. Which of the following would not promote trust in the nurse-patient relationship? *(ESIC 2019)*

a. Examining a wound without providing privacy
b. Fulfilling promises
c. Returning at the stated time
d. Maintaining confidentiality

Explanation: The client may experience the exploitation of privacy if wound examination is done without providing privacy. This feeling may result in lack of trust in the nurse-patient relationship. Other given actions are the measures to promote trust in nurse-patient relationship.

828. The following are the barriers of Therapeutic relationships: *New Q (AIIMS Raipur Grade II 2017)*

I. Too many questions II. Assertive style
II. Stereotyping IV. Patronizing

a. I, II, III
b. II, III, IV
c. I, III, IV
d. I, II, III, IV

Explanation: The barriers of therapeutic relationship include Physiological barriers, environmental barriers, psychological barriers, social barriers, cultural barriers, semantic barriers, Organizational barriers and communication process related barriers.

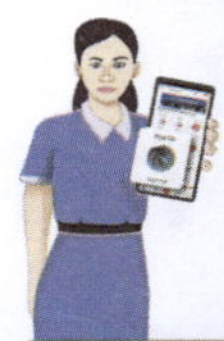

829. The principles of communication in the workplace include: *New Q (AIIMS Raipur Grade II 2017)*

I. Use language that is easily understood
II. Do not repeat phrases
III. Do not use indirect mode of communication
IV. Encourage feedback

a. I, II, III
b. II, III, IV
c. I, III, IV
d. I, II, III, IV

Explanation: Repeating phrases or rephrasing key points can sometimes be helpful in ensuring that the message is clearly understood by the recipient. So, "do not repeat phrases" is not the principle of communication in workplace. All other given options (I, III, IV) are principles of communication in workplace.

830. Providing health education about the environmental hygiene to the community people is an example of: *(AIIMS Raipur Grade II 2017)*

a. Social communication
b. Structural communication
c. Therapeutic communication
d. Formal communication

Ans.

817. d
818. c
819. d
820. a
821. a
822. a
823. c
824. c
825. d
826. d
827. a
828. c
829. c
830. b

Explanation:

Structural communication is an instructional approach that provides a simulated dialogue between an author of instructional materials and the students. In this context, it can indeed be applied to community health education.

Providing health education about environmental hygiene to the community people through structural communication would involve creating instructional materials that simulate a dialogue between the author (educator) and the community members (students).

Social communication or pragmatics is the way in which children use language within social situations. **Social communication** often occurs in informal settings, and its primary goal is to build relationships, share personal experiences, and opinions.

Therapeutic communication is a collection of techniques that prioritize the physical, mental, and emotional well-being of patients that open a new window.

The **Formal communication** is the exchange of official information that flows along the different levels of the organizational hierarchy and conforms to the professional rules, policy, standards, processes and regulations of the organization.

831. Which phase of the nurse - patient relationship focuses to develop clarity about the patient's preconceptions and expectations of nurses and develop acceptance of each other and respond to people who can offer help?

(AIIMS Raipur Grade II 2017)

a. Orientation phase b. Working phase
c. Exploitation phase d. Termination phase

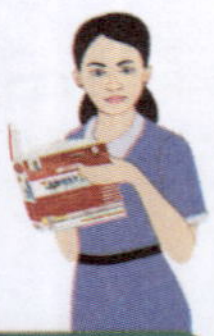

Explanation: In orientation stage, therapeutic environment is established, trust develops, roles, goals, rules and limitations are defined. In working/exploration/identification stage the client's problems are identified and solutions are explored, applied and evaluated. In termination stage/resolution stage relationship is terminated when the mutually agreed goals are met, the patient is discharged or transferred there than in the usual plan.

832. A strategy commonly used to improve therapeutic communication skills is called: *(AIIMS Raipur Grade II 2017)*

a. Active listening
b. Restating and clarifying
c. Validating
d. Process recording

Explanation: Active Listening is to be attentive what client is saying verbally and non-verbally. Clarifying is to check whether understanding is accurate or to understand better. The nurses restate an unclear or ambiguous message to clarify sender's meaning. Restating is repeating the main idea in different words. Validating is searching for mutual understanding, for accord in the meaning of words.

833. Which is the example of one-way communication?

(AIIMS Raipur Staff Nurse Grade I-2018)

a. Class lecture b. Group discussion
c. Conference d. Workshop

Explanation: Class lecture is an example of one-way communication. Here teacher will take class and students will listen. In all other methods both speaker and listener will actively interact, so all other methods are examples of two-way communication.

834. Which is the most important factor in a therapeutic relationship?

a. Trust b. Knowledge
c. Respect d. Motivating

Explanation: Trust is the most important factor in therapeutic relationship as it is very important to build rapport between patient and nurse.

835. Response from a receiver to sender is known as:

(AIIMS Raipur Staff Nurse Grade I-2018)

a. Message b. Context
c. Feedback d. Stimulus

Explanation: Information sent by sender to receiver is a message and from receiver to sender is feedback.

836. Following radiation therapy nurse is providing health education to a client. Which of the following is not included in the health teaching?

a. Protect the skin from direct sunlight, chlorine, and extreme temperature
b. Wear loose-fitting cloths
c. Shave with an electric razor only
d. Avoid foods which are rich in protein

Explanation: Healthy eating tips for a client undergoing radiation therapy are as follows:

- Eat slowly, eat small meals several times a day
- Eat food high in protein and calories
- Drink plenty of water and other fluids
- Consult the doctor before taking any OTC medications or vitamin supplements

837. Which of the following questioning techniques provides opportunity to discuss:

a. Restating b. Probing
c. Closed-ended questions d. Open-ended questions

838. "How do you describe your experience of being alone?" This is an example of:

a. Probing
b. Close-ended question
c. Open-ended question
d. Structured question

839. "Do you feel discomfort now?" This is an example of:

a. Open ended question
b. Close-ended question
c. Probing
d. Restating

840. Cultural barrier of communication includes:

a. Knowledge b. Language
c. Anxiety d. Fear

841. The most important characteristic of a verbal communication is:

a. Appearance b. Clarity
c. Eye contact d. Posture

842. Which strategy is effective while communicating with a client having hearing impairment?

a. Speak slowly and allow the client to do lip reading
b. Face the patient when speaking
c. Speak slower and in a normal pace
d. All of the above

Ans.

831.	b
832.	d
833.	a
834.	a
835.	c
836.	d
837.	d
838.	c
839.	b
840.	b
841.	b
842.	d

843. During the orientation phase of the relationship, what would the nurse talk to a patient who is awaiting for amputation of foot?
- a. Summarize previous sessions
- b. Talk with him about his favorite hobbies
- c. Allow him to express his feelings
- d. Review his medical record

Explanation: Considering the options provided and the context of the orientation phase, the most appropriate action would be: 'Talk with him about his favorite hobbies'.

Talking about the patient's favorite hobbies helps establish a connection and rapport, making the patient feel more comfortable and at ease with the nurse. While allowing the patient to express their feelings is also important, initially discussing lighter topics, such as hobbies, can help create a foundation of trust before delving into deeper emotions related to the amputation.

844. Communication means:
- a. Sharing ideas
- b. Sharing beliefs
- c. Sharing thought
- d. All of these

845. All are the elements of communication process; EXCEPT:
- a. Source
- b. Message
- c. Channel
- d. Physical barrier

846. All are physical barriers of communication; EXCEPT:
- a. Noise
- b. Attention
- c. Environment
- d. Visibility

847. Which of the following is an examples of non-verbal communication:
- a. Facial expression
- b. Posture
- c. Gesture
- d. All of these

848. All are therapeutic communication techniques; EXCEPT:
- a. Silence
- b. Accepting
- c. Offering self
- d. Feedback

Explanation: While feedback can be a part of the communication process, it is not considered a therapeutic communication technique in the same way as the other options. Therapeutic communication techniques are strategies specifically designed to facilitate open and supportive communication between healthcare providers and their patients. Silence, accepting, and offering self are all techniques that promote understanding, empathy, and trust in the therapeutic relationship.

MISCELLANEOUS

849. Largest immunoglobulin is
- a. IgG
- b. IgA
- c. IgM
- d. IgE

Explanation: IgM is the largest immunoglobulin. It is also known as Macro-immunoglobulin.

850. The theme of World Health Day 2023 is: *New Q*
- a. Depression: Let's talk
- b. Support nurses and midwives
- c. Health for all
- d. Healthy heartbeat, Healthy blood pressure

Explanation:

Themes of World Health Day from 2012 to 2023

2023	:	**Health for all**
2022	:	**Our Planet, Our Health**
2021	:	Building a Fairer and Healthier World for Everyone
2020	:	Support Nurses and Midwives
2019	:	Universal Health Coverage: Everyone, everywhere
2018	:	Universal Health Coverage: Everyone, everywhere
2017	:	Depression: Let's talk
2016	:	Halt the rise: Beat diabetes
2015	:	Food safety
2014	:	Vector-borne diseases: Small bite, big threat
2013	:	Healthy heartbeat, Healthy blood pressure
2012	:	Good health adds life to years

851. A plaster cast applied to the trunk of the body and one or both legs:
- a. Hip spica
- b. Thumb spica
- c. Body spica
- d. None of these

852. Backflow of content from stomach to mouth is called as:
- a. Vomiting
- b. Nausea
- c. Regurgitation
- d. Reflex

853. Identify correct statements in relation to hiccups:
- a. It is also known as diaphragmatic breathing
- b. 3-10% carbon dioxide is the management
- c. Both a and b
- d. None of the above

854. Identify the wound healing phases among the following:
- a. Inflammatory phase
- b. Proliferative phase
- c. Maturation phase
- d. All of these

855. Universal recipient blood group is:
- a. O
- b. AB
- c. A
- d. B

Explanation: Blood group AB individuals have both A and B antigens on the surface of their RBCs, and their blood plasma does not contain any antibodies against either A or B antigen. Therefore, an individual with type AB blood can receive blood from any group (with AB being preferable), but cannot donate blood to any group other than AB. They are known as universal recipients. Blood group O is known as universal donor.

856. Laparoscopy is:
- a. Visualization of the abdominal organs through the opening in the abdominal wall
- b. Visualization of the stomach
- c. Visualization of the pelvic organs through the vaginal wall
- d. Visualization of urinary bladder

Explanation: Option a is laparoscopy, option b is gastroscopy, option c is Culdoscopy and option d is cystoscopy.

857. Recording of electrical activity of skeletal muscle is known as:
- a. Electromyography
- b. Electroencephalography
- c. Electrocardiography
- d. Electro convulsive therapy

Explanation: Option a is the correct answer. Option b is recording electrical activity of brain, option c is recording electrical activity of heart and option d is a treatment modality used in severely depressed client.

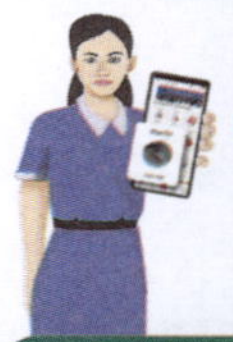

Ans.

843. b
844. d
845. d
846. b
847. d
848. d
849. c
850. c
851. a
852. c
853. c
854. d
855. b
856. a
857. a

"It is health that is real wealth and not pieces of gold and silver."
—Mahatma Gandhi

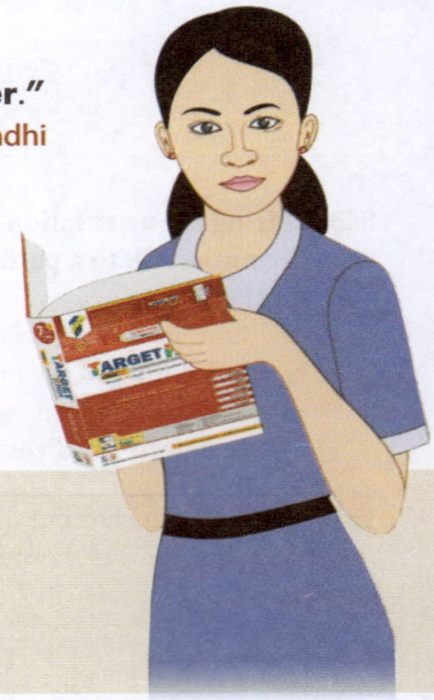

CHAPTER 2

MEDICAL SURGICAL NURSING/ ADULT HEALTH NURSING

SYNOPSIS

INFLAMMATION AND WOUND HEALING

INFLAMMATION

Definition: Inflammation is a localized reaction intended to neutralize, control or eliminate the offending agent to prepare the site for repair.

Five Cardinal Signs of Inflammation

1. Redness
2. Warmth (Heat)
3. Swelling
4. Pain
5. Loss of function

Chemical Mediators

a. Histamine released by mast cells at the site of injury causes vasodilation and vascular permeability.
b. Kinins are responsible to attract neutrophils.
c. Prostaglandins cause increased vascular permeability.

Three Phases of Inflammation

Phase 1: **Inflammatory response (3–5 days)**

a. Transient vasoconstriction occurs immediately after injury followed by vasodilation and increased capillary permeability which results in redness, swelling and warmth.
b. Exudate consists of plasma, plasma proteins, solutes, WBCs, etc., migrate into tissues resulting in pressure of fluid on nerve endings (*pain and loss of function*).
c. Leukocytes are responsible for engulfing offending organisms and for removing cellular debris. (*phagocytosis by macrophages*).

Phase 2: **Repair and Regeneration (2–8 weeks)**

a. It is characterized by new collagen formation.
b. These fibers are laid down in disorganized manner to make scar but the link between fibers is weak. Thus new tissue is susceptible to disruption on aggressive activity.

Phase 3: **Remodeling and Maturation (Months to years)**

a. In this phase, tissue continues to remodel, strengthen and improve its cellular organization.
b. Increase in organization of collagen fibers and bonds become stronger.

> **Exudate**
>
> The fluid involved in inflammatory edema is known as exudate.
>
> a. **Serous exudate:** Water-like exudate; seen in minor injury
> b. **Fibrinous exudate:** Contains fibrin
> c. **Purulent exudate (pus):** Creamy white exudate from dead neutrophils; seen in bacterial infection
> d. **Hemorrhagic exudate:** Bloody red exudate

WOUND HEALING

Definition: Wound healing is a complex and dynamic process of replacing devitalized and missing cellular structures and tissue layers.

Types of Wounds

- **Acute wound:** Heals without many complications within expected time frame, e.g., surgical wounds and trauma wounds.
- **Chronic wound:** Underlying pathology or infection causes wound or interferes with the healing process. For example, diabetic ulcer and pressure ulcer.

> **POINT TO REMEMBER**
>
> Fever is systemic response of inflammation.

> **Recent Questions**
> **(NORCET 2020)**
>
> **1. Which of the following is incorrect about bedsore?**
> a. Mobilization will affect bedsore?
> b. Moisture will affect bedsore
> c. Friction force will affect bedsore
> d. Nutritional status does not affect bedsore
>
> **Ans. (d) Nutritional status does not affect bedsore...**
>
> **2. A 65-year-old patient admitted in a long-term care facility has developed pressure ulcer. On assessment, the nurse found that the bone is visible and palpable on the wound site. The nurse knows that the stage of the pressure ulcer is:**
> a. Stage-I
> b. Stage-II
> c. Stage-III
> d. Stage-IV
>
> **Ans. (d) Stage-IV**

Wound Healing Process

- **Healing by primary intention:** No or little scar tissue. For example, surgical wounds.
- **Healing by secondary intention:** Marked loss of tissue. Edges of the wound are too far and wound gets closed naturally through granulation and epithelialization. For example, lacerated wounds, pressure ulcers, and traumatic injuries.
- **Healing by tertiary intention:** Characterized by delayed wound closure. This results in granulation of wound edges. Characterized by edema, infection, exudates from wound and excessive scar formation.

Stages of Wound Healing

The following are four stages of wound healing:

1. **Hemostasis:** Causes coagulation
2. **Inflammation:** Destroys bacteria and removes debris
3. **Proliferation:** Fills and covers the wound
4. **Maturation:** Tissue gains strength and flexibility

Wound healing can progress backward or forward depending on internal and external patient conditions.

Hemostasis

(*A brief period of vasoconstriction as an attempt to stop the bleeding*).

- Begins at the onset of injury and its objective is to stop bleeding.
- Blood vessels constrict to restrict the blood flow.
- Platelets stick together and adhere to sub-endothelium surface of epithelial wall of blood vessel in order to seal the break.
- After this, first fibrin strand begins to adhere in about 60 seconds.
- As the fibrin mesh begins, blood is transformed from liquid to gel through coagulation.

Inflammatory Phase

(*Starts immediately after injury and lasts for 2–6 hours*)

- Injured blood vessels leak exudate (neutrophils, water, salt and proteins) and cause localized swelling.
- Increased capillary permeability and blood flow to the site of injury assists phagocytosis.
- During this phase, damaged cells, pathogens and bacteria are removed from wound area.
- Swelling, redness and pain in the injured/affected area are common in this phase.

Proliferation

This stage has three distinct phases:

1. Filling the wound
2. Contraction of wound margins
3. Covering the wound (Epithelialization)
   - It is a phase of rebuilding of new tissues made up of collagen and extracellular matrix.
   - Formation of granulation tissue (pink-to-red moist tissue) followed by epithelialization (migration of epithelial cells across wound surface).
   - New network of blood vessels is constructed for sufficient supply of oxygen and nutrients to granulation tissue.

Maturation Phase

(*Remodeling stage*)

- Strengthening and reorganization of collagen occurs (remodeling of Collagen).
- Cells that had been used to repair the wound but no longer needed are removed by apoptosis.
- Scar thickness reduces and makes the area stronger.
- The process takes months to year. It takes 2–3 weeks to regain 50% of strength.
- Only 70–75% of its original strength will be regained at the end of wound healing process.

Recent Question
(CNCI 2021)

3. While assessing Mr. Gupta with Braden Scale, the score attained was 8 which indicates that the risk of developing pressure sore for Mr. Gupta is ________

a. Mild
b. Moderate
c. High
d. Very High

Ans. (d) Very High

KEY POINTS

- Blood vessels constrict to restrict the blood flow during **hemostasis stage** of wound healing.
- The **inflammatory/exudative phase of wound healing** is from onset of wound (day 1 to day 4).
- Contraction of wound margins and covering (epithelialization) occurs during **proliferation stage** of wound healing.
- **Surgical wound** is an example of healing with primary intention.
- Lacerated wounds, pressure ulcers and traumatic injuries are the examples of healing with secondary intention.

KEY POINTS

- Cellulitis: Inflammation of subcutaneous connective tissue (inner layer of the skin)
- Colonization: Presence of proliferating bacteria without causing systemic or local infections (without a host response to presence of bacteria)
- Dehiscence: Wound ruptures along (splitting) a surgical line
- Full thickness wound: Wound indicates that damage extends below all layers of the skin into the subcutaneous tissue or beyond (i.e., muscle, tendons, bone or other adjacent structures)
- Maceration: Softening and breaking down of skin surrounding the wound due to prolonged contact with moisture.
- Partial thickness wound: Loss of epidermis with involvement of all or part of dermis layer of the skin.
- Sloughing: Process of shedding necrotic (dead) tissues from the wound or skin.

Types of Wound Debridement

Goal of debridement is to remove all the devitalized tissues from the wound bed to promote wound healing. The five methods of debridement are given below:

1. **Mechanical debridement:** It is the process of removal of damaged tissues or foreign objects from a wound by physical force
2. **Chemical or enzymatic debridement:** Topical application of proteolytic substance (e.g., Enzymes) can assist in removal of devitalized tissues from wound.
3. **Sharp debridement:** Sharp instrument (e.g., Scissors, scalpel) is used in the removal of necrotic or foreign material from the wound.
4. **Autolytic debridement:** Useful in pressure ulcers. Synthetic dressings (e.g., Transparent adhesives, hydrogel) are used to cover the wound. This facilitates the naturally available enzymes in wound to digest devitalized tissue itself.
5. **Biologic debridement or Maggot debridement therapy:** Introduction of live, disinfected maggots (fly larvae) into the non-healing skin and soft tissue of a human for the purpose of cleaning out the necrotic tissues within a wound.

KEY POINTS

- Healthy granulation tissue is pink or red and uneven in texture.
- Dark granulation tissue can be a sign of poor perfusion or infection.
- Stages of wound care can be speeded up by keeping wounds clean and moist.
- Factors that lead to chronic wounds are: Venous disease, infection, diabetes, metabolic deficiencies.

GANGRENE

- Gangrene is a type of tissue death due to lack of blood supply and oxygen.
- Gangrene is usually external affecting extremities but it can also affect internal tissues.

Types of Gangrene

Table 1: Types of gangrene

Dry Gangrene	Wet Gangrene
• Begins in the distal part of the limb due to ischemia and spreads upward. • Most commonly affects limbs • Commonly due to arterial occlusion, e.g., Raynaud's disease, Buerger's disease • Organ is dry, shrink and black in color • Bacteria fail to survive	• Affects naturally moist tissues such as oral cavity, bowel, cervix, lungs, etc. • More commonly affects bowel • Commonly due to blockage of venous supply and less commonly due to blockage of arterial supply, e.g., Diabetic foot, bedsore, gas gangrene • Organ is moist, soft, swollen, rotten and dark • This gangrene favors bacterial growth.
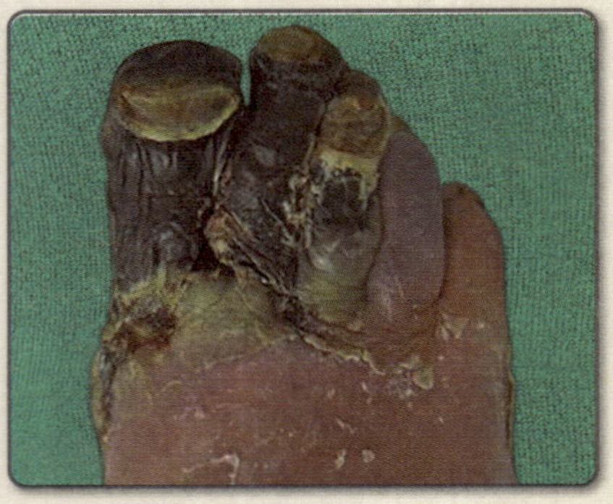 Dry gangrene	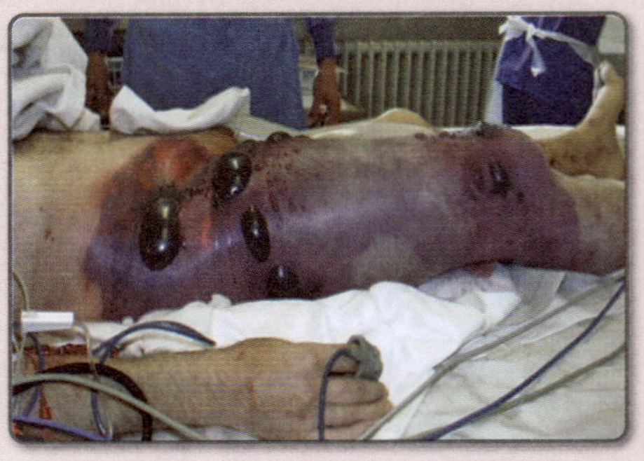 Wet Gangrene (gas gangrene)

A special form of wet gangrene caused by Gram-positive anaerobic bacteria of *Clostridium* species is known as gas gangrene.

Golden Points to Remember

- Kinins are plasma-derived chemical mediators of acute inflammation.
- **Nociception** is the physiologic process by which information about tissue damage is communicated to the Central Nervous System (CNS).
- **Prostaglandins** increase the sensitivity of pain receptors by enhancing the pain-provoking effect of bradykinin.
- **Endorphins** interact with the opiate receptors in the brain to reduce our perception of **pain** and act similarly to drugs such as morphine and codeine.
- **Nociceptor** is a sensory neuron that responds to damaging or potentially damaging stimuli by sending "possible threat" signals (pain) to the spinal cord and the brain.
- **Dehiscence** is the separation and disruption of previously-joined wound edges.
- **Hyperbaric oxygen** therapy means delivery of O_2 at increased atmospheric pressure, that accelerates granulation tissue formation and wound healing.
- Primary leukocyte that responds during inflammation is Neutrophil.
- Increase in immature neutrophils is known as '**left shift**.'
- Most common cause of altered inflammatory response is **Neutropenia**.
- Phagocytosis is also known as opsonization. This is used to neutralize foreign molecules.
- **Increased Erythrocyte Sedimentation Rate (ESR)** indicates inflammatory process.
- **Eosinophilic response** is seen in allergy, parasitic infection and cancer.
- In the first 24 hours of Inflammation process, Ischemic cell injury and infiltration of neutrophils occur.
- During 24 to 48 hours to inflammatory process, **Macrophages** become dominant.
- Increased capillary permeability and blood flow to the site of injury occur during **inflammatory phase** of wound healing.
- Healthy granulation tissue is pink or red and uneven in texture.
- Dark granulation tissue can be a sign of poor perfusion or infection.
- **Position change every 2 hours** is the most effective method of prevention of pressure ulcer in a bedridden patient.
- **Norton or Braden scales** are valid risk assessment tools for the assessment of pressure ulcers.
- **Waterlow scale or score** is used for risk assessment of pressure ulcer.
- **Movement of the affected area** is one of the important factors that delays wound healing. Age, blood flow, nutrient, moisture are some of the other factors that affect the wound healing process.
- Gangrene is a type of tissue death due to lack of blood supply and oxygen.
- Dry gangrene mostly affects limbs.
- Moist gangrene mostly affects bowel.

"He who has health has hope; and he who has hope has everything."
—Arabian proverb

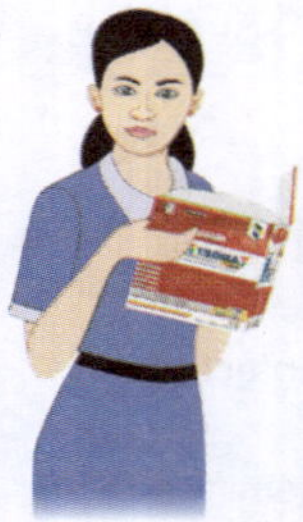

MULTIPLE CHOICE QUESTIONS
(Including Explained and Practice Questions)

INFLAMMATION AND WOUND HEALING

INFLAMMATION

1. Severe generalized edema is called: *(Safdarjung NO 2018)*
a. Myxedema b. Pitting edema
c. Anasarca d. Dependent edema

Explanation:

- When Edema is massive and generalized, it is called anasarca. It is caused by a variety of clinical conditions, like heart failure, renal failure, liver failure, or problems with the lymphatic system.
- The swelling is mainly caused by abnormal retention of body fluids in extracellular space and body tissues. Due to this, Anasarca is also known as dropsy, massive edema or generalized edema. In Anasarca the inflammation is widespread throughout the whole body.

2. Which of the following is NOT a plasma-derived chemical mediators?
a. Cytokines
b. Complement components
c. Kinins
d. Coagulation proteins

3. Cytokines are secreted by:
a. Neutrophils
b. B-Lymphocytes
c. Endothelial cells
d. All of the above

4. Which of the following increases vascular permeability during acute inflammation?
a. Histamine b. Cytokines
c. AFP d. Both A and B

5. Mechanism behind the characteristic feature of acute inflammation is:
a. Redness and pain
b. Pancytopenia
c. Vasodilatation and increased vascular permeability
d. Spongy bone marrow

6. The classical substances that increase the sensitivity of pain receptors by enhancing the pain-provoking effect of bradykinin is *(ESIC 2019)*
a. Nociceptor b. Endorphins
c. Prostaglandins d. Encephalin

Explanation:

- High levels of prostaglandins are produced in response to injury or infection and cause inflammation, which is associated with the symptoms of redness, swelling, pain and fever. This is an important part of the body's normal healing process.
- **In contrast,** Endorphins – causes analgesic effect.

7. Which of the following is a substance that decreases pain transmission and causes an inflammatory response? *(AIIMS-BBS SNO 2019)*
a. Substance P b. Endorphin
c. Prostaglandin d. Histamine

8. All of the following are evidences of an infection, Except
a. Elevated WBC b. Purulent drainage
c. Primary intention d. Increased leukocytes

9. Hemorrhage with collection of blood in the soft tissue is called
a. Contusion b. Purpura
c. Ecchymoses d. Hematoma

10. Thick yellow drainage from the wound is known as: *(AIIMS 2016)*
a. Sanguineous b. Serous-sanguineous
c. Serous d. Purulent

Explanation: Clear and watery drainage is serous. Sanguineous drainage is fresh blood that is prevalent among deep wounds of full and partial thickness. Serous-sanguineous leakage is thin and watery, and it's pink in color. Purulent drainage is when the leakage from wound appears milky. It's generally gray, green or yellow.

11. Which of the following types of exudates contains fibrin?
a. Hemmorhagic exudate b. Serous exudate
c. Fibrinous exudate d. Purulent exudate

WOUND HEALING

12. An opening of surgical wound edges is called: *(AIIMS Nagpur NO 2018)*
a. Wound evisceration b. Wound rupture
c. Wound approximation d. Wound dehiscence

Explanation:

- *Wound dehiscence* is a surgical complication in which a wound ruptures along a surgical incision. It may be due to too tight suturing or loose improper suturing, sneezing, and coughing.
- Wound evisceration - surgical incision opens (dehiscence) and the abdominal organs protrude or come out of the incision.

13. Diffuse, purulent inflammation of a tissue is called _____. *(AIIMS Nagpur NO 2018)*
a. Abscess b. Cellulitis
c. Boils d. Ulcers

Explanation:

- **Cellulitis** is a bacterial infection of underlying layers of the skin and the site of infection turns red with swelling and pain. It can be purulent (presence of pus) or non-purulent.
- **Key point:** Cellulitis is diffused whereas abscess is localized.

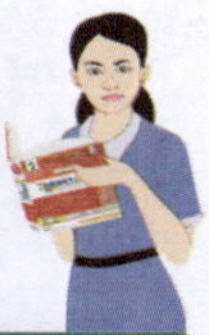

Ans.

1.	c
2.	a
3.	d
4.	d
5.	c
6.	c
7.	b
8.	c
9.	d
10.	d
11.	c
12.	d
13.	b

14. First process in wound healing:
a. Collagen fibril will form
b. Granulation tissue will appear
c. First intentional healing will take place
d. Neutrophils line the wound edge

15. The inflammatory/exudative phase of wound healing will last for: *(ESIC 2019)*
a. 1 year
b. 1-4 days
c. 21 days to a month
d. 5-20 days.

Explanation: The inflammatory/exudative phase of wound healing is from onset of wound (day 1) to Day 4. **Healing actions in this stage include** Clot formation to arrest bleeding, migration of inflammatory cells to the site of wound, neutralization of bacteria by macrophages and WBC and secretion of growth factors and cytokines.

16. If the incisional area of an abdominal surgery is weak, what is possible to happen when abdominal muscles contract and increases intra abdominal pressure?
a. Evisceration
b. Dehiscence
c. Laceration
d. Shearing

17. Stab wound for a drainage system is known as
a. Incision
b. Puncture
c. Cautery
d. Laceration

18. In which of the following, the phases of wound healing is arranged in sequence?
a. Inflammatory phase, hemostasis, reconstruction, maturation
b. Hemostasis, reconstruction, maturation, inflammatory phase
c. Hemostasis, inflammatory phase, reconstruction, maturation
d. Hemostasis, maturation, inflammatory phase, reconstruction

19. Which of the following is in the blood clot helps hold the wound together during hemostasis phase of wound healing?
a. Granulation
b. Neutrophil
c. Fibrin
d. Leucocytes

20. Wound dehiscence primarily takes place during which phase of wound healing?
a. Maturation phase
b. Homeostasis
c. Inflammatory phase
d. Reconstruction phase

21. Overgrowth of a collagenous scar tissue at the site of the wound is known as:
a. Granulation
b. Keloid
c. Hematoma
d. Celluloid

22. The term applied for the fluid, cells, or other substances that are slowly discharged, from cells or blood through small pores or breaks in cell membranes is:
a. Exudate
b. Pus
c. Infiltrates
d. Secretion

23. Soft, pink, fleshy projections consisting of capillaries surrounded by fibrous collagen:
a. Keloid
b. Granulation tissue
c. Cellulitis
d. Collagen

24. Which of the following factors is most likely to inhibit wound healing by interfering with the mechanisms that release oxygen to tissues and reducing the amount of functional hemoglobin in blood?
a. Obesity
b. Smoking
c. Radiation
d. None of the above

25. All of the following factors lead to impaired wound healing process; EXCEPT:
a. Impaired oxygenation, obesity and smoking
b. Drugs, diabetes mellitus and wound stress
c. Height, weight and body mass
d. Radiation, malnutrition and age

26. Complications of wound healing is:
a. Infection and suppuration
b. Hypertrophied scar or keloid formation
c. Contracture
d. All of the above

27. The dressings over closed wound usually are removed on the
a. Day after surgery
b. Next of surgery
c. On the third day
d. When the Doctor gives the order

28. How often would you inspect the dressings during the first day after surgery?
a. Every hour for the first 24 hours
b. Two to four hours for the first 24 hours
c. Two to four hours for first 12 hours
d. Every 6 to 8 hours for the first 24 hours

29. Correct about healing by primary intention is:
a. It is seen in healthy wound
b. Epithelial layer damage is there
c. Minimal granulation tissue formation
d. All of the above

30. Correct about healing by secondary intention is:
a. Seen in extensive tissue damage
b. Wound contraction will be there
c. Abundant granulation tissue and scarring can be seen
d. All of the above

31. Healing of a laceration can be promoted by:
a. Antibiotics
b. Daily dressing
c. Pressure dressing and ROM
d. Pressure dressing and dry cold application

32. Edema develops if plasma albumin falls below: *New Q*
a. 2.5 g/dL
b. 3.5 g/dL
c. 4.5 g/dL
d. 5.0 g/dL

Explanation: The normal plasma level of albumin in an adult is 3.5 to 5.5 grams per deciliter (g/dL). It is responsible for most of the osmotic pressure of blood. The osmotic pressure of blood helps to keep water from leaving the blood vessels and leaking into the tissues. If the albumin level falls below 2.5 g/dL, the osmotic pressure of blood will decrease, and water will leak into the tissues, causing edema.

33. What is the most appropriate nursing intervention while treating a laceration? *(ISRO)*
a. Monitor blood pressure
b. Elevate the body part
c. Apply pressure dressing and heat
d. Apply pressure dressing and ice pack

Ref: https://www.drugs.com/cg/laceration-aftercare-instructions.html

Explanation: For the management of Laceration, Apply direct pressure over the wound to stop bleeding and apply ice on the wound every 15 to 20 min. Ice helps prevent tissue damage and decreases swelling and pain.

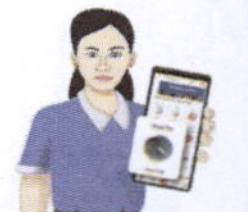

Ans.
14. d
15. b
16. b
17. b
18. c
19. c
20. d
21. b
22. a
23. b
24. b
25. c
26. d
27. c
28. b
29. d
30. d
31. d
32. a
33. d

34. In order to cease bleeding from an open wound, indirect pressure is applied to the affected artery which is:

a. Distal to the wound b. Proximal to the wound
c. Lateral to the wound d. Medial to the wound

35. Type of healing occurs in a decubitus ulcer which is treated with debridement and moist gauze dressing is:

a. Tertiary intention b. Secondary intention
c. Regeneration of cells d. Remodeling of tissues

WOUND DEBRIDEMENT

36. Surgically creating an opening into an organ or space in the body by a sharp instrument is known as:

a. Laceration b. Abrasion
c. Puncture d. Incision

37. Removal of nonviable tissue from an open wound to promote healing is known as:

a. Debridement b. Dressing
c. Cleansing d. Excision

38. Sharp removal of tissue at the wound margin or at the wound base until viable tissue is removed is known as:

a. Selective debridement b. Excisional debridement
c. Cleansing d. Dressing

39. Components of granulation tissue is:

a. Angiogenesis
b. Fibroblasts
c. Chronic inflammatory cells
d. All of the above

40. Which of the following type of debridement involves Introduction of live maggots into the soft tissue of the wound for the purpose of cleaning the necrotic tissue?

a. Autolytic debridement b. Biologic debridement
c. Enzymatic debridement d. Mechanical debridement

Explanation: Biological Debridement - Biological debridement (maggot therapy), also known as larval therapy, uses sterile larvae of the *Lucilia sericata* species of the green bottle fly. It is an effective mode of debridement, particularly appropriate in large wounds where a painless removal of necrotic tissue is needed.

41. Which of the following type of debridement refers to the process of removal of damage tissue or foreign objects from a wound by physical force?

a. Sharp debridement b. Mechanical debridement
c. Autolytic debridement d. Enzymatic debridement

Explanation: Mechanical Debridement - Mechanical debridement is a nonselective type of debridement, meaning that it will remove both devitalized tissue and debris as well as viable tissues. It is usually carried using mechanical force: wet-to-dry, pulsatile lavage, or wound irrigation. It is indicated for both acute and chronic wounds with moderate to large amounts of necrotic tissue, regardless of the presence of an active infection.

GANGRENE

42. Characteristic of wet gangrene is:

a. Venous obstruction is there
b. It is invariably followed by bacterial infection
c. It is most commonly seen in the bowel
d. All of the above

43. Dry gangrene most commonly affects the

a. Bowel b. Limbs
c. Lungs d. Cervix

44. Dry gangrene commonly occurs due to:

a. Blockage of the venous supply
b. Arterial occlusion
c. Excessive blood supply to the limbs
d. Blockage of arterial supply

45. Meleney's synergistic gangrene is caused by:

a. Staphylococcus aureus b. Streptococcus aureus
c. Streptococcus anginosus d. Streptococcus bovis

46. Which of the following condition may lead to dry gangrene?

a. Buerger's disease
b. Diabetic foot ulcer
c. Bed sore
d. None of the above

47. Which of the following type of gangrene affects the genital region of the body?

a. Wet gangrene b. Dry gangrene
c. Fournier's gangrene d. Meleney's gangrene

PREVENTION & MANAGEMENT OF PRESSURE ULCER

48. All of the following scales are used to assess risk for pressures sore in patients; EXCEPT:

a. Waterlow scale b. Broset scale
c. Norton scale d. Braden's scale

49. The Braden Scale score of a client is 16. Most appropriate nursing action is:

a. Change position every 2 hours
b. High fowlers position
c. Apply moisturizer on the affected skin
d. Administer oxygen via mask

Explanation: A Braden Scale score of 16 indicates a moderate risk for developing pressure ulcers. Clients at moderate risk for pressure ulcers require regular repositioning to relieve pressure on vulnerable areas. Changing the client's position every 2 hours helps to redistribute pressure and reduce the risk of developing pressure ulcers.

50. Decubitus ulcer on scapula measures 1 × 2 × 0.8 cm and pink subcutaneous tissue is completely visible on the wound bed, identify the stage:

a. Stage I b. Stage II
c. Stage III d. Stage IV

51. To properly stage a pressure ulcer: *(ESIC 2019)*

a. The patient must be supine
b. The skin must be completely dry
c. Natural light must be used
d. Eschar must be removed

Explanation: For assessment of stage of pressure ulcer, the eschar and slough must be removed before assessment. Position of the patient depends upon the site of pressure ulcer (not necessarily supine). A completely dry skin is not expected before assessing for staging. Day light may be preferred but not mandatory.

Ans.

34.	b
35.	b
36.	d
37.	a
38.	b
39.	d
40.	b
41.	b
42.	d
43.	b
44.	b
45.	a
46.	a
47.	c
48.	b
49.	a
50.	c
51.	d

IMMUNE SYSTEM

OVERVIEW OF IMMUNE SYSTEM

Lymphatic System

- Lymphatic system is a major part of the immune system which contains lymphatic vessels that carry lymph- a clear fluid.
- Lymph contains lymphocytes, other WBCs, waste products and debris from other organs.
- Group of lymphocytes are seen in lymph node.
- Spleen and thymus are the lymphoid organs.

Immunity

Immunity is the ability of a body to fight against infectious agents and other foreign materials.

Types of Immunity

There are two types:
1. Innate immunity
2. Acquired immunity/adaptive

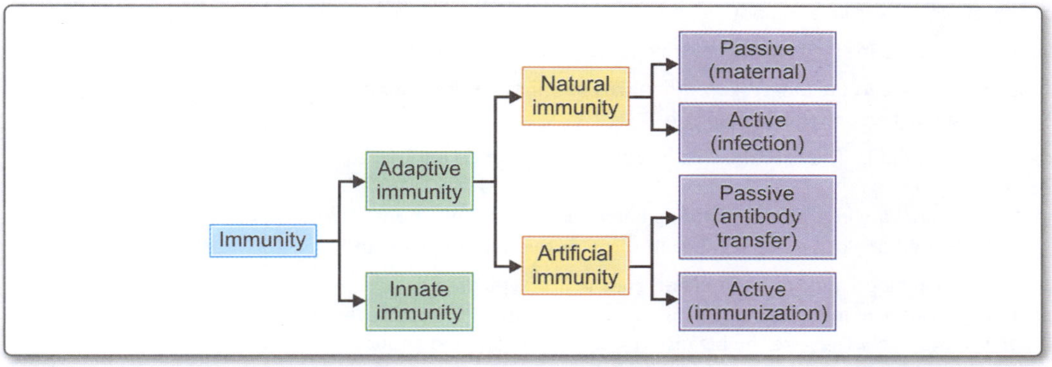

Figure 1: Types of immunity

Innate Immunity

- Immune system is activated immediately after the exposure to antigen.
- It is nonspecific type.
- External components of innate immunity - Skin, mucosal barrier, body secretions such as saliva, tears, HCl in the stomach, normal flora of the body
- Internal components of innate immunity – Inflammatory response, phagocytic cells, natural killer cells, etc.

Acquired Immunity or Adaptive Immunity

- Immunity developed by an individual during its life time.
- This has two components:
  - **Humoral immunity:** Antibody mediated immunity-B-lymphocyte is responsible.
  - **Cell mediated immunity:** T lymphocytes are responsible.

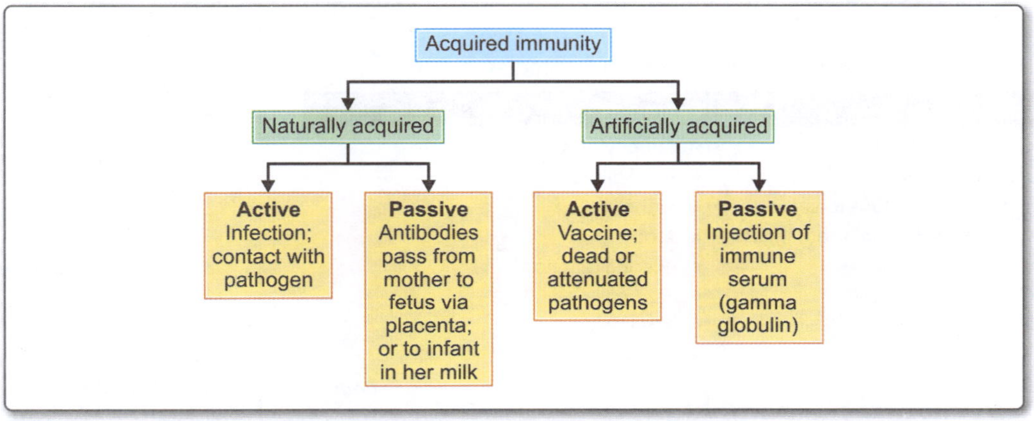

Figure 2: Classification of acquired immunity

KEY POINTS

- Antibodies are produced by B lymphocytes. They function in the humoral immunity.
- T lymphocytes are associated with cell mediated immunity.
- Breastfeeding is natural passive immunity which is obtained by immunoglobulins in mother's breast milk.
- Artificial active immunity may be produced by vaccination.
- Artificial passive immunity is through the parenteral administration of antibodies.
- Herd immunity is the overall resistance in a community.

Practice Questions

1. Which component of innate immunity is responsible for antibody-mediated immunity?
   a. Natural killer cells
   b. Phagocytic cells
   c. B-lymphocytes
   d. T-lymphocytes

Ans. (c) B-lymphocytes

2. Breastfeeding provides which type of immunity?
   a. Artificial active immunity
   b. Natural passive immunity
   c. Artificial passive immunity
   d. Innate immunity

Ans. (b) Natural passive immunity

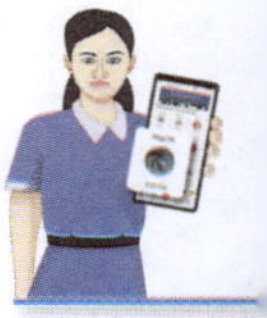

Table 2: Differences between innate and acquired immunity

Innate immunity	Acquired immunity
No time lag, action is immediate	There is a lag period
Not antigen specific	Antigen specific
No memory	Development of memory

IMMUNOGLOBULINS

Table 3: Summarized description of different types of immunoglobulins

Name	Description
Immunoglobulin A	• About 10–15% of the antibodies present in the body are IgA antibodies • Found in areas of the body such as nose, breathing passages, digestive tract, ears, eyes, and vagina • IgA is present in colostrum and body secretions.
Immunoglobulin D	• Antibodies are found in small amounts in the tissues that line the belly or chest
Immunoglobulin E	• Antibodies are found in the lungs, skin, and mucus membranes. IgE antibody levels are often high in people with allergies
Immunoglobulin G	• Found in all body fluids. They are the smallest but most common antibodies (75–80%). • IgG antibodies are very important in fighting bacterial and viral infections. • **IgG** is the only antibody class that significantly crosses the **human placenta**.
Immunoglobulin M	• They are found in blood and lymph fluid and are the first type of antibody made in response to an infection. IgM antibodies are about 5–10% of all the antibodies in the body. They are the biggest in size, so called macro antibody.

BLOOD PRODUCTS, STORAGE TEMPERATURE, SHELF LIFE AND COMPATIBILITY

Table 4: Different components, storage temperature, shelf life and compatibility of blood products

Component	Storage temp	Shelf life	Compatibility
Packed red cells	2 to 6°C	35/42 days	ABO, Rh, Cross-match
Fresh frozen plasma	–30°C or below	1 year	ABO
Platelet concentrate	22 to 24°C	5 days	Preferably ABO, but can be given without regard to ABO
Cryoprecipitate	–30°C or below	1 year	Any group

TYPES OF TRANSFUSION REACTIONS

Table 5: Different types of transfusion reactions along with description and examples

Type	Description	Examples
Type 1 (immediate hypersensitivity reaction)	• IgE and mast cell mediated • It occurs in minutes • Provoked by re-exposure to same antigen by contact, inhalation, ingestion, or injection) • It can be local or systemic	• Anaphylaxis • Food allergy • Asthma • Atopy • Allergic reaction • Eczema • Hay fever • Hives

Contd...

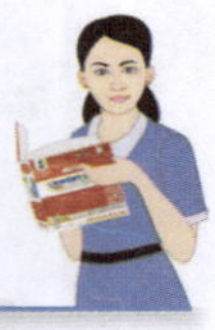

KEY POINTS

- The major class of immunoglobulin present in human serum is **IgG**.
- **IgE** is associated with allergic reactions.
- **IgG** is the most abundant immunoglobulin (75%) found in all body fluids (Remember G-greatest).
- **IgM** is the largest (size) immunoglobulin (Remember – M-Macro).
- The average risk of HIV infection after needlestick injury to HIV-infected blood is 1 in 300.
- The average risk after exposure of nose, eye, or mouth to HIV-infected blood is 0.1% (1 per 1,000).
- Persistent generalized lymphadenopathy is caused by HIV infection.

Practice Question

3. The order of the total immunoglobulin percentage in serum, from highest to lowest, is as follows:

a. IgM, IgG, IgA, IgD, IgE
b. IgM, IgA, IgG, IgE, IgD
c. IgG, IgM, IgA, IgE, IgD
d. IgG, IgA, IgM, IgD, IgE

Ans. (d) IgG, IgA, IgM, IgD, IgE

IgG (75-80%) is the most abundant immunoglobulin in serum, followed by IgA (15%), IgM (5%), IgD (0.2%), and IgE (0.002%).

Type	Description	Examples
Type 2 (antibody dependent)	• Type 2 hypersensitivity is IgG /IgM mediated • Type 2 hypersensitivity can lead to tissue damage by direct cellular destruction, inflammation or disrupting cellular function	• Autoimmune hemolytic anemia • Immune thrombocytopenia • Goodpasture syndrome • Acute rheumatic fever • Myasthenia gravis • Graves' disease • Blood transfusion reactions • Erythroblastosis fetalis
Type 3 (immune complex)	• Occurs because of the excess production of immune complexes or impaired clearance of them	• Serum sickness • Systemic lupus erythematosus • Post-streptococcal glomerulonephritis. • Arthus reaction
Type 4 (cell mediated/ delayed type)	• It is mediated by T cells and macrophages	• Multiple sclerosis • Contact dermatitis • Tubercular lesion • Graft rejection

Practice Question

4. Which type of hypersensitivity reaction is mediated by IgE and mast cells?
a. Type 1
b. Type 2
c. Type 3
d. Type 4

Ans. (a) Type 1

IMMUNOLOGICAL DISORDER

Acquired Immunodeficiency Syndrome (AIDS)

- AIDS is caused by HIV (Human Immunodeficiency virus).
- HIV is a retro virus and has RNA as genetic material (makes DNA from RNA).
- HIV/AIDS is characterized by reduced CD4 + (T-helper cells). It also affects monocytes, macrophages, dendritic cells (skin), microglial cells (CNS).
- Normal life span of CD4+ T cells is 100 days but HIV infected CD4 cell dies within 2 days.
- Normal value of CD4+ T cells is from 500 to 1200 cells/ micro-liters.
- As the disease progresses, CD4+ T cells count decreases.
- Immune system remains healthy when CD4+ T cells > 500 cells/microliters.
- Problems related to immune system arise when CD4+ T cells count ranges from 200 to 500 cells/ microliters.
- Immune system becomes severely compromised when CD4+ T cells count is less than 200 cells/ microliters.
- **Normal CD4 to CD8 ratio is 2:1.** This ratio decreases with the progression of disease.
- HIV infection leads to immune-compromise and opportunistic infections increase in the affected person.
- **HIV virus infects and destroys helper T cells.**

Transmission of HIV/AIDS

- Sexual intercourse with infected person
- Exposure to blood or blood products of infected person.
- Perinatal transmission or vertical transmission (During delivery or through breastfeeding)
- Exposure to body fluids (Semen, vaginal secretions, saliva, CSF, tears)
- Sharing of needles.

Recent Question (NORCET 2020)

4. A nurse caring for an HIV positive patient got an accidental needle stick injury. Which of the following is an appropriate immediate action following needle stick injury?
a. Squeeze the wound to bleed it
b. Wash the wound and surrounding skin with soap and rinse
c. Use Bleach or alcohol to clean the wound
d. Put the pricked finger in mouth

Ans. (b) Wash the wound and surrounding skin with soap and rinse

Table 6: WHO clinical staging of HIV/AIDS for adults and adolescents

Stages	Clinical manifestations
Primary HIV infection	• Acute retroviral syndrome • Asymptomatic
Clinical stage 1	• Asymptomatic • Persistent generalized lymphadenopathy (PGL)
Clinical stage 2	• Moderate unexplained weight loss (<10% of measured body weight) • Recurrent oral ulcerations • Recurrent respiratory tract infections • Herpes zoster • Angular cheilitis and papular pruritic eruptions • Seborrheic dermatitis • Fungal nail infections

Contd...

Practice Question

5. AIDS is the last and most severe stage of HIV infection. It is diagnosed if the CD4+ cell count is less than:
a. 800 cells/ microliters
b. 600 cells/ microliters
c. 500 cells/ microliters
d. 200 cells/ microliters

Ans. (d) 200 cells/ microliters

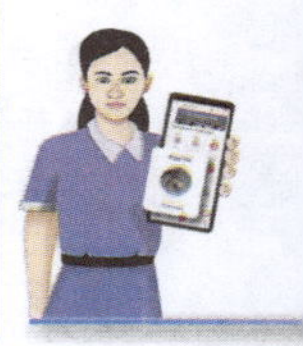

Stages	Clinical manifestations
Clinical stage 3	• Unexpected severe weight loss (>10% of presumed or measured body weight) • Unexplained chronic diarrhea for more than one month • Unexplained persistent fever (for more than one month) • Oral candidiasis • Oral hairy leukoplakia • Pulmonary tuberculosis (TB) diagnosed in last two years • Severe presumed bacterial infections • Acute necrotizing ulcerative stomatitis, gingivitis or periodontitis • Unexplained anemia (<8 g/dL), and or neutropenia (<500/mm3) and or thrombocytopenia (<50,000/ mm3) for more than one month
Clinical stage 4	• **HIV wasting syndrome** • Pneumocystis pneumonia • **Kaposi's sarcoma** • Recurrent severe or radiological bacterial pneumonia • Chronic herpes simplex infection (orolabial, genital or anorectal of more than one month's duration) • Esophageal candidiasis • **HIV encephalopathy** • **Extrapulmonary TB** • Central nervous system (CNS) toxoplasmosis • Extrapulmonary cryptococcosis including meningitis • Cytomegalovirus (CMV) infection (retinitis or of an organ other than liver, spleen or lymph nodes) • Atypical disseminated leishmaniasis • Disseminated mycosis

Source: WHO (2007) clinical staging of HIV/AIDS

Diagnostics Tests for HIV and AIDS

- **ELISA Test (Enzyme-Linked Immunosorbent Assay):** This test is sensitive in chronic HIV infection but less sensitive for recent infection. If ELISA test is positive, the Western blot test is usually administered to confirm the diagnosis.
- **Western Blot:** This is a very sensitive blood test used as confirmatory test for HIV infection.
- **Viral Load Test:** This test measures the amount of HIV in the blood. It is used to monitor progress of treatment or to detect early HIV infection.
- **CD4 cell count** test is useful for monitoring progress of the disease.

Management

Antiretroviral Drugs (ART)

- **Nucleoside reverse transcriptase inhibitors (NRTIs):** Abacavir (ABC), Didanosine (DDI), Emtricitabine (FTC), Lamivudine (3TC), Stavudine (d4T), Tenofovir alafenamide (TAF), Tenofovir disoproxil fumarate (TDF), Zidovudine (ZDV)
- **Non-nucleoside reverse transcriptase inhibitors (NNRTIs):** Delavirdine (DLV), Doravirine (DOR), Efavirenz (EFV), Etravirine (ETR), Nevirapine (NVP), Rilpivirine (RPV)
- **Protease inhibitors (PIs):** Atazanavir (ATV), Darunavir (DRV), Forsamprenavir (FPV), Indinavir (IDV), Nelfinavir (NFV), Ritonavir (RTV), Tipranavir (TPV), Saquinavir (SQV)
- **Fusion inhibitors:** Enfuvirtide (ENF)
- **C-C Chemokine Receptor type 5 Antagonists (CCR5 antagonist):** Maraviroc (MVC)

Recent Question
(NORCET 2022)

5. Mantoux test is done on a patient who has been suffering from HIV. What value of induration indicates the TB infection in the patient?

a. 5 b. 7
c. 11 d. 15

Ans. (a) 5

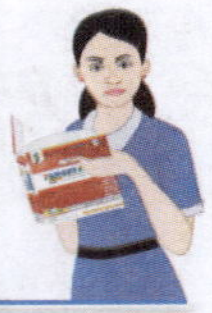

Practice Question

6. What is the criteria to start Anti-retro viral (ART) therapy in adults/ adolescents:

a. CD4 ≤ 200 in Clinical stage I & II
b. CD4 ≤ 500 in Clinical stage I & II
c. CD4 ≤ 200 in Clinical stage III & IV
d. CD4 ≤ 500 in Clinical stage III & IV

Ans. (b) CD4 ≤ 500 in Clinical stage I & II

KEY POINTS

Key Points to Remember in Nursing Care of HIV Patient

- Maintain confidentiality
- Explain side-effects of medications
- Provide counseling and psychological support

KEY POINT

Life span of **CD4+ T** cells is 100 days, but in HIV infected patients, it is only 2 days that causes immunodeficiency in patients.

POINT TO REMEMBER

WHO has recommended the use of the newer HIV drug "Dolutegravir (DTG)" as the preferred first-line and second-line treatment for HIV patients.

When to Start Antiretroviral Therapy (ART)

Table 7: Time for initiation of ART

WHO clinical staging	Recommendations
HIV Infected Adults and Adolescents	
Clinical Stage I and II	Start ART if CD4 ≤ 500
Clinical Stage III and IV	Start ART irrespective of CD4 count
All Pregnant/Breastfeeding Women	
All clinical Stages	Start ART irrespective of CD4 count
HIV-TB Co-Infected Patients	
Patients with HIV and TB co-infection (Pulmonary or Extra Pulmonary)	• Start ART irrespective of CD4 count • Start ATT first, initiate ART as early as possible between 2 weeks -2 months. • For patients with CD4 below 50, ART might be initiated simultaneously with ATT with strict clinical and laboratory monitoring

Source: National AIDS Control Organization (NACO Guidelines)

Table 8: Dosing schedules for ART of pregnant women

Clinical scenario	ARV prophylaxis and dosing	Antepartum	Intrapartum	Postpartum
Pregnant women requiring ART	Tenofovir (TDF)- 300 mg OD, Lamivudine (3TC) – 300 mg OD, Efavirenz (EFV) - 600 mg OD	Start ART as soon as possible	Continue ART	Continue ART life-long

National AIDS Control Program (NACP)

- The National AIDS Control Program (NACP) is a government-funded program in India that aims to prevent and control HIV/AIDS.
- The NACP has been running since 1992 and has gone through five phases.

Phases of National AIDS Control Program

Table 9: Different phases of NACP along with their periods and focus areas

Phase	Period	Focus
First phase	1992–1999	Awareness generation and blood safety
Second phase	1999–2007	Direct interventions across the prevention-detection-treatment continuum with capacity building of States on program management
Third phase	2007–2012	Scale-up with program management decentralized up to the district level
Fourth phase	2012–2017	Consolidation and enhanced Government funding
Fifth and current phase	2017–2026	Reduce annual new HIV infections and AIDS-related mortalities by 80% by 2025–26 from the baseline value of 2010

Golden Points to Remember

- Contact dermatitis occurs due to delayed hypersensitivity (Type IV) type of reaction.
- **Corticosteroids** block the action of **phospholipase**, thereby reducing the production of both prostaglandin and leukotrienes.
- Administration of corticosteroids diminishes the activity of the immune system, so they may mask some usual symptoms of infection.
- **Psychoneuroimmunology (PNI)** is an interdisciplinary science that seeks to understand the reactions among psychology, neurologic and immune responses.
- **Cytokines cause fever** by their ability to initiate metabolic changes in the temperature regulating center.
- The **cardinal signs** of inflammation include **redness, heat, pain, swelling** and **loss of function**.
- **Sirolimus** is an immunosuppressive agent used in renal transplant recipient in combination with corticosteroids and cyclosporine.
- **Kaposi sarcoma** is a tumor caused by human herpes virus 8, it is commonly associated with human immunodeficiency virus.
- Drugs commonly used in **antiretroviral therapy (ART)** are Zidovudine (ZDV), also known as azidothymidine (AZT), Nevirapine and Stavudine.

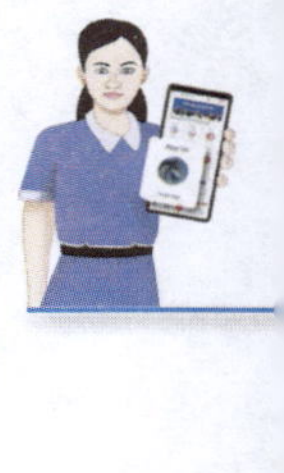

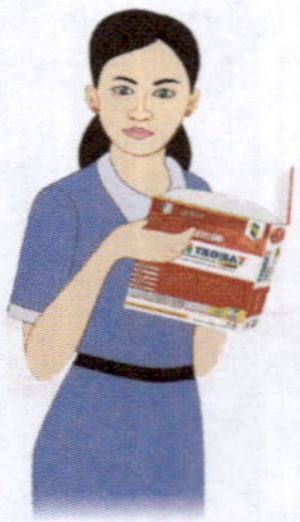

"He who has health has hope; and he who has hope has everything."

—Arabian proverb

MULTIPLE CHOICE QUESTIONS

(Including Explained and Practice Questions)

IMMUNE SYSTEM

LYMPHATIC SYSTEM

52. Antibodies are produced by: *New Q* *(JIPMER 2012)*

a. Plasma cells
b. T-helper cells
c. Neutrophils
d. Basophills

Explanation: Plasma cells are differentiated B-lymphocytes that is capable of secreting immunoglobulin or antibodies. When an antigen binds to a B-lymphocytes, it will divide and differentiate into a plasma cells. The plasma cell will then produce antibodies that are specific to the antigen.

53. Plasma cells are formed from:

a. T cells
b. B cells
c. RBC
d. WBC

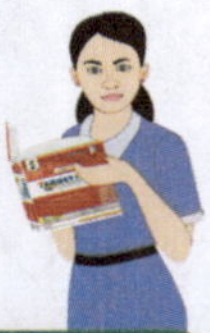

54. All of the following are organs of the lymphatic system; EXCEPT: *(AIIMS Raipur Staff Nurse Grade I-2018)*

a. Tonsils
b. Thymus
c. Spleen
d. Pancreas

Ans.

52. a
53. b
54. d
55. c
56. a
57. c
58. a
59. a

Explanation: Lymphatic system is a network of very small tubes that drain lymph fluid from all part of the body. The major parts of lymph tissue are located in bone marrow, spleen, thymus, lymph nodes and tonsils.

55. How to palpate lymph nodes?

a. With pressure and tip of fingers
b. Apply pressure while palpating the lymph nodes
c. Palpate superficial lymph nodes with the pads of the fingers.
d. Use palm of hand while palpating the lymph nodes

56. When a B-cell is exposed to an antigen for the first time:

a. The primary response occurs
b. The primary response takes 1-3 hours to become effective
c. The B-cell divides to form plasma cells and T-helper cells
d. The B-memory cells produce antibodies

57. The following statements are TRUE in reference to endotoxins; EXCEPT: *(AIIMS Raipur Grade II 2017)*

a. They are lipopolysaccharides in nature
b. They are released from the bacterial surface by natural lysis
c. They are heat liable proteins
d. Their toxicity depends in the lipid component

Explanation:

Characteristics	Exotoxins	Endotoxins
Source	Living gram positive and gram negative bacteria	Lysed gram negative bacteria
Location	Released from the cell	Part of cell
Chemical Composition	Protein	Lipopolysaccharide
Heat Sensitivity	Liable (6°-8°C)	Stable (25°C)
Immune Reactions	Strong	Weak
Conversion to Toxoids	Possible	Not possible
Fever	No	Yes
Enzyme Activity	It has mostly enzymatic activity.	It has no enzymatic activity.
Molecular Weight	Its molecular weight is 10 KDa.	Its molecular weight is 50-1000 KDa.
Denaturing	On boiling it get denatured.	On boiling it cannot be denatured.
Specificity	Specific to particular bacterial strain	Non specific
Antigenicity	High	Poor
Examples	Staphylococcus aureus, Bacillus cereus, Streptococcus pyogenes, Vibrio cholera, Bacillus anthracis.	E. coli, Salmonella typhi, Shigella.

58. Payers patches are found in:

a. Wall of the small intestine
b. Inner lining of esophagus
c. Buccal cavity
d. Wall of the stomach

Explanation: **Peyer's patches** are small masses of lymphatic tissue found throughout the ileum region of thesmall intestine. Also known as aggregated lymphoid nodules, they form an important part of the immune system by monitoring intestinal bacteria populations and preventing the growth of pathogenic bacteria in the intestines.

59. Perforins are produced by?

a. Natural killer cells
b. Chief cells
c. B cells
d. T cells

Explanation: **Perforin** is a cytolytic mediator **produced** by killer lymphocytes, and is stored in and released by cytoplasmic granules.

60. A process by which certain cells engulf and destroy foreign particles or microorganisms is known as:
a. Cytolysis b. Phagocytosis
c. Apoptosis d. All of the above

61. Phagocytosis is considered as a ________ against infection.
a. First line defense b. Second line defense
c. Third line defense d. Fourth line defense

TYPES OF IMMUNITY

62. Humoral immunity is provided by:
a. T-lymphocytes b. B- lymphocytes
c. Immunoglobulin d. Interferon

63. Humoral immunity is also known as:
a. Cell mediated b. Antibody mediated
c. Natural d. Interferon mediated

64. T cell immunity is:
a. Cell mediated b. Antibody mediated
c. Natural d. Interferon mediated

65. Occurrence of certain disease or subclinical infection provides .... Immunity.
a. Natural active b. Natural passive
c. Active artificial d. Passive artificial

66. Vaccination provides .... immunity.
a. Natural active b. Natural passive
c. Active artificial d. Passive artificial

67. Type of hypersensitivity reaction occurs during transfusion and erythroblastosis fetalis are:
a. Type I b. Type II
c. Type III d. Type IV

68. Lifelong immunity developed after the occurrence of disease is known as:
a. Natural passive immunity b. Artificial passive immunity
c. Natural active immunity d. Artificial active immunity

69. Cell mediated immunity is carried out by:
a. B lymphocytes b. T lymphocytes
c. Monocytes d. CD4 cells

70. Which of the following type of hypersensitivity is known as delayed type hypersensitivity and is carried out by T-lymphocytes?
a. Type I b. Type II
c. Type III d. Type IV

71. Identify the correct statement related to type I hypersensitivity:
a. Immunoglobulin responsible for type I hypersensitivity reaction is IgE
b. Mast cells are important cells in type I hypersensitivity
c. Immunoglobulin responsible for type I hypersensitivity reaction is IgG
d. Both A and B

72. Immediate treatment of Anaphylaxis is: *(NCFL 2019)*
a. Adrenaline b. Benzyl penicillin
c. Hydrocortisone d. Atropine

Explanation: Adrenaline or epinephrine is the immediate treatment of anaphylaxis. It will stimulate the alpha adrenoceptors and thereby it increases peripheral vascular resistance that leads to the improvement of blood pressure, reversing of peripheral vasodilation, coronary perfusion and it decreases angioedema.

73. During blood transfusion therapy, patient developed wheezing and her skin becomes flushed with hives. These are the characteristics of:
a. Hemolytic reaction b. Allergic reaction
c. Transfusion reaction d. Thrombotic crisis

74. Identify the transfusion reactions among the following:
a. Hemolytic transfusion reactions—immediate or delayed
b. Infections
c. Allergic reactions
d. All of the above

75. Identify autoimmune diseases among the following:
a. SLE b. Grave's disease
c. Myasthenia gravis d. All of the above

76. The nurse is caring for a child who is taking corticosteroids for systemic lupus erythematosus. The nurse carefully monitors child's condition because the nurse is aware that corticosteroids can have what major action?
a. They increase liver enzymes *(AIIMS Raipur NO 2019)*
b. They can mask signs of infection
c. They cause bone marrow suppression
d. They decrease renal function

Explanation: Corticosteroids suppress the immune system, so the immune response to infection is diminished. It may mask or hide some signs and symptoms of infection.

77. HLA elevates in .... condition.
a. Congenital malformation b. Malignant tumor
c. Hepatic disorders d. Autoimmune disorders

78. A rise of an existing antibody level in response to irrelevant stimulus is called: *(AIIMS Raipur Grade II 2017)*
a. Anaphylactic reaction b. Anamnestic reaction
c. Agglutination reaction d. Precipitation reaction

Explanation: Anamnestic reaction, also known as booster response, is a delayed immunologic response. Exposure to antigen in a sensitized individual results in massive production of existing antibody. Agglutination reaction is the process that occurs if an antigen is mixed with corresponding antibody. Anaphylactic reaction are life threatening reactions which exhibit symptoms such as generalized itching and hives, swelling, wheezing and difficulty breathing, fainting, and/or other allergy symptoms. Precipitation reaction refers to the formation of an insoluble salt when two solutions containing soluble salts are combined.

79. Which of the following is a priority in planning care for a client with a diagnosis of immune deficiency?
a. Providing emotional support to decrease anxiety
b. Identifying factors that decreased the immune function
c. Encouraging discussion about lifestyle changes
d. Protecting the client from infection

Explanation: Immunodeficiency is state of diminished or absence of immune response that increases susceptibility to infection. Protecting the client from the infection is the priority while planning the care of patient with compromised immunity.

80. Delayed hypersensitivity reaction can be managed with:
a. Adrenaline b. Dopamine
c. IV fluid d. Corticosteroids

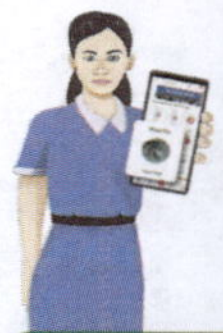

Ans.

60.	b
61.	b
62.	b
63.	b
64.	a
65.	a
66.	c
67.	b
68.	c
69.	b
70.	d
71.	d
72.	a
73.	b
74.	d
75.	d
76.	b
77.	d
78.	b
79.	d
80.	d

81. The aim of immunosuppressive therapy is to:

a. Stimulate the antibody production against foreign antigens
b. Suppress the production of antibodies against foreign antigens
c. Promote phagocytosis
d. All of the above

Explanation: The purpose of immunosuppressive therapy is to reduce the immune response to foreign antigens (infections) by suppressing the production of antibodies against it.

82. Corticosteroid suppresses the function of:

a. Sympathetic response
b. Parasympathetic
c. Immune response
d. Cardiac system

83. Nurse needs to suspect anaphylactic reaction following the IM administration of streptomycin if the patient is complaining of:

a. Edema and itching at the injection site
b. Increases in induration
c. Increase in body temperature
d. Vertigo

84. Secondary immunodeficiency is most commonly due to:

a. Drugs b. Anxiety
c. Malnutrition d. Infection

85. Following traumatic injury and infection a patient is receiving high-dose corticosteroids and broad-spectrum antibiotics. The suspected condition is:

a. Candidiasis b. CMV
c. Shigella d. Plasmodium

86. Which of the following viral infection causes Kaposi`s sarcoma?

a. Human herpes virus 8 (HHV8)
b. Cytomegalo virus
c. Rota virus
d. Human papilloma virus

Explanation: Kaposi sarcoma (KS) is a tumor caused by infection with a virus called the Kaposi sarcoma associated herpesvirus (KSHV), also known as human herpesvirus 8 (HHV8). KSHV is in the same family as Epstein-Barr virus (EBV), the virus that causes infectious mononucleosis (mono) and is linked to several types of cancer.

87. About Kawasaki disease all are true; EXCEPT:

a. Seen in children
b. Coronary artery is involved
c. Mucocutaneous lesions
d. Suppurative lymphadenopathy

88. Strawberry tongue is seen in:

a. PAN b. Kawasaki disease
c. MPA d. Wegener's

IMMUNOGLOBULINS

89. Immunoglobulin increased during secondary response is:

a. IgD b. IgG
c. IgM d. IgA

90. Secondary immune response is mediated by:

a. IgA b. IgG
c. IgM d. IgE

91. Which of the following immunoglobulin secreted in the mucous membrane of the respiratory tract?

a. IgA b. Igd
c. IgE d. IgM

92. Which of the following immunoglobulin first produced and expressed after an exposure to the infectious agent?

a. IgG b. IgM
c. IgE d. IgD

93. Which is the only immunoglobulin made by the fetus at 5 months?

a. IgA b. IgM
c. IgE d. IgG

94. Which of the following immunoglobulin is very important in fighting bacterial and viral infections?

a. IgA b. IgM
c. IgE d. IgG

95. Which type of immunoglobulin is associated with allergic reaction?

a. IgA b. IgM
c. IgE d. IgG

96. Which of the following immunoglobulin is the most abundant isotype in the blood?

a. IgA b. IgM
c. IgE d. IgG

97. Immunoglobulins are proteins that are produced by or present on the surface of:

a. B cells b. T cells
c. Chief cells d. Parietal cells

98. Which immunoglobulin is present in the mucus and helps in protecting against bacteria and virus?

a. IgA b. IgM
c. IgE d. IgG

HIV AND AIDS

99. Which immunity is affected by HIV infection?

a. Natural immunity b. Active immunity
c. Cellular immunity d. Humoral immunity

Explanation: HIV attacks and destroys the T helper lymphocytes, or T-cells, which are crucial to the immune system and immune response. CD4 T cells will be affected which is responsible for cellular immunity.

100. HIV affects :

a. B-cells b. Helper T cells
c. Neutrophil d. Lymphocyte

101. While screening for HIV, blood is tested for:

a. P24 antigen b. HIV DNA plasma
c. HIV antibodies d. Presence of HIV RNA

102. Which of the following diagnostic test is considered as a gold standard for confirmation of HIV infection?

a. ELISA test
b. Tri-dot test
c. Western blot test
d. Polymerase Chain Reaction (PCR test)

Explanation: Western blot is often used as a follow-up test to confirm the presence of an antibody of HIV virus. This test is considered to be the gold standard for confirmation of HIV infection.

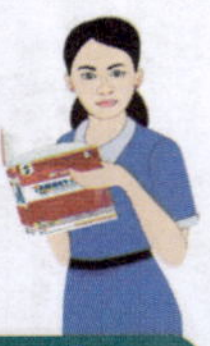

Ans.

81. b
82. c
83. a
84. a
85. a
86. a
87. d
88. b
89. b
90. b
91. a
92. b
93. b
94. d
95. c
96. d
97. a
98. a
99. c
100. b
101. c
102. c

103. Which among the following is the most appropriate intervention to prevent the progression of HIV to AIDS?
- a. Monthly plasmapheresis
- b. Abstinence
- c. Compliance with complete therapeutic regimen
- d. Monthly blood test

104. Risk for vertical transmission of HIV is more during:
- a. Antenatal period
- b. Intranatal period
- c. Postnatal period
- d. Breast feeding

105. Which of the following statement is false? *(LNJP H D 2012)*
- a. Untreated HIV infection can remain in the early chronic stage for a decade or more
- b. Infection with HIV results in a chronic disease with acute exacerbations
- c. Late stage detection is called AIDS
- d. Opportunistic disease occurs more often when the CD4 T cells count is high and viral load is low

106. The diagnosis of HIV AIDS is made based on:
- a. CD4+ T cell count
- b. Sudden weight loss
- c. Diarrhea
- d. Persistent fever

107. Which of the following is an indicator of AIDS? (DSSSB 2013)
- a. CD4 count lower than 1000 cells/mm^3
- b. CD4 count lower than 600 cells/mm^3
- c. CD4 count lower than 400 cells/mm^3
- d. CD4 count less than 200 cells/mm^3

Explanation: According to the CDC disease staging system, the definition of AIDS includes all HIV-infected individuals with CD4 counts of <200 cells/μL (or CD4 percentage <14%) as well as those with certain HIV-related conditions and symptoms.

108. The clinical symptoms of wasting syndrome in AIDS include: *(AIIMS Raipur Grade II 2017)*
- a. Involuntary weight loss
- b. Chronic diarrhea
- c. Protein - energy malnutrition
- d. Oesophageal candidiasis

- a. A, B, C
- b. B, C, D
- c. A, B, D
- d. A, B, C, D

Explanation: The symptoms of wasting syndrome in AIDS include involuntary weight loss, diarrhea for at least a month, protein energy malnutrition, extreme weakness and fever that's not related to infection. Esophageal candidiasis is an opportunistic infection of oesophagus by candida albicans.

109. Organism responsible for pneumonia in AIDS patient is:
- a. Cytomegalo virus
- b. Fungi
- c. Pneumocystis carinii
- d. Mycoplasma

110. Which of the following condition is associated with AIDS?
- a. Invasive cervical cancer
- b. Kaposi's sarcoma
- c. Burkitt's lymphoma
- d. All of the above

111. Find out the malignancies associated with HIV AIDS:
- a. Kaposi's Sarcoma
- b. Non Hodgkin's lymphoma
- c. Cervical cancer
- d. All of the above

112. Which is the most common cancer associated with AIDS? *(Kerala PSC, Nov 2014)*
- a. Leukemia
- b. Adenocarcinoma
- c. Osteosarcoma
- d. Kaposi's sarcoma

Explanation: Kaposi sarcoma (KS) is one of the first conditions recognized as an opportunistic sequela of HIV infection, and remains the most common AIDS-associated neoplasm. Non-Hodgkin lymphoma (NHL) is the second most common AIDS related cancer.

113. While providing oral care to a retro positive client, nurse should:
- a. Use special mouth care solution
- b. Use soft tooth brush
- c. Isolate the client
- d. Wear gloves

114. While taking temperature of HIV positive client nurse should:
- a. Wear all PPE
- b. Wear mask and gloves
- c. Use 1% hypochlorite solution
- d. Wash hands before and after the procedure

115. Which among the following food item need to be avoided by an immunocompromised person who is experiencing frequent diarrhea?
- a. Milk
- b. Rice water
- c. Fruits
- d. Curd

Explanation: Parasites may be the most common etiology for enteritis, especially in patients who are greatly immunosuppressed. Feed intolerance is common in immunosuppressed patients and is usually manifested by vomiting and diarrhea. In these patients, bulking agents, lactose-free diets, and antidiarrheal medications like diphenoxylate with atropine or loperamide are beneficial in treating diarrheal symptoms.

116. Opportunistic diseases:
- a. Can be sudden in onset
- b. Can occur at any point of time
- c. Occur during immunosuppression
- d. Can be treated with oral antibiotics

117. Rapidly progressive dementia is seen in:
- a. Alzheimer's disease
- b. Vascular dementia
- c. HIV Dementia
- d. Parkinson's disease

ANTIRETROVIRAL THERAPY

118. ART stands for:
- a. Antiretroviral Therapy
- b. Antiretroviral Treatment
- c. Anti rhesus Treatment
- d. All retroviral Therapy

119. Antiretroviral drugs help to:
- a. Treat HIV infection
- b. Decrease viral RNA levels
- c. Control pneumocystis carinii pneumonia
- d. Decrease pain and diarrhea

120. Which of the following anti-retroviral drug is newly introduced by NACO for the treatment of HIV positive patients?
- a. Tenofovir Disoproxil fumarate
- b. Lopinavir
- c. Lamivudine
- d. Dolutegravir

Explanation: Based on new evidence assessing benefits and risks, the WHO recommends the use of the HIV drug dolutegravir (DTG) as the preferred first-line and second-line treatment for all populations, including pregnant women and those of childbearing potential. NACO introduced dolutegravir on February 2020 in India.

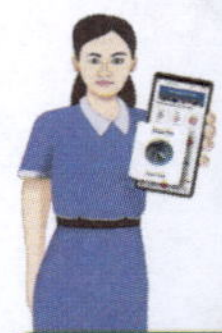

Ans.

103. c
104. b
105. d
106. a
107. d
108. a
109. c
110. d
111. d
112. d
113. d
114. d
115. a
116. c
117. c
118. a
119. b
120. d

MUSCULOSKELETAL SYSTEM

ANATOMY AND PHYSIOLOGY OF MUSCULOSKELETAL SYSTEM

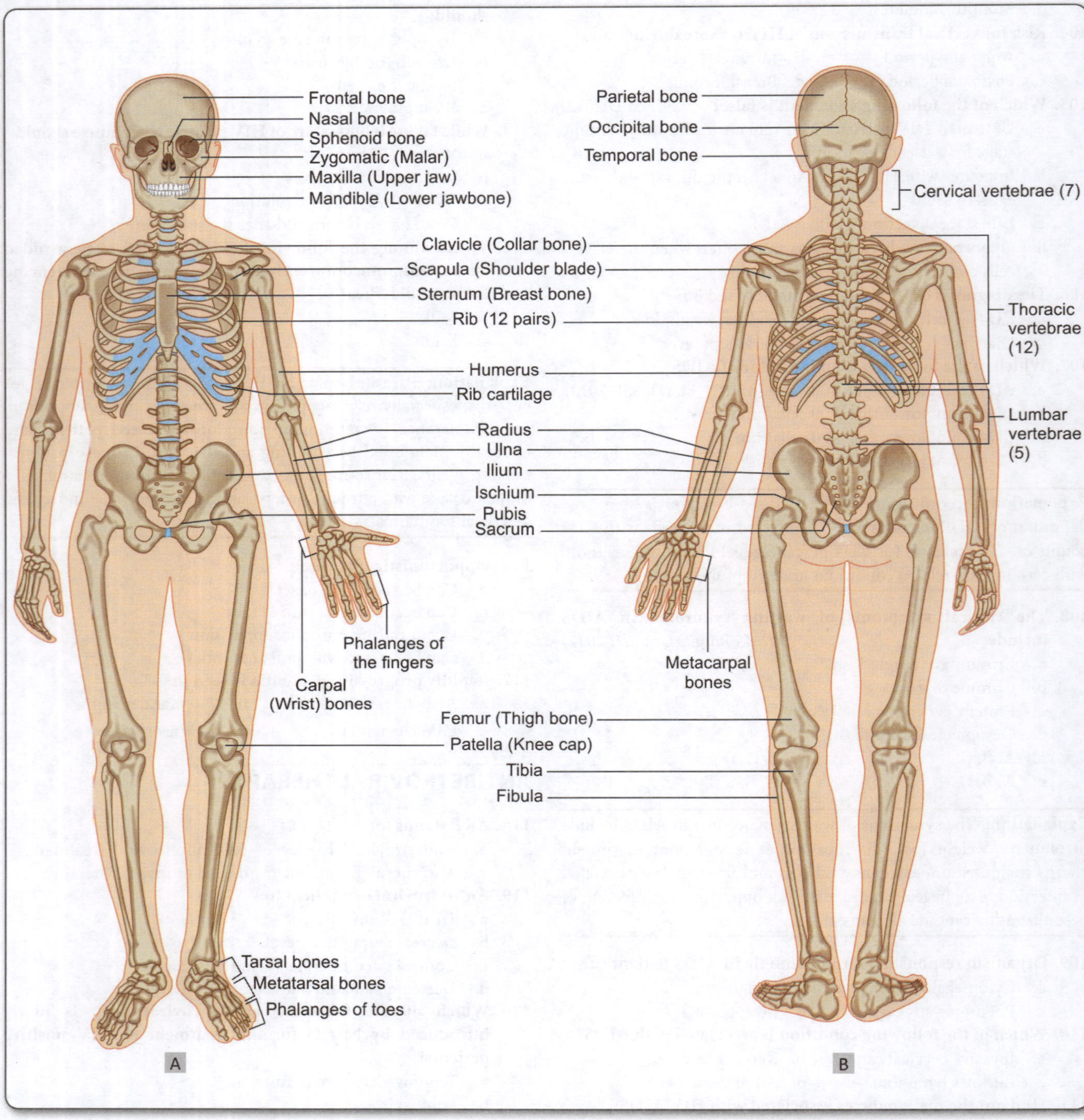

Figures 3A and B: Skeletal system of human body: (A) Anterior view; (B) Posterior view

CLASSIFICATION OF BONES

Table 10: Classification of bones with their numbers in human body

S.No.	Name	Number	Bone
		Axial skeleton (80 bones)	
1	• Cranial bones	8	Frontal bone-1 Parietal bones-2 Temporal bones-2 Occipital bone-1 Ethmoid bone-1 Sphenoid bone-1
	• Facial bones	14	Zygomatic bones-2 Maxilla bones-2 Nasal bones-2 Lacrimal bones-2 Vomer bone-1 Palatine bones-2 Inferior nasal conchae-2 Mandible-1
2	Hyoid bone	01	Hyoid bone-1
3	Auditory ossicles	06	Malleus-2 Incus-2 Stapes-2
4	Rib cage	25	Ribs-24 Sternum-01
5	Vertebral column	26	Cervical vertebrae-7 Thoracic vertebrae-12 Lumbar vertebrae-5 Sacrum vertebra-1 Coccyx vertebra-1
Total			**80 bones**
		Appendicular skeleton (126 bones)	
1	Shoulder girdle	4	Scapulae-2, Clavicle-2
2	Upper extremity	60	Humerus-2 (1 + 1) Radius-2 (1 + 1) Ulna-2 (1 + 1) Carpals-16 (8 + 8) Metacarpals-10 (5 + 5) Phalanges-28 (14 + 14)
3	Pelvic girdle	02	Innominate bones-2
4	Lower extremity	60	Femur-2 (1 + 1) Tibia-2 (1 + 1) Fibula 2 (1 + 1) Patella-2 (1 + 1) Tarsals-14 (7 + 7) Metatarsals-10 (5 + 5) Phalanges-28 (14 + 14)
Total bones			**80 (Axial) + 126 (Appendicular) = 206**

- There are 206 bones in human body.
- Among 206 bones, 80 bones are the part of axial skeleton which comprise skull, vertebral column and thorax.
- 126 bones are the part of appendicular skeleton system.
- Based upon the shape, bones in the human body are classified into four categories which is shown in Table 11.

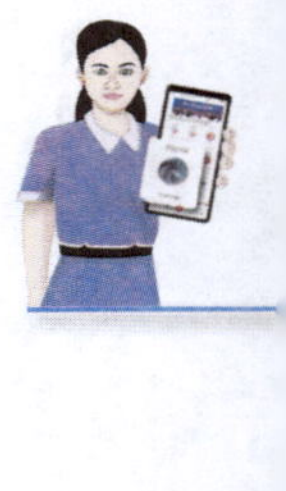

Table 11: Types of bones on the basis of shape

Category	Description with example
Long bones	These are shaped like rods or shaft with rounded end, e.g., humerus, radius, ulna, femur, tibia, fibula, etc.
Short bones	They do not have long axis, they are cubical, e.g., carpals, tarsals
Flat bones	They protect the underlying structure and provide surface area for muscle attachment, e.g., sternum, skull
Irregular bones	These bones are having various shapes, e.g., vertebral column, ear ossicles, facial bone, pelvic bone

REVIEW POINTS

- Osteoblasts vs osteoclasts vs osteocytes
  - Osteoblasts = stem cells that give rise to osteocytes = build bone.
  - Osteocytes = mature bone cells = reside in bones for housekeeping.
  - Osteoclasts = large cells that break down bone = cells that absorb old bone.
- Bones are classified as **long bones, short bones, flat bones and irregular bones.**
- Long bones include femur, tibia, fibula, radius, ulna, and humerus. They consist of a long, thin part called the **diaphysis, or shaft,** and two bulbous-type ends called the **epiphysis.**
- **Short bones are basically** cube-shaped as wide as they are long. For example, bones found in the wrist and ankle.
- **Flat bones** are thin and generally flat. Examples of flat bones are the cranial bones, which protect the brain, and the scapula (shoulder blade).
- **Irregular bones** include many of the bones that do not fall into the other three categories. They have complex shapes and include bones like the vertebrae.
- Bones are composed of **spongy and compact bone, periosteum and endosteum,** and a **medullary cavity.**
- The **periosteum** is a dense, white, fibrous sheath that covers the surface of the bone where muscles and tendons are attached.
- The **medullary** cavity of the bone is a cavity in the center of the bone filled with yellow, and fatty marrow.
- The **endosteum** is the layer of cells that lines the medullary cavity.
- The human skeleton consists of **206 bones** and is divided into two parts.
- **Joints** are classified as **immovable, slightly movable, or freely movable.**
- The **vertebral column**, or backbone of the human skeleton, is typically made up of **26 bones (33 bones if sacrum and coccyx are considered 5 and 4 respectively)**
- Cervical spine contains 7 smaller vertebrae.
- Thoracic spine consists of **12** midsized vertebrae.
- Lumbar spine consists of **5** large vertebrae.
- Sacrum, which is one bone made up of **5 fused sacral vertebrae.**
- The coccyx, or tailbone, is made up of **four vertebrae fused** into one or two bones.
- **Acetabulum:** Concave surface of the pelvis. It is socket of pelvis in which head of femur fits.
- **Acromion:** It is a bony process on the scapula (shoulder blade).
- **Knee cap:** Patella
- **Collar bone**: Clavicle
- **Example of Pivot Joint**: Proximal radioulnar joint, distal radioulnar joint, median atlanto-axial joint
- **Example of hinge joint**: Knee joint, elbow joint and ankle joint
- **Example of ball and socket joint:** Shoulder joint, hip joint
- **Example of gliding joint:** Wrist joint.
- **Coronal suture:** Unites the frontal bone with the parietal bones.
- **Sagittal suture:** Unites the 2 parietal bones in the midline.
- **Lambdoid suture:** Unites the parietal bones with the occipital bone.
- **Squamosal suture:** Unites the squamous portion of the temporal bone with the parietal bones.
- **Metopic suture:** (if present) Unites the 2 frontal bones
- **Tendons**: Tendons are tough bands of connective tissue found in the joints. **They connect muscles to bones.**
- **Ligaments**: Ligaments connect the bones to each other, and are designed to help stabilize the joints and provide a structure for the bones.

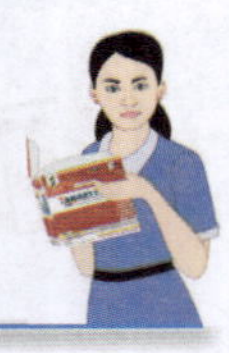

KEY POINTS

- **Largest bone:** Femur
- **Smallest bone:** Stapes (Bone in the middle ear)
- **Total number of ribs:** 12 pairs
- **Most mobile joint:** Ball and socket joint. For example, shoulder joint.
- **Least stable joint:** Ball and socket joint.
- **Smallest vertebra:** Cervical
- **Only movable bone of the skull:** Mandible bone
- **Most prominent cartilage of the larynx:** Thyroid cartilage

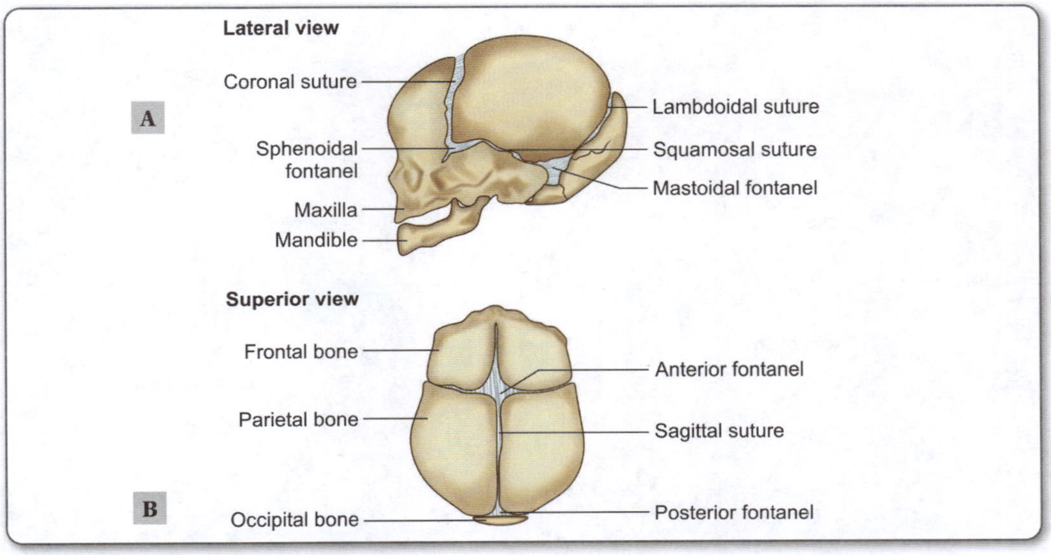

Figures 4A and B: (A) Lateral view of newborn skull; (B) Superior view of newborn skull

- Voluntary muscles = you can control = skeletal muscles, e.g., Biceps.
- Involuntary muscles = you cannot control = smooth (e.g., gut) and cardiac (heart) muscles.
- Total number of intercostals muscles = 11 pairs.
- **Site of intramuscular injection**
  - Infants below 18 months – Vastus lateralis muscle
  - Children – Deltoid, ventrogluteal, dorsogluteal (not recommended for <3 years), vastus lateralis muscle
  - Adult (>18 years) – Deltoid, ventrogluteal, dorsogluteal, vastus lateralis muscle
- **Anatomical terms of motion**
  - **Flexion and extension:** *Flexion* describes bending movement that *decreases* the angle between a segment and its proximal segment. *Extension* is the opposite of flexion.
  - **Abduction and adduction:** *Abduction* refers to a motion that pulls a structure or part *away from* the midline of the body. *Adduction* refers to a motion that pulls a structure or part *toward* the midline of the body.
  - **Elevation and depression:** The terms elevation and depression refer to movement above and below the horizontal.
  - **Rotation:** Internal rotation (or medial rotation) refers to rotation towards the axis of the body. External rotation (or lateral rotation) refers to rotation away from the center of the body.
  - **Pronation and supination:** Pronation and supination refer to rotation of the forearm or foot so that in the anatomical position, the palm or sole is facing anteriorly (supination) or posteriorly (pronation).
- Diaphragm is a dome-shaped muscular structure which separates the thoracic cavity and abdominal cavity. Diaphragm helps in respiration.

KEY POINTS

- **Total number of muscles – 639.**
- **Longest muscle – Sartorius**
- **Shortest muscle – Stapedius muscle**
- **Strongest muscle – Masseter (helps in mastication)**

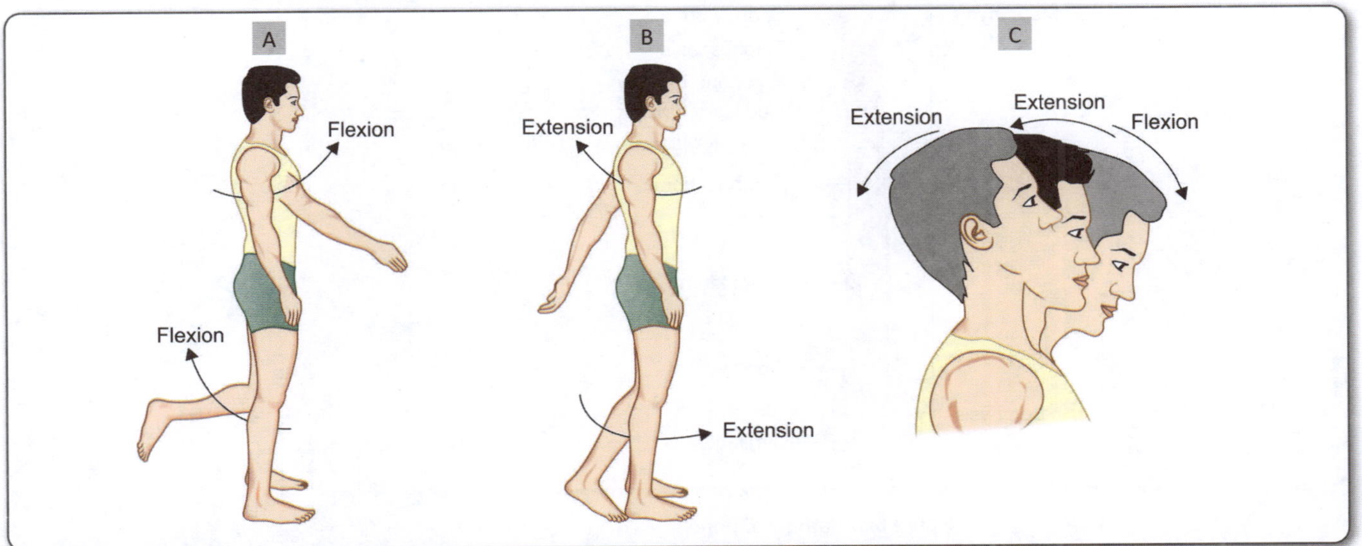

Figures 5A to C:

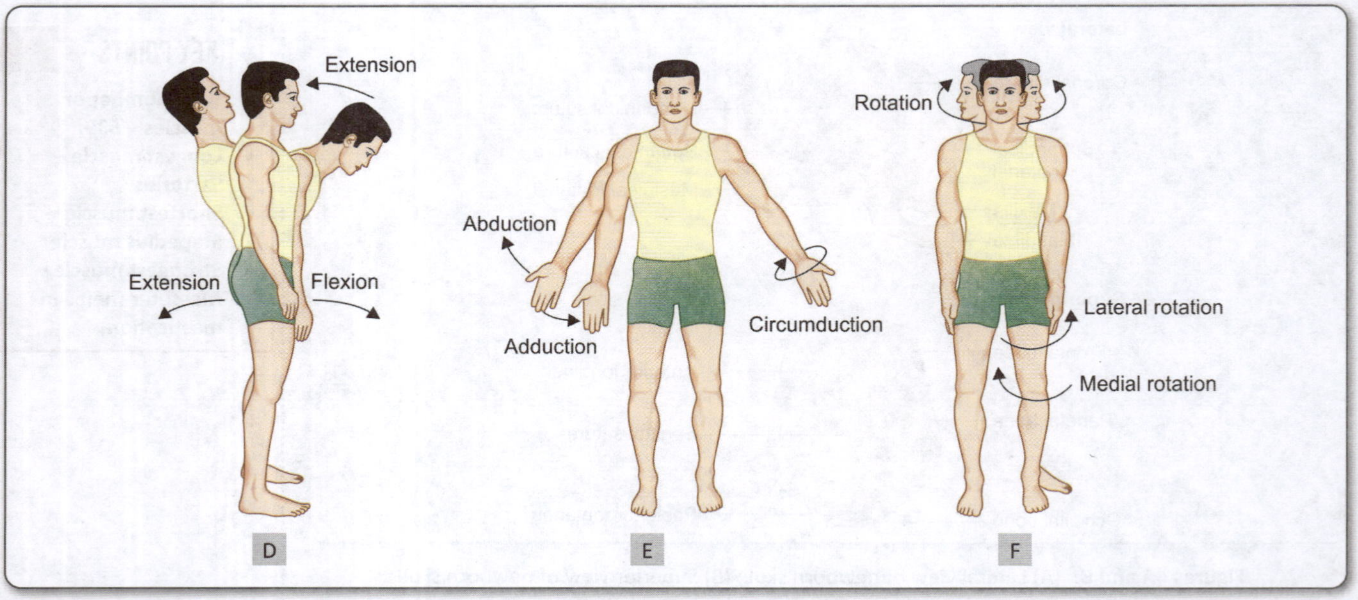

Figures 5A to F: Angular movements: (A and B) Flexion and extension at the shoulder and knees; (C) Extension and flexion of the head and neck; (D) Angular movements: Flexion and extension of the vertebral column; (E) Abduction, adduction and circumduction of the upper limb at the shoulder; (F) Rotation of the head, neck and lower limb

ANATOMY OF BONE

- Long bone has a shaft called diaphysis.
- Diaphysis is a hollow cylinder that covers the bone marrow.
- The two ends of long bones are called proximal and distal epiphyses
- In children, epiphyses are separated from diaphysis by epiphyseal plate.
- Epiphyseal plate or cartilage is the site for bone growth, once the bone growth is complete, this cartilage is replaced with bone and it will be joined to the diaphysis.
- Fracture to the epiphyseal cartilage results in retreated bone growth and limb shortening in children.
- Bone is covered with an outer layer known as periosteum, which has good blood and nerve supply.

KEY POINTS

- Both proximal and distal ends of bone are called epiphysis.
- Primary function of epiphysis is to connect adjacent bones to form joints.
- The epiphyseal plate is the area of growth in a long bone.

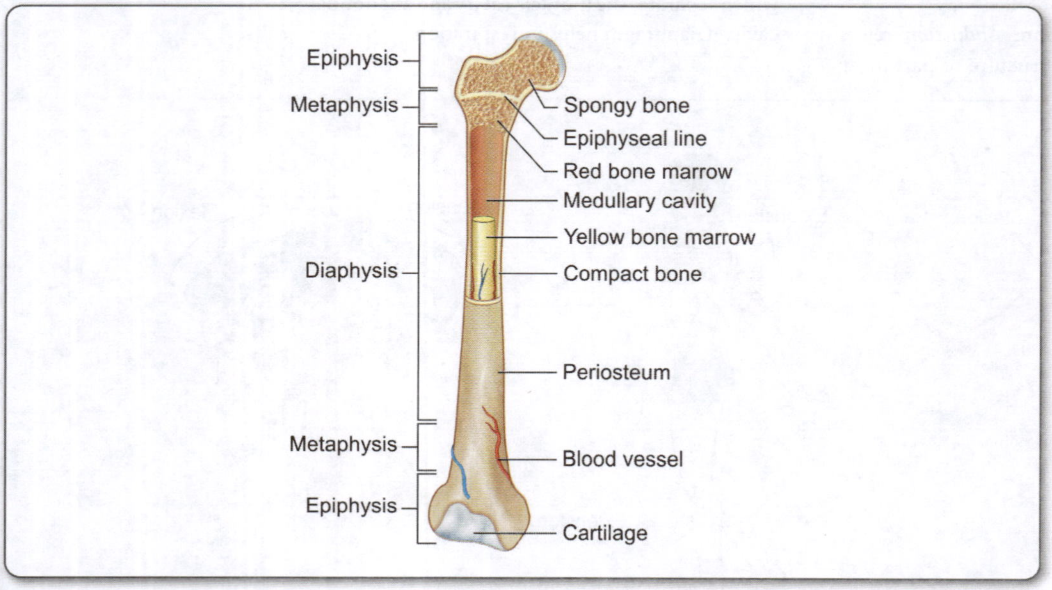

Figure 6: Anatomy of bone

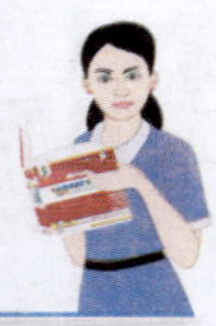

Microscopic Anatomy of Long Bone

- Fundamental functional unit of a compact bone is known as Haversian system or osteon.
- Haversian system contains vessels in the central part known as Haversian canal.
- Around the Haversian canal, there are concentric, circular layers called lamellae.
- Space between the lamellae is known as lacunae.
- Osteocytes are present in the lacunae.
- Canaliculi are small channels for blood vessels through which blood flows into the bone and back from the bone with nutrient and waste products.

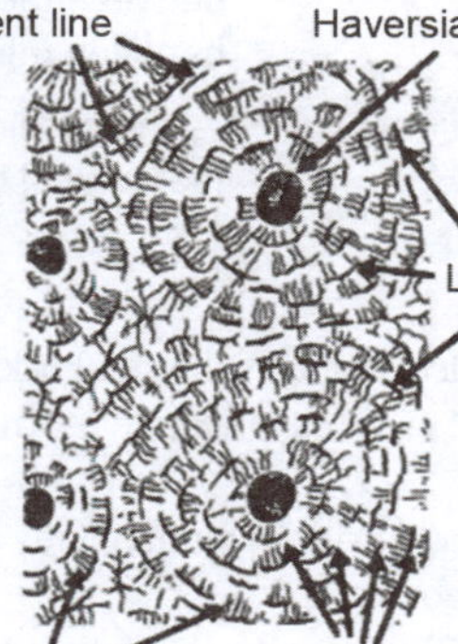

Figure 7: Microscopic anatomy of long bone

Composition of Bone

- Bone is made up of collagen and it provides strength to the bone; and inorganic salts like calcium and phosphate allow bone to withstand compression.
- Bone has three types of cells and these are osteoblast, osteocyte and osteoclast.
  - **Osteoblast:** Bone forming cells
  - **Osteocyte:** Mature form of osteoblast found in the bone matrix
  - **Osteoclast:** Bone removing cells.

KEY POINTS

- Periosteum is a dense layer of vascular connective tissue enveloping the bones except at the surfaces of the joints.
- Haversian canals are a series of microscopic tubes in the outermost region of bone called cortical bone.
- Spongy (cancellous) bone is lighter and less dense than compact bone.
- Flat bone, irregular shaped bone, short bone, and epiphysis of long bones contain mostly spongy bone.

TYPES OF JOINTS IN HUMAN BODY

Table 12: Types of joints in human body with their description and examples

Name of the joints	Description	Examples
Fibrous joints	These joints are linked with tough, fibrous material and they do not permit movement	Joints between the skull bones called sutures
Cartilaginous joints	These are connected entirely by cartilage (fibrocartilage or hyaline). These joints allow more movement between the bone than a fibrous joint but less than highly mobile synovial joint	• Between the manubrium and sternum • Between the vertebra • Symphysis pubis • Epiphyseal plates
Synovial joints	These are characterized by the presence of space or capsule between the articulating bones. The end of the bones are held together by fibrous tissue and capsule is lubricated with small amount of fluid called synovial fluid and it permits range of motion	
Types of Synovial Joints		
Ball and socket joints	The head of one bone is ball-shaped and articulates with a cup-shaped socket of another. The joint allows wide range of movement, including flexion, extension, adduction, abduction, rotation and circumduction	Hip joint, shoulder joint
Hinge joint	Articulating surface of bone forms an arrangement like hinge on a door and movement is restricted to flexion and extension	Elbow, knee, ankle, interphalangeal

Contd...

Name of the joints	Description	Examples
Gliding joint	Surface is flat or curved, gliding one over another, but the amount of movement is very restricted	Carpals and tarsal bone, intervertebral joint
Pivot joint	In this type of joint, one bone fits into a hoop-shaped ligament that holds it close to another bone and allows it to rotate in ring form	Head, radioulnar joint
Condyloid joint	Joint sits within a cup-shaped depression of another bone	Condylar process of mandible and temporal bone, between metacarpal and phalanges of hand, between metatarsals and phalanges of foot
Saddle joint	The articulating surface of bone fits together like a man sitting on a saddle	At the base of thumb, between trapezium and first metacarpal bone

VERTEBRAL COLUMN

- Vertebral column consists of 33 vertebrae, which are divided as follows:
  - Cervical -7
  - Thoracic-12
  - Lumbar-5
  - Sacral- 5 fused vertebral
  - Coccyx – 4 fused vertebrae
- Vertebrae are separated by disc except at first and second cervical, the sacrum and at the coccyx.
- C1 vertebra which supports the skull is known as atlas and the C2 vertebra which pivots the atlas is known as axis.
- There are 12 pairs of ribs in human body attached to thoracic vertebrae.
- First 7 pairs (1–7) - **true ribs** (Directly attached to sternum with costal cartilage)
- Ribs 8–12 - **False ribs** (costal cartilages are attached to the cartilage of the next higher rib)
- Last 2 pairs (11–12) - **Floating ribs** (Attached only to vertebrae. Do not attach to sternum)

KEY POINTS

- An injury to the joint ligament and joint capsule is termed **Sprain.**
- The largest synovial joint in the human body is **knee joint**.
- The average length of the vertebral column: Male - 71 cm; Female - 61 cm
- One sacrum consists of five fused vertebrae
- One Coccyx consists of four fused vertebrae

DIAGNOSTIC EVALUATION

Table 13: Commonly used diagnostic tests in orthopedic conditions

Name of the test	Description
Arthrography	• To find out joint pain or to assess the progression of a joint disease. • Contrast injected into the joint and then joint is put on range of motion exercises and series of X-rays are taken to find out the problem. • **Nursing Responsibility:** Assess the allergy toward contrast agent
Bone densitometry	• To assess the bone mineral density. • This study helps us to find out the risk or progression of osteoporosis.
Bone scan	• To find out or to assess the progression of a bone tumor or a degenerative disease. • Radio isotope is injected via IV route and scan is performed 2–3 hours later. • Increased uptake of isotope can be seen in bone diseases such as osteosarcoma, osteomyelitis and metastatic bone disease.
Arthroscopy	• Direct visualization of a joint through fibro optic endoscope. • This procedure is done under strict aseptic technique along with local or general anesthesia. • After the procedure, joint is covered with compression dressing to control bleeding. • **Joint is elevated to reduce swelling** • **Ice pack may be applied to enhance the comfort of the client**
Arthrocentesis	• This procedure is performed to remove excessive synovial fluid from the joint for examination • Anti-inflammatory medications may be injected into the joint • Informed consent needs to be obtained • Apply elastic compression dressing after the procedure

Contd...

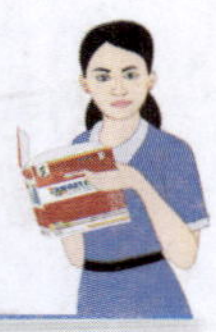

Name of the test	Description
Electromyography	• Electrical potential of muscles and nerves leading them, is studied • Needle electrodes are inserted into selected muscles and responses are recorded on an oscilloscope. • Contraindicated in patients receiving anticoagulants and in patients with active skin infection. • Patient has to be instructed not to use any cream or lotion on the day of test.
Biopsy	• Test is performed to assess the composition and structure of bone marrow, bone, muscles or synovium. • Analgesics need to be given and assess the biopsy site for edema, pain, and bleeding and hematoma formation is assessed.

DISORDERS OF MUSCULOSKELETAL SYSTEM

Fractures

- A **fracture** is defined as a complete or incomplete damage in the continuity of a ***bone***.
- A **traumatic fracture** is caused by some type of accident, fall, or other kind of force.
- A **pathologic fracture** is a broken bone caused by disease. For example, osteoporosis, bone cyst.

Types of Fracture

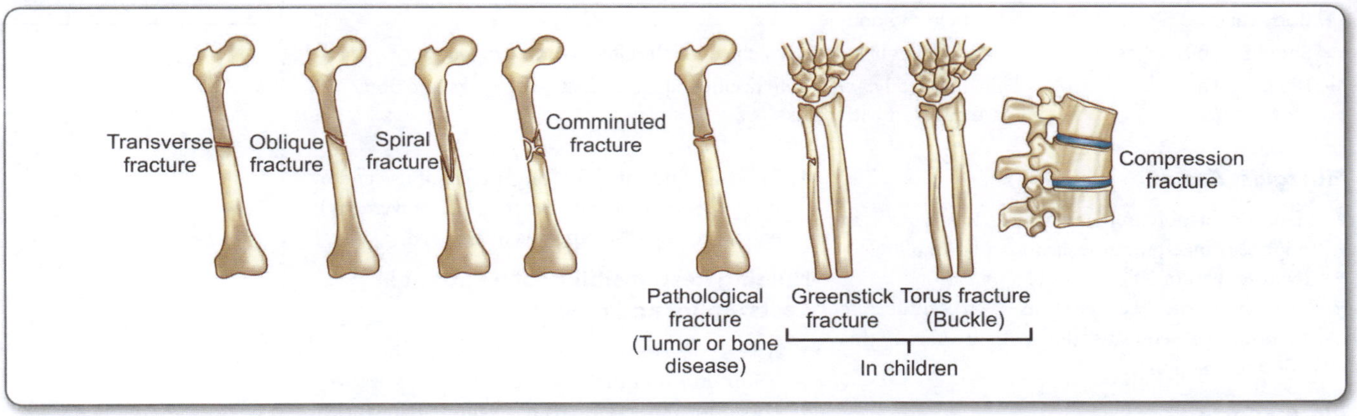

Figure 8: Types of fracture

- **Complete fracture:** Bone is broken completely into two separate parts
- **Incomplete fracture:** Bone is broken but doesn't completely break
- **Comminuted fracture:** Bone is broken into several small parts
- **Greenstick fracture:** One side of bone surface is broken and another is only bend (most commonly in children)
- **Simple fracture (closed):** Bone is broken under the skin and no change in skin texture/continuity
- **Compound fracture (open):** Bone is broken along with skin and sometimes bone comes out of skin

Clinical Findings

- Pain at fracture site
- **Crepitus sound when fractured limb is moved**
- Shortening of extremity
- Five Ps (pain, pulselessness, pallor, paresthesia, paralysis)

Key Nursing Interventions

- Assess for shock because there may be significant blood loss.
- Assess for signs of fat embolism (confusion, dyspnea, hypotension, tachycardia, tachypnea).
- Apply cold packs at fracture sites (it helps to decrease bleeding and edema).
- Notify the health care provider about any sign of **fat emboli, dyspnea, chest pain, decreased saturation and diaphoresis**
- **Provide diet high in protein, vitamin C to help in quick healing**
- **Diet with high calcium content is usually not indicated in prolonged bedridden patient because decalcification is already there and it can cause further calculi in renal.**
- Maintain hydration
- Isometric exercise
- **Positioning frequently or every 2 hours**
- Teach about three-point (non-weight bearing) and four-point gait (weight bearing)

KEY POINTS

- **Colles' fracture** refers to the fracture of Radius. It is a type of fracture of the distal forearm.
- Colles' fracture is commonly described as a **dinner fork deformity.**
- **Monteggia fracture** is a fracture of the proximal third of the ulna with dislocation of the radius.
- Tripod fracture is seen in Zygomatic bone.
- Provide a **diet high in protein and vitamin C** to the patient with fracture.

Stages of Bone Healing

- **Inflammatory phase** (48 hours after the injury); hematoma is formed
- **Repairing phase** (lasts for 2–3 weeks); develops new tissue and cartilage known as callus
- **Bone remodeling**; also called final phase, solid bone replaces spongy bone

Casts

Care of Patient with Casts

- Casts are rigid immobilizing agents applied externally to a body part to immobilize that part.
- They are used following the fracture to immobilize that part.

Table 14: Types of casts

Types of casts	Description
• Short arm casts	Cast is extending from below the elbow to palmar crease and is secured around the thumb
• Thumb spica or gauntlet cast	Cast extends from below the elbow and covers thumb
• Long arm casts	Extending from axilla to palmar crease, elbow is immobilized at right angle.
• Short leg casts	Extending below knee to base of toe
• Long leg casts	Tending from the junction of thigh to the base of toe
• Walking casts	Short or long leg casts reinforced for strength
• Body casts	Encircle the body
• Shoulder spica casts	Body jacket like casts which cover shoulder, trunk and elbow
• Hip spica casts	Encircle body and leg. In double hip spica casts, both legs and body are covered with casts.

Fiberglass Casts

- Made up of polyurethane resins. It is lighter in weight, stronger, water resistant and durable.
- It will set within 30 minutes of application
- Application of this cast causes an exothermic reaction. So, educate the patient about this expected reaction.

Plaster Casts

- It is made up of plaster of paris
- Less costly, heavy, not water resistant and can take up to 24–72 hours to set
- Application of plaster is an exothermic reaction
- A freshly applied cast should be exposed to air and supported on a firm surface
- Elevation of the applied part is needed to reduce the swelling.

Splint

- Splint is used to support and immobilize a body part in functional position.
- It is easy to apply and does not cover the entire part so circulation is not compromised.
- It can be easily removed so visualization of injured part can be easily done.
- Protect the open wound with sterile dressing before splinting.

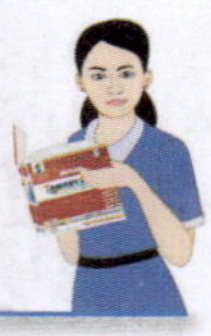

Braces

- Used to support, control movement and to prevent additional injury.
- These are indicated for longer term of use and by using braces deformity is corrected, movement is enhanced and discomfort is minimized.

Nursing Responsibility of a Patient in Casts, Splint and Braces

- Assess the neurovascular status of the client before and after the procedure
- Look for five Ps (pain, pallor, paresthesia, pulselessness and paralysis)
- In the first 24–48 hours after the application, make sure that extremity is above the level of heart to decrease edema
- Monitor for complications such as compartment syndrome, pressure ulcer, disuse syndrome.

Compartment Syndrome

- Increased pressure in a particular area compromises the circulation and decreases the tissue perfusion. It will lead to ischemia and irreversible neuromuscular damage.
- Manifestations: Dusky pale appearance of the extremity, cool skin, increased capillary refill time, paresthesia and unrelieved pain.
- If the casts, splint or braces are tight, loosen them or remove them.
- Fasciotomy can be done to relieve pressure within the compartment.

Pressure Ulcer

- Inappropriately applied casts can cause pressure on tissue leading to tissue hypoxia.

KEY POINTS

- Diet with high calcium content is usually **not indicated** to prolonged bedridden patient with fracture.
- Handle the cast with palm not with finger as it could cause **pressure area** within the cast.
- Cast should **not be covered** until it is dry. Use fan to circulate air.
- Elevate the casted limb on pillow but not amputated limb as it creates **contracture**.

- Pressure necrosis happens when the patient reports hot spot and tightness under the casts.
- To assess the area, physician may remove or cut an area (window) in the casts.

Disuse Syndrome

- Immobilization of a part leads to muscle atrophy and loss of strength.
- To prevent this, nurse must educate the client to tense and contract muscles without moving bones
- Isometric exercises help to prevent this complication.

Patient with External Fixator

- External fixator is used to treat complex open fracture with soft tissue damage.
- In external fixator, pins are inserted into the bones and these pins are attached to an external metal apparatus to provide proper alignment
- Immediate fracture stabilization, minimal blood loss as compared to internal fixation, improved wound care, increased patient comfort are the advantages of external fixator.
- Most common complication associated with external fixator is pin site infection.

Pain around the pin site, warmth, redness, swelling, purulent discharge indicate pin site infection which can develop as osteomyelitis.

KEY POINTS

- Prevent the cast from any kind of damage until it dries.
- Never let the wet cast to rest on a flat surface because it causes pressure within the cast.
- Check and compare the pulse on both sides of body; it should be equal.
- **Perform blanching (capillary refill) test**
- Educate the patient to notify the health-care provider if any sign of infection is present **(increased temperature, foul smell from cast)**

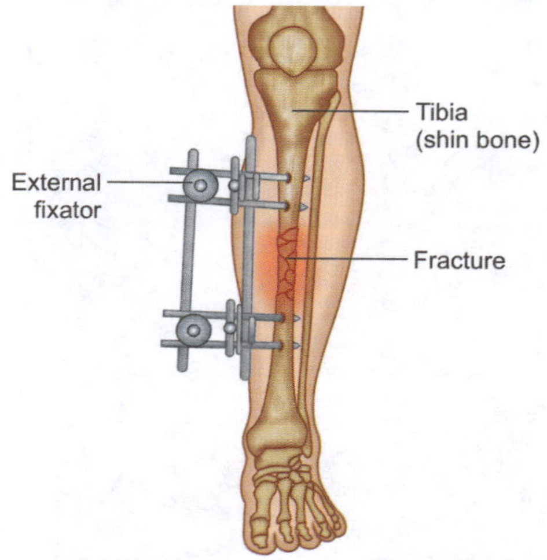

Figure 9: External fixation

Traction

- Traction uses pulling force to align injured body part.
- **Purposes**
  - To eliminate muscles spasm
  - To relieve pressure on nerve
  - To prevent further deformities
  - To regain normal alignment of bone

Table 15: Description of different types of traction

Types of traction	Description
Straight and running traction (For example: Buck's extension traction)	Traction in straight line with body part resting on the bed. Counter traction is provided by patient's weight
Balanced suspension traction	It supports the affected extremity off the bed and allows some movements. Counter traction is given by slings or splints
Skin traction For example: • Buck traction for lower extremity • Chin Halter Strap for neck pain • Pelvic belt (lower back pain) • Hamilton Russell traction (femur) • Bryant's traction (femur) • Dunlop's traction (upper arm, recommended for not more than 20 minutes)	**Traction is applied to the skin.** **Weight for traction used on** • **Extremity – 2 to 3.5 kg** • **Pelvis – 4.5 to 9 kg**
Skeletal traction For example: Halo traction (skull traction)	**Weight is put on** pins/wires/screws which are attached surgically to the **bone.** Most commonly used for femur. (e.g., Thomas Splint with Pearson attachment) Preferred when continuous traction is needed.

Care after traction:

- **T–** Temperature may be from infection or fractured extremities
- **R–** Rope of traction should be hanged freely
- **A–** Alignment should be maintained (counter traction needed)
- **C–** Circulation should be checked with 5 Ps (pain, pallor, paresthesia, pulselessness and paralysis)
- **T–** Type and location of fracture
- **I–** Increase fluid intake
- **O–** Overhead trapeze use
- **N–** Never touch the weight to bed as well as to floor

The tractions used in different types of fractures have been shown in the following figure.

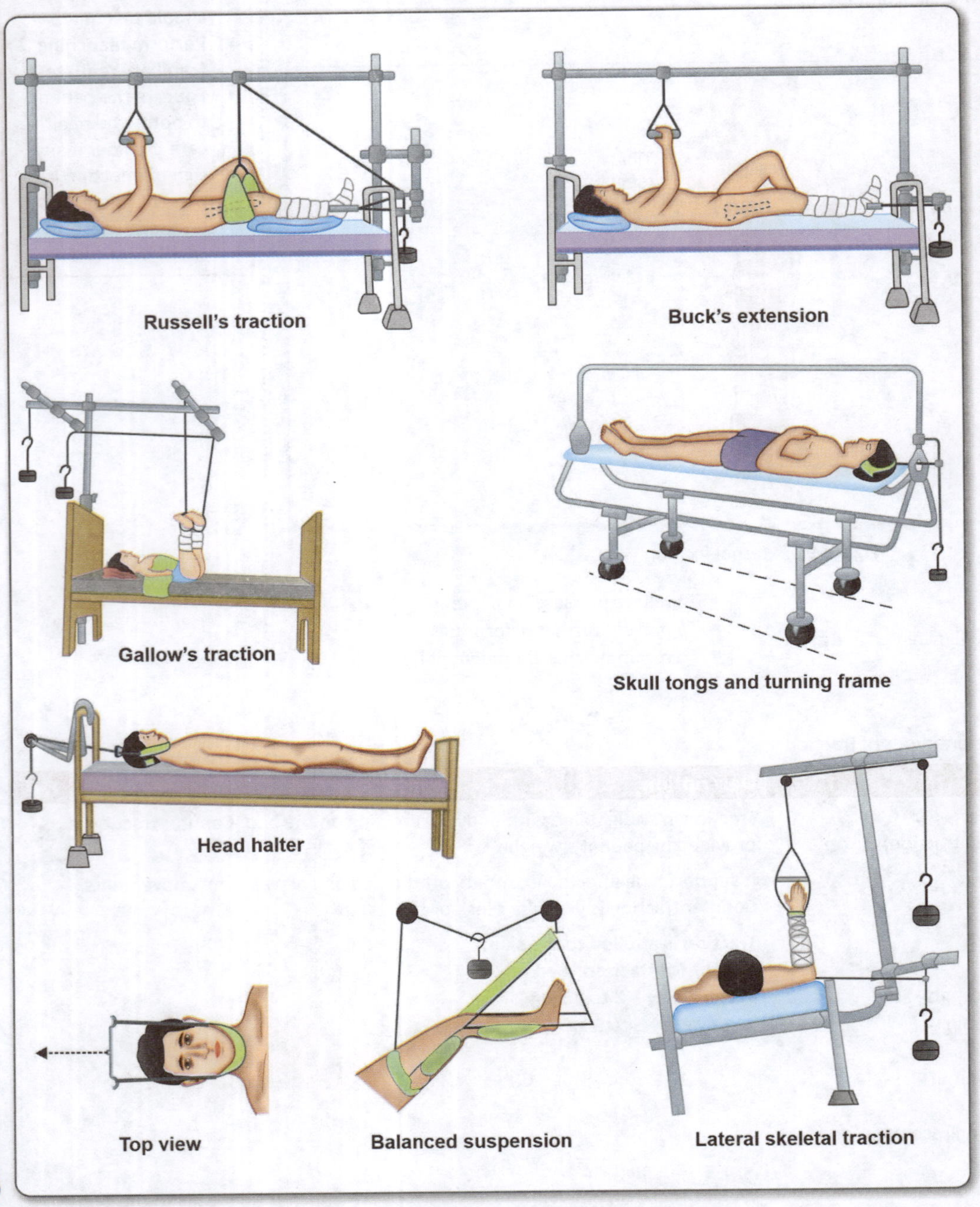

Figure 10: Types of traction

KEY POINTS

- **In a client with traction,** neurovascular assessment is the priority nursing intervention
- **In a client with skin traction,** dorsiflexion of the foot indicates functioning of peroneal nerve; plantarflexion of the foot indicates functioning of the tibial nerve
- **In a client with skeletal traction,** nurse should not remove weight from the traction unless a life threatening emergency.
- **Buck's skin traction** is used to treat knee injuries.
- **Gallows/Bryant's traction** is used in the fracture of shaft of femur.
- **Russel's traction** is used in trochanteric fracture.

ORTHOPEDIC SURGERIES

- **Open Reduction with Internal Fixation (ORIF):** It is a surgical procedure to fix a bone using surgical plates, screws, nails, or pins
- **Closed Reduction with Internal Fixation (CRIF):** It is reduction without any open surgery, followed by internal fixation.

Joint Replacement

Total Knee Replacement (TKR) or Total Knee Arthroplasty

- **Indications**
  - Osteoarthritis, Rheumatoid arthritis or Trauma (fracture of surrounding bones)
  - Best age for TKR: 50 to 80 years
- **Common complication**
  - Pain and swelling of legs
  - Chest pain and sudden breathlessness (risk of fat embolism)
- **Nursing management**
  - Compression bandage postoperatively
  - Ice or cold packs over the affected knee to arrest edema and bleeding

Total Hip Replacement (THR) or Total Hip Arthroplasty

- Replacement of severely damaged hip joint with prosthesis (artificial joint)
- **Indications**
  - Osteoarthritis, Rheumatoid arthritis, Femoral neck fracture
- Points to remember for care of Patient with Posterior or Posteriolateral approach for THR
- **Don'ts**
  - Do not cross operated legs past the midline
  - Do not sit with crossed legs
  - Do not sit in low height chair
  - Avoid hip flexion more than 90°
  - Patient should not turn to the operative side

> **KEY POINTS**
>
> **Positions after Hip Surgery:**
> - Patient should sleep on his/her back with a pillow between knees after Hip replacement surgery.
> - Patient should always sit on a high chair.
> - Avoid crossing legs
> - Avoid hip flexion more than 90°

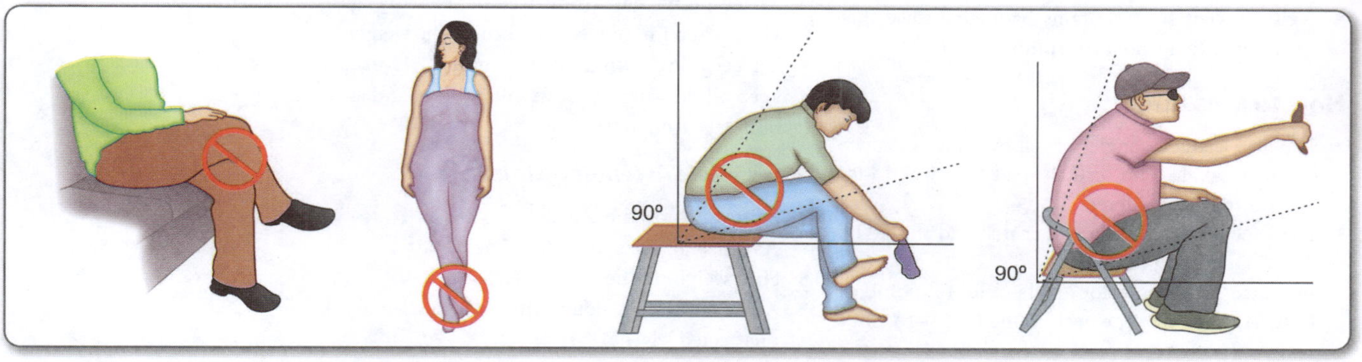

Figure 11: Don'ts for the patient with total hip replacement

- **Do's**
  - Use high toilet
  - Use pillow between legs while sleeping (abduction pillow)
  - Use long device to grab the things instead of bending past 90°
  - Always sit on high chair with comfort/padded arms (hip should be higher than knee while seated)
  - Promote use of trapeze (horizontal bar hung by ropes)
  - Use antiembolic stocking to prevent DVT
  - Maintain alignment of fractured leg

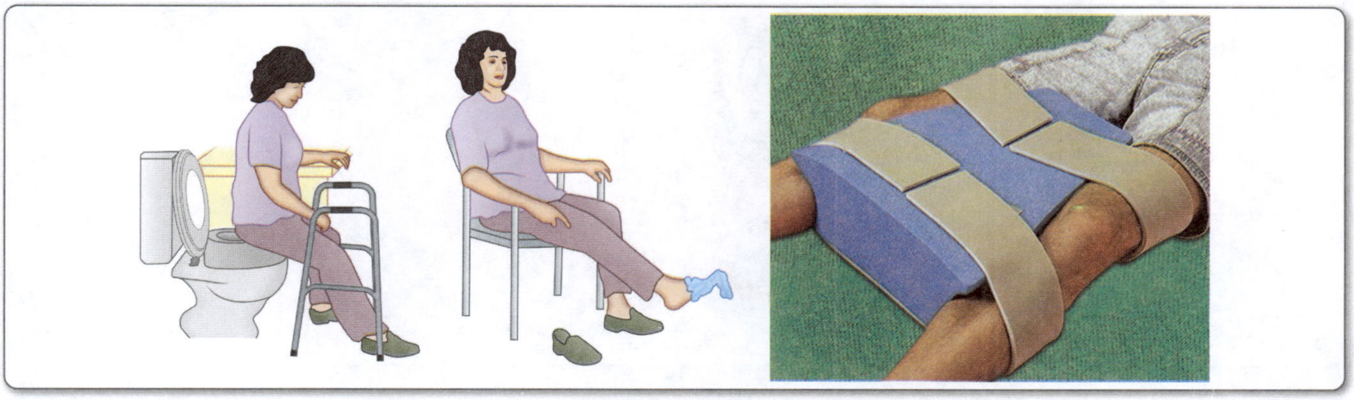

Figure 12: Do's for the patient with total hip replacement

- **Signs and symptoms of hip prosthesis dislocation**
    - Shortening of the affected limb
    - Abnormal internal or external rotation of the affected limb
    - Intense pain, swelling and immobilization of affected hip
    - Popping (sound) sensation in hip

CRUTCHES

- **Temporary crutch:** Used when ligament of knee is damaged
- **Permanent crutch:** Used in paralysis of the lower extremities
- One crutch can bear 80% and two can bear 100% of body weight.

Types

- **Forearm crutch:** It contains metal band and hand grip which fits around forearm
- **Axillary crutch:** It contains padded surface that fits in the axilla **(most commonly used)**

How to Measure

- Patient's height, angle of elbow and distance between axilla and crutch pad are important aspects to be considered
- Distance between axilla and crutch pad should be **2–4 finger** width **(4–5 cm)**
- Distance from anterior axilla fold to point of crutch or lateral to the heel should be **15–16 cm.**

Points to be Considered

- Never put whole body weight on axilla because it damages brachial plexus that can cause paralysis of arm **(crutch palsy).**
- Always support weight by the help of flexed elbow **(flexion angle should be 25–30° and verify with the help of Goniometer)**.
- Wear flat shoes to provide a good base of support.
- Exercise to strengthen upper arm, triceps and elbow is important
- For wide base of support, tripod position along with erect vertebra, neck and head is very important.
- Don't look down while crutch walking.
- **Hunching shoulder** if patient uses too long crutch and **stooping shoulder** if uses too short crutch

Crutch Walking (GAIT)

Types

- **Four-point gait (weight bearing gait):** Most commonly used when both legs are in a weakened condition.
- **Three-point gait (non-weight bearing gait):** Used when injured legs can bear some weight.
- **Three-point swing through gait:** It is used to keep all pressure off from injured legs and swing both legs trough.

Steps While Ascending Stairs

- Shift weight to the crutches
- Advance unaffected leg up to next stair
- Shift weight to the unaffected leg
- Advance crutch along with affected leg to the unaffected leg (next stair)

KEY POINTS

- Nurse should stand on the affected side while ambulating the client
- **Swing-to-gait:** The patient will move both crutches forward and then swing both legs forward, **to the point of crutches.**
- **Swing-through-gait:** The patient will move both crutches forward and then swing both legs forward, **past the crutches.**

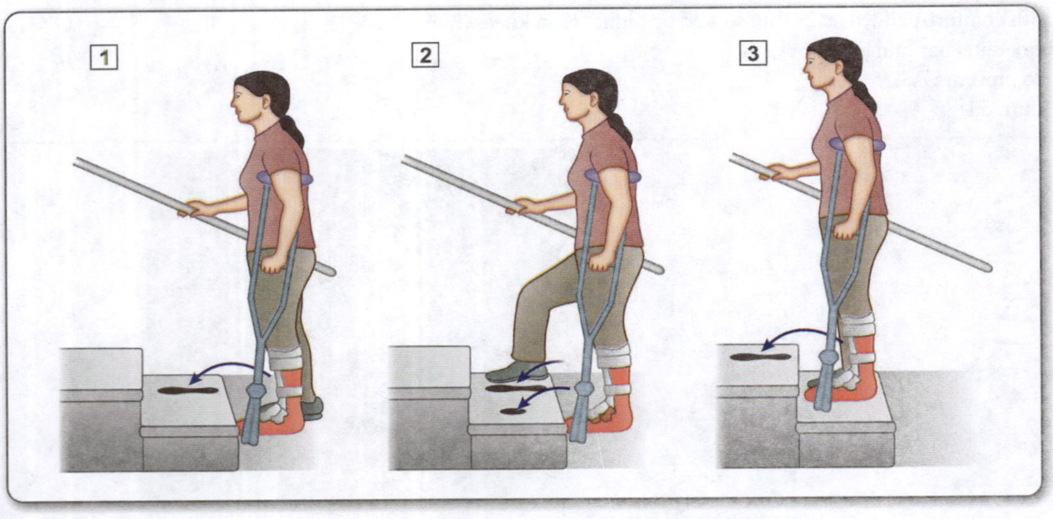

Figure 13: Steps while ascending stairs—Crutch walking

Steps While Descending Stairs

- Shift weight to unaffected leg
- Advance affected leg along with crutch down the stair
- Shift weight to the crutch
- Advance unaffected leg down to the stair

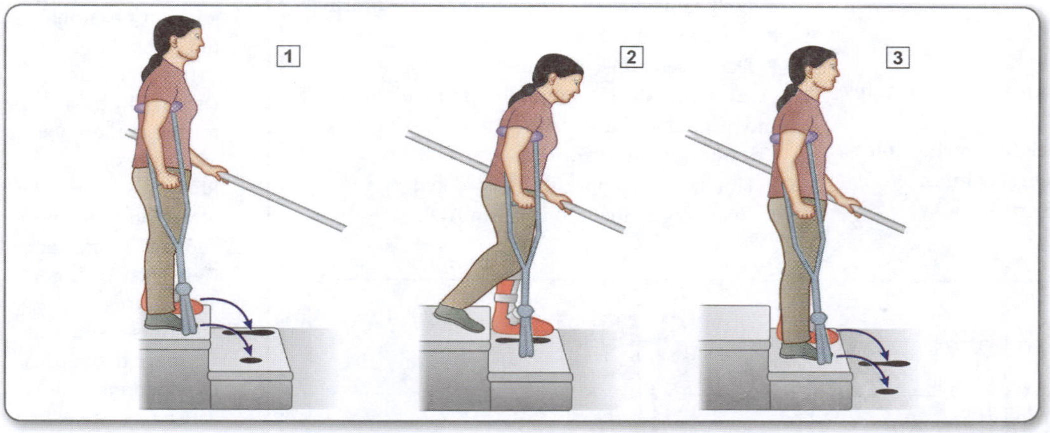

Figure 14: Steps while descending stairs - Crutch walking

Sitting in Chair with Crutches

- Position the posterior surface of the unaffected leg against the front of the chair
- Move the crutches in hand of affected side
- Hold the arm of the chair with the unaffected hand
- Flex the unaffected leg and lower into chair
- Keep the affected leg straight in front of the chair
- Patient who wants to stand, reverse the steps and walk

GOUT

- Gout is an inflammatory arthritis caused by deposition of uric acid crystals in joint
- **Causes of primary gout include:**
  - Reduced excretion of uric acid by kidney
  - Abnormality with purine metabolism
  - Over production of uric acid
  - Starvation
  - Consumption of seafood, red meat and organ meats
  - More consumption of beer.
- Reasons for secondary gout
  - Some medications such as cyclosporine and thiazide diuretics
  - Hypertension
  - Diabetes mellitus
  - Leukopenia
  - Polycythemia
  - Myeloma
  - Truncal obesity
  - High cholesterol
  - Renal disease
- **Clinical manifestation**
  - Acutely painful joints with swelling and redness
  - Commonly affects great toe, mid foot and ankle
- **Diagnosis**
  - Increased serum uric acid level
  - Elevated WBC count
  - Needle aspiration of synovial fluid shows needle like intracellular crystals.
- **Treatment**
  - Nonsteroidal anti-inflammatory drug (NSAID) (indomethacin)
  - **Allopurinol is the drug of choice to treat gout**
  - Other drugs include sulfinpyrazone and probenecid
  - **Dietary restrictions: Avoid alcohol, limited intake of purine-rich foods (liver and sardines), increase intake of fluid**
  - Corticosteroid may be used
  - **Colchicine is used to stop acute attacks.**
- **Key nursing interventions:**
  - Bed rest; pain relief; comfort measures
  - Dietary restrictions
  - Family teaching.

TENDINITIS

- **Tendinitis (also tendonitis), means inflammation of a tendon. It affects tendon and tendon muscle attachments.**
- **Achilles' tendon, hip, elbow, knee and shoulder rotator cuff are the most commonly affected parts.**
- **Causes:** Hypermobility in calcific tendinitis, abnormal body development, postural malalignment and trauma.

BURSITIS

- Bursitis is a painful inflammation of a bursa.
- Commonly affected parts are subdeltoid, olecranon, trochanteric, and subacromial bursae.

POINT TO REMEMBER

If both lower limbs are paralyzed and supported with braces, then hold the crutches in hand of patient's stronger side.

KEY POINTS

- Gout most classically affects the joint in the base of the big toe.
- Allopurinol is a drug of choice to treat chronic gout or prevent gout.
- Colchicine is used to treat acute gout attack.

POINT TO REMEMBER

Incidence of primary gout is more among men than in women.

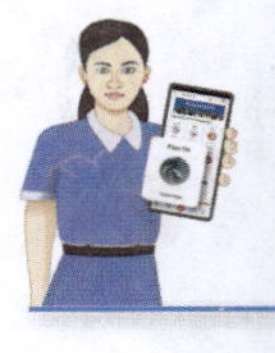

- **Types:** Acute, chronic, septic, calcific
- **Signs and symptoms:** Pain on palpation of affected area, warmth and restricted movement
- **Treatment:** Rest and symptomatic treatment. NSAID for pain and antibiotics for infection.

OSTEOARTHRITIS

- Osteoarthritis is a non-inflammatory degenerative joint disease
- **Most commonly affects weight bearing joints, e.g., Hip, Knee, Lower vertebral column**
- **Most common form of arthritis**
- Associated with aging and obesity
- **Signs and symptoms**
  - **Presence Heberden's nodes or Bouchard's nodes**
  - Joint stiffness and soreness of the joint
  - Dull pain which increases with weight bearing
  - Rest may relieve pain
  - Decreased range of motion
- **Treatment:** NSAID, salicylates, muscle relaxants and intra-articular steroids.
- **Key nursing interventions**
  - Hot or cold compression as ordered
  - Encourage patient to perform ADL

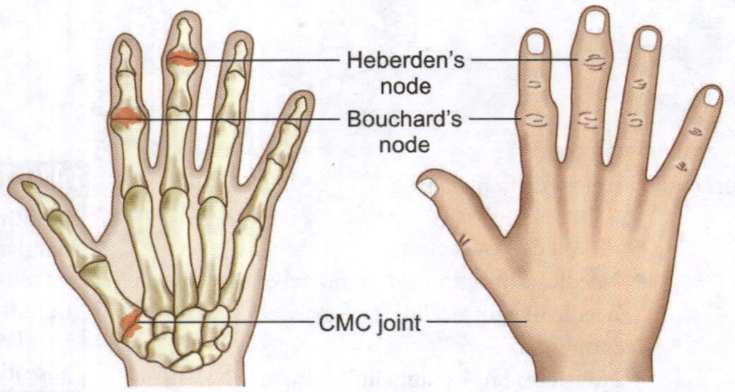

Figure 15: Heberden's nodes or Bouchard's nodes

RHEUMATOID ARTHRITIS

- Rheumatoid arthritis is an inflammatory condition affecting connective tissue and synovial membrane of the joint
- **Manifestations:** Tenderness, stiffness of the joint (morning stiffness lasting for 30 mins), and decreased Range of Motion
- **Rheumatoid arthritis is the most common cause of Swan Neck Deformity** of fingers
- **Diagnosis:** Elevated ESR and Rheumatoid factor
- **Medical Management:** NSAIDs, Antirheumatic drugs (e.g., Methotrexate, Hydroxychloroquine, Sulfasalazine), Glucocorticoids.
- **Surgical Management:** Synovectomy, arthrodesis and joint replacement

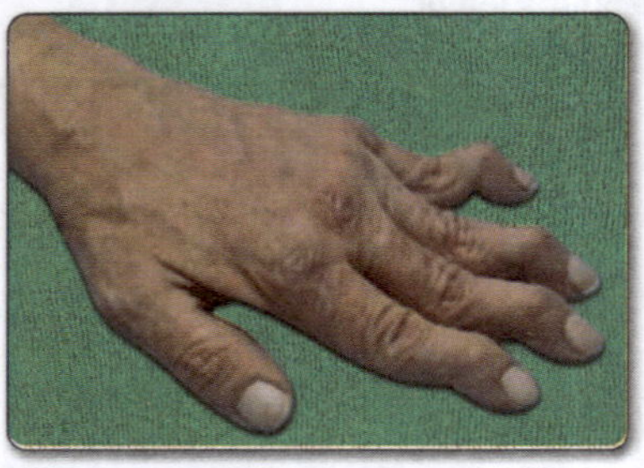

Figure 16: Swan neck deformity

OSTEOMYELITIS

- Osteomyelitis is the infection and inflammation of bone and bone marrow.
- It can occur because of direct bone injury (gunshot wound, bone surgery), through hematogenous route from other site of infection.
- **More than 50% of infections are caused by *Staphylococcus aureus.***
- *Other infections include pseudomonas, enterococci and streptococci.*
- **Management**
  - Antibiotic therapy
  - Surgical debridement of bone.
- **Key nursing interventions**
  - Relieving pain
  - Improve physical mobility
  - Control infectious process
  - Patient teaching regarding mobility and exercise.

OSTEOPOROSIS

- Osteoporosis is defined as decreased bone mass and bone density. Bone becomes weak and brittle.
- **Osteoporosis is the most prevalent bone disease in the world.**

KEY POINTS

- Osteoarthritis most commonly affects weight-bearing joints, for example, hip, knee, lower vertebral column.
- Osteoarthritis is most common type of arthritis.
- Rheumatoid arthritis is the most common cause of **Swan Neck Deformity** of fingers.
- Staphylococcus aureus is responsible for more than 50% of infections that cause osteomyelitis.

Practice Question

7. Osteoarthritis in spine may possibly lead to:

a. Damages to the cartilage
b. Damages to the joints in the spine
c. Both a and b
d. None of the above

Ans. (c) Both a and b

- The condition is a result of imbalance between bone resorption and bone formation.
- It increases the risk of fracture.
- **Usual onset of age is 30 years. Rapid progression is seen in postmenopausal women.**
- **Etiological factors include:**
  - Menopause
  - Prolonged use of corticosteroids
  - Deficiency of vitamin D and calcium
  - Smoking and alcohol
- **Clinical manifestation:**
  - Tingling and numbness
  - Lower backache
  - Kyphosis
- **Treatment:**
  - Calcium intake is increased to 1,500 mg/day
  - Hormone replacement therapy (estrogen and progesterone)
  - Calcitonin and biphosphonates to prevent bone resorption.
- **Key nursing interventions:**
  - Teach about dietary sources of calcium (Milk, yogurt, cheese, seafood, legumes, etc.)
  - Encourage modification of lifestyle (avoid smoking and alcohol; increase mobility, etc.)

OSTEOMALACIA

- Softening of the bone due to impaired bone metabolism. It is primarily due to inadequate calcium, phosphate, and vitamin D or because of resorption of calcium
- The bones are **porous and brittle in osteoporosis**, whereas in **osteomalacia** the bones are soft
- **Management:** Vitamin D and Calcium supplements, exposure to sunlight

PAGET'S DISEASE

- Paget's disease is a disorder of bone remodeling process.
- Body absorbs old bones and forms abnormal new bone.
- Paget's disease of bone most commonly occurs in the pelvis, skull and legs.

RHABDOMYOLYSIS

- Rhabdomyolysis refers to the breakdown of the muscle tissue due to muscle trauma which may result in myoglobinuria (presence of myoglobin in urine). Accumulated myoglobin may even lead to renal failure if left untreated.
- **Signs and symptoms:** Muscle weakness, tenderness and swelling. Dark, reddish brown urine.
- **Treatment**
  - IV crystalloids to increase GFR.
  - Diuretics and or dialysis may be required
  - If compartment syndrome develops, immediate fasciotomy and debridement may be necessary.

SPINAL COLUMN DEFORMITIES

Scoliosis: Lateral curvature of the spine
Kyphosis: Outward curvature of thoracic spine. It is also known as **humpback** or **Dowager's hump.**
Lordosis: Inward curvature of the lumbar spine. Seen in pregnant women and obese persons.

Practice Questions

8. Which of the following age groups is most commonly affected by Paget's disease?
a. Children under age 12
b. Adolescents
c. Adults under 30
d. Adults over 45

Ans. (a) Children under age 12

9. Often, the symptoms of Paget's disease are confused with:
a. Arthritis
b. Hypocalcemia
c. Wilson's disease
d. Bone cysts

Ans. (a) Arthritis

10. An abnormal increase in the thoracic curvature of the vertebral column is called:
a. Spondylosis
b. Lordosis
c. Kyphosis
d. Paget's disease

Ans. (c) Kyphosis

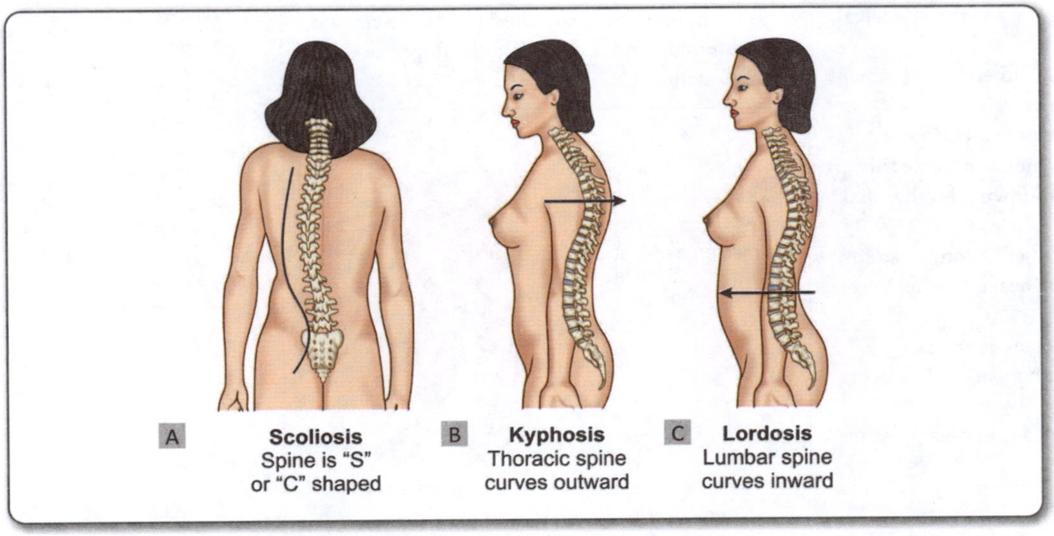

Figures 17A to C: **A.** Scoliosis; **B.** Kyphosis; **C.** Lordosis

PROLAPSED INTERVERTEBRAL DISK

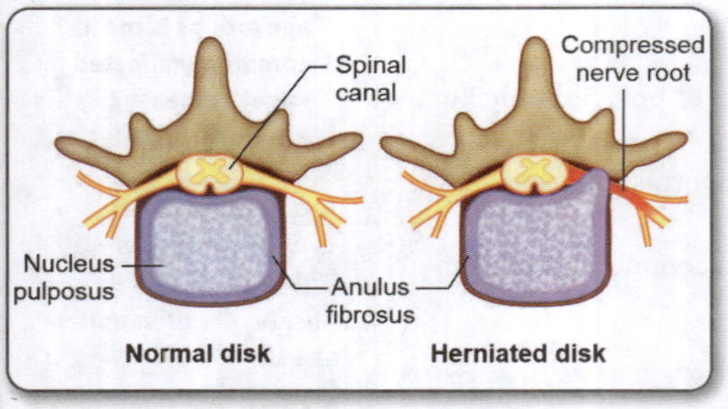

Figure 18: Top views of vertebrae showing herniated disk

- Nucleus of the disk protrudes into the annulus and causes nerve compression.
- **Manifestation**
  - Numbness, pain or tingling in one or both arms or legs
  - Pain behind the shoulder blades or in the buttocks
  - In severe cases - Loss of bladder and/or bowel control, numbness in the genital area, and impotence (in men)
  - Location of symptoms depends on location of prolapse
- **Management**
  - Bed rest, maintain head and spine in alignment
  - Avoid prolonged sitting, avoid flexion, extension and rotation of the joint
  - Cervical collar
  - Analgesics, anti-inflammatory and sedatives
  - Exercises regimen to strengthen the muscles
  - Surgery if conservative treatment fails
- **Client is advised to sleep on one side with hip and knee flexed and a pillow between legs**
- **Postoperative Monitoring Following Cervical Disc Surgery**
  - **Assess respiratory status and encourage deep breathing and coughing exercises**
  - **Look for laryngeal nerve damage: Hoarseness of voice and inability to cough indicate this.**
- **Postoperative monitoring following lumbar disk surgery**
  - **Assess movement, sensation, color, temperature and paraesthesia in the lower extremities.**
  - **Assess bowel and bladder movements.**
  - **Client has to be in supine position following surgery**
  - **Avoid prolonged sitting as it causes pressure in the surgical site**

AMPUTATION OF THE LOWER EXTREMITY

- Removal of a limb or part of limb is known as amputation.
- **Complications:** Bleeding, infection, ghost pain (phantom limb pain), flexion contracture
- **Phantom limb pain (ghost pain):** Pain experienced by the patient following amputation from the part of limb that is no longer existing. The pain experienced is real.
- **Nursing Management**
  - Prone position may be recommended following amputation
  - Stump should not be elevated on a pillow because it can lead to flexion contracture. If physician recommended, then the foot end of the bed can be elevated.
  - **Above knee amputation:** Prevent the external rotation of stump by using sand bag.
  - **Below knee amputation:** Discourage prolonged sitting and hanging the stump while sitting
  - Reinforce surgical dressing and elastic compression dressing which shrink the stump, reduce edema and prepare the stump for prosthesis.

POTT'S DISEASE

- TB of the spine which can cause kyphosis and paraplegia
- Anti-tubercular drugs are the treatment of choice.

CARPEL TUNNEL SYNDROME

- Compression of the median nerve causes this condition
- Pain, numbness, paresthesia and weakness over thumb, index and middle finger are the manifestations.

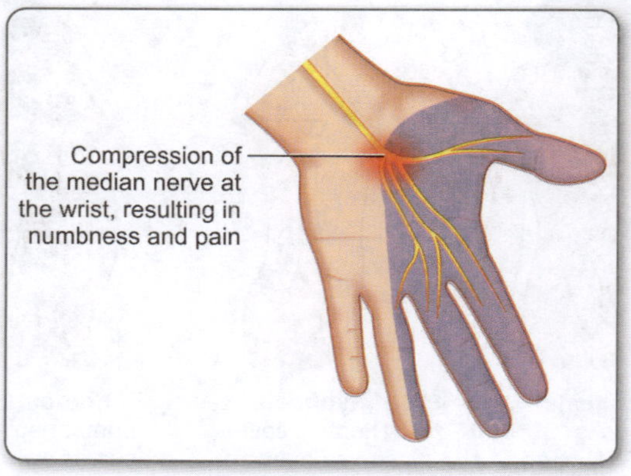

Figure 19: Carpel tunnel syndrome

KEY POINTS

- C5-C6 and C6-C7 are the most common sites for cervical vertebrae prolapse
- L4-L5 and L5-S1 are the most common sites for lumbar vertebrae prolapse.

Recent Question (NORCET 2020)

6. Amputation that includes all levels of thigh amputations from the hip to the knee joint is known as:

a. Transfemoral amputations
b. Transtibial amputations
c. Lower limb amputation
d. Hip Disarticulation Amputation

Ans. (a) Transfemoral amputations

DISORDERS OF LOWER LIMB

Table 16: Disorders of lower limb

Conditions with their description					
Genu-valgum (Knock-knee) Both knees are touching each other when the leg is straightened.	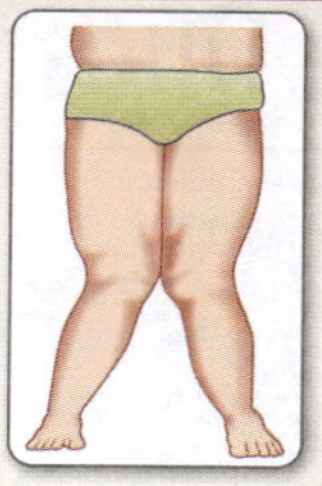	**Genu-varum (Bowlegged)** Angular deformity of proximal tibia in which child appears bow legged	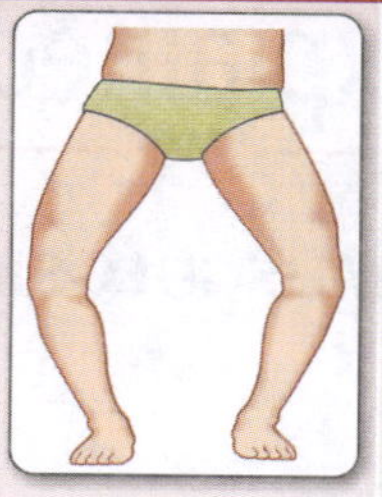	**Genu recurvatum** Due to abnormal intra uterine position which may recover spontaneously	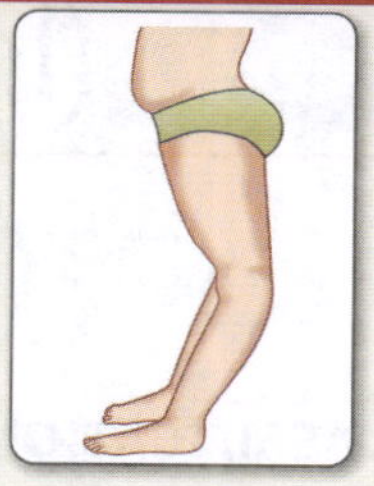

Golden Points to Remember

- There are four muscle tendons that connect to the shoulder to make up the rotator cuff muscle. These muscles are: 1) Supraspinatus, 2) Infraspinatus, 3) Teres minor, 4) Subscapularis
- The extensor muscle of the elbow joint is called **Triceps brachii**
- The three main flexor muscles of the elbow joint are the **biceps brachii, the brachioradialis, and the brachialis.**
- The type of joint found between the skull bones is fibrous joint
- The hammer-shaped bone of the middle ear which contacts with the tympanic membrane is malleus.
- **Osteoporosis** is the most prevalent bone disease in the world.
- Oral corticosteroids can cause secondary osteoporosis.
- Fracture of the distal radius is called **Colle's fracture**.
- **Compartment syndrome** is a complication of fracture in this increased pressure within the myofascial compartment.
- Compartment syndrome is a serious complication of casting and splinting. It occurs when there is an increased pressure within a confined space which compromises blood flow, and low tissue perfusion occurs.
- **Osteoporosis** (porosity and brittleness of bone) is caused by deficiency of Vitamin D.
- Vitamin D deficiency in adults leads to Osteomalacia.
- Cardinal symptoms of rickets are craniotabes (thinning of skull bones), rachitic rosary (rib beading), pigeon breast (pectus carinatum), bowing of legs, waddling gait and short stature.
- **Rachitic rosary** can be frequently seen in Rickets. It is a classic beading of osteochondral junction of ribs.
- **Carpopedal spasm** indicates hypocalcemia.
- Significant elevation of ESR and C Reactive Protein (CRP) is seen during actual phase of Rheumatoid Arthritis (RA).
- Carpal tunnel syndrome is caused by the compression of the **median nerve**.
- Cubital tunnel syndrome occurs when the **ulnar nerve** in the arm becomes compressed or irritated.
- **Foot drop** is caused by an injury to the common peroneal nerve.
- Pain around the pin site, warmth, redness, swelling, purulent discharge is indicative of pin-site infection which can develop as **osteomyelitis**.
- Nurse should stand on the affected side while **ambulating the client**.
- **Four-point gait or weight-bearing gait is** most commonly used when both legs are in a weakened condition.
- **Three-point gait or non-weight bearing gait** is used when injured legs can bear some weight.
- **Three-point swing through gait** is used to keep all pressure off from injured legs and swing both legs through.
- **Gout** is a syndrome of acute attacks of arthritis caused by **hyperuricemia**.
- Incidence of **primary gout** is more among men than in women.
- Limited intake of purine-rich food (e.g., liver and sardines) is advised for the patient with gout.
- Paget's disease is a disorder of bone remodeling process.
- **Scoliosis** is a lateral curvature of the spine.
- Kyphosis is outward curvature of the thoracic spine. It is also known as **humpback**.
- Lordosis is inward curvature of the lumbar spine.
- Patient with prolapsed intervertebral disk is advised to sleep on one side with hip and knee flexed and a pillow between legs.
- C5-C6 and C6-C7 are the most common sites for cervical vertebrae prolapse.
- L4-L5 and L5-S1 are the most common sites for lumbar vertebrae prolapse.
  - Prone position may be recommended following amputation of lower limb.
  - In lower limb amputation, stump should not be elevated on a pillow because it can lead to flexion contracture. If physician recommended, then the foot end of the bed can be elevated.
  - In above knee amputation, prevent the external rotation of stump by using sand bag.
  - In below knee amputation, discourage prolonged sitting and hanging the stump while sitting.
- Amputation that includes all levels of thigh amputations from the hip to the knee joint is known as **Transfemoral amputation**

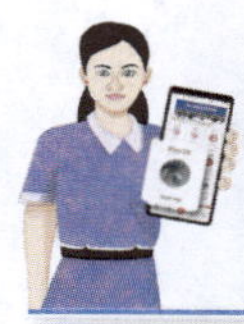

"He who has health has hope; and he who has hope has everything."
—Arabian proverb

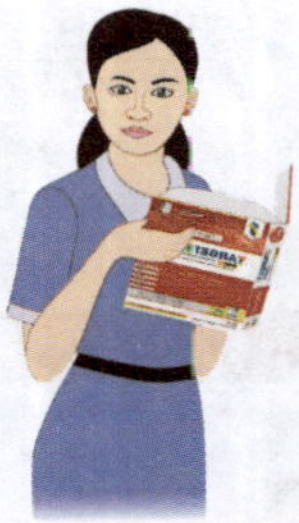

MULTIPLE CHOICE QUESTIONS
(Including Explained and Practice Questions)

MUSCULOSKELETAL SYSTEM

CLASSIFICATION OF BONES

121. In an adult, the skeleton comprises around: *(ESIC Chennai May 2012)*
a. 40–50% of the total body weight
b. 30–40% of the total body weight
c. 60–70% of the total body weight
d. 10–20% of the total body weight

122. Total number of bones in human body: *(ESIC Chennai May 2012; RRB Feb 2012; LNJP H D 2012)*
a. 206 b. 213
c. 209 d. 300

123. Total number of facial bones: *(RRB Feb 2012)*
a. 12 b. 10
c. 14 d. 16

124. Number of bones in the skull is:
a. 22 b. 24
c. 26 d. 28

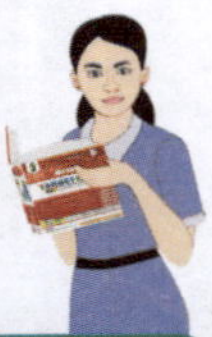

125. Which of the following vertebral bone consists of 5 fused bones?
a. Atlas b. Axis
c. Coccyx d. Sacrum

126. There are ________ pairs of ribs present in human body:
a. 10 pairs b. 11 pairs
c. 12 pairs d. 13 pairs

127. How many pairs of true ribs are there?
a. 7 b. 8
c. 10 d. 12

128. Number of floating ribs is:
a. 2 pairs b. 3 pairs
c. 4 pairs d. 5 pairs

129. False rib is:
a. 1st rib b. 2nd rib
c. 7th rib d. 10th rib

130. True ribs are (pair or number):
a. 7th rib b. 8th rib
c. 10th rib d. 12th rib

131. Total number of metatarsal bones in human body is:
a. 8 b. 10
c. 14 d. 16

132. Total number of carpal bones in human body is:
a. 8 b. 10
c. 14 d. 16

133. Total number of intercostal muscles is:
a. 9 pairs b. 10 pairs
c. 11 pairs d. 12 pairs

ANATOMY OF BONE

134. Winging of scapula is caused due to injury to which of the following parts? *(AIIMS BBS NO 2018)*
a. Ulnar nerve
b. Thoracodorsal nerve
c. Long thoracic nerve of bell
d. Dorsal scapular nerve

Explanation: Injury to the long thoracic nerve causes serratus anterior. Paralysis is the most common cause for Winging of Scapula. Winging of scapula (or scapula alata) is a musculoskeletal disorder characterized by the protrusion of shoulder blade, or shoulder bone, from a person's back in an abnormal position.

135. Muscle of thigh present in anterior aspect: *(Safdarjung NO 2018)*
a. Rectus femoris b. Hamstring
c. Deltoid d. Tibialis anterior

Explanation: The muscles present in the anterior aspect of the thigh are Sartorius, Quadriceps femoris, Rectus femoris and Articularis genu.
Hamstring muscles are present at the back of thigh and knee. **Deltoid muscle** is the muscle of the scapular region and upper limb. **Tibialis anterior** is the muscle of the anterior compartment of the leg.

136. Identify the hip bone from the following: *(DSSSB PHN, 2015)*
a. Femur b. Humerus
c. Innominate d. Sacrum

137. The muscle covers the shoulder and the back of the neck is: *(Kerala PSC, Nov 2014)*
a. Trapezius b. Masseter
c. Biceps d. Temporalis

138. Which bone is the largest bone in human body? *(ESIC Chennai May 2012)*
a. Tibia b. Radius
c. Femur d. Humerus

139. Contraction of the abdominal muscles is important in: (ESIC Chennai May 2012)
a. Normal (quiet) expiration
b. Forced (maximum) expiration
c. Normal (quiet) inspiration
d. Forced (maximum) inspiration

140. Which answer best explains the location of the humerus?
a. Knee to ankle
b. Elbow to wrist (on the pinky side)
c. Elbow to wrist (on the thumb side)
d. Shoulder to elbow

Ans.
121. d
122. a
123. c
124. a
125. d
126. c
127. a
128. a
129. d
130. a
131. b
132. d
133. c
134. c
135. a
136. c
137. a
138. c
139. b
140. d

141. The elbow is ______ to the wrist: *(PGIMER 2000)*
a. Distal b. Anterior
c. Posterior d. Proximal

Explanation: The elbow before the wrist, means it is proximal to the wrist.

142. The basic structural and functional unit of the skeletal muscle is the:
a. Fasciculus b. Fiber
c. Myofibril d. Sarcomere

143. The trapezius muscle is located in the:
a. Lower leg b. Back
c. Forearm d. Buttocks

144. Osteoclasts are known as:
a. Bone forming cells
b. Bone destroying cells
c. Bone repairing cells
d. All of the above

145. Which of the following is known as bone forming cells?
a. Fibrinoblasts
b. Osteocytes
c. Osteoclasts
d. Osteoblasts

146. Site of growth in length of a long bone is:
a. Diaphysis
b. Epiphyseal plate
c. Bone marrow
d. Periosteum

147. Covering of the bone is:
a. Diaphysis
b. Epiphyseal plate
c. Bone marrow
d. Periosteum

148. True regarding isometric contraction is:
a. Shortening of muscle fiber
b. Lengthening of muscle fiber
c. Length of muscle fiber remains the same
d. Pressure of the muscle remain unchanged

149. True regarding concentric isotonic contraction is:
a. Shortening of muscle fiber
b. Lengthening of muscle fiber
c. Length of muscle fiber remains the same
d. Pressure of the muscle remain unchanged

150. Thin filament is:
a. Actin b. Troponin
c. Tropomyosin d. All of the above

151. The maintenance of posture in a normal adult human being depends upon:
a. Integrity of reflex arc
b. Muscle power
c. Type of muscle fibers
d. Joint movements in physiological range

152. Major constituent of bone is:
a. Calcium sulphate b. Calcium phosphate
c. Magnesium sulphate d. Sodium chloride

153. Vitamin essential for a healthy skeletal system is:
a. Vitamin A b. Vitamin D
c. Vitamin E d. Vitamin K

154. Osteocytes are located in:
a. Lamellae b. Haversian canals
c. Canaliculi d. Lacunae

155. True regarding intramembranous ossification is:
a. In the bones of the roof of the skull
b. As a process that produces most of the skeletal system
c. When ones develop from cartilage models
d. When osteoblasts invade the spaces left by dying cartilage cells

156. Bones in the axial skeleton include:
a. Skull b. Ribs
c. Sternum d. All of the above

157. Smallest bone is:
a. Malleus b. Incus
c. Stapes d. Phalangenes

158. Relationships between biceps brachii and triceps brachii muscles are:
a. Synergists
b. Antagonists
c. Both flex the forearm
d. Both extend the forearm

159. Main abductor muscle of the upper limb is:
a. Latissimus dorsi
b. Deltoid
c. Pectoralis major
d. Pectoralis minor

160. Haversian canal together with the lamellae and surrounding is known as:
a. Haversian system
b. Canaliculi
c. Cancellous bone
d. Medullary cavity

161. Ossification starts with ......bone:
a. Fontanel b. Clavicle
c. Humerus d. Femur

162. Ossification of Posterior fontanels completes at:
a. 1½ months
b. 3 months
c. 6 months
d. 18 months

163. Ossification of anterior fontanels completes at:
a. 3 months b. 6 months
c. 12 months d. 18 months

164. Anterior fontanel is formed by all; EXCEPT:
a. Coronal suture
b. Frontal bone
c. Lambdoid suture
d. Sagittal suture

165. The one and only mobile or movable bone in the skull is:
a. Maxilla
b. Mandible
c. Ear ossicle
d. Frontal

166. Sinuses means:
a. Cavities in the bones
b. Nasal cavity
c. Nasal blockage
d. Space between tissues

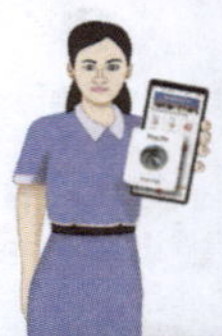

Ans.
141. d
142. d
143. b
144. b
145. d
146. b
147. d
148. c
149. a
150. d
151. a
152. b
153. b
154. d
155. a
156. d
157. c
158. b
159. b
160. a
161. b
162. a
163. d
164. c
165. b
166. a

167. Teeth are located in .... bone.

a. Maxilla and mandible
b. ethmoid and sphenoid
c. Maxilla and frontal bone
d. Zygomatic and vomer

168. The structures of ear are encased in:

a. Temporal bone b. Parietal bone
c. Ethmoid bone d. Frontal bone

169. Forgotten muscle is:

a. Supraspinatus b. Infraspinatus
c. Subscapularis d. Teres minor

170. The epithelial tissue that lines the urinary bladder is:

a. Simple b. Stratified
c. Transitional d. Squamous

171. First bone of the vertebral column is called:

a. Atlas b. Axis
c. Clavicle d. Hyoid

172. Second vertebral bone is also known as:

a. Atlas b. Axis
c. Sacrum d. Coccyx

173. Ear ossicles are made of:

a. Hyaline cartilage b. Fibrocartilage
c. Elastic cartilage d. None of the above

174. Bone without medullary cavity is:

a. Fibula b. Clavicle
c. Femur d. Humerus

175. Collar bone is:

a. Atlas b. Axis bone
c. Clavicle d. Scapula

176. Most commonly fractured carpal bone:

a. Hamate b. Lunate
c. Scaphoid d. Capitates

177. Which of the following is NOT a long bone?

a. Humerus b. Sternum
c. Tibia d. Ulnar

178. Location of the humerus is ....?

a. Knee to ankle b. Knee to hip
c. Elbow to wrist d. Shoulder to elbow

179. Knee is supplied by .... artery.

a. Great saphenous b. Popliteal
c. Dorsalis pedis d. Posterior tibial

180. Ilium is the part of:

a. Shoulder girdle b. Pelvis
c. Spine d. Upper extremity

181. The part of the bone that enters into the formation of a joint is called: *(AIIMS Raipur Grade II 2017)*

a. Articulating surface b. Bony sinus
c. Condyle d. Facet

Explanation: Sinus refers to any of the cavities in the skull that are connected with nasal activity. Condyle is a round prominence at the end of bone, mostly a part of joint which articulates with another bone. A facet is a small smooth area on a bone, usually an articular surface.

182. Strongest muscle in the human body based on its weight is:

a. Triceps b. Biceps
c. Masseter d. Deltoid

183. Which of the following is a connective tissue?

a. Blood
b. Cartilage
c. Bone
d. All of the above

184. Longest muscle in the body:

a. Biceps b. Triceps
c. Sartorius d. Quadriceps

185. Division of joints fibrous in nature permitting no movement is: *New Q*

a. Diarthrosis
b. Synarthroses
c. Tendons and tibia
d. Ligaments and femur

Explanation: Synarthroses are joints that are fibrous in nature and permit no movement. They are the least movable type of joint. Some examples of synarthroses include the sutures between the bones of the skull and the joints between the teeth and the jawbone.

186. Which of the following is the largest cavity is human body?

a. Abdominopelvic cavity
b. Cranial cavity
c. Thoracic cavity
d. Pelvic cavity

187. Smallest abdominal muscle is: *New Q*

a. External oblique
b. Internal oblique
c. Pyramidalis
d. Rectus abdominis

Explanation: The pyramidalis muscle is the smallest abdominal muscle. However, pyramidalis muscle is not present in everyone, as its presence can vary among individuals. The pyramidalis muscle is absent in about 20% of people.

External oblique is the largest abdominal muscle.

188. Elevation of the ribs during passive/normal inspiration is caused by:

a. Diaphragm
b. External intercostals
c. Internal intercostal
d. Sternocleidomastoid

189. The anterior hip muscle that flexes the thigh is the:

a. Iliopsoas
b. Gluteus medius
c. Tensor fascia latae
d. Glute maximus

190. The anterior thigh muscle that extends the leg is the:

a. Sartorius
b. Quadriceps femoris
c. Hamstring muscles
d. Iliopsoas

191. Function of superior oblique muscle is:

a. Intorsion, adduction and depression
b. Intorsion, abduction and elevation
c. Intorsion, abduction and depression
d. Extorsion, abduction and depression

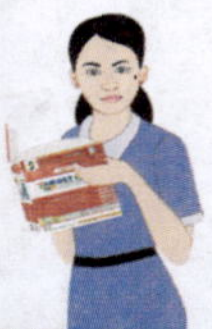

Ans.

167.	a
168.	a
169.	c
170.	c
171.	a
172.	b
173.	c
174.	b
175.	c
176.	c
177.	b
178.	d
179.	b
180.	b
181.	a
182.	c
183.	d
184.	c
185.	b
186.	a
187.	c
188.	b
189.	a
190.	b
191.	c

192. Insertion of pectoralis major is at:

a. Humerus b. Femur
c. Knee d. Clavicle

193. All of the following muscles are composite muscle; EXCEPT:

a. Pectineus b. Rectus femoris
c. Adductor magnus d. Biceps femoris

194. Protein synthesis occurs in:

a. Ribosome b. Lysosomes
c. Endosomes d. Golgi apparatus

195. Site of injection in gluteus:

a. Inferomedial b. Superomedial
c. Superolateral d. Superomedial

196. Which of the following statements about muscle tissue is true?

a. Smooth muscle is striated
b. Skeletal muscle is non-striated
c. Smooth muscle is involuntary
d. Cardiac muscle is not-striated

197. Resorption of bone tissue is done by:

a. Osteoids b. Osteocytes
c. Osteoclasts d. Osteoblasts

198. A nurse is working in an outpatient orthopedic clinic. During the patient's history the patient reports, "I tore 3 of my 4 rotator cuff muscles in the past." Which of the following muscles cannot be considered possibly being torn? *New Q*

a. Supraspinatus b. Infraspinatus
c. Teres major d. Teres minor

Explanation: The teres major muscle cannot be considered possibly being torn in this case. The teres major muscle is not part of the rotator cuff muscles. The rotator cuff muscles consist of four muscles that help stabilize and move the shoulder joint. These muscles are the supraspinatus, infraspinatus, teres minor, and subscapularis.

TYPES OF JOINTS

199. The number of cervical vertebrae in a normal adult is: *(AIIMS Bhopal Nursing Officer, 2018)*

a. 11 b. 9
c. 5 d. 7

Explanation:

Cervical	7
Thoracic	12
Lumbar	5

200. Total number of vertebrae is:

a. 25 b. 27
c. 29 d. 33

201. Which among the following is the largest vertebra?

a. Cervical b. Lumbar
c. Thoracic d. Sacrum

202. Which among the following is the smallest vertebra?

a. Axis b. Cervical
c. Lumbar d. Thoracic

203. Which of the following sections of vertebral column is matched with its correct number of vertebrae?

a. Thoracic - 7 vertebrae b. Cervical - 12 vertebrae
c. Sacral - 3 fused vertebrae d. Lumbar - 5 vertebrae

204. Largest joint of the human body is:

a. Ankle joint b. Elbow joint
c. Knee joint d. Wrist joint

205. Which is a hinge joint?

a. Knee b. Elbow
c. Atlanto Axial d. Both A and B

206. Which of the following is an example of saddle joint?

a. Carpometacarpal joint of the thumb
b. Elbow joint
c. Ankle joint
d. Knee joint

207. Example for ellipsoid joint is:

a. Wrist b. Knee
c. Ankle d. Shoulder

208. Type of joint in symphysis pubis is:

a. Primary cartilaginous b. Secondary cartilaginous
c. Synovial d. Syndesmosis

209. A strong weight bearing synovial joints with irregular elevations and depressions that produce interlocking of the bones is called: *(AIIMS Raipur Grade II 2017)*

a. Vestigial tail b. Symphysis pubis
c. Sacroiliac joints d. Sacrococcygeal joint

Explanation: The true vestigial tail of humans arises from distal remnant of the embryonic tail. It contains adipose and connective tissue, central bundles of striated muscle, blood vessels, and nerves which is covered by skin and does not contain Bone, cartilage, notochord, and spinal cord. The pubic symphysis is a cartilaginous joint that sits between and joins left and right the superior rami of the pubic bones which is located in front of and below the urinary bladder. The sacrococcygeal joint is an amphiarthrodial joint formed between the oval surface at the apex of the sacrum and the base of the coccyx.

210. 'Knee Joint' is the example of which of the following joints? *(AIIMS Bhopal Nursing officer, 2018)*

a. Ball and socket joint b. Hinge joint
c. Pivot joint d. Saddle joint

Explanation:

Joint	Definition
Ball and socket joint	The ball and socket joint (or spheroid joint) is a type of synovial joint in which the ball-shaped surface of one rounded bone fits into the cup-like depression of another bone. E.g.: hip joint, shoulder joint.
Hinge joint	a joint between bones that permits motion in only one plane. E.g.: ankle, elbow, and knee.
Pivot joint	a freely moveable joint that allows only rotary movement around a single axis. E.g.: Proximal radioulnar joint, Distal radioulnar joint, Median atlanto-axial joint.
Saddle joint	A saddle joint is a synovial joint where one of the bones forming the joint is shaped like a saddle with the other bone resting on it like a rider on a horse. E.g.: Carpometacarpal joint of the thumb, between the malleus and incus in the middle ear.

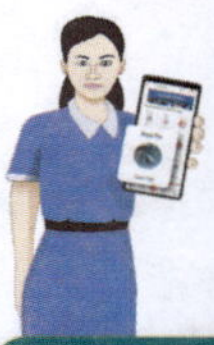

Ans.

192.	a
193.	b
194.	a
195.	c
196.	c
197.	c
198.	c
199.	d
200.	d
201.	b
202.	b
203.	d
204.	c
205.	d
206.	a
207.	a
208.	b
209.	c
210.	b

211. Surgical fusion of a joint is known as: *(JIPMER 2012)*
a. Arthrodesis b. Arthroplasty
c. Arthrotomy d. Nailing

212. The presence of synovial fluid in joints reduces: *(JIPMER 2012)*
a. Efficiency b. Workload
c. Friction in joints d. Speed of movements

213. Movement of a body part away from the midline is:
a. Abduction b. Adduction
c. Extension d. Flexion

214. Movement of a body part towards the midline is:
a. Abduction b. Adduction
c. Extension d. Flexion

215. The type of joint present between ear ossicles is:
a. Primary cartilaginous b. Secondary cartilaginous
c. Synovial d. Fibrous

216. Fibrous joints between the bones of the skull are called:
a. Fossa b. Sutures
c. Synovial joints d. Cartilaginous joints

217. Knee cap is:
a. Femur b. Fibula
c. Patella d. Tibia

218. Patella completely ossifies by the age of:
a. 6 yrs b. 10 yrs
c. 14 yrs d. 21 yrs

219. Type of cartilage seen at temporo-mandibular joint is:
a. Hyaline cartilage b. Fibrocartilage
c. Elastic cartilage d. All of the above

220. Which is the most prominent cartilage found in larynx?
a. Cricoid b. Thyroid
c. Hyoid d. Epiglottis

221. The strongest ligament in the body is:
a. Iliofemoral ligament b. Lacunar ligament
c. Ligamentum flavum d. Inguinal ligament

222. Posterior dislocation of the femur on the tibia is prevented by:
a. Anterior cruciate ligament b. Posterior cruciate ligament
c. Medial collateral ligament d. Lateral collateral ligament

223. Which of these structures has no cartilage in it?
a. Epiglottis b. Trachea
c. Bronchi d. Bronchiole

224. Correct regarding Tendon is:
a. It connects bone to muscle
b. It connects bone to bone
c. It connects muscle to muscle
d. All of the above

225. Correct regarding ligament is:
a. It connects bone to muscle
b. It connects bone to bone
c. It connects muscle to muscle
d. All of the above

226. The repair and reconstruction of the joint is called: *(AIIMS Raipur Grade II 2017)*
a. Arthrodesis b. Arthrotomy
c. Arthroplasty d. Amputation

Explanation: Arthrotomy is creation of an opening in joint. Arthrodesis is surgical immobilization of joint by fusion of bones. Amputation is the removal of limb by trauma, illness or surgery.

227. Overstress and stretching of ligament lead to:
a. Strains b. Sprains
c. Contracture d. Dislocation

VERTEBRAL COLUMN

228. Abnormal lateral deviation of vertebral column is: *(DSSSB PHN, 2015)*
a. Lordosis b. Kyphosis
c. Scoliosis d. Osteoporosis

229. Subarachnoid space ends at the level of:
a. S1 b. S2
c. L2 d. C7

230. Which of the following statement is false?
a. Sacrum consists of 6 fused vertebrae
b. Coccyx consists of 4 fused vertebrae
c. Vertebral column consists of 33 vertebrae
d. There are 7 cervical vertebrae present

231. The vertebral column bones are classified as which type of bone?
a. Long bones b. Short bones
c. Irregular bones d. Flat bones

DIAGNOSTIC EVALUATIONS IN MUSCULOSKELETAL DISORDERS

232. In electromyogram (EMG):
a. Insert needle into 4th or 5th ICS
b. Insertion of small needles into certain muscles
c. Placement of electrodes over the chest
d. Placement of catheter into the ventricles of brain

233. In rheumatoid arthritis, during the acute phase the values which are significant are: *(ESIC 2019)*
a. ESR and C reactive Protein (CRP) elevation
b. RFT elevation (renal Function Test)
c. CBC elevation (Complete Blood Count)
d. LFT elevation (Liver Function Test)

Explanation: Abnormal values of the tests for evaluation of systemic inflammation are the most typical humoral features of Rheumatoid Arthritis. These includes erythrocyte sedimentation rate/ESR, acute phase proteins (such as C-Reactive protein) and plasma viscosity.

234. Important nursing intervention after bone biopsy include:
a. NPO
b. Send samples to the laboratory
c. Monitor the site for bleeding, swelling and hematoma formation
d. Analgesics

Explanation: Monitoring the site for complications takes priority in the immediate post-biopsy period. After a bone biopsy, it is crucial to closely monitor the site for any signs of complications, such as bleeding, swelling, or hematoma formation.

235. Muscle strength 3/5 indicates:
a. Active movement against resistance
b. No active movement at all
c. Active movement against gravity and resistance
d. Active movement against gravity but not against resistance

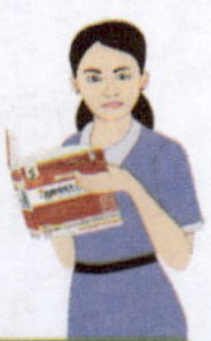

Ans.

211. a
212. c
213. a
214. b
215. c
216. b
217. c
218. c
219. b
220. b
221. a
222. a
223. d
224. a
225. b
226. c
227. b
228. c
229. b
230. a
231. c
232. b
233. a
234. c
235. d

236. All are abnormal findings in musculoskeletal system; EXCEPT:
a. No deformity or crepitus
b. Positive ortolani sign
c. Ulnar deviation and subluxation
d. Swan neck deformity

237. Kyphosis is the deformity of:
a. Lower limbs b. Spine
c. Ribs d. Upper limbs

238. After arthrocentesis procedure client reports pain in the joint after administering corticosteroids. Which of the following action by the nurse is most appropriate?
a. Report to the physician
b. Avoid the client behaviour
c. Provide further pain medication
d. Tell the client it is a normal finding

239. Which of the following test which measures electrical potential associated with the skeletal muscle contraction?
a. Bone densitometry b. Biopsy
c. Electromyography d. Arthrography

240. Which of the following intervention is most important after the injection of radioisotope during the procedure of bone scan?
a. Advise the client to drink more water if not contraindicated
d. Advise the client to elevate the legs
c. Advise the client not to drink water
d. Advise the client to take rest

241. Which of the following procedure involves the aspiration of synovial fluid by means of inserting a needle into the joints?
a. Bone scan b. Electromyography
c. Arthrocentesis d. Arthroscopy

FRACTURES & TYPES OF FRACTURES

242. The long-term effects of a prolonged diet that contains too little calcium would include:
a. Increased calcitonin secretion
b. Increased thyroid hormone secretion
c. Decreased bone thickness
d. Acromegaly

243. The clinical manifestations of fractures include:
a. Fever, heaviness, weakness
b. Edema, pallor, ecchymosis
c. Pain, pallor, paresthesia
d. Pain, coolness, loss of pulse

244. Fracture occurs at the distal end of the fibula: *(Kerala PSC, Nov 2014)*
a. Colles' fracture
b. Oblique fracture
c. Spiral fracture
d. Pott's fracture

245. Which of the following is a fracture in which bone is shattered into numerous fragments? *(Staff Nurse G II 2014)*
a. Displaced fracture
b. Avulsion fracture
c. Comminuted fracture
d. Spiral fracture

246. A bone fracture resulting in an open wound through which bone fragments usually protrude is known as:
a. Simple fracture b. Buckled fracture
c. Compound fracture d. Complete fracture

247. All of the following are the causes of pathological fracture; EXCEPT?
a. Osteoporosis
b. Osteomyelitis
c. Primary Hyperparathyroidism
d. Multiple sclerosis

248. Complications of fracture healing include:
a. Fibrous union b. Nonunion
c. Pseudo arthrosis d. All of the above

249. What type of fracture is green stick fracture?
a. Complete fracture b. Incomplete fracture
c. Complicated d. Penetrating

250. Impacted fracture is also known as:
a. Buckled fracture b. Complicated fracture
c. Communicated fracture d. Green stick fracture

251. Which of the following term is used for the fracture in which the broken bone causes damage to other organs or structures?
a. Communicated fracture b. Complicated fracture
c. Buckled fracture d. Complete fracture

252. Colle's fracture refers to the injury of: *(DSSSB PHN, 2015)*
a. Shoulder joint b. Knee joint
c. Wrist joint d. Elbow joint

253. Colle's fracture refers to the fracture of: *(Daman and Diu NO 2018)*
a. Ulna b. Humerus
c. Radius d. Olecranon

Explanation: A Colle's fracture is a type of complete fracture of the radius bone of the distal forearm close to the wrist resulting in an upward (posterior) displacement of the radius and obvious deformity. The clinical presentation of Colle's fracture is commonly described as a **dinner fork deformity** along with inability to grasp objects.

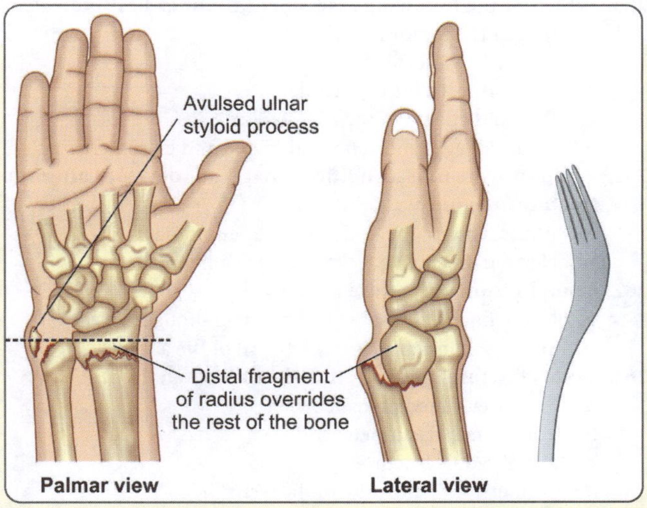

254. Fracture of the distal radius is called: *(DSSSB 2013)*
a. Hume fracture b. Monteggia fracture
c. Galeazzi fracture d. Colles' fracture

255. Hangman's fracture refers to:
a. Fracture of median radius
b. Fracture of metacarpal bones
c. Fracture of clavicle bone
d. C2-C3 traumatic spondylolisthesis

Ans.
236. a
237. b
238. d
239. c
240. a
241. c
242. c
243. c
244. d
245. c
246. c
247. d
248. d
249. b
250. a
251. b
252. c
253. c
254. d
255. d

256. Which of the following statement describes pathological fracture?
a. Break or splinter of the bone into more than two fragments
b. A bone fracture accompanied by damage to regional organs and/or neurovascular bundles
c. Ends of the bone are driven into each other
d. Fracture is caused by a disease that weakens the bones

257. Older adults are more prone to develop hip fracture because of:
a. Decreased bone density b. Sedentary lifestyle
c. Weakness in them d. Age

Explanation: Hip fracture is more common among older adults because their bone density decreases, becomes thinner and weaker due to calcium loss.

258. Elderly women are more prone to develop hip fracture because:
a. Decreased estrogen secretion
b. Increased bone density
c. Increased calcium absorption
d. Sedentary lifestyle

Explanation: Estrogen withdrawal among elderly women leads to osteoporosis and decreased bone density, so they are more prone to develop hip fracture.

259. A 30-year-old male patient was admitted with a fractured femur. A nurse would assess for sign of circulatory impairment in this client by asking him to:
a. Turn himself in bed
b. Cough and deep breathe
c. Perform biceps exercise
d. Twist his toes

260. Which of the following assessment findings best indicates a fracture of the femoral neck?
a. Pain in the affected leg
b. Hematoma in the affected leg
c. Pain and edema in the affected leg
d. Affected leg is shortened, adducted and extremely rotated

261. A life-threatening condition that can develop after the fracture of femur is:
a. Atelectasis b. Pneumonia
c. Nerve damage d. Fat embolism

262. Complication of fracture is:
a. Nerve injury b. Fat embolism
c. Soft tissue injury d. All of the above

263. Colle's fracture refers to all of the following; EXCEPT:
a. Fracture of medial malleolus
b. Transverse wrist fracture
c. Distal radius fracture
d. Dinner-fork deformity of the wrist

264. Fracture of malleoli or lower end of the fibula is known as
a. Colles' fracture b. Pott's fracture
c. Jone's fracture d. Jefferson's fracture

265. Fracture of the base of the first metacarpal bone which extends into the carpometacarpal (CMC) joint is known as:
a. Hangman's fracture
b. Jone's fracture
c. Bennet fracture
d. Boxer's fracture

Explanation:
- Bennet fracture, an intra-articular fracture, is the most common type of fracture of the thumb.
- Boxer's fracture refers to fracture of 5th Metacarpal bones.
- Hangman's fracture is a fracture of the axis in the cervical region. It is often seen with people who tries to hang themselves.
- Jones fracture is a fracture between the base and middle part of the fifth metatarsal of the foot.

266. Parameter need to be monitored in a client with fracture of the pelvis is:
a. Changes in urine output b. Lower limb sensation
c. Femoral pulse d. Pain

267. Which nerve is most likely to be injured in fracture of shaft of humerus?
a. Median nerve b. Musculocutaneous nerve
c. Radial nerve d. Dinar nerve

268. Manual manipulation of dislocated shoulder joint is known as:
a. A Close reduction b. An open reduction
c. Internal fixation d. External fixation

269. Healing following fracture to the distal shaft of the humerus is indicated by:
a. Formation of callus b. Formation of keloids
c. Formation of scar d. Presence of contracture

270. Correct regarding open reduction and internal fixation (ORIF) is:
a. Fast method of recovery
b. Can use in all patients
c. Adequate alignment is not obtained from CRIF then ORIF will use
d. Plaster of Paris can be used instead of ORIF

271. Neurovascular problem following fracture is indicated by:
a. Pain
b. Pulselessness distal to the injury
c. Pallor
d. Loss of movement

272. Diet of a fracture patient should be rich in:
a. Calcium b. Potassium
c. Vitamin C d. Sodium

273. Bandage indicated in collar bone fracture is:
a. Cap line b. Spiral
c. Figure of eight splint d. Splint

STAGES OF BONE HEALING

274. In which of the following stages of bone healing, the bleeding occurs around the edges of the fractured bones and a hematoma develops:
a. Stage one b. Stage two
c. Stage four d. Stage three.

275. Bony callus formation take place in which stage of the bone healing?
a. Stage one b. Stage two
c. Stage four d. Stage three

276. Lamellar bone deposition takes place in which stages of the bone healing?
a. Stage one b. Stage two
c. Stage four d. Stage three

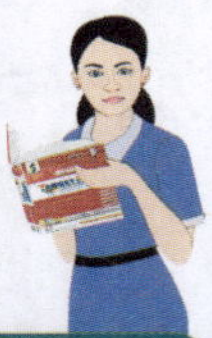

Ans.

256.	d
257.	a
258.	a
259.	d
260.	d
261.	d
262.	d
263.	a
264.	b
265.	c
266.	a
267.	c
268.	a
269.	a
270.	c
271.	b
272.	a
273.	c
274.	a
275.	d
276.	c

277. During bone healing process after a fracture, bone remodeling begins approximately at:
a. 7 days b. 14 days
c. 18 days d. 28 days

278. In the bone healing process, granulation tissue formation take place in:
a. Stage one b. Stage two
c. Stage three d. Stage four

Explanation: Following the fracture of a bone, secondary healing begins, which consists of four steps:

- Stage 1: Hematoma formation (days 1 to 5)
- Stage 2: Fibrocartilaginous callus formation (days 5 to 11)
- Stage 3: Bony callus formation (Days 11 to 28)
- Stage 4: Bone remodeling (Day 18 onwards)

CASTS, SPLINTS & BRACES

279. A patient is lying in a supine position. External rotation of the lower extremity can be prevented in this patient by using:
a. Foot board below the extremity
b. Sandbag on the foot
c. Trochanter roll to the knee
d. Trochanter roll to the thigh

280. Infection needs to be suspected in a casted extremity if there is:
a. Pain b. No pulse
c. Paranesthesia d. Hot spot

281. Spica cast is used for: *(ISRO)*
a. Arm b. Leg
c. Foot d. Hip

282. An 8-year-old girl was diagnosed with a closed fracture of the radius at approximately 2 PM. The fracture was reduced in the emergency room and her arm placed in a cast. At 11 PM her mother brought her back to the emergency room due to unrelenting pain that has not been relieved by the prescribed narcotics. What should the nurse do first? *(AIIMS Raipur NO 2019)*
a. Notify the doctor immediately
b. Apply ice
c. Elevate the arm
d. Give additional pain medication as ordered

Explanation: Compartment syndrome is a serious complication of casting and splinting. Ischemia and irreversible neuromuscular damage can occur. The first action should be to notify the physician. Applying ice and elevating the arm will worsen the condition further.

283. A plaster cast takes how many hours to dry completely?
a. 12 to 24 hrs b. 6 to 12 hrs
c. 24 to 72 hrs d. None of the above

284. Synthetic casts dry in:
a. 10 mins b. 15 mins
c. 20 mins d. 40 mins

285. What type of reaction takes place in the application of plaster?
a. Endothermic reaction
b. Exothermic reaction
c. Isothermic reaction
d. Mesothermic reaction

Explanation: When plaster of Paris and water are mixed, there is a chemical reaction and heat is released. A reaction that gives off energy like heat is called an exothermic reaction.

286. Which of the following cast is also called as gauntlet cast?
a. Thumb spica b. Long arm cast
c. Short arm cast d. Shoulder spica cast

287. Which of the following does not comes under 5 p's?
a. Pulseness b. Pallor
c. Paralysis d. Palpitation

288. Turn buckle cast is used for:
a. Cervical spine injury b. Scoliosis
c. Fracture shaft humerus d. Fracture shaft femur

EXTERNAL FIXATOR

289. What is the most common complication associated with external fixator?
a. Numbness b. Necrosis
c. Gangrene d. Pin site infection

290. A client with external fixator who complains of redness, swelling and purulent discharge around the pain site are the indicative of:
a. Pin site infection b. Gangrene
c. Necrosis d. Foot ulcer

291. What is the essential care for a client with Ilizarov external fixator?
a. Check the clients vital signs on the regular basis
b. Discourage the client not to do strenuous activities
c. Clean the pin sites with sterile saline twice a day
d. Provide proper positioning

292. The Hoffmann external fixator has proved to be an effective means of stabilizing:
a. Femoral fracture b. Tibial fracture
c. Shoulder dislocation d. Patellar fracture

TRACTION

293. Purposes of traction include:
a. Used in the treatment of fracture
b. It helps to reduce muscle spasm and contracture
c. Helps in internal reduction
d. Both a and b

294. Bryant's traction is indicated in: *(Kerala PSC, Nov 2014)*
a. Fractures of femur b. Fractures of humerus
c. Spinal fractures d. Fractures of radius

295. Identify skin traction among the following:
a. Buck's extension traction b. Russell's traction
c. Dunlop's traction d. All of the above

Explanation: Skin traction is one of two basic types of traction used for the treatment of fractured bones. It works by applying weight to tape, sponge rubber, or canvas materials which have been attached to the skin surrounding the damaged body structure. Buck's traction is a form of traction where pull is exerted in one plane. It is used when partial or temporary immobilization is required, and it is used to provide comfort following injury while awaiting surgical fixation, especially in hip and femur injuries. Russell's Traction can be used for fractures of the tibial plateau, it works by supporting the flexed knee in a sling and applying a horizontal pulling force by use of traction tape and elastic bandage attached to the lower leg.

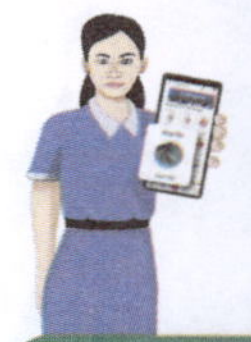

Ans.

277. c
278. b
279. d
280. d
281. d
282. a
283. c
284. c
285. b
286. a
287. d
288. b
289. d
290. a
291. c
292. a
293. d
294. a
295. d

Dunlop's Traction is used for fractures of the upper extremities. It works in the form of horizontal traction which is applied to the abducted humorous, while vertical traction is applied to the flexed forearm.

296. In an immobilized patient with traction, muscle atrophy can be prevented by:

a. ROM exercises b. Stretc.hing exercises
c. Isotonic contractions d. Isometric contractions

297. Foot drop is caused by an injury to: *(AIIMS-BBS SNO 2019)*

a. The tibial nerve
b. The common peroneal nerve
c. The obturator nerve
d. The sciatic nerve

298. Which of the following intervention is most appropriate to prevent foot drop in a client with buck's traction?

a. Provide proper positioning for the patient
b. Keep pillows under patient's heels
c. Teach the patient isometric exercise
d. All of the above

Explanation: Mobility and muscle tone can be improved through isometric exercise. Hence teaching isometric exercise to patient can prevent foot drop. Use of foot board effective in foot drop prevention.

299. When a client is with traction, which of the following is the priority nursing intervention?

a. Neurovascular assessment
b. Temperature assessment
c. Fracture site inspection
d. Client hygienic status

Explanation: Neurovascular assessment is the priority nursing intervention when a client is in traction. Traction can exert pressure on the surrounding tissues and compromise circulation and nerve function. Therefore, regular neurovascular assessments are essential to monitor for any signs of neurovascular compromise, such as decreased sensation, changes in motor function, pallor, coolness, or delayed capillary refill.

300. What is the average weight should be used for traction on extremity?

a. 1 to 1.5 kg b. 2 to 3.5 kg
c. 4 to 5 kg d. 5 to 5.5 kg

301. What is the average weight should be used for traction on pelvis?

a. 2 to 3.5 kg b. 4.5 to 9 kg
c. 4 to 5 kg d. 5 to 6 kg

302. In a client with skin traction dorsiflexion of the foot indicates the functioning of which nerve?

a. Peroneal nerve b. Tibial nerve
c. Radial nerve d. Facial nerve

ORTHOPEDIC SURGERIES

303. Total hip arthroplasty means:

a. Fuse the joint
b. Replace the hip joint
c. Fixation of femur with rod
d. Remove the cartilage tissue

304. After total hip replacement the precautions to be taken to avoid dislocation of prosthesis include:

a. Avoid crossing your legs and bending your hip past a right angle
b. Avoid low chair
c. Sleep with a pillow between legs for 6 weeks
d. All of the above

Explanation: All of the above management is indicated to prevent hip prosthesis dislocation. Avoid bending over to pick things up is also recommended.

305. Identify the statement that indicates a lack of understanding in the client regarding immediate post-operative management following total hip replacement. *New Q*

a. I need to avoid bending over
b. I need to avoid crossing legs
c. Need to avoid sleep on the operative side.
d. Analgesic IM injections can be taken in the operated hip.

Explanation: Option D is correct answer because the surgical site needs time to heal, and unnecessary injections into the hip joint can increase the risk of infection or damage to the newly replaced joint.

Bending over and crossing legs may result in hip dislocation. So the client statement about avoiding it shows correct understanding. Sleeping on the operative side result in pressure in operated area. So this need to be avoided.

306. Which of the following position is appropriate for a patient who is on first postoperative day after total hip replacement?

a. Supine with abduction pillow
b. Prone with abduction pillow
c. Semi Fowler's position
d. Trendelenburg position

307. A patient is scheduled for a right total hip replacement. The nurse should teach which of the following postoperative leg positions? *(RAK MSc 2018)*

a. Maintain legs in adduction
b. Maintain legs in abduction
c. Maintain internal leg rotation
d. Maintain >90° hip flexion

Explanation:

- The reason for maintaining legs in abduction following the right hip replacement is to maintain the alignment of legs with the hip. Abduction means to move the legs away from the midline, doing so, it prevents internal rotation of legs and displacement of the replaced hip bone.
- **Maintaining leg adduction, doing internal rotation and keeping the legs at an angle >90°** will interfere with the alignment of the newly replaced hip bone.

308. Health education after total ankle replacement includes:

a. Avoid walking for 6 weeks
b. Elevate the leg always
c. Wear elastic stockings always
d. Non-weight bearing for 6 weeks

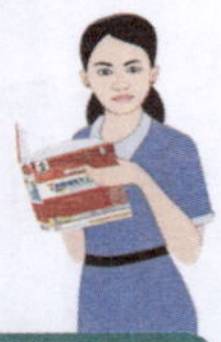

Ans.

296. d
297. b
298. c
299. a
300. b
301. b
302. a
303. b
304. d
305. d
306. a
307. b
308. d

309. The surgical procedure done to relieve pressure in compartment syndrome is: *(DSSSB 2013)*
- a. Open reduction with internal fixation (ORIF)
- b. Meniscectomy
- c. Fasciotomy
- d. Arthroplasty

Explanation: Fasciotomy or fasciectomy is a surgical procedure where the fascia is cut to relieve tension or pressure commonly to treat the resulting loss of circulation to an area of tissue or muscle. Fasciotomy is a limb-saving procedure when used to treat acute compartment syndrome.

310. A nurse is caring for a patient who has had hip replacement (THR). Which of the following findings are of paramount importance? *(AIIMS Bhopal Nursing officer, 2018)*
- a. Complaints of pain during repositioning
- b. Scant bloody discharge on the surgical dressing
- c. Complaints of pain following physical therapy
- d. Temperature of 101.8°F (38.7°C)

Explanation: Except option D others are normal findings following THR. Increased temperature indicates risk for infection.

311. Chemotherapy before the surgical resection of osteosarcoma will help to:
- a. Avoid the need for surgery
- b. Reduce the tumor size
- c. Kill the tumor cell and prevent blood supply
- d. All of the above

312. Watson jones anterolateral approach is performed for:
- a. Muscle paralysis
- b. Valgus deformity
- c. Neglected club foot
- d. Hip replacement

CRUTCHES

313. Nurse Ramya is observing a patient who is practicing Swing-through crutch gait. In this method, the patient needs to move both crutches forward, leans on the crutches and then lift and swing both legs to place it:
- a. Before reaching the crutch tips
- b. At the Level with the crutch tips
- c. Past the crutch tips
- d. At either before or at the level of crutch tips

Explanation: During the swing-through gait, the client advances both crutches, leans on the crutches, and then lifts and swings both legs past the crutch tips.

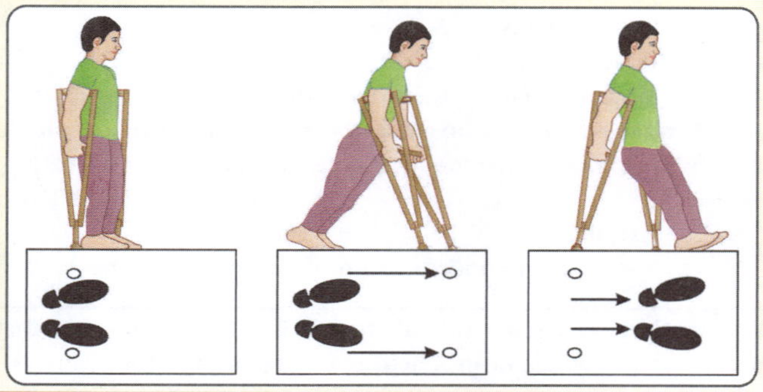

314. Which of the following assistive device would be most appropriate for a patient who needs only minimal assistance with ambulation?
- a. A cane
- b. A walker without wheels
- c. A wheeled walker
- d. Axillary crutch

Explanation: A general standard cane, is used with patients who requires only minimal assistance with ambulation. A walker has four wide-placed legs and is the assistive device that provides the greatest support for ambulation. Crutches are used to remove weight from a lower extremity by transferring the weight to the upper extremities. Hence A cane is appropriate assistive device for these client.

315. An adult patient using the crutches with a moves of both crutches forward and then moves both legs forward to the level of placement of crutch tips. This kind of moving and using a crutches would be referred as:
- a. Two-point gait
- b. Three point gait
- c. Swing-to-gait
- d. Swing-through gait

Explanation: The given description refers the swing-to-gait. The key word to let you know the answer is **'swing-to'**. This indicates that the patient moves both legs **to** the placement of the crutches. It would have been the swing-through-gait if both legs moved forward past the point of the crutch placement.

316. Sequentially arrange the following steps of moving downward staircase with the help of crutches?
- i. Place the unaffected leg forward and down
- ii. Place affected leg forward and down
- iii. Put the crutches on step below first
- a. i, ii, iii
- b. ii, I, iii
- c. iii, ii, i
- d. iii, i, ii

Explanation: (C) When moving down the stairs with the help of crutches, the patient will move the crutches down first onto the step and then followed by moving the affected (weak) leg and then the patient will move the non-injured leg down. This action can be reversed when the patient is supposed to climb up the stairs.

GOUT

317. Gout is a disorder of:
- a. Pyrimidine metabolism
- b. Purine metabolism
- c. Amino acid transport defect
- d. Mismatch repair of DNA

318. Gout is a type of arthritis that occurs due to the accumulation of:
- a. Purines
- b. Creatinine
- c. Uric acid
- d. Bilirubin

319. Needle-like crystals forms around the joints that cause severe pain is a feature of:
- a. Gout arthritis
- b. Rheumatoid arthritis
- c. Ankylosis
- d. All of the above

320. Gout tends to start at which of the following site?
- a. Elbow
- b. Knee joint
- c. Index finger or thumb
- d. Big toe

321. Drug used to treat acute gout attack:
- a. Allopurinol
- b. Sulfinpyrazone
- c. Colchicine
- d. Probenacid

Ans.

309. c
310. d
311. b
312. d
313. c
314. a
315. c
316. c
317. b
318. c
319. a
320. d
321. c

322. Drug of choice for gout is:

a. Phenytoin
b. Allopurinal
c. Diazepam
d. Methyl prednisolone

Explanation: Allopurinol is an antihyperuricemic which prevents the production of uric acid. So Allopurinol is used to prevent gout attacks. NSAIDs and Colchicine are best for treating the inflammation and pain during a gout attack.

323. What is the priority nursing intervention for a client with acute gout?

a. Provide adequate fluids
b. Explain the client about the dietary habits
c. Promote bed rest
d. Administer prescribed analgesics

Explanation: Acute gout is characterized by severe pain and inflammation in the affected joint(s). The priority nursing intervention is to provide relief from pain and discomfort. Administering prescribed analgesics, such as nonsteroidal anti-inflammatory drugs (NSAIDs) can help alleviate the pain associated with acute gout.

324. Which of the following dietary pattern is best for the client with gout?

a. Low purine diet
b. High protein diet
c. Fiber rich foods
d. Low carbohydrate diet

325. Which of the following instruction the nurse should give when a client is taking allopurinol?

a. Drink 10 glasses of water every day
b. Take pain medication double if you feel more pain
c. Add excessive protein to the diet
d. Avoid fiber in the diet

326. Incidence of primary gout is more common in:

a. Children
b. Adults
c. Men
d. Women

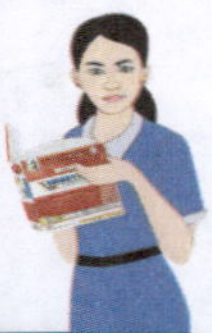

Ans.

322. b
323. d
324. a
325. a
326. c
327. a
328. b
329. b
330. a
331. d
332. a
333. b
334. d
335. c
336. b

TENDINITIS & BURSITIS

327. Which of the following is the most common cause of bursitis?

a. Repetitive action on a joint
b. Fracture
c. Injury
d. Genetic

328. The most common affected part in tendinitis is?

a. Interphalangeal joint
b. Achille's tendon
c. Intervertebral joint
d. Trapezium

329. The arm position for the client with supraspinatus tendinitis:

a. Arm should be elevated high
b. Arm fully extended & internally rotated
c. Abduct the arms
d. Adduction over the abdomen

330. The inflammation of the fluid filled sac that cushion the bone, tendon and muscles:

a. Bursitis
b. Tendonitis
c. Osteomyelitis
d. Enchondroma

331. The human bursa contains:

a. Endolymph
b. CSF fluid
c. Vitreous humor
d. Synovial fluid

332. From among the following persons, who is having highest of developing bursitis?

a. 27-year-old Carpenter
b. 30-year-old nurse
c. 28-year-old software engineer
d. 10-year-old school child

Explanation: Bursitis is usually caused by repeated pressure on an area or by using a joint too much. High-risk activities include gardening, raking, carpentry, shoveling, painting, scrubbing, tennis, golf, skiing, and throwing where a particular action is repeated. From given options above, the carpenter is at high-risk to develop bursitis than others.

333. Which of the following is NOT recommended for the management of bursitis?

a. Inj. Corticosteroid
b. Allopurinol
c. NSAIDs
d. Isometric exercises

Explanation: Management of bursitis includes rest of the affected joint, ice packages, NSAIDs (analgesics), and injection with steroid agents. Resting the affected joint does not mean immobilizing, and a graduate increase in isometric exercises and activities is recommended. Allopurinol used in the treatment of gout arthritis, not in bursitis.

334. Which of the following is not the signs and symptoms of Bursitis?

a. Warmth
b. Pain
c. Restricted movement
d. Heberdens node

Explanation: Bursitis is a painful condition that refers to the inflammation of the bursae (a small, fluid-filled sacs) that provides cushion to the bones, tendons and muscles near the joints. Redness, warmth, pain and restricted range of motion are features of bursitis. **Heberden's nodes** are hard bony lumps in the joints of your fingers. They are typically a symptom of osteoarthritis.

ARTHRITIS

335. A client is complaining of fatigue, weight loss, and a low-grade fever and pain in fingers, elbows, and ankles. These symptoms are suggestive of:

a. Bone pain
b. Osteoarthritis
c. Rheumatoid arthritis
d. Systemic lupus erythematosus (SLE)

336. A nurse is caring for an old lady with osteoarthritis and all the following facts are true regarding osteoarthritis; EXCEPT: *(NCFL 2019)*

a. Crepitus
b. Tophi
c. Subcutaneous nodes
d. Pain on moving the joint

Explanation: A **tophus** (plural: **tophi**) is symptom of gout that occurs when crystals of **uric acid** builds up around the joints. All other given features are associated with osteoarthritis.

337. Heberden nodes is seen in:
a. Rheumatoid arthritis b. Osteoarthritis
c. Spondylosis d. Tendinitis

338. Clinical manifestation of ankylosing spondylitis includes:
a. Fever and headache
b. Fatigue and night sweats
c. Low back pain
d. Urinary incontinence

339. Risk for developing rheumatoid arthritis is more in:
a. A 30-year-old woman b. A 30-year-old man
c. A 65-year-old woman d. A 65-year-old man

340. First line drug of choice for a client recently diagnosed with rheumatoid arthritis is:
a. NSAIDs b. Opioid analgesics
c. Local anesthetics d. All of the above

341. Main goal of treatment in rheumatoid arthritis is to:
a. To treat the disease completely
b. To prevent osteoporosis
c. To control inflammation
d. To maintain ROM

342. All of the following tests are used in diagnosis of Rheumatoid Arthritis; EXCEPT:
a. AFP level
b. Erythrocyte Sedimentation Rate (ESR)
c. Anti-cyclic citrullinated peptide (Anti-CCP)
d. C reactive protein (CRP)

343. Which of the following condition improves with pregnancy?
a. Rheumatoid arthritis b. SLE
c. Myasthenia gravis d. Multiple sclerosis

344. Pathogens responsible for septic arthritis are:
a. Streptococci b. Staphylococci
c. Haemophilus influenzae d. All of the above

345. Least priority nursing care in a client with rheumatoid arthritis is:
a. Prevent joint deformity
b. Maintaining usual ways of accomplishing task
c. Relieving pain
d. Preserving joint function

346. Which among the following needs to be assessed by the nurse in a postoperative patient who underwent spinal fusion surgery?
a. Lower extremity sensation and mobility
b. Urinary control
c. Urine out put
d. Pain level in patient

347. NSAID drug of choice to treat uncomplicated rheumatoid arthritis is:
a. Aspirin b. Dexamethasone
c. Ibuprofen d. Diclofenac sodium

348. Main side effect of allopurinol is:
a. Maculopapular rash b. Nasal congestion
c. Headache d. Neutropenia

349. Patient with which of the following disease condition often gets relief through complementary therapies?
a. Ulcers
b. Chronic pain and arthritis
c. Myocardial infraction
d. Diabetes

OSTEOMYELITIS

350. Organism responsible for pyogenic osteomyelitis is:
a. Staphylococcus aureus b. Salmonella
c. Pseudomonas d. Pneumococci

351. For which disease condition there is no genetic cause for the disease?
a. Spina bifida b. Bursitis
c. Tics disease d. Osteomyelitis

352. Most common causative organism of osteomyelitis?
a. Staphylococcus aureus
b. Streptococcus aureus
c. Staphylococcus epidermidis
d. Staphylococcus saphrophyticus

353. What is the most common organism causing osteomyelitis in drug abusers?
a. E. coli
b. Klebsiella
c. Staphylococcus aureus
d. Pseudomonas

354. What is the surgical choice for osteomyelitis?
a. Sequesterectomy
b. Fasciotomy
c. Episiotomy
d. Escharatomy

Explanation: Sequesterum is a dead bone. As a result of any bone disease or injury the fragment of dead bone will come out from the normal healthy bone. The surgical removal of sequesterum is called sequesterectomy.

355. Which organism causing osteomyelitis in sickle cell anemia?
a. E. coli
b. H. influenza
c. Staphylococcus
d. Salmonella

356. Which of the following vital sign reading is abnormal in a patient diagnosed with osteomyelitis?
a. Blood pressure 130/80
b. Heart rate 90 beats per min
c. Respiratory rate 24 breaths per min
d. Temperature 100°F

357. Which of the following intervention is most important for a client diagnosed with osteomyelitis of fever who is admitted for initiation of antibiotic infusion?
a. Immobilization of leg
b. Range of motion exercise
c. Avoid NSAID's
d. Monitoring of vital signs

Explanation: Immobilization of leg will help to reduce the pain and reduce the risk of pathological fractures.

358. Sequestrum refers to:
a. a bone with poor blood supply
b. a dead bone surrounded by infected tissue
c. a dead bone with necrotic tissue
d. a dead tissue

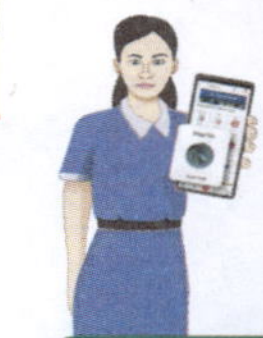

Ans.
337. b
338. c
339. c
340. a
341. c
342. a
343. a
344. d
345. b
346. a
347. c
348. a
349. b
350. a
351. d
352. a
353. c
354. a
355. d
356. d
357. a
358. b

OSTEOPOROSIS & OSTEOMALACIA

Bone Pathology

359. Correct regarding osteoporosis is:
- a. High risk in elderly and postmenopausal woman.
- b. Leads to reduction of bone tissue mass
- c. There is normal levels of serum calcium and inorganic phosphorus
- d. All of the above

360. Risk factor for osteoporosis is:
- a. Hyperthyroidism
- b. Hypoparathyroidism
- c. Prolonged use of glucocorticoids
- d. Consumption of milk

361. Risk factors of osteoporosis include all; EXCEPT:
- a. Hypothyroidism
- b. Hyperparathyroidism
- c. Post menopausal women
- d. Vitamin D deficiency

362. Abnormal hardening of bone and an elevation in bone density is known as:
- a. Osteoporosis
- b. Osteopetrosis
- c. Osteomalecia
- d. Arthritis

Explanation:
- Osteopetrosis is a bone disease that makes bones abnormally dense and hard that is susceptible to fracture.
- Osteoporosis - decreased bone density (weakening).
- Otosclerosis - abnormality in ear ossicles which leads to deafness.
- Osteomalecia - softening of the bones caused by impaired bone metabolism.

363. Causes of osteomalacia include:
- a. Calcium deficiency
- b. Vitamin D deficiency
- c. Both a and b
- d. Exposure to sunlight

364. The rapid progression of osteoporosis is seen in: *New Q*
- a. Young women
- b. Middle aged men
- c. Post-menopausal women
- d. Middle-aged pre-menopausal women

Explanation: Osteoporosis is a condition in which the bones become weak and brittle. The rapid progression of osteoporosis is seen in post-menopausal women because of the decrease in the production of estrogen after menopause. Estrogen helps to keep bones strong, so when its level decreases, the risk of osteoporosis increases.

365. Which of the following should be monitored when a client is taking calcitonin for osteoporosis?
- a. Hypocalcemia
- b. Hypercalcemia
- c. Hyperkalemia
- d. Hypophosphotemia

Explanation: Calcitonin decreases the blood calcium levels by two mechanisms:
- Osteoclasts are responsible for breaking down the bone which releases the bone from calcium into blood. Calcitonin inhibits the osteoclast activity that leads to reduction in the amount of calcium released into bone.
- In addition, calcitonin decreases the resorption of calcium in the kidney which leads to hypocalcemia.
- NOTE: In contrast to calcitonin, Parathyroid Hormone (PTH) increases blood calcium levels by stimulating osteoclasts.

366. What is the priority nursing diagnosis for a client diagnosed with a history of osteoporosis and severe kyphosis?
- a. Limit the mobility
- b. Knowledge deficit related to disease condition
- c. Risk for fall
- d. Sleep pattern disturbance

Explanation: The patient is at risk for fall due to severe kyphosis and it will be the priority nursing diagnosis.

367. Windswept deformity is seen in which of the following disease condition?
- a. Rickets
- b. Scurvy
- c. Ankylosing spondylitis
- d. Achondroplasia

Explanation: Windswept deformity, which is valgus deformity in one knee and varus deformity in the other, is the most common deformity encountered in patients with hypophosphataemic rickets.

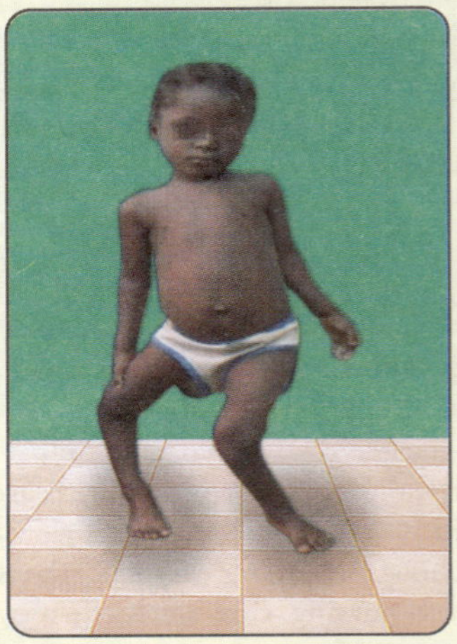

PAGET'S DISEASE & POTT'S DISEASE

368. Pott's disease is:
- a. TB meningitis
- b. TB spine
- c. TB bone
- d. TB lung

369. The other name of Paget's disease is:
- a. Osteitis deformans
- b. Osteitis endorfans
- c. Hansen disease
- d. Baedows disease

370. Which of the bone physiology process is very high and abnormal in Paget's disease:
- a. Osteoblast
- b. Osteoclast
- c. Osteocyte
- d. Osteocyst

Explanation: Paget's disease is a disorder of bone remodeling that typically begins with excessive bone resorption followed by an increase in bone formation. This **osteoclastic overactivity** followed by **compensatory osteoblastic activity** leads to a structurally disorganized mosaic of bone, which is weaker, larger, less compact, more vascular, and more susceptible to fracture.

371. The major complication of the Paget disease would be:
- a. Altered level of consciousness
- b. Tetany
- c. Severe hypocalcemia
- d. Pathological fracture

Ans.

359.	d
360.	c
361.	a
362.	b
363.	c
364.	c
365.	a
366.	c
367.	a
368.	b
369.	a
370.	b
371.	d

372. Calcitonin is useful in the condition of Paget's disease because it inhibits:
a. Osteoblast activity
b. Osteoclast activity
c. Osteocyte activity
d. Osteocyst activity

373. The expansion of 'POTS' would be:
a. Postural orthostatic tachycardia syndrome
b. Post orthostatic tachycardia syndrome
c. Postural orthostatic tibial syndrome
d. Postural orthopenic tachycardia syndrome

RHABDOMYOLYSIS

Muscular System

374. Rhabdomyosarcoma in children originates in:
a. Cerebrum b. Kidney
c. Striated muscles d. Tendons

375. A child is diagnosed with pheochromocytoma. Which of the following post-manifestation will indicate that the child is in crisis?
a. Diastolic blood pressure 75 mm Hg
b. Heart rate of 98 beats per min
c. Rhabdomyolysis
d. Urine output of 30 mL/hr

Explanation: A pheochromocytoma is a rare, usually noncancerous (benign) tumor that develops in an adrenal gland. Complications of pheochromocytoma include rhabdomyolysis and acute renal failure. Rhabdomyolysis is a potentially life-threatening syndrome resulting from the breakdown of skeletal muscle fibers with leakage of muscle contents into the circulation. So the nurse should be alert and assess for the complications of rhabdomyolysis.

376. Which laboratory findings indicate the presence of rhabdomyolysis?
a. Elevation in creatinine kinase
b. Elevation of bleeding time
c. Increased PT
d. Decreased PT

Explanation: The most reliable test in the diagnosis of rhabdomyolysis is the level of creatine kinase (CK) in the blood. This enzyme is released by damaged muscle, and levels are seen above 1000 U/L.

377. What is the most common life-threatening complication of rhabdomyolysis?
a. Acute kidney injury b. Flapping tremor
c. Tinnitus d. Hemorrhage

Explanation: Acute kidney injury is the most life-threatening complication due to the accumulation of myoglobin which is nephrotoxic.

378. What is the color of urine for a client with rhabdomyolysis?
a. Red b. Brown
c. Straw color d. Orange

Explanation: Client with rhabdomyolysis had brown color urine due to the excretion of myoglobin in the urine (myoglobinuria).

379. The acute necrosis of the skeletal muscle fibers that leads to the leakage of cellular content in the actual circulation is called:
a. Agranulocytosis b. Wilson disease
c. Rhabdomyolysis d. Paget disease

380. Following are the intracellular content dumped in the circulation while the person is suffering from rhabdomyolysis; EXCEPT:
a. Myoglobin, CK b. Bence jones protein
c. Lactate dehydrogenase d. Aspartate aminotransferase

Explanation: Bence Jones protein is made by plasma cells and is found in the urine of most people with multiple myeloma. It is not associated with rhabdomyolysis.

381. The most sensitive and reliable indicator for the condition of muscle injury would be:
a. Elevated serum CK b. Bence jones protein
c. Lactate dehydrogenase d. Aspartate aminotransferase

Explanation: Creatine kinase (CK) is present in the highest concentrations in serum in response to muscle injury. CK is the most sensitive indicator of muscle injury, and is the best measure of the course of muscle injury.

382. The client got admitted to the ER with the diagnosis of Rhabdomyolysis. The nursing priority action would be:
a. Check the patient weight
b. Whole body physical examination
c. Measure the abdominal circumference
d. Initiate Rehydration therapy

Explanation: Fluid therapy (rehydration) aimed at increasing urine output is a commonly employed strategy to prevent acute kidney injury (AKI) in critically ill patients with rhabdomyolysis.The ideal fluid regimen for patients with rhabdomyolysis consists of half isotonic saline (0.45%), to which 75 mmol/L sodium bicarbonate is added.

383. The development of rhabdomyolysis with the clinical feature of muscle tenderness or myalgia is an adverse reaction to:
a. ACE inhibitor b. Statin drugs
c. Calcium channel blocker d. Hormonal therapy

Explanation: Rhabdomyolysis is a well-documented side effect of statin therapy. This risk is increased with concurrent use of medications that inhibit cytochrome, such as macrolide antibiotics. Simvastatin is the most common statin reported in association with rhabdomyolysis.

SPINAL COLUMN DEFORMITIES

384. Pain and muscle spasm associated with disc herniation can be managed with:
a. Lie down in supine position
b. Teach muscle strengthening exercises
c. Always wear belt
d. Use of cold and hot compresses along with analgesics

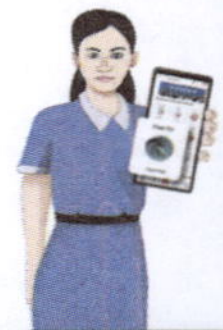

Ans.
372. b
373. a
374. c
375. c
376. a
377. a
378. b
379. c
380. b
381. a
382. d
383. b
384. d

385. Anterior curvature of the spine is called:
a. Lordosis b. Kyphosis
c. Scoliosis d. Osteomalacia

386. Posterior curvature of the spine is called:
a. Lordosis b. Kyphosis
c. Scoliosis d. Osteomalacia

387. Lateral curvature of spine is called:
a. Lordosis b. Kyphosis
c. Scoliosis d. Osteomalacia

388. What is the main goal of therapy a nurse should explain the parent that his child is diagnosed with scoliosis?
a. Prepare the surgery required for scoliosis
b. Restrict the development of curvature
c. Reduce the complication from immobilization
d. Prepare the pain management protocol

Explanation: The main goal is to limit the progression of the curve. Not all the client required surgery for scoliosis.

389. A young child with exaggerated lumbar curve is diagnosed as:
a. Scoliosis b. Lordosis
c. Kyphosis d. Kyphoscoliosis

Explanation: Lordosis involves lumbar curve, scoliosis involves lateral curve, kyphoscoliosis involves both curve in a same individual, kyphosis involves thoracic curve.

390. Lordosis is common in the children before the age of:
a. 2 years b. 4 years
c. 5 years d. 6 years

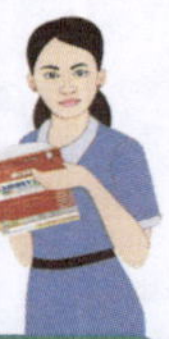

CARPAL TUNNEL SYNDROME

391. Carpal tunnel syndrome is caused by the compression of: *(AIIMS-BBS SNO 2019, JIPMER 2012)*
a. The median nerve b. The radial nerve
c. The ulnar nerve d. The femoral nerve

392. Which of the following test is used for the identification of carpal tunnel syndrome?
a. Allen's test b. Phalen's test
c. Spurling test d. Trendelenburg test

Explanation: Phalen's maneuver is positive when flexing the wrist to 90 degrees for 1 minute elicits symptoms in the median nerve distribution.

393. Tinel's sign test is used to diagnose which disease?
a. Carpal tunnel syndrome b. Buerger's disease
c. Varicose vein d. Deep vein thrombosis

Explanation: Phalen's test and Tinel's test are used as part of a comprehensive evaluation to assist in the diagnosis of nerve-related conditions, and the results are interpreted in conjunction with other clinical findings and diagnostic tests. Both these tests are used to diagnose carpal tunnel syndrome.

394. Which of the following drug may cause carpal tunnel syndrome?
a. Acetazolamide b. Anastrozole
c. Letrozole d. Exemestane

395. Carpal tunnel syndrome is more commonly in:
a. Adult b. Children
c. Men d. Women

396. All of the following persons are prone to develop carpel tunnel syndrome; EXCEPT:
a. Massage therapist b. Waver workers
c. Computer workers d. Security guard

397. All of the following are appropriate interventions to treat patients with carpel tunnel syndrome; EXCEPT:
a. NSAIDS b. Cryosurgery
c. Wrist splint d. Corticosteroids

Explanation: Non-pharmacological Interventions for carpal tunnel syndrome include wrist splinting, NSAIDs, corticosteroids and cryotherapy (ice packs), not cryosurgery.

398. The following are the clinical features seen in Carpel tunnel syndrome; EXCEPT:
a. Pain b. Tingling
c. Numbness d. Contusion

399. Comparatively which gender is more prevalent to develop carpel tunnel syndrome?
a. Male b. Female
c. Equal ratio
d. There is no sufficient data to conclude

Explanation: Women are three times more likely to develop carpal tunnel syndrome than men. In large part, it's due to anatomical differences; the average woman's carpal tunnel (wrist) is simply narrower than men.

AMPUTATION OF THE LOWER EXTREMITIES

400. The nurse is caring for a patient immediately after a below-knee amputation. Which of these assessments should the nurse consider a priority? *(RAK MSc 2018)*
a. Sacral edema b. Mobility
c. Stump dressing d. Blood sugar level

Explanation: The priority intervention would be stump dressing as if it is not done periodically or ignored may cause change in shape of stump, edema or interferes with shrinking of stump that later creates a problem for making a properly fitted prosthesis.

401. The nurse is caring for a patient who underwent above-knee amputation 48 hours before. The nurse is aware that the edema in the stump can be managed by: *New Q*
a. Keeping abduction pillow in between
b. Providing Trendelenburg position
c. Keeping the remaining limb elevated on a pillow
d. Rewraping the elastic bandage as necessary

Explanation: After above-knee amputation, elevating the limb is generally not recommended after 24 hours of postoperative period. Elevating the limb can indeed lead to contractures and should be avoided. Rewrapping the elastic bandage as necessary is a better option to manage edema after an amputation. This will help to drain the fluid from the tissues and prevent it from accumulating.

402. For the first 24 hours after surgery, above-knee amputation stump should be elevated.
a. To prevent edema
b. To prevent hip flexion contractures
c. To promote hemostasis
d. To promote healing

Ans.

385.	a
386.	b
387.	c
388.	b
389.	b
390.	c
391.	a
392.	b
393.	a
394.	b
395.	d
396.	d
397.	b
398.	d
399.	b
400.	c
401.	d
402.	a

Explanation: For the first 24 hours after surgery, keep the residual limb raised on one to two pillows to prevent edema. After 24 hours, keep the residual limb flat on the bed to prevent hip flexion contractures (tightening).

403. A patient who recently underwent amputation of a leg complains of pain in the amputated part. The nurse should explain to the patient which of the following?

(AIIMS Bhopal Grade-I 2018)

a. The patient is experiencing central pain syndrome
b. The pain cannot exist because the leg has been amputated
c. The pain is a phenomenon known as "ghost pain"
d. The pain is a real experience for the patient

Explanation: Ghost pain (Phantom pain) sensations are described as perceptions that an individual experiences relating to an limb or an organ that is not physically a part of the body (amputation or limb loss).

DISORDERS OF LOWER LIMB

404. A painful condition that occurs when pressure within the muscles builds to dangerous levels that decreases the blood flow is known as:
a. Compartment syndrome
b. Myasthenia gravis
c. Parkinsonism
d. Neuroleptic malignant syndrome

405. In adolescents, Osgood-Schlatter disease is a common cause of pain and swelling in the:
a. Lateral aspect of ankle
b. Inferior aspect of knee
c. Dorsal aspect of foot
d. Proximal aspect of humerous

406. Foot drop is caused by damage to:
a. Interosseous nerve
b. Superficial peroneal nerve
c. Deep peroneal nerve
d. Deltoid ligament of the ankle joint

407. Pain in the calf with dorsiflexion of the foot is known as:
a. Homan's sign b. Trousseau sign
c. Chvostek sign d. Kernig's sign

Explanation: Pain in the calf with dorsiflexion of the foot is known as Homan's sign. Homan's sign indicates thrombophlebitis or thrombosis or deep vein thrombosis (DVT).

408. Which of the following structure is not usually visualized during the arthroscopy of the knee?
a. Meniscus b. Cruciate ligament
c. Collateral ligament d. Patella articular surface

409. Cotton's fracture involves:
a. Knee b. Spine
c. Ankle d. Foot

410. Cobra plating is used to stabilize fracture of:
a. Patellar fracture b. Hip fracture
c. Tibia Fracture d. Calcaneal fracture

411. What is the classical example of muscular violence?
a. Fracture of clavicle b. Fracture of fibula
c. Fracture of Patella d. Fracture of pelvis

412. Haglund deformity is associated with?
a. Wrist b. Elbow
c. Knee d. Ankle

Explanation: Prominence of posterosuperior portion of calcaneus leading to heel pain is called Haglund deformity.

413. A 35-year-old male patient comes with a complaint of lower limb weakness. During physical examination, the patient is placed in a supine position. The examiner places one hand under the patient heel and patient is then asked to raise his other leg against downward resistance. What is the test being performed?
a. Waddell's test b. McBride test
c. Hoover's test d. O'donoghue's test

Explanation: The purpose of the Hoover's test is to differentiate between functional (no definitive neurological pathology) or organic paresis (identifiable cause). The patient is placed in supine position. The examiner's hand is placed under the non-paralyzed heel, and the patient is asked to elevate the paralyzed leg. In organic paresis the examiner feels a downward pressure under the non-paralyzed heel; in malingering no pressure is felt.

414. Which of the following traction is not used in lower limb?
a. Gallow's traction b. Bryant traction
c. Perkin traction d. Dunlop traction

CONGENITAL DEFORMITIES

415. Most common congenital anomaly of face is:
a. Cleft lip with or without palate
b. Cleft palate only
c. Cleft lip with cleft palate
d. Submucous cleft palate

416. Cleft lip is due to non-fusion of:
a. Maxillary process with lateral nasal process
b. Maxillary process with medial nasal process
c. Maxillary process with mandibular process
d. All of the above

417. What is the talocalcaneal angle in club foot?
a. 15 to 35 degree b. Less than 15 degree
c. More than 35 degree d. None of the above

418. What is the name of the splint used for club foot?
a. Denis browne splint b. Milwaukee brace
c. Cock up splint d. Thomas splint

Explanation:

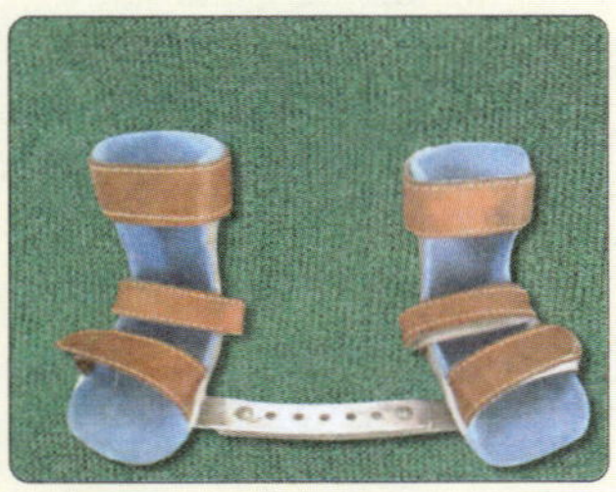

The Denis Browne Bar, also known as the Denis Browne Splint or foot abduction orthosis, is a medical device used in the treatment of club foot.

Ans.

403. c
404. a
405. b
406. c
407. a
408. c
409. c
410. b
411. c
412. d
413. c
414. d
415. a
416. b
417. b
418. a

GASTROINTESTINAL AND HEPATOBILIARY SYSTEM

GASTROINTESTINAL SYSTEM

Anatomy and Physiology of Gastrointestinal System

- Gastrointestinal (GI) system extends from mouth to anus and the total length is 23–26 feet.
- Part of GI system includes mouth, pharynx, esophagus, stomach, small intestine, large intestine, rectum and anus.

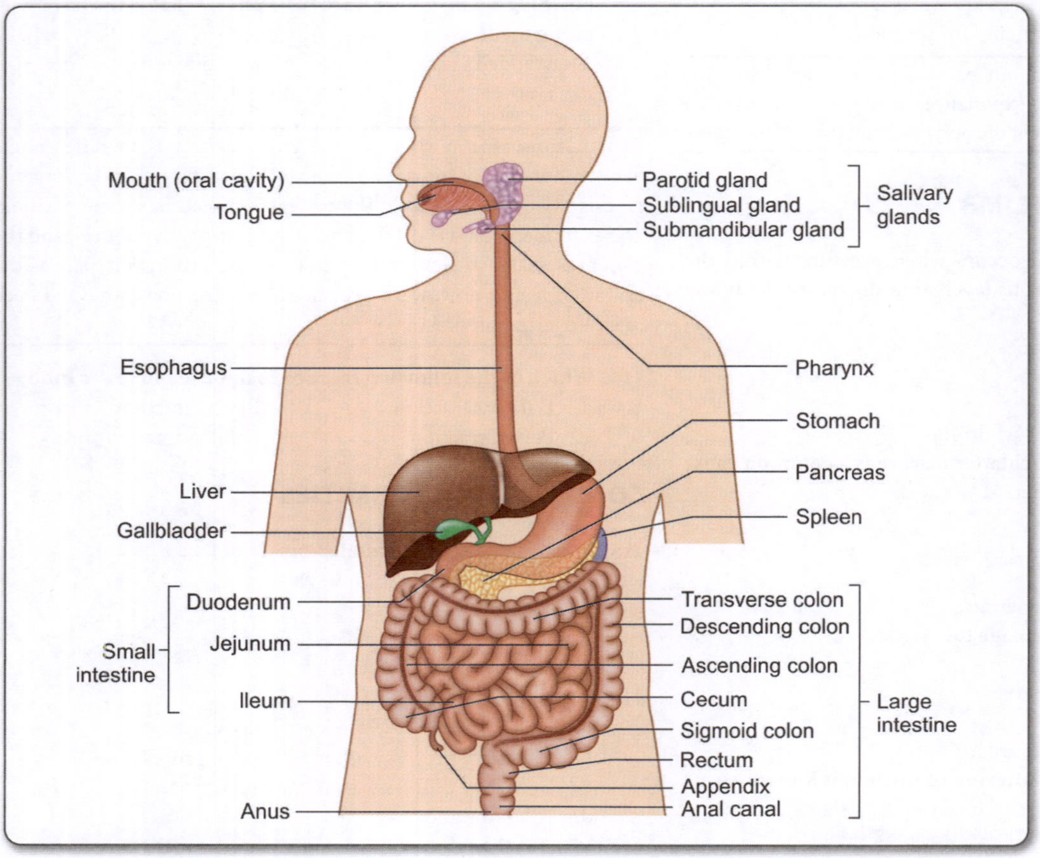

Figure 20: Gastrointestinal system

Mouth

- Mouth is the first site of digestion.
- Three pairs of salivary glands are named as:
  - Parotid
  - Submaxillary (submandibular), and
  - Sublingual glands secrete saliva to the oral cavity.
- Approximately 1.5 L of saliva is secreted daily.

KEY POINT

Average length of Gastrointestinal tract—7–9 meters (23–30 feet)

Recent Questions (NORCET 2020)

7. Which of the following vitamin deficiency leads to bleeding gums?
  a. Vitamin C
  b. Vitamin A
  c. Vitamin B
  d. Vitamin K

Ans. (a) Vitamin C

8. Oral white patches commonly seen in infants which bleed on touching are:
  a. Pancytopenia
  b. Leukoplakia
  c. Leucopenia
  d. Myeloma

Ans. (b) Leukoplakia

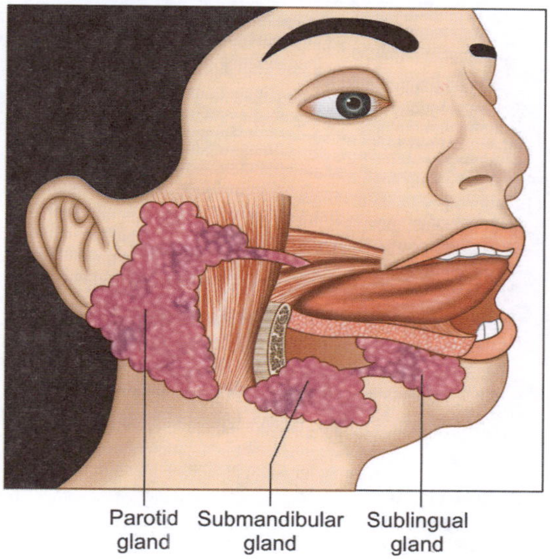

Figure 21: Salivary glands

- Parotid is the largest salivary gland
- Mumps (Viral infection) affects parotid gland
- Submaxillary gland is the gland with the longest duct

Esophagus

- Esophagus a collapsible tube of **25 cm length**
- Located in the mediastinum of thoracic cavity
- It is located anterior to the spine and posterior to the trachea and heart.
- It passes through the diaphragm at an opening called the **diaphragmatic hiatus**.
- Upper esophageal sphincter prevents the entry of air into the esophagus; lower esophageal sphincter prevents gastroesophageal reflux disease (GERD).

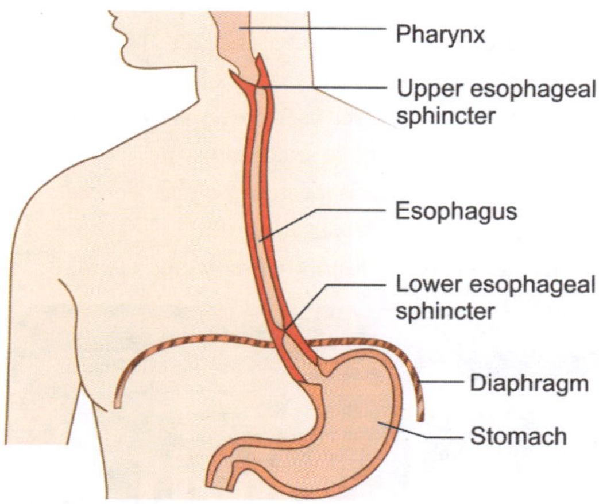

Figure 22: Esophagus

- If lower esophageal sphincter fails to close properly, it leads to GERD and then to Barrett's esophagus.
- Upper portion of esophagus and the external sphincter of the anus are under voluntary control; and remaining portions are involuntary in control

KEY POINTS

- Hard palate - Anterior part of palate formed by maxilla and palatine bone.
- Soft palate - Posterior part of palate.
- Odynophagia refers to pain with swallowing, typically in the chest.
- Lactobacillus acidophilus is the common normal flora of oral cavity
- The **cardiac sphincter** (lower esophageal sphincter) located at the junction of the esophagus and the stomach prevents the regurgitation of food and acids back into the esophagus.
- **Upper esophageal sphincter (UES) or Cricopharyngeus sphincter** is located in the upper part of esophagus and the stomach prevents the reflux of foods from the esophagus into the throat.
- **Achalasia** - Failure of the lower esophageal sphincter to relax

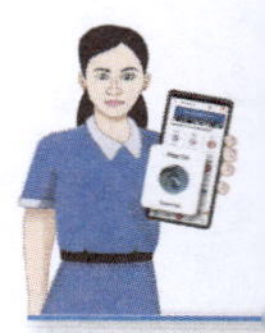

Stomach

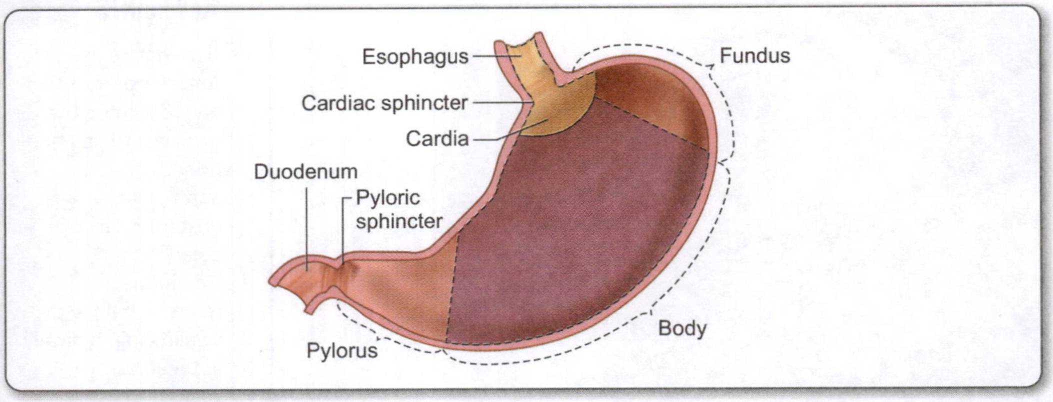

Figure 23: Stomach

- Stomach is a distensible pouch located left to the midline just under the left diaphragm.
- Capacity - 1500 mL.
- The inlet of esophagus into the stomach is known as **esophagogastric junction**
- Esophagogastric junction is surrounded by a ring of smooth muscle known as lower esophageal sphincter or **cardiac sphincter**
- Stomach is divided into four anatomic regions:
  - Cardiac (entrance),
  - Fundus
  - Body
  - Pylorus (outlet)
- Circular muscle in the wall of pylorus becomes the pyloric sphincter.
- **Pyloric sphincter controls the opening between the stomach and small intestine.**
- **Stomach produces 2.4 L of gastric juice per day.**
- **Gastric chief cells** (zymogenic cells/peptic cells) **secrete pepsinogen** which helps in digestion of protein
- **Parietal cells (oxyntic cells/delomorphous) secrete HCl and intrinsic factor.**
- Intrinsic factor is essential for the absorption of Vit B12.

Small Intestine

- The longest segment of the GI system
- It is divided into three parts:
  - Duodenum (25 cm); shortest part of small intestine
  - Jejunum (8 feet)
  - Ileum (12 feet)
- Absorption of Vit B12 takes place in ileum
- The common bile duct allows the passage of both bile and pancreatic secretion.
- Common bile duct empties into the duodenum at **ampulla of Vater** and this opening is surrounded by sphincter of Oddi.
- **Sphincter of Oddi** contains three sphincters.
- Junction between small intestine and the large intestine is the cecum which is located in the right lower quadrant, ileocecal valve is located here.
- **Ileocecal valve** controls the entry of content into the large intestine as well as it **prevents the reflex of bacteria from large to small intestine**.
- **Vermiform appendix** is located near the ileocecal junction in the right lower quadrant.
- Deficiency of vit B12 results in pernicious anemia.

KEY POINTS

- Body is the central, largest part of the stomach.
- The semifluid mass of partly digested food expelled by the stomach into the duodenum is known as "Chyme".
- **Pyloric stenosis** refers to narrowing of pyloric sphincter.
- Parietal cells produce gastric hydrochloric acid and intrinsic factor.
- Intrinsic factor is essential for the absorption of vitamin B12.
- Chief cells secrete pepsinogen.
- The pH of gastric juice is 1.5 to 3.5.

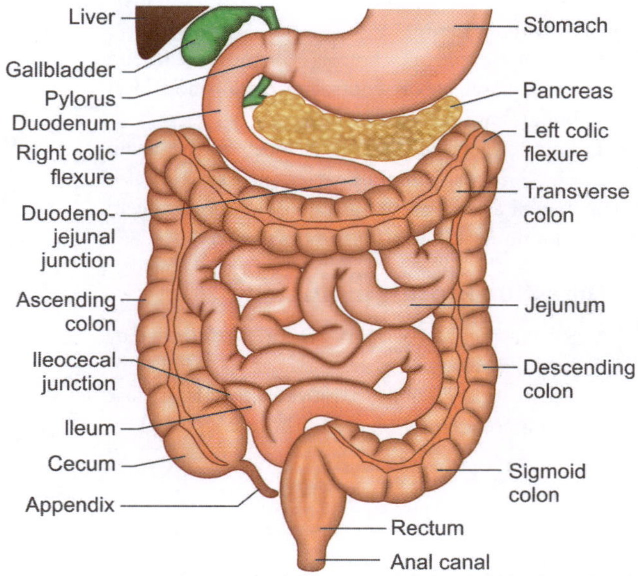

Figure 24: Small intestine and large intestine

Large Intestine

- Total length of large intestine is approximately 1.5 meter and is divided in three parts cecum, colon and rectum.
- Colon is further divided into:
  - Ascending colon (shortest portion of colon)
  - Transverse colon
  - Descending colon
  - Sigmoid colon.
- Rectum continues in an external opening called anus.
- Network of striated muscles forms both internal and external anal sphincters.

Layers of Digestive System

- Layers of digestive system from inner to outer are mucosa, submucosa, muscularis and serosa/adventitia. The description has been summarized as follows:

Table 17: Layers of digestive system

Layer	Description
Mucosa	• Inner most layer contains many of the goblet cells which secrete mucus. • Mucosal layer also contains villi in some of the parts to increase the area of absorption
Submucosa	• Contains nerves including the submucosal plexus (Meissner's plexus), blood vessels and elastic fibers with collagen.
Muscularis	• Comprises both longitudinal and circular smooth muscles which help with continued peristalsis.
Serosa/adventitia	• Outermost layer • Made up of loose connective tissues and coated in mucus so as to prevent any frictional damage from the intestine rubbing against other tissues.

Blood Supply to the GI System

- GI system – Supplied by arteries originating from abdominal and thoracic aorta.
- Stomach – Supplied by gastric artery which is a branch of splenic artery.
- Small Intestine – Superior mesenteric artery branches.
- Colon – Superior mesenteric artery (right colic and middle colic branches) and inferior mesenteric artery (left colic and sigmoid branches)

KEY POINTS

- Ileum (12 feet) is the longest part of small intestine.
- Duodenum (25 cm) is the shortest part of small intestine.
- Blood supply to small intestine: the celiac trunk, superior mesenteric artery, and inferior mesenteric artery.
- Peyer's patches are small masses of lymphatic tissue found throughout the ileum region of the small intestine.
- Tiny projections called villi and microvilli increase the total area for absorption in the small intestine.
- The transverse colon (40–50 cm) is the most mobile and longest part of the large intestine.
- **Blood supply:** The superior mesenteric artery (SMA) and the inferior mesenteric artery (IMA) provide blood supply to the colon.
- The **myenteric plexus (Auerbach's plexus)** is located between the longitudinal and circular muscle layers of the GI tract.
- The **submucosal plexus** (Meissner's plexus) is situated in the submucosal region between the circular muscle and mucosa.

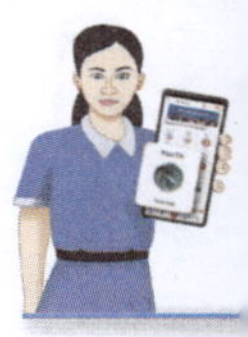

- Venous drainage of the GI system is unique, because the venous blood from the GI organs merges to form large vessel called portal vein. Nutrient rich blood in the **portal vein** enters the liver and undergoes detoxification process before it enters into the general circulation.

Nerve Supply to the GI System

- Both sympathetic and parasympathetic nervous system supply the GI system
- Sympathetic nervous system exerts inhibitory action on GI system, i.e., it decreases gastric secretion, motility and constriction of sphincter and blood vessels
- Sympathetic nervous system slows down GI activity; and parasympathetic nervous system speeds up the GI activity.
- GI system has its own nerve supply called enteric nervous system. It's also known as **intrinsic nervous system**.
- Myenteric plexus controls GI movement and submucosal plexus controls secretion and local blood flow.
- Enteric nervous system is one of the main divisions of autonomic nervous system also known as second brain. Enteric nervous system communicates with CNS via vagus nerve.

Digestion Process in Human

- Swallowing is a voluntary act and is controlled by medulla oblongata
- Pancreatic secretions have an alkaline pH because of high concentration of bicarbonate.

Recent Question (CNCI 2021)

9. A 60-year-old man suffering from left colon cancer presented with acute left colonic obstruction and the treatment is__________.
a. Primary resection and Hartman procedure
b. Defunctioning colostomy
c. Right hemicolectomy
d. Resection and end to end anastomosis

Ans. (a) Primary resection and Hartman procedure

Table 18: Enzymes secreted in digestion process in human

Part of the digestive system	Enzyme secreted	Digestion
Mouth	Salivary glands in the mouth secrete saliva which contains **ptyalin or salivary amylase**	• Starch (carbohydrate) digestion begins at mouth. • 30% of starch hydrolyzed by the action of salivary amylase • Starch + salivary amylase give maltose
Pharynx and esophagus	Helps in swallowing and to carry food from mouth to stomach	
Stomach	HCl, intrinsic factor, pepsinogen and pepsin	• Intrinsic factor combines with Vit B12 and helps in its absorption • The mass of food that is semi-digested, acidic and pulpy in the stomach is called the chyme • HCl converts inactive form of pepsinogen to pepsin • Pepsin converts protein into peptones and proteoses. • Prorenin (proenzyme) is converted into renin by HCl. • Casein (milk protein) is converted into peptides by renin.
Small intestine	**Pancreatic juice** trypsinogen, chymotrypsinogen, elastase, carboxypeptidase, pancreatic lipase, and amylase. **Bile and bile salts**	• Enterokinase converts trypsinogen into trypsin • Trypsin converts proteins into dipeptides • Trypsin converts chymotrypsinogen into chymotrypsin. • Chymotrypsin converts peptones into dipeptides. • Fats $\rightarrow$ fatty acids and glycerol with the help of pancreatic lipase and bile salts. • Carbohydrates $\rightarrow$ simple sugars/ monosaccharides with the help of pancreatic amylase.

Waste Products of Digestion

- The brown color of the fecal matter is due to the breakdown of bile by intestinal bacteria.
- Chemicals formed by intestinal bacteria such as **indole and skatole are responsible for fecal odor.**
- Internal anal sphincter is under autonomic nervous system control
- External anal sphincter is under voluntary control of somatic motor neurons (exit spinal cord at S2-S4).

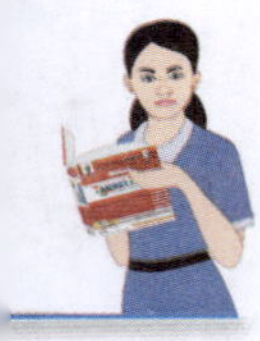

Abdominal Quadrants and Organs

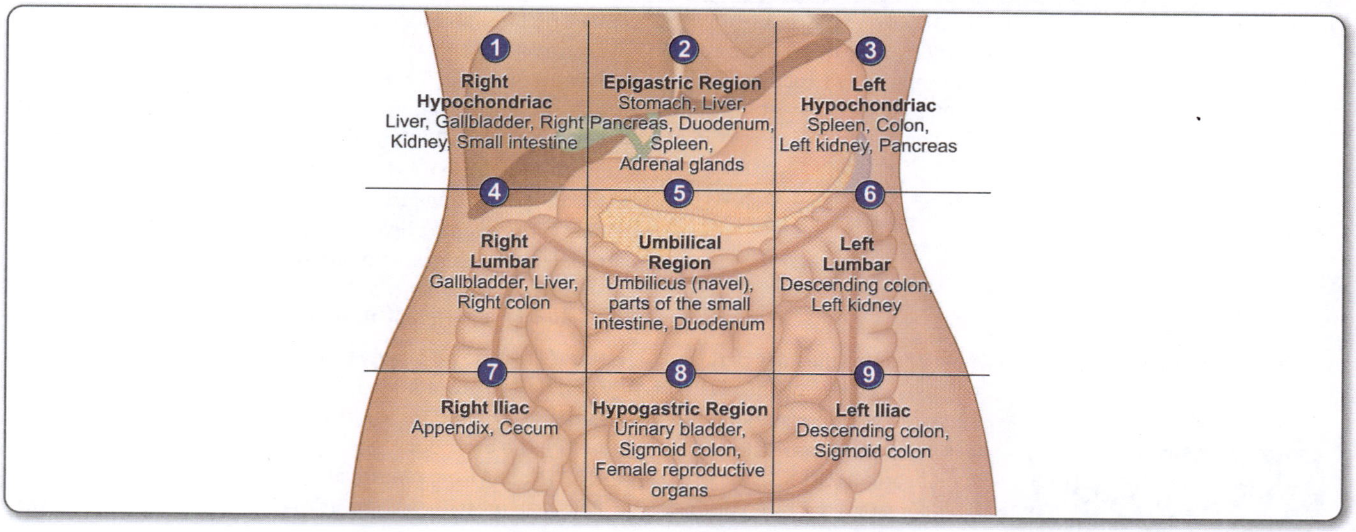

Figure 25: Abdominal quadrants and organs

Diagnostic Evaluation in GI System

Table 19: Diagnostic evaluation

Name of the procedure	Description	Important points to remember
Stool test • Inspecting stool specimen for consistency and color • Stool for occult blood	Stool specimens are collected on random basis unless it's a quantitative study	• Random sample should be sent to the lab immediately • Quantitative specimen should be refrigerated until they are taken to the laboratory. • Stool for occult blood is a screening test to detect colon cancer in the early stage. • In stool, occult blood testing is done to detect heme, the iron containing pigment of hemoglobin. • This test is contraindicated in a patient with hemorrhoidal bleeding • False positive test result can occur in occult blood test if patient has eaten meat, liver, poultry, turnips, broccoli, cauliflower, sardines, within seven days before testing • Medications such as aspirin, ibuprofen, indomethacin, corticosteroids, anti-coagulants, cancer chemotherapeutic agents can cause false positive stool for occult blood result.
Hydrogen breath test	This test determines the amount of hydrogen expelled in breath after it has been produced in colon and absorbed into the blood	• This test is used to evaluate carbohydrate absorption • This test is also helpful to evaluate bacterial overgrowth in the intestine and short bowel syndrome.
Urea breath test	To detect *H. pylori*. Patient is given capsule of carbon labeled urea and then a breath sample is taken after 10–20 minutes. *H. pylori* metabolizes urea rapidly and the labeled carbon gets absorbed quickly. It can be determined by measuring carbon dioxide in the expired air.	**Patient is instructed to avoid:** • **Antibiotics and loperamide:** For one month before the test • **Sucralfate and omeprazole:** For one week before the test • Cimetidine, ranitidine, famotidine and nizatidine - 24 hours before the test

Contd...

Name of the procedure	Description	Important points to remember
Abdominal ultrasonography	In ultrasonogram (USG), high frequency sound waves are passed into internal body structures and ultrasonic echoes are recorded in an oscilloscope.	• USG requires non-ionizing radiation and there is no noticeable side effect. • **Disadvantage:** USG can't examine the structures lying behind bony tissue • Patient fasts for 8–12 hours before the test to decrease gas in the bowel. • If USG is to be done to study gallbladder conditions, **fat free diet in the evening before procedure is advised** • If USG and barium studies are planned on same day, then USG has to be conducted before barium study, otherwise barium will interfere with sound wave transmission.
Upper GI tract study Or Barium swallow 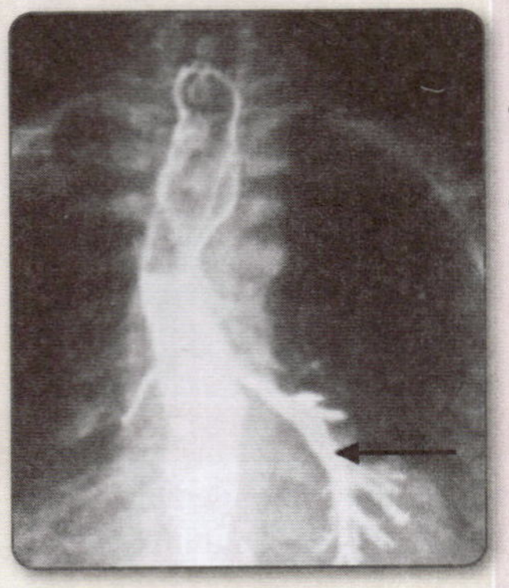	• A radiopaque liquid like barium sulfate is ingested by the client. • It's tasteless, odorless, non-granular, completely insoluble and non-absorbable liquid. • Multiple X-rays are taken during the procedures. • In double contrast study, first a thick barium suspension is given to outline the GI tract following that a tablet which releases carbon dioxide in presence of water is given.	• **Assess for known allergy toward iodine, shelly fish or sea food before procedure** • Patient is advised to maintain low residue diet several days before the procedure • NPO (Noting from mouth) after midnight before the test • Physician prescribes laxatives to clean the GI tract before the procedure • Ask patient to refrain from smoking in the morning before the examination • Withhold all medications which have influence on GI system • After the procedure, fluids are encouraged to eliminate contrast agent from the tract. • **Stool color will be changed to chalky white while barium sulfate is getting eliminated.** • If patient is getting T. metformin, this needs to be withheld and alternative medicines need to be taken as it can cause lactic acidosis by combining with contrast agent.
Capsule endoscopy 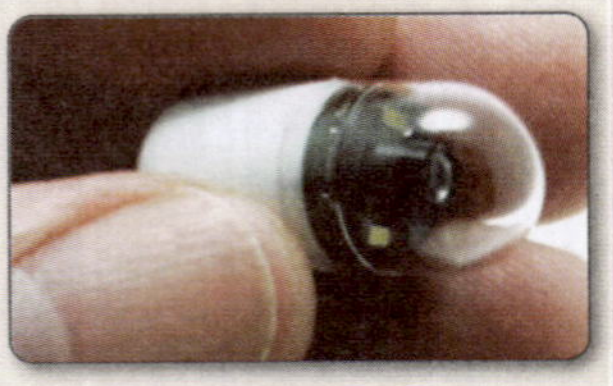	• A small camera which looks like a capsule will be swallowed and it will take series of pictures of GI cavity and it will send to externally worn source. • After 8–72 hours, this capsule will be eliminated from the body, naturally.	• NPO after midnight before the procedure • Bowel preparation with laxatives before the procedure
Lower GI tract study Or Barium enema 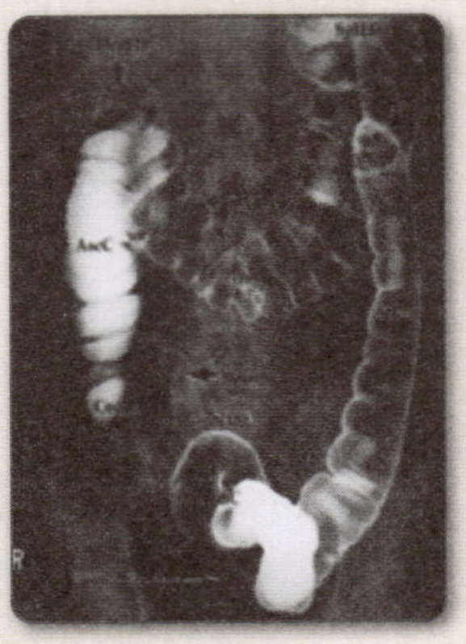	When barium is instilled via rectum to visualize GI tract, it's known as barium enema. In double contrast or air contrast enema, air will be instilled following barium. In this study, air will be filled in the lumen which is lined with barium and allows easy detection of small lesions.	• The purpose of barium enema is to detect polyps, tumors and other lesions in the GI tract. • Bowel preparation is necessary before the procedure • Assess known allergy toward iodine, shelly fish or sea food before procedure. • Cramping and discomfort are expected in double contrast enema • Low residue diet two days before the procedure • Clear liquid diet and laxatives in the evening before the procedure • NPO after midnight • Cleansing enema in the morning on the day of procedure • **If upper GI study is also there, it has to be done following lower GI study** • **Barium enema study is contraindicated in clients with perforation, obstruction and active GI bleeding.** • Fluids are encouraged after the study to eliminate contrast. • Stool color will be changed to chalky white while barium sulfate is getting eliminated. • If patient is getting T. metformin, this needs to be withheld as it can cause lactic acidosis by combining with contrast agent.

Contd...

Name of the procedure	Description	Important points to remember
Computed tomography	Cross-sectional images of abdominal organ and structures are taken.	• NPO 6–8 hours before the procedure • If CT scan is performed with contrast agent, allergy needs to be assessed. • If barium study is also there, it has to be scheduled after CT scan
MRI	• Non-invasive technique which uses magnetic field and radio waves to produce image. • It's useful in evaluating abdominal soft tissue and blood vessels.	• MRI is contraindicated in patients with permanent pacemaker, artificial heart valve, implantable defibrillator, implanted insulin pumps and metal device • NPO 6–8 hours before the procedure • Remove all the jewelry and metallic things from body before the procedure • Client with claustrophobia may require sedation before the procedure • Inform the client that knocking sound may be heard during the procedure
Gastrointestinal motility studies	Liquid and solid component of food mixed with radionuclide markers.	• After ingestion of food, the patient is placed under scintiscanner. This measures the rate of passage of radioactive food out of the stomach • This procedure is done to study the gastric emptying and colonic passage time
Upper gastrointestinal fibroscopy Or Esophagogastroduodenoscopy	• Fibroscope is flexible tube with fibro optic lenses which allow the visualization of esophagus, stomach and duodenum.	• It can be used as both therapeutic and diagnostic purposes • After patient is sedated, fibroscope is lubricated with jelly and slowly passed through the mouth. • Patient wears a mouth guard to protect the scope from biting. • NPO 6–12 hours before the procedure • Atropine may be administered to decrease the secretions • Sometimes glucagon may be given to relax sphincters • Left lateral position will be given during and after the procedure. • After the procedure, patient will be advised to eat or drink after the return of gag reflex. • Post procedure complications include perforation, bleeding, elevated temperature and difficulty in swallowing
Endoscopic retrograde cholangiopancreatography (ERCP)	• Side viewing flexible endoscope is used to view common bile duct, hepatic duct and pancreatic duct through ampulla of Vater in the duodenum.	
Anoscopy, proctoscopy and sigmoidoscopy	• Anoscope used for visualization of anus and rectum • Proctoscope for the visualization of rectum • Sigmoidoscope is used for the visualization of sigmoid colon	• Patient is positioned in knee chest position and the back of the table is inclined about 45° • During the procedure, patient feels an urge to have bowel movement • Enema before the procedure until the returns are clear. • After the procedure, observe the patient for bleeding and signs of intestinal perforation (fever, rectal drainage, abdominal distention and pain).
Fiberoptic colonoscopy	Direct visualization of colon and cecum	• This can be diagnostic and therapeutic • Patient positioned initially on left side with legs drawn toward the chest • Patient's position is kept on changing during the procedure • Enema before the procedure • Limit the intake of fluids 24–72 hours before the procedure • Patient is advised to maintain clear liquid diet at noon, the day before the procedure • NPO after mid night

Disorders of Gastrointestinal System

Disorders of Lips, Mouth and Gums

The disorders of lips, mouth and gums have been discussed here as follows:

Table 20: Disorders of lip, mouth and gum

Name of the condition	Description	Intervention
Chancre 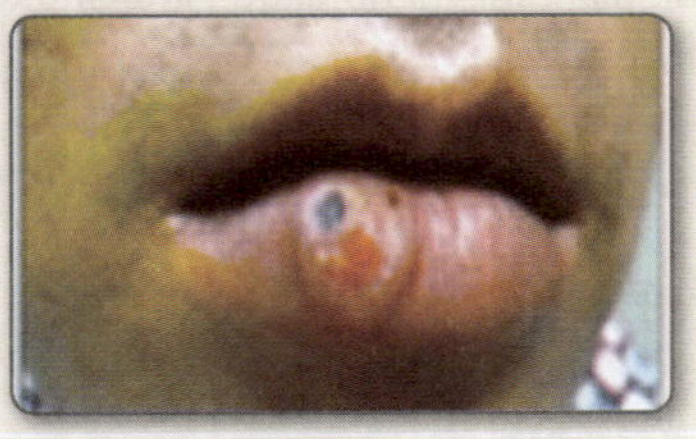	• Reddened circumscribed lesions that ulcerates and become crusted • It is the primary lesion of syphilis and is contagious.	• Cold soak to lips and mouth care • Antibiotic
Leukoplakia 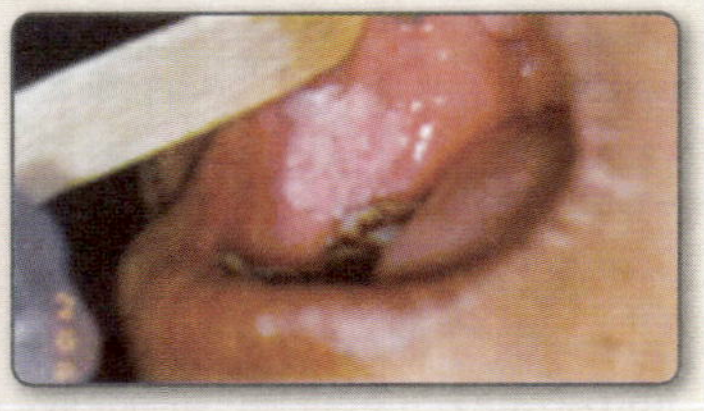	White patches in the buccal mucosa which are usually painless	Instruct patient to consult doctor if it is persisting for more than two weeks
Hairy leukoplakia 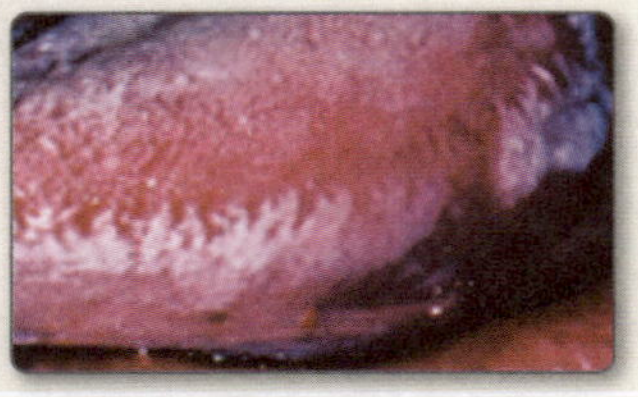	• White patches with hair-like projections most commonly occur along the lateral borders of tongue. • Often seen among HIV patients and patient with tobacco use.	Valaciclovir Gentian violet
Oral Lichen planus 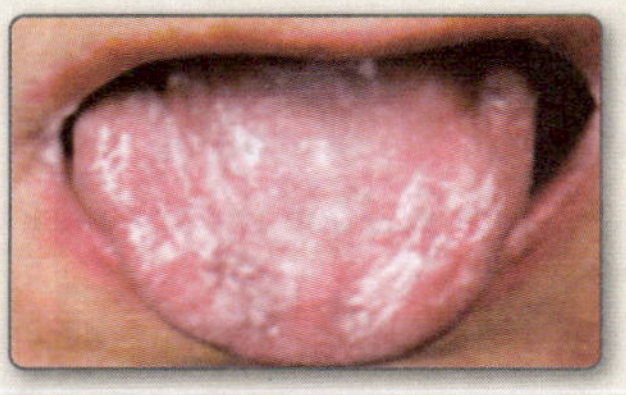	White papules which are painful and usually ulcerated. It may develop as malignancy.	• Corticosteroid administration • Avoidance of irritating substance
Candidiasis 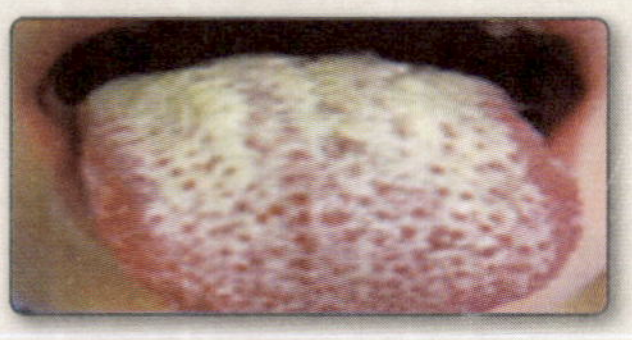	• Cheesy white plaque that looks like milk curd. If rubbed, it will bleed. • Causative organism is *Candida albicans* (fungus)	Antifungal medications
Kaposi sarcoma 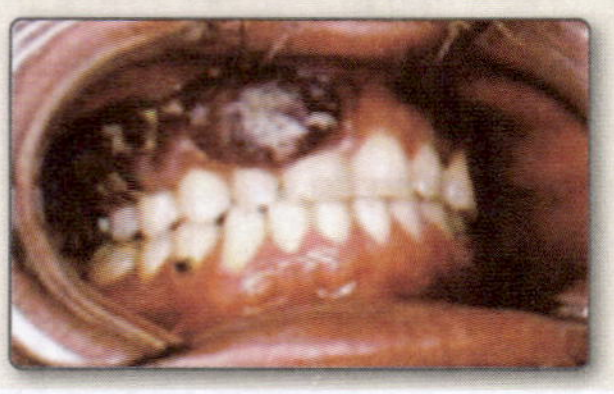	• Appears first in the oral mucosa as red, purple or blue lesions • Seen in patient with HIV infection	Radiation therapy Chemotherapy Surgical excision

Contd...

Name of the condition	Description	Intervention
Gingivitis 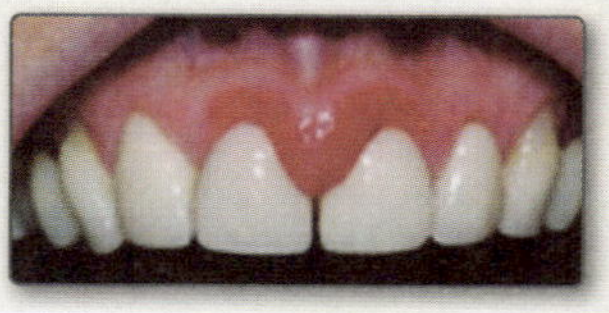	Inflammation of gums	Follow good oral hygiene
Dental plaque 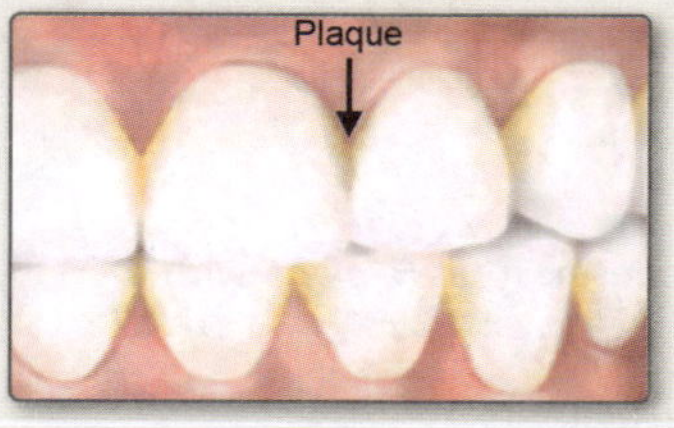	Gel-like substance adheres to the teeth	Effective mouth care
Periapical abscess 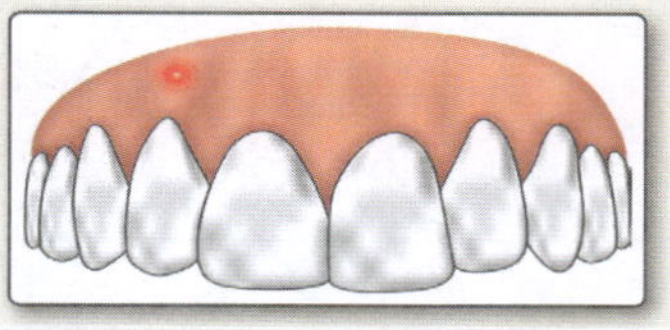	Abscessed tooth with collection of pus in the apical dental periosteum	Aspiration of pus by dental surgeon
Parotiditis 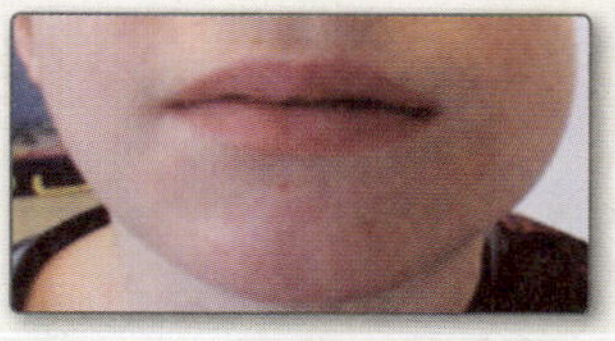	• Inflammation of parotid salivary gland • Most common organism is *Staphylococcus aureus* (except mumps).	• Good oral hygiene • Discontinue the medications which diminish salivation • Antibiotics and analgesics are also necessary • Parotidectomy is the surgery of choice
Sialadenitis	Inflammation of salivary gland	• Good oral hygiene • Discontinue the medications which diminish salivation • Antibiotics and analgesics • Surgical drainage and excision of the gland and its duct
Sialolithiasis	• Salivary calculi • Most commonly affecting submandibular gland. • Calculi are formed mainly from calcium and phosphate.	Lithotripsy is the procedure of choice
Xerostomia	Dry mouth	• Avoid irritating food and fluids • Increase the fluid intake
Stomatitis 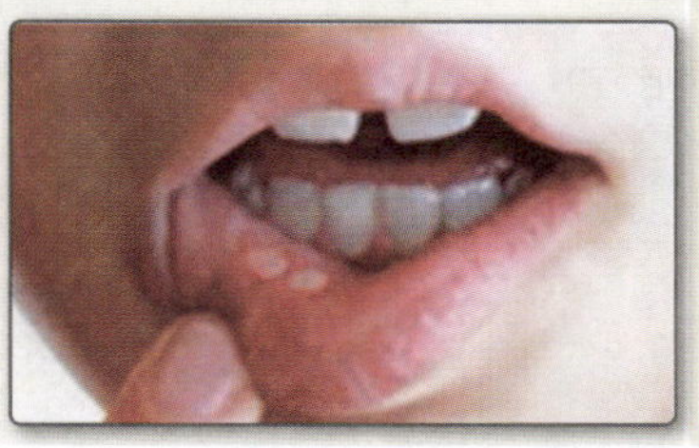	Inflammation of oral/buccal mucosa	Periodic mouth care

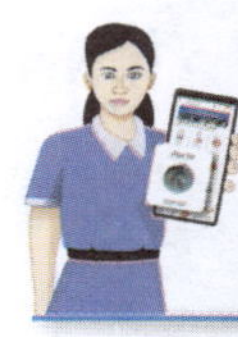

Vincent's Infection

- Vincent's infection is also known as **trench mouth.**
- Vincent's infection is a bacterial infection that affects the gums.
- It is caused by a combination of bacteria, including Fusobacterium nucleatum and Borrelia vincentii.
- The infection is characterized by bleeding gums, bad breath, and painful ulcers in the mouth.

Disorders of Esophagus

Table 21: Disorders of esophagus

Condition	Description	Intervention
Dysphagia	Difficulty in swallowing	
Odynophagia	Painful swallowing	
Dyspepsia	Indigestion Involves discomfort or pain in the upper abdomen	**Functional dyspepsia:** Treat *H. pylori* with antibiotics
Achalasia	Ineffective peristalsis in the distal esophagus and failure of esophageal sphincter to relax	Calcium channel blockers Small frequent feeding and soft diet

Hiatal Hernia

Esophagus enters into the stomach through an opening in the diaphragm known as hiatus.

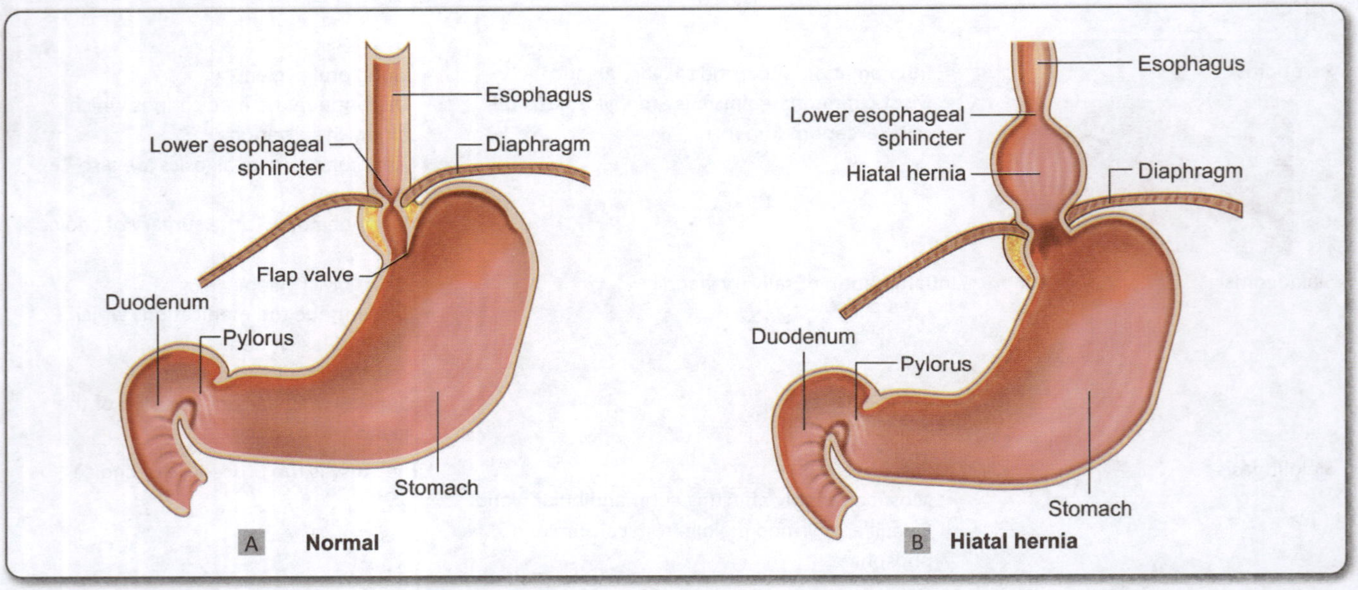

Figures 26A and B: (A) Normal stomach; (B) Hiatal hernia

In hiatal hernia, this opening becomes larger and upper portion of the stomach moves into lower thorax.

Two types are there:

- **Type 1 or sliding:** Upper portion of the stomach and gastro-esophageal junction are displaced and move in and out of the thorax.
- **Type 2 or paraesophageal:** All parts of the stomach move beside the esophagus.

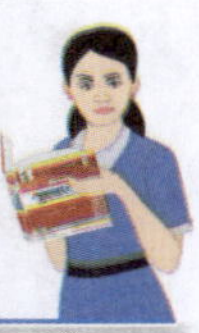

Clinical manifestation

- Heart burn, regurgitation, dysphagia
- Reflux is more commonly seen in sliding type while sense of fullness is seen in paraesophageal type.

Assessment and diagnostic findings

- X-ray, barium study and fluoroscopy

Management

- **Sliding hernia:** Elevation of head end of the bed during and after feeding is needed.
- Surgery is needed for permanent correction of sliding hernia.
- **Paraesophageal hernia:** Emergency surgery is needed to correct torsion.

KEY POINTS

- **Hernia** is a condition in which part of an organ is displaced and protrudes through the wall of the cavity.
- Surgical repair of hernia is known as **herniorrhaphy**.

Esophageal Diverticulum

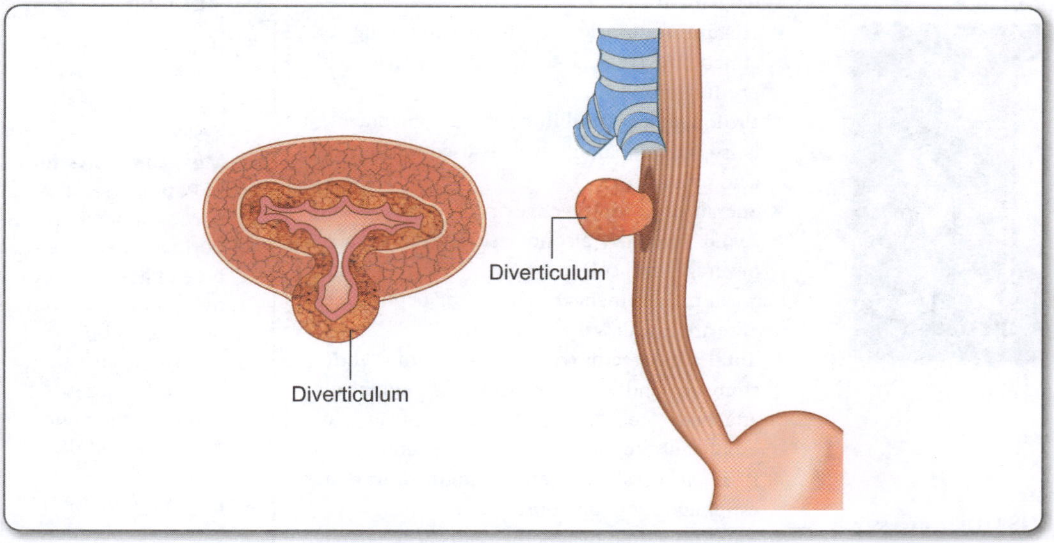

Figure 27: Esophageal diverticulum

- Outpouching of mucosal and submucosal layer through the weak muscularis portion
- **Zenker's diverticulum** or paraesophageal diverticulum: Most commonly seen in the upper portion of the esophagus.
- **Epiphrenic diverticulum:** Largest diverticulum which is seen in the lower portion of the esophagus just above the diaphragm

Clinical manifestation

- **In paraesophageal diverticulum** difficulty in swallowing, fullness in the neck, regurgitation of undigested food.
- Halitosis (bad breath) and sore taste in the mouth are common because of the decomposition of the food retained in the diverticulum.

Assessment and diagnosis

- Barium study
- **Esophageal manometry:** To rule out motion disorders
- **Esophagoscopy is contraindicated** because of the risk of perforation.

Management

- Diverticulectomy is the surgery of choice

Gastroesophageal Reflux Disease (GERD)

- Back flow of gastric or duodenal content into the esophagus

Causes

- Incompetent lower esophageal sphincter (cardiac sphincter), pyloric stenosis or due to a motility disorder.

Clinical manifestation

- Heartburn (pyrosis), dyspepsia, dysphagia, odynophagia, esophagitis

Assessment and diagnostic findings

- **Endoscopy and Barium swallow** to evaluate the damage to mucosa
- Scintigraphy (to assess gastric emptying)
- Ambulatory esophageal pH monitoring: To evaluate degree of acid reflux

Management

- **Dietary modification:** Encourage low fat diet; avoid caffeine, tobacco, beer, carbonated beverages and milk
- Avoid eating and drinking 2 hours before the bed time
- Maintain normal body weight
- Avoid tight fitting clothes
- Elevate head end of the bed and elevate upper part of the body over a pillow
- **Pharmacological Management:**
  - H_2 histamine receptor antagonists (decrease acidity) - Reduce gastric acidity: Ranitidine.
  - Proton pump inhibitors (decrease acidity and increase lower esophageal sphincter tone): Pantoprazole and Omeprazole.
  - **Gastric emptying:** Prokinetic agents: Reglan.
- **Surgery: Nissen fundoplication:** Wrapping of the gastric fundus around the sphincter area of the esophagus

Benign and Malignant Tumor of Esophagus

- Leiomyoma is the most common type of benign esophageal tumor
- Adenocarcinoma is the most common type of malignant tumor of esophagus
- **Dysphagia is the initial symptom** of esophageal cancer

KEY POINTS

- Patient is advised to avoid gas forming food or food containing seeds, nuts or roughage because these food items may be trapped in diverticulum and cause diverticulitis.
- **Meckel's diverticulum** is an outpouching or bulge in the lower part of the small intestine. The bulge is congenital (present at birth) and is a leftover of the umbilical cord.
- Meckel's diverticulum occurs when the **Vitelline duct,** a small tube that connects the fetus's umbilical cord to its small intestine does not fully close during development.
- Complications of gastroesophageal reflux disease include esophagitis, esophageal strictures, aspiration of gastric contents and aspiration pneumonia.

- Characteristic X-ray in cancer of esophagus is bird beak appearance or rat tail appearance

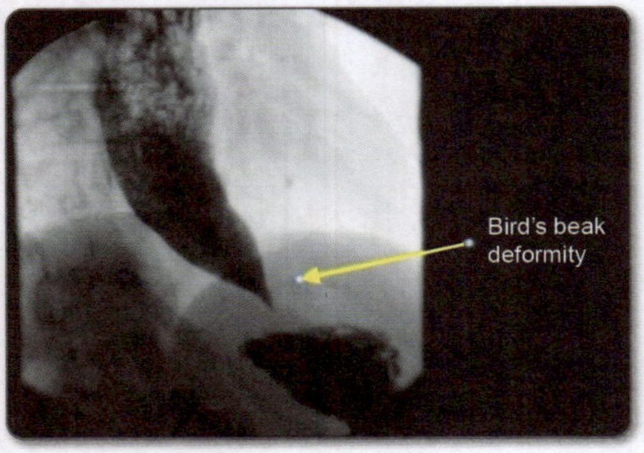

Figure 28: Tumor of esophagus

Gastritis

- Inflammation of gastric mucosa.
- Causes: use of aspirin, NSAIDs, excessive alcohol intake, radiation therapy, bile reflux and microorganism such as *H. pylori*.
- Gastric mucosa becomes edematous, hyperemic and undergoes erosion.

Peptic Ulcer Disease

- Peptic ulcer disease is the erosion of the mucosal wall of stomach, duodenum or in esophagus.
- Based upon the location, it is also called esophageal ulcer, gastric ulcer or duodenal ulcer.
- **Peptic ulcer is more commonly seen in duodenum.**
- Abdominal pain with burning sensation is the **most common symptom** of peptic ulcer
- **Causes: *Helicobacter* pylori (*H. pylori*); NSAID**
- **Management**
  - **Histamine blocker** such as ranitidine or cimetidine is used to decrease gastric acid production.
  - **Proton pump inhibitor** such as omeprazole, lansoprazole, pantoprazole is used to suppress acid production.
  - Sucralfate (cytoprotective drug)
  - Avoid smoking, alcohol use and caffeinated beverages and coffee
- Surgical managements of choice for peptic ulcer disease are as follows:
  - **Total gastrectomy:** Removal of entire stomach and some portion of esophagus attached to it and anastomosis of esophagus to jejunum or duodenum. So it is also called **esophagojejunostomy or esophagoduodenostomy**
  - **Vagotomy:** Removal of the vagus nerve supply to stomach and thereby decreases the stimuli for gastric acid secretion
  - **Gastric resection:** Removal of the lower portion of the stomach usually along with vagotomy. It is also called **antrectomy**.
  - **Billroth I:** Partial gastrectomy and anastomosis of remaining stomach to duodenum. It is also called **gastroduodenostomy**.
  - **Billroth II:** Reconstruction after a partial gastrectomy, the duodenal stump is closed and a **gastrojejunostomy** is created.
  - **Pyloroplasty:** Enlargement of pylorus to prevent or decrease pyloric obstruction and thereby enhancing gastric emptying.

KEY POINTS

- **Helicobacter pylori** is the causative agent for chronic gastritis.
- **Most common site of Peptic ulcer:** First part of duodenum
- **Curling's ulcer** is a type of gastroduodenal ulcer due to complication of **burn**. It is due to stress induced decrease in mucus secretion and increased HCl secretion
- **Dumping syndrome** is the complication of **subtotal gastrectomy**.
- **Billroth I Surgery** - Gastroduodenostomy
- **Billroth II Surgery** - Gastrojejunostomy
- **HCl secretion is increased** with the use of milk, caffeinated beverages, smoking and alcohol use.

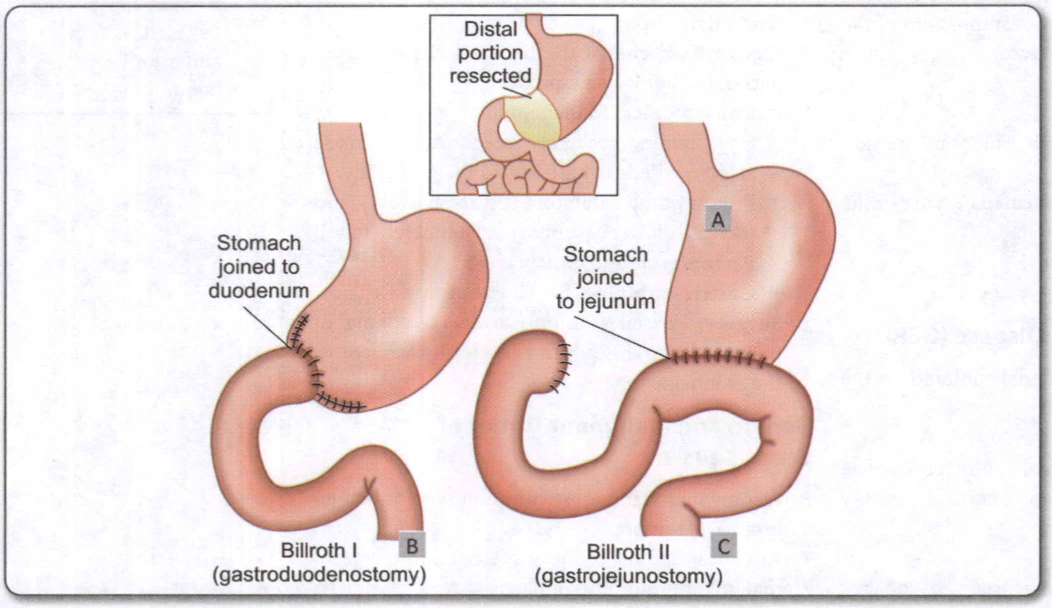

Figures 29A to C: **A.** Resection of distal portion of stomach; **B.** Billroth I; **C.** Billroth II

Table 22: Comparison between gastric and duodenal ulcers

Characteristic	Gastric ulcer	Duodenal ulcer
Incidence Age Male: female	 50 or more 1:1	 30–60 years 2–3:1
Clinical manifestations	• Normal or hypo-secretion of HCl • Weight loss • Pain occurs 30–60 min. after a meal. • **Pain relieved by vomiting** • **Ingestion of food may increase the pain** • Vomiting and hematemesis are seen	• Hyper secretion of HCl • May have weight gain • Pain occur 2–3 hours of eating • Wakes up in the night due to pain • **Ingestion of food may decrease pain** • Vomiting is uncommon • Melena is common • Chances of perforation are more • Rare possibility of malignancy

Gastrointestinal Bleeding

- Bleeding from any part of the GI system is known as GI bleed.
- **Causes:** Peptic ulcer disease, esophageal varices, diverticular disease, ulcerative colitis and tumors.
- **Signs and symptoms**
  - Coffee-ground vomitus
  - Bloody, maroon-colored, or black and tarry stools
  - Anemia in case of chronic GI bleeding.
- **Treatment**
  - Treatment depends on location
  - Gastric lavage
  - A **Sengstaken-Blakemore** tube to control bleeding from esophageal varices
  - Cauterization or endoscopic injection sclerotherapy.

Dumping Syndrome

- Also called rapid gastric emptying.
- Occurs when food moves from stomach to intestine too quickly.
- It is one of the major complications of patients who underwent partial or complete resection of stomach.
- The symptoms occur because of the rapid distention of jejunal loop anastomosed to stomach.
- Hypertonic content in the intestine draw fluids from extracellular circulating volume to dilute the contents in it.
- **Manifestations:** Sensation of fullness, weakness, faint, dizziness, palpitation, diaphoresis, cramping pain, diarrhea and borborygmi (loud gurgles indicating hyperperistalsis)

Patient education to prevent dumping syndrome

- Avoid sugar, salt and milk
- Eat high protein, high fat, low carbohydrate food items
- Eat small meals and avoid consuming fluids along with meal.
- Lie down after eating

Appendicitis

- Appendix is a small finger-like projection attached to cecum below ileocecal valve. Inflammation of this projection is known as appendicitis.
- Fecalith is the most common cause of appendicitis.
- Most commonly occur in adolescents

Clinical Manifestations

- Low grade fever, nausea and vomiting
- **Rebounding tenderness on palpation at McBurney's point.** (it is a point 2/3rd of the way umbilicus to Anterior Superior Iliac Spine)
- **Rovsing sign:** Palpation of left lower quadrant paradoxically elicits pain in the right lower quadrant.

Recent Question
(NORCET 2023)

11. A 32-year-old woman presents in emergency with ruptured gall bladder. Emergency open cholecystectomy surgery performed in the hospital. On the second postop day, she begins to complain of cramping abdominal pain without vomiting. She has a temperature of 99.6 °F, blood pressure is 128/84 mmHg, and pulse is 82/min. Her physical exam reveals absent bowel sounds, a mildly distended abdomen with mild diffuse tenderness without rebound or guarding. Which of the following would most likely the suspected complication associated with this clinical finding?

a. Peritonitis
b. Gastritis
c. Evisceration
d. Dehiscence

Ans. (a) Peritonitis

KEY POINTS

- *H. pylori* is the only bacteria classified as Class I carcinogen by WHO.
- **Gastric balloon is the first inflating balloon** in Sengstaken-Blakemore tube and esophageal balloon is the first deflating balloon.
- The patient with appendicitis usually exhibits the **Rebound tenderness at the McBurney's Point,** it is also called Blumberg's sign.
- **Rovsing's sign** is elicited by palpation of the left lower quadrant, causing pain to be felt in the right lower quadrant. Positive Rovsing's sign is associated with appendicitis.

Recent Question
(CNCI 2021)

10. What is the most common cause of upper GI bleeding?

a. Gastric ulcer
b. Esophageal varices
c. Gastritis
d. Carcinoma stomach

Ans. (a) Gastric ulcer

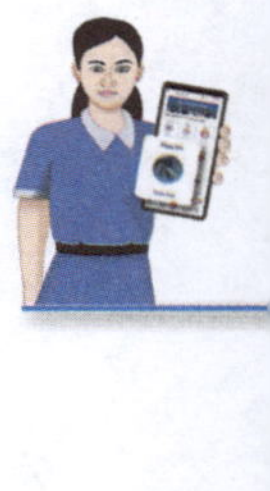

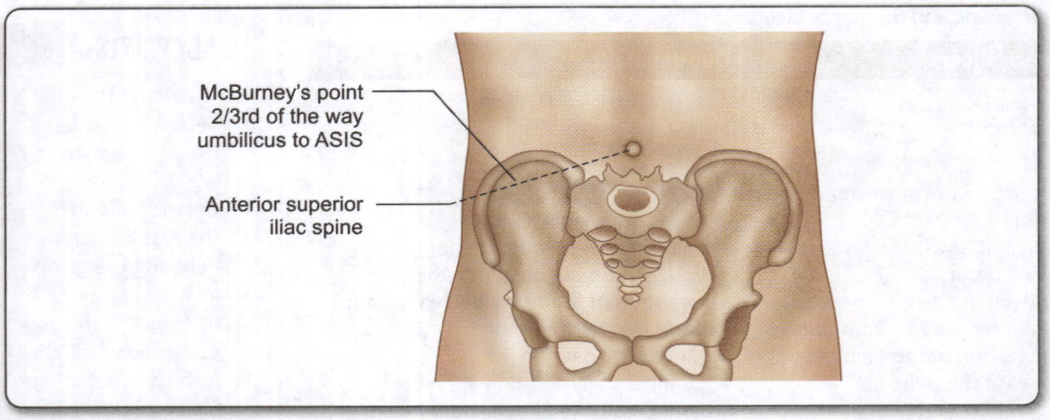

Figure 30: McBurney's point

Assessment and diagnosis
- **Blood test:** Elevation of WBCs
- Abdominal X-ray, USG, CT

Complication
- Perforation of appendix which leads to peritonitis

Management
- Appendectomy

Peritonitis

- **Inflammation of peritoneum,** the serous membrane covering the abdominal cavity.
- Content of abdominal organ leaks into the abdominal cavity as a result of trauma, perforation, infection, or inflammation
- Immediate response of intestinal tract in peritonitis is **hyper motility** followed by **paralytic ileus**.
- **Manifestation:**
    - Diffused pain in the abdomen which becomes constant and localized.
    - Movement may aggravate the pain.
    - Rebound tenderness and paralytic ileus may be present.
    - Elevated leukocyte count and electrolyte abnormalities.
    - Rigid board like abdomen (abdominal rigidity)
- **Diagnosis**
    - X-ray shows air and fluid levels and distended bowel loops.
    - Culture and sensitivity of peritoneal fluid to identify the cause.
- **Management**
    - Fluid, colloid and electrolyte replacement is the major focus of management.
    - **Lung expansion is compromised** due to the compression of intra-abdominal fluid over the lung. So oxygen therapy or intubation is often necessary for airway management.
    - **Massive antibiotic therapy.**
    - **Surgical management** is needed if peritonitis occurred as a result of appendicitis, perforation etc.
    - **Peritonitis patients placed on side with knee flexed. This position will reduce the tension on the abdominal organs.**

Inflammatory Bowel Disease (IBD)

IBD mainly refers to two disease conditions:
1. Regional enteritis (Crohn's disease or granulomatous colitis)
2. Ulcerative colitis.

These two diseases have been summarized as follows:

KEY POINTS
- **Enema, laxatives and hot applications are contraindicated** in case of appendicitis. It may lead to rupture of appendix and peritonitis.
- Fowler's position to minimize pain.
- **After surgery**, place the client in a **semi-Fowler's position.** This will help to reduce tension in suture and abdominal organ.
- **Inflammatory bowel disease (IBD)** is an autoimmune disease which includes Crohn's disease and ulcerative colitis.
- **Ulcerative colitis** is a disease of colon and rectum.
- **Crohn's disease** involves all layers of the bowel wall and can occur anywhere in the GI tract from mouth to the anus.

Recent Question
(NORCET 2020)

12. Pain in the McBurney's point is a characteristic feature of:
a. Cholelithiasis
b. Appendicitis
c. Urolithiasis
d. Nephrolithiasis

Ans. (b) Appendicitis

Table 23: Comparison of regional enteritis and ulcerative colitis

Regional enteritis (Crohn's disease or granulomatous colitis)	Ulcerative colitis
Commonly occurs among adolescents and young adults. But can occur at any age.	Peak incidence age is 30–50 years.
It can occur anywhere along the GI tract, but **most commonly affecting ileum and colon.**	Disease process **starts at rectum and affects continuously the entire colon.**
Lesions or ulcers occurring in Crohn's disease are not in continuance (Separated by normal tissue). It's also known as cobblestone appearance	Lesions or ulcers are continuous and occur one after another
Rectal involvement, bleeding and diarrhea are less	Rectal involvement, bleeding and diarrhea are common.
Patients with Crohn's disease are **at increased risk of colon cancer.**	**Risk of colon cancer is as** less compared to Crohn's disease.

Management of IBD

- ***Nutritional therapy: Low residue, high protein, high calorie diet with supplementary vitamin and iron therapy.*** Food items contributing to diarrhea are often avoided.
- ***Pharmacological therapy: Sedatives, anti-diarrheal and anti-peristaltic to give rest to the inflamed bowel.***
- Aminosalicylate and sulfasalazine to manage inflammation
- Corticosteroid preparations are used to manage inflammation

Surgical management

- **Strictureplasty:** Blocked narrowed section of the bowel is widened, leaving intact.
- **Total colectomy with ileostomy:** Colon is completely removed and an opening is created in the ileum as a stoma on the abdominal wall.
- **Total colectomy with continent ileostomy:** Colon is completely removed and ileal reservoir (kock pouch) is created. Need for external reservoir is eliminated. 30 cm of the ileum is created as pouch with nipple valve. A catheter is inserted via nipple valve to empty the pouch.
- **Total colectomy with ileoanal anastomosis:** Colon is completely removed and ileum is connected to anus. No external stoma. Voluntary defecation is preserved through intact anus.

Intestinal Obstruction

Intestinal obstruction is the blockage or obstruction in the intestinal tract which prevents the normal flow of content via intestine.

Two types of obstruction can be there as follows:

- **Mechanical obstruction:** Intraluminal obstruction due to pressure on the intestinal wall, e.g., tumor, adhesions, stricture, stenosis, intussusception, etc.
- **Functional obstruction:** Intestinal musculature cannot propel the content through the bowel.

KEY POINTS

Colostomy Care

- Output from the colostomy is known as **effluent**.
- Skin barrier and colostomy pouch should be of right size to fit the stoma well.
- Small opening may obstruct and make the stoma swell, and large opening may cause leakage of effluent.
- Try to perform colostomy irrigation at that time when the patient usually had bowel movement before colostomy surgery
- Colostomy irrigation works well if performed after a hot drink.
- Colostomy irrigation is preferably performed at the same time every day.
- Avoid food items producing gas such as eggs, broccoli, cabbage, onion, fish, beans, milk, cheese, carbonated drinks, and alcohol.
- Food items causing odor to be avoided, e.g., eggs, cabbage, cheese, cucumber, onion, garlic, fish, dairy foods, and coffee.

Table 24: Mechanical causes of intestinal obstruction

Type	Description
Adhesions	Loops of intestine adhere to a slowly healing area or scar after the abdominal surgery
Intussusceptions	Telescopic movement of one part of intestine to another part of intestine which is located below
Volvulus	Bowel twist and turn around itself
Hernia	Protrusion of intestine through a weakened area of abdominal wall

KEY POINT

In patients with ulcerative colitis, use of cathartics is contraindicated because it may lead to megacolon, perforation and death.

POINT TO REMEMBER

After colostomy or creation of stoma, purple black color of the stoma indicate compromised blood supply and it needs immediate attention.

Clinical Corner

CASE SCENARIO 1:

Following a class on inflammatory bowel disease, which among the following signs identified by the student regarding ulcerative colitis shows that class was effective?

a. Lesion throughout the GI system
b. Cobblestone appearance
c. Strictures and fissures are present
d. Profuse diarrhea

Ans. (d) Profuse diarrhea

KEY POINTS

- A retracted colostomy stoma has a concave, bowl-shaped appearance.
- Retraction causes a poor pouching surface, leading to frequent peristomal skin complications.
- A healthy stoma is **pinkish-red and moist.**
- A narrowed or constricted or flattened stoma is a **sign of stenosis.**
- Narrowing of the stoma is a **late complication of a stoma.**
- A dry and reddish-purple stoma **indicates ischemia.**

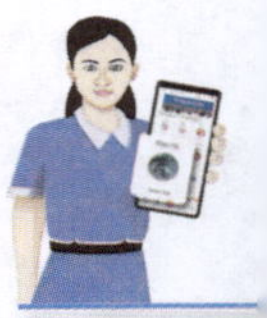

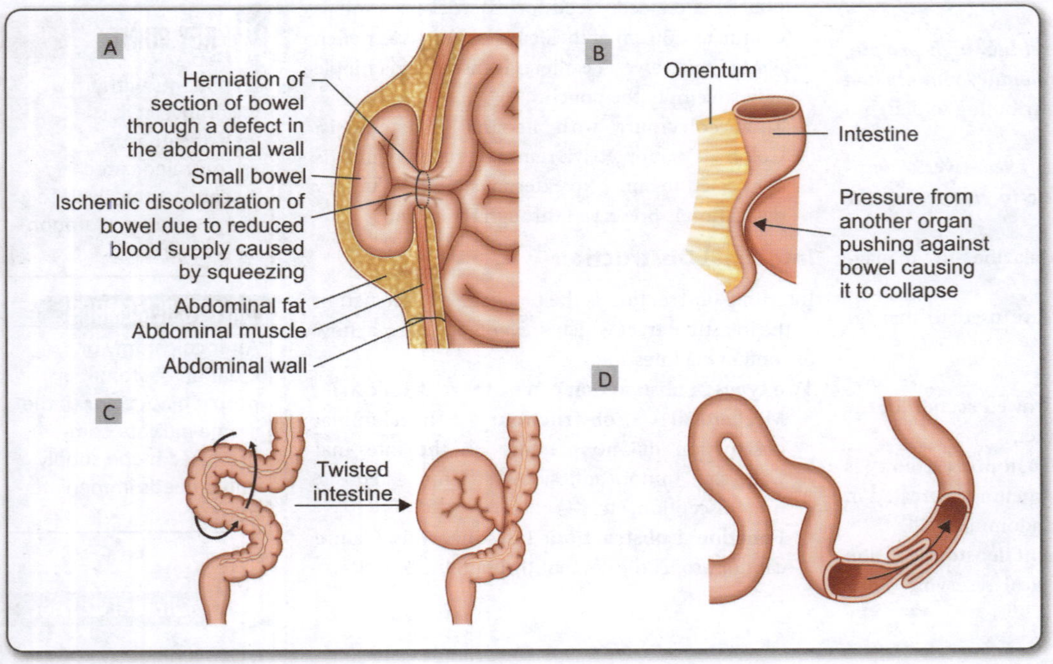

Figures 31A to D: A. Anatomy of hernia; **B.** Compression of bowel by other organ; **C.** Volvulus; **D.** Intussusception

Hernia

Protrusion of an organ through weakened wall containing it.

Table 25: Types of hernia

Type	Description
Reducible	Content in the hernia sac can be pushed back
Irreducible	Content in the hernia sac can't be pushed back
Incarcerated	Adhesion between hernia sac and its content. Reduction is difficult. There is no obstruction of blood supply.
Obstructed	Herniation leads to obstruction of the bowel. Blood supply remains intact.
Strangulated	Blood supply to the hernia sac is compromised. If surgical repair is not done, hernia sac will become gangrenous.
Inguinal hernia	Content in the abdominal cavity protrude through the inguinal canal (abdominal wall).
Femoral hernia	Content protrudes through the weak portion in the inner thigh.
Umbilical hernia	Protrusion of content occurs at the umbilicus.

Bariatric Surgery

Bariatric surgery is a surgery performed to reduce gastric capacity and thereby it helps in weight loss among clients with morbid obesity.

Two types of surgeries are there:

- **Gastric restrictive surgery:** Vertical banded gastroplasty or Circumgastric banding. This allows normal digestion without any risk for nutritional deficiency.
- **Gastric restriction combined with malabsorption:** Stomach is stapled to reduce the capacity. Duodenum and a portion of ileum are bypassed to reduce the calories absorbed.

Dietary education to client following bariatric surgery

- Avoid food high in protein, fat and sugar.
- Eat slowly and chew well
- Take nutritional supplements such as calcium, iron, multivitamin and Vitamin B12 as prescribed.

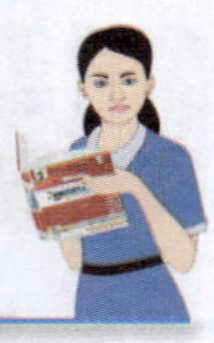

Practice Questions

11. Which of the following instruction must be included in discharge teaching of a patient who is treated for umbilical hernia?
   a. Maintain bed rest
   b. Restrict analgesic
   c. Avoid coughing
   d. Irrigation of the drain

Ans. (c) Avoid coughing

Explanation: Coughing should be avoided following umbilical hernia repair to prevent disruption of tissue integrity.

12. Which of the following intervention helps in reduction of postoperative swelling in a patient after inguinal hernia repair?
   a. Limit fluid intake
   b. Heat application on abdomen
   c. Elevate scrotum
   d. Low-fiber diet

Ans. (c) Elevate scrotum

13. A 60-year-old male patient has underwent bariatric surgery a few months back. Now the patient expressed to the nurse that his skin is hanging and may need cosmetic surgery. Which of the following response by the nurse would be the most appropriate?
   a. "You need to discuss with a counselor about your body image"
   b. "Cosmetic surgery is possible after your weight is stabilized"
   c. "The skinfolds will disappear with time"
   d. "Cosmetic surgery is unnecessary as you are improving already"

Ans. (b) "Cosmetic surgery is possible after your weight is stabilized"

Hemorrhoids

Hemorrhoids are swollen veins in the anal canal caused by chronic excess pressure from straining during a bowel movement, persistent diarrhea, or pregnancy.

Types

There are two types of hemorrhoids: Internal and external

- **Internal hemorrhoids:** Internal hemorrhoids are usually painless. There may be bright red rectal bleeding during or following a bowel movement. The fresh blood typically covers the stool (a condition known as hematochezia), is on the toilet paper, or drips into the toilet bowl.
  - **Treatment**
    - Avoiding constipation, not straining during bowel movements, using elastic bands to pull the internal hemorrhoids back into the rectum.
    - Surgery is needed only for a small number of patients with very large, painful, and persistent hemorrhoids.
- **External hemorrhoids:** External hemorrhoids are veins that lie just under the skin, on the outside of the anus. When thrombosed, hemorrhoids may be very painful.
  - **Treatment**
    - Removing the clot in vein under local anesthesia known as hemorrhoidectomy.
    - Assist the client to assume prone or side lying position following surgery to minimize the bleeding.

It is the gastric outlet (pyloric) obstruction that occurs as a result of hypertrophy and hyperplasia of the muscular layers of the pylorus.

> **KEY POINTS**
> - After hemorrhoidectomy, Sitz baths should be done 3 times a day and after every bowel movement.
> - Non-bilious **projectile vomiting** and **Olive like mass on palpation** of right upper quadrant of the abdomen are the characteristic features of Hyper-pyloric stenosis.

> **Recent Question** (NORCET 2023)
>
> **13. A 30-year-old male patient presented to Surgery OPD with complaint of bleeding per rectum. History is suggestive of hemorrhoids. What will be the confirmatory test in OPD?**
> a. Proctoscopy
> b. Sigmoidoscopy
> c. Digital rectal examination
> d. USG whole abdomen
>
> Ans. **(c) Digital rectal examination**

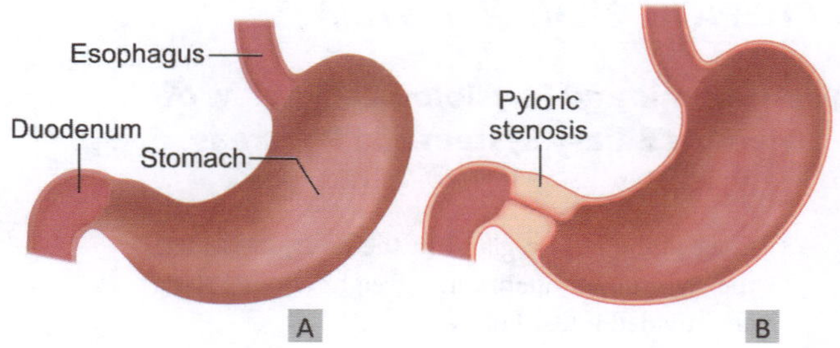

Figures 32A and B: (A) Normal anatomy; (B) Pyloric stenosis

Hyper-pyloric Stenosis

- **Major clinical manifestation**
  - Non-bilious **projectile vomiting**
  - Dehydration and electrolyte imbalance
  - **Olive like mass on palpation** of right upper quadrant of the abdomen
  - **Left to right peristaltic movement** across the abdomen
- **Investigations**
  - Physical examination and radiological investigations (USG, X-ray)
  - X-ray film of patient with hyper-pyloric stenosis shows string sign in the X-ray.
- **Management**
  - **Pyloromyotomy known as Ramstedt's procedure:** Dividing the muscle of the pylorus to open up the gastric outlet.

Diverticular Disease

- Pouch-like bulging in the GI tract is known as diverticular disease and is more commonly found in sigmoid colon.
- Surgical resection of the affected part is the management.
- Colostomy is the temporary management of the condition.

Clinical Manifestation

- Lower abdominal pain
- Bleeding per rectum

Complications

- Abscess formation
- Peritonitis
- Perforation
- Stricture formation
- Fistula
- Bleeding
- Diverticulitis

Treatment

- Consume diet high in fiber, fruits, vegetables and limit red meat.
- Surgical resection of the affected part
- Colostomy is the temporary management

> **KEY POINT**
> In diverticular disease, avoid food items which all are hard to digest such as nuts, corn, pop corn and seeds because these items may get stuck in diverticula and can cause inflammation

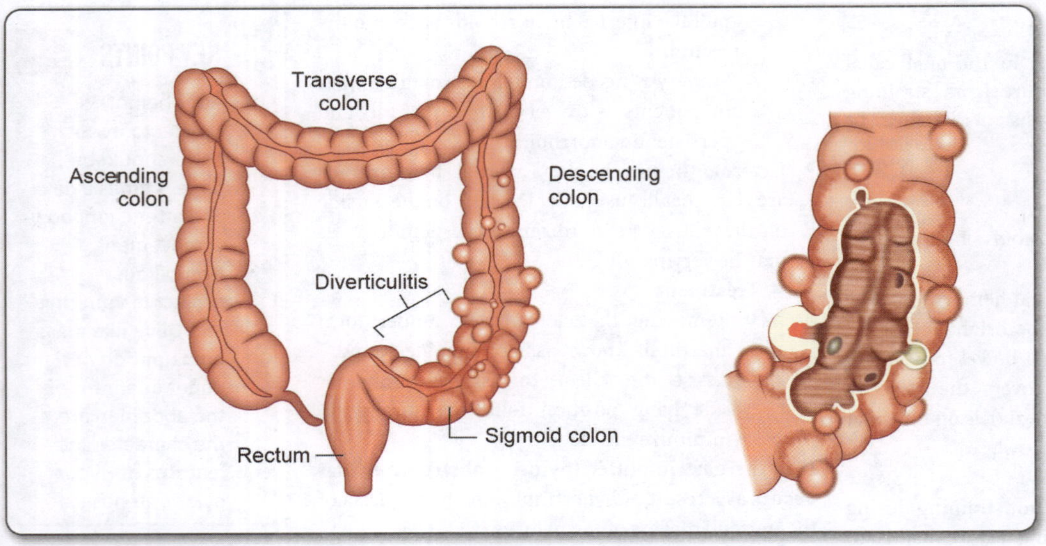

Figure 33: Diverticular disease

Colorectal Cancer

- It is a type of adenocarcinoma.
- It affects more than twice as many people as rectal cancer.
- **Clinical manifestation** includes bowel pattern changes and malena
- **Diagnosis:** Abdominal and rectal examination. Biopsy, barium enema or cytology smears.
- **Treatment**
  - Supportive therapy includes chemotherapy, radiation therapy, immunotherapy
  - Surgery is the primary treatment
  - Bowel resection with anastomosis and possible temporary or permanent colostomy or ileostomy.

HEPATIC BILIARY SYSTEM

Anatomic and Physiological Review of Hepatic Biliary System and Pancreas

Liver

- Liver is the largest gland in the body, located in the right upper quadrant. It weighs about 1500 g and divided into 4 Lobes
- Lobes are further divided into lobules.
- Kupffer cells are the phagocytic cells present in the liver.
- Smallest bile duct called canaliculi are located between the lobules of liver.
- Canaliculi carry bile secreted by hepatocytes to larger bile duct, which eventually become hepatic duct.
- Hepatic duct from liver and cystic duct from gallbladder join to form common bile duct which empties bile into the duodenum of small intestine.

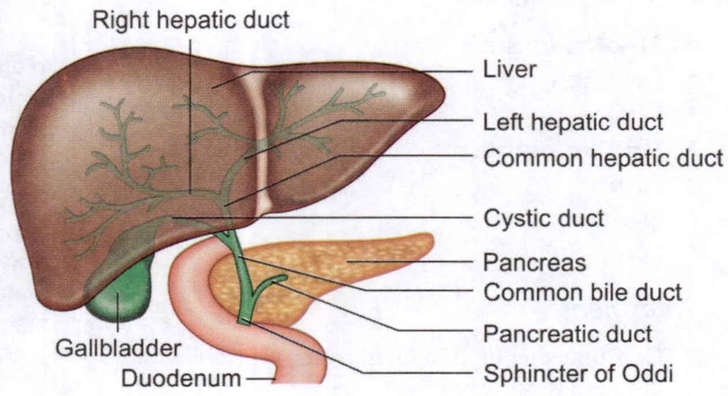

Figure 34: Biliary tree

Clinical Corner

CASE SCENARIO 2:

A nurse in the ED is assessing a patient who had a fiberoptic colonoscopy 18 hours ago. The patient complains of worsening abdominal pain, fever, and chills. Among the following conditions, which one should the nurse prioritize as the most immediate concern?

a. Colon cancer
b. Bowel perforation
c. Viral gastroenteritis
d. Diverticulitis

Ans. (b) Bowel perforation

Bowel perforation is a serious complication of colonoscopy that can occur when the colonoscope is inserted too forcefully or when a polyp is removed. Symptoms of bowel perforation include abdominal pain, fever, chills, and nausea and vomiting.

KEY POINTS

- The liver is situated mainly at **right hypochondrium**, extending through the epigastrium and reaching the left hypochondrium.
- **Kupffer cells** are specialized macrophages located in the liver.
- **In the liver**, bacteria that found their way into portal circulation are destroyed by **Kupffer cells.**
- Bile secretion - 500 to 1000 mL/day
- Bile is called pseudodigestive juice because it does not contain any digestive enzymes.

Functions of Liver

- **Glucose metabolism:** After digestion, glucose is converted to glycogen and whenever the body requires, glycogen is converted to glucose:
  - **Glycogenesis:** Glucose is converted and stored as glycogen
  - **Glycolysis:** Glycogen is converted back to glucose
  - **Gluconeogenesis:** Glucose is synthesized from non-carbohydrate substances such as protein and amino acids.
- **Ammonia conversion:** Protein and amino acid metabolism leads to ammonia generation. Liver converts this highly toxic ammonia to urea for excretion.
- **Protein metabolism:** Liver synthesizes all plasma protein **(except gamma globulin)** such as albumin, alpha and beta globulins.
- **Fat metabolism:** When glucose is not available, fatty acids are broken down for the production of energy.
- **Vitamin and iron storage:** Liver stores large amount of vit A, D, E, K and vit. B12 and it also stores iron and copper.
- **Drug metabolism:** Liver is a major site for drug metabolism
- **Bile formation:** Hepatocytes synthesize bile and stores in gallbladder. Bile salts are formed from cholesterol

Enterohepatic Bilirubin Circulation

- Bilirubin is released from the breakdown of RBCs at reticuloendothelial system
- Hepatocytes convert this bilirubin (unconjugated) to conjugated bilirubin by mixing it with glucuronic acid which is more soluble in aqueous solution.
- Later conjugated bilirubin in the hepatocytes will be secreted along with bile into the duodenum.
- In the small intestine, bilirubin is converted as urobilinogen.
- A part of urobilinogen is excreted via feces, another part is reabsorbed in the small intestine. It reaches the liver via portal vein and the remaining part enters the systemic circulation and is excreted via kidneys in urine.

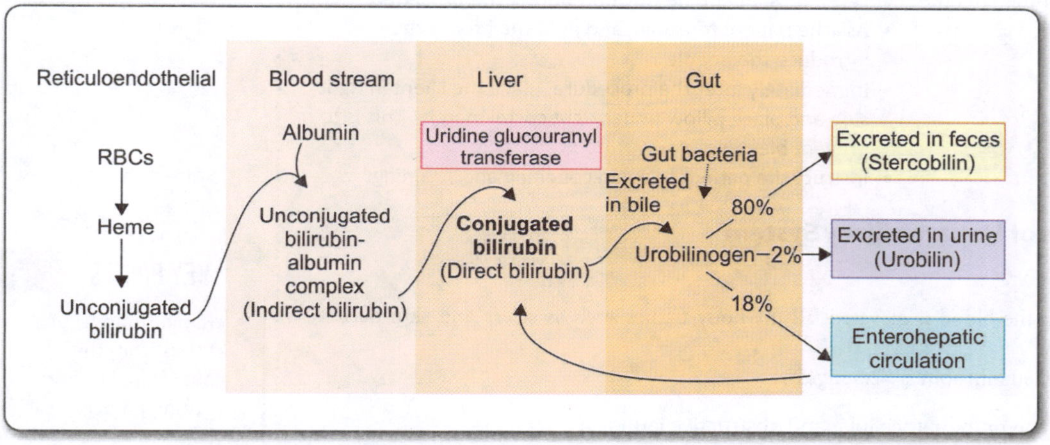

Figure 35: Production and enterohepatic circulation of bilirubin

Gallbladder

- It is a pear shaped organ of 7.5–10 cm in size.
- Capacity of gallbladder is 30–50 mL.
- Gallbladder is connected to common bile duct by the cystic duct.
- Functions of gallbladder are:
  - To store bile
  - Water content of the bile is absorbed by gallbladder wall during storage and the bile becomes 5–10 times concentrated.

Pancreas

- It has both endocrine as well as exocrine functions in the body.
- Secretion of pancreatic juice via pancreatic duct represents exocrine function
- Alpha cells of pancreas produce **glucagon** and beta cells of pancreatic islets produce **Insulin.**
- Pancreatic enzymes are given as follows:

KEY POINTS

- Pancreas is both endocrine and exocrine gland (995 exocrine and 1% endocrine).
- Beta cells of Islets of Langerhans concentrated in tail portion of pancreas secret insulin.
- The opening of the pancreatic duct into the duodenum is at the ampulla of Vater.
- Majority of the **pancreatic cancer** arises at the head of the pancreas.

Table 26: Pancreatic enzymes

Pancreatic enzyme	Substrate
Trypsin, Chymotrypsin Carboxy Peptidase	Protein
Pancreatic amylase	Carbohydrate
Pancreatic lipase, Cholesterol esterase, Phospholipase	Fats

Diagnostic Tests

Table 27: Description of diagnostic tests

Name of the tests	Description	Points to keep in mind
Liver function test (LFT) (Please refer Synopsis of FON for normal ranges of LFT)	It is a blood serum test which assesses liver functions in terms of serum enzymatic activity	• Serum enzymes monitored are: ▪ Alkaline phosphate ▪ Lactic dehydrogenase ▪ Serum aminotransferase • Albumin • Globulin • Bilirubin • Ammonia
Liver biopsy	Removal of small amount of liver tissue, usually through needle aspiration	• Coagulation study has to be obtained before biopsy • Informed written consent • **Left lateral or supine position during the procedure** • Ask the patient to exhale and hold the breath then introduce the needle • Immediately after the procedure, place the client in right side and place pillow under right costal margin. This is to prevent bleeding. • Instruct the patient to avoid coughing and straining.

Disorders and Diseases of Hepatobiliary System

Jaundice

- When the bilirubin level in the blood is elevated, all the body tissues such as sclera and skin become yellowish or greenish yellow.
- This discoloration occurs when bilirubin is >2.5 mg/dL.

Table 28: Comparison of hemolytic, hepatocellular and obstructive jaundice

Hemolytic jaundice (Prehepatic)	Hepatocellular jaundice	Obstructive jaundice (Post hepatic)
• Hemolysis (destruction of RBCs) results in increased bilirubin in the blood • Liver is unable to conjugate excessive bilirubin from hemolysis • **Elevated unconjugated bilirubin is seen in serum** • It is seen in patients with hemolytic transfusion reaction and other hemolytic disease • Normal prothrombin time	• Damaged hepatic cells can't clear the bilirubin in the blood. • **Both conjugated and unconjugated bilirubin elevated.** • Abnormal prothrombin time; not corrected with Vit K.	• Impaired excretion of bilirubin due to mechanical obstruction of biliary tract • Extrahepatic obstruction occurs as a result of occlusion of the bile duct by gall stone. • Intrahepatic obstruction resulting from stasis of bile within the canaliculi. • **Mainly (>50%) elevated levels of Conjugated bilirubin is seen in serum.** • Abnormal prothrombin time; corrected with Vit K.

Recent Question
(NORCET 2022)

14. What is the complication of liver biopsy in children?
a. Bleeding
b. Bile leak
c. Pneumothorax
d. Prolonged drainage of ascitic fluid

Ans. (a) Bleeding

KEY POINTS

- Rapid removal of fluids from the abdominal cavity during paracentesis leads to decreased abdominal pressure which can cause vasodilation and shock.
- **Icterus (jaundice)** is a sign that is present if a patient is experiencing hepatic coma.
- **Clay-colored stools** is the sign of obstructive jaundice
- Variceal hemorrhage is the most common complication associated with portal hypertension.

Portal Hypertension

- Obstructed blood flow through the liver resulting in increased blood pressure is known as portal hypertension.
- Normal range of portal venous pressure is 5–8 mm Hg
- Splenomegaly is a common manifestation in portal hypertension.
- Consequences of portal hypertension include ascites and varices.

Ascites

- Fluid accumulates in the abdominal cavity.
- Fluid moves from vascular system into peritoneal space due to
  - Sodium and water retention
  - Increased intravascular blood volume
  - Decreased albumin synthesis
- **Signs and symptoms**
  - Increased abdominal girth
  - Rapid weight gain
  - Shortness of breath
  - Striae (stretch marks) and distended veins

Shifting dullness test: In a patient with ascites, area of dullness gets shifted to the dependent area. This is the positive shifting dullness test for ascites.

- **Management**
  - Sodium restriction
  - Diuretics
  - **Paracentesis:** Needle is inserted into peritoneal cavity to remove fluid from the abdominal cavity.
    - Patient is placed in supine position during procedure
    - Slightly rotated to the side of the procedure (to minimize the risk of perforation)
    - Left lateral approach is preferred (cecum is relatively fixed on right)

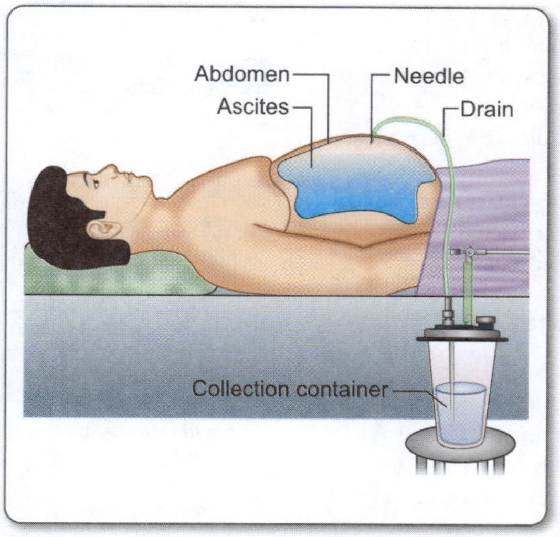

Figure 36: Paracentesis

Esophageal Varices

- Esophageal varices are dilated tortuous veins usually found in submucosal layer of lower esophagus.
- **Cause**
  - Liver disease
  - In case of portal obstruction, blood from intestinal tract and spleen seek a new pathway via esophageal plexus.
  - Esophageal plexus is not elastic so it becomes tortuous, fragile and bleed easily.
- **Clinical manifestation**
  - Hematemesis, melena and symptoms of shock are the common manifestations.
- **Management**
  - Vasopressin, somatostatin, octreotide are the drug of choice to decrease the bleeding.
  - **Balloon tamponade: It is done with sengstaken-blackemore tube.**
  - **Endoscopic sclerotherapy:** Sclerosing agent is injected into the bleeding varices to promote healing.
  - **Esophageal banding therapy/variceal band ligation:** Elastic rubber band is slipped over (through endoscope) the bleeding varices, which causes necrosis of the bleeding varices.
  - **Transjugular intrahepatic portosystemic shunt (TIPS):** Intrahepatic shunt is created between portal circulation and hepatic vein.
  - **Surgical management:** Surgical ligation of bleeding varices and esophageal transection and devascularization.
  - **Surgical bypass procedures:** These procedures help to drain a portion of portal blood and thereby help to reduce portal pressure.
  - Spleno-renal shunt, Mesocaval shunt and Portocaval shunt

Sengstaken-Blakemore tube

- Sengstaken-Blakemore tube has got 3 lumens (ports for gastric and esophageal balloon and gastric aspiration)
- Minnesota tube has 4 lumens and two balloon (has an esophageal aspiration port in addition to the gastric aspiration port).
- Purpose of lumens are gastric aspiration, esophageal aspiration, gastric balloon inflation, esophageal balloon inflation.
- Stomach balloon is inflated with 100–200 mL of air. X-ray confirms the position of gastric balloon. Then gastric balloon is pulled against cardiac part of stomach.
- Irrigation of the tube is done to detect bleeding. If return from irrigation is clear, esophageal balloon will not be inflated.
- If bleeding is present, then esophageal balloon will be inflated.

Recent Question (CNCI 2021)

15. The most likely cause of fluctuating jaundice in a middle aged/elderly man is

a. Periampullary cancer
b. Liver fluke infestation
c. Choledochal cyst
d. Carcinoma head of pancreas

Ans. (a) Periampullary cancer

Practice Question

14. The patient has a Sengstaken-Blakemore Tube inserted to stop bleeding in the stomach. Which of the following statement about this tubing is NOT true?

a. It is a four-lumen gastric tube
b. Irrigation of the tube is done to detect bleeding
c. It is used to stop bleeding in patients with esophageal varices
d. Scissors is kept at the bedside for emergency use with this tubing type

Ans. (a) It is a four-lumen gastric tube

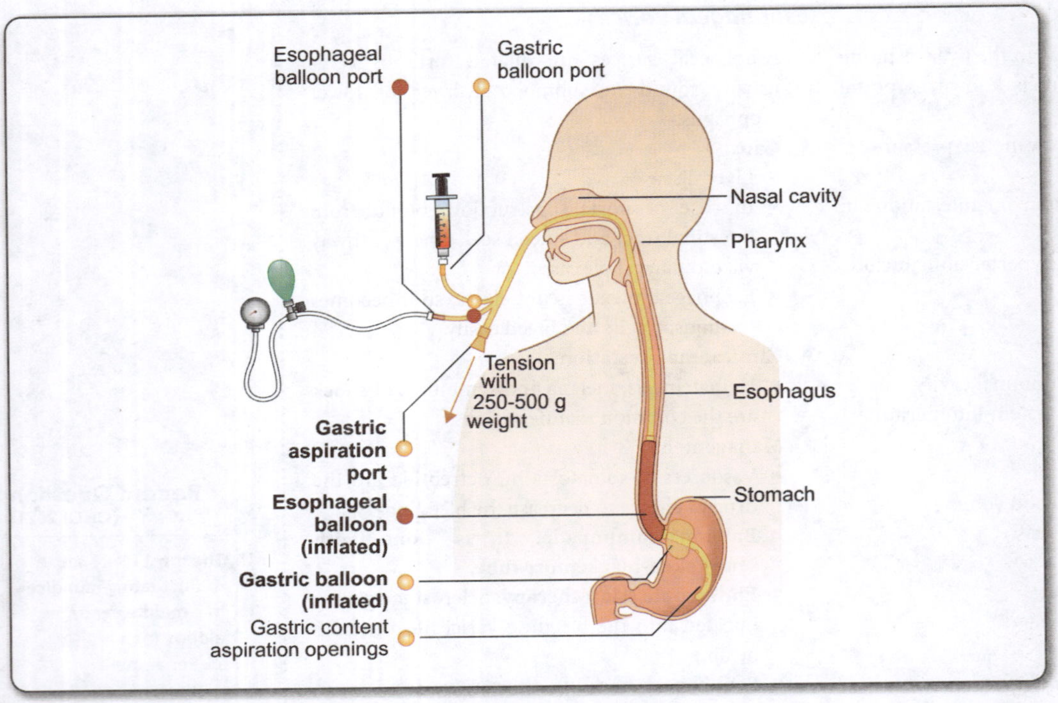

Figure 37: Sengstaken-Blakemore tube

- Pressure in the esophageal balloon is – 25 mm Hg
- Pressure in gastric balloon is – 40 mm Hg.
- Once the bleeding varices stop, first esophageal balloon will be deflated. After several hours without bleeding, gastric balloon will be deflated.
- If several bleeding free hours are there, then the tube will be removed.

Liver Abscess

- **Pyogenic and amebic abscesses are the most common type of abscess**
- Amebic abscess is caused by ***entamoeba histolytica***
- **Clinical manifestation:** Fever, right upper quadrant pain, anorexia, nausea, vomiting, hepatomegaly, jaundice
- **Diagnosis:** CT, MRI, aspiration and analysis of liver abscess under CT and MRI guidance.
- **Management:** Antibiotics, drainage of cyst.

Hepatic Encephalopathy and Coma

- Failed liver cells are unable to convert ammonia to urea, as a result ammonia accumulates in the blood stream.
- Hepatic encephalopathy occurs due to accumulation of ammonia (toxic to brain cells) and other metabolites in the blood.
- Hepatic coma is the most advanced stage of hepatic encephalopathy.
- **Earliest symptoms of hepatic encephalopathy**
  - Minor mental changes and motor disturbances
- **Asterixis** flapping tremors of the hands occur in this condition and simple tasks like writing becomes difficult.
- **Inability to reproduce a simple image is known as constructional apraxia.**
- In the initial stage of hepatic encephalopathy, deep tendon reflexes are hyperactive and with the worsening of disease, these reflexes disappear and extremity becomes flaccid.
- **Fetor hepaticus:** A sweet, slightly fecal odor of the breath can be there which is intestinal in origin.
- **Management**
  - Lactulose is administered to reduce serum ammonia level. It helps in excretion of ammonia through bowel.
  - Eliminate protein from diet to reduce serum ammonia.
  - Administration of neomycin sulfate reduces the number of intestinal bacteria which are capable of converting urea to ammonia.

The Model for End-stage Liver Disease (MELD) Score

- MELD score is a tool used to predict the risk of death in patients with liver disease.
- The MELD score was developed in 2002 by **Dr. Ronald W. Busuttil** and colleagues at the University of Pittsburgh Medical Center.

KEY POINTS

- Esophageal varices are common in patients with Liver disease due to portal hypertension.
- **Scissors is an emergency bedside article** needs to be kept with a client with **Sengstaken-Blakemore tube** because rupture of balloon or migration of balloon to the oropharynx can cause life-threatening airway obstruction and asphyxiation.

Recent Question (NORCET 2022)

16. Lactulose is prescribed for the patient suffering from Liver cirrhosis so as to:
a. Prevent hepatic encephalopathy
b. Decrease production of bilirubin
c. Increase lactulose level in blood
d. Increase breakdown of bilirubin

Ans. (a) Prevent hepatic encephalopathy

Recent Question (NORCET 2020)

17. Which of the following is not transmitted by needle stick injury?
a. HIV
b. Hepatitis B
c. Scrub Typhus
d. Hepatitis C

Ans. (c) Scrub Typhus

- It is calculated using three laboratory values:
  1. Serum bilirubin
  2. Serum creatinine
  3. International Normalized Ratio (INR)
- The MELD score ranges from 6 to 40, with higher scores indicating a higher risk of death.
- Patients with a MELD score of 15 or higher are considered to be candidates for liver transplantation.

Viral Hepatitis

The viruses which are responsible for viral hepatitis and their modes of remission have been tabulated as:

Table 29: Types of virus hepatitis

Types of hepatitis	Types of virus	Incubation period	Mode of transmission
Hepatitis A (Infectious hepatitis)	RNA Virus	15–45 days	Fecal-oral route
Hepatitis B (Serum hepatitis)	DNA Virus	28–180 days	Parenteral, serum, saliva, semen and vaginal secretion
Hepatitis C	RNA Virus	15–160 days	Parenteral Commonly associated with Blood Transfusion.
Hepatitis D	RNA Virus	28–180 days	Parenteral. It requires Hep B surface antigen for its replication. So it is seen in only those who are affected with Hep B
Hepatitis E	RNA virus	14–63 days	Fecal-oral route

- **Investigations**
  - **Hepatitis A:** Antibody, IgM
  - **Hepatitis B:** IgM and HBSAg
  - **Hepatitis C:** Antibody
- **Management**
  - Supplementation of vitamins
  - Fat digestion will be affected so need to have diet control
  - Antiviral drugs are used in treatment of this condition.

Hepatic Cirrhosis

- Replacement of normal liver tissue with fibrotic tissue that disrupts normal structure and function of liver. It can be classified as:
  - **Alcoholic cirrhosis (micronodular):** Chronic consumption of alcohol leads to cirrhosis and is the **most common type of cirrhosis**
  - **Post-necrotic cirrhosis (macronodular):** Cirrhosis occurs as a result of any infection or inflammation to liver such as hepatitis
  - **Biliary necrosis:** Scarring occurs around the bile duct. As a result of chronic biliary obstruction and infection
  - **Cardiac:** Caused by right-sided heart failure
- **Incidence**
  - It is twice as common in men as compared to women, peak incidence at 40 – 60 years of age.
- **Signs and symptoms**
  - Anorexia, nausea, vomiting, weight loss, constipation or diarrhea
  - Jaundice and hepatic encephalopathy may occur
  - **Complications:** Ascites, esophageal varices, portal hyper-tension and peripheral edema may occur
  - Decreased synthesis of bile affects the absorption of fat soluble vitamins.
  - **Coagulation abnormalities** due to deficiency of vitamin K and clotting factors II, VII, IX and X.
- **Treatment**
  - Paracentesis to remove ascetic fluid (if present); Peritoneovenous shunt may be used
  - Potassium-sparing diuretic to treat ascites and peripheral edema
  - Vitamin K—to reduce bleeding tendency
  - Lactulose—to treat hepatic encephalopathy
  - Vasopressin—to treat bleeding esophageal varices
  - Blood transfusions may be required if excessive bleeding exists.

Cholecystitis

- Inflammation of gallbladder
- **Most common cause** is stone in the biliary tract.
- **Clinical Manifestation**
  - Right upper quadrant pain mainly after the ingestion of fatty food
  - Acute pain, tenderness and rigidity over Right Upper Quadrant associated with mid-sternal and right shoulder pain.

Recent Questions
(CNCI 2021)

18. While providing care to a patient with Hepatitis, the nursing officer should take special precautions to __________.
a. Prevent droplet spread of infection
b. Use caution when bringing food for PT
c. Wear mask and gown before entering the room
d. Use gloves when removing the patient's bed pan

Ans. (d) Use gloves when removing the patient's bed pan

19. Kernicterus, which may occur as a complication of jaundice is a pathological condition of:
a. Liver
b. Brain
c. Kidney
d. Heart

Ans. (b) Brain

KEY POINTS

- Low fat diet is recommended for the patients of cholelithiasis.
- **Pain in the right upper quadrant** of the abdomen which is radiating to back and right shoulder suggestive of **cholecystitis.**
- **Murphy's sign** → acute cholecystitis

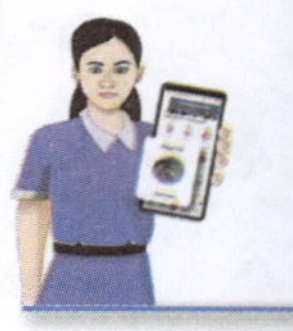

- **Positive Murphy's sign:** Patient can't take deep breath when examiner's hand passes below the hepatic margin because of the pain (painful inspiration).
- Chronic cholecystitis occurs because of the inefficient emptying of gallbladder and gallbladder muscle wall disease
- Acalculous cholecystitis occurs in the absence of gallstone disease and is caused by bacterial invasion via lymphatic and vascular system.
- Dark orange and foamy urine
- Steatorrhea, clay colored stool and pruritus.
- **Management**
  - Anticholinergic to decrease the spasm of the bile duct
  - Analgesics for pain control
  - Gallbladder and gallstones are surgically removed if pain persists.
  - Cholecystectomy is the surgical procedure performed to remove gallbladder.
  - **Choledocholithotomy:** Requires incision in the common bile duct to remove stone.

Cholelithiasis

- Calculi or stones are formed in the gallbladder from the solid constituents of the bile.
- **There are two types of stones:**
  - **Pigment stone:** Unconjugated pigment in the bile precipitate to form stone. It can't be dissolved. Surgical removal is the treatment of choice.
  - **Cholesterol stone:** Cholesterol is a natural component of bile. Its solubility depends upon bile acid and lecithin. Cholesterol precipitates to form stones when bile acid synthesis is less than cholesterol synthesis.
- **Signs and symptoms**
  - Pain in the right upper quadrant, radiating to back and right shoulder (biliary colic).
  - Obstructive jaundice
  - Color of the urine becomes dark and **stool becomes clay colored.**
  - Bleeding manifestation
- **Investigation**
  - **Abdominal X-ray:** USG, cholescintigraphy, cholecystography, ERCP and percutaneous transhepatic cholangiography
- **Management**
  - **Ursodeoxycholic acid (UDCA) and chenodeoxycholic acid** (CDCA) to dissolve cholesterol stones.
  - **Dissolving gall stones:** Solvent such as **mono-octanoin or methyl tertiary butyl ether** is infused into gallbladder through a catheter.
  - **Stone removal by instrumentation:** A catheter and an instrument with basket threaded through T-tube, or through a fistula is created and stones are removed.
  - **Extracorporeal shock wave lithotripsy:** Non-invasive procedure
  - **Intracorporeal shock wave lithotripsy:** Under fluoroscopy, laser pulse is directed towards gallbladder and stones are fragmented.
  - **Laparoscopic cholecystectomy:** Removal of gallbladder through a small incision in the umbilicus
  - **Cholecystectomy:** Gallbladder is removed via an abdominal incision
  - **Choledochostomy:** Incision in the common bile duct to remove stone

Pancreatitis

- Inflammation of pancreas. It is often described as auto digestion of pancreas.
- **Causes**
  - **More common:** Obstruction of biliary tract, long-term alcohol use.
  - **Less common:** Viral or bacterial infections.
- **Types**
  - **Acute pancreatitis**
    - It occurs suddenly as one attack or recurrent with resolutions.
    - Sudden onset of abdominal pain or left upper quadrant pain radiating to the back.
    - **Pain is aggravated by alcohol or a fatty meal**
    - Abdominal tenderness, guarding, decreased bowel sounds, elevated WBCs, glucose, bilirubin, alkaline phosphatase, and urinary amylase.
    - Elevated **serum amylase and lipase level** are seen.
  - **Chronic pancreatitis**
    - It's continuous inflammation and destruction of pancreas with scar tissue replacing the pancreatic tissue.
    - Abdominal pain and tenderness, steatorrhea, weight loss, sign and symptoms of diabetes mellitus.
- **Diagnosis**
  - Increased pancreatic hormones such as serum amylase, lipase, glucose and bilirubin.
  - Increase in the count of white blood cells because of infection.
  - Cullen's sign and Grey Turner's sign are the characteristics of this condition.

Recent Question (NORCET 2020)

20. Murphy's sign is seen in which of the following disease condition?

a. Liver abscess
b. Splenomegaly
c. Peritonitis
d. Acute cholecystitis

Ans. (d) Acute cholecystitis

Recent Questions (CNCI 2021)

21. Which maneuver is done to temporarily stop inadvertent bleeding during cholecystectomy

a. Patey
b. Pringle
c. Kocher
d. Billroth

Ans. (b) Pringle

Explanation: The Pringle maneuver is one technique that enables surgeons to halt hemorrhage and find the source of bleeding, allowing time for repair of the vessel.

22. After Cholecystectomy, there was 50 mL bile output from the drain on the first postoperative day management is ________.

a. Intrabiliary stent
b. Immediate exploration
c. T-tube drainage
d. Observation

Ans. (d) Observation

Cullen's Sign and Turner's Sign

- **Cullen's sign** is superficial edema and bruising in the subcutaneous fatty tissue around the umbilicus. It is a sign of intraperitoneal hemorrhage. It is also a sign of rupture of fallopian tube or ectopic pregnancy.
- **Grey Turner's** sign refers to bruising of the flanks, the part of the body between the last rib and the top of the hip. It is a sign of retroperitoneal hemorrhage, or bleeding behind the peritoneum.

Grey turner's sign (flank ecchymosis) may also be seen in rupture of aneurysm.

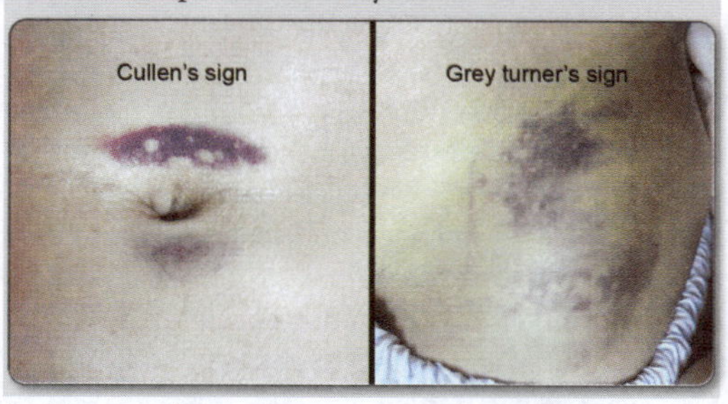

- **Signs and symptoms**
  - Severe epigastric pain that worsens after meals
  - Fever and malaise
  - Bulky, fatty and foul-smelling stool
  - Abdominal tenderness and distension.
- **Management**
  - Limit fat and protein intake, avoid alcohol, and heavy meals.
  - **Acute Pancreatitis: NPO; Total Parenteral Nutrition (TPN)**
  - Administer pancreatic enzyme as prescribed to aid in digestion
  - **Surgical Interventions:**
    - **Pancreaticojejunostomy:** Anastomosis of pancreatic duct to jejunum.
    - **Whipple resection** (Pancreaticoduodenectomy)
      - The head of the pancreas, the first part of the small intestine (duodenum), the gallbladder and the bile duct will be removed. The remaining organs are reattached to allow digestion of food normally after surgery.

Pancreatic Enzyme Replacement Therapy (PERT)

- PERT is a method of treating exocrine pancreatic deficiency. It is useful for treating many conditions such as pancreatic cancer, cystic fibrosis, chronic pancreatitis.
- Fecal elastase-1 level helps to diagnose pancreatic enzyme deficiency. If it is decreased in stool, this means person has pancreatic enzyme deficiency.
- PERT should be taken as divided dose throughout the meal.

Wilsons's Disease

- It is a disorder of copper metabolism
- Characterized by deposition of Copper in liver, brain and other tissues (known as Hepatolenticular degeneration)
- Copper gets deposited in basal ganglia leading to tremors, chorea, dystonia and rigidity
- ***Kayser - Fleischer ring*** *(brownish color ring on sclera-corneal junction of eye) and* ***sunflower cataract*** *are seen in this condition.*
- **Management:**
  - Lifelong zinc and penicillamine/trientine
  - Ammonium tetrathiomolybdate is a chelating drug used as initial treatment

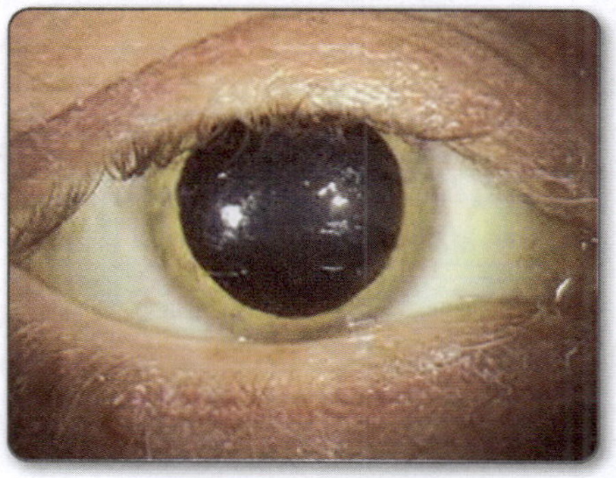

Figure 38: Kayser–Fleischer ring

KEY POINTS

- **Morphine** causes spasm of **Sphincter of oddi** so it is **contraindicated** in patients with **cholecystitis** and **pancreatitis.**
- Elevated serums amylase and lipase are suggestive of pancreatitis.
- **Cullen's sign** is discoloration of abdomen and periumbilical area visible in pancreatitis.
- **Turner's sign** is bluish discoloration of the flank visible in pancreatitis.

Recent Question (CNCI 2021)

23. The following anastomosis are done in Whipple procedure except ________?

a. Hepatico-jejunostomy
b. Pancreato gastrectomy
c. Gastro jejunostomy
d. Jejuno-jejunostomy

Ans. (d) Jejuno-jejunostomy

Recent Question (NORCET 2022)

24. In assessing the nature of the stool of a client who has cystic fibrosis, what would the nurse expect to see?

a. Clay-colored stools
b. Steatorrhea stools
c. Dark brown stools
d. Blood-tinged stools

Ans. (b) Steatorrhea stools

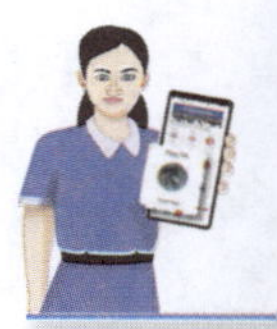

Golden Points to Remember

- The average distance from the incisor teeth to the top of the stomach is 38 to 40 cm in men and 36 to 38 cm in women.
- The microorganism closely associated with dental cavities is Streptococcus sanguis.
- **Parotid** is the largest salivary gland.
- **Submaxillary gland** is the gland with longest duct.
- **Glossitis** is inflammation of the tongue.
- **Vincent's infection** is characterized by bleeding gums, bad breath and painful ulcers in the mouth.
- Inflammation of mouth is called **Stomatitis**.
- **Iron absorption** occurs in **duodenum**.
- **Leiomyoma** is the most common type of benign esophageal tumor.
- **Adenocarcinoma** is the most common type of malignant tumor of esophagus.
- Strongest layer of gut is **Submucosa**.
- **Caecum** is the thinnest muscular wall; most vulnerable for perforation; least vulnerable for obstruction.
- Caecum is the widest portion of the colon.
- Narrowest part of large intestine is Sigmoid colon.
- Ascending colon is the shortest part of colon.
- Area of colon least visualized by barium studies is Sigmoid colon.
- First organ to be affected in CA stomach is Liver.
- H. pylori is a risk factor for intestinal type of CA stomach.
- Urea breath test in exhaled breath is used to detect the presence of **Helicobacter pylori**.
- **Cullen's sign** → hemorrhagic pancreatitis
- **Mirizzi's syndrome:** gallstone gets impacted in the cystic duct or neck of the gallbladder and causes compression of the Common Bile Duct.
- **Hematemesis** is blood in vomitus.
- SGOT/SGPT (AST) ratio >3:1 is highly suggestive of alcoholic liver disease.
- AST > ALT is seen in Cirrhosis.
- The parasitic organism that causes hydatid cyst of the liver is Echinococcus granulosus, a tapeworm that is found in dogs and other animals.
- Esophageal varices are common in patients with liver disease (especially cirrhosis) due to portal hypertension.
- **CAGE** questionnaire is used in the clinical diagnosis of alcohol dependence and abuse.
- **Normal portal vein pressure is:** 5–10 mm Hg or 10–15 cm of water.
- Ground glass hepatocytes are seen in Chronic viral hepatitis.
- Wilson's disease is a disorder of copper metabolism.
- Hemochromatosis refers to abnormal accumulation of iron in various organs.
- Waist to hip ratio <0.8 is normal, if greater, it indicates high risk or obesity.
- **Curling's ulcer** is a complication of **burn**. It is a type of gastroduodenal ulcer caused by a generalized stress response resulting in decreased production of mucus and increased gastric acid secretion.
- Catheter is placed in subclavian and jugular vein for providing parenteral nutrition.
- The complication of GERD is **Barrett's esophagus**. It is considered precancerous lesion for esophageal cancer.
- Distended abdomen and absence of bowel sound after abdominal surgery indicate **paralytic ileus**.
- **Nissen** and **Toupet fundoplications** are common surgical procedures for the treatment of GERD.
- **Halitosis** is foul smelling of breath.
- **McBurney's** point is located in right lower quadrant of abdomen. It is situated at one-third of the distance from the anterior superior iliac spine to the umbilicus (navel).
- Heartburn regurgitation and dysphagia are classical signs of GERD (gastroesophageal reflex disease).
- **Zollinger-Ellison syndrome** is rare condition characterized by severe peptic ulceration, gastric acid hyper secretion, elevated gastrin level and gastrinoma of pancreas.
- Antacid neutralizes the hydrochloric acid secreted in stomach.
- **Billroth I Surgery (Gastroduodenostomy)** involves partial gastrectomy with removal of the distal two-third of the stomach and anastomosis of the gastric stump to the duodenum.
- **Billroth II surgery (Gastrojejunostomy)** involves partial gastrectomy with removal of the distal two-third of the stomach and anastomosis of the gastric stump to the jejunum.
- Pernicious anemia is a long-term complication of total gastrectomy.
- **Inflammatory bowel disease (IBD)** is an autoimmune disease includes Crohn's disease and ulcerative colitis.
- **Ulcerative colitis** is a disease of colon and rectum, it starts in the rectum and moves in a continual fashion toward the cecum.
- **Crohn's disease** involves all layer of the bowel wall and can occur anywhere in the GI tract from mouth to the anus.
- **Hematochezia** is passage of fresh blood through rectum.
- **Malena** is dark tarry stools containing occult blood. It is associated with upper GI bleeding.
- **Oral erythromycin** and **neomycin** are given in preoperative time of gastric surgery to reduce the number of bacteria and prevent post-operative complication.
- A barium enema is used to determine narrowing or obstruction of the colonic lumen.
- Clinical manifestation of fat malabsorption is **Steatorrhea**. It is a bulky, foul smelling, yellow, gray, greasy stools with putty-like consistency.
- Some of the most common causes of malabsorption syndrome include Celiac disease, Crohn's disease, Pancreatic insufficiency, bile duct obstruction, Giardia infection, Whipple's disease.

Contd...

- The digestion of carbohydrates takes place mainly in the small intestine
- Celiac disease is treated with lifelong avoidance of dietary **gluten**.
- The hallmark of **Wilson** disease is corneal **Kayser–Fleischer rings**.
- **Grey Turner sign** and **Cullen's sign** are signs of pancreatitis.
- **Whipple procedure** (radical pancreaticoduodenectomy) is classic surgery for pancreatic cancer.
- **Rapid removal of fluids** from the abdominal cavity during **paracentesis** leads to decreased abdominal pressure which can cause **vasodilation** and **shock**.
- In case of airway obstruction tube needs to be cut to relieve pressure in the oropharynx.
- Patient receiving lactulose for the management of hepatic encephalopathy and coma should be closely monitored for watery stool which indicates medication overdose.
- Hepatitis B is caused by **DNA virus** and all other hepatitis is caused by RNA virus.
- **Murphy's sign:** Patient can't take deep breath when examiner's hand passed below the hepatic margin because of the pain the patient felt in cholecystitis.
- **Adhesion** is the union of two opposing tissue surfaces.
- **Volvulus** refers to abnormal twisting of a part of the large or small intestine.
- **Intussusception** is a condition in which one segment of intestine slips into another portion located below it, just like telescope.
- Currant jelly-like stools are feature of **Intussusception** (intestine telescopes into itself).
- **Hirschsprung's disease** is an **aganglionic disease**. It is a congenital defect of the intestinal tract which causes inadequate motility.
- **Phenylketonuria (PKU)** is an inborn error of metabolism that results in decreased metabolism of the amino acid phenylalanine.
- Low-residue, low-fiber diet is recommended for a patient with **ulcerative colitis.**

Most Common

- Most common cause of Portal HTN in Adults**: Cirrhosis**
- Most common cause of Cirrhosis: **Alcoholic liver disease**
- Most common cause of diarrhea in children of age 6–24 months: **Rotavirus**
- Most common pathogenic parasitic infection in the human: **Giardia**
- Most common site for Amoebiasis: **Caecum**
- Most common site of intestinal TB: **Ileum**
- Most common symptom CA pancreas: **Painless jaundice**
- Most common site of CA Stomach: **Antrum**
- Most common site of Peptic ulcer: **First part of duodenum**
- Most common symptom of peptic ulcer: Abdominal pain with burning sensation
- Most common site of Typhoid ulcer: **Terminal ileum**
- Most common site of Amoebic colitis: **Sigmoid colon**
- Most common site of Colonic diverticula: **Sigmoid colon**
- Most common site of Ulcerative colitis: **Rectum**
- Most common site of Hirschsprung disorders: **Rectum**
- Women who have had any type of bariatric surgery should supplement their diets with vitamin B12, folate, iron, and calcium because the surgery decreases the absorption of these vitamins and minerals.

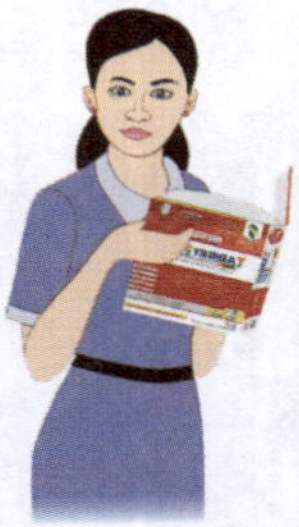

"Three things in life – your health, your mission, and the people you love.... That's it."

—Naval Ravikant

MULTIPLE CHOICE QUESTIONS
(Including Explained and Practice Questions)

GASTROINTESTINAL AND HEPATOBILIARY SYSTEM

GENERAL ANATOMY OF GASTROINTESTINAL SYSTEM

419. Gallbladder is located: *(ESIC Chennai May 2012)*
- a. Upper right part of abdomen
- b. On right side of liver
- c. On the left side of liver
- d. Below the liver

420. Which of these parts in the digestive system constitute the gastrointestinal or alimentary tract?
- a. Salivary glands
- b. Gallbladder
- c. Pancreas
- d. Anal canal

421. The flow of pancreatic juice into the duodenum is controlled by the:
- a. Ampulla of Vater
- b. Duct of Wirsung
- c. Sphincter of Oddi
- d. Pyloric antrum

422. All the following enzymes are secreted by gastrointestinal system; EXCEPT:
- a. Ptyalin
- b. Pepsinogen
- c. Gastric lipase
- d. Angiotensin

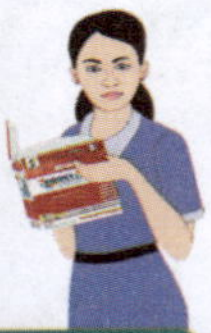

ANATOMY & PHYSIOLOGY OF MOUTH

423. Go through the following statements regarding salivary glands and identify the correct statement:
- a. Parotid glands are located on each side of the face just below the external acoustic meatus
- b. Parotid, sublingual and submandibular are the various types of salivary glands
- c. Parotid is the largest salivary gland
- d. All of the above

424. The presence of amylase in the saliva serves the purpose of:
- a. Washing away food particles to cleanse the mouth
- b. Lubricating the food to minimize friction with oral mucosal
- c. Destroying harmful bacteria to prevent oral infection
- d. Catalyzing the chemical reaction for the digestion of starch

425. The structure that is located near the laryngopharynx to prevent a food bolus from entering the airway during deglutition is the:
- a. Cricoid
- b. Epiglottis
- c. Palate
- d. Tongue

426. Which of the following taste buds is NOT correctly matched with the area of the tongue where it is most abundant?
- a. Sweet-tip of the tongue
- b. Bitter-back of the tongue
- c. Salty-posterior side of the tongue
- d. Sour-side of the tongue

427. Which of the following is NOT one of the four primary taste sensations?
- a. Bitter
- b. Sour
- c. Salty
- d. Spice

428. Which part of the tongue senses bitterness?
- a. Anterior one-third of the tongue
- b. Lateral aspect of the tongue
- c. Posterior one-third of the tongue
- d. All of the above

429. Safety muscle of tongue is:
- a. Styloglossus
- b. Genioglossus
- c. Hyoglossus
- d. Palatoglossus

430. Which of the following cranial nerve supplies the taste buds in the anterior two third of the tongue?
- a. Facial nerve (CN VII)
- b. Trigeminal nerve (CN V)
- c. Glossopharyngeal nerve (CN IX)
- d. Hypoglossal nerve (CN XII)

431. Taste sensation form tongue is carried out by all of the following cranial nerves; EXCEPT:
- a. V
- b. VII
- c. IX
- d. X

432. The anterior roof of the mouth is formed by:
- a. Soft palate
- b. Hard Palate
- c. Uvula
- d. Tonsil

433. The posterior roof of the oral cavity is made up of:
- a. Hard palate
- b. Tonsil
- c. Soft palate
- d. Frenulum

434. The structure of Uvula present on the deeper portion of the oral cavity is an extension of:
- a. Tonsil
- b. Soft palate
- c. Hard palate
- d. Nasopharynx

435. The action of lysosome in the oral cavity is to:
- a. Destroy the bacteria
- b. Breaks down the food material
- c. Digest the fat material
- d. Emulsify the fat.

436. Among the given parts of teeth, which of the following comprises the nerve and blood supply:
- a. Pulp
- b. Cementum
- c. Dentin
- d. Enamel

ANATOMY & PHYSIOLOGY OF ESOPHAGUS

437. Cardiac sphincter is situated at:
- a. Heart
- b. Cardiam
- c. End of esophagus
- d. End of stomach

438. Length of esophagus in adults is:
- a. 25 cm
- b. 10 cm
- c. 15 cm
- d. 20 cm

Ans.

419.	d
420.	d
421.	c
422.	d
423.	d
424.	d
425.	b
426.	c
427.	d
428.	c
429.	b
430.	a
431.	a
432.	b
433.	c
434.	b
435.	a
436.	c
437.	c
438.	a

439. Narrowest part of the esophagus is:
a. Cricopharynx
b. Esophagogastric junction
c. At the level of arch of aorta
d. Level of tracheal bifurcation

440. Esophagus enters through:
a. Central tendon of diaphragm
b. Along aortic opening
c. Muscular part of diaphragm
d. Right crus

441. The esophagus of the digestive system is located .... to the trachea?
a. Anterior b. Posterior
c. Lateral d. Ventral

442. The esophagus begins at the level of lower border of:
a. Cricoid cartilage
b. Hyaline cartilage
c. 4th cervical vertebra
d. 2nd thoracic vertebra

Explanation: The **esophagus** extends from the lower border of the cricoid cartilage (at the level of the sixth cervical vertebra) to the cardiac orifice of the stomach at the side of the body of the 11th thoracic vertebra.

443. Which of the following part in the digestive system allows the esophagus to connect with stomach region?
a. Diaphragmatic hiatus b. Esophageal hiatus
c. Cardiac sphincter d. Pyloric sphincter

444. When a person swallows a food material, which part of the digestive system allows food from mouth to esophagus, by closing the tracheal opening?
a. Pharyngeal rings b. Cricoid process
c. Epiglottis d. Glottis

445. The length of the Esophagus in a typical adult would be:
a. 3 inches long b. 5 inches long
c. 6 inches long d. 10 inches long

446. Which of the following physiology is taken place in Esophagus to conduct and transfer the food from mouth to the stomach region?
a. Ciliary movement
b. Peristalsis movement
c. Pump and dump
d. Active movement.

447. The peristalsis movement takes place in the esophageal region is a (an)
a. Voluntary action
b. Involuntary action
c. Depends (either voluntary or Involuntary)
d. None of the above

448. The vertebral level of the esophageal region would be:
a. C6 – T11 b. C2 – C3
c. C4 – T1 d. T6 – T 11

ANATOMY & PHYSIOLOGY OF STOMACH

449. The process of taking food into the digestive system is: *(RRB SSNE 2015)*
a. Ingestion b. Propulsion
c. Digestion d. Elimination

450. Mr Hari was complaining about the pain at his right hypochondriac region which refers to a region of the:
a. Head b. Thorax
c. Abdomen d. Upper limb

451. The secretion and motility of the stomach can be stimulated by this hormone:
a. Secretin b. Cholecystokinin
c. Gastrin d. Gastric gelatinase

452. Capacity of stomach of newborn:
a. 20 mL b. 30 mL
c. 50 mL d. 100 mL

453. Where is cardiac sphincter located? *(Staff Nurse GII 2014)*
a. Lungs b. Liver
c. Stomach d. Heart

454. Hydrochloric acid that enhances the digestion process in the stomach is secreted by:
a. Chief cells b. Parietal cell
c. Globin cells d. Chyme cells

455. The convex lateral surface of the stomach is referred to as which structure:
a. Greater curvature b. Medial Curvature
c. Lesser Curvature d. Lateral curvature

456. The structure present over the concave medial portion of the stomach is:
a. Greater Curvature b. Medial Curvature
c. Lesser Curvature d. Anterior Curvature

457. The gastric secretion inside the stomach can be inhibited by which of the following hormone?
a. Glucocorticoid b. Androgen
c. Somatostatin d. Gastrin

458. Which part of the stomach structure allows the processed food material to reach the intestinal region?
a. Pyloric sphincter b. Diaphragmatic Sphincter
c. Stomach fundus d. Jejunum

459. The term that refers to the folds present on the mucosal membrane which forms the covering layer of the stomach is:
a. Rugae b. Sulci
c. Sphincter d. Polyps

460. The structure present on the superior portion of the opening of the stomach is:
a. Pylorus b. Fundus
c. Cardia d. Omentum

ANATOMY & PHYSIOLOGY OF SMALL AND LARGE INTESTINE

461. Which one of the following structures holds the small intestine in its position?
a. Mesentery b. Mesocolon
c. Lesser omentum d. Greater omentum

462. The group of nerves that is located in the submucosal layer to regulate the secretory activities of the intestine is called:
a. Meissner's plexus b. Auerbach's plexus
c. Vagal nerve d. Sympathetic nerve

463. The surface area for absorption is enlarged by the following structures of the small intestine; EXCEPT:
a. Crypts of Lieberkuhn
b. Plicae circularis
c. Villus
d. Microvillus

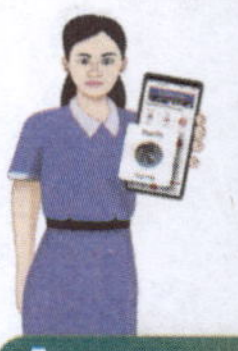

Ans.

439.	a
440.	c
441.	b
442.	a
443.	a
444.	c
445.	d
446.	b
447.	b
448.	a
449.	a
450.	c
451.	c
452.	b
453.	c
454.	b
455.	a
456.	c
457.	c
458.	a
459.	a
460.	c
461.	a
462.	a
463.	a

464. Which type of gastrointestinal motility thoroughly mixes the chyme in the small intestine?
a. Propulsion b. Churning
c. Segmentation d. Peristalsis

465. The part of the large intestine that is joined to the rectum is called:
a. Ascending colon b. Transverse colon
c. Descending colon d. Sigmoid colon

466. Pouch of Douglas is placed between:
a. Rectum and Sacrum
b. Uterus and Urinary bladder
c. Bladder and pubis symphysis
d. Rectum and Uterus

467. Meckel's diverticulum arises from:
a. The foregut b. Caecum
c. Colon d. Ileum

468. Sphincter of Oddi consists of:
a. 2 sphincters b. 3 sphincters
c. 4 sphincters d. 5 sphincters

469. Commonest position of appendix:
a. Pelvic b. Retrocecal
c. Subcecal d. Promontoric

470. The length of the large intestine is about:
a. 1.5 meters b. 3 meters
c. 4.5 meters d. 6 meters

471. Foramen of Morgagni refers to an opening in:
a. The brain b. The lesser omentum
c. The skull d. The diaphragm

472. The narrowest part of the small intestine:
a. 60 cm proximal to ileocecal valve
b. 60 inches proximal to ileocecal valve
c. 90 cm proximal to ileocecal valve
d. 90 inches proximal to ileocecal valve

473. The levator ani is composed of all; EXCEPT:
a. Pubococcygeus b. Puborectalis
c. Iliococcygeus d. Transverse peronei

474. Branch of internal iliac artery:
a. Ovarian artery b. Testicular artery
c. Superior vesical artery d. None

475. Shortest part of colon:
a. Ascending colon b. Transverse colon
c. Descending colon d. Sigmoid colon

476. Gland of Brunner's is found in:
a. Jejunum b. Duodenum
c. Ileum d. All

477. Peyer's patches are present in:
a. Jejunum b. Ileum
c. Colon d. Duodenum

478. Iron is absorbed almost entirely in:
a. Stomach b. Duodenum
c. Jejunum d. Ileum

479. Which among the following is a part of small intestine?
a. Cardia b. Duodenum
c. Transverse colon d. Sigmoid colon

LAYERS OF DIGESTIVE SYSTEM

480. The serous membrane that lines the organs of the digestive system is called:
a. Parietal peritoneum b. Visceral peritoneum
c. Abdominal peritoneum d. Pelvic peritoneum

481. The basic general layout of the gastrointestinal tract wall from inside to outside follows this sequence:
a. Submucosa → mucosa → muscular → serosa
b. Muscular → serosa → mucosa → submucosa
c. Mucosa → submucosa → muscular → serosa
d. Serosa → muscular → submucosa → mucosa

482. The chief cells of the gastric glands secrete:
a. Pepsinogen b. Trypsinogen
c. Intrinsic factors d. Hydrochloric acid

483. Abdominoplasty is:
a. Removal of the larger skin wrinkles and folds from the face and neck
b. Removal of excess abdominal skin and fat
c. Smoother appearance of photo-damaged and wrinkled skin
d. Improve the appearance of photo damaged and acne scarring

484. Which of the following layer is the first and the Innermost layer of the stomach?
a. Serosa b. Subserosa
c. Mucosa d. Endothelium

485. Among the major layer of the stomach and the intestinal region, which of the following would be regarded as outermost and the last covering layer:
a. Serosa b. Mucosa
c. Epithelium d. Exothelium

486. Which of the following layer is present in between the sub mucosa and serosa:
a. Muscularis Externa b. Subserosa
c. Mucosa d. None of the above

487. The layer between the mucosa and muscularis externa would be referred to as:
a. Submucosa b. Submuscularis
c. Serosa d. Subserosa

Explanation:

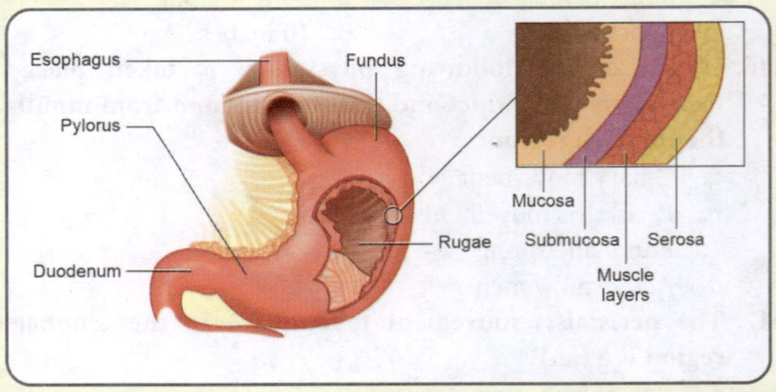

Figure: Layers of stomach

488. Which of the following layers of the stomach would churn out the food material and cause them to move within the stomach:
a. Mucosa b. Muscularis
c. Serosa d. Submucosa

489. The type of epithelium present on the mucosal layer of the stomach and intestine would be:
a. Transitional epithelium
b. Stratified epithelium
c. Squamous epithelium
d. Simple Columnar epithelium

Ans.

464.	c
465.	d
466.	d
467.	d
468.	b
469.	b
470.	a
471.	d
472.	a
473.	d
474.	c
475.	a
476.	b
477.	b
478.	b
479.	b
480.	b
481.	c
482.	a
483.	b
484.	c
485.	a
486.	a
487.	a
488.	b
489.	d

490. What type of epithelium is present on the mucosal layer of the mouth and pharynx:
a. Transitional epithelium
b. Stratified epithelium
c. Squamous epithelium
d. Stratified squamous epithelium

491. The major function of the submucosal layer would be:
a. To provide cushion to stomach
b. To contain major blood vessel & nerve for stomach function
c. To help the food material to breaks down and in peristalsis
d. To act as layer of filtrating waste material

492. How many days does a cell remain present in the GI tract to get renewed approximately:
a. At least 10 days
b. Every 2 days
c. 2 months once
d. 4 to 5 days

493. What kind of nerve system present on the stomach mucosal layer that controls and innervates the muscular movement and its action:
a. Mesenteric plexus
b. Submucosal plexus
c. Muscularis plexus
d. Peritonial plexus

BLOOD AND NERVE SUPPLY OF GI SYSTEM

494. Short gastric arteries are branches of:
a. Celiac artery
b. Splenic artery
c. Left gastroepiploic artery
d. Right gastroepiploic artery

495. Portal vein is formed by splenic vein and:
a. Superior mesenteric vein
b. Portal vein
c. Inferior mesenteric vein
d. Hepatic vein

496. Superior rectal vein drains into:
a. Superior mesenteric vein
b. Inferior mesenteric vein
c. Inferior vena cava
d. Portal vein

497. Veins draining into portal vein are all; EXCEPT:
a. Renal vein
b. Splenic vein
c. Left gastric vein
d. Superior mesenteric vein

498. The right suprarenal vein drains into:
a. Left renal vein
b. Right renal vein
c. Inferior vena cava
d. Right phrenic vein

499. Which of the following is correct regarding portal vein?
a. Formed by the superior mesenteric vein
b. Formed by the splenic vein
c. Formed at the level of 2nd lumbar vertebra
d. All of the above

500. Which statement about absorption from the gastrointestinal (GI) tract is accurate? *New Q*
a. The absorption of glucose is associated with sodium uptake.
b. Glucose is more rapidly absorbed than galactose when administered separately.
c. Fructose is more rapidly absorbed than glucose.
d. The majority of water absorption along the GI tract occurs in the Large intestine.

Explanation: Glucose is absorbed in the small intestine by a process called **facilitated diffusion**. This process requires the presence of sodium ions. When glucose molecules bind to the transporter, sodium ions are also transported into the cell. This helps to drive the absorption of glucose.

Glucose is typically absorbed more rapidly than fructose in the small intestine.

Glucose and galactose are absorbed at similar rates in the small intestine. They both utilize the same transporter, SGLT1, for absorption.

The majority of water absorption along the GI tract occurs in the small intestine, particularly the jejunum and ileum

501. Portal vein supplies:
a. Spleen
b. Liver
c. Pancreas
d. Colon

502. Blood supply of Hindgut:
a. Coeliac trunk
b. Splenic artery
c. Superior mesenteric artery
d. Inferior mesenteric artery

503. Venous blood of liver is drained by:
a. Portal vein
b. Hepatic artery
c. Sinusoids
d. Hepatic veins

504. Posterior gastric artery is a branch of:
a. Left gastric artery
b. Right gastric artery
c. Splenic artery
d. Hepatic artery

505. Blood supply to the proximal large intestine is supplied by: *(AIIMS Bhopal Grade-I 2018)*
a. Inferior mesenteric
b. Celiac trunk
c. Superior mesenteric
d. Anterior mesenteric

Explanation: Unlike the other branches of abdominal aorta, there are three unpaired branched arteries that supply the intestine. Superior mesenteric artery supplies the whole small intestine and proximal large intestine, whereas the branched celiac trunk supplies the spleen by splenic (lineal) artery, stomach by gastric artery (further branched as gastroduodenal arteries supplies blood to pylorus and duodenum of small intestine) and liver by common hepatic artery. Inferior mesenteric artery is responsible for supplying blood to the descending colon and sigmoid colon.

506. Which of the following is false about portal vein?
a. Formed behind the neck of pancreas
b. Bile duct lies anterior and right to it
c. Gastro duodenal artery lies to the left and anterior to it
d. Ascends behind the 2nd part of duodenum

507. Inferior mesenteric artery is a branch of:
a. Internal iliac artery
b. External iliac artery
c. Abdominal aorta
d. Superior mesenteric artery

DIGESTION PROCESS IN HUMAN

508. Stimulation of the parasympathetic nerve on the digestive system results in:
a. Decreased gastrointestinal motility
b. Decreased dilatation of portal veins branches
c. Increased gastrointestinal secretions
d. Increased tone of anal sphincters

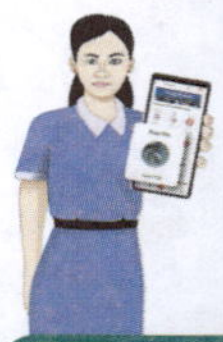

Ans.
490. d
491. b
492. d
493. b
494. b
495. a
496. d
497. a
498. c
499. d
500. a
501. b
502. d
503. d
504. c
505. c
506. d
507. c
508. c

509. Defecation reflexes are set by:
a. The gastro-ileal reflex
b. The stretch receptors in the wall of the rectum
c. The relaxation of the external anal sphincter.
d. Release of gastrin

510. One of the end products of carbohydrate digestion in the small intestine is:
a. Sucrose b. Maltose
c. Lactose d. Fructose

511. Which of these substances hydrolyzes the dietary proteins into amino adds?
a. Amylase b. Trypsin
c. Lipase d. Bile

512. Most of the absorption of fats occur in the:
a. Duodenum b. Jejunum
c. Ileum d. Caecum

513. In intestinal absorption, the chylomicron is transferred to the lymph capillaries of the villus by:
a. Reverse osmosis
b. Facilitated transport
c. Active transport
d. Passive diffusion

514. The main source of body fuel is:
a. Carbohydrates
b. Amino acids
c. Proteins
d. Fat

515. Encik Ali is at risk of diuretic-induced hypokalaemia. Which of the following food that has the highest content of potassium would you advise him to consume?
a. Chicken b. Potatoes
c. Banana d. Soya milk

516. The rate of a reaction catalyzed by an enzyme will reach its optimum level in the human body when:
a. Blood pH is between 10 and 12
b. There is an enzyme antagonist
c. The body temperature reaches 32°C
d. The enzyme activator acts on the enzyme precursor

517. The energy exchange molecule that stores and releases energy as required by the body is the:
a. Nicotinamide-adenine dinucleotide
b. Flavin-adenine dinucleotide
c. Adenosine triphosphate
d. Adenosine diphosphate

518. The breakdown of glycogen storage for more glucose occurs in a biochemical process called:
a. Glycolysis
b. Glycogenolysis
c. Gluconeogenesis
d. Glycogenesis

519. Lactose intolerance is a condition that occurs because of the deficiency of enzyme known as:
a. Lactase b. Maltase
c. Gluten d. Pepsin

Explanation: In lactose, intolerance inability to tolerate the sugar found in dairy products as a result of an absence or deficiency of lactase.

520. One of the key molecules in the metabolism of carbohydrates, proteins and fats to produce energy output is:
a. Pyruvic acid
b. Citric acid
c. Keto acids
d. Fatty acids

521. The catabolic reaction of proteins to produce energy is called:
a. Transamination
b. Deamination
c. Beta oxidation
d. Oxidative phosphorylation

522. Order of using stored energy sources during starvation is:
a. Carbohydrate, Amino acids, and Lipoproteins
b. Glycogen, fat and skeletal protein
c. Glycogen, Skeletal protein, and fat
d. Protein, fat, and glycogen

523. Normal pH of gastric HCl is:
a. 0.2–1.5 b. 1.5–3.5
c. 3.5–5.5 d. 5.5–6.5

524. All of the following stimulate secretion from parietal cells in stomach; EXCEPT:
a. Acetylcholine b. Somatostatin
c. Gastrin d. Histamine

525. Vitamin K synthesis is done by:
a. Liver b. Colonic bacteria
c. Skin d. Blood vessels

526. Iron absorption is increased by:
a. Vitamin-C b. Phytic acid
c. Fiber diet d. Phosphates

527. Intrinsic factor is secreted by:
a. Chief cells
b. Delta cells
c. Parietal cells
d. Enterochromaffin-like cells

528. In the stomach, H^+ are secreted in exchange for:
a. Na^+ b. K^+
c. Ca^+ d. Cl^-

529. Gastric motility is increased in:
a. Increased cortisol level
b. High fiber diet
c. Opioid drugs
d. Gastroparesis

530. Salivary amylase is activated by:
a. Sodium Ion
b. Chlorine Ion
c. Potassium Ion
d. Bicarbonate Ion

531. Intestinal motility is increased by:
a. Secretin
b. Gastrin
c. Cholecystokinin
d. None

532. Intrinsic factor in stomach is secreted by:
a. Parietal cells b. Chief cells
c. Zymogen cells d. Enterochromaffin cells

533. Vitamin B_{12} is absorbed in:
a. Duodenum b. Jejunum
c. Ileum d. Colon

Ans.

509.	b
510.	d
511.	b
512.	b
513.	d
514.	a
515.	c
516.	d
517.	c
518.	b
519.	a
520.	a
521.	b
522.	b
523.	b
524.	b
525.	b
526.	a
527.	c
528.	b
529.	b
530.	b
531.	c
532.	a
533.	c

534. Pepsinogen is secreted by:
a. Parietal cells b. Mucus cells
c. Chief cells d. Oxyntic cells

535. A man cannot digest carbohydrate. The enzyme deficient is:
a. Lipase b. Amylase
c. Pepsin d. Trypsin

536. Iron absorption takes place in which part of intestine?
a. Duodenum b. Ileum
c. Jejunum d. Colon

537. Chyme is formed by:
a. Esophagus b. Stomach
c. Duodenum d. Jejunum

538. Stimulation for gastric emptying:
a. Secretin b. CCK
c. Gastrin d. Distension

539. Diet devoid of carbohydrates causes:
a. Ketosis b. DM
c. No effect d. Obesity

540. Gastric acid secretion phase includes:
a. Cephalic phase b. Gastric phase
c. Intestinal phase d. All of the above

541. Content in gastric secretion includes:
a. HCl b. Pepsinogen
c. Mucus d. All of the above

542. Which artery supplies oxygenated blood to the stomach? *(RRB SSNE 2015)*
a. Carotid artery b. Gastric artery
c. Celiac artery d. Cephalic artery

543. All of the following factors increase gastric motility; EXCEPT: *(DSSSB 2006)*
a. Abdominal distension b. Fear
c. Stress d. Vagotomy

Explanation: Fear, anger, stress and vagotomy increase peristalsis (gastric motility). Abdominal distension diminishes peristalsis.

544. Decrease in the production of HCl acid in the stomach is known as:
a. Achlorhydria b. Hypochlorhydria
c. Hyperchlorhydria d. Anaplasia

545. Absence in the production of HCl acid in the stomach is known as:
a. Achlorhydria b. Hypochlorhydria
c. Insomnia d. Anaplasia

Explanation: Achlorhydria is absence of HCl. Hypochlorhydria means decreased amount of acid secretion. Hyperchlorhydria is high level of acid.

546. Activation of .... leads to increase in peristalsis.
a. Sympathetic stimulation
b. Parasympathetic stimulation
c. RAAS activation
d. ACE inhibition

547. Identify clear fluid diet among the following:
a. Black tea or black coffee
b. Apple juice
c. Gelatin
d. All of the above

548. Gastric acid is neutralized in the intestine due to the action of:
a. Pepsinogen b. Bicarbonate
c. Erythropoietin d. Calcium carbonate

549. Richest source of energy among the following is:
a. Cereals
b. Rice
c. Glass of orange juice
d. Glass of milk

550. Which of the following is considered to be a clear liquid diet?
a. Pasteurized milk b. Ice cream
c. Plain gelatins d. Fresh orange juice

Explanation: Milk, ice cream (contains milk) and freshly squeezed orange juices are not considered to be clear liquid diet. Plain gelatins (Jello) can be given to a patient who is on a clear liquid diet.

ABOMINAL QUADRANTS AND ORGANS

551. While palpating a male client's right upper quadrant (RUQ), the nurse can palpate:
a. Spleen b. Liver
c. Kidney d. Appendix

552. The jejunum and the proximal ileum is located on the which part of the abdominal quadrants?
a. Right upper quadrant
b. Right lower quadrant
c. Left upper quadrant
d. Left lower quadrant

553. The appendix and the most part of the ileum is present on the which side of abdominal quadrants?
a. Right lower quadrant b. Right upper quadrant
c. Left lower quadrant d. Left Upper quadrant

554. In the classification of the abdominal quadrants, sigmoid colon comes under the:
a. Left upper quadrant b. Left lower quadrant
c. Right upper quadrant d. Right lower quadrant

555. The spleen is present on the which quadrant of the abdominal region?
a. Left hypochondriac region
b. Umbilical region
c. Left lumbar region
d. Right lumbar region

556. Most part of the small intestine is present on the which part of the abdominal quadrants?
a. Right lumbar region
b. Left lumbar region
c. Left hypochondriac region
d. Umbilical region

557. The Urinary bladder is located at which of the abdominal quadrants?
a. Umbilical region b. Hypogastric region
c. Epigastric region d. Left lumbar region

558. The location of gallbladder in the abdominal quadrant would be:
a. Right lumbar region
b. Right hypochondriac region
c. Epigastric region
d. Left lumbar region

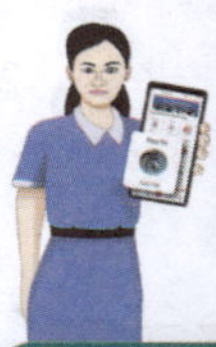

Ans.
534. c
535. b
536. a
537. b
538. c
539. a
540. d
541. d
542. c
543. a
544. b
545. a
546. b
547. d
548. b
549. c
550. c
551. b
552. c
553. a
554. b
555. a
556. d
557. b
558. a

559. The anatomical part of the liver is present on the which portion of the abdominal quadrants?
a. Right lumbar region
b. Umbilical region
c. Right hypochondriac region
d. Left hypochondriac region

DIAGNOSITIC EVALUATION IN GI SYSTEM

560. Normal GI system findings in adults include:
a. Non-palpable liver and spleen
b. Liver in the right upper quadrant
c. Tenderness over McBurney's point
d. Both a and b

561. Diagnostic test for pancreatitis is:
a. Serum amylase b. Serum lipase
c. Ultrasound d. All of the above

562. Microscopic stool examination techniques involve:
a. Saline mount causes
b. Iodine mount
c. Concentration techniques
d. All of the above

563. In a client with dark complexion icterus will be checking at:
a. Nasal bridge
b. Hard palate of the mouth
c. Nail beds
d. Skin

564. Most accurate method for confirming the NG tube placement is:
a. X-ray
b. Auscultation
c. Observing patient for coughing aspiration of content and pH monitoring
d. Dip in a bowel of water

565. Invertogram is one of the diagnostic tests in: *(JIPMER 2012)*
a. Pyloric stenosis b. Intussusception
c. Anorectal anomalies d. Diverticulum

566. Which of the following diagnostic tests would be used initially to assess a client with acute upper GI bleeding?
a. Upper GI series b. Barium X-ray
c. Endoscopy d. Arteriography

567. Which of the following diagnostic test is useful in diagnosis of diverticulosis?
a. Endoscopy b. Barium swallow
c. Barium enema d. USG abdomen

568. Pre-procedural preparation for sigmoidoscopy is:
a. NPO
b. Enema before the procedure
c. Insertion of NG tube
d. Ask about iodine allergy

Explanation: Enema before the procedure helps to clean the colon, NPO is required for upper GI procedure. In this, there is no use of dye, so question related to iodine allergy is least important.

569. Sigmoidoscopy is done in which position? *(Safdarjung NO 2018)*
a. Lithotomy position
b. Jack knife position
c. Fowler's position
d. Knee chest position

Explanation: Sigmoidoscopy is done in knee chest or left sims position. These positions aid in easy movement of sigmoidoscope in the colon, and better visualization.

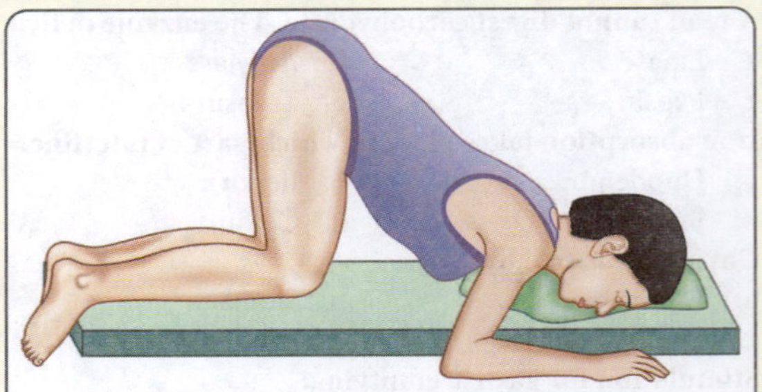

For a sigmoidoscopy, the nurse should place the patient in the knee-chest position or Sims' position, depending on the physician's preference.

570. Double bubble sign in the X-ray is the characteristic of which disease condition?
a. Pyloric stenosis b. Duodenal atresia
c. Hirschsprung's disease d. Trachea esophageal fistula

Explanation: Radiography shows a distended stomach and distended duodenum, which are separated by the pyloric valve, a finding described as the double-bubble sign.

571. Priority nursing intervention in the immediate post-gastroscopy period will be:
a. Administer oxygen
b. Assess gag reflex prior to administration of fluids
c. Administer ordered fluid and drugs
d. Replace NG drainage every 2 hourly

Explanation: Gag reflex assessment before the administration of fluid is the priority nursing intervention. Usually these patients are conscious and not have any respiratory difficulty.

572. Best disinfectant for endoscope is: *(AIIMS Bhuvneshwar LP 2017)*
a. Hypochlorite b. Formaldehyde
c. Glutaraldehyde d. Chlorohexidine

Explanation: Glutaraldehyde is used to disinfect the endoscope.

573. Which of the following diagnostic test is NOT used to investigate dysphagia?
a. Laryngoscopy b. Manometry
c. Barium swallow d. Colonoscopy

Explanation: A colonoscopy is a visual examination of the entire large intestine (colon) using a lighted, flexible colonoscope. It is not used to investigate dysphagia which is associated with upper GI. Barium swallow, esophageal manometry and laryngoscopy are used to investigate dysphagia as these procedures helps in visualization of upper GI structures.

574. Patient with abdominal trauma presents with hypotension, tachycardia, pallor and restlessness which among the following organ is most likely to be ruptured?
a. Liver b. Spleen
c. Intestine d. Gallbladder

Ans.
559. c
560. d
561. d
562. d
563. b
564. a
565. c
566. c
567. c
568. b
569. d
570. b
571. b
572. c
573. d
574. b

575. Following fiberoptic colonoscopy patient reports increasing abdominal pain, fever, and chills, which among the following complication need to suspect by the nurse?

a. Bowel perforation b. Pneumoperitoneum
c. Paralytic ileus d. Diverticulitis.

576. Correct information regarding colonoscopy is:

a. Informed consent is necessary
b. Sedation may be used during the procedure.
c. NPO status is needed d. All of the above

577. Dark ground illumination technique is used in the diagnosis of:

a. Tetani b. S. typhi
c. Treponema pallidum d. Herpes

578. Position used while inserting NG tube is:

a. Supine b. High Fowler's
c. Low Fowler's d. Orthopneic

Explanation: High Fowler's position facilitates the entry of tube easily. So it is the indicated position.

579. Nurse is about to insert Ryle's Tube for a patient. Before this act, she must be aware of the distance between incisor teeth and gastro esophageal junction. Which of the following is correct distance? *(NCFL 2019)*

a. 30 cm b. 40 cm
c. 50 cm d. 60 cm

Explanation: Measurements obtained during endoscopic examination reveal the average distance from the incisor teeth to the gastroesophageal junction to be 38 to 40 cm in men and 36 to 38 cm in women. 40 cm is the closest answer to both the ranges.

580. A 45-year-old male patient is on total parenteral nutrition (TPN). Which of the following assessment is important for this patient?

a. Assess the bowel sound
b. Assess the peripheral IV site for extravasation injury
c. Confirmation that the tube is in the stomach
d. Fluid and electrolyte monitoring

Explanation: Total parenteral nutrition (TPN) is a method of feeding that bypasses the gastrointestinal tract. Fluids are given into a vein to provide most of the nutrients the body needs. Because of the nutritional composition of TPN, it is important to monitor the client's fluid status, electrolytes, blood glucose and weight.

581. What is meant by Dysphagia?

a. Difficulty in breathing
b. Difficulty in voiding
c. Difficulty in swallowing
d. Difficulty in speaking

582. Which of the following diagnostic test helps to identify whether the patient has bleeding from the GI tract?

a. Complete blood court b. Abdominal girth
c. Abdominal palpation d. Guaiac test

583. Difficulty in swallowing is known as:

a. Dyspepsia b. Nausea
c. Dysphagia d. Phagitis

ANATOMY & PHYSIOLOGY HEPATOBILIARY SYSTEM

584. The synthesis of bile occurs in the:

a. Liver b. Gallbladder
c. Pancreas d. Duodenum

585. Bilirubin conjugation occurs in:

a. Liver b. Duodenum
c. Spleen d. Pancreas

586. Nutmeg liver is seen in:

a. Chronic venous congestion liver
b. Infarction of liver
c. Amyloidosis
d. Budd Chiari syndrome

587. The liver is kept in position by:

a. Hepatic veins b. Intra-abdominal pressure
c. Hepatic artery d. a and b

588. Bile duct opens into:

a. Second part of duodenum
b. Third part of duodenum
c. Pyloric end of stomach
d. Ileocecal junction

589. Entero-hepatic circulation is necessary for the secretion of:

a. Bile b. Intestinal juice
c. Pancreatic juice d. Gastric juice

590. Unconjugated hyperbilirubinemia is seen in:

a. Neonatal hepatitis
b. Gilbert syndrome
c. Dubin-Johnson syndrome
d. Rotor syndrome

591. The average size and weight of a adult liver is:

a. 5-8 cm long/3000 g b. 5-8 cm long/3500 g
c. 13–15 cm long/1500 g c. 13–15 cm long/600 g

592. Which type of cells form the functional unit of the liver? *New Q*

a. Kupffer cells b. Hepatic cells
c. Neuronal cells d. Chief cells

Explanation: The functional unit of the liver is called the hepatic lobule, and it is primarily composed of **hepatic cells**, also known as hepatocytes.

Kupffer cells (option a) are a type of specialized macrophage found in the liver. They play a role in immune function and are involved in filtering and phagocytosing foreign substances in the liver.

Neuronal cells (option c) are not the primary cell type of the liver.

Chief cells (option d) are typically associated with the gastric glands of the stomach and are responsible for producing pepsinogen.

593. The layer that covers the liver region would be:

a. Peritoneal layer b. Glisson's capsule
c. Kupffer shell d. Pseudo epithelium

594. The ligamentum that separates the left and the caudate lobes would be:

a. Ligamentum granulosum b. Ligamentum serosum
c. Ligamentum Venosum d. Ligamentum falciform

595. What type of ligament connects the ventral wall abdomen with the anterior part of the liver?

a. Ligamentum granulosum b. Ligamentum serosum
c. Ligamentum Venosum d. Ligamentum falciform

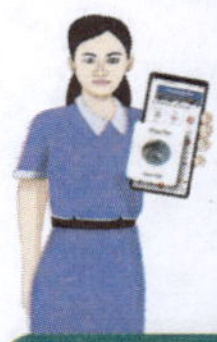

Ans.

575. a
576. d
577. c
578. b
579. b
580. d
581. c
582. d
583. c
584. a
585. a
586. a
587. d
588. a
589. a
590. b
591. c
592. b
593. b
594. c
595. d

596. The substance that gets released during the time of RBC break down:

a. Bilirubin pigment b. Hemoglobin pigment
c. Centrosome d. Ferratin

597. If person's body experiences poor dietary sugar, the person liver converts the:

a. Glucagon into glucose
b. Glucose to glucagon
c. Glycogen to glucose
d. Glucose to glycogen

598. Which type of protein that a liver produces abundantly for the intercellular homeostasis?

a. Globlin b. Albumin
c. Fibrinogen d. Keratin

599. The amount of bile that the gallbladder normally stores is:

a. 20–25 mL b. 10–15 mL
c. 30–50 mL d. 80–120 mL

DIAGNOSTIC TESTS IN HEPATOBILIARY SYSTEM

600. Direct serum bilirubin range is:

a. 0.1–0.4 mg/dL b. 0.2–0.8 mg/dL
c. 0.3–1.6 mg/dL d. 0.4–0.8 mg/dL

601. Indirect serum bilirubin level is:

a. 0.1–0.6 mg/dL b. 0.2–0.8 mg/dL
c. 0.3–1.2 mg/dL d. 0.4–1.4 mg/dL

602. Which among the following is a basic diagnostic test to assess the liver function?

a. Serum bilirubin b. ALT enzyme
c. Serum proteins d. All of the above

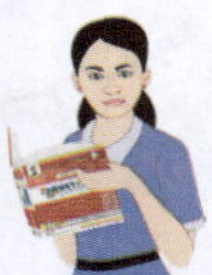

603. Preprocedural investigation required for a client who is scheduled for ERCP is:

a. Bilirubin level b. Hemoglobin level
c. Bile amount d. Lipase level

604. Which is the best test for detecting Liver dysfunction? *(RRB SSNE 2015)*

a. Serum albumin b. Serum bilirubin
c. SGPT d. Prothrombin time

605. Right side lying position given to a client following liver biopsy is:

a. For hemostasis b. For comfort
c. To decrease pain d. For observing easily

606. 3 L of fluid is obtained via paracentesis in a client, what is the immediate complication expected in this client?

a. Vascular collapse b. Peritonitis
c. Respiratory arrest d. Cardiac arrest

Explanation:

- Ascites is one of the most common complications of cirrhosis of liver. Ascites refers to accumulation of fluid in the peritoneal cavity.
- Abdominal paracentesis is a procedure in which fluid from peritoneal cavity is removed by inserting a needle. The rapid decrease in abdominal pressure during the procedure may lead to vasodilation and vascular collapse (distributive shock).
- Peritonitis due to infection is also an expected complication but not an immediate complication.
- Respiratory arrest and cardiac arrest may be possible but are secondary to vascular collapse.

607. Among the given imaging studies which of the following are the most specific and accurate methods to rule out and or diagnose the acute pancreatitis?

1. CT
2. SPECT
3. Sonography

a. 1 only c. 1 and 2 only
b. 2 only d. 1 and 3 only

608. Which of the following diagnostic test is most preferred for a client with right upper quadrant pain related with biliary system?

a. Sonogram
b. Radiography
c. Nuclear medicine with contrast
d. CT without contrast

609. Aspartate Aminotransferase is also known as:

a. Serum glutamic-oxaloacetic transaminase
b. Serum glutathione oxalate transaminase
c. Sodium glutamic-oxaloacetic transferase
d. Sodium glutamic-oxaloacetic transaminase

610. The normal range for ALT test results in men would be found in between:

a. 10–40 IU/L b. 40–70 IU/L
c. 50–80 IU/L d. 70–100 IU/L

Explanation: **Serum** alanine aminotransferase (ALT) is the most common and economical screening test for the assessment of asymptomatic liver disease. Most laboratories in **India** mention the upper limit of **normal** for **ALT** as 30–40 IU/L.

611. The normal range for AST is:

a. 5–10 U/L b. 10–42 U/L
c. 30–60 U/L d. 90–110 U/ L

DISORDERS OF MOUTH AND GUMS

612. Inflammation of salivary gland is:

a. Salpingitis b. Sialadenitis
c. Oophoritis d. Rhinitis

613. Inflammation of oral cavity is:

a. Stomatitis b. Gastritis
c. Glossitis d. Gingivitis

614. Inflammation of gum is:

a. Stomatitis b. Gastritis
c. Glossitis d. Gingivitis

615. Stone in the salivary gland is known as:

a. Cholelithiasis b. Sialolithiasis
c. Nephrolithiasis d. Xanthelasma

616. A canker sore of the oral soft tissues is known as:

a. Aphthous stomatitis b. Angular stomatitis
c. Infectious stomatitis d. Oral thrush

Explanation: Aphthous stomatitis is a common condition characterized by the repeated formation of benign and non-contagious mouth ulcers (aphthae or canker sore) in otherwise healthy individuals.

617. Carcinoma of acinic cell is associated with:

a. Parathyroid gland b. Salivary gland
c. Lacrimal duct d. Sebaceous gland

Ans.

596. a
597. c
598. b
599. c
600. a
601. b
602. d
603. a
604. c
605. a
606. a
607. d
608. a
609. a
610. a
611. b
612. b
613. a
614. d
615. b
616. a
617. b

618. The term that refers the Irritation of lips along with signs of scaling and the crusting over lips is:
a. Actinic cheilitis b. Chancre
c. Lichen planus d. Aphthous stomatitis

619. The Red color patch seen on the oral mucus membrane is known as:
a. Erythema b. Erythroplakia
c. Chancre d. Erythrochelitis

620. A Serious gum infection that can even lead to loosening of teeth is:
a. Stomatitis b. Gingivitis
c. Periodontitis d. Cheilitis

621. The pathological term that refers the bad breath would be:
a. Halosis b. Gingivitis
c. Cheilitis d. Halitosis

622. Risk factors of gingivitis include:
a. Diabetes b. Smoking
c. Certain Drugs d. All of the above

623. Inflammation of the tongue is known as: *(DSSSB 2013)*
a. Gingivitis b. Glossitis
c. Parotitis d. Stomatitis

Explanation: Glossitis is an inflammation of the tongue. Gingivitis is inflammation of gum. Parotitis is an inflammation of one or both parotid glands. Stomatitis is the inflammation of the oral mucosa.

HIATAL HERNIA

624. Which of the following are the two types of hiatal hernia?
a. Primary and secondary
b. Sliding and paraesophageal
c. Obstructive and contractive
d. Acute and chronic

625. While standing up the stomach moves into the thoracic cavity while supine gets into the abdominal cavity is referreds to as:
a. Sliding Hiatal hernia b. Paraesophageal hernia
c. Rolling hernia d. Obstructive hernia

626. The fundus and greater curvature of the stomach moves up through the diaphragm where the esophageal junction remains in the constant place:
a. Sliding Hiatal hernia
b. Paraesophageal hiatal hernia
c. Esotracheal hiatal hernia
d. Obstructive hernia

627. The following are the major complications of Hiatal hernia; EXCEPT:
a. Esophagitis b. GERD
c. Portal hypertension b. Hemorrhage with erosion

628. All are used as a surgical intervention for the client with hiatal hernia; EXCEPT:
a. Herniotomy b. Pyeloplasty
c. Herniography d. Antireflux procedure

ESOPHAGEAL DIVERTICULUM

629. The most common type of esophageal diverticulum:
a. Traction diverticula b. Zenker's Diverticula
c. Epiphrenic Diverticula d. Fundus Diverticula

630. In which portion of the esophagus, the abnormality takes place in the Zenker's Diverticula?
a. Upper 1/3 of esophagus
b. Mid-esophagus
c. Lower 1/3 of esophagus
d. Lateral side of esophagus

631. Traction diverticulum has an abnormality over the:
a. Upper 1/3 of esophagus
b. Mid-esophagus
c. Lower 1/3 of esophagus
d. Lateral side of esophagus

632. Epiphrenic diverticula has a herniation over the:
a. Upper 1/3 of esophagus b. Midesophagus
c. Lower 1/3 of esophagus d. Lateral side of esophagus

633. The following are interventions given in the esophageal diverticulum; EXCEPT:
a. Applying pressure at the point on neck
b. Endoscopic surgery
c. Blenderized Diet
d. Splint over the cervical region

Explanation: Blenderized foods are pureed foods that are thinned with additional liquid so that they can be consumed without chewing. Applying pressure at the point on neck and endoscopic surgery also used as an intervention in diverticulum. Splint over the cervical region is not an appropriate intervention for esophageal diverticulum.

GASTROESOPHAGEAL REFLUX DISEASE (GERD)

634. Frequent vomiting put the patient at risk of:
a. Metabolic acidosis with hyperkalemia
b. Metabolic acidosis with hypokalemia
c. Metabolic alkalosis with hyperkalemia
d. Metabolic alkalosis with hypokalemia

Explanation: Excessive vomiting results in expulsion of gastric acid and potassium form gastric content which leads to metabolic alkalosis and hypokalemia.

635. Identify the correct statements about gastroesophageal reflux disease (GERD)
a. GERD often involves relaxation of the lower esophageal sphincter
b. Nissen's fundoplication is the surgical management for the condition
c. Lying in supine position is helpful
d. Both a and b

636. Health education to a client with GERD includes:
a. Avoid lying down immediately after food
b. Avoiding heavy lifting
c. Have small frequent meal
d. All of the above

637. All are the nursing management for a person who is suffering from gastroesophageal reflex disease; EXCEPT:
a. Provide supine position after feeding
b. Burp in between
c. Use thickened feed
d. Serve small frequent diet

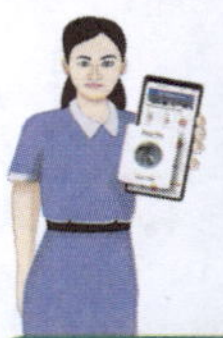

Ans.

618.	a
619.	b
620.	c
621.	d
622.	d
623.	b
624.	b
625.	a
626.	b
627.	c
628.	b
629.	b
630.	a
631.	b
632.	c
633.	d
634.	d
635.	d
636.	d
637.	a

Explanation: The cardiac sphincter and lower portion of the esophagus are weak, allowing regurgitation of gastric contents back into the esophagus. Except option A, all other managements indicated in a person who is suffering from GERD because all these measures reduce the chance of GERD. Neissan Fundoplication is the surgical management of choice for a child who is suffering from GERD.

638. Gastric aspiration can lead to:
a. Water and electrolytes imbalances
b. Bicarbonate imbalance
c. Protein and fat imbalances
d. Micronutrient deficiency

OTHER DISORDERS OF ESOPHAGUS

639. Meaning of Barrett's esophagus is:
a. Lower esophagus lined by columnar epithelium
b. Upper esophagus lined by columnar epithelium
c. Lower esophagus lined by cuboidal epithelium
d. Upper esophagus lined by cuboidal epithelium

640. Heart burn refers to an uneasy burning sensation in the: *(RRB Feb 2012)*
a. Jejunum b. Duodenum
c. Esophagus d. Stomach

641. Dysphagia for fluids but not for solids is seen in:
a. Carcinoma oesophagus
b. Achalasia
c. Reflux oesopagitis
d. Stricture

642. Postoperatively after the initiation of feed following esophagectomy client develops increasing pain, fever and dyspnea. These are suggestive of:
a. Feed intolerance
b. Anastomosis leakage into mediastinum
c. Gastritis
d. GERD

643. In a patient with decreased or absent gag reflex, side lying position is given to:
a. Prevent aspiration b. Prevent bed sore
c. Stimulate gag reflex d. Maintain nutritional status

GASTRITIS

644. Inflammation of stomach is:
a. Stomatitis b. Gastritis
c. Glossitis d. Gingivitis

645. Causes of gastritis is:
a. H. Pylori infection b. Over use of NSAIDs
c. Alcohol and smoking d. All of the above

646. Most common viral cause of gastritis:
a. H. pylori
b. CMV
c. Hepatitis A
d. Enterovirus

647. Identify the cause of gastritis among the following:
a. Over use of aspirin and NSAIDs
b. Excessive alcohol intake
c. Infection by H. pylori
d. All of the above

648. Contraindicated medication in a patient with acute gastritis is:
a. Naproxen sodium b. Calcium carbonate
c. Azithromycin d. Furosemide

649. GI irritability increase with the use of:
a. Sugar products b. Dairy products
c. Cola drink and coffee d. Both b and c

650. The following are the risk factors that cause gastritis; EXCEPT:
a. Alcohol use b. Long-term steroid use
c. High caloric intake d. Emotional stress.

651. One of the prominent signs and symptoms of Acute gastritis is:
a. Epigastric pain, hematemesis
b. Projectile vomiting
c. Grey turner sign
d. Psoas sign

652. The term that refers to the passage of black and tarry stools:
a. Hematochezia b. Hematemesis
c. Melena d. Hyperemesis

653. The most regarded gold standard diagnostic test for gastritis:
a. Endoscopy b. Gastroscopy
c. Colonoscopy
d. Esophagogastroduodenoscopy (EGD)

654. Major complication of gastritis would be:
a. Hemorrhage & Pernicious anemia
b. Pyloric stenosis
c. Dumping syndrome
d. Gastric cancer

655. All of the following are the important pharmacological management of gastritis; EXCEPT:
a. Antacid b. Inj. B_{12}
c. H_2 receptor agonists
d. Proton pump Inhibitor drugs

656. The surgical intervention where the diseased part of the stomach is removed is:
a. Vagotomy b. Gastrectomy
c. Gastrotomy d. Pyloroplasty

657. Following are the commonly used proton pump Inhibitors for the gastritis; EXCEPT:
a. Omeprazole b. Ranitidine
c. Pantaprazole d. Lanzoprazole

PEPTIC ULCER DISEASE

658. Urea breath test in exhaled breath is used to detect the presence of: *(AIIMS BBS NO 2018)*
a. Escherichia coli
b. Streptococcus
c. Helicobacter pylori
d. Staphylococcus

Explanation: Helicobacter pylori bacteria produce enzyme called Urease. In Urea breath test, a tablet containing urea is given to patient to swallow. If patient having infection of H pylori in stomach, it breaks urea into ammonia and carbon dioxide with presence of enzyme urease. Carbon dioxide is measured after swallowing the tablet. If patient is infected there will be rise in carbon dioxide level. If patient is not infected, urea will be excreted by kidneys.

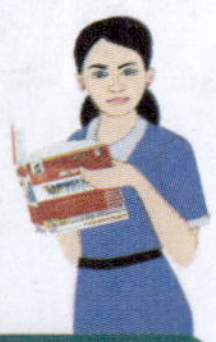

Ans.
638. a
639. a
640. c
641. b
642. b
643. a
644. b
645. d
646. b
647. d
648. a
649. d
650. c
651. a
652. c
653. d
654. a
655. c
656. b
657. b
658. c

659. Which medical diagnosis can the nurse expect when collecting a health history from a client who is scheduled for antrectomy? *(RAK MSc 2018)*

a. Cataract
b. Gastric ulcers
c. Otosclerosis
d. Trigeminal neuralgia

Explanation:
- The nurse expects a client to have Gastric ulcer when collecting a health history from a client who is scheduled for antrectomy. Stomach ulcers, also known as gastric ulcers, are common in lesser curvature near incisura and antrum of the stomach.
- An antrectomy is the resection, or surgical removal, of a part of the stomach is known as the antrum.

660. The erosion of mucosal layer of stomach is termed: *(DSSSB PHN, 2015)*

a. Duodenal ulcer
b. Gastric ulcer
c. Chron's disease
d. Diverticulitis

661. Which of the following is NOT true regarding gastric ulcer?

a. Long-term use of NSAIDs causes gastric ulcer
b. Intake of spicy food causes gastric ulcer
c. Food may cause pain and vomiting may relieve it
d. Helicobacter pylori infection causes gastric ulcer

662. Risk factors for peptic ulcer include:

a. Taking NSAIDs
b. Smoking
c. Alcohol consumption
d. All of the above

663. Which of the following statement is NOT true about peptic ulcer disease?

a. Peptic ulcer is more likely to occur in the first part of duodenum than in the stomach
b. Gram negative H-pylori bacteria causes peptic ulcer
c. Avoid food items like coffee and caffeinated beverages
d. Consumption of milk and cream is encouraged

664. The most common site of occurring peptic ulcers in stomach: *(JIPMER 2012)*

a. Pyloric portion
b. Cardiac portion
c. Esophageal junction
d. Body of the stomach

665. Most common site/location of peptic ulcer is:

a. At gastroesophageal junction
b. Gastric antrum
c. 1st part of duodenum
d. Lesser curvature of stomach

666. The main action of ranitidine in treating peptic ulcer is: *(JIPMER 2012)*

a. Increase gastric motility
b. Neutralize gastric acidity
c. Inhibit gastric acid secretion
d. Increase histamine release

667. A major causative organism for peptic ulcer is: *(DSSSB 2013, ESIC Chennai May 2012)*

a. Escherichia coli
b. Streptococci
c. Staphylococci
d. Helicobacter pylori

Explanation: H. pylori is gram-negative bacteria that grow in the digestive tract and have a tendency to attack the lining of the stomach. Individuals infected with H. pylori have a 10–20% lifetime risk of developing peptic ulcers and a 1–2% risk of acquiring stomach cancer.

668. Best test for determining eradication of H. pylori infection:

a. Urease test
b. Serum ELISA
c. Tissue biopsy
d. Breath urea test

669. Peptic ulcer caused by helicobacter pylori is treated with:

a. Ranitidine and antibiotics
b. Ranitidine and omeprazole
c. Ranitidine and pantoprazole
d. Surgical intervention

Explanation: Anti H. pylori therapy to treat gastric ulcer consists of combination of antimicrobials, like amoxycillin or clarithromycin and nitroimidazoles (Metronidazole, Tinidazole and Ornidazole). Eradication of H. pylori concurrently with H_2 blocker (ranitidine) has been associated with faster ulcer healing and lower relapse rate.

670. Raju is suffering from peptic ulcer disease and during his discharge counseling educate him to avoid:

a. Coffee and cola
b. Alcohol
c. Milk
d. All of these

Explanation: Peptic ulcer disease refers to painful sores or ulcers in the lining of the stomach or first part of the small intestine, called the duodenum. Frequent milk ingestion as previously prescribed is not encouraged. This is owing to the transient buffering effect and significant gastric acid secretion effect of milk. Currently, studies indicate that it is prudent to avoid alcohol. This is especially true for the concentrated forms, such as 40% alcohol. Coffee should be avoided on the basis of its strong acid secretagogue property. Some fiber-containing foods may possess factors that are protective against ulcer disease.

671. Gastric ulcer occurs due to:

a. GERD
b. Hyperacidity
c. Decreased mucosal resistance
d. Microorganisms

672. Common site for stress induced gastric ulcer is:

a. Greater curvature
b. Antrum
c. Lesser curvature
d. Anywhere in stomach

Explanation: The gastric body and fundus is a common location for stress ulcerations but can also be seen in antrum and duodenum.

673. Most common site of Curling's ulcer:

a. Proximal Duodenum
b. Esophagus
c. D. jejunum
d. Distal duodenum

Explanation: Curling's ulcer is an acute gastric erosion resulting as a complication from severe burns when reduced plasma volume leads to ischemia and cell necrosis (sloughing) of the gastric mucosa. It commonly occurs in proximal duodenum.

674. Identify the clinical manifestation of duodenal ulcer among the following:

a. Hematemesis will be present
b. Patient is generally malnourished
c. Pain occurs 1-2 hours after eating
d. Food may relieve pain

675. Which of the following is the initial symptom of perforated duodenal ulcer?

a. Hyperpyrexia
b. Mid-epigastric pain
c. Projectile vomiting
d. Heart burn

Explanation: A hole that goes all the way through the duodenum is called a perforated duodenal ulcer. A perforation is a medical emergency. Sudden, sharp pain, begins mid-epigastric is the initial symptom of perforation.

Ans.

659. b
660. b
661. b
662. d
663. d
664. a
665. c
666. c
667. d
668. d
669. a
670. d
671. c
672. d
673. a
674. d
675. b

676. Correct option regarding a tuberculous ulcer is:
a. Transverse orientation
b. Stricture formation
c. Presence of caseous necrosis on cut surface
d. All of the above

677. Which among the following diet will be helpful for maintaining positive nitrogen balance?
a. High-protein, high-carbohydrate, low-fat diet
b. High-calorie low protein diet
c. Low-calorie low protein and low fat diet
d. High-calorie low protein and high fat diet

678. Combination of omeprazole, clarithromycin and metronidazole regimen is the treatment of choice for:
a. Food poison
b. Irritable bowel syndrome
c. Helicobacter pylori infection
d. Celiac disease

679. In Zollinger-Ellison Syndrome, the main manifestation is:
a. Peptic ulceration b. Watery diarrhea
c. Hyperglycemia d. Hypocalcemic tetany

GASTROINTESTINAL BLEEDING

680. Hematemesis is:
a. Blood in vomitus b. Blood in sputum
c. Fresh blood in stool d. Occult blood in stool

681. Hemoptysis is:
a. Blood in vomitus b. Blood in sputum
c. Fresh blood in stool d. Occult blood in stool

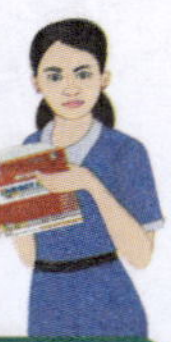

682. The passage of bloody stools, where the blood appears fresh and red to maroon in color is known as:
a. Melena b. Hematochezia
c. Hemorrhoid d. Hematemesis

683. Hematochezia is seen in all; EXCEPT:
a. Piles b. Anal fissure
c. Upper Gi bleeding d. Lower GI bleeding

684. Melena is black, tarry stool and typically indicates:
a. Upper GI bleeding
b. Lower GI bleeding
c. Bleeding from hemorrhoids
d. Bleeding from anal fissures

685. Which of the following is the appropriate diet plan for first 24 hours for a patient with active upper GI bleeding?
a. Regular diet b. Bland diet
c. Clear liquids d. NPO

Explanation: Bleeding must be brought under control before oral intake of food.

686. Which of the following is most appropriate diet for a patient with active upper GI bleeding in the first 24 hours of admission?
a. Regular diet b. Bland diet
c. BRAT diet d. Nothing by mouth

687. In gastrointestinal perforation nurse need to suspect:
a. Paralytic ileus
b. McBurney's point pain
c. Sudden, severe abdominal pain
d. Diarrhea

688. Hematochezia may result from all of the following; EXCEPT:
a. Lower GI bleeding b. Massive upper GI bleeding
c. Over intake of antacids d. Diverticulitis

Explanation: Hematochezia refers to appearance of bright red blood in the stool. It is usually from lower gastrointestinal tract (colon or rectum). The common causes include hemorrhoids, diverticulitis, anal fissures, colon cancer, ischemic colitis, inflammatory bowel disease. Hematochezia may also result from massive upper GI bleeding.

689. The test to detect the bleeding present on the stool would be:
a. Transit test b. Psoas test
c. Guaiac test d. Melanil test

690. Mallory-Weis tears refers to the tear present on the:
a. Esophagus
b. Greater curvature of stomach
c. Esophagogastric junction
d. Pyloric junction

691. The following are major root source for the upper GI bleeding; EXCEPT:
a. Peptic ulcer disease b. Mallory-Weis tears
c. Erosive gastritis d. Pernicious Anemia

DUMPING SYNDROME

692. Dumping syndrome is characterized by which one of the following symptoms?
a. Hypertension b. Hypervolemia
c. Hyperglycemia
d. Generalized weakness dizziness and sweating after meals

693. Cause of dumping syndrome includes:
a. Gastrectomy b. Esophagectomy
c. Both a and b d. None of the above

694. Dumping syndrome is a complication of: *(DSSSB 2013)*
a. Nephrectomy b. Subtotal gastrectomy
c. Ileostomy d. Hysterectomy

Explanation: Dumping syndrome is common after gastric surgery. It is a group of symptoms, including weakness, abdominal discomfort, and sometimes abnormally rapid bowel evacuation, occurring after meals in some patients who have undergone gastric surgery.

695. Important management of diarrhea is:
a. More intake of liquids b. Start metronidazole
c. Isolate the client
d. Start antibiotic based on stool culture and sensitivity

696. The onset of the early dumping syndrome is usually within .... after eating.
a. 30 minutes b. 45 minutes
c. 60 minutes d. 90 minutes

Explanation: With **dumping syndrome**, food moves too quickly from stomach into the intestine. Symptoms of **early dumping syndrome occur within 30 minutes after a meal**, while symptoms of **late dumping syndrome occur 1 to 3 hours after a meal**. The most common cause of rapid gastric emptying and dumping syndrome is surgery of the stomach or esophagus. Early dumping syndrome is caused by sudden arrival of large quantity of food in the stomach. This leads to the rapid movement of fluid into the intestine, **which causes** discomfort, bloating, and diarrhea. Late dumping syndrome occurs due to release of a large amount of insulin.

Ans.
676. d
677. a
678. c
679. a
680. a
681. b
682. b
683. c
684. a
685. d
686. d
687. c
688. c
689. c
690. c
691. d
692. d
693. c
694. b
695. a
696. a

697. What would be the goal of management in dumping syndrome?

a. To help the stomach to excrete
b. To reduce the digestion process
c. To dilate the intestinal length
d. To delay gastric emptying process

698. What kind of bowel sound is auscultated with a patient with early dumping syndrome?

a. Hypoactive sound b. Borborygmi sound
c. Rigor sound d. Ronchi sound

Explanation: **Borborygmi** refers to a loud, hyperactive bowel sound (growling and rumbling sounds) that the stomach and intestines make as food, fluids, and gas pass through them.

699. Which type of diet should be avoided with a person who has dumping syndrome?

a. Milk and sweet product b. Low carbs
c. High protein d. Green vegetables.

Explanation: Refined sugars rapidly absorb water from the body, **causing** symptoms. Symptoms may also happen after eating dairy products and certain fats or fried foods. Foods to avoid: candy, sweet drinks, cakes, cookies, pastries, sweetened breads, dairy products and fried foods.

Foods to eat: Complex carbohydrates, fiber supplements, vegetables, whole-wheat bread.

700. The cause of late dumping syndrome seen in elderly patient is:

a. Narrowing of the small intestine
b. Excessive release of fatty acid
c. Excessive release of insulin
d. Jejunum receiving food bolus

701. The primary cause of dumping syndrome would be considered as:

a. Diarrheal disorder
b. Pyloric stenosis
c. Reduced abdominal capacity
d. Presence of hypertonic content in small intestine.

702. All of the given clinical manifestation are seen in dumping syndrome; EXCEPT:

a. Epigastric fullness b. Hyperglycemia
c. Colic pain d. Tremors and giddiness.

703. All of the following are recommended interventions for dumping syndrome; EXCEPT:

a. Eat small and frequent meals
b. Eat simple sugars (carbohydrates)
c. Take high protein diet
d. Increase fiber intake

APPENDICITIS

704. Vermiform appendix is the part of which organ?

a. Duodenum b. Ileum
c. Cecum d. Ascending colon

705. Which of the following is the most common cause of acute appendicitis?

a. Fecalith b. Tumor of the appendix
c. Bowel kinking d. Foreign body

706. McBurney's point is associated with: *(Kerala PSC, Nov 2014)*

a. Appendix b. Stomach
c. Spleen d. Larynx

707. Location of McBurney's point is:

a. Midway between umbilicus and anterior superior iliac spine on right side
b. Midway between umbilicus and anterior superior iliac spine on left side
c. Midway between umbilicus and pubic symphysis
d. Midway between umbilicus and coccyx

Explanation: McBurney's point is the name given to the point over the right side of the abdomen that is one-third of the distance from the anterior superior iliac spine to the umbilicus (navel). This point roughly corresponds to the most common location of the base of the appendix where it is attached to the cecum.

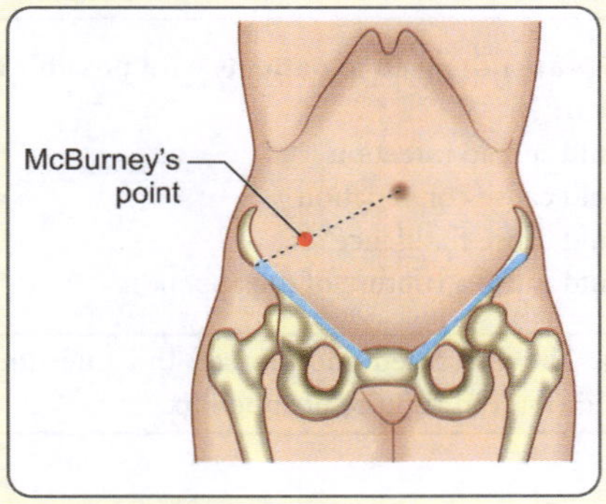

Figure: McBurney's point

708. The patient with appendicitis usually exhibits the following clinical manifestations. *(ESIC 2019)*

a. Rebound tenderness at the McBurney's Point
b. Pain occurs immediately after eating
c. Heartburn regurgitation and dysphagia
d. Hematemesis or melena

Explanation: The patient with appendicitis usually exhibits the **Rebound tenderness at the McBurney's Point**, it is also called as Blumberg's sign or rebound tenderness. It refers to pain upon removal of pressure rather than application of pressure to the abdomen. It is positive in appendicitis.

709. All are correct regarding appendicitis; EXCEPT:

a. Pain at McBurney's point is an important symptom of appendicitis
b. Positive Homan's sign suggest appendicitis
c. Rovsing's sign is the characteristic sign of appendicitis
d. Appendix is usually located in the lower right quadrant of the abdomen

710. A 45-year-old patient with the complaints of pain in the right lower quadrant of abdomen was admitted in the ward. Assessment findings revealed tenderness on palpation at McBurney's point. Which one of the following additional laboratory findings is suggestive of appendicitis in this patient?

a. WBC of 13, 000 b. RBC of 4. 7 million
c. Platelet count of 250,000 d. All of these

Explanation: In appendicitis, WBC count is elevated. The RBC and Platelet values given above are within normal limits.

Ans.

697. d
698. b
699. a
700. c
701. d
702. b
703. b
704. c
705. a
706. a
707. a
708. a
709. b
710. a

711. Clinical sign in which pressure on the left lower quadrant of the abdomen causes pain in the right lower quadrant is known as:

a. Rovsing's sign b. Cullen sign
c. Homan's sign d. Kerning's sign

712. Preoperative preparation for appendectomy NOT includes:

a. Enema STAT b. Consent (DSSSB 2013)
c. Skin preparation d. Removal of jewelries

Explanation: Administration of enema causes increased pressure in the colon, which may lead to rupture of appendix and infection such as peritonitis. So enema is contraindicated in a person who is suffering from appendicitis. Hot application is also contraindicated in this condition as it leads to inflammation and rupture of appendix.

713. Laxatives are not given to patients with possible appendicitis because it:

a. Could spread infection
b. Could cause constipation
c. Could cause flatulence
d. Could cause a rupture of the appendix

Explanation: The increased motility of the intestine caused by laxatives could result in rupture of appendix.

PERITONITIS

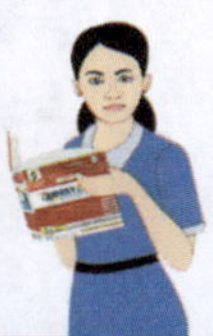

714. Finding suggestive of peritonitis is:

a. Rebound abdominal pain b. Pain at McBurney's point
c. Guarding of abdomen d. Cullen's sign

715. Which among the following is a clinical manifestation of peritonitis?

a. Icterus
b. Abdominal rigidity
c. Umbilical hernia
d. Increased bowel sounds

716. The membranes that line the walls of the abdomen and provide protection to the cavity region is:

a. Visceral layer b. Parietal layer
c. Squamous layer d. Epicardial layer

717. Which of the following substance is produced by the mesothelial layer that allows organ to glide easily?

a. Intrinsic factor b. Mucus
c. Serous fluid d. Endolymph

718. Peritonitis results in the inflammatory response which leads to:

a. Melana b. Constipation
c. Massive fluid shift (edema) d. Coolness of the muscles

719. All the given symptoms are seen in peritonitis; EXCEPT:

a. Muscular rigidity b. Grey turner sign
c. Rebound tenderness d. Abdominal distension.

720. The most common risk factors for primary spontaneous peritonitis include:

a. Liver disease with cirrhosis
b. Pancreatitis
c. Diverticulitis
d. Perforated colon

INFLAMMATORY BOWEL DISEASE (IBD)

721. Inflammatory bowel disease results in:

a. Perforation b. Stricture
c. Obstruction d. Paralytic ileus

722. Pain associated with irritable bowel disease can be treated with:

a. Paracetamol b. Opioids
c. Laxatives d. Buscopan

723. A client is admitted to the hospital with a bowel obstruction. Which of the following is the priority nursing diagnosis?

a. Fluid volume deficit
b. Deficient knowledge
c. Ineffective tissue perfusion
d. Pain related to abdominal distention

Explanation: Bowel obstruction results in accumulation of feces, fluid and gas above the obstructed part. This causes decreased fluid absorption, hence fluid volume deficit.

724. Patient complaining of pain in lower abdomen with malaise, semi-solid stools with an offensive odor, blood and mucous, organism responsible for this is:

a. Hook worm
b. Entamoeba histolytica
c. Tape worm
d. Plasmodium

725. Which of the following statement is NOT TRUE regarding Taenia solium infestation?

a. It is also known as round worm
b. Transmitted by eating improperly cooked pork
c. Adults worms are big in length and eggs are passed in feces
d. Adults worms have hooks and suckers

726. Which of the following is correct regarding hookworm infestation?

a. Adults are found in small intestine
b. Causes iron-deficiency anemia
c. Larvae pass through blood circulation
d. All of the above

727. All are true about Giardia lamblia infection; EXCEPT:

a. It is a type of gram-positive bacteria
b. Water-borne infection
c. Pear-shaped trophozoites are seen
d. Causes watery diarrhea

Explanation: Giardia lamblia, also known as Giardia intestinalis, is a flagellated parasitic microorganism. G. lamblia trophozoites are pear-shaped cells and motile by way of four pairs of flagella. It causes the diarrheal illness known as Giardiasis.

728. Travelers diarrhea is most commonly caused by:

a. Enterotoxigenic *E. coli* b. Exogenic *E. coli*
c. EIEC d. Shigella

729. Most common cause for diarrhea in adults associated with intake of Shell fish?

a. Norwalk virus b. Calicivirus
c. Rotavirus d. Filovirus

730. Vitamin deficiency seen in short bowel syndrome is?

a. Vitamin A b. Vitamin B_{12}
c. Vitamin D d. All of these

Ans.

711. a
712. a
713. d
714. a
715. b
716. b
717. c
718. c
719. b
720. a
721. a
722. d
723. a
724. b
725. a
726. d
727. a
728. a
729. a
730. d

INTESTINAL OBSTRUCTION

731. Which of the following is a manifestation of pyloric stenosis? *(DSSSB 2013)*
a. Projectile vomiting
b. Regurgitation
c. Steatorrhea
d. Tenesmus

Explanation: Vomiting with the material ejected with great force; seen commonly in congenital pyloric obstruction.

732. All the following are causes of constipation; EXCEPT: (AIIMS BBS NO 2018)
a. Inadequate fiber intake
b. Decreased fluid intake
c. Laxative abuse
d. Decreased gastrointestinal motility

Explanation: Laxatives (e.g. Bisacodyl, liquid paraffin) are drugs that **relieve constipation** by loosening stools or inducing a bowel movement. It does not cause constipation. All other given factors are associated with constipation.

733. Aganglionic disease of the intestinal tract which causes inadequate motility is termed as: *(ESIC 2019)*
a. Ulcerative colitis
b. Crohn's disease.
c. Hirschsprung's disease
d. Diverticular disease

Explanation: Aganglionic disease is a congenital defect of the intestinal tract which causes inadequate motility. It is termed as **Hirschsprung's disease**. The nerve supply is absent from parts of the intestine, therefore called aganglionic. **The most common symptom** is failure to pass meconium followed by 24-48 after birth.

734. The corrective surgery for Hirschsprung's Disease is: *(Staff Nurse G II 2014)*
a. Pyloroplasty
b. Kasai procedure
c. Duhamel procedure
d. Pyeloplasty

735. Currant jelly stool is a manifestation of: *(Staff Nurse G II 2014)*
a. Trachea esophageal fistula
b. Intussusception
c. Oesophageal atresia
d. Anorectal malformation

736. To perform colostomy irrigation, the catheter should be inserted into the stoma up to: *(Safdarjung NO 2018)*
a. 5 cm
b. 10 cm
c. 15 cm
d. 20 cm

Explanation: To perform colostomy irrigation, insert catheter gently 2" to 4" (5 cm to 10 cm) into the bowel to instill the irrigant fluid. So the catheter can be inserted up to 10 cm.

737. Most common site for intestinal obstruction is:
a. Duodenum
b. Ileum
c. Jejunum
d. Cecum

738. Which among the following is a treatment option for intestinal obstruction?
a. Decompress the bowel
b. Resection and anastomosis
c. Both a and b
d. None of the above

739. Leading cause of small intestinal obstruction is.
a. Volvulus
b. Intussusception
c. Adhesions secondary to previous pelvic surgery
d. Congenital causes

740. While doing colostomy irrigation, the irrigation bag should be hung .... above the level of the stoma:
a. 8–12 inches
b. 12–18 inches
c. 18–24 inches
d. 24–36 inches

Explanation: The irrigation bag should be hung 12–18 inches. Irrigation bag above this level can create increased pressure and sudden intestinal distention to the patient.

741. There is no drainage from colostomy after 24 hours of its creation. Nurse should be aware that it is because of:
a. Absence of gastrointestinal motility
b. GERD
c. Low fluid intake
d. Enema

742. Maximum normal functioning of the bowel will be present in ....colostomy.
a. Sigmoid colostomy
b. Ascending colon
c. Descending colon
d. Transverse colon

743. Solution of choice for colostomy irrigation is:
a. Distilled water
b. Lactated Ringer's
c. Luke warm water
d. Tap water

744. Among the following which must be there in the discharge teaching plan of a permanent colostomy client:
a. Diet restriction
b. Frequent emptying of stoma bag
c. Importance of stool softeners
d. Dilation of the stoma

745. Patient with colostomy should be advised to eat:
a. Bland diet so that the intestines do not become irritated
b. Everything they ate before the surgery but will avoid those foods that produce gas
c. Food low in fiber
d. Soft foods that are more easily digested

Explanation: Patient with colostomy can eat a regular diet. There is no special dietary restrictions, however, the patient is advised to avoid gas-forming foods which in turn can cause distention and discomfort.

746. Side effect of omeprazole is:
a. Heart burn
b. Constipation
c. Itching
d. Icterus

HERNIA

747. Hiatal hernia present with:
a. Dysphasia
b. Regurgitation
c. Heart burn and chest pain
d. All of the above

748. Main clinical symptom of hiatal hernia is:
a. Heartburn
b. Vomiting
c. Abdominal distention
d. Dysuria

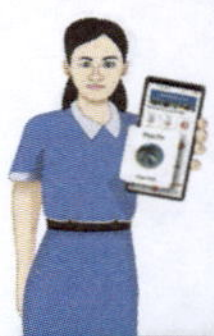

Ans.

731. a
732. c
733. c
734. c
735. b
736. b
737. b
738. c
739. c
740. b
741. a
742. a
743. d
744. d
745. b
746. b
747. d
748. a

749. The type of hernia that is more prone to become strangulated is:

a. Inguinal hernia b. Femoral hernia
c. Hiatal hernia d. Umbilical hernia

750. The following inguinal herniorrhaphy scrotal edema can be reduced by:

a. Providing Trendelenburg position
b. Hot water fomentation
c. Restrict fluid intake
d. Scrotal support with ice bag

BARIATRIC SURGERY

751. Which among the following complication will be present in a client following gastrectomy?

a. Anemia
b. Deficiency of fat soluble vitamin
c. Peptic ulcer
d. Pancytopenia

752. Gastroenterostomy is creation of connection between:

a. Stomach and the jejunum
b. Stomach and distal ileum
c. Stomach and proximal ileum
d. Esophagus and duodenum

753. In which surgery part of stomach is removed and remaining portion is anastomosed to duodenum? *(LNJP H D 2012)*

a. Gastrectomy
b. Endoscopic mucosal resection
c. Gastrojejunostomy
d. Gastroduodenostomy

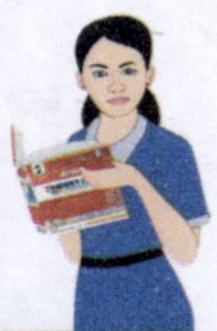

754. Best position that can be given to a client after gastrectomy is:

a. Lateral b. Low fowlers
c. Supine d. Prone

755. Vitamin supplementation needed after gastrostomy is:

a. Vit B_{12} b. Vit A
c. Vit D d. Vit E

756. Absence of bowel sounds and abdominal distension after abdominal surgery indicates: *(DSSSB 2013)*

a. Hemorrhage b. Paralytic Ileus
c. Intussusception d. Flatulence

Explanation: Paralytic ileus is the occurrence of intestinal blockage in the absence of an actual physical obstruction. A temporary paralysis of a portion of the intestines occurs typically after an abdominal surgery.

HEMORRHOIDS

757. Hematochezia is:

a. Blood in vomitus b. Blood in sputum
c. Fresh blood in stool d. Occult blood in stool

758. Melena is:

a. Blood in vomitus b. Blood in sputum
c. Fresh blood in stool d. Occult blood in stool

759. Melena suggests which of the following? *(AIIMS BPL SNO 2018)*

a. Head injury
b. Injury to the upper bowel
c. Miscarriage
d. Injury to the lower bowel

Explanation: Melena is the presence of digested blood pigments in feces, causing a dark, tarry appearance and a foul odor as a consequence of oxidized iron derived from hemoglobin which usually occurs as a result of upper gastrointestinal bleeding.

760. Dark red/black color stool can be seen after:

a. Beet roots and Blueberries
b. Bleeding
c. Iron supplements
d. All of the above

761. A client is scheduled for a hemorrhoidectomy. The nurse should observe the client for the presence of which common clinical indicator associated with hemorrhoids:

a. Pruritis b. Flatulence (RAK MSc 2018)
c. Anal stenosis d. Rectal bleeding

Explanation: The nurse should observe for rectal bleeding in case of hemorrhoids. Hemorrhoids are perianal varicose vein which are characterized by bleeding and prolapse of the engorged veins. These engorged veins may rupture and produce bright red blood. So, it is important to observe for rectal bleeding in a client posted for hemorrhoidectomy.

762. Clinical manifestation of hemorrhoids includes:

a. Rectal bleedings
b. Extreme itching around the anus
c. A painful bowel movement
d. All of the above

763. Correct regarding hemorrhoids is:

a. Swollen blood vessels of the rectum.
b. Hemorrhoidal veins are located in the lowest area of the rectum and the anus
c. Internal hemorrhoids "prolapse", or enlarge and protrude outside the anal sphincter
d. All of the above

764. Straining during defecation cause:

a. Polyps b. Diarrhea
c. Hemorrhoids d. Constipation

HYPER-PYLORIC STENOSIS & DIVERTICULAR DISEASE

765. Which of the following statement regarding diverticulitis is TRUE:

a. Abdominal pain, fever, nausea and a change in bowel habits are the sign and symptoms
b. Diverticulitis is most common in Sigmoid colon
c. Treatment can include rest, a liquid or high-fiber diet and antibiotics
d. All of the above

766. As compared to diverticulitis, patient with diverticulosis has:

a. Rectal bleeding
b. No symptoms
c. Localized cramping pain
d. Abdominal distention

767. An abnormal sac or pouch formed at a weak point in the wall of the alimentary tract is:

a. Aneurysm b. Diverticulum
c. Hernia d. Protrusion

Ans.

749. b
750. d
751. a
752. a
753. d
754. b
755. a
756. b
757. c
758. d
759. b
760. d
761. d
762. d
763. d
764. c
765. d
766. b
767. b

768. The development of diverticulitis is associated with which of the following type of diet?

a. High-fiber diet
b. Low-fiber diet
c. Low-fat diet
d. Protein rich diet

COLORECTAL CANCER

769. Which of these patient's dietary habits does the nurse understand may increase the risk for development of colon cancer? *(RAK MSc 2018)*

a. High fat, low fiber intake
b. High intake of milk and milk products
c. Low meat and protein intake
d. Low fat, high carbohydrate intake

Explanation:

- Colon cancer is cancer of the large intestine. High fat, low fiber intake may contribute to an increased risk of colorectal cancer.
- The levels of *Fusobacterium nucleatum*, a bacteria that predisposes to cause colon cancer by inducing inflammation or irritating the colon tissue. This mechanism increases if an individual switches from a low-fat, high fiber diet to a high-fat, low-fiber diet, which is usually characterized by a high intake of red and processed meats.

770. Nurse Ramya is providing care for a patient who is newly confirmed with colon cancer. The patient has become withdrawn from his family members. Which of the following nursing action is most appropriate for this patient?

a. Approach the doctor and recommend a psychiatric consultation for the client.
b. Motivate the client to verbalize feelings about what he feels internally.
c. Give health education regarding available new treatment with successful outcomes.
d. Ask family and friends to visit the patient and enhance emotional support.

Explanation: A newly diagnosed patient with cancer may experience a range of emotions, including fear, anxiety, and sadness. It is important for the nurse to create a supportive environment and encourage the patient to express their feelings and concerns. By motivating the client to verbalize their emotions, the nurse can help facilitate open communication and provide emotional support.

Option (a) may be considered if the patient's withdrawal and emotional state persist or worsen over time.

771. Nurse was checking the reports of a male patient who is taking 5-fluorouracil chemotherapy IV for the treatment of colon cancer. Which of the following finding should alert the nurse to contact the physician?

a. WBC count of 1800/mm^3
b. Platelet count of 150000/mm^3
c. Hemoglobin 9.5 g/dL
d. Hematocrit 42%

Explanation: Chemotherapy, such as 5-fluorouracil, can have significant effects on blood cell counts. A low white blood cell (WBC) count, known as leukopenia, can increase the risk of infection. A WBC count of 1800/mm^3 is considered significantly low, and it puts the patient at an increased risk of developing infections. It is important to promptly notify the physician to ensure appropriate evaluation and management of the low WBC count.

772. Nurse Ramya was performing abdominal examination of a patient with colorectal cancer. Auscultation findings revealed high-pitched bowel sounds and presence of clear peristaltic waves. Which action should the nurse take?

a. Check that the client is having pain at the right shoulder
b. Perform the digital rectal examination and check for polyps
c. Approach the doctor and recommend for CT
d. Provide a laxative to increase bowel movement activity

Explanation: The auscultation findings of high-pitched bowel sounds indicate a partial obstruction due to the cancer. Hence the further investigation is needed to rule out the condition.

773. A patient diagnosed with colon cancer had a new colostomy. The patient states, "I need someone to talk who had experienced what I'm experiencing now." Which of the following response by the nurse would be most appropriate?

a. I know a patient with a colostomy who would be willing to have a conversation with you.
b. The enterostomal therapist will be respond all your doubts.
c. I will arrange a referral to the Ostomy Associations of India.
d. Don't worry, you will get to know everything by yourself as the time progress.

Explanation: The patient's statement indicates a desire for support and connection with someone who has gone through a similar experience. Referring the patient to an ostomy association or support group can provide the opportunity to connect with others who have colostomies and can share their experiences and provide emotional support.

774. A nurse is preparing to provide health education to a client who is healing from a recent colon resection. Which of the following statement should the nurse include in the plan of care?

a. You may have nausea and vomiting for the first few days.
b. Carbonated beverages can help minimize acid reflux from anastomosis sites.
c. Provide stool softener to make easy of their defecation process.
d. You may be able to do your daily routines, including weight lifting workouts.

Explanation: After a colon resection, the client may experience changes in bowel habits, including temporary constipation or difficulty with bowel movements. Providing stool softeners can help prevent constipation. This is important in promoting optimal bowel function and preventing complications such as straining or discomfort during bowel movements.

775. A client with late-stage colon cancer had metastasis spread to the spine. Which of the following nursing action is appropriate to address a priority issue?

a. Provide five small meals and snacks daily.
b. Give the client prune juice twice a day.
c. Allow to have adequate rest.
d. Give the pain drugs at regular interval.

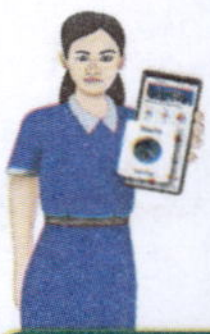

Ans.

768. b
769. a
770. b
771. a
772. c
773. c
774. c
775. d

Explanation: Metastasis to the spine can cause severe pain for the client. Managing pain is a priority in this situation to ensure the client's comfort and quality of life. The nurse should administer pain medications as prescribed and at regular intervals to maintain adequate pain control. Regular administration of pain medication helps to prevent breakthrough pain and maintain a consistent level of pain relief.

776. Nurse Ramya is preparing a patient for a colonoscopy scheduled the next day. The patient states that the fecal occult blood test was negative for colon cancer as per the information provided by the physician and expressed that it is not necessary to go for colonoscopy. The patient further insists on canceling the coloscopy procedure. What should be the most appropriate response by the nurse to this patient? *New Q*

a. Your doctor should not have shared this information with you.
b. The colonoscopy is essential as per hospital protocol.
c. A negative fecal occult blood test does not rule out or confirm the colon cancer.
d. I will approach your doctor so that you can discuss with him.

Explanation: A negative fecal occult blood test does not completely rule out the presence of colon cancer. While it is a useful screening test, it has limitations, including false negatives. The colonoscopy procedure is considered the gold standard for detecting colon cancer and other abnormalities in the colon. It allows for direct visualization and biopsy if necessary.

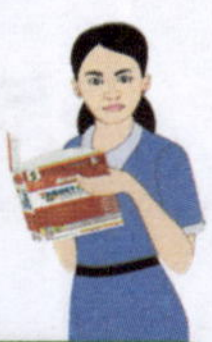

ANATOMY & PHYSIOLOGY OF LIVER

777. In the liver, bacteria that found their way into portal circulation is destroyed by______ *(ESIC 2019)*

a. Cilia b. Hydrochloric acid
c. Leukocytosis d. Kupffer cells

Explanation: **Kupffer cells** are also known as stellate macrophages Kupffer-Browicz cells. They are specialized **macrophages located in the liver**, lining the walls of the sinusoids. It helps in clearance of blood bacteria which enter from guts into the portal circulation.

778. Function of Kupffer cells in liver is:

a. Phagocytic
b. Lytic
c. Secretory
d. Excretory

779. Kupffer cells are a type of:

a. Dendritic cells b. Macrophages
c. B cells d. T cells

780. Kupffer cells are seen in:

a. Duodenum b. Gastric mucosa
c. Liver d. Spleen

781. Epinephrine action in liver:

a. Glycogenolysis
b. Gluconeogenesis
c. Glycolysis
d. Lipolysis

JAUNDICE

782. The nurse is collecting data for a patient who develops jaundice and dark, amber-colored urine. The nurse recognizes that which of the following is most likely the cause of these manifestations? *(RAK MSc 2018)*

a. Encephalopathy b. Pancreatitis
c. Bile duct obstruction d. Cholecystitis

Explanation:

- When one or more of the *ducts* that transport *bile* become blocked, it is known as a *bile duct obstruction*. It is also commonly referred to as *biliary obstruction*.
- When the bile ducts get blocked, bile builds up in the liver and the symptoms such as jaundice and amber-colored urine develops because of increasing level of bilirubin in the blood. The other clinical manifestation includes itching, abdominal pain usually in the upper right side.

783. Which of the below-mentioned sign indicates obstructive jaundice? *(Daman and Diu NO 2018)*

a. Straw-colored urine b. Clay-colored stools
c. Reduced hematocrit d. Elevated urobilinogen in urine

Explanation: Obstructive jaundice occurs due to the intra and extra hepatic obstruction of bile ducts. The liver releases bile salts into the stool, giving it a normal brown color. In obstructive jaundice, conjugated bilirubin does not reach the gut, no stercobilin or urobilin and the stools are devoid of yellow color. This makes the stool **pale, white, or look like clay or putty.**

784. Increased level of unconjugated bilirubin is because of the problem with ……organ:

a. Liver b. Small intestine
c. Bone marrow d. Spleen

785. Which is not prehepatic jaundice?

a. Hemolysis b. Ineffective erythropoiesis
c. Obstructive jaundice d. Both a and b

786. Most common cause of obstructive jaundice in children:

a. Biliary atresia b. Crigler-Najjar syndrome
c. Byler disease d. Caroli cyst

787. Vitamin to be corrected in obstructive jaundice is:

a. Vitamin K b. Vitamin B12
c. Vitamin D d. Vitamin C

PORTAL HYPERTENSION (INCLUDING ASCITIS & ESOPHAGEAL VARICES)

788. Cause of esophageal varices is:

a. Change in oncotic pressure
b. Damage to the vein valves
c. GERD
d. Portal hypertension

789. Achalasia cardia results in absence of:

a. Esophageal peristalsis
b. Gastric acid
c. Cardiac sphincter of stomach
d. Pyloric sphincter

Ans.

776. c
777. d
778. a
779. b
780. c
781. a
782. c
783. b
784. a
785. c
786. a
787. a
788. d
789. a

790. A patient who has Sengstaken-Blakemore tube inserted, suddenly experiences difficulty in breathing. Which of the following actions should the nurse take first? *(DSSSB 2013)*
a. Administer oxygen with oxygen mask
b. Cut and remove the tube
c. Elevate the head end of the bed
d. Listen to the client's lung sound

Explanation: A Sengstaken–Blakemore tube is a medical device inserted through the nose or mouth and used occasionally in the management of upper gastrointestinal hemorrhage due to esophageal varices. Difficulty in breathing is an indication of airway obstruction in the oropharynx caused by inflated balloon of the Sengstaken-Blakemore tube. The immediate action is to cut and remove the tube.

791. Dietary management of ascites is:
a. Restrict water intake b. Restrict sodium intake
c. Both a & b d. None of these

792. Peritoneovenous shunt move fluid from:
a. Abdomen to peritoneum
b. Peritoneum to abdomen
c. Peritoneum to veins
d. Pulmonary vein to peritoneum

LIVER ABSCESS

793. Common location of liver abscess is:
a. Right lobe of liver b. Left lobe of liver
c. Middle lobe d. All the lobes

794. The following are causes of the pyogenic liver abscess; EXCEPT:
a. Biliary obstruction
b. SIADH
c. Portal vein mesenteric infection
d. Liver tumor/cyst

795. All of the following are the significant clinical features of the liver abscess; EXCEPT:
a. Fever
b. Hepatomegaly
c. Dark brown-colored stools
d. Right upper quadrant pain

796. The organism that causes amoebic liver abscess is:
a. Entamoeba histolytica b. Staph aureus
c. E. coli d. H. pylori

797. Common site for the presence of amoebic liver abscess is:
a. Left lobe b. Right lobe
c. All over the liver d. Both a and b

798. Which organism is responsible for causing hydatid cyst:
a. Entamoeba histolytica
b. Staph aureus
c. Echinococcus granulosus
d. H. pylori

HEPATIC ENCEPHALOPATHY & COMA

799. Hepatic coma is manifested by all the following; EXCEPT:
a. Respiratory alkalosis
b. EEG abnormalities
c. Elevation of blood ammonia
d. Flapping tremor

800. Use of lactulose in hepatic encephalopathy is to:
a. Increase lactase level in the blood
b. Decrease serum ammonia level
c. Increase the breakdown of bilirubin
d. Decrease the production of bilirubin

Explanation: The presence of a carbohydrate and the acidic environment caused by the production of organic acids also act to reduce the breakdown of other nitrogen-containing compounds to ammonia and other potential cerebral toxins. The administration of lactulose to humans causes an increase in fecal nitrogen, but very little increase in ammonia nitrogen. Most of the nitrogen is contained in the fecal bacterial and the soluble fractions of stool. The administration of lactulose causes a reduction in the urea production rate consistent with a reduced entry of ammonia into portal blood.

801. Food item needs to be avoided in a client with hepatic dysfunction to prevent hepatic coma is:
a. Carbohydrate b. Protein
c. Vitamins d. Minerals

VIRAL HEPATITIS

802. Which hepatitis is often seen as outbreaks in camps and institutions? *(AIIMS-BBS SNO 2019)*
a. Hepatitis A b. Hepatitis C
c. Hepatitis D d. Hepatitis B

Explanation: The *hepatitis A* virus (HAV) is transmitted through feco-oral route. Contaminated food and water are the major sources of infection. This is the reason why it is often seen as outbreaks in camps and institutions.

803. The common route of transmission of Hepatitis-A is: *(Safdarjung NO 2018; NCFL 2019)*
a. By blood transfusion b. Oro-fecal
c. By sexual intercourse d. By droplet

Explanation: The common route of transmission of Hepatitis-A is orofecal route. Hepatitis A and hepatitis E spreads through oral-fecal route. Hepatitis C, hepatitis B and hepatitis D spreads through blood and blood products, sexual intercourse and needle prick incidences.

804. Identify DNA virus among the following:
a. Hepatitis A virus b. Hepatitis B virus
c. Hepatitis D virus d. Hepatitis G virus

805. In which hepatitis ground glass appearance of the hepatocytes can be seen?
a. Hepatitis A virus b. Hepatitis B virus
c. Hepatitis D virus d. Hepatitis G virus

806. Hepatitis is highly infectious during ....
a. Convalescent period b. Remission period
c. Incubation period d. Relapse period

807. Risk of .... is more after blood transfusion:
a. Hepatitis A b. Hepatitis B
c. Hepatitis C d. Hepatitis D

808. Mode of transmission of hepatitis A is:
a. Sexual contact b. Contaminated food
c. Blood transfusion d. Mosquito bite

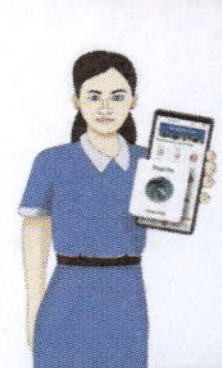

Ans.
790. b
791. c
792. c
793. a
794. b
795. c
796. a
797. b
798. c
799. a
800. b
801. b
802. a
803. b
804. b
805. b
806. c
807. c
808. b

809. Hepatitis-A mostly occurs among:
- a. Immunocompromised person
- b. Children between 3 and 12 years
- c. Teenagers
- d. Older adult

810. Identify the type of Hepatitis that is transmitted through non-parenteral route:
- a. Hepatitis A
- b. Hepatitis B
- c. Hepatitis E
- d. Hepatitis A and E

811. Identify the type of Hepatitis that is transmitted through parenteral route:
- a. Hepatitis A
- b. Hepatitis E
- c. Hepatitis A and Hepatitis E
- d. Hepatitis B

812. Mode of transmission of Hepatitis E virus is: *(AIIMS Bhopal Grade-I 2018)*
- a. Sexual
- b. Blood transfusion
- c. Injections
- d. Fecal–oral

Explanation: Mode of transmission of different types of hepatitis is as follows:

Type of hepatitis	Mode of trans-mission	Source of virus
Hepatitis A	Fecal-oral	Feces
Hepatitis B	Percutaneous, permucosal	Blood/blood derived body fluids
Hepatitis C	Percutaneous, permucosal	Blood/blood derived body fluids
Hepatitis D	Percutaneous, permucosal	Blood/blood derived body fluids
Hepatitis E	Fecal-oral	Feces

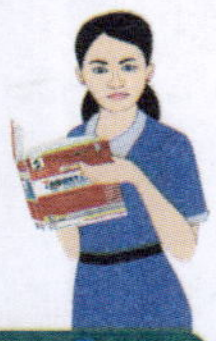

813. Which among the following condition has highest levels of serum transaminases?
- a. Acute hepatitis
- b. Chronic hepatitis
- c. Acute pancreatitis
- d. Chronic pancreatitis

814. Hepatitis-B Virus carrier stage duration is:
- a. 3 months
- b. 6 months
- c. 9 months
- d. 12 months

815. Common problem in the acute phase of hepatitis A:
- a. Pruritis
- b. Nutritional deficiency
- c. Steatorrhea
- d. Melena

816. Which of the following is a complication of acute hepatitis?
- a. Fulminant hepatic failure
- b. Cirrhosis
- c. Both a and b
- d. None of the above

817. Discharge teaching to a client with hepatitis B is:
- a. Use lotions to get relieve from itching
- b. Practice safe sex with condom
- c. Take hepatitis B vaccination
- d. Follow low carbohydrate, low protein and low fat diet

818. In a Hepatitis-B patient which activity order would the nurse expect to be prescribed:
- a. Bed rest
- b. Encourage ambulation
- c. Strenuous activity
- d. Sedentary activity

HEPATIC CIRRHOSIS

819. Mallory's degeneration seen in alcoholic liver disease is a form of: *(Safdarjung NO 2018)*
- a. Hyaline degeneration
- b. Amyloid degeneration
- c. Hydropic degeneration
- d. Fatty degeneration

Explanation: Mallory's degeneration seen in alcoholic liver disease is a form of Hyaline degeneration. Histologically, Mallory bodies are irregular, rope-like amorphous eosinophilic intracytoplasmic structures found in hepatocytes.

820. The nurse is planning care for a patient with cirrhosis. For which condition would the nurse place the patient on bleeding precautions? *(RAK MSc 2018)*
- a. Encephalopathy
- b. Low vitamin K
- c. Elevated liver enzymes
- d. Hepatorenal syndrome

Explanation:
- One of the factors implicated in the pathogenesis of the coagulopathy of liver disease is vitamin K deficiency. Vitamin K is an essential fat-soluble vitamin that is important in maintaining normal coagulation. The body stores of vitamin K are not high, and its absorption is highly dependent upon bile.
- For these reasons, patients with cholestatic liver disease, cirrhosis and small bowel malabsorption may develop vitamin K deficiency. Insufficient vitamin K can lead to excessive bleeding and easy bruising.

821. Hepatic cirrhosis is characterized by:
- a. Atrophy of hepatic cell
- b. Degeneration and destruction of liver cells
- c. Necrosis of hepatic cell
- d. Stricture in hepatic cell

822. The inflammation and degeneration of liver parenchyma is referred to as: *(DSSSB PHN, 2015)*
- a. Cirrhosis
- b. Jaundice
- c. Colitis
- d. Cystitis

823. Pathophysiology behind edema in cirrhosis is:
- a. Liver is unable to neutralize the toxic substance
- b. Fall in oncotic pressure due to low albumin and portal hypertension
- c. Due to paralytic ileus
- d. More blood volume causes edema

824. Which among the following sign will be present in a client who is suffering from cirrhosis of liver and hepatic coma?
- a. Elevated creatinine level
- b. Decreased SGOT/SGPT
- c. Icterus
- d. Hypervitaminosis

825. When the nurse is assessing a patient who has cirrhosis of the liver, which of the following findings would indicate that the patient's condition is worsening? *(LNJP HD 2012)*
- a. Positive Babinski sign
- b. Bilateral basal lung creps
- c. Visual field loss
- d. Flapping hand tremors

826. In a cirrhosis patient administration of neomycin helps to prevent the formation of:
- a. Urea
- b. Ammonia
- c. Creatinine
- d. Ketone

Ans.

809.	b
810.	d
811.	d
812.	d
813.	a
814.	c
815.	a
816.	c
817.	b
818.	a
819.	a
820.	b
821.	b
822.	a
823.	b
824.	c
825.	d
826.	b

827. Mr. Ravi, a 45-year-old male was admitted into HDU with liver failure due to chronic alcohol abuse. Close monitoring of the blood pressure was advised. Which change that is associated with liver failure affects the blood pressure of this patient?
   a. Increased capillary permeability
   b. Peripheral vasodilation
   c. Increased renin release from kidney
   d. Hypoalbuminemia

Explanation: Albumin maintains oncotic pressure of the plasma. Hypoalbuminemia is one of the characteristics of liver failure. So blood pressure decreases as the body is unable to maintain normal oncotic pressure due to hypoalbuminemia which necessitate close monitoring of BP.

CHOLECYSTITIS

828. Organism most commonly responsible for cholecystitis is:
   a. Meningococci b. Klebsiella
   c. Staphylococci d. Pneumococci

829. One of the major causes for Cirrhosis of liver is:
   a. Alcohol abuse b. Drug abuse (DSSSB 2013)
   c. Smoking d. Hepatitis A

Explanation: Alcohol is reported as the most common cause of cirrhosis of liver in India. The other common etiologies include Hepatitis B and C infections, autoimmune, and non-alcoholic fatty liver.

830. Which of the following is considered as the major cause for developing cholecystitis:
   a. Alcohol consumption b. Gall stones
   c. Obesity d. Aging

831. The following are some significant risk factors for developing cholecystitis; EXCEPT:
   a. Rapid weight loss b. High fat diet
   c. Being a male d. Genetics and older people

Explanation: Women are more likely to develop cholesterol gallstones than men, especially during their reproductive years, when the incidence of gallstones in women is two to three times that of men. The difference is mainly due to to estrogen, which increases biliary cholesterol secretion.

832. The fatty stools that is seen in a patient with cholecystitis would be referred to as:
   a. Hematochezia b. Steatorrhea
   c. Hematemesis d. Melena

833. The best dietary recommendation for the person who is experiencing cholecystitis is:
   a. Low fat diet
   b. Diet rich in fat
   c. High carbohydrate diet
   d. Low carbohydrate diet

834. All of the following are the gas forming food material that should be avoided in a person with cholecystitis; EXCEPT:
   a. Cauliflower
   b. Brocolli
   c. Carrot
   d. Beans

CHOLELITHIASIS

835. Major types of galls stones include:
   a. Cholesterol and calcium stone
   b. Pigmental and calcium stone
   c. Cholesterol and pigmental stone
   d. Pigmental and xanthine stone

836. Choledocholithiasis is:
   a. Stone in pancreatic duct
   b. Stone in common biliary duct
   c. Stone in cystic duct
   d. Stone In urethra

837. Stone in the bile duct is known as:
   a. Choledocholithiasis b. Cholelithiasis
   c. Cholangitis d. Jaundice

838. Identify the risk factor for cholelithiasis:
   a. Obesity b. Change in weight
   c. Hormonal therapies d. All of the above

839. Clinical manifestation of Choledocholithiasis is:
   a. Icterus b. Obstructive jaundice
   c. Clay colored stools d. All of these

PANCREATITIS

840. Bluish discoloration or ecchymosis around the umbilicus is known as:
   a. Homan's sign b. Kernig's sign
   c. Cullen's sign d. Osiander sign

841. Which of the following is a cause of acute pancreatitis?
   a. Alcohol consumption b. Gall-stones
   c. High triglyceride levels d. All of the above

842. Most common cause of Chronic Pancreatitis:
   a. Gallstones b. Alcoholism
   c. Trauma d. ERCP

Explanation: Heavy alcohol consumption is the most common cause of chronic pancreatitis (70% to 80% of cases).

- However, only 3% to 7% of heavy drinkers develop chronic pancreatitis suggests that alcohol is only a cofactor and that other factors are required for development of this complication.
- Mutations in the cationic trypsinogen gene, also known as protease serine 1 *(PRSS1)* gene, are common in hereditary chronic pancreatitis. *PRSS1* is located on chromosome 7
- In up to 20% of patients, a clear cause cannot be documented and cases are considered to be idiopathic.
- *Ref: Sabiston 20th page 1532*

843. Most common cause of Viral pancreatitis:
   a. Coxsackie virus b. Mumps
   c. CMV d. HIV

844. Which of the following laboratory findings is a primary indicator of pancreatitis?
   a. Elevated AST b. Elevated ALT
   c. Elevated serum lipase d. Elevated BUN

845. Elevation of which of the following laboratory value indicates the presence of pancreatitis? *(DSSSB 2013)*
   a. Serum amylase
   b. Serum lipase
   c. Aspartate aminotransferase (AST)
   d. Both a and b

Ans.

827. d
828. c
829. a
830. b
831. c
832. b
833. a
834. c
835. c
836. b
837. a
838. d
839. d
840. c
841. d
842. b
843. b
844. c
845. d

Explanation: A normal serum lipase level is 0–160 U/L. A normal blood amylase level is 23–85 U/L. Pancreatitis—also known as inflammation of the pancreas, can cause amylase and lipase levels to be increased up to 3 times normal. Both values should be increased, in order to carry the diagnosis of pancreatitis.

846. Grey Turner's sign is seen in:
a. Myocarditis b. Cholecystitis
c. Pancreatitis d. Pleural effusion

847. All of the following are the complications of acute pancreatitis; EXCEPT:
a. Irritable bowel syndrome b. Pseudocyst
c. Colitis d. Splenic vein thrombosis

848. Which of the following is NOT a complication of acute pancreatitis?
a. Increased ICP b. Ascites
c. Splenic vein thrombosis d. Renal dysfunction

849. Fluid volume deficit is most likely associated with which of the following conditions?
a. Pancreatitis b. Congestive heart failure
c. Gastritis d. Appendicitis

Explanation: Pancreatitis can lead to inflammation and leakage of fluid into the peritoneal cavity, causing a shift of fluid from the intravascular space (blood vessels) to the third space (interstitial spaces). This fluid shift can result in reduced circulating blood volume and contribute to fluid volume deficit.

In CHF, fluid volume excess is evident.

850. Nursing management of the patient with acute pancreatitis includes:
a. Assess for hypocalcaemia
b. Treat hyperglycemia based on insulin sliding scale
c. Both a and b
d. Provide enzyme replacement

851. Complication of chronic pancreatitis includes the following:
a. Deficiency of fat soluble vitamin
b. Pseudocyst
c. Diabetes mellitus d. All of these

852. Pancreatitis client manifest with:
a. Midepigastric pain b. Abdominal blotting
c. Nausea and vomiting d. All of these

853. Drug of choice for pain control in acute pancreatitis?
a. Morphine b. Diclofenac sodium
c. Meperidine d. Indomethacin

Explanation: Meperidine (Demerol) is the drug of choice for pain control in acute pancreatitis. Diclofenac and indomethacin are NSAID and less efficient to control severe pain caused by irritation and edema of the inflamed pancreas. Morphine also an effective analgesic but likely to cause spasm of sphincter of oddi.

854. Purpose of continuous low NG drainage in a client with pancreatitis is to prevent:
a. GERD b. Abdominal distention
c. Pancreatic stimulation d. Intestinal obstruction

855. Which among the following food type needs to be restricted in a client with pancreatitis?
a. Carbohydrate b. Fat
c. Protein d. Vitamins and mineral

WILSON'S DISEASE

856. Wilson's disease is diagnosed by?
a. Increased serum ceruloplasmin
b. Decreased liver copper
c. Increased urinary copper excretion
d. Decreased urine copper excretion

857. Correct option regarding Wilson's disease is:
a. Kayser-Fleischer rings are present in this condition
b. An autosomal recessive genetic disorder
c. Copper accumulation manifests as neurological symptoms and liver disease
d. All of the above

858. Wilson's disease as a genetic disorder comes under the classification of:
a. Autosomal recessive b. Autosomal dominant
c. Xlinked recessive d. Xlinked dominant

859. A client is experiencing Wilson's disease. The nurse need to have knowledge that these condition will lead the client's liver, kidney and cornea to have abnormal accumulation of:
a. Iron b. Lead
c. Copper d. Bile

860. The actual site for absorption of copper in a normal person would be:
a. Proximal ileum b. Terminal ileum
c. Stomach and duodenum d. Liver

Explanation: The copper is absorbed in the stomach and duodenum and then it is transported to the liver.

861. The copper gets primarily excreted through:
a. Renal excretion
b. Sloughing of intestinal mucosal
c. Liver sulphation
d. Biliary excretion

862. The following are the true about Kayser-Fleischer rings; EXCEPT:
a. It won't interfere the vision
b. Sunflower cataract is related to this condition
c. It leads to chemical induced psychosis
d. It encircle the iris of the eye.

OTHER GI DISORDERS

863. Obesity is one of the risk factors for:
a. Esophageal adenocarcinoma
b. Renal carcinoma
c. Endometrial carcinoma d. All of the above

864. Weight loss is seen in:
a. Hyperthyroidism b. Anorexia nervosa
c. Pulmonary TB d. All of these

865. Particular smell of fecal matter is due to:
a. Hydrogen sulfide b. Indole
c. Biliverdin d. Both a and b

866. Condition in which excess gas accumulates in the gastrointestinal tract and causes abdominal distension is known as:
a. Flatulence b. Infestation
c. Meteorism d. Bloating

Ans.
846. c
847. a
848. a
849. a
850. c
851. d
852. d
853. c
854. c
855. b
856. c
857. d
858. a
859. c
860. c
861. d
862. c
863. d
864. d
865. d
866. c

867. Tenesmus is:

a. A rumbling or gurgling noise made by the movement of fluid and gas in the intestines
b. Difficulty in passing stool
c. Fat in stool
d. Ineffectual straining of stool

Explanation: Option d is the correct answer. Option a is the definition of Borborygmus, option b is the definition of constipation and option c is the definition of Steatorrhea.

868. Which of the following characteristics indicates protein deficiency in a client?

a. Spoon-shaped nails
b. Increased bleeding time
c. Negative nitrogen balance
d. Positive nitrogen balance

Explanation: Negative nitrogen balance indicates that there is more protein catabolism than anabolism. This indicates output exceeds intake (negative nitrogen balance).

869. Malabsorption syndrome features include all; EXCEPT:

a. Anemia b. Constipation
c. Tetany d. Steatorrhea

870. Increased gastrin is seen in:

a. Zollinger-Ellison syndrome
b. Iron deficiency anemia
c. Duodenal ulcer
d. Gastric cancer

871. Which of the following is correct regarding Zollinger-Ellison syndrome?

a. Increased secretion of gastrin
b. Increased production of gastric acid
c. Gastric and duodenal ulcer formation
d. All of the above

872. Cystic fibrosis leads to:

a. Poor nutrition
b. Infertility
c. Lack of fat soluble vitamin
d. All of the above

Explanation: Cystic fibrosis is an inherited disorder that causes severe damage to the lungs, digestive system and other organs in the body. Cystic fibrosis affects the cells that produce mucus, sweat and digestive juices. Clients with cystic fibrosis have impaired fat digestion and iron absorption. This leads to fatigue, susceptible for infection and shorter life span

873. Thiamine deficiency cause:

a. Beriberi b. Pellagra
c. Dermatitis d. Scurvy

874. Which of the following is a complication of splenectomy? *(DSSSB 2013)*

a. Cholecystitis b. Pancreatitis
c. Appendicitis d. Gastritis

Explanation: Bleeding, blood clots, infection, injury to nearby organs, including stomach, pancreas and colon are the complications of splenectomy. Pancreatitis is the complication associated with splenectomy.

875. The nurse is reinforcing patient teaching. Which of the following foods should the nurse avoid while enforcing food to the patient of ulcerative colitis? (RAK MSc 2018)

a. Fresh fruits b. White bread
c. Sweet desert d. Meat

Explanation:

- Fresh fruits are high in fiber and notable for causing gas which further causes diarrhea and abdominal pain; so, the patient with ulcerative colitis should avoid fresh fruits and vegetables.
- White bread is not rich in fiber so it can be taken. Sweet desert doesn't aggravate the sign and symptom of ulcerative colitis. Meat in less quantity can be taken by the patient with ulcerative colitis.

876. After a surgery for an ileal conduit a nurse should closely evaluate client for which complication?

a. Peritonitis b. Infection
c. Thrombophlebitis d. Hematuria

877. Currant jelly-like stools containing mucous among 3 months to 3-year-old child is suspected to have: *(ESIC 2019)*

a. Hirschsprung's disease
b. Abdominal hernia
c. Meckel's diverticulum
d. Intussusception

Explanation: Currant jelly-like stools is a feature of intussusception. It is a condition in which part of the intestine telescopes into itself. Later signs of intussusception include rectal bleeding often with 'red currant jelly' stool (stool mixed with blood and mucus) and lethargy.

878. Crohn's Disease most commonly affects the:

a. Stomach
b. Rectum
c. Ileum
d. Duodenum

879. Which of the following is earliest manifestation of Crohn's disease?

a. Deep ulcers involving GI mucosa
b. Aphthous ulcers
c. Cobblestone appearance
d. Discontinuous involvement of ileum

Explanation: The earliest gross manifestations of Crohn's disease are the development of small mucosal ulcerations call aphthous ulcers.

880. Which of the following bowel disorder is commonly associated with fistulas?

a. Diverticulitis b. Appendicitis
c. Irritable bowel syndrome d. Crohn's disease

881. A 55-year-old male is admitted with a diagnosis of Crohn's disease. The nurse knows that the most common location of digestive tract affected by Crohn's disease is:

a. Jejunum b. Terminal Ileum
c. Ascending column d. Sigmoid column

882. Which of the following symptoms is likely to be exhibited by a patient with Crohn's disease?

a. Ribbon-like stools b. Steatorrhea
c. Hematochezia d. Malena

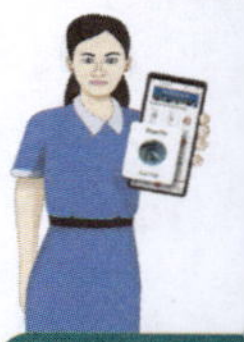

Ans.

867.	d
868.	c
869.	b
870.	a
871.	d
872.	d
873.	a
874.	b
875.	a
876.	b
877.	d
878.	c
879.	b
880.	d
881.	b
882.	b

883. Rectal bleeding is the predominant symptom in which of the following conditions?

a. Crohn's disease
b. Ulcerative colitis
c. Appendicitis
d. Diverticulitis

884. Purpose of ileostomy in ulcerative colitis is:

a. To prevent possible perforation from colitis
b. To prevent fecal impaction
c. To decrease abdominal distention
d. To prevent peritonitis

885. The nurse is aware that the most common assessment finding in a child with ulcerative colitis is:

a. Intense abdominal cramps
b. Profuse diarrhea
c. Anal fissures
d. Abdominal distention

886. All are true about ulcerative colitis; EXCEPT:

a. Smoking may prevent the disease
b. Male: female ratio is 1:1
c. Presents with bloody diarrhea
d. Highly associated with infertility

887. Which of the following is not true about ulcerative colitis?

a. Lesions are continuous and superficial and limited colon and rectum
b. Anal lesions are less
c. Risk for cancer is more
d. Rectal bleeding is less as compared to Crohn's disease

Explanation: Ulcerative colitis and Crohn's disease are two type of inflammatory bowel disease (IBD). Crohn's disease is a chronic inflammatory process of any part of GI from the mouth to anus but most often affects the terminal ileum. Ulcerative colitis is a disease characterized by remitting and relapsing inflammation of the large intestine. The inflammation is limited to colon and rectum. Rectal bleeding is more common in ulcerative colitis as compared to Crohn's disease. So the statement mentioned in D is not true

888. What is NOT true about prevention or control of flare-ups in ulcerative colitis? *New Q*

a. High-fiber diet should be avoided during flare-up
b. Nuts, raw vegetables or fruits are encouraged to prevent flare-ups.
c. Sulfasalazine is advised to prevent flare-ups.
d. Low-fiber and high-protein diet prevent/control flare-ups.

Explanation: In ulcerative colitis, a flare-up is characterized by inflammation and increased sensitivity of the intestinal lining. During flare-ups, certain dietary modifications are often recommended to help manage symptoms and reduce inflammation. However, high-fiber foods, including nuts, raw vegetables, and certain fruits, are generally advised to be avoided during flare-ups as they can worsen symptoms and irritate the inflamed intestines.

Option b is not true because Raw vegetables and fruits are high-fiber foods that is to be avoided.

889. Which of the following statement is NOT true regarding typhoid fever?

a. Rose spots, leucopenia, fever and diarrhea are the important features
b. Low grade fever
c. Ceftriaxone is the drug of choice for treatment of typhoid fever
d. Widal test is used to diagnose the condition

890. Correct option regarding a typhoid ulcer is:

a. Terminal ileum will be affected
b. Longitudinal orientation
c. Bleeding
d. All of these

891. Hypoalbuminemia is present in:

a. Cirrhosis
b. Malnutrition
c. Nephrotic syndrome
d. All of these

892. In Gluten Intolerance, the following is not recommended: *(Safdarjung NO 2018)*

a. Wheat
b. Rye
c. Oats
d. All of these

Explanation: In Gluten intolerance, wheat, rye, oats are not recommended to eat, as all these have gluten protein. The person can consume rice, millets, legumes (beans, lentils, peas, peanuts), nuts and seeds, red meat (fresh beef, pork, lamb, bison), poultry (fresh chicken, turkey), seafood (fresh fish, scallops, shellfish) and traditional soy foods (tofu etc.).

893. The nurse is caring for a patient who is receiving a parenteral nutrition infusion. The nurse should perform blood glucose monitoring every 6 hours to detect which complication? *(RAK MSc 2018)*

a. Hyponatremia
b. Hyperkalemia
c. Hypocalcemia
d. Hyperglycemia

Explanation: Elevation of blood glucose occurs as the result of increased hepatic glucose production and reduced glucose utilization by peripheral tissues during the stress of hospitalization. Also, excessive delivery of glucose and gluconeogenic substrates via enteral or parenteral route in hospitalized patients also contributes to hyperglycemia. Hence the nurse should **measure blood glucose levels every 6 hours.**

894. A low-residue diet contains all; EXCEPT:

a. Roast beef
b. Fresh peas
c. Mashed potatoes
d. Baked chicken

Explanation: Fresh peas is high residue all others are low residue diet. A low residue diet is a diet designed to reduce the frequency and volume of stools while prolonging intestinal transit time. It is similar to a low-fiber diet, but typically includes restrictions on foods that increase bowel activity, such as milk, milk products, and prune juice.

895. Rapid effect of antacid medication will be there if they are taken:

a. At bedtime
b. On an empty stomach
c. After food
d. Every 4 hourly

896. All of the following activities promotes Valsalva's maneuver; EXCEPT:

a. Enema administration
b. Gagging while toothbrushing
c. Lifting heavy objects
d. Use of stool softeners

Explanation: Stool softeners prevent constipation and straining at stool and prevents the patient to perform Valsalva maneuver. Gargling while tooth brushing, and lifting heavy objects as well as enema administration promote Valsalva's maneuver.

897. Best vein for total parenteral nutrition is:

a. Subclavian vein
b. Femoral vein
c. Brachial vein
d. Saphenous vein

Explanation: Subclavian vein is commonly used to administer Total Parenteral Nutrition (TPN) through Peripherally Inserted Central Catheter (PICC) line.

Ans.

883. b
884. a
885. b
886. d
887. d
888. b
889. b
890. d
891. d
892. d
893. d
894. b
895. b
896. d
897. a

ENT SYSTEM

ANATOMY OF EAR

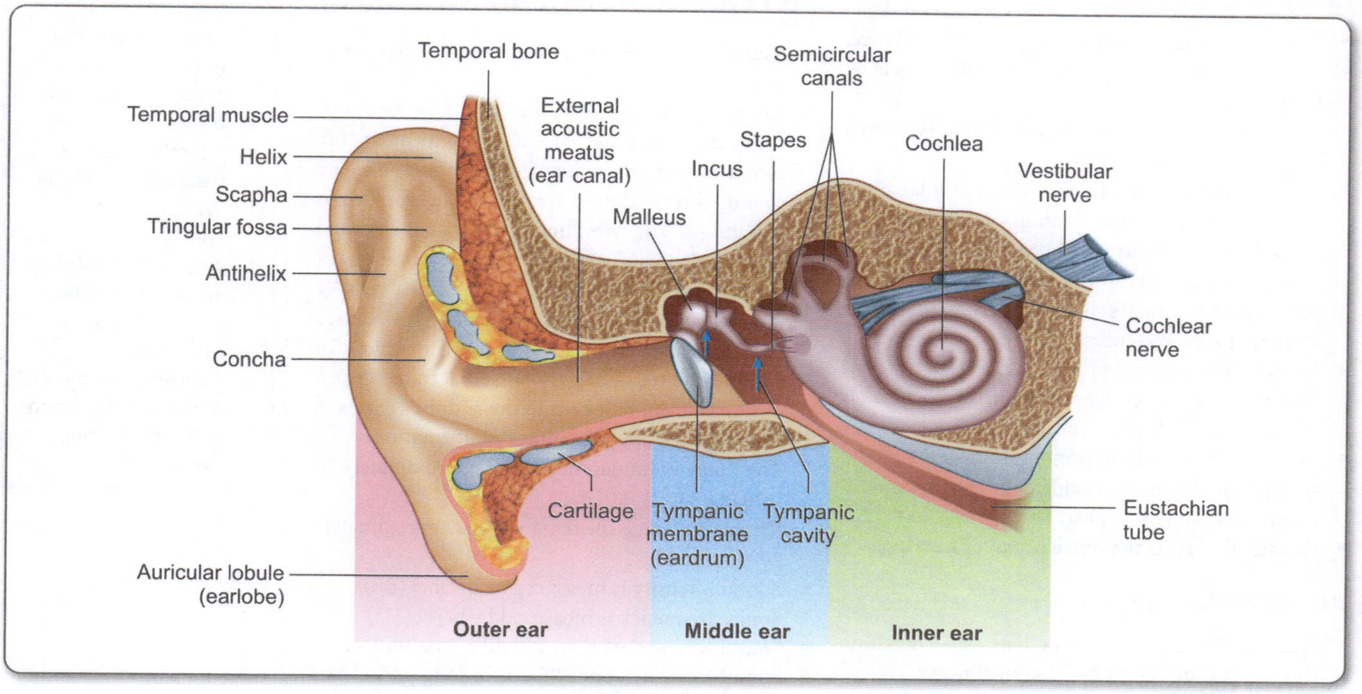

Figure 39: Anatomy of ear

- Ear is an organ of hearing and equilibrium.
- Three divisions of ear are:
  1. Outer (external) ear
  2. Middle
  3. Inner (Internal) ear
- Nerve supply to ear: acoustic nerve (8th CN)
- Blood supply: major blood supply by posterior auricular artery which is a branch of external carotid artery.

Outer (External) Ear

- Consists of pinna (auricle) and the external auditory meatus
- Pinna is made up of fibro-elastic cartilages.
- Pinna collects and reflects the sound waves into external auditory canal.
- **Tragus** is the cartilaginous projection in front of external auditory tube, main purpose is to direct sound toward the eardrum
- External auditory meatus extends from pinna to the tympanic membrane. Its length is about 2.5 cm and 0.7 cm in diameter.
- It secretes wax from the ceruminous glands and oil from sebaceous glands.

Middle Ear

- It is also known as tympanic cavity
- It includes:
  - Tympanic membrane
  - Eustachian tube
  - Ear ossicles
  - Windows and muscles
- Tympanic membrane is a cave shaped structure. Concavity is directed towards the external auditory meatus.
- Eustachian tube connects the middle ear with pharynx. It is approximately 35 mm long and 3 mm in diameter.
- There are three ear ossicles:
  1. **Malleus** (Connected to inner surface of the tympanic membrane) hammer shaped
  2. **Incus** (Middle ossicle; articulates with head of Malleus) Anvil shaped.
  3. **Stapes** (Smallest bone of the body; head articulates with incus; oval footplate contacts the membrane of the oval window of cochlea) stirrup shaped.
- **Windows**
  - Oval window (fesnestra vestibule) is present above; it transmits the sound vibrations of ossicles to the perilymph.
  - Round window is present in the lower part. It accommodates the pressure waves transmitted to the perilymph.

KEY POINTS

- The organ most damaged in bomb explosion is **Ear.**
- Most common cause of hearing loss is Impacted wax.
- **Otoscope** – device to examine the ear

- **Muscles:** Middle ear consists of two muscles:
  - Tensor tympani and Stapedius.
  - Stapedius is the smallest muscle of the body

Inner (Internal) Ear

- It contains organs of sense of hearing and balance.
- It consists of the bony labyrinth. Three parts of bony labyrinth are:
  1. The vestibule : Oval shaped. Consists of two sacs; utricle and saccule
  2. The semicircular canals: There are total three semicircular canals. Ampulla is ending part of the canal. **Both vestibule and semicircular canal contain receptors of balance.**
  3. The cochlea: Snail's shell shaped. Organ of corti contains the receptors of hearing.
- Perilymph is the fluid present in the scala tympani and scala vestibule compartments of cochlea. It resembles ECF (high in Na^+ and low in K^+).
- Endolymph is the fluid present in the scala media or the membranous cochlea. It resembles ICF (High in K^+ and low in Na^+).
- **Organ of Corti is the sense organ of hearing.**

Auditory Pathways

- Afferent fibers supplying the hair cells constitute the cochlear division of VIII cranial nerve.
- The cochlear nerve ends in the cochlear nuclei in medulla.
- Major areas constituting auditory cortex present in the temporal lobes are:
  - Primary auditory cortex (Areas 41 and 42)
  - Auditory association areas (Areas 20, 21, and 22)

PHYSIOLOGY OF HEARING

- Sound waves are the stimuli for the receptors of sound waves.
- External ear captures the sound waves and conducts (via external auditory meatus) the sound waves to tympanic membrane → The sound waves cause Tympanic membrane to vibrate → The vibrating tympanic membrane causes ear ossicles to vibrate → vibration of basilar membrane → Stimulation of hair cells → movement of hair cells of organ of corti causes their depolarization leading to generation of action potential in neuron → Neural transmission of signals from hair cells to the auditory cortex → Neural processing of Auditory information
- The range of human hearing is approximately 20 – 20,000 Hz.
- Range of average speaking voice is approximately 2000 – 5000 Hz.
- Sound intensity is measured by decibel (dB).
- Sound frequency is measured by hertz (Hz).
- Sound waves more than 140 dB are painful.
- Sound intensity above 85 dB for long period can cause deafness.
- Loud noise above 120 dB can cause immediate deafness.

KEY POINTS

- **Myringotomy** is a surgical incision of tympanic membrane. Commonly done to drain pus present in the middle ear
- **Otosclerosis:** Bony fusion between the foot plate of the stapes and the margins of the fenestra vestibule. This leads to loss of hearing (deafness)
- **Acoustic neuroma** is a tumor of Schwann cells of VIII cranial nerve.

Diagnostic Tests

Table 30: Description of diagnostic tests for ear disorders

Name of the test	Description	Points to remember
Otoscopic examination	• Examiner holds otoscope in the right hand and the pinna with left hand • The color of the healthy tympanic membrane is pearly grey. • It is positioned obliquely at the base of canal.	• To straighten the external auditory canal • **In adult:** Pinna has to be grasped upward and backward • **In children:** Pinna has to be grasped downward and backward
Whisper test	• One ear is tested at a time, the untested ear is covered with palm of hand • Examiner stands 1–2 feet away from the patient and stay outside the visual field. • The examiner whispers in the ear to be tested. • A person with normal hearing can repeat what examiner said.	
Weber test	• It is a bone conduction test to assess lateralization of sound. • Examiner vibrates a tuning fork and places it on the forehead or head of the patient. • A person with normal hearing will hear sound equally in both ears or says that sound originates from the center of head.	• **Conductive hearing loss:** Patient will hear better in the affected ear. This is because the affected side will be free from external noises, so it will hear the bone conduction loudly than the normal ear. • **Sensorineural hearing loss:** Hearing is better in the unaffected ear or in the ear with least problem.

Contd...

Name of the test	Description	Points to remember
Rinne test	• Vibrating tuning fork is placed in the mastoid bone (bone conduction) of the patient. When no longer the sound is audible, it will be taken two inches from the opening of ear canal (air conduction). • In a normal person, when tuning fork is taken to the front of ear canal, usually sound will be audible. • This test helps to **differentiate between conductive hearing loss and sensory neural hearing loss.**	• **Conductive hearing loss:** Longer duration (or equal) of sound conduction when the tuning fork is placed behind the ear at mastoid process than tuning fork in the front of ear. • **Sensory-neural hearing loss:** Longer duration of sound conduction when the tuning fork is in front of the ear than at the mastoid process. • In a person with normal hearing ear, air conduction sound is louder than bone conduction.
Audiometry	• Most important test in determining hearing loss. • Two types of sounds are used (1) Pure or musical tone (2) Speech • Frequency, pitch and intensity are assessed • Normal human ear can perceive **frequency ranging from 20–20,000 Hz.**	• Audiometric evaluation needs to be done in sound proof room. • Response plotted in a graph is known as audiogram.
Tympanogram Or Impedance audiometry	A graphic representation of the relationship between the air pressure in the ear canal and the movement of tympanic membrane, and the tiny bones in the middle ear.	
Electronystagmography	• Measurement of electrical potential evoked by eye movements • Occulomotor and vestibular system and its interaction is also assessed.	Used to **diagnose Meniere's disease**, internal auditory canal tumor and posterior fossa tumors.
Platform posturography	To analyze the postural control capabilities	Patient may be exposed to stationary platform and moving screen, moving screen and moving platform, etc.

Weber's and Rinne's test are the tests done to assess hearing loss. The interpretation of the tests is:

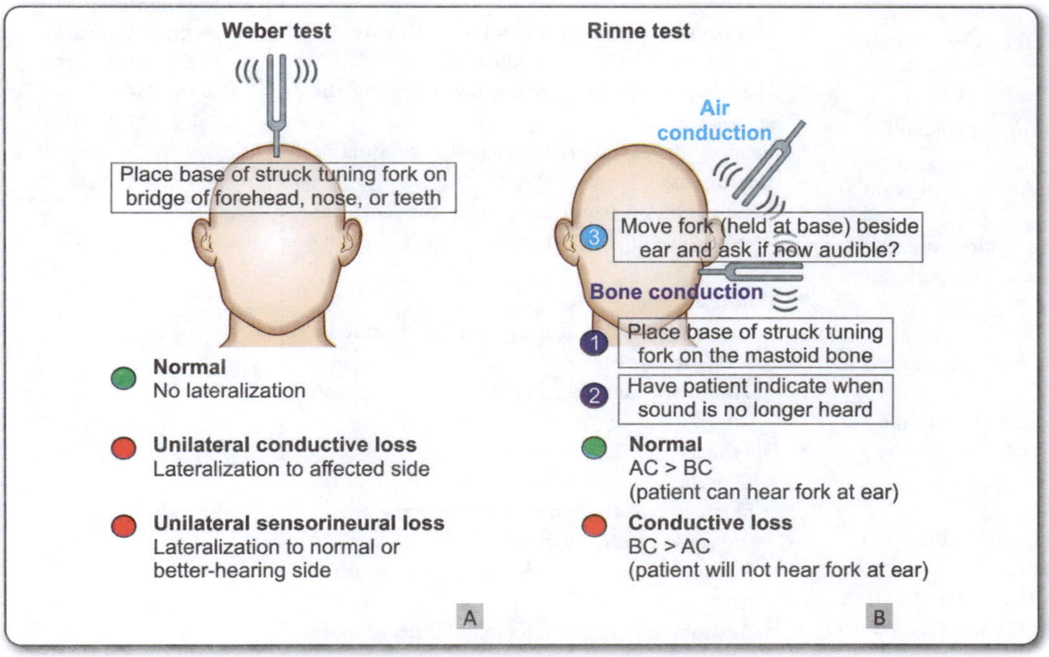

Figures 40A and B: A. Weber Test; **B.** Rinne's Test

Recent Question (NORCET 2023)

25. What is the Frequency of tuning fork used in the clinical setting?
- a. 256 Hz
- b. 512 Hz
- c. 1024 Hz
- d. 3048 Hz

Ans. (b) 512 Hz

Interpretation of Weber's and Rinne's tests is as follows:

Table 31: Interpretation of Weber's and Rinne's tests

	Normal	Conductive hearing loss	Sensorineural hearing loss
Rinne	AC > BC Rinne +ve	BC > AC Rinne -ve	AC > BC Rinne +ve
Weber	«	Lateralized to poor ear	Lateralized to better ear

Abbreviations: BC, bone conduction; AC, air conduction; Snhl, sensorineural hearing loss

DISORDERS OF EAR

Otitis Media

- Inflammatory disease of the middle ear
- **Types**
  - **Acute otitis media (AOM):** Less than 3 weeks
  - **Sub-acute otitis media:** 3 weeks to 3 months
  - **Chronic otitis media:** 3 months or longer
- **Causes**
  - *Streptococcus pneumoniae, Moraxella catarrhalis, and non-typeable Haemophilus influenzae.*
  - Respiratory infection by RSV (respiratory syncytial virus) is the most common viral cause.
- **Acute suppurative otitis media**
  - Common among children due to shorter Eustachian tube
  - **Signs and symptoms:** Heaviness in the ear, severe ear pain at night, tinnitus, cart wheel appearance of ear drum and deafness
  - Otorrhea with mucopurulent discharge occurs during suppurative stage
  - Pulsatile discharge occurs (lighthouse sign)
  - Pneumatic otoscopy is the gold standard diagnostic test
- **Treatment**
  - Tetracycline, erythromycin, penicillin or ampicillin for 6 days
  - Glycerin carbolic ear drops or warm olive oil to reduce pain
  - Antibiotic drops such as Chloramphenicol, spirit boric drops (to be used after perforation of tympanic membrane)
- **Surgical interventions**
  - **Myringotomy:** TM is incised to drain the middle ear cavity.
  - **Myringo-puncture:** Puncture the middle ear with a long needle to aspirate the middle ear contents
- **Chronic otitis media (COM)**
  - Chronic infection of middle ear cleft mucosa
  - Three types of COM include:

    1. **Chronic suppurative otitis media (CSOM):** Most common type; intermittent or continuous otorrhea present
    2. **Chronic nonsuppurative otitis media (CNSOM):** No otorrhea
    3. **Chronic specific otitis media:** TB OM or Syphilitic OM

External Otitis

- External otitis is more common in children and swimmers.
- It causes infection and inflammation of external auditory canal.
- Also called swimmer's ear.
- Manifestations – edematous, pain, redness, itchy

Treatment

- Antibiotic ear drops (bacterial infection) - Ciprofloxacin
- Corticosteroid ear drops (reduce swelling) - dexamethasone
- Antifungal ear drops
- Acidic ear drops (kill bacteria)
- Complication can be **conductive hearing loss.**

Otosclerosis

- **Autosomal dominant hereditary disorder** of labyrinthine capsule of middle ear
- Characterized by **bony overgrowth around the ear ossicles.**
- Fixation of ear ossicles leads to **conductive hearing loss**
- If the condition is affecting inner ear (cochlear sclerosis) it will lead to sensory-neural hearing loss.
- **Manifestation**
  - Gradual onset of hearing loss which may be severe in one ear.
  - Tinnitus, a constant ringing in the ears with no external source.
- **Diagnosis**
  - Otoscopy shows **Schwartze's sign** (reddish blue color of the tympanic membrane which suggests vascular changes).
  - Pneumo otoscopy to rule out other reasons for hearing loss.
  - **Audiometry**, Weber test (sound is heard more in the ear with conductive hearing loss), Rinne test (negative)

KEY POINTS

- Tubercular Otitis Media® Painless otorrhea, fails to respond to usual antimicrobial, multiple TM perforation, pale granulation tissue present.
- **Cholesteatoma** is a complication of chronic otitis media. It is a mass of epithelial cells and cholesterol in the middle ear.
- Stapedectomy/ Stapedotomy is the surgical management of otosclerosis.
- **Flamingo pink sign** or Schwartz sign is visible in **otosclerosis.**
- **Schwartz's sign** is reddish bluish of tympanum mainly present in **otosclerosis.**
- **Myringotomy** involves an incision in the tympanum to release the increased pressure and exudates from the middle ear.

- **Management**
  - Removal of bony overgrowth surrounding the ear ossicles
  - A partial or complete stapedectomy with prosthesis (fenestration).
- **Postoperative care following fenestration**
  - Inform the patient that initially hearing will be poor and it will be improved as edema resolves
  - Assist the patient in ambulation as there is a chance of vertigo
  - Instruct the patient to slowly move the head in order to prevent vertigo.
  - Instruct the patient to avoid sneezing, coughing, sudden change in position, nose blowing, straining and high altitude because these may increase the pressure in the middle ear and cause prosthesis dislodgement

Tympanic Membrane Perforation

- Rupture or perforation of tympanic membrane is caused by infection or trauma.
- **Causes:** Foreign body such as pointed objects, skull fracture, trauma, removal of ear wax
- **Manifestations:** Otalgia, fullness, discomfort, blood stained discharge from ear, hearing loss, vertigo, tinnitus.
- **Diagnosis:** Otoscopy, tympanogram, audiometry
- **Management:**
  - Usually perforated tympanic membrane heals spontaneously
  - Lesions which do not heal need to be treated surgically with tympanoplasty.

Meniere Disease (Meniere Syndrome or Idiopathic Endolymphatic Hydrops)

- Malabsorption of the endolymphatic fluid causes inner ear fluid imbalance.
- **Clinical manifestation:** Hearing loss, tinnitus, vertigo along with nausea and vomiting, pressure in the ear
- **Diagnosis:** Audiogram shows ear with sensory neural hearing loss, Weber test will report that sound is better heard in the unaffected ear.
- **Management**
  - Sodium restriction helps to control the fluid balance in endolymphatic sac
  - Symptomatic management for nausea, vomiting and vertigo.
- **Surgical management:** Endolymphatic sac decompression, infusion of ototoxic medication to inner and middle ear, vestibular nerve dissection, intraotologic catheter.

Labyrinthitis

- Bacterial or viral inflammation of the inner ear
- **Clinical manifestation:** Hearing loss, tinnitus, vertigo, nausea and vomiting
- **Management:** Antibiotic therapy for bacterial labyrinthitis, viral labyrinthitis need symptomatic management.

Hearing Aids

- An electro-acoustical device that amplifies sound. The four primary types of devices are as follows:
  1. Behind-the-ear (BTE)
  2. In-the-canal (ITC)
  3. In-the-ear (ITE)
  4. Receiver-in-canal (RIC)

Cochlear Implants

- Mostly used for sensorineural hearing loss.
- An electrical device that is implanted in cochlea helps in receiving sound and transmitting the signal.
- These are lifelong implants.

DISORDERS OF NOSE

Epistaxis

- It is also known as nose bleed
- Anterior septum is the most common site of nose bleed.
- **Causes:** Nasal blowing, trauma, insertion of any object, etc.
- **First aid management**
  - Pinch the nose and apply direct pressure over the area to control bleeding
  - Ask the client to attain sitting position with leaning forward to avoid secretions to not to go down the throat.
- **Treatment**
  - Vasoconstrictor medications are the drug of choice, **e.g., adrenaline 1:1000, phenylephrine,** etc.

Rhinitis

- Inflammation of nasal mucosa is caused by bacteria, virus or allergen
- **Clinical manifestation:** Running nose, sneezing, nasal congestion, headache
- **Management**
  - **Viral rhinitis:** Symptomatic management
  - **Allergic rhinitis:** Anti-histamine are the drug of choice.
  - **Bacterial rhinitis:** Anti-microbial therapy
  - Nasal decongestant may also be prescribed.

KEY POINTS

- Ensuring patient safety and environment safety is the priority nursing intervention while caring for a patient with Meniere's disease.
- Meniere's disease **(Endolymphatic hydrops)** is a disease of the inner ear characterized by recurring episodes of vertigo, tinnitus and deafness.
- Fluctuating deafness is seen in Meniere's disease.
- To stop nose bleed, firmly pinch the entire soft part of the nose just above the nostrils, sit and lean forward.
- Most of the nasal bleed occur from Kiesselbach's plexus or little area of the nose

Recent Question (CNCI 2021)

26. Meniere's disease is related to__________.

a. Eye
b. Ear
c. Respiratory system
d. Digestive system

Ans. (b) Ear

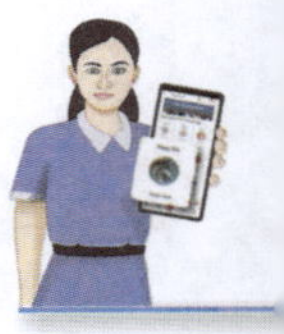

Sinusitis

- Inflammation of paranasal sinus caused by bacteria, virus or allergens
- **Clinical manifestation:** Fever, headache, nasal congestion, purulent nasal discharge, otalgia, and facial pain
- **Management:** Antimicrobial therapy and nasal decongestant are the drugs of choice
- **Complication:** Meningitis, abscess, ischemic infraction, osteo-myelitis

Nasal Obstruction

- Obstruction of nasal passage due to polyp like growth, deviated nasal septum, neoplasm, turbinate hypertrophy, congenital obstruction (choanal atresia), etc.
- Obstruction cause difficulty in passage of air through one or both nostrils.
- **Management**
    - Often surgery is required to remove the obstruction.
- **Nursing responsibility following surgery**
    - Provide upright position to promote drainage
    - Provide frequent mouth care to prevent dryness of oral mucosa.

Deviated Nasal Septum

- Deviated nasal septum is a condition in which nasal septum deviates to one side and makes the air flow through the passage more difficult.

Nasal Polyps

- Non-cancerous growth on the nasal mucosa and sinus which leads to loss of sense of smell and frequent infection.

DISORDERS OF THROAT

Pharyngitis

- Inflammation of pharynx
- **Causes:** Bacteria or virus. If caused by group a beta hemolytic streptococci then it will be known as strep-throat.
- **Clinical manifestation:** Fever, red swollen pharynx, sore throat
- **Viral pharyngitis:** Only symptomatic management.
- **Pharyngitis caused by bacteria:** Penicillin or erythromycin. If allergic or resistant to these drugs then **cephalosporin** group is needed.
- **Complication associated with step-throat** are rheumatic fever, nephritis, otitis media, mastoiditis.

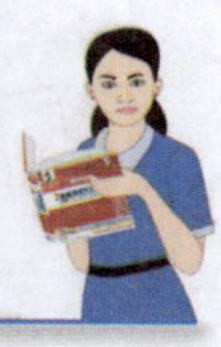

Tonsillitis

- Tonsils are the lymphatic tissue
- Inflammation of tonsils is known as tonsillitis
- **Clinical manifestation:** Red swollen tonsils, fever, dysphagia and sore throat
- Tonsillectomy is the surgical treatment of choice in case of recurrent infection and fails to respond to antibiotic therapy.

Adenoiditis

- Adenoid is the lymphatic tissue
- Inflammation of adenoid is known as adenoiditis.
- **Clinical manifestation:** Mouth breathing, snoring, foul smell in the mouth, fever
- **Complications:** Otitis media and mastoiditis.
- **Adenoidectomy** is the surgical treatment of choice in case of recurrent infection and fails to respond to antibiotic therapy.

Postoperative care following tonsillectomy and adenoidectomy

- Place the client in prone position to promote drainage of secretion from the oral cavity and to prevent aspiration
- Observe the patient for major complications associated with the surgery, i.e., hemorrhage. Frequent swallowing among the patients indicates hemorrhage.
- Repeated bright red color vomiting indicates hemorrhage
- Patient should avoid activities which cause strain in surgical site such as coughing, gargling and vigorous brushing
- Patient should avoid food items which are spicy, hot, acidic, milk and milk products.

Peri-Tonsillar Abscess

- It is also known as **quinsy**
- Collection of pus in the peri-tonsillar space
- It occurs as a complication of tonsillitis
- **Clinical manifestation:** Fever, malaise, odynophagia, dysphagia, dyspnea, dysphonia, severe throat pain, bad odor from mouth
- **Management:** Antibiotic therapy, analgesics and oral hygiene.
- **Surgical management** involves incision and drainage of abscess.

Laryngitis

- Inflammation of larynx is characterized by hoarseness of voice or aphonia.
- **Causes:** Exposure to smoke, dust, allergens and other pollutants.
- **Management:** Antibiotic therapy, voice rest and avoid agents such as smoke, chemical, dust, etc.

KEY POINTS

- Increased fluid intake and warm humidified environment is recommended to loosen the secretions in these patients.
- Frequent swallowing is a sign of hemorrhage in a child who underwent tonsillectomy.

Golden Points to Remember

- The part of the ear that helps in maintaining balance is vestibule.
- Normal hearing frequency of child and adult is **16–20,000 Hz.**
- **Acoustic Neuroma or Vestibular Schwannoma** is a benign tumor that occurs where the acoustic nerve (CN VIII) enters the internal auditory canal.
- Normal hearing is **0–15 dB** range; the profound deafness occurs due to the sound level reaches above 91 dB.
- Normal conversation sound level is 60 dB.
- Permissible level of noise in industries in India.
- 90 dB for 8 hours a day × 5 days a week.
- Syringing is done in Posterosuperior direction to remove wax.
- Ototoxicity is due to damage to Outer hair cells of cochlea.
- Least toxic aminoglycoside is Natilmycin.
- Viral infections associated with hearing loss is MMR.
- Average length of male vocal cord is 18–23 mm.
- Average length of female vocal cord is 16–17 mm.
- All muscles of larynx are supplied by recurrent laryngeal nerve (except cricothyroid which is supplied by external division of SLN).
- A nurse caring for a patient subjected to total laryngectomy should plan for **alternate communication method**.
- **Mulberry mucosa** is seen in Hypertrophic rhinitis.
- The beta-2 transferrin assay is the test of choice for **Confirmatory test to identify the CSF leak in body fluids.**
- Most of the nasal bleeds occur from Kiesselbach's plexus or little's area of the nose.
- Weber's and Rinne's test are the tests done to assess hearing loss.
- In **Rinne's test**, bone conduction if better than air conduction indicates conductive hearing loss.
- In **Weber's test**, lateralization of sound to affected side indicates unilateral conductive hearing loss.
- In **Weber's test**, lateralization of sound to normal or better-hearing side indicates unilateral sensorineural loss.

Most Common

- Most common cause of hearing loss is **Impacted wax**.
- Most common cause of hearing loss in children is **Secretory otitis media**.
- Most common complication of Chronic Suppurative Otitis Media (CSOM) is **Mastoiditis**.
- Most common tumor of middle ear is **Glomus tumor**.
- Most common histopathological variety of CA larynx is **Squamous cell carcinoma.**
- Most common sinusitis in children is **Ethmoid**.
- Most common sinusitis in Adult is **Maxillary**.
- Most common benign tumor of sinus is **Osteoma**.
- Most common fracture of bone of face is **Nasal bone**.

"The human body is the best picture of the human soul."
—Tony Robbins

MULTIPLE CHOICE QUESTIONS
(Including Explained and Practice Questions)

ENT SYSTEM

ANATOMY OF EAR

898. All are sinuses and belong to paranasal sinuses; EXCEPT: *(Safdarjung NO 2018)*

a. Maxillary b. Ethmoid
c. Sphenoid d. Mastoid

Ref: BD Chaurasia's, Human Anatomy, 7th edition, 2016, Vol. 3, PP. 254–255

Explanation: Mastoid is a bone present in the ear. The remaining others are paranasal sinuses. Paranasal sinuses are a group of air-filled spaces that surround the nasal cavity. There are four paranasal sinuses named after the bone where it is located.

Ethmoidal: Located between the eyes
- **Sphenoidal:** Located behind the eyes
- **Maxillary:** Located under the eyes
- **Frontal:** Located above the eyes

The functions of the sinuses are:
- Lighten the skull
- Improve our voices
- Sinuses produce mucus that moisturizes the nose from the inside. This mucus layer protects the nose from pollutants, microorganisms, dust and dirt.

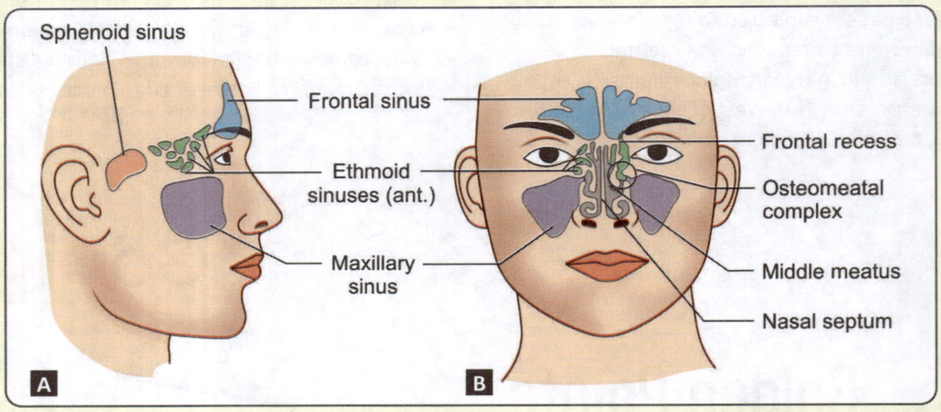

Figure: Paranasal sinuses

Ans.
898. d
899. a
900. d
901. c
902. b
903. c
904. d
905. d
906. c

899. Ear pinna develops from:

a. Ectoderm b. Endoderm
c. Mesoderm d. All

Explanation:

Development of Ear
- Developmentally, the internal ear appears first from an ectodermal vesicle, the otocyst.
- The middle ear develops next from the endoderm of the tubotympanic recess.
- The external ear appears last from the ectodermal first branchial cleft.

900. Which of the following attains adult size before birth?

a. Parietal bone b. Mastoid
c. Maxilla d. Ear ossicles

901. Function of ear ossicles is:

a. Amplification b. Equilibrium
c. Impedance matching d. None of these

902. Type of joint between the ear ossicles:

a. Primary cartilaginous b. Synovial joint
c. Secondary cartilaginous d. Fibrous joint

903. Nerve supply of the tympanic membrane is by:

a. Lesser occipital b. Parasympathetic ganglion
c. Auriculotemporal d. Greater occipital

904. Concha present in the nasal cavity helps to:

a. Divide the nose into right and left
b. Helps in immunological reaction
c. Filter the air and dust in the inhaled air
d. They increase the surface area

905. All of the following are blood supply of tonsils; EXCEPT:

a. Facial artery b. Maxillary artery
c. Lingual artery d. Middle meningeal artery

906. Primary auditory area is:

a. Inferior temporal gyrus
b. Occipital cortex
c. Superior temporal gyrus
d. Frontal cortex

907. Ear structure is enclosed by ....bone:
a. Frontal b. Parietal
c. Occipital d. Temporal

908. Length of tympanic membrane:
a. 10 mm b. 8 mm
c. 6 mm d. 4 mm

909. The length of Eustachian tube is:
a. 16 mm b. 24 mm
c. 36 mm d. 40 mm

910. Cranial Nerve VIII exits through which of the following?
a. Foramen ovale
b. Foramen rotundum
c. Internal acoustic meatus
d. Stylomastoid foramen

911. Number of muscles in middle ear:
a. 1 b. 2
c. 3 d. 4

912. Ear lobule is made-up of:
a. Elastic cartilage
b. Hyaline cartilage
c. Fibrocartilage
d. All of the above

913. The auditory ossicles are:
a. The malleus, incus and stapes
b. Located in the inner ear
c. Structures that decrease the vibrations from the tympanic membrane
d. Connected to the round window

914. Auditory tube is also known as:
a. Middle ear
b. External ear
c. Inner ear
d. Eustachian tube

915. The structure that opens into the pharynx and enables air pressure to be equalized between the middle ear and the outside is the:
a. Oval window
b. Round window
c. Eustachian tube
d. Auditory ossicles

916. Auditory tube opens into:
a. Oropharynx
b. Nasopharynx
c. Trachea
d. Esophagus

917. Nasopharynx is lined by which epithelium?
a. Ciliated columnar
b. Stratified squamous keratinized
c. Stratified squamous nonkeratinized
d. Cuboidal

918. VIII cranial nerve affects:
a. Taste b. Equilibrium
c. Touch d. Smell

919. Labyrinth is also known as:
a. Ear pinna b. Middle ear
c. Inner ear d. Semicircular canal

920. Oval window is adjacent to ....ear ossicle.
a. Malleus b. Incus
c. Cochlea d. Stapes

921. The organ of Corti is:
a. Located in the scala tympani
b. Made up of specialized sensory cells with hair-like projections
c. Located in the Eustachian tube
d. Afferent nerve fibers that form the tectorial nerve

922. Semicircular canals are present in:
a. Outer ear
b. Middle ear
c. Cochlea
d. Inner ear

923. Tonsils reach their maximum size by:
a. 1 years b. 3 years
c. 5 years d. 12 years

924. Nerve supply of tonsil is:
a. Facial nerve
b. Hypoglossal nerve
c. Glossopharyngeal nerve
d. Vagus nerve

925. The ear bones that transmit the vibrations to cochlea are situated in: *(JIPMER 2012)*
a. Middle ear b. Inner ear
c. Outer ear d. Eustachian tube

PHYSIOLOGY OF HEARING

926. The portion of the inner ear that involved with hearing is:
a. Semicircular canal
b. Vesitubular canal
c. Stapes
d. Cochlea

927. Which of the following acts as a "Transducer" that converts sound energy into other form of energy that are relevant to the nervous system?
a. Cochlea
b. Utricle
c. Saccule
d. Vestibular canal

928. The ear contains the receptor of both:
a. Hearing and understanding
b. Hearing and feeling
c. Hearing and balancing
d. Hearing and sensing

929. For what purpose the auditory tube gets opened while swallowing or yawing:
a. Pressure equalization on either side of ear drum
b. Attain body balance
c. Prevent airway obstruction
d. To accumulate the external air

930. The ossicles of the middle ear are connected by:
a. Fibrous joint
b. Cartilaginous joint
c. Synovial joint
d. Sesamoid joint

931. Which of the ear ossicle helps to check during when a person experiences large vibration from loud noise?
a. Malleus b. Incus
c. Stapes d. Saccule

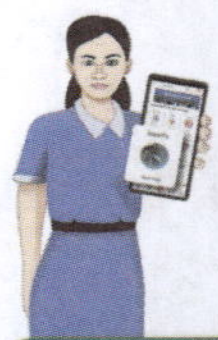

Ans.
907. d
908. a
909. c
910. c
911. b
912. a
913. a
914. d
915. c
916. b
917. a
918. b
919. c
920. d
921. b
922. d
923. d
924. c
925. a
926. d
927. a
928. c
929. a
930. c
931. c

932. The fluid present in the bony labyrinth which is critical for physiology of hearing is known as:
a. Synolymph
b. Endolymph
c. Perilymph
d. Exolymph

933. The membranous labyrinth which is covered by epithelium and filled with:
a. Synolymph
b. Endolymph
c. Perilymph
d. Exolymph

934. The organ of hearing that present and rest over the basilar membrane is known as:
a. Organ of Corti
b. Organ of caudal
c. Organ of synole
d. Organ of tympanium

935. What would be frequency of the sound waves?
a. Warts
b. Pitch
c. Rhythm
d. Tempo

DIAGNOSTIC TESTS IN ENT

936. Examination of external ear and tympanic membrane is done with the help of:
a. Otoscope
b. Ophthalmoscope
c. Proctoscope
d. Tuning fork

937. Which of the following is an unexpected finding during an otoscopic examination of the ear? *(AIIMS-BBS SNO 2019)*
a. Malleus visible behind the tympanic membrane
b. Pearl grey tympanic membrane
c. Flaky skin in the external canal near the tympanic membrane
d. Black cerumen occluding the tympanic membrane

Explanation: Normally tympanic membrane is pearly grey and shiny. Cerumen (ear wax) is normally of yellow to brown color. Black colored cerumen is not present normally, it indicates abnormality.

938. How to hold pinna in children younger than 3 years of age while observing the ear canal?
a. Pull the pinna downward and backward
b. Pull the pinna upward and backward
c. Pull pinna backward
d. Pull pinna upward

939. While instilling ear drops to an adult client, the ear canal is straightened by pulling the pinna: *(DSSSB 2013)*
a. Straight backward
b. Downwards and backwards
c. Straight downward
d. Upwards and backwards

Explanation: With the non-dominant hand, straighten the external ear canal by gently pulling up and back on the ear for an adult, or down and back for a child.

940. Test used to compare the bilateral hearing of a client is:
a. Allen's test
b. Weber's test
c. Rinne's test
d. Romberg's test

941. Test used to check whether air conduction or bone conduction is more:
a. Allen's test
b. Weber's test
c. Rinne's test
d. Romberg's test

942. Test used to assess whether the patient will be able to maintain equilibrium even after the eyes are closed is known as:
a. Allen's test
b. Weber's test
c. Rinne's test
d. Romberg's test

943. In Weber's test, lateralization of sound to diseased ear indicates: *(AIIMS BBS NO 2018)*
a. Conductive deafness
b. Sensorineural deafness
c. Tympanic deafness
d. Combination of both sensorineural deafness and conductive deafness

Explanation:

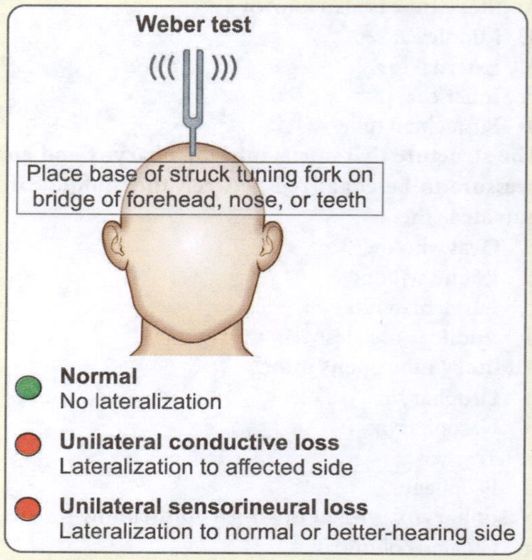

OTITIS MEDIA

944. Infection of middle ear is called: *(LNJP H D 2012)*
a. Otitis media
b. Labyrinthitis
c. Sinusitis
d. Mastoiditis

945. All of the following conditions are contraindicated for irrigation of ear; EXCEPT:
a. Otitis externa
b. Tympanic membrane perforation
c. History of middle ear infection before 6 months
d. Repaired cleft palate

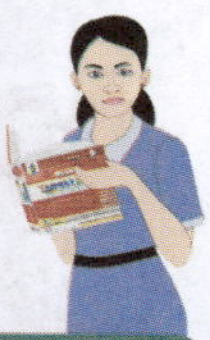

Ans.
932. c
933. b
934. a
935. b
936. a
937. d
938. a
939. d
940. b
941. c
942. d
943. a
944. a
945. c

Explanation: Contraindications for irrrigation of ear includes:
- Complications following previous ear irrigation
- A current ear infection or an infection within the last 6 weeks
- Any previous ear surgery (apart from grommets which have come out 18 months ago)
- Grommets in situ
- A current perforation or history of ear perforation
- A cleft palate (even if it has been repaired)
- Recurrent otitis externa

946. Method of choice to remove ear wax is:
a. Mineral oils
b. Cotton swab applicator
c. Warm normal saline irrigation
d. Otoscope

947. A client has painless purulent exudate, along with nausea, vomiting and dizziness, the nurse suspects the following condition:
a. Chronic otitis media b. Otorrhea
c. Meniere's disease d. Tympanic perforation

948. Complications of chronic suppurative otitis media (CSOM) is:
a. Cholesteatoma b. Meningitis
c. Both a and b d. Conductive hearing loss

949. Commonest intracranial complication of CSOM is:
a. Conductive deafness b. Cholesteatoma
c. Temporal lobe abscess d. Meningitis

950. Blue ear drum is seen in:
a. Serous otitis media b. CSOM
c. Perforation d. None

951. Hemorrhagic otitis externa is caused by:
a. Influenza b. Streptococcus
c. Staphylococcus aureus d. Proteus

952. Malignant otitis externa is caused by:
a. Staphylococcus aureus
b. Pseudomonas
c. Staphylococcus epidermidis
d. Klebsiella

Explanation:

Malignant otitis externa

Malignant otitis externa (MOE) is an aggressive and potentially life-threatening infection of the soft tissues of the external ear and surrounding structures, quickly spreading to involve the periosteum and bone of the skull base.
- Pseudomonas aeruginosa is the most common pathogen and is responsible in >95% of cases of MOE.
- The treatment of choice for MOE is systemic anti-Pseudomonas antibiotics.

OTOSCELEROSIS

953. Otosclerosis is also known as:
a. Otofibrosis b. Otospongiosis
c. Otophysis d. Otorrhea

954. Otosclerosis commonly presents with?
a. Fluctuating hearing loss b. Conductive deafness
c. Mixed hearing loss d. Sensorineural deafness

955. Which of the following procedure is used to correct otosclerosis? *(Staff Nurse G II 2014)*
a. Myringotomy b. Mastoidectomy
c. Stapedectomy d. Myringoplasty

TYMPANIC MEMBRANE PERFORATION

956. Vertigo is due to problem in: *(Daman and Diu NO 2018)*
a. External ear b. Tympanic membrane
c. Inner ear d. Middle ear

Explanation: Vertigo refers to a sense of spinning dizziness. Vertigo that is caused by problems in the inner ear is known as peripheral vertigo, or problems in the brain or nervous system is known as central vertigo. External ear, tympanic membrane and middle are not the causes of vertigo.

957. Which among the following needs to include in the nursing health teaching plan following tympanoplasty?
a. Maintain NPO
b. Ask the patient to walk around
c. Provide fowlers position
d. Avoid forceful nose blowing

958. A condition caused by calcification of tissues in the middle ear, sometimes resulting in a detrimental effect to hearing is known as:
a. CSOM b. Otosclerosis
c. Tympanosclerosis d. Meniere's disease

959. Tympanosclerosis is also known as:
a. Myringosclerosis b. Otosclerosis
c. Meniere's disease d. CSOM

MENIERE DISEASE & LABYRINTHITIS

960. Which of the following diet is suitable for a patient with Meniere's syndrome?
a. High-fiber diet b. Low sodium diet
c. High-protein diet d. Iodine rich diet

961. Risk associated with long-term use of Lasix (frusemide) is:
a. Renal failure b. Tinnitus and hearing loss
c. Hypervolemia d. Hyperkalemia

962. Meniere's disease affects:
a. Stomach b. Ear
c. Liver d. Lungs

963. Clinical manifestation of Meniere's disease is:
a. Vertigo b. Tinnitus
c. Deafness d. All of these

964. Drugs used in relieving symptoms of Meniere's disease includes all; EXCEPT:
a. Antiemetics b. Diuretics
c. Atropine d. Diazepam

965. Excess endolymph in the vestibular and semicircular canal will lead to:
a. CSOM b. Tympanitis
c. Meniere's disease d. Vertigo

966. Selective low frequency sensorineural hearing loss occurs in:
a. BPPV b. Glomus tumor
c. Schwannoma d. Meniere's disease

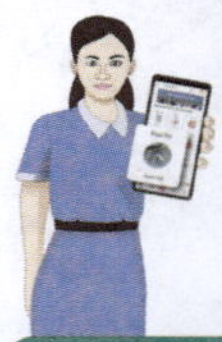

Ans.

946. c
947. a
948. c
949. d
950. a
951. a
952. b
953. b
954. b
955. c
956. c
957. d
958. c
959. a
960. b
961. b
962. b
963. d
964. c
965. c
966. d

967. Fluctuating deafness is seen in:
a. Meniere's disease b. Otosclerosis
c. CSOM d. ASOM

968. The most common complaint of patients with disorder in the inner ear is:
a. Hearing loss b. Burning of the ear
c. Pruritis d. Tinnitus

969. Characteristic symptom in Meniere's disease is:
a. Epistaxis
b. Otalgia
c. Sensory neural hearing loss
d. Tinnitus

DISORDERS OF NOSE

970. Epistaxis management includes the following actions; EXCEPT: *(AIIMS BBS NO 2018)*
a. Applying pressure by pinching the nose
b. Applying ice over the nose
c. Allowing the patient to sneeze
d. Keeping the patient in sitting position with the neck flexed

Explanation: Allowing the patient to sneeze as may worsen the bleeding. All other interventions are recommended in the management of epistaxis.

971. Pansinusitis refers to inflammation of:
a. All sinuses on only one side of the nose
b. All sinuses on both sides of the nose
c. All sinuses on one or both sides of the nose
d. Only one sinus on either side of the nose

972. Acute hemorrhage (bleeding) from the nasal cavity is termed as *(DSSSB 2013)*
a. Epistaxis b. Hemoptysis
c. Hematemesis d. Rhinorrhea

Explanation: Epistaxis is defined as acute hemorrhage from the nostril, nasal cavity, or nasopharynx. It is otherwise known as nose bleed. There are two types: Anterior (the most common), and posterior (less common, more likely to require medical attention). The vast majority of nose bleeds occur in the anterior (front) part of the nose from the nasal septum. This area is richly endowed with blood vessels (Kiesselbach's plexus). This region is also known as Little's area.

973. The most common cause of epistaxis is associated with: *(AIIMS Jodhpur Nursing Tutor 2016)*
a. Rhinorrhea b. Infection
c. Sinusitis d. Little's area

Explanation: The vast majority of nose bleeds occur in the anterior (front) part of the nose from the nasal septum. This area is richly endowed with blood vessels (Kiesselbach's plexus). This region is also known as Little's area.

974. Most common site of nose bleed in a child:
a. Little's area b. Woodruff area
c. Brown area d. None

975. Epistaxis in elderly person is commonly due to:
a. Allergic rhinitis b. Foreign body
c. Hypertension d. Nasopharyngeal carcinoma

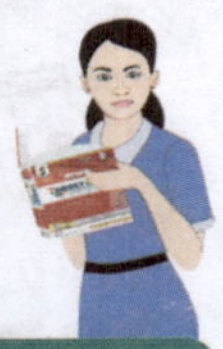

Ans.
967. a
968. d
969. d
970. c
971. c
972. a
973. d
974. a
975. c
976. d
977. d
978. b
979. c
980. a
981. c
982. b
983. c

976. Commonest cause of epistaxis in children is:
a. Enlarged adenosis b. Foreign body
c. Nasal diphtheria d. Trauma

977. Watery otorrhea is seen in:
a. CSOM
b. Glomus tympanicum
c. Otitis media with effusion
d. Fracture of temporal bone

978. Loss of sense of smell is called:
a. Anhedonia b. Anosmia
c. Anoxia d. Aphasia

979. The nasal cavity is divided into right and left sides by the:
a. Conchae b. Paranasal sinuses
c. Nasal septum d. Hard palate

980. Bleeding from the nose is known as: *(DSSSB 2013, DSSSB PHN, 2015)*
a. Epistaxis b. Hemoptysis
c. Hematemesis d. Hematuria

Explanation: Epistaxis, or bleeding from the nose. Epistaxis can be divided into 2 categories, anterior bleeds and posterior bleeds, on the basis of the site where the bleeding originates.

DISORDERS OF THROAT

981. A nurse is caring for a 9-year-old child who underwent tonsillectomy. Which of the following observation by the nurse is most concerned?
a. 30 mL of dark brown secretions
b. A heart rate of 90 beats per minute
c. Expectorating bright red secretions
d. Infrequent swallowing

Explanation: Spitting out bright red secretions by the child indicates active bleeding. Frequent swallowing also indicates of bleeding.

982. Which of the following nursing intervention is appropriate while caring for child postoperatively after tonsillectomy and adenoidectomy?
a. Allow the child to drink through a straw
b. Observe swallowing patterns
c. Offer ice cream every 2 hours
d. Place the child in a supine position

Explanation: Observing swallowing pattern of the child will help to determine if there is active bleeding from site of surgery. The more the child swallows the more bleeding happens.

983. The bacterial infection of the submandibular space would be:
a. Pectoralis angina b. Prinz metal angina
c. Ludwig angina d. Mandibulitis.

Explanation: *Ludwig's angina* is a bilateral infection of the *submandibular space* that consists of two compartments in the floor of the mouth, the sublingual space (under the tongue) and submaxillary space. It often develops after an infection of the roots of the teeth (such as tooth abscess) or a mouth injury.

984. The 3 Ds of epiglottitis would be:
- a. Dysphagia, drooling, distress
- b. Dyspepsia, drooling, distress
- c. Dysphagia, draught, distress
- d. Dysphagia, drooling, difficulty digestion.

985. Following are the classical symptoms of croup; EXCEPT: *New Q*
- a. Stridor
- b. Hoarseness
- c. Hemorrhage
- d. Seal bark cough

Explanation: Croup is a viral infection that causes inflammation of the larynx and trachea. It is most common in children under the age of 5 years. The classic symptoms of croup include: Stridor, Hoarseness, Seal bark cough, and difficulty breathing.

986. The most common bacteria that cause throat infection are:
- a. Streptococcus
- b. Mycobacterium
- c. Staphylococcus
- d. Corynebacterium

ANY OTHER ENT DISORDERS

987. Age-related hearing loss is known as: *(AIIMS-BBS SNO 2019)*
- a. Otosclerosis
- b. Otitis media
- c. Presbycusis
- d. Presbyopia

Explanation: **Presbycusis** is the hearing loss that gradually occurs in older people. It is the most common type of sensorineural hearing loss caused by natural aging of the auditory system.

988. Profound hearing loss is described as greater than: *(AIIMS BBS NO 2018)*
- a. 20 dB
- b. 60 dB
- c. 80 dB
- d. 40 dB

Explanation:

Degree of hearing	Decibels (dBs)
Normal hearing	0-20 dB
Mild hearing loss	24-39 dB
Moderate hearing loss	40-69 dB
Severe hearing loss	70-89 dB
Profound deafness	90 dB+

The options which is closest to profound hearing loss is 80 db.

989. Maximum audible tolerance is:
- a. 90 db for 6 hours
- b. 90 db for 8 hours
- c. 85 db for 6 hours
- d. 85 db for 8 hours

Explanation:
- Permissible exposure in cases of continuous noise or a number of short term exposures. [Government of India, Ministry of Labour, Model Rules under Factories Act 1948 (corrected up to 31.3.87)]
- Noise level* (dBA) Permitted daily exposure (hours).

Nose level (dB)	Permitted daily exposure (hours)
90	8 hours
92	6 hours
95	4 hours
97	2 hours
100	2 hours
102	1½ hours
105	1 hours
110	30 minutes
115	15 minutes

Contd...

5 dB rule of time-intensity states that "any rise of 5 dB noise level will reduce the permitted noise exposure time to half".

990. Conductive hearing loss is caused by all; EXCEPT:
- a. Foreign body obstruction in auditory canal
- b. Perforation of the tympanic membrane
- c. Freezing of the ossicles
- d. Damage to 8th cranial nerve

991. Which among the following is a cause for sensorineural hearing loss?
- a. Foreign body obstruction in auditory canal
- b. Perforation of the tympanic membrane
- c. Freezing of the ossicles
- d. Damage to 8th cranial nerve

992. The risk factors of sensorineural impairment include the following: *(AIIMS Raipur Grade II 2017)*
- a. Family history of sensorineural impairment
- b. Congenital malformations of the cranial structures
- c. Chronic exposure to loud noise
- d. Recurrent ear infection
- a. A, B, C
- b. B, C, D
- c. A, B, D
- d. A, C, D

Explanation: The risk factors include ototoxic medication, hyperbilirubinemia, in utero infections (including CMV, rubella, syphilis, herpes, and toxoplasmosis), craniofacial anomalies, syndromes associated with Sensory neural hearing loss, low birth weight (<1, 500 g), low Apgar score, mechanical ventilation lasting for 5 days or longer, bacterial meningitis, family history of hereditary childhood SNHL, endocranial hemorrhage, hypoxic ischemic encephalopathy, convulsions, and sepsis.

993. The patient who has a conductive hearing loss:
- a. Hears better in a noisy environment
- b. Hears murmur
- c. Often speaks loudly because his or her own voice seems low.
- d. Hear sounds less than 30 db

994. Which among the following techniques can be used by a nurse while communicating with a client who has hearing impairment?
- a. Do face to face conversation
- b. Speak normally and slowly
- c. Use non-verbal clues
- d. All of the above

995. Postoperative position given after stapedectomy is:
- a. The affected side
- b. The unaffected side
- c. Prone
- d. Lateral

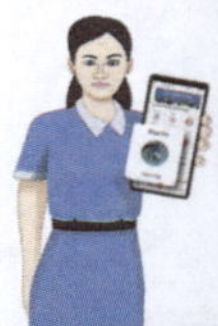

Ans.

984. a
985. c
986. a
987. c
988. c
989. b
990. d
991. d
992. c
993. a
994. d
995. b

OPHTHALMOLOGY

ANATOMY AND PHYSIOLOGY OF EYE

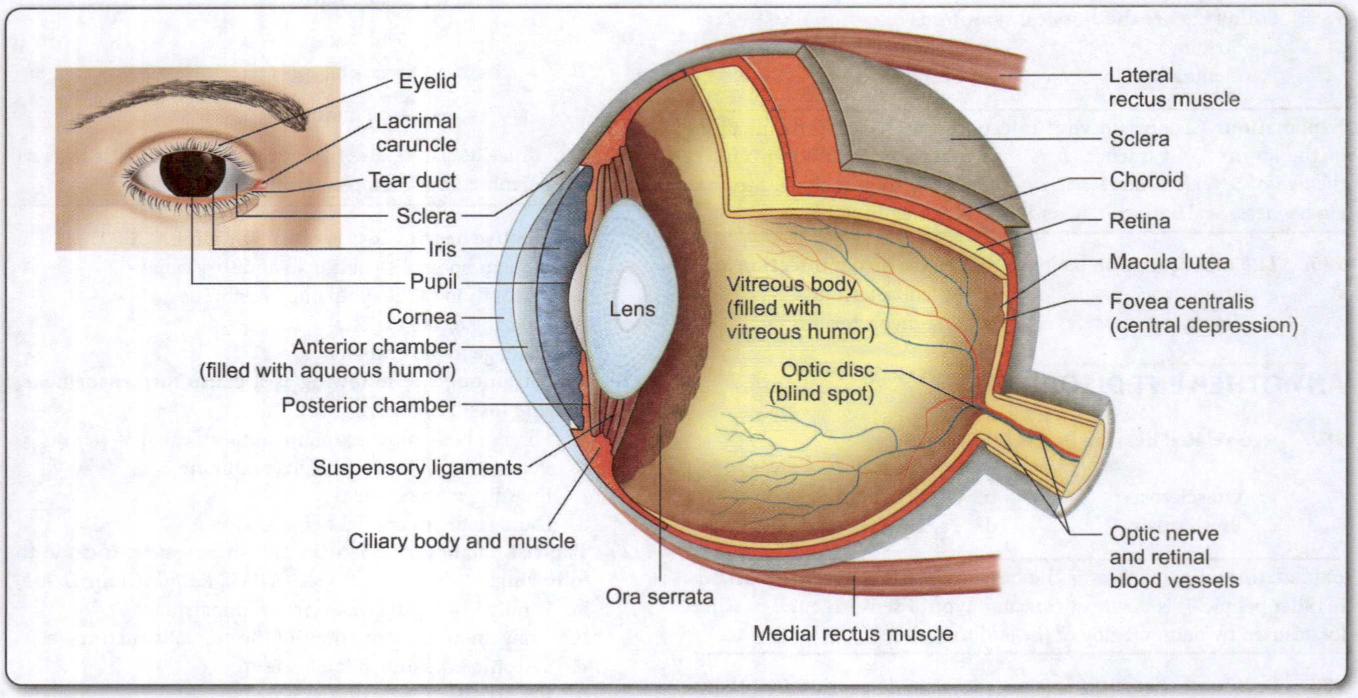

Figure 41: Anatomy of eye

Extraocular Structures

a. Eye orbit

- It is the bony socket (4 cm in diameter) of skull and protects the eye by pads of fat.

b. Eye lids

- These are composed of thin elastic skin and are responsible to protect anterior portion of eye. Eyelids are covered by palpebral conjunctiva.
- Lid margins contain meibomian glands (responsible to provide lipoid component to tears) and eye lashes.
- **Upper eyelid movement** is controlled by a muscle called levator palpebrae superioris which is innervated by **cranial nerve-III** (Occulomotor nerve).

c. Conjunctiva

- Composed of non-keratinized, stratified squamous epithelium.

It is a thin transparent mucous membrane that nourishes the eye. It is of two types:

1. **Bulbar conjunctiva:** It covers sclera.
2. **Palpebral conjunctiva:** It covers the inner surface of eyelids.

d. Lacrimal glands

- It is an almond shaped exocrine gland.
- Situated in upper and lateral region of each orbit in frontal bone's fossa.
- Responsible to produce tears (Tear has 3 components—mucoid, Lipoid and aqueous).
- Tears produced by lacrimal glands wash sclera, cornea and flows through lacrimal canal → Lacrimal sac → Nasolacrimal duct.
- Contains lysosomes and Ig A
- Inflammation of the lacrimal glands is called **dacryoadenitis.**
- It is stimulated by parasympathetic nerve of CN VII
- 5–12 small ducts are open.

e. Extra ocular muscles

- There are 6 extra ocular muscles and these muscles are innervated by three cranial nerves.
- These muscles are responsible to move eyeball.

Recent Question (NORCET 2020)

27. After death of a person, how long cornea can be preserved for transplantation?

a. 2 hours
b. 6 hours
c. 8 hours
d. 12 hours

Ans. (b) 6 hours

Recent Question (CNCI 2021)

28. The term Aphakia means?

a. Inflammation of lens
b. Absence of lens
c. Enhancement of lens
d. Lens disease

Ans. (b) Absence of lens

POINTS TO REMEMBER

- **Blepharitis** – inflammation of eyelids
- **Chalazion** – cyst on eyelids due to blockage of tarsal glands
- **Stye**- also called hordeolum, acute painful modular infection of sebaceous or meibomian glands

Table 32: Nerve supply to eye muscles

Cranial nerve-III (Occulomotor nerve)	• Innervates all the extrinsic muscles **except** superior oblique and lateral rectus
Cranial nerve-IV (Trochlear nerve)	• Superior oblique muscle
Cranial nerve-VI (Abducent nerve)	• Lateral rectus muscle

Ocular Structures

a. **Eye ball**
   - It is 1 inch (2.5 cm) in diameter and is located in orbit.
   - It consists of three layers:
     1. External layer (sclera and cornea)
     2. Middle layer (Uveal tract)
     3. Inner layer (Retina)

b. **Layers of Eye**
   - **External layer (Sclera and Cornea)**
     - **Sclera** is the white part of eye comprising posterior 5/6 of external layer of eye.
     - **Cornea** is the anterior 1/6 part of external layer of eye. It is transparent, avascular and dome like structure. It contains three layers – outer is stratified squamous epithelium, middle lined collagen fiber and inner is simple squamous epithelium.
   - **Middle layer (Uveal tract)**
     - Uveal tract consists of choroid, ciliary body and iris.

- **Choroid**
  - Choroid is the vascular layer (1mm thick) and lies between retina and sclera.
  - Choroid provides nourishment to outer layer of retina
- **Ciliary body**
  - Ciliary body consists of ciliary muscles and ciliary process and it connects the choroid and iris.
  - It has two functions: **Production of aqueous humor and Accommodation reflex.**
  - **Accommodation** is a process of adjustment of lens thickness as per the distance of the object from eye.
  - **For focusing on closer objects:** Ciliary muscles contract → lens convexity increases (controlled by **parasympathetic nervous system**).
  - **For focus on distant objects:** Ciliary muscles relax → flattens the lens (controlled by **sympathetic nervous system**).
- **Iris**
  - It is colored, highly vascularized part of eye behind cornea. Color of iris depends on amount of melanin pigment present
  - Pupil is a space through which light enters into eye. It dilates and constricts in response to light (**Pupillary reflex**).
  - Bright light → stimulates sphincter muscles of iris → pupils constrict (controlled by **parasympathetic nervous system**).
  - Dim light → stimulates dilator muscles of iris → pupils dilate (controlled by **sympathetic nervous system**).
- **Inner layer (Retina)**
  - It is the innermost layer of eye and contains photoreceptors – **Cones and Rods**
  - **Cone cells:** Responsible for central, night and color vision, functions in bright light
  - **Rod cells:** Responsible for peripheral vision, functions in dim light.
  - Rod cells contain only single type of rhodopsin photopigment.
  - Cone cells contain three types-
    - Porphyropsin (response to red light)
    - Cyanopsin (response to blue light)
    - Iodopsin (response to green light)
  - It is the layer which converts light into nerve impulses.
  - Optic pathway starts from retina and ends with occipital lobe of cerebrum.
  - **Optic disk:** This is where the optic nerve enters the eyeball. It is also known as **blind spot** because it does not contain any photoreceptors.

KEY POINTS

- Three **cranial nerves** that are related to eye movements are Oculomotor, Trochlear and Abducens.
- **Pupil** contracts in response to bright light and dilates in dim light.
- **Anisocoria** is unequal pupil size.
- Color blindness is due to problem with cones, genetic X linked.
- Night blindness is due to deficiency of vit. A, which is essential for rod cells.
- Most common type is red-green color blindness.

Recent Question
(CNCI 2021)

29. Munson's sign is a characteristic of advanced cases of:

a. Keratoconus
b. Cataract
c. Strabismus
d. Diabetic Retinopathy

Ans. (a) Keratoconus

Explanation: Keratoconus is an eye disease that affects the structure of the cornea, resulting in loss of vision.

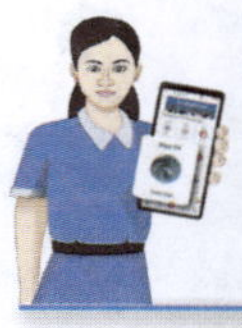

c. Segments and chambers

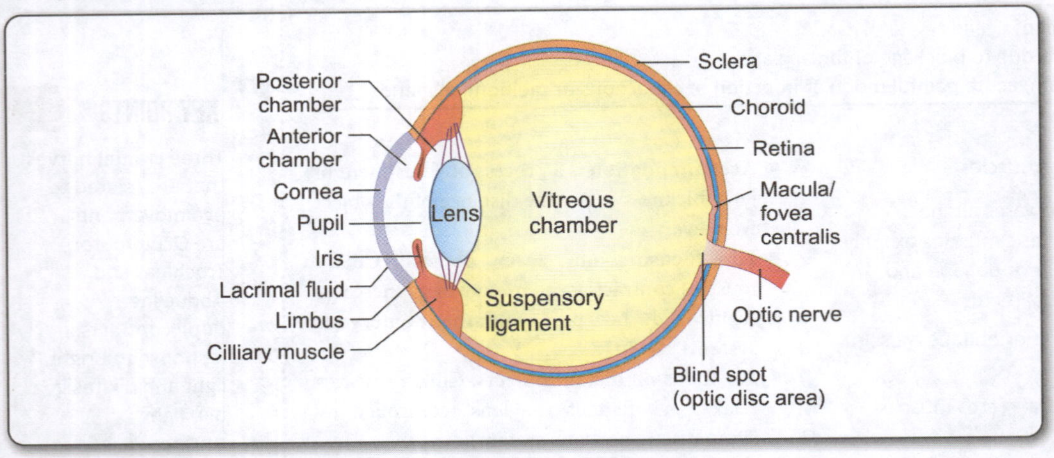

Figure 42: Segments and chambers of eye

- Eye is divided into anterior and posterior segments.
- **Anterior segment** (contains aqueous humor) is a cavity between cornea and lens which is further divided into anterior and posterior chambers.
- Anterior chamber is a space between cornea and iris.
- Posterior chamber is a space between iris and lens.
- **Aqueous humor is secreted by ciliary body** in posterior chamber and it enters into anterior chamber through pupil.
- **Aqueous humor is a transparent watery fluid similar to plasma.** It provides nourishment to cornea and lens, maintains intraocular pressure **(10–21 mm Hg).**

- Aqueous humor is replaced in every 90 minutes
  - **Posterior segment** (contains vitreous body) is a cavity between lens and retina.
  - Vitreous body is a transparent, colorless, gelatinous mass which makes up 4/5th volume of eye ball and helps to **maintain shape of eye.**
  - Vitreous humor is not replaced in lifetime. It is considered one of refractory media.

d. Lens

- It is colorless, transparent, biconvex structure
- Lens contains protein known as Crystallin
- It is held in position by **zonular fibers** and lies behind iris and pupil.
- Lens has no blood and nervous supply.
- It provides refractive power to eye (**20 diopter**)

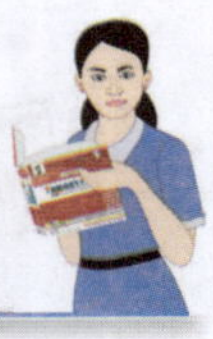

Dark Adaptation

- Dark adaptation refers to how the eye recovers its sensitivity when entering in the dark room after exposure to bright lights.
- Maximum time for adaptation is 20 -30 min

Visible Light or Vision Spectrum

- White color reflects all visible light wavelengths and black absorbs all wavelengths.
- Visible spectrum color is VIBGYOR (violet, indigo, blue, green, yellow, orange, red)

Normal eye can see between 10 cm near point vision to 6 m far point of vision.

ASSESSMENT AND DIAGNOSTIC TESTS

External Eye Examination

Patient is examined for:

- **Ptosis:** Drooping eyelid
- **Ectropion:** Outward turning of eyelid
- **Entropion:** Inward turning of eyelid
- **Nystagmus:** Oscillating movement of eyeball
- **PERRLA:** Pupils Equally Round and Reactive to Light and Accommodation
- Intactness of extraocular muscles is assessed by following the examiner's finger in six cardinal positions of gaze.

Visual Acuity

a. Snellen chart

- It is used to test distance vision from 20 feet or 6 meters and is composed of series of progressively smaller rows of letters.
- If the patient is able to read all the lines then visual acuity (VA) is recorded as 6/6 or 20/20.
- **Abbreviations used**
  - **OD (Ocular dexter):** Right eye
  - **OS (Ocular sinister):** Left eye
  - **OU (Ocular uterque):** Both eyes.

- If the patient is unable to read the largest letter, patient should be moved toward the chart till a distance of 3 m and if still unable to read, examiner should determine if patient can count fingers (CF) at 1 m.

Practice Questions

15. The presence of Kayser Fleischer ring is seen in
a. Kernicterus
b. Lowe's syndrome
c. Wilson's disease
d. Siderosis

Ans. (c) Wilson's disease

16. Which of the following is the earliest symptom to occur in corneal ulcer?
a. Pain
b. Photophobia
c. Blurred vision
d. Diminished vision

Ans. (a) Pain

17. Diagnostic tests useful in evaluating a patient with a retained magnetic intraocular foreign body is all, except:
a. Perimetry
b. Computed tomography
c. Slip lamp exam
d. Magnetic resonance imaging (MRI)

Ans. (d) Magnetic resonance imaging (MRI)

- If patient cannot count fingers then vision can be determined by hand movement (HM).
- A patient who can perceive only light is described as having light perception (LP). Unable to perceive light is documented as no light perception (NLP).
- Near vision is assessed by a hand held card at a distance of 14 inches (35 cm).
- **Legal blindness:** It is defined as the visual acuity in better eye as 20/200 or less or visual field 20 degrees or less

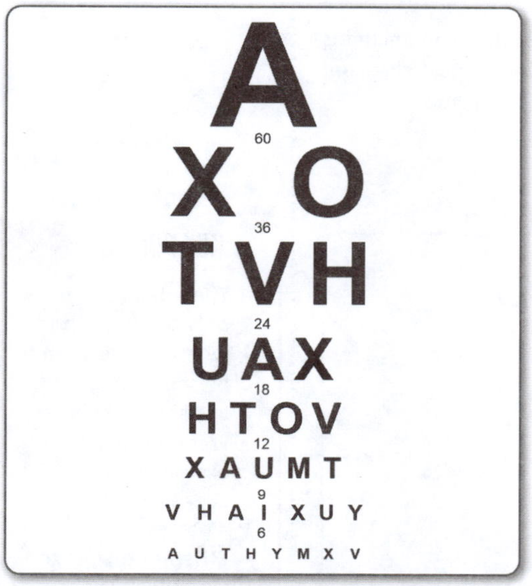

Figure 43: Snellen chart

Confrontation Test

- Confrontation test measures the peripheral vision.
- Examiner compares the normal vision with client's vision.

Ishihara Chart for Color Vision

- This test consists of a booklet with number of colored plates (38 plates).
- Only 3 sec are given to answer.

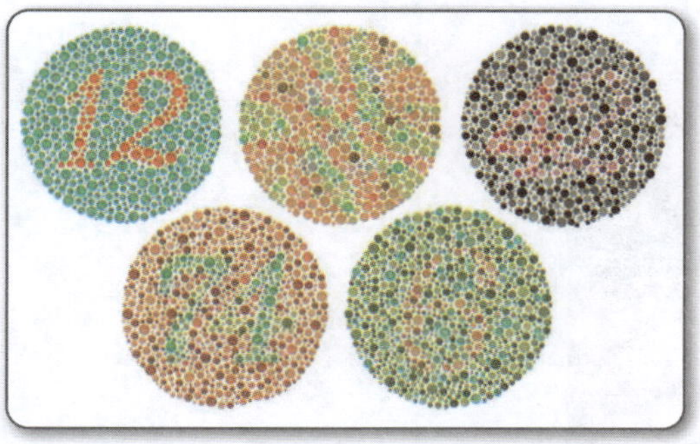

Figure 44: Ishihara chart for color vision

Perimetry

- It measures the visual field and helps to identify scotomas (blind areas in visual field).
- Average extent of visual field in a healthy eye during its primary gaze is 65 degrees upward, 75 downward, 60 inward and 95 outward.

Ophthalmoscopy (Fundoscopy)

Direct Ophthalmoscopy

- It is a hand held instrument with various plus and minus lenses.
  - Examiner holds the ophthalmoscope in right hand and visualizes right eye of patient with his right eye and vice versa.
  - Dilation of pupil (Mydriasis by 1–2 drops of Tropicamide 0.5%) is done before doing this test for proper visualization.
  - This test should be performed in dark room and examiner uses red reflex (red light) through pupil, lens and focuses on retina.

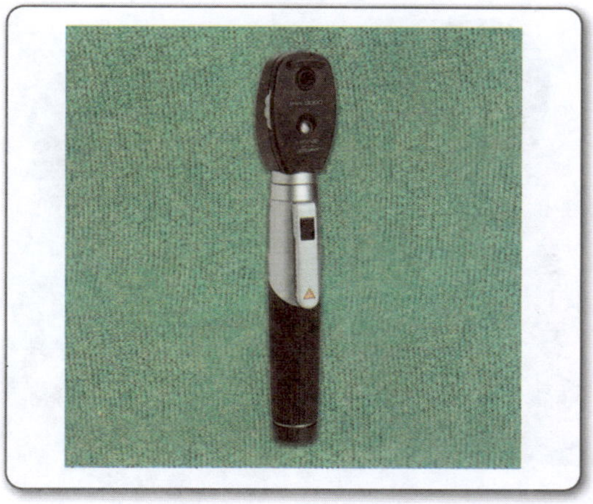

Figure 45: Direct ophthalmoscope

  - Macula should be examined in the last because it is highly sensitive to light.
  - **Inferences**
    - Papilledema (swelling in optic disc) indicates raised intracranial pressure.
    - Cupped optic disc (Optic cupping) indicates glaucoma (raised intraocular pressure).
    - Flame-shaped red smudges can be a manifestation of hypertension.
    - Cotton wool spots (caused by micro-infarcts) may indicate diabetic retinopathy, or hypertension.
    - Drusen (tiny, yellowish spots) indicates macular degeneration

KEY POINT

Color blindness is due to the problem with **cones**.

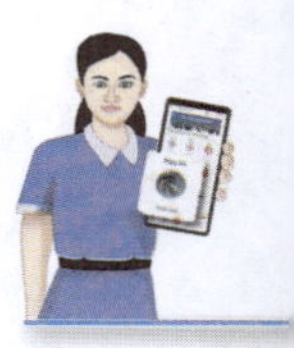

Indirect Ophthalmoscopy

- This test should be performed in dark room

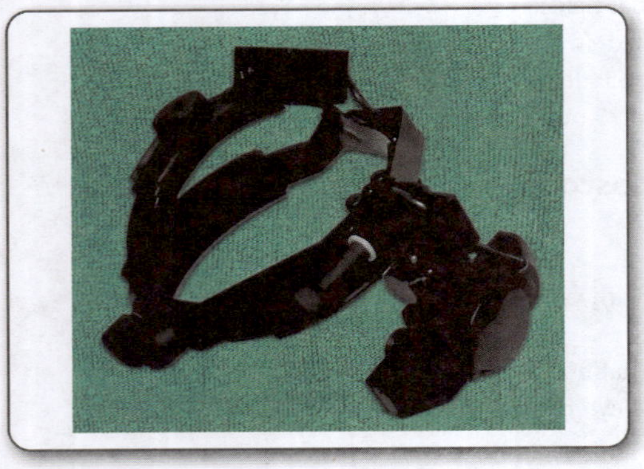

Figure 46: Indirect ophthalmoscope

  - Ophthalmoscope consists of a light source, which is affixed with a pair of binocular lenses, mounted on examiner's head with a hand held 20 diopter lens.

Slit-lamp Examination

- Slit lamp is a binocular microscope mounted on a table.
- Patient is asked to place the chin in chin rest and forehead against the forehead band to keep the head steady.
- This is used to assess scleritis, conjunctivitis (pink eye), corneal dystrophy, corneal abrasion, cataract, retinal detachment, and glaucoma.

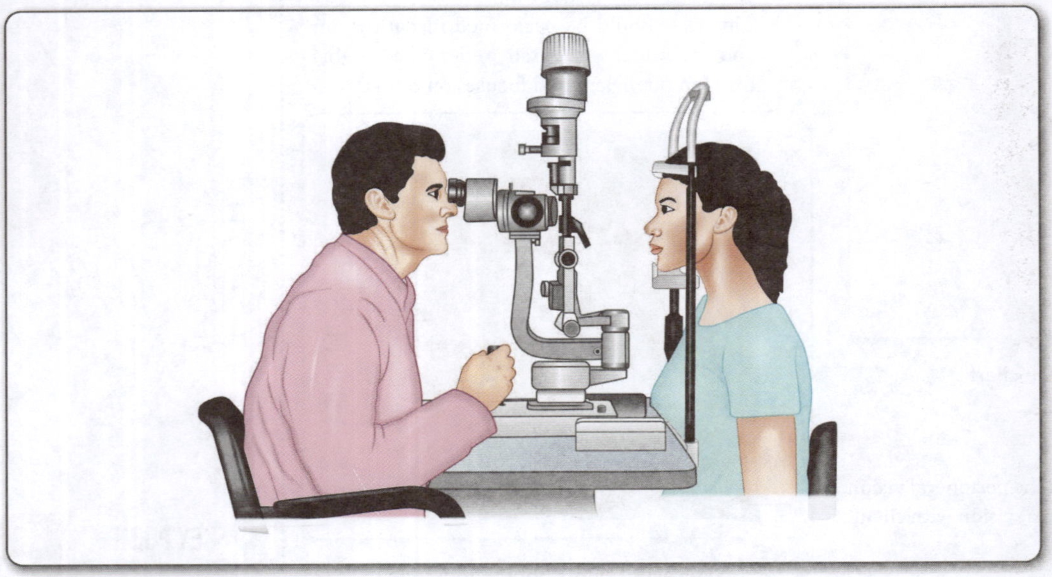

Figure 47: Slit lamp examination

Tonometry

- Tonometry is done to measure intraocular pressure (IOP) and is of two types:
  - **Contact tonometry:** Done with the help of slit lamp, hand held prism and indentation tonometry. Local topical anesthetic and fluorescein dye are instilled into the eye before the test.
  - **Non-contact tonometry (NCT):** Air-puff tonometry; helps to calculate IOP by using rapid air to flatten the cornea

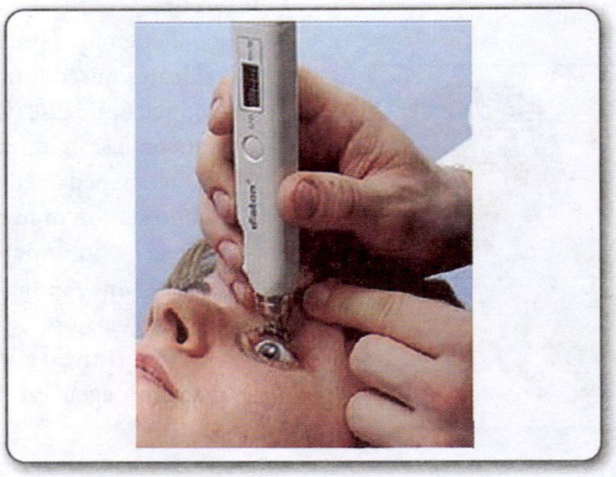

Figure 48: Ocular tonometry

KEY POINTS

- The retina is the only site in the body where arteries can be seen without invasive techniques.
- Frequent visual examination is suggested for a patient on **Ethambutol** due to the risk of ocular toxicity (decreased red-green color discrimination).

Gonioscopy

- It is performed by using slit lamp and special contact lens prism.
- It visualizes the angle between cornea and iris for the proper drainage of aqueous humor.

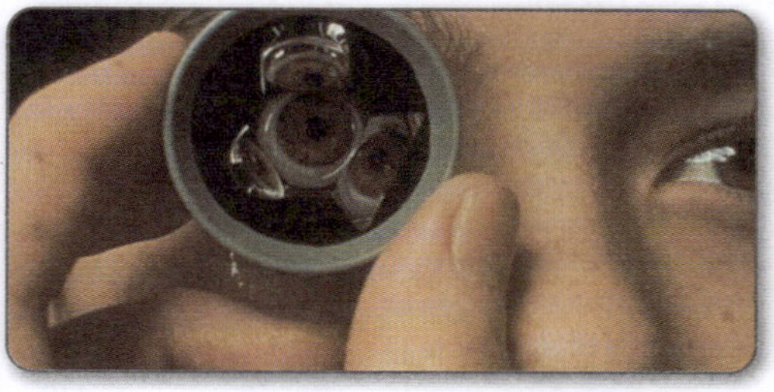

Figure 49: Gonioscopy

Amsler Grid

- Used to screen macular degeneration.

Corneal Staining

- It is done to detect corneal abrasions or lesions.
- A piece of blotting paper containing fluorescein (orange) dye is touched to surface of eye and then the patient is instructed to blink which spreads the dye.
- Cornea is looked for any abrasion (appear in green color) by shining a blue light.

Fluorescein Angiography

- It is done to visualize retinal vasculature by taking a series of photographs after administering fluorescein dye into a vein.
- Patient is assessed for any allergy and mydriatic eye drops are administered 1 hour before the test.
- Dye may cause yellowish discoloration of skin, urine and patient may experience nausea, vomiting, weakness of tongue and pain at injection site.
- Reaction to dye is rare but is usually manifested as hives on skin.
- Encourage fluid intake after the procedure for elimination of dye.

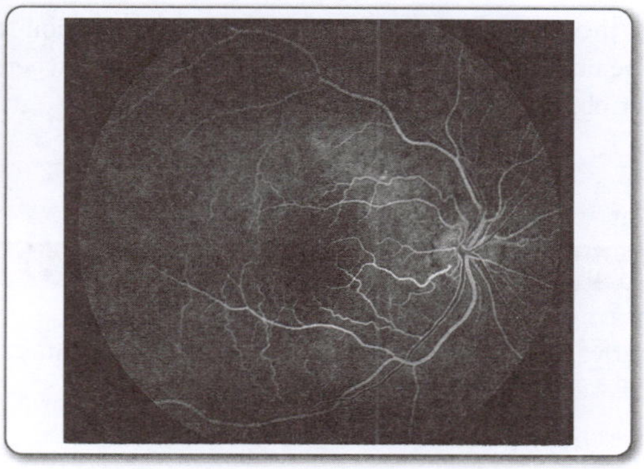

Figure 50: Fluorescein angiography

DISORDERS OF EYE

Refractive Errors

Refraction is the bending of light rays by cornea and lens, so that the image is formed on the retina (emmetropia).

Myopia (Near Sightedness)

- In this condition, convexity of the lens increases, which increases the refractive power of lens and hence the image falls in front of retina.
- These patients can see the near objects clearly, but distant vision is impaired.

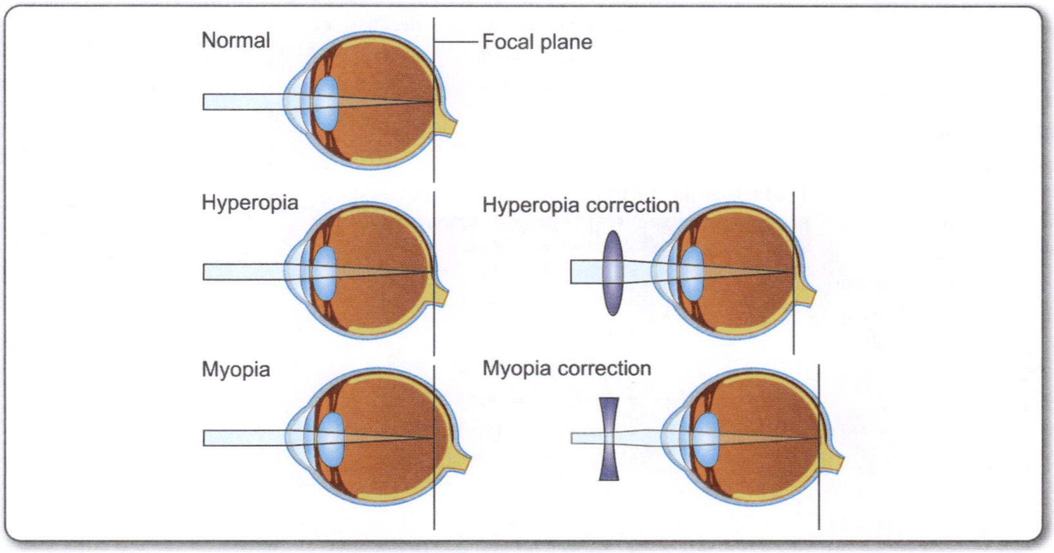

Figure 51: Refractive errors

Hyperopia (Far Sightedness)

- In this condition, convexity of the lens decreases, which decreases the refractive power of lens and hence the image falls behind the retina.
- These patients can see the far objects clearly, but near vision is impaired.

Presbyopia

- This condition is age related, there is loss of lens elasticity and the image falls behind the retina.
- These patients can see the far objects clearly, but near vision is impaired.

Astigmatism

- It occurs because of irregular curvature of cornea.
- Acuity of distance and near vision can be decreased.

Assessment and Diagnostic Tests for Refractive Errors

Refractive errors are assessed by Snellen chart for myopia and by near vision test card at a distance of 14 inches or 35 cm for hyperopia.

KEY POINTS

- **Presbyopia** is a form of hyperopia, or farsightedness that occurs as a normal process of aging, usually around 40.
- **Presbycusis** is the most common type of sensorineural hearing loss caused by natural aging of the auditory system.

Table 33: Medical management

Condition	Management
Myopia	• Concave eye glasses or contact lenses. • Negative number (e.g., –2 diopter) of glasses or contact lenses in order to decrease the refractive power of lens.
Hyperopia	• Convex eye glasses or contact lenses. • Positive number (e.g., +2 diopter) of glasses or contact lenses in order to supplement the refractive power of lens.
Astigmatism	• Eyeglasses with cylindrical correction.
Presbyopia	• Biconvex lens used for correction

Surgical Interventions

Indications: Age >18 years, stable number.
Contraindications: Autoimmune disorders, keratoconus, herpes simplex infection

a. **LASIK (Laser in situ keratomileusis)**
   - A very thin flap is created and lifted in central part of cornea with laser.
   - Underlying cornea is reshaped according to the refractive error.

b. **PRK (Photorefractive keratomy)**
   - Corneal surface is reshaped with the help of laser.

Glaucoma

- It is a group of ocular conditions characterized by optic nerve damage due to raised IOP (more than 21 mm Hg).
- Normal IOP (10 to 21 mm Hg) is maintained by aqueous humor in anterior segment of eye.
- There is a 45 degree angle present between cornea and iris where trabecular meshwork is present and hence drainage of aqueous humor takes place from anterior chamber → Trabecular meshwork → canal of schlemm → Episcleral veins.
- Over-production or inhibition of drainage of aqueous humor leads to raised IOP which can damage optic disk.
- **Glaucoma has two types:** Open angle glaucoma and Close angle glaucoma.
   - **Open angle glaucoma:**
     - Open angle glaucoma occurs due to occlusion of flow of aqueous humor because of clogging of trabecular meshwork.
     - It is the **most common type**, also called **silent glaucoma (80%).**
     - Common symptoms: Tunnel vision and painless
   - **Close angle glaucoma:**
     - Close angle glaucoma is an ocular emergency and occurs due to occlusion of flow of aqueous humor because of narrowing of angle between cornea and iris.
     - Also caused by dilation of lens or pupil due to drug overdose.
     - Most serious type of glaucoma

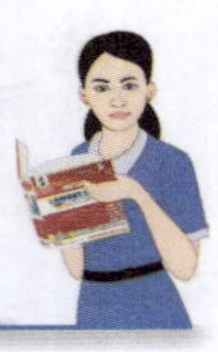

Table 34: Clinical manifestations of glaucoma

Condition	Clinical manifestations
Open angle glaucoma	• Blurred vision • Loss of peripheral visual field • Headache • Halos around light
Close angle glaucoma	• Periocular pain • Hyperemia (Red eye) • Nausea/Vomiting • Bradycardia • Profuse sweating • Pupils fixed and semi dilated • Pupils non-reactive to light • Loss of accommodation

KEY POINTS

Lens for Refractive errors:

- Myopia - Concave eye glasses
- Hyperopia - Convex eye glasses
- Astigmatism - Eyeglasses with cylindrical correction

Table 35: Diagnostic tests

Diagnostic test	Purpose	Findings of Glaucoma
Perimetry	To assess visual field	Peripheral visual field loss or localized areas of visual loss (scotomas)
Ophthalmoscopy	To assess optic disc	Pallor and cupping of optic disc
Tonometry	To assess IOP	Raised IOP
Gonioscopy	To assess angle between cornea and iris	

Medical Management

- Mitotic (e.g., Pilocarpine) works by increasing the drainage of intraocular fluid.
- B-blocker like timolol can be used.
- Carbonic anhydrase inhibitors (e.g., acetazolamide) work by decreasing the production of intraocular fluid.
- Instruct the patients not to take anticholinergics.

Surgical Management

- **Laser trabeculoplasty:** It opens the intra-trabecular spaces and widen the canal of schelmn and hence increases the outflow of aqueous humor.
- **Trabeculectomy:** Part of trabecular meshwork of canal of schlemm is removed to reduce IOP. Opening is made through sclera.
- **Peripheral iridectomy:** Removal of peripheral tissue from iris to reduce pressure
- **Laser Iridotomy:** An opening is made in the iris.
- **Drainage implants or shunts:** Open tubes are implanted between anterior chamber to conjuctival space.

Cataract

- Cataract is a condition of lens opacity and cloudiness. Cloudiness of lens is due to changes in crystalline protein.
- It is usually manifested as three types-
  - Nuclear (Opacity at center of lens)
  - Cortical (Opacity at periphery of lens)
  - Posterior subcapsular (front of posterior capsule).
- Slit lamp examination is used to establish the degree of cataract.

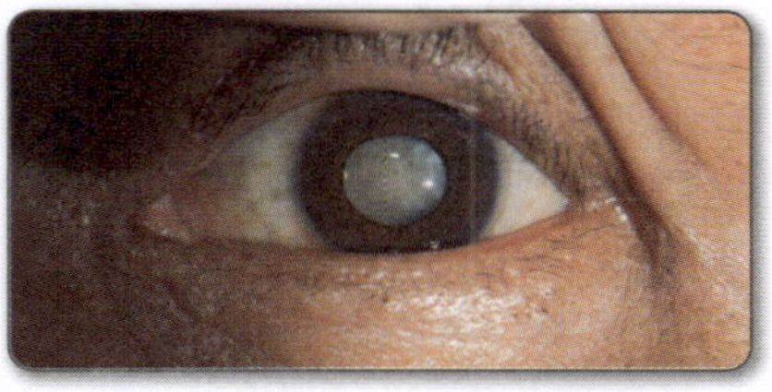

Figure 52: Cataract of eye

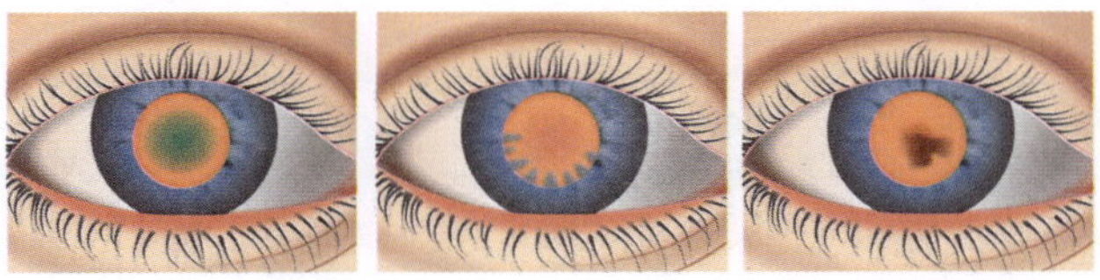

Figure 53: Types of cataracts

Table 36: Risk factors and clinical manifestation of cataract

Risk factors	Clinical manifestation
• Aging (senile cataract, most common risk factor) • Hereditary (congenital cataract) • Myopia • Retinal detachment • Long-term use of corticosteroids • Ultraviolet radiations • Diabetes Mellitus	• Blurred vision and Decreased color perception (Earliest sign) • Opacity is a late sign for cataract • Reduced visual acuity • Sensitivity to glare • Diplopia in affected eye • Absence of red reflex during ophthalmoscopy

Practice Question

18. Pilocarpine reduces the elevated intraocular pressure in glaucoma by
a. Inhibiting the production of aqueous humor
b. Decreasing the outflow of the aqueous humor
c. Increasing the outflow of the aqueous humor
d. Relaxing the ciliary muscles

Ans. (c) Increasing the outflow of the aqueous humor

KEY POINTS

- Normal intraocular pressure is 12–21 mm Hg.
- Painless peripheral loss of vision in an elderly diabetic patient is associated with **Open-angle glaucoma**.
- Most common cause of blindness in India is Cataract (62%) followed by refractive errors (20%).

KEY POINTS

- The patient should be instructed not to bend over knees at least for the first week after cataract surgery.
- Major signs of retinal detachment are **photopsia (light flash), floater sand and hairnet.**

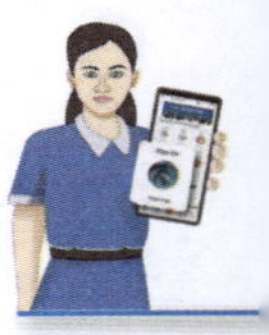

Surgical Management

- Lens replacement is the surgery of choice. Lens is made of polymethyl methacrylate, acrylic or silicone.
- **Intracapsular cataract extraction (ICCE):** The entire lens (nucleus, cortex and capsule) is removed.
- **Extra-capsular cataract extraction (ECCE):** In this surgery nucleus, cortex and portion of anterior capsule is removed. Posterior capsule and zonular fibers are kept intact.
- **Phacoemulsification:** This method liquefies and suctions the nucleus and cortex of lens with the help of ultrasonic device.
- **Lens replacement:** Insertion of Intraocular lens (IOL) is done during cataract surgery. After ICCE, surgeon usually puts anterior chamber IOL (in front of iris).

Nursing Management

- To avoid retro-bulbar hemorrhage anticoagulant therapy should be stopped before surgery.
- Prescribed mydriatics should be administered before surgery.
- Elevate the bed 30–45°
- Take measures to prevent constipation

Instructions for patients after surgery:

- Wear eye shield/glasses.
- Wash hands before touching the operated eye and clean eye from inner to outer canthus.
- Do not lie down on affected eye.
- Do not do any activity which can increase IOP (lifting, pushing, pulling, bending, stooping,vigorous coughing or sneezing, rubbing eye, tight closing of eye, valsalva maneuver, constipation).
- Follow the prescribed topical medications regimen- Antibiotics, Corticosteroids, NSAIDs.

Retinal Detachment

Retinal detachment is a condition of separation of Retinal pigment epithelium(RPE) from sensory epithelium. It has 4 types:

- **Rhegmatogenous detachment:** A tear develops in sensory retina and vitreous fluid seeps through tear and separates it from RPE.
- **Traction detachment:** Pulling force is responsible for detachment.
- **Rhegmatogenous and traction detachment:** Combination of first two types.
- **Exudative detachment:** Conditions like uveitis cause the production of fluid which can cause detachment.

Table 37: Diagnostic tests

Signs and symptoms	Diagnostic test
• Sensation of shade or curtain • Cobwebs • Flashing lights • Floaters • Usually painless	• Indirect ophthalmoscopy • Slit lamp examination • Fluorescein angiography • Eye ultrasound • Optical coherence tomography

Surgical Management

- **Scleral buckle:** Sclera is compressed with the help of scleral buckle to hold sclera, choroid and retina.
- **Pneumatic Retinopexy:** A gas bubble or silicon oil is injected into vitreous cavity which pushes the retina against RPE.
- **Cryo-surgery/Laser therapy/Diathermy:** These procedures help to initiate inflammatory response and scar formation to seal the retinal tears.

Immediate Nursing Management

- Cover both eyes to minimize stress, further detachment and damage.
- Prevent the patient from any jerky movements of head.

Postoperative Nursing Management

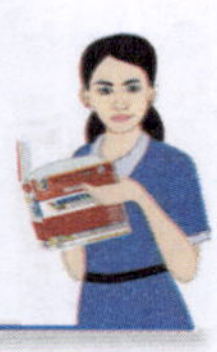

- Provide bed rest, dark glasses (for day time) eye patches (for night time) and assist with daily activities.
- Monitor for bleeding, sudden eye pain and notify to physician.
- After pneumatic retinopexy, provide prone position to allow the gas bubble act as a tamponade for the retina.
- Reading, watching television or computer is limited for 3 to 5 weeks.
- Restrict patient from any activity, which can increase IOP (lifting, pushing, pulling, bending, stooping, vigorous coughing or sneezing, rubbing eye, tight closing of eye, valsalva maneuver, constipation).

Age Related Macular Degeneration (AMD)

- It is a condition of deterioration of macula and has two types-
  1. **Dry AMD:** It occurs due to clogging of arteries/capillaries supplying to macula (ischemia) and it becomes thin.
  2. **Wet AMD:** Blood vessels grow under retina (Choroidal neovascularization-CNV) and leak at macula.

KEY POINT

Macular degeneration is the most common cause of irreversible central vision loss.

Table 38: Age related macular degeneration

Signs and symptoms	Risk factors	Diagnostic test
• Central vision loss (central scotomas) • Difficulty in adapting to low light. • Difficulty in recognizing faces. • Decreased ability to recognize colors. • Straight lines look wavy (earliest sign). • Missing letters in words	• Age • Family history and genetics • Smoking • Obesity • Cardio-vascular disease. • Hypertension	• Amsler grid- wavy lines • Ophthalmoscopy- Drusen • Optical coherence tomography

Management

a. **Photodynamic therapy**
   - A photo-sensitive dye (verteporfin) is infused IV which is retained by abnormal blood vessels under retina and then diode laser (for 83 seconds) is used. This dye takes up/activates by the energy from laser and abnormal vessels get closed.
   - Instruct the patient to bring dark sunglasses, hat, full sleeved shirt, gloves, socks and avoid exposure to sunlight, bright light for 5 days which can cause blisters and sun burn.

b. **Macular translocation:** Retinal detachment of 360 degrees is surgically created and retina is gently lifted and replaced by moving macula away from CNV.

Orbital and Ocular Trauma

Table 39: Orbital and ocular trauma

Type of injury	Signs and symptoms	Management
Soft tissue Injury	• Ecchymosis • Lid swelling • Tenderness • Black eye • Pain • Photophobia	• Cold compress in early phase followed by warm compress. • Complete eye examination.
Foreign bodies	• Redness • Irritation • Discomfort • Blurred vision	• Use a cotton applicator dipped in NS to remove foreign body if it is superficial and blunt. • Slit lamp or indirect ophthalmoscope may be needed to visualize the foreign body. • Surgical assistance may be required.
Penetrating object	• Visible penetrating object into the eye	• Do not try to remove the object. • Limit patient's movement. • Cover the affected eye with a paper or plastic cup. • Notify the physician immediately • Prepare the patient for radiological examination-X-rays/CT scan (MRI may be contraindicated due to metallic nature of penetrating object). • If cornea is perforated, Inj TT and antibiotics should be given.
Hyphema (Hemorrhage within anterior chamber)	• Blurred vision • Signs and symptoms of raised IOP.	• Hospitalization and activity limitation may be required. • Provide eye shield and instruct the patient to avoid sudden eye movements.
Chemical burns (Acid/ Alkali/ Active organic substance)	• Spotty or complete damage of cornea • Subconjunctival hemorrhage	• Check pH of eye and assess for the type of chemical splashed. • Immediately flush the eye (irrigation from inner to outer canthus) with water/NS/RL for 20 minutes. • Check pH of eye after irrigation (should be between 6 and 7). • If pH is not attained, irrigation should be continued.

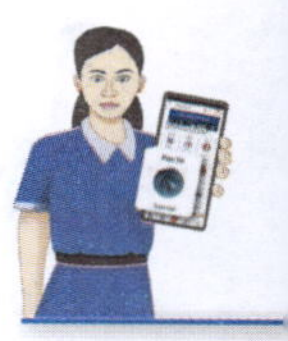

Infectious and Inflammatory Conditions

Conjunctivitis

Table 40: Various causes of conjunctivitis

Causes	Signs and symptoms	Management
Bacterial- Streptococcus pneumonia, Hemophilus influenza, staphylococcus aureus	• Redness of eye • Burning • Discharge (exudate)	• Topical Antibiotics
Chlamydial conjunctivitis (Trachoma)	• Purulent exudate • Ocular pain • Periauricular lymphadenopathy • Trichiasis (Inward turning of hair follicles) • Entropian • Corneal erosion and ulceration.	• Broad spectrum antibiotics. • Surgical correction of trichiasis • Assessment and treatment of genital chlamydial infection.
Viral-Adenovirus, Herpes simplex	• Watery discharge • Extreme tearing • Discomfort • Lid edema • Photophobia	• Cold compress for 10 minutes (5 times in a day) • Frequent hand hygiene. • Do not share towels, eye drops. • May use artificial tears (lubricants). • Do not visit public places till redness or discharge is cleared. • Every time use new tissue to wipe the eyes. • Do not apply makeup till symptoms subside. • Wear dark glasses.
Allergic	• Rhinitis • Itching • Excessive tearing	• Lubricants • Corticosteroids

Enucleation, Evisceration, Exenteration

- **Enucleation:** It is a surgical procedure of removal of entire eye and part of optic nerve.
- **Evisceration:** Removal of ocular contents but sclera,optic nerve, extra-ocular muscles are kept intact.
- **Exenteration:** Entire orbital contents and soft tissue are removed.

Indications

- Severe injury

Intraocular tumors (Ocular melanoma, Retinoblastoma, etc.)

A disfigured, deformed eye.

Ocular Prostheses

- After enucleation, a conformer (shell) is placed to prevent contracture of eye socket.
- After 4 to 8 weeks of surgery, patients are referred to ocularist for prosthetic fitting.

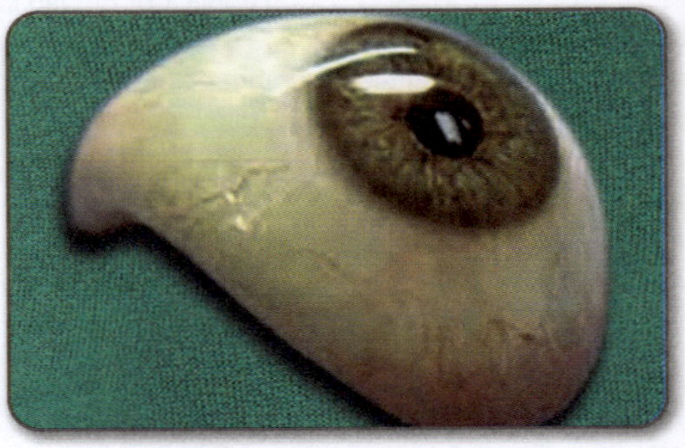

Figure 54: Ocular prosthesis

KEY POINT

Most common type of bacterial conjunctivitis is Acute Mucopurulent conjunctivitis. Most common cause is *S. aureus*

Table 41: Insertion and removal of prosthesis

Steps of insertion of prosthesis	Steps of removal of prosthesis
• Clean eyes with NS dipped gauze. • Moisten the prosthesis with NS. • Hold prosthesis b/w thumb and fore-finger with indentation uppermost and convex surface outermost. • Lift upper eyelid with other hand. • Insert upper part of prosthesis in upward, backward and inward direction. • Remove hand from upper eyelid and pull lower eyelid. • Slip lower part of prosthesis inside lower eyelid. • Eyelids closure should be comfortable after insertion.	• Clean eyes with NS dipped gauze. • Pull down the lower eyelid to see the edges of prosthesis. • Gently push the eyelid under prosthesis and exert fingertip pressure on upper eyelid. • Prosthesis slips out into cupped hand. • Place it in NS.

Administration of Eye Medications

- Wash hands, read label and shake the suspension
- Do not touch the tip of medication dropper in the eye.
- By putting gentle pressure on cheek bone, pull lower lid down with the help of a finger.
- Instill eye drops (if prescribed) before administration of ointment.
- Apply ointment (as half inch ribbon) in lower conjunctival sac.
- Ask the patient to keep eyelids closed and gently put pressure on inner canthus for 1 min.
- Use clean tissues to remove excess medicine or tears.

Golden Points to Remember

- **Function of the iris** is to regulate the size of pupil and allow light to pass only through the center of the lens, which is optically most effective part.
- **Ptosis** is dropping of eyelids.
- **Amblyopia** is reduced vision in the affected eye.
- **LASIK** (Laser assisted in situ keratomileusis) is the treatment for myopia, hyperopia and astigmatism.
- **Hordeolum (stye)** is an infection of the sebaceous glands in the lid margin.
- **Keratoconjunctivitis** is the inflammation of cornea and conjunctiva.
- **Keratoconjunctivitis sicca** is otherwise known as dry eye.
- **Enucleation** is the removal of eye. Indications are blind patient and painful eye.
- Emmetropia is a condition in which the eye is relaxed and focused on an object more than 6 meters or 20 feet away.
- **Arcus senilis** is a sign of high cholesterol, manifested by presence of a white or gray opaque ring in corneal margin.
- **Macropsia** is an illusion in which objects appear larger than their actual size.
- **Fleischer rings** are pigmented rings in the peripheral cornea, due to iron deposition.
- **Proptosis** is a bulging of the eye anteriorly out of the orbit.
- Complication—**Marginal corneal ulcer**
- **Ethambutol** causes impairment of Red and Green color vision.
- Most common cause of Acute Hemorrhagic Conjunctivitis—**Enterovirus (70%).**
- Most common cause of cataract is Senility (age related).

"A few germs never hurt anyone."
—unknown

MULTIPLE CHOICE QUESTIONS
(Including Explained and Practice Questions)

OPHTHALMOLOGY

ANATOMY OF EYE (DIAGRAM)

996. Thinnest part of lens is?
a. Anterior pole b. Apex
c. Posterior capsule d. Posterior pole

997. Which part of the eye acts as a hole space that allows light to enters in:
a. Lens b. Retina
c. Choroid d. Pupil

998. Shape of Eye lens gets varies according to the light it received for a proper focusing of image is enhanced by:
a. Cornea b. Choroid
c. Pupil d. Ciliary muscles

999. The fluid substance present on the anterior part of the eye:
a. Aqueous Humor b. Vitreous humor
c. Perilymph d. Endolymph

1000. The fluid that is critical to maintain the eye shape and attach the retina to its place:
a. Aqueous Humor b. Vitreous humor
c. Perilymph d. Endolymph

1001. Which of the following structure contains cells which are referred as photoreceptor that respond to light:
a. Choroid b. Retina
c. Iris d. Macula

1002. The small tiny central area present on the retina which are responsible for fine working and reading is known as:
a. Ovoid b. Macula
c. Lens d. Sclera

1003. These are photoreceptor cells which are responsible for color and bright vision:
a. Cilia b. Rods
c. Cones d. Retinal cells

1004. One of the photoreceptor cells that dim and low light condition:
a. Cilia b. Rods
c. Cones d. Retinal cells

EXTRAOCULAR STRUCTURES

1005. A thin, transparent mucous membrane that covers the inner surface of the eyelids and the anterior surface of the eye is the:
a. Sclera b. Conjunctiva
c. Choroid d. Glabella

1006. Cranial nerve responsible for sensation of smell is:
a. Facial nerve b. Hypoglossal nerve
c. Olfactory nerve d. Trigeminal nerve

1007. The smallest cranial nerve is:
a. Olfactory b. Oculomotor
c. Trochlear d. Accessary

1008. Number of extrinsic muscles involved in movement of the eyeball is:
a. 4 b. 6
c. 7 d. 9

1009. Hypoglossal nerve is:
a. 6th nerve b. 7th nerve
c. 12th nerve d. 9th nerve

1010. Eye ball movements are controlled by all of the following cranial nerves; EXCEPT:
a. Optic nerve b. Abducens nerve
c. Trochlear nerve d. Oculomotor nerve

1011. Ophthalmic artery is a branch of: *New Q*
a. Vertebral artery
b. Basilar artery
c. Internal carotid artery
d. External carotid artery

Explanation: The ophthalmic artery is a branch of the internal carotid artery. It arises from the ophthalmic segment of the internal carotid artery within the cranial cavity.

OCULAR STRUCTURES

1012. Color blindness is due to the problem with:
(Daman and Diu NO 2018)
a. Lens b. Aqueous humor
c. Cones d. Rods

Explanation: Cones are photoreceptor cells in the retina that respond differently to light of different wavelengths and are thus responsible for color vision and function best in relatively bright light, as opposed to rod cells, which work better in dim light. So color blindness is due to problems with cones.

1013. The anterior transparent part of the eye is:
(DSSSB PHN, 2015)
a. Pupil b. Conjunctiva
c. Cornea d. Sclera

1014. Muscles of the eye are supplied by all of the following cranial nerves; EXCEPT?
a. Abducent nerve b. Hypoglossal nerve
c. Oculomotor nerve d. Trochlear nerve

1015. Which of the following artery supplies the eye?
a. Internal carotid artery
b. External carotid
c. Facial artery
d. Right and left subclavian artery

Ans.

996.	d
997.	d
998.	d
999.	a
1000.	b
1001.	b
1002.	b
1003.	c
1004.	b
1005.	b
1006.	c
1007.	c
1008.	b
1009.	c
1010.	a
1011.	c
1012.	c
1013.	c
1014.	b
1015.	a

1016. Which cranial nerve is responsible for movement of eye ball?
a. Oculomotor b. Vagus
c. Trigeminal d. Olfactory

1017. The fluid found in posterior segment of eye is known as:
a. Aqueous fluid b. ICF
c. ECF d. Vitreous body

1018. The firm, opaque and white outer connective tissue layers of the posterior five-sixths of the eye is the:
a. Sclera b. Cornea
c. Vascular tunic d. Choroid

1019. The anterior segment of eye is filled with:
a. Aqueous fluid b. ECF
c. Ocular fluid d. Vitreous body

1020. All among the following are different types of color blindness; except: *New Q*
a. Protanomaly b. Astigmatism
c. Monochromacy d. Deuteranomaly

Explanation: Astigmatism is not a type of color blindness; it is a refractive error of the eye. Astigmatism occurs when the cornea or lens of the eye has an irregular shape, causing blurred or distorted vision at all distances.

- Protanomaly: Protanomaly is a type of red-green color blindness
- Monochromacy: Monochromacy, also known as achromatopsia, is a severe form of color blindness where individuals have difficulty perceiving any color at all.

Individuals with deuteranomaly have difficulty differentiating between red and green shades. Less severe than protanomaly.

1021. The blind spot of eye is known as:
a. Cons b. Rods
c. Pupil d. Optic Disc

1022. Rod cells and con cells are associated with .... sensation:
a. Smell b. Vision
c. Hearing d. Touching

1023. To focus on objects closer than 20 feet:
a. The lens must become flatter
b. The ciliary muscles must contract
c. The suspensory ligaments must increase tension on the lens
d. The cornea must move inward

1024. Rod cells are:
a. More sensitive to light than cone cells
b. Able to produce sharper images than cone cells
c. Sensitive to red, blue and green colors
d. Found in greatest quantity in the fovea centralis

1025. The light-sensitive and pigmented layer of tissue in the eye is known as: *(Karnataka PSC 2001)*
a. Lens b. Retina
c. Cornea d. Iris

Explanation: The retina is a light-sensitive layer at the back of the eye that covers about 65% of its interior surface. Photosensitive cells called rods and cones in the retina convert incident light energy into signals that are carried to the brain by the optic nerve.

1026. Which of the following structure alters the size of the pupil?
a. Ciliary muscle b. Iris
c. Cornea d. Lens

Explanation: The iris is a thin, circular structure in the eye, responsible for controlling the diameter and size of the pupil and thus controls the amount of light reaching the back of eye.

1027. The size of which part of the eye contributes to the controlling the amount of light entering the eye. *(ESIC 2019)*
a. Pupil b. Lens
c. Optic disc d. Macula lutea

Explanation: The size of pupil of the eye contributes to the controlling the amount of light entering the eye, pupil contracts in response to bright light and it relaxes in dim light.

1028. Which of the following structures control the amount of light rays entering the eye? *(RRB 2002)*
a. Pupil b. Iris
c. Lens d. Both a and b

Explanation: The iris and the pupil control how much light to let into the back of the eye. When it is very dark, our pupils are very large, letting in more light. The pupil size is controlled by the dilator and sphincter muscles of the iris.

1029. The process of automatic adjustment of retinal sensitivity when a person moves from light to dark is known as:
a. Dark adaptation b. Light adaptation
c. Dark accommodation d. Light accommodation

Explanation: Adaptation is an automatic adjustment of retinal sensitivity to the amount of light present when a person moves from dark to light or lit to dark. Dark adaptation occurs when going from a well-lit area to a dark area, rods become active. Light adaptation occurs when we move from dark to light, cones become active.

1030. Enophthalmos is due to palsy of:
a. Levator palpebrae superioris
b. Superior tarsal muscle
c. Orbitalis muscle
d. Inferior tarsal muscle

1031. Ptosis results from trauma to which nerve?
a. III b. VI
c. VII d. VIII

1032. Vitamin important for the normal functioning of eye is:
a. Vitamin A b. Vitamin D
c. Vitamin E d. Vitamin K

1033. Hypervitaminosis of .... cause sign and symptoms such as headache, vomiting, vertigo, diplopia and skin desquamation:
a. Vitamin A b. Vitamin D
c. Vitamin E d. Vitamin K

1034. Xanthelasma refers to:
a. Dryness of conjunctiva
b. Dry mouth
c. Yellowish plaques that occur most commonly near the inner canthus of the eyelid
d. Fatty growths develop underneath the skin

1035. Aphakia is:
a. Absence of ciliary body
b. Absence of the lens
c. Absence of conjunctiva
d. Absence of pinna

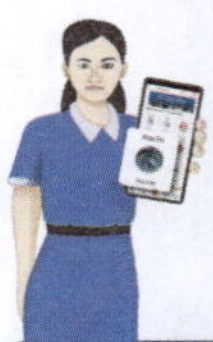

Ans.
1016. a
1017. d
1018. a
1019. a
1020. b
1021. d
1022. b
1023. b
1024. a
1025. b
1026. b
1027. a
1028. d
1029. a
1030. c
1031. a
1032. a
1033. a
1034. c
1035. b

1036. Keratitis is the inflammation of:

a. Retina b. Cornea
c. Conjunctiva d. Keratin

1037. In posterior cavity hemorrhage of the eye, blood accumulates between:

a. The lens and conjunctiva
b. The lens and the retina
c. Between the cornea and the lens
d. Lens and optic disc

1038. Copper deposition in cornea leads to:

a. Keratoglobus
b. Siderosis
c. Kayser-Fleischer ring (KF ring)
d. Keratoconus

1039. Golden period of eye donation:

a. 6 hours
b. 12 hours
c. 18 hours
d. 24 hours

ASSESSMENT AND DIAGNOSITIC TESTS IN OPHTHALMOLOGY

1040. Tonometry is the method of measuring: *(ISRO)*

a. Blood pressure in children
b. Blood pressure in elderly
c. Foot pressure
d. Intraocular pressure

1041. Which of the following test is used to assess distance (long-sightedness) vision? *(DSSSB 2013)*

a. Rinne's test b. Hirschbergs test
c. Optometry d. Snellen chart

Explanation: A Snellen chart is an eye chart that can be used to measure visual acuity. Snellen charts are named after the Dutch ophthalmologist Herman Snellen who developed the chart.

1042. First assessment needs to be done in a client with ophthalmic problem is:

a. Visual acuity
b. Intraocular pressure
c. Intraocular hemorrhage
d. Opacity of lens

1043. Fluorescein angiography (FA) of eye allows study of the circulation of the:

a. Choroid b. Retina
c. Both a & b d. Iris

REFRACTIVE ERRORS

1044. Myopia is a condition in which:

a. The image is focused behind the retina
b. The cornea or lens is not uniformly curved
c. There is a decrease in the ability of the eye to accommodate for near vision
d. Correction is possible with a concave lens

1045. The most common cause of myopia is:

a. The viscosity of aqueous humor is increased
b. The thickness of lens is increased
c. The viscosity of vitreous humor is increased
d. Antero-posterior diameter is increased

1046. The refractive error caused by the differences in the curvature of the cornea and lens is called: *(AIIMS Raipur Grade II 2017)*

a. Emmetropia b. Astigmatism
c. Myopia d. Hypermetropia

Explanation: Astigmatism is a type of refractive error in which the eye does not focus light evenly on the retina which results in distorted or blurred vision. Emmetropia is a state in which the eye is relaxed and focused on an object more than 6 meters or 20 feet away. Near-sightedness or myopia is a condition of the eye where light focuses in front of instead of on the retina. Hypermetropia is a defect of vision that causes the impossibility for rays of light to be focused on the retina, but behind it.

1047. Presbyopia occurs because of:

a. Lens becomes elongated
b. The lens becomes inflexible
c. Lens becomes opaque
d. Retinal curvature will vary

1048. Treatment of presbyopia:

a. Radial Keratotomy b. LASIK
c. Convex lens d. Both b and c

Explanation:

- Both presbyopic LASIK and convex lens are used for correction of presbyopia.
- Apart from this multifocal IOL implant, multifocal contact lens and surgically implanted corneal inlays can be used to correct presbyopia.

1049. Myopia is corrected by: *(AIIMS Nagpur NO 2018)*

a. Bifocal lens b. Biconvex lens
c. Cylindrical lens d. Biconcave lens

Explanation:

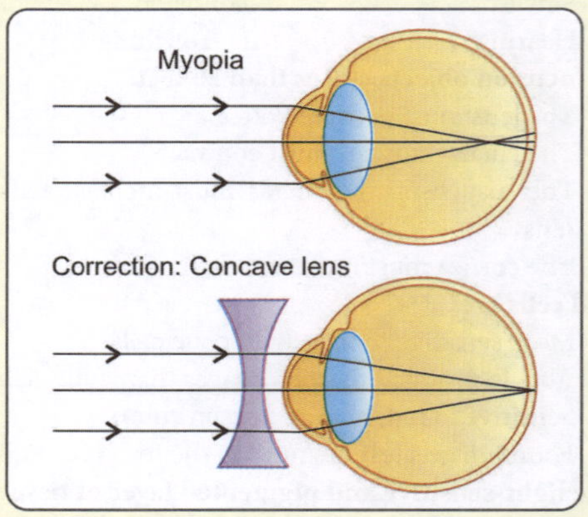

Figure: Myopia and its correction

1050. Trachoma is a disease related to: *(NCFL 2019)*

a. Eyes b. Ears
c. Nose d. Throat

Explanation: **Trachoma** is contagious disease caused by Chlamydia trachomatis and affects the conjunctiva of the eye, cornea and eyelids. It occurs due to poor hygiene primarily. It is preventable as well as curable.

Ans.

1036. b
1037. b
1038. c
1039. a
1040. d
1041. d
1042. a
1043. c
1044. d
1045. d
1046. b
1047. b
1048. d
1049. d
1050. a

1051. Drug of choice for mass treatment of trachoma is:
a. Sulfonamide
b. Chloramphenicol
c. Tetracycline
d. Penicillin

1052. The inability to read small words held at usual distance is a primary feature of: *(DSSSB PHN, 2015; ISRO)*
a. Myopia b. Astigmatism
c. Presbyopia d. Cataract

1053. Which of the following is true regarding macular degeneration? *(AIIMS-BBS SNO 2019)*
a. It is the central loss of vision
b. Wet macular degeneration is more common in this
c. Dry macular degeneration is less common in this
d. It affects the cornea of the eye

Explanation: Macular degeneration is the most common cause of irreversible central vision loss. It is of two types: (1) dry and (2) wet type. Dry type is the more common type and it is a slowly progressive and painless vision loss. Wet macular degeneration is rapid in onset.
Strategy: Eliminate Options b and c as both are essentially same statement. If wet macular degeneration is more, then dry has to be less. So both are similar statements. So use the strategy, "if two options are similar then both cannot be the answer".

1054. Risk for retinal detachment is more among patients with:
a. Refractive error like myopia
b. Diabetic retinopathy
c. Previous cataract surgery
d. All of the above

GLAUCOMA

1055. Which statement about glaucoma is true and accurate? *(Safdarjung NO 2018)*
a. Acute angle-closure glaucoma is an ocular emergency
b. Bubbles are implanted to protect the retina from the glaucoma
c. Acute angle-closure glaucoma results in loss of peripheral vision and tunnel vision
d. Primary open-angle glaucoma leads to eye pain, nausea and vomiting, blurry vision and halos

Explanation:
- Acute angle-closure glaucoma is an ocular emergency, characterized by opposition of iris to the trabecular meshwork, which results in raised intra ocular pressure. It causes sudden dramatic onset of symptoms as blurred vision, red eye, pain, headache, nausea and vomiting, sudden elevations in the IOP that may lead to optic nerve damage.
- Compressive gonioscopy is done to push down the cornea and then easing upon it.

1056. Normal range of IOP is:
a. 8-10 mm Hg b. 10-12 mm Hg
c. 12-22 mm Hg d. 15-15 mm Hg

1057. Which of the following condition is associated with increased intraocular pressure? *(DSSSB 2013)*
a. Cataract b. Conjunctivitis
c. Retinitis d. Glaucoma

Explanation: Intraocular pressure (IOP) is the fluid pressure inside the eye. Elevated intraocular pressure is an important risk factor for glaucoma. Normal Intraocular Pressure (IOP) ranges from 10 mm Hg to 21 mm Hg. Tonometry is the method eye care professionals use to determine this. The two main types of glaucoma are open-angle and angle-closure glaucoma.

1058. An aged client with diabetes mellitus complaining of a painless peripheral loss of vision is at risk for: *(AIIMS-BBS SNO 2019)*
a. Cataract b. Uveitis
c. Angle-closure glaucoma d. Open-angle glaucoma

Explanation:
- **Open angle glaucoma** means that the angle where the iris meets the cornea is as wide and open as it should be. Loss of peripheral or side vision is usually the first sign of glaucoma.
- **Angle-closure glaucoma** presents with eye pain with nausea and sudden visual disturbance.

1059. The first-line treatment of open angle glaucoma is:
a. Pilocarpine b. Carbonic anhydrase inhibitor
c. Timolol d. Epinephrine

1060. Drug of choice for acute congestive glaucoma is:
a. Atropine b. Timolol
c. Levobunonol d. 1–2% pilocarpine

1061. Management of angle closure glaucoma is: *New Q*
a. Laser iridotomy b. Phacoemulsification
c. Scleral bulking d. Corrective lense.

Explanation: Laser iridotomy is a procedure that creates a small opening in the iris, which allows the aqueous humor to flow out of the eye and prevent the pressure from rising. It is one of the common treatment for angle closure glaucoma.

Phacoemulsification is a surgery that removes the cloudy lens in the eye and replaces it with a plastic lens. It is used to treat cataracts.

Scleral bulking is a procedure that involves injecting a material under the sclera. It is used to treat corneal ectopia.

Corrective lens is a lens that is used to correct vision problems due to refractive errors.

1062. Clinical manifestation of glaucoma includes:
a. Blurred and loss of vision
b. Headache
c. Halos around lights
d. All of the above

1063. Earliest sign of glaucoma is:
a. Double vision b. Halos around lights
c. Blurred vision d. Headache

1064. Commonest type of glaucoma is:
a. Primary open angle glaucoma
b. Secondary open angle glaucoma
c. Primary angle closure glaucoma
d. Secondary angle closure glaucoma

1065. Glaucoma management focuses upon:
a. Increase inflow of aqueous humor
b. Increase outflow of aqueous humor
c. Increase production of aqueous humor
d. Increase the production and inflow of aqueous humor

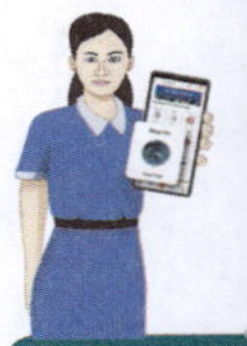

Ans.
1051. c
1052. c
1053. a
1054. d
1055. a
1056. c
1057. d
1058. d
1059. c
1060. d
1061. a
1062. d
1063. b
1064. a
1065. b

1066. Characteristic findings in a client with acute angle-closure glaucoma includes:
a. Severe pain
b. Decreased vision with halos around lights
c. Erythematous conjunctiva
d. All of the above

1067. Narrow angle glaucoma management medications include:
a. Miotics b. Topical beta blockers
c. Oral carbonic anhydrase inhibitors
d. All of the above

1068. Action of miotics in narrow angle glaucoma is:
a. Constriction of pupils
b. Increase the production of aqueous humor
c. Increase the inflow of aqueous humor
d. Decrease the outflow of aqueous humor

1069. Medications used during open angle glaucoma include all; Except: *New Q*
a. Prostaglandin analogues
b. Cycloplegic agent
c. Beta blockers
d. Carbonic anhydrase inhibitors

Explanation: Drugs that reduce IOP in open angle glaucoma are:
- **Prostaglandin analogues:** Increase aqueous outflow
- **Beta blockers:** Decrease aqueous production
- **Carbonic anhydrase inhibitors:** Decrease aqueous production.
- **Parasympathomimetic:** Increase aqueous outflow.
- **Sympathomimetic:** Increase aqueous outflow.

However, Cycloplegics cause significant IOP elevation in 2% of the normal population and up to 23% of patients with primary open angle glaucoma.

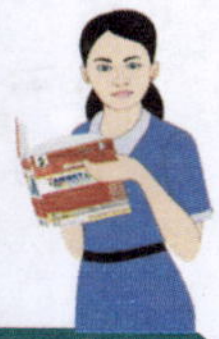

1070. Management of glaucoma includes all; EXCEPT:
a. Laser trabeculoplasty b. Trabeculectomy
c. Iridectomy d. Scleral buckling

1071. All of the following are the causes of increased Intra Ocular Pressure (IOP); EXCEPT:
a. Poor drainage of aqueous humor
b. Decreased reabsorption of aqueous humor
c. Use of beta-blockers
d. Increased production of aqueous humor

CATARACT

1072. Diabetic cataract occurs due to accumulation of:
a. Fructose b. Galactitol
c. Glucose d. Sorbitol

1073. Typical appearance of diabetic cataract is:
a. Sunflower type
b. Polychromatic lustuer
c. Breadcrumb type
d. Snow flake appearance

1074. Most common cause of blindness in India is: *(NCFL 2019)*
a. Cataract b. Glaucoma
c. Refractive index d. Vitamin A deficiency

Explanation: As per the National Programme for control of Blindness in India, the leading causes of blindness in India include cataract (62%), refractive errors (20%), glaucoma (6%), surgical complications/corneal opacities(1%) and others (10%).

1075. A cataract is: *(JIPMER 2012)*
a. Crystallization of the pupil
b. Opacity of lens
c. Thin film over the cornea
d. Opacity of conjunctiva

1076. After cataract surgery, the nurse should notify the physician if the client is complaining of:
a. Headache b. Eye pain
c. Lacrimation d. Edema

1077. Discharge teaching given to client following cataract surgery is:
a. Wear sunglass to protect eyes from sun light
b. Avoid vigorous brushing of teeth and hair
c. Both a and b d. None of these

1078. Following cataract surgery how long sunglass need to be used?
a. 4 weeks after operation b. 6 weeks after operation
c. 8 weeks after operation d. 10 weeks after operation

1079. Causes of cataract include:
a. Exposure to ultraviolet light
b. People who work in bright sunlight
c. Welders without eye protection
d. All of the above

1080. Management of cataract include all; EXCEPT:
a. Intra capsular cataract extraction
b. Extra capsular cataract extraction
c. Phacoemulsification d. Scleral buckling

1081. Correct option regarding intracapsular cataract extraction is:
a. Removing the lens including the lens capsule
b. Removing the lens and the anterior portion of the lens
c. Enucleation of eyes
d. Removing the lens of the eye

1082. Correct option regarding extracapsular cataract extraction is:
a. Removing the lens including the lens capsule
b. Removing the lens and leaving the elastic capsule partially intact
c. Enucleation of eyes
d. Removing the lens of the eye

1083. Complications related to cataract extraction include:
a. Secondary glaucoma b. Infection
c. Bleeding d. All of these

RETINAL DETACHMENT

1084. Important intervention to a client with retinal detachment is:
a. Admitting him to the hospital and strict bed rest
b. Patching both of his eyes
c. Use sunglass
d. Use topical antibiotic and analgesics

1085. Priority nursing management after the surgery for retinal detachment is:
a. Prevent increase in IOP b. Decrease pain
c. Promote rest d. Maintain nutritional status

1086. Main symptom associated with retinal detachment is:
a. Flashing lights and floaters
b. Pain and tenderness
c. Increased IOP
d. Ptosis

Ans.
1066. d
1067. d
1068. a
1069. b
1070. d
1071. c
1072. d
1073. d
1074. a
1075. b
1076. b
1077. c
1078. b
1079. d
1080. d
1081. a
1082. b
1083. d
1084. a
1085. a
1086. a

1087. Surgical management related to retinal detachment is all; EXCEPT:
a. Cryopexy
b. Scleral buckling
c. Intraocular injection of air or SF6
d. Phacoemulsification

AGE RELATED MACULAR DEGENERATION (AMD)

1088. Which of the following assessment finding can be seen in macular degeneration?
a. Halos around the vision
b. Decline in the central vision
c. Night blindness
d. Increased IOP

1089. Which among the following is the management for macular degeneration?
a. Scleral buckling b. Laser therapy
c. Cryosurgery d. Extracapsular extraction

1090. Which among the following age group is at highest risk for macular degeneration?
a. Age over 20 years b. Age over 35 years
c. Age over 55 years d. Age over 60 years

1091. Which among the following is a major risk factor for macular degeneration?
a. Smoking b. Hypotension
c. Diabetes mellitus d. Migraine

1092. Macular degeneration is:
a. Increased in IOP
b. Irregular curvature of cornea
c. Loss of lens elasticity
d. Deterioration of macula

ORBITAL AND OCULAR TRAUMA

1093. Pinpoint pupil is a characteristic of: *(AIIMS BBS NO 2018)*
a. Barbiturate poisoning b. Pontine hemorrhage
c. Glaucoma d. Cocaine abuse

Explanation: Pinpoint pupil (or miosis) is contraction of pupil under normal lighting conditions. Barbiturate poisoning and cocaine abuse leads to dilation of pupil. Glaucoma alone does not affect pupil size. Pontine hemorrhage causes pinpoint pupil which was due to a disorder of the sympathetic pupillary pathways in the pontine tegmentum.
Strategy: Use the elimination rules to find the correct answer.

1094. Which of the following statement by the client indicates orbital fracture?
a. Vertical movements of the eye
b. Epistaxis
c. Tinnitus
d. Halos around the vision

1095. Which type of orbital fracture is dangerous and may lead to potential complication to the brain?
a. Zygomatic fracture b. Orbital roof fracture
c. Maxillary fracture d. Midfacial Fracture

1096. Which of the following diagnostic test is contraindicated in intraocular foreign body exposure?
a. CT b. X-ray
c. MRI d. Both a and b

Explanation: MRI is contraindicated because most foreign bodies are metallic and magnetic.

1097. A client had a metallic object stuck in his eye during a car accident which of the following intervention should not be done in this situation?
a. Try to remove the metallic object
b. Apply pressure in the injured area
c. Both a and b
d. The eye must be protected

1098. The irrigation of eye should be done for a client affected by chemical ocular burn until the pH of conjunctiva within a range between:
a. 7.3 and 7.6 b. 5.0–5.6
c. 4.5–5.0 d. 6.2–7.0

CONJUNCTIVITIS

1099. Most common form of conjunctivitis in newborn at birth is caused by:
a. Chlamydia b. Neisseria
c. Streptococci d. Staphylococci

Explanation:
Ophthalmia Neonatorum
- Ophthalmia neonatorum is a purulent conjunctivitis occurring during the first four weeks of life.
- Also called neonatal conjunctivitis
  - Chlamydial ophthalmia (caused by **Chlamydia trachomatis**) is the most common bacterial cause; it accounts for up to 40% of conjunctivitis in neonates <4 weeks of age.
  - Hyperacute cases are usually caused by Neisseria gonorrhoeae or N. meningitidis.

1100. Which of the following refers to dryness of conjunctiva?
a. Xerophthalmia b. Xanthelasma
c. Xanthoma d. Xerostomia

Explanation:
- Xerophthalmia-Dryness of Conjunctiva
- Xanthelasma-Yellowish plaques that occur most commonly near inner canthus of the eye lid
- Xanthoma-Fatty growths develop underneath the skin
- Xerostomia-Dryness of mouth

1101. Which of the following is NOT a symptom of conjunctivitis?
a. Itching b. Partial vision loss
c. Redness d. Tearing of eyes

1102. Which among the following is a highly contagious eye condition?
a. Conjunctivitis b. Open angle glaucoma
c. Astigmatis d. Cataract

1103. Which among the following is a treatment of choice for allergic conjunctivitis?
a. Cholinergic agonists b. Anti histamines
c. Antibiotic eye drop d. Corticosteroids

1104. Treatment of choice for bacterial conjunctivitis is:
a. Cycloplegics b. Anticholinergics
c. Antibiotic eye drops d. Antiseptic ointments

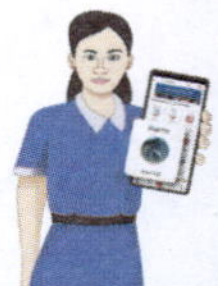

Ans.
1087. d
1088. b
1089. b
1090. d
1091. a
1092. d
1093. b
1094. a
1095. b
1096. c
1097. c
1098. a
1099. a
1100. a
1101. b
1102. a
1103. b
1104. c

INTEGUMENTARY SYSTEM AND BURNS

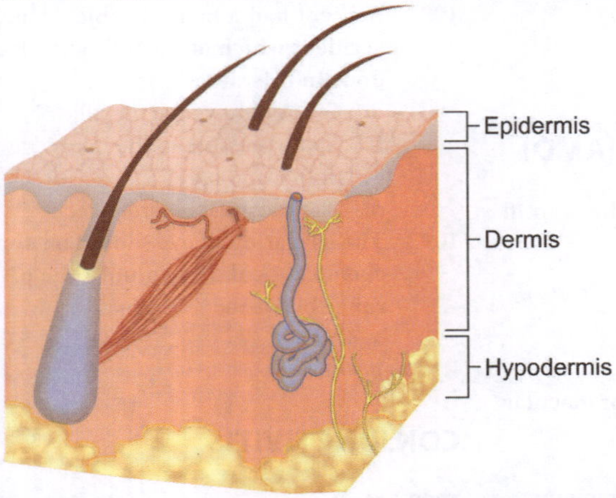

Figure 55: Skin

INTEGUMENTARY SYSTEM

Anatomy and Physiology

- Largest organ of the body
- Surface area: 15–20 sq. ft
- Weight = 4 kg or 9 pounds (approx)
- It is composed of epidermis, dermis and subcutaneous tissue

Epidermis

- Outermost layer of the skin
- Composed predominantly of keratocytes.
- Four layers of epidermis from outer to inner are:

Table 42: Layers of epidermis with their thickness and description

Layer	Thickness	Description
Stratum corneum	25–30 rows	Dead keratinocytes (corneocytes), can replaced by germinative layers (complete 40 days).
Stratum lucidum	3–5 rows	**Present only in thick skin of soles and palms**
Stratum granulosum	3–5 rows	Contains precursor of keratin (keratohyalin granules)
Stratum germinativum	Single row	Deepest layer, single row with cuboidal or columnar keratinocytes contains melanocytes, similar to stem cell

- **Epidermis** is thickest over palms of hands and soles of feet
- The junction between epidermis and dermis is known as **rete ridges**.
- The interlocking rete ridges produce ripples on the surface of skin (finger prints).

Table 43: Different types of cells in the epidermis and their functions

Cell Type	Function
Keratinocytes	Responsible for producing the protein keratin
Melanocytes	Produce a pigment called melanin, which is responsible for the color of the skin, hair, and eyes.
Merkel cells	Responsible for detecting and transmitting the sense of touch to the nervous system.
Langerhans cells	Specialized immune cells found in the epidermis.

Dermis

- It is the largest part of the skin and is often called true skin.
- It is made up of two layers:
  - Papillary dermis (dermis beneath the epidermis)
  - Reticular dermis

KEY POINTS

- **Melanocyte** in epidermis produces the pigment melanin.
- **Melanin** is the substance responsible for color of the skin and hair
- An area of hard thickened skin on foot or between the toes is called "Corn"
- ***Staphylococcus epidermidis*** is normal skin commensal (normal flora)
- Arrector pili is the muscle responsible for "Goose bumps"
- Langerhans cells are responsible for cell mediated immunity in dermis of the skin
- Skin accounts for 7% of total body weight
- **Thinnest skin**- eyelids or glans penis (0.5 mm)
- **Thickest** – palms of hands and heels of feet

KEY POINTS

- **Vitiligo /Leukoderma** – Partial or complete **loss of melanocyte** from skin
- **Albinism – inability to produce melanin pigment** due to lack of tyrosinase enzyme

- Dermis has its own blood supply, nerve, lymph, sweat, sebaceous and hair root.
- Contains collagen and elastic fibers.
- These layers have blood supply, nerve ending (Meissner's corpuscle sensitive to touch), receptors like proprioceptors (balance and position) and nociceptors (pain receptors).

Subcutaneous Tissue/Hypodermis

- It is also known as hypodermis and is made up of fat.
- It produces cushion between skin layers, muscles and bones.

Epidermal Appendages

- These are the down growth of epidermis into the dermis - **glands, nails and hair**

Glands

Glands consist of mainly sweat glands, sebaceous glands and ceruminous glands.

Sweat glands or sudoriferous glands – (3–4 million)

Two types – Apocrine and eccrine glands

- **Eccrine gland**
  - These are sweat producing glands found all over the body except at lips, nail bed, ears, penis and labia minora.
  - Highest density of eccrine glands is found on palms and soles of the body.
  - Eccrine glands exit the body independently on hair shaft
  - Eccrine glands help in regulation of body temperature, whereas apocrine glands can't.
  - Sweat contains urea, fatty substances and sodium chloride.
- **Apocrine glands**
  - Seen in axillae, breast, anal region, ear canal and labia majora.
  - Apocrine gland becomes active on puberty.
  - Activity of apocrine gland needs high output of sex hormones
- **Sebaceous Gland**
  - Found abundantly in face, scalp, upper back and chest
  - Sebaceous glands are absent over palms and soles.
  - Secretion of sebaceous gland is known as sebum.
  - Lipids of sebum prevent heat loss from body
  - **Ceruminous glands** – These are a modified sweat glands in external ear, produce wax.

Nail

- Hard transparent plate of keratin covers the dorsal surface of fingers on hands and feet.
- Nail roots are covered by a thin layer of skin called **cuticle**.
- Average growth of nail is **0.1 mm per day** and it grows throughout the life.
- Finger nail grows faster than toe nail, complete renewal of finger nail takes 170 days where as toe nail takes 12–18 months.
- The crescent-shaped whitish area at proximal of nail is called lunula.

Hair

- Hair are distributed all over the body except palms and soles.
- Hair follicles usually occur along with sebaceous gland and together they contribute to **pilosebaceous unit**.
- **Arrector pili** are the muscles attached to hair follicles and are responsible for goosebumps.
- **Hair color is determined by melanin** present in the hair shaft.
- Male pattern baldness in male is due to Testosterone hormone.
- Replacement of melanin by air bubble = white hair
- Normal hair loss per day = 70–100 hairs
- Hair grow 1cm per month

Functions of Skin

- Protection
- Homeostasis
- Thermoregulation
- Sensory function
- Vitamin D production

Recent Question (CNCI 2021)

30. Inflammation of tissues surrounding the nail is known as?

a. Clubbing
b. Koilonychia
c. Paronychia
d. Onycholysis

Ans. (c) Paronychia

KEY POINTS

- A thicker layer containing collagen and elastic fibers to support the epidermis is known as "Dermis".
- **Onycholysis** – loosening of nail from nail bed
- **Paronychia** – infection of tissue surrounding the nail
- **Koilonychia** (spooning of fingernails, concave shaped, seen in iron deficiency anemia

Diagnostic Evaluation

Table 44: Diagnostic tests

Name of the test	Description
Skin biopsy	• Skin biopsy is obtained through scalpel excision or through punch biopsy. • Biopsy is performed over skin nodule, plaque, blisters and other skin lesions
Immunofluorescence	• This test combines antigen or antibody with fluorochrome dye • Antibody can be conjugated to fluorochrome by attracting them to the dye • Direct immunofluorescence tests on the skin are techniques to detect autoantibodies directed against portion of the skin • Indirect immunofluorescence test detects specific antibodies in patient's serum

Contd...

Name of the test	Description
Patch testing	• This test is to determine substance to which the patient has allergy • In this, selected allergens are applied over the skin as patches • Patient wears the patches for 48 hours and skin is assessed after 72 hours. • Redness, fine elevation and itching over the skin is considered as mild reaction • Fine blisters, papules and severe itching is considered as moderate reaction • Blisters, pain and ulceration indicates severe reaction.
Skin scrapings	• Suspected fungal lesions are scraped with oil moistened scalpel blade and then transferred to a glass slide covered with cover clip and examined microscopically for fungal growth
Tzanck smear	• This smear test is to examine the blistering skin condition such as herpes, varicella and all forms of pemphigus. • The secretions from the suspected lesion are applied over a slide, stained and then examined.
Wood's light examination	• It's a special lamp which produces long wave ultraviolet rays which become blue to dark purple in color • These lights can be well seen in darkened room • These lights help to differentiate hyperpigmented skin lesions from normal skin. • The lesion that contains melanin will disappear under light and lesion without melanin can be well seen in the light • Reassure the client that light is not harmful for eyes and skin

Disorders of Skin

Table 45: Primary and secondary skin lesions

Lesion	Description
Macule	Skin color changes without elevation, e.g., vitilgo
Papule	Elevated solid lesion of skin less than 1 cm
Plaque	Raised lesion formed by merging papules.
Nodule	Larger than papule. Raised skin lesion extends into dermis. A large nodule is called as tumor.
Wheal	Elevations on the skin that are irregularly shaped
Vesicle	Elevated lesion usually containing fluid and is less than 1 cm
Bulla	Elevated fluid filled lesion usually more than 1 cm
Cyst	Elevated thick walled lesion containing fluid or semi-solid matter
Pustule	Elevated lesions less than 1 cm containing purulent material
Scale	Dried fragments of epidermal layers, irregular in shape white, tan, yellow or silver in color
Erosion	Moist, demarcated depressed area due to partial or full thickness loss of epidermis
Deep ulcer	Irregularly shaped exudate, depressed lesion in which all epidermis and all or part of dermis is lost
Scar	Mark left on the skin after healing
Excoriation	Superficial linear abrasion of epidermis is visible sign of itching caused by rubbing or scratching
Fissure	Deep linear split through epidermis and extends into dermis
Keloid	Irregularly shaped elevated progressively enlarging scar extends beyond the boundaries of wound.

Pruritus

- In common man's term it is known as itching.
- Most common symptom in patient with dermatological problem.
- Antipruritic agents are useful to manage the condition.

Seborrheic Dermatoses

- **Seborrhea:** Excessive production of sebum
- **Seborrheic dermatitis:** Inflammatory disease of the skin in which bacterial counts are more in the area with large amount of sebaceous gland secretion.
- It can be of two forms, oily and dry:
  1. Oily form appears moist and greasy and appear over forehead, nasolabial fold, beard area, scalp, etc.
  2. Dry form appears like flaky desquamation of the scalp with profuse amount of white, fine, powdery scales.

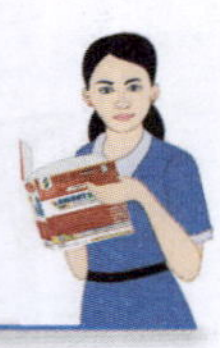

Acne Vulgaris

- It is a condition affecting susceptible hair follicles.
- Most commonly seen over face, neck and upper trunk.
- This condition is characterized by comedones, both opened and closed, papules, pustules, nodules and cyst.
- During puberty, under the influence of androgen sebaceous gland produces more amount of sebum and this sebum will plug the pilosebaceous gland and cause acne.
- Comedones are the major clinical manifestations for this condition.
- Salicylic acid and benzyl peroxide preparations are effective against acne.
- Vitamin A preparations are also useful for removing keratin plug. Patient should be cautioned that these preparations are sensitive to sunlight, so avoid exposure to sun.

Impetigo

- Superficial infection of the skin
- Caused by Staphylococci, Streptococci or other bacteria
- Bullous impetigo is caused by *Staphylococcus* aureus.
  - Characterized by bullae.
- Exposed areas of the body are most commonly affected (face, neck and extremities)
- It is contagious and can spread via sharing towels, touching skin of the patients, etc.
- Impetigo is a risk factor for **glomerulonephritis**.
- **Treatment**
  - **For small lesions:** Topical antimicrobial agents (e.g., Mupirocin, Retapamulin)
  - **Wide spread lesions:** Systemic antibiotics (e.g., Augmentin, Cloxacillin)

Herpes Zoster (Shingles)

- It is a viral infection of skin caused by Varicella-zoster virus Type 3 (same virus that causes chickenpox)
- Type I causes cold sores and fever blister on lips
- Type II caused genital herpes
- Incubation period 7–21 days
- Infect on nerve root ganglion of sensory nerve of peripheral nervous system.
- **Major manifestation:** Painful vesicular eruption along the area of distribution of the sensory nerves.
- **Treatment:** Antiviral agents (e.g., Acyclovir, Valacyclovir), isolate the patient, assess for CN VIIth for Bell's palsy complication.

KEY POINTS

- Tzanck test is used for microscopic assessment of fluids and cells from vesicles and bullae.
- Tzanck test or Tzanck smear is scraping of an ulcer base to screen for Tzanck cells.
- Tzanck cells are found in herpes simplex, varicella and herpes zoster.

Table 46: Summarized content of herpes zoster

Phases of manifestations	Duration	Manifestations
Preeruptive phase	1 to 10 days	Pain, pruritis and paresthesia
Eruptive phase	10 to 15 days	Unilateral patchy erythematous areas, vesicles develops
Postherpetic neuralgia	Variable (30 days to 60 days)	Residual and itching

Pediculosis

Table 47: Summarized description of pediculosis

Condition	Description
Pediculosis capitis	• Infestation of scalp with louse. • Head lice are seen behind the back and ears. Bite of the insect causes intense itching.
Pediculosis corporis	• Infestation of the body by the louse. • Body lice are seen in the area of skin that comes in close contact with the underclothings (neck, trunk and thighs). • It bites and causes characteristic minute hemorrhagic points.
Pediculosis pubis	• Infestation is in the genital area and is transmitted chiefly by sexual contact. • Pruritus especially at night is the characteristic. • Reddish-brown dust can be seen in patient's underclothing.

Treatment

- Washing the affected area with shampoo which contains pyrethrin and piperonyl butoxide.
- All co-habitants should take the medicine on same day and avoid sharing combs, brushes and hats.

Scabies

- Infestation of skin with an itch mite called *Sarcoptes scabiei*.
- Seen among people who live in unhygienic condition and people who all are sexually active
- Infestation is commonly seen in fingers and therefore hand contact may cause spread of infection.
- Intense itching is the complaint by the client
- Spread of infection is mostly seen among institutional population like school and hostel
- Incubation period – one month
- Magnifying glass and pen light examination show small raised burrows created by itch mites.
- Classic sign of scabies is increased itching during overnight because of the hyperactivity of the mite due to increased body temperature.
- Skin scrapings from the area of itching are placed on a slide and examined under microscope.
- 5% permethrin is the medicine of choice.
- Other scabicides – benzyl benzoate, lindane etc. 6% precipitated sulfur in petrolatum should be used for pregnant women and for infant less than two months of age.
- Instruct the client to take a warm soapy shower to remove scaling and debris then pat dry the skin and allow it cool and then apply the scabicide.
- Patient is instructed to apply scabicide all over the body except over face and scalp and let it be there for 24–48 hours. Usually one application may be effective but it is advisable to repeat it after 1 week.
- Patient is instructed to clean all clothing and to dryclean them.

Psoriasis

- Psoriasis is a chronic, non-infectious skin inflammation that involves keratin synthesis.
  - Silvery scales are found over elbow, knee, scalp, buttock and lower back
  - Psoriasis vulgaris being most common.
  - Koebner phenomenon is development of psoriasis lesions at the site of injury, like sunburn area
- **Management**
  - Gentle removal of the scales is the main management
  - Taking bath with added oils (olive oil, mineral oil) and use of soft brush.
  - Application of alpha hydroxyl acid and salicylic acid after bathing helps to soften the thick scales.
  - Topical corticosteroid along with occlusive dressing.
  - **Phototherapy** for clients who are not responding to topical therapy. Psoralen and ultraviolet A (PUVA) is effective treatment.
  - **Methotrexate and cyclosporine** are useful systemic corticosteroids/cytotoxic preparations but side effects associated with each therapy are more.

Pemphigus Vulgaris

- It is an autoimmune disease
- IgG antibodies are directed against specific cell surface antigen on epidermis
- **Manifestation**
  - Characterized by varying sizes of bullae on the skin and mucous membrane.
  - Oral lesions are of irregular shape which, bleed easily and heal slowly and are painful.
  - Specimen from blisters and surrounding skin shows acantholysis (separation of epidermal cells from each other).
- **Management**
  - Corticosteroid and immunosuppressive agents

Stevens Johnson Syndrome (SJS) and Toxic Epidermal Necrolysis (TEN)

- Both are potentially fatal skin conditions
- Characterized by widespread erythema and macule formation with blistering resulting in epidermal detachment.
- TEN is more severe than SJS.
- **Cause**: Adverse reaction to drug in use
- In Children, SJS is usually triggered by viral infections, e.g., Mumps, flu, Coxsackie virus, Herpes-simplex virus, Epstein-Barr virus.
- **Management**
  - Immediate management is discontinuation of drug
  - Treatment has to be provided similar to that of burn [discussed later in this chapter].

Practice Question

19. Which of the following body parts are commonly affected by psoriasis

a. Elbows
b. Scalp
c. Chest
d. Back and abdomen

Ans. (a) Elbows

Recent Question (CNCI 2021)

31. As a staff nurse you are caring a patient with Psoriasis. Salicylic acid is prescribed to the patient. Which finding indicates that presence of systemic toxicity from this medication?

a. Respiration decreased
b. Tinnitus
c. Constipation
d. Diarrhea

Ans. (b) Tinnitus

Skin Tumors

Benign Tumors of Skin

Table 48: Benign tumors of skin

Condition	Description
Cyst	• Epithelium lined cavities that contain fluid or solid material. • Epidermal cyst most frequently occur over face, neck, upper chest and back.
Seborrheic and actinic keratosis	• Benign warts like lesion of varied size and color vary from light to dark. • Excision is the treatment of choice
Warts	• These are caused by **infection with HPV virus** (DNA virus). • **Treatment:** Laser, liquid nitrogen, salicylic and electro-dessication.
Angiomas	• Benign vascular tumors involving skin and subcutaneous tissue. • They present at birth as patches or raised bright red, nodular lesions.
Pigmented nevi-mole	• Moles are of varying size and shape ranging from yellowish brown to black. • It can be flat or elevated and occasionally containing hair.
Keloids	• Fibrous tissue that grow over the site of scar or trauma. • They are harmless but cause cosmetic concern
Dermato-fibroma	• Benign tumor of connective tissue occurs predominately on extremities. • Excisional biopsy is the treatment of choice

Malignant Skin Tumors

- Exposure to the sun is a **leading cause for skin cancer**.

Basal Cell Carcinoma (BCC)

- Most common type of skin cancer
- It appears over the area of sun exposure
- Frequently appear over the areas of face.
- Metastasis is rare but recurrence is common.
- **Management:** Excision of the tumor

Squamous Cell Carcinoma (SCC)

- Malignant proliferation arising from epidermis
- It can occur in sun damaged area, in a normal skin or a skin with previous lesion
- SCC can metastasis by blood and lymphatic system.
- **Management:** Excision of the tumor

Melanoma

- Neoplastic melanocytes are present in the epidermis and dermis
- It is the most lethal skin cancer
- **Diagnosis:** Biopsy results confirm the melanoma
- **Treatment:** Surgery and chemotherapy

Skin Grafts

- Skin graft is a technique in which skin is detached from its own blood supply and transferred to other (recipient) site.
- **Auto graft**: Tissue is obtained from patient's own skin
- Isograft/syngraft – identical twins
- **Homograft / Allograft**: Tissue is obtained from donor of the same species.
- **Xenograft/heterograft:** Skin tissue is obtained from other species.

Graft Application

- Recipient site must have adequate blood supply
- Recipient site must be in close contact with its bed to avoid accumulation of blood
- Graft must fix firmly so that it remains in place

Flap

In this type, one end of the tissue remains attached with its own blood supply and the other end moves to cover the wound.

Hair Loss/Alopecia

- Most common type of alopecia is male pattern of alopecia (androgenic alopecia).
- It is associated with aging, hereditary and androgen
- Hair loss starts at frontal temporal area and gradual thinning and complete loss of hair over the scalp.
- **Drug of choice:** Minoxidil and finasteride

Irritant Contact Dermatitis

- It is also known as eczema.
- It is the inflammatory reaction of the skin to physical, chemical and biological agents.
- **Primary cause** of contact dermatitis is **allergy**.
- **Manifestation:** Pruritus, burning, erythema, edema, papules, vesicles
- **Management**: Cool and wet dressing, thin layer of cream containing corticosteroids

KEY POINTS

- Substance used to smoothen or soften the skin is known as "Emolients"
- A syndrome caused by the accumulation of homogentisic acid in connective tissues is called "Ochronosis".
- Albinism is a rare group of genetic disorders that cause the skin, hair, or eyes to have little or no color.
- Albinism is a defect of melanin production.

Recent Question
(NORCET 2023)

32. In Split thickness skin grafting, what all layers of skin are present?

a. Epidermis only
b. Epidermis and entire dermis
c. Epidermis and superficial dermis
d. Tissue and cartilage

Ans. (c) Epidermis and superficial dermis

Split-thickness skin grafts (STSGs) are a type of skin graft that consists of the epidermis and a portion of the dermis. The thickness of the dermis that is included in the graft can vary, but it is typically 0.15 to 0.45 mm.

POINT TO REMEMBER

Melanoma is the most lethal skin cancer.

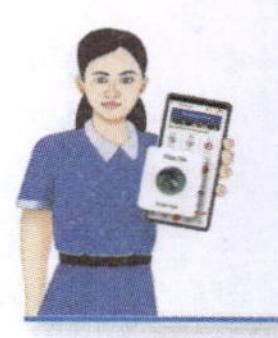

Systemic Lupus Erythematous (SLE)

- It is an autoimmune disease.
- **Discoid lupus**: Affects face
- **Drug induced lupus:** Affects kidney or brain
- **Neonatal lupus:** It passes into newborn during delivery
- SLE affects almost all systems of the body.
- **Causes:** Immunological factor, genetic factor, environmental factor
- **Characteristic feature:** Butterfly shaped erythematous, patches.
- **Other manifestation:** Alopecia, splinter hemorrhage, Raynaud's phenomenon, arthralgia/ osteoarthritis, joint swelling and tenderness.
- **Diagnosis**: Antinuclear antibody test
- **Management:** NSAIDs, corticosteroids, anti-malarial agents are the drug of choice.

KEY POINTS

- Characteristic feature of SLE is Butterfly-shaped emphysematous, patches.
- **Antinuclear antibody test** is the diagnostic test for SLE.

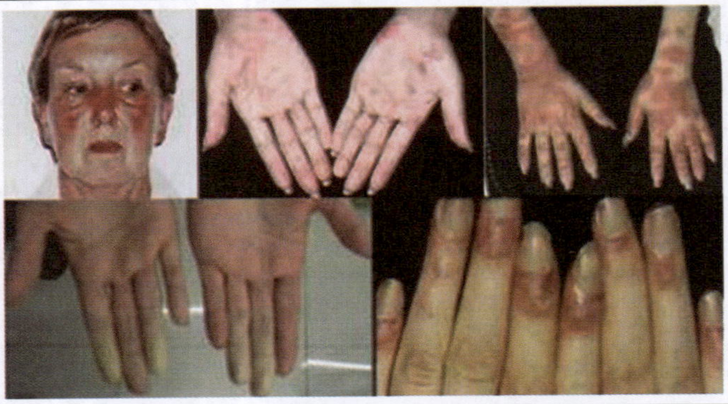

Figure 56: Systemic lupus erythematous

Cellulitis

- Suppurative inflammation of dermis and subcutaneous layer.
- Bacteria invades and releases toxin into the subcutaneous tissue
- Commonly caused by Streptococcus Pyogen.
- **Manifestation:** Local edema, redness and pain
- **Management:**
  - Local and systemic
  - Elevation of the affected area and warm moist pack application
  - Universal precaution
  - Penicillin antibiotic is commonly used

Fungal Infections

- Can occur in any part of the body
- Characterized by scaling, itching, painful lesion
- Types –
  - **Tinea pedis or athlete's foot**- between toes
  - **Tinea cruris or jock itch** – between skinfold of groin
  - **Tinea capitis** – infection on scalp
  - **Tinea unguium** – infection on nails

Frostbite

- Prolonged exposure to cold causes severe damage to tissues and cells.
- Commonly affects fingers, toes, nose and ears
- S/S- pain, numbness, paresthesia, erythema
- Management – warm the affected area with warm water for 15–20 min
- Complications – gangrene, necrosis, compartment syndrome

BURNS

It is the transfer of energy from one source to another which leads to tissue damage, destruction, protein denaturalization and ionization of content.

Classification of Burn Injury Based upon the Depth

- **First degree burns (Superficial partial-thickness burns)**
  - Mainly involves epidermis layer of the skin, e.g., sun burn
    - Pink in color
    - Painful
- **Second degree burns (Deep partial-thickness burns)**
  - Epidermis along with upper and deeper portion of the dermis e.g., Scald
    - White to pink or red in color
    - Very painful
- **Third degree burns (Full-thickness burns):**
  - Epidermis, dermis, subcutaneous tissue and even deeper tissue will be affected. It is painless because nerves are completely destroyed, e.g., burn from flame and electric burn.
    - White to charred
    - Little or no pain

Extent of Body Surface Area Burned

- **Rule of Nines:** A method used to estimate the total body surface area of burn by assigning percentages in multiples of nine to major body surfaces.

Recent Question (NORCET 2020)

33. Most painful type of burns is

a. First degree burns
b. Second degree burns
c. Third degree burns
d. Fourth degree burns

Ans. (b) Second degree burns

Recent Question (NORCET 2022)

34. A patient admitted in emergency department with burn on one upper limb and full back. According to rule of 9, calculate the burn area:

a. 18%
b. 27%
c. 9%
d. 36%

Ans. (b) 27%

One upper arm = 9%

Full back=18%.

Total=27%

Table 49: Percentage of body surface area burnt

Adult body area	%
Arm x 2 x 9%	18%
Head	9%
Groin	1%
Leg x 2	36%
Anterior trunk	18%
Posterior trunk	18%

Rule of Nines

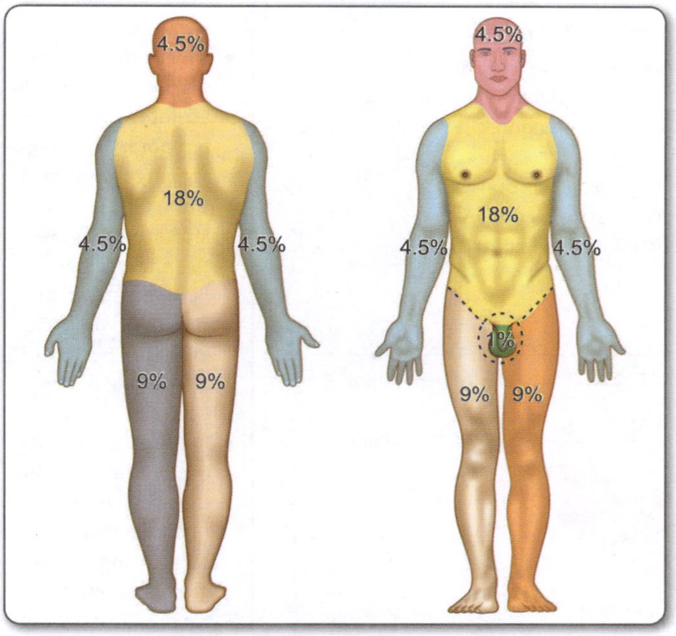

Figure 57: Rule of nines for an adult

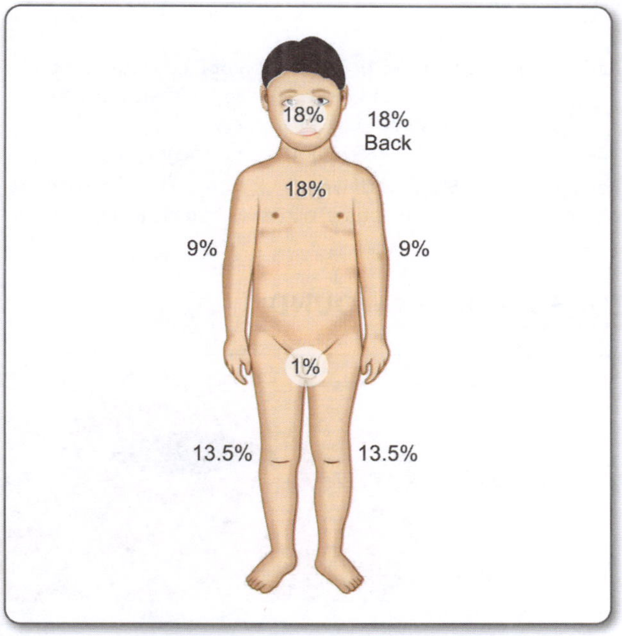

Figure 58: Rule of nines for a child

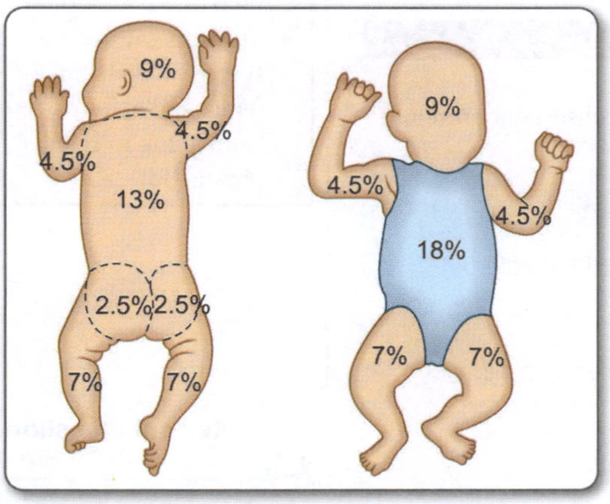

Figure 59: Rule of nines for an infant

Lund and Browder Chart

The chart, if used correctly, is the most accurate method to assess burned area. It compensates for the variation in body shape with age and therefore can give precise estimation of body surface area burned.

Palmar Method

Palmar method in a patient with scattered burn is useful. Patient's own palm is considered as 1% of the total body surface area.

Body Response to Burn Injury

- Because of hypovolemia, there is significant decrease in cardiac output and f**all in BP occurs**.
- Loss of capillary integrity leads to shift of fluid and **edema around the burn injuries**.
- In case of circumferential burn, edema causes pressure on small blood vessels and nerves which obstruct the blood flow to distal part and is known as **compartment syndrome**.
- **Escharotomy** is the surgical procedure of choice to maintain blood supply.
- Due to tissue death, serum **potassium will be elevated** and **sodium level will fall**.
- Due to hypovolemia and blood loss, **hematocrit value will be elevated**.

- Due to decreased blood flow to the kidney, **urine output will be reduced**.
- Loss of skin integrity leads to **impaired thermoregulation.**

Phases of Burn Care

Table 50: Phases of burn

Phase	Duration	Priority care
Emergent phase or resuscitative phase	Onset of injury to completion of fluid resuscitation Usually last for 36–48 hours.	• First aid • Patent airway • Prevent hypovolemia and shock. • Initial wound assessment and care • Prevent electrolyte imbalance. • Main goal is to maintain vital organ function and perfusion
Acute phase	Starts with completion of fluid resuscitation (start with diuresis) and ends with wound closure. Begins 48 -72 hours after the injury.	• Wound care and closure • Provide adequate nutrition • Prevent infection
Rehabilitation phase	Starts with wound closure to return of patient to the optimal activities of daily living	• Psychological counseling • Cosmetic surgeries • Prevention of contracture

ZONES OF BURN WOUND

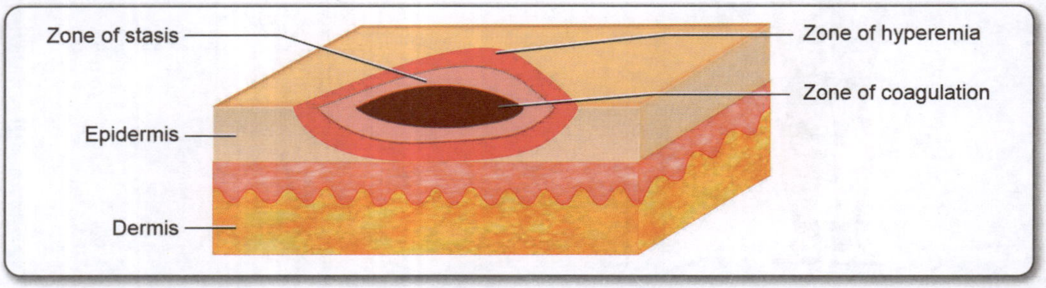

Figure 60: Zones of burn wound

Table 51: Three zones of burn wound and their description

Zone	Description
Zone of coagulation	• Area with maximum tissue damage. • Irreversible tissue damage occurs due to coagulation of the constituent proteins.
Zone of stasis	• Area surrounding the zone of coagulation. • Characterized by decreased tissue perfusion. • Tissue in this zone is potentially salvageable. • Aim of burn care is to increase tissue perfusion of this area and prevent permanent tissue damage.
Zone of hyperemia	• Outermost zone with increased tissue perfusion. • Tissue here will invariably recover unless there is severe sepsis or prolonged hypoperfusion.

Formulas for Fluid Replacement in Burn Victim

Consensus Formula

- **RL solution:** 2–4 mL × body weight in kilogram × percentage of total body surface area burned
- Half of the fluid has to be given in 8 hours and remaining half in 16 hours

Evans Formula

- **Colloids:** 1 mL × body weight in kilogram × percentage of total body surface area burned
- **Electrolyte (saline):** 1 mL × body weight in kilogram × percentage of total body surface area burned
- **Glucose (5% in water):** 2000 mL for insensible water loss

KEY POINTS

- Urine output of 0.5 mL/kg or about 30–50 mL/hr in adults and 0.5–1.0 mL/kg/hr in children less than 30 kg is a good target for adequate fluid resuscitation
- **Silver nitrate:** Produce stains, mafenide acetate–may cause temporary burning or stinging sensation.
- Urine output is the indicator to assess the effectiveness of fluid resuscitation
- Don't give IM or SC injection, because of decreased absorption.
- Hyperglycemia can occur after burn due to excessive secretion of corticosteroids, catecholamine and glycogenolysis.
- Severe burn patient may gain weight of 10–20 kg after initial fluid resuscitation.
- In emergent phase, there will be hypokalemia and hypernatremia due to cellular destruction

Recent Question (NORCET 2020)

35. Antimicrobial dressing composed of which of the following metal?

a. Copper
b. Zinc
c. Sodium
d. Silver

Ans. (d) Silver

- **Day 1:** Half of the fluid has to be given in 8 hours and remaining half in 16 hours
- **Day 2:** Half of the previous day's electrolyte and colloids and all of the insensible water loss

Brooke Army Formula

- **Colloids:** 0.5 mL × body weight in kilogram × percentage of total burned surface area
- **Electrolyte (RL):** 1.5 mL × body weight in kilogram × percentage of total body surface area burned
- **Glucose (5% water):** 2000 mL for insensible water loss
- **Day1:** Half of the fluid has to be given in 8 hours and remaining half in 16 hours
- **Day 2:** Half of the previous day's electrolyte and colloids and all of the insensible water loss

Parkland/Baxter Formula

- **Ringer lactate:** 4 mL × body weight in kilogram × percentage of total body surface area burned
- **Day 1:** Half of the fluid has to be given in 8 hours and remaining half in 16 hours
- **Day 2:** Varies, colloid is added

Complications of Burn

- Curling ulcers (acute gastric erosion due to ischemia and cell necrosis) can occur if TBSA is more than 30%
- Intestinal ileus (loss of bowl motility)
- Compartment syndrome (escharotomy and fasciotomy can be used to relieve the pressure)
- Skin contracture

Wound Debridement

- It means removal of devitalized tissue and dead tissue, removal of bacteria and other foreign bodies.

Types

- **Natural debridement:** Dead tissue gets separated from underlying viable tissue by the action of natural proteolytic enzyme.
- **Mechanical debridement:** Dead tissues are removed with the help of scissors and forceps.
- **Surgical debridement:** Surgical excision of the devitalized tissue.

Recent Question (NORCET 2022)

36. A patient with circumferential burn comes to the emergency. The patient should be assessed for which complication?

a. Absent peripheral pulse
b. Fluid status
c. Urine output
d. Engorged neck veins

Ans. (a) Absent peripheral pulse

Golden Points to Remember

- Stratum lucidum layer of the epidermis is present only in **thick skin** of soles and palms.
- The junction between epidermis and dermis is known as **rete ridge**.
- **Vitiligo/Leukoderma** refers to partial or complete **loss of melanocyte** from skin.
- **Albinism- inability to produce melanin pigment** due to lack of tyrosinase enzyme
- The most common type of albinism is oculocutaneous albinism (OCA), which affects the skin, hair, and eyes.
- Carotenemia (carotenosis) is yellow discoloration of skin most noticeable on palms and soles, no yellowing of sclera, caused by increased intake of vegetable containing carotene.
- Methods used for determining the extent of burn are **Rule of Nines** and **Lund Browder method**.
- The **Brook** and **Parkland** formulas are used for fluid calculation of burn patient.
- **Hypovolemia** is the major cause of shock in severe burn patients.
- Curling ulcers can occur if total burn surface area is more than 30%
- IM or SC injection is not recommended in burn patients because of decreased absorption.
- Hyperglycemia can occur after burn due to excessive secretion of corticosteroids, catecholamine and glycogenolysis.
- In emergent phase, there will be hypokalemia and hypernatremia due to cellular destruction.
- **Ceruminous glands** are modified sweat glands in external ear that produce wax.
- **Dapsone** is used in treatment of leprosy, pneumocystis pneumonia, and dermatitis herpetiformis.
- **Butterfly rash** is a sign of systemic lupus erythematosus.
- **EUSOL** (Edinburgh University Solution of lime Composition): Antiseptic solution contains 12.5 g boric acid +12.5 g bleaching powder in 100 mL of water; used in treating wound and burn area.
- **Erythromelalgia** is caused by an increased platelet count that results in formation of tiny clots in vessels of the extremity. It is characterized by sudden severe pain in hand and feet with reddish or bluish coloration of skin.
- **Erythromelalgia** is a classic symptom of **polycythemia vera**.
- **Hamartoma** is an excess of normal tissue in a normal situation, e.g., **birth mark on skin**.
- **Pachyderma** means thick skin caused by dysregulation of mesenchymal cells.
- Basal cell carcinoma (BCC) is the most common type of skin cancer.
- For assessment of stage of pressure ulcer, the eschar and slough must be removed before assessment.
- Dapsone or Diaminodiphenylsulfone is drug of choice for **Leprosy**.
- Herpes Zoster (Shingles) is caused by the Varicella-zoster virus Type 3 (same virus that causes chickenpox).
- Tzanck cells are found in herpes simplex, varicella and herpes zoster.
- 5% permethrin is the drug of choice to treat Scabies.
- Management of psoriasis includes gentle removal of the scales, bathing with added oils, application of alpha hydroxyl acid and salicylic acid after bathing and topical corticosteroids with occlusive dressing.

"A man with a cough cannot conceal himself."
—African proverb

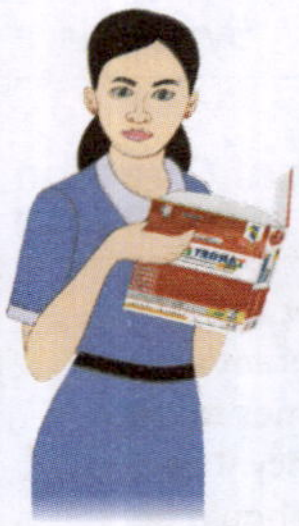

MULTIPLE CHOICE QUESTIONS (Including Explained and Practice Questions)

INTEGUMENTARY SYSTEM AND BURNS

ANATOMY AND PHYSIOLOGY OF INTEGUMENTARY SYSTEM

1105. Primary function of the skin is:
a. Vit D synthesis b. Protection
c. Sensation d. Temperature regulation

1106. Tunica adventitia is a layer of: *(Staff Nurse GII 2014)*
a. Blood vessels b. Uterus
c. Testis d. Lungs

1107. The outermost layer of the skin is known as:
a. Cutaneous b. Subcutaneous
c. Dermis d. Epidermis

1108. The layers of epidermis from outer side to inner side is:
a. Corneum – granulosum – germinative – lucidum
b. Corneum – lucidum – germinative – granulosum
c. Corneum – lucidum – granulosum – germinative
d. Lucidum – Corneum – granulosum – germinative

1109. Sweating is mediated by:
a. Norepinephrine b. Epinephrine
c. Acetylcholine d. Histamine

1110. Insensible water loss per day is:
a. 100 mL b. 300 mL
c. 700 mL d. 100 mL

1111. The Eccrine gland secrets:
a. Sebum b. Sweat
c. Melanine d. Hormones

1112. Skin color is given by the pigment known as:
a. Sebum b. Carotenes
c. Melanin d. Keratin

1113. Melanocytes secretes:
a. Sebum b. Melanin
c. Sweat d. All of the above

1114. Diaphoresis means:
a. Excessive production of sebum
b. Excessive production of sweat
c. Excessive skin shedding
d. Excessive production of tears

1115. Healthy hair receives a good blood supply from the:
a. Hair follicle
b. Hair shaft
c. Hair papillae
d. Hair bulb

1116. Which vitamin is synthesized when skin exposed to the ultraviolet rays of the sun?
a. Vitamin A b. Vitamin B
c. Vitamin C d. Vitamin D

1117. When one is having fever, the excessive heat is removed by the:
a. Constriction of skin blood vessel
b. Active production of sweat
c. Contraction of arrector pili
d. Erection of the hair shaft

1118. Sebaceous glands are NOT found in:
a. Palm of the hand b. Sole of the feet
c. Back of the hand d. Option A and B

1119. Receptors for touch is:
a. Meissner's b. Merkel's disc
c. Free nerve terminal d. All of the above

1120. Non-shivering thermogenesis in adults is due to:
a. Thyroid hormone
b. Brown fat between the shoulders
c. Noradrenaline
d. Muscle metabolism

1121. Main mechanism in thermoregulation-heat loss is:
a. Radiation b. Evaporation
c. Conduction d. Convection

1122. Vasoconstriction in skin is ______ function.
a. Sympathetic b. Parasympathetic
c. Wheal and flare d. Warm climate

1123. Functions of epithelial tissue include:
a. Absorption b. Protection
c. Secretion d. All of the above

1124. Aldosterone directly regulates the concentration of:
a. Sodium b. Potassium
c. Calcium d. Phosphate

1125. Which of these layers has shedding of cells occurring continuously due to wear and tear?
a. Stratum corneum b. Stratum lucidum
c. Stratum granulosum d. Stratum spinosum

1126. Glands present in the skin is:
a. Sebaceous gland b. Apocrine gland
c. Sweat gland d. All of the above

1127. Skin glands activated by increase in temperature is:
a. Sebaceous gland b. Apocrine glands
c. Sweat glands d. Bartholin's glands

1128. Which among the following is the characteristic of protective epithelium?
a. Regeneration of membrane
b. Melanin production
c. Thinness d. Phagocytic vesicle

1129. In human, skin accounts for approximately ______ percentage of an adult's total body weight? *(RML 1998)*
a. 7% b. 9%
c. 12% d. 14%

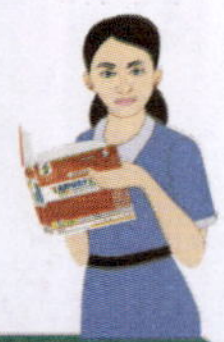

Ans.
1105. b
1106. a
1107. d
1108. c
1109. c
1110. c
1111. b
1112. c
1113. b
1114. b
1115. c
1116. d
1117. b
1118. d
1119. d
1120. a
1121. a
1122. a
1123. d
1124. a
1125. a
1126. d
1127. c
1128. a
1129. a

Explanation: In humans, the skin accounts for about 7% of the total body weight.

ASSESSMENT AND DIAGNOSTIC EVALUATION

1130. Rule of nine is ____________:
a. A tool used to assess eye sight of a person
b. An allergy identification test
c. A chart used to assess the area of body burned
d. A tool used to assess nutritional deficiency

1131. The procedure for collecting sample of skin for biological examination is called:
a. Surgical shave b. Biopsy
c. Aspiration d. Injection

1132. All the following are various types of skin biopsy; EXCEPT:
a. Punch biopsy b. Excisional biopsy
c. Shave biopsy d. Gross biopsy

1133. A client underwent skin biopsy reported to the nurse regarding excessive drainage and redness, what is the appropriate nursing action?
a. Record the findings
b. Advise the client that it is a normal finding
c. Inform the physician
d. Flush the site with normal saline

1134. Viral culture media should be transported on:
a. Ice b. Room temperature
c. Hot air oven d. Incubator

1135. Tzanck smear helps to identify which among the following organism?
a. Erysipelas b. MRSA
c. Herpes zoster d. Leukemia

1136. Koebner phenomenon is associated with: *New Q*
a. Psoriasis
b. Acne vulgaris
c. Stevens Johnson syndrome
d. Cellulitis

Explanation: The Koebner phenomenon, also known as the Koebner response or isomorphic response, refers to the development or worsening of skin lesions in response to injury or trauma to the skin. Psoriatic rashes appear around an injury such as cut or burn.

1137. Which test confirms the presence of MRSA?
a. Culture and sensitivity test
b. Woods light examination
c. Tzanck smear
d. Diascopy

PRIMARY AND SECONDARY SKIN LESIONS

1138. Which of the following is considered as primary prevention strategy?
a. Early identification
b. Reduction of disability
c. Control of spread of disease
d. Early treatment of disease

1139. Bluish discoloration of skin is termed as:
a. Pallor b. Cyanosis
c. Erythema d. Chromatosis

1140. A secondary skin lesion occurs due to constant rubbing or scratching and is characterized by hyperpigmentation, thickening of the skin and exaggerated skin lines is known as:
a. Papule b. Fissure
c. Atrophy d. Lichenification

1141. A circumscribed area of skin which is not swollen or elevated is called as:
a. Atrophy b. Flat
c. Vesicle d. Blister

1142. Excess scar tissue caused by excessive collagen during wound healing is known as:
a. Crust b. Macule
c. Keloids d. Scar

1143. Dry wrinkled skin surface leads to wasting of skin due to loss of collagen is called:
a. Atrophy b. Macule
c. Blister d. Fissure

PRURITIS AND SEBORRHEIC DERMATOSES

1144. A common site for the lesions associated with atopic dermatitis is:
a. Buttocks b. Shoulder
c. Antecubital space d. Thigh

1145. Skin manifestation commonly seen after 2 days of radiotherapy is:
a. Atrophy b. Dermatitis
c. Erythema d. Hyperpigmentation

1146. Which of the following is not advised for a patient with pruritus?
a. Daily baths with scented soap
b. Wearing cloths made of 100% cotton
c. Increasing fluid intake
d. Apply moisturizer after bath

Explanation: Use of scented soap (with aromatic oils) lead to dryness of skin. This may cause aggravation of pruritus.

1147. Which among the following is the medication of choice for a patient with red and irritated skin following diarrheal episode: *(AIIMS Raipur Staff Nurse Grade I-2018)*
a. Silver sulfadiazine b. Zinc oxide
c. Mafenide acetate d. Actiot

Explanation: Zinc oxide is the medication of choice for a patient with red and irritated skin following diarrheal episode.

ACNE VULGARIS

1148. Which among the following is a skin lesion with whiteheads and non-inflamed lesions:
a. Open comedones
b. Closed comedones
c. Pustules
d. Papules

Ans.
1130. c
1131. b
1132. d
1133. c
1134. a
1135. c
1136. a
1137. a
1138. c
1139. b
1140. d
1141. b
1142. c
1143. a
1144. c
1145. c
1146. a
1147. b
1148. b

1149. Which among the following statement is correct regarding acne vulgaris?
a. Instruct the client not to take topical or oral medications
b. Instruct the client not to squeeze the lesions
c. Instruct the client to pick the lesion
d. Advise the client to use oil-based formulas.

1150. Which type of lesion is NOT seen in acne vulgaris?
a. Pustule b. Comedones
c. Lichensification d. Nodules

1151. Acne vulgaris usually more common among:
a. Young males b. Young females
c. Middle aged males d. Middle aged females

1152. Most common causative agent of acne vulgaris is:
a. Propionibacterium acnes b. Varicella zoster
c. Trypanosoma cruzi d. Borrelia burgdorferi

IMPETIGO

1153. What is the most common causative agent for impetigo?
a. Staphylococcus aureus b. Streptococcus sanguis
c. Viridans streptococci d. Streptococcus sobrinus

1154. Impetigo is also called as:
a. Rosacea b. Hives
c. School sores d. Acne

1155. Which of the following condition is contagious?
a. Vitiligo b. Psoriasis
c. Cellulitis d. Impetigo

1156. Early sign of impetigo is:
a. Painless itching b. Reddish sore on the skin
c. Hardening of the skin d. Wrinkles on skin

1157. Which of the following statement is correct regarding impetigo?
a. Restriction of participation in contact sports
b. Take fresh sea foods
c. Promote physical contact sports
d. Advice the client to withhold other medications

HERPES ZOSTER (SHINGLES)

1158. What medication is most likely to be administered to the client with diagnosis of herpes zoster?
a. Penicillin b. Acyclovir
c. Doxycycline d. Fluconazole

Explanation: Herpes zoster is usually treated with orally administered acyclovir, an antiviral agent. Adults with herpes zoster can be treated with oral acyclovir at a dose of 800 mg five times daily. Other antiviral medications include famciclovir and valacyclovir.

1159. What is the main complication of shingles?
a. Bell's palsy b. vision impairment
c. Phantom limb pain d. Tinnitus

1160. Which of the following disease is NOT contagious?
a. Herpes zoster b. Impetigo
c. Psoriasis d. None of these

1161. Causation of Shingles is:
a. Skin to skin contact
b. Varicella zoster virus
c. Herpes virus
d. Exposure to excessive sun light

1162. Drug of choice for shingles ?
a. Anti-bacterial drugs b. Anti-fungal drugs
c. Anti-viral drugs d. Anti-protozoan drugs

1163. Which of the following lesion is caused by Herpes simplex virus type-1?
a. Cold sore on the lips b. Redness of lips
c. Crust d. Papule

PEDICULOSIS

1164. Pediculosis is caused due to the infestation of:
a. Lice b. Botfly
c. Flea d. Tsetse fly

1165. Which of the following is not the type of pediculosis?
a. Pediculosis pubis b. Pediculosis capitis
c. Pediculosis carporis d. Pediculosis cruris

1166. The type of pediculosis which commonly affects the human head is:
a. Pediculosis carporis b. Pediculosis capitis
c. Pediculosis pubis d. Pediculosis cruris

1167. Which age group are highly affected with head-lice infestation?
a. Children aged 3 – 10 years
b. Age 11 to 18 years
c. female 21 to 31 years
d. Male 21 to 31 years

1168. Which of the following is the effective treatment for pediculosis?
a. Acetretin b. Infliximab
c. Permethrine lotion d. Ingenol mebutate

1169. Pediculosis can be treated with all of the following; EXCEPT:
a. Lindane b. Ivermectin
c. Permethrin 1% d. Benzyl Alcohol 70%

Explanation: Permethrin crème, malation (0.5%) lotion, lindane lotion, and Ivermectin lotion are used in the treatment of pediculosis. Benzyl alcohol 5% is used in treatment of pediculosis.

SCABIES

1170. Clinical manifestation of scabies includes all; EXCEPT:
a. Severe itching usually worse at morning
b. Presence of burrows
c. Erythematous papules
d. Irregular burrow tracks made up of tiny blisters

1171. In scabies, burrows are present over:
a. Interdigital webs b. Flexor surface of wrist
c. Anterior axillary fold d. All of the above

1172. Drug of choice to treat scabies is:
a. Permethrin b. Calamine lotion
c. Tincture benzoate d. Povidone iodine

PSORIASIS, PEMPHIGUS VULGARIS

1173. Silvery scales plaques that are mildly itchy on the patient's knees and elbows are known as:
a. Scabies b. Vitiligo
c. Impetigo d. Psoriasis

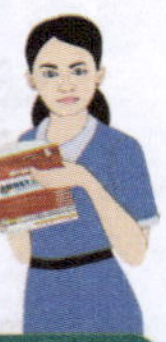

Ans.
1149. b
1150. c
1151. a
1152. a
1153. a
1154. c
1155. d
1156. b
1157. a
1158. b
1159. a
1160. c
1161. b
1162. c
1163. a
1164. a
1165. d
1166. b
1167. a
1168. c
1169. d
1170. a
1171. d
1172. a
1173. d

1174. Which of the following statement is correct about psoriasis?
- a. Showering with antiseptic soap will prevent transmission to other family members
- b. Washing clothes separately from the rest of the family are necessary
- c. Psoriasis is not contagious, so no special precautions are necessary
- d. Psoriasis is transmitted primarily by direct contact with the skin

Explanation: Psoriasis is a skin condition that causes red, flaky, crusty patches of skin covered with silvery scales. Psoriasis is not contagious so it will not spread from one person to other person.

1175. Psoriasis affects:
- a. Scalp, knees and elbows b. Nails
- c. Joints d. All of these

SYSTEMIC LUPUS ERYTHEMATOUS (SLE)

1176. What is the hallmark sign of systemic lupus erythematous?
- a. Malar rashes b. Buffalo hump
- c. Severe abdominal pain d. Petechiae

1177. SLE is a/an:
- a. Congenital disorder b. Auto immune disease
- c. Genetic disorder d. x–linked disorder

1178. All of the following can cause drug induced SLE; EXCEPT:
- a. Phenytoin b. Isoniazid
- c. Procainamide d. Clomiphine citrate

1179. Type of hypersensitivity reaction is seen in SLE is:
- a. Type I hypersensitivity
- b. Type II hypersensitivity
- c. Type III hypersensitivity
- d. Type IV hypersensitivity

1180. Autoantibody production occurs in SLE is due to:
- a. Hyperreactivity of cellular immune response
- b. Hyperactivity of humoral immune response
- c. Hyper reaction of T cell
- d. None of the above

STEVENS-JOHNSON SYNDROME (SJS) AND TOXIC EPIDERMAL NECROLYSIS (TEN)

1181. The complications of Steven - Johnson Syndrome include:
(AIIMS Raipur Grade II 2017)
- A. Untreated sepsis B. Keratoconjunctivitis
- C. Conjunctival retraction D. Corneal lesions
- a. A, B, C b. B, C, D
- c. A, C, D d. A, B, C, D

Explanation: Steven Johnson syndrome is a disorder of skin and mucus membrane. The signs and symptoms include fever, unexplained widespread skin pain, a red or purple skin rash that spreads, blisters on skin and the mucous membranes of mouth, nose, eyes and genitals and shedding of skin within days after blisters form. The complications include cellulitis, sepsis, eye problems, lung involvement and permanent skin damage. The drugs which cause this syndrome include allopurinol, penicillin, pain relievers like acetaminophen, ibuprofen and naproxen sodium, anticonvulsants and antipsychotics.

1182. Systemic lupus erythematosus (SLE) affects:
- a. Connective tissue b. Liver
- c. Kidney d. Retina

1183. Most common and life-threatening complication of SLE is:
- a. Arthralgia b. Nephritis
- c. Butterfly rashes d. Sydenham's chorea

1184. Clinical manifestation related to neurological involvement of SLE is:
- a. Delirium b. Psychosis
- c. Anxiety d. Convulsion

1185. Most appropriate medication for treating SLE is:
- a. Fentanyl b. Prednisolone
- c. Hydroxychloroquine d. Adrenaline

Explanation: Antimalarial remains the first-line treatment for SLE along with NSAIDs. The two types of antimalarials most often prescribed today for SLE are hydroxychloroquine and chloroquine. Antimalarials combined

1186. All of the following are the clinical features of systemic lupus erythematosus (SLE); EXCEPT:
- a. Arthralgia b. Butterfly rashes
- c. Portal hypertension d. Myalgia

1187. Blood dyscrasias present in a client with systemic lupus erythematosus (SLE) is:
- a. Disseminated intra vascular coagulopathy
- b. Polycythemia
- c. Essential thrombocytopenia
- d. Thalassemia

SKIN TUMORS

1188. Majority of melanomas are caused by:
- a. Exposure to ultraviolet ray
- b. Excess fatty tissues
- c. Lack of exposure to sunlight
- d. Lack of vitamin D

1189. Commonest form of skin cancer is:
- a. Basal cell carcinoma
- b. Squamous cell carcinoma
- c. Malignant melanoma
- d. Hemangioma

1190. Which of the following information should be included in a health teaching regarding 'how to reduce the risk of skin cancer'?
- a. Avoid prolonged exposure to the sun
- b. After being in the woods or in tall grass, check for ticks
- c. Avoid strong deodorants, perfumes and body lotions
- d. Shower immediately after being outdoors

Explanation: Prolonged exposure to ultraviolet rays is the major risk factor for skin cancer.

SKIN GRAFTS

1191. Graft from identical twin is:
- a. Allograft b. Isograft
- c. Xenograft d. Autograft

1192. Autograft is between:
- a. Different species b. Same individual
- c. Twins d. Same species

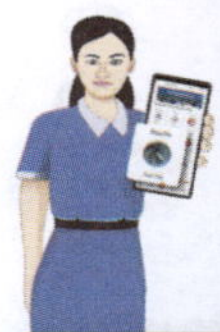

Ans.

1174. c
1175. d
1176. a
1177. b
1178. d
1179. c
1180. b
1181. d
1182. a
1183. b
1184. b
1185. c
1186. c
1187. c
1188. a
1189. a
1190. a
1191. b
1192. b

1193. Xenograft is between:
a. Different species b. Same individual
c. Twins d. Same species

HAIR LOSS/ALOPECIA

1194. Thinning of hair is called:
a. Alopecia areata b. Hypotrichosis
c. Telogen effluvium d. Anagen effluvium

1195. Which of the following is the major cause of thinning of hair (telogen effluvium):
a. Hypothyroidism
b. Physical or psychological stress events
c. Chemotherapy
d. Trichotillomania

1196. What is the approximate rate of hair fall per day?
a. 100–150 hairs per day
b. 20–50 hairs per day
c. 50–100 hairs per day
d. 200–250 hairs per day

1197. Which of the following is not the phase of hair growth?
a. Anagen b. Catagen
c. Endogen d. Exogen

1198. The other name of scarring alopecia is:
a. Cicatricial alopecia b. Alopecia areta
c. Telogen effluvium d. Anagen effluvium

Explanation: Primary cicatricial alopecia refers to a disorder that destroy the hair follicle, replace it with scar tissue, and cause permanent hair loss. Hair loss can be gradual, without symptoms, and unnoticed for long periods.

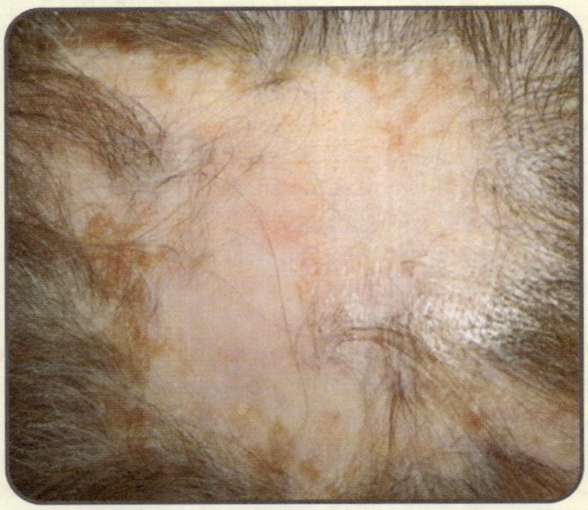

IRRITANT CONTACT DERMATITIS

1199. The two major types of contact dermatitis are:
a. Primary and secondary
b. Sensitive and Non-sensitive
c. Allergic & Irritant Mediated
d. Acute and chronic

1200. The nurse is explaining a middle-aged client about risk factors that cause allergic skin reactions. Which among the following should not be included in her teaching:
a. Dry environment b. Exposure to plants
c. Exposure to soap d. Exposure to perfume

1201. Which of the following treatment plan is expected to be ordered by the dermatologist for a patient with a severe case of allergic contact dermatitis, which covers 45% of the client's body?
a. Applying wet dressings
b. Providing oral corticosteroids
c. Giving topical antibiotics
d. Antipruritic medication

1202. Patient with allergic contact dermatitis is planned for a skin test in which small amounts of an allergen will be injected into the skin on the person's body. Which of the following test the nurse teach the patient to be prepared for:
a. Patch test on skin b. Scratch test biopsy
c. IgE antibody screening d. Intradermal test

1203. Nurse Ramya is performing physical examination in an adult male patient. On inspection, she finds a skin lesion due to contact dermatitis. Besides inspection, what other method that the nurse applies to diagnose the condition accurately:
a. Percussion b. Palpation
c. Skin Biopsy d. Stethoscope Auscultation

CELLULITIS

1204. The most common causative organism of cellulitis is:
a. Staphylococcus aureus b. Streptococcus aureus
b. Streptococcus pyogens d. Epstein Barr virus

1205. The following clinical features are seen in cellulitis; EXCEPT:
a. Redness and tenderness b. Cold clammy skin
c. Warmth d. Edematous skin

1206. An adult person develop cellulitis mostly on the:
a. Scalp and back region
b. Groin region
c. Facial and the lower extremity
d. Chest region

1207. Untreated cellulitis may lead to which of the following conditions?
a. Septicemia/septic shock b. Wound injury
c. Evisceration d. Loss of body surface area

1208. Client is diagnosed with cellulitis on his lower extremity. He should know the best way to assess the spreading of the disease would be:
a. Physical examination
b. Asking patient feeling
c. Drawing line around the border
d. Appling bandage to the affected area

BURNS AND CLASSIFICATION OF BURN INJURY

1209. Eschar refers to:
a. Loss of skin elasticity
b. A dry scab or slough formed on the skin as a result of burn
c. An area of red skin
d. Excessive sweating

1210. Characteristic features of skin in a dehydrated patient include:
a. Warm and dry b. Loss of elasticity
c. Pigmented skin d. Both a and b

Ans.
1193. a
1194. c
1195. b
1196. c
1197. c
1198. a
1199. c
1200. a
1201. b
1202. d
1203. b
1204. a
1205. c
1206. c
1207. a
1208. c
1209. b
1210. d

1211. If a patient has severe burns on the upper torso, which would be a primary concern: *(Safdarjung NO 2018)*
  a. Administering antibiotics
  b. Debriding and covering the wounds
  c. Frequently observing for hoarseness, stridor and dyspnea
  d. Establishing a patent IV line for fluid replacement

Explanation: Burns on the upper torso may have inhalational burns. Upper torso burns have a potential threat to burns in upper respiratory tract that necessitates, the frequent monitoring of respiratory function and sounds. So, the primary concern is to frequently observe for hoarseness, stridor and dyspnea. The patient may need early intubation and ventilatory support.

Antibiotics and wound debridement are common for all kind of burns. If upper torso is burnt, central venous access can be taken through femoral vein.

1212. Which type of burn is painless? *(LNJP H D 2012)*
  a. Third degree b. Second degree
  c. First degree d. None of these

1213. Which among the following burn is characterized by no pain? *(AIIMS Raipur staff nurse grade I-2018)*
  a. Superficial partial thickness
  b. Deep partial thickness
  c. Full thickness burn
  d. All of the above

Explanation: In full thickness burn, nerve endings are also damaged and patient will not perceive pain.

1214. First degree partial thickness burn is characterized by:
  a. Involvement of epidermis and dermis
  b. Burn site appears red, blistered
  c. Superficial and painful burn
  d. Surface of the wound is leathery and may be brown

1215. Which of the following observation best describes the characteristics of a second-degree partial thickness burn?
  a. Redness in the skin without blisters
  b. Redness in the skin with clear blister
  c. Stiff and white/brown skin
  d. All of the above

1216. Third degree full thickness burn is characterized by:
  a. Epidermis dermis and subcutaneous tissue is affected
  b. Painless burn
  c. Appears dry and may be black and white
  d. All of the above

1217. A patient is admitted with burns on his right lower extremity. Client states that he has minimal pain. The burned area appeared as white and leather-like. Observation showed no blister or bleeding. This burn injury is categorized as:
  a. Full thickness
  b. Partial thickness-deep
  c. Partial thickness-superficial
  d. Superficial

Explanation: White skin (also black/brown or yellow) and no or minimal pain are the characteristic of full thickness burn.

1218. Least risk for full thickness burn is associated with:
  a. Sunburn b. Thermal injury
  c. Chemical burn d. Electrical injury

1219. Most common type of burn injury is:
  a. Chemical b. Electrical
  c. Thermal d. Inhalation

1220. A patient with burn injury will be always complaining of some amount of pain and is known as:
  a. Resting pain b. Procedural pain
  c. Break through pain d. Severe pain

1221. A patient with burn injury will be complaining of pain during dressing change. This is known as:
  a. Resting pain b. Procedural pain
  c. Break through pain d. Severe pain

1222. A patient with burn injury will always be complaining of some amount of pain as the level of analgesics decreased in the blood and is known as:
  a. Resting pain b. Procedural pan
  c. Break through pain d. Severe pain

1223. Burn over which part of the body causes risk of life-threatening complications?
  a. Lower extremities b. Hands and feet
  c. Perineum d. Upper part of the body

Explanation: Burn injury to the upper part of the body causes risk of life-threatening complications due to frequent respiratory involvement.

1224. Which of the following is not a possible systemic clinical manifestation of severe burns?
  a. Insulin resistance b. Hypermetabolism
  c. Sepsis d. Systemic hypertension

1225. Mechanism behind the development of edema in burn patient is:
  a. Increased capillary permeability
  b. Due to renal failure
  c. Increased IV fluid administration
  d. Decreased urine output

Explanation: Increased capillary permeability leads to fluid shift from the circulation into burned tissue because of a moderate increase in capillary permeability to fluid and macromolecules and a modest increase in hydrostatic pressure inside the perfusing microvessels.

1226. Best blood test to assess the fluid status in a burn patient is:
  a. Electrolyte level b. Creatinine level
  c. Hematocrit d. Hemoglobin level

1227. What type of room is appropriate to shift a severely burned client from emergency department?
  a. General ward with a noninfectious clients
  b. A semi-private room with a postoperative client
  c. A private room with a private bath
  d. An isolation room

Explanation: Burn victims are highly susceptible for infection. They should be preferably kept in an isolation room to protect from infection.

EXTENT OF BODY SURFACE AREA BURNED

1228. Burn severity is assessed with:
  a. Burned surface area b. Depth
  c. Body parts affected d. All of these

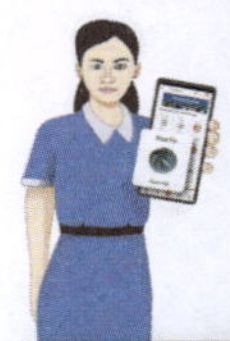

Ans.

1211. c
1212. a
1213. c
1214. c
1215. b
1216. d
1217. a
1218. a
1219. c
1220. a
1221. b
1222. c
1223. d
1224. d
1225. a
1226. c
1227. d
1228. d

1229. Burn injury to which of the following area considered to be largest area as per rule of nine? *(AIIMS Staff Nurse 2016)*
a. Anterior upper chest b. Face and neck
c. Right leg d. Left arm

1230. A client is admitted with a burn injury to both of his upper extremities. What is the total body surface area (TBSA) affected for this patient, according to rule of nine?
a. 9% b. 18%
c. 36% d. 27%

Explanation: As per rule of nines, each of the upper limbs is considered 9%. As the patient has burn injury to both of his limbs, the burn affected percentage is 18%.

1231. A 25-year-old male patient sustained severe burns of the right lower extremity. Using the rule of nines, which is the best estimate of total body-surface area burned?
a. 18% b. 22%
c. 31% d. 40%

Explanation: Please refer to the explanation of next question.

1232. A patient is admitted with burn injury to entire anterior chest and abdomen. The nurse calculates the total body surface area affected by burn using the rule of nine as:
a. 9% b. 18%
c. 27% d. 36%

Explanation: Rule of nines a method of estimating the extent of burns. The following image illustrates the calculation of body surface area of burn using rule of nines.

Surface area of affected area:
9 (anterior chest) + 9 (anterior abdomen) = 18%

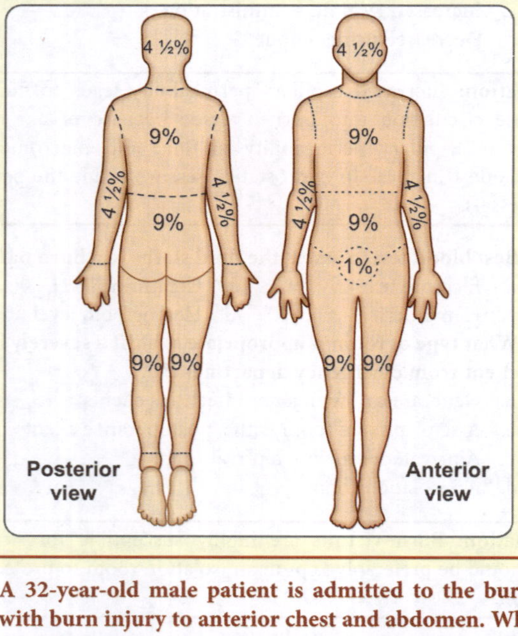

1233. A 32-year-old male patient is admitted to the burn unit with burn injury to anterior chest and abdomen. Which of the following assessment is most important for this client in first 48 hours?
a. Assessment of skin color and capillary refill
b. Hourly urine output measurement
c. Hourly blood pressure measurement
d. Frequent assessment for pain

Explanation: Hourly measurement of urine output is necessary to manage fluid replacement therapy. Though other observations also important, measurement of urine output is the priority.

1234. All of the following methods are used to assess the area of burn injury; EXCEPT:
a. Lund Browder Chart b. Rule of nines
c. Parkland formula d. Palmar method

Explanation: Parkland formula for burns is used to calculate fluid requirements for burn patients in 24-hr period. Other three given methods are used to calculate the area of burn injury. Wallace rule of nines is a good quick method for estimation of medium to large burn in adults. Lund and Browder method is an age specific chart and most accurate method. Palmar surface can be used to estimate relatively small burns (<15%) or very large burns (>85%).

BODY RESPONSE TO BURN INJURY

1235. In post-burn patient, true is:
a. Hypokalemic alkalosis b. Hyperkalemic alkalosis
c. Hyperkalemic acidosis d. Hypokalemic acidosis

Explanation: Hyperkalemic acidosis is seen in acute burns. The combination of potassium shift out of cells and diminished urine K^+ excretion causes hyperkalemia. Tissue destruction also releases K^+ into circulation.

1236. Following a burn injury the capillary permeability will:
a. Increase b. Decrease
c. Not change d. Fluctuate

1237. Which of the following electrolyte imbalance is seen in burn injury?
a. Hyponatremia b. Hypokalemia
c. Hypernatremia d. None of these

1238. The normalization of capillary permeability after burn injury will take up to:
a. 1–2 weeks b. 2–3 weeks
c. 7 days d. 14 days

1239. Following a burn injury the hematocrit level will:
a. Increase b. Decrease
c. Not change d. Fluctuate

1240. Which of the following is not a major complication after burn injury?
a. Intestinal ileus b. Infection
c. Pulmonary hypertension d. Bradycardia

Explanation: Cardiac stress, mediated by increased catecholamines, is the hallmark of severe burn injury typified by marked tachycardia, increased myocardial oxygen demand, and increased cardiac output. So bradycardia is not a complication of burn injury. Other given complications are seen in burn injury.

CARE OF PATIENT WITH BURN INJURY

1241. Lindane is a: *(NCFL 2019)*
a. DDT
b. BHC
c. Malathion
d. Fenthion

Ans.

1229. c
1230. b
1231. a
1232. b
1233. b
1234. c
1235. c
1236. a
1237. a
1238. b
1239. a
1240. d
1241. b

Explanation: Lindane, also known as gamma-hexachlorocyclohexane, and sometimes incorrectly called benzene hexachloride (BHC) is widely used in the control of pests of agricultural crops. It is used as a second-line pharmaceutical treatment for lice and scabies though it has an adverse effect on human health.

1242. Which among the following is the medication of choice for a patient with red and irritated skin following diarrheal episode?

a. Silver sulfadiazine b. Zinc oxide
c. Mafenide acetate d. Actiot

1243. Health education to a client after chemical peeling is:

a. Avoidance of sun exposure
b. Drink plenty of water
c. Use cold application at the site
d. Use scrubber while taking bath

1244. Hypertrophic scar in a burn victim can be prevented by:

a. Massaging the body with moisturizer
b. Applying pressure garments
c. Change position every hourly
d. Dressing the wound properly

1245. First nursing intervention while seeing a burn client is:

a. Stop further burn
b. Make the client in a safe place
c. Ensure ABC
d. Shift to hospital

1246. Which of the following nursing intervention is necessary for a client who has silver nitrate dressings applied to his burns?

a. Restrict fluid intake
b. Change the dressings every two hours
c. Keep the dressings wet
d. Frequently observe for black discoloration

Explanation: Silver nitrate dressings must always be kept wet to be effective. Silver nitrate does cause black discoloration, but this is incidental and not a major nursing consideration.

1247. Silver nitrate dressings may cause:

a. Abnormality in blood gases
b. Abnormal blood count
c. Depletion of sodium and potassium
d. Increased blood urea nitrogen (BUN)

Explanation: Silver nitrate can cause depletion of potassium, sodium, and chloride; therefore, assessment of serum electrolytes is essential when the patient has silver nitrate dressings.

1248. The best indicator of adequate fluid balance in a client with burn, especially in the first 48 hours of care is:

a. Change in level of consciousness
b. Elevated hematocrit levels.
c. Urine output of 30–50 mL/hr
d. Weight of the patient

Explanation: Urine output of 30 mL 50 mL/hr is the best indicator for adequate fluid balance. Urine output of at least 30 mL/hr ensures adequate tissue perfusion to vital organs such as kidney, heart and brain.

1249. Cimetidine is administered 6 hourly to client with burn in order to:

a. Prevent secondary infection
b. Maintain fluid-electrolyte balance
c. Promote GFR
d. Prevent Curling's ulcer

Explanation: Stress ulcers (Curling's ulcer) occur frequently in burn victims. Cimetidine is a histamine blocker that reduces gastric acid and helps to prevent the development of gastric ulcers.

1250. A severely burned woman had her last tetanus shot a couple of years before. Which of the following should be administered for this patient?

a. DPT booster
b. Tetanus antitoxin
c. Tetanus toxoid booster
d. Hyperimmune human tetanus globulin

Explanation: DPT is not given after the age of six years. Tetanus toxoid booster is required for this patient as the patient had her last tetanus dose two years ago. Tetanus antitoxin is administered if considerable time has elapsed from the time of injury. Hyperimmune tetanus globulin is given when the person has not had prior tetanus immunization.

1251. Indwelling catheter is inserted in a severely burned client. The major purpose is to:

a. Maintain the bladder tonicity
b. Measure hourly urine output
c. Prevent urinary tract infection
d. Prevent contamination of burned areas

Explanation: Fluid replacement is based on measurement of urine output and it is a high priority for a client with burn injury.

1252. Diet advised to a burn victim is:

a. High calorie diet
b. High fat diet
c. High calorie and low protein diet
d. High protein and high calorie diet

FORMULAS FOR FLUID REPLACEMENT IN BURN VICTIM

1253. Which type of solution is commonly used for the fluid replacement in burns?

a. Hartmann solution b. Normal saline
c. 5% dextrose d. 5% dextrose in normal saline

Explanation: Hartmann solution contains Sodium, Potassium, Calcium, Chloride and Lactate. It is useful in resuscitation of burn patient. Risk of causing metabolic acidosis (due to high Na and low Cl concentration of Hartmann solution) if being used as the sole fluid.

1254. All of the following formulas are used for fluid replacement in burn injury except?

a. Modified Brookes formula
b. Modified parkland formula
c. Baxter formula
d. Mostellar formula

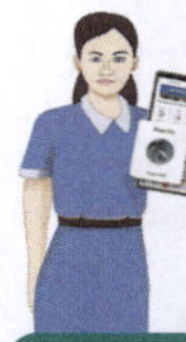

Ans.

1242. b
1243. a
1244. b
1245. a
1246. c
1247. c
1248. c
1249. d
1250. c
1251. b
1252. d
1253. a
1254. d

Explanation: Mosteller formula is used to calculate Body Surface Area (BSA). All other formulas are used in calculation of fluid replacement in burn injury.

1255. An adult patient is receiving treatment for burn injury. The urinary output is recorded in excess of 50 ml/hr. It indicates:

a. IV fluid administration can be decreased
b. IV fluid administration has to be increased
c. No change is required in IV fluid administration
d. None of the above

Explanation: Urine output of 0.5 mL/kg or about 30–50 mL/hr in adults and 0.5-1.0 mL/kg/hr in children less than 30 kg is a good target for adequate fluid resuscitation. Since the urine output is in excess of 50 ml/hr the volume of IV fluid administration/flow rate has to decrease.

1256. What is the normal duration of resuscitation/emergent phase in phases of management of burns?

a. 1–6 hours b. 6–12 hours
c. 12–24 hours d. 48–72 hours

1257. The following are the phases of management of burns injury except?

a. Emergent phase b. Resuscitative phase
c. Chronic phase d. Rehabilitative phase

WOUND DEBRIDEMENT

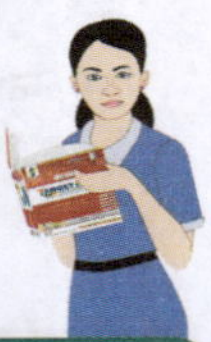

1258. Which type of wound debridement method is also called Maggot debridement therapy?

a. Biological debridement b. Mechanical debridement
c. Sharp debridement d. Autolytic debridement

1259. The main purpose of wet to dry dressing is:

a. To decrease the pain b. To prevent the infection
c. To keep the wound clean d. To debride the wound

Explanation: It is a type of mechanical debridement. Wet to dry dressing is used to remove drainage and dead tissue from **wounds.** This **form of debridement** is the removal of tissue using a **dressing** that is changed regularly. It consists of **moist gauze** being applied to a wound that requires **debridement**, which is then covered with a sterile **bandage**.

1260. The type of debridement method that removes both necrotic tissue and the healthy tissue is:

a. Selective method b. Non selective method
c. Total method d. Missed method

1261. In which of the following method of debridement, the health care provider only removes the necrotized tissue and leaving the normal tissue on intact while doing wound debridement.

a. Selective method b. Non selective method
c. Total method d. Missed method

1262. All of the following observation indicates the need for wound debridement procedure; EXCEPT:

a. Necrotic tissue
b. Debris
c. Pink reddish tissue formation
d. Blister and calluses possibility

Ans.

1255. a
1256. d
1257. c
1258. a
1259. d
1260. b
1261. a
1262. c
1263. b
1264. a
1265. c
1266. d
1267. d
1268. d
1269. b

1263. Following are the primary and general contraindication for the wound debridement procedure; EXCEPT:

a. Debris b. Red, granular wounds
c. Necrotic tissue d. Blister formation

1264. Among the given method of debridement the most aggressive and fastest method of wound debridement would be:

a. Sharp b. Enzymatic
c. Autolytic d. Biologic

OTHER SKIN DISORDERS

1265. Which of the following term refers to a fungal infection of the foot (Athlete's foot):

a. Impetigo b. Acne vulgaris
c. Tinea pedis d. Scabies

1266. Inflammation of tissues surrounding the nail is known as: *(DSSSB 2013)*

a. Clubbing b. Koilonychia
c. Onycholysis d. Paronychia

Explanation: An infection that develops along the edge of the fingernail or toenail is called a paronychia. More specifically, it is a superficial infection of epithelium lateral to the nail plate that begins as cellulitis.

Tips: Use the key word "Para" (side of beside) from option D which will help you to connect the key term in the stem "tissues surrounding".

1267. Lyme's disease produces a characteristic annular or circular rash known as:

a. Plaques b. Papules
c. Bullae d. Bull's eye rash

1268. Xanthoma refers to:

a. Dryness of conjunctiva
b. Dry mouth
c. Yellowish plaques near the inner canthus of the eyelid
d. Fatty growths develop underneath the skin

1269. The benign changes in elderly skin include the following; EXCEPT: *(AIIMS Raipur Grade II 2017)*

a. Cherry angiomas b. Telangiectasis
c. Spider angiomas d. Pseudoxantoma elasticum

Explanation: Telangiectases are dilated capillaries that appear as red linear stellate or punctate lesions. Telangiectasia may represent a benign condition or a marker of a much more serious internal or cutaneous malignancy.

All other given conditions are benign skin conditions. Spider angioma, also known as spider naevus or spider telangiectasia, is a vascular lesion characterized by anomalous dilatation of end vasculature found just beneath the skin surface. Spider angiomas are seen in young adults, pregnant women and in patients with cirrhosis, alcoholic hepatitis, and hepatopulmonary syndrome. Spider angioma are more likely in older persons because ageing causes value in veins to weaken.

Cherry hemangiomas, also known as Campbell de Morgan spots and senile angiomas, are found commonly in elderly patients.

Pseudoxanthoma elasticum (PXE) is a progressive disorder that is characterized by the accumulation of deposits of calcium and other minerals (mineralization) in elastic fibers. In PXE, mineralization can affect elastic fibers in the skin, eyes, and blood vessels.

RESPIRATORY SYSTEM

ANATOMY AND PHYSIOLOGY

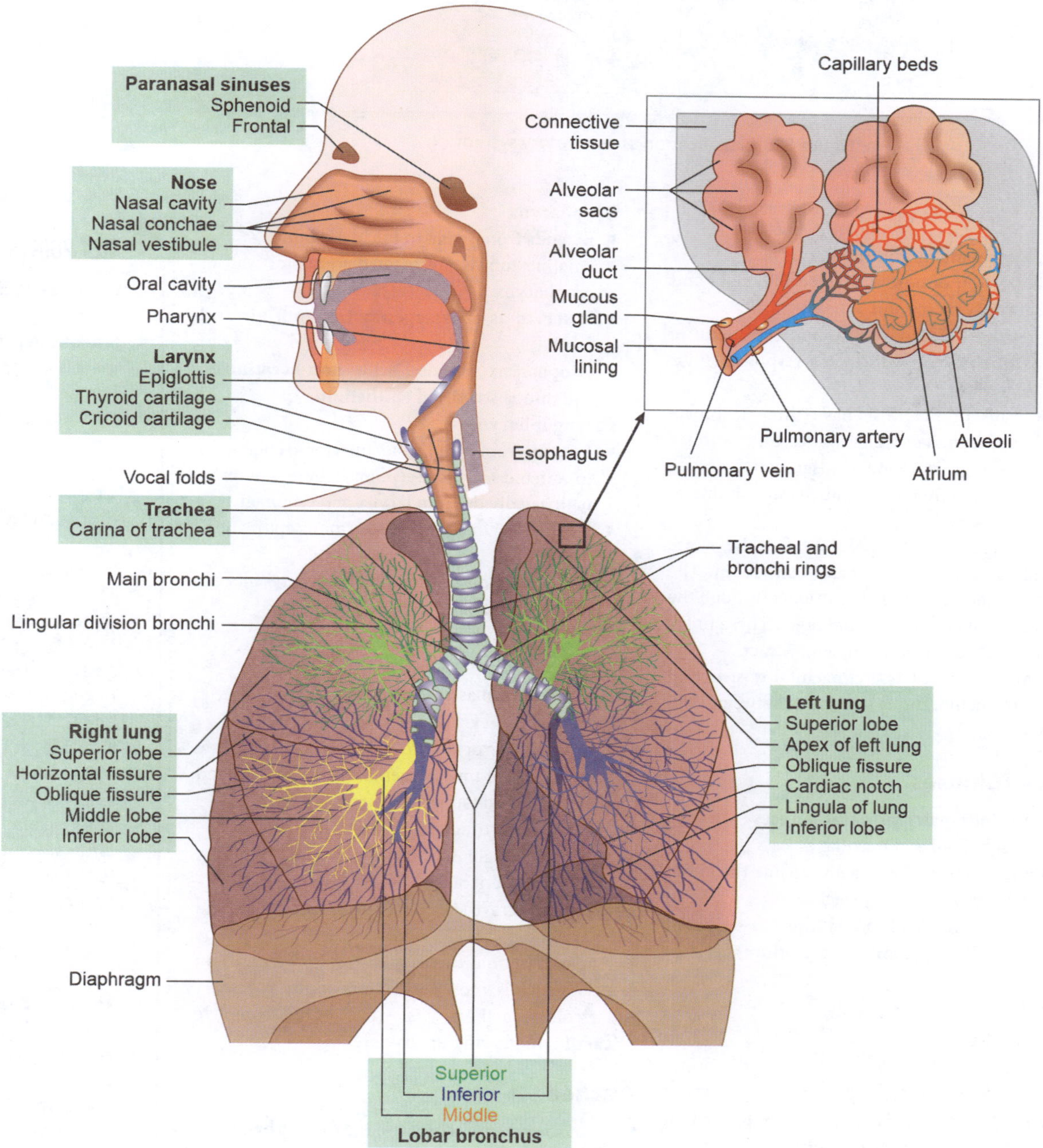

Figure 61: Respiratory system and an enlarged cross-section of lungs

CLASSIFICATION OF RESPIRATORY SYSTEM

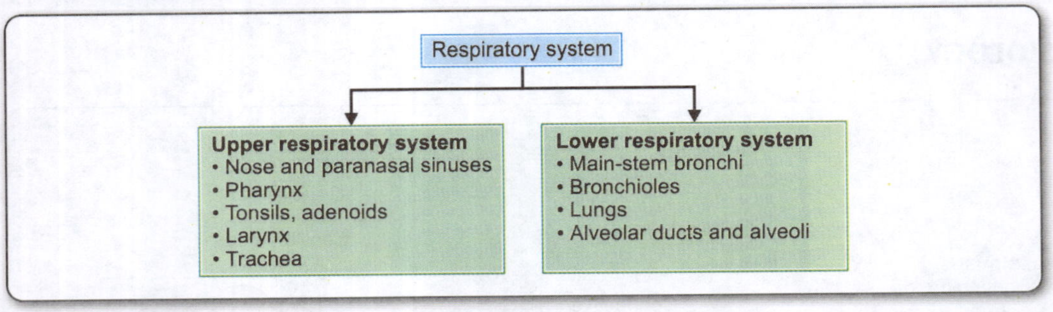

Figure 62: Classification of respiratory system

Nose

- Filters, warms and humidifies the air.
- Internal portion of nose is divided into right and left nasal cavity by septum.
- Lined with **ciliated columnar epithelium,** contains goblet cells which are responsible for mucus secretion.
- Lateral walls of the nose have three turbinate bones called **conchae** which increase the surface area of mucous membrane of nasal cavity.
- **Rhinitis** – inflammation of mucus membrane of nose
- Olfactory receptors, responsible for the sense of smell, are found in the nasal epithelium. The olfactory receptors extend their fibers through the cribriform plate of the ethmoid bone. These fibers come together to form the olfactory tract.
- **Choanal atresia** – it is a congenital obstruction by bony or membranous structures between nose and pharynx.

Paranasal Sinuses

- There are **four pairs of nasal sinuses** - frontal, ethmoid, sphenoid and maxillary.
- Nasal sinuses are hollow cavities inside the bones and help in resonation of speech.
- Sinuses are lined with nasal mucosa (**ciliated pseudo-stratified columnar epithelium**).

Pharynx

- **Nasopharynx**
  - Extends from base of the skull to the upper surface of soft palate.
  - Adenoids (pharangeal tonsils) are located in nasopharyngeal posterior wall.
  - **Eustachian tube starts from middle ear and opens into nasopharynx.**
  - Nasopharynx is lined with respiratory epithelium (**ciliated pseudo-stratified columnar epithelium**).
- **Oropharynx**
  - Extends from uvula to the hyoid bone.
  - Palatine tonsils are located in lateral wall of oropharynx.
  - **It serves as a passageway for both air and food.**
  - Oropharynx is lined with **non-keratinized squamous stratified epithelium**
- **Laryngopharynx**
  - Extends from hyoid bone (inferior to epiglottis) to cricoid cartilage (point where common pathway divides into larynx and esophagus).
  - It is lined with stratified squamous epithelium.
- **Tonsil**
  - Collection of lymphoid tissue presents in pharynx and base of the tongue

Larynx

- It is also known as **voice box.**
- It extends from **C4** to **C6**
- Two types of vocal cord - True vocal cord (the inferior fold of mucus membrane of larynx) and false vocal cord (superior pairs fold)
- **Total nine cartilages** are present in larynx –
  - Three Single cartilage (3), i.e., thyroid, epiglottis, cricoids
  - Three Pairs (6) i.e., cuneiform, corniculate and arytenoid.
- Angle of thyroid cartilage forms a protrusion on neck which is known as **Adam's apple.**
- **Cricoid cartilage** is the only complete **cartilaginous ring** in larynx.

Trachea

- It is also known as **windpipe** and formed by 16–20 incomplete hyaline cartilage (C-shaped rings) which are posteriorly incomplete.
- Diameter – 2.5 cm.
- The adult trachea begins at the lower edge of cricoid cartilage (at the level of C6 vertebra).

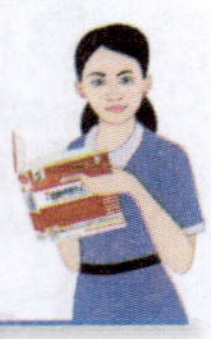

KEY POINTS

- Larynx extends from C4 to C6
- Size of the Larynx in male is larger than female.
- On average, the length of the trachea is 11.8 cm with a normal range of 10–13 cm in males.
- The trachea tends to be shorter in females.
- The adult trachea begins at the lower edge of cricoid cartilage, at the level of sixth cervical vertebra (C6).
- The trachea bifurcates into the left and right main bronchus, at the level of the sternal angle and of the T4-T5
- The cricoid cartilage is a ring of hyaline cartilage located at the inferior aspect of the larynx and is the only complete ring of cartilage around the trachea.

- The trachea branches into left and right main bronchi., at the level of sternal angle (T4-T5) vertebra.
- It extends from larynx and branches into two main stem bronchi.
- Carina of trachea – the point where the trachea gets divided into two bronchi

Lungs

- Lungs are the paired structures in thoracic cage.
- Right lung is divided into three lobes- upper, middle and lower.
- Left lung is divided into two lobes- upper and lower.
- Two main bronchi (left and right main bronchus) enter the lung through an opening called **hilum**.

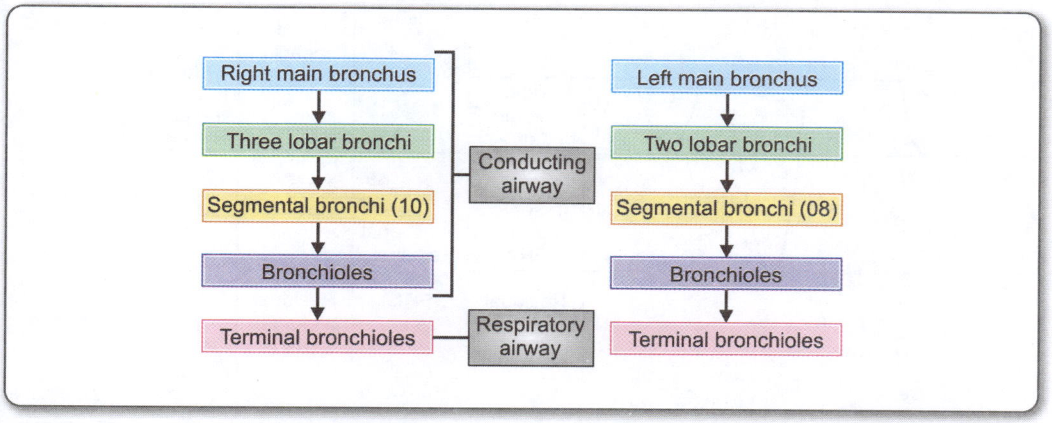

Figure 63: Schematic diagram of left and right lung

- Bronchi and bronchioles are lined with cilia which help in removing secretions and foreign particles from lungs toward upper respiratory tract.
- Conducting airway contains 150 mL of air which does not participate in gas exchange (**physiological dead space**).
- Each lung contains approximately **300 million alveoli** with a surface area of 50 to 100 m^2.
- Alveolar cells have three types:
  - **Type-I:** These cells make up the alveolar epithelium
  - **Type-II:** These cells produce surfactant (which reduces the surface tension and prevents alveoli from collapsing).
  - **Type-III:** Alveolar macrophages.
- Lungs are covered by pleural cavity which contains small amount of pleural fluid between visceral and parietal pleura.
- Respiration occurs due to excitation of respiratory muscles by **phrenic nerve**.
- **Apneustic** and **pneumotaxic center** present in **pons and medulla** control respiration.
- Central chemoreceptors in medulla respond to chemical changes (pH).
- Peripheral chemoreceptors in carotid arteries and aorta respond to PaO_2 and $PaCO_2$.
- **Respiration** – Two types – external respiration and internal respiration
  - **External respiration** = exchange of gases between lungs and blood
  - **Internal respiration** = exchange of gases between blood and cells/tissues
- **Breathing** –
  - Process of taking air into and flush out carbon dioxide.
  - Two phases – inhalation and exhalation
- **Inhalation/inspiration/breathing in** –
  - Active process
  - Primary inspiratory muscle – Diaphragm (contraction, 75% air into) and external intercostal muscle (elevates the ribs, 25% air into). When the diaphragm contracts, it moves downward, increasing the vertical dimension of the thoracic cavity and creating space for the lungs to expand.
  - Creates negative pressure inside thoracic cavity
  - **Accessory inspiratory muscles** - sternocleidomastoid, pectoralis and trapezius, and Scalene muscle.
- **Exhalation/expiration/breathing out** –
  - Passive process
  - Primary expiratory muscle – diaphragm
  - **Accessory expiratory muscle** – abdomen muscle and internal intercostal muscle.

KEY POINTS

- Alveoli are the sites of gas exchange in the lungs
- The walls of the alveoli are lined with simple squamous epithelial cells known as alveolar cells.
- Type I alveolar cells (95%) - Squamous and extremely thin. Involved in gas exchange.
- Type II alveolar cells (5%) - Granular and roughly cuboidal. It secretes surfactant.
- **Hyaline membrane disease/ Respiratory Distress Syndrome** – absence of surfactant in infant

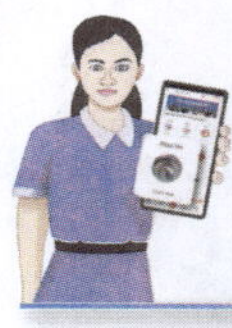

Lung Volumes and Capacities

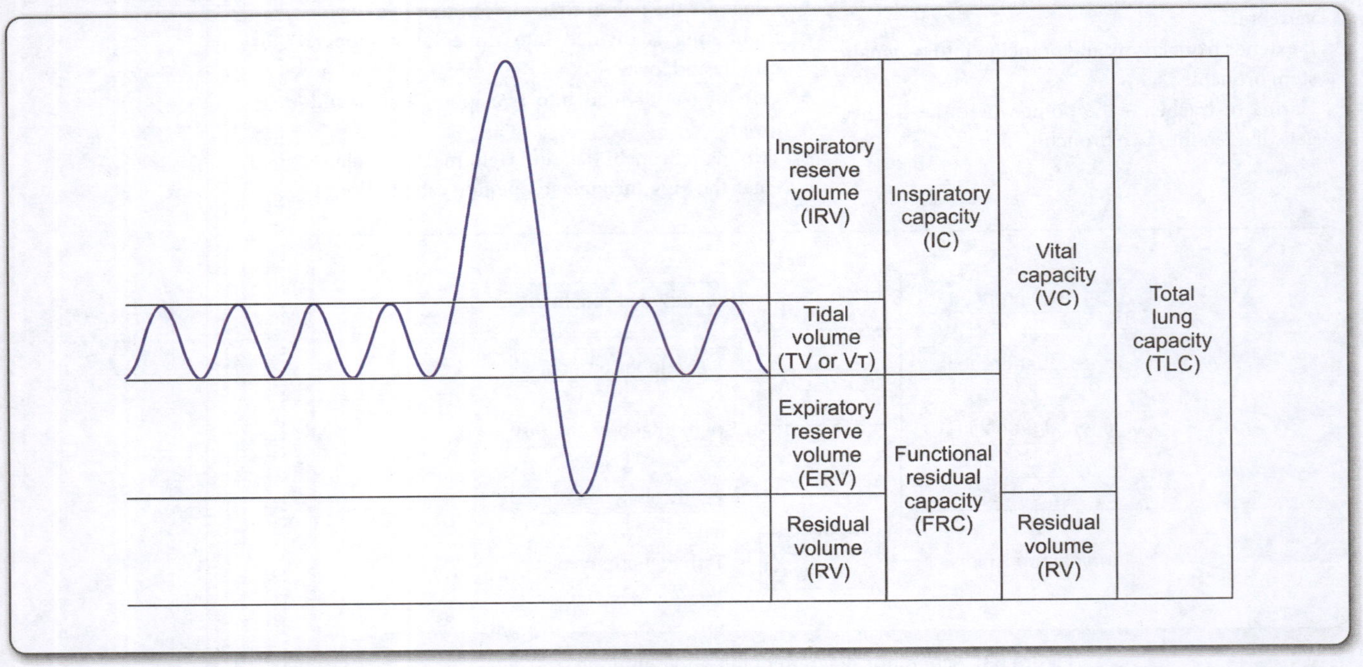

Figure 64: Lung volume and capacities

Lung Volume Along with Normal Values

Table 52: Lung volume along with normal volumes

Lung volume	Description	Normal Volume
Tidal volume (TV)	Amount of air inhaled during a normal, relaxed breathing.	500 mL
Inspiratory reserve volume (IRV)	Quantity of the air that can be forcibly inspired after a normal tidal inspiration	3,000 mL
Expiratory reserve volume (ERV)	Quantity of air that can be forcibly exhaled after a normal tidal expiration	1,100 mL
Residual volume (RV)	Amount of air that is still left in the lungs after the expiratory reserve volume is exhaled	1,200 mL

Lung Capacities

Table 53: Lung capacities

Name	Volume	Definition
Total lung capacity (TLC)	6,000 mL	Quantity of air that can fill the lungs (TLC = TV + IRV + ERV + RV).
Vital capacity (VC)	4,800 mL	Quantity of air that can be expired after fully inhaling (VC = TV + IRV + ERV = approximately 80% TLC). The value varies according to age and body size.
Inspiratory capacity (IC)	3,600 mL	It is the maximum quantity of air that can be inspired (IC = TV + IRV).
Functional residual capacity (FRC)	2,400 mL	It is the amount of air left in the lungs after a normal expiration (FRC = RV + ERV).

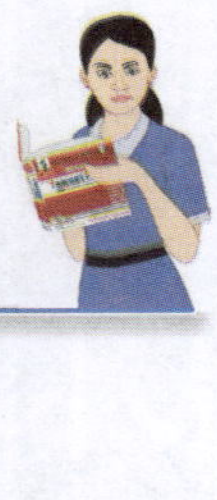

Pulmonary Pressure

- Systolic blood pressure in pulmonary artery is 20 to 30 mm Hg.
- Diastolic blood pressure in pulmonary artery is 5 to 15 mm Hg.

Ventilation/Perfusion Ratio (V/Q)

- Normal ratio- 1:1
- Low Ventilation perfusion ratio (V/Q): <1
  - Perfusion exceeds ventilation.
  - Occurs in conditions of obstruction of distal airways (**pneumonia, atelectasis,** etc.)
- High Ventilation perfusion ratio (V/Q): >1
  - Ventilation exceeds perfusion which leads to dead space.
  - Occurs in conditions like pulmonary embolism, pulmonary infraction, cardiogenic shock.
- **Silent unit**
  - It occurs when there is limited ventilation and perfusion.
  - It occurs in conditions like pneumothorax and ARDS (Acute respiratory distress syndrome).

Partial Pressure of Gases

Table 54: Atmospheric air versus alveoli air

Atmospheric air	Alveoli air
Total pressure is 760 mm Hg at sea level. • Nitrogen (78.6% = 597 mm Hg) • Oxygen (21% = 158 mm Hg) • Water vapor (0.05%)	**Total pressure is 760 mm Hg** • Nitrogen (74.9% = 569 mm Hg) • Oxygen (13.6% = 104 mm Hg) • CO_2 (5.3% = 40 mm Hg) • Water vapor (47 mm Hg)

Effect of Pressure on Oxygen Transport

- **PaO_2** (partial pressure of arterial oxygen): It represents the volume of oxygen dissolved in plasma.
- At PaO_2 100 mm Hg, each 100 mL of arterial blood carries-
  - 20 mL of oxygen by oxy-hemoglobin.
  - 0.3 mL of oxygen dissolved in plasma.
- Amount of oxygen combines with hemoglobin is measured as saturation (**SpO_2**)
- At **PaO_2** of 100 mm Hg, 97% of Hb is saturated with oxygen.
- When **PaO_2** is 150 mm Hg, then Hb is fully saturated with oxygen (100%).
- When Hb is fully saturated, then 1 g of Hb combines with 1.34 mL of O_2.

ASSESSMENT AND DIAGNOSTIC TESTS

- **Clubbing of Nails**
  - It is a change in normal nail bed. It is present in chronic hypoxic conditions.
  - Schamroth's window is absent.
- **Cyanosis**
  - It is the bluish discoloration of skin
  - It is determined by deoxygenated hemoglobin in blood. It is manifested when at least 5 g/dL of blood gets deoxygenated.
  - **Central cyanosis** is observed in **lips and tongue**.
  - Peripheral cyanosis is **NOT** a reliable indicator of hypoxia.
- **Chest Configuration**
  - Normal ratio of antero-posterior to lateral diameter of thorax is 1:2.
  - **Barrel chest**- Sign of **Chronic obstructive pulmonary disease (COPD)** and **emphysema**. Antero-posterior to lateral diameter of thorax is 1:1.
  - **Funnel chest** (Pectus excavatum)- In this, there is a depression in lower part of sternum that compresses heart and great vessels. It occurs in rickets or **Marfan's syndrome**.
  - **Pigeon chest** (Pectus Carinatum)- It occurs due to displacement of sternum anteriorly which increases antero-posterior diameter.

KEY POINTS

- During inspiration, the **diaphragm and external intercostal muscles contract**, causing the rib cage to expand and expanding the thoracic cavity and lung volume.
- During expiration, the diaphragm and intercostal muscle relax.

KEY POINTS

- Nail clubbing occurs when the tips of the fingers enlarge and the nails curve around the fingertips.
- Clubbing often occurs in heart and lung diseases that reduce the amount of oxygen in the blood.

KEY POINTS

- **Barrel chest:** Sign of Chronic obstructive pulmonary disease (COPD) and emphysema.
- Funnel chest (Pectus Excavatum) is seen in Rickets or Marfan's syndrome
- Central cyanosis is observed in lips and tongue.

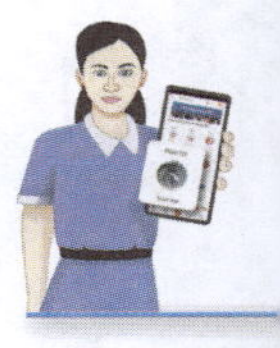

Breathing Patterns

Table 55: Various breathing patterns

Condition	Assessment	Associated with
Normal respiratory rate in an adult	12–20 breaths/min	
Bradypnea	<10 breaths/min	Raised ICP, brain injury.
Tachypnea	>24 breaths/min	Pneumonia, metabolic acidosis, hypoxia.
Hyperpnea	Deep breathing	During and after exercise, High altitude, severe sepsis
Hypoventilation	Shallow breathing	Muscle weakness, decrease in ventilator drive
Hyperventilation (Kussmaul's respiration)	Increased rate and depth of breathing	Decreased $PaCO_2$, anxiety, metabolic acidosis
Apnea	Transient cessation of breathing	
Obstructive sleep apnea	Pause of breathing during sleep with transient upper airway obstruction.	Most common cause is excess weight and obesity
Cheyne Stokes	Rate and depth of breathing increase and then decrease until apnea	Usually associated with heart failure or stroke 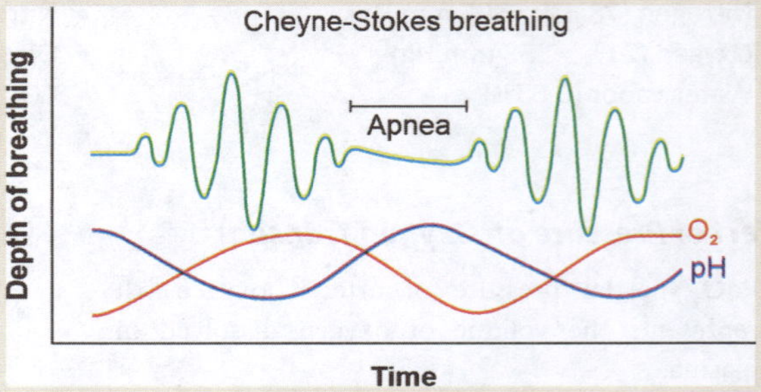

- **Pulmonary Function Tests (PFTs) are Performed with the Help of Spirometer**

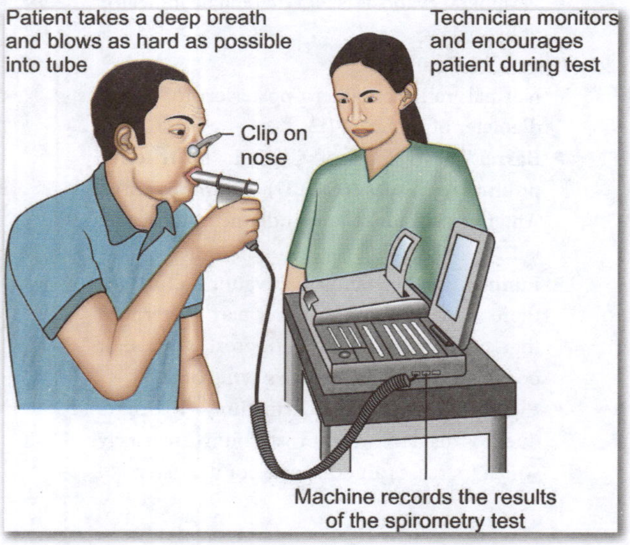

Figure 65: Pulmonary function test

Recent Question (CNCI 2021)

37. Increased depth of breathing with normal respiratory rate is called?
a. Kussmaul's breathing
b. Bradypnea
c. Orthopnea
d. Hyperpnea

Ans. (d) Hyperpnea

- **Pulmonary angiography**
  - It is a procedure to visualize pulmonary vasculature
  - Informed consent should be taken
  - Assess the patient for allergy to radio-opaque dye
  - Keep patient NPO for 6 to 8 hours before investigation.
  - Inform patient about warm, flushed feeling after insertion of dye.
  - After procedure, closely monitor vital signs, SaO_2, bleeding, hematoma at puncture site.
- **Ventilation/Perfusion Scan**
  - It is performed to assess Ventilation/Perfusion (V/Q) ratio with the help of radioactive agent.
  - Perfusion to the lungs is assessed by administering radioactive agent through peripheral vein with a mask fitted over nose of the patient.
  - It is followed by ventilation scan by asking the patient to take a deep breath of mixture of oxygen and radioactive gas.
- **Bronchoscopy**
  - It is the direct visualization of tracheobronchial tree by flexible fiberoptic bronchoscope or rigid bronchoscope.
  - Purposes:
    - To directly visualize the extent or location of lesion, tumor, etc.
    - To collect secretions for diagnosis.
    - To assess site of bleeding (Hemoptysis).
    - To take biopsy
    - To remove foreign body.
  - Nursing responsibilities:
    - Obtain informed consent.
    - Keep patient NPO 4–8 hours before the test.
    - Remove dentures or any oral prosthesis.
    - Administer topical lidocaine spray over the posterior wall of pharynx.
    - After procedure, keep the patient NPO until gag reflex appears.
    - Start with ice chips followed by clear fluids.
    - Monitor patient for hypoxia, tachycardia, dyspnea, hemoptysis, etc.
- **VATS (Video assisted thoracoscopy)**
  - A fiberoptic mediastinoscope is inserted into pleural cavity which is visualized on a screen.
- **Thoracocentesis/thoraccentesis**
  - It is the procedure of aspiration of fluid or air from pleural cavity.
  - Nursing responsibilities
    - Obtain informed consent.
    - Inform patient to remain immobile during procedure. Ask the patient to refrain from coughing during procedure.
    - Obtain baseline chest X-ray, vital signs, pain level and SaO_2.
    - **Position:** Sitting on edge of bed with arms supported on padded cardiac table/Sitting on chair with arms and head resting on back of chair/lying on unaffected side either 30 to 45 degrees elevated head end.
    - For **pneumothorax location** for needle insertion is **2nd or 3rd intercostal space in mid-clavicular line**.
    - Strict aseptic precautions should be taken during the procedure.
    - Post-procedure X-ray should be obtained.
    - Closely monitor vital signs, pain level and SaO_2 after procedure.

DISORDERS OF RESPIRATORY SYSTEM

Acute Respiratory Distress Syndrome (ARDS)

- Also called as shock lung, wet lung, etc.
- Acute respiratory distress syndrome (ARDS) is a severe form of acute lung injury characterized by sudden and progressive pulmonary edema, hypoxemia unresponsive to oxygen supplementation, and the absence of an elevated left atrial pressure.
- ARDS occurs due to diffuse alveolar damage and lung capillary endothelial injury.
- Lungs fail to maintain balance between oxygen and carbon dioxide.
- Neutrophils play a key role in the pathogenesis of ARDS, as suggested by BAL
- ARDS was recognized as the most severe form of acute lung injury (ALI)
- **Signs and symptoms:** Tachycardia, tachypnea, increased blood pressure, accessory muscle use for respiration, crepitus, diminished breath sounds, cyanosis, diaphoresis, bibasilar crackles, dyspnea, and hypoxia.
- **Management**
  - Mechanical ventilation may be necessary
  - Vasopressors and diuretics as ordered.

Acute Respiratory Failure

- Respiratory failure is called when
  - PaO_2 <60 mm Hg
  - $PaCO_2$ >50 mm Hg
- **Etiology**
  - Collection of secretion in the lungs due to cough suppression, bronchospasm, and airway irritants
  - Central nervous system depression, disorders of respiratory muscles, peripheral nervous system, and chest wall
  - Endocrine or metabolic disorders
  - Heart failure, gas exchange failure, MI, and pulmonary embolism

KEY POINTS

- Tidal volume - 500 mL
- Inspiratory reserve volume (IRV) - 3000 mL
- Expiratory reserve volume (ERV) - 1100 mL
- Residual volume (RV) - 1200 mL
- Total lung capacity = TV + IRV + ERV + RV = 5,800 mL
- Patient has to be kept NPO for 6 to 8 hours before pulmonary angiography.
- Inform patient about warm, flushed feeling during pulmonary angiography after injection of dye.
- Patient should be instructed to drink plenty of water (if not contraindicated) after pulmonary angiography procedure to facilitate elimination of contrast dye.

- **Signs and symptoms**
  - Absent breath sounds
  - Rhonchi, Crackles, and Wheezes
  - Yawning and use of accessory muscles for breathing.
- **Treatment:** Oxygen therapy, mechanical ventilation.
- Bronchodilators such as terbutaline, albuterol, theophylline and ipratropium bromide.

Asthma

- Asthma is a chronic disease characterized by recurrent attacks of breathlessness and wheezing, shortness of breath, and chest tightness.
- During an asthma attack, the lining of the bronchial tubes (airways) swells, causing the airways to narrow, turn more sensitive to irritants in the environment, and thus reducing the flow of air into and out of the lungs.
- It is probably caused by interplay of hereditary and environmental factors like an inherited tendency to develop allergies, called atopy.
- Children with eczema or food allergy are more likely to develop asthma than other children.

  Two types of asthma – allergic and nonallergic
  - **Allergic asthma** - IgE mediated or extrinsic asthma, causes are dust, dust, pollution etc
  - **Nonallergic-** Intrinsic asthma or non-IgE mediated, causes are drugs like aspirin, esercises, respiratory tract infection.
- **Diagnosis:** Medical history, chest X-ray, physical examination, Liver Function Tests (LFTs) and lab tests, Radioallergosorbent test (RAST) – To test the specific allergen in blood.
- **Salbutamol, levo-salbutamol and terbutaline** are utilized in stopping asthma attacks.
- Short courses of corticosteroid and other drugs (oral or injectable) may be required during acute attacks and are to be used after medical advice only.

Acute Severe Asthma/Status Asthmaticus

- **Acute severe asthma (Status asthmaticus)** is an acute exacerbation of asthma that remains unresponsive to initial treatment with bronchodilators.
- Manifestation: Tachypnea and significant wheezing.
- Normally, the difference in SBP between inspiration and expiration does not exceed 15 mm Hg. In patients with severe asthma, a difference of greater than 25 mm Hg may be noted which is known as pulsus paradoxus.
- **First line treatment**: Bronchodilator treatment with a β2-agonist, typically salbutamol. The inhaled route is most effective.
- **Anticholinergic agents:** Ipratropium bromide does not cross the blood-brain barrier and is the recommended agent of choice.
- **Glucocorticoids** are the most important treatment for status asthmaticus. Action usually requires at least 4–6 hours to occur because protein synthesis is required before the initiation of its anti-inflammatory effects.

Bronchitis

- Bronchitis is an inflammation of the mucous membranes of the bronchi.
- Bronchitis can be divided into: Acute and Chronic
  - **Acute bronchitis** is characterized by the feeling of cough or small sensation in the back of the throat. It can be with or without the sputum. **Acute bronchitis is one of the most common types of lung infection.** It can occur at any age.
  - **Chronic bronchitis** is a type of COPD, which involves a cough that produces sputum for 3 months for 2 consecutive years.
- **Main symptom:** Bronchitis is persistent cough with thick yellow gray mucous, though it may not always be present.
- **Other symptoms of bronchitis may include:** A tight feeling in chest, breathlessness, wheezing, sore throat, slight fever and chills, headache, blocked nose and sinuses, body ache and pains.
- **Causes**: Virus or bacteria; **viral bronchitis** is much more common.
- Bronchitis can also be caused by breathing irritant substances, such as smog, chemicals in household products or tobacco smoke.
- **For managing acute bronchitis:** Advise the patients to take rest, drink plenty of fluids. Headaches and body aches can be treated with pain relievers like paracetamol or ibuprofen. Stop smoking or inhaling irritant.
- **For managing chronic bronchitis:** There is no cure for chronic obstructive pulmonary disease (COPD), but management can help slow the progression of the condition and reduce the symptoms. Smoking should be stopped to avoid further damage to lungs.

Chronic Obstructive Pulmonary Disease (COPD)

COPD is a life threatening lung disease. It causes chronic obstruction of airway in the lungs.

In some cases, the air sacs (alveoli) get damaged gradually leading to a condition called emphysema **(pink puffers)**. In other cases, the airways get, inflammed (irritation) leading to a condition called chronic bronchitis **(blue bloaters)**.

KEY POINTS

- **Stridor** is a high-pitched, wheezing sound caused by disrupted airflow.
- Stridor may also be called musical breathing or **extra thoracic airway obstruction**.
- **Single largest risk factor for Asthma:** Atopy/Hereditary
- **Asthma triad** includes nasal **polyps, asthma**, and sensitivity to **aspirin** and **NSAIDs**.
- Drug of Choice for chronic asthma: Inhaled corticosteroid + Long Acting Beta Agonists (LABA)
- Drug of Choice for acute, severe asthma: Inhaled Short Acting Beta Agonists (SABA) + Systemic steroids
- Bronchodilator of choice in COPD: Anticholinergics

Recent Question (NORCET 2022)

38. All of the following are included in the ventilator associated pneumonia bundle care, EXCEPT:

a. Head elevated at 30°
b. Sedation vacation
c. Antibiotic prophylaxis
d. Supraglottic suctioning

Ans. (c) Antibiotic prophylaxis

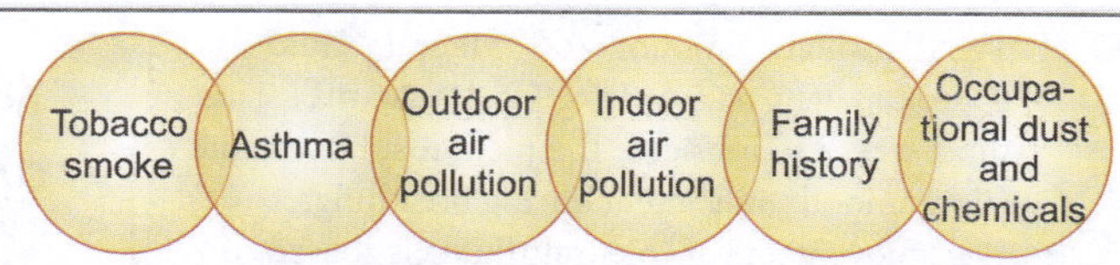

Tobacco smoke
Asthma
Outdoor air pollution
Indoor air pollution
Family history
Occupa-tional dust and chemicals

Figure 66: Risk factors of COPD

- **Symptoms of COPD:** Shortness of breath (Dyspnea), wheezing (Whistling sound while breathing), chest tightness, cough with mucus often called smoker's cough, Unintended weight loss (in later stages)
- **Diagnosis:** Detailed history, chest X-ray and pulmonary function tests. In ABG, patient will have **respiratory acidosis**.
- **Management:** Inhaled bronchodilators, nebulization and inhaled or oral steroids; antibiotics, oxygen therapy, steam inhalations, chest physiotherapy and pulmonary rehabilitation program.
- **Chest physiotherapy (CPT) given in morning is the best,** can also be given 1 hour before meal and 2- 3 hours after food.
- Management – Bronchodilators, mucolytics, corticosteroids, antibiotics.
- **Complications:** Respiratory infections such as cold, flu and pneumonia; high blood pressure, heart problems including heart attack, right sided heart failure (cor pulmonale), lung cancer, depression, etc.

Pneumonia

- Pneumonia is inflammation (swelling) of tissue in one or both lungs.
- It is a condition which primarily affects the lung parenchyma (Alveoli, alveolar ducts and bronchioles).
- **Causes:** infection with viruses or bacteria and less commonly other microorganisms, certain drugs. **Most common cause is *Streptococcus pneumonia.***
- **Types:**
  - **Hospital acquired pneumonia:** Developed 48–72 hours after admission into hospital
  - **Community acquired pneumonia:** Most commonly occurring
- **Risk factors:** Previous flu or cold, weakened immunity (elderly or immunosuppressant therapy), COPD, Cough depression (post-op), immobility, etc.
- **Common symptoms: Difficulty in breathing, tachycardia**, fever, sweating and shivering, loss of appetite, pain in chest. Person may also have hemoptysis, headache, fatigue, nausea or vomiting.
- **Diagnosis:** Auscultation may reveal coarse crackles, rhonchi. Chest X-ray and sputum culture.
- Physical examination may sometimes reveal **low blood pressure and low oxygen saturation.** Increased **respiratory rate and heart rate** may be found.
- **Management**: Simple painkillers (analgesics) like ibuprofen, and antibiotics.
- **Complications associated** with pneumonia are pleurisy and septicemia.

Sputum Color

Note

Color of sputum	Agent
Rusty brown	Pneumococcal
Red currant jelly	Klebsiella
Green	Pseudomonas
Black	Allergic Bronchopulmonary Aspergillosis (ABPA)

Swine Flu

- Swine flu also known as swine influenza or pandemic influenza is a respiratory disease.
- Cause: **H1N1 virus** (introduced in 2009). This virus infects the wind pipe (respiratory tract) of pigs and later it gets transmitted to human beings.
- **Manifestation**: Nasal secretions, cough, decreased appetite, and restless behavior.
- **Incubation period:** 1–4 days.
- **Symptoms:** Similar to influenza (flu). Fever, headache, running nose, sore throat, shortness of breath or cough, loss of appetite, diarrhea or vomiting.
- Swine flu can spread to others up to about 6 feet away. The flu viruses are spread mainly by droplets when people with flu cough, sneeze or talk.
- **Diagnosis**: Through patient's history and symptoms.
- **Confirmatory test:** Reverse transcription polymerase chain reaction (RT-PCR).
- **Management**: **Zanamivir** (Relenza) and **oseltamivir** (Tamiflu).

KEY POINTS

- **Pink puffers:** Puffing to breathe (hyperventilation) and pink complexion (maintain oxygen level with rapid breathing)
- **Blue bloaters:** Cyanosis (blue) and edema (bloating) due to chronic bronchitis
- **Signs and Symptoms:** Remember LUNG DAMAGE
  - **L –** Lack of energy
  - **U –** Unable to tolerate (shortness of breath)
  - **N –** Nutrition poor (weight loss due to energy utilized for breathing effort particularly in emphysema)
  - **G –** Gases abnormal (Low PO_2 and High PCO_2)
- Teach the patient about pursed-lip and diaphragmatic breathing to manage shortness of breath
- Low amount of oxygen delivery is advised (1–2 L/min)
- Maintain oxygen saturation at 88–93% (Low oxygen is the respiratory stimulant in patients with COPD....Not CO_2)

Recent Question

(NORCET 2022)

39. Most infectious disease leading to mortality in children world-wide:

a. Diarrhea
b. Pneumonia
c. Acute epiglottitis
d. CROUP

Ans. (b) Pneumonia

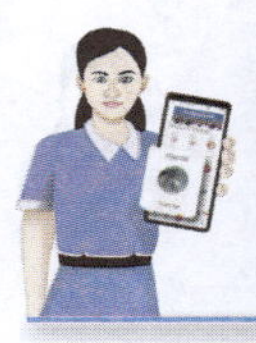

- The most effective way to prevent the spread of infections is to practice good hygiene. Vaccination against influenza also has some role.

Atelectasis

- **Atelectasis:** A collapsed or airless state of the lung, which maybe acute or chronic and may involve all or part of the lung
- It may be from imperfect expansion of pulmonary alveoli at birth (congenital) or as the result of disease or injury
- **Features:** Crackles, tachycardia, tachypnea and fever
- **Management**: Bronchodilator and antibiotics are used for treatment.

Emphysema

- The abnormal presence of air in tissues or cavities of the body.
- **Pulmonary emphysema:** A chronic disease of the lungs. Distension of alveoli causes intervening walls to break down and bullae to form on the lung surface. It also causes distension of the bronchioles and eventual loss of elasticity so that inspired air cannot be expired, making breathing difficult.
- **Surgical emphysema:** The presence of air or any other gas in the subcutaneous tissues, introduced through a wound and evidenced by crepitation on pressure.

Cor pulmonale

- Cor pulmonale is defined as an alteration in the structure and function of the right ventricle caused by a primary disorder of the respiratory system.
- Pulmonary hypertension is common link between lung dysfunction and the heart in Cor pulmonale.
- Cor pulmonale usually presents chronically, but 2 main conditions can cause acute Cor pulmonale: pulmonary embolism (more common) and acute respiratory distress syndrome (ARDS).

Influenza

- ***Condition caused by RNA virus and is commonly called as flu.***
- There are 3 types of influenza virus that can all infect humans: Influenza A, influenza B, and influenza C.
- **Signs and symptoms:** Cold and cough, muscle pain, respiratory distress.

Pleural Effusion

- A pleural effusion is the abnormal accumulation of fluid in the pleural space.
- Accumulation of blood is known as hemothorax and accumulation of air is known as pneumothorax.

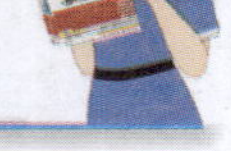

- The normal amount of pleural fluid is approximately 0.25 mL/kg or 10–20 mL. This fluid serves to lubricate the pleural surfaces and allow smooth movement during breathing.
- The movement of pleural fluid is based on **Starling's principle**, which involves the balance of hydrostatic and oncotic pressures across the capillaries and pleural membranes.
- If the amount of fluid exceeds 250 mL, it can cause a mediastinal shift, which refers to the displacement of mediastinal structures toward the unaffected lung.

Two types of pleural effusion –

1. **Exudative effusion** – caused by obstruction of blood vessel of lymph nodes, infection, inflammation, tumors. **High concentration of protein, Yellow in color**
2. **Transudative effusion** – caused by non – inflammatory conditions like heart failure, liver or renal disease, **low protein count, clear in appearance.**
   - Thoracocentesis is the management for pleural effusion which is usually performed in between 7th and 8th ribs.
   - **1000–1200 mL** fluid can be removed at one time.

Pneumothorax

- Accumulation of air in pleural space
- Normally, pleural space remains negative (4mm/hg) but during pneumothorax it becomes positive.
- Most common cause – **Blunt trauma causes Flail chest.**
- **Paradoxical respiration** – inward movement of ribs during inspiration and outward movement during expiration is one of the common clinical manifestations of Flial chest.
- Types of pneumothorax –
  - **Tension pneumothorax** – air entry to pleural space but cannot escape.
  - **Open pneumothorax** – air entry during inspiration and move out during expiration. It is also known as sucking chest wound.
  - **Closed pneumothorax** – air entry to pleural space and some amount got trapped.
- 2nd rib is the site for needle aspiration for tension pneumothorax.
- **Posterior mid-scapular line** is the preferred site for thoracentesis procedure performed in the upright or seated position

Pulmonary Edema

- Excess of fluid in the lungs and alveoli
- **Causes:** Left-sided heart failure, mitral stenosis, ARDS, fluid overload, Myocardial infarction, or pulmonary emboli.

KEY POINTS

- *CURB -65* is used as a predictor of severity of pneumonia
  - **C:** Confusion
  - **U:** BUN >20 mg%
  - **R:** RR >30
  - **B:** SBP <90; DBP <60
  - **65:** Age >65
- Productive cough and pleuritic pain is characteristic feature
- Abnormal breath sounds (coarse crackles, rhonchi) in peripheral lung fields
- Encourage incentive spirometer for deep breathing
- Encourage coughing and deep breathing
- 2–3 L of fluid intake (except patients with heart failure)

Recent Question (CNCI 2021)

40. A 17-year-old student has a long history of bronchial asthma and has experienced several severe asthmatic attacks during the school year. The school nurse is required to administer 0.2 mL of 1/1000 solution of epinephrine SC during an asthma attack. How does the school nurse evaluate the effectiveness of this intervention?

a. Increased pulse rate
b. Increased expectorate of secretions
c. Decreased inspiratory difficulty
d. Increased respiratory rate

Ans. (c) Decreased inspiratory difficulty

Pulmonary Embolism (PE)

- **Definition:** Obstruction of pulmonary artery or its branches by thrombus, tumor, air or fat that originated elsewhere in the body
- **Acute PE:** In massive PE, there is reduction of BP below 90/40 in less than 15 minutes
- **Saddle PE:** Embolus lodges at the main pulmonary artery bifurcation
- **Signs and Symptoms:** Tachypnea, tachycardia, crackles, loud second heart sound (S2), Raised Jugular venous pressure (JVP), Dyspnea at rest or with exertion, pleuritic pain, calf or thigh pain, cough, orthopnea, wheezing
- **Management**: Anticoagulation (Heparin), Warfarin

Tuberculosis (TB)

- Tuberculosis, or TB, is an infectious bacterial disease caused by ***Mycobacterium tuberculosis***, which most commonly affects the lungs.
- It is transmitted from person to person via droplets from the throat and lungs of people with the active respiratory disease.
- **Risk factors:** Immunosuppression, HIV infection, alcoholism, living in crowded areas, malnutrition, lower socio economic status, and older adults
- **Mode of spread:** Droplets
- **Incubation period:** 2–12 weeks
- Active TB infection occurs years after the exposure or when the person becomes immune compromised is known as latent infection.
- **Clinical manifestation**
  - Cough, fever, increased weight loss, night sweat and hemoptysis
  - Anorexia, weight loss, chills, fever, chest pain
- **Diagnosis:**
  - **Mantoux TB skin test:** A standard dose of 5 tuberculin units is injected intradermally. The reaction is read (48–72 hours later) by measuring the diameter of induration (palpable, raised, hardened area).
  - Chest X-ray (but not a confirmatory test)
  - Sputum smear for acid fast bacilli
  - A positive culture of *M. Tuberculosis*
- **Treatment:** (Refer Community Health Nursing synopsis for details on ATT drugs)
  - Post exposure prophylaxis is done with isoniazid for 9–12 months
  - Inactive TB case, isoniazid with rifampicin is usually the first choice; other antituberculotics include ethambutol, and pyrazinamide.

Lung Abscess

- Aspiration or entry of infectious material in the lung causes collection of purulent material in the lung parenchyma and leads to cavity formation
- **Causes:** Aspiration, following pneumonia, chest trauma
- In a bedridden patient lung abscess most commonly occurs in the posterior segment of upper lobe and superior part of the lower lobe.
- **Clinical manifestation:** Productive cough, foul smelling sputum, fever, anorexia, weakness, weight loss
- **Diagnosis:** CT, X-ray, physical assessment show pleural friction rub, crackles
- **Management:** Antibiotic therapy, chest physiotherapy and postural drainage, lobectomy is the surgery of choice.

Chest Injuries

- Blunt or penetrating injury to chest, lung, ribs, heart, great vessels, trachea and esophagus.
- Rib fracture, hemothorax, flail chest, pulmonary contusion and cardiac tamponade are different types of chest injuries.

Rib Fracture

- Most common type of chest injury which causes pneumothorax and pulmonary contusion.
- **Clinical manifestation:** Splinting of chest. Pain increases with inspiration, shallow respiration, and tenderness at injury site.
- **Management:** Pain management, Fowler's position to the client

Hemothorax

- Blood in the pleural space
- Chest tube insertion is the management

Flail Chest

- Occurs as a result of chest trauma, one portion of the chest loses its connection with remaining part of rib cage.
- Paradoxical respiration can be seen in this condition, which means the detached segment moves inward during inspiration and move outward during expiration and interfere with normal breathing process.
- **Clinical manifestation:** Severe pain, dyspnea, cyanosis, tachycardia, hypotension
- **Management:** Fowler's position, oxygen administration, respiratory support if needed, pain management.

Pulmonary Contusion

- Leakage of blood and fluid into alveoli and interstitial space.
- **Clinical manifestation:** Decreased breath sound, dyspnea, hypoxemia, hemoptysis, restlessness
- **Management:** Fowler's position, oxygen administration

Recent Questions (NORCET 2020)

41. Which of the following drug causes red color urine?
a. Streptomycin
b. Rifampicin
c. Ethambutol
d. Isoniazid

Ans. (b) Rifampicin

42. Diminished lung sound and pain during inspiration is a classical sign of
a. Hemothorax
b. Pneumothorax
c. Pyothorax
d. Chylothorax

Ans. (b) Pneumothorax

Recent Questions (CNCI 2021)

43. Which anti-tuberculosis drug causes poor vision and difficulty in color perception?
a. Streptomycin
b. Ethambutol
c. Rifampicin
d. Pyrazinamide

Ans. (b) Ethambutol

44. A 30-year-old pregnant woman is diagnosed with pulmonary tuberculosis. Which of the following anti tuberculosis drug should not be given?
a. INH
b. Rifampicin
c. Streptomycin
d. Ethambutol

Ans. (c) Streptomycin

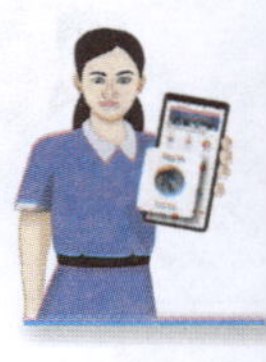

Pneumothorax

- Trapping of atmospheric air in the pleural space which leads to increased intra-thoracic pressure and decreased vital capacity
- **Management:** Fowler's position, oxygen administration, chest tube insertion.

KEY POINTS

Management of Chest Tube/ICD

- Never lift the chest drain (under water seal) drainage bottles above the level of chest
- Never clamp the ICD unless it is ordered by the physician because clamping causes tension pneumothorax.
- ICD tubing and bottles should be below the level of patient to facilitate drainage
- Tubing should be unobstructed and without kink.
- Suction is not needed always, if needed it should be prescribed by medical staff. If suction is applied, it will cause light bubbling in the suction chamber.
- Milking of the ICD should not be done without written order because it will create negative pressure—further trauma.
- Intermittent bubbling (during exhalation and cough) is expected in a client with ICD for pneumothorax. Continuous bubbling indicates, air leakage. In this case, check the tubing for disconnection and inform the physician.
- Oscillation or swing of the water is a normal finding in a client with ICD. As the pneumothorax resolves, swing will also reduce. Unexpected cessation of the oscillation or swing of water indicates kink or blockage of tubes.
- If accidental disconnection of the system occurs then clean it and reconnect the drain.
- If accidental dislodgement of chest tube occurs, then the nurse should cover the insertion site with sterile pressure dressing.
- ICD can be removed if there is no more air leakage. In case of pneumothorax there is diminished amount of secretions. X-ray shows expansion of lungs.
- While removing ICD ask the client to exhale and hold the breath.

Recent Question
(NORCET 2022)

45. A patient presents with tension pneumothorax. What will be the priority nursing intervention?
a. Wide bore needle in 2nd mid clavicular space followed by chest tube drainage
b. Providing prone position
c. Giving chest physiotherapy
d. Providing pain medication

Ans. (a) Wide bore needle in 2nd mid clavicular space followed by chest tube drainage

Occupational Lung Diseases

Table 56: Occupational lung diseases

Types of dusts	Disease
Organic dust	
Cotton dust	Byssinosis
Sugarcane dust	Bagossosis
Grain dust or Hay	Farmer's lung
Tobacco	Tobacossis
Infested wheat	Wheat weevil
Inorganic dust	
Silica	Silicosis
Asbestos	Asbestosis
Iron	Siderosis
Coal dust	Anthracosis

Recent Question
(NORCET 2023)

46. Identify the condition shown in the given image of X-ray?

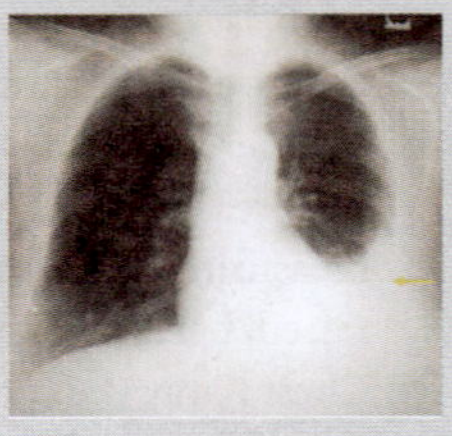

a. Pneumothorax
b. Pleural effusion
c. Pleurisy
d. Pulmonary infarction

Ans. (b) Pleural effusion

Golden Points to Remember

- **Epistaxis (nosebleed)** is bleeding from the nose.
- The amount of air passing into and out of the lungs during each cycle of breathing is referred to as **Tidal volume**. It is 500 mL for adult.
- **Total lung capacity**: The maximum amount of air contained in lungs after a maximum inspiratory effort is 6000 mL in normal adult.
- **Vital Capacity:** The maximum amount of air that can be expired after a maximum inspiratory effort is 4800 mL in normal adult.
- **Cheyne-Stokes respiration:** Progressively deeper, and sometimes faster, breathing followed by a gradual decrease that results in a temporary stop in breathing is called apnea.
- The **trachea** is a cylindrical tube about 5 inches long and 1 inch in diameter.
- **Surfactant** is a lipoprotein that lowers the surface tension in the alveoli and decreases the tendency of the alveoli to collapse. Deficiency of surfactant leads to alveolar collapse.
- **Most Important risk factor for COPD:** Cigarette smoking
- **Obstructive lung disease:** Decreased expiratory flow rates
- **Restrictive lung disease:** Decreased in lung volumes
- **Atelectasis refers** to collapsed alveoli, postoperative patient is at risk for atelectasis because of effect of anesthesia and restricted breathing with pain.
- **Hering-Breuer reflex:** As the lung inflates, pulmonary stretc.h receptors activate the inspiratory center to inhibit further lung expansion.
- **Cordectomy** is partial removal of one vocal cord.
- **Pneumocystis jiroveci** is an opportunistic pathogen which causes Pneumocystis jiroveci pneumonia in AIDS patient.
- **Tuberculin skin test (Mantoux test):** In this test purified protein derivative (PPD) is used to diagnose TB infection.
- A positive tuberculin test is indicated by induration of **10 mm or more in diameter.**
- Ethambutol causes **retrobulbar neuritis** and can result in red-green blindness.
- **Pneumoconiosis** is a group of lung disease caused by inhalation and retention of dust particle.
- **Hemothorax** is the accumulation of blood in the intrapleural space.
- **Pleurodesis** is the artificial production of adhesions between the parietal and visceral pleura, usually done with a chemical sclerosing agent.
- **Flail chest** results from a multiple rib fracture.
- The ratio of anteroposterior to transverse diameter is 1:2 in a normal adult.
- In barrel chest, the ratio of anterioposterior to transverse diameter is 1:1.
- Barrel chest is seen in **emphysema**.
- Chest tube is inserted in **sitting and lying position** with the affected side elevated.
- Posterior mid-scapular line is the preferred site for thoracentesis procedure performed in the upright or seated position.
- Hyperresonance of chest during percussion indicates pneumothorax.
- "Tracheostomy" is usually performed between the **second** and **third** cartilage rings of trachea.
- **Thoracotomy** is a surgical opening into the thoracic cavity. There are two types of thoracic incision:
  - Median sternotomy used for surgery involving the heart.
  - Lateral thoracotomy used for surgery related to lungs.
- **Pneumonia** is acute inflammation of lung tissue caused by bacteria, viruses, fungi, chemical and other factors.
- **Empyema** is pleural effusion that contains pus.
- **Emboli** are mobile clots that generally do not stop moving until they are lodged at a narrowed part of the circulatory system.
- Common symptoms of **pulmonary embolism** are anxiety, sudden onset of unexplained dyspnea, tachypnea and tachycardia.
- **D-dimer test** is done if pulmonary embolism is suspected, its level is increased 8 times in venous thromboembolism.
- **Tidal volume (TV):** It is the amount of air (500 mL) inspired during normal, relaxed breathing.
- **Treprostinil**, a prostacyclin, is used as a continuous subcutaneous injection, which causes vasodilation of the pulmonary arterial system and inhibits platelets aggregation.
- **COPD** is a chronic obstructive pulmonary disease that includes chronic bronchitis and emphysema.
- **Surgical treatment for COPD** includes lung volume reduction therapy, bullectomy and lung transplantation.
- Bronchodilator of choice in COPD: Anticholinergics
- Treatment of Choice in Bronchiectasis: postural drainage
- **Chest physiotherapy (CPT)** has no role and is not recommended for asthma because it is too stressful for breathless patient.
- **Pursed lip breathing (PLB)** is effective in acute state of asthma it keeps the airway open by maintaining positive pressure.
- **Cigarette smoking** is the major risk factor for developing COPD.
- Environmental tobacco smoke or second-hand smoke is the exposure of nonsmoker to cigarette smoke.
- **α1–Antitrypsin (AAT)** deficiency is the genetic risk factor that leads to COPD.
- Removal of an entire lung is called pneumonectomy.
- **Pulmonary Function Test (PFT)** is the confirmatory test for COPD.
- For detection of air under diaphragm most suitable X-ray is chest PA view.
- High concentration of O_2 can be delivered through non-rebreather mask.
- Pursed lip breathing is to prolong exhalation and thereby prevent bronchiolar collapse and air trapping.
- **CPT** consists of percussion, vibration and postural drainage.
- Postural drainage uses the **principle of gravity** to assist in bronchial drainage.

Contd...

- There are 18 segments in the lungs so **18 positions** are used for drainage.
- **Morphine** is contraindicated in bronchial asthma and pancreatitis.
- **Cystic fibrosis** is an autosomal recessive multisystem disease characterized by altered function of the exocrine glands, involving lungs, pancreas, and sweat glands.
- **Sweat chloride test** is performed to diagnose cystic fibrosis, sweat chloride is found four times higher than normal.
- The hallmark of **bronchiectasis** is persistent or recurrent cough with production of a large amount of purulent sputum that may exceed 500 mL/day.
- The most appropriate time for the nurse to obtain a sputum specimen for culture is **early in the morning**.
- Venturi mask is a medical device used to deliver known oxygen concentration to patient on controlled oxygen therapy.
- Venturi mask is invented by **Moran Campbell**.
- β-lactam or macrolide antibiotics are the Drug of Choice for Pneumococcal Pneumonia.
- If the chest tube dislodges, immediately it should be reconnected to the water seal. Pressure should be applied over the chest tube insertion site.
- Rifampicin leads to reddish discoloration of urine.
- Culture and Sensitivity test determines whether the prescribed antibiotics will be effective.

Most Common

- Most common agent to cause drug induced asthma: **Aspirin**
- Most common pneumothorax: **COPD**
- Most common fetal response to acute hypoxia: **Bradycardia**
- Most common site of primary TB: **Middle lobe**

"A merry heart doeth good like a medicine, but a broken spirit drieth the bones."
—Proverbs

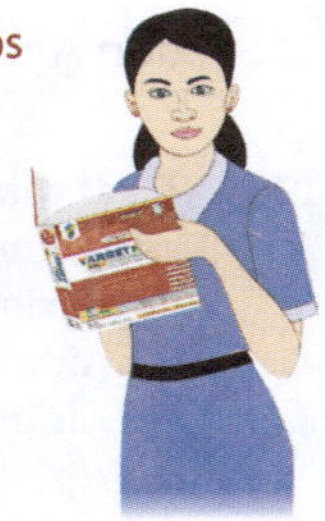

MULTIPLE CHOICE QUESTIONS
(Including Explained and Practice Questions)

RESPIRATORY SYSTEM

ANATOMY AND PHYSIOLOGY OF UPPER RESPIRATORY SYSTEM

1270. Normally respiratory center is stimulated by: *(JIPMER 2012)*
a. Oxygen b. HCO_3^-
c. Carbon Dioxide d. Lactic Acid

1271. The chemoreceptors in the medulla oblongata increases the breathing rate in response to increase in blood concentration of:
a. Oxygen b. Carbon dioxide
c. H+ d. Carbon Dioxide and H+

1272. Carina is situated at which level of .... in adult:
a. T3 b. T4
c. T6 d. T9

1273. Trachea is lined by:
a. Stratified squamous epithelium
b. Cuboidal epithelium
c. Simple columnar epithelium
d. Pseudostratified columnar epithelium

1274. The length of an adult trachea is:
a. 6–8 cm b. 10–11 cm
c. 14–15 cm d. 16–20 cm

1275. Tracheal bifurcation occurs at level:
a. T1-T2 b. T3-T4
c. T4-T5 d. None

1276. Sinuses are:
a. Cavities in nasal bone
b. Chamber containing vitreous humor in eye
c. Chamber producing ear wax
d. All of the above

1277. The cartilage that completely encircles the larynx with the narrow part anteriorly and the broadpart posteriorly is called: *(AIIMS Raipur Grade II 2017)*
a. Thyroid cartilage b. Cricoid cartilage
c. Arytenoid cartilage d. Epiglottis

Explanation: The thyroid cartilage is a hyaline cartilage structure that sits in front of the larynx and above the thyroid gland. The arytenoid cartilages are a pair of small three-sided pyramids which form part of the larynx to which the vocal folds (vocal cords) are attached. The epiglottis is a flap in the throat which keeps food from entering the windpipe and the lungs.

1278. "Tracheostomy" is usually performed between the tracheal rings of cartilage of: *(AIIMS Raipur NO 2019)*
a. Second and third b. Third and fourth
c. Fourth and fifth d. All of these

1279. Trachea starts at the level of:
a. 4th cervical vertebra b. 5th Cervical vertebra
c. 6th Cervical vertebra d. 7th Cervical vertebra

ANATOMY AND PHYSIOLOGY OF LOWER RESPIRATORY SYSTEM

1280. Muscles used in respiration are all; EXCEPT:
a. Internal intercostal muscles
b. External Intercostal Muscles
c. Diaphragm
d. Sternocleidomastoid muscles

1281. The nerve which supplies the diaphragm is:
a. Diaphragmatic b. Phrenic
c. Radial d. Sciatic

1282. Blood supply of lungs are:
a. Pulmonary artery b. Pulmonary vein
c. Bronchial artery d. All of these

1283. Which among the following activity helps in the production of surfactant?
a. Taking deep breaths b. Coughing exercises
c. Strenuous exercises d. ROM exercises

1284. The artery that supply blood to the diaphragm is called: *(AIIMS Raipur Grade II 2017)*
a. Inferior mesenteric arteryb. Suprarenal arteries
c. Inferior phrenic arteries d. Coeliac arteries

Explanation: Inferior mesenteric artery supplies large intestine and upper part of rectum. Suprarenal arteries refers to Superior, middle and inferior suprarenal arteries which supplies adrenal gland. Celiac artery supplies oxygenated blood to liver, stomach, abdominal oesophagus, spleen and superior half of both duodenum and pancreas.

LUNG VOLUME AND CAPACITIES (NORMAL VALUES)

1285. Normal Tidal Volume in adult is about:
a. 300 mL b. 500 mL
c. 1200 mL d. 3600 mL

1286. Which of the following lung volume is the base of functioning of Heimlich maneuver (abdominal thrust)?
a. Tidal volume b. Inspiratory reserve volume
c. Residual volume d. Total lung capacity

Explanation: Residual volume (RV) is a lung volume representing the amount of air left in the lungs after a forced exhalation; this volume cannot be measured, only calculated. This volume is the base of functioning of abdominal thrust.

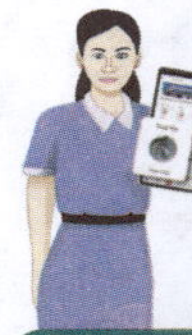

Ans.
1270. c
1271. d
1272. b
1273. d
1274. b
1275. c
1276. a
1277. b
1278. a
1279. c
1280. d
1281. b
1282. d
1283. a
1284. c
1285. b
1286. c

1287. Tidal volume is:
- a. Normal amount of air move into and out of the lung during respiration
- b. Air exhaled after normal inspiration
- c. Air inhaled after normal exhalation
- d. Air remaining in the lung after forceful exhalation

Explanation: Tidal volume is the lung volume representing the normal volume of air displaced between normal inhalation and exhalation when extra effort is not applied. In a healthy, young human adult, tidal volume is approximately 500 mL per inspiration or 7 mL/kg of body mass.

1288. All the following lung volumes can be measured by a simple spirometer; EXCEPT:
- a. Vital capacity
- b. Residual volume
- c. Tidal volume
- d. Forced vital capacity

1289. Advantage of a Venturi mask over other oxygen administration method is:
- a. Deliver 100% oxygen
- b. Prevent mucosal drying
- c. Deliver a precise concentration O_2
- d. Encourage activity

1290. Highest oxygen concentration will be delivered by:
- a. Nasal catheter
- b. Nasal cannula
- c. Partial non-rebreather mask
- d. Simple oxygen mask

Explanation: Partial masks are designed to capture the first 150 mL of the exhaled breath into the reservoir bag for inhalation during the subsequent breath. This portion of the breath was initially delivered at the end of inhalation and was therefore delivered to the "deadspace" anatomy where gas exchange did not occur. Therefore, there would be neither the depletion of oxygen nor the gain of carbon dioxide during the rebreathing component. It delivers the highest oxygen concentration from 95% to 100%.

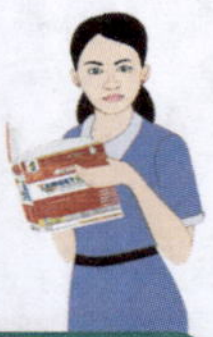

Ans.

1287. a
1288. b
1289. c
1290. c
1291. b
1292. b
1293. d
1294. d
1295. b
1296. c
1297. c
1298. d
1299. c
1300. b

ASSESSMENT AND DIAGNOSITIC TESTS

1291. A client is admitted with suspected atelectasis. Which clinical indicator does the nurse expect to identify during the assessment of client? *(RAK MSc 2018)*
- a. Slow, deep respirations
- b. Diminished breath sounds
- c. A dry, unproductive cough
- d. A normal oral temperature

Explanation: Atelectasis is a condition in which the alveoli collapses or is filled with fluid, as a result there are diminished breath sounds.

1292. Which of the following assessment findings does the nurse expect in the patient with emphysema? *(RAK MSc 2018)*
- a. Purulent sputum
- b. Diminished breath sounds
- c. Generalized edema
- d. Dull chest pain

Explanation: Emphysema, a lung disease is an irreversible, progressive condition characterized by inflammation and reduced airflow in the lungs. Diminished breath sounds are found in patient with emphysema. The reduction in the generation of sounds is due to the accompanying airflow limitation or because of poor transmission of sounds due to destruction of parenchyma.

1293. Which laboratory result should alert the nurse to perform further assessment on a patient admitted with respiratory distress? *(RAK MSc 2018)*
- a. $PaCO_2$<50 mm Hg
- b. HCO_3<27 mEq/L
- c. PaO_2<90 mm Hg
- d. SPO_2 <90%

Explanation: The laboratory result which should alert the nurse to perform further assessment on a patient admitted with respiratory distress is **SPO_2 less than 90%.**

$PaCO_2$< 50 mm Hg (normal: 35-45 mm Hg), PaO_2< 90 mm Hg (normal: 75 – 100 mm Hg) and HCO_3 < 27 mEq/L are within normal ranges.

1294. The largest volume of air, which can be expelled from the lungs during maximal expiration is called: *(AIIMS Raipur Grade II 2017)*
- a. Tidal volume
- b. Residual volume
- c. Inspiratory reserve volume
- d. Expiratory reserve volume

Explanation: Tidal volume is the measure of amount of air a person inhales during a normal breath. Tidal volume is 500 mL. Residual volume is the amount of air that remains in a person's lung after maximum exhalation. Residual volume is 1200 mL. Inspiratory reserve volume is maximum amount of additional air that can be drawn into lungs. Inspiratory reserve volume is 3100 ml. Expiratory reserve volume is about 1200 mL.

1295. The normal mean pulmonary artery pressure is: *(DSSSB 2013)*
- a. 5–10 mm Hg
- b. 10–20 mm Hg
- c. 20–30 mm Hg
- d. 30–40 mm Hg

Explanation: Pulmonary blood pressure is normally a lot lower than systemic blood pressure. Normal Pulmonary artery pressure is about 8-20 mm Hg at rest. If the pressure in the pulmonary artery is greater than 25 mm Hg at rest and 30 mm Hg during exercise, it is abnormally high and is called pulmonary hypertension.

1296. While auscultating lung field of a client with respiratory distress best method of auscultation is:
- a. Listen to the apex
- b. Begin listening at the lung bases
- c. Listen side to side from top to bottom
- d. Anterior chest then posterior chest

1297. Test used to assess the arterial oxygen status is:
- a. VBG
- b. SPO_2
- c. ABG
- d. Incentive spirometry

1298. Which among the following is the most accurate method of determining oxygen demand in a COPD client?
- a. Check respiratory rate
- b. SPO_2
- c. X-ray
- d. Blood gas analysis

1299. SPO_2 indicate:
- a. Percentage of oxygen in blood
- b. Percentage of free hemoglobin
- c. Percentage of oxyhemoglobin
- d. Respiratory rate

1300. What is indicated if pH is abnormal along with abnormal $PaCO_2$ and HCO_3^-?
- a. Compensated condition
- b. Partially compensated
- c. Uncompensated
- d. Equilibrium

1301. What is FiO_2?
a. Fraction of inspired O_2 delivered on inspiration to the patient
b. Fraction of O_2 delivered during inspiration and expiration
c. Fraction of O_2 delivered on expiration to the patient
d. Fraction of O_2 needed by the patient

1302. Characteristic respiratory sound in pulmonary edema is:
a. Crackles b. Tracheobronchial
c. Bronchial d. Adventitious

1303. Breath sound auscultated over the lung periphery except over the scapula is:
a. Vesicular b. Bronchovesicular
c. Bronchial d. Tracheal

1304. Breath sound auscultated posteriorly between the scapula and anteriorly over bronchioles lateral to sternum over 1 and 2 ICS:
a. Vesicular
b. Bronchovesicular
c. Bronchial
d. Tracheal

1305. Breath sound auscultated over the trachea is:
a. Vesicular b. Bronchovesicular
c. Bronchial d. Tracheal

1306. Chest auscultation findings in a client with pleural effusion is:
a. Wheezing
b. Vesicular
c. Diminished breath sounds
d. Grunting

1307. When is the best time for the nurse to collect the sputum specimen?
a. In the morning right after the client awakens
b. Immediately after breakfast
c. Two hours after eating
d. Shortly before the patient retires for the evening

Explanation: Early morning is the best time to collect a sputum specimen because the patient has not yet cleared the respiratory passages. The sputum is most concentrated early in the morning.

1308. Parameter needs to be monitored in a client receiving morphine injection is:
a. Deep tendon reflexes b. Respiratory rate
c. Pulse rate d. Temperature

1309. The last physiologic function that the client loses during the induction of anesthesia is:
a. Consciousness b. Cough reflex
c. Respiratory movement d. Voluntary muscle control

1310. Following bronchoscopy and biopsy which among the following sign is of immediate concern?
a. Hemoptysis b. Bronchospasm
c. Hematemesis d. Pyuria

1311. Paradoxical respiration can be seen in the following condition:
a. Phrenic nerve damage b. Flail chest
c. Rib fracture d. All of these

1312. Types of auscultating sound present over the area of consolidation?
a. Bronchovesicular b. Adventitious
c. Bronchial d. Vesicular

1313. Confirmatory test for pneumonia to determine the extent and location of the infection is:
a. Bronchoscopy
b. Chest X-ray
c. Blood cultures
d. Sputum culture and sensitivity

1314. A client with left lobar pneumonia is ready to discharge if:
a. Grunting present
b. Fever of 104°F
c. Productive cough
d. Breath sounds are present in left side

1315. Mantoux test read after 72 hours shows 3 mm induration and red color. Then the result is:
a. Risk b. Need to do the test again
c. Negative d. Positive

1316. Well-functioning of an ICD indicated by:
a. No tingling movement in the water column
b. Ensure that the drainage system is kept at the chest level.
c. Clamp the ICD every 5th hourly
d. Fluctuation of the fluid level in the water seal chamber.

1317. Laryngospasm is seen in:
a. Hyper responsiveness of air way to varying stimuli
b. Repeated traumatic attempts of endotracheal intubation
c. After GA
d. All of the above

1318. Definitive diagnostic method for pulmonary embolism is:
a. Pulmonary angiography
b. Pulmonary function test
c. Pulse oximetry
d. Ventilation-Perfusion scan

1319. A patient with shortness of breath is being tested for lung cancer. Which of the following diagnostic test will be most conclusive? *(RAK MSc 2018)*
a. Chest X-ray b. MRI
c. Sputum culture d. Biopsy

Explanation: Biopsy is the most conclusive test in the diagnosis of lung cancer. It is helpful in determining the type of lung cancer as well as the molecular or genetic profile of the tumor, whereas other tests detects the physical variations in the lung.

Chest X-ray and sputum culture are not confirmatory test for diagnosis of lung cancer. Instead of MRI, CT scan is a reliable test for diagnosis of lung cancer

1320. Which of the following finding during auscultation suggests a right pneumothorax?
a. Absence of breaths sound in the right thorax
b. Bilateral Rhonchi
c. Bilateral inspiratory crackles
d. All of the above

1321. Confirmatory diagnostic test for pneumothorax is:
a. Auscultating breath sounds
b. Sputum culture
c. Chest X-ray
d. Bronchoscopy

1322. Mantoux test is the sensitivity test for: *(Staff Nurse G II 2014)*
a. AIDS
b. Bronchial asthma
c. Allergic disorders
d. Tuberculosis

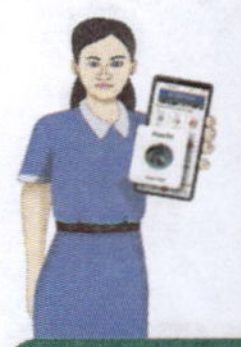

Ans.

1301. a
1302. a
1303. a
1304. b
1305. d
1306. c
1307. a
1308. b
1309. c
1310. b
1311. d
1312. c
1313. b
1314. d
1315. c
1316. d
1317. d
1318. a
1319. d
1320. a
1321. c
1322. d

1323. A positive tuberculin test is indicated by induration of:
a. 1-3 mm in diameter b. 10 mm or more in diameter
c. 7-9 mm in diameter d. 4-6 mm in diameter

Explanation: Tuberculin skin test is one of the important and widely used tests for the diagnosis of Tuberculosis (TB). One ml of Purified Protein Derivative (PPD) will be injected intradermally and will read 48 to 72 hours later. The result will be depending upon the medical risk factors and sites of induration.

5 mm or more is positive in:
- HIV positive person
- Recent contact with active TB cases
- Person with nodular or fibrotic changes in chest X-ray
- Organ transplant recipients and other immunosuppressed patients.
- Patient on long-term systemic corticosteroid therapy
- Patient on long-term systemic corticosteroid therapy
- End Stage Renal Disease

10 mm is positive in
- Recent arrival from high prevalence country
- IV drug abusers
- Residence and employers of high-risk congregate settings
- Mycobacterial lab personnel
- Person with clinical conditions that place them high risk, e.g., diabetes, leukemia, LBW, ESRD.
- Children less than 4 years of age.

15 mm or more is positive in:
- Person with no known risk for TB

1324. The purpose of chest X-ray in a Mantoux positive client is:
a. Determine the category
b. To confirm the diagnosis
c. Determine the extent of lesions
d. Determine the duration of treatment

1325. Mantoux test performed in a nurse who is working in TB clinic will be:
a. Negative skin test b. Suffering from TB
c. Need hospitalization d. A positive skin test

1326. Definitive diagnostic test for TB is:
a. Chest X-ray b. Mantoux test
c. Sputum culture d. Thoracentesis

BREATHING PATTERNS

1327. Atmospheric pressure is important for:
a. Blood Flow b. Micturition
c. Reproduction d. Breathing

1328. Which substance forms approximately 20% of air?
a. Oxygen b. Carbon dioxide
c. Nitrous Oxide d. Carbon monoxide

1329. Relaxation of internal intercostals muscles causes:
a. Inspiration b. Expiration
c. No effect on respiration d. Both a and b

1330. Relaxation of external intercostal muscles causes:
a. Inspiration b. Expiration
c. No effect on respiration d. Both a and b

1331. The actual gas exchange with blood occurs in the:
a. Bronchi
b. Respiratory bronchioles
c. Terminal bronchioles
d. Alveolar ducts and alveoli

1332. Which of the following statements concerning ventilation is NOT correct?
a. During inspiration, the pressure in the alveoli is less than atmospheric pressure.
b. When the diaphragm contracts, the thoracic cavity volume increases.
c. Contraction of the external intercostal muscles decreases the volume of the thoracic cavity.
d. During quiet breathing, passive recoil of the lung and thoracic wall causes expiration.

1333. Which one of the following factors does NOT influence the exchange of gases across the respiratory membrane?
a. The thickness of the membrane
b. The total surface area of the membrane
c. The size of the pores in the alveoli
d. The concentration gradient for gases across the membrane

1334. Most carbon dioxide is transported:
a. As bicarbonate ions in the blood
b. In dissolved form in the plasma
c. In combination with blood proteins
d. In combination with sodium ions in the blood

1335. When carbon dioxide level in the blood increases:
a. pH of the blood increases
b. The blood becomes more acidic
c. The number of hydrogen ions decreases
d. All of the above occur

1336. Normal Inspiration: Expiration time ratio at rest is:
a. 1:1 b. 2:1
c. 1:2 d. 1:3

1337. External respiration is:
a. Exchange of gases between the blood and lungs
b. Exchange of gases between the blood and the cells
c. Transportation of oxygen from lung tissues to hemoglobin
d. Combining oxygen with RBCs to form oxyhemoglobin

1338. Internal respiration is:
a. Exchange of gases between the blood and lungs
b. Exchange of gases between the blood and the cells
c. Transportation of oxygen from lungs to tissues
d. Combining oxygen with RBCs to form oxyhemoglobin

1339. Stimulation of chemoreceptors occur if:
a. Partial pressure of CO_2 decreases
b. Partial pressure of CO_2 increases
c. Partial pressure of O_2 is normal
d. Partial pressure of O_2 decreases

1340. During exercise, the respiration rate increases primarily because of:
a. Increased blood carbon dioxide levels
b. Decreased blood oxygen levels
c. Decreased blood pH levels
d. Limb movements and input from the cerebrum

1341. Maximum CO_2 is carried in the blood in which form?
a. Plasma b. Hemoglobin
c. Bicarbonate d. Lactate

1342. Hyperventilation of lungs leads to:
a. Respiratory acidosis b. Respiratory alkalosis
c. Metabolic acidosis d. Metabolic alkalosis

1343. Which of the following does not cause hyperventilation?
a. Anxiety b. Psychotic illness
c. Pulmonary hypertension d. High altitude

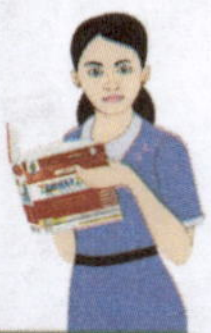

Ans.
1323. b
1324. c
1325. d
1326. c
1327. d
1328. a
1329. a
1330. b
1331. d
1332. c
1333. c
1334. a
1335. b
1336. c
1337. a
1338. b
1339. b
1340. b
1341. c
1342. b
1343. c

1344. Correct option regarding breathing exercise is:
a. Helps to reduce pulmonary complications
b. Use pursed lip breathing techniques
c. Place hand on the abdomen and feel its rise
d. All of the above

1345. Correct option regarding deep breathing exercise is:
a. Place hands on abdomen while performing
b. Take deep breaths
c. Exhale in pursed lip manner
d. All of the above

1346. Difficulty in breathing is:
a. Dyspnea
b. Dysphagia
c. Dyspepsia
d. Dysphonia

Explanation: Option A is the correct answer, option B indicates difficulty in swallowing, C indicates difficulty in digestion and D indicates difficulty in speaking.

ACUTE RESPIRATORY DISTRESS SYNDROME (ARDS)

1347. Early sign and symptom of hypoxia is:
a. Cyanosis
b. Apprehension and restlessness
c. Convulsion
d. Altered level of consciousness

1348. Most common early clinical manifestations of ARDS are:
a. Dyspnea and tachypnea
b. Restlessness and grunting
c. Bradypnea and tachycardia
d. Cyanosis

1349. Which among the following is necessary for the maintenance of fluid balance in the patient with ARDS?
a. Hydration using hypertonic solution
b. Provide humidified oxygen
c. Fluid restriction and diuretics
d. Daily electrolyte monitoring

1350. Identify the correct statement regarding acute respiratory distress syndrome (ARDS):
a. Alveoli are over expanded
b. Alveoli lost elasticity
c. Alveolar spaces are filled with fluid
d. Alveoli are collapsed

1351. Which of the following is NOT a sign of respiratory distress in a newborn? *(AIIMS-BBS SNO 2019)*
a. Cyanosis
b. Expiratory grunting
c. Sternal retractions
d. Respiratory rate varying according to the newborn's activity

Explanation: Respiratory rate normally varies with newborn's activity. So, it is not a sign of respiratory distress.

ACUTE RESPIRATORY FAILURE

1352. Which of the following is the earliest sign of poor respiratory function? *(ESIC Chennai May 2012)*
a. Fast thready pulse
b. Restlessness
c. Cyanosis
d. Faintness

1353. The highest risk for respiratory failure is present in:
a. A client with asthma
b. A client with COPD
c. A client with pericarditis
d. A client with Guillain-Barre syndrome

1354. All of the following are the possible causes of type I respiratory failure; EXCEPT?
a. Pneumonia
b. Pulmonary embolism
c. Pulmonary edema
d. Guillain-Barre syndrome

Explanation: Respiratory failure is classified according to blood gases abnormalities into type 1 and type 2. Type 1 (hypoxemic) respiratory failure has a P_aO_2 < 60 mm Hg with normal or subnormal P_aCO_2. Type 2 (hypercapnic) respiratory failure has a P_aCO_2 >50 mm Hg. Hypoxemia is common, and it is due to respiratory pump failure. Respiratory muscle and chest wall weakness as in cases of Guillian-Barre syndrome and myasthenia gravis are likely cause of type II respiratory failure. All other given conditions are associated with type I respiratory failure.

1355. An emergency treatment for an acute asthmatic attack is:
a. Adrenaline 1:100
b. Adrenaline 1:1000
c. Betamethasone
d. Hydrocortisone

Explanation: Acute asthmatic attack is characterized by severe bronchospasm. An emergency treatment for an acute asthmatic attack is Adrenaline 1:1000 given intradermally relax the bronchial smooth muscle.

1356. Type II respiratory failure may occur as a result of:
a. Ventilation perfusion mismatch
b. Poor respiratory effect
c. Right to left cardiac shunt
d. Fluid in the alveoli

1357. Complication associated with tracheostomy is:
a. Damage to the laryngeal nerve
b. Bronchoconstriction
c. Pneumonia
d. Excessive secretions

1358. An adult patient is scheduled for a tracheostomy. Which of the following nursing action is the priority for this client?
a. Insert a Foley catheter
b. Establish a means of communication
c. Prepare the bowel by administering enemas until clear
d. Start an IV line

Explanation: Preoperatively, the priority nursing action for the patient who is undergoing tracheostomy is to establish a means of communication because the patient will not be able to speak after the tracheostomy is performed.

1359. The priority nursing diagnosis for the client with tracheostomy is: *(Bihar PSC 2010)*
a. Pain related to tracheostomy
b. Impaired verbal communication related to tracheostomy procedure
c. Ineffective airway clearance related to increased tracheobronchial secretions
d. Risk for impaired skin integrity related to tracheostomy incision

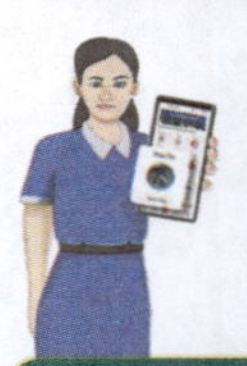

Ans.

1344. d
1345. d
1346. a
1347. b
1348. a
1349. c
1350. c
1351. d
1352. b
1353. d
1354. d
1355. b
1356. b
1357. a
1358. b
1359. c

Explanation: Ineffective airway clearance is the priority nursing diagnosis for the patient with tracheostomy tube in place because it is important to maintain airway clear from tracheobronchial secretions. The ABC (airway, breathing and circulation) protocol assists the nurse to prioritize airway clearance.

1360. An adult man has a tracheostomy tube in place. Which of the following actions is appropriate for the nurse to take when suctioning the tracheostomy?

a. Use a sterile tube each time and suction for 20 seconds
b. Use sterile technique and turn the suction off as the catheter is introduced
c. Use clean technique and suction for 15 seconds
d. Discard the catheter at the end of every shift

Explanation: Suctioning should be done under sterile technique for no more than 10 seconds. The suction should be off as the tube is inserted and applied intermittently as it is withdrawn.

1361. Nursing action while doing tracheostomy suction includes:

a. Pre-oxygenate the client
b. Strict aseptic technique while doing suctioning
c. Assessing the patient's oxygenation saturation before, during, and after suctioning
d. All of the above

1362. When suctioning the tracheostomy tube we must limit the suctioning to a maximum of:

a. 5 sec b. 10 sec
c. 15 sec d. 20 sec

1363. A patient, with portex tracheostomy tube, develops sudden complete blockage of the tube. Which of the following is the best intervention to prevent complication?

(AIIMS Bhopal Grade-I 2018)

a. Ausculate for breath sounds
b. Deflate the tracheostomy cuff and supply high flow oxygen
c. Suction of tube with normal saline
d. Immediate removal of the tracheostomy tube

Explanation: The best intervention to prevent the complication is **immediate removal of the tracheostomy tube** because the most frequent cause of blockage is plugging of the tracheostomy tube with a crust or mucous plug. These plugs can also be aspirated and lead to atelectasis or lung abscess. Deflation of the tracheostomy tube is not appropriate because that will not clear the plug material of the tube.

1364. What happens if the cuff pressure of ET tube exceeds the normal limit?

a. ET tube dislodge
b. Air leak occurs
c. Mucosal damage occurs
d. Secretions will pool off around the cuff

1365. Parts of a tracheostomy tube include:

a. Outer cannula with cuff
b. Inner cannula
c. Obturator
d. All of the above

1366. Non-traumatic insertion of tracheostomy tube is achieved with the help of:

a. Outer cannula with cuff b. Inner cannula
c. Obturator d. All of these

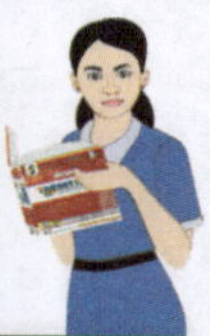

Ans.

1360. b
1361. d
1362. b
1363. d
1364. c
1365. d
1366. c
1367. c
1368. b
1369. d
1370. d
1371. b
1372. c
1373. a
1374. d

ASTHMA

1367. Characteristic sign of asthma:

a. Cyanosis b. Grunting
c. Wheezing d. Cough

1368. In which condition Charcot-Leyden crystals are seen in sputum?

a. TB b. Bronchial asthma
c. Pneumonia d. Empyema

1369. Advantage of using spacer in MDI is:

a. Easier for medication to reach the lungs
b. Less medication gets deposited in the mouth and throat
c. Helps to coordinate breathing in and activating an MDI
d. All of the above

Explanation: A **spacer (Asthma spacer)** is a device used to increase the ease of administering aerosolized medication from a metered-dose inhaler (**MDI**). It adds space in the form of a tube or "chamber" between the mouth and canister of medication. Spacers can make it easier for medication to reach the lungs, and also mean less medication gets deposited in the mouth and throat, where it can lead to irritation and mild infections.

1370. Best for treatment of Exercise induced asthma?

a. Montelukast b. Salbutamol
c. Ipratropium
d. Low dose Inhaled corticosteroids

1371. Main drug of choice to treat asthma is:

a. Antibiotics b. Bronchodilators
c. Anticholinergics d. Muscle relaxant

1372. Which of the following conditions is NOT commonly associated with long-standing, uncontrolled asthma?

a. COPD b. Emphysema **New Q**
c. Atelectasis d. Pneumonia

Explanation: Long-standing, uncontrolled asthma (chronic asthma) can indeed be associated with certain respiratory conditions such as COPD and emphysema. Chronic inflammation and ongoing damage to the airways in asthma can contribute to the development of these conditions over time.

Individuals with chronic asthma are also more prone to developing lung infections, including pneumonia.

Atelectasis is the collapse of a lung. It is not commonly associated with asthma because the inflammation and narrowing of the airways that are characteristic of asthma do not typically lead to the collapse of a lung.

1373. Highest nursing priority for a client with status asthmatics is:

a. Avoiding intubation
b. Adherence to treatment
c. Monitor respiratory status
d. Prevent complications

1374. Nurse Ramya is suctioning a tracheostomy tube of an adult patient. During the procedure, the catheter appears to attach to the tracheal wall and creates a pulling sensation. What is the best action for the nurse to take?

a. Continue suctioning until the obstruction removed
b. Increase the pressure of suction
c. Insert the tube deeper and apply more pressure
d. Release the suction by opening the vent

Explanation: Suction should not be applied as the suction tube is inserted, because this will cause the suction tube to appear to attach to the tracheal wall and create a pulling sensation. If pulling sensation is created during suction, release the suction by opening the vent.

BRONCHITIS

1375. Permanent abnormal dilation and destruction of bronchi and bronchioles is known as:
a. Atelectasis b. Asthma
c. Emphysema d. Bronchiectasis

1376. Complication of bronchiectasis is .... *(JIPMER 2001)*
a. Cerebral abscess b. Lung abscess
c. Amyloidosis d. All of these

1377. Which of the following findings is expected in chronic bronchitis?
a. Barrel chest b. Rales
c. Stridor d. Hyperpnea

1378. Which of the following health teaching is essential for a client diagnosed with chronic bronchitis?
a. Increase fluid intake b. Restrict the fluid intake
c. Strenuous exercise d. None of these

Explanation: Increasing fluid intake is a crucial recommendation for individuals with chronic bronchitis. Adequate hydration helps to thin the mucus in the airways, making it easier to clear and reducing the risk of mucus plugs and exacerbations. It also helps to keep the airways moist and can ease coughing and promote comfort.

Strenuous exercise, may not be appropriate for all individuals with chronic bronchitis.

1379. Oral terbutaline drug should be used in caution for the persons who has:
a. Strabismus b. Hyperthroidism
c. Hypothyroidim d. Diabetes insipidus

1380. Which of the following is the priority nursing diagnosis for the client with bronchitis?
a. Sleep pattern disturbance
b. Impaired skin integration
c. Ineffective breathing pattern
d. Knowledge deficit

1381. A student nurse has conducted a health talk for a patient diagnosed with bronchitis. Which of the following statement made by the patient after the health talk indicates that the student nurse has given an effective health talk to this patient?
a. I should stop smoking
b. I will able to take hot and spicy foods
c. I must restrict fluid intake
d. If the symptoms are present, then I can stop the medications

CHRONIC OBSTRUCTIVE PULMONARY DISEASE (COPD)

1382. Classic barrel-shaped chest is seen in patients with: *(Staff Nurse G II 2014)*
a. Congestive cardiac failure
b. COPD
c. Bronchiectasis
d. Pulmonary effusion

1383. Which term should be used to document the musical sounds generated by airflow through narrowed airways? *(RAK MSc 2018)*
a. Crackles b. Wheezes
c. Friction rub d. Stridor

Explanation: Wheezes are musical sounds caused by air movement through constricted small airways, such as bronchioles. This high-pitched whistling noise happens during breathing in or out. Stridor is a high-pitched sound originating from the upper airway and occurring on inspiration. Like wheezes, stridor is produced by airway narrowing, but only in the upper airways.

1384. The two main forms of COPD are:
a. Asthma and chronic bronchitis
b. Asthma and Emphysema
c. Chronic bronchitis and atelectasis
d. Chronic bronchitis and emphysema

1385. Respiratory drive is maintained in a COPD client by:
a. Oxygen b. Carbon dioxide
c. Nitrogen d. Oxyhemoglobin

1386. Respiratory drive in COPD patient is:
a. Oxygen b. Carbon dioxide
c. PO_2 d. pH of the blood

Explanation: The hypoxic drive is a form of respiratory drive in which the body uses oxygen chemoreceptors instead of carbon dioxide receptors to regulate the respiratory cycle. Hypoxic stimuli is the respiratory drive in COPD patient. When there is an increase in oxygen levels the body will decrease the rate of respiration. To maintain this respiratory drive in patient with COPD Oxygen at 1–2 L/min is given.

1387. Long-term outcome of COPD includes:
a. Hypoxemia b. Hypercapnia
c. Leukopenia d. All of these

1388. Nursing care for a COPD client include:
a. High flow rate of O_2
b. Cholinergic agents
c. Use spacer
d. Breathing exercise such as pursed-lip breathing that focus on exhalation

1389. In a patient with COPD, best management option is:
a. Quit smoking b. Bronchodilators
c. Low flow oxygen d. Mucolytics

1390. A 52-year-old male client is admitted with chronic obstructive pulmonary disease (COPD). The nurse notes that he has neck vein distention and slight peripheral edema. These signs indicate the onset of:
a. Cardiogenic shock b. Cor pulmonale
c. Left-sided heart failure d. Pneumothorax

Explanation: Cor pulmonale is a condition that causes the right side of the heart to fail. It is manifested by jugular venous distention (distended neck vein) and peripheral edema.

1391. Blue bloater is known as:
a. COPD
b. ARDS
c. Chronic obstructive bronchitis
d. Emphysema

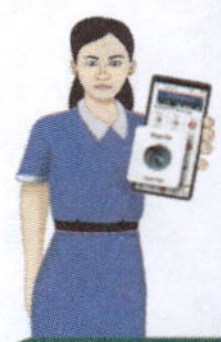

Ans.
1375. d
1376. d
1377. a
1378. a
1379. b
1380. c
1381. a
1382. b
1383. b
1384. d
1385. a
1386. a
1387. d
1388. d
1389. c
1390. b
1391. c

1392. Which is a high pitched lung sound? *(NORCET 2021)*

a. Wheezes b. Rhonchi
c. Rales d. Coarse crackles

1393. Most important nursing intervention while caring a person with artificial airway is:

a. Maintain the patency of the tube
b. Administer antibiotic as ordered
c. Monitor ventilator parameter
d. Monitor SPO_2

1394. Which of the following is most suitable method for long-term management of airway:

a. Endotracheal intubation
b. Tracheostomy
c. Nasal prongs
d. Oxygen mask

1395. Which among the following devices assists a critical patient in breathing? *(AIIMS Raipur staff nurse grade I-2018)*

a. Gamco machine
b. Ventilator machine
c. Defibrillator machine
d. Oxygen humidifier

Explanation: Ventilator is the mechanical device which assist a person in breathing. Defibrillator is the mechanical device used to treat life-threatening cardiac dysrhythmias. Oxygen humidifier is a device used to humidify oxygen before supplying to patient.

1396. Which among the following is present in a client receiving positive end-expiratory pressure (PEEP) therapy?

a. Bradypnea b. Tachycardia
c. Hypertension d. Reduced cardiac output

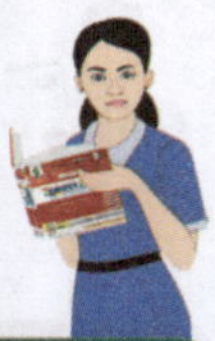

1397. Which of the following artificial ventilation mode is best suitable for a patient with respiratory arrest? *(AIIMS Raipur Grade II 2017)*

a. Continuous positive airway pressure
b. Continuous mandatory ventilation
c. Assistant-controlled mandatory ventilation
d. Non-invasive positive pressure ventilation

Explanation: Continuous Mandatory Ventilation (CMV) is a mode of mechanical ventilation in which breaths are delivered based on set variables which is preferred in respiratory arrest.

Continuous positive airway pressure is used in patients with complex underlying respiratory diseases.

Non-invasive positive pressure ventilation is used in patients with COPD who are having exacerbations and patients with hypercapnic respiratory distress.

RESPIRATORY INFECTIONS

1398. Upper airway illness that results from swelling of the epiglottis and larynx is broadly called: *(AIIMS BPL NO 2018)*

a. Measles b. Rubella
c. Croup d. Whooping cough

Explanation: Croup, also known as laryngotracheobronchitis, is a type of upper airway infection that is usually caused by a Parainfluenza virus. Obstruction of airway causes a characteristic barking cough.

1399. All are upper respiratory tract infection; EXCEPT:

a. Rhinitis b. Coryza
c. Bronchiolitis d. Laryngitis

1400. Expected color of the drainage in acute rhinitis is:

a. Clear b. Green
c. Yellow d. Greyish

Explanation: The color of nasal drainage in acute rhinitis is normally clear. The drainage will be yellow or green when there is an infection to the sinuses. Gray drainage is a sign of secondary infection.

1401. Greenish tinge sputum is seen in .... infection.

a. Streptococci b. Staphylococci
c. Plasmodium d. Pseudomonas

1402. The nutritional management of patient with acute pharyngitis includes: *(AIIMS Raipur Grade II 2017)*

a. Advice for liquid or soft diet
b. Administer IV fluids for hydration
c. Advice to avoid cool beverages and ice creams
d. Advice to drink more fluids.

a. a, b, c b. b, c, d
c. a, c, d d. a, b, c, d

Explanation: The nutritional management includes administration of salt water, honey , warm soups and soft foods. Avoid foods such as Dry/fried foods, citrus foods, pickled foods, foods having vinegar, spicy foods, alcohol and caffeine.

1403. Which among the following is a risk factor for pneumonia?

a. Seasonal change b. Living in crowded place
c. Mosquito d. Malnutrition

1404. Which of the following nursing diagnosis is a priority for a patient diagnosed with pneumonia?

a. Fluid volume deficit
b. Impaired gas exchange
c. Ineffective coping
d. Risk for infection

Explanation: Pneumonia is an inflammation of the lung parenchyma, associated with alveolar edema and congestion that impair gas exchange.

1405. A 65-year-old male client is admitted to the hospital with a diagnosis of pneumococcal pneumonia. The client has dyspnea. The client's temperature is 101°F, respirations are 34, and pulse is 94. Bed rest is ordered for this client primarily to:

a. Decrease metabolic needs
b. Prevent the development of atelectasis
c. Prevent pneumothorax
d. Promote postural drainage

Explanation: The client is having difficulty in breathing and meeting the oxygen needs. Providing bed rest will reduce the metabolic needs of the client, so reduced oxygen need.

1406. A client who smokes two packs of cigarettes per day is most at risk postoperatively for: *(AIIMS Raipur Staff Nurse Grade I-2018)*

a. Infection b. Pneumonia
c. Hypotension d. Cardiac dysrhythmias

Ans.

1392. a
1393. a
1394. b
1395. b
1396. d
1397. b
1398. c
1399. c
1400. a
1401. d
1402. c
1403. b
1404. b
1405. a
1406. b

Explanation: Smoking affects lungs and respiration, so post operatively client is at risk for developing respiratory complications, so from the given options client is at risk for developing pneumonia.

1407. First stage of pneumonia is:
a. Congestion b. Red hepatization
c. Gray hepatization d. Resolution

1408. Final stage of pneumonia is:
a. Congestion b. Red hepatization
c. Gray hepatization d. Resolution

1409. The common cause for bacterial sore throat is: *(DSSSB PHN, 2015)*
a. Beta-hemolytic streptococcus
b. Mycoplasma pneumonia
c. Corynebacterium
d. Mycobacterium

1410. Most commonly seen organism in tonsillitis is:
a. Streptococci b. Shigella
c. Flagella d. Staphylococci

1411. Commonest complication of measles in children is:
a. Septicemia b. Otitis media
c. Meningitis d. Bronchopneumonia

1412. Complication of mumps infection in male is:
a. Pancreatitis b. Laryngitis
c. Orchitis d. Glomerulonephritis

1413. Organism responsible for community-acquired pneumonia is:
a. Gonococci
b. E. coli
c. Streptococcus pneumonia
d. Shigella

1414. Major cause of nosocomial pneumonia is:
a. Gram +ve bacilli b. Gram –ve bacilli
c. Gram +ve cocci d. Gram –ve cocci

1415. A factor predisposing a person to nosocomial pneumonia is: *(AIIMS Bhopal Grade-I 2018)*
a. Oropharyngeal colonization due to mouth breathing
b. Use of nasogastric tube
c. Endotracheal intubation
d. Use of H_2 antagonist

Explanation: Nosocomial Pneumonia remains a common complication in patients treated with endotracheal intubation and mechanical ventilation due to various reasons like endotracheal tube has direct effect on the airway that results in reduction in local host defense mechanism and mucosal injury can reduce the mucociliary function which further reduces effectiveness of the cough.

1416. A client is suspected to be suffering from histoplasmosis. Which of the following factor is associated with the diagnosis of histoplasmosis?
a. He drinks raw cow milk
b. He walks bare footed in field
c. He handles fertilizer frequently
d. He cleans chicken houses

Explanation: Histoplasmosis is a disease caused by the fungus histoplasma capsulatum. This fungus grows in chicken and pigeon manure. Person who cleans chicken house is at risk of infection with histoplasma capsulatum.

1417. Which of the following drug is prescribed for the treatment of histoplasmosis?
a. Penicillin b. Chloromycetin
c. Streptomycin d. Amphotericin B

Explanation: Histoplasmosis is a fungal infection caused by histoplasma capsulatum. Amphotericin B is an antifungal agent and drug of choice to treats histoplasmosis. Other three drugs are antibiotics.

1418. Causative agent of Farmer's lung is:
a. Thermophilus actinomycetes
b. Penicillium glabrum
c. Rhizopus
d. Aspergillus

1419. Ventilator-associated pneumonia is defined as pneumonia that occur ____ or after ET intubation.
a. 12 hours b. 24 hours
c. 36 hours d. 48 hours

1420. Immediate treatment of tension pneumothorax involves insertion of needle into ______ intercostals space.
a. 6th b. 5th
c. 3rd d. 2nd

1421. The priority treatment for a client with spontaneous pneumothorax is:
a. High fowlers position b. Activity restriction
c. Chest tube placement d. Hyperbaric chamber

ATELECTASIS

1422. Collapse of lung is called:
a. Atelectasis b. Emphysema
c. Bronchitis d. Bronchiectasis

1423. Collapse of the alveoli is:
a. Atelectasis b. Asthma
c. Emphysema d. Bronchiectasis

1424. Identify the clinical manifestation of atelectasis among the following?
a. Diminished breaths sound
b. Rapid and shallow respiration
c. Loose productive cough
d. All of the above

Explanation: Atelectasis is the collapse or closure of a lung resulting in reduced or absent gas exchange. It may affect part or all of a lung.

1425. What is the priority intervention for a client diagnosed with atelectasis?
a. Monitor the oxygen saturation level
b. Monitor the vital signs
c. Use incentive spirometer every hour
d. Assess the pain level

1426. Nurse Ramya is assessing a client having history of smoking for past 18 years. Assessment findings revealed that the client had diminished breath sound, decreased oxygen saturation level and achieve 500 ml only on incentive spirometer. What is the appropriate interpretation of the findings?
a. Atelectasis b. COPD
c. Emphysema d. Empyema

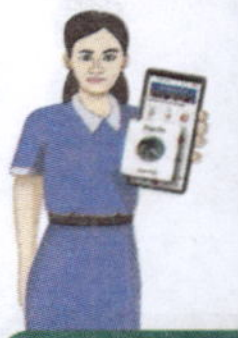

Ans.
1407. a
1408. d
1409. a
1410. a
1411. b
1412. c
1413. c
1414. b
1415. c
1416. d
1417. d
1418. a
1419. d
1420. d
1421. c
1422. a
1423. a
1424. d
1425. c
1426. a

1427. Which of the following respiratory complication is most common after surgery?

a. Pulmonary embolism b. Empyema
c. Atelectasis d. Pulmonary edema

1428. Which of the following is not the type of atelectasis?

a. Obstructive b. Restrictive
c. Compressive d. Adhesive

EMPHYSEMA

1429. Barrel chest is seen in: *(Daman and Diu NO 2018)*

a. Pneumonia b. Rickets
c. Kyphoscoliosis d. Emphysema

Explanation: In a normal adult chest, the ratio of anteroposterior to transverse diameter is 1:2, whereas in barrel chest, it is 1:1 due to the enlargement of anteroposterior diameter. Barrel chest is most often associated with **Emphysema.** It occurs because the lungs are chronically overinflated with air, so the rib cage stays partially expanded all the time.

1430. The destruction of alveolar walls is called: *(RRB SSNE 2015)*

a. Empyema b. Bronchitis
c. Emphysema d. Lung abscess

1431. Pink puffer is known as:

a. COPD
b. ARDS
c. Chronic obstructive bronchitis
d. Emphysema

1432. A 65-year-old male patient with emphysema and acute upper respiratory infection is admitted. Oxygen is ordered at 2 L/min. The reason for low-flow oxygen is to:

a. Compensate for airway resistance
b. Facilitate oxygen diffusion
c. Prevent depression of the respiratory drive
d. Prevent excessive drying of secretions

Explanation: The stimulus to breathe in a person with COPD is a low oxygen level rather than a high carbon dioxide level, as in normal persons. If high-flow oxygen were given, the oxygen level would increase, and the respiratory drive would cease.

1433. The nurse administers oxygen at 5 L/min via nasal cannula to a client with emphysema. For which clinical indicators should the nurse closely observe the client? *(RAK MSc 2018)*

a. Cyanosis and lethargy
b. Anxiety and tachycardia
c. Drowsiness and decreased respirations
d. Hyperemia and increased respirations

Explanation:

- Emphysema is a type of COPD where alveoli are damaged and are unable to receive enough oxygen unless provided in a higher concentration on a long-term basis. As stated above that nasal cannulas are used, they are capable of delivering 24%–44% of oxygen at 1–6 L/min.
- Administering oxygen for long-term around 12–15 hours a day may also cause a complication called hypercapnia, i.e. carbon dioxide retention due to oxygen toxicity. These causes symptoms such as drowsiness, decreased respirations, headache and sometimes death.

PULMONARY EDEMA AND PLEURAL EFFUSION

1434. Management of pleural effusion is:

a. Paracentesis b. Thoracentesis
c. Lumbar puncture d. Ventriculopleural shunt

1435. Expected finding in a client with right lung pleural effusion is:

a. Tracheal deviation
b. Absence of breath sound in the right side of lung
c. Wheezing
d. Subcutaneous emphysema

1436. Which among the following blood gas value is most suggestive of pulmonary edema?

a. Decrease in oxygen
b. Increase in oxygen
c. Decrease in carbon dioxide
d. Increases in carbon dioxide

1437. Typical sign of pleurisy is:

a. Sharp stabbing pain when breathing
b. Hemoptysis
c. Hematemesis
d. Dyspnea

1438. Identify correct statement regarding pleural fluid?

a. Very minimal amount is present
b. Helps to reduce friction between visceral and parietal pleura
c. Act as a lubricant
d. All of the above

1439. Pleural effusion is present in all of the following; EXCEPT:

a. Congestive heart failure b. Cirrhosis
c. Nephrotic syndrome d. Angina Pectoris

1440. What nursing action will most help a client obtain maximum benefits after postural drainage? *(RAK MSc 2018)*

a. Administer PRN oxygen
b. Place the client in a sitting position
c. Encourage the client to cough deeply
d. Encourage the client to rest for 30 minutes

Explanation: Postural drainage is an airway clearance technique that helps people clear mucus from their lungs. Postural drainage helps to dislodge and loosen the secretions. It uses gravity and percussion (clapping on the chest and/or back) to loosen the thick, sticky mucus in the lungs so it can be removed by coughing. Therefore, patient is encouraged to **cough deeply** so that the loosened secretions are easily removed.

1441. Chest tube inserted into 2nd or 3rd intercostal space suggestive of:

a. Pneumothorax b. Hemothorax
c. Pyothorax d. Emphysema

1442. Chest tube inserted into 4th or 5th intercostal space suggestive of:

a. Pneumothorax b. Hemothorax
c. Pyothorax d. Emphysema

1443. Clamping of chest tube will lead to:

a. Atelectasis b. Tension pneumothorax
c. Emphysema d. Pneumonia

1444. Which among the following finding indicates correct chest tube placement?

a. Respiratory sounds are absent
b. Vesicular sounds heard over upper lung fields
c. Bronchovesicular sounds heard over both lung fields
d. Crackles heard on the affected side

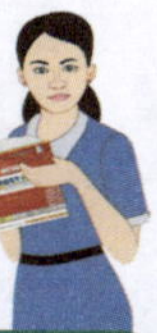

Ans.

1427. c
1428. b
1429. d
1430. c
1431. d
1432. c
1433. c
1434. b
1435. b
1436. d
1437. a
1438. d
1439. d
1440. c
1441. a
1442. b
1443. b
1444. c

1445. In a client with chest tube lack of fluctuation of water in a water seal chamber occurs because of:

a. Kinking of tube
b. Re-expansion of lung
c. Both a and b
d. None of these

Explanation: Fluctuation of water will stop in two conditions, either because of kinking or obstruction in the tube or because of chest re-expansion is completed.

1446. A patient had chest tubes on his right chest which were connected to the water seal, during ambulation, the tubes got dislodged from the water seal. Which of the following actions by the nurse would be appropriate? *(AIIMS Bhopal Grade-I 2018)*

a. Instruct the patient to cough forcibly several times
b. Assess the lung sound of the patient
c. Place the patient on bed and provide oxygenation
d. Reconnect the tubes to water seal

Explanation: During ambulation if chest tubes got dislodged from the water seal, the primary step is to reconnect the tubes to the water seal. This is to prevent any entry of air accidentally into the chest cavity, after that assist the client to ambulate back to the bed and auscultate breathing sounds bilaterally to determine any type of air entry. Client is never be instructed to cough when chest tubes gets dislodged because it promotes air entry into the chest cavity.

1447. How do you know that intercostal drainage tube is functioning? *(RAK MSc 2018)*

a. Continuous bubbling in water seal bottle
b. Continuous bubbling from suction tube
c. Oscillation of water column in drainage bottle
d. No bubbling in the drainage bottle

Explanation:

- The functioning of intercostal drainage tube is confirmed by observing oscillation of water column in drainage bottle which occurs due to change in pressure during respiration. The intrapleural pressure is decreased during inspiration and it increases during expiration.
- Continuous bubbling in water seal bottle and suction tube is considered abnormal as it is due to air passing out of the pleural space.
- No bubbling in the drainage bottle indicates that the intercostal drainage tube is not functioning properly or if its patency is endangered.

1448. Deep vein thrombosis renders a person at a risk of: *(AIIMS Nagpur NO 2018)*

a. Shock
b. Pulmonary embolism
c. Heart attack
d. Stroke

Explanation: Deep vein thrombosis (DVT) occurs when a blood clot (thrombus) forms in one or more of the deep veins in body, usually in legs. Thrombus dislodged from legs can travel to the lungs, which obstructs the pulmonary artery and produces **pulmonary embolism (PE)**.

1449. Principles used in closed chest drainage: *(AIIMS Nagpur NO 2018)*

a. Gravity, positive pressure, suction
b. Gravity, negative pressure, suction
c. Ambulation
d. Posture

Explanation: In closed chest drainage the chest tube is connected to a closed chest drainage system, which allows for air or fluid to be drained, and prevents air or fluid from entering the pleural space. Emphysema, traumatic pneumothorax, pleural effusion, thoracic surgeries are common indications for closed chest drainage. Principles used to drain are gravity, negative pressure and suction.

1450. What should the nurse do while preparing the client for thoracentesis?

a. Administer anticholinergics as ordered
b. Keep the patient NPO for six hours
c. Explain the procedure to him
d. Prepare him to go to the operating room

Explanation: The nurse should explain the procedure to the patient to gets informed consent. The procedure is usually done at bedside not at operating room. Keeping the patient NPO is not necessary this procedure. Anticholinergics or analgesics are not ordered for thoracentesis.

1451. A thoracentesis was performed on an adult client. After the procedure, the client has hemoptysis and a pulse of 80, respirations of 28, and temperature of 99°F. Which of these is of greatest concern to the nurse?

a. Hemoptysis
b. Pulse of 80
c. Temperature of 99°F
d. Respirations of 28

Explanation: Hemoptysis is the only abnormal finding. All of the others are within normal range for someone who has undergone an invasive procedure.

1452. Thoracocentesis is contra indicated in ....client.

a. Bleeding and clotting disorder
b. Uncooperative patient
c. Cardiac problems
d. All of the above

1453. Appropriate position given to a client experiencing acute pulmonary edema is:

a. Supine
b. Prone
c. High Fowler's position
d. Left lateral

1454. ICD is inserted into a client with pneumothorax, but accidentally ICD is malpositioned, which among the following is a serious complication associated with malpositioned ICD?

a. Subcutaneous emphysema
b. Worsening of pneumothorax
c. Pneumo-peritoneum
d. Both a and b

1455. The functioning of the ICD chest tube is assessed by:

a. Seeing for continuous air bubbles coming out of the underwater drain
b. Seeing the movement of air water column in the tube during respiration
c. Taking X-ray chest repeatedly
d. Auscultation

Explanation:

- Functioning of the Tube can be confirmed by seeing the column of water in the Chest tube moving up and down during respiration.
- Underwater drainage tube if fails to expand a lung of Open pneumothorax we will use 5 cm water low pressure suction.
- Heimlich valve is a special valve used instead of underwater drain only for Pneumothorax cases.

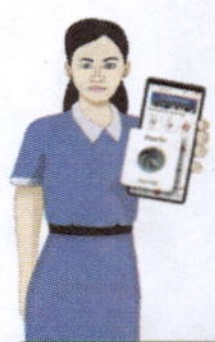

Ans.

1445. c
1446. d
1447. c
1448. b
1449. b
1450. c
1451. a
1452. d
1453. c
1454. d
1455. b

PULMONARY EMBOLISM (PE)

1456. Most common clinical sign of pulmonary embolism is:
a. Tachypnea b. Tachycardia
c. Cyanosis d. Sweating

1457. For the prevention of further pulmonary embolism, which of the following is the correct maintenance infusion dose of intravenous heparin? *(AIIMS Bhopal Nursing officer, 2018)*
a. 48 m/kg/hr
b. 18 m/kg/hr
c. 28 m/kg/hr
d. 38 m/kg/hr

Explanation: In pulmonary embolism one or more pulmonary vessel is occluded with blood clot. Fibrinolytic or anticoagulant therapy is needed in this condition. The maintenance infusion dose of intravenous heparin in this condition is 18 m/kg/hr.

1458. Identify correct statement regarding transudates?
a. Produced because of increased hydrostatic pressure
b. Produced because of reduced oncotic pressure
c. Clear in appearance with Proteins <3 g/dL
d. All of the above

1459. Identify correct statement regarding exudates?
a. Produced due to increased capillary permeability occur because of infection
b. Cloudy in appearance with proteins >3 g/dL
c. Specific gravity >1.020
d. All of the above

1460. DVT emboli most commonly lodges in:
a. Heart b. Lung
c. Kidney d. Brain

1461. Common cause of pulmonary embolism is:
a. Fat emboli b. Air emboli
c. Septic thrombi d. Venous thrombi

1462. Drug ordered in pulmonary embolism is:
a. Warfarin b. Heparin
c. Streptokinase d. Vitamin K

1463. Identify the signs of pulmonary consolidation among the following:
a. Dullness b. Increased fremitus
c. Crackles d. All of these

Explanation: A pulmonary consolidation is a region of (normally compressible) lung tissue that has filled with liquid, a condition marked by induration (swelling or hardening of normally soft tissue) of a normally aerated lung. All of the above-mentioned signs will be present in that condition.

1464. Postoperative pulmonary thromboembolism chances are more in:
a. Hormonal replacement therapy and obesity
b. Immobility
c. Pregnant women
d. All of the above

1465. A 65-kg patient with a pulmonary embolism is ordered to receive heparin 10 units/kg/hour by I.V. infusion. How many units of heparin should he receive each hour?
a. 500 b. 550
c. 600 d. 650

Explanation:
- Patient has to receive 10 units/kg/hr
- Patient weight = 65 kg
- Dose required per hour = 65 × 10 = 650 units/hr

TUBERCULOSIS (TB)

1466. Typical signs of TB include:
a. Night sweats b. Hemoptysis
c. Fever d. All of these

1467. Ghon's foci is seen in:
a. Rheumatic fever b. Measles
c. Renal tumor d. Tuberculosis

Explanation: In case of tuberculosis, the inhaled bacilli implant in distal airspaces of lower part of upper lobe or upper part of lower lobe usually close to the pleura and emerge as consolidation of 1 to 1.5 cm Gray-white color. It is known as Ghon's foci.

1468. A client with past history of TB infection presently becomes immunocompromised and suffering from TB, it is known as:
a. Latent infection b. Nosocomial infection
c. Opportunistic infection d. Tertiary infection

1469. Characteristic clinical features of TB include:
a. Cough and chest pain
b. Weight loss, fever, night sweats, and hemoptysis
c. Cough, nausea and vomiting
d. Headache fever and diarrhea

1470. In TB hospitalization is to:
a. Provide health education
b. Adhere to treatment regimen
c. Prevent spread of the disease
d. Teach proper sputum disposal

1471. Sites of primary tuberculosis is:
a. Skin b. Lung
c. Gastrointestinal tract d. All of these

1472. Intestinal TB affects ....part of the intestine.
a. Duodenum b. Ileum
c. Ascending colon d. Sigmoid colon

1473. For the treatment of tuberculosis, chemotherapy must be continued for:
a. 1–3 months b. 6–12 months
c. 3–5 months d. 2 years or more

Explanation: Tuberculosis is caused by tubercle bacilli. Treatment with combination of multiple drugs including rifampicin, isoniazid, pyrazinamide, ethambutol and streptomycin for at least 6 months is essential to eradicate tubercle bacilli.

1474. Which of the following drug in DOTS therapy can cause deafness? *(AIIMS Raipur Staff Nurse Grade I-2018)*
a. Ethambutol b. Isoniazid
c. Rifampicin d. Streptomycin

Explanation: Streptomycin is ototoxic and can cause deafness. Side effect of ethambutol is commonly related to visual changes such as blurred vision/ decreased vision or color blindness or it may be related to liver disease. Rifampicin causes secretions such as urine, saliva, etc. in red-orange color. Side effect related to isoniazid include peripheral neuropathy, pellagra, like symptoms and pyridoxine deficiency.

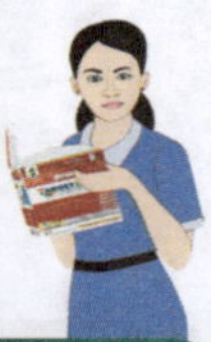

Ans.
1456. a
1457. b
1458. d
1459. d
1460. b
1461. d
1462. b
1463. d
1464. d
1465. d
1466. d
1467. d
1468. c
1469. b
1470. c
1471. d
1472. b
1473. b
1474. d

1475. Frequent visual examination is suggested for a patient on: *(AIIMS Raipur NO 2019)*
a. Rifampicin b. INH
c. Ethambutol d. Dapsone

Explanation: The patient on ethambutol has increased risk of ocular toxicity (decreased red-green color discrimination), so it is recommended to monitor visual acuity and color discrimination regularly.

1476. Which of the following is seen in sarcoidosis?
a. Hypercalcemia b. Hypocalcemia
c. Hyperphosphatemia d. Hypophosphatemia

Explanation: Sarcoidosis is an inflammatory disease that affects multiple organs in the body, but mostly the lungs and lymph glands. Hypercalcemia is a highly prevalent complication of sarcoidosis. Hypercalcemia in sarcoidosis is due to the uncontrolled synthesis of Vitamin D3 by macrophages.

1477. Which of the following is the confirmatory test for the diagnosis of tuberculosis?
a. Bronchoscopy b. Saline test
c. Tuberculin test d. Sputum culture

LUNG ABSCESS

1478. Causes of lung abscess is:
a. Aspiration of gastric contents
b. Aspiration of infective materials
c. Complication of pneumonia
d. All of the above

1479. Most common cause of Lung abscess:
a. *Staph aureus*
b. *Pneumococcus*
c. Aerobic and anaerobic streptococci
d. *E. coli*

1480. Most common cause of lung abscess in comatose patient:
a. Staph aureus b. Oral anaerobes
c. Klebsiella d. Tuberculosis

1481. The most common area where lung abscess is found:
a. Anterior segment of the upper lobe
b. Posterior segment of the upper lobe
c. Apical segment of the lower lobe
d. Both b and c

1482. Most common organism responsible for lung abscess is:
a. *Klebsiella* b. *Pseudomonas*
c. *E. coli* d. *Salmonella*

1483. Which of the following diagnostic test is not used in lung abscess?
a. X-ray b. Sputum culture
c. Fiberoptic bronchoscopy d. Pulmonary Function Test

1484. Which diet is highly preferred in the clients with lung abscess?
a. High calorie and high protein diet
b. Low calorie and low protein diet
c. Low fiber diet
d. High carbohydrate diet

Explanation: High calorie and high protein diet will facilitate healing.

1485. Which of the following is the most common cause of lung abscess?
a. Aspiration
b. Increased alveolar fluid
c. Pertussis
d. Pneumonia

CHEST INJURIES

1486. A wound through which the air passes during inspiration and expiration resulted in:
a. Pneumothorax
b. Flail chest
c. Hemothorax
d. Blunt chest trauma

1487. Emergency nurse observed paradoxical chest rise in a client. Which among the following procedure she should anticipate in this client?
a. Extra-ventricular drainage
b. Intubation
c. Defibrillation
d. Chest compression

1488. While caring for a client with ICD drainage nurse observed dyspnea, respiratory rate 42, blood pressure of 80/60 and left side of chest is not expanding. Which among the following is the appropriate nursing action?
a. Check the ICD tubing for its patency
b. Notify the physician
c. Observe the findings
d. Provide appropriate medication as per the physician order

1489. Paradoxical respiration is observed in which among the following condition?
a. Flail chest b. Blunt chest trauma
c. Pneumothorax d. Hemothorax

1490. The condition in which sudden impact to the chest which may cause sudden death without having any cardiac damage is called:
a. Commotio cordis b. algor mortis
c. Cardiac tamponade d. Concussion

OCCUPATIONAL LUNG DISEASES

1491. Asbestos-related diseases include:
a. Diffuse pleural fibrosis
b. Bronchogenic carcinoma
c. Mesothelioma
d. All of the above

1492. Monday fever is the other name for: *(AIIMS BPL NO 2018)*
a. Asbestosis b. Byssinosis
c. Silicosis d. Anthracosis

Explanation: Byssinosis, also called "brown lung disease" or "Monday fever", is an occupational lung disease caused by exposure to cotton dust in inadequately ventilated working environments.

1493. Bagassosis is caused by inhalation of: *(Kerala PSC, Nov 2014)*
a. Sugarcane dust b. Cotton dust
c. Coal dust d. Silica dust

1494. Asbestosis gets inhaled and settled down in:
a. Middle lung zone b. Lower lung zone
c. Upper lung zone d. Throughout entire lung

Ans.
1475. c
1476. a
1477. d
1478. d
1479. c
1480. b
1481. d
1482. a
1483. d
1484. a
1485. a
1486. a
1487. b
1488. a
1489. a
1490. a
1491. d
1492. b
1493. a
1494. b

1495. Bagassosis is acquired by the inhalation of which form of dust?

a. Sugarcane b. Cotton
c. Bicarbonate d. Asbestos

1496. The farmer lung is developed by the inhalation of:

a. Sugarcane
b. Grain dust
c. Cotton fiber
d. Silicon dust

1497. Byssinosis is acquired by the inhalation of which form of dust:

a. Sugarcane b. Grain dust
c. Cotton fiber d. Silicon dust

1498. The Lung disease that occurs as the result of inhaling iron containing material:

a. Bagassosis b. Siderosis
c. Anthracosis d. Asbestosis

1499. The Lung disease that occurs as the result of inhaling coal dust is known as:

a. Bagassosis
b. Siderosis
c. Anthracosis
d. Asbestosis

1500. The Lung disease that occurs as the result of inhaling asbestos:

a. Silicosis
b. Siderosis
c. Anthracosis
d. Asbestosis

1501. The characteristic features of asbestosis on chest radiographs include:

a. Ground-glass appearance
b. Snow-storm appearance
c. Both a & b
d. None of the above

Explanation:

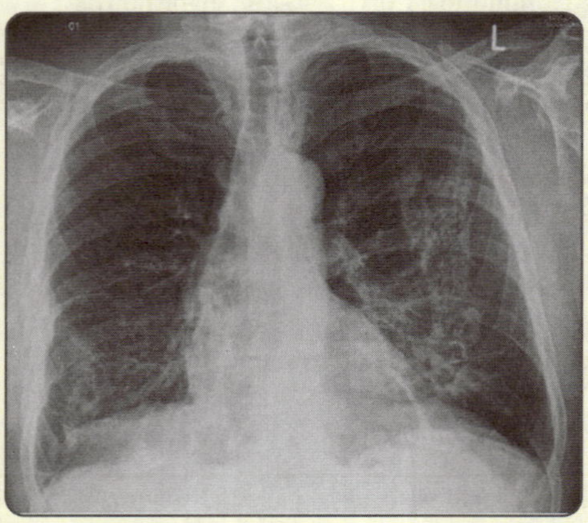

Figure: Ground-glass appearance of lungs as seen in asbestosis

1502. Snow-storm appearance in lung X-ray is seen in which of the following occupational disease?

a. Asbestosis b. Silicosis
c. Siderosis d. Anthracosis

Explanation:

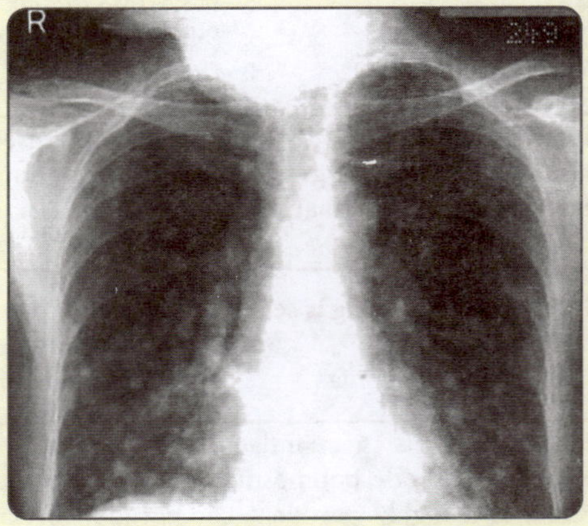

Figure: Snow-storm appearance of lungs as seen in silicosis

1503. The hypersensitivity pneumoconiosis caused by tobacco:

a. Tobacossis b. siderosis
c. Anthracosis d. Hay lung disease

1504. The inhalation of barium containing dust in the industrial area leads to:

a. Chalicosis b. Chelosis
c. Baritosis d. Bariumtis

1505. The chalicosis is found largely on the people who work as:

a. Coal worker b. Wood cutter
c. Stone cutter d. Iron maker

OTHER RESPIRATORY DISEASES

1506. Most common type of diaphragmatic hernia is:

a. Bochdalek hernia
b. Morgagni's hernia
c. Hernia through the dome
d. Hiatus hernia

1507. Protrusion of mucous membrane of nose and para nasal sinus is known as:

a. Nasal polyp b. Nasal proliferation
c. Coryza d. Mucosal hypertrophy

1508. Appropriate position to a person with epistaxis is:

a. Sitting up b. Trendelenburg's position
c. Lying down d. Lateral position

1509. A client comes to the clinic with a bleeding nose. Which of the following instruction to the client is most appropriate?

a. "Sit up with your head tilted forward. Grasp the soft part of your nose firmly between your thumb and forefinger"
b. "Lay down and tilt your head backward. Grasp the end of your nose between your fingers"
c. "Sit up and lean backwards. Put pressure on the side of your nose with your hand"
d. "Lay down and tilt your head to one side and put pressure on the side of your nose with your hand"

Explanation: This position will help to stop bleeding without causing aspiration of any blood dripping down the back of the throat.

Ans.

1495. a
1496. b
1497. c
1498. b
1499. c
1500. d
1501. a
1502. b
1503. a
1504. c
1505. c
1506. d
1507. a
1508. a
1509. a

CARDIOVASCULAR SYSTEM

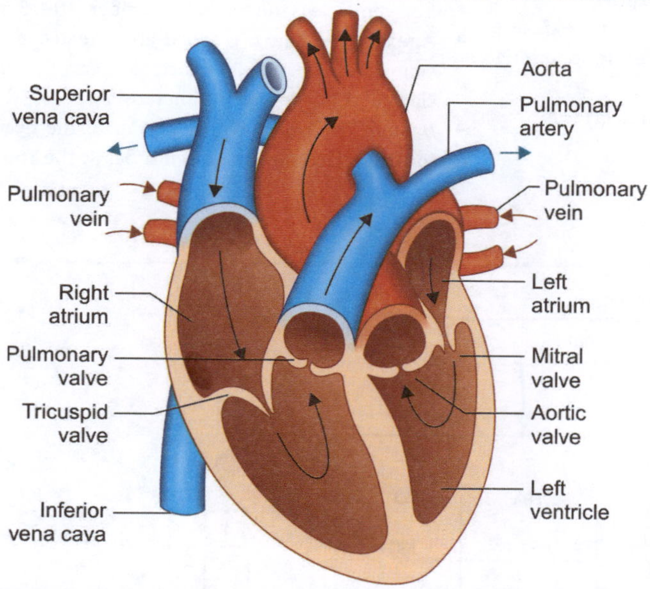

Figure 67: Anatomy of heart

ANATOMIC AND PHYSIOLOGIC OVERVIEW OF HEART

- Heart is a cone shaped, hollow muscular organ located in the mediastinal space between the lungs and rests on the diaphragm.
- **Size:** 12 cm long × 8 cm width × 6 cm thickness
- **Weight:** About 300 g

Layers of Heart

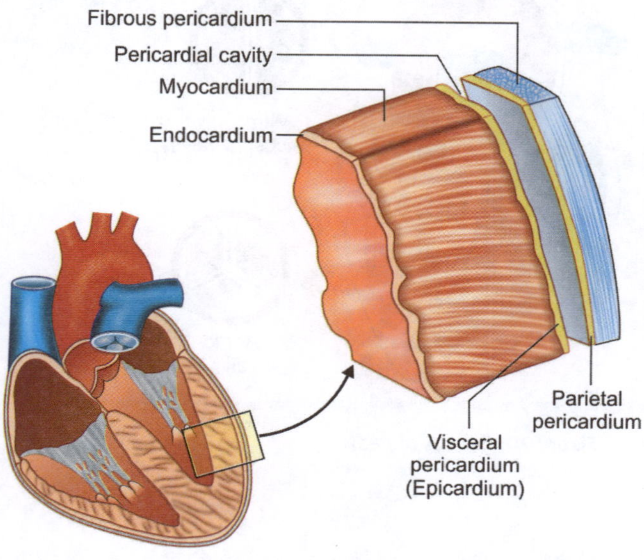

Figure 68: Cross-section of heart showing its layers

- **Pericardium:** Outer most layer of heart; covering of heart; consists of 3 layers:
  - Fibrous pericardium (outermost layer)
  - Parietal pericardium (middle layer)
  - Visceral pericardium (Epicardium)
- **Myocardium:** Middle layer of heart wall. Thickest layer of the heart wall. It is responsible for pumping action.
- **Endocardium:** Inner most layer of heart wall.

Heart Chambers

- It has four chambers:
  - 2 Atrium (Right atrium and Left atrium)
  - 2 Ventricle (Right ventricle and Left ventricle)
- Left ventricle is the thickest chamber (10–15 mm)
- **Apex of the heart:** Conical area created by left ventricle. The apex is located near the mid-clavicular line in the 5th intercostal space.
- **Base of the heart:** Upper border of the heart is formed by left atrium. Lies just below the 2nd rib.

POINT TO REMEMBER

Between visceral and parietal pericardium there is pericardial space and it contains approximately 30 mL of pericardial fluid.

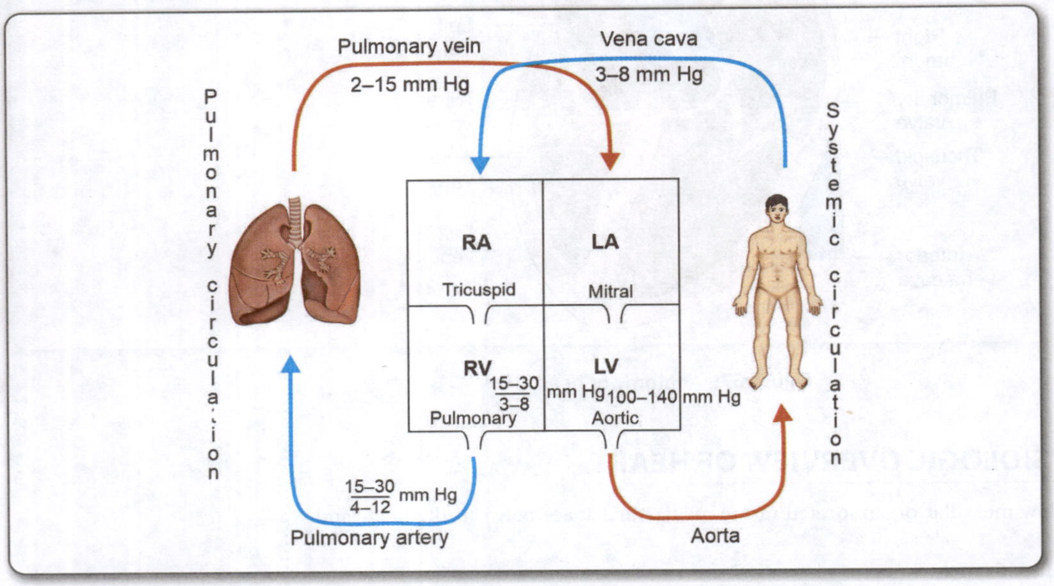

Figure 69: Schematic diagram of blood circulation in the heart

POINT TO REMEMBER

Right atrium receives blood from superior vena cava (from head, neck and upper extremities), inferior vena cava (from trunk and lower extremities) and coronary sinus.

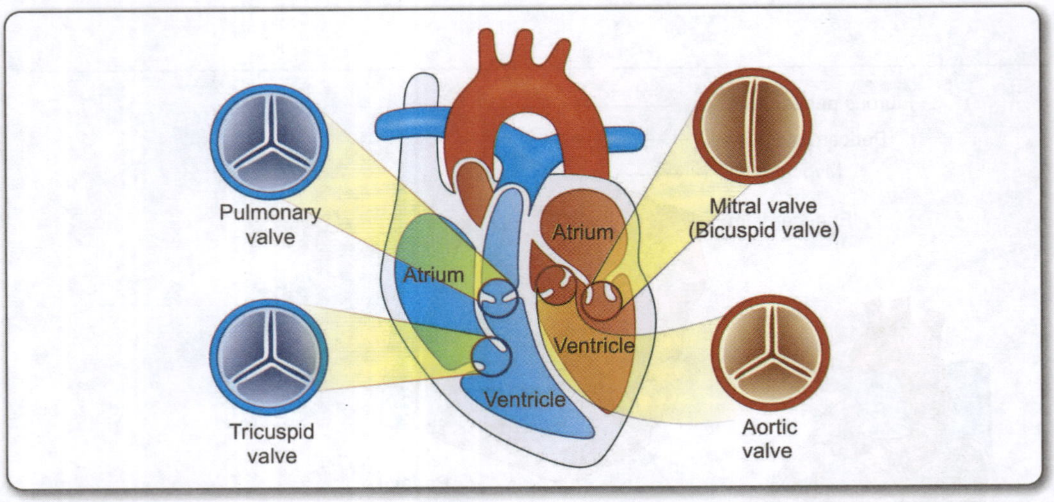

Figure 70: Valves of heart

KEY POINT

Closure of **AV** valves gives rise to first-heart sound **(lub)** and closure of **SV** valve gives rise to second-heart sound **(dub)**.

Heart Valves

- **Two Atrio-Ventricular (AV) valves**
  - **Bicuspid valve (Mitral valve):** Between left atrium and left ventricle
  - **Tricuspid valve:** Between right atrium and right ventricle
- **Two Semi-lunar valves** (half-moon shaped leaflet)
  - **Pulmonary valve:** Between pulmonary artery and right ventricle
  - **Aortic valve:** Between aorta and left ventricle

Coronary Arteries

- Left and right coronary arteries and their branches supply arterial blood to the heart.
- These arteries arise from aorta just above the aortic leaflet.
- Coronary arteries receive blood supply during diastole.
- Left coronary artery has three branches:
  - Left main coronary artery
  - Left anterior descending artery (supply anterior wall of the heart)
  - Circumflex artery (supply lateral wall of the heart).
- Right side of heart receives blood supply from right coronary artery.
- Posterior wall of the heart receives blood from posterior descending artery.
- Venous supply from the heart returns blood to the right atrium via coronary sinus located behind the right atrium.

Cardiac Conduction System

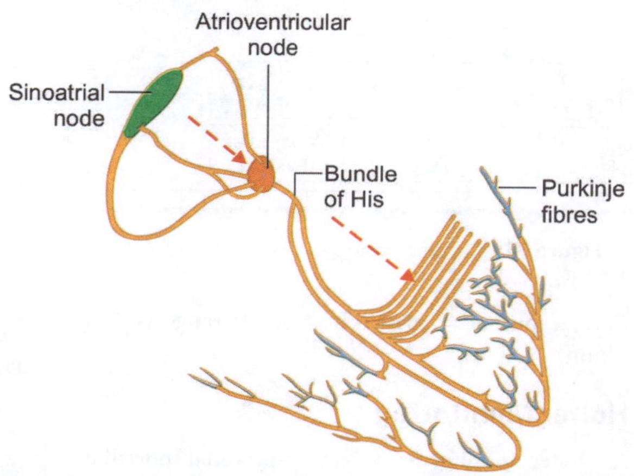

Figure 71: Cardiac conduction system

- Characteristics of cardiac conduction include:
  - **Automaticity:** Ability to initiate an electrical impulse
  - **Excitability:** Ability to respond to an electrical impulse
  - **Conductivity:** Ability to transmit electrical impulse from one cell to another.
- **SA node (Sino-Atrial node)**
  - It is the primary pacemaker of the heart
  - Located at the junction between superior vena cava and right atrium
  - SA node generates impulse at a rate of 60–100 per minute.
  - Electrical impulse is generated at SA node and conducted to AV node via inter nodal pathway.
- **AV node** (Atrio-Ventricular node)
  - Located in the right atrial wall near tricuspid valve
  - AV node coordinates the incoming impulse from SA node
  - After a slight delay, relays the impulses to ventricles.
- **Bundle of His**
  - Present in the septum between right and left ventricle
  - It conducts the impulses received from AV node to purkinje fibers
  - It is divided into right and left bundle branch.
- **Purkinje fibers**
  - Terminal part of conduction system
  - Myocardial cells are stimulated causing cardiac contraction.

KEY POINTS

- **Rheumatic fever** is the most common cause of **mitral valve** stenosis.
- Valves are affected due to Rheumatic fever in the following order- **M**itral, **A**ortic, **T**ricuspid and **P**ulmonic (Remember MAT-P)
- ***Streptococcus pyogenes*** **or Group A beta hemolytic streptococci** are the causative organisms for Rheumatic fever.
- Left Anterior Descending Artery (LAD) is the most commonly occluded artery due to atherosclerosis
- Heart attack due to 100% Occlusion of LAD is often called **'widowmaker heart attack'**
- Conduction of electrical impulse is fastest in purkinje system (4 m/sec)

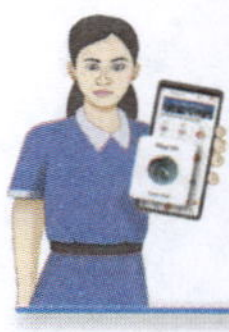

Cardiac Cycle

- Normal duration of each cardiac cycle = 0.8 sec

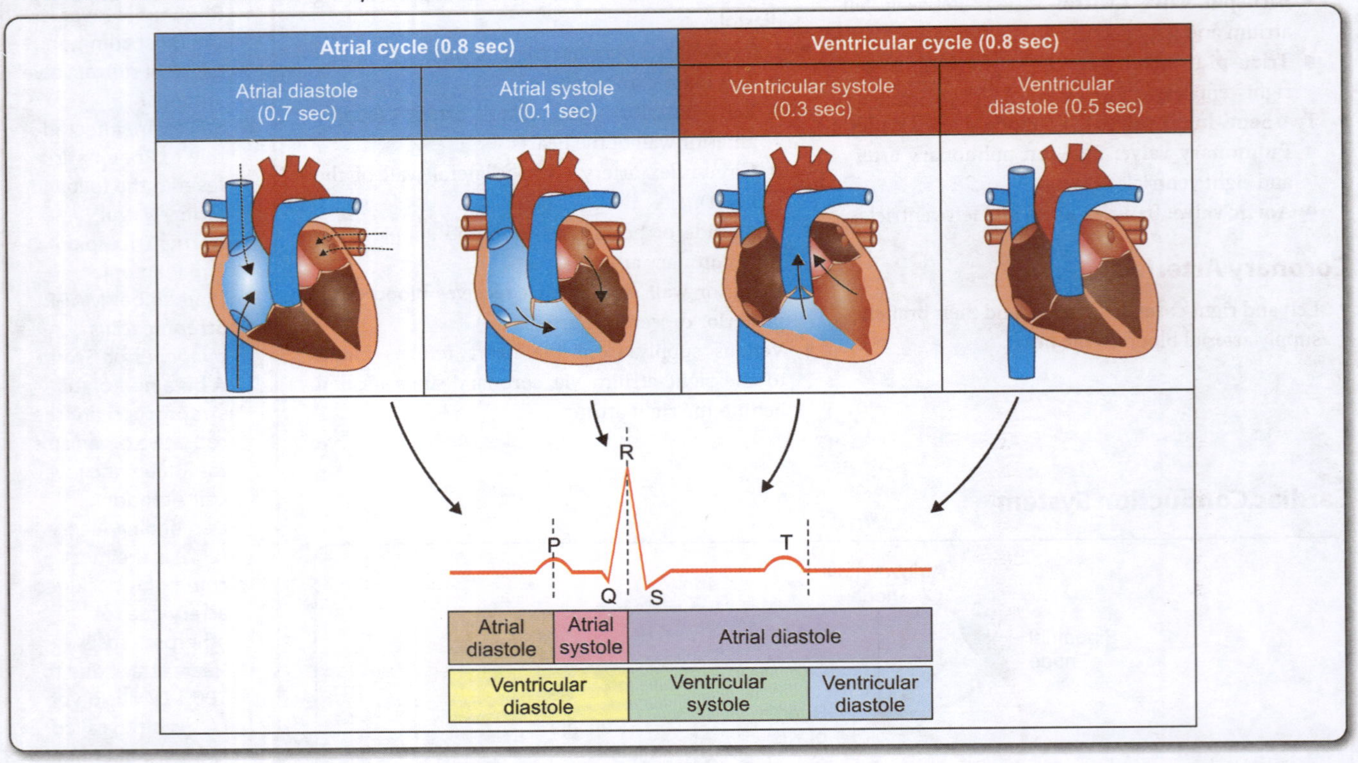

Figure 72: Cardiac cycle

Cardiac Output

- Each ventricle ejects approximately 70 mL of blood per beat.
- **Stroke volume (SV):** Volume of blood pumped from the left ventricle per beat. Normal stroke volume is 70 mL.
- **Cardiac output** = Stroke volume (SV) × Heart Rate (HR)

  = 70 × 72

Cardiac output = 5040 mL (Normal range is 4–8 L/min)

Holter Monitoring

A Holter monitor is a battery-powered portable device that records patient's Cardiac activity (ECG) continuously for 24 to 48 hours or longer depending on the type of monitoring used.

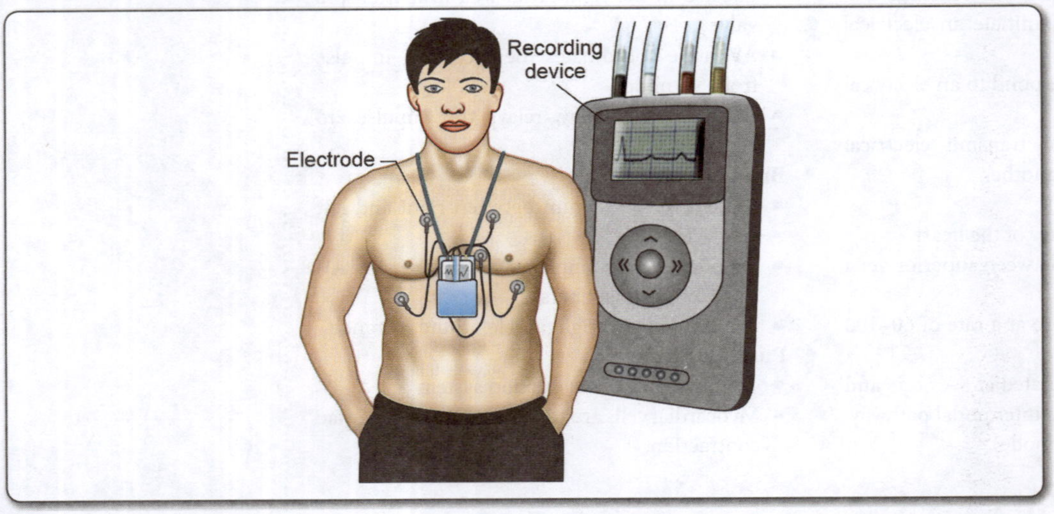

Figure 73: Holter monitor

Recent Question (NORCET 2020)

47. Dicrotic notch of the arterial wave form indicates ....

a. Increased resistance to blood flow
b. Sudden fall in blood pressure
c. Opening of aortic valve
d. Closure of aortic valve

Ans. (d) Closure of aortic valve

KEY POINTS

- **Cardiac index** is cardiac output divided by the body mass index.
- Cardiac output is usually normal in **Circulatory/ Distributive Shock**.

Heart Sounds

Normal heart sounds

- **S1 (First Heart sound-LUBB):** Produced by closure of AV valves (Tricuspid and Mitral)
- **S2 (Second Heart sound-DUBB):** Produced by closure of Semilunar valves (Aortic and Pulmonic valve)

Abnormal heart sounds

- **S3** (Third heart sound): Also known as **ventricular gallop**. It corresponds to early ventricular filling (passive filling) when mitral valve opens. It is often associated with **Heart failure**.
- **S4** (Fourth heart sound): Also known as Atrial gallop

Blood Vessels

- Arteries and veins have three layers:
  - Tunica intima (inner layer)
  - Tunica media (middle layer)
  - Tunica adventitia (outer layer)
- Thickest layer of artery is tunica media
- Thickest layer of vein is tunica adventitia
- **Largest artery in the body is Aorta**
- Largest vein in the body is Inferior vena cava

KEY POINTS

- Left ventricle is responsible for apex beat. Point of maximum impulse can be auscultated in the **mid-clavicular line in the 5th intercostal space.**
- S3 corresponds with early ventricular filling and S4 corresponds with late ventricular filling.
- The gap between S1 and S2 indicates time for systole.
- The gap between S2 and S1 indicates time for diastole.
- While assessing blood pressure use of:
  - Small/narrow cuff leads to → Falsely high BP
  - Large/wide cuff leads to → Falsely lower BP

Table 57: Differences between arteries and veins

Characteristics	Artery	Vein
Direction of blood flow	Heart to the body	Body to the heart
Oxygen concentration	Carry oxygenated blood (except pulmonary artery and umbilical artery)	Carry de-oxygenated blood (except pulmonary vein and umbilical vein)
Anatomy	Thicker walls Narrow lumen	Thinner walls Large lumen
Valve	Absent	Present
Pressure	High	Low

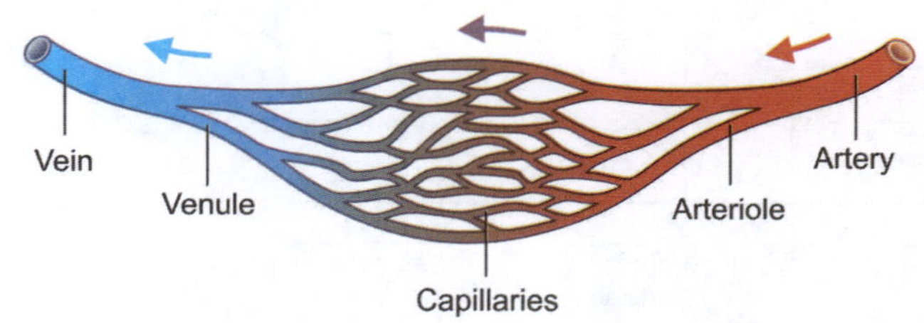

Figure 74: Exchange of blood between arterioles and venules

- Arterioles – Resistant vessels
- Capillaries – Exchange vessels
- Venules – Smallest veins

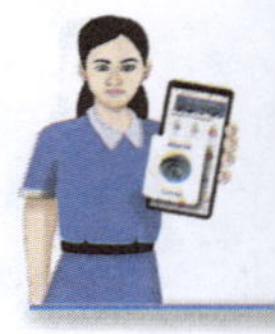

Branches of Aorta

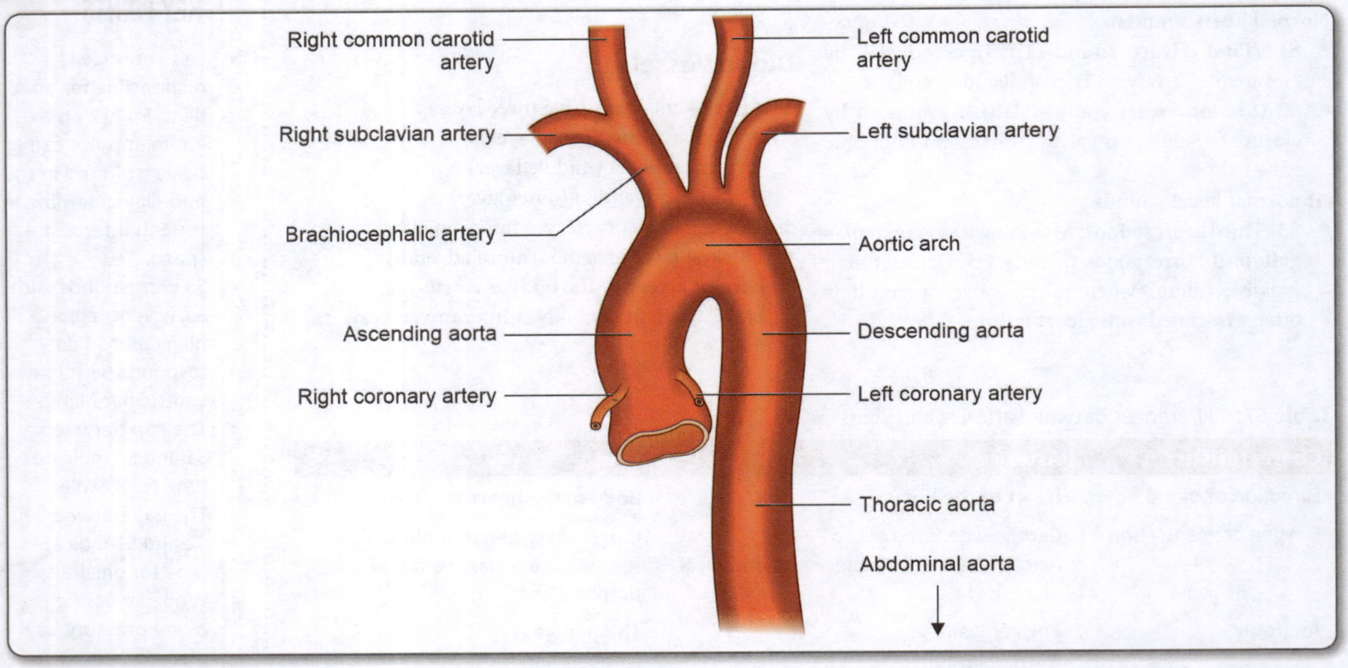

Figure 75: Branches of aorta

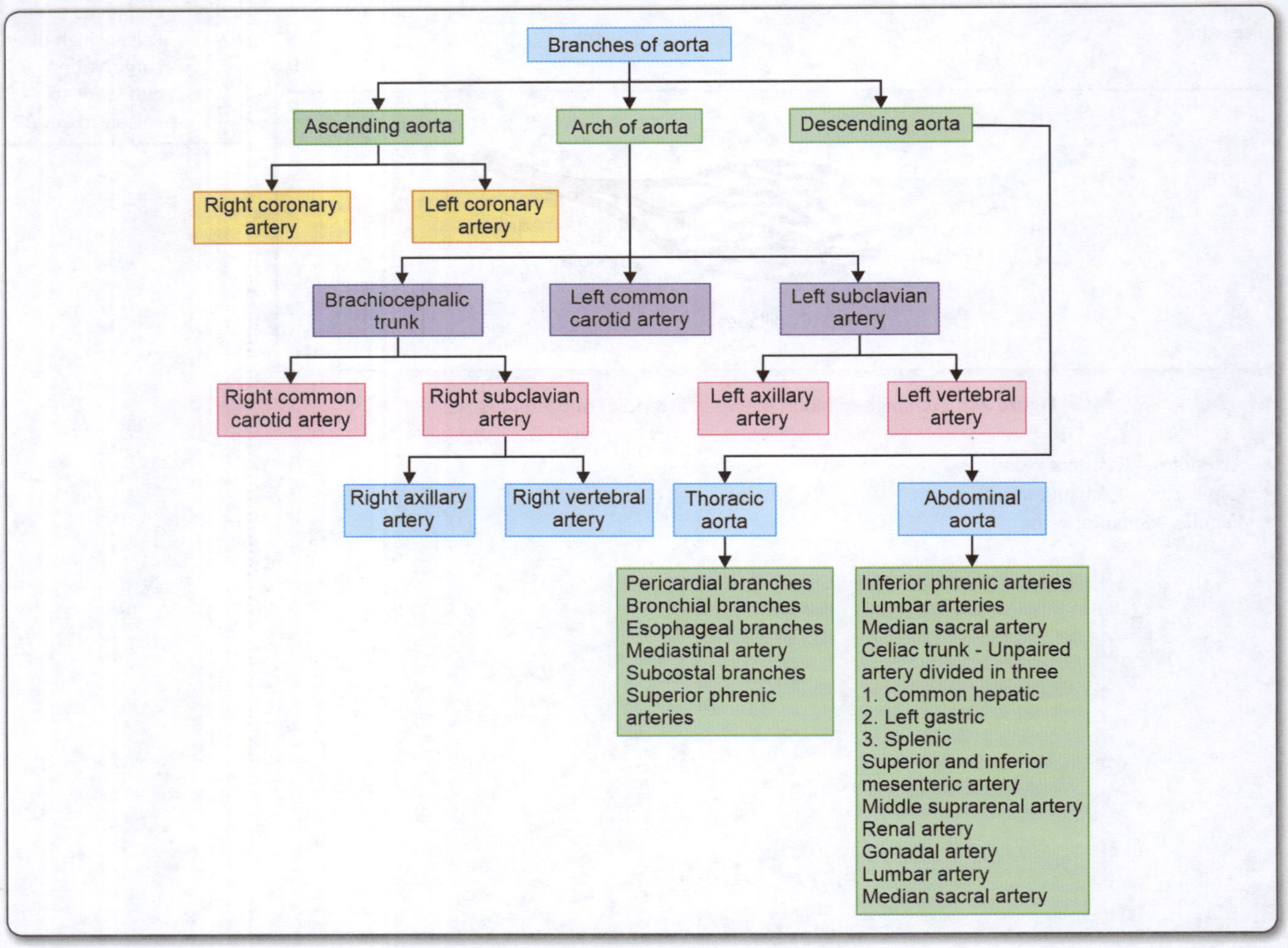

Figure 76: Detailed classification of branches of aorta

Table 58: Arteries and the areas supplied by arterial

Name of artery	Area which is supplied by artery
Right and left coronary artery	Myocardium layers
Right common carotid artery	Right side of head and neck
Right axillary artery	Right upper arm
Right vertebral artery	Right side of head and neck
Left common carotid artery	Left side of head and neck
Left axillary artery	Left upper arm
Left vertebral artery	Left side of head and neck
Pericardial branches	Pericardium layer of heart
Bronchial branches	Right branch supplies right bronchus, bronchopulmonary lymph nodes, pericardium and esophagus. Two left branches supply left side of bronchial tree.
Esophageal branches	Supply to esophagus
Mediastinal branches	Supply to posterior mediastinum's lymph node, vessels, nerve and tissue
Posterior intercostal artery	Nine pairs of arteries supply to the intercostal spaces
Subcostal arteries	Run inferior to the 12th rib and supply subcostal area
Superior phrenic arteries	Supply posterior site of mediastinum's superior surface
Inferior phrenic arteries	Inferior diaphragm
Celiac trunk	Esophagus's abdominal part, liver, stomach, gallbladder, proximal duodenum, pancreas, and spleen
Superior mesenteric artery	Small intestine, cecum, appendix, ascending colon, and first $2/3^{rd}$ of transverse colon.
Inferior mesenteric artery	Distal $1/3^{rd}$ of transverse colon, descending colon, sigmoid colon, rectum, and some portion of anal canal
Middle suprarenal artery	Supply to suprarenal glands
Renal artery	Both kidneys
Gonadal artery	In male: testicular artery supplies testes In female: ovarian artery supplies ovaries
Lumbar arteries	Spinal cord and posterior abdomen wall
Median sacral artery	Supply Lumbar vertebrae and sacrum

Blood Pressure

- Normal range of systolic blood pressure (SBP) – 90–140 mm Hg
- Normal range of diastolic blood pressure (DBP) – 60–90 mm Hg
- **Pulse Pressure:** Difference between SBP and DBP is known as pulse pressure. The normal range is 30–40 mm Hg.

Practice Question

20. Which of the following pairs, linking an artery with its supplied area, is incorrect?

a. Celiac trunk - Liver and gallbladder
b. Phrenic arteries - Diaphragm
c. Inferior mesenteric artery - Distal 1/3 of transverse colon
d. Superior mesenteric artery - Stomach

Ans. (d) Superior mesenteric artery - Stomach

Clinical Corner

CASE SCENARIO 3:

A 50-year-old patient visits the clinic for a routine check-up. Their blood pressure reading is recorded as 130/80 mm Hg. Based on the provided blood pressure reading, what is the calculated pulse pressure for this patient, and how is it interpreted?

a. Pulse pressure is 50 mm Hg, which is within the normal range.
b. Pulse pressure is 105 mm Hg, which is above the normal range.
c. Pulse pressure is 50 mm Hg, which is below the normal range.
d. Pulse pressure is 50 mm Hg, which is above the normal range.

Ans. (d) Pulse pressure is 50 mm Hg, which is above the normal range.

The pulse pressure is calculated by subtracting the diastolic blood pressure (DBP) from the systolic blood pressure (SBP).

In this case, SBP is 130 mm Hg and DBP is 80 mm Hg.

Pulse Pressure = SBP - DBP = 130 - 80 = 45 mm Hg.

The normal range for pulse pressure is 30–40 mm Hg. Since the calculated pulse pressure (50 mm Hg) falls above the normal range.

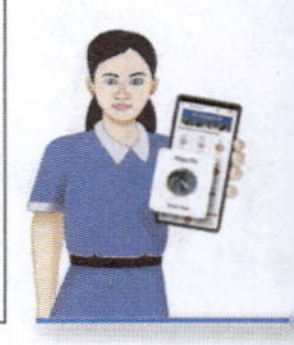

Auscultation Sites for Different Areas of Heart

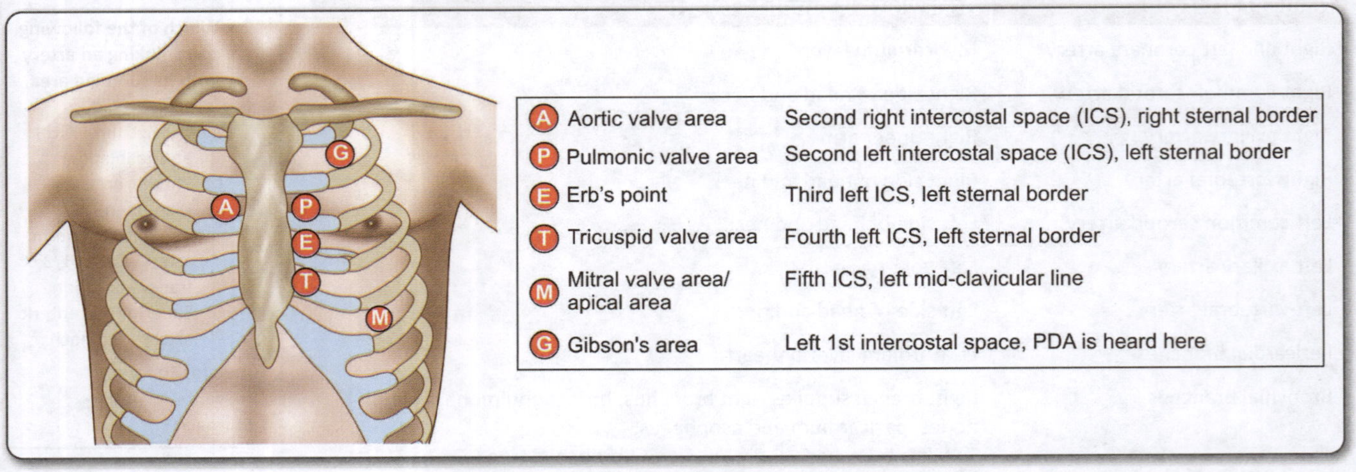

Figure 77: Auscultation sites for different areas of heart

Common Sites for Assessment of Pulse

Table 59: Common sites for assessment of pulse

Pulse site	Commonly used for/significance
Carotid	During CPR
Apical	Assessed with Stethoscope
Brachial	For assessment of Blood pressure
Radial	To count pulse
Femoral	For assessment
Popliteal	For assessment
Dorsalis pedis	Used to evaluate the arteriosclerotic diseases

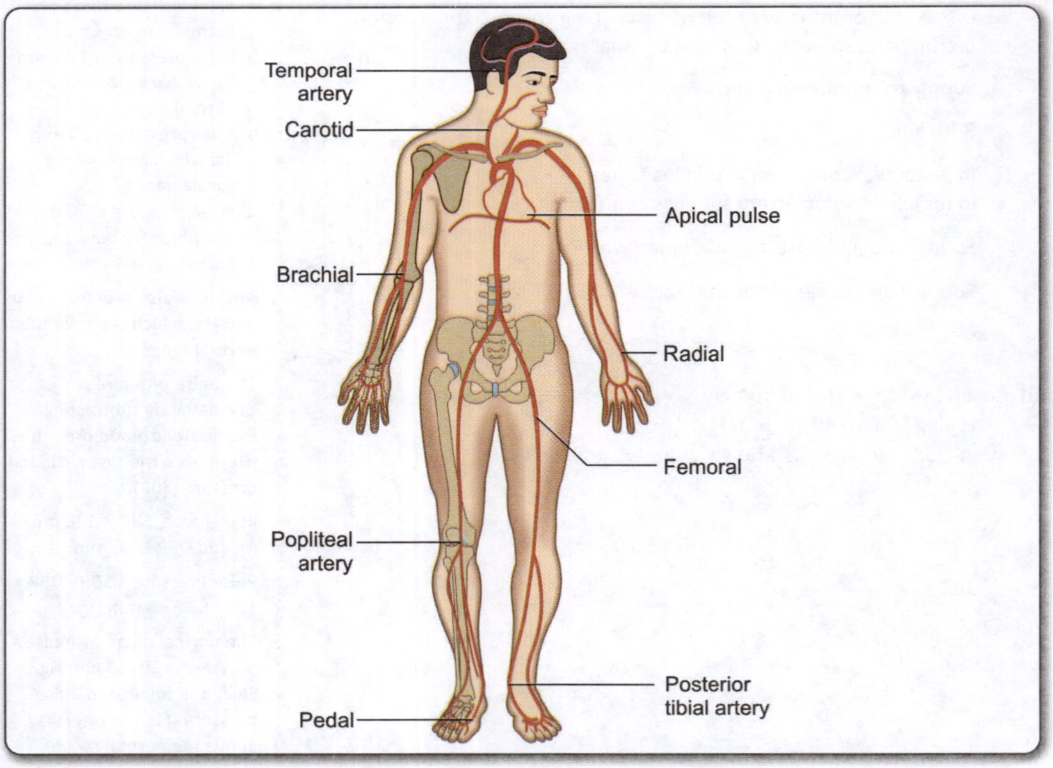

Figure 78: Sites for assessment of pulse

KEY POINTS

- Bobbing head with each pulse is seen in patient with Aortic regurgitation.
- Water hammer pulse is a feature of Aortic regurgitation.
- When a pulse rate is irregular, it is best to count the Apical pulse for a full minute.
- Apical pulse can be auscultated in the mid-clavicular line in the 5th intercostal space.

POINT TO REMEMBER

Pulse deficit refers to the difference between apical pulse and radial pulse.

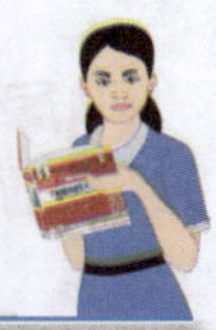

Pulse difference
- The difference between apical and radial pulse is known as pulse difference. Normally pulse difference is ZERO.
- Pulse difference usually occurs in conditions like atrial fibrillation, atrial flutter, premature ventricular contraction and varying degree of heart block.

DIAGNOSTIC TESTS

Table 60: Diagnostic test

Name of the test	Description
Cardiac enzyme (CK-MB)	Elevated value indicates myocardial damage. Usually elevation occurs within hours and peaks at 18 hours.
Lactate dehydrogenase (LDH)	Usually elevation occurs in 24 hours following MI and peaks at 48–72 hours. Normally LDH1 is higher than LDH2. The normal ratio of LDH1 to LDH2 is 2:1. If this is reversed, it indicates severe myocardial necrosis.
Troponin	Troponin is composed of three proteins troponin I, troponin C and troponin T. Troponin I has highest affinity towards myocardial damage. It rises three hours after injury and remains persistent up to 7–10 days.
Myoglobin	The level rises for two hours after MI and declines after 7 hours. It is non-specific marker.

Cardiac Markers in MI

Table 61: Cardiac markers and time of elevation and peaks

Cardiac markers	Time of elevation	Peaks	Normalize
Myoglobin	1–4 hrs	8–10 hrs	24 hrs
Troponin I/T	4–6 hrs	12 hrs	3–10 days
CK-MB	4–8 hrs	12–24 hrs	2–3 days

Treadmill Test/ Exercise Tolerance Test/Stress Test

- A treadmill stress test is used to diagnose a variety of cardiovascular disorders.
- Complete vital signs with ECG are recorded before the patient is allowed to walk or run on the treadmill and according to **Bruce protocol,** every 3 minutes the speed and slope are increased.
- The patient's vital signs and ECG are checked during the procedure.
- If any abnormality in patients or monitor is seen the procedure has to be stopped.
- The crash cart has to be made ready for this procedure.

HEMODYNAMIC MONITORING

Table 62: Various hemodynamic parameters

Parameter	Normal range
CVP (Central Venous Pressure)/ Right Atrial Pressure	2–6 mm Hg
Right Ventricular Pressure • Systolic • Diastolic	 • 15–30 mm Hg • 2–8 mm Hg
JVP (Jugular Venous Pressure)	6–8 cm H_2O
Portal Venous Pressure	8–12 mm Hg
PAWP (Pulmonary Artery Wedge Pressure)	6–12 mm Hg
PAP (Pulmonary Artery Pressure) • Systolic • Diastolic	 • 15–30 mm Hg • 8–15 mm Hg
MAP (Mean Arterial Pressure)	70–105 mm Hg

Contd...

KEY POINTS
- Do not palpate carotid artery and temporal artery simultaneously because it may reduce cerebral blood flow
- 1 mm Hg = 13.6 mm of H_2O or 1.36 CM of H_2O
- 1 cm of H_2O = 0.74 mm Hg

POINT TO REMEMBER

Myoglobin (nonspecific) is the early marker for MI but **Troponin is the most sensitive** (superior) marker.

Recent Question (NORCET 2020)

48. What is the normal CVP pressure?
a. 1–2 mm Hg
b. 2–6 mm Hg
c. 3–8 mm Hg
d. 5–8 mm Hg

Ans. (b) 2–6 mm Hg

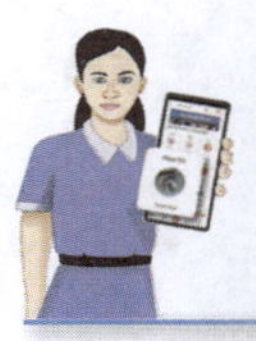

Parameter	Normal range
Arterial PO_2	100 mm Hg
Arterial Oxygen Saturation (SaO_2)	95–100%
Central Venous Saturation ($ScvO_2$)	70%
Cardiac output	4–8 L

Central Venous Pressure

- The central venous pressure (CVP) is the pressure measured in the central veins close to the heart.
- It is also known as right atrial pressure.
- CVP reflects the amount of blood returning to the heart and the ability of the heart to pump the blood into the arterial system.

Measurement of CVP

- The CVP can be measured either manually using a manometer or electronically using a transducer.
- It is measured by connecting the patient's central venous catheter to a special infusion set which is connected to a small diameter water column.
- In either case, the CVP must be 'zeroed' at the level of the right atrium.
- The phlebostatic axis is the reference point for zeroing the hemodynamic monitoring device.
- Phlebostatic axis is a point located by drawing an imaginary line from the fourth intercostal space at the sternum and finding its intersection with an imaginary line drawn down the center of the chest below the axillae.

Electrocardiogram (ECG)

Electrocardiography (ECG or EKG) is the process of recording the electrical activity of the heart over a period of time using electrodes placed on a patient's body.

Table 63: Placement of electrodes and leads

Electrode name	Electrode placement
V_1	4th intercostal space to the right of the sternum
V_2	4th intercostal space to the left of the sternum
V_3	Directly between leads V_2 and V_4.
V_4	5th intercostal space at left midclavicular line
V_5	Level with lead V_4 at left anterior axillary line
V_6	Level with lead V_5 at left midaxillary line
RA	On the right arm
LA	On the left arm (similar location to RA)
RL	On the right leg
LL	On the left leg (similar location to RL)

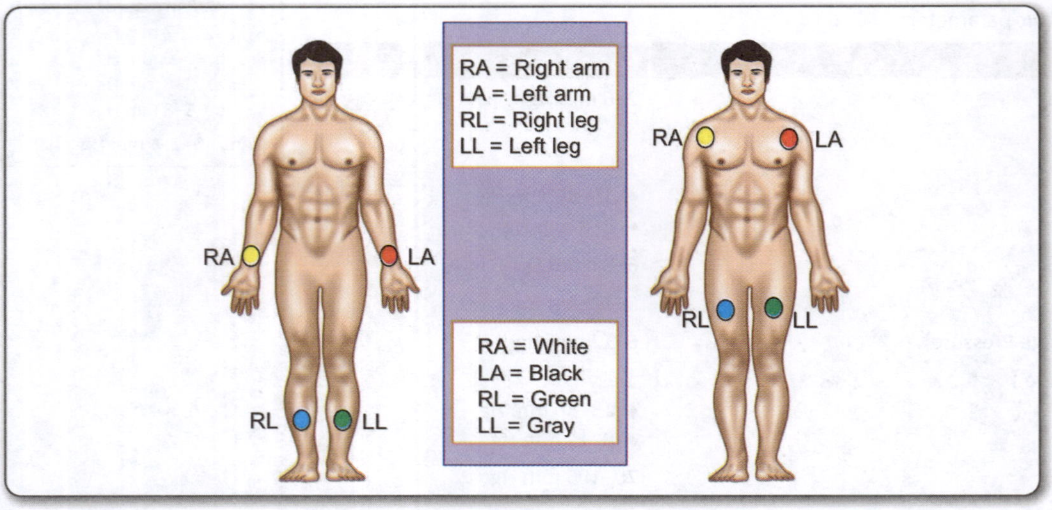

Figure 79: Electrode placement for ECG

KEY POINTS

- CVP is measured at the end of expiration.
- Phlebostatic axis is regarded as the anatomical point that corresponds to the right atrium and most accurately reflects a patient's hemodynamic status
- Phlebostatic axis is located at the 4th intercostal space at the mid-anterior-posterior diameter of the chest wall.

Recent Question (CNCI 2021)

49. Phlebostatic axis is the point at intersection of:

a. Mid-axillary line and line drawn through fourth intercostal space
b. Anterior axillary line and sixth intercostal space
c. Posterior axillary line and fifth intercostal space
d. Anterior axillary line and sixth intercostal space

Ans. (a) Mid-axillary line and line drawn through fourth intercostal space

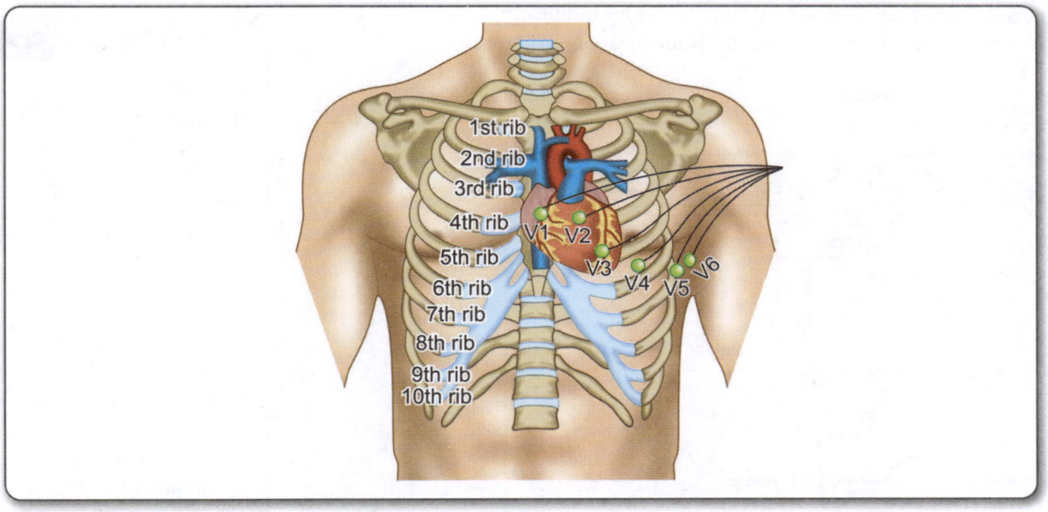

Figure 80: Electrode placement for ECG

POINT TO REMEMBER

Assess the client's chest for areas of irritation, skin breakdown, or excessive hair growth that may interfere with the electrode placement.

Horizontal Plane (Transverse Leads)

- Six chest electrodes (V1, V2, V3, V4, V5, and V6) provide information about the heart's horizontal plane.

Vertical plane (Frontal Leads)

- The **Einthoven's triangle** explains how these 4 limb electrodes provide 6 frontal leads.

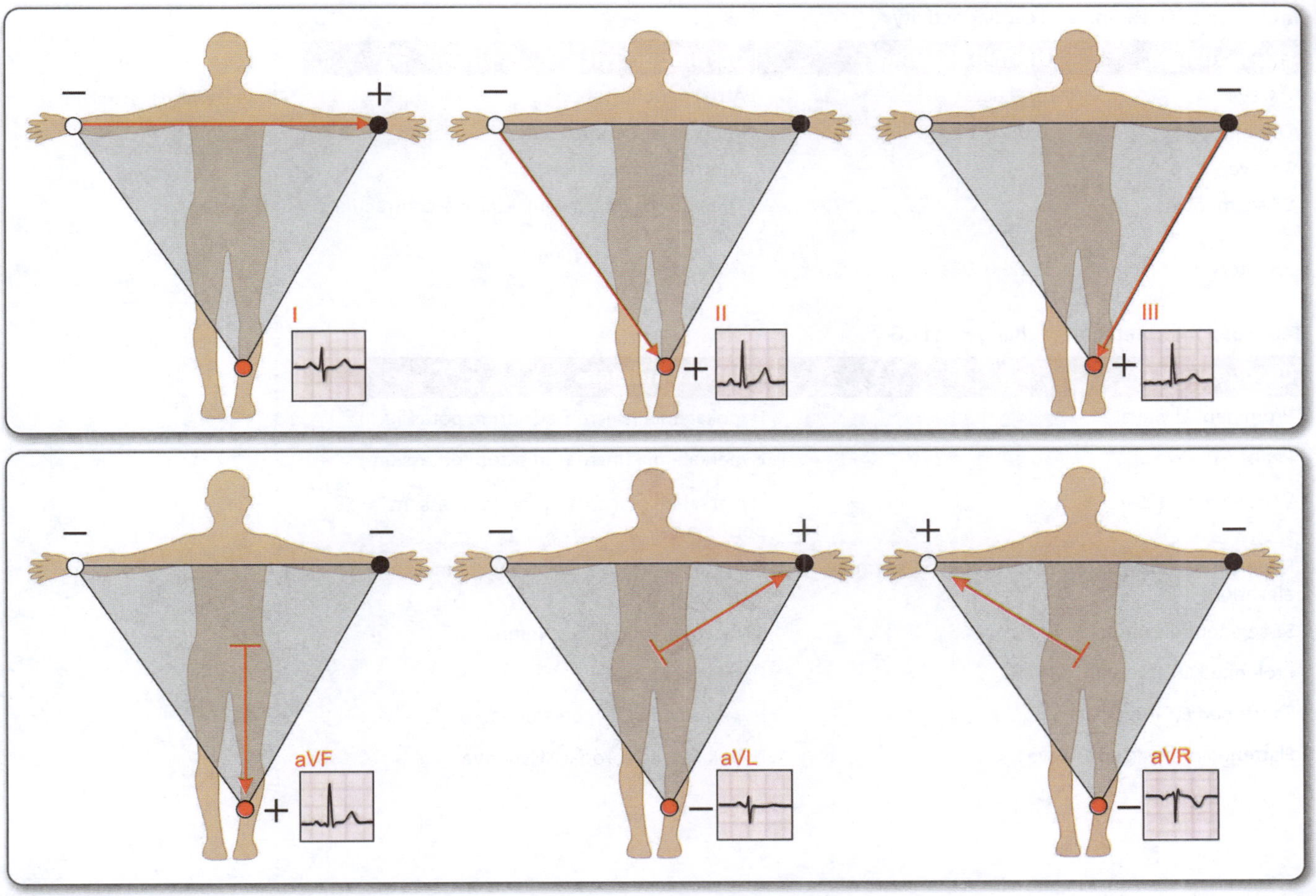

Figure 81: Einthoven's triangle

- Leads I, II, and III require a negative and positive electrode (bipolarity) for monitoring.
- aVR, aVL, and aVF are unipolar and require only a positive electrode for monitoring.

Normal ECG Pattern

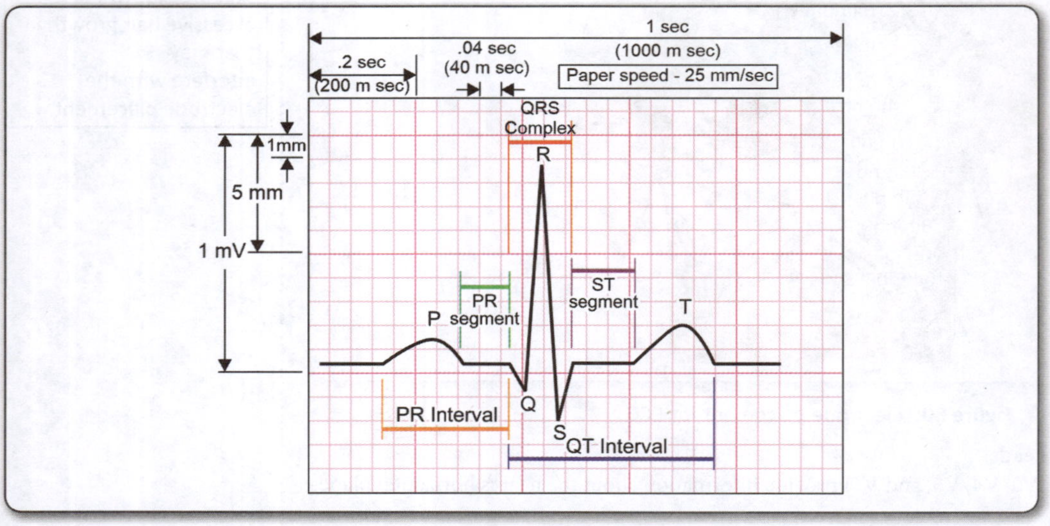

Figure 82: Normal ECG pattern

Table 64: ECG reading and cardiac activity

ECG reading	Normal duration	Cardiac activity
P wave	0.11 sec	Atrial depolarization
QRS complex	0.08–0.12 sec	Ventricular depolarization
T wave		Ventricular repolarization
ST segment		Time during which ventricles are contracting and emptying
PR interval	0.12–0.20 sec	AV Nodal delay

Table 65: Interpretation of changes in ECG

Changes in ECG	Related conditions
Prominent U waves	Hypokalemia (Decreased serum potassium)
Peaked T wave or	Hyperkalemia (Increased serum potassium)
Widening of QRS	Hyperkalemia or tricyclic antidepressant poisoning
Hyperacute T waves (usually precedes ST segment elevation)	Coronary artery occlusion (Acute myocardial infarction)
ST segment elevation	Myocardial ischemia or infarction
Prolonged QT interval	Hypocalcemia
Shortened QT interval	Hypercalcemia, hyperkalemia
Flattened or inverted T waves	Hypokalemia, coronary ischemia

KEY POINTS

Calculation of heart rate using ECG

Rate = 300/No. of large square between consecutive R waves

- ECG: On the horizontal axis, each large box = 0.2 seconds & each smaller box = 0.04 seconds.
- On the vertical axis, each small box is 1 mm in height; 10 mm = 1 mV

Recent Question
(NORCET 2020)

50. Which electrolyte causes atrial depolarization?

a. Sodium
b. Potassium
c. Calcium
d. Phosphate

Ans. (a) Sodium

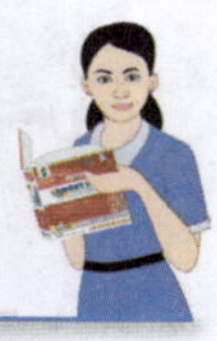

Coronary Angiography

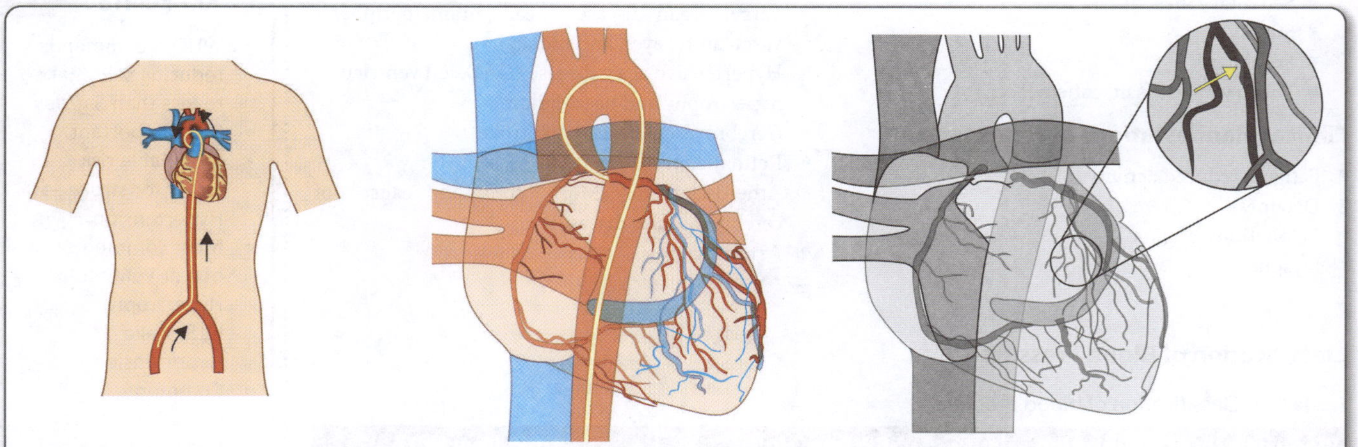

Figure 83: Coronary angiography

- Coronary angiography is performed to visualize coronary arteries, branches, vessel bifurcations, anomalies and specific lesions.
- It is performed for the diagnosis of Coronary Artery Disease and to determine patency of CABG.
- **Contraindications**
  - **Coagulopathy**, decompensated congestive heart failure, **renal failure**, uncontrolled hypertension, **CVA**, pregnancy, active infection, and allergy to contrast medium
- **Before procedure**
  - Blood tests must be done including PTT, INR, BUN, Creatinine, insulin/sugar levels
- **During procedure**
  - Two 500 mL bags of saline is infused with 2 cc (2000 units) of heparin each for flushing tubings
  - Lidocaine is used as local anesthesia
  - Puncture is generally done via femoral artery; radial and brachial arteries are alternative sites
  - Access is easiest from right side of the patient
  - Movement of catheter is monitored under fluoroscopy
  - **Contrast media:** Usually, right coronary artery is filled with 3–5 mL and left coronary artery is filled with 6–8 mL of contrast (320–370 mg of iodine/mg).
  - **Possible complications**
    - Dissection of femoral/iliac artery or aorta
    - Hematoma, coronary embolus
    - Embolus to head and neck vessels
    - Arrhythmia due to catheter wedging.
- **Post procedure:**
  - **Manual pressure** must be applied to site of puncture **for 15 minutes**
  - Patient must lie flat and **supine for minimum of two hours.**

DISORDERS OF CARDIOVASCULAR SYSTEM

Hypertension

- Systolic Blood Pressure (SBP) ≥140 mm Hg and/or Diastolic Blood Pressure (DBP) ≥90 mm Hg.
- ***Blood Pressure Classification*** *(According to the criteria of the Joint National Committee on detection, evaluation and treatment of High Blood Pressure).*
- It can be classified as:
  - Essential or idiopathic hypertension (cause is unknown)
  - Secondary hypertension (secondary to renal, vascular diseases, and pregnancy)
  - Malignant hypertension (Diastolic pressure ≥140 mm Hg)

Risk Factors

- Non-Modifiable Risk factors for primary or essential hypertension
  - Family history
  - Male > Female
  - Obesity
  - Age
  - Ethnicity

KEY POINTS

- After coronary angiography procedure, **Manual pressure** must be applied to site of puncture **for 15 minutes to prevent bleeding**.
- Hypertension is also called **silent killer** because it is frequently asymptomatic until it becomes severe.
- Essential hypertension is the most prevalent form of hypertension accounting for 90 percent of all cases of hypertension.

- **Modifiable Risk factors**
  - Sedentary lifestyle
  - Stress
  - Smoking
  - Dietary habits (salt, caffeine, etc.)

Clinical Manifestations of Hypertension

- Fatigue, reduced activity tolerance
- Dizziness
- Palpitations, angina
- Dyspnea

Complications

- Target organ diseases (heart, brain, peripheral vasculature, eyes, and kidney)
- Hypertensive heart disease (CAD, left ventricular hypertrophy and heart failure)
- Cerebrovascular disease (Stroke)
- Retinal damage
- Atherosclerosis (Most common cause of cerebrovascular disease)
- Arteriosclerosis

Classification of Blood Pressure

Table 66: Classification of blood pressure

Blood pressure classification	SBP[a] (mm Hg)	DBP[b] (mm Hg)
Normal	120 and	80
Prehypertension	120–139 or	80–89
Hypertension	≥140 or	≥90
Stage 1	140–159 or	90–99
Stage 2	≥160 or	≥100
Hypertensive crisis	>180	>110

[a]SBP: Systolic blood pressure, [b]DBP: Diastolic blood pressure

Types

Postural (Orthostatic Hypotension)

- BP falls significantly after assuming an upright position.
- 15 mm Hg fall in systolic BP and 10 mm Hg fall in diastolic BP is termed as postural hypotension.

White Coat Hypertension

- BP rises when assessed by healthcare personnel due to anxiety in a normal individual.

Malignant Hypertension

- Blood pressure rises rapidly. **Diastolic BP > 120 mm Hg.**
- It is a medical emergency. Untreated malignant hypertension causes target organ damage and death.

Hypertensive Crisis

Abrupt increases in blood pressure more than 180/120 mm Hg which may result in end organ damage.

It includes -

- **Hypertensive urgency:** High blood pressure (BP > 180/120 mm Hg) without any organ damage.
- **Hypertensive emergency:** High blood pressure (BP > 180/120 mm Hg) with evidence of end organ damage.

Management of Hypertensive Crisis – Sodium Nitroprusside is drug of choice.

Nonpharmacological management of hypertension:

- ***Diet modification:***
  - DASH (Dietary approach to stop hypertension) diet has to be followed which includes high proteins, free or low-fat dairy products (2 or 3 servings per day), low sodium (1.5 g/day), and more fruits and vegetables.
  - No smoking and do not consume alcohol
  - Restricted intake of tea and coffee.
- ***Exercises, meditation, and yoga***
- ***Stress management*** with biofeedback

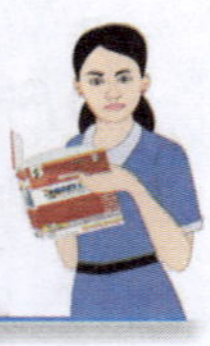

KEY POINTS

- WHO recommends reducing salt intake to less than 5 g/day
- Most important modifiable risk factor for stroke → Hypertension
- Most common cause of Left Ventricular Hypertrophy is: Systolic Hypertension
- Common complications of hypertension are cerebrovascular disease, peripheral vascular disease, nephrosclerosis, and retinal damage.

Recent Question (NORCET 2020)

51. Clonidine is used to

a. Increase low BP
b. Decrease high BP
c. Increase pulse rate
d. Decrease pulse rate

Ans. (b) Decrease high BP

Cardiac Arrhythmias

Table 67: Description of cardiac arrhythmias

Types of rhythm	Description
Normal sinus rhythm	• Atrial or ventricular rate 60–90 beats per minute 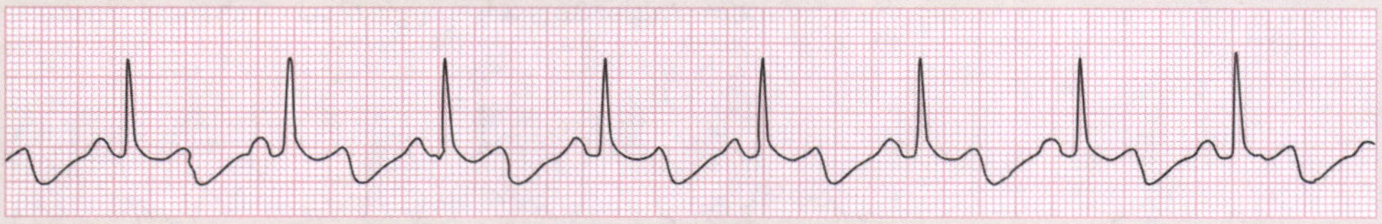
Sinus bradycardia	• HR < 60 BPM. Each P wave is followed by QRS complex • **Management:** Dopamine, Atropine I.V. (Epinephrine if atropine is not effective) and transcutaneous pacemakers. 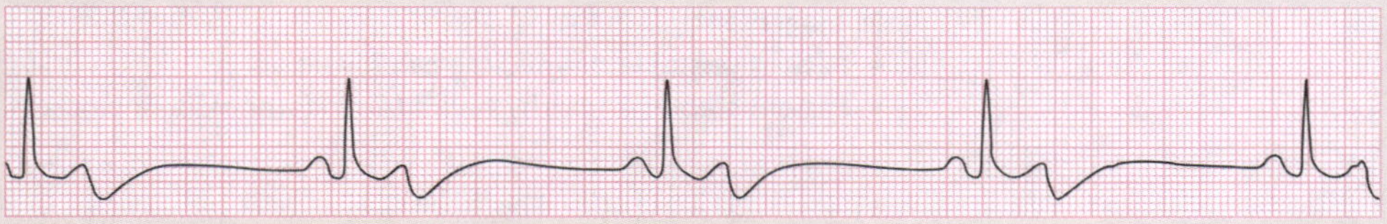
Sinus tachycardia	• HR > 100 bpm. Every QRS complex is followed by P wave. • **Management:** Calcium-channel blocker and beta blockers 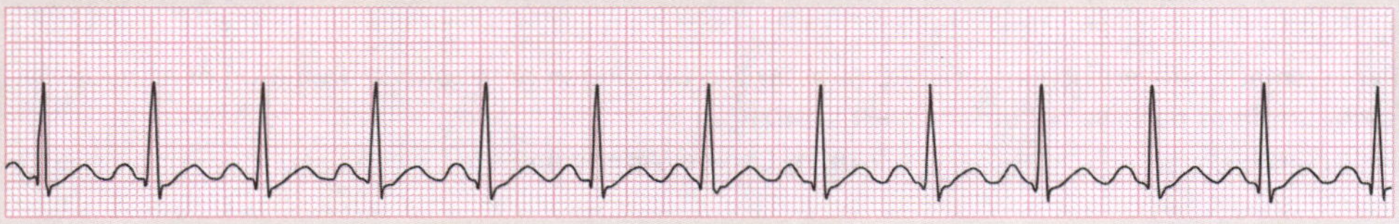
Ventricular tachycardia (VT)	• Ventricular heart rate 100 to 220 BPM. The rate may be regular. • Generally no visible P wave present • Irregular and wide QRS complex, p wave appears as erratic, irregular waves. • **Management:** ▪ CPR and ACLS in pulseless VT ▪ Defibrillation, Vasopressin or IV epinephrine. 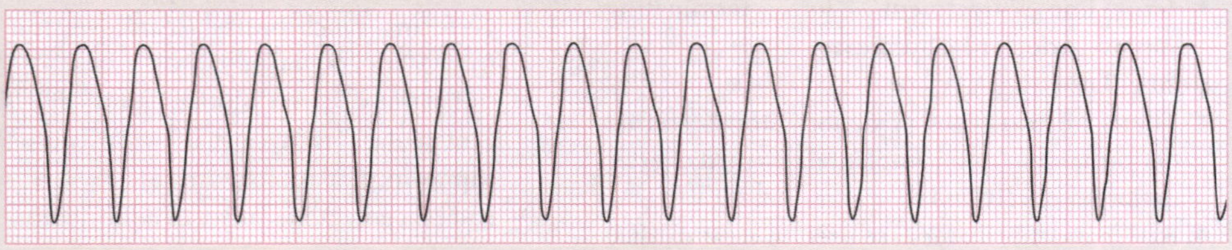
Ventricular fibrillation (VF)	• Rapid ventricular rhythm. • There is no visible P wave or QRS complex. • **Management:** CPR following ACLS ▪ Epinephrine, amiodarone, vasopressin, or lidocaine are used for management ▪ Defibrillation 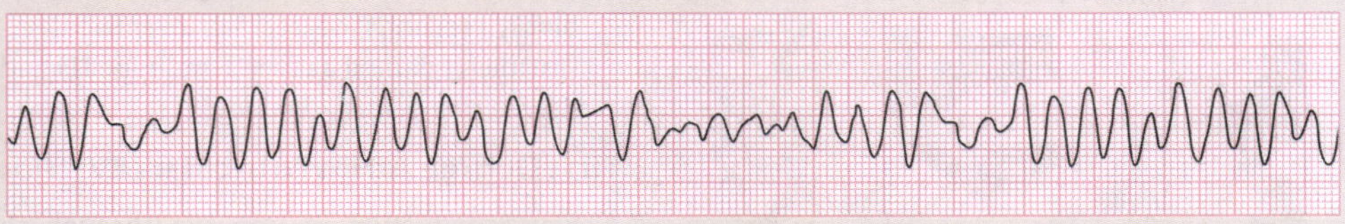

Contd...

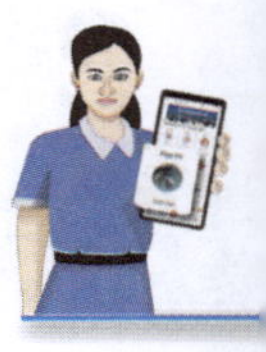

Types of rhythm	Description
Atrial fibrillation	• Atrial rate will be usually above 400 beats per minute and ventricular rate vary. • Uniform QRS complex at irregular interval. • **Management** ▪ **Patient unstable:** Immediate cardioversion ▪ **Patient stable:** Beta adrenergic blocker, channel blockers, or antiarrhythmics (Amiodarone). 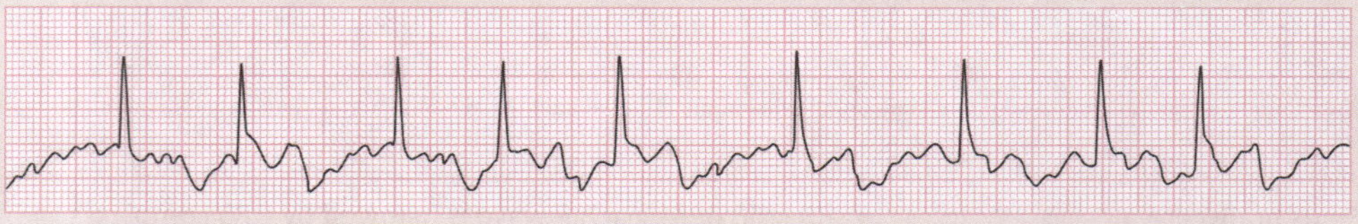
Atrial flutter	Atrial rate is regular but the rate varies from 250 to 400 beats per minute Typically irregular but **uniform QRS complex** **Management:** • **Patient unstable:** Immediate cardioversion • **Patient stable:** Antiarrhythmics (Amiodarone), beta blockers, channel blockers 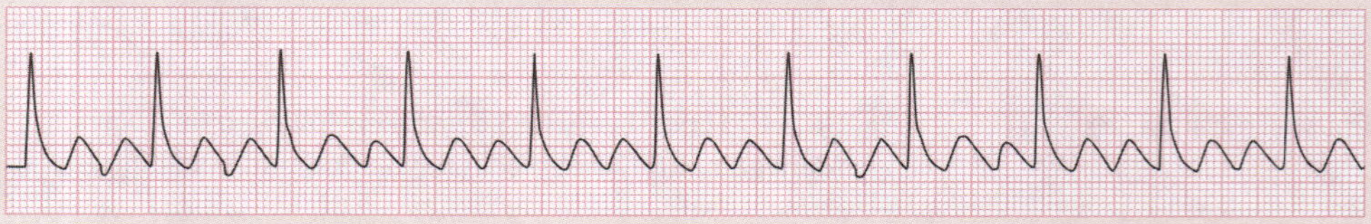
Paroxysmal supraventricular tachycardia or paroxysmal atrial tachycardia	Characterized by sudden onset and termination of arrhythmia. HR > 140 bpm **Drug of Choice: Adenosine**

Management of Arrhythmias

- **Vagal maneuver:**
  - Parasympathetic nerve system activation by carotid sinus massage, straining or bearing down, gagging, coughing etc.
  - 1st line treatment for terminating supraventricular tachycardia
- **Defibrillator**
  - There are two types of defibrillators: external defibrillators and implantable cardioverter defibrillators (ICDs).
  - External defibrillators are used to treat cardiac arrest, while ICDs are used to prevent cardiac arrest.
  - For biphasic defibrillators, the initial energy level is typically between 120 and 200 joules
  - For monophasic defibrillators, the initial energy level is typically 360 joules.

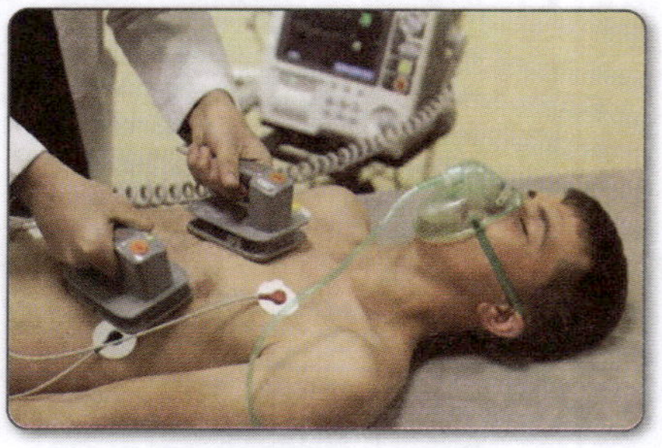

Figure 84: Defibrillator

- **Cardioversion**
  - The shock is delivered with synchronization of QRS complex.
  - Very low energy about 50 Joules shock is given at first.
  - The recommended energy levels used to perform synchronized cardioversion vary from 50 to 200 joules
  - Indications: atrial flutter, atrial fibrillation, ventricular tachycardia with pulse, and supraventricular tachycardia
  - Pad placement is similar to defibrillator.

Heart Block

- It occurs as a result of delay in conduction of electrical impulses through the conduction pathway.
- It is classified as first degree atrioventricular block, second degree atrioventricular block (further classified as type I and type II) and third degree atrioventricular block.

First Degree Atrioventricular (AV) Block

- Slow conduction of impulses through the AV node, which leads to PR interval > 0.2 seconds.
- Ratio of P: QRS complex is 1:1.
- Usually it is asymptomatic.
- No treatment required.

Recent Questions
(NORCET 2020)

52. Lignocaine is used to treat
a. MI
b. Angina
c. CAD
d. Arrhythmia

Ans. (d) Arrhythmia

53. Use of epinephrine will cause which of the following symptoms?
a. Bradycardia
b. Tachycardia
c. Increased BP
d. Tachypnea

Ans. (b) Tachycardia

Second Degree AV Block

Second degree type I

- Also called as Mobitz type I or Wenkebach's phenomenon.
- Here AV node is fatigued and fails to conduct an impulse into the ventricles.
- PR interval is progressively lengthened and then one QRS complex is missed.

Second degree type II

- Also called Mobitz Type II
- In this type intermittently AV node does not respond to the impulse from SA node, as a result some of the p waves are not followed by a QRS complex
- QRS complexes are randomly dropped. There is no pattern in the conduction blockade.
- PR interval is constant. There is no progressive lengthening of PR interval.

Third Degree AV Block

- Also known as complete heart block.
- None of the electrical impulses are conducted to the ventricles through the AV node. No relation between atria and ventricles.
- Ventricles make its own impulses at a slower rate.
- All RR interval will be equal and all PP interval are equal.
- Permanent pacemaker is the treatment of choice.

Cor Pulmonale

- Lung disorders such as pulmonary artery hypertension which leads to structural and functional alteration of right ventricle is known as cor pulmonale.
- **Clinical manifestation:** Dyspnea, fatigue, peripheral edema, ascites, enlarged neck vein, pleural effusion
- **Management:** Focuses on reducing pulmonary artery hypertension by providing supplemental oxygen, bronchodilators, bed rest, sodium and water restriction

CORONARY ARTERY DISEASES

Arteriosclerosis

- It refers to hardening of the arteries.
- It is one of the most common diseases of arteries.

Atherosclerosis

- It refers to accumulation of lipids in the blood vessels.
- Atherosclerosis mainly affects tunica intima (innermost layer) of the medium-sized and large arteries.
- **Risk factors:** High fat intake, obesity, diabetes, tobacco use, hypertension, sedentary lifestyle with minimum exercises and stress.

Angina Pectoris

- Angina pectoris is a condition characterized by pain (often retrosternal) in the anterior chest wall due to insufficient coronary blood flow.
- **Pain often radiates to the shoulders, arms, neck and jaw.**
- Pain is relieved by rest or nitroglycerine.
- **Atherosclerosis** is the most common predisposing factor for angina pectoris.
- Resolving the predisposing factors subsides pain.

KEY POINTS

- Most important modifiable risk factor for atherosclerosis is smoking
- **Most common cause of aortic aneurysm is:** Atherosclerosis
- The coronary artery most commonly involved in atherosclerosis is Left Anterior Descending Artery (LAD).
- Infective agent causing atherosclerosis is *Chlamydia pneumoniae*
- Elevated Low Density Lipoprotein (LDL) is a risk factor for atherosclerosis.
- High Density Lipoprotein (HDL) prevents formation of atheroscelerosis
- Rest and nitroglycerine will relieve the angina pain but not in myocardial infarction (MI).
- In angina, cardiac enzymes level do not rise

Table 68: Types of angina pectoris

Stable angina	Variant angina	Unstable angina
Experienced during exercise or increased workload; relieved by rest or nitroglycerin	Unrelated to physical activity. Caused by coronary artery spasm. Rare and episodic. Relieved by nitroglycerin, vasodilators, Ca^+ channel blockers	Caused by acute plaque change; occurs with increased frequency, intensity and duration. Occurs at lower level of physical activity or rest. It is warning sign for Acute MI

Myocardial Infarction (MI)

- Myocardial tissue of heart dies (ischemia) from lack of blood supply.
- **Causes**
  - **Most common:** Blockage (thrombus or lipid) of coronary artery from Coronary artery disease.
  - Most common site of blockage is Left Anterior Descending Artery (LAD).
  - **LAD blockage cause worst damage** because it supplies left ventricle.
  - **Other causes:** Vasospasm of coronary artery, decreased oxygen supply and increased demand for oxygen
- **Clinical manifestations: (Remember – CRUSHING)**
  - **C:** Chest Pain (severe intensity)
  - **R:** Radiating chest pain that moves to left arm, jaw and back
  - **U: Unrelieved pain by rest or nitroglycerin (Hallmark of MI)**
  - **S:** Sweating
  - **H:** Hard to breathe (Shortness of breath)
  - **I:** Increased and irregular Heart Rate, Increased blood pressure.
  - **N:** Nausea and vomiting
  - **G:** Going to be anxious

Recent Question (NORCET 2022)

54. This is the classic ECG change in Myocardial infarction:

a. ST-segment elevation
b. Negative T-waves
c. Development of an abnormal Q wave
d. All of these

Ans. (d) All of these

Recent Question (NORCET 2020)

55. Silent MI is commonly seen in

a. CKD
b. HTN
c. Diabetes mellitus
d. COPD

Ans. (c) Diabetes mellitus

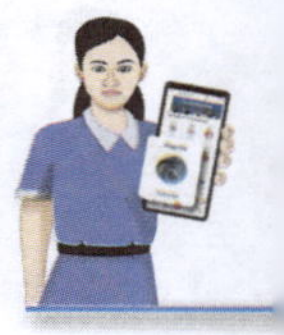

- **Assessment/diagnosis**
  - Patient history
  - ECG within 10 minutes of arrival in emergency room
  - Echocardiography
- **Cardiac enzyme and biomarkers**
  - Elevated levels of Troponins (highest sensitivity), CK-MB, Myoglobin and Lactate Dehrogenase (LDH).
  - Detailed parameters regarding biomarkers are provided in the beginning of this chapter.

Electrocardiography Changes

- **STEMI:** New or presumed new ST elevation at the J point in two anatomically contiguous leads using the following diagnostic thresholds:
  - ≥0.1 mV (1 mm) in all leads other than V2–V3.
- **NSTEMI:** New or presumed new horizontal or down-sloping ST depression ≥0.05 mV (0.5 mm) in two anatomically contiguous leads **and/or** T wave inversion ≥0.1 mV (1 mm) in two anatomically contiguous leads with prominent R wave.
  - **Q wave** on ECG indicates an old MI
- **Management**
  - **To treat suspected acute MI**

    M – Morphine **O – Oxygen**

    N – Nitroglycerin **A – Aspirin**

Management of Heart Failure

- High fowler's position to reduce breathing difficulty.
- If patient is in shock, administer the inotropic agents (dopamine, dobutamine, amrinone, etc.)
- If heart rate < 60 beats/minute, digoxin should be withheld
- Continuous ABG monitoring

Monitor intake and output and restrict fluid according to that

- **Reperfusion:** Thrombolytic medications (Actilyse, Strepto-kinase) or percutaneous coronary interventions.
- Reduce myocardial oxygen demand and increase oxygen supply
- Coronary artery bypass graft (CABG).
- **Other Pharmacological therapy:**
  - Anticoagulators (heparin and warfarin) and Aspirin (anti-platelet)
  - ACE (Angiotensin-converting enzyme inhibitors)

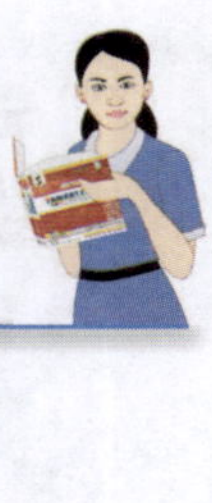

Intervention for a suspected heart attack (Myocardial infarction/mg)

M — Morphine
O — Oxygen
N — Nitroglycerin
A — Aspirin

Percutaneous Transluminal Coronary Angioplasty (PTCA)

- PTCA is performed to open narrowed or blocked coronary arteries caused by coronary artery disease.
- The catheter has a tiny balloon at the tip and the balloon is inflated once the catheter is placed into the narrowed artery area.
- Stent placement: A tiny, expandable metal coil is expanded at the newly opened site of the coronary artery to prevent closing again.

Intra Aortic Balloon Pump (IABP)

- IABP is a volume displacement device (counterpulsation system)
- The balloon must be inflated at the onset of diastole
- Inflation of IABP results in increased coronary perfusion pressure and systemic perfusion pressure
- Balloon deflation occurs during systole
- Deflation – To reduce left ventricular workload. It results in reduction of afterload.
- **Purposes**
  - Cardiac support for hemodynamically challenged patients
  - Post-surgical myocardial dysfunction
  - For maintenance of graft patency in post CABG client
  - Cardiac support after surgical correction of anatomical defects
  - Support for weaning from cardiopulmonary bypass
- **Insertion technique**
  - Percutaneous (Sheath less)
  - Surgical incision (Femoral cut down or Trans-thoracic)
- **Positioning of balloon**
  - The tip is approximately 1–2 cm below the origin of the left subclavian artery and above the renal arteries
  - On chest X-ray the tip should be visible in the **2nd or 3rd intercostal space.**

NURSING CARE OF PATIENT UNDERGOING CABG (CORONARY ARTERY BYPASS GRAFT)

- **Preoperative Care**
  - Obtain history of allergy and hypersensitivity to specific drugs
  - Teach the patient and family about surgery and immediate postoperative period.
- **Intraoperative Care**
  - Patient is placed on a cardiopulmonary bypass machine (Heart lung machine).
  - Bypass graft is usually harvested from **saphenous vein in the leg or internal mammary artery.**

KEY POINTS

- Hallmark of MI is pain unrelieved by rest or medication (nitroglycerine)
- **Myoglobin is the early marker** for MI but **Troponin is the most sensitive** (superior) marker.

Recent Questions (CNCI 2021)

56. Which assessment indicates the nurse about development of cardiogenic shock in M.I. patient in I.C.U.?

a. Bradycardia
b. Increased blood pressure
c. Oliguria
d. Warm & flushed skin

Ans. (c) Oliguria

57. Medical treatment of coronary artery disease includes which of the following procedures?

a. Cardiac catheterization
b. Oral medication administration
c. Coronary artery bypass grafting
d. Percutaneous transluminal coronary angioplasty

Ans. (b) Oral medication administration

- **Postoperative Care**
  - Hemodynamic monitoring (cardiac output, central venous pressure, etc.).
  - ECG evaluations
  - **Swan-Ganz catheterization** is a type of pulmonary artery catheterization procedure (right heart catheterization). It is used to determine whether any hemodynamic abnormalities exist in the heart and lungs.
  - **Change the position 2 hourly** to promote **venous drainage.**
  - Drainage cessation or sudden red-colored discharge that lasts more than a minute need to be informed to the physician.
  - Inform physician if patient does not wake up 1–3 hours after surgery.

Heart Failure

- Heart is no longer able to pump the blood needed to meet the body's requirement.
- Coronary Artery Disease (CAD) is the most common cause of Heart Failure.
- **Types of heart failures:**
  1. **Left Sided Heart Failure:** Left ventricle is unable to pump out enough blood to the body
     a. Systolic failure (reduced ejection fraction)
     b. Diastolic failure (preserved ejection fraction)
  2. **Right Sided Heart Failure:** Right ventricle is unable to pump enough blood into lungs

Recent Question (NORCET 2020)

58. Which electrolyte is closely monitored in digoxin administration?
a. Sodium
b. Calcium
c. Potassium
d. Phosphate

Ans. (c) Potassium

Table 69: Differences between left-sided and right-sided heart failure

	Left-sided heart failure	Right-sided heart failure
Cause	Ventricular septal defect Cardiomyopathy Anterior wall myocardial infarction (MI) Cardiac tamponade Constrictive pericarditis Mitral stenosis and insufficiency Aortic stenosis and insufficiency Hypervolemia	Left-sided heart failure Atrial septal defect Right ventricular myocardial infarction Pulmonary hypertension (cor pulmonale) Sodium retention and hypervolemia Pulmonary embolism, mitral stenosis Pulmonary outflow stenosis COPD, or thyrotoxicosis
Clinical manifestation	Dyspnea on exertion, cheyne-stokes respirations, **rhonchi, crackles,** orthopnea, hypoxia, respiratory acidosis, peripheral cyanosis, and abnormal heart sounds (S3 and S4)	Splenomegaly, hepatomegaly, Ascites, Weight gain, anorexia, bounding peripheral pulses, **hepatojugular reflex, Kussmaul's respirations**
	Shortness of breath, chest discomfort, peripheral edema, bloating, paroxysmal nocturnal dyspnea, distended jugular veins, and reduced urine output	
Management	Oxygen administration, activity restriction, **Drug of Choice: Digoxin** **Other Drugs:** ACE inhibitors, diuretics, and beta blockers	

OTHER DISEASES OF HEART

For management of Acute Heart Failure or a CHF exacerbation (i.e., a patient presenting with acute pulmonary edema).

LMNOP
- **L**asix (Furosemide)/Loop diuretic
- **M**orphine (narcotic analgesic)
- **N**itroglycerin (Vasodilators)
- **O**xygen
- **P**osition: Upright

Myocarditis

- Inflammation of myocardium is known as myocarditis.
- It is classified into acute and chronic myocarditis.
- It can lead to congestive heart failure and sudden cardiac death.

Pericarditis

- It refers to inflammation of pericardium which is a protective layer covering the heart.
- Chest pain from pericarditis is referred to by: **Phrenic nerve**
- Most common cause of constrictive pericarditis in, India →TB
- Most common cause of endocarditis: *S. aureus*
- **Dukes Criteria** is used for diagnosis of pericarditis

Cardiac Tamponade

- Clinical syndrome caused by accumulation of fluid in the pericardial space.
- It leads to reduced ventricular filling.
- **15 to 50 mL is the normal pericardial fluid volume in adult.**
- **Beck's triad** is a collection of 3 signs associated with Cardiac Tamponade.

Recent Question (NORCET 2023)

59. When performing a cardiovascular assessment, the nurse notes that patient needs to sit upright to breathe. This behavior is most indicative of:
a. Pericarditis
b. Anxiety
c. Congestive heart failure
d. Angina

Ans. (c) Congestive heart failure

- Hypotension with narrowed pulse pressure
- Jugular venous distension
- Muffled Heart Sounds

Pulmonary Edema

- It is a life-threatening condition that occurs because of the accumulation of fluid in the lungs (alveoli and interstitial space).
- **Clinical manifestation:** Dyspnea, cyanosis, agitation, anxious, tachycardia, tachypnea, crackles over the lung field during auscultation.
- Pink frothy sputum is the characteristic of pulmonary edema.

Acute Rheumatic Fever

Acute rheumatic fever's etiology, age preference, sex preference, clinical manifestations and management have been given in a summarized table.

Table 70: Acute rheumatic fever

Acute rheumatic fever	
Etiology	• Caused by Group-A beta hemolytic streptococci
Sex	• Female > Male
Age group	• 5–15 years
Clinical Manifestations	• Joint pain and swelling (Most common feature) • **Aschoff's bodies** (On microscopic examination) • **Sydenham Chorea:** Uncoordinated jerky movements of the face and limbs • **Erythema marginatum** (rare symptom)
Management	• Single dose of Inj. Benzathine Penicillin OR Procaine penicillin BD for 10 days • Steroids for 12 weeks (If Carditis present) • Erythromycin for Penicillin allergic patient • DOC for prophylaxis: Benzathine Penicillin/Erythromycin (in allergic patient)

Cardiomyopathy

It is a disorder of the myocardium which causes myocardial dysfunction that results in poor cardiac performance.

- **Hypertrophic Cardiomyopathy**
  - In hypertrophic cardiomyopathy, the myocardium becomes hypertrophied (thickened), resulting in diastolic dysfunction (impaired relaxation of the ventricles) and smaller ventricular size.
  - There are two subtypes:
    1. Obstructive hypertrophic cardiomyopathy - septal hypertrophy obstructs the ventricular outlet
    2. Nonobstructive hypertrophic cardiomyopathy.
  - Hypertrophic cardiomyopathy is considered normal for certain group of people like athletes, pregnant women, and younger age groups.
- **Dilated Cardiomyopathy**
  - In dilated cardiomyopathy, one or both ventricles become pathologically dilated (enlarged).
  - This condition is characterized by systolic dysfunction, where the heart has difficulty in contracting effectively.
- **Restrictive Cardiomyopathy**
  - Restrictive cardiomyopathy involves ventricular dysfunction without significant dilation or hypertrophy.
  - The ventricle loses its flexibility due to infiltration of substances like amyloid protein or other substances.
  - Both systolic and diastolic dysfunction can occur in this type.

Management

- Definitive management is heart transplantation

Table 71: Left heart obstructive lesions and right heart obstructive lesions

Left heart obstructive lesions	Right heart obstructive lesions
• Aortic stenosis • Aortic regurgitation • Hypertrophic cardiomyopathy • Coarctation of the aorta • Mitral stenosis • Mitral regurgitation	• Pulmonary stenosis • Pulmonary regurgitation • Ebstein's anomaly • Tricuspid atresia • Tetralogy of Fallot • Transposition of the great arteries

ARTERIAL DISEASES

Aortic Aneurysm

- It is a sac like projection or dilation in the weak wall of the aorta. **(Ballooning of Artery)**
- Saccular and fusiform aneurysm are the most common types.
- Abdominal aortic aneurysm is most commonly seen in older persons.

KEY POINTS

- **Left ventricular failure results in blood backing into the pulmonary circulation. This causes PULMONARY EDEMA, a medical emergency.** It is manifested by extreme dyspnea and cough, may lead to Pulmonary edema, a life-threatening condition.
- **Management:** High Fowler Position with legs in dependent position and High concentration Oxygen delivery through mask or nasal cannula
- Globular or Flask or Pear-Shaped heart is seen in cardiac tamponade

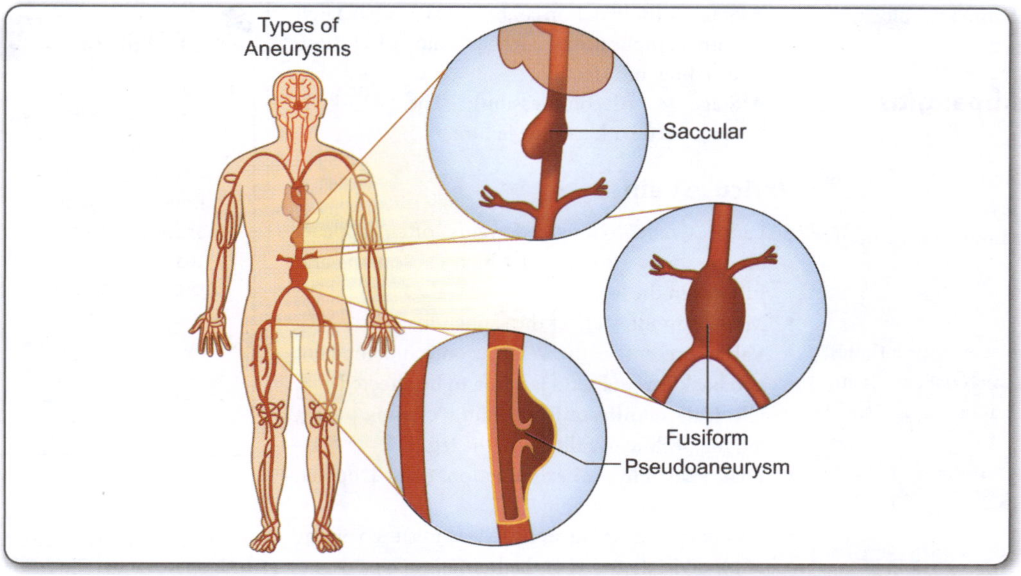

Figure 85: Types of aneurysms

Thoracic Aneurysm

- Pain in the jaw, neck, chest or upper back.
- Wheezing, coughing, or shortness of breath as a result of pressure on the trachea (windpipe)
- Hoarseness as a result of pressure on the vocal cords and trouble in swallowing due to pressure on the esophagus.

Abdominal Aneurysm

- Pulsatile abdominal mass, tenderness and ecchymosis (if aneurysm ruptured).
- Usually painless if the size is increased the surrounding organ is compressed that result in flank and groin pain.

Nursing Management

- Instruct patient for smoking cessation.
- Instruct patient to avoid heavy lifting and stretching activity.
- Avoid deep palpation.

Aortic Stenosis

- Narrowing of the aortic valve orifice located between left ventricle and aorta.
- Rheumatic endocarditis or degenerative calcifications are the most common causes of aortic stenosis.
- Heart muscles increase in size in response to obstruction.
- Heart failure occurs when compensatory mechanisms fail to compensate.

Manifestations: (Remember SAD)
- **S:** Syncope
- **A:** Angina Pectoris
- **D:** Dyspnea (exertional dyspnea)

Arterial Embolism

- An **arterial embolism** may be caused by one or more clots. The clots can get stuck in an artery and block blood flow.
- **Emboli (moving clot)** arises most commonly from thrombi that develop in the chambers of the heart.
- The immediate effect is cessation of distal blood flow.
- Emboli tend to lodge at arterial bifurcations and areas of atherosclerotic narrowing (cerebral, mesenteric, renal, and coronary arteries).
- Acute thrombosis frequently occurs in patients with pre-existing ischemic symptoms.
- **Management:**
  - Heparin therapy
  - Emergency embolectomy only if the involved extremity is viable.
  - Intra-arterial thrombolytic therapy (streptokinase, urokinase or staphylokinase).

Raynaud's Disease (Raynaud's Phenomenon)

- Vasospasm of the small peripheral arteries and arterioles of limbs in response to severe cold or emotional stress. This results in excessively reduced blood flow to the extremities.
- **Causes:** Cold temperature, stress, blood vessels in spasm, scleroderma, Sjögren disease, Carpal tunnel syndrome.
- **Clinical manifestation:** Blanching and cyanosis in the skin of fingers, tingling, and numbness.
- **Investigation:** Cold stimulation test, Nailfold capillaroscopy, C-reactive protein test, ESR

KEY POINTS

- Elevated ASO (Anti streptolysin 'O') Titre is evident in streptococcal infection. Can be seen in Rheumatic fever/Rheumatic Heart Disease/ Glomerulonephritis.
- **Jones criteria** is used for diagnosis of Rheumatic fever (Refer Pediatric Nursing Synopsis for explanation).
- **Atherosclerosis** is the most common cause of Aortic aneurysm.
- The presence of a pulsating mass in the abdomen indicates abdominal aortic aneurysm.
- Marfan syndrome is a genetic disorder of the connective tissue. It may result in premature loss of elasticity of blood vessels and Aneurysm.
- Aortic dissection most commonly occurs in thoracic aorta.

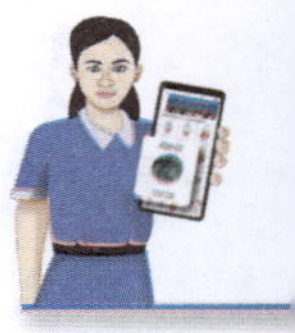

- **Treatment:** Calcium channel blockers, vasodilators, alpha blockers

Buerger's Disease (Thromboangitis Obliterans)

- Inflammatory occlusive vascular disorder affecting small and medium sized arteries and veins.
- Distal part of lower and upper limbs is commonly affected.

Intermittent Claudication

- Muscle pain (cramp, numbness, or fatigue), especially in the calf muscle, which occurs during exercise, such as walking, and is relieved by a short period of rest.
- **Common Cause:** Arterial insufficiency due to atherosclerotic blockage

Thrombophlebitis

- The formation of blood clots or thrombus in the blood vessels results inflammation of blood vessels.
- The pathophysiology behind this disease is venous stasis, endothelium damage, hypercoagulability (OCP use) long-term immobility.
- It occurs both in superficial and deep veins.

Nursing Management of Thrombophlebitis

- Avoid rubbing or massaging the affected leg.
- Avoid pressure behind the knee and constrictive clothing.
- Give anti-inflammatory and analgesic if the pain is present.
- Use elastic stocking.
- Monitor for signs and symptoms of pulmonary embolism.
- Instruct the patient not to cross the legs during sitting.

Arteriovenous Malformation

- An arteriovenous malformation (AVM) is a tangle of blood vessels that connects arteries and veins directly, bypassing the capillaries
- AVMs can occur anywhere in the body, but they are most common in the brain and spinal cord.
- **The Schöbinger staging system** is a clinical classification system used to grade the severity of AVMs.
- **The four stages are as follows:**
  - Stage 1 (quiescence): The AVM is small and asymptomatic. There may be a visible cutaneous blush or warmth, but no other symptoms.
  - Stage 2 (expansion): The AVM is larger and may be associated with symptoms such as bruit, palpable thrill, or expanding lesion.
  - Stage 3 (destruction): The AVM is associated with complications such as pain, ulceration, bleeding, or infection.
  - Stage 4 (decompression): The AVM is associated with cardiac failure.

Varicose Vein

- Large swollen elongated veins often appears on the lower extremities which cause pain and fullness in the leg.
- Most commonly affect the saphenous vein
- Valves present in the vein become incompetent and backflow of blood is going to be affected.
- **Clinical manifestation:** Pain, cramps, ache, fatigue, feeling of fullness in the leg
- **Diagnosis:** Physical examination, color Doppler, duplex ultrasonography.
- **Venous plethysmography:** Measures the volume of blood in the veins of the legs
- **Complication:** Bleeding, thrombophlebitis, leg ulcer
- Avoid prolonged standing, elevate leg, use of elastic bandage from toe to thigh which promote venous return.
- **Surgical management:** Sclerotherapy, ligation and stripping of vein and laser ablation.
- **Foam sclerotherapy:** By injecting sclerosant into a varicose vein, destroy its endothelium in that area, and thus induce an aseptic thrombosis which organizes and closes the vein.
- **Contraindications:** Pregnancy, pelvic tumor, DVT, previous history of reaction to sclerosant.

Immediate Postoperative Care

- Maintenance of firm elastic pressure over limb
- Regular movement and exercise of legs
- Elevation of foot of the bed 6–9 inches
- Patient is not allowed more than 2 pillows
- The original firm crepe bandage put on at the operation should remain untouched for 7 days
- Stitches are removed after 7 days
- A firm webbing elastic bandage from ankle to knee should be worn throughout the day for 2 weeks

Postoperative Complications

- Hematoma and Bruising
- Lymphoma
- Wound sepsis
- Postoperative saphenous neuritis
- Lymphedema
- DVT and embolism
- Induration of stripper tract

KEY POINTS

- Calcium channel blockers **(nifidipine)** is first line drug therapy for patient with Raynaud disease.
- **Trendelenburg's test** is used to assess the competency of the valves in the superficial and deep veins of the legs in patients with **varicose veins.**

Recent Questions (NORCET 2020)

60. Bandaging of lower legs should be started from

a. Ankle
b. Foot
c. Knees
d. Fingers

Ans. (b) Foot

61. While giving CPR what is the correct position of hand?

a. Above the chest
b. Above the nipples
c. Just below the nipple
d. Lower half of the sternum

Ans. (d) Lower half of the sternum

Table 72: Drug of choice for cardiac diseases

Cardiac disease/abnormality	Drug of choice
Angina Pectoris	Sublingual Nitroglycerin
Acute Ventricular Tachycardia (when refractory to cardioversion shock)	Amiodarone
Supraventricular Tachycardia	Adenosine or Verapamil
Cardiogenic shock	Dopamine
Heart Failure	Digoxin
Hypertensive emergency/malignant hypertension	Sodium nitroprusside

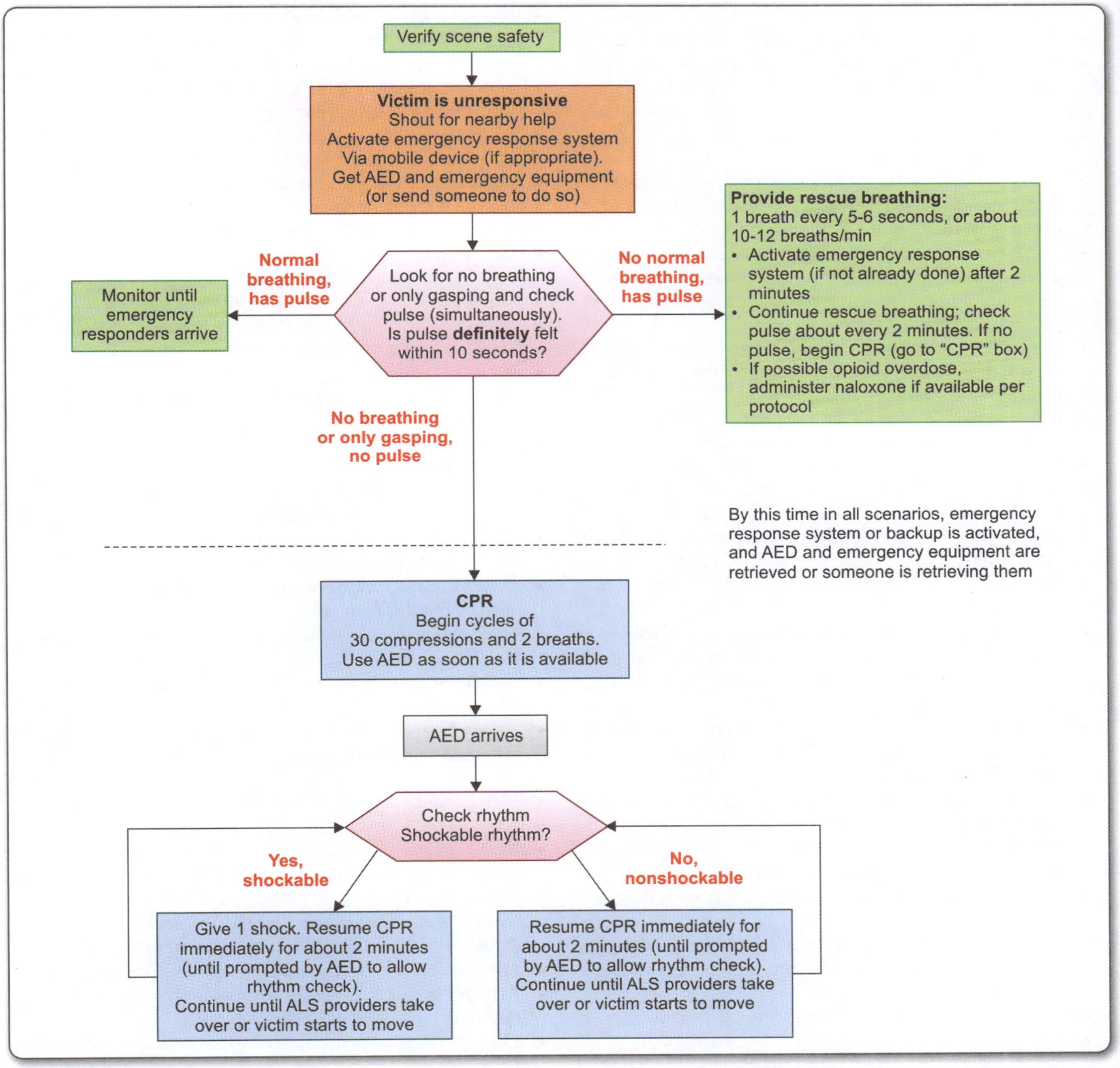

Figure 86: Cardiopulmonary resuscitation algorithm — 2015 update

Golden Points to Remember

- As per WHO data (2015) Coronary artery disease causes most deaths world-wide (8.8 Million deaths) followed by Stroke (6.2 Million deaths).
- High Homocysteine level (**>12–15 mmol/L**) damages the inner lining of the blood vessel and causes atherosclerosis.
- Orthostatic hypotension is defined as a decrease in **systolic blood pressure** of 20 mm Hg or a decrease in **diastolic blood pressure** of 10 mm Hg within three minutes of standing when compared with blood pressure from the sitting or supine position.
- Outpouching or dilation of arterial wall is called **aneurysm**.
- Pulmonary hypertension increases the workload of the right ventricle and causes right ventricular hypertrophy also known as **cor pulmonale**.
- **Dyspnea** on exertion and **fatigue** are classic symptom of **pulmonary hypertension**.
- World Health Organization recommends a reduction to <2 g/day sodium (5 g/day salt) in adults to reduce the risk of hypertension and cardiovascular disease.
- Postural hypotension (orthostatic hypotension) refers to fall in SBP over 20 mm Hg or DBP over 10 mm Hg when standing up or lying down after sitting (i.e., when there is a change in posture).
- The artificial cardiac pacemaker is an electronic device used to pace the heart when the normal conduction pathway is damaged or diseased.
- Common cause of infective endocarditis are **Staphylococcus aureus** and **Streptococcus viridians, and bacterial**.
- **Dukes Criteria** is used for diagnosis of pericarditis.
- **Roth's spots** are hemorrhagic retinal lesion revealed by fundoscopic examination in infective endocarditis.
- Inadequately treated streptococcal throat might cause **Rheumatic fever**.
- The most common causative agent of rheumatic fever is **streptococcus pyogens**.
- According to **Jones (1944) criteria** the presence of **two major criteria** or **one major and two minor criteria** plus evidence of group A streptococcal infection indicates a high probability of acute rheumatic fever.
- Classic symptom of peripheral arterial disease is intermittent claudication pain that occurs after considerable level of exercise and relieved by rest.
- Clinical manifestation of acute arterial ischemia includes the **six Ps:** Pain, Pulselessness, Paresthesia, Paralysis, Pallor and Poikilothermia.
- **Boot-shaped heart** is seen in Fallot's teratology disease.
- **Pear-shaped/flask-shaped** heart is seen in pericardial effusion.
- Right ventricle is the most common site of injury from blunt chest trauma. It is because of the proximity of right ventricle to sternum.
- Dressler syndrome is also known as **late pericarditis**.
- **Pain nature** in pericarditis is progressive, sharp pleuritic in nature, radiates to neck arm and can be relieved by sitting.
- **Hallmark sign of MI** includes severe pain which is not relieved by rest, position change, or nitrate administration.

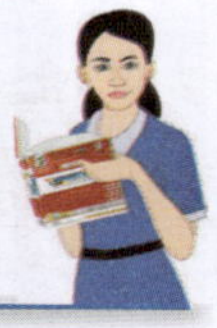

- **Cardiogenic shock** occurs when inadequate oxygen and nutrients are supplied to the tissue because of left ventricular failure.
- **Cyanosis** and **pallor** are signs of poor perfusion.
- **Assessing the weight of the patient** is the accurate indicator of health status in **heart failure patient who is on diuretics**.
- Major evidence of ischemia is drop in systolic BP of **>20 mm Hg** from baseline BP despite an increase in workload.
- Chest pain can be reduced by administering nitroglyecerin, morphin sulfate, and supplemental oxygen.
- **Digitalis** is a positive inotropic agent that improves left ventricular function (increase the force of contraction of left ventricle).
- **Inotropic agents** are the drugs that increase the force of contraction and exert a positive effect.
- **Hypokalemia**, secondary to diuretics, is one of the most common causes of digitalis toxicity.
- **Digitalis toxicity** results in **hyperkalemia**.
- **Digoxin** is contraindicated if apical pulse is below 60 beats per minute because it further decreases heart rate.
- Early symptoms of **digitalis toxicity** include anorexia, nausea, vomiting and visual disturbance.
- Method: HR = number of R waves in a 6 second strip x 10
- Most lethal arrhythmia – Ventricular Fibrillation
- Stimulation of **Vagus Nerve** → Decrease in **Heart Rate**
- **Sinus bradycardia** is seen in athletes.
- Most common site of Myocardial Infarction (MI) is Anterior wall of left ventricle.
- The coronary artery most commonly involved in atherosclerosis is Left Anterior Descending Artery (LAD).
- 'Transportation of triglycerides from liver to adipose tissues' is the function of Very Low Density Lipoproteins (VLDL).
- Person with serum cholesterol level **>200 mg/dL** is at high risk for development of CAD.
- **Osler's nodes** (small, painful nodes in fingers and toes) are seen in **infective endocarditis**.
- The most common direct cause of sudden death is Coronary Artery Disease.
- **Aspirin** in Coronary Artery Disease is used primarily to **inhibit platelet adhesion**.
- **Hemorrhage** and **falling Blood Pressure** are potential complications in the initial 12 hours after cardiac catheterization procedure.
- Most common cause of Intermittent claudication is **atherosclerosis**.
- Most common cardiac anomaly among infants of diabetic mothers is **Transposition of great arteries**.
- **Transfusion** of one unit of Whole Blood/PRBC can increase **Hb by 1 g/dL** and **Hematocrit by 3%** in an adult.
- **Flushed cheeks** are seen in patients with **Mitral stenosis**.
- **Rheumatic fever** is associated with **Valvular heart disease**.
- **Aschoff's bodies** are found in myocardium in rheumatic heart disease.
- Elevated levels of antistreptolysin O are seen in **rheumatic fever**.
- Most common site of **Atherosclerotic plaques is Lower Abdominal Aorta**.

Contd...

- Most common clinical manifestation of **Pulmonary embolism is Dyspnea**.
- Most dangerous complication of venous thrombus is **Pulmonary embolism**.
- **In patient with DVT** – blood clot travels to heart and gets **lodged in lungs** resulting in **pulmonary embolism**.
- Oxygen therapy followed by High Fowler's position is the priority nursing intervention for patient with Pulmonary edema.
- While measuring Central Venous Pressure (CVP), the transducer is zeroed at the level of the **4th intercostal space** (corresponds to level of right atrium) **in the mid-axillary line** on a supine patient.
- Central Venous Pressure (CVP) is measured at the end of expiration.
- Location of placement of **Permanent Pacemaker** is **subcutaneous tissue below the clavicle**.
- **Atrial Natriuretic Peptide (ANP)** is a hormone secreted by Right Atrium.
- Management of Cyanotic spell – Knee-Chest Position (increases preload and SVR).
- **Great Sephanous vein and Left Internal Mammary Artery (LIMA)** are the commonly used vein grafts in CABG.
- **Endarterectomy** is a surgical procedure to remove the atheromatous plaque material, or blockage, from the arterial wall.
- Kawasaki Disease is an acute inflammatory disease. It causes inflammation in the medium-sized arteries. It most commonly affects infants and young children.
- **Orthostatic hypotension** is a complication of all nitrates.
- Nitroglycerin is given sublingually to relieve from chest pain due to angina pectoris.
- **Raynaud's disease** is spasm of digital arteries caused by abnormal response of sympathetic nervous system to cold or emotional stress.
- Hallmark finding in acute **pericarditis** is the **pericardial friction rub**.
- The causative agent for pericarditis is **coxsackievirus B group**.
- The corrective procedure for Ebstein anomaly is Starnes procedure.
- The corrective procedure for TGA - transposition of great arteries is Jantene's repair
- Egg on end appearance or Egg-on-a-string sign is seen in TGA (Transposition of great artery)
- Reverse three sign on barium meal is seen in COA (Coarctation of aorta)
- Vitum's sign is seen in Tricuspid regurgitation. In Vitum's sign, the murmur of tricuspid regurgitation may increase with compression of liver.
- Osborn wave is seen in Hypercalcemia. Osborn waves or J waves are positive deflections occurring at junction between QRS and ST segment.
- Wellen's syndrome is seen with unstable angina. Wellen's syndrome is a pattern of deeply inverted or biphasic T waves.
- ROSE questionnaire is used to evaluate the subjective severity of ischemic heart pain and intermittent claudication in patients with coronary artery disease.
- Mc Callum's patch is found in deep layers of endocardium in patients with Rheumatic endocarditis.
- High density lipoprotein helps decrease the development of atherosclerosis.
- Normally, heart sounds aren't heard in the midaxillary line or the seventh intercostal space in the midclavicular line.
- Abnormalities of the pulmonic valve are auscultated at the second left intercostal space along the left sternal border.
- Mitral valve abnormalities are heard at the fifth intercostal space in the midclavicular line.
- In aortic valve regurgitation, some blood leaks back to Left Ventricle
- Rheumatic fever is caused by group A beta hemolytic streptococci infection.
- An ECG is the most common diagnostic tool used to evaluate MI.
- Beta-adrenergic blockers work by blocking beta receptors in the myocardium, reducing the response to catecholamines and sympathetic nerve stimulation.
- Calcium channel blockers reduce the workload of the heart by decreasing the heart rate.
- Staphylococcus aureus is a Gram-positive cocci associated with infective endocarditis in IV drug users.
- The most accurate area on the body to assess dependent edema in a bedridden client is the sacral area.
- **Intraoperative blood salvage (IOS)**, also known as **cell salvage,** is a specific type of autologous blood transfusion. It is done by suctioning blood directly from a surgical incision. It is then filtered, washed, and returned to the patient.
- Pulmonic sounds can be auscultated at the left second intercostal space in the midclavicular line.
- Hypertrophic obstructive cardiomyopathy is an abnormal symmetry of the ventricles.
- PCI (Percutaneous coronary intervention) should be done within 90 minutes of arrival at emergency department.
- The normal homocysteine level is 0.54 to 1.9 mg/L.
- Pain is frequently the first indicator of postoperative graft occlusion.
- Before defibrillating a client, make sure that the oxygen supply is off to prevent the hazard of fire.
- The recommended energy levels used to perform synchronized cardioversion vary from **50 to 200 joules**
- Metformin needs to be withheld 24 hrs. before and for 48 hrs. after cardiac catheterization because of the injection of contrast medium during the procedure.
- The only definitive treatment for cardiomyopathy that can't be controlled medically is a heart transplant.
- Nifedipine is a calcium channel blocker primarily used to decrease coronary artery spasm, as in variant angina.
- Metoprolol is a beta-adrenergic blocker that slows heart rate and lowers blood pressure; So it is contraindicated **in patients with hypotension or cardiogenic shock**
- A pulmonary artery catheter is used to give accurate pressure measurements within the heart.
- The mitral valve is best heard with the bell of the stethoscope at the fifth intercostal space, left midclavicular line.
- Right-sided heart failure produces venous congestion in the systemic circulation resulting in Jugular Venous Distension (JVD) and ascites.
- Milrinone is used in short-term treatment of congestive heart failure unresponsive to conventional therapy with digoxin, diuretics, and vasodilators.

"Adapt the remedy to the disease."
—Chinese Proverb

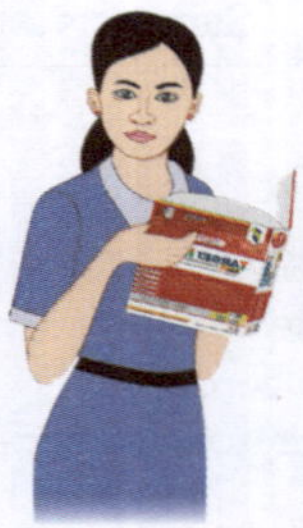

MULTIPLE CHOICE QUESTIONS
(Including Explained and Practice Questions)

CARDIOVASCULAR SYSTEM

ANATOMY OF HEART

1510. Specialized cardiac muscles are present in .... layer of the heart.
a. Epicardium b. Myocardium
c. Endocardium d. Pericardium

1511. One of the organs located in the mediastinum is the:
a. Cerebellum b. Heart
c. Stomach d. Uterus

1512. Posterior surface of heart is formed by:
a. RA b. LA
c. LV d. RV

1513. Coronary sinus opens into:
a. Inferior vena cava b. Right atrium
c. Left atrium d. Great cardiac vein

1514. What is the normal amount of pericardial fluid?
a. 5–10 mL b. 20–50 mL
c. 50–100 mL d. 100–200 mL

HEART VALVES

1515. Cardiac muscle differs from skeletal muscle by:
a. It is an involuntary muscle
b. It has automaticity
c. It has conductivity
d. All of the above

1516. The heart valves are lined by .... layer of the heart.
a. Epicardium b. Myocardium
c. Endocardium d. Pericardium

1517. Valve between left atrium and left ventricle is:
a. Bicuspid valve b. Tricuspid valve
c. Tetracuspid valve d. Monocuspid valve

1518. Valve between right atrium and right ventricle is:
a. Bicuspid valve b. Tricuspid valve
c. Tetracuspid valve d. Monocuspid valve

1519. Mitral valve is also known as:
a. Bicuspid valve b. Tricuspid valve
c. Tetracuspid valve d. Monocuspid valve

1520. Which valve prevents backward flow of blood into the left atrium? *(RRB SSNE 2015)*
a. Aortic valve
b. Pulmonary valve
c. Tricuspid valve
d. Mitral valve

1521. Tricuspid valve is located between:
a. Aorta and right atrium
b. Left atrium and left ventricle
c. Right atrium and right ventricle
d. Right ventricle and pulmonary artery

1522. Valve responsible for murmurs which auscultates at the second left intercostal space along the left sternal border is:
a. Aortic b. Bicuspid
c. Pulmonic d. Tricuspid

1523. The closure of the aortic valve in the arterial waveform is denoted by:
a. Anaerobic notch b. Dicrotic notch
c. Systolic notch d. End diastolic point

1524. Coronary sinus is guarded by:
a. Crista terminalis b. Thebesian valve
c. Mitral valve d. Spiral valve

CORONARY ARTERIES

1525. The arteries that supply the heart muscles are branches of the:
a. Abdominal aorta b. Thoracic aorta
c. Aortic arch d. Ascending aorta

1526. "Potential anastomosis" seen in:
a. Labial branch of facial artery
b. Intercostal artery
c. Coronary artery
d. Arterial arcades of mesentery

1527. Identify the artery that carries deoxygenated blood:
a. Umbilical artery b. Pulmonary artery
c. Both a and b d. Carotid artery

1528. Blood supply to the heart is maintained by:
a. Pulmonary b. Coronary
c. Aorta d. Myocardial

1529. Posterior communicating artery is branch of:
a. Internal carotid artery b. External carotid artery
c. Middle cerebral artery d. Posterior cerebral artery

1530. Which of the following is not a branch of first part of maxillary artery?
a. Greater palatine artery b. Middle meningeal artery
c. Deep auricular artery d. Inferior alveolar artery

1531. Left coronary artery supplies all; EXCEPT:
a. Anterior 2/3 of interventricular septum
b. Posterior 1/3 of interventricular septum
c. Left ventricle
d. Apex of heart

1532. Right coronary artery supplies all; EXCEPT:
a. Apex of heart b. Intraventricular septum
c. Inter atrial septum d. SA mode

CARDIAC CONDUCTION SYSTEM

1533. Pacemaker of heart is: *(JIPMER 2012)*
a. AV Node b. SA node
c. Purkinje fibers d. Parasympathetic system

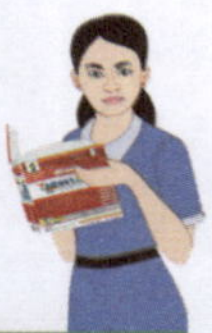

Ans.
1510. b
1511. b
1512. b
1513. b
1514. b
1515. d
1516. c
1517. a
1518. b
1519. a
1520. d
1521. c
1522. c
1523. b
1524. b
1525. d
1526. c
1527. c
1528. b
1529. a
1530. a
1531. b
1532. a
1533. b

1534. Which of the statements is TRUE regarding heart contraction?
- a. The intercalated discs allow the atria and ventricles to contract together simultaneously.
- b. The sudden influx of potassium into myocytes triggers depolarization.
- c. The pressure and volume changes in the heart stimulate heart contraction.
- d. Ventricular systole occurs following depolarization of the ventricles

1535. The pacemaker of the heart is the:
- a. Purkinje fibers
- b. Atrioventricular bundle (bundle of His)
- c. Atrioventricular node
- d. Sinoatrial node

1536. SA node is located in:
- a. In the wall of right atrium
- b. In the wall of left atrium
- c. In the wall of atrioventricular septum
- d. In the wall of ventricular septum

1537. Slowest conduction is in:
- a. SA node
- b. Purkinje fibers
- c. AV node
- d. Bundle of His

1538. Distention and recoil of blood vessel during systole and diastole is achieved through the .... property of blood vessel.
- a. Peripheral vascular resistance
- b. Elasticity
- c. Diameter
- d. Smooth muscle contraction

1539. Vasoconstriction leading to increased blood pressure is triggered by the following situation:
- a. Stimulation of the parasympathetic nerve supply.
- b. Stimulation of the cardioinhibitory center in the medulla.
- c. Increased levels of angiotensin II in the blood.
- d. Increased level of carbon dioxide in the blood.

1540. Baroreceptors help in:
- a. Stimulating respiration
- b. Stimulating sweating
- c. Maintaining BP
- d. Stimulating thirst

1541. Arterial supply to SA node is by:
- a. Left anterior descending coronary artery
- b. Posterior interventricular (descending) artery
- c. Left coronary artery
- d. Right coronary artery

1542. Sympathetic supply to heart:
- a. C5-C7
- b. T1-T4
- c. C1-C4
- d. T5-T9

1543. The coronary sinus:
- a. Lies in anterior part of the coronary sulcus
- b. Ends in right atrium
- c. Has venae cordis minimae as its tributaries
- d. Develops from right anterior cardinal vein

1544. The arterial supply of the bundle of His is:
- a. Interventricular branch of left coronary
- b. Atrioventricular branch of right coronary artery
- c. Marginal
- d. Right aortic sinus

1545. Which is true about arch of aorta?
- a. Starts at 3rd right ICS and ends at left 3rd ICS
- b. Left vagus arches over it
- c. Lies behind body of sternum
- d. It is closely related to parietal pleura

1546. Stimulation of vagus nerve results in: *(JIPMER 2012)*
- a. Increase in heart rate
- b. Decrease in heart rate
- c. Dilatation of bronchioles
- d. Dilatation of coronary artery

1547. Most common cause of hypertension is?
- a. Renal artery stenosis
- b. Essential hypertension
- c. Pheochromocytoma
- d. Chronic Glomerulonephritis

CARDIAC CYCLE AND CARDIAC OUTPUT

1548. Normal Cardiac Output in a healthy adult is:
- a. 1 L/ min
- b. 3 L/ min
- c. 5 L/min
- d. 7 L/min

1549. Time duration of cardiac cycle is:
- a. 0.5 sec
- b. 0.8 sec
- c. 1 sec
- d. 2 sec

1550. The blood circulation that is responsible for gas exchange between alveoli and capillaries resulting in the oxygenation of blood is the:
- a. Coronary circulation
- b. Hepatic circulation
- c. Pulmonary circulation
- d. Systemic circulation

1551. Blood from the right side of the heart flows into the:
- a. Superior vena cava
- b. Pulmonary trunk (artery)
- c. Pulmonary veins
- d. Aorta

1552. The amount of blood that is ejected from the left ventricle in one contraction is called the:
- a. Cardiac output
- b. Stroke volume
- c. Preload
- d. Afterload

1553. Cardiac Output can be calculated using:
- a. CO = tidal volume X heart rate
- b. CO = tidal volume X peripheral vascular resistance
- c. CO = peripheral vascular resistance X-heart rate
- d. CO = stroke volume X-heart rate

1554. What is the source that you might suspect if bright red blood is back-flowing into the tubing of an intravenous drip?
- a. Capillary blood
- b. Venous blood
- c. Arterial blood
- d. Peripheral blood

1555. The venous blood from organs of the digestive system such as the stomach and intestines will drain into the:
- a. Portal vein
- b. Mesenteric veins
- c. Internal iliac veins
- d. Lumbar veins

1556. Oxygen is carried by blood after it is combining with:
- a. Albumin
- b. WBC
- c. Hemoglobin
- d. Platelet

1557. Baro-receptors control:
- a. Blood pressure
- b. Arterial oxygen tension
- c. SPO_2
- d. Stroke volume

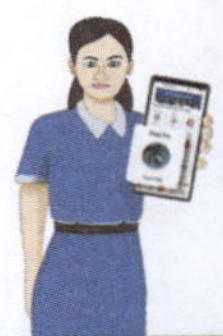

Ans.

1534. d
1535. d
1536. a
1537. c
1538. b
1539. c
1540. c
1541. d
1542. b
1543. b
1544. b
1545. d
1546. b
1547. b
1548. c
1549. b
1550. c
1551. b
1552. b
1553. d
1554. c
1555. a
1556. c
1557. a

1558. Normal cardiac output is:

a. 1–2 L/min b. 3–4 L/min
c. 5–6 L/min d. 7–8 L/min

Explanation: Cardiac output = Stroke volume × Heart Rate
Stroke volume is approximately 70 mL
Normal heart rate is 72 beats per minute.
Cardiac output = 70 × 72
= 5040 mL
This is in the range of 5–6 L

1559. What is preload?

a. Pressure in the ventricle at the end of systole
b. Pressure in the ventricle at the end of diastole
c. Pressure in the aorta at the end of systole
d. Pressure in the atria at the end of systole

1560. The formula for ejection fraction is:

a. $EF = \frac{\text{Stroke Volume}}{\text{End Diastolic Volume}}$

b. $EF = \frac{\text{Stroke Volume}}{\text{CO} \times \text{Heart Rate}}$

c. $EF = \frac{\text{Diastolic Volume}}{\text{CO} \times \text{Heart Rate}}$

d. $EF = \frac{\text{End systolic Volume}}{\text{Stroke Volume}}$

1561. Most common sign associated with decreased cardiac output is:

a. Shortness of breath
b. Peripheral edema
c. Cardiac murmurs
d. Arthritis

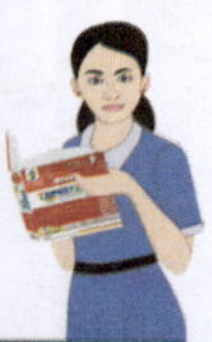

HEART SOUNDS

1562. Heart sounds are the result of: *(LNJP H D 2012)*

a. Movement of blood into the heart form the aorta
b. Blood flow through the heart
c. Closure of the heart valves
d. Contraction of the cardiac muscle

1563. When listening to heart sound, you can best hear sound, at the:

a. Base of the heart
b. Apex of heart
c. Aortic area
d. IInd ICS to the left of sternum

1564. Ventricular gallop:

a. S1 b. S2
c. S3 d. S4

1565. S1 heart sound corresponds to:

a. Closure of the aortic and pulmonic valve
b. Closure of the aortic valve
c. Closure of the mitral and tricuspid valve
d. Closure of the mitral valve

1566. S2 heart sound corresponds to:

a. Closure of the aortic and pulmonic valve
b. Closure of the aortic valve
c. Closure of the mitral and tricuspid valve
d. Closure of the mitral valve

Explanation

Normal heart sounds:

- S1 (First Heart sound-LUBB) produced by closure of AV valves (Tricuspid and mitral)
- S2 (Second Heart sound-DUBB) produced by closure of Semilunar valves (aortic and pulmonic valve)

Abnormal heart sounds:

- **S3** (Third heart sound) Also known as **ventricular gallop.** It corresponds to early ventricular filling (passive filling) when mitral valve opens. It is often associated with **Heart failure.**
- **S4** (Fourth heart sound) Also known as Atrial gallop.

BLOOD VESSELS

1567. Which is the longest vein in the human body? *(AIIMS Nagpur NO 2018)*

a. Great saphenous b. Popliteal
c. Iliac d. Femoral

Explanation: The great (long) saphenous veins is the longest veins in the body. It ascends from the foot to the groin.

1568. Largest vein is:

a. Superior vena cava b. Saphenous
c. Inferior vena cava d. Jugular

1569. Connection between artery and vein is known as:

a. Capillaries b. Arterioles
c. Venules d. Lymph

1570. The network between the arteries that supplying to a particular area is known as:

a. Collateral arteries b. Anastomoses
c. Capillary networks d. Vena-caval junction

1571. The largest artery of human body is: *(DSSSB PHN, 2015)*

a. Aorta b. Carotid artery
c. Subclavian artery d. Pulmonary artery

1572. Artery in anatomical snuff box is:

a. Radial b. Brachial
c. Ulnar d. Interosseous

1573. Identify the blood vessel which carry blood into right atrium:

a. Inferior vena cava b. Superior vena cava
c. Pulmonary vein d. Both a and b

1574. Identify the blood vessel which carries blood into left atrium:

a. Inferior vena cava b. Superior vena cava
c. Pulmonary vein d. Both a and b

1575. Largest artery is:

a. Aorta b. Carotid
c. Coronary d. Femoral

1576. Largest branch of vertebral artery is:

a. Middle cerebral b. Posterior cerebral
c. Posterior inferior cerebellar
d. Post. superior cerebellar

1577. Posterior cerebral artery is a branch of which of these?

a. Vertebral artery b. Basilar artery
c. Posterior cerebral artery d. Posterior choroidal artery

1578. Terminal branch of Internal Carotid Artery:

a. Anterior choroidal artery
b. Anterior cerebral artery
c. Ophthalmic artery
d. Inferior hypophyseal artery

Ans.

1558. c
1559. b
1560. a
1561. a
1562. c
1563. b
1564. c
1565. c
1566. a
1567. a
1568. c
1569. a
1570. a
1571. a
1572. a
1573. d
1574. c
1575. a
1576. c
1577. b
1578. b

1579. Not a branch of external carotid artery:
a. Inferior thyroid artery b. Facial artery
c. Superior thyroid artery d. Maxillary artery

1580. Smallest vein is:
a. Venules b. Capillaries
c. Lymph d. Arterioles

1581. Smallest artery is:
a. Arterioles b. Venules
c. Capillaries d. Lymph

1582. Vein used in bypass surgery:
a. Great saphenous vein b. Short saphenous vein
c. Femoral vein d. Brachial vein

1583. Which of the following is an artery of the forearm?
a. Brachial artery
b. Axillary artery
c. Ulnar artery
d. Femoral artery

1584. Great saphenous vein is present in .... body part.
a. Trunk b. Spinal cord
c. Abdomen d. Legs

1585. The inner most layer of blood vessels is:
a. Tunica media
b. Tunica adventitia
c. Tunica intima
d. Tunica mucosa

1586. Base of the heart is formed mainly by:
a. Right atrium b. Left atrium
c. Right ventricle d. Left ventricle

1587. Major part of the myocardium is drained by:
a. Coronary sinus
b. Great cardiac vein
c. Anterior cardiac veins
d. Venae cordis minimae (Thebesian veins)

1588. The left subclavian artery is a branch of:
a. Brachiocephalic trunk
b. Ascending aorta
c. Arch of aorta
d. Left common carotid

1589. Posterior communicating artery a branch of:
a. Posterior superior cerebellar artery
b. External carotid artery
c. Middle cerebral artery
d. Internal carotid artery

1590. Branches of brachial artery are all; EXCEPT:
a. Profunda brachii
b. Superior ulnar collateral
c. Inferior ulnar collateral
d. Radial collateral

1591. Cephalic vein drains into:
a. Brachial vein
b. Subclavian
c. Axillary vein
d. Inferior Vena Cava

1592. Right common carotid artery arises from:
a. Right axillary artery
b. Arch of aorta
c. Brachiocephalic artery
d. Left subclavian artery

1593. Branches of left coronary artery are all of the following; EXCEPT:
a. Anterior interventricular branch
b. Left diagonal artery
c. Left atrial artery
d. Posterior interventricular branch

1594. All of the following drain into coronary sinus; EXCEPT:
a. Great cardiac vein
b. Small cardiac vein
c. Middle cardiac vein
d. Anterior cardiac vein

1595. Azygous vein opens into:
a. Inferior vena cava
b. Superior vena cava
c. Right brachiocephalic vein
d. Left brachiocephalic vein

1596. Femoral ring is bounded by all; EXCEPT:
a. Inguinal ligament
b. Superior ramus of pubis
c. Femoral artery
d. Femoral vein

1597. All are branches of Internal Iliac artery; EXCEPT:
a. Ovarian artery
b. Superior vesical artery
c. Middle rectal artery
d. Inferior vesical artery

1598. All of the following veins in the body lack valves; EXCEPT:
a. Femoral vein b. Portal vein
c. IVC d. Dural venous sinuses

1599. Which of the following is valveless?
a. Portal system veins
b. Saphenous vein
c. Popliteal vein
d. Ulnar vein

1600. Veins are an example of:
a. Conducting vessels
b. Distributing vessels
c. Resistance vessels
d. Capacitance vessels

1601. True about valves in portal venous system:
a. Present at the junction of superior mesenteric artery with the splenic artery
b. Within the portal vein only
c. Whole system is valveless
d. In the intrahepatic portion of portal vein

1602. IV infusion is avoided in:
a. Long saphenous vein
b. Cephalic vein
c. External Jugular vein
d. Internal Jugular vein

1603. Aneurysm affects which layer of the artery?
a. Tunica intima
b. Tunica media
c. Tunica adventitia
d. All of the above

Explanation: Muscular layer of the artery, i.e. tunica media is most commonly affected with aneurysm.

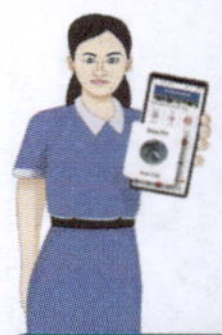

Ans.

1579. a
1580. a
1581. a
1582. a
1583. c
1584. d
1585. c
1586. b
1587. a
1588. c
1589. d
1590. d
1591. c
1592. c
1593. d
1594. d
1595. b
1596. c
1597. a
1598. a
1599. a
1600. d
1601. c
1602. a
1603. b

AUSCULTATION SITES

1604. The breath sound that can be found anteriorly and posteriorly in the lung field is called?
a. Bronchial b. Vesicular
c. Wheezes d. Crackles

1605. Bronchial breath sound should be assessed in:
a. Tracheal area b. Clavicular area
c. Mid axillary area d. None of these

1606. The apex of the lungs is auscultated at:
a. 7th intercoastal space mid clavicular line
b. 5th intercoastal space mid axillary line
c. Slightly above the clavicle
d. 4th intercoastal space mid clavicular line

Explanation: Chest auscultation refers to listening to the internal sounds of trachea and bronchial tree as the air flow through them. The apical zone is auscultated just above the clavicle. The bell of the stethoscope is usually used to detect high-pitched sounds (at the apex). The diaphragm of the stethoscope is used to detect low-pitched sounds (rest of the chest).

1607. The right middle lobe of the lung is auscultated at:
a. Anterior to the 4th intercoastal space
b. posterior to the 4th intercoastal space
c. Between c7 and t5
d. Between t3 and t7

Explanation:

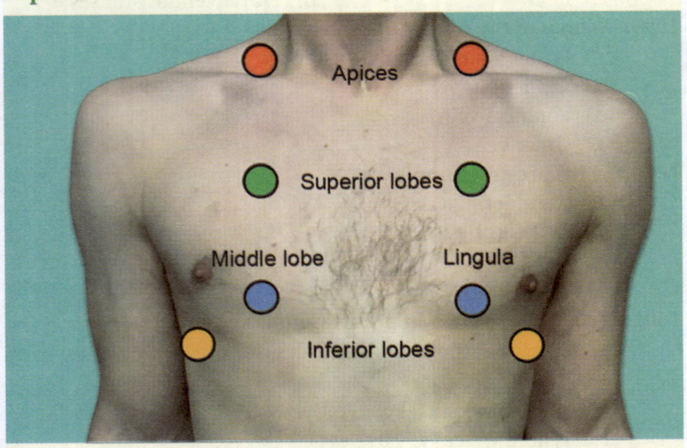

Figure: Location in the chest for auscultation of different part of lungs

1608. High-pitched harsh sound during inspiration is called:
a. Rales b. Rhonchi
c. Stridor d. Wheezes

SITES FOR ASSESSMENT OF PULSE

1609. Apical pulse is auscultated at:
a. Fourth intercostal in the left side on mid axillary line
b. Fourth intercostal in the right side on mid axillary line
c. Fifth intercostal space in the left side on mid-clavicular line
d. Fifth intercostal space in the right side on mid-clavicular line

Explanation: 5th intercostal space in the mid clavicular line is the closer area to the apex of the heart as shown in the following figure.

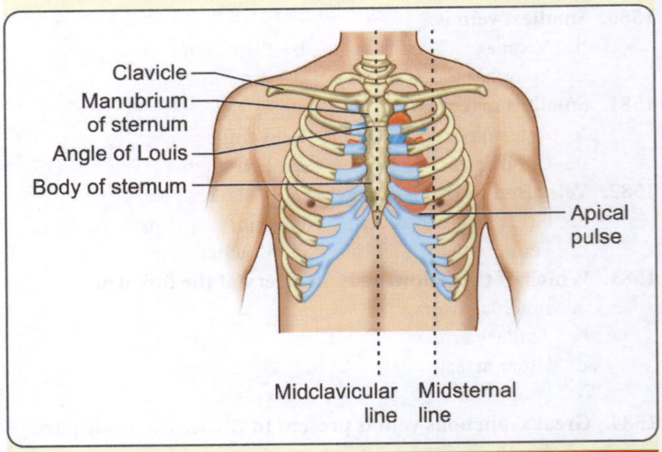

1610. During the resuscitation of a patient, the palpable artery in the neck used to assess the patient's cardiovascular status is the:
a. Brachiocephalic artery b. Subclavian artery
c. Common carotid artery d. Temporal artery

1611. Where should you attempt to perform a pulse check in a child from one year of age to puberty?
a. Carotid or femoral artery b. Temporal artery
c. Ulnar artery d. Brachial artery

Explanation: As per American Heart Association (AHA) guidelines, pulse should be checked either in carotid artery or femoral artery for children aged one year until puberty. The brachial artery located on the upper arm is used in infants below 1-year-old.

1612. The pulse which is located on the arm just above the elbow is known as:
a. Radial pulse b. Brachial pulse
c. Ulnar pulse d. Femoral pulse

1613. The pulse that is feeble at the lateral part of the wrist is referred to as:
a. Radial pulse b. Brachial pulse
c. Ulnar pulse d. Femoral pulse

1614. The pulse that can be located on the medial and inner part of the wrist is:
a. Radial pulse b. Brachial pulse
c. Ulnar pulse d. Femoral pulse

1615. The pulse which is located on the pelvis area, i.e. midway between the pubic bone and the anterior iliac crest is:
a. Radial pulse b. Brachial pulse
c. Ulnar pulse d. Femoral pulse

1616. The pulse that can be assessed from behind the knee is known as:
a. Popliteal pulse b. Dorsalis pedis pulse
c. Posterior tibial pulse d. Temporal pulse

1617. Pulse located on the top portion of the foot:
a. Popliteal pulse b. Dorsalis pedis
c. Posterior tibial d. Temporal

1618. This pulse can be identified behind the ankle of the lower limbs:
a. Popliteal b. Dorsalis pedis
c. Posterior tibial d. Temporal

Ans.
1604. b
1605. a
1606. c
1607. a
1608. c
1609. c
1610. c
1611. a
1612. b
1613. a
1614. c
1615. d
1616. a
1617. b
1618. c

1619. The only pulse that we can listen through stethoscope is:
a. Carotid pulse b. Apical pulse
c. Arterial pulse d. Radial pulse

1620. The pulse which can be located over person's neck region:
a. Temporal pulse b. Carotid pulse
c. Apical pulse d. Cervical pulse

ASSESSMENT AND DIAGNOSTIC TESTS

1621. The pH of blood is: *(DSSSB PHN, 2015)*
a. 6.4 b. 7.4
c. 7.8 d. 6.8

1622. The average Hb content of human blood is: *(DSSSB PHN, 2015)*
a. 18-23 g/dL b. 14-16 g/dL
c. 8-10 g/dL d. 16-20 g/dL

1623. What is the effect of an extremely rapid pulse rate of 200/ minute on blood pressure?
a. The blood pressure remains unchanged
b. The blood pressure will fall
c. The blood pressure will be raised
d. The blood pressure will fluctuate constantly

1624. Which among the following is a modifiable risk factors?
a. Age b. Smoking
c. Genetics d. Previous history of disease

1625. Which one of the following is a nonmodifiable risk factors for atherosclerosis? *(Banaras HU 2015)*
a. Cigarette smoking
b. Hyperlipidemia
c. Female over 55 years of age
d. Sedentary lifestyle

1626. Holter monitoring means:
a. Ambulatory BP b. Ambulatory ECG
c. ECG monitoring while sleeping
d. Hourly BP monitoring

1627. All of the following statements are correct regarding Holter monitoring; EXCEPT:
a. The patient should keep a diary of what activities he does while wearing the monitor
b. Holter monitor continuously records the heart's rhythms
c. It is also known as ambulatory electrocardiography
d. Holter monitoring is an invasive procedure

Explanation: A Holter monitor is a device that records the client's heart beats. It contains electrodes, wires, and a small machine that attaches to the portable device. It is a noninvasive procedure.

1628. Which among the following diagnostic test is preferred to determine the location of myocardial damage?
a. Troponin - I b. CK-MB
c. Electrocardiogram d. Echocardiogram

1629. In an adult patient, arterial function of the lower extremity can be determined by assessing the:
a. Allen's test b. Homan's sign
c. Pedal pulse d. Cullen's sign

1630. Auscultation over the left mid-clavicular line at the level of the fifth intercostal space is the area for S1. It indicates .... heart valve.
a. Aortic b. Bicuspid
c. Tricuspid d. Semilunar

1631. CVP catheter is inserted to estimate all of the following; EXCEPT:
a. Mean right atrial pressure
b. Pulmonary capillary wedge pressure
c. Pressure in SVC
d. Right ventricular preload

1632. Normal CVP is .... *(Safdarjung NO 2018; AIIMS Rishikesh Senior Nursing Officer 2018)*
a. 5 and 10 cm H_2O b. 10 and 15 cm H_2O
c. 15 and 20 cm H_2O d. 20 and 30 cm H_2O

1633. Zeroing point in CVP monitoring is known as:
a. Midclavicular line b. Mid axillary line
c. Phlebostatic axis d. At the level of atrium

1634. For effective measurement of CVP the transducer must be leveled to the reference point of:
a. Phlebostatic axis b. Pneumostatic axis
c. Intercostal axis d. Coronal axis

1635. Complication of faulty/incorrect insertion of CVP line is:
a. Pleural effusion b. Pneumothorax
c. Cardiac tamponade d. Subcutaneous emphysema

1636. Internal jugular vein pressure determines pressure of:
a. RA b. RV
c. LA d. LV

1637. Elevation in jugular venous pressure is observed in all of the following conditions; EXCEPT: *(AIIMS Raipur Grade II 2017)*:*
a. Right sided heart failure b. Cardiac tamponade
c. Constrictive pericarditis d. Myocarditis

Explanation: Increased jugular venous pressure is seen in right sided heart failure, pulmonary hypertension, tricuspid valve stenosis, superior vena cava obstruction, constructive pericarditis, and cardiac tamponade. Myocarditis does not cause elevation of JVP.

**The original question from the AIIMS Raipur Grade II has been modified due to multiple correct answers.*

1638. Position used for assessing jugular vein distention is:
a. High Fowler's b. Trendelenburg
c. Raised 30 degrees d. Side lying

1639. Kussmaul sign is:
a. Rise of jugular venous pressure on inspiration
b. Rise of jugular venous pressure on expiration
c. Visible carotid pulsation during inspiration
d. Visible carotid pulsation during expiration

Explanation: Kussmaul's sign is the rise of jugular venous pressure during inspiration usually due to condition that limits filling of right ventricle or right ventricular dysfunction.

1640. The diagnostic study to assess left ventricular dysfunction is: *(JIPMER 2012)*
a. Angiogram b. Catheterization
c. ECG d. Echocardiography

1641. What is a desirable total cholesterol level?
a. 200–239 b. Less than 200
c. Greater than 240 d. None of these

Explanation: Total cholesterol should be less than 200 mg.

1642. Which of the following is known as "good cholesterol"?
a. LDL b. VLDL
c. HDL d. Triglycerides

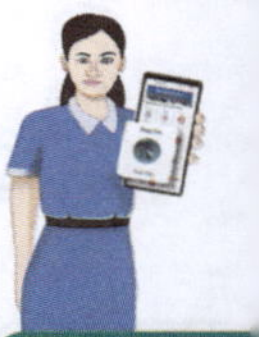

Ans.
1619. b
1620. b
1621. b
1622. b
1623. b
1624. b
1625. c
1626. b
1627. d
1628. c
1629. c
1630. b
1631. b
1632. a
1633. c
1634. a
1635. b
1636. a
1637. d
1638. c
1639. a
1640. a
1641. b
1642. c

Explanation: Lipoproteins are those molecules that transport cholesterol in the blood. High Density Lipoprotein (HDL) transports excess of cholesterol back to liver to be excreted as bile. Since it is beneficial and protective, the HDL is known as Good Cholesterol. Low Density Lipoprotein (LDL) is known as BAD Cholesterol as it is associated with increased risk of cardiovascular disease. [Tips to Remember: GOOD and HIGH is 4 letters; LOW and BAD is 3 letters each]

1643. Boot-shaped heart in a chest X-ray is commonly associated with *(ISRO)*
a. Mitral stenosis b. Rheumatic Fever
c. Aortic regurgitation d. Fallot's Tetralogy

1644. Differentiation of various cardiomyopathy is done with the help of ....diagnostic test.
a. Echocardiography b. ECG
c. Cardiac enzyme study d. Endomyocardial biopsy

1645. The drug that is used for stress test is:
a. Atropine b. Adrenaline
c. Dobutamine d. Thallium

1646. Transesophageal echocardiography (TCE) combines ultrasonography with which other procedure?
a. Electro cardiogram b. Endoscopy
c. Sigmoidoscopy d. Endoscopic cholangiogram

1647. Criteria for diagnosing infective endocarditis is:
a. Jones criteria b. Dukes criteria
c. Fallot criteria d. Bernard criteria

1648. Bobbing of head with each pulse can be seen in Patient with?
a. Tricuspid regurgitation b. Aortic regurgitation
c. Aortic stenosis d. Mitral regurgitation

1649. The normal jugular venous pressure is:
a. <9 cm of H_2O
b. <15 cm of H_2O
c. <12 cm of H_2O
d. <3 cm of H_2O

1650. Cardiac enzyme levels are monitored in the patient with chest pain because:
a. Serial measurement of enzyme level reveals the extent of cardiac damage and helps to monitor healing progress
b. It helps to identify area of myocardial injury
c. It reveals if the patient is truly having chest pain
d. Decreasing enzyme level helps to estimate the recovery time for the Patient with MI

1651. The enzyme level which is found elevated after myocardial infarction is: *(DSSSB PHN, 2015)*
a. Serum creatinine b. Alkaline phosphatase
c. Phosphokinase d. Creatine kinase

1652. Which of the following lab tests is most indicative of myocardial damage?
a. Lactic acid level b. Lactate dehydrogenase
c. Creatine Kinase d. Troponin I

Explanation: Troponin is the most sensitive and specific cardiac marker of myocardial damage. Troponin has increased specificity compared with CK-MB.

1653. Origin of a knifelike chest pain that increases in intensity with inspiration is:
a. Cardiac b. Hepatic
c. Hematological d. Pulmonary

1654. Which among the following needs to be monitored before administering digoxin?
a. Apical pulse b. Pulse deficit
c. Radial pulse d. Pulse pressure

HEMODYNAMIC MONITORING

1655. Lack of oxygen in the blood stream is: *(Kerala PSC, Nov 2014)*
a. Apnea b. Cyanosis
c. Anoxia d. Hypoxemia

1656. History needs to be obtained from a client by the nurse prior to cardiac catheterization is:
a. BMI
b. Allergy to iodine or shellfish
c. Family history of the problem
d. Informed consent

1657. Left sided cardiac catheterization is done through .... blood vessel.
a. Femoral artery b. Femoral vein
c. Jugular vein d. Carotid

1658. Right sided cardiac catheterization is done through .... blood vessel.
a. Femoral artery b. Femoral vein
c. Brachial artery d. Carotid

1659. Nurse received patient from Cath lab following cardiac catheterization, which among the following is the priority nursing action?
a. Assess the pain
b. Administer ordered medication and IV fluids
c. Check distal site for pulsation
d. Check the level of consciousness

Explanation: Immediate nursing action directed towards assessing the catheterized site for bleeding and distal site for pulsation. If bleeding or absence of pulse is observed, report to the physician immediately.

ELECTROCARDIOGRAM (ECG)

1660. Which of these planes does the chest leads of a 12-leaded ECG (electrocardiograph) record the heart electrical activity?
a. Sagittal b. Coronal
c. Transverse d. Horizontal

1661. The 'p' wave on the electrocardiogram corresponds to: *(RRB SSNE 2015; JIPMER 2012)*
a. Atrial depolarization
b. Atrial repolarization
c. Ventricular depolarization
d. Ventricular repolarization

1662. P wave of ECG represents:
a. SA node and repolarizing the atria
b. SA node and depolarizing the atria
c. AV node and depolarizing the atria
d. Impulse travelling from SA node to AV node

1663. 'T' wave in an ECG represents:
a. Ventricular depolarization
b. Ventricular repolarization
c. Atrial depolarization
d. Atrial repolarization

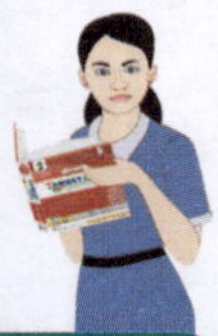

Ans.
1643. d
1644. a
1645. c
1646. b
1647. b
1648. b
1649. a
1650. a
1651. d
1652. d
1653. d
1654. a
1655. d
1656. b
1657. a
1658. b
1659. c
1660. d
1661. a
1662. b
1663. b

1664. U wave is seen in which of the following conditions:

a. Hypotension b. Hypokalemia
c. Hyperkalemia d. Hypertension

Explanation: Prominent 'U' wave in ECG is the characteristic of hypokalemia. "U" wave represents repolarization of the Purkinje fibers. Peaked T wave is seen in Hyperkalemia.

1665. Which of the following ECG findings indicates hypokalemia? *(DSSSB 2013)*

a. Tented T wave
b. ST segment depression
c. Widening of QRS complex
d. Prolonged PR interval

Explanation: The earliest electrocardiogram (ECG) change associated with hypokalemia is a decrease in the T-wave amplitude. As potassium levels decline further, ST-segment depression and T-wave inversions are seen

1666. T-wave inversion on the ECG are seen in following conditions; EXCEPT:

a. Hyperkalemia
b. Myocardial infarction
c. Myocarditis
d. Subarachnoid hemorrhage

Explanation: Tall T-wave (>5 mV in standard leads and 10 mV in chest leads) is seen in hyperkalemia. All the other condition causes T-wave inversion.

1667. Normal PR interval in ECG is: *(Kerala PSC, Nov 2014)*

a. 0.20-0.35 sec b. 0.30-0.45 sec
c. 0.35-0.40 sec d. 0.12-0.20 sec

1668. Hyperkalemia leads to what changes in ECG? *(DSSSB PHN, 2015)*

a. Inverted T waves b. Tall T waves
c. Prolonged QT interval d. Wide QRS complex

1669. QRS complex in ECG represents:

a. Atrial depolarization
b. Ventricular depolarization
c. Ventricular repolarization
d. Atrial repolarization

1670. ST depression in ECG represents:

a. Myocardial ischemia b. Angina
c. Hyperkalemia d. Hypercalcemia

1671. Which of the following ECG findings indicates myocardial infarction? *(DSSSB 2013)*

a. ST segment elevation b. Wide QRS complex
c. Presence of U wave d. T wave inversion

Explanation: The most important cause of ST segment abnormality (elevation or depression) is myocardial ischemia/infarction. Both ST segment elevation and depression are seen in MI. STEMI: ST-elevation myocardial infarction; STDMI: ST-depression myocardial infarction. Hypokalemia causes U wave presence.

1672. A client is suspected to have cardiac tamponade. Which of the following findings in QRS complex of a lead II ECG will support the suspicion?

a. Amplitude increase b. Amplitude decrease
c. Narrowing complex d. Widening complex

Explanation: Peaked P waves, decrease of QRS complex voltage, left axis deviation of the QRS complex, deep T wave inversions, and ST segment change are present in cardiac tamponade. Fluid accumulated in the pericardium suppresses the amplitude of the QRS complex on the ECG.

1673. Affected blood vessel, if ECG shows ST elevation in leads V2?

a. Marginal artery
b. Circumflex artery
c. Left anterior descending artery
d. Right coronary artery

1674. In myocardial ischemia, ECG looks like:

a. Prolonged PR interval b. Spiky T wave
c. T-wave inversion d. Abnormal U wave

1675. ECG changes in Digoxin toxicity are:

a. Prolonged QT interval
b. Prolonged PR interval
c. ST segment elevation
d. Tall T-waves

CORONARY ANGIOGRAPHY

1676. Correct option regarding angiogenesis is:

a. New blood vessels will form
b. Repair by connective tissues
c. Formation of the blood clot
d. All of the above

1677. Two days after the coronary angiography, the client reports increased pain and discomfort at the catheter site, what should the nurse do?

a. Explain the client that it is normal after coronary angiography
b. Assess the signs for infection
c. Elevate the affected extremity
d. Give massage to the pain site

1678. Coronary Angiogram helps to find out the following; EXCEPT?

a. Blockage of coronary artery
b. Perfusion of lungs
c. Blood supply to the heart
d. Detect the blocked blood vessels

1679. Which of the following assessment findings is not normal after a person is returned from coronary angiogram procedure?

a. Blood pressure of 135/85
b. Ecchymosis
c. Apical pulse of 130 beats/min
d. Pedal pulses palpable at +1

Explanation: Dysrhythmia is a common complication after the coronary angiogram so client should be placed on a cardiac monitor to detect the abnormality.

1680. Which among the following is the best diagnostic procedure for coronary atherosclerosis?

a. Chest X-ray
b. Cardiac catheterization
c. MRI
d. Doppler

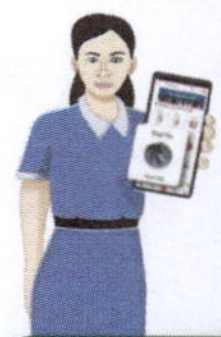

Ans.

1664. b
1665. b
1666. a
1667. d
1668. b
1669. b
1670. a
1671. a
1672. b
1673. c
1674. c
1675. b
1676. a
1677. b
1678. b
1679. b
1680. b

1681. Before the coronary angiography procedure the INR level should be at the level of?

a. <4.5
b. <4.0
c. <1.5
d. <2.0

HYPERTENSION

1682. What will be the change in the BP of a person if peripheral vascular resistance decreases?

a. Decrease
b. Increase
c. No change
d. Slightly increase then come to the normal value

1683. When blood pressure rises, the arterial baroreceptor inhibits the sympathetic nervous system which leads to:

a. Vasodilation   b. Vasoconstriction
c. Tachycardia   d. Tachypnea

1684. Risk factors of hypertension is:

a. Hyperlipidemia   b. Cardiovascular problems
c. Family history   d. All of these

1685. In elderly, increased peripheral resistance and decreased vascular elasticity causes:

a. Dementia
b. Cardiac arrhythmias
c. Increased blood pressure
d. Decreased blood pressure

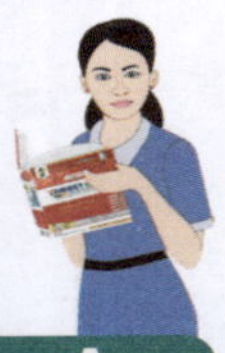

Explanation: Blood pressure elevates in response to hardening and thickening of arteries and veins. In addition, the increased peripheral resistance results in increased systemic vascular resistance contribute to elevated blood pressure.

1686. BP 142/90 mm Hg is interpreted as:

a. Prehypertension   b. Stage 1 hypertension
c. Stage 2 hypertension   d. Stage 3 hypertension

1687. Persistently elevated blood pressure with an unknown cause is known as:

a. Stage 1 hypertension   b. Malignant hypertension
c. Primary hypertension   d. Chronic hypertension

1688. Unchecked rapid rise in diastolic BP above 110–120 mm Hg is:

a. Malignant hypertension   b. Hypertensive crisis
c. Hypertensive emergency   d. White coat hypertension

Explanation: Malignant hypertension is rapid uncheck rise in diastolic above 110–120 mm Hg.

Hypertensive emergency (crisis) is characterized by a severe elevation in blood pressure (>180/120 mm Hg) complicated by progressive organ dysfunction.

White coat hypertension—hypertensive when the BP is measured by a health care professional.

1689. Postural hypertension is defined as a fall in systolic blood pressure by ------mm Hg or diastolic by-----mm Hg within 3 minutes of standing from a supine or sitting position:

a. 20, 10
b. 10, 20
c. 10, 10
d. 20, 20

Explanation: Postural hypertension or orthostatic hypotension is defined as a decrease in systolic pressure by 20 mm Hg or a decrease in diastolic pressure by 10 mm Hg within 3 minutes of changing posture from a sitting or lying down posture to standing posture.

1690. According to the Joint National Guidelines (JNG) 8 pharmacological therapy is started at a BP reading of:

a. >120/80   b. >130/90
c. >140/90   d. >150/90

Explanation: JNG8 recommends to start pharmacological therapy for hypertension at a BP reading of >140/90

1691. Prehypertension is usually treated with:

a. Diuretics   b. Lifestyle modification
c. β-blockers   d. ACE inhibitors

1692. Hypertension may be controlled by the use of medications, but it can also be improved by:

a. Weight loss
b. Exercise
c. Low sodium diet
d. All of the above

Explanation: All of the above are nonpharmacological methods to control hypertension.

1693. Essential hypertension can be managed with:

a. A diuretic agent
b. ACE inhibitors
c. Beta blockers
d. Diet, exercise and weight reduction program

1694. The full form of DASH diet is:

a. Dietary allowances to stop hypertension
b. Dietary aids to stop hypertension
c. Dietary approaches to stop hypertension
d. Dietary assistance to stop hypertension

Explanation: DASH (Dietary Approaches to Stop Hypertension) Diet modification is effective treatment to reduce blood pressure especially in stage 1 HTN.

1695. With aging blood pressure is often higher due to: *(LNJP H D 2012)*

a. Decreased peripheral resistance
b. Decreased elasticity in arterial walls
c. Loss of muscle mass
d. Changes in exercise and diet

1696. Most common cause of aortic dissection:

a. Syphilis
b. Hypertension
c. Marfan syndrome
d. Cystic medial necrosis

1697. Which of the following complications can occur due to untreated hypertension?

a. Renal failure, hydatidiform mole , angina
b. Asthma, cardiac tamponade, angina
c. Aortic dissection, renal failure, stroke
d. Pneumothorax, pleural effusion, cardiac tamponade

Explanation: Hypertensive cardiovascular disease, Hypertensive cerebrovascular disease (stroke), hypertensive renal disease (renal failure), aortic dissection, and atherosclerotic dissection are the complications of untreated hypertension.

Ans.

1681. c
1682. a
1683. a
1684. d
1685. c
1686. b
1687. c
1688. a
1689. a
1690. c
1691. b
1692. d
1693. d
1694. c
1695. b
1696. b
1697. c

1698. Calcium channel blockers help to reduce BP through:
a. Vasodilation
b. Volume depletion
c. Beta receptor block
d. None of the above

1699. Which among the followings drugs has the side effect as hypertension?
a. Oral contraceptives
b. Cocaine use
c. Corticosteroids
d. All of the above

1700. Cough is a side effect of which of the following antihypertensive medications?
a. Calcium channel blocker
b. Beta blockers
c. ACE inhibitors
d. Diuretics

Explanation: ACE inhibitors are associated with a dry, persistent cough in 5-35% of patients. ACE inhibitors prevent the breakdown of bradykinin and substance P, resulting in an accumulation of these protussive mediators in the respiratory tract.

1701. Treatment of choice for hypertension includes:
a. Weight reduction
b. Sodium restriction
c. Exercise
d. All of these

1702. Severe hypertensive client is experiencing increased workload of the heart due to:
a. Increased afterload
b. Increased cardiac output
c. Decreased peripheral vascular resistance
d. Decreased blood volume

1703. Action of angiotensin-converting enzyme (ACE) inhibitor is:
a. Promote sodium retention
b. Increase contractility
c. Decrease contractility
d. Reduce blood pressure

1704. Antihypertensives should be used cautiously in clients taking:
a. Aspirin
b. Diclofenac
c. Thioridazine
d. Warfarin

1705. A hypertensive patient has been admitted in a ward for observation. He mentions the attending nurse about squeezing pain in the chest even at rest. Which of the following actions is necessary for this patient? *(Banaras HU 2015)*
a. Give ibuprofen tablet to reduce pain
b. Advise the patient to move out for fresh air
c. Rest to the patient and call the attending doctor
d. Inform the patient that he is fine nothing to worry

1706. The most common presentation in portal hypertension is: *(DSSSB 2013)*
a. Asterixis
b. Hematemesis
c. Elevated blood pressure
d. Confusion

Explanation: Portal hypertension is an increase in the blood pressure within a system of veins called the portal venous system. Veins coming from the stomach, intestine, spleen, and pancreas merge into the portal vein, which then branches into smaller vessels and travels through the liver. They may develop life-threatening hemorrhage, with hematemesis or malena. Hematemesis is the commonest presentation in portal hypertension. Melena without hematemesis may result from bleeding varices.

CARDIAC ARRHYTHMIAS

1707. Fever with relative bradycardia is seen in: *(Banaras HU 2015)*
a. Malaria
b. Typhoid
c. Filaria
d. Diphtheria

1708. Blood pressure is difficult to measure in a patient with:
a. Mitral stenosis
b. Aortic stenosis
c. Complete heart block
d. Atrial fibrillation

1709. Sinus Bradycardia is defined as heart rate of:
a. <40/min
b. <50/min
c. <60/min
d. <70/min

1710. Which is the most lethal arrhythmia? *(Staff Nurse G II 2014)*
a. Atrial fibrillation
b. Ventricular fibrillation
c. Ventricular tachycardia
d. Sinus arrhythmia

1711. A nurse is watching the cardiac monitor and notices that the rhythm suddenly changes, there are no P waves, the QRS complexes are wide and the ventricular rate is regular but over 100, the nurse determines that the patient is experiencing: *(LNJP H D 2012)*
a. Ventricular tachycardia
b. Ventricular fibrillation
c. Premature ventricular contractions
d. Sinus tachycardia

1712. The response to hyperstimulation of vagus nerve is:
a. Skeletal muscle relaxation
b. Skeletal muscle contraction
c. Tachyarrhythmia
d. Bradyarrhythmia

Explanation: Vagus nerve or the Xth cranial nerve innervates with the parasympathetic fibers of heart, lungs and GI tract. Hyperstimulation promotes bradyarrhythmias. When hyperstimulated, the left vagal branch predisposes the heart to conduction block at the atrioventricular node.

1713. In atrial flutter, the key consideration in determining the treatment is:
a. Atrial rate
b. PR interval
c. Ventricular rate
d. P wave

1714. Which of the following is a cause of embolic brain injury?
a. Persistent hypertension
b. Supraventricular tachycardia
c. Atrial fibrillation
d. Skull fracture

1715. Which of the following statements regarding ventricular tachycardia (ventricular dysrhythmia) is true?
a. Electrocardiography (ECG) is the criterion standard for the diagnosis of VT
b. Lidocaine hydrochloride (xylocaine) is the drug of choice
c. Hypokalemia, hypomagnesemia, and hypocalcemia may predispose patients to VT
d. All of the above

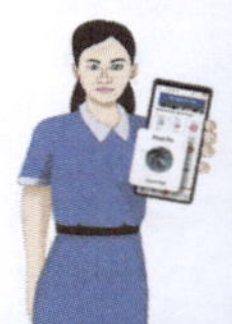

Ans.

1698. a
1699. d
1700. c
1701. d
1702. a
1703. d
1704. c
1705. c
1706. b
1707. b
1708. b
1709. c
1710. b
1711. a
1712. d
1713. c
1714. c
1715. d

1716. A patient in ventricular fibrillation is about to be defibrillated with biphasic defibrillator. A nurse knows that to convert this rhythm effectively, the machine should be set at which of the following energy levels for the best delivery? *(LNJP H D 2012)*

a. 200 Joules b. 360 Joules
c. 50 Joules d. 100 Joules

1717. Identify the irregular cardiac rhythm which can be converted to regular rhythm by using cardioversion?

a. Atrial fibrillation
b. Supraventricular tachycardia
c. Ventricular tachycardia with pulse
d. All of the above

Explanation: Cardioversion is a medical procedure by which an abnormally fast heart rate (tachycardia) or cardiac arrhythmia is converted to a normal rhythm using electricity or drugs. Synchronized electrical cardioversion uses a therapeutic dose of electric current to the heart at a specific moment in the cardiac cycle. In this, electrical current is delivered in synchronization with R wave to interrupt heart rate.

1718. Defibrillation should be given when patient is having:

a. SVT (supraventricular tachycardia)
b. Ventricular tachycardia
c. PEA (pulseless electric activity)
d. Atrial fibrillations

HEART BLOCK

1719. Which of the following types of fats is considered to be harmful to the body?

a. Cis fat b. Trans fat
c. Poly unsaturated fatty acids
d. Omega 3 fatty acids

Explanation: Monounsaturated fatty acids are of two types, i.e., cis fatty acids and trans fatty acids. Trans fatty acids have markedly adverse effects on serum lipids by raising levels of the lipoprotein LDL (so-called "bad cholesterol"), lowering levels of the lipoprotein HDL ("good cholesterol").

1720. Any disturbance that blocks the transmission of nerve impulse from SA node downwards is known as: *(DSSSB PHN, 2015)*

a. Heart block b. Heart attack
c. Nerve block d. Cardiac arrhythmias

1721. Wenckebach pattern is also known as:

a. 1st degree heart block b. Mobitz type II
c. Mobitz type I d. Complete heart block

1722. The most common cause of new onset complete heart block is:

a. Myocardial infarction b. Hyperkalemia
c. Atrial fibrillation d. Infective endocarditis

Explanation: A complete heart block may occur due to occlusion of the right coronary artery.

1723. Which of the following statements by the client is an indication that he/she is at risk of atherosclerosis?

a. I had mid-hypogastric pain during intake of food
b. I had bilateral calf pain while walking
c. I had swelling of legs
d. I didn't have normal sleep time

Explanation: Intermittent claudication is pain affecting the calf, and less commonly the thigh and buttock, that is induced by exercise and relieved by rest. Intermittent claudication is a suspect for atherosclerosis that can lead to heart block/coronary artery disease.

1724. The coronary artery which supplies blood to the left atrium and left ventricle is:

a. Right coronary artery b. Sinoatrial nodal artery
c. Left circumflex artery d. Acute marginal artery

Explanation: The circumflex artery, a branch of left coronary artery, is responsible for blood supply to the left atrium and the posterior-lateral aspect of the left ventricle. Left circumflex artery which is a branch of Acute marginal artery and sinoatrial nodal artery (supplies SA node) are branches of right coronary artery which supplies primarily the right atrium and right ventricle.

1725. Which of the following is not the surgical procedure of coronary artery disease?

a. PTCA
b. Laser angioplasty
c. Atherectomy
d. TIPS

1726. Drugs to be preferred for the clients with coronary artery disease?

a. Nitrates
b. Cholinergic drugs
c. ACE inhibitors
d. Opioids

1727. Wenckebach Heart Blocks are also known as:

a. First degree heart block
b. Mobitz type 1 heart block
c. Second degree heart block
c. Both b & c

COR PULMONALE

1728. Clinical manifestation involved in right side heart failure is:

a. Ascites b. Pedal edema
c. Oliguria d. All of these

1729. Which of the following is the most common cause of cor pulmonale?

a. Cyanosis b. Severe COPD
c. Hypotension d. Septal defect

1730. Which of the following etiology is observed in the patient with cor pulmonale?

a. Obstructive sleep apnea b. Increased appetite
c. Dysphagia d. Tremors

1731. Most common clinical manifestation seen in cor pulmonale?

a. Lethargy
b. Dyspnea on exertion
c. Syncope
d. Fatigue

1732. What is the confirmatory test for the diagnosis of cor pulmonale?

a. CT scan
b. MRI
c. Echocardiogram
d. Right heart catheterization

Ans.

1716. a
1717. d
1718. b
1719. b
1720. a
1721. c
1722. a
1723. b
1724. c
1725. d
1726. a
1727. c
1728. d
1729. b
1730. a
1731. b
1732. d

ARTERIOSCLEROSIS AND ATHEROSCLEROSIS

1733. Which of the following is high in saturated fatty acids?
- a. Fatty fish, walnuts and green leafy vegetables
- b. Poultry skin, full fat milk products and tropical oils
- c. Canola oil, flaxseeds and olive oil
- d. Wild game, low fat milk and yogurt

Explanation: Saturated fatty acids are chiefly found in animal fats.

1734. Hyperlipidemia is seen in:
- a. Hypothyroidism
- b. Nephrotic syndrome
- c. Metabolic syndrome
- d. All of the above

1735. Which among the following is not a manifestation of hyperlipidemia?
- a. Corneal Arcus
- b. Xanthelasma
- c. Xanthoma
- d. Erythema marginatum

Explanation:
- Corneal Arcus-grayish white ring around cornea due to lipid infiltration.
- Xanthelasma-yellowish deposition of fat under the skin usually around the eyelids.
- Xanthoma-deposition of cholesterol in tendon or other body parts.
- Erythema marginatum non-itchy red rings on extensor surfaces commonly seen in rheumatic fever.

1736. Hereditary risk factor for developing CAD is:
- a. Family history of heart disease
- b. High cholesterol level
- c. Smoking
- d. Oral contraceptive use

1737. All among the following are non-modifiable risk factor for Coronary Artery Disease; EXCEPT:
- a. Obesity
- b. Heredity
- c. Gender
- d. Age

1738. Which of the following statements by the client to the nurse indicates a modifiable risk factor for coronary artery disease?
- a. I exercise every other day
- b. My father died of myocardial infarction
- c. My cholesterol is 180
- d. I smoke 2 packs of cigarettes per day

Explanation: Cigarette smoking is considered as one of the major modifiable risk factors for CAD. Family history of death due to myocardial infarction is a non-modifiable risk factor while option a and c is not considered to be a risk factor for coronary artery disease.

1739. An amino acid that increases the risk for CAD is:
- a. Homocysteine
- b. Alanine transaminase
- c. Glutamic acid
- d. L-proline

Explanation: High levels of homocysteine causes endothelial damage, inflammation and subsequent atherogenesis.

1740. The most common direct cause of sudden death is:
- a. Cardiomyopathy
- b. Pulmonary hypertension
- c. Heart failure
- d. CAD

1741. Coronary arteries primarily receive blood supply during:
- a. Inspiration
- b. Expiration
- c. Diastole
- d. Systole

1742. Health education given to a client with CAD is effective, if the client states that:
- a. Blood pressure need to be kept in normal limit
- b. Decrease the intake of saturated fat
- c. Avoid smoking and alcoholism
- d. All of the above

1743. Which among the following values is the risk factor for CAD?
- a. HDL: 90 mg/dL
- b. LDL = 130 mg/dL
- c. VLDL = 24%
- d. Total cholesterol = 250 mg/dL

1744. Priority nursing intervention in a client with CAD is:
- a. Decrease activity
- b. Enhance myocardial oxygenation
- c. Plan for surgery
- d. Carry out lab investigations

1745. Immediate management in a client with aortic dissection is:
- a. Maintain perfusion to the organ
- b. Control blood pressure
- c. Monitor peripheral pulse
- d. Maintain cardiac output

1746. Atherosclerosis is a:
- a. Chronic inflammatory and immune disease
- b. Acute inflammatory and immune disease
- c. Acute tissue response
- d. Atrophy of epithelial tissue

1747. Which among the following is the modifiable risk factor of atherosclerosis?
- a. Obesity
- b. Male gender
- c. Advanced age
- d. Family history

1748. Following are the modifiable risk factor of atherosclerosis; EXCEPT:
- a. Physical inactivity
- b. Family history
- c. Diabetes
- d. Hypertension

1749. Atherosclerotic plaques are most commonly seen in:
- a. Abdominal aorta
- b. Arch of aorta
- c. Descending aorta
- d. Ascending aorta

1750. The coronary artery most commonly involved in atherosclerosis is:
- a. Left anterior descending artery
- b. Left main coronary artery
- c. Right coronary artery
- d. Circumflex coronary artery

1751. Which of the following is a risk factor for the development of atherosclerosis and Peripheral Vascular Disease (PVD)?
- a. Low levels of triglycerides concentration
- b. Low levels of low density lipoprotein (LDL)
- c. High levels of low-density lipoprotein (LDL)
- d. High levels of high-density lipoprotein (HDL)

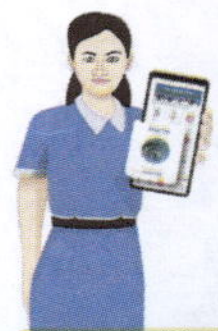

Ans.

1733. b
1734. d
1735. d
1736. a
1737. a
1738. d
1739. a
1740. d
1741. c
1742. d
1743. d
1744. b
1745. b
1746. a
1747. a
1748. b
1749. a
1750. a
1751. c

Explanation: Increased level of serum low density lipoprotein (LDL) cholesterol is considered as a risk factor for the development of atherosclerosis. LDL cholesterol is not broken down into the liver but is deposited into the wall of the blood vessels.

1752. Complications associated with atherosclerosis is:
- a. Embolism
- b. Hemorrhage
- c. Decreased blood supply
- d. All of these

1753. Infective agent causing atherosclerosis:
- a. Clostridium Diphtheriae
- b. Chlamydia Pneumoniae
- c. Hemophilus influenza
- d. Mycobacterium Pneumoniae

ANGINA PECTORIS

1754. Angina is:
- a. Back pain
- b. Chest pain
- c. Leg pain
- d. Headache

1755. In angina pectoris, pain occurs due to:
- a. Accumulation of HCl
- b. Lack of oxygen supply
- c. Accumulation of Lactose Dehydrogenase
- d. Movement of thrombus

1756. What is the main reason for angina pectoris? *(RRB SSNE 2015)*
- a. Neurological disease
- b. Gastric disease
- c. Respiratory disease
- d. Cardiac disease

1757. Pathophysiology behind angina pectoris is:
- a. Increased preload
- b. Decreased afterload
- c. Thrombi in coronary artery
- d. Inadequate oxygen supply to the myocardium

1758. Which condition is associated with a predictable level of pain that occurs as a result of physical or emotional stress?
- a. Prinzmetal angina
- b. Stable angina
- c. Unstable angina
- d. Variant angina

Explanation:
- Angina is chest discomfort or pain due to poor blood flow through the blood vessels in the heart.
- Anginal pain occurring at rest is an instance of unstable angina.
- Stable angina occurs with activity or emotional stress.
- Prinzmetal or variant angina-occurs in cycles during rest due to coronary artery spasm.

1759. Identify correct statement regarding Angina Pectoris:
- a. Radiates to the left arm
- b. Lasts less than 15 minutes
- c. Is relieved by rest and nitroglycerin
- d. All of the above

1760. Identify correct statement regarding stable angina:
- a. Cause is coronary atherosclerosis
- b. It is precipitated by physical activity.
- c. Managed with nitroglycerin.
- d. All of the above

1761. Which among the following is caused due to spasm of the coronary artery?
- a. Stable angina
- b. Variant angina
- c. Unstable angina
- d. Myocardial infarction

Explanation: Variant angina, or Prinzmetal's angina, is prolonged and severe and occurs at the same time each day, most often at rest. Stable angina is induced by exercise and relieved by rest or nitroglycerin tablets. Unstable angina occurs at lower and lower levels of activity or at rest, is less predictable, and is often a precursor of myocardial infarction.

1762. Reversible ST segment elevation is seen in:
- a. Unstable angina
- b. Variant angina
- c. Refractory angina
- d. Silent ischemia

1763. Which type of angina is also called prinzmetal angina?
- a. Variant angina
- b. Stable angina
- c. Refractory angina
- d. Silent ischemia

1764. If unstable angina is left untreated it can lead to:
- a. Atherosclerosis
- b. Stable angina
- c. Arrthymias
- d. Variant angina

1765. Which of the following is the most dangerous complication of angina pectoris?
- a. Heart failure
- b. Patent ductus arteriosus
- c. Coarctation of aorta
- d. Tetralogy of Fallot

1766. Which of the following is NOT true about angina pectoris? *New Q*
- a. Inadequate coronary blood flow
- b. Increased myocardial oxygen demand
- c. Reduced pulmonary artery pressure
- d. Relieved by rest or nitroglycerin administration

Explanation: In angina pectoris, the pulmonary artery pressure is not necessarily reduced. Angina pectoris is primarily caused by inadequate coronary blood flow (option a) and increased myocardial oxygen demand (option b). The symptoms of angina pectoris are typically relieved by rest or nitroglycerin administration (option d). However, reduced pulmonary artery pressure is not a characteristic feature of angina pectoris.

MYOCARDIAL INFARCTION (MI)

1767. The lack of oxygen supply to myocardium of heart leads to: *(DSSSB PHN, 2015)*
- a. Fibrillation
- b. Heart failure
- c. Angina
- d. Infarction

1768. First elevating enzyme following MI is:
- a. CPK-MB
- b. Troponin-I
- c. Myoglobin
- d. Troponin-T

Explanation: Myoglobin is the first elevating enzyme after myocardial injury but is less specific for myocardial necrosis, especially, in the presence of skeletal muscle injury or renal insufficiency.

1769. The enzyme study that is most specific to Myocardial Infarction is:
- a. CPK-MB
- b. LDH
- c. SGOT
- d. SGPT

1770. Which enzyme is found only in myocardium?
- a. Troponin-T
- b. Troponin-I
- c. Myoglobin
- d. Lactate dehydrogenase

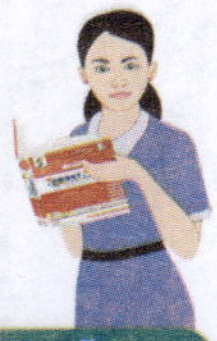

Ans.

1752. a
1753. b
1754. b
1755. b
1756. d
1757. d
1758. b
1759. d
1760. d
1761. b
1762. b
1763. a
1764. c
1765. a
1766. c
1767. d
1768. c
1769. a
1770. b

1771. The most sensitive biochemical marker in a patient with 7 days old Myocardial Infarction is:
a. Troponin I, T b. LDH
c. Myoglobin d. CPK MB

1772. Which among the following is the most specific marker for the diagnosis of acute myocardial infarction?
a. Troponin b. Creatinine kinase
c. LDH d. Myoglobin

1773. Chest pain is described as pleuritic when it:
a. Resolves with sublingual NTG
b. Increases with deep inspiration and decreases when the patient sits up and leans forward
c. Occurs only during sitting
d. Resolves with a deep breath

1774. Which among the following statements is FALSE regarding risk factors for ischemic heart disease:
a. Regular aerobic exercise protects against ischemic heart disease
b. Elevated serum homocysteine is an independent risk factor
c. Blood pressure lowering reduces the risk for ischemic cardiac events
d. Women on hormone replacement therapy are at risk for ischemic heart disease

Explanation:
- A minimum of 150 minutes of moderate exercise per week has been recommended by American Heart Association as measure to lower blood cholesterol.
- Homocysteine is an amino acid that is related to early development of CAD.
- Elevated blood pressure damages the intima of blood vessel.
- Hormone replacement therapy in women is beneficial in preventing atherosclerosis. Estrogen lyses fat from the body.
- Aneurysm, Atherosclerosis and Arteriosclerosis

1775. Type of angina experienced by a client with an impending myocardial infarction (MI) is:
a. Variant angina b. Stable angina
c. Micro vascular angina d. Unstable angina

1776. Myocardial infarction (MI) commonly known is:
a. Angina b. Heart attack
c. Dysrhythmias d. Heart block

1777. Most common site of myocardial infarction is:
a. Anterior wall of left ventricle
b. Inferior wall of left ventricle
c. Posterior wall of right ventricle
d. Posterior wall of left ventricle

1778. Which among the following is NOT suggestive of acute myocardial infarction:
a. A sudden onset severe central chest pain
b. A sudden onset burning hypogastric pain
c. A new onset complete heart block
d. Sudden death

Explanation: Burning hypogastric pain is often due to gastritis or Gastroesophageal Reflux Disease (GERD). All other signs are associated with myocardial infarction.

1779. Risk of myocardial infarction (MI) increases with:
a. Using oral contraceptive pills
b. Hyperlipidemia
c. Elevated serum iron level
d. All of the above

1780. Irreversible injury in myocardium occurs after:
a. 15 minutes b. 30 minutes
c. 45 minutes d. 60 minutes

1781. Occlusion of which of the following blood vessels causes inferior wall myocardial infarction (MI)?
a. Right coronary artery
b. Left anterior descending artery
c. Interventricular artery
d. Nodal branch

Explanation: Approximately 40% of all MIs involve the inferior wall. Inferior wall myocardial infarctions are due to ischemia and infarction to the inferior region of the heart. In 80% of patients, the inferior wall of the heart is supplied by the right coronary artery via the posterior descending artery (PDA). In the other 20% of patients, the PDA is a branch of the circumflex artery.

1782. Parameters increase as myocardial oxygen consumption increases are:
a. Preload, afterload, and peripheral vascular resistance
b. Preload, afterload, and stroke volume
c. Preload, afterload, contractility, and heart rate
d. Preload, afterload, peripheral vascular resistance and stroke volume

1783. Occlusion of circumflex branch of coronary artery causes:
a. Inferior wall infarction b. Anterior wall
c. Lateral wall infarction d. Septal infarction

1784. Signs and symptoms of MI include:
a. Radiating pain b. Tachycardia
c. Dyspnea d. All of these

1785. Early complications of acute myocardial infarction include:
a. Arrhythmias b. Contractile dysfunction
c. Myocardial rupture d. All of these

1786. Which of the following complications occur within 24 hours after sustaining an MI?
a. Left ventricular aneurysm
b. Ventricular septal rupture
c. Cardiogenic shock
d. Atrial septal rupture

Explanation: Cardiogenic shock after AMI develops within 6 hours in about 50% of patients and within 24 hours in about 75% of patients. Other given complications are mechanical complications that can occur as early as within 48 hours or two weeks post-infarction.

1787. Which of the following is the priority intervention for a patient experiencing myocardial infarction?
a. Obtain ECG
b. Administer sublingual nitroglycerin
c. Administer oxygen
d. Administer Aspirin

1788. Among the following drugs, which is to be given first to client with acute MI is:
a. Lovastatin b. Amlodipine
c. Aspirin d. Beta blockers

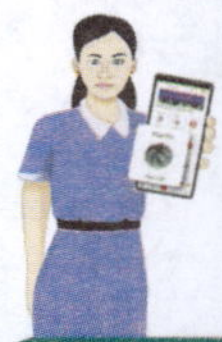

Ans.
1771. a
1772. a
1773. b
1774. d
1775. d
1776. b
1777. a
1778. b
1779. d
1780. b
1781. a
1782. c
1783. c
1784. d
1785. d
1786. c
1787. c
1788. c

1789. A client with myocardial infarction suddenly becomes tachycardiac, shows signs of air hunger, and begins coughing frothy, pink-tinged sputum. Initial nursing interventions should be:

a. Lasix, oxygen, nitrates, morphine, propped up position
b. Morphine, oxygen, nitrates, aspirin
c. Oxygen, thrombolytic, aspirin, aminophylline, inotropes
d. Oxygen, aspirin, beta blockers, nitrates

Explanation: Pulmonary edema is characterized by extreme breathlessness, dyspnea, air hunger, and the production of frothy, pink-tinged sputum. Auscultation of the lungs reveals crackles. Initial nursing intervention is to administer Lasix, morphine, nitrates, oxygen, and to give propped up position (LMNOP)

1790. Which measures should be performed immediately following CABG?

a. Ambulation, 12 lead ECG, clear liquid diet
b. Vital signs, cardiac rhythm, pulse oximetry
c. Vital signs, cardiac rhythm, clear liquid diet
d. 12-lead ECG, vitals, ambulation

1791. Cause of shock in a client with MI is:

a. Decrease in cardiac output
b. Less blood volume
c. Vasodilation
d. Pulmonary edema

1792. Which of the following conditions can decrease oxygen demand on the heart?

a. Thyrotoxicosis b. Treatment with diltiazem
c. Pregnancy d. Aortic stenosis

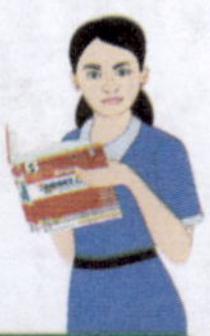

Explanation: Diltiazem is a calcium channel blocker. Cardioselective Calcium Channel Blockers (Diltiazem and Verapamil) decrease heart rate and contractility, which leads to a reduction in myocardial oxygen demand, which makes them excellent antianginal drugs

1793. Following MI client is advised to do leg exercises and ambulation to prevent .... complication.

a. Lymphadenopathy
b. Pressure ulcers
c. Deep vein thrombosis
d. Air embolism

1794. Common complication following myocardial infarction (MI) is:

a. Cardiac tamponade b. Cardiomyopathy
c. Arrhythmias d. Endocarditis

1795. Post MI client complaining of chest pain while taking deep breaths, appropriate nursing action is:

a. Give NTG tablets
b. Auscultate pericardial friction rub
c. Give oxygen
d. Administer analgesics

1796. In myocardial infarction, morphine helps in all of the following EXCEPT:

a. Decrease pain
b. Dissolve the infarction
c. Decrease the client's anxiety
d. Decrease oxygen demand of myocardium

1797. All are used for secondary prevention of MI; EXCEPT:

a. Aspirin b. Beta blockers
c. Warfarin d. Statins

1798. Dose of streptokinase to be used in MI is:

a. 0.15 Million units b. 1.5 Million units
c. 15 Million units d. 150 Million units

1799. A 60-year-old male patient had myocardial infarction one month ago. He is currently undergoing cardiac rehabilitation sessions at the gym. This is considered as __________ prevention:

a. Primordial b. Primary
c. Secondary d. Tertiary

INTRA-AORTIC BALLOON PUMP (IABP)

1800. When caring for a client after cardiac catheterization, which nursing action is most important? *(RAK MSc 2018)*

a. Administer oxygen
b. Provide rest
c. Check the ECG every 5–15 minutes
d. Check a pulse distal to the insertion site

Explanation: The pulse distal to the insertion site is assessed to prevent complications like hypotension, cardiac tamponade or any coronary artery dissection/perforation. The distal pulse is preferred over proximal pulse because the artery used for cardiac catheterization needs a week to gets completely healed.

1801. All of the following are potential complication in the initial 24 hours after cardiac catheterization procedure; EXCEPT:

a. Hemorrhage of the insertion site
b. Falling blood pressure
c. Formation of thrombus in the coronary arteries
d. Angina at rest

1802. The gas used for inflating IABP balloon:

a. Hydrogen b. CO_2
c. Neon d. Helium

CORONARY ARTERY BYPASS GRAFT (CABG)

1803. Which of the following is expected from a patient who had coronary artery bypass graft (CABG) with mammary artery graft a week before? *(ESI 2007)*

a. Ankle edema b. Depression
c. Dizziness d. Memory lapses

Explanation: Following CABG clients commonly experience depression, fatigue, incisional chest discomfort, dyspnea, and anorexia. Depression typically resolves on its own and does not require medical intervention.

1804. Which of the following techniques is used to support circulation during a cardiac surgery?

a. Intra-aortic balloon pump
b. Cardiopulmonary bypass machine
c. Positive pressure ventilation
d. Negative pressure ventilation

Explanation: Cardiopulmonary bypass (heart lung machine) is a technique that maintains the circulation of the blood and oxygen content of the body by taking over the function of the heart and the lungs during surgery.

Ans.

1789. a
1790. b
1791. a
1792. b
1793. c
1794. c
1795. b
1796. b
1797. c
1798. b
1799. d
1800. d
1801. d
1802. d
1803. b
1804. b

1805. Mr. Siddappa has been received from operation room by the PICU nurse after the coronary artery bypass grafting procedure. Which of the following intervention would be appropriate to prevent early complications?

(AIIMS Bhopal Grade-I 2018)

a. Employing leg exercises and turning him in bed every 2 hours
b. Keeping him from ambulating until the day after surgery
c. Keeping him cool with light patient body cover to prevent elevated temperature
d. Positioning him in bed with pillows placed under his knees to improve venous return

Explanation: After CABG procedure, lower leg edema may occur after removal of the saphenous vein (which is most commonly used graft in CABG). So, employing leg exercises and turning the patient in bed every 2 hours is very important to be followed. It also facilitates the recovery.

1806. The complication that needs to be suspected in a client who has paradoxical pulses following CABG surgery is:

a. Cardiomyopathy b. Pericarditis
c. Aortic dissection d. Pericardial tamponade

HEART FAILURE

1807. Sudden cardiac death is due to the dysfunction of:

a. Right atrium b. Mitral valve
c. Left ventricle d. Coronary artery

1808. Most common cause of left sided heart failure is:

(Kerala PSC, Nov 2014)

a. Septal defect
b. Congenital heart disease
c. Coronary Artery Diseases (CAD)
d. Hypertension

Explanation: Coronary Artery Diseases (CAD) is the most common cause of heart failure.

Other causes include Cardiomyopathy, Congenital heart defect, heart valve disease, Hypertension, emphysema, etc.

1809. Clinical signs of left sided heart failure:

a. Dyspnea and bradycardia
b. Dyspnea and tachycardia
c. Tachycardia and restlessness
d. Restlessness and coughs

1810. Auscultation of crackles in the lungs is present in .... condition.

a. Pulmonic valve malfunction
b. Tricuspid valve malfunction
c. Left-sided heart failure
d. Right-sided heart failure

1811. The edema in congestive heart failure is due to:

a. Change in oncotic pressure
b. Renal failure
c. Liver failure
d. Venous stasis

1812. Cheyne stokes breathing is seen in:

a. Intracranial hypotension b. Congestive heart failure
c. Left atrial myxoma d. Pickwickian syndrome

1813. Weight gain, nausea, and a decrease in urine output are the manifestation of:

a. Myocardial infarction
b. Pericarditis
c. Right-sided heart failure
d. Left-sided heart failure

1814. Which of the following tests can be used for the diagnosis and assessment of the severity of heart failure:

a. BNP b. PSA
c. Troponin d. ANA

Explanation: Brain natriuretic peptide or B-type natriuretic peptide (BNP) secreted by the ventricles in response to excessive stretc.hing of heart muscle cells.

1815. Right ventricular hypertrophy is a complication of:

a. Cor pulmonale b. Pneumonia
c. Hemothorax d. Peritonitis

1816. Drug of choice to improve the cardiac performance is:

a. Beta-adrenergic blockers b. Nitroglycerin
c. Opioids d. Inotropic agents

1817. The dietary management of a patient with congestive cardiac failure includes:

a. Fat restricted diet b. Sodium and water rich diet
c. Rich fiber content diet d. Salt restricted diet

1818. A client with chronic heart failure placed on a sodium restricted diet. Which among the following food items needs to be avoided by the client?

a. Eggs b. Canned Sardines
c. Plain nuts d. Whole milk

Explanation: Canned sardines (sea food) are generally rich in sodium content. One can of Sardines in oil contain 500 mg of sodium (approx).

1819. Among the following identify the food group with least level of sodium:

a. Milk b. Meat
c. Vegetables d. Fruits

1820. Priority intervention in a heart failure patient secondary to dilated cardiomyopathy is:

a. Cardiac enzyme study
b. Rehabilitate the client
c. Check response to prescribed medications
d. Monitor blood level of medication

1821. Final treatment for cardiomyopathy if the medical management fails is:

a. Valve replacement b. Pacemaker
c. Heart transplantation d. Cardio version

1822. Identify the correct statement regarding pacemaker:

a. Asynchronous mode pacemaker has a set rate
b. Synchronous mode pacemaker works on demand to maintain normal heart rate
c. In asynchronous pacemaker pulse rate more or less than the set rate is considered as malfunctioning
d. All of the above

Explanation: All of the above statements are correct in relation to pacemaker. In synchronous pacemaker, pacing starts when the pulse rate falls below the preset rate. The pulse generator is internal in permanent pacemakers (subcutaneously or submuscularly) and external in temporary pacing.

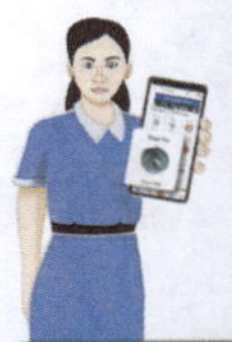

Ans.

1805. a
1806. d
1807. c
1808. c
1809. b
1810. c
1811. d
1812. b
1813. c
1814. a
1815. a
1816. d
1817. d
1818. b
1819. d
1820. c
1821. c
1822. d

1823. Health education after pacemaker implantation includes:
a. Change the battery daily
b. Avoid use of lift
c. Check blood pressure every day
d. Check the pulse every day for one full minute at the same time

1824. Health education regarding pacemaker includes:
a. Do not raise your arm above the level of your heart for the first few weeks
b. Gently wash the incision site, but do not put lotion or powder on it
c. Do not lift, push, or pull anything that weighs more than 5 pounds for one to two months
d. All of the above

Explanation: All of the above should be included in the health teaching and the client also needs to avoid the use of cellular phones. Client will be also asked to avoid magnetic checking file which will interfere with the pacemaker activity.

1825. The nurse is providing discharge teaching to an adult patient who had a permanent artificial pacemaker implanted. Which of the following information given by the nurse is inappropriate?
a. The client may be allowed to use household electrical appliances
b. The client should check the pulse rate once a day, in the morning upon awakening
c. The client should have regular follow up care
d. The client may engage in contact sports

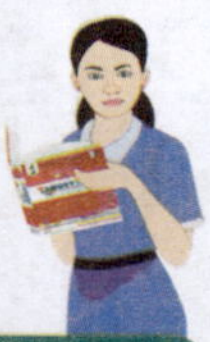

Explanation: Contact sports such as football, basketball, and cricket should be avoided as this may cause trauma to the area of pacemaker implantation. Using household electrical appliances are generally safe for patient implanted with pacemaker provided the appliances are in good working condition.

MYOCARDITIS AND PERICARDITIS

1826. A client is suffering from constrictive pericarditis, which among the following findings reveals the serious complication associated with that?
a. Activity intolerance
b. Pitting edema over the legs
c. Jugular venous distention
d. Hypertrophy of pericardium in echo

1827. What type of inflammation is bread and butter pericarditis?
a. Erythematous
b. Fibrinous
c. Connective tissue
d. Purulent

1828. All of the following statements are correct regarding pericarditis pain; EXCEPT:
a. Chest pain is almost always present, may be felt in the neck, shoulder, back, or abdomen
b. Pain may increase with coughing and swallowing
c. Pain is worst in the supine position
d. Exertion can increase the pain

Explanation: In pericarditis, exertion does not change the pain whereas in myocardial infarction, exertion can increase the pain. Sharp, pleuritic, retro-sternal pain, radiates to trapezius ridge or no radiation, worsening pain in the supine position and sudden onset of pain are the features of pericarditis pain.

1829. Focal or diffuse inflammation of the cardiac muscle is:
a. Endocarditis
b. Myocarditis
c. Pericarditis
d. Myocardial infarction

1830. Most important nursing responsibility while caring a client with myocarditis is:
a. Isolation technique
b. Antibiotic prophylaxis
c. Activity restriction
d. Oxygenation and ventilation

1831. Small painful nodes on fingers and toes called Osler's nodes are seen in: *(Staff Nurse G II 2014)*
a. Cardiomyopathy
b. Pericarditis
c. Infective endocarditis
d. Myocarditis

1832. Infective endocarditis client developed sudden left leg pain with pallor, paresthesia, and a loss of peripheral pulses. Priority nursing action is:
a. Elevate the leg to promote venous return.
b. Apply constrictive elastic bandage
c. Notify the physician
d. Use blood blocks to elevate foot end

CARDIAC TAMPONADE

1833. Which among the following conditions is accompanied by distant, muffled heart sounds and prominent neck vessels?
a. Cardiogenic shock
b. Cardiac tamponade
c. Pulmonary embolism
d. Dissecting thoracic aortic aneurysm

Explanation:

- Cardiogenic shock occurs with severe damage (more than 40%) to the left ventricle. Classic signs of cardiogenic shock include hypotension, a rapid pulse that becomes weaker, decreased urine output, and cool, clammy skin.
- Cardiac tamponade is characterized by distant, muffled heart sounds and prominent neck vessels.
- Pulmonary embolism has a sudden presentation of severe dyspnea accompanying the chest pain.
- Dissecting aortic aneurysms usually are accompanied by back pain.

1834. What is the immediate goal of treatment for cardiac tamponade?
a. Relieving pain
b. Alleviating anxiety
c. Improving mobility
d. Relieving intra-pericardial pressure

Ans.
1823. d
1824. d
1825. d
1826. c
1827. b
1828. d
1829. b
1830. d
1831. c
1832. c
1833. b
1834. d

1835. The triad of signs/symptoms seen in cardiac tamponade is:
a. Tachycardia, tachypnea, tender hepatomegaly
b. Muffled heart sound, distended neck veins, hypotension
c. Stasis, hypercoagulability, vessel injury
d. Chest pain, heart failure, syncope

Explanation: Muffled heart sound, distended neck veins, and hypotension (**Becks triad**) are signs of cardiac tamponade. Symptoms include anxiety, restlessness, light-headedness, palpitations, swelling of legs and abdomen, etc.

1836. Which among the following parameter suggests that pericardiocentesis was effective?
a. Increased JVP
b. Increase in pulse paradoxical
c. Increased blood pressure
d. Muffled heart sounds

PULMONARY EDEMA

1837. Damage to .... heart chamber causes acute pulmonary edema:
a. Left atrium b. Right atrium
c. Left ventricle d. Right ventricle

1838. In pulmonary edema, crackles of the lungs are especially seen in:
a. Anterior bases b. Posterior base
c. Superior base d. Inferior region

1839. Pulmonary edema is defined as:
a. Damage of the alveoli
b. Inflammation of bronchi
c. Inflammation of alveoli
d. Abnormal accumulation of fluid in the lung tissue

1840. Which of the following is the confirmatory test for pulmonary edema?
a. Chest X-ray
b. MRI
c. Incentive spirometry
d. Blood culture

1841. Crackles are formed due to the:
a. Movement of air through the alveolar fluid
b. Damaging of the pleural cavity
c. Inflammation of the peritoneal cavity
d. Decreased blood supply to the lungs

ACUTE RHEUMATIC FEVER

1842. Name the microorganism which is most commonly responsible for rheumatic fever, scarlet fever, glomerulonephritis etc. is:
a. Staphylococci b. Streptococci
c. H. influenza d. Meningococci

1843. Elevated levels of antistreptolysin O are seen in: *(AIIMS BPL NO 2018)*
a. Subacute endocarditis b. Ventricular septal defect
c. Rheumatic fever d. Cardiomyopathy

Explanation: Elevated levels of antistreptolysin O are seen in **rheumatic fever**.
- Positive titer: >200 IU/mL
- Rises to peak: 4–6 weeks
- Remain elevated for 1 year
- **Subacute Endocarditis**: ESR is elevated

1844. Important feature of rheumatic heart disease:
a. Valvular disease b. Angina
c. Myocardial infarction d. Cardiomyopathy

1845. Streptococcal throat infection can later lead to: *(NCFL 2019)*
a. Tuberculosis b. Leprosy
c. Rheumatic heart disease d. Malaria

Explanation: Streptococcal throat infection can later lead to Rheumatic heart disease. Inadequately treated streptococcal throat might cause Rheumatic fever. Rheumatic fever causes permanent damage to heart valves and leads to heart failure (Rheumatic Heart Disease)

1846. Rheumatic heart disease is caused by:
a. Meningococci
b. Group A β-hemolytic staphylococci
c. Group A β-hemolytic streptococci
d. Pneumococci

1847. The guidelines for the clinical diagnosis of acute rheumatic fever was suggested by: *(Safdarjung NO 2018)*
a. Dr T. Duckett Jones b. Robert Koch
c. Landsteiner d. Michael Smith

Explanation: The guidelines for the clinical diagnosis of acute rheumatic fever was suggested by Dr T. Duckett Jones. That includes Major and minor criteria.

1848. Jones criteria guides in the diagnosis of:
a. Infective endocarditis b. Rheumatic fever
c. Congestive heart failure d. Congenital heart disease

Explanation: Jones criteria guides in the diagnosis of rheumatic fever.

Jones criteria
- **Major Criteria**
  - Carditis
  - Polyarthritis
  - Subcutaneous nodules
  - Chorea (Sydenham Chorea, St Vitus dance)
  - Erythema Marginatum
- **Minor criteria**
  - Fever
  - Arthralgia
  - Increased ASO titer
  - Prolonged PR interval

1849. All the following are major Jones criteria for rheumatic fever; EXCEPT: *(AIIMS BBS NO 2018)*
a. Carditis b. Migratory polyarthritis
c. Fever d. Erythema marginatum

Explanation: **Fever** comes under Jones minor criteria for rheumatic fever. All other given signs are under Major Jones criteria.

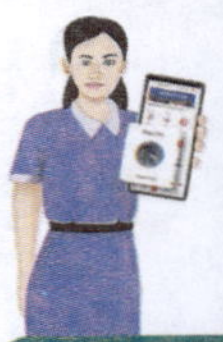

Ans.
1835. b
1836. c
1837. c
1838. b
1839. d
1840. a
1841. a
1842. b
1843. c
1844. a
1845. c
1846. c
1847. a
1848. b
1849. c

1850. Most common symptom of acute rheumatic fever in adults:
a. Migratory polyarthritis b. Carditis
c. Chorea d. Rash

1851. Which is not a major criterion for diagnosis of rheumatic fever?
a. Carditis b. Arthritis
c. Increased ASO titer d. Subcutaneous nodules

1852. Effect of repeated attack of rheumatic fever is:
a. Valvular heart disease
b. Arthritis
c. Mediastinal mass
d. Cardiomegaly

1853. Mc Callum's patch is diagnostic of:
a. Tetralogy of Fallot (ToF)
b. Rheumatic endocarditis
c. Infective endocarditis
d. Myocardial infarction

Explanation: Mc Callum's Patch is seen on posterior wall of Left atrium above the mitral valve, it often forms nidus for endocarditis. It is very specific for Rheumatic Endocarditis.

1854. Management of rheumatic fever is:
a. Antibiotics b. Valve replacement
c. Corticosteroids d. Cardiac catheterization

AORTIC ANEURYSM AND STENOSIS

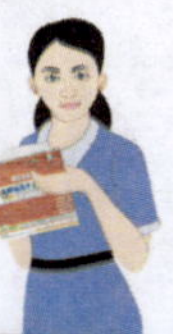

1855. The abnormal dilatation of the wall of an artery is referred to as: *(DSSSB PHN, 2015)*
a. Aneurysm b. Hernia
c. Atherosclerosis d. Phlebitis

1856. Most common site of aortic aneurysm is:
a. Ascending aorta
b. Descending thoracic aorta
c. Aortic arch
d. Abdominal aorta

1857. Which among the following genetic disorder is a risk factor for aneurysm?
a. Down syndrome
b. Neurofibromatosis
c. Marfan's syndrome
d. Fanconi anemia

1858. Pulsating abdominal mass on palpation is the clinical manifestation of:
a. Abdominal aortic aneurysm
b. Wilms tumor
c. Anastomosis
d. Paralytic ileus

1859. Site for palpating abdominal aortic aneurysm is:
a. Right upper quadrant of abdomen
b. Right lower quadrant
c. Middle lower abdomen to the left of the midline
d. Middle lower abdomen to the right of the midline

1860. Definitive diagnostic test for abdominal aortic aneurysm is:
a. MRI
b. Aortogram
c. Computed tomography (CT) scan
d. Contrast studies

1861. Localized enlargement of an artery caused by weakness in the arterial wall is:
a. Aneurysm b. Diverticulum
c. Hernia d. Protrusion

1862. Common cause of aneurysm or aortic aneurysm is:
a. Syphilis
b. Atherosclerosis
c. Congenital
d. Trauma

1863. Aneurysm leads to:
a. Compression on adjacent structures
b. Thrombosis
c. Rupture and hemorrhage
d. All of the above

1864. Leading cause of aortic aneurysm is:
a. Loss of elasticity b. Trauma
c. Atherosclerosis d. Septicemia

ARTERIAL EMBOLISM

1865. Which of the following is not the risk factor for the arterial embolism?
a. Damage to the arterial wall
b. Atrial fibrillation
c. Increased blood supply
d. Hemophilia A

1866. Which of the following condition may cause arterial embolism?
a. Endocarditis
b. Mitral stenosis
c. Both a and b
d. None of the above

1867. Most common occluded sites of arterial embolism is:
a. Lungs and feet
b. Kidney
c. Eyes
d. None of the above

1868. Which of the following is not the preventive measure of arterial embolism?
a. Physical exercise
b. Smoking cessation
c. Dieting
d. Prophylactic medication

RAYNAUD'S DISEASE (RAYNAUD'S PHENOMENON)

1869. The person with Raynaud's disease would develop following complication; EXCEPT:
a. Ischemia b. Cancer cell formation
c. Hematoma d. Amputation

1870. The primary and the most important lifestyle modification that the nurse needs to educate the client with Raynaud's disease would be:
a. Avoid red meats
b. Avoid high calorie food
c. Smoking cessation
d. Frequent hand washing and hygiene

Ans.
1850. a
1851. c
1852. a
1853. b
1854. a
1855. a
1856. d
1857. c
1858. a
1859. c
1860. b
1861. a
1862. b
1863. d
1864. c
1865. d
1866. c
1867. a
1868. d
1869. b
1870. c

1871. All of the following are the treatment option for the client experiencing Raynaud's disease; EXCEPT:
- a. Debridement
- b. Amputation
- c. Sympathectomy
- d. Suturing

1872. All of the following are the possible nursing diagnosis for a patient with Raynaud's disease; EXCEPT:
- a. Impaired skin integrity
- b. Ineffective breathing pattern
- c. Acute pain
- d. Ineffective role performance

1873. The other name of Reynaud's disease would be:
- a. Blue white red disease
- b. Hand foot syndrome
- c. Palmer erythema
- d. Thromboangitis obliterans

BUERGER'S DISEASE (THROMBOANGITIS OBLITERANS)

1874. A condition in which cramping pain in the leg is induced by exercise, typically caused by obstruction of the arteries is known as:
- a. Arthritis
- b. Arthralgia
- c. Intermittent claudication
- d. Myasthenia gravis

1875. All of the following are the characteristics of intermittent claudication; EXCEPT:
- a. It occurs as a result of muscle ischemia during exercise
- b. It is commonly caused by atherosclerosis
- c. It is characterized by pain in the calf induced by exercise and relieved by rest
- d. It is due to neuromuscular disorder that causes weakness in the skeletal muscles

DRUGS OF CHOICE FOR CARDIAC DISEASES

1876. The drug of choice for supraventricular tachycardia is:
- a. Adenosine
- b. Diluter
- c. Carvedilol
- d. Amiodarone

1877. Emergency management of angina is:
- a. Aspirin
- b. Adrenaline
- c. Nitroglycerin
- d. Dopamine

1878. Nitroglycerine belongs to .... Group of drugs:
- a. Vasodilator
- b. Beta blocker
- c. Calcium channel blocker
- d. ACE inhibitors

1879. Common side effects of nitroglycerin include:
- a. High blood pressure
- b. Headache
- c. Shortness of breath
- d. Constipation

Explanation: Nitroglycerine is used in treating high blood pressure. Nitroglycerin is a nitrate. It works by relaxing (widening) blood vessels. Chest pain occurs when the heart needs more oxygen than it can get. Relaxing blood vessels allow blood to flow more easily. This reduces the heart's workload and the amount of oxygen needed by the heart. Vasodilatory effect of NTG causes headache, hypotension and dizziness

1880. Medication likely to be prescribed to reduce the risk of coronary artery spasms in a client with Prinzmetal's angina is:
- a. Thiazide diuretics
- b. Digoxin
- c. Lidocaine
- d. Calcium channel blocker

1881. Which among the following is the correct way to administer nitroglycerin for chest pain?
- a. One tablet or spray every three minutes, up to five times; then drive yourself to the ER
- b. Take as many tablets or sprays as necessary to relieve pain; if the pain persists, it is probably not your heart
- c. One tablet or spray every five minutes, up to three times; call 101 or 112 if the pain is not completely relieved
- d. Take one tablet or spray and call the Heart Clinic

1882. Which among the following is FALSE regarding the drug nitroglycerine:
- a. Before taking the drug drink sips of water
- b. The drug is administered sublingually or as sprays in angina
- c. Nitroglycerine is a vasoconstrictor
- d. The drug is photosensitive

Explanation: Nitroglycerine is a vasodilator. So Vasoconstrictor (option c) is the wrong answer. All other statements are true about nitroglycerine.

1883. Nurse should recognize that a patient has coronary artery disease is receiving acetylsalicylic acid (aspirin) to: *(LNJP H D 2012)*
- a. Relieve pain
- b. Decrease platelet adhesion
- c. Reduce fever
- d. Diminish inflammation

1884. Patient is on enalapril and diuretic therapy for heart failure. Nurse should notify the physician that the therapy is not effective when she finds: *(NCFL 2019)*
- a. Dry cough
- b. Skin rash
- c. Edema in legs
- d. Postural fall in B.P.

Explanation: Diuretics are administered to relieve water retention. Edema (fluid accumulation) in the legs indicates that the therapy is not effective. Postural fall in BP, dry cough and skin rash are most likely to be the sign of excessive water loss rather than water accumulation.

1885. Commonly using drug for the management of cardiomyopathy?
- a. Decongestants
- b. Beta-adrenergic blockers
- c. Dobutamine
- d. Nitroglycerine

1886. The drug of choice in the treatment of congestive cardiac failure is:
- a. Digoxin
- b. Adrenaline
- c. Diazepam
- d. Atenolol

1887. Digoxin is a/an: *(AIIMS Bhopal Grade-I 2018)*
- a. Calcium channel blockers
- b. Cardiac glycosides
- c. Thrombolytic agent
- d. Anti-angina drug

Explanation: Cardiac glycosides are the class of organic compounds that increase the force of contraction of the heart but decrease the rate of contraction. Digoxin (Brand name: Lanoxin) is a cardiac glycoside which is mainly used in the treatment of Congestive Heart Failure, atrial fibrillation and atrial flutter

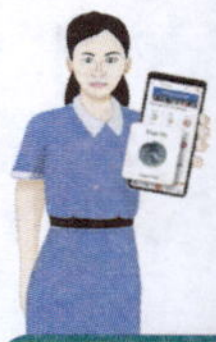

Ans.

1871. d
1872. b
1873. a
1874. c
1875. d
1876. a
1877. c
1878. a
1879. b
1880. d
1881. c
1882. c
1883. b
1884. c
1885. b
1886. a
1887. b

1888. All of the following statements are correct about Digoxin; EXCEPT:

a. It has positive inotropic and negative chronotropic effects
b. Withhold the drug if the pulse rate is less than 60 per minute
c. Toxicity can occur more easily in the presence of hypokalemia
d. The positive inotropic effect will decrease urine output

Explanation: Digoxin is a positive inotropic agent used to treat congestive heart failure and to slow the heart rate in patients with atrial fibrillation. It increases the force of contraction of heart. Positive inotropic effect promotes diuresis by increasing cardiac output

1889. Normal therapeutic range of serum digoxin is:

a. 0. 2–0. 5 ng/mL b. 0. 5–2. 2 ng/mL
c. 2. 2–3 ng/mL d. 3–4 ng/mL

1890. Which of the following therapeutic effects is expected with digoxin administration:

a. Positive dromotropic, negative inotropic, positive chronotropic
b. Negative dromotropic, positive inotropic, positive chronotropic
c. Negative dromotropic, positive inotropic, negative chronotropic
d. Positive dromotropic, positive inotropic, negative chronotropic

Explanation: Digoxin increases cardiac contractility (positive inotropic effect), decreases heart rate (negative chronotropic effect), and decreases conductivity (negative dromotropic effect).

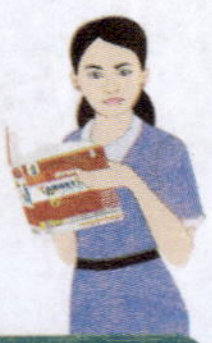

Ans.

1888. d
1889. b
1890. c
1891. a
1892. a
1893. d
1894. b
1895. c
1896. a
1897. d
1898. c
1899. d
1900. b

1891. Which of the following electrolyte value can potentiate digoxin toxicity:

a. Hypokalemia
b. Hyperkalemia
c. Hypocalcemia
d. Hypercalcemia

Explanation: In states of hypokalemia, digoxin toxicity is actually worsened because digoxin normally binds to the ATPase pump on the same site as potassium. When potassium levels are low, digoxin can more easily bind to the ATPase pump, exerting the inhibitory effects.

1892. Digoxin toxicity cause which of the following electrolyte imbalance?

a. Hyperkalemia b. Hypokalemia
c. Hypernatremia d. Hyponatremia

Explanation: Digoxin toxicity causes hyperkalemia (high potassium). The sodium/potassium ATPase pump normally causes sodium to leave cells and potassium to enter cells. Blocking this mechanism results in higher serum potassium levels.

Digoxin toxicity is worsened in states of hypokalemia (low potassium) since digoxin normally binds to the ATPase pump on the same site as potassium. When potassium levels are low, digoxin can more easily bind to the ATPase pump exerting the inhibitory effects.
Note: Hypokalemic condition can potentiate digoxin toxicity. On the other hand, Digoxin toxicity can cause hyperkalemia.

1893. Signs and symptoms of digoxin toxicity include all; EXCEPT:

a. Anorexia, nausea and vomiting
b. Blurred or yellow vision
c. Dizziness and mental confusion
d. Tachycardia

1894. In a child, digoxin needs to withheld if the apical pulse rate is less than:

a. 60 beats/min b. 70 beats /min
c. 90 beats/min d. 100 beats/min

1895. In an adult patient digoxin will be withheld if the pulse rate is below:

a. 40 bpm b. 50 bpm
c. 60 bpm d. 70 bpm

1896. Which of the following drug is withheld if the patient's pulse is less than 60/min? *(DSSSB 2013)*

a. Digoxin b. Dobutamine
c. Dopamine d. Phenytoin

Explanation: Digoxin is a positive inotropic agent (cardiac glycoside) which is used in the treatment of congestive heart failure. It increases the force of contraction of heart. Digoxin causes bradycardia. Hence the drug should be withheld if the pulse rate of the patient is less than 60 beats/minute. Pulse rate less than 60 beats/min indicates digoxin toxicity.

1897. Side-effect of digoxin is/are:

a. Visual disturbance b. GI disturbance
c. Bradycardia d. All of these

1898. Which among the following electrolyte value reveals that a client who was on digoxin therapy is at risk of developing toxicity?

a. Sodium level 140 mEq/L
b. Potassium level 5 mEq/L
c. Potassium level 2 mEq/L
d. Sodium level 120 mEq/L

1899. How soon after symptom onset must a person who has had a stroke receive thrombolytic treatment? *(RAK MSc 2018)*

a. 30 minutes b. 1 hour
c. 2 hours d. 4.5 hours

Explanation: As per the guidelines of American Stroke Association and European Stroke Organization—A person who had a stroke must receive thrombolytic treatment within 4.5 hours.

1900. Immediate treatment of choice for ventricular fibrillation is: *(AIIMS MSc (N) Entrance 2008)*

a. Administer adrenaline 0.1 mg/kg
b. Defibrillate with 360 joules
c. Cardioversion
d. Administer anti arrhythmic drugs

Explanation: Ventricular fibrillation is the most serious cardiac rhythm disturbance. The heart's electrical activity becomes disordered. When this happens, the heart's lower (pumping) chambers contract in a rapid, unsynchronized way. Ventricular fibrillation can be stopped with a defibrillator, which gives an electrical shock to the heart.

1901. An example of alpha-adrenergic blocking drug is:

a. Phentolamine b. Carvedilol
c. Lasix d. Acebutolol

1902. The following drugs are calcium channel blockers; EXCEPT:

a. Amlodipine b. Verapamil
c. Ramipril d. Diltiazem

1903. The following drugs are ACE inhibitors except one:

a. Ramipril b. Verapamil
c. Enalapril d. Benazepril

1904. Drug that protects the ischemic myocardium by blocking catecholamines and sympathetic nerve stimulation is:

a. Calcium channel blockers
b. Beta-adrenergic blockers
c. Cardiac glycosides
d. Nitroglycerines

1905. Which of the following is a desired effect on heart rate while a patient is on beta blockers?

a. Heart rate greater than 100 beats/min
b. A heart rate less than 60 beats/min
c. Heart rate between 60-70 beats/min
d. Beta blockers have no effect on heart rate

Explanation: Betablockers antagonize beta receptors inhibiting the actions of the sympathetic nervous system reducing heart rate, contractility and blood pressure thus significantly decreasing oxygen demand for optimal relief from angina symptoms titration to achieve a heart rate of about 60 beats/min is frequently required.

1906. Which of the following medications should be withheld a week before cardiac surgery?

a. Ramipril b. Metiprolol
c. Furosemide d. Clopidogrel

Explanation: Clopidogrel is an antiplatelet agent withheld to prevent perioperative hemorrhage.

1907. Antidote for heparin is:

a. Calcium gluconate b. Magnesium sulfate
c. Protamine sulphate d. Vitamin K

Explanation: Intravenous protamine sulfate can rapidly reverse the anticoagulant effects of heparin. One milligram of protamine sulfate neutralizes approximately 100 units of heparin. Vitamin K is an antidote for warfarin.

1908. Drug likely to be ordered by physician in a client with transient ischemic attack secondary to atrial fibrillation is:

a. Dopamine
b. Amiodarone
c. Warfarin
d. Lorazepam

1909. Oral medication of choice to prevent further thrombus formation is:

a. Warfarin b. Heparin
c. Streptokinase d. Vit K

1910. Which among the following medication needs to be withheld by the physician one day prior to superior vena cava filter insertion procedure?

a. Thyroxine b. Warfarin
c. Frusemide d. KCl

1911. An alternate to aspirin for the prevention of acute coronary syndrome in a patient allergic to aspirin is:

a. Stop aspirin as it is not necessary
b. Take any other NSAIDS instead of aspirin
c. Take clopidogrel instead of aspirin
d. Take ticlopidine instead of aspirin

Explanation: Aspirin is a non-steroidal anti-inflammatory drug but unlike other NSAIDS, aspirin has additional antiplatelet activity thereby decreasing platelet aggregation and thrombus formation. Clopidogrel is another antiplatelet drug that can be used instead of aspirin.

1912. An active male patient who weighs 81.65 kg has undergone dietary instruction. The patient reports that his current diet consists of 60 g of fat, 200 mg of cholesterol, 5 g of sodium per day. What does a nurse advise the patient to do? *(NCFL 2019)*

a. Increase cholesterol b. Increase sodium
c. Decrease cholesterol d. Decrease sodium

Explanation: Recommended sodium intake is less than 2g/day that is equal to 5 g of salt (sodium chloride) per day. Hence, the given option is more than double the recommended amount and it needs to be reduced. WHO recommends that reduced sodium intake will reduce the risk of hypertension, stroke and cardiovascular diseases in adults.

CARDIOPULMONARY RESUSCITATION (CPR) ALGORITHM

1913. Grape juice needs to be avoided in a patient who is on:

a. Warfarin b. Heparin
c. Cyclosporine d. Penicillin

1914. For giving CPR, after ascertaining unresponsiveness one should: *(JIPMER 2012)*

a. Call for help b. Establish an airway
c. Check the carotid pulse d. Give chest compression

1915. A patient becomes unconscious and unresponsive to the stimuli, next action is:

a. Activate the resuscitation team
b. Inform the physician
c. Give adrenaline
d. Perform suction

1916. A nurse finds the patient unconscious on his bed in the ward. She assessed and found that there was no pulse or respirations. As per the new AHA (American Heart Association 2010), the first action she should take after calling for help is:

a. Establish airway
b. Obtain a crash cart
c. Initiate high quality chest compressions
d. Establish a peripheral IV line

1917. Which method is used to open airway when the victim is suspected to have cervical injury?

a. Jaw thrust maneuver
b. Head tilt chin lift method
c. Both a and b
d. Nose pinch technique

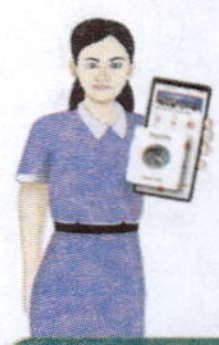

Ans.

1901. a
1902. c
1903. b
1904. b
1905. c
1906. d
1907. c
1908. c
1909. a
1910. b
1911. c
1912. d
1913. c
1914. a
1915. a
1916. c
1917. a

1918. Which one of following is the recommended order for resuscitation?

a. A–B–C b. C-A-B
c. C–B–A d. B–C–A

1919. Which one of following option is correct regarding compression?

a. Use palm of hand
b. Use heel of the hand
c. Compression depth of at least 5 inches
d. Check ECG at the end of each compression

1920. Correct position of hand placement during chest compression is:

a. Anywhere along the sternum
b. Upper portion of the sternum
c. Middle portion of the sternum
d. Lower portion of the sternum

Explanation: Good quality compressions are with arms extended, elbows locked, shoulders directly over the victim's chest and heel of the palm on the lower half of the sternum.

The rescuer pushes hard and fast, compressing 4–6 cm deep for adults at 100–120 compressions per minute with complete chest recoil.

1921. What is the recommended rate of chest compression?

a. 90 per minute b. At least 100/min
c. Between 100–120/min d. >120/min

1922. What should be the depth of chest compression in adult?

a. 3 inches b. >2.4 inches
c. At least 5 cm d. At least 7 cm

1923. What is the ratio of chest compressions to ventilations when one rescuer performs cardiopulmonary resuscitation (CPR) on an adult?

a. 30:1 b. 30:2
c. 15:1 d. 15:2

1924. What is the ratio of chest compressions to ventilations when two rescuers perform cardiopulmonary resuscitation (CPR) on an adult?

a. 30:1 b. 30:2
c. 15:1 d. 15:2

1925. Compression to ventilation ratio during 2-rescuer Child/infant CPR is:

a. 15:1 b. 15:2
c. 30:1 d. 30:2

1926. Compression to ventilation ratio during 1-rescuer Child/infant CPR is: *New Q*

a. 15:1 b. 15:2
c. 30:1 d. 30:2

1927. When 2 or more rescuers are available for resuscitation, rescuer can be changed:

a. Every 2 min b. Every 2 cycles
c. Every 5 min d. Every 6 min

1928. AED stands for: *(LNJP H D 2012)*

a. Arrhythmia eliminating device
b. Advanced emergency defibrillator
c. Authorised emergency defibrillator
d. Automated external defibrillator

1929. Which among the following statements is correct?

a. Each shock should be followed by CPR
b. CPR is not mandatory after each shock
c. Defibrillation is indicated in pulseless electrical activity
d. Compress the heart during defibrillation

VALVULAR HEART DISEASE

1930. Mitral regurgitation is seen during:

a. Ventricular diastole
b. Ventricular systole
c. Atrial diastole
d. Atrial systole

1931. Turner syndrome is associated with?

a. Aortic regurgitation b. Pulmonic stenosis
c. Coarctation of aorta d. Aortic dissection

1932. Displacement of cardiac apex to left and downwards indicates?

a. Right ventricular hypertrophy
b. Left ventricular hypertrophy
c. Right atrial hypertrophy
d. Left atrial hypertrophy

1933. Vegetation on the heart valves result from:

a. Bacterial invasion b. Poor diet
c. Hypertension d. Diabetes mellitus

1934. Causes behind cardiac valve disorders include all; EXCEPT:

a. Rheumatic fever
b. Infection endocarditis
c. Connective tissue abnormalities
d. Congestive heart failure

1935. Water hammer pulse is a feature of:

a. Aortic stenosis b. Aortic regurgitation
c. Mitral regurgitation d. Aortic aneurysm

1936. Flushed cheeks can be seen in patients with:

a. Mitral stenosis b. Aortic stenosis
c. Mitral regurgitation d. Tricuspid regurgitation

1937. Commonest cause of mitral valve stenosis in Indian patients?

a. Rheumatic fever
b. Rheumatic endocarditis
c. Cyanotic heart disease
d. Infective endocarditis

1938. Inflammation of the valves and inner layer of the heart is known as:

a. Endocarditis b. Myocarditis
c. Pericarditis d. Epicarditis

1939. Organism responsible for bacterial endocarditis is:

a. α-Hemolytic streptococci
b. β-Hemolytic streptococci
c. Staphylococcus aureus
d. Pneumococci

1940. Which type of valve is porcine heart valve?

a. Xenogeneic b. Allogeneic
c. Autologous d. Metallic

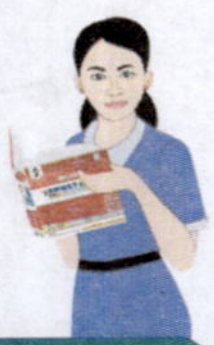

Ans.

1918. b
1919. b
1920. d
1921. c
1922. c
1923. b
1924. b
1925. b
1926. d
1927. a
1928. d
1929. a
1930. b
1931. c
1932. b
1933. a
1934. d
1935. b
1936. a
1937. b
1938. a
1939. b
1940. a

HEMATOLOGY

ANATOMY AND PHYSIOLOGY OF HEMATOLOGIC SYSTEM

- **Bone Marrow**
  - Aggregate weight of bone marrow in an adult is 3000 g.
  - Based upon the visual appearance it is divided as red and yellow
  - Red marrow is actively involved in hematopoiesis, while yellow marrow is less active in hematopoiesis.
  - **Functions of bone marrow**
    - Maintenance of pluripotent stem cells from which blood cells are derived
    - Origination and maturation of blood cells
    - Storage of large number of RBCs and neutrophils
    - Maturation of B-lymphocyte
    - Antibody production
- **Spleen**
  - Oval-shaped, dark red organ, largest lymphoid organ in the body.
  - 100–300 mL blood (approximately 4% of whole-body blood) contains in splenic circulation. During sympathetic system, stimulation, the splenic vessels constrict and eject the blood into circulation.
  - **Location:** Left upper quadrant of abdomen behind rib and above stomach.
  - Spleen is known as the graveyard of red blood cells
  - Acts as a site for humoral immune response to blood borne antigen.
  - Damage to the spleen increases the risk for infection.
  - Functions
    - Helps in recycling iron from destroyed RBCs by capturing hemoglobin
    - Removal of particles from RBCs without destroying it.
- **Formation of Blood Cells**
  - Hematopoiesis is the process of formation of blood cells
  - It starts in early embryonic period and persist throughout the life
  - Major sites for hematopoiesis in adults are flat bones of sternum, ilium, ribs and vertebrae.
- **Blood**
  - Blood contains many types of cells such as RBCs, WBCs and platelets suspended in plasma.
  - 8% of body weight is of blood
  - **Arterial blood is bright red in color** because of oxygen carrying hemoglobin and **venous blood is dark red in color** because of lack of oxygen
  - **Specific gravity of blood is 1.048–1.066**
  - **pH of blood is 7.35–7.45**
- **Plasma**
  - Liquid portion of the blood
  - Plasma = Blood – Cellular components
  - Serum = Plasma – Clotting factors
  - Straw-colored
  - Plasma is composed of 92% water, 7% protein and less than 1% nutrient and metabolic waste.
- Major plasma protein is **albumin** which helps to maintain oncotic pressure of blood.
- Total protein concentrations in plasma is **6–8 g/dL**
- Liver cells synthesize all plasma proteins except gamma globulin.

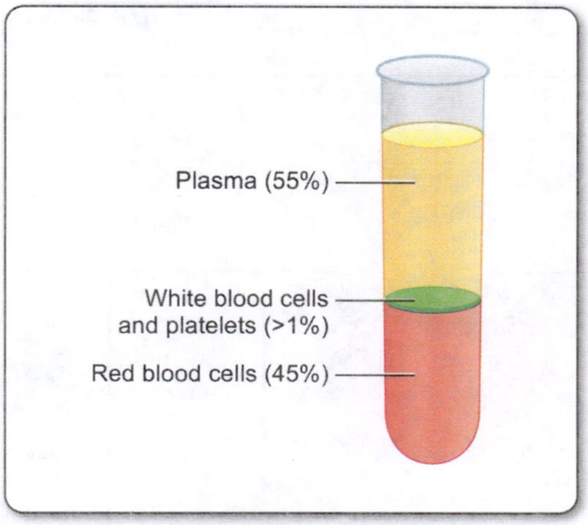

Figure 87: Components of blood

Hematocrit/Packed Cell Volume

- If a tube of blood is allowed to stand or centrifuged, blood cells settle down at the bottom. The term hematocrit or PCV is used to express the volume or percentage of RBCs in that sample.
- Normal hematocrit is 35%–45%.
- Hematocrit increases if plasma is less or RBCs are more, e.g., dehydration, increased RBC production (polycythemia)
- Hematocrit decreases if plasma is more or RBCs are less, e.g., overhydration, enhanced RBC loss, anemia

KEY POINTS

- Red marrow is actively involved in hematopoiesis, while yellow marrow is less active in hematopoiesis.
- Plasma = Blood – Cellular components
- Serum = Plasma – Clotting factors
- Major plasma protein is **albumin** which helps to maintain oncotic pressure of blood
- Total protein concentrations in plasma is **6–8 g/dL**
- Spleen is the graveyard of the Red Blood Cells

KEY POINTS

- Hematocrit is the percentage of red blood cells in the blood.
- Normal levels of hematocrit:
  Male - 41% to 50%.
  Female - 36% to 48%.

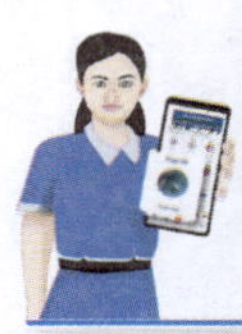

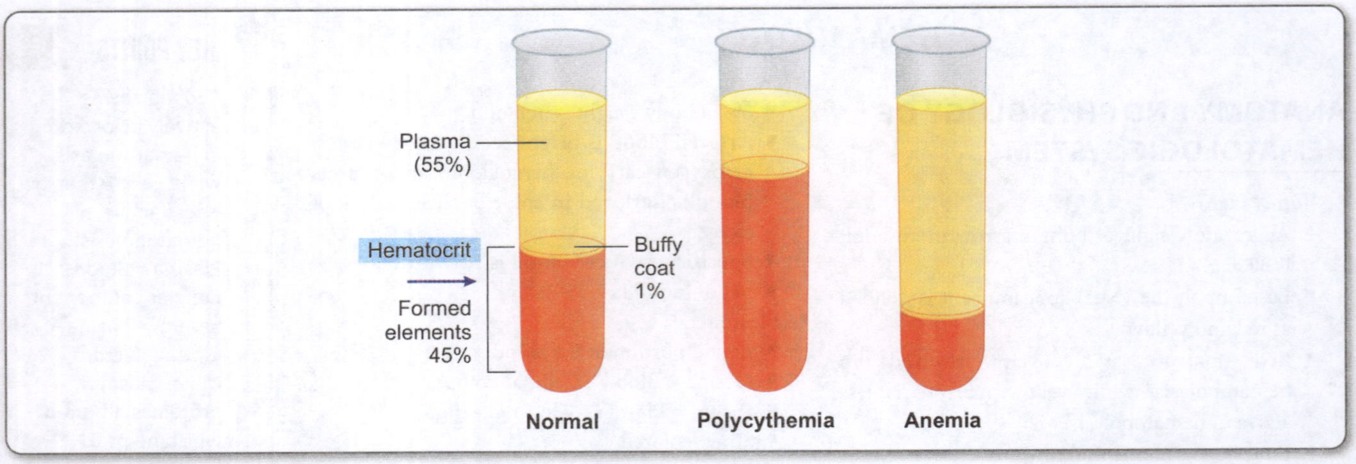

Figure 88: Hematocrit

Hematopoiesis

Bone marrow contains pluripotent stem cells which give rise to different forms of blood cells.

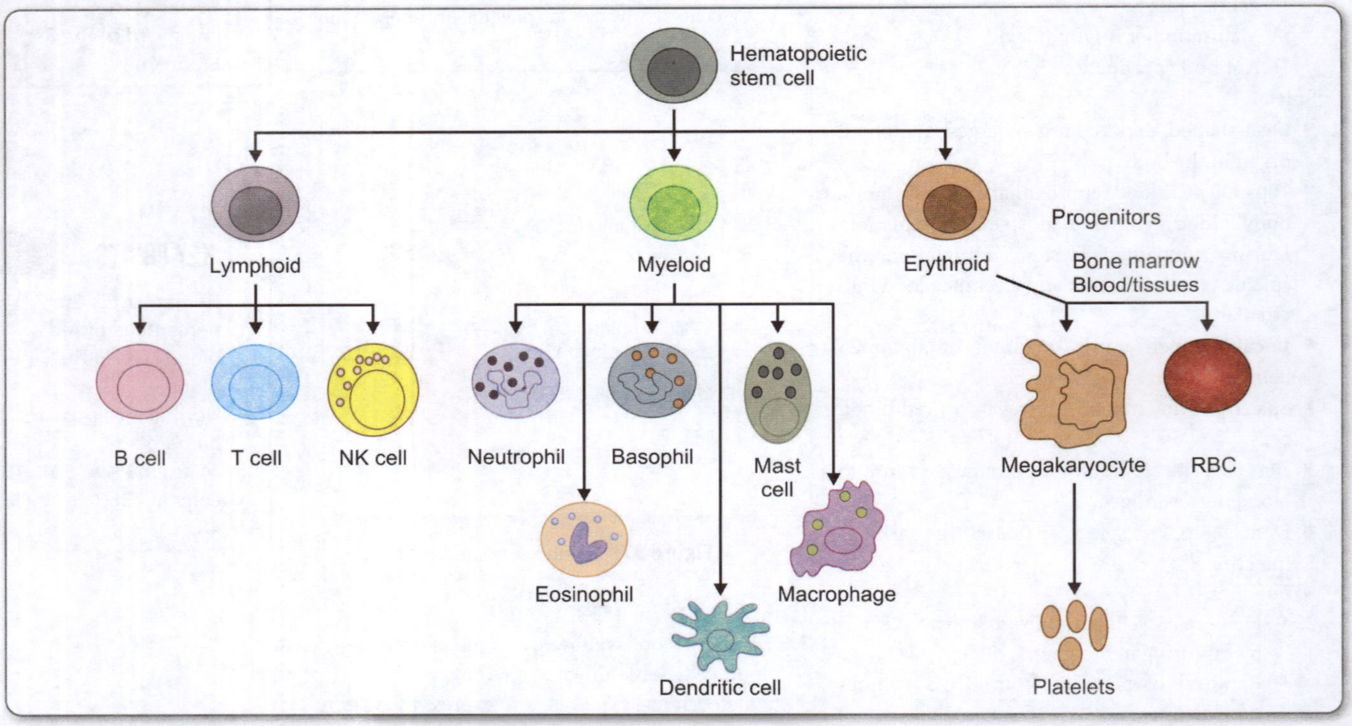

Figure 89: Process of hematopoiesis

- **RBCs/Erythrocyte**
  - They are oxygen carrying cells in the blood and they carry carbon dioxide back to the lung
  - Mature RBC has no nucleus
  - **Shape:** Bi-concave shape which increases the surface area of RBCs.
- Hemoglobin = 4 heme groups + one globin groups
- Heme: One porphyrin ring and a central iron. Oxygen attaches with iron. So, each hemoglobin can attach 4 molecules of oxygen.
- Globin: 4 chains [Adults: two α + two β; Fetus: two α + two γ
- Oxygen carrying capacity of fully saturated hemoglobin is 1.34 mL/g

KEY POINTS

- The most abundant type of blood cells is erythrocyte.
- **Monocyte** is the largest white blood cell with finely granulated chromatin dispersed throughout the nucleus.
- **The lifespan of RBCs is about 120 days.**

- **Functions**
  - Carry oxygen and nutrients towards cells
  - Assist in excretion of waste products from tissue through lungs, kidneys and skin
  - Transporting hormones to the target site of action
  - Protecting body from harmful substance/organism
  - Hemostasis
  - Homeostasis

Hematocrit

- It is also known as packed cell volume (PCV), erythrocyte volume fraction (EVF), or volume of packed red cells (VPRC).
- Packed cell volume/hematocrit is the volume of RBC per liter of whole blood.
- Hematocrit value = (RBCs volume/Blood volume) × 100
- Hematocrit value 40% means 40% of volume of whole blood consist of RBCs.
- Normal value is
  - Adult male: 42–52%
  - Adult female: 37–47%
  - Infant/child: 30–43%
  - Neonate: 53–65%
- **Hematocrit value low - Anemia (30%):** Causes are hemolysis, bleeding,renal failure, etc.
- **Hematocrit value high - polycythemia:** Causes are dehydration, diarhhea, burns, smoking, high altitude etc.
- **Polycythemia vera:** Primary polycythemia
- Venous blood is collected in EDTA anticoagulant vial as a sample for hematocrit and then it is centrifuged within 6 hours of specimen collection.

Erythrocyte Sedimentation Rate (ESR)

- It is measured how fast RBCs are settled down at the bottom of a vertical sample tube (anticoagulated blood with EDTA, heparin, sodium citrate) in millimeters (mm) per hour
- During sickle cell crisis, ESR increases but during symptomatic stage it is normal or decreases.
- In any type of inflammation, ESR increases but it is not a single most confirmatory test of any disease.
- After 24–48 hours of the onset of inflammation, the ESR level begins to rise.
- **ESR depends on** globulin, plasma fibrinogen, settling of RBCs, size and shape of RBCs, mechanical and technical factors, and rouleaux formation (Aggregation of RBCs in a chain that looks like stacks of coin).
- **Megakaryocytes/platelets**
  - Hemostasis is the major function.
  - Time needed for the formation of platelet is **5 days**.
  - Hemostasis occurs in three stages:
    1. Vasoconstriction
    2. Formation of platelet plug
    3. Formation of fibrin clot
- **White blood cells/leukocytes**
  - Five types of WBCs.
  - Based upon the presence of granules in the cytoplasm they are classified as granulocytes and agranulocytes
    - **Granulocytes:** Neutrophil, eosinophil and basophils
    - **Agranulocytes:** Monocyte and lymphocyte

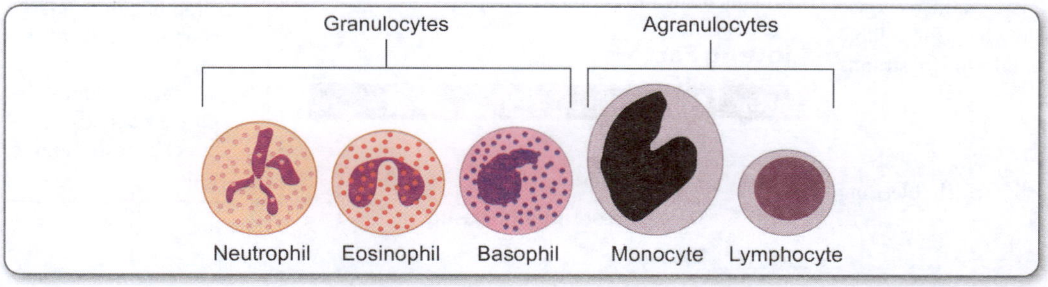

Figure 90: White blood cells

- **Granulocytes**
  - **Neutrophils**
    - Also known as polymorphonuclear leukocytes
    - These are the primary cells which respond during inflammation.
    - 90% of mature neutrophils remain in the bone marrow so that they can easily release into the circulation whenever any inflammation occurs.
    - Lifespan of neutrophil is hours to three days.

KEY POINTS

- Neutrophils and monocyte have **phagocytic action**.
- The first cells attracted to a site of injury are neutrophils.
- Increase in immature neutrophils is known as **'left shift.'**
- Most common cause of altered inflammatory response is **Neutropenia**.
- **Universal donor** is blood group O **Negative** and universal recipient is blood group **AB positive**.

- **Eosinophils**
  - These cells contain large granules in the cytoplasm.
  - They are needed against parasitic infection and IgE mediated allergic response
  - The lifespan is hours to three days.
- **Basophils**
  - Basophils are the least common of the granulocytes (0.5–1.0%).

- **Agranulocytes**
  - **Monocyte**
    - They are transformed to form macrophages with full phagocytic action
  - Lymphocytes
    - Lymphocytes that mature at thymus are T lymphocytes and which mature at bone marrow are B lymphocytes.
    - Some lymphocytes not classified as B or T lymphocyte are known as natural killer cells
    - B-cell mediate antibody mediated immune response
    - T-cells mediate cell mediated immune response.

BLOOD GROUPS AND BLOOD TYPING

Blood Groups

- Important blood groups are A, B, AB and O.
- Blood is grouped according to the antigen found on RBC and antibody found in plasma.

KEY POINTS

- Universal donors are those with an O negative blood type
- Universal recipients are those with AB positive blood type
- Rh positive patients can receive BOTH negative and positive blood
- Rh negative patients can receive ONLY negative blood.
- Agglutination occurs when the same antigens found on the RBCs from the donor come into contact with its corresponding antibody (found in the recipient's plasma surrounding the RBCs).

Table 73: Blood groups

Blood group	Antigen on RBC	Antibody on plasma
A	A	Anti-B
B	B	Anti-A
AB	A and B	None
O	None	Anti-A and Anti-B

The Rh System

- Rh system determines whether a person has positive or negative blood group.
- If D antigen is present then that person is said to be Rh positive.
- If D antigen is absent then that person is said to be Rh negative.

BLOOD COAGULATION

Blood clotting, or coagulation, is a rapid response to tissue damage. It is a process in which the soluble fibrinogen is converted to insoluble fibrin strands (blood clot).

Hemostasis

It is the physiological process by which bleeding stops.

Four stages of hemostasis

1. **Vasoconstriction:**
   - Within 30 minutes of injury, the blood vessels spasm start.
   - Extracellular matrix (ECM) or collagen exposed to blood cells at the injury site
2. **Temporary "platelet plug" formation**
   - "Platelet plug" is formed by the inflammatory mediators and cytokines of ECM which causes aggregation of the platelet.
   - There are various proteins and receptors involved such as VWF, glycoprotein receptors, etc.
   - Adhered platelets undergo very particular conformational changes and more platelets are adhered at the injured endothelial site resulting in a primary platelet plug.
3. **Coagulation pathway activation:** Shown in figure 86
4. **"Fibrin plug" formation:** The last step in the coagulation pathway. Formation of fibrin monomers from fibrinogen and then it polymerizes to form mesh of fibrin polymer that finally form a fibrin plug.

Clotting Factors

Factor	Synonym
I	Fibrinogen
II	Prothrombin
III	Tissue factor thromboplastin
IV	Calcium
V	Proaccelerin, labile factor
VI	—
VII	Proconvertin, stable factor
VIII	Antihemophilic factor
IX	Christmas factor
X	Stuart-Prower factor
XI	Plasma thromboplastin antecedent
XII	Hageman factor
XIII	Fibrin-stabilizing factor, transglutaminase

KEY POINTS

- The role of vitamin K is to stimulate the production or the release of certain coagulation factors.
- Warfarin inhibits activation of the vitamin K dependent **coagulation factor II, VII, IX, X.**
- Warfarin requires **48–72** hours to affect prothrombin time.

Coagulation Pathway

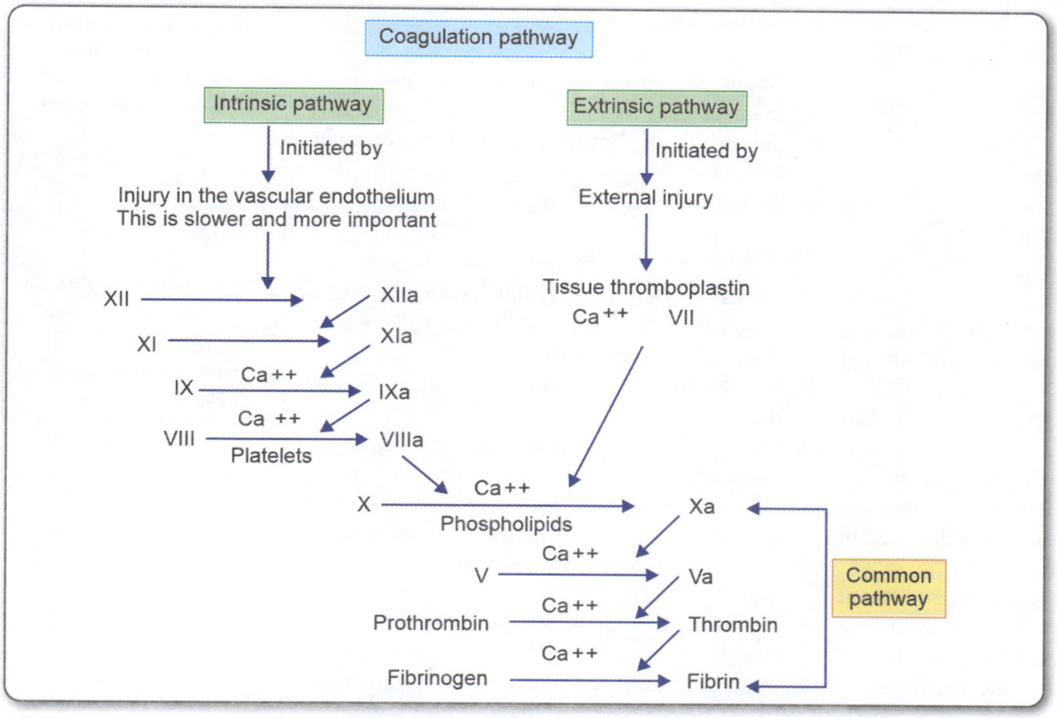

Figure 91: Coagulation pathway

DIAGNOSTIC TESTS

(Kindly refer to Target High Appendices and Fundamentals of Nursing for normal value table of Hemoglobin, Coagulation studies and Arterial blood gas).

Role of vitamin K

- Clotting *factor II, VII, IX and X* are synthesized by vitamin K in hepatocytes.
- Bacteria of large intestine produces vitamin k
- Vitamin k is an antidote of warfarin and its level is measured by prothrombin time and clotting time.

HEMATOLOGICAL DISEASES AND DISORDERS

Anemia

- **According to WHO,** Anemia is defined in children (below 5 years) and pregnant women as Hb level <11 mg/dL, in nonpregnant women as Hb <12 mg/dL, and <13 mg/dL in male.
- Classification of Anemia:
  - Mild – Hb < 10 – 10.9 mg/dL
  - Moderate – Hb< 9.9 – 7 mg/dL
  - Severe – Hb< 6.9 – 4 mg/dL
  - Very severe – Hb< 4 mg/dL
- It is a clinical condition resulting from decrease in healthy RBCs, decreased packed cell volume/ hematocrit or due to decreased hemoglobin.
- RBCs carry oxygen to various cells, so anemia results in hypoxia.

Table 74: Main causes of anemia

Decreased production of healthy RBCs	Increased RBC destruction	Blood loss
• Folic acid deficiency • Vitamin B12 deficiency • Iron deficiency • Thalassemia • Aplastic anemia • Anemia in chronic condition such as renal failure	• Sickle cell anemia • G6PD deficiency	• Trauma • Blood vessel rupture

KEY POINT

Anemia is a deficiency in the number of erythrocyte, the quantity of hemoglobin and the volume of packed RBCs.

Recent Questions (NORCET 2020)

62. Premature destruction of RBC's were seen in which of the following condition?
a. Sickle cell anemia
b. G6PD Deficiency
c. Systemic lupus erythematosus
d. Guillain-Barre Syndrome

Ans. (b) G6PD Deficiency

63. Which of the following vitamin deficiencies will cause pernicious anemia?
a. Vitamin B12
b. Folic acid deficiency
c. Serum Iron deficiency
d. Calcium deficiency

Ans. (a) Vitamin B12

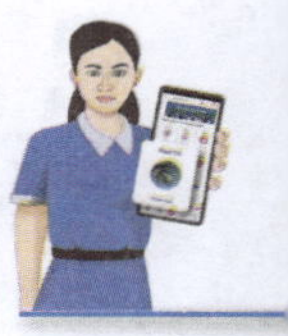

- **Manifestations:** Dyspnea, palpitation and diaphoresis are the major clinical manifestations.
- **Management**
  - Iron supplement, nutritional supplements
  - Control hemorrhage
  - Spleenectomy
  - Removal of toxic agents
  - Bone marrow transplantation
  - Corticosteroid therapy
  - Immunosuppressive therapy

Iron Deficiency Anemia

- Lack of iron resulting in inadequate hemoglobin storage in RBC and thus it affects oxygen carrying capacity
- RBCs are microcytic hypochromic in this condition
- Blood loss is the most common etiological factor
- **Manifestations:** Fatigue, dyspnea, palpitation, diaphoresis, headache, pallor in face, hands, nail bed and mucous membrane.
- **Foods rich in iron:** Almond, beans, carrot, cauliflower, egg yolk, spinach, soybean, whole wheat, beef, cabbage, cucumber, mushroom, orange, peanut, peas, potato, pineapple, tomato.
- Iron supplements have to be taken with or after food.
- Vitamin C increases the absorption of iron.
- Side effects of iron therapy include constipation, nausea and vomiting, dark tarry stool.
- Avoid antacid and milk with iron tablet

Megaloblastic Anemia

- It occurs because of defective DNA synthesis which results in abnormally large RBC.
- **Causes:** Vitamin B12 deficiency and folic acid deficiency is the reason.

Vitamin B12 Deficiency/Cobalamine Deficiency/Pernicious Anemia

- Due to deficiency of intrinsic factor in gastric juice which affects absorption of vitamin B12.
- **Diagnosis:** Schilling test is the confirmatory laboratory test
  - **Schilling test:** It measures the absorption of orally administered radioactive Vitamin B12 before and after parenteral administration of intrinsic factor.
- Client with pernicious anemia need **lifelong supplement of vitamin B12.**
- Macrocytic, normochromic is seen in this

Folic Acid Deficiency Anemia

- Folic acid deficiency occurs due to lack of food items which contain folic acid (green leafy vegetables, citrus fruit, liver, grain and yeast).

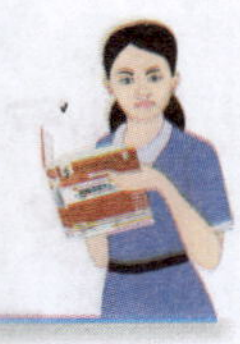

- FA deficiency is common with chronic alcoholic client, client on hemodialysis and client with malabsorption syndrome such as celiac disease, and steatorrhea.
- **Diagnosis:** Blood smear and bone marrow examination
- **Serum folate level appear low (normal 7–20 ng/mL).**
- **Treatment:** Folic acid supplement.

Hemolytic Anemia

- Premature destruction of RBC due to hereditary disorders or hemolytic conditions (e.g., Malaria, drug-induced, hemolysis).
- Bone marrow fails to replace RBC at the rate of their destruction.
- **Extrinsic hemolysis (most common):** Hemolysis due to toxin, mechanical injury, etc.
- **Intrinsic hemolysis:** Damage to RBC itself. For example, Sickle cell anemia, G6PD deficiency, etc.
- Intravascular hemolysis occurs in the circulation itself.
- **Extravascular hemolysis** occurs in liver and spleen.
- **Manifestations:** Hemochromatosis (bronze skin tone), hemoglobinuria (dark urine), jaundice, hepatomegaly, spleenomegaly, renal failure (due to increased work load with RBC break down product).
- **Treatment:** Treat the underlying cause of hemolysis.

Sickle Cell Anemia

- It is an autosomal recessive condition.
- Sickle hemoglobin gene is inherited.
- When sickle hemoglobin is exposed to low oxygen concentration, RBC looses its normal shape and property and becomes sickle in shape.
- Sickle RBC adhere together in small blood vessels and obstruct the blood flow to organ and cause ischemia or infarction.
- Cold can aggravate the condition.
- **Manifestations: Enlargement of the facial and skull bones**, tachycardia, cardiac murmur, pain, swelling and fever
- **Sickle cell crisis:** Three types of crisis are there. They are vaso-occlusive crisis, aplastic crisis, sequestration crisis.
- **Vasoocclusive crisis:** Entrapment of RBC and WBC in micro blood vessel leading to lack of perfusion to an organ which causes tissue hypoxia and necrosis. Good hydration is the management
- **Aplastic crisis:** Fall in hemoglobin and decreased production of RBCs, as bone marrow is not able to produce RBC

Recent Question (CNCI 2021)

64. How should a nurse administer an iron injection to an adult?

a. Intradermal in the forearm
b. Subcutaneous in the arm
c. Z track intramuscular in the gluteal
d. Intramuscular in the deltoid

Ans. (c) Z track intramuscular in the gluteal

KEY POINTS

- Presence of Dark urine and increased serum bilirubin are seen in hemolysis.
- Aplastic anemia decreases the bone marrow production of RBCs, WBCs, and Platelets. The client is at increased risk for infection, bruising and bleeding tendencies.
- Sickle cell anemia is an autosomal recessive condition
- Prevention of injury and hemorrhage is the primary focus while caring for a patient with coagulation disorder.
- The **Schilling test** is a diagnostic test that is used to evaluate **vitamin B12 absorption.**
- Megaloblastic anemia is due to deficiency of vitamin b12 and folic acid

- **Sequestration crisis:** When other organ pooled with sickle cell. In children - most commonly spleen is affected. In adult - Liver and lungs are affected.
- **Acute chest syndrome:** Sickling of small blood vessels in the lung causes acute chest syndrome, characterized by fever, cough and respiratory distress
- **Diagnosis:**
  - Low hematocrit and sickled cells on smear.
  - Hemoglobin electrophoresis is the diagnostic method
- **Management:**
  - Hydroxyurea is effective in reducing sickled Hb and increasing fetal Hb.
  - Hematopoietic stem cell transplantation is also treatment of choice.
  - RBC transfusion is also useful.

Polycythemia Vera

- Increased production of RBC, WBC and platelet is caused by excessive activation of pluripotent stem cells in the bone marrow.
- Blood viscosity and volume increase. Severe blood congestion in tissue and organ occurs.
- **Manifestations:** Hypoxia, dizziness, headache, vertigo, tinnitus, visual disturbance and angina, hypertension, cardiac failure, increased chances of stroke due to increased clotting, hepatomegaly, splenomegaly.

Hemochromatosis

- Increased iron level in blood due to the increased absorption of iron from GI tract.
- Iron gets deposited in liver, heart and pancreas and can damage the vital organs.
- **Manifestations:**
  - Joint pain is the most common manifestation.
  - Fatigue, lack of energy, irritability, depression, abdominal pain, loss of body hair are other manifestations.
  - **Management:** Phlebotomy is the management along with iron restriction.

Agranulocytosis/Granulocytopenia/ Malignant Neutropenia

- Reduced number of granulocytes in the blood
- 93% of granulocytes are made up of neutrophils so it is often called as neutropenia.
- Neutrophils are the first cells to respond to an infection.
- Neutropenia can lead to fatigue, weakness, sore throat, ulceration of pharyngeal and buccal mucosa, dysphagia, and fever.
- **Management**
  - Bone Marrow Transplantation (BMT) is the treatment of choice

Aplastic Anemia

- Bone marrow is damaged and unable to produce blood cells.
- RBC deficiency leads to anemic manifestations.
- WBC deficiency leads to infection.
- Platelet deficiency leads to bleeding manifestations.
- **Diagnosis:** Bone marrow aspiration shows hypoplastic or aplastic bone marrow.
- **Management:** Immunosuppressive therapy and bone marrow transplantation

Thalassemia

- Autosomal recessive condition
- Synthesis of one or more of the globulin chain within the hemoglobin is affected.
- Thalassemia is further classified as alpha and beta based upon the chain affected.
  - In alpha thalassemia, alpha chain of the hemoglobin is affected and often has no symptoms.
  - In beta thalassemia, beta chain of the hemoglobin is affected, it produces mild to severe symptoms
- **Thalassemia major/Cooley's anemia:** Severe deficiency or complete lack of beta chain of hemoglobin. Here both genes are abnormal
- **Thalassemia minor:** One gene is defective, it causes mild to moderate anemia.
- **Manifestations:** Paleness, failure to thrive, frequent infection, loss of appetite, jaundice, enlarged forehead and jaw
- **Management:**
  - Blood transfusion. Frequent blood transfusion causes iron overload which can be treated with chelation therapy (Deferoxamine)
  - **Bone marrow transplant and spleenectomy** are also treatment options.

Glucose-6-Phosphate Dehydrogenase (G6PD) Deficiency

- It is an X-linked recessive disorder
- Normally, G6PD gene in RBC produce an enzyme which is necessary for membrane stability.
- In G6PD deficiency, client has inherited a defective enzyme which causes hemolysis of the RBC.
- It most commonly affects male whereas majority of the females are carrier.
- **Manifestations:** Paleness, extreme tiredness or dizziness, fast heartbeat, fast breathing or shortness of breath, jaundice, spleenomegaly dark, tea-colored urine

Purpura

- It is characterized by the appearance of purple or red spots or patches on the skin.

KEY POINTS

- Fetal hemoglobin is a protective factor against sickling process.
- A sickle cell crisis is a type of pain that begins suddenly and lasts for several hours to several days.
- Hair-on-end appearance of the skull is a characteristic feature of chronic hemolysis usually seen in patients with **thalassemia and sickle cell anemia.**

KEY POINTS

- **A characteristic of X-linked inheritance is that fathers cannot pass X-linked traits to their sons.**
- Thalassemia Major or Cooley's Anemia is the most severe form of beta thalassemia in which the complete lack of beta protein in the hemoglobin causes a life-threatening anemia that requires regular blood transfusions.
- Treatment of choice for thalassemia major is **blood transfusion and desferrioxamine.**

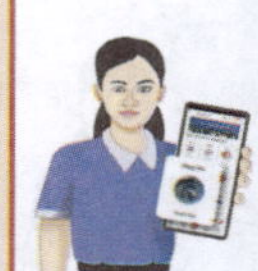

- These spots are caused by bleeding under the skin or mucous membranes, resulting from the leakage of blood from small blood vessels called capillaries.
- Purpura spots do not blanch or fade when pressure is applied to them.
- ***Causes:*** Platelet disorders, coagulation disease, vascular disorder (vasculitis) etc

Thrombocytopenic Purpura

- Low level of platelet occurs as a result of decreased production, increased consumption or due to increased destruction of platelet.

Nonthrombocytopenic Purpura

- Platelet level does not decrease
- Blood clotting disorders, long-term sun exposure or older age, steroids or other drugs etc cause ***weakened blood vessels*** which leads to bleeding.
- **Manifestations:** Bleeding and petechiae are common.
- **Diagnosis:** Bone marrow aspiration and biopsy

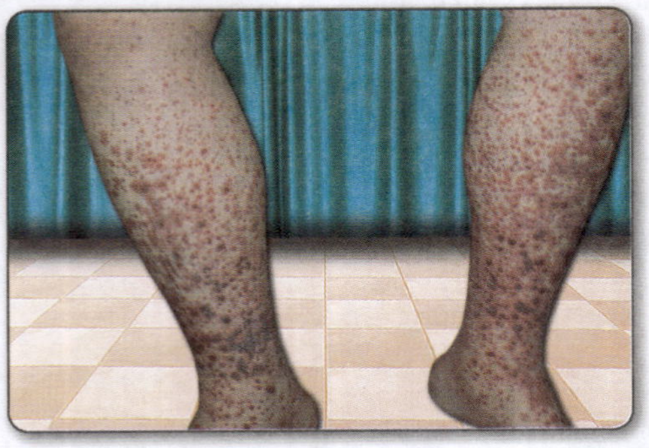

Figure 92: Purpura

Idiopathic (or immune) Thrombocytopenic Purpura (ITP)

- Abnormal reduction in platelet counts due to unknown cause.
- In ITP, platelets are destroyed earlier (less than 7–10 days).
- **Two types:**
  1. ***Acute thrombocytopenic purpura:***
     - **Young children** (two to six years) get affected most commonly.
     - Sudden onset but last <6 months (commonly within one week).
     - Occur commonly following a viral disease, e.g., chicken pox.
     - Does not reoccur
  2. ***Chronic thrombocytopenic purpura:***
     - **Adults are most commonly** affected and adolescent as well.
     - Last minimum of 6 month to many years.
     - Does reoccur and for that a continue follow-up is required.

Manifestation

- Petechiae: Purple spot < 3 mm
- Bleeding: Gingival bleeding, epistaxis (nasal bleeding), GI bleeding, menorrhagia etc.
- Ecchymosis – larger spot

Diagnosis

- Platelet count reduced
- Antiplatelet antibodies
- Clotting time will be normal (Presence of all clotting factors) but increased bleeding time.
- Bone marrow aspiration and biopsy

Management

- For thrombocytopenic purpura, Platelet count below 20,000 require treatment

  Tx –
  - Steroids (prednisolone)—suppress the immunity response.
  - Immunosuppressive treatment with cyclophosphamide, azathioprine, methotrexate, vinblastine etc.
  - Transfusion of platelets and IVIG
  - Splenectomy may be required.

Hemophilia

- X-linked recessive disorder
- It occurs due to deficiency of:
  - Clotting factor VIII (hemophilia A or classic hemophilia) and
  - Clotting factor IX (hemophilia B or Christmas disease)
- Hemophilia gene is located in X chromosome, so usually females are carrier and males are affected.
  - **Father with Hemophilia:** Daughters are carriers, Sons are normal.
  - **Mother with hemophilia gene (carrier):** Sons - 50:50 - normal: affected; Daughters - 50:50 -normal: carriers.
- **Hemorrhage is the most common manifestation.**
- Majority of the bleeding occurs in the joints
- Bleeding can be internal (manifested as hematuria, blood in stool) or external.
- **Management:**
  - Factor concentrates are available to transfuse
  - Avoid IM injection and contact sports among hemophilic patients.
- Fresh frozen plasma which consists of concentrated clotting factors.
- To produce more clotting factor VIII, DDAVP (1-deamino-8-D-arginine vasopressin) can be given.
- No anticoagulant
- Avoid sharp or traumatic injury

KEY POINTS

- In Idiopathic Thrombocytopenic Purpura (ITP), platelets are destroyed earlier (less than 7-10 days)
- Hemophilia is an X-linked recessive disorder.
- Hemophilia A, also known as classical hemophilia, is caused by deficiency of clotting factor VIII
- Hemophilia B, also known as Christmas disease is caused by deficiency of clotting factor IX.
- Advise to avoid contact sports for children with hemophilia.
- Advise low-impact sport such as Swimming for children with Hemophilia

Table 75: Types of hemophilia and deficiency factors

Disease	Deficiency factor	Inheritance type
Hemophilia A	VIII	X-linked recessive
Hemophilia B	IX	X-linked recessive
Hemophilia C	XI	Autosomal recessive
Von Willebrand disease	VIII; vW	Autosomal dominant
Parahemophilia (Owren's disease)	V	Autosomal recessive

Von Willebrand Disease

- Condition occurs due to deficiency of Von Willebrand factor which is necessary for factor VIII activity.
- Manifestations: Prolonged bleeding time, Normal platelet count, and slightly prolonged APTT.
- **Management:**
  - Goal of treatment is to replace the deficient factor.
  - Desmopressin can be used before surgery or dental procedure to control bleeding.

Disseminated Intravascular Coagulation (DIC)

- Coagulation proteins are activated and coagulation occurs in micro circulation which prevents blood supply to organs, resulting in organ dysfunction.
- Consumption of clotting factors can lead to life threatening hemorrhage in the client.
- All kinds of hemorrhagic manifestations occur, e.g., purpura, petechiae, ecchymosis, intracerebral bleeding, GI bleed, severe uncontrolled bleeding after surgery and child birth, etc.
- **Lab findings:** Prolonged PT, prolonged APTT, very low platelet count, reduced fibrinogen level, prolonged clotting time
- **Confirmatory test:** Presence of fibrinogen degradation products such as D-dimer.
- **Management:** Transfusion of platelet and specific clotting substances such as fibrinogen or cryoprecipitate or fresh frozen plasma.

Thrombophlebitis

- It is the inflammation of venous wall resulting in thrombus formation. It can occur in superficial as well as deep veins.
- The thrombus will move and can lead to occlusion of blood vessel.
- **Signs and symptoms**
  - **Superficial vein thrombophlebitis:** Warmth, pain or tenderness which increases on applying pressure; swelling, and induration.
  - **Deep vein thrombophlebitis:** Positive Homan's sign, edema, cramping pain, fever, tenderness to touch, malaise and chills.
- **Management**
  - **Superficial vein thrombophlebitis:** May not require specific therapy. It requires treatment for symptoms.
  - **Deep vein thrombophlebitis:** Anticoagulant therapy or thrombolytic therapy.
  - Drug of choice for anticoagulant therapy includes heparin (Intravenous) and warfarin (oral).
  - **Acute vein thrombophlebitis:** Thrombolytic therapy is required.

Homan's Sign

1. The examiner should support the client's thigh with one hand and his foot with the other hand.
2. With the knee in the flexed position, forcibly dorsiflex the ankle.
3. Pain in the calf with maneuver. This maneuver indicates a positive Homan's sign.
4. Positive Homan's sign suggest deep vein thrombosis (DVT).

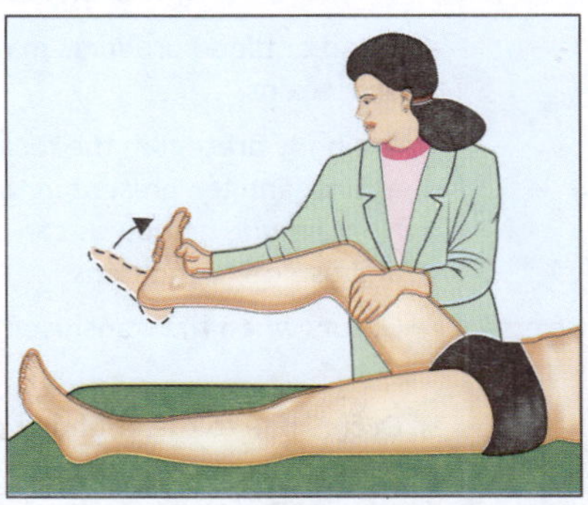

Figure 93: Homan's sign

Recent Question (NORCET 2020)

65. Diagnostic test used for DIC
a. PT
b. INR
c. PT, aPTT
d. DCT, ICT

Ans. (c) PT, aPTT

Recent Questions (NORCET 2020)

66. Which snake venom causes rapid DIC?
a. Cobra
b. Krait
c. Viper
d. Bandy-Bandy

Ans. (c) Viper

67. Which blood group is known as universal recipients?
a. O Negative
b. O Positive
c. AB Positive
d. AB Negative

Ans. (c) AB Positive

KEY POINTS

- If a patient develops chills and headache during blood transfusion, the immediate action is to **stop the transfusion.**
- **Transfusion** of one unit of Whole Blood/PRBC can increase **Hb by 1 g/dL** and **Hematocrit by 3%** in an adult.

BLOOD TRANSFUSION

Table 76: Blood transfusion compatibility chart

Blood type	Donate blood to	Receive blood from
A+	A+ AB+	A+ A– O+ O–
O+	O+ A+ B+ AB+	O+ O–
B+	B+ AB+	B+ B- O+ O-
AB+	AB+	Everyone
A–	A+ A- AB+ AB-	A– O–
O–	Everyone	O–
B–	B+ B– AB+ AB–	B– O–
AB–	AB+ AB–	AB– A– B– O–

Blood Products

Table 77: Uses of various blood products and their indications

Product	Description	Indication
Whole blood	• Deficient in factor V and VII • Stored at 2–4°C	• Acute blood loss • Exchange transfusion
Packed RBC	1 unit should raise Hct by 3%	• In acute and chronic blood loss
Platelet concentrate	• PCs may be stored for up to 5 days at +20°C to +24°C	• Thrombocytopenia (<10,000) • Major Surgery (<50,000) • Spontaneous hemorrhage • C/I in ITP and TTP
FFP	• Stored at –18°C to –20°C	• Clotting factor replacement • Emergency reversal of warfarin
Cryo precipitate	• Contains ▪ Fibrinogen ▪ vWF ▪ VIII, XIII	• Fibrinogen deficiency • vWD • Hemophilia A

Recent Question
(NORCET 2020)

68. Which of the following IV fluid is administered with packed RBC?
a. 3% NaCl
b. 5% Dextrose
c. RL
d. Normal Saline

Ans. (d) Normal Saline

Recent Question
(NORCET 2023)

69. After starting blood transfusion patient develops chills after 30 minutes. What is first nursing action?
a. Stop the transfusion.
b. Slow the transfusion.
c. Administer antihistaminic
d. Inform the doctor.

Ans. (a) Stop the transfusion.

Table 78: Acute transfusion reaction

Type	Sign and symptoms	Description
Mild allergic reaction	Urticaria (hives) and/or itching	Occurs due to the foreign protein in the donor blood products
Anaphylactic reaction	Urticaria (hives) and/or itching Hypotension	More severe than allergic reaction. Sometimes it can occur in patient with IgA deficiency, who receive a blood product contain IgA.
Febrile nonhemolytic	Fever/Chills	Generally thought to be caused by cytokines released from donor blood WBCs.
Septic	Fever/Chills Hypotension	Blood or blood products may be contaminated with bacteria or bacterial endotoxins.
Acute hemolytic transfusion reactions	Fever/Chills Hypotension	Antibody present in the recipient blood may cause immune-mediated reaction against antigen present in the donor blood. Nonimmune hemolysis can occur before transfusion because of incorrect heat and osmotic conditions.
Transfusion associated circulatory overload	Respiratory distress/ Dyspnea	Occurs when the transfused blood cause circulatory overload.
Transfusion-related acute lung injury	Respiratory distress/ Dyspnea hypotension	Occurs due to the antibody present in the donor blood which reacts with the antigen present in the recipient. Thus, recipient body releases mediators which result in pulmonary edema.

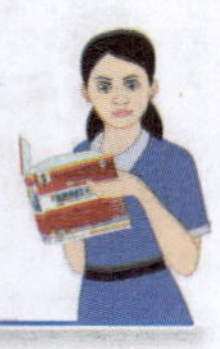

Contd...

Type	Sign and symptoms	Description
Delayed hemolytic transfusion reaction	5–10 days after transfusion, Fever Anemia Jaundice	Anamnestic response to a foreign antigen causes this condition. Recipient exposed to this antigen previously through blood transfusion or surgery.
Transfusion-associated graft-versus-host disease	10–12 days after transfusion Fever Rash and desquamation Diarrhea Hepatitis Pancytopenia	It occurs due to the engraftment of donor lymphocyte in an immunocompromised patient's bone marrow. Donor lymphocytes identify patient as foreign and react to it. This condition is rare but fatal.

NOTE: Topping the transfusion immediately is the immediate intervention if there is an acute transfusion reaction.

Hypocalcemia

- Caused by citrate content of large infusion of blood
- **Manifestations:** Hypotension, arrhythmias, seizures, muscle cramps and prolongation of QT interval.
- **Management**
  - Calcium gluconate IV
  - ECG monitoring

Golden Points to Remember

- Blood transfusion is contraindicated in congestive cardiac failure.
- Normal life span of RBCs is **80–120** days.
- **Schistocytes** are fragmented red blood cells.
- When fully saturated, 1 g of hemoglobin contains **1.39 mL of oxygen**
- Absorption of dietary nonheme iron is enhanced by **Vitamin C.**
- Clinical symptoms of chronic iron deficiency include pallor skin, glossitis, and cheilitis.
- **Pernicious anemia** is a disease in which gastric mucosa is not secreting intrinsic factor, that is needed for cobalamin absorption.
- The preferred method to give iron is **Z-Track Method**.
- **Apheresis** is a procedure used to separate components of blood, followed by the removal of one or more of these components.
- The dosage of **heparin** is adjusted according to the activated partial thromboplastin time **(aPTT)**, while **warfarin** dose is determined by the International Normalized Ratio **(INR)**.
- Reticulocytes is an immature RBCs which is nucleated.
- **Erythropoiesis** is regulated by cellular oxygen requirement and controlled by erythropoietin.
- **Pancytopenia** refers to decreased number of RBCs, WBCs and platelets.
- **Cobalamin** absorption occurs in **distal ileum**.
- **Schilling test** is done for assessing parietal cell function in case of B12 deficiency.
- **Direct coombs test detects:** Antibody attached to RBC surface.
- **Indirect coombs test detects:** Antibody in the serum.
- **Ecchymosis:** Large purplish lesion is caused by hemorrhage.
- **Hemophilia A** (Classical hemophilia) is caused by deficiency of factor VIII (Anti-Hemophilic Factor).
- **Hemophilia B** (Christmas disease) is caused by deficiency/absence of Factor IX.
- In hemophilia, Hepatitis C infection is common due to repeated blood transfusion.
- Hepatitis C is the most common type of post blood transfusion Hepatitis.
- Activated partial thromboplastin time (APTT) is prolonged in Hemophilia.
- **Myelodysplastic syndrome** is a group of related hematologic disorder characterized by a change in quantity and quality of bone marrow elements.
- **Azacitidine** is the first effective treatment for patient with MDS.
- **Virchow's triad** includes venous stasis, damage of the endothelium and hypercoagulability of blood which are causes of venous thrombosis.
- **Homan's sign** (pain on forced dorsiflexion of the foot when the leg is raised) is classic but unreliable sign of Deep Venous Thrombosis (DVT).
- Treatment of DVT involves bed rest, elevation of the extremity and anticoagulant therapy.
- **Telangiectasias (spider vein)** <1 cm in diameter that appears bluish purple or red.
- **Lead poisoning leads to** Sideroblastic anemia/Microcytic-Hypochromic anemia, Hemolysis
- **Oral manifestation of vitamin B12 deficiency includes** Atrophic glossitis, Beefy tongue, Macroglossia.

Most Common

Most common cause of vitamin B_{12} deficiency	Malabsorption
Thalassemia major	Thalassemia or Cooley's anemia
Most common manifestation of Hemophilia A	Recurrent hemarthrosis
Most common transfusion association Viral Hepatitis	Hepatitis C virus

"After dinner rest a while; after supper walk a mile."
—T. Cogan

MULTIPLE CHOICE QUESTIONS
(Including Explained and Practice Questions)

HEMATOLOGY

ANATOMY AND PHYSIOLOGY OF HEMATOLOGIC SYSTEM

Anatomy and Physiology

1941. The spleen lies against: *(Safdarjung NO 2018)*
a. 6th, 7th and 8th ribs
b. 7th, 8th and 9th ribs
c. 8th, 9th and 10th ribs
d. 9th, 10th and 11th ribs

(Ref: Gray's Anatomy for Students, 3rd edition, 2015, PP. 338)

Explanation:
- Spleen lies in the area of 9th to 11th ribs. It is in the left upper quadrant of the abdomen or in the left hypochondriac region of the abdomen.
- The spleen is the largest organ in the lymphatic system. Spleen is soft and generally looks purple.

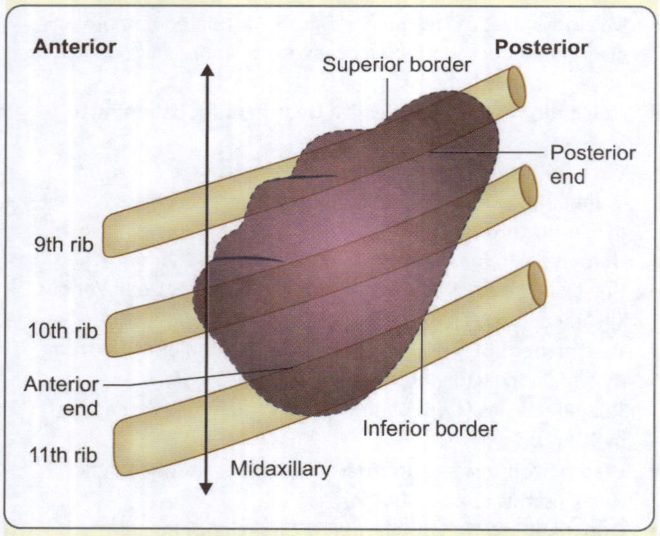

Figure: Position of spleen in the human body

1942. Blood without blood cell is:
a. Serum
b. Plasma protein
c. Plasma
d. Coagulation factors

1943. Part of the blood without cells and protein is known as:
a. Serum b. Plasma
c. Blood d. None

1944. True regarding plasma is:
a. Sedimentation of uncoagulated blood gives plasma
b. Fibrinogen and other clotting factors are present
c. Both a and b
d. None of the above

1945. Which of these statements is TRUE regarding blood?
a. Generally, there are four types of blood cells
b. Plasma constitutes 55% of the blood volume
c. The normal pH of blood is between the ranges of 7.2 and 7.5
d. The blood volume in an average adult is about 4% of the body weight

1946. Blood cells are formed at .... organ:
a. Liver b. Thymus
c. Red bone marrow d. Spleen

1947. The functions of the lymphatic system include all of the following; EXCEPT:
a. Maintaining tissue fluid balance
b. Functioning as body's defence system
c. Absorbing fat and other substances from the digestive system
d. Producing red blood cells

1948. The process that assists in the transport of lymph includes:
a. Gravity
b. Blood moving through the arteries
c. Blood moving through the veins
d. Contraction of the surrounding skeletal muscles

1949. Substances that stimulate an acquired immunity response are called:
a. Antigens b. Antibodies
c. Complements d. Histamines

1950. Antibody-mediated immunity is effective against:
a. Bacteria b. Viruses
c. Toxins d. All of these

1951. "Prothrombin time" of plasma is prolonged by administration of:
a. Vitamin K b. Dicoumarol
c. Calcium and vitamins d. Proteins and minerals

1952. Maximum reservoir of blood:
a. Veins b. Aorta
c. Heart d. Capillaries

1953. Biconcave shape of RBC's is helpful because:
a. Easily passage through capillaries
b. Increased surface area for a given diameter
c. Both a and b
d. None of the above

1954. The largest group of axillary lymph nodes is:
a. Central b. Lateral
c. Apical d. Medial

Ans.
1941. d
1942. c
1943. a
1944. c
1945. b
1946. c
1947. d
1948. d
1949. a
1950. d
1951. b
1952. a
1953. c
1954. a

1955. Branch of science that studies the diseases of blood and approach to their diagnosis is:
a. Hematopathology
b. Forensic pathology
c. Transfusion medicine
d. Clinical pathology

1956. Which among the following suggests problem with hematological system?
(AIIMS Raipur staff nurse grade I-2018)
a. Jaundice b. Asthma
c. Renal Calculi d. None of these

Explanation: If there is any problem with hematological system, increased RBC break down can occur and pigment will be released into the blood stream and can lead to jaundice. Asthma and renal calculi are unrelated to hematological system.

1957. Blood coagulation requires:
a. Vit. K b. Calcium
c. Fibrinogen d. All of these

1958. Vitamin required for maintaining blood circulation and coagulation is:
a. Vit. A b. Vit. D
c. Vit. E d. Vit. K

1959. Macrophages are responsible for:
a. Phagocytosis
b. Pinocytosis
c. Apoptosis
d. Endocytosis

1960. Neutrophils are responsible for:
a. Apoptosis b. Pinocytosis
c. Phagocytosis d. Endocytosis

HEMATOPOIESIS

1961. The last product in the process of blood coagulation is:
(LNJP H D 2012)
a. Thromboplastin
b. Prothrombin
c. Fibrin
d. Thrombin

1962. Leukocytes consists of all; EXCEPT:
a. Neutrophils
b. Eosinophil
c. Basophil
d. Thrombocytes

1963. Granulocytes are:
a. Neutrophil b. Eosinophil
c. Basophil d. All of these

1964. Agranulocyte is/are:
a. Neutrophil
b. Monocyte
c. Lymphocyte
d. Both b and c

1965. All statements are correct regarding lymphocytes; EXCEPT:
a. Comprise 25-40% of white cell population
b. Small and large types can be seen
c. It belongs to agranulocyte
d. T lymphocytes matures in Thyroid gland

1966. All are true regarding monocytes; EXCEPT:
a. Largest leukocytes can be seen
b. Abundant blue gray cytoplasm
c. Perform phagocytic action
d. It belongs to granulocyte category

1967. Identify correct statement regarding Eosinophil:
a. 1-6% of total leukocyte count
b. Larger than neutrophils
c. Count will elevate during allergic reaction
d. All of the above

1968. Which among the following is required for the production of RBCs?
a. Vitamin A b. Folic acid
c. Vitamin D d. Vitamin E

1969. What is the function of thymus gland?
a. Store melanin
b. Store blood cells until they mature
c. Maintain circadian rhythm
d. Kill pathogens

1970. True about macrophage is:
a. Macrophages are found in Late phase of inflammation
b. Histocytes, Kupffer cells, Osteoclasts are the examples of macrophages
c. Both a and b
d. None of the above

1971. Blood cells that defend against bacterial and fungal infection:
a. Eosinophil
b. Neutrophil
c. T-lymphocytes
d. B-Lymphocytes

1972. Myeloid stem cells give rise to all; EXCEPT:
a. Neutrophils b. Eosinophil
c. Basophils d. Lymphocyte

1973. Bone marrow components are:
a. Erythroid cells b. Myeloid cells
c. Lymphoid cells d. All of these

1974. Highest number of bone marrow cells are:
a. Promyelocytes
b. Myeloid stem cells
c. Erythroid cells
d. Precursor

1975. Biconcave shape of RBC is maintained by ....protein:
a. Albumin b. Spectrin
c. Globulin d. Microfilament

1976. Hematopoietic site in fetus is:
a. Liver b. Spleen
c. Bone marrow d. Thymus

1977. Color of hemosiderin is:
a. Black b. Brown
c. Ash d. Red

1978. Schistocytes are:
a. Material parasite
b. It indicates increased hemolysis
c. Fragmented RBC
d. Both b and c

1979. Hemoglobin metabolism release all; EXCEPT:
a. Biliverdin b. Bilirubin
c. Interferon d. Urobilinogen

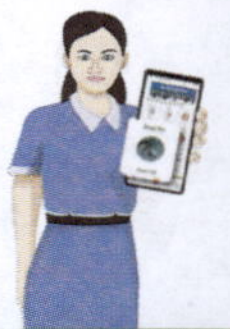

Ans.
1955. a
1956. a
1957. d
1958. d
1959. a
1960. c
1961. c
1962. d
1963. d
1964. d
1965. d
1966. d
1967. d
1968. b
1969. b
1970. c
1971. b
1972. d
1973. d
1974. c
1975. b
1976. a
1977. b
1978. d
1979. c

1980. Most sensitive cells to hypoxia is:
a. Myocardial cells
b. Neurons
c. Nephrons
d. Skeletal muscles

1981. Chemical causing vasoconstriction is:
a. Endothelium releasing substance
b. Thromboxane A2
c. AFP
d. PGE2

1982. Chemical causing platelet aggregation is:
a. Endothelium releasing substance
b. Thromboxane A2
c. AFP
d. PGE2

1983. Immediate hemostatic mechanism just following the injury is:
a. Collagen formation
b. Vasoconstriction
c. Pro-thrombin will convert to thrombin
d. Fibrin deposition

1984. The insufficiency of this substance in the blood may lead to edema of the body:
a. Albumin
b. Hormones
c. Electrolytes
d. Gases

1985. Which of these types of plasma protein plays an important role in the formation of blood clots?
a. Albumin
b. Fibrinogen
c. Glycoprotein
d. Immunoglobulins

1986. Blood cell which is responsible for coagulation is:
a. RBC
b. WBC
c. Platelet
d. Neutrophil

1987. In coagulation, the platelets:
a. Activate the soluble fibrinogen to insoluble fibrin
b. Neutralize any free radicals circulating in the blood
c. Aggregate and become adhesive to the damaged vessel wall
d. Attract migration of fibroblasts to form fibrous connective tissues

1988. The following are the essential requirements for efficient haemostasis; EXCEPT:
a. Intrinsic factor
b. Clotting factors
c. Calcium
d. Vitamin K

1989. Plasma protein which present in highest concentration is:
a. Albumin
b. Globulin
c. Thromboplastin
d. Fibrin

1990. The main function of haemoglobin is to:
a. Maintain a normal erythrocyte sedimentation rate
b. Neutralize any free radicals circulating in the blood
c. Bind to oxygen and transport it to the tissues
d. Absorb heat generated as a by-product of cell metabolism

1991. Excessive haemolysis may accumulate this substance in the body:
a. Bilirubin
b. Globulin
c. Haem
d. Mineral

1992. The primary stimulus to increase the rate of erythropoiesis is:
a. Hypoxia
b. Hypokalemia
c. Hyperthermia
d. Hypercapnia

1993. When a patient has a bacterial infection, which of these blood cells will play an immediate and major role in combating the invading pathogens?
a. Lymphocytes
b. Thrombocytes
c. Basophils
d. Neutrophils

1994. The leucocytes which contain heparin and histamine in their granules and enter tissues as mast cells are:
a. Lymphocytes
b. Monocytes
c. Basophils
d. Neutrophils

1995. Which of the following statements is true about hemopoiesis?
a. The megaloblast undergoes a series of differentiation in thrombopoiesis.
b. All blood cells originate from multipotent stem cells
c. The formation of platelets is called neutropenia.
d. Vitamin K is essential for erythropoiesis.

1996. Helper and cytotoxic cells belong to:
a. T cells
b. B cells
c. Monocytes
d. Macrophages

1997. Identify correct statement regarding hemoglobin:
a. One Hb molecule contain 4 globulin chain
b. One Hb molecule can form bond with 4 oxygen molecule at a time
c. Oxygen is carried in the form of oxyhemoglobin
d. All of these

1998. Oncotic pressure of plasma is due to:
a. Albumin
b. Preabumin
c. Electrolytes
d. Fibrinogen

1999. Heme is converted to bilirubin mainly in:
a. Kidney
b. Liver
c. Spleen
d. Bone marrow

2000. Absence of lymph nodes is characteristic of:
a. Brain
b. Liver
c. Lung
d. Placenta

2001. All of the following have no lymphatics; EXCEPT:
a. Brain
b. Internal ear
c. Comea
d. Liver

2002. Cell with a horse-shoe shaped nucleus and abundant cytoplasm in a peripheral blood smear is: *(Banaras HU 2015)*
a. Neutrophil
b. Monocyte
c. Lymphocyte
d. Eosinophil

2003. Infectious mononucleosis invades................cells.
a. B-cells
b. T-cells
c. Neutrophil
d. Lymphocyte

BLOOD GROUPS AND BLOOD TYPING

2004. A person with one of the following blood groups is considered a universal recipient: *(LNJP H D 2012)*
a. A negative
b. AB positive
c. O negative
d. B positive

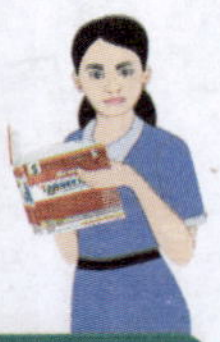

Ans.
1980. b
1981. b
1982. b
1983. b
1984. a
1985. b
1986. c
1987. c
1988. a
1989. a
1990. c
1991. a
1992. a
1993. d
1994. c
1995. b
1996. a
1997. d
1998. a
1999. c
2000. a
2001. d
2002. b
2003. a
2004. b

2005. Universal donor blood group is:
a. O negative b. O positive
c. AB negative d. AB positive

2006. Which chromosome contain ABO locus on its long arm (q arm)?
a. 7th b. 8th
c. 9th d. 10th

2007. Technique used for blood grouping is:
a. Immunochromatographic cartridge
b. Card agglutination
c. Gel card technique
d. All of these

DIAGNOSTIC TESTS

2008. Prolonged stay in space will lead to all of the following changes in the body; EXCEPT: *(Safdarjung NO 2018)*
a. Decreased blood volume
b. Decreased hematocrit
c. Decreased cardiac output
d. Decreased muscle strength

Explanation: There will be increased hematocrit after a prolonged stay in space due to increased RBC concentrations.

An astronaut in space can lose up to 22% of blood volume after only two or three days. The cardiac output of the heart decreases in space. Astronauts experience up to a 20 percent loss of muscle mass on spaceflights lasting five to 11 days.

2009. Blood drawn for complete blood count (CBC) is collected in: *(Banaras HU 2015)*
a. EDTA vial b. Plain vial
c. Citrate vial d. Chloride vial

2010. Anti-coagulant used in blood sugar vial is:
a. EDTA
b. Heparin
c. Potassium oxalate
d. Potassium oxalate + Sodium fluoride

2011. Anticoagulant appropriate for hematological test is:
a. EDTA b. Sodium fluoride
c. Heparin d. Clexane

2012. Supravital staining is used for?
a. Nucleated RBC's b. Reticulocytes
c. Myeloblasts d. Basophils

Explanation:

Stain	Blood cell
Wright's stain	RBC, WBC (differential count)
Supravital stain	Reticulocyte [stain used New methylene blue or Brilliant cresyl blue]

2013. Diagnostic test for anemia is:
a. Hematogram and hematocrit
b. History and examination
c. Peripheral blood smear examination
d. All of these

2014. Test used to find out Vitamin B12 deficiency is:
a. Schilling test b. Widal test
c. Ortolani's test d. Benedict's test

2015. Total serum protein range is:
a. 4.0–6.2 g/dL b. 5.5–6.5 g/dL
c. 6.0–8.2 g/dL d. 7.0–9.1 g/dL

2016. What is the INR value for patient with mechanical prosthetic heart valve?
a. 1.5–2.5 b. 2–3
c. 3–4 d. 2.5–3.5

2017. Another name for cardiac blood pool image is:
a. MUGA scan b. Cardiac MRI
c. Thallium scans d. Cardiac PET

2018. Capillary refill time is normally:
a. 1–6 sec b. 1–3 sec
c. 2–5 sec d. Less than 10 sec

2019. All of the following statements are true regarding serological tests; EXCEPT:
a. They are type of in-vivo test
b. They are used for identification and quantification of antigens and antibodies
c. Environmental factors like pH, salt concentration and temperature interfere these tests
d. Agglutination reaction and precipitation reactions are examples for serological test

2020. Which is a true statement regarding direct agglutination tests?
a. Detect presence of antibodies in serum
b. Use known antigens present on coated cells
c. Can be used for leishmaniasis and for diagnosing typhoid
d. All of these

2021. Bone marrow examination is used in:
a. Megaloblastic anemia
b. Leukemia
c. Myelodysplastic syndrome
d. All of the above

2022. Hemolytic disease of the new born is diagnosed with ......:
a. Amniocentesis b. Direct Coombs' test
c. Indirect Coombs test d. Plasmapheresis

2023. Supra vital staining and Brilliant cresyl blue technique is used for .... cells:
a. Lymphocyte b. Reticulocytes
c. Neutrophil d. Monocyte

2024. Which one of the following cause hemoglobin curve to shift to right?
a. Decrease in pH b. Increase in pH
c. Decrease in temperature d. ↓ in 2, 3–DPG

2025. A pulse oximeter continuously measures the level of oxygen saturation of haemoglobin in the:
a. Venous blood b. Arterial blood
c. Alveolar capillaries d. Peripheral veins

2026. Which among the following lab findings is expected in a patient with deficiency of Von Willebrand factor?
a. Increased PT, Increased- aPTT
b. Decreased.PT, decreased apTT
c. Decreased PT, increased aPTT
d. Normal PT, Increased aPTT

2027. The nurse is caring for a client who had a splenectomy. In the immediate postoperative period, for which complication should the nurse specifically assess in this client? *(RAK MSc 2018)*
a. Infection b. Peritonitis
c. Intestinal obstruction d. Abdominal distention

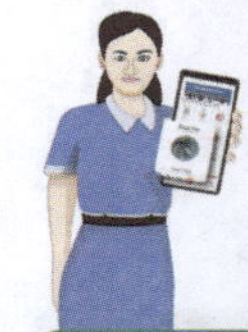

Ans.

2005. a
2006. c
2007. d
2008. b
2009. a
2010. d
2011. a
2012. b
2013. d
2014. a
2015. c
2016. d
2017. a
2018. b
2019. a
2020. d
2021. d
2022. b
2023. b
2024. a
2025. b
2026. d
2027. d

Explanation:

- As splenectomy is a procedure that involves surgical removal of spleen and though a person can survive without it but as its function is to filter blood as a part of immune system, the immunity is highly compromised, making the patient more vulnerable to infections. Though overwhelming post splenectomy infection is common, it is considered to be a long-term complication. In a immediate postoperative client with splenectomy, assessment for abdominal distension is more important.

2028. During the time of any infection what will happen to the WBC count?

a. Increased b. Decreased
c. Remain unchanged d. Fluctuating

2029. The cells involved in inflammatory reactions are called: *(Kerala PSC, Nov 2014)*

a. Neutrophils b. Lymphocytes
c. Basophils d. All of these

Explanation: Blood cells involved in inflammatory reactions are Basophils, which are granulocyte type of WBCs. When basophils are encountered with allergin they release histamine which causes increased blood flow to damaged tissues, resulting in swelling and inflammation.

2030. Eosinophilia causes all; EXCEPT:

a. Allergic disorders b. Psoriasis
c. Atopic dermatitis d. Asthma

2031. Bone marrow aspiration site is:

a. Sternum b. Posterior superior iliac spine
c. Lumbar vertebrae d. All of these

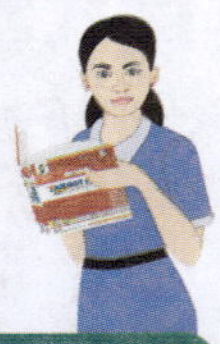

2032. The preferred site for bone marrow biopsy in adult is: (ISRO 2018, AIIMS Rishikesh Senior Nursing Officer 2018)

a. Posterior iliac crest b. Anterior iliac crest
c. Lumbar spinous process d. All of these

2033. Site for bone marrow biopsy in an infant is:

a. Tibia b. Fibula
c. Femur d. Iliac crest

2034. Complications of bone marrow aspiration include:

a. Local infections
b. Bleeding and discomfort at the biopsy site
c. Sternal plate puncture
d. All of these

2035. Nursing intervention for a client who is having procedural anxiety related to bone marrow biopsy and aspiration is:

a. Restrain the patient
b. Administer GA
c. Teach relaxation techniques
d. Postpone the procedure.

2036. Nursing care following bone marrow biopsy and aspiration include:

a. Give pain killers
b. Pressure dressing
c. Look for bleeding and monitor vitals
d. All of these

2037. The confirmative test for the diagnosis of multiple myeloma is:

a. Bone marrow biopsy b. Differential count of WBC
c. Serum calcium d. PET

Explanation: Blood test, Urine test, X-rays, PET, CT scans, and MRI are useful in diagnosis of multiple myeloma but the definitive confirmation of multiple myeloma can be made only through a bone marrow biopsy.

2038. Which of the following actions should the nurse prioritize when taking care of a patient with a platelet count of 23,000/mm? *(RAK MSc 2018)*

a. Request an order for an anticoagulant
b. Protect the patient from injury
c. Encourage the patient to drink plenty of fluids
d. No action is necessary

Explanation: The normal value of platelets is 150,000-400.000/mm^3. In the above-mentioned situation, the number of platelets is 23,000/mm^3, therefore, such patients are at risk of uncontrolled bleeding if injured. So, the priority nursing intervention would be to **protect the patient from injury.**

2039. Which of the following is affected by platelet count?

a. Bleeding time
b. Thrombin time
c. Prothrombin time
d. Partial thromboplastin time

2040. Which test helps us to assess the platelet function?

a. PT b. aPTT
c. C-reactive protein d. Bleeding time

2041. Bleeding time range using Duke Method is:

a. 30 sec–1 min b. 0–1 min
c. 1–3 min d. 2–5 min

Explanation: There are two methods of Bleeding time assessment.

- Normal range in Duke method is 1-3 m.
- Normal range in Ivy method is 2-9 m.

2042. Clotting time range is:

a. 30 sec -1minute b. 0-1 minutes
c. 1-3 minutes d. 2-6 minutes

2043. Prolonged Prothrombin time (PT) can be seen in all; EXCEPT:

a. Disseminated intravascular coagulation (DIC)
b. Warfarin therapy
c. Low level of vitamin K
d. Defective factor VIII

Explanation: Prothrombin time (PT) is prolonged in Liver disease, vitamin K insufficiency, decreased or defective factor I, II, V, VII or X, chronic low-grade disseminated intravascular coagulation (DIC), anticoagulation drug (warfarin) therapy.

PT is normal in decreased or defective factor VIII, IX, XI, or XII, von Willebrand disease (severe type), presence of lupus anticoagulant, autoantibody against a specific factor (e.g., factor VIII).

ANEMIA

2044. Iron chelating agent is: *(AIIMS Bhopal Senior Nursing Officer 2018)*

a. Charcoal b. Deferoxamine
c. Calcium gluconate d. Alum

2045. Blood cell decreased in case of anemia is:

a. Erythrocytes b. Lymphocytes
c. Leukocytes d. Thrombocytes

Ans.

2028. a
2029. c
2030. b
2031. d
2032. a
2033. a
2034. d
2035. c
2036. d
2037. a
2038. b
2039. a
2040. d
2041. c
2042. d
2043. d
2044. b
2045. a

2046. Commonest cause of anemia is:
a. Lack of dietary iron b. B12 deficiency
c. Bleeding disorders d. Hook worm infestation

2047. Chief storage form of iron in human body is:
a. Elementary iron
b. Serum ferritin
c. Iron hemoglobin complex
d. Serum dextran

2048. Which of the following statement is not true regarding iron absorption?
a. Iron is absorbed better in presence of Vitamin C
b. Citrus fruits promote iron absorption
c. Iron taken on empty stomach enhances its absorption
d. Calcium containing foods including milk promotes iron absorption

2049. Iron deficiency anemia is present in:
a. CRF b. Thalassemia
c. Sickle cell anemia d. DIC

2050. Cause of iron deficiency anemia in CRF is:
a. Iron absorption is not taking place
b. Unable to convert iron to transferrin form
c. Decreased erythropoietin secretion
d. Increased RBC destruction

2051. Correct about iron deficiency anemia is:
a. Reduced hemoglobin and packed cell volume
b. Reduced mean corpuscular volume
c. Microcytic hypochromic cells on peripheral smear
d. All of the above

2052. Which among the following blood test reflects the iron deficiency anemia correctly?
a. Hb level b. MCH
c. MCHC d. ESR

Explanation: MCHC stands for Mean Corpuscular Hemoglobin Concentration. These parameters reflect the size and hemoglobin content of the RBC.

2053. All of the followings statements are true regarding iron deficiency anemia; EXCEPT:
a. Iron is stored in the form of ferritin
b. Initial management is iron rich food and oral iron supplements
c. High MCV
d. Low MCHC

Explanation: Complete Blood Count (CBC) results in iron deficiency anemia include the following: Low mean corpuscular volume (MCV), Low mean corpuscular hemoglobin concentration (MCHC) and Elevated platelet count (>450,000/μL) in most cases.

2054. Microcytic, hypochromic anemia is the characteristic of .... anemia:
a. Vit B_{12} b. Iron deficiency
c. Folic acid deficient d. Hemorrhagic

2055. Macrocytic anemia is the characteristic of all; EXCEPT:
a. Liver disease b. Iron deficiency anemia
c. Thiamine deficiency d. Vitamin B12 deficiency

2056. Megaloblastic anemia is present in:
a. Ileal resection b. Crohn's disease
c. Appendicitis d. Cirrhosis

2057. Type of anemia present in hemolytic uremic syndrome is:
a. Microangiopathic b. Macroangiopathic
c. Microcytic d. Normochromic

2058. A Nurse is caring for an anemic patient. What finding should suggests her that it is acute blood loss anaemia? *(NCFL 2019)*
a. Exertional dyspnea b. Easy Fatigue on exertion
c. Bradycardia at rest d. Postural hypotension

Explanation: The question is interpreted as "what finding (except anemia) among given options is associated with acute blood loss?". Acute blood loss and dehydration are the major causes of acute postural hypotension. So postural hypotension is the correct answer.

2059. All of the following are signs of anaemia in a patient EXCEPT *(Banaras HU 2015)*
a. Yellowness of the skin b. Tachycardia
c. Dyspnoea on exertion d. Lethargy

2060. Priority nursing diagnosis for a client with iron deficiency anemia?
a. Impaired gas exchange b. Activity intolerance
c. Imbalanced nutrition d. Knowledge deficit

2061. What is the expected findings during liquid iron therapy?
a. Patients teeth are stained
b. Stool is black in color
c. Complaining of constipation and leg cramps
d. All of the above

Explanation: All of the above-mentioned findings are expected during iron therapy. These signs and symptoms help to find out the compliance with the therapy.

2062. Actual impact of anemia is:
a. Decreased oxygen carrying capacity
b. Low immunity
c. Prolong bleeding
d. Coagulation abnormality

2063. Risk factor for developing anemia is:
a. Gastric suction b. NG drainage
c. Gastrectomy d. Gastrostomy feeding

2064. Chances of occurrence of sickle cell anemia among children whose parents are affected with the condition:
a. 25% b. 50%
c. 75% d. 100%

2065. Hb electrophoresis shows .... number of bands in sickle cell trait:
a. 1 b. 2
c. 3 d. 4

2066. Correct regarding Sickle cell anemia is:
a. Low hemoglobin level and sickled RBC
b. Cause for hemolytic anemia
c. Fetal Hb is a protective factor
d. All of these

2067. Which of the following statement is not correct about Sickle Cell Anemia?
a. Highest prevalence is seen in Africa
b. It is an autosomal recessive disorder
c. Fetal Hemoglobin is a protective factor
d. High oxygen tension promotes sickling of RBC

2068. All of the following are characteristics of sickle cell anemia; EXCEPT:
a. It is an inherited form of anemia
b. RBC has life span of 60-90 days
c. Acute chest syndrome
d. Fetal Hb is a protective factor

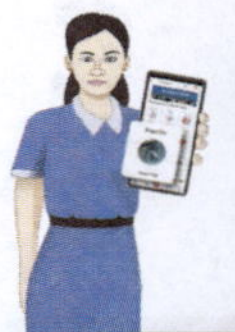

Ans.
2046. a
2047. b
2048. d
2049. a
2050. c
2051. d
2052. c
2053. c
2054. b
2055. b
2056. a
2057. a
2058. d
2059. c
2060. c
2061. d
2062. a
2063. c
2064. d
2065. b
2066. d
2067. d
2068. b

2069. Which of the following parameter would be increased in a child having sickle cell anemia?

a. Leukocyte level b. Hemoglobin level
c. Hematocrit level d. Reticulocyte level

2070. Sickle cell anemia gives protection against:

a. Dengue b. Kala-azar
c. Malaria d. Chikungunya

2071. Hb chain affected in sickle cell anemia is:

a. α-chain b. β-chain
c. Gamma chain d. All the chain

2072. Auto splenectomy is seen in………….. condition:

a. Iron deficiency anemia b. Thalassemia
c. Sickle cell anemia d. Hemophilia

2073. Hemolytic anemias are characterized by:

a. Shortened red cell survival
b. Bone marrow shows erythroid hyperplasia
c. Reticulocyte count and unconjugated bilirubin level will be elevated
d. All of the above

2074. All of the following are types of hemolytic anemia; EXCEPT:

a. Sickle cell anemia
b. G6PD deficiency
c. Thalassemia
d. Megaloblastic anemia

2075. Which of the following lab findings is expected in a patient with pernicious anemia?

a. Hemoglobin >12.5 g%
b. ESR, 17 mm/hr
c. Intrinsic factor, absent
d. Microcytic hypochromic RBCs

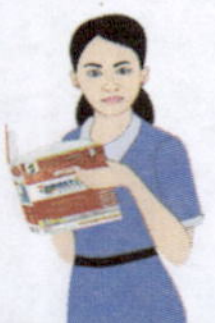

2076. Vitamin B_{12} deficiency is rare in:

a. Non-vegetarians b. Strict vegetarians
c. Elderly d. None of the above

2077. Which among the following is the richest source of vitamin B12?

a. Meats and dairy products
b. Grains
c. Green leafy vegetables
d. Mushroom

2078. All are true in relation to schilling test; EXCEPT:

a. The Schilling test is used to determine whether the body absorbs vitamin B12
b. 24-hour urine sample is required for the test
c. Test is performed in four stages
d. NPO is not required for the procedure

Explanation: The Schilling test is a medical investigation used for patients with vitamin B12 (cobalamin) deficiency. The purpose of the test is to determine whether the patient has pernicious anemia. This test is performed in four stages and patient preparation like NPO is required for this procedure.

2079. A patient with pernicious anemia is receiving Vitamin B_{12} injection. The client asks to the nurse how long I will receive the therapy. The best nursing response is:

a. Till blood level of B12 become normal
b. Till your hemoglobin level improves
c. Life long
d. For 1 month

Explanation: Injections of vitamin B12 will be necessary because without intrinsic factor vitamin B12 absorption would not take place. So, the person need B12 injection lifelong.

2080. A patient with hemoglobin of 10 g/dl likely to present with:

a. Pallor
b. Palpitations
c. Shortness of breath
d. No clinical signs

2081. Nutritional education given to a client with Hb 10 g/dL is:

a. Prepare food in iron containing vessels
b. Use green leafy vegetables and legumes
c. Take deworming tablets
d. All of the above

POLYCYTHEMIA VERA AND HEMOCHROMATOSIS

2082. Preservation used for storing blood for transfusion is:

a. Heparin + dextrose
b. Citrate + glucose
c. CPDA (citrate phosphate dextrose adenine)
d. EDTA

2083. Increased RBC's count is known as:

a. Anemia b. Leukemia
c. Polycythemia d. Thalassemia

2084. Causes of relative polycythemia includes all of the following; EXCEPT:

a. Dehydration b. Haemorrhagic fever
c. High altitude d. Gaisbock syndrome

Explanation: People living at high altitudes have absolute polycythemia due to increased erythropoietin synthesis (not relative polycythemia).

2085. Relative and absolute polycythemia can be differentiated by:

a. Measuring red cell mass and plasma volume
b. Peripheral smearing
c. Agglutination test
d. All of the above

Explanation: In relative polycythemia, the Hemoglobin and RBC is abnormally high due to an increased concentration of blood (e.g., dehydration, vomiting, diarrhea, etc.). Absolute polycythemia is due to increase in the number of RBC.

Relative polycythemia – loss of plasma volume

Absolute polycythemia – increased RBC in circulation

So, relative and absolute polycythemia can be differentiated by measuring red cell mass and plasma volume.

2086. Correct regarding polycythemia vera is:

a. Maintain adequate oxygenation
b. Phlebotomies need to be done to decrease the blood volume
c. Activities must be initiated to decrease the thrombus formation
d. All of the above

2087. Which of the following is late symptom of polycythemia vera?

a. Shortness of breath b. Dizziness and headache
c. Nausea and vomiting d. Pruritis

Ans.

2069. d
2070. c
2071. b
2072. c
2073. d
2074. d
2075. c
2076. a
2077. a
2078. d
2079. c
2080. d
2081. d
2082. c
2083. c
2084. c
2085. a
2086. d
2087. d

AGRANULOCYTOSIS/GRANULOCYTOPENIA/ MALIGNANT NEUTROPENIA

2088. All of the following conditions cause neutropenia; EXCEPT:
a. Typhoid b. Viral infections
c. Cancer chemotherapy d. Granulocyte transfusion

2089. The causes of neutropenia include: *(AIIMS Raipur Grade II 2017)*
a. Metastatic cancer and lymphoma
b. Cyanotic spell and lymphoma
c. Hypersplenism and chemotherapy
d. Infectious hepatitis and radiation therapy
a. a, b, c b. b, c, d
c. a, b, d d. a, c, d

Explanation: The specific causes of neutropenia includes chemotherapy, chronic idiopathic neutropenia in adults, Kostmann's syndrome, Leukemia, myelodysplastic syndrome, myelofibrosis, Myelokathexis, Radiation therapy and vitamin deficiencies. Certain infections which cause neutropenia include Hepatitis A, B, C, AIDS, Malaria, Lyme disease, Salmonella infection, Sepsis, Hypersplenism and Rheumatoid arthritis and other immune disorders.

2090. Patient with which of the following condition is at higher risk of pseudomonas infection?
a. Neutropenia b. Eosinophilia
c. Thrombopenia d. Leukocytosis

2091. Important nursing action while caring for a neutropenia client is:
a. Pain management b. Infection prevention
c. Prevent fatigue d. Maintain mobility

2092. Laboratory result expected in a client with infection is:
a. Pancytopenia b. Leukocytosis
c. Thrombocytopenia d. Anemia

2093. Patient is susceptible for febrile neutropenia after:
a. 3 days of chemotherapy b. 5 days of chemotherapy
c. 7 days of chemotherapy d. 2 weeks of chemotherapy

2094. Which of the following should be instituted to a patient to prevent febrile neutropenia?
a. Antibiotic prophylaxis b. Chlorhexidine mouth wash
c. Sitz bath d. Steam inhalation

Explanation: Antibiotic prophylaxis decrease febrile neutropenia. Antibiotic prophylaxis to patients receiving chemotherapy for acute leukemia and high dose chemotherapy for solid tumors is recommended. It should also be offered to those receiving moderately myelosuppressive chemotherapy for solid tumors and lymphomas during the first cycle of chemotherapy.

APLASTIC ANEMIA

2095. Which among the following is the most probable diagnosis if RBC, WBC and platelet count is depressed?
a. Lymphoma b. Aplastic anemia
c. DIC d. Thalassemia

2096. Pancytopenia is present in:
a. Aplastic anemia
b. Hemolytic anemia
c. Pernicious anemia
d. Sickle cell anemia

2097. Aplastic anemia can progress to:
a. AML b. ALL
c. Lymphoma d. All of these

2098. The change associated with aplastic anemia is:
a. Bowel function
b. Bleeding tendencies
c. Fluid deficit
d. Bladder function

Explanation: Aplastic anemia affects the bone marrow which in turn affect all type of blood cells and it cause bleeding tendencies.

2099. The symptoms of congenital aplastic anemia include: *(AIIMS Raipur Grade II 2017)*
a. Purpura b. Petechia
c. Neutropenia d. Thalassemia
a. a, b, c b. b, c, d
c. a, c, d d. a, b, c, d

Explanation: The symptoms of congenital aplastic anemia are pallor, headache, palpitations, dyspnea, fatigue, foot swelling, gingival bleeding, petechial. In aplastic anemia, bone marrow and hematopoietic stem cells are damaged and cannot produce new blood cells. So, deficiency symptoms related to RBC, WBC and platelet will be there.

2100. In aplastic anemia, lab value will be:
a. Increased proliferation of macrophages
b. Decreased levels of white blood cells (WBCs), red blood cells (RBCs), and platelets
c. Hyper cellular bone marrow
d. Leukopenia

2101. Vitamin B12 deficiency causes:
a. Aplastic anemia b. Iron deficiency anemia
c. Pernicious anemia d. Hemolytic anemia

THALASSEMIA

2102. Defect in which of the following is seen in thalassemia:
a. Hemoglobin b. Plasma proteins
c. Platelets d. Coagulation proteins

2103. All of the following are true regarding thalassemia; EXCEPT:
a. Thalassemia minor is also known as Cooley's anemia
b. Hb electrophoresis and DNA analysis are useful for diagnosing
c. It can affect alpha or beta chain of Hb
d. Thalassemia major is transfusion-dependent.

Explanation: Thalassemia major is also known as Cooley's anemia. All other statements are true regarding thalassemia.

2104. All of the following statement regarding Beta thalassemia is true; EXCEPT:
a. Reduced or absent synthesis of beta chains of hemoglobin
b. It results in macrocytic hypochromic anemia
c. Patients with thalassemia major have hepatosplenomegaly
d. Treatment includes regular blood transfusion and reducing transfusion iron overload

2105. The thalassemia is referred to as:
a. Autosomal dominant disease
b. Autosomal recessive disease
c. X-linked dominant
d. X-linked recessive

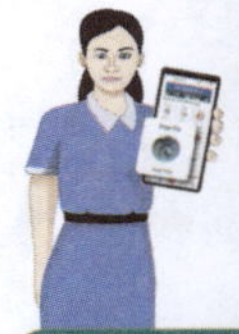

Ans.
2088. d
2089. d
2090. a
2091. b
2092. b
2093. c
2094. a
2095. b
2096. a
2097. a
2098. b
2099. a
2100. b
2101. c
2102. a
2103. a
2104. b
2105. b

2106. The defect in globin chain synthesis that is essential for the hemoglobin functioning is defined as:
a. Hemolytic anemia
b. Thromboplastic anemia
c. Thalassemia
d. Megaloblastic anemia

2107. Thalassemia is characterized by the defect in the synthesis of:
a. Beta globulin b. Alpha globulin
c. Gamma globulin d. Delta globulin

2108. Severe form of beta thalassemia major is referred as:
a. Hemolytic anemia b. Cooley's anemia
c. Pernicious anemia d. Beta defects

GLUCOSE-6-PHOSPHATE DEHYDROGENASE (G6PD) DEFICIENCY

2109. Hereditary pattern of G6PD deficiency is:
a. Autosomal dominant trait
b. Autosomal recessive trait
c. X-linked recessive trait
d. X-linked dominant trait

2110. Which of the following is true regarding G6PD deficiency?
a. X linked recessive disorder
b. It is a cause for hemolytic anemia
c. Both intravascular and extravascular hemolysis is seen
d. All of the above

2111. Drug that is safe in G6PD deficiency:
a. Primaquine b. Acetanilide
c. Quinidine d. Dapsone

2112. Drug causing maximum hemolysis in G6PD deficiency is:
a. Primaquine b. Chloroquine
c. Ciprofloxacin d. Gatifloxacin

2113. Individuals having G6PD deficiency can be poisoned by:
a. Fava beans b. Soya beans
c. Khesari dhal d. Maize

THROMBOCYTOPENIA

2114. Thrombocytopenia stands for: *(Banaras HU 2015)*
a. Weakness of platelet aggregation
b. Reduced platelet count
c. Increased platelet count
d. Normal platelet count

2115. Thrombocytopenia is a clinical manifestation of:
a. Dengue hemorrhagic fever
b. Idiopathic thrombocytopenic purpura
c. Leukemia
d. All of the above

2116. Expected clinical manifestation in a thrombocytopenic client is:
a. Spontaneous bleeding b. Activity intolerance
c. Frequent infection d. Nutritional imbalances

2117. Which among the following symptom is the major complaint of a client with thrombocytopenia?
a. Weakness and fatigue
b. Frequent fever attack
c. Bruising and hemorrhage
d. Nausea and vomiting

2118. Care instruction to a patient with thrombocytopenia includes all; EXCEPT:
a. Do not perform ROM exercise
b. While shaving, do not use razor blade.
c. Avoid forceful nasal blowing
d. Avoid medication like aspirin

2119. Drug that can induce thrombocytopenia:
a. Heparin b. Dapsone
c. Streptomycin d. Adrenaline

2120. Which of the following vitamin is affected by oral antibiotic therapy that may lead to hypoprothrombinemia?
a. Vitamin A b. Vitamin D
c. Vitamin E d. Vitamin K

2121. Drug of choice to improve platelet count in a patient with idiopathic thrombocytopenic purpura is:
a. Salicylic acid b. Corticosteroids
c. Allopurinol d. Vitamin K

2122. All of the following statement regarding Idiopathic Thrombocytopenic Purpura (ITP) are true; EXCEPT:
a. Patients suffer from bruising
b. Nosebleeds and bleeding gums may occur
c. Shortened bleeding time
d. It is an autoimmune disorder

2123. Which of the following statement is not correct about immune thrombocytopenic purpura (ITP)?
a. It is an autoimmune disorder
b. Immune mediated destruction of platelets occurs
c. Anti-platelet antibodies will not cross the placenta in a pregnant woman
d. Spontaneous resolution of Acute form of ITP within two months

HEMOPHILIA AND VON WILLEBRAND DISEASE

2124. Bone marrow examination is contraindicated in:
a. Hemophilia b. Leukemia
c. Anemia d. None of these

2125. Bone marrow transplantation is a treatment option for......:
a. Thalassemia b. Leukemia
c. Aplastic anaemia d. All of these

2126. Reduced number of platelets is found in all the conditions EXCEPT: *(Safdarjung NO 2018)*
a. Disseminated intravascular coagulation
b. Aplastic anemia
c. Acute myeloid leukemia
d. Von Willebrand disease

Explanation:

- Von Willebrand disease (vWD) is an inherited hemorrhagic disorder caused by a deficiency or dysfunction of the protein termed von Willebrand factor (vWF). Consequently, defective vWF interaction between platelets and the vessel wall impairs primary hemostasis. The number of platelets is not reduced.
- Reduced platelet count is seen in all other given conditions.

2127. Composition of blood transfused to hemophilia patient is: *(AIIMS Nagpur NO 2018)*
a. Plasma b. Packed cells
c. Cryoprecipitate d. Platelets

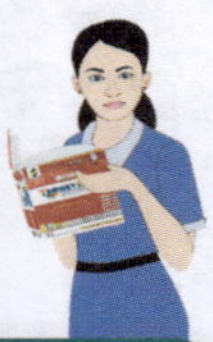

Ans.

2106. c
2107. a
2108. b
2109. c
2110. d
2111. c
2112. a
2113. a
2114. b
2115. d
2116. a
2117. c
2118. a
2119. a
2120. d
2121. b
2122. c
2123. c
2124. a
2125. d
2126. d
2127. c

Explanation: Hemophilia is a condition in which there is lack of sufficient blood clotting proteins in the blood. Cryoprecipitate is prepared from plasma and contains fibrinogen, von Willebrand factor, factor VIII, factor XIII and fibronectin.

2128. Bleeding time is more in:
a. Von Willebrand disease b. Thrombocytopenia
c. Both a and b d. DIC

2129. Clotting time is more in:
a. Severe hemophilia b. Afibrinogenemia
c. DIC d. All of these

2130. Increase in coagulation time is the characteristic of:
a. Hemophilia b. Von Willebrand disease
c. Christmas disease d. All of these

2131. Hemophilia is associated with:
a. X chromosome b. Y chromosome
c. Chromosome 11 d. Chromosome 21

2132. If a cross is made between hemophilic man and normal woman, chance of the progeny in the subsequent generation is: *(Kerala PSC, Nov 2014)*
a. Hemophilic male b. Hemophilic female
c. Carrier male d. Carrier female

2133. Production site for Von Willebrand factor is:
a. Vascular endothelium b. Platelet
c. Liver d. RBCs

2134. The best screening test for hemophilia:
a. Bleeding time b. Clotting time
c. PTT d. All of these

2135. A patient with von Willebrand (vWF) deficiency undergoing surgery, this patient needs to be treated with ....along with vWF:
a. Thrombin b. Factor VII
c. Factor VIII d. Factor IX

DISSEMINATED INTRAVASCULAR COAGULATION (DIC)

2136. Laboratory value findings in a client with disseminated intravascular coagulation (DIC)?
a. Thrombocytopenia
b. High fibrinogen levels
c. Low levels of fibrin degradation products
d. Reduced prothrombin time (PT)

2137. The purpose of anti-embolism stockings is to:
a. Promote warmth in the legs (Daman and Diu NO 2018)
b. Decrease the arterial circulation to the legs
c. Prevent deep vein thrombosis
d. Prevent foot drop

Explanation: Stockings are applied to prevent venous stasis and usually is applied in the bedridden patients so as to prevent the development of deep vein thrombus, reducing the edema.

2138. The laboratory results of a patient with disseminated intravascular coagulation are likely to include:
a. Prolonged prothrombin and partial thromboplastin times
b. Increased platelet counts
c. Increased levels of fibrinogen
d. Decreased levels of fibrin split products.

2139. Important observation for a patient on anticoagulant therapy includes: *(JIPMER 2012)*
a. Headache b. Chest pain
c. Epistaxis d. Hypotension

2140. Warfarin should be withheld ___________ before any invasive procedure?
a. 5 hours b. 18 hours
c. 10 hours d. 24 hours

2141. The drug that act by dissolving the blood clot is:
a. Aspirin b. Heparin
c. Streptokinase d. Vitamin-K

2142. True about heparin therapy is that heparin:
a. Prolongs the blood clotting time
b. Prolongs the bleeding time
c. Decreases the clotting time
d. Decreases blood viscosity

2143. Heparin acts by:
a. Interfering with vitamin K absorption
b. Dissolving existing thrombi
c. Inactivating thrombin that forms and dissolves existing thrombi
d. Preventing conversion of factors that are needed in the formation of clots

Explanation: Once active thrombosis has developed, larger amounts of heparin can inhibit further coagulation by inactivating thrombin and preventing the conversion of fibrinogen to fibrin. Heparin also prevents the formation of a stable fibrin clot in inhibiting the activation of the fibrin stabilizing factor.

2144. Increased Prothrombin time is/are seen when Patient:
a. Is on oral anticoagulant
b. Has liver disease and Vitamin K deficiency
c. Factor VII and X deficiency
d. All of the above

2145. International normalized ratio (INR) is a laboratory test used to:
a. Assess the effect of oral anticoagulant
b. A measure of the number of polymorphonuclear cells in the blood
c. Is a relative amount of albumin to globulin
d. To differentiate various causes of liver damage

Explanation: The international normalised ratio (INR) is a laboratory measurement of how long it takes blood to form a clot. It is used to determine the effects of oral anticoagulants on the clotting system.

2146. Warfarin interferes with:
a. Calcium metabolism b. Fibrin formation
c. Vitamin K cycle d. Collagen formation

2147. The choice of coagulation study for a person who is in warfarin therapy is:
a. PT b. INR
c. APTT d. Platelet count

Explanation: International normalized ratio (INR) is a calculation made to standardize prothrombin time. INR is based on the ratio of the patient's prothrombin time and the normal mean prothrombin time. Prothrombin time is a test to learn how fast the blood clots in patients receiving oral anticoagulant medication. APTT is used to evaluate the effect of heparin.

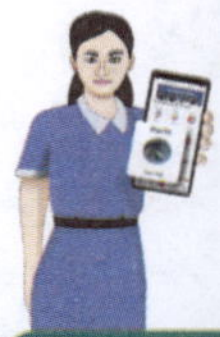

Ans.
2128. c
2129. d
2130. d
2131. a
2132. d
2133. a
2134. c
2135. c
2136. a
2137. c
2138. a
2139. c
2140. d
2141. c
2142. a
2143. d
2144. d
2145. a
2146. c
2147. b

2148. Recommended value of international normalization ratio (INR) during warfarin therapy?
a. 1–2 b. 1–3
c. 2–3 d. 2–4

2149. In a client with bleeding disorder, all of the following signs and symptoms suggest internal bleeding; EXCEPT:
a. Unexplained nosebleeds
b. Melena
c. Hypertension
d. Bruising

2150. Which of the following statement regarding DIC is not true?
a. Thrombocytopenia occurs
b. Depleted clotting factors
c. Increased prothrombin time
d. Lab investigation shows decreased d-dimer level

2151. DIC can occur in all of the following; EXCEPT:
a. Snake bite b. Placenta praevia
c. Falciparum malaria d. Hemophilia

2152. Blood coagulating faster than normal, causing thrombin and other clotting factors to multiply is known as:
a. DIC b. Hypercoagulability
c. Hemophilia d. Thalassemia

2153. Calf muscle pain due to sharp dorsiflexion of the foot is known as:
a. Chovstek sign b. Trousseau's sign
c. Positive Babinski's reflex d. Positive Homans' sign

2154. Health education to a client on anticoagulant therapy includes:
a. Report any signs of bleeding
b. Do lab studies such as PT, INR as ordered
c. Both a and b
d. None of the above

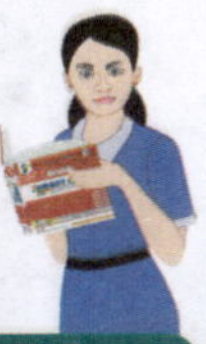

THROMBOPHLEBITIS

2155. Most dangerous complication of venous thrombus is: *(LNJP H D 2012)*
a. Chronic occlusion of the vein
b. Pulmonary embolism
c. Formation of venous ulcers
d. Gangrenous development of veins

2156. A major complication associated with thrombolytic therapy is:
a. Clot expansion b. Air embolism
c. Cerebral hemorrhage d. All of these

2157. Most commonly thrombosis occurs in:
a. Vein b. Artery
c. Lymph d. Capillary

2158. Thrombolytic therapy used in myocardial infarction is:
a. Heparin b. T-PA
c. Nitroglycerine d. Streptokinase

2159. Clinical manifestations of thromboembolism?
a. Edema b. Swelling
c. Redness d. All of these

2160. Risk factor for Deep Vein Thrombosis (DVT) among the following is:
a. Oral contraceptive pills b. Hypertension
c. Myocardial infarction d. All of these

2161. Classic symptoms of deep vein thrombosis (DVT) include all of the following; EXCEPT: *(DSSSB 2013)*
a. Homans sign b. Muscle pain
c. Cyanosis d. Swelling

Explanation: Classic symptoms of DVT includes: Leg pain, including tenderness to the touch, that may worsen when standing or walking, swelling of the affected leg, skin discoloration and warmth and redness of the skin.

2162. Client with DVT experiencing dyspnea, chest pain, and diminished breath sounds. Possible diagnosis will be:
a. Pericarditis
b. Pneumothorax
c. Pulmonary embolism
d. Mediastinal tumor

2163. Characteristic pain in newly diagnosed DVT is:
a. Stabbing pain b. Shooting pain
c. Sudden onset d. Tingling

2164. In DVT client pain can be managed by:
a. Elastic stockings
b. Leg elevation
c. ROM exercises
d. Hot application

2165. Pressure on the popliteal space can lead to .... complication:
a. Pulmonary embolism b. Air embolism
c. Pulmonary edema d. Deep vein thrombosis

Explanation: Popliteal vein thrombosis is a condition in which a blood clot develops in the popliteal vein. Popliteal vein thrombosis is a type of venous thromboembolism (VTE), which is also called deep vein thrombosis (DVT). It is potentially life-threatening because the thrombus that can move and travels to the lungs and cause pulmonary embolism (PE).

2166. Which term best describes the findings on cautious palpation of the vein in typical superficial thrombophlebitis?
a. Dilated b. Knotty
c. Smooth d. Tortuous

2167. Nursing management for a client with thrombolytic agent include:
a. Avoid puncture wounds
b. Monitor potassium levels
c. Avoid swimming
d. Activity restriction

2168. An emboli is:
a. Movable blood clot b. Movable debris
c. Movable pus d. Movable air bubble

BLOOD TRANSFUSION COMPATIBILITY

2169. Most Alicia's blood group is A negative. She may receive a blood transfusion from an individual whose blood group is:
a. A positive c. AB positive
c. B negative d. O negative

2170. Which among the following blood group is safe for an AB negative client?
a. AB positive b. B positive
c. B Negative d. O positive

Ans.

2148. c
2149. c
2150. d
2151. d
2152. b
2153. d
2154. c
2155. b
2156. c
2157. a
2158. d
2159. d
2160. d
2161. c
2162. c
2163. c
2164. b
2165. a
2166. b
2167. a
2168. a
2169. d
2170. c

2171. Blood group which is not likely to be present in a baby born to mother with O positive and father with A negative blood group?
a. A positive b. A negative
c. O positive d. AB positive

2172. Most accurate statement regarding blood transfusion is:
a. Double checking is required before blood transfusion
b. Use large bore cannula of 16-18 G for blood transfusion
c. In the initial 15 min timing nurse should remain with the client
d. All of the above

2173. A severe anemic client prescribed to undergo blood transfusion. The total duration of the treatment would be:
a. No longer than 4 hours b. 6 hours
c. 8 hours d. 10 hours

BLOOD PRODUCTS AND THEIR INDICATIONS

2174. Lifespan of Neutrophil:
a. 120 days b. 2-5 days
c. 24 hours d. 4-6 hours

2175. Life span of platelets are:
a. 8–12 days b. 20–30 days
c. 30–60 days d. 60–70 days

2176. Life span of RBCs is: *(DSSSB PHN, 2015)*
a. 120 days b. 80 days
c. 200 days d. 60 days

2177. The life-span of the average RBC in a new-born is:
a. 100 days b. 120 days
c. 160 days d. 60 days

2178. Which of the following components of WBC has longest lifespan?
a. T-Lymphocyte b. Eosinophil
c. Neutrophil d. Monocyte

2179. Fresh frozen plasma contains:
a. Plasma proteins and clotting factors
b. RBCs
c. Platelets
d. None of the above

2180. Platelets are stored at:
a. −40 to −50°C b. −30°C
c. 4°C d. 20-24°C

2181. In which of the following condition is blood transfusion contraindicated? *(AIIMS BPL SNO 2018)*
a. Bleeding Hemorrhoids
b. Hemorrhage
c. Congestive cardiac failure
d. Hemophilia

Explanation: Congestive cardiac failure patients are not usually given blood transfusion as the pumping action of heart in congestive cardiac failure is highly compromised. Blood transfusion will result in fluid overload. Bleeding hemorrhoids, Hemorrhage and Hemophilia are indications for blood transfusion because there is excessive blood loss.

2182. During blood donation at a time single donor can donate ……..mL:
a. 100–200 mL b. 200–250 mL
c. 250–300 mL d. 350–450 mL

2183. Types of blood products that can be prepared from one unit of blood is:
a. Packed red cells
b. Platelet concentrate
c. Fresh plasma
d. All of the above

2184. Platelets can be stored at:
a. 20–24°C for 5 days
b. 20–24°C for 8 days
c. 4–8°C for 5 days
d. 4–8°C for 8 days

Explanation: All platelets are stored at room temperature (20–21°C) for 5 days from date of collection.

2185. Normal Hb range in adult is:
a. 8-10 g/dL b. 10-12 g/dL
c. 12-16 g/dL d. 14-18 g/dL

2186. After the transfusion of one unit whole blood expected increase in hemoglobin level is:
a. 0.5 g% b. 1 g%
c. 1.5 g% d. 2 g%

2187. Normal hematocrit value in male is:
a. 10-24% b. 20-34%
c. 30-48% d. 40-54%

2188. Characteristic RBC in Chronic Renal Failure is:
a. Microcytic b. Hypochromic
c. Normocytic d. Macrocytic

2189. In high altitude individual RBC count is more because:
a. Variation in pressure cause increased RBC production
b. Erythropoiesis will be stimulated because of atmospheric hypoxia
c. RBC destruction is more in high altitude
d. Bone marrow become more active

2190. The major function of platelets is to:
a. Carry oxygen
b. Assist phagocytosis
c. Prevent bleeding
d. Maintain oncotic pressure

2191. Platelet count is normal in patient with:
a. DIC
b. Shaken baby syndrome
c. Aplastic anemia
d. Thrombocytopenia

TRANSFUSION REACTIONS

2192. Complication associated with blood transfusion includes:
a. Hyperkalemia
b. Air embolism
c. Thrombocytopenia
d. All of these

2193. During blood transfusion therapy patient developed symptoms like increased temperature, chills and pain in the kidney region. These symptoms indicate ……. reaction:
a. Hemolytic transfusion reaction
b. Anaphylactic transfusion reaction
c. Septic transfusion reaction
d. Thrombotic crisis

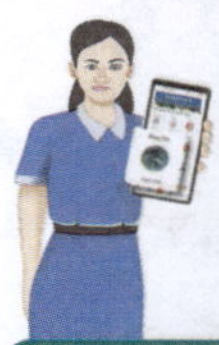

Ans.

2171. d
2172. d
2173. a
2174. b
2175. a
2176. a
2177. d
2178. a
2179. a
2180. d
2181. c
2182. d
2183. d
2184. a
2185. c
2186. b
2187. d
2188. c
2189. b
2190. c
2191. b
2192. d
2193. a

2194. While receiving blood transfusion the patient develops chills and headache. What should be the nurse's initial action? *(NCFL 2019)*

a. Notify the physician STAT
b. Stop the transfusion immediately
c. Cover the patient with a blanket and administer ordered acetaminophen.
d. Slow the blood flow to keep vein open

Explanation: While receiving blood transfusion, the patient develops chills and headache is the sign of early adverse reaction (febrile reaction). Nurses initial action is to stop the transfusion immediately because it helps to prevent the further life-threatening situations.

2195. Anti-Rh antibody can be seen after:

a. Pregnancy b. Blood transfusion
c. DIC d. Both a and b

2196. Intra vascular hemolysis can be seen in:

a. Falciparum malaria
b. Acute G6PD deficiency
c. Incompatible blood transfusion
d. All of the above

2197. Extravascular hemolysis occurs in:

a. Thalassemia b. Hereditary spherocytosis
c. Sickle cell disease d. All of these

OTHER HEMATOLOGICAL DISORDERS

2198. Which among the following suggest problem with hematological system?

a. Uremia b. Polycythemia vera
c. Gout d. Renal calculi

2199. Multiple myeloma occurs due to uncontrolled proliferation of:

a. B-lymphocyte b. T-lymphocyte
c. Basophil d. Plasma cell

2200. Most common cause of traumatic splenic rupture is:

a. Blunt abdominal blows
b. Sharp injury to abdomen
c. Lymphoma
d. Rib fracture

2201. Most common cause of non-traumatic splenic rupture is:

a. Malaria b. Cirrhosis
c. Thalassemia d. ITP

2202. Expected laboratory finding after splenectomy is:

a. Decreased WBC count
b. Increased hemoglobin
c. Decreased hemoglobin
d. Increased thrombocyte count

2203. Splenomegaly is evident in:

a. Malaria b. Kala azar
c. Hemolytic anemia d. All of these

CLOTTING FACTORS

2204. Total no. of blood clotting factors are:

a. 12 b. 13
c. 14 d. 15

2205. Which of the following is not a clotting factor? *(AIIMS Bhopal Nursing officer, 2018)*

a. Fibrinogen b. Prothrombin
c. Calcium d. Sodium

Explanation: Sodium is not involved in clotting process.

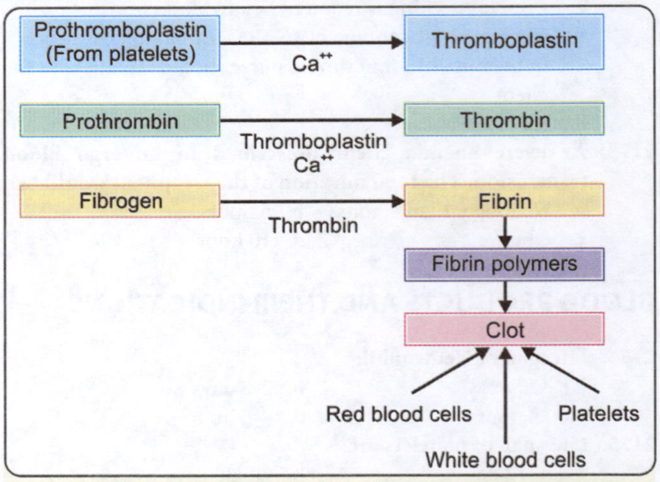

2206. Vitamin required for blood clotting is:

a. Vitamin – A b. Vitamin – D
c. Vitamin – E d. Vitamin – K

2207. Electrolyte required for blood clotting is:

a. Na b. K
c. Ca d. P

2208. Antihemophilic factor – B is:

a. Factor 7 b. Factor 8
c. Factor 9 d. Factor 10

2209. Antihaemophilic factor – A is:

a. Factor 7 b. Factor 8
c. Factor 9 d. Factor 10

2210. Factor 9 is also known as:

a. Stuart Prower factor b. Hageman factor
c. Christmas factor d. Thromboplastin

2211. Von Willebrand factor is secreted by:

a. Liver b. Kidney
c. Vascular endothelium d. Adrenals

2212. Coagulation factor VII is:

a. Thromboplastins b. Accelerin
c. Proconvertin d. Antihemophilic factor

2213. Vitamin K dependent factor is:

a. Factor XII b. Factor IV
c. Prothrombin d. Factor V

2214. All of the following clotting factors are Vitamin K dependent; EXCEPT:

a. Factor II b. Factor VII
c. Factor VIII d. Protein IX

Explanation: The key vitamin K-dependent proteins include:
- **Coagulation proteins:** Factors II (prothrombin), VII, IX and X
- **Anticoagulation proteins:** Proteins C, S and Z
- **Others:** Osteocalcin and matrix-Gla protein, and certain ribosomal proteins

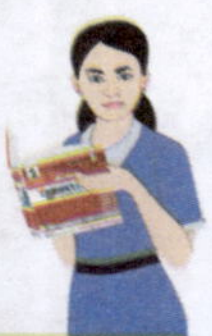

Ans.

2194. b
2195. d
2196. d
2197. b
2198. b
2199. d
2200. a
2201. a
2202. d
2203. d
2204. b
2205. d
2206. d
2207. c
2208. c
2209. b
2210. c
2211. c
2212. c
2213. c
2214. c

2215. All of the following are platelet associated coagulation factors; EXCEPT:
a. Von Willebrand Factor b. Factor IX
c. Factor XI d. Factor XIII

2216. Feature of factor XIII deficiency is:
a. Early solubilization of clot
b. Fibrinogen to fibrin conversion will not be there
c. Activation of platelet will be delayed
d. Small clot fragments

2217. Hemophilia A is caused by lack of clotting factor:
a. VII b. VIII
c. IX d. X

2218. Hemophilia B is caused by lack of clotting factor:
a. VII b. VIII
c. IX d. X

2219. Which of the following coagulation disorder is an autosomal dominant disease?
a. Hemophilia A b. Hemophilia B
c. Von Willebrand Disease d. All of these

LEUKEMIA

2220. Laboratory results of a client with leukemia indicates elevated blood urea nitrogen (BUN) and uric acid levels. These laboratory results indicates:
a. Lymphadenopathy b. Thrombocytopenia
c. Hepatic encephalopathy d. Hypermetabolic state

Explanation: The hypermetabolic (increased rate of metabolism) state related to leukemia causes increased production of urea and uric acid (end products of metabolism). The end products get accumulated in the blood.

2221. Philadelphia chromosome can be seen in:
a. Cancer of breast
b. Chronic myeloid leukemia
c. Burkitt lymphoma
d. Hodgkin's lymphoma

2222. Acute lymphocytic leukemia (ALL) is commonly seen in people of which age group?
a. 4–12 years b. 20–30 years
c. 30–45 years d. 50–70 years

Explanation: The highest incidence of acute lymphocytic leukemia (ALL) is in children of 4–12 years of age.

2223. Which of the following is NOT a common clinical manifestation of Acute Lymphocytic Leukemia (ALL)? *New Q*
a. Bone and joint pain b. Night sweats
c. Petechiae d. Weight gain

Explanation: Easy bruising, signs of bleeding (petechiae), bone and joint pain, anorexia, weight loss, paleness, pain, lymphadenopathy and night sweats are the common symptoms of ALL. Anorexia and weight loss is common not weight gain.

2224. Malignancy affecting the granulocytic cells lead to:
a. Fatigue b. Anemia
c. Bleeding d. Infection

2225. Bone marrow biopsy is useful in the diagnosis of:
a. CML b. ALL
c. Hodgkin's lymphoma d. All of these

2226. Most common childhood malignancy is:
a. ALL b. AML
c. Wilms tumor d. Retinoblastoma

2227. Commonly seen leukemia in older adult is:
a. Acute myelocytic leukemia (AML)
b. Acute lymphocytic leukemia (ALL)
c. Chronic myelocytic leukemia (CML)
d. Chronic lymphocytic leukemia (CLL)

2228. Leukemia and lymphoma are treated with combination of chemotherapeutic drug because:
a. Minimize the side effect
b. Tackle the problem of drug resistance
c. Maximize the effect of therapy
d. Both b and c

2229. Platelet count of patient suffers from leukemia is 19,000/mm³. Which will be appropriate nursing action?
a. Check the platelet count again
b. Isolate the patient
c. Use soft toothbrush
d. Monitor for signs of infection

Explanation: Patient has chances for bleeding from decreased platelet count. So, bleeding precautions should be initiated which includes using soft toothbrush to prevent gum bleeding.

2230. A client has been admitted with a diagnosis of acute lymphoblastic leukemia and receiving chemotherapy. Which of the following should be monitored to assess the patient for the development of life-threatening thrombocytopenia? *(DSSSB 2006)*
a. Diarrhea b. Intermittent fever
c. Headache d. Hematuria

Explanation: Thrombocytes (platelets) play a major role in blood clotting. Thrombocytopenia (decreased platelet count) leads to decreased coagulability of blood and results in hematuria (blood in urine).

2231. Which type of leukemia commonly affects the persons younger than 15 years?
a. Acute myelogenous leukemia
b. Acute Lymphocytic leukemia
c. Chronic Myelogenous leukemia
d. Chronic Lymphocytic leukemia

2232. A client is diagnosed with acute myeloid leukemia. The priority nursing care for this client is the management of:
a. Weakness and fatigue b. Pain
c. Ecchymosis d. Hypertension

2233. Which of the following medication is used to prevent graft versus host disease?
a. Cyclosporin b. Cisplatin
c. Doxorubicin d. Filgrastim

2234. What is the primary action of the drug Allopurinol?
a. It decreases the production of uric acid
b. It decreases the pain level
c. It reduces the inflammation
d. It helps in excretion of uric acid

Explanation: **Allopurinol** is the first-line drug for **urate**-lowering therapy. It is a **purine** analogue which competitively inhibits xanthine oxidase, reducing the production of **uric acid**. It does not have role in excretion of uric acid. It is neither an anti-inflammatory nor an analgesic.

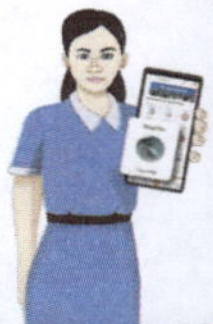

Ans.
2215. b
2216. a
2217. b
2218. c
2219. c
2220. d
2221. b
2222. a
2223. d
2224. d
2225. d
2226. a
2227. d
2228. d
2229. c
2230. d
2231. b
2232. b
2233. a
2234. a

RENAL SYSTEM

ANATOMY AND PHYSIOLOGY OF RENAL SYSTEM

Kidney

- Paired brownish red structures located retroperitoneally
- **Location:** T12-L3 (in Adult)
- **Weight:** 120–170 g
- **Dimension:** 12 cm long × 6 cm wide × 2.5 cm thick
- Kidney has two distinct regions (Renal parenchyma and renal pelvis)
- The left kidney is slightly higher located behind the 11th rib and the right kidney is located behind the 12th rib because of the liver position

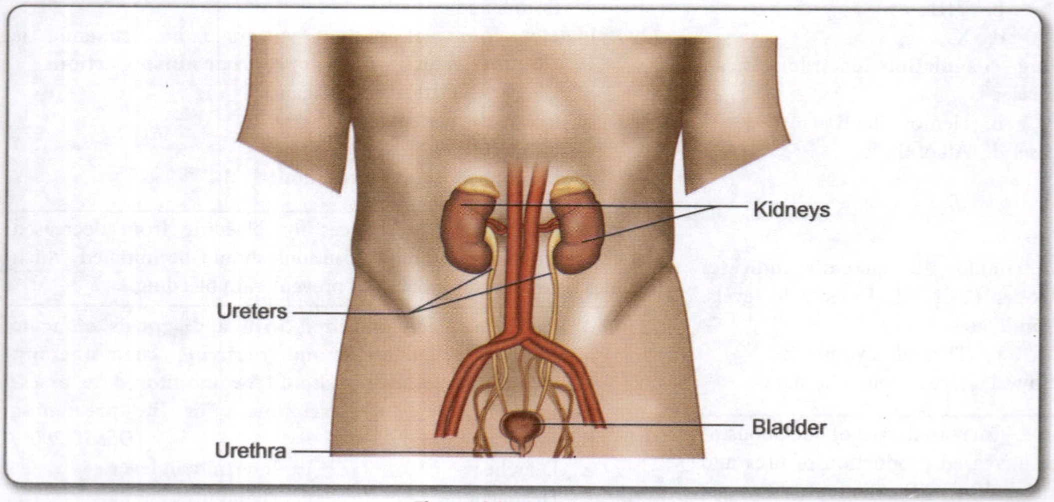

Figure 94: Renal system

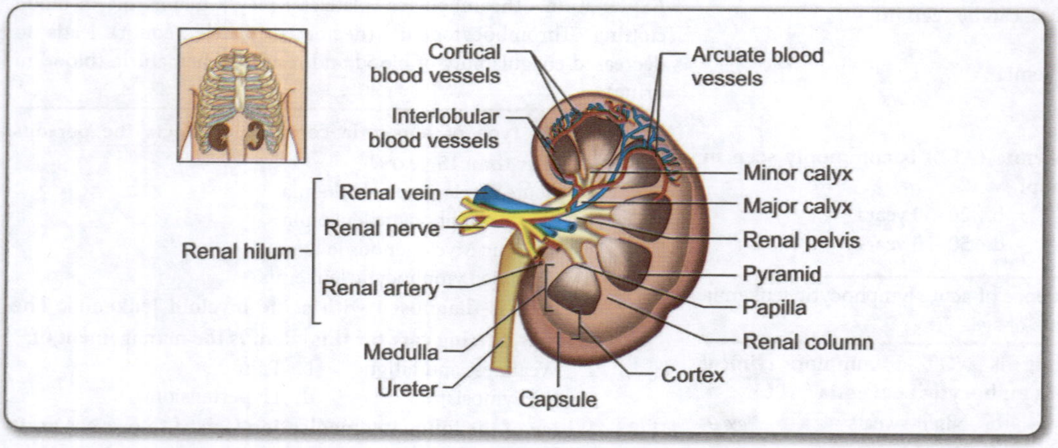

Figure 95: Cross section of kidney

- **Renal parenchyma**
  - It is further divided into cortex and medulla.
  - Cortex contains glomeruli, proximal and distal tubules and cortical collecting duct.
  - Renal medulla contains pyramids.
- **Renal pelvis**
  - **Renal pelvis or hilum:** Area through which artery, veins and nerves enter and leave kidney.

- **Glomerulus**
  - Renal artery is a branch of abdominal aorta.
  - Renal artery divides into smaller vessels and form glomerulus.
  - Glomerulus is the capillary bed responsible for filtration:
    - **Afferent arterioles:** Blood enters into the glomerulus through it (**Remember:** A before E – Entry before exit)
    - **Efferent arterioles:** Blood leaves the glomerulus through it.
  - **Normal GFR: 90–120 mL/min**

KEY POINTS

- Nephron is the structural and functional unit of Kidney.
- The kidneys lie retroperitoneally (behind the peritoneum) in the abdomen, either side of the vertebral column.
- The left kidney is located at about the **T12 to L3 vertebrae,** whereas the right is lower due to slight displacement by the liver.
- The renal cortex, renal medulla, and renal pelvis are the three main internal regions found in a kidney.
- The renal parenchyma is the functional part of the kidney that includes the renal cortex and the renal medulla
- Renal cortex - Outer region of the kidney.
- Renal medulla - Inner- most region of the kidney.

POINT TO REMEMBER

Most tubular re-absorption occurs at the **Proximal convoluted tubule.**

- **Nephrons**
  - Functional units of kidney
  - Each nephron consists of
    - **Renal corpuscle:** It is made up of glomerulus with Bowman's capsule and it helps in the filtration of blood plasma.
    - **Renal tubules:** It is made up of proximal convoluted tubule, Loop of Henle, distal convoluted tubules, and collecting duct and these structures help in reabsorption and carrying away the filtrate.
  - Collecting duct empties into minor calyx then to major calyx and it opens to renal pelvis.
  - Two types of nephrons are there:
    - Cortical nephron - Found in the cortex of kidney
    - Juxtamedullary nephron - Seen adjacent to medulla

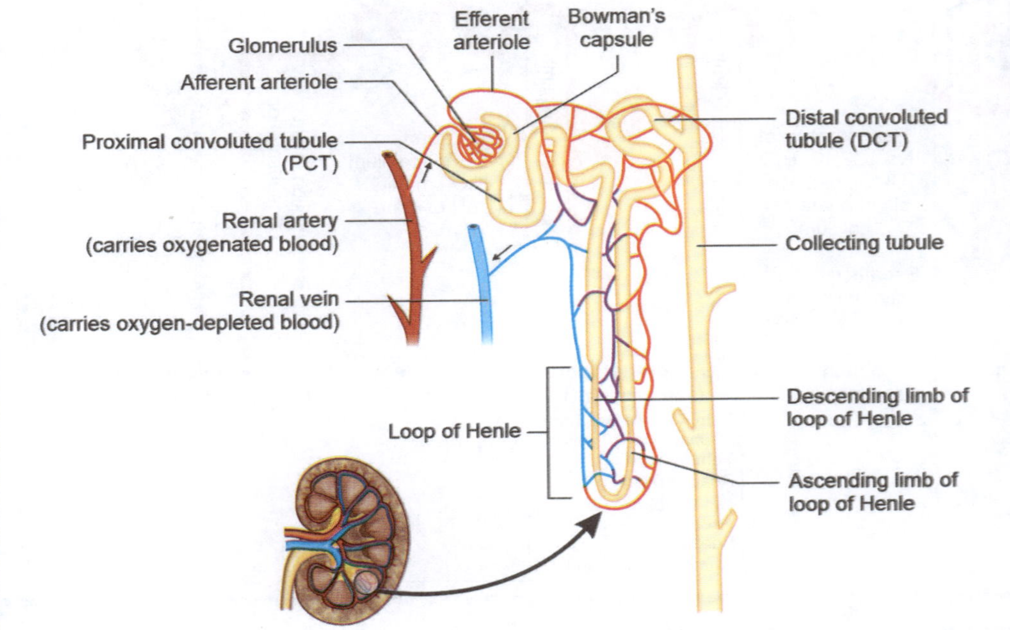

Figure 96: Structure of nephron

Bowman's capsule

- Double-walled capsule that surrounds glomerulus.
- Glomerular filtrate filtered into Bowman's space.
- Made up of simple squamous epithelium.

Proximal convoluted tubule

- Receives glomerular filtrate from Bowman's capsule.
- Reabsorbs water and electrolyte through active and passive transport.
- Made up of cuboidal epithelium with brush border microvilli to increase surface area.

Descending loop of Henle

- Passively reabsorbs water
- Thin part made up of simple squamous cells
- Loop diuretics work in this area

Ascending loop of Henle

- Passively reabsorbs sodium and chlorine.
- Thick part made up of simple cuboidal cells.
- Fluid received from descending loop of Henle is rich in salt and urea.
- Salt is reabsorbed to the surrounding from the thin part of ascending loop of Henle.
- Thick part removes salt against the concentration gradient with an active process.

Distal convoluted tubule

- Actively and passively removes sodium and water
- ADH makes DCT and collecting duct permeable to water.
- Shortest segment, length 5 mm.
- Made up of single layer of simple cuboidal epithelium.
- Principal cells of this part **regulate water reabsorption by ADH.**
- At the ascending loop of Henle and early DCT the osmolarity decreases to 100 mOsm/L due to ion reabsorption and these two segments together are known as **'diluting segment.**

KEY POINTS

- ADH acts upon the **distal convoluted tubules** (greatest effect) and **collecting ducts** of nephrons to increase water reabsorption.
- ADH is normally released by the pituitary in response to increase in blood osmolality or decrease in blood volume.
- Normal range of GFR in adult is 90 to 120 mL/min/1.73 m^2
- The two kidneys together filter 180 L of fluid every 24 hours.

NORCET 2023

Normal urine output—800 mL to 2000 mL/day.

KEY POINTS

- Nephron is the structural and functional unit of Kidney.
- The kidneys lie retroperitoneally (behind the peritoneum) in the abdomen, either side of the vertebral column.
- The left kidney is located at about the **T12 to L3 vertebrae,** whereas the right is lower due to slight displacement by the liver.
- The renal cortex, renal medulla, and renal pelvis are the three main internal regions found in a kidney.
- The renal parenchyma is the functional part of the kidney that includes the renal cortex and the renal medulla.

- Also reabsorbs sodium, secretes potassium, and regulates calcium and magnesium level.
- Helps in the homeostasis process.

Collecting duct

- The collecting duct system is made up of connecting tubules and collecting ducts.
- Approximately 6 nephrons connect with a single collecting duct.
- 20 large collecting ducts form the papillary of Bellini and this opens into the papilla.
- This papilla opens into the minor calyx. 8–18 minor calyces are present in one kidney.

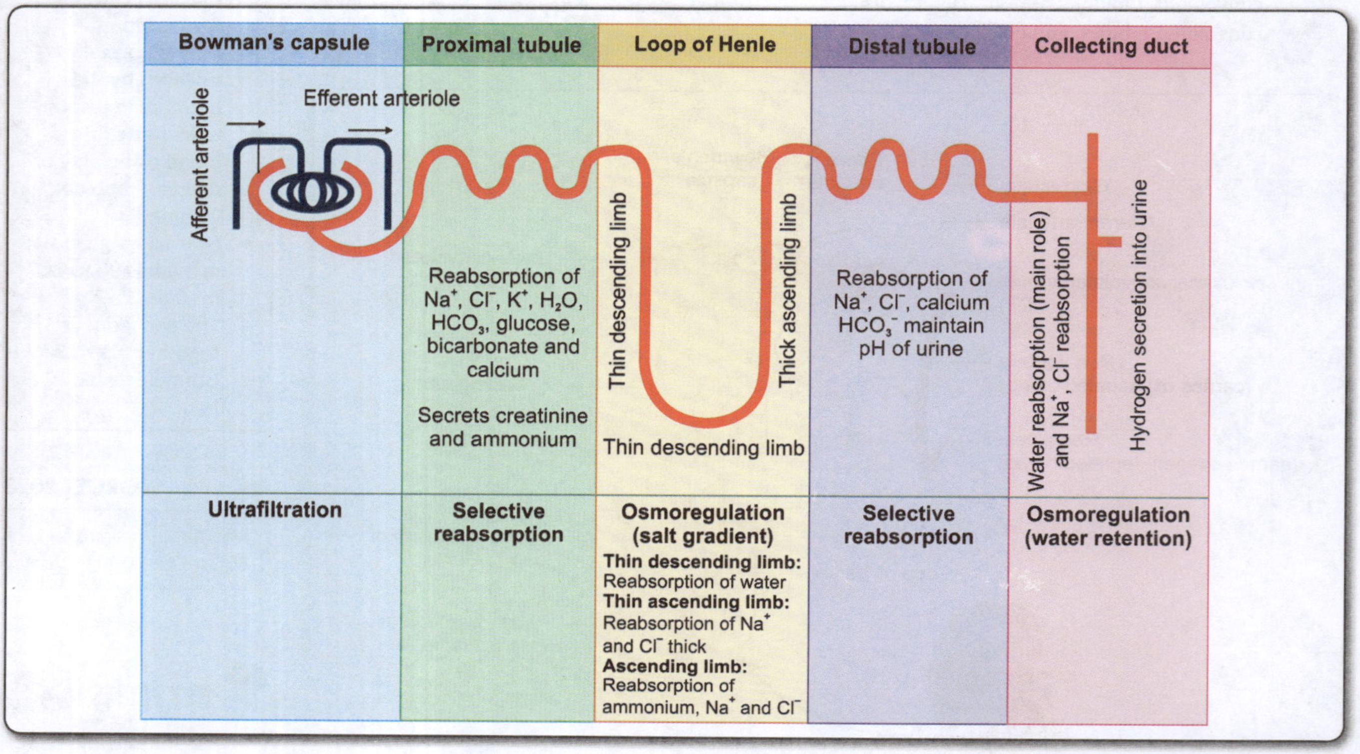

Figure 97: Ultrafiltration, selective reabsorption and osmoregulation by kidney

Ureter

- Fibromuscular tube which connects kidney and bladder.
- Urine formed in the nephron drains into ureter.
- 24–30 cm in length; 3–4 mm in diameter
- Originates in the lower portion of renal pelvis and terminates at trigone of bladder.
- **Right ureter is slightly shorter than the left** (due to position of the kidney)
- Ureter is lined with transitional epithelium.
- It has three narrowed portions:
  - Ureteropelvic junction
  - Ureteral part near sacroiliac segment
  - Ureterovesical junction
- Narrowed portions of the ureter are more prone to develop stricture and calculi.

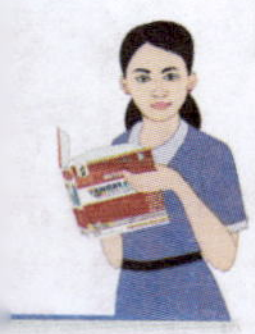

Three layers of Ureter –

- **Mucosa:** It is the inner layer, made up of transitional epithelium.
- **Muscular layer:** Middle muscular layer consists of two longitudinal layers with a middle circular layer. This layer generates ureteric peristaltic motion.
- **Adventitia:** Consists of elastic fibers and dense collagen.

Urinary Bladder

- Muscular hollow organ located behind pubic bone.
- Four layers (from inside to outside):
  - Mucosa (innermost)
  - Submucosa
  - Muscularis
  - Serosa or adventitia (outermost)
- In infancy, bladder is an abdominal organ. Later it descends into the pelvic cavity.
- **Capacity:** 300–600 mL of urine in adult
- Bladder is lined with **transitional epithelium.**
- In adult, bladder filling and emptying is mediated by sympathetic and parasympathetic nervous system while in an infant it is controlled by the micturition center located in the pons area of brain stem.

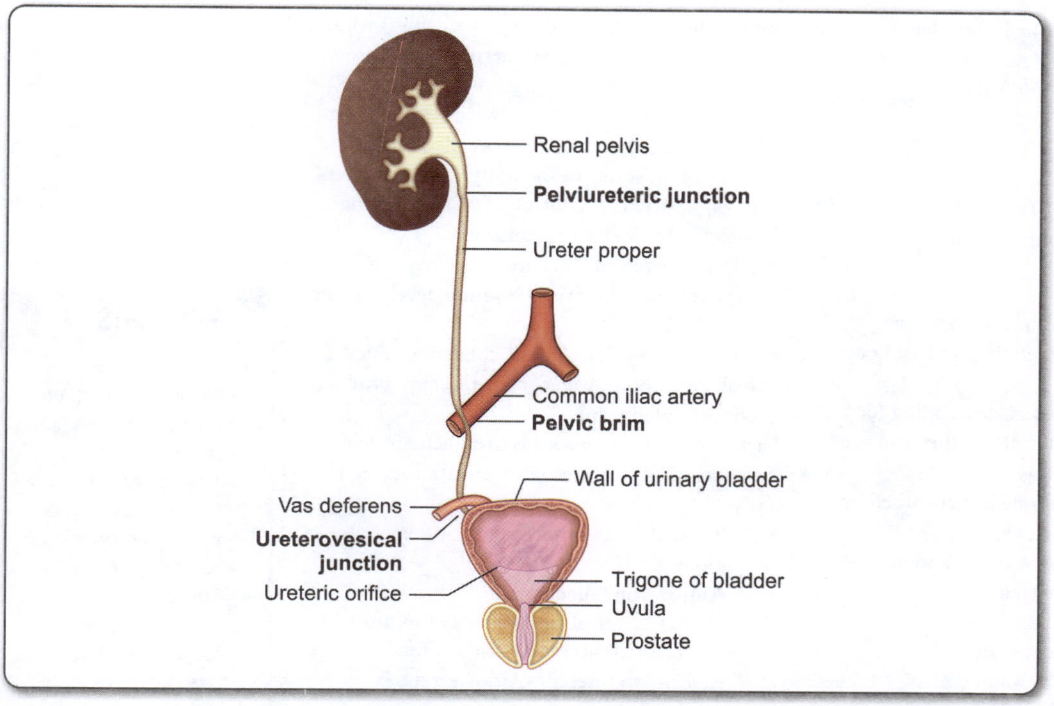

Figure 98: Renal system– anatomical view

Urethra

- In males, it passes through penis while in female it opens just anterior to vagina.
- **Female:** 4 – 5 cm long; Urethra is only for urinating.
- **Male:** 20 cm long; common for urination and ejaculation
- Urethritis is more common among females than male.
- **Hypospadias:** Urethra opens on the underside (ventral surface) of penis.
- **Epispadias:** Urethra opens on the topside (dorsum) of penis.

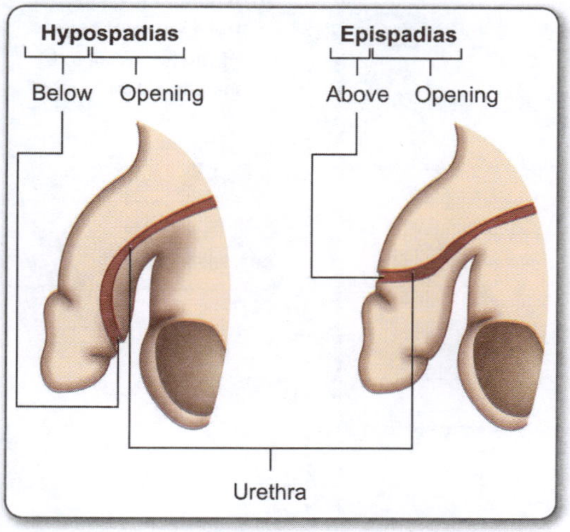

Figure 99: Hypospadias and epispadias

Three regions of the male urethra:

- ***Prostatic Urethra:*** It is 2–3 cm long which runs between prostate gland.
- ***Membranous Urethra:*** It is 1 cm long that goes through pelvic floor and enters into penis. This is the external urethral sphincter and most common place for stricture formation of urethra due to instrumentation.
- ***Spongy or penile:*** It is 15–16 cm long runs through penis.

FUNCTIONS OF KIDNEY

Urine Formation

Urine is formed in the nephrons through three steps:

1. Glomerular filtration
2. Tubular reabsorption
3. Tubular secretion

Glomerular Filtration

- It is also known as ultra-filtration as the minute particles are also can pass through it.
- Except blood cells and plasma proteins all can pass through it.
- The afferent arterioles carry the blood toward glomerular and efferent arterioles carry the blood away from it.
- The efferent arterioles' diameter is narrower than afferent which generates ***hydrostatic pressure.***
- With the help of this pressure, the blood filtrate through glomerulus.

KEY POINTS

- The trigone of the bladder originates from the meso-derm-derived Wolffian ducts while the remain-der of the bladder originates from the endoderm-derived urogenital sinus.
- The point where the ureter joins the urinary bladder is called the urete-ro-vesical junction and is the narrowest part of ureter.
- Narrowed portion of the ureter are more prone to develop stricture and urine stones.
- Right ureter is slightly shorter than the left.
- Most common cause of urethritis is **C. trachomatis**.

Practice Question

21. Which of the following areas of the kidney secretes renin into the blood?

a. Bowman's capsule
b. Distal convoluted tubule
c. Juxtaglomerular cells
d. Cortical nephron

Ans. (c) Juxtaglomerular cells

- **Net filtration pressure (NFP)**= 10 mm Hg
- **Filtration fraction** = (GFR/ Renal Plasma Flow)
  = (125 / 650) mL/minute
  = 19.2%
- **Filtration fraction** = (GFR/ Net filtration pressure)
  = (125 mL / 10 mm of Hg)
  = 12.5 mL / mm of Hg

Tubular Reabsorption

- Water is majorly reabsorbed through osmosis.
- Na^+ actively reabsorbed at ascending limb of Loop of Henle.
- Water is passively reabsorbed at descending loop of Henle and collecting duct along the osmotic gradient.
- Approximately 60–70% of filtrate is reabsorbed by PCT and 15–20% only goes to DCT.
- Reabsorption of Glucose, vitamins and amino acids also absorbed by active transport.
- Positive charge—reabsorbed actively
- Negative charge—reabsorbed passively
- Small protein—reabsorbed by pinocytosis
- Blood glucose level more than 180 mg/dL is the renal threshold for glucose.

Tubular Secretion or Excretion

- At PCT, H^+ is secreted which maintains blood pH and cells of DCT secrete K^+ with the exchange.
- Some drugs or substances (e.g., Penicillin) which are not filtered through glomerulus, are secreted into convoluted tubules.
- The final product of filtration, absorption, and secretion is hypertonic which is called urine.
- **Regulation of water in the body**
  - It is under the control of ADH hormone secreted by posterior pituitary.
  - ADH secretion occurs in response to hypovolemia, increased sodium level and in dehydration.
  - ADH makes DCT and collecting duct to reabsorb more water and thereby produce concentrated urine.

  Lack of ADH hormone leads to diabetes insipidus.
- **Regulation of sodium and Potassium in the body**
  - Controlled by two hormones; Aldosterone & Angiotensin II
    - **Aldosterone mechanism**
      - Retention of potassium is the most life threatening complication of renal failure.
    - **Renin-Angiotensin-Aldosterone mechanism**
      - Increased sodium and water reabsorption leads to increased blood volume and BP.

KEY POINTS

- Renin acts on Angiotensinogen to convert into Angiotensin I.
- The targets of angiotensin II are blood vessels and Adrenal cortex.
- The action of aldosterone is to increase Sodium reabsorption.
- The kidney secretes Erythropoietin to stimulate bone marrow activity.

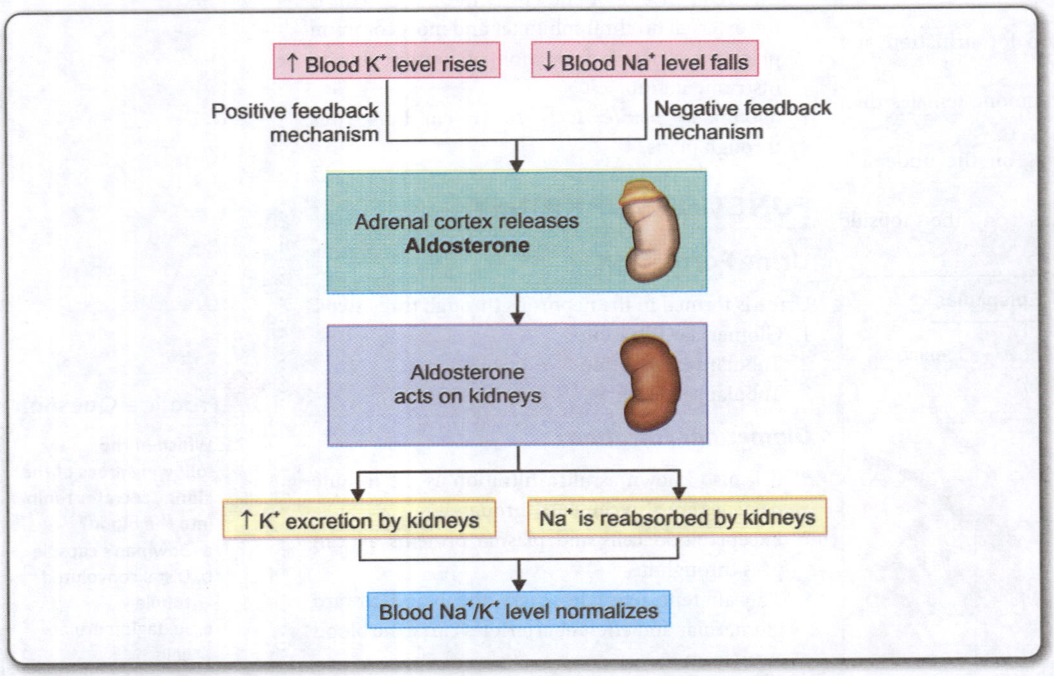

Figure 100: Sodium and potassium regulation by aldosterone

Recent Question (NORCET 2020)

70. A patient is taking furosemide. Which of the following to be included in the diet of the patient?
a. Nuts
b. Vegetable soups
c. Raw vegetables
d. Banana

Ans. (d) Banana

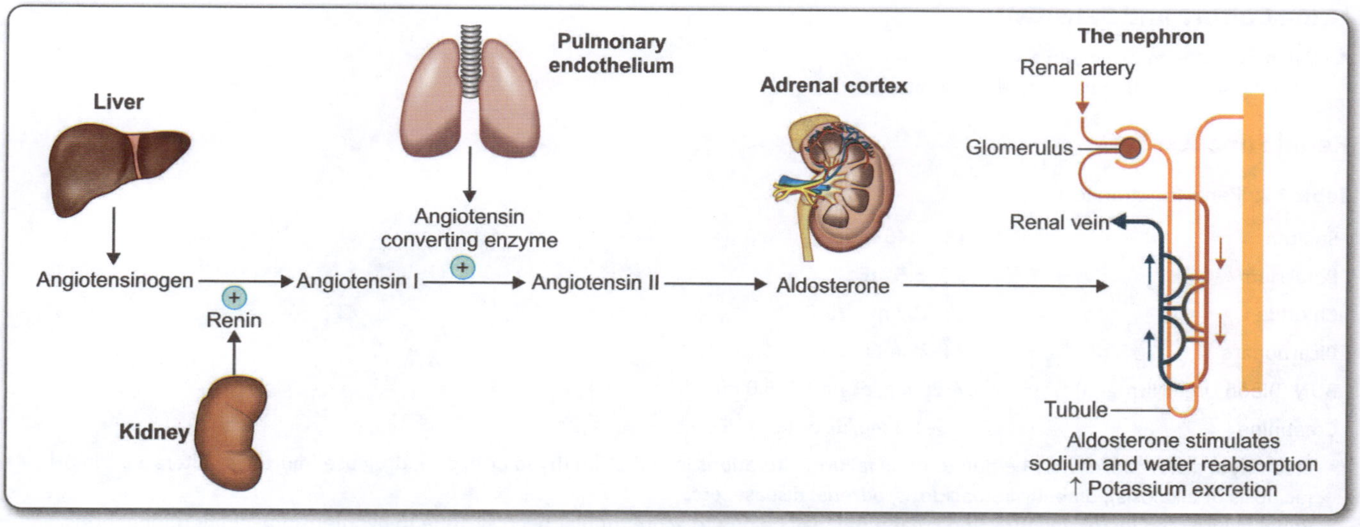

Figure 101: Renin-Angiotensin-Aldosterone mechanism

- **Regulation of blood pH**
  - Blood pH is controlled through buffer system
  - Carbonic acid and Sodium-bi-carbonate are blood buffers to maintain its pH.
  - Concentration of carbonic acid – Under the control of respiratory system
  - Concentration of bicarbonate - Under the control of kidney.
- Sodium is reabsorbed in DCT in exchange for hydrogen or potassium ion.
- **Regulation of RBC production**
  - When there is decreased oxygen tension in the renal blood flow kidney produces erythropoietin hormone which stimulates RBC production.
- **Vitamin D synthesis**
  - Kidneys are also responsible for final conversion of inactive form of vitamin D to its active form 1, 25 dihydroxy-cholecalciferol.

INVESTIGATIONS

Urine Specific Gravity

- Normal value: 1.010–1.030
- **Methods of assessment:** Multiple dipstick test, urinometer and refractometer

Urinalysis

- Catch early morning voiding sample.
- In case of a female patient with menstruation, indicate it in the form.

Table 79: Urinalysis values

Color	Straw
Specific gravity	1.005 to 1.030
pH	4.6–8.0
Na	40–220 mEq/24 hrs
K	25–125 mEq/24 hrs
Cl	80–250 mEq/day
Total Nitrogen	10–20 g/24 hrs
Creatinine	1.0 – 2.0 g/24 hrs
Calcium	0.1 – 0.7 g/24 hrs
Protein	1–15 mg/dL
Osmolality	80–1300 mOsm/L
Urine bilirubin	Negative
Urine blood	Negative
Urine ketone	Negative
Urine leukocytes	Negative
RBC's	0–2/HPF
WBC's	0–2/HPF
RBC casts	0/HPF

KEY POINTS

- Specific gravity increases in concentrated urine (with less fluid intake, dehydration, etc.)
- Specific gravity decreases in diluted urine (polyuria, diabetes insipidus, etc.)
- Uric acid results from purine metabolism.
- Eating large amounts of meat will increase the levels of urea in the blood.
- A decreased creatinine clearance is a sensitive indicator of a reduced GFR.

POINT TO REMEMBER

Inulin clearance Test: Gold standard test to estimate GFR (Creatinine clearance can overestimate GFR as it is also secreted into the proximal tubules).

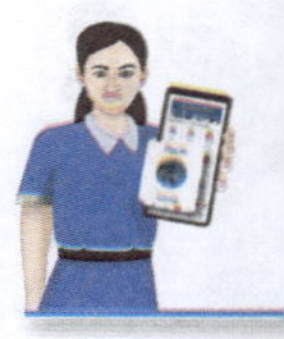

Urine Culture and Sensitivity

- Catch mid-stream urine into a sterile container
- Send the sample immediately to the laboratory.

Renal Function Test

Table 80: Renal function tests

Sodium	135–145 mEq/L
Potassium	3.5–5.5 mEq/L
Chloride	98–107 mEq/L
Bicarbonate	24–28 mEq/L
BUN (Blood Urea Nitrogen)	7–20 mg/dL or 2.5–8.0 mmol/L
Creatinine	0.6–1.2 mg/dL or 60–125 umol/L

- Electrolyte disturbances may be due to renal failure, alterations in hydration (hypo or hyper), drug use (diuretics), alterations in pH (acidosis or alkalosis), diabetic ketoacidosis, adrenal disease, etc.
- Renal failure (and increasing BUN and creatinine) may be due to acute tubular necrosis (due to hypotension), glomerulonephritis, diabetic nephropathy, urinary tract infection, etc.

KEY POINTS

Name of the procedure	Points to remember
Intravenous pyelography: After the injection with a dye, X-ray is taken to assess the renal system functioning.	**Pre-Procedure** • Informed consent • Assess allergy to dye, iodine and sea food • NPO after midnight • Inform the client about warm, salty, metallic taste after the injection of dye. **Post-procedure** • Increase the fluid intake if not contraindicated • Assess the puncture site for bleeding
Vanillylmandelic acid (VMA) test: 24 hr urine collection to diagnose pheochromocytoma.	• Instruct client to avoid foods such as coffee, cola, vanilla, cheese, gelatin and fruits before the test. • Instruct to avoid stress • Encourage adequate food and fluid intake
Renal angiography: Dye is injected through a catheter inserted in the axillary or femoral artery to examine renal vein and artery.	**Before procedure** • Informed consent • Assess allergy to dye, iodine and sea food. • NPO after midnight • Inform the client about warm, salty, metallic taste after the injection of dye. • Instruct client to void immediately before the procedure. **Post-procedure** • Observe the injection site for bleeding and hematoma. • If axillary artery is used, BP has to be taken on the opposite arm • Assess peripheral pulse distal to the puncture site to assess the circulation. • After the procedure client has to lie in **supine position with legs straight**.
Renal biopsy	**Before procedure** • Informed consent • Obtain coagulation studies • Position the client in a prone with pillow under abdomen and shoulder • NPO after midnight • Contraindications to biopsy are uncontrolled hypertension, solitary kidney and bleeding tendencies. **During procedure** • While inserting the needle client is instructed to **breathe in and hold the breath** to prevent kidney from moving. **Post-procedure** • Monitor for hypotension and tachycardia which indicates bleeding. • Apply pressure at puncture site • After biopsy, place client in supine position and on bed rest.

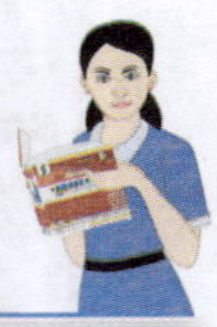

DISORDERS OF RENAL SYSTEM

Urethral Strictures

- Narrowing of the urethra as a result of contraction or scar.
- Gradual dilatation and surgery (internal urethrotomy) are the management.

Urolithiasis

- **Urolithiasis:** Stone anywhere in the urinary tract
- **Renal calculi or nephrolithiasis:** stone in the kidney
- **Causes:** Dehydration, presence of crystal forming substances, and absence of substances that inhibit crystallization of urine
- **Crystal forming substances:** Calcium, phosphate, Oxalate, Uric acid, cysteine
- **Crystallization preventing substances:** Magnesium, citrate, nephrocalcin and osteopontin
- **Predisposing factors:** Immobility, dehydration, increased calcium concentration in blood and urine
- **Pain in renal calculi:** Originates in lumbar region and radiates around the testicle in man and bladder in women.
- **Pain in urethral colic** will be radiating towards the genital area and thigh.
- **Uric acid stone**
  - Seen in patient with gout and myeloproliferative disease.
  - **Low purine diet** (restrict organ meat, mushroom and shellfish) is advised
  - **Treatment:** Allopurinol
  - **Alkaline-ash diet** is recommended (because it is acidic stone).
- **Oxalate stone**
  - Stone formation occurs in patient with inflammatory bowel disease, ileostomy or bowel resection because more oxalate will be absorbed in these patients.
  - Decrease intake of oxalate containing food items such as spinach, chocolate, almond, wheat bran, tea and peanut.
  - Acid-ash diet is recommended
  - It is produced by urinary tract infection (UTI) as this bacteria breakdown urea to ammonia which makes the urine more alkaline. Eg: Pseudomonas, E. Coli, Proteus, Staphylococcus, Klebsiella and Mycoplasma.
- **Struvite stone**
  - Also known as infection stone
  - Formed due to persistently alkaline and ammonia rich urine.
  - Composed of magnesium and ammonium phosphate.
  - Acid-ash diet is recommended.
- **Cystic stone**
  - Formed in patient with rare hereditary disorder of cysteine absorption
  - Client is instructed to avoid milk, meats, eggs and cheese
  - Alkaline ash and low methionine diet (as it converts to cysteine) is recommended.
- **Treatment of urolithiasis**

  General treatment
  - Primary goal – Pain relief
  - More fluid intake – up to 3 L/day
  - Stone size <5 mm – Treat with adequate hydration and diet.
  - **Cystoscopy:** For stones in lower ureter or bladder

Table 81: Differences between acid-ash diet and alkaline-ash diet

Acid-ash diet	Alkaline-ash diet
• Decreases the urinary pH • Foods to be included: ▪ Bread, cereal, whole grain, cheese, eggs, corn, legumes, plumes, tomato, meat, fish, poultry	• Increases urine pH • Foods to be included: ▪ Fruits except tomato, cranberry, plums, and prunes. ▪ Milk, most of the vegetables

  - **Extracorporeal shock wave lithotripsy (ESWL)**
    - Non-invasive method
    - Ultrasonic waves are used to crush the stone into pieces and it is excreted via urine
    - Fluoroscopy helps in visualizing stones.
    - Suitable for stones in upper ureter or kidney
    - **Before procedure:** Keep the patient NPO 8 hours before procedure
    - **Post procedure**
      - Monitor the client for bleeding
      - Maintain intake-output chart
      - Increase fluid intake
      - Ambulation helps in removal of stones
  - **Percutaneous lithotripsy**
    - Invasive method
    - Under fluoroscopy guidance, guide wire is inserted and ultrasonic waves are delivered to break the stone.
    - Used for ureter, bladder or kidney stones
- After surgery 3–4 L/day hydration is recommended to excrete out fragmented stone.

KEY POINTS

- More than 75% of urinary stones are calcium based. Calcium restriction along with increased fluid intake and thiazide diuretics are recommended.
- Low purine diet for uric acid stone
- Acid-ash diet is recommended for Oxalate and Struvite stone
- Alkaline-ash diet is recommended for Uric acid and cystic stone.
- **Stones formed in** Acidic urine: Uric acid stones and cystine stone.
- **Stones formed in** Alkaline urine: Struvite and phosphate.
- Acid-ash diet foods: fish, shellfish, meats, eggs, cheese and grains.
- Alkaline-ash diet foods: fruits and vegetables, soybeans and tofu, and some nuts, seeds, and legumes.
- **High oxalate diet** – Tea, almond, chocolate, cashew, nuts, spinach, almond, tomatoes, spinach etc.
- **High methionine diet** – Egg, meat, milk, and cheese.
- **Calcium-rich diet** – Milk, yogurt, cheese, fish (along with fishbone), dried fruits, nuts, beans (other than green beans).
- **Phosphate rich diet** – Whole grains, dairy products and meats.
- **High purine diet** – Sardines, red wines, gravies and organ meats.

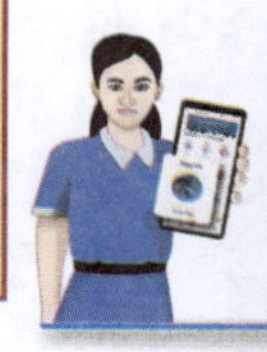

Ureteroscopy lithotripsy:

- By inserting a ureteroscope through urethra, a laser beam is directly targeted at stone and break it down. Average time needed is 30 minutes.
  - **Ureterolithotomy**
    - Open surgical procedure to remove stones in the ureter.

Glomerulonephritis

- Inflammation of glomeruli due to infection or autoimmune reactions in the body.
- Antigen-antibody reaction leads to inflammation of glomeruli
- **Causes**
  - Group A beta hemolytic streptococci
  - Immunological or autoimmune diseases
  - Autoimmune diseases such as systemic lupus erythematosus (SLE).

Types

- Acute – Develop within 2–3 weeks after streptococcal infection.
- Chronic – Develop slowly over may years.
- This can occur following a throat infection (strep throat) or impetigo
- **Clinical Manifestations**
  - Gross hematuria (blood is visible in urine)
  - Proteinuria
  - Dark smoky cola colored urine
  - Low urine pH
  - Increased C- reactive protein (CRP).
  - Increased specific gravity of urine
  - Increased BUN and serum creatinine
  - Oliguria or anuria
- **Increased ASO titer** can be seen

Management

- No potassium during oliguria
- Daily weight monitoring
- Antibiotic treatment (penicillin for streptococcal infection)
- High calorie, low sodium, low potassium, low protein diet is advised.

Complications

- Renal failure
- Hypertensive encephalopathy
- Pulmonary edema
- Heart failure

Nephrotic Syndrome

- Characterized by triad of symptoms such as heavy proteinuria (>1 g/m²/day), hypoalbuminemia (serum albumin <2.5 mg/dL) and edema.
- Monitor vital signs mainly BP for hypertension and hypotension due to fluid shift.
- Strict intake and output monitoring and abdominal girth monitoring.
- Assess daily weight on same time in minimal clothing.
- Edema first appears around the eyes and then it spreads to other body parts.
- Hypercoagulability is a well known complication due to loss of clotting factor which results in thromboembolism
- ***Anemia*** – Loss of transferrin protein through renal system.
- **Management**
  - Diuretics, corticosteroids
  - Low sodium and low to moderate protein diet.
  - Provides sufficient carbohydrate and calorie-rich food

KEY POINTS

- Most common cause of nephrotic syndrome in adults is Diabetes Mellitus.
- Nephrotic syndrome is more common in male children aged between 2 and 6 years.
- The hallmark of nephrotic syndrome is heavy **proteinuria**, and the most common presenting sign is edema.
- **Nephritic syndrome** is a condition involving **hematuria**, mild to moderate proteinuria (typically less than 3.5 g/L/day), hypertension, oliguria and red cell casts in the urine.
- Most common type of Acute Renal Failure (ARF) is prerenal failure.

Table 82: Comparison of nephritic syndrome and nephrotic syndrome

Nephritic syndrome	Nephrotic syndrome
• Hematuria • Azotemia • Proteinuria (<3.5 g/day) • Oliguria • Edema • Hypertension	• Proteinuria (>3.5 g/day) • Hypoalbuminemia • Hyperlipidemia • Lipiduria • Edema

KEY POINTS

- **Increased ASO titer** can be seen in Glomerulonephritis.
- High calorie, low sodium, low potassium, low protein diet is advised in Glomerulonephritis.
- Low sodium and low to moderate protein diet is advised in Nephrotic syndrome.

Acute Renal Failure (ARF)

- Rapid loss of kidney function from renal cell damage.
- Causes of renal failure

Table 83: Causes of renal failure

Pre-renal cause	Intra-renal cause	Post-renal cause
Impaired renal blood flow leads to hypo perfusion in the kidney	Glomeruli damage lead to impaired filtration	Obstruction beyond kidney
Volume depletion Heart failure Sepsis Anaphylaxis	Burns Renal trauma Infection Nephrotoxic drug	Bladder neck obstruction Bladder cancer Calculi Post renal infection

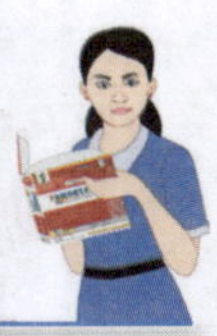

Phases of Renal Failure

1. Initiation
• Start with initial insult till the development of oliguria
2. Oliguria
• Urine output less than 400 mL/day • Signs of excess fluid volume such as hypertension, pleural effusion, pericardial effusion, edema, CHF • Signs of metabolic acidosis including Kussmaul's respiration • Hypervolemia, hyperkalemia and hypernatremia
3. Diuresis
• Urine output slowly rises • Gradual decline in BUN level and creatinine level. • Hyponatremia and hypovolemia can occur.
4. Recovery
Improvement in GFR

- **Nursing Management**
  - Strict intake and output monitoring
  - Daily weight on same scale at same time in minimal clothing

Chronic Renal Failure (End Stage Renal Disease)

- Progressive and irreversible loss of renal function which leads to azotemia and uremia.
- Uremic syndrome causes varying symptoms in the body and it will affect almost all systems of the body.

Uremic syndrome: Refers to accumulation of nitrogenous waste in the body due to the inability of kidneys to filter them in ARF and CRF.

- **Clinical manifestations**
  - Hypertension (due to sodium and water accumulation)
  - Pulmonary edema (due to fluid overload)
  - Pericarditis (due to uremic toxins)
  - Pruritus, uremic frost (due to uremic toxins)
  - Weakness, fatigue, confusion, tremors, seizure, disorientation
  - Crackles, pleuritic pain, Kussmaul respiration
  - Uremic fetor (ammonia odor to breathe), metallic taste, nausea, vomiting
  - Anemia, thrombocytopenia, hyperkalemia

Stages of CKD

Stage 1
• 40–75% of nephrons are damaged. • Patient remains asymptomatic as the remaining nephrons overwork
Stage 2
• 75–90% of the nephrons lost their function. • Serum BUN and creatinine rise. • Polyuria and nocturia occur in patient.
Stage 3 (End Stage Renal Disease)
• Less than 10% of the nephrons are functioning. • Dialysis is needed immediately

Hemodialysis

- Removal of uremic and nitrogenous waste from the body with the help of a machine.
- A dialyzer or artificial kidney serves as a semi-permeable membrane in place of renal glomeruli.
- Principles used in Hemodialysis:
  - **Diffusion:** Toxins and waste products move from area of higher concentration to area of lower concentration, i.e., from blood to dialysate.
  - **Osmosis:** Water moves from area of higher solute concentration to area of lower solute concentration.
  - **Ultrafiltration:** Water moving from area of higher pressure to area of lower pressure. More efficient method in removing water than osmosis. This can be achieved by applying negative pressure or suction to dialysate membrane.
    - Bicarbonate or acetate is used in dialysate bath preparation.
- **Dialyzer**
  - Flat plate or hollow fiber dialyzers are available. Semipermeable membrane is made up of cellophane tubules.

KEY POINTS

- Daily weight on same scale at same time is the best method to monitor fluid balance.
- CKD patients are at risk for life threatening arrhythmia due to hyperkalemia. Need to be continuously monitored.
- Injection erythropoietin is needed by CKD client to stimulate erythropoiesis.
- Peritoneal dialysate contains higher glucose concentration than hemodialysis.
- Client with femoral catheter should not sit at more than 45 degree angle because it may lead to catheter displacement.

KEY POINTS

- Oliguria refers to Urine output less than 400 mL/day.
- Daily weight on same scale at same time in minimal clothing is an important nursing assessment for patient with Acute renal failure.
- Principles used in Hemodialysis are diffusion, osmosis and ultrafiltration.

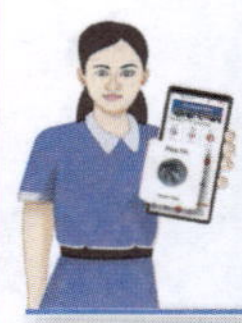

- **Dialysate**
  - The fluid medium passed in a dialysis filter (membrane) to exchange solutes with the blood is known as dialysate.
  - The composition of dialysate includes Sodium, Potassium, Chloride, Calcium, Magnesium, Acetate, Bicarbonate, Lactate and Glucose.
  - Dialysate flow rate of 500–800 mL/min will produce an efficient dialysis

Vascular Access in Hemodialysis

- **Subclavian/Internal jugular/Femoral**
  - Insert double lumen or multiple lumen catheter into the desired vein to establish vascular access.
  - Assess site for bleeding, hematoma, infection and thrombus formation.
  - Between dialysis treatments, catheter should be filled with heparin and cap it to maintain patency of the line.
- **Fistula**
  - Anastomosing an artery and vein either side to side or end to side
  - Arterial segment is for outflow and venous segment is for inflow.
  - **Maturity** of the fistula will take **4–6 weeks**.
  - **Squeezing of a ball** exercise helps the fistula to mature.

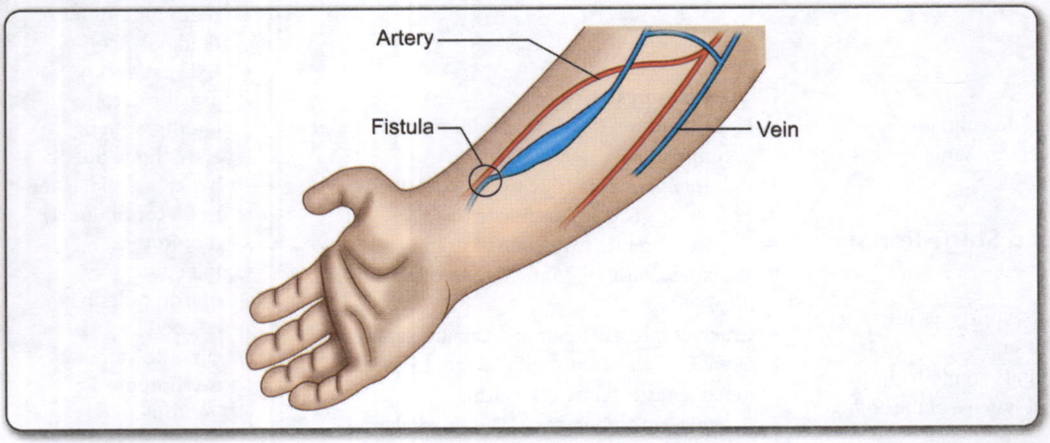

Figure 102: Fistula

- **Graft**
  - It is created by placing a biological or semi-biological or synthetic material between artery and vein.
  - This is used when fistula is not possible.
  - **Complications:** Thrombosis and infection are the most common complications
  - Graft can be **used after 2 weeks** of creation.

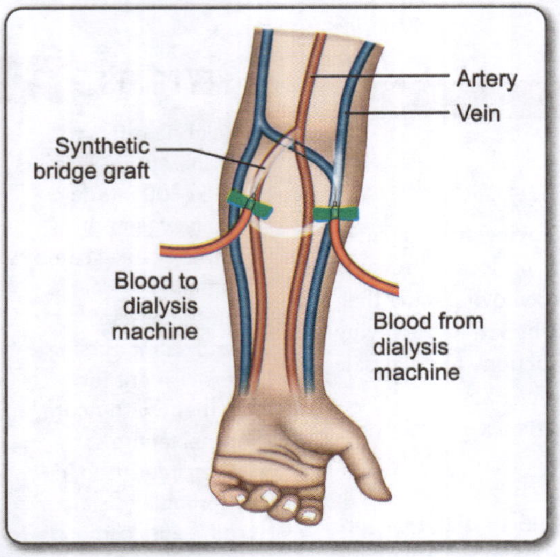

Figure 103: Vascular access

Complications of Hemodialysis

- **Hypotension:** A client may be asked to skip anti-hypertensive drug dosage before hemodialysis.
- **Muscle cramps** due to the movement of electrolyte from extracellular space.
- **Dysrhythmia** due to fluid and electrolyte changes.
- Air embolism.
- **Disequilibrium syndrome:** During hemodialysis, solutes are removed faster from ECF, as compared to CSF. This causes fluid shift into the brain and cerebral edema.
- Dialysis encephalopathy – It is caused by toxicity of Aluminium of dialysate
- **Management:** Stop dialysis and reduce the duration of dialysis. Administer Hypertonic solution, Albumin and mannitol.

Management of air embolism during hemodialysis

- Stop hemodialysis
- Place client in left lateral position with head down (to trap the emboli in right side of the heart and prevent its movement toward lung.)
- Administer oxygen
- Assess vital sign and record the event.

KEY POINTS

- Disequilibrium syndrome is a rare but potentially serious complication that can occur after the first session of hemodialysis.
- Early signs of Disequilibrium syndrome include nausea, headache, vomiting, and restlessness. More serious symptoms can result in seizures and coma.

KEY POINTS

- **Arterial steal syndrome** can happen in case of fistula or graft because too much of blood is diverted into the venous end and it can even lead to Congestive Heart Failure.

Points to remember while caring a client with graft or fistula are:

- **Extremity with graft or fistula** should not be used for BP monitoring, IV line insertion, drawing blood sample or giving injections.
- Normally a **thrill can be palpated** and a **bruit can be auscultated** over graft or fistula site.
- Palpate the pulse distal to fistula or graft to ensure tissue perfusion.

Drugs used in Hemodialysis

- **Heparin:** Dialysis machine tubing is first flushed with heparinized saline to prevent clotting of the blood in the circuit.
- **Erythropoietin injection:** Subcutaneous erythropoietin injection is given to client on hemodialysis to stimulate RBC production.

Peritoneal Dialysis (PD)

- Peritoneum acts as a semipermeable membrane.
- Osmosis and diffusion are the major principles.
- Water removal is achieved through ultrafiltration which is created using higher glucose concentration in the dialysate fluid.

PD catheter insertion

- Informed consent
- Empty the bladder to avoid injury to the bladder
- Catheter is inserted 3–5 cm below the umbilicus as this area is free of any major blood vessels.
- Usual PD catheters are swanz, tenkoff, and cruz made up of silicon material which is radio-opaque.

Performing PD Exchange/Cycle

- PD contains many exchanges or cycle.
- One exchange or cycle consists of infusion, dwell and drainage.
  - **Infusion:** Flowing of PD fluid into the abdominal cavity under the influence of gravity.
  - **Dwell:** Withholding the dialysate fluid in the abdominal cavity for prescribed period of time.

Do not extent the dwell time beyond prescribed as it increases the risk for hyperglycemia.

  - **Drainage:** Once the dwell time is over, drainage will be started by unclamping the catheter under the influence of gravity.

Normally PD drainage is colorless or straw colored. If the drainage is cloudy, peritonitis need to be suspected in the patient.

- Heparin, potassium and antibiotics may be added to PD fluid.

In a PD patient, excessive water is removed by adding glucose/dextrose to the dialysate fluid to make it hypertonic.

KEY POINTS

- Monitor base line vitals and laboratory values before and after HD.
- After HD, patient's temperature may be slightly elevated due to the warming of blood by dialysis machine.
- Weight of the client has to be taken before and after HD to calculate fluid loss.

Recent Question (NORCET 2020)

71. **Arteriovenous fistula is assessed for**
    a. giving IV medication
    b. blood sampling
    c. arterial BP
    d. patency

Ans. (d) patency

POINT TO REMEMBER

Peritonitis is the most common complication associated with Peritoneal dialysis.

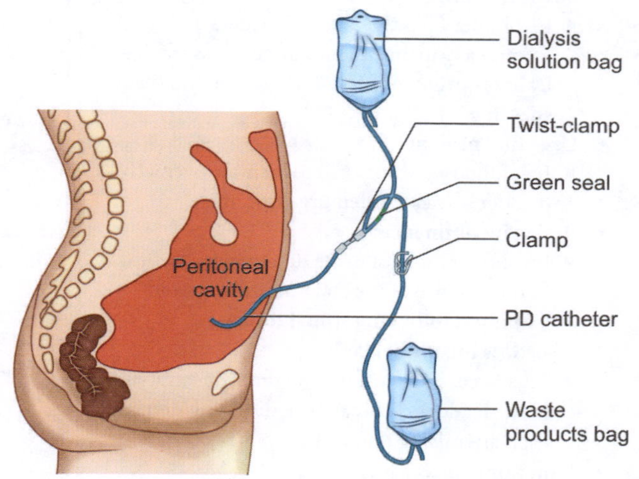

Figure 104: Peritoneal dialysis

Complications of PD

- **Peritonitis:** Most common complication of PD is characterized by cloudy outflow, rebound tenderness and abdominal pain.
- **Leakage**
- **Bleeding:** During bleeding, more frequent exchange is needed to avoid clot formation in the PD catheter.
- **Long-term complications:** Hypertriglyceridemia, abdominal hernia, aggravation of hemorrhoids, lower backache and anorexia.

Types of Peritoneal Dialysis

- **Acute intermittent PD**
  - Treatment of choice for hemodynamically unstable patient.
  - PD is performed with the help of PD machine. It removes fluid gradually.
- **Continuous ambulatory PD**
  - After infusion of dialysate, patient fold back the bags, clamp the catheter and move around. Patient is ambulatory during dwell time.
  - Once dwell time is over patient lies down and drainage will be initiated.

- **Continuous cyclic PD**
  - Dialysis is done with the help of machine.
  - Usually 3 cycles are done at night and one cycle with long dwell time of 8 hours is done in the morning.

RENAL TRANSPLANT

- Transplantation of kidney from a living/cadaver donor to a client with End Stage Renal Disease.
- **Donor Screened for:** ABO incompatibility, tissue specific antigen, histocompatibility and communicable disease.
- **Cold ischemic time:** Time gap between cessation of blood flow to kidney and the time required to anastomosis the kidney to the recipient.
- **Preoperative**
  - Immunosuppressive therapy
  - Completion of hemodialysis 24 hours before the transplantation
  - Strict aseptic technique. Recipient must be free from infection.
- **Postoperative**
  - Urine output may be established immediately in living donor kidney and may be delayed in cadaveric donor kidney.
  - Hemodialysis is needed until the adequate renal function is established.
  - Monitor urine output hourly.
  - Daily weight monitoring.

Graft Rejection

- **Hyper acute rejection:** Rejection occurs within minutes to hours
- **Acute rejection:** Usually occurs within 6 weeks post-operatively
- **Chronic rejection:** Occurs in months to years after the transplantation

Oliguria, edema, fever, increased BP, weight gain, swelling and tenderness over the transplanted site are the symptoms of rejection.

MISCELLANEOUS URINARY DISEASES

Urinary Tract Infections

- UTI is caused by pathogenic organism in the urinary tract.
- Upper UTI includes:
  - Pyelonephritis (inflammation of renal pelvis)
  - Interstitial nephritis (inflammation of the kidney)
- Lower UTI includes:
  - Cystitis (inflammation of urinary bladder)
  - Prostatitis (inflammation of prostate gland)
  - Urethritis (inflammation of urethra)
- **Manifestations:** Frequent pain and burning micturition, frequency, urgency, nocturia, incontinence, fever, chills, flank or lower back ache, and **tenderness in costovertebral angle**.
- Colony count of at least **1,000,000/mL of urine** is the major criteria for UTI.
- **Hematuria:** More than 4 RBC per high power field
- **Pyuria:** More than 4 WBC per high power field.
- **Diagnosis:** Urine culture and sensitivity.

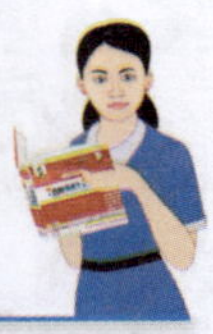

Management

- Antibiotic treatment with nitrofurantoin, sulfa drugs, quinolones, or cephalosporins.
- Increased fluid intake
- Acid-ash diet
- Perineal care for female
- Urinate after every intercourse.

Pyelonephritis

- Repeated attack of UTI leads to chronic pyelonephritis.
- *E. coli* is the most common causative organism.

Urinary Incontinence

- Unplanned involuntary loss of urine
- **Stress incontinence**
  - Involuntary passage of urine occurs as a result of increase in intra-abdominal pressure, e.g., leak of urine occurs during coughing and sneezing.
- **Urge incontinence**
  - Involuntary loss of urine when an overactive bladder causes sudden urge to urinate.
- **Reflex incontinence**
  - Involuntary loss of urine due to hyper-reflexia in the absence of normal sensation to void.
  - **Common following spinal injury.**
- **Overflow incontinence**
  - This occurs as a result of incomplete emptying of the bladder. There will be dribbling of urine even after using the washroom.
- **Functional incontinence**
  - Normal lower urinary tract. Cognitive and physical impairment makes it difficult to void.
- **Iatrogenic incontinence**
  - Incontinence occurs as a result of external medical factors such as medication.
- **Management:** Behavioral therapy, anti-cholinergic agents and surgical management (if any anatomical problem present).

Urinary Retention

- Inability to empty bladder completely during voiding
- This leads to overflow incontinence
- **Causes:** Diabetes mellitus, prostate enlargement, pregnancy, trauma to pelvic floor
- **Complications:** Infection, calculi and pyelonephritis.

KEY POINTS

- High protein loss occurs during peritoneal dialysis (PD), so the client is advised to consume high protein diet and low carbohydrate diet.
- Most common viral infection after renal transplant is CMV

KEY POINTS

- Most common agent associated with catheter associated UTI → E. coli
- Urinary tract is the most common site for nosocomial infection.
- UTIs are common among women than men because of their shorter urethra and proximity of the urethra to the rectum

Practice Question

22. The best indicator of renal function in a postoperative patient is

a. Level of consciousness
b. Hemoglobin level
c. Urine output
d. Thirst

Ans. (c) Urine output

Neurogenic Bladder

- Bladder dysfunction due to lesion in the nervous system.
- It can occur following spinal cord injury, prolapsed inter vertebral disc, spinal tumor, multiple sclerosis, spina bifida, etc.
- There are two types of neurogenic bladders:
  - **Spastic neurogenic bladder**
    - Injury on upper motor neuron
    - No conscious sensation of voiding
    - Bladder emptied on reflex (reflex incontinence)
  - **Flaccid neurogenic bladder**
    - Injury on lower motor neuron
    - Bladder won't contract forcefully. Leads to overflow incontinence.
  - **Complications:** UTI, renal calculi, Vesicoureteral Reflux (VUR), renal failure
  - **Management**: Catheterization and adequate fluid intake.

Vesicoureteral Reflex

- Retrograde or back flow of urine from bladder to ureter even sometimes to kidney is known as VUR.
- **Features of recurrent VUR:** UTI, palpable renal mass, and renal failure
- **Diagnosis:** Voiding cystourethrogram, uroflometry.

Golden Points to Remember

- **Length of male urethra:** 18 to 20 cm
- **Length of Female urethra:** 4 to 5 cm
- **Normal weight of prostate gland:** 20 g
- **Significant post void residual volume:** >50 mL
- The renal artery first divides into segmental arteries, followed by further branching to form **multiple interlobar arteries** that pass through the renal columns to reach the renal cortex.
- **Interlobar veins from kidney drains into inferior vena cava.**
- **Microalbuminuria:** Urinary albumin excretion of 30–300 mg/day.
- Neonatal kidney achieves concentrating ability equivalent to adult kidney around the age of 1 year.
- Infant kidney achieves GFR as of adult values around 2 years of age.
- Stress urinary incontinence is more common in women.
- **Tear drop bladder** on Intravenous Pyelogram (IVP) suggest: Pelvic hematoma
- **Spider leg appearance** in IVP is suggestive of: Renal cyst
- Water deprivation test is used to access the function of distal tubule.
- **Aminoglycoside antibiotics** (e.g. amikacin, gentamycin) are nephrotoxic drugs.
- **Lasix** competes with aspirin for renal excretion sites and may cause **aspirin toxicity**.
- Chronic glomerulonephritis is a syndrome characterized by proteinuria, hematuria and slow development of uremia.
- **Hyperkalemia** is one of the serious complications of acute renal failure, it can cause life-threatening cardiac dyserhythmias.
- Syndrome of Inappropriate Antidiuretic Hormone (SIADH) causes increased urine osmolarity, increased urine sodium concentration and decreased plasma osmolarity
- Cystine stones are very rare and occur due to an inborn congenital disorder
- Nail and half nail sign are seen in Renal failure.
- Dialysis in initiated when **GFR (or creatinine clearance)** is less than 15 mL/minute.
- **Ham test:** Blood test to diagnose paroxysmal nocturnal hemoglobinuria (PNH).
- Furosemide (Loop diuretics) acts on the thick **ascending loop of Henle.**
- Thiazides and potassium sparing diuretics act in the early **distal tubule**.
- Osmotic diuretics acts in **Descending limb of the loop of Henle.**

Most Common

- **Most common cause of neurogenic bladder in children:** Spina bifida
- Most common renal calculus is calcium oxalate dihydrate.
- Most common hospital acquired infection is UTI.
- Most common agent associated with catheter associated UTI is E. coli.
- Most common cause of complicated UTI is E. coli.
- Most common viral infection after renal transplant is CMV.
- Most common cause of Nephrotic syndrome in adults is Diabetes Mellitus.
- Most common type of ARF is Prerenal.

"An ounce of prevention is worth a pound of cure."
—Unknown

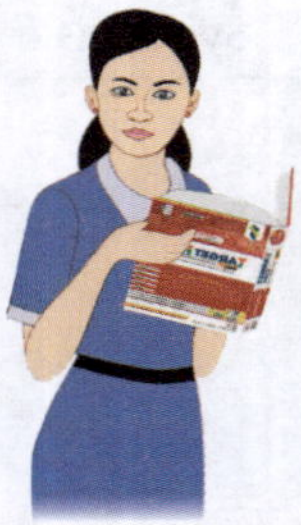

MULTIPLE CHOICE QUESTIONS
(Including Explained and Practice Questions)

RENAL SYSTEM

ANATOMY AND PHYSIOLOGY OF KIDNEY

2235. The main function of kidney is to: *(RRB SSNE 2015)*
- a. Eliminate oxygen
- b. Regulate fluid balance and removing waste products
- c. Metabolize vitamins
- d. Eliminate carbon dioxide

2236. Weight of kidney is:
- a. 150 g
- b. 100 g
- c. 200 g
- d. 80 g

2237. Excretory unit of kidney is: *(LNJP H D 2012)*
- a. Nephron
- b. Henle's loop
- c. Bowman's capsule
- d. Glomerulus

2238. The organs of the excretory system consist of the following; EXCEPT:
- a. Blood vessels
- b. Skin
- c. Liver
- d. Kidneys

2239. The interstitium of kidney tissue that has the highest osmolality is the:
- a. Outer cortex
- b. Outer medulla
- c. Inner cortex
- d. Inner medulla

2240. The functional unit of kidney is called:
- a. Bowman's Capsule
- b. Malpighian corpuscles
- c. Pyramid
- d. Nephron

2241. Renal vein is .... to superior mesenteric artery:
- a. Posterior and inferior
- b. Posterior and superior
- c. Anterior and inferior
- d. Anterior and superior

2242. Countercurrent mechanism in the kidney is responsible for:
- a. Absorption of glucose
- b. Maintenance of blood flow
- c. Osmotic gradient in medulla
- d. Secretion of uric acid

2243. Diaphragm is supplied by which nerve:
- a. Phrenic nerve
- b. Intercostal
- c. Peroneal
- d. Vagus

2244. Thirst is activated by:
- a. Increased Angiotensin II level
- b. Extracellular hyperosmolarity
- c. Increased ANP levels
- d. Increased Renin levels

2245. Right kidney is lower than the left kidney because:
- a. In right side liver is occupying considerable space
- b. Right kidney is larger in size
- c. Pulling force exerted by renal ligament on right side
- d. Left kidney is smaller in size

2246. How the kidneys help normalizes blood pressure in a hypotensive patient?
- a. Retain sodium and excrete water
- b. Retain sodium and water
- c. Excrete sodium and retain water
- d. Excrete sodium and water

2247. The three regions of kidney are:
- a. Cortex, medulla, peritoneum
- b. Cortex, medulla, pelvis
- c. Cortex, mediastinum, pelvis
- d. Omentum medulla, pelvis

2248. Each kidney consist is of:
- a. Ten thousand nephrons
- b. 1 billion nephrons
- c. 1 million nephrons
- d. Thousand nephrons

2249. Structures involved in blood pH regulation is:
- a. Kidney
- b. Blood plasma
- c. Lungs
- d. All of these

2250. Which of the following is TRUE regarding Renin-Angiotensin-Aldosterone System (RAAS) mechanism?
- a. Decreased urine output, increased reabsorption of sodium and water
- b. Decreased urine output, decreased reabsorption of sodium and water
- c. Increased urine output, increased reabsorption of sodium and water
- d. Increased urine output, decreased reabsorption of sodium and water

2251. The hormone which regulate the blood pressure and is primarily secreted by the kidney is:
- a. Angiotensinogen
- b. Erythropoietin
- c. Renin
- d. Aldosterone

2252. Hydronephrosis means:
- a. Dilation of renal pelvis
- b. Constriction of renal pelvis
- c. Narrowing of renal pelvis
- d. Atrophy of renal pelvis

ANATOMY AND PHYSIOLOGY OF URETER AND BLADDER

2253. Length of ureters:
- a. 8–12 cm
- b. 25–30 cm
- c. 40–50 cm
- d. 10–20 cm

2254. Normal range of glomerular filtration rate is: *(JIPMER 2012)*
- a. 90 –120 mL/m
- b. 120–150 mL/m
- c. 60–90 mL/hr
- d. 30–50 mL/hr

2255. The blood vessels entering the glomerulus is known as:
- a. Afferent
- b. Efferent
- c. Renal artery
- d. Renal vein

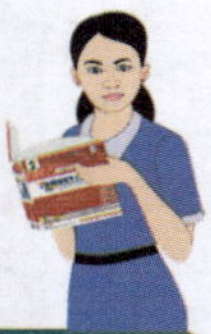

Ans.

2235. b
2236. a
2237. a
2238. a
2239. d
2240. d
2241. a
2242. c
2243. a
2244. b
2245. a
2246. b
2247. b
2248. c
2249. d
2250. a
2251. c
2252. a
2253. b
2254. a
2255. a

2256. The blood vessels leaving the glomerulus is known as:
a. Afferent b. Efferent
c. Renal artery d. Renal vein

2257. The immediate structure that channels urine to the ureters is the:
a. Renal pyramids b. Renal Calyces
c. Renal Pelvis d. Renal hilum

2258. Which part of the nephron is relatively impermeable to water?
a. Descending loop of Henle
b. Ascending loop of Henle
c. Distal convoluted tubule
d. Collecting duct

2259. The formation of filtrate in the Bowman's capsule across the glomerulus occurs by a process called:
a. Ultrafiltration b. Active transport
c. Osmosis d. Diffusion

2260. Payer's patches are found in:
a. Stomach b. Liver
c. Small intestine d. Large intestine

2261. GFR is increased by:
a. ANP b. Vasopressin
c. Histamine d. Endothelium

2262. Best measure for GFR:
a. Serum creatinine b. Urine output
c. BUN d. PAN

2263. Potassium is maximally absorbed in which part of nephron:
a. Proximal convoluted tubules
b. DCT
c. Collecting ducts
d. Loop of Henle

2264. Amount of blood filtered in renal capsule per minute is known as:
a. Glomerular filtration rate
b. Urine per minute
c. Tidal volume
d. Blood flow per minute

Explanation: Glomerular filtration rate (GFR) is a test used to check how well the kidneys are working. Specifically, it estimates how much blood passes through the glomeruli each minute. Glomeruli are the tiny filters in the kidneys that filter waste from the blood. According to the National Kidney Foundation, normal results range from 90 to 120 mL/min/1.73 m^2. Older people will have lower than normal GFR levels, because GFR decreases with age.

2265. Polyuria is seen in:
a. Diabetes insipidus b. Diabetes mellitus
c. Chronic renal failure d. All of these

2266. In a patient who is complaining of intra-abdominal pressure nurse is suspecting certain mass like structure above the pubis symphysis, that is:
a. Appendix
b. Cholelithiasis
c. Nephrolithiasis
d. Urinary bladder

2267. Oliguria and decreased creatinine clearance indicate problem with:
a. Tubular secretion
b. Glomerular filtration
c. Tubular reabsorption
d. Counter current mechanism

2268. How Furosemide (Lasix) helps to control BP?
a. It dilates renal blood vessels
b. It deactivates sympathetic nervous system
c. Activate RAAS mechanism
d. Decreases reabsorption of sodium and water in the loop of Henle

ANATOMY AND PHYSIOLOGY OF URETHRA

2269. Length of female urethra is:
a. 2 cm b.. 3 cm
c. 4 cm d. 6 cm

2270. The urethra connects the bladder to the:
a. Kidney
b. Renal pelvis
c. Urethral orifice
d. Uterus

2271. The internal urethral sphincter is made of:
a. Smooth involuntary muscles
b. Skeletal voluntary muscle
c. Smooth voluntary muscles
d. Skeletal Involuntary muscles

2272. The external urethral sphincter is made up of:
a. Smooth involuntary muscles
b. Skeletal voluntary muscle
c. Smooth voluntary muscles
d. Skeletal Involuntary muscles

PHYSIOLOGY OF URINE FORMATION

2273. Urine formation is most likely reduced in this condition:
a. Pulse rate of 100–110/minute
b. Pulse rate of 60–70/minute
c. Blood pressure of 70/40 mm Hg
d. Blood pressure of 90/40 mm Hg

2274. A patient weighing 50 kg would be suspected of oliguria if the hourly urine output is:
a. 15 mL b 25 mL
c. 35 mL d. 45 mL

2275. Voluntary micturition will occur when the:
a. Detrusor contracts
b. Detrusor muscle relaxes
c. External sphincter contracts
d. External sphincter relaxes

2276. Which of the following physiological response is expected in a client with hypernatremia?
a. Diminished action of ADH
b. Increased secretion of ADH
c. Secretion of aldosterone
d. Decreased reabsorption of water in the renal system

Explanation: Normal defenses against hypernatremia are thirst and the secretion of ADH. ADH plays a role in lowering osmolarity (reducing sodium concentration) by increasing water reabsorption in the kidneys, thus helping to dilute bodily fluids.

2277. Glycosuria is the manifestation of all of the following; EXCEPT:
a. Diabetes mellitus b. Cushing's syndrome
c. Hyperthyroidism d. SIADH

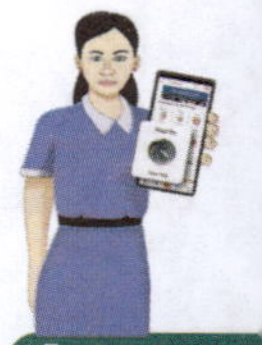

Ans.
2256. b
2257. c
2258. b
2259. a
2260. c
2261. a
2262. a
2263. a
2264. a
2265. d
2266. d
2267. b
2268. d
2269. c
2270. c
2271. a
2272. b
2273. c
2274. a
2275. d
2276. b
2277. d

2278. Anuria means:
a. More urine at night time
b. Urine output of less than 100 mL in 24 hours
c. Urine output of at least 100 mL in 2 hours
d. Urine output less than 400 mL in 24 hours

2279. Oliguria means:
a. More urine at night time
b. Urine output of less than 100 mL in 24 hours
c. Urine output of at least 100 mL in 2 hours
d. Urine output less than 400 mL in 24 hours

2280. All the food item cause color to the urine; EXCEPT: *(IHBAS 2002)*
a. Berries b. Beets
c. Carrot d. Food coloring agents

Explanation: Option c is the correct answer except carrot all the given food items cause red color to the urine.

2281. Frequency of urination at night is called:
a. Dysuria b. Nocturia
c. Oliguria d. Anuria

2282. The highest concentration of HIV virus is found in:
a. Saliva b. CSF
c. Blood d. Semen

2283. Disease like chromosomal abnormalities, hemophilia and thalassemia are of _________:
a. Infectious origin b. Hereditary origin
c. Developmental origin d. Psychological origin

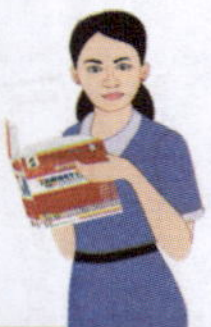

ASSESSMENT AND DIAGNOSTIC TEST

2284. The secretion of aldosterone would be inhibited in this situation:
a. Serum urea of 5.0 mmol/L
b. Serum creatinine of 100 mmol/L
c. Serum potassium of 4.0 mmol/L
d. Serum sodium of 160 mmol/L

2285. Best method to collect urine for culture in children under 2 years is:
a. Midstream voiding b. Bag aspiration
c. Catheter aspiration d. Suprapubic aspiration

2286. Way to obtain sterile urine specimen from an indwelling urinary catheter is:
a. Clamp the catheter above the bifurcation and aspirate
b. Disconnect the tubing and collect
c. From the urinary bag
d. All of these

2287. BUN used for kidney function tests stand for: *(Banaras HU 2015)*
a. Blood urine nitrogen b. Blood uric acid nitrogen
c. Blood uracil nitrogen d. Blood urea nitrogen

2288. Identify the change that does not occur in a urine sample after prolonged time?
a. Decrease in specific gravity
b. Loss of ketone bodies
c. Bacterial growth
d. Disintegration of casts

2289. Instrument used for measuring urinary specific gravity is all; EXCEPT:
a. Urinometer b. Refractometer
c. Reagent strips d. Densitometry

Explanation: Densitometry is the quantitative measurement of optical density in light-sensitive materials. All other instruments are used for measuring specific gravity.

2290. Normal specific gravity of urine is:
a. 1.010–1.030
b. 1.001–1.50
c. 1.05–1.5
d. 1.05–1.8

2291. Random urine test contain .... amount of protein.
a. 30-40 mg/dL
b. 0–20 mg/dL
c. 50–60 mg/dL
d. 60–120 mg/dL

2292. Normal serum creatinine level:
a. 0.5–1.1 mg/dL b. 0.6–2 mg/dL
c. 0.1 –0.6 mg/dL d. 0.8–2 mg/dL

2293. Creatinine clearance is measured as the amount of creatinine the kidneys are able to clear in a _____ period.
a. 12 hours b. 18 hours
c. 24 hours d. 36 hours

2294. Normal GFR level: *(AIIMS Bhopal Senior Nursing Officer 2018)*
a. 60 mL/min b. 80 mL/min
c. 120 mL/min d. 180 mL/min

2295. Normal range of pH of urine is:
a. 4.5–8.0 b. 4.0– 6.0
c. 6.0–7.0 d. 7.0–8.0

2296. PH of normal urine is:
a. Slightly alkaline b. Slightly acidic
c. Highly alkaline d. Highly acidic

2297. Normal level of urea in the blood is:
a. 2-15 mg/dL
b. 7-20 mg/dL
c. 15-40 mg/dL
d. 20-50 mg/dL

2298. Normal urine output per day in an adult is:
a. 500-1000 mL/day
b. 800 to 2000 mL/day
c. 1000-2500 mL/day
d. 1500-3000 mL/day

2299. Which of the following is normally found in urine?
a. Glucose b. Protein
c. RBC d. Creatinine

2300. A patient is scheduled for an IVP using a radio-opaque dye, which of the following assessment is most critical before the procedure: *(LNJP H D 2012)*
a. Measurement of baseline peripheral pulse rates
b. History of intake and output
c. History of allergy to iodine
d. Measurement of heights and weight

2301. Renal blood flow, glomerular filtration, tubular function, and excretion can be assessed with the help of:
a. IVP b. VCUG
c. Renal scan d. Ultrasonography

2302. In a dehydrated client urinary specific gravity will be:
a. Elevated
b. Decreased
c. Normal
d. Unpredictable

Ans.
2278. b
2279. d
2280. c
2281. b
2282. c
2283. b
2284. d
2285. d
2286. a
2287. d
2288. a
2289. d
2290. a
2291. b
2292. a
2293. c
2294. c
2295. a
2296. b
2297. b
2298. b
2299. d
2300. c
2301. c
2302. a

2303. In a client with diabetes insipidus urine specific gravity will:

a. Elevated b. Decreased
c. Normal d. Cannot measure

2304. Which of the following should be immediately noted by a nurse in a client who had undergone renal biopsy?

a. Sweating
b. Increased urination
c. Pain at the abdomen, back of shoulder or chest
d. Pain at biopsy site

Explanation: Localized pain at biopsy site is normal after the procedure. Pain at the back of shoulder, abdomen or chest should be immediately reported. Pain in the abdomen after the procedure is a sign of internal bleeding.

2305. Types of ketones present in blood/urine is:

a. Acetone b. Acetoacetic acid
c. Both a and b d. None of these

2306. Presence of bilirubin in urine can be checked with: *New Q*

a. Fouchet's test b. Gmelin's test
c. Reagent strip test d. All of these

2307. Radiographic study which is commonly used to evaluate the structure & function of ureters, bladder and kidney is:

a. Intravenous pyelogram b. Cystoscopy
c. Ureteroscopy d. Ultrasound

2308. Types of bile salts present in the urine include:

a. Cholic acid b. Deoxycholic acid
c. Chenodeoxycholic acid d. All of these

2309. Excess of nitrogenous substance in feces and urine is known as:

a. Azotorrhea b. Azotemia
c. Steatorrhea d. Malena

2310. Increase in urine specific gravity occurs with all of the following conditions; EXCEPT:

a. High protein diet b. Dehydration
c. Decrease renal perfusion d. Diabetes insipidus

2311. Increased nitrogenous substance in blood:

a. Azotorrhea b. Azotemia
c. Steatorrhoea d. Malena

2312. Tetrad of hematuria include all; EXCEPT: *(PGIMER 2007)*

a. Purpura b. Arthritis
c. Granulomatosis d. Abdominal pain

Explanation: Purpura, arthritis, kidney disease and abdominal pain are in tetrad of hematuria.

2313. Blood in urine: *(RRB Feb 2012)*

a. Hemosiderosis b. Hematopoiesis
c. Hematuria d. None of these

2314. Pus in urine is called: *(Safdarjung NO 2018)*

a. Pyuria b. Polyuria
c. Pusuria d. Dysuria

2315. A client is complaining of urinary urgency and frequency. Clean-voided urine sample appears to be cloudy. Most probable diagnosis will be:

a. Cystitis b. Dysuria
c. Nephrotic syndrome d. Hematuria

2316. Inability to urinate despite of desire is known as:

a. Incontinence b. Retention
c. Enuresis d. Encopresis

2317. Involuntary passing of urine is called as:

a. Incontinence b. Retention
c. Enuresis d. Encopresis

2318. Sudden loss of urine while straining is called as:

a. Stress incontinence b. Urge incontinence
c. Overflow incontinence d. Functional incontinence

2319. Involuntary loss of urine preceded by strong desire to void is:

a. Stress incontinence b. Urge incontinence
c. Overflow incontinence d. Functional incontinence

2320. Leakage of urine due to weak bladder muscle or to blockage- when the bladder becomes over distended is known as:

a. Stress incontinence
b. Urge incontinence
c. Overflow incontinence
d. Functional incontinence

2321. Lower urinary tract is intact while other factors leads to incontinence such as immobility is:

a. Stress incontinence
b. Urge incontinence
c. Overflow incontinence
d. Functional incontinence

2322. Passage of gas or air from urethra during or after voiding is called as:

a. Pneumaturia b. Uremia
c. Dysuria d. Strangury

2323. Slow and painful urination is called as:

a. Pneumaturia b. Uraemia
c. Dysuria d. Stranguary

UROLITHIASIS

2324. Risk factor for urinary calculi is:

a. Hyperthyroidism b. Hypothyroidism
c. Hyperparathyroidism d. Both b and c

2325. Risk factors for urinary stone include:

a. Dehydration
b. High-protein, salt, or glucose diet
c. Hyperparathyroid condition
d. All of these

2326. The nurse sends the renal calculi specimen to laboratory for analyzing ....:

a. Composition of calculi b. Infectious organism
c. Size of calculi d. Blood presence in stone

2327. Which of the following is an incorrect statement regarding urinary stone? *New Q*

a. Found mostly in women with urinary tract infections
b. Cystine stones are rare
c. Cystine is an acid that occurs naturally in the body
d. Alkaline-ash diet is recommended for client with cystine stone

Explanation: Urinary stones can affect both men and women, and they are not necessarily more prevalent in women with urinary tract infections.

Urinary tract infections are more common in women than men, but they do not cause urinary stones.

Other statements about cystine stone are correct.

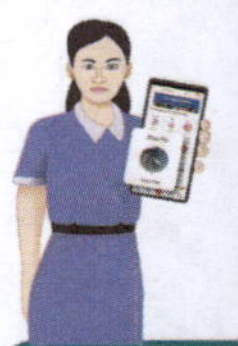

Ans.

2303. b
2304. c
2305. c
2306. d
2307. a
2308. d
2309. a
2310. d
2311. b
2312. c
2313. c
2314. a
2315. a
2316. b
2317. a
2318. a
2319. b
2320. c
2321. d
2322. a
2323. d
2324. d
2325. d
2326. a
2327. a

2328. The diet prescribed for a patient with cysteine renal stone:
a. High protein
b. Moderate protein
c. Low protein
d. Protein in diet is not considered

2329. Correct regarding uric acid stone is:
a. This type of stone develops when urine is too acidic
b. A diet rich in purines can increase urine's acidic level
c. Purine is present in animal proteins, such as fish, shellfish, and meats
d. All of the above

2330. Dietary modification for a client with several uric acid renal stones include:
a. Increase food rich in sodium
b. Decrease intake of calcium rich food
c. Restrict food rich in purine
d. Increased intake of spinach, strawberry and peanuts

2331. Which of the following intervention is appropriate for the patient with renal calculi?
a. Restrict fluids b. Increase dietary purines
c. Maintain bed rest d. Strain all urine

2332. Which of the following fruit is a rich source of oxalate which has to be avoided in a patient with oxalate renal calculi?
a. Citrus fruits b. Pears
c. Strawberries d. Apples

2333. Stones associated with urinary tract infections are:
a. Oxalate stones b. Pyruvate stones
c. Mixed struvite stones d. Cystine stone

2334. Renal stone in the pelvic portion of kidney:
a. Block to afferent arterioles
b. Block to efferent arterioles
c. Affect drainage of urine from kidney
d. Prevent urine concentration capacity

2335. Common type of stones seen in kidney is:
a. Calcium stones b. Oxalate stones
c. Pyruvate stones d. Mixed struvite stones

2336. Commonest type of urinary stone is:
a. Calcium b. Atruvite
c. Cystine d. Pyruvate

2337. Which among the following is the most common calcium substance responsible for stone?
a. Calcium oxalate b. Calcium pyruvate
c. Calcium malate d. Calcium carbonate

2338. Cause of pain in urolithiasis is:
a. Pressure exerted by the stone
b. Movement of stone
c. Decreased water intake
d. Disintegration of stone

2339. High oxalate containing food items include:
a. Potato chips
b. Pea nut
c. Chocolate
d. All of the above

2340. Which among the following patient is at risk for developing uric acid stone?
a. People with gout
b. People with chemotherapy
c. Both a and b
d. None of the above

2341. Clinical manifestation related to renal calculi include:
a. Hematuria
b. Frequent need to urinate
c. Urinating small amounts of urine
d. All of the above

2342. Patient develops small stones in the renal system. In order to promote the passage of these stones in the urine patient is advised to ....:
a. Increase the fluid intake b. Ambulate.
c. Both a and b d. Avoid activities

Explanation: Increased fluid intake and mobilization will help to increase the chance of passage of stone via urine.

2343. Stag-horn calculi are made up of:
a. Calcium oxalate b. Cholesterol
c. Purine
d. Magnesium ammonium phosphate

2344. Diet recommended for calcium phosphate stone is called:
a. Alkali-ash food b. Acid –ash food
c. High calcium rich food d. Both a and b

2345. Which among the following intervention is important for a patient with urolithiasis?
a. Strict bed rest b. Strain all urine
c. High purine diet d. Decrease fluid intake

2346. ESWL is contraindicated in which of the following stones:
a. Cysteine stones b. Urate Stones
c. Oxalate Stones d. Phospate Stones

2347. Dietary education to a patient with cholesterol stone includes:
a. Take low calorie diet b. Well-balanced diet
c. Limit sugar intake d. Limit fatty foods

2348. Severe renal colic can be managed with:
a. Opioids as prescribed b. Increase water intake
c. Insert Foley's catheter d. Ambulation of patient

GLOMERULONEPHRITIS

2349. Hematuria is the manifestation of:
a. Acute glomerulonephritis
b. Bladder tumors
c. Renal stones
d. All of the above

2350. Glomerulonephritis means:
a. Inflammation of renal pelvis
b. Inflammation of glomerulus of nephron
c. Inflammation of afferent arterioles
d. Inflammation of efferent arterioles

2351. Clinical features of acute glomerulonephritis includes all; EXCEPT:
a. Oliguria
b. Hematuria
c. Sudden onset of hypotension
d. Proteinuria

2352. In a patient hospitalized with acute glomerulonephritis, nursing care include all of the following; EXCEPT:
a. Recording vital signs every 4 hourly *(Banaras HU 2015)*
b. Recording the weight of the patient twice weekly
c. Recording fluid intake and output every 8 hourly
d. Recording BP 4 hourly

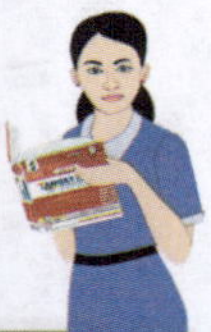

Ans.
2328. c
2329. d
2330. c
2331. d
2332. c
2333. c
2334. c
2335. a
2336. a
2337. a
2338. b
2339. d
2340. c
2341. d
2342. c
2343. d
2344. b
2345. b
2346. a
2347. d
2348. a
2349. d
2350. b
2351. c
2352. b

2353. Clinical manifestation of post-streptococcal glomerulonephritis include:

a. Oliguria b. Smoky urine
c. Proteinuria d. All of these

2354. Clinical manifestations of acute glomerulonephritis includes all of the following; EXCEPT:

a. Hematuria and proteinuria
b. Azotemia
c. Sudden onset of hypertension
d. Polyuria

2355. The main cause of glomerulonephritis:

a. Group A beta-hemolytic streptococcal infection
b. Staphylococcal infection
c. E.coli infection
d. Clostridium infection

2356. Glomerulonephritis which affects the entire glomerulus is....:

a. Focal glomerulonephritis
b. Global glomerulonephritis
c. Proliferative glomerulonephritis
d. Rapidly progressive glomerulonephritis

2357. Diet recommended for patient with glomerulonephritis:

a. High protein, low calorie
b. Low protein, high calorie
c. Low protein, high sodium, potassium
d. High calorie, high protein

2358. Clinical manifestations of glomerular injury is:

a. Proteinuria b. Hematuria
c. Hypertension d. All of these

2359. Proteinuria is a sign of:

a. A diet with lot of protein b. Damaged nephrons
c. Healthy muscles d. Taking less water

2360. Polyuria with low fixed specific gravity urine is seen in:

a. Potomania
b. Diabetes mellitus
c. Chronic glomerulonephritis
d. Diabetes insipidus

Explanation: Low specific gravity (<1.005) is characteristic of diabetes insipidus, nephrogenic diabetes insipidus, acute tubular necrosis, or pyelonephritis. Fixed low specific gravity, in which values remain 1.010 regardless of fluid intake, occurs in chronic glomerulonephritis with severe renal damage.

2361. A patient with glomerulonephritis is complaining of thirst. The nurse should offer:

a. Juice b. Water
c. Tea d. Hard candy

PYELONEPHRITIS

2362. The clinical manifestations of pyelonephritis includes:
(AIIMS Raipur Grade II 2017)

a. Abdominal or suprapubic pain
b. Costovertebral angle tenderness
c. Persistent vomiting
d. Severe dehydration

a. a, b, c b. b, c, d
c. a, c, d d. a, b, c, d

Explanation: The symptoms of pyelonephritis include a sudden onset of chills, fever (body temperature of 38°C or greater), and unilateral or bilateral flank pain with costovertebral tenderness, dysuria, urinary frequency and urgency.

2363. The most common microorganism that cause pyelonephritis in human is:

a. H. pylori b. E. coli
c. S. aureus d. HPV

2364. Which of the following assessment is important to be checked on daily basis for the client with pyelonephritis?

a. Weight check b. Abdominal circumference
c. Skin integrity d. CVP

2365. Which of the following is one of the best preventive measure for pyelonephritis?

a. Drinking water regularly b. Proper exercise
c. Prevention from UTI d. Prophylactic antibiotics

2366. The inflammation of the renal pelvis, tubules and interstitium is known as:

a. Raynaud's disease b. Wilson disease
c. Pyelonephritis d. Cystitis

2367. All of the following are the major clinical features of the patient with pyelonephritis; EXCEPT:

a. Dysuria b. Hematuria and urgency
c. Periumbilical pain d. Flank pain

NEPHROTIC SYNDROME

Nephritis, Nephrotic Syndrome, Nephritic Syndrome

2368. Risk/causative factor for nephrotic syndrome is:

a. Amyloidosis b. Diabetes mellitus
c. Glomerulonephritis d. All of these

2369. Triad of symptoms in nephrotic syndrome include all; EXCEPT:

a. Proteinuria b. Hypoalbuminemia
c. Edema d. Weight loss

Explanation: Nephrotic syndrome is defined by a triad of clinical features: oedema, substantial proteinuria (>3.5 g/24 hours) and hypoalbuminaemia (<30 g/L). It is often associated with hyperlipidaemia, thromboembolism and an increased risk of infection. Weight gain occurs due to fluid retention.

2370. Causes of nephrotic syndrome include:

a. Diabetes mellitus. b. Idiopathic
c. SLE d. All of these

2371. Reason behind edema in nephrotic syndrome:

a. Proteinuria b. Hypoalbuminemia
c. Hyperlipidemia d. Hematuria

2372. In nephrotic syndrome edema first appear:

a. Around the eyes b. Lower leg
c. Abdomen d. All over the body

2373. Priority nursing intervention for edema in a child with nephrotic syndrome is: *New Q*

a. Provide meticulous skin care
b. Maintain intake output
c. Administer diuretics
d. Administer corticosteroids

Explanation: The priority nursing intervention for managing edema in a client with nephrotic syndrome involves accurate monitoring and documentation of intake and output. It is important to consistently weigh the child at the same time every day, using the same scale and

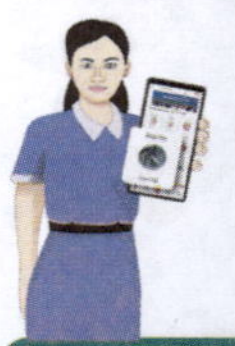

Ans.

2353. d
2354. d
2355. a
2356. b
2357. b
2358. d
2359. b
2360. c
2361. d
2362. b
2363. b
2364. a
2365. c
2366. c
2367. c
2368. d
2369. d
2370. d
2371. b
2372. a
2373. b

clothing. Additionally, daily measurement of the child's abdomen at the level of the umbilicus is necessary to track changes in abdominal girth.

While options such as meticulous skin care and administering corticosteroids are important aspects of care, the fluid balance takes priority over other care needs.

2374. Prolonged steroid therapy to treat nephrotic syndrome can leads to:

a. Cushingoid appearance b. Hypoaldosteronism
c. Cryptorchidism d. Oliguria

2375. Which of the following characteristic defines nephritic syndrome?

a. Fatty casts in urine
b. Polyuria & hypotension
c. Proteinuria (<3.5 g/dL) and Hematuria
d. RBC casts in urine with a decreased BUN & creatinine

2376. Lipid casts are seen in:

a. Cytomegalic inclusion disease
b. Acute tubular necrosis
c. Nephrotic syndrome
d. None of the above

2377. The cause of edema in Nephritic syndrome is:

a. Decreased in plasma protein concentration
b. Reduced plasma osmotic pressure
c. Increased in plasma protein concentration
d. Sodium and water retention

(Ref: Harsh Mohan 4th/e pg. 644, 645)

Explanation:

- The heavy proteinuria depletes serum albumin levels in patients with nephrotic syndrome. This results in generalized edema as a consequence of ↓ed colloid osmotic pressure. Sodium & water retention is also seen which aggravates the edema.
- However, in Nephritic syndrome damage to glomeruli causes a fall in GFR and eventually produces uremic symptoms with salt & water retention, leading to edema and hypertension.

2378. Proteinuria is seen in:

a. Nephrotic syndrome b. Nephritic syndrome
c. Multiple myeloma d. All of these

RENAL FAILURE (ARF AND ESRD)

2379. The most important cause of kidney failure is:

a. Accidents b. Type 2 diabetes
c. Heart disease d. Pneumonia

2380. When the kidneys fail, the body fills with extra fluid & waste products. This condition is called:

a. Uremia b. Hypertension
c. Anemia d. Diabetes

2381. Risk factor associated with renal disorder:

a. High sodium diet b. Hypertension
c. Diabetes mellitus d. All of these

2382. Acute Renal failure is defined as:

a. 15% or greater increase in serum creatinine above baseline
b. 20% or greater increase in serum creatinine above baseline
c. 30% or greater increase in serum creatinine above baseline
d. 50% or greater increase in serum creatinine above baseline

2383. Parameter helpful to assess the renal failure as early as possible:

a. BUN b. Urine output
c. Creatinine clearance d. GFR

2384. In chronic renal failure all the following are noticed; EXCEPT: *(DSSSB PHN, 2015)*

a. Anemia b. Hypocalcemia
c. Metabolic acidosis d. Hypokalemia

2385. Acute renal failure results in:

a. Hypokalemia acidosis b. Hyperkalemia alkalosis
c. Hyperkalemic acidosis d. Hypokalemic acidosis

2386. CRF is associated with?

a. Respiratory acidosis b. Metabolic alkalosis
c. Metabolic acidosis d. Respiratory alkalosis

2387. Expected laboratory findings in a person with renal failure is: *(AIIMS 2010)*

a. BUN 35 mg/dL, potassium 4.0 mEq/L
b. Blood pH 7.2, potassium 6.5 mEq/L
c. BUN 15 mg/dL, increased serum calcium, creatinine 1.0 mg/dL
d. BUN 45 mg/dL, potassium 3.5 mEq/L

Explanation: Because of accumulation of uremic waste blood ph become acidic and lack of kidney function leads to accumulation of potassium.

2388. All of the following electrolyte imbalances are seen in patient with Chronic Renal Failure (CRF); EXCEPT:

a. Hypocalcemia b. Hyperkalemia
c. Hyponatremia d. Hypophosphatemia

2389. The cause of pruritus in CKD patients:

a. Hyperkalemia b. Uremia
c. Hyperphosphatemia d. Hypernatremia

2390. The cause of acidosis in CKD:

a. Inability of kidney tubules to excrete ammonia
b. Inability to reabsorb sodium bicarbonate
c. Decreased excretion of phosphate & organic acids
d. All of these

2391. The GFR value of patients with stage V CKD is:

a. 15–29 mL/min/1.73 m^2 b. 30–59 mL/min/1.73 m^2
c. <15 mL/min/1.73 m^2 d. 15–20 mL/min/1.73 m^2

2392. The amount of protein intake to be maintained during renal failure is: *(DSSSB PHN, 2015)*

a. 0.6–0.8 g/kg/day b. 0.8-1.0 g/kg/day
c. 1.0-1.5 g/kg/day d. 1.5-2.0 g/kg/day

2393. The most important nursing diagnosis for a patient in end-stage renal disease is:

a. Risk for injury
b. Activity intolerance
c. Fluid volume excess
d. Altered nutrition less than body requirement

2394. Patient with chronic renal failure need to avoid:

a. Banana
b. Yogurt
c. Dark green leafy vegetables
d. All of the above

Explanation: All of the above-mentioned food items are potassium rich and a patient with chronic renal failure need to avoid all these items. High potassium foods include beans, dark leafy greens, potatoes, squash, yogurt, fish, avocados, mushrooms, and bananas.

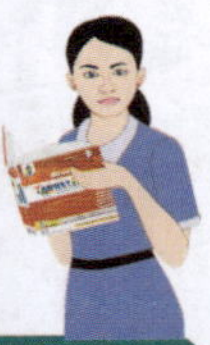

Ans.

2374. a
2375. c
2376. c
2377. d
2378. d
2379. b
2380. a
2381. d
2382. d
2383. c
2384. d
2385. c
2386. c
2387. b
2388. d
2389. b
2390. d
2391. c
2392. a
2393. c
2394. d

2395. Electrolyte abnormality need to be closely monitored in the diuretic phase of renal failure is:
a. Hyperkalemia and hyponatremia
b. Hyperkalemia and hypernatremia
c. Hypokalemia and hyponatremia
d. Hypokalemia and hypernatremia

2396. Which of the following is the cause of pre-renal failure?
a. Interference with renal perfusion
b. Interference with renal function
c. Obstruction in urine flow
d. All of the above

2397. Acute renal failure (ARF) secondary to cardiogenic shock is considered as:
a. Prerenal b. Intrinsic
c. Postrenal d. Idiopathic

2398. Major electrolyte elevated in the oliguric phase of renal failure is:
a. Sodium b. Potassium
c. Calcium d. Phosphorus

2399. Which of the following is the cause of intra-renal failure?
a. Interference with renal perfusion
b. Interference with renal function
c. Obstruction in urine flow
d. All of the above

2400. Which of the following is the cause of post-renal failure?
a. Interference with renal perfusion
b. Interference with renal function
c. Obstruction in urine flow
d. All of the above

2401. Which among the following is the most common cause of intra-renal failure?
a. Glomerulonephritis b. Acute tubular necrosis
c. Wilms tumor d. Nephrotic syndrome

2402. Low erythropoietin level is seen in:
a. Aplastic anemic b. Renal failure
c. Obesity d. Hematoma

2403. In ESRD, GFR will be:
a. $<15/1.73\ m^2$ b. $<15–29/1.73\ m^2$
c. $<30–34/1.73\ m^2$ d. $<35–59/1.73\ m^2$

2404. Furosemide acts on which part of the nephron? *(NCFL 2019)*
a. Proximal tubule
b. Descending limb of the loop of Henle
c. Ascending limb of the loop of Henle
d. Distal tubule

Explanation: Furosemide (Loop diuretics) acts on the thick **ascending loop of Henle.** It blocks the sodium, chloride and potassium co-transporter and it increases sodium, chloride and potassium excretion. Thereby, it increases the rate of urine flow.

HEMODIALYSIS

2405. When receiving hemodialysis, the complication of the removal of too much sodium may occur. Therefore, the nurse should assess the client for: *(RAK MSc 2018)*
a. Chvostek's sign b. Cardiac dysrhythmias
c. Muscle cramps d. Increased temperature

Explanation: If sodium levels are too low, the client will experience muscle cramps and hypotension due to changes in concentration between intracellular and extracellular compartments.

2406. The nurse is checking patency of a new right arm AV fistula. What should be the action of the nurse in this condition?
a. Auscultate the right brachial pulse *(RAK MSc 2018)*
b. Auscultate and palpate the right radial pulse
c. Measure blood pressure in the right arm
d. Palpate for thrill and auscultate bruit over the fistula

Explanation: AV fistulas are artificial passage made between a vein and an artery for purpose such as hemodialysis treatment. It is usually made on the dominant side of the patient, i.e., right, hence called right hand AV fistula. For assessing the patency of right arm AV fistula, the nurse has to palpate thrill and auscultate bruit, these are the vascular sounds heard as a result of turbulence made by blood. In case of an AV fistula, these sounds serve as an indicator for its patency.

2407. Hemodialysis is a process of:
a. Adding O_2 to the blood
b. Extracting nitrogenous wastes from the blood
c. Extracting antibodies from the blood
d. Mixing blood with essential nutrients

2408. Among the following which is not the principle of hemodialysis:
a. Ultrafiltration b. Osmosis
c. Inhibition d. Diffusion

2409. For a patient on hemodialysis, increased fluid intake may cause:
a. Sinus problems, bad breath, ringing in the ears, body odour
b. Headache, hearing problem
c. Swelling, trouble breathing, heart damage, hypertension
d. Weight loss, slurred speech, uncontrolled sneezing

2410. Which among the following parameter is helpful for assessing the effectiveness of hemodialysis?
a. Electrolyte value such as potassium
b. Low serum creatinine level
c. Blood pressure
d. Urine output

2411. A synthetic semi-permeable membrane that is used in hemodialysis is known as:
a. Dialysate b. Dialyzer
c. Shunt d. Extracorporeal tubing

2412. Which mineral must be limited for a person on hemodialysis?
a. Potassium b. Iron
c. Zinc d. Molybdenum

2413. Hemodialysis removes harmful wastes from the body. It also removes:
a. Extra protein b. Extra water
c. Extra insulin d. All of these

2414. Common side effect of hemodialysis:
a. Muscle cramps and weakness
b. Dizziness
c. Nausea
d. All of these

2415. Which of the following is not a likely cause of muscle cramps during hemodialysis?
a. Hypernatremia b. Excess fluid removal
c. Hypercalcemia d. Hypokalemia

Ans.
2395. c
2396. a
2397. a
2398. b
2399. b
2400. c
2401. b
2402. b
2403. a
2404. c
2405. c
2406. d
2407. b
2408. c
2409. c
2410. b
2411. b
2412. a
2413. b
2414. d
2415. c

2416. The HD access that is surgically created by anastomosing an artery to vein either side to side or end to side is known as:

a. AV graft b. AV fistula
c. AV shunt d. Catheter

2417. The complication that occurs during hemodialysis as a result of cerebral fluid shift is:

a. Hypotension b. Dysrhythmia
c. Disequilibrium d. Chest pain

2418. The access used for short term hemodialysis is:

a. Fistula b. Graft
c. Catheter d. Shunt

2419. The amount of protein recommended for a patient on hemodialysis is:

a. 1.2–1.3 g/kg of body wt/day
b. 4–6 g/kg of body wt/day
c. 1.6–2 g/kg of body wt/day
d. 5–8 g/kg of body wt/day

2420. Bruit in the fistula can be checked by monitoring its:

a. Color b. Small
c. Sound d. Feel

2421. The thrill in the fistula can be checked by monitoring its:

a. Color b. Smell
c. Sound d. Feel

2422. Dementia in patient of chronic renal failure with chronic hemodialysis is due to:

a. Aluminium toxicity b. Uremia
c. A Beta amyloid d. A Beta amyloid deposition

PERITONEAL DIALYSIS (PD)

2423. The purpose of peritoneal dialysis is to: *(JIPMER 2012)*

a. Clean the peritoneal cavity
b. Re-establish kidney function
c. Remove the toxins and metabolic waste
d. Provide fluid

2424. Advice given to a client before the insertion of peritoneal dialysis catheter is:

a. Empty the bladder
b. Instruction regarding the venous access created
c. Types of diet need to be followed
d. All of these

2425. Peritoneal dialysis uses ______ as the access for treatment.

a. Catheter b. Fistula
c. Graft d. Dialysis machine

2426. The process of infusing dialysate, dwell drainage of the dialysate is called:

a. Replacement b. Exchange
c. Hemo sterilizing d. Equilibration

2427. The semi permeable membrane used in peritoneal dialysis is:

a. Pleural membrane b. Peritoneum
c. Osseous membrane d. Pericardium

2428. The substance is dialysate fluid that causes ultra-filtration through an osmotic gradient is:

a. Protein
b. Electrolytes
c. Glucose
d. All of the above

2429. The most common serious complication of peritoneal dialysis is:

a. Leakage b. Bleeding
c. Peritonitis d. Hypertriglyceridemia

2430. Common complication associated with peritoneal dialysis is:

a. Over flow problem b. Bleeding
c. Peritonitis d. Back ache

RENAL TRANSPLANT

2431. Kidney transplantation is an:

a. Allograft b. Isograft
c. Xenograft d. Synergic graft

Explanation:

- **Allograft:** An organ or tissue transplanted from one individual to another individual of same species
- **Alloantigen:** Transplant antigen
- **Alloantibody:** Transplant antibodies

ADD:

- **Xenograft:** A tissue graft or organ transplant from a donor of a different species from the recipient.

2432. Which among the following is an absolute exclusion criteria for living kidney donors?

a. Obesity
b. Border line urinary abnormalities
c. Cancer
d. H/o Gestational diabetes

2433. First sign/symptom of renal graft rejection is:

a. Tenderness b. Fever
c. Increased creatinine d. Rash

Explanation: In case of transplant rejection, clinical evidence in the form of fever, swelling and tenderness over the auograft is rarely appreciated. Rise in serum creatinine may be the only initial evidence which may or may not present with a reduction in urine volume.

2434. Chronic rejection in renal transplantation usually occur after:

a. 1 week b. 2 weeks
c. 4 weeks d. 12 weeks

Explanation:

- Hyperacute Rejection - Minutes to Hours
- Acute rejection - 10 days to 30 days
- Chronic rejection - Months to years

2435. In the immediate post renal transplant period which condition a physician should be noted immediately?

a. Pain
b. Urine output <30 mL/h
c. Hematuria
d. Bleeding from surgical site

2436. Mr. Rahul has undergone renal transplantation. Which of the following assessment indicates the possibility of organ rejection?

a. Sudden weight loss
b. Shock
c. Hypertension
d. Polyuria

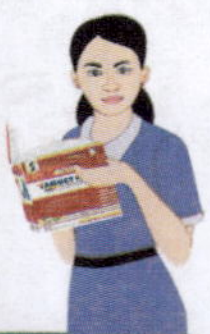

Ans.

2416. b
2417. c
2418. c
2419. a
2420. c
2421. d
2422. a
2423. c
2424. a
2425. a
2426. b
2427. b
2428. c
2429. c
2430. c
2431. a
2432. c
2433. c
2434. d
2435. d
2436. c

2437. Clinical manifestation for transplanted kidney rejection include:
a. Diminished urine output
b. Hypoxemia
c. Malaise
d. Pain at the incision sites

2438. Immunosuppressant therapy following renal transplantation is required:
a. For 36 hours
b. For 1 week
c. Until serum creatinine becomes normal
d. For life long

2439. Which lab result indicate an adverse effect of cyclosporine prescribed for a renal transplant patient?
a. Increase in Hb level
b. Decrease cellulite want
c. Increase in BUN
d. Decrease in urea level

2440. Which among the following is the main side effect of corticosteroids?
a. Hair loss
b. Increased blood glucose
c. Increased creatinine level
d. Darkening of skin

2441. The most common ocular infection after renal transplantation is by:
a. Cytomegalovirus
b. Toxoplasma
c. Herpes virus
d. EB virus

URINARY TRACT INFECTIONS (UTI)

2442. Benign Prostatic hypertrophy results in obstruction of urinary tract. Specific condition is associated with enlargement of:
a. Entire prostate gland
b. Lateral lobes
c. Median lobe
d. Posterior lobes

2443. The most common lower urinary tract infection is:
a. Prostatitis
b. Cystitis
c. Urethritis
d. Renal & peri renal abscess

2444. Characteristics of urinary system that helps in maintaining its sterility includes all; EXCEPT:
a. Adequate urine volume
b. Complete bladder emptying
c. Ureterovesical junction
d. Alkaline urine

2445. Married women comes to the clinic with frequent history of UTI, nurse need to educate the client to:
a. Take sitz bath
b. Urinate before and after sexual intercourse
c. Clean the area with luke-warm water and apply topical antibiotic creams
d. Take acid-ash diet

2446. Which of following causes majority of UTI in hospitalized patients? *(AIIMS Rishikesh Senior Nursing Officer 2018)*
a. Decrease fluid intake
b. Invasive procedures
c. Inadequate self-care
d. Immunosuppressant

2447. Who among the following is at a risk of developing UTI?
a. A woman with otitis media
b. A post-menopausal woman
c. A woman with pneumonia
d. A woman with fracture in upper extremity

2448. Discharge teaching for a patient taking pyridium for the management of UTI include:
a. Take this drug along with food
b. Stop this drug if you develop abdominal pain
c. Urine become bright orange
d. Take drug at bed time

2449. Which of following juices is recommended for a patient with UTI?
a. Apple juice
b. Lemon juice
c. Cranberry juice
d. Grape juice

2450. Which of the following is not a common cause of UTI among men?
a. Prostate enlargement
b. Erectile dysfunction
c. Renal stone
d. Indwelling catheter

URINARY INCONTINENCE AND NEUROGENIC BLADDER

2451. Christmas tree appearance of urinary bladder is seen in:
a. Enuresis
b. Stress incontinence
c. Neurogenic bladder
d. Autonomous bladder

2452. Urine urge occurs at what bladder capacity?
a. 50 mL
b. 150 mL
c. 250 mL
d. 400 mL

2453. Involuntary loss of urine which result from sudden increases in abdominal pressure such as coughing/ sneezing is known as:
a. Functional incontinence
b. Stress incontinence
c. Reflex incontinence
d. Total incontinence

2454. Which among the following help to increase the bladder control in an incontinence client?
a. Frequent micturition
b. Intermittent self-catheterization
c. Kegel exercises
d. Douching

2455. Enuresis is:
a. Involuntary passage of urine
b. Painful urination
c. Involuntary passage of urine during night
d. Excessive urination at night

2456. Amphetamine is indicated in:
a. Attention deficit hyperkinetic disorder in children
b. Enuresis
c. Obesity
d. All of the above

OTHER RENAL DISEASES

2457. Hardening of the renal arteries are called as:
a. Nephrosclerosis
b. Nephritis
c. Nephrotic syndrome
d. Arteriosis

2458. When the posterior bladder wall protrudes downward through the anterior vaginal wall. It is known as: *(AIIMS-BBS SNO 2019)*
a. Rectocele
b. Pyocele
c. Cystocele
d. Bubonocoele

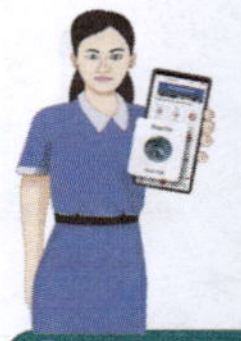

Ans.

2437. a
2438. d
2439. c
2440. b
2441. a
2442. c
2443. b
2444. d
2445. b
2446. b
2447. b
2448. c
2449. c
2450. b
2451. c
2452. b
2453. b
2454. c
2455. c
2456. d
2457. a
2458. c

Explanation: When the posterior bladder wall protrudes downward through the anterior vaginal wall. It is known as cystocele. It is also called prolapsed or dropped bladder, is the bulging or dropping of the bladder into the vagina. **Note:** Use of keyword **'bladder'** leads to the answer '**cysto**cele'

2459. Distension of renal pelvis caused by obstruction to normal urine flow: *(AIIMS Nagpur NO 2018)*

a. Renal failure b. Renal calculi
c. Hydronephrosis d. Polycystic kidney

Explanation: Hydronephrosis is swelling of one or both kidneys. It occurs when urine cannot drain from a kidney and builds up in the kidney as a result. This can occur from a blockage in the tubes that drain urine from the kidneys (ureters) or from an anatomical defect that doesn't allow urine to drain properly.

2460. Clinical feature of CKD includes:

a. Hypertension b. Anemia
c. Hyperkalemia d. All of these

2461. Early sign of renal carcinoma is:

a. Dysuria b. Flank pain
c. Pyuria d. Hematuria

Explanation: Hematuria is the classical and early sign of renal carcinoma. The presence of blood in urine is known as hematuria

2462. Clinical manifestations of cystitis are:

a. Persistent urge to urinate
b. Burning sensation when urinating
c. Hematuria
d. All of these

2463. Positive dipstick for RBC with Red color urine and clear supernatant after centrifugation is due to:

a. Porphyria b. Hematuria
c. Hemolysis d. Rhabdomyolysis

2464. Micro-organism responsible for renal candidiasis is:

a. Bacterial b. Viral
c. Protozoal d. Fungi

2465. A patient with heart failure is on diuretics. Which of the following is the accurate indicator of such patient's health status? *(Daman & Diu NO 2018)*

a. Vital signs
b. Urine-specific gravity
c. Fluid intake and output
d. Weight

Explanation: Assessing the weight is the accurate indicator of health status in heart failure patient who is on diuretics. Measuring weight daily helps to detect hypervolemia before symptoms develop and may prevent full exacerbations.

2466. Surgery involving renal pelvis is: *(JIPMER 2012)*

a. Pyloroplasty
b. Urethroplasty
c. Lithotripsy
d. Pyeloplasty

2467. A client has a ureteral catheter in place after renal surgery. The nurse should:

a. Clamp catheter every 2 hours
b. Irrigate catheter with NS every day
c. Ensure that catheter is draining freely
d. All of the above

2468. Correct regarding urinary catheter irrigation is:

a. Use sterile equipment
b. Follow strict surgical asepsis
c. Both a and b
d. None of the above

2469. Which of the following findings is anticipated from a patient who has been taking furosemide for the last one week?

a. Edema of the foot
b. Anorexia
c. Gastric irritation
d. Weight gain of 2 kg

2470. Radiation therapy to treat the cancer of kidney can cause damage to:

a. Liver
b. Spleen
c. Adrenal glands
d. Intestine

2471. Correct regarding steroid therapy is:

a. Complication associated with long-term use of topical steroid is Glaucoma
b. Common complication of systemic steroid therapy is Cataract
c. Steroid therapy cause hyperglycemia
d. All of these

2472. A client with ileal conduit is advised to empty the pouch frequently, so as to prevent:

a. Interruption of urine production
b. Damage to ileal conduit
c. Development odor
d. Separation of appliance from skin

2473. A client with ileal conduit complained presence of moderate amount of mucus in urine. Which among the following is most appropriate action?

a. Notify physician immediately
b. Encourage excess of fluid intake
c. Change the pouch
d. Change the position of patient

2474. The nurse should teach the client with ileal conduit to wash the reusable appliance with:

a. Soap and water
b. Sprit
c. Hydrogen peroxide
d. Only with water

2475. Wilms tumor is associated with: *(Kerala PSC, Nov 2014)*

a. Polycystic kidney
b. Renal dysplasia
c. Renal Hypoplasia
d. Horse-shoe kidney

2476. The polycystic kidney disease is first identified by:

a. Lower abdominal pain
b. Upper abdominal pain
c. Flank pain
d. Both a and b

2477. Renal bone disease occurs when phosphorous in the blood pulls ____ mineral from the bone?

a. Zinc
b. Calcium
c. Iron
d. Potassium

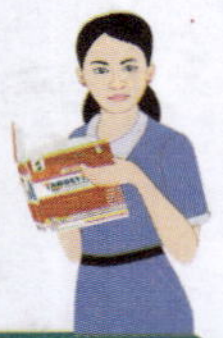

Ans.

2459. c
2460. d
2461. d
2462. d
2463. d
2464. d
2465. d
2466. d
2467. c
2468. c
2469. b
2470. c
2471. d
2472. d
2473. b
2474. a
2475. b
2476. c
2477. b

ENDOCRINE SYSTEM

ANATOMY AND PHYSIOLOGY OF ENDOCRINE SYSTEM

- Endocrine glands are ductless glands.
- Their secretions are known as hormones and these are secreted directly into the blood.
- Hormones are of different categories:
  - Steroids (corticosteroid hormones)
  - Peptide (insulin)
  - Amino acid derivatives (tyrosine, epinephrine, norepinephrine).

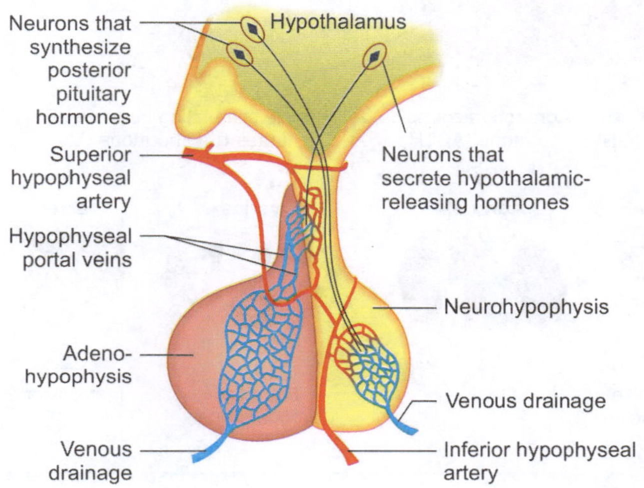

Figure 105: Anatomy of endocrine gland

Hypothalamus

- Hypothalamus regulates pituitary function.
- Specialized neuron clusters called neurosecretory cells in the hypothalamus produce ADH and oxytocin
- ADH and oxytocin are stored in posterior pituitary.

Pituitary Gland

- It is known as the **master gland** in the body.
- It is also called as **hypophysis**.
- It is situated in the **dorsal surface of hypothalamus** and is connected to hypothalamus with hypophyseal stalk.
- It has three lobes:
  1. Anterior pituitary (adenohypophysis)
  2. Posterior pituitary (neurohypophysis)
  3. Intermediate lobe

KEY POINTS

- Endocrine glands are ductless glands.
- Hormones are chemical messengers that are secreted directly into the blood, which carries them to organs and tissues of the body to exert their functions.
- The **hypothalamus** is considered to be a link structure between the nervous and the endocrine system.
- The main function of hypothalamus is to maintain the homeostasis of the body.
- Hunger, sleep, thirst, temperature control and sexual response are under the control of hypothalamus.

Recent Question (CNCI 2021)

72. The heat regulatory center of the body is located at:
a. Medulla oblongata
b. Thalamus
c. Limbic system
d. Hypothalamus

Ans. (d) Hypothalamus

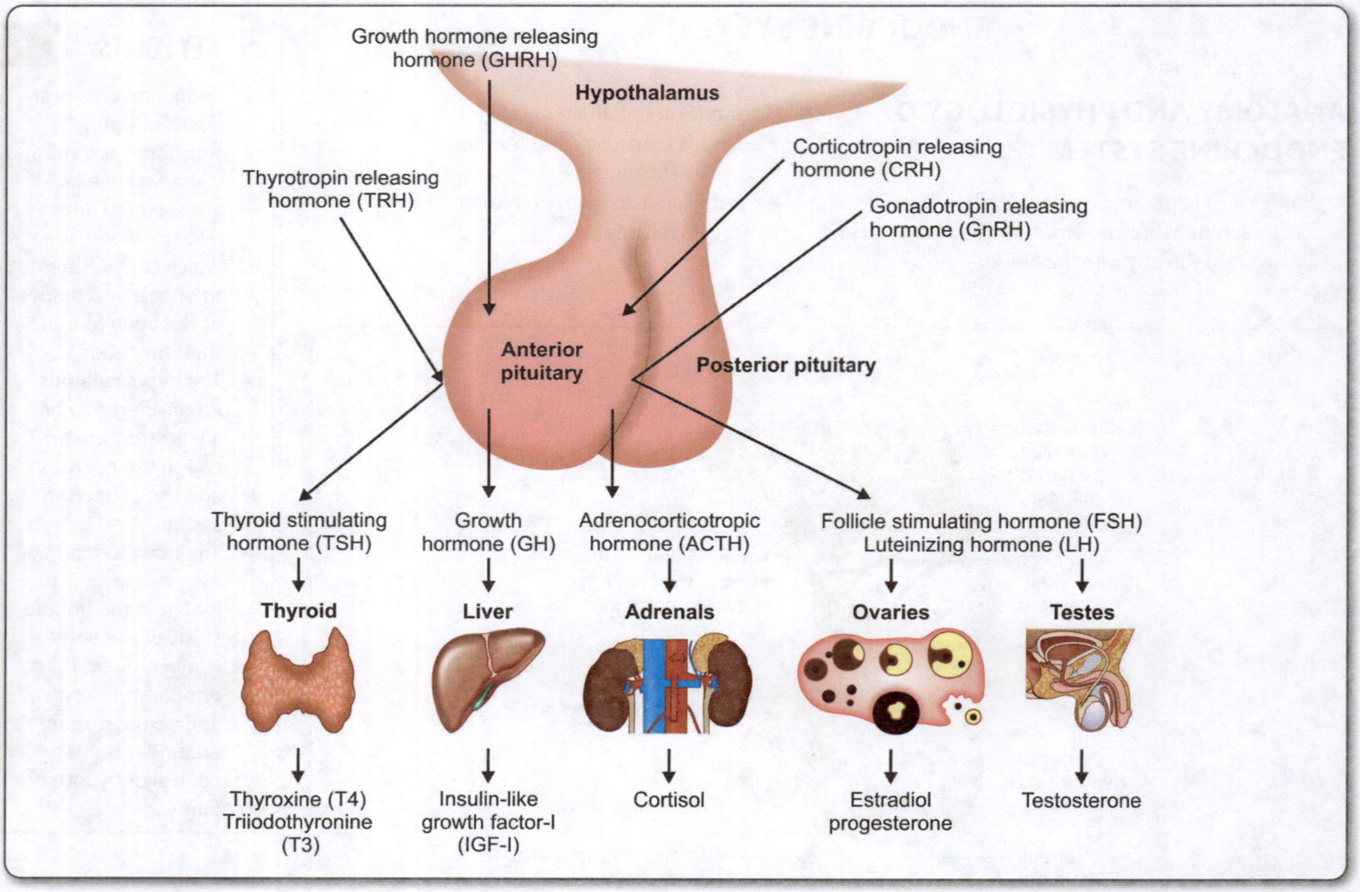

Figure 106: Anterior pituitary hormones and their functions

Anterior lobe of the pituitary

- Anterior lobe of the pituitary secretes stimulating hormone in response to releasing hormone from the hypothalamus.
- This lobe secretes and stores hormones such as:
  - Growth hormone (GH) } Hormones
  - Prolactin
  - Adrenocorticotropic (stimulating) hormone (ACTH) } Stimulating Hormones
  - Follicle stimulating hormone (FSH)
  - Thyroid stimulating hormone (TSH)
  - Luteinizing hormone (LH)
- Except Growth hormone and prolactin, anterior pituitary hormones are stimulating hormones (Functions mentioned in the figure)

Growth hormone (somatotropin)

- It is secreted by anterior pituitary.
- Stimulates growth of all tissues by hypertrophy (increase in cell size) and hyperplasia (increase in number of cells).

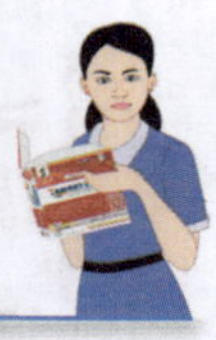

Prolactin

- **Anterior pituitary** produces prolactin.
- Lactotrophs cells of anterior pituitary secret prolactin
- Sucking reflex promotes prolactin secretion and thereby milk production.

Melanocyte stimulating hormone.

- Corticotroph cells of the anterior pituitary secret it.
- Target cells are melanocytes.
- It stimulates melanin production in skin, hair, and eyes which protects the skin from UV radiation.

Simmonds disease, also known as panhypopituitarism or pituitary cachexia, is a condition characterized by the atrophy or destruction of the entire anterior pituitary lobe. This leads to a significant decrease in the secretion of all hormones normally produced by the anterior pituitary gland.

Posterior Lobe of the Pituitary

- This lobe stores the hormones secreted by hypothalamus.
- Hormones stored include ADH (vasopressin) and Oxytocin.

KEY POINTS

- Hyposecretion of growth hormone in children results in **Dwarfism.**
- Hypersecretion of growth hormone in adults results in **acromegaly**.
- Enlargement of pituitary tumor after adrenalectomy is called Nelson's syndrome.

Antidiuretic Hormone (ADH)/ Vasopressin

- It decreases urine production.
- ADH acts on the kidneys to increase water reabsorption in the distal tubules and collecting ducts.
- Release of ADH is primarily regulated by the osmolarity of the blood and the volume.
- When the body senses high osmolarity or low blood volume, such as during dehydration or increased salt intake, ADH secretion is increased. This helps to conserve water by reducing urine production and preventing excessive water loss.

Oxytocin

- It is synthesized by the paraventricular nucleus of hypothalamus.
- It causes milk ejection from mammary gland and uterine contraction

Intermediate lobe

- It has little physiological significance in human.

Pineal Gland

- Small and secretory endocrine organ situated at the center of brain outside the blood-brain barrier.
- Melatonin is secreted from pinealocytes
- Weight: 100–150 g.

Functions

- Regulates the circadian rhythm.
- Promotes sexual maturation and puberty.

Thymus Gland

- Retrosternal organ located in the superior mediastinum.
- Bilobed organ fused together.
- It develops during fetal life, matures during early postnatal life and shrinks as people age.
- T-lymphocyte is differentiated in thymus.
- Hormones secreted: ***Thymopoietin, Thymulin and thymosin, Thymic humoral factor.***
- Resection of thymus gland is known as ***thymectomy*** and it does not affect his/her immune system.

Thyroid Gland

- Thyroid gland is located in the neck just below the cricoid cartilage.
- It is a butterfly shaped gland.
- Lobes of the thyroid gland lie on the sides of trachea and lobes are connected with the help of stalk called **isthmus.**
- Thyroid is the only gland which synthesizes and stores its own secretion and secretes it into the blood whenever needed.
- Secretions of thyroid glands **are triiodothyroxine (T3), thyroxine (T4) and thyrocalcitonin**

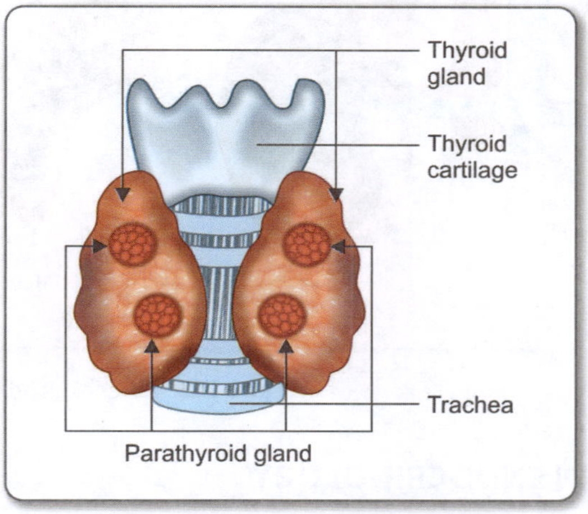

Figure 107: Thyroid and parathyroid glands

Parathyroid Gland

- There are four parathyroid glands.
- They are seen near or embedded in thyroid gland.
- Hormone secreted by parathyroid gland is parathyroid hormone or parathormone.

Pancreas

- Endocrine system of pancreas is known as islets of Langerhans.
- Pancreas secrete three types of hormone which control the blood glucose level
- Alpha cells of pancreas secrete **glucagon**, beta cells secrete **insulin** and delta cells secrete **somatostatin**.

Adrenal Gland

- Paired endocrine gland located above the kidney like a cap
- Outer region of the gland is known as cortex and inner region is known as medulla.
- Adrenal cortex has three regions such as:
  - **Zona glomerulosa** which secretes mineralocorticoids (aldosterone) and corticosterone.
  - **Zona fasciculata** and **zona reticularis** which secrete glucocorticoid (cortisol), corticosterone and androgen sex hormones.
- Adrenal medulla secretes **catecholamine** such as **epinephrine** and **norepinephrine**.

Recent Question (NORCET 2020)

73. Which hormone regulates calcium and phosphate?
a. Parathyroid Hormone
b. TSH
c. FSH
d. LH
Ans. (a) Parathyroid

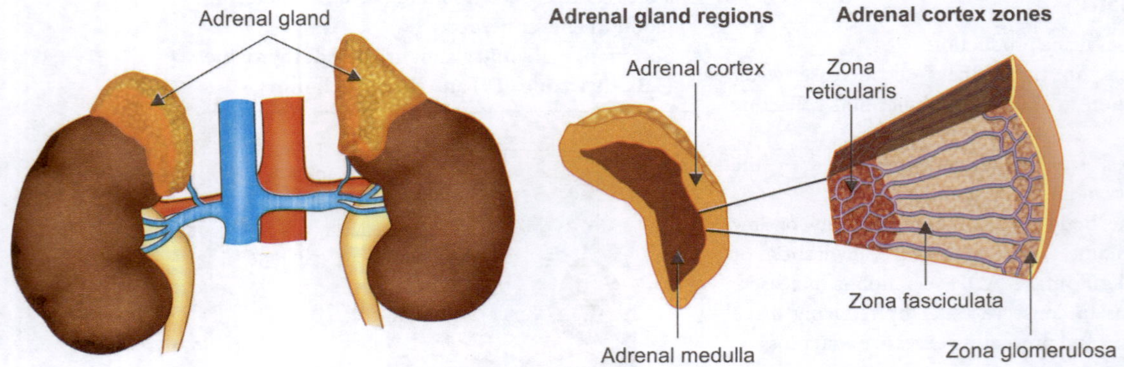

Figure 108: Adrenal gland

DIAGNOSTIC TESTS IN ENDOCRINOLOGY

Table 84: Description of diagnostic tests in endocrinology

Diagnostic test	Description	Points to remember
Thyroid function test (TFT)	• To determine primary and secondary hypothyroidism • **Primary hypothyroidism:** TSH is elevated • **Secondary hypothyroidism:** TSH is low or undetectable	Early morning fasting blood sample is needed
Anti-thyroid antibodies	• To diagnose autoimmune diseases of thyroid gland • Serological test will be performed	
Glycosylated hemoglobin (HbA1C)	• It reflects the blood glucose level over 2–3 months. • **Normal value:** Less than **6.5%**	

DISORDERS OF ENDOCRINE SYSTEM

Hyperpituitarism

- Excessive secretion of one or more of the pituitary hormones.
- Growth hormone and prolactin are the two major hormones overproduced by anterior pituitary.
- Overstimulation of other endocrine gland through excessive production of stimulating hormone can also be seen.
- Overproduction of prolactin causes hyper-prolactinemia.
- Overproduction of growth hormone in children causes gigantism and in adult it causes acromegaly.

Gigantism

- Overproduction of growth hormone in children causes this condition.
- Gigantism occurs before the closure of epiphyseal plates of the bone.
- Skeletal growth velocity will be increased but with little bony deformity.
- **Cause:** Most commonly due to pituitary adenoma
- **Management**
  - Resection of the tumor
  - GH analogue octreotide is very effective in reducing GH level.
  - Pituitary radiation

Acromegaly

- Overproduction of GH in adult causes acromegaly.
- It occurs after the closure of epiphyseal plate, so **transverse growth** can be observed.
- Large hands and feet, thick lips, coarse facial features, protruding forehead and enlarged jaw, widely spaced teeth are the clinical manifestations.
- **Management:** Similar to gigantism.

Hyperprolactinemia

- Increased level of prolactin in the blood is known as hyperprolactinemia
- **Cause:** Tumor in the pituitary
- **Manifestations**
  - Infertility, decreased sex drive and bone loss in both sexes
  - In males: erectile dysfunction and gynecomastia

POINT TO REMEMBER

Elevated levels of prolactin after delivery is normal.

- In females: vaginal dryness, irregular or absence of menstruation, production of milk in non-pregnant and non-nursing mothers.
- **Diagnosis**
  - Serum hormonal assay
  - CT and MRI of brain
- **Management**
  - Bromocriptine and cabergoline decreases the prolactin level.
  - Surgery and radiation therapy may also be useful in case of tumor.

Hypopituitarism

- Deficiency of anterior lobe pituitary hormones is named as hypopituitarism.
- Failure of both anterior and posterior pituitary lobes to secrete hormone is called as **panhypopituitarism**.
- **Short stature**
  - Stunted growth resulting from absence or deficient growth hormone.
- **Sexual and reproductive disorders**
  - Deficiencies of gonadotropins (FSH and LH) lead to sterility, decreased sex drive and decreased secondary sexual characters.
- Hypothyroidism
- Secondary adrenocortical insufficiency
- Prolactin deficiency

Posterior Pituitary Disorders/ Neurohypophyseal Disorders

- Posterior pituitary disorders are rare, even if damaged, because posterior lobe is only storing the hormones produced by hypothalamus.
- If the hypothalamus is damaged then even if there is a healthy pituitary, disorders are going to occur.
- Posterior lobe of the pituitary stores **ADH** and **oxytocin**.
- **Antidiuretic hormone (ADH)/vasopressin**
  - Hormone produced by hypothalamus and stored in posterior pituitary
  - Water balance of the body is under the control of this hormone.
  - Deficiency of ADH causes **diabetes insipidus**.
  - Excessive secretion of ADH causes syndrome of inappropriate anti-diuretic hormone (SIADH).
- **Oxytocin**
  - Hypothalamus produces, oxytocin and posterior pituitary stores and releases it.
  - It promotes uterine contraction during delivery.
  - It causes ejection of milk from the breast tissue following sucking, so this is the hormone responsible for **let down reflex**.

Diabetes Insipidus (DI)

- **Deficiency of ADH** leads to inability to conserve water.
- It can be central/neurogenic or nephrogenic.
  - **Central/neurogenic:** DI occurs as a result of problem with CNS or posterior pituitary.
  - **Nephrogenic:** DI occurs as a result of inability of distal tubules of the kidney to respond to ADH.
- **Risk factors for neurogenic DI:** Head injury, neurosurgery, CNS infection, pituitary tumors, etc.
- In this condition, water won't be absorbed back from distal tubules, resulting in loss of large amount of water via urine.
- **Characteristic feature:** Large quantity of dilute urine with **low urine specific gravity**
- **Other Manifestations**
  - Skin and mucous membrane become dry; tachycardia can be seen in cardiovascular system.
  - Hypovolemia, hypotension and shock can occur.
  - Serum sodium level increases and urinary sodium decreases.
- **Water deprivation test:** Client with DI continues to eliminate large quantity of urine even if water intake is restricted and there is a weight loss. It is confirmatory test for DI.
- **Management:** ADH replacement and removal of tumors are the management.

Syndrome of Inappropriate Antidiuretic Hormone (SIADH)

- **Large amount of Antidiuretic hormone (ADH)** from posterior pituitary causes SIADH.
- **Causes:** Ectopic tumors such as bronchogenic cancer, lymphoma of the duodenum, brain, bladder and pancreatic cancer secrete ADH like substance and causes SIADH.
- **Manifestations**
  - Water retention, hyponatremia and hypo-osmolality
  - Increased extra cellular fluid volume.
  - Physical manifestation related to hyponatremia such as decreased deep tendon reflex, fatigue, headache, seizure, anorexia, nausea and change in mental status.
  - Weight gain related to water retention, jugular venous distention, tachycardia and tachypnea can be seen.
- **Management:** Fluid restriction and hypertonic saline.

KEY POINT

Manifestations of Diabetes insipidus: Polyuria (up to 8 L/day), constant thirst, and an unusually high oral intake of fluids.

Recent Question (NORCET 2023)

74. Identify the Procedure in which the following image given below is used?

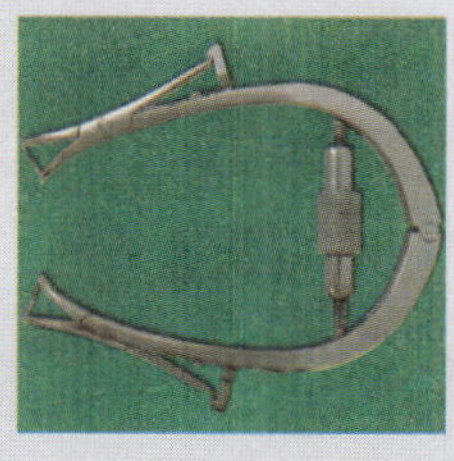

a. Abdominal surgery
b. Thyroidectomy
c. Whipple Surgery
d. Orthopaedic surgery

Ans. (c) Decreased inspiratory difficulty

THYROID GLAND

- **Euthyroidism:** Normal thyroid gland
- **Hyperthyroidism:** Increased secretion of thyroid hormone
- **Hypothyroidism:** Decreased secretion of thyroid hormones

Thyroid Hormone

- T3 (triiodothyronine) and T4 (thyroxine) are thyroid hormones.
- They are lipid soluble and found in plasma by binding with thyroid binding globulin.
- T3 has rapid effect than T4.
- These hormones increase the metabolism and heat production.
- They promote growth in children.

Disorders of Thyroid Gland

Goiter

- Enlargement of the thyroid gland
- **Causes:** Deficiency of iodine, inflammation or benign/malignant changes
- It can be seen in both hyperthyroidism and hypothyroidism.
- **Endemic goiter:** Due to nutritional iodine deficiency and is seen in people living in iodine deficient regions.
  - In India, the **Himalayan** region is **often** termed the 'goiter belt'.
- **Sporadic goiter:** Due to faulty iodine metabolism (genetic issue), people who consume more food items (cabbage, soybeans or spinach) which inhibit T4 and cause goiter. Ingestion of certain medications such as dopamine, glucocorticoids and lithium also causes sporadic goiter. It is not related to iodine deficiency.
- **Treatment:** Iodine and thyroid hormones supplements. A strong iodine solution such as Lugol's solution or potassium iodide can be given.
- Educate the client to consume iodine rich food and switch to iodized salt.

Hypothyroidism

- Decreased production of thyroid hormone → decreased tissue metabolism, decreased heat production and decreased oxygen consumption by the tissues.
- It can be either due to primary thyroid gland dysfunction or secondary to anterior lobe of pituitary dysfunction.

Primary hypothyroidism

- Thyroid gland is unable to produce sufficient amounts of thyroid hormone.
- Low thyroid hormones and High (TSH) Thyroid stimulating hormone level
- Pituitary tries to overcome the under production of thyroid hormone.
- **Autoimmune**: This is also known as **Hashimoto's disease.**
- Most common cause is iodine deficiency.
- ***Cretinism:*** Decrease thyroid hormone production due to congenital defects.

Secondary hypothyroidism

- Low secretion of TSH from the pituitary
- It occurs because of the problem with the pituitary or due to peripheral resistance to thyroid hormone.
- Both TSH and thyroid hormones are in low range.

Tertiary or central hypothyroidism

- Inadequate secretion of (TRH) thyrotropin releasing hormone from the hypothalamus
- Low level of TSH and thyroid hormones in serum.

- **Manifestations**
  - Decreased body metabolism, decreased heat production, decreased body temperature.
  - Cold, lethargy, dry skin, forgetfulness, depression, weight gain can be seen
  - **Myxedema:** When a person with hypothyroidism faces stressful situation such as infection, trauma or surgery, he may not be able to cope up with the situation. It is characterized by skin changes such as puffiness and swollen skin.
- **Management**
  - Thyroid hormone supplement such levothyroxine sodium.

Myxedema coma: It is a medical emergency triggered by stressful situations in life and is characterized by hypothermia, hypoventilation, respiratory acidosis and hypotension.

T4 supplement to an **older client** has the risk of development of ischemic heart disease evidenced by angina. So client should be closely monitored for blood level of drug and also pulse needs to be recorded.

Practice Questions

23. A female client with hypothyroidism is on oral levothyroxine, 25 mcg daily. Which of the following is an adverse effect of levothyroxine?
a. Bradycardia
b. Leg cramps
c. Tachycardia
d. Double vision

Ans. (c) Tachycardia

24. Which of the following interventions is appropriate for a patient with syndrome of inappropriate antidiuretic hormone (SIADH)?
a. Fluid restriction
b. Encourage plenty of oral fluid
c. Infuse Dextrose 5% as ordered
d. Infuse IV fluids rapidly as ordered

Ans. (a) Fluid restriction

Explanation: Patient with SIADH will have fluid retention. Fluid must be restricted to reduce the fluid retention.

POINT TO REMEMBER

To prevent excessive pressure on the surgical incision after subtotal thyroidectomy, the patient should be advised to **avoid hyperextending the neck**

Recent Question (NORCET 2023)

75. A patient presented with swelling in front of neck in midline which moves on deglutition. Which among the following will be the LESS likely diagnosis?
a. Thyroglossal Cyst
b. Solitary thyroid nodule in isthmus
c. Subhyoid bursitis
d. Lipoma

Ans. (d) Lipoma

Congenital Hypothyroidism

- Most common cause is thyroid dysgenesis (75 - 80%)
- **Significant Clinical features**
  - Asymptomatic at birth (due to maternal T4)
  - **Wide and open posterior fontanel**
  - Macroglossia (Large tongue)
  - Prolongation of physiological jaundice
  - Edematous face
  - Hoarse cry
  - Growth retardation
  - Mental retardation within 2 years of age
  - **Delayed dentition**
- Neonatal Screening for TSH and T4 can be done at postnatal day 2 – 4 by filter paper method
- **Treatment:** Replacement therapy with Thyroxine T4

Hyperthyroidism

- Excessive secretion of TSH
- Hyperthyroidism is more common in females than males.
- Most common form of hyperthyroidism is **Grave's disease** characterized by hyperthyroidism, goiter and exophthalmos.
- **Assessment**
  - Thyroid gland is enlarged
  - Bruit heard over thyroid arteries
  - Low serum TSH, high free T4
  - Increased radioactive iodine intake
- **Manifestations**
  - Client appears extremely irritated and agitated
  - Tremors at rest, weight loss despite of increased hunger and food intake
  - Heat intolerance, diaphoresis, tachycardia
  - Warm, smooth and moist skin
  - Hair appear thin and soft
  - Mood swings are common from mild euphoria to hyperactivity.

Thyroid storm is the complication associated with Grave's disease.

- **Thyroid storm/ thyrotoxicosis/ thyroid crisis:** It is a fatal condition characterized by high fever, hyper-reflexia, severe tachycardia, delirium, dehydration, hypertension and extreme irritability.
- **Treatment for Grave's disease:** Anti-thyroid medication, Radioactive iodine therapy [I^{131}], and thyroidectomy.
- **Antithyroid medications** - Propylthiouracil and methimazole.

Agranulocytosis is the side effect of propylthiouracil.

- Most common complication associated with radio iodine therapy is development of hypothyroidism in later life.
- Surgical management – Total or partial Thyroidectomy
- Lifelong replacement of thyroid hormone is necessary in total thyroidectomy.
- In subtotal thyroidectomy, one sixth of the gland remains intact and is able to produce thyroid hormone. Hormone replacement may not be necessary.
  - Total thyroidectomy: The whole gland is removed. Life-long replacement is required.
  - Sub-total thyroidectomy: The 1/6th of the gland remains intact and is able to produce thyroid hormone. Hormone replacement may not be necessary.
  - Thyroid lobectomy: A whole lobe is removed.

Post-thyroidectomy care

- Keep a tracheostomy tray at the bedside with oxygen and suction tray.
- Avoid hyperextension and flexion of the neck. Maintain a neutral position of the head in a semi-fowler position.
- Monitor for tetany which results from low calcium level because of accidental resection of the parathyroid gland.

Thyroiditis

- Inflammation of the thyroid gland
- Most commonly caused by *Streptococcus pyogenes, S.aureus and Pneumococcus pneumoniae.*

PARATHYROID GLAND

Parathyroid Hormone

- Role of parathyroid gland is to maintain normal blood calcium level.
- Fall in serum calcium level promotes the production of parathyroid hormone.
- Parathormone increases the release of calcium from bone to blood and increases the GI absorption of calcium.
- At distal convoluted tubule of kidney, the vitamin D or calcitriol is activated by PTH which stimulates absorption of calcium from GI tract.
- In kidney it will prevent the urinary loss of calcium.

Disorders of Parathyroid Gland

Hyperparathyroidism

- Overactivity of one or more of the parathyroid gland
- In hyperparathyroidism, more calcium will be mobilized from bone to blood, that leads to bone damage, hypercalcemia and kidney damage.

KEY POINTS

- **Pre-operative preparation for thyroidectomy -** Administer anti-thyroid drugs and iodine supplements to achieve euthyroid state and to decrease the size and vascularity of the gland.
- **Complications of thyroidectomy -** Hemorrhage, laryngeal edema, infection, vocal cord injury and thyroid storm.
- Accidental removal of parathyroid gland is very common during thyroidectomy. So closely monitor the client for calcium imbalances.
- **Thyroid storm** (thyrotoxic crisis) is an acute, life-threatening complication of hyperthyroidism.
- Thyroid crisis usually occurs in the first 12 hours after thyroidectomy and causes exaggerated signs of hyperthyroidism.
- Severe hypothyroidism in adults may result in myxedema coma. It is characterized by drastic drop in the metabolic rate, decreased vital signs, hypoventilation, and edema.

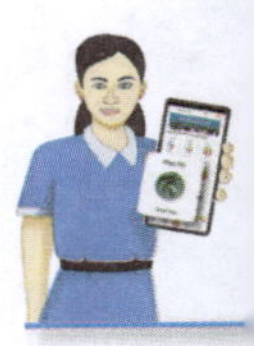

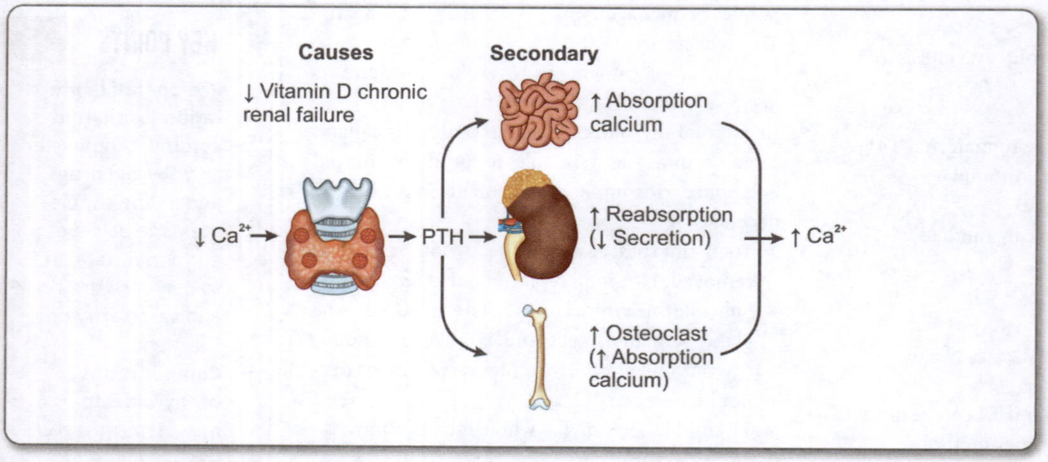

Figure 109: Hyperparathyroidism

- **Manifestations**
  - Bone pain, backache, pathological fracture, in long standing it may cause bone bending.
  - Nephrolithiasis and urine may contain sand, gravel or stone.
- **Management**
  - Drug that inhibits bone resorption such as plicamycin, calcitonin, gallium nitrate, etc.
  - Increases the hydration and achieve calciuria with the help of frusemide
  - Parathyroidectomy is the permanent surgical management for the condition.

Hypoparathyroidism

- Under-secretion of parathyroid hormone causes abnormally low serum calcium level, increased phosphate level and manifestation of tetany.
- Because of decreased serum calcium level, calcium may deposit in various body tissues and can lead to brain stem calcification and cataract formation.
- **Manifestations:** Chvostek's sign, trousseau's sign, hyperactive deep tendon reflex, circumoral paresthesia, numbness and tingling in the fingers are the common manifestations.
- **Medical management:** Increase the serum calcium level by administering 10% calcium gluconte.

ENDOCRINE-PANCREAS

- Pancreas is a **digestive exocrine gland** and a **hormone-producing endocrine gland.**
- Endocrine pancreas produces Insulin, Glucagon and Somatostatin.
  - **Insulin**
    - Insulin is secreted by Beta cells in the islets of Langerhans of pancreas.
    - Insulin decreases blood sugar level by increasing the storage, use and uptake of glucose and by promoting glycogenesis, lipogenesis and inhibiting gluconeogenesis.
  - **Glucagon**
    - Glucagon is secreted by Alpha cells in islets of Langerhans.
    - Glucagon increases the blood sugar level by acting on the liver.
  - **Somatostatin**
    - Somatostatin is secreted by Delta cells in islets of Langerhans.
    - Usually it releases after the intake of food.
    - It inhibits the release of insulin and glucagon.
    - It delays the nutrient absorption by prolonging the intestinal duration of food.
- **Counter-regulatory hormone:** The hormones ***glucagon, adrenaline, cortisol, and growth hormone*** have insulin-antagonistic effect during hypoglycemia or other stress condition.

Disorder of Pancreas

Diabetes Mellitus

- Diabetes mellitus is a group of metabolic disorders characterized by elevated levels of blood glucose (hyperglycemia) resulting from defects in insulin secretion, insulin action, or both.

Types

- **Type 1 diabetes mellitus (insulin-dependent)**
  - Deficiency of insulin secretion and it may be hereditary
  - 5–10% of patients with diabetes have type I
- **Type 2 diabetes mellitus (Non-insulin dependent)**
  - In this condition insulin production is there in the body but the body receptors are unable to respond to that insulin.
  - 90–95% of patients with diabetes have type II
- **Gestational Diabetes Mellitus**
  - Any degree of glucose intolerance with onset during pregnancy. It usually disappears after delivery.

KEY POINTS

- Respiratory distress either related to bleeding or due to damage to laryngeal nerve is common following parathyroidectomy.
- After the removal of the gland, client needs supplements such as calcium and vitamin D.
- Untreated hypothyroidism may cause laryngeal spasm and respiratory obstruction due to tetany.
- Patient is instructed to inhale CO_2 by exhaling into a paper bag while administering calcium gluconate to manage hypocalcemia. This is because CO_2 causes respiratory acidosis and increases the ionized calcium level in the blood.

Recent Question
(NORCET 2022)

76. A patient who has undergone thyroidectomy shows the symptoms of carpopedal spasm. Which medication is to be administered to this patient?

a. Calcium carbonate
b. Calcium gluconate
c. Calcium lactate
d. Calcium citrate

Ans. (b) Calcium gluconate

POINT TO REMEMBER

Anatomy of Pancreas has been discussed in the unit 'Gastrointestinal System'

Clinical Manifestations

- Classic signs: Polyuria, polydipsia, and polyphagia
- Sudden vision changes, fatigue, somnolence, wounds or skin lesions that are slow to heal.

Diagnosis

- Glucose tolerance test (GTT)
- Fasting plasma glucose levels above 125 mg/dL
- Random and postprandial (2 hours) blood sugar levels more than 200 mg/dL
- Other tests include glycosylated hemoglobin which helps to assess the blood sugar level in the last three months.

Complications of Diabetes Mellitus

- **Acute:** Hypoglycemia, **hyperglycemic hyperosmolar nonketotic syndrome** (HHNS) and **Diabetic Ketoacidosis (DKA)**
- **Chronic**
  - Macrovascular disease, affects coronary artery disease, cerebrovascular accident, diabetic foot due to peripheral neuropathy.
  - Microvascular disease affects eyes (retinopathy) and kidneys (nephropathy)
  - Neuropathic disease affects sensory motor and autonomic nerves which leads to impotence and foot ulcers.

Diabetic Ketoacidosis (DKA)

- It results from insufficient insulin, which prevents glucose from entering cells and causes it to accumulate in the blood.
- Liver increases the biosynthesis of glucose from noncarbohydrate substance such as protein and fat.
- Use of fat resulting in generation of ketone bodies, accumulation of ketone bodies results in ketosis and ketonuria.
- Accumulation of ketone bodies causes metabolic acidosis and results in DKA.
- **Management:** DKA is treated with regular IV insulin, IV fluids to supplement intravascular volume, potassium replacement, and sodium bicarbonate if the pH is less than 6.9.
- **Complications**
  - Body attempts to eliminate ketone and glucose via urine. This will result in increased urine output and dehydration.
  - Because of metabolic acidosis, hydrogen ion moves into the cells and potassium ion moves out of the cell which causes **intracellular potassium depletion.**

Hyperglycemic Hyperosmolar Nonketotic Syndrome (HHNS)

- In this condition some amount of insulin is there, so there would not be any fat breakdown so there is no ketone body release.
- This condition is characterized by extreme hyperglycemia, dehydration, hyperosmolarity and mild or undetectable ketonuria.
- Commonly seen in older clients with type 2 DM.
- Important electrolyte that needs to be replaced in this condition is potassium

Treatment

- Type I DM: Insulin
- Type II DM
  - Weight reduction
  - Exercise is important in enhancing the effectiveness of insulin.
  - Oral hypoglycemic agents if exercise is not effective
  - Change of lifestyle.

Nutritional Management

- Diet is planned for individual patient based on their metabolic and nutritional requirements.
- **Recommended diet restriction**
  - Fat intake should equal 20–30% of total calories
  - Protein intake, 10–20% of total calories
  - Carbohydrate intake, 50–60% of calories
  - Cholesterol intake, 300 mg or less
  - Fiber intake, 20–30 g daily
  - Sodium intake, 2–3 g daily.
- Simple sugar (monosaccharide and disaccharide) should be limited for DM patients.
- Diet should be included with soluble fibers that reduce blood glucose level and cholesterol and insoluble fibers which prevent constipation.

Exercise

- It improves insulin resistance of cells, glucose tolerance and also reduce weight and cholesterol level.
- Blood glucose level should be checked before and after exercises.
- If blood glucose level is >250 mg/dL or below normal value, exercises should not be done.
- Diabetic patients should do aerobic exercises and brisk walking minimum 150 min/ week or 3 days/week but maximum 2 consecutive days between periods of aerobic activity.

KEY POINTS

- Rate and depth of respiration increases in DKA and is known as kussmaul's respiration. The breath has fruity or acetone like odor.
- In hyperglycemia, urine osmolarity increases as glucose particles move into the urine. Increased osmolarity is an indication of fluid volume deficit.

Practice Question

25. Nurse Ramya is educating a patient regarding diet management to a female client with hypoglycemia. Which of the following should be recommended to control hypoglycemic episodes?

a. Vitamin B and iron supplements
b. Increased saturated fat intake
c. Consume low-carbohydrate and high protein diet
d. Eat a sugar candy if light-headedness occurs

Ans. (c) Consume low...

Recent Question (NORCET 2022)

77. A patient with Diabetes Mellitus is on regular insulin and insulin was administered a 9:00 am. How much time will it take to reach its peak level?

a. 10:30 am
b. 12:00 noon
c. 04:00 pm
d. 10:30 am

Ans. (b) 12:00 noon

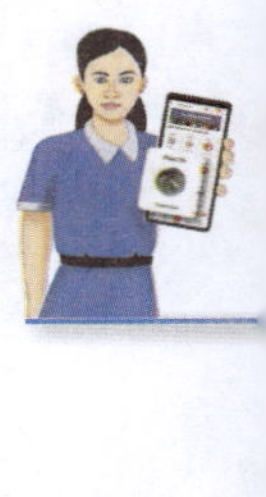

Table 85: Types of insulin used in the treatment of diabetes mellitus

Types of insulin	Onset of action	Peak action	Duration of action
Regular insulin	30–60 minutes	1–5 hours	6–10 hours
Rapid-acting insulins lispro (Humalog) and aspart (Novolog)	5–25 minutes	30–90 minutes	2–5 hours
Intermediate-acting insulin (Neutral protamine Hagedorn (NPH) or Lente insulin)	1–4 hours,	6–12 hours	12–24 hours
Long acting insulins (Protamine zinc or Ultralente insulin)	4–8 hours	16–18 hours	Up to 30 hours

Adverse Effects of Insulin

Insulin lipodystrophy

- It is swelling at injection site due to insulin's direct anabolic effect that leads to protein and fat synthesis.
- Change the injection site. Do not use a single site more than one time in a period of 14–21 days.

Dawn phenomenon

- Rise in blood glucose levels during the early morning hours, typically between 4 am and 8 am, without any preceding hypoglycemia.
- During the night, various hormonal changes occur in the body, including an increase in the secretion of growth hormone, cortisol, and adrenaline. These hormones work in combination to stimulate glucose production in the liver (gluconeogenesis) and decrease insulin sensitivity, leading to an increase in blood glucose levels.

Somogyi effect

- Rebound hyperglycemia
- In late-night, because of the night dose of insulin the patient will have hypoglycemia which activated the counter-regulatory hormone such as thyroxin, glucagon, cortisol, and adrenaline that leads to elevation of blood sugar level in the morning.
- The difference between the dawn phenomenon and the Somogyi effect is that in the dawn phenomenon there will be no history of hypoglycemia in night where as in Somogyi effect there will be a late-night hypoglycemia.

ADRENAL CORTEX

- **Aldosterone**
  - It is the **mineralocorticoid** hormone of the **adrenal cortex.**
  - It promotes the sodium absorption in kidneys and increases the potassium excretion in distal convoluted tubule.
  - It helps to prevents acidosis by helping in the excretion of H+ ions through urine.
- **Cortisol**
  - It is the **glucocorticoid** hormone of the **adrenal cortex.**
  - It increases metabolism and increases the blood glucose level.
  - It is also known as stress hormone.
  - It has anti-inflammatory action (it prevents vasodilation, decreases vascular permeability, and prevents leukocyte migration to the inflamed site).
  - It has antiallergy and immunosuppressive action.
  - It delays the wound healing in chronic stress state of the body.
  - Its secretion exhibits diurnal rhythm, so secretion is highest in the early morning and lowest in the evening.

Sex Hormones

- Major sex hormone secreted from adrenal cortex is androgen.
- Androgens are ***dehydroepiandrosterone (DHEA), androstenedione, and testosterone.***
- Most active androgen is DHEA.
- Masculine feature of the body results from androgen secretion.

Virilism: The male feature in the female body such as hirsutism, beard, enlarged clitoris, atrophied breast, deep voice, and more muscle as a result of increased androgen secretion in female.

Disorders of Adrenal Glands

Adrenal Insufficiency/Addison's Disease

- Hypo-functioning of the adrenal cortex is termed as adrenal insufficiency.
- **Primary adrenal insufficiency:** Due to impairment of adrenal gland which causes hypo function.

Causes

- Auto-immunity is the most common cause.

KEY POINTS

- The acid-base imbalance seen in Cushing's syndrome is metabolic alkalosis
- Osteoporosis and hypercortisolism are the common complications of management with glucocorticoids.
- Cortisol is known as stress hormone. Secretion of cortisol is highest in the early morning and lowest in the evening.
- **Addison's disease** is caused by deficiency of corticosteroid hormone.
- An adrenal adenoma is the most common cause of hyperaldosteronism.

Recent Question (NORCET 2022)

78. Skin of a patient with Addison's disease appears:

a. Yellow
b. Bronze
c. Black
d. Gray

Ans. (b) Bronze

- X-linked or autosomal recessive
- Drugs—Ketoconazole, mitotane, rifampicin, phenytoin, etc.

- **Secondary adrenal insufficiency:** Due to problem with hypothalmo-pituitary axis
- **Manifestations:** Fatigue, irritability, weight loss, nausea, vomiting and postural hypotension.
- **Diagnosis**
  - Low level of plasma cortisol and increased level of adrenocorticotropic hormone (ACTH)
  - **High** serum **potassium** and **low** serum **sodium**
- **Management**
  - Replacement of glucocorticoids and mineralocorticoids.
  - Hypoglycemia needs to be corrected.

Addison's Crisis

- A person who is with adrenal insufficiency with no adequate hormone replacement, when faces a stressor in life such as infection, surgery, pregnancy, etc. may show sudden pain in the back, abdomen, legs, volume depletion, hypotension, loss of consciousness and shock.
  - In a client with Addison's crisis, hypotension and electrolyte imbalance need to be corrected quickly. Ensure adequate rehydration of the client.

Adrenocortical Hyperfunction

Hyperfunction of the adrenal cortex results in increased secretion of glucocorticoids, mineralocorticoids and androgen.

Hypercortisolism/Cushing's Syndrome

- Characterized by **excessive secretion of glucocorticoids**.
- It is of two types:
  - **ACTH Independent**
    - Functioning adrenocortical tumor (85% in children <7 years, girls: boys ratio 3:1)
    - Primary pigmented nodular adrenocortical disease
    - Nodular hyperplasia, adenoma (Mccune-Albright syndrome)
  - **ACTH Dependent**
    - Bilateral adrenal hyperplasia (older children, boys = girls)
    - Pituitary adenoma (Cushing's disease)
    - Ectopic ACTH production - rare in children
- **Causes**
  - Iatrogenic administration of steroids
  - Hypersecretion of cortisol by cortisol secreting adrenal tumor
  - Hyperplasia of adrenal gland
- **Clinical manifestation**
  - Persistent hyperglycemia or steroid diabetes
  - Muscle wasting and weakness, capillary fragility which cause ecchymosis
  - **Osteoporosis** → compression fracture in spinal cord causes kyphosis
  - Loss of height
  - Sodium and water retention causes hypertension and edema.
  - **Hypernatremia and hypokalemia** are the electrolyte imbalances seen in this condition.
  - **Moon shaped face, buffalo hump, truncal obesity** with thin limbs
  - Pink purple striae appear over breast, abdomen, axilla and legs because of the thinning of skin
  - Susceptibility to infection and poor wound healing
  - Hirsutism and masculine characters in women
- **Management:** Bilateral adrenelectomy. Lifelong replacement with glucocorticoids and mineralocorticoids is needed after bilateral adrenelectomy.

Hyperaldosteronism

Primary Hyperaldosteronism

- Lesion in the adrenal gland results in **excessive secretion of aldosterone.**
- Sodium and water retention → hypertension and excessive loss of potassium (hypokalemia)
- This condition is also known as **Conn's syndrome.**

Secondary Hyperaldosteronism

- It occurs **not** because of the adrenal cortex issue but because of other conditions, e.g., sodium wasting renal disease, diuretic usage, etc.
- **Manifestations:** Hypernatremia, hypokalemia, water retention, hypertension
- **Management:** Unilateral or bilateral adrenelectomy

ADRENAL MEDULLA

- It is composed of chromaffin cells which secrete epinephrine and norepinephrine.
- It also secretes small amount of dopamine which is a precursor of norepinephrine.
- Actions of this hormone mimics sympathetic nervous system.
- These hormones are known as emergency hormones.
- Both these hormones increase the metabolism
- All the hormones secrete from the adrenal medulla is commonly called as catecholamines.

Disorders of Adrenal Medulla

- Main two types of tumors of adrenal medulla are **pheochromocytoma** and **neuroblastoma**.

Pheochromocytoma

- Catecholamine secreting tumor of the chromaffin cells of the adrenal medulla.

KEY POINTS

- Adrenal Insufficiency/Addison's Disease is an X-linked or autosomal recessive disease.
- Hyperkalemia (high potassium) and Hyponatremia (low sodium) is seen in Adrenal Insufficiency/Addison's Disease.
- Hypernatremia and hypokalemia are the electrolyte imbalances seen in Cushing syndrome.
- Moon shaped face, buffalo hump, truncal obesity with thin limbs are the features of Cushing syndrome.
- Addison crisis, also known as acute adrenal insufficiency, is a life-threatening emergency, characterized by hypotension, hypoglycemia, hyperkalemia, and hyponatremia.

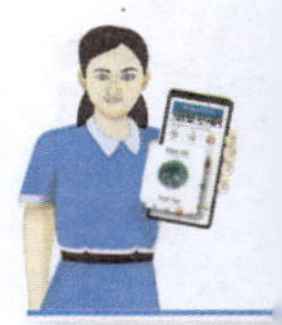

- Catecholamine release occurs at various frequencies and intensities known as paroxysm.
- **Manifestations:** Diabetes mellitus and glycosuria, hypertension, hyperthyroidism and psychoneurosis.
- **Management:** Unilateral or bilateral adrenelectomy

Neuroblastoma

- Tumor found on the top of the adrenal glands.
- **Symptoms**
  - Fatigue, loss of appetite and fever
  - Lump or compression of tissues in the affected area.
- **Management:** Surgery, chemotherapy and radiotherapy.

GONADS

Testosterone

- Male sex hormones produced by gonads.
- This is the primary steroid abused by athletes.
- It has anabolic action.

Estrogen

- Female sex hormones produced by gonads.
- Puberty related growth and initiation of menstruation are linked with the increased release of estrogen and progesterone.

KEY POINT

Manipulation of tumor during surgery for pheochromocytoma causes release of hormones into the blood and results in rapid rise in BP. Following surgery, withdrawal of hormone can cause fall in BP.

Golden Points to Remember

- Increased parathyroid hormone (PTH) results in hypercalcemia
- Maximum level of ACTH and cortisol is at the time of early morning.
- In secondary adrenal insufficiency: Aldosterone secretion is not affected therefore electrolytes are usually normal.
- Midline facial defect, single central incisor micro penis, hypoglycemia are the features seen in the deficiency of **Growth hormone**.
- Earliest manifestation of Cushing's syndrome: Loss of diurnal variation.
- 1st sign of pubertal changes in boys: Enlargement of testis.
- 1st sign of pubertal changes in girls: Thelarche.
- Testis starts producing testosterone under the influence of: Placental hCG.
- Normal consonance of puberty is:
  - Girls → Thelarche → Pubarche → Menarche
  - Boys → Gonadarche → Pubarche → Spermarche
- **Hashimoto's thyroditis**: It is progressive autoimmune disease of the thyroid gland with degeneration of its epithelial elements and replacement by lymphoid and fibrous tissue.
- Cretinism is the endocrine disorder that can lead to **mental retardation**.
- The sign of Cushing syndrome is moon face appearance, and buffalo hump.
- The classic symptoms of DM are **polyuria** (frequent urination), **polydipsia** (increased thirst) and **polyphagia** (increased hunger).
- Calcitonin is secreted by the thyroid gland and inhibits osteoclastic bone resorption by directly interacting with active osteoclast.
- **Diabetic insipidus** occurs due to the deficiency of Antidiuretic hormone.
- **Whipple's triad visible** in Insulinoma and other conditions cause hypoglycemia.
- Symptoms of hypoglycemia is low plasma glucose levels.
- Relief of symptoms after plasma glucose is raised.
- HbA1c indicates post serum glucose levels over previous 3 months' period.
- Exercise increases insulin receptor sites in the tissue and can have a direct effect on lowering blood glucose levels.
- The onset of Glargine is 1 hour and it lasts for 24 hours. Glargine lowers the blood glucose by promoting the conversion of glucose to glycogen.

"**Before healing others, heal yourself.**"
—Gambian (on health and wellness)

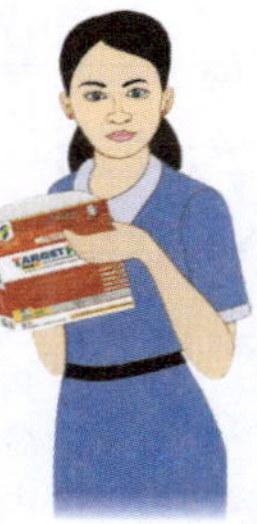

MULTIPLE CHOICE QUESTIONS
(Including Explained and Practice Questions)

ENDOCRINE SYSTEM

HYPOTHALAMUS AND PITUITARY GLAND

2478. The gland that is located below Hypophyseal Fossa of Sphenoid bone is: *(DSSSB PHN, 2015)*
a. Adrenal gland b. Thyroid gland
c. Pituitary gland d. Thymus

2479. The effect of Antidiuretic Hormone (ADH) is: *(DSSSB PHN, 2015)*
a. Oliguria b. Anuria
c. Increased urine output d. Decreased urine output

2480. The hormone secreted by Posterior Pituitary gland:
a. Insulin b. Glucagon
c. Corticotrophin d. Oxytocin

2481. Pituitary gland releases all of the following hormones; EXCEPT:
a. ACTH b. Oxytocin
c. TSH d. Cortisol

Explanation: Cortisol is released from the adrenal cortex. Other hormones are released from pituitary.

2482. ADH secretion increases when there is:
a. Hyperkalemia b. Hypokalemia
c. Hypernatremia d. Hyponatremia

2483. Hormone responsible for fluid and electrolyte balance is:
a. Antidiuretic hormone b. Angiotensin
c. Aldosterone d. Rennin

2484. All the following hormones are secreted by anterior pituitary; EXCEPT:
a. GH b. TSH
c. ADH d. ACTH

2485. Posterior pituitary secretes:
a. Growth hormone b. Prolactin
c. TSH d. Oxytocin

2486. The hormone secreted by anterior pituitary gland includes:
a. Antidiuretic hormone b. Adrenocorticotropin
c. Cortisol d. Oxytocin

Explanation: Adrenocorticotropin is secreted by the anterior pituitary gland. Antidiuretic hormone (vasopressin) and oxytocin are secreted by posterior pituitary gland. Cortisol is secreted by the adrenal gland.

2487. Ovarian reserve is best indicated by:
a. FSH b. LH: FSH ratio
c. LH d. Estrogen

2488. GH secretion decrease in which of the following conditions:
a. Sleep b. Hyperglycemia
c. Surgical stress d. Glucagon

2489. All are true about Melatonin; EXCEPT:
a. Secreted by Pineal gland
b. Maintains sleep-wake cycle
c. Increase in melatonin cause awakening
d. Secretion decrease in light

2490. Pineal gland located at:
a. Thalamus b. Epithalamus
c. Hypothalamus d. Telencephalon

2491. Catecholamines are synthesized from:
a. Tyrosine b. Insulin
c. Glucagon d. Alanine

2492. Gonadotrophin releasing factor is secreted by:
a. Adenohypophysis b. Neurohypophysis
c. Hypothalamus d. Basal ganglion

2493. Major stress hormone is:
a. Epinephrine b. Norepinephrine
c. Thyroxine d. Cortisol

2494. Hormone increased in post menopausal women:
a. FSH b. LH
c. HCG d. Prolactin

2495. Milk ejecting hormone is:
a. Prolactin b. Oxytocin
c. Progesterone d. Estrogen

2496. Let down reflex is the responsibility of ……… hormone:
a. Prolactin b. Oxytocin
c. Progesterone d. Estrogen

2497. Milk producing hormone is:
a. Prolactin b. Oxytocin
c. Progesterone d. Estrogen

2498. Hormones from anterior pituitary are all; EXCEPT:
a. Growth Hormone b. Prolactin
c. Luteinizing Hormone d. Oxytocin

2499. Anterior pituitary is also known as:
a. Adenohypophysis b. Neurohypophysis
c. Corpus callosum d. Arachnoid villi

2500. Posterior pituitary is also known as:
a. Adenohypophysis
b. Neurohypophysis
c. Corpus calosum
d. Arachnoid villi

2501. ACTH level is highest during:
a. Early morning b. Evening
c. Afternoon d. Night

2502. Serotonin is secreted by:
a. Argentaffin cells b. Adrenal medulla
c. Adrenal cortex d. Thyroid

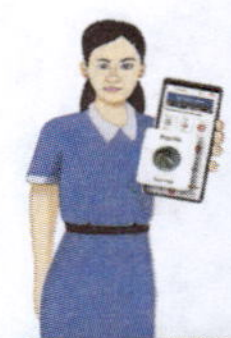

Ans.

2478. c
2479. d
2480. d
2481. d
2482. c
2483. a
2484. c
2485. d
2486. b
2487. a
2488. b
2489. c
2490. b
2491. a
2492. c
2493. d
2494. a
2495. b
2496. b
2497. a
2498. d
2499. a
2500. b
2501. a
2502. a

2503. All of the following hormones are secreted by anterior pituitary; EXCEPT:
a. Growth hormone
b. Oxytocin
c. Prolactin
d. Gonadotropin

2504. Which of the following stimulates the release of ADH from posterior pituitary gland?
a. Increased sodium level in blood
b. Decreased sodium level in blood
c. Increased glucose level in blood
d. Decreased glucose level in blood

2505. Vasopressin is synthesized in:
a. Renal cortex b. Anterior pituitary gland
c. Posterior pituitary gland d. Hypothalamus

2506. FSH is produced by:
a. Chromophobes b. Acidophiles
c. Basophils d. All of these

2507. Melatonin is secreted by:
a. Pineal gland b. Thyroid gland
c. Anterior Pituitary d. Pancreas

2508. Hormones secreted by the placenta include:
a. Progesterone
b. Human chorionic gonadotropin
c. Estradiol
d. All of these

2509. Action of ADH:
a. Reabsorption of NN in DCT
b. Reabsorption of water in DCT
c. Reabsorption of Glucose in DCT
d. Reabsorption of HCO_3 in DCT

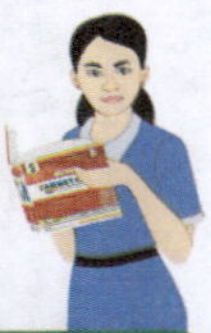

2510. Site of action of ADH is:
I. Distal Convoluted tubules
II. Collecting Duct
III. Proximal convoluted tubules
IV. Loop of Henle
a. II and III b. II and IV
c. I and II d. I and III

2511. Diabetes insipidus is related to deficiency of:
a. Oxytocin b. Insulin
c. Vasopressin d. Prolactin

2512. The hormone from the anterior pituitary gland that stimulates ovulation is called:
a. Follicle-stimulating hormone
b. Luteinizing hormone
c. Adrenocorticoid trophic hormone
d. Progesterone

2513. The functions of the placenta include the production of:
a. FSH b. LH
c. HCG d. TSH

2514. The suckling reflex occurs in response to:
a. Prolactin
b. Progesterone
c. Oxytocin
d. Estrogen

2515. A drug that would stop the production of milk in the breast after a few days probably has the effect of:
a. Inhibiting prolactin secretion
b. Inhibiting oxytocin secretion
c. Increasing prolactin secretion
d. Increasing oxytocin secretion

2516. Adrenocorticotrophic hormone (ACTH) stimulates the:
a. Thyroid gland b. Ovaries and testes
c. Hypothalamus d. Adrenal cortex

2517. The hormone from the posterior pituitary that increases water reabsorption in the kidney tubules is:
a. Antidiuretic hormone b. Prolactin
c. Oxytocin d. Aldosterone

2518. The hormone that acts to increase the permeability of renal tubules to water in order to produce less urine output is:
a. Rennin b. Aldosterone
c. Antidiuretic hormone d. Atrial natriuretic hormone

2519. Excessive secretion of growth hormone leads to:
a. Gigantism before the closure of epiphyseal plate
b. Acromegaly after the closure of epiphyseal plate
c. Both a and b
d. Cretinism

2520. Aldosterone directly regulate the concentration of:
a. Calcium b. Potassium
c. Sodium d. Phosphorous

2521. Hyperpigmentation is seen with which hormone?
a. FSH b. LH
c. ACTH d. TSH

2522. Growth hormone is secreted by: *(Kerala PSC, Nov 2014)*
a. Neurohypophysis b. Adrenal cortex
c. Adenohypophysis d. Adrenal medulla

2523. Identify the lobes of pituitary gland:
a. Adenohypophysis
b. Intermediate lobe of the pituitary
c. Neurohypophysis
d. All of the above

Explanation: All of the above are the lobes of pituitary. It has 3 lobe anterior lobe (adenohypophysis), posterior lobe (neurohypophysis) and intermediate lobe.

2524. Thirst control center is located in:
a. Cerebrum b. Hypothalamus
c. Cerebellum d. Medulla oblongata

2525. Which of the following hormones is secreted by anterior pituitary?
a. Prolactin b. TSH
c. GH d. All of these

2526. Which of the following hormone is secreted by posterior pituitary?
a. ACTH b. LH
c. FSH d. ADH

2527. The serological reaction, which sensitizes bacteria for phagocytosis is called: *(AIIMS Raipur Grade II 2017)*
a. Co-agglutination
b. Neutralization
c. Opsonization
d. Complement fixation

Explanation: Coagglutination is the process of aggregation of particulate antigens bound with agglutinins of more than one specificity. Neutralization is a chemical reaction in which acid and base react quantitatively with each other. Complement fixation test is immunological test that can be used to detect either specific antibody or specific antigen in a patients serum based on occurrence of complement fixation.

Ans.
2503. b
2504. a
2505. d
2506. c
2507. a
2508. d
2509. b
2510. c
2511. c
2512. b
2513. c
2514. c
2515. a
2516. d
2517. a
2518. c
2519. c
2520. c
2521. c
2522. c
2523. d
2524. b
2525. d
2526. d
2527. c

THYROID AND PARATHYROID GLANDS

2528. Thyroid gland is present in: *(ESIC Chennai May 2012)*
- a. Chest
- b. Back
- c. Abdomen
- d. Neck

2529. Which among the following hormone has intracellular receptors in all the organ?
- a. Parathyroid hormone
- b. Estrogen
- c. Growth hormone
- d. Thyroid hormone

2530. Complications of total thyroidectomy are all; EXCEPT:
- a. Hypocalcaemia
- b. Hypercalcemia
- c. Hoarseness of voice
- d. Parathyroid loss

2531. Parathyroid hormone acts on kidney causing:
- a. Calcium retention, phosphate loss
- b. Calcium loss, phosphate retention
- c. Loss of both calcium and phosphate
- d. Retention of calcium and phosphate

2532. Calcitonin is secreted by:
- a. Thyroid gland
- b. Parathyroid gland
- c. Both a and b
- d. None of these

2533. Role of calcitonin is:
- a. Decrease Ca level
- b. Increase Ca level
- c. Increase PO_4
- d. None of these

2534. Not required for absorption of calcium:
- a. Parathyroid hormone
- b. Calcitonin
- c. Bile salts
- d. Vitamin D

2535. Number of parathyroid gland in human body is/are:
- a. 1
- b. 2
- c. 3
- d. 4

2536. Thyroid-binding globulin increases in:
- a. Diabetes mellitus
- b. Pregnancy
- c. Grave's disease
- d. Nephrotic syndrome

2537. Which of the following is the primary function of the parathyroid gland?
- a. Regulates serum calcium levels
- b. Maintains BMR
- c. Receive hormonal signals from hypothalamus
- d. Send hormonal signals to other endocrine glands

2538. The main function of parathyroid hormone is to:
- a. Increase the calcium level in the blood
- b. Inhibit the formation of vitamin D in the kidneys
- c. Decrease the rate of bone breakdown
- d. Decrease the blood calcium level

2539. Mechanism of action of parathyroid hormone:
- a. Decreases Calcitriol
- b. Decreases Phosphate excretion
- c. Increases Calcium absorption
- d. Act an osteoclast

2540. The only endocrine gland which can store its hormone is:
- a. Pituitary
- b. Pancreas
- c. Thyroid
- d. Adrenal gland

Explanation: Thyroid is the only endocrine gland which can store its hormonal secretion and can secrete it into the blood whenever the body is in need. Pituitary stores the hormones which are secreted by hypothalamus.

2541. Thyroid releasing hormone is secreted by:
- a. Thyroid gland
- b. Hypothalamus
- c. Parathyroid gland
- d. Anterior pituitary gland

Explanation: Hypothalamus secretes releasing hormones including Thyrotropin-releasing hormone, Growth-releasing hormone, Gonadotropin-releasing hormone, and Corticotropin-releasing hormone.

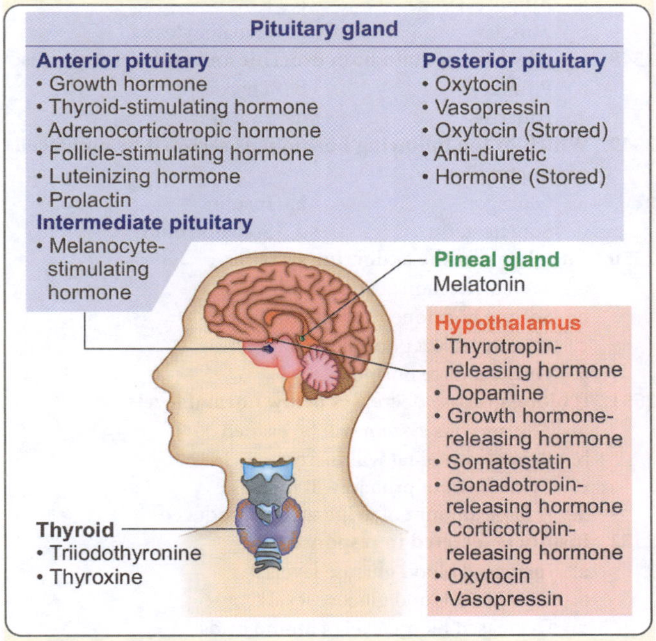

PANCREAS (ENDOCRINE PANCREAS)

2542. Insulin increases the entry of glucose into:
- a. All tissues
- b. Renal tubular cells
- c. Mucosa of the small intestine
- d. Skeletal muscle

2543. Insulin acts by stimulation of:
- a. Ionotropic receptor
- b. Enzymatic receptor
- c. Metabotropic receptor
- d. Nuclear receptor

2544. All of the following are features of diabetes insipidus include all the following; EXCEPT:
- a. Low specific gravity of urine
- b. Increased serum sodium
- c. Increased osmolality
- d. Hyperkalemia

2545. Insulin is essential for entry of glucose in:
- a. Most neurons in cerebral cortex
- b. Renal tubular cells
- c. Skeletal muscles
- d. Mucosa of small intestine

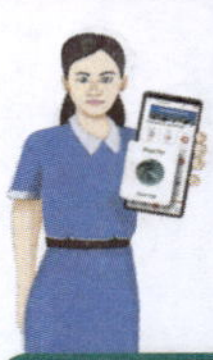

Ans.

2528. d
2529. d
2530. b
2531. a
2532. a
2533. a
2534. c
2535. d
2536. b
2537. a
2538. a
2539. c
2540. c
2541. b
2542. d
2543. b
2544. d
2545. c

2546. Which of the following hormones helps in increasing the blood glucose level?

a. Insulin b. Estrogen
c. Glucagon d. Progesterone

Explanation: Glucagon helps in increasing the blood glucose level by activating gluconeogenesis. Gluconeogenesis refers to synthesis of glucose from non-carbohydrate sources such as protein and fat.

2547. Insulin promotes transport of glucose in all of the following; EXCEPT:

a. Adipose Tissue b. RBC
c. Muscles d. Hepatocytes

2548. Gland which contain both exocrine and endocrine part is:

a. Pituitary b. Thyroid
c. Pancreas d. Uterus

2549. Which of the following hormone is secreted by alpha cells of pancreas?

a. Glucagon b. Insulin
c. Somatostatin d. Somatotropin

2550. The glands of the endocrine system:

a. Secrete hormones into blood
b. Secrete hormones into ducts
c. Usually have a poor blood supply
d. Only produce hormones

2551. If blood glucose decreases below normal levels:

a. The nervous system will be excited
b. Breakdown of fat will increase
c. Breakdown of protein will increase
d. A large amount of urine will be produced

2552. Insulin is secreted in response to:

a. Increased blood glucose levels
b. Decreased blood glucose levels
c. Decreased blood level of amino acids
d. Decreased parasympathetic stimulation

2553. The major target tissue for glucagon is the:

a. Heart b. Brain
c. Liver d. Stomach

2554. The hormone that increases blood glucose levels and lipid breakdown, but slows, protein breakdown is:

a. Glucagon
b. Insulin
c. Glucocorticoid
d. Growth hormone

2555. Hormones are secreted into the blood stream by:

a. Unicellular glands
b. Multicellular glands
c. Endocrine glands
d. Exocrine glands

2556. Hypoglycemia is present in:

a. Addison's disease
b. Hepatocellular failure
c. Glucose-6 phosphatase defect
d. All of the above

2557. Hyperglycemia is the manifestation of:

a. Diabetes mellitus
b. Cushing syndrome
c. Hyperthyroidism
d. All of the above

ADRENAL GLAND

2558. Corticosteroid is naturally produced by:
(ESIC Chennai May 2012)

a. Thalamus b. Ovary
c. Thyroid gland d. Adrenal glands

2559. Which inhibits glucagon secretion?

a. Secretin b. Beta agonist
c. Exercise d. Aminoacids

2560. Which hormone is released from zona glomerulosa?
(AIIMS Bhopal Grade-I 2018)

a. Oestrogen b. Aldosterone
c. Adrenalin d. Cortisol

Explanation: The zona glomerulosa of the adrenal gland is the most superficial layer of the adrenal cortex, lying directly beneath the renal capsule. Aldosterone is mineralocorticoid hormone expressed in the zona glomerulosa.

2561. Stress hormone is:

a. Gonadotrophins
b. Insulin
c. Cortisol
d. Growth hormone

DIAGNOSTIC TESTS IN ENDOCRINOLGY

2562. Glycated hemoglobin (HbA1c) tests, mean glucose levels:
(RAK MSc 2018)

a. Over 2 days b. Over 15 days
c. Over 90 days d. Over 30 days

Explanation: HbA1c also called hemoglobin A1c (HbA1c), glycated hemoglobin or glycosylated hemoglobin. It is a blood test that is used to help diagnose and monitor people with diabetes.

The HbA1c test tells average level of blood glucose over the past 3 months (90 days) in the body. The HbA1c test measures how much glucose is bound to RBC.

2563. Normal random blood sugar level is:

a. 30–60 mg/dL b. 60–90 mg/dL
c. 80–110 mg/dL d. 180–210 mg/dL

2564. In normal person, the percentage of glycosylated haemoglobin is:
(ESIC Chennai May 2012)

a. <5.7 b. >5.7
c. Both a and b d. None of these

2565. Impaired glucose tolerance is said when:

a. Fasting blood sugar >100 mg%
b. Fasting blood sugar is normal and PP blood is 100–140 mg%
c. Fasting blood sugar is normal and PP blood is 140–200 mg%
d. Fasting blood sugar is 100-120 mg% and PP blood is >200 mg%

2566. Fasting blood sugar is 120 mg/dL and 2 hours post prandial sugar after 75 g of oral glucose administration is 180 mg/dL. Diagnosis is:

a. Normal individual
b. Impaired glucose tolerance
c. Pre-diabetes
d. Diabetes mellitus

Ans.

2546. c
2547. b
2548. c
2549. a
2550. a
2551. b
2552. a
2553. c
2554. d
2555. c
2556. d
2557. d
2558. d
2559. a
2560. b
2561. c
2562. c
2563. c
2564. a
2565. c
2566. c

2567. In a person with hypocalcaemia parathyroid dysfunction is suspected, the confirmatory diagnostic test shows:
a. Decreased parathormone
b. Increased parathormone
c. Decreased calcitonin
d. Increased serum calcium

2568. Diagnostic test specific to Cushing syndrome is:
a. Urine cortisol level
b. Dexamethasone suppression test
c. Plasma cortisol level
d. All of these

2569. Levodopa test is used to detect:
a. LH
b. ACTH
c. FSH
d. GH reserve

2570. Most sensitive method to diagnose thyroid function is:
a. T3
b. T4
c. TSH
d. Thyroglobulin

Explanation:
- Most sensitive and specific test to detect hypothyroidism and hyperthyroidism is **TSH** Assay.
  - **Total T4:** Reflects output from thyroid gland.
  - **Total T3:** More indicative of peripheral thyroid metabolism, hence, not useful for screening.

HYPERPITUITARISM

2571. Gigantism is seen in:
a. Hyperpituitarism
b. Hypopituitarism
c. Hyperthyroidism
d. Hypothyroidism

2572. Short stature, secondary to growth hormone deficiency is associated with:
a. Height age is equal to Bone age
b. Normal body proportion
c. Low birth weight
d. Normal epiphyseal development

Explanation:

Growth Hormone deficiency
- GHD babies are born AGA (not SGA)
- They have maintained body proportions, i.e., - proportionate short stature
- Disproportionate SS is seen in following (Upper segment: lower segment)
  - US > LS → Richets & Achondroplasia
  - US < LS → Spondylo epiphyseal dysplasia
  - GHD — Children have significantly delayed bone age - but which is appropriate for height age, i.e., CA > HA = BA

2573. The hyper secretion of growth hormone leads to:
(DSSSB PHN, 2015)
a. Cretinism
b. Myxedema
c. Acromegaly
d. Grave's diseases

2574. Excessive secretion of growth hormone by anterior pituitary in prepubertal children causes:
a. Addison's disease
b. Cushing's disease
c. Gigantism
d. Adenomegaly

HYPOPITUITARISM

2575. Lack of thyroid hormone in children leads to:
a. Cretinism
b. Gigantism
c. Acromegaly
d. Grave's disease

2576. Which of the following is the most common cause of hypopituitarism?
a. Congenital adenoma
b. Pituitary adenoma
c. Craniopharyngioma
d. None of the above

2577. Panhypopituitarism is also called:
a. Simmond's disease
b. Sheehan's syndrome
c. Kahler's disease
d. Basedow's disease

2578. After a hypophysectomy procedure, which of the following statement by the client represents best understanding of the health education?
a. Thyroid hormone replacement therapy is the essential one
b. My menstruation will be ceased
c. I may had infertility
d. All of the above

2579. The syndrome which commonly occur in women with severe blood loss at the time of delivery is called:
a. Sheehan's syndrome
b. Cushings disease
c. Turner syndrome
d. Simmonds disease

Explanation: Sheehan's syndrome (SS) is postpartum hypopituitarism caused by necrosis of the pituitary gland. It is usually the result of severe hypotension or shock caused by massive hemorrhage during or after delivery.

2580. Which type of tumor in the pituitary gland may cause gigantism?
a. Eosinophilic tumor
b. Basophilic tumor
c. Monophilic tumor
d. Chromophobic tumor

POSTERIOR PITUITARY DISORDERS/ NEUROHYPOPHYSEAL DISORDERS

2581. Increased blood sugar level is the characteristic feature of all of the following; EXCEPT:
a. Diabetes mellitus
b. Corticosteroid therapy
c. Pancreatitis
d. SIADH

2582. Clinical manifestation of SIADH includes:
a. Increased urine Na^+
b. Decreased serum Na^+
c. Increased urine osmolality
d. All of the above

2583. The Hypofunction of the anterior pituitary gland that rarely affects the posterior lobe leading to:
(AIIMS Raipur Grade II 2017)
a. Grave's disease
b. Simmond's disease
c. Frohlick's Syndrome
d. Levi Syndrome

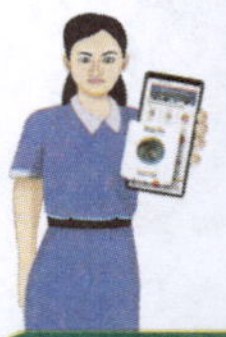

Ans.

2567. a
2568. d
2569. d
2570. c
2571. a
2572. b
2573. c
2574. c
2575. a
2576. b
2577. a
2578. d
2579. a
2580. a
2581. d
2582. d
2583. b

Explanation: Simmonds disease is characterized by pan-hypopituitarism that causes progressive emaciation, atrophy of the gonads, thyroid, and adrenal cortex, and loss of body hair that results from atrophy or destruction of the anterior lobe of the pituitary gland.

Fröhlich's syndrome/Adiposogenital Dystrophy is a metabolic disorder characterized by obesity, growth retardation, and retarded development of the genital organs associated with tumours of the hypothalamus, causing increased appetite and depressed secretion of gonadotropin.

Roussy–Lévy syndrome/Roussy–Lévy hereditary areflexic dystasia is a rare genetic disorder of humans that results in progressive muscle wasting which is caused by mutations in the genes.

Graves' disease/toxic diffuse goiter is an autoimmune disease which is a common cause of hyperthyroidism.

2584. Twelve hours after a transsphenoidal hypophysectomy, the client keeps clearing his throat and complains of a drip in his mouth. To accurately assess this, the nurse should test the fluid for:

a. Glucose b. Protein
c. Bacteria d. Blood

Explanation: Dripping in the back of the throat after a transsphenoidal hypophysectomy may be cerebrospinal fluid. CSF contains glucose. Testing for glucose will confirm if CSF present in the fluid. Saliva and mucus do not contain glucose.

Diabetes Insipidus and SIADH

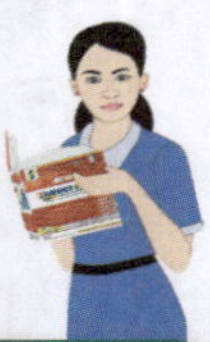

2585. Diabetes insipidus is caused by the deficiency of:

(DSSSB 2013)

a. Antidiuretic hormone b. Insulin
c. Glucagon d. Renin

Explanation: Diabetes insipidus (DI) is a condition caused by inadequate output of the pituitary hormone ADH (antidiuretic hormone). It is characterized by excessive thirst and excretion of large amounts of diluted urine.

2586. Clinical manifestation expected in a client with diabetes insipidus is:

a. Polyuria and hyponatremia
b. Polyuria and hypernatremia
c. Low urine output and hyponatremia
d. Low urine output and hypernatremia

2587. In a client with diabetes insipidus, the serum sodium level:

a. Increases
b. Decreases
c. Within the normal range
d. Fluctuating

2588. Water deprivation test is used for the diagnosis of:

a. Diabetic mellitus b. Diabetic insipidus
c. SIADH d. Diabetic ketoacidosis

Explanation: In diabetic insipidus water intake will be restricted in the person, following that, if urine output increases and weight loss occurs in a person, then the person is diagnosed as diabetes insipidus.

2589. Causes of nephrogenic diabetes insipidus include:

(DSSSB 2001, AIIMS Raipur staff nurse grade I-2018)

a. Idiopathic b. Genetic
c. Head injury d. Histiocytosis X

Explanation: Nephrogenic diabetes insipidus (NDI) is characterized by inability to concentrate the urine, which results in polyuria (excessive urine production) and polydipsia. Cause of Nephrogenic diabetes insipidus is either acquired or hereditary (genetic). Options a, c and d are causes of cranial diabetes insipidus. Genetic is the most common cause for nephrogenic diabetes insipidus.

2590. Priority nursing management in a client with Diabetes insipidus is:

a. Hourly urine output
b. Hourly blood glucose
c. Hourly head circumference
d. Hourly abdominal circumference

2591. What should be included in the nursing care plan of a client with diabetes insipidus?

a. Measure blood pressure every hour
b. Glucose monitoring four times a day
c. Maintain strict intake and output
d. Monitor urine for ketone bodies

Explanation: Diabetes insipidus is excessive and severely diluted urine excretion due to insufficient antidiuretic hormone. Because of the excessive urine output, it is necessary to monitor intake and output.

2592. Following the resection of craniopharyngioma important nursing intervention is measurement of:

a. Hourly urine specific gravity
b. Hourly blood sugar
c. Hourly abdominal girth
d. Hourly head circumference

Explanation: Surgery can cause damage to hypothalamus

2593. Cause of SIADH:

a. Excess of ADH b. Deficiency of aldosterone
c. Deficiency of ADH d. Excess of aldosterone

2594. In a client with SIADH, serum sodium level:

a. Increases b. Decreases
c. Remain in normal range d. Fluctuates

2595. Clinical manifestation expected in a client with SIADH is:

a. Polyuria and hyponatremia
b. Polyuria and hypernatremia
c. Low urine output and hyponatremia
d. Low urine output and hypernatremia

GOITER AND THYROIDITIS

2596. Cause of goiter is:

a. Iodine deficiency b. Excess iodine
c. Thyroiditis d. Thyroidectomy

2597. Most common cause of goiter in India is:

a. Diffuse Endemic Goiter
b. Hashimoto's Thyroiditis
c. Papillary carcinoma
d. Toxic Multinodular

2598. Which of the following is not correct about Hashimoto's disease?

a. Chronic lymphocytic thyroiditis
b. An autoimmune disorder
c. Treated by oral levothyroxine
d. Characterized by severe weight loss

Ans.

2584. a
2585. a
2586. b
2587. a
2588. b
2589. b
2590. a
2591. c
2592. a
2593. a
2594. b
2595. c
2596. a
2597. a
2598. d

2599. The most common cause of hypothyroidism in adults is:
- a. Myxedema coma
- b. Hashimoto's thyroiditis
- c. Sub acute thyroiditis
- b. Both a and c

2600. What is the most common causative agent for acute thyroiditis?
- a. Staphylococcus aureus
- b. Streptococcus aureus
- c. Salmonella species
- d. Plasmodium species

2601. Painless thyroiditis most often occurs in:
- a. Pregnancy women
- b. Postpartum women
- c. Nulliparous women
- d. Multiparous women

Explanation: **Postpartum thyroiditis** is the term used for patients who develop **painless thyroiditis** in the **postpartum** period. It usually occurs within six months after delivery and runs a clinical course similar to that of **painless thyroiditis** occurring without relation to pregnancy.

2602. Which of the following symptom is not present in hyperthyroidism?
- a. Tachycardia
- b. Bradycardia
- c. Heat intolerance
- d. Hypertension

2603. Which of the following symptom is not present in hypothyroidism?
- a. Cold intolerance
- b. Heat intolerance
- c. Constipation
- d. Lethargy

HYPOTHYROIDISM

2604. Under production of thyroxine leads to: *(JIPMER 2012)*
- a. Myxedema
- b. Grave's disease
- c. Cushing's disease
- d. Acromegaly

2605. Deficiency of thyroxin in adults leads to a condition called: *(Safdarjung NO 2018)*
- a. Tetani
- b. Cretinism
- c. Myxedema
- d. Graves' disease

Explanation: Deficiency of thyroxin in adults leads to a condition called myxedema. Deficiency of thyroxine in infant and children causes cretinism that is associated with mental retardation and edema. Excessive thyroxine hormones in adults may leads to graves' disease that is hypermetabolic state.

2606. Hormone elevated in a client with hypothyroidism is:
- a. T3
- b. T4
- c. TSH
- d. Thyroxine

2607. Most reliable investigation for hypothyroidism is:
- a. T3 and T4 levels
- b. TRH level
- c. TSH level
- d. Iodine level

2608. A life-threatening clinical condition that represents severe hypothyroidism with physiological decompensation is known as:
- a. Myxedema crisis
- b. Hypertensive crisis
- c. Delirium tremens
- d. Thyroid storm

2609. Clinical manifestations of grave's disease includes:
- a. Metabolic rate will increases and weight loss will be there
- b. Exophthalmos is a clinical manifestation of this condition
- c. Over production of thyroid hormone
- d. All of the above

2610. Clinical manifestation related to hypothyroidism is:
- a. Weight loss
- b. Shivering hands
- c. Tachycardia
- d. Weight gain

2611. Which of the following signs and symptoms are expected from a client with diagnosis of hypothyroidism?
- a. Elevated blood pressure
- b. Moist and coarse hair
- c. Tachycardia and weight gain
- d. Hypothermia and constipation

Explanation: Hypothyroidism is a condition which slows the metabolic rate and peristalsis, leading to hypothermia and constipation respectively.

2612. Drug of choice for hypothyroidism is:
- a. Propylthiouracil (PTU)
- b. Methimazole
- c. Levothyroxine sodium
- d. Both a and b

2613. An adult patient with myxedema is started on thyroid replacement therapy. Which of the following is considered to be an expected adverse reaction to the medication?
- a. Angina pectoris
- b. Bradycardia
- c. Severe cramps
- d. Weight gain

Explanation: Thyroxine will increase the heart rate, and the heart will require more oxygen. Angina is a likely and serious complication that can occur as result of thyroid replacement therapy.

2614. A patient who is on oral levothyroxine should be advised to take the medication at what time of the day:
- a. Morning
- b. In between meals
- c. Evening
- d. At bedtime

HYPERTHYROIDISM

2615. Clinical features of congenital hypothyroidism is:
- a. Large anterior fontanelle
- b. Poor feeding
- c. Macroglossia
- d. All of the aboves

2616. Congenital hypothyroidism is:
- a. Graves disease
- b. Cretinism
- c. Myxedema
- d. Acromegaly

2617. Cretinism/myxedema develops due to:
- a. Hypothyroidism
- b. Hyperthyroidism
- c. Hypopituitarism
- d. Hyperpituitarism

2618. Nursing management of a client with hyperthyroidism is:
- a. Provide cool environment
- b. Provide a restful environment
- c. Both a and b
- d. Provide small meals

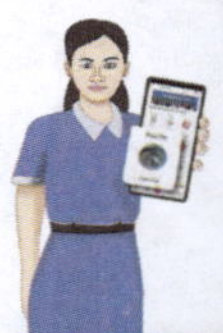

Ans.

2599. b
2600. a
2601. b
2602. b
2603. b
2604. a
2605. c
2606. c
2607. c
2608. a
2609. d
2610. d
2611. d
2612. c
2613. a
2614. a
2615. d
2616. b
2617. a
2618. c

2619. Hyperthyroidism leads to:
a. Weight loss b. Sweating
c. Irritability d. All of these

2620. All of the following are clinical manifestations of thyroid storm; EXCEPT:
a. High fever b. Tachycardia
c. Hypertension d. Severe constipation

2621. Which of the following is the priority nursing care for a client with severe hyperthyroidism?
a. Assess for emotional trauma
b. Encourage range-of-motion exercises
c. Provide diversionary activity
d. Provide a calm and non-stimulating environment

Explanation: Distractible over activity and exaggerated sensitivity to noise are characteristic features of hyperthyroidism. A calm environment is important to reduce activity.

2622. Drug of choice for hyperthyroidism is:
a. Propylthiouracil (PTU) b. Methimazole
c. Levothyroxine sodium d. Both a and b

2623. Which of the following complication is most likely to develop if hyperthyroidism remains untreated?
a. Respiratory failure b. Cerebro vascular accident
c. Heart failure d. Pulmonary embolism

Explanation: Some of the most serious complications of hyperthyroidism involve the heart. These include a rapid heart rate, a heart rhythm disorder called atrial fibrillation and congestive heart failure.

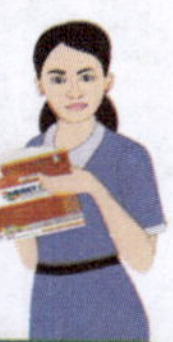

2624. Exophthalmos of the eyes is a characteristic sign of: *(LNJP H D 2012)*
a. Grave's disease b. Cushing's disease
c. Myxedema d. Cretinism

2625. Which of the following nursing intervention is essential for client with exophthalmos? *New Q*
a. Administer artificial tears
b. Encourage the client to wear spectacle
c. Promote bed rest
d. Monitor pulse rate q4h

Explanation: Exophthalmos (protrusion of the eyes) may be so severe that the eyelids cannot close. The most essential measure is to keep the eyes moist. Hence, artificial tears keep the eyes moist so that abrasions do not occur.

2626. Electrolyte imbalance seen in hyperthyroidism is:
a. Hypocalcemia
b. Hypercalcemia
c. Hypernatremia
d. Hyperkalemia

Explanation:

Causes of Hypocalcemia
- Hypoparathyroidism
- Deficiency of vitamin D

Causes of Hypercalcemia
- Hyperparathyroidism
- Hyperthyroidism

Hyperthyroidism is reported to be associated with mild to moderate hypercalcemia in approximately 20% of total patients

2627. Which among the following intervention is most appropriate in a client who is experiencing hemorrhage following thyroidectomy?
a. Intubate the client b. Prepare for tracheostomy
c. Lateral position d. Start IV fluids

2628. A 45-year-old female patient underwent subtotal thyroidectomy in the morning. On the same day evening, she complains of nausea. Assessment found that her temperature is 104°F, tachycardia and restlessness. This nurse understands that the most likely cause of these signs and symptoms is:
a. Hypoglycemia b. Thyroid crisis
c. DKA d. Hypocalcemia

2629. Which of the following is the best method to assess for hemorrhage in a client who underwent thyroidectomy?
a. Check blood pressure hourly
b. Assess the client for frequent swallowing
c. Roll the client to side and check for bleeding
d. Place a hand under the client's neck and shoulders to feel bed linens

Explanation: Client will be in semi-sitting position so drainage would go to the back of the neck. So, the right method to assess bleeding is to place a hand under the client's neck and shoulders to feel bed linens. Blood trickling down the throat is seen in patients with tonsillectomy.

2630. A patient who has just had a thyroidectomy returns to the unit in a stable condition. Which of the following equipment is important for the nurse to have readily available?
a. Dressing set b. Thoracotomy tray
c. Tracheostomy set d. Ice collar

Explanation: Thyroidectomy is subject to complications in the first 48 hours after surgery. Inflammation of operative site may cause airway obstruction. The nurse should have a tracheostomy set and oxygen at the bedside for 48 hours after thyroidectomy.

2631. During early post-operative period after thyroidectomy, which of the following findings is a cause of concern?
a. A sore throat
b. Complaints of pain in the area of the surgical incision
c. Carpal spasm when the blood pressure is taken
d. Temperature of 101°F

Explanation: Carpal spasm is a sign of tetany and is known as Trousseau sign. Trousseau sign of latent tetany is a medical sign observed in patients with low calcium. Inadvertent removal of parathyroid glands causes hypocalcemia which leads to tetany.

2632. After thyroid surgery (thyroidectomy) patient shows carpopedal spasm. This sign indicates *(Banaras HU 2015)*
a. Severe post-operative bleeding
b. Very low thyroid hormone levels
c. Decreased metabolism and hypothermia
d. Hypocalcemic tetany

DISORDERS OF PARATHYROID GLAND

2633. Which of the following is associated with hypercalcemia?
a. Tetany b. Urinary calculi
c. Petechiae d. T wave inversion in ECG

2634. Hormones involved in calcium homeostasis is:
a. Calcitonin b. Parathormone
c. Adrenaline d. Both a and b

Ans.
2619. d
2620. d
2621. d
2622. d
2623. c
2624. a
2625. a
2626. b
2627. b
2628. b
2629. d
2630. c
2631. c
2632. d
2633. b
2634. d

2635. Which among the following is an expected lab finding in client with primary hyperparathyroidism?
a. Elevated serum calcium
b. Low level of serum calcium
c. Increased bone density
d. Low urine calcium

2636. All are features of hyper-parathyroidism; EXCEPT:
a. Increase serum calcium
b. Decreased serum phosphate
c. Diarrhea d. Nephrocalcinosis

2637. Clinical manifestations of hypoparathyroidism includes:
a. Muscle weakness b. Positive Chvostek's sign
c. Positive trousseau's sign d. All of these

2638. Which of the following is caused by hypoparathyroidism?
a. High serum calcium b. Low serum calcium
c. High serum potassium d. Low serum potassium

Explanation: Hypoparathyroidism is a condition characterized by decreased blood levels of parathyroid hormone. Parathyroid along with vitamin D and dietary phosphorous regulates calcium level in the body. Decreased parathyroid hormone leads to hypocalcemia (low calcium).

2639. Electrolyte imbalance seen in hyperparathyroidism is:
a. Hypocalcemia b. Hypercalcemia
c. Hypernatremia d. Hyperkalemia

2640. Electrolyte imbalance seen in hypoparathyroidism is:
a. Hypocalcemia b. Hypercalcemia
c. Hypernatremia d. Hyperkalemia

2641. Secretion of parathyroid hormone is stimulated by: *(Kerala PSC, Nov 2014)*
a. Hypokalemia b. Hypercalcemia
c. Hyperkalemia d. Hypocalcemia

2642. The causes of hypoparathyroidism include: *(AIIMS Raipur Grade II 2017)*
a. Damage of glands during thyroidectomy
B. Congenital anomaly of the gland
C. Fractured base of skull
D. Development of antibodies to parathyroid cells
a. A, B, C b. B, C, D
c. A, B, D d. A, B, C, D

Explanation: The causes of hypoparathyroidism include injury to or removal of parathyroid glands, DiGeorge syndrome, genetics, autoimmune diseases, cancer radiation treatments and low magnesium levels.

2643. Which of the following laboratory value is expected in patient diagnosed with hyperparathyroidism?
a. Elevated serum vitamin D b. Elevated serum calcium
c. Low urine calcium d. All of these

2644. Which of the following hormone antagonize the action of parathyroid hormone?
a. Insulin b. Glucagon
c. Calcitonin d. Triiodothyronine

2645. After thyroidectomy accidental removal of parathyroid gland need to suspect if:
a. Easily fracture following a minor fall injury
b. Renal calculi occurred
c. Hypertension and difficulty swallowing
d. Laryngospasms and tingling in the hand and feet

DIABETES MELLITUS

2646. Which meal plan is best for the patient with reactive hypoglycemia? *(Kerala PSC, Nov 2014)*
a. Avoidance of fats and proteins
b. Small frequent meals
c. Low fiber, high carbohydrate diet
d. Avoid fats, complex carbohydrates and proteins

2647. Glipizide, an oral hypoglycemic agent should be administered:
a. With breakfast b. Before lunch
c. After dinner d. At bed time

2648. World diabetes day is celebrated on: *(Safdarjung NO 2018)*
a. 14th September b. 14th August
c. 14th November d. 24th January

Explanation: World diabetes day is celebrated on 14 November. It is observed by International Diabetes Federation in response to creating awareness about rising threats from diabetes.
Tips to Remember: Children's day and Diabetes day are on 14th November.

2649. Symptoms of diabetes mellitus include:
a. Weight gain b. Increased appetite
c. High energy level d. Limited urine output

2650. Hypertriglyceridemia can be seen in:
a. Obesity b. Diabetes
c. Cushing syndrome d. Both a and b

2651. Risk factors for autoimmune thyroiditis (hashimoto disease) is:
a. DM b. Myasthenia gravis
c. SLE d. All of these

2652. The most rapid absorption of insulin occurs in: *(Safdarjung NO 2018)*
a. Abdomen b. Arms
c. Thigh d. Buttocks

Explanation: The most rapid absorption of insulin occurs through abdomen. More subcutaneous tissue is present in abdomen area than arms, thighs and buttocks for better absorption of insulin.

2653. Other name for type-I diabetes mellitus (DM) is:
a. Juvenile diabetes
b. Adult onset diabetes mellitus
c. Gestational diabetes
d. DM with infection

2654. Type II diabetes mellitus is also known as:
a. Juvenile diabetes
b. Adult onset diabetes mellitus
c. Gestational diabetes
d. DM with infection

2655. Which among the following DM is characterized by resistance of the cells to insulin:
a. Type 1 b. Type 2
c. Gestational d. All of these

2656. Which among the following DM is characterized by damage to beta cell?
a. Type 1 b. Type 2
c. Gestational d. All of these

2657. Ps of diabetes mellitus are all; EXCEPT:
a. Polyuria b. Polyphagia
c. Polydipsia d. Polyarthria

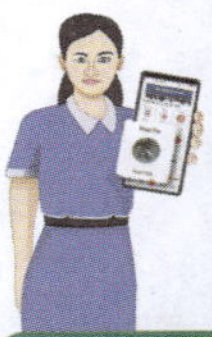

Ans.
2635. a
2636. c
2637. d
2638. b
2639. b
2640. a
2641. d
2642. c
2643. b
2644. c
2645. d
2646. b
2647. a
2648. c
2649. b
2650. d
2651. a
2652. a
2653. a
2654. b
2655. b
2656. a
2657. d

2658. Patient with diabetes mellitus complaining of irritability, sweating and thirst. These are suggestive of:

a. Hypoglycemia b. Dawn phenomenon
c. DKA d. HHNKS

2659. All of the following are the clinical manifestation of diabetes mellitus; EXCEPT: *(DSSSB 2013)*

a. Glycosuria b. Hyperglycemia
c. Hypoglycemia d. Polyuria

Explanation: The most common diabetes signs and symptoms include frequent urination (polyuria), presence of glucose in urine (glycosuria), increased blood sugar (hyperglycemia), intense thirst and hunger, weight gain, unusual weight loss, fatigue, cuts and bruises that do not heal, male sexual dysfunction, numbness and tingling in hands and feet. Hypoglycemia is not feature of diabetes mellitus.

2660. Mechanism behind polyuria and polydipsia in diabetes mellitus is:

a. Fat metabolism leads to ketone release
b. Hyperglycemia cause osmotic imbalance
c. Renal threshold of the kidney for glucose will exceeds
d. Decreased erythropoietin secretion

2661. A patient with diabetes mellitus is complaining of irritability, sweating and thirst. The priority nursing action is:

a. Ask the patient to lie down
b. Check urine for ketone bodies
c. Check the patient's blood glucose level
d. Assess for other neurologic symptoms

2662. The complaint of Insulin secretion is noticed in: *(DSSSB PHN, 2015)*

a. Type I diabetes b. Type II diabetes
c. Secondary diabetes d. Diabetes insipidus

2663. SGL 2 Inhibitors are the new group of drugs used in treatment of: *(ISRO)*

a. Diabetes Mellitus b. Dyslipidemia
c. Hyperthyroidism d. Chronic renal failure

2664. Complication of diabetes mellitus include:

a. Hyperglycemic hyperosmolar non-ketotic syndrome
b. Diabetic ketoacidosis
c. Microvascular complication
d. All of these

2665. While preparing a patient for surgery who has diabetes mellitus, the nurse should be aware of which of the following potential surgical risks associated with this disease? *(AIIMS Bhopal Grade-I 2018)*

a. Altered metabolism and excretion of drugs
b. Fluid and electrolyte imbalance
c. Respiratory depression from anesthesia
d. Poor wound healing

Explanation: The patients with diabetes mellitus have high blood glucose level which contributes to the formation of fatty deposits in blood vessels wall. Overtime, it leads to hardening and narrowing of the blood vessels which restricts the blood flow to peripheral areas or wound. Also an elevated blood sugar level decreases the function of RBC's that carry nutrients to the tissues, this lowers the efficiency of WBC's to fight with infection. So, the nurse should be aware that poor wound healing is potential surgical risk associated with diabetes.

2666. Rotation of injection site while administering insulin prevents:

a. Insulin resistance b. Anaphylactic reactions
c. Edema d. Lipodystrophy

2667. Which of the following insulin has the most rapid action?

a. Lente b. Ultralente
c. Lispro d. Humulin N

2668. Most common cause for insulin resistance is:

a. Over-weight b. Postreceptor defects
c. Damage to beta cell d. Pancreatic dysfunction

2669. Characteristic respiration present in diabetic ketoacidosis is:

a. Kussmaul respiration
b. Chyne-stroke respiration
c. Hyperventilation
d. Apnea

2670. Electrolyte needs to be replaced in DKA is:

a. Sodium b. Potassium
c. Calcium d. Phosphorous

2671. How exercise helps a diabetes patient?

a. Reduce insulin need by reducing blood glucose level
b. Use stored fat to meet the energy requirement
c. Sweating control the electrolyte imbalances
d. None of the above

2672. Diabetic foot care teaching plan include:

a. Apply a moisturizing lotion to dry feet but not between the toes
b. Use mirror to check the foot
c. Use shoe of appropriate size
d. All of the above

2673. All of the following are included in diabetic teaching plan; EXCEPT:

a. Change position frequently to increase circulation
b. Inspect feet and legs daily for any changes
c. Keep the unused insulin in the refrigerator
d. Keep legs elevated on 2 pillows while sleeping

Explanation: In a diabetic patient, there is impaired blood circulation to distal part of the extremities. Elevation of legs during sleep will further decrease the circulation.

2674. The nurse is teaching a client to self-administer insulin. The instructions should include teaching the client to:

a. Inject the needle at 45° angle into the muscle
b. Rotate injection sites
c. Vigorously massage the area after injection
d. All of these

Explanation: Injection sites should be rotated to prevent tissue damage or lipodystrophy. Insulin is injected at 90° angle into the deep subcutaneous tissue, not 45° angle into the muscle. Vigorously massaging the injection site is not advised.

2675. Which of the following tests is most sensitive for detecting early diabetic nephropathy?

a. Serum Creatinine b. Ultra sonography
c. Microalbuminuria d. Creatinine clearance

2676. Most common oral infection in diabetes mellitus:

a. Candida b. Staphylococcus
c. Streptococcus d. Aspergilius

2677. Incorrect about gestational diabetes mellitus?

a. Congenital malformations
b. Metformin is used
c. Prolonged labour
d. Large for date baby

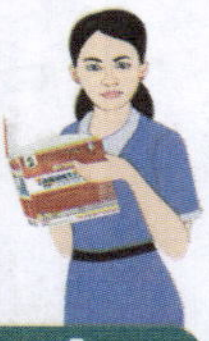

Ans.

2658. a
2659. c
2660. b
2661. c
2662. a
2663. a
2664. d
2665. d
2666. d
2667. c
2668. b
2669. a
2670. b
2671. a
2672. d
2673. d
2674. b
2675. c
2676. a
2677. a

2678. Which of the macrovascular complication of Diabetes occurs first?
a. Diabetic neuropathy b. Diabetic nephropathy
c. Diabetic. retinopathy d. CAD

2679. Niacin is contraindicated in diabetes patient because:
a. It increases insulin resistance
b. It increases metabolism of anti diabetic drugs
c. It causes scleroderma which leads to loss of injection sites
d. It causes hypoglycemia

2680. Oral anti-diabetic drug safe in renal failure is:
a. Glyburide b. Chlorporamide
c. Repaglinide d. Metformin

Explanation: Repaglinide is excreted through bile and is independent of renal function.

2681. Female with blood sugar of 600 mg% and sodium of 110 mEq. Insulin was given, what will happen to serum sodium levels?
a. Sodium increase b. Sodium decrease
c. Sodium unaffected d. Relative sodium deficiency

Explanation: Insulin stimulates reabsorption of sodium for DCT

2682. The most effective correction of acidosis in diabetic ketoacidosis is by:
a. IV bicarbonate b. IV saline
c. IV insulin d. Oral bicarbonate

ADRENAL CORTEX AND MEDULLA

2683. Emergency or acute stress hormones are released from:
a. Adrenal cortex b. Adrenal medulla
c. Pituitary d. Thyroid

Explanation: Stress hormones (Epinephrine, norepinephrine) stimulate sympathetic nervous system. They are secreted by Adrenal medulla.
Adrenal **Cor**tex secretes **cor**tisols and aldosterone.

2684. Increased adrenal cortex hormone secretion leads to:
a. Cushing's syndrome b. Addison's syndrome
c. Pheochromocytoma d. Adrenal insufficiency

2685. Decreased adrenal cortex hormone secretion leads to:
a. Cushing's syndrome b. Addison's syndrome
c. Pheochromocytoma d. Wilms tumor

2686. Which of the following hormone is called a "Stress" hormone? *(Kerala PSC, Nov 2014)*
a. Calcitonin b. Vasopressin
c. Cortisol d. Prolactin

2687. Adrenal medulla hormone include:
a. Epinephrine b. Norepinephrine
c. Both a and b d. None of these

2688. Which of the following hormone is not a steroid hormone?
a. Mineralocorticoids b. Glucocorticoids
c. Sex hormones d. Epinephrine

2689. Adrenal cortex hormone include:
a. Corticosteroids b. Androgens
c. Mineralocorticoids d. All of these

2690. Angiotensin-II increases which of the following? *(Kerala PSC, Nov 2014)*
a. Vasodilation and ADH secretion
b. Vasoconstriction and aldosterone secretion
c. Venous flow from the extremity
d. Arterial flow to the extremity

DISORDERS OF ADRENAL GLANDS

2691. Weight gain is the feature of:
a. Hyperthyroidism b. Steroid therapy
c. Cushing's syndrome d. Both b and c

2692. All are seen in Addison's disease; EXCEPT?
a. Hypotension b. Hyponatremia
c. Hyperkalemia d. Metabolic alkalosis

2693. Glucose fever is related with:
a. Glucagon b. Parathyroid
c. Cortisol d. GH

Explanation: Patient with Addison's disease may develop high grade fever following glucose infusion. This is what is caused as Glucose fever and is linked to lack of cortisol. Following the fever patient may develop adrenal crisis.

2694. Electrolyte abnormality seen in Cushing syndrome is:
a. Hypokalemia b. Hypernatremia
c. Both a and b d. None of these

2695. What are the signs and symptoms of Cushing's syndrome other than obesity? *(DSSSB 2010)*
a. Abdominal striae and ankle enlargement
b. Large thighs and upper arms
c. Posterior neck fat pad and thin extremities
d. Flabby abdomen and large hips

Explanation: Common signs and symptoms of Cushing's syndrome involve progressive obesity and skin changes, such as weight gain and fatty tissue deposits, particularly around the midsection and upper back, in the face (moon face), and between the shoulders (buffalo hump).

2696. Not seen in Cushing's syndrome:
a. Hypoglycemia b. Hypertension
c. Frank psychosis d. Hypokalemia

2697. Principal hormone high in Cushing syndrome is:
a. Glucocorticoids b. Mineralocorticoids
c. Aldosterone d. Androgens

2698. Causes of Cushing's syndrome is:
a. Prolonged administration of corticosteroids
b. ACTH secreting pituitary tumor
c. Cortisol secreting neoplasm
d. All of these

2699. Moon face with central obesity is noticed in: *(DSSSB PHN, 2015)*
a. Addison's disease b. Cushing's syndrome
c. Down's syndrome d. Turner's syndrome

2700. Moon face, hirsutism and truncal obesity are the characteristic of:
a. Addison's disease b. Cushing's syndrome
c. Pheochromocytoma d. Renal blastoma

2701. Which of the following feature is not related to Cushing's triad? *(JIPMER 2012)*
a. ↑ systolic BP b. Hypothermia
c. Bradycardia d. Widening pulse pressure

2702. Which of the following is not true regarding pheochromocytoma is:
a. Catecholamine secreting tumor found in adrenal medulla
b. Client will be having hypertension
c. Pounding headache and profuse sweating are the clinical manifestations
d. Bradycardia is present

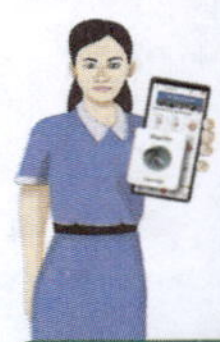

Ans.
2678. d
2679. a
2680. c
2681. a
2682. c
2683. b
2684. a
2685. b
2686. c
2687. c
2688. d
2689. d
2690. b
2691. d
2692. d
2693. c
2694. c
2695. c
2696. a
2697. a
2698. d
2699. b
2700. b
2701. b
2702. d

Explanation: Tachycardia and profuse sweating are the clinical manifestations of pheochromocytoma. So, presence of bradycardia is incorrect regarding pheochromocytoma.

2703. A 40-year-old lady comes with pheochromocytoma. Most characteristic symptom is:
a. Orthostatic hypotension
b. Weight loss
c. Sweating attacks
d. Paroxysmal hypertension

2704. Drug given to diminish the catecholamine production is:
a. Metyrosine b. Phenoxybenzamine
c. Prazosin d. All of these

2705. Which among the following is an expected pre-operative preparative order for a patient with adrenalectomy for hyperaldosteronism?
a. Monitor catecholamine level
b. Measure urinary catecholamine level
c. Administer potassium-sparing diuretics
d. Enema

2706. One of the interventions associated to manage the side effects of corticosteroid therapy is:
a. Increase calcium intake to 1500 mg/day
b. Perform Kegel exercises
c. Get all immunization to control infection
d. Stop the drug if you feel better

2707. Electrolyte abnormality seen in Addison's disease is:
a. Hyperkalemia b. Hyponatremia
c. Both a and b d. None of these

Explanation: Addison's disease is caused by inadequate secretion of adrenal gland. Aldosterone (secreted by adrenal cortex) regulates blood pressure and electrolytes. Aldosterone enhances excretion of potassium and increases reabsorption of sodium. Hence, hypoaldosteronism can be associated with hyperkalemia and hyponatremia.

2708. Management of Addison's disease include all; EXCEPT:
a. Salt restriction
b. Replacement therapy with hydrocortisone
c. Minerelocorticoid supplementation
d. Oral corticosteroids such as hydrocortisone

2709. Symptoms of Addison's diseases includes all; EXCEPT:
a. Weight gain
b. Bronze or hyperpigmentation of the face, neck
c. Cramping and abdominal pain
d. Postural hypotension

2710. Best time to have the corticosteroids replacement therapy is:
a. Night before going to the bed
b. Any time every alternative day
c. After waking up or in the late afternoon
d. Every 4 hourly

2711. Which of the following diet is not appropriate for a patient diagnosed with Addison's disease?
a. Sodium restricted diet
b. High protein diet
c. Diet with adequate calorie intake
d. Diet high in complex carbohydrates

2712. All of the following are the complication associated with long-term use of corticosteroid therapy; EXCEPT:
a. Hypolipidemia
b. Osteoporosis
c. Cushingoid appearance
d. Adrenal insufficiency

Explanation: Long-term corticosteroid use is associated with **hyperlipidemia**, osteoporosis, aseptic joint necrosis, adrenal insufficiency, gastrointestinal, hepatic, and ophthalmologic effects, growth suppression, and possible congenital malformations. So, hypolipidemia is incorrect.

2713. All of the following are the complication associated with short term use of corticosteroid therapy; EXCEPT:
a. Hypertension b. Immunosuppression
c. Hypoglycemia d. Electrolyte abnormalities

Explanation: Short-term corticosteroid use is associated with generally mild side effects, including hyperglycemia, hypertension, electrolyte abnormalities, pancreatitis, cutaneous effects, hematologic, immunologic, and neuropsychologic effects.

2714. A client is getting inj. Prednisolone as continuous IV infusion. Important nursing management is:
a. Hourly urine specific gravity
b. Hourly blood sugar
c. Hourly abdominal girth
d. Hourly head circumference

GONADS

2715. Production of estrogen by a mature ovarian follicle leads to:
a. Negative inhibition to estrogen production
b. Increased production of progesterone
c. Release of GnRH and increased secretion of LH
d. Oogenesis

2716. Human chorionic gonadotropin is produced by:
a. Placenta b. Ovary
c. Pituitary d. Gonads

2717. Which part of the reproductive organ functions as gonads in male?
a. Scrotum b. Prostate gland
c. Testis d. Glans penis

2718. Which part of the reproductive organ functions as gonads in females:
a. Ovary
b. Uterus
c. Fallopian tube
d. Ampulla

2719. Gonad is a reproductive organ that make:
a. Fertilized egg b. Gametes
c. Semen d. Albicans

2720. Which type of germ cell is seen on the product of gametes?
a. Haploid b. Diploid
c. Monoploid d. Gamaploid

2721. The gonadotropin releasing hormone is present in the:
a. Anterior pituitary b. Posterior pituitary
c. Hypothalamus d. Medulla oblongata

Ans.
2703. d
2704. a
2705. c
2706. a
2707. c
2708. a
2709. a
2710. c
2711. a
2712. a
2713. c
2714. b
2715. c
2716. a
2717. c
2718. a
2719. b
2720. a
2721. c

NERVOUS SYSTEM

ANATOMY AND PHYSIOLOGY OF NERVOUS SYSTEM

Neuron

- Basic functional unit of the nervous system.

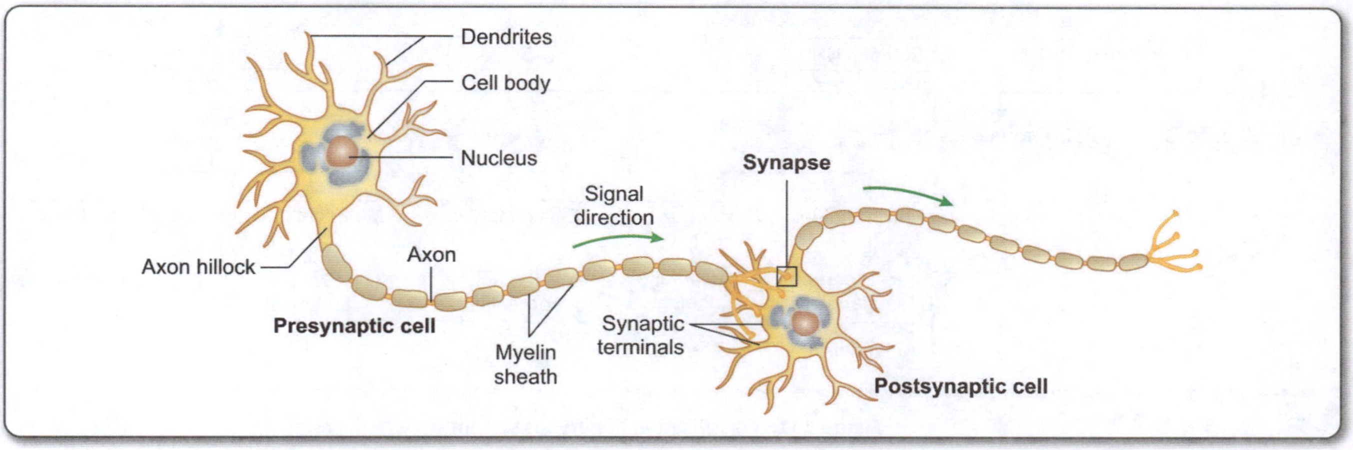

Figure 110: Structure of a Neuron

- **Dendrite:** A branch-like structure for receiving electrochemical message.
- **Axon:** Long projections which carry impulses away from cell body.
- **Synapse:** It is the specialized junction between neurons.
- **Myelin:** A fatty material that acts as an insulator and conductor to speed up the process of communication.
- **Synaptic cleft/synaptic gap:** It is the space between neurons at which nerve impulses are transmitted by neurotransmitters.
- Nerve cells are different from other cells—no centrosome and presence of processes.
- Due to absence of centrosome, nerve cells cannot multiply.
- Nissl bodies (tigroid substance) help in synthesis of protein as ribosome is present.
- Axon—the longest axon is about 1 meter.
- Nodes of ranveir—myelin sheath are absent at regular interval. The interval is called Nodes of Ranveir.
- Myelinogenesis of PNS starts from 4th month of intrauterine life and completed by 2nd year after birth.
- Synaptic cleft space is about 20–50 nm

Neuroglia

Neuroglia and glia cells are the supporting cells of nerve. It includes:

- Oligodendrocytes—for formation and maintenance of myelin sheath around CNS nerves.
- Astrocytes—for making BBB, largest and most abundantly present
- Microglia—functions same as macrophages in CNS system.
- Schwann cells—formation and maintenance of myelin sheath in PNS
- Satellite cells—enclose the cell bodies in sensory neurons of PNS.

Neurotransmitter

- Neurotransmitter helps to communicate information between two neurons. The chemical substances help in transmission of impulse from one nerve to other through synapses
- Neurotransmitters are synthesized and stored in synaptic vesicles.

Types

- Inhibiting neurotransmitters: These are responsible for inhibiting the conduction of impulse.
  For example- Dopamine, GABA, serotonin
- Excitatory neurotransmitters: Responsible to increase/initiate the conduction of impulse.
  For example- acetylcholine, noradrenalin, glutamine

Recent Question (CNCI 2021)

79. Name of the receptor on epidermis that transmits stimuli to the axon through a chemical synapse.
a. Langerhans's cells
b. Merkel cells
c. Woodzer cells
d. Berger cells

Ans. (b) Merkel cells

CLASSIFICATION OF NERVOUS SYSTEM

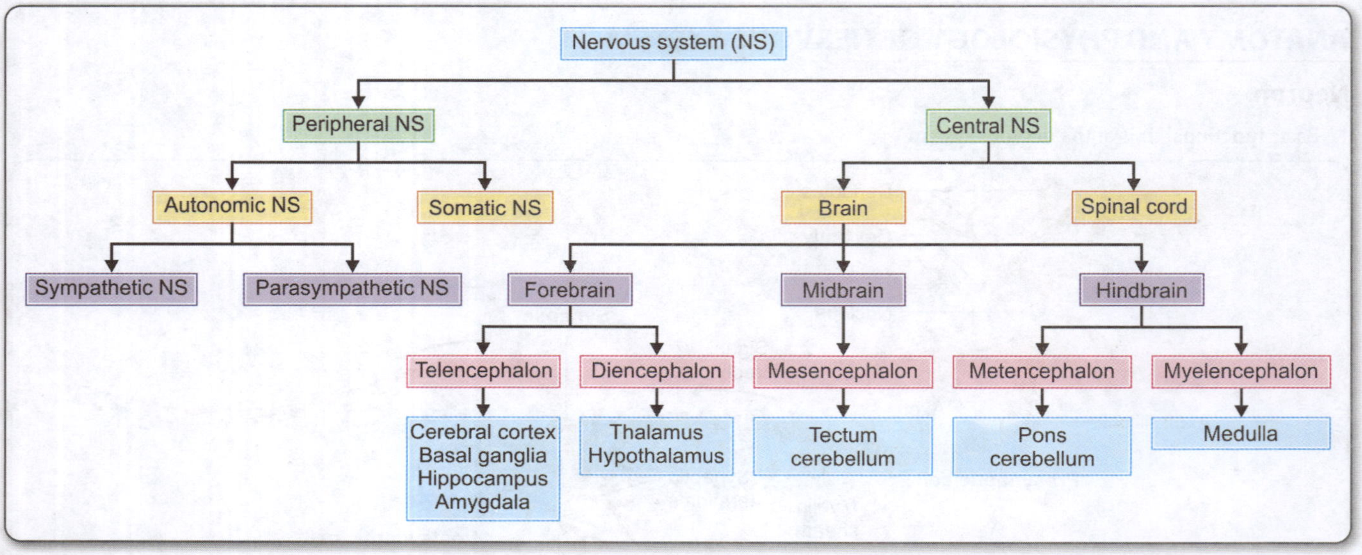

Figure 111: Classification of nervous system

Brain

- Brain is divided into three major areas:
  - **Cerebrum** – Composed of two hemispheres, thalamus, hypothalamus and basal ganglia
  - **Cerebellum** – Located under cerebrum and behind the brain stem
  - **Brain stem** – Includes midbrain, pons and medulla

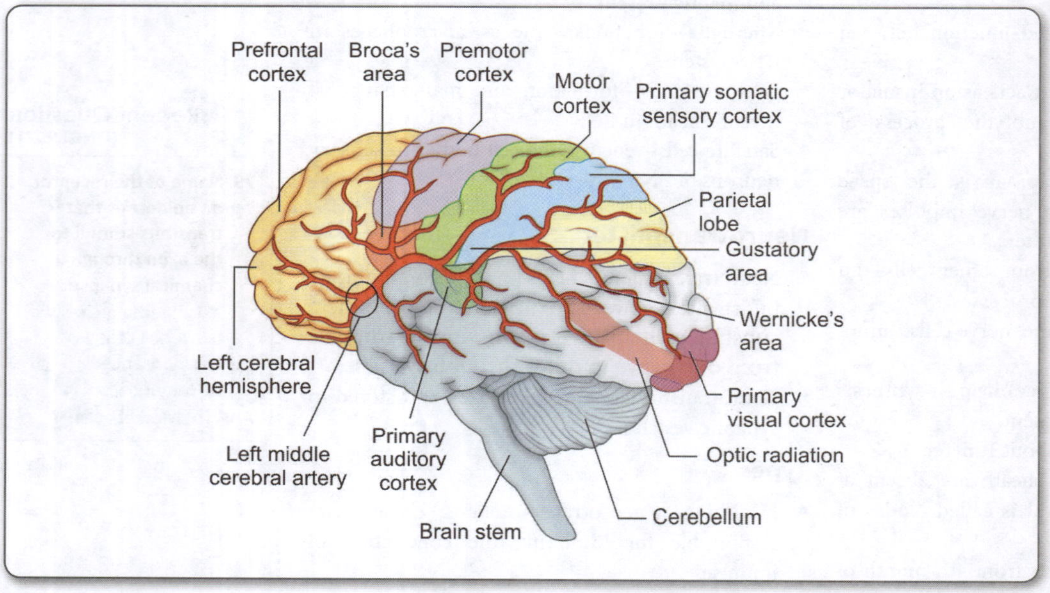

Figure 112: Brain structures

KEY POINTS

- Auditory lobe is found in **temporal lobe**.
- Wernicke's area (temporal lobe) of the brain is involved in the understanding of meaning.
- The temporal lobe regulate memory and learning problems because of the integration of the **hippocampus.**
- Visual area is found in **occipital lobe**.
- Broca's area of speech (production of speech) is located in the **frontal lobe.**
- Hypothalamus contains temperature control center of the body.

Cerebrum

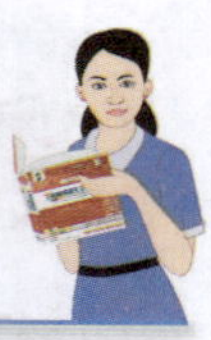

- It is the largest part of brain consists of two hemispheres, right and left hemispheres.
- It is also called seat of intelligence
- Right-handed persons are having dominant left hemisphere which is responsible for linguistic, verbal, calculating, arithmetic, and analytical functions.

- Non-dominant hemisphere is for geometric, visual, spatial, pattern and musical function.
- Corpus callosum connects both hemispheres.
- **Gyri** - Outside wrinkled (folded) appearance of cerebral hemisphere. This folded appearance increases the surface area of brain.
- External surface or cerebral cortex is made up of grey matter, i.e., cell bodies.
- Inner surface or white matter is made up of nerve fibers.
- Function of cerebrum is mainly mental activities, sensory and control of voluntarily muscles.
- Sensory perception area is present in cerebrum are as follows:
  - **Primary visual area** located in occipital lobe.
  - **Primary auditory area** located in temporal lobe.
  - **Primary olfactory area** located in temporal lobe.
  - **Primary gustatory area** located in parietal lobe
  - **Thalamus**
    - It lies on either side of the third ventricle.
    - It is the relay center for all information except smell.
    - Pain gate and reticuloendothelial system (RES) is also the part of this lobe.
  - **Hypothalamus**
    - Lies inferior and anterior to thalamus
    - It contains **optic chiasm** (point at which two optic nerves intersect) and mammillary bodies (involved in olfactory reflex and emotional response to odors)
    - Hypothalamus connects to the pituitary via infundibulum and plays an important role in endocrine regulation and fluid regulation
    - Involved in **temperature regulation**
    - **Hunger center** is located in hypothalamus.
  - **Basal ganglia**
    - Located deep in cerebral hemisphere
    - It is responsible for fine motor movements of upper and lower extremities
  - **Limbic system**
    - It is a group of brain structures interconnected which includes hippocampus, amygdala, cingulate gyrus, gyrus fornicates, the archicortex.
    - It is responsible for memory, emotion and motivational behavior.
- The cerebral hemispheres are divided into frontal, parietal, temporal and occipital lobes.

Recent Question (CNCI 2021)

80. The space between arachnoid & pia mater is called________?
a. Epidural
b. Subdural
c. Subarachnoid
d. Extradural
Ans. (c) Subarachnoid

Table 86: The functions of each lobe of cerebral hemisphere

Lobe	Function
Frontal lobe	• Largest lobe • Concentration, abstract thought, information storage, memory, motor function, affect, personality and inhibitions. • Broca's area of speech (production of speech) is located in this lobe
Parietal lobe	• Sensory cortex is present in this lobe • Helps in individual's awareness of the body in perception of taste, space, orientation and spatial relationship.
Temporal lobe	• Auditory receptive area • Wernicke's area for language development is in this lobe
Occipital lobe	• Visual interpretation

Cerebellum

- Cerebellum is separated from cerebrum by tentorium cerebelli.
- It has **excitatory and inhibitory action**.
- It is responsible for coordination of movement, balance and equilibrium of the body.

Brain Stem

- It consists of **mid brain, pons and medulla oblongata**.
- **Midbrain** connects pons and cerebrum.
- **Medulla oblongata:** Most inferior region of the brain stem. It becomes the spinal cord at the level of the foramen magnum. Medulla oblongata is regulatory center for Respiratory, cardiac, deglutition, vomiting.

Protective Structures of Brain

- Brain is covered by rigid skull bone.
- Meninges are fibrous connective tissues which cover brain and spinal cord.
- Layers of meninges are:
  - **Dura mater:** Outermost cover of brain and spinal cord
  - **Arachnoid mater:** It has no blood supply. This layer contains **choroid plexus** which produces CSF. This membrane also has finger like projections called arachnoid villi which reabsorb CSF.
  - **Pia mater:** Innermost layer.

KEY POINTS

- The brain region which is responsible for coordination of voluntary muscular movement, posture and balance is **cerebellum**.
- The neurons of motor pathway control voluntary muscles.
- The medulla oblongata is a portion of the hindbrain that controls autonomic functions such as breathing, digestion, heart and blood vessel function, swallowing, and sneezing.
- Parkinson's disease is caused by the degeneration of neurons in the substantia nigra.

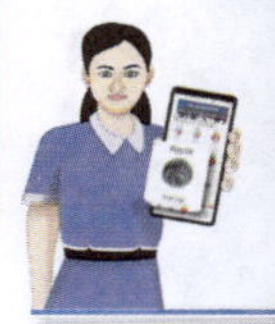

Production and Circulation of CSF

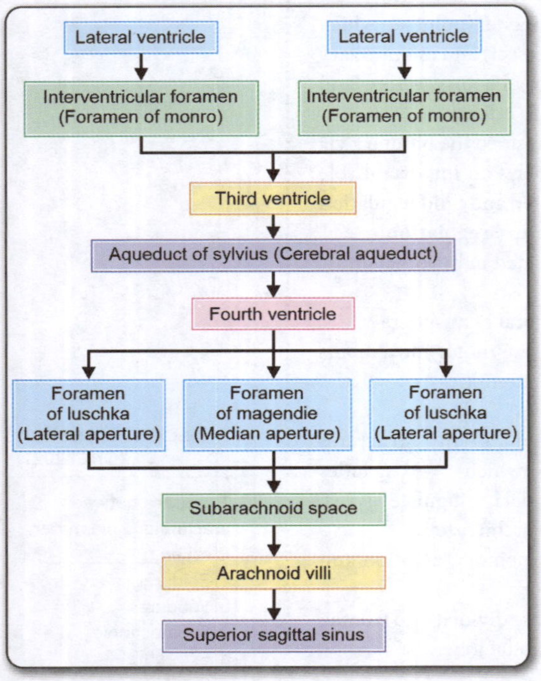

Figure 113: Production and circulation of CSF

Cerebral Circulation

- Brain receives 15% of cardiac output.
- Brain has high metabolic demand and it requires high blood flow.
- Blood flow to the brain is against gravity.
- Brain has good collateral circulation.
- Arterial Supply to the Brain:
  - Two internal carotid arteries and two vertebral arteries provide blood supply to the brain.
  - Internal carotid artery arises from common carotid artery.
  - Vertebral artery is a branch of subclavian artery that enters the cranium through foramen magnum.
  - Vertebral artery joins to form basilar artery at the level of brain stem.
  - At the base of the brain, internal carotid artery and vertebral artery form rings of arteries known as circle of Willis.
  - Arteries in the circle of Willis provide collateral circulation if one or more of the arteries are ligated or occluded.
  - The arteries along with the circle of Willis are the frequent sites for aneurysm.
- **Venous Drainage from the Brain**
  - Network of sinus (dural sinus) carries venous blood from the brain and empties into internal jugular vein returning blood to the heart.
  - Unlike other veins cerebral vein does not have valves. It depends on gravity and blood pressure.

POINTS TO REMEMBER

- The CSF is produced by specialized **ependymal cells** in the **choroid plexuses** of the ventricles of the brain
- CSF is absorbed into the blood by **arachnoid villi.**
- Normal ICP (CSF pressure) is 5–15 mm Hg.
- Lumbar puncture done at L3-L4 or L4-L5
- Specific gravity of CSF – 1.005

KEY POINT

Middle cerebral artery is the largest branch of the internal carotid artery.

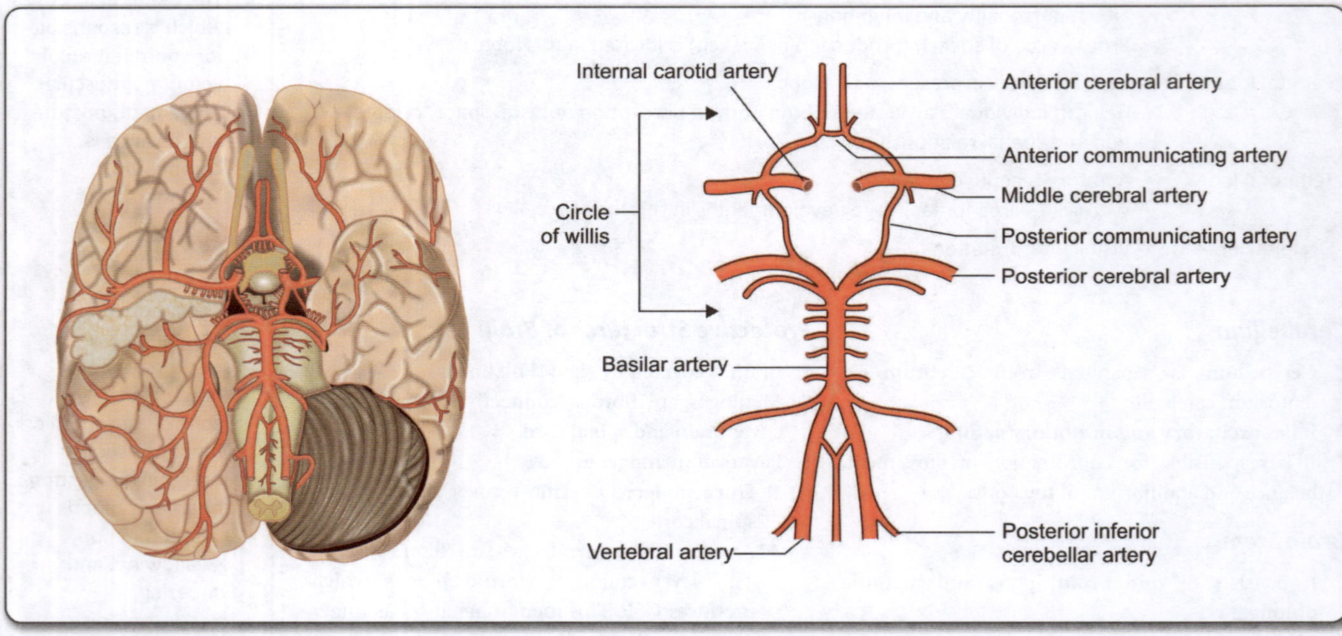

Figure 114: Arterial supply to brain

Blood Brain Barrier

- All the substances entering in the brain will be filtered by endothelial cells and astrocytes (blood brain barrier).
- This property helps in proper neuronal function and also protects the neural tissue from toxins and pathogens.

Spinal Cord

- It is approximately **45 cm long**.
- It is H-shaped structure that extends from foramen magnum at the base of the skull to lower border of the first lumbar vertebra.
- **Grey matter** (Ascending tract) is in the center and is surrounded by the **white matter** (Descending tract).
- There are **31 pairs of spinal nerves**.

Vertebral Column

- It consists of 33 vertebrae which are divided as follows:
  - Cervical -7
  - Thoracic-12
  - Lumbar-5
  - Sacral- Five fused vertebrae
  - Coccyx – Four fused vertebrae
- Vertebrae are separated by discs except at first and second cervical, the sacrum and at the coccyx.
- C1 vertebra which supports the skull is known as atlas and the C2 vertebra which pivots the atlas is known as axis.

The Peripheral Nervous System

- It consists of cranial nerves (12 pairs), spinal nerves (31 pairs) and autonomic nervous system.

KEY POINTS

- The Circle of Willis is the joining area of several arteries at the bottom (inferior) side of the brain.
- The structure of the circle of Willis includes:
  - Left and right internal carotid arteries
  - Left and right anterior cerebral arteries
  - Left and right posterior cerebral arteries
  - Left and right posterior communicating arteries
  - Basilar artery
  - Anterior communicating artery

Cranial Nerves and its Functions

Table 87: Cranial nerves with their functions

Cranial nerve	Fibers	Structures innervated	Functions	Brainstem nucleus
I Olfactory	**Sensory**	Olfactory epithelium (via olfactory bulb)	Olfaction	
II Optic	**Sensory**	Retina	Vision	
III Oculomotor	**Motor**	Superior/middle/inferior rectus, inferior oblique, levator palpebrae	Movement of eyeball	Oculomotor nucleus
	Parasympathetic	Pupillary constrictor, ciliary muscle of eyeball. Both via the ciliary ganglion	Pupillary constriction and accommodation	Oculomotor nucleus
IV Trochlear	**Motor**	Superior oblique	Movement of eyeball	Trochlear nucleus
V Trigeminal	**Sensory**	Face, scalp, cornea, nasal and oral cavities, cranial dura mater.	General sensation	Trigeminal sensory nucleus
	Motor	Muscles of mastication	Opening/closing mouth	Trigeminal motor nucleus
		Tensor tympani muscle	Tension of tympanic membrane	Trigeminal motor nucleus
VI Abducens	**Motor**	Lateral rectus	Movement of eyeball	Abducens nucleus
VII Facial	**Sensory**	Anterior 2/3 of tongue	Taste	Nucleus solitarius
	Motor	Muscles of facial expression	Facial movement	Facial motor nucleus
		Stapedius muscle	Tension of ossicles	Facial motor nucleus
	Parasympathetic	Salivary and lacrimal glands via submandibular and pterygopalatine ganglia	Salivation and lacrimation	Superior salivatory nucleus

Contd...

Cranial nerve	Fibers	Structures innervated	Functions	Brainstem nucleus
VIII Vestibulocochlear	**Sensory**	Cochlea	Hearing	Cochlear nucleus
		Vestibular apparatus	Proprioception of head, balance.	Vestibular nucleus
IX Glossopharyngeal	**Sensory**	Eustachian tube, middle ear	General sensation	Trigeminal sensory nucleus
		Carotid Body, and sinus	Chemo/baroreception	
		Pharynx, posterior 1/3 of tongue	Taste	Nucleus solitarius
	Motor	Stylopharyngeus	Swallowing	
	Parasympathetic	Salivary glands via the otic ganglion	Salivation	Inferior salivatory nucleus
X Vagus	**Sensory**	Pharynx, larynx, esophagus, external ear	General sensation	Trigeminal sensory nucleus
		Aortic bodies and arch	Chemo/baroreception	
		Thoracic and abdominal viscera	Visceral sensation	Nucleus solitarus
	Motor	Soft palate, larynx, pharynx, upper esophagus	Speech, swallowing	Nucleus ambiguus
	Parasympathetic	Cardiovascular, respiratory and gastrointestinal systems	Control of these systems	Dorsal motor nucleus of vagus
XI Accessory	**Motor**	Sternomastoid, trapezius	Movement of head and shoulders	Nucleus ambiguus, cranial nerves
XII Hypoglossal	**Motor**	Intrinsic and extrinsic muscles of tongue	Movement of tongue	Hypoglossal nucleus

Spinal Nerves

- There are 31 pairs of spinal nerves (8 cervical, 12 thoracic, 5 lumbar, 5 sacral and 1 coccyx).
- Each spinal nerve has a dorsal root and ventral root.
- Dorsal root carries sensory information from body parts through dorsal ganglia.
- Ventral roots carry information from spinal cord to body parts.

Autonomic Nervous System

- **Function** - Maintenance of internal environment
- It has two divisions namely **sympathetic and para-sympathetic**
    - **Sympathetic nervous system** (adrenergic) is mainly excitatory and responsible for **fight or flight response.**
    - **Para-sympathetic nervous system** is cholinergic and is responsible rest-and-digest or feed-and-breed activities.
- Sympathetic stimuli are mediated by nor-epinephrine.
- Parasympathetic impulses are mediated by acetylcholine.
- Sympathetic and parasympathetic systems are antagonistic with each other.

KEY POINTS

- There are 31 pairs of spinal nerves
- Sympathetic nervous system - Fight flight response
- Parasympathetic nervous system - rest and bread.

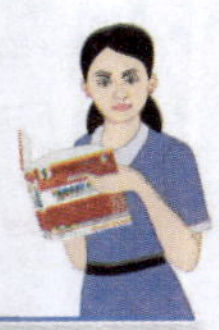

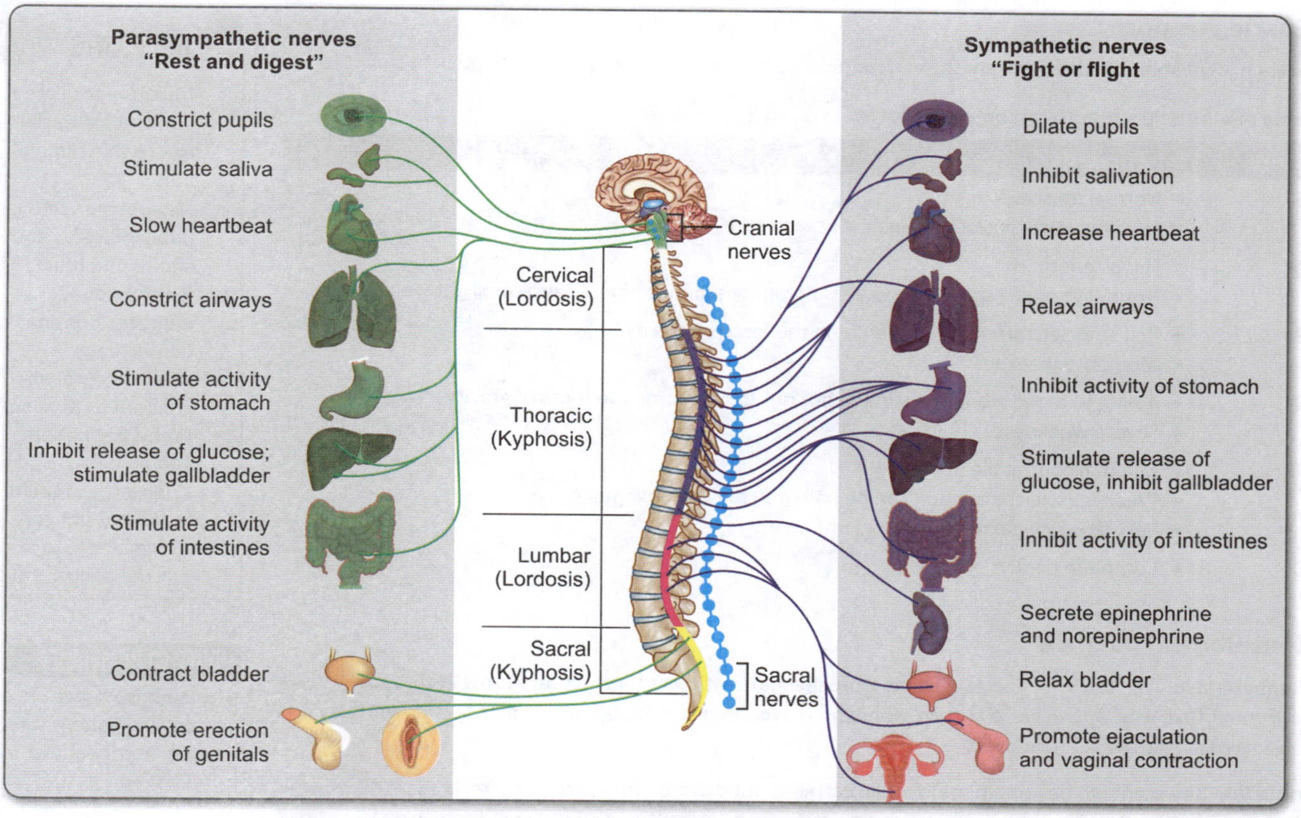

Figure 115: Autonomic nervous system

ASSESSMENT AND DIAGNOSTIC TESTS

Table 88: Assessment of cranial nerves

Cranial nerve	Type	Assessment
Olfactory	Sensory	Smell – Coffee, peppermint, gloves
Optic	Sensory	Visual acuity – Snellen chart; test for visual field; ophthalmoscope
Oculomotor	Motor and Sensory	Move eye ball up and down; Test for accommodation; pupillary constriction
Trochlear Abducens	Motor and Sensory	Lateral and inferior movement of eye
Trigeminal	Sensory and Motor	Assess corneal reflex; Sensation in skin of the face with cotton wisp; chewing, biting, lateral jaw movements
Facial	Sensory and Motor	Taste – anterior 2/3rd of tongue; (sweet, salt and sour)
Vestibulocochlear	Sensory	Hearing, balance (Weber and Rinne test), Romberg test
Glossopharyngeal	Sensory and Motor	Swallowing; Taste – Posterior 1/3rd of tongue (bitter)
Vagus	Sensory and Motor	Assess Gag reflex, Swallowing, and sensation of posterior 1/3rd of tongue. Assess movement of Uvula
Spinal Accessory	Motor and Sensory	Shoulder Shrug, Shoulder movement, head rotation.
Hypoglossal	Motor and sensory	Tongue movement (protrude tongue, Push tongue into the cheek)

Muscle Strength

Assess patient ability to flex or extent the extremities against resistance test muscle strength.

Table 89: Muscle strength is scored as follows:

Score	Interpretation
5	• Normal muscle strength • Full power of contraction against gravity and resistance
4	• Fair strength • Not full strength against gravity or moderate amount of resistance or slight weakness
3	• Just sufficient strength to overcome the force of gravity • Moderate weakness
2	• Ability to move along the surface but not to overcome the force of gravity • Severe weakness
1	• Minimal contractile power • Weak muscle contraction can be palpated but no movement • Very severe weakness
0	• Complete paralysis

Neurological Balance

Romberg test: This test is to check balance. Patient stands with feet together and arms at the side. This is performed first with open eyes and then with closed eye. If patient loses balance and falls down then it is considered as positive Romberg test.

Table 90: Key points to be kept in mind while carrying out diagnostic neurological tests

Name of the diagnostic test	Description	Points to remember
Cerebral angiography	• X-ray study of the cerebral circulation with the help of a dye injected into selected artery • This is a valuable test to find out aneurysm, arterio-venous malformation.	• Instruct the client that a warmth and metallic taste may be felt in the mouth while injecting dye. • Observe the site of dye injection following procedure for bleeding and hematoma. • Monitor pulse, distal to the puncture site.
Myelography	• It is the X-ray of the spinal arachnoid space after the injection of a contrast agent. • This test helps to find out tumors, cyst, herniated intervertebral disc or other lesions.	After myelography patient lies in the bed with 30–40° head end elevation Advise the patient to take large amount of fluids after the procedure for rehydration and to replace CSF and thereby to avoid post lumbar puncture headache.
Electroencephalography (EEG)	• It records the cerebral activity through the electrodes placed over scalp or micro-electrodes placed inside the brain tissue. • Useful for diagnosing seizure disorder, coma or organic brain syndrome	• Sometimes to increase the chances of electrical activity patient may be deprived of sleep one night before procedure. • Sedatives, Stimulants, Anti-seizures, tranquillizers, types of drugs may be withheld 24–48 hours before the procedure. • Coffee, tea, cola and chocolate are omitted from diet • Sleep EEG needs collodion based glue for electrode application

Contd...

KEY POINTS

- Unilaterally dilated pupil indicates damage to third cranial nerve
- Mid position or fixed pupil indicates damage to mid brain
- Pinpoint pupil indicates pontine hemorrhage
- After Cerebral angiogram or Myelography, the patient should be advised to drink large amount of fluid (if not contraindicated) to flush out the contrast dye.

POINT TO REMEMBER

Nurse should give priority to patient safety during Romberg test to prevent fall.

Recent Question (NORCET 2023)

81. A patient can move her extremities in normal manner but she can't move against resistance. What is her muscle strength testing score?

a. 1
b. 2
c. 3
d. 4

Ans. (c) 3

Name of the diagnostic test	Description	Points to remember
Evoked potential studies	• In visual evoked response, patient is exposed to visual stimuli and transit time from retina to the occipital areas is measured. • In auditory evoked response, auditory stimulus is given and transit time from brain stem to cortex is measured. • In somatosensory evoked response, peripheral nerves are stimulated through skin electrodes and transit time from spinal cord to cortex is measured.	
Electromyography	• Electrodes are introduced into skeletal muscles to measure change in electrical potential of the muscles • Useful for diagnosing neuromuscular disorders and myopathies.	
Lumbar puncture	• Lumbar puncture or spinal tap is performed to withdraw CSF from subarachnoid space. • Needle is inserted between L3-L4 or L4-L5.	• Collected specimen should be sent to the laboratory immediately • Post lumbar puncture headache can be reduced by making the patient lie down and increasing the fluid intake. • Complications: Herniation of intracranial content, epidural abscess, hematoma and meningitis

KEY POINT

Lumbar puncture is contraindicated in patients with a known or suspected intracranial mass or suspicion of highly elevated ICP.

KEY POINTS

GCS:
- Maximum score of GCS is 15.
- Minimum score of GCS is 3.
- GCS score 8 - Coma (severe injury)
- GCS score 9–12 - moderate injury
- GCS score 13–15 - minor injury

Glasgow Coma Scale (GCS)

The **Glasgow Coma Scale** is the most common scoring system used to describe the level of consciousness in a person following a traumatic brain injury.

Table 91: Glasgow Coma Scale

Behavior	Response	Score
Eye opening response	Spontaneously To speech To pain No response	4 3 2 1
Best verbal response	Oriented to time, place and person Confused Inappropriate words Incomprehensible sounds No response	5 4 3 2 1
Best motor response	Obeys command Moves to localized pain Flexion withdrawal from pain Abnormal flexion (decorticate) Abnormal extension (decerebrate) No response	6 5 4 3 2 1
Total score	Best responses Comatose client Totally unresponsive	15 8 or less 3

Recent Question (CNCI 2021)

82. Which position to be provided to an unconscious patient while performing mouth care?
a. Fowler's position
b. Knee chest
c. Supine
d. Side lying

Ans. (d) Side lying

Altered Level of Consciousness

- It is apparent in patient who is not oriented, does not follow command or needs persistent stimuli to achieve alertness.
- **Coma** is a clinical stage in which patient is not aware about self and environment for prolonged period of time.
- **Akinetic mutism**: A state of unresponsiveness to the environment in which patient makes no movement or sound but opens the eyes.
- **Decorticate positioning**: Involves adduction and flexion of upper extremities, internal rotation of the lower extremities and plantar flexion of the feet

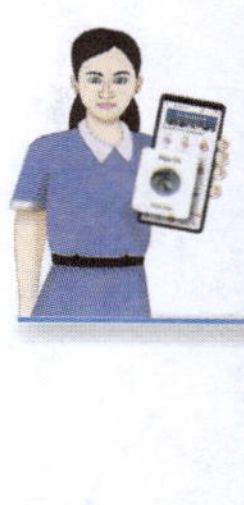

- **Decerebrate positioning:** Involves extension and outward rotation of upper extremities and plantar flexion of the feet.

In an unconscious patient, taking temperature *via* oral route is contraindicated because of the risk for bite.

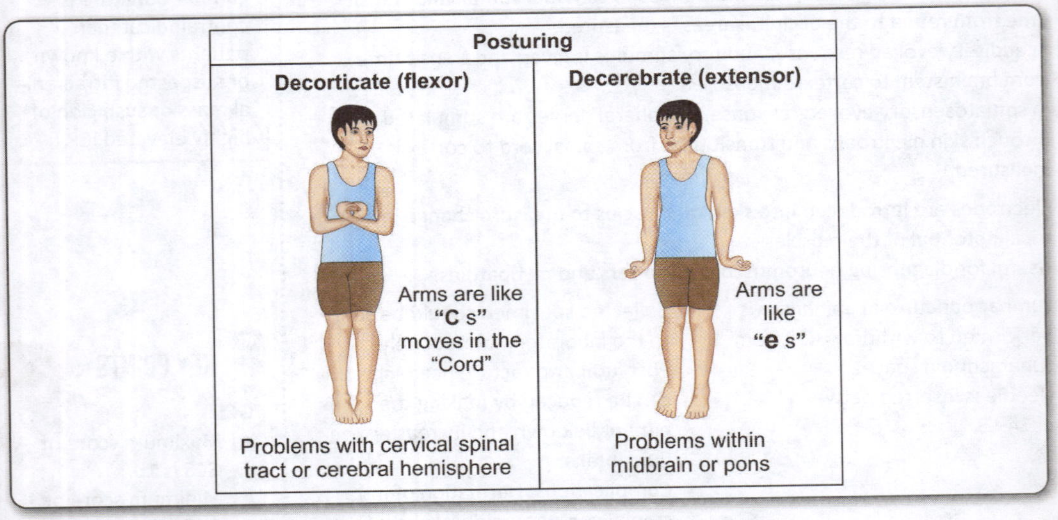

Figure 116: Decorticate and decerebrate positioning

Increased Intracranial Pressure (ICP)

- **Intracranial pressure (ICP)** is the pressure inside the cranial cavity.
  - **Normal:** 5–15 mm Hg
  - **Mild elevation:** 16–20 mm Hg
  - **Moderate elevation:** 21–30 mm Hg
  - **Severe elevation:** More than 30 mm Hg
- Cerebral perfusion pressure (CPP) is the net pressure that causes cerebral blood flow to the brain cells;
- CPP = Mean Arterial Pressure (MAP) – Intracranial Pressure (ICP)
- Normal range of CPP is 70–100 mm Hg
- **Causes:** Cerebral edema, intracranial or subarachnoid bleeding, brain tumor, interstitial cerebral edema.
- **Signs and symptoms**
  - Altered loss of consciousness is usually the **earliest sign of increased ICP**.
  - Cushing's triad is a late sign of increased ICP. It includes **bradypnea, bradycardia, and hypertension.**
  - Partial or complete loss of sensory or motor function may occur.
- Complications of increased ICP include brain stem herniation, diabetes insipidus, and syndrome of inappropriate anti-diuretic hormone (SIADH).
- **Diagnosis:** CT scan, skull X-ray, ICP monitoring
- **Treatment:** Treatment goal is to normalize ICP and avoid complications:
  - Surgical placement of shunts to correct CSF blockage
  - Surgical removal of tumor or hematoma
  - Burr holes or craniotomy for decompression
  - Hyperventilation therapy to decrease the partial pressure of CO_2
  - Osmotic diuretics such as mannitol to withdraw the fluids from brain tissue
  - Fever control and avoidance of shivering
  - Slight elevation of head end of bed to increased venous return from the brain.
  - **Lumbar puncture is contraindicated in increased ICP** because of the chances of brain stem herniation.

Intracranial Surgery

Cranial surgeries are used to open the skull and to gain access to intracranial content. There can be different types of approaches and they are:

- **Supratentorial:** These are the parts of brain located above the tentorium cerebelli. After this approach client has to be placed in 30–45° head elevation with neck in neutral alignment
- **Infratentorial:** These are the parts of brain located below the tentorium cerebelli. After surgery, maintain neck in neutral position and place the client on either side.
- **Transsphenoidal:** In this, incision is made below the upper lip through the mouth and nasal cavity to gain access to pituitary gland.
  - Advise the client to avoid blowing through nose.
  - Keep the head end of the bed elevated to promote venous drainage from the brain.

KEY POINTS

- The earliest sign of increase in ICP is change in level of consciousness.
- Projectile vomiting may occur in a client with increased ICP.
- When ICP is monitored, the fluid system and transducer is calibrated at 2.5 cm above the ear when the patient is in supine position and this point is correspondence to foramen of monro in the brain.
- A client who is on ventilator and is having increased ICP suction should not be longer than 15 seconds.
- High level of PEEP (Positive end expiratory pressure) needs to be avoided among these patients as it will increase the intra thoracic pressure.
- Increased urine output is an indication that the mannitol is effective.

Recent Question
(NORCET 2020)

83. What is the cerebral tissue perfusion pressure if Blood Pressure is 90/60 and ICP is 18?

a. 42 mm Hg
b. 52 mm Hg
c. 60 mm Hg
d. 72 mm Hg

Ans. (b) 52 mm Hg

Explanation:

CPP = MAP – ICP
MAP = [SBP + 2(DBP)]/3
MAP = [90 + 2(60)//3
= 210/3
MAP = 70 mm Hg
CPP = MAP – ICP
= 70 – 18
= 52 mm Hg

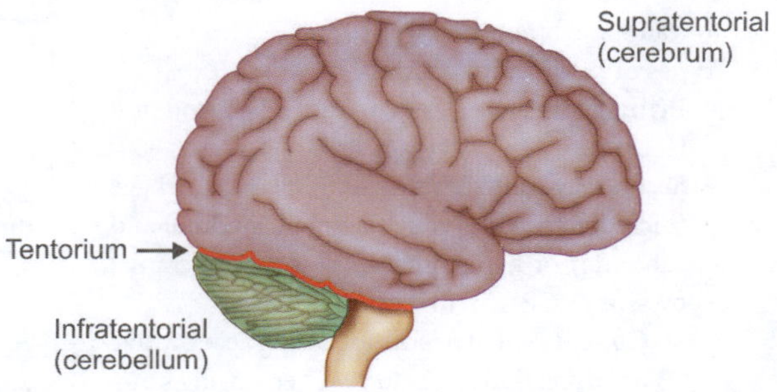

Figure 117: Tentorium cerebelli

SEIZURE DISORDERS

- A **seizure** is a sudden disruption of the brain's normal electrical activity accompanied by altered consciousness and/or other neurological and behavioral manifestations.
- **Epilepsy** is a condition characterized by recurrent seizures that may include repetitive muscle jerking called convulsions.
- **Causes:** Electrolyte imbalances, toxic state, tumors, anorexia, increased ICP, CNS inflammation or idiopathic
- **Types:** Seizures are classified into two main categories:
  - **Partial seizures** involve a part of the brain. They can be:
    - **Simple partial seizures:** Symptoms may include involuntary twitching of the muscles or arms and legs; changes in vision; vertigo; and having unusual tastes or smells. The person does not lose consciousness.
    - **Complex partial seizures:** Symptoms may be like those of partial seizures, but the person does lose awareness for a time.
  - **Generalized seizures** involve much more or all of the brain. They can be:
    - **Absence seizures (petit mal):** Characterized by a short period of blanking out or "absent" stare.
    - **Myoclonic seizures:** Characterized by jerking or twitching of the limbs on both sides of the body.
    - **Tonic-clonic seizures (grand mal):** Symptoms include jerking or shaking of the body, LOC (Loss of consciousness) and loss of bladder control. The person may have an aura before the seizure starts. Tonic-clonic seizures may last for 1–3 minutes. A tonic-clonic seizure that lasts longer than 5 minutes is considered as Medical Emergency.
- **Diagnosis:** Medical history, neurological examination, CT scan, cerebral angiography, electroencephalogram (EEG), and MRI
- **Treatment:** Anticonvulsants (e.g., Carbamazepine, sodium valproate). If brain tumor is involved, it should be surgically removed.
- **Key nursing interventions**
  - Prevent injury
  - Do not force tongue blade during an episode of seizure (it may injure tooth)
  - Loosen tight clothes
  - If possible, place the client on the side which prevents falling back of tongue and to facilitate drainage of secretions.
  - Note prodromal signs and time of onset after a seizure occurs.

Status epilepticus: Series or chain of seizure attacks, between each seizure attack patient won't gain full recovery of consciousness.

STROKE

- **Stroke**, also known as **cerebrovascular accident (CVA)** is a disruption in cerebral perfusion causing neurological deficit.

Three main types of strokes are:

1. **Ischemic stroke:** It happens when the artery that supplies blood to the brain is blocked. Blood clots (thrombus) often cause the blockages.
2. **Hemorrhagic stroke:** An artery in the brain ruptures or leaks blood. High blood pressure and aneurysms are the common causes.
3. **Transient ischemic attack (mini stroke):** Blood flow to the brain is blocked for a short time (not more than 5 mins). It is a warning sign of future stroke.
    - Most of the intracerebral hemorrhages are arterial in origin.
    - Severe **explosive headache** is the characteristic of hemorrhagic shock.

- **Signs and symptoms** depend on the affected artery and severity of the damage.
  - **Motor symptoms**
    - **Hemiplegia:** Paralysis of one side of the body.
    - **Hemiparesis:** Weakness in one side of the body

Recent Question
(NORCET 2020)

84. All of the following signs and symptoms are indicative of increased intracranial pressure in children, EXCEPT
a. Nausea
b. Vomiting
c. Extreme irritability
d. Decreased Pulse pressure

Ans. (d) Decreased...

KEY POINTS

- The types of seizures that involve both sides of brain are called **generalized seizures**.
- Focal (or partial) seizures occur when seizure activity is limited to a part of **one brain hemisphere**.
- The type of seizure that involves one side of brain is called **partial seizure**.
- **Ischemic stroke** is the most common type.
- Embolism **is the most common cause** of ischemic strokes.
- **Intracerebral hemorrhage** is the most common type of hemorrhagic stroke.
- **Subarachnoid hemorrhage** (less common type) refers to bleeding into the space surrounding the brain.
- Uncontrolled hypertension is a risk factor for hemorrhagic stroke (most common cause of hemorrhagic stroke).

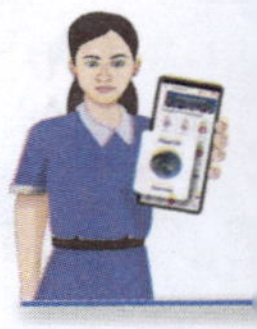

- **Paraplegia:** Paralysis of lower extremities
- **Quadriplegia:** Paralysis of all four limbs of the body
- **Ataxia:** Unsteady gait

- **Communication disturbance**
  - **Dysarthria**: Difficulty in speaking
  - **Dysphasia or aphasia:** Defective speech or loss of speech. It can be expressive, receptive or mixed
  - **Expressive aphasia:** It is due to damage to broca's area of speech, here client can understand what others are communicating but can't communicate back.
  - **Receptive aphasia**: Wernicke's area in the temporal lobe is affected. In this condition, client is unable to understand spoken or written word.
  - **Apraxia:** It is the inability to perform previously learned activities.
- **Perceptual problems**
  - **Hemianopsia:** Loss of half of the visual field
  - **Diplopia:** Double vision
- **Agnosia:** Inability to recognize familiar object or person.

- **Treatment**
  - Anticoagulants are contraindicated in patients with hemorrhagic stroke but useful in nonhemorrhagic stroke.
  - The only fibrinolytic agent that has been shown benefit in selected patients with acute ischemic stroke is tissue plasminogen activator (t-PA).
  - NIH stroke scale/score (NIHSS) is done to ascertain the need of thrombolysis.
  - Surgical evacuation of clot or hematoma relieves increased ICP.
  - Carotid endarterectomy removes plaques.
  - Anticonvulsants to prevent seizure. Analgesics to control pain.
- **Key nursing interventions**
  - Assess LOC
  - Monitor ICP and vital signs
  - Bleeding is the most common side effect of t-PA. So closely monitor the client.
  - Speak slowly and simply to patient.
  - Monitor fluid input and output hourly.
  - Positioning of the patient to prevent deformity.
  - Physical therapy to prevent contractures.

Unilateral neglect or neglect syndrome: Seen in stroke patient who is unaware about the existence of paralyzed part.

HEAD TRAUMA/HEAD INJURY

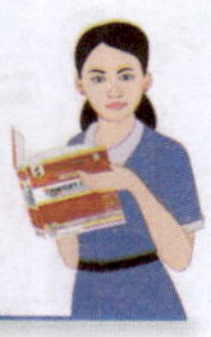

- Head trauma/head injury refers to any trauma to scalp, skull or brain.
- Head trauma may be ranging from minor bruise to traumatic brain injury.
- **Types of head trauma/injury**
  - **Primary injuries:** Concussion, contusion and laceration.
  - **Secondary injuries:** Intracranial hemorrhage (including cerebral, subarachnoid, epidural and subdural) or hematoma, increased intracranial pressure (ICP), herniation of brain.
    - **Concussion**: It occurs following accelerative or decelerative injury. There will be a transient loss of consciousness which may last over 3 min.
    - **Contusion**: Closed brain injury which leads to bruising of the tissue within the local area. If the injury occurs at the site of impact, it is called as coup and if it occurs on opposite side away from injury is known as contrecoup.

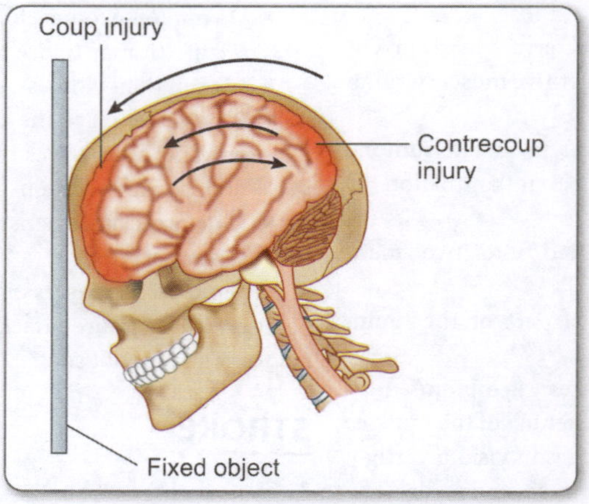

Figure 118: Contusion

    - **Laceration:** It involves tearing of blood vessel due to penetrating trauma or injury. It is associated with bleeding.
- **Signs and symptoms**
  - Loss of consciousness (LOC)
  - Increased ICP
  - Motor and sensory changes, seizures
  - Frequent swallowing, rhinorrhea and otorrhea may manifest, if CSF leakage occurs.
- Bulging fontanel and increase of head circumference is the 1st sign of ICP in infant.
- **Late sign of increase ICP-**
  - **Cushing triad** – Increase BP, bradycardia and bradypnea.
  - **Decorticate posture**
  - Decerebrate posture
- **Battle's sign:** Area of ecchymosis or bruising over temporal bone. It indicates basilar skull fracture. CSF otorrhea and CSF rhinorrhea are the major manifestations.

POINT TO REMEMBER

Patients with **epilepsy** are advised to avoid taking showers in bathtub due to risk of drowning if seizure occurs during shower.

Recent Question (CNCI 2021)

85. Name the neurological disorder characterized by the loss of the ability to execute or carry out skilled movements and gestures, despite having the desire and the physical ability to perform them?

a. Anhedonia
b. Apraxia
c. Apathy
d. Amnesia

Ans. (b) Apraxia

KEY POINTS

- Assessment of Pupil size and pupillary response is the priority nursing assessment in the first 24 hours after a thrombotic stroke.
- The time of onset of stroke to administration of Tissue plasminogen activator (tPA) is critical.
- Administration of tPA within 3 hours of onset of stroke has better outcomes.
- The primary nursing goal is to control blood pressure in first 24 hours of tPA therapy.
- The earliest symptom of elevated ICP is a change in mental status (restless and confusion).
- A patient with stroke should be positioned on the side (lateral position) while providing oral care to minimize the risk of aspiration.

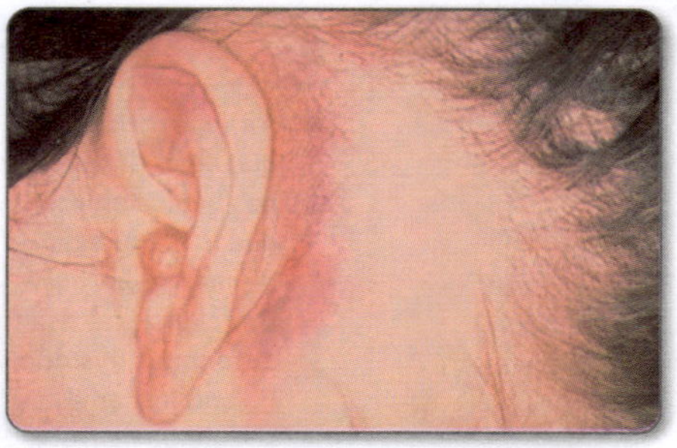

Figure 119: Battle's sign

- **Racoon eyes:** Periorbital ecchymosis following orbital fracture is known as raccoon eyes.

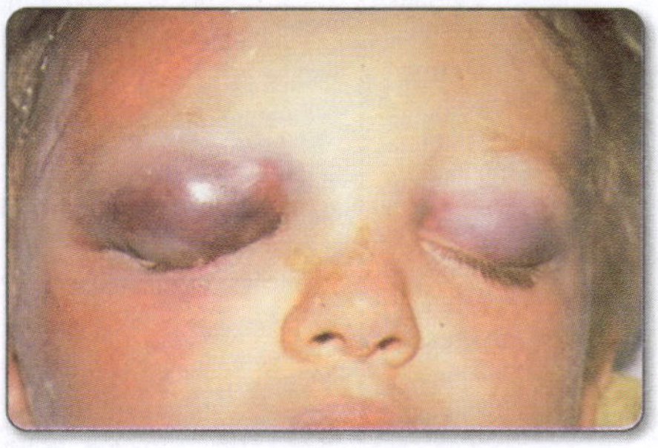

Figure 120: Racoon eyes

- **Halo sign:** It is also known as ring sign, double-ring sign. It indicates CSF leakage. Drainage from the nose is collected over a white paper or filter paper that produces characteristic halo sign, i.e., following the ring of blood another concentric yellow colored ring will be formed by CSF.

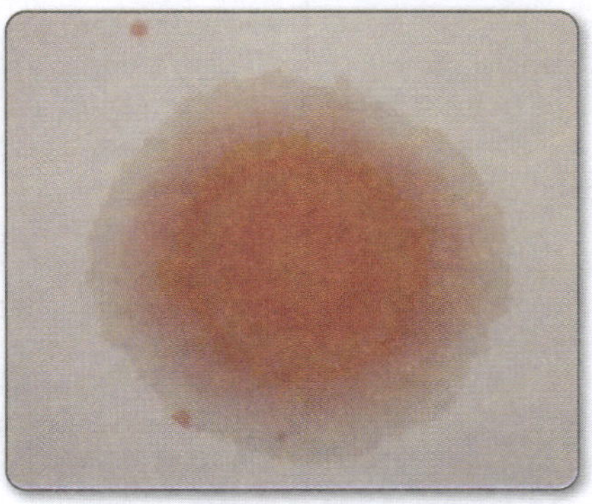

Figure 121: Halo sign

- **Diagnosis:** Skull X-ray, CT scan, MRI, lumbar puncture, cerebral angiography and EEG.
- **Treatment:** (Depends on severity and location)
  - Drug therapy for increased ICP
  - Intubation and mechanical ventilation
  - Invasive hemodynamic monitoring
  - Invasive ICP monitoring
- Don't allow patient to flex the neck and hip, avoid trendelenberg's position.
- Fluid intake is usually limited to 1200 mL/day

INTRACRANIAL/BRAIN HERNIATION

- Intracranial herniation is a medical emergency that occurs when brain tissue is displaced from its normal position in the skull.
- **Causes:** Head injury, stroke, brain tumor, or infection
- **Common symptoms:** Headache, vomiting, seizure, altered consciousness, visual disturbances, loss of balance and coordination

Table 92: Types of brain herniation

Type of Brain Herniation	Description
Subfalcine herniation	Brain tissue is displaced **under the falx cerebri**
Transtentorial herniation	A mass in the cerebrum pushes the medial temporal lobe **under the tentorium cerebelli.**
Central herniation	Both temporal lobes are pushed through **the tentorial notch.**
Tonsillar herniation	The cerebellar tonsils are pushed through the **foramen magnum.**
Upward herniation	An infratentorial mass compresses the brainstem.

SPINAL CORD INJURIES

Injury to the spinal cord resulting in total disruption of the neuronal pathway.

Complications are respiratory failure, autonomic dysreflexia and spinal shock.

Table 93: Associated motor loss according to level of spinal injury

Level of spinal injury	Associated motor loss
C1–C4	Loss of respiratory function and Quadriplegia
C4–C5	Quadriplegia Respiratory function may be affected if phrenic nerve is damaged by edema
C5–C6	Quadriplegia Loss of intercostal muscle innervations
C6–C7	Quadriplegia Weakened thumb grasp Intact diaphragmatic breathing

Contd...

Recent Question (NORCET 2022)

86. You have received a victim with a history of fall from 3rd floor and on examination the victim is unresponsive. Which method the nurse will use to assess the airway in this victim?

a. Jaw thrust maneuver
b. Head-tilt-chin lift maneuver
c. Heimlich maneuver
d. None of the above

Ans. (a) Jaw thrust maneuver

KEY POINTS

- Battle's sign indicates basilar skull fracture
- Raccoon eyes (peri-orbital ecchymosis) is a sign of orbital fracture
- Halo sign (ring sign) indicates CSF leakage.
- Diagnosing a CSF leak includes an analysis of the nasal fluid for a protein called **beta-2 transferrin** which is only found in cerebrospinal fluid.
- Other tests to diagnose the CSF leak are **CT cisternogram** and a **pledget study.**
- **CT cisternogram** assists to determine the exact **location of the CSF leak.**
- Pledget study involves placing a small cotton pads (pledget) into the nose before injecting radioactive material. The pledget will be removed later to analyze the radioactivity.

Level of spinal injury	Associated motor loss
C7–C8	Quadriplegia Loss of intercostal muscle innervations Intact diaphragmatic breathing
T1 and L1– L2	Paraplegia Loss of some intercostal muscle innervations Intact voluntary motor function of the arms
Cauda equina	Loss of sensory and motor functions Loss of bladder and bowel functions Loss of sexual function
Sacral spinal nerves	Loss of bladder, bowel and sexual functions

Cervical Spine Injuries

- Injury to C1 and C2 is fatal.
- C4 provides supply to diaphragm via phrenic nerve. So C4 injury leads to respiratory difficulty.

Thoracic Spine Injuries

- Loss of movement and sensation in chest, trunk, lower extremities, bowel and bladder can happen.
- **Autonomic dysreflexia**
  - Spinal cord injury at T6 or above leads to this condition. Any stimuli (signal) that occurs below the spinal cord injury is blocked at spinal cord injury site and it is not possible to correct it. It leads to hypertension, vasodilation, bradycardia, sweating and stiff neck.
  - It can be caused by a full bladder and bowel.
  - This condition calls for emergency and is fatal.
  - **Immediate management includes:** Provide Fowler's position, empty bowel and bladder, provide anti-hypertensive drugs and loosen the tight clothes.

Lumbar and Sacral Injuries

- Loss of sensation and movement of the lower extremities.
- S2 and S3 are centers of micturition, so below this level bladder can't empty. This is called as neurogenic bladder.

Management of Spinal Cord Injury

- Immobilize the client in a spinal back board with head in neutral position.
- Log roll the client
- Skull tongs and halo traction are used to immobilize the cervical spine.
- Assess and support respiratory status of the client.

Spinal shock or neurogenic shock: Complete loss of reflex below the level of injury is known as spinal shock.

MENINGITIS

- Inflammation of the meninges that is covering brain and spinal cord.
- **Septic meningitis:** Caused by bacteria, e.g., *Neisseria meningitides*
- The most common cause of Bacterial Meningitis in adults: ***Streptococcus pneumoniae***
- **Aseptic meningitis:** Caused by virus, abscess, lymphoma or leukemia
- **Manifestations:** Fever, headache, nuchal rigidity (early sign) and photophobia are some of the manifestations.
  - **Kernig's sign:** When patient lies in supine position and legs flexed to abdomen, the legs cannot be extended.
  - **Brudzinski's sign:** When patient's neck is flexed, flexion of knees and hips also occur.
- Transmission of meningitis is via droplet and direct contact.
- Rashes over the body (Red maculopapular rashes) are one of the features of meningitis caused by *Neisseria meningitides*.
- Isolation is priority in case of a client with meningitis.

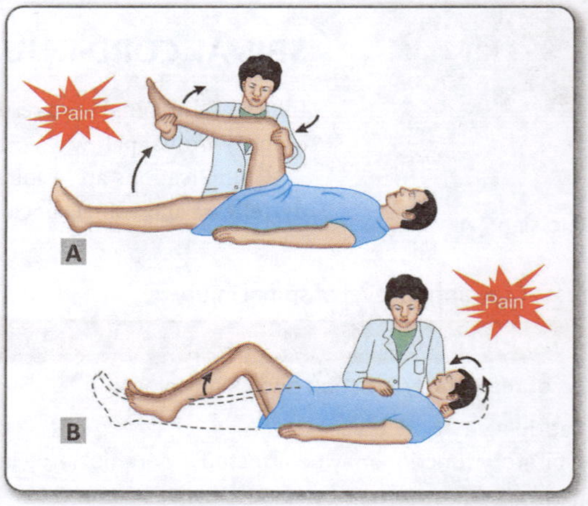

Figures 122A and B: (A) Kernig's sign; (B) Brudzinski sign

Recent Question (NORCET 2023)

87. A client with a diagnosis of C-4 injury has been stabilized and is ready for discharge. Because this client is at risk for autonomic dysreflexia, he and his family should be instructed to assess for and report:

a. Dizziness and tachypnea
b. Circumoral pallor and lightheadedness
c. Headache and facial flushing
d. Pallor and itching of the face and neck

Ans. (c) Headache and facial flushing

KEY POINTS

- The **classic triad** of diagnostic signs of meningitis consists of nuchal rigidity, sudden high fever, and altered mental status.
- Positive Kernig's sign, Brudzinski's sign and nuchal rigidity are signs of meningitis.
- **Brudzinski's sign:** Hips and knees to flex when the neck is flexed.
- **Kernig's sign:** Inability to straighten the leg when the hip is flexed to 90°.
- Common signs and symptoms of viral meningitis include fever, nuchal rigidity, irritability and photophobia
- Most common cause of **viral meningoencephalitis:** Herpes Simplex Virus.

Table 94: Comparison of CSF analysis in bacterial meningitis v/s viral meningitis

Bacterial meningitis	Viral meningitis
Low glucose	Normal glucose
High protein level	Normal or high protein level
Polymorphonuclear cells > 300/mm^3	Mononucleate cells <300/mm^3

ENCEPHALITIS

- Defined as an acute inflammation of brain, caused by infection or allergic reaction.
- **Causes**
  - **Viral encephalitis:** Enteroviruses (e.g., Polio), adenoviruses, mumps and measles viruses, HIV, herpes virus, and arboviruses.
  - **Bacterial and other:** Amebic infection, toxoplasmosis, malaria and mycoplasma (in a person with compromised immune system)
- **Signs and symptoms:** Acute onset of fever, headache, confusion, nausea, vomiting, absent superficial reflexes, exaggerated deep tendon reflexes, paralysis of the extremities, **positive Brudzinski's sign, positive Kernig's sign and nuchal rigidity.**
- **Diagnosis:** CSF culture; CSF may contain elevated protein, WBC and decreased glucose
- **Treatment** focuses on treating underlying cause.

BRAIN ABSCESS

- It is the collection of infectious material within the brain tissue.
- It occurs either due to direct invasion (intracranial trauma or surgery) of brain tissue by infectious organism or via spread from nearby sites such as paranasal sinus, ear, teeth, etc.

MULTIPLE SCLEROSIS

It is the demyelinating disorders of the CNS which cause demyelination of brain and spinal cord.

- **Signs and symptoms**
  - Sensory and visual problems
  - Diplopia, blurred vision, nystagmus, optic neuritis and ophthalmoplegia
  - Muscular dysfunction includes gait ataxia, hyperreflexia, weakness of muscle, spasticity and paralysis of extremities.
- **Treatment:** Corticosteroids and muscle relaxants
- **Key nursing interventions:** Encourage physical therapy, bowel and bladder training and family education.
- Demyelination of the nerves in the CNS, which leads to impaired impulse transmission.
- Most frequently affected parts are optic nerve, chiasm and tract, cerebrum, brain stem and cerebellum.
- **Causes:** Autoimmune disease, viral disease, and allergic reaction to infection.
- Diagnosis by **McDonald criteria**
  - MRI → **Dawson finger** appearance
  - CSF → Oligoclonal bands and Intrathecal IgG production
- **Manifestations**
  - Early symptoms are visual problems such as diplopia, blurring of vision and patchy blindness, nystagmus, ophthalmoplegia, optic neuritis.
  - Other symptoms include fatigue, weakness, ataxia, vertigo, tremors and spasticity of lower extremities, paresthesia, emotional changes, hyperreflexia or absent reflex.
- **Treatment:** Beta interferons, corticosteroids and muscle relaxants.
- **Nursing Management**
  - Management of bowel and bladder dysfunction involves use of toileting regime, continence management, teaching self-catheterization and education.

MYASTHENIA GRAVIS

- It is a chronic autoimmune neuromuscular disorder marked by muscular weakness without atrophy.
- It is characterized by abnormal muscle weakness during activity which is usually relieved by rest.
- **Cause:** Acetylcholine deficiency or defect of postsynaptic receptor site.
- In Myasthenia Gravis, antibodies are bound to the acetylcholine receptors, so only few receptors are available for acetylcholine to bind which impair impulse transmission and cause muscle weakness.
- **Manifestations:** Ptosis (drooping of the eyelid), diplopia, weakness of facial muscles results in bland facial expression, laryngeal involvement causes dysphonia and increased risk for choking and aspiration.
- It may affect the respiratory muscle and cause respiratory failure.
- MG is purely a motor disorder and has no effect on sensation and coordination
- **Diagnosis**
  - **Edrophonium chloride or tensilon test:** I/V Edrophonium is given to the client. If there is improvement in facial weakness and ptosis for about 5 min, diagnosis of MG is confirmed as positive Edrophonium test.

Recent Question
(NORCET 2022)

88. Which sign is the most indicative of myasthenia gravis?
a. Propulsive gait
b. Drooping of one or both eyelids
c. Waddling gait
d. Pill-rolling tremor

Ans. (b) Drooping of one or both eyelids

KEY POINTS

- Multiple sclerosis (MS) is the **most common demyelinating disease** of the central nervous system.
- In MS, immune system attacks myelin sheath in CNS.
- MS affects women more than men and age of onset is 20–40 years.
- The myelin sheath, which is made up of Schwann cells, is damaged along the axon.
- Triad signs of multiple sclerosis include **ataxia (unsteady gait), nystagmus, and tremor.**
- Ptosis or drooping eyelid is the earliest sign of Myasthenia Gravis.
- Edrophonium chloride or Tensilon test is used to diagnose Myasthenia Gravis.
- Edrophonium test places the client at risk for ventricular fibrillation and cardiac arrest.

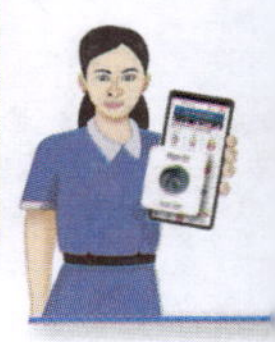

- If there is no improvement of symptoms after the administration of Edrophonium, it indicates negative test and the antidote (atropine sulfate) has to be given.

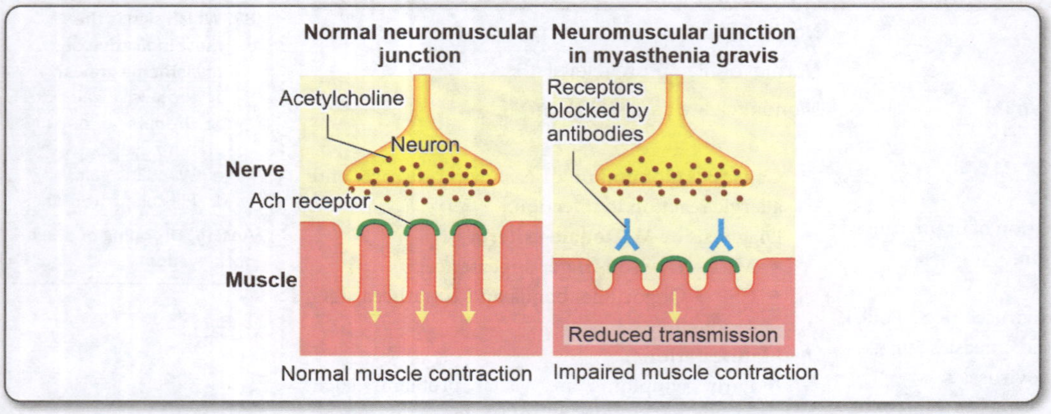

Figure 123: Neuromuscular junction in myasthenia gravis

- **Treatment:** Anticholinesterase alleviates symptoms. Corticosteroid, immunosuppressive therapy and thymectomy.
- **Key nursing interventions**
  - Maintain patent airway; use oral or endotracheal suction.
  - Schedule activity 20–30 minutes after medication is given.

GUILLAIN-BARRE SYNDROME

- It is an autoimmune disease which causes demyelination of the peripheral nerves.
- **Typical Characteristics:** It causes **ascending weakness.**
- It begins with weakness and diminished reflexes in the lower limbs
- Weakness and hyporeflexia results in quadriplegia.
- **Guillain-Barré syndrome** is the most common cause of **acute flaccid paralysis.**
- It can also cause respiratory muscle paralysis.
- Treatment includes supportive hemodynamic measures including plasmapheresis.

TRIGIMINAL NEURALGIA

- Sudden, recurrent severe pain in the area supplied by fifth cranial nerve is known as trigeminal neuralgia.
- Pain is described as unilateral, shooting and stabbing sensation.
- **Manifestations**
  - Washing of the face, brushing teeth, shaving, eating, drinking, a draft of cold air and direct pressure against nerve trunk can cause pain.
  - Client may complain of pain around gums, lips, and nose and across cheek.
- **Management**
  - Carbamazepine relieves pain in most of the patients.
  - Microvascular decompression and percutaneous radiofrequency trigeminal gangliolysis are the surgical management.
  - Educate the client to chew on the unaffected side and to avoid hot or cold foods.

BELL'S PALSY

- It is also called as facial paralysis which affects seventh cranial nerve.
- It can occur as a result of infection, trauma, meningitis or tumor.
- This condition may result in **unilateral paralysis of the face**.
- **Manifestations**: Flaccid paralysis of facial muscles, inability to raise eyebrows, frown smile, puffing out of the cheeks, upward movement of the eyes when trying to close the eyelid and loss of taste.
- **Management**: Encourage facial exercise, prevent dryness of the eyes and frequent oral care are the management.

PARKINSON'S DISEASE

- It is a chronic, progressive degenerative disease of the nervous system marked by tremor, muscular rigidity and slow movement (bradykinesia).
- It is associated with degeneration of substantia nigra, basal ganglia, and corpus striatum of the brain.
- Shortage of dopamine causes imbalance between excitatory (Acetylcholine) and inhibitory (dopamine) neurotransmitters which lead to movement problems.
- **Signs and symptoms**
  - Cardinal symptoms of Parkinson's disease are tremors, rigidity and bradykinesia. (abnormally slow movement).
  - Pill rolling tremor of the fingers, arms and hands that may also affect the chin, lips, legs and the trunk.

Recent Question (NORCET 2022)

89. Which among the following is seen in Multiple Sclerosis?

a. Bradykinesia
b. Loss of consciousness
c. Rhythmic shaking
d. Speech changes

Ans. (d) Speech changes

POINT TO REMEMBER

Breathing difficulty is one of the major concerns in GBS, so closely monitor the respiratory status of the client.

KEY POINTS

- Signs and symptoms in Guillain-Barré Syndrome (GBS) will most likely start in the lower extremities, be symmetrical, and will gradually spread upward (ascending) to the head.
- In GBS, Characteristic findings on CSF analysis include high protein (>0.55 g/L) with normal WBC.
- Plasmapheresis and immunoglobin therapies are treatment options available for GBS. Treatment is most effective if given within 2 weeks from onset of symptoms.
- **Trigeminal nerve has three branches:** ophthalmic, maxillary and mandibular.

- **Postural instability** or impaired balance and coordination
- Micrographia (shrinking, slow hand writing), mask like face (expression less face) and frequency of eye blinking also decreases.
- Dysphonia (soft, slurred low-pitched voice), dysphagia, drooling and risk for choking and aspiration.

- **Treatment:** Carbidopa/levodopa, dopamine receptor agonists (Bromocriptine, pergolide, ropinirole) and Selegline (MAOI)
- **Key nursing interventions**
  - Patient and family teaching about safety; install hand rail, remove loose carpeting, elevate toilet seat, etc.
  - Encourage physical therapy.
  - Instruct the client to avoid food high in vitamin B_6 because they block the effect of antiparkinsonian drug.
  - Monoamine oxidase inhibitor (MAOI) are contraindicated. It may precipitate hypertensive crisis.

ALZHEIMER'S DISEASE

- Alzheimer's disease (AD) is one of the most common forms of dementia seen in old age people.
- AD is a progressive, irreversible, degenerative neurologic disease that **begins insidiously** and is characterized **by gradual loss of cognitive function** and disturbances in behavior and effect.
- AD is the most common cause of cortical dementia.
- **Dementia:** Loss of memory, reasoning, language and judgment which is going to affect day to day activities of a person.
- Old age and genetics are the two main factors contributing to dementia.
- **Stages of Alzheimer's disease**
  - **Early stage:** Recent memory loss, personality changes, difficulty in finding words and mood swings.
  - **Intermediate stage:** Reduced ability to remember past events, wandering, agitation, hostility, incontinence and disorientation to place and time.
  - **End stage:** Total incontinence, recent and remote memory loss, and inability to walk, eat and swallow.
- **Clinical manifestations**
  - Forgetfulness and subtle memory loss
  - Conversation becomes difficult with word finding difficulties
  - Cognitive impairment
  - Personality changes
  - Dysphagia as the disease progresses
  - As the disease progresses, patient needs assistance for all activities of daily living.
- **Diagnostic findings**
  - Functional ability assessment (MMSE; mini mental status examination) and health history
  - EEG, CT and MRI
  - Laboratory examination of CSF
  - Decrease in Ach levels
- **Medical management**
  - Treatment relies on management of cognitive symptoms
    - Cholinesterase inhibitors (Donepezil, rivastigmine, galantamine and tacrine)

HUNTINGTON'S DISEASE

- It is also known as Huntington's chorea.
- Autosomal dominant neurodegenerative disease. It results in death of brain cells and consequently dementia.
- **Age of onset:** Between 25 and 45 years
- An affected person has 50% chance to pass the disease to their offspring.
- Condition is characterized by **chorea** (involuntary body movements), intellectual decline, emotional disturbance and difficulty in chewing and swallowing.
- Death typically occurs within 10–15 years after the onset of the illness

AMYOTROPHIC LATERAL SCLEROSIS (ALS)

- ALS (Lou Gehrig's disease or Charcot's disease)) is a specific disorder of unknown cause that involves loss of motor neurons that control voluntary muscles.
- In specific, it is due to the loss of motor neurons in the lower brainstem and anterior horns of the spinal cord.
- Commonly manifested by fatigue, progressive muscle weakness, cramps, muscle twitching, and incoordination.
- No specific treatment available. Symptomatic treatment is given based on symptoms.

BRAIN TUMOR

- Brain tumor can be malignant or benign.
- It compresses the adjacent tissue that results in destruction of neurons, increased ICP and displacement of brain structures.
- Meningiomas and gliomas are the most common types of primary brain tumors.
- **Signs and symptoms**
  - Symptoms of increased ICP (altered LOC, bradycardia, impaired temperature regulation, nausea and vomiting, etc.).

Clinical Corner

CASE SCENARIO 4:

A 28-year-old male client presents to the Emergency Department with unexplained paralysis from the hip downwards. Further assessment and investigations revealed that the patient has Guillain-Barré Syndrome (GBS). Which of the following assessment findings requires immediate nursing action?

a. Diminished reflexes in the lower extremities
b. Persistent head ache
c. The patient has a weak cough
d. Paraesthesia in the upper limbs

Ans. (c) The patient

Explanation: GBS can cause respiratory muscle paralysis. Therefore, the nurse should assess for any signs and symptoms of respiratory muscle weakness. Findings such as weak cough, shortness of breath, dyspnea need to be reported immediately to the physician for further intervention (e.g., Mechanical ventilation).

KEY POINTS

- The most common cause of dementia is Alzheimer's disease.
- The five "A's" of Alzheimer's disease refers to the five common cognitive disabilities in all types of dementia — Amnesia, Aphasia, Apraxia, Agnosia and Anomia
- **Key points to remember in nursing care of patient with Alzheimer disease**
  - Supporting cognitive functions
  - Promote physical safety of the patient
  - Promote independence in self-care activities

Contd...

- **Temporal tumors:** Seizures
- **Occipital tumors:** Visual disturbances or blindness
- **Frontal tumors:** Memory loss, personality changes
- **Acoustic tumors:** Impaired hearing
- **Tumor near the optic tract:** Visual disturbances
- **Pituitary tumors:** Disrupted hormonal functions

- **Diagnosis**: X-ray of skull, MRI, EEG, and CT scan
- **Treatment:** Surgery and radiation depends on histologic type and size of the tumor.

NEUROCYSTICERCOSIS

- It is the infection of CNS caused by larvae of ***Taenia solium***.
- It is the most common parasitic disease of CNS and is the leading cause of adult onset disease
- Consumption of infected pork with cysticercosis is the risk factor.

- Reduce anxiety and agitation in patient
- Improve communication and socialization
- Adequate nutrition and balancing activity

- **Most common type of brain tumor is glioma.**

Golden Points to Remember

- Tumors within Sella turcica and small adenomas of the pituitary glands can be removed through **transsphenoidal approach**.
- **Glasgow Coma Scale (GCS):** The lowest possible score is 3, and the highest possible score is 15.
- A patient whose GCS score is 8 or less is said to be in coma.
- **The biceps and brachioradialis** reflexes are mediated by the C5 and C6 nerve root.
- **The triceps** reflex is mediated by the **C6 and C7** nerve root, mainly by C7 nerve root.
- The knee jerk reflex is mediated by the **L3 and L4** nerve roots, mainly L4.
- **Wernicke's encephalopathy** is inflammatory, hemorrhagic, degenerative condition of brain caused by **thiamine deficiency**. It is common with **chronic alcoholic patients**.
- Corticosteroids (e.g., methylprednisolone) are used to reduce brain swelling and inflammation.
- Ascending paralysis is seen in Guillain–Barré syndrome.
- Compression of facial nerve in the temporal bone will lead to **Bell's palsy**.
- **Vagus nerve** has the highest number of branches.
- Trigeminal nerve is the largest cranial nerve.
- **Trigeminal neuralgia (tic douloureux):** In this sensory or afferent branch primarily the maxillary and mandibular branches are involved.
- The first-line therapy for trigeminal neuralgia **carbamazepine, phenytoin** and **valproate**.
- Parkinson's disease is characterized by tremor and rigidity of limbs.
- Contusion is the bruising of the brain tissue within a focal area without altering the integrity of pia mater and arachnoid layer.
- Signs of meningitis include positive Kerning's sign, Brudzinski sign, stiff neck, bulging fontanel (in infants), fever, bradycardia and increased ICP.
- **Cold caloric test** is performed to assess function of brain stem.
- **Amyotrophic lateral sclerosis** is a progressive neurodegenerative disease that affects nerve cells in the brain and spinal cord.
- Main cause of peripheral neuropathy is Diabetes Mellitus.
- Tubercular Meningitis is most commonly seen between 6–24 months of age.
- Kernicterus (bilirubin deposition in Basal Ganglia) can lead to Choriothetoid/Dystonic Cerebral palsy.
- Basal ganglia is affected in dyskinetic cerebral palsy.
- **Negri bodies** are found in Rabies.
- **Lewy bodies** are found in Parkinson's disease.
- Pinpoint pupil is a characteristic of Pontine hemorrhage (a form of intracranial hemorrhage).
- **Babinski reflex** is one of the normal reflexes in infants up to 2 years of age.
- Babinski reflex is an **abnormal reflex** action in adults.
- The patellar reflex or knee-jerk is a stretch reflex which tests the L2, L3, and L4 segments of the **spinal cord**.
- A client with high cervical injury (C1-C4) is at greatest risk for **respiratory compromise**.
- Cervical injuries above the level of C4 may cause total **loss of respiratory muscle (diaphragm) function**.
- **Altered level of consciousness** is most sensitive and earliest indicator of Increased Intracranial Pressure (ICP).
- Patients with a left-brain stroke have right hemiplegia and right brain stroke have left hemiplegia.
- **Anosmia** refers to loss of sense of smell.
- Guillain-Barré syndrome (GBS) is a rare neurological disorder in which the immune system of body mistakenly attacks part of its own **peripheral nervous system**.
- **Tay-Sachs** disease is a genetic disorder that results in the destruction of nerve cells in the brain and spinal cord.
- While performing Romberg test a nurse must ensure patient's safety to prevent a fall during examination.

Most Common

- Most Common cause of viral meningoencephalitis: Herpes Simplex Virus
- Most common site of Neural Tube Defect: Lumbosacral region
- Most common location of Myelomeningocoele: Lumbosacral region
- Most common genetic cause of MR: Down's syndrome
- Most common cerebrovascular diseases/stroke: ischemic stroke
- Most common cause of ischemic stroke is embolism
- Most common site of hemorrhagic CVA is Brain parenchyma
- Most common cause of hemorrhagic CVA is Hypertension

"When you are sick of your sickness, you are no longer sick."
—Chinese Proverb

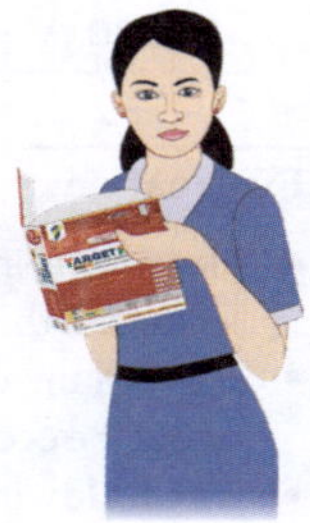

MULTIPLE CHOICE QUESTIONS
(Including Explained and Practice Questions)

NERVOUS SYSTEM

ANATOMY AND PHYSIOLOGY OF NEURON

2722. Cell most sensitive to hypoxia is?
a. Neuron b. Liver cell
c. Stem cell d. Muscle

2723. Damage to nervous tissue is repaired by which cells of CNS:
a. Neuroglia b. Axons
c. Microglia d. Fibroblasts

2724. In a neuron, the cell processes that receive information and carry it to the cell body are called:
a. Dendrites b. Axons
c. Tracts d. Projections

2725. The gaps between the segments of oligodendrocytes or between individual Schwann cells are called:
a. Nodes of Ranvier b. Synapse
c. Synaptic cleft d. Sulci

2726. Identify the correct statement regarding neurons:
I. Synaptic vesicles contains neurotransmitters
II. Dendrites typically carry signals toward the cell body
III. Schwann cells forms myelin sheath
IV. Nodes of Ranvier are found in dendrite
a. I, II, III, IV b. I, III, IV only
c. I, II, IV only d. I, II, III only

2727. Clusters of nerve cell bodies located in the peripheral nervous system are called:
a. Nuclei b. Ganglia
c. Nerve tracts d. Nerves

2728. The presynaptic terminal is separated from the postsynaptic terminal by:
a. Vesicles b. Action potential
c. Synaptic cleft d. Synaptic terminal

2729. An action potential occurs when:
a. The membrane potential reaches a threshold value
b. Negative proteins and ions rapidly enter the cell
c. The inside of the cell becomes negative compared to the outside
d. There is repolarization

2730. The action potential relies on movement of:
a. Calcium and magnesium
b. Iron and iodide
c. Sodium and magnesium
d. Sodium and potassium

2731. Depolarization of axolemma during nerve conduction takes place because *(DSSSB 2010)*
a. More Na^+ outside
b. Equal amount of Na^+ and K^+ move out across axolemma
c. Na^+ move inside and K^+ move more outside
d. None of the above

Explanation: The axolemma is the cell membrane surrounding an axon. Sodium channels open when the threshold potential is reached, facilitating a rapid influx of sodium into the axolemma interior and producing depolarization. Option c refers to sodium influx (move inside).

2732. All of the following are neurotransmitters; EXCEPT:
a. Dopamine b. GABA
c. Serotonin d. Troponin

Explanation: Dopamine, GABA (Gamma Amino Benzoic Acid), Serotonin (5-HT) are neurotransmitters. Troponins are specific proteins found in heart muscles. It is considered as a biomarker in diagnosis of myocardial infarction (MI).

2733. Which one of the following is not a neurotransmitter? *(PGIMER 2007)*
a. Cortisone b. Acetylcholine
c. Epinephrine d. Norepinephrine

Explanation: Cortisone is a steroid (glucocorticoid) while others function as neurotransmitters.

2734. Which of these is an example of a neurotransmitter? *(RRB SSNE 2015)*
a. Dopamine b. Norepinephrine
c. Acetylcholine d. All of these

2735. Which of the following is not an essential component of reflex arc?
a. Afferent neuron b. Efferent neuron
c. Spinal pathway d. Effector organ

ANATOMY AND PHYSIOLOGY OF BRAIN

2736. The parts of brain stem are: *(Safdarjung NO 2018)*
a. Mid brain, pons and medulla
b. Pons and Medulla
c. Midbrain and Medulla
d. Pons, cerebellum and medulla

Explanation: Brainstem is the area at the base of the brain that connects the cerebrum with the spinal cord. It includes mid brain (mesencephalon), pons (part of metencephalon) and medulla oblongata (myelencephalon). The brainstem regulates vital cardiac and respiratory functions and acts as a vehicle for sensory information.

2737. Function of cerebellum is all; EXCEPT:
a. Maintenance of muscle tone (Safdarjung NO 2018)
b. Maintenance of posture
c. Equilibrium
d. Hearing

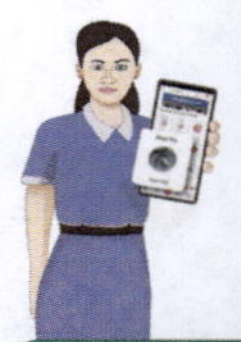

Ans.
2722. a
2723. a
2724. a
2725. a
2726. d
2727. b
2728. c
2729. a
2730. d
2731. c
2732. d
2733. a
2734. d
2735. c
2736. a
2737. d

Explanation:

- Hearing is not a function of cerebellum. The auditory cortex located at the temporal lobe of the brain is responsible for hearing.
- Cerebellum also called "little brain" is located at the back of the brain, under the occipital and temporal lobes of the cerebral cortex.
- **The following are the functions of Cerebellum:**
  - Coordinates voluntary movements
  - Controls tone, posture and equilibrium
  - Controls movement of eyeballs
  - Plays a role in cognition
  - Helps in learning of special motor skills
  - Maintenance of muscle tone and posture.

2738. The white matter of the nervous system is formed by the:
a. Nerve cell bodies and their dendrites
b. Nerve tracts
c. Nuclei
d. Sulci

2739. Outermost layer of meninges is:
a. Duramater b. Piamater
c. Arachnoid matter d. Choroid plexuses

2740. The middle layer of meninges is: *(DSSSB PHN, 2015)*
a. Dura mater b. Pia mater
c. Arachnoid mater d. Choroid Plexus

2741. Inner most layer of meninges is:
a. Duramater b. Piamater
c. Arachnoid matter d. Choroid plexuses

2742. The space between the duramater and vertebral wall is known as:
a. Cavity b. Epidural
c. Subdural d. Subarachnoid

2743. CSF is contained in:
a. Extradural space b. Subdural space
c. Subarachnoid space d. Subpial space

2744. Folded appearance on the surface of cerebrum is known as:
a. Sulci b. Gyri
c. Both a and b d. Corpus callosum

2745. Number of pairs of spinal nerves that exit from the spinal cord are: *(ESIC Chennai May 2012)*
a. 31 b. 33
c. 24 d. 30

Explanation: In humans there are 31 pairs of spinal nerves. This includes 8 cervical, 12 thoracic, 5 lumbar, 5 sacral, and 1 coccygeal. Each pair connects the spinal cord with a specific region of the body. The spinal nerves are named according to where it emerges.

2746. The lobe of the brain that can decode and interpret visual information: *(Staff Nurse GII 2014)*
a. Temporal b. Frontal
c. Parietal d. Occipital

2747. A client with C4 spinal cord injury is at greatest risk for: *(AIIMS-BBS SNO 2019)*
a. Neurogenic shock b. Respiratory compromise
c. Paralytic ileus d. Stress ulcer

Explanation: Cervical injuries above the level of C4 present special problems because of the total loss of respiratory muscle function. The fourth cervical vertebra is the level where nerves run to the diaphragm, the main muscle that allows us to breathe.

2748. The Broca's areas are situated in the:
a. Temporal lobe
b. Occipital calcarine fissure
c. Inferior frontal gyrus
d. Mammillary body region

2749. Respiratory center is located at: *(JIPMER 2012, Kerala PSC, Nov 2014)*
a. Cerebrum b. Pons
c. Medulla oblongata d. Spinal cord

2750. The part of the brainstem that regulates heart rate, breathing, swallowing, coughing and sneezing is the:
a. Cerebellum b. Medulla oblongata
c. Pons d. Midbrain

2751. The part of brain, which is responsible for the co-ordination of movement is: *(LNJP H D 2012)*
a. Brain stem b. Thalamus
c. Cerebellum d. Hypothalamus

2752. The group of nuclei scattered throughout the brainstem that play role in arousing and maintaining consciousness is the:
a. Reticular formation b. Pons
c. Colliculi d. Pyramids

2753. CSF is secreted from:
a. Choroid plexuses b. Arachnoid villi
c. Base of lateral ventricle d. Aqueduct

2754. Drainage of CSF from lateral to third ventricle is through:
a. Foramen of Monro
b. Foramen of Luschka
c. Foramen of Magendie
d. Aqueduct of Sylvius

2755. CSF pressure depends primarily on:
a. Rate of CSF absorption
b. Rate of formation from the choroid plexus
c. Cerebral blood flow
d. Blood pressure

2756. Which is not true about CSF?
a. It is clear, colorless, odorless fluid
b. Present in ventricles, spinal canal, and around the brain
c. Arachnoid villi produce CSF
d. CSF contains glucose, protein and WBC

2757. Aqueous humor is secreted by ....:
a. Choroid plexus b. Papillary muscles
c. Arachnoid villi d. Ciliary body

2758. Which one of the following brain area regulates body temperature? *(Staff Nurse GII 2014, Banaras HU 2015)*
a. Cerebrum
b. Cerebellum
c. Hypothalamus
d. Hippocampus

2759. Normal CSF contain all among the following; EXCEPT:
a. Red blood cells
b. White blood cells
c. Insulin
d. Protein

2760. Normal level of glucose in CSF is:
a. 10–20 mg/dL b. 20–40 mg/dL
c. 45–80 mg/dL d. 75–85 mg/dL

2761. Normal level of protein in CSF is:
a. 5–12 mg/dL b. 15–45 mg/dL
c. 45–80 mg/dL d. 75–85 mg/dL

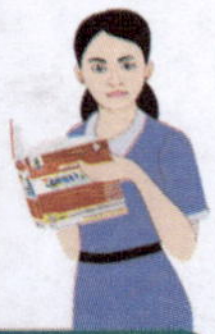

Ans.
2738. b
2739. a
2740. c
2741. b
2742. b
2743. c
2744. c
2745. a
2746. d
2747. b
2748. c
2749. c
2750. b
2751. c
2752. a
2753. a
2754. a
2755. a
2756. c
2757. d
2758. c
2759. a
2760. c
2761. b

ANATOMY & PHYSIOLOGY OF SPINAL CORD

2762. Malformation of the spine in which the posterior portion of the lamina of one or more vertebrae fails to fuse, with or without defective development of the spinal cord is called:- *(AIIMS Raipur Grade II 2017)*

a. Rachischisis b. Encephalocele
c. Spina bifida d. Anencephaly

Explanation: Rachischisis and spina bifida are both terms used to describe certain types of spinal cord malformations, but they differ in specific characteristics.

Spina bifida refers to the failure of the closure of the dorsal aspect of the vertebral foramen of one or a few vertebrae.

Rachischisis is a more severe form of spina bifida, in which the spinal cord and meninges are exposed. In this, many adjacent vertebrae are involved. This results in a cleft along the entire length of the spine, exposing the spinal cord and its surrounding tissues directly to the outside environment.

2763. The posterior (dorsal) horns of the spinal cord contain:

a. Sensory neurons b. Motor neurons
c. Nerve tracts d. White matter

2764. Largest branch of Lumbar plexus:

a. Sciatic nerve b. Femoral nerve
c. Obturator nerve d. Pudendal nerve

2765. Most sensory input that ascends through the spinal cord and brainstem projects to the:

a. Pineal body b. Hypothalamus
c. Thalamus d. Mamillary bodies

2766. True about spinal cord is/are:

a. In adults spinal cord ends at lower border of L1 vertebra
b. In newborn may extend up to L3
c. Cauda equina extends from lumbar vertebra to coccyx
d. All of the above

2767. The extension of the spinal cord take place from which bone of the skull:

a. Parietal bone
b. Occipital bone
c. Temporal bone
d. Root originate from frontal bone

2768. Which spinal plexuses innervate and control the head and neck region?

a. Cervical plexus b. Brachial plexus
c. Lumbar plexus d. Thoracic plexus

2769. Which is referred as bundle of nerve fibers present below the spinal cord?

a. Conus medullaris
b. Fasciculi
c. Cauda Equina
d. Dermatomes

2770. The bundles of the fibers or the tract present on the white matter of the spinal cord:

a. Conus medullaris
b. Fasciculi
c. Cauda Equina
d. Dermatomes

2771. In human being, the spinal cord opening begins at:

a. Foramen magnum b. Foramen ovale
c. Foramen monro d. Foramen rotundum

2772. All of the following are the functions of spinal cord; EXCEPT:

a. Carrying out reflexes
b. Sensory and motor tract
c. Memory and comprehension
d. Transport message to and from brain

2773. In which of the following part the nerves from arm enter and get exited?

a. Cervical enlargement
b. Lumbrosacral enlargement
c. Central canal
d. Cauda equina

2774. In which of the following part the nerves from leg enter and get exited?

a. Cervical enlargement
b. Lumbrosacral enlargement
c. Central canal
d. Cauda equine

2775. The Cerebrospinal fluid-filled ependymal space present on the spinal cord is known as:

a. Cervical enlargement b. Lumbrosacral enlargement
c. Central canal d. Cauda equina

PERIPHERAL NERVOUS SYSTEM (CRANIAL AND SPINAL NERVES)

2776. The number of pairs of cranial nerves are: *(ESIC Chennai May 2012)*

a. 14 b. 16
c. 10 d. 12

2777. The 10th cranial nerve is: *(DSSSB PHN, 2015)*

a. Abducent b. Vagus
c. Facial d. Hypoglossal

2778. Which of the following is the 5th cranial nerve? *(Kerala PSC, Nov 2014)*

a. Trochlear b. Trigeminal
c. Abducent d. Facial

2779. Which is the largest cranial nerve?

a. Vagus nerve
b. Trigeminal nerve
c. Facial nerve
d. Abducent nerve

2780. The smallest cranial nerve in terms of the number of axons it contains is:

a. Olfactory nerve
b. Oculomotor nerve
c. Trochlear nerve
d. Accessory nerve

Explanation:

- Largest cranial nerve: Trigeminal
- Smallest cranial nerve: Trochlear
- Shortest cranial nerve: Olfactory

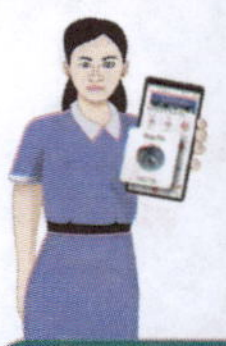

Ans.

2762. c
2763. a
2764. b
2765. c
2766. d
2767. b
2768. a
2769. c
2770. b
2771. a
2772. c
2773. a
2774. b
2775. c
2776. d
2777. b
2778. b
2779. b
2780. c

2781. The cranial nerve which regulates heart rate is:

a. VII b. VIII
c. IX d. X

Explanation: The vagus nerve (X nerve) mediates important homeostatic reflexes such as heart rate, blood pressure, and respiration.

2782. Pupillary constriction is controlled by …….. cranial nerve:

a. I b. III
c. V d. VII

2783. Cranial nerve first to be affected by increased intracranial pressure:

a. II b. III
c. IV d. VI

2784. Largest nerve in human body is:

a. Sciatic nerve b. Femoral nerve
c. Obturator nerve d. Pudendal nerve

2785. Medulla oblongata is also called:

a. Prosencephalon b. Mesencephalon
c. Myeloncephalon d. Metencephalon

2786. Circle of Willis is formed by all; EXCEPT:

a. Anterior communicating artery
b. Posterior inferior cerebellar artery
c. Anterior cerebral artery
d. Posterior communicating artery

2787. Middle meningeal artery is a branch of:

a. Middle cerebral artery
b. Maxillary artery
c. Superficial temporal artery
d. Vertebral artery

2788. The following nerves supply to the muscles of the forearm EXCEPT:

a. Musculocutaneous nerve
b. Radial nerve
c. Median nerve
d. Ulnar nerve

Explanation: The major peripheral nerve of upper arm is musculocutaneous nerve which innervates the anterior compartment muscles (brachialis, bicep brachii and coracobrachialis) of upper arm and gives rise to lateral cutaneous nerve of forearm which innervate lateral surfaces of the forearm. But the muscles of forearm (Flexor carpi ulnaris, Flexor carpi radialis, pronator teres, etc.) innervated by radial nerve, ulnar nerve and median nerve. PS: The question is about muscle innervations (not cutaneous innervations). Cutaneous innervations of forearm is supplied by musculocutaneous nerve.

2789. Ulnar nerve severed above elbow causes all; EXCEPT:

a. Complete loss of sensation in 4th and 5th fingers
b. Paralysis of all lumbricals
c. Paralysis of flexor carpi ulnaris
d. Paralysis of flexor profundus

2790. Triceps is supplied by………..nerve:

a. Axillary b. Ulnar
c. Radial d. Musculocutaneous

2791. Nerve supply to hypothenar muscles is from:

a. Ulnar nerve b. Median nerve
c. Radial nerve d. Musculocutaneous nerve

2792. The cubital fossa is bounded by the:

a. Biceps b. Triceps
c. Brachioradialis d. Coracobrachialis

2793. Ulnar nerve paralysis causes:

a. Ape thumb deformity b. Wrist drop
c. Claw finger deformity d. Madelung deformity

2794. The plexus that supply nerves to the skin and muscles of the upper limbs and some of the chest muscles is: *(AIIMS Raipur Grade II 2017)*

a. Cervical plexus b. Brachial plexus
c. Lumbar plexus d. Sacral plexus

Explanation: Cervical plexus supply nerves to the back of the head and some neck muscles. Lumbar plexus supply nerves to the vascular lacuna near the saphenous hiatus and supplies the skin below the inguinal ligament. Sacral plexus supply nerves to the skin and muscles of the pelvis and lower limb.

2795. The nerve fibers which carry impulses from the receptors to the central nervous system are known as:

a. Afferent b. Efferent
c. Synapse d. Nodes of Ranvier

Explanation: The afferent neurons are also known as the sensory neurons they bring the stimuli from the sensors (e.g., skin, eyes, ears) to the CNS. The efferent neurons are also known as motor neurons they bring the responses from the brain to the muscles and the glands.

2796. Sixth cranial nerve (Abducens) controls:

a. Movement of the eyeball
b. Taste perception
c. Closure of epiglottis
d. Movement of the tongue

Explanation: Movement of the eyeball is controlled by three cranial nerves, i.e., oculomotor (III), trochlear (IV) and abducens nerve (VI). The abducens nerve supplies the lateral rectus muscle of the eye.

2797. Monro-Kellies hypothesis is about:

a. Equilibrium of cranial content
b. Affected mental function
c. Increasing intracranial pressure
d. Unresponsive to environment

Explanation: The pressure-volume relationship between ICP, volume of CSF, blood, and brain tissue, and cerebral perfusion pressure (CPP) is known as the Monro-Kellie doctrine or the Monro-Kellie hypothesis. The Monro-Kellie hypothesis states that because of the limited space for expansion within the skull, an increase in any one of the components causes a change in the volume of the others. Because brain tissue has limited space to change, compensation typically is accomplished by displacing or shifting CSF, increasing the absorption of CSF, or decreasing cerebral blood volume. Without such changes, ICP will begin to rise.

2798. Labourer's nerve is another name for which nerve?

a. Median nerve b. Radial nerve
c. Ulnar nerve d. Axillary nerve

2799. As a part of the assessment of the cranial nerves, the nurse asks the patient to arise the eyebrows, smile and show the teeth, these actions provide information about which cranial nerve? *(LNJP H D 2012)*

a. Facial b. Vagus
c. Olfactory d. Optic

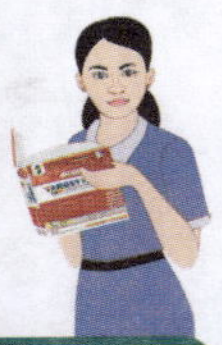

Ans.

2781. d
2782. b
2783. d
2784. a
2785. c
2786. b
2787. b
2788. a
2789. b
2790. c
2791. a
2792. c
2793. c
2794. b
2795. a
2796. a
2797. a
2798. a
2799. a

AUTONOMIC NERVOUS SYSTEM (SYMPATHETIC AND PARASYMPATHETIC NERVES)

2800. Most important nerve in parasympathetic nervous system is:

a. Olfactory b. Abducent
c. Vagus d. Spinal accessory

2801. Which of the following function is not likely to be affected by vagus nerve?

a. Tongue movements b. Peristaltic movements
c. Pancreatic secretion d. Heart rate

Explanation: Movement of the tongue is controlled by 12th cranial nerve (Hypoglossal nerve). All other functions (option b, c, and d) are controlled by vagus nerve.

2802. Which of the following activity is increased by sympathetic nervous system?

a. Heart rate b. Secretion of digestive juices
c. Secretion of saliva d. All of these

Explanation: Activation of sympathetic nervous system leads to increase in heart rate, widening of airways (bronchioles) in the lungs, and dilation of pupils. It also results in slowing down of digestive activity by inhibiting secretion of digestive juices and saliva.

2803. Vasoconstriction in skin is due to:

a. Sympathetic b. Parasympathetic
c. Wheal and flare d. Warm climate

2804. Which division of the nervous system initiates a response known as fight or flight? *(RRB SSNE 2015)*

a. The parasympathetic nervous system
b. The sympathetic nervous system
c. The somatic nervous system
d. None of these

2805. The autonomic nervous system regulates visceral activities such as *(ESIC Chennai May 2012)*

a. Respiration
b. Contraction of smooth muscles
c. Gastrointestinal motility
d. All of the above

2806. Which of the following is a function of parasympathetic nervous system?

a. Contraction of arrector pili
b. Stimulation of sweat glands
c. Acceleration of heart rate
d. Constriction of pupil

Explanation: Stimulation of the parasympathetic nervous system leads to constriction of pupil. Option a, b and c are associated with sympathetic nervous system functions.

2807. Which of the following function is influenced by autonomous nervous system?

a. Knee-jerk response
b. Pupillary reflex
c. Peristalsis of the intestine
d. Blinking of eye

Explanation: The digestive system is under control of the autonomic nervous system (ANS). Autonomic nervous system (sympathetic and parasympathetic nervous system) is involved in peristalsis of the intestine. Option a, b and d are somatic reflexes.

2808. The emergency room nurse is assessing an adult patient who was brought in following a road traffic accident. Which of the following manifestations could have resulted from sympathetic nervous system stimulation?

a. Increased awareness and attention
b. Decreased physiologic functioning
c. Increased salivation
d. A rapid pulse and increased respiratory rate

Explanation: Activation of sympathetic nervous system leads to increase in heart rate, widening of airways (bronchioles) in the lungs, and dilation of pupils. This is similar to fight or flight response facilitated by sympathetic nervous system. Increased cardiac and respiratory activity facilitates survival.

ASSESSMENT AND DIAGNOSTIC TESTS

2809. Injury to radial nerve at wrist leads to:

a. Wrist drop
b. Sensory loss on adjacent sides of IIIrd and IVth fingers
c. Paralysis of adductor pollucis
d. Loss of supination in extended position

2810. Policeman's tip hand is seen in:

a. Erb's palsy b. Klumpke's paralysi
c. Axillary nerve injury d. None of these

2811. The commonest cause for neuralgic pain in foot is:

a. Compression of communication between medial and lateral plantar nerves
b. Exaggeration of longitudinal arches
c. Injury to deltoid ligament
d. Shortening of planter aponeurosis

2812. The injury of which nerve leads to Wrist Drop'? *(DSSSB PHN, 2015)*

a. Axillary nerve b. Median nerve
c. Radial nerve d. Ulnar nerve

2813. Functions affected in anterior cerebral artery obstruction is:

a. Language comprehension
b. Balance and coordination
c. Judgment, insight, and reasoning
d. Visual and auditory

2814. Nerve involved in Carpal tunnel syndrome is:

a. Peroneal nerve b. Ulnar nerve
c. Brachial plexuses d. Median nerve

2815. Foot drop result as a result of injury to:

a. Deep peroneal nerve b. Superficial peroneal nerve
c. Tibial nerve d. Deltoid ligament

2816. Which assessment finding is specific in client having neurological deficit involving limbic system?

a. Affect is flat
b. Recall deficit
c. Disoriented to time and place
d. Inability to add and subtract

Explanation: Limbic system is responsible for affect.

2817. Two point discrimination test exhibits maximum sensitivity in?

a. Shin b. Soles
c. Toes d. Finger pads

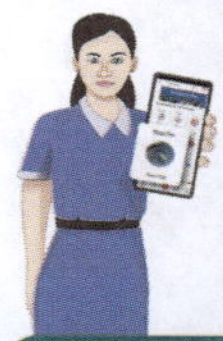

Ans.

2800. c
2801. a
2802. a
2803. a
2804. b
2805. d
2806. d
2807. c
2808. d
2809. a
2810. a
2811. a
2812. c
2813. c
2814. d
2815. a
2816. a
2817. d

2818. Which of the following is not a test for integrity of 7th and 9th nerve:

a. Taste
b. Palate symmetry
c. Tongue protrusion
d. Position of uvula

2819. While performing Romberg test nurse must ensure patients *(AIIMS Raipur NO 2019)*

a. Gait b. Posture
c. Safety d. Closing of Eyes

Explanation: Romberg test is used to assess neurological function for balance. The standing patient is asked to close eyes. It is positive if there is actual loss of balance and patient falls while the eyes are closed. Gait, posture and closing of eyes are observed during exam but the priority is to ensure the patient's safety during examination.

2820. In adult, the reflex action of the toes that is indicative of abnormalities in the motor control pathway leading from cerebral cortex is known as. *(ESIC 2019)*

a. Romberg test b. Patellar reflex
c. Babinski reflex d. Achilles reflex

Explanation: Babinski sign occurs when stimulation of lateral plantar aspect of the foot leads to extension (dorsiflexion or upward movement) of the big toe (hallux). Also, there may be fanning of the other toes. Babinski reflex is an abnormal reflex action in adults while it is normal in infants up to 2 years of age.

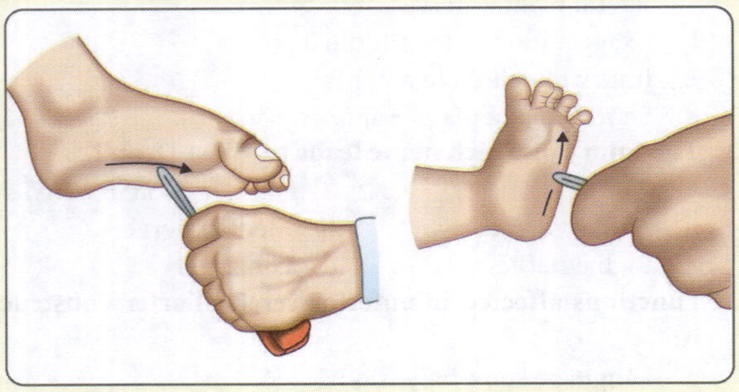

Figures A and B: A. Plantar reflex; **B.** Babinski sign

2821. While assessing an unconscious client who was brought into emergency room after a road traffic accident, the nurse would be most concerned if the assessment revealed:

a. An elevated temperature
b. An increased blood pressure
c. Bleeding from ears
d. All of the above

Explanation: Nurse should thoroughly assess for signs that could indicate increased intracranial pressures, fractures and bleeding. Bleeding from the ears occurs only with basal skull fractures that can easily lead to raise in intracranial pressure and brain herniation.

2822. Complaints of pain by the elderly patient is to be carefully assessed because older people:

a. Have increased tactile perception
b. Often experience chronic pain
c. Have a decreased pain threshold
d. Have reduced sensory perception

Explanation: Age-related degenerative changes in the elderly causes decreased sensory perception. This may result in altered pain perception in older persons. So it is essential to carefully assess any complaints of pain by elderly because pain has an impact on quality of life.

2823. A 42-year-old male client is to undergo lumbar puncture. Which of the following is the least important information about lumbar puncture (LP)?

a. It may be used to withdraw CSF for diagnostic purpose.
b. Specimens obtained to be labeled in their proper sequence.
c. Force fluids before and after the procedure
d. Assess movements and sensation in the lower extremities after the procedure

Explanation: The client is advised to increased fluid intake to 3L (if not contraindicated) for 24-48 hours after the procedure (to facilitate CSF production). There is no instruction to increased fluid intake before the procedure.

- Lumbar puncture involves insertion of a needle into spinal cord to withdraw CSF or inject drugs into spinal cord.
- Specimens obtained to be labeled.
- Assessment of sensation in lower extremities after the procedure is important to rule out nerve injury.

2824. A patient with cerebral thrombosis is scheduled for cerebral angiography. Which of the following nursing care is appropriate for this client?

a. Inform the client that a warm, flushed feeling and a salty taste may occur
b. Avoid applying a pressure dressing over the site of puncture
c. Keep the extremity used as puncture site flexed to prevent bleeding
d. All of the above

Explanation: Angiography is imaging technique that uses an injection of a liquid dye to make the arteries easily visible on X-rays. During the procedure contrast (dye) is injected into the bloodstream to make the blood vessels visible on X-rays. When the contrast is injected the client may feel flushing sensation, a salty or metallic taste in the mouth, nausea, and/or a brief headache. These effects usually last for only a few moments. The nurse must inform about this to patient before undergoing the procedure. Also the nurse must apply a pressure dressing over the site of puncture to prevent bleeding. Keeping the extremity used as puncture site flexed will increase chance of thrombus formation so it is to be avoided.

2825. Which of the following is the most important assessment during the acute stage of an unconscious patient?

a. Coherence and sense of hearing
b. Level of awareness and response to pain
c. Pupillary reflexes and response to sensory stimuli
d. Patency of airway and adequacy of respiration

Explanation: Checking airway, breathing and circulation is the priority assessment for the unconscious patient. At all levels of care, the ABC (Airway, Breathing and Circulation) protocol exists to remind the person delivering treatment of the importance of airway, breathing, and circulation to the maintenance.

Ans.

2818. c
2819. c
2820. c
2821. c
2822. d
2823. c
2824. a
2825. d

2826. Which of the following diagnostic procedure involves the injection of radioisotopes into the body?
a. CT imaging b. MRI
c. PET d. X-ray

Explanation: A positron emission tomography (PET) an imaging test that helps reveal how the tissues and organs are functioning. A PET scan uses a radioactive drug (tracer) to show this activity. The tracer may be injected, swallowed or inhaled, depending on which organ or tissue is being studied by the PET scan.

2827. What must the nurse do when preparing a client for a computed tomography (CT) scan?
a. Administer a laxative preparation
b. Encourage fluid intake
c. Administer a radioisotope
d. Explain the procedure

Explanation: The client is not given a radioisotope. Fluids are not pushed prior to the procedure.
Tips: Use elimination technique to eliminate inappropriate answers.

2828. Electroencephalogram is: *(ESIC Chennai May 2012)*
a. Recording of brain wave activity
b. Recording of peristalsis
c. Recording of heart activity
d. None of the above

2829. The most common site of rupture of a cerebral aneurysm with resulting subarachnoid hemorrhage is:
a. Anterior communicating artery
b. Posterior communicating artery
c. Middle cerebral artery
d. Internal carotid artery

2830. In case of delay in transportation of cerebrospinal fluid (CSF) sample, it should be *(Banaras HU 2015)*
a. Kept at room temperature
b. Refrigerated at 4°C
c. Kept at – 20°C
d. Kept in ice bucket

2831. All among the following investigation can be performed in a patient with brain tumor; EXCEPT:
a. CT scan
b. MRI
c. Doppler
d. Lumbar puncture

2832. Contraindications of Lumbar Puncture include all; EXCEPT:
a. Raised intracranial pressure
b. Suspected CNS infection
c. Infected skin over the puncture site
d. Trauma or mass to lumbar vertebrae

Explanation: Suspected CNS infection (e.g., meningitis) is one of the indication for LP. All other conditions are contraindications of LP.

2833. Optic nerve damage can be assessed through: ***New Q***
a. Ophthalmoscopy
b. Slit lamp examination
c. Perimetry
d. Goniometer

Explanation: Optic nerve damage can be assessed through ophthalmoscopy, also known as fundoscopy. Ophthalmoscopy is a procedure that allows a doctor to see the inside of the eye, including the optic nerve. This procedure is performed with a handheld instrument called an ophthalmoscope. The doctor shines a light into the eye and uses the ophthalmoscope to look at the retina, the optic nerve, and other structures at the back of the eye.
Slit lamp examination is primarily used to examine the anterior segment of the eye, such as the cornea, iris, and lens. **Perimetry** is a test to assess the visual field and may indirectly provide information about optic nerve function. **A goniometer** is a device used to measure angles and is not directly related to assessing optic nerve damage.

2834. A lethargic patient who has fever, vomiting, headache and the nurse has to prepare him for which one of the following procedures? *(RAK MSc 2018)*
a. Blood culture b. Lumbar puncture
c. CAT scan d. Ultrasound scan

Explanation: A lethargic patient with fever, vomiting and headache may be the manifestations of injury or infection of brain or spinal cord which can only be confirmed by analyzing the CSF. CSF samples can be obtained by performing lumbar puncture. Hence the nurse may prepare the patient for Lumbar puncture. Lumbar puncture, also known as a spinal tap, is a medical procedure in which a needle is inserted into the spinal canal, most commonly to collect cerebrospinal fluid for diagnostic testing.

2835. Which of these is true regarding lumbar puncture method?
a. Also known as spinal tap
b. Needle passed between 3rd and 4th or 4th and 5th lumbar vertebrae
c. Knee chest position will be given to client
d. All of the above

2836. Site for lumbar puncture is:
a. L1-L2 b. L2-L3
c. L2-L4 d. L3-L4

2837. Which of the following is the diagnostic indication of lumbar puncture?
a. Intra cranial infection b. Meningeal leukemia
c. Neoplasms of brain d. All of these

2838. Complications of LP include:
a. Infection b. Brain stem herniation
c. Hematoma d. All of these

2839. Trendelenburg test is positive due to injury to which of the following nerve:
a. Obturator b. Sciatic
c. Superior Gluteal d. Inferior Gluteal

2840. Unilateral trigeminal nerve injury is tested by:
a. Elevation and lowering of jaw
b. Inability to tense the jaw
c. Blinking of eye
d. Corneal reflex

2841. Pre-procedural preparation for MRI include:
a. Enema
b. Prostheses or a pacemaker
c. Any known allergy to antibiotics
d. Vitals monitoring

2842. Neurological examination of a client shows that client is unable to perceive pain, so the examiner need to avoid:
a. Balancing test b. Hearing test
c. Temperature perception d. Rombers's test

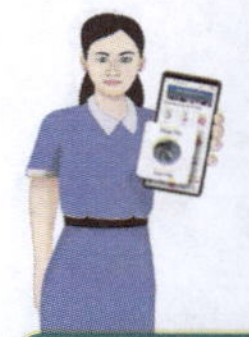

Ans.
2826. c
2827. d
2828. a
2829. a
2830. a
2831. d
2832. b
2833. a
2834. b
2835. d
2836. d
2837. d
2838. d
2839. c
2840. a
2841. b
2842. c

2843. Allen's test is used for:
a. Integrity of palmar arch
b. Ulnar nerve function
c. Median nerve compression
d. None of the above

2844. Which of the following is a feature of extrapyramidal tract involvement:
a. Positive Babinsky Sign
b. Increased Muscular Tone
c. Exaggerated Deep tendon reflexes
d. Paralysis

2845. All of the following are metabolic causes of headache; EXCEPT:
a. Hyperglycemia
b. Hyponatremia
c. Hypercapnia
d. Hypoxia

2846. Which of the following function will be affected due to an obstruction of the anterior cerebral arteries?
a. Auditory perception
b. Judgement, insight, and reasoning
c. Balance and coordination
d. Visual integration from language comprehension

Explanation: The medial and anterior portions of the frontal lobes are supplied by the anterior cerebral arteries. The anterior portion of the frontal lobe controls higher mental functions such as judgement, insight and reasoning. Hence, the obstruction of blood supply to anterior portion of the frontal lobe results in impairment of judgement, insight and reasoning.

2847. Which of the following term is used to describe edema of the optic nerve?
a. Angioneurotic edema
b. Papilledema
c. Glaucoma
d. Lymphedema

Explanation: Papilledema (or papilloedema) is optic disc swelling that is caused by increased intracranial pressure. The swelling is usually bilateral and can occur over a period of hours to weeks.

2848. Aphasia refers to: *(Banaras HU 2015)*
a. Increased rate of speech
b. Inability to speak
c. Loud speech
d. High pitch speech

2849. Immediate chief complaint following cerebral aneurysm rupture is:
a. Photophobia
b. Explosive headache
c. Otorrhea
d. Epistasis

2850. Patient is complaining of drainage from nose and ear, which among the following sign suggest that drainage is CSF?
a. Halo sign
b. Goodle's sign
c. Hagar's sign
d. Chadwick sign

2851. Involuntary, jerking, rhythmic movement of the eyes is known as:
a. Diplopia
b. Double vision
c. Nystagmus
d. Ptosis

2852. Cushing's triad is seen in: *(ISRO)*
a. Cushing's Syndrome
b. Hypothyroidism
c. Increased intracranial tension
d. Hyperthermia

2853. Ice pack test is done for:
a. Myasthenia Gravis
b. Hypokalemic periodic paralysis
c. Hyperparathyroidism
d. Multiple system atrophy

2854. ________ bladder is expected when a patient is experiencing spinal shock *(AIIMS 2006)*
a. Atonic
b. Normal
c. Spastic
d. Uncontrolled

Explanation: Atonic, or sometimes 'flaccid', bladder sees the organ dilate as usual but fail to empty. This is often due to the brain sending incorrect signals to the bladder usually stemming from some kind of spinal cord injury or a condition such as multiple sclerosis.

2855. Cold calorie test used to check the functioning of ......:
a. Heart
b. Hypothalamus
c. Brain stem
d. Pons

Explanation: Caloric stimulation is a test that uses differences in temperature to diagnose damage to the acoustic nerve. This is the nerve that is involved in hearing and balance. The test also checks for damage to the brain stem.

2856. Cold calorie test is interpreted as normal if:
a. Rapid, side-to-side eye movements occur when cold or warm water is placed into the ear
b. Eye movements are similar on both sides when cold or warm water is placed into the ear
c. Rapid, side-to-side eye movements do not occur even after ice cold water is given
d. Both a and b

Explanation: Rapid, side-to-side eye movements should occur when cold or warm water is placed into the ear. The eye movements should be similar on both sides. If the rapid, side-to-side eye movements do not occur even after ice cold water is given, there may be damage to the:
- Nerve of the inner ear
- Balance sensors of the inner ear
- Brain

GLASGOW COMA SCALE (GCS)

2857. A person present in emergency. On examination he is found to open eyes only on painful stimuli, he says inappropriate words and moves his limbs on commands. His GCS is:
a. 11
b. 10
c. 9
d. 13

Explanation: Based on GCS table,
- Eye opening on painful stimuli-2 points
- Inappropriate words-3 points
- Obeys commands to motor response-6 points

2858. Which of the following score indicates coma in an adult patient as per Glasgow Coma Scale?
a. 0
b. 5
c. 9
d. 12

Ans.
2843. a
2844. b
2845. a
2846. b
2847. b
2848. b
2849. b
2850. a
2851. c
2852. c
2853. a
2854. a
2855. c
2856. d
2857. a
2858. b

Explanation: A score below 8 in Glasgow Coma Scale indicates Coma. 15 is the maximum score and 3 is the minimum achievable score. Zero score is not applicable as per GCS.

2859. Glasgow coma scale has all; EXCEPT: *(LNJP H D 2012)*
a. Sensory response b. Eye opening
c. Verbal response d. Motor response

2860. What is the minimum score in Glasgow coma scale?
a. 0 b. 1
c. 2 d. 3

ALTERED LEVEL OF CONSCIOUSNESS

2861. The nurse is aware that the early indicator of hypoxia in an unconscious patient is:
a. Cyanosis of extremities b. Altered respirations
c. Hypertension d. Restlessness

Explanation: If the patient is unconscious but shows restlessness, attention should be given to the possibility of cerebral hypoxia.

2862. While monitoring an unconscious child admitted with a history of fall, nurse notices that the child suddenly has a fixed and dilated pupil. This indicates *(Banaras HU 2015)*
a. Eye trauma
b. Neurosurgical emergency
c. Increased parasympathetic activity
d. Indication of brain death

2863. When caring for an unconscious patient, which of the following nursing intervention would be of highest priority to maintain the patient in a stable condition?
a. Measuring the urine output
b. Maintaining a patent airway
c. Putting a nasogastric (NG) tube in place
d. Monitoring intake and output

Explanation: Maintaining airway is always the first priority. Other interventions also important but the maintenance of airway is a priority over others. The nursing interventions can be prioritized using ABC (Airway, Breathing, and Circulation) principle.

2864. Which of the following respiratory pattern indicates that the patient is experiencing increased ICP?
a. Slow, irregular respirations
b. Rapid, deep respirations
c. Symmetric chest excursion
d. Nasal flaring and red eyes

2865. A patient with altered level of consciousness has an increased ICP of 22 mmHg. The nurse should take which of the following action first:
a. Provide the client a warming blanket
b. Give High-dose barbiturates
c. Direct the client to take deep breaths to hyperventilate
d. Stop the fluid administration

Explanation: Hyperventilation is one of the method of rapidly lowering ICP. Cerebral blood flow is largely dependent on $PaCO_2$. Hyperventilation causes decreased $PaCO_2$ which subsequently leads to arterial vasoconstriction thus, lowering cerebral blood flow (CBF), cerebral blood volume, and ICP.

2866. If a client shows no observable signs or symptoms to the external stimuli, then the client is on the state of:
a. Lethargy b. Confused
c. Comatose d. Semiconscious

2867. A client who is on the state of drowsy, and needs certain verbal or touch stimulation to initiate response. This indicates that the client is in the state of:
a. Lethargy b. Confused
c. Comatose d. Semiconscious

INCREASED INTRACRANIAL PRESSURE (ICP)

2868. Normal range of ICP is:
(AIIMS Rishikesh Senior Nursing Officer 2018)
a. 0–5 mm Hg b. 5–10 mm Hg
c. 5–15 mm Hg d. 15–20 mm Hg

2869. Normal range of cerebral perfusion pressure is:
a. 10–35 mm Hg b. 40–80 mm Hg
c. 50–100 mm Hg d. 60–140 mm Hg

2870. CPP (cerebral perfusion pressure) can be calculated using:
a. MAP–ICP b. SBP–ICP
c. ICP–MAP d. DBP–ICP

2871. Which of the following is considered to be the earliest sign of increased ICP?
a. Ipsilateral dilation of the pupils
b. Contralateral hemiparesis
c. Progression from restlessness to confusion and disorientation to lethargy
d. Widening of pulse pressure

Explanation: Increasing ICP decreases the cerebral perfusion causing hypoxia of brain cells. It produces a progressive alteration in the loss of consciousness. Alternation in LOC is initially manifested by restlessness.

2872. Raised intra cranial pressure (ICP) is seen in all; EXCEPT:
a. Inspiration
b. Mechanical ventilation
c. Coughing
d. Valsalva maneuver

2873. Flapping hand tremors is seen in which of the following conditions?
a. Uremic syndrome b. Chronic renal failure
c. Hepatic encephalopathy d. All of these

Explanation: Asterixis (also called the flapping tremor, or liver flap) is a tremor of the hand when the wrist is extended, sometimes said to resemble a bird flapping its wings. Chronic renal failure and hepatic encephalopathy results in uremia (uremic syndrome) which is a major cause of flapping hand tremors. It can be seen in any metabolic encephalopathy, e.g., chronic renal failure, severe congestive heart failure, acute respiratory failure and commonly in decompensated liver failure.

2874. Which of the following is a symptom of increasing intracranial pressure that should be reported immediately to the health care provider? *(RAK MSc 2018)*
a. Constricted pupils
b. Tachycardia
c. Narrowing pulse pressure
d. Bradypnea

Ans.
2859. a
2860. d
2861. d
2862. b
2863. b
2864. a
2865. c
2866. c
2867. a
2868. c
2869. d
2870. a
2871. c
2872. b
2873. d
2874. d

Explanation:

- Cushing's triad is the presentation of three clinical manifestations as they relate to decompensated responses to increasing intracranial pressure (ICP) widening pulse pressure with hypertension (increasing systolic BP), bradycardia, and irregular respirations (most commonly **bradypnea**).
- Dilated pupil and widened pulse pressure are expected in increased ICP.

2875. Increased ICP is shown by?

a. Miosis b. Reduction in GCS
c. Tachycardia d. Systemic hypotension

2876. Increased intra-cranial pressure is related to:

a. Hypotension and tachycardia
b. Hypertension and bradycardia
c. Hypertension and tachycardia
d. Hypotension and bradycardia

2877. Later signs of increased Intracranial pressure (ICP) includes which of the following?

a. Narrow pulse pressure b. Increased diastolic BP
c. Decreased pulse rate d. Projectile vomiting

Explanation: Projectile vomiting is an early sign of increased ICP. Later sign of ICP is cushing triad and its components are increased systolic BP, bradycardia and bradypnea. Increased pulse pressure is also seen as later sign

2878. Which of the following is not an expected finding in the assessment of a client having increased intracranial pressure? *(AIIMS-BBS SNO 2019)*

a. Unequal pupils
b. Clear consciousness
c. Irritability
d. Headache

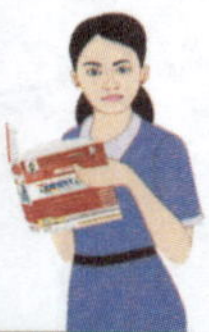

Explanation: Clear consciousness is NOT an expected finding in the assessment of a client having increased ICP. **Loss of consciousness** is most sensitive and reliable indicator of increased ICP. So, change in consciousness is a sign of increased ICP..

2879. A nurse is monitoring an adult male patient 8 hours after a road traffic accident, which of the following findings by a nurse suggest increasing intracranial pressure (ICP)?

a. Blood pressure is decreased from 150/90 to 110/70
b. The patient is oriented when aroused from sleep, and fall asleep immediately
c. Pulse is increased from 80 to 92
d. The client refuses dinner because of anorexia

Explanation: Change in LOC is one of the major indication of increased ICP. Oriented immediately after arousal from sleep and going back to sleep immediately is the indication that the patient's consciousness is decreasing.

2880. Medical management for increased intracranial pressure (ICP) includes: *(DSSSB 2013)*

a. Administer half strength saline
b. Administer plasma volume expanders
c. Administer mannitol
d. Reduce the number of breaths in the ventilator

Explanation: Management of increased ICP includes sedation, drainage of cerebrospinal fluid, and hyperosmolar therapy (Mannitol or hypertonic saline). Other interventions do not reduce ICP.

2881. Which one of the following is not true for increased intracranial pressure (ICP) in infants? *(Banaras HU 2015)*

a. Drowsiness b. Increased blood pressure
c. Bulging fontanelle d. Vomiting

2882. Benign intracranial hypertension is found in *(ISRO)*

a. Vit. C toxicity b. Vit. D toxicity
c. Vit. K toxicity d. Vit. A toxicity

2883. Which among the following is the management for increased ICP?

a. Provide semi fowler's position
b. Minimum stimuli to the patient
c. Administer ICP lowering agents as ordered
d. All of the above

2884. Position given to a client with increased intracranial pressure is:

a. Supine position
b. Elevate the head of the bed to 30 degrees
c. High fowler's position
d. Knee chest position

2885. All of the following nursing procedures increases ICP of the patient; EXCEPT:

a. Application of suction
b. Elevation of head end of bed to 30°
c. Repositioning of patient
d. Neurological assessment

2886. Management of increased intracranial pressure (ICP) resulting from traumatic brain injury (TBI) includes all; EXCEPT:

a. Corticosteroids
b. Elevation of head end of bed
c. Mannitol
d. Sedation

Explanation: Medical management of increased ICP include sedation, drainage of CSF, and osmotherapy with either mannitol or hypertonic saline. For ICP refractory to initial medical management, barbiturate coma, hypothermia, or decompressive craniectomy should be considered. **Steroids are not indicated** and may be harmful in the treatment of increased ICP resulting from TBI.

2887. First sign and symptom following head injury which indicative of increased ICP is:

a. Bradycardia
b. Vomiting
c. Restlessness and confusion
d. Blurred vision

2888. What should be the initial action of a medical-surgical nurse if a patient develops 'slurred speech and disorientation to time and place' who sustained a head injury 24 hours ago?

a. Recheck the patient's neurologic status in 15 minutes
b. Prepare the patient for emergency surgery
c. Continue to hourly neurologic assessments
d. Inform the neurosurgeon of the patient's status

Explanation: Change in the level of consciousness need to be informed the concerned doctor first.

2889. Clinical manifestation of increased ICP includes:

a. Vomiting
b. Headache
c. Blurring of vision
d. All of the above

Ans.

2875. b
2876. b
2877. c
2878. b
2879. b
2880. c
2881. b
2882. d
2883. d
2884. b
2885. b
2886. a
2887. c
2888. d
2889. d

Explanation: Drowsiness, separated sutures on the skull, bulging of the soft spot on top of the head (bulging fontanelle), vomiting.

Older children and adults: Behavior changes, decreased consciousness, headache, lethargy, neurological symptoms, including weakness, numbness, eye movement problems, and double vision, seizures, vomiting.

INTRACRANIAL SURGERY

2890. An adult male client has undergone spinal surgery. Which of the following intervention is appropriate for this client? *(ESI 2009)*

a. Assess the client's feet for sensation and circulation
b. Encourage client to drink plenty of fluids
c. Log-roll the client to prone position
d. Observe the client's bowel movement and voiding patterns

Explanation: The client's feet must be assessed for any alteration in sensation and circulation. Altered sensation and circulation to feet indicates damage to the spinal cord, if these occurs notify the physician immediately.

2891. What is the site of surgery in transphenoidal approach?

a. Above the tentorium b. Below the brain stem
c. Sella turcica d. None of these

2892. Which of the following is cranial surgery approach?

a. Supratentorium b. Infratentorium
c. Transphenoidal approach d. All of these

2893. After cranial surgery, the nurse should assess the client for any CSF leakage is present or not. Which of the following characteristic of CSF would assist in differentiation of CSF and mucus?

a. CSF contains glucose b. CSF is vicious and dark fluid
c. Mucus contains glucose d. Mucus contain protein

2894. What is the post-operative position for a client who had cranial surgery with supratentorial cranial approach?

a. On the back side b. On the non-operative side
c. On the operative side d. Both a and b

2895. What is the preferred post-operative position for a client who had cranial surgery with infratentorial cranial approach?

a. Head of the bed flat b. Fowler's position
c. Prone position d. Low-fowlers position

SEIZURE DISORDERS

2896. Neurological manifestation of Whipple's disease is:

a. Encephalopathy
b. Cerebellar ataxia
c. Focal neurological deficits
d. Seizures

2897. A 23-year-old client is admitted with tonic-clonic seizure. The nurse knows that the most common cause of tonic-clonic seizure for this age group is:

a. Stroke
b. Electrolyte imbalance
c. Head trauma
d. Congenital defect in brain

Explanation: Head injury is the most commonly known cause in young adults. For middle-age individuals, strokes, tumors and injuries are more frequent catalysts. In people age 65 and older, stroke is the most common known cause, followed by degenerative conditions such as Alzheimer's disease. Often, seizures do not begin immediately after a person has an injury to the brain. Instead, a seizure may occur many months later.

2898. Which of the following action is contraindicated in epileptic patient?

a. Loosen the clothes
b. Restrain client's limbs
c. Raising padded side rails
d. Give side lying position

Explanation: Limbs are never restrained because the strong muscle contractions could cause harm.

2899. Which of the following is not a triggering factor for seizures and epilepsies? *(AIIMS-BBS SNO 2019)*

a. Acute alcohol ingestion
b. Exposure to flashing lights
c. Hyperventilation
d. Decreased physical activity

Explanation: Alcohol intake or drug use, exposure to flashing light, hyperventilation, non-compliance to medication and sleep deprivation are common triggers for seizures, whereas decreased physical activity is a positive activity that usually do not trigger seizures.

2900. What should the nurse do first when a male client is having a tonic-clonic seizure? *(AIIMS Bhopal Nursing Officer, 2018)*

a. Restrain the client's arms and legs
b. Elevate the head of the bed
c. Place a tongue blade in the client's mouth
d. Take measures to prevent injury

Explanation: If any person is experiencing tonic clonic seizure most appropriate nursing intervention is to ensure measures to prevent injury.

2901. Which of the following diagnostic investigation is useful to detect seizure? *(DSSSB 2013)*

a. CT scan b. EEG
c. MRI scan d. X-ray

Explanation: Electroencephalography (EEG) is a test that detects electrical activity of the brain through electrodes attached to scalp. EEG is most often used to diagnose epilepsy, which causes obvious abnormalities in EEG readings.

2902. Which action should the nurse implement to prevent aspiration in patient who is experiencing seizure in bed?

a. Elevate the head
b. Loosen restrictive clothing
c. Position the client on the side with head flexed forward
d. Use tongue depressor between teeth

Explanation: Positioning patient in side lateral position prevent aspiration. Other interventions also useful in the management of patient with seizure but does not prevent aspiration.

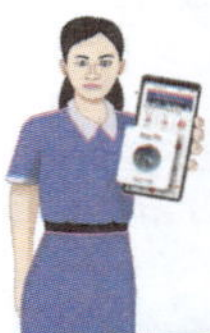

Ans.

2890. a
2891. c
2892. d
2893. a
2894. d
2895. a
2896. d
2897. c
2898. b
2899. d
2900. d
2901. b
2902. c

2903. Mr. Santosh 18-years-old student, is admitted to the ward with a diagnosis of epilepsy. He tells the nurse that he is experiencing a generalized tingling sensation and smell of roses. These complaints indicate *(Banaras HU 2015)*

a. Acute neuritis
b. Acute cerebrovascular accident
c. An aura
d. An olfactory hallucination

2904. Most common type of seizure in early childhood period is:

a. Intra cranial infection b. Febrile illness
c. Intra cranial malignancy d. Electrolyte imbalance

2905. Absence seizure is treated with:

a. Clonazepam
b. Valproate
c. Phenytoin
d. Midazolam

2906. Complex partial seizure can be managed with:

a. Midazolam
b. Sodium valproate
c. Lorazepam
d. Carbamazepine

2907. Important nursing intervention for a client having a tonic-clonic seizure?

a. Maintaining a patent airway
b. Restrain the client
c. Intubate the client
d. Insert Foley's catheter

2908. Drug of choice for status epilepticus is/are ....:

a. IM Midazolam
b. IV Lorazepam
c. IV Diazepam
d. All of the above

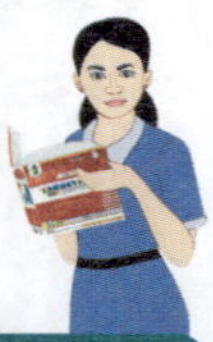

Explanation: The benzodiazepines are the most effective drugs in the treatment of acute seizures and status epilepticus (SE). The benzodiazepines most commonly used to treat status epilepticus are diazepam, lorazepam, and midazolam. Intravenous lorazepam or intramuscular midazolam effectively control early SE in around two thirds of patients. IV diazepam remains the drug of choice for short-term control of seizures.

2909. A client recalls headache and unusual sensation before seizure attack. It is known as:

a. Atonic seizure b. Aura
c. Tonic d. Clonic

2910. Seizure in a meningitis client can be controlled by all of the following interventions; EXCEPT:

a. Administration of phenytoin
b. Side lying position
c. Control of fever
d. Minimal environmental stimuli

2911. The key instruction to be given to the patient and the caregiver with epilepsy is as follows; EXCEPT: *(ESIC 2019)*

a. Take medications daily
b. Maintain medication and seizure chart
c. Avoid alcohol, smoking, hypoglycemia
d. Take showers in bathtubs

Explanation: Taking showers in bathstub is not advised because it is a high-risk activity for a patient with epilepsy. If seizure occurs while bathing in tub then drowning can occur and client may die.

2912. Drug of Choice for Generalized Tonic-Clonic Seizure (GTCS) in pregnancy is:

a. Lamotrigine b. Valproate
c. Levetiracetam d. CBZ

2913. Best drug for photosensitive epilepsy:

a. Topiramate b. Valproate
c. Zonisamide d. Ethosuximide

2914. Health education to a client on phenytoin therapy include:

a. Report for blood monitoring as ordered to avoid toxicity
b. Use soft bristle brush to avoid injury to oral mucosa
c. Quit the habit of consuming alcohol
d. All of the above

2915. Which among the following is correct regarding phenytoin and alcohol interaction?

a. Alcohol increases effectiveness of phenytoin activity
b. Alcohol decreases seizure threshold
c. Alcohol has no interaction with phenytoin
d. Alcohol decreases the effectiveness of phenytoin

2916. Common side effect of drug phenytoin is:

a. Gingival hyperplasia b. Hirsutism
c. Cushingoid appearances d. Bleeding gum

2917. Correct regarding IV phenytoin is:

a. Administer via IV push
b. Stop the drug if there is no sign and symptoms
c. Mixing the drug with saline solution only
d. Flushing the IV catheter with dextrose solution

STROKE (CEREBROVASCULAR ACCIDENT)

2918. Which of the following condition most commonly causes ischemic stroke?

a. AV malformation
b. Cocaine use
c. Head trauma
d. Rupture of aneurysm

Explanation: Cocaine is a potent vasoconstrictor and may result in a life-threatening reaction.

2919. Lower motor neuron lesions cause:

a. Flaccid muscle paralysis
b. Hyperactive and abnormal reflexes
c. Increased muscle tone
d. Hypertrophy of muscle

Explanation: A lower motor neuron lesion is a lesion which affects nerve fibers traveling from the ventral horn or anterior grey column of the spinal cord to the relevant muscles. Hence, lower motor neuron lesions cause flaccid muscle paralysis, muscle atrophy, decreased muscle tone and loss of voluntary control.

2920. Upper motor neuron lesions causes all; EXCEPT:

a. Flaccid muscle paralysis b. Hyperactive reflexes
c. Spastic muscle paralysis d. Loss of voluntary control

Explanation: Upper motor neuron lesions do not cause muscle atrophy but do cause loss of voluntary control.

2921. Leading cause of cerebrovascular accident (C.V.A) is:

a. Embolism b. Hypertension
c. Aneurysm d. Blunt trauma

Ans.

2903. c
2904. b
2905. b
2906. d
2907. a
2908. d
2909. b
2910. b
2911. d
2912. a
2913. b
2914. d
2915. d
2916. a
2917. c
2918. b
2919. a
2920. a
2921. a

Explanation: Cerebrovascular Accident is also known as stroke. The three main types of stroke are Ischemic stroke, hemorrhagic stroke and transient ischemic attack (mini stroke). More than 80% of strokes are Ischemic strokes. An ischemic stroke happens when blood flow through the artery that supplies oxygen-rich blood to the brain becomes blocked. Blood clots (emboli) often cause the blockages that lead to ischemic strokes.

2922. Which among the following client is at maximum risk for stroke?
- a. Obese 45-year-old man
- b. 35-year-old men with alcohol intake
- c. 32-year-old woman with DM
- d. 65-year-old man with hypertension

2923. A client is admitted with thrombotic cerebrovascular accident (CVA). Which of the following is the priority nursing assessment in the first 24 hours after admission?
- a. Bowel sounds
- b. Electroencephalogram
- c. Electromyogram
- d. Pupil size and pupillary response

Explanation: Pupil size and papillary response indicate changes around the cranial nerves. In the first 24 hours, it is vital to monitor for pupil size and response.

2924. Hemiplegia involves: *(JIPMER 2012)*
- a. Paresis of both lower extremities
- b. Paralysis of one side of the body
- c. Paralysis of both lower extremities
- d. Paresis of upper and lower extremities

2925. Which among the following is most commonly seen in a client with C6 injury?
- a. Paralysis
- b. Hemiparesis
- c. Paraplegia
- d. Quadriplegia

2926. If both lower limbs are paralyzed then it is known as:
- a. Quadriparesis
- b. Paraplegia
- c. Hemiparesis
- d. Quadriplegia

2927. If all the four limbs are paralyzed then it is known as:
- a. Quadriplegia
- b. Paraplegia
- c. Hemiplegia
- d. Paralysis

2928. If half of the body is paralyzed then it is known as:
- a. Quadriplegia
- b. Paraplegia
- c. Hemiplegia
- d. Paralysis

2929. Symptom helps to differentiate between hemorrhagic stroke from a thrombotic stroke is:
- a. Loss of consciousness
- b. Recent memory
- c. Muscle weakness
- d. Sudden onset of severe headache

2930. Which of the following will not be observed in a client with a right hemispheric stroke? *(AIIMS-BBS SNO 2019)*
- a. Impulse control difficulty
- b. Loss of depth perception
- c. Right hemiplegia
- d. Lack of awareness

Explanation: Patients with a right-brain stroke have left hemiplegia and left-brain stroke will have right hemiplegia.

2931. Left sided hemiplegia and aphasia occur because of the involvement of:
- a. Carotid artery
- b. Vertebral artery
- c. Left middle cerebral artery
- d. Right middle cerebral artery

2932. A male patient is experiencing urinary incontinence after a stroke. Bladder training for this patient includes all; EXCEPT:
- a. Kegel exercises
- b. Intermittent self-catheterization
- c. Assisting the patient to stand to void
- d. Continuous urinary drainage

2933. Leading risk factor of hemorrhagic stroke is:
- a. CAD
- b. Atherosclerosis
- c. Hypertension
- d. Aneurysm

2934. Nurse has to insert a nasogastric tube to a stroke client and understands that the best position for the insertion is: *(AIIMS Raipur NO 2019)*
- a. Low Fowlers position
- b. Sims position
- c. High Fowler's position
- d. Trendelenburg position

Explanation: Patient with stroke is also associated with dysphagia, therefore, the insertion of NG tube become more difficult. High Fowler's position eases the insertion of NG tube and reduces the risk of aspiration. Semi Fowler's or Low Fowler's position prevents the risk of aspiration especially in comatose patients.

2935. Long-term treatment for thrombotic stroke is:
- a. Acetaminophen
- b. Tissue Plasminogen Activator
- c. Aspirin
- d. Warfarin

2936. Long-term treatment for embolic stroke is:
- a. Acetaminophen
- b. Tissue Plasminogen Activator
- c. Aspirin
- d. Warfarin

2937. Most effective treatment for ischemic stroke is:
- a. Acetaminophen
- b. Tissue Plasminogen Activator
- c. Aspirin
- d. Warfarin

2938. Which of the following pharmacological management is inappropriate regarding medical management of a client with CVA?
- a. Osmotic diuretics are given to decrease cerebral edema
- b. Aspirin is used in the acute management of a completed stroke
- c. Corticosteroids are given to decrease cerebral edema
- d. Thrombolytics are most useful within three hours of an occlusive CVA

Explanation: Aspirin is a platelet deaggregator used in the prevention of recurrent or embolic stroke but is not used in the acute management of completed stroke as it may lead to bleeding.

2939. The paralysis of both upper and lower extremities is known as: *(DSSSB PHN, 2015)*
- a. Hemiplegia
- b. Paraplegia
- c. Monoplegia
- d. Quadriplegia

Ans.

2922. d
2923. d
2924. b
2925. d
2926. b
2927. a
2928. c
2929. d
2930. c
2931. d
2932. c
2933. c
2934. c
2935. c
2936. d
2937. b
2938. b
2939. d

HEAD INJURY/HEAD TRAUMA

2940. Uncoordinated movement of the extremities in a patient with a traumatic brain injury is termed as:

a. Ataxia b. Apraxia
c. Dystonia d. Dyskinesia

Explanation: The word 'ataxia' means without coordination. The ataxia is often used to describe symptoms of incoordination which can be associated with infections, injuries, other diseases, or degenerative changes in the central nervous system. Clients with ataxia have problems with coordination because parts of the nervous system that control movement and balance are affected. Ataxia may affect the fingers, hands, arms, legs, body, speech, and eye movements.

2941. Which of the following symptoms is commonly reported by the patients immediately following cerebral aneurysm rupture?

a. Explosive headache
b. Photophobia
c. Hemiparesis
d. Seizures

Explanation: An intracranial (cerebral) aneurysm is a dilation of the walls of a cerebral artery that causes explosive headache. An explosive headache is often the first presenting symptom of a bleeding cerebral aneurysm. Photophobia, seizures, and hemiparesis may occur later.

2942. Which of the following terms refers to weakness of both legs and lower part of the trunk?

a. Paraparesis
b. Quadriparesis
c. Hemiplegia
d. Tetraplegia

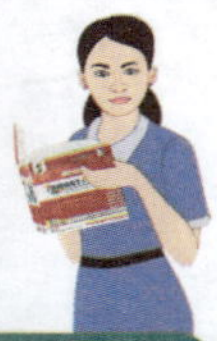

Ans.

2940. a
2941. a
2942. a
2943. a
2944. d
2945. d
2946. a
2947. b
2948. b
2949. c
2950. b
2951. a

Explanation: Paraparesis (paraplegia) refers to partial (-paresis) or complete (-plegia) loss of voluntary motor function in the pelvic limbs. Similar involvement of all four limbs is termed tetraparesis (tetraplegia) of Quadriparesis (Quadriplegia). Hemiplegia refers to paralysis of one side of the body.

2943. If a nurse notes colorless drainage on dressing after surgery of brain tumor, then which of the following is the prompt nursing action?

a. Notify the physician
b. Elevate the head of bed
c. Documentation
d. Monitor the patient continuously

Explanation: Colorless drainage on dressing after surgery of brain tumor shows presence of cerebrospinal fluid, so it should be reported to doctor immediately.

2944. Which option shows the presence of cerebrospinal fluid leakage from nose after basilar skull fracture, if the fluid:

a. Shows negative for glucose
b. Is clear
c. Clumps on dressing
d. Shows positive for glucose

Explanation: Cerebrospinal fluid always test positive for glucose.

2945. Most common type of intracranial hemorrhage is:

a. Subdural hemorrhage
b. Subarachnoid hemorrhage
c. Extradural hemorrhage
d. Intracerebral hemorrhage

2946. Priority nursing intervention for a client admitted with head injury is:

a. Patency of airway
b. Peripheral perfusion
c. Nutritional balance
d. Hydration

2947. A 35-year-old male patient is brought into emergency room with a head injury following a road traffic accident. Patient is confused, drowsy and has unequal pupils. Which of the following nursing diagnosis is given priority in this condition?

a. Altered cognition
b. Altered cerebral tissue perfusion
c. High risk for injury
d. Altered sensory perception

Explanation: Maintaining cerebral perfusion is essential to prevent further brain damage. Hence, restoration of cerebral perfusion is the priority intervention at this time.

TIPS: Use ABC (Airway, Breathing and Circulation) principle to locate the answer. Here altered cerebral perfusion is related to circulation and there are no other nursing diagnosis related to airway or breathing.

2948. A patient was brought to the emergency department after a head injury. The nurse noticed that there is a clear drainage from the nose. Which of the following test is useful and most reliable to determine if the drainage is a cerebrospinal fluid (CSF)?

a. pH test b. Test for Beta2-transferrin
c. Test for glucose d. Test for chlorides

Explanation: The CSF contains a large amount of glucose. A rapid but highly unreliable test is glucose-content determination with the use of glucose oxidase paper. This method of detecting cerebrospinal fluid (CSF) in rhinorrhea is no longer reliable screening or confirmatory test. Due to the presence of reducing substance in the lacrimal-gland secretions, it can lead to false positive results. Test for beta 2-transferrin is a most reliable test to determine whether the nasal drainage is CSF because the substance is only present in CSF.

2949. All of the following are symptoms of head injury EXCEPT *(Banaras HU 2015)*

a. Sleepiness b. Vomiting
c. Sweating d. Headache

2950. Position given to a patient with multiple injury over the face and neck is:

a. Supine position b. Semiprone position
c. Side lying d. Trendelenburg

Explanation: Vomiting and risk of aspiration are high when patients are in supine position. Semiprone or sims position facilitates drainage from the mouth and prevents aspiration of fluids.

2951. Drainage of CSF via nose suggestive of:

a. Basilar skull fracture b. Frontal fracture
c. Temporal fracture d. Nasal septal fracture

2952. Leading cause of subarachnoid hemorrhage is:
a. Embolism b. Hypertension
c. Aneurysm d. Blunt trauma

2953. Intracranial hemorrhage most commonly occur in:
a. Cerebellum b. Cerebrum
c. Medulla oblongata d. Pons

2954. Priority nursing intervention after craniotomy is:
a. GCS assessment
b. Neutral position
c. Prevent infection
d. Prevention of increase in ICP

2955. Type of bandage used in head injury is:
a. Spira b. Figure of eight
c. Capline d. Sling

SPINAL CORD INJURIES

2956. Speech center is: *(JIPMER 2012)*
a. Broca's area b. Premotor area
c. Frontal area d. Postcentral area

2957. Which of the following substance can lead to neurological injury in a newborn known as kernicterus?
a. Bile salt b. Conjugated bilirubin
c. Unconjugated bilirubin d. Biliverdin

Explanation: Unbound, unconjugated, circulating bilirubin crosses the blood-brain barrier, and because it is lipid soluble, it penetrates neuronal and glial membranes. Unconjugated hyperbilirubinemia in a newborn can lead to accumulation of bilirubin in certain brain regions (particularly the basal nuclei) with consequent irreversible damage to these areas manifesting as various neurological deficits, seizures, abnormal reflexes and eye movements. This type of neurological injury in newborn is known as kernicterus.

2958. Cause of autonomic dysreflexia is:
a. Hypertension b. Noxious stimuli
c. Head injury d. Neurogenic shock

2959. A client with a spinal cord injury has paraplegia. The nurse assesses for which major problem the client may experience early in the recovery period. *(RAK MSc 2018)*
a. Bladder control b. Nutritional intake
c. Quadriceps setting d. Use of aids for ambulation

Explanation:

- Client with spinal cord injury with paraplegia experience issues related to bladder control in the recovery period which is a major concern.
- The sacral spinal cord segments, i.e., S2-S4 segments is the place from which the spinal nerves travel to innervate the bladder. In case of spinal injury, this route of communication between bladder musculature and brain is compromised resulting in impaired bladder control.

2960. The most common and early symptom of a spinal cord injury is:
a. Urinary incontinence
b. Back pain that worsens with activity
c. Bowel incontinence
d. Absence of cough and gag reflex

2961. Following spinal cord injury patient is experiencing falling blood pressure with bradycardia, it indicates:
a. Hypovolemia
b. Cardiac injury
c. Neuronal injury
d. Neurogenic shock from massive vasodilation

2962. Client at risk for autonomic dysreflexia is:
a. Head injury
b. Neurogenic bladder
c. A client with a high cervical spine injury
d. Femur fracture

2963. Which among the following indicate improvement after spinal shock?
a. Cough and gag reflex
b. Return of reflexes below the injury
c. Spontaneous respirations
d. Urinary incontinence

2964. Which of the following assessment indicates that spinal shock persists following spinal cord injury?
a. Overactive reflexes
b. Normal reflexes
c. Flaccid paralysis
d. Unconciousness

Explanation: Flaccid paralysis shows the presence of spinal shock.

2965. A 35-year-old male client has undergone spinal anesthesia. The nurse should immediately position the client in which of the following position?
a. Flat in a supine position
b. Left lateral position
c. Prone position with the head turned to the side
d. Knee chest position

Explanation: The client should be kept in flat in a supine position for approximately 4–12 hours post-operatively to prevent the complication of a painful spinal headache. Leakage of CSF from the puncture site is believed to be the cause of headaches. By keeping the client in supine position, pressure of CSF is equalized, which prevents trauma to the neurons.

2966. Doctor has advised the nurse to prepare the room for a patient with a spinal cord injury (at C7 level). Which one of the following is most essential to be kept ready for this patient? *(Banaras HU 2015)*
a. The halo brace device b. A catheterization tray
c. A ventilator on stand by d. The spinal kinetic bed

2967. Nursing intervention for a client who had undergone a L4-L5 laminectomy?
a. Encourage the client to be out of in bed the first post-operative day
b. Adhere to the treatment regimen
c. Maintain ROM of all joints
d. Health education and discharge teaching

2968. Following laminectomy a client is experiencing frequent voiding of small amounts of urine. The problem experienced by the patient is:
a. Urinary incontinence
b. Diabetes insipidus
c. Urine retention
d. Neurogenic bladder

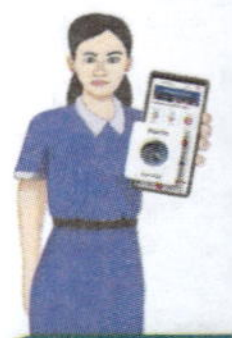

Ans.
2952. c
2953. b
2954. d
2955. c
2956. a
2957. c
2958. b
2959. a
2960. b
2961. d
2962. c
2963. b
2964. c
2965. a
2966. c
2967. a
2968. c

MENINGITIS

2969. A 36-year-old female complains of headache and neck pain, examination by a nurse reveals painful flexion of the neck to the chest (nuchal rigidity). This could be due to: *(Banaras HU 2015)*

a. Brain tumor
b. Meningitis
c. Cerebrovascular accident
d. Subdural hematoma

2970. Decreased glucose in CSF suggestive of:

a. Bacterial meningitis b. Viral meningitis
c. Brain abscess d. Encephalitis

2971. A mother brings her 8-year-old child to the clinic with the complains of severe headache, vomiting and fever. While performing physical examination for the signs of meningitis, the inability of the child to extend the legs fully when lying supine is known as:

a. Positive Homan's sign
b. Positive Brudzinski sign
c. Positive Kernig's sign
d. Positive Cullen's sign

2972. CSF findings in bacterial meningitis is:

a. Increased protein and decreased sugar
b. Increased protein and increased sugar
c. Decreased protein and increased sugar
d. Decreased protein and decreased sugar

2973. CSF laboratory findings in bacterial meningitis shows:

a. CSF protein level elevated
b. CSF glucose level decreases
c. WBC level increases
d. All of the above

2974. Which of the following shows presence of meningitis?

a. Glasgow Coma Scale score of 15
b. Positive Brudzinski sign
c. Negative Kernig sign
d. Nil nuchal rigidity

Explanation: In meningitis, patient shows positive brudzinski sign, positive Kernig sign and nuchal rigidity.

2975. Which of the following signs in a child with meningitis is characterised by pain or resistance on extending the legs at the knee when the child is lying supine? *(AIIMS Bhopal Grade-I 2018)*

a. Brudzinski b. Kernig's
c. Macewen d. Chvostek's

Explanation: Meningitis is an inflammation of the meninges, is a life-threatening illness. Kernig's sign (flexing the patient's hip 90 degree then extending the patients knee causes pain) and Brudzinski's sign (flexing the patient's neck causes flexion of the patient's hips and knees) are clinical signs facilitate the diagnosis of meningitis.

2976. Fever, headache and nuchal rigidity are classic symptoms seen in: *(DSSSB 2013)*

a. Alzheimer's disease b. Brain abscess
c. Meningitis d. Parkinson's disease

Explanation: Classic symptoms of meningitis include nuchal rigidity (neck stiffness), sudden high fever, and head-ache. This is known as classic triad of diagnostic signs of meningitis.

2977. Brudzinski's sign and Kernig's sign are diagnostic signs of: *(AIIMS Nagpur NO 2018)*

a. Tetanus
b. Meningitis
c. Encephalitis
d. Kernicterus

Explanation: Positive Kernig's sign and Brudzinski's sign are observed in **Meningitis.**

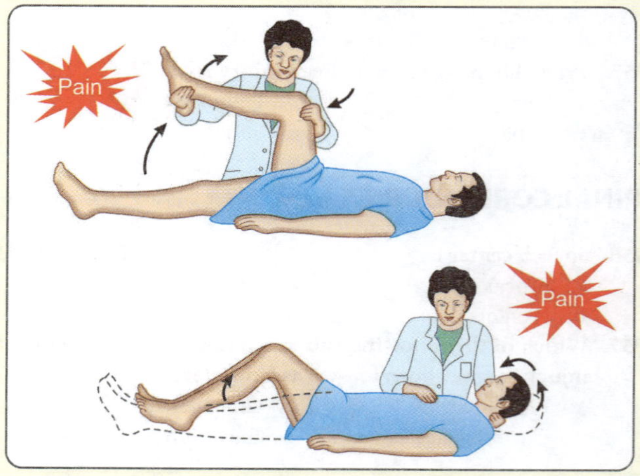

2978. Positive Kernig's sign is observed in: *(Daman & Diu NO 2018; DSSSB PHN, 2015)*

a. Cholecystitis b. Nephritis
c. Meningitis d. Appendicitis

2979. Painful extension of knee when the thigh is flexed at the hip and knee at 90 degree angle is known as:

a. Positive Kernig's sign b. Positive Brudzinski's sign
c. Positive Babinski's sign d. Positive Homan's sign

2980. If the bending of patient's neck produces flexion of the knee and hip, it is known as:

a. Positive Cullen's sign b. Positive Brudzinski's sign
c. Positive Babinski's sign d. Positive Homan's sign

2981. Basic nursing measures in the care of patient with viral encephalitis is:

a. Providing comfort measure
b. Monitoring cardiac output
c. Administer narcotics
d. Administer amphotericin B

Explanation: Providing comfort measures directed at the headache, include dimmed lights, limited noise and analgesics are basic nursing measures in the care of patient with viral encephalitis. Amphotericin B is an antifungal agent which is not useful in viral encephalitis.

2982. The most common complication of Tuberculous meningitis is: *(Kerala PSC, Nov 2014)*

a. Encephalitis b. Subdural empyema
c. Hydrocephalus d. Brain abscess

2983. Meningitis is: *(ESIC Chennai May 2012)*

a. Inflammation of the membranes that surround the liver
b. Inflammation of the membranes that surround the brain and the spinal cord
c. Inflammation of the membranes that surround the heart
d. Inflammation of the membranes that surround the kidney

Ans.

2969. b
2970. a
2971. c
2972. a
2973. d
2974. b
2975. b
2976. c
2977. b
2978. c
2979. a
2980. b
2981. a
2982. c
2983. b

2984. Correct regarding pyogenic meningitis (bacterial meningitis) is:
a. Haemophilus influenzae, Streptococcus pneumonia and Neisseria meningitides are the main organisms
b. Markedly decreased CSF glucose and increase in CSF protein is present
c. CT and MRI shows thin and linear leptomeningeal enhancement
d. All of the above

2985. Most common complication of tubercular meningitis is:
a. Lymphoma b. Tuberculoma
c. Lymphadenopathy d. Aneurysm

2986. Important nursing intervention in a client with meningitis is.........:
a. Check for Kernig's sign, Brudzinski's sign and nuchal rigidity
b. Isolate the child immediately
c. Prepare for lumbar puncture
d. Give prophylactic antibiotic to family members

2987. Which among the following is the sign of meningitis?
a. Battle sign
b. Brudzinski sign
c. Cullen's sign
d. Ring sign

2988. Inflammation of pia arachnoid is:
a. Nuchal rigidity b. Leptomeningitis
c. Meningismus d. TB meningitis

2989. CSF of acute pyogenic meningitis shows:
a. Cloudy/frankly turbid CSF
b. Elevated CSF pressure (above 180 mm water)
c. Presence of polymorphs (10-10,000/ul)
d. All of the above

2990. CSF findings in tubercular meningitis includes:
a. Mild turbidity; may form fibrin web on standing
b. Mononuclear leukocytosis
c. Increased protein
d. All of the above

ENCEPHALITIS & BRAIN ABSCESS

2991. Subdural empyema is caused by:
a. Pneumococci
b. Gonococci
c. Streptococcus pneumonia
d. Staphylococcus aureus

2992. All of the following are correct regarding poliomyelitis; EXCEPT:
a. Caused by RNA virus
b. The virus belongs to enterovirus family with three subtypes
c. Affects the motor neurons of spinal cord and brainstem
d. Route of transmission is fecal–oral route

2993. VP shunt is the surgical management for: *(JIPMER 2012)*
a. Spina bifida b. Brain tumor
c. Hydrocephalus d. ASD

2994. Significant complication associated with thrombolytic therapy is:
a. Ischemia b. Cerebral hemorrhage
c. Microthrombi d. Resolution of the clot

2995. Purpose of carotid endarterectomy for a patient with TIA is to:
a. Decrease cerebral edema
b. Reduce cerebral ischemia
c. Prevent a stroke by removing atherosclerotic plaques that is blocking cerebral blood flow
d. Provide a circulatory bypass around thrombotic plaques obstructing cranial circulation

2996. An assessment specific to safe administration of IV mannitol is: *(RRB 2005)*
a. Vital signs q4h b. Weighing daily
c. Hourly urine output d. Level of consciousness q8h

Explanation: Mannitol is an osmotic diuretic which increases the urine excretion. Hence, the urine output must be carefully monitored (hourly) to prevent any fluid imbalance.

2997. In CSF pathway obstruction at aqueduct of sylvius cause enlargement of:
a. Lateral ventricle b. Third ventricle
c. Fourth ventricle d. Both a and b

2998. How can we differentiate between hydrocephalus due to aqueductal stenosis and Dandy walker malformation?
a. Third ventricle size b. Posterior fossa volume
c. Lateral ventricular size d. Fourth ventricle size

2999. The commonest cause of primary hydrocephalus is:
a. Obstruction to flow of CSF
b. Overproduction of CSF
c. Decreased reabsorption of CSF
d. Congenital malformation

3000. All of the following measures are used to decrease brain edema; EXCEPT: *(AIIMS Bhopal Grade-I 2018)*
a. Hydrocortisone b. Hyperventilation
c. Dextrose infusion d. Mannitol infusion

Explanation: Movement of the water between the brain and intravascular space is dependent on osmotic gradients. Mannitol, a hypertonic crystalloid solution is commonly used to reduce the ICP. But the hypo-osmolar solutions like 5% dextrose in water reduce serum sodium, and increases brain water and ICP.

AUTOIMMUNE NEUROLOGICAL DISORDERS

3001. Surgery done for myasthenia gravis is: *(JIPMER 2012)*
a. Pallidotomy b. Hypophysectomy
c. Sympathectomy d. Thymectomy

3002. All of the following are the autoimmune neurological disorders; EXCEPT:
a. Multiple sclerosis
b. Myasthenia gravis
c. Guillain bare syndrome
d. Neurocysticercosis

Explanation: Neurocysticercosis is a preventable parasitic infection caused by larval cysts of the pork tapeworm (Taenia solium). The larval cysts can infect various parts of the body causing a condition known as cysticercosis. In developing countries, **neurocysticercosis** is the **most common** parasitic disease of the nervous system and is the main **cause** of acquired epilepsy.

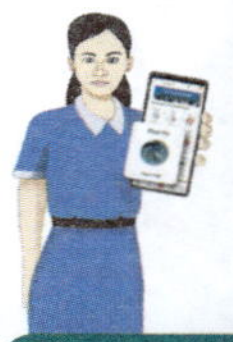

Ans.
2984. d
2985. b
2986. b
2987. b
2988. b
2989. d
2990. d
2991. c
2992. a
2993. c
2994. b
2995. c
2996. c
2997. d
2998. b
2999. a
3000. c
3001. d
3002. d

3003. Multiple sclerosis most commonly affects the age group of:

a. 20 to 40 years b. 40 to 50 years
c. Below 20 years d. Above 50 years

3004. For a client with multiple sclerosis, what are the abnormal findings noted in lumbar puncture?

a. Decreased gamma globulin level
d. Increased gamma globulin level
c. Normal serum globulin level
d. Decreased IgG index

3005. Which medication is essential during tensilon test?

a. N-Acetyl cysteine b. Flumazenil
c. Atropine sulfate d. Nalaxone

Explanation: A tensilon (edrophonium) test is a diagnostic test used to diagnose myasthenia gravis. Edrophonium prevents the breakdown of acetylcholine that increases acetylcholine levels in the neuromuscular junction and improves the strength. Atropine is prepared for immediate use in case cholinergic crisis occurs.

3006. Which of the following is the major concern in Guillain-barre syndrome?

a. Pain level b. Respiratory status
c. Knowledge deficit d. None of these

TERMINAL NEURALGIA & BELL'S PALSY

3007. Ipsilateral facial palsy with contralateral hemiplegia is seen in lesions of:

a. Medulla b. Pons
c. Tegmentum d. Mid brain

3008. Which of the cranial nerve disorder causes Bell's palsy?

a. Facial (VII)
b. Trigeminal (V)
c. Vagus (X)
d. Vestibulocochlear (VIII)

Explanation: Bell's palsy is characterized by facial dysfunction, weakness and paralysis. Bell's palsy is a condition whereby the inner ear becomes inflamed, resulting in pressure on the facial nerve, which in turn causes facial paralysis on the affected side.

3009. Bell's Palsy is due to the injury of which cranial nerve? *(DSSSB PHN, 2015)*

a. Trigeminal b. Facial
c. Trochlear d. Hypoglossal

3010. Which one of the following is the most appropriate additions to the care plan for the patient with Bell's palsy? *(LNJP H D 2012)*

a. Inspect the buccal pouch for food after eating
b. Advise the patient to drink liquids from a cup
c. Discourage the patient from looking in a mirror
d. Reduce the amount of light with in the room

NEURODEGENERATIVE DISEASES

3011. Correct option regarding amyotrophic lateral sclerosis is:

a. It is a progressing disease
b. It eventually results in permanent paralysis
c. Person will not lose any cognitive function
d. All of the above

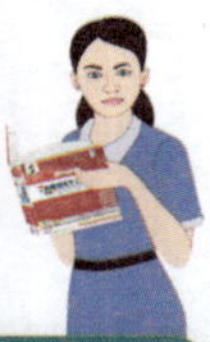

Ans.

3003. a
3004. d
3005. c
3006. b
3007. b
3008. a
3009. b
3010. a
3011. d
3012. c
3013. b
3014. c
3015. b

3012. Which among the following condition is characterized by gradual loss of ability to speak and/or understand what others are saying?

a. Agnosia
b. Apraxia
c. Primary progressive aphasia
d. Echopraxia

Explanation: Primary progressive aphasia (PPA) is a condition that results from damage to areas of the brain that control speech and language. Persons with PPA experience a gradual loss in their ability to speak, write, read, and/or understand what others are saying.

There are three subtypes of PPA

1. **Progressive nonfluent/agrammatic aphasia** - People with this subtype have difficulty speaking
2. **Semantic variant primary progressive aphasia** - People with this subtype lose the meaning of words (comprehension)
3. **Logopenic aphasia (progressive fluent aphasia)** - People with this subtype have difficulty finding the right words when they are speaking. But they know the meaning of words.

Inability (or impaired ability) to understand or produce speech, as a result of brain damage is called as Aphasia. Agnosia means inability to interpret sensations. Apraxia is a motor disorder and insomnia refers to sleep disturbances.

3013. The patient may suffer from Guillain Barre Syndrome, if he has shown the symptoms of:

a. Encephalitis
b. Gastrointestinal and respiratory infection in first 4 weeks
c. Trauma to Brain
d. Spinal Cord Injury

Explanation: Recent history of gastrointestinal and respiratory infection are predisposing factors of Guillain Barre Syndrome

3014. When caring for a patient admitted with Guillain-Barre syndrome, which nursing diagnosis should take priority? *(RAK MSc 2018)*

a. Anxiety
b. Imbalanced nutrition
c. Impaired gas exchange
d. Impaired mobility

Explanation: Guillain-Barre syndrome is an autoimmune disorder resulting in progressive muscle weakness due to damaged nerves. Impaired gas exchange is related to skeletal muscle weakness. Diaphragmatic weakness due to phrenic nerve involvement is also common. Approximately one-third of hospitalized GBS patients require mechanical ventilation because of respiratory muscle or oropharyngeal weakness.

3015. Damage to which of the following leads to Gullain-Barré syndrome?

a. Brain parenchyma
b. Peripheral nervous system
c. Spinal cord
d. Thyroid glands

Explanation: Guillain-Barré syndrome (GBS) is a rapid-onset muscle weakness caused by the immune system damaging the peripheral nervous system. This autoimmune disease is caused by the body's immune system mistakenly attacking the peripheral nerves and damaging their myelin insulation. Sometimes this immune dysfunction is triggered by an infection. The diagnosis is usually made based on the signs and symptoms, through the exclusion of alternative causes, and supported by tests such as nerve conduction studies and examination of the cerebrospinal fluid.

3016. True about Gullain-Barre syndrome is all; EXCEPT:

a. Inflammatory
b. Plasmapheresis can be done
c. Descending paralysis
d. Demyelinating

Explanation:

- GBS is an acute inflammatory demyelinating polyradiculo-neuropathy (AIDP) that presents within 2-4 weeks of a respiratory or GI infection.
- It presents as ascending weakness with areflexia.
- CSF picture is of normal cell counts with raised proteins.
- Treatment consist of IVIG or plasmapheresis.

3017. CSF finding in Gullian Barre syndrome:

a. Normal cells with increased protein
b. Normal cells and normal protein
c. Increased cells with low sugar
d. Increased protein with increased cells

3018. A nurse is caring for a patient with myasthenia gravis. Which of the following nursing diagnosis is a priority which needs immediate intervention?

a. High risk for injury related to muscle weakness
b. Ineffective coping related to illness
c. Ineffective airway clearance related to muscle weakness
d. Pain related to muscle weakness

Explanation: Ineffective airway clearance is a priority nursing diagnosis which needs immediate intervention by a nurse. Weakness of respiratory muscles decreases airflow, causing a gradual decline in vital capacity making breathing and clearing the airway through coughing difficult.

3019. Which of the following conditions is an early symptom of myasthenia gravis? *(AIIMS Staff Nurse 2016; RML 2007)*

a. Dysphagia
b. Fatigue improving in the evening
c. Ptosis
d. Respiratory distress

Explanation: In more than half the people who develop myasthenia gravis, their first signs and symptoms involve eye problems, such as drooping of one or both eyelids (ptosis), double vision (diplopia), which may be horizontal or vertical, and improves or resolves when one eye is closed.

3020. Immunosuppressive therapy is effective in patient with myasthenia gravis because it:

a. Decreases the production of auto antibodies that damage the acetylcholine receptors
b. Increases the production of acetylcholine
c. Inhibits the breakdown of acetylcholine
d. Removes antibodies that impair the transmission of impulses

Explanation: Immunosuppressant medications work to decrease the production of auto antibodies. This results in decreased immune system response at the neuromuscular junction (NMJ) and limits muscle fatigue A combination of corticosteroids (prednisone or prednisolone) and azathioprine remains the first-choice immunosuppressive drug alternative for most MG patients.

3021. Degenerative neurological disorders include which of the following:

a. Huntington's disease b. Glioma
c. Paget's disease d. Osteomalacia

Explanation: Huntington's disease is a chronic, progressive, degenerative neurological hereditary disease of nervous system that results in involuntary choreiform movement and dementia.

3022. In multiple myeloma neurological complication usually involve:

a. Brain
b. Spinal column
c. Cranial nerves
d. Autonomic nervous system

3023. Earliest sign of myasthenia gravis is:

a. Pill rolling movements of the hand
b. Fatigue improving at the end of the day
c. Ptosis
d. Respiratory distress

3024. Which among the following lab test is reliable for diagnosing autoimmune myasthenia gravis?

a. C-Reactive protein
b. Anti–acetylcholine receptor (AChR) antibody test
c. Anti-cyclic citrullinated peptide (anti-CCP) test
d. Anti-nuclear antibody

3025. Correct option regarding Huntington's disease is:

a. Progressive breakdown (degeneration) of nerve cells in the brain
b. Chorea, Intellectual decline and Emotional disturbances are the clinical manifestations
c. Treatments cannot prevent the physical, mental and behavioral decline associated with the condition.
d. All of the above

3026. Effectiveness of levodopa in a myasthenia gravis client will be evaluated through:

a. No ptosis
b. Fatigue improving at the end of the day
c. Reduction in short-term memory
d. Lessened rigidity and tremor

3027. Earliest symptoms of multiple sclerosis is:

a. Ptosis b. Diplopia
c. Pill rolling movement d. Dementia

Explanation:

- Problems with vision, including diplopia, can be an early symptom of multiple sclerosis. Damage to nerve pathways that controls eye movements are damaged in MS.
- Ptosis (drooping of one of both eyelids) - Earliest sign of **Myasthenia Gravis.**
- Pill rolling movements are seen **Parkinsonism.**
- Most common cause of Dementia is **Alzheimer's disease.**

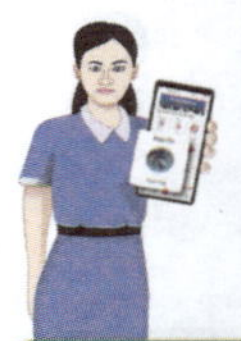

Ans.

3016. c
3017. a
3018. c
3019. c
3020. a
3021. a
3022. b
3023. c
3024. b
3025. d
3026. d
3027. b

3028. Guillain-Barre syndrome affects:
a. Brain b. Cranial nerve
c. Peripheral nerve d. Spinal cord

3029. In Guillain-Barre syndrome, respiratory distress occurs because of:
a. Elevated protein levels in the CSF
b. Respiratory infection
c. Absence of gag and cough reflex
d. Paralysis ascending to the nerves that stimulate the thoracic area

3030. Guillain-Barré syndrome is manifested with: *(Kerala PSC, Nov 2014)*
a. Muscle atrophy and persistent reflexes
b. Symmetric muscle weakness, diminished reflexes and paresthesia
c. Muscle atrophy convulsions and behavioral problems
d. Symmetric muscle weakness, increased tone and persistent reflexes

3031. A patient with multiple sclerosis was advised to undergo an exercise program. While teaching this patient about the exercise program, the nurse should caution to avoid activities that:
a. Are aerobic b. Increases the heart rate
c. Leads to dehydration d. All of these

3032. Which is the earliest symptoms of Parkinsonism?
a. Tremors
b. Rigidity
c. Bradykinesia
d. Chorea

3033. Element causing Parkinsonism?
a. Copper b. Zinc
c. Iron d. Manganese

3034. Which of the following is not a physical assessment finding in Parkinson's disease? *(AIIMS-BBS SNO 2019)*
a. Absence of cognitive impairment
b. Mask-like expression
c. Dysarthria
d. Pill rolling tremors of the fingers

Explanation:
- Cognitive impairment is a significant non-motor symptom of Parkinson's disease (PD). So, cognitive impairment is likely to be a finding in a patient with Parkinson's disease. So, absence of cognitive impairment is not a correct answer.
- All other given symptoms are present in Parkinson's disease.
- **Note**: Question has 'negative stem' with a key word "not a finding" and the answer also has a negative key word "absence of cognitive impairment".

3035. Which of the following lobe of the brain is affected earliest in most of the cases of Alzheimer's disease?
a. Temporal lobe b. Parietal lobe
c. Frontal lobe d. Occipital lobe

Explanation: Alzheimer's disease (AD) is a progressive, degenerative brain disease that slowly erodes memory and thinking skills, and eventually even the ability to carry out simple tasks. It is the most common cause of dementia. The **hippocampus** in the temporal lobe is one of the earliest affected brain regions in Alzheimer's disease (AD) and its dysfunction is believed to underline the core feature of the disease-memory impairment.

3036. Parkinson's disease is caused by deficiency of which of the following neurotransmitter?
a. Acetylcholine b. Dopamine
c. GABA d. Serotonin

Explanation: Parkinson's disease is a degenerative disorder of the central nervous system mainly affecting the motor system. Parkinson's disease is primarily caused by low and falling dopamine levels.

3037. Which of the following is the earliest sign of Parkinson's disease?
a. Disturbed vision b. Forgetfulness
c. Tremors d. Muscle atrophy

Explanation: The three cardinal signs of Parkinson's disease are tremor, rigidity, and bradykinesia. Tremor is the most apparent and well-known symptom. It is also the most common and earliest sign of Parkinson's disease.

3038. Mr. Prem has been diagnosed to have Parkinson's disease. He complains that the resting tremors he is experiencing in his right hand are very frustrating. What advice to be given to him by the attending nurse? *(Banaras HU 2015)*
a. To take a warm bath
b. To hold an object
c. To practice deep breathing
d. To give diazepam as needed

3039. Which among the following area in the brain is affected earliest in Alzheimer's disease?
a. Occipital lobe b. Hippocampus
c. Broca's area d. Wernicke's area

3040. Earliest sign in Parkinson's disease?
a. Akinesia
b. Ptosis
c. Dementia
d. Pill rolling movements of the hand

3041. Mask like facies is the clinical feature of:
a. Guillain-Barre syndrome b. Multiple sclerosis
c. Parkinson disease d. Mental retardation

3042. Which antiparkinsonian drug cause tolerance or toxicity if taken for too long?
a. Amantadine b. Carbidopa-levodopa
c. Imipramine d. Sertraline

3043. The nurse administers levodopa to a client with Parkinson's disease. Which therapeutic effect does the nurse expect the medication to produce? *(RAK MSc 2018)*
a. Increase in acetylcholine production
b. Replacement of the neurotransmitter in brain
c. Regeneration of injured thalamic cells
d. Improvement in myelination of neurons

Explanation: Levodopa is converted to dopamine in the basal ganglia producing symptom relief. It acts by reducing the excessive influence of excitatory cholinergic neurons on the extrapyramidal tract.

3044. True regarding dementia is:
a. Cognitive dysfunction is there
b. Loss of memory is also present
c. Both a and b
d. None of the above

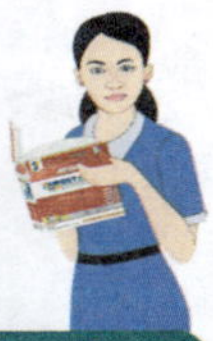

Ans.
3028. c
3029. d
3030. b
3031. c
3032. a
3033. d
3034. a
3035. a
3036. b
3037. c
3038. b
3039. b
3040. d
3041. c
3042. b
3043. b
3044. c

3045. Vascular dementia occurs because of:
a. Aneurysm rupture
b. Intra cranial infection
c. Cerebral ischemia
d. All of the above

3046. Dementia is diagnosed on the basis of:
a. CT/MRI
b. Doppler study
c. EEG
d. Patient history and cognitive assessment

3047. Earliest feature of Alzheimer Disease is:
a. Somnambulism
b. Memory problems and mild confusion
c. Nocturia
d. Mood disorder

3048. Main nursing intervention to a client with Alzheimer Disease is:
a. Maintain patient safety
b. Maintain nutritional status
c. Maintain normal activity level
d. Meet elimination needs

3049. Bromocriptine is indicated in:
a. Prolactinoma
b. Parkinson's disease
c. Infertility
d. All of the above

BRAIN TUMOR & NEUROCYSTICERCOSIS

3050. The most common type of brain neoplasm is:
a. Acoustic neuroma b. Neuroma
c. Glioma d. Angioma

Explanation: Gliomas is a malignant tumor of the glial tissue of the nervous system. It is the most common brain neoplasm, accounting for 45% of all brain tumors.

3051. Most common intracranial tumor is:
a. Glioma
b. Craniopharyngioma
c. Meningioma
d. Retinoblastoma

3052. Most common site from which brain metastasis occur is:
a. Neck
b. Lung
c. Breast
d. Oral cavity

3053. Location of brain tumor in a client with signs and symptoms include memory deficits, visual disturbances, weakness of right upper and lower extremities, and personality changes is:
a. Frontal lobe
b. Parietal lobe
c. Occipital lobe
d. Temporal lobe

3054. An adult patient diagnosed with brain tumor was scheduled for craniotomy. Which of the following class of drugs are useful in prevention and management of Increased Intracranial Pressure (ICP) after surgery?
a. Antihypertensives b. Loop diuretics
c. Osmotic diuretics d. Antihistamines

Explanation: Osmotherapy has been the mainstay of pharmacologic therapy in the prevention and management of incrased ICP. Mannitol and hypertonic saline (HS) are the most commonly used osmotic agents.

OTHER DISORDERS OF NERVOUS SYSTEM

3055. Which of the following is a neural tube defect? *(Staff Nurse G II 2014)*
a. Meningitis
b. Meningocele
c. Scoliosis
d. Encephalitis

3056. The following factor is most important in preventing fetal open neural tube defects: *(Staff Nurse G II 2014)*
a. Zinc
b. Folic Acid
c. Vitamin–D
d. Vitamin–A

3057. All are present in Dandy- Walker syndrome; EXCEPT:
a. Hydrocephalus
b. Arnold Chiari malformation
c. Posterior fossa cyst
d. Cerebellar vermis deficiency

3058. Inability to carryout normal activities despite intact motor function is: *(AIIMS Raipur Grade II 2017)*
a. Anhedonia b. Apraxia
c. Apathy d. Amnesia

Explanation: Anhedonia is inability to experience pleasure. Apathy is a state of indifference or suppression of emotions. Amnesia is deficit in memory caused by brain damage or disease and psychological trauma. Apraxia is inability to execute complete coordinated movement without muscular or sensory impairment. It occurs because of the underlying brain damage.

3059. Willis-Ekbom syndrome is also known as *(AIIMS BPL SNO 2018)*
a. Kleine-Levin syndrome b. Dhat syndrome
c. Restless legs syndrome d. Ganser syndrome

Explanation: Willis Ekbom Syndrome is also known as Restless legs syndrome. It is a chronic neurosensory disorder that is characterized by a strong urge to move, accompanied by an uncomfortable paresthesia in the legs.

3060. Vitamin E deficiency causes:
a. Ataxia
b. Megaloblastic anemia
c. Hemorrhagic stroke
d. Cardiac failure

3061. Muscular hypertonicity with increased resistance to stretc.h is called as:
a. Atonicity
b. Spasticity
c. Jerking movements
d. Reflexes

Explanation: Spasticity is a condition in which there is an abnormal increase in muscle tone (hypertonicity) or stiffness of muscle, which might interfere with movement or be associated with discomfort or pain.

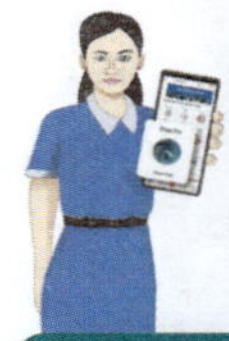

Ans.
3045. c
3046. d
3047. b
3048. a
3049. d
3050. c
3051. a
3052. b
3053. a
3054. c
3055. b
3056. b
3057. b
3058. b
3059. c
3060. a
3061. b

3062. Macewen's sign is an indication of *(JIPMER 2012)*

a. Cerebral Palsy
b. Mental Retardation
c. Hydrocephalus
d. Meningitis

3063. Extra pyramidal symptoms occur because:

a. Nerve damage
b. Drug toxicity
c. Integration of somatic and special sensory inputs.
d. Loss of automatic movements associated with skeletal muscle activitysssw

3064. Creutzfeldt-Jakob disease is characterized by:

a. Memory loss
b. Memory impairment, muscle jerks, and blindness
c. Remission and relapse
d. Increased ICP and cognitive impairment

3065. The neural tube defect among new born can be prevented by providing:

a. Folic acid to the mother in first trimester
b. Vitamin K to the mother in first trimester
c. Iron and folic acid throughout pregnancy
d. Iron to the mother in 3rd trimester

3066. Arsenic poisoning causes

a. Mononeuritis multiplex
b. Myelopathy
c. Radiculopathy
d. Polyneuritis

Ans.

3062. c
3063. d
3064. b
3065. a
3066. d

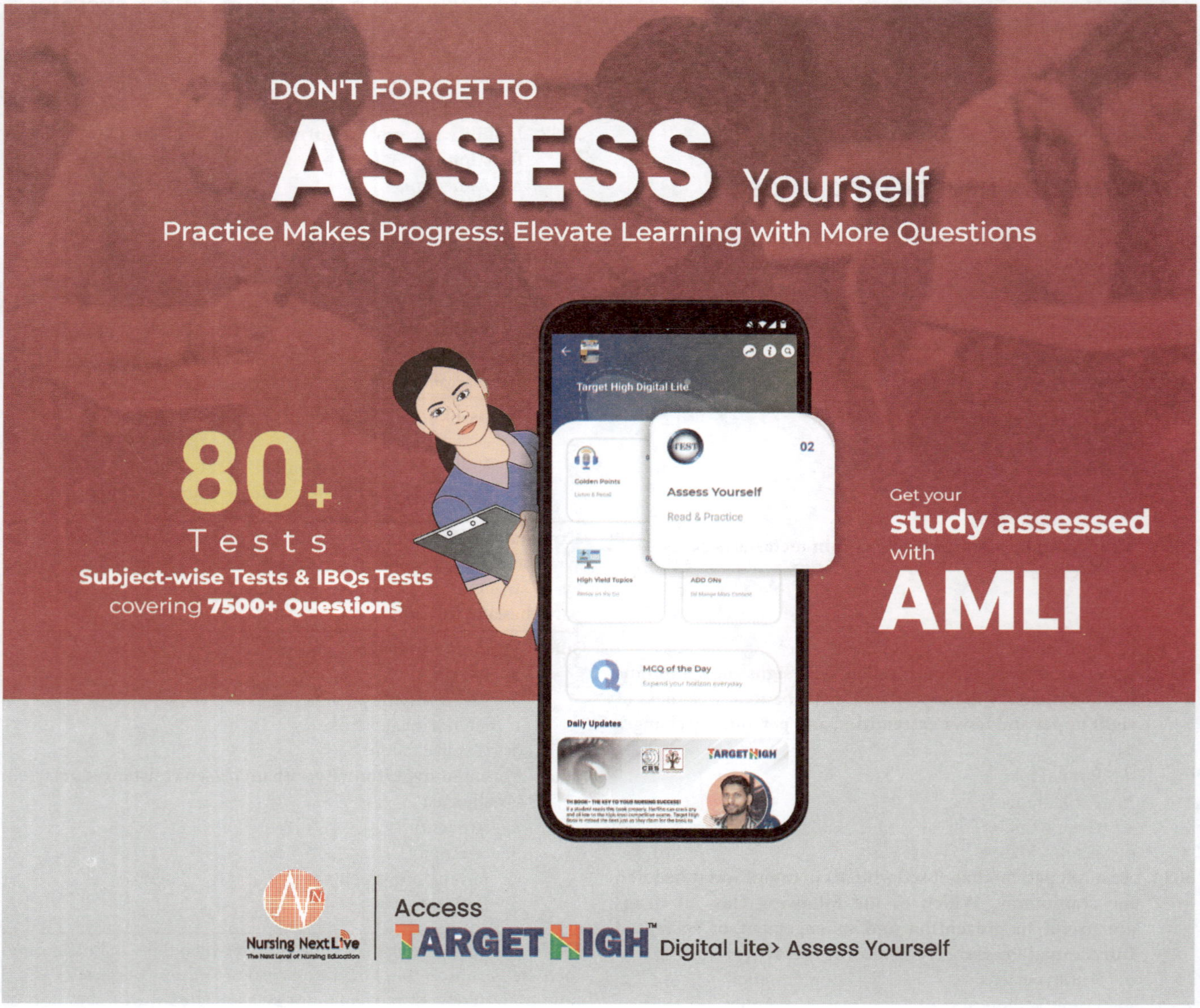

ONCOLOGY

CANCER

- Cancer is considered as chronic disease requiring ongoing management, rather than terminal illness.
- **Risk factors**
  - Age
  - Tobacco
  - Carcinogen exposure
  - UV rays
  - Genes
- **Metastasis**
  - Cancer cells move from their original location to other site.
  - **Hematogenous spread** is the most common route of spread of cancer.

Table 95: Infections and viruses associated with an increased risk of certain forms of cancer

Infection	Increased risk of certain forms of cancer
HPV	Cervical cancer, anal cancer, upper airway cancer
Epstein-Barr virus	Lymphoma, nasopharyngeal cancer, gastric cancer, Kaposi sarcoma
Cytomegalovirus	Kaposi sarcoma, colon cancer
Hepatitis B & C	Hepatocellular cancer

Screening Test for Cancer

- **Breast cancer**
  - Breast self-examination – 3 to 5 days after the period starts every month. After menopause, one day of every month or any fixed day in a month.
  - **Clinical breast examination:** Preferably every 3 year
  - **Mammography**: After the age of 40 years
- **Cervical cancer**
  - Women ≥ 21 years: Pap test is done
- **Colon cancer**
  - Fecal Occult Blood Test, Guaiac based test.
- **Prostate cancer**
  - Prostate specific antigen (PSA)

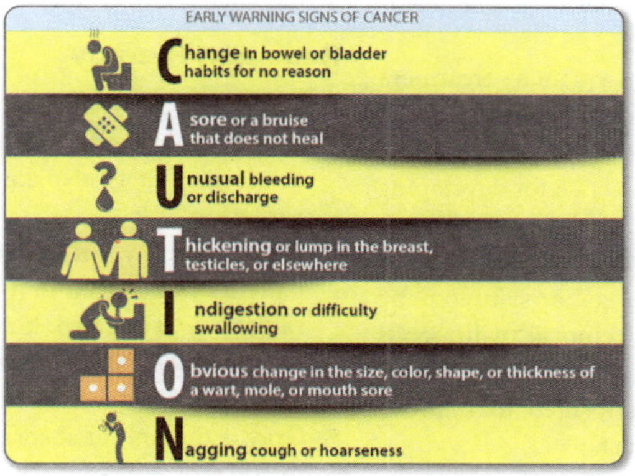

Figure 124: Early warning signs of cancer

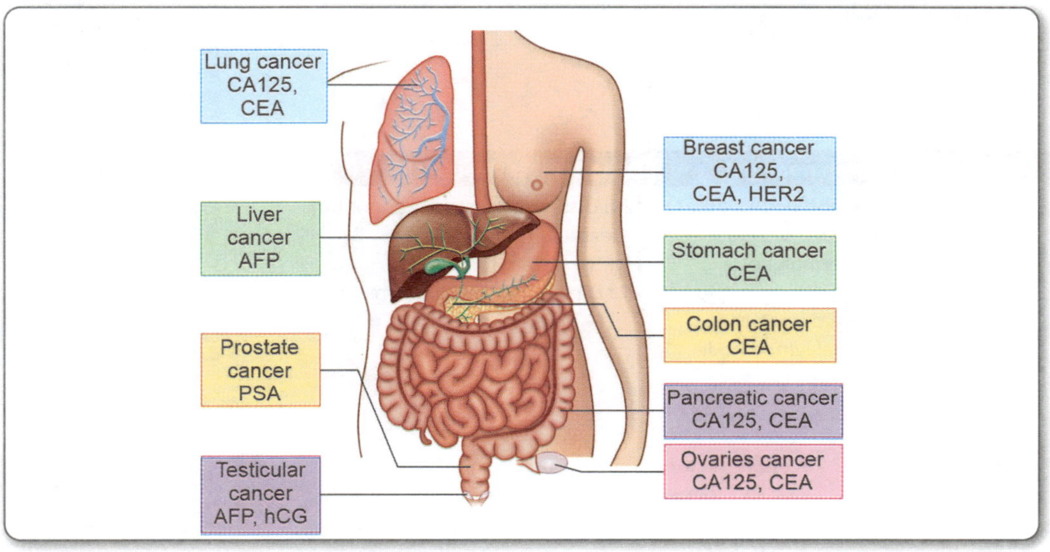

Figure 125: Types of cancer and its tumor markers

KEY POINT

World Cancer Day – February 4. World Cancer Day 2021 is led by the theme "I Am and I Will"

Recent Questions (CNCI 2021)

90. Kaposi's sarcoma is the type of cancer which is common in people with?
a. Kidney failure
b. Liver cirrhosis
c. Kangri cancer
d. HIV

Ans. (d) HIV

91. Which type of cancer has poorest prognosis given below?
a. Leukemia
b. Breast cancer
c. Pancreatic cancer
d. Lymphoma

Ans. (c) Pancreatic...

92. All are recognized tumor markers except ________?
a. Beta HCG
b. Beta-2-microglobulin
c. Alpha fetoprotein
d. Acid phosphatase

Ans. (d) Acid...

Recent Question (NORCET 2020)

93. Which of the following is primary prevention in skin cancer?
a. Applying sunscreen creams and lotions while going out
b. Professional skin examination and self-skin examination
c. Early diagnosis and initiation of treatment for skin cancer
d. Health education regarding treatment compliance of chemotherapy

Ans. (a) Applying...

Table 96: Types of cancer and its tumor markers

Tumor markers	Type of cancers
CEA	Colorectal, breast, lung cancer
Total PSA	Prostate cancer
Free PSA	Distinguish prostate cancer from BPH
hCG	Germ cell and trophoblastic tumors
NMP 22	Bladder cancer
CA 125	Ovarian cancer
CA 15–3	Breast cancer
AFP	Germ cell tumors, liver cancer

Cancer Treatment Modalities

Surgical Management

- Surgical management for cancer consists of diagnostic surgery (biopsy), surgery as primary treatment, prophylactic surgery, palliative surgery and reconstructive surgery.
- **Biopsy**: It can be incisional, excisional and needle method.
- When surgery is considered as a primary treatment option, **debulking surgery** will be performed.
- **Prophylactic surgery:** Removal of non-vital tissue or organ which are at increased risk for developing cancer.
- **Palliative surgery:** Surgeries performed to improve quality of life as a symptomatic management when surgical removal of tumor is not possible.
- **Reconstructive surgery:** Performed to improve functions or for cosmetic effect.

Chemotherapy

- **Adjuvant**: Use of systemic treatment following surgery and radiation
- **Neoadjuvant**: Use of systemic treatment prior to primary surgery or radiation
- **Nadirs**: Period of Lowest blood cell and platelet count as a side effect of chemotherapy is known as Nadirs.
- Chemotherapy usually affects hair, skin, mucous, etc.
- Fatigue, alopecia, nausea, vomiting, anemia, thrombocytopenia and leucopoenia are expected during chemotherapy.

Radiation Therapy

- **Teletherapy**: Radiation source is external to patient's body. Delivered through linear accelerator. It is also known as **external beam radiation.**
- **Brachytherapy**: Radiation sources is inside patient's body. Seed or wires are used to deliver radiation. It is also known as **internal beam of radiation. Patient emits radiation that is considered hazardous to others.**
- Gray is the unit of absorbed radiation dose equal to 100 rads.

TNM Classification

T: Extent of primary Tumor
N: Lymph Node involvement
M: Distant Metastasis.

Table 97: TNM classification

Primary tumor (T)	Regional lymph node (N)	Distant metastasis (M)
Tx: Primary tumor cannot be assessed. **T_0:** no evidence of primary tumor **Tis:** Carcinoma in situ **T1, T2, T3, T4:** Increasing size or local extent of the primary tumor.	**Nx:** regional lymph node cannot be assessed. **N_0:** no regional lymph node involvement **N1, N2, N3:** based upon the extent of regional lymph node	**Mx:** Distant metastasis cannot be assessed. **M_0:** No distant metastasis **M_1:** Distant metastasis is present.

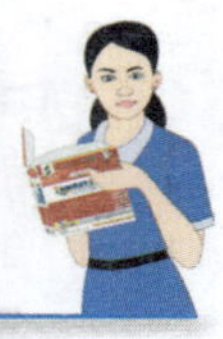

FEW COMMON CANCERS

Oral Cancer

- **Most common type of oral cancer** - Squamous cell carcinoma
- **Risk factors:** Tobacco use, alcohol, virus (HPV, EBV, herpes simplex), poor dental hygiene, exposure to radiation and malnutrition
- Most of the time clients present with non-healing ulcer with varying degree of pain and bleeding.

Recent Questions (CNCI 2021)

94. Administration of Mesna with a chemotherapy agent helps in ______?
a. Favoring the destruction of cancer cells
b. Protecting the cells
c. Preventing formation of uric cells
d. Increasing production of WBC

Ans. (b) Protecting...

95. Your patient complains of dry mouth with swallowing difficulty. Which among the following drugs can produce these side effects when administered in the above condition?
a. Dicyclomine
b. Pyrantel Pamoate
c. Griseofulvin
d. Naloxone

Ans. (a) Dicyclomine

96. The patient with cancer is receiving chemotherapy and develops thrombocytopenia. The nurse identifies which intervention as the highest priority in the nursing plan of care?
a. Ambulation three times a day
b. Monitoring a platelet count
c. Monitoring temperature
d. Monitoring for pathological factors

Ans. (b) Monitoring a...

97. Skin reactions are common in radiation therapy. Nursing responsibilities on promoting skin integrity should be promoted apart from?
a. Avoiding the use of ointments, powders and lotion to the area
b. Using soft cotton fabrics for clothing
c. Washing the area with a mild soap and water and patting it dry, not rubbing it
d. Avoiding direct sunlight or cold

Ans. (c) Washing the...

KEY POINT

Lip/Oral cavity cancer is the most common cancer among male in India.

Laryngeal Cancer

- It is the malignant growth in the larynx.
- Based upon the anatomic location, laryngeal cancer is divided as supraglottic, glottic and subglottic.
- **Glottic is the most common type** followed by supraglottic and then subglottic.
- **Risk factors:** Smoking, alcohol, exposure to chemical such as sulphuric acid, mist and asbestos
- **Clinical Manifestations**
  - **Early symptoms:** Hoarseness of voice and change in quality of voice
  - Painless lump in the throat, dysphagia, dyspnea, weight loss, weakness, and hemoptysis
- Chemotherapy and radiation therapy can be used as treatment modality.
- Laryngectomy is the surgery of choice.
- Nursing responsibility following laryngectomy:
  - Assess the client for respiratory complications and ensure a patent airway.
  - Fowler's position to client for better gas exchange
  - Establish an alternative way of communication. It includes:
    - Speech therapy
    - Esophageal speech
    - Electric larynx
    - Transesophageal puncture

Cancer of Lung

- Malignant growth in the bronchi and peripheral lung tissue.
- **Histological classification**
  - Small cell carcinoma
  - Non-small cell carcinoma
    - Squamous cell carcinoma
    - Adenocarcinoma
    - Large cell carcinoma
- **Risk factors:** Smoking (active and passive), exposure to chemicals such as silica, coal, mustard gas.
- **Clinical manifestations:** Cough, wheezing, dyspnea, hoarseness, hemoptysis, chest pain, anorexia, and weight loss.
- **Management**: Chemotherapy, radiation therapy and surgery
  - **Pneumonectomy**: Surgical removal of one entire lung
  - **Lobectomy**: Surgical removal of one lobe of the lung
  - **Segmental resection:** Surgical removal of a lobe segment
- **Nursing Management**
  - Provide fowler's position to the client
  - Provide humidified oxygen

Often drainage tube is not inserted after pneumonectomy. The serous fluid accumulates over the space of removed lung and it prevents the shift of mediastinum, heart and the other lung.

Cancer of Stomach (Gastric Carcinoma)

- It is the invasion of cancer in the inner cell lining of the stomach.
- **Risk factors:** Spicy food, smoked food, salty food, low-fruit and vegetables in diet, *H-pylori* infection, smoking, alcohol, and family history
- **Clinical manifestations**
  - **Early symptoms:** Indigestion, abdominal discomfort, and fullness in the stomach
  - **Others**: Nausea, Vomiting, Anorexia, weight loss, abdominal pain, fatigue, dysphagia, iron deficiency anemia, palpable abdominal mass
- **Diagnosis:** Endoscopy with biopsy
- **Treatment of choice**: Tumor resection and partial or complete gastric resection
- **Subtotal gastrectomy**
  - Part of stomach will be removed. It is of two types:
    1. **Billroth I:** It is also known as gastroduodenostomy. Stomach is partially resected and remaining portion is anastomosed to duodenum.
    2. **Billroth II:** It is also known as gastrojejunostomy. Stomach is partially resected and remaining portion is anastomosed to jejunum.
- **Total gastrectomy**
  - Complete excision of stomach followed by anastomosis of esophagus either to duodenum or to jejunum.

Recent Questions (CNCI 2021)

103. Warning signs of lung cancer include persistent cough, bloody sputum, dyspnea and which of the other following symptoms?

a. Dizziness
b. Generalized weakness
c. Hypotension
d. Recurrent pleural effusion

Ans. (d) Recurrent pleural effusion

104. In the patient with terminal lung cancer, the focus of nursing care is on which of the following nursing interventions?

a. Prepare the patient's will
b. Provide nutritional support
c. Provide emotional support
d. Provide pain control

Ans. (d) Provide pain control

Recent Questions (CNCI 2021)

98. In staging and grading neoplasm TNM system is used. TNM stands for:

a. Time, neoplasm, mode of growth
b. Tumor, node, metastasis
c. Tumor, neoplasm, mode of growth
d. Time, node, metastasis

Ans. (b) Tumor, node,...

99. Common cancer of oral cavity is __________?

a. Adenocarcinoma
b. Squamous cell carcinoma
c. Sarcoma
d. Melanoma

Ans. (b) Squamous...

100. A male patient is receiving external radiation to the neck for cancer of the larynx. The most likely side effect to be expected is________?

a. Dyspnea
b. Diarrhea
c. Sore Throat
d. Constipation

Ans. (c) Sore Throat

101. In which of the following head/neck cancers is lymph node metastasis least common?

a. Tongue
b. Buccal Mucosa
c. Hard Palate
d. Lower alveolus

Ans. (c) Hard Palate

102. Least amenable to screening is

a. Breast
b. Cervix
c. Oral cavity
d. Lung

Ans. (d) Lung

KEY POINTS

- Majority of the gastric carcinomas are **adenocarcinoma.**
- Most common type of lung cancer is **adenocarcinoma.**
- Lung cancer is the most common cancer among males worldwide.
- Lung cancer is the most common cancer death in India and world.

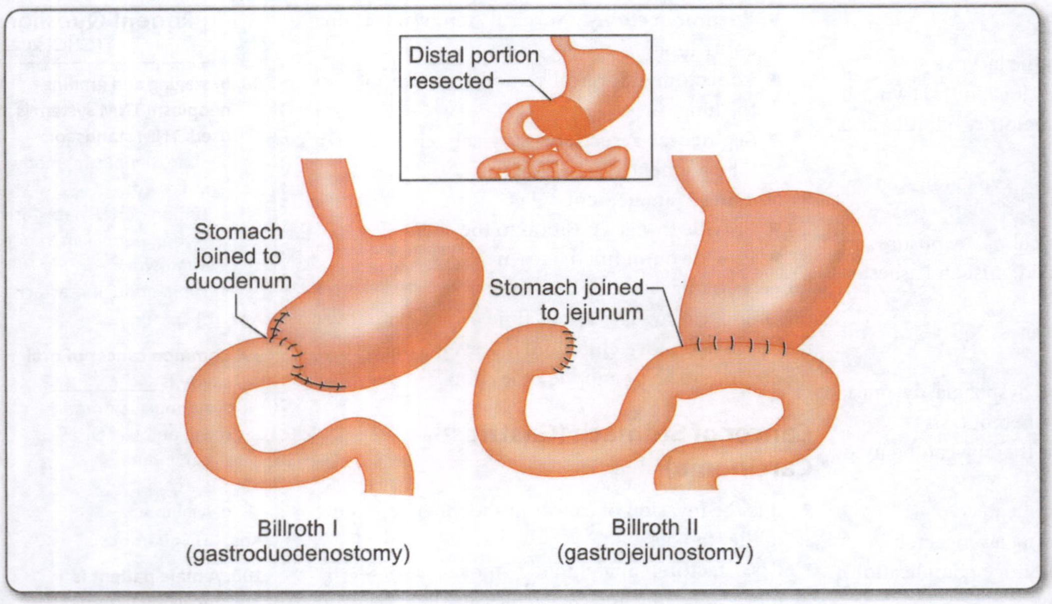

Figure 126: Billroth I & II procedure

KEY POINTS

- Billroth I procedure— Creation of an anastomosis between the duodenum and the gastric remnant.
- Billroth II procedure - The proximal remnant of the stomach is anastomosed to the proximal jejunum.
- The nurse should never irrigate or reposition the gastric tube after Billroth II procedure unless specifically ordered by the physician.
- Increased levels of Ala-fetoprotein (AFP) is seen in Primary Hepatocellular Carcinoma.
- A normal healthy stoma is moist and pink or red-colored.

Carcinoma of Liver (Hepatocellular Carcinoma)

- **Risk factors:** Hepatitis B & C infection, cirrhosis of liver, smoking, alcohol intake
- Males are at increased risk than females.
- **Common presenting symptoms**: Right upper quadrant mass, pain and weight loss
- **Diagnosis**: Biopsy, Blood test, CT, MRI
- Primary hepatocellular carcinoma: Increased levels of alpha-fetoprotein is seen.
- **Treatment**: Hepatic resection, liver transplantation, percutaneous ablation, chemotherapy, radiation therapy, chemoembolization

Colon Cancer

- **Most common type** of colon cancer is **adenocarcinoma**.
- **Risk factors:** Inflammatory bowel disease, family history, decreased fiber intake, increased red meat and fat in diet, **age > 50 years**
- **Diagnosis**: Fecal occult blood test, sigmoidoscopy, colonoscopy, air contrast barium enema, carcinogenic embryonic antigen
- **Diagnostic colonoscopy along with biopsy** is considered as **gold standard** tool for diagnosing cancer of colon.
- **Clinical manifestations:** Hematochezia, melena, change in bowel pattern, weakness, anemia, palpable abdominal mass
- **Treatment:** Surgical resection of cancerous cells along with regional lymph nodes and anastomosis, chemotherapy and radiation therapy
- Colostomy and ileostomy may be in place after the surgery for colon cancer.
- In ileal, stoma there is a great risk associated with fluid and electrolyte imbalance.
- **Complications of colostomy:** Peritonitis, abscess, fistula formation, hemorrhage, intestinal obstruction.

Table 98: Location of stoma in colostomy and appearance of stool

Location of stoma in colostomy	Appearance of stool
• Ileal stoma	• Initially green in color. • Yellow once patient starts to eat.
• Ascending colon	• Liquid form
• Transverse colon	• Semisolid form
• Descending colon	• Close to normal stool
• Sigmoid colon	• Close to normal stool

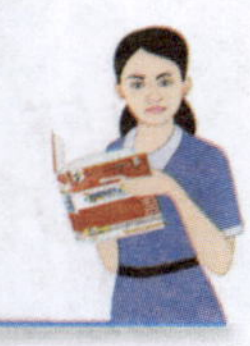

Breast Cancer

- Breast cancer is the **most common cancer** in women (India & World)
- **Invasive ductal carcinoma** is the most common type of breast cancer.
- **Upper outer quadrant of the breast tissue** is most commonly affected area.
- **Risk factors**
  - Early menarche, late menopause
  - Late first child birth or nulliparity
  - Family history
  - Obesity
  - Exposure to radiation
  - Previous history of cancer to ovary, breast and uterus
  - Women who are not lactated
  - Increased use of OCP and hormonal replacement
  - Alcohol consumption
- **Clinical manifestations**
  - New lump or mass in the breast
  - Irritation or dimpling in the breast skin
  - Secretion other than milk from nipple
  - Change in shape of the breast
- **Diagnosis**: Needle biopsy, mammogram, ultrasound, PET, MRI, breast self-examination
- **Treatment**: Chemotherapy, hormonal therapy (only for those women who have estrogen receptor positive tumor), radiation therapy and surgical management.
- **Metastasis**
  - **Most common site for metastasis** is **bone** followed by lungs.
  - Liver and skull are also the sites of metastasis.
- **Surgeries**
  - **Lumpectomy**: Tumor cells are removed. Breast tissue conserving surgery. Additional incision for removal of lymph nodes.
  - **Simple mastectomy:** Nipple and breast tissue are removed, lymph nodes are left intact.
  - **Modified radical mastectomy:** Breast tissue, nipples and lymph nodes are removed. **Muscles are left intact.**
- **Post-operative care**
  - Semi-fowler's position
  - Position the head on the back or unaffected side
  - Elevate the upper extremity on the side of surgery on a pillow to reduce lymphedema
  - If drainage is in situ, maintain adequate suction and record the amount and color of drainage.

Cancer of Cervix

- It is the malignant tumor deriving from the cells of cervix.
- Second most common cancer among women in India
- **Most common type of cervical cancer** is squamous cell carcinoma.
- **Risk factors:** HPV infection, younger age at first intercourse, multiple sexual partners, multiparity with poor birth spacing, STD, OCP use, smoking, poor personal hygiene and poor socio-economic status.
- **Clinical manifestations:** Post-coital bleeding or discharge (clear or foul smelling), post-menopausal bleeding, heavier and larger menstrual period, discomfort while urinating, pelvic pain, leg pain, weight loss and fatigue.
- **Diagnosis:** Pap smear, colposcopy, biopsy,
- **Site for metastasis:** lungs, extra pelvic nodes, liver and bone.
- **Treatment**: Chemotherapy, surgery, cryotherapy, laser therapy and radiation therapy.

Table 99: Procedures in case of cancer of cervix

Procedure	Description
Loop electrocautery excision procedure (LEEP)	A thin wire loop with laser is used to remove the cancerous cervical tissue.
Cone biopsy (conization)	Removal of cone shaped portion of the cervix.
Total hysterectomy	Removal of uterus, cervix and ovaries
Radical hysterectomy	Removal of uterus, ovaries, fallopian tube, proximal vagina and bilateral lymph nodes via **abdominal approach or via vaginal approach**.
Bilateral pelvic lymphadenectomy	Removal of lymphatic vessels and nodes
Pelvic exenteration	Removal of pelvic organ including bladder, rectum, and pelvic lymph nodes and construction of diversional conduit, colostomy and vagina
Radical trachelectomy	Removal of cervix and selected lymph nodes to preserve child bearing capacity of the women.

Recent Questions
(CNCI 2021)

105. A nurse is teaching a patient who suspects that she has a lump in her breast. The nurse instructs the patient that a diagnosis of breast cancer is confirmed by_______?

a. Breast self-examination
b. Mammography
c. Chest X-ray
d. Fine needle aspiration

Ans. (d) Fine needle...

106. Mrs. Sharma with advanced breast cancer is prescribed tamoxifen (Nolvadex). When teaching the patient about this drug, the nurse should emphasize the importance of reporting which adverse reaction immediately?

a. Hearing loss
b. Headache
c. Vision changes
d. Anorexia

Ans. (c) Vision changes

107. A 25-year-old patient is inquiring about the method or ways to detect cancer earlier. The nurse least likely identifies this method by stating:

a. Annual chest X-ray
b. Annual pap smear for sexually active women only
c. Annual digital rectal examination for persons over age of 40
d. Yearly physical and blood examination

Ans. (c) Annual digital...

KEY POINTS

- Avoid BP monitoring, IV injections and other interventions in the arm on the side of mastectomy as it increases the risk for lymphedema.
- Breast Cancer is the **most common cancer** in women (India and World).

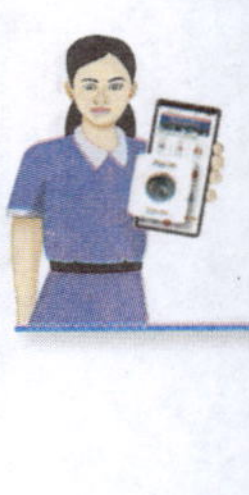

Cancer of Ovary

- These are the invasive tumors which originate in the ovary.
- Most common type is **epithelial ovarian cancer**.
- **Risk factors: Early menarche, late menopause**, family history, old age, obesity
- **Clinical manifestations:** Increased abdominal girth, pelvic pressure, bloating, back pain, constipation, abdominal pain, urinary urgency, indigestion, flatulence, increased waist size, leg pain and pelvic pain
- **Diagnosis:** MRI, transvaginal and pelvic ultrasound, chest X-ray, blood test for CA-125., abdominal CT with or without contrast
- **Treatment:** Chemotherapy, radiation therapy and surgery.
- **Surgical management**
  - Bilateral salpingo-oopherectomy and omentectomy (removal of ovaries, fallopian tube and omentum),
  - Total abdominal hysterectomy

Uterine Cancer (Endometrial Cancer)

- These are the tumors of endometrial mucosal lining of the uterus.
- **Risk factors:** Exposure to estrogen therapy, early menarche, late menopause, nulliparity, anovulation, family history, infertility, diabetes.
- **Clinical manifestations:** Abnormal bleeding, vaginal discharge, low back ache, pelvic pain, abdominal pain, enlarged uterus.
- Radiation therapy, chemotherapy and surgery are the treatment modalities.
- **Surgical management**
  - **Total hysterectomy:** Removal of uterus, cervix and ovaries
  - **Radical hysterectomy:** Uterus, ovaries, fallopian tube, proximal vagina and bilateral lymph nodes are removed. It can be done via abdominal approach or via vaginal approach.
  - **Bilateral salpingo-oophorectomy:** Removal of the ovaries and fallopian tube.

Bladder Cancer

- **Risk factors:** Smoking, exposure to environmental **carcinogen (rubber, dye, leather, ink or paint), recurrent UTI**, bladder stone, pelvic radiation therapy
- **Metastasis to**: Liver, bone and lung
- **Clinical manifestations:** Gross or microscopic painless hematuria **(most common sign)**, frequency, urgency, dysuria.
- **Diagnosis**: Urine cytological studies, tumor marker analysis, Intravenous Pyelogram (IVP), ultrasound, CT, MRI, bladder wash specimen and biopsy.

Management

- **Radiation therapy** is useful for decreasing the tumor size to relieve symptoms.
- **Chemotherapy**: Chemotherapeutic agents are instilled into bladder and then client's position is changed every 15–30 minutes. After 2 hours client voids in sitting position.

  → Instruct the client to increase the fluid intake to clear the bladder

  → The urine excreted by the patient is a biohazard.
- Transurethral resection of bladder tumor, partial cystectomy (removal of up to half of bladder)
- Cystectomy and urinary diversion is the other method of surgery. In this, complete removal of bladder and the creation of urinary diversion technique will be there.
  - **Ileal conduit (Bricker's procedure):** It is also known as ureteroileostomy. Ureters are attached to a portion of ileum and one part of the ileum is taken to the abdominal wall as stoma. Continuous leakage of urine will be there. Client has to wear any appliance over stoma.
  - **Kock pouch (continent ileostomy):** Part of ileum and ascending colon is used to create urinary pouch. Ureters are implanted on the side of pouch. It has nipple valve that helps the patient to be continent (unlike ileal conduit). Patient is to be educated about intermittent self-catheterization to empty the bladder.
  - **Indiana pouch:** Pouch is created using terminal ileum and ascending colon which provide a pouch with higher capacity than kock pouch.
  - **Neobladder**: Segment of intestine is used to create internal pouch and ureters are connected to the pouch. The reservoir is connected to urethra. So client can void via natural orifice by increasing abdominal pressure or by intermittent-self catheterization.
  - **Nephrostomy**: Stoma is created over kidney and urine is drained with the help of tube.
  - **Ureterostomy**: Ureters are brought over the abdomen to drain urine.
  - **Vesicostomy**: Stoma is created over bladder and urine is drained.

Prostate Cancer

- Most common type of cancer of prostate is adenocarcinoma
- **Risk factors:** Increase in age, family history, excessive red meat and dairy products in diet, hormones such androgen and estrogen
- **Clinical manifestations**
  - Asymptomatic at early stages
  - Urinary obstruction in advanced stage (due to obstruction of bladder neck by prostate tumor)

Recent Questions
(CNCI 2021)

108. A patient has undergone external radiation therapy. The expected side effects include the following apart from?

a. Hair loss
b. Ulceration of oral mucous membranes
c. Constipation
d. Headache

Ans. (c) Constipation

109. Radiation protection is very important to implement when performing nursing procedures. When the nurse is not performing any nursing procedures, what distance should be maintained from the patient?

a. 1 feet
b. 2 feet
c. 2.5 feet
d. 3 feet

Ans. (d) 3 feet

110. Which of the following is suggested surgical intervention for Ca Prostate?

a. Radical prostatectomy
b. Bilateral orchiectomy
c. Transurethral resection of prostate (T.U.R.P)
d. Transurethral resection of bladder tumor (T.U.R.B.T)

Ans. (a) Radical...

111. Which of the following is a diagnostic test for the diagnosis of prostate cancer?

a. Digital rectal examination
b. Prostate specific antigen (PSA)
c. Prostate biopsy
d. All of the above

Ans. (d) All of the above

- Painful ejaculation, Blood in urine and semen
- Sexual dysfunction usually occurs before diagnosis is made.

- **Diagnosis**: Pea-sized, hard nodule is palpated on Digital Rectal Examination (DRE). Prostate Specific Antigen, Transrectal Ultrasound (TRUS) with biopsy. **Histological examination** is confirmatory test.
- **Gleason score** is the most commonly used tumor grading system
- **Metastasis to:** Mainly bone, lungs, liver and kidney.
- **Treatment**
  - **Radical prostatectomy – first line treatment.** Prostate, seminal vesicles, tip of vas deferens and surrounding blood vessels and fat is removed.
  - **Transurethral Resection of the Prostate (TURP)** is the most commonly used surgical procedure.
    - Chemotherapy, Brachytherapy and Teletherapy.
  - **Hormonal therapy: Androgen deprivation therapy**

Gliomas

- Most common type of brain tumors among adults.
- These originate from glial cells.
- Astrocytoma are the most common type of glioma.
- **Risk factor:** Exposure to ionizing radiation
- **Clinical manifestations:** Signs and symptoms related to increased ICP such as headache, vomiting, visual disturbance, seizure, mental status changes
- **Diagnosis:** CT, MRI, cerebral angiography, EEG, cytological studies of CSF
- **Management:** Chemotherapy, radiation therapy and surgical resection of tumor.

Osteosarcoma

- Most common and fatal malignant bone tumor.
- **Risk factor:** Paget's disease, exposure to radiation
- **Clinical manifestations:** Pain, swelling, limited motion, weight loss, bony mass may be palpable, tender and fixed.
- **Diagnosis:** CT, MRI, bone scan, myelography, biopsy and blood serum shows elevated alkaline phosphate level.
- **Management:** Surgical excision, radiotherapy and chemotherapy.

KEY POINTS

- Hemorrhage is the most common complication after TURP.
- Continuous bladder irrigation is recommended after TURP to prevent obstruction of catheter by blood clot.
- Hyponatremia is a possible complication due to bladder irrigation
- A feeling of urge to void is normal after prostatectomy
- Sterility may occur after prostatectomy

Recent Question
(CNCI 2021)

112. Which of the following is a malignant tumor of the connective tissue?
a. Sarcoma
b. Carcinoma
c. Osteoma
d. Glaucoma

Ans. (a) Sarcoma

Oncological Emergencies

Table 100: Management of oncological emergencies

Condition	Description	Clinical manifestations	Management
Superior vena cava syndrome	• Obstruction of superior vena cava by tumor obstruct the venous drainage from head, neck arm and thorax. • Most commonly seen in lung cancer • If it is left untreated oxygenated blood supply to brain will be affected resulting in tissue anoxia and death of person.	• Swelling over the face • Swelling over arm, neck and thorax • Dysphagia and dyspnea • Enlarged jugular vein and temporal vein • Increased ICP and related headache, visual disturbance, altered mental status.	• Chemotherapy or radiation therapy to shrink the tumor size. • Thrombolytic therapy if thrombus is in the blood vessel. • Vena cava bypass surgeries • Assist the client with breathing support • Monitor fluid volume status of the client and administer fluid carefully.
Tumor lysis syndrome	Due to the destruction of rapidly growing tumor cells by radiation therapy or chemotherapy, the intracellular content is released into the blood and it leads to electrolyte imbalances such as hyperkalemia, hyperuricemia, hypocalcemia and hyperphosphatemia.	**Neurological:** Seizure, fatigue, weakness, altered mental status, cramps, muscle pain, tetany, and paresthesia.	• Ensure good hydration before chemotherapy itself. Good hydration helps to increase urine volume and thereby eliminates uric acid and electrolyte released into the blood following chemotherapy. • Adding sodium bicarbonate helps to alkalize urine and thereby prevents kidney failure secondary to uric acid. • Diuretics therapy with carbonic anhydrase inhibitor or acetazolamide therapy alkalizes urine and helps to prevent renal damage.

Contd...

Condition	Description	Clinical manifestations	Management
		Cardiovascular: Elevated BP, prolonged QT interval, wide QRS complex, dysrhythmia, cardiac failure. **GI:** Cramps, nausea, vomiting, anorexia. **Renal:** Oliguria, anuria, renal failure, pain in the flank region.	• Administration of sodium polystyrene sulfonate helps to remove potassium through bowel. • Giving hypertonic dextrose with saline helps to shift potassium into the cells. • Administration of aluminium hydroxide helps to remove excessive phosphate through bowel. • Hemodialysis is also a treatment of choice • Assess urine pH to confirm the alkalization of urine.
Spinal cord compression	Compression of spinal cord from tumor, lymphoma, intervertebral disc prolapse or tumor metastasized from breast, lung, kidney, prostate, myeloma and lymphoma cause this. It will lead to permanent neurological damage and mortality.	Local inflammation, edema, venous stasis, pain along the affected nerve root, neurological dysfunction (motor and sensory), weakness and flaccid paralysis, bowel and bladder dysfunction.	• Radiation therapy and chemotherapy to reduce the size of tumor and to relieve compression. • Corticosteroid therapy to lessen the inflammation • Surgery may be required to remove tumor.
Hypercalcemia	• A life-threatening condition among patients with cancer because of release of calcium from bones more than in amount which can be eliminated by kidney. It occurs because of: ▪ Destruction of bone by cancer cells ▪ Some tumors release parathyroid hormone like substance which leads to demineralization of bones ▪ Release of prostaglandin and osteoclast like substances which activate bone demineralization. ▪ Excessive use of vitamins and minerals and other conditions like dehydration, hyperparathyroidism, renal impairment, use of diuretics, etc.	Fatigue, weakness, fracture, hyporeflexia, hyporesponsiveness, polyuria, polydipsia, dehydration, dysrhythmias.	• Encourage fluid intake among the clients • Use laxatives and stool softeners to treat constipation. • Promote mobility and emphasize its importance in preventing demineralization and breakdown of bone.

Leukemia

- It is the malignancy of the blood forming cells.
- Leukemia is the uncontrolled proliferation of leukocyte which causes bone marrow to be replaced by immature and undifferentiated cells.
- Immature blast cell proliferation will result in proliferation of blood cells which leads to deficiency of healthy RBC, WBC and Platelets.

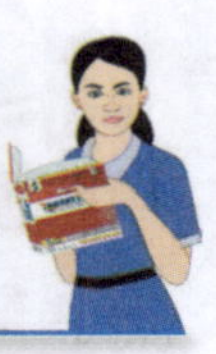

Acute Lymphoid Leukemia (ALL)

- Uncontrolled proliferation of immature cells from lymphoid stem cell is known as ALL.
- Infiltration of leukemic cells in the liver and spleen cause enlarged liver and spleen. CNS manifestations also seen.
- **Management**
  - Chemotherapy is the treatment of choice

Recent Question (CNCI 2021)

113. Which of the following is a malignant tumor of the bone?
a. Fibrosarcoma
b. Lipoma
c. Osteogenic sarcoma
d. Osteoma

Ans. (c) Osteogenic...

- **Stages of chemotherapy:** Induction, consolidation/intensification, maintenance, CNS prophylaxis.

Chronic Lymphoid Leukemia (CLL)

- **It is the most common malignancy seen among older adults.**
- Pancytopenia and related manifestations can be seen.
- Clients with CLL develops B symptoms such as fever, drenching sweats and unintentional weight loss

Acute Myeloid Leukemia (AML)

- It is the malignancy of myeloid stem cell.
- Pancytopenia and related manifestations can be seen.
- **Manifestations:** Enlarged spleen and liver, Lymphadenopathy can be also seen
- **Diagnosis:** CBC and bone marrow aspiration are the diagnostic tests
- **Management:**
  - Chemotherapy and hematopoietic stem cell transplantation

Chronic Myeloid Leukemia (CML)

- Uncontrolled proliferation of blast cells from myeloid stem cell.
- Pancytopenia related symptoms and lymphadenopathy can be seen.
- **Diagnosis:** CBC and bone marrow aspiration
- **Management:** Chemotherapy and bone marrow transplantation
- This condition is associated with Philadelphia chromosome—Chromosome 9 (ABL1 gene) and 22 (BCR gene) translocation which form BCR-ABL1, a mutated gene.

Lymphoma

- These are the neoplasms of the lymphoid origin.
- Classified as Hodgkin lymphoma and Non-Hodgkin lymphoma.

Hodgkin Lymphoma

- It originates in a single lymph node and spreads along the lymphatic system.
- Malignant cells in HL are **Reed Sternberg cells**.
- Most common site for lymphadenopathy are cervical, supraclavicular and mediastinal.
- B-symptoms are the characteristics of HL and they include fever without chills, drenching sweats and unintentional weight loss.
- Hodgkin lymphoma has high prevalence in two distinct age groups: one in young adulthood (20–40 years) and another in older adulthood (50 years and above). In both age groups, men are affected more than women.
- **Risk factors:**
  - Epstein-Barr virus infection or mononucleosis
  - Patient taking chemotherapy, immunosuppressive therapy etc.
  - Age and gender
  - Family history
  - Weak immune system – AIDS patient
- **Diagnosis:** Excisional lymph node biopsy shows **Reed Sternberg cell.**
- **Management:** Chemotherapy and radiation therapy
- Good prognosis

Non-Hodgkin Lymphoma

- Neoplastic growth of the lymphoid tissue which involves **malignant B lymphocyte**.
- Peak age of incidence is more than 50 years and is condition with poor prognosis.
- **Lymphadenopathy** is one of the clinical manifestations.
- One third of the client will be having **B symptoms**.
- **Management**: Chemotherapy, radiation therapy or combination of both.

Multiple Myeloma

- Malignancy of plasma B cells
- These malignant plasma B cells infiltrate bone marrow and cause destruction.
- The infiltrated B cells produce excessive amount of immunoglobulin (myeloma protein)
- Accumulation of myeloma protein affects hematopoiesis and leads to anemia, increased chance for infection and bleeding tendencies.
- **Most common presenting complaint is bone pain.**
- Cell destruction leads to hypercalcemia and renal stone.
- **Diagnosis**: Radiographic studies, bone marrow examination, blood and urine studies.
- Bence-Jones protein: Immunoglobulin light chain or globulin protein (monoclonal) found in urine of patients with multiple myeloma.

CRAB Criteria for diagnosis of Multiple Myeloma

- **Calcium elevation (C):** Serum calcium levels greater than 2.75 mmol/L or 11 mg/dL. Hypercalcemia can occur in multiple myeloma due to the release of calcium from damaged bones.
- **Renal insufficiency (R):** Elevated levels of creatinine (>2 mg/dL) or reduced creatinine clearance (<40 mL/min). Impaired kidney function is often due to the accumulation of abnormal proteins in the kidneys.

KEY POINT

Acute Lymphoid Leukemia (ALL) is most common in young children; boys are affected more than girls.

Recent Questions (CNCI 2021)

114. The patient with leukemia is receiving busulfan (Myleran) and allopurinol (Zyloprim). The nurse tells the patient that the purpose of the allopurinol is to prevent________?

a. Alopecia
b. Hyperuricemia
c. Vomiting
d. Nausea

Ans. (b) Hyperuricemia

115. At the time of diagnosis of Hodgkin's lymphoma, which of the following area is often involved?

a. Back b. Neck
c. Chest d. Groin

Ans. (b) Neck

116. A 36-year-old man with lymphoma presents with signs of impending septic shock 9 days after chemotherapy. The nurse could expect which of the following to be present?

a. Flushing, decreased oxygen saturation, mild hypotension
b. Low grade fever, chills, tachycardia
c. Elevated temperature, oliguria, hypotension
d. High grade fever, normal blood pressure, increased respirations

Ans. (b) Low grade...

- **Anemia (A):** Hemoglobin levels below 10 g/dL. Anemia can develop due to decreased production of red blood cells or their destruction in multiple myeloma.
- **Bone lesions (B):** Presence of one or more round, punched-out, and radiolucent osteolytic bone lesions seen on imaging studies such as CT, PET-CT, or radiography.

At least one of the above criteria along with abnormal plasma cell in bone-marrow is considered diagnostic criteria for multiple myeloma.

- **Management**: Autologous bone marrow and peripheral blood stem cell transplantation and high dose chemotherapy

BONE MARROW TRANSPLANTATION (BMT)

- BMT helps to replace unhealthy blood forming cells with healthy ones.
- Hips, breast bone, spine, ribs, and skull are usually the sites of choice for bone marrow aspiration.
- **Autologous bone marrow transplant:** Bone marrow is taken from one person and transfused back to the same person.
- **Allogeneic bone marrow transplant:** Bone marrow is taken from one person and transfused to another person of same species.
- **Umbilical Cord Blood Transplant:** Umbilical cord blood is harvested immediately after delivery and this blood has the capacity to provide stem cells and can be used in future if child needs.
- Human leukocyte antigen (HLA) needs to be checked before BMT.

KEY POINTS

- **Hodgkin's lymphoma** is a malignant condition characterized by proliferation of abnormal giant, multinucleated cells, called **Reed-Sternberg cells**.
- **Triad of B-symptoms of Hodgkin's lymphoma:** Fever, night sweats and weight loss
- **Pel-Ebstein Fever** is characteristic feature of Hodgkin's lymphoma.

Recent Questions
(CNCI 2021)

117. The presence of which protein in urine is suggestive of the diagnosis for multiple myeloma?

a. Fibronectin
b. Elastin
c. Bence-Jones proteins
d. Collagen

Ans. (c) Bence-Jones proteins

118. A patient is taking cyclophosphamide for the treatment of the lymphoma. The nurse is very cautious while administering the medication because this drug poses the fatal side effect of ______?

a. Alopecia
b. Myeloma
c. CNS toxicity
d. Hemorrhagic cystitis

Ans. (d) Hemorrhagic cystitis

Golden Points to Remember

- Cancer that forms in bones and soft tissues, including muscle, fat, blood vessels, lymph vessels, and fibrous tissue is called Sarcoma (Cancers that develop in connective tissues).
- Carcinomas are cancers that develop in epithelial cells, which are the cells that line the surface of the body's organs and tissues.
- Benign tumors are confined to a specific, localized area (Encapsulation) and does not metastasize (spread).
- Cell division is uncontrolled and abnormal in malignant tumors (cancer).
- Malignant tumors are not encapsulated.
- Malignant tumors metastasize to surrounding area via blood stream or lymphatic system.
- A **1 cm** tumor that is detectable by palpation contains 1 billion cancer cells.
- A **0.5 cm** tumor is the smallest that can be detected by MRI.
- **Asthenia** is abnormal physical weakness or lack of energy.
- Most common type of prostate CA is **Adenocarcinoma**.
- Most common site of metastasis from prostrate CA is **Vertebrae**.
- Most common tumor to metastasize to bone:
  - Males → CA prostate (osteoblastic secondaries)
  - Females → CA breast (osteoblastic secondaries)
- Radiation dose was expressed in units called **rads** (radiation absorbed doses).
- Radiation can be delivered externally (**teletherapy**), and internally (**brachytherapy**).
- Most radiosensitive cell in the blood: **Lymphocyte**.
- Least radiosensitive cell in the blood: **Platelet**.
- Least radiosensitive cell of the body: **Neurons**.
- **Xerostomia** means dry mouth. It is a common side-effect of head and neck radiation therapy.

Contd...

- Palmar–plantar erythrodyesthesia (PPE) or hand foot syndrome is a cutaneous toxicity that occurs mainly due to targeted chemotherapy.
- Temporary hair loss occurs at 30 GY, and permanent at 55 Gy of radiation exposure.
- The **four hallmark signs** of tumor lysis syndrome are **hyperuricemia, hyperphosphatemia, hyperkalemia** and **hypocalcemia**.
- **Chemotherapy** is the first treatment recommended for multiple myeloma. Common regimen is VAD—vincristin, doxorubicin, and dexamethasone.
- Common side-effect of chemotherapy is **nausea**.
- **CRAB criteria** are used to distinguish smoldering myeloma and monoclonal gammopathies of undetermined.
- Screening for CA prostrate is commonly done by: Digital Rectal Examination+ PSA.
- Normal level of PSA in male: <4 ng /mL.
- Palliative surgery is performed to reduce the intensity of illness by debulking tumors so as to relieve several symptoms.
- Opioid analgesics are commonly used for the pain management of cancer patients with severe pain.
- Topoisomerase inhibitors are the Chemotherapeutic agents that is essential to maintain the Topology of the DNA.
- Adjuvant therapy is given after the primary treatment, such as surgery or radiation therapy, to help kill any remaining cancer cells
- Neoadjuvant therapy is given before the primary treatment, to shrink the tumor and make it easier to remove.
- Most common type of colon cancer is **adenocarcinoma**.
- **Pancreatic cancer** has the poorest prognosis. It usually does not show early symptoms and diagnosed at late stage. Survival rate is only 8% (Source: American Cancer Society).
- Whenever a biopsy is taken it should be kept in 10% buffered formalin
- Cadmium exposure can predispose to prostate cancer
- For Fine needle aspiration cytology, 23 – 30 Gauge needle is used
- For Trucut/core needle biopsy, 8 – 18-gauge needle is used
- 18-Fluorodeoxy glucose (18- FDG) is used for positron emission tomography (PET)
- Six hours NPO is essential for PET- CT.
- BI – RADS is a scoring system where radiologists used to describe mammogram results.
- Mosteller formula is used for chemo drug calculation.
- **Grafeel Injection** is used to prevent infections after chemotherapy. It is a growth factor that stimulates the bone marrow to produce white blood cells.
- Chemoport catheter inserted in internal jugular vein or subclavian vein.
- Pressure bandage should not be done on the entire arm for the chemotherapy extravasation.
- Iridium 192 is the isotope which is commonly used for brachytherapy.
- For external beam radiation therapy previously cobalt 60 was used, now LINAC linear accelerator is used.
- Lung cancer has the maximum risk of brain metastasis.
- Drug busulfan can increase the uric acid level.
- Drug etoposide can lead to orthostatic hypotension.
- Chemo drugs should be prepared in chemohood.
- National cancer control program in India was launched in 1975 and revised on 1984-1985.
- A chemo port is a small, implantable reservoir with a thin silicone tube that attaches to a vein. The advantage of this device is that chemotherapy medications can be delivered directly into the port rather than a vein. The port can be used for 3 to 5 years.

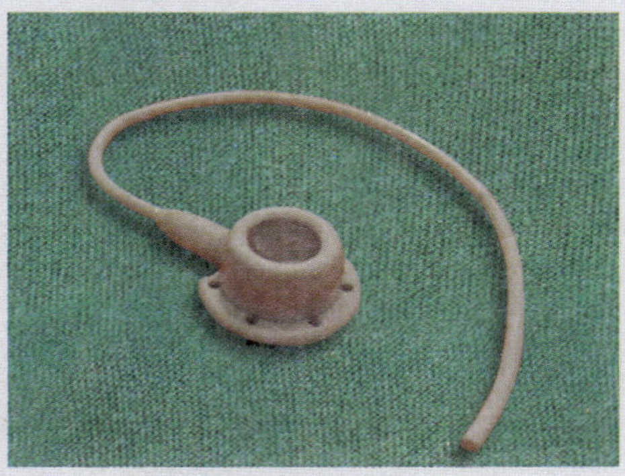

Figure 127: Chemoport

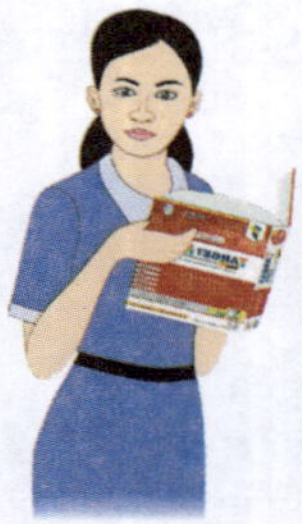

"Better ten times ill than one time dead."
—Yiddish

MULTIPLE CHOICE QUESTIONS
(Including Explained and Practice Questions)

ONCOLOGY

CANCER: DEFINITION AND TNM CLASSIFICATION

3067. Increase in number of cells in a tissue is called: *(Banaras HU 2015)*
a. Hypertrophy b. Hyperplasia
c. Aplasia d. Hypoplasia

3068. Hypertrophy is:
a. Increase in number of cells
b. Increase in size of cells
c. Uncontrolled multiplication
d. Spreading to other site

3069. Qualitative alteration of differentiation of cells is known as:
a. Anaplasia b. Metaplasia
c. Hypoplasia d. Aplasia

3070. Transformation of one type of differentiated cell type to another differentiated cell type is known as:
a. Anaplasia b. Metaplasia
c. Hypoplasia d. Aplasia

3071. The most important characteristics of malignant tumor as compared to a benign tumor is:
a. Hyperplasia b. Metastasis
c. Hypertrophy d. Poor differentiation

3072. Energy deriving process that take place in cancer cell is:
a. Glycolysis
b. Krebs cycle
c. HMP shunt
d. Pentose phosphate pathway

3073. Any deformity in the organ or structure is termed as:
a. Malformation b. Mutation
c. Amputation d. Association

3074. All among the following are cellular adaptations except-:
a. Hypertrophy b. Hyperplasia
c. Neoplasia d. Metaplasia

3075. Difference between benign and malignant neoplasm is:
a. Extent of tissue invasiveness
b. Metastasis
c. Both a and b
d. None of the above

3076. Which is not cancer? *(ESIC Chennai May 2012)*
a. Glaucoma b. Leukaemia
c. Carcinoma d. Sarcoma

3077. Absence of differentiation among the cell is known as:
a. Anaplasia b. Metaplasia
c. Mutation d. Hypertrophy

3078. Malignant tumor of fibrous tissue is:
a. Primitive cell tumor b. Myoma
c. Lymphoma d. Fibrosarcoma

3079. Which of the following is not a typical difference factor between benign and malignant tumors? *(ESIC 2019)*
a. Growth rate b. Encapsulation
c. Cell differentiation d. Size of the tumor

Explanation: Size of the tumor is not a typical difference factor, whereas characteristics such as growth rate, encapsulation, cell differentiation, morphology of cells and treatment differs.

Table: Key features of benign and malignant tumors

Benign tumors	Malignant tumor
Cells tend not to spread	Cells can spread
Rate of cell division is slow (Cell differentiation)	Cell division is uncontrolled and abnormal.
The tumor confined to a specific, localized area (Encapsulation)	Mostly, malignant tumors are not encapsulated.
Do not metastasize (spread) to other parts of the body	Often invade basal membrane that surrounds nearby healthy tissue. Can spread via bloodstream or lymphatic system
Shape, chromosomes, and DNA of cells appear normal	Cells have abnormal chromosomes and DNA characterized by large, dark nuclei; may have abnormal shape
Do not secrete hormones or other substances (except pheochromocytomas)	Can secrete substances that cause fatigue and weight loss (paraneoplastic syndrome)

3080. Major difference between benign and malignant neoplasms is:
a. Rate of hyperplasia
b. Incidence rate
c. Complicity of diagnosis
d. Characteristic of tissue invasiveness

3081. Benign tumor of fat is:
a. Primitive cell tumor b. Myoma
c. Lymphoma d. Lipoma

3082. Spread of malignant cells from one part to other part of the body is known as:
a. Invasion b. Spreading
c. Metastasis d. Seeding

3083. In which phase of cell cycle is DNA replicated?
a. C1 phase b. S phase
c. G2 phase d. M phase

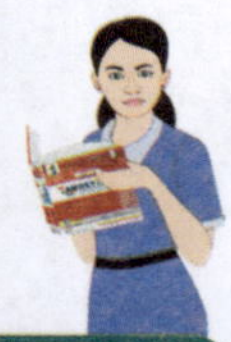

Ans.
3067. b
3068. b
3069. a
3070. b
3071. b
3072. a
3073. a
3074. c
3075. c
3076. a
3077. a
3078. d
3079. d
3080. d
3081. d
3082. c
3083. b

3084. During metaphase of mitosis, chromosomes:
a. Undergo coiling
b. Move towards the poles
c. Line up at the equator
d. Break & disintegrate

3085. UV rays commonly damages:
a. Heart
b. Liver
c. Pancreas
d. Skin

3086. Identify tumor suppressor gene among the following:
a. APC
b. NF1
c. RB
d. All of these

3087. Which of the following statement regarding epithelial dysplasia is not true?
a. Nuclear hyperchromatism
b. Enlarged nucleoli
c. Cellular pleomorphism
d. Decreased normal and abnormal mitosis

3088. All are the examples of malignant tumor; EXCEPT:
a. Leukemia
b. Fibrosarcoma
c. Leiomyoma
d. Lymphoma

3089. The tumor of the hyaline cartilage is called *(AIIMS Raipur Grade-II)*
a. Osteochondroma
b. Osteosarcoma
c. Enchondroma
d. Chondrosarcoma

Explanation: An enchondroma is a type of non-cancerous bone tumor that begins in cartilage. Osteochondroma is an overgrowth of cartilage and bone that happens at the end of the bone near the growth plate. Osteosarcoma (OS) or osteogenic sarcoma (OGS) is a cancerous tumor that arises from primitive transformed cells of mesenchymal origin which exhibits osteoblastic differentiation and produces malignant osteoid. Chondrosarcoma is a cancer composed of cells derived from transformed cells that produce cartilage

3090. The severe weight loss accompanied by progressive weakness, loss of appetite and anemia that is usually associated with advanced cancer is called: *(AIIMS Raipur Grade II 2017)*
a. Carcinomatosis
b. Cachexia
c. Anaplasia
d. Dysplasia

Explanation: Cachexia is loss of weight, muscle atrophy, fatigue, weakness and significant loss of appetite in someone who is not actively trying to lose weight. Carcinomatosis is a condition in which cancer is widespread in the body. Anaplasia is a condition of cells with poor cellular differentiation. Dysplasia is an abnormality of development or epithelial anomaly of growth and differentiation.

3091. Identify the features of malignant tumors among the following:
a. Poor prognosis
b. Metastasize easily
c. They do not show encapsulation
d. All of the above

3092. Identify the feature of benign tumor among the following:
a. They are invasive and destructive
b. Their constituent cells shows anaplasia
c. They are usually well circumscribed
d. They are usually not encapsulated

3093. Most common route of initial metastasis for carcinomas is:
a. Direct invasion
b. Lymphatic spread
c. Hematogenous spread
d. None of these

SCREENING TESTS FOR CANCER

3094. Taking out a small piece of tissue for diagnostic purpose is known as:
a. Biopsy
b. Dissection
c. Reconstruction
d. Extraction

3095. Which among the following is diagnosed based on Reed Sternberg cell type? *(AIIMS Bhopal Grade-I 2018)*
a. Hodgkin's disease
b. Non-Hodgkin's disease
c. Nephroblastoma
d. Hepatoblastoma

Explanation: Reed Sternberg cells are large, abnormal lymphocytes that may contain more than one nucleus and are essential to the diagnosis of Hodgkin's lymphoma

3096. Which of the following tumors causes elevated carcino-embryonic antigen (CEA) levels?
a. Breast
b. Gastric
c. Lung
d. All of the above

3097. The most useful circulating marker for patient with hepatocellular carcinoma is:
a. CA 50
b. Level of Vit. B12
c. CEA
d. AFP

3098. In patients with colorectal cancer serum CEA level is clinically useful for all of the following reasons; EXCEPT:
a. Prognosis
b. Detection of recurrence
c. Guiding treatment response
d. Early diagnosis

3099. Identify example of tumor markers:
a. Alpha-fetoprotein
b. Thyroglobulin
c. β2-microglobulin
d. All of the above

3100. Which of the following is not the definition of possible neutropenia?
a. Fever 2 consecutive readings >38.0°C for 2 hours
b. ANC count = 500
c. ANC count <500
d. Single reading of 100.4°F

3101. Which among the following parameter shows abnormal value in the lab test in a person recently diagnosed with multiple myeloma?
a. Immunoglobulin
b. Electrolytes
c. White Blood Cells (WBCs)
d. All of the above

Ans.
3084. c
3085. d
3086. d
3087. d
3088. c
3089. c
3090. b
3091. d
3092. c
3093. b
3094. a
3095. a
3096. d
3097. d
3098. d
3099. d
3100. d
3101. d

COMMON CANCER TREATMENT MODALITIES

3102. Match the following regarding types of cancer treatment:

I. Primary treatment	A. Treatment as a first step to shrink a tumor before main treatment
II. Adjuvant treatment	B. Aimed at relief of symptoms, and improve quality of life
III. Neo-adjuvant treatment	C. Radiation therapy is the main treatment
IV. Palliative treatment	D. Surgery followed by chemo- or radiotherapy to prevent recurrence

	I	II	III	IV
a.	C	D	A	B
b.	C	A	B	D
c.	D	C	B	A
d.	A	B	C	D

Explanation:
- **Primary treatment:** When radiation is the main treatment for the cancer
- **Adjuvant treatment:** Surgery followed by chemo- or radiotherapy to help decrease the risk of the cancer recurring
- **Neo-adjuvant treatment:** Treatment given as a first step to shrink a tumor before the main treatment
- **Palliative treatment:** Designed to relieve symptoms, and improve the quality of life

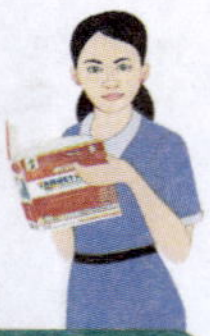

3103. Palliative treatment is *(AIIMS Raipur NO 2019)*
a. Radiation therapy used to treat cancer
b. Surgery followed by chemo and radiation
c. Given as a first step to shrink the tumor before giving main treatment
d. Relieve symptom and improves quality of life

Explanation: Palliative care is an interdisciplinary approach focuses on providing relief from the symptoms, pain, physical stress, and mental stress at any stage of illness.

3104. Radio sensitive tissue is minimum in........... tissue:
a. Blood b. Bone
c. Lung d. Thyroid

3105. Least affected by radiation therapy is:
a. Thymus gland b. Gonads
c. Nerve cells d. Lymphocytes

3106. Radioisotope used for cancer treatment is:
a. Strontium-89
b. Samarium-153
c. Radium-223
d. All of the above

3107. Insertion of radioactive implants directly into the tissue is known as:
a. Teletherapy b. Brachytherapy
c. Chemotherapy d. Microwave therapy

3108. Most common side effect associated with radiation therapy to the neck is:
a. Alopecia
b. Dermatitis
c. Hemoptysis
d. Sore throat

3109. An external source of ionizing radiation is pointed at a particular part of the body is known as:
a. Teletherapy b. Brachytherapy
c. Chemotherapy d. Microwave therapy

3110. Nursing responsibilities for either external or internal radiation therapy include: *(ESIC Chennai May 2012)*
a. Assist in documenting the results of therapy
b. Carefully assess and manage any complications, in collaboration with the radiation oncologist
c. Provide emotional support
d. All of the above

3111. Priority nursing intervention while caring for a terminally ill client is:
a. Provide psychological support
b. Maintain nutritional status
c. Provide pain control
d. Maintain hydration

3112. After a radical mastectomy with lymph node removal, which of the following measures help to prevent lymphoedema?
a. Warm moist heat application (Staff Nurse G II 2014)
b. Restricting all movements of the arm
c. Raising arm above heart on pillows
d. Placing arm close to body in sling

3113. Post-operative teaching points to decrease lymphedema in a mastectomy client includes:
a. Avoid wearing tight elastic or jewellery on the affected arm
b. Sleep on back or non-surgical side
c. Avoid lifting heavy objects during the first 4 to 6 weeks after surgery
d. All of the above

3114. A nurse is caring for a 45-year-old female patient who undergone mastectomy. Which of the following intervention is appropriate to prevent the lymphedema as a post-operative complication?
a. Ensuring patency of wound drainage tube
b. Frequently elevating the arm of the affected side above the level of the heart
c. Placing the arm on the affected side in a dependent position
d. Restricting movement of the affected arm

Explanation: Elevation of the affected arm above the level of the heart promotes lymphatic drainage and venous return thus, preventing chances of lymphedema.

3115. Correct regarding cryosurgery is:
a. Use of extreme cold to destroy abnormal cells, such as tumor cells
b. Often involves the use of liquid nitrogen, although carbon dioxide and argon may also be used
c. It is also called as cryotherapy
d. All of the above

3116. For a patient getting methotrexate, what should be the specific nursing intervention?
a. Use soft bristle tooth brush
b. Teach how to check urine pH
c. Avoid IM injection
d. Teach hand washing

3117. For administering methotrexate urine pH should be:
a. <6 b. 7
c. 8 d. >9

Ans.
3102. a
3103. d
3104. b
3105. c
3106. d
3107. b
3108. d
3109. a
3110. d
3111. c
3112. c
3113. d
3114. b
3115. d
3116. b
3117. c

3118. Dosage of chemo drugs is calculated based on:
a. Height
b. Weight
c. BMI
d. BSA

3119. Which of the following formula can be helpful for calculating Body Surface Area (BSA)?
a. $\frac{\text{Wt (kg)}}{\text{Ht (m}^2\text{)}}$
b. $\sqrt{\frac{\text{Height (cm)} \times \text{weight (kg)}}{3600}}$
c. $\sqrt{\frac{\text{W (kg)} \times 6}{\text{Ht (m}^2\text{)}}}$
d. W (kg) × Ht (m) × 60

3120. A chemo drug which can be administered intrathecally is:
a. Cytarabine
b. Vincristine
c. Vinblastine
d. 5-Flurouracil

3121. Chemo port is used to administer chemo drugs in case of:
a. Drug to be administered to artery
b. Lung cancer patients
c. Long-term use
d. All of the above

3122. Chemo drugs will attack which of the following tissues/ cells in our body?
a. Bone marrow
b. Skin
c. Nails
d. Blood vessel

3123. Most effective and safe way to administer chemotherapy drug is by:
a. Enteral
b. Any parenteral route
c. Intra osseous
d. Central venous catheter

3124. Following chemotherapy, which instruction needs to be given to the client:
a. Avoid direct sun exposure
b. Perform activity as tolerated
c. Avoid crowded places
d. All of the above

3125. Most common complication that requires alterations of planned chemo regimen is:
a. Pulmonary fibrosis
b. GI ulcerations
c. Hematologic suppression
d. Hepatotoxicity

3126. Allopurinol and well hydration given to a client before chemotherapy for:
a. Pneumocystis carinii pneumonia
b. Coagulopathy
c. Tumor lysis syndrome
d. Vena cava syndrome

3127. Which among the following assessments need to be performed by the nurse before administering chemotherapy?
a. Back flow in the central line
b. Concurrent infection
c. Anthropometric measurement
d. All of the above

3128. The most serious long-term side effect of bleomycin therapy is:
a. Pulmonary fibrosis
b. Cataract formation
c. Cardiomyopathy
d. Aplastic anemia

3129. Which of the following interventions is effective to treat breathlessness in end-stage cancer patients?
a. Fanning the face
b. Morphine administration
c. Inhaled furosemide
d. All of the above

3130. Most common radioisotope used in brachytherapy is:
a. 125I
b. 14C
c. 3 H
d. 34 P

3131. Interval which is required for PICC line dressing:
a. 1 day
b. 2 day
c. Weekly
d. Bi weekly

3132. Management of tumor lysis syndrome is:
a. Antidotes
b. IV hydration
c. Blood transfusion
d. Calcium gluconate

3133. Drug of choice to treat cancer pain is:
a. NSAID
b. Opioids
c. Diclofenac sodium
d. Diversion therapy

3134. Which of the following is not a chemotherapeutic drug?
a. Doxorubicin
b. Etoposide
c. Rasburicase
d. Cisplatin

3135. Which of the following should be avoided by patients taking cyclosporine?
a. Grape juice
b. Orange juice
c. Apple juice
d. Banana

3136. Which among the following is not an adverse effect of cyclosporine?
a. Gum hyperplasia
b. Anorexia
c. Flushing
d. Hypoglycemia

3137. All among the following hormones are used in chemotherapy to treat cancer; EXCEPT:
a. Glucocorticoids
b. Estrogens
c. Progesterone
d. Thyroxin

3138. Examples for glucocorticoids hormones used in chemotherapy include:
a. Prednisone
b. Methyl prednisolone
c. Dexamethasone
d. All of the above

3139. Permanent management of retinoblastoma is:
a. Teletherapy
b. Brachy therapy
c. Enucleation
d. Chemotherapy

3140. Respite care refers to: *(AIIMS BPL NO 2018)*
a. Palliative care
b. Rehabilitation
c. Part-time supervision of patients with chronic conditions
d. End-of-life care

Explanation: Respite care is the short-term or temporary care of the sick or disabled for a few hours or weeks.

3141. The treatment that uses light and energy aimed at an exact tissue location and depth to vaporize cancer cells is:- *(AIIMS Raipur Grade II 2017)*
a. En bloc dissections
b. Photoablation
c. Debulking
d. Diathermy

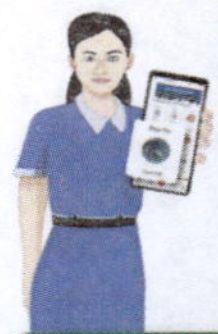

Ans.
3118. d
3119. b
3120. a
3121. c
3122. a
3123. d
3124. d
3125. c
3126. c
3127. a
3128. a
3129. d
3130. a
3131. c
3132. b
3133. b
3134. c
3135. a
3136. d
3137. d
3138. d
3139. c
3140. c
3141. b

Explanation: Laser ablation or photoablation is the process of removing material from a solid (or occasionally liquid) surface by irradiating it using high energy UV photons. En bloc dissections are autopsy techniques in which visceral organs are removed in large bulk. Debulking is the process of reducing the volume of tumour as much as possible. Diathermy is the use of high-frequency electromagnetic currents as a form of physical or occupational therapy and in surgical procedures

3142. Palliative surgery is done: *(AIIMS BBS NO 2018)*
a. To improve self-concept
b. To reduce the intensity of illness
c. To confirm the diagnosis
d. To remove the disease

Explanation: Palliative surgery is surgical intervention targeted to make a patient's symptoms less severe, thus make the patient's quality of life better despite negligible impact on the patient's survival. It is done by debulking tumors so as to relieve several symptoms because of excessive large tumor.

ORAL AND LARYNGEAL CANCER

3143. Predisposing factors for development of oral carcinoma is:
a. Smoking b. Alcohol
c. Syphilis d. All of these

Explanation: Predisposing factors for development of oral carcinoma inculde:

- Tobacco use (Smoking)
- Alcohol
- Prolong sun exposure
- HPV infection
- Male gender
- Fare skin
- Measured age
- Poor oral hygiene
- Marijuana use
- Weak immune system

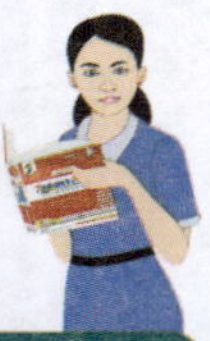

Ans.
3142. b
3143. d
3144. d
3145. d
3146. d
3147. c
3148. a
3149. d
3150. d
3151. b
3152. b
3153. b
3154. a

3144. Most common part of oral cavity affected with oral cancer is: *New Q*
a. Hard palate b. Lower lips
c. Soft palate d. Tongue

Explanation: The most common part of the oral cavity affected by oral cancer is the tongue. This is because the tongue is made up of thin, non-keratinized tissue, which is more susceptible to cancer than thicker, keratinized tissue.

3145. Risk factor for the development of cancer of the tongue is:
a. Poor oral hygiene
b. Oral candidiasis
c. Consumption of preserved food items
d. Consumption of alcohol

3146. Persistent hoarseness of voice is indicative of:
a. Laryngitis b. Tonsillitis
c. Cancer esophagus d. Laryngeal cancer

3147. The most common early symptom of laryngeal cancer is:
a. Dysphagia b. Airway obstruction
c. Hoarseness of voice d. Pneumothorax

Explanation: Persistent hoarseness of voice that is lasting more than two weeks should be evaluated because it is one of the most common warning signs of laryngeal cancer.

3148. Most common cancer in India among men is:
a. Cancer of oral cavity b. Cancer of lung
c. Breast cancer d. Cervical cancer

Explanation:

Table: Cancer Statistics in India/World

Gender	Category	India	World
Both sexes (overall)	Most common cancer	Breast	Lung
	Second most common cancer	Cervix	Breast
	Most common cancer deaths	Breast	Lung
Men	Most common cancer	Lip/Oral Cavity	Lung
	Second most common cancer	Lung	Prostate
	Most common cancer deaths	Lung	Lung
Women	Most common cancer	Breast	Breast
	Second most common cancer	Cervix/ Uterus	Colorectum
	Most common cancer deaths	Breast	Breast

Source: ICMR–National Institute of Cancer Prevention and Research, 2012 and World Cancer Research Fund International, 2012 and GLOBOCAN 2012.

CANCER OF LUNGS

3149. Smoking causes:
a. Chronic bronchitis b. Lung cancer
c. Emphysema d. All of these

3150. Most common cause of lung cancer is:
a. Family history b. Mine workers
c. Air pollution d. Smoking cigarettes

3151. Most common cancer in the world among male population is:
a. Prostate cancer b. Lung cancer
c. Colorectal cancer d. Oral cavity cancer

3152. Leading causes of cancer death among men is:
a. Prostate cancer b. Lung cancer
c. Colorectal cancer d. Oral cavity cancer

3153. Early sign of cancer of lung is:
a. Hemoptysis
b. Persistent cough
c. Hoarseness of voice
d. Chest indrawing

3154. Which of the following is a common symptom of lung cancer?
a. Cough or change in a chronic cough
b. Wheezing sound on inspiration
c. Foamy, blood-tinged sputum
d. Dyspnea on exertion

Explanation: Smoke and the carcinogen irritate the respiratory mucosa which in turn lead to cough and change in chronic cough.

3155. Asbestos exposure can cause:

a. Carcinoma of lung b. Carcinoma of esophagus
c. Gastric carcinoma d. All of the above

3156. Of the following, which is the most common site for metastasis in lung cancer? *(RRB SSNE 2015)*

a. Kidney b. Stomach
c. Liver d. Spleen

3157. Which of the following statement is true about lung cancer?

a. 75% of the lung cancers are small cell in type
b. 80% of the lung cancers are due to smoking
c. Routine screening has proved beneficial
d. 25% of lung cancers are large cell anaplastic

3158. Which of the following symptoms is the most common characteristic of a patient with a cancer of the lung?

a. Air hunger *(Banaras HU 2015)*
b. Exertional dyspnea
c. Cough with night sweats
d. Persistent or intense coughing

3159. All of the following statement regarding squamous cell carcinoma are true; EXCEPT:

a. It is the most common type of lung cancer
b. It is more common in males
c. It has a strong association with smoking
d. Exposure to asbestos increases the risk of developing this condition

3160. Identify correct statement regarding bronchioloalveolar carcinoma:

a. It affects terminal bronchioles and alveolar region
b. It may present only as single nodule
c. Second most common type of lung cancer
d. Tumor destructs alveolar architecture

3161. Most common site of metastasis is:

a. Lung b. Bone
c. Liver d. Uterus

3162. Removal of an entire lung is called as: *(DSSSB 2013)*

a. Lobectomy b. Pneumonectomy
c. Segmental resection d. Wedge resection

Explanation: Pneumonectomy (or pneumectomy) is a surgical procedure to remove a lung. Removal of just one lobe of the lung is specifically referred to as a lobectomy, and that of a segment of the lung as a wedge resection (or segmentectomy).

CANCER OF STOMACH

3163. Metastasis to the left supraclavicular lymph node (Virchow's node) is commonly seen in:

a. Carcinoma stomach b. Carcinoma of lung
c. Wilms tumor d. Leukemia

3164. Which of the following is not a risk factor for gastric carcinoma?

a. Chronic gastritis
b. H. Pylori infection
c. Higher socioeconomic class
d. Hereditary Nonpolyposis colon cancer syndrome

3165. Risk for gastric carcinoma includes all; EXCEPT: *New Q*

a. Chronic gastritis and undergone surgery for gastric ulcer
b. Consuming preserved and smoked food
c. Cigarette smoking
d. Increased consumption of citrus fruits

Explanation: Chronic gastritis, especially when caused by Helicobacter pylori infection, is a risk factor for gastric carcinoma.

The consumption of preserved and smoked foods, such as salted, cured, or smoked meats and fish, has been linked to an increased risk of gastric carcinoma.

Smoking cigarettes is a well-established risk factor for several types of cancer, including gastric carcinoma.

There is no evidence linking increased consumption of citrus fruits to an increased risk of gastric carcinoma. In fact, certain components of citrus fruits, such as vitamin C and other antioxidants, have a protective effect against development of stomach cancer.

3166. Helicobacter pylori is most commonly associated with:

a. Squamous cell carcinoma b. MALT lymphoma
c. Adenocarcinoma d. Angiosacroma

3167. From the following option which is the most common site for stomach cancer:

a. Fundus b. Cardia
c. Antrum d. Greater curvature

3168. What is the most common site for gastrointestinal stromal tumor?

a. Liver b. Duodenum
c. Stomach d. Colon

3169. Which of the following is not the early assessment finding of the gastric cancer?

a. Indigestion b. Epigastric pain
c. Vomiting d. Abdominal discomfort

3170. Which of the following manifestation is found commonly in patient with advanced stages of gastric cancer and less likely in early stages of cancer?

a. Blood in stool
b. Bloated feeling after meal
c. Heartburn
d. Loss of appetite

Explanation:

Symptoms in the early stages of stomach cancer:	Symptoms in more advanced stages of stomach cancer:
• Indigestion and stomach discomfort • A bloated feeling after meal • Mild nausea • Heartburn (epigastric pain) • Loss of appetite	• Blood in the stool • Vomiting • Weight loss • Jaundice • Ascites • Dysphagia • Stomach pain

3171. Following the gastrectomy, the drainage from the nasogastric tube appears bloody. What is the appropriate nursing responsibility in this scenario?

a. Inform the physician immediately
b. It is a normal finding
c. Change the position of the client
d. Assess the surgical site for any infection

3172. Which vitamin deficiency is seen in after gastrectomy for gastric cancer?

a. Vitamin A b. Vitamin B6
c. Vitamin B12 d. Vitamin B1

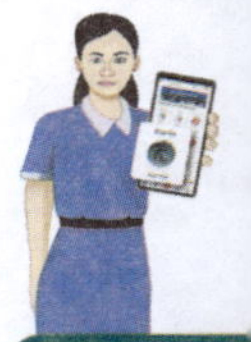

Ans.

3155. d
3156. c
3157. b
3158. d
3159. a
3160. a
3161. a
3162. b
3163. a
3164. c
3165. d
3166. b
3167. c
3168. c
3169. c
3170. a
3171. b
3172. c

Explanation: The stomach is the only site of secretion of intrinsic factor. **Following** total **gastrectomy**, the human would be expected to have trouble in the absorption of **vitamin** B_{12} due to absence of intrinsic factor and eventually develops **vitamin** B_{12} **deficiency.**

3173. Approximately, how long NPO should be maintained after gastrectomy surgery?

a. 0–1 day b. 1–3 days
c. 1–4 days d. 2–5 days

CARCINOMA OF LIVER

3174. The most common cause of hepatocellular carcinoma (HCC) in India is:

a. Hepatitis B infection b. Hepatitis C infection
c. Alcohol abuse d. HIV infection

3175. Hepatitis-B infection is associated with which of the following malignancy?

a. Burkitt's lymphoma b. Esophageal cancer
c. Hepatocellular cancer d. Gastric cancer

3176. Occupational exposure to which of the following material is one of the risk factor for angiosarcoma of liver?

a. Benzene
b. Asbestos
c. Sugarcane
d. Vinyl chloride

3177. Which of the following virus is responsible for the cause of hepatocellular carcinoma?

a. Rota virus
b. Hepatitis B
c. Herpes simplex virus
d. Varicella zoster virus

3178. The best diagnostic measure for liver tumor is:

a. PET scan
b. X-ray
c. MRI
d. CT scan

Explanation: The diagnostic efficacy of MRI in the diagnosis of small hepatocellular carcinoma (HCC) is better than that of CT scan screening. When CT screening is not sufficient to accurately determine liver tumor lesions, MRI can provide a more precise imaging basis.

3179. The malignant condition which is associated with liver cirrhosis?

a. Squamous cell carcinoma
b. Hepatocellular carcinoma
c. Adenocarcinoma
d. Hemangioma

3180. Exposure to the drug aflatoxin may cause:

a. Stomach cancer
b. Lung fibrosis
c. Hemangioma
d. Hepatocellular carcinoma

Explanation: Dietary exposure to **aflatoxins** is among the major risk factors of hepatocellular carcinoma (HCC). **Aflatoxin** B1, which is a genotoxic hepatocarcinogen, which presumptively **causes cancer** by inducing DNA adducts leading to genetic changes in target **liver** cells.

3181. What is the most common type of liver cancer?

a. Hepatocellular carcinoma
b. Hepatoblastoma
c. Cholangiocarcinoma
d. None of the above

3182. Which of the following is not the risk factor of liver cancer?

a. Excessive alcohol consumption
b. Hepatitis-B infection
c. Age of below 20
d. Exposure to aflatoxins

3183. What is the confirmatory test for liver cancer?

a. MRI scan b. CT scan
c. Liver biopsy d. X-ray

Explanation: A biopsy means removing a sample of cells or tissue and looking at it under a microscope. The only clear way to tell the difference between a malignant or benign growth is to examine it by removing a sample of tissue and reviewing it under a microscope. There is no single imaging technique (CT, MRI, USG, etc. that will correctly identify all hepatocellular carcinoma.

3184. The presence of high levels of alpha feto protein (AFP) is seen in which of the following cancer?

a. Breast cancer
b. Liver cancer
c. Prostate cancer
d. Pancreatic cancer

Explanation: AFP is produced whenever liver cells are regenerating. With chronic liver diseases, such as hepatitis and cirrhosis, AFP may be chronically elevated. Very high concentrations of AFP may be produced by certain tumors. High levels of AFP can be a sign of liver cancer or cancer of the ovaries or testicles. High AFP levels don't always mean cancer, and normal levels don't always rule out cancer.

3185. Which of the following type of liver cancer spreads more rapidly?

a. Hemangiosarcoma
b. Adenocarcinoma
c. Hepatocellular cancer
d. Squamous cell carcinoma

COLON CANCER

3186. Risk factor of colonic cancer includes all; EXCEPT:

a. Altered intestinal bacterial flora
b. High-intake of refined carbohydrate
c. Intake of red meat
d. Intake of high-fiber diet

3187. Constipation and early obstructive symptoms are the typical clinical presentation of:

a. Right-sided colonic cancer
b. Left-sided colonic cancer
c. Both a and b
d. None of the above

3188. Earliest symptom of colorectal cancer is:

a. Blood in the stools
b. Change in the bowel habit
c. Flatulence
d. Stetorrhea

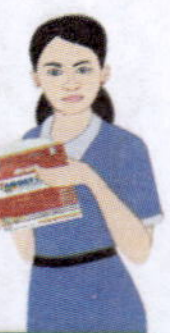

Ans.

3173. b
3174. a
3175. c
3176. d
3177. b
3178. c
3179. b
3180. d
3181. a
3182. c
3183. c
3184. b
3185. a
3186. d
3187. b
3188. b

3189. **Which of the following is one of the risk factors associated with colorectal cancer?**
a. Low intake of dietary fiber
b. Low intake of red meat
c. Irritable bowel syndrome
d. Aspirin therapy

3190. **Risk factor associated with colorectal cancer includes:**
a. Irritable bowel syndrome
b. Low intake of dietary fiber
c. Low intake of red meat
d. Low intake of Aspirin

3191. **Which of the following conditions is a risk factor associated with colon cancer?**
a. Gastric ulcer b. Anal fissures
c. Hemorrhoids d. Ulcerative colitis

BREAST CANCER

3192. **Paget's disease is characterized by:**
a. Hypocalcemia b. Hypernatremia
c. Hyperkalemia d. Hypercalcemia

3193. **Correct regarding Paget's disease of breast is:**
a. It is a rare form of ductal carcinoma
b. It leads to fissuring and ulceration of skin of nipple and areola
c. The histological hallmark is involvement of epidermis by malignant cells
d. All of the above

3194. **BRCA-1 mutation is associated with which cancer?**
a. Nerve b. Breast
c. Leukemia d. Lymphoma

3195. **Risk factors for breast cancer include?**
a. Young age b. Young age at menopause
c. Young age at first births d. Young age at menarche

3196. **Which of the following is a good prognostic factor in breast cancer?**
a. Estrogens receptor positivity
b. Grade III tumor
c. HER 2 receptor over expressions
d. Lymph node involvement

3197. **Which of the following is a risk factor for development of breast cancer?** *(Staff Nurse G II 2014)*
a. Late menarche b. Early menopause
c. No pregnancies d. Early first pregnancy

3198. **Which of the following statement is true about breast cancer?**
a. Life time risk for a woman of developing breast cancer is 1/9
b. A specific cause of the breast cancer is known for each case
c. Incidence of breast cancer is decreasing in the last one decade
d. Prognosis is worse in women of higher socioeconomic status

3199. **Which of the following is one of the risk factors for breast cancer?**
a. Young age at menopause
b. Young age at menarche
c. Young age at first child
d. Young age at first pregnancy

3200. **All of the following assessments may be necessary for a patient who first presents with a breast lump; EXCEPT:**
a. Fine Needle Aspiration (FNA)
b. Examination of axillary lymph nodes
c. Examination of breasts in supine position
d. Chest X-ray

3201. **Risk factor for breast cancer is:**
a. Early menarche
b. Going through menopause after age 55
c. Radiation exposure
d. All of the above

3202. **In breast self-examination palpation of breast tissue and axillary lymph node is there along with:**
a. Inspection of bilateral breast
b. Mammography
c. Percussion of breast tissue for any dullness
d. Palpation of cervical lymph node

3203. **Which of the following is not a screening examination for breast cancer?** *(AIIMS Bhopal Nursing Officer, 2018)*
a. Breast imaging
b. Intravenous pyelography
c. Breast biopsy
d. Clinical breast examination

Explanation: Except intravenous pyelography all others are the screening examination for breast cancer. An intravenous pyelogram (IVP) is an X-ray examination of the kidneys, ureters and urinary bladder

3204. **Most accurate test to diagnose cancer of breast is:**
a. MRI b. Mammography
c. Breast self-examination d. Myelography

3205. **The commonest carcinoma among women is:**
a. Carcinoma of cervix b. Carcinoma of breast
c. Carcinoma of oral cavity d. Carcinoma of lung

3206. **Most common site for breast cancer metastasis:**
a. Brain b. Liver
c. Bone d. Kidney

3207. **Which among the following is a rare site of breast cancer metastases?**
a. Kidney b. Brain
c. Bone d. Liver

3208. **Which among the following intervention is appropriate for restoring the normal functioning of arm on the affected site after mastectomy?**
a. Sleep on the affected side
b. Place daily ice packs to minimize the risk of lymphedema
c. Teach passive exercises with the affected arm in a dependent position
d. Do post mastectomy exercises to increase range of motion

3209. **Correct statement regarding fibroadenoma is:**
a. Commonest benign neoplasm of the breast
b. Thought to be due to increased estrogen activity.
c. It is a biphasic tumor of stromal origin
d. All of the above

3210. **Carcinoma breast is more commonly seen in .... quadrant of the breast:**
a. Lower inner quadrant
b. Upper outer quadrant
c. Upper inner quadrant
d. Lower outer quadrant

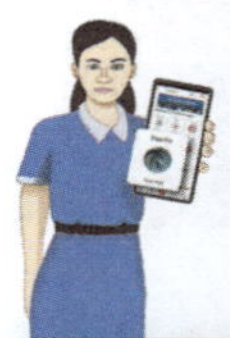

Ans.
3189. a
3190. b
3191. d
3192. d
3193. d
3194. b
3195. d
3196. a
3197. c
3198. a
3199. b
3200. d
3201. d
3202. a
3203. b
3204. b
3205. b
3206. c
3207. a
3208. d
3209. d
3210. b

3211. The commonest type of breast cancer is:
a. Ductal carcinoma b. Lobular carcinoma
c. Nodular carcinoma d. Segmental carcinoma

3212. Risk factors of breast carcinoma includes:
a. Mutation in BRCA1 gene
b. Family history of breast cancer
c. Nulliparous women
d. All of the above

3213. Most common histological subtype of cancer of breast is:
a. Ductal carcinoma b. Medullary carcinoma.
c. Lobular carcinoma d. Mucinous carcinoma.

3214. Factors contributing to poor prognosis of carcinoma breast include:
a. Lymphovascular invasion
b. Poorly differentiated tumor
c. Distant metastasis
d. All of the above

3215. Which of the following chemotherapeutic agents are used in the treatment of breast cancer?
a. 5 – fluorouracil
b. Cyclophosphamide
c. Doxorubicin
d. All of the above

3216. Psychological need of a women who is scheduled for mastectomy can be achieved through:
a. Explain about the pre-operative preparations
b. Explain the surgical process
c. Promote an environment for expression of feelings
d. Teach her how to do BSE

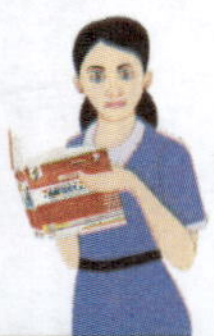

CANCER OF CERVIX

3217. Which of the following action by a women who was diagnosed as having cancer of cervix indicates that she is using an emotion-focused coping process?
a. Denying the diagnosis
b. Discuss with family members
c. Joins a support group for women with breast cancer
d. Doing further tests to diagnose the condition

3218. Most common germ cell tumor is:
a. Choriocarcinoma
b. Small cell carcinoma
c. Squamous cell carcinoma
d. Yolk sac tumor

3219. Most common invasive malignancy of the female genital tract is:
a. Endometrial carcinoma
b. Carcinoma ovary
c. Cancer of cervix
d. Cancer of uterus

3220. Risk factors for endometrial cancer include:
a. Increased amount of circulating estrogen
b. Early menarche
c. Presence of other reproductive organ cancer
d. All of the above

3221. Risk factor for endometrial carcinoma type 1 includes:
a. Unopposed estrogen therapy
b. Obesity
c. Hypertension
d. All of the above

3222. Nursing intervention for a patient receiving brachytherapy for endometrial cancer is:
a. Maintaining absolute bed rest
b. Can use common toilet
c. Visitors are allowed daily for 1 hour
d. Limiting direct nurse-to-patient contact to 30 minutes per shift

3223. Nursing advice to a client during brachytherapy for cancer of cervix is:
a. Minimize the visitors
b. Need to take radioactive precautions while providing care
c. Both a and b
d. She may experience itching and burning sensation

3224. Organism responsible for Cancer Cervix is:
a. Myxovirus b. Papilloma virus
c. Rhino virus d. Rota virus

3225. Diagnostic test for Cancer Cervix is:
a. Pap smear b. Blood test
c. Endometrial biopsy d. PV ultrasonography

3226. Confirmatory diagnosis of cervical cancer is:
(AIIMS Rishikesh & Bhopal 2018 SNO)
a. Mammography b. Biopsy
c. Colposcopy d. Pap's smear

3227. Serum marker elevated during choriocarcinoma is:
a. PSA b. AFP
c. Beta HCG d. CK/MB

3228. Most common histologic type of cancer of cervix is:
a. Squamous cell carcinoma
b. Ductal cell carcinoma
c. Epithelial cell carcinoma
d. Full thickness carcinoma

3229. Which among the following is the risk factor for cervical cancer?
a. Low socio-economic status
b. Early sexual intercourse
c. Both a and b
d. Nulliparity

3230. All of the following are the clinical features of carcinoma of cervix; EXCEPT:
a. Bleeding in between periods
b. Offensive vaginal discharge
c. Low back pain
d. Missed periods

3231. Which among the following is the surgical intervention for cervical cancer?
a. Cryosurgery b. Conization
c. Hysterectomy d. All of these

CANCER OF OVARY AND UTERINE CANCER

3232. A patient is receiving external beam radiation for treatment of metastatic endometrial cancer. The treatment field includes the entire pelvis. Which of the following tissues within this radiation field is most radiosensitive?
(Banaras HU 2015)
a. Vagina b. Ovary
c. Rectovaginal septum d. Bladder

3233. Risk factor for ovarian cancer include:
a. Young age b. Nulliparity
c. Multiple pregnancies d. Prolonged use of OCP

Ans.
3211. a
3212. d
3213. a
3214. d
3215. d
3216. c
3217. a
3218. a
3219. a
3220. d
3221. d
3222. a
3223. c
3224. b
3225. a
3226. b
3227. c
3228. a
3229. c
3230. d
3231. d
3232. b
3233. b

3234. All of the following treatment are beneficial for locally advanced epithelial ovarian cancer; EXCEPT:
a. Radiation therapy
b. Standard IV chemotherapy
c. Intraperitoneal chemotherapy
d. Surgery

3235. All of the following are the side effects of hormone replacement therapy with estrogen; EXCEPT:
a. Breast tenderness
b. Indigestion
c. Vaginal bleeding
d. Increased risk for osteoporosis

3236. Correct regarding uterine fibroid is:
a. Heavy menstrual bleeding
b. Malignant transformation is rare
c. It causes menorrhagia
d. All of the above

BLADDER CANCER

3237. Common clinical feature of renal carcinoma is:
a. Dysuria b. Pain less haematuria
c. Urgency d. Erythema

3238. Which of following is a risk factor for bladder cancer?
a. High fat diet b. Prolonged bed rest
c. Exposure to dyes and paints
d. High fiber diet

3239. Which among the following is a risk factor for renal and bladder cancer?
a. Certain drugs b. Tobacco use
c. Obesity d. Oral contraceptives

3240. First and common symptom of cancer bladder:
a. Painless hematuria b. Oliguria
c. Back pain d. Hesitancy

3241. Prognosis of Wilms tumor depends upon:
a. Histopathology b. Metastasis
c. Age < 1 year d. Treatment taken

3242. WT1 gene is associated with:
a. Wilms' tumor b. Rhabdomyosarcoma
c. Osteo sarcoma d. Retinoblastoma

PROSTATE CANCER

3243. Painless gross hematuria is the most common clinical manifestation of:
a. Cancer of prostate
b. Renal blastoma
c. Carcinoma-urinary bladder
d. Acute kidney injury

3244. Most commonly seen carcinoma in elderly male is:
a. Oral
b. Lung
c. Tongue
d. Prostate

3245. Risk factor for prostate cancer include:
a. Removal of testicles before 40 years of age
b. Black race
c. Asian race
d. Young age

3246. All of the following are useful in diagnosing carcinoma of prostate; EXCEPT:
a. Free Prostate Specific Antigen
b. Total prostate specific antigen
c. Carcinoembryonic antigen
d. Prostatic Acid Phosphatase

3247. Which of the following is correct about the diagnosis of prostate cancer?
a. Digital Rectal Examination (DRE) is performed for the diagnosis of prostate cancer
b. Most patient with PSA >40 ng/mL will have prostate cancer
c. Urinary obstructive symptoms are highly suggestive
d. It is diagnosed with biopsy by FNA

3248. All of the following statements regarding prostate cancer is true; EXCEPT:
a. It usually affects men over 50 years of age
b. In 70-80% of cases, it arises in the peripheral zone
c. Burning or pain during urination is an early sign of prostate cancer
d. Low serum calcium levels in advanced stage of prostate cancer

3249. Most specific indicator marker for diagnosing prostate cancer:
a. AFP b. CA-125
c. CEA d. PSA

Explanation: The PSA test (prostate-specific antigen) is a blood test used primarily to screen for prostate cancer. PSA is a protein produced by both cancerous and non-cancerous tissue in the prostate. The PSA test can detect high levels of PSA that may indicate the presence of prostate cancer. However, the confirmatory test to diagnose prostate cancer is biopsy.

3250. Risk for prostatic cancer is:
a. Older than 65 years
b. Fat rich diet
c. BPH
d. Previous history of urinary stones

3251. Ca prostate develops in which region of the prostate?
a. Transition zone b. Peripheral zone
c. Central zone d. Both a & c

3252. Treatment of cancer of prostate includes:
a. Bilateral orchiectomy
b. Luteinizing hormone releasing hormone agonists
c. Antiandrogen drugs
d. All of the above

3253. Which one of the following cancers does not metastasize commonly to liver? *(NCFL 2019)*
a. Breast
b. Lung
c. Colon
d. Prostate

Explanation: Prostate Cancer does not commonly metastasize to liver. It commonly metastasizes to bone.

3254. Principle behind hormonal therapy in prostate cancer is:
a. Reduce testosterone production
b. Improve testosterone production
c. Improve 5 alpha reductase production
d. Reduce 5 alpha reductase production

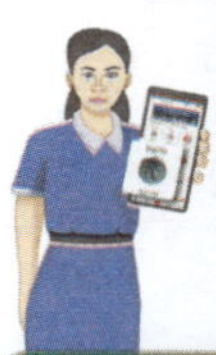

Ans.
3234. a
3235. d
3236. d
3237. b
3238. c
3239. b
3240. a
3241. a
3242. a
3243. c
3244. d
3245. b
3246. c
3247. a
3248. d
3249. d
3250. a
3251. b
3252. d
3253. d
3254. a

3255. Hormonal therapy used in cancer of prostate is also known as:
a. Androgen deprivation therapy
b. Testosterone therapy
c. Estrogen therapy
d. Antagonizing therapy

3256. Testicular cancer is often presented with:
a. Dysuria
b. Cryptorchidism
c. Dyspareunia
d. Painless mass and heaviness sensation over the scrotal sac

3257. Earliest sign in testicular cancer is:
a. Frequency of urine
b. Painless enlargement of testes
c. Urgency
d. Dysuria

3258. True about penile carcinoma is:
a. Most of the penile cancers are squamous in origin.
b. Total incidence is less than 1% of all cancers in male.
c. Chance is more with HPV
d. All of the above

GLIOMAS (BRAIN TUMOR)

3259. Tumor of blood vessel of brain is:
a. Glioma b. Meningioma
c. Hemangioma d. Astrocytoma

3260. The commonest tumor associated with type I neurofibromatosis is:
a. Optic nerve glioma b. Meningioma
c. Schwannoma d. Oligodendroglioma

3261. Most commonly seen meningeal tumor is:
a. Meningioma b. Glioma
c. Schwannoma d. Neurofibroma.

3262. Following are the type of gliomas; EXCEPT:
a. Astrocytomas
b. Oligodendrogliomas
c. Ependymoma
d. Ostoblastoma

3263. The cell that act as a support, insulate and metabolically assist the neural tissue is known as:
a. Neural cells
b. Glial cells
c. Malila cells
d. Meninges cells

3264. The patient's MRI shows the presence of a brain tumor. The nurse expect which of the following treatment modality is suitable for the patient?
a. Surgical procedure
b. Chemotherapy
c. Radiation therapy
d. Biologic drugs administration

OSTEOSARCOMA

3265. Benign tumor of bone is:
a. Osteoma
b. Ewing's sarcoma
c. Rhabdomyosarcoma
d. Osteogenic sarcoma

3266. Codman's triangle is typically seen in which of the following tumors:
a. Rhabdomyosarcoma b. Osteosarcoma
c. Neuroblastoma d. Ewing's sarcoma

3267. Correct option regarding primary bone tumors is:
a. Commonly seen in the first three decades of life and benign tumors are more
b. Leads to osteoporosis
c. Easily metastasis to adjacent bone
d. All of the above

3268. Malignant tumor of bone is:
a. Osteoma b. Ewing's sarcoma
c. Rhabdomyosarcoma d. Osteogenic sarcoma

3269. "Onion-skin" appearance is present in:
a. Ewing's sarcoma b. Rhabdomyosarcoma
c. Primitive cell tumor d. Wilms tumor

ONCOLOGICAL EMERGENCIES

3270. Which of the following electrolyte imbalance is not seen in tumor lysis syndrome?
a. Hyperkalemia
b. Hyperphosphatemia
c. Hyperurecemia
d. Hypercalcemia

Explanation: **Tumor lysis syndrome** (TLS) is a condition that occurs when a large number of cancer cells die within a short period, releasing their contents in to the blood. **Tumor lysis syndrome** is characterized by hyperkalemia hyperphosphatemia, **hypocalcemia,** hyperuricemia, and elevated blood urea nitrogen (BUN) and other nitrogen-containing compounds (azotemia).

3271. Stokes sign is seen in:
a. Tumor lysis syndrome
b. Superior vena cava syndrome
c. SIADH
d. Spinal cord compression

Explanation: Superior vena cava syndrome (SVCS) happens when the superior vena cava is partially blocked or compressed. Cancer is usually the main cause of SVCS. Edema of the neck, called the collar of Stokes, light headedness, facial swelling, migraines, difficulty breathing cough, and upper limb edema are commonly seen in SVCS.

3272. What is the life threating sign of superior vena cava syndrome?
a. Cyanosis
b. Erythema of the upper arm
c. Swelling of the veins
d. Epistaxis

3273. What is the early sign or symptom of superior vena cava syndrome?
a. Periorbital edema b. Arm edema
c. Ecchymosis d. Dysphagia

3274. Which of the following ECG changes is seen in hypercalcemia?
a. Shortening of QT interval
b. Shortening of ST segment
c. Both a and b
d. Prolongation of QT interval

Ans.
3255. a
3256. d
3257. b
3258. d
3259. c
3260. a
3261. a
3262. d
3263. b
3264. a
3265. a
3266. b
3267. d
3268. d
3269. a
3270. d
3271. b
3272. a
3273. a
3274. c

Explanation: In Hypercalcemia, short QT interval is the most common finding, and this is contributed mainly by the shortening of ST segment.

3275. Which of the following nursing diagnosis is a priority for a patient with superior vena cava syndrome?
a. Ineffective tissue perfusion
b. Sleep pattern disturbance
c. Ineffective breathing pattern
d. Impaired skin integrity

3276. All of the following are oncological metabolic emergency; EXCEPT:
a. Febrile neutropenia
b. Tumor lysis syndrome
c. SIADH
d. Hypercalcemia of malignancy

Explanation:

- Metabolic emergencies include tumor lysis syndrome, hypercalcemia of malignancy, and syndrome of inappropriate antidiuretic hormone (SIADH)
- Tumor lysis syndrome is a metabolic emergency that presents as severe electrolyte abnormalities.
- The leading cause of hyponatremia in patients with cancer is syndrome of inappropriate antidiuretic hormone secretion (SIADH). This oncologic emergency requires immediate intervention. Hyponatremia may result in serious and life-threatening consequences including seizure, coma and respiratory arrest if not corrected.
- Hypercalcemia of malignancy is a common finding typically in patients with advanced stage cancers. It occurs in approximately 20% of all cancer patients.
- **Febrile neutropenia** is a hematologic emergency that usually requires inpatient therapy with broad-spectrum antibiotics. Episodes of febrile neutropenia are considered an oncologic emergency.

3277. Which of the following electrolyte imbalance is seen in SIADH?
a. Hyponatremia
b. Hypernatremia
c. Hyperkalemia
d. Hypokalemia

Explanation: SIADH is characterized by impaired water excretion leading to hyponatremia with hypervolemia or euvolemia.

3278. Which of the following electrolyte imbalance observed in SIADH?
a. Sodium level 120 mEq/L
b. Potassium 3.6 mEq/L
c. Magnesium 2.0 mg/dL
d. Calcium 9.0 mg/dL

Explanation: The syndrome of inappropriate secretion of antidiuretic hormone (**SIADH**) is a disorder of impaired water excretion caused by the inability to suppress the secretion of antidiuretic hormone (ADH). If water intake exceeds the reduced urine output, the ensuing water retention **leads** to the development of **hyponatremia** with concomitant hypo-osmolality and high urine osmolality that are the hallmark of SIADH.

3279. Which of the following drug is used to decrease the uric acid level for the client diagnosed with tumor lysis syndrome?
a. Allopurinol
b. Tamoxifen
c. Cisplatin
d. Doxorubicin

Explanation: **Allopurinol**, a xanthine oxidase inhibitor, reduces the conversion of nucleic **acid** byproducts to **uric acid**, in this way preventing **urate** nephropathy and subsequent oliguric renal failure.

LEUKEMIA

3280. Philadelphia chromosome associated with which type of cancer:
a. Leukemia b. Nerve
c. Thyroid d. Breast

LYMPHOMA

Hematology and Lymphatic

3281. Which of the following is characteristic of Hodgkin's disease?
a. Excessive vomiting
b. Anorexia
c. Weight loss
d. Painless, movable adenopathy in cervical area

Explanation: Hodgkin's disease is associated with painless adenopathy. Other three options are common in every disease.

3282. B symptoms of Hodgkin's disease includes:
a. Fever b. Night sweats
c. Weight loss d. All of these

3283. Most commonly initiation of Hodgkin's lymphoma occur from *(AIIMS Rishikesh 2017)*
a. Mediastinum b. Axillary
c. Abdomen d. Neck

3284. Most common Non Hodgkin lymphoma is:
a. B cell lymphoma b. T cell lymphoma
c. Ductal d. Burket's

3285. Major difference between Hodgkin's lymphoma and non-Hodgkin's lymphoma is that:
a. Hodgkin's lymphoma occurs only in young adults
b. Hodgkin's lymphoma multicentric in origin
c. Non-Hodgkin's lymphoma can manifest in multiple organs
d. Non-Hodgkin's lymphoma is treated only with radiation therapy

3286. A client comes to the clinic complaining of fever, drenching night sweats, and unexplained weight loss and single enlarged supraclavicular lymph node, most probable diagnosis will be:
a. Lymphadenopathy b. Thalassemia
c. Wilms' tumor d. Hodgkin's disease

3287. Patient with AIDS are at higher risk of developing:
a. Meningioma
b. Hepatocellular cancer
c. Kaposi's sarcoma
d. Colorectal cancer

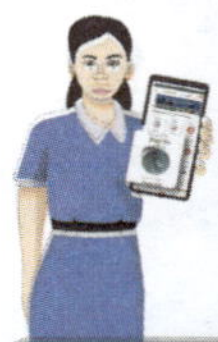

Ans.
3275. c
3276. a
3277. a
3278. a
3279. a
3280. a
3281. d
3282. d
3283. d
3284. a
3285. c
3286. d
3287. c

MULTIPLE MYELOMA

3288. The presence of bence jonce protein in the urine indicates which type of cancer?
- a. Leukemia
- b. Multiple myeloma
- c. Hodgkins disease
- d. Non hodgkins disease

Explanation: The presence of Bence-Jones proteins in urine can be a sign of multiple myeloma or another rare condition called Waldenstrom macroglobulinemia. About 50% to 80% of people with multiple myeloma have Bence-Jones proteins in their urine.

3289. Multiple myeloma is also called:
- a. Honey syrup disease
- b. Basedow's disease
- c. Kahler's disease
- d. Wilsons disease

3290. Which of the following electrolyte imbalance is seen in multiple myeloma?
- a. Hypocalcemia
- b. Hypercalcemia
- c. Hypokalemia
- d. Hyperkalemia

Explanation: **Multiple myeloma** is associated with excessive tumor-induced, osteoclast-mediated bone destruction. This leads to release of calcium from bone to blood stream. This results in **hypercalcemia.**

3291. Which of the following intervention helps to reduce the calcium level?
- a. Encourage the consumption of fluids
- b. Provide adequate range of motion exercise
- c. Give fiber-rich foods
- d. Radiation therapy

3292. Multiple myeloma commonly affects the age group of:
- a. Younger than 15 years
- b. Between 15 to 40
- c. Between 30 to 40
- d. Above 60 years

3293. The client with multiple myeloma is at the risk of:
- a. Pathological fractures
- b. Dysuria
- c. Hematuria
- d. Night sweats

3294. Which of the following lab findings is not seen in patient with multiple myeloma?
- a. Hypercalcemia
- b. Hypocalcemia
- c. Hyperurecemia
- d. Thrombocytopenia

3295. Which of the following drug therapy is necessary to slow down the bone damage and reduce the pain in patients with multiple myeloma?
- a. Bisphosphonate
- b. Analgesics
- c. Calcium channel blockers
- d. ACE inhibitors

Explanation: **Bisphosphonates** are specific inhibitors of osteoclastic activity and are used in the **treatment** of patients with **multiple myeloma** (MM). It is also found to be effective in reducing pain and vertebral pain.

3296. Which of the following statement is correct regarding multiple myeloma?
- a. It is due to the excessive numbers of abnormal plasma cells invade the bone marrow
- b. It is due to the demyelination of myelin sheaths
- c. It is due to the overproduction of leukocytes
- d. It is due to the increased destruction of Blood cells

3297. Which of the following lab tests helps to find out the abnormal number of immature plasma cells?
- a. Complete blood test
- b. Bone marrow aspiration
- c. CSF analysis
- d. Urine analysis

BONE MARROW TRANSPLANTATION

3298. The bone marrow engraftment process takes upto:
- a. 1 to 2 weeks
- b. 1 to 4 weeks
- c. 2 to 5 weeks
- d. 6 to 10 weeks

3299. Which site is best for bone marrow transplantation for adults?
- a. Iliac crest
- b. Femur
- c. Sternum
- d. Tibia

3300. The stem cell which is taken from an identical twin is called:
- a. Allogenic
- b. Autologous
- c. Syngenic
- d. None of these

3301. PBSCT stands for:
- a. Peripheral blood stem cell transplantation
- b. Pulmonary blood stem cell transplantation
- c. Peripheral body stem cell transplantation
- d. Pulmonary breast stem cell transplantation

3302. The stem cells used in the Peripheral blood stem cell transplantation (PBSCT) should come from the process of: *New Q*
- a. Dialysis
- b. Apheresis
- c. Leukapheresis
- d. Both b and c

Explanation: The stem cells used in PBSCT come from the bloodstream. PBSCs for transplantation is obtained through a process called apheresis or leukapheresis. For 4 or 5 days before apheresis, the donor may be given a medication to increase the number of stem cells released into the bloodstream. (Source: National Cancer Institute. Ref: www.cancer.gov)

3303. Which type of donor stem cell is most common?
- a. Allogenic
- b. Autologous
- c. Syngenic
- d. None of these

3304. Which type of donar marrow should be transplanted immediately?
- a. Allogenic
- b. syngenic
- c. Autologous
- d. Xenologous

3305. Which type of bone marrow is frozen for the later use?
- a. Allogenic
- b. syngenic
- c. Autologous
- d. Xenologous

3306. All of the following are the common signs and symptoms of acute graft versus host disease; EXCEPT:
- a. Dermatitis
- b. Rashes
- c. Hepatitis
- d. Vision changes

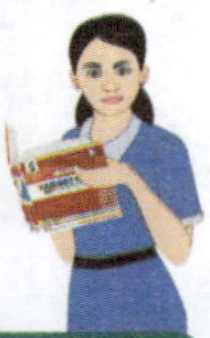

Ans.

3288. b
3289. c
3290. b
3291. a
3292. d
3293. a
3294. b
3295. a
3296. a
3297. b
3298. c
3299. a
3300. c
3301. a
3302. d
3303. b
3304. a
3305. c
3306. d

Explanation: Graft versus host disease (GVHD) are multisystem disorders that can be a life-threatening complication of allogenic hematopoietic cell transplant. Acute GVHD typically occurs within 100 days after the stem cell transplantation. Symptoms of acute GVHD includes dermatitis, itching, rashes, hepatitis, jaundice, enteritis, nausea and vomiting, abdominal pain, blood in stool, etc.

Chronic GVHD usually begins after the first 100 days following a transplant. Signs and symptoms of chronic GVHD includes dryness of eys, vision changes, mouth pain, white patches in mouth, dysphagia, hair loss, wheezing, shortness of breath, joint pain, fatigue, loss of appetite, weight loss, etc.

OTHER CANCERS

3307. Which among the following is not present in tumor lysis syndrome?

a. Hyperkalemia b. Hyperphosphatemia
c. Hyperuricemia d. Hypercalcemia

3308. Which type of cancer has the poorest prognosis? *(NCFL 2019)*

a. Squamous cell carcinoma
b. Breast cancer
c. Pancreatic cancer
d. Gastric cancer

Explanation:

- As per the data of National Cancer Institute's Surveillance, Epidemiology & End Results program as well as **American Cancer Society (ACS).** Type of cancer has the poorest prognosis are arranged in order as follows:
- **Pancreatic cancer**
- **Liver and intrahepatic bile duct cancer**
- **Lung and bronchus cancer**
- **Esophageal cancer**
- **Stomach cancer (or) Gastric cancer**

3309. Glandular tissue cancer is known as:

a. Adenocarcinoma
b. Liposarcoma
c. Neuroblastoma
d. Osteogenic sarcoma

3310. Which of the following is used for the treatment of thyroid cancer?

a. I131 b. 99m Tc
c. 32P d. 1311–MIB2

3311. Calcitonin is used as a marker in ....cancer:

a. Prostate cancer b. Cancer of thyroid
c. Cancer of lung d. Cancer of oral cavity

3312. Barrett's esophagus represents which of the following findings?

a. Cellular hyperplasia b. Cellular hypertrophy
c. Metaplasia d. Carcinoma in situ

3313. Tylosis is associated with which cancer:

a. Pancreas b. Esophagus
c. AML d. ALL

3314. Commonly seen carcinoma in the middle 1/3rd of the esophagus:

a. Adeno carcinoma b. Squamous cell carcinoma
c. Meningioma d. Leiomyoma

3315. Risk factor for Ca. esophagus is:

a. Chronic Achalasia b. Achalasia cardia
c. Smoking d. All of these

3316. Which part of the pancreas is at risk for developing cancer the most?

a. Head b. Body
c. Tail d. Equal chance in all part

3317. Which among the following is the most radio sensitive cancer?

a. Leukemia
b. Renal cell carcinoma
c. Colorectal cancer
d. Adenocarcinoma

3318. Which of the following is a feature of Lynch syndrome?

a. Predominantly left-sided colon cancer
b. Autosomal dominant inherited
c. Multiple polyps beginning in adolescence
d. All of the above

Explanation: Lynch syndrome is also known as hereditary non polyposis colorectal cancer (HNPCC). Lynch syndrome is an autosomal dominant genetic condition that is associated with a high risk of colon cancer. Lynch syndrome (LS) accounts for 2-4% of all diagnosed cases of colorectal cancer (CRC). It is characterized by a relatively young age of onset (45 years) and predominantly right-sided colon cancer.

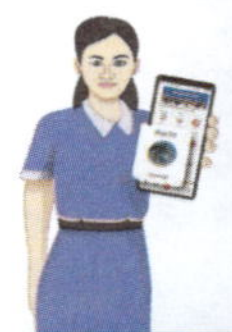

Ans.

3307. d
3308. c
3309. a
3310. a
3311. b
3312. c
3313. b
3314. b
3315. d
3316. a
3317. a
3318. b

MALE REPRODUCTIVE SYSTEM

ANATOMY AND PHYSIOLOGY OF MALE REPRODUCTIVE SYSTEM

- Male reproductive organs consist of:
  - Paired testicles in the scrotum
  - Epididymis
  - Vas deferens (seminal duct)
  - Spermatic cord
  - Seminal vesicles
  - Ejaculatory ducts
  - Cowper's gland (bulbourethral glands)
  - Prostate gland
  - Penis
- Among the male reproductive structures only scrotum and penis are external and other structures are internal.
- Male perineum is the area between scrotum and anus.

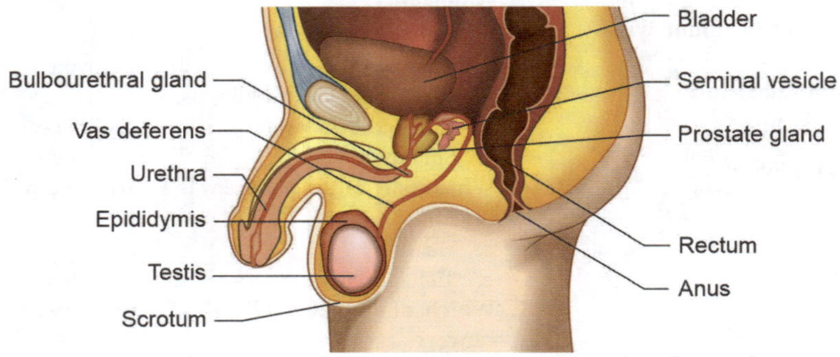

Figure 128: Male reproductive organs

Penis

- It is both sexual organ as well as organ for urination.
- Portion of the penis between its attachment to the pubic bone and to the head of the penis is known as shaft.
- External opening of the urethra is in the glans and is covered by foreskin or prepuce.
- Penis is homologous to female clitoris
- Penis is flaccid but during the time of erection it becomes rigid because corpora cavernosa fills with blood.
- Three erectile tissue—Two corpus cavernosa at dorsolateral site and one midventral tissue, corpus spongiosum
- Following ejaculation blood leaves the penis and it becomes flaccid.

Scrotum and Testes

- Scrotum is a double pouch hanging at the base of penis.
- It consists of two types of muscles –
  1. Dartos muscle: It made septum that separates two sacks of the scrotum.
  2. Cremaster muscle: This paired muscle made spermatic cord that connects testis to the inguinal ring.
- These two muscles contract to bring the scrotum close to the body cavity according to body temperature.
- Sperm production needs 2–3 degrees less temperature than core body temperature.
- Each half of the scrotum contains testicle with its epididymis and part of spermatic cord is held together by spermatic fascia.
- Vas deferens is the excretory duct of the testicle, and is the target in vasectomy
- Vas deferens is the continuation of epididymis and it continues with the ejaculatory duct and that conveys semen into urethra.
- Sperms are produced at seminiferous tubules and stored in epididymis.
- Length – 4.5–5.2 cm
- Weight – 10.5–14 g each
- By 33rd weeks of gestation the testes descend into the scrotum sac.
- Testes produce androgen as an endocrine gland and produce spermatozoa as an exocrine gland.
- Testicles produce male hormone testosterone and sperm.
- Three layers of testis (from inner to outer): Tunica Vasculosa, Tunica Albuginea, Tunica Vaginalis

Epididymis

- The epididymis is a crescent-shaped organ located at the posterior surface of each testis.
- It is approximately 4 cm long.
- The epididymis is divided into three parts: head, body, and tail.
- The head is the uppermost and largest part while tail is the smallest part of the epididymis.
- Inside the head of the epididymis, there is a highly coiled duct called the ductus epididymidis, which is about 4–5 cm in length.
- The tail of the epididymis continues as the vas deferens, which is a tubular structure that transports sperm from the epididymis to the ejaculatory duct.

Vas Deferens

- Length—45 cm
- Known as ductus deferens or sperm duct or spermatic deferens.
- It consists of pseudostratified columnar epithelium.

Sperm

- They are mature male sex cells.
- Sperms have self-propelling capacity with the help of flagella.
- A normal sperm has oval-shaped flattened head with nucleus, middle piece or protoplasmic neck and a tail.
- During fertilization, sperm head penetrates the ovum and tail part is lost.

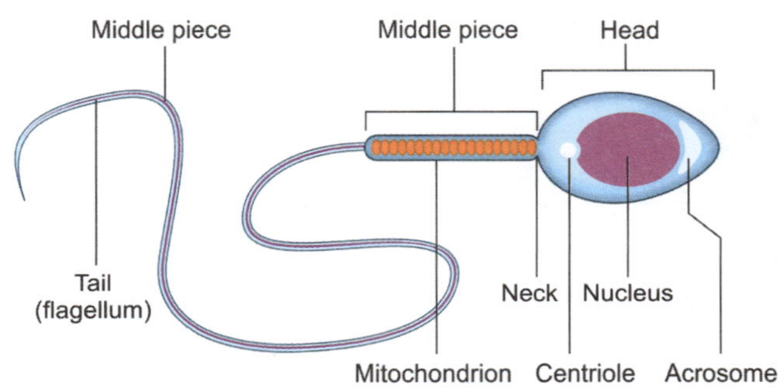

Figure 129: Structure of sperm

ACCESSORY SEX GLANDS

Seminal Vesicle

- The seminal vesicle is a gland located between the posterior part of the bladder and the rectum.
- It is responsible for providing up to 85% of the seminal plasma, which is the fluid that combines with sperm to form semen.
- The fluid secreted by the seminal vesicle is viscid (thick and sticky), alkaline (with a pH of 7.2–8), and yellow in color.
- The secretion of the seminal vesicle contains various components, including fructose, proteins, and prostaglandins.
- Fructose serves as an energy source (ATP) for the sperm cells.
- Prostaglandins are substances that play a role in smooth muscle contraction, which helps in ejaculation and sperm motility.

Prostate and Related Structures

- Prostate gland surrounds male urethra and urinary bladder.
- Adult prostate gland weighs 15–20 g and is 4–6 cm long.
- Posterior surface of the prostate is in close contact with rectal wall, and is the surface available for digital examination.
- Portion of urethra that passes through the prostate is known as prostatic urethra.

Cowper's Gland (Bulbourethral gland)

- The Cowper's gland is a paired gland located below each side of the prostate gland.
- It is homologous to the female Bartholin's gland.
- The secretion from the Cowper's gland is a clear, mucus-like fluid called pre-ejaculate or pre-cum.
- The pre-ejaculate serves multiple functions—Lubrication, neutralization of acidity and cleansing of the urethra before ejaculation.

MALE SEXUAL DEVELOPMENT AND FUNCTION

- Development of male genitalia requires two hormones:
  - Mullerian duct inhibitory factor secreted by sertoli cells
  - Testosterone secreted by Leydig cells.

Recent Question (NORCET 2022)

119. Male infertility is common complication of:
a. Measles
b. Chickenpox
c. Mumps
d. Rubella

Ans. (c) Please provide Answer

KEY POINTS

- The **temperature** in human testis is **2°-3°C** less than that of body providing a suitable environment for sperm production.
- The production of mature sperm from spermatogonia takes 74 days.

- Hypothalamus secretes GNRH which stimulates pituitary gland to produce LH and FSH.
  - LH stimulates leydig cells to produce testosterone.
  - Testosterone and FSH stimulate sertoli cells to start and complete spermatogenesis.
- Inhibin released from sertoli cells gives negative feedback to anterior pituitary.

Spermatogenesis

- Production and maturation of sperm in the seminiferous tubules is known as spermatogenesis.
- This process starts at puberty because of stimuli from anterior pituitary.
- Spermatogonia are the germinal cells and a portion continues to develop as sperm.
- During 24 days, when they are in contact with sertoli cells spermatogonia change and enlarge to form primary spermatocytes.
  - Primary spermatocyte divides and forms two secondary spermatocytes each with half number of chromosomes.
  - Secondary spermatocyte undergo next division after 2–3 days and become four spermatids each with half number of chromosome.

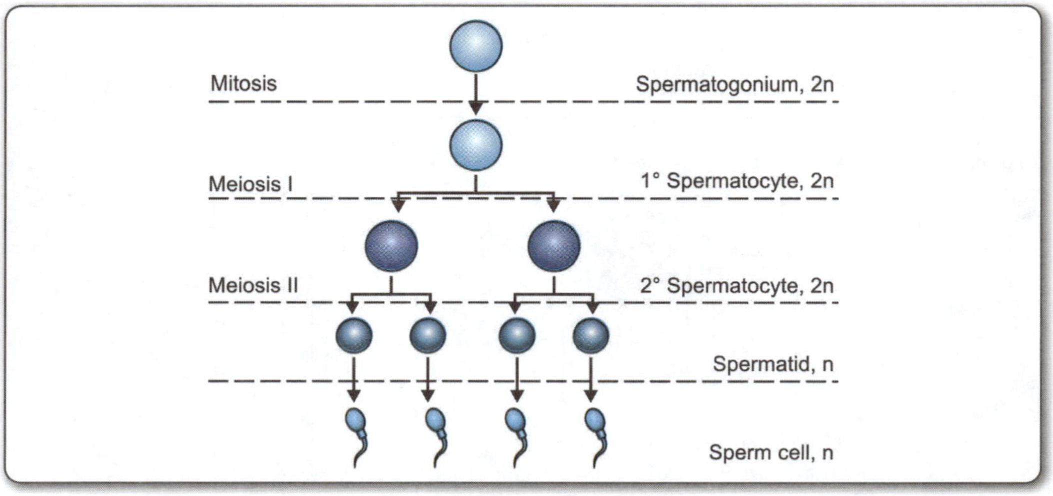

Figure 130: Spermatogenesis

Maturation in the Epididymis

- Sperms are produced in seminiferous tubules, these sperms are then stored in epididymis.
- After spending 24 hours in epididymis they become motile and capable of fertilization.
- Sperms can be stored up to a month.

Prostatic Fluid

- Prostate gland secretes milky fluid that forms the part of semen.
- This fluid keeps the sperm alive supplying nutrition to them.

Semen

- It is the thick secretion discharged by males at the end of sexual activity or orgasm.
- It contains both sperms and other secretions.
- It is slightly alkaline with a pH of about 7.5.
- Sperms live in the vagina for about 24–48 hours after the ejaculation.

KEY POINTS

- Prostate Specific Antigen (PSA) and Digital Rectal Examination are the screening test for Prostate Cancer.
- After TURP, continuous irrigation is needed.
- Irrigant of choice in Transurethral Resection of Prostate (TURP): **1.5% glycine**.
- Irrigant of choice in TURP with Bipolar cautery (plasmakinetics): **Normal saline (NS)**.

DIAGNOSTIC TESTS

Table 101: Diagnostic tests

Diagnosis	Description	Points to remember
Prostate specific antigen	• Screening test for cancer of prostate. • Normal PSA levels are less than 0.2–4 ng/mL. • PSA can be elevated during BPH and prostatitis.	• Prostatic massage, urethral instrumentation, ejaculation or rectal examination within 48 hours before assay can cause elevated PSA level.

Contd...

Diagnosis	Description	Points to remember
Digital rectal examination	Helps to assess size, shape and consistency of prostate gland. Helps to screen for prostate cancer.	
Semen analysis	Normal semen analysis shows following values Volume : 1.5–2 mL Concentration > 20 million sperm/mL Total sperm count>50–60 million Motility 60% grade 2 or higher Morphology 60% normal	

DISORDERS OF MALE REPRODUCTIVE SYSTEM

Benign Prostatic Hyperplasia (BPH)

- It is the benign enlargement of prostate gland.
- The enlargement of prostate gland is sufficient to obstruct the urethra and to cause lower urinary tract symptoms, urinary tract infection, and hematuria or compromized urinary tract function.
- In the prostate, testosterone is converted as dihydrotestosterone (DHT) by 5 alpha reductase. DHT suppresses the prostate growth and development throughout the life.
- In a person with BPH, the balance between DHT and 5 alpha reductase is lost.
- Man with BPH complains urinary symptoms such as nocturia, increased day time urinary frequency, urgency, hesitancy, decline in force of urinary stream, incomplete bladder emptying.
- Urinary obstruction leads to urinary retention and client may complain of dribbling of urine.
- Digital rectal examination is performed to differentiate between benign enlargement of prostate from prostatitis or adenocarcinoma.
- Urine test to rule out other conditions such as infection which may cause similar symptoms.
- **Prostate specific antigen:** PSA values are elevated in a person with BPH.
- **Urinary flow test:** To measure the strength and amount of urinary flow
- **Post void residual volume test:** To measure the amount of urine in bladder after voiding.
- Medications such as alpha blockers (these medications relax bladder neck muscles and make urination easier), 5 alpha reductase inhibitors (these medications shrink the size of prostate gland preventing the hormonal change)
- **Surgery Transurethral resection of the prostate (TURP):** Through the bladder, scope is inserted and prostate is removed. Soon after the removal, client may have a stronger urinary flow.
- **Transurethral incision of the prostate (TUIP):** Two small incisions or cuts given in prostate gland after it is accessed via urethra.
- **Suprapubic prostatectomy:** An abdominal incision is made to remove the prostate through the bladder.
- **Retropubic prostatectomy:** Without opening the bladder, by doing a low abdominal incision the prostate is removed. Erectile dysfunction and urinary incontinence may develop.
- **Perineal prostatectomy:** By an incision between anus and scrotum, the prostate is removed.

Transurethral Resection Syndrome

- It occurs when the irrigating fluid used during the procedure is absorbed into the bloodstream, causing fluid and electrolyte imbalances.
- During TURP, the fluid is irrigated in the closed space which leads to fluid and electrolytes shifting during the perioperative period and developing TURP syndrome.
- Due to fluid absorption (≥ 2 L), hyponatremia (Na <120 mmol/L) is developed that leads to ***bradycardia, confusion and hypertension.***

PROSTATE CANCER

- Carcinoma of the prostate gland which can spread to other body tissues such as bones and lymph nodes.
- Exact cause of prostate cancer is not known, but family history is believed as a risk factor.
- Digital rectal examination and prostate specific antigen have 50% accuracy in diagnosing this condition.
- Transrectal ultrasound and biopsy is also useful for diagnosing the condition.
- Radical prostatectomy is the treatment of choice for client with localized prostate cancer. Radical surgery involves removal of entire prostate gland, its outer capsule, the seminal vesicle, sections of vas deferens, adjacent lymph nodes and in many cases bladder neck.

Recent Question (CNCI 2021)

120. Which of the following is the feature of benign tumor?
a. Infiltrative type of growth
b. Metastasis is present
c. Contained within a capsule
d. Grows rapidly
Ans. (c) Contained within...

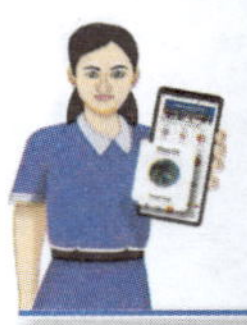

- **Cryosurgical ablation:** In this, surgeon inserts cryoprobes under transrectal ultrasound guidance, then freeze and destroy the tissue.

Testicular Cancer

- Cancerous growth in the testicle.
- Family history, exogenous estrogen and cryptorchidism are the known risk factors.
- Most common clinical manifestation is painless enlargement noted as heaviness in the testicle described as dragging sensation.
- Pain is rarely felt in this condition.
- Metastasis can occur to retroperitoneal lymph nodes and lungs.
- Alpha fetoprotein, beta human chorionic gonadotropin and lactic acid dehydrogenase are the tumor markers to detect testicular cancer.
- Radical orchiectomy is the surgery of choice in which testis, epididymis and vas deferens are removed.
- Retroperitoneal lymph node dissection will be done if there is lymph node involvement.

Testicular Torsion

- It occurs when the testicle is mobile and spermatic cord twists which causes cutting off blood supply.
- Acute scrotal swelling and severe pain are the manifestations.
- Testicular scan and Doppler ultrasonography are useful diagnostic tests.
- If torsion happens, emergency surgery is needed to untwist spermatic cord and immobilize testicle in scrotal sac by suturing them.
- Without emergency, surgery testicle may be atrophied or abscess can develop.

Orchitis

- Inflammation of testicle caused by viral infection.
- Mumps orchitis is developed by man who had mumps infection after puberty and usually both testicles are affected.
- Clinical manifestations include fever, reddened scrotal skin, extremely tender testicle and prostration
- Management includes bedrest, scrotal support, local heat application, and symptomatic management for pain, fever and infection.
- Permanent sterility can occur if both testicles are affected.

Epididymitis

- Inflammation of epididymis is known as epididymitis.
- Most often caused by bacteria.
- Warm, red and swollen scrotum, discharge from penis, painful urination or urge to urinate

Hydrocele: Painless collection of clear, yellow fluid in the scrotum

Hematocele: collection of blood in the tunica vaginalis caused by trauma.

Spermatocele: Cystic dilation of part of epididymis that contains a milky fluid and dead spermatozoa

Varicocele

- Dilation of network of vein (pampiniform plexus) supplying the testicle within the scrotum
- Most commonly it is seen in left side than right side because in the left side spermatic vein enters the renal vein at 90°.
- Right sided varicocele suggests tumor or retroperitoneal fibrosis.
- Pain is there and is relieved by masturbation, or sexual intercourse.
- Palpation of varicocele done with man in standing. On palpation, varicocele feels like a mass above and posterior to testicle.

Vasectomy

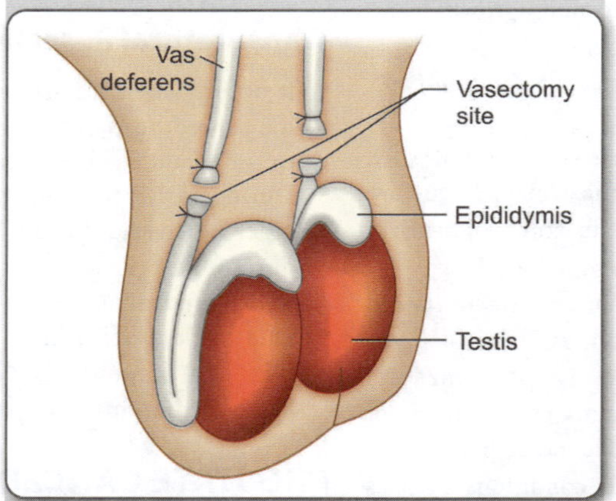

Figure 131: Vasectomy

- It is the permanent method of contraception among men.
- Cutting of vas deferens is done in the surgery. After cutting, tips are ligated or tucked into the adjacent tissue to prevent reanastomosis.
- Slight pain, swelling and bruising occurs post operatively and these symptoms can be controlled with ice packs and mild analgesics.
- Scrotal support also helps to provide comfort to the client.
- Client can resume sexual activities and heavy lifting after two weeks of surgery.

KEY POINTS

- Immediate post-operative period after prostatectomy, red-colored urine is anticipated. But if it becomes brisk bleeding or passage of clots, promptly contact the physician.
- **Varicocele** is predominantly seen on: Left side.
- Testicular torsion is treated with orchiopexy, in which the testis is anchored to the scrotal wall.

KEY POINTS

- After vasectomy, the client must practice alternative contraceptive methods until the semen analysis shows azoospermia.
- Vasovasostomy is the surgical reversal of vasectomy. It is expensive and fertility is not guaranteed.
- Cryptorchidism (undescended testes) occurs when one or both testicles do not descend into the scrotum.
- Orchiopexy (orchidopexy) or orchiorrhaphy is a surgery to move an undescended testicle into the scrotum and fix it there.

Undescended or Malpositioned Testis

- Testes descend from abdomen into the scrotum before birth.
- Undescended testis is known as cryptorchidism.
- A retractile testis descend into the scrotum and pull back into the inguinal canal because of hyperactive cremasteric reflex.

Infertility

- It means pregnancy doesn't occur even after having regular unprotected sex over 12 months period.
- **Pre-testicular cause:** Problem is with hormone. For example, some problems with pituitary or adrenal cortex.
- **Testicular:** Problem with testicles itself such as varicocele, torsion, etc.
- **Post-testicular:** Problem with structures distal to testis such as congenital blockage of vas deferens.
- Certain infection, exposure to certain chemicals, faulty intercourse practices are also responsible for infertility.

Phimosis

- Retraction of foreskin is impossible or difficult.
- Edema, erythema, tenderness, purulent discharge are the manifestations.
- Circumcision is the surgical management of choice.

Paraphimosis

- Tight foreskin once retracted cannot return to the normal position.
- Circulation may be affected causing edema and swelling rapidly.
- Condition is painful.
- Surgical incision over the foreskin is the management.

Posthitis

- Inflammation of the foreskin
- Good hygiene is recommended to prevent the condition

Balanitis

- Inflammation of the glans penis and mucous membrane beneath it
- Good hygiene is the preventive measure.

Priapism

- Prolonged persistent erection of penis without sexual desire
- Condition is painful.
- Occur, as a result of self-injection of medication such as papaverine (to treat impotence), use of certain medications such as phenothiazine, anticoagulants, etc.
- Two types are there, first high flow arterial priapism (less common and less painful) second veno-occlusive priapism (more common and painful).

Erectile Dysfunction

- Inability to achieve and maintain erection sufficient for sexual activities.
- Psychological factors like performance, anxiety, stress, fatigue, low-self-esteem, depression and change in relationship can cause this.
- Physiological factors like decrease in testosterone level, increase in estrogen and prolactin levels, reduced libido can also contribute to this.

Golden Points to Remember

- **Spironolactone** is the drug causing **gynecomastia** by decreasing testosterone production.
- Orchitis is the complication of mumps.
- Most common zone of origin for CA Prostate: **Peripheral zone.**
- Most common lobe involved in CA prostrate: **Posterior lobe.**
- Earliest symptoms of prostatism: **Nocturia.**
- Irrigant of choice in Transurethral Resection of Prostate (TURP): **1.5% glycine**.
- Irrigant of choice in TURP with Bipolar cautery (plasmakinetics): **Normal saline (NS).**
- Most common complication after TURP: Retrograde ejaculation OR Dry ejaculation.
- **Undescended testes** are more common on: **R**ight side [**Mn:** RUN]
- Congenital hydrocele is best treated by **Herniotomy**.
- Absence of fructose in semen indicates obstruction to seminal vesicle.
- Most common cause of urethritis is **C. trachomatis**.
- Absence of living spermatozoa in semen is called **Azoospermia**.
- Inability to retract the prepuce to reveal the glans penis is called **Phimosis.**
- **Descent of the testes** into the scrotum normally occurs before birth.
- **Cryptorchidism** is a condition in which one or both the testicles do not descend into the scrotum.
- The main cause of **genital warts** (Condylomata Acuminata) is human papilloma virus (HPV).

"Eat to live, not live to eat"
—Socrates

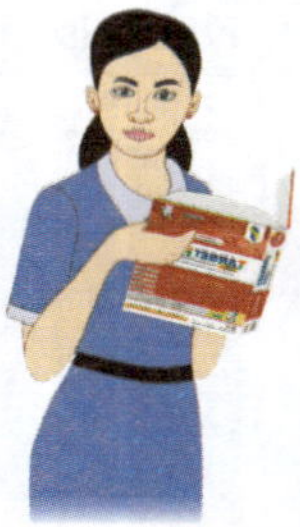

MULTIPLE CHOICE QUESTIONS
(Including Explained and Practice Questions)

MALE REPRODUCTIVE SYSTEM

ANATOMY OF MALE REPRODUCTIVE SYSTEM

3319. In male individuals, testosterone is normally produced by:
a. The Sertoli cells *(AIIMS-BBS SNO 2019)*
b. The interstitial cells of Leydig
c. The vas deferens
d. The epididymis

3320. What is the WHO criterion for minimum sperm count in normal semen? *(RAK MSc 2018)*
a. 60 Million b. 15 Million
c. 20 Million d. 30 Million

Explanation: A normal sperm count is at least 15 million sperm per milliliter of semen.

3321. Find out the correct statement regarding Bartholin's glands:
a. Homologous to bulbourethral glad in males
b. Found posteriorly and to right and left of the opening of vagina
c. They secrete mucous
d. All of the above

3322. Of the 46 chromosomes in the human cells, __________ are autosomes, and __________ are sex chromosomes.
a. 40, 6 b. 42, 4
c. 43, 3 d. 44, 2

3323. Males are determined by:
a. The presence of only one type of X chromosome
b. The presence of a Y chromosome
c. A gene carried on chromosome pair number 21
d. A gene carried on chromosome pair number 1

3324. The testes are located in the scrotum outside the body cavity because they:
a. Are closer to the penis than they would be in the body cavity
b. Are originally developed in the scrotum
c. Must be at a lower temperature than the body cavity for sperm production
d. Are pushed out because there is no room in the body cavity

3325. Erection of the penis occurs as a result of:
a. Contraction of the bulbourethral muscles
b. Movement of internal bones
c. Accumulation of lymphatic fluid
d. Engorgement of erectile tissue with blood

3326. The forceful expulsion of semen from the urethra caused by the contraction of the smooth muscle in the urethra and skeletal muscle surrounding the base of the penis is called:
a. Ejaculation b. Emission
c. Climax d. Neutralization

3327. The size of a prostate is about the size of:
a. Pea b. Lime
c. Walnut d. Grape

3328. Function of prostate gland:
a. Makes fluid that nourishes sperm
b. Sterilizes urine in men
c. Filters urine in men
d. Backup storage for sperm

3329. The testes are suspended in the scrotum in order to:
a. Protect the sperm from high abdominal temperature
b. Protect the testes from traumatic injuries
c. Facilitate blood flow to testes during embryonic period
d. All of the above

3330. Abnormal communication between the urinary and genital tract is called genitourinary: *(RRB SSNE 2015)*
a. Fistula b. Tumor
c. Atresia d. Prolapse

3331. Length of male urethra is:
a. 4 cm b. 10 cm
c. 15 cm d. 20 cm

Explanation: length of male urethra is 20 cm and that of female is 4 cm.

3332. Ejaculatory duct opens into:
a. Membranous urethra
b. Prostatic urethra
c. Penile urethra
d. Seminal vesicles

3333. Fructose, a source of energy for spermatozoa, is found primarily in secretions from:
a. Bulbourethral glands b. Epididymus
c. Prostrate d. Seminal vesicles

3334. Which among the following is present in male with hypospadias:
a. Unable to produce healthy sperm
b. Sperm count will decreases
c. Hematuria
d. Unable to deposit sperms high in vagina

3335. The narrowest part of male urethra is the:
a. Prostatic part
b. Membranous part
c. External urethral meatus
d. Internal urethral orifice

3336. During intra-uterine life of fetal development majority of testicles descend into the scrotum by:
a. 24 weeks b. 26 weeks
c. 28 weeks d. 30 weeks

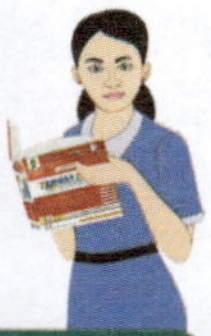

Ans.
3319. b
3320. b
3321. d
3322. d
3323. b
3324. c
3325. d
3326. a
3327. c
3328. a
3329. a
3330. a
3331. d
3332. b
3333. d
3334. d
3335. c
3336. c

MALE SEXUAL DEVELOPMENT & FUNCTION

3337. All of the following enzymes are present in Leydig cells except: *(Safdarjung NO 2018)*

a. CYPscc b. 17-alpha hydroxylase
c. 17, 20 lyase d. 21- hydroxylase

Explanation:

- CYPscc is not present in Leydig cells
- The biosynthesis of testosterone requires the activities of four enzymes, cholesterol side-chain cleavage enzyme (P450, c), 3-hydroxysteroid dehydrogenase/A5 -A4 isomerase (3PHSD), 17alpha-hydroxylase/ 17-20 lyase (P45017), Steroid **21-hydroxylase**, also called steroid **21**-monooxygenase and 17-ketosteroid reductase.

3338. Normal pH of Semen is:

a. Acidic
b. Alkaline
c. Neutral
d. Some-times acidic and some-time alkaline

3339. Capacitance of sperm takes place in:

a. Vas deferens b. Uterus
c. Epididymis d. Testis

3340. The process of maturation of sperm is referred as:

a. Spermatogenesis b. Oogenesis
c. Orthogenesis d. Ovogenesis

3341. Correct order of spermatogenesis?

a. Germ cells → spermatogonia → primary spermatocyte → secondary spermatocyte → spermatids
b. Germ cells → primary spermatocytes → secondary spermatocytes → sperms
c. Germ cells → primary spermatocytes → spermatogonia → secondary spermatocytes → sperms
d. Germ cells → primary spermatocytes → secondary spermatocytes → sperms → spermatogonia

3342. Capacitation of sperm means:

a. They become motile
b. Able to fertilize secondary oocyte
c. They can penetrate the cervical mucosa
d. All of the above

3343. Time duration for maturation of spermatogonia to mature spermatozoa:

a. 14 days b. 28 days
c. 61 days d. 280 days

3344. Sperms are produced by the process of:

a. Spermatogenesis b. Ovulation
c. Oogenesis d. Gestational

ASSESSMENT & DIAGNOSTIC TESTS

3345. Most commonly performed test for assessing the adequacy of sperm is:

a. Sperm morphology b. Sperm motility
c. Sperm count d. Semen volume

Explanation: Sperm motility is the most significant criterion when assessing male infertility. As per WHO 1 mL of semen contain 15 million sperm.

3346. Huhner test is used for:

a. To determine the number, motility and activity of sperm
b. To determine ABO incompatibility reaction between mother and newborn
c. To assess the respiratory maturity of newborn
d. To assess the respiratory distress of newborn baby

Explanation: It is a test used in sterility studies that involves postcoital examination of fluid aspirated from the vagina and cervix to determine the presence or survival of sperm in these areas.

3347. Semen collection technique include:

a. Coitus interruptus b. Condom collection
c. Epididymal extraction d. All of these

3348. Correct regarding semen collection include:

a. Provide a fresh sample
b. Sample should be refrigerated
c. Patient can continue with sexual activity, no need of any abstinence
d. All of the above

3349. Gross examination of semen does include:

a. Volume b. Color
c. Viscosity d. All of these

3350. Which of the following is not a microscopic examination of semen?

a. Counting b. Motility
c. pH d. Viability

3351. Semen pH level is:

a. 3.2-4.8 b. 4.2-5.8
c. 5.2-6.8 d. 7.2-7.8

3352. Solution used for bladder irrigation during TURP is:

a. NS b. RL
c. Glycine d. Sterile water

Explanation: 1.5% Glycine Irrigation is used as a urologic irrigating fluid with endoscopic instruments during transurethral procedures requiring distension, irrigation, and lavage of the urinary bladder. It may be used for lavage of an indwelling catheter to maintain patency.

3353. Normal level of PSA is:

a. 5–8 ng/ml b. 0.3–0.8 ng/ml
c. 1–4 ng/ml d. 4–5 ng/ml

3354. Congenital factor related to male that is responsible for infertility includes:

a. Undescended testes b. Hypospadias
c. Kartagener syndrome d. All of the above

3355. All among the following are characterized by raised scrotal temperature; EXCEPT:

a. Varicocele
b. Big hydrocele
c. Filariasis
d. BPH

BENIGN PROSTATIC HYPERPLASIA (BPH)

3356. Education to a client who is undergoing antibiotic therapy for chronic bacterial prostatitis include:

a. Surgery is needed
b. Prolonged hospital stay is recommended
c. Long-term therapy may be indicated in immune-compromised client
d. It can lead to BPH

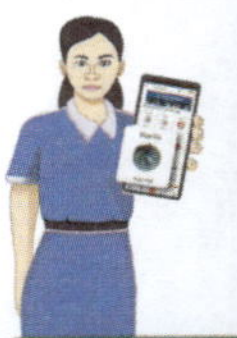

Ans.

3337. a
3338. b
3339. b
3340. a
3341. a
3342. b
3343. c
3344. a
3345. b
3346. a
3347. d
3348. a
3349. d
3350. c
3351. d
3352. c
3353. c
3354. d
3355. d
3356. c

3357. Early clinical manifestations of Nodular Hyperplasia of Prostate (NHP) include:
a. Frequency of urine
b. Nocturia.
c. Overflow dribbling
d. All of these

3358. BPH is:
a. Hyperplasia of stromal cells
b. Hyperplasia of epithelial cells
c. Hyperplasia of endothelial cells
d. Both a and b

3359. BPH develops from which zone of prostate gland?
a. Peripheral zone
b. Transition zone
c. Central zone
d. Both a and c

3360. Hormonal cause behind BPH is:
a. Oestrogen
b. Testosterone
c. Dihydrotestosterone
d. Progesterone

3361. Which of the following drug can aggravate BPH?
a. Inhalational Ipratropium
b. Timolol
c. Oral hypoglycemic agents
d. Calcium channel blockers

3362. Which among the following sign and symptom can be seen in BPH?
a. Difficulty in initiating voiding
b. Incomplete bladder emptying
c. Dribbling at the end of urination
d. All of the above

3363. In BPH difficulty in initiating voiding and a feeling of incomplete bladder emptying is because of:
a. Urethral obstruction
b. Inflammation of the prostate
c. Low bladder tone
d. VUR

3364. Which of the following statement regarding relationship between prostate cancer and BPH is true?
a. Prostate cancer is caused by BPH
b. BPH and prostate cancer are unrelated
c. BPH is a symptom of prostate cancer
d. None of the above

3365. Which of the following is true about benign prostatic hypertrophy (BPH)?
a. It causes urethral obstruction
b. Hydronephrosis and renal failure are its complication
c. Digital rectal examination is used for diagnosing this condition
d. All of the above

3366. Aim of medical management of benign prostate hyperplasia (BPH) is:
a. Improve symptoms and relief obstruction
b. Improve bladder emptying
c. Prevent UTIs and avoid renal insult
d. All of the above

3367. Patients who have been operated for BPH:
a. Require routine rectal examination to detect development of ca prostate
b. Do not require prostate examination
c. Have lesser incidence of ca prostate
d. Have a greater incidence of Ca prostate

3368. The following are the important preoperative nursing care for a patient with benign prostatic hypertrophy; EXCEPT:
a. Hormonal therapy *(ESIC 2019)*
b. Assure nutrition and correct fluid and electrolyte balance.
c. Promoting urinary drainage
d. Acid-ash diet to treat infection

Explanation: Hormone therapy is not advised for a client with benign prostatic hypertrophy, it can further increase the growth of prostatic cells.

CANCER OF PROSTATE AND TESTIS

3369. Major clinical finding in prostatic enlargement is:
a. Red blood cell casts in urine
b. Pain in the groin
c. Increased urinary frequency in an old man
d. General malaise

3370. Which of the following test is used to assess size, shape and consistency of prostate?
a. PSA
b. DRE
c. TURP
d. Proctoscope

Explanation: In a male patient, Digital Rectal Examination (DRE) is used to examine prostate for its size, shape and consistency by palpating the prostate through rectal wall as shown in the picture below.

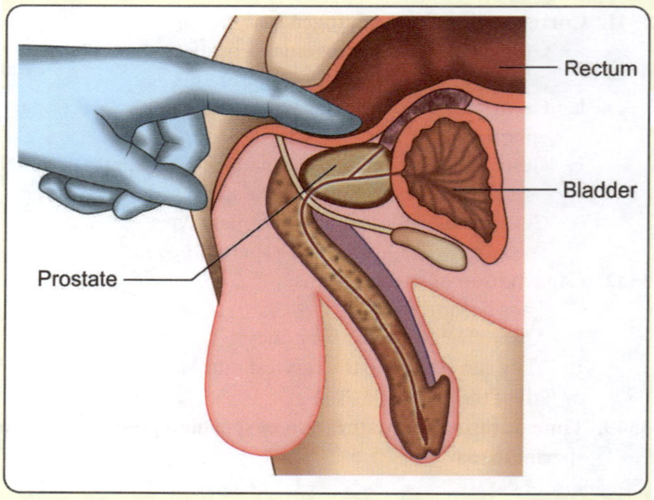

3371. Surgical removal of prostate through an endoscope is called:
a. TUNA
b. TURP
c. PVP
d. PUJO

3372. Important nursing management following transurethral resection of prostate is: *(AIIMS 1996)*
a. Assess the surgical site for signs of infection
b. Assess the vital signs
c. Maintaining patency of a three-way Foleys catheter for hemostasis
d. Administer ordered analgesics

Explanation: Catheter provides decompression to the bladder and it prevent bladder distention and bleeding and thus, promote hemostasis.

Ans.

3357. d
3358. d
3359. b
3360. c
3361. a
3362. d
3363. a
3364. b
3365. d
3366. d
3367. a
3368. a
3369. c
3370. b
3371. b
3372. c

3373. Which among the following will be affected in a client with prostatectomy?
a. Erection function
b. Spermatogenesis
c. Production of seminal fluid
d. Ejaculatory function

3374. Which of the following complication require immediate attention in a patient who underwent prostatectomy?
a. Abdominal pain
b. Hemorrhage
c. Oliguria
d. Urinary incontinence

3375. During bladder irrigation with a three-way urinary catheter following prostatectomy client complains of bladder spasms with the catheter in place. The best nursing advice is:
a. Remove the catheter
b. Insert new catheter
c. Educate Kegel exercises
d. This feeling is normal and he should not try to urinate around the catheter

OTHER DISORDERS OF MALE REPRODUCTIVE SYSTEM

3376. Vaccination against mumps can prevent: *(AIIMS Nagpur NO 2018)*
a. Hydrocele b. Orchitis
c. Varicocele d. Undescended testes

Explanation: Most common cause of viral orchitis is the mumps. Vaccination against mumps can prevent orchitis.

3377. Complete absence of seminal fluid upon ejaculation is known as:
a. Aspermia b. Azoospermia
c. Asthenospermia d. Teratozoospermia

3378. Absence of sperm in the ejaculate is known as:
a. Aspermia b. Azoospermia
c. Asthenospermia d. Teratozoospermia

Explanation: Azoospermia is a condition in which there is no sperm in the ejaculate. A patient has azoospermia if microscopic examination of two separate concentrated semen samples reveals no sperm. Aspermia is the complete absence of seminal fluid upon ejaculation.

3379. Presence of sperm with abnormal morphology that affects fertility in males:
a. Azoospermia
b. Teratozoospermia
c. Asthenospermia
d. Aspermia

3380. Asthenospermia is:
a. Failure to produce semen
b. Absence of sperms from the semen
c. Reduced sperm motility
d. Presence of sperm with abnormal morphology

3381. Necrospermia refers to:
a. Absence of sperm b. Dead sperm
c. Immotile sperm d. Low sperm count

3382. Causes of infertility in males include:
a. Defective spermatogenesis
b. Sexual dysfunction
c. Obstruction of the efferent ducts
d. All of the above

3383. Hydrocele is:
a. Collection of clear yellow fluid in scrotum
b. Collection of blood in the tunica vaginalis layer of testes
c. Dilation and varicosity of the network of veins supplying the testicles
d. All of the above

3384. Hematocele is:
a. Collection of clear yellow fluid in scrotum
b. Collection of blood in the tunica vaginalis layer of testes
c. Dilation and varicosity of the network of veins supplying the testicles
d. All of the above

3385. Dilatation of the pampiniform venous plexus and the internal spermatic vein is known as:
a. Varicose veins b. Varicosities
c. Varicocele d. Hematocele

3386. "Bag of worms" feel in testis is characterstic of:
a. Varicocele b. Hydrocele
c. Rotation of testis d. Testicular malignancy

3387. Varicocele is most commonly seen in:
a. Left side
b. Right side
c. Always occurs on both side together
d. Equally on left and right side

Explanation: Most varicoceles occur on the left side as a result of the left spermatic vein draining into the left renal vein at a 90-degree angle, compared to the right spermatic vein, which drains more directly into the inferior vena cava.

3388. What is the common complication of varicocele? *(Kerala PSC, Nov 2014)*
a. Phimosis b. Erectile dysfunction
c. Infertility d. Cancer

3389. Infertility is defined as pregnancy doesn't occur even after having regular unprotected sex over the period of:
a. Six months b. Nine months
c. Twelve months d. Eighteen months

3390. Post-testicular cause of infertility includes:
a. Hormonal problems
b. Testicular torsion
c. Congenital blockage of vas deferens
d. Varicocele

Explanation: Post-testicular cause of infertility in male includes problem with structures distal to testis such as congenital blockage of vas deference. Hormonal problems are pretesticular, varicocele and testicular torsion are testicular cause of infertility.

3391. In vasectomy, which of the following structure is cut:
a. Epididymis b. Pampiniform plexus
c. Vas deferens d. Ejaculatory duct

Explanation: Cutting of vas deference is done in the surgery after cutting tips are ligated or tucking into the adjacent tissue to prevent re anastomosis.

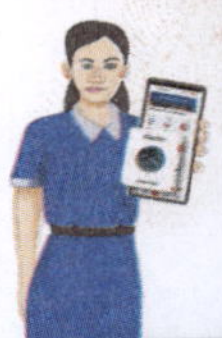

Ans.
3373. c
3374. b
3375. d
3376. b
3377. a
3378. b
3379. b
3380. c
3381. b
3382. d
3383. a
3384. b
3385. c
3386. a
3387. a
3388. c
3389. c
3390. c
3391. c

3392. The nurse should explain to the patient who underwent vasectomy that:
a. Immediately after the surgery you are sterile
b. No need to use any other contraceptive methods
c. Normal erection and ejaculation functions will be there
d. An alternative form of contraception will be necessary for 6–8 weeks

3393. Undescended testes are known as:
a. Cushingoid appearance b. Hypoaldosteronism
c. Cryptorchidism d. Phimosis

3394. Which of the following is true about cryptorchidism:
a. It is also known as undescended testes
b. In most of the cases testes lie at inguinal ring
c. Orchidopexy is the surgical management
d. All of the above

3395. Testicular atrophy is caused by:
a. Atherosclerotic narrowing of testicular blood vessels
b. Testicular inflammation
c. Poor nutrition
d. All of the above

3396. Most common location of undescended testes is:
a. Retro-peritoneum b. Inguinal ring
c. Upper scrotum d. Inguinal canal

3397. Twisting of spermatic cord which leads to cutting off blood supply to testicle is known as:
a. Varicosities b. Testicular torsion
c. Orchitis d. Cryptorchidism

3398. Best indication of testicular biopsy is:
a. Oligospermia b. Azoospermia
c. Dyspareunia d. BPH

3399. Retraction of foreskin is difficult or impossible is known as:
a. Cushingoid appearance b. Hypoaldosteronism
c. Cryptorchidism d. Phimosis

3400. Foreskin cannot be returned to its normal position, once retracted is known as:
a. Balanitis b. Paraphimosis
c. Posthitis d. Cryptorchidism

3401. Surgery of phimosis is:
a. Orchidopexy b. Circumcision
c. Shunting surgery d. Dilatation

3402. The urethra which opens on the dorsal surface of the penis is termed: *(DSSSB PHN, 2015)*
a. Epispadias b. Hypospadias
c. Cryptorchidism d. Anorchidism

3403. Inflammation of glans penis is:
a. Balanitis b. Paraphimosis
c. Posthitis d. Cryptorchidism

3404. Inflammation of foreskin of penis is:
a. Balanitis b. Paraphimosis
c. Posthitis d. Cryptorchidism

3405. Persistent and prolonged penile erection without sexual desire is known as:
a. Phimosis b. Paraphimosis
c. Cryptorchidism d. Priapism

3406. Management for scrotal edema following penile implant is:
a. Cold application
b. Trendelenburg position
c. Maintain strict I/O chart and report to physician
d. Elevate the scrotum using a soft support

Explanation: Scrotal elevation using soft support will help us to reduce the edema. T-bandage is commonly used.

3407. Genetic condition characterized by azoospermic male is:
a. Down's Syndrome
b. Edward syndrome
c. Klinefelter's Syndrome
d. Neurofibromatosis

3408. Male intersex is:
a. Male gonads with female external genitalia
b. Female gonads with male external genitalia
c. Sex between two males
d. Sex between one male and one female

3409. Gonadotropin deficiency leads to testicular failure is known as:
a. Exstrophy bladder
b. Kallmann Syndrome
c. Male pseudohermaphroditism
d. Bloom syndrome

3410. Gynecomastia is present in:
a. Altered ratio of estrogens to androgens
b. Klinefelter's syndrome
c. Increase in estrogen production
d. All of the above

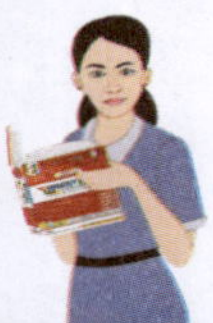

Ans.
3392. d
3393. c
3394. d
3395. d
3396. d
3397. b
3398. b
3399. d
3400. b
3401. b
3402. a
3403. a
3404. c
3405. d
3406. d
3407. c
3408. a
3409. b
3410. d

PERIOPERATIVE NURSING CARE

INTRODUCTION

- Perioperative nursing consists the roles and responsibilities during the three phases of surgery (preoperative, intra-operative and post-operative) of the patients.
  - **Preoperative:** This phase starts from the decision of surgery till the time the patient reaches on OT table.
  - **Intraoperative:** Starts from the time when the patient is brought inside OT till the time patient is transferred to the recovery area.
  - **Postoperative:** Begins when the patient is transferred to recovery area till the time patient undergoes a follow-up check up either in hospital setting or at home.
    - **Immediate postoperative stage:** 1–4 hours after surgery
    - **Intermediate postoperative stage:** 4–24 hours after surgery
    - **Extended postoperative stages:** 1–4 days after surgery
- Metformin is usually held 48 hours before surgery and restarted when full food and fluid intake has restarted and normal renal function has been resumed.
- **Deep breathing and coughing exercises** in the pre-operative and post-operative period help to reduce respiratory complications in the client.

TYPES OF SURGERIES

- **Emergent**: Delay can be fatal, e.g., Head-injury, intestinal obstruction, heavy bleeding, Gunshot injury, etc.
- **Urgent**: Surgery can be delayed only up to 24 hrs. e.g., Ureteral stones, appendicitis, etc.
- **Elective**: Surgery can be planned, e.g., Gall bladder stones, Total hip replacement, cataract, etc.
- **Optional**: Decision to undergo surgery is optional, e.g., Cosmetic surgeries

SURGICAL APPROACHES

- **Curative:** Treats disease/disorder
- **Ambulatory:** Patient gets discharged within 24 hours after surgery
- **Palliative:** Relieves symptoms only
- **Laparoscopic:** Uses small incisions and fiberoptic instruments.
- **Robotic:** Provides 3D view. Requires laparoscopic cameras, computer and robotic instruments. High quality of precision.

PREOPERATIVE NURSING CARE

Table 102: Nursing responsibility in preoperative period

Preoperative nursing care	Description
Informed consent	• Obtaining informed consent is a surgeon's responsibility • Nurse has to verify that informed consent is taken • Nurse must ensure that patient has understood all aspects of surgery. • Minors, elderly, psychiatric patients may need a legal guardian to provide consent.
Preoperative Assessment	• Perform thorough physical examination and notify physician for any peculiar findings. • Take thorough history to assess any allergy to latex, rubber items, food substance, iodine, any medication, etc.
Nutrition/ Elimination	• Check physician's orders for NPO status. • Withhold solid foods 6 hours before general anesthesia and 3 hours before local anesthesia. • Insert a large I/V cannula to administer fluids or blood products in case of emergency or for subsequent use. • Check physician's orders for bowel preparation especially in case of abdominal surgeries. • Administer laxatives/enema as per the hospital policy. • Document last meal or drinks taken along with time.

Contd...

KEY POINT

Incentive spirometry is contraindicated in some surgeries such as **craniotomy, eye, ear surgery**.

Recent Question (NORCET 2023)

121. Surgical check list includes all except:
a. Time in
b. Time out
c. Sign in
d. Sign out
Ans. (a) Time in

Recent Question (NORCET 2022)

122. Which gas is used in laparoscopy procedure?
a. CO2
b. CO
c. Oxygen
d. Nitrogen
Ans. (a) CO2

(NORCET 2022)

Requires insufflation of body cavity with CO_2.

Recent Questions (NORCET 2020)

123. Patients scheduled for surgery are instructed to remove nail polish. What is the reason for removing nail polish before surgery?
a. To observe clubbing of fingers
b. To detect cyanosis caused by low oxygen level
c. Both A and B
d. None of the above
Ans. (b) To detect...

124. Surgical glove will be discarded in which color biomedical bag?
a. Yellow
b. Black
c. Green
d. Red
Ans. (d) Red

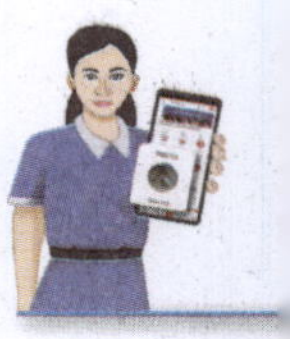

Preoperative nursing care	Description
Preparation of Patient and Surgical site	• Instruct patient to remove nail-polish, jewellery, dentures, contact lenses (if any), pins, any metal item. • Assess patient for any history of metal implant, pacemaker, prostheses, etc. • Surgical site should be shaved and cleaned with anti-septic solution one day before surgery. • Put an identification band over patient's wrist. • Obtain all lab reports, ECGs, X-rays, CT scan, etc. and attach with patient's file. • Administer pre-operative medication/ perform sensitivity test as prescribed by surgeon before shifting the patient to OT.
Patient centered teaching	• Teach deep breathing and coughing exercises • Teach diaphragmatic breathing. • **Incentive spirometry** ▪ Place mouthpiece tightly inside mouth. ▪ Inhale gently and try to lift all three balls/flow rate indicator from 600 to 900. ▪ Try to hold balls for at least 5 sec. ▪ Breathe out through pursed lips. • **Leg exercises** ▪ Gastrocnemius (calf—muscles) exercise- Point your toes up and down. ▪ Quadriceps (Thigh-muscles) exercise – Press and relax the back of the knee against bed alternatively. ▪ **Foot exercise:** Rotate foot in circle (clockwise and anti-clock wise). • **Pain management** ▪ Inform patient about pain-medications, side-effects, use of opioids. ▪ Demonstrate the use of patient controlled analgesia (PCA), if preferred.

PREOPERATIVE PERIOD: NURSING RESPONSIBILITY

- Ensure NPO status of the client
- Assist the surgeon while getting informed written consent
- Ask about any known allergy
- Ask about previous and current medical history
- Collect current medication history such as anti-hypertensive, hypoglycemic agents, anti-coagulants, etc.
- Make sure that ordered investigations are done for the clients such as coagulation profile, CBC, etc.
- Confirm the identification of patient before receiving him/her on the OT table.

INTRAOPERATIVE PERIOD: NURSING RESPONSIBILITY

Scrub Nurse

- Ensure surgical asepsis
- Provide all the instruments and materials required by surgical team for the surgery.
- Keep a count of instruments, sutures, needles and sponge used during surgery
- Coordinate with circulatory nurse

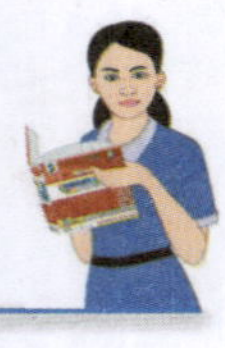

Circulatory Nurse

- Arrange, supply and articles needed by surgical team
- Communicate the progress about the surgery to patient's relatives and recovery room staff.

PAIN

- Pain is defined as an unpleasant sensory perception caused by injury or illness.
- Pain is the fifth vital sign (although it is a symptom; not a sign)
- **Pain theories**
  - **The specificity theory:** There are specific pain receptors and pathways which exist to transmit pain signals to pain center in the brain.
  - **The pattern theory:** This theory asserts the existence of rapid and slow conduction pathway which conducts pain signal to the brain through spinal cord.
  - **The gate control theory:** This theory emphasizes that non-painful signal (input) closes the gates to painful signal (input). This prevents pain information from travelling to CNS. Hence non-painful stimulus can suppress the pain perception. This theory forms the basis for some non-pharmacological pain management techniques, i.e., distraction, acupressure and cutaneous stimulation, etc.
- **Pain assessment**
  - Wong-baker Pain Rating Scale

Recent Questions (NORCET 2020)

125. Use of vaporizers in OT is to:
a. Maintain required humidity in OT
b. Make sure required air exchange occurred in OT
c. Deliver given concentration of volatile anesthetic agent.
d. Disinfect environmental air in OT

Ans. (c) Deliver given...

126. Therapeutic use of paracetamol is:
a. Prevent nausea and vomiting
b. Pain relief
c. Motion sickness
d. All of the above

Ans. (b) Pain relief

127. The primary action of injection paracetamol is
a. Antiemetic
b. Anti-motility
c. Anti-Inflammatory
d. Antipyretic

Ans. (d) Antipyretic

128. Surgical complications that result from foreign materials such as surgical sponge or gauze piece accidentally left inside patient's body is known as:
a. Surgical hemostatic syndrome
b. Gossypiboma
c. Idiopathic necrosis
d. Gossypium hirsutum

Ans. (b) Gossypiboma

129. Jackson Pratt drain was used in all of the following surgery, EXCEPT
a. Thoracic surgery
b. Head and neck surgery
c. Abdominal surgery
d. Breast reduction and breast reconstruction surgery

Ans. (b) Head and neck...

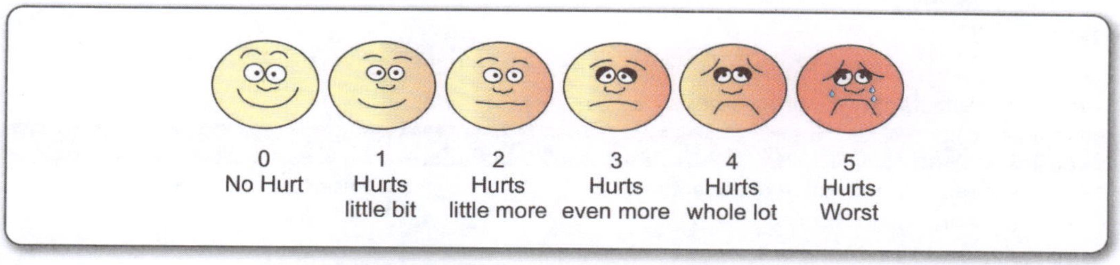

0
No Hurt
1
Hurts
little bit
2
Hurts
little more
3
Hurts
even more
4
Hurts
whole lot
5
Hurts
Worst

Figure 132: Wong-Baker pain rating scale

- Used in children aged more than three years to rate pain severity
  - Numerical rating scale

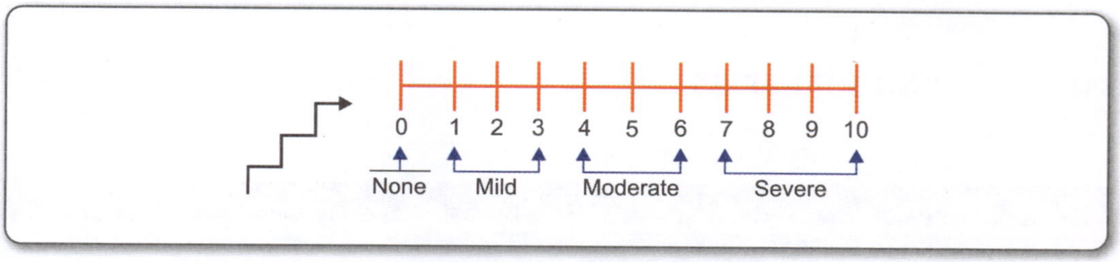

Figure 133: Numerical rating scale

- Used among children and adult aged more than 10 years.

Dolorimeter: It is the instrument used to measure pain threshold and pain tolerance.

  - Visual analogue scale
- This pain rating scale consists of a straight line between two extreme sensations of pain, i.e., no pain at all to the most severe pain.

No
pain
Pain as bad
as it could
possible be

Figure 134: Visual analogue scale

Pain Management

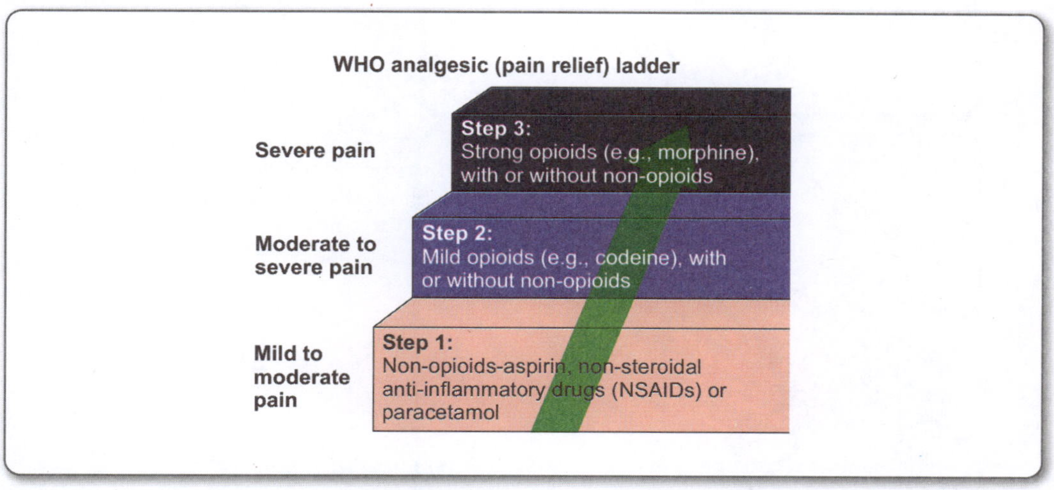

Figure 135: WHO pain ladder

KEY POINT

Patient-controlled analgesia (PCA) is a method of pain control that gives patients the power to control their pain

Recent Question
(NORCET 2023)

130. As per the schedule OT list nurse Reena has to scrub for the next laparoscopic cholecystectomy surgery. Arrange the given below activity in ascending order which the nurse reena will perform to get ready for the surgery?

a. Wear gloves
B. Scrubbing
C. Wear gown
D. Arrange and count instrument

a. D, B, A, C
b. B, A, C, D
c. B, C, A, D
d. D, A, B, C

Ans. (c) B, C, A, D

Recent Question
(NORCET 2020)

131. Which of the following gases is most pungent smelling?

a. Sevoflurane
b. Isoflurane
c. Both are equally pungent
d. Benzene

Ans. (b) Isoflurane

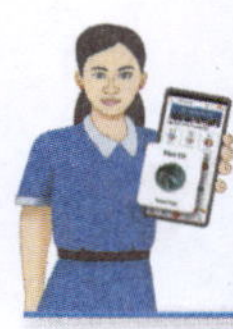

TYPES OF ANESTHESIA

Table 103: Methods of administration and effects of types of anesthesia

Types of anesthesia	Effects	Methods of administration
General anesthesia	• Loss of sensory perception of the entire body • Produce unconsciousness	IV infusion or inhalation
Regional anesthesia or nerve block anesthesia	• Loss of sensation over specific region of the body • No unconsciousness	• Spinal block • Epidural block • Regional block
Local anesthesia	• Loss of sensation over a small/limited area of the body • No unconsciousness	Topical application or infiltration

COMMON POSITIONS USED DURING SURGERIES

Table 104: Common positions used during surgeries

Position	Picture	Surgeries used for
Supine/Dorsal position	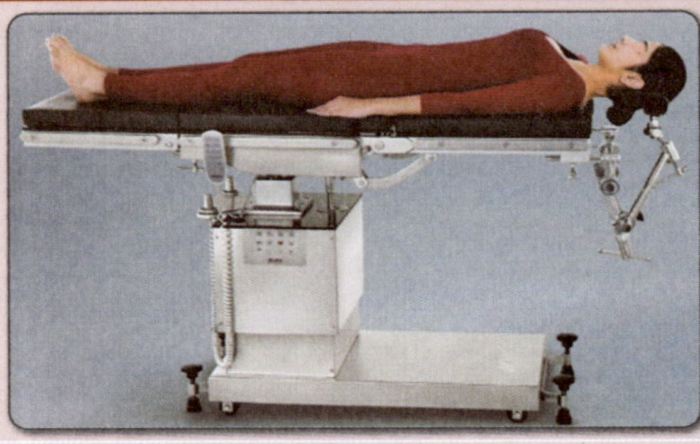	Most common operative position, e.g., Laparotomy, certain Gynecological and Orthopedic cases.
Prone	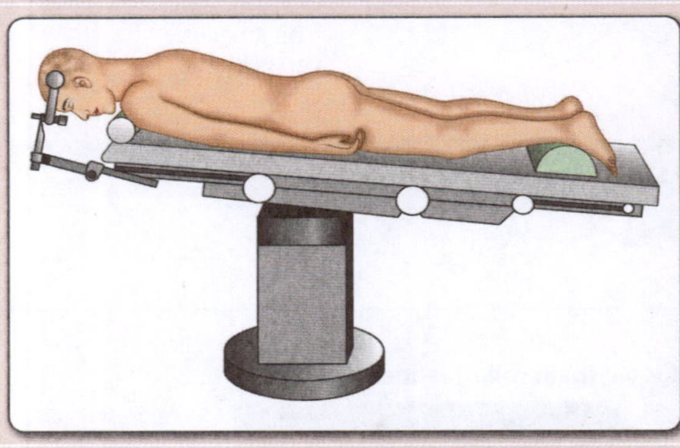	Laminectomy, rectal surgery, surgery involves cervical spine, back and dorsal extremities
Trendelenburg Position (Head tilted down 15 degree)	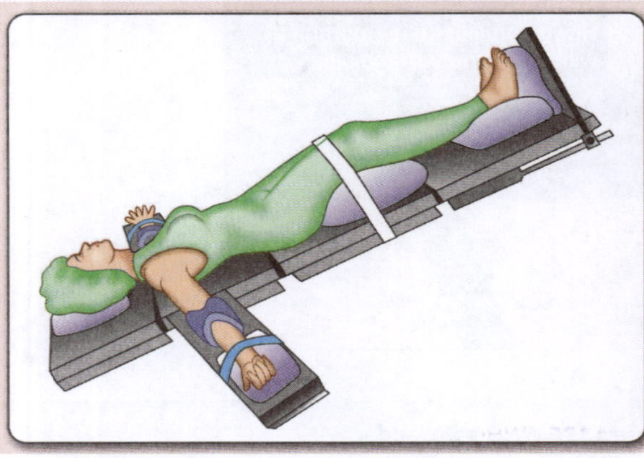	Common position for laparoscopic surgery in pelvic or lower abdominal region

Contd...

Position	Picture	Surgeries used for
Reverse Trendelenburg Position	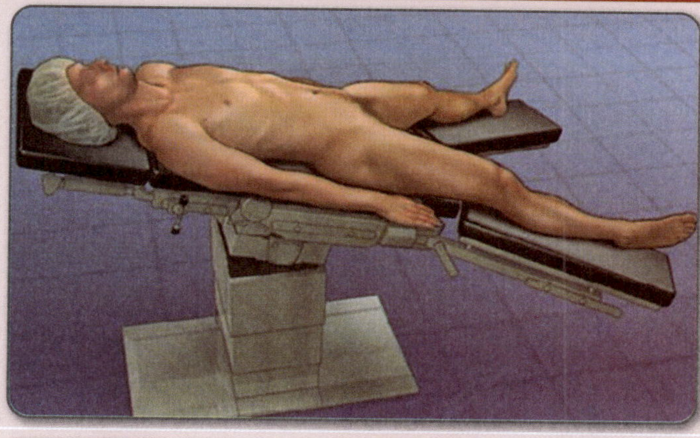	Used for Head and Neck surgery to reduce venous congestion
Lateral of Kidney position	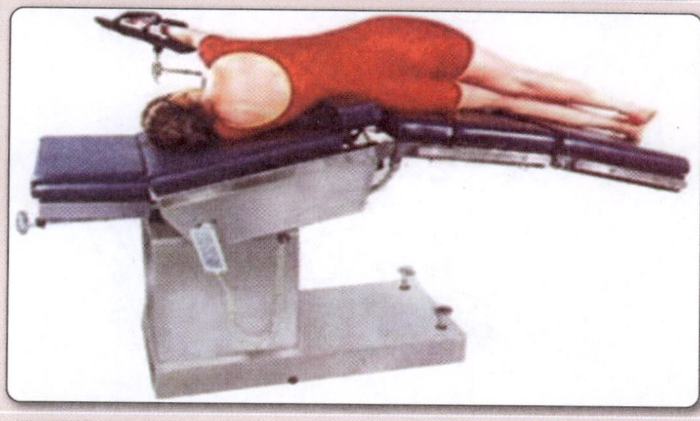	Renal surgery
Lithotomy	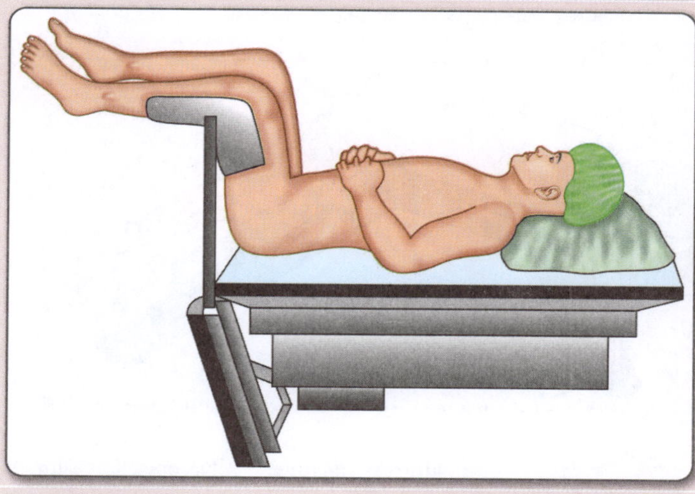	Vaginal surgery, vaginal delivery, perineal or rectal surgeries
Fracture Position (Supine with the pelvis stabilized against well-padded vertical perineal post)	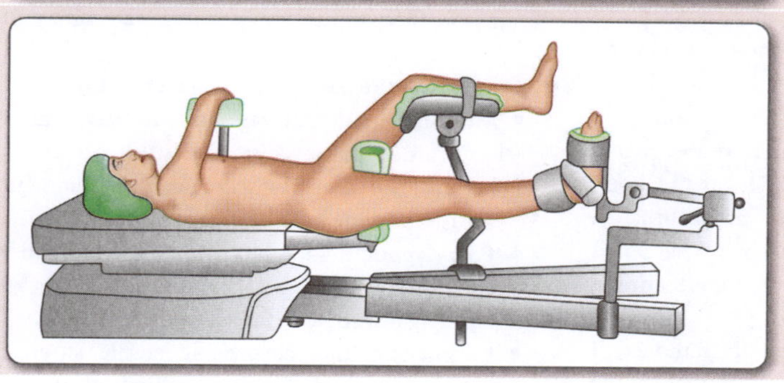	Common position for ORIF of hip or closed femoral nailing

Contd...

Position	Picture	Surgeries used for
Knee-Chest Position	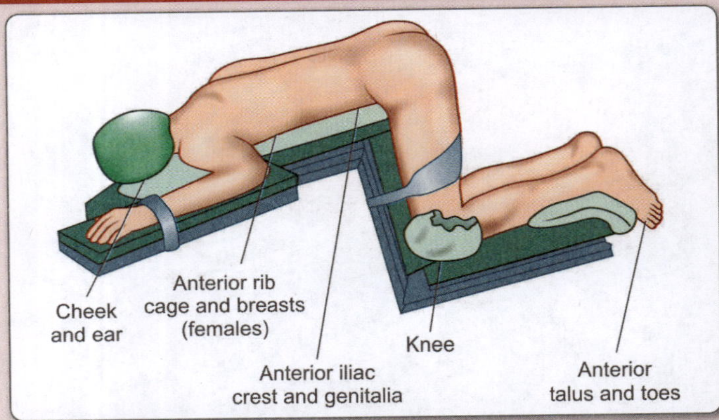	Sigmoidoscopy and laminectomy procedure
Semi-Fowler's & Fowler's positions	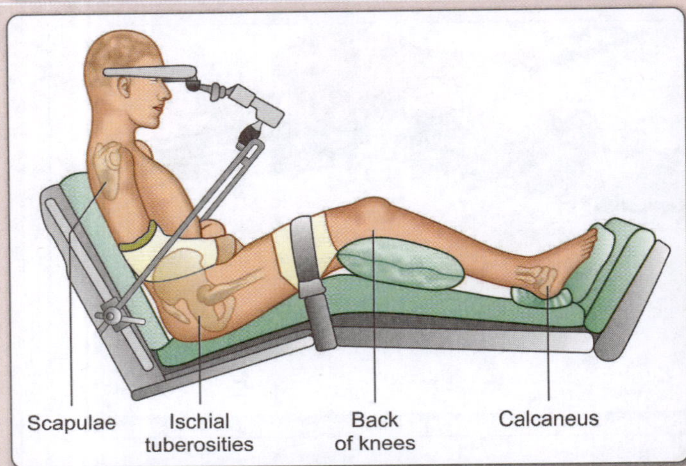	Craniotomies, Shoulder or breast reconstruction, ENT surgeries
Jackknife position	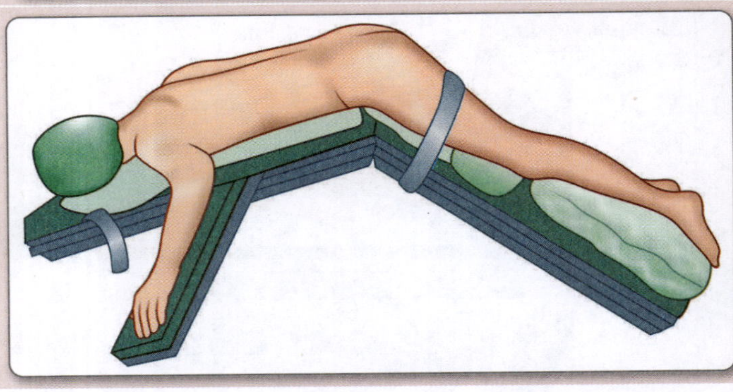	Common position for Hemorrhoidectomy or pilonidal sinus procedures.

SUTURES

- **Sutures or stitches:** As a method for closing cutaneous wounds.
- **Type A: According to nature of absorption**
  - **Absorbable suture:** Those which are absorbable and will break down harmlessly in the body within 60 days are known as absorbable. **Absorbable sutures include:** Polyglycolic acid sutures, Polyglactin 910, Catgut, Poliglecaprone 25 and Polydioxanone sutures.
  - **Nonabsorbable suture:** Manually removed if they are not left indefinitely. **Non-absorbable sutures include:** Polypropylene sutures, nylon (polyamide), polyester, PVDF, silk and stainless steel sutures.
- **Type B: On the basis of material structure**
  - **Monofilament** sutures and **multifilament** or **braided** sutures. Braided sutures provide better knot security whereas monofilament sutures provide better passage through tissues.
  - **Polyglycolic** acid is known for high quality and undoubted performance. Made-up of braided and coated 100% polyglycolic acid.
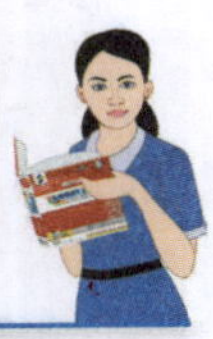

  - **Catgut** is pliable, absorbable, sterile, surgical suture composed of highly purified connective

KEY POINTS

- Catgut is derived from the submucosa of the sheep intestine (YELLOW color). Lasts for 7 to 10 days
- Plain catgut is mixed with chromic salts to derive chromic catgut (BROWN color). Lasts for 15 to 25 days

tissue. Chromic catgut lasts for 2–3 weeks and is used for ligatures and tissue suture.

- **Braided suture** is usually made of natural products (silk, linen or cotton). It is acceptable in many situations, but is contraindicated in a wound that is, or may be, contaminated.
- **Poliglecaprone** suture is a fast absorbing suture made of a synthetic absorbable monofilament composed of glycolide and epsilon-caprolactone copolymer (usually called PGCL suture). It comes as both dyed (violet) and undyed (clear), and is a monofilament suture.

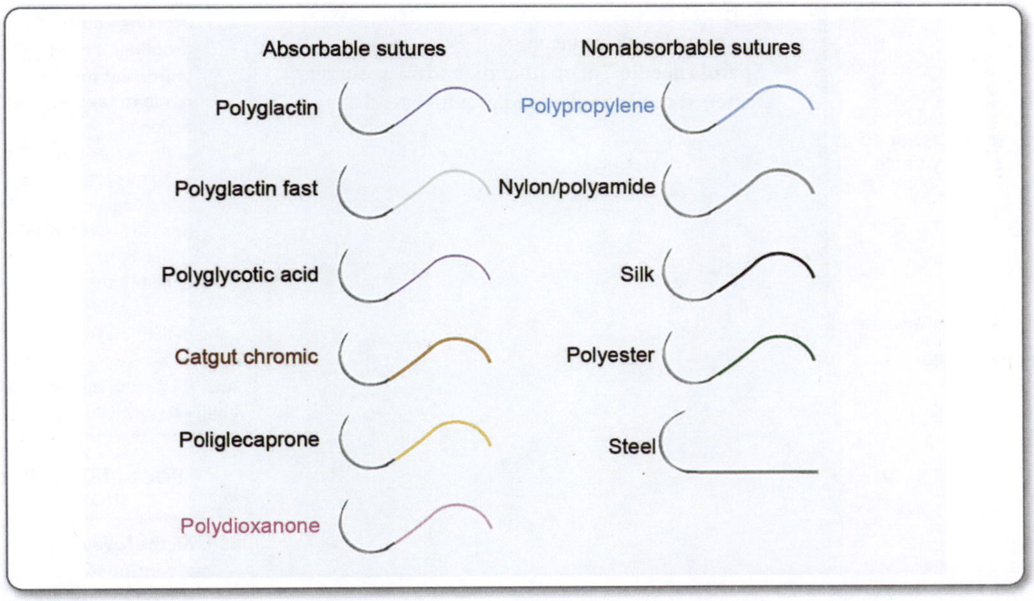

Figure 136: Absorbable and non-absorbable sutures

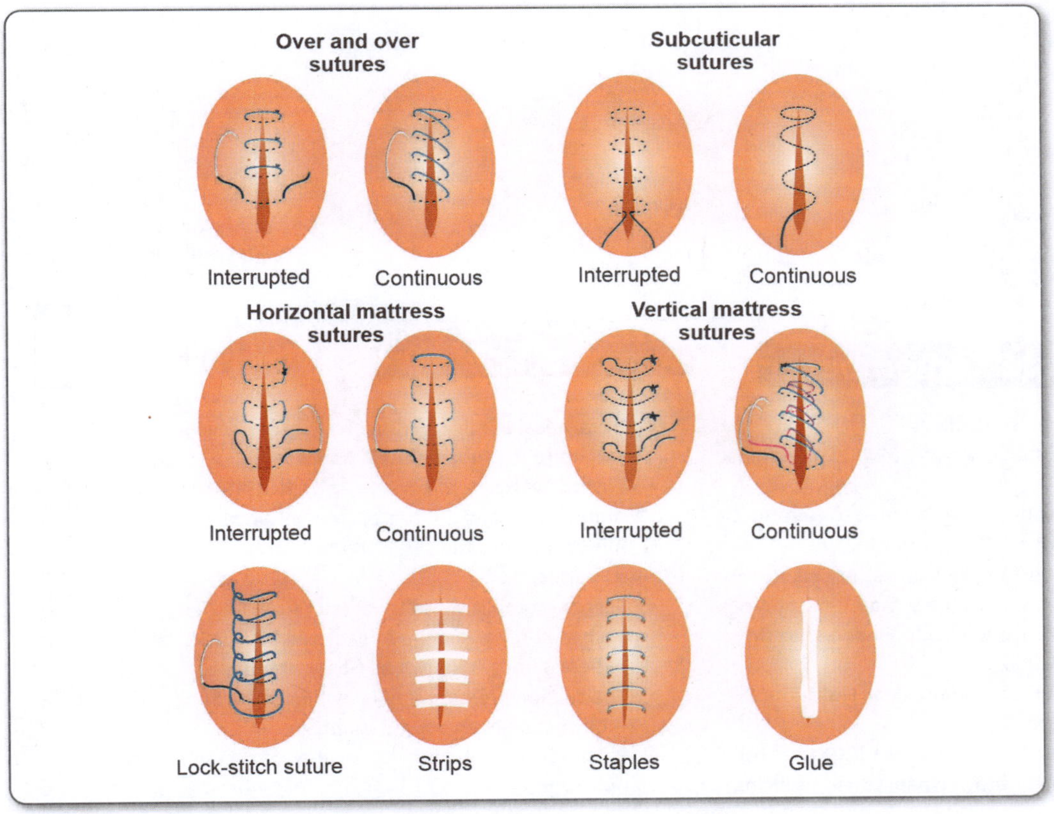

Figure 137: Types of surgical sutures

KEY POINT

Vicryl (Polyglactin) is a synthetic and absorbable suture (VIOLET color)

Recent Question
(NORCET 2022)

132. Which is Non-absorbable suture?
a. Chromic catgut
b. Polyglactin
c. Polypropylene
d. Monocry

Ans. (c) Polypropylene

Recent Questions
(NORCET 2020)

133. PDS suture is an example of
a. Natural absorbable suture
b. Synthetic absorbable suture
c. Synthetic Non absorbable suture
d. Natural Non absorbable suture

Ans. (b) Synthetic...

134. Catgut is banned in Europe and Japan. The reason for the ban is due to concern over the risk of developing
a. Cancer due to carcinogenic ingredients
b. Bovine spongiform encephalopathy (BSE)
c. Necrotic lesions
d. None of the above

Ans. (b) Bovine...

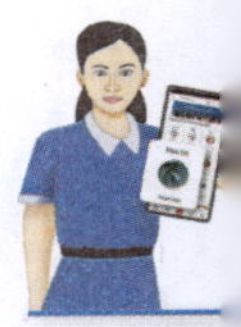

SURGICAL NEEDLES

All surgical needles have three basic components:
- Eye (or Swage)
- Body
- Point

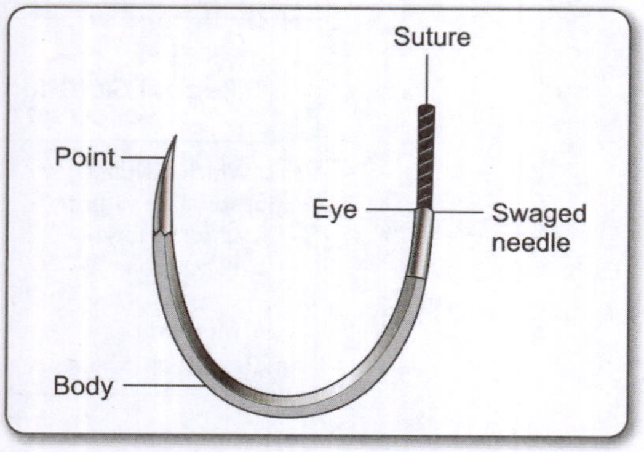

Figure 138: Basic needle design

- **Round-bodied:** For soft (subcutaneous) tissues such as muscle, fascia, mucous membrane. The middle of the needle is flat for better seating in the needle holder and easy entry.
- **Cutting:** For firm tissue, sclerotic vessels and prostheses.
- **Trocar:** Trocar needles have a sharp tip but a round body. They are useful necessary to perforate tough tissue.
- **Spatula needle:** For ophthalmic and microsurgery flattened needle body hand ground lateral.

Recent Question (NORCET 2022)

135. A client undergoes mastoidectomy. When the client returns to the unit postoperatively, the client has difficulty drinking without drooling. It is most important for the nurse to take which action?

a. Re-assure patent as this is a normal finding
b. Assess patient's ability to whistle
c. Notify the physician.
d. Suction the secretions

Ans. (b) Assess patient's ability to whistle

Recent Question (NORCET 2022)

136. All the following are included in the surgical safety checklist, EXCEPT:

a. Name of the surgeon and anesthetic
b. Confirm the site
c. Confirm the specimen labelling for transport biopsy
d. Confirm the patient blood group

Ans. (d) Confirm the patient blood group

Golden Points to Remember

- **Synalgia** is also called referred pain.
- The most common preventable complication of abdominal surgery is **Atelectasis.**
- Aspirin has a prolonged anti-platelet activity; therefore, it should be stopped for at least 7 days prior to surgery.
- A common physiologic effect of spinal anesthesia is **Hypotension**, primarily due to blockade of the sympathetic nervous system causing arterial and venous vasodilation with subsequent "functional" hypovolemia.
- Postoperatively, a patient is started on **Clear Fluids** once bowel sounds can be heard.
- **NSAIDs** block the action of **Cyclooxygenase (COX)**, thereby interfering the production of prostaglandins and reducing pain.
- **Intrathecal** administration of analgesics involves insertion of catheter into **Subarachnoid Space**.
- **Eutectic Mixture of Local Anesthetics (EMLA)** (a combination of prilocaine and lidocaine) cream is applied to the site 30–60 minutes before the surgical procedure. It is used in minor surgeries.
- Surgical complications that result from foreign materials such as surgical sponge or gauze piece accidentally left inside patient's body is known as **Gossypiboma.**
- The suction pressure applied while performing endotracheal tube suction in an adult patient.
- Patients scheduled for surgery are instructed to remove nail polish.

"Feed a cold and starve a fever."
—C. Morley

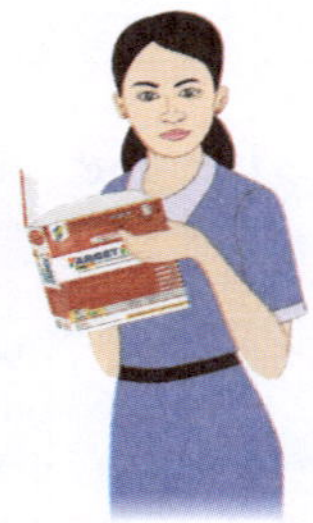

MULTIPLE CHOICE QUESTIONS
(Including Explained and Practice Questions)

PERIOPERATIVE NURSING

INTRODUCTION TO PERIOPERATIVE NURSING

3411. A perioperative nurse is leading a patient for the treatment of spleen that ruptured. The nurse should anticipate that this type of surgery belongs in what category?
a. Minor, diagnostic
b. Minor, selective
c. Major, emergency
d. Major, palliative

3412. A 64-year-old female who is planned for a hip replacement is taking several medications on a routine basis. Which of the following classes of drug might create a surgical risk for this patient?
a. Anticoagulants b. Antacids
c. Diuretics d. Sedatives

3413. A nurse is preparing for an obese patient who has had operative procedure. The nurse assesses this patient for what post-operative complication?
a. Anesthetic agent interactions
b. Impaired wound healing
c. Hemorrhage
d. Gas pains

3414. A client had an operative procedure over the thoracic incision. The nurse expects that he will have a higher risk for post-operative complications involving which body system?
a. Respiratory system
b. Circulatory system
c. Gastrointestinal system
d. Central Nervous system

3415. When a patient is in the Post Anesthesia Care Unit (PACU), a nurse finds extra wound drainage, dizziness, a decreased BP, and a higher pulse rate. The nurse interprets these findings as most likely indicating:
a. Increased ICP
b. Lung Atelectasis
c. Infection
d. Hemorrhage

TYPES OF SURGERIES AND SURGICAL APPROACHES

3416. The most common, preventable complication of abdominal surgery is:
a. Thrombophlebitis
b. Fluid and electrolyte imbalance
c. Urinary retention
d. Atelectasis

Explanation: Atelectasis refers to a partial collapse of the small airways. The majority of post-operative patients will develop some degree of atelectasis, resulting in abnormal alterations in lung function or compromise to the lung's immune defense. Current theories suggest that airway collapse is due to a combination of airway compression, alveolar gas resorption intraoperatively and impairment of surfactant production. General anesthesia is another common cause of atelectasis.

3417. The surgery to remove the gallbladder entirely is referred as:
a. Cholelithiasis
b. Cholecystectomy
c. Colectomy
d. Gallectomy

3418. The surgery performed to remove entire breast along with surrounding muscles and lymph nodes:
a. Radical mastectomy
b. Simple mastectomy
c. Mastectomy with lymphadenectomy
d. Lumpectomy

3419. Anatomic sublobar resection is also known as ..... *New Q*
a. Lobectomy b. Segmentectomy
c. Pneumectomy d. Sleeve resection

Explanation: Anatomic sublobar resection is also known as segmentectomy. It involves the surgical removal of a specific segment of a lung lobe while preserving the remaining healthy lung tissue.

This procedure is often performed when a smaller portion of the lung needs to be removed, such as in cases of early-stage lung cancer or certain lung infections.

3420. The whipple procedure is referred as:
a. Pancreaticojejunostomy
b. Illeopancreatomy
c. Gastrojejunostomy
d. Pancreaticoduodenectomy

3421. One of the noted surgeries for the Hirschsprung disease:
a. Nissen fundoplication
b. Pyloromyotomy
c. Duhamel procedure
d. Conization

Explanation: In Duhamel procedure, The aganglionic colon is resected to the rectum and the normal proximal colon and rectum are brought together in an end-to-side anastomosis.

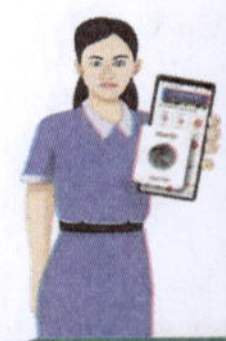

Ans.
3411. c
3412. a
3413. b
3414. a
3415. d
3416. d
3417. b
3418. a
3419. b
3420. d
3421. c

3422. The surgical step taken to treat the client with Gastroesophageal reflux disease:
a. Nissen fundoplication
b. Pyloromyotomy
c. Duhamel procedure
d. Conization

3423. The best surgical intervention to treat pyloric stenosis is:
a. Nissen fundoplication
b. Pyloromyotomy
c. Duhamel procedure
d. Conization

3424. A short surgical procedure in which certain tissue portion which are affected by malignant cells in the cervix are removed; This procedure is known as:
a. Nissen fundoplication
b. Pyloromyotomy
c. Duhamel procedure
d. Conization

3425. A new surgical technique to treat the patient with cancer cells on lower rectum:
a. Extra levator abdominal perineal excision
b. Transurethral resection
c. Anterior peritoneal resection
d. Pull through procedure

3426. The surgical procedure to remove the ovaries present in the pelvic cavity is known as:
a. Hysterectomy
b. Salpingectomy
c. Oophorectomy
d. Vulvectomy

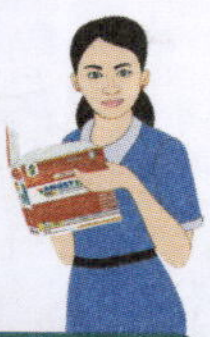

PREOPERATIVE NURSING CARE

3427. Pre-operative instructions to the client would include the following; EXCEPT: *(AIIMS Bhopal Grade-I 2018)*
a. Deep breathing and coughing exercise
b. Continue anticoagulants
c. Lower limb exercises
d. Reassuring the client

3428. The reason why lipstick and nail-polish is removed before surgery is: *(RRB SSNE 2015)*
a. Surgery becomes easier
b. Surgery becomes more successful
c. Psychological benefits to the patient
d. Cyanosis is checked

3429. Which among the following pre-operative order is the most important order one day prior to the surgery?
a. Inform the family
b. Informed consent form
c. Physical examination
d. Respiratory exercises

3430. First nursing intervention while implementing pre-operative teaching to a client is:
a. Assess the client's basic knowledge regarding the surgical procedure
b. Provide premedications
c. Assist the doctor for performing PAC
d. Get informed consent from the client

3431. All among the following are the components of pre-operative check list; EXCEPT:
a. NPO status
b. Checking for allergy
c. Part preparation
d. Completion of history and physical examination

3432. The last pre-operative assessment of a client going for elective splenectomy will be:
a. Name band
b. Signed consent
c. Empty bladder
d. Vital signs

Explanation: Elective surgical procedure is planned and scheduled in advance. Checking of name band, obtaining consent and emptying bladder will be completed ahead of time. Vital signs assessment will be the last and final assessment before the surgery commences in elective procedure.

3433. The important nursing intervention prior to administration of pre-anesthetic medication is: *(ESIC Chennai May 2012)*
a. Ask patient to empty the bladder
b. Do deep breathing and coughing exercises
c. Shave the skin
d. Regulate IVF accurately

3434. Nursing intervention to manage fear and anxiety associated with post-operative pain in pre-operative period is:
a. Teach diversion activity
b. Allow the patient to communicate with another patient who underwent for the same procedure
c. Explain the procedures associated with pain assessment and management
d. Help the patient to ventilate the feeling

3435. Which among the following history increases the risk during surgical procedure?
a. Drug abuse
b. Previous surgery
c. Daily taking thyroxin
d. All of these

3436. Atropine is a premedication given to the patient before surgery. Which among the following is the expected actions of atropine?
a. Reduce secretions
b. Prevent bradycardia
c. Prevent hypotension
d. All of these

INTRAOPERATIVE NURSING CARE

3437. While scrubbing, nurse should:
a. Scrub from hands to elbow
b. Scrub with mechanical friction.
c. Hold the hands higher than the elbows.
d. All of the above

3438. Who is responsible for coordinating all the activities with the surgical team and family while the surgery is going on?
a. Scrub nurse
b. Circulatory nurse
c. Anesthetist
d. Surgeon

3439. Which of the following procedure always requires surgical asepsis? *(Staff Nurse G II 2014)*
a. Colostomy irrigation
b. Vaginal irrigation
c. Urinary catheterization
d. Nasogastric tube insertion

Ans.
3422. a
3423. b
3424. d
3425. a
3426. c
3427. b
3428. d
3429. b
3430. a
3431. d
3432. d
3433. a
3434. c
3435. a
3436. d
3437. d
3438. b
3439. c

TYPES OF ANESTHESIA

3440. To decrease the likelihood of bradyarrhythmias in children during endotracheal intubation, succinylcholine (Anectine) is used with which of the following agents?
- a. Epinephrine (Adrenaline)
- b. Isoproterenol (Isuprel)
- c. Atropine sulfate
- d. Lidocaine hydrochloride (Xylocaine)

3441. In the pre-anesthetic orders a patient is to receive 6 mg of morphine sulphate, the ampoule contains 15 mg/mL. The nurse should administer approximately how much amount?
- a. 0. 3 mL
- b. 0. 4 mL
- c. 0. 5 mL
- d. 0. 6 mL

Explanation: Amount to be administered (A) – (desired dose/ dose in hand)*amount in which the drug comes A = (6 mg/15 mg) *1 mL = 0. 4 mL

3442. Intravenous induction for general anesthesia is more commonly practiced because:
- a. Easy to administer
- b. Cost effective
- c. Induction is rapid and pleasant
- d. Last for long time with fewer complications

3443. Dissociative anesthesia produced by:
- a. Haloperidol
- b. Imipramine
- c. Ketamine
- d. Formaldehyde

3444. In regional anesthesia, patient:
- a. Become unconscious rapidly
- b. Is conscious
- c. Is able to recognize pain
- d. Is having long-term effects of anesthesia

Explanation: Regional anesthesia is the use of local anesthetics to block sensations of pain from a large area of the body, such as an arm or leg or the abdomen. Regional anesthesia allows a procedure to be done on a region of the body without being unconscious.

3445. Spinal anesthesia is given at:
- a. L1-L2
- b. L2-L3
- c. L3-L4
- d. L4-L5

Explanation: Spinal needle is introduced at L3-L4 because the spinal cord ends before this level which helps to avoid injury to spinal cord.

3446. Which of the following is most dangerous complication during induction of spinal anesthesia? (ESIC Chennai May 2012)
- a. Hyperthermia
- b. Bradypnea
- c. Tachycardia
- d. Hypotension

3447. Common complications associated with spinal anesthesia includes all; EXCEPT:
- a. Hypotension
- b. Hypothermia
- c. Headache
- d. Urinary incontinence

3448. Which of the following would the nurse assess following assessment of vital signs in a patient who has undergone epidural anesthesia? *(ESI 2009)*
- a. Ability to move legs sideways
- b. Bladder distension
- c. Dizziness
- d. Headache

Explanation: After epidural anesthesia, perineal area is the last area to return to sensation. So the nurse should monitor the patient for distended bladder to determine if the sensation is returned.

COMMON POSITIONS DURING SURGERIES

3449. Patient recovering from general anaesthesia should be positioned in: *(JIPMER 2012)*
- a. Supine position
- b. Fowler's position
- c. Trendelenburg position
- d. Side lying position

3450. Which of the following position is appropriate during a liver biopsy procedure?
- a. High Fowler's
- b. Semi-Fowler's
- c. Supine with right arm raised and extended behind head
- d. Left lateral position with right arm raised above head

Explanation: The patient should be supine, with his or her right side near the edge of the bed. The patient's right arm should be above the head. The feet should be angled across the bed to expand the intercostal space as much as possible.

3451. Which of the following position should be provided to the patient immediately after percutaneous liver biopsy?
- a. Semi-Fowler's
- b. Left-lateral position
- c. Right lateral position
- d. Supine position

Explanation: The most serious complication after liver biopsy is bleeding. In the right-lateral position, there will be direct pressure on the puncture site which will prevent hemorrahge.

3452. Which of the following position is provided to the patient for the next 8 to 12 hours after the angiogram procedure?
- a. High Fowler's with leg extended
- b. Left lateral
- c. Semi-Fowler's with leg flexed
- d. Supine with leg extended

Explanation: In supine position with leg extended, the circulation will not be affected because the leg is at the level of heart and is straight.

3453. Which of the following patient would benefit if the head end of the bed is elevated?
- a. Patient who underwent lumbar puncture
- b. Patient with above-knee amputation
- c. Patient with burns of the face and head
- d. Patient who underwent hemorroidectomy

Explanation: Head end of the bed needs to be elevated while caring for a patient with burns to head and face in order to prevent edema in the trachea which can lead to respiratory arrest.

3454. The position used for the anal surgery and excision in which the patient is on prone with head and feet at a lower level:
- a. Frog leg position
- b. Beach chair position
- c. Jackknife position
- d. Reverse Trendelenburg

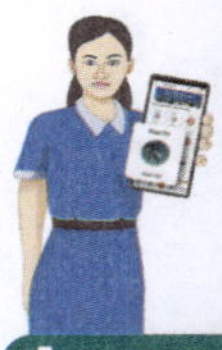

Ans.

3440. c
3441. b
3442. c
3443. c
3444. b
3445. c
3446. d
3447. d
3448. b
3449. d
3450. c
3451. c
3452. d
3453. c
3454. c

Explanation:

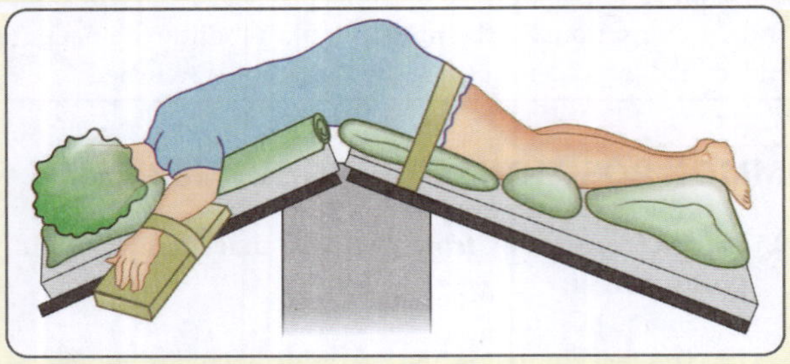

Jackknife position is also known as Kraske. A position in which the patient lies on the back, shoulders elevated, legs flexed on thighs, thighs at right angles to the abdomen. It is often used for colorectal surgeries. This position places extreme pressure on the knees. While positioning, the operation theatre nurse should place extra padding for the knee area.

3455. The position given for the orthopedic shoulder anthroscopy would be:

a. Frog leg position
b. Beach chair position
c. Jackknife position
d. Reverse Trendelenburg

Explanation: The beach chair (barbershop) position was developed in the 1980s for orthopedic shoulder arthroscopy procedures. Patient sit up at angles varying from 30-90° above the horizontal plane with appropriate padding and with the head secured in a headrest.

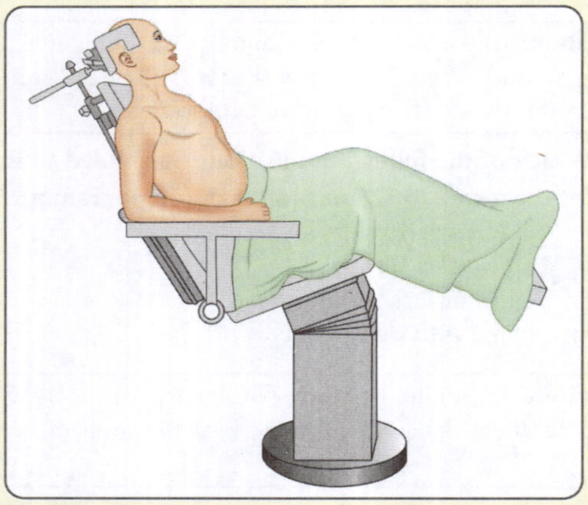

3456. The surgical position often used in the head and neck surgery for the reduction of venous congestion is:

a. Frog leg position
b. Beach chair position
c. Jackknife position
d. Reverse Trendelenburg

3457. The position usually used to perform Foley's catheterization In OT room:

a. Frog leg position
b. Beach chair position
c. Jackknife position
d. Reverse Trendelenburg

3458. Which of the following is the modified prone and knee chest position for spinal surgeries?

a. Wilson spinal position
b. Horizontal Knee chest position
c. Modified Fowler position
d. Beach chair sitting

Explanation:

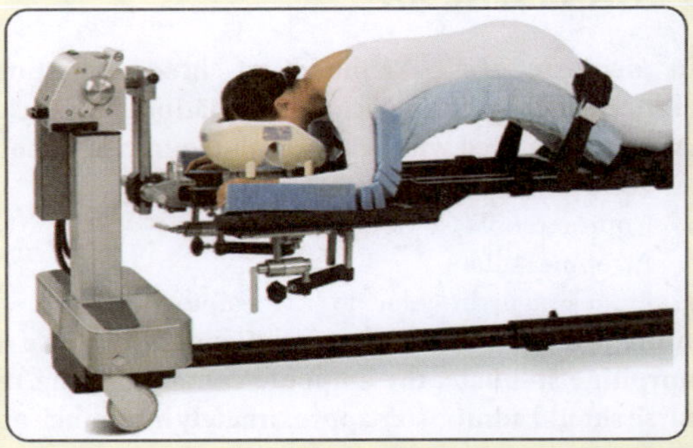

The **Wilson** supporting frame provides a convenient and stable method of maintaining patients in a flexed **position** for **spinal** surgery.

3459. The surgical position which is involved in the sigmoidoscopy and lumbar laminectomy is:

a. Hamelton position
b. Knee chest position
c. Modified Fowler position
d. Beach chair sitting

3460. The suggested position to facilitate surgical access to the cranium, neck, or shoulder and to have drainage from the surgical site:

a. Wilson spinal position
b. Horizontal Knee chest position
c. Modified Fowler position
d. Beach chair sitting

3461. The excessive arm abduction and the external rotation during the surgical procedure and the compression will affect the:

a. Brachial nerve
b. Ulnar nerve
c. Peroneal nerve
d. Medial nerve

3462. The term neuropraxia is involved in the assessment after the surgical position. Neuropraxia refers to:

a. Nervous dysfunction
b. Peripheral nerve injury
c. Nerve bulging
d. Nerve weakness

3463. During lithotomy position the nerve compression over the fibula will affect:

a. Brachial nerve
b. Ulnar nerve
c. Peroneal nerve
d. Medial nerve

SUTURES & SURGICAL NEEDLES

3464. Alternative for skin closure rather than suture is:

a. Glue
b. Staple
c. Dressing
d. Acticoat

3465. The disadvantages of using a braided suture (multifilament) material are:

a. High risk of infection and highly unstable
b. High risk of infection and high failure rate
c. High risk of infection and reactivity
d. Highly unstable and high failure rate

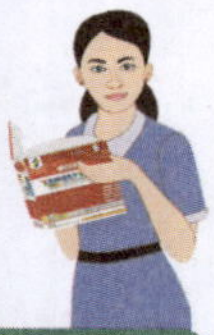

Ans.

3455. b
3456. d
3457. a
3458. a
3459. b
3460. c
3461. a
3462. b
3463. c
3464. b
3465. c

3466. The advantages of using a monofilament suture material are:
a. Low risk of infection and minimal tissue reactive
b. Low risk of infection and good knot security
c. Good knot security and minimal tissue reactive
d. None of the above

3467. Which of the following statement regarding plain Catgut is NOT true?
a. Catgut is derived from the submucosa of the sheep intestine
b. Color of plain catgut is yellow
c. It lasts 14–28 days
d. It is a monofilament suture material

Explanation: Plain catgut lasts about 7 to 10 days, hence its use is minimal. All other statements about plain catgut are correct. It can be used to put subcutaneous fat stitches.

3468. All of the statements regarding chromic catgut is true; EXCEPT:?
a. Color of chromic catgut is blue
b. It lasts about 15–25 days
c. Plain catgut is mixed with chromic salts to obtain chromic catgut
d. The chromic catgut is preserved in 70% alcohol

Explanation: The color of the chromic catgut is brown. Other statements are true about chromic catgut. Chromic catgut is biological, absorbable and monofilament suture material. It is used in intestinal anastomosis, closure of urinary bladder, closure of bile duct, etc.

3469. Vicryl rapide is a:
a. Synthetic absorbable suture
b. Synthetic non-absorbable suture
c. Natural absorbable suture
d. Natural nonabsorbable suture

3470. What type of material that monocryl suture would be:
a. Braided
b. Monofilament
c. Threads
d. Silicone

3471. Suture ethilon is a/an:
a. Absorbable suture
b. Nonabsorbable suture
c. Semi absorbable
d. Not a suture material

3472. The suture variety Chromic gut is a/an: *New Q*
a. Absorbable monofilament
b. Nonabsorbable suture
c. Absorbable Braided
d. Not a suture material

3473. Ethibond suture is an a/an:
a. Absorbable suture
b. Nonabsorbable Monofilament
c. Semi absorbable
d. Non absorbable braided

POST-OPERATIVE NURSING CARE

3474. Which of the parameter indicates infection in a post-operative patient? *(Daman & Diu NO 2018)*
a. White blood count of 6,000 cells/cu.mm
b. Presence of an indwelling urinary catheter
c. Rectal temperature of 37.8°C
d. Red, warm and tender incision site

Explanation:

- Surgical site infections (SSI) are most commonly caused by Staphylococcus aureus. Red, warm and tender incision site indicates infection in a post-operative patient. Any SSI may cause redness, delayed healing, fever, pain, tenderness, warmth, or swelling.
- WBC > 11000 indicates infection. Rectal temperature > 38°C is an indication for infection. Presence of urinary catheter is unrelated to surgical site infection.

3475. Which among the following parameter of a patient in post-operative unit requires immediates attention?
a. Oxygen saturation of 85%
b. Respiratory rate of 14/min
c. Temperature of 980 F (38°C)
d. Blood pressure of 110/80 mm Hg

3476. In the immediate post-operative period nursing interventions are directed to prevent which of the following respiratory complication?
a. Atelectasis b. Emphysema
c. COPD d. ARDS

3477. Which among the following is the most appropriate intervention in the post-operative client to prevent respiratory complications?
a. Deep breathing and coughing
b. Use of an incentive spirometer
c. Both a and b
d. Oxygen administration

3478. How frequent should the nurse monitor the vital signs of the patient in the recovery room? *(ESIC Chennai May 2012)*
a. Every 15 minutes b. Every 60 minutes
c. Every 30 minutes d. Every 45 minutes

Explanation: Every 15 minutes the vitals need to monitor to find out the occurrence of any complication as early as possible.

3479. On the first post-operative day of a patient with abdominal resection procedure has been ordered opioid for pain relief. Which of the following critical aspects has to be considered before administration of an opioid injection to prevent respiratory depression? *(AIIMS Bhopal Grade-I 2018)*
a. Bowel movements
b. Postsurgical blood loss
c. Level of consciousness
d. Oxygen saturation

Explanation: Opioid induced respiratory depression is potentially life-threatening and the cause of substantial morbidity and mortality. So, before administering opioid, patient's oxygen saturation level should be monitored to assess the level of oxygenation or to prevent the complications due to respiratory depression.

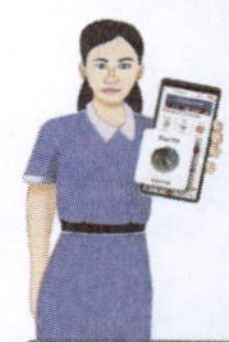

Ans.

3466. a
3467. c
3468. a
3469. a
3470. b
3471. b
3472. a
3473. d
3474. d
3475. a
3476. a
3477. c
3478. a
3479. d

3480. A child in post-operative ward under observation after tonsillectomy is suspected to have postoperative hemorrhage when the child: *(Banaras HU 2015)*

a. Snores noisily
b. Becomes pale
c. Complains of thirst
d. Swallows frequently

3481. A patient has just returned from the post anesthesia care unit (PACU) after hemorrhoidectomy. His postoperative order includes sitz bath every morning. The nurse understand that sitz bath is necessary for *(Banaras HU 2015)*

a. Relieving tension
b. Promote healing
c. Lower body temperature
d. Reduce pain

Explanation: Anticoagulants may increase the risk of bleeding post-operatively. Preoperatively client is advised based on type of anticoagulant he/she used or about the associated risks. Example, if warfarin is used by the patient it should be discontinued 5 days before the surgery because of its long acting effect.

3482. The most important factor in the prevention of post-operative infection is: *(ESIC Chennai May 2012)*

a. Frequent change of wound dressings
b. Proper administration of antibiotics
c. Fluid intake of 2-3 L/day
d. Practice of strict aseptic techniques

3483. Most important post-operative teaching for a client scheduled for a vaginal hysterectomy?

a. Deep breathing and leg exercises
b. Kegel exercises
c. Vaginal pessaries
d. Sitz bath

3484. In the recovery room patient is shivering uncontrollably. The first nursing intervention is:

a. Provide blanket and continue oxygen
b. Take temperature of the patient
c. Provide warm IVF
d. Inform the surgeon

3485. Following surgery gas can be expelled out through:

a. Ambulation and moving around
b. Insertion of flatus tube
c. Bearing down
d. Taking bed rest

3486. Which of the following is a function of prostaglandin I_2 or prostacyclin *(PGI2)*

a. Vasoconstriction
b. Inhibition of platelet aggregation
c. Helps in wound healing
d. Piloconstriction

3487. Risk factors for deep vein thrombosis (DVT) are:

a. Prolonged surgery
b. Overweight and obesity
c. Hormonal contraceptive
d. All of the above

3488. After a child returns from post anesthesia care unit after surgery. Which of the following would the nurse assess first? *(RAK MSc 2018)*

a. The intravenous fluid access site
b. The child's level of pain
c. Surgical site dressing
d. Functioning of the nasogastric tube

Explanation:

- After Surgery, the child will be shifted to post anesthesia care unit or recovery Room. When assessing the post-operative patient, it is vital that the patient is observed for signs of hemorrhage, shock, sepsis and the effects of analgesia and anesthesia. So, the priority is to check the surgical site dressing for bleeding and drainage.
- While a child returns from post anesthesia care unit after surgery usually fluids are running.
- Level of pain can assess by pain scale when the child came out from anesthesia.
- While a child received with nasogastric tube after surgery usually X-ray is done for confirmation of nasogastric tube on site.

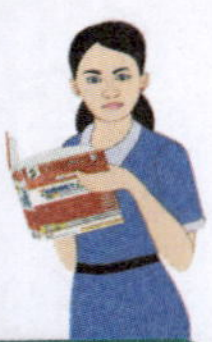

Ans.

3480. d
3481. b
3482. d
3483. a
3484. a
3485. a
3486. b
3487. d
3488. c

HOMEOSTASIS, EMERGENCY AND CRITICAL CARE NURSING

STRESS

- It is a physical or psychological reaction to real or perceived threat.
- Stress reaction increases cortisol (glucocorticoids and mineralocorticoids) levels in the blood.
- Prolonged physiologic stress responses may contribute to gastric ulcers, decreased immunity, infections, renal failure and result in damage to the body, resulting in problems such as kidney failure, gastric ulcers, and aggravation of an existing illness.
- The term "stress" was first used by the endocrinologist ***Hans Selye (1930s)***.
- General adaptation syndrome is a three-stage response that the body has to stress.

General Adaptation Syndrome (GAS)

There are three stages of GAS:

1. **Alarm stage**
   - It is the emergency response of the body in response to the stressor
   - There is a flight or fight response.
   - Mainly mediated by sympathetic nervous system
     - Anxiety or fear; sorrow or depression; shock or confusion
2. **Resistance stage**
   - If continuous stressor is present, body tries to resist the effects
   - Hormonal responses of the body come to play (adrenocorticotropic-ACTH- axis)
     - Cortisol secretion
   - But high level of Cortisol in the blood for longer time causes immune suppression, high BP
3. **Exhaustion stage**
   - Inability to defend against stressors
   - Body's capacity to respond to stressors is been seriously compromised.
   - Person may become ill or can even die (due to the high Cortisol)

SHOCK

- Shock is a condition in which the systemic blood pressure is inadequate to deliver oxygen and nutrients to cellular function and vital organs.
- It is an acute medical condition associated with reduced perfusion to body tissues.

Stages of Shock

1. **Initial stage**
   - Decreased cardiac output results in reduced mean arterial pressure.
   - Increase in heart rate due to stimulation of sympathetic nervous system
   - Characterized by increased heart rate, decreased blood pressure, thirst, pale, cool, moist skin over the face.
2. **Compensatory stage**
   - Stimulation of sympathetic nervous system releases epinephrine and norepinephrine to maintain homeostasis.
   - Peripheral vasoconstriction caused by stimulation of α_1 adrenergic fibers assures more blood available for heart and brain.
   - Coronary and cerebral artery dilation occurs due to stimulation of beta adrenergic fibers. This results in increased cardiac output.
   - Increased renal sodium and water reabsorption results in increased cardiac output.
3. **Progressive stage**
   - Compensatory mechanisms become ineffective.
   - Impaired perfusion results in anaerobic metabolism and cellular hypoxia
   - Renal ischemia stimulates renin-angiotensin-aldosterone system which further causes vasoconstriction.
4. **Irreversible stage**
   - Compensatory mechanisms are ineffective.
   - Coronary and cerebral tissue perfusion drops, and organ systems fail.

Classification of Shock Based on Etiology

- Hypovolemic shock
- Cardiogenic shock
- Circulatory or Disruptive shock

KEY POINTS

- Elevated serum lactate demonstrates that the patient's cells are using anaerobic metabolism.
- When the body is attempting to compensate for shock the adrenal cortex will release aldosterone due to the presence of angiotensin II.
- Release of aldosterone causes an increase in sodium and water reabsorption into the blood stream resulting in increased blood volume.
- During compensatory stage of shock, **sympathetic nervous system releases epinephrine** and norepinephrine to maintain homeostatic.

Recent Question
(NORCET 2023)

137. Cause of decrease peripheral vascular resistance:
a. Cardiogenic shock,
b. Hypovolemic shock,
c. Neurogenic shock
d. Pulmonary embolism

Ans. (c) Neurogenic shock

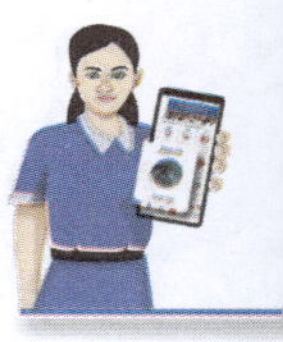

Table 105: Description of different types of shocks and their management

Types of shocks	Description	Management
Hypovolemic shock	**Occurs because of low blood volume** **Causes** • **External fluid loss** such as vomiting, diarrhea, diuresis, Diabetes Insipidus, Trauma, surgery. • **Internal fluid shift** such as hemorrhage, burns, ascites, peritonitis and dehydration **Manifestations** • Rapid, irregular, and thready pulse. • Urine output less than 20 mL/hr or 480 mL/24 hrs.	**Crystalloids:** RL and NS are commonly used for fluid replacement **Colloids:** Albumin, Dextran and Hectastarch can also be used to replace fluid volume. Blood transfusion, if the cause is hemorrhagic shock **Position:** Trendelenburg is preferred because it promotes venous return **Medication:** Vasoactive drugs, e.g., Dobutamine, Dopamine, Epinephrine, Norepinephrine, Vasopressin, Amrinone.
Cardiogenic shock	Heart is not able to perform its function. **Causes:** Myocardial infarction, cardiomyopathy, valve disease, cardiac tamponade, arrhythmia **Manifestations** • Anginal pain • Dysrhythmia • Cyanotic skin • Jugular vein distension • Pulmonary crackles	Supplemental oxygen Pain management Selected fluid support Vasoactive medications, e.g., Dobutamine, Nitroglycerine, Dopamine, Epinephrine, Norepinephrine, Vasopressin, Amrinone and antiarrhythmic drugs. ***Cardiac supportive measures such as*** *pacemaker, ventricular assistive devices, Intra-aortic balloon pump (IABP), or Extracorporeal cardiopulmonary bypass*
Circulatory or Distributive shock (It includes septic shock, anaphylactic shock, neurogenic shock and hypodynamic shock)	• Results from excessive vasodilation and impaired distribution of blood flow. • Cardiac output is usually normal. • **Septic shock is the most common cause of disruptive shock.** • **Other causes:** Systemic inflammatory response syndrome (SIRS) • **Other non-infectious causes** include toxic shock syndrome, anaphylaxis, insect bites, transfusion reaction, etc.	
	Septic shock: Occurs because of infection. Manifestation include rapid heart rate, warm, pink extremities and widening pulse pressure	Treat the underlying cause by administering broad spectrum antibiotics
	Anaphylactic shock: Occurs because of allergic reaction. Manifestation include feeling warm, abdominal pain, diarrhea, flushing, pruritus, urticaria.	Remove the causative antigen Epinephrine to restore vasoconstrictive action Diphenhydramine Albuterol (if histamine induced bronchospasm present)
	Neurogenic shock: Dilation of blood vessels because of the damage to sympathetic nervous system controlling it. Signs and symptoms include **bradycardia**, hypotension, hypothermia, dry warm skin.	Treatment of the underlying cause and restore sympathetic tone
	Hypodynamic shock: Narrowing pulse pressure, oliguria, cold extremities.	

POINT TO REMEMBER

Calculation of Mean Arterial Pressure

There are two methods:

Method 1

Mean Arterial Pressure (MAP) = DBP + 1/3 (SBP – DBP)

Where, SBP – Systolic Blood Pressure and DBP – Diastolic Blood Pressure.

For e.g., if the SBP = 120 mm Hg and DBP = 75 mm Hg, the MAP is:

$$\begin{aligned} \text{MAP} &= 75 + 1/3\,(120 - 75) \\ &= 75 + 45/3 \\ &= 75 + 15 \\ &= 90 \end{aligned}$$

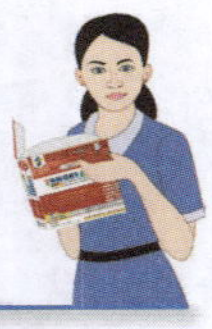

KEY POINT

If the cause for hypovolemic shock is hemorrhage, then the use of Dextran is contraindicated because it interferes with the platelet aggregation.

POINT TO REMEMBER

Method 2

$$\text{Mean Arterial Pressure (MAP)} = \frac{\text{SBP} + (2 \times \text{DBP})}{3}$$

e.g., if the SBP = 120 mm Hg and DBP = 75 mm Hg, the MAP is

$$\text{MAP} = \frac{120 + (2 \times 75)}{3}$$
$$= (120 + 150)/3$$
$$= 270/3$$
$$\text{MAP} = 90$$

ANAPHYLAXIS

- Anaphylaxis is an acute allergic (immunologic) reaction to an antigen.
- **Release of IgE mediated chemicals** trigger rapid immune response.
- **Causes**
  - Common substances that cause anaphylaxis include food, medications, contrast dyes, insect stings and latex.
  - Peanuts, shellfish, fish, milk, soy, wheat and eggs are common food stuffs that causes anaphylactic reactions
- **Mild reactions:** Symptoms begin within 2 hours of exposure. Characterized by fullness in the mouth, a warm sensation, sweating, clammy skin, peripheral tingling, nasal congestion, sneezing, pruritus, periorbital swelling, and teary eyes.
- **Moderate reactions:** In addition to milder symptoms, itching, anxiety, warmth, and flushing may occur.
- **Severe reactions: Abrupt onset**. Symptom proceeds with bronchial spasm, laryngeal edema, dyspnea, cyanosis, and fall in blood pressure. Cardiac arrest and coma may follow.
- **Treatment**
  - Epinephrine, antihistamines, and corticosteroids
  - **IV fluids**: Vasopressor agents and volume expanders to maintain blood pressure.
  - Corticosteroids and aminophylline to improve airway patency.
- **Management**
  - Establish patent airway and maintain ventilation
  - Maintain patent IV access and administer **epinephrine**
  - **Antihistamines** to counter the effect of histamine
  - **Aminophylline** and **Albuterol** to reverse bronchospasm and wheezing
  - **Vasoactive drugs: Dopamine** to improve cardiac output
  - **Corticosterioids**
  - Vital signs monitoring
  - Teach the patient and family about specific allergen which caused anaphylaxis.

FLUID IMBALANCES

(Basics of Fluid and electrolyte balance have been discussed under Fundamentals of Nursing)

Types of Parenteral Solutions

Table 106: Types of solutions and their indications

Type of solution	Example	Indications
Isotonic solution	Normal saline (NS) or 0.9% sodium chloride lactated Ringer's solution (RL) 5% dextrose in water	• To increase extracellular fluid volume • To treat hypovolemia for electrolyte replacement
Hypotonic solution	Half-normal saline (0.45% sodium Chloride)	To expand the intracellular fluid compartment
Hypertonic solution	Dextrose 5% in normal saline solution (DNS) 10% dextrose in water 3% sodium chloride	• To correct severe hyponatremia • To treat hypoglycemia

EDEMA

- Edema refers to excess fluid in the body tissues mainly in the ECF, may also present in ICF.
- It is an accumulation of fluid in interstitial space.
- Generalized edema is called anasarca.
- **Grading of edema**
  - 0+ : No pitting edema
  - 1+ : Mild pitting edema. 2 mm depression
  - 2+ : Moderate pitting edema. 4 mm depression
  - 3+ : Moderate severe pitting edema. 6 mm depression
  - 4+ : Severe pitting edema, 8 mm depression

KEY POINTS

- **IgE mediated chemicals** are associated with **Anaphylactic** reaction.
- The commonest drug which is administered during an anaphylactic reaction is injection **Epinephrine/ Adrenaline**.
- Isotonic crystalloid solutions are typically given for intravascular repletion during shock and hypovolemia.
- Crystalloid solutions are the resuscitative fluid of choice for patients with sepsis and septic shock.

Recent Question (NORCET 2022)

138. In clinical setup KCL bolus is contraindicated because:

a. It may lead to cardiac arrest and sudden death.

b. It leads to hypotension.

c. It may damage the veins of the patient.

d. It may lead to thrombobhlebitis

Ans. (a) It may lead to cardiac arrest and sudden death.

UNDERSTANDING ACID-BASE IMBALANCE

Table 107: Normal ABG values

Analyze	Normal value	Normal range
pH	7.40	7.35–7.45
$PaCO_2$ (mm Hg)	40	35–45
HCO_3^- (mmol/L)	24	21–28
PaO_2 (mm Hg)	100	80–110

Interpretation of ABG Values

The following chart explains how to interpret the lab results of ABG analysis:

Table 108: Interpretation of ABG values

Acid-base disorders	pH	Primary change	Compensatory change
Metabolic acidosis	↓	HCO_3↓	$PaCO_2$↓
Respiratory acidosis	↓	$PaCO_2$↑	HCO_3↑
Metabolic alkalosis	↑	HCO_3↑	$PaCO_2$↑
Respiratory alkalosis	↑	$PaCO_2$↓	HCO_3↓

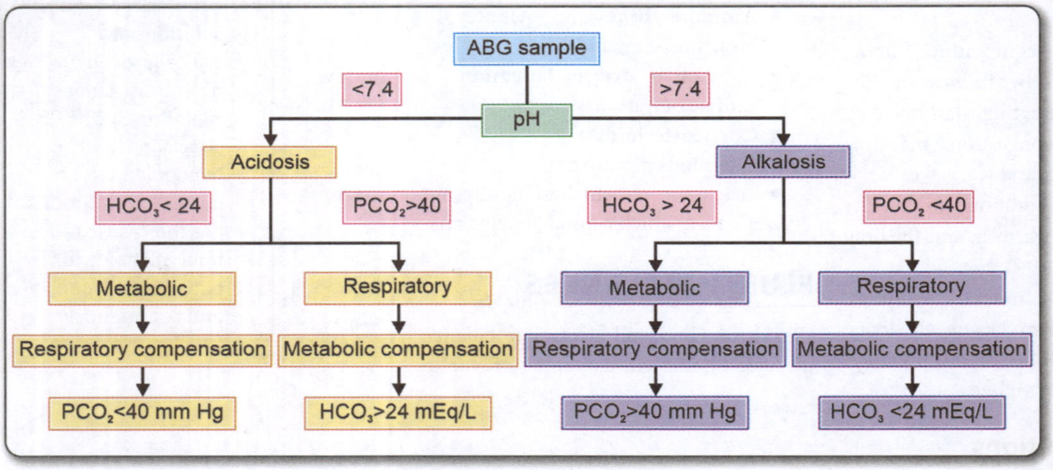

Figure 139: ABG analysis

Clinical Corner

ABG Analysis Practice: Interpret acid-base disorder from the following ABG values:

CASE 1:

pH 7.55, P_aO_2 85 mm Hg, P_aCO_2 40 mm Hg, and HCO_3 35 mmol/L

a. Respiratory alkalosis, uncompensated
b. Metabolic alkalosis, uncompensated
c. Respiratory alkalosis, partially compensated
d. Metabolic alkalosis, partially compensated

Ans. (b) Metabolic alka...

CASE 2:

pH 7.38, P_aCO_2 28 mm Hg, and HCO_3 18 mEq/L

a. Respiratory acidosis, uncompensated
b. Metabolic acidosis, uncompensated
c. Respiratory acidosis, fully compensated
d. Metabolic acidosis, fully compensated

Ans. (d) Metabolic...

CASE 3:

pH 7.2, P_aCO_2 72 mm Hg, and HCO_3 24 mEq/L.

a. Respiratory acidosis, uncompensated
b. Respiratory acidosis, compensated
c. Metabolic acidosis, uncompensated
d. Metabolic acidosis, compensated.

Ans. (a) Respiratory...

ROME – Respiratory Opposite; Metabolic Equal (relationship between pH and other parameters)

CAUSES OF OTHER ACID-BASE DISORDERS

Table 109: Acid-base disorders and their causes

Metabolic acidosis	Metabolic alkalosis	Respiratory acidosis	Respiratory alkalosis
• GI loss of HCO_3 ▪ Diarrhea, Cholera, Fistula • Renal loss of HCO_3 • Pancreatitis • Ureterosigmoidostomy • Ileostomy fluid loss • Metabolic disorders ▪ Lactic acidosis ▪ DKA ▪ Alcoholic ketoacidosis	• **Vomiting/gastric suction** • Pyloric stenosis • Diuretics • Hyperaldosteronism/ Conn's syndrome • **Cushing syndrome** • Bartter syndrome • **Hypokalemia** • $NaHCO_3$ infusion • **Multiple blood transfusion**	• **Asthma** • **COPD** • **ARDS** • Obesity • **Hypoventilation** • Myasthenia • Pneumothorax • Pulmonary edema	• **Normal pregnancy** • **High altitude residence** • CHF • **Hyperventilation syndrome** • Hepatic failure • Salicylate intoxication

ELECTROLYTES

Table 110: Electrolytes, their functions, effects of their deficit and excess

Electrolyte (Normal range)	Functions	Deficit leads to	Excess leads to
Sodium (135–145 mEq/L)	• Osmotic balance maintenance • Regulation of acid base balance. • Normal muscle irritability • Initiates and maintains heartbeat	**Hyponatremia** **Causes** • Low sodium consumption • Increased loss of sodium • Overhydration • Use of diuretics • Increased ADH hormone • Addison's disease • Hypoaldosteronism. **Signs and symptoms** • Confusion, drowsiness, muscle weakness, seizure	**Hypernatremia** **Causes** • Dehydration • Diabetes insipidus • Cushing syndrome • Hyperaldosteronism ▪ *Prolonged cortisone use.* **Signs and Symptoms** • Thirst • Confusion • Neuromuscular excitability • Hyperreflexia Seizures • Coma
Potassium (3.5 – 5 mEq/L)	• Maintains intracellular osmotic pressure • Transmission of nerve impulse • Cardiac muscle activity • Regulation of acid-base balance.	**Hypokalemia** **Causes** • Cushing syndrome • Prolonged cortisone use • Diuretics • Diarrhea • Vomiting. **Signs and symptoms** • Fatigue • Confusion • Cramps • Paralysis • Muscle weakness • Arrhythmia • ST wave depression and abnormal U wave.	**Hyperkalemia** **Causes** • Kidney failure • Potassium sparing diuretics • Burn wound • Tissue injury • Addison's disease. **Signs and symptoms** • Prolonged PR interval, spiked/peaked T wave.
Calcium (8.5–10.5 mg/dL).	• Development of bones and teeth • Nerve impulse transmission • Important role in muscle contraction	**Hypocalcemia** **Causes** • Deficiency of vitamin D • Hypoparathyroidism **Signs and symptoms** • Tetany • Positive **Chvostek sign** • Positive Trousseau's sign • Cramps • Neuromuscular irritability • Numbness • Spasm • Convulsion • Seizure • Osteoporosis	**Hypercalcemia** **Causes** • Bone cancer (Paget's disease) • Hyperparathyroidism • Hyperthyroidism • Sarcoidosis • Hypervitaminosis D **Signs and symptoms** • Excess urination • Dehydration • Nausea and vomiting • Muscle cramps and weakness • Flank pain • Bone pain • Confusion and coma (severe cases)

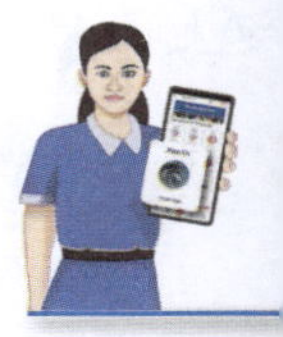

HEMORRHAGE

- Hemorrhage, also known as bleeding, refers to escape of blood from circulatory system through damaged blood vessels
- Most common cause of Hypovolemic shock
- **Manifestation**
  - Cool and moist skin, fall in BP, tachycardia, increased capillary refill time and decreased urinary output
- **Management**
  - Control of external hemorrhage
    - Direct pressure over bleeding area
    - Injured part is elevated to arrest venous and capillary bleeding
    - **Tourniquet** is to be used only when all other methods fail to control bleeding (**as a last resort**)
  - Control of Internal bleeding
  - Fluid and blood volume replacement
  - Packed RBC is administered in case of severe blood loss.

POINT TO REMEMBER

Use packed RBC in emergency situation when same group RBC is not available or cross matching is not possible

Table 111: Age/gender criteria for PRBCs

Age/Gender criteria	Group of packed RBC
All patients under 16 years of age	Type O, Rh negative RBC's
Female of child bearing age (<50 years)	Type O, Rh negative RBC's
Male (>16 years) and Female (post menopausal)	Type O, Rh positive*

*Used only in life-threatening emergencies; there is a positive D-Immunization if When Rh-positive RBC's are used in an Rh-negative patient.

Recent Question (CNCI 2021)

139. Which of the following is not an isotonic fluid?
a. 0.9%
b. RL
c. Dextrose 5% in water
d. Dextrose 5% in normal saline

Ans. (d) Dextrose 5% in...

Recent Question (NORCET 2020)

140. Heimlich maneuver is used as an intervention in which of the following conditions?
a. Lower airway obstruction
b. Nasal Obstruction
c. Tracheal Obstruction
d. Upper airway obstruction

Ans. (d) Upper airway...

EMERGENCY NURSING - PRIORITIZATION OF CARE

- Airway with cervical spine protection
- Breathing and ventilation
- Circulation with hemorrhage control
- Disability–GCS
- Exposure, event and hypothermia

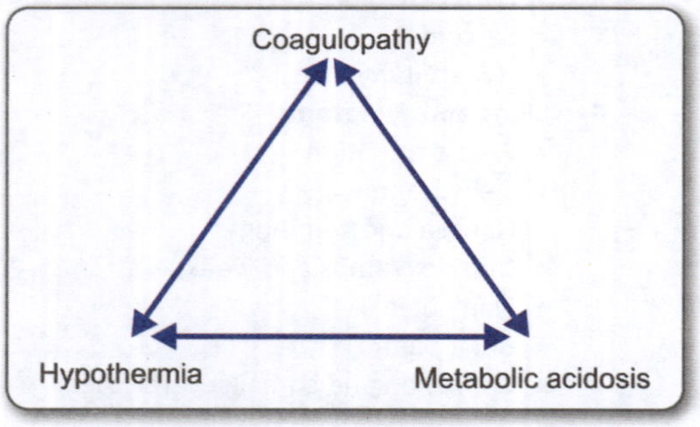

Figure 140: Triad of trauma death

PRIORITIES OF CARE AND TRIAGE CATEGORIES

Level 1: Resuscitation (immediate clinical assessment)
Level 2: Emergent
Level 3: Urgent (time critical)/potential life threatening
Level 4: Semiurgent/situational urgency
Level 5: Less/nonurgent

- The patient who has been resuscitated is at risk for another episode of cardiac arrest.
- Orogastric tube is inserted if basilar skull fracture is expected.
- Antidotes generally have a shorter half-life, repeated dosing is often necessary.

Compartment syndrome is a painful, limb-threatening event. Do not elevate limb above the level of heart. Emergency fasciotomy is often required.

Clinical Corner

CASE SCENARIO 5:

A 25-year-old male client who suffered multiple injuries from a road traffic accident is brought to the emergency room. Which of the following assessments should take the highest priority?
a. Unequal pupils
b. Tachycardia
c. A deviated trachea
d. Ecchymosis in the umbilical region

Ans. (c) A deviated...

Explanation: A deviated trachea is a symptom of tension pneumothorax, which may result in respiratory distress if left untreated.

Strategy: Use Airway Breathing Circulation (ABC) principle to prioritize the nursing care.

COMMON EQUIPMENT IN CRITICAL CARE AREA

Ventilator

It is a machine designed to provide artificial respiration to patients who are unable to breathe themselves.

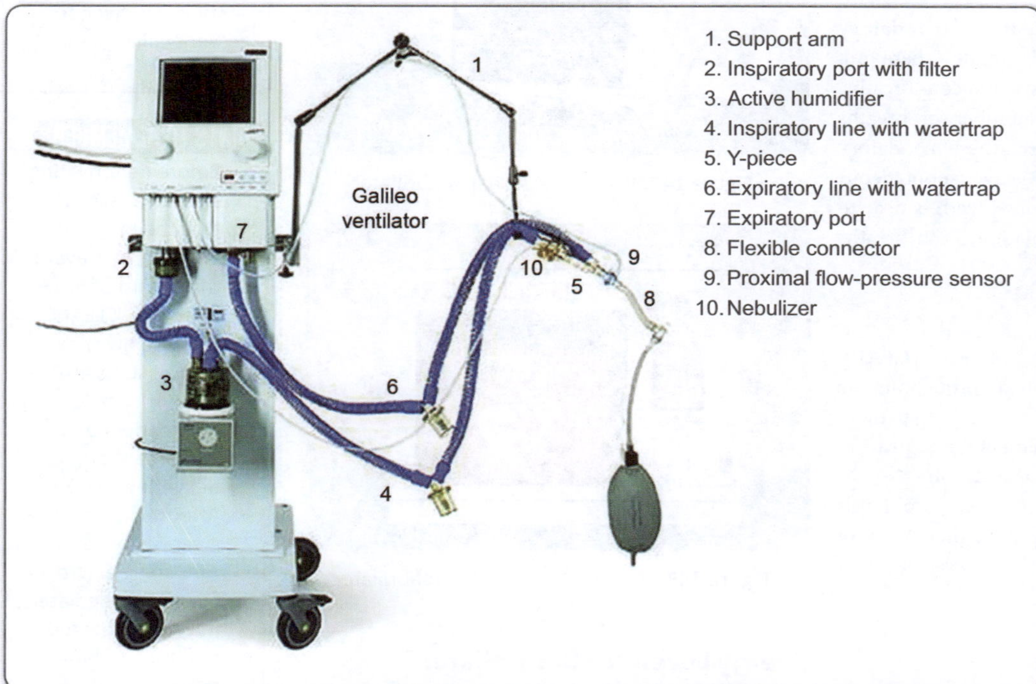

Figure 141: A mechanical ventilator for intensive care, with the external circuit

Types of Ventilators

- **Transport ventilators:** They are small ventilators that run with the help of AC or DC and the main purpose of this ventilator is to shift or transport patient from one area of hospital to another or to a different hospital.
- **Intensive care ventilators:** They are large sophisticated equipment with greater control over parameters.
- **Neonatal ventilators:** These are the ventilators designed for small preterm babies to provide precise amount volume, pressure, etc. as needed by the baby.

Forms of Mechanical Ventilation

Positive Pressure Ventilator

- These ventilators achieve positive pressure in the airway of client through ET or tracheostomy tube.
- Positive pressure allows the air to flow into the lungs.

Negative Pressure Ventilator

This type of ventilator creates negative pressure around patient's trunk and helps in breathing.

High Frequency Oscillatory Ventilation

These types of ventilators provide respiratory rate four times that of the normal.

Terminologies Related to Ventilator

Fraction of inspired oxygen (FiO_2): Concentration of oxygen in the inspired air. Atmospheric air contains 21% of oxygen.

Tidal volume: Volume of air delivered to patient during each breath.

Respiratory rate/frequency: Number of breaths per minute.

Minute volume: Total volume of air moved into the lung in a minute. It is the product of multiplication of tidal volume and respiratory rate /frequency.

Exhaled tidal volume: Volume of air coming out of patient's lung during exhalation.

Positive end expiratory pressure (PEEP): Positive pressure maintained in the airway at the end of expiration.

Modes of Ventilation

Volume Modes

- **Controlled mandatory ventilation (CMV):** Ventilator delivers set number of breaths at set volume which is independent of patient's effort.

Recent Question (CNCI 2021)

141. A nurse enters a room and finds a patient lying on the floor. Which action should the nurse perform first?
a. Assist the patient back to bed
b. Establish whether the patient is responsive
c. Ask the patient what happened
d. Call for help to get the patient back in bed

Ans. (b) Establish...

Recent Questions (NORCET 2020)

142. While performing an endotracheal tube (ET) suction, the nurse observed that the client is having sudden severe tachycardia. Which of the following should be the immediate response of the nurse?
a. Continue the suction
b. Stop suction and perform re-oxygenation
c. Hyperoxygenate before suctioning
d. Call the physician

Ans. (b) Stop suction and...

143. What is the suction pressure applied while performing endotracheal tube suction in an adult patient?
a. 40–60 mm Hg
b. 50–75 mm Hg
c. 60–100 mm Hg
d. 100–120 mm Hg

Ans. (d) 100–120 mm Hg

- **Assist/controlled ventilation (ACV)**: Ventilator provides pre-set number of breaths at pre-set volume. When the patient initiates breathing effort, ventilator will provide pre-set volume of assisted breath.
- **Synchronized intermittent mandatory ventilation (SIMV)**: In this mode, there are mandatory breaths as well as spontaneous breaths. Ventilator provides pre-set number of breaths with pre-set volume. In between these mandatory breaths, patient will try to have spontaneous breaths. If patient's spontaneous breath is near to the time of mandatory ventilation, both breaths will be synchronized.

Pressure Modes

Continuous positive airway pressure (CPAP): Positive airway pressure is applied throughout the respiratory cycle of a spontaneous breathing patient. **Positive pressure applied at the end of the expiration helps to prevent the collapse of the alveoli.**

Bi-level positive airway pressure: Two levels of airway pressure is applied. A higher level of inspiratory airway pressure and a lower level of expiratory airway pressure.

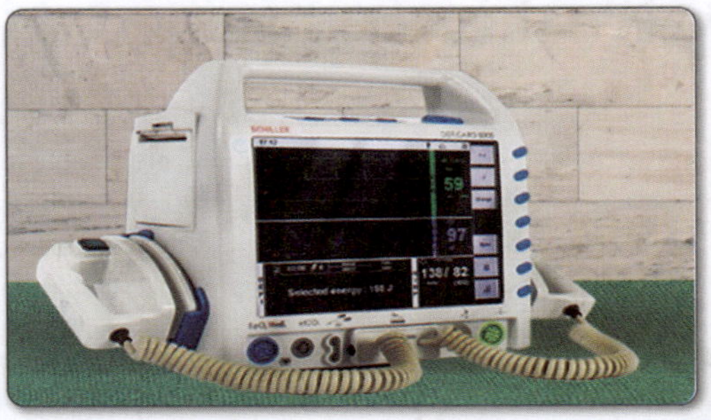

Figure 142: Manual external defibrillator

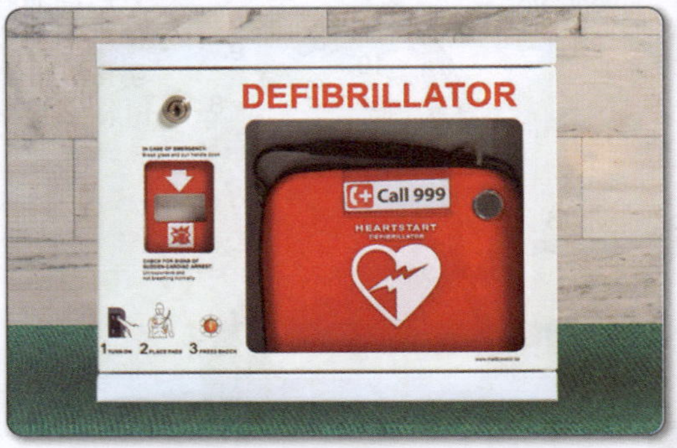

Figure 143: Automated external defibrillator (AED)

DEFIBRILLATOR

- Application of pre-set electrical current to myocardium which converts dysrhythmia to normal rhythm.
- **Indication**: Definitive treatment for ventricular fibrillation, pulseless ventricular tachycardia.

Types

- Manual external defibrillator
- Automated external defibrillator
- Implantable cardiac defibrillator

Energy Levels for Defibrillator

- Monophasic: 360 J
- Biphasic: 120–200 J

Electrodes Placement

- **Anteroapical:** One pad/paddle is placed to the right of the sternum just below the clavicle, and the other is centered lateral to the normal cardiac apex in the anterior or midaxillary line (V5–6)
- **Anteroposterior:** The anterior pad/paddle is placed over the precordium or apex, and the posterior pad/paddle is placed on the back in the left or right infrascapular region.

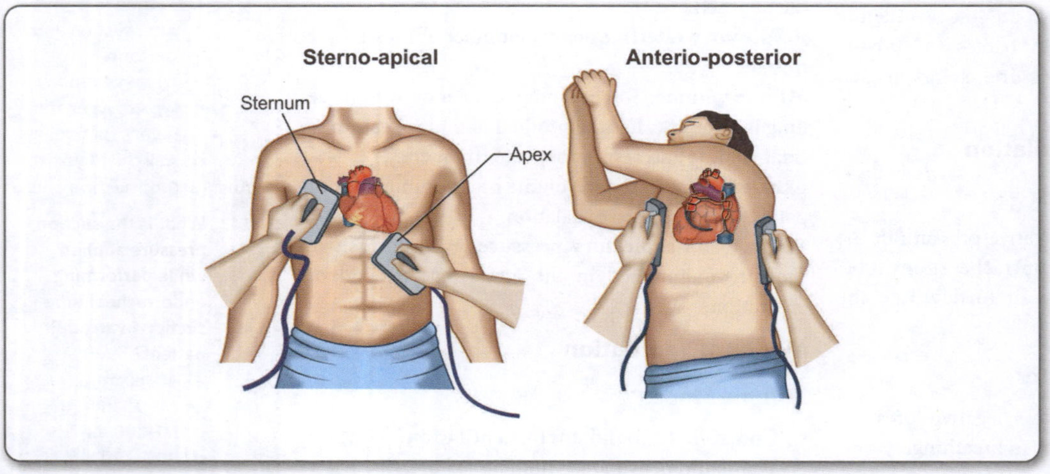

Figure 144: Placement of electrodes

KEY POINT

Positive-End-Expiratory Pressure (PEEP) in ventilator is given to prevent collapse of alveoli.

POINTS TO REMEMBER

- Before defibrillating a client, make sure that the oxygen supply is off to prevent the hazard of fire.
- State "ALL CLEAR" and visually check that all staffs are clear of contact with bed, patient and equipment before delivering shock.
- After the procedure, clear defibrillator of remaining electrical current immediately; never set charged defibrillator paddles down

Recent Question (NORCET 2023)

144. The nurse provides care for a patient with an endotracheal tube and positive pressure mechanical ventilation. Which of the following observation requires intervention by the nurse?

a. The intern nurse drains ventilator tubing condensation towards the endotracheal tube connection
b. The patient gags and bites the endotracheal tube
c. The intern nurse reports that the patient's weight has increased 1.3 kg over past 72 hours
d. The endotracheal tube cuff pressure is 22 cm H_2O

Ans. (b) The patient gags and bites the endotracheal tube

STAGES OF DEATH AND DYING (KUBBLER ROSS STAGES OF DYING)

Stages (DABDA)

- **Denial (D):** Shock, doubt and disbelief about the loss are the primary response.
- **Anger (A):** Characterized by anger often towards others. This stage is often very short-lived.
- **Bargaining (B):** When denial and anger fail to work, people make an effort to bargain for a better outcome rather than a current situation.
- **Depression (D):** When it becomes obvious that the loss/death is obvious, people feel depressed characterized by persistent sadness. This stage is important one to go through. If a person is able to complete the stage of depression successfully, the acceptance will follow.
- **Acceptance (A):** In this stage, the person gradually and peacefully accepts death. He quietly accepts the arrival of death.

Nursing Management

- Assist the client make final plans towards death.
- Encourage reminiscence
- Help the client in validation of self-image.
- Use touch as a communication tool if it is acceptable to the client.
- Provide spiritual support.

Golden Points to Remember

- **General Adaptation Syndrome (GAS)** is composed of three stages (in sequence):
  1. Alarm reaction
  2. Stage of resistance
  3. Stage of exhaustion
- An increased metabolic rate intensifies water loss. There is a **7%** increase in metabolism for every **1°F** increase in temperature above **100°F** or a **13%** increase for every **1°C** increase.
- Causes of **Hypokalemia** include vomiting, diarrhea, prolonged GI suction and prolonged IV therapy.
- **Hypokalemia** is deficiency of potassium in blood.
- **Signs of Hypocalcemia:** Trousseau's sign/carpopedal spasm, Chvostek's sign.
- **Trousseau's Sign** is a sign of tetany in which carpal spasm can be elicited by compressing the upper arm and causing ischemia to the nerves distally.
- **Sulkowitch Test** is used to measure the calcium content in urine mainly in hypocalcemia.
- Do not use sterile water to flush the NG tube, as it has a pH of **4.5** and could cause **Metabolic Acidosis**.
- **Perineal Hematoma** after trauma occurs due to Rupture of bulbar urethra.
- **IgE mediated chemicals** are associated with **Anaphylactic** reaction.
- **Alarm reaction, Resistance and Exhaustion** (in same sequence) are the three stages of General Adaptation Syndrome (GAS) of stress.
- Sympathetic nervous system is responsible for **Fight of Flight response**.
- Cardiac output is usually normal in **Circulatory/Distributive Shock**.
- Most frequently encountered acid base disorder is **Respiratory Alkalosis**.
- Acid base disorder seen in normal pregnancy is **Respiratory Alkalosis**.
- Fever of >41.5°C (>106.7°F) is called hyperpyrexia.
- The pathway through which a cell produces the maximum number of ATP molecules is **TCA cycle.** It produces 38 ATPs in total (34 from oxidative phosphorylation + 4 from substrate level phosphorylation).
- **Atropine** is the antidote for **organophosphorus poisoning**.
- The antidote for atropine positioning is **Physostigmine**.
- A food item commonly associated with Bacillus cereus food poisoning is **Fried Rice**.
- K bind is given for patients with **Hyperkalemia** to reduce the serum potassium level.
- **The Revised Trauma Score (RTS)** is made up of a combination of results from three categories: Glasgow coma scale, systolic blood pressure, and respiratory rate.
- A 25-year-old male presents with road traffic accidents with a BP of 100/80 mm Hg and a pulse of 84/min. Best fluid for resuscitation is Crystalloid.
- In Salicylates (Aspirin) overdose there is metabolic acidosis with respiratory alkalosis.
- **Capnography** is a noninvasive method for monitoring the level of CO_2 in exhaled breath to assess a patient's ventilatory status. The CO_2 detector should change color from purple to yellow.
- The elderly individual is at greater risk for **Dehydration** because the compensatory mechanism works less efficiently in old age.
- In a stroke patient, the best position for the insertion of NG tube is **High Fowler's position**.

Contd...

- **Pulse pressure** is the difference between the systolic and diastolic blood pressure. Normal is 30–50 mm Hg.
- **Assessment of Client's Response** is the first step when a nurse finds a collapsed patient.
- **For Adult CPR:** Chest compression to ventilations ratio is 30:2. (single or two rescuer)
- **For Child CPR:** Chest compression to ventilations ratio is 30:2 for single rescuer. 15:2 for two rescuers.
- **Positive End-Expiratory Pressure (PEEP)** is the positive pressure that will remain in the airways at the end of the respiratory cycle (end of exhalation) that is greater than the atmospheric pressure in **Mechanically Ventilated Patients**.
- **Normal Intracranial Pressure** (ICP) is 5–15 mm Hg.
- **Morphine** is contraindicated in a patient with head injury. Morphine should only be used in head injury patients if it is extremely essential.
- Symptoms of "**Opioid Overdose Triad**" is pinpoint pupils, respiratory depression and unconsciousness.
- Drastic drop in blood pressure may be seen in **Neurogenic Shock**.
- Increased heart rate or pulse rate is the early sign of **Hemorrhagic Shock**. It happens as a compensatory mechanism due to the release of epinephrine.
- Protecting the client from injury is the immediate priority during a **Seizure**.
- The McGill Pain Questionnaire (MPQ) is a multi-dimensional pain assessment tool which assesses sensory intensity, the cognitive evaluation of pain and the emotional impact of pain.

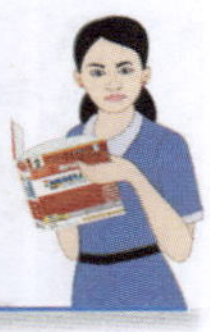

"If you would live long, open your heart."
—Bulgarian

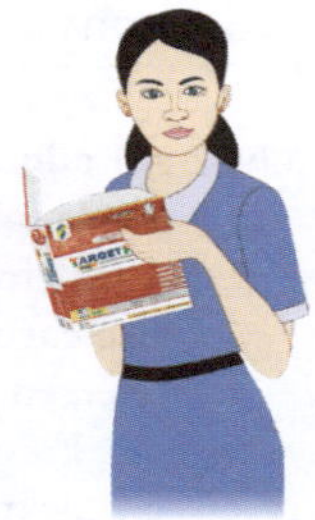

MULTIPLE CHOICE QUESTIONS
(Including Explained and Practice Questions)

HOMEOSTASIS, EMERGENCY AND CRITICAL CARE NURSING

STRESS AND ADAPTATION

3489. Which of the following response to stress is due to negative feedback mechanism?
- a. Neurophysiological response
- b. Hypothermia
- c. Hyperventilation
- d. Altered level of consciousness

3490. An adolescent boy who is shifting to a different school expresses anxiety over changing his school. Voicing anxiety is an act of:
- a. Reaction
- b. Evaluation
- c. Adaptation
- d. Resistance

3491. Which of the following physiological response is experienced during alarm stage of general adaptation syndrome (GAS)?
- a. Decreased blood pressure
- b. Vasodilation
- c. Decreased mental alertness
- d. Initiation of neuroendocrine activity

Explanation: The alarm stage of GAS is often accompanied by increased mental alertness, initiation of endocrine activity and vasoconstriction. Exhaustion stage is often accompanied by decreased blood pressure and vasodilation.

3492. Which of the following nursing diagnosis in an anxious patient may require a short-term pharmacological therapy?
- a. Defensive coping
- b. Disturbed sleep pattern
- c. Disturbed thought process
- d. Ambivalence

Explanation: Disturbed sleep patterns are often treated with appropriate sedative and hypnotics. Defensive coping, ambivalence and disturbed through process (eg., Delusion) are less amenable to short-term pharmacological treatment.

3493. Cortisol is involved in all of the following biological functions; EXCEPT:
- a. Immune suppression
- b. Hyperglycemia
- c. Increased inflammatory response
- d. Lypolysis

3494. Which of the following brain areas is affected by the stress hormone (cortisol), and results in impaired memory function?
- a. Hippocampus
- b. Parietal lobe
- c. Hypothalamus
- d. Frontal lobe

3495. Which of the following hormone released from the hypothalamus stimulates the anterior pituitary to release adrenocorticotropic hormone (ACTH)?
- a. GnRH
- b. CRH
- c. ADH
- d. Growth Hormone

Explanation: The anterior pituitary produces ACTH. Corticotropin releasing hormone (CRH) is released from the hypothalamus which stimulates the anterior pituitary to release adrenocorticotropic hormone (ACTH). ACTH then acts on its target organ, the adrenal cortex.

3496. All of the following manifestation may be the effect of excessive stress, excessive cortisol levels, or Cushing's disorder:
- a. Moon face
- b. Hypoglycemia
- c. Diminished inflammatory response
- d. None of the above

3497. Which of the following substance is released in response to alarm reaction and promotes the sense of well-being?
- a. Aldosterone
- b. Thyroid-stimulating hormone
- c. Endorphins
- d. Adrenocorticotropic hormone

Explanation: Endorphins are released in response to pain or stress. Since endorphins act on the opiate receptors in our brains, they reduce pain and boost pleasure, resulting in a feeling of well-being.

3498. A Client says that she is having a vague mind, uneasy feeling of dread, and had a raised heart rate. Which nursing diagnosis is appropriate for treating this patient:
- a. Anger
- b. Fear
- c. Anxiety
- d. Hopelessness

3499. What is the Role of antidiuretic hormone when released in the alarm stage of the Generalized Anxiety Syndrome:
- a. Enhance fluid retention by reabsorption of water
- b. Enhance fluid excretion by decreasing resorption of water
- c. Increase energy by means of fat conservation
- d. Release the endorphin hormone to alleviate the stress

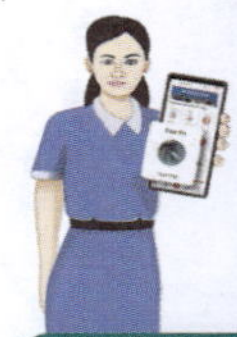

Ans.

3489. a
3490. c
3491. d
3492. b
3493. c
3494. a
3495. b
3496. b
3497. c
3498. c
3499. a

3500. An adult woman's father has passed away, and her mom needs physical and emotional help due to disabilities. Apart from working fulltime in a workshop, the woman also caring for two school going children. All of the factors referred are known as:

a. Stressors b. Demands
c. Sickness d. Stimuli

Explanation: Stressors are external events or circumstances that can trigger a stress response in an individual. They can be physical, psychological, or social in nature and can vary widely depending on the individual's perception and ability to cope.

SHOCK

3501. Vasoconstrictors should not be used in:

a. Neurogenic shock *(Safdarjung NO 2018)*
b. Hemorrhagic shock
c. Secondary shock
d. Hypotension due to spinal anesthesia

Explanation:

- Vasoconstrictors should not be used in hemorrhagic shock as it may lead to severe arteriolar vasoconstriction causing tissue ischemia. In hemorrhagic shock, the body's normal response is vasoconstriction to divert blood toward the vital organs, severe vasoconstriction may cause the tissue hypoxia and anaerobic respiration and death.
- While in other shocks, vasoconstrictors are recommended to combat the hypotension.

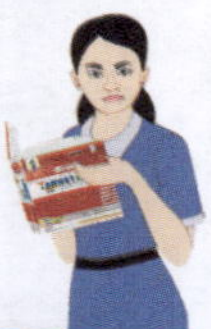

3502. In shock primarily, there is:

a. Metabolic waste accumulates
b. Poor perfusion of tissues
c. Decreased cardiac contraction
d. Skeletal muscles become fatigue

3503. Shock resulting from severe allergic reaction is:

a. Septic shock
b. Anaphylactic shock
c. Neurogenic shock
d. Traumatic shock

3504. Shock due to overwhelming infection is known as:

a. Anaphylactic shock
b. Cardiogenic
c. Neurogenic shock
d. Septic shock

3505. Shock due to spinal cord injury is known as:

a. Anaphylactic shock b. Cardiogenic
c. Neurogenic shock d. Septic shock

3506. After falling from a 10 feet ladder, a patient is brought to the emergency department. The patient is alert, reports back pain, and difficulty moving the lower extremities. Which additional observation is an indication the patient may be experiencing neurogenic shock? *(NCFL 2019)*

a. Cool and pale skin
b. Bradycardia
c. Poor skin turgor
d. Increased systolic blood pressure

Explanation:

- Neurogenic shock is an emergency situation caused by impaired blood circulation due to trauma of spine. It leads to the drastic **drop in blood pressure**. Symptoms include fainting, nausea, vomiting, increased sweating, anxiety, pale skin, dizziness, etc. In severe patients – **bradycardia, hypotension**, hypothermia, feeble pulse and cyanosis is seen.
- Bradycardia is seen in neurogenic shock because the blood vessels are relaxed and so the heart doesn't beat fast.
- Skin remains warm in the neurogenic shock.

3507. Drug of choice in anaphylactic shock is:

a. Atropine b. Adrenaline
c. Amiodarone d. Propofol

3508. Important nursing responsibility during anaphylactic reaction is:

a. Administering oxygen b. Administer adrenaline
c. Provide antidote d. Monitor vitals

3509. Mediator of Anaphylactic shock is:

a. Histamine b. Cytokines
c. Dopamine d. Adrenaline

3510. Most important nursing intervention in a client who is experiencing anaphylactic reaction following antibiotic administration is:

a. Administer antidote b. Maintain a patent airway
c. Provide RL d. Record the reaction

Explanation: Anaphylactic reactions are severe and potentially life-threatening hypersensitivity reactions that can occur in response to certain medications, including antibiotics. The priority nursing intervention in anaphylaxis is to ensure a patent airway to support adequate oxygenation and ventilation.

Strategy: Use ABC principle to solve the question. Airway is the priority.

3511. Emergency treatment of hypovolemic shock includes:

a. Relief of pain
b. Administration of vasodilators
c. Administration of IV fluids or blood product
d. Administration of antibiotics

3512. Position given to a client experiencing shock is:

a. Fowler's position b. Trendelenburg
c. Prone position d. Supine position

3513. Which among the following is present in the patho-physiology of septic Shock?

a. Vasodilatation
b. Decreased cardiac output
c. Increased capillary permeability
d. All of the above

3514. The acid-base imbalance which commonly accompanies shock is:

a. Respiratory acidosis b. Respiratory alkalosis
c. Metabolic acidosis d. Metabolic alkalosis

3515. True about shock:

a. In early stage cardiac output and BP are maintained
b. Perfusion to the cells is inadequate to supply oxygen and nutrient
c. Activation of sympathetic nervous system
d. All of the above

Ans.

3500. a
3501. b
3502. b
3503. b
3504. d
3505. c
3506. b
3507. b
3508. a
3509. a
3510. b
3511. c
3512. b
3513. d
3514. c
3515. d

3516. Which among the following parameters need to monitor in a client at risk for shock?

a. Temperature b. Pulse
c. Respiration d. Blood pressure

3517. Systolic BP is ....in cardiac shock:

a. <60 mm Hg b. <70 mm Hg
c. <80 mm Hg d. <90 mm Hg

3518. Type of shock seen in burns cases:

a. Hypovolemic b. Cardiogenic
c. Neurogenic d. None of these

Explanation: Causes of hypovolemic shock: (the most common form of Shock)

Hemorrhagic	Nonhemorrhagic
Trauma	Dehydration Vomiting Diarrhea Diabetes having urinary loss **Evaporation in Burns** Third space loss pancreatitis, bowel obstruction

3519. In stage 3 hypovolemic shock, the patient will have blood loss of:

a. 10-20% b. 20-30%
c. 30-40% d. 40-50%

3520. Ms. Babita is in the emergency room after being involved in a traffic accident. What would be an early sign of hemorrhagic shock? *(NCFL 2019)*

a. Increased blood pressure b. Pallor
c. Increased heart rate d. Deep breathing

Explanation: Hemorrhagic shock is a sudden circulatory shock happens because of the huge blood loss. Increased heart rate or pulse rate is the early sign of hemorrhagic shock. It happens as a compensatory mechanism due to the release of epinephrine which makes the heart to beat faster and also promotes vasoconstriction.

3521. Which among the following is the management modality for cardiogenic shock?

a. Dobutamine to increase the heart's pumping capacity
b. Antibiotics to treat the infection
c. Colloids to increase the blood volume
d. NTG to dilate coronary blood vessels

Explanation: In cardiogenic shock, the goal of treatment is to improve cardiac function and restore tissue perfusion.

Dobutamine is a catecholamine with β-1 and β-2 adrenergic agonist properties which help improve myocardial contractility. In patients with cardiogenic shock due to decompensated heart failure, dobutamine decreases left ventricular end-diastolic pressure and raises blood pressure by increasing cardiac output.

3522. Client is experiencing tachycardia, decreased blood pressure, weak thready pulse, and cool skin. Assessment found crackles and tachypnea. These manifestation suggests:

a. Anaphylactic shock
b. Cardiogenic shock
c. Hypovolemic shock
d. Septic shock

Explanation: Cardiogenic shock is a condition characterized by inadequate cardiac output due to a severe impairment in the heart's ability to pump effectively. The manifestations described, such as tachycardia, decreased blood pressure, weak thready pulse, cool skin, and crackles, can be consistent with the signs of cardiogenic shock. Tachypnea may also be present as a compensatory response to maintain oxygenation.

The presence of crackles suggests the accumulation of fluid in the lungs, which can occur in cardiogenic shock due to impaired cardiac function and fluid backup in the pulmonary circulation.

3523. Which among the following clients is at risk for developing cardiogenic shock?

a. Acute myocardial infarction (MI)
b. Coronary artery disease (CAD)
c. Pulmonary edema
d. Microvascular thrombi

Explanation: Myocardial infarction can result in significant damage to the heart muscle, impairing its ability to pump effectively and increasing the risk of developing cardiogenic shock.

While options b (coronary artery disease), c (pulmonary edema), and d (microvascular thrombi) are associated with cardiovascular issues, they may not directly lead to cardiogenic shock.

3524. Earliest sign of cardiogenic shock is:

a. Peripheral vascular resistance
b. Altered level of consciousness
c. Pitting edema
d. Heart murmurs

Explanation: Cardiogenic shock occurs when the heart is unable to pump enough blood to meet the body's demands. It is a severe condition that can be life-threatening. The earliest sign of cardiogenic shock is often a change in the level of consciousness, which can range from mild confusion to severe lethargy or loss of consciousness. This change in mental status reflects the inadequate perfusion of oxygen and nutrients to the brain due to reduced cardiac output.

While options a, c, and d may be present in individuals with cardiogenic shock, they are not the earliest signs.

3525. Drug of choice to treat cardiogenic shock is:

a. Dopamine b. Adrenaline
c. NTG d. Lidocaine

3526. ....is the diagnostic and monitoring tool for determining the severity of a shock state:

a. CVP line b. Indwelling urinary catheter
c. IABP d. Pulmonary artery catheter

3527. Adequacy of fluid replacement in hypovolemic shock can be assessed through:

a. Skin turgor b. Urine output
c. Blood pressure d. Distal pulse

Explanation: Most accurate information regarding the fluid replacement adequacy will be given by the urine output in the person.

3528. The nurse suspect the patient is in shock after craniotomy. Which would be the appropriate nursing action?

a. Inform the physician
b. Increase intravenous fluids
c. Give Trendelenburg's position
d. Monitor vital signs continuously

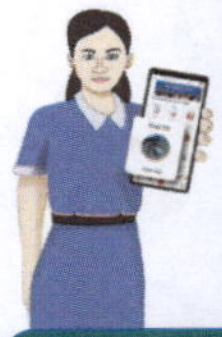

Ans.

3516. b
3517. d
3518. a
3519. c
3520. c
3521. a
3522. b
3523. a
3524. b
3525. a
3526. d
3527. b
3528. a

Explanation: Nurse should inform the physician immediately because she should not give intravenous fluids without doctor's prescription. Trendelenburg's position may increase intracranial pressure and monitoring vital signs will not alleviate shock.

ANAPHYLAXIS

3529. All of the following effects on the body are mediated by the release of histamine during anaphylactic shock; EXCEPT:
- a. Constriction of airways
- b. Vasodilation
- c. Decreased capillary permeability
- d. Decreased heart rate

Explanation: During anaphylactic shock the mast cells and basophils release large amount of histamine. Release of histamine results in increased capillary permeability by shifting intravascular fluid to the interstitial space. It causes edema, hypotension, vasodilation, decreased heart rate, constriction of airways, etc.

3530. Intramuscular Adrenaline or Epinephrine is administered to treat anaphylactic reaction. Which of the following effects does epinephrine have on the body?
- a. Bronchodilation
- b. Vasodilation
- c. Hypotension
- d. Bradycardia

3531. If a patient develops anaphylactic reaction to an IV medication, which of the following should be the immediate response of a nurse? *New Q*
- a. Call for emergency help
- b. Stop the medication administration immediately
- c. Administer IM Epinephrine
- d. Start CPR

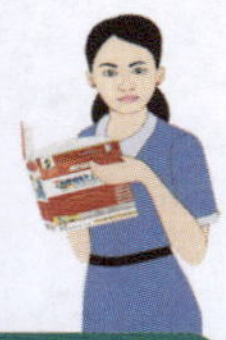

Explanation: The immediate response of the nurse should be removing the allergen (stopping IV medication in this case). The next step is to call rapid response and start basic life support (BLS/CPR) until the help arrives.

3532. Which of the following position is most appropriate for a patient in anaphylactic shock?
- a. High-Fowler's
- b. Left lateral
- c. Supine with legs elevated
- d. Prone

Explanation: Supine with legs elevated position will promote venous return to the heart that helps in increased cardiac output and blood pressure.

FLUID IMBALANCES

3533. In healthy individuals, plasma osmolality ranges from: *(AIIMS-BBS SNO 2019)*
- a. 300-310 mOsm/kg of H_2O
- b. 270-280 mOsm/kg of H_2O
- c. 280-295 mOsm/kg of H_2O
- d. 320-325 mOsm/kg of H_2O

3534. Physiological process which is responsible for maintaining fluid balance across the intracellular and extracellular compartments mainly is:
- a. Osmosis
- b. Facilitated diffusion
- c. Simple diffusion
- d. Active transport

3535. The percentage of water in human body is: *(Jipmer 2012)*
- a. 60%
- b. 80%
- c. 35%
- d. None of these

3536. Fluid compartment of blood is:
- a. Lymph
- b. Plasma
- c. Intracellular fluid
- d. Extracellular fluid

3537. Which of these statements is TRUE regarding total body water?
- a. The intracellular fluid compartment constitutes ½ of the total body water.
- b. The ECF compartment comprises about 40% of the body weight.
- c. About 10% of ECF compartment is comprised of plasma.
- d. The interstitial fluid constitutes about ¾ of the ECF compartment.

3538. All the following systems are involved in maintaining fluid and electrolyte balance; EXCEPT:
- a. Muscle system
- b. Urinary system
- c. Integumentary system
- d. Digestive system

3539. Movement across fluid compartments is controlled by:
- a. ATP
- b. Sodium
- c. Osmatic and hydrostatic pressures
- d. Potassium

3540. Active transport requires:
- a. ATP
- b. ADP
- c. Electrolyte
- d. Buffer system

3541. The ability of an organism to maintain internal stability to compensate for environmental changes is termed as:
- a. Adaptation
- b. Homeostasis
- c. Tolerance
- d. Survival

Explanation: The tendency of the body to maintain a condition of balance or equilibrium within its internal environment, even when faced with external changes. A simple example of homeostasis is the body's ability to maintain an internal temperature around 98. 6°F, whatever the temperature outside.

3542. Diffusion of water from a hypotonic solution into a hypertonic solution across and selectively permeable membrane is referred to as:
- a. Active transport
- b. Osmosis
- c. Diffusion
- d. Filtration

3543. Administration of 3 L of 5% dextrose solution will provide:
- a. 400 kilocalories
- b. 600 kilocalories
- c. 900 kilocalories
- d. 1200 kilocalories

Explanation: 1 L of 5% dextrose contains 50 g of glucose. Each gram of glucose (carbohydrate) provides 4 kcal. Therefore 3 L × 50 g × 4 kcal = 600 kcal.

3544. The IV fluid of choice in a patient with severe dehydration: (ISRO)
- a. 5% Dextrose
- b. Dextrose Normal Saline (DNS)
- c. IV albumin
- d. Ringer Lactate

3545. Which of the following is the best guide for fluid administration?
- a. Urine output
- b. CVP
- c. HR
- d. Blood pressure

Ref: S Pandya 2/e, P. 47

Ans.

3529. c
3530. a
3531. b
3532. c
3533. c
3534. a
3535. a
3536. b
3537. d
3538. a
3539. c
3540. a
3541. b
3542. b
3543. b
3544. d
3545. a

Explanation:

- The best single indicator of adequate fluid resuscitation is the urine output on an hourly basis. Adequate end-organ perfusion is best indicated by urine output of > 0.5 to 1 mL/kg/h.
- Hypotension is a late finding in hypovolemic shock; so, pulse rate is a much more sensitive monitoring parameter than arterial blood pressure.

3546. Which type of solution causes water to shift from the cells into the plasma?
a. Hypertonic b. Hypotonic
c. Isotonic d. Alkaline

3547. Hypotonic solution among the following is:
a. 0.45 NS b. 0.9% NS
c. 10% Dextrose d. 25% Dextrose

3548. Isotonic solution among the following is:
a. 0.33% NS b. 0.9% NS
c. Dextran d. 50% Dextrose

3549. Hypertonic solution among the following is:
a. 0.33% NS b. 0.9% NS
c. 5% Dextran d. 50% Dextrose

3550. Colloid solution among the following is:
a. 0.33% NS b. 0.9% NS
c. Dextran d. 50% Dextrose

3551. Nurse Hema is totaling the intake and output for a patient. The patient diagnosed with septicemia who is on a clear liquid diet. The client intakes 4 oz of orange juice, 900 mL of water, 8 oz mL of soup, and 1000 mL of half-normal saline solution and outputs 1,400 mL of urine during the shift. How many milliliters should the nurse document as the patient's intake:
a. 2160 mL b. 2260 mL
c. 2500 mL d. 2380 mL

Explanation: 1 oz = 30 mL

Total input:	
4 oz of Orange juice	= 120 mL
8 oz of soup	= 240 mL
Water	= 900 mL
Half NS	= 1000 mL
Total	**= 2260 mL**

3552. Fluid loss first occurs from:
a. Intracellular b. Intravascular
c. Extravascular d. Interstitial

3553. Insensible losses of water per day are:
a. 400 mL/day
b. 1200 mL/day
c. 800 mL/day
d. 1500 mL/day

3554. In an adult, fever increases water losses by .... mL/day/°C:
a. 70 b. 175
c. 350 d. 600

Explanation: With fever, each degree rise in temperature above 98.6°F (37°C) adds 2.5 mL/kg/day to normal insensible water loss. Average weight of an adult is 70 kg. So 70 × 2.5 = 175 mL. Normal daily insensible water loss is nearly 600-900 mL.

3555. Abrupt stoppage of vasoactive medication will lead to:
a. Hemodynamic instability
b. Increase in cardiac output
c. Anaphylactic reaction
d. All of the above

3556. Mr. Amit is on fluid replacement therapy. Which of the following assessments findings by the nurse indicates adequate tissue perfusion to vital organs?
a. Blood pressure readings from 50/30 to 80/50 in an hour
b. Central venous pressure reading of 2 cm H_2O
c. Pulse rate of 120 and 110 in a 15 minute period
d. Urinary output is 30 mL in an hour

Explanation: Urinary output of 30 mL/hr or more is one of the key indicators of adequacy of blood flow to vital organs such as heart, brain and kidney.

3557. Ideal fluid to provide in fluid volume deficit is:
a. DNS b. 0.45% saline
c. Lactated Ringer's d. 5% dextrose in 0.45% saline

EDEMA

3558. One among the following is the reason for developing edema that is:
a. Dehydration b. Excessive water intake
c. Hyponatremia d. Lymphatic blockage

3559. Which complication of IV infusion can cause pulmonary edema or heart failure? *(RRB SSNE 2015)*
a. Infiltration b. Circulatory overload
c. Infection d. Pyrogenic reactions

3560. Non-inflammatory edema occurs due to:
a. Raise in intravascular hydrostatic pressure
b. Decreased plasma oncotic pressure
c. Obstruction in the lymphatic flow channels
d. All of the above

3561. All of the following are the manifestation of Deep Vein Thrombosis; EXCEPT:
a. Pitting edema in the affected leg
b. Cool and clammy skin in the affected leg
c. Redness
d. Tenderness

3562. Generalized edema is not a common manifestation in one of the following conditions associated with hypoproteinemia:
a. Nephrotic syndrome b. Cirrhosis of liver
c. Malnutrition d. Renal failure

Explanation: Edema in legs, feet and ankle and ascites is more common in liver cirrhosis and, or liver failure. Generalized edema is not a common presentation in patients with liver cirrhosis.

ACID-BASE IMBALANCE

3563. Regulation of pH within the body is done by: *(AIIMS Nagpur NO 2018)*
a. Spleen b. Liver
c. Heart d. Kidney

Explanation: *Kidneys* help control acid-base balance by excreting hydrogen ions and generating bicarbonate that helps to *maintain* blood plasma *pH* within a normal range.

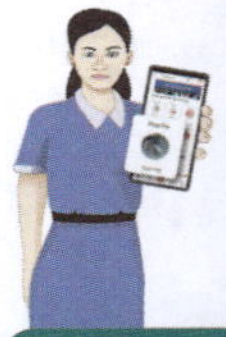

Ans.
3546. a
3547. a
3548. b
3549. d
3550. c
3551. b
3552. b
3553. c
3554. b
3555. d
3556. d
3557. c
3558. d
3559. b
3560. d
3561. b
3562. b
3563. d

3564. What is the normal pH of blood? *(Kerala PSC, Nov 2014)*

a. 6.65-6.45 b. 5.35-6.0
c. 7.35-7.45 d. 6.35-7.0

3565. Most abundant buffer in blood is:

a. Bicarbonates b. Hemoglobin
c. Protein d. Phosphate

3566. Which lab test is useful to find out the blood pH:

a. Arterial blood gas (ABG) levels
b. X-ray
c. Ventilation perfusion match
d. Blood electrolyte

3567. Features of metabolic acidosis?

a. Low plasma bicarbonate
b. High plasma CO_2
c. pH above 7.45
d. Both a and b

3568. ABG values pH: 7.6 $PaCO_2$: 30 mm Hg, HCO_3: 24 mEq and normal PaO_2 suggests:

a. Respiratory acidosis b. Respiratory alkalosis
c. Metabolic acidosis d. Metabolic alkalosis

3569. ABG analysis of an adult patient is as follows: pH = 7. 29, $PaCO_2$ = 47, and HCO_3 = 24. This can be interpreted as:

a. Metabolic acidosis b. Metabolic alkalosis
c. Respiratory acidosis d. Respiratory alkalosis

Explanation: pH below 7.35 indicates acidosis. An elevated $PaCO_2$ indicates the acidosis is due to respiratory problem. So the condition is respiratory acidosis.

3570. pH = 7.55, pCO_2 = 32, HCO_3 = 33, what is the primary abnormality:

a. Respiratory alkalosis b. Metabolic acidosis
c. Respiratory acidosis d. Mixed alkalosis

(Ref: Harrison's 19th ed. pg. 322)

Explanation:

- Interpretation of ABG
  - pH = 7.55 Alkalosis (>7.4)
  - PCO_2 = 32 Low (<35) → Hence alkalosis
  - HCO_3 = 33 High (>26) → Hence alkalosis
- Thus, this ABG shows mixed acid base disorder with both respiratory and metabolic alkalosis [Hint: Think of mixed disorder when "Same direction rule" does not follow]

3571. Which of the following nursing interventions is the most appropriate for the client who has developed respiratory alkalosis due to hyperventilation?

a. Encourage slow, deep breath
b. Start low-flow oxygen therapy
c. Administer Sodiumbicarbonate
d. Administer Ringer Lactate solution

Explanation: The carbon dioxide level of hyperventilated patient is low that leads to respiratory alkalosis. In order to increase the carbon-dioxide concentration, the patient should be encouraged to slow, deep breath which will retain carbondioxide and reverse alkalosis.

3572. The cause for respiratory acidosis among the following is: *(AIIMS BPL NO 2018)*

a. Hyperventilation b. Excessive vomiting
c. Respiratory obstruction d. Diabetic ketoacidosis

Explanation: Respiratory acidosis develops when the lungs do not expel carbon dioxide adequately (inadequate ventilation), a problem that can occur in disorders that severely affect the lungs (such as chronic obstructive pulmonary disease, severe pneumonia, and asthma).

3573. Reason behind metabolic alkalosis after massive blood transfusion is:

a. Anticoagulant sodium citrate will be metabolized to sodium bicarbonate
b. Because of hemolysis of RBCs
c. Electrolyte imbalance in potassium will cause this
d. All of the above

3574. Which among the following metabolic abnormality is seen in a client with vomiting?

a. Metabolic acidosis
b. Metabolic alkalosis
c. Hypokalemia
d. Both b and c

3575. Interpret the following lab report of ABG analysis: pH = 7.27, HCO_3^- = 10 mEq/dl pCO_2 = 23 mm Hg:

a. Respiratory alkalosis
b. Metabolic alkalosis
c. Respiratory acidosis
d. Metabolic acidosis

3576. Best for management of respiratory alkalosis?

a. Mechanical ventilation
b. IPPV
c. Normal saline
d. Rebreathing in paper bag

(Ref: Harrison's 19th/e pg. 324)

Explanation:

Treatment	Metabolic Acidosis	Bicarbonate administration
		Correction of hydration and electrolytes
	Metabolic Alkalosis	Correction of hydration and electrolytes
		H_2 blocker/Proton pump inhibitor
		IV isotonic saline/KCl (avoid Ringer lactate)
		Dilute HCl (rarely)
		Dialysis
	Respiratory Acidosis	Patent airway and adequate oxygenation
		Mechanical ventilation
		Alkali therapy
		O_2 supplementation
	Respiratory Alkalosis	Rebreathing in paper bag
		Pretreatment with acetazolamide before going to high altitude.

3577. When Allen's test is performed?

a. Before venous line insertion
b. Before CVP line insertion
c. Before femoral arterial line insertion
d. Before ABG sampling

Ans.

3564. c
3565. a
3566. a
3567. a
3568. b
3569. c
3570. d
3571. a
3572. c
3573. a
3574. d
3575. d
3576. d
3577. d

ELECTROLYTE IMBALANCE

3578. Which of the following is the function of sodium in the body? *(Kerala PSC, Nov 2014)*
a. Formation of bones
b. Functioning of skeletal muscle
c. Functioning of cardiac muscle
d. Maintenance of serum osmolarity

3579. Hyperkalemia refers to:
a. High chloride b. High potassium
c. High calcium d. High sodium

3580. Aldosterone is directly regulating the concentration of ……….. electrolyte:
a. Calcium b. Potassium
c. Sodium d. Chlorine

3581. Movement of particles (ions or molecules) from an area of higher concentration to an area of lower concentration is referred to as:
a. Inhibition b. Ultrafiltration
c. Diffusion d. Osmosis

3582. Potassium intake is restricted in: *(Staff Nurse G II 2014)*
a. Cardiac failure b. Liver failure
c. Renal failure d. Lung failure

3583. Parenteral preparation of potassium should be administered slowly to prevent: *(JIPMER 2012)*
a. Acidosis b. Cardiac arrest
c. Respiratory arrest d. Over load

3584. In hypoalbuminemia there is:
a. Increase in extra cellular fluid
b. Decrease in extra cellular fluid
c. Increase in intracellular fluid
d. Decrease in intracellular fluid

3585. Poorly controlled diabetes with blood sugar of 450 mg% is associated with:
a. Hyponatremia b. Hypernatremia
c. Hypokalemia d. Hypomagnesemia

Explanation: Glucose produces a drop in the serum sodium concentration by a factor of 1.6 mEq/L–2.4 mEq/L for each 100mg/dL increase in serum glucose greater than 100 mg/dL. [Ref: Harrison's 19th/e pg. 299]

3586. Hypokalemia causes death due to:
a. Diastolic arrest b. Bidirectional Tachycardia
c. Respiratory insufficiency d. Systolic arrest

3587. Important nursing intervention while caring for a client with dilutional hyponatremia includes:
a. Fluid restriction
b. Provide isotonic saline
c. Administer potassium as ordered by physician
d. Provide NG feed

3588. All are used for management of hypernatremia; except:
a. 5% dextrose in water b. Indomethacin
c. Nil by mouth d. N/2 in 5% dextrose

3589. Most common cause of hypernatremia?
a. Sweating b. Carcinoid syndrome
c. Primary hypodipsia d. Renal losses

3590. A convulsion during diarrhea is because of?
a. Hypokalemia b. Hyponatremia
c. Hyperkalemia d. Hypernatremia

3591. In hyperphosphatemia, the electrolyte that needs to be provided is:
a. Potassium b. Calcium
c. Sodium d. Magnesium

3592. Hypokalemia is seen in all; EXCEPT:
a. Vomiting
b. Hyperaldosteronism
c. Administration of loop diuretics
d. Rhabdomyolysis

3593. Which among the following signs need to be reported to the physician of a client receiving loop diuretic?
a. Restlessness and agitation
b. Irregular cardiac rhythm
c. Weak, irregular pulse and poor muscle tone
d. Chvostek's sign

3594. Electrolyte needs to be replaced in a client receiving furosemide (Lasix) is:
a. Sodium b. Potassium
c. Chlorine d. Magnesium

3595. Identify the electrolyte imbalance which is responsible for weakness, vertigo and convulsions?
a. Hypomagnesemia
b. Hypocalcemia
c. Hypokalemia
d. Hypophosphatemia

3596. Hypercalcemia can cause all; EXCEPT:
a. Confusion
b. Muscle weakness
c. Oliguria
d. Loss of appetite

3597. Hypercalcemia can cause:
a. Fracture b. Muscle spasms
c. Renal insufficiency d. Seizure

3598. Cause of hypercalcemia:
a. Hypoparathyroidism
b. Renal tubular acidosis
c. Less intake of vit D
d. Increased calcitriol

3599. Select the cause of hypercalcemia from the following:
a. Primary hyper parathyroidism
b. Excess vitamin D
c. Acute pancreatitis
d. Both a and b

3600. Signs related to hypocalcemia is:
a. Chvostek's sign
b. Trousseau's sign
c. Tenderness at McBurney's point
d. Both a and b

3601. Twitching of the facial muscles in response to tapping over the area of the facial nerve:
a. Chvostek's sign
b. Trousseau's sign
c. Tenderness at McBurney's point
d. Allen's test

3602. Carpopedal spasm caused by inflating the blood-pressure cuff to a level above systolic pressure for 3 minutes:
a. Chvostek's sign
b. Trousseau's sign
c. Mac Burney's point pain
d. Allen's test

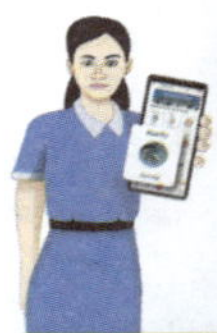

Ans.
3578. d
3579. b
3580. c
3581. c
3582. c
3583. b
3584. a
3585. a
3586. c
3587. a
3588. c
3589. d
3590. b
3591. b
3592. d
3593. c
3594. b
3595. a
3596. c
3597. c
3598. b
3599. d
3600. d
3601. a
3602. b

3603. Positive Chvostek's and Trousseau's signs are early indication of: *(Kerala PSC, Nov 2014)*
a. Rickets b. Addison's disease
c. Tetany d. Cushing's syndrome

3604. Hyperkalemia is caused due to all of the following EXCEPT:
a. Addisons disease b. Acute renal failure
c. Excess hemolysis d. Alkalosis

3605. Hyperkalemia can be managed with:
a. Sodium b. Dextrose with insulin
c. Dextrose with calcium d. Sodium nitroprusside

3606. K Bind is given for patients with: *(Daman & Diu NO 2018)*
a. Hypernatremia b. Hypokalemia
c. Hyperkalemia d. Hyponatremia

Explanation: K Bind Sachet contains Calcium Polystyrene Sulfonate as an active ingredient. K Bind Sachet works by swapping calcium for potassium in large intestine. It is used for the treatment of hyperkalemia (high potassium levels) associated with kidney conditions.

3607. Which of the following electrolyte is most frequently administered in conjunction with furosemide?
a. Sodium b. Chloride
c. Calcium d. Potassium

3608. Which among the following electrolyte imbalance manifest with confusion and lethargy?
a. Hyperkalemia b. Hypermagnesemia
c. Hypercalcemia d. Hypocalcemia

3609. The electrolyte imbalance that needs to be suspected in a client receiving furosemide is:
a. Hyperkalemia b. Hyperphosphatemia
c. Hypokalemia d. Hypernatremia

3610. Phosphorus binders are administered:
a. 1 hour after food b. 1 hour before food
c. With food d. Bed time

3611. Choose phosphate binder drug from following:
a. Calcium carbonate
b. Calcium acetate
c. Sevelamer hydrochloride
d. All of the above

HEMORRHAGE

3612. Which can be given in hemorrhagic stroke?
a. Isotonic fluids b. Colloids
c. Blood transfusion d. Packed RBC

3613. Which of the following symptoms is NOT considered to be compensatory mechanism associated with hypovolemia due to hemorrhage?
a. Tachycardia b. Tachypnea
c. Oliguria d. Hypertension

Explanation: In hypovolemia, activation of the sympathetic nervous system increases the respiratory rate (tachypnea) and pulse rate (tachycardia) and help restore the BP to maintain tissue perfusion but does not cause a hypertension. SNS stimulation also play a role in decreased glomerular filtration and increased reabsorption of water and sodium which leads to oliguria.

3614. Bleeding time is prolonged in all of the following conditions; EXCEPT:
a. DIC
b. Von-Willebrand disease
c. Hemophilia-A
d. Idiopathic thrombocytopenia

3615. Which of the following blood cells performs an important role in blood clotting?
a. Lymphocytes b. Thrombocytes
c. Erythrocytes d. T-cells

3616. Natural anticoagulant present in human body is:
a. Fibrinogen b. Heparin
c. Warfarin d. Enoxaparin

3617. Which of the following is the most common inherited bleeding disorder?
a. Hemolytic anemia b. Von Willebrand's disease
c. Hemophilia A d. Hemophilia B

Explanation: Von Willebrand disease is the most common inherited bleeding disorder. Von Willebrand factor helps platelets to clump together and stick to vessel wall, which is necessary for blood clotting. A lack of the von Willebrand factor prevents the blood from clotting properly. Von Willebrand disease affects both males and females and is generally milder than hemophilia.

3618. Presence of delayed epistaxis after maxillofacial trauma should raise suspicion on:
a. Chronic bacterial infection in nasal mucosa
b. Untreated deviated nasal septum
c. Arterial aneurysm
d. Continued traumatic insult to nasal mucosa

3619. In which of the following type of bleeding bright red blood spurts with each heartbeat?
a. Arterial bleeding b. Capillary bleeding
c. Venous bleeding d. In all type of hemorrhage

3620. The most commonly used and appropriate technique to stop bleeding of wounds in extremities is to:
a. Apply direct pressure with cloth
b. Position the client on his/her left side
c. Flex the extremity at nearest point of bleeding
d. Apply a tourniquet.

EMERGENCY NURSING

3621. Calculate set rate in an infusion pump to administer 100 mL of NS over 2 hours?
a. 20 mL/hr b. 40 mL/hr
c. 50 mL/hr d. 100 mL/hr

3622. After IV fluid administration balance between intracellular and extracellular fluid is established through .... process:
a. Osmosis b. Diffusion
c. Active transport d. All of these

3623. The Maximum concentration of potassium delivered via central vein is?
a. 20 mmol/hr b. 40 mmol/hr
c. 60 mmol/hr d. 100 mmol/hr

(Ref: Harrison's 19th ed. pg. 307)

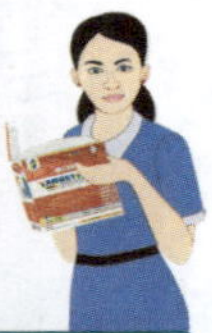

Ans.
3603. c
3604. d
3605. b
3606. c
3607. d
3608. c
3609. c
3610. c
3611. d
3612. a
3613. d
3614. c
3615. b
3616. b
3617. b
3618. c
3619. a
3620. a
3621. c
3622. a
3623. a

Explanation:
- IV potassium therapy:
  - Via peripheral vein = 20-40 mEq of KCI per liter.
  - Via central vein = 10–20 mEq of KCI per hour

3624. Immediate management of choice to restore B.P. and peripheral circulation is:
a. Trendelenburg position
b. Ringer lactate
c. Colloids
d. Inotropes

3625. When administering large volume of colloids nurse need to monitor for:
a. Adventitious respiratory sounds
b. Interstitial edema
c. Hypotension
d. Both a and b

3626. What should the initial action of a medical-surgical nurse be if a patient develops slurred speech and disorientation to time and place' who sustained a head injury 24 hours ago? *(AIIMS BPL SNO 2018)*
a. Recheck the patient's neurologic status in 15 minutes
b. Prepare the patient for emergency surgery
c. Continue the hourly neurologic assessments
d. Inform the neurosurgeon of the patient's status

Explanation: Slurred speech and disorientation to time and place reflects the sign of concussion which should be treated as early as possible, so the neurosurgeon should be notified soon. Prepare the patient for emergency surgery only if neurosurgeon orders.

3627. The process of assessing patients who come to emergency department and determining the management priorities is called? *(RAK MSc 2018)*
a. Mirage b. Triage
c. Lavage d. Collage

Explanation:
- Triage is the sorting of patients by priority for treatment, evacuation or transport. Conventionally, casualties are divided into the categories.
- **Immediate category:** These casualties require immediate life-saving treatment.
- **Urgent category:** These casualties require significant intervention as soon as possible.
- **Delayed category:** These patients will require medical intervention, but not with any urgency.

3628. Which can be safely given in hemorrhagic stroke?
a. Normal Saline
b. Hypertonic fluids
c. Colloids
d. Blood transfusion

3629. The most common cause of embolic stroke:
a. Paradoxical embolism
b. Carotid artery atherosclerosis
c. Non rheumatic atrial fibrillation
d. LV aneurysm

3630. Commonest cause of cerebrovascular accident:
a. Hemorrhage b. Aortic dissection
c. Embolism d. Infarction

3631. Which among the following is a priority nursing intervention in a client experiencing stroke?
a. Maintain airway
b. Range of motion (ROM) exercises
c. Maintain tissue perfusion
d. Nutritional maintenance

3632. A client is admitted to neuro emergency with brain stem infarction. The important nursing intervention is to assess for:
a. Aphonia b. Bradypnea
c. Cushing triad d. Weakness

3633. Following C5 injury, which among the following is the important nursing intervention?
a. Patent airway
b. Peripheral circulation
c. Skin cared
d. Bladder distention

3634. Release of which of the following chemical causes pain at injury site:
a. Prostaglandins
b. Serotonins
c. Norepinephrine
d. Endorphins

3635. Appropriate non-opioid analgesics for mild pain is:
a. Oxycodone b. Ibuprofen
c. Lorazepam d. Tramadol

3636. Most common side effect associated with morphine administration is:
a. Cardiac arrest b. Coma
c. Paralytic ileus d. Respiratory arrest

3637. A patient presenting to the ED with complains of chest pain aggravated by coughing and relieved by sitting upright may have additional physical examination finding of:
a. Pericardial friction rub
b. Pulses paradoxes
c. Crackles
d. Wheezing

Explanation: This may be due to pericardial effusion or pericarditis. Pericardial friction rub can be auscultated in these conditions.

3638. Which of the following is not a cause/risk factor for cardiac arrest?
a. Hyperkalemia b. Hyperglycemia
c. Hypovolemia d. Hypoxia

Explanation: Hypoglycemia is one of the risk factors for cardiac arrest, not hyperglycemia.

Potential causes to consider cardiac arrest (6H's and 6T's) are:
- Hyper/hypokalemia
- Hypoglycemia
- Hypovolemia
- Hypoxia
- Hydrogen ion (acidosis)
- Hypothermia
- Toxin
- Thrombosis (coronary or pulmonary)
- Tension pneumothorax
- Tamponade
- Tablets (overdose or ingestion)
- Trauma

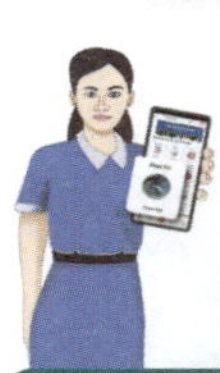

Ans.
3624. b
3625. d
3626. d
3627. b
3628. a
3629. c
3630. c
3631. a
3632. b
3633. a
3634. a
3635. b
3636. d
3637. a
3638. b

3639. The most important finding which causes concern during examination of a patient in the emergency department: (ISRO)

a. Difficulty in arousing the patient
b. Oxygen saturation at room air of 89%
c. Respiratory rate of 12/minute
d. Peripheral cyanosis

3640. Which of the following CANNOT cause a low pulse oximetry reading in a patient with respiratory distress? *(AIIMS-BBS SNO 2019)*

a. Inadequate peripheral circulation
b. Edema
c. Hyperthermia
d. Nail polish

Explanation: **Inadequate peripheral circulation** is the principal cause for failure to obtain a satisfactory signal by the probe attached to finger tips. Edema or venous congestion of the limb can also interfere with readings of pulse oximetry. Nail polish of black, blue and green color disturbs the sensor in the probe, hence lower oximeter readings.

Hyperthermia will not affect readings of pulse oximeter.

3641. The first priority in the management of trauma patient is: *(AIIMS Bhopal Grade-I 2018)*

a. Maintenance of an adequate airway
b. Control of hemorrhage
c. Maintenance of adequate arterial blood pressure
d. Ruling out a spinal injury

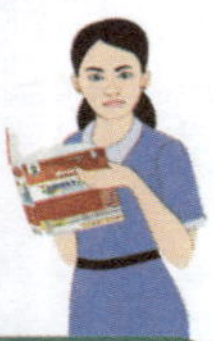

Explanation: The airway is the most important priority in the management of the severely injured patients. It is essential to open and clear the airways to allow free access of air to the distal endotracheal tree. Once the airway is maintained, it is important to ensure adequate oxygenation and ventilation through the airways.

3642. During intubation administration of succinylcholine can cause bradycardia. Which of the following agents used to overcome this effect?

a. Adrenaline
b. Lidocaine
c. Calcium gluconate
d. Atropine

Explanation: Use of Succinylcholine can result in Bradycardia, especially in children. Atropine is the drug of choice in treating succinylcholine-induced bradycardia. Lidocaine is used in adults only.

3643. Which of the following is NOT an essential finding for brain death:

a. Loss of pupillary reflex
b. Loss of brain stem function
c. Negative Apnea test
d. Loss of deep tendon reflexes

3644. Compression of bleeding carotid artery immediately leads to: *(AIIMS BPL SNO 2018)*

a. Vomiting
b. Stroke
c. Blindness
d. Loss of sense of smell

Explanation: The compression of bleeding carotid artery leads to failure of brain perfusion due to thromboembolic events leading to devastating **stroke.** Vomiting, blindness and loss of sense of smell is not present in the patient with carotid artery injury.

3645. Nurse giving oxygen therapy should know that it has to be humidified because: *(NCFL 2019)*

a. Oxygen is a hot air and it may burn trachea
b. Oxygen is a dry gas and thickens the mucus
c. Oxygen gets cleaned of pathogens by humidification
d. Oxygen is easily absorbed because humidification adds H-ion to it

Explanation: Oxygen has a drying effect on mucus membrane that results in damage to the airways, secretions may become thick and difficult to clear. Oxygen is humidified before administration by flowing through a humidifier.

3646. What is the full explanation of ATLS?

a. Advanced trauma life support
b. Advanced tertiary life support
c. Advanced trauma life salvage
d. Advanced tertiary long-term safety

Explanation: ATLS- Advanced Trauma Life Support is followed in all cases in management of trauma.

3647. Prakash, a 32-year-old male has been admitted to the intensive care unit following a motor vehicle accident. Assessment found a positive Cullen' sign. What does this indicate?

a. Pelvic fracture
b. Skull fracture
c. Retroperitoneal hemorrhage
d. Hemothorax

3648. The Heimlich maneuver (abdominal thrust), for acute airway obstruction, attempts to: *(Kerala PSC 1992)*

a. Force air out of the lungs
b. Induce emptying of the stomach
c. Put pressure on the apex of the heart
d. All of the above

Explanation: The Heimlich maneuver (abdominal thrust) is an emergency technique for preventing suffocation when a person's airway (windpipe) becomes blocked by a piece of food or other object. The pressure from thrusts lifts the diaphragm and forces enough air from the lungs that expels the aspirated material.

3649. Most Common injury in blunt abdominal trauma:

a. Kidney
b. Liver
c. Bladder
d. Spleen

Explanation: Spleen is the most commonly injured organ in abdominal trauma.

The small intestine takes up a large part of the abdomen and is likely to be damaged in penetrating injury.

3650. Saleema 25-year-old male has been admitted to the intensive care unit following a motor vehicle accident. Bowel sounds are audible while auscultating Saleem's lungs. This indicates:

a. Ruptured Liver
b. Ruptured lungs
c. Diaphragmatic injury
d. Ruptured Aorta

3651. When an elderly patient complains of pain, the attending nurse should be careful because (ISRO)

a. Elderly patients are expected to experience chronic pain
b. Elderly patients experience reduced sensory perception
c. Elderly patients have indifferent pain threshold
d. Elderly patients have altered mental function

Ans.

3639. b
3640. c
3641. a
3642. d
3643. d
3644. b
3645. b
3646. a
3647. c
3648. a
3649. d
3650. c
3651. b

3652. What is the effect of atherosclerosis on arterial waveform?
a. Increase in systolic waveform
b. Decrease in the size of diastolic wave
c. Decrease in the size of dicrotic notch
d. All of the above

3653. What is the area under arterial pressure waveform denotes?
a. Systolic pressure b. Coronary artery pressure
c. End diastolic pressure d. Mean arterial pressure

3654. ROSE questionnaire is used for?
a. Alcohol addiction
b. Sex addiction
c. Angina assessment
d. Deep Vein thrombosis Assessment

(Ref: Braunwald 8th edn Ch 57)

Explanation: ROSE Questionnaire is used to evaluate the subjective severity of ischemic heart pain and intermittent claudication in patients with Coronary Artery Disease.

3655. A patient received Atropine sulphate as a premedication 30 minutes ago and is now complaining of dry mouth. On assessment the nurse found the pulse rate is higher, than before Atropine was administered. The nurse understands that this is:
a. An allergic reaction to Atropine
b. Due to higher dose of Atropine
c. Due to anxiety of patient about upcoming surgery
d. Normal side effect of Atropine

Explanation: Atropine is an anticholinergic drug with expected side effects of dryness mouth and tachycardia. So complains of dry mouth and increased pulse rate is considered to be normal and expected after a dose of Atropine sulphate.

3656. Client receiving TPN via CVP complains of chest pain and dyspnea, tachycardia and hypertension. Which among the following complications nurse need to suspect in this client?
a. Hypoglycemia b. Electrolyte imbalances
c. Sepsis d. Air embolism

3657. Important nursing intervention for a client who has been sexually assaulted is:
a. Treat urgent medical problems
b. Inform the NGO
c. Psychological support to the client
d. Recording and reporting

Poisoning/Overdose/Toxicity

3658. An emergency room nurse is assessing a 22-year-old male who has been using opioids. What symptoms indicate that the client has over dosed? *(NCFL 2019)*
a. Constricted pupils and hypotension
b. Vomiting and Tachypnea
c. Pupillary dilatation and hypertensive crisis
d. Tremors and ataxia

Explanation:

- Symptoms of "opioid overdose triad" is pinpoint pupils, respiratory depression and unconsciousness. Acute intoxification symptoms of opioids are hypothermia, hypotension, bradycardia apathy, Pinpoint Pupil, delay in reflexes and coma
- Nausea and Vomiting may be present, but it is not a typical symptom of opioid overdose.

3659. Antidote of opioid is:
a. Administer adrenaline b. Administer IV naloxone
c. Maintain hydration d. Give charcoal

3660. Antidote to benzodiazepine poisoning is:
a. N-Acetylcysteine b. Naltrexone
c. Flumazenil d. Barbiturates

3661. The drug used in paracetamol (acetaminophen) poisoning is:
a. Naloxone b. Acetyl salicylic acid
c. Flumazenil d. N-Acetylcysteine

3662. Symptoms of Central nervous system depression, cardiac depression and optic nerve atrophy in methanol poisoning is due to:
a. Acetic acid b. Acetaldehyde
c. Pyridine
d. Formaldehyde and formic acid

3663. The most useful bedside diagnostic test to suggest snake bite envenomation is:
a. Platelet count
b. Bleeding time
c. International normalized ratio
d. 20 minutes whole blood clotting time

3664. Antidote for anticholinergic poisoning is:
a. Atropine b. Physostigmine
c. Pyridoxine d. Beta blockers

3665. Deferoxamine is an antidote of:
a. Lead b. Iron
c. Calcium d. Magnesium

3666. Clinical manifestation of cocaine overdose includes:
a. Lacrimation, restlessness, and irritability.
b. Agitation, cardiac dysrhythmias, and seizures.
c. Euphoria, nausea and vomiting.
d. Altered respirations; hyporeflexia and blurred vision.

3667. A 12-year-old child was brought to the emergency department 30 minutes after accidental ingestion of 12 tablets of Paracetamol 650 mg. Which of the following intervention is the priority for this child?
a. Administer N-Acetylcysteine
b. Administer activated charcoal
c. Perform gastric lavage
d. Administer 5% dextrose in half normal saline

Explanation: Treatment guidelines for oral Paracetamol (acetaminophen) ingestion in Children

- Less than 4 **hours** after ingestion - Consider activated charcoal if dose is >150 mg/kg (activated charcoal is not advised if the ingested dose is unknown)
- **4 to 24 hours** – Obtain plasma acetaminophen level as soon as possible. Start with N-Acetylcysteine (NAC) administration.
- **Longer than 24 hours** – NAC administration

3668. Warfarin (Coumadin) toxicity can be treated with:
a. Phytonadione (vitamin K)
b. Protamine sulfate
c. Acetyl cysteine
d. Heparin

Explanation: Vitamin K is an antidote of warfarin. Since warfarin has a much longer duration of action than vitamin K, vitamin K may need to be re-administered in patients with massive warfarin overdose or ongoing bleeding.

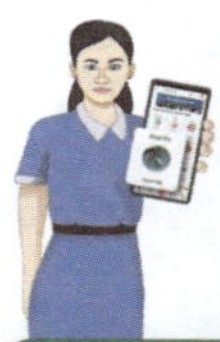

Ans.

3652. d
3653. d
3654. c
3655. d
3656. d
3657. a
3658. a
3659. b
3660. c
3661. d
3662. d
3663. d
3664. b
3665. b
3666. b
3667. b
3668. a

3669. Which of the following poisoning form a strong bond with hemoglobin and creates a functional anemia?
a. Carbon monoxide poisoning
b. Atropine poisoning
c. Organophosphorus poisoning
d. Arsenic poisoning

EQUIPMENT IN CRITICAL CARE AREA

3670. CPAP stands for:
a. Continuous Permanent Airway Pressure
b. Continuous Positive Airway Pressure
c. Continuous Prolonged Airway Pressure
d. Continuous Passive Airway Pressure

3671. PEEP in ventilator helps to:
a. Prevent collapse of alveoli (AIIMS Raipur NO 2019)
b. Prevent oxygen toxicity
c. Prevent ventilator fighting
d. Avoid over ventilation

3672. All of the following is true about positive-end expiratory pressure (PEEP); EXCEPT: *(AIIMS-BBS SNO 2019)*
a. It reduces venous return
b. It improves alveolar gas exchange
c. It prevents alveolar collapse
d. It decreases mean airway pressure

Explanation: Positive end-expiratory pressure (PEEP) is the positive pressure that will remain in the airways at the end of the respiratory cycle (end of exhalation) that is greater than the atmospheric pressure in mechanically ventilated patients. PEEP is applied to recruit lung volumes, elevate mean airway pressure, and improve oxygenation.

3673. Which among the following is a non-invasive ventilation method?
a. SIMV b. Bi PAP
c. Laryngeal mask airway d. Pressure support ventilation

3674. Which one of these is not a weaning mode?
a. CMV b. C-PAP
c. BiPAP d. PSV

3675. Patient's fighting with the ventilator is called:
a. Bucking
b. Weaning
c. Kinking
d. Distress

3676. Why pressurized bag is used in arterial line monitoring?
a. To prevent the backflow of blood in the tubing
b. To prevent blood leakage
c. To maintain the shape of saline bag
d. To provide bolus dose

3677. Which of these can provide 100% O_2?
a. Bag value mask alone
b. Bag value mask with supplemental O_2
c. Oxygen via facemask
d. Partial rebreather mask

3678. C wave in the CVP waveform denotes:
a. Onset of atrial systole
b. Onset of Ventricular diastole
c. Onset of ventricular systole
d. Onset of arterial diastole

STAGES OF DEATH & DYING

3679. Which among the following is a criterion to classify a death as brain death? *(AIIMS BPL NO 2018)*
a. Presence of EEG activity b. Cessation of breathing
c. Responsive to deep pain d. Hypothermia

Explanation: Brain death is defined as the irreversible loss of all functions of the brain, including the brainstem. The three essential findings in brain death are coma, absence of brainstem reflexes, and apnea.

3680. The suction of the internal fluids, of the corpse and the injection of embalming chemicals into body cavities, using an aspirator and trocar is the method of: *(AIIMS Raipur Grade II 2017)*
a. Surface embalming b. Cavity embalming
c. Hypodermic embalming d. Arterial embalming

Explanation: Surface embalming involves application of embalming fluid to the skin of the deceased body to preserve damage suffered during autopsy, the removal of organs for donation, or disease. Arterial embalming involves injecting the embalming fluid into the carotid artery using a centrifugal pump to displace the blood, which drains through the right jugular vein. Hypodermic embalming refers to the injection of embalming chemicals into tissue with a hypodermic needle and syringe, which is used to treat areas where arterial fluid has not been successfully distributed during the main arterial injection.

3681. In which of the following stages of Kubler-Ross' grief process, the individual postpones awareness of reality as though the loss can be prevented?
a. Denial b. Anger
c. Bargaining d. Depression

3682. In which of the following stages of Kubler-Ross' grief process, the individual acts as though nothing has happened and may refuse to believe or understand the loss has occurred?
a. Denial b. Anger
c. Bargaining d. Depression

Explanation:

- **Kubler**-Ross' stages of dying:
- **Denial**: Individual acts as though nothing has happened and may refuse to believe or understand loss has occurred
- **Anger**: Individual resists the loss and may strike out at everyone and everything
- **Bargaining**: Individual postpones awareness of reality as though the loss can be prevented
- **Depression**: Individual feels overwhelmingly lonely and withdraws from interpersonal interaction
- **Acceptance**: Individual accepts the loss and looks to the future

3683. An individual in which of the following age group will have an attitude toward death that is influenced by religious and cultural beliefs?
a. 5–10 years b. 9–12 years
c. 12–18 years d. 18–45 years

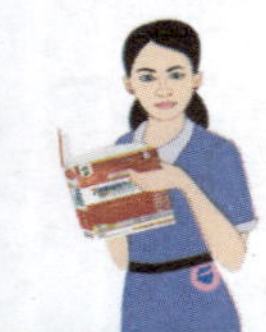

Ans.

3669. a
3670. b
3671. a
3672. d
3673. b
3674. a
3675. a
3676. a
3677. b
3678. c
3679. b
3680. b
3681. c
3682. a
3683. d

Explanation:

Age group	Concept of death
Infancy to 5 years	Does not understand concept of death
5–9 years	Understands that death is final
9–12 years	Understands death as the inevitable end of life
12–18 years	Fears an enduring or lingering death
18–45 years	Attitude toward death influenced by religious and cultural beliefs

3684. A 75-year-old woman has never gotten over the death of her daughter 15 years ago. She reports that she always feels sad and never again able to enjoy life as before. Which of the following type of grief is being experienced by this woman?
a. Anticipatory grief b. Dysfunctional grief
c. Cumulative grief d. Inhibited grief

3685. All of the following are the manifestation of brain death; EXCEPT:
a. Diabetes insipidus
b. Pupils do not respond to light
c. Pulse rate unresponsive to atropine
d. EEG shows only delta waves

Explanation: Delta waves in Electroencephalogram (EEG) are usually associated with the deep stage 3 of NREM sleep (also known as slow-wave sleep). In case of brain death, EEG shows no brain activity at all.

- Signs of brain death include:
  - Pupils do not respond to light
  - No reaction to pain
  - Absence of corneal reflex
  - Absence of oculocephalic reflex (eyes do not move when head is moved)
  - Absence of oculovestibular reflex (Eyes do not move when ice water is poured into the ear)
  - Absence of gagging reflex
  - Absence of breath when the ventilator is switched off.
  - No brain activity in EEG.

MISCELLANEOUS

3686. The blood contains: *(LNJP H D 2012)*
a. 95% of water b. 60% of water
c. 90% of water d. 80% of water

3687. Pain is:
a. Unpleasant experience b. Subjective in nature
c. Both a and b d. Maladaptive behavior

3688. Hydrophobia is seen in:
a. Scorpion bite b. Dog bite
c. Snake bite d. Spider bite

3689. Branch of science that determines the cause and manner of death is:
a. Immunopathology b. Hematopathology
c. Forensic pathology d. Histopathology

3690. Substances poorly absorbed by activated charcoal include all; EXCEPT:
a. Lead b. Lithium
c. Cyanide d. Phenobarbital

Explanation:

- Substances poorly absorbed by Activated charcoal include
  - **Heavy metals:** Iron, Lead, Lithium, Mercury
  - **Chemicals: Petroleum distillates,** Ethanol, Methanol, Mercury, Ethylene glycol, Cyanide, Saline cathartics,
  - **Corrosive chemicals:** Acids, Alkalis
  - Gastric lavage is contraindicated in poisoning with ingestion of Acids, Alkalis, and Petroleum distillates.

3691. Lead poisoning is also known as: *(DSSSB 2013)*
a. Asterixis
b. Plumbism
c. Plummer-Vinson syndrome
d. Prader-Willi syndrome

Explanation: Lead poisoning is a type of metal poisoning and a medical condition in humans and other vertebrates caused by increased levels of the heavy metal lead in the body. Lead poisoning is also known as plumbism, colicapictonum, saturnism, Devon colic, or painter's colic.

3692. Pus formation in the socket of teeth is:
a. Periodontal disease b. Halitosis
c. Cheilosis d. Sordes

3693. Cracking of lips especially at the angle of mouth is:
a. Periodontal disease b. Halitosis
c. Angular Cheilitis d. Sordes

3694. Increase in number of stool and the passage of liquid, unformed feces is termed as:
a. Diarrhea b. Constipation
c. Encopresis d. Incontinence

3695. Decrease in frequency of bowel movement associated with difficulty in passage of hard stool is:
a. Diarrhea b. Constipation
c. Encopresis d. Incontinence

3696. Varicose vein at or near anus is:
a. Flatulence b. Hemorrhoids
c. Impaction d. Dangling

3697. Blood in sputum is:
a. Hemoptysis b. Hematemesis
c. Hemothorax d. Hematochezia

3698. Blood in vomitus is:
a. Hemoptysis b. Hematemesis
c. Hemothorax d. Hematochezia

Ans.
3684. b
3685. d
3686. d
3687. c
3688. b
3689. c
3690. d
3691. b
3692. a
3693. c
3694. a
3695. b
3696. b
3697. a
3698. b

"He who has health has hope; and he who has hope has everything."
—Arabian proverb

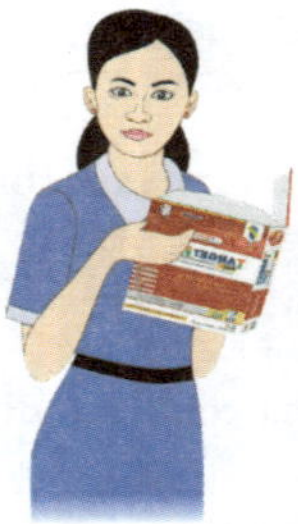

CLINICAL CASE-BASED QUESTIONS
(Including All Topics)

1

A patient was admitted in surgery ward as a case of abdominal Koch. After the laparotomy surgery, the wound edges are not surgically approximated so that doctor has applied packing over the wound and left for healing. The integumentary continuity is restored by which type of wound healing method?

a. Primary intentional wound healing
b. Second intentional wound healing
c. Third intentional wound healing
d. First intentional wound healing

Ans. (b) Second intentional wound healing

Explanation: In the scenario described, where the wound edges are not surgically approximated after a laparotomy surgery and packing is applied, the healing process that occurs is known as second intentional wound healing. This type of wound healing involves allowing the wound to heal by granulation tissue formation from the base of the wound, gradually filling it in and restoring integumentary continuity. The wound is left open and allowed to heal by secondary intention.

2

Vikas, 38-year-old, was admitted in surgical floor with wound over sacral region. The nurse when doing the dressing of the wound observed the bloody drainage. While documenting the procedure the term used by the nurse to denote for bloody discharge:

a. Serous
b. Sanguineous
c. Serosanguineous
d. Purulent

Ans. (b) Sanguineous

Explanation: Sanguineous drainage refers to the presence of blood in the wound discharge. It typically has a bright red color and indicates active bleeding. This type of drainage is commonly seen in fresh wounds or wounds with active bleeding.

3

You have received a patient from the OT who has had general anesthesia for major surgery is in the post-operative unit. The patient became conscious and said that he wants to drink some water. Which is the appropriate nursing action?

a. Check the respiratory rate first
b. Check the lung sounds
c. Check the gag reflex
d. Check the deep tendon reflex

Ans. (c) Check the gag reflex

Explanation: After general anesthesia, patients may have a decreased gag reflex. This means that they may not be able to protect their airway from aspiration. Before giving a patient anything to drink, it is important to check their gag reflex. This can be done by touching the back of the patient's throat with a tongue depressor. If the patient gags, then they have a gag reflex and it is safe to give them water.

4

While performing the systemic health assessment the nurse has to auscultate the heart sound. Identify which among the following statement is incorrect related to the auscultation point location.

a. Apical pulse: 5th Intercostal space (ICS) mid-clavicular line left side
b. Erb's Point: Right of sternal border in 2nd ICS
c. Aortic: Right of the sternal border in 2nd ICS
d. Pulmonic: Left of the sternal border in 2nd ICS

Ans. (b) Erb's Point: Right of sternal border in 2nd ICS

Explanation: "Erb's point" of auscultation for the heart exam, located in the left third intercostal space close to the sternum.

5

A nurse has started the infusion of sodium nitroprusside antihypertensive drug intravenously to a patient for control of severe hypertension. The patient's blood pressure (BP) is unstable and 160/94 mmHg before the infusion. Ten minutes after the infusion, the nurse recorded the blood pressure again and found the patient's BP increases to 180/100 mmHg. Identify the type of response.

a. Synergistic
b. Hypersusceptibility
c. Allergic
d. Paradoxical

Ans. (d) Paradoxical

Explanation: A paradoxical response refers to a reaction or outcome that is contrary to what is expected or intended. In this case, the patient's blood pressure increased after the infusion of Sodium nitroprusside, which is an antihypertensive drug used to lower blood pressure.

6

Ravi, a registered nurse, is having his evening duty in cardiac ICU. The team leader has assigned a patient of congestive heart failure (CHF) with history of hypothyroidism to nurse Ravi. While taking the handover from the morning staff nurse Ravi noticed that attended doctor's has mentioned on the patient's file not to take the temperature from the rectal route. Ravi ask to the morning staff the reason of not taking the temperature from rectal in this patient. What statement made by the morning staff is considered to be correct?

a. Checking rectal temperature in this case will cause increase in heart rate.
b. Checking rectal temperature in this case will cause decrease in heart rate.
c. Checking rectal temperature in this case will cause increase in blood pressure.
d. Checking rectal temperature in this case will cause increase in pulse rate.

Ans. (b) Checking rectal temperature in this case will cause decrease in heart rate.

Explanation: Checking the temperature via the rectal route can stimulate the vagus nerve, leading to vagal stimulation. Vagal stimulation can result in a decrease in heart rate, which can be detrimental for patients with CHF.

7

You are working as a day care nurse and posted in the endoscopy room where you have a patient shifted from the nephrology department for the procedure of PEG tube insertion. Select the most appropriate statement related to the insertion of PEG tube.

a. PEG tube is inserted into the jejunum through the endoscope.
b. A PEG tube exits from the right upper quadrant of the abdomen.
c. A PEG tube is inserted with the help of an endoscope through the nose and held in abdomen for feeding purpose.
d. A PEG tube is inserted with the help of an endoscope through the mouth and then with the help of guide wire the gastrostomy tube is placed.

Ans. (d) A PEG tube is inserted with the help of an endoscope through the mouth and then with the help of guide wire the gastrostomy tube is placed.

8

A group of nursing students are discussing the case file of the patient in ICU. The students are going through the doctor's progress notes to identify the nutritional status of the patient. They have found one terminology PEG-J under nutritional management. They asked the senior nurse present at nursing station about the full form of PEG-J. Select the best response from the following.

a. Percutaneous endoscopic transgastric jejunostomy
b. Percutaneous extension gastrostomy and jejunostomy
c. Percutaneous entero gastric jejunostomy
d. Permanent entero gastric jejunostomy

Ans. (a) Percutaneous endoscopic transgastric jejunostomy

Explanation: Percutaneous endoscopic transgastric jejunostomy (PEG-J) using large-bore jejunal tubes may help by by-passing gastric passage during enteral nutrition and improving drainage of gastric secretions.

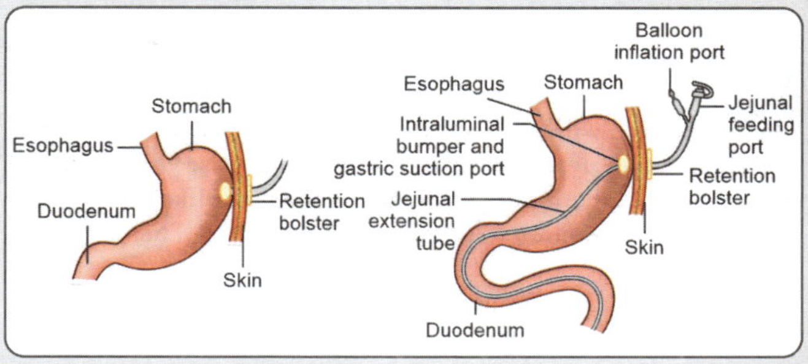

9

Nurse Ramya has assigned to provide care to her patient who is with a chest tube catheter. On assessment of the drainage system, the nurse has observed that there is bubbling in the water seal chamber when the patient breaths. Which among the following is the primary nursing action to be applied by the nurse Rose?

a. Inform to the doctor immediately as it is considered as an abnormal finding.
b. Check the drainage system for any air leakage.
c. Continue to monitor as this is considered as a normal finding.
d. Check the drainage system for any tube kink or obstruction.

Ans. (c) Continue to monitor as this is considered a normal finding.

Explanation: Bubbling in the water seal chamber when the patient breathes is generally considered a normal finding. It indicates that the chest tube is functioning as intended and allows air to escape from the pleural space during expiration. This bubbling is known as tidaling and is expected to occur with respiratory movements.

10

While taking the nursing round you have noticed that one of the patient's chest tube drainage system has disconnected from the chest tube catheter and fallen onto the floor. While the chest tube catheter is secured with sutures and hanging in the air, what would be your priority nursing action?

a. Inform the team leader immediately.
b. Insert the chest tube catheter tubing 1 inch into a bottle of sterile water and obtain a new system.
c. Clamp the chest tube catheter and inform to the doctor.
d. Remove the chest tube catheter from the insertion site to reduce the risk of infection.

Ans. (b) Insert the chest tube catheter tubing 1 inch into a bottle of sterile water and obtain a new system.

Explanation: When a chest tube drainage system becomes disconnected, it is important to maintain a closed system to prevent air from entering the pleural space. By inserting the chest tube catheter tubing into a bottle of sterile water, a temporary seal is created to prevent air from entering the chest cavity. After that, obtaining a new chest tube drainage system will be necessary to ensure proper drainage and functioning.

Clamping the chest tube catheter may lead to tension pneumothorax.

11

You are assigned to provide care to the patient admitted in medicine ward with diabetes mellitus and planned for Humulin NPH insulin daily morning. As an assigned nurse you are giving instruction to the nurse intern about the most likely time for a hypoglycemic reaction to occur in this patient will be:

a. 1–2 hours after administration
b. 4–12 hours after administration
c. 16–18 hours after administration
d. 24 hours after administration

Ans. (b) 4–12 hours after administration

Explanation: Humulin NPH insulin is an intermediate-acting insulin that typically peaks in its action 4–12 hours after administration. This means that during this time frame, there is a higher risk of experiencing a hypoglycemic reaction due to the insulin's maximum effect on lowering blood sugar levels.

12

A patient is intubated with endotracheal tube and to confirm the placement of the tube the bedside chest X-ray is recommended by the doctor. The tube is correctly placed if, it is how many centimeters above the carina?

a. 1–2 cm   b. 2–4 cm
c. 4–6 cm   d. 6–10 cm

Ans. (a) 1–2 cm

Explanation: The optimal placement of an endotracheal tube is 1-2 cm above the carina. The carina is the point where the trachea divides into the right and left mainstem bronchi. If the tube is placed too high, it can enter the right mainstem bronchus and block the left lung. If the tube is placed too low, it can enter the right or left bronchus and block both lungs. A bedside chest X-ray is the best way to confirm the placement of an endotracheal tube.

13

A 22-year-old alcoholic malnourished patient presented to hospital with respiratory distress. His pulse was 110/minute. Patient had edema, hypertension, and systolic murmur along the left sternal edge. Bilateral crepitations were left in the lungs. A diagnosis of congestive high output cardiac failure was made. Which vitamin is deficiency?

a. Vitamin B_1 b. Vitamin C
c. Vitamin B_2 d. Vitamin B_6

Ans. (a) Vitamin B_1

Explanation: Thiamine (Vitamin B_1) is an essential vitamin that plays a crucial role in energy metabolism, particularly in the utilization of glucose by the body. The clinical presentation described in the scenario is consistent with Wernicke-Korsakoff syndrome, which is caused by thiamine deficiency.

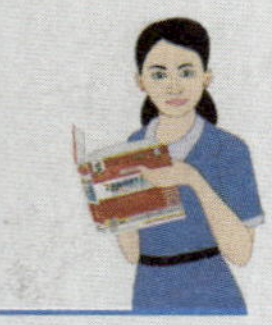

14

Which of the following stage of anesthesia is characterized by stage of surgical anesthesia, eyes roll, then become fixed and the corneal and laryngeal reflexes are lost?

a. Stage 1   b. Stage 2
c. Stage 3   d. Stage 4

Ans. (c) Stage 3

Explanation: Stage 3 is the stage of surgical anesthesia. The patient is unconscious and unresponsive to verbal or painful stimuli. The eyes are rolled back and fixed, and the corneal and laryngeal reflexes are lost. The patient's breathing is regular and slow.

- Stage 1 is the stage of analgesia (induction).
- Stage 2 is the stage of excitement or delirium.
- Stage 4 is the stage of medullary depression.

15

A 75-year-old patient with Alzheimer's disease is brought to the hospital by her family. They report that she has been having trouble performing her activities of daily living, including brushing her teeth. When you observe the patient, you see that she is having difficulty holding the toothbrush and making the appropriate movements to brush her teeth. Which of the following neurological disorders is the patient most likely experiencing?

a. Agnosia   b. Apraxia
c. Anomia   d. Aphasia

Ans. (b) Apraxia

Explanation: Apraxia is a neurological disorder that affects a person's ability to perform learned motor skills. In the case of the patient with Alzheimer's disease, the patient is having trouble performing the movements needed to use her toothbrush. This is an example of ideomotor apraxia, which is a type of apraxia that affects the ability to perform purposeful movements.

- Agnosia is a neurological disorder that affects a person's ability to recognize objects or people.
- Anomia is a neurological disorder that affects a person's ability to name objects or people.
- Aphasia is a neurological disorder that affects a person's ability to communicate.

16

A 62-year-old male patient with a long history of cardiovascular disease is admitted to the hospital with worsening ventricular arrhythmias. The healthcare provider suspects that a medication might be causing the arrhythmias. Which of the following medications is most likely responsible for the development of the arrhythmias?

a. Dobutamine   b. Quinidine
c. Methyldopa   d. Propranolol

Ans. (b) Quinidine

Explanation: Quinidine is an antiarrhythmic medication that is used to treat various types of arrhythmias. However, it can also have proarrhythmic effects, meaning it can actually worsen or induce new arrhythmias in some cases. This risk is particularly significant in patients with pre-existing cardiovascular disease. Quinidine works by blocking sodium channels in the heart. This can lead to a prolongation of the QT interval, which increases the risk of ventricular arrhythmias, such as ventricular tachycardia and ventricular fibrillation.

17

A 52-year-old man is hospitalized for treatment of adrenal crisis. On the morning rotation, the nurse is evaluating the care provided to the patient for his treatment. Which of the following changes would indicate the nurse that the patient is responding favorably to medical and nursing treatment?

a. The patient has experienced weight loss
b. The patient's urinary output has increased
c. The patient's peripheral edema has decreased
d. The patient's blood pressure has increased

Ans. (d) The patient's blood pressure has increased

Explanation: Adrenal crisis is typically associated with low blood pressure (hypotension) due to the deficiency of cortisol and other adrenal hormones. Treatment for adrenal crisis involves prompt administration of glucocorticoid medications to restore hormone levels and stabilize the patient. An increase in blood pressure is a positive sign indicating that the body is responding favorably to the treatment for adrenal crisis.

18

The nurse is performing an initial postoperative assessment on a patient who has a chest tube attached to a water seal drainage system. The nurse should immediately intervene for which of the following observations?

a. Water seal drainage system is above patient's chest.
b. There are no dependent loops in the chest tube.
c. Fluid level in water seal chamber is at 2 cm.
d. The chest tube remains unclamped.

Ans. (a) Water seal drainage system is above patient's chest.

Explanation: Having the water seal drainage system positioned above the patient's chest can impede the proper functioning of the system. It prevents gravity from assisting in the drainage of fluid and can potentially lead to backflow of fluid into the patient's chest. To allow proper drainage, the water seal drainage system should be positioned below the patient's chest, typically kept on the floor or at an appropriate level.

19

A patient with a diagnosis of chronic lymphocytic leukemia is admitted to the hospital for management of hemolytic anemia. Which intervention included in the nursing care plan best meets the patient's needs?

a. Encourage activities with other patients in the ward.
b. Vitamin C supplementation.
c. Maintain a quite environment to promote adequate rest.
d. Isolate the patient to prevent infection.

Ans. (c) Maintain a quite environment to promote adequate rest.

Explanation: Patients with chronic lymphocytic leukemia often have compromised immune systems and are susceptible to infections. Patient is currently admitted for the treatment of hemolytic anemia which increases the risk of fatigue and weakness. Providing a quiet environment promotes adequate rest, which is essential for the patient's recovery and overall well-being.

20

A patient arrives at the emergency department with the complaint of chest pain. The nurse performs an assessment. Which of the following symptoms would be most characteristic of an acute myocardial infarction?

a. Severe substernal pain radiating down the left arm
b. Intermittent, localized epigastric pain
c. Sharp, burning chest pain moving from place to place
d. Sharp, localized, unilateral chest pain

Ans. (a) Severe substernal pain radiating down the left arm

Explanation: The most common symptom of an Acute Myocardial Infarction is chest pain, which is often described as a severe, crushing pain that radiates down the left arm. The pain may also be accompanied by other symptoms, such as shortness of breath, nausea, vomiting, and sweating.

21

A 40-year-old female with previous case history of fever, fatigue, weight loss, polyarthralgia. The radiological findings given below, what may be your diagnosis?

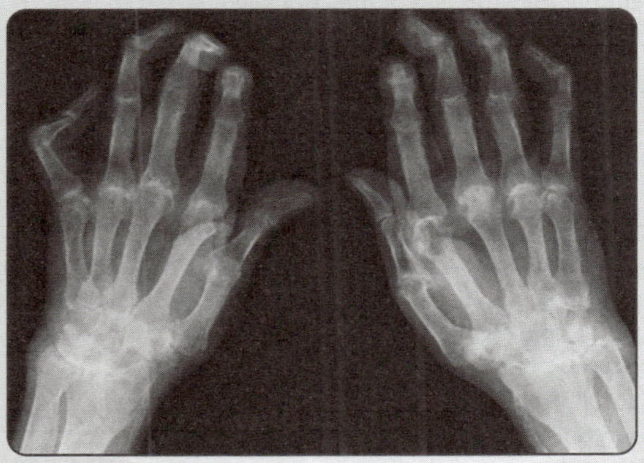

a. Osteoarthritis
b. Rheumatoid arthritis
c. Gout
d. Psoriatic arthritis

Ans. (b) Rheumatoid arthritis

Explanation: The X-ray shown image depicts swan-neck deformity which is characteristic feature of Rheumatoid Arthritis. RA can lead to swan-neck deformities (and boutonniere deformity) over time.

22

The nurse suspects a patient has meningitis. The nurse places the patient in a dorsal recumbent position, places the hands behind the patients' neck, and bends it forward. The nurse knows that pain and resistance may indicate neck injury or arthritis, but if the patient also flexes the hips and knee, this positive response is which of the following?

a. Brudzinski's sign
b. Chovstek's sign
c. Homan's sign
d. Trousseau's sign

Ans. (a) Brudzinski's sign

Explanation: Brudzinski's sign is a clinical sign that is used to assess for meningitis. It is elicited by passively flexing the neck of a supine patient. If the patient also flexes the hips and knees, this is a positive Brudzinski's sign.

23

In a postoperative unit, a patient developed a wound infection, and later, three other patients in the same unit also developed infections. What is the most optimal method to prevent the transmission of infection?

a. Wash OT instrument with 1% perchlorate
b. Give IV antibiotics to all patients in the ward
c. Fumigation of the ward
d. Proper hand washing of all ward personnel

Ans. (d) Proper hand washing of all ward personnel

Explanation: Proper hand hygiene, including thorough hand washing with soap and water or the use of alcohol-based hand sanitizers, is one of the most important and effective measures to prevent the transmission of infections.

24

A 20-year-old female is brought to the emergency department by her parents. Her blood pressure is 220/136 mmHg, heart rate 142 beats/minute, and respiratory rate 20 breaths/minute. She is responsive only to deep pain. Her parents say she has been trying to lose weight and has been taking "these pills she gets over the Internet." What will the nurse consider as the most likely cause for this patient's symptoms?

a. Cardiac arrest
b. Food poisoning
c. Hemorrhagic stroke
d. Pregnancy-induced hypertension

Ans. (c) Hemorrhagic stroke

Explanation: The patient's presentation with severely elevated blood pressure (220/136 mmHg), tachycardia (heart rate of 142 beats/minute), altered mental status (responsive only to deep pain), and a history of taking unidentified weight-loss pills obtained from the Internet raises concerns for a potential hemorrhagic stroke.

Hemorrhagic stroke occurs when there is bleeding in the brain, often due to a ruptured blood vessel.

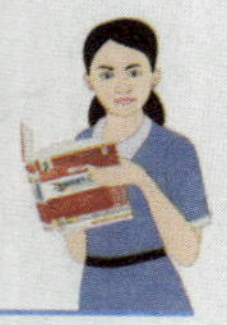

25

A 44-year-old female cook presents with a 1-year history of dyspnea, episodic cough, and wheeze, shortness of breath and chest tightness. What is the best way to diagnose bronchial asthma in this patient?

a. Wheeze
b. Dyspnea
c. FEV1 values
d. Vital Capacity

Ans. (c) FEV1 values

Explanation: FEV1, or forced expiratory volume in 1 second, is a measure of how much air a person can forcefully exhale in one second. It is a good indicator of how well the lungs are functioning. In people with asthma, FEV1 values are typically lower than normal.

26

Ramesh was rushed to hospital owing to vomiting and reduced consciousness. Patient shows slow and deep breathing and is lethargic and irritable. Appears dehydrated with sunken eyes and dry mucous membrane. He has a history of polydipsia, polyuria and weight loss since 2 weeks. Measurement of arterial blood gas shows: pH - 7.2; PaO_2 - 90 mmHg; $PaCO_2$ - 23 mmHg, and HCO_3 - 12 mmol/L; What is your interpretation?

a. Respiratory acidosis, uncompensated
b. Respiratory acidosis, partially compensated
c. Metabolic alkalosis, uncompensated
d. Metabolic acidosis, partially compensated

Ans. (d) Metabolic acidosis, partially compensated

Explanation: The pH is 7.2, which is below the normal range of 7.35–7.45. This indicates acidosis.

The HCO_3 is 12 mmol/L, which is below the normal range of 22–26 mmol/L. This indicates that the acidosis is due to decreased bicarbonate (metabolic acidosis).

The $PaCO_2$ is 23 mmHg, which is below the normal range of 35–45 mmHg. This indicates the respiratory system is attempting to remove CO_2 to compensate for the acidosis. However, the pH remains acidic.

So, the answer is metabolic acidosis, partially compensated.

TIPS: Use the mnemonic technique ROME to analyse ABG values.

ROME – Respiratory Opposite, Metabolic Equal.

- **Respiratory Opposite:** If the pH and PCO_2 values move on opposite direction from its normal value – It is due to respiratory cause. For example, if pH is 7.2 (below normal) and PCO_2 is 50 (above normal), it is respiratory acidosis. If pH is 7.5 (above normal) and PCO_2 is 30 (below normal), it is respiratory alkalosis.
- **Metabolic Equal:** If the pH and HCO_3 values move on same direction from its normal value- It is due to metabolic cause. For example, if pH is 7.2 (below normal) and HCO_3 is 20 (below normal), it is metabolic acidosis. If pH is 7.5 (above normal) and HCO_3 is 28 (above normal), it is metabolic alkalosis.
- Once the respiratory and metabolic components of acid-base balance have been identified, then use the following method to determine whether it is compensated, uncompensated or partially compensated.

- Fully compensated – the pH is within normal limits but both the PCO_2 and HCO_3 are deranged.
- Partially compensated – pH is deranged; both PCO_2 and HCO_3 are also deranged.
- Uncompensated- pH is deranged; either PCO_2 or HCO_3 only deranged.

27

Mr Ramaswamy is a 55-year-old male with a history of chronic obstructive pulmonary disease. He was taken to the emergency department with complaint of shortness of breath, pyrexia, and a productive cough with yellow-green sputum. He has difficulty communicating because of his inability to complete a sentence. His wife says he has been unwell for three days. Upon examination, crackles and wheezes can be heard in the lower lobes; with tachycardia and a bounding pulse. Measurement of arterial blood gas shows:

- **pH - 7.3,**
- **$PaCO_2$ - 68 mmHg,**
- **HCO_3 - 28 mmol/L, and**
- **PaO_2 - 60 mmHg.**

What would be your interpretation?

a. Respiratory acidosis, uncompensated
b. Respiratory acidosis, partially compensated
c. Metabolic alkalosis, uncompensated
d. Metabolic acidosis, partially compensated

Ans. (b) Respiratory acidosis, partially compensated

Explanation:

- The pH is 7.3, which is below the normal range of 7.35–7.45. This indicates acidosis.
- The $PaCO_2$ is 68 mmHg (normal is 35–45), which indicates it is respiratory acidosis.
- The HCO_3 is 28 mmol/L (normal 22–28). This indicates that the kidneys have attempted to compensate for the acidosis by retaining bicarbonate. However, the pH is still acidic. So, the correct answer is "respiratory acidosis, partially compensated".

28

Approximately 30–60 minutes after being bitten by a "bug", a 30-year-old man noticed a localized swelling and erythema in the affected area. The edema is most likely the result of:

a. Altered plasma oncotic pressure
b. Increased arterial hydrostatic pressure
c. Increased vascular permeability
d. Lymphatic obstruction

Ans. (c) Increased vascular permeability

Explanation: Edema is most likely the result of increased vascular permeability. This is because the bug's bite releases histamine, which causes the blood vessels in the area to dilate. This increased vascular permeability allows fluid to leak out of the blood vessels and into the tissues, resulting in edema.

29

A 35-year-old female presented with a swelling in the neck for the past 2 months. She received radiation to the neck when she was 20 years old. Clinical examination also revealed a single node in the left side of the neck, which moves with deglutition. This condition is:

a. Anaplastic carcinoma
b. Follicular carcinoma
c. Medullary carcinoma
d. Papillary carcinoma

Ans. (d) Papillary carcinoma

Explanation: Papillary carcinoma is the most common type of thyroid cancer, and it usually presents as a subtle, commonly slow-growing, painless thyroid mass or a solitary nodule in the neck. Papillary thyroid carcinoma occurs predominantly in middle-aged adults with a 3 to 1 female-to-male ratio. Radiation exposure, particularly during childhood or adolescence, is a known risk factor for the development of papillary carcinoma.

30

A 26-year-old lady comes with right upper abdominal pain and vomiting since 1 day. Patient had a similar episode 2 months back. On examination, there is tenderness in the right hypochondrium. What is the investigation of choice to confirm the diagnosis?

a. USG
b. MRCP
c. ERCp
d. CECT

Ans. (a) USG

Explanation: USG (Ultrasonography) is the initial imaging modality of choice for evaluating abdominal pain and diagnosing various conditions, including those affecting the liver, gallbladder, and biliary tract. In this case, the symptoms, such as right upper abdominal pain and tenderness, along with the history of a similar episode in the past, suggest a possible biliary cause, such as gallstones or cholecystitis.

31

A man is brought to the emergency after he fell into a man hole and injured his perineum. He feels the urge to micturate but is unable to pass urine and there is blood at the tip of the meatus with extensive swelling of the penis and scrotum. What is the location of the injury?

a. Bulbar urethra
b. Prostatic urethra
c. Bladder
d. Membranous urethra

Ans. (a) Bulbar urethra

Explanation: Injuries to the urethra are commonly classified as anterior or posterior based on their location. The presentation of urinary retention, blood at the meatus, and extensive swelling of the penis and scrotum suggests significant trauma to the bulbar urethra, leading to obstruction of urine flow and blood extravasation.

32

The nurse is providing indwelling catheter care to her assigned male patient. After cleaning the glans penis, the nurse noticed that the foreskin retracted behind the glans penis and cannot be pulled back forward. On documentation, the nurse will use which terminology to express this condition?

a. Phimosis
b. Paraphimosis
c. Hypospadias
d. Circumcision

Ans. (b) Paraphimosis

Explanation: Paraphimosis is a condition in which the foreskin becomes trapped behind the glans and cannot be returned to its normal position. It occurs when the foreskin is retracted behind the glans and then becomes stuck in that position. On the other hand, phimosis refers to a condition in which the foreskin of the penis is tight and cannot be easily retracted over the glans.

33

The nurse is caring for a patient diagnosed with an acute MI. The patient has severe, uncontrolled hypertension. The BP is 190/110 mm of Hg. The nurse should question which of the following cardiologist prescriptions?

a. Give thrombolytic therapy
b. Limit physical activity for 12 hours
c. Provide supplemental oxygen therapy
d. Administer IV nitroglycerin

Ans. (a) Give thrombolytic therapy

Explanation: Thrombolytic therapy is contraindicated in patients with a systolic blood pressure greater than 185 mmHg or diastolic blood pressure greater than 110 mmHg. The American Heart Association and American Stroke Association advise against the use of tPA when systolic BP reaches above 185 mmHg.

34

A patient with a history of myasthenia gravis is admitted to the medical-surgical unit. All of the following tests should the nurse expect to prescribe for the patient; except:

a. Electroencephalogram (EEG)
b. Electromyograph (EMG)
c. Tensilon test
d. Nerve conduction studies

Ans. (a) Electroencephalogram (EEG)

Explanation: An EEG is a test that records electrical activity in the brain. It is not typically used to diagnose myasthenia gravis. The other tests listed are all used to diagnose myasthenia gravis.

35

A 50-year-old male comes with complaints of progressive weakness worsening in the evening. He is diagnosed with myasthenia gravis. What is the drug of choice for this patient?

a. Edrophonium
b. Prednisone
c. Intravenous immunoglobulin (IVIG)
d. Pyridostigmine

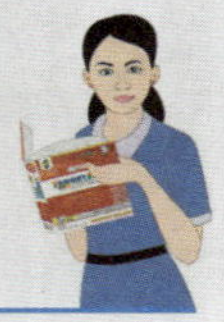

Ans. (d) Pyridostigmine

Explanation: Pyridostigmine is a cholinesterase inhibitor and is the primary medication used for symptomatic treatment of myasthenia gravis. It works by increasing the amount of acetylcholine available at the neuromuscular junction, enhancing muscle strength and reducing muscle weakness.

36

The nurse is providing care for a client following hypophysectomy and observes the presence of clear drainage from the client's nostril. What should be the nurse's initial course of action in response to this observation?

a. Obtain a culture of the drainage
b. Lower the head of the bed
c. Test the drainage for glucose
d. Continue to observe the drainage

Ans. (c) Test the drainage for glucose

Explanation: After a hypophysectomy, which involves the surgical removal of the pituitary gland, clear nasal drainage is expected. In the immediate postoperative period, it is important to observe the drainage to confirm if it is CSF. CSF rhinorrhea is usually clear and watery, and it can be tested for glucose to confirm its composition.

37

A patient is being evaluated for a possible myocardial infarction. The nurse is checking for increases in which of the following isoenzyme values that are associated with the creatine kinase level?

a. MB
b. BB
c. MM
d. MK

Ans. (a) MB

Explanation: Creatine kinase (CK) is an enzyme found in various tissues, including skeletal muscle, brain tissue, and the heart. It exists in different forms or isoenzymes, with CK-MB being specific to cardiac muscle.

38

The nurse is caring for a 62-year-old male patient diagnosed with Alzheimer's disease, who is currently displaying agitation and engaging in pulling behaviors. What is the most appropriate action for the nurse to take when providing care for this patient?

a. Place the patient in a room with several other patients.
b. Provide the patient with therapeutic sensory devices
c. Leave the patient alone and set limits
d. Allot room for the patient along with another agitated patient.

Ans. (b) Provide the patient with therapeutic sensory devices

Explanation: Alzheimer's disease is a progressive neurodegenerative disorder that affects cognitive function, including memory, thinking, and behavior. Agitation is a common behavioral manifestation in patients with Alzheimer's disease. Therapeutic sensory devices, such as fidget pillow, stress balls, or textured objects, can help provide sensory stimulation and a sense of calm for patients with Alzheimer's disease who are agitated.

39

The patient is admitted to the emergency department with symptoms of respiratory, vasomotor, and cardiac dysfunction. Which specific region of the brain is involved in causing these manifestations?

a. Parietal lobe
b. Medulla
c. Cerebellum
d. Wernicke's area

Ans. (b) Medulla

Explanation: The medulla, specifically the medulla oblongata (lowest part of brainstem), is located in the brainstem and plays a vital role in regulating many autonomic functions, including respiratory rhythm, blood pressure control, and cardiac function.

40

A nurse in the outpatient clinic is assessing the Mantoux test of a patient who has a history of being treated for an AIDS-related infection in the past year. The nurse should document a positive reaction if there is an area of induration that measures what size?

a. 1 mm
b. 3 mm
c. 6 mm
d. 10 mm

Ans. (c) 6 mm

Explanation: CDC recommends that HIV-positives with tuberculin test reaction of 5 mm or more are at greater risk of developing tuberculosis and hence, they should be administered prophylactic treatment. For individuals with HIV infection, recent close contact with a person with active TB, or other immunocompromised conditions, a positive reaction is considered when the area of induration measures 5 mm or greater.

41

As a patient is being discharged from the clinic with a new prescription for Lisinopril, what advice can the nurse provide to minimize one of the primary side effects of the medication?

a. Eat fruits and vegetables high in iron
b. Rise slowly from a lying to a sitting position
c. Increase fluid intake
d. Avoid aspirin-containing drugs

Ans. (b) Rise slowly from a lying to a sitting position

Explanation: Lisinopril is an ACE inhibitor, which means it works by blocking the action of angiotensin-converting enzyme (ACE). One of the side effects of ACE inhibitors is orthostatic hypotension, which is a sudden drop in blood pressure when you stand up from a lying or sitting position. This can cause dizziness or lightheadedness. To minimize the risk of orthostatic hypotension, the nurse should advise the patient to rise slowly from a lying or sitting position.

42

A nurse administers IV furosemide to a patient admitted with congestive heart failure. The patient is not expected to experience.

a. Increased urinary output
b. Decreased edema
c. Decreased pain
d. Decreased blood pressure

Ans. (c) Decreased pain

Explanation: Furosemide is a loop diuretic commonly used to treat conditions such as congestive heart failure and edema by promoting diuresis (increased urine output) and reducing fluid volume overload. This may result in decreased blood pressure too. However, furosemide is not specifically indicated for pain relief.

43

During an assessment in the emergency department, a nurse evaluates a patient who has been on long-term corticosteroid therapy for renal disease. Which of the following is a common adverse effect associated with corticosteroid treatment?

i. Hypertension
ii. Cushingoid features
iii. Low serum albumin
iv. Hyponatremia

a. Only i, ii and iii are correct
b. Only i and iii are correct
c. Only ii and iv are correct
d. All four (i, ii, iii and iv) are correct

Ans. (a) Only i, ii and iii are correct

Explanation: Corticosteroids can indeed cause a range of side effects, and the ones listed in options (i) Hypertension, (ii) Cushingoid features, and (iii) Low serum albumin are generally associated with long-term corticosteroid treatment. Corticosteroids generally cause sodium retention and can lead to hypernatremia (high sodium levels) rather than hyponatremia.

44

The nurse is providing instructions to a male patient on how to correctly use crutches for his right ankle injury. The patient will need to avoid putting weight on the affected leg for a period of 4 to 6 weeks. Which crutch gait should the nurse teach the patient to ensure safe mobility?

a. The two-point gait
b. The three-point gait
c. The four-point gait
d. None, there is no special gait for crutch training

Ans. (b) The three-point gait

Explanation: Three-point gait is used when one of the lower extremities is unable to fully bear weight due to injury or fracture.

In the three-point gait, the patient bears weight on only one leg while using crutches. The sequence is as follows:

I. The patient moves both crutches forward.
II. The patient swings the injured leg forward, keeping it off the ground.
III. The patient places weight on the unaffected leg and moves it forward.

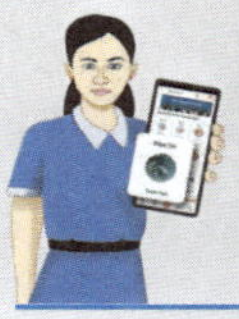

45

A patient is hospitalized with a diagnosis of primary hyperparathyroidism. When reviewing the patient's laboratory results, the nurse would anticipate which of the following alterations in the lab findings?

a. Elevated serum calcium
b. Low serum parathyroid hormone (PTH)
c. Elevated serum vitamin D
d. Low urine calcium

Ans. (a) Elevated serum calcium

Explanation: Primary hyperparathyroidism is a disorder characterized by excessive production of parathyroid hormone (PTH) by the parathyroid glands. The excessive PTH production results in increased release of calcium from bones, increased calcium reabsorption from the kidneys, and increased absorption of calcium from the gastrointestinal tract. This leads to elevated serum calcium level, which is a hallmark finding in primary hyperparathyroidism.

46

The nurse in an outpatient clinic has the opportunity to provide education to a patient who is dependent on insulin. Which of the following topics would be the most suitable for the nurse to include when discussing personal hygiene?

a. Oral care is not a major concern.
b. Hair care is the most important part of personal hygiene for the diabetic patient.
c. It is most important to keep skin clean and dry, especially the feet.
d. Personal hygiene is not addressed in diabetic education because it is an individual choice.

Ans. (c) It is most important to keep skin clean and dry, especially the feet

Explanation: Proper care of the skin, particularly the feet, is crucial due to the increased risk of foot problems in people with diabetes. High blood sugar levels can affect the nerves and blood vessels, leading to reduced sensation and circulation in the feet. Therefore, it is essential to keep the feet clean and dry to prevent infections, ulcers, and other foot-related complications.

47

A patient who has recently begun hemodialysis expresses curiosity about how the treatment will replace the function of their kidneys. The nurse's explanation is grounded in the understanding that hemodialysis functions by:

a. Passing water through a dialyzing membrane
b. Filtering waste through a dialyzing membrane
c. Eliminating plasma proteins from the blood
d. Balancing the pH by removing nonvolatile acids

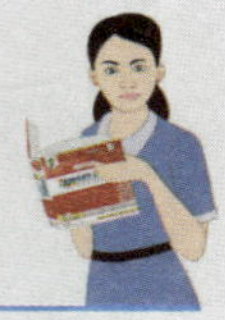

Ans. (b) Filtering waste through a dialyzing membrane

Explanation: During hemodialysis, the patient's blood is circulated outside of the body through a dialysis machine. The machine pumps the blood through a dialyzer, which contains a semipermeable membrane.

As blood flows through the dialyzer, waste products, toxins, and excess fluid pass through the membrane, while essential substances such as red blood cells and proteins remain in the blood.

48

A nurse who is responsible for multiple patients on the cardiac unit is informed that one of them is scheduled to undergo implantation of an automatic internal cardioverter-defibrillator. Which of the following patients is most likely to undergo this procedure?

a. A patient admitted for myocardial infarction without cardiac muscle damage
b. A patient with a history of ventricular tachycardia and syncopal episodes
c. A post-op CABG patient, recovering on schedule
d. A patient with a history of atrial tachycardia and fatigue

Ans. (b) A patient with a history of ventricular tachycardia and syncopal episodes

Explanation: An automatic internal cardioverter-defibrillator (AICD) is a device implanted in patients at high risk for life-threatening ventricular arrhythmias, such as ventricular tachycardia or ventricular fibrillation. A patient with a history of ventricular tachycardia and syncopal episodes is the most likely candidate for an AICD implantation due to their higher risk of life-threatening ventricular arrhythmias.

49

A young adult patient who met a car accident is brought to the emergency department (ED) with unconsciousness and severe hypotension. The patient is suspected to have multiple fractures in the pelvis and legs. Considering the patient's current condition, which of the following intravenous fluids would be the most appropriate choice?

a. Fresh frozen plasma
b. Packed red blood cells
c. 0.9% sodium chloride solution
d. Lactated Ringer's solution

Ans. (b) Packed red blood cells

Explanation: Based on the clinical presentation of severe hypotension, the patient is likely experiencing hypovolemic shock due to significant blood loss from the trauma. In this situation, the priority is to restore circulating blood volume and provide oxygen-carrying capacity to the tissues.

Packed red blood cells (PRBCs) are specifically indicated for patients with significant blood loss or anemia. They contain concentrated red blood cells, which can effectively increase the oxygen-carrying capacity of the blood. PRBCs are the most appropriate choice to address the potential hemorrhage and improve tissue perfusion in this patient.

50

A patient presents to the emergency department with abdominal pain. Further assessment reveals the presence of an abdominal aortic aneurysm that is rapidly increasing in size. What should the nurse anticipate as the next course of action for the patient?

a. The patient will be admitted to the medicine unit for monitoring and administration of medication.
b. The patient will be admitted to the surgical unit and resection will be scheduled.
c. The patient will be admitted to the day surgery unit for sclerotherapy treatment.
d. The patient will be discharged home to follow-up with his cardiologist in 24 hours.

Ans. (b) The patient will be admitted to the surgical unit and resection will be scheduled.

Explanation: An abdominal aortic aneurysm (AAA) is a serious condition where the wall of the aorta in the abdomen weakens and bulges, increasing the risk of rupture. Rapid enlargement of the AAA is a critical situation that requires immediate medical attention and intervention.

Given the potential life-threatening nature of a rapidly enlarging AAA, the patient would typically be admitted to the surgical unit.

51

A patient who is hospitalized with MRSA (methicillin-resistant Staphylococcus aureus) is placed on contact precautions. Which statement accurately describes the precautions for infections transmitted through contact?

a. The patient should be placed in a room equipped with negative pressure.
b. Infection transmission requires close contact, therefore, the door to remain open.
c. Transmission is highly probable, necessitating the patient to wear a mask constantly.
d. Infection requires skin-to-skin contact and is prevented by hand washing, gloves and a gown.

Ans. (d) Infection requires skin-to-skin contact and is prevented by hand washing, gloves and a gown.

Explanation: Contact precautions are implemented to prevent the transmission of infections that are spread through direct contact with the patient or their environment. In the case of MRSA, the bacteria can be present on the patient's skin or contaminated surfaces. To prevent the spread of MRSA, healthcare providers should practice good hand hygiene, wearing gloves and a gown.

52

The nurse is observing a patient after undergoing a lung resection. The chest tube has recorded an hourly output of 300 mL. What should be the nurse's priority action at this time?

a. Turning the patient to the left side
b. Milking the tube to ensure patency
c. Slowing the intravenous infusion
d. Notifying the physician

Ans. (d) Notifying the physician

Explanation: An hourly output of 300 mL from a chest tube following a lung resection is excessive. It may indicate that there is active bleeding or an increased risk of complications such as hemothorax or pneumothorax. The nurse should notify the physician immediately so that the patient can be evaluated and treated.

53

A patient who was admitted to the intensive care unit (ICU) five days ago for severe pneumonia now exhibits a sudden inability to recognize his relatives and is under the false belief that he is in jail, as mentioned by the doctor. The patient is experiencing an altered level of consciousness.

a. Acute dementia
b. Brief psychotic reaction
c. ICU Psychosis
d. Acute paranoia

Ans. (c) ICU Psychosis

Explanation: ICU psychosis, also known as ICU delirium or intensive care unit delirium, is a common condition characterized by an acute onset of confusion, disorientation, altered consciousness, and perceptual disturbances in patients who are critically ill and admitted to the intensive care unit (ICU). Patients with ICU psychosis may experience hallucinations, delusions, and difficulty with attention, memory, and cognition.

54

Nurse Ramya is caring for a client with chronic obstructive pulmonary disease (COPD). Ramya noticed that the patient has a nasal cannula delivering oxygen at a flow rate of 6 liters per minute. The client's skin color appears pink and the respirations are measured at 9 breaths per minute and are shallow. What should be the nurse's first course of action in this situation?

a. Take heart rate and blood pressure
b. Lower the oxygen rate
c. Position the client in a Fowler's position
d. Call the physician

Ans. (b) Lower the oxygen rate

Explanation: The client's oxygen is running at a high flow rate of 6 L per minute, which may contribute to hypoventilation by decreasing the client's respiratory drive. Lowering the oxygen rate to a more appropriate level is necessary to avoid suppressing the client's respiratory drive further. This will allow the client to maintain a more normal respiratory rate and depth.

55

In developing a care plan for a patient with advanced AIDS and impaired memory due to neurologic changes, what should the nurse prioritize as the most important aspect of care?

a. Maintain a safe patient environment
b. Provide a quiet, non-stressful environment to avoid overstimulation
c. Use memory cues such as clocks to promote orientation
d. Provide written instructions of directions to promote orientation

Ans. (a) Maintain a safe patient environment

Explanation: While planning a nursing care plan, the safety is the top priority.

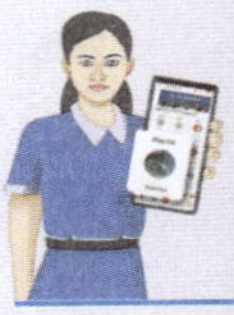

56

A 30-year-old female presents to the emergency department (ED) with hyperventilation. Initially, her respiratory rate is 27 breaths per minute and her oxygen saturation is 100% on room air. She complains of difficulty breathing and experiencing cramping in her hands and feet. The patient denies any history of trauma, past medical conditions, or illicit drug use. Auscultation of her chest reveals clear breath sounds bilaterally. A subsequent chest X-ray shows no abnormalities. After reassessment, the patient reports improved breathing, with a respiratory rate of 14 breaths per minute and an oxygen saturation of 100% on room air. What is the most likely cause of this patient's symptoms?

a. Pneumothorax b. Hemopneumothorax
c. Pleural effusion d. Anxiety attack

Ans. (d) Anxiety attack

Explanation: The patient's symptoms of hyperventilation, chest tightness, and tingling in the hands and feet are classic symptoms of an anxiety attack. The chest radiograph is normal, which rules out any underlying medical conditions.

57

A 24-year-old burn patient weighing 60 kg presents with involvement of face, neck, anterior chest wall and abdominal wall and both arms circumferential burns. Calculate the fluid to be given in the first 8 hours using Parkland formula:

a. 4.9 L b. 5.8 L
c. 6.4 L d. 7.2 L

Ans. (a) 4.9 L

Explanation: To calculate fluid requirement, we need to calculate Total Body Surface Area (TBSA) of burn.
Using rule of nine, the TBSA of affected area is as follows:
Face – 4.5%
Anterior chest wall- 9%
Anterior abdominal wall – 9%
Both arms – 9+9 = 18%
Total TBSA affected = 40.5
Now, use the Parkland formula to calculate fluid requirement for 24 hours:
Fluid requirement = 4 mL × body weight (kg) × TBSA
= 4 mL × 60 × 40.5
= 9720 mL
As per Parkland formula, 50% of the fluid need to be infused in first 8 hours.
So, 9720/2 = 4860 ml = 4.86 L.
So the answer is a. 4.9 L in first 8 hours.

58

A 60-year-old woman presents with a severe drug-induced reaction. Within a few days, the skin begins to blister and peel after a flu-like symptoms. The insulting drug was carbamazepine (Tegretol). On examination, extensive necrosis and detachment of the epidermis, which involves skin and mucosal surfaces (genitals, eyes, and mouth) were assessed. Identify the condition of this patient.

a. Dermatitis herpetiformis b. Stevens-Johnson syndrome
c. Keloid d. Herpes gestationis

Ans. (b) Stevens-Johnson syndrome

Explanation: Stevens-Johnson syndrome (SJS) is a severe, life-threatening skin reaction that is often triggered by certain medications, including carbamazepine (Tegretol). It is characterized by a widespread rash that can involve the skin and mucous membranes. The rash typically starts with flu-like symptoms, followed by the development of blisters that break open and leave the skin raw and painful.

59

After receiving an intramuscular injection of penicillin in the gluteus maximus, a patient experiences dyspnea and weakness within minutes. What other assessment findings suggest that the patient is experiencing an anaphylactoid reaction?

i. Hypertension ii. Wheezing
iii. Rash on arms iv. Feeling of impending doom

a. Only i, ii and iii are correct
b. Only i and iii are correct
c. Only ii and iv are correct
d. If all four (i, ii, iii and iv) are correct

Ans. (c) Only ii and iv are correct

Explanation: Wheezing is a common symptom of bronchoconstriction, which can occur in an anaphylactoid reaction due to the release of inflammatory mediators. A feeling of impending doom is a subjective sense of extreme unease, anxiety, or fear that can be experienced during an anaphylactoid reaction. Hypertension and rash on the arms are not specific to anaphylactoid reactions and can occur in various other conditions.

60

The given procedure in the image is performed for the patient with acute pericarditis. Postoperatively what complication should the nurse monitor the patient for?

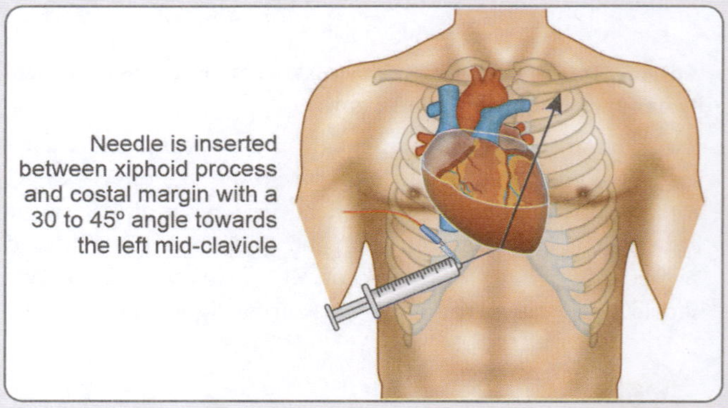

a. Pneumonia b. Pneumothorax
c. Myocardial infarction (MI)
d. Cerebrovascular accident (CVA)

Ans. (b) Pneumothorax

Explanation: Pneumothorax is a complication that can occur during or after pericardiocentesis. It is a condition in which air enters the space between the lung and the chest wall. This can cause the lung to collapse, which can lead to shortness of breath, chest pain, and difficulty breathing.

61

Which of the following nursing interventions would be inappropriate for a patient admitted to the emergency department with a lacerated liver due to blunt abdominal trauma?

a. Monitor for respiratory distress
b. Monitor for coagulation studies
c. Administer pain medications as ordered
d. Administer normal saline, crystalloids as per order

Ans. (c) Administer pain medications as ordered

Explanation: Administering pain medications, especially opioids, can potentially mask important signs and symptoms of worsening internal bleeding or other complications. It also interferes with the assessment of neurologic status of the patient.

62

A female patient with chronic skin lesions on her face and arms expresses feelings of extreme dissatisfaction with her appearance and avoidance of looking at herself in the mirror. The nurse recognizes this as indicative of which nursing diagnosis?

a. Anxiety related to Skin lesions
b. Disturbed body image related to perception of unappealing lesions
c. Social isolation related to decreased activities as a result of poor self-image
d. Ineffective self-care management related to lack of knowledge of coping mechanism

Ans. (b) Disturbed body image related to perception of unappealing lesions

Explanation: The patient's statement about not being able to stand looking at herself in the mirror due to her appearance indicates a disturbance in body image. Body image refers to one's perception and feelings about their own physical appearance. In this case, the patient's chronic skin lesions on the face and arms are negatively impacting her body image and causing distress.

63

Ravi, a patient with diabetes, is presenting with alternating periods of nocturnal hypoglycemia and hyperglycemia in the morning. Which of the following conditions is most likely contributing to these symptoms?

a. Poorly controlled diabetes
b. Somogyi phenomenon
c. Brittle diabetes
d. Diabetes insipidus

Ans. (b) Somogyi phenomenon

Explanation: The Somogyi phenomenon, also known as rebound hyperglycemia, is characterized by a pattern of nocturnal hypoglycemia followed by morning hyperglycemia. This occurs as a result of the body's response to low blood glucose levels during sleep. In response to hypoglycemia, counterregulatory hormones are released, leading to increased glucose production by the liver. However, this rebound response can lead to excessive glucose production, resulting in hyperglycemia in the morning.

64

The patient with advanced cancer is struggling to manage her pain and expresses concern about developing an addiction to opioids. What is the initial action the nurse should take in response to this patient's concerns?

a. Advise the patient to maintain a pain diary to record the medicine use history.
b. Assess the patient's vital signs and behavior to determine the appropriate drug.
c. Administer NSAID for pain control.
d. Obtain a detailed pain history including quality, location, intensity, duration and type of pain.

Ans. (d) Obtain a detailed pain history including quality, location, intensity, duration and type of pain.

Explanation: The first thing the nurse should do for the patient is to obtain a detailed pain history including quality, location, intensity, duration, and type of pain (Option d). This will help the nurse assess the nature of the pain and develop an appropriate pain management plan.

65

The nurse is caring for a patient with infective endocarditis involving a prosthetic mitral valve who presents with left hemiparesis and visual changes. Which intervention should the nurse anticipate as part of the collaborative management?

a. Removal of the embolus
b. Replacement of the prosthetic valve through surgery
c. Initiation of anticoagulant therapy
d. Administration of higher than usual doses of antibiotics

Ans. (b) Replacement of the prosthetic valve through surgery.

Explanation: In this case, the patient's left hemiparesis and visual changes suggest the presence of an embolus in the brain, which requires immediate intervention.

Surgical valve replacement may be necessary to remove the infected prosthetic valve and replace it with a new valve. This is done to remove the source of infection and prevent further embolization.

66

The nurse is preparing to care for a patient scheduled for surgical repair of a 5.5 cm abdominal aortic aneurysm (AAA). What assessment findings should the nurse anticipate in this patient?

a. Hoarseness and difficulty swallowing
b. Severe back pain with bruising on the flank
c. Presence of a bruit in the periumbilical area
d. Progressive weakness in the lower extremities leading to paraplegia

Ans. (c) Presence of a bruit in the periumbilical area

Explanation: An abdominal aortic aneurysm (AAA) is a localized dilation of the abdominal aorta. The most common assessment finding in a patient with an AAA is the presence of a bruit, which is an abnormal vascular sound caused by turbulent blood flow through the dilated vessel. The bruit is typically heard in the periumbilical area.

67

During the emergent phase in a patient with a full-thickness burn over the lower half of the body, what is one clinical manifestation the nurse would expect to find?

a. Elevated body temperature
b. Shivering
c. Intense pain at the burn site
d. Loss of consciousness

Ans. (b) Shivering

Explanation: Burn patients are at an increased risk for hypothermia due to the loss of the protective barrier provided by the skin, which leads to increased heat loss. Shivering is a physiological response to generate heat and maintain body temperature. Full-thickness burns are usually anesthetic or hypoesthetic. So, pain is not likely.

68

A 40-year-old female patient has been admitted with a new diagnosis of Cushing's syndrome, which is characterized by elevated serum and urine cortisol levels. Which assessment findings should the nurse anticipate in this patient?

a. Thinning hair and moon face
b. Weight loss and hirsutism
c. Decreased muscle mass and thick skin
d. Increased blood pressure and hyperglycemia

Ans. (d) Increased blood pressure and hyperglycemia

Explanation: Since, the patient has been newly diagnosed with Cushing's syndrome, the focus would be on the acute manifestations and immediate effects of elevated cortisol levels. Long-term symptoms and physical changes such as weight gain, hirsutism, and muscle wasting may develop over time with chronic exposure to excess cortisol.

69

A patient is receiving 1000 mL of parenteral nutrition solution over 24 hours. When it is time to change the solution, there is still 100 mL remaining in the bottle. What should the nurse do?

a. Infuse the remaining solution rapidly through the IV line
b. Notify the physician for instructions on the infusion rate
c. Hang the new solution and discard the unused solution
d. Delay changing the solution until the remaining solution infuses at the prescribed rate

Ans. (c) Hang the new solution and discard the unused solution

Explanation: TPN solutions hung, but not infused, shall be discarded after 24 hours.

70

A patient with AIDS is receiving a combination therapy of zidovudine, lamivudine, and indinavir. The patient develops pulmonary tuberculosis and begins treatment for it. Which of the following should be contraindicated for this patient?

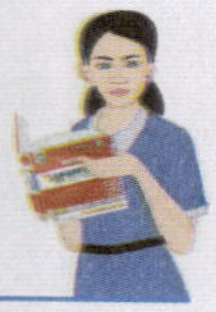

a. INH
b. Ethambutol
c. Pyrazinamide
d. Rifampicin

Ans. (d) Rifampicin

Explanation: The protease inhibitor indinavir is primarily metabolized by CYP3A4 and is also a P-glycoprotein substrate. This makes treatment of tuberculosis with rifampin in HIV-infected patients receiving indinavir complicated because of markedly diminished indinavir concentrations.

71

A 24-year-old female patient presents to her family physician with persistent hiccups that have been difficult to control. The physician recommends a technique of breathing in and out of a bag to rebreathe exhaled carbon dioxide (CO_2). In the bloodstream, the majority of CO_2 is transported in which form?

a. Carbaminohemoglobin
b. Bicarbonate
c. Carboxyhemoglobin
d. Carbonic acid

Ans. (b) Bicarbonate

Explanation: Carbon dioxide (CO_2) is transported in the blood primarily in the form of bicarbonate (HCO_3^-) ions. When CO_2 combines with water (H_2O) in the presence of the enzyme carbonic anhydrase, it forms carbonic acid (H_2CO_3), which rapidly dissociates into hydrogen ions (H+) and bicarbonate ions (HCO_3^-). The bicarbonate ions are then transported in the plasma to the lungs, where they are converted back into CO_2 for elimination from the body.

72

A 56-year-old woman has come with complaints of hand tremors which worsens while reaching out for objects. In the absence of any stimulus, what would her resting membrane potential be in the ulnar nerve of right hand?

a. -90 mV
b. -110 mV
c. +50 mV
d. -70 mV

Ans. (d) -70 mV

Explanation: The resting membrane potential of neurons is typically around -70 mV. This is the electrical charge difference between the inside and outside of the cell when the cell is at rest and not receiving any signals or stimuli.

73

A 35-year-old female complains of forgetfulness, loss of hair and cold intolerance. Her TSH levels are high and free T3 and T4 are low. What would be the effect of this disease on Basal Metabolic Rate (BMR)?

a. Normal BMR
b. BMR increases
c. BMR decreases
d. There is initial rise with a subsequent fall

Ans. (c) BMR decreases

Explanation: The described symptoms and laboratory findings are consistent with hypothyroidism, which is characterized by low levels of thyroid hormones. In hypothyroidism, the metabolic rate of the body decreases, leading to a decrease in Basal Metabolic Rate (BMR).

74

A 35-year-old male patient suffering from epilepsy, deep vein thrombosis, and rheumatoid arthritis comes to Emergency Department with multiple bruises on his body. Which probable drug interaction the nurse should think about?

a. Aspirin and warfarin
b. Phenytoin and Ibuprofen
c. Warfarin and propranolol
d. Ibuprofen and valproate

Ans. (a) Aspirin and warfarin

Explanation: Aspirin and warfarin both have anticoagulant properties, meaning they can increase the risk of bleeding. When taken together, they can potentiate the anticoagulant effect, further increasing the risk of bleeding and bruising. Therefore, the nurse should consider the interaction between aspirin and warfarin as a potential cause of the patient's multiple bruises.

75

A patient was started on antileprosy drugs. Which of the following could have caused the side-effects seen in picture?

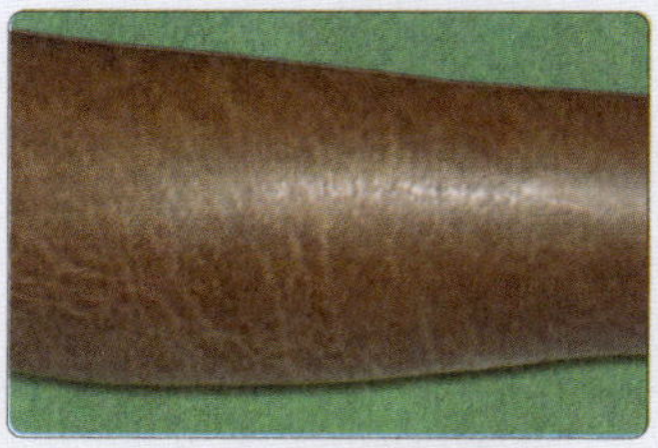

a. Rifampicin
b. Dapsone
c. Clofazimine
d. Ofloxacin

Ans. (c) Clofazimine

Explanation: Some frequent skin-related side effects of clofazimine include:

- Skin discoloration: reddish to brownish-black color, particularly in fair-skinned patients at sites exposed to light.
- Scaly and dry skin (acquired ichthyosis). The image shown here resembles ichthyosis.

76

An unconscious kid was brought to the emergency in a PHC with history of consumption of a thorny fruit given in the picture. What kind of poisoning should the nurse anticipate?

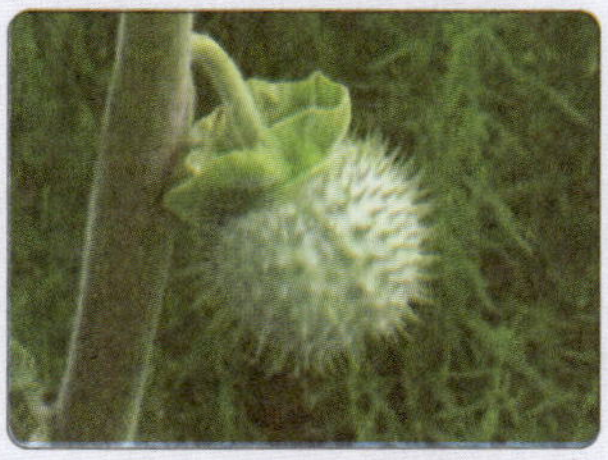

a. Cholinergic
b. Anticholinergic
c. Sympathomimetic
d. Sympatholytic

Ans. (b) Anticholinergic

Explanation: Datura poisoning is classified as an anticholinergic poisoning. Datura plants contain tropane alkaloids, including atropine, hyoscyamine, and scopolamine, which exert anticholinergic effects on the body.

77

A patient with asthma wants to know how albuterol inhaler works to improve his breathing. Which explanation by the nurse best describes the action of the medication?

a. It is a beta blocking agent that causes bronchodilation.
b. It is an anticholinergic agent and causes bronchodilation.
c. It is a beta agonist that causes bronchodilation.
d. It is a beta agonist that decreases bronchial secretions.

Ans. (c) It is a beta agonist that causes bronchodilation.

78

A patient arrives at the clinic complaining of a swollen face and tongue, difficulty breathing, and audible wheezing immediately after consuming a peanut butter sandwich. What should be the nurse's initial action in this situation?

a. Ensure airway patency.
b. Obtain an electrocardiogram.
c. Administer 1 mg of 1:1000 epinephrine subcutaneously.
d. Initiate an intravenous infusion of normal saline.

Ans. (a) Ensure airway patency.

Explanation: The patient's symptoms suggest a severe allergic reaction, possibly anaphylaxis. The priority in this situation is to ensure that the patient's airway is open and unobstructed to maintain adequate breathing. TIPS: Use the ABC principle to solve the question.

79

A patient who has undergone major surgery is experiencing difficulty sleeping despite nonpharmacologic measures. Which medication does the nurse anticipate may be prescribed?

a. Flumazenil
b. Phenobarbital
c. Clomipramine
d. Zolpidem

Ans. (d) Zolpidem

Explanation: Zolpidem is a sedative-hypnotic medication commonly prescribed for the short-term treatment of insomnia. Flumazenil is a medication used for the reversal of benzodiazepine overdose. Phenobarbital is a barbiturate that is not typically used for insomnia management. Clomipramine is an antidepressant medication

80

A 65-year-old patient is experiencing cardiac arrest with refractory ventricular fibrillation that has not responded to other treatments. Which medication is the preferred choice when other agents have been ineffective?

a. Amiodarone
b. Atropine
c. Acebutolol HCl
d. Propafenone HCl

Ans. (a) Amiodarone

Explanation: Amiodarone is considered the drug of choice for treating ventricular fibrillation that is unresponsive to initial therapies. It has antiarrhythmic properties and can help restore normal cardiac rhythm.

81

A patient in the ward has been prescribed promethazine for the management of nausea and vomiting. The patient is curious about how the medication exerts its effects. How should the nurse best explain the mechanism of action?

a. It inhibits the D2 receptors in the brain.
b. It blocks the H1 receptors in the chemoreceptor trigger zone (CTZ).
c. It inhibits the M1 receptors in the gastrointestinal tract.
d. It blocks the 5HT-3 receptors in the central nervous system.

Ans. (b) It blocks the H1 receptors in the chemoreceptor trigger zone (CTZ).

Explanation: Promethazine is an antihistamine medication that works by blocking the H1 receptor sites in the chemoreceptor trigger zone (CTZ) of the brain. The CTZ is responsible for triggering the sensation of nausea and vomiting. By blocking these receptors, promethazine helps to alleviate nausea and vomiting symptoms.

82

A patient is given reteplase for thromboembolic stroke. His blood pressure suddenly begins to fall because of hemorrhage. What medication does the nurse anticipate which will potentially be used as treatment for this hemorrhage?

a. Streptokinase
b. Aminocaproic acid
c. Calcium gluconate
d. Protamine sulfate

Ans. (b) Aminocaproic acid

Explanation: Aminocaproic acid, an antifibrinolytic agent, is a medication used to manage and treat acute bleeding disorders. Protamine sulfate is used to counteract the effect of heparin, not to control bleeding.

83

A 35-year-old patient presents to the clinic with complaints of red and irritated skin following a recent episode of diarrhea. The patient reports discomfort and itching in the affected area. Based on the patient's symptoms and assessment findings, which medication would be the most appropriate choice to alleviate the patient's skin irritation?

a. Silver sulfadiazine
b. Zinc oxide
c. Mafenide acetate
d. Action

Ans. (b) Zinc oxide

Explanation: Zinc oxide is commonly used as a topical agent to soothe and protect irritated skin. It provides a barrier against moisture and can help reduce inflammation and itching.

84

A 62-year-old patient with pneumonia is receiving Gentamicin. It would be most important for a nurse to monitor which of the following laboratory values in this patient?

a. Hemoglobin and hematocrit
b. Blood urea nitrogen and creatinine
c. Platelet count and clotting time
d. Sodium and potassium

Ans. (b) Blood urea nitrogen and creatinine

Explanation: Gentamicin, an aminoglycoside, is an antibiotic known to have potential nephrotoxic effects. Monitoring BUN and creatinine levels is crucial to assess renal function and detect any signs of kidney damage or impaired renal clearance.

85

A patient suffering from histoplasmosis has been prescribed Topical Ketoconazole (Nizoral). What advice the nurse will give to the patient while taking the medication?

a. Avoid sunlight exposure
b. Limit alcohol to 2 ounces daily
c. Take medicine empty stomach
d. Take medicine with an antacid

Ans. (a) Avoid sunlight exposure

Explanation: Ketoconazole can increase the sensitivity of the skin to sunlight, leading to an increased risk of sunburn.

86

A patient is on warfarin for prevention of deep vein thrombosis. He develops depression and is started on fluoxetine, which is highly protein-bound. What interaction might be seen?

a. Increased protein binding of warfarin
b. Decreased protein binding of warfarin
c. Cannot comment on protein binding
d. No change in protein binding

Ans. (b) Decreased protein binding of warfarin

Explanation: Fluoxetine, sertraline and paroxetine are highly bound to plasma proteins and therefore can displace other protein-bound drugs such as warfarin which may lead to increased therapeutic response and toxicity of warfarin.

87

A patient was prescribed aspirin for treatment of rheumatoid arthritis. When patient asked about, how it acts, the answer given by nurse should be:

a. Aspirin is a LOX inhibitor
b. Aspirin is a nonselective COX inhibitor
c. Aspirin is an opioid analgesic
d. Aspirin selectively inhibits COX-2

Ans. (b) Aspirin is a nonselective COX inhibitor

Explanation: Aspirin (acetylsalicylic acid) acetylates a serine residue in the active sites for both COX-1 and COX-2, which irreversibly inhibits these enzymes.

88

A female patient comes to OPD with complaints of white vaginal discharge and pruritus. She is taking ampicillin for last 7 days for treatment of upper respiratory infection. What causes the nurse should think about the patient's symptoms?

a. Cystitis
b. Urinary tract infection
c. Dysbacteriosis
d. Candidiasis

Ans. (d) Candidiasis

Explanation: The symptoms of white vaginal discharge and pruritus in this patient suggest a possible vaginal yeast infection, also known as candidiasis. Ampicillin is an antibiotic that can disrupt the normal balance of microorganisms in the body, including the natural protective bacteria in the vagina. This disruption can lead to an overgrowth of *Candida*, a type of yeast that commonly causes vaginal yeast infections.

89

A patient was started on antibiotic recently for treatment of Traveler's diarrhea. After 2 days, he developed pain in ankle. The nurse should think about which antibiotic in this case?

a. Amikacin
b. Ampicillin
c. Erythromycin
d. Ciprofloxacin

Ans. (d) Ciprofloxacin

Explanation: Ciprofloxacin is a fluoroquinolone antibiotic commonly used to treat Traveler's diarrhea caused by enterotoxigenic *E. coli*. However, a known side effect of fluoroquinolone antibiotics is the risk of tendonitis and tendon rupture, particularly in the Achilles tendon. Therefore, the development of ankle pain in a patient recently started on ciprofloxacin raises concern for a potential adverse effect of ciprofloxacin.

90

A patient reports a change in urine color and attributes it to medication. Which of the following medications is least likely to cause urine discoloration?

a. Sulfasalazine
b. Amitriptyline
c. Chloroquine
d. Aspirin

Ans. (d) Aspirin

Explanation: Medications such as sulfasalazine, amitriptyline, and chloroquine are known to cause urine discoloration. Sulfasalazine can cause an orange-yellow discoloration, amitriptyline can cause a blue or green discoloration, and chloroquine can cause a brown or black discoloration of the urine. However, aspirin is not typically associated with urine discoloration.

91

You are responsible for reviewing the nursing unit's refrigerator. If you found the following drug in the refrigerator, which should be removed from the refrigerator's contents?

a. Nadolol
b. Humulin injection
c. Urokinase
d. Epogen injection

Ans. (a) Nadolol

Explanation: Nadolol tablets should be stored in tight, light-resistant containers at room temperature. Other given drugs need to be refrigerated.

92

A patient visiting the clinic has been diagnosed with acute gastritis. Which of the following medications would the nurse consider contraindicated for this patient?

a. Naproxen sodium
b. Calcium carbonate
c. Clarithromycin
d. Furosemide

Ans. (a) Naproxen sodium

Explanation: Acute gastritis involves inflammation of the stomach lining, which can be exacerbated by nonsteroidal anti-inflammatory drugs (NSAIDs) like naproxen sodium. NSAIDs can further irritate the stomach lining and increase the risk of gastrointestinal bleeding.

93

Injection morphine is given into thecal space during procedure for pain relief after the procedure. After procedure which of the following analgesic you will not administer?

a. Paracetamol
b. Diclofenac
c. Tramadol
d. Fentanyl

Ans. (d) Fentanyl

Explanation: Injecting morphine into the thecal space provides localized pain relief, and administering additional systemic opioids such as fentanyl may result in an excessive analgesic effect and increased risk of adverse effects, including respiratory depression. Therefore, fentanyl would not be administered after the procedure to avoid potential opioid overdose.

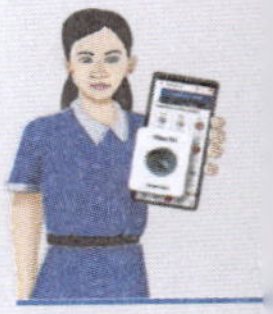

94

How do drugs such as methotrexate, hydroxychloroquine, or penicillamine differ from typical NSAIDs in managing rheumatoid arthritis that is not adequately controlled?

a. Neutralize inflammatory mediators
b. Are remarkably free from serious toxicities
c. Slow, stop, possibly reverse joint pathology in rheumatoid arthritis
d. Provide much quicker relief of arthritis signs and symptoms

Ans. (c) Slow, stop, possibly reverse joint pathology in rheumatoid arthritis

Explanation: Methotrexate, hydroxychloroquine, and penicillamine are disease-modifying antirheumatic drugs (DMARDs) commonly used in the management of rheumatoid arthritis. Unlike typical nonsteroidal anti-inflammatory drugs (NSAIDs), which primarily provide symptomatic relief by reducing pain and inflammation, DMARDs have the ability to slow down or stop the progression of joint damage caused by rheumatoid arthritis.

95

After ingesting an excessive dose of theophylline, a patient develops symptoms of drug toxicity. Which of the following is the most likely manifestation of theophylline toxicity?

a. Bradycardia
b. Drowsiness progressing to sleep and then coma
c. Hepatotoxicity
d. Seizures

Ans. (d) Seizures

Explanation: One of the most common consequences of theophylline toxicity is the development of seizures. Theophylline has a stimulatory effect on the central nervous system, and at toxic levels, it can lead to hyperexcitability and seizures.

96

A patient with deep partial-thickness burns covering 45% of his trunk and legs is scheduled for debridement in the cart shower 48-hours post-burn. The nurse anticipates the need for pharmacological pain management during the procedure. Which medication would be the most appropriate choice to control the patient's pain?

a. IV morphine
b. Midazolam
c. IM meperidine
d. Long-acting oral morphine

Ans. (a) IV morphine

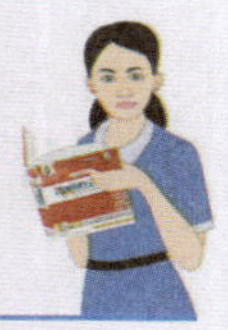

Explanation: IV morphine is the drug of choice to control pain during debridement in a patient with deep partial-thickness burns. Morphine is a potent opioid analgesic that provides effective pain relief. Intravenous administration allows for rapid onset of action, ensuring prompt pain control during the procedure.

97

A physician prescribes furosemide (Lasix) for a client. What should the nurse inform the client to expect if the medication is achieving the desired outcome?

a. Increased heart rate
b. Increased frequency of urination
c. Elevated blood pressure
d. Decreased nocturnal urination

Ans. (b) Increased frequency of urination

Explanation: Furosemide is an antidiuretic agent. The client should be informed to expect increased urine frequency if the drug is effective.

98

What is one of the primary considerations in determining the initiation of antiretroviral therapy in a patient diagnosed with HIV infection?

a. Presence of elevated levels of HIV antibodies in the patient
b. Verification of the patient's HIV infection status
c. The patient's willingness to adhere to a lifelong and challenging medication regimen
d. Availability of a support system to assist the patient in managing the financial burden

Ans. (c) The patient's willingness to adhere to a lifelong and challenging medication regimen

Explanation: The initiation of antiretroviral therapy in patients with HIV infection requires careful consideration of various factors. One of the most significant factors is the patient's willingness and readiness to commit to the lifelong and demanding drug regimen. Adherence to the medication regimen is crucial for successful treatment outcomes and preventing the development of drug resistance. In this case, the HIV status of the patient is already known, therefore, option (b) is not applicable.

99

A patient with diabetes expresses resistance to change his eating habits because he is not overweight. What should be the action of nurse at this stage of the transtheoretical model of behavior change?

a. Help the patient prioritize managing his diabetes
b. Arrange appointment with the dietitian to discuss what dietary changes are needed
c. Explain that dietary changes can help prevent long-term complications of diabetes
d. Emphasize that he must change behaviors if he is going to control his blood glucose levels

Ans. (c) Explain that dietary changes can help prevent long-term complications of diabetes

Explanation: At this stage of the transtheoretical model of behavior change, the nurse should explain to the patient that dietary changes can help prevent long-term complications of diabetes. This is because the patient is expressing resistance to changing his eating habits due to not being overweight. By highlighting the long-term benefits and potential complications of diabetes, the nurse can provide the patient with a better understanding of the importance of dietary changes for managing their condition effectively.

100

In an 85-year-old male patient with pneumonia in the ICU for treatment, the nurse observes a decline in cognitive function. What is the primary potential cause that the nurse should consider for this change?

a. Fatigue
b. Infection
c. ICU psychosis
d. Medication allergy

Ans. (b) Infection

Explanation: Infections, including pneumonia, can lead to systemic inflammation and affect the brain, resulting in cognitive changes.

101

A 75-year-old female patient is admitted to the hospital with a hemoglobin level of 7.0 g/dL and is presenting with ataxia and confusion. Which of the following nursing intervention is the priority for this patient?

a. Ensure the patient is in a dimly lit and calm environment.
b. Keep the top rails of the bed raised and place the call bell within easy reach.
c. Encourage the presence of family members at the bedside.
d. Inquire with the patient about potential causes of anemia.

Ans. (b) Keep the top rails of the bed raised and place the call bell within easy reach.

Explanation: The patient's presentation of ataxia and confusion, along with a low hemoglobin level, indicates a risk of falls and compromised mobility. Keeping the top bedside rails up and ensuring the call bell is within close reach promotes patient safety by preventing falls and providing easy access for assistance. **TIPS:** Use the patient safety first principle to solve this question.

102

A 45-year-old woman undergoing radiation therapy for breast cancer expreses to nurse that she finds it difficult to vocalize her anxieties and worries about her treatment. Which alternative or complementary therapy would be the most appropriate for the nurse to teach the patient to deal with this situation?

a. Journaling
b. Yoga therapy
c. Herbal therapy
d. Chiropractic therapy

Ans. (a) Journaling

Explanation: Journaling is a form of expressive writing that can be helpful for people who are struggling to express their emotions. It can be a way to process thoughts and feelings, and it can also be a way to track progress and see how one is feeling over time.

103

A patient with sickle cell anemia inquires why the sickling crisis does not resolve upon initiation of oxygen therapy. How should the nurse best explain this to the patient?

a. Sickling occurs in response to decreased blood viscosity
b. When RBCs sickle, they occlude small vessels, which causes more local hypoxia and more sickling
c. Destruction of the abnormal cells results in fewer RBCs to carry oxygen
d. All of the above

Ans. (b) When RBCs sickle, they occlude small vessels, which causes more local hypoxia and more sickling

Explanation: The nurse should explain to the patient that the sickling crisis does not resolve upon initiation of oxygen therapy because when red blood cells (RBCs) sickle, they occlude small blood vessels. This occlusion leads to more local hypoxia (lack of oxygen supply) and further sickling of RBCs. Option a and option c do not fully explain the mechanism behind the persistence of the sickling crisis despite oxygen therapy.

104

While providing care for a female patient with Alzheimer's disease and her husband who is the primary caregiver, the nurse observes that the patient's husband is experiencing an increase in asthma symptoms. What is a potential explanation for this observation?

a. Age-related deterioration leads to progressive worsening of asthma symptoms.
b. The husband may be smoking more as a coping mechanism to deal with the challenges of caring for his wife.
c. Chronic and intense stress can contribute to the exacerbation of immune-related conditions.
d. The husband's inadequate coping mechanisms may result in forgetting to take his prescribed medications.

Ans. (c) Chronic and intense stress can contribute to the exacerbation of immune-related conditions.

Explanation: Chronic and intense stress can have a negative impact on the immune system and can trigger exacerbations of immune-related diseases, including asthma.

105

The nurse Rosy noticed the positive sign demonstrated in the image in a patient. The nurse would anticipate the IV administration of which medication?

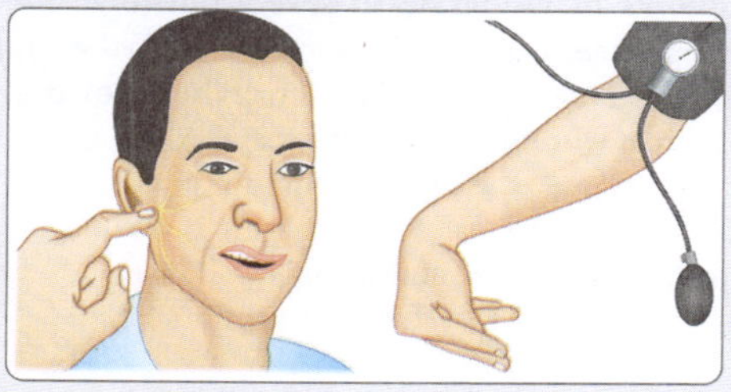

a. Calcitonin
b. Vitamin D
c. Loop diuretics
d. Calcium gluconate

Ans. (d) Calcium gluconate

Explanation: The sign shown in the image is Chvostek sign and Trousseau's sign. It is a clinical finding associated with hypocalcemia, or low levels of calcium in the blood. Administering calcium gluconate intravenously is the appropriate intervention for treating hypocalcemia.

106

A patient in the terminal stage of life is experiencing dyspnea and a feeling of suffocation. According to practice guidelines, what should be the nurse's primary intervention?

a. Use any methods that comfort the patient
b. Administer supplemental oxygen
c. Administer bronchodilator medications
d. Administer antianxiety agents

Ans. (a) Use any methods that comfort the patient

Explanation: Dyspnea is a common symptom in the terminal stage of life, and it can be very distressing for patients. The primary goal of the nurse should be to comfort the patients and to make them feel as comfortable as possible. This may involve using any methods that the patient finds helpful, such as positioning, massaging, providing reassurances, relaxation technique, or administering medications such as opioids or sedatives.

107

After a patient with a stroke develops a fever and abnormal lung sounds, the physician writes several orders. Which order should the nurse prioritize and implement first?

a. CBC with white blood cell (WBC) count and differential
b. Anterior/posterior chest X-rays
c. Start IV levofloxacin 250 mg every 12 hours
d. Sputum specimen for Gram stain and culture and sensitivity

Ans. (d) Sputum specimen for Gram stain and culture and sensitivity

Explanation: The nurse should implement the order for a sputum specimen for Gram stain and culture and sensitivity first (option d). This will allow for identification of the specific pathogen causing the infection and guide appropriate antibiotic therapy. The other orders can be implemented subsequently to further assess the patient's condition and provide appropriate treatment.

108

Nurse Ramya is caring for a patient with trigeminal neuralgia with symptoms of moderate to severe burning and shooting pain. The patient asks the nurse about the appropriate pharmacological management. Which of the following responses by nurse Ramya would be appropriate?

a. Treatment includes the use of corticosteroids.
b. Anticonvulsants such as carbamazepine is useful.
c. Require long-term treatment with NSAIDs.
d. Responds to around-the-clock doses of oral opioids.

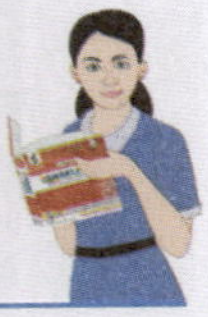

Ans. (b) Anticonvulsants such as carbamazepine is useful.

Explanation: The anticonvulsant drug most commonly prescribed for trigeminal neuralgia is carbamazepine (Tegretol), which can provide at least partial pain relief for up to 80–90% of patients. Both NSAIDs (nonsteroidal anti-inflammatories) and corticosteroids provide very little to no relief for trigeminal neuralgia. Because both of these types of drugs can have serious side effects from long-term use, they are not recommended for trigeminal nerve pain.

109

Ritu, working in emergency trauma center, received a patient with a history of motor vehicle accidents. On arrival, the nurse has to assess the level of consciousness, by using AVPU assessment. Select which of the following statement are true related to AVPU assessment:

a. Awake, voice, pupils, unresponsive
b. Alert, voice, pupils, unavailable
c. Awake, vision, pressure, unresponsive
d. Alert, voice, pain, unresponsive

Ans. (d) Alert, voice, pain, unresponsive

Explanation: The AVPU assessment is a simple and commonly used method to assess a patient's level of consciousness. It stands for:

- A - Alert
- V - Voice
- P - Pain
- U - Unresponsive

The nurse would start by assessing the patient's level of alertness. If the patient is alert, he will be able to answer questions appropriately and follow commands. If the patient is not alert, the nurse would assess his response to voice. If the patient does not respond to voice, the nurse would assess his response to pain. If the patient does not respond to pain, he would be considered unresponsive.

110

An adult client with HIV infection has been given a treatment with efavirenz. The Nurse expects this drug to be given along with emtricitabine and tenofovir as a combination (Atripla). The reason for administering this combination is to:

a. Prevent development of psychiatric comorbidities.
b. Avoid dizziness, sedation, and nightmares.
c. Reduce viral resistance.
d. Control severe rash and hepatotoxicity.

Ans. (c) Reduce viral resistance

Explanation: Atripla is a fixed-dose combination tablet containing efavirenz, emtricitabine, and tenofovir. The actual reason for using combination products is to reduce viral resistance. Atripla is not approved for the treatment of chronic hepatitis B virus (HBV) infection.

111

A 35-year-old male patient complains of abdominal discomfort and bloating. On examination, the nurse found leakage of watery stool from his rectum. The nurse is aware that this could be a possible sign of:

a. Intussusception
b. Bowel incontinence
c. Fecal impaction
d. Constipation

Ans. (c) Fecal impaction

Explanation: Fecal impaction is a severe bowel condition in which a hard, dry mass of stool gets stuck in the colon or rectum. Fecal impaction can be serious. Fecal impaction can cause a range of symptoms, which include liquid stool leaking from the rectum, pain or discomfort in the abdomen, nausea or vomiting, abdominal bloating and feeling of a need to push.

112

A patient is diagnosed with Crohn's disease and colostomy was performed as an intervention. While assessing the new stoma, the nurse suspects that the stoma has retracted. Which of the following findings by the nurse would suggest that the stoma has retracted?

a. Narrowed and flattened stoma
b. Stoma appears pinkish red and moist
c. Concave and bowl-shaped stoma
d. Stoma appears reddish purple and dry

Ans. (c) Concave and bowl-shaped stoma

Explanation: A retracted stoma has a concave, bowl-shaped appearance. Retraction causes a poor pouching surface, leading to frequent peristomal skin complications. A healthy stoma is pinkish-red and moist. A narrowed or constricted or flattened stoma is a sign of stenosis. Narrowing of the stoma is a late complication of a stoma. A dry and reddish-purple stoma indicates ischemia.

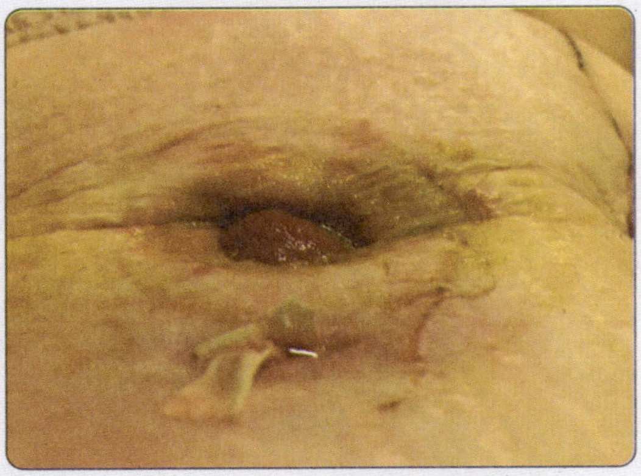

113

Nurse Ramya is preparing a 45-year-old male client for gastrectomy surgery. The patient apprehensively asked the nurse about the possible complications of gastrectomy. Which of the following responses by the nurse is appropriate?

a. Dumping syndrome
b. Clay-colored stool
c. Ribbon-like stool
d. Jaundice

Ans. (a) Dumping syndrome

Explanation: In dumping syndrome, the stomach empties its contents into the small intestine (duodenum) faster than normal. Dumping syndrome is also known as rapid gastric emptying. The sudden influx of food into the intestine causes a lot of fluid to move from bloodstream into intestine. This extra fluid causes diarrhea and bloating.

114

A 45-year-old patient with frequent GI disturbances is apprehensive about developing a colorectal cancer. He approached a nurse regarding dietary recommendation. Which of the following dietary recommendations is recommended to reduce the risk of developing colon cancer?

a. Take low-fiber and low-residual foods regularly
b. Avoid whole grain in the diet
c. Add more green vegetables such as broccoli and cauliflower in the diet.
d. Take diet which is high in red meat

Ans. (c) Add more green vegetables such as broccoli and cauliflower in the diet.

Explanation: High-fiber diets that include lots of vegetables, fruits, and whole grains have been linked with a decreased risk of colon or rectal cancer. Increased consumption of red meat (lamb, beef and pork) is associated with risk of colorectal cancer.

115A

Mr Raj Kumar is a chronic alcoholic who comes to the outpatient department with complaints of weakness and anorexia. His physical assessment shows abdominal distention, dull pain in the right upper quadrant, pale conjunctiva, and hepatomegaly. The nurse understands which of the following tests is not required for Mr Raj Kumar?

a. Ultrasonography
b. Biopsy
c. Blood biochemistry
d. Colonoscopy

Ans. (d) Colonoscopy

Explanation: The patient shows the clinical features related to liver disease, hence to confirm the condition USG, Biopsy and Blood testing are relevant, whereas the colonoscopy is not relevant to diagnose the liver condition rather it is used to rule out the problems related to the large intestine.

115B

The patient was diagnosed with Stage II liver cancer. The priority nursing diagnosis for this patient is:

a. Fluid volume excess
b. Imbalanced nutrition
c. Impaired skin integrity
d. Disturbed body image

Ans. (b) Imbalanced nutrition

Explanation: A client with this condition is not able to digest and process the food materials and absorb the nutrient, hence he/she experiences weight loss and poor muscle tone. Thus, the priority nursing care plan should be focused on imbalanced nutrition which is less than the body requirements.

116

Mrs Ruma, a 27-year-old, female has fever and pain in the right upper quadrant that increases on eating fatty food and anorexia. She is recently diagnosed with cholelithiasis on abdominal ultrasound. The nurse explains to the patient food which she should avoid taking is:

a. Potato
b. Rice
c. Bread
d. Cheese

Ans. (d) Cheese

Explanation: The patients with cholelithiasis are advised not to take food with high fat content such as dairy products like butter, cheese and ghee and should avoid fried foods. This is because these fatty foods will further worsen the condition and result in severe pain to the patient. Other listed food items are appropriate for the client to consume.

117

A male patient is admitted with Addison's disease. Laboratory test report reveals low aldosterone. The patient is on high doses of corticosteroids. The nurse is planning for a health teaching on dietary modifications. The nurse is aware that the following dietary modifications is NOT recommended for this patient:

a. High carbohydrate diet
b. Calcium rich food
c. Food rich in vitamin-D
d. Sodium restricted diet

Ans. (d) Sodium restricted diet

Explanation: Sodium should not be restricted in patient with low aldosterone levels. A patient with Addison's disease (adrenal insufficiency) needs to take adequate sodium to prevent excess fluid loss and to maintain electrolyte balance. High doses of corticosteroids are linked to a higher risk of osteoporosis, so calcium and vitamin-D rich diet is recommended. The patient should be instructed to have diet rich in complex carbohydrates and protein.

118

A 58-year-old male patient with Chronic Renal Failure (CRF) is on hemodialysis. He is advised to do peritoneal dialysis at home. While teaching the patient about how to perform peritoneal dialysis, the nurse instructs to warm the dialyzing solution to 37°C. The primary reason behind warming the dialyzing solution is to:

a. Remove the waste materials from body cells
b. Relax the abdominal muscles
c. Dilate peritoneal blood vessels
d. Maintain a constant body temperature

Ans. (c) Dilate peritoneal blood vessels

Explanation: Warming the dialyzing solution to 37°C helps in the dilation of peritoneal blood vessels, which improves the rate of urea clearance. Warmed solution also helps in prevention of cold sensations and maintains body temperature, however, the primary reason is to dilate peritoneal blood vessels.

119A

A 60-year-old female patient who is admitted for more than two weeks in Intensive Care Unit has developed a pressure ulcer on the sacral region. The nurse assessed the site of pressure ulcer and observed that the wound extends through the dermis into fatty subcutaneous tissue but the bone and tendons are not visible. Which of the following stages will the nurse assign this pressure ulcer?

a. Stage-I
b. Stage-II
c. Stage-III
d. Stage-IV

Ans. (c) Stage-III

Explanation: Signs of stage-III wound: The wound extends through the dermis (second layer of skin) into the fatty subcutaneous (below the skin) tissue. Bone, tendon and muscle are not visible. Possible signs of infection include redness around the edge of the sore, pus, odor, fever, or greenish drainage from the sore and possible necrosis (black, dead tissue).

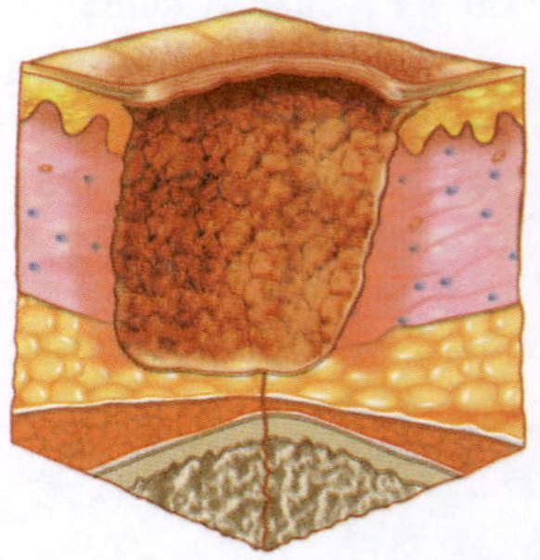

119B

Ms. Rajni, a 30-year-old female, suffered with deep partial thickness burns on the front and back of both legs, and anterior trunk. Calculate the burn area using the 'Rule of nine'.

a. 27%
b. 36%
c. 45%
d. 54%

Ans. (d) 54%

Explanation: In the given patient, the burns had occurred over the front and back of the both legs, according to the Rule of nine, each complete leg occupies 18%; hence, for the both legs, it would be 36% and for the anterior trunk, it covers 18%; hence, the total burned area would be 36 + 18 = 54%.

119C

Which type of fluid should the nurse expect to prepare and administer as fluid resuscitation during the emergent phase of burn recovery?

a. Colloids
b. Crystalloids
c. Fresh-frozen plasma
d. Packed red blood cells

Ans. (b) Crystalloids

Explanation: The person undergone burn injury needs a priority action of fluid resuscitation rather than providing blood products, Hence the crystalloids such as Ringer's lactate and NS should be administered for fluid resuscitation and the blood products like colloid are not appropriate for the fluid management.

119D

The weight of Ms. Rajni is 63 kg using the Parkland Formula, the nurse calculates the total amount of Ringer's Lactate that will be given over the next 24 hours is:

a. 13, 608 mL
b. 12200 mL
c. 8625 mL
d. 6789 mL

Ans. (a) 13, 608 mL

Explanation: Here, the client's weight is 63 kg, therefore, according to the Parkland Formula, 4 mL should be multiplied with the percentage of burned surface area (BSA) and the weight of the client, here the calculated BSA is 54% and the weight is 63 kg. Therefore, it would be $4 \times 54 \times 63$ = 13,608 mL fluid should be administered over next 24 hours. Out of this, half of the fluid needs to be administered in the first 8 hours and remaining half in the next 16 hours.

120

A 42-year-old woman with cancer of breast underwent mastectomy. A Jackson-Pratt drain is placed to help empty excess fluid from the wound site. After emptying a Jackson-Pratt bulb, the nurse needs to re-establish the negative pressure in the system. Which of the following actions is required to re-establish negative pressure?

a. Place the bulb lower than chest level
b. Fill the bulb with normal saline
c. Compress the bulb and open the valve
d. Compress the bulb and close the valve

Ans. (d) Compress the bulb and close the valve

Explanation: A Jackson-Pratt drain (also called a JP drain) is a closed-suction medical device that is commonly used as a post-operative drain for collecting bodily fluids from surgical sites. Jackson-Pratt drain has a soft plastic bulb with a valve (stopper) and a flexible tube attached to it. The drainage end of the tubing (flat white part) is placed into surgical site through a small opening near incision. A suture will hold it in place. The rest of the tube will extend outside the body and will be attached to the bulb.

The nurse has to squeeze the bulb when the stopper is open and then close the valve. When the bulb is compressed (squeezed) with the valve (stopper) closed, a constant gentle suction is created. The bulb should be compressed at all times, except when the drainage is being emptied.

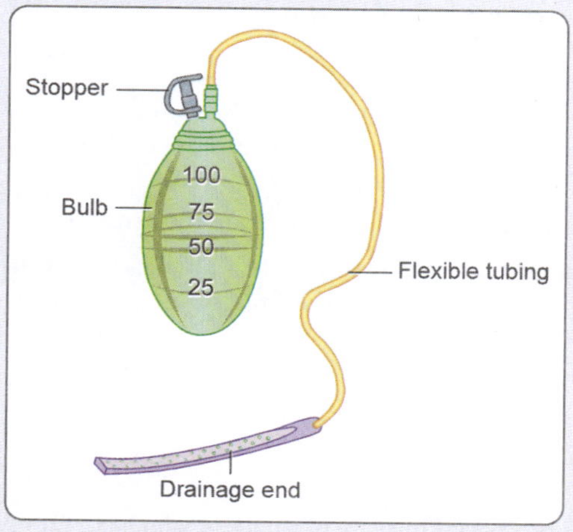

121

A 42-year-old woman with cancer of breast underwent mastectomy. A Jackson-Pratt drain is placed to help empty excess fluid from the wound site. The nurse is aware that the Jackson-Pratt drain is usually removed when the 24-hours drainage volume is equal to or less than:

a. 20 mL
b. 30 mL
c. 50 mL
d. 60 mL

Ans. (b) 30 mL

Explanation: How long the Jackson-Pratt drain has to be inserted depends on the surgery and the amount of drainage. The Jackson-Pratt drain is usually removed when the drainage is 30 mL or less than 24 hours.

122

Nurse Ramya, a palliative care nurse, is providing nursing care to a terminally ill patient during the dying and grieving process. She is aware that the least important goal of nursing intervention in this client is:

a. Providing comfort measures
b. Promotion of rest and sleep
c. Increase self-esteem through cosmetic improvement
d. Pain management

Ans. (c) Increase self-esteem through cosmetic improvement

Explanation: The nursing interventions should target pain management through pain-reduction techniques and analgesia, providing comfort measures, promotion of sleep and rest, and energy conservation for this patient. Though dying with dignity and self-esteem is important, increase of self-esteem through cosmetic improvement is not important for this client.

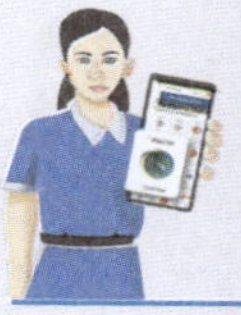

123

A 42-year-old woman is recovering from mastectomy. The patient has to be positioned to promote the lymphatic fluid return. Which of the following positions is inappropriate to promote lymphatic fluid return?

a. Semi-Fowler's position
b. Placing the affected arm on the pillow
c. Side-lying position on the unaffected side
d. Turn the patient on the prone position on the affected side every 2 hours

Ans. (c) Side-lying position on the unaffected side

Explanation: Semi-Fowler's position (head of the bed 30 degrees) with the affected arm placed on the pillow promotes lymphatic fluid return. Side-lying position on the unaffected side will not promote lymphatic fluid return.

124

Nurse Ramya is taking care of a patient who has a family history of colon cancer. The patient is anxious and afraid that she may develop a colon cancer. The patient states "My elder sister and father had colon cancer. What would be chance that I will get colon cancer in near future?" Which of the following would be the best response by the nurse?

a. Take low-residual and low-fiber diet, then the chances will get decreased.
b. You do not need to worry as this is an autosomal recessive disorder.
c. Prophylactic chemotherapy and surgery may be required to prevent you from developing colon cancer
d. You should have colonoscopy done more frequently to find abnormal polyps early.

Ans. (d) You should have colonoscopy done more frequently to find abnormal polyps early.

Explanation: People with history of colorectal cancer in first-degree relative (parent, siblings or child) are at higher risk of developing colorectal cancer. So, it is recommended to have frequent colonoscopy to find any abnormal polyps. This will help in early diagnosis. Recommendation of low-fiber and low-residual diet will increase the risk of colorectal cancer. False assurances such as "you do not need to worry" should be avoided. Prophylactic surgery is not performed to prevent cancer. It is a curative intervention.

125

A nurse is providing health education to a patient receiving external beam radiation. Which of the following is not included in the health teaching?

a. Protect the skin from direct sunlight, chlorine, and extreme temperature
b. Shave with an electric razor only
c. Apply good scented cream to moisturize the skin
d. Wear loose-fitting clothes

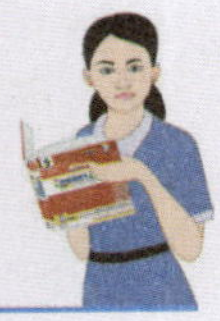

Ans. (c) Apply good scented cream to moisturize the skin

Explanation: After external radiation therapy, patients are not allowed to have direct contact with UV light and to use any creams or lotion or liquid over their skin. Hence, the nurse should not educate applying of any manual cream over their skin. Other statements are appropriate for teaching this client.

126

A long-term hemodialysis is planned for a 60-year-old male patient with end stage renal disease. He opted for an arteriovenous fistula for hemodialysis. Following surgical creation of AV fistula, how long the patient has to wait to use it for hemodialysis?

a. 2–3 weeks
b. 3–4 weeks
c. 2–3 months
d. 4–6 months

Ans. (c) 2–3 months

Explanation: The arteriovenous fistula (AVF) remains the 'gold standard' access to hemodialysis, showing better survival and lower complication rates than graft and catheters. However, fistulae are not readily usable after creation. The current guidelines suggest a minimum of 1 month and preferably 2–3 months before utilization of an AV fistula.

127

A factory worker is admitted with a fractured femur after a fall from first floor. A full leg plaster cast is applied. The nurse provides discharge instructions for the patient. All of the following instructions are appropriate for this patient; except:

a. Keep the limb raised on a soft surface, such as pillow
b. Put an ice pack over the cast to avoid itching
c. Walk around on your cast as soon as you get home
d. Call your doctor if toes become numb or turn blue

Ans. (c) Walk around on your cast as soon as you get home

Explanation:

Client instructions include:

1. Keep the plastered body part raised to prevent swelling, especially for the first 48 hours.
2. Keep the cast clean and dry.
3. Check for cracks or breaks in the cast.
4. Apply ice pack over the cast to avoid itching. Do not scratch the skin under the cast by putting objects inside the cast.
5. Immediately report any pain, tingling, or numbness, or if the toes turn blue or white.

128

A client reported that he had foul smell from the cast. Which of the following actions by the nurse is most appropriate?

a. Advise the client to elevate the casted limb on pillow
b. Check pulse on casted limb
c. Perform blanching test
d. Notify the physician

Ans. (d) Notify the physician

Explanation: Strong or persistent unpleasant odor may be a sign of a skin infection. This must be notified to the physician to determine if the cast should be changed.

129

After arthroscopy procedure, client reports increased knee pain for more than 3 days. Which of the following actions by the nurse is most appropriate?

a. Notify the physician
b. Advise the client to elevate the legs
c. Apply ice package on the site of pain
d. Explain the client that it is normal finding

Ans. (a) Notify the physician

Explanation: One complication that has been linked to knee arthroscopy is a condition called spontaneous osteonecrosis of the knee, or SONK. After their surgery, they develop persistent pain, typically along the inner (medial) side of the knee. SONK is a condition that causes inflammation within the bone. This needs to be notified to the physician for further treatment.

130

A 54-year-old woman who is on treatment for her osteoporosis is prescribed alendronate. The nurse is providing health education regarding self-administration of alendronate for this client. Which of the following instructions has to be included in the health teaching of this client?

a. Take the drug on an empty stomach with full glass of milk
b. Always take the drug with food
c. Take the drug on an empty stomach with full glass of water and stay upright for 30 minutes
d. Take the drug after breakfast

Ans. (c) Take the drug on an empty stomach with full glass of water and stay upright for 30 minutes

Explanation: The drug alendronate will cause GI upset, so, always administer this medication with full glass of water. The patient should take this drug on empty stomach in the morning at least 30 minutes before any food and stay upright for 30 minutes that will help in absorption of alendronate.

131A

Mr Rajan, 42-year-old male, is experiencing weakness in lower limbs and bladder dysfunction due to prolapsed L1-L2 disk. The student nurse checks the doctor's chart and found which surgery is planned to correct the prolapsed disk?

a. Burr hole
b. Laminectomy
c. Septoplasty
d. Decompressive hemicraniectomy

Ans. (b) Laminectomy

Explanation: The patient is diagnosed with prolapsed lumbar disk and the doctor has planned to have a surgical intervention to correct the prolapse. Laminectomy is the surgical method to remove a certain part or whole lamina (vertebral bone) to relieve the pressure on the spinal cord and to treat the client condition.

131B

Which of the following interventions by the nurse is essential in the management of the patient after laminectomy?

a. Insertion of Ryle's tube to start feeding and maintain nutrition
b. Arterial line insertion to assess arterial BP
c. Foley's catheter insertion
d. Central line insertion to guide IV fluids in view of cardiac problems

Ans. (c) Foley's catheter insertion

Explanation: After laminectomy, the client should be placed in an appropriate position to restrict the common movements like bending or stooping or lifting anything that cause pressure to the back for several weeks. Hence, the HCP will plan to have Foley's catheter to prevent the unwanted movements and protect the operated sites. Although other interventions are necessary, the nurse would give priority care to the Foley's catheterization.

132

A strong, healthy patient with a lower leg cast is learning to move and mobilize with axillary crutches. Which of the following gaits is most appropriate for this type of patient in this scenario?

a. Two-point gait
b. Three-point gait
c. Four-point gait
d. Any gait can be applied

Ans. (c) Four-point gait

Explanation: The four-point gait enables a normal step pattern, and requires low energy expenditure. The patient must be able to bear weight on both feet. Patients are often taught the four-point gait as the first gait and then faster gaits are taught when this one is mastered.

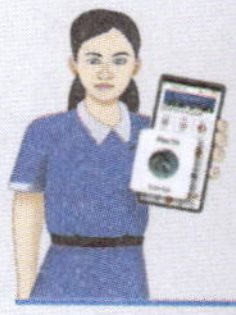

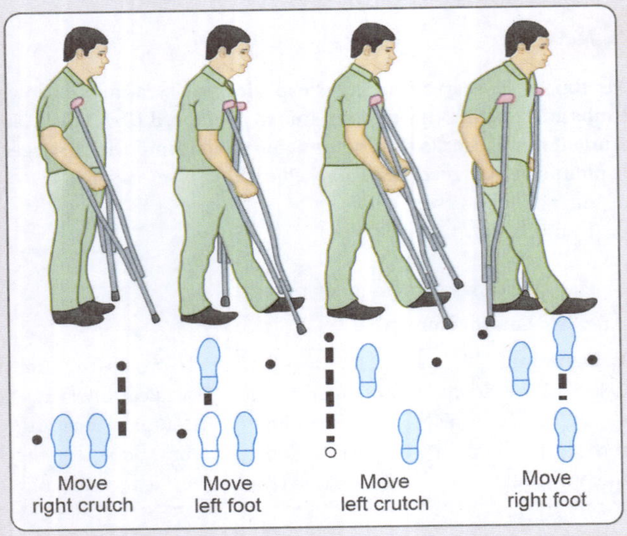

The three-point gait is the least stable pattern and requires balance, coordination, and strength. This pattern is tiring but allows for rapid ambulation. The two-point pattern is used when additional gait stability is needed. Therefore, the four-point gait must be applied for this patient.

133

A 35-year-old male patient is recovering from an orthopedic surgery in lower leg and is practising swing-to crutch gait. In this method, the patient needs to move both crutches forward, leans on the crutches and then lift and swing both legs to place it.

a. Before reaching the crutch tips
b. At the level with the crutch tips
c. Past the crutch tips
d. At either before or at the level of crutch tips

Ans. (b) At the level with the crutch tips

Explanation: During the swing-to-gait, the patient advances both crutches, leans on the crutches, and then lift and swing both legs to the same point as crutch tips. In swing-through crutch gait, the patient swings both legs past the crutch tips.

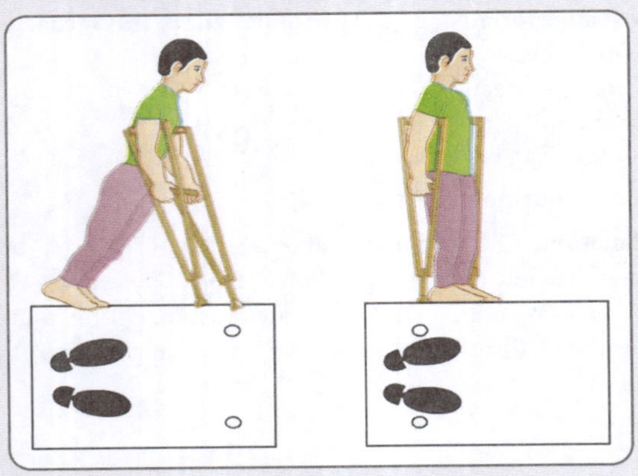

134

The nurse is instructing a patient who has crutches how to sit down on a chair while holding the crutches. While doing this action, the patient should hold both crutches in the:

a. Dominant hand
b. Nondominant hand
c. Hand on the affected side
d. Hand on the unaffected side

Ans. (c) Hand on the affected side

Explanation: Steps while sitting down on a chair with crutches:

1. Back up until you feel the chair with the back of your leg.
2. Hold both crutches in the hand on the affected side.
3. Grab the armrest or the side of the chair with the free hand.
4. Lower yourself onto the front of the chair, then slide back.
5. To get up, reverse the 4 steps.

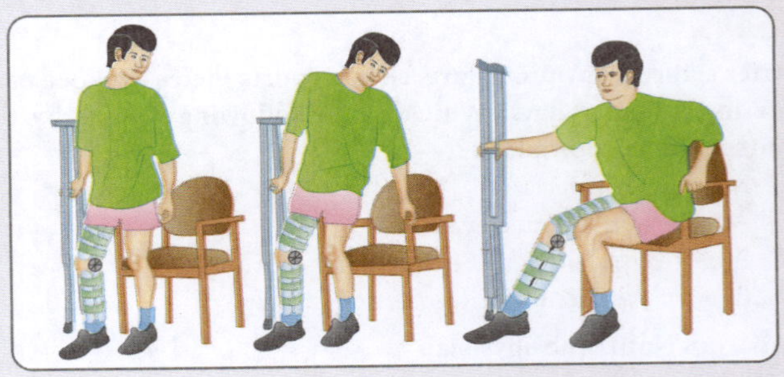

135

A 35-year-old male patient is brought to the emergency room after he sustained multiple injuries from a road traffic accident. Which of the following assessments should take the highest priority to take?

a. Grey Turner's sign in the flank
b. Irregular pulse
c. Pupils unequal
d. A deviated trachea

Ans. (d) A deviated trachea

Explanation: A deviated trachea is a sign of tension pneumothorax that indicates chest injury. If untreated, this will result in respiratory distress. NOTE: Use the ABC technique. Airway comes first while prioritizing intervention.

136

Nurse Ramya is working in emergency room as a triage nurse. A 45-year-old male patient is brought to the emergency room with complaint of dizziness, diaphoresis, and mid-sternal chest pain. Which of the following nursing interventions is the priority action for this client?

a. Notify the physician
b. Attach ECG leads and put on ECG monitoring
c. Collect complete history
d. Administer oxygen via nasal cannula

Ans. (d) Administer oxygen via nasal cannula

Explanation: The priority action in this scenario is to start oxygen through nasal cannula to increase myocardial oxygenation. Other given interventions are also important but that can be given after starting oxygen therapy. NOTE: Use ABC strategy to solve the question.

137

Nurse Ramya is educating a patient allergic to pollen about signs and symptoms of anaphylactic shock. She is aware that all of the following signs and symptoms are associated with anaphylactic shock; except:

a. Feeling dizzy
b. Itching
c. Hypertension
d. Dyspnea

Ans. (c) Hypertension

Explanation: In anaphylactic shock, the signs and symptoms are associated with the effects of histamine. Histamine affects cardiac, GI, respiratory system and skin. The patient in anaphylactic shock may have dyspnea, wheezing, swelling of upper airway, coughing, difficulty in speaking, watery eyes, stuffy nose, tachycardia, hypotension, loss of consciousness, dizziness, nausea and vomiting, itching, etc.

138

A patient admitted in the ward has developed a sudden anaphylactic reaction while administering an IV medication. The nurse responds by immediately stopping the medication. Assessment of vitals revealed blood pressure 80/50, heart rate 124, and SpO_2 88%. Redness on face, swelling and wheezing are noted. The nurse is aware that the most appropriate initial treatment for this condition is:

a. IV Chlorpheniramine
b. IV Normal Saline Bolus
c. IM Adrenaline
d. Budecort nebulization

Ans. (c) IM Adrenaline

Explanation: IM or subcutaneous Adrenaline/Epinephrine is the first-line treatment to treat anaphylactic reaction. Adrenaline/Epinephrine will increase blood pressure (vasoconstriction effect) and dilation of airways (bronchodilation effect). Hence, IM Adrenaline is the appropriate drug to administer in this situation.

139

Nurse Ramya is caring for a patient who is in anaphylactic shock. While checking the prescription order before administering medication, she found an inappropriate drug is ordered and asked for an order clarification from the treating doctor. Which of the following drugs is most likely the inappropriate drug for this patient?

a. Adrenaline
b. Corticosteroids
c. IV furosemide
d. Isotonic IV fluids

Ans. (c) IV furosemide

Explanation: Furosemide, a loop-diuretic, removes extra fluid from the blood volume while the patient in anaphylactic shock need fluids because of shift of fluid from intravascular space to interstitial space. All other medications are appropriate to treat a patient in anaphylactic shock.

140

A 52-year-old postmenopausal woman presented to the emergency department with 24-hour history of right leg pain, redness, warmth and tenderness. Which of the following is the most likely diagnosis of this client?

a. Muscle strain
b. Deep vein thrombosis
c. Nephrotic syndrome
d. Chronic venous insufficiency

Ans. (b) Deep vein thrombosis

Explanation: Swelling (edema) in the affected leg (rarely, there is swelling in both legs), tenderness, redness, and a feeling of warmth in the affected leg are the manifestations of deep vein thrombosis.

141A

A 30-year-old laborer, Ram Lal is admitted to hospital with high degree of fever, maculopapular rash and joint pain from last 4 days. The patient shows typical symptoms of:

a. Dengue shock syndrome
b. Dengue hemorrhagic fever
c. Classical dengue fever
d. Malaria

Ans. (c) Classical dengue fever

Explanation: The major significant symptoms of the classical dengue fever are the high-degree fever, frontal headache, measles like rashes especially over the chest and upper limbs, joint pains and painful limbs. Hence, Ram Lal shows all the positive signs of classical dengue fever. The nurse would confirm the diagnosis as the other conditions are not relevant to the client's symptoms.

141B

Next day, the nurse assesses increase in abdominal girth, distention and shifting dullness. The nurse suspects ascites in this patient because of:

a. Decrease platelet count
b. Increase in capillary permeability
c. Increase in hydrostatic pressure
d. Liver involvement

Ans. (b) Increase in capillary permeability

Explanation: Decrease in the oncotic pressure or the increased capillary permeability will allow the excess of fluid movements into the interstitial space. In this case, the fluid gets shifted to the peritoneal space that results in the development of ascites.

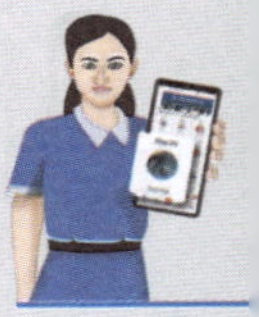

142

Mr. Jagdeep, 47-year-old male, is admitted in ortho ward with a fracture of right leg, suddenly complains of chest pain and dyspnea. His BP is 85/50 mm of Hg, PR- 124 beats/min and RR- 24 breaths/min. Which of the following initial assessments should a nurse perform to diagnose the condition?

a. Take a sample for ABG analysis
b. Obtain a chest X-ray
c. Auscultate the lung and heart sound
d. Prepare the patient for pulmonary angiography

Ans. (d) Prepare the patient for pulmonary angiography

Explanation: From the given clinical scenario and manifestations, client is experiencing pulmonary embolism as a complication of fracture. The best diagnostic test for pulmonary embolism is pulmonary angiography.

143

A student nurse is caring for a patient with DVT. Which action by the student nurse should be corrected by the duty nurse?

a. Elevating the legs of the patient
b. Applying warm packs
c. Applying compression pumps
d. Applying pressure after IM injection

Ans. (c) Applying compression pumps

Explanation: Compression devices are used to prevent the blood clot and thus prevent the occurrence of DVT, whereas in this case the client is already diagnosed with DVT, hence sequential compression pump or device is not appropriate or contraindicated to this client. Other interventions given in the options are relevant to the client with DVT.

144

A 45-year-old woman is admitted with generalized edema and suspected heart failure. The nurse expects which of the following diagnostic tests to be ordered by the physician in addition to standard blood tests?

a. D-dimer
b. Serum ferritin
c. Serum albumin
d. Serum brain natriuretic peptide level

Ans. (d) Serum brain natriuretic peptide level

Explanation: Brain natriuretic peptide (BNP) test measures levels of a protein called BNP that is made by the heart and blood vessels. BNP levels are higher than normal in case of heart failure.

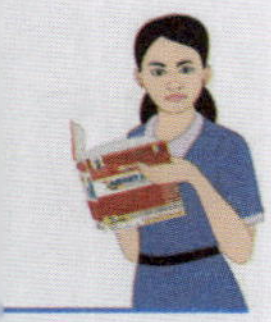

145A

Nurse Ramya is providing care to a patient who acutely experiences a cardiac arrest. As the nurse is in the emergency situation, which substance in the nurse's body will be secreted in huge amounts to help the nurse respond to this situation?

a. Aldosterone
b. Thyroid-stimulating hormone
c. Epinephrine
d. ACTH

Ans. (c) Epinephrine

Explanation: Adrenaline or Epinephrine hormone is known as the emergency hormone because it initiates a rapid reaction that helps the person think rapidly and respond to stress. It raises the rate of metabolism, dilating the blood vessels going into the heart and brain.

145B

The patient needs to be shifted for a CT scan. What mandatory precaution the duty nurse should take before shifting Mr. Rajesh?

a. Philadelphia collar for neck stabilization
b. Insert a Ryle's tube to decompress the stomach
c. Perform oral and nasal suctioning
d. Insert an arterial line to accurately measure BP

Ans. (a) Philadelphia collar for neck stabilization

Explanation: After head injury, the patient's head movement should be restricted to prevent the further complications. Hence, attaching Philadelphia collar will prevent the head or neck movement while shifting the patient from one place to another.

145C

The CT scan shows a subdural hematoma with radiological signs of increased intracranial pressure. Which of the following actions by the nurse will be helpful in preventing further increase in intracranial pressure?

a. Placing the patient in lateral position
b. Raising head end of bed by 30 degrees
c. Keeping the neck flexed
d. Doing a lumbar puncture

Ans. (b) Raising head end of bed by 30 degrees

Explanation: In semi-Fowler's position, the gravity pulls and works against the circulation, hence the flow of blood to the cranial region will be compromised and the raise of the Intracranial pressure level can be prevented. But in the supine it will raise up the ICP level.

145D

After about one hour of the injury, the nurse assesses the patient again. Which of the following would alert her toward the worsening status of the patient?

a. Pupils reactive to light
b. Headache
c. Decrease in GCS score
d. Hypertension

Ans. (c) Decrease in GCS score

Explanation: By measuring the Glasgow Come Scale (GCS), the nurse can find alertness and the level of consciousness of the patient. With the total score of 15, the highest range of score expresses the client's good level of consciousness and the decreased range of (GSC) score shows the deterioration of conscious level and the nurse needs to provide immediate intervention to the client.

146A

Mr. Sanjay, 57-year-old male, is admitted in emergency with complaints of chest pain, shortness of breath and dyspnea. The nurse administers oxygen and nitroglycerin to the patient as prescribed. She understands the rationale behind this intervention:

a. To decrease the workload of lung and heart
b. To prevent hypoxia of body tissue
c. To increase the cardiac output
d. To meet the oxygen demand of cardiac muscles

Ans. (d) To meet the oxygen demand of cardiac muscles

Explanation: The main indication for giving nitroglycerin is to dilate the coronary blood vessels and relax the smooth muscles which will decrease the chest pain and improve the oxygen supply. Along with this drug, the oxygen administration will help to manage the client with coronary artery disease.

146B

A relative standing in the waiting room suddenly falls on the floor. List the order for the actions that the duty nurse must perform.

1. Call for help and activate the code team.
2. Start compressions
3. Give breaths
4. Establish unresponsiveness.

a. 4, 1, 2, 3
b. 3, 1, 2,4
c. 1, 2, 3, 4
d. 4, 3, 2, 1

Ans. (a) 4, 1, 2, 3

Explanation: According to the Basic Life Support (BLS) guidelines, if someone is found unresponsive, the rescuer should first look the scene safety and check the response of the victim. Then immediately call for help or activate the emergency response team. Then the compression and rescue breath should be followed. These are the orders to be followed by the rescuer during emergency condition.

147A

Mr. Ramu, carpenter by profession, has come to emergency 1 hour back with severe nonproductive cough, difficulty breathing, and shortness of breath. He has an allergic history of wood dust. Which of the following lung sounds a nurse may expect while auscultating the lungs of Mr. Ramu?

a. Rhonchi
b. Wheezing
c. Pleural friction rub
d. Stridor

Ans. (b) Wheezing

Explanation: In the given scenario, the client's signs and symptoms show that he is experiencing occupational asthma, due to the inhalation of wood dust in his workplace. The clinical features of occupational asthma would be same as asthma, hence the nurse would anticipate the sound of wheezing while auscultating his lung.

147B

The vital signs of a 30-year-old patient are Pulse- 110/min, RR-26/min, SpO_2- 94%. What priority action the nurse should take to manage this patient in emergency?

a. Deep breathing and coughing exercise
b. Give sedation
c. Intubate the patient
d. Nebulize the patient

Ans. (d) Nebulize the patient

Explanation: The patient under respiratory disorder often experiences airway obstruction or narrowing that leads to decreased saturation level and increased heart rate. Hence, the primary intervention should focus on dilating the airways rather than providing oxygen. Hence, the priority action should be taken to nebulize the patient.

148A

Ms. Madhu, a 50-year-old female, admitted in ICU due to mitral valve stenosis, developed pulmonary edema. The nurse understands the reason to it is:

a. Decreased filling of left ventricle
b. Increased pulmonary venous pressure
c. Decreased pulmonary vascular resistances
d. Increased lung compliance

Ans. (b) Increased pulmonary venous pressure

Explanation: In mitral valve stenosis, there would be no adequate path for the blood flow from the left atrium to the ventricle, hence, the pressure gets raised in the left atrium, that leads to pulmonary venous congestion which may result in pulmonary hypertension and edema.

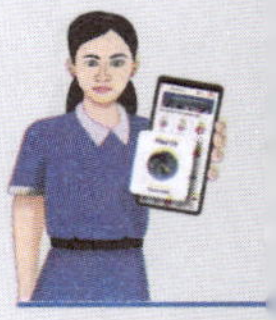

148B

On assessment of Mrs. Madhu, nurse found that patient is coughing sputum. The sputum characteristics are:

a. Thick and green-colored
b. Frothy and pink-tinged
c. Mucoid and transparent
d. Sticky and yellow-colored

Ans. (b) Frothy and pink-tinged

Explanation: In pulmonary edema, there would be leakage of fluids into the alveolar capillaries that mix up with the small amount of blood. On clinical manifestation, the patient shows hemoptysis or there would be sputum that is pink and frothy in nature.

149A

Anshu, 14-year-old girl, is nearly drowned during her swimming session at school. Which of the following signs indicates that patient has respiratory arrest?

a. No pulse
b. Absent lung sound
c. Pulsus paradoxus
d. Cyanosis

Ans. (b) Absent lung sound

Explanation: The child drowned in the water experienced excess of fluid intake that covered the child's lung with fluids. Hence, auscultation shows flat or decreased lung sound. On the respiratory arrest, the auscultation reveals absence of lung sounds because of the fluid build-up in and around the lungs.

149B

Anshu's coach gave her rescue breaths after checking her pulse. The purpose of giving rescue breaths in respiratory arrest is to:

a. Artificially contract the lungs
b. Provide oxygen to victim's lungs
c. Push the diaphragm to remove water
d. Create a negative pressure in the chest

Ans. (b) Provide oxygen to victim's lungs

Explanation: During respiratory arrest, the person's lungs stop functioning and they cannot breathe normally that leads to an oxygen depletion. Hence, by providing external breath by another person with cardiac compression, it is possible to retrieve the victim.

149C

How many rescue breaths per minute the coach should give to Anshu in this case (As per AHA guidelines)?

a. 2–3 breaths
b. 5–6 breaths
c. 10–12 breaths
d. 18–20 breaths

Ans. (c) 10-12 breaths

Explanation: According to AHA guidelines, it is suggested to provide 10 to 12 rescue breaths within a minute or we should need to provide 1 breath for every 5 to 6 seconds. Hence, giving 10 to 12 breaths to Anshu by her coach is appropriate.

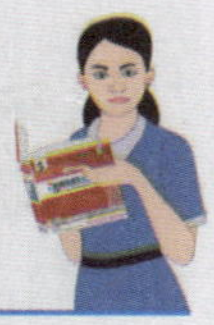

150A

Mr. Sajan, 40-year-old patient, presented in emergency with sudden onset of left side facial drooping, left arm weakness and slurred speech. His BP- 220/100 mm of Hg, Pulse-98 beats/min and pupils are equal. What is the likely diagnosis?

a. Myocardial infarction
b. Bell's palsy
c. Stroke
d. Raised intracranial pressure

Ans. (c) Stroke

Explanation: In the given scenario, the client has the clinical features of facial drooping, upper limb weakness, slurred speech and hypertension. These manifestation reveal that the client had undergone cerebrovascular accident or the stroke. Other given conditions in the options are not related to the client's clinical features.

150B

The nurse explains the relative that which of the following risk factors of stroke may be responsible for the brain attack in the patient mentioned in previous question?

a. Anemia
b. Oral contraceptives
c. Hypertension
d. Age

Ans. (c) Hypertension

Explanation: One of the most prevalent risk factors for a person to develop stroke is the high blood pressure, because it damages, the inner lining of the walls of the blood vessels that may lead to the narrowing and blocking of the blood vessels and interfering the systemic circulation and results in poor blood supply to the brain and the person experiences stroke.

150C

Which famous mneumonic best describes the warning signs of the above mentioned disease?

a. RICE
b. APGAR
c. ABC
d. FAST

Ans. (c) FAST

Explanation: This acronym easily detects the person with stroke and fastens the second person to take action and provide intervention as soon as possible, that are facial drooping for F, Arm weakness for A, speech difficulty for S and Time for T.

150D

Mr. Sajan was brought to ER within 1.5 hours of the appearance of first symptom of ischemic stroke. The nurse understands the patient is within the window period and is eligible for getting:

a. Anticoagulants
b. Thrombolytics
c. Antihypertensives
d. Steroids

Ans. (b) Thrombolytics

Explanation: Here Mr. Sajan is in the window period of ischemic stroke. It is beneficial and treatable with thrombolytic agents that break down and destroy the blood clots present in the circulation, but it is useful only when it is provided within 3 hours of the first symptoms of ischemic stroke. Therefore, it is appropriate for this patient.

150E

The nurse explains the student nurses that the rationale behind administering Recombinant tissue plasminogen therapy to Mr. Sajan is:

a. Preventing formation of new clots
b. Preventing conversion of thrombi into emboli
c. Breaking already existing clots
d. Increasing plasma level in the blood

Ans. (c) Breaking already existing clots

Explanation: This drug contains certain amount of protein that as a nature of breaking formed clots, hence for Mr. Sajan with already developed clots it is appropriate to provide tissue plasminogen therapy. Other given statements are not relevant to the mechanism action of tPA.

151A

A 14-year-old boy had fever for 5 days which is not responding to over the counter medicines. He has headache, vomiting and is not accepting orally. His vitals are pulse rate 108/min, SpO_2 is 97% on room air and T- 38 C. Which of the following tests a nurse should perform during the assessment to establish a provisional diagnosis?

a. Corneal reflex
b. Weber's test
c. Cold Caloric test
d. Kernig's sign

Ans. (d) Kernig's sign

Explanation: The nurse should perform the physical examination and assess the child's range of motion. While on examining, the nurse may find strong stiffness in the hamstring muscle of the child (which is called Kernig's sign) and this sign indicates that the child has infection or inflammation in his meninges layer.

151B

The patient undergoes a contrast CT scan and it does not show any evidence of increased intracranial pressure. Which test is likely to be done next to establish a diagnosis?

a. Electronystagmography
b. Lumbar puncture
c. Intracranial pressure monitoring
d. Digital subtraction angiography

Ans. (b) Lumbar puncture

Explanation: For an accurate and definitive diagnosis of the meningitis and to analyze the etiology behind the alteration of ICP level, it is recommended to have spinal tap or lumbar puncture to collect the CSF fluid, it may show increased WBC level and decreased glucose level which are confirmative for the meningitis.

151C

The nurse positions the head in neutral position. She understands that it is important to:

a. Reduce neck movements to prevent vomiting
b. Reduce neck pain and headache
c. Facilitate venous drainage from brain
d. Monitor jugular venous pressure

Ans. (c) Facilitate venous drainage from brain

Explanation: The neutral or the supine position facilitates the venous drainage from the vein especially through the internal jugular veins, hence the nurse should keep in mind that the venous drainage will be improved by keeping the client in the neutral position by enhancing the IJV.

152A

A 30-year-old female patient presented with a history of fall at home. She was not able to move her lower limbs after the fall. She has normal power in upper limbs. The patient had a pacemaker inserted 4 years back and is on antiplatelets. She is conscious and hemodynamically stable. The nurse suspects injury to which part of the spine?

a. Cervical spine
b. Coccyx
c. Dorsal spine
d. Sacral spine

Ans. (c) Dorsal spine

Explanation: The patient falls and had an injury over the thoracic or dorsal spine region. The injury over or the lower thoracic region or to the lumbar region affects the movement of the legs, torso, bowel and bladder function, whereas the upper limb gets affected if a person had injury over the cervical spine. Hence, the nurse should expect injury over the dorsal spine.

152B

After 3 days of admission, nurse assesses a 4 × 3 cms reddish discoloration over the sacral area. She suspects that this discoloration is the:

a. Bruise from the fall
b. Tinea versicolor, a fungal infection
c. Pressure sore
d. Erythema nodosum

Ans. (c) Pressure sore

Explanation: The bedridden patient with lack of positional change for every 2 to 3 hours develop the pressure sore or bed sore due to the compression of bony region especially over the sacral spine. Hence, the reddish discoloration shows the initial stage of pressure ulcer and the nurse needs to provide immediate intervention to this issue.

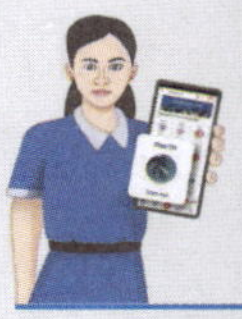

152C

The nurse is preparing the patient for discharge. Which of the following statements by the patient reflects that the patient understood the discharge teaching?

a. I will perform ROM exercise of my legs with the help of my upper extremities
b. I will take twice the energy requirements for wound healing
c. I will take steroids whenever I feel pain and inflammation
d. I can resume driving for long distance

Ans. (a) I will perform ROM exercise of my legs with the help of my upper extremities

Explanation: After spinal injury the patient would experience weakness of the upper or lower limbs depending upon the site of the spinal injury. Hence there is need for long term ROM exercise to gain the strength over their affected limbs. The nurse should teach the appropriate ROM exercise to perform regularly in the home with the supervision of other person.

153A

A 36-year-old male patient has been experiencing progressively worsening headaches in morning associated with vomiting for 2 weeks. He has become forgetful but can take care of his daily needs. As a nurse you suspect raised intracranial pressure. What clinical test would help you to establish raised intracranial pressure?

a. Pupillary asymmetry
b. GCS score below 8
c. Corneal reflex
d. Fundus examination for papilledema

Ans. (d) Fundus examination for papilledema

Explanation: Due to the impaired CSF absorption or due to the blockage of CSF outflow, the increased protein level present in the CSF would result in raised ICP and papilledema, which are seen in the condition of brain tumor and Guillain-Barre syndrome. Hence the fundal examination that shows papilledema is a diagnostic method to rule out the increased ICP.

153B

In case of headaches associated with raised intracranial pressure, the following association with vomiting is observed

a. Vomiting follows headache and makes it worse
b. Vomiting follows headache and relieves it
c. No relation between headache and vomiting
d. Headache starts after projectile vomiting

Ans. (b) Vomiting follows headache and relieves it

Explanation: Most common and earliest signs of increased ICP are headache, vomiting and papilledema. But in most cases, after a certain period of headache, if the patient had a projectile or sudden vomiting, it would relieve the severity of headaches and the patient feels relieved from the ache rather it will not worsen or increase the level of the headache.

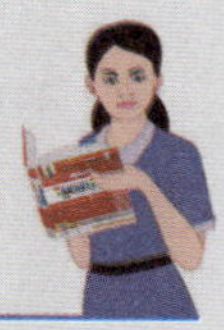

153C

The nurse expects which one of the following medication will be prescribed for reducing high intracranial pressure?

a. Mannitol
b. Dilantin sodium
c. Lorazepam
d. Syndopa

Ans. (a) Mannitol

Explanation: The drug mannitol will reduce the ICP level by two aspects in the cerebral region. It will generate osmotic gradient over the blood brain barrier, thus moves the water from the parenchyma tissue to intravascular space that results in decreased brain tissue volume. It also decreases the blood viscosity and expands the size of plasma and causes cerebral vasoconstriction to drain out the cerebral blood volume. Hence through this physiology the increased ICP would be reduced.

153D

The child became unresponsive and started showing abnormal hand and leg movements with up rolling of eye balls and tongue bite. Which of the following actions by the relative should be stopped by the nurse?

a. Turning the patient on one side
b. Protecting the patient by keeping side rails up
c. Inserting a rubber object between teeth to prevent tongue bite
d. Loosening the clothes of the child

Ans. (c) Inserting a rubber object between teeth to prevent tongue bite

Explanation: In the given scenario, the child is experiencing the seizure activity and has already bitten his/her tongue. During Seizure movement it is not allowed to put any object inside the mouth and it is impossible for a person to swallow his own tongue. Other statement given in the options are recommended to be performed while having seizure activity except the answer.

154A

Mrs. Sheela is suffering from severe hypertension from past 10 years. She was found unconscious in bathroom. Her assessment in ER reveals she can open her eyes only on painful stimuli, is confused, and move her limbs away on painful stimuli. The duty nurse assesses the Glasgow Coma Scale (GCS) of this patient and found it to be:

a. 5
b. 8
c. 10
d. 13

Ans. (c) 10

Explanation: According to the GCS parameters, the score for opened eyes on painful stimulation would be 2 and the score for the confused state would be 4 and the score for moving limbs on painful stimuli would be 4. Hence the total GCS score would be 10.

154B

The nurse understands that the kind of response recorded in GCS is the:

a. The worst response
b. The best response
c. The average response of 3 examinations
d. Both the best and worst response

Ans. (b) The best response

Explanation: GCS score explains the actual level of consciousness and alertness of the patient. The GCS score of 15 would be best score, the score of less than or equal to 8 refers to the comatose state of the client and the score of 3 refers to the unresponsive state.

155A

A nurse is caring for a patient with corneal transplant. Which of the following indicates need for more education, if patient of corneal transplant say that he is allowed to:

a. Wear eye patch
b. Lift heavy weight
c. Avoid sun exposure
d. Put eye drops in the operated eye

Ans. (b) Lift heavy weight

Explanation: In the postoperative period of corneal transplant, client is advised not to rub or squeeze their eyes and they are restricted to lift weight because it will lead to strain in the eyes and further complication.

155B

The nurse is giving health education to community regarding eye donation. Which of the following patients are ineligible to donate eyes?

a. Diabetes
b. Syphilis
c. Refractive errors
d. Anemia

Ans. (b) Syphilis

Explanation: A person with Syphilis (sexually transmitted disease) is not eligible to donate eyes, other than that, patient with HIV, hepatitis B and C and other communicable disease are not eligible to donate eyes. Persons with diabetes and other noncommunicable diseases are eligible to donate their eyes.

156

Ms Riya is 45-year-old and was diagnosed with diabetes 12 years ago. She recently started complaining of floaters and sensation of curtain falling in her visual field. The nurse doing her assessment suspects patient to be suffering from which complication of diabetes?

a. Glaucoma
b. Cataract
c. Retinal Detachment
d. Presbyopia

Ans. (c) Retinal Detachment

Explanation: The major complications for the client with chronic diabetes who do not control their blood glucose level are neuropathy, nephropathy, retinopathy and diabetic foot ulcer and even certain cardiovascular disorder. The clinical feature in the given scenario shows that client had issue with the retina and hence the nurse should suspect retinal detachment.

157

What is important for the nurse to include in the postoperative care of the patient following tympanoplasty?

a. Avoid flight travel
b. Encouraging the patient to bathe next day after surgery.
c. Avoid changing the cotton padding.
d. Instruct patient to forcefully blow the nose.

Ans. (a) Avoid flight travel

Explanation: After tympanoplasty surgery, the client should not be allowed to take bath for a certain period of weeks, patient should be advised not to blow their nose forcefully, dressing should be changed at regular intervals and patient should be advised not to have any flight travel because it increases the internal pressure within the ear and causes further damage to the operated site.

158A

A 65-year-old man is experiencing sensorineural hearing loss associated with presbycusis. What is the priority nursing diagnosis for this patient?

a. Disturbed body image
b. Impaired verbal communication
c. Ineffective coping
d. Disturbed sleep pattern

Ans. (b) Impaired verbal communication

Explanation: The most common nursing diagnosis for the client with hearing disorder would be the communication problem with the other person. Presbycusis is a kind of hearing loss related to the person aging. Other nursing diagnoses are not related to the given condition.

158B

The student nurse is checking the surgical notes of a patient operated for otosclerosis. She learns that the surgery done to correct otosclerosis is called:

a. Myringoplasty
b. Stapedectomy
c. Myringotomy
d. Mastoidectomy

Ans. (b) Stapedectomy

Explanation: In otosclerosis, there will be an abnormal tissue growth over the bone present in the middle ear, especially over the stapes bone, hence the surgical procedure should be used to remove the stapes bone which is known as stapedotomy. Other mentioned surgeries are not relevant to treat the otosclerosis.

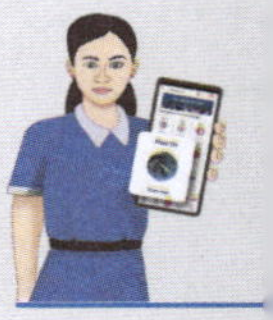

Image-Based Questions (Including All Topics)

1. Identify the disease condition of the GI system shown in the image

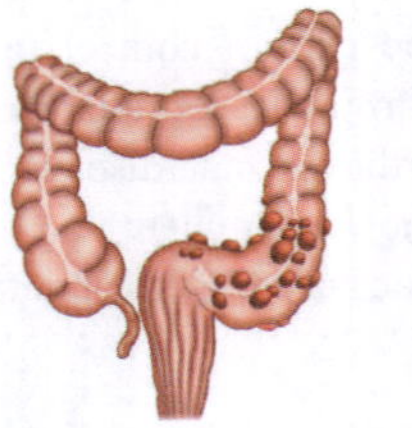

a. Crohn's disease
b. Colon cancer
c. Diverticular disease
d. Inflammatory Bowel Disease

2. Identify the type of drain used in this image

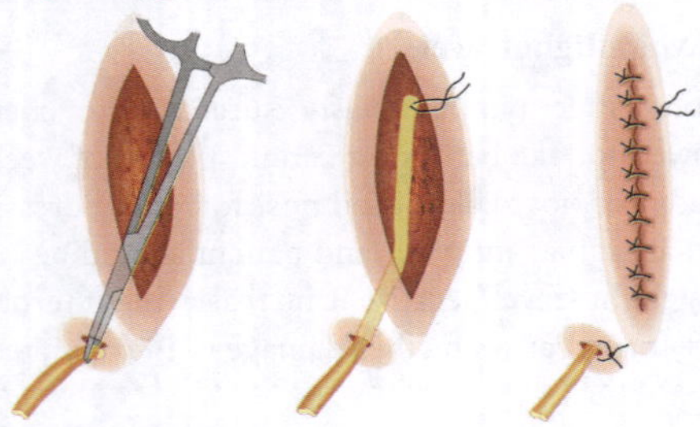

a. Tube drain
b. Penrose drain
c. Jackson-Pratt drain
d. Hemovac drain

3. Identify the sign shown in the picture

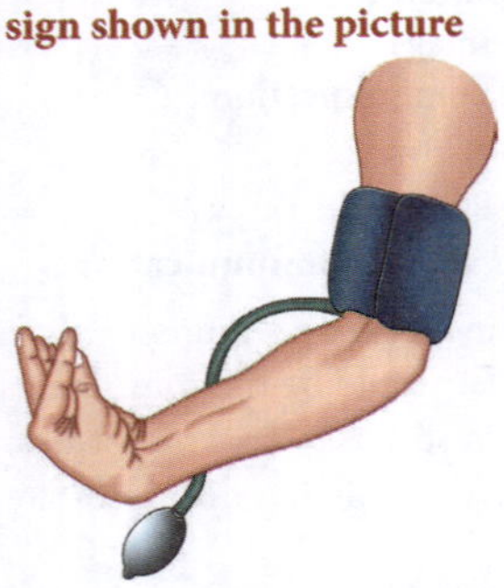

a. Allen's sign
b. Chvostek's sign
c. Trousseau's sign
d. Tetany

4. Identify the sign that is being elicited to assess for hypocalcemia in this picture

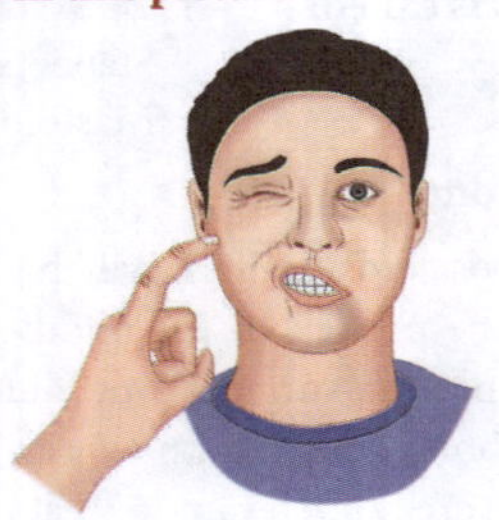

a. Allen's sign
b. Chvostek's sign
c. Trousseau's sign
d. Tetany

5. Identify the condition shown in the image

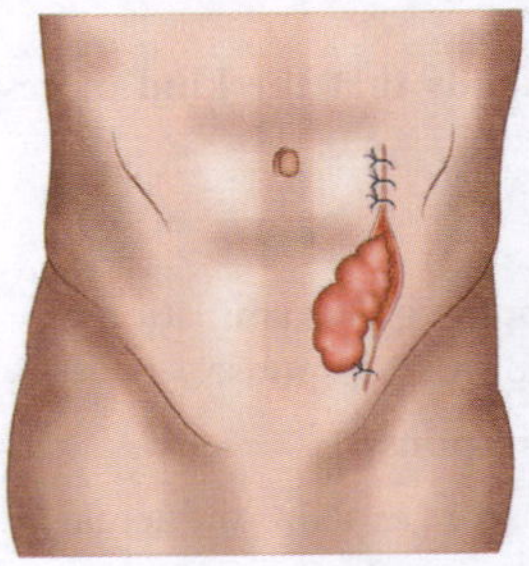

a. Dehiscence
b. Enucleation
c. Evisceration
d. Extenteration

6. Identify the type of laceration shown in the image

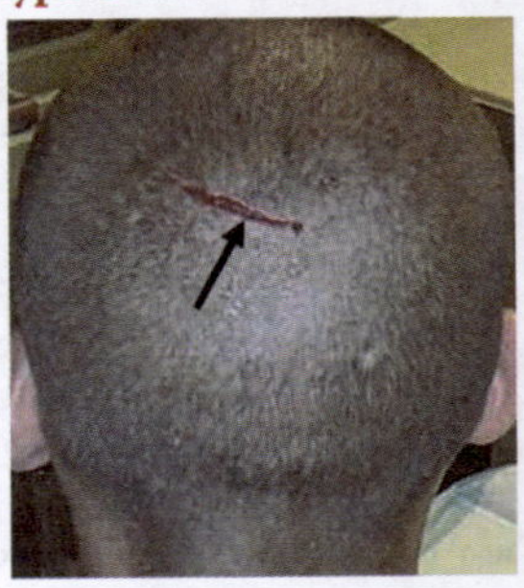

a. Stretch laceration
b. Split laceration
c. Incision tear
d. Tear laceration

7. Identify the type of suture shown in the image below

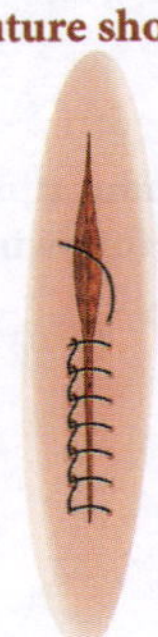

a. Cushing suture
b. Halsted suture
c. Lock-Stitch stuture
d. Everting suture

8. Identify the device used to cover the patient.

(Refer explanation at the end)

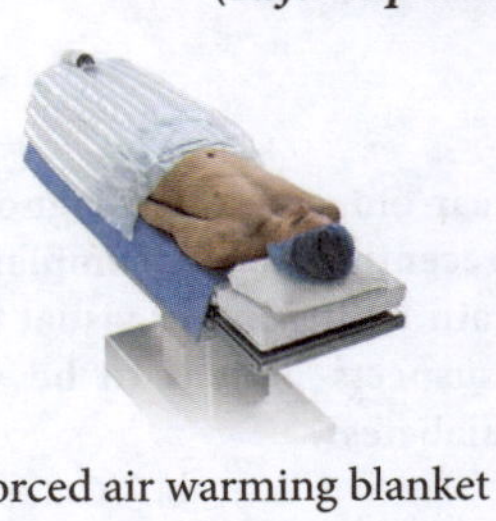

a. Bair hugger forced air warming blanket
b. Alpha blanket
c. Thermal insulation blanket
d. Top thermal blanket

Ans.

1. c
2. b
3. c
4. b
5. c
6. b
7. c
8. a

[*Courtesy*: PHOTON-20® 3th ed. by Vivek Jain, CBS Publishers and Distributors Pvt Ltd]

9. Identify the device shown in the image
(Refer explanation at the end)

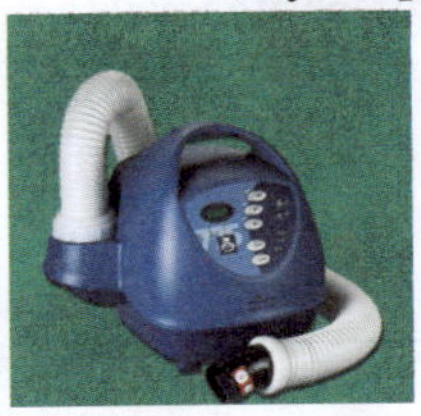

a. Portable ventilator device
b. Bair Hugger warming unit
c. Vacuum clearner
d. Alpha bed controller

10. Identify the device shown in the image
(Refer explanation at the end)

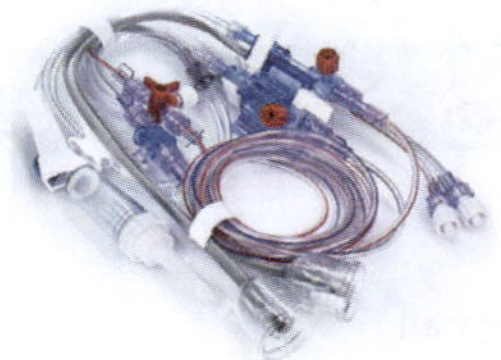

a. Hemodialysis catheter
b. Disposable Blood Pressure Transducer
c. Arterial line Catheter
d. Double lumen catheter kit

11. Identify the device shown in the image

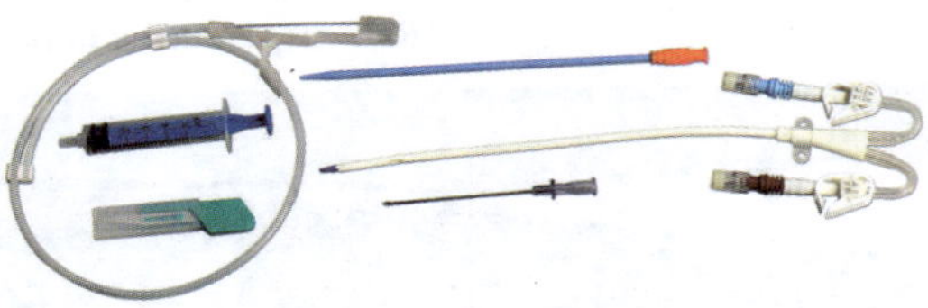

a. Peritoneal dialysis kit
b. Blood Pressure Transducer
c. Hemodialysis catheter kit
d. Double lumen catheter kit

12. Identify the device shown in the image
(Refer explanation at the end)

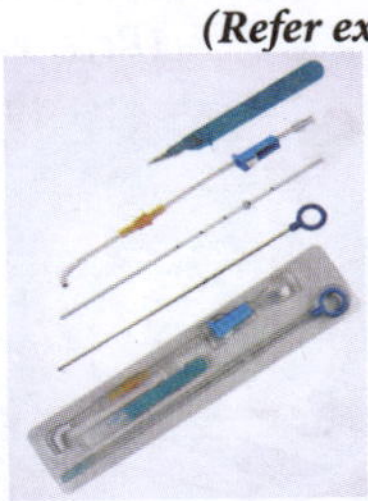

a. Peritoneal dialysis kit
b. Lumbar Puncture Kit
c. Biopsy kit
d. Chest drainage insertion kit

13. Identify the device shown in the image
(Refer explanation at the end)

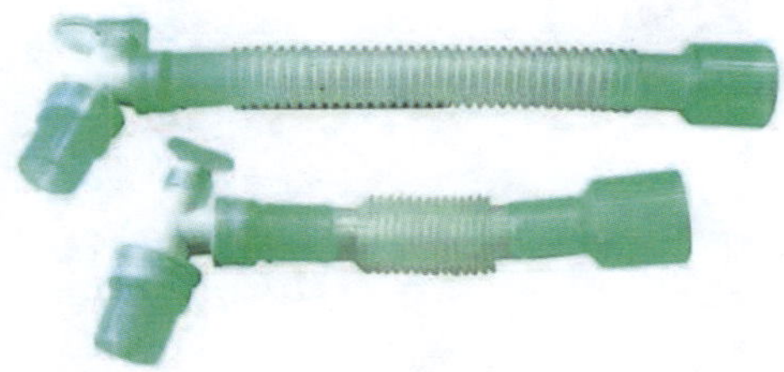

a. Ventilator circuit
b. Ventilator tube
c. HME filter
d. Catheter mount

14. Identify the device shown in the image
(Refer explanation at the end)

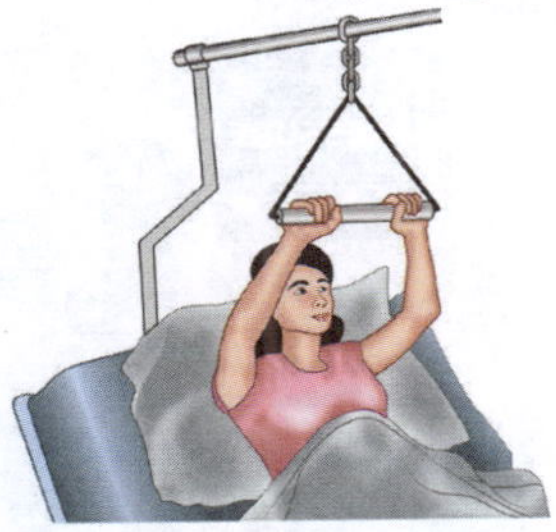

a. Overhead patient lift
b. Overhead Trapeze
c. Over head arm support
d. Ceiling lift

15. Identify the instrument shown in the image
(Refer explanation at the end)

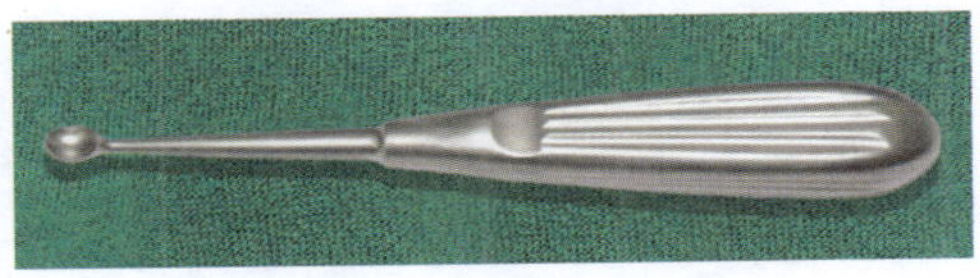

a. Adenoid curette
b. Bone curette
c. Universal curette
d. Periodontal curette

16. Identify the name of the equipment shown in the image

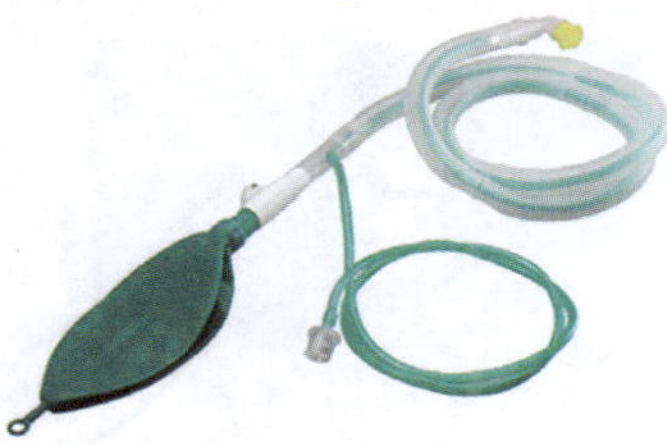

a. Bain breathing circuit
b. Mapleson-C circuit
c. McKesson breathing circuit
d. Y-type corrugated breathing unit

Ans.

9. b
10. b
11. c
12. a
13. d
14. b
15. b
16. a

17. Type of mask used for the patient shown in the image is

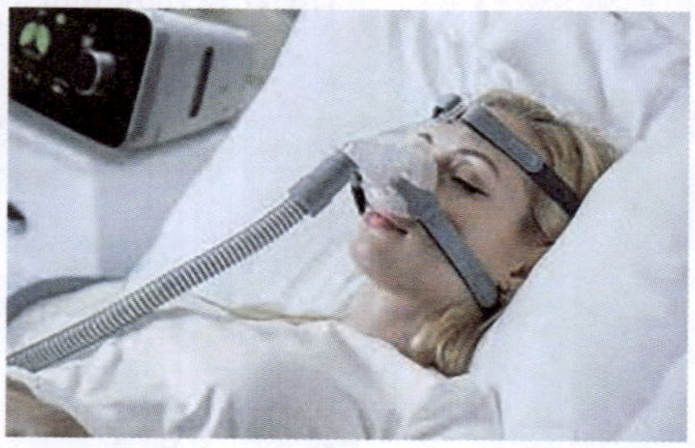

a. Rebreather mask
b. Bi-Pap mask
c. Venturi mask
d. Simple face mask

18. The image below illustrates which type of positive airway pressure?

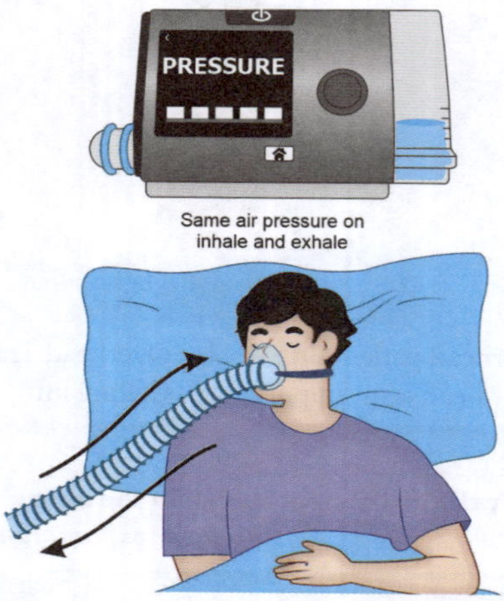

a. CPAP
b. BiPAP
c. VPAP
d. Autotitrating pressure device

19. The image below illustrates which type of positive airway pressure? ***(Refer explanation at the end)***

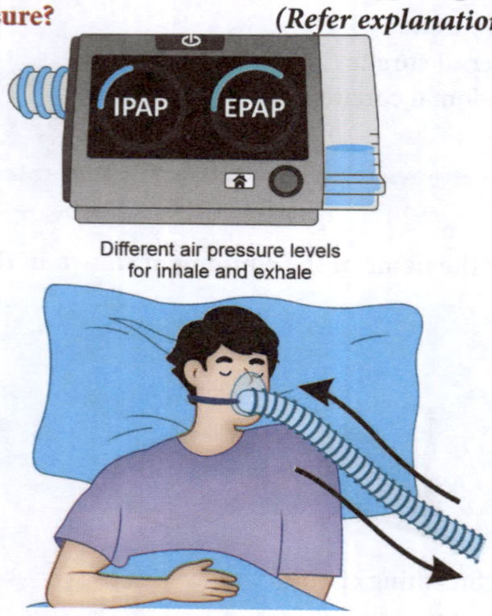

a. CPAP
b. BiPAP
c. VPAP
d. Autotitrating pressure device

20. A foot morphology characterized by high arch of the foot that does not flatten with weightbearing as shown below is known as ***(Refer explanation at the end)***

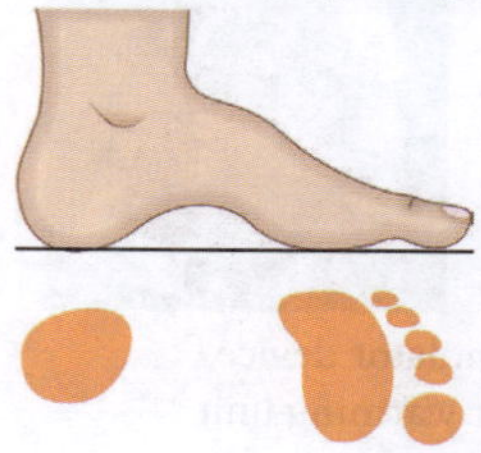

a. Flat foot
b. Pes Cavus
c. Fallen arch
d. Splayed foot

21. Identify the device used in orthopedic surgery ***(Refer explanation at the end)***

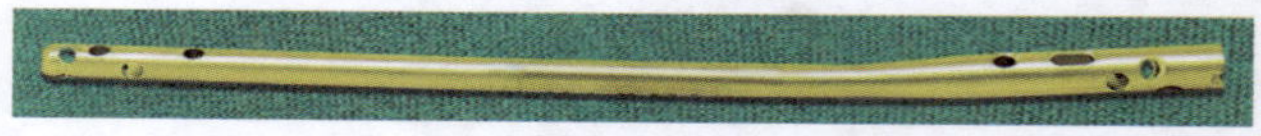

a. Osteotome
b. Interlocking nail
c. Bone lever
d. Gouges

22. Identify the device used in orthopedic surgery ***(Refer explanation at the end)***

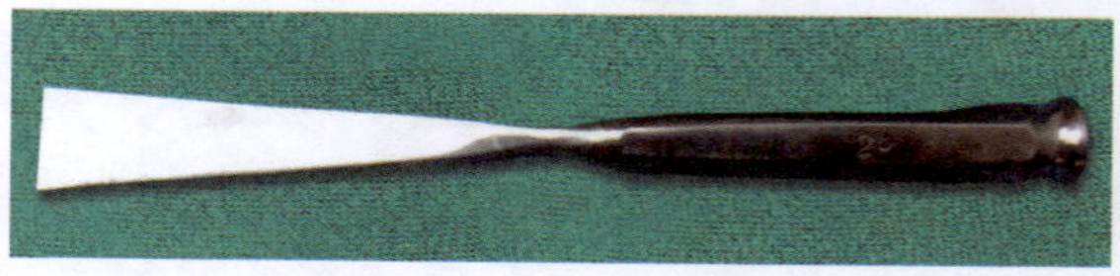

a. Osteotome
b. Impactor
c. Driver
d. Chisel

23. Identify the Device used in ophthalmology for diagnostic purpose ***(Refer explanation at the end)***

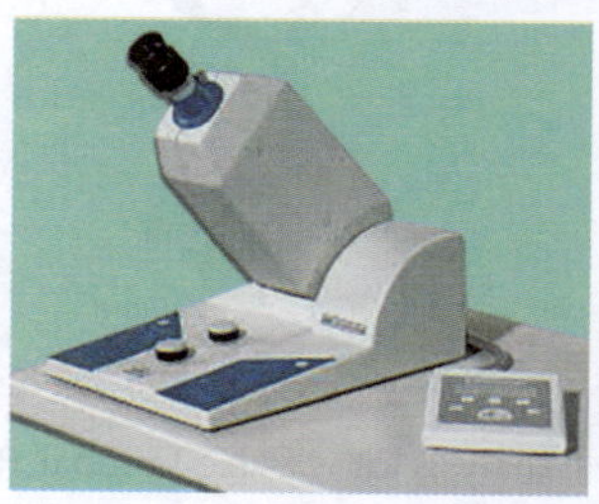

a. Anomaloscope
b. Ophthalmoscope
c. Retinoscope
d. Retinal camera

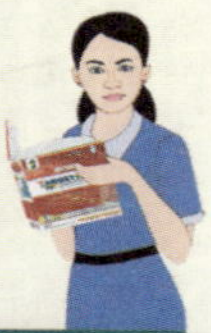

Ans.

17.	b
18.	a
19.	b
20.	b
21.	b
22.	a
23.	a

24. Identify the Device used in ophthalmology for diagnostic purpose ***(Refer explanation at the end)***

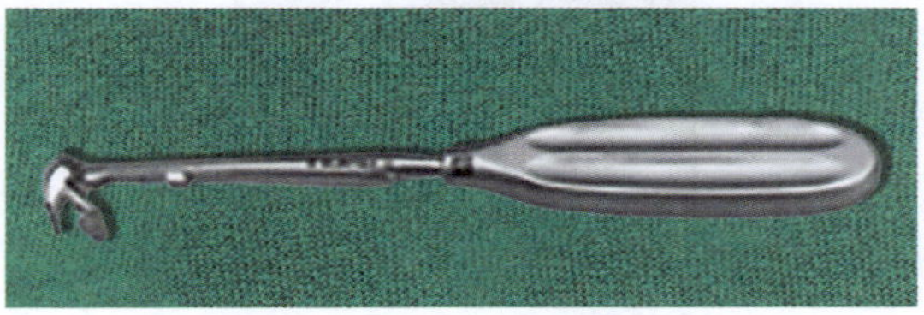

a. Periodontol curete
b. Bond curette
c. Adenoid curette
d. Uterine curette

25. Identify the device shown here which is used for the therapeutic purposes in dermatology? ***(Refer explanation at the end)***

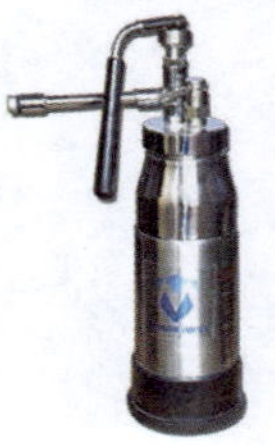

a. Mini cryogun
b. Cryogenic tank
c. Nitrogen dewar
d. Vacuum chamber

26. Identify the device shown here

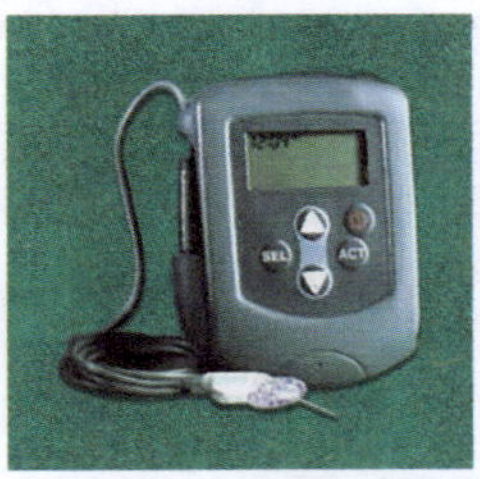

a. Continuous Glucose Monitoring System (CGSM)
b. Holter moniter
c. Insulin pump
d. Patient Controlled Analgesia pump

27. Identify the device shown in the image

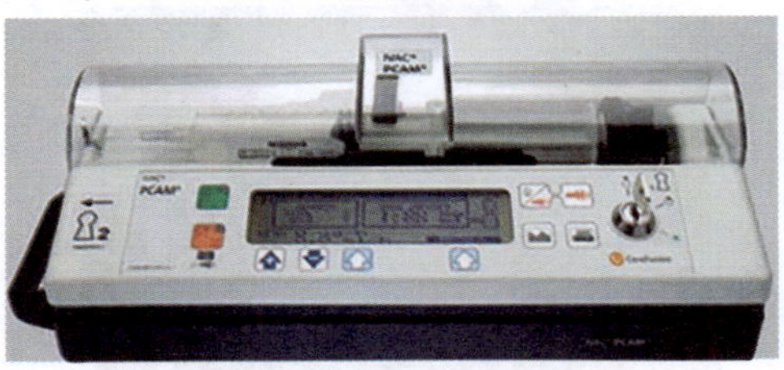

a. Holter monitor
b. Patient controlled analgesia pump
c. DVT pump
d. Volumetric infusion pump

28. Identify the device shown in the image

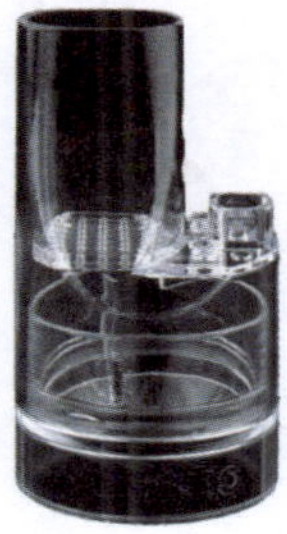

a. Metered dose inhaler
b. Rotahaler
c. Spacer
d. Spirometer

29. Identify the device shown in the image

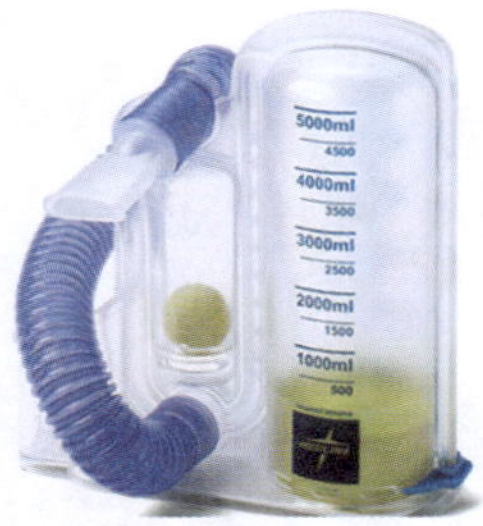

a. Flow based spirometer
b. Volume based spirometer
c. Ultrasonic spirometer
d. Differential pressure spirometer

30. Identify the device shown in the image

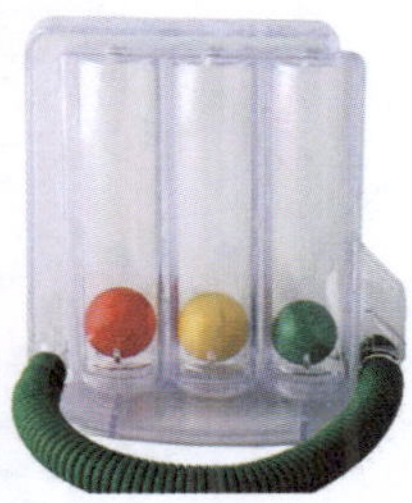

a. Flow based spirometer
b. Volume based spirometer
c. Ultrasonic spirometer
d. Differential pressure spirometer

31. A clinical sign that is being examined in this image is ***(Refer explanation at the end)***

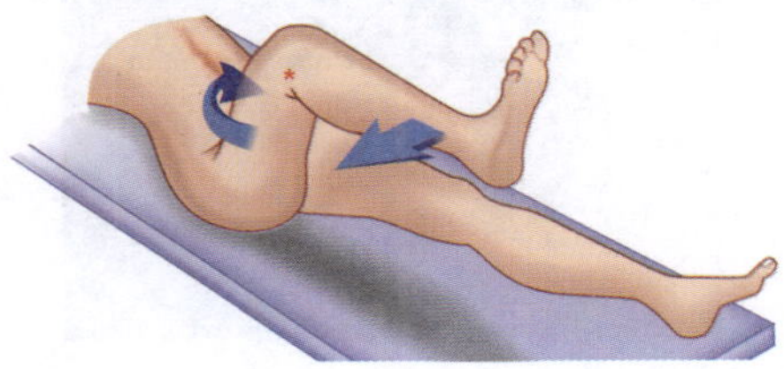

a. Obturator sign
b. Brudzinski's sign
c. Psoas sign
d. Kernig's sign

Ans.

24. c
25. a
26. a
27. b
28. b
29. b
30. a
31. a

32. A clinical sign that is being examined in this image is
(Refer explanation at the end)

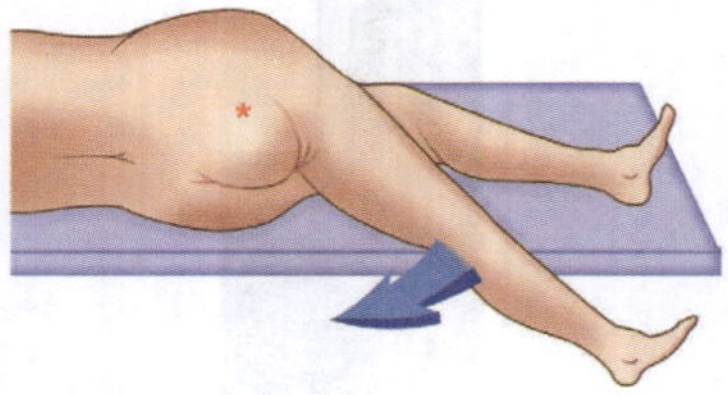

a. Obturator sign
b. Brudzinski's sign
c. Psoas sign
d. Kernig's sign

33. What is the name of heart valve indicated by the arrow mark

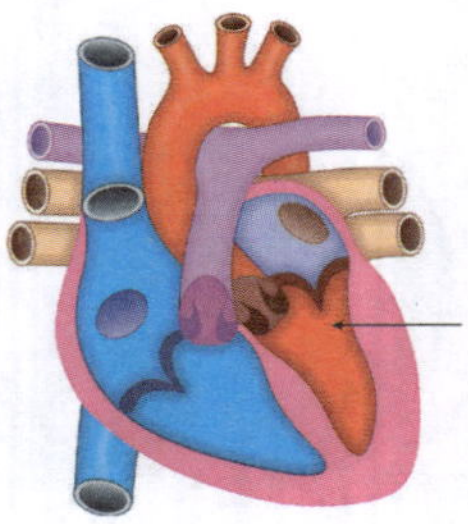

a. Tricuspid valve
b. Mitral valve
c. Aortic valve
d. Pulmonary valve

34. Identify the refractive error.
(Refer explanation at the end)

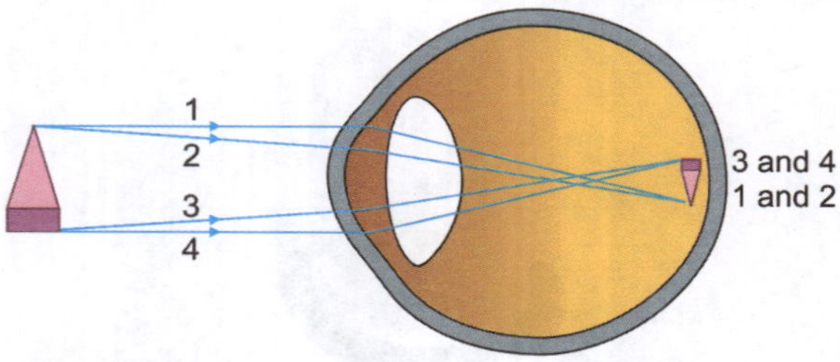

a. Myopia
b. Hypermetropia
c. Presbyopia
d. Astigmatism

35. Identify the type of cataract depicted in the image.

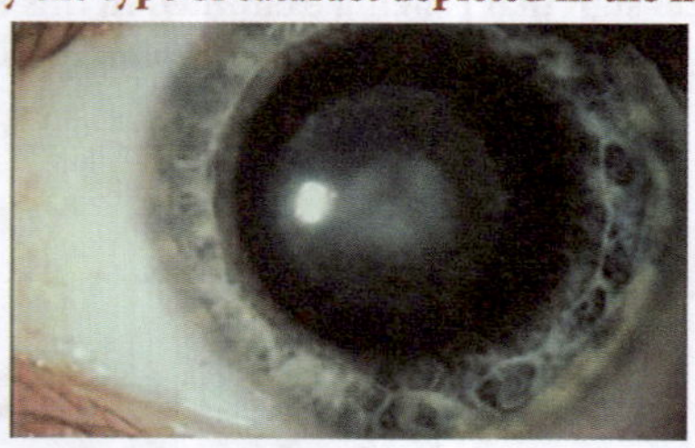

a. Posterior polar cataract
b. Blue dot cataract
c. Coronary cataract
d. Zonular cataract

36. Identify the pathology depicted in the given image.

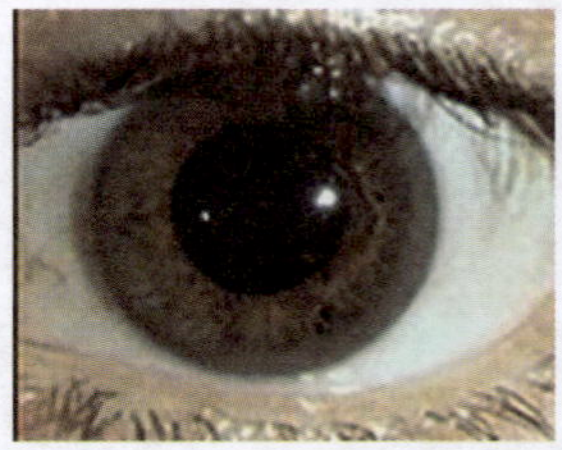

a. Corneal ulcer
b. Aniridia
c. Circumcorneal congestion
d. Kayser-Fleischer ring

37. The following picture exhibits which cranial nerve palsy?
(Refer explanation at the end)

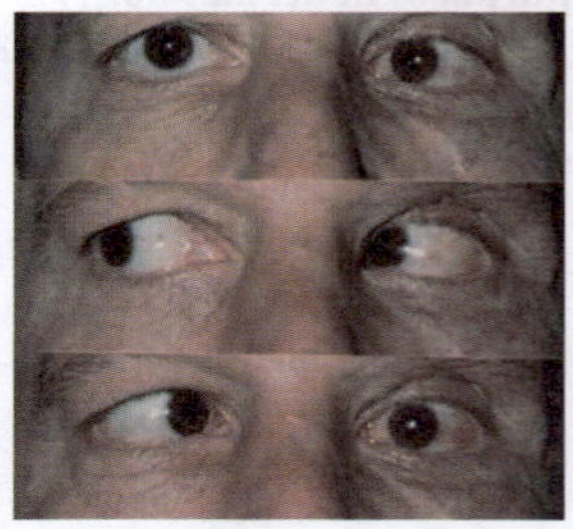

a. Oculomotor nerve
b. Trochlear nerve
c. Abducent nerve
d. Vestibulocochlear nerve

38. A patient was suffering from ptosis and hypotropia. After giving an IV drug to the patient, in 6 minutes his ptosis & hypotropia improved. What is the probable diagnosis?

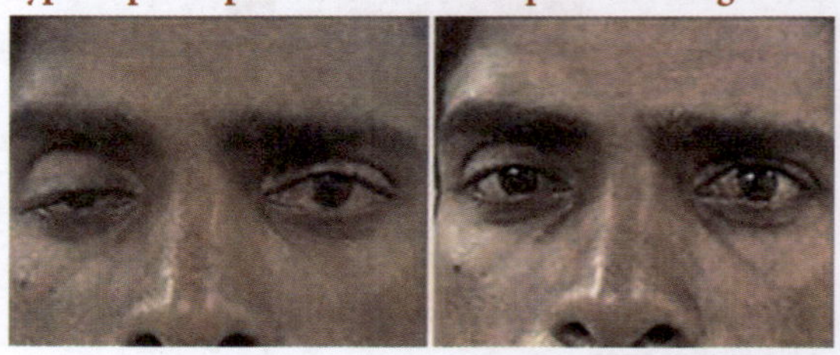

a. 6th nerve palsy
b. Tolosa-Hunt syndrome
c. Third nerve palsy
d. Myasthenia gravis

39. Identify the pathology depicted in the image.

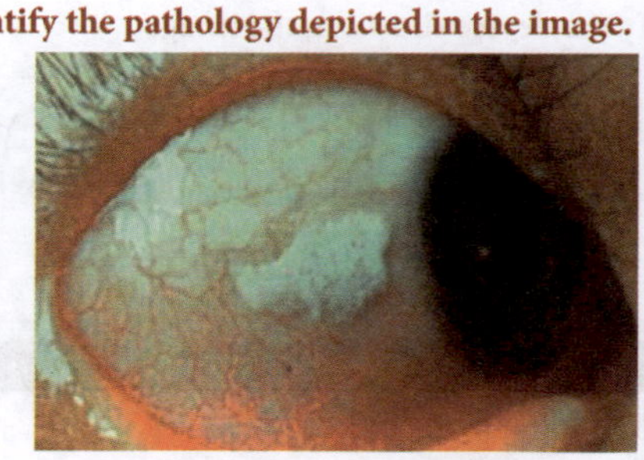

a. Foreign body
b. Anterior staphyloma
c. Bitot's spots
d. Normal anatomical variant

Ans.

32.	c
33.	b
34.	a
35.	d
36.	d
37.	c
38.	d
39.	c

40. Identify the instrument given in the image.

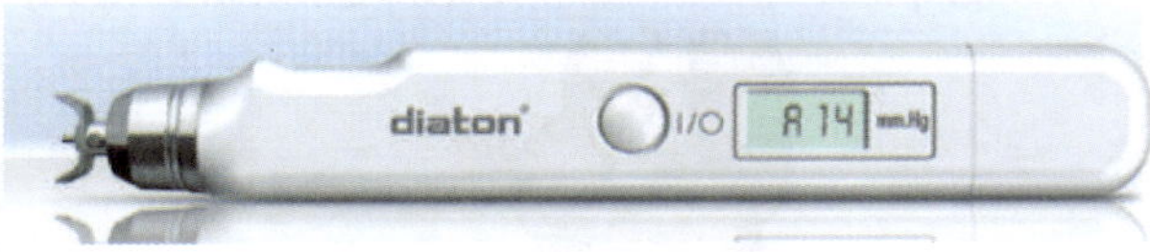

a. Tonometer
b. Pachymeter
c. Keratometer
d. Ophthalmometer

41. The following CXR shows:

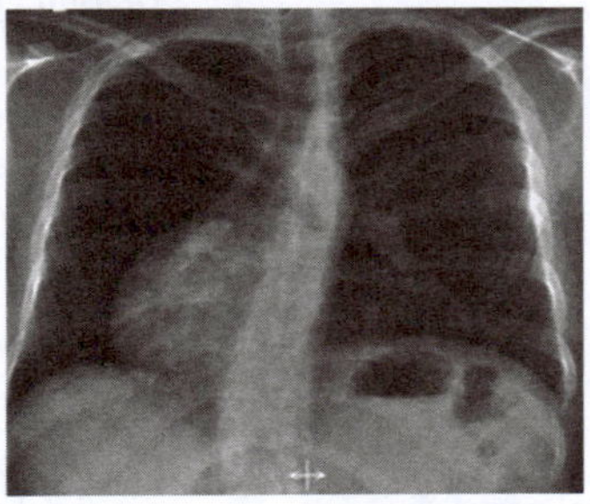

a. Dextrocardia
b. Pneumothorax
c. Pneumomediastinum
d. Pulmonary hamartoma

42. ECG given below is of:

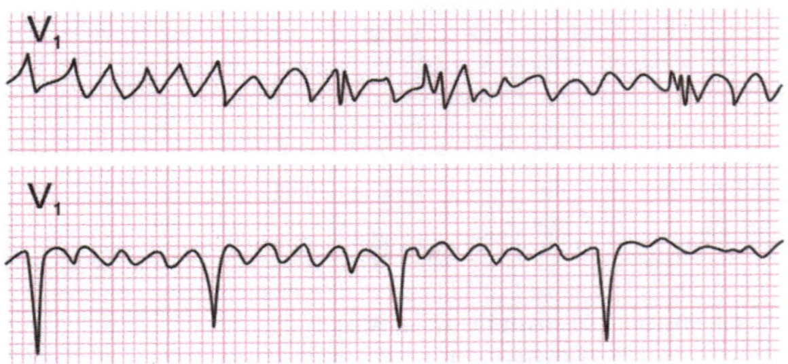

a. Atrial fibrillation
b. Atrial flutter
c. Sinus tachycardia
d. PSVT

43. Procedure shown below is:

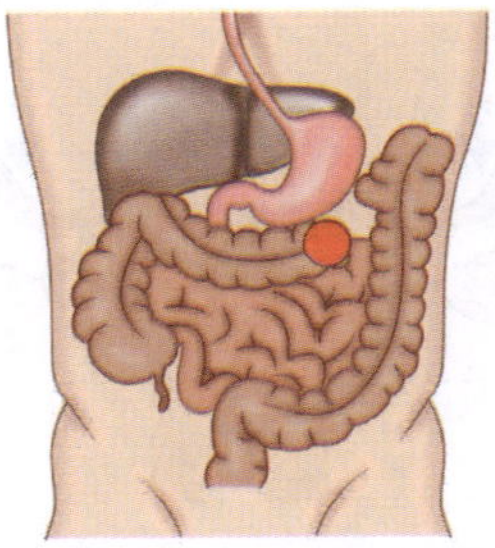

a. Transverse colostomy
b. Hartman procedure
c. Ileostomy
d. Descending colostomy

44. Radio image shows technique of:

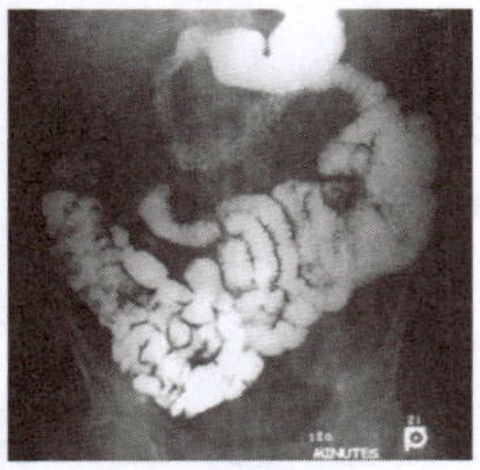

a. Barium meal follow through
b. Enteroclysis
c. Barium enema
d. Barium swallow

45. A patient of ESRD is being performed hemodialysis. Central dialysis catheter is placed at which site?

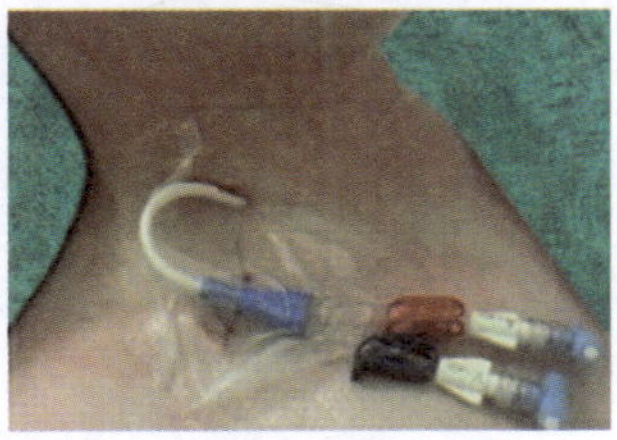

a. Right internal jugular vein
b. Left internal jugular vein
c. Right subclavian vein
d. Right subclavian artery

46. Peripheral smear is suggestive of which anemia?

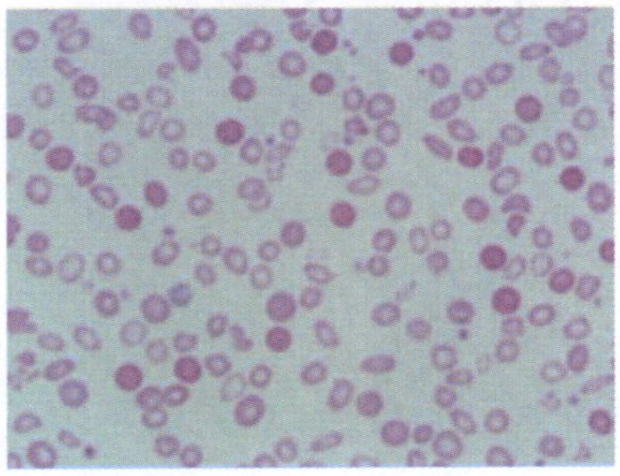

a. Iron deficiency anemia
b. Macrocytic anemia
c. HUS
d. Hereditary spherocytosis

47. Lady presents with joint pain in both knees and low grade fever off and on. On examination she has a rash on sun exposed parts. Image shown below. What is the clinical diagnosis?

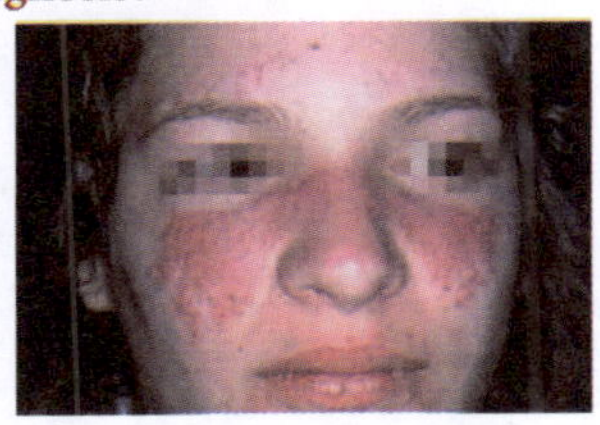

a. Lupus vulgaris
b. SLE
c. Photodermatitis
d. CREST syndrome

Ans.

40. a
41. a
42. a
43. a
44. a
45. a
46. a
47. b

48. Inheritance shown in diagram depicts:

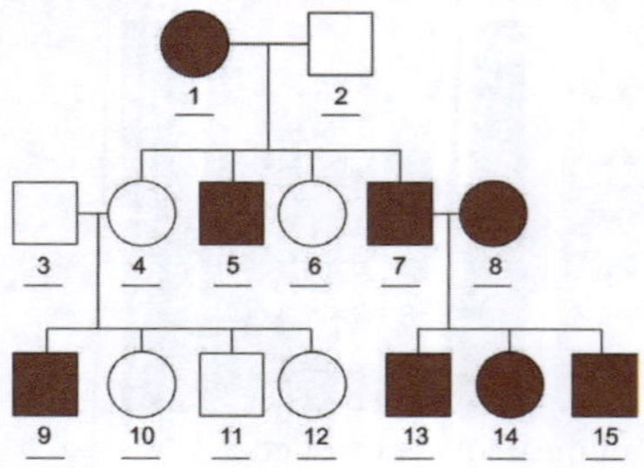

a. X linked dominant
b. X linked recessive
c. Autosomal dominant
d. Autosomal recessive

49. Sign shown in the photograph occurs due to injury of: ***[Recent Question 2017, 2014, 2012]***

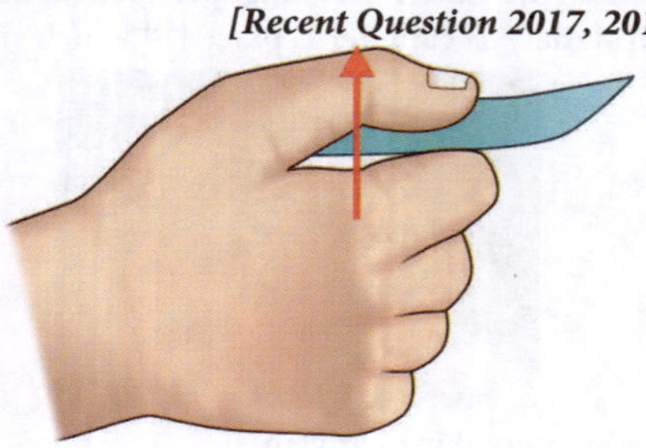

a. Radial nerve
b. Median nerve
c. Ulnar nerve
d. Axillary nerve

50. Artery (Arrow) shown in photograph supplies all of the following EXCEPT:

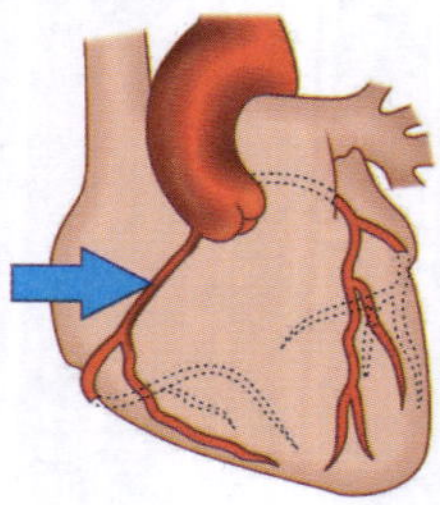

a. SA node
b. AV node
c. AV bundle
d. Right bundle branch

51. Lymph nodes (encircled) shown in photograph are:

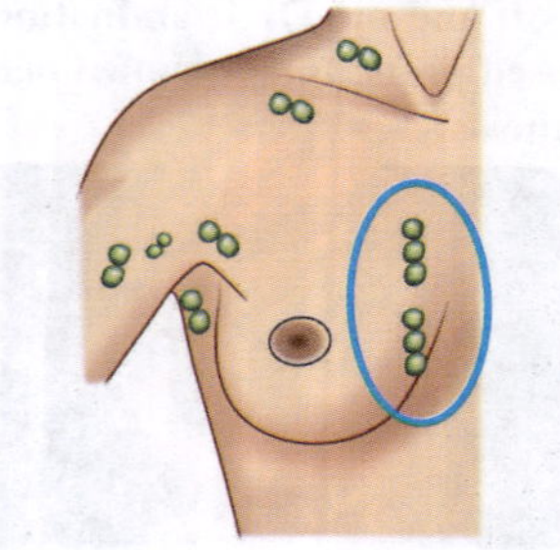

a. Supraclavicular LN
b. Anterior axillary LN
c. Apical LN
d. Internal mammary LN

52. Most common position of organ (Encircled) shown in photograph is: ***[Recent Question 2013-14]***

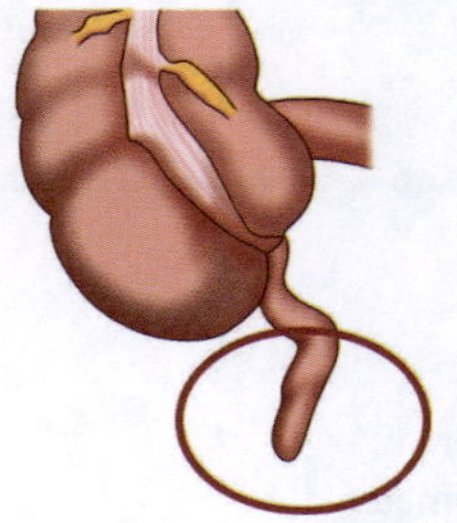

a. Pelvic
b. Retrocecal
c. Preileal
d. Postileal

53. Nerve supplying the area (arrow) shown in photograph is: ***[Recent Question 2012]***

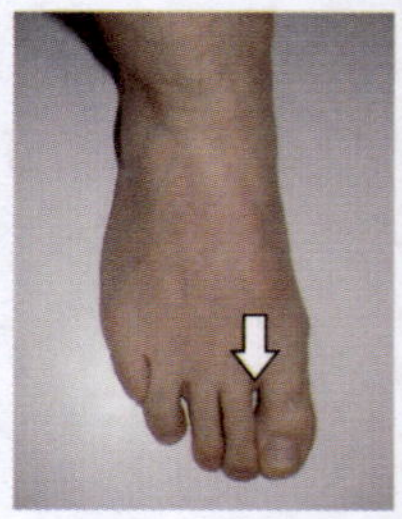

a. Femoral nerve
b. Superficial peroneal nerve
c. Deep peroneal nerve
d. Saphenous nerve

54. Epithelial lining of structure (Box) shown in photograph is:

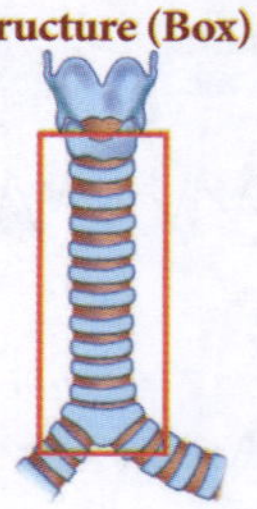

a. Simple columnar epithelium
b. Pseudostratified columnar epithelium
c. Stratified squamous epithelium
d. Ciliated columnar epithelium

55. Type of epithelium seen in parts (arrows) of organ shown in photograph is:

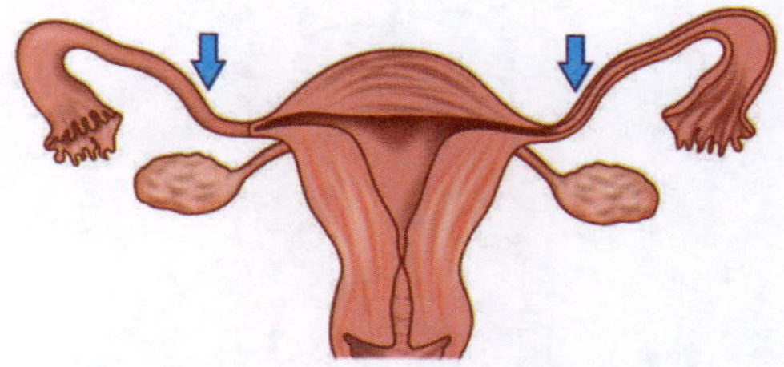

a. Simple columnar
b. Ciliated columnar
c. Pseudostratified columnar
d. Simple cuboidal

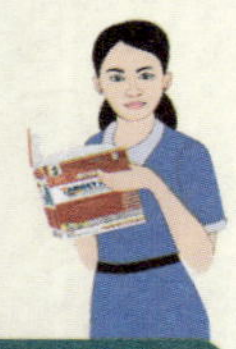

Ans.

48.	b
49.	c
50.	d
51.	d
52.	b
53.	c
54.	b
55.	b

56. Length of organ (arrow) shown in photograph is: *[Recent Question 2012]*

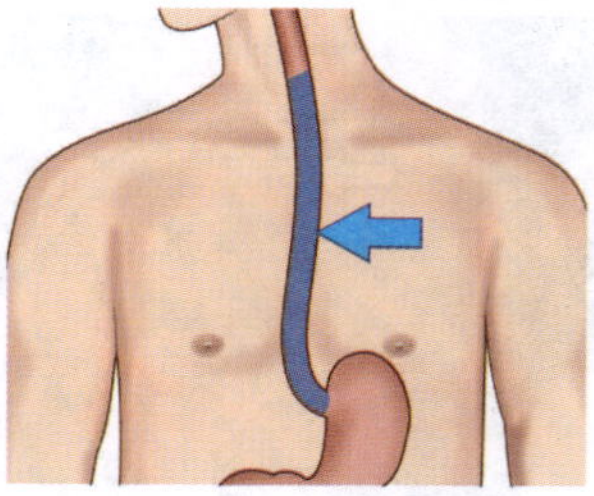

a. 10 cm
b. 15 cm
c. 25 cm
d. 40 cm

57. Level of angle (encircled) shown in photograph is:

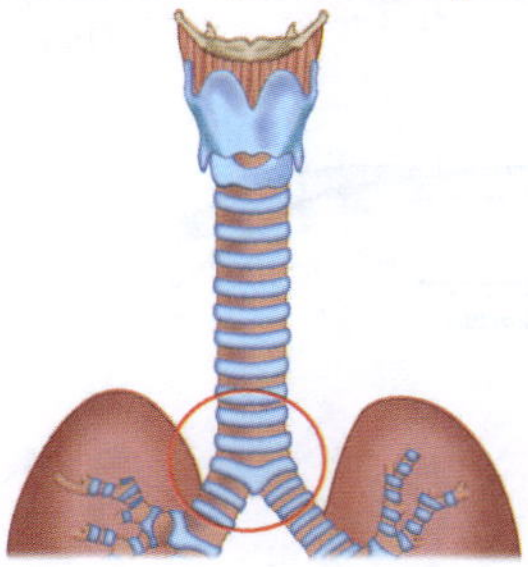

a. T3
b. T4
c. T6
d. T9

58. Condition of the hand (photograph) is due to ......nerve palsy. *[Recent Question 2015]*

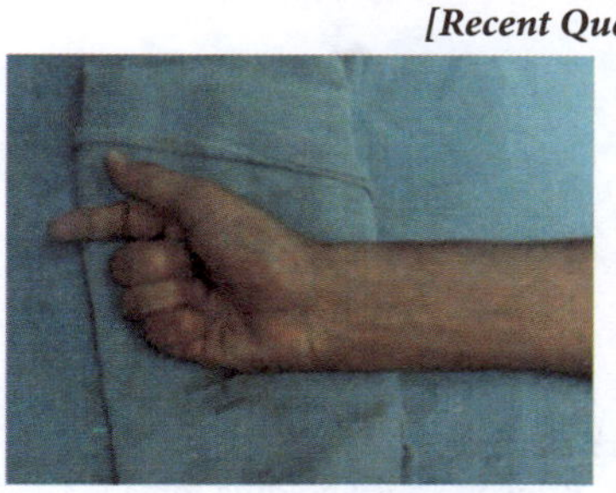

a. Radial N
b. Ulnar N
c. Axillary N
d. Median N

59. Injury to .... nerve results in deformity (encircled) as shown in photograph:

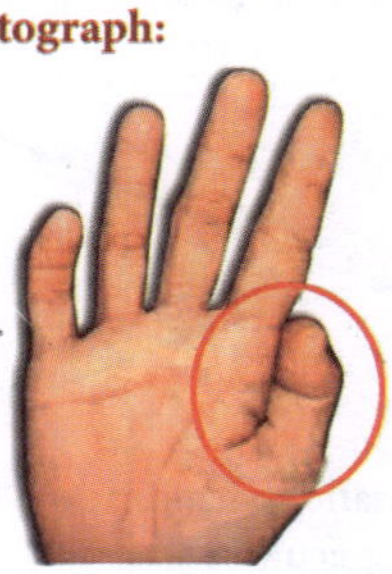

a. Radial
b. Ulnar
c. Median
d. Axillary

60. Identify the nails disorder as shown in the photograph:

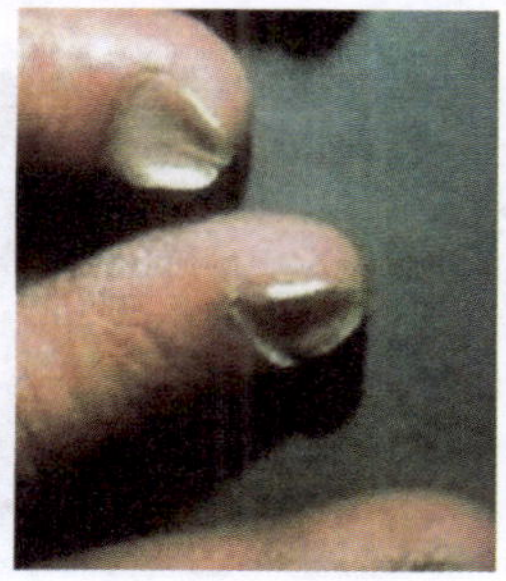

a. Anonychia
b. Koilonychia
c. Leukonychia
d. Paronychia

61. Condition shown in photograph occur due to: *[Recent Question 2013]*

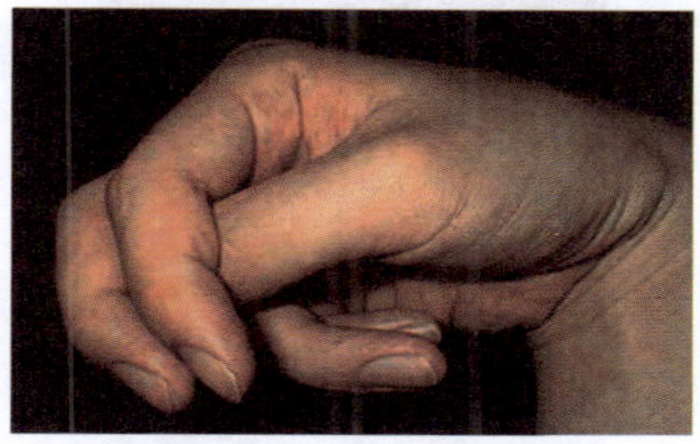

a. Low levels of potassium
b. Hypermagnesemia
c. Hypocalcemia
d. Hypophosphatemia

62. Identify the worm shown in the photograph:

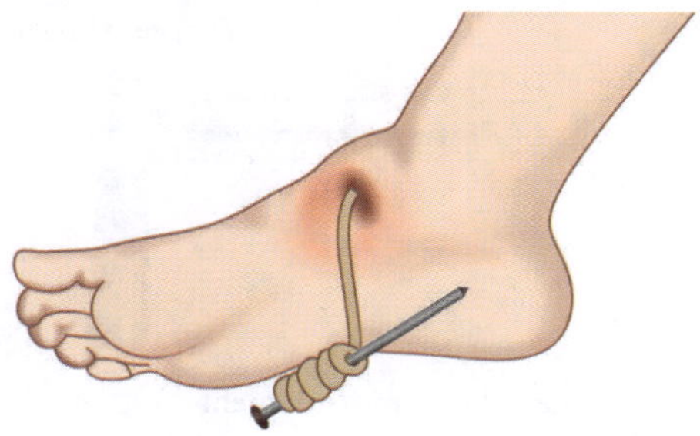

a. Round worm
b. Hook worm
c. Tape worm
d. Guinea worm

63. Type of venom produced by snake shown in photograph is:

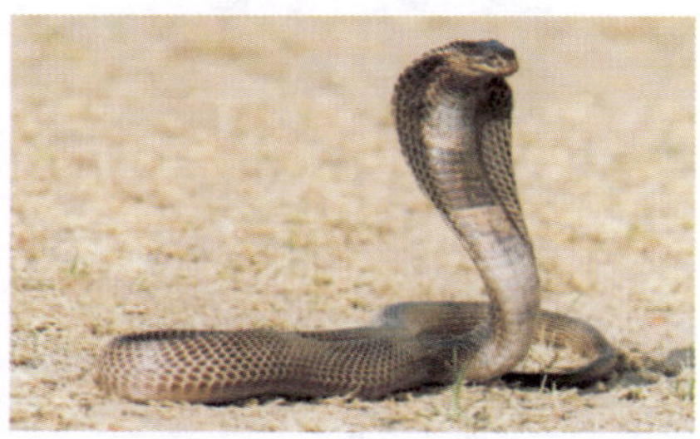

a. Myotoxic
b. Neurotoxic
c. Hemolytic
d. Proteolytic

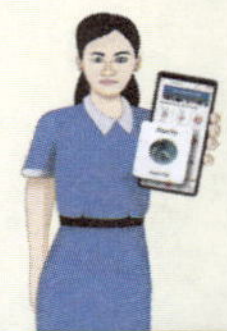

Ans.

56.	c
57.	b
58.	d
59.	c
60.	b
61.	c
62.	d
63.	b

64. Type of venom produced by snake shown in photograph is:

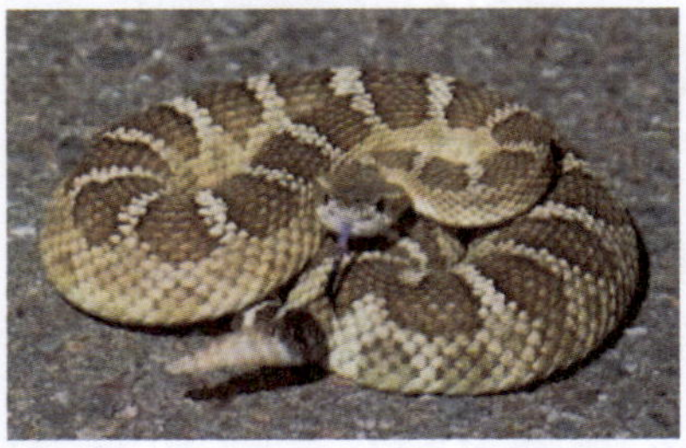

a. Myotoxic
b. Neurotoxic
c. Hemolytic
d. Proteolytic

65. Mask shown in photograph was used for prevention of:

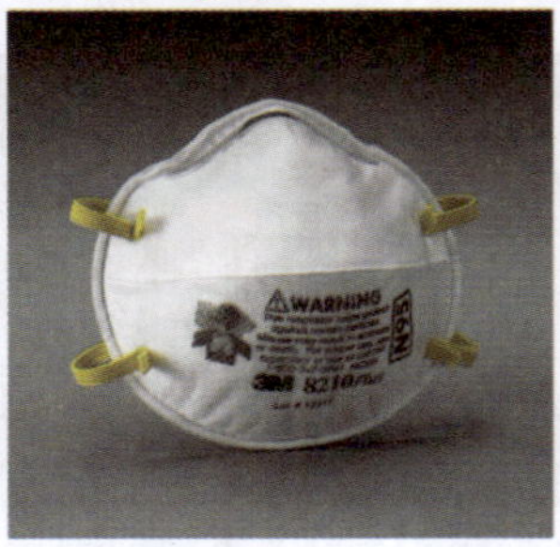

a. Tuberculosis
b. Covid 19
c. Pneumonia
d. Typhoid

66. Instrument shown in photograph is used to assess:
[Recent Question 2016]

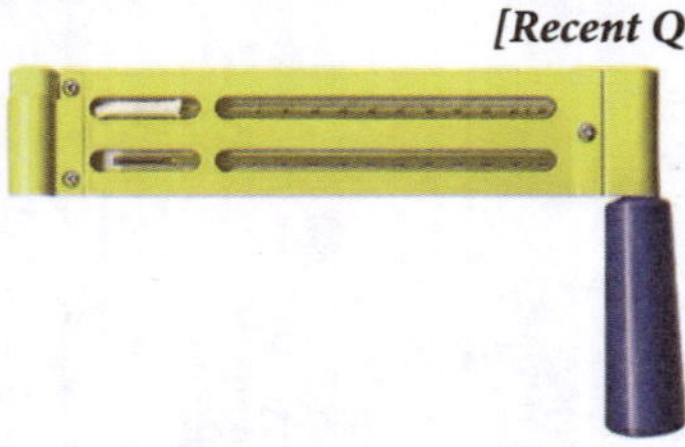

a. Environmental heat measurement
b. Cooling power of air
c. Mean radiant temperature of surroundings
d. Relative humidity of air

67. Test of color vision shown in photograph is known as:

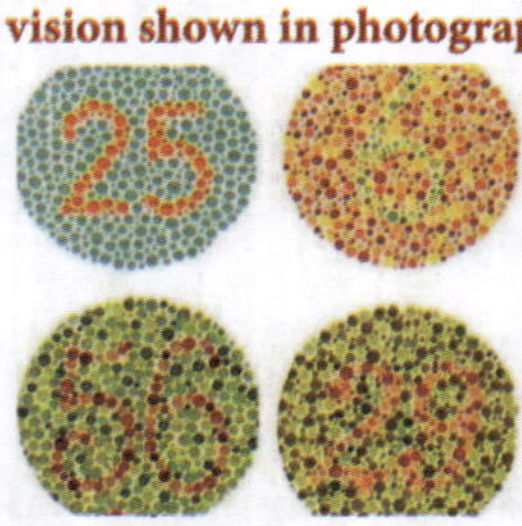

a. Ishihara plates
b. Edridge Green lantern test
c. Farnsworth-Munsell 100 hue test
d. Nagel's anomaloscope

68. Identify the paranasal sinus being tested by technique as shown in photograph:

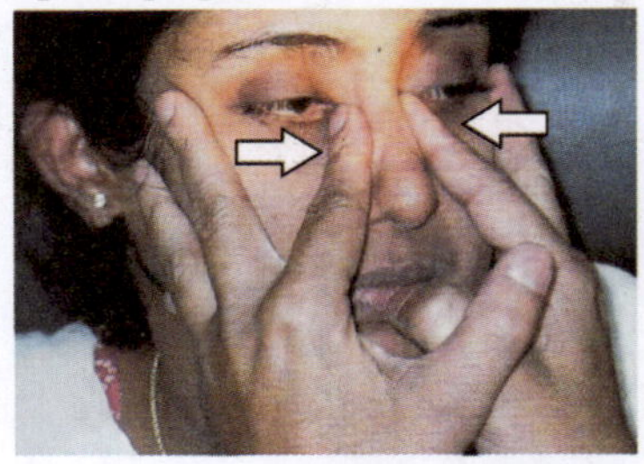

a. Frontal sinus
b. Maxillary sinus
c. Ethmoid sinus
d. Sphenoid sinus

69. Identify the instrument shown in the photograph:
[Recent Question 2016]

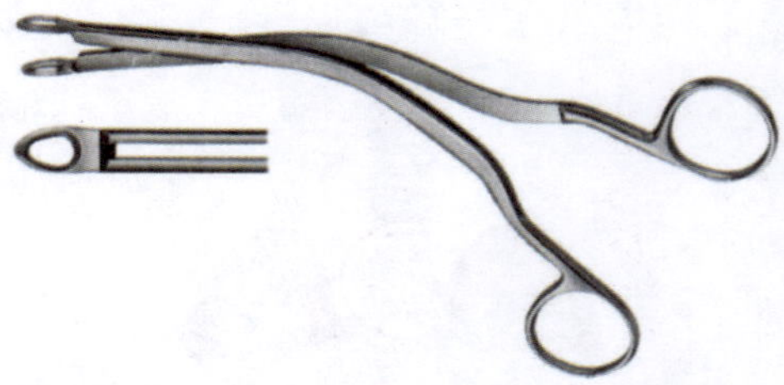

a. Hazek's punch forceps
b. Irwin Moore's forceps
c. Asch's septum forceps
d. Luc's forceps

70. Identify instrument shown in photograph:

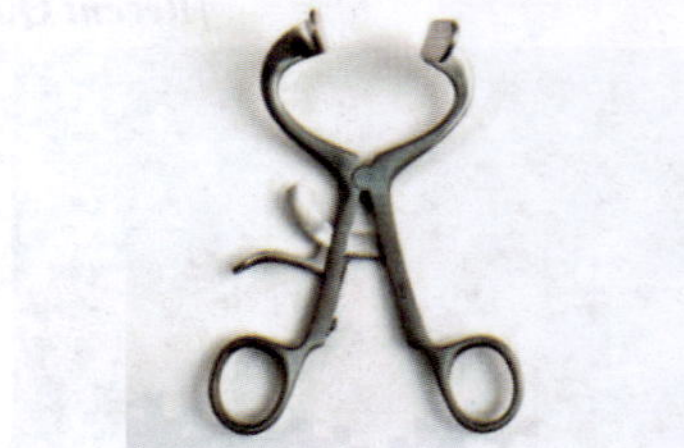

a. Freer's elevator
b. Denis Browne Tonsil holding forceps
c. Doyen's mouth gag
d. Hagen's Cheek retractor

71. Identify the instrument shown in the photograph:
[Recent Question 2014]

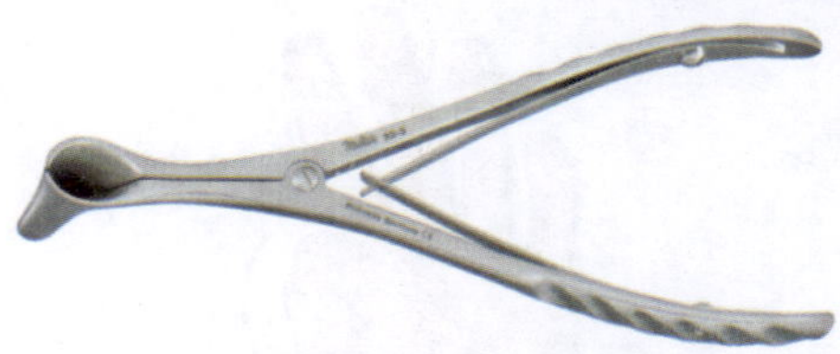

a. Siegel's pneumatic speculum
b. Vienna nasal speculum
c. Thudicum nasal speculum
d. Beckmann nasal speculum

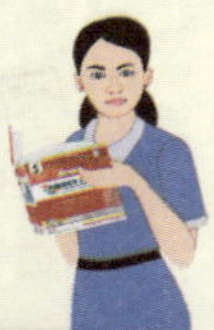

Ans.

64.	d
65.	b
66.	d
67.	a
68.	c
69.	d
70.	c
71.	b

72. Identify the instrument shown in the photograph:

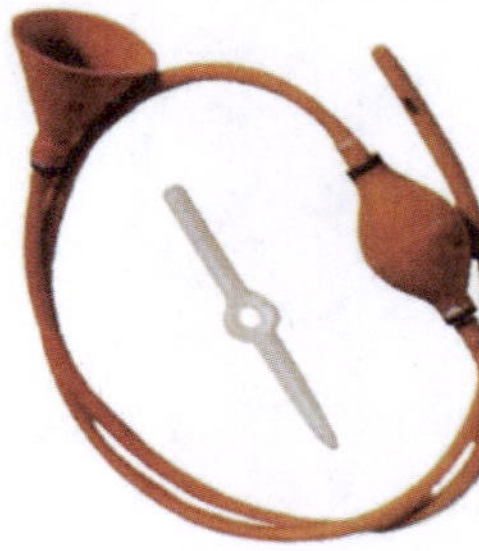

a. Foley's catheter
b. Nasogastric tube
c. Malecot catheter
d. Stomach tube

73. Nerve tested by using clinical test shown in photograph: ***[Recent Question 2013]***

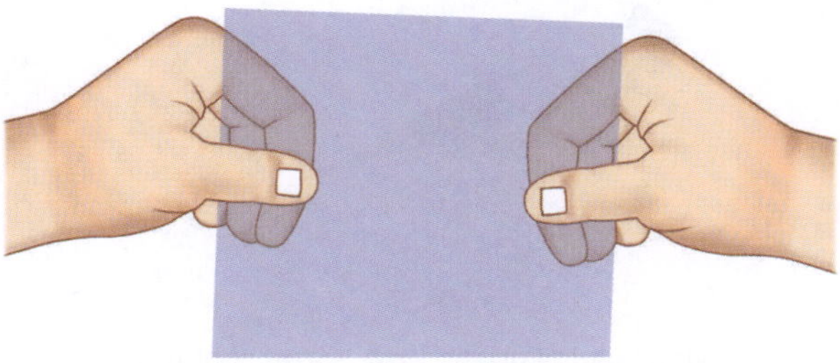

a. Median nerve
b. Radial nerve
c. Axillary nerve
d. Ulnar nerve

74. Identify the condition (arrow) as shown in photograph: ***[Recent Question 2013]***

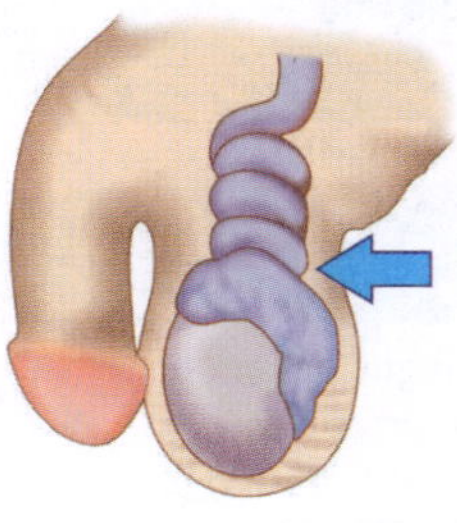

a. Testicular hematoma
b. Testicular torsion
c. Testicular hydrocele
d. Testicular carcinoma

75. Identify the nerve being tested in maneuver shown in the photograph is: ***[Recent Question 2015]***

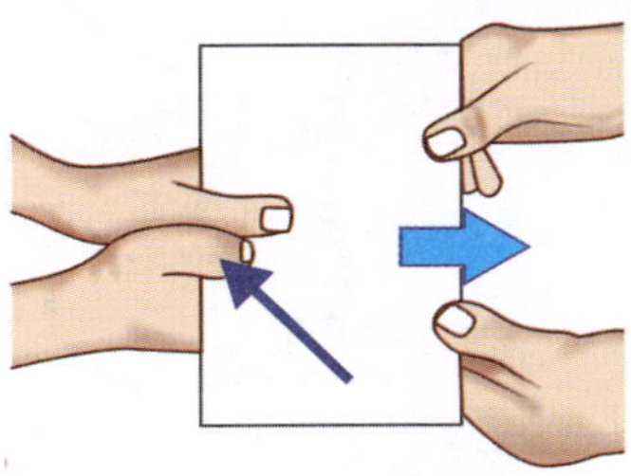

a. Radial nerve
b. Ulnar nerve
c. Median nerve
d. Musculocutaneous nerve

76. Underlying nail disorder shown in the photograph is:

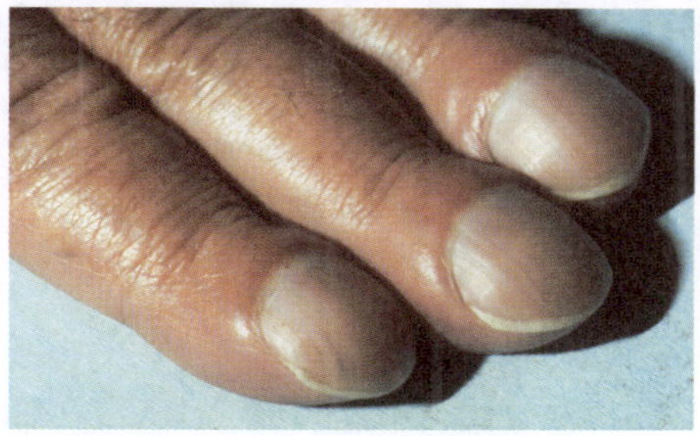

a. Leukonychia
b. Melanonychia
c. Clubbing
d. Koilonychia

77. Chief cells are mainly found in ....part of organ shown in photograph. ***[Recent Question 2013]***

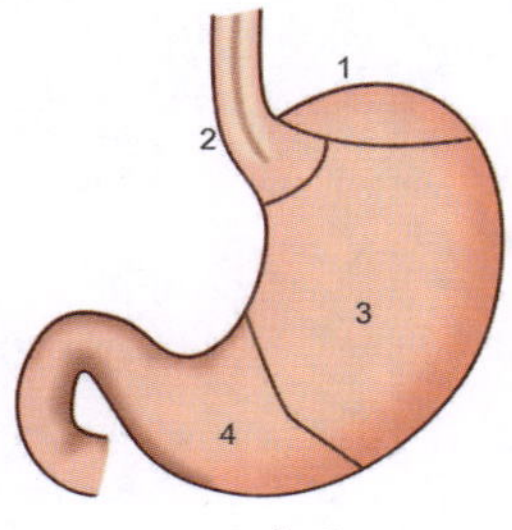

a. 1
b. 2
c. 3
d. 4

78. Type of joint seen in region of pelvis (encircled) in the photograph is: ***[Recent Question 2013]***

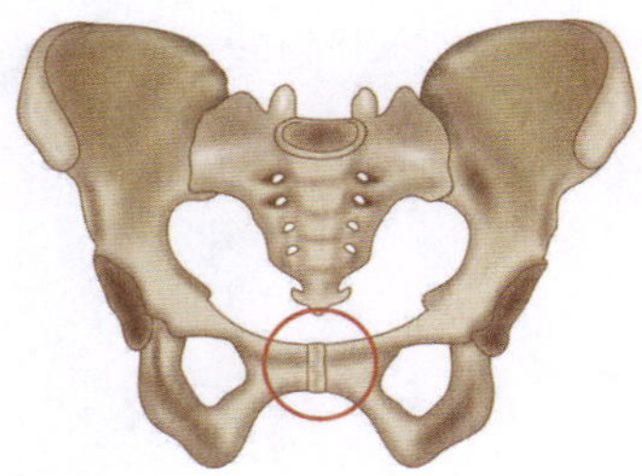

a. Fibrous
b. Cartilaginous
c. Synovial
d. Gomphosis

79. Movement of thumb (arrow) as shown in photograph is lost in injury to: ***[Recent Question 2014]***

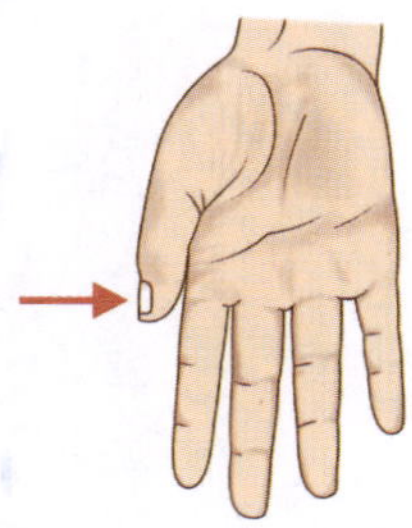

a. Median nerve
b. Radial nerve
c. Ulnar nerve
d. Axillary nerve

Ans.

72.	d
73.	d
74.	b
75.	b
76.	c
77.	a
78.	b
79.	c

80. The solution shown in the picture is used for disinfection of instruments in hospitals. Dry instruments should be soaked for .... at 20°C for effective disinfection.
(Refer explanation at the end)

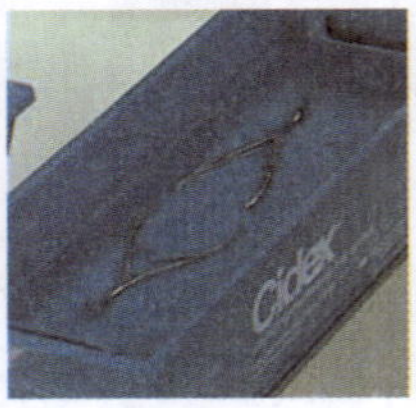

a. 3 minutes
b. 12 minutes
c. 20 minutes
d. 30 minutes

81. What is the purpose of blue color thread present in the gauze swab?

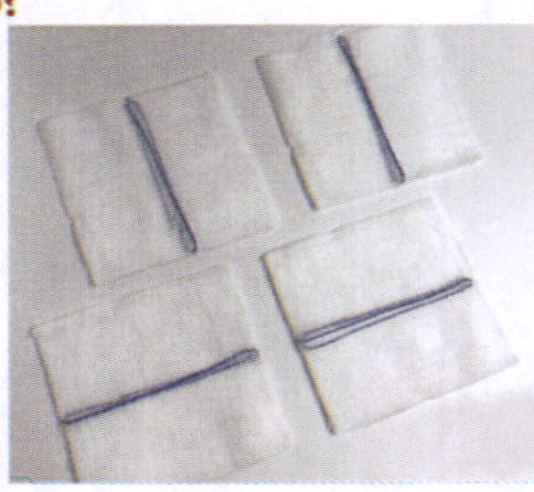

a. It is radiopaque
b. For easy counting
c. Easy visibility when soaked in blood
d. For designing purpose

82. Severe pain in the area shown in the picture indicates:

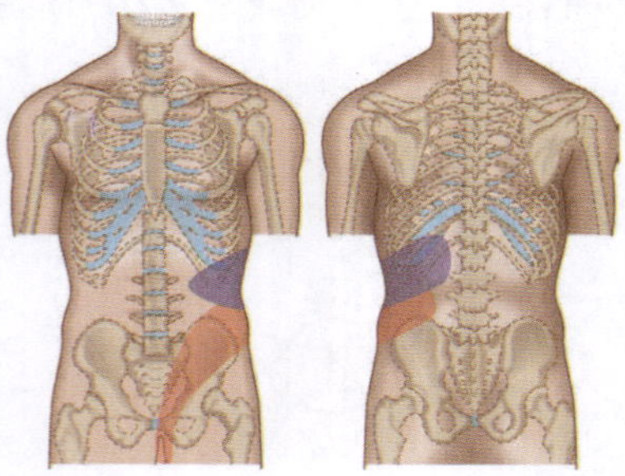

a. Appendicitis
b. Ureteral colic
c. Hydrocele
d. Renal colic

83. Severe pain in the area indicated by arrow mark indicates:

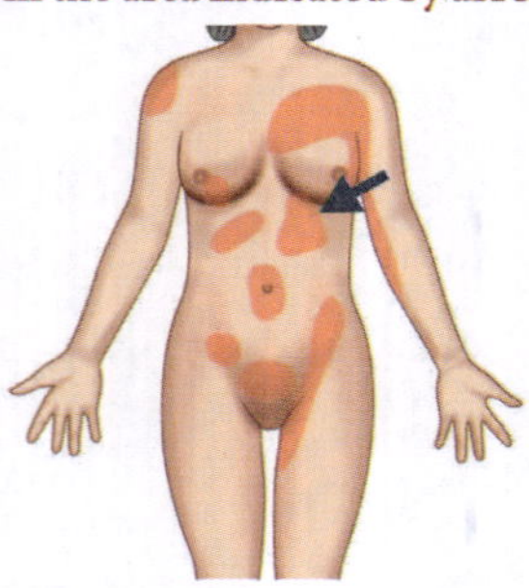

a. Appendicitis
b. Ureteral colic
c. Hydrocele
d. Renal colic

84. Severe pain in the area indicated by arrow mark indicates problem with:

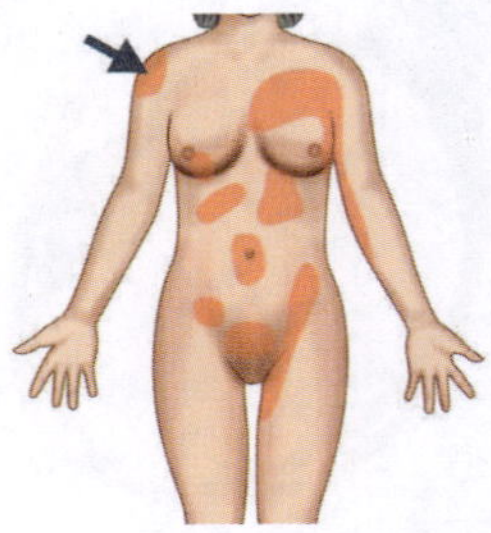

a. Lungs
b. Liver and gallbladder
c. Heart
d. Duodenum

85. Identify following instrument which is used in diagnostic procedures.

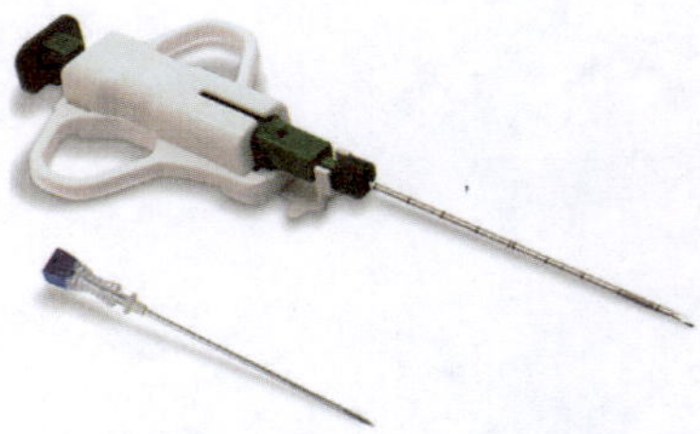

a. Pleural tapping needle
b. Tru-cut biopsy needle
c. Punch biopsy
d. Lumbar puncture needle

86. Identify the equipment given in the image.

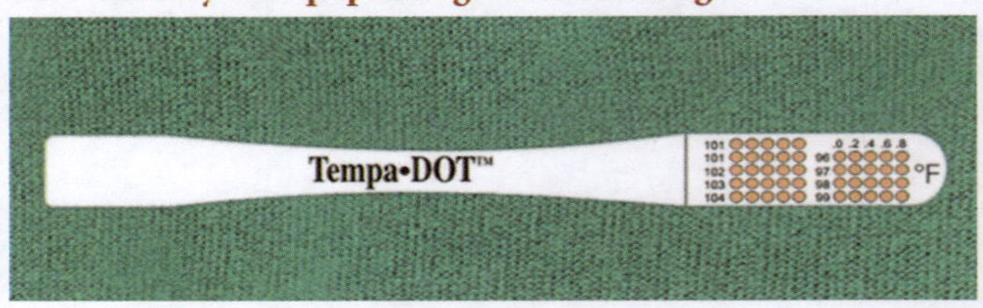

a. Single use tongue depressor
b. Disposable thermometer
c. Percutaneous Bilirubin meter
d. Disposable SpO_2 probe

87. Type of dressing shown in the picture is:
(Refer explanation at the end)

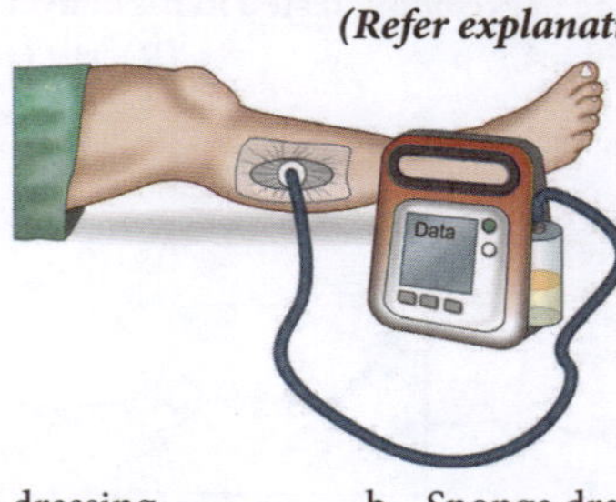

a. Foam dressing
b. Sponge dressing
c. Positive pressure dressing
d. Negative pressure dressing

Ans.

80.	b
81.	a
82.	b
83.	d
84.	b
85.	b
86.	b
87.	d

88. The medication given in the picture is used for: ***(Refer explanation at the end)***

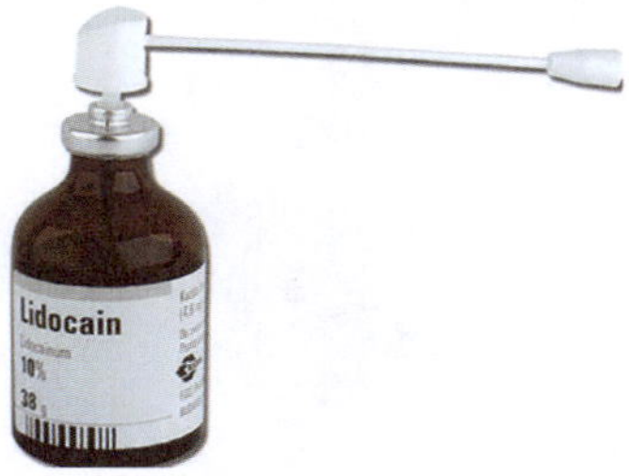

a. Endotracheal intubation
b. NG tube insertion
c. Oral procedures
d. All of these

89. Identify this instrument.

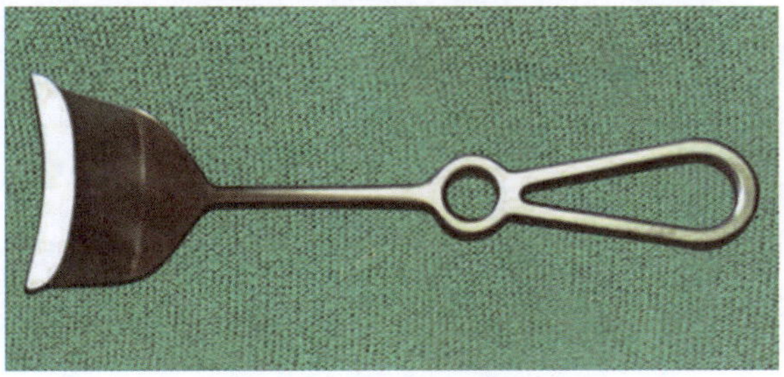

a. Jolly's retractor
b. Morris retractor
c. Langenback retractor
d. Thompson liver retractor

90. Identify the name of the tube.

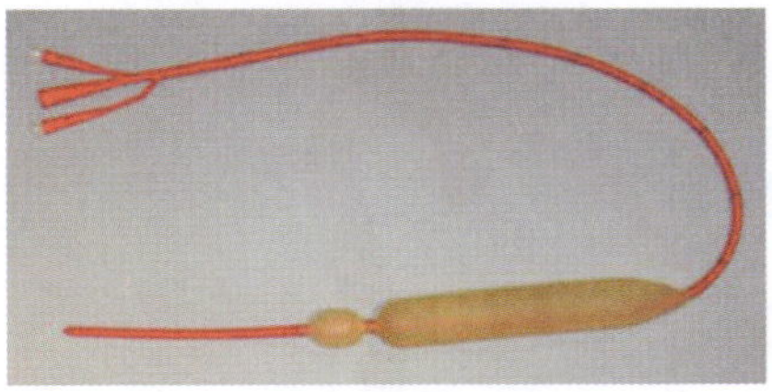

a. Freka tube
b. Nasogastric tube
c. Sengstaken Blakemore tube
d. Linton Blakmore tube

91. Identify the equipment.

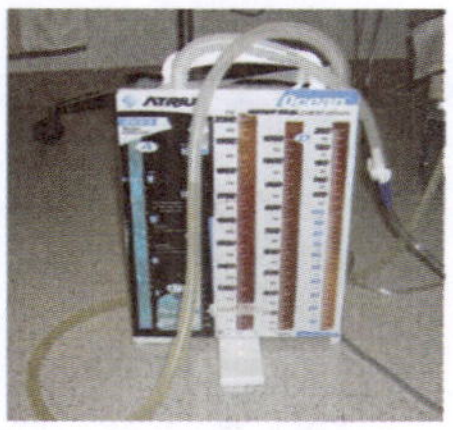

a. Chest tube drainage system
b. Penrose drainage system
c. Surgery wound drainage
d. Tru-close drainage system

92. Identify the PR interval in the given ECG strip.

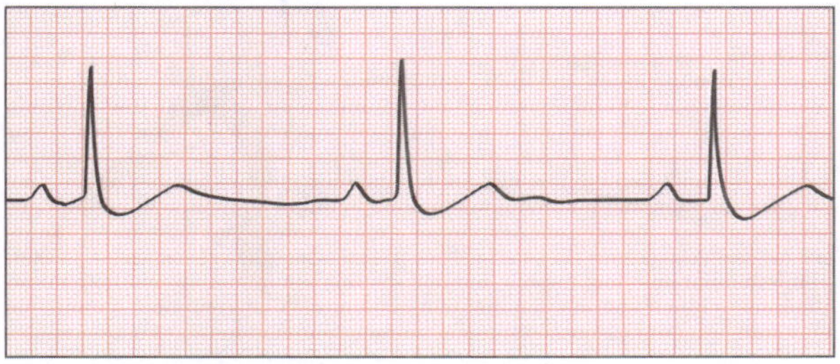

a. 0.12
b. 0.18
c. 0.24
d. 0.40

93. What is the name of this catheter?

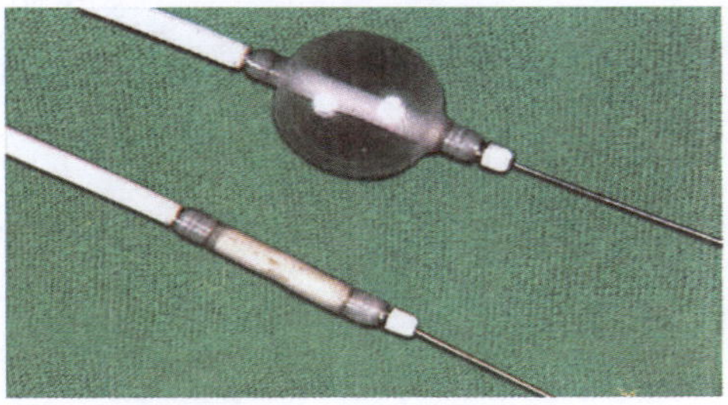

a. Foley
b. Malecot
c. Seldinger
d. Fogarty

94. Identify the procedure performed in the given picture: ***(Refer explanation at the end)***

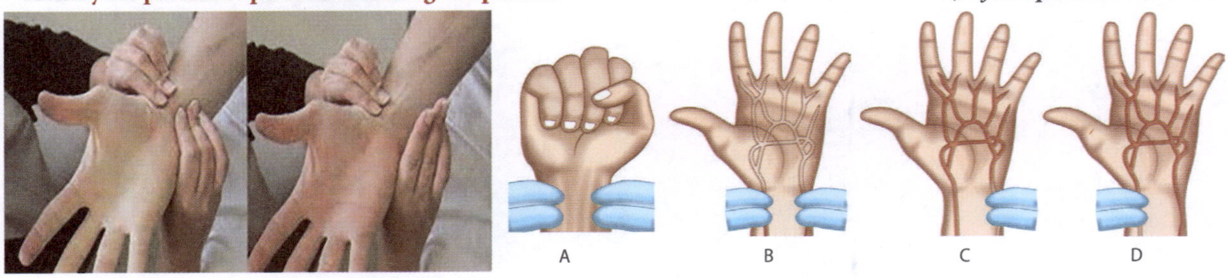

a. Perfusion index test
b. Allen's test
c. LEAT test
d. None of these

Ans.

88.	d
89.	b
90.	c
91.	a
92.	d
93.	d
94.	b

95. Identify the procedure.

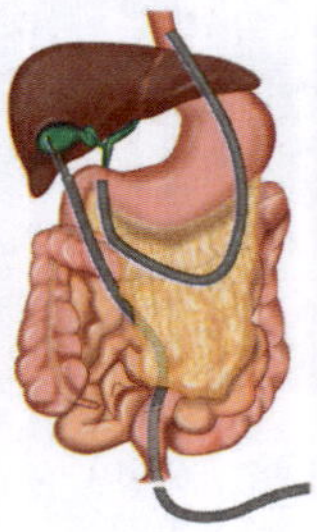

a. Endoscopy
b. Laparoscopy
c. NOTES
d. VATS

99. Identify the testicular structure (arrow) shown in the photograph:

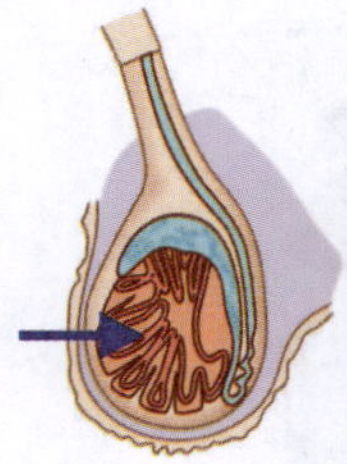

a. Vas deferens
b. Rete testes
c. Seminiferous tubules
d. Epididymis

96. Use of instrument shown in the photograph is:

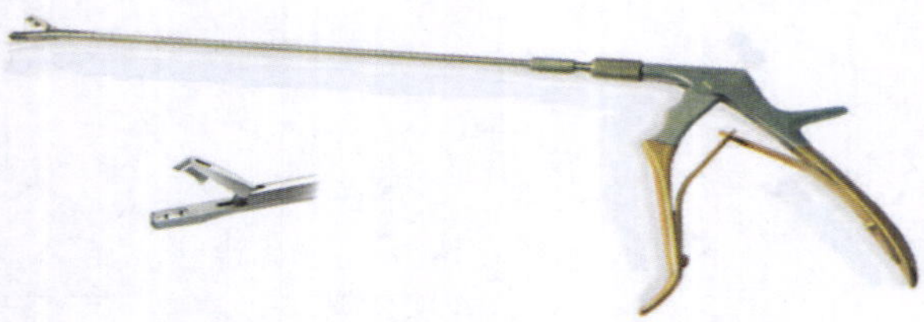

a. Pap smear
b. Cervical dilation
c. Punch biopsy
d. Curetting

100. Condition (arrow) shown in photograph is due to:

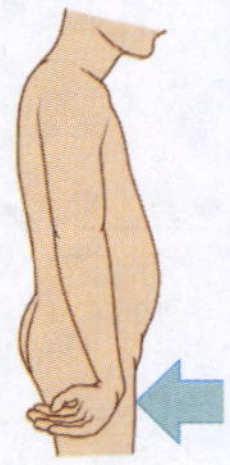

a. Klumpke's paralysis
b. Erb's palsy
c. Long thoracic nerve palsy
d. Thoracic outlet syndrome

97. Identify the device/instrument shown in the photograph:

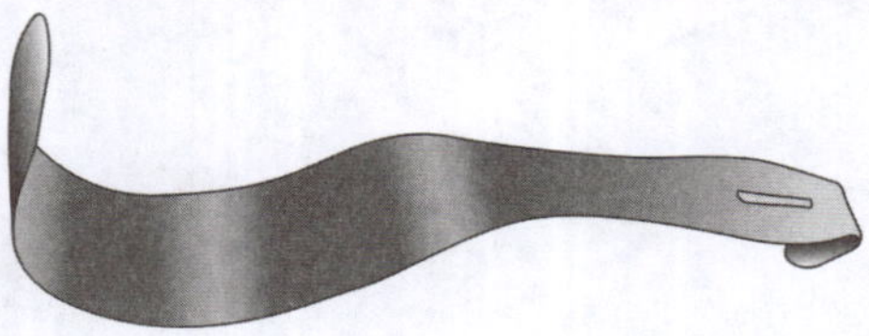

a. Doyen's retractor
b. Deaver retractor
c. Anterior vaginal wall retractor
d. HSG cannula

101. Identify the blood vessel (arrow) shown in photograph:

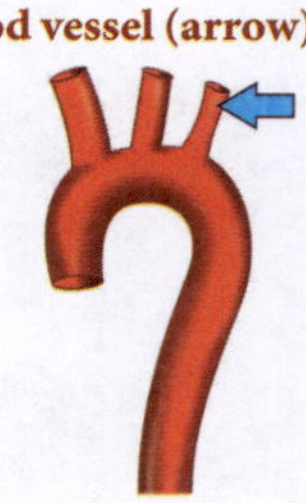

a. Brachiocephalic artery
b. Left common carotid artery
c. Left subclavian artery
d. Right subclavian artery

98. Identify the device/instrument shown in the photograph:

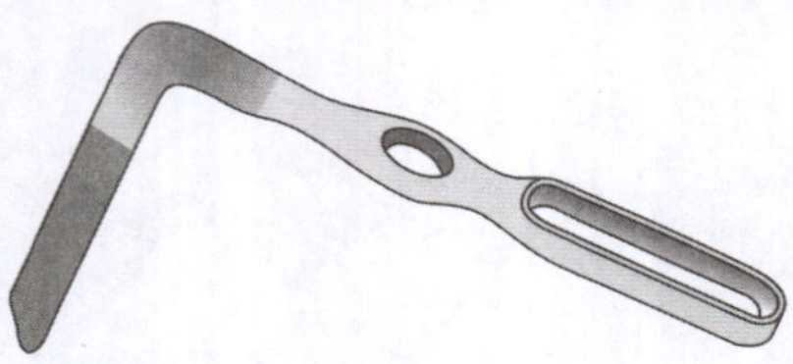

a. Doyen's retractor
b. Landon's retractor
c. Anterior vaginal wall retractor
d. Carman's suction cannula

102. Weight of Organ (Blue arrow) as shown in photograph is:

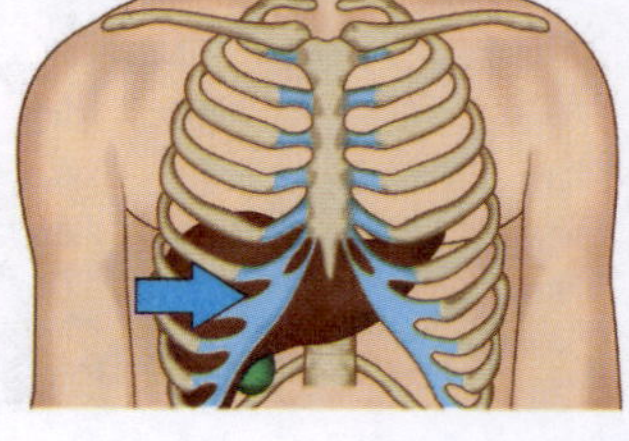

a. 600 – 800 grams
b. 1000 – 1200 grams
c. 1400 – 1600 grams
d. 1800 – 2000 grams

Ans.

95. c
96. c
97. b
98. b
99. c
100. b
101. c
102. c

103. Structure (Box) shown in photograph develops from:

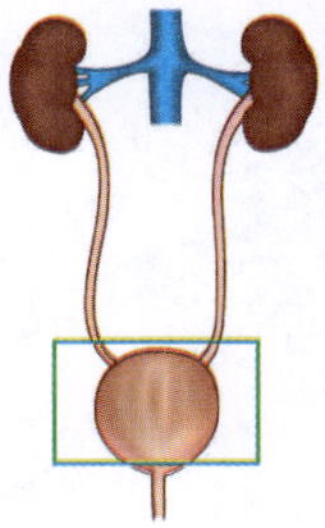

a. Endoderm b. Ectoderm
c. Tubule cell d. Neural crest cells

104. Structure shown in photograph develops from:

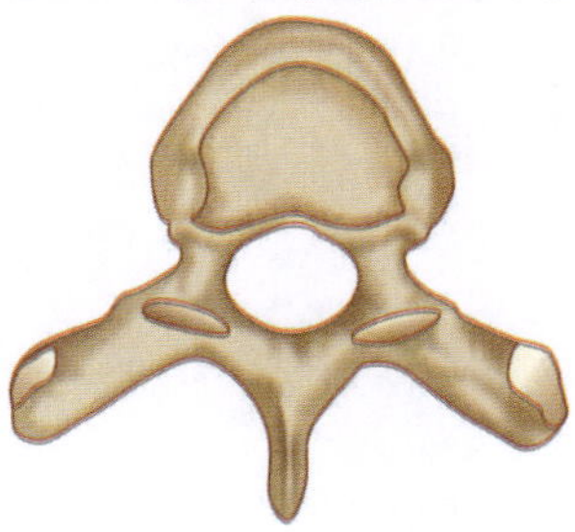

a. Endoderm b. Ectoderm
c. Somite d. None

105. The name of the bones which is shaded red in the image is:

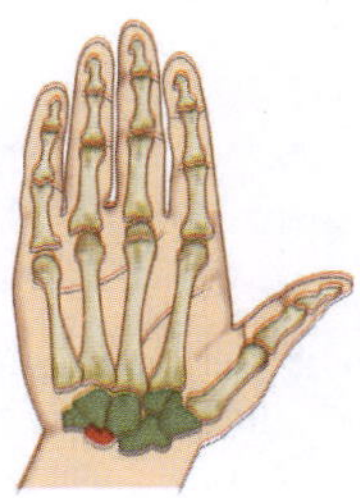

a. Scaphoid b. Lunate
c. Hamate d. Capitate

106. Complex shown in the photograph is due to:

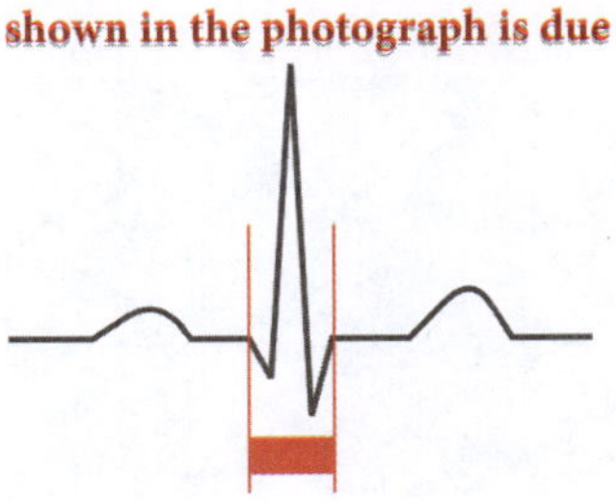

a. Atrial depolarization
b. Conduction through AV node
c. Ventricular depolarization
d. Ventricular repolarization

107. S2 shown in the photograph is due to:

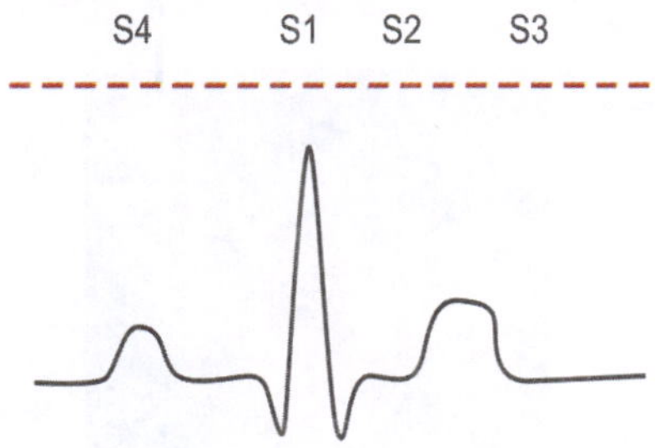

a. Atrial contraction b. Right ventricular filling
c. Inthrushing of blood d. Closure of Aortic valve

108. Atrial depolarization in ECG is represented by:

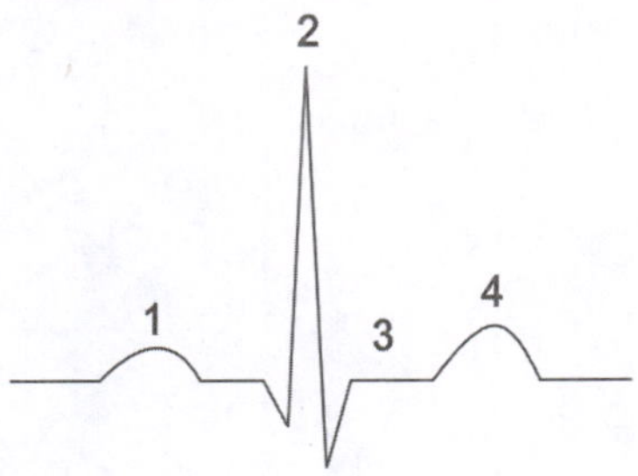

a. 1 b. 2
c. 3 d. 4

109. Normal value of interval shown in the photograph is:

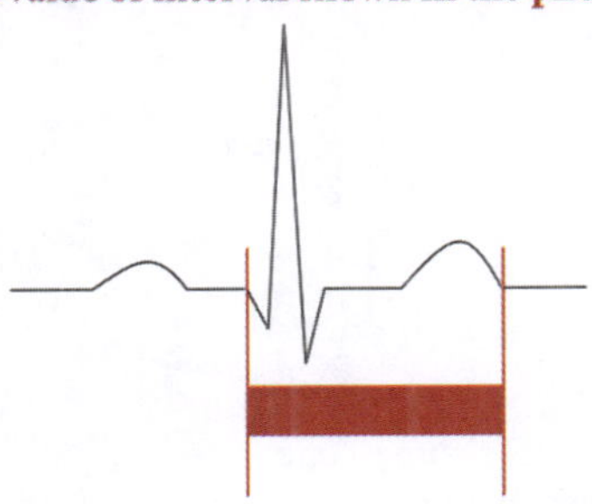

a. 0.12 – 0.20 seconds b. 0.08 – 0.12 seconds
c. 0.40 – 0.45 seconds d. 0.80 – 0.95 seconds

110. In the photograph of organ shown, arrows represent sites of:

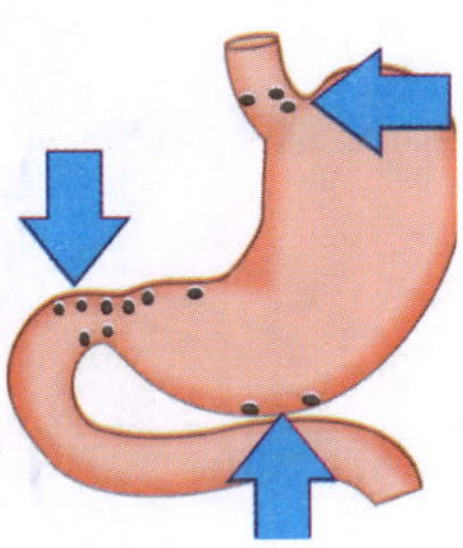

a. Gastric carcinoma b. Gastric ulceration
c. Fat absorption d. Pepsin production

Ans.

103. a
104. c
105. b
106. c
107. d
108. a
109. c
110. b

111. Deficiency causing manifestation (arrows) shown in photograph:

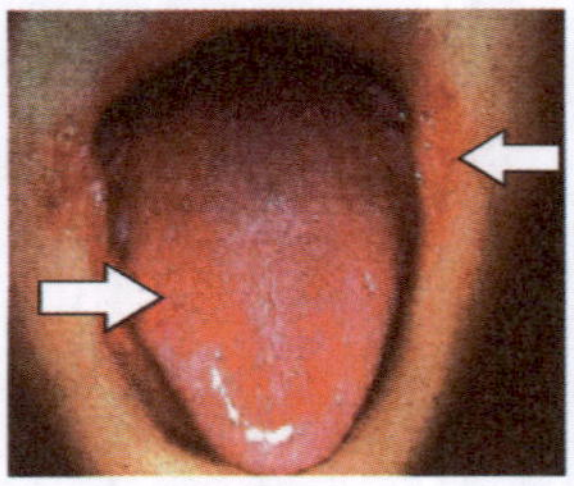

a. Vitamin Thiamine
b. Vitamin Riboflavin
c. Vitamin Niacin
d. Vitamin Ascorbic acid

112. The skin condition shown in the image is known as:

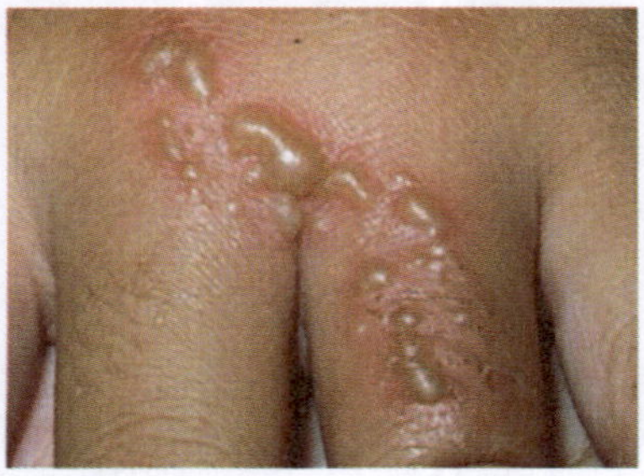

a. Ecchymosis
b. Blisters
c. Psoriasis
d. Warts

113. Identify the instrument shown in the photograph:

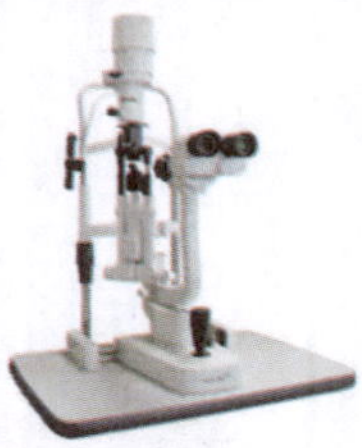

a. Direct Ophthalmoscope
b. Indirect Ophthalmoscope
c. Retinoscope
d. Slit lamp

114. Identify the instrument shown in the photograph:

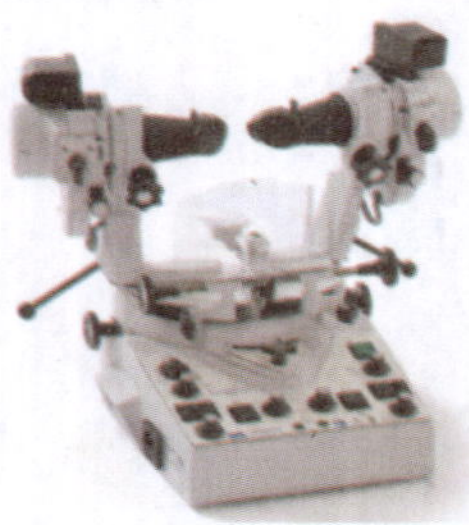

a. Slit lamp microscopy
b. Synoptophore
c. Indirect ophthalmoscope
d. Hess screen

115. Instrument shown in the photograph is used for measurement of:

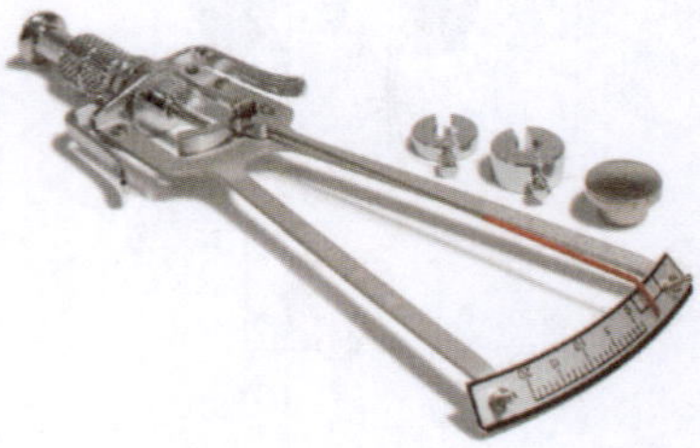

a. Corneal diameter
b. Visual field
c. Visual acuity
d. Intraocular pressure

116. Identify the instrument shown in the photograph:

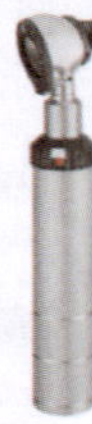

a. Siegel's pneumatic speculum
b. Rhinoscope
c. Otoscope
d. Laryngoscope

117. Identify the instrument shown in the photograph:

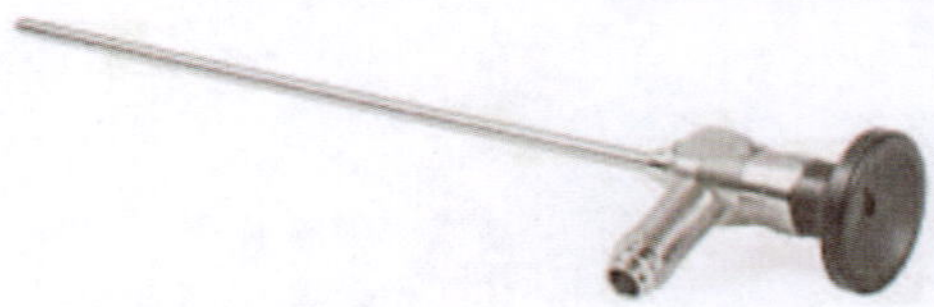

a. Frazier's straight Suction tube
b. Nasal Hopkin endoscope
c. Atomizer
d. Tilley antral trocar and cannula

118. Device shown in the image is used for:

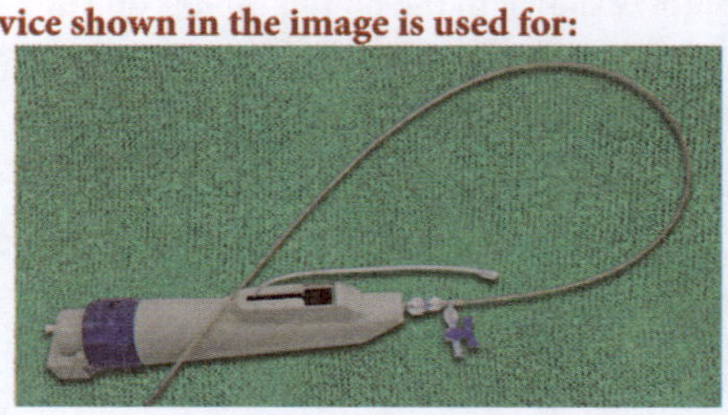

a. Stomach irrigation
b. Angiogram
c. Thrombectomy
d. Insertion of cardiac pacemaker

Ans.

111. b
112. b
113. d
114. b
115. d
116. c
117. b
118. c

119. Identify the type of hearing aid device shown in photograph:

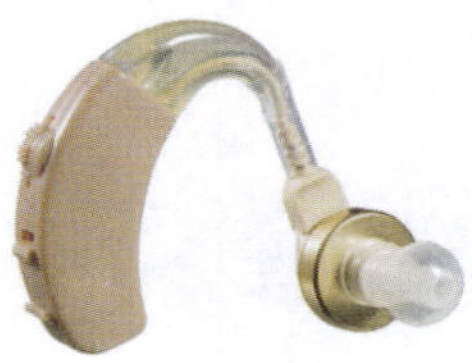

a. Body-worn hearing aid
b. Behind-the-ear hearing aid
c. Eyeglass integrated hearing aid
d. In-the-ear hearing aid

120. Identify the condition of oral cavity shown in the photograph:

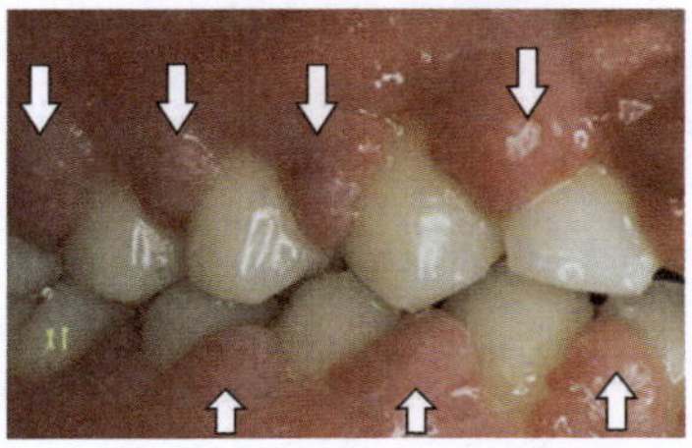

a. Reparative granuloma
b. Gingival hyperplasia
c. Hemangioma
d. Papilloma

121. Diagnose the underlying medical disorder by ECG change in photograph:

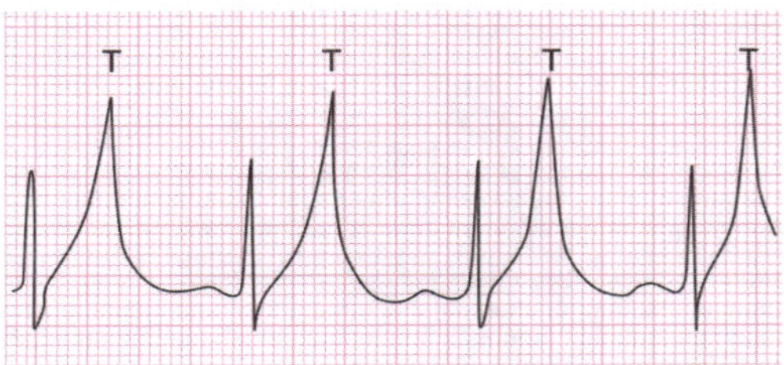

a. Hypokalemia
b. Hyperkalemia
c. Hypercalcemia
d. Hypocalcemia

122. Diagnose the underlying medical disorder by ECG change in photograph:

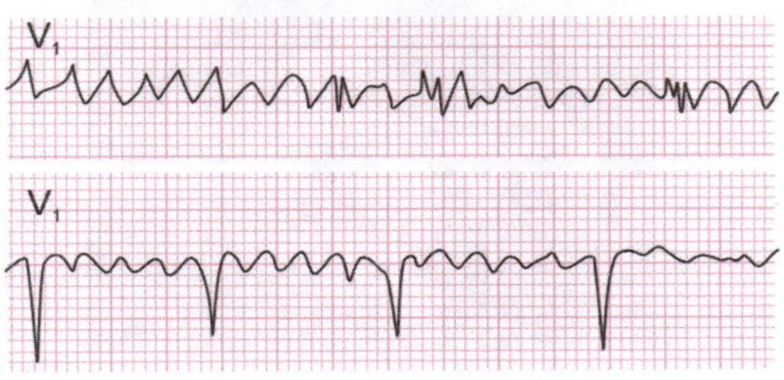

a. Sinus arrhythmia
b. Atrial flutter
c. Atrial fibrillation
d. AV block

123. Diagnose the underlying medical disorder by ECG change in photograph:

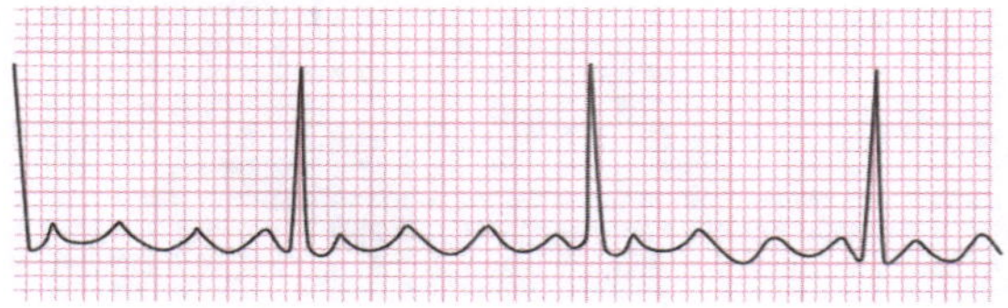

a. Sinus arrhythmia
b. Atrial flutter
c. Atrial fibrillation
d. AV block

124. Identify the ECG type shown in the photograph:

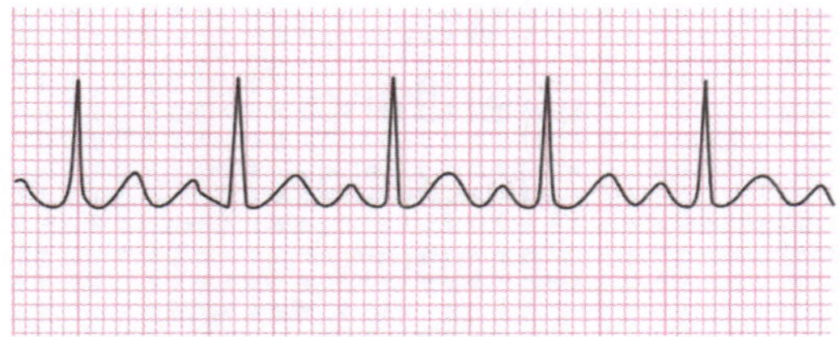

a. P-mitrale
b. Sinus tachycardia
c. Atrial ectopics
d. PSVT

125. Best line of management of condition shown in photograph is:

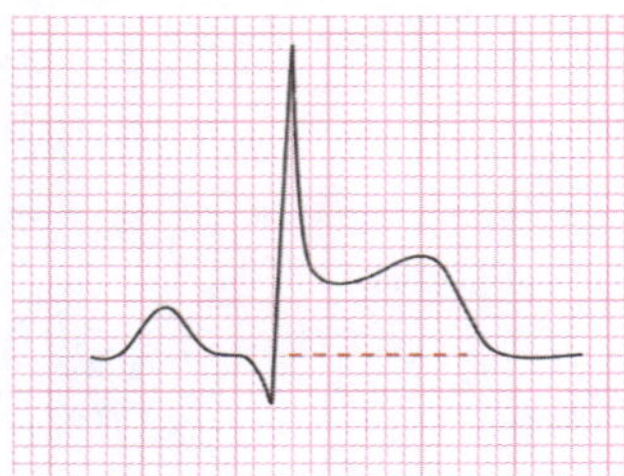

a. IABP
b. Vasopressors
c. Reperfusion therapy
d. Thrombolysis

126. Most common cause of the Aortic condition as shown in the photograph is:

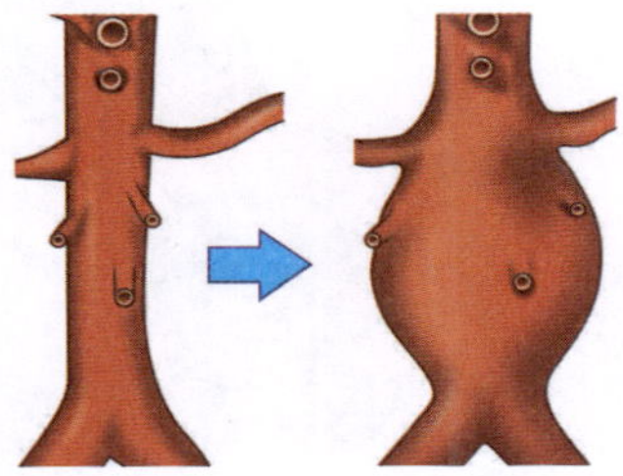

a. Idiopathic
b. Trauma
c. Atherosclerosis
d. Arteriosclerosis

Ans.

119. b
120. b
121. b
122. c
123. b
124. b
125. c
126. c

127. Contraindication for procedure shown in the photograph:

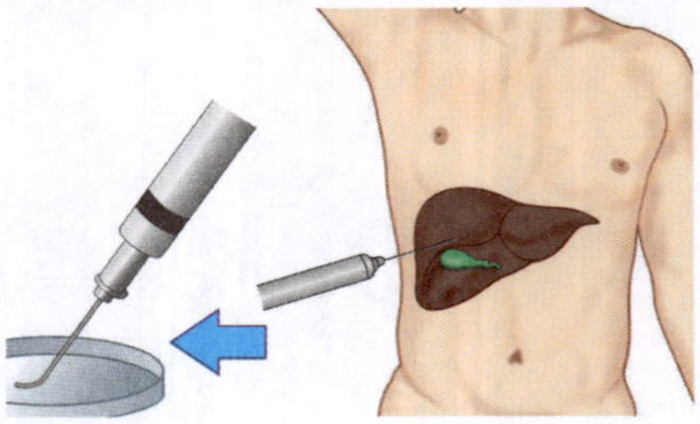

a. Wilson's disease b. Autoimmune Hepatitis
c. Hemangioma d. Chronic Hepatitis B & C

128. Primary survey shown in photograph is mainly used for:

Airway
Breathing
Circulation
Disability
Exposure

a. Post-operative care b. Pre-operative care
c. Trauma care d. Immunization care

129. Identify the condition shown in the photograph:

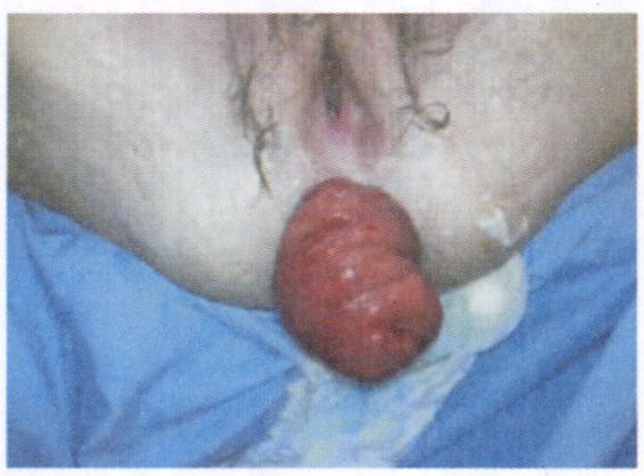

a. Perianal abscess b. Fistula in ano
c. Rectal prolapse d. Rectal cancer

130. Identify the surgical procedure shown in photograph:

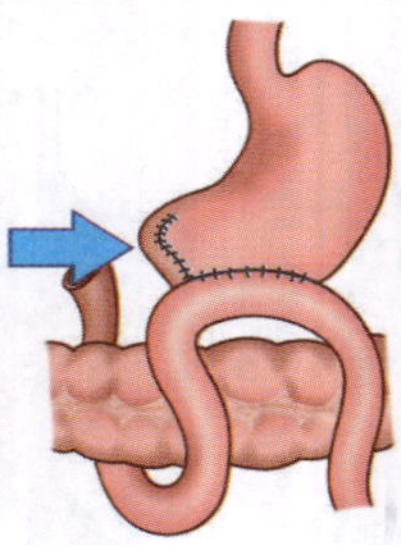

a. Billroth I gastrectomy b. Billroth II gastrectomy
c. Gastroenterostomy d. Truncal vagotomy

131. Identify the device shown in the photograph:

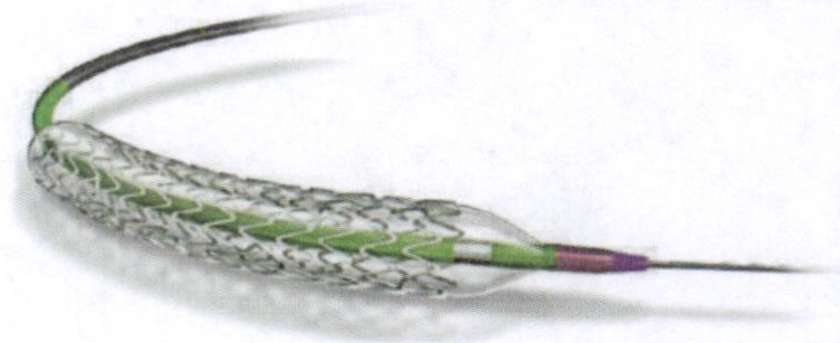

a. Vascular ring connector
b. Cardiac pacemaker
c. Cardiac shunt
d. Coronary stent

132. Identify the type of traction shown in the photograph:

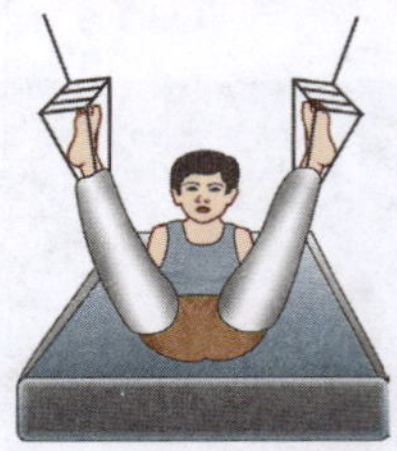

a. Hamilton Russell traction
b. Gallows traction
c. Buck's traction
d. Balanced skeletal traction

133. Identify the type of traction shown in the photograph:

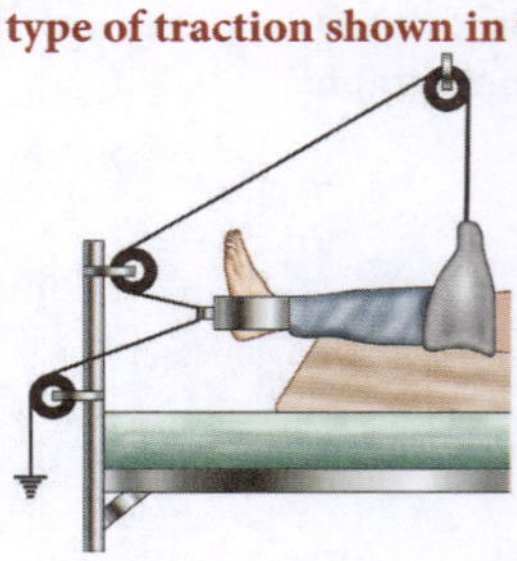

a. Hamilton Russell traction b. Gallows traction
c. Buck's traction
d. Balanced skeletal traction

134. Deformity shown in photograph is characteristic of:

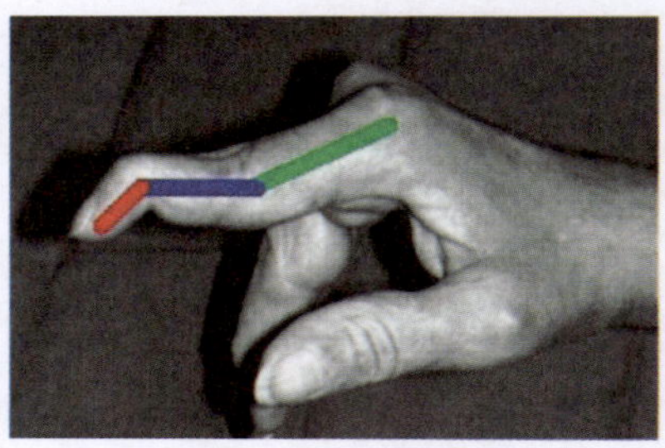

a. Osteoarthritis b. Rheumatoid arthritis
c. Ankylosing spondylitis d. Psoriatic arthritis

Ans.

127. c
128. c
129. c
130. b
131. d
132. b
133. a
134. b

135. The condition shown in the image is known as:

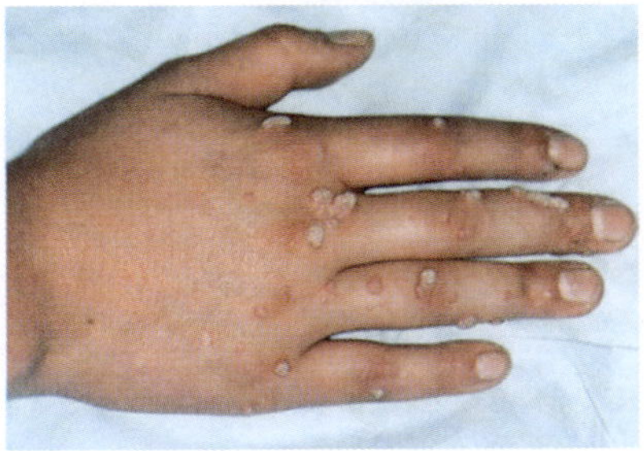

a. Warts
b. Psoriasis
c. Blisters
d. Mole

136. What is the use of the instrument shown below?

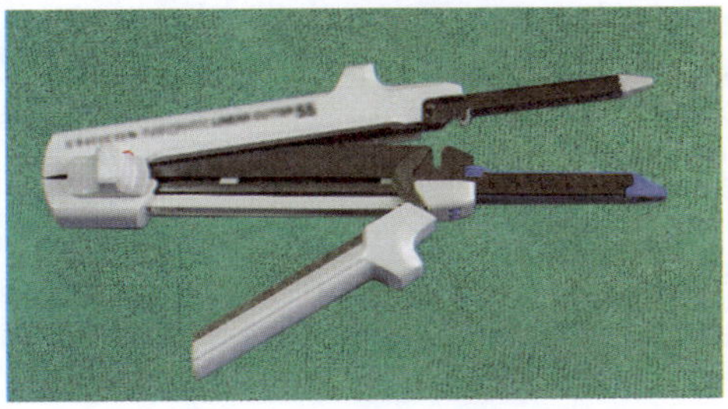

a. Intestinal anastomosis
b. Vascular anastomosis
c. Neurosurgery
d. Urology surgery

137. What is the instrument shown below?

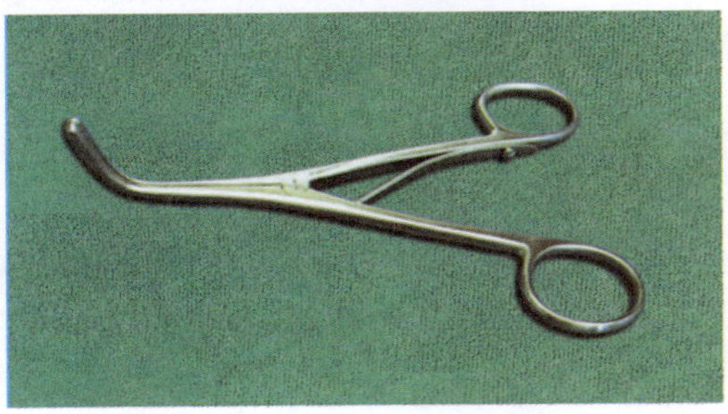

a. Urethral dilator
b. Tracheal dilator
c. Aneurysm needle
d. Urethral dilator

138. What is the instrument shown below?

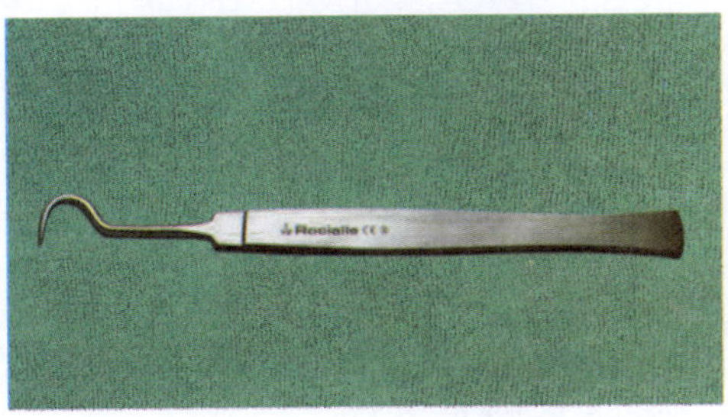

a. Aneurysm needle
b. Veress needle
c. Trucut biopsy needle
d. Cobbler needle

139. What is the use of the instrument shown here?

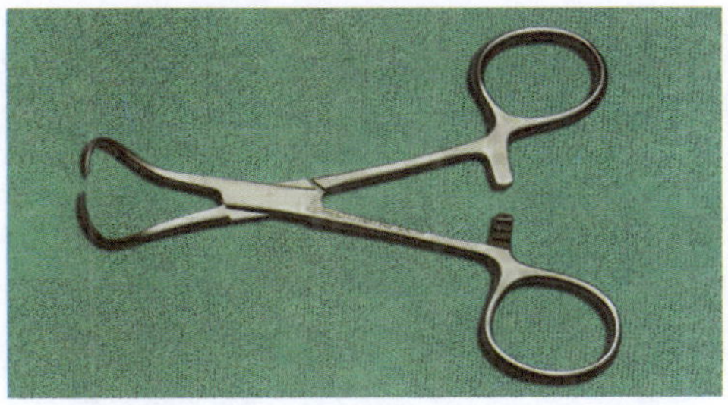

a. To catch bleeding artery
b. Occlude bowel
c. Vascular clamp
d. Clip the towel

140. What is the use of the clamp shown in the image below?

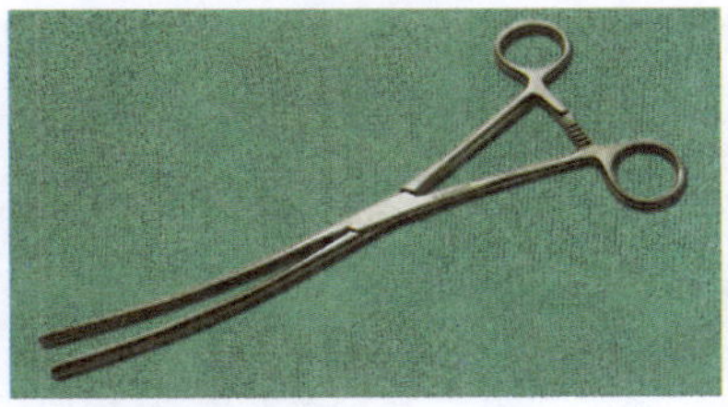

a. Soft occlusion of bowel
b. Crush occlusion of bowel
c. Used to stop bleeding vessels
d. Used to retract

141. The skin condition shown in the picture is known as:

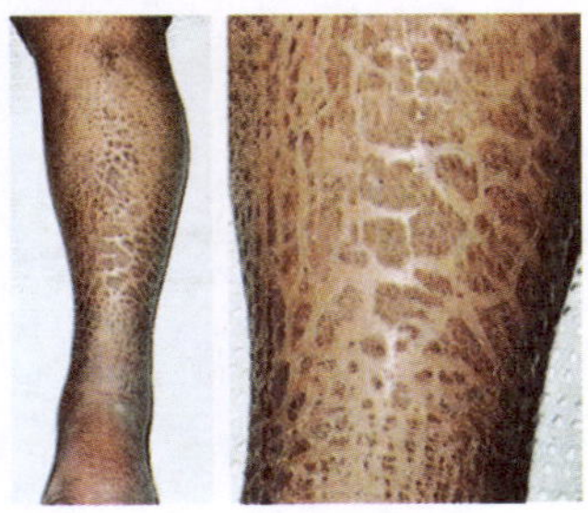

a. Ecchymosis
b. Ichthyosis
c. Warts
d. Petechiae

142. Identify the instrument/device shown in photograph:

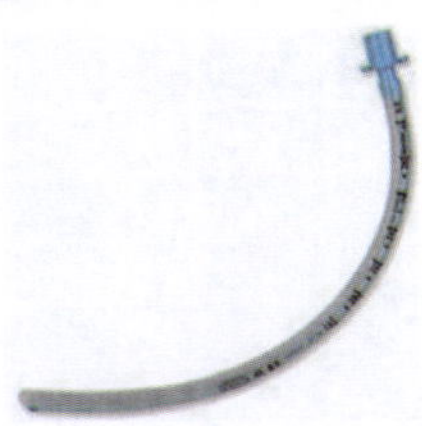

a. Uncuffed Endotracheal tube
b. Cuffed Endotracheal tube
c. Endotracheal tube Double lumen
d. Water's airway

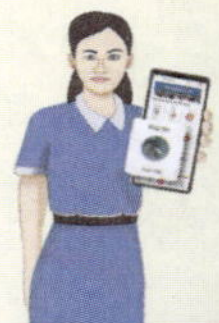

Ans.

135. a
136. a
137. b
138. a
139. d
140. a
141. b
142. a

143. Identify the instrument:

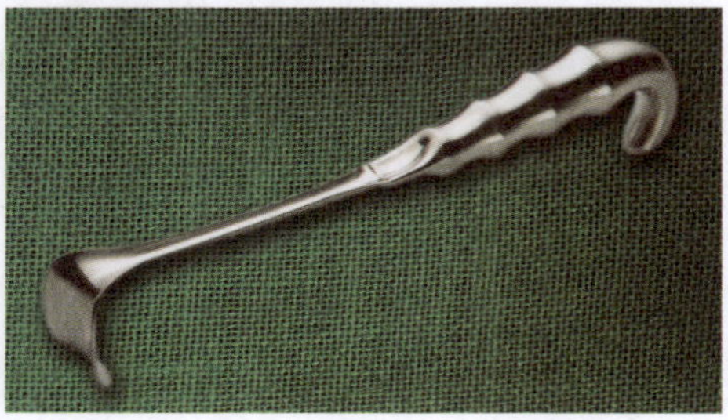

a. Kelly retractor
b. Doyen retractor
c. Deaver retractor
d. Harrington retractor

144. Identify the instrument:

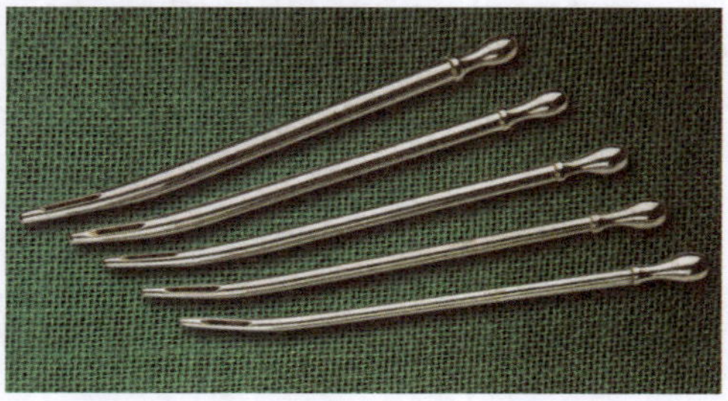

a. Female urethral sound
b. Hang dilators
c. Hegar dilators
d. Uterine dilators

145. The given instrument is commonly used for:

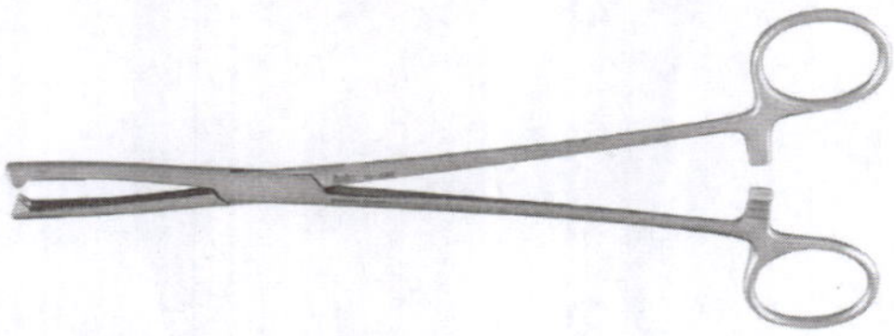

a. D & C
b. Vaginal hysterectomy
c. Both
d. None of the above

146. The given instruments are used during:

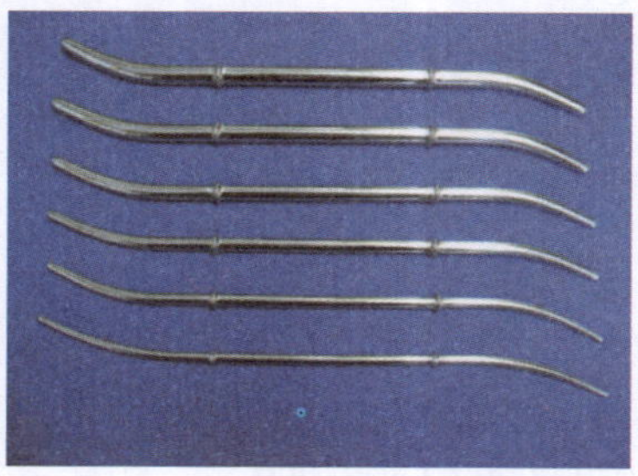

a. D & C
b. S & C
c. D & E
d. All of the above

147. Identify the given instrument:

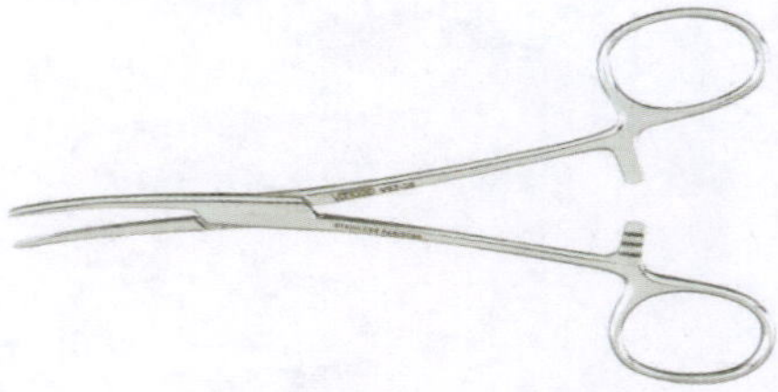

a. Halstead head forceps
b. Kelly forceps
c. Crile forceps
d. None of the above

148. The given instrument is commonly used to hold:

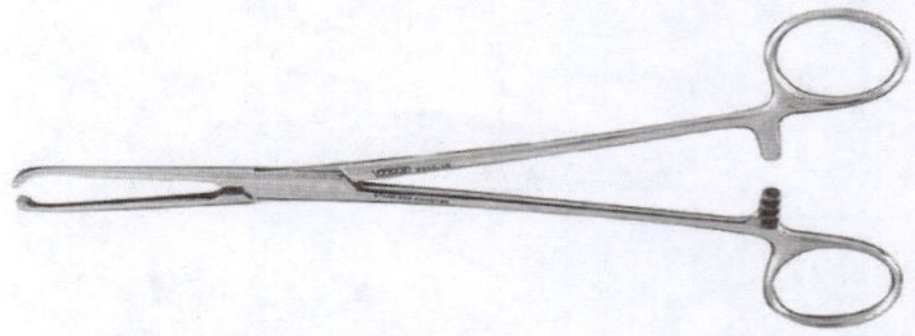

a. Tonsils
b. Ovaries
c. Ureters
d. Appendix

149. The given instrument is used for providing exposure for visualization of:

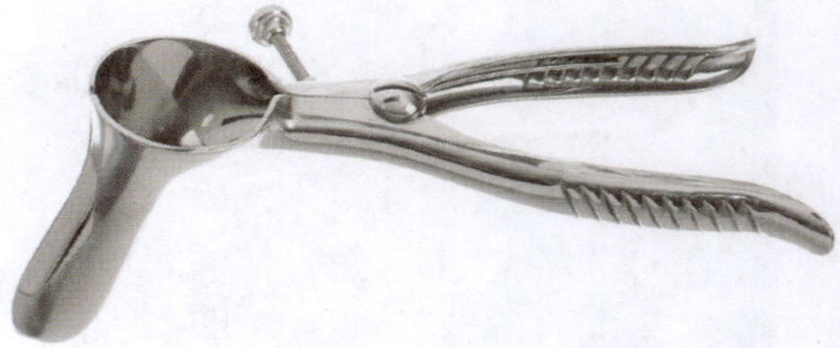

a. Vagina
b. Uterus
c. Rectum
d. None of the above

150. What does the following ECG indicates?

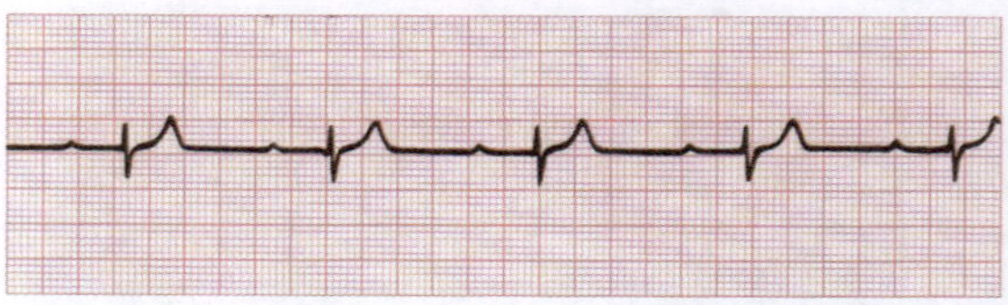

a. Complete heart block
b. First degree heart block
c. Second degree heart block
d. Third degree heart block

Ans.

143. a
144. a
145. c
146. d
147. b
148. a
149. a
150. b

151. What does the following ECG indicate?

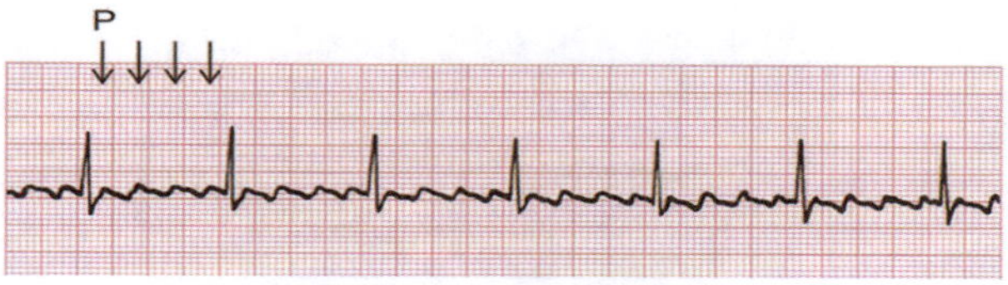

a. Atrial flutter
b. Atrial tachycardia
c. Ventricular tachycardia
d. Functional tachycardia

152. Interpret the following ECG.

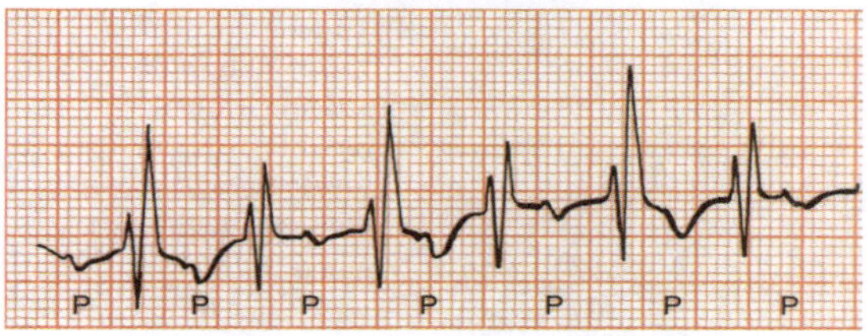

a. Paroxysmal atrial tachycardia
b. Multifocal atrial tachycardia
c. Atrial flutter
d. PSVT

153. Interpret the following ECG.

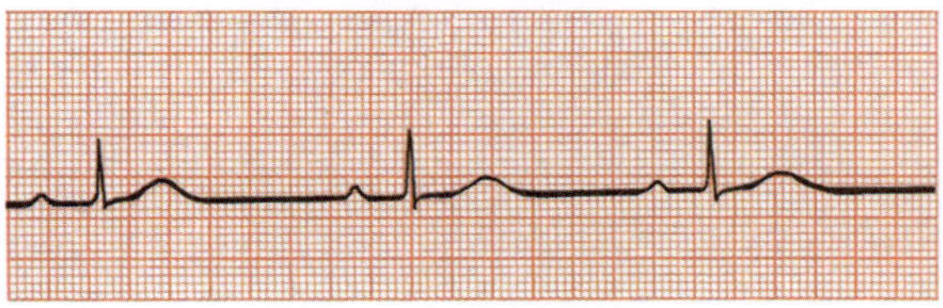

a. Sinus arrest
b. Normal sinus rhythm
c. Sinus tachycardia
d. Sinus bradycardia

154. What does ST elevation suggest?

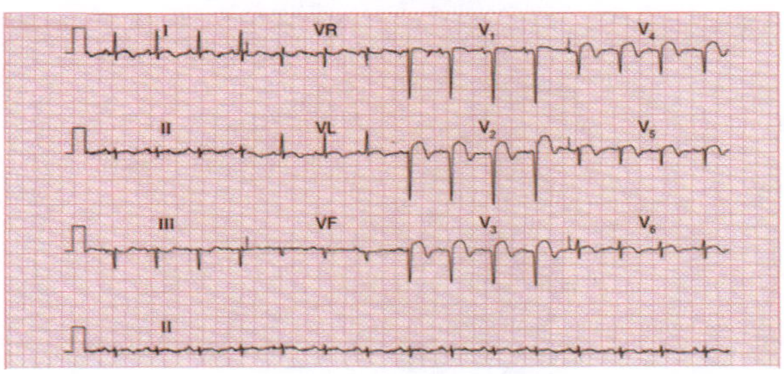

a. Bundle branch block
b. Myocardial infarction
c. Heat murmur
d. Heart block-Mobitz type

155. Most common Fracture site of the bone shown in photograph is:

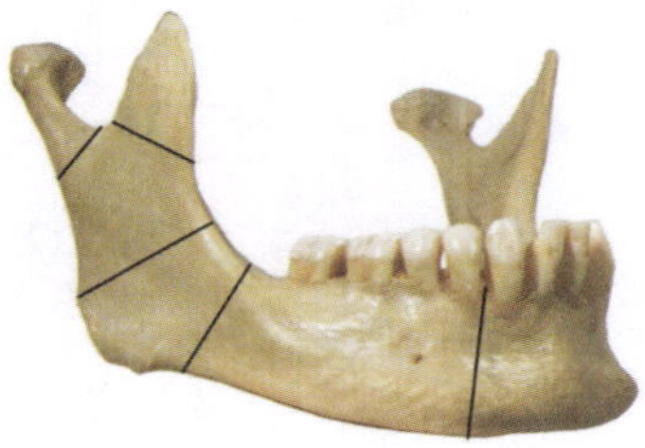

a. Condyle
b. Angle
c. Mandible
d. Coronoid process

156. Type of Graft shown in photograph is:

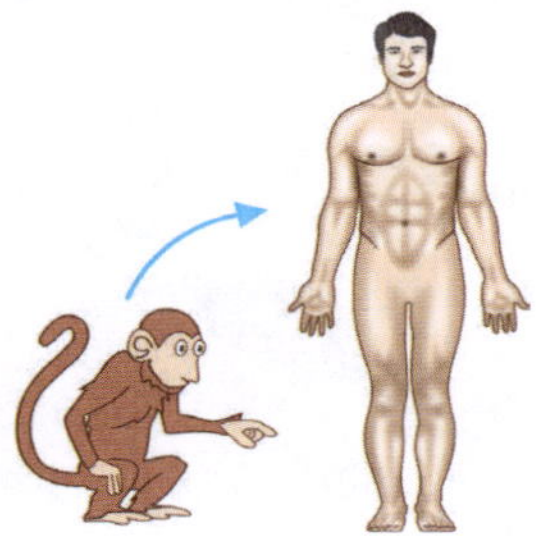

a. Isograft
b. Autograft
c. Allograft
d. Xenograft

157. Identify the fluid bag shown here:

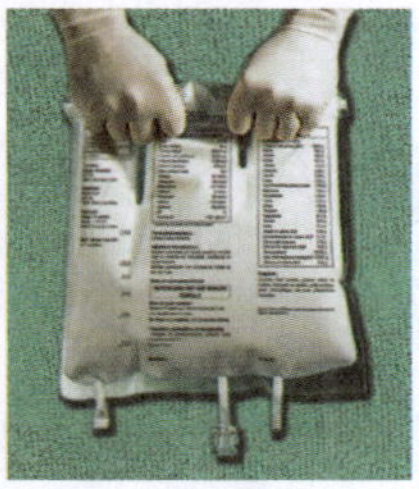

a. Jejunostomy bag with milk
b. Albumin
c. TPN
d. Astymin

158. Identify the condition depicted in the figure:

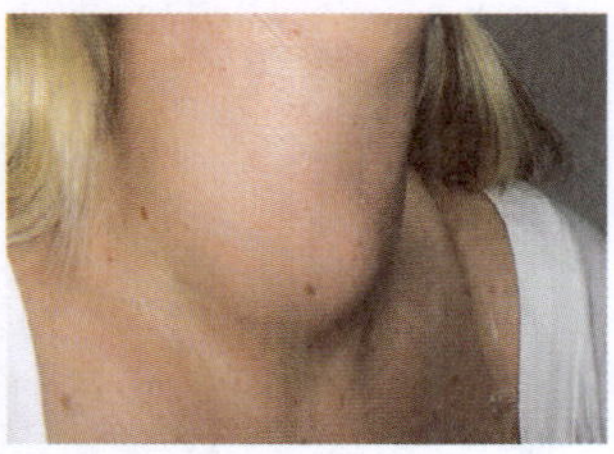

a. Goiter
b. Submandibular lymph node enlargement
c. Ludwig's angina
d. Hyoid bone displacement

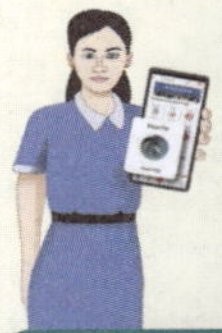

Ans.

151. a
152. a
153. d
154. b
155. a
156. d
157. c
158. a

159. Identify the use of the tube shown here:
(Refer explanation at the end)

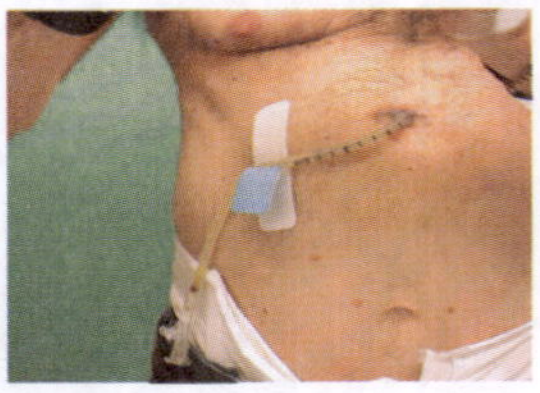

a. Venous cannulation
b. Feeding Gastrostomy by surgery
c. PEG
d. Feeding jejunostomy

160. A 55-year-old male came with complaints of bleeding per rectum, diagnosed to be Carcinoma colon underwent right hemicolectomy. Identify the instrument in the given picture: *(AIIMS Nov 2016)*
(Refer explanation at the end)

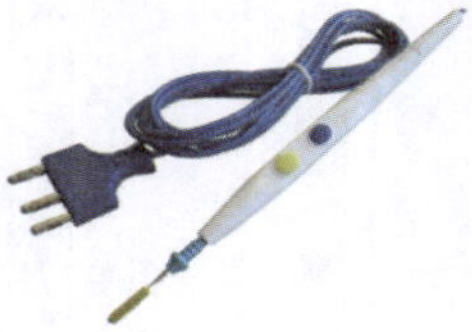

a. Hyfrecator
b. Ligasure vessel ligator
c. Harmonic scalpel
d. Monopolar cautery

161. A patient admitted in casualty after RTA- shows bruising behind the mastoid- This sign is known as:
(Refer explanation at the end)

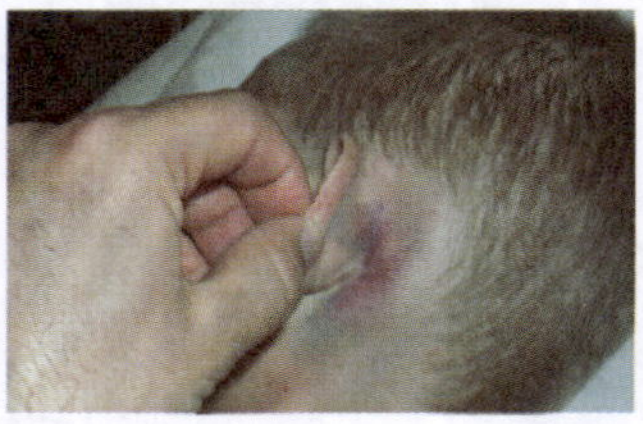

a. Prehn sign
b. Battle sign
c. Catel Sign
d. Dietel's sign

162. Use of the tube shown here:
(Refer explanation at the end)

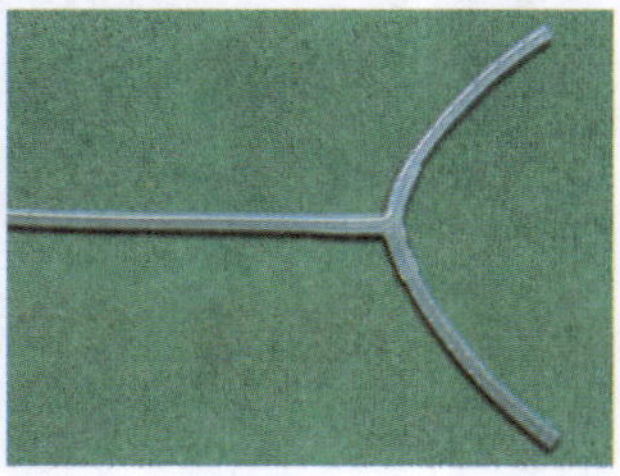

a. CBD drainage
b. Drainage of stomach
c. Feeding jejunostomy
d. Pelvic drain

163. What is the name of this catheter?
(Refer explanation at the end)

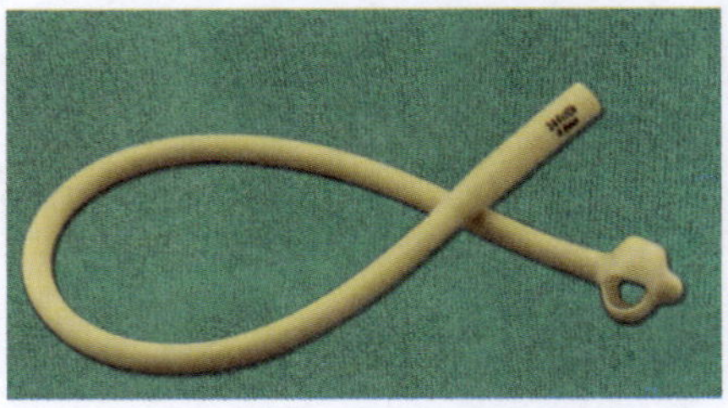

a. Malecot's
b. Foleys
c. Sengstaken
d. Hudd's

164. What is this? *(Refer explanation at the end)*

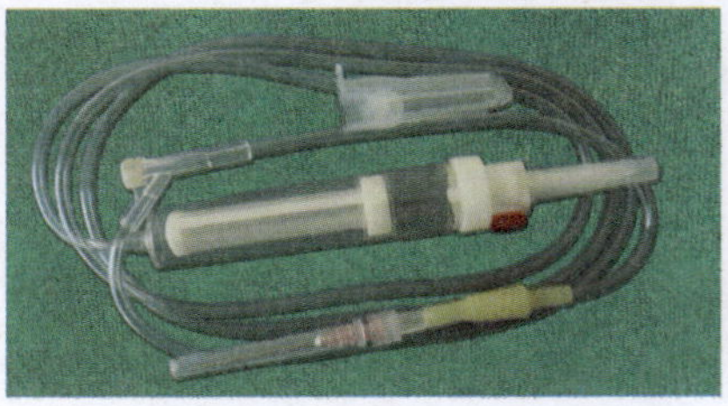

a. Intravenous fluid infusion set
b. Blood set
c. Arterial line
d. CVP line

165. Identify the type of fracture shown in the photograph:
(Refer explanation at the end)

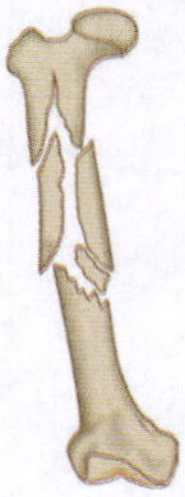

a. Transverse
b. Spiral
c. Oblique
d. Comminuted

166. Identify the deformity shown in the picture:
(Refer explanation at the end)

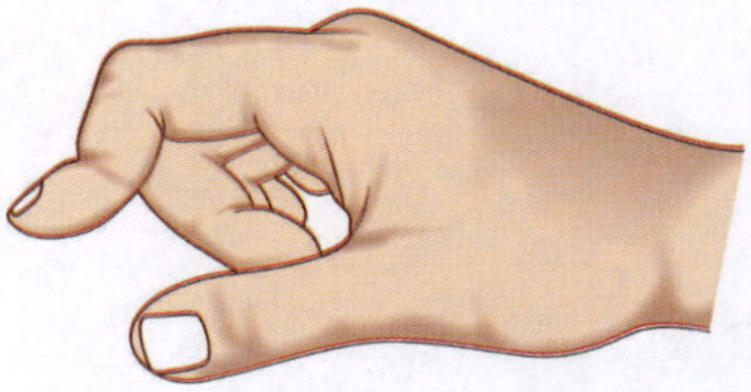

a. Trigger finger
b. Mallet finger
c. Boutonniere deformity
d. Swan neck deformity

Ans.

159. c
160. d
161. b
162. a
163. a
164. b
165. d
166. c

167. Identify the Instrument/device shown in photograph: *(Refer explanation at the end)*

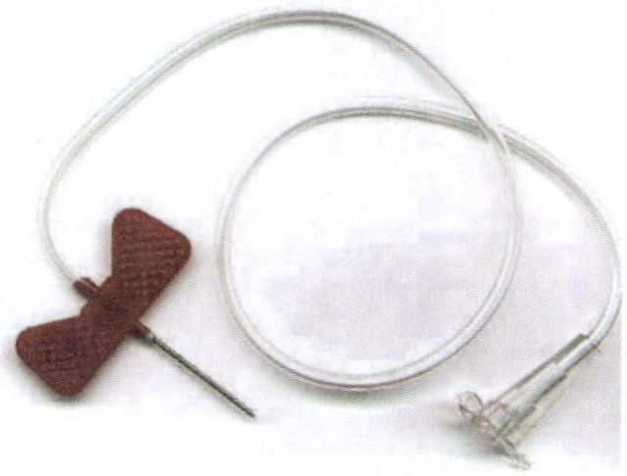

a. IV transfusion set b. IV cannula
c. Scalp vein d. Ryle's tube

168. Sign shown in photograph is pathognomonic of: *(Refer explanation at the end)*

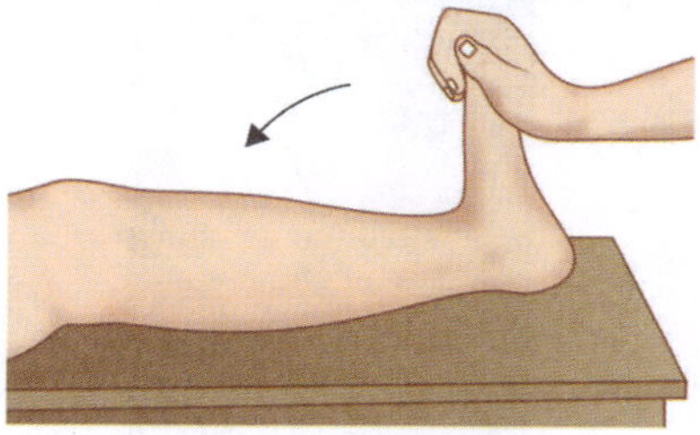

a. Spondylolisthesis b. Spondylosis
c. Deep vein thrombosis d. Peroneal nerve injury

169. Diagnose the knee deformity as shown in the photograph: *(Refer explanation at the end)*

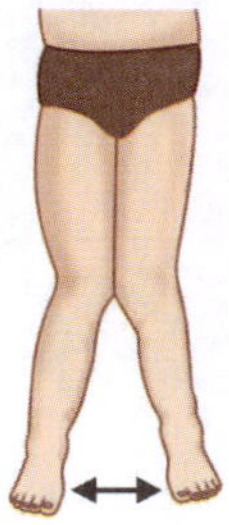

a. Genu varum b. Genu valgum
c. Genu recurvatum d. Clergyman's knee

170. Identify the procedure performed on a patient as shown in photograph: *(Refer explanation at the end)*

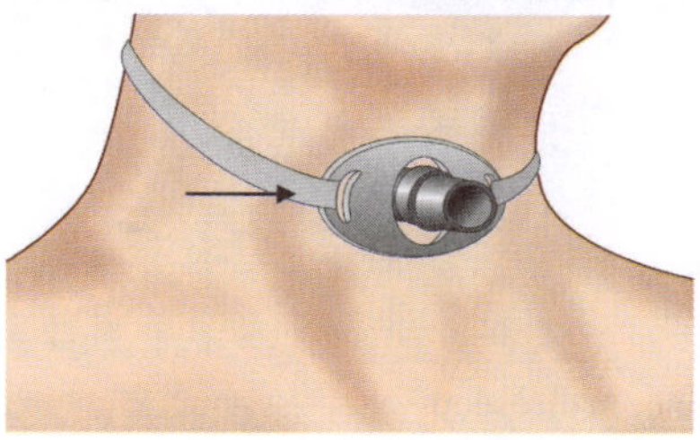

a. Cricothyroidotomy b. Tracheostomy
c. Intubation d. Hyodotomy

171. Identify the refractive error based on the image given below.

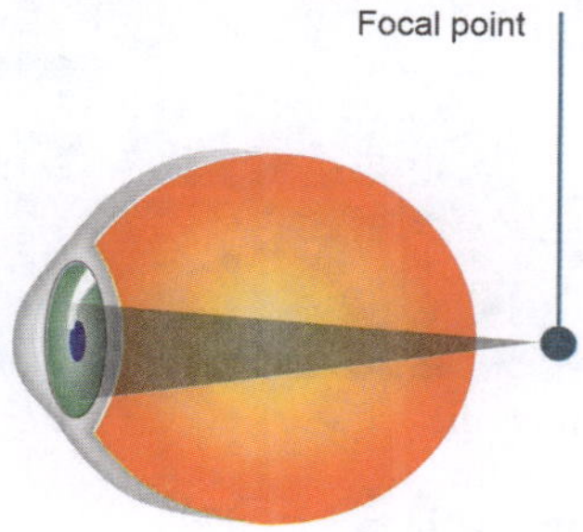

a. Myopia b. Hypermetropia
c. Presbyopia d. Astigmatism

172. Identify the device shown in the picture:

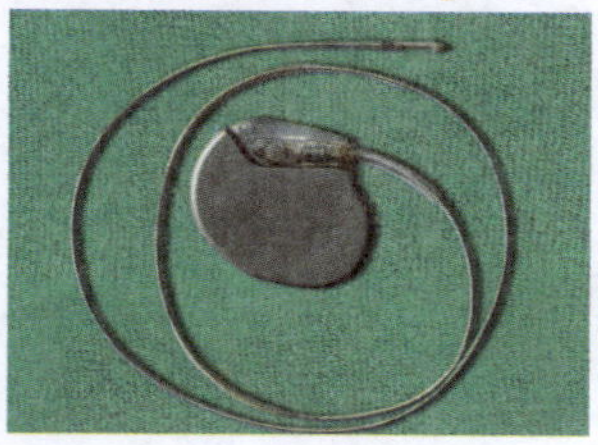

a. Automated External Defibrillator
b. Holter monitor
c. Sustained release drug device
d. Cardiac pacemaker

173. Identify the type of mattress used in this bed:

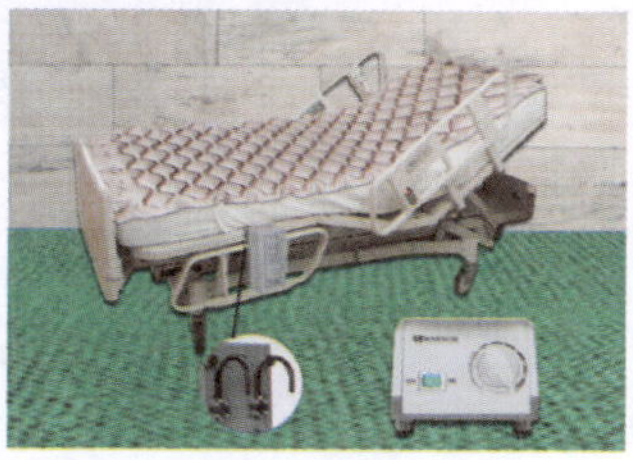

a. Alternating pressure mattress
b. Ripple mattress
c. Alpha mattress
d. All of the above

174. Name the adhesive material placed on the skin:

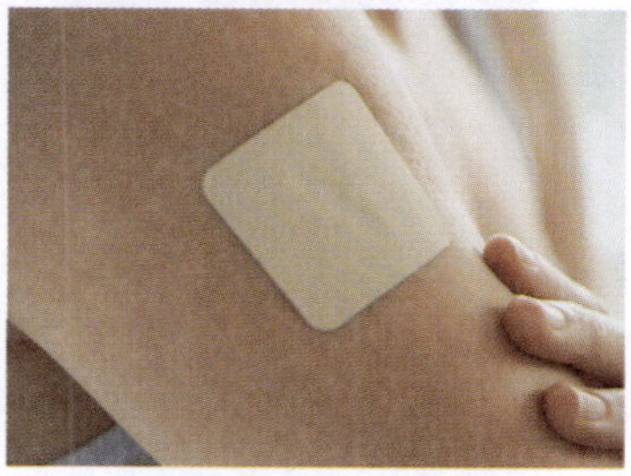

a. Transdermal patch b. Intradermal patch
c. Hair removal patch d. Percutaneous patch

Ans.

167. c
168. c
169. b
170. b
171. c
172. d
173. d
174. a

175. Identify the instrument shown in the image:

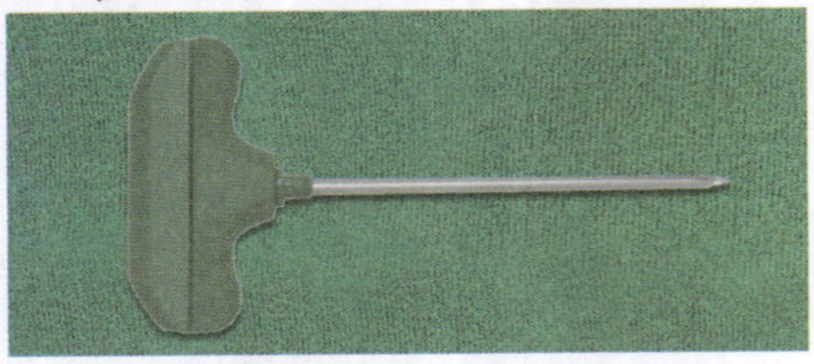

a. Tru-cut needle
b. Chiba needle
c. Bone marrow biopsy needle
d. Core Needle

176. Identify the instrument shown in the image:

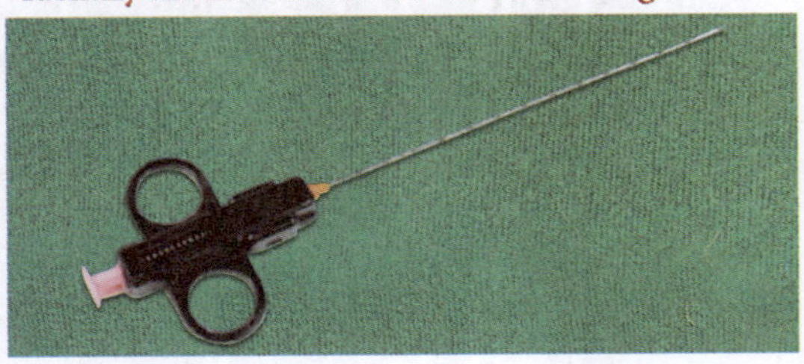

a. Tru-cut needle
b. Chiba needle
c. Bone marrow biopsy needle
d. Core Needle

177. Name of the device shown in the image is:

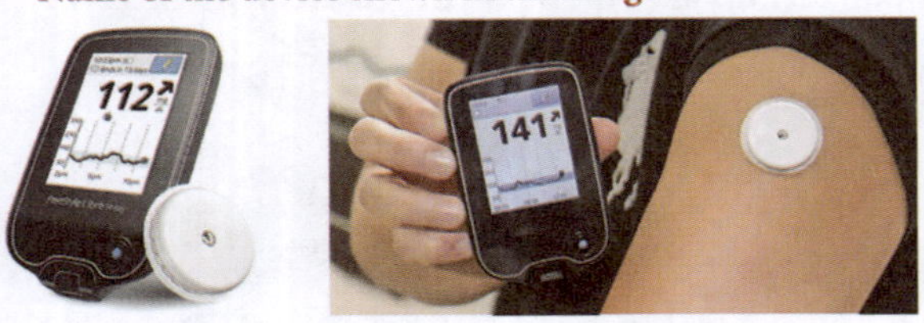

a. Glucometer
b. CGM meter
c. Invasive glucometer
d. Automatic insulin delivery device

178. Which of the following reflex is being examined?

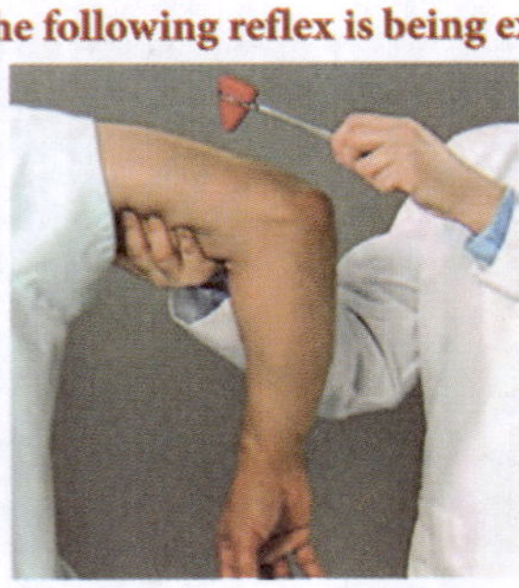

a. Biceps reflex
b. Triceps reflex
c. Elbow reflex
d. Plantar reflex

179. Identify the following bowel disease:

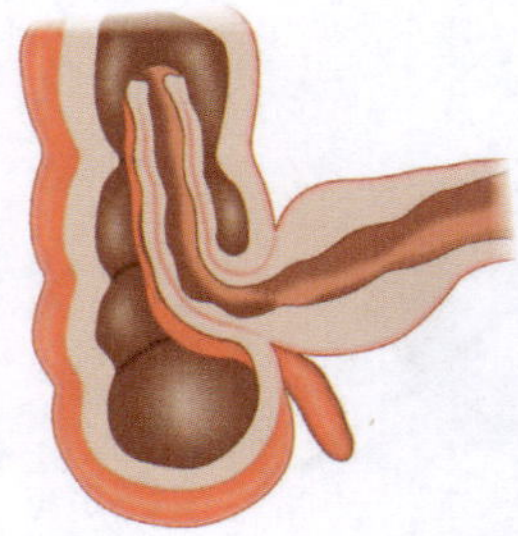

a. Intussusception
b. Hirschsprung disease
c. Crohn's disease
d. Intestinal obstruction

180. Barium enema findings of a one-year-old baby suggests.

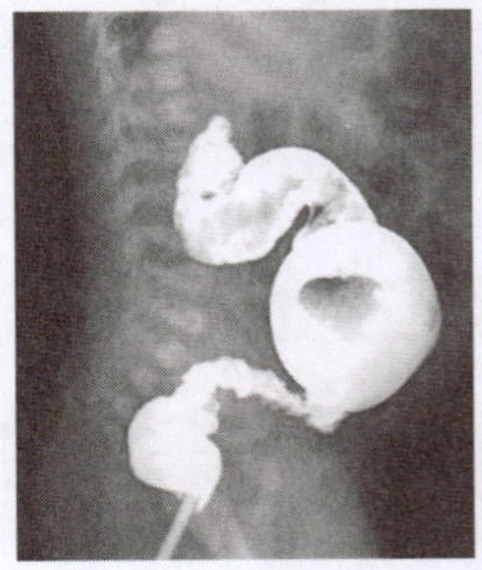

a. Intussusception
b. Hirschsprung disease
c. Crohn's disease
d. Intestinal obstruction

181. The procedure that is being performed in the picture is:

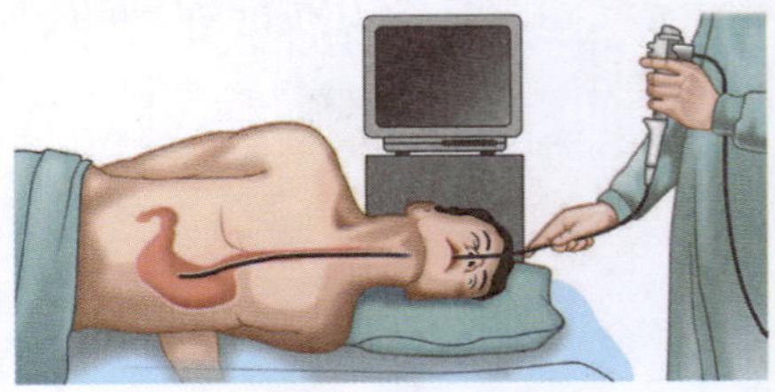

a. Arthroscopy
b. Endoscopy
c. Gastric lavage
d. Gastric gavage

182. The procedure that is being performed in the picture is:

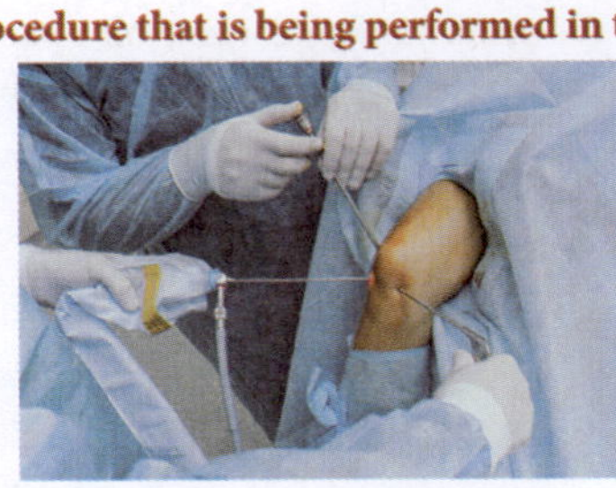

a. Knee arthroscopy
b. Total knee replacement surgery
c. Partial knee replacement surgery
d. Lachman procedure

Ans.

175.	c
176.	a
177.	b
178.	b
179.	a
180.	b
181.	b
182.	a

183. Name the maneuver being performed to open the airway in the unconscious patient:

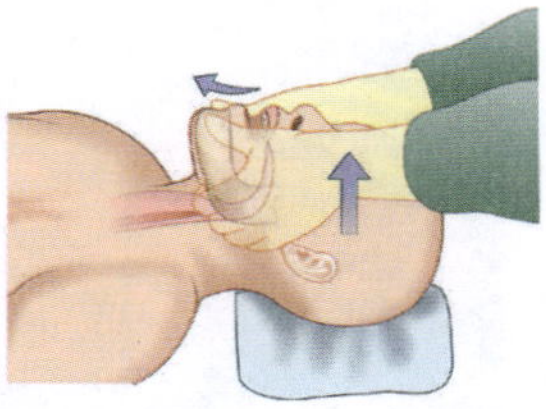

a. Head tilt-Chin Lift
b. Modified jaw thrust maneuver
c. Heimlich maneuver
d. Triple airway maneuver

184. Identify the device shown in the picture:

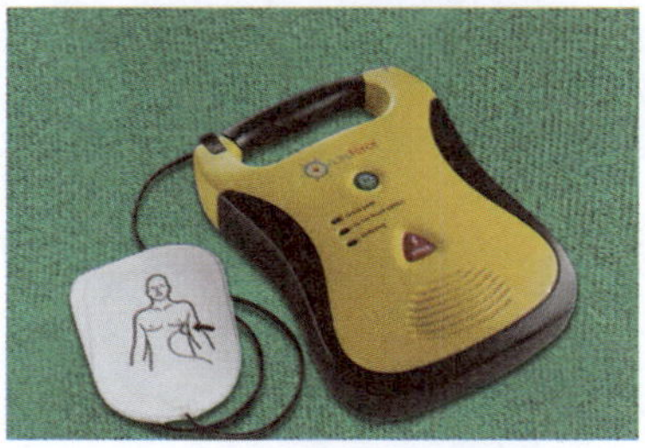

a. AED
b. ICDs
c. WCDs
d. External Pacemaker

185. Identify the condition in which the following phenomena is seen:

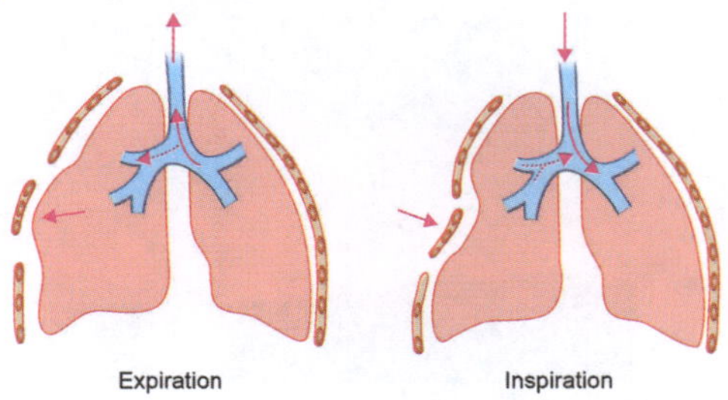

a. Pneumothorax
b. Hemothorax
c. Flail chest
d. Pigeon chest

186. Identify the type of splint used in this picture:

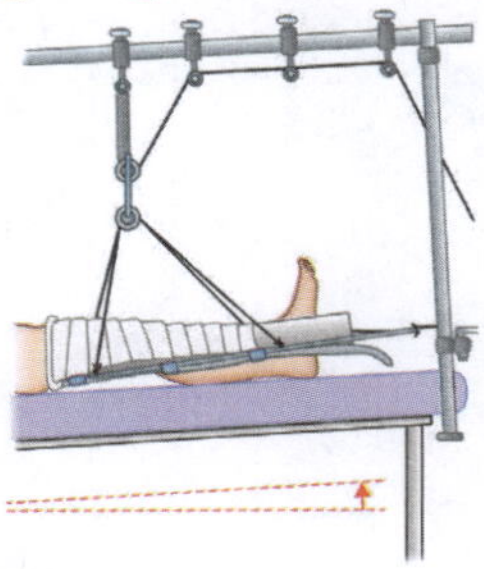

a. Cock-up splint
b. Kendrick traction device
c. Thomas splint
d. Donway traction splint

187. Identify the type of splint used in this picture:

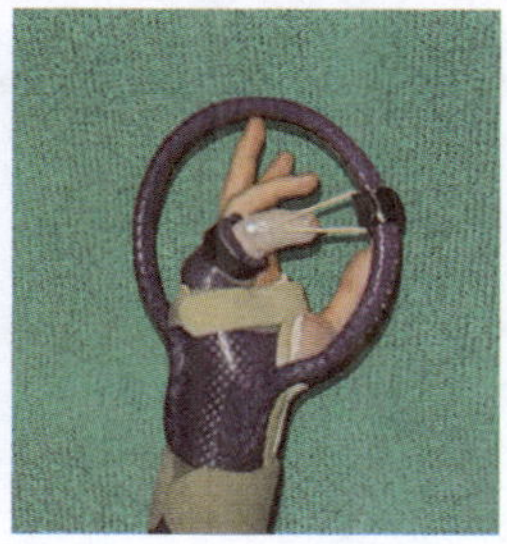

a. Cock-up splint
b. Kendrick traction device
c. Thomas splint
d. Dynamic traction splint

188. Identify the instrument shown in the image:

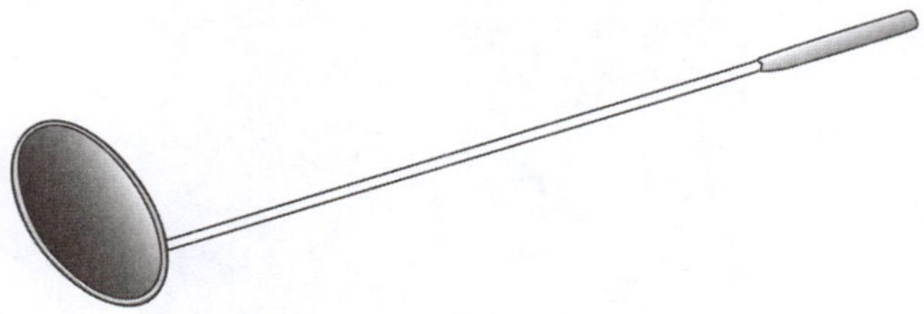

a. Uterine sound
b. Laryngeal mirror
c. Richardson retractor
d. Curettage

189. Identify the instrument shown in the image:
(Refer explanation at the end)

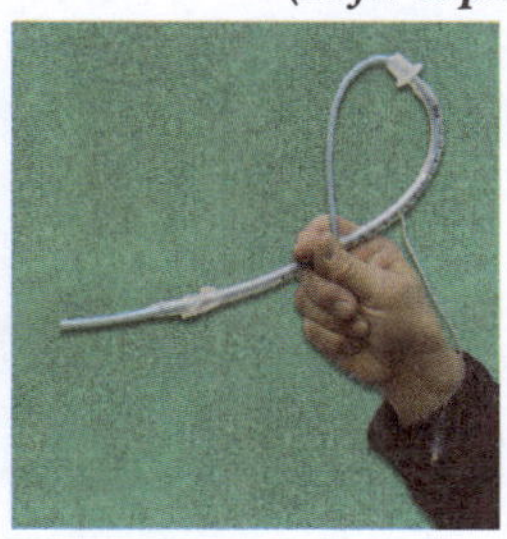

a. Ryle's tube
b. Bougie
c. Uterine sound
d. Tube stylet

190. Identify the catheter shown in the picture:

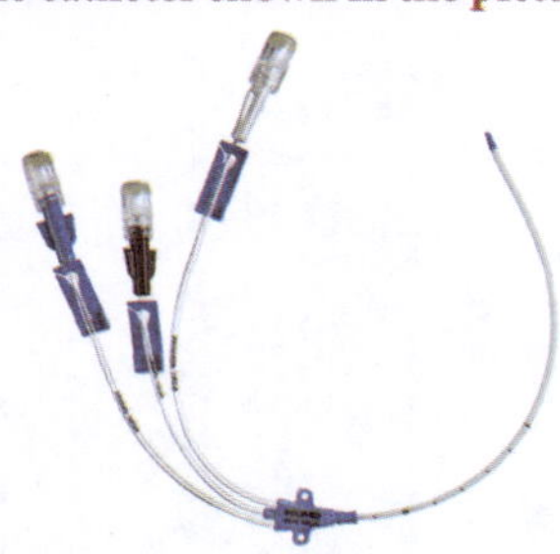

a. PICC line
b. Pressure monitoring line
c. Central venous catheter
d. Mallecot catheter

Ans.

183. b
184. a
185. c
186. c
187. d
188. b
189. b
190. c

191. Identify the catheter shown in the picture:

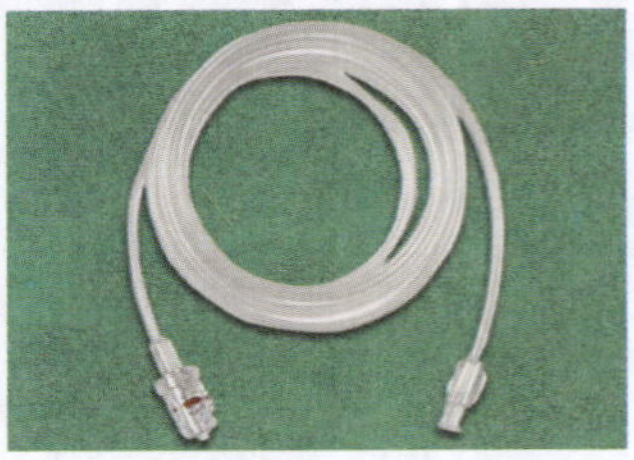

a. PICC line
b. Pressure monitoring line
c. Central venous catheter
d. Mallecot catheter

192. Identify the catheter shown in the picture:

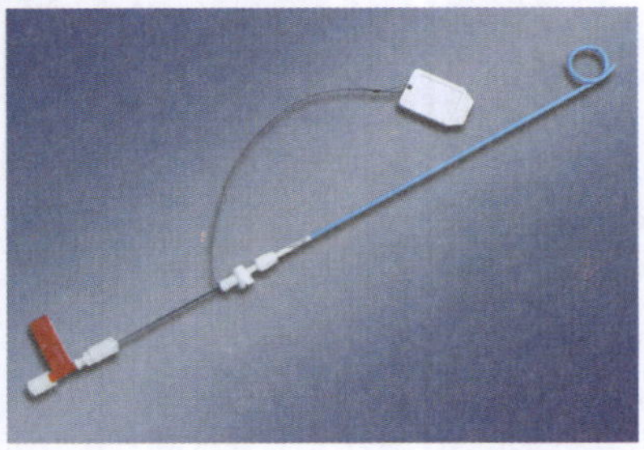

a. Suction catheter
b. Pigtail catheter
c. Mallecot catheter
d. AV Shunt catheter

193. Identify the traction shown in the picture:
(Refer explanation at the end)

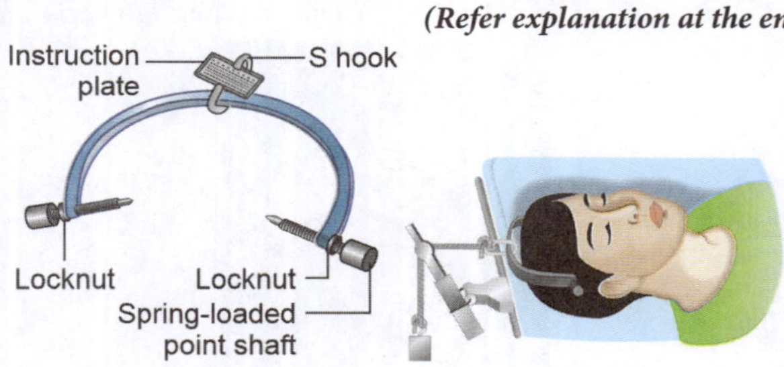

a. Russel's traction
b. Bryant's traction
c. Gardner well tongs
d. Axial traction

194. Identify the name of the device shown in the picture:

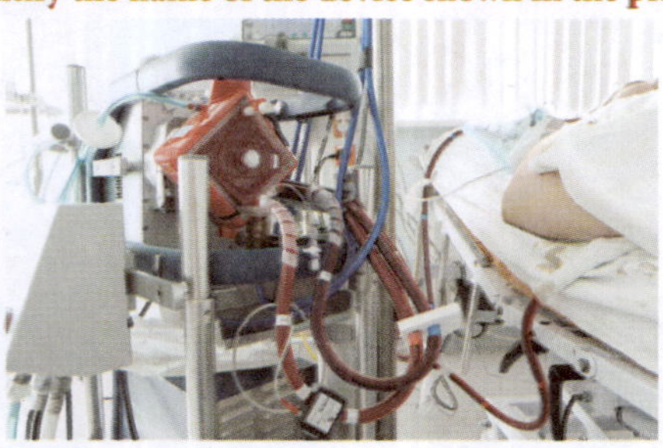

a. Hemodialysis machine
b. ECMO machine
c. Heart-Lung machine
d. Defibrillator

195. Identify the investigation procedure depicted below.
(Refer explanation at the end)

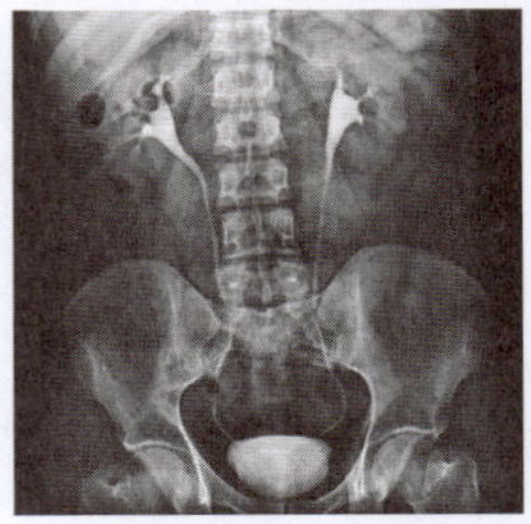

a. Pelvic X-ray
b. Barium scan
c. KUB X-ray
d. Intravenous pyelogram

196. The man in the picture is most likely suffering from:

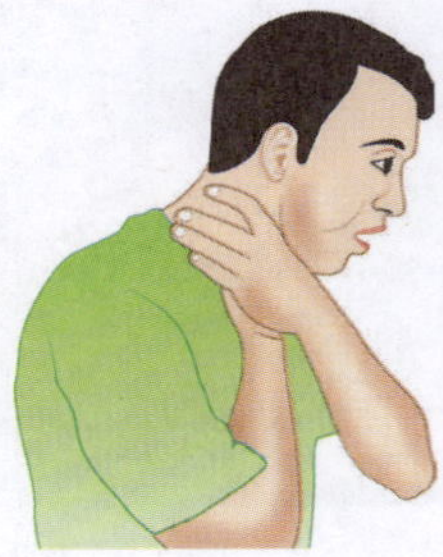

a. Cardiac arrest
b. Chocking
c. Throat pain
d. GERD

197. In Tuberculosis, Test shown in Photograph is a type of .... hypersensitivity. ***[Recent Question 2014]***

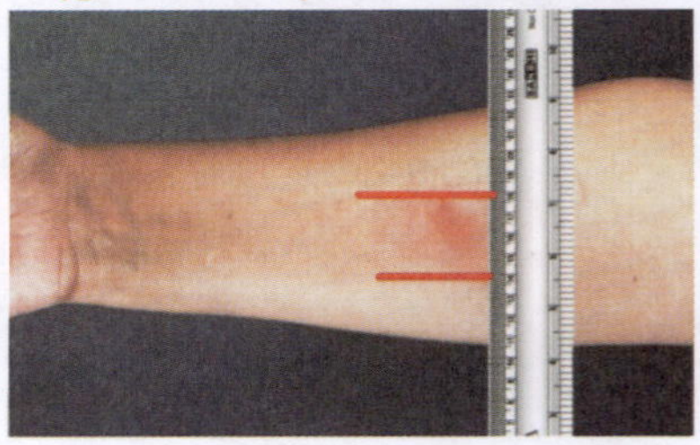

a. I
b. II
c. III
d. IV

198. Autoimmune Neuromuscular disorder shown in Photograph is associated with: ***[Recent Question 2013]***

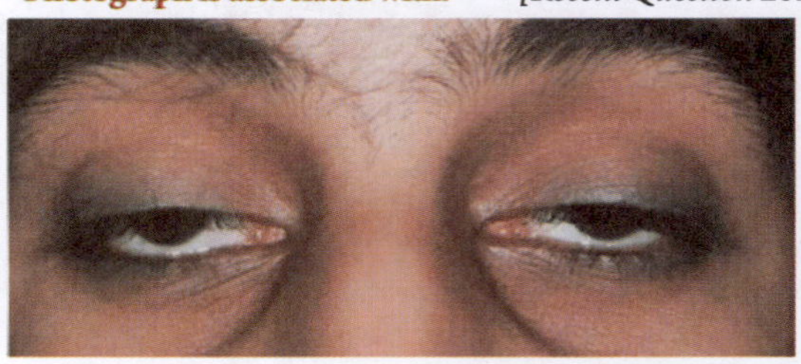

a. Thymoma
b. Thymic carcinoma
c. Thyroid hyperplasia
d. Lymphoma

Ans.

191.	b
192.	b
193.	c
194.	b
195.	d
196.	b
197.	d
198.	a

199. Disease condition shown in Photograph is a type of ………… hypersensitivity:

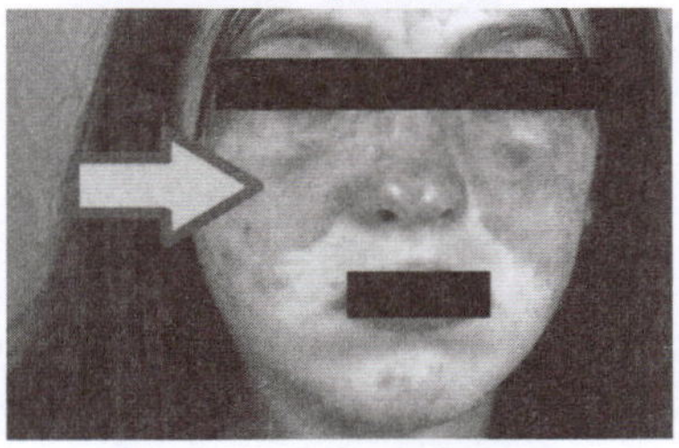

a. I b. II
c. III d. IV

200. Most common site of Disease shown in Photograph is ……….. artery.

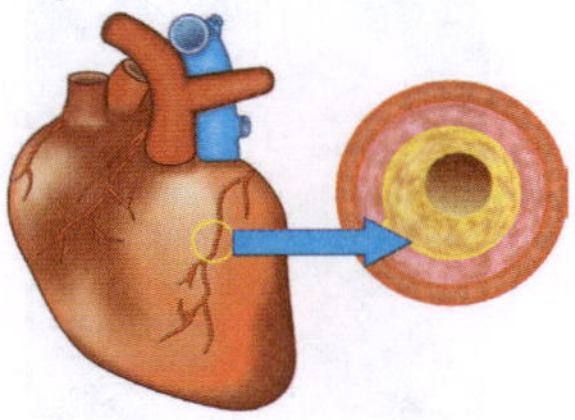

a. Left anterior descending artery
b. Right coronary artery
c. Left circumflex artery
d. Diagonal branch of LAD

201. False regarding Fluid portion of human blood shown in Photograph is:

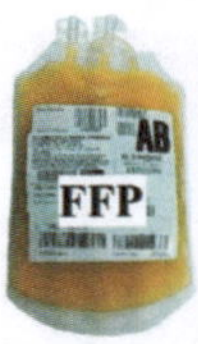

a. Supplies major coagulation factors
b. ABO match not required
c. Should be used in replacement of factors in DIC/ trauma
d. Use within 30 minutes of trauma

202. Type of Graft shown in Photograph is:

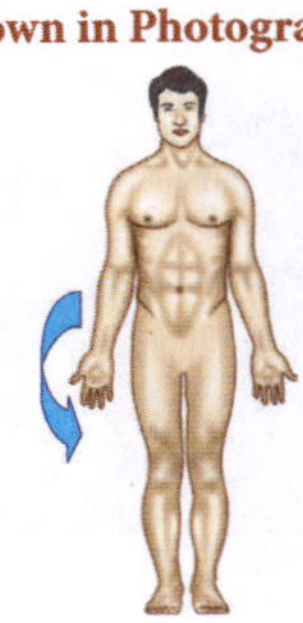

a. Isograft b. Autograft
c. Allograft d. Xenograft

203. Method shown in Photograph is Contraindicated in: ***[Recent Question 2012]***

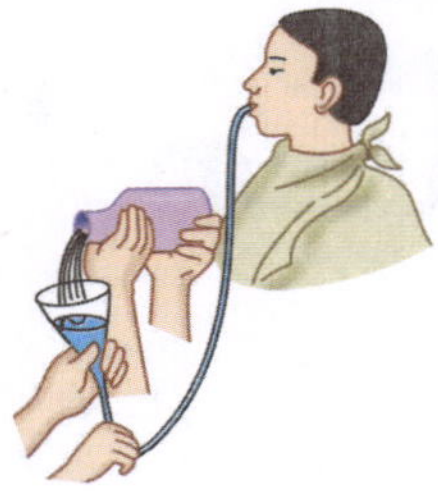

a. Cyanide poisoning b. Morphine poisoning
c. Barbiturate poisoning d. Kerosene poisoning

204. Identify the Congenital disorder of Eyelid shown in Photograph:

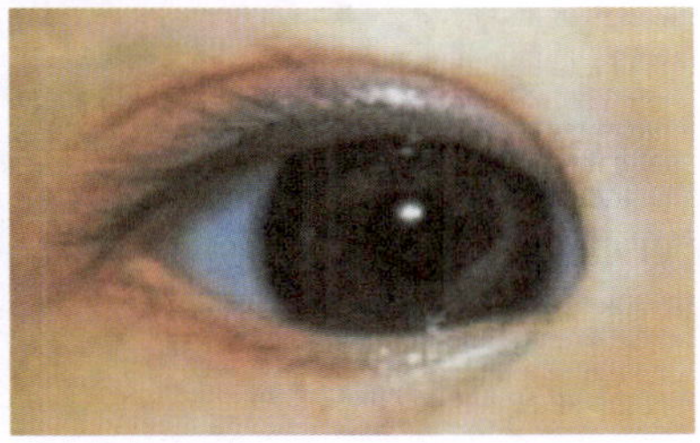

a. Congenital ptosis b. Congenital coloboma
c. Epicanthus d. Cryptophthalmos

205. Identify the Congenital disorder of Eyelid shown in Photograph:

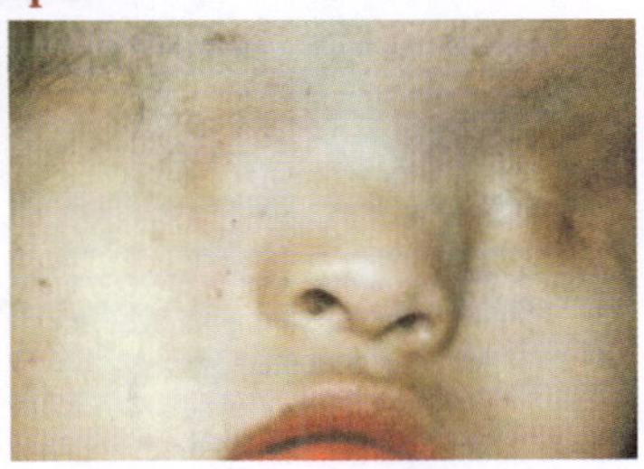

a. Congenital ptosis b. Congenital coloboma
c. Epicanthus d. Cryptophthalmos

206. Part (Arrow) in Visual pathway as shown in Photograph is:

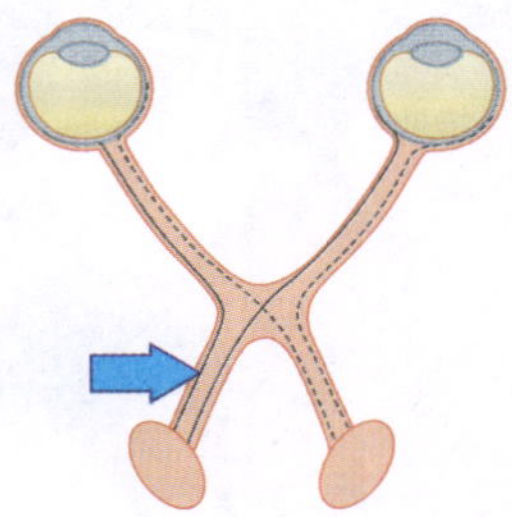

a. Optic nerve b. Optic chiasma
c. Optic tract d. Optic radiations

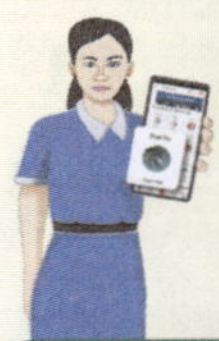

Ans.

199. c
200. a
201. d
202. b
203. d
204. c
205. d
206. c

207. Instrument shown in the Photograph is used for measurement of:

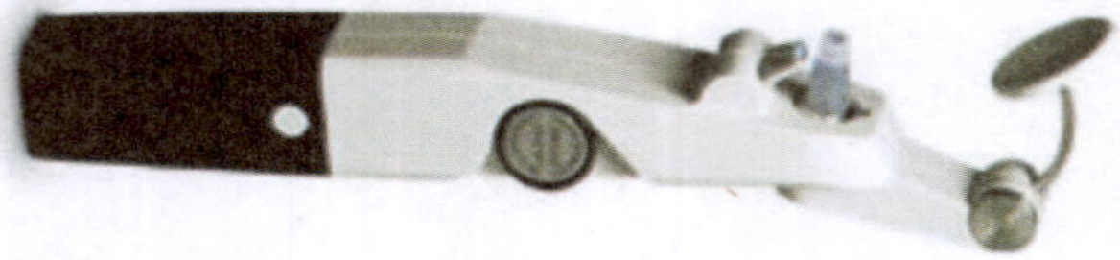

a. Intraocular pressure
b. Visual field
c. Visual acuity
d. Corneal diameter

208. Identify the Clinical test shown in the Photograph:

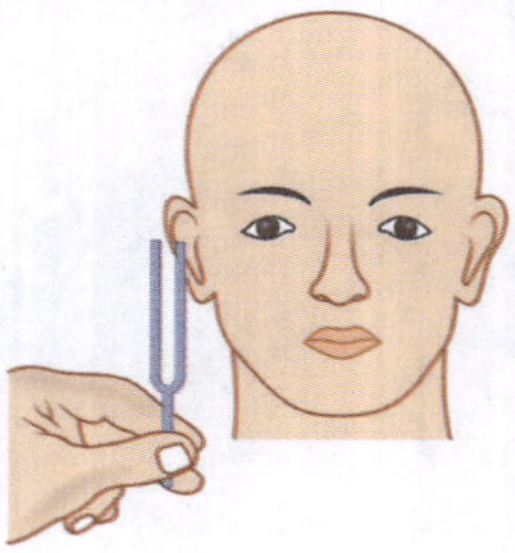

a. Rinne's test
b. Weber's test
c. Modified Schwabach's test
d. Gelle's test

209. Identify the Instrument/device shown in the Photograph:

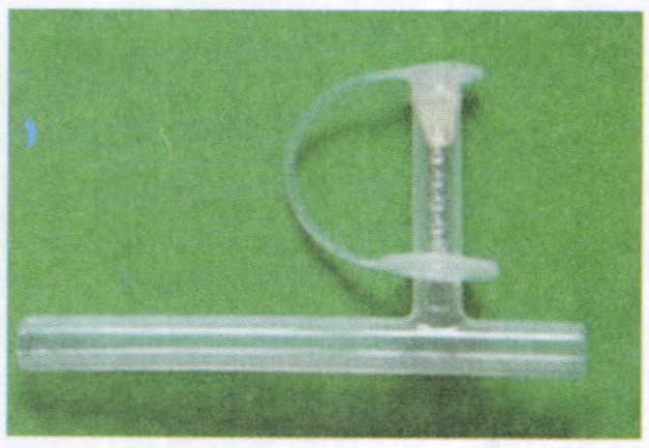

a. Nitinol stent
b. Endocracheal tube
c. Montogomery T tube
d. Suspension laryngoscope

210. Identify the test shown in the Photograph:

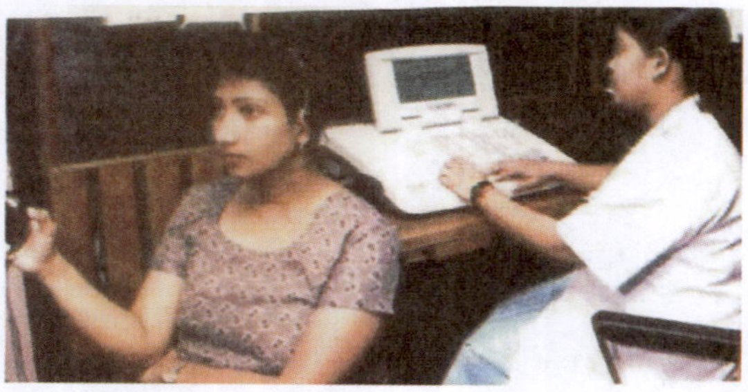

a. Bing test
b. Gelle's test
c. BERA test
d. Pure tone audiometry

211. Diagnose the Pinna swelling as shown in the Photograph:

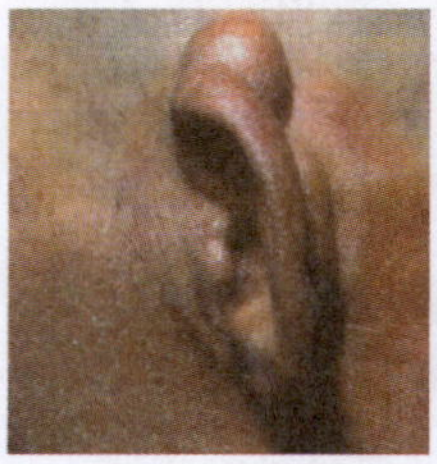

a. Preauricular sinus
b. Inclusion cyst of pinna
c. Perichondritis pinna
d. Rhandomyosarcoma pinna

212. Pinna swelling as shown in Photograph:

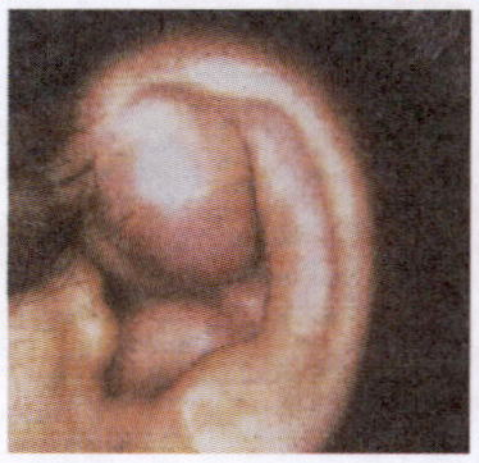

a. Preauricular sinus
b. Inclusion cyst of pinna
c. Pseudocyst pinna
d. Squamous cell carcinoma pinna

213. Identify the Condition of Oral cavity shown in the Photograph:

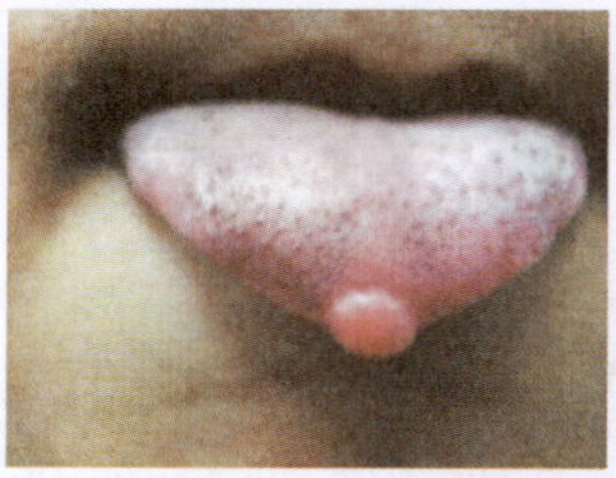

a. Epulis
b. Hemangioma
c. Papilloma
d. Gumma

214. Clinical test shown in Photograph is used to assess:

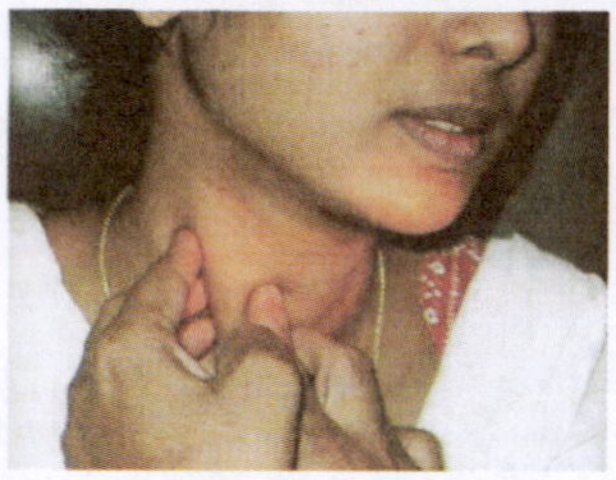

a. Thyroid gland
b. Hyoid bone
c. Sternocleidomastoid muscle
d. Carotid triangle

Ans.

207.	a
208.	a
209.	c
210.	d
211.	b
212.	c
213.	c
214.	a

215. Diagnose the Underlying disorder that appears on Valsalva maneuver (Photograph):

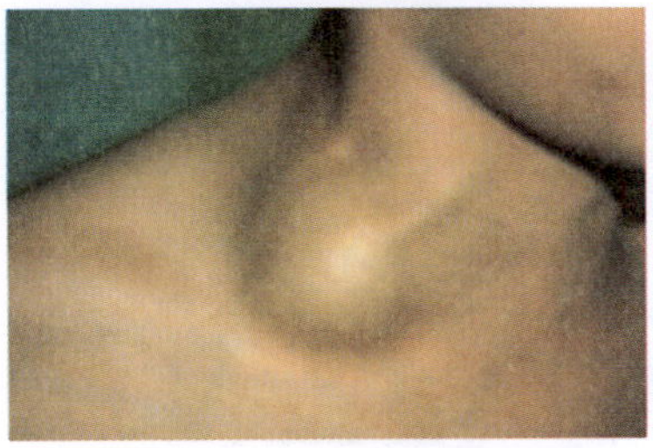

a. Cystic hygroma
b. Laryngocele
c. AV malformation
d. Thyroglossal cyst

216. Anatomical landmark of Bifurcation (Box) shown in Photograph: ***[Recent Question 2014]***

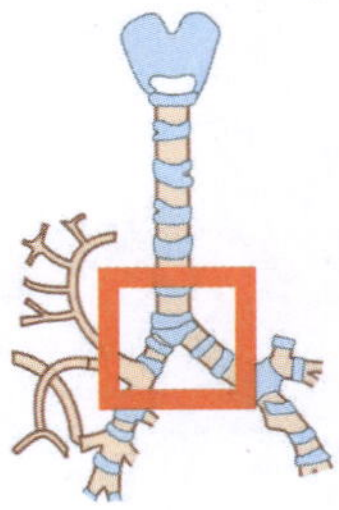

a. C3-C4
b. C6-C7
c. T4-T5
d. T10-T11

217. MC cause of Unilateral condition of foot shown in Photograph is: ***[Recent Question 2014]***

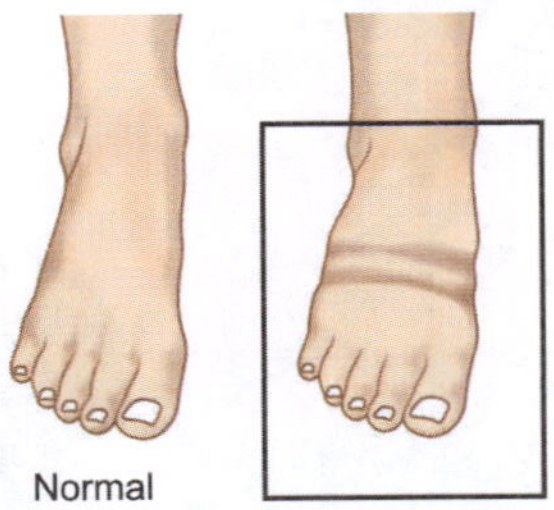

a. Pregnancy
b. Lymphedema
c. Venous insufficiency
d. Milroy disease

218. Wave (Arrow) shown in Photograph is characteristic of: ***[Recent Question 2014]***

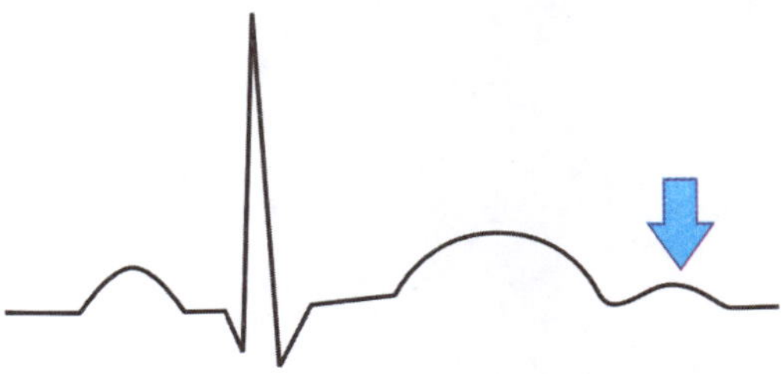

a. Hypocalcemia
b. Hyponatremia
c. Hypomagnesemia
d. Hypokalemia

219. Method (Box) shown in photograph is used for:

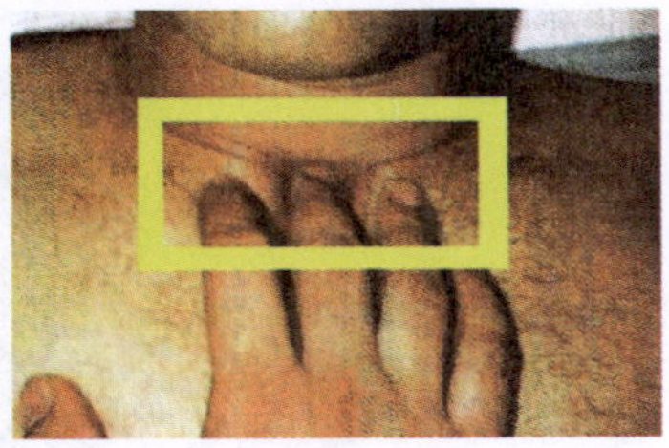

a. Palpation of thyroid gland
b. Palpation of trachea
c. Palpation of Carotid pulse
d. Palpation of hyoid bone

220. Characteristic appearance (Arrows) of Colon in Photograph is seen for: ***[Recent Question 2014]***

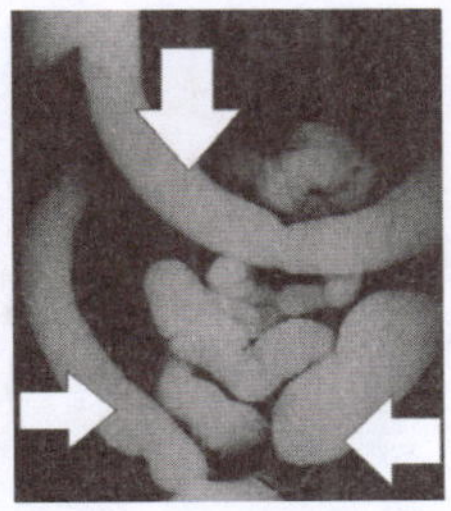

a. Crohn's disease
b. Ulcerative colitis
c. Tuberculosis of colon
d. Carcinoma colon

221. Clinical maneuver shown in Photograph is used for:

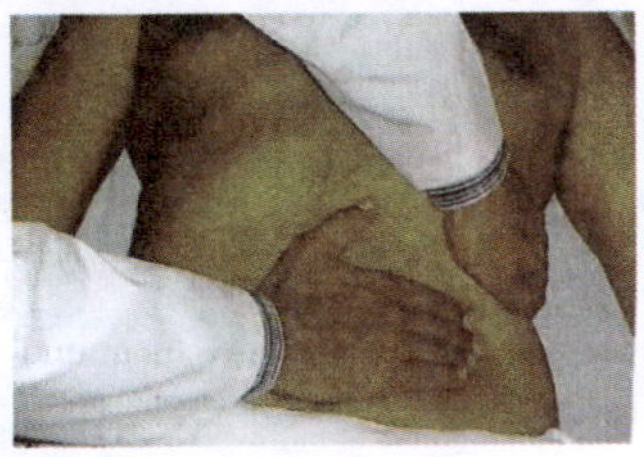

a. Palpation of Left kidney
b. Presence of ascites
c. Palpation of Spleen
d. Tenderness in Appendicular mass

222. Acute failure of Organ shown in Photograph results in: ***[Recent Question 2014]***

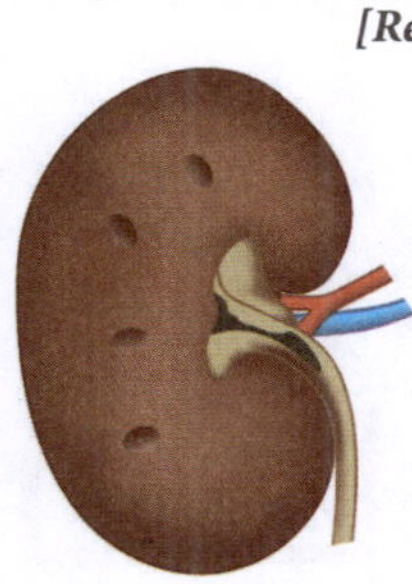

a. Hyperkalemic alkalosis
b. Hypokalemic alkalosis
c. Hyperkalemic acidosis
d. Hypokalemic acidosis

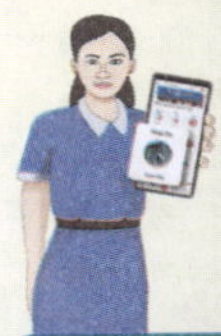

Ans.

215. c
216. c
217. c
218. d
219. b
220. b
221. c
222. c

223. Condition shown in Photograph is NOT seen in:
[Recent Question 2012]

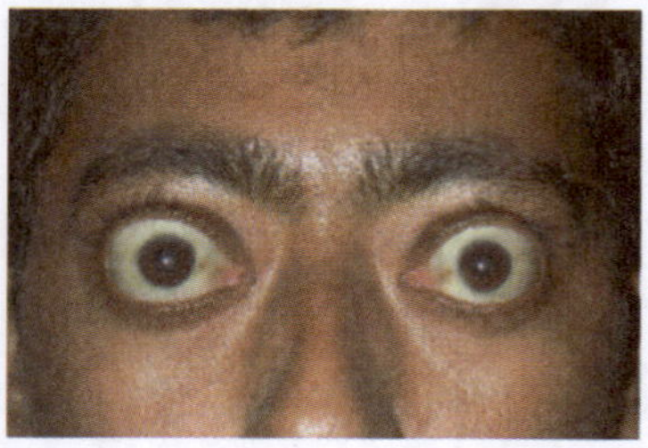

a. Grave's disease b. Sarcoidosis
c. Myxedema d. Pituitary adenoma

224. A 35-year-old Smoker presents with Condition shown in Photograph. Most likely diagnosis is:
[Recent Question 2013]

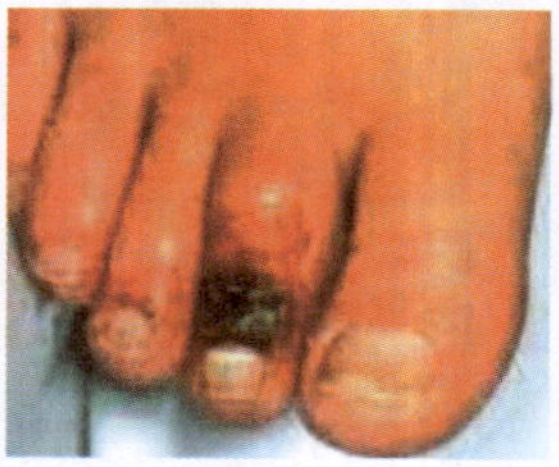

a. Diabetic gangrene b. Buerger's disease
c. Atherosclerotic plaque d. Septic foot

225. Sign elicited (Arrow) as shown in Photograph indicate:

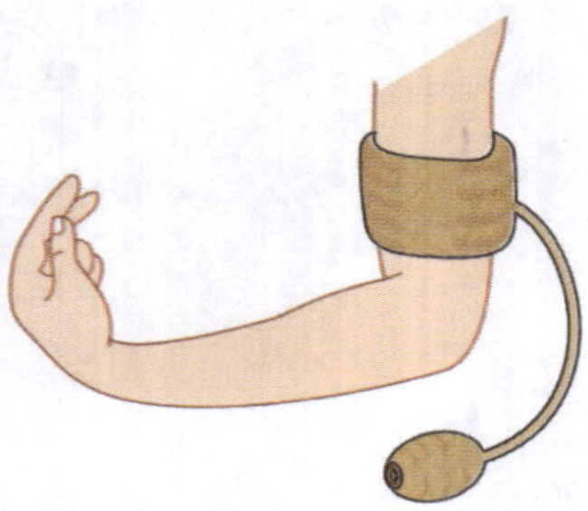

a. Hypercalcemia b. Hypocalcemia
c. Hypernatremia d. Hyponatremia

226. Best Investigation for Function of part (Box in Photograph):
[Recent Question 2013]

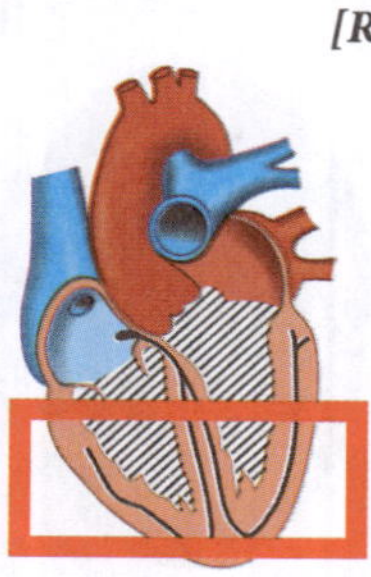

a. ECHO b. MRI
c. Nuclear scan d. Multi-slice CT scan

227. Site (Arrow) shown in the Photograph is used for:

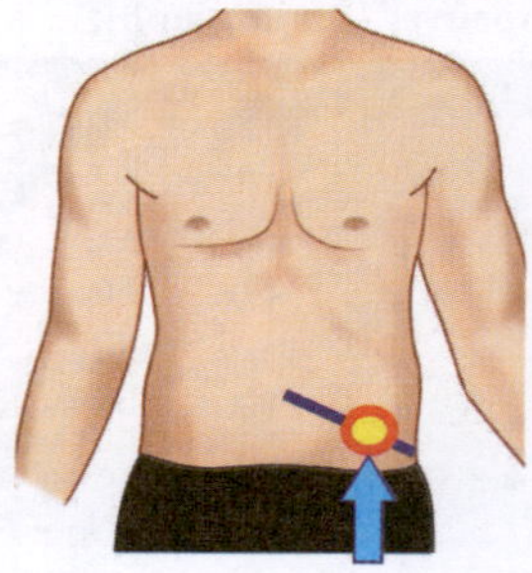

a. Pleural fluid aspiration b. Bone marrow biopsy
c. Ascitic tap d. McBurney's incision

228. Site (Arrow) shown in the Photograph is used for:

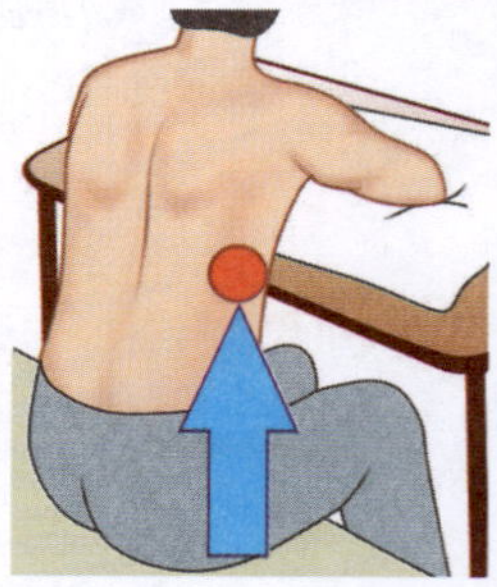

a. Pleural fluid aspiration b. Bone marrow biopsy
c. Ascitic tap d. Liver biopsy

229. Site (Arrow) shown in the Photograph is used for:

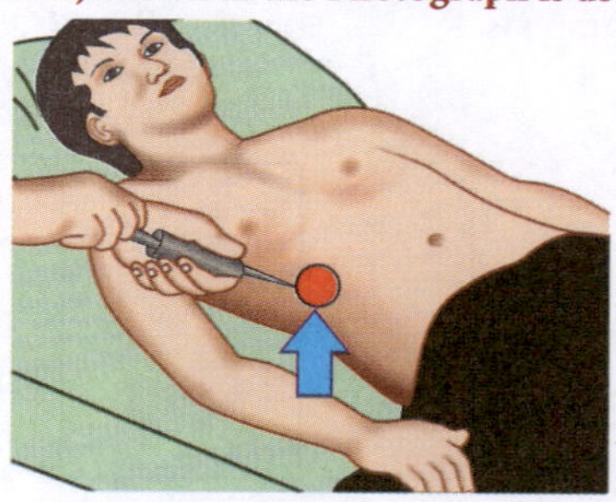

a. Pleural fluid aspiration b. Ascitic tap
c. Bone marrow aspiration d. Liver biopsy

230. Sensory loss (Shaded area) shown in Photograph indicate palsy of:

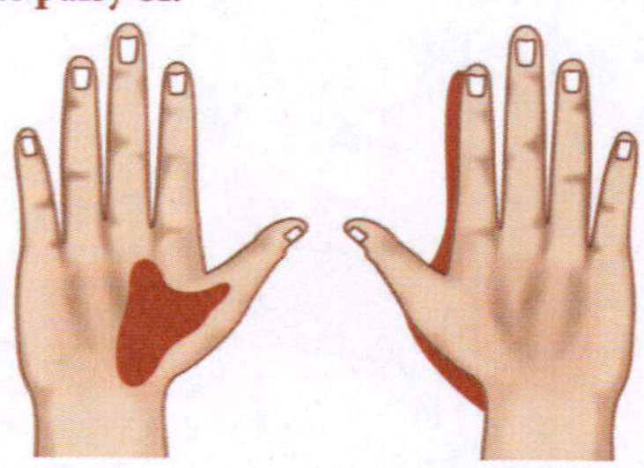

a. Radial nerve b. Ulnar nerve
c. Median nerve d. Axillary nerve

Ans.

223. c
224. b
225. b
226. a
227. c
228. a
229. d
230. a

231. Sign shown in Photograph is generally characteristic of:

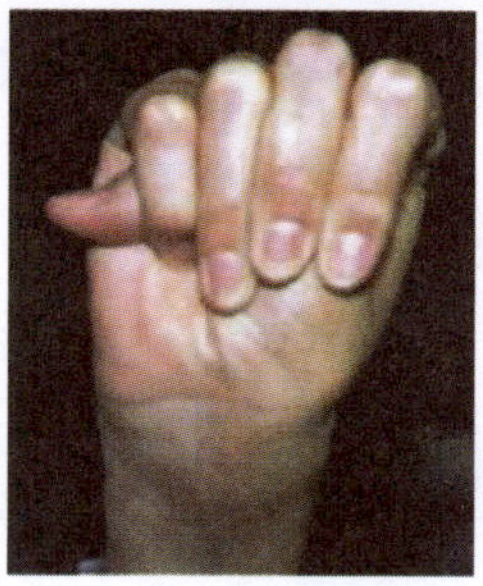

a. Down' syndrome
b. Klinefelter's syndrome
c. Turner's syndrome
d. Marfans' syndrome

232. Underlying genetic disorder shown in Photograph:

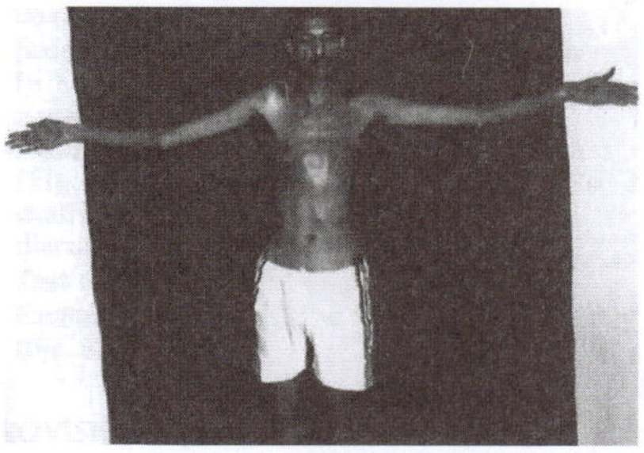

a. Down' syndrome
b. Klinefelter's syndrome
c. Turner's syndrome
d. Marfans' syndrome

233. Underlying genetic disorder shown in Photograph:

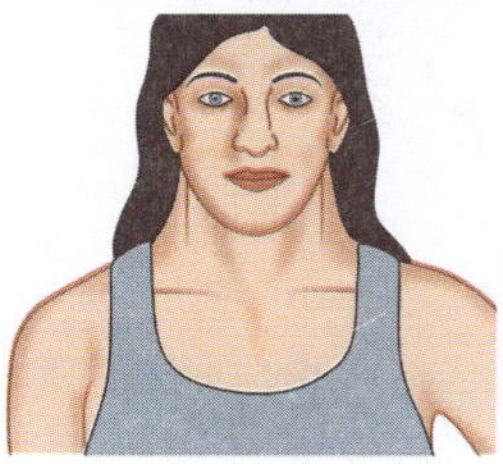

a. Down' syndrome
b. Klinefelter's syndrome
c. Turner's syndrome
d. Marfans' syndrome

234. In Emergency wing, a 16-year-old boy presented with history of fever and abdominal pain. On examination, febrile and pulse rate 104/min was recorded. Doctor on dutyelicited the sign shown in Photograph. Identify the sign. *[AIIMS May 2017]*

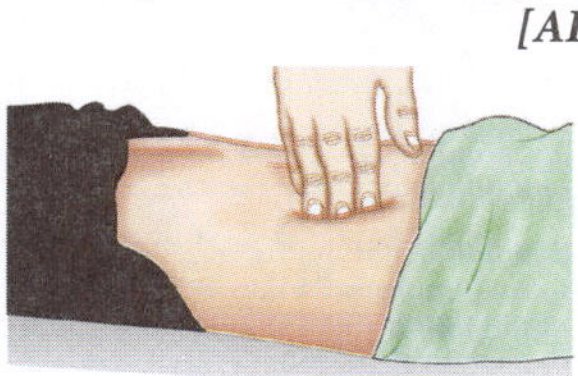

a. Psoas sign
b. Ballance sign
c. Blumberg sign
d. Rovsing's sign

235. Most commonly used preservative for suture shown in Photograph is: *[Recent Question 2017]*

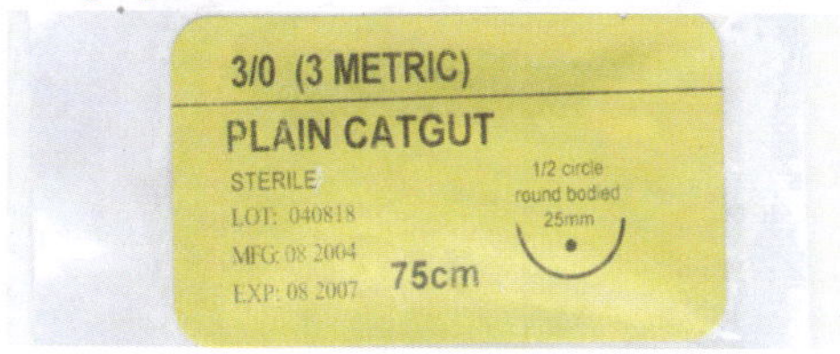

a. Iodine
b. Glutaraldehyde
c. Isopropyl alcohol
d. Cetrimide

236. Identify the diagnostic technique shown in Photograph: *[Recent Question 2013]*

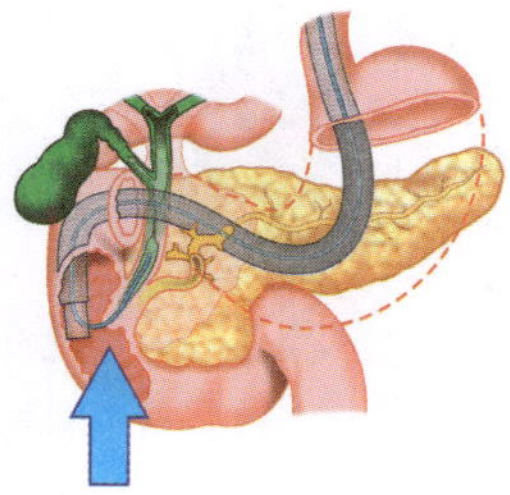

a. ERCP
b. MRCP
c. Colonoscopy
d. Sigmoid colonoscopy

237. Instrument shown in Photograph is used for:

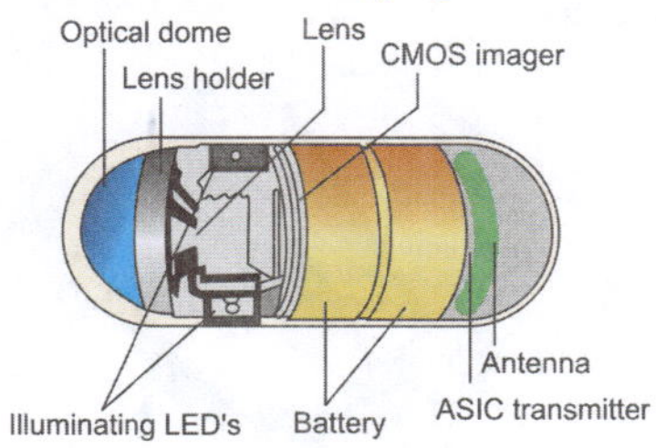

a. Single balloon enteroscopy
b. Double balloon enteroscopy
c. Capsule endoscopy
d. ERCP

238. Type of Knot used in Surgery shown in Photograph is:

a. Reef knot
b. Surgeon's knot
c. Half hitch knot
d. Granny knot

Ans.

231. d
232. b
233. c
234. c
235. c
236. a
237. c
238. b

239. Type of Fracture shown in Photograph is:

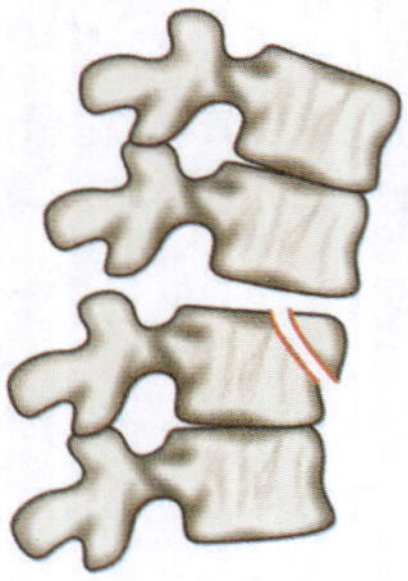

a. Compression b. Angulation
c. Burst d. Translational

240. Surgical procedure shown in Photograph is: ***[Recent Question 2013]***

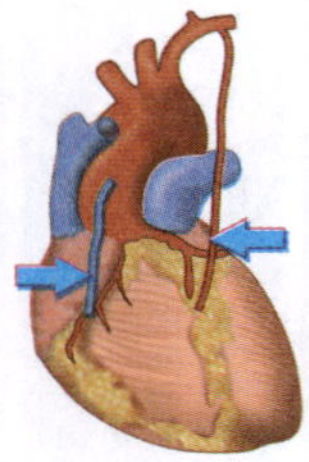

a. Angioplasty
b. Coronary artery bypass grafting
c. Coronary stenting d. Bentall procedure

241. Identify the Type of Prosthetic heart valve shown in the Photograph:

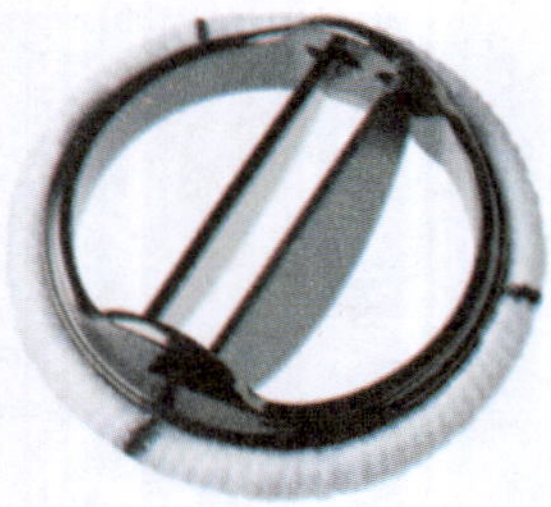

a. Bi-leaflet mechanical b. Tri-leaflet mechanical
c. Ball and cage mechanical d. Tilting disc mechanical

242. Identify the Type of Prosthetic heart valve shown in the Photograph:

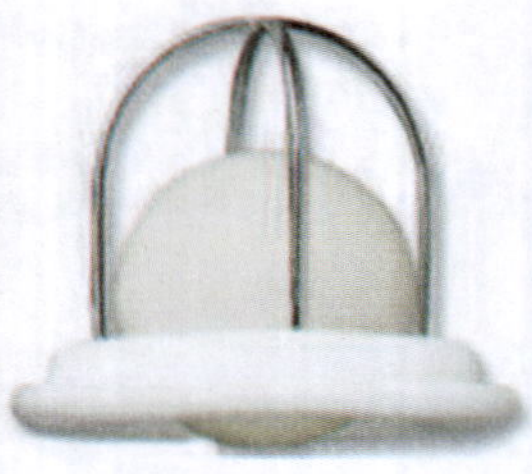

a. Bi-leaflet mechanical b. Tri-leaflet mechanical
c. Ball and cage mechanical
d. Tilting disc mechanical

243. Identify the Valvular condition shown in the Photograph: ***[Recent Question 2012]***

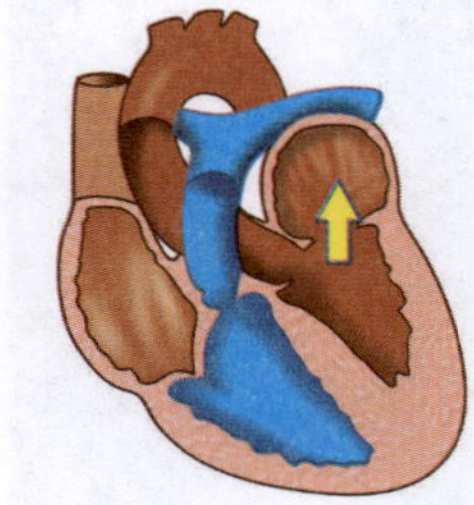

a. Mitral regurgitation b. Aortic regurgitation
c. Mitral stenosis d. Aortic stenosis

244. Procedure shown in Photograph is:

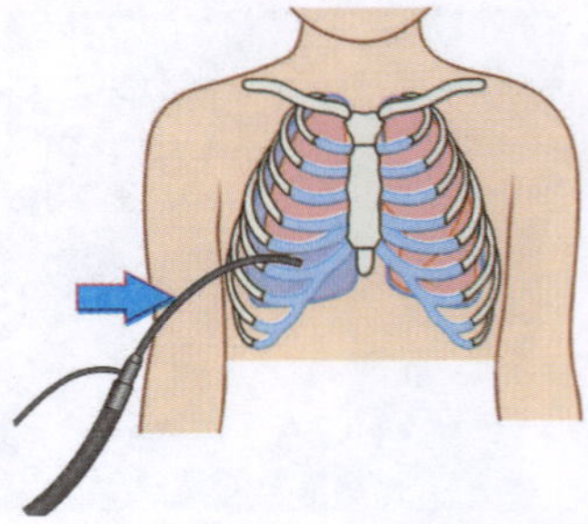

a. Chest tube drainage b. Pericardial aspiration
c. Pleural aspiration d. ECG

245. Identify the Hernia type shown in Photograph: ***[Recent Question 2012]***

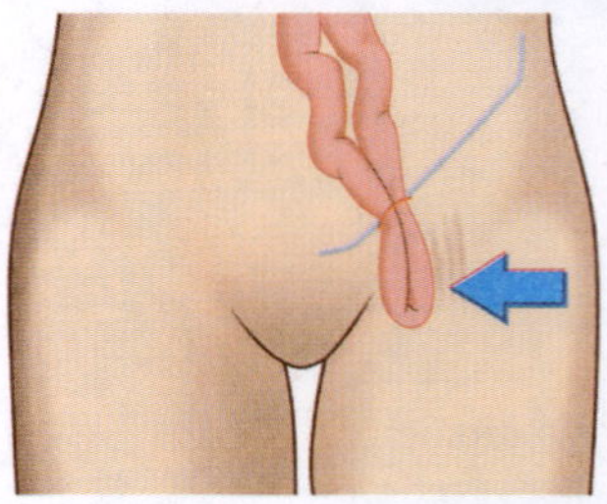

a. Direct inguinal b. Indirect inguinal
c. Femoral d. Umbilical

246. Most common carcinoma type seen at site depicted (Arrow) in Photograph:

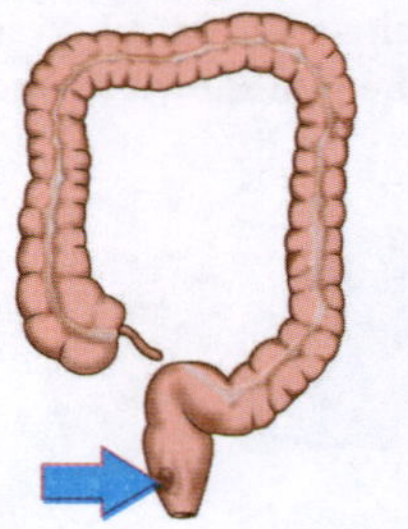

a. Squamous cell b. Basal cell
c. Cuboidal d. Cloacogenic

Ans.

239. d
240. b
241. a
242. c
243. a
244. a
245. c
246. a

247. Identify the Sign shown in Photograph: *[Recent Question 2013, 2012]*

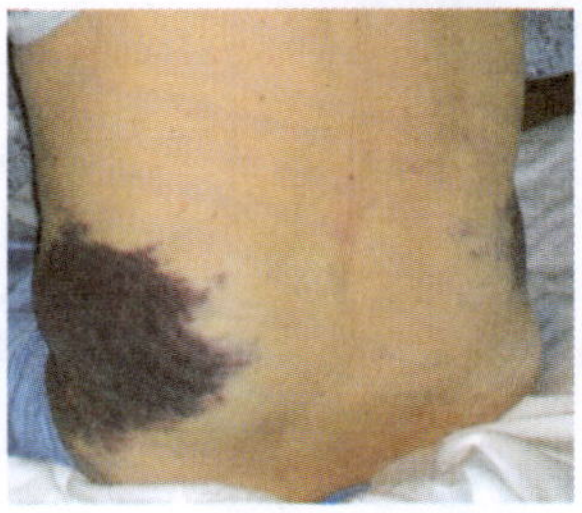

a. Cullen's sign b. Grey turner sign
c. Trousseau sign d. Fothergill sign

248. Identify the Abnormality shown (Arrow) in the Photograph: *[Recent Question 2016]*

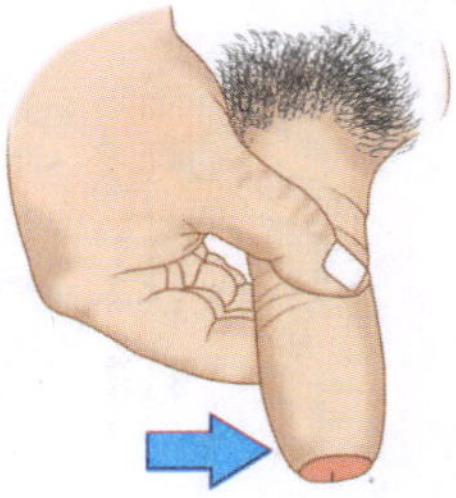

a. Epispadias b. Hypospadias
c. Phimosis d. Circumcision

249. Orthopedic device shown in Photograph is: *[Recent Question 2012, 2016]*

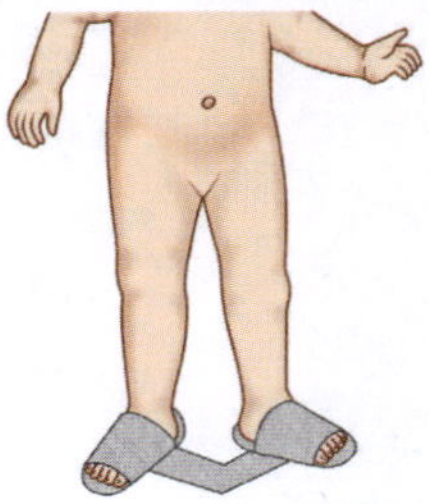

a. CTEV shoes b. Below knee calipers
c. Denis Browne splint d. Phelps brace

250. Splint in Orthopedics as shown in Photograph is used for management of:

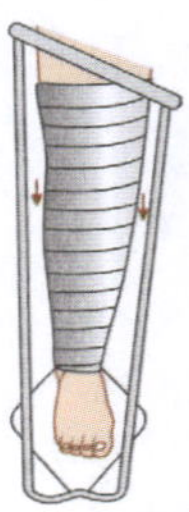

a. Fracture hip b. Fracture shaft femur
c. Fracture tibia d. Fracture fibula

251. Identify the Type of Splint shown in the Photograph: *[Recent Question 2012]*

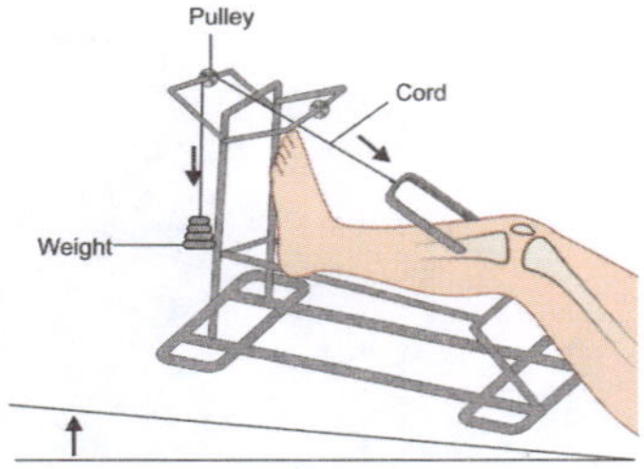

a. Thomas splint b. Bohler Braun splint
c. Von Rosen splint d. Aeroplane splint

252. Identify the orthopedic prosthesis shown in Photograph:

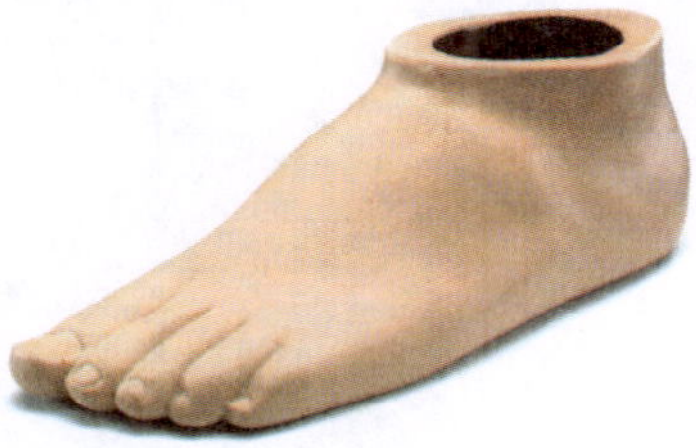

a. CTEV shoes b. SACH foot
c. Jaipur foot d. Syme's prosthesis

253. Identify the orthopedic prosthesis shown in photograph:

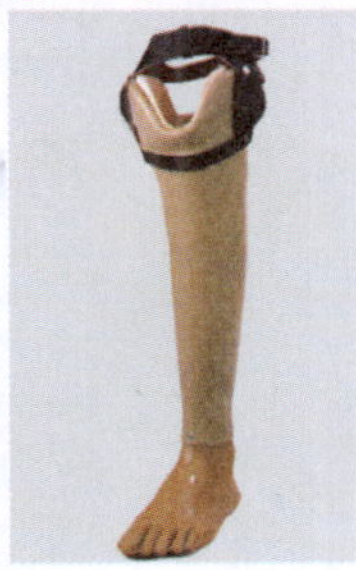

a. CTEV shoes b. SACH foot
c. Jaipur foot d. Syme's prosthesis

254. Identify the Orthopedic device shown in Photograph:

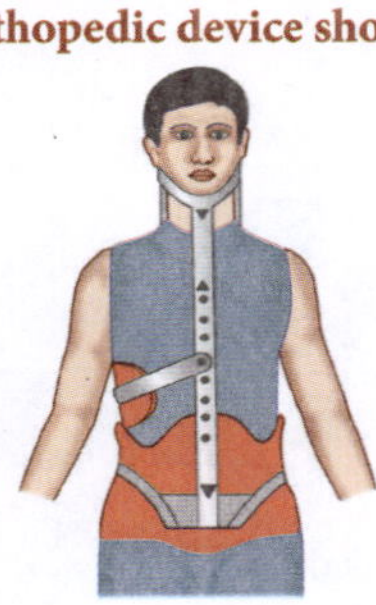

a. SOMI brace b. Halo-body orthosis
c. Lumbo-sacral belt d. Milwaukee brace

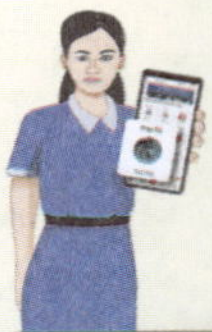

Ans.

247. b
248. c
249. c
250. b
251. b
252. b
253. c
254. d

255. Identify the Clinical test shown in Photograph:

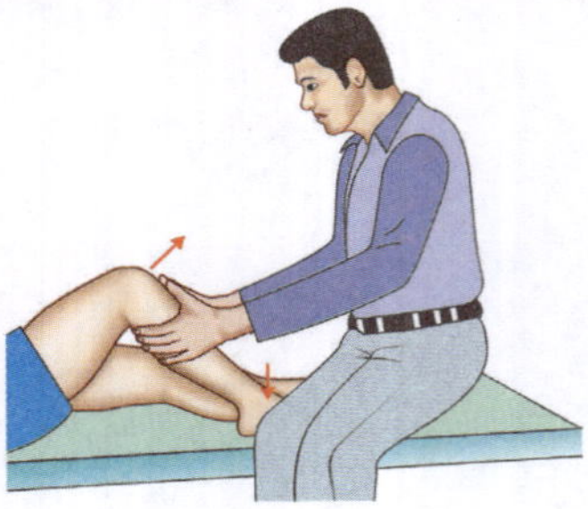

a. Lachmann test
b. Apley's test
c. Anterior drawer test
d. McMurray' test

256. Orthopedic device shown in Photograph is:
[Recent Question 2013]

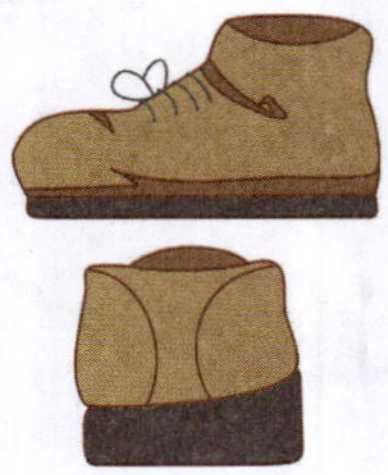

a. CTEV shoes
b. Below knee calipers
c. Denis Browne splint
d. Phelps brace

257. Bandage shown in Photograph is used in Fracture of:
[Recent Question 2012, 2014]

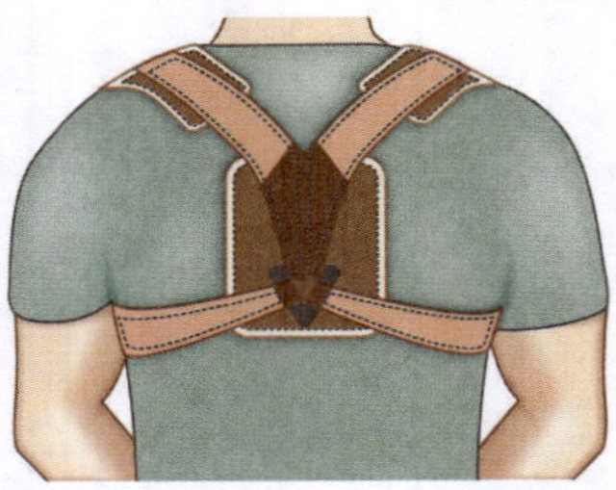

a. Humerus
b. Scapula
c. Clavicle
d. Cervical spine

258. Mechanism of Spine injury shown in Photograph is:

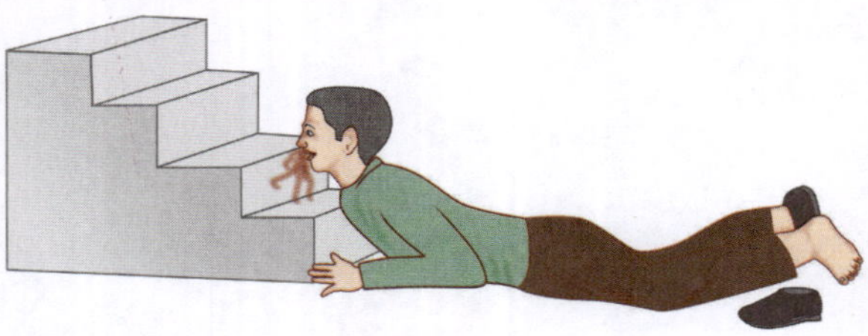

a. Flexion extension injury
b. Hyperextension injury
c. Flexion rotation injury
d. Flexion injury

259. Identify the Type of deformity shown in Photograph:

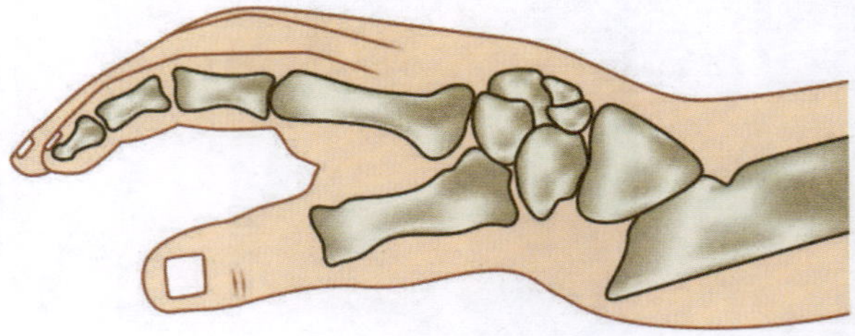

a. Boutonniere deformity
b. Swan neck deformity
c. Dinner fork deformity
d. Gun-stock deformity

260. Splint (Arrow) shown in Photograph is known as:

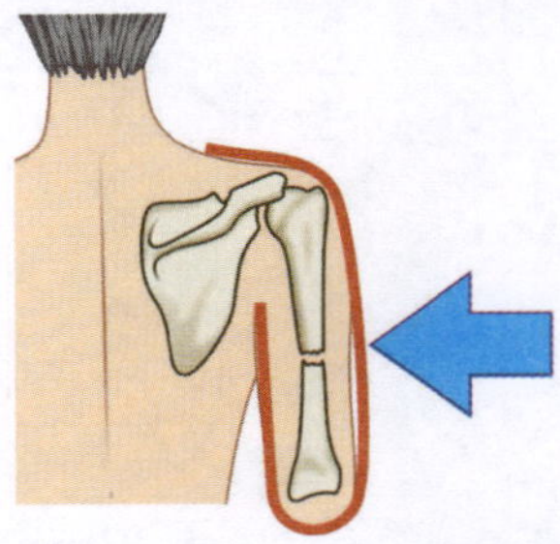

a. Von Rosen splint
b. Hanging cast
c. Functional cast brace
d. U-slab

261. Cast shown in Photograph is used for:

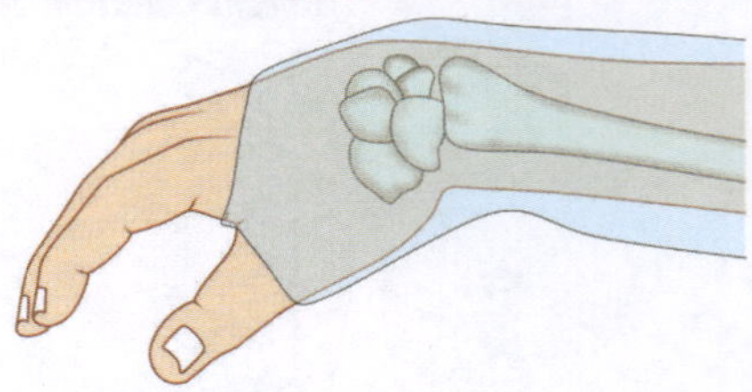

a. Fracture Colles'
b. Fracture Scaphoid
c. Fracture Lunate
d. Fracture Olecranon

262. Cast shown in Photograph is used for:

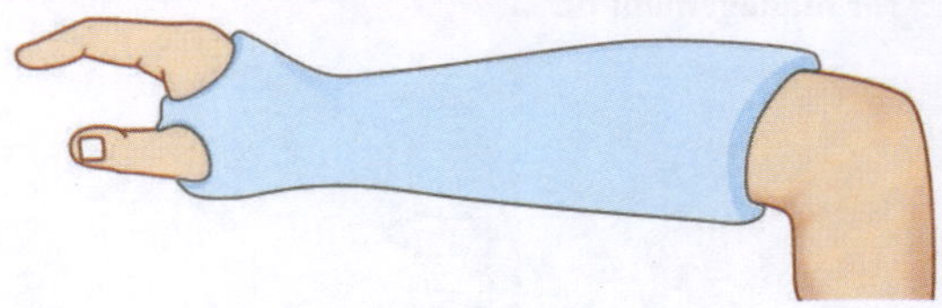

a. Fracture Colles'
b. Fracture Scaphoid
c. Fracture Lunate
d. Fracture Olecranon

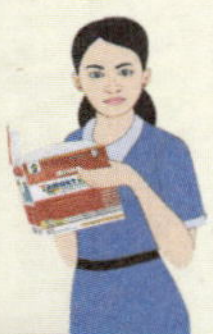

Ans.

255. c
256. a
257. c
258. b
259. c
260. d
261. a
262. b

263. Identify the abnormality shown in Photograph: *[AIIMS November 2015]*

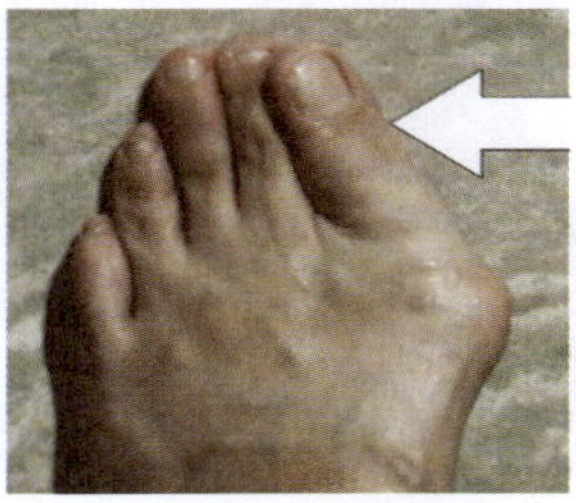

a. Hallux valgus b. Hallux varus
c. Rheumatoid nodule d. Subcutaneous nodule

264. In Syndrome shown in Photograph, pain occurs in range of:

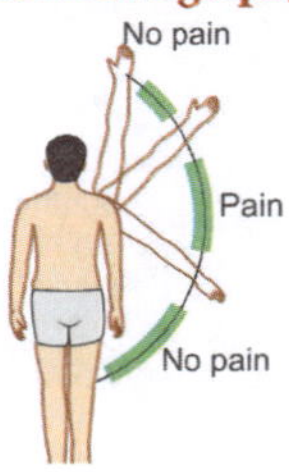

a. 0 – 30 degrees of abduction
b. 30 – 60 degrees of abduction
c. 60 – 120 degrees of abduction
d. 120 – 180 degrees of abduction

265. Condition shown in Photograph is present from birth. Diagnose: *[AIIMS May 2017]*

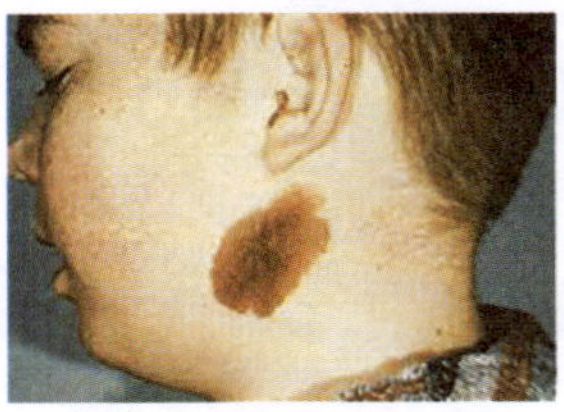

a. Melanoacanthoma
b. Malignant melanoma
c. Congenital nevus
d. Epidermal verrucous nevus

266. Dermatological test shown in the Photograph is:

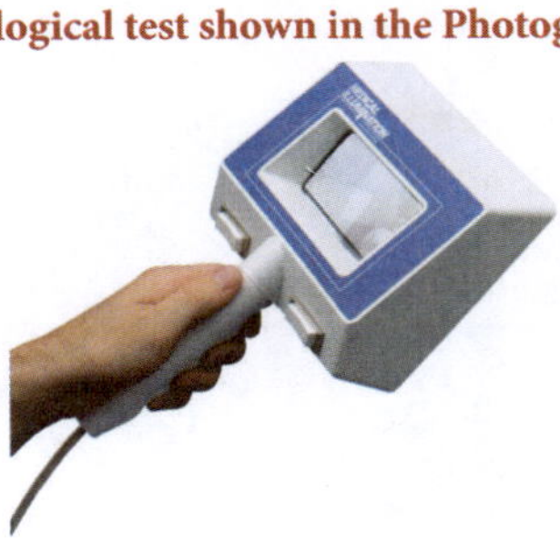

a. Wood lamp examination b. Patch testing
c. Diascopy d. Blanch test

267. Organism causing Condition shown in Photograph is:

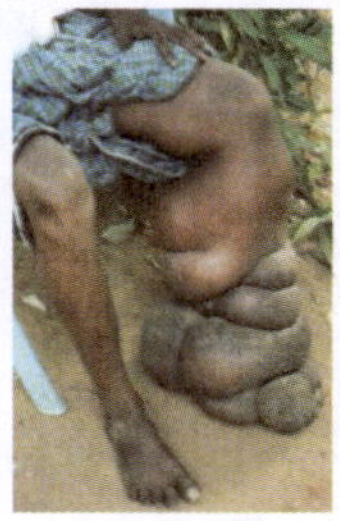

a. Mycobacterium tuberculosis
b. Mycobacterium leprae c. Wuchereria bancrofti
d. HIV

268. Identify the Dermatological test shown in Photograph: *[Recent Question 2013]*

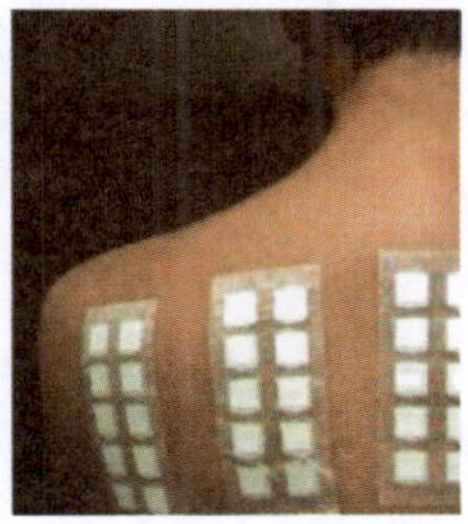

a. Dermascopy b. Diascopy
c. Skin biopsy d. Patch test

269. Identify the Dermatological test shown in Photograph:

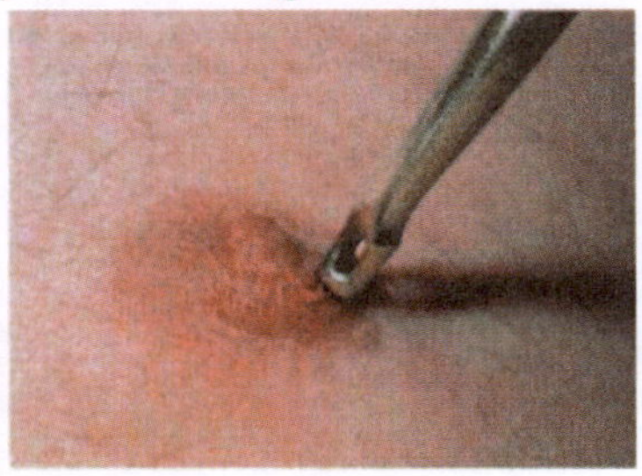

a. Dermascopy b. Photo-patch test
c. Skin biopsy d. Patch test

270. Identify the Skin disorder as shown in Photograph: *[Recent Question 2013, 2012]*

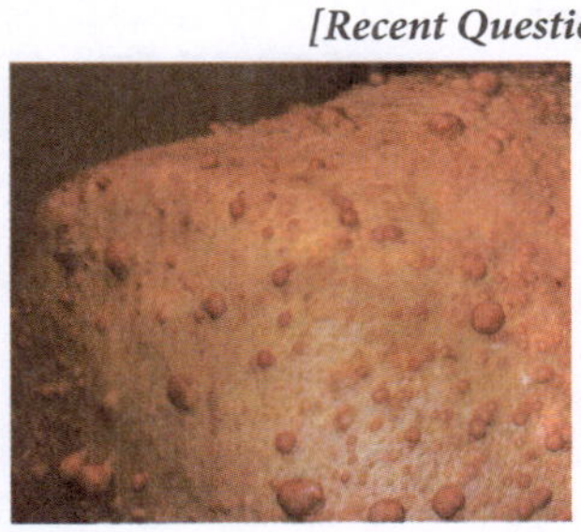

a. Angiofibroma b. Neurofibromatosis
c. Xeroderma pigmentosum d. Acanthosis nigricans

Ans.

263. a
264. c
265. c
266. a
267. c
268. d
269. c
270. b

271. Distribution of disease shown in the Photograph:

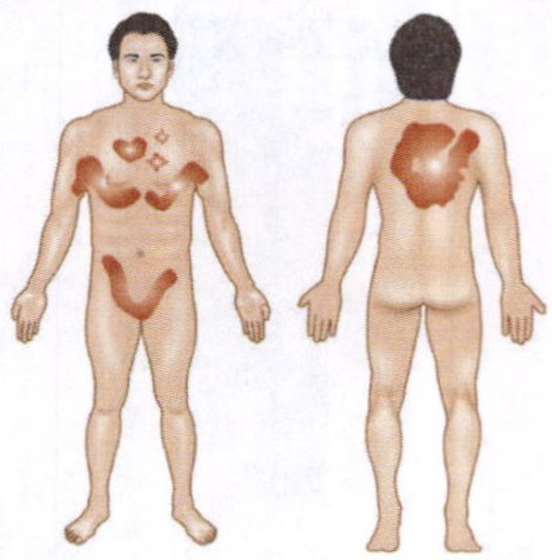

a. Pemphigus vulgaris
b. Contact dermatitis
c. Seborrheic dermatitis
d. Bullous pemphigoid

272. Distribution of disease shown in the Photograph:

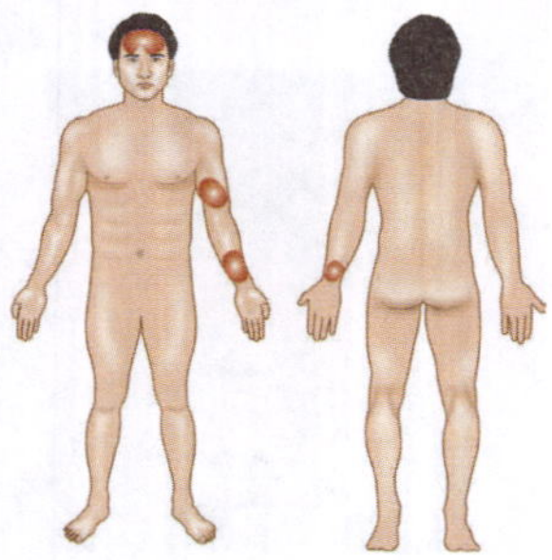

a. Atopic dermatitis
b. Seborrheic dermatitis
c. Allergic contact dermatitis
d. Stasis eczema

273. Identify the Infective disorder of skin as shown in Photograph:

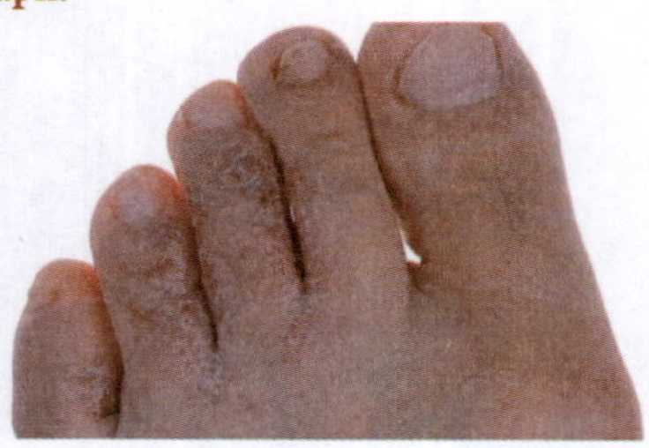

a. Tinea capitis
b. Tinea corporis
c. Kerion
d. Tinea pedis

274. Diagnose the Causative organism shown in the Photograph: ***[Recent Question 2013, 2017]***

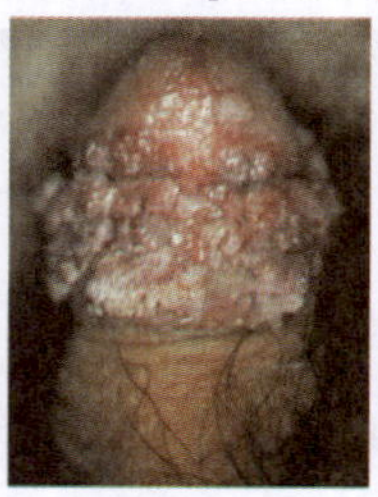

a. HIV
b. HBV
c. Herpes
d. HPV

275. Identify the Skin disorder shown in the Photograph:

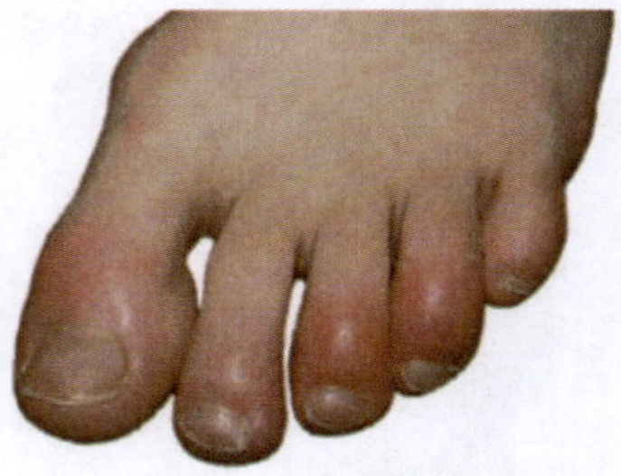

a. Chillblains
b. Acrocyanosis
c. Angioedema
d. Sunburn

276. Identify the Disease distribution as shown in the Photograph:

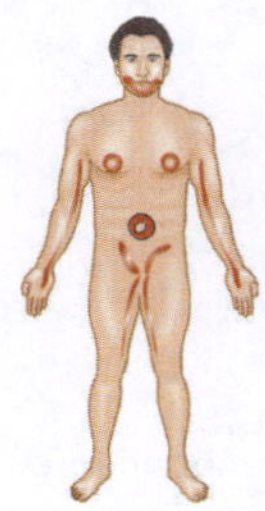

a. Scabies
b. Myiasis
c. Pediculus corporis
d. Cysticercosis

277. Machine shown in photograph is used in hospitals for:

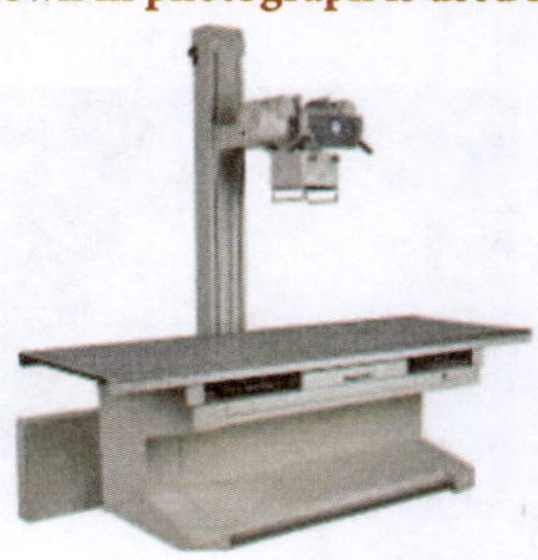

a. X-rays
b. CT scan
c. MRI
d. PET scan

278. Condition shown in Photograph is seen in all EXCEPT: ***[Recent Question 2012]***

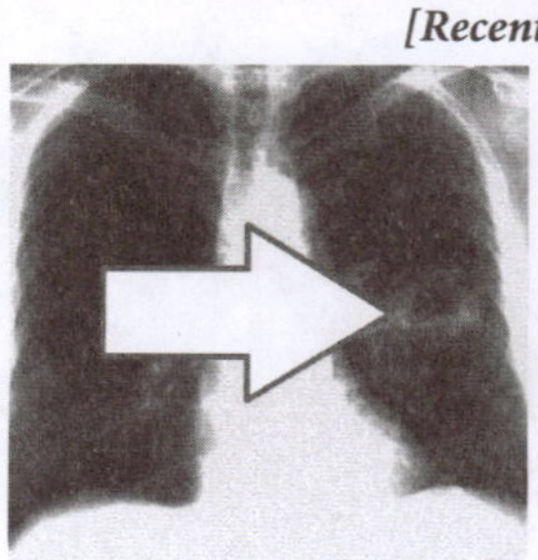

a. Lung abscess
b. Lung hamartoma
c. Tuberculosis
d. Emphysematous bulla

Ans.

271. c
272. c
273. d
274. d
275. a
276. a
277. a
278. b

279. Most commonly involved segment of Lungs in Foreign body aspiration (Supine position):

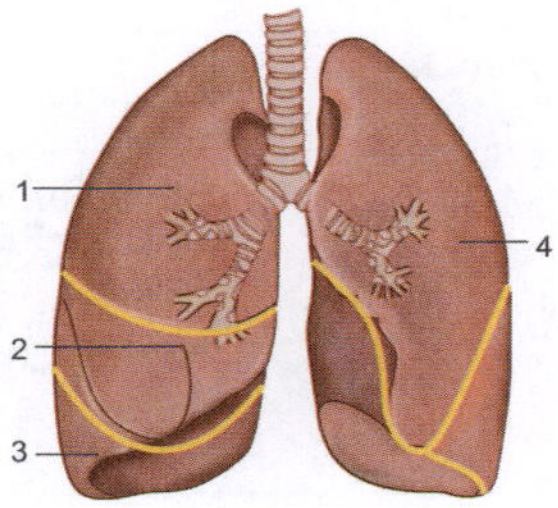

a. 1
b. 2
c. 3
d. 4

282. Identify the Instrument/ device shown in Photograph:

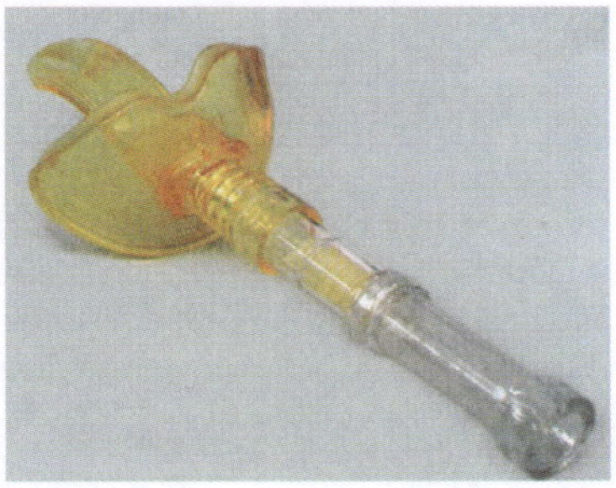

a. Brook airway
b. Water airway
c. Safar airway
d. Guedel airway

280. Identify the Instrument/ device shown in Photograph:

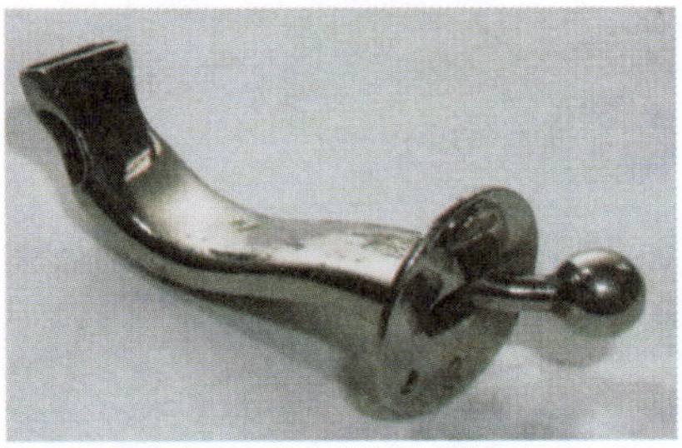

a. Brook airway
b. Water's airway
c. Safar airway
d. Guedel airway

283. Identify the Instrument/ device shown in Photograph:

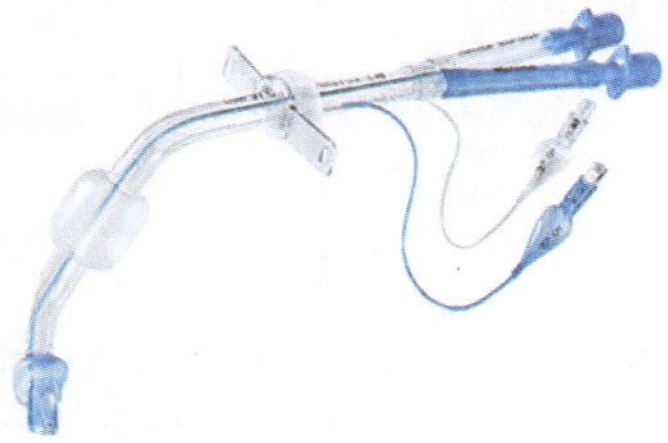

a. Endotracheal tube
b. Endotracheal tube Double lumen
c. Laryngeal mask airway
d. Guedel airway

281. Identify the Instrument/ device shown in Photograph:

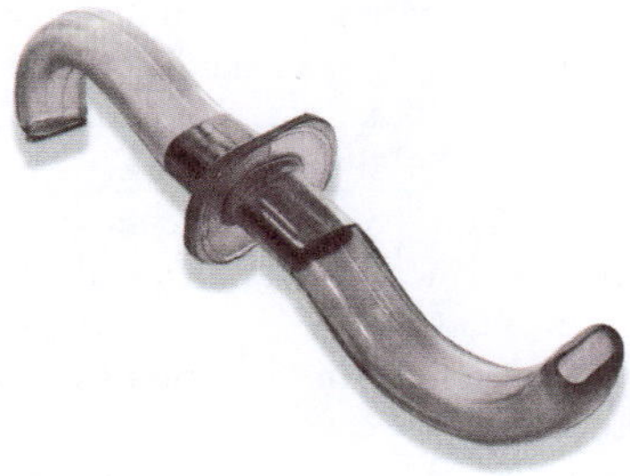

a. Brook airway
b. Water airway
c. Safar airway
d. Guedel airway

284. Identify Parts of Endotracheal tube:

[Recent Question 2015, 2016]

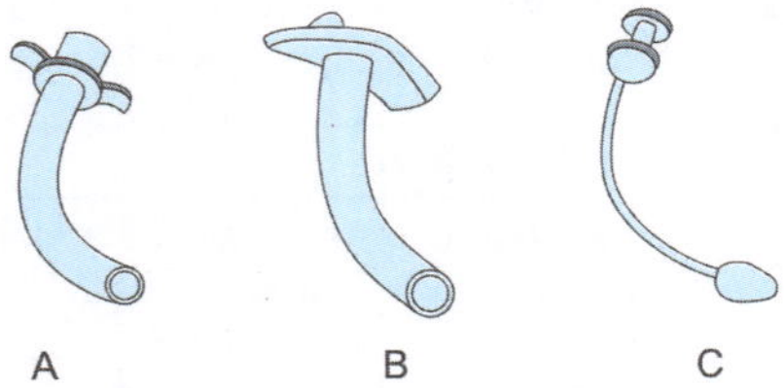

a. A–Outer cannula, B–Inner cannula, C–Obturator
b. A–Obturator, B–Outer cannula, C–Inner cannula
c. A–Obturator, B–Inner cannula, C–Outer cannula
d. A–Inner cannula, B–Outer cannula, C–Obturator

285. Name the following external fixator:

(Refer explanation at the end)

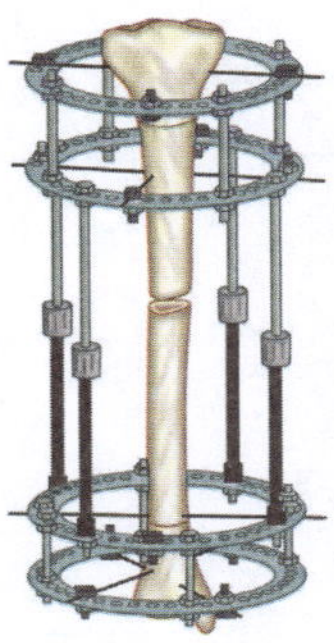

a. Ilizarov external fixator
b. Monolateral external fixator
c. Taylor spatial frame
d. Hoffman external fixator

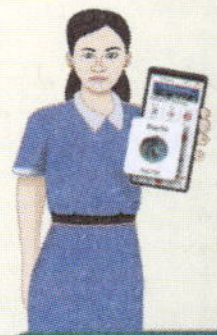

Ans.

279. c
280. b
281. c
282. a
283. b
284. d
285. a

Explanations of Image-Based Questions

8. Ans. (a) Bair Hugger Forced Air Warming Blanket

The Bair Hugger system is a convective temperature management system used in a hospital or surgery center to maintain a patient's core body temperature. The Bair Hugger system consists of a reusable warming unit and single-use disposable warming blankets for use before, during and after surgery.

9. Ans. (b) Bair Hugger warming unit

The Bair Hugger system consists of a warming unit and a disposable blanket. The image shown here is a warming unit. The warming unit is a compact device that delivers temperature-controlled air through a flexible hose. The air is then distributed evenly throughout the disposable blanket, which is placed over the patient.

10. Ans. (b) Disposable blood pressure transducer

A Disposable Pressure Transducer (DPT) is indicated for pressure sensing during clinical invasive procedures without interfering with the patient's blood flow and /or blood pressure. Disposable Blood Pressure Transducer is used in the ICU and Anesthesiology intended for pressure monitoring in arterial and venous vessels.

12. Ans. (a) Peritoneal dialysis kit

Peritoneal dialysis kit consists: Stainless steel trocar, Multi hole smooth tip catheter, Junction unit with control clamp and Scalpel.

13. Ans. (d) Catheter mount

Catheter mounts with swivel connectors are used to attach the endotracheal tube to the ventilator circuit.

14. Ans. (b) Overhead Trapeze

An overhead trapeze is a triangle-shaped metal bar. It hangs from a metal frame, which is attached to the headboard and footboard of the bed. Overhead trapeze is helpful to move in bed when the patient is weak, injured, or cannot move easily.

15. Ans. (b) Bone curette

With a small spoon on the end of the tool similar to that of an ice-cream scoop, a curette allows the surgeon to scrape away bone. The spoon of the bone curette has durable, sharp edges. Its handle may be large and thick, taking up the entire hand, or small and thin.

19. Ans. (b) BiPAP

- BiPAP stands for bilevel positive airway pressure. A BiPAP machine delivers pressurized air that can keep the airway to the lungs open.
- CPAP machine generally releases air at a single pressure. A BiPAP machine pumps air at two different air pressure levels, one for breathing in and another for breathing out.

20. Ans. (b) Pes Cavus

Pes Cavus is defined primarily by the elevation of the longitudinal arch of the foot: a high arched foot.

21. Ans. (b) Interlocking nail

Interlocking Nails are the preferred mode of treatment for fractures of long bones viz. femur, tibia and humerus. Interlocking Nail is a nail placed within the medullary cavity of a long bone secured in position by proximal and distal transfixing screws to provide axial, bending and torsional stability.

22. Ans. (a) Osteotome

An osteotome is an orthopedic instrument that is typically used for cutting bone. A chisel is used for shaping bone. Functionally, the primary difference is that a chisel has one beveled, while an osteotome has two beveled edges (as shown below).

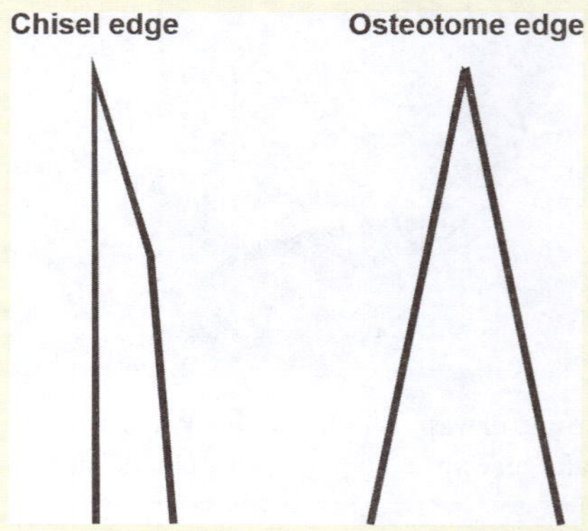

23. Ans. (a) Anomaloscope

The Nagel anomaloscope is used for diagnosing red-green color vision deficiencies (protan and deutan)

24. Ans. (c) Adenoid curette

Hospitime St. Clair Thompson Adenoid Curette has a rectangular curette blade with a cage to retain the adenoid tissue. Hospitime Adenoid Curette is a standard operating instrument which is used to remove the adenoid tissues in adenoidectomy (ENT) procedures.

25. Ans. (a) Mini cryogun

Cryotherapy is a minimally-invasive treatment that uses extreme cold to destroy abnormal tissue. It is often used to treat skin lesions, such as warts, moles, and actinic keratosis. Liquid nitrogen is the most common substance used for cryotherapy. The cryogun is a device that is used to spray liquid nitrogen directly onto the skin.

31. Ans. (a) Obturator sign

The obturator sign can be elicited in an individual by flexing their right knee to a 90 degree angle while a clinician internally rotates the hip by moving the ankle away from the body. Pain associated with this maneuver can be indicative of an inflamed appendix.

32. Ans. (c) Psoas sign

Positive psoas sign refers to Pain on passive extension of the right thigh. It is present when the inflamed appendix is retrocecal and overlying the right psoas muscle.

34. Ans. (a) Myopia

Myopia (Near-sightedness/short-sightedness), is a dioptric condition of the eye where light focuses in front of, instead of, on the retina.

37. Ans. (c) Abducent nerve

- 6th cranial nerve (abducent nerve) palsy leads to abduction of the eyeball as it supplies LR muscle.

To Summarize

- 6th nerve palsy – failure of lateral gaze
- 3rd nerve palsy – eyeball down and out, dilated pupil, ptosis
- 4th nerve palsy – vertical diplopia on looking down – difficulty in going downstairs, reading book

80. Ans. (b) 12 minutes

- **Soak instruments** in Cidex solution for 12 minutes at 20°C **to** achieve high-level disinfection.
- The solution is reusable for up to 14 days.

87. Ans. (d) Negative pressure dressing

- **Negative-pressure wound therapy** (NPWT), also known as a vacuum dressing or vacuum assisted closure, is a therapeutic technique using a suction **dressing** to remove excess exudation and promote **healing** in acute or chronic **wounds** and second- and third-degree burns.

88. Ans. (d) All of these

- **Lidocaine spray** is used to numbs the lining of the **mouth, nasal cavity** and **throat** before certain medical procedure (e.g., intubation).
- It is a local anesthetic that numbs the lining of the mouth and throat 1-2 minutes after application. It also helps prevent the urge to close the throat (gag reflex), which might make the procedure more difficult.

94. Ans. (b) Allen's test

- The **Allen test** is a first line standard **test** used to assess the arterial blood supply of the hand.
- A **positive Allen test** means that the patient does not have an adequate dual blood supply to the hand which would be a negative indication for catheterization, removal of the radial artery or any procedure which may result in occlusion of the vessel (e.g., sample collection for ABG)

159. Ans. (c) PEG

- PEG – percutaneous endoscopic gastrostomy is an endoscopic method of inserting gastrostomy tube for patients who cannot take oral diet.
- For those who need Ryle's tube for more than 4 weeks we will put PEG tube.
- Infection around the PEG tube is a common complication.

160. Ans. (d) Monopolar cautery

Ref: Bailey and Love Page 47

- This is the monopolar diathermy handle- Blue color is for coagulation and Yellow for cutting of tissues

Bipolar Diathermy Handle:

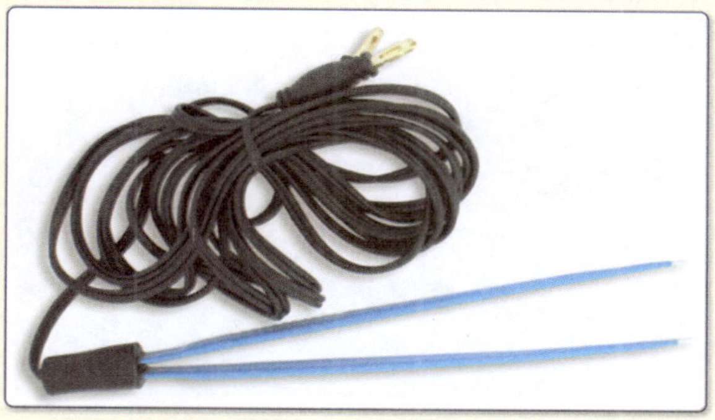

- Bipolar is used for coagulating only, any vessel in between the two limbs gets coagulated.
- No earth plate needed for bipolar.

161. Ans. (b) Battle sign

- Battle sign is due to Fracture of base of skull*
- **Middle cranial fossa fracture**** is associated with Battle sign*

162. Ans. (a) CBD drainage

- This is T –Tube.
- Used to drain Bile after CBD Exploration.
- T Tube cholangiogram done on 7th POD and if Normal Tube can be removed.
- T- tube tract matured for 6 weeks to remove the Stone via T- tube tract is BURHENNE TECHNIQUE**

163. Ans. (a) Malecot's

- This is self-retaining Malecot's catheter.
- Used to drain the abscess
- It has capacity to get retained once placed in a cavity
- It has also been used for feeding purpose*

Other catheters:

Foley's catheter:

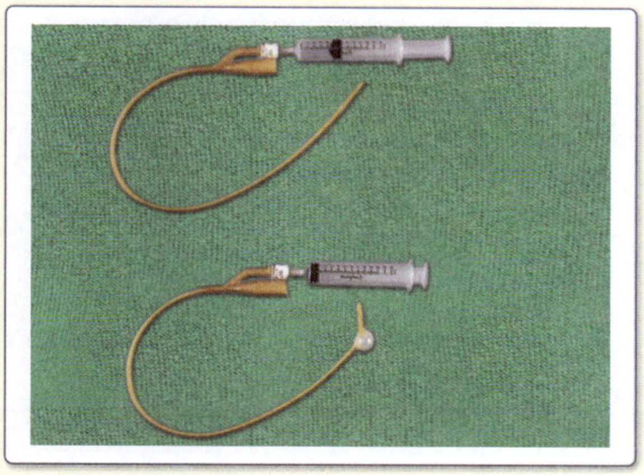

- Foley's catheter- Used to drain urine.
- The Balloon when inflated gets retained in the Bladder*

Central Venous catheter:

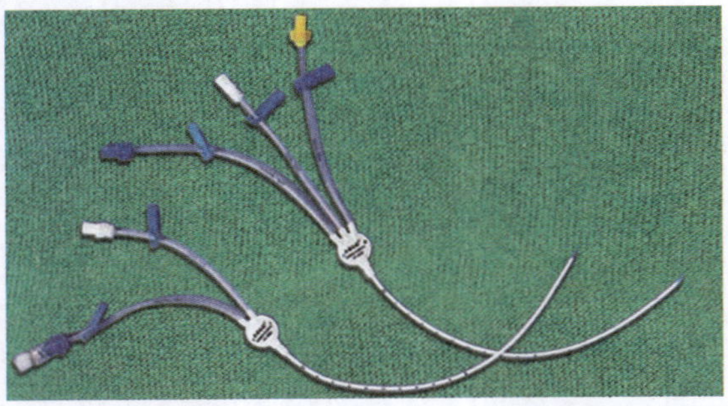

- Central venous Catheter is inserted via Subclavian or IJV for giving Total parenteral nutrition.
- Separate channels are used for IV fluids, Antibiotics and TPN.

164. Ans. (b) Blood set

- This is blood transfusion set with Filter seen inside the IV set collector and the needle is red color in Blood set.

165. Ans. (d) Comminuted

Multiple fractured fragments are present.

166. Ans. (c) Boutenniere deformity

Flexion at PIP joint and extension at DIP joint is Buttonhole or Boutenniere deformity.

167. Ans. (c) Scalp vein

[Ref. Pediatric Emergency Procedures by King, 1/e p734]

- A winged infusion set also known as butterfly or scalp vein **(Photograph)** set is a device specialized for venipuncture, i.e., For accessing a superficial vein for either intravenous injection or phlebotomy
- Consists, from front to rear, of a hypodermic needle, two bilateral flexible wings, flexible small-bore transparent tubing (20–35 cm long), and lastly a connector (female Luer); this connector attaches to syringe / another device

168. Ans. (c) Deep vein thrombosis

[Ref. Maheshwari, 5/e p44]

Homan's Sign

- Pathognomonic of DVT
- Leg swelling and calf tenderness are usual signs
- The calf tenderness may get exaggerated by passive dorsiflexion of the ankle this is called as Homan's sign **(Photograph)**

169. Ans. (b) Genu valgum

[Ref. Maheshwari, 5/e p324, 301]

- Knock-knee deformity (genu valgum) **(Photograph)**: This is a condition where the knees are abnormally approximated and the ankles abnormally divergent

Topper's edge

- Bow legs (Genu Varum) This is a condition where the knees are abnormally divergent (bow like) and the ankles abnormally approximated.
- Genu recurvatum: hyperextension at the knee joint. It may be congenital or acquired. Polio is the commonest cause of acquired genu recurvatum.
- Clergyman's knee: Infrapatellar bursitis

170. Ans. (b) Tracheostomy

- A tracheostomy is a surgical procedure to create an opening through the neck into the trachea (windpipe)
- A tube is usually placed through this opening to provide an airway and to remove secretions from the lungs
- This tube is called a tracheostomy tube or trach tube

189. (b) Bougie

- **Bougies** are long, stiff plastic wands inserted into the trachea through the glottis during direct laryngoscopy (DL), providing a "guidewire" over which an **endotracheal (ET) tube** can then be more easily advanced into the trachea.

193. (c) Gardner well tongs

- Gardner-Wells tongs are U- shaped tongs used for spinal traction, having pressure--controlled pins that are inserted into the skull at opposite ends to permit application of a longitudinal force to the axis of the spinal column.

195. (d) Intravenous pyelogram

- Kidneys, ureters, and bladder **X-ray (KUB)** is a plain (noncontrast) radiograph. An intravenous pyelogram (IVP) uses contrast to highlight the urinary tract.

285. (a) Ilizarov external fixator

- Ilizarov external fixator (Ilizarov frame) is a ring-like brace. The frame is applied to the outside of the limb and connected through the unbroken part of the bone inside the limb. An Ilizarov frame is used to help heal complex fractures, severe skin or tissue loss, lengthen long bones if too much bone has been lost at the time of accident, and correct congenital or traumatic deformity of the bones.

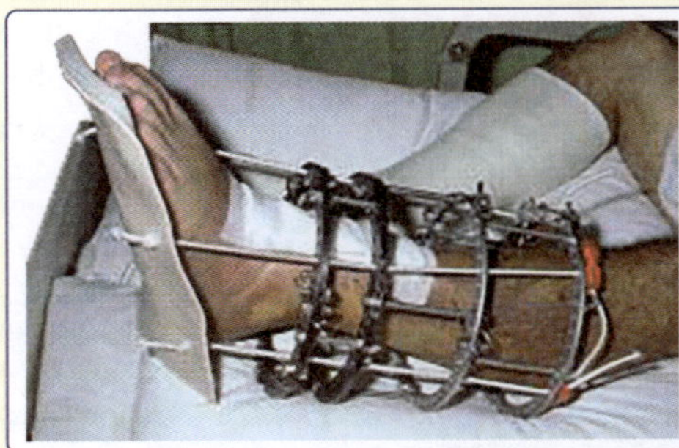

"It is health that is real wealth and not pieces of gold and silver."
—Mahatma Gandhi

CHAPTER 3

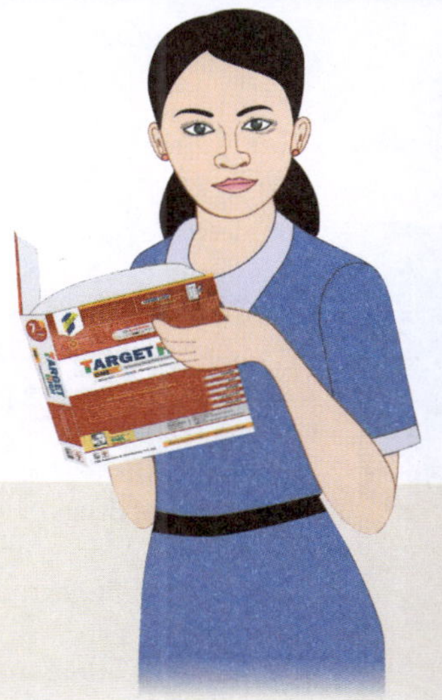

PHARMACOLOGY

SYNOPSIS

KEY TERMINOLOGIES

- **Pharmacology**: It is derived from Greek words 'pharmacon' which means drugs and 'logos' which means study or knowledge. It is the scientific study of the origin, nature, chemistry, effects and uses of drugs.
- **Drug/medications:** Any chemical substance which affects living systems. French word 'drogue' means 'dry herb.' – used for treatment of disease, for the prevention of illness of pathologic states and for diagnosing disease condition.
- **Chemotherapy: Therapeutic treatment of various local or systemic infections or malignancies by using various drugs or chemicals is called chemotherapy.**
- **Pharmacognosy**: The branch of pharmacology dealing with the economic, biological and chemical aspects of natural drugs and their constituents. Study of the sources of drugs and the physical characteristics of crude or unrefined drugs, e.g., plants.
- **Pharmacodynamics** is the effect that drugs have on the body (what drug does to the body).
- **Pharmacokinetics** is the study of the way in which drugs move through the body during **absorption, distribution, metabolism** and **excretion** (what body does to the drug).
- **Absorption**
  - Physiological considerations in absorption: **Blood flow**, **total surface area**, **time of arrival of the drug** and **time of drug at absorption site**.
  - Other considerations for absorption: **Solubility**, **chemical stability** and solubility of drug in **lipids**.
- **Distribution**
  - Drugs are distributed, into major body fluids (e.g., plasma).
  - Drug distribution is affected by the extent that the drug binds to plasma proteins and barriers.
- **Biotransformation**
  - It is a process of metabolizing drugs in the body.
  - Occurs mainly in liver**.**
  - Prodrugs are only activated by the hepatic metabolism **e.g., Levodopa.**
- **Excretion:** Excretion includes renal (by active glomerular filtration and fecal elimination).
- The time of the onset of drug action is determined by the time taken by the drug to reach to the site of action. It is largely controlled by:
  - Route of administration
  - Rate of absorption
  - Manner of distribution.
- **Bioavailability:** It is a measure of fraction of administered drug that reaches the systemic circulation in the unchanged form.
- **First Pass Metabolism**: It is the metabolism of a drug at the site of absorption during its passage from the site of absorption into the systemic circulation. All orally administered drugs undergo first pass metabolism. Drugs administered through sublingual, transdermal and parenteral routes do not undergo first pass metabolism (bypasses portal circulation)
- **Agonist**: These are the drugs which bind to the receptor and produce same biological effect as that of the receptor.
- **Antagonist**: These are the drugs which oppose the action of the receptor or an agonists.
- **Antidote**: A drug which can counteract a form of poisoning, e.g., Atropine is an antidote to organophosphorus poisoning.
- **Lethal Dose 50 (LD50):** Standard measure of the toxicity of a drug/substance that will kill half of the sample population of a specific test animal in a specific period.
- **Pharmacovigilance**: The science and activities relating to the detection, assessment,

KEY POINTS

- Father of Pharmacology - Oswald Schmiedeberg
- Pharmacokinetics - What the body does to the drug?
- Pharmacodynamics - What the drug does to the body?
- Bioavailability of Intravenous (IV) route is 100%.
- Lipophilic drugs (barbiturates, benzodiazepines) are better absorbed in intestine than hydrophilic drugs.
- The liver is the main drug metabolizing organ in the body.
- The first-pass effect can occur in the gastrointestinal tract, the liver and lung.

understanding and prevention of adverse effects, or any other drug related problem.

- **Teratogenicity**: It is the ability of a drug to produce harmful effect of drugs on fetus when administered during pregnancy.
- **Anaphylaxis**: It is a severe allergic reaction (hypersensitive reaction), which occurs due to ingestion of drugs or any foreign protein material.
- **Antidote**: A drug or chemical substance which counteracts the harmful effects of other drug or chemical.
- **Contraindication**: Any condition or factor, which prevents or withholds the use of a medicine or drug.
- **Emulsion**: It is the mixture of two or more liquids that are normally immiscible (e.g., Mixture of water and oil). Milk is a natural emulsion.
- **Half-life**: It is the period of time required for the concentration of drug in body (usually plasma) to be reduced to one-half. It is one of the major factor influences the duration of action of a drug.
- **Iatrogenic**: Refers to condition or illness, occurs due to the action of physician or therapy. It is the result of diagnostic and or therapeutic procedures undertaken on a patient.
- **Idiosyncrasy**: It is genetically determined abnormal reactivity to a drug.
- **Loading dose:** Administering a drug at a dose higher than the routinely used dose is called as loading dose.
- **Synergism:** Drugs are said to be synergistic when the action of one drug is potentiated or increased by the other. It can be additive or superadditive.
  - **Additive:** Effect of drugs A + B = Effect of drug A + Effect of Drug B. e.g., 1 + 1 = 2
  - **Superadditive:** Effect of drugs A + B > Effect of drug A + Effect of Drug B. e.g., 1 + 1 = 10
- **Antagonism:** Drugs are said to be antagonistic when one drug decreases or abolishes the action of another drug.
- **Pharmacopoeia:** It is the official publication which contains all details about established drugs, being in a particular country, e.g., Indian Pharmacopoeia (IP), British Pharmacopoeia (BP), United States Pharmacopoeia (USP)

PRODRUGS

- A prodrug is a medication or compound, which is inactive, that needs to converted in the body into pharmacologically active drug.

  List of prodrugs and their active forms are as follows:

Table 1: Active form of prodrug

Prodrug	Active form
Acyclovir	Acyclovir triphosphate
Fluorouracil	Fluorouridine monophosphate
Bacampicillin	Ampicillin
Prednisone	Prednisolone
Sulindac	Sulfide metabolite
Enalapril	Enalaprilat
Alfa-Methyldopa	Alpha-methyl norepinephrine
Fosphenytoin	Phenytoin

THERAPEUTIC INDEX (TI)

- It is also called safety margin of a drug. It refers to the ratio between the dosage of a drug that causes **a lethal effect** and the dosage that causes a **therapeutic** effect.
- Therapeutic Index (TI) = LD50/ED50

  Where LD 50: Lethal Dose 50 and ED: Effective dose 50
- For the drugs with narrow therapeutic index: Slight deviation from the prescribed dose can be harmful to patients. **Plasma level monitoring is required.**
- For drugs with wide therapeutic index: Usually deviation from prescribed dosage may not be harmful for the patient.

Practice Question

1. Prodrugs with two active compounds are known as ________

a. Mixed prodrugs
b. Mutual prodrugs
c. Dual prodrugs
d. Pro-prodrugs

Ans. (b) Mutual prodrugs

Rationale: Pro-drugs contains two active pharmacological agents coupled together to form a single product e.g., benorylate prodrug for NSAIDs and paracetamol.

KEY POINTS

- Prontosil (prodrug for sulfanamide) was the earliest prodrug discovered accidentally.
- A drug which gets bio-transformed rapidly is known as a **'soft drug'**.
- Antibiotics such as Aminoglycosides and vancomycin have a narrow therapeutic index, and toxicity may be severe and irreversible.
- Digoxin has a therapeutic index value of 2. This means 2 doses of digoxin taken at one time have a 50:50 chance of developing toxic side effects.

Table 2: Therapeutic indices of some common drugs

Very narrow therapeutic index	Narrow therapeutic index	Wide therapeutic index
• Vancomycin • Amphotericin • B Polymyxin	• Warfarin • Levothyroxine • Carbamazepine • Lithium Carbonate • Digoxin • Phenytoin • Theophylline • Morphine	• Almost all Antibiotics • NSAIDS • Hypnotics/Sedatives • Beta-blockers • Benzodiazepines

DIFFERENT ROUTES OF ADMINISTRATION, ITS ADVANTAGES AND DISADVANTAGES

Table 3: Advantages and disadvantages of different routes

Route	Advantages	Disadvantages
Oral route	Easy to take No professional assistance required Economical	Gastric acid may decrease the drug efficiency It causes GI irritation Variable rate of absorption will occur
Sublingual route	This helps to avoid the first pass metabolism and interaction with gastric acid	Not suitable for all the preparation
Rectal route	This helps to avoid the first pass metabolism and interaction with gastric acid	Not suitable for all the preparation Administration may affect the dignity of the patient.
Parenteral (refers to IV, IM and SC) Routes		
Intravenous	Fast action and 100% bioavailability	Lack of aseptic technique may lead to sepsis. Danger of extravasation. Phlebitis can occur if irritant drugs are administered
Intramuscular	Rapid absorption	Painful, increased risk for tissue damage
Subcutaneous	Provide drug over a period of time, i.e., it promotes slow absorption of drug	Absorption rate will be varying
Intradermal route	Absorption is slow, so useful for testing allergies	Amount of drug administered must be small
Inhaled drug	Large absorption area	

SPECIAL DRUG DELIVERY SYSTEM

- **Dermojet:** This is painless and needleless method of drug administration. A high velocity jet of drug solution is projected through a micro-fine orifice using a gun-like device. The drug will get deposited in the subcutaneous tissue.
- **Pellet implantation:** The drug is in the form of solid pellet. It is introduced surgically with the help of trocar and cannula. The drug will be released from the solid pellet for weeks and month, e.g., DOCA, testosterone.
- **Implants:** Drug packed in tube or capsule is implanted under the skin. Uniform and slow release of drug occurs for months together.
- **Liposomes:** Minute vesicles made of phospholipids into which the drug is incorporated. It is used for targeted delivery, e.g., Amphotericin B and Anticancer drugs.
- **Monoclonal antibodies:** These are antibodies which selectively react with specific antigen, e.g., Rituximab, cetuximab.

Table 4: Drugs and their deposition in the various body tissues

Body tissues where deposition occurs	Drugs
Bone and teeth	Tetracycline, heavy metals
Skeletal muscle and heart	Digoxin, emetine (bound to muscle proteins)
Liver	Chloroquine, tetracycline, emetine, digoxin
Kidney	Digoxin, chloroquine, emetine
Thyroid	Iodine
Retina	Chloroquine (bound to nucleoproteins)

KEY POINTS

- Intradermal route is used for testing allergies (test dose) and BCG vaccination.
- Angles for injections:
  - Intradermal - 10 to 15 degree
  - Intravenous - 25 degree
  - Subcutaneous - 45 degree
  - Intramuscular - 90 degree
- Subcutaneous route is not useful for emergency due to slow absorption rate.
- Intravenous administration is useful for large volume administration and for emergency.
- Sustained/Controlled release tablets reduce the dosing frequency especially in chronic diseases. There is less chance of over dosage.
- Transdermal drug delivery system is a form that delivers the drug at a constant rate to systemic circulation, e.g., Transdermal patch & Ointment.
- Implantable insulin pumps implanted in subcutaneous tissue delivers insulin depends on plasma glucose level.

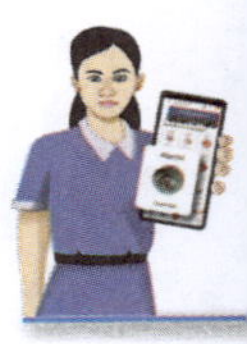

Commonly used Abbreviations in Prescriptions

- **R_x:** The symbol R is an abbreviation for the Latin word RECIPE, which means take thou or you take. The line on the foot of R is set to designate an invocation to Jupiter, the God of Knowledge, learning and healing.
- **Tab:** Tablet
- **Cap:** Capsule
- **Inj:** Injection
- **IM:** Intramuscular
- **IV:** Intravenous
- **SC:** Subcutaneous
- **I/D:** Intradermal
- **OD:** Once in a day
- **BD/BID:** Bis in die (Twice a day)
- **TDS:** Ter in die sumendum (To be taken thrice a day)
- **TID:** Ter in die (Three times a day)
- **QID:** Quarter in die (Four times a day)
- **HS:** Hora somni (At bed time)
- **Stat:** Stain (Immediately)
- **Rept:** Repetatur (Repeat)
- **Non rept:** Non repetatur (Non repeat)
- **AC:** Ante cibum (Before meals)
- **PC:** Post cibum (After meals)
- **NPO:** Nil per orally (Nothing to taken by mouth)
- **BBF:** Before breakfast
- **AD:** After dinner
- **SOS:** As and when required

CONVERSION EQUIVALENCE OF WEIGHT

Table 5: Conversion equivalence of weight

Unit	Symbol	Equivalent
1 kilogram	kg	1,000 grams (g)
1 kilogram	Kg	2.2 pounds (lb)
1 gram	g	1,000 milligrams (mg)
1 milligram	mg	1,000 micrograms (μg)
1 microgram	μg	1,000 nanograms (ng)
1 ounce	oz	28.35 g
1 pound	Lb	454 g
1 gram	g	15.432 grains

CONVERSION EQUIVALENCE OF VOLUME

Table 6: Conversion equivalence of volume

Unit	Equivalent
1 drop (gtt)	0.05 mL
1 mL	20 drops
1 teaspoon full	5 mL
1 Tablespoon full	15 mL
1 mL	16.23 minims
1 minim	0.06 mL
1 pint	473 mL
1 quart	949 mL
1 gallon	3745 mL

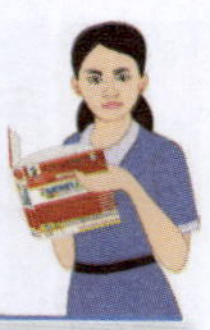

DRUG CALCULATION

- To convert a smaller unit (e.g., a gram) into a larger unit (e.g., a kilogram), divide by 1000, so
  - 3000 g ÷ 1000 = 3 kg
- To convert a larger unit (e.g., a kg) into a smaller unit (e.g., a gram), multiply by 1000, so:
  - 3 kg × 1000 = 3000 g

Basic Formula

There is more than one way to do a drug calculation, but the simplest and most widely used method is the basic formula shown here:

$$\frac{(D \times Q)}{H} = X$$

D = desired dose

H = strength available

Q = quantity or unit of measure (for tablets Q = 1, for liquids Q can vary)

X = dose to be determined/amount to be given

Practice Question

2. Nurse Ramya has to infuse 500 mL DNS solution in over 6 h Drop factor is 20 gtt/mL. What flow rate (drops/min) will nurse Ramya on the IV infusion pump?

Explanation:

Formula:

Drop/min = (Total infusion volume (in mL) x drop factor)/infusion time (in minutes)

$$= \frac{(500 \times 20)}{360}$$

$$= \frac{10,000}{360}$$

= 27.7 (rounded off to 28 drops/min)

POINT TO REMEMBER

While calculating for tablets Q = 1; for liquids, usually Q is the no. of mL given. In this case 5 mL)

Some Examples

1. The doctor orders a dose of 100 mg to be given orally. You have 25 mg tablets. How many tablets should you give?

   $$\frac{(100 \times 1)}{25} = X$$

   X = 4 tablets
2. The patient requires 800 mg of liquid to be given orally. You have 250 mg in 5 mL of solution. What volume of drug should be given? Applying the same formula given above

   $$\frac{(800 \times 5)}{250} = X$$

   400/25 = 16 mL
3. The patient needs 270 mg of drug D by injection. 150 mg in 5 mL of liquid is available. How many mL will you administer?

   $$\frac{(270 \times 5)}{150} = X$$

   X = 9 mL

ANTIMICROBIAL AGENTS

Table 7: Antibiotics, antifungals and antivirals with their examples, therapeutic uses and side effects

Class of drugs	Examples	Therapeutic uses	Side effects
Penicillins	**Natural penicillin** • Penicillin G (Acid-labile) • Penicillin V (Acid-resistant) Penicillinase-resistant agent • Oxacillin • Cloxacillin Aminopenicillins • Ampicillin • Amoxicillin β-lactamase inhibitors • Clavulanic acid • Sulbactam • Tazobactam	• Streptococcal infection • Gonococcal and syphilis • *Pseudomonas aeruginosa* • *Haemophilus influenzae*	• Hypersensitivity. • Skin rash to anaphylactic shock (penicillin allergy) • It is more common with parenteral administration of penicillin
Cephalosporins	**First generation** • Cefazolin • Cefadroxil • Cefalexin **Second generation** • Cefuroxime • Cefoxitin • Cefaclor • Cefprozil **Third generation** • Cefixime • Cefotaxime • Ceftriaxone **Fourth generation (parenteral)** • Cefepime • Cefpirome **Fifth generation (parenteral)** • Ceftobiprole • Ceftaroline	• Urinary Tract infection (UTI) • Pneumonia • Serious bacterial infections • Soft tissue infection	• Minor gastrointestinal complaints • Nephrotoxicity • Thrombophlebitis on IV (intravenous) administration
Aminoglycosides	Streptomycin, Amikacin, Gentamicin, Neomycin, Kanamycin, Tobramycin	• Gram negative pneumonias • Pseudomonas infections	• Nephrotoxicity • Ototoxicity • Neuromuscular blockage
Tetracyclines	Tetracycline, Doxycycline, oxytetracycline, Minocycline and Demeclocycline.	• Atypical pneumonias • Mycoplasma infection	• **Tooth discoloration in children** • **Growth retardation** • Bone marrow depression • Hypersensitivity • Oral and vaginal candidiasis

Contd...

KEY POINTS

- Alexander Fleming discovered Penicillin in 1928.
- Penicillin was the first antibiotic used clinically in 1941.
- Cephalosporins are chemically similar to penicillins.
- Tetracyclines is contraindicated in pregnancy and in young children.
- Tooth discoloration and growth retardation are the major side effects of Tetracyclines.
- **Gray baby syndrome** is an adverse reaction to chloramphenicol that is characterized by abdominal distention, hemodynamic collapse, and ashen-gray skin discoloration in neonates.
- As per the WHO guidelines, ciprofloxacin or ofloxacin is recommended for fully sensitive typhoid cases.
- Neomycine and Soframicine are topically used Aminoglycosides.
- Ototoxicity and Nephrotoxicity are the major side effects of Amnioglycosides.

Recent Question (NORCET 2023)

1. **Administration of which antibiotic does not require a sensitivity test?**
   a. Metronizadole
   b. Amoxicillin
   c. Cefoparazone
   d. Merepenem

Ans. **(a) Metronizadole**

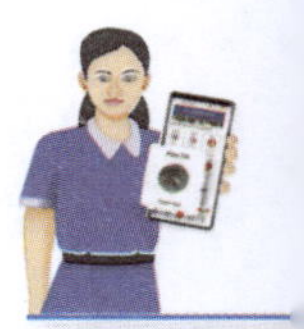

Class of drugs	Examples	Therapeutic uses	Side effects
Fluoroquinolones	**First generation** • Ciprofloxacin • Ofloxacin • Norfloxacin **Second generation** • Levofloxacin • Moxifloxacin	• Chronic bronchitis • Cystic fibrosis • Effective against *H. influenzae,* P. pneumonia, *N. meningitides,* Pertussis, Pseudomonas	• Ciprofloxacin contraindicated for children (below age 21).
Macrolide antibiotics	Erythromycin Azithromycin Clarithromycin Roxithromycin	• Respiratory infection • Genital, GI and soft tissue infections. • Drug of choice for mycoplasma	• GI upset • Anorexia • Diarrhea
Sulfonamides	Trimethoprim Sulfamethoxazole (Cotrimoxazole: Combination of above two drugs)	• UTI • *Pneumocystis carinii* pneumonia • Pneumonia	• Leukopenia • Rash • Fever
Antifungal agents	Amphotericin B	Severe fungal infections (systemic antifungal)	• Nephrotoxicity • Hypotension
	Nystatin Ketoconazole Fluconazole	(Oral and topical) • Oral thrush • *Candida albicans*	• Allergic reaction • Itching, burning sensation and redness on local application
Antiviral	Acyclovir Ganciclovir Amantadine Rimantadine **Antiretroviral** • Lamivudine • Zidovudine • Stavudine	• Herpes simplex virus • Herpes zoster • Cytomegalovirus • HIV infection	• Dizziness, nausea, vomiting, stomach pain and joint pain
Antimalarial	Quinine Chloroquine Primaquine Mefloquine	• Treatment of malaria • Chloroquine use is safe in pregnant women.	• Stomach upset • Blurred vision

CARDIAC DRUGS

Cardiac Glycosides (Digitoxin)

- Cardiac glycosides are effective drugs for treatment of Congestive Heart Failure (CHF).
- **Drugs:** Digitoxin (0.05–0.3 mg/day), Digoxin (0.4-0.6 mg followed by 0.05–0.35 mg once or twice daily).
- **They increase the force of myocardial contractions** (positive inotropic).
- Increases the release of **Ca^{++}** ions in the myocardial cells.
- Used to treat cardiac **arrhythmia** because they decrease heart rate.
- **Pulse should be assessed before Digoxin administration and it should not be administered if heart rate (pulse) is below 60 b/min.**
- **Indications: CHF, cardiac arrhythmia** (atrial fibrillation, atrial flutter and sinus tachycardia).

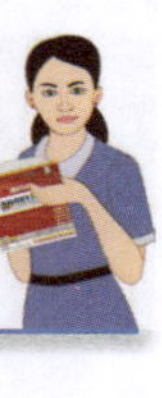

- **Side effects:** Cardiac arrhythmia such as bradycardia (below 60 beat/minute), ventricular fibrillation (which may lead to cardiac arrest and death) and bigeminal rhythm and skin rashes. Vision changes including **blurring of vision, blind spots, diplopia** and **white halos.**
- **Digoxin and Potassium: H**ypokalemia in the body can increase the risk of digitalis toxicity. On the other hand, digoxin toxicity causes hyperkalemia.

Nitrates/Nitrites

- Treatment of chronic angina pectoris and hypertension associated with MI or CHF
- **Nitroglycerin ointment** for treatment of **Raynaud's disease.**
- **Dose: Sublingual–5 mg PRN; Oral–20–40 mg twice a day.**

KEY POINTS

- Co-trimoxazole is a combination drug of trimethoprim (TMP) and sulfamethoxazole (SMX) in a 1:5 ratio.
- Antifungals such as Amphotericin B, Posaconazole, or Isavuconazole are used in the treatment of Mucormycosis.
- Antiretroviral drugs are used in the treatment of HIV/AIDS.
- Protease inhibitors affect replication of HIV at different stages than nucleoside analogs.
- Monotherapy for treatment of HIV disease cause rapid drug resistance.
- Hypokalemia increases the risk of digoxin toxicity.
- Digoxin toxicity leads to hyperkalemia.
- Digoxin should be withheld if the pulse is below 60 bpm in adults.

Recent Question (NORCET 2022)

2. To ensure proper client education, the nurse should teach the client taking sublingual nitroglycerine to expect which of the following responses with administration?

a. Stinging, burning when placed under the tongue
b. Temporary blurring of vision
c. Generalized urticaria with prolonged use
d. Urinary frequency

Ans. (a) Stinging, burning...

POINT TO REMEMBER

If one dose of Digoxin is missed, take the next dose at usual time. Do not take a double dose to make up for the missed dose.

- **Side effects:** Headache, syncope, dizziness, postural hypotension, transient flushing and palpitation. Topical application may lead to dermatitis.

Calcium Channel Blockers

- Diltiazem, Nifedipine, Amlodipine besylate, Verapamil
- Reduce myocardial contractility
- Inhibit spasm of coronary arteries
- Peripheral vasodilation

Antihypertensive Drugs

Antihypertensive agents are initiated when systolic blood pressure more than 140 mm Hg and diastolic blood pressure is higher than 90 mm Hg.

Angiotensin-Converting Enzyme Inhibitors (ACE Inhibitor)

E.g., Captopril, Enalapril maleate.

- **Indications:**
  - Hypertension
  - In combination with diuretics and digitalis in the treatment of CHF
  - Most common side effect is dry cough.
- **Side effects:** Skin rash, loss of taste, neutropenia, nausea, vomiting, hypotension, proteinuria, renal failure and hyperkalemia.
- **Dose:** 12.5 mg 2–3 times per day (captopril).

Beta-Adrenergic Blocking Agents

E.g., Atenolol, Sotalol, Propranolol, Metoprolol, Timolol.

- **Action:** It combines with beta-adrenergic receptors to block the response to sympathetic nerve impulses, circulating catecholamines or adrenergic drugs.
- **Uses:** Hypertension, angina pectoris, cardiac arrhythmias, myocardial infarction, prophylaxis of migraine.
- **Side Effects:** Bradycardia, CHF, hypotension, cold extremities, edema, dyspnea, shortness of breath, nausea, vomiting, hepatomegaly and bronchospasm.

Centrally Acting Agents

- These agents are used for treatment of chronic hypertension, since it affects CNS.
  E.g., Clonidine hydrochloride, Methyldopa.
- **Uses:**
  - **Clonidine:** Mild to moderate hypertension.
  - **Methyldopa:** Hypertension and hypertensive crisis (parenteral).
- **Side effects:** Drowsiness, headache, malaise, dry mouth, **bradycardia** and constipation.

Agents that Act Directly on Vascular Smooth Muscles

E.g., Hydralazine hydrochloride.

- **Uses:** These agents are used with combination therapy to treat hypertension. Given **parenterally** in hypertension emergencies.
- **Side effects:** Orthostatic hypotension, tachycardia, nausea, vomiting, headache, dizziness, constipation and male impotence.

KEY POINTS

- **Sodium Nitroprusside** is used predominantly to treat hypertensive emergencies, such as to lower blood pressure during acute aortic dissection or to improve cardiac output in severe congestive heart failure.
- Hydralazine can cause an SLE type syndrome in up to 10 – 20% of patients.
- Spironolactone and or potassium supplements combined with ACE inhibitors can cause dangerous hyperkalaemia.
- Longest acting beta blocker: **Nadolol**
- Shortest acting beta bloker: **Esmolol**

Table 8: Antihypertensive drugs with their examples and action

Category	Examples	Action
Diuretics	• Chlorothiazide • Hydrochlorothiazide • Furosemide • Amiloride	Thiazide diuretics are the 1st line drug in mild to moderate hypertension
β-Blockers	• Propranolol • Atenolol • Labetalol • Esmolol • Nadolol	• Block β-receptors thereby ↓Heart rate and CO.
Calcium channel blockers	• Nifedipine • Nicardipine • Amlodipine • Nimodipine • Verapamil • Diltiazem	• Prevent entry of calcium • Causing relaxation of blood vessels • ↓Myocardial contractions.
ACE inhibitors	• Captopril • Enalapril	• Inhibit conversion of Angiotensin I to Angiotensin II (Angiotensin II cause vasoconstriction and increased BP)
Vasodilators	• Hydralazine • Sodium nitroprusside	• Dilate blood vessels

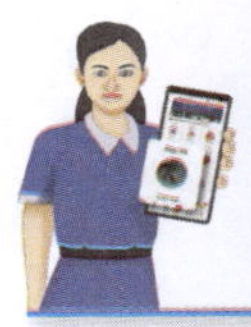

Antiarrhythmic Agents

- **Amiodarone hydrochloride (200–400 mg/day):** Reserved for life threatening ventricular arrhythmias which don't respond to other therapy
- **Lidocaine hydrochloride:** Used in acute ventricular arrhythmias which follows MI or cardiac surgeries.
  - **Loading dose:** IV bolus 50–100 mg, followed by intravenous **Infusion**: 20–50 mg/kg at a rate of 1–4 mg/m.
- **Procainamide:** Used in ventricular tachycardia, atrial fibrillation, digitalis intoxication.
- **Propranolol**
- **Verapamil.**

DRUGS ACTING ON CENTRAL NERVOUS SYSTEM

General Anesthetics

These are group of drugs which bring about a reversible loss of pain, sensation and consciousness.

Classification

- **Inhalational anesthetics**
  - Gases
    - Nitrous oxide (70–80% with other agents) (used as an adjuvant with other anesthetic agents).
    - Cyclopropane (5–25%)
  - Volatile Liquids
    - Ether (Diethyl ether) 3–10%
    - Trichloroethylene (0.25–0.75%)
    - Halothane (0.5–2.0%)
    - Methoxyflurane (0.1–0.3%)
    - Enflurane (1–3%)
    - Isoflurane (0.8–2.0% or not)
- **Intravenous Anesthetics**
  - Ultra-short acting barbiturates
    - Hexobarbitone
    - Thiopentone sodium (3–5 mg/kg)
    - Methohexital sodium (1–3 mg/kg)
  - Non-barbiturate intravenous anesthetics
    - Propofol
    - Ketamine
    - Diazepam
    - Lorazepam
    - Midazolam
- Nitrous oxide is also called **"Laughing gas".**
- The usual concentration used is 70% nitrous oxide + 30% oxygen with some muscle relaxants.
- **Cyclopropane** may produce a variety of **cardiac irregularities** such as **tachycardia and fibrillation.**

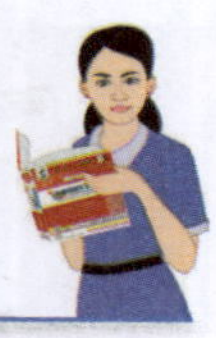

- **Ether was the first substance to be used for general anesthesia (1846).**
- **Halothane** causes relatively greater **respiratory depression.**
- **Methoxyflurane** is the most potent inhalational anesthetic. It also produces respiratory and cardiovascular depression like **Halothane** but **bradycardia** is more prominent.
- After thiopentone injection, **blood pressure falls** immediately but recovers rapidly.
- **Ketamine is a new non-barbiturate anesthetic agent. IV ketamine produces unconsciousness and analgesia within 30 seconds. It acts on cerebral cortex and subcortical areas.**
- **Fentanyl-droperidol combination** is recommended for endoscopies, angiographies, burn dressings, etc.
- **Chlorpromazine (25 mg), triflupromazine (10 mg) or haloperidol (2-4 mg) IM are used as preanesthetic medication.**

SEDATIVE AND HYPNOTICS

Classification

- Barbiturates
  - Phenobarbitone
  - Butobarbitone
  - Pentobarbitone
  - Secobarbitone
- Benzodiazepines
  - Used as hypnotics
    - Diazepam
    - Nitrazepam
    - Midazolam
  - Used as antianxiety agents
    - Diazepam (long acting)
    - Chlordiazepoxide (long acting)
    - Lorazepam (short acting)
    - Alprazolam (short acting)
    - Oxazepam
  - **Newer nonbenzodiazepines hypnotics**
    - Zopiclone
    - Zolpidem
- Manifestations of **Barbiturate poisoning** includes respiratory depression, circulatory shock, initially constriction of pupil and then dilated, hypothermia, renal failure and pulmonary edema.
- **Treatment of acute barbiturate poisoning:** Gastric lavage, mechanical ventilation, forced diuresis and dialysis.
- **Benzodiazepines** act by potentiating neural **inhibition in CNS** which is mediated by **GABA** (GABA facilitator).
- **Antidote** → Flumazenil

KEY POINTS

- Adverse effects of thiopentone include laryngospasm, shivering and delirium.
- Alprazolam is effective in managing panic disorder.
- Triazolam is the shortest acting benzodiazepine.
- **Diazepam and Clonazepam are also used as antiepileptic agents also in emergency like status epilepticus.**
- **Barbiturates** produce CNS depression.
- **Phenobarbital is drug of choice for convulsion.** It is also used as preanesthetic medication.
- Prolonged administration of nitrous oxide as in cases of tetanus, may cause bone marrow depression and agranulocytosis.
- Flumazenil is an antidote for Benzodiazepines.

Table 9: Sympathetic and parasympathetic mediated actions on different organs

Site	Action of sympathetic	Action of parasympathetic
Heart	Stimulates HR (heart rate), conduction	Depress (↓es, HR, ↓es conduction)
Bronchus	Relaxes (bronchodilation)	Stimulates (broncho-constriction)
GIT	Relaxes (↓es movements)	Stimulates (movements)
Bladder	Relaxes (↓es urine flow)	Stimulates (↑es urine flow)
Pupil	Relax (mydriasis)	Stimulates (miosis)
Glands	Depress (secretions except sweating)	Stimulates (secretions except sweating)

KEY POINT

In schizophrenia, Clozapine is more effective than haloperidol against social withdrawal symptoms.

ANTIPSYCHOTIC DRUGS

Classification

Typical Antipsychotics

- **Phenothiazines**
  - Chlorpromazine: 40–800 mg
  - Perphenazine: 12–64 mg
  - Fluphenazine: 1–10 mg
  - Thioridazine: 100–400 mg
- **Thioxanthenes**
  - Thiothixene: 6–30 mg
- **Butyrophenones**
  - Haloperidol: 1–20 mg
- **Dibenzothiazepine**

Atypical Antipsychotics

- Clozapine: 100–300 mg
- Risperidone: 2–8 mg
- Olanzapine: 5–20 mg
- Quetiapine: 50–400 mg
- Aripiprazole: 15-30 mg/day

Indications

- Acute and chronic psychosis.
- Selected agents used as antiemetics (chlorpromazine, prochlorperazine).
- Intractable hiccoughs (chlorpromazine, perphenazine)
- Tics and vocal utterances in Tourette's disorder (haloperidol, pimozide).
- Doc for Tourette Syndrome → ARIPIPRAZOLE

Action

Acts by blocking postsynaptic dopamine receptors in the basal ganglia, hypothalamus, limbic system, brainstem and medulla.

Contraindications

- Blood dyscrasias
- Parkinson' disease
- Liver/renal/cardiac insufficiencies.

Side Effects

- **Anticholinergic effects**
  - Dry mouth, Blurred vision, constipation, urinary retention.
- Nausea, skin rash, sedation
- Orthostatic hypotension
- Photosensitivity
- **Hormonal effects**
  - Decreased libido, retrograde ejaculation, gynecomastia, amenorrhea, weight gain.
- **ECG changes:** Prolongation of the QT interval, are possible with most of the antipsychotics.
- Reduction of seizure threshold.
- **Agranulocytosis**:
  - Clozapine: Weekly/biweekly blood investigation. Hypersalivation **(clozapine).**
- **Extrapyramidal Symptoms (EPS) mainly with typicals**
  - Pseudoparkinsonism
    - Tremor, shuffling gait, drooling, rigidity.
    - 5–30 days after initiation of antipsychotics.
  - Akinesia
  - Akathisia (5–60 days after initiation of therapy).
  - Dystonia: Men; <25 years of age. Earliest onset EPS
  - **Oculogyric crisis**
    - Treated as emergency
    - Physician should be contacted immediately
    - Management: IV benztropine mesylate
  - Tardive dyskinesia.
- **Neuroleptic Malignant Syndrome (NMS)**
  - Severe parkinsonian muscle rigidity
  - Up to 107°C, tachycardia, tachypnea
  - Fluctuations in blood pressure, diaphoresis and rapid deterioration of mental status to stupor and coma
  - This is rare but potentially fatal complication of treatment with neuroleptic drugs
  - It may precipitate within hours to years after drug initiation.
  - Discontinue neuroleptic immediately
  - Management: Bromocriptine (Antidote)
  - Dantrolene

Practice Question

3. A 19-year-old female patient diagnosed with schizophrenia was prescribed Fluphenazine. She developed high fever and lead-pipe rigidity three days after starting Fluphenazine. The most appropriate treatment for this patient would be:

a. Continue Fluphenazine and add anticholinergic
b. Discontinue Fluphenazine and administer Haloperidol
c. Discontinue Fluphenazine and administer Dantrolene
d. Continue Fluphenazine and add Diazepam

Ans. (c) Discontinue Fluphenazine and administer Dantrolene

Rationale: Neuroleptic malignant syndrome (NMS) is a life-threatening idiosyncratic reaction to antipsychotic drugs characterized by fever, altered mental status, muscle rigidity, and autonomic dysfunction. Medications prescribed as treatment may include skeletal muscle relaxants, such as dantrolene. Dantrolene sodium directly relaxes muscles by inhibiting calcium release from the sarcoplasmic reticulum.

ANTIDEPRESSANTS

Classification

Monoamine Oxidase Inhibitors (MAOI)
• **Moclobemide, Clorgyline**
Tricyclic Antidepressants (TCAs)
• NA + 5-HT reuptake inhibitors ▪ Imipramine, Amitriptyline, Trimipramine, Doxepin, Dothiepin, Clomipramine • Predominantly NA reuptake inhibitors ▪ Desipramine, Nortriptyline, Amoxapine
Selective Serotonin Reuptake inhibitors (SSRIs)
• Fluoxetine, Fluvoxamine, Paroxetine, Sertraline, Citalopram
Atypical Antidepressants
• Trazodone, Mianserin, Mirtazapine, Venlafaxine, Tianeptine, Amineptine, Bupropion.

Monoamine Oxidase Inhibitors (MAOI)

- Mood elevating effect develops **after 3–4 weeks.**
- Excitement and hypomania may be produced even in nondepressed individuals.
- **Side Effects:**
  - They produce a variety of **CNS and autonomic side effects.**
  - Agitation, hallucinations, mania, peripheral neuropathy and hepatocellular damage are serious toxic effects.
  - **Cheese reaction**. Avoid consuming cheese containing foods. When taking MAOIs, food high in tyramine needs to be avoided because these items can cause high increase in blood pressure. E.g., Aged cheese, cured meats, fermented cabbage, soy sauce, and fish sauce.

Tricyclic Antidepressants (TCAs)

- The TCAs inhibit monoamine uptake and interact with a variety of receptors (muscarinic, alpha adrenergic, histamine H1, 5-HT1, 5-HT2 and occasionally dopamine D2).
- **After 2–3 weeks** of continuous treatment the mood is gradually elevated.
- **Adverse effects:**
  - Dry mouth, bad taste, constipation, epigastric distress, urinary retention, blurred vision, palpitation, sedation, mental confusion and weight gain
  - Some patients may switch to hypomania or mania
  - Sweating and fine tremors are relatively common
  - Seizure threshold is lowered-**fits may be precipitated**
  - **Postural hypotension**, especially in older patients.

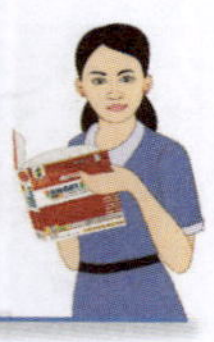

Selective Serotonin Reuptake Inhibitors (SSRI)

- Their relative safety and better acceptability has made them **first line drugs in depression** and allowed their extensive use in **anxiety**, **phobias**, **OCD** and related disorders.
- SSRIs are preferred for **prophylaxis of recurrent depression.**
- **Side Effects:** Nervousness, restlessness, insomnia, anorexia, dyskinesia, headache and diarrhea is associated with them, but patient acceptability is good.

MOOD STABILIZERS

Classification

- **Anticonvulsant mood stabilizers**
  - Valproic acid (Depakene) and sodium valproate (Depacon, Epilim)
  - Lamotrigine (Lamictal)
  - Carbamazepine (Tegretol)
  - Gabapentin (Neurontin)
- **Other mood stabilizers**
  - Lithium carbonate
- **Calcium Channel Blocker**
  - Verapamil

Lithium

- Lithium is used to treat the manic episodes of manic depression.
- Lithium may enhance reuptake of norepinephrine decreasing the levels in the body, resulting in decreased hyperactivity
- **Indications**
  - Prevention and treatment of manic episodes of bipolar disorder.
  - Also used for bipolar depression
- **Contraindications:**
  - Cardiac or renal disease
  - Dehydration
  - Sodium depletion
  - Brain damage
  - Pregnancy and lactation

POINT TO REMEMBER

Dangerous hypertensive crisis with excitement and hallucinations have occurred when TCAs are given with selective serotonin reuptake inhibitors (SSRI).

KEY POINTS

- It takes about 1–3 weeks for lithium to show the effects and remission of symptoms.
- Patient on lithium should be advised to take 6–8 large glasses of water and maintain normal sodium intake in the diet.
- Lithium is contraindicated in pregnancy and lactation.

Side effects of Lithium (LITH)
L - Leucocytosis
I - Insipidus (Nephrogenic Diabetes Insipidus)
T - Tremer/Teratogenic (Ebstein's anomaly)
H - Hypothyroidism

Practice Question

4. All of the following interventions are used in the treatment of lithium toxicity, except

a. Using an antagonist
b. Ingestion of polystyrene sulfonate
c. Treating dehydration
d. Hemodialysis

Ans. (a) Using an antagonist

Table 10: Descriptions of clinical condition and dose

Clinical condition	Dose
Acute mania **Maintenance**	1200–2400 mg 300–1200 mg
Therapeutic plasma range	**Dose**
Acute mania Maintenance	1.0–1.5 mEq/L 0.6–1.2 mEq/L

- **Side Effects**
  - **Adverse reactions:** Below 1.5 mEq/ L.
    - CNS problem including lethargy, muscle weakness, and fine tremor; polyuria (renal toxicity); Beginning of GI toxicity, with nausea, vomiting and diarrhea; weight gain
  - **Mild to moderate adverse reactions:** 1.5–2.5 mEq/L
    - Intensification of all the reaction as mentioned above, with ECG changes.
    - At 2–2.5 mEq/L level, there will be possible CNS effects such as ataxia, clonic movements, hyperreflexia, and seizures; ECG changes, hypotension and polyuria (diluted urine) and dehydration; fatalities secondary to pulmonary edema
  - **Severe reactions:** 2.5 mEq/L and above.
    - Complex multi-organ toxicity, with a significant risk of death
  - **EEG Changes**: Diffuse slowing, widening of the frequency spectrum.
  - **ECG Changes:** Reversible flattening, isoelectricity or inversion of T-waves.
- **Client/Family Education**
  - **Not to drive or operate dangerous machinery** until lithium levels are stabilized.
  - The client should drink **6–8 large glasses of water** each day and avoid excessive use of beverages containing caffeine.
  - Notify the physician if **vomiting or diarrhea** occurs. These symptoms can result in **sodium loss and an increased risk of toxicity**.
  - Includes **adequate sodium** and other nutrients while decreasing number of calories.
  - **Be aware of risks of becoming pregnant** while receiving lithium therapy.

Carbamazepine

- Carbamazepine (CBZ) is an **anticonvulsant** and **mood stabilizing drug** used primarily in the treatment of **epilepsy** and **bipolar disorder**.
- It is also used to treat **Attention Deficit Disorder (ADD), Attention Deficit Hyperactive Disorder (ADHD), schizophrenia, phantom limb syndrome** and **trigeminal neuralgia**.
- **Daily Dose**: 400–1200 mg for mania. (Plasma level 6–12 μg/mL).

Valproic Acid

- Valproic acid (VPA) has found clinical use as an **anticonvulsant** and **mood-stabilizing drug.**
- It is also used to treat **migraine headaches** and **schizophrenia.**
- Valproate is believed to affect the function of the **neurotransmitter GABA.**
- **Daily adult dosage:** 500–1500 mg (plasma range: 50–100 ug/mL).

DEADDICTION DRUGS

Phases in Treatment of Substance Abuse

- **Withdrawal phase:** Treatment of withdrawal symptoms
- **Maintenance phase**

Agents Used to Treat the Withdrawal Phase

- **Opioid withdrawal:** Buprenorphine, dextropropoxyphene, clonidine.
- **Alcohol withdrawal:** Long acting benzodiazepines (chlordiazepoxide/diazepam).
- **Benzodiazepine withdrawal:** Shift to long acting benzodiazepines.
- **Nicotine withdrawal:** Nicotine gums and nicotine transdermal patch.
- **General management during withdrawal:** Analgesics/sedatives/antiemetics and anti-diarrheals.

Maintenance Phase

For Alcohol Use Disorders

- **Deterrent**: Disulfiram, calcium carbamide, metronidazole.
- **Anti-craving**: Acamprosate, naltrexone, Fluoxetine.

For Opioid Use Disorders

- Opioid agonist substitution: **Methadone, buprenorphine, morphine.**
- Antagonist therapy:
  NALTREXONE—in maintenance phase
  NALOXONE — in acute positioning

Disulfiram

- Disulfiram irreversibly inhibits the activity of a particular enzyme (**aldehyde dehydrogenase**) in the body. This leads to disulfiram ethanol reaction (DER).
- Usually patient experiences nausea, vomiting, headache, redness, flushing, fall in BP and even coma may occur.

KEY POINTS

- **Varenicline** is a prescription medication that can help reduce cravings for tobacco and control nicotine withdrawal symptoms.
- Nicotine replacement therapy (NRT) in the form of gum, patches, sprays, inhalers, or lozenges is used to treat nicotine dependence.

Recent Question (NORCET 2021)

3. An alcoholic patient is given disulfiram. This dose can cause DRE for how many days?
a. 96 hours
b. 1 week
c. 36 hours
d. 24 hours
Ans. (b) 1 week

KEY POINTS

Disulfiram therapy
- Liver function test every 3 months and ophthalmology checkup every year is recommended.
- All patients need to be monitored in regular 3 months for liver function tests and once a year ophthalmology checkup for rate ophthalmologic side effects.
- **Use of alcohol containing products** by patients is strictly prohibited, e.g., cough syrup, perfumes, etc.
- Patient must remain abstinent from alcohol for **2 weeks** from last dose of disulfiram.

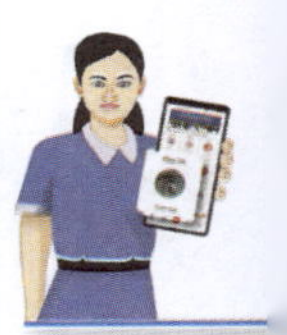

- **Dose**: 250 mg tab (**1–2 doses/day).**
- **Side effects**: Drowsiness, hepatotoxicity, peripheral neuropathy, skin reactions and psychosis.

ANTICONVULSANTS

- **Phenytoin**
    - Used in chronic epilepsy, premature ventricular contractions and tachycardia.
    - **Side effects:** Gingival hyperplasia, hirsutism and ataxia, fetal hydantoin syndrome
- **Ethosuximide**
    - Depress motor cortex and raise the threshold of the CNS to convulsive stimuli
    - **Uses:** Primarily, **petit mal seizure**
    - **Side effect:** Nausea, vomiting, anorexia, dizziness, drowsiness, fatigue, lethargy.
- **Acetazolamide**
    - Anticonvulsant, diuretic
    - Act as an anticonvulsant by inhibition of carbonic anhydrase in the CNS
    - **Uses:** Absence seizure (petit mal), grand-mal (tonic-clonic) seizure and glaucoma, mountain sickness
- **Carbamazepine** [**Drug of choice (DOC) for partial seizure**]
    - Anticonvulsant, antimanic, anticholinergic and antipsychotic effects
    - **Uses:** Epilepsy, tonic-clonic seizures, alcohol-withdrawal, resistant schizophrenia, trigeminal neuralgia.
    - **Side effects:** Photosensitivity, drowsiness, dizziness, unsteadiness, blurring of vision and aplastic anemia.
    - **Contraindication:** Bone marrow depression, **patient taking MAO Inhibitors**
- **Diazepam:** Discussed under sedatives hypnotics
- **Paraldehyde**
    - Emergency treatment of seizure
    - Delirium tremens
- **Valproic acid**
    - Anticonvulsant, used for the treatment of **epilepsy.**
    - **Side effects:** Sedation, depression, bone marrow depression, skin rashes, transient alopecia, hepatotoxicity.
    - **Dose:** Initially 5–10 mg/kg/day, increased at one week.
- **Other drugs:**
    - Lamotrigine
    - Gabapentin
    - Vigabatrin
    - Topiramate
    - Levetiracetam

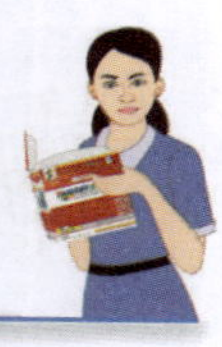

ANALGESICS

- **Non-narcotic or Nonsteroidal anti-inflammatory drugs (NSAIDS)**
    - **Nonselective COX inhibitors:** Aspirin, Ibuprofen, Naproxen, Mefenamic acid, Piroxicam, Ketorolac, Indomethacin, Phenylbutazone
    - **Preferential COX-2 inhibitors:** Nimesulide, Diclofenac, Meloxicam
    - **Selective COX-2 inhibitors:** Celecoxib, Etoricoxib, Parecoxib. Analgesic-antipyretics with poor anti-inflammatory action: Paracetamol (acetaminophen), metamizole.
- **Narcotic Analgesics**
    - **Examples:** Natural opium Alkaloids: morphine, codeine.
        - **Semisynthetic opioids:** Diacetylmorphine (Heroin), Ethyl-morphine, Oxycodone, Hydrocodone
        - **Synthetic opioids:** Pethidine, fentanyl, methadone, tramadol.
    - **Contraindications of Narcotic analgesics: Children less than age of 6 months, hepatic cirrhosis, Addison's disease, myxedema, emphysema, asthmatic conditions and convulsions.**
    - **Side effects of Opioid analgesics:** Respiratory depression, apnea, dizziness, euphoria headache, mental clouding, insomnia nausea, vomiting, constipation, dry mouth, skin rashes, laryngospasm, urinary retention and decreased libido.

ANTI-GOUT AGENTS

- **Allopurinol is the drug of choice for chronic gouty arthritis (not useful for treatment of acute gout)**
- **Allopurinol** is contraindicated in **hemochromatosis and children (except those with neoplastic disease)**
- **Side effects** include skin rash, alopecia, fever leucopenia, arthralgia, nausea, vomiting
- Administer **allopurinol with food** to avoid gastric irritation.
- NSAIDs and Colchicine are used for prophylaxis and treatment of acute attacks of gout
- **Prolong administration** of colchicine may lead to bone marrow depression.

KEY POINT

Misoprostol is a prostaglandin that is used to reduce the risk of stomach ulcers in patients treated with NSAIDs.

POINTS TO REMEMBER

- The benzodiazepines are the most effective drugs in the treatment of acute seizures and status epilepticus.
- The benzodiazepines most commonly used to treat status epilepticus are diazepam, lorazepam, and midazolam.

KEY POINTS

- **NSAIDs** are **contraindicated** in peptic ulcer disease **(Except paracetamol)**
- Oral N-acetylcysteine (mucomyst) is used for the treatment of paracetamol overdose/toxicity.
- The anti-inflammatory effects of **Aspirin** decreases **prostaglandin synthesis.**
- **Aspirin** also produces **inhibition of platelet aggregation.**
- **Aspirin** is contraindicated in Vitamin K deficiency, chickenpox, influenza, pregnancy and lactation.

SYMPATHOMIMETIC (ADRENERGIC) DRUGS

- **Alpha receptors**
  - **Alpha 1-adrenergic receptors** (vasoconstriction, decon-gestion, dilation of eye pupil, contraction of urinary bladder sphincters)
  - **Alpha 2-adrenergic receptors** (decrease insulin secretion, decrease motility and secretion of GIT)
- **Beta receptors**
  - **Beta 1-adrenergic** (myocardial contraction, regulate heart rate, improves impulse, increases lipolysis and gluconeogenesis)
  - **Beta 2-adrenergic** (skeletal and coronary vasodilation, bronchial dilation, decreases renin secretion, decreases gastric motility.)
- **Albuterol (salbutamol):** Sympathomimetic agent. It stimulates **β2 receptors** of the bronchi leading to bronchodilation. Used in the treatment of bronchial asthma and status epilepticus (parenteral administration)
- **Dopamine Hydrochloride (adrenergic agent):** It produces direct stimulation of β1 receptors resulting in **increasing myocardial contraction, cardiac output** as well as **increase renal blood flow** and **sodium excretion.**
- **Dopamine is used in cardiogenic shock, hypotension due to poor cardiac output and cardiomyopathy**.
- **Contraindications for dopamine include** pheochromocytoma, uncorrected tachycardia and arrhythmias.
- **Epinephrine:** Commonly known as Adrenaline, a natural hormone produced from adrenal medulla, induce marked stimulation of alpha, β1 + β2 receptors causing cardiac stimulation, bronchodilation and decongestion.
- **Epinephrine** is used to get relief from respiratory distress due to bronchospasm and rapid relief from hypersensitivity reactions.
- **Nursing responsibility during epinephrine administration:**
  - Never administer 1:100 solution IV
  - Use 1: 10,000 solution For IV use.
  - Use tuberculine (1 cc) syringe to measure adrenaline/epinephrine.
  - In anaphylactic shock, adrenaline is given by intra muscular (IM) route (1:1000)

CHOLINERGIC DRUGS

- Acetylcholine, Methacholine, Carbachol, Bethanechol, Muscarine, Pilocarpine and Arecoline are **Cholinergic agonists.**
- **Pyridostigmine bromide and neostigmine bromide (Reversible anticholinesterases):** Used in the treatment of Myasthenia Gravis
- Carbachol, physostigmine salicylate and pilocarpine nitrate **(miotic agents):** treatment of glaucoma
- Irreversible anticholinesterases are used as insecticides (e.g. Malathion, Carbaryl, Diazinon, etc.)

Cholinergic Blocking (Parasympatholytic) Drugs

- **Atropine sulfate:** Cholinergic blocking agent. Used in the treatment of irritable bowel syndrome, treatment of spastic disorders of biliary tract, parkinsonism.
  - During anesthesia to control salivation and bronchial secretions
  - Used as prophylaxis and treatment of toxicity due to cholinesterase inhibitor including organophosphate pesticides.
  - Antiarrhythmic (prophylaxis) and ophthalmologic treatment of uveitis
- **Management of Organophosphorus poisoning:** Give Atropine 2-4 mg IV initially then 2 mg every 5-10 minutes until muscarinic symptoms disappear and signs of atropine toxicity begins to appear like dilation of pupils, flushing of face and tachycardia.

DRUGS AFFECTING THE RESPIRATORY SYSTEM

Antiasthmatic Drugs

- **Aminophylline** (theophylline + ethylenediamine): Relaxes smooth muscles of bronchi causing bronchodilation and increasing vital capacity of the lungs. It is also used in the treatment of neonatal apnea and bradycardia.
- Sympathomimetics such as salbutamol and salmeterol.
- Anticholinergics such as ipratropium bromide, tiotropium bromide.
- Corticosteroids such as hydrocortisone, prednisolone, budesonide, etc. are also used in the treatment of asthma.

Antitussives

- **Expectorants:** Expectorants liquefy mucus and facilitate its removal from the lungs through coughing, e.g., Guaifenesin.
- **Acetylcysteine (Mucolytic):** Reduces the viscosity of purulent and nonpurulent pulmonary secretion and facilitate its removal.

KEY POINTS

- Salbutamol is preferred over Adrenaline in an asthmatic because of its (salbutamol) beta-2 selective agonist action.
- Intramuscular Adrenaline (epinephrine) is the recommended first line treatment for patients with anaphylaxis.
- 1:1000 concentration is recommended for adult patient.
- 1:10000 is recommended for children.
- Dopamine is a potent drug. It must be diluted before administration to the patient. It can be diluted with NS, DNS or RL.
- Most common dose related side effect of salbutamol is tremors.

Recent Question (NORCET 2023)

4. Atropine can use topically except in

a. catract
b. corneal ulcer
c. uveitis
d. Acute congestive glaucoma

Ans. (d) Acute congestive glaucoma

Atropine is an anticholinergic medication commonly used in ophthalmology to dilate the pupil (mydriasis) and temporarily paralyze the accommodation reflex (cycloplegia). However, it is contraindicated in cases of acute congestive glaucoma because it can exacerbate the condition by further increasing intraocular pressure.

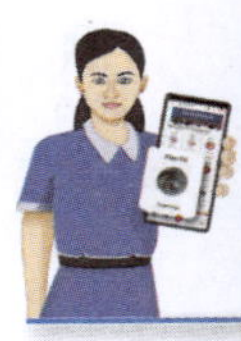

- **Used** along with treatment of chronic bronchitis, emphysema, tuberculosis, pneumonia, bronchiectasis and atelectasis.

Antihistamines

- **Drugs:** Astemizole, brompheniramine maleate, chlorpheniramine maleate, promethazine HCL.
- Antihistamines are used for the treatment of allergic conditions (e.g., Cetirizine) are referred to as H1-receptor blockers while those used for treatment of GI disorders as peptic ulcer are referred as H_2-receptor blockers (e.g., Ranitidine).
- **Contraindicated** in pregnancy, glaucoma, CNS depression, bone marrow depression.
- **Side effects include** sedation, deep sleep, dizziness, epigastric distress, paradoxical excitation, tremors, euphoria, hallucination, disorientation and convulsion.

DRUGS ACTING ON GASTROINTESTINAL TRACT

Antacids

- **Aluminum hydroxide gel, calcium carbonate, magnesium hydroxide, sodium bicarbonate.**
- Antacids act by neutralizing or reducing gastric acidity, thus increasing the pH of the stomach and relieving hyperacidity
- If the **pH is increased to 4**, the activity of pepsin is inhibited.
- **Used in the treatment of** hyperacidity, peptic ulcer, duodenal ulcer and gastroesophageal reflux disease (GERD).
- **Contraindicated** in children less than 6 years of age, CHF, hypertension and pregnancy.
- **Systemic antacids:** Highly water soluble and rapidly absorbed from the gut. Rapidly neutralize the acid in the stomach, e.g., sodium bicarbonate, sodium citrate.
- **Non-systemic antacids**: Insoluble basic compounds and neutralize acid in the stomach, e.g., magnesium hydroxide, magnesium trisilicate, aluminum hydroxide gel, magaldrate, and calcium carbonate.

Antiulcer Drugs

- **Cimetidine, ranitidine (H_2 receptor blockers):** Decreases the acidity of the stomach by blocking the action of histamine which is involved in triggering gastric acid secretion
- **Omeprazole, pantoprazole (Proton pump inhibitors):** Inhibits activity of acid (proton) pump and binds to hydrogen-potassium adenosine triphosphatase at secretory surface of gastric parietal cells to block formation of gastric acid.

Laxatives

Table 11: Types of laxatives used in the treatment of constipation

Types of laxative	Action	Examples
Bulk forming laxatives	These are not digested but absorb liquid in the intestines and swell to **form** a soft and bulky stool	Psyllium, methylcellulose, polycarbophil
Stool-softeners	An emollient laxative	Docusate, glycerin, mineral oil
Osmotic laxatives (saline laxatives)	**Act** by increasing fluid in the small intestine	Magnesium oxide, sorbitol, lactulose, magnesium citrate, sodium phosphate, polyethylene glycol
Stimulant	Fastest-acting; Act by increasing peristalsis in the intestines	Bisacodyl (dulcolax), mineral oil (liquid paraffin), aloe, senna, cascara, castor oil
Chloride channel activator	Activates **chloride channels** in the intestine and increases secretion of intestinal fluid	Lubiprostone (used in constipation in inflammatory bowel disease), linaclotide

Digestants

- **Pancreatin:** This mixture of enzymes (pancreatin, lipase, and amylase) is obtained from hog pancreas. The preparation increases digestion of food.
  - **Indications**: Pancreatic deficiency as pancreatitis, cystic fibrosis and pancreatectomy.
- **Emetics:** Used in cases of acute poisoning to induce vomiting
  - **Apomorphine HCl:** Synthetic derivative of morphine which produces vomiting by stimulating the CTZ.
  - **Ipecac syrup:** Alkaloid extracted from Brazil root, acts both locally on the gastric mucosa and centrally on the CTZ.

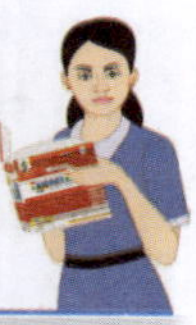

KEY POINTS

- Antacids containing **magnesium** have a **laxative** effect
- Opioid analgesics such as Morhpine and Codeine causes Constipation.
- Absolute contraindication to Laxatives is fecal impaction, and gastrointestinal obstruction.
- Laxatives increase peristaltic activity

POINT TO REMEMBER

Laxatives decrease the pharmacological effect of poorly absorbed drugs, delayed acting drugs, and sustained/extended release drugs.

POINT TO REMEMBER

Ipecac syrup must not be confused with **ipecac fluid** extract which is 14 times as potent.

Antiemetics

- **Metoclopramide HCl:** It is dopamine receptor antagonist acts both centrally (CTZ) and peripherally (stimulation of upper GIT motility)
    - **Indications:** Nausea and vomiting as in chemotherapy. Facilitate diagnostic procedure such as barium meal. GIT pain, dyspepsia and regurgitation in peptic ulcer, reflux esophagitis and post-anesthetic vomiting.

INSULIN

- **Type I diabetes:** Insulin dependent diabetes mellitus
- **Type II diabetes:** Noninsulin dependent diabetes mellitus
- Insulin cannot be given by oral route as proteolytic enzymes will destroy it.
- Insulin is administered by subcutaneous (SC) route in routine and by IV route in case of emergency
- Insulin is broken down into amino acids and these amino acids are recycled and reutilized
- Adverse effects of insulin
    - Hypoglycemia is the most common and serious side effect
    - Lipodystrophy, weight gain and injection site reactions
- Insulin delivery devices
    - Insulin syringes, pen devices, inhaled insulin (available in USA and Europe only), Insulin pump and implantable insulin pump

Table 12: Class, onset of action and duration of action of insulin

Class	Drugs	Onset of action	Duration of action
Ultra short or rapid acting insulin	Lispro- Insulin	0.2–0.3 hours	3–5 hours
	Aspart- Insulin	0.2–0.3 hours	3–5 hours
	Glulisine - Insulin	0.2–0.4 hours	3–5 hours
Short acting insulin	Regular soluble insulin	0.5–1 hours	5–8 hours
	Semilente	1–2 hours	12–14 hours
Intermediate acting insulin	Insulin zinc or Lente	1–2 hours	20–24 hours
	Neutral protamine hagedorn or isophane insulin	1–2 hours	20–24 hours
Long acting insulin	Insulin detemir	1–4 hours	20–24 hours
	Insulin glargine	2–4 hours	24 hours
Ultra-long acting insulin	Degludec	30–90 minutes	24–40 hours
	Ultralente	6 hours	20–36 hours

ORAL HYPOGLYCEMIC (ANTIDIABETIC) AGENTS

- These agents are used for patients with noninsulin dependent diabetes (Type II).
- **Second-generation oral hypoglycemic agents** are more lipophilic and have greater hypoglycemic potency (200 times) than first generation.
- **Classification**
    - **First: Generation sulfonylureas compounds**
        - Tolbutamide
        - Chlorpropamide
    - **Second-generation sulfonylureas compounds**
        - Glibenclamide
        - Glyburide
    - **Other drugs**
        - Metformin, phenformin, acarbose.
- Oral hypoglycemic agents act by increasing the sensitivity of pancreatic islet cells and insulin secretion. The peripheral tissues become more sensitive to insulin.
- Contraindicated in Type I of DM, renal and liver disease, and in recurrent episodes of ketoacidosis.

ADRENOCORTICOSTEROIDS AND ANALOGUES

- These are natural hormones produced by the adrenal cortex.
- **Glucocorticoids,** e.g., cortisone and hydrocortisone, betamethasone.
- **Dexamethasone:** Regulate the metabolism of carbohydrates, protein and fat.
- **Mineralocorticoids** e.g., aldosterone and fludrocortisone acetate
- **Deoxycorticosterone:** Increases reabsorption of Na^+ (+water) and excretion of potassium and hydrogen.

POINT TO REMEMBER

The preferred site for insulin injection is abdomen (around umbilicus). Insulin is absorbed more quickly and predictably from this site.

POINTS TO REMEMBER

- When you mix regular insulin with another type of insulin, always draw the regular insulin into the syringe first.
- When you mix two types of insulin other than regular insulin, the order of withdrawal does not matter.

POINT TO REMEMBER

Oral hypoglycemic drugs are used only in the treatment of type II diabetes which is a disorder involving resistance to secreted insulin.

Recent Questions (NORCET 2023)

5. **Which of the following is a longest acting basal insulin?**
    a. Lispro
    b. Aspart
    c. Glargin
    d. Degludec

Ans. (d) Degludec

6. **A patient with type I DM came in ED in condition of DKA. His RBS is 550 mg/dl. What is the priority nursing action?**
    a. Start Regular Insulin Infusion with Normal saline
    b. Start NPH Insulin
    c. Give Sweet juice
    d. Start Dextrose 50%

Ans. (a) Start Regular Insulin Infusion with Normal saline

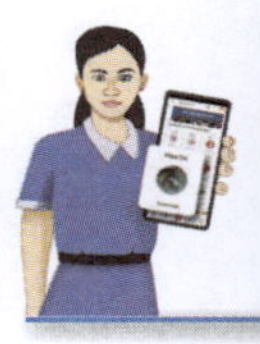

- **Prednisone** is a synthetic adrenocorticosteroid.
- **Uses:**
  - **Replacement therapy**: Adrenal insufficiency (Addison's disease).
  - **Rheumatic disorders**: Rheumatoid arthritis and osteoarthritis.
  - **Collagen diseases:** Systemic lupus erythematosus, rheumatic cardiac disease.
  - **Allergic diseases**: Drug hypersensitivity, urticarial transfusion reaction.
  - **Respiratory diseases**: Bronchial asthma, rhinitis.
  - **Malignancies**: Leukemia, lymphoma
  - Nephrotic syndrome, Hematologic diseases, Septic shock, liver cirrhosis.
- **Contraindications**:
  - Peptic ulcer, acute glomerulonephritis, Cushing's syndrome, hyperlipidemia.

POSTERIOR PITUITARY HORMONES

Methylergonovine Maleate (Methergine)

- Oxytocic agent. It is a synthetic agent which stimulates the rate, tone and amplitude of uterine contractions.
- **Uses:**
  - Management and prevention of **postpartum hemorrhage** by producing firm contraction and decrease uterine bleeding.
    - Incomplete abortion.
    - Migraine headache
- **Contraindicated** in **pregnancy** and prior to **delivery of placenta.**

Oxytocin

- It has uterine stimulant, vasopressin and antidiuretic properties.
- Mimics uterine contractions of normal labor.
- Facilitates ejection of milk from the breasts by stimulating smooth muscles.
- **Uses**:
  - Antepartum induction or stimulation of labor.
  - Uterine inertia (hypotonic contractions).
  - To hasten uterine involution.
  - Intranasally for postpartum hemorrhage and uterine atony.
- **Preparation:** IV infusion is prepared by adding 10 Units (1 mL) of Oxytocin in 1000 mL of normal saline or RL. This solution contains 10 mU of oxytocin per mL.
- **Administration:**
  - Initial dose: 0.5–1.0 mU/min (equal to 3–6 mL of diluted solution per hour)
  - At 30 – 60 minutes: 1–2 mU/min

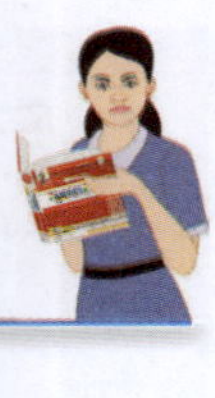

- **Precautions**:
  - Discontinue the infusion immediately in the event of uterine hyperactivity or fetal distress.
  - Except unusual circumstances, oxytocin should not be administered in case of fetal distress, partial placenta previa, hydramnios, borderline cephalopelvic disproportion, prematurity and any other condition which predisposes uterine rupture.

Vasopressin Tannate or Antidiuretic Hormone (ADH)

- **Used in** neurogenic diabetes insipidus.

CALCITONIN AND CALCIUM SALTS

- Maintenance of **extracellular calcium** levels is controlled by **parathyroid hormone** utilizing a feedback mechanism similar to that of other hormones.
- **Calcitonin**: Calcium regulator.
  - Used in the treatment of hypercalcemia, postmenopausal osteoporosis (with calcium and Vitamin D), hyperpara-thyroidism, moderate to severe Paget's disease, vitamin D intoxication.
- **Calcium salts**: (Calcium carbonate, calcium gluconate)
  - **Uses (IV):** Acute hypocalcemic tetany (IV) due to renal failure, hypoparathyroidism. During cardiac resuscitation.
  - **IM or IV**: To reduce spasm, to get, relief from sensitivity reactions due to insect bites.
  - **Oral:** Chronic hypoparathyroidism, osteoporosis, osteo malacia, rickets, myasthenia gravis.

THYROID DRUGS

- The thyroid manufactures 2 active hormones, **thyroxine** and **triiodothyronine**, both contain iodine.
- **Hypothyroidism:** Cretinism in infancy and early life, myxedema in adult.
- **Hyperthyroidism:** Graves' disease characterized by protruding eyes and extreme nervousness.
- **Thyroid hormone preparations**
  - Levothyroxine sodium (T_4)
  - Liothyronine sodium (T_3)
  - Liotrix (Mixture of T_4+ T_3)
- **Uses**
  - Replacement therapy in primary and secondary myxedema, nontoxic goiter and chronic thyroiditis.
  - Used with antithyroid drugs for thyrotoxicosis to prevent hypothyroidism.
  - Surgical removal of thyroid gland.

KEY POINTS

- Prednisone (if OD dose) is preferably taken in the morning with breakfast.
- The morning is best to take prednisone as it mimics the timing of body's own production of cortisone.
- Taking prednisone too late in the evening may cause sleeping difficulty.

KEY POINTS

- Oxytocin should **never be given IV undiluted** in high concentration.
- Calcitonin inhibits bone resorption while Parathormone increase it.

Practice Question

5. An adult patient who complains of recent weight gain, chronic fatigue, cold intolerance, and myxedema is diagnosed with hypothyroidism. Which of the following is the most appropriate treatment for this patient?

a. Methimazole
b. Iodide salts
c. Levothyroxine (T4)
d. Triiodothyroxine (T3)

Ans. (c) Levothyroxine (T4)

Rationale: T4 has a half life of approximately 1 week, and is converted to T3 intracellularly in peripheral tissues. It is preferred over T3 for chronic therapy because it is less cardiotoxic, it does not have to be taken more frequently, and is easier to monitor with conventional lab tests.

- **Contraindications**: MI, uncorrected adrenal insufficiency.
- **Side effects:** Arrhythmias, palpitations, angina pectoris, dyspnea and hypertension, abdominal cramps, appetite changes, diarrhea and loss of weight, menstrual irregularities.

ANTITHYROID DRUGS

E.g., Methimazole, propylthiouracil (PTU).

- **Used** in hyperthyroidism and in preparing the patient who is undergoing surgery or radioactive iodine therapy.
- **Contraindication:** Lactation and pregnancy

Sodium Iodide I^{131}: Radioactive Agent

- **Indications**: Hyperthyroidism in **thyroid cancer.**
- **Contraindications:** Lactation, Patients under 30 years of age.
- **Side effects:** Bone marrow depression, pain in swallowing, sore throat, sickness, and alopecia.

DIURETICS

- **Carbonic anhydrase inhibitor diuretics:** Acetazolamide
  - Anticonvulsant, diuretic.
  - Limited use as a diuretic. Used in glaucoma.
- **Loop diuretics:** Furosemide (Lasix)
  - Inhibits the reabsorption of sodium and chloride in the ascending loop of Henle that results in the excretion of sodium, chloride and to a lesser degree potassium and bicarbonate ions.
  - It has a slight antihypertensive effect.
  - **Uses**: Edema associated with congestive heart failure, liver cirrhosis, nephrotic syndrome. Acute pulmonary edema and Hypertension.
  - **Contraindications**: Anuria, hepatic coma, severe renal diseases.
  - **Side effects**: Hypokalemia, dehydration, hypovolemia, hypo-natremia, hyperglycemia.
- **Osmotic diuretics:** Mannitol, glycerol, isosorbide
  - Decrease the reabsorption of water while increasing the excretion of sodium and chloride.
  - Increases the osmolarity of the plasma.
  - **Uses**: Acute renal failure. Cerebral edema. Glaucoma and to decrease intracranial pressure.
  - **Side effects:** Hypernatremia, electrolyte imbalance, acidosis, dehydration, dry mouth, thirst, edema, hypotension, blurring of vision, headache, dizziness.
- **Potassium-sparing diuretics:** Spironolactone, eplerenone
  - Inhibit sodium exchange for potassium which results in increased secretion of sodium and water and **conservation of potassium**.
  - It is also an **aldosterone antagonist.**
  - It also **interferes** with synthesis of **testosterone.**
  - **Uses**: Edema due to congestive heart failure, liver cirrhosis, nephrotic syndrome, essential hypertension, primary hyperaldosteronism and hypokalemia.
  - **Contraindication**: Acute renal failure hyperkalemia.
  - **Protect drug from light**. Avoid food high in potassium.
- **Thiazides and related diuretics:** Hydrochlorothiazide
  - Promote diuresis by decreasing the rate at which sodium and chloride are reabsorbed by the distal renal tubules of the kidney.
  - **Uses**: Hypertension, Edema due to congestive heart failure, nephrosis, liver cirrhosis and renal failure.

POINT TO REMEMBER

Use of Oxytocin during labor may result in **uterine tetany with rupture, cervical laceration**, embolism of amniotic fluid and **intracranial hemorrhage in infant.**

KEY POINTS

- Spironolactone has anti-androgen effect.
- Spironolactone is contraindicated with Enalapril.
- Furosemide is a high-ceiling diuretic.
- Furosemide is used in the treatment of Pulmonary edema.
- Furosemide should not be administered with NSAIDs because it inhibits prostacyclin synthesis.
- Ethacrynic acid causes increased concentration of Na+ & Cl- in urine.
- Potassium. supplements are given with Thiazide diuretics.
- Acetazolamide is used in the treatment of Glaucoma.

ANTITUBERCULAR DRUGS

Table 13: Categories of TB cases and treatment regimens under RNTCP

Category	Characteristic of TB patient	Treatment regimen		Total duration
		Intensive phase	Continuation phase	
Category I (Red color box) Daily dose	New sputum smear-positive Seriously ill, sputum smear-negative Seriously ill, extrapulmonary	2 $(HRZE)_3$	4 $(HR)_3$	6 months
Category II (Blue color box)	Relapse Treatment failure Treatment after default	2 $(SHRZE)_3$ + 1 $(HRZE)_3$	5 $(HRE)_3$	8 months

Note: According to latest guideline category III is no longer followed

POINTS TO REMEMBER

- A prefix number denotes number of months; suffix denotes number of times a week.
- R-Rifampicin, H-Isoniazid, E-Ethambutol, S-streptomycin, Z-Pyrazinamide

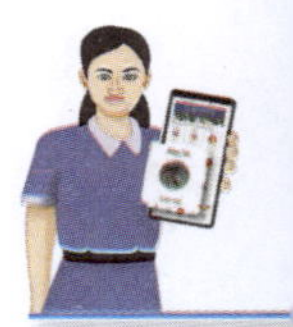

Side Effects of Antitubercular Drugs

Table 14: Major side effects of antitubercular drug

Antitubercular drug	Major side effects
Streptomycin	Ototoxicity (hearing loss), vestibular damage. It is contraindicated in pregnancy.
Ethambutol	**E:** Eye toxicity (Ocular toxicity) **T:** Toxicity dose and duration dependent **H:** Hyperuricemia **Others:** Blurring and red green color blindness
Rifampicin	**R:** Red discoloration of urine **I:** Induction of liver enzyme **F:** Flu-like symptoms **A:** Abdominal symptoms (nausea, vomiting, saliva, abdominal cramps) **M:** Malaise
Isoniazid	**I:** Insanity (mental disturbance) **N:** Neuritis (peripheral neuropathy) **H:** Hepatitis Others: Skin rash, pellagra like syndrome
Pyrazinamide	**Py:** Problem in liver (hepatitis) **R:** Rashes **A:** Arthralgia **I:** Increase in uric acid levels.

KEY POINTS

- Coumadin should be stopped 4–5 days before an elected surgery.
- Vitamin K is an antidote to Coumadin.
- It is recommended to stop Aspirin 7 to 10 days before an elective surgery.

ANTICANCER DRUGS

The anticancer drug either kills cancer cells or modify their growth.

Classification of Anticancer Agents

Drugs Acting Directly on Cells (Cytotoxic Drugs)

E.g., cyclophosphamide, chlorambucil, methotrexate, 6-mercaptopurine, thioguanine, azathioprine, vinca alkaloids (vincristine, vinblastine), actinomycin D, doxorubicin, cisplatin, carboplatin.

Drug Altering Hormonal Milieu

E.g., Prednisone, fosfestrol, ethinylestradiol, toremifene, fulvestrant, letrozole, flutamide.

Toxicity Associated with Anticancer Drugs

- Bone marrow depression
- Lymphocytopenia
- Stomatitis
- Nausea, vomiting (most prominent with cytotoxic drugs), diarrhea
- Alopecia
- **Oligozoospermia** and impotency in males. **Inhibition of ovulation and amenorrhea** are common in females
- Abortion, fetal death, teratogenesis
- **Hyperuricemia:** Gout and urate stones in the urinary tract may develop.

ANTICOAGULANTS

E.g., Heparin, Low molecular weight heparin, warfarin, etc.

- **Uses:**
  - For venous thrombus and embolus
  - Treatment and prophylaxis of deep vein thrombosis
  - In disseminated intravascular coagulation
- **Antidotes:**
  - Antidote of **warfarin** (oral anticoagulant) is vitamin K
  - Antidote of **heparin** is protamine sulfate

THROMBOLYTIC MEDICATIONS

- **Drugs**: Streptokinase, tissue plasminogen activator (tPA), alteplase, urokinase, etc.
- Thrombolytic medications are the drugs which help in breaking of thrombus.
- **Indication:** Early course of myocardial infarctions etc.
- **Contraindications**: active internal bleeding, history of cerebrovascular accident.

ANTIPLATELET DRUG

E.g., Aspirin, clopidogrel, dipyridamole, abciximab.

- **Indications**: To prevent the adverse clinical sequel of thrombosis in atherosclerotic arteries to heart, brain, limbs, etc.

POINTS TO REMEMBER

In vitro anticoagulants (used outside body):
- Heparin
- Sodium Citrate
- Sodium Oxalate
- Sodium edetate

In vivo anticoagulants:
- Parenteral: Heparin, Low molecular weight Heparin (eg., Enoxoparin, Dalteparin)
- Oral: Warfarin

KEY POINT

Streptase, Streptokinase, is indicated for use in the management of acute myocardial infarction (AMI) in adults, for the lysis of intracoronary thrombi.

SPECIFIC ANTIDOTES AGAINST POISONING

Table 15: Descriptions of drug overdose/poisoning and antidote

Drug overdose/poisoning	Antidote
Arsenic	Dimercaprol
Atropine	Physostigmine
Barbiturate/Benzodiazepine	Flumazenil
Beta-blockers	Glucagon (IV)
Cisplatin	Mannitol
Copper	D-penicillamine
Heparin	Protamine sulfate
Insulin	Glucose/fruit juice
Iodine	Sodium thiosulfate
Iron	Deferoxamine
Lead	Dimercaprol (Ca-EDTA)
Magnesium sulfate	Inj. calcium gluconate 10% IV
Morphine, opioids	Naloxone (Narcan)
Mushroom : Poisoning	Atropine
Neostigmine bromide (used in myasthenia gravis)	Atropine sulfate
Organophosphorus poisoning	Atropine sulfate
Paracetamol	N-acetyl cysteine
Salicylate (Aspirin)	Frusemide + Vit K + $NaHCO_3$/ forced alkaline diuresis with $NaHCO_3$
Warfarin	Vitamin K+ fresh blood

DISEASE AND DRUG OF CHOICES

Table 16: Disease condition and drug of choice

Disease condition	Drug of choice (First line drug)
Acute dystonia	Promethazine/Atropine
Alopecia	Minoxidil (topical), biotin (oral)
Amebiasis	Metronidazole, tinidazole, ornidazole
Anaphylactic shock	Adrenaline
Anginal pain	Nitroglycerin
Anorexia	Cyproheptadine
Anxiety	Alprazolam, etizolam
Anthrax Listeria and leptospirosis Pasteurella Actinomycosis Syphilis	Penicillin

Contd...

Practice Questions

6. All of the following effects are seen in Organophosphate poisoning, except
a. CNS effects
b. Nicotinic effects
c. Muscarinic effects
d. Adrenergic effects

Ans. (d) Adrenergic effects

Rationale:
Organophosphates inhibit cholinesterase, an enzyme in the human nervous system that breaks down acetylcholine. This leads to increased acetylcholine in the body. acute OP poisoning has centered on receptor specific effects on muscarinic, nicotinic and central nervous system (CNS) receptors that result in diverse signs and symptoms.

7. Marquis test is used in the diagnosis of which of the following poisoning?
a. Lead poisoning
b. Organophosphate poisoning
c. Opium poisoning
d. Arsenic poisoning

Ans. (c) Opium poisoning

Rationale: Marquis (reagent) test is used to identify the presence of opioid substance.

Recent Question (NORCET 2023)

7. The child with iron poisoning is given IV deferoxamine mesylate (Desferal). Following administration, the child suffers hypotension, facial flushing, and urticaria. The initial nursing intervention would be to:
a. Discontinue the IV
b. Stop the medication, and begin a normal saline infusion
c. Take all vital signs, and report to the physician
d. Assess urinary output, and if it is 30 mL an hour, maintain current treatment

Ans. (b) Stop the...

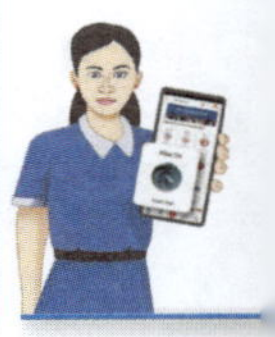

Disease condition	Drug of choice (First line drug)
Atypical pneumonia Brucellosis Cholera Plague Relapsing fever Rickettsial infections	Tetracyclines
Bacillary dysentery	Ciprofloxacin, norfloxacin, ofloxacin
Bacterial meningitis	Benzyl penicillin
Bacterial vaginosis	Metronidazole
Bell's palsy	Prednisolone
Campylobacter enterocolitis	Erythromycin
Chancroid	Azithromycin
Chlamydia	Azithromycin
Cholera	Tetracycline or doxycycline
Closure of ductus arteriosus	Indomethacin
Conjunctivitis	Chloramphenicol
Crohn's disease	Steroids
Diabetes insipidus	Vasopressin
Diabetes insipidus (Lithium induced)	Thiazide
Delirium Tremens	Diazepam
Depression phase of bipolar disorder (BPD)	Lamotrigine
Dysmenorrhea	Mefenamic acid + dicyclomine
Emergency contraception	Levonorgestrel
Erectile dysfunction	Sildenafil citrate (Viagra)
Filariasis	Diethylcarbamazine citrate (DEC)
Leprosy	Dapsone
Manic phase of BPD	Lithium
Rapid cycling BPD	Sodium valproate
Diagnostic test for myasthenia gravis	Edrophonium
Drug induced parkinsonism	Benzhexol
Febrile seizures	Rectal diazepam
Giardiasis	Ornidazole
Gonorrhea	Ceftriaxone and azithromycin
Gout (Acute)	NSAIDs, Colchicine

Contd...

Recent Question (NORCET 2023)

8. What you will do to increase absorption of percutaneous nitroglycerin.

a. Apply near heart.
b. Apply in non-hairy area.
c. Apply over bony prominence
d. Apply on abdomen.

Ans. (b) Apply in non-hairy area.

The drug is absorbed more effectively through the skin when applied to areas where the skin is smooth and hair-free.

9. A long acting NTG drug must be administered at what time for patient with nocturnal angina?

a. Noon
b. Evening
c. Early morning
d. Bedtime

Ans. (b) Evening

10. Patient with digoxin should be checked for which electrolyte?

a. Potassium
b. Calcium
c. Magnesium
d. Sodium

Ans. (a) Potassium

Disease condition	Drug of choice (First line drug)
Gout (Chronic)	Allopurinol, febuxostat
Huntington's chorea Acute schizophrenia Tourette syndrome Sydenham chorea	Haloperidol
Lithium induced neuropathy	Amiloride
Malaria Malaria in pregnancy	Chloroquine
MRSA (Methicillin-Resistant *Staphylococcus aureus*)	Vancomycin
Neonatal herpes simplex	Acyclovir
Nocturnal enuresis	Desmopressin/Imipramine
Otitis media	Amoxicillin
Partial seizures	Carbamazepine
Pharyngitis	Amoxicillin
Pelvic Inflammatory disease (PID)	Ceftriaxone
Pertussis	Azithromycin
Pneumonia (adult)	Amoxicillin
Pyelonephritis (acute)	Co-trimoxazole
Renal failure with oliguria	Furosemide
Rheumatic fever	Aspirin, amoxicillin, PPF
Rheumatic heart disease	Benzathine penicillin
Salmonella enterocolitis	Ciprofloxacin
Scabies	Ivermectin (oral), permethrin (topical)
Sjogren's syndrome/radiation induced xerosis	Pilocarpine and cevimeline
Trichomoniasis	Metronidazole
Typhoid	Ciprofloxacin & 3rd generation cephalosporins
Ulcerative colitis	Sulfasalazine (if no response, steroids)
Urinary tract infection (UTI)-adult	Trimethoprim or nitrofurantoin.
Urinary tract infection (UTI)-child	Co-trimoxazole.
Vaginal Candidiasis	Cotrimoxazole (local vaginal pessaries) Fluconazole
Vertigo	Cinnarizine
Worm infestation	Albendazole + ivermectin
Xeropthalmia	Vitamin A
Zollinger Ellison syndrome	Lansoprazole, levosulpiride

Recent Question
(NORCET 2023)

11. Patient has BP of 155/88. Pulse 86 and respiration 20. You administered nitroglycerin by IV route. Which of the following is expected response of the drug.?

a. BP 160/70, pulse 98, RR 20
b. BP 90/60, pulse 48, RR 24
c. BP 88/56, pulse 92, RR 20
d. BP 170/82, pulse 60, RR 24

Ans. (c) BP 88/56 , pulse 92, RR 20

Vasodilators like nitroglycerin cause relaxation of blood vessels, leading to a decrease in blood pressure. Option C shows a decrease in BP to 88/56, which indicates the expected vasodilatory effect. The increase in pulse rate (pulse 92) is a compensatory response known as reflex tachycardia, which can occur when the blood pressure falls rapidly due to vasodilation. The respiratory rate remains stable at 20.

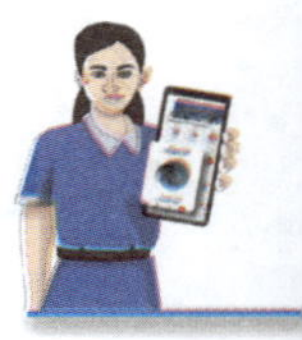

ADVERSE EFFECTS OF SOME COMMON DRUGS

Table 17: Adverse effects of some common drugs

Drug	Adverse effects
Alpha Blockers (E.g., Prazosin, Terazosin, Silodosin, etc.)	Postural hypotension
Amantadine	Ankle edema + livedo reticularis (mottled discoloration of the skin)
Amiodarone	**P**ulmonary fibrosis **P**eripheral neuropathy **P**hotosensitivity **L**iver damage **T**hyroid dysfunction **C**orneal deposits
Amphotericin B	Nephrotoxicity
Ampicillin	Diarrhea
Bleomycin	Pulmonary fibrosis Mucocutaneous fibrosis
Bromocriptine	Psychosis and mental confusion, pleuro–pulmonary fibrosis
Carbenicillin	Platelet dysfunction at high doses
Clonidine	Mental depression
Clozapine	**My**ocarditis **C**holestatic jaundice **A**granulocytosis (most dangerous) **P**illow wet syndrome (Hypersalivation)
Cyclophosphamide	Hemorrhagic cystitis
Heparin	Heparin induced thrombocytopenia (HIT)
Lignocaine	Circumoral paresthesia, convulsion
Methicillin	Interstitial nephritis
Methyldopa	Hemolysis in mother
Nitrates	Monday morning headache
Oxacillin	Hepatitis
Phenytoin	Gingival hyperplasia; gum bleeding
Quetiapine	Cataract Priapism
Quinidine	Ventricular tachycardia
Sildenafil citrate (Viagra)	Blue vision defects
Tetracyclines	Tooth discoloration; liver failure in mother
Thalidomide	Potentially teratogenic drug Constipation
Valproate (Valproic acid) [A HOT TEA]	**A**lopecia, allergy **H**yperammonemia **O**besity **T**remors **T**eratogenicity **E**levated liver enzymes **A**cute pancreatitis, polycystic ovarian disease (PCOD)
Vancomycin	Red man syndrome
Warfarin	**D**ermal vascular necrosis **P**urple toe syndrome **T**eratogenicity

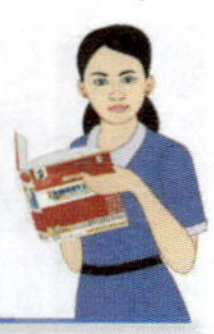

DRUG SAFETY DURING PREGNANCY

Table 18: FDA pregnancy category of drugs

Category	Interpretation
A	Controlled studies show no risk.
B	No evidence of risk in humans.
C	Risk cannot be ruled out. A drug gets this category if there is insufficient data on its use during pregnancy. It could be safe or probably safe, or it could be potentially harmful.
D	Positive evidence of risk. Investigational or post-marketing data show risk to the fetus. Nevertheless, potential benefits may outweigh risks.
X	Contraindicated in pregnancy. Potential fetal risk that clearly outweigh any benefits.

Table 19: Drugs contraindicated in pregnancy

Category X (Contraindicated)		Category D (Positive evidence of risk in pregnancy)	
Thalidomide	Triazolam	Tetracycline	Chlordiazepoxide
Methotrexate	Estazolam	Doxycycline	Chlorthiazide
Ribavirin	Warfarin	Streptomycin	Co-trimaxazole
Griseofulvin	Clomiphene	Amikacin	Fluconazole
Aminopterin	Nicotine	Gentamycin	Primaquine
Busulfan	Alcohol	Tobramycin	Phenytoin
Chlorambucil	Diethylstilbesterol	Phenobarbital	Atenolol
Cyclophosphamide	Norinyl	Pentobarbital	Amiodarone
Phenytoin	Oxytocin	Valporic acid	Aspirin
		Lithium	Warfarin (first trimester)
		Diazepam	Penicillamine
		Lorazepam	Ibuprofen
		Alprazolam	Tamoxifen

DRUG SAFETY DURING BREASTFEEDING

Table 20: Safe and contraindicated drugs during breastfeeding

Safe during breastfeeding		Contraindicated during breastfeeding	
Propylthiouracil	Warfarin	Antithyroid drugs and radioiodine	Phenindione
Insulin	Digoxin	Lithium	Ergotamine, gold salt
Erythromycin, cephalosporin	Antacids	Tetracycline	Anticancer/cytotoxic drugs, e.g., methotrexate, cyclophosphamide

Practice Questions

8. A women in a first trimester pregnancy is having impaired left ventricular function. Which of the following drugs is safe to be ordered in the first trimester pregnancy?

a. Enalapril
b. Metoprolol
c. Warfarin
d. ACE inhibitors

Ans. (b) Metoprolol

9. Which of the following drug is contraindicated in pregnancy due to its teratogenic effect?

a. Isoniazid
b. Heparin
c. Retinol
d. Penicillin

Ans. (c) Retinol

Also Know

*(**Source:** Pathania J.S. Textbook of Pharmacology, CBS Publishers and Distributors Pvt. Ltd.)*

- **Pin-point pupil seen in**
  O – Opium, organophosphate poisoning
  C – Carbamate and carbolic acid poisoning
  P – Pontine hemorrhage
- **Clinical uses of atropine**
  A: As mydriatic-cycloplegic
  T: Traveler's diarrhea
  R: Rapid onset mushroom poisoning
  O: Organophosphate poisoning
  P: Preanesthetic medication
  A: Arrhythmias
- **Atropine side effects (Remember DHATURA)**
  D: Dry mouth
  H: Hypotension
  A: Accommodation paralysis
  T: Tachycardia
  U: Urinary retention
  R: Respiratory depression
  A: Ataxia, acute congestive glaucoma
- **Clinical symptoms of organophosphate poisoning (remember SLUDGE syndrome)**
  S: Salivation
  L: Lacrimation
  U: Urination
  D: Diaphoresis
  G: GI symptoms
  E: Emesis
- **Clinical use of adrenaline**
  A: Anaphylactic shock
  B: Bronchial asthma
  C: Cardiac resuscitation
  D: Duration prolongation of Local anesthetics
  E: Epistaxis control by local action
- **Side effects of lithium (remember LITHIUM)**
  LI: Leukocytosis (increased leukocytes)
  T: Tremors and thirst increased
  H: Hypothyroidism

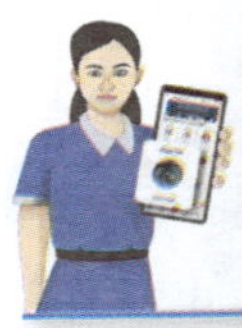

Contd...

IU: Increased Urine output
M: Mother to child (Teratogenicity causing fatal goiter and cardiac anomalies)

- **Side effects of Phenytoin (remember PHENYTOIN)**
  P: Plasma level monitoring is required
  H: Hypertrophy of gum and hypersensitivity
  E: Enzyme inducer, epigastric pain
  N: Neutropenia
  Y: Younger patients (hirsutism and acne may occur)
  T: Teratogenicity
  O: Osteomalacia
  I: IV injection causes hypotension and cardiac arrhythmia
  N: Neurological manifestations (ataxia, vertigo and nystagmus)
- **Side effects of opioids (remember BAD-AMERICANS)**
  B: Bradycardia and hypotension
  A: Anorexia
  D: Depression of respiratory and vasomotor center
  A: Apnea of newborn
  M: Mental clouding, miosis
  E: Euphoria
  R: Respiratory depression
  I: Increase smooth muscle activity
  C: Constipation
  A: Ameliorate cough reflex
  N: Nausea and vomiting
  S: Sedation
- **Uses of benzodiazepines (remember AC-DIAZEPAM)**
  A: Alcohol withdrawal syndrome
  C: Conscious sedation
  D: Diagnostic and minor operative procedure
  I: Insomnia
  A: Adjuvant to antiemetic
  Z: Zia-zag movements of tardive dyskinesia
  E: Epilepsy
  P: Preanesthetic medication
  A: Antianxiety
  M: Muscles relaxant
- **Drugs increasing potassium levels (remember K-BANK)**
  K: K^+ sparing diuretics (E.g., Spironolactone)
  B: Beta-blocker
  A: ACE inhibitors
  N: NSAIDs
  K: K^+ supplement
- **Drugs used in CHF**
  D: Digitalis (digoxin and digitoxin)
  D: Dopamine and dobutamine
  D: Dilators of arterioles and venules (ACE inhibitors and nitrates)
  D: Diuretics
  D: Diesterase, amrinone, milrinone

Golden Points to Remember

- Oswald Schmiedeberg (1838–1921) is generally recognized as the founder of modern *pharmacology.*
- *Pharmacology* is a branch of science that deals with the study of drugs and their actions on living systems.
- The study of poisons, their actions, detection, prevention and the treatment of poisoning is known as toxicology.
- Pharmacopoeia is a book containing formulas and information that provide a standard for preparation and dispensation of drugs.
- Pharmacokinetics is the study of what the body does to the drug. It includes absorption, distribution, metabolism and excretion.
- Pharmacodynamics is the study of what the drug does to the body. It includes receptor, enzymes, ion channels, immune system, etc.
- Protein binding of a drug helps in prolonging half-life, distribution and limiting metabolism
- An **enteric coating** is a polymer barrier applied to oral medication that prevents its dissolution or disintegration in the gastric environment.
- Film coatings **are** very thin layers of a safe ingredient placed around the **tablet to** again protect the tongue from the flavor of the contents and protect the contents from moisture and light.
- **An aqueous solution of sucrose containing added medicinal substances is known as syrup**
- **A liquid consisting of undissolved particles of one or more medicinal agents mixed with a liquid vehicle for oral administration, is known as suspension. Shake well before use**
- **A liquid containing a drug with syrup, glycerine, or alcohol added to mask its unpleasant taste is known as Elixir.**
- Essential medicines are those that satisfy the priority health care needs of the population.

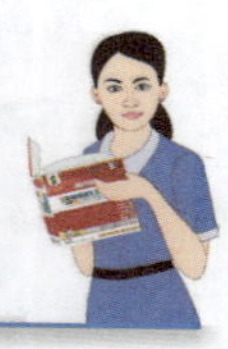

- Inactive drug which gets activated in the body to an active form is known as 'Prodrug.'
- Drugs mostly cross biological membranes by passive diffusion.
- *Bioavailability* is defined as the fraction (percentage) of an administered dose of unchanged medicine that reaches the systemic circulation.
- Drugs given by *intravenous route* have 100% bioavailability since they avoid the hepatic *first-pass effect*.
- Drugs administered through sublingual, transdermal and parenteral routes do not undergo first pass metabolism (bypasses portal circulation).
- Oral route of administration has high first pass metabolism than other routes.
- BCG, Mantoux and Drug sensitivity tests are administered intradermally. The needle is inserted at 15-degree angle.
- **Appropriate site for administering iron injection (Dextran) is Dorsogluteal muscle**
- **The maximum volume of a drug that can be injected through intramuscular injection is 5 ml.**
- Hydrophilic substances can permeate membranes by active transport and not by passive diffusion.
- **The most important route of excretion of drugs is through Kidney.**
- *Orphan drugs* are medications or other medicinal products used to treat rare diseases or disorders.
- An agonist is a drug that binds to the receptor, producing a similar response to the intended chemical and receptor.
- An antagonist does the opposite of an agonist. It binds to receptors, and stops the receptor from producing a desired response.
- Additive interaction means the effect of two drugs is equal to the sum of the effect of the two drugs taken separately.

Contd...

- A combination of drugs is synergistic when the combined effect is larger than the additive effect of each individual drug.
- Secobarbital and Ethanol given together show additive sedative action.
- Alcohol should not be given with Metronidazole (Flagyl).
- Drugs that can be sold to the patient without the need for a doctor's prescription are known as Over the Counter (OTC) drugs.
- **Naloxone** is an opioid receptor antagonist used to rapidly reverse an opioid overdose.
- Teratogenicity refers to the ability of a drug to produce harmful effect of drugs on fetus when administered during pregnancy.
- Antidotes are drugs or chemical substances which counteracts the harmful effects of other drug or chemical.
- Idiosyncrasy is genetically determined abnormal reactivity to a drug.
- Therapeutic index refers to the ratio between the dosage of a drug that causes a lethal effect and the dosage that causes a therapeutic effect.
- For drugs with narrow therapeutic index, slight deviation from the prescribed dose can be harmful to patients. Plasma level monitoring is required for these drugs.
- Examples for drugs with very narrow therapeutic index are Vancomycin, Amphotericin, B Polymyxin.
- Examples for drugs with narrow therapeutic index are Warfarin, Lithium, Digoxin, Levothyroxine, Phenytoin, Morphine.
- Positive inotropic agents increase the force of myocardial contractions. Example: Digoxin
- Pulse should be assessed before Digoxin administration and it should not be administered if heart rate (pulse) is below 60 b/min in adults.
- Hypokalemia in the body can increase the risk of digitalis toxicity. On the other hand, digoxin toxicity causes hyperkalemia.
- Side effects of digoxin include bradycardia, ventricular fibrillation, blurring of vision, blind spots, diplopia and white halos.
- Dobutamine is a cardiac inotrope useful in the acute treatment of congestive heart failure. Dobutamine can only be administered intravenously.
- Nitrates are used to treat chronic angina pectoris and hypertension, associated with Myocardial infarction or congestive heart failure.
- Nitroglycerin ointment is used in the treatment of Raynaud's disease.
- Calcium channel blockers reduce myocardial contractility, inhibit spasm of coronary artery and cause peripheral vasodilation.
- Sodium nitroprusside is the drug of choice for therapy of hypertensive emergencies or hypertensive crisis.
- Lidocaine acts as local anesthetic as well as anti-arrpythmic agent.
- Benzodiazepines act by potentiating neural inhibition in CNS which is mediated by GABA
- Antidote to benzodiazepines is Flumazenil
- The benzodiazepines most commonly used to treat status epilepticus are diazepam, lorazepam, and midazolam.
- Phenobarbitone is effective in preventing the recurrence of simple febrile seizures in children.
- Phenytoin is the drug of choice for Grand mal epilepsy.
- Chlorpromazine was the first conventional antipsychotic developed and is still in wide use for treatment of schizophrenia.
- **Barbiturates are contraindicated in older persons because it causes delirium.**
- First-generation antipsychotics are also known as Typical antipsychotics.
- Second generation antipsychotics (newer) are also known as atypical antipsychotics.
- Typical antipsychotics produce more EPS-related side effects in comparison to atypical antipsychotics.
- Atypical antipsychotics can result in metabolic syndrome with problems related to weight gain, diabetes, and dyslipidemia, often resulting in cardiovascular disease.
- Hypersalivation is a significant side effect affecting about one-third of patients treated with clozapine.
- A *rare but potentially fatal* adverse effect associated with Clozapine is *Agranulocytosis.*
- For the first 18 weeks after initiation of Clozpine, patients require routine *weekly* blood tests to detect emergent *agranulocytosis* or *neutropenia.*
- Oculogyric crisis is a **potential side effect of antipsychotic** medications and can be treated with Intravenous Benztropine mesylate.
- Neuroleptic Malignant Syndrome (NMS) is rare but potentially fatal complication of treatment with neuroleptic drugs. It is manifested by fever up to 107 degree Fahrenheit, tachycardia, tachypnea and severe parkinsonian muscle rigidity.
- The two most frequently used medications to treat Neuroleptic Malignant Syndrome are **bromocriptine mesylate** and **dantrolene sodium.**
- When taking Monoamine Oxidase Inhibitors (MAOIs), food high in tyramine needs to be avoided because these items can cause high increase in blood pressure. For example, aged cheese, cured meats, fermented cabbage, soy sauce, and fish sauce.
- Tricyclic antidepressants lower seizure threshold. F**its may be precipitated.**
- The therapeutic serum drug value of lithium is 0.6-1.2 mEq/L (maintenance). During acute phase: 1.0-1.5 mEq/L.
- It takes about 1 to 3 weeks for lithium to show the effects and remission of symptoms.
- Patient on lithium should be advised to take 6 to 8 large glasses of water and maintain normal sodium intake in the diet.
- Lithium in contraindicated in pregnancy and lactation.
- lithium treatment during pregnancy has been associated with cardiovascular malformations, including Ebstein anomaly.
- Ebstein anomaly is a congenital malformation characterised by an abnormal development of the tricuspid valve and the right ventricle.
- Client on lithium should be advised n**ot to drive or operate dangerous machinery** until lithium levels are stabilized.
- Client on lithium should be advised to include **adequate sodium** and other nutrients in the diet while decreasing number of calories.
- Disulfiram is a deterrent agent. It is used in the maintenance phase of the treatment of alcohol dependence syndrome.

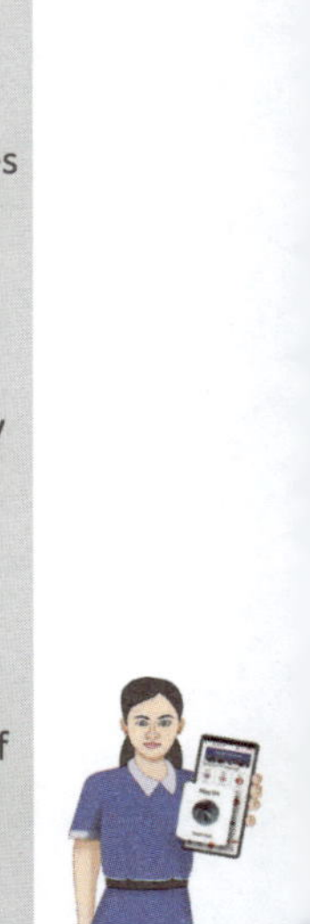

and many more

Image-Based Questions

1. Which of the following is incorrect regarding the device in the picture? ***(Refer explanation at the end)***

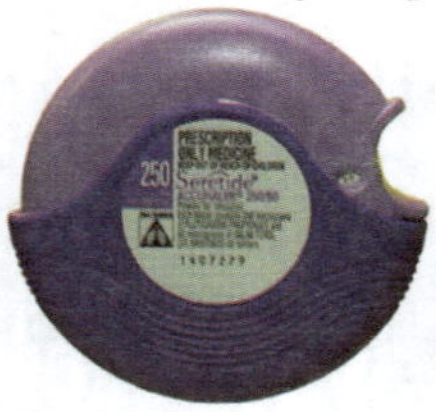

a. Requires coordination with inspiration
b. Easier to maneuver
c. Known as dry powder inhaler
d. Insulin can be used

2. The most important component of the anesthetic machine component given in the picture is: ***(Refer explanation at the end)***

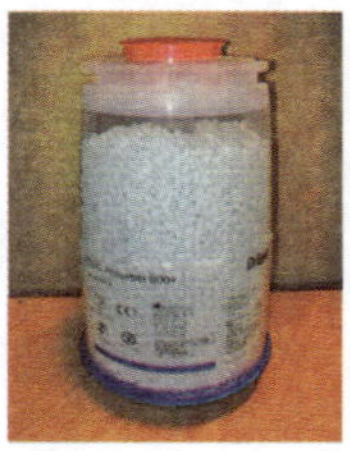

a. Calcium hydroxide
b. Potassium hydroxide
c. Sodium hydroxide
d. Water

3. The test done in the picture is to test the patency of: ***(Refer explanation at the end)***

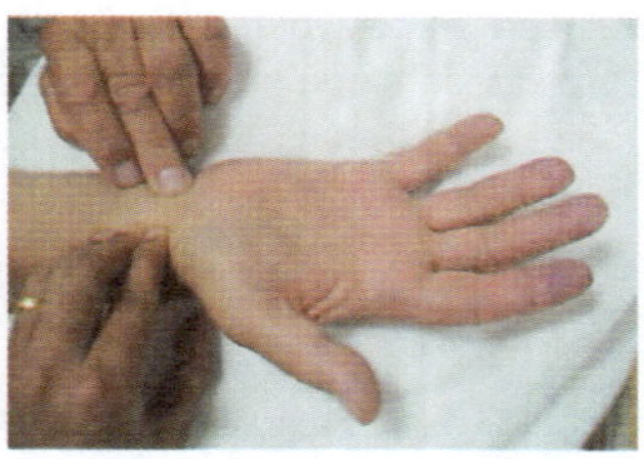

a. Ulnar artery
b. Radial artery
c. Ulnar vein
d. Radial vein

4. DOC for Poisoning due to Food item shown in the Photograph is: ***[Recent Question 2014]***

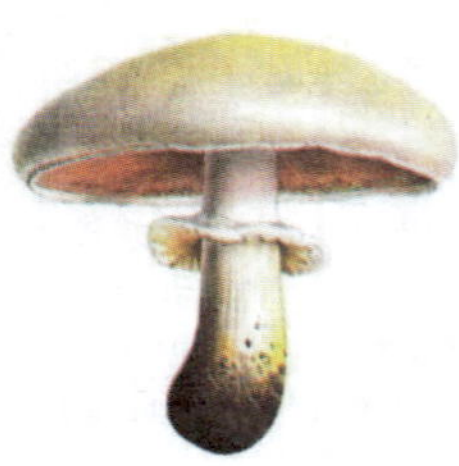

a. Hyoscine
b. Propranolol
c. Phenylepherine
d. Atropine

5. DOC for Poisoning due to Substance produced by Plant shown in Photograph is: ***[Recent Question 2013]***

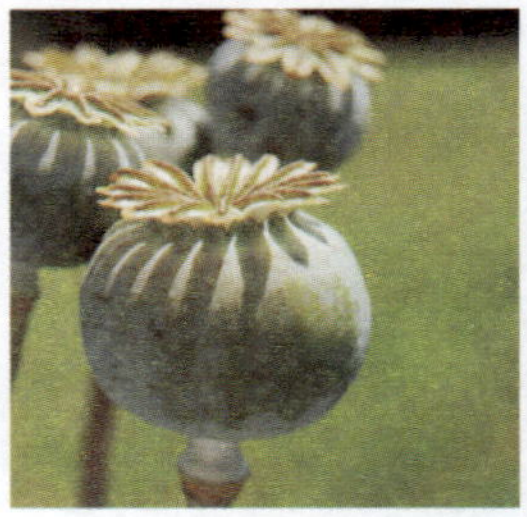

a. Pyridoxine
b. N-acetylcysteine
c. Prazosin
d. Naloxone

6. DOC for Poisoning due to Sting of Arthropod animal shown in Photograph is:

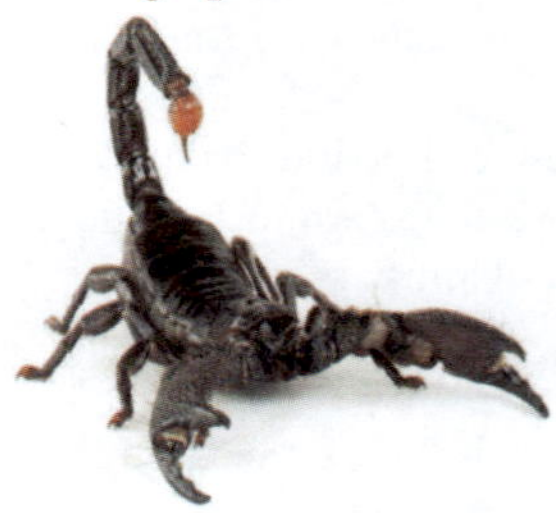

a. Esmolol
b. Adrenaline
c. N-acetyl cysteine
d. Prazosin

7. DOC for Congenital condition (Arrow) shown in the Photograph is:

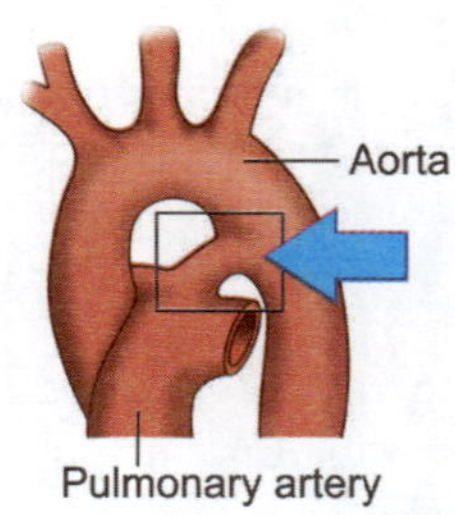

a. Aspirin
b. Indomethacin
c. Nimesulide
d. Propranolol

8. Muscle relaxant of choice for Use for instrument shown in Photograph is:

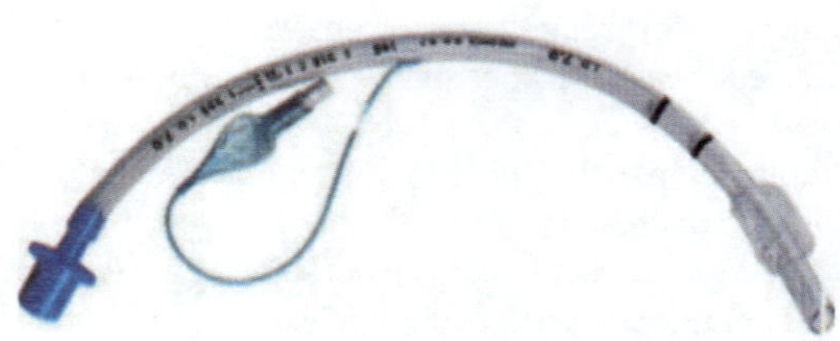

a. Pancuronium
b. Roxacuronium
c. Succinylcholine
d. Atracurium

Ans.

1.	a
2.	a
3.	a
4.	d
5.	d
6.	d
7.	b
8.	c

[*Courtesy*: PHOTON-20® 3th ed. by Vivek Jain, CBS Publishers and Distributors Pvt Ltd]

"He who has health has hope; and he who has hope has everything."

—Arabian proverb

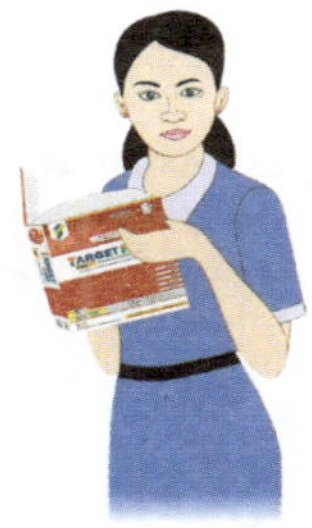

MULTIPLE CHOICE QUESTIONS
(Including Explained and Practice Questions)

KEY TERMINOLOGIES IN PHARMACOLOGY

1. Unwanted but unavoidable pharmacodynamic effects of a drug at therapeutic dose is known as:

a. Hypersensitivity b. Toxic effects
c. Side effects d. Idiosyncrasy

Explanation: Side effects are undesired but often unavoidable pharmacodynamic effects that occur at therapeutic dose. Idiosyncrasy refers to individual's peculiar sensitivity to a drug. Drug intolerance is defined as a lower threshold to the normal pharmacologic action of a drug.

2. A drug can: *(ESIC Chennai May 2012)*

a. Diagnose disease b. Cure disease
c. Prevent disease d. All of these

3. Pharmacodynamic includes:

a. Drug elimination b. Drug excretion
c. Drug absorption d. Mechanism of action

4. Loading dose of a drug is given:

a. To achieve high concentration in short time
b. For rapid onset of action
c. To avoid complication
d. To minimize side effects

Explanation: Loading doses of drugs are typically administered to achieve a high concentration of the drug in the body quickly. This is done to attain rapidly a therapeutic level of the drug, especially in cases where immediate action or relief is required. By providing a larger initial dose, the drug quickly reaches the desired concentration in the body, ensuring a more rapid onset of action.

5. The maximum effect of a drug is defined by:

a. Therapeutic index b. Potency
c. Efficacy d. Adversity

6. Drugs used for rare disease are known as:

a. Orphan drugs b. Rare drugs
c. Over the counter drugs d. Emergency drugs

7. Which of the following is true of placebo?

a. Placebo is a dummy medication
b. Placebo is the inert material added to drug for making
c. Placebo is an additive added with the drug during manufacturing
d. All patients respond to placebo

Explanation: A placebo is an inactive substance or treatment that is designed to resemble a real medication or intervention. It does not contain any active ingredients that directly treat the condition or symptoms being addressed. Placebos are commonly used in medical research as a control group to assess the efficacy of a new treatment.

8. The substances derived from living organisms that are used to kill or prevent the growth of bacteria is known as:

a. Antibiotics b. Antidotes
c. Antihistamines d. Antipyretics

9. Drugs used to reduce the increased temperature of the body are called as:

a. Antibiotics b. Analgesics
c. Antipyretics d. Antihistamines

10. Drugs used to relieve pain are known as:

a. Antibiotics b. Analgesics
c. Antipyretics d. Antihistamines

11. Drugs which increase urinary excretion is known as:

a. Antidiuretics b. Diuretics
c. Laxatives d. Vasopressin

12. Which of the following is an example of urinary antiseptic?

a. Cresol b. Furosemide
c. Nitrofurantoin d. Hypochlorite

13. Drug used to treat itching is known as:

a. Analgesic b. Anti-infective
c. Antispasmodic d. Antipruritic

14. Severe allergic reaction to a drug is known as:

a. Anaphylaxis b. Adverse effect
c. Drug interaction d. Toxicity

Explanation: Anaphylaxis is an allergic reaction to an antigen (e.g., an antibiotic) to which the body has become hypersensitive. It typically causes a number of symptoms including an itchy rash, throat swelling and low blood pressure.

15. Substances used to counteract the effects of poison are called as:

a. Antibiotics b. Anticholinergics
c. Antiemetics d. Antidotes

16. The ability of the drug to cause foetal damage is called as:

a. Amniotic b. Fetotoxic
c. Ototoxic d. Teratogenicity

17. Teratogenicity refers to:

a. Toxic action on the liver
b. Toxic action on fetus
c. Toxic action on blood system
d. Toxic action on kidneys

Explanation: Teratogenic drugs crosses placental barrier and cause damage to the growth and development of fetus.

18. Cholagogues are drugs used to:

a. Increase the amount of secretion of bile
b. Increases peristalsis
c. Treat flatulence on tissues and arrest secretions
d. Inhibit peristalsis

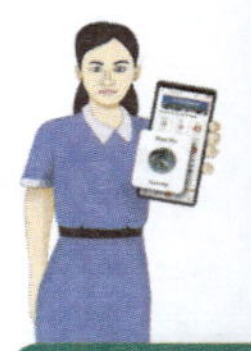

Ans.

1. c
2. d
3. d
4. a
5. c
6. a
7. a
8. a
9. c
10. b
11. b
12. c
13. d
14. a
15. d
16. d
17. b
18. a

19. Astringents are drugs used:

a. As cosmetics
b. Reduce bleeding from minor abrasions
c. To arrest secretions
d. All of the above

DOSAGE FORMS

20. Glucose is added in ORS to:

a. Improve taste
b. Decrease bacterial colonization of GIT
c. Increase the stability
d. Increase the absorption of sodium

Explanation: Glucose is added to ORS to increase the absorption of sodium. This is because glucose and sodium are absorbed together in the small intestine through a process called cotransport. When glucose is present, it helps to pull sodium into the bloodstream, which helps to rehydrate the body.

21. Age-appropriate dosage form for a 7-year-old boy to administer antibiotic as the treatment for his ear infection is:

a. Tablet
b. Capsule
c. I.M Injection with 20 g needle
d. Oral suspension

Explanation:

- Oral suspensions are a liquid form of medication that is easy to swallow and can be flavored to make it more palatable for children. They are also a good choice for children who have difficulty in swallowing tablets or capsules.
- Tablets and capsules may be difficult for young children to swallow, especially if they have not yet developed the necessary coordination and swallowing skills.
- Injections with a 20 g needle are typically administered intramuscularly (IM) and are generally not the preferred route especially if oral alternatives are available.

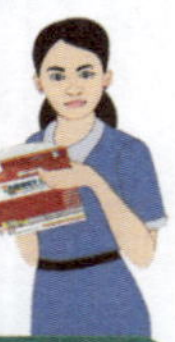

Ans.

19. d
20. d
21. d
22. c
23. c
24. c
25. a
26. c
27. b
28. b
29. c

22. Which of the following dosage form does not dissolve in the stomach?

a. Hard capsule
b. Soft capsule
c. Enteric coated tablet
d. Film coated tablet

Explanation: An **enteric coating** is a polymer barrier applied to oral medication that prevents its dissolution or disintegration in the gastric environment. Film coatings **are** very thin layers of a safe ingredient placed around the **tablet to** again protect the tongue from the flavor of the contents and protect the contents from moisture and light. Due to its large size, sugar coatings are largely replaced by film coating to mask the unpleasant odor/taste of the drug.

23. Which of the following dosage form is best suitable in a medical emergency where a centrally acting rapid action is required?

a. S.C. injection
b. Transdermal patch
c. I.V. Injection
d. I.M. Injection

Explanation: IV route of administration is the fastest route and bypasses absorption barriers and first-pass metabolism. It is used when a rapid effect is required in continuous administration and in large volumes.

24. A liquid containing a drug with syrup, glycerine, or alcohol added to mask its unpleasant taste is known as:

a. Lotion
b. Syrup
c. Elixir
d. Suspension

25. A liquid consisting of undissolved particles of one or more medicinal agents mixed with a liquid vehicle for oral administration is known as:

a. Suspension
b. Elixir
c. Syrup
d. Lotion

26. An aqueous solution of sucrose containing added medicinal substances is known as:

a. Elixir
b. Suspension
c. Syrup
d. Lotion

Explanation:

Syrup	Elixir	Suspension
• Syrup is concentrated, viscous, aqueous solution of sugar or a sugar substitute with or without medicinal substances (Drug) • Syrups are thicker and vicious than Elixirs	• Elixirs are clear and pleasantly flavored solution with or without medicinal substance (drug) • Primary solvents are alcohol and water	• Suspensions are liquid dosage forms containing finely divided insoluble materials • **Shake well before use**

PRODRUGS

27. A medication which is metabolized and converted into a pharmacologically active drug after administration is known as:

a. Active drug
b. Prodrug
c. Premetabolite
d. Placebo

28. Which of the following is a prodrug?

a. Captopril
b. Enalapril
c. Phenytoin
d. Ampicillin

Explanation: A prodrug is a medication or compound that, after administration, is metabolized into a pharmacologically active drug. Enalapril maleate is a prodrug which when administered orally is hydrolysed to release the active converting enzyme inhibitor enalaprilat. Enalapril maleate is 60% absorbed and 40% bioavailable as enalaprilat.

29. All of the following are prodrugs; EXCEPT:

a. Allopurinol
b. Levodopa
c. Oxazepam
d. Prednisone

Explanation: Some of the commonly used prodrugs and its active form of drug (metabolite) is given below:

Prodrug	Active drug
Allopurinol	Oxypurinol
Levodopa	Dopamine
Prednisone	Prednisolone
Diazepam	Oxazepam
Aspirin	Salicylic acid
Enalapril	Enalaprilat
Ramipril	Ramiprilat
Valacyclovir	Acyclovir
Simvastatin	Beta Hydroxy Acid derivative
Talampicillin	Ampicillin
Protonsil	Sulfanilamide
Cortisone	Hydrocortisone
Azidothymidine	Zidovudine triphosphate
Dipivefrin	Adrenaline

30. Which of the following is the earliest discovered prodrug?
a. Enalapril b. Prontosil
c. Diazepam d. Levodopa

31. Which of the following statement regarding prodrug is incorrect?
a. Prodrug is chemically drug precursor
b. Pro-drugs comprising of 2 pharmacologically active agents are known as 'mutual prodrug'
c. A hard drug is a biologically active compound which gets bio-transformed rapidly in vivo
d. Aspirin is the prodrug of salicylic acid used to minimize gastric irritation

Explanation: A **soft drug** is a biologically active compound which gets bio-transformed rapidly in vivo and begins the pharmacological action. So, the statement C is incorrect.
All other statements regarding prodrug are correct.

32. Which one of the following antiplatelets is a prodrug?
a. Aspirin b. Dipyridamole
c. Ticlopidine d. Abciximab

THERAPEUTIC INDEX

33. Therapeutic serum level of phenytoin in the treatment of seizure is:
a. Below 5 mcg/mL b. 10-20 mcg/mL
c. 25-35 mcg/mL d. 40-50 mcg/mL

Explanation: In the treatment of seizure, serum therapeutic level of phenytoin must be maintained around between 10 and 20 mcg/mL for effectiveness.

34. Therapeutic serum level of digoxin is:
a. 0.25 to 0.5 ng/mL b. 0.5 to 2 ng/mL
c. 1.5 to 3.0 ng/mL d. 2.0-3.5 ng/mL

35. Therapeutic plasma level of digoxin:
a. 0.1 – 0.3 ng/mL b. 0.8 – 1.5 ng/mL
c. 1.2 – 2 ng/mL d. >2.4 ng/mL

36. The therapeutic level of serum lithium is:
a. 0.25-0.5 mEq/L b. 0.6-1.2 mEq/L
c. 1.5-2.5 mEq/L d. 2.0-3.0 mEq/L

Explanation: The therapeutic serum drug value of lithium is 0.6-1.2 mEq/L (maintenance). During acute phase: 1.0-1.5 mEq/L.

ROUTES OF ADMINISTRATION

37. Which of the following route of drug administration is most likely to lead to the first-pass effect?
a. Sublingual b. Oral
c. Intravenous d. Intramuscular

Explanation: Orally administered drugs are absorbed in the intestine and enter portal circulation. This leads to first-pass effect in the liver.

38. Which of the following factor may affect the drug absorption rate from IM injection site?
a. Muscle tone
b. Muscle strength
c. Amount of body fat at injection site
d. Blood flow to the injection site

Explanation: Amount of blood flow to the site of injection determines the rate of absorption of drug into the circulation. Amount of body fat may determine the size of the needle to be used. Muscle tone and strength do not have any effect on drug absorption.

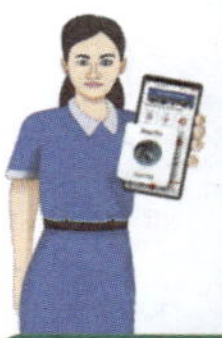

39. Which of the following site must be avoided while giving I. M. injection to a 2-year-old child?
a. Deltoid muscle b. Dorsogluteal muscle
c. Ventrogluteal muscle d. Vastus lateralis muscle

Explanation: Dorsogluteal muscle is not sufficiently developed to be safe injection site for infants and small children. Other mentioned sites are safe for I.M injection in a 2-year-old child.

40. Route of administration of BCG vaccine is:
a. Intradermal b. Subcutaneous
c. Intramuscular d. Oral

Explanation: BCG, Mantoux and Drug sensitivity test are administered intradermally. The needle is inserted at 15 degree angle.

41. All are local routes of drug administration; EXCEPT:
a. Topical b. Intra-articular
c. Oral d. Intra-vaginal

42. Which of the following is the most preferred route of administration in an unconscious patient?
a. Inhalation route b. Enteral route
c. Oral route d. Parenteral route

43. Injection of a drug directly into joints is termed as:
a. Intra-articular b. Intra-arterial
c. Intraossicular d. Intramedullary

44. Administration of drug into the spinal cavity is termed as ______ route:
a. Intra-articular b. Intra medullary
c. Intra osseous d. Intrathecal

Ans.
30. b
31. c
32. c
33. b
34. b
35. b
36. b
37. b
38. d
39. b
40. a
41. c
42. d
43. a
44. d

45. Which of the following route of administration refers to introduction of drug directly into the bone marrow? *[ESI Staff Nurse Exam 2010]:*

a. Intra articular b. Intramedullary
c. Intra peritoneal d. Intrathecal

46. Application of a drug on the skin with friction is known as:

a. Inhalation b. Infiltration
c. Infusion d. Inunction

47. Administration of a drug in liquid form into a body cavity or body orifice is known as:

a. Inhalation b. Infiltration
c. Insertion d. Instillation

48. Test dose of penicillin is administered through ______ route:

a. Intradermal b. Intramuscular
c. Intravenous d. Subcutaneous

49. Which one of the following drugs is administered sublingually for the management of angina pectoris? *(DSSSB 2013)*

a. Aspirin b. Nitroglycerine
c. Atenolol d. Warfarin

Explanation: Sublingual administration bypasses the first-pass metabolism of the drug in the liver. Sublingual nitroglycerine is rapidly absorbed into circulation through blood vessels in sublingual mucosa and is useful for the management of angina pectoris.

50. The route of administration of nitroglycerine is:

a. Inhalation b. Intramuscular
c. Subcutaneous d. Sublingual

51. Appropriate site for administering iron injection (Dextran) is:

a. Anterior thigh
b. Dorsogluteal muscle
c. Ventrogluteal muscle
d. All of the above

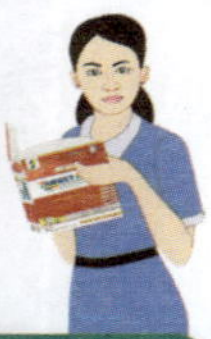

52. What is the best reason for the nurse in instructing the patient to rotate injection sites for insulin?

a. Lipodystrophy can result and is extremely painful
b. Poor rotation technique can cause superficial hemorrhaging
c. Lipodystrophic areas can result, causing erratic insulin absorption
d. Injection sites can never be reused

Explanation: Lipodystrophy refers to changes in the fatty tissue beneath the skin, which can occur as a result of repeated injections of insulin in the same site or sites. Lipodystrophic areas can manifest as either hypertrophy (thickening of the fatty tissue) or atrophy (thinning of the fatty tissue).

When lipodystrophic areas develop, they can affect the absorption of insulin, leading to erratic blood glucose control. If insulin is injected into a lipodystrophic area, it may be absorbed more slowly or inconsistently, resulting in unpredictable insulin action and potentially poor glucose management.

53. Sensitivity or allergic reaction to the drug is tested by administering the drug:

a. Intradermally b. Subcutaneously
c. Intramuscularly d. Intravenously

Explanation: Sensitivity or allergic reaction to drug is tested by administering the drug intradermally usually with a very minimal dose (0.01-0.1 mL).

ABBREVIATIONS USED IN PHARMACOLOGY/ PRESCRIPTION

54. The abbreviation hs means:

a. At bed time b. Early morning
c. After meals d. Before meals

55. 'gtt' means:

a. A drop b. mL
c. An ounce d. gallon

56. Which of the following combination acronym and its meaning is incorrect?

a. prn – as needed
b. npo – Nothing by mouth
c. pc – after meals
d. OS – Right eye

Explanation: OS means Left eye; OD – Right eye; OU-both eyes

57. Which of the following combination acronym and its meaning is incorrect?

a. qd – 4 times a day b. bid – 2 times a day
c. qh – every hour d. hs – bed time

Explanation: qd means every day; qid means 4 times a day.

58. The physician medication order reads as "Lasix 40 mg I.M. Stat". Which of the following is the correct interpretation of prescription by the nurse?

a. Intramuscular injection of 40 mg Lasix to be administered immediately
b. Intramuscular injection of 40 mg Lasix to be administered as a single dose as and when the patient needed
c. Intramuscular injection of 40 mg Lasix to be administered after meals
d. Intramuscular injection of 40 mg Lasix to be administered before bedtime

WEIGHTS AND MEASURES OF DRUGS

59. The maximum volume of a drug that can be injected through intramuscular injection is:

a. 2 mL b. 5 mL
c. 10 mL d. 20 mL

60. One tablespoon is equal to:

a. 5 mL b. 15 mL
c. 25 mL d. 30 mL

61. Two teaspoonful is equal to:

a. 6 mL b. 10 mL
c. 20 mL d. 30 mL

62. One pint =

a. 250 mL b. 300 mL
c. 500 mL d. 750 mL

63. Dose of acetyl salicylic acid is: *(JIPMER 2012)*

a. 10 mg/kg/dose
b. 500 mg/dose
c. 100 mg/kg/dose
d. 50 mg/kg/dose

Ans.

45.	b
46.	d
47.	d
48.	a
49.	b
50.	d
51.	b
52.	c
53.	a
54.	a
55.	a
56.	d
57.	a
58.	a
59.	b
60.	b
61.	b
62.	c
63.	a

DRUG/DOSE CALCULATION

64. Physician prescribes an infusion of 1800 mL of IV Fluid over 24 hours, with half of this amount to be infused over first 10 hours. The client should receive how many milliliters of IV Fluid per hour during the first 10 hours?

a. 60 mL b. 90 mL
c. 100 mL d. 120 mL

Explanation:

- 1800 mL in 24 hours
- Determine how many mL in 10 hours.
- 1800/2 = 900 mL
- 900 mL in 10 hours
- 900/10 = 90 mL in one hour.

65. The physician medication order reads as "Paracetamol 500 mg". The available dose in hand is Paracetamol 200 mg in 5 mL. How many ml of drug has to be administered to achieve the desired dose?

a. 5 mL b. 7.5 mL
c. 10 mL d. 12.5 mL

Explanation:

Calculation:
Desired dose (D = 500 mg
On hand (H) = 200 mg
Vehicle (V) = 5 mL
Formula:
The amount to be administered=Desired (D. x Vehicle (V)/on Hand (H)
Applying to the given scenario
The amount (ml) to be administered = 500 × 5/200
= 12.5 mL

66. The nurse need to administer 0.25 mg Digoxin orally. The available dose in hand is 0.5 mg. How many tablet has to be administered to achieve the desired dose?

a. ½ tablet b. 1 tablet
c. 1½ tablet d. 2 tablet

Explanation:

Calculation:
Desired dose (D) = 0.25 mg
On hand (H) = 0.5 mg
Vehicle (V) = 1 tablet
Formula:
The amount to be administered = Desired (D) × Vehicle (V)/on Hand (H)
Applying to the given scenario
The amount to be administered = 0.25 × 1/0.5
= ½ tablet

67. A community health nurse is providing care for a patient at home. The patient has to take 15 ml Lactulose before bedtime every day. Which of the following instruction to patient regarding measurement of Lactulose 15 ml for oral administration is correct?

a. 1 teaspoon b. 1 tablespoon
c. 2 teaspoon d. Half a cup

68. A patient has a bottle of Levothyroxine (Eltroxin) 50 mcg scored tablets. The doctor has ordered 75 mcg/day. How many tablets should the patient take?

a. ½ tablet
b. 1 ½ tablet
c. 2 tablet
d. 2 ½ tablet

Explanation:

Calculation:
Formula:
The amount to be administered=Desired (D. x Vehicle (V)/on Hand (H)
Applying to the given scenario
The amount to be administered = 75 × 1/50
= 1.5 tablet

69. Dexamethasone 8 mg in 100 ml of NS to be infused over 60 minutes. The tubing has a drip factor of 15 gtt/ml. How many drops per minute has to be set in the infusion pump?

a. 15 gtts/min
b. 21 gtts/min
c. 25 gtts/min
d. 30 gtts/min

Explanation:

Calculation:

$$\text{Drops per minute (gtts/min)} = \frac{\text{Total in fusion volume} \times \text{drop factor}}{\text{Total time of infusion in minutes}}$$

Apply values into the formula:
Drops per minute = 100 mL × 15/60
= 1500/60
= 25 gtts/min

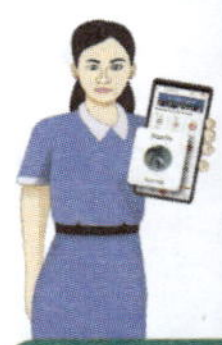

PHARMACOKINETICS

70. Which route of drug administration provides a rapid response in a patient? *(Daman and Diu NO 2018)*

a. Oral b. Intramuscular
c. Sublingual d. Subcutaneous

Explanation:

- Sublingual route offers better dissolution and increased bioavailability. Drugs given by sublingual route bypass hepatic metabolism (first pass metabolism), hence can directly enter the systemic circulation and yield a quick response.
- **Routes of drug administration arranged in order of time until effect:** Intravenous > Intraosseous > Endotracheal > Inhalation > Sublingual > Intramuscular > Subcutaneous > Rectal > Oral > Transdermal

71. The study of absorption, distribution, metabolism and excretion of drugs is referred as:

a. Pharmacology b. Pharmacokinetics
c. Pharmacodynamics d. Pharmaceutics

Explanation: Pharmacokinetics refers to what body does to the drug. It facilitates the movement of drug in the body.

Ans.

64.	b
65.	d
66.	a
67.	b
68.	b
69.	c
70.	c
71.	b

72. What kind of substances cannot permeate membranes by passive diffusion?

a. Lipid-soluble
b. Non-ionized substances
c. Hydrophobic substances
d. Hydrophilic substances

Explanation: Hydrophilic substances can permeate membranes by active transport and not by passive diffusion. Other mentioned substances can permeate through passive diffusion.

73. The most important route of excretion of drugs:

a. Through kidney b. Saliva and sweat
c. Exhaled air d. Feces

74. The rate of drug absorption is greatest in the: *(RRB SSNE, 2015)*

a. Large intestine b. Stomach
c. Gallbladder d. Small intestine

75. Maximum Na^+ reabsorption occurs at:

a. Proximal tubule b. Loop of Henle
c. Distal tubule d. Collecting duct

76. The client on Coumarin therapy should be instructed to avoid which of the following over-the-counter medication?

a. NSAID
b. Cough medicines
c. Histamine blockers
d. Laxatives containing Magnesium salts

77. Atropine is useful in organophosphate poisoning because it:

a. Reactivates acetyl cholinesterase
b. Competes with acetylcholine release
c. Binds with both nicotinic and muscarinic acetylcholine receptors
d. Is a competitive antagonist of acetylcholine

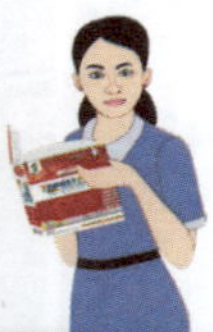

Explanation: Organophosphates are acetylcholinesterase inhibitors, which means that they block the breakdown of acetylcholine. This leads to an accumulation of acetylcholine, which can cause a variety of symptoms, including sweating, salivation, bronchoconstriction, and bradycardia. Atropine is a muscarinic receptor antagonist. It blocks the binding of acetylcholine to muscarinic receptors, which helps to relieve the symptoms of organophosphate poisoning.

CHEMOTHERAPEUTIC AGENTS/ANTIBIOTICS/ ANTIMICROBIALS

78. Which test result should a nurse review to determine if the antibiotic prescribed for the patient will be effective? *(NCFL 2019)*:

a. Serologic test
b. Sensitivity test
c. Serum osmolality
d. Sedimentation rate

Explanation: A sensitivity test or culture and sensitivity test will determine the "sensitivity" of bacteria to antibiotics and also determines the ability of the antibiotics to kill the bacteria. The results obtained from this test can help to explore which drugs are more effective in treating the infection.

79. Which of the following statement is NOT correct about cephalosporins?

a. They are bacteriostatics
b. They are β-lactam group of antibiotics
c. They have wider spectrum of activity than penicillins
d. Cephalosporins work by interfering with the synthesis of the bacterial cell wall

Explanation:

- The statement that cephalosporins are bacteriostatics is not correct. Cephalosporins are actually bactericidal antibiotics, meaning they work by killing bacteria.
- They achieve their bactericidal effect by interfering with the synthesis of the bacterial cell wall, leading to the lysis and death of the bacteria.
- Cephalosporins belong to the β-lactam group of antibiotics, which also includes penicillins and carbapenems.
- Cephalosporins are effective against a wide range of bacteria, including gram-positive and gram-negative bacteria.

80. Which of the following aminoglycoside antibiotic has the broadest spectrum of antibacterial action?

a. Amikacin b. Gentamicin
c. Neomycin d. Streptomycin

Explanation: Amikacin has the broadest spectrum (coverage) against bacterias among aminoglycosides because it is resistant to aminoglycoside inactivating enzymes.

81. Which of the following tetracycline antibiotic does not require dose reduction in patients with renal failure?

a. Doxycycline b. Meclocyline
c. Tetracycline d. Methacycline

Explanation: Doxycycline primarily excreted in bile to feces. So, renal failure does not lead to toxicity of doxycycline.

82. Metronidazole is effective antibacterial agent against all of the following; EXCEPT:

a. H. pylori eradication
b. Pseudomembranous colitis
c. Streptococcal pneumonia
d. Ulcerative gingivitis

Explanation: Metronidazole is an antimicrobial agent and is not active against Streptococcal pneumonia. Beta-lactam antibiotic (e.g., Cephalosporins) is the drug of choice in this condition.

83. Which of the following aminoglycoside drug has the maximum potential for ototoxicity?

a. Amikacin b. Kanamycin
c. Gentamycin d. Streptomycin

Explanation: Amikacin has the highest potential to cause ototoxicity among aminoglycoside antibiotics. Neomycin has the maximum potential to cause nephrotoxicity.

84. Which of the following drug may cause "Gray baby syndrome"? *(ESI 2009)*

a. Chloramphenicol b. Penicillin
c. Doxycycline d. Kanamycin

Ans.

72. d
73. a
74. d
75. a
76. a
77. d
78. b
79. a
80. a
81. a
82. c
83. a
84. a

Explanation: Gray baby syndrome is a rare but serious side effect that occurs in newborn infants (especially premature infants) following the intravenous administration of chloramphenicol, an antimicrobial agent.

85. All of the following antibiotics acts by inhibiting protein synthesis in bacteria; EXCEPT:
a. Amikacin b. Gentamycin
c. Clindamycin d. Cefotaxime

86. Cotrimoxazole is a combination of which of the following two drugs:
a. Sulphonamide and penicillin
b. Ciprofloxacin and methoxazole
c. Trimethoprim and Sulpamethoxazole
d. Tetracycline and carbaxazole

87. Drug contraindicated in infants:
a. Ciprofloxacin b. Barbiturate
c. Theophylline d. Chloroquine

88. Which among the following penicillin has the longest duration of action?
a. Potassium phenethicillin
b. Benzathine penicillin
c. Procaine penicillin -G
d. Benethamine penicillin

89. Which of the following is not a natural penicillin?
a. Ampicillin
b. Benzyl penicillin - G
c. Benzathine penicillin
d. Procaine penicillin - G

90. Which of the following antimicrobial agent is most useful in the treatment of amoebic dysentery?
a. Cefotaxime b. Ciprofloxacin
c. Metronidazole d. Ofloxacin

91. Drugs useful against bacteria resistant to penicillin include:
a. Cephalosporin b. Erythromycins
c. Amoxyicillin d. Both a and b

92. Anticipatory nausea and vomiting occurs:
a. One week after chemotherapy
b. Before chemotherapy administration
c. During chemotherapy administration
d. Within the first few hours after chemotherapy

Explanation:
- Anticipatory nausea and vomiting associated with chemotherapy occurs prior to administration of chemotherapy.
- **Tips:** Note the key word "anticipatory". Understanding the meaning of anticipation leads to option B

93. Ondansetron administered before chemotherapy is to prevent:
a. Alopecia b. Anemia
c. Pain d. Vomiting

Explanation: Ondansetron is an antiemetic agent which prevents nausea and vomiting.

94. Methotrexate acts by inhibition of:
a. Aldose dehydrogenase
b. Aldehyde dehydrogenase
c. Dihydrofolate reductase
d. Sterol synthesis

Explanation: Methotrexate acts by inhibition of folate metabolism, blocking dihydrofolic acid reductase, thereby inhibiting synthesis of purines and pyrimidines and decreasing DNA and RNA synthesis.

95. Which of the following anticancer drug causes 'Hand and foot syndrome' as a side effect?
a. Vincristine b. Vinblastine
c. Capecitabine d. Methotrexate

Explanation: One of the side effects of treatment with capecitabine is hand-foot syndrome.

96. Anticancer drug of plant source: *(AIIMS, Rishikesh 2015)*
a. Vincristine b. Isotretinoin
c. bleomycin d. Methotrexate

97. What is the effect of cyclosporine in a patient undergone renal transplantation? *(Recent Question 2019)*
a. Immunosuppressant b. Anti-inflammatory
c. Antibacterial d. Diuretic

ANTISEPTICS AND DISINFECTANTS

98. Which of the following solution is used as an antimicrobial cleanser to clean the skin site before surgery?
a. Chlorhexidine 0.5%
b. Glutaraldehyde >2%
c. Hydrogen peroxide 7.5%
d. Hypochlorite 650-675 ppm

Explanation: Glutaraldehyde (≥2.0%), hydrogen peroxide (7.5%), and hypochlorite (650–675 ppm) are high-level disinfectants used for disinfection of surfaces and equipment/instruments. Chlorhexidine 0.5% is used as an antimicrobial cleanser to prepare the skin site before surgery in order to prevent surgical site infection.

99. Which of the following is used on live tissues to prevent infection?
a. Disinfectant b. Antiseptic
c. Lotion d. Sterile water

100. Which of the following category of drug prevents the growth of molds and yeasts?
a. Bacteriostatic
b. Fungistatic
c. Fungicidal
d. Antiprotozoal

101. Iodophores belongs to which of the following chemical family?
a. Halogens
b. Aldehydes
c. Phenols
d. Ammonium compounds

Explanation: Iodophores are combinations of iodine with surface-active agents such as non-ionic detergents. They are non-staining and non-irritant, and are effective as **antiseptics** and as surface disinfectants.

102. The duration required for alcohol to be in wet contact with an item to achieve disinfection is:
a. 30 seconds
b. 1–2 m
c. 2–3 m
d. 5–10 m

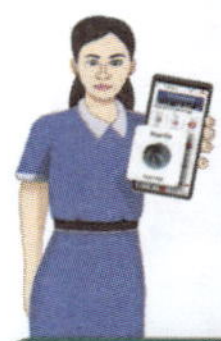

Ans.

85. d
86. c
87. a
88. b
89. a
90. c
91. d
92. b
93. d
94. c
95. c
96. a
97. a
98. a
99. b
100. b
101. a
102. d

DRUGS ACTING ON GI SYSTEM

103. Lansoprazole is not used in which of the following cases? *(Safdarjung NO 2018)*

a. Gastritis
b. Peptic Ulcers
c. Zollinger-Ellison syndrome
d. Thalamus hypertrophy

Explanation:

- Lansoprazole is a proton pump inhibitor (PPI). It Inhibits gastric acid secretion from the stomach. PPIs are used to treat Peptic ulcer disease, Gastroesophageal reflux disease (GERD), Stress ulcers, Zollinger-Ellison syndrome (ZES) and Aspiration pneumonia.
- **Dose:** 15 mg and 30 mg.

104. Which of the following food enhances the absorption of an iron supplement? *(Safdarjung NO 2018)*

a. Baked potato b. Orange juice
c. Green beans d. Fortified Milk

Explanation:

- Orange juice contains vitamin C (ascorbic acid). Ascorbic acid enhances iron absorption by two ways:
  1. Prevents formation of insoluble and non-absorbable iron compounds
  2. Reduces ferric to ferrous iron. This is required for the iron uptake into the mucosal cells.

Factors that increase absorption of an iron supplement:
1. Acid and reducing substances
2. Vitamin C
3. Meat (increase HCL acid and facilitate absorption)
4. Empty stomach.

Factors that interfere with absorption of an iron supplement:
1. Alkalis (antacids)
2. Phosphates (egg yolk)
3. Phytates (most plant sources, maize, wheat)
4. Tetracycline
5. Food in stomach.

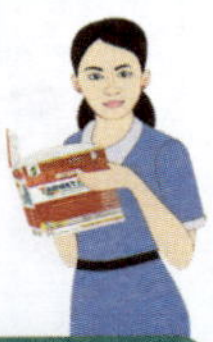

Ans.
103. d
104. b
105. a
106. c
107. a
108. b
109. b
110. b
111. a
112. a
113. b
114. d
115. c
116. a
117. d
118. c
119. d
120. b

105. Which of the following drug is an example of proton pump inhibitor?

a. Pantoprazole
b. Famotidine
c. Ranitidine
d. Sucralfate

Explanation: Pantoprazole and omeprazole are proton pump inhibitors (PPI) which inhibits the production of hydrochloric acid in the stomach.

106. The drug used for prevention and treatment of nausea and vomiting is known as: *(DSSSB 2013)*

a. Antitussives b. Antibiotics
c. Antiemetics d. Antipyretics

Explanation: An antiemetic is a drug that is effective against vomiting and nausea. Antiemetics are typically used to treat motion sickness and the side effects of opioid analgesics, general anesthetics, and chemotherapy directed against cancer.

107. The drug used in the treatment of hook worm infestation is: *(DSSSB 2008)*

a. Albendazole
b. Bephenium hydroxynaphthoate
c. Mebendazole
d. Piperazine citrate

Explanation: Albendazole is the treatment of choice for hook worm infestation. Single dose of 400 mg orally is effective.

108. Misoprostol, a prostaglandin analogue is useful as:

a. Uterine relaxant b. Antiulcer
c. Bronchodilator d. Vasodilator

109. Drugs used to prevent or relieve nausea and vomiting are known as:

a. Antacids b. Antiemetics
c. Antitussives d. Emetics

110. Drugs used in the treatment of worm infestations are known as:

a. Antibiotics b. Anthelmintics
c. Antimicrobials d. Antiprotozoal

111. Out of the following, which medicines are used for intestinal evacuation? *(RRB SSNE, 2015)*

a. Cathartics b. Carminatives
c. Astringents d. Antimycotics

112. If gut motility is increased then: *(RRB SSNE, 2015)*

a. Drug absorption is decreased
b. Drug absorption is increased
c. Drug absorption is not affected
d. Nothing definite can be said

113. Iron is absorbed actively in the:

a. Stomach b. Duodenum
c. Terminal ileum d. Proximal ileum

114. Which of the following drug is a proton pump inhibitor?

a. Ranitidine b. Cimetidine
c. Cetirizine d. Omeprazole

115. Sucralfate is useful in the treatment of:

a. Fluid deficit b. Fluid overload
c. Peptic ulcer d. Peritonitis

116. Vitamin D causes:

a. ↑ Intestinal absorption of calcium
b. ↓ Intestinal absorption of calcium
c. ↓ Intestinal absorption of phosphate
d. ↓ Renal absorption of calcium

117. All are uses of antihistaminic; EXCEPT:

a. Urticaria b. Motion sickness
c. Pruritus d. Glaucoma

118. Antihistaminic used in motion sickness is:

a. Cetirizine b. Meclizine
c. Diphenhydramine d. Fexofenadine

119. Anti-emetics with least CNS side effect is:

a. Metoclopramide b. Chlorpromazine
c. Prochlorperazine d. Ondansetrone

DRUGS ACTING ON RESPIRATORY SYSTEM

120. The action of the drug pseudoephedrine is: *(ESI 2009)*

a. Antimanic b. Decongestant
c. Antihistamine d. Antiemetic

Explanation: Pseudoephedrine is a sympathomimetic drug which acts as a stimulant and decongestant. It is used to treat nasal and sinus congestion.

121. Which of the following drug is not available as metered dose inhaler (MDI)? *(LNJP H D 2012)*
a. Albuterol b. Salbutamol
c. Aminophylline d. Terbutaline

122. Most common dose related side effects of salbutamol is:
a. Nervousness b. Palpitations
c. Restlessness d. Tremors

123. Most common effect of inhalational beclomethasone is:
a. Adrenal suppression b. Oropharyngeal candidiasis
c. Bronchoconstriction d. Hepatitis

124. Which of the following is bronchodilator?
a. Corticosteroids b. Salmeterol
c. Ketotifen d. Sodium cromoglycate

125. Which of the following drug is an example of mucolytics:
a. Bromhexine b. Codeine phosphate
c. Levocetirizine d. Pheniramine maleate

126. The administration of histamine in man can produce:
a. Bronchodilation
b. Vasodilation
c. Negative chronotropic action
d. Reduced secretion of intrinsic factors

DRUGS USED IN TREATMENT OF CARDIOVASCULAR SYSTEM AND BLOOD DISORDERS

127. Digoxin is not given when heart rate is: *(AIIMS 2011)*
a. Below 50 b. Below 60
c. Above 70 d. Above 80

Explanation: Digoxin should not be given if the heart rate is below 60 beats per minute because digoxin further reduces the heart rate and it could be dangerous.

128. Dopamine is preferred in the management of shock because it:
a. Decreases cardiac output
b. Has prolonged action
c. Has peripheral vasoconstriction effect
d. Has renal vasodilatory effect

Explanation: Dopamine at low doses acts on D1 receptors which causes renal vasodilation which improves renal perfusion and saves it from damage due to shock.

129. Which of the following drugs should be first administered in a patient admitted with a diagnosis of acute myocardial infarction? *(RPSC NG-II, 2007)*
a. ACE inhibitor b. Aspirin
c. Calcium channel blocker d. Statin

Explanation: Aspirin is a powerful antiplatelet agent, with a rapid onset of action, which reduces mortality by 20%. All patients with a suspected myocardial infarction should be given aspirin. Aspirin, 150-300 mg, should be swallowed as early as possible. General practitioners should give aspirin or advise the patient to take an aspirin when they are called by a patient who may be suffering a myocardial infarction. There is no need to wait for an electrocardiograph (ECG). If the patient has not already taken aspirin, it should be given in the ambulance or emergency room.

130. Which electrolyte imbalance may predispose the patients to digitalis toxicity?
a. Hypercalcemia b. Hypermagnesemia
c. Hypokalemia d. Hypernatremia

Explanation: Conditions that may predispose a patient to digitalis toxicity include hypokalemia, hypomagnesemia, hypothyroidism, hypoxemia, myocardial disease, myocardial ischemia, and altered autonomic tone.

131. Calcium channel blockers which are used in the treatment of hypertension include:
a. Prazosin b. Enalapril
c. Captopril d. Nifedipine

Explanation: Nifedipine is a calcium channel blocker used in the treatment of hypertension. Prazosin is an alpha blocker. Enalapril and Captopril belongs to ACE inhibitors.

132. Which of the following receptor is activated by low doses of dopamine?
a. Dopaminergic b. Beta 1
c. Beta 2 d. Alpha

Explanation: Dopamine activates dopaminergic receptor only at low doses. At normal or high doses, it activates alpha and beta 1 receptors.

133. The main drug of choice for Heart Failure is: *(DSSSB PHN, 2015)*
a. Decadron b. Digoxin
c. Morphine d. Efcorlin

134. The procedure which involves giving a synchronized counter-shock to convert an undesirable rhythm to stable rhythm is: *(DSSSB PHN, 2015)*
a. Defibrillation b. Cardiac stimulator
c. Pacemaker d. Cardioversion

135. Identify the calcium channel blocker from the following: *(DSSSB PHN, 2015)*
a. Nifedipine b. Atenolol
c. Lasix d. Mannitol

136. Which among the following medicines is used for the pharmacologic closure of patent ductus arteriosus? *(Kerala PSC, Nov 2014)*
a. Methoxamine b. Ecosprin
c. Indomethacin d. Prostaglandin

137. A patient can become toxic on a normal dose of digitalis when ---------- is present. *(Kerala PSC, Nov 2014)*
a. Hyperkalemia b. Hypertension
c. Hypokalemia d. Hypotension

138. Verapamil is: *(JIPMER 2012)*
a. Beta adrenergic Blocker b. H_2 receptor antagonist
c. Cardiac glycoside d. Calcium channel blocker

139. Dobutamine causes:
a. Increased cardiac output
b. Marked increase in HR
c. Increased total peripheral resistance
d. Marked increase in BP

140. A 53-year-old male patient is brought into emergency room with acute myocardial infarction. Which of the following drug should be administered first?
a. ACE inhibitor b. Aspirin
c. Calcium channel blocker d. Statin

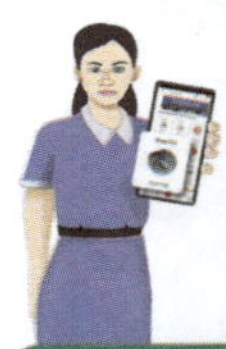

Ans.
121. c
122. d
123. b
124. b
125. a
126. b
127. b
128. d
129. b
130. c
131. d
132. a
133. b
134. d
135. a
136. c
137. c
138. d
139. a
140. b

141. Which of the following instruction is appropriate in regard to nitroglycerine (NTG) for a patient with angina pectoris?

a. To take it before meals
b. To take with a glass of water
c. To store in amber colored bottle and keep it away from sunlight
d. None of the above

142. Which of the following is an early indication of digitalis toxicity?

a. Visual aberration b. Fatigue
c. Seizures d. Headache

143. Atenolol is a/an:

a. α-adrenergic blocker b. β-blocker
c. Anticholinergic agent
d. Cholinergic agent

144. Which of the following is not indicated in digitalis poisoning?

a. Potassium b. Hemodialysis
c. Phenytoin d. Lidocaine

145. Which of the following is a protective lipoprotein?

a. LDL b. IDL
c. VLDL d. HDL

146. The action of cardiotonics is to:

a. Decrease the force of contraction of heart
b. Increase the force of contraction of heart
c. Treat rheumatic heart disease
d. Treat primary hypertension

147. Which of the following drug would be least effective in lowering a client's serum potassium level?

a. Glucose and insulin b. Polystyrene sulfonate
c. Calcium gluconate d. Aluminum hydroxide

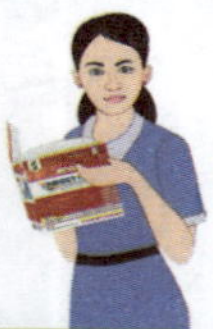

CARDIAC GLYCOSIDES AND NITRATES

148. The side-effect of nitroglycerin is: *(Safdarjung NO 2018)*

a. Vomiting b. Diarrhea
c. Headache d. Constipation

Explanation: Nitroglycerin acts as a vasodilator due to its smooth muscle relaxant action. They reduce both after and preload with coronary blood flow redistribution.

Side effects of Nitroglycerin

- Throbbing **headache**, fullness of head.
- Postural hypotension.
- Methemoglobinemia
- Skin rashes
- Tachyphylaxis → Tolerance (to prevent this, everyday nitrate free interval is indicated).
- Dependence → Sudden withdrawal leads to vascular spasm → Myocardial infarction and Sudden death.

149. The drug that increases both systolic and diastolic blood pressure for prolonged period is:

a. Dopamine b. Ephedrine
c. Epinephrine d. Dobutamine

Explanation: The mechanism of action of ephedrine relies on its indirect stimulation of the adrenergic receptor system by increasing the activity of norepinephrine at the postsynaptic α and β receptors. It increases BP by direct and indirect action and has longer duration of action than epinephrine.

150. The inotropic agent that can only be administered intravenously for heart failure is:

a. Digoxin b. Dobutamine
c. Nifedipine d. Atenolol

Explanation: Dobutamine is a cardiac inotrope useful in the acute treatment of congestive heart failure. Dobutamine can only be administered IV. Digoxin and Nifedipine can be administered orally. Atenolol is not an inotropic agent.

151. Digoxin (Digitalis) is the drug of choice for:

a. Angina pectoris b. Congestive heart failure
c. Hypertension d. Myocardial infarction

Explanation: Digoxin, a cardiac glycoside used in the treatment of congestive heart failure. It acts by increasing the force of contraction ventricle.

152. A client with heart failure has digoxin ordered. What would the nurse expect to find when evaluating for the therapeutic effectiveness of this drug?

a. Diaphoresis with decreased urinary output
b. Increased heart rate with increase respirations
c. Improved respiratory status and increased urinary output
d. Decreased chest pain and decreased blood pressure

Explanation: Digoxin is a medication commonly used in the treatment of heart failure. Digoxin works by increasing the force of the heart's contractions and slowing the heart rate. This can help to improve the heart's ability to pump blood and reduce the symptoms of heart failure, such as shortness of breath and fatigue.

One of the ways that digoxin is evaluated for therapeutic effectiveness is by monitoring the patient's respiratory status and urinary output.

153. Digoxin acts by:

a. Increasing myocardial contractility
b. Decreasing myocardial contractility
c. Increasing heart rate
d. Increasing preload

154. Antidote for digoxin toxicity is:

a. Digoxin immune FAb b. Dobutamine
c. Flumazenil d. Adrenaline

ANTIHYPERTENSIVE DRUGS

155. A drug ending in the suffix (pril) is considered a: *(Safdarjung NO 2018)*

a. Antidepressant b. ACE inhibitor
c. Antifungal d. Beta agonist

Explanation: ACE inhibitors include drugs like Captopril, Enalapril, Lisinopril, Ramipril, Fosinopril, Quinapril, Trandolapril, imidapril, perindopril. Angiotensin-converting enzyme (ACE) inhibitors are drugs often used to treat high blood pressure.

156. Which of the following drug is used as an antihypertensive?

a. Anticholinergics
b. Mydriatics
c. Vasodilators
d. Vasopressin

Ans.

141. c
142. a
143. b
144. b
145. d
146. b
147. d
148. c
149. b
150. b
151. b
152. c
153. a
154. a
155. b
156. c

157. Propranolol can be used to allay anxiety associated with: *(Safdarjung NO 2018)*

a. Chronic neurotic disorder
b. Schizophrenia
c. Short-term stressful situations
d. Endogenous depression

Explanation:

- Beta-blocker like propranolol is useful in short-term stressful situation (performance or situational anxiety). It does not affect psychological symptoms like worry, fear, etc.
- Usually not administered on a chronic basis for treating anxiety, rather before stressful events, for example, public speaking or acting.

158. Which of the following drug crosses blood-brain barrier?

a. Glycopyrrolate
b. Dopamine
c. Streptomycin
d. Propranolol

Explanation: Propranolol crosses blood-brain barrier. Dopamine, streptomycin and glycopyrrolate do not cross blood-brain barrier.

159. All of the following drugs has to be avoided in combination with ACE inhibitors; EXCEPT:

a. Ibuprofen
b. Potassium supplements
c. Spironolactone
d. Theophylline

Explanation: NSAIDs such as Ibuprofen decreased the effectiveness of ACE inhibitors. Higher levels of potassium intake may increase the risk of hyperkalemia during the use of ACE inhibitors. The diuretic spironolactone can cause dangerous hyperkalemia in patients who are also taking angiotensin converting enzyme (ACE) inhibitors. Theophylline is useful in preventing ACE inhibitor-induced cough.

160. Which of the following statement regarding propranolol is not true?

a. It is a B1 receptor specific blocker
b. It causes prominent postural hypotension
c. Has a very short half-life of 6 h
d. It has no effect on plasma

Explanation: Propranolol has a half-life of 12 h

161. Which of the following antihypertensive drug is contraindicated in the treatment of preeclampsia?

a. Magnesium sulfate
b. Labetalol
c. Nifedipine
d. ACE inhibitors

162. Which of the following adverse effect is associated with the drug Prazosin?

a. Sexual dysfunction
b. Dry mouth
c. Bradycardia
d. Both a and b

Explanation: Prazosin (Minipress) is an alpha blocker used as antihypertensive. The adverse effects include sexual dysfunction, dry mouth, orthostatic hypotension, palpitation, tachycardia, difficulty in breathing, depression, edema of extremities and allergic reaction.

163. All of the following adverse effects are associated with the use of labetalol; EXCEPT:

a. Bronchospasm
b. Urinary retention
c. Priopism
d. Orthostatic hypotension

ANTIARRHYTHMIC AGENTS

164. Which of the following increases the risk of digoxin induced arrhythmias? :

a. Hyperkalemia
b. Hypercalcemia
c. Hypermagnesaemia
d. Hypernatraemia

Explanation: Increased intracellular calcium seen with digitalis use may lead to premature contractions of the myocytes (cardiac muscle cells). Repolarization time for atria and ventricles are reduced. This decreased refractory period leads to increased automaticity and the induction of arrhythmias.

165. Which of the following drug is effective in acute termination of supraventricular tachyarrhythmias (SVT)?

a. Adenosine
b. Verapamil
c. Hydroxyzine
d. Both a and b

Explanation: Intravenous adenosine, verapamil, and diltiazem are effective in acute termination of SVT (first-line treatment). Beta blockers (metoprolol, atenolol, propranolol, and esmolol) are also effective in acute termination of SVT.

166. Which of the following is the Class II antiarrhythmic agent?

a. Lidocaine
b. Diltiazem
c. Amiodarone
d. Esmolol

167. Which of the following is the class IV antiarrhythmic agent?

a. Verapamil
b. Amiodarone
c. Adenosine
d. Magnesium Sulfate.

168. Class III antiarrhythmic agents act as:

a. Sodium channel blockers
b. Beta-adrenoreceptor blockers
c. Potassium channel blockers
d. Calcium channel blockers

Explanation:

Class of Antiarrhythmic drugs	Mechanism	Example
Class I	Sodium channel blockers	Lignocaine, Lidocaine, Procainamide, Quinidine
Class II	Beta-adrenoreceptor blockers	Propranolol, Esmolol, Atenolol
Class III	Potassium Channel blockers	Amiodarone, Sotalol
Class IV	Calcium Channel Blockers	Verapamil, Diltiazem
Class V	Other, unknown mechanism	Magnesium Sulfate, Digoxin

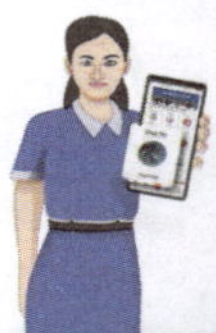

Ans.

157. c
158. d
159. d
160. c
161. d
162. d
163. c
164. b
165. d
166. d
167. a
168. c

DRUGS USED IN TREATMENT OF BLOOD DISORDERS

169. Which of the following drug is used to prevent blood clotting during hemodialysis procedure?

a. Aspirin b. Heparin
c. Protamine sulfate d. Coumadin

Explanation: Anticoagulation in routine hemodialysis consists of a standard dose of heparin given as a bolus at the start of the dialysis treatment with a mid-treatment dose to maintain suitable anticoagulation.

170. Warfarin acts as an anticoagulant by blocking the synthesis of: *(DSSSB PHN, 2015)*

a. RBC's b. Vitamin E
c. Hemoglobin d. Vitamin K

171. Which of the following is not a direct acting anti-platelet agent?

a. Aspirin b. Clopidogrel
c. Atorvastatin d. Ticlopidine

172. Heparin is the most widely used antithrombotic agent. It acts by activating:

a. Plasmin b. Antithrombin III
c. Fibrinolysin d. Factor X

173. Which of the following is vitamin K-dependent clotting factors?

a. Factor VII b. Factor I
c. Factor XI d. Factor XII

174. Which of the following is not an oral anticoagulant?

a. Warfarin b. Dicumarol
c. Phenindione d. Heparin

175. Aspirin is contraindicated in a patient who in on treatment with:

a. Prednisolone b. Warfarin
c. Theophylline d. Oral contraceptives

176. A client is being maintained on heparin therapy for deep vein thrombosis. The nurse must closely monitor which of the following laboratory values?

a. Bleeding time
b. Platelet count
c. Activated PTT
d. Clotting time

Explanation: The aPTT test measures the time it takes for blood to clot in the presence of heparin. By monitoring the aPTT, healthcare professionals can adjust the dosage of heparin to ensure therapeutic anticoagulation. The goal is to maintain the aPTT within a target range specific to the client's condition and the prescribed heparin regimen.

177. Which of the following drug is used to prevent blood clotting during hemodialysis?

a. Coumarin
b. Heparin
c. Protomine Sulfate
d. Warfarin

CORTICOSTEROIDS AND IMMUNOSUPPRESANTS

178. Immune suppressive therapy is effective in patient with myasthenia gravis because it:

a. Promotes the removal of antibodies
b. Stimulates the production of Ach at the synoptic cleft
c. Decreases the production of autoantibodies that attack the acetylcholine
d. Inhibits the breakdown of acetylcholine at the NMJ.

179. Which of the following corticosteroid is produced naturally by the body?

a. Dexamethasone
b. Hydrocortisone
c. Prednisone
d. Methylprednisolone

180. All of the following are true about Glucocorticoids; EXCEPT:

a. Glucocorticoids are secreted by zona fasciculata of cortex
b. Secretions are under the control of renin-angiotensin system
c. They are anti-inflammatory and antiallergic
d. They reduce pain

Explanation: Secretion of glucocorticoids are under the control of ACTH of adenohypophysis. Mineralocorticoids secretion is under the control of renin-angiotensin system. All other statements regarding glucocorticoids are true.

181. All of the following are inhaled corticosteroids; EXCEPT:

a. Beclomethasone
b. Budesonide
c. Fluticasone
d. Methylprednisolone

182. Which of the following is the side effect of long-term corticosteroid therapy?

a. Exogenous Cushing's syndrome
b. Endogenous Cushing's syndrome
c. SIADH
d. Diabetes insipidus

183. Which of the following controls the section of adrenocortical steroids? :

a. Vasopressin
b. ACTH
c. Renin
d. Angiotensin

184. A patient is prescribed prednisone once a day. Which of the following instruction regarding prednisone administration should be included in the discharge teaching?

a. Take the medication before bed time
b. Take the medication in the evening
c. Take the medication in the morning with breakfast
d. Take the medication between two meals

Explanation: Prednisone should be taken in the morning with breakfast. The morning is best as it mimics the timing of production of cortisone in the body. Taking the dose of prednisone too late in the evening may cause difficulty in sleeping.

Ans.

169. b
170. d
171. c
172. b
173. a
174. d
175. b
176. c
177. b
178. c
179. b
180. b
181. d
182. a
183. b
184. c

INSULIN AND ORAL HYPOGLYCEMICS

185. An insulin drip is initiated for a patient with 40 U of insulin in 100 mL of normal saline solution. The IV is being infused via an infusion pump and the pump is currently set at 20 mL/h. How many units of insulin is infused each hour?

a. 4 U b. 8 U
c. 0.4 U d. 0.8 U

Explanation:

- 100 mL normal saline contains = 40 U of insulin
- 1 mL normal saline contains = 40/100 = 0.4 U
- 20 mL normal saline contains = 0.4 × 20 = 8 U

186. Which of the following action is correct in regard to insulin administration?

a. Inject insulin at an angle of 45° into deltoid muscle
b. Take insulin after the first meal of the day
c. Draw up clear insulin first when mixing two types of insulin in one syringe
d. Shake the insulin vial vigorously before withdrawing medication.

Explanation: When mixing two types of insulin, the clear (regular) insulin should be drawn first into syringe. Insulin typically administered before first meal of the day. Insulin vial must be gently (in case of NPH) rolled in between palms before withdrawing medication. It should not be vigorously shaked.

187. Which of the following drugs has reducing effect on proteinuria in a normotensive diabetic patient?

a. Beta blockers b. ACE inhibitors
c. Loop diuretics d. Osmotic diuretics

Explanation: ACE stands for 'angiotensin-converting enzyme'. ACE inhibitors are a group of medicines that are used for two reasons: to treat high blood pressure and to reduce protein in the urine (proteinuria). They are used in various illnesses, including heart failure, kidney problems and diabetes.

188. Which of the following type of insulin is prescribed for a client with diabetic ketoacidosis?

a. Long acting insulin b. Human Regular insulin
c. Lente insulin d. Human NPH insulin

Explanation: Regular insulin acts rapidly and should be used for diabetic coma and diabetic ketoacidosis to achieve immediate action.

189. Which of the following anti-diabetic drugs can cause vitamin B12 deficiency?

a. Glipizide b. Acarbose
c. Metformin d. Pioglitazone

190. Insulin causes all of the following; EXCEPT:

a. Glycogenesis b. Glycolysis
c. Lipogenesis d. Ketogenesis

191. All are used in diabetic ketoacidosis; EXCEPT:

a. Insulin b. I.V. fluids
c. Sodium bicarbonate d. Glucagon

192. Which of the following is a rapid acting insulin?

a. Regular insulin b. Humalog Novolog
c. Lente insulin d. Semilente insulin

193. Which of the following is a short acting insulin?

a. Regular insulin b. NPH
c. Lente insulin d. Semilente insulin

194. Insulin causes:

a. Na^+ entry into cells b. K^+ exit from cells
c. Na^+ exit/K^+ entry d. K^+ entry into cells

195. Insulin overdose can be treated by administration of:

a. 50% dextrose IV
b. 5% dextrose in Normal Saline IV
c. Oral hypoglycemic agents
d. Ringer lactate solution IV

196. Indications of newer insulin include all; EXCEPT:

a. Insulin resistance b. Lipodystrophy
c. Pregnancy d. Diabetic kidney disease

197. Which of the following type of insulin can be administered through intravenous route (IV) in emergency conditions?

a. Humulin lente b. Humulin ultralente
c. Insulin semilente d. Regular insulin

HORMONES

198. Increased suicidal tendency is associated with:

a. Low levels of serotonin b. High levels of serotonin
c. Low levels of dopamine d. High levels of dopamine

Explanation: Low levels of serotonin (5-HT) in brain are associated with depression and suicidal behavior. High level of serotonin is associated with anxiety.

199. Deficiency of which of the following neurotransmitter is associated with depression?

a. Acetylcholine b. Norepinephrine
c. Dopamine d. Serotonin

Explanation: Low serotonin (5-HT) levels are found to be the cause of many cases of mild to severe depression

200. Major neurotransmitter in parasympathetic:

a. Acetylcholine b. Adrenaline
c. Noradrenaline d. Dopamine

201. Organophosphate inhibits:

a. Anionic site of AChEs b. Esteric site of AChEs
c. ACh d. None of these

202. The pharmacological action of adrenaline includes: *(ESI 2009)*

a. Vasoconstriction b. Increase in heart rate
c. Vasodilation d. Both a and b

Explanation: Epinephrine (Adrenaline) reaction with α receptors causes vasoconstriction while reaction with β1 receptor causes increase in heart rate and cardiac output.

203. Epinephrine reacts with which of the following receptors?

a. Adrenergic receptors b. Cholinergic receptors
c. Muscarinic receptors d. Nicotinic receptors

Explanation: Epinephrine (also known as Adrenaline) has adrenergic effect. Adrenergic receptors respond to sympathetic stimulation and blood-borne epinephrine. Epinephrine release is a vital component of the fight-or-flight response of the sympathetic nervous system.

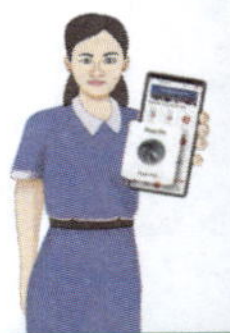

Ans.

185. b
186. c
187. b
188. b
189. c
190. d
191. d
192. b
193. a
194. d
195. a
196. d
197. d
198. a
199. d
200. a
201. b
202. d
203. a

204. Corticosteroids suppresses:
a. Baroreceptors
b. Pain receptors
c. Immune response
d. Neural transmission

Explanation: Corticosteroids suppresses immune response in the body. Other physiological processes include stress response, regulation of inflammation, carbohydrate metabolism, and protein catabolism.

205. Mifepristone is an example of:
a. Progesterone antagonist
b. Estrogen antagonist
c. Progesterone agonist
d. Estrogen supplement

Explanation: Mifepristone is a progesterone antagonist, also known as RU-486, is a medication typically used with misoprostol to bring about Medical Termination of Pregnancy (Abortion).

206. For a client with hyperthyroidism, treatment is most likely to include:
a. A thyroid hormone antagonist
b. Thyroid extract
c. A synthetic thyroid hormone
d. Emollient lotions

Explanation: Thyroid hormone antagonists block thyroid hormone synthesis and reduce increased production of thyroid hormone.

207. Which of the following action is not caused by oxytocin?
a. Lactogenesis
b. Ejection of breast milk
c. Contraction of myoepithelial cells
d. Uterine contraction

Explanation: Prolactin is a hormone responsible for lactogenesis (milk production). Other actions are caused by oxytocin.

208. In which of the following condition, the drug epinephrine is not used?
a. Anaphylaxis
b. Local homeostasis
c. Chronic bronchial asthma
d. All of the above

209. Mineralocorticoid causes:
a. Na^+ reabsorption
b. Glycogen synthesis
c. Gluconeogenesis
d. Lipolysis

210. Prolactin secretion is inhibited by:
a. Dopamine antagonist
b. GABA
c. Neurophysin
d. Bromocriptine

211. All are released from pituitary; EXCEPT:
a. GH
b. Prolactin
c. ADH
d. Glucagon

212. Growth hormone release is controlled by:
a. GHRH
b. Dopamine
c. FSH
d. CRH

213. Thyroxine is synthesized from:
a. Cysteine
b. Arginine
c. Tyrosine
d. Alanine

214. L-thyroxine is used in:
a. Thyroid storm
b. Cretinism
c. Endemic goiter
d. Graves' disease

215. Which is fastest calcium lowering agents?
a. Calcitonin
b. Plicamycin
c. Etidronate
d. Zoledronate

216. Estrogen therapy is contraindicated in patient with:
a. Pelvic inflammatory disease
b. Dysmenorrhea
c. Cervical cancer
d. Liver disease

217. Which of the following drug induces ovulation?
a. Clomiphene citrate
b. Mifepristone
c. Misoprostol
d. Ritodrine

218. Mifepristone is an example of:
a. Prostaglandin
b. Vasodilator
c. Estrogen antagonist
d. Progesterone antagonist

219. Corticosteroid which is given by inhalation route is:
a. Prednisolone
b. Beclomethasone
c. Dexamethasone
d. Hydrocortisone

220. All are side effects of steroids; EXCEPT:
a. Diabetes
b. Osteoporosis
c. Fragile skin
d. Hypotension

221. Which of the following is the side effect of steroids due to its mineralocorticoid component?
a. Skin striae
b. Hypertension
c. Osteoporosis
d. Moon face

222. Prolonged testosterone treatment to a man results in:
a. Increased spermatogenesis
b. Increased sperm motility
c. Azoospermia
d. Increased gonadotropins

223. Somatostatin secreted by which type of cells in pancreas?
a. Gamma cells
b. Delta cells
c. Alpha cells
d. Beta cells

224. Complications of aerosol steroids use includes:
a. Oral candidiasis
b. Cushing's syndrome
c. Decreased ACTH
d. Systemic complications

225. One of the following is not true about melatonin:
a. Induces sleep
b. Used in treatment of jet lag syndrome
c. Is secreted by pituitary
d. Is a pineal hormone

226. ADH acts on:
a. Proximal convoluted tubule
b. Distal convoluted tubule
c. Loop of Henle
d. Collecting duct

DRUGS USED IN TREATMENT OF INTEGUMENTARY SYSTEM

227. Clotrimazole is: *(ESIC Chennai May 2012)*
a. Antiprotozoal drug
b. Antibacterial drug
c. Antiviral drug
d. Antifungal drug

228. Which of the following is not an antifungal agent?
a. Fluconazole
b. Ketoconazole
c. Tinidazole
d. Clotrimazole

229. Liniments should not be applied on the:
a. Normal skin
b. Painful skin
c. Broken skin
d. Swollen skin

Explanation: Liniments are applied with rubbing or massaged into the skin as counter irritating or stimulating agents to the affected area. Liniment should not be applied to the bruised or broken because they would cause irritation especially if alcohol is used as solvent.

Ans.

204. c
205. a
206. a
207. a
208. c
209. a
210. d
211. d
212. a
213. c
214. b
215. a
216. d
217. a
218. d
219. b
220. d
221. b
222. c
223. b
224. a
225. c
226. d
227. d
228. c
229. c

230. A patient with Systemic Lupus Erythematosus (SLE) is being assessed to start hydroxychloroquine therapy. Which of the following pre-existing condition is a contraindication to start hydroxychloroquine?

a. Maculopathy b. Rheumatoid arthritis
c. Asthma d. Pregnancy

Explanation: Patients with a history of retinopathy or pre-existing maculopathy should not be treated with hydroxychloroquine because the drug hydroxychloroquine is associated with macular edema and retinopathy.

231. Amphotericin B is a:

a. Azole b. Benzofuran
c. Fungicidal d. Fungistatic

DRUGS USED IN TREATMENT OF COMMUNICABLE DISEASES

232. Which of the following drug is recommended along with intravenous administration of quinine sulfate for treatment of malaria? *(RPSC NG-II, 2007)*

a. Calcium gluconate b. Hydrocortisone
c. Multivitamin d. Glucose

Explanation: Quinine sulfate administration may cause low blood sugar (hypoglycemia). So, glucose has to be administered to counter hypoglycaemic effect of quinine.

233. Which of the following antimalarial drug is safe for a child with GPD (glucose-6-phosphate dehydrogenase) deficiency?

a. Methoquine b. Quinine
c. Mefloquine d. Chloroquin

Explanation: Mefloquine is considered to be a safe drug to be used in children with glucose–6 phosphate dehydrogenase deficiency. Other drugs given above are contraindicated to use in this condition.

234. Chloroquine is a/an ______ drug.

a. Antimalarial b. Antimicrobial
c. Antiviral d. Antiamoebic

235. Primaquine is contraindicated in deficiency of:

a. Glucose-6-Phosphate
b. Glucose-6-phosphate dehydrogenase
c. Alpha ketoglutarate dehydrogenase
d. Pyruvate kinase

236. The drug of choice in the management of preeclamsia is:

a. Magnesium sulfate b. Calcium gluconate
c. Sodium bicarbonate d. Sodium nitroprusside

Explanation: Magnesium sulfate ($MgSO_4$) is the agent most commonly used for treatment of eclampsia and prophylaxis of eclampsia in patients with severe preeclampsia.

237. Which of the following drugs is implicated in the causation of osteomalacia of the bone?

a. Phenytoin b. Steroids
c. Heparin d. Estrogen

238. Drug of choice for status epilepticus is:

a. Carbamazepine b. Diazepam
c. Phenytoin sodium d. Valporic acid

239. Which of the following antiepileptic is preferred when an epileptic patient is not responding to phenytoin?

a. Carbamazepine b. Clonazepam
c. Diazepam d. Sodium Valproate

240. Intravenous phenytoin should not be infused rapidly because it can cause:

a. Hypertension and Syncope
b. Hypotension and cardiac dysrhythmia
c. Hypertension and atrial fibrillation
d. Hypotension and hypoglycemia

241. Medications used for pediculosis treatment includes:

a. DDT 5%-10%
b. Carbolic lotion 1: 40
c. Kerosene coconut oil 1:1 ratio
d. All of the above

ANTITUBERCULAR DRUGS

242. Which of the following is a common side effect of streptomycin? *(ESI-2010)*

a. Damage to facial nerve
b. Damage to 8th cranial nerve
c. Bone marrow depression
d. Hypersensitivity

Explanation: Antibiotics in the aminoglycoside class (Streptomycin, Gentamicin, tobramycin) may cause damage to 8th cranial nerve which results in loss of hearing, balancing problems, neuromuscular blockage, peripheral neuropathy, dizziness and vomiting.

243. Which of the following antitubercular drug causes red orange discoloration of urine?
[Bhopal Memorial Hospital Nursing Tutor, 2013]

a. Isoniazid b. Ethambutol
c. Streptomycin d. Rifampicin

Explanation: Rifampicin causes red orange discoloration of urine

244. All of the following antitubercular drugs crosses blood-brain barrier; EXCEPT:

a. Isoniazid b. Rifampicin
c. Pyrazinamide d. Streptomycin

Explanation: Each antitubercular drug differs in its ability to cross the blood-brain barrier and achieve sufficient intracerebral concentrations to kill bacilli. Isoniazid and pyrazinamide pass freely into the cerebrospinal fluid (CSF), whereas CSF concentrations of rifampicin are probably <10% of serum concentrations. Streptomycin and Ethambutol, the other first-line treatment agents, probably only penetrate the blood-brain barrier in the presence of inflammation during the early stages of treatment.
Remember: Streptomycin is no longer considered as an ATT drug.

245. Which of the following antitubercular drug causes peripheral neuropathy?

a. Isoniazid b. Pyrazinamide
c. Rifampicin d. Dapsone

Explanation: Prolonged use of Isoniazid (INH) leads to deficiency of pyridoxine hence, causes peripheral neuropathy.

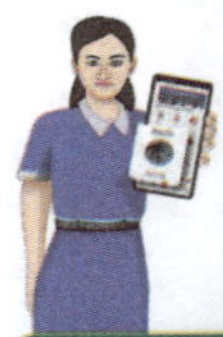

Ans.

230. a
231. c
232. d
233. c
234. a
235. b
236. a
237. a
238. b
239. a
240. b
241. d
242. b
243. d
244. d
245. a

246. Prolonged use of isoniazid (INH) leads to deficiency of:

a. Niacin b. Cyanocobalamin
c. Folic acid d. Pyridoxine

Explanation: Prolonged treatment with the drug Isoniazid (INH) will cause deficiency of pyridoxine which leads to peripheral neuropathy.

247. The drug of choice for prophylaxis of tuberculosis is:

a. Streptomycin b. Ethambutol
c. Isoniazid (INH) d. Rifampicin

Explanation: Isoniazid (INH) is the drug of choice for chemoprophylaxis. All of the other drugs listed can be used in the treatment of tuberculosis.

248. The purpose of combination drug therapy in the treatment of tuberculosis is to reduce:

a. The duration of treatment
b. Adverse effects of the drugs
c. Dosage of drugs
d. Drug resistance

Explanation: Use of combination of drugs reduces the risk of drug resistance by infective organism.

249. Retrobulbar neuritis is a side effect of which of the following drug?

a. Ethambutol b. Isoniazid
c. Streptomycin d. Pyrazinamide

Explanation: Ethambutol causes optic neuropathy (retrobulbar neuritis) in 1-5% of patients using the antituberculosis drugs.

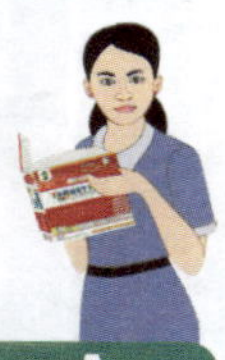

250. Rifampicin is used for prophylaxis of: *(Recent Question 2012)*

a. Gonorrhea b. Malaria
c. Leprosy d. Meningococcal meningitis

251. Which of the following antitubercular drug is an amino-glycoside?

a. Rifampicin b. Isoniazid
c. Ethambutol d. Streptomycin

252. Streptomycin is not administered orally because:

a. It gets deactivated during first-pass metabolism
b. It can cause gastric ulcer
c. It can cause gastric bleeding
d. It is not absorbed orally

253. Which of the following antitubercular drugs is associated with red green color blindness?

a. Cycloserine b. Isoniazid
c. Pyrazinamide d. Ethambutol

254. INH induced peripheral neuropathy results from deficiency of:

a. B1 b. B2
c. B6 d. B12

255. Peripheral neuritis is a side effect of which antitubercular drug:

a. Rifampicin b. Isoniazid
c. Streptomycin d. Ethambutol

256. Peripheral neuritis caused by isoniazid can be prevented by providing:

a. Niacin b. Aspirin
c. Pyridoxine d. Thiamine

257. Bacteriostatic antitubercular drug is:

a. Isoniazid b. Rifampin
c. Streptomycin d. Ethambutol

258. All of the following are the side effects of Rifampicin; EXCEPT:

a. Anorexia b. Dizziness
c. Orange colored urine d. Hypertension

259. Which of the following laboratory test must be ordered before the patient started on isoniazid (INH) therapy?

a. Bleeding time and Coagulation time
b. Liver Function test
c. Renal Function Test
d. Serum electrolytes

DRUGS USED IN OPHTHALMOLOGY AND ENT

260. All of the following are the actions of acetylcholine; EXCEPT:

a. Contraction of detrusor muscle
b. Decrease in heart rate
c. Dilatation of pupil
d. Increased salivation

Explanation: Acetylcholine is a miotic agent thus, causes constriction of pupil. Mydriatic agents (Atropine) causes dilation of pupil.

261. Which of the following class of drugs constricts the pupil?

a. Mydriatics
b. Miotics
c. Both mydriatics and miotics
d. None of the above

262. The action of mydriatics is:

a. Contraction of arteries b. Constriction of the pupil
c. Dilation of arteries d. Dilation of the pupil

263. Which of the following drug likely to cause macular toxicity when administered intravitreally?

a. Cefotaxime b. Vancomycin
c. Gentamycin d. Dexamethasone

264. All of the following drugs are used topically to treat open angle glaucoma; EXCEPT:

a. Dorzolamide
b. Acetazolamide
c. Latanoprost
d. Brinzolamide

DIURETICS

265. Which of the following medication is used in the management of raised ICP? *(RPSC NG-II, 2007)*

a. Diazepam b. Phenytoin
c. Mannitol d. Furosemide

Explanation: Mannitol is an osmotic diuretic agent. Its osmotic properties take effect in 15–30 minutes when it sets up an osmotic gradient and draws water out of neurons. Mannitol is therefore, best used by bolus administration where an acute reduction in ICP is necessary.

266. Mannitol decreases the intraocular pressure by:

a. Withdrawing water from vitreous
b. Increasing uveoscleral outflow
c. Increasing aqueous through trabecular meshwork
d. Inhibiting the enzyme anhydrase in the ciliary body

Ans.

246. d
247. c
248. d
249. a
250. d
251. d
252. d
253. d
254. c
255. b
256. c
257. d
258. d
259. b
260. c
261. b
262. d
263. c
264. b
265. c
266. a

267. Which of the following drug is administered to reduce the elevated intracranial pressure?

a. Hydralazine
b. Mannitol
c. Nitrofurantoin
d. Sodium nitroprusside

268. Which of the following is an osmotic diuretic? *(JIPMER 2012)*

a. Lasix
b. Spironolactone
c. Aldactone
d. Mannitol

269. Which of the following is not an osmotic diuretic?

a. Furosemide
b. Glycerol
c. Isosorbide
d. Mannitol

Explanation: Furosemide is a loop diuretic. All other drugs given above are osmotic diuretics.

270. The diuretics should be administered early in the morning to:

a. Prevent drug-food interaction
b. Prevent nausea and vomiting
c. To avoid nocturia
d. To promote absorption

Explanation: Diuretics increases the urine excretion. If the drug is administered in the evening/night, it may result in nocturia. Nocturia is a condition in which the patient need to get up many times during the night to urinate. So, it is recommended to administer diuretics early in the morning.

271. When administering loop diuretic to a client, the nurse anticipates that the client may develop which electrolyte imbalance?

a. Hyperkalemia
b. Hypernatremia
c. Hypokalemia
d. Hypervolemia

Explanation: Loop diuretic inhibits the reabsorption of sodium and chloride in the ascending loop of Henle resulting in the excretion of sodium, chloride and to a lesser degree potassium and bicarbonate ions.

272. The diuretic used in the treatment of open angle glaucoma is:

a. Furosemide
b. Acetazolamide
c. Spironolactone
d. Mannitol

273. Potassium sparing diuretics is:

a. Spironolactone
b. Triamterene
c. Amiloride
d. All of these

274. The nurse must take the following precaution when the patient is receiving furosemide:

a. Advise the patient to quit smoking
b. Advise the patient to do regular aerobic exercises
c. Advise the patient for low calorie diet
d. Check blood sugar and urine sugar of the patient

Explanation: Hyperglycemia is a well known adverse effect of therapy with diuretics. In adipose tissue, hydrochlorothiazide and furosemide inhibit the rate of glucose transport. In skeletal muscle, furosemide decreases the rate of glucose phosphorylation and glycolysis. This may result in hyperglycemia. So the blood glucose and urine sugar should be monitored.

GENERAL ANESTHETICS

275. Which of the following is a contraindication for spinal anesthesia?

a. Diabetes
b. Children
c. Elderly patients
d. Sepsis

276. Which of the following drug in combination with catecholamines given during surgery likely to cause arrhythmias?

a. Lidocaine
b. Halothane
c. Propofol
d. Digoxine

277. A patient underwent surgical procedure under general anesthesia and being shifted to postanesthesia care unit (PACU). While receiving the patient in PACU, which of the following assessment is most important?

a. Vital signs
b. Level of patients
c. Respiratory status
d. Consciousness level

Explanation: When receiving a patient in the postanesthesia care unit (PACU) following a surgical procedure under general anesthesia, the most important assessment is the patient's respiratory status. General anesthesia can depress the respiratory drive and suppress the normal protective reflexes, such as coughing and gag reflex. It is crucial to monitor the patient's breathing, airway patency, and oxygen saturation to ensure adequate ventilation and oxygenation.

Assessing Vital signs and Level of consciousness are also significant assessments, but they may be influenced by the residual effects of anesthesia and medications. The respiratory assessment is the priority.

278. During induction of general anesthesia, the patient becomes extremely anxious, hyperactive and physically resists the treatment. Which of the following intervention is required in this situation? *New Q*

a. Need to reschedule the surgery
b. Anesthesia should be discontinued
c. An IV drug to be administered to calm down the patient
d. Do nothing as it is a normal reaction

Explanation: During the induction of general anesthesia, the patient may become anxious, hyperactive, and physically resist the treatment. This is a common reaction, and it is usually caused by fear or anxiety about the surgery. In this situation, it is important to calm the patient down and administer an IV drug to sedate them.

279. Nurse Ramya is preparing a patient who is scheduled for a surgery under general anesthesia. Which of the following preoperative instruction is appropriate for this patient?

a. Eat light breakfast on the day of surgery
b. Urinary incontinence is expected postoperatively
c. Nausea, vomiting, shivering are expected postoperatively
d. Take all the medications due of the day in the morning itself

Explanation: The appropriate preoperative instruction for a patient scheduled for surgery under general anesthesia is to inform them that postoperative symptoms such as nausea, vomiting, and shivering are expected. This information helps set realistic expectations for the patient and reduces anxiety or confusion if these symptoms occur after the surgery.

Options a, b, and d are not appropriate preoperative instructions for this situation.

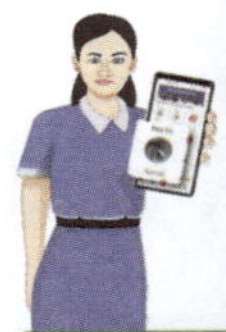

Ans.

267. b
268. d
269. a
270. c
271. c
272. b
273. d
274. d
275. d
276. b
277. c
278. c
279. c

280. Common adverse effects of thiopental include:
a. Nausea and vomiting
b. Headache
c. Emergence delirium
d. Hemiparesis

Explanation: Emergence delirium (ED) is an abnormal mental state that develops as a result of anesthesia administration during the transition from unconsciousness to complete wakefulness. It is characterized by hallucination, confusion, and excitability.

SEDATIVE AND HYPNOTICS

281. All of the following drugs belong to sedative and hypnotics group; EXCEPT:
a. Diazepam b. Nitrazepam
c. Clozapine d. Lorazepam

Explanation: All of the above given drugs belongs to benzodiazepines. However, clozapine is primarily an antipsychotic drug. All other given drugs belong to sedative and hypnotics.

282. Which of the following drug is not an example of benzodiazepines?
a. Alprazolam b. Chlordiazepoxide
c. Clorazepate d. Phenytoin

283. Benzodiazepines acts by amplifying which of the following neurotransmitter in the body?
a. Epinephrine b. Acetylcholine
c. GABA d. Serotonin

284. Benzodiazepines are useful in the treatment of all the following conditions; EXCEPT:
a. Insomnia b. Epilepsy
c. Alzheimer's disease d. Anxiety disorders

285. Antidote of benzodiazepines is:
a. Flumazenil b. Naloxone
c. Atropine sulphate d. Acetylcysteine

ANTICONVULSANTS

286. Which of the following drugs is associated with the reaction of Stevens-Johnson syndrome? *(Safdarjung NO 2018)*
a. Valproic acid b. Quinidine
c. Isoniazid d. Procainamide

Explanation:
- Stevens-Johnson syndrome (SJS) is one of the most severe adverse drug reactions occurring in pediatric population. It is a type III reaction (Retarded, Arthus).
- Many drugs including antibiotics, NSAIDs, and anticonvulsants can cause SJS. However, anticonvulsants (e.g., Valproic acid) are the commonest group of drugs causing Stevens–Johnson syndrome (SJS) and toxic epidermal necrolysis (TEN).

287. Phenytoin is used in the treatment of:
a. Petit mal epilepsy b. Grand mal epilepsy
c. Myoclonic seizures d. All of these

Explanation: Phenytoin is the drug of choice for Grand mal epilepsy.

288. Magnesium sulfate is administered to a client with preeclampsia to:
a. Increase diuresis b. Prevent seizures
c. Reduce blood pressure d. Slow the process of labor

Explanation: Chemically, magnesium is similar to that of calcium and, therefore magnesium will act like calcium in the body. So, magnesium will block seizure activity by interfering with signal transmission at the neural musculature junction.

289. Megaloblastic anemia is caused by:
a. Phenytoin toxicity b. Long term aspirin use
c. NSAIDs d. Opioid analgesics

Explanation: Phenytoin (dilantin) causes megaloblastic anemia due to decreased folate absorption.

290. Best prophylaxis for a 3-year-child with febrile seizures:
a. Benzodiazepines
b. Paracetamol q6h
c. Paracetamol and nitrazepam
d. Phenobarbitone

Explanation: Phenobarbitone is effective in preventing the recurrence of simple febrile seizures in children.

291. All of the following are the side effects of Phenytoin; EXCEPT: *(AIIMS Rishikesh 2015)*
a. Ataxia b. Hirsutism
c. Hypoglycemia d. Gum Hypertrophy

Explanation: Side effects of Phenytoin includes gingival hyperplasia, Hirsutism, and ataxia. It can cause Hyperglycemic.

292. Neural tube defect is due to:
a. Valproate b. Phenytoin
c. Diazoxide d. None of these

ANALGESICS

293. Withdrawal symptoms do not usually occur in case of which of the following medications? *(AIIMS-BBS SNO 2019)*
a. Monoamine oxidase inhibitors
b. Non-steroidal anti-inflammatory drugs
c. Selective serotonin reuptake inhibitors
d. Tetracyclic anti-depressants

Explanation: Withdrawal symptoms do not usually occur in case of Non-steroidal anti-inflammatory drugs (NSAIDs. All other given drugs are antidepressants with a side effect of withdrawal symptoms o abrupt discontinuation of drug.

294. Which of the following analgesic is preferred in elderly patients? *(AIIMS-2011)*
a. Aspirin b. Morphine
c. Diclofenac sodium d. Ampicillin

Explanation: Diclofenac sodium is a non-steroidal anti-inflammatory drug (NSAID). It is recommended for old age people because of its analgesic effect with less side effects. Ampicillin (option d) is an antibiotic, so not correct. Aspirin is risky in old age people as it increases the chances of gastric ulcer.

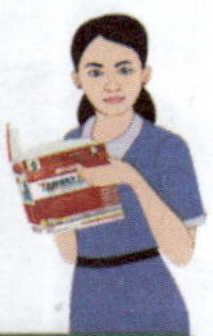

Ans.

280. c
281. c
282. d
283. c
284. c
285. a
286. a
287. b
288. b
289. a
290. d
291. c
292. a
293. b
294. c

295. Morphine is contraindicated in which of the following condition? *(ESI 2010)*
a. Angina
b. Bronchial asthma
c. Appendicitis
d. Myocardial infarction

Explanation: Morphine is an opioid derivative that causes respiratory depression. So, it is contraindicated in patients with Bronchial asthma.

296. Paracetamol is an: *(RPSC NG-II, 2010)*
a. Antipyretic b. Antitussives
c. Antibiotic d. Antiemetic

Explanation: Paracetamol (acetaminophen) is an antipyretic (reduce fever) and analgesic (reduce pain) agent.

297. A client receiving morphine sulfate should be observed for: *(Kerala PSC, Nov 2014)*
a. Respiratory depression b. Blood dyscrasias
c. Gastritis d. Jaundice

298. Opioids are obtained from: *(Staff Nurse G II 2014)*
a. Erythroxylum coca b. Claviceps purpurea
c. Cannabis sativa d. Papaver somniferum

299. NSAIDs are used in all; EXCEPT:
a. As analgesic b. In peptic ulcer
c. Rheumatoid arthritis d. Osteoarthritis

300. Which of the following drug is an example of Synthetic opioid analgesic?
a. Aspirin b. Morphine
c. Fentanyl d. Indomethacin

301. Analgesics are prescribed to: *(RPSC NG-II, 2010)*
a. Induce sleep b. Give rest
c. Relieve pain d. Kill pathogens

302. Contraindications to aspirin are all; EXCEPT:
a. Peptic ulcer b. Bleeding tendencies
c. Chicken pox d. Rheumatoid Arthritis

303. Which one of the following is aspirin?
a. Methyl salicylate
b. Para amino benzoic acid
c. Para amino salicylic acid
d. Acetyl salicylic acid

304. Tramadol is:
a. Antiflatulent b. Antireflux drug
c. Beta blocker d. Opioid analgesic

LOCAL ANESTHETICS

305. The nurse has applied EMLA cream as ordered. How does the nurse assess that cream has achieved its purpose? *(AIIMS Raipur NO 2019)*:
a. Assess the skin for redness
b. Note any blanching of the skin
c. Lightly tap the area where the cream is applied
d. Gently poke the individual with a needle

Explanation: Eutectic mixture of local anesthetics (EMLA) is a combination of prilocaine and lidocaine. Lightly tapping the area where the cream is applied is the correct way to assess whether the cream has achieved its purpose or not.

306. Which of the following local anesthetic agent has shorter duration of action?
a. Lidocaine b. Procaine
c. Bupivacaine d. Ropivacaine

Explanation: Procaine exerts shorter local anesthetic action. Procaine is preferred local anesthetic agent in patient with liver disease. It is not used these days.

307. The local anesthetic which also acts as an antiarrhythmic agent:
a. Cocaine b. Lidocaine
c. Bupivacaine d. Ropivacaine

Explanation: Lidocaine acts as local anesthetic as well as anti-arrpythmic agent.

308. The local anesthetics primarily acts on:
a. Inactivated K^+ channels b. Inactivated Na^+ channels
c. Activated Ca^+ channels d. Resting K^+ channels

309. The most cardiotoxic local anesthetic among given drugs is:
a. Procaine b. Lidocaine
c. Bupivacaine d. Lignocaine

310. The purpose of adding a vasoconstrictor to a local anesthetic drug is:
a. To increase the duration of local anesthetic effect
b. For rapid action of local anesthetic
c. To minimize the allergic reaction
d. To enhance the affinity to Na^+ channels

Explanation: Addition of a vasoconstrictor to a local anesthetic has the following benefits:
- Decrease in the peak plasma concentration of local anesthetic (LA)
- Increase in the duration of LA effect (by reducing the absorption into the circulation)
- Reduction in minimum concentration of LA required for nerve block.
- Decrease of blood loss during surgery.

311. A higher dose of local anesthetic agent was inadvertently administered through Intravenous route. Which of the following system is most likely involved in the toxic effect?
a. Cardiovascular system
b. Immune system
c. Gastrointestinal system
d. Respiratory system

MUSCLE RELAXANTS

312. Barbiturates are contraindicated in older persons because it cause:
a. Convulsions b. Delirium
c. Panic attack d. Urinary incontinence

313. Which of the following drug is used to reverse the muscle relaxant effect of tubocurarine?
a. Succinylcholine b. Neostigmine
c. Dantrolene d. Baclofen

314. Which of the following skeletal muscle relaxant has the lowest duration of action?
a. Vecuronium b. Succinylcholine
c. Dantrolene d. Tubocurarine

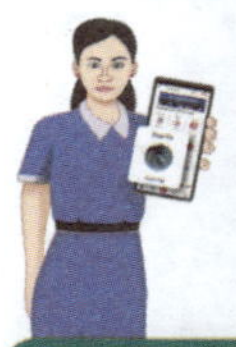

Ans.

295.	b
296.	a
297.	a
298.	d
299.	b
300.	c
301.	c
302.	d
303.	d
304.	d
305.	c
306.	b
307.	b
308.	b
309.	c
310.	a
311.	a
312.	b
313.	b
314.	b

315. Which of the following muscle relaxant is used to treat spasticity and malignant hyperthermia of neuroleptic malignant syndrome?

a. Vecuronium b. Dantrolene
c. Neostigmine d. Baclofen

316. A patient scheduled for a mastectomy surgery has a 10 year history of COPD. Which of the following muscle relaxant is contraindicated in this patient during the surgery?

a. Clonidine b. Vecuronium
c. Tubocurarine d. Succinylcholine

Explanation: Tubocurarine may lead to release of histamine from mast cells which in turn cause bronchoconstriction. Hence tubocurarine should not be used in a patient with COPD or asthma.

ANTI-GOUT AGENTS

317. Which of the following drug acts by decreasing uric acid levels in blood and urine?

a. Colchicine b. Indomethacin
c. Allopurinol d. Aspirin

Explanation: Allopurinol is a xanthine oxidase inhibitor. It acts by reducing the uric acid production in the body. Allopurinol is used to prevent gout attacks, not to treat them once they occur.

318. Which of the following drug acts by decreasing swelling and lessoning the deposition of uric acid crystals in the affected joints?

a. Allopurinol b. Colchicine
c. Indomethacin d. Aspirin

319. Which of the following drug inhibits cyclooxygenase irreversibly to prevent the production of pain causing prostaglandins?

a. Colchicine b. Allopurinol
c. Aspirin d. Paracetamol

320. Which of the following immunosuppressant drug is used in the treatment of rheumatoid arthritis?

a. Indomethacin b. Azathioprine
c. Ibuprofen d. Colchicine

Explanation: The immunosuppressants used in the treatment of rheumatoid arthritis are nitrogen mustard, azathioprine, methotrexate, Chlorambucil, 6-mercaptopurine, and cyclophosphamide.

321. Which of the following is an antimalarial drug which is used widely for the treatment of rheumatoid arthritis?

a. Naproxen
b. Artimisinin
c. Hydroxychloroquine
d. Mefloquine

322. All of the following drugs are useful in the treatment of gout arthritis; EXCEPT:

a. Allopurinol b. Colchicine
c. Probenecid d. Acetazolamide

323. Drug useful for gout:

a. Pyrazinamide
b. Rifampicin
c. Allopurinol
d. Naloxone

SYMPATHOMIMITIC (ADRENERGIC) DRUGS

324. Which of the following food item is avoided in patients who is on MAO inhibitors such as phenelzine?

a. Grapes b. Banana
c. Strawberry d. Red wine and Cheese

325. Which of the following drug is a beta-1 selective agonist which is used to increase stroke volume in patients with cardiogenic shock?

a. Epinephrine b. Dobutamine
c. Dopamine d. Norepinephrine

326. An 18-year-old patient suffering from anaphylactic reaction is brought to the emergency room. The patient is having severe dyspnea and urticaria and lower blood pressure. Which of the following is the most suitable drug to treat this patient's life-threating condition?

a. Terbutaline b. Phenylephrine
c. Epinephrine d. Dobutamine

Explanation: Beta-2 effects of epinephrine produces bronchodilation and decreased release of inflammatory mediators from mast cells and basophils. So, parenterally administered epinephrine is a drug of choice for treating anaphylactic reactions.

CHOLINERGIC AND ANTICHOLINERGIC DRUGS

327. Atropine does not cause:

a. Increase bowel sound b. Decrease bowel sound
c. Hypotension d. Tachycardia

328. Atropine is commonly used prior to administration of inhalant anesthetics to reduce:

a. Muscle tone b. Secretions
c. Nausea and vomiting d. All of these

Explanation: Atropine is an anticholinergic agent which reduces secretions in respiratory tract.

329. Atropine is most sensitive to:

a. Mucous and pharyngeal secretions
b. Heart
c. Pupil
d. GI Tract motility

330. Which one of the following acts commonly both on parasympathetic and sympathetic division?

a. Atropine b. Pilocarpine
c. Acetylcholine d. Adrenaline

331. Acetylcholine is not used commercially because:

a. Long duration of action
b. Costly
c. Rapidly destroyed in the body
d. Crosses blood brain barrier

ANTIPSYCHOTICS

332. Extrapyramidal symptoms (EPS) are associated with:

a. Anxiolytics b. Antipsychotic
c. Antidepressants d. Antimanics

Explanation: Extrapyramidal symptoms (EPS) are one of the major complication of using Antipsychotic drug.

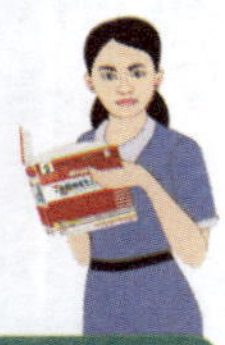

Ans.

315. b
316. c
317. c
318. b
319. c
320. b
321. c
322. d
323. c
324. d
325. b
326. c
327. a
328. b
329. a
330. c
331. c
332. b

333. An irreversible side effect of antipsychotics is: *(Recent Question 2012)*

a. Akathisia b. Tardive dyskinesia
c. Tremor d. Sleeplessness

334. All of the following may be seen with neuroleptic malignant syndrome; EXCEPT:

a. Hypothermia b. Altered consciousness
c. Muscle rigidity d. Involuntary movements

335. Clozapine is an example of:

a. Antipsychotic b. Antidepressant
c. Mood stabilizer d. Anxiolytic

336. Schizophrenia is treated by:

a. Antidepressants b. Antipsychotics
c. Antiepileptics d. Mood stabilizers

337. Neuroleptic malignant syndrome is characterized by:

a. Hypothermia b. Labile blood pressure
c. Bradycardia d. Flaccidity

338. Drug-induced Parkinsonism is treated by:

a. Anticholinergics b. Anticholinesterases
c. Cholinergic drugs d. Hydralazine

Explanation: Drug induced parkinsonism is treated with anticholinergic drugs. For example, trihexyphenidyl, benztropine, amantadine, etc.

ANTIDEPRESSANTS

339. Imipramine is an antidepressant of _______ group. *(RML 2002)*

a. Tricyclic antidepressant (TCA)
b. Selective serotonin reuptake inhibitor (SSRI)
c. Monoamine oxidase inhibitor (MAOI)
d. Non-selective serotonin reuptake inhibitor

Explanation: Imipramine is a tricyclic antidepressant (TCA) of the dibenzazepine group. Imipramine is mainly used in the treatment of major depression and enuresis (inability to control urination).

340. Dry mouth during antidepressant therapy is caused by blockade of:

a. Muscarinic acetylcholine receptors
b. Dopaminergic receptors
c. GABA receptors
d. Serotonergic receptors

Explanation: Antidepressants causes blockage of the muscarinic acetylcholine receptors which interferes with the salivary secretion.

341. Anxiolytic drug with antidepressant action is:

a. Lorazepam b. Diazepam
c. Alprazolam d. Triazolam

342. Which of the following drug is an example of Tricyclic Antidepressant (TCA)?

a. Imipramine b. Sertraline
c. Hydralazine d. Fluoxetine

343. Which of the following antidepressants cause urine retention:

a. Imipramine
b. Fluoxetine
c. Dothiepin
d. Risperidone

344. Anti-depressant drug that can safely be used in children is:

a. Imipramine b. Fluoxetine
c. Dothiepin d. Chlorpromazine

MOOD STABILIZERS

345. Which of the following is excreted in saliva?

a. Tetracycline b. Ampicillin
c. Lithium d. Choloramphenicol

346. Frequent serum level monitoring is required when the patient is on:

a. Amitriptyline b. Haloperidol
c. Lithium d. Lorazepam

Explanation: Lithium has very low therapeutic index. The therapeutic range for lithium is 0.6 - 1.2 mmol/L. Within this range, most people will respond to the drug without symptoms of toxicity. Below this range, it will not produce therapeutic effect, whereas lithium level above this range leads to toxic effects on patients. So, it is essential to regularly monitor serum level of lithium to ensure that it remains within therapeutic range.

347. Lithium is used in a pregnant woman. Which of the following congenital anomaly occurs in fetus?

a. Tetralogy of Fallot
b. Tricuspid atresia
c. Ebstein's anomaly
d. Pulmonary stenosis

348. Long term use of lithium causes:

a. Peripheral neuropathy
b. Hypothyroidism
c. Anemia
d. Jaundice

349. The therapeutic serum level of lithium is:

a. 0.3-0.6 mEq/L b. 0.6-1.2 mEq/L
c. 1.2-1.8 mEq/L d. 1.8-2.5 mEq/L

350. Treatment of choice of bipolar mood disorder:

a. Fluoxetine b. Imipramine
c. Lithium d. Chlorpromazine

351. Lithium monitoring is done because of:

a. Low therapeutic efficacy
b. Very low therapeutic index
c. Adverse effects
d. Long half-life

352. Therapeutic drug monitoring must be done for:

a. Penicillin b. Lithium
c. Erythromycin d. Lignocaine

353. Lithium therapy during pregnancy increases the chance of _______ in fetus.

a. Anencephaly
b. Neural tube defects
c. Defects in extremities
d. Cardiac malformations

Explanation: Women treated with lithium during pregnancy are at risk for Ebstein's anomaly of the fetus. Ebstein's anomaly is a congenital malformation of the heart.

354. Drug of choice for prophylaxis of mania is:

a. Lithium b. Haloperidol
c. Clozapine d. Carbamazepine

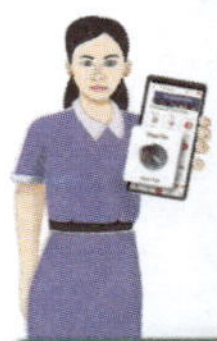

Ans.

333. b
334. a
335. a
336. b
337. b
338. a
339. a
340. a
341. c
342. a
343. a
344. a
345. c
346. c
347. c
348. b
349. b
350. c
351. b
352. b
353. d
354. a

355. Drug which causes hypothyroidism is:
a. Carbamazepine b. Lithium
c. Sulphur d. Methotrexate

DRUGS USED FOR DEADDICTION

356. Disulfiram, an antabuse drug used in Alcohol Dependence Syndrome acts by deactivating:
a. Acetaldehyde dehydrogenase
b. GABA
c. Acetylcholine
d. Choline-esterase

Explanation: Alcohol is broken down by the enzyme alcohol dehydrogenase to acetaldehyde, which is then converted by the enzyme acetaldehyde dehydrogenase to the harmless acetate (acetic acid). Disulfiram irreversibly deactivates the enzyme acetaldehyde dehydrogenase that leads to accumulation of acetaldehyde. This is termed as Disulfiram Ethanol Reaction (DER). This manifests with unpleasant symptoms.

357. A patient with substance use disorder presents with increased lacrimation, abdominal cramping, agitation, and rhinorrhea. These symptoms indicate withdrawal of:
a. Opioid b. Cocaine
c. Nicotine d. Marijuana

Explanation: Withdrawal symptoms of opioid includes sweating, lacrimation, diarrhea, abdominal cramping, muscle aches, yawning, rhinorrhea, fever, agitation, goose bumps, and insomnia.

358. Disulfiram (antabuse) is used in:
a. Withdrawal phase of Alcohol Dependence Syndrome
b. Maintenance phase of Alcohol Dependence Syndrome
c. Treatment of alcohol intoxication
d. All of the above

Explanation: Benzodiazepines is used during withdrawal phase of treatment of Alcohol Dependence Syndrome (ADS). Disulfiram is a deterrent agent used during the maintenance phase of the treatment.

359. Which among the following drugs is used in the treatment of alcohol dependence? *(Kerala PSC, Nov 2014)*
a. Disulfiram b. Lithium
c. Carbamazepine d. Verapamil

360. The drug which is used to create aversion in Alcohol Dependence:
a. Apomorphine b. Propranolol
c. Diazepam d. Disulfiram

361. Drug used in uncomplicated alcohol withdrawal:
a. Diazepam b. Clonidine
c. Propranolol d. Methadone

362. Disulfiram inhibits:
a. Alcohol dehydrogenase
b. Aldehyde dehydrogenase
c. G6PD
d. Acetate dehydrogenase

363. Ethanol is given in methyl alcohol poisoning because:
a. It inhibits aldehyde dehydrogenase
b. It inhibits aldehyde synthetase
c. It binds to alcohol dehydrogenase stronger than methanol
d. None of the above

364. Which of the following is most commonly used worldwide for maintenance therapy of opioid dependence?
a. LAMA b. Methadone
c. Naloxone d. Pethidine

365. With barbiturate and benzodiazepine abuse and dependency, sedative intoxication is generally associated with: *(LNJP H D 2012)*
a. Slurred speech
b. Impairment in attention and speech
c. Uncoordinated motor movements
d. All of the above

366. Flumazenil is:
a. Diazepam inverse agonist
b. Diazepam antagonist
c. Opioid antagonist
d. Opioid inverse agonist

ORAL CONTRACEPTIVES

367. A client reported that she has missed a single dose of her combined oral contraceptive pills (OCP). Which of the following advice is appropriate for this patient?
a. Take 2 pills the next day and continue with the course
b. Take 2 pills every day for the remaining part of the course
c. Discontinue the course and use barrier method for the rest of the cycle
d. Continue with the course without regard to the missed dose

Explanation: If one tablet is missed, it should be taken as soon as it is remembered, alternatively 2 tablets can be taken the following day.

368. Use of oral contraceptive pills by women reduces the risk of:
a. Breast cancer b. Ovarian cancer
c. Cervical cancer d. Uterine cancer

Explanation: Use of oral contraceptive pills protects the women against ovarian cancer.

369. Which of the following drug may cause contraceptive failure if taken along with oral contraceptive?
a. Isoniazid b. Ethambutol
c. Rifampicin d. Pyrazinamide

Explanation: Rifampicin enhances metabolism of oral contraceptives causing contraceptive failure.

370. OCPs can cause all; EXCEPT:
a. Mastalgia b. Dysmenorrhea
c. Chloasma d. Breakthrough bleeding

371. Mala- N contains:
a. Ethinyl estradiol 0.3 mg b. Norethisterone 1 mg
c. D-norgestrel 0.5 mg d. D-norgestrel 0.3 mg

372. Ergometrine is used in:
a. Postpartum hemorrhage
b. Induction of labor
c. Breast engorgement
d. Contraception

373. Side effect of oral contraceptives are all; EXCEPT:
a. Irregular bleeding
b. Headache
c. Venous thrombosis
d. Increased risk of ovarian cancer

Ans.
355. b
356. a
357. a
358. b
359. a
360. d
361. a
362. b
363. c
364. b
365. d
366. b
367. a
368. b
369. c
370. b
371. b
372. a
373. d

374. "Oral contraceptive pills" protect against:
a. Thrombosis
b. Ovarian cancer
c. Cancer cervix
d. Hepatocellular adenoma

375. Adverse effects of oral contraceptive pills include all; EXCEPT:
a. Swelling of ankles and feet
b. Tenderness of breast
c. Abdominal cramping
d. Weight loss

376. Failure of oral contraceptives occur when used with any of these; EXCEPT:
a. Aspirin b. Tetracycline
c. Phenytoin d. Rifampicin

377. The progesterone only emergency contraceptive pills act by all of the following; EXCEPT:
a. Altered cervical secretion
b. Inhibition of ovulation
c. Anti-implantation effect
d. Inhibition of LH secretion

UTERINE STIMULANTS AND RELAXANTS

378. By which of the following mechanism the ergometrine controls the postpartum hemorrhage?
a. By enhancing blood clotting activity
b. By increasing the tone of uterine muscles
c. By enhancing platelet aggregation
d. By stimulating vasocontriction

379. Which of the following drug is used to suppress premature labor?
a. Ritodrine b. Clonidine
c. Oxytocin d. Epinephrine

380. Which of the following hormone is known as milk ejection hormone?
a. Prolactin b. Oxytocin
c. Progesterone d. Estrogen

381. A patient in the second stage of labor is given which of the following injections to improve uterine contractions?
a. Diazepam b. Methergine
c. Phenergan d. Oxytocin

Explanation: Oxytocin mimics uterine contractions of normal labor. It is used for antepartum induction or stimulation of labor.

VITAMIN SUPPLEMENTATION

382. The reason for deep IM injection of iron preparation is to:
a. Enhance absorption of the medication
b. Ensure higher bioavailability
c. Provide more even distribution of the drug.
d. Prevent the drug from tissue irritation

383. Which of the following vitamin is known as anti-sterility vitamin?
a. Thiamine b. Niacin
c. Vitamin D d. Vitamin E

384. Which of the following vitamin is a water soluble vitamin?
a. Vitamin A b. Vitamin C
c. Vitamin D d. Vitamin K

385. The daily recommended dietary allowances (RDAs) of thiamine in adult men is:
a. 1.2 mg b. 3.0 mg
c. 5.0 mg d. 7.5 mg

Explanation: The recommended **daily** amount of **thiamine** for adult men is 1.2 milligrams and for adult women is 1.1 milligrams.

386. Excessive intake of Vitamin D will lead to:
a. Hypercalcemia b. Hypocalcemia
c. Urinary retention d. Hypophosphatemia

387. What is the dose of prophylactic vitamin given at the age of 9 months?
a. 60,000 IU b. 1,00,000 IU
c. 1,50,000 IU d. 2,00,000 IU

Explanation:

Prophylactic Vitamin A as per the following dosage schedule:
- 100,000 IU at 9 months with measles immunization
- 200,000 IU at 16-18 months, with DPT booster
- 200,000 IU every 6 months, up to the age of 5 years.

Thus, a total of 9 mega doses are to be given from 9 months of age up to 5 years.

388. World Health Organization (WHO) recommends initiation of folic acid supplementation as early as possible in the pregnancy. What is the WHO recommended daily dose of folic acid supplementation in pregnant women?
a. 100 mcg
b. 200 mcg
c. 400 mcg
d. 600 mcg

DRUGS USED FOR PREGNANT WOMEN (ANTENATAL/INTRANATAL/POSTNATAL)

389. Which of the following antimalarial drug is safe during pregnancy?
a. Chloramphenical b. Quinine
c. Chloroquine d. Primaquine

Explanation: Chloroquine or hydroxychloroquine are considered safe to use in all trimesters of pregnancy. Chloramphenical is not an antimalarial drug. Quinine and primaquine are avoided during pregnancy.

390. Drug of choice for epilepsy in pregnancy is:
a. Lamotrigine b. Sodium valproate
c. Phenobarbitone d. Phenytoin

391. A client is receiving IV calcium gluconate for pregnancy induced hypertension (PIH). Plan of care throughout injection of the drug must include:
a. ECG monitoring b. CVP readings
c. Ventilator assistance d. Continuous CPR

Explanation: ECG monitoring is required when calcium is administered by intravenous injection because the potential side effect of calcium gluconate administration is cardiac arrest.

392. Drug of choice of hypertension in pregnancy is:
a. Methyldopa b. Thiazide
c. Nifedipine d. Labetalol

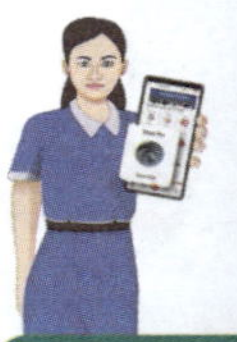

Ans.
374. b
375. d
376. a
377. c
378. b
379. a
380. b
381. d
382. d
383. d
384. b
385. a
386. a
387. b
388. c
389. c
390. a
391. a
392. a

EMERGENCY DRUGS

393. Which of the following action is exerted by inotropic agents?

a. Increase heart rate
b. Decrease afterload
c. Increase ICP
d. Increase force of contraction

394. What is the outcome if the nitrates are administered early to the client with acute myocardial infarction?

a. Reduced mortality b. Reduced morbidity
c. Bradycardia d. Hypertension

Explanation: Research evidences suggest that the nitrate administration early into the acute MI attack results in reduced mortality, size of infarct and infarct extension. Reduced morbidity is not applicable as morbidity already occurred. Administration of nitrates results in hypotension and a likely tachycardia.

395. Which of the following antidote is used to heparin to control bleeding related to heparin overdose?

a. Vitamin K b. Protamine sulphate
c. Fibrinogen d. Naproxen

396. The most effective benzodiazepine for treating status epilepticus and is the treatment of choice for controlling seizures acutely?

a. Nitrazepam b. Oxazepam
c. Flurazepam d. Lorazepam

397. The dilution required for intravenous administration of adrenaline for anaphylactic shock in an adult patient is:

a. 1: 100 b. 1: 1000
c. 1: 10,000 d. 1: 100,000

398. Intervention for a patient who has swallowed an acid includes all of the following; EXCEPT:

a. Stimulation of vomiting
b. Aspirating secretions from the pharynx if respirations are affected
c. Neutralizing the chemical with alkaline solution
d. Washing the esophagus with large volumes of water via gastric lavage

399. The drug administered during acute anaphylactic reaction is *(AIIMS 2011)*

a. Adrenaline b. Aminophylline
c. Atropine d. Furosemide

Explanation: Injection of epinephrine (Adrenaline) is the first-aid medication of choice for anaphylaxis, as recommended in all anaphylaxis guidelines. Adrenaline helps to relieve the symptoms of anaphylaxis by causing vasoconstriction, and opening up airways. This prevents the blood pressure from dropping and makes breathing easier.

IV FLUIDS AND ELECTROLYTES REPLACEMENT

400. Which of the following parameter is the most reliable indicator of adequate IV infusion?

a. Blood pressure of 120/80 mm Hg
b. Normal skin turgor
c. Pulse rate – 70-80/m
d. Urine output of 30 mL/h

401. Deficiency of which of the following cation may cause amphotericin B toxicity when the drug is administered?

a. Magnesium b. Calcium
c. Sodium d. Potassium

Explanation: If amphotericin B is administered when the patient is hyopkalemic, it may cause toxicity of amphotericin B.

402. Which of the following drugs is not a plasma expander?

a. Dextran b. Mannitol
c. Human albumin d. Hexa starch

Explanation: Dextran, Human albumin and Hexa starch are plasma expanders. Mannitol is an osmotic diuretic.

403. Plasma expanders are used in:

a. Severe anemia b. Circulatory shock
c. Chronic renal failure d. Congestive Heart Failure

Explanation: Plasma expanders are used in circulatory shock. Plasma volume expanders increase the oncotic pressure in the intravascular space.

ANTIDOTES

404. Antidote for overdose of Warfarin is: *(AIIMS, 2010)*

a. Protamine sulfate b. Heparin
c. Atropine sulfate d. Vitamin K

Explanation: Vitamin K is an antidote of warfarin. Protamine sulfate is an antidote to heparin. Atropine sulfate is an anti-cholinergic agent.

405. Antidote for organophosphorous poisoning is: *(RPSC NG-II, 2007)*

a. D- Penicillamine b. Atropine
c. Magnesium sulfate d. Physostigmine

Explanation:

- Organophosphorus (OP) poisoning commonly results from exposure to pesticides. OP inhibits acetylcholinesterase, leading to accumulation of acetylcholine in the body. Atropine sulfate, an anticholinergic agent is used to counter the cholinergic effects produced by accumulated acetylcholine.
- Protocol to administer Atropine in case of OP poisoning:

Inject 1.8-3 mg (3-5 mL) of atropine bolus.

- Check pulse, blood pressure and chest crackles after 5 minutes.
- Aim for heart rate >80 beats per minute, SBP >80 mm Hg, and a clear chest (atropine won't dry focal areas of aspiration).
- Double the atropine dose at every five minutes if the objectives are not achieved
- Review patient at every 5 minutes.
- Once these parameters start improving, repeat last same or smaller dose of atropine.
- If improvement in these parameters is persistent and satisfactory after 5 minutes, now atropine infusion can be planned.
- Ignore pupils—they take time to dilate.

406. Antidote for Heparin is:

a. Vitamin K b. Protamine Sulfate
c. Vitamin d. Coumadin

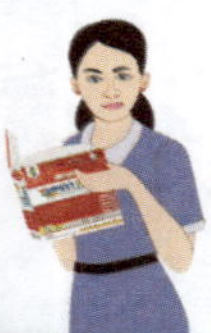

Ans.

393. d
394. a
395. b
396. d
397. c
398. a
399. a
400. d
401. d
402. b
403. b
404. d
405. b
406. b

Explanation: Protamine sulfate is an antidote to heparin which reverses the anticoagulant effects of heparin by binding to it. Dose: 1.0-1.5 mg per 100 units of heparin that had been administered in last 4 hours. PTT should be monitored at 5–15 minutes after dose then in 2–8 hours afterward.

407. The antidote for paracetamol poisoning is:
a. Atropine b. Naloxone
c. Vitamin K d. N-Acetylcysteine

Explanation: N-Acetylcysteine is an antidote for paracetamol poisoning.

408. Antidote for benzodiazepines:
a. Flumazenil b. N-Acetylcysteine
c. Naloxone d. Atropine

Explanation: Flumazenil is the antidote for benzodiazepines. It is the drug of choice for benzodiazepine overdose/poisoning.

409. The antidote to warfarin is: *(Kerala PSC, Nov 2014)*
a. Heparin b. Vitamin K
c. Vitamin B12 d. Iron

410. The antidote of organophosphorus poisoning is: *(Staff Nurse G II 2014)*
a. Adrenaline b. Atropine
c. Sodium bicarbonate d. Dopamine

411. The antidote of heparin is:
a. Coumarin b. Protamine sulfate
c. Vitamin-K d. Aspirin

412. Antidote for organophosphorus poisoning is:
a. Atropine b. Neostigmine
c. Succinylcholine d. D-Tubocurarine

413. Following are the name of drugs and its antidotes. Which of the following combination is not correct?
a. Benzodiazepines – Flumazenil
b. Paracetamol – Acetyl Cystine
c. Warfarin – Protamine sulfate
d. Opioid - Naloxone

Explanation: The combination of warfarin and protamine sulfate as an antidote is not correct. Warfarin is an oral anticoagulant medication used to prevent blood clot formation. The reversal agent or antidote for warfarin is vitamin K, not protamine sulfate.

Protamine sulfate, on the other hand, is used as an antidote for heparin.

414. Following are the types of poisoning and its antidotes. Which of the following combination is not correct?
a. Organophosphorus poisoning – Atropine sulfate
b. Heavy metal poisoning – Chelating agents
c. Methanol poisoning - Ethanol
d. Mushroom poisoning - Dopamine

415. Antidote for opioids is:
a. Atropine sulfate b. Flumazenil
c. Neostigmine d. Naloxone

DISEASES AND DRUG OF CHOICES

416. Simple herpes virus infection is treated with:
a. Stavudine b. Ganciclovir
c. Acyclovir d. Lamivudine

Explanation: Acyclovir is the drug of choice in treating simple herpes virus infection.

417. The drug used by Health workers in the management of Acute respiratory illness is:
a. Cotrimoxazole b. Chloramphenicol
c. Benzyl Penicillin d. Gentamycin

418. Drug of choice for rheumatic fever is: *(Recent Question 2012)*
a. Cephalosporin b. Penicillin
c. Streptomycin d. Gentamycin

419. Drug of choice for syphilis is:
a. Ciprofloxacin b. Cotrimoxazole
c. Doxycycline d. Penicillin

420. Drug of choice for syphilis in a pregnant lady is:
a. Penicillin b. Azithromycin
c. Tetracycline d. Ceftriaxone

421. Drug of choice in treatment of typhoid fever is:
a. Ampicillin b. Ceftriaxone
c. Ciprofloxacin d. Methicillin

422. Drug of choice for primary syphilis is:
a. Ampicillin b. Benzathine penicillin
c. Erythromycin d. Tetracycline

423. Drug of choice for chemoprophylaxis against rheumatic fever is:
a. Penicillin V b. Erythromycin
c. Benzathine penicillin d. Procaine penicillin

424. Drug of choice for prophylaxis of meningococcal meningitis is:
a. Penicillin b. Erythromycin
c. Septran d. Rifampicin

425. In leprosy, the best bactericidal agent is:
a. Clofazimine b. Dapsone
c. Rifampicin d. Ethionamide

426. Drug of choice for malaria during pregnancy is:
a. Chloroquine b. Quinine
c. Primaquine d. Mefloquine

427. Tetracycline is used for prophylaxis of: *(AIIMS 2003)*
a. Leptospirosis b. Cholera
c. Meningitis d. Brucellosis

428. Treatment of drug resistant malaria is:
a. Quinine b. Pyrimethamine
c. Mefloquine d. All of these

429. The drug of choice for partial seizures is:
a. Carbamazepine
b. Barbiturates
c. Diazepam
d. Lamotrigine

Explanation: Carbamazepine is the drug of choice for the treatment of partial seizures. It is also used as an antimanic drug.

430. Drug of choice in treatment of partial complex seizures:
a. Carbamazepine b. Sodium valproate
c. Ethosuximide d. Phenytoin

431. Drug of choice in acute central anticholinergic syndrome is:
a. Neostigmine b. Physostigmine
c. Tacrine d. 4-amino pyridine

432. Drug used for postoperative reversal of muscular paralysis:
a. Neostigmine b. Pyridostigmine
c. Physostigmine d. D tubocurarine

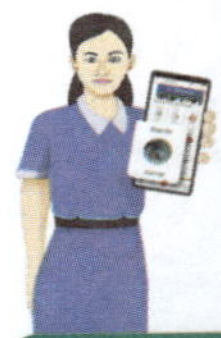

Ans.

407. d
408. a
409. b
410. b
411. b
412. a
413. c
414. d
415. d
416. c
417. a
418. b
419. d
420. a
421. b
422. b
423. c
424. d
425. c
426. a
427. b
428. a
429. a
430. a
431. b
432. a

433. Drug of choice in treatment of myasthenia gravis is:
a. d-tubocurarine b. Hexamethonium
c. Pyridostigmine d. Gallamine

434. Drug of choice in nocturnal enuresis is:
a. Imipramine b. Diazepam
c. Amoxapine d. Desmopressin

435. Drug used in the treatment of Attention Deficit Hyperactivity Disorder (ADHD) is:
a. Carbamazepine b. Levodopa
c. Methylphenidate d. Diazepam

436. Drug of choice in theophylline poisoning:
a. Cortisone b. Propranolol
c. Thyroxine d. Phenytoin

437. Drug of choice for ascariasis:
a. Piperazine citrate
b. Bephenium hydroxynaphthoate
c. Mebendazole
d. Albendazole

438. Drug of choice for Zollinger-Ellison syndrome:
a. Antihistaminics
b. Proton pump inhibitors
c. Dopamine agonists
d. Antacids

439. The drug of choice for the treatment of thyrotoxicosis during pregnancy is:
a. Carbimazole
b. Iodine therapy
c. Propylthiouracil
d. Methimazole

440. Drug of choice for acute adrenal insufficiency is:
a. Oral prednisone b. IV hydrocortisone
c. IV betamethasone d. IV dexamethasone

441. Drug of choice in breast carcinoma is:
a. Fluorouracil b. Tamoxifen citrate
c. Vincristine d. Vinblastine

442. The drug of choice in mushroom poisoning is:
a. Atropine b. Neostigmine
c. Physostigmine d. Epinephrine

Explanation: In mushroom poisoning that produces primarily muscarinic effects, atropine is the drug of choice.

443. Treatment of atropine toxicity:
a. 2-Pralidoxime b. Naloxone
c. Flumazenil d. Physostigmine

444. Drug of choice for anaphylactic shock:
a. Adrenaline b. Antihistaminic
c. Glucocorticoids d. Epinephrine

445. First drug to be used in anaphylactic shock is:
a. Intramuscular adrenaline
b. I.V. corticosteroid
c. Theophylline
d. Antihistaminic

446. Drug of choice to treat drug induced anaphylactic shock is:
a. Adrenaline
b. Betamethasone
c. Dopamine
d. Noradrenaline

ADVERSE EFFECTS OF COMMON DRUGS

447. Which of the following drugs can cause cartilage damage in children?
a. Cotrimoxazole b. Penicillin
c. Ciprofloxacin d. Metronidazole

448. One of the major side effect of sulphonamides is:
a. Ototoxicity b. Renal calculi
c. Tinnitus d. Vertigo

449. Ototoxicity is maximum with:
a. Streptomycin b. Kanamycin
c. Tobramycin d. Amikacin

450. Which of the following group of drug causes ototoxicity and nephrotoxicity?
a. Aminoglycosides b. Fluoroquinolones
c. Penicillins d. Sulfonamides

451. Cocaine intoxication causes:
a. Visual sensations b. Tactile sensations
c. Olfactory sensations d. Kinetic sensations

Explanation: Cocaine toxicity causes tactile stimulations.

452. Pin point pupil suggests poisoning with:
a. DDT b. Opiates
c. Belladonna d. Barbiturates

453. All of the following drugs can cause neuroleptic malignant syndrome; EXCEPT:
a. Amantadine b. Domperidone
c. Haloperidol d. Metoclopramide

454. Oculogyric crisis is known to be produced by all of the following; EXCEPT:
a. Trifluoperazine b. Atropine
c. Prochlorperazine d. Perphenazine

455. Features of opioid intake are all of the following; EXCEPT:
a. Feeling of relaxation
b. Euphoria
c. Analgesia
d. Dilated pupils

456. Which of the following is not an adverse effect of morphine? *(AIIMS-BBS SNO 2019)*
a. Euphoria b. Respiratory stimulation
c. Nausea d. Histamine release

Explanation: Morphine belongs to opioid analgesics. Respiratory depression is an expected adverse effect of opioids (morphine). So, respiratory stimulation is not an expected adverse effect. Other side effects include Low blood pressure, nausea, vomiting, constipation, euphoria and drowsiness.

457. Long term use of omeprazole can cause:
a. Vitamin B12 Deficiency
b. Folic acid deficiency
c. Iron deficiency anemia
d. Thiamine deficiency

458. Which of the following adverse effect is not likely to be caused by insulin therapy?
a. Allergic reactions b. Hyperglycemia
c. Lipodystrophy d. Blurred vision

Explanation: Insulin causes hypoglycemia not hyperglycemia.

Ans.
433. c
434. d
435. c
436. b
437. d
438. b
439. c
440. b
441. b
442. a
443. d
444. a
445. a
446. a
447. c
448. b
449. d
450. a
451. b
452. b
453. a
454. b
455. d
456. b
457. a
458. b

459. Lactic acidosis is a side effect of:
a. Acarbose b. Metformin
c. Chlorpropamide d. Glibenclamide

460. Which of the following can cause lactic acidosis?
a. Biguanides b. Glibenclamtide
c. tolbutamide d. Chlorpropamide

461. A serious adverse effects of the drug oxytocin is:
a. Hypertension b. Uterine rupture
c. Fluid deficit d. Convulsion

462. All are side effects of steroids, given in anti-inflammatory dosages; EXCEPT:
a. Diabetes mellitus b. Hyperkalemia
c. Osteoporosis d. Na^+ and water retention

463. Gynecomastia is one of the side effect of:
a. Spironolactone b. Rifampicin
c. Penicillin d. Bumetanide

Explanation: Spironolactone (potassium sparing diuretic) causes gynecomastia as a side effect.

464. In patient with chronic renal failure, all of the following drugs likely to cause raise in potassium level; EXCEPT:
a. ACE inhibitors b. Beta blockers
c. Lasix (Furosemide) d. Spironolactone

Explanation: Lasix (furosemide) causes balanced excretion of potassium through kidney hence, the chances of causing hyperkalemia is less. Spironolactone is a potassium sparing diuretic hence, retains potassium.

465. Side effects of thiazides may include:
a. Hypokalemia b. Hyperuricemia
c. Hyperglycemia d. All of these

466. Side effect of diuretic administration includes all; EXCEPT:
a. Hypotension b. Postural hypotension
c. Dehydration d. Hypernatremia

467. Use of aspirin in the children with viral disease is associated with:
a. Hematuria b. Reye's syndrome
c. Metabolic acidosis d. Renal tubular acidosis

Explanation: Reye's syndrome seems to be triggered by using aspirin to treat a viral illness or infection—particularly flu (influenza and chicken pox—in children and teenagers who have an underlying fatty acid oxidation.

468. Patient who is allergic to intravenous contrast media are also usually allergic to:
a. Eggs b. Latex
c. Milk d. Shellfish

Explanation: Shellfish and contrast media both contains iodine. Patients are frequently asked about iodine or seafood (shellfish) allergy before IV contrast media is injected. Person who is allergic to shellfish is likely to be allergic to contrast media.

469. Early features of aspirin poisoning is/are:
a. Throbbing headache
b. Rash
c. Ringing sensation in ear
d. Metabolic acidosis

470. Which of the following drug increases the risk of gastro-intestinal bleeding?
a. Aspirin b. Acetaminophen
c. Tranexamic acid d. Dextran

DRUGS CONTRAINDICATED IN PREGNANCY AND BREASTFEEDING

471. Which of the following antimalarial drug is not safe to prescribe to a pregnant woman?
a. Chloroquine b. Primaquine
c. Quinine d. Quinidine

472. Which of the following anti tubercular drugs is contraindicated in a pregnant woman?
a. Pyrazinamide b. Isoniazid
c. Rifampicin d. Streptomycin

Explanation: Streptomycin can cause fetal harm (8th cranial nerve damage to fetus) when administered to a pregnant woman. So use of streptomycin during pregnancy is absolutely contraindicated.

473. Which of the following drug is not contraindicated in a lactating mother?
a. Bromocriptine b. Amiodarone
c. Ibuprofen d. Retinoids

Explanation: Bromocriptine inhibits lactation. Amiodarone has a long half-life, iodine-containing molecule, and may affect thyroid function in infant. Retinoids are potential for serious adverse effects. Ibuprofen is safe during lactation.

474. Consumption of which of the following drug by a mother during pregnancy may cause phocomelia to the fetus?
a. Tetracycline b. Thalidomide
c. Warfarin d. Doxycycline

Explanation: Even a single dose of thalidomide taken during pregnancy can cause severe birth defects including phocomelia or death of the unborn baby. Phocomelia is a birth defect in which the hands and feet are attached to abbreviated arms and legs.

475. Which of the following drug is contraindicated in pregnancy?
a. ACE inhibitors b. Beta blockers
c. Heparin d. Hydralazine

Explanation: ACE inhibitors are contraindicated in pregnancy due to its potential for teratogenicity.

476. Which of the following drug is contraindicated in pregnancy?
a. Methyl dopa b. Clonidine
c. Amlodipine d. Enalapril

Explanation: Diuretic like ACEI and ARB inhibitors are teratogenic, hence contraindicated in pregnancy.

AYUSH DRUGS

477. International Yoga Day is celebrated on:
a. April 7 b. May 21
c. June 21 d. June 25

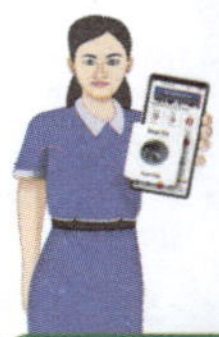

Ans.

459. b
460. a
461. b
462. b
463. a
464. c
465. d
466. d
467. b
468. d
469. c
470. a
471. b
472. d
473. c
474. b
475. a
476. d
477. c

"A person cannot accumulate a fortune very well when he is sick."
—P. T. Barnum

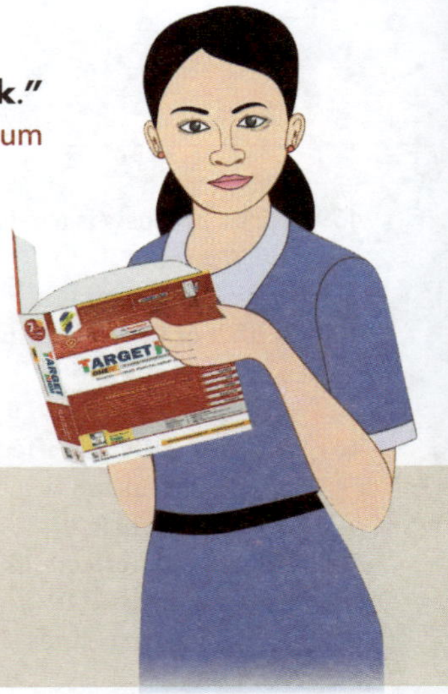

CHAPTER 4

COMMUNITY HEALTH NURSING

SYNOPSIS

Community: A group of people with diverse characteristics who are linked by social ties, share common perspectives, and engage in joint action in geographical locations or settings.

Community health nursing: Community health nursing is a synthesis of nursing practices and public health practices applied in promoting and preserving the health of population.

CONCEPTS AND DETERMINANTS OF HEALTH AND WELL-BEING

Concepts of Health

Health: It is a state of complete physical, mental and social well-being and not merely an absence of disease or infirmity (WHO 1948).

Following are the changing concepts of health:

- **Biomedical concept:** This has been viewed that health is an absence of disease and if one was free from disease then the person was considered as healthy. This concept has its basis in germ theory.
- **Ecological concept:** This has been viewed that health is a dynamic equilibrium between man and his environment and disease is maladjustment of the human being to the environment.
- **Psychosocial concept:** According to this concept health is influenced by social, psychological, cultural, economic and the political factors.
- **Holistic concept:** This model is a synthesis of all the above concepts. It recognizes the strength of social, economic, political and environmental influences on health. This approach implies that all sectors of society have an impact on health.

Dimensions of Health

- Physical dimension
- Mental dimension
- Social dimension
- Spiritual dimension

Concept of Disease

- A condition in which body function is impaired.
- A maladjustment of human to the environment.

Causes

- Supernatural causes and karma
- Theory of humors (fluid)
- Theory of contagion
- Germ theory
- Epidemiological triad
- Multi-factorial causation
- Web of causation

Disease: Biological concept-physiological/ psychological dysfunction

Illness: Socio–pathological concept-subjective feeling of not being well.

Sickness: Biological concept of social dysfunction

Determinants of Health

Table 1: Factors of determinants of health

Determinants	Factors
Biological	Genetic make-up, Growth and Development
Behavioral and sociocultural conditions	Life style, personal habit (smoking, drinking), nutritional status, sleep pattern, physical activity

Contd...

KEY POINTS

- The three features of a community are **location**, **population** and **social system.**
- England is the first country to start Concept of Healthcare and Public health.
- In 1861, Louis Pasteur published his germ theory which proved that bacteria caused diseases.
- The father of modern public health is 'John Snow' for his pioneering investigations on Cholera epidemics.
- Fastigium stage is the highest point of disease or illness.

KEY POINT

Public health science Era (1950-75): Integration of social science and public health sciences took place. It is being called era of Community-centered approach.

Determinants	Factors
Environment	**Internal environment:** Each and every body tissue and its functioning **External environment (macro environment):** All that external to the individual and can be divided as physical, biological, chemical and psychosocial **Domestic environment (micro environment):** Way of living and lifestyle such as eating habits, smoking, drinking, use of drugs, etc.
Socioeconomic conditions	Per capita GNP, education, nutrition, employment, housing, political system of country and occupation
Health services	Affordability, Accessibility and Availability of healthcare services, e.g., Access to and availability of vaccination
Aging of the population	Major concern of rapid population aging is the increased prevalence of chronic diseases and disabilities
Gender	Many programs have been established for female empowerment that focus on nutritional and reproductive health among females
Other factors	Factors such as revolution in information and communication also help us to access good health

Concept of Well-Being

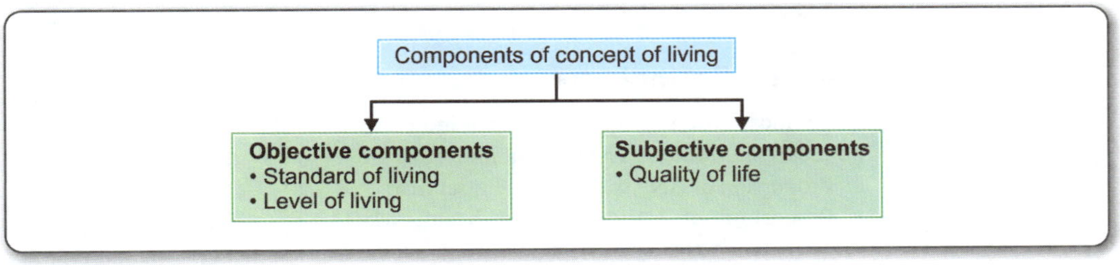

Figure 1: Concept of well-being

PQLI: Physical quality of life index
HDI: Human development index

Three indicators of human development index:
1. Life expectancy index
2. Education index
3. CNI index.

INDICATORS OF HEALTH

Indicators of Health or (Health Index/Indices)

Indicators are required not only to measure the health status of the community but also to compare the health status of one country with that of another, for the assessment of healthcare needs, for allocation of scarce resources and for monitoring and evaluation of health service activities and programs.

- **Health Indices:** It is a pleural form of health index (indicator)

Mortality and Morbidity Indicators

Mortality indicators	• Crude Birth Rate • Crude Death Rate • Maternal Mortality Rate • Neonatal Mortality Rate • Infant Mortality Rate • Under-five mortality Rate • General fertility rate • Life expectancy at birth • Age specific death rates • Under 5 proportionate mortality rate • Disease specific death rate • Case fatality rate • Year of potential life lost
Morbidity indicators	• Incidence • Prevalence • Notification rate • Admission, Discharge or Readmission rate • Attendance rate of OPD of health center • Duration of stay in the hospital • Absence from work or duty

Recent Question (NORCET 2022)

1. **PQLI (The Physical Quality of Life Index) is all, except:**
   a. Life expectancy at one year of age
   b. Literary rate
   c. IMR
   d. Income

Ans. (d) Income

KEY POINTS

- Barometer of social welfare is 'Tuberculosis'
- Disability Adjusted Life Years (DALY) = Years of life lived with disability (YLD) + Years of Life Lost due to disability (YLL)
- Sullivan's index = Life expectancy - years of life lived with disability (YLD) = Expectation of Life free of disability

IMR = the number of deaths in the first year of life/the number of live births in the same year X 1000.

POINT TO REMEMBER

Infant Mortality Rate (IMR) is the most universally accepted indicator of health status of the whole population

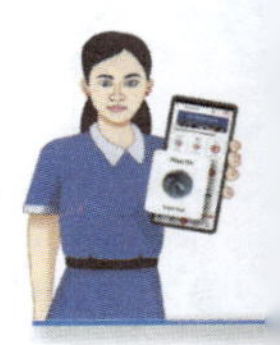

Disability Rate

Commonly used disability rates fall into two categories: Event type indicators and person type indicators.

Event Type Indicators

- Number of days of restricted activity.
- Disability leading to confinement to bed.
- Workless days within a specific period.

Person Type Indicators

- **Limitation of mobility:** For example confined to bed, confined to house, special aid in getting around either inside or outside.
- **Limitation of activity:** Limitations to perform the basic activities of daily living.

Sullivan's index: Expectation of life free of disability. It is computed by subtracting from the life expectancy from the probable duration of bed disability and inability to perform major activities.

Nutritional Status Indicators

It is a positive health indicator and other three important indicators are as follows:

- Anthropometric measurement of preschool children (height, weight and mid upper arm circumference).
- Heights of children at school entry.
- Prevalence of low birth weight.

Healthcare Delivery Indicators

- Doctor-population ratio
- Doctor-nurse ratio
- Population-bed ratio
- Population per health subcenter
- Population per traditional birth attendant.

Utilization Rate

In order to obtain additional information on health status, the extent of use of health services is often calculated.

- Proportion of children who are fully immunized against 6 vaccine preventable diseases.
- Proportion of women who receive antenatal care
- Percentage of population using various family planning method
- Bed-occupancy rate
- Average length of stay
- Bed turnover ratio.

Indicators of Social and Mental Health

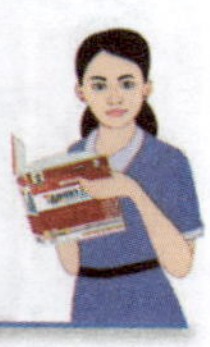

It includes information regarding suicide, homicide, other act of violence and other crime, road traffic accidents, juvenile delinquency, alcohol and drug abuse, smoking, consumption of tranquillizer, obesity, etc. These indicators provide a guide to social action for improving the health of people.

Environmental Indicators

It reflects to the quality of physical and biological environment in which diseases occurs and in which people live. For example, pollution of air and water, radiation, solid waste, noise, exposure to toxic substance in food or drink. Among these most useful indicators are those measuring the proportion of population having access to safe water and sanitation facility.

Socioeconomic Indicators

They do not directly measure health. It includes:

- Rate of population increase
- Per capita GNP (Gross National Product)
- Level of unemployment
- Dependency ratio
- Literacy (especially female literacy)
- Family size
- **Housing:** Number of persons per room
- Per capita calorie availability.

Health Policy Indicators

Single most indicator of health policy indicators is political commitment. The relevant indicators are:

- Proportion of GNP spent on health services
- Proportion of GNP spent on health related activities (water, sanitation, housing, nutrition and community development)
- Proportion of total health resources devoted to primary health-care.

LEVELS OF HEALTHCARE AND HEALTH FOR ALL

- **Primary healthcare:**
    - This is the first level of contact between individual and health system where essential healthcare is provided
    - A majority of prevailing problems can be satisfactorily dealt at this level.
    - This level of healthcare is closest to the people.
    - In India, Primary healthcare is provided by
        - Primary health centers (phc)
        - Sub centers with community participation.
- **Secondary healthcare**
    - This level deals with more complex problems
    - This level serves as the **first referral unit (FRU) in the health system.**
    - Care comprises essentially curative services and is provided by
        - District hospital
        - Community health centers.
- **Tertiary healthcare**
    - This level offers super-specialist care.
    - Care is provided by regional teaching hospitals and central level institutions.

KEY POINTS

- The modified Kuppuswamy scale is commonly used to measure SES in urban and rural areas.
- The Modified Kuppuswamy scale consists of a composite score which includes the **education** and **occupation of the Family Head, income per month of the family, which yields a score of 3–29.**
- Alma–Ata declaration statement is placing **"people's health in people's hands".**

KEY POINTS

Facts on Literacy (2021):

- Current Literacy rate of India is 74.04%
- Most Literate State - Kerala (94%)
- Most Literate UT - Lakshadweep (91.85%)
- Least Literate State - Bihar (64%)
- Least Literate UT - Dadra & Nagar Haveli (77.24)

- These institutions along with specialized care are also providing planning and managerial skills and teaching for specialized staff.
- Examples include
  - Super specialty hospital
  - Regional hospital
  - Medical College hospital
  - Central institutes such as AIIMS, PGIMER, JIPMER, NIMHANS etc. (these are also known as Institutions of National Importance or INIs)

Health for All

- In **May 1977,** WHO assembly decided that the main goal of government and WHO in the coming years should be attainment of health by all people of the world by 2000 AD, that will permit them to lead a socially and economically productive life.
- The essential principle of health for all is the concept of equity in health, that is all people should have an opportunity to enjoy good health.

MILLENNIUM DEVELOPMENT GOAL AND SUSTAINABLE DEVELOPMENT GOAL

Millennium Development Goal

- Declaration was on **September 2000**
- Government set date of **2015** to meet the millennium development goal, previously

Goals

- Eradicate extreme poverty and hunger
- Achieve universal primary education
- Promote gender equality and empower women
- Reduce child mortality
- Improve maternal health
- Combat HIV/AIDS, malaria and other diseases
- Ensure environmental sustainability
- Develop a global partnership for development

Sustainable Development Goals (SDG)

- It has **17 goals** and **169 targets set by United Nations in 2015** for the year 2030.
- "Global **Goals** for **Sustainable Development**" is another name used.
- Universal call to action to end poverty, protect the planet and ensures that all people enjoy peace and prosperity
- In relation to health, third goal is "to be active" and it has 13 targets.
- 13 targets are focusing the following areas:
  1. Reduce MMR (70 per 100,000 live births)
  2. Newborn and under 5 children
  3. End the epidemic of HIV/AIDS, TB, malaria
  4. Non communicable disease and mental health
  5. Road traffic accidents
  6. Universal access to sexual and reproductive healthcare services
  7. Substance abuse
  8. Universal health coverage
  9. Environmental pollution
  10. Tobacco control
  11. Research on vaccines for Communicable and Non-communicable diseases
  12. Health financing for health work force
  13. Strengthen the capacity of developing countries to manage global health risks.

POINT TO REMEMBER

Beti Bachao, Beti Padhao is the latest initiative taken by Government of India to save and educate the girl child in India. It was launched in Panipat, Haryana for the first time.

KEY POINTS

- MDG-1 is to eradicate extreme poverty and hunger. United Nations currently define living on less than US$ 1.90 a day (from 2015) as a global poverty line.
- Ghana was the first country to achieve the goal of having extreme poverty.
- MDG-6 is to combat HIV/AIDS, malaria and other diseases
- SDG encourage the promotion of health, well-being, and education for all, at all ages.

LEVELS OF PREVENTION

Table 2: Levels of prevention and mode of intervention

Levels of prevention	Definition and concept	Mode of intervention	Stage of the disease
Primordial prevention (Normal individual)	Prevention of development of risk factors. Consist of actions and measures that inhibit the emergence of risk factors in the form of • Environment • Economic conditions • Social conditions • Behavioral conditions • Cultural patterns	• Individual and Mass Education • Life style adaptation from childhood	Life time
Primary prevention ↓ Before the disease occurrence	Action taken prior to the onset of disease • Focus on positive health • Promote wellbeing and quality of life	Health promotion and specific protection. **Approaches:** • Population strategy • High risk strategy	Pre-pathogenesis phase

Contd...

Levels of prevention	Definition and concept	Mode of intervention	Stage of the disease
Secondary prevention ↓ during disease process	• Actions halt the disease progress and prevents complications	Early Diagnosis and treatment • Screening test • Case findings	Pathogenesis phase (early)
Tertiary prevention ↓ (after)	• Used when the disease process has advanced beyond its early stages • Defined as all measures available to limit impairments and disabilities and to promote the patient's adjustment to irremediable conditions	• Disability limitation • Rehabilitation	Late Pathogenesis phase

- **Rehabilitation:** Combined and coordinated use of medical, social, educational and vocational measures for training and retreating the individual to the highest possible level of functional ability
- **Population (mass) strategy:** This approach is directed towards population irrespective of individual risk level.
- **High risk strategy:** This is aimed at preventive care to individual at high risk.

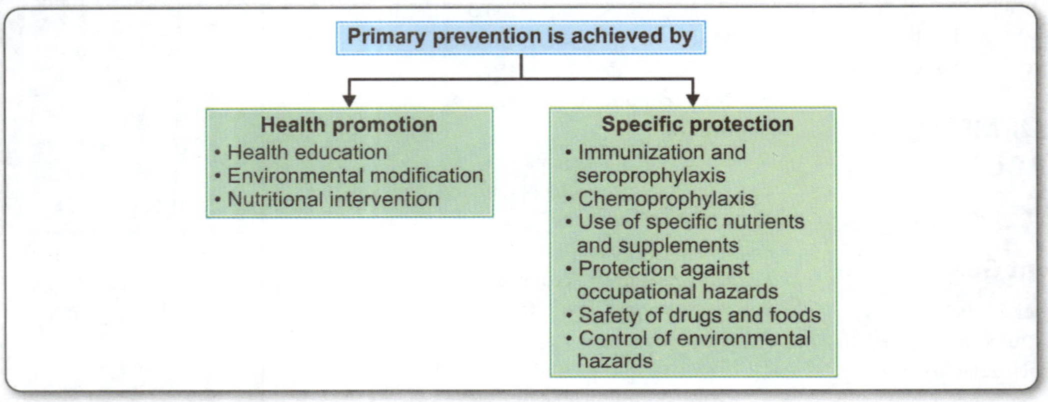

Figure 2: Types of primary prevention

- **Health promotion:** It is the process of enabling people to increase control over the determinants of health and there by improve their health.

Some Common Examples for Each Level of Prevention

Levels of prevention	Examples (Commonly asked Question)
Primordial prevention	• Increasing taxes on cigarettes • Decreasing advertisement of tobacco • Access to safe walking paths • Access to stores with healthy food options • Prevention of bad food habits and to prevent smoking/alcoholism.
Primary prevention	• **Vaccination/ immunization against various disease conditions.** • **Infection control measures such as hand washing** • Tobacco Cessation Programs • Micro-Nutrient Supplementation Programs (Vit A prophylaxis, iodine supplementation) • Environmental modification (avoid waterlogging in nearby area to prevent mosquito breeding) • **Avoid smoking** • Water purification and sanitation • Maintain ideal body weight and good personal hygiene • Contraceptive methods to prevent STDs • Quarantine for communicable diseases • Pasteurization of milk. • Wearing helmet and seat belt while driving

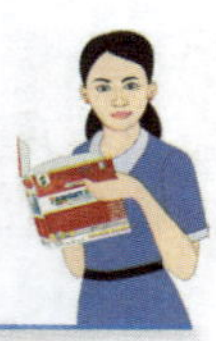

KEY POINTS

- The study of distribution and determinants of the disease is called epidemiology
- Father of Modern Epidemiology - John Snow
- Rate, Ratio and Proportion are the tools of measurement in Epidemiology
- Chain of infection includes agent, susceptible host, portal of entry, mode of transmission, portal of exit and reservoir.
- Portal of entry is the site through which microorganisms enter the susceptible host.

KEY POINTS

- Primordial prevention focus on whole population.
- Primary prevention- target population is healthy individual.
- Secondary prevention-focuses on individual who are at risk.
- Tertiary prevention- focuses on individual with already diagnosed condition.

Levels of prevention	Examples (Commonly asked Question)
Secondary prevention	• Papanicolaou (Pap) smear for early detection of cervical cancer • Mammography, for early detection of breast cancer • Colonoscopies, for early detection of colon cancer • Blood Pressure Screening • Breast self-examination. • Isolation for communicable diseases • School health check-up.
Tertiary prevention	• Rehabilitation efforts. • Occupational and physical therapy in burn patients • Cardiac rehab in post-myocardial infarction patients • Diabetic foot care • Palliative and hospice care.

INTRODUCTION TO EPIDEMIOLOGY

It is the branch of medicine, which deals with the incidence, distribution, and possible control of diseases and other factors relating to health.

Focus Area

- Disease frequency
- Distribution of diseases
- Determinants of diseases

Tools of Measurement

- Rate
- Ratio
- Proportions

Key Words

- **Endemic:** Constant presence of disease in a particular geo-graphical area
  - **Hyperendemic:** Disease affects high proportion of the population
  - **Mesoendemic:** Disease affects moderate proportion of population
  - **Hypoendemic:** Disease affects small proportion of population
  - **Haloendemic:** A disease is **haloendemic** when essentially every individual in a population is infected.
- **Epidemic**: Unusual occurrence of a disease. Excess of its normally expected frequency of occurrence
- **Pandemic** (worldwide): Usually affecting large proportion of the population. It may involve several countries or continents.
- **Sporadic**: It means scattered about. Disease occurs in an irregular pattern in a community.
- **Exotic**: A disease is imported into a country. Unusual presence of a disease in a country.
- **Zoonosis**: A communicable disease transmitted from a vertebrate animal to man, e.g., Rabies, Bovine Tuberculosis, Plague.
  - **Anthropozoonoses**: Infection transmitted from vertebrate animals to men
  - **Zooanthroponoses**: Infection transmitted from men to vertebrate animal.
  - **Amphixenoses**: Infection transmitted in a mixed direction, i.e., man animal
- **Epizootic**: It is an outbreak (epidemic) of disease in an animal population
- **Enzootic**: It is an endemic occurring in animals
- **Epornithic**: Outbreak of disease in Bird population
- **Infection**: Entry and development (or multiplication) of an infectious agent in the body of man (animals).
- **Contamination**: Presence of an infectious agent on a body surface, clothes, etc.
- **Infestation**: Lodgment, development and reproduction of arthropods
- **Contagious disease**: Transmitted through contact
- **Host**: Person or animal that affords place to an infectious agent under normal condition.
  - **Obligate host:** All stages of development of organism occurs in same host
  - **Definitive host:** Maturation and sexual stage development of organism occurs in host
  - **Intermediate host:** Larva stage (or asexual state)
  - **Transport host:** Acts as carrier but no development of organism occurs in transport host.
- **Vector of infection**: An insect or any living carrier that transports an infectious agent is known as vector.

Recent Question (NORCET 2022)

2. The Endemic Disease that occurs every 4 years of interval is called:
a. Secular Trend
b. Time trend
c. Periodic trend
d. Cyclic trend

Ans. (d) Cyclic trend

Practice Questions

1. In the definition of epidemiology, the term "determinants" generally refers to all of the following, except
a. Agents
b. Sources
c. Modes of transmission
d. Control measures

Ans. (d) Control measures

Determinants generally includes the causes (including agents), risk factors (including exposure to sources), and modes of transmission, but does not include the resulting public health action (control measures).

2. Which of the following is the hallmark feature of an analytic epidemiologic study?
a. Use of an appropriate comparison group
b. Laboratory confirmation of the diagnosis
c. Publication in a peer-reviewed journal
d. Statistical analysis using regression methods

Ans. (a) Use of an appropriate...

Practice Question

3. Which level of prevention involves restoring an individual's functional capacity and reducing the impact of a disease or injury to promote the highest possible quality of life?
a. Primordial prevention
b. Primary prevention
c. Secondary prevention
d. Tertiary prevention

Ans. (d) Tertiary prevention

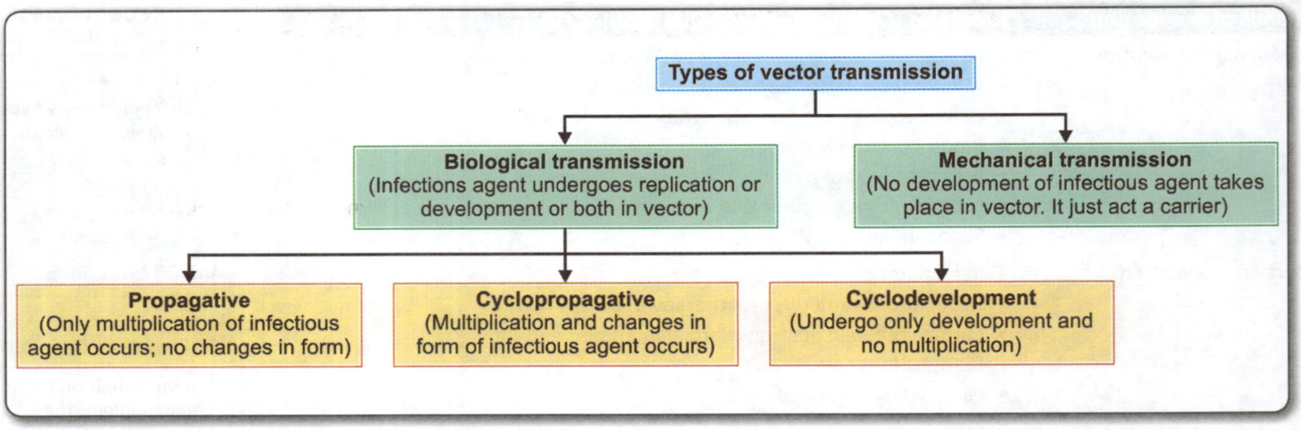

Figure 3: Types of vector transmission

- **Reservoir**: Any person, animal, arthropod or plant in which an infectious agent normally lives and multiplies.
- **Virulence**: It is the degree of pathogenicity of a infectious agent. It is the proportion of clinical cases resulting in severe clinical manifestation.
- **Pathogenicity**: It is the ability to induce clinically apparent illness.
- **Incubation period**: time from exposure to development of disease or appearance of the first sign of symptom
- **Latent period**: The period between exposure and onset infectiousness.
- **Communicable period** (infectious period): Length of time a person can transmit a disease.
- **Incidence**: Number of new cases
- **Prevalence**: Number of new cases and old cases
- **Epidemic curve**: A histogram that shows the course of an epidemic by plotting the number of cases by time of onset.
- **Nosocomial infection** (Hospital acquired infection): Infection in patient which originates in a hospital setting.
- **Opportunistic infection:** Infection occurs due to defect in host defense.
- **Iatrogenic infection**: Physician induced infection due to diagnostic or therapeutic procedures.
- **Eradication:** Termination of infection from the route cause, e.g., Small pox
- **Elimination:** Refers to the reduction to zero new cases in defined geographical area.
- **Control:** the reduction of disease incidence, prevalence, morbidity, or mortality to a locally acceptable level.
- **Extinction: The specific infectious agent no longer exists in nature or laboratory.**

Practice Questions

4. An example of mechanical transmission of disease by vector is

a. Flies carrying shigella
b. Chagas disease
c. Avian influenza
d. Scrub typhus

Ans. (a) Flies carrying shigella

5. A mosquito bites a person who subsequently develops a fever. What type of transmission would this be?

a. Mechanical vector transmission
b. Biological vector transmission
c. Direct contact transmission
d. Airborne transmission

Ans. (b) Biological vector transmission

MORTALITY RATE AND RATIOS

Table 3: Mortality rates and ratios its definitions and formulas

Mortality rate and ratios	Definition	Formula
Crude death rate	The number of death (from all causes) per 1000 estimated mid-year population in 1 year, in a given place.	$\frac{\text{Number of deaths}}{\text{Mild year population}} \times 1000$
Case fatality ratio	It represents the killing power of a disease. It is simply the ratio of death to the cases. It is closely related to virulence.	$\frac{\text{Total number of deaths due to particular disease}}{\text{Total number of cases due to same disease}} \times 1000$

Contd...

Mortality rate and ratios	Definition	Formula
Proportional mortality rate	It is sometimes useful to know what proportion of total death is due to a particular disease or a cause.	$\frac{\text{Number of deaths from the specific disease in a year}}{\text{Total deaths from all cause}} \times 1000$
Under five proportionate mortality rate		$\frac{\text{Number of deaths under 5 years of age in the given year}}{\text{Total number of death during the same period}} \times 1000$
Proportional mortality rate for aged above 50 years		$\frac{\text{Number of deaths of person above 50 years}}{\text{Total deaths of all age group in that year}} \times 1000$
Survival rate	It is the proportion of survivors in a group, (e.g., Patients) studied and followed over a period	$\frac{\text{Total no. of patients alive after a particular time period}}{\text{Total number of patients diagnosed or treated}} \times 1000$
Maternal Mortality Rate (MMR)	It is the number of female deaths in a year per 100,000 live births due to birth or pregnancy-related complications	$\frac{\text{Number of maternal deaths}}{\text{Total number of live births during the same year}} \times 100{,}000$
Infant Mortality Rate (IMR)	Number of deaths of children under one year of age per 1,000 live births.	$\frac{\text{Deaths among children} < 1 \text{ year}}{\text{Number of live births}} \times 1{,}000$

INCIDENCE AND PREVALENCE OF DISEASE

- **Incidence:** It is the number of new cases occurring in a defined population during a specified period of time.

$$\textbf{Incidence} = \frac{\text{Number of new cases of specific disease during a given period of time in the given year}}{\text{Population of risk during that period}} \times 1000$$

- **Prevalence:** It refers to all current cases (old and new) existing at a given point of time, or over a period of time in a given population. It is mainly of two types. They are point prevalence and period prevalence.
- **Point prevalence:** Number of all current cases (old and new) of a disease at one point of time, in relation to defined population.

$$\textbf{Point Prevalence} = \frac{\text{Number of all current cases (old and new) of a specified disease existing at a given point of time}}{\text{Estimated population at the same point of time}} \times 100$$

- **Period prevalence**: It measures the frequency of all cases (old and new) existing during a defined period of time expressed in relation to a defined population

$$\textbf{Period prevalence} = \frac{\text{Number of existing cases (old and new) of a specified disease during a given period of time}}{\text{Estimated mid interval population at risk}} \times 100$$

Practice Questions

6. Which of the following is the denominator of the formula to calculate Maternal Mortality Rate (MMR)?

a. Total number of pregnancy during the year
b. Total number of live births during the year
c. Number of maternal deaths in a year
d. Total number of Live births + still births during the year

Ans. (b) Total number of live births during the year

7. Infant Mortality Rate (IMR) is expressed in terms of number of deaths of children under one year age per

a. 100 live births
b. 1,000 live births
c. 10,000 live births
d. 1,00,000 live births

Ans. (b) 1,000 live births

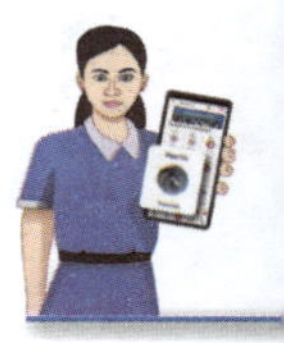

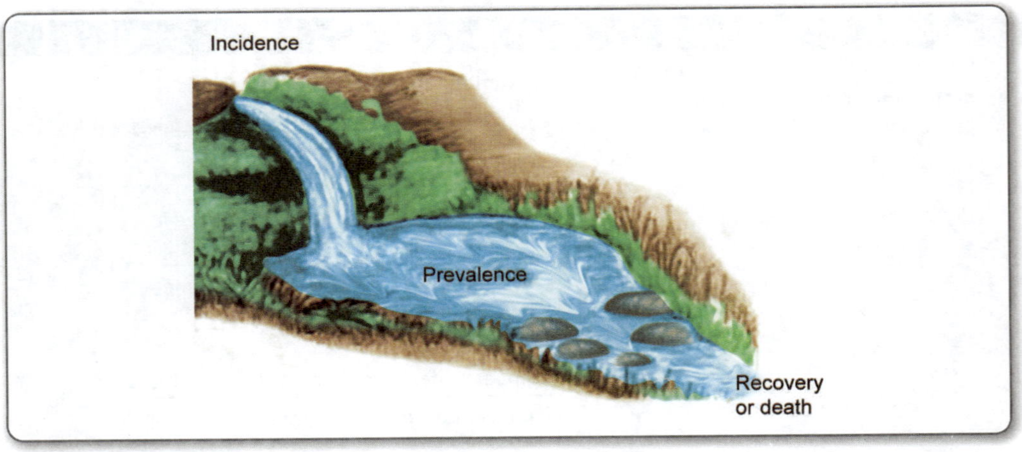

Figure 4: Incidence and prevalence of disease

Relationship between Prevalence and Incidence

Prevalence depends upon two factors, **the incidence and duration of illness**. Given the assumption that the population is stable and incidence and duration of illness are unchanging, the relationship between incidence and prevalence can be expressed as:

P = I × D

P = Prevalence

I = Incidence

D = Duration of illness

EPIDEMIOLOGICAL METHOD

1. Observational studies	
• Descriptive study	
• Analytical studies	
• Ecological/correlational	With population as a unit of study
• Cross sectional/prevalence	With individual as a unit of study
• Case control/case reference	With individual as a unit of study
• Cohort/follow-up	With individual as a unit of study
2. Experimental studies/interventional studies	
• Randomized controlled trials/clinical trial	With patients as a unit of study
• Field trials/community interventional studies	With healthy people as unit of study
• Community trials	With community as unit of study

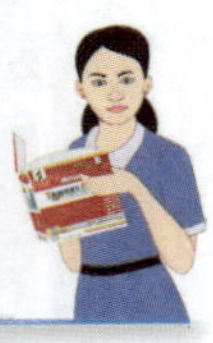

Observational Studies

Descriptive Studies

These are usually the first phase of an investigation. These studies are concerned with observing the distribution of disease or health related characteristics in human populations and identifying the characteristic with which the disease in question seems to be associated.

Phases of Descriptive Study

1. Defining the population to be studied
2. Defining the disease under the study
3. Describing the disease by:
    - Time
    - Place
    - Person
4. Measurement of disease
5. Comparing with known indices
6. Formulation of an **etiological** hypothesis

Analytical Studies

Analytical Epidemiology

This is the second most major type of epidemiological studies. In contrast to descriptive study that looks at entire population, in analytical studies the subject of interest is the individual within the population. The object is not to formulate but to test hypothesis.

Case Control Study

These are often called as retrospective studies and are common approaches to test casual hypothesis. This method has three distinct features:

1. Both exposure and outcome have occurred before the start of the study
2. The study proceeds backward from effect to cause
3. It uses a control or comparison group to support or refute an inference.
4. It is also known **prevalence study.**

Practice Question

8. For a disease which is highly fatal (e.g., Ebola) and of short duration, which of the following statements is correct?

a. Incidence rate will be much higher than mortality rate

b. Mortality rate will be much higher than incidence rate

c. Incidence rate and mortality rate will be nearly similar.

d. Incidence rate will have no association with mortality rate

Ans. (c) Incidence rate and mortality rate will be nearly similar.

KEY POINTS

- The two most common types of observational studies are cohort studies and case-control studies; a third type is cross-sectional studies.
- A case-control study is always **retrospective** because it starts with an outcome (case) then traces back to investigate exposures (cause).

Practice Question

9. A pediatric nurse researcher wants to study the association between use of tap water for drinking and diarrhoea. The researcher enrolls children suffering from diarrhea and same aged healthy children in the study. The children were questioned about their practice of drinking tap water. The association is determined using the measured data. What type of study is this?

a. Case-control study

b. Cohort study

c. Prospective study

d. Cross-sectional study

Ans. (a) Case-control study

Cohort Study

It is another type of analytical study, usually undertaken to obtain additional evidences to support the existence of an association between suspected cause and disease. This study is known by other names also such as prospective study, longitudinal study, incidence study and forward looking study.

Distinguishing features of these methods:

- The cohorts are identified before the appearance of the disease under investigation.
- The study group so defined is observed over a period of time to determine the frequency of disease among them.
- The study proceeds from cause to effect.

Elements of Cohort Study

- Selection of study subjects
- Obtaining data on exposure
- Selection of comparison group
- Follow-up
- Analysis.

Experimental/Interventional Studies

Randomized Control Trial (RCT)

- It is really an epidemiological experiment
- To assess the new programs or new therapies
- RCT is not the method of evaluation.

Steps

- Drawing up a protocol
- Selecting references and experimental populations
- Randomization
- Manipulation or intervention
- Follow-up
- Assessment of outcome

Blinding

- **Single blind trial**: Researcher knows which subjects are receiving treatment or placebo, whereas the subjects are not aware.
- **Double blind trial:** Neither the researcher nor the subjects know what the subjects are receiving (placebo or treatment)
- **Triple blind trial:** Neither the subject, nor the person administering treatment, nor the evaluator of outcome are aware which subjects are receiving treatment or placebo.

Relative Risk (Risk Ratio)

It is the incidence of disease or death among exposed and non-exposed.

Relative risk =

$$\frac{\text{Incidence of disease among the exposed}}{\text{Incidence of death or disease among the non-exposed}}$$

Attributed Risk

It is the difference in the incidence rate of disease or death between an exposed group and non-exposed group.

Attributed risk =

$$\frac{\text{(Incidence of disease rate among the exposed—incidence of disease rate among the non-exposed)}}{\text{Incidence rate among the exposed}} \times 100$$

Practice Question

10. In a clinical trial, Group A consists of 100 participants who received a new medication, and Group B consists of 100 participants who received a placebo. After the trial, it is found that 10 participants in Group A and 20 participants in Group B developed the targeted disease. What is the relative risk of developing the disease between Group A and Group B?

a. 0.5
b. 1.0
c. 2.0
d. 0.2

Ans. (a) 0.5

Practice Question

11. A public health researcher takes a sample of healthy adults, records their ongoing solar exposure, and correlate that to the subsequent occurrence of cataract in the same group. Which type of study is this?

a. Case-control study
b. Cohort study
c. Retrospective study
d. Cross-sectional study

Ans. (b) Cohort study

EPIDEMIOLOGICAL TRIAD

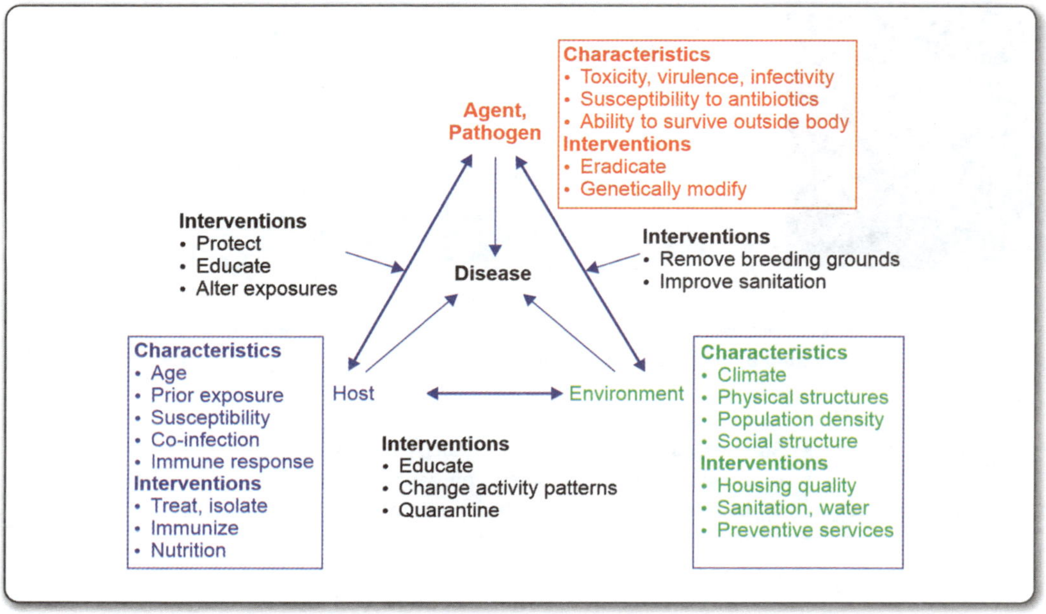

Figure 5: Epidemiological triad

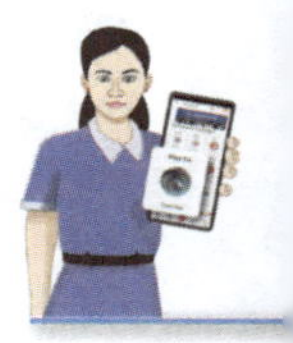

SURVEILLANCE AND MONITORING FOR DISEASE

- **Screening:** It is the search for unrecognized disease or defect by means of rapid application of test, examinations or other procedures in apparently healthy individuals.
- **Quarantine**: It is a strict isolation imposed to prevent the spread of disease. Isolation/restriction of a person or domestic animal exposed to communicable disease for a period of time not longer than usual incubation period of the disease.
- **Monitoring:** Performance and analysis of routine measurement to detect changes in the environment and health status of population, e.g., monitoring of air pollution, ongoing measurement of performance of health service.
- **Surveillance:** To watch over with great attention. Continuous screening of the factors that determine the occurrence and distribution of diseases.

Types of Surveillance

- **Passive surveillance:** Regular reporting of disease data by all institutions that see patients and are part of reporting network is known as passive surveillance.
- **Active surveillance:** Systematic collection of data (agency initiated), e.g., field surveys.
- **Sentinel surveillance:** Reporting by specified units from defined area. A method of identifying missing cases.
- **Syndromic surveillance: Surveillance** using health-related data that precede diagnosis and signal a sufficient probability of a case or an outbreak to warrant further public health response.
- **Sensitivity:** It is defined as the ability of a test to identify correctly all cases those who have the disease that is true positive. A 90% sensitivity means that 90% of the diseased people screened by this test will be identified as positive and 10% of patients who have the disease will be identified as negative.
- **Specificity:** It is the ability of a test to correctly identify those who do not have disease that is true negative. A 90% specificity means 90% of the non-diseased person will give true negative result. 10% of non-diseased people screened by this test will be wrongly classified as diseased when they are not actually negative.

KEY POINTS

- International Health Regulation (IHR) came into force from 15th June 2007. It requires 176 member countries to report certain disease outbreaks and public health events to WHO.
- The term sensitivity was introduced by **Yerushamly**.

KEY POINT

Sensitivity = True positive
Specificity = True negative
Type I error = False positive
Type II error = False negative

ICEBERG PHENOMENON

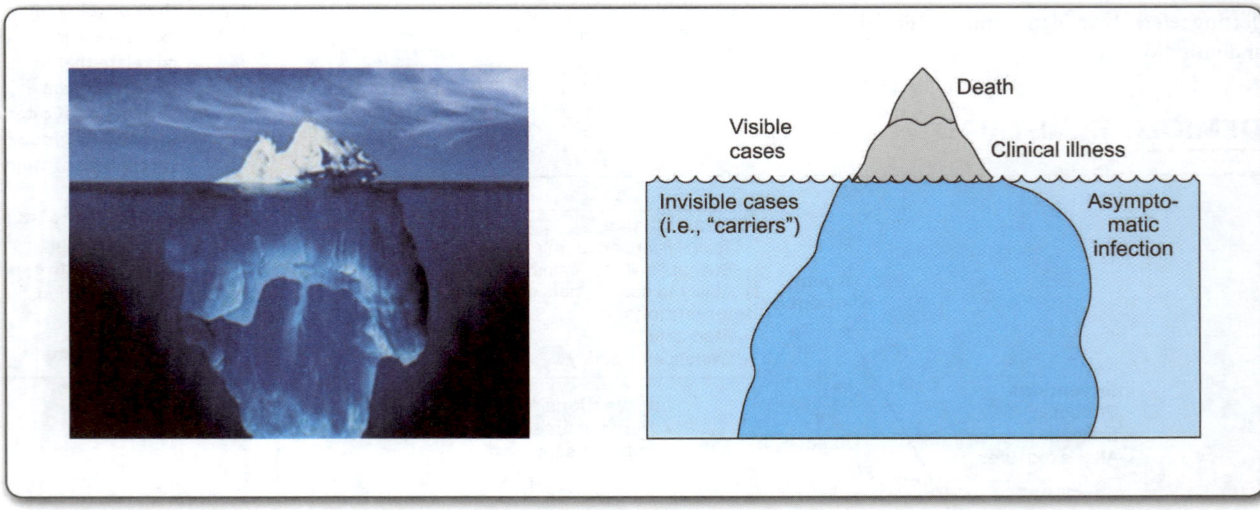

Figure 6: Iceberg phenomenon

- Disease in the community is compared with an Ice-berg.
- **Floating tip:** Physician can see disease in the community (clinical cases).
- **Submerged portion:** Invisible (hidden part) cases of disease - latent, unapparent, presymptomatic, undiagnosed and carrier in the community.
- **Water line:** Between apparent and subclinical cases or unapparent disease (subclinical cases).

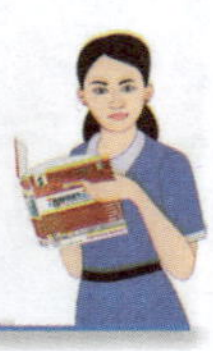

IMMUNITY

- Immunity is the ability of an organism fight against a disease.

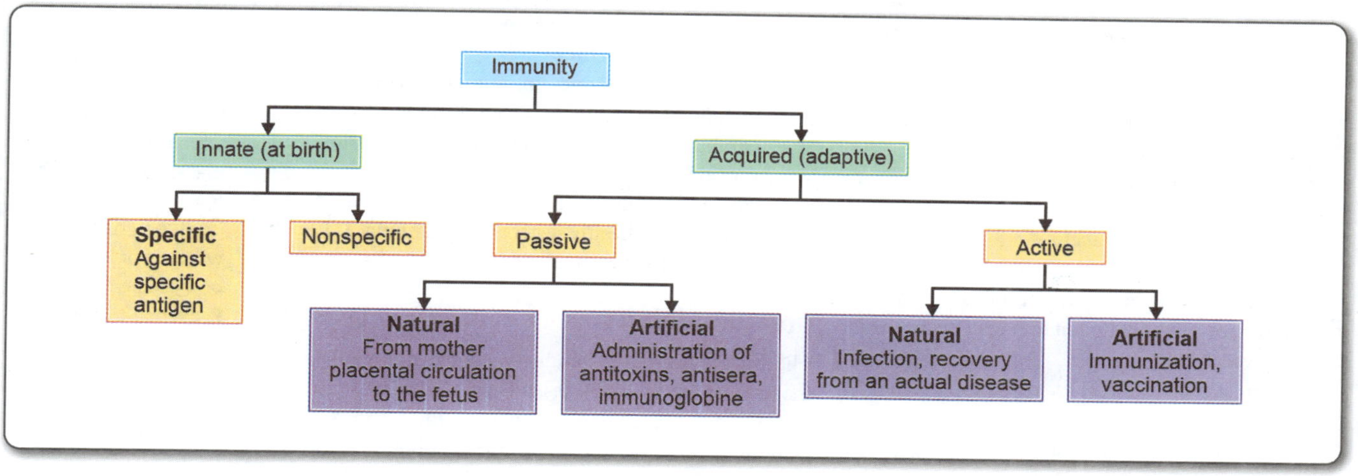

Figure 7: Types of immunity

- **Active immunity:** It is the immunity which an individual develops as a result of an infection or by specific immunization and is usually associated with presence of antibodies or cells having a specific action on the micro-organism concerned with a particular infectious disease or its own toxin. It can be acquired in three ways:
  1. Following clinical infection for example, chicken pox, rubella and measles.
  2. Following subclinical or inapparent infection, e.g., polio, diphtheria.
  3. Following immunization with an antigen which may be a killed vaccine or a live attenuated vaccine.

Humoral immunity, cellular immunity and combination of above two also comes under active immunity.

- **Humoral immunity:** It comes from B cell which proliferates and manufacture specific antibodies after antigen presen-tation by macrophages. The antibodies are located in the immunoglobulin fraction of serum and are of five main types, they are **IgG, IgM, IgA, IgD and IgE.**
- **Cellular immunity:** Although antibodies are quiet effective in combating most infectious disease, humoral immunity does not cover all the situation that one finds in infectious disease. Some pathogens such as ***M. leprae, M. tuberculosis*** and ***S. typhi*** escapes the bactericidal action of leukocyte. Here the **activate T cell** perform phagocytic action.

- **Passive immunity:** When antibodies produced in one body are transferred to another to induce protection against disease, it is known as passive immunity. Here the body does not produce its own antibodies but depends upon ready-made antibodies. Passive immunity can be induced:
  - By administration of an antibody containing preparation (immunoglobulin or antiserum).
  - By transfer of maternal antibodies across the placenta. Human milk also contains protective antibodies (IgA).
  - By transfer of lymphocytes to induce passive cellular immunity.
- **Herd immunity:** It is the level of resistance of a community or a group of people to a particular disease.

Immunizing Agents

These agents can be mainly classified as vaccines, immunoglobulin, and antisera.

Vaccines

It is an immune biological substance, designed to produce specific protection against a given disease. It stimulates the production of protective antibodies and other immune mechanisms.

- **Live vaccines**
  - These type of vaccines are prepared from live organisms. These organisms lost their capacity to produce a full blown disease but retain their immunogenicity.
  - Live vaccines should not be administered to an individual with immunodeficiency, immune suppression, malignancy or on therapy with corticosteroids, alkylating agents, antimetabolite or on radiation.

KEY POINTS

- Artificially acquired immunity is obtained by immunization with antibody response; antibodies are administered, not produced by the body.
- **Artificial active immunity** may be produced by vaccination.
- **Artificial passive immunity** is through the parenteral administration of antibodies.
- Breastfeeding is natural passive immunity which is obtained by immunoglobins in mothers breast milk.
- **Herd immunity** is the overall resistance in a community.
- Edward Jenner developed the first human vaccine (smallpox vaccine) and coined the term 'Vaccination'
- Louis Pasteur developed the first vaccine for Anthrax & Rabies

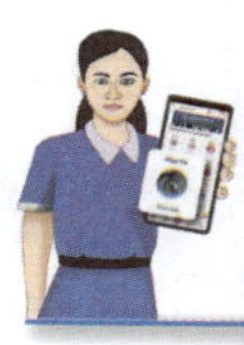

- When two live vaccines need to be administered either administer them simultaneously at two different sites or maintain a gap of four weeks between the administrations of two vaccines.
- Live vaccines will achieve its immunization with single dose, **exception is polio vaccines** which require three or more doses at spaced interval to produce effective immunity.
- Live vaccines must be stored properly to maintain its potency.

- **Inactivated or killed vaccines**
  - Organisms killed by heat or chemicals when infected into the body stimulate immunity. They are usually safe but are less effective than live vaccines.
  - In most cases these kinds of vaccines require a booster dose.
  - The duration of immunity following killed vaccines vary from months to many years.
  - The only absolute contraindication against killed vaccines are severe general or local reaction to the previous dose.
- **Toxoid**
  - Certain organisms produce exotoxins (diphtheria, tetanus). The toxins produced by these organisms are detoxified and used in the preparation of vaccines.
- **Cellular fractions**
  - In certain instances, vaccines are prepared from extracted cellular fractions. For example, meningococcal, pneumococcal.
- **Combinations vaccines**
  - If more than one immunizing agent is included in a single vaccine they are called as combination vaccines. The aim of combination vaccine is to simplify administration, reduce cost and minimize the number of contact of patient with health system. For example, **DT, DPT, MMR. Pentavalent vaccine.**

Immunoglobulin

The human immunoglobulin system composed of major five immunoglobulins, IgG, IgA, IgD, IgM, IgE.

- **IgG:** Major immunoglobulin in serum. It consists of 85% of total serum immunoglobulin. It is the only immunoglobulin which can cross the placenta.
- **IgM:** Accounts for 10% serum immunoglobulin. It represents the antibody that promptly formed with exposure to antigen. Its presence may be indicative of recent infection.
- **IgA:** About 15% of total serum immunoglobulin. It is found relatively in larger quantities in body secretions.

Table 4: Immunizing agents

Types of vaccines	Examples
Live attenuated (Mnemonic: MY ROME TRIP)	M — Mumps Y — Yellow fever R — Rubella O — Oral Polio; Oral Typhoid M — Measles E — Endemic Typhus T — TB Vaccine (BCG) R — Rubella I — Influenza P — Plague
Inactivated/killed vaccines	Typhoid Cholera Pertussis CS meningitis Plague Rabies Salk (polio vaccine) Influenza Hepatitis A Hepatitis B Japanese encephalitis
Toxoids	Diphtheria Tetanus

Contd...

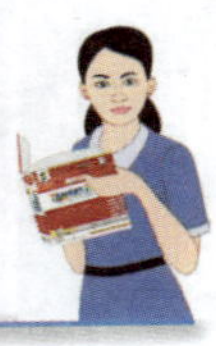

KEY POINTS

- **IgG** is the major serum immunoglobulin and is the only immunoglobulin which can cross the placenta.
- **IgA** is the main immunoglobulin which is present in body secretions.
- **Presence of IgM** antibody in the serum of a newborn baby suggestive of congenital infection.
- **IgE** mediate type-1 hypersensitivity reactions.
- **IgM** is the macro immunoglobulin.
- Immune response of Killed vaccine is relatively poor in comparison to live vaccines
- Killed vaccines are safer than live vaccines.
- Adjuvants required in Killed vaccine

Practice Questions

12. All of the following vaccines are inactivated or attenuated whole pathogen, except

a. Salk
b. Rabies
c. Hepatitis A
d. Tetanus

Ans. (d) Tetanus

Explanation: Tetanus vaccine, also known as tetanus toxoid (TT), is a toxoid vaccine used to prevent tetanus.

Rabies and Hepatitis A are inactivated/killed vaccine whereas Sabin (oral polio) is a live attenuated vaccine.

13. The first ever recombinant vaccine approved for human use is

a. DPT vaccine
b. Hepatitis B vaccine
c. Polio vaccine
d. Influenza vaccine

Ans. (b) Hepatitis B...

Types of vaccines	Examples
Immunoglobulin	
Human immunoglobulin	Hepatitis A Measles Rabies Tetanus Mumps Hepatitis B Varicella Diphtheria
Non-human	Diphtheria Tetanus Gas gangrene Botulism Rabies

Table 5: Comparison between live and killed vaccines

Characteristics	Killed vaccine	Live vaccine
Number of doses	Multiple	Single
Need for adjuvant	Yes	No
Duration of immunity	Shorter	Longer
Effectiveness of protection	Lower	Greater
Immunoglobulin produced	IgG	IgA and IgG
Mucosal immunity produced	Poor	Yes
Cell-mediated immunity produced	Poor	Yes
Residual virulent virus in vaccine	Possible	No
Reversion to virulence	No	Possible
Excretion of vaccine and transmission to non-immune contact	No	Possible
Interference by other virus in the host	No	Possible
Stability at room temperature	High	Low

COLD CHAIN

- Cold chain is a system of storage and transport of vaccines at low temperature from the manufacturer to the actual vaccination site. The cold chain system is necessary because vaccine failure may occur due to failure of storage and transport under strict temperature controls.
- Vaccine stored in the freezer compartment are **polio and measles.**
- Vaccine which must be stored in the cold part and never allowed to freeze are **BCG, DPT, DT, TT, typhoid and diluents.**
- Vaccines must be protected from sunlight and prevented from contact with antiseptics.
- At health center most of the vaccine (except polio) can be stored up to 5 weeks, if refrigerator temperature is strictly kept between 4°C and 8°C.
- Storage of opened vial:
  With preservatives: up to **three hours**
  Without preservatives: up to **one hour**

The Cold Chain Equipment

- Walk in cold room
- Deep freezer
- Small deep freezer
- Cold boxes
- Vaccine carrier
- Day carrier
- Ice packs.

Ice-lined Refrigeration: (ILR)

- Important in the cold chain link
- Maintains temp between +2°C and +8°C
- Small size ILR in PHC level
- ILR is divided into two parts
  - **Upper part:** Storing for freeze sensitive vaccines, e.g., DPT, TT, hepB, IPV, Pentavalent
  - **Lower part:** OPV, BCG, measles, Ig

VVM

- Vaccine viral monitoring
  It is a label containing a heat–sensitive material to check the status of vaccines viability.

POINT TO REMEMBER

Rabies Immune Globulin (RIG) - RIG always should be used in conjunction with rabies vaccine in previously unvaccinated persons.

KEY POINTS

Intensified Mission Indradhanush (IMI) 3.0:
- The scheme has rolled out to cover children and pregnant women who missed routine immunisation during the Covid-19 pandemic.
- **Provides vaccination against 12 Vaccine-Preventable Diseases (VPD):**
  - Diphtheria
  - Whooping cough
  - Tetanus
  - Polio
  - Tuberculosis
  - Hepatitis B
  - Meningitis and pneumonia
  - Haemophilus influenzae type B infections,
  - Japanese encephalitis (JE)
  - Rotavirus vaccine
  - Pneumococcal conjugate vaccine (PCV) and
  - Measles-rubella (MR).

KEY POINTS

- Minimum Interval between two live vaccines is 4 weeks.
- Post exposure immunisation is given in
  - M - Measles
  - T -Tetanus
  - R - Rabies
  - M - Meningococcal meningitis
  - C - Chicken pox
  - H - Hepatitis

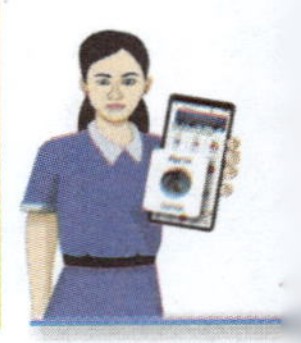

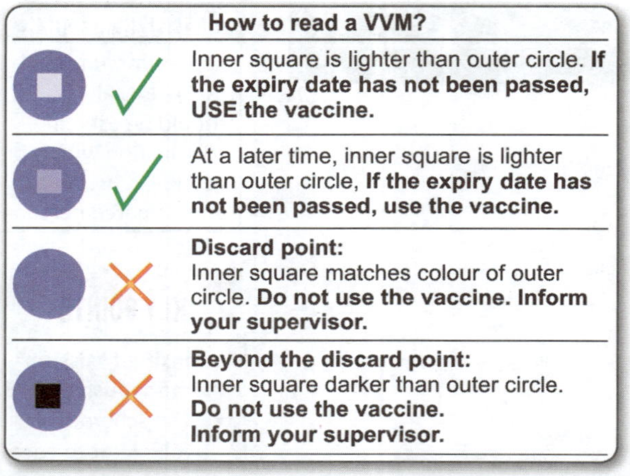

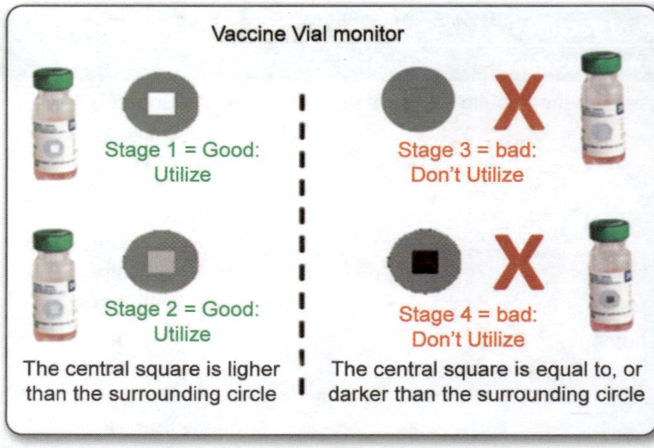

Vaccine Storage

Do's

- Keep the equipment in cold room away from direct sunlight and at least 10 cm away from wall.
- Keep the equipment through voltage stabilizer.
- Keep vaccines neatly with space between stacks for circulation of air.
- Keep the equipment locked and open only when it is necessary.
- Defrost periodically.
- Supervise the temperature record.
- If vaccines are in carton make holes on side of the carton for cold air circulations.

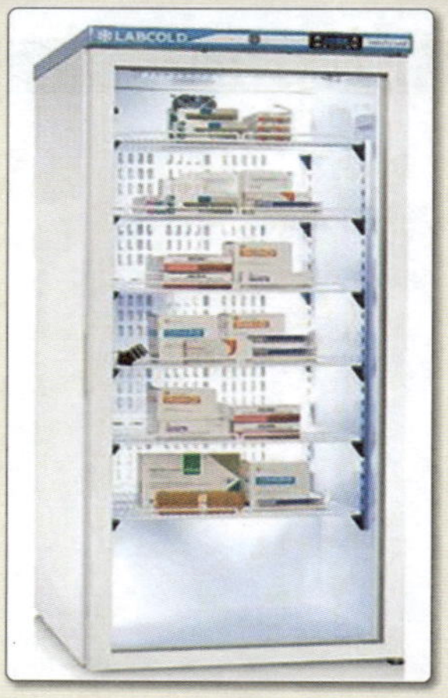

Don'ts

- Do not keep any other things other than vaccine in these boxes.
- Do not store any other drug.
- Do not keep drinking water or food in them.
- Do not keep more than 1 month requirements in PHC
- Do not keep expired date vaccines.

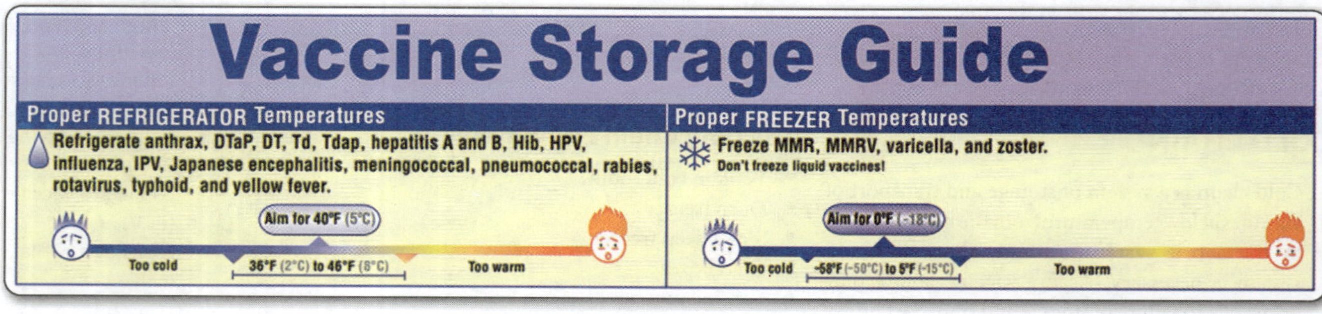

ADVERSE EVENTS FOLLOWING IMMUNIZATION

Classification of Adverse Events following Immunization

Table 6: Types of immunization reactions

Type of reaction	Explanation
Vaccine reaction	Event caused or precipitated by the vaccine when given correctly, caused by inherent properties of vaccine
Program error	Event caused by an error in the vaccine preparation, handling or administration
Coincidental	Events that happens after immunization but not caused by the vaccine-a chance of association
Injection reaction	Events from anxiety about or pain from the injection itself rather than the vaccine
Unknown	Events cause cannot be determined

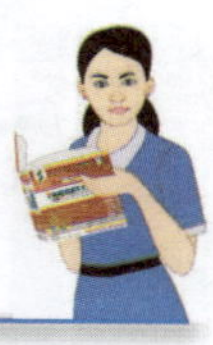

Common Minor Vaccine Reactions

Table 7: Various vaccines and their common minor reactions

Vaccine	Possible minor reactions
BCG	Local reaction (pain, redness and swelling)
Cholera	Oral presentation-none
DTP	Local reaction (pain, redness and swelling), fever
Hepatitis A	Local reaction (pain, redness and swelling)
Hepatitis B	Local reaction (pain, redness and swelling), fever
Hib	Local reaction (pain, redness and swelling), fever
Japanese encephalitis	Local reactions, low grade fever, myalgia, GI upset
Measles/MMR	Local reaction (pain, redness and swelling), irritability, malaise and non-specific symptoms, fever
Pneumococcal	Local reaction (pain, redness and swelling)
OPV	None
IPV (poliomyelitis)	None
Rabies	Local or general reaction
Meningococcal disease	Mild local reaction
TT	Local reaction (pain, redness and swelling), malaise, non-specific symptoms
Tick borne encephalitis	Local reaction (pain, redness and swelling)
Yellow fever	Headache, influenza like symptoms, Local reaction (pain, redness and swelling)

Rare Vaccine Reactions

Table 8: Vaccines and their rare reactions

Vaccine	Reaction
BCG	Suppurative lymphadenitis, BCG osteitis, disseminated BCG infection
Hib	None
Hepatitis B	Anaphylaxis
Measles/MMR	Febrile seizure, thrombocytopenia, severe allergic reaction, encephalopathy
OPV	Vaccine associated poliomyelitis
TT	Brachial neuritis, anaphylaxis
DT	Same as that of TT
Pertussis/DPT	Inconsolable screaming, seizure, hypotonic or hypo responsive episode, anaphylaxis, encephalopathy

Contraindication to Vaccination

Table 9: Vaccines and their contraindications

Vaccine	Contraindication
All	An anaphylactic reaction following previous dose of vaccine is a true contraindication to further immunization with the antigen concerned
Live vaccines (MMR, BCG, yellow fever)	Pregnancy, total body radiation
Yellow fever	Egg allergy, immunodeficiency
BCG	Symptomatic HIV infection
Influenza, yellow fever	History of anaphylaxis reaction following egg allergy
Pertussis	Anaphylactic reaction to previous dose Evolving neurological disease

Recent Question
(NORCET 2022)

3. Which test is used to check whether freeze-sensitive vaccines have been damaged by exposure to temperatures below 0 °C?

a. Stick test
b. Shake test
c. Shick test
d. Shock test

Ans. (b) Shake test

Practice Question

14. Which of the following is an example of a systemic reaction to a vaccine?

a. Mild soreness at the injection site
b. Redness and swelling at the injection site
c. High fever and bodyaches
d. Itching and hives at the injection site

Ans. (c) High fever and bodyaches

KEY POINTS

- Inactivated polio vaccine is known as **SALK**
- Oral polio vaccine is known as **SABIN**
- **Hepatitis B** virus was discovered by **Blumberg**
- **Hepatitis C** virus was identified in the year of **1989**
- **First major epidemic** because of **hepatitis E** was reported in **New Delhi in winter 1995–1996.**
- A vast international campaign was held by WHO between **1967** and **1979** led to eradication of smallpox.
- On **5 July 1975** India was proclaimed to be no longer a smallpox endemic country.

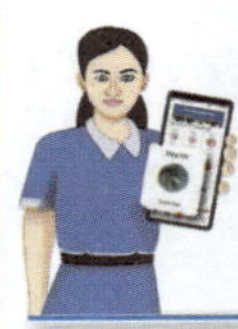

NATIONAL IMMUNIZATION SCHEDULE/UNIVERSAL IMMUNIZATION PROGRAM

National Immunization Schedule (NIS)

- Under Universal Immunization Program (UIP), Government of India is providing vaccination to prevent seven vaccine preventable diseases, Diphtheria, Pertussis, Tetanus, Polio, Measles, Hepatitis B and Tuberculosis.

National Immunization Schedule is provided in Pediatric Nursing Synopsis

POINT TO REMEMBER

A Detailed National Immunization Schedule with Dose, Diluents, Routes and sites is given in Appendices

COMMUNICABLE DISEASES

Table 10: Communicable disease — a summary

Disease	Causative agent	Incubation period	Mode of transmission	Sign and symptoms	Complications
Smallpox	Variola virus		Respiratory	Fever, typical rash occur in centrifugal distribution	
Chicken pox	Varicella-zoster	14–16 days	Person to person by droplet	Vesicular rashes; Pleomorphism is a characteristic feature of the rash in chicken pox fever, malaise	**Reye's syndrome:** occurs during recovery from viral disease. Disseminated Intravascular Coagulation (DIC) may occur
Measles (Rubeola)	Myxoviruses	10–14 days	Droplet	Fever, coryza, nasal discharge, cough, redness of eyes, lacrimation, vomiting, diarrhea, **Koplik's spot**, maculopapular rashes begins behind the ear and spread rapidly in few hours over face and neck and extend down to the body taking 2–3 days to progress to the lower extremities.	Otitis media Conjunctivitis Pneumonia
Rubella (germen measles)	RNA virus of toga virus family.	2–3 weeks Average 18 days	Droplet	Coryza, sore throat, low grade fever, lymphadenopathy, rash	Arthralgia Thrombocytopenic purpura
Mumps	Genus rubulavirus of the family paramyxoviridae	2–3 weeks usually 18 days	Droplet	Pain and swelling in either or both parotid gland but may also involve sublingual and submandibular glands, ear ache, pain and stiffness on opening the mouth	Orchitis Ovaritis and oophoritis Pancreatitis (children)
Influenza	Type A, Type B, Type C viruses in the orthomyxoviridae family	18–72 hours	Droplet	Inflammation and necrosis of superficial epithelium of respiratory tract, fever, chills, aches, pain, cough, generalized weakness	Reye's syndrome Pneumonia Acute sinusitis and bronchitis
Diphtheria	Corynebacterium diphtheria	2–6 days	Droplet infection	Sore throat, difficulty swallowing, low grade fever, throat may show mild erythema, localized exudate, pseudo membrane, difficulty with vision, speech and swallowing, toxins produced by the bacteria may cause nerve damage resulting in often paralysis of soft palate, eye muscles and extremities	Neurological problems (encephalopathy, convulsions), infantile spasms

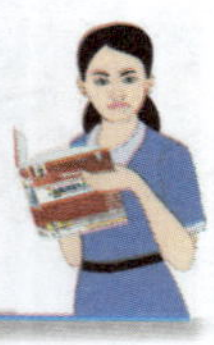

Contd...

Disease	Causative agent	Incubation period	Mode of transmission	Sign and symptoms	Complications
Pertussis (whooping cough)	*B. pertussis*	7–14 days	Droplet and direct contact	Lacrimation, sneezing, coryza, anorexia, malaise, hacking night cough, deep high pitched inspiration (whoop), vomiting, cyanosis, apnea, hemorrhage, epistaxis, hemoptysis, cerebral hemorrhage, convulsions, coma.	Bronchitis (common), Bronchiectasis, epistaxis and hemoptysis, Subconjunctival hemorrhage
Meningococcal meningitis	*N. meningitidis*	3–4 days	Droplet	Headache, vomiting, stiff neck, photophobia, various neurological sign	Total hearing loss, Balance and coordination problems, Septicemia, Arthritis
Severe acute respiratory syndrome (SARS)	New strain of coronavirus	2–7 days	Close contact with the patients infected material	Fever, malaise, chills, headache, myalgia, dizziness, cough, sore throat, running nose.	Pulmonary decompensation, ARDS
Tuberculosis	*M. tuberculosis*	3–6 weeks	Droplet infection	Persistent Cough of about 3–4 weeks duration, weight loss, fever, hemoptysis	Spinal pain, Cardiac temponade, Hemoptysis, Lung abscess
Poliomyelitis	Polio virus	7–14 days	Primary mode: Fecal-oral route. Less commonly through droplet	Fever, malaise, anorexia, nausea, vomiting, signs of meningeal irritation, child finds difficulty in sitting, descending paralysis, muscle strength vary in different muscle, cranial nerve involvement is present in bulbar and bulbospinal forms of paralytic poliomyelitis	Pneumonia, Edema, mycocarditis, corpulmonale, soft tissue and bone deformities
Hepatitis A (formerly known as infectious hepatitis, epidemic jaundice)	Hepatitis A virus	10–50 days	Feco-oral route	Nonspecific symptoms such as nausea, vomiting, anorexia, mild fever, jaundice, generalized weakness, aches and pain	Hepatic encephalopathy, Cirrhosis, Liver failure, Fulminant Hepatic failure
Hepatitis B (serum hepatitis B)	Hepatitis B virus	50–180 days	Parenteral route Perinatal transmission Sexual transmission	Jaundice, flu-like sign and symptoms, chronic hepatitis and can lead to complications like, liver cancer, cirrhosis, etc.	
Hepatitis C	Hepatitis C virus	6–7 weeks	Parenteral transmission	Chronic hepatitis, liver cirrhosis, liver cancer	
Hepatitis E (enterically transmitted hepatitis non A non B	Hepatitis E virus	2–9 weeks	Water borne disease (feco-oral route)	Initial phase of mild fever, anorexia, nausea and vomiting, abdominal pain, itching without skin lesions, skin rash, or joint pain Jaundice Hepatomegaly	
Hepatitis D	Hepatitis D virus	2–12 weeks	Parenteral route	Mild-to-severe or even **fulminant hepatitis**	
Hepatitis G	Hepatitis G virus				
Diarrhea	Virus and bacteria		Fecal oral route	Passage of watery stools leading to dehydration which shows signs of sunken eyes, skin pinch goes back slowly, etc.	Acidosis

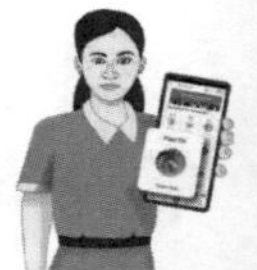

Contd...

Disease	Causative agent	Incubation period	Mode of transmission	Sign and symptoms	Complications
Cholera	*V. cholera*	Hours to 5 days	Fecally contaminated water, contaminated food and drinks Direct contact	Profuse painless watery diarrhea, vomiting, rice water stool leading to dehydration symptoms presenting as sunken eyes, hollow cheeks, scaphoid abdomen, sub-normal temperature, **washerman's hand and feet,** absent pulse, unrecordable BP, loss of skin elasticity	Severe dehydration, Shock, Renal failure
Typhoid fever (enteric fever)	*S. typhi*	10–14 days	Fecal-oral route or urine-oral route	Malaise, headache, sore throat, cough, abdominal pain, constipation, constipation is present either in the early stage or pea soup diarrhea, fever, abdominal distention, rose spot rashes	Intestinal hemorrhage, Intestinal perforation, Shock
COVID-19	SARS Cov-2	1-14 days	Contact, droplet, airborne, fomite, fecal-oral, blood borne, mother to child, animal to human	Cough, breathing difficulty, fever, body ache, bilateral infiltrates on chest imaging	Respiratory failure, Septic shock, Pneumonia, Pulmonary embolism

EBOLA VIRUS

- Ebola Virus Disease (EVD) is a rare and deadly disease in people and nonhuman primates caused by *Zaire ebolavirus*.
- People can get EVD through direct contact with an infected animal (bat or nonhuman primate) or a sick or dead person infected with Ebola virus.
- Incubation period : 2-21 days
- **Symptoms:** Fever, Fatigue, Muscle pain, Headache, Sore throat followed by: Vomiting, Diarrhea, Rash, Symptoms of impaired kidney and liver function, in some cases, both internal and external bleeding (for example, oozing from the gums, or blood in the stools), Laboratory findings include low white blood cell and platelet counts and elevated liver enzymes.

Diagnosis

- Antibody-capture enzyme-linked immunosorbent assay (ELISA)
- Antigen-capture detection tests
- Serum neutralization test
- Reverse transcriptase polymerase chain reaction (RT-PCR) assay
- Electron microscopy
- Virus isolation by cell culture.

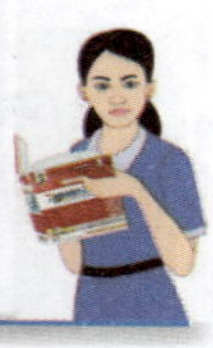

Prevention

- Avoid contact with blood and body fluids of people who all are infected
- Avoid contact with items that may have come in contact with an infected person's blood or body fluids
- Avoid funeral or burial practices that involve touching the body of someone who died from EVD or suspect EVD.
- Avoid contact with bats, forest antelopes, and nonhuman primates (such as monkeys and chimpanzees) blood, fluids, or raw meat prepared from these or unknown animals (bushmeat).

Vaccine

- The U.S. Food and Drug Administration (FDA) approved the Ebola vaccine rVSV-ZEBOV (called Ervebo®) on December 19, 2019. This is the first FDA-approved vaccine for Ebola.
- This vaccine is given as a single dose vaccine and has been found to be safe and protective against *Zaire ebolavirus*, which has caused the largest and most deadly Ebola outbreaks to date.

KEY POINTS

- The Ebola virus is transmitted to people from wild animals and spreads in the human population through human-to-human transmission.
- Ebola is contagious only when someone has symptoms
- Ebola virus lives on something outside the body up to 6 days
- Early supportive care with rehydration, symptomatic treatment improves survival.
- Two monoclonal antibodies (Inmazeb and Ebanga) were approved for the treatment of Ebolavirus infection in adults and children by the US Food and Drug Administration in late 2020.

COVID-19 (REFER TO ANNEXURE FOR DETAILED NOTE OF COVID-19)

- COVID-19 is the infectious disease caused by corona virus. This new virus and disease were unknown before the outbreak began in Wuhan, China, in December 2019.
- Signs and symptoms: fever, tiredness, and dry cough, aches and pains, nasal congestion, runny nose, sore throat or diarrhea.
- Transmission: Main route of transmission is droplet.
- Incubation period: 1-14 days
- Diagnosis
  - **PCR test.** Also called a molecular test, this COVID-19 test detects genetic material of the virus using a lab technique called polymerase chain reaction (PCR)
  - **Antigen test.** This COVID-19 test detects certain proteins in the virus. Using a long nasal swab to get a fluid sample, some antigen tests can produce results in minutes.
- Prevention
  - Regularly wash your hands with soap and water or alcohol-based hand rub
  - Maintain 3 feet distance between people
  - Avoid frequent touching of eyes, nose and mouth.
  - Follow respiratory hygiene. This means covering your mouth and nose with your bent elbow or tissue when you cough or sneeze. Then dispose of the used tissue immediately.
  - Stay home if you feel unwell or any symptoms
  - Always wear mask while going outside

NIPAH VIRUS INFECTION

- Nipah virus (NiV) infection is an emerging zoonotic disease which was first recognized in a large outbreak in Malaysia and Singapore from September 1998 to May 1999.
- In India, three outbreaks in humans were reported from Siliguri (2001), Nadia (2007) in West Bengal and Kozhikode (2018) in Kerala.
- Fruit bats of *Pteropus* genus are the natural reservoir of Nipah Virus (paramyxovirus)
- Transmission to humans occurs after direct contact with infected bats, pigs or from human being.
- Incubation period: 4–21 days

Clinical Features

- Moderate to high grade fever, headache, vomiting, cough, breathlessness, change in sensorium, seizures, myalgia, fatigue
- Treatment is limited to supportive care.

GASTROINTESTINAL DISORDERS

Acute Diarrheal Disease

Diarrhea: Passage of watery stools more than 3 times a day. However recent changes indicated that it is the consistency of the stool which is more important than the number of stool per day.

Table 11: Organisms causing diarrhea

Viruses	• Rotaviruses (Most common cause of diarrhea in infants and children) • Astroviruses • Adenoviruses • Calciviruses • Coronaviruses • Norwalk group viruses • Enteroviruses
Bacteria	*Campylobacter jejuni* *E. coli* *Shigella* *Salmonella* *V. cholera* *V. parahaemolyticus* *Bacillus cereus*
Others	*E. histolytica* *Giardia intestinalis* *Trichuriasis* *Cryptosporidium* Spp Intestinal worms

KEY POINTS

COVID Vaccination:
INDIA:
- India began administration of COVID-19 vaccines on 16 January 2021.
- As of 13 August 2021, India has administered over 529 million doses overall.
- **Covishield** (AstraZeneca's vaccine manufactured by Serum Institute of India) & **Covaxin** (manufactured by Bharat Biotech Limited) were granted emergency use authorization by the Central Drugs Standard Control Organization (CDSCO).
- Sputnik - V has been granted Emergency Use Authorization in the month of April 2021.

USA:
- Only one shot of Johnson & Johnson's Janssen (J&J/Janssen) COVID-19 Vaccine is sufficient to get the complete protection
- The **Pfizer-BioNTech COVID-19 Vaccine** and **Moderna COVID-19 Vaccine** both need 2 shots in order to get the complete protection.

KEY POINT

- Nipah virus infection is an emerging public health concern, particularly in the South East Asian region.

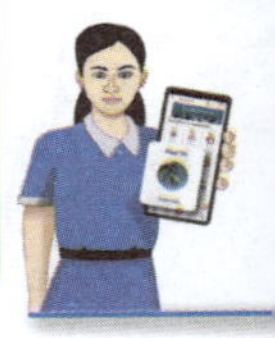

Composition of Reduced Osmolarity ORS (WHO Recommended)

Table 12: Reduced osmolarity ORS composition

Reduced osmolarity ORS	g/L
Sodium chloride	2.6
Glucose anhydrous	13.5
Potassium chloride	1.5
Trisodium citrate, dihydrate	2.9
Total weight	**20.5**

Reduced osmolarity ORS	Mol/L
Sodium	75
Potassium	20
Chloride	65
Glucose anhydrase	75
Citrate	10
Total osmolarity	**245**

Advantages of Reduced Osmolarity ORS

Reduced osmolarity ORS is more stable and results in less stool output, probably because of direct effect of **trisodium citrate** in increasing the water and salt absorption in intestine.

When zinc is supplied during an acute episode of diarrhea, it reduces episodes, duration and severity.

FOOD POISONING

Food poisoning is the ingestion of food or drinks contaminated either with living bacteria or their toxins or inorganic chemical substance derived from plants and animals.

Types of Food Poisoning

Bacterial and non-bacterial

- **Bacterial:** Caused by ingestion of food contaminated with living bacteria or their toxins.
- **Non-bacterial:** Caused by chemicals such as arsenic, certain plant and sea food.

KEY POINTS

- Initial fluid of choice for diarrhea in infant is ORS.
- The content of one ORS pocket has to be dissolved in one liter of Water and to be used within 24 hours.
- Molar ratio of sodium and Glucose in WHO ORS is 1:1
- Bacillus cereus is a toxin-producing bacteria that causes food poisoning, also called "fried rice syndrome."

Practice Question

15. The main advantage of using reduced osmolarity ORS compared to the standard ORS in the treatment of dehydration is that the reduced osmolarity ORS

a. Has a better taste, making it more palatable for children.
b. Contains additional nutrients.
c. Reduces the volume of stool output during diarrhea.
d. Facilitates faster absorption, hence more effective in rehydration.

Ans. (d) Facilitates faster absorption, hence more effective in rehydration

Bacterial Food Poisoning

Table 13: Summary of bacterial food poisoning

Agent	Source	Incubation period	Mechanism of food poisoning	Signs and symptoms
Salmonella typhimurium *S. choleraesuis* *S. enteritidis*	Primarily disease of animal and men gets infection from farm animal and poultry	12–24 hours	The organism after ingestion multiply and gives rise to acute enteritis and colitis	Fever, chills, vomiting, nausea, profuse watery diarrhea
Staphylococcal food poisoning	*S. aureus* are ubiquitous in nature and found on the skin and in the throat and nose of men and animals. Cows suffering from mastitis have been reasonable for the outbreak of disease	1–6 hours	Food poisoning occurs from the cooking of food on which bacteria have grown. Since the toxin is heat resistant it can remain in the food after organism have died. The toxin act directly on the CNS and intestine	Vomiting, abdominal cramps, diarrhea, blood and mucus may appear in severe cases It rarely causes fever

Contd...

Agent	Source	Incubation period	Mechanism of food poisoning	Signs and symptoms
Botulism *Clostridium botulinum*	The organism widely distributed in soil and dust and intestinal tract of animal and enter in food as spores	12–36 hours	The toxin is prepared in food under suitable anaerobic conditions. Toxin act on the parasympathetic nervous system Antidote for botulism poisoning is Guanidine hydrochloride	Dysphagia, diplopia, ptosis, dysarthria, blurring of vision, muscle weakness, quadriplegia
Cl. Perfringens (Welchii)	It has been found in the faces of animals, soil, water and air, majority of the outbreaks occurred because of the ingestion of meat, meat dishes and poultry. The usual story is that food has been prepared 24 hours or more before consumption	6–24 hours	The spores are able to survive cooking, if the cooked meat and poultry are not cooled enough they will germinate and produce toxins as alpha toxins and theta toxins	Diarrhea, abdominal cramps, little or no fever, nausea vomiting are rare
Cereus food poisoning *Bacillus cereus*	It is ubiquitous in soil and in raw dried and processed foods. The spores can survive cooking and germinate and multiply when the food is held at favorable temperature	Emetic form 1–6 hours Diarrheal form 12–24 hours	Two forms of disease are there one is emetic form and other is diarrheal form	**Emetic form:** Upper GI sign and symptoms **Diarrheal form:** Diarrhea, abdominal pain, nausea with little or no vomiting, no fever

PARASITIC INFECTIONS

Amebiasis

- It is cause by the **protozoan parasite *Entamoeba histolytica.***
- Man is the only reservoir of infection.
- Period of communicability is as long as the cysts are excreted.
- Amebiasis is closely related to poor sanitation and socio economic status.
- Mode of transmission are fecal oral route, sexual transmission (oral-rectal contact) and vectors (such as flies, cockroaches and rodents are capable of carrying cyst and contaminating food and drink).
- Prevention measures are proper sanitation, water supply, food hygiene and health education.

Ascariasis

- It is an infection of the intestinal tract of adult caused by *Ascaris lumbricoides.*
- Mode of transmission is fecal-oral route.
- Preventive measure is proper sanitary, disposal of human excreta.

Hookworm (Infective Larvae)

- This can be defined as any infection caused by ***Ancylostoma duodenale* and *Necator americanus.*** Worms are mainly attached to the jejunum of intestine.
- Hook worm enter the body usually by penetrating the skin of feet.
- Mainly recommended antithelminthic agents for hook worm infestation are Albendazole, Mebendazole, Levimisole and Pyrantel.
- **Preventing measure:** To avoid walking bare foot.

Dracunculiasis

- It is also known as **guinea worm** disease.
- It is a vector borne parasitic disease mainly of subcutaneous tissue (usually leg and foot).
- Once the agent enters in the body, the gravid female makes its own way down to the infected person's lower limb and cause subsequent blister formation.
- Once this blister comes in contact with water it breaks and release up to 1 million parasites. These parasites are ingested by Cyclops. When person drink this contaminated water with cyclops, it can lead to the development of the disease, i.e., Cyclops dies in the stomach due to acid reaction and parasites are released into the gut.
- Mode of transmission is water, the person who drinks the contaminated water will develop the disease.

Practice Question

16. All of the following statements regarding hookworm infection is true, except:
a. Hookworm infection can cause pneumonia
b. Infective larvae enter the body by penetrating the skin
c. Hookworm infection is caused by Necator americanus
d. Hookworm infestation is diagnosed by finding the trophozoite in the stool

Ans. (d) Hookworm infestation is diagnosed by finding the trophozoite in the stool

Recent Question (NORCET 2022)

4. The antilarval method includes:
a. Rosemary
b. Citronella Geranium
c. Gambusia affinis
d. Malathion

Ans. (c) Gambusia affinis

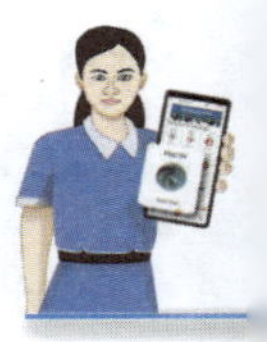

ARTHROPOD-BORNE INFECTIONS

Table 14: Diseases caused by arthropods

Arthropod	Disease transmitted
Mosquito	Malaria, filaria, viral encephalitis, dengue fever, West Nile, viral hemorrhagic fever (yellow fever, dengue)
Housefly	Typhoid and paratyphoid fever, diarrhea, dysentery, cholera, gastroenteritis, amebiasis, helminthic infestation, polio, conjunctivitis, trachoma, anthrax, yaw
Sandfly	Kala-azar, oriental sore, sandfly fever, oraya fever
Tsetse fly	Sleeping sickness
Louse	Epidemic typhus, relapsing fever, trench fever, pediculosis
Rat flea	Bubonic plague, endemic typhus, chiggerosis, *Hymenolepis diminuta*
Blackfly	Onchocerciasis
Reduviid bug	Chagas disease
Hard tick	Tick typhus, viral encephalitis, viral fever, viral hemorrhagic fever (kyasanur forest disease) tularemia, tick paralysis, human babesiosis
Soft tick	Q fever, relapsing fever
Trombiculid mite	Scrub typhus, rickettsial-pox
Itch mite	Scabies
Cyclops	Guinea worm disease, fish tapeworm
Cockroaches	Enteric pathogen

Dengue

The Dengue Syndrome

- **Classical dengue** or break bone fever is an acute viral infection caused by four serotypes (1, 2, 3 and 4) of dengue viruses.
- Mode of transmission is via ***Aedes aegypti* mosquito.**
- Reservoir of infection is both men and mosquito and transmission cycle is man-mosquito-man.
- The signs and symptoms are chills with high fever, intense headache, muscle and joint pain, retro-orbital pain, photophobia, extreme weakness, anorexia, constipation, altered taste sensation, abdominal tenderness, dragging pain in inguinal region, sore throat.

Dengue Hemorrhagic Fever (DHF)

This is a severe form of disease in which **person is affected with more than one type of dengue viruses.**

- It is also transmitted by ***Aedes aegypti.***
- **Sign and symptoms** are mainly high grade fever, facial flushing, headache, anorexia, vomiting, epigastric discomfort, tenderness in the right costal margin, generalized abdominal pain are common.

  Leucopenia: WBC ≤5000 cells/mm^3

  Thrombocytopenia: Platelet count <150000 cells/mm^3

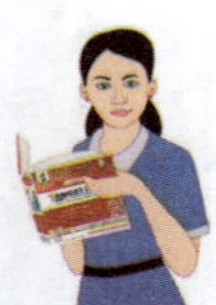

- The major pathological changes occur during DHF is plasma leakage and abnormal hemostasis manifested by raising hematocrit value and moderate to marked thrombocytopenia.

Clinical Criteria for Diagnosing DHF

- **Fever:** Acute, high, continuous lasting for 2–7 days.
- **Hemorrhagic manifestations:** Positive tourniquet test (more than 20 petachiae per 2.5 cm), petachiae, purpura, ecchymosis, epistaxis, gum bleeding, hematemesis, melena.
- **Enlargement of liver.**

Laboratory Findings

- Thrombocytopenia
- Hemoconcentration.

Dengue Shock Syndrome (DSS)

All the above clinical criteria and manifestation of shock such as rapid weak pulse, hypotension, presence of cold clammy skin and restlessness.

Treatment

Management is symptomatic and supportive. Bed rest, antipyretics, fluid and electrolyte maintenance are advised. Fluid replacement should be based on vitals monitoring and hematocrit values. Plasma transfusion is indicated.

Malaria

- Malaria is a protozoan infection caused by an organism known as ***Plasmodium.***

KEY POINTS

- Dengue viruses are spread to people through the bites of infected Aedes species mosquitoes (Ae. aegypti or Ae. albopictus).
- Thrombocytopenia is a common laboratory finding in dengue infection
- Severe Dengue is characterized by bleeding tendencies, organ dysfunction and capillary leakage.

Practice Question

17. Signs and symptoms manifested by a patient in the febrile phase of Dengue Fever is all, except:

a. Petechiae
b. High fever
c. Severe GI bleeding
d. Muscle aches

Ans. (c) Severe GI bleeding

- The vector of this condition is **female mosquito Anopheles.**
- Three distinct stages of infection are present in this case, they are **cold stage, hot stage** and **sweating stage.**
- **Agent:** *Plasmodium vivax, Plasmodium falciparum, Plasmodium malariae* and *Plasmodium ovale.*
- Malarial parasite undergoes two distinct stages of development, they are asexual cycle (human being) and sexual cycle (mosquito). Man is the intermediate host and mosquito is the definitive host.
- **Asexual life cycle (schizogony) in human being** has got phases, they are hepatic phase, erythrocyte phase and gametogany.
- Sexual life cycle is also known as **sporogony**.
- Newborn infant has high resistance to *P. falciparum* infection because of the high concentration of fetal hemoglobin.
- Individual with sickle cell trait has milder form of disease as compared to a person with normal hemoglobin.
- **Modes of transmission** are vector borne (transmitted by female anopheles mosquito), direct transmission (hypodermic intramuscular and intravenous injection of blood or plasma) and congenital malaria (newborn affected with malaria but it is very rare).
- **Incubation period** vary from species to species, *P. falciparum* [12 (9–14) days], *P. vivax* [14 (8–17) days], quartan malaria [28 (18–40) days] and for *P. ovale* [17 (16-18) days].
- **Cold stage (1/4 to 1 hour) sign and symptoms:** Headache, nausea, chilly sensation, vomiting, skin feels cold in the early part of disease. In hot stage (2–6 hour) patient feels burning hot spot, skin is dry to touch, headache, nausea, pulse and respiration become rapid. In **sweating stage (2–4 hours)** fever comes down, profuse sweating, skin is cool and moist, patient feel relieved and often falls asleep.
- **Complication associated with *P. falciparum* infection** are cerebral malaria, acute renal failure, liver damage, GI symptoms, dehydration, collapse, anemia, blackwater fever, etc.
- **Complications associated with *P. vivax, P. ovale, P. malariae*** are anemia, splenomegaly, enlargement of liver, herpes, renal complication etc.
- **Diagnosis** is based on blood film examination. **Thick and thin film.** Thick film is more reliable in searching for parasite, while thin film is more valuable in identifying the species.
- All fever cases should be investigated for malaria either by microscopy or by rapid diagnostic kit **(RDK)**
- First line **treatment** for malaria is choloroquine. In choloroquine resistant *P. falciparum* cases first line of treatment is **Artesunate combination therapy consisting of artesunate + sulphadoxine/sulphalene + pyrimethamine.** In case of resistant to all these drugs and to treat severe complicated cases **quinine** is the drug of choice.
- Chloroquine has fewer side effects such as nausea, vomiting, blurring of vision and headache. Person who all are exposed to large cumulative dose have been reported with retinal damage.

API → Annual parasite index

$$\text{API} = \frac{\text{Conformed cases during one year}}{\text{Population under surveillance}} \times 1000$$

Lymphatic Filariasis

- It means **infection caused by three nematodes namely W. bancrofti, B. malayi and B. timori.** All three infections are transmitted to man by the bite of infective mosquitoes.
- Microfilariae deposited near the site of puncture and they finally reach the lymphatic system.
- The objective of any lymphatic filariasis disability prevention program should be increased to access is hydrocelectomy.
- **Diethylcarbamazine (DEC)** is safe and effective and is the most widely accepted treatment of choice especially for Bancroftian filariasis.

Yellow Fever

- It is **caused** by an agent known as **Flavivirus fibricus** formerly classified as **group B arbovirus.**
- In forest region monkeys and forest mosquito act as reservoir of infection. In urban region the reservoir of infection is man and ***Aedes aegypti*** mosquitoes.
- Control of yellow fever in jungle region is not possible, virus maintain itself in the animal kingdom.
- Yellow fever in urban region can be controlled through rapid immunization of population at risk as well as vector control.

ZOONOSES

Rabies

- It is also known as **hydrophobia** affecting CNS and caused by **Lyssavirus type 1.**
- It is transmitted to man by bite or lick of animals.
- **Classical hydrophobia** is clinically characterized by long and variable incubation period, a short period of illness and encephalitis resulting in death of the person.

POINT TO REMEMBER

API ≥ per 1000 population per year have been classified as high risk areas in India, and eligible for vector control

KEY POINTS

- Chloroquine should not be given empty stomach.
- The life cycle of Plasmodium can be divided into two distinct phases: the asexual cycle in humans and the sexual cycle in mosquitoes.
- Blackwater fever (BWF) is a severe clinical manifestation of malaria, characterized by hemoglobinuria, intravascular hemolysis, and acute renal failure caused by *P. falciparum* infestation.
- Crescent-shaped or banana-shaped gametocytes are seen in infection with *P. falciparum*

KEY POINTS

Rabies is commonly known as hydrophobia because it induces a fear of water in the infected person. Those afflicted with rabies experience difficulties in drinking water due to this aversion.

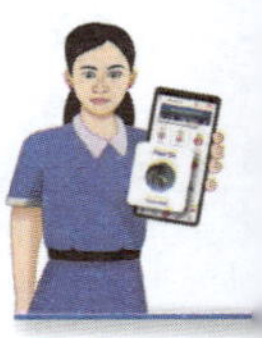

- All **warm** blooded animals including man are susceptible for disease.
- **Mode of transmission** are animal bite, licks, aerosols and person to person contact.
- Usual **incubation period** is 3–8 weeks following exposure.
- Rabies virus replicate at the site of introduction, connective tissue or muscles and enter the peripheral nerves and ascends towards CNS. Invasion of salivary gland is crucial for disease transmission of virus to another person.
- **Sign and symptoms** include headache, malaise, sore throat, slight fever, patient is intolerant to noise, bright light or a cold drought of air, aerophobia, spasm of pharyngeal and neck muscles, dilatation of pupil, increased perspiration, salivation, lacrimation, swallowing liquid become unsuccessful.

Currently we are using three type of vaccines and these are:

- **Nervous tissue vaccine:** It is developed from fixed virus grown in the brain of adult sheep or other animals.
- **Duck embryo vaccine:** Attempt is made to develop this vaccine in order to eliminate the neuroparalytic factors contained in the brain tissue vaccine.
- **Cell culture vaccine:** These are more potent and much safer than conventional brain tissue vaccine. Further immunization requires injection of smaller volume with relatively few side effects. These are of two type they are **human diploid cell vaccine** and second **generation tissue culture vaccine.**

Intramuscular Rabies Vaccine Schedule Recommended by WHO

The vaccine schedule recommended consists of 6 doses 1 mL each on day 0, 3, 7, 14 and 28. Booster dose is recommended on day 90. Injections are given intramuscularly on deltoid region not to be given in buttocks.

Reduced Multisite Intramuscular Regimen (2-1-1)

In this schedule first dose is given on right arm and left arm on day followed by one dose in the deltoid region via I/M route on day 7 and day 21.

Intradermal schedule: Two intradermal regimen are there, they are 2 site intradermal regimen and 8 site intradermal regimen.

2 Site Intradermal Regimen

This regimen endorsed by WHO expert committee on rabies. It consists of one dose (0.1 mL or 0.2 mL) of vaccine given at each of two sites on day 0, 3, 7 and one site on day 28 and 90.

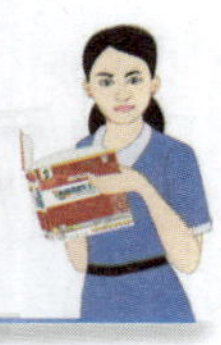

8 Site Intradermal Method

After reconstitution of vaccine 0.1 mL of reconstituted vaccine is given at each of 8 site using content of whole vial. Inject intradermally over deltoid, lateral thigh, suprascapular region and lower quadrant of abdomen. On day 7, 0.1 mL of vaccine is given at each of the 4 site over deltoid and thighs. On day 28 and 90, 0.1 mL of vaccine is given at one site over deltoid.

Brucellosis

- It is also known as **undulant fever**. It is occasionally transmitted to man by direct or indirect contact with infected animals.
- **Condition** is characterized by profuse sweating, arthritis and enlarged spleen.
- Causative organism is *B. meltensis*, *B. abortus*, *B. suis* and *B. canis*.
- **Main reservoir** of human infection are cattle, sheep, goats, swine, buffalo, horse and dogs.
- **Mode of transmission** are direct contact, food borne infection, air borne infection.
- **Incubation period** vary from 1–3 weeks.
- **Clinical manifestation** includes swinging pyrexia, sweating, arthralgia, lower back pain, headache, insomnia, splenomegaly, hepatomegaly, and leukopenia.

Leptospirosis

- It is considered as the most wide spread disease transmitted from animal to man.
- **Causative agent** is leptospira, it is excreted from the urine of infected animal for a long period of time.
- The organism is visible by dark field illumination and silver staining.
- Mode of transmission are direct contact, indirect contact and droplet infection.
- Diagnosis made by isolating the organism from blood and urine of infected person.
- Agglutination, indirect hemagglutination, Immunofluorescent antibody and ELISA **tests** are also available.
- Penicillin is the **drug of choice.**

LEPROSY (HANSEN'S DISEASE)

- Chronic infective disease caused by organism called as ***M. leprae.*** It affects mainly the **peripheral nerves** and also affects the skin, muscles, bones, testis and internal organ.
- **Two polar forms** of disease are lepromatous leprosy and tuberculoid leprosy.
- **Lazarine Leprosy:** Seen in association with **HIV**
- **Clinical characteristics** are hypopigmented patches, partial or total loss of cutaneous sensation, presence of thickened nerves, presence of acid fast bacilli in the skin and nasal smears.

KEY POINTS

- Death rate in Rabies is highest in children with 40% under the age of 15 years.
- Rabies vaccine is an inactivated vaccine, usually from the Wistar rabies strain.
- Adverse effect of Rabies vaccination are local redness, pain, headache and fever.
- Mass vaccination programs for Dogs is an effective public health measure. By vaccinating 70% of dogs actually breaks the transmission cycle.

Practice Question

18. All of the following statements regarding leptospirosis are correct, except:

a. It is zoonotic disease
b. Man is an accidental host
c. It is treated with doxycycline or penicillin
d. Bed bugs act as reservoirs of infection

Ans. (d) Bed bugs act as reservoirs of infection

KEY POINTS

- **Leprosy** is also known as **Hansen's disease**
- Multibacillary leprosy is diagnosed when there are more than 5 skin patches.
- New case detection rate is an indicator for incidence of leprosy
- **Dapsone** was the **first drug** discovered to treat **leprosy**.
- National Leprosy Control Program (NLCP) was launched by the Govt. of India in 1954-55.
- National Leprosy Eradication Program (NLEP) was introduced in 1983.

- The **signs** of advance disease include presence of nodules or lumps especially in the skin of face and ears; plantar ulcers, loss of fingers and toes, nasal depression, foot drop, claw toe and other deformities.
- **Agent:** *M. leprae*, an acid fast bacilli and occur in human host both intracellularly and extracellularly.
- **Sources of infection:** Man and wild animals.
- **Portal of exit:** Nose is the major portal of exit. Millions of *M. leprae* leased when patient sneeze or blow the nose.
- **Mode of transmission:** Droplet infection; contact transmission; other routes (transmitted by insect vector or by tattooing needles).
- **Incubation period:** 3–5 years or more for lepromatous cases.
- **Diagnosis:** Clinical examination (presence of hypopigmented patch with partial or total loss of sensation) bacteriological examination (skin smear, nasal smear or blow, nasal scraping).
- **Lepromin test**
  - 0.1 mL of lepromin into the inner aspect of the forearm
  - Read reaction at 48 hours and 21 days' interval. **Early Fernandez reaction** (leprosy) or **late Mitsuda reaction** (in tuberculoid form of leprosy) occurs in positive cases.
- **Treatment** is multidrug therapy. Till recently chemotherapy for leprosy has relied on **dapsone**.
- At present only small number of **drugs** are available and are Rifampicin, Dapsone, Clofazimine, Ethionamide and Prothionamide, quinolones, minocycline, clarithromycin.

TETANUS

- **Causative agent:** *Clostridium tetani,* gram positive aerobic, spore bearing organism.
- The spores are terminal and give organism a drum stick appearance.
- **Reservoir** of organism is soil and dust.
- **Incubation period** is 6–10 days.
- Tetanus bacilli produce exotoxin with astounding lethal capacity, it affects motor end plate of skeletal system, spinal cord, brain and sympathetic system.
- Infection is acquired by contamination of wound by spores.
- **Types of tetanus**
  - **Traumatic:** Major cause of tetanus.
  - **Puerperal:** Tetanus following abortion more frequently than normal labor.
  - **Otogenic:** It is a rare portal of entry, introduction of foreign material such as pencils, matches and beads may introduce infection.
  - **Idiopathic**: There is no definite history of any injury.
  - **Tetanus neonatorum:** The common route of infection is umbilical stem after birth. First symptom being seen by 7th day of life. Clean delivery and cord care will help to reduce the incidence of tetanus neonatorum in newborn baby.
  - **Prevention:** Active immunization with tetanus toxoid.

SEXUALLY TRANSMITTED DISEASES (STDs)

Table 15: Common sexually transmitted diseases and their pathogens

Pathogen	Disease or syndrome
Neisseria gonorrhoeae	Gonorrhea, urethritis, cervicitis, epididymitis, salpingitis, PID, neonatal conjunctivitis
Treponema pallidum	Syphilis
Haemophilus ducreyi	Chancroid
Chlamydia trachomatis	LGV, urethritis, cervicitis, proctitis, epididymitis, infant pneumonia, Reiter's syndrome, PID, neonatal conjunctivitis
Calymmatobacterium granulomatis	Donovanosis
Herpes simplex virus	Genital herpes
Hepatitis B virus	Acute and chronic hepatitis
Human papilloma virus	Genital and anal warts
HIV	AIDS
Molluscum contagiosum	Genital *Molluscum contagiosum*
Candida albicans	Vaginitis
Trichomonas vaginalis	Vaginitis

POINT TO REMEMBER

Only two states/UTs are yet to achieve Elimination of Leprosy - Chhattisgarh and Dadra and Nagar Haveli.

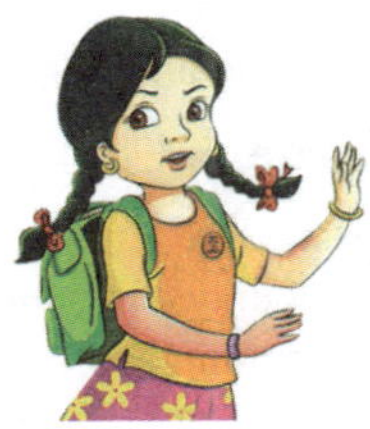

KEY POINTS

Recent Update on NLEP:

- **2019:** Convergence of leprosy screening with Rashtriya Bal Swasthya Karyakram (RBSK) to screen children (0-18 years) at Anganwadi Centers and Govt. schools.
- **2020:** Convergence of NLEP with Rashtriya Kishore Swasthya Karyakaram (RKSK) for counseling the children of teen age group (13-19 yrs) about leprosy at Adolescent Friendly Clinics
- **"Sapna"** is a concept (mascot) designed and developed using a common girl living in community, who will help spread awareness in the community about Leprosy, through key IEC messages. Sapna can be local school-going girl who is willing to be 'Sapna'. There can be any number of Sapnas in a village.

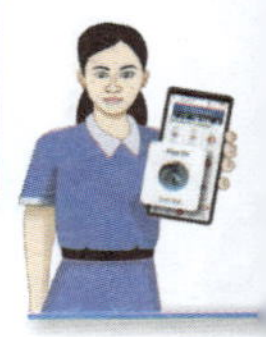

PURIFICATION OF WATER

Water purification can be done on large scale or small scale.

Purification of Water on Large Scale

Components include:

- Storage
- Filtration
- Disinfection.

Storage

- Water is drawn out from the source and impounded in natural or artificial reservoirs.
- Optimum period of storage: **10–14 days**
- **Advantages:** Storage provides a reserve of water from which further pollution is excluded.
- By mere storage, about 90% of suspended impurities settle down in 24 hours by gravity, the water becomes clear allowing penetration of light.
- Aerobic bacteria oxidize organic matter present in the water with the aid of dissolved oxygen. Free ammonia and nitrates drop.
- Pathogenic organisms eventually die out.
- Decrease in bacterial count by 90% within 5–7 days.
- If water is stored for long periods there is likelihood of development of algae which imparts foul odor and color to water.

Filtration

- Slow sand filters
- Rapid sand filters

Slow Sand Filters or Biological Filters

They consist of:

- Supernatant (raw) water
- A bed of graded sand
- An under-drainage system
- A system of filter control valves.

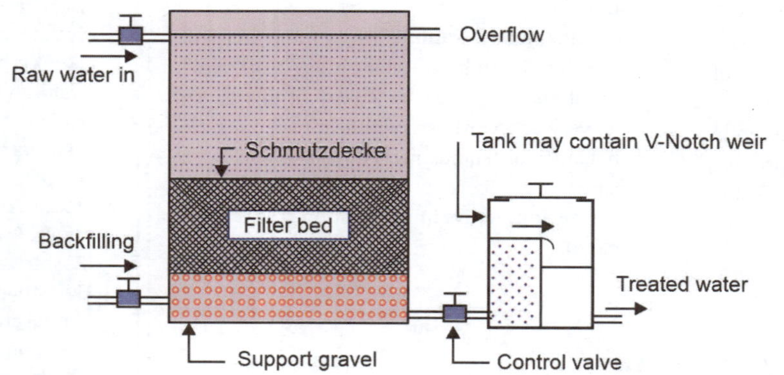

Figure 8: Slow sand filter

Supernatant water

- Depth: 1–1.5 meter
- Provides waiting period (3–12 hours) for raw water to undergo purification by sedimentation, oxidation and particle agglomeration.
- Level of supernatant is kept constant.

Sand bed

- Thickness: 1 meter
- Sand grains: Preferably rounded and have an effective diameter between 0.2 and 0.3 mm. Should be clean
- Sand bed is supported by layer of graded gravel. (30–40 cm deep)
- Water percolates slowly.
- Purification processes: mechanical straining, sedimentation, adsorption, oxidation, bacterial action.
- Rate of filtration: 0.1–0.4 m^3/h/sq. meter of sand bed surface.

KEY POINTS

- WHO recommended water requirement per capita per day is 50-100 liters.
- As per Ministry of Housing and Urban Affairs, India, **135 liter per capita per day** (lpcd) has been suggested as the benchmark for urban water supply.
- For rural areas, a minimum service delivery of 55 lpcd has been fixed under Jal Jeevan Mission.
- The nitrate concentration in domestic water supplies, is generally limited to 45 ppm.
- The hardness of natural water is generally caused by the bicarbonates and sulphates of calcium and magnesium
- Alum is a coagulant used to remove turbidity, color, and some bacteria from water.

Practice Question

19. The process of adding chlorine at intermediate points, usually at service reservoirs and booster pumping stations in water supply distribution is commonly referred to as:

a. Pre-chlorination
b. Post-chlorination
c. Re-chlorination
d. De-chlorination reservoirs of infection

Ans. (c) Re-chlorination

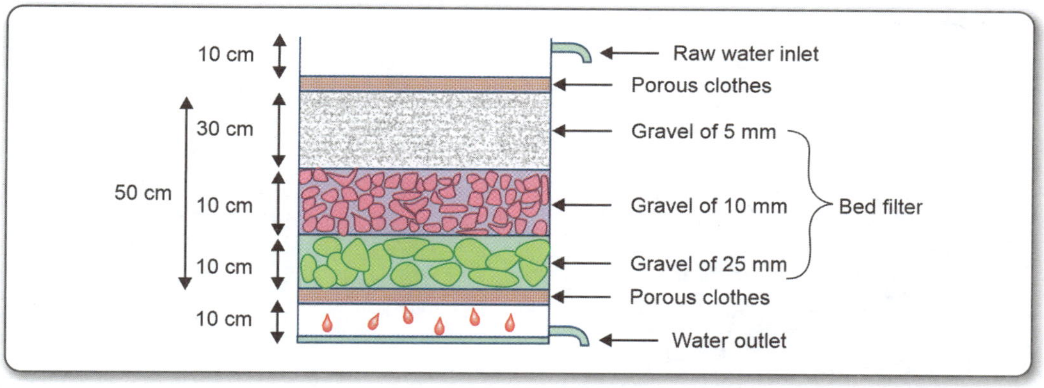

Figure 9: Sand bed

Vital Layer

- Schmutzdecke, zoogleal layer or biological layer
- Contains threadlike algae and numerous lifeforms like plankton, diatoms and bacteria.
- Process of formation called ripening of the filter. It takes several days to form.
- Extends 2–3 cm into top portion of sand bed.
- Removes organic matter, holds back bacteria, and oxidizes ammoniacal nitrogen into nitrates.

Under-drainage system

- Located at bottom of filter bed
- Consists of porous or perforated pipes.

Filter box

- Rectangular open box 2.5 to 4 m deep built wholly or partly below the ground.
- Supernatant water—1.5 m, Sand Bed—1.2 m, Gravel support—0.30 m, Filter Bottom—0.16 m

Filter control

- Venturi meter
- Measures bed resistance or "loss of head"
- When loss of head exceeds 1.3 meter, it is uneconomical to run the filter.

Advantages

- Simple to construct and operate
- Cost of operation is cheap
- Quality of filtered water is high
- Known to reduce bacterial counts by 99.9–99.99%

Rapid Sand Filters or Mechanical Filters

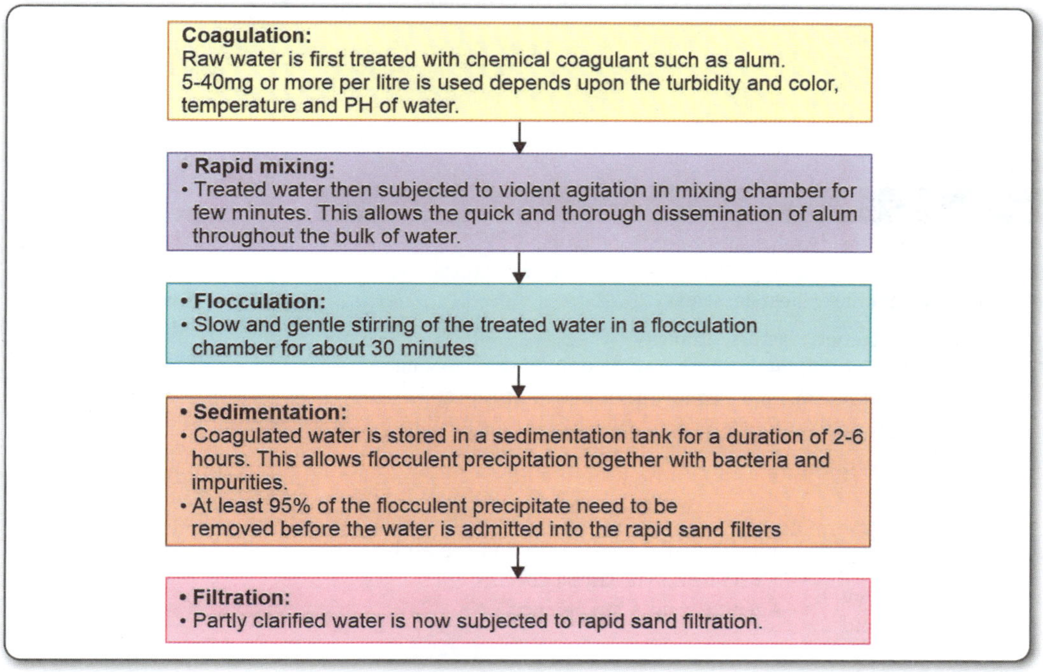

Figure 10: Steps of rapid sand filter

KEY POINTS

- **CO_2** dissolved in water is the most common cause of acidity in water.
- **Slow sand filter** removes about 98 to 99% of Bacteria.
- **Slow sand filter** removes turbidity to the extent of 50 PPM.
- **Filtration** is used to separate the solids from water. It does not disinfect the water.
- **Amount of chlorine** required for water disinfection is around **1–16 micrograms** per liter of water.
- **Zero hardness of water** is achieved by ion exchange method.
- **Ferric chloride, Aluminium chloride, Aluminium chlorohydrate, and Ferric and Ferrous sulfate** are the coagulants used for **sewage treatment**.
- Alum, Ferrous sulphate, Sodium aluminate, and Chlorinated ferrous sulfate are coagulants used for **water treatment**.

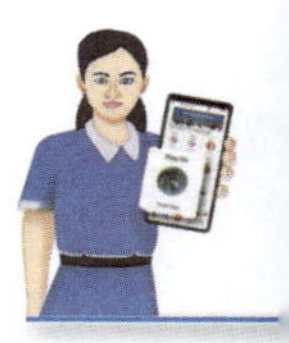

Steps Involved in Rapid Sand Filters

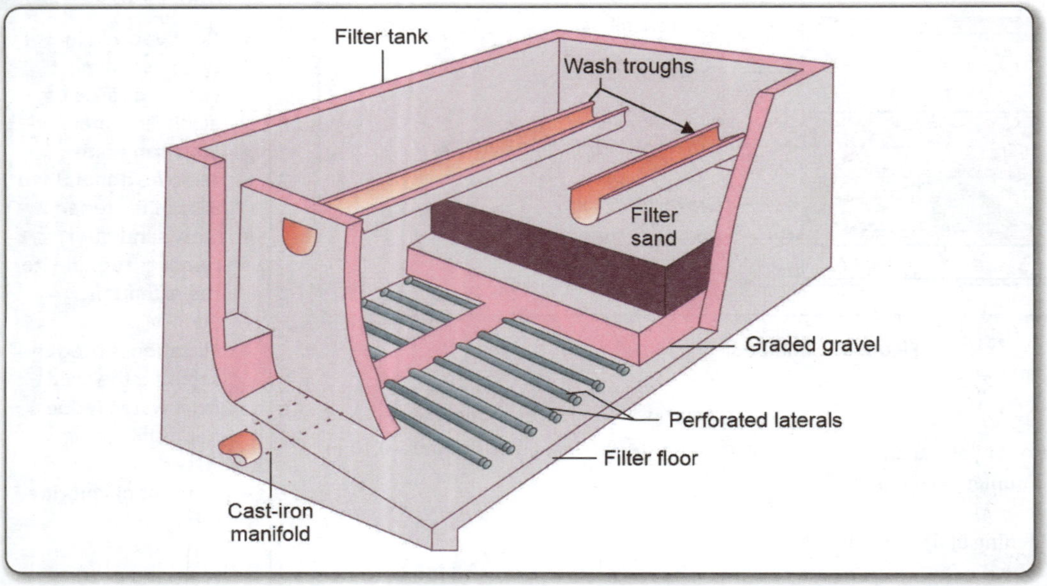

Figure 11: Rapid sand filter

Advantages of rapid sand filters:

- Can deal with raw water directly. No preliminary storage required
- Filter beds occupy less space
- **Filtration is rapid**: 40 – 50 times that of a slow sand filter
- Washing of filter is easy

Disinfection

Principles of Chlorination

- Water to be chlorinated should be free of turbidity
- Chlorine demand should be estimated: Chlorine demand = Amount of chlorine added – residual chlorine
- Point at which chlorine demand is met is called **break point chlorination**
- Contact period of at least one hour
- Minimum recommended concentration of free chlorine: 0.5 mg/L for one hour
- The sum of chlorine demand of specific water plus the free residual chlorine of 0.5 mg/L constitutes the correct dose of chlorine to be added.

> **KEY POINTS**
>
> **Chlorination:**
> - Hypochlorous acid & Hypochlorite ion are responsible for disinfectant action.
> - Recommended Free residual chlorine
>   0.5 ppm - Normally
>   0.7 ppm - Post disaster
>   1.0 ppm - Swimming pool
>   5.0 ppm - To prevent guinea worm infestation.
> - Chloroscope - Instrument used for measuring free residual chlorine.
> - Chloronome - Instrument used for disinfecting with chlorine gas
> - Horrock's Apparatus - For estimating chlorine demand.

> **KEY POINTS**
>
> - High amount of fluoride causes dental and skeletal fluorosis. The water safety limit is from 0.1 to 1.0 ppm.
> - The steps of large scale water purifications: **Storage → Filtration → Disinfection**
> - Residual Chlorine after chlorination of water should be greater than or equal to 0.5 mg/L (0.5 ppm) after 1 hour

NONCOMMUNICABLE DISEASE

Table 16: Few noncommunicable diseases

Disease	Risk factors
Coronary heart disease	**Non-modifiable:** Age, sex, family history, genetic factors, **Modifiable:** Cigarette smoking, high BP, elevated serum cholesterol level, diabetes, obesity, sedentary lifestyle, stress
Hypertension	**Non-modifiable:** Sex, genetic factors, ethnicity **Modifiable:** Obesity, high salt intake, increased amount of saturated fat, decreased dietary fiber intake, high alcohol intake, sedentary life style
Stroke	Hypertension, cardiac abnormality, diabetes, elevated blood lipid, glucose intolerance, obesity, smoking

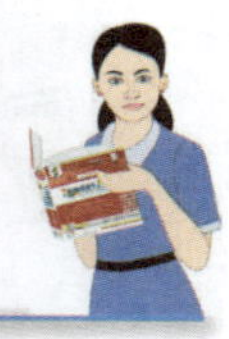

Rheumatic Heart Disease

- **Rheumatic fever:** It is a febrile disease affecting the connective tissue particularly in heart and joints initiated by the infection caused by group A beta hemolytic streptococci.
- **Agent:** Group A streptococci.

Clinical Manifestation

- **Major manifestations:** Carditis, polyarthritis, chorea, erythema marginatum, subcutaneous nodule.
- **Minor manifestations:** Fever, arthralgia, increased ESR and leukocyte count.
- **Lab studies:** Rising antistreptolysin O, streptococcal antibody, positive throat culture, recent scarlet fever.
- **ECG changes:** Prolonged PR interval.
- **Treatment:** Antibiotic management with penicillin group of drugs. If patient is having allergy to penicillin, then erythromycin is the drug of choice.

Cancer

- Cancer can be defined as uncontrolled growth of cells with the ability to invade adjacent tissues and even organ.
- **Causes of cancer**
  - **Environmental factors:** Tobacco, alcohol, dietary factors, occupational exposure, viruses, parasites (schistomiasis), custom habit and life style, others (sunlight, radiation, air and water pollution, medications)
  - **Genetic factors**
- **Treatment:** It is multi-modality approach, including radiation therapy, chemotherapy, surgical removal, etc.

Table 17: Cancer statistics in India/World

Gender	Category	India	World
Both sexes (overall)	**Most common cancer**	**Breast**	**Lung**
	Second most common cancer	**Cervix**	**Breast**
	Most common cancer deaths	**Breast**	**Lung**
Men	**Most common cancer**	**Lip/ Oral Cavity**	**Lung**
	Second most common cancer	**Lung**	**Prostate**
	Most common cancer deaths	**Lung**	**Lung**
Women	**Most common cancer**	**Breast**	**Breast**
	Second most common cancer	**Cervix/Uterus**	**Colorectum**
	Most common cancer deaths	Breast	Breast

Source: ICMR–National Institute of Cancer Prevention and Research, 2012 & World Cancer Research Fund International, 2012 and GLOBOCAN 2012.

Diabetes Mellitus

It is a heterogeneous group of disease characterized by hyperglycemia. The characteristic signs include 3Ps, i.e., Polyuria, Polydipsia and Polyphagia.

WHO Classification of Diabetes Mellitus

Diabetes mellitus (DM)

- Insulin dependent DM (IDDM)
- Non-insulin dependent DM (NIDDM)
- Malnutrition related DM (MRDM)
- Gestational DM (GDM)
- Other type (secondary to pancreatic, hormonal drug-induced, genetic and other abnormalities)
- Impaired glucose tolerance (IGT)

Table 18: Differences between Type I and Type II DM

Characteristics	Type 1 (IDDM)	Type 2 (NIDDM)
Age	<20 years	>45 years
Onset	Abrupt	Gradual
Sex	Male > female	Female > male
Family history	Sometimes	Frequently
Leukocyte antigen	Present	Not present
Presenting sign and symptoms	3P's (Polyuria, Polydipsia, Polyphagia)	Related to long-term complication
Weight	Underweight	Overweight
Serum insulin	Low to absent	High or low

Contd...

KEY POINTS

- Cancer is the **second leading cause of death globally**; nearly 1 in 6 deaths is caused due to cancer
- Freedom from cancer pain is now considered a right of cancer patient.
- Breast Cancer is the most common cancer in women (India and World).
- Lung cancer is the most common cancer among male worldwide.
- Lip/Oral cavity cancer is the most common cancer among male in India.
- Lung cancer is the most common cancer death in India and world.

KEY POINTS

The HbA1c test evaluates an individual's glucose control by showing the average blood sugar level over the past 90 days, presented as a percentage.

- **Normal:** Below 5.7%
- **Pre-diabetes:** 5.7%-6.4%
- **Diabetes:** 6.5% or higher

KEY POINTS

- Rotation of sites for insulin injection should be done every week or two.
- The injection site should be separated from one another by 2.5 cm (1 inch)

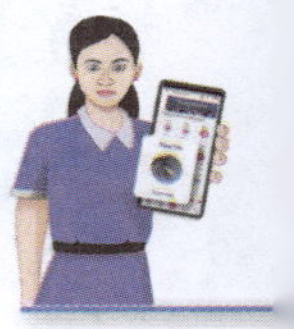

Characteristics	Type 1 (IDDM)	Type 2 (NIDDM)
Islet cell antibody	80–85%	<5%
Insulin need	Always	Sometimes
Oral hypoglycemic agent	Ineffective	Effective
Diet	Ineffective	Effective
Ketoacidosis	Common	Infrequent
Micro vascular complications	Rare at diagnosis	Present at the time of diagnosis

KEY POINT

Benedict's Test is a qualitative test that distinguishes between reducing and nonreducing carbohydrates. The reaction between benedict reagent and reducing sugar (glucose) in urine produces brick red color precipitation.

Urine Test for Diabetes Mellitus in Community

Benedict's Test

- Benedict's test is used to test for presence of glucose in Urine sample.
- Components of Benedict's solution: Anhydrous Sodium Carbonate, Sodium citrate, and Copper sulfate pentahydrate. The solution is **blue** in color.
- **Procedure:** 1 mL (8 drops) of urine sample is mixed with 5 mL of Benedict's solution in a test tube. The mixed solution is heated for 3 to 5 mins. Observe the color change in the solution of test tubes.
- **Interpretation**

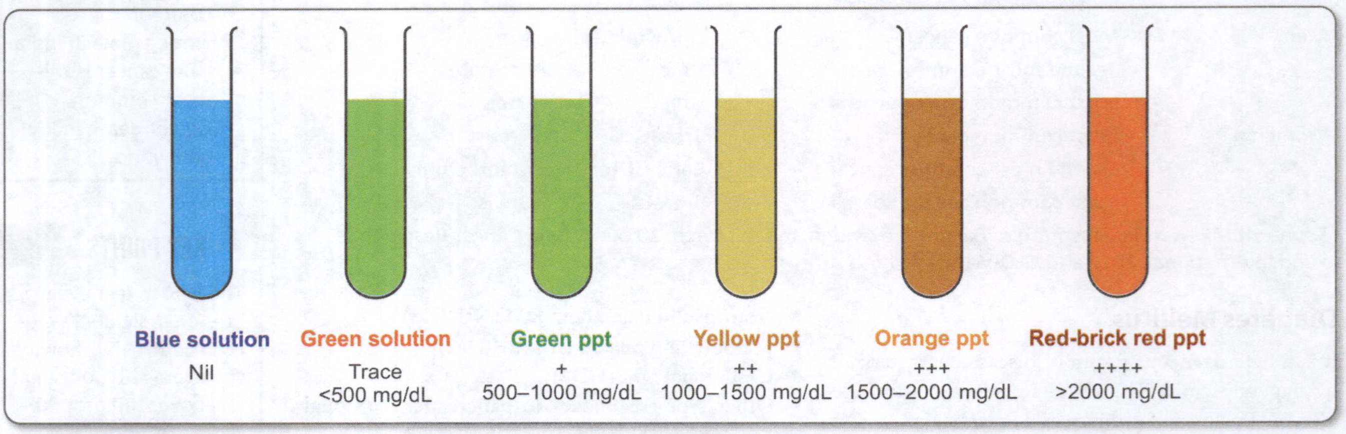

Figure 12: Benedict's test
(*Abbreviation*—ppt: precipitation)

Obesity

It is the abnormal growth of adipose tissue or an increase in fat cell number. Obesity is often expressed in terms of BMI.

BMI = weight in kilogram/(height in meter)^2

WHO Classification of BMI for Adult

Table 19: WHO classification of BMI for adult

Classification	BMI
Underweight	<18.50
Normal range	18.50–24.99
Overweight	≥25.00
Pre-obese	25.00-29.99
Obese class 1	30.00-34.99
Obese class 2	35.00-39.99
Obese class 3	≥40.00

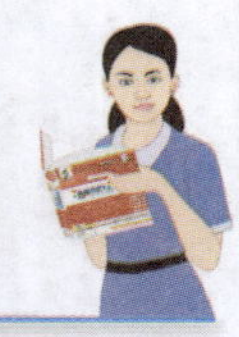

Broca Index (BI)

Broca Index is an estimation of ideal body weight using height measurement only.

BI = Height (cm) – 100

Blindness

Epidemiological Determinants

- **Age:** About 30% of the blind in India lost their vision before they reach the age of 20. Among these, majority are under 5 age-children.
- **Primary eye care:** Wide range of conditions can be treated or prevent at grass route level by locally trained primary healthcare workers. For this purpose, they are provided with essential drugs, topical tertracycline, vitamin A, eye bandages, shields etc.

KEY POINT

INDIA is the first country to start Blindness Control Program.

- **Secondary care:** Definitive management of common blindness causing conditions such as cataract, trichiasis, glaucoma, etc. This care is provided at PHC or district hospital where eye centers or eye clinics are established.
- **Tertiary care:** They provide sophisticated eye care such as retinal detachment surgery, corneal grafting, and other complex forms of care.

Specific Health Programs to Combat Blindness

- **Trachoma control:** Mass campaigns with topical tetracycline and improvement of socioeconomic conditions have markedly reduced the incidence severity of trachoma and associated bacterial conjunctival infection. The trachoma control program was launched in 1963 and later merged with national program for control of blindness.
- **School eye health services:** Students are taught about the importance of good posture, good lighting, avoidance of glare, proper distance and angle between books and eyes.
- **Vitamin A prophylaxis**
  - 1st Dose (1 mL or 1 lakh IU orally) is given at the completion of 9 months (with measles)
  - 2nd dose at 18 months (2 mL or 2 lakh IU orally)
  - 3rd dose to 9th dose: once every six months up to the age of 5 years (i.e., at 24, 30, 36, 42 and 48, 54, 60 months)
- **Occupational health services:** To prevent occupational eye hazards.

HEALTH PROGRAMS IN INDIA

Refer Appendices

DEMOGRAPHIC TRENDS IN INDIA

Sex ratio: The number of females per 1000 male.

Dependency ratio: Persons above 65 years of age and children below 15 years of age are considered as **dependent population.**

The dependency ratio can be further classified as **younger age (0–15) dependency ratio** and **older age (>65 years) dependency ratio.**

Density of population: Number of persons living per square kilometer.

Family size: It refer to the total number of persons in the family.

Life expectancy (expectation of life): At a given age it can be defined as the average number of years which a person of that age may expect to live, according to the mortality pattern prevalent in that country.

Fertility: It means the actual bearing of the children. Some demographers use the word natality instead of fertility.

KEY POINTS

- Census is done on 1st March at sunrise time.
- Sample registration system started in the Mid-1960s.

KEY POINT

Life expectancy for a child born in 2021 in India:
India's life expectancy is 69 years and 4 months. It is less than the world's average lifespan of 72.81 years.

POINT TO REMEMBER

Refer to Appendices for recent statistics

Demographic Cycle

Table 20: Five stages of demographic cycle

Stage	Birth Rate	Death Rate	Effect on population
First stage (High stationary)	**High**	**High**	Population stationary (India until 1920)
Second stage (Early expanding)	**Unchanged**	**Decline**	Population expands (Many Asian countries in this stage now)
Third stage (Late expanding)	**Begins to decline**	**Further declines**	Population Expands (slower than 2nd stage) (Currently, India is at this stage)
Fourth stage (Low stationary)	**Low**	**Low**	Stationary (European countries, e.g., Sweden, Belgium, Denmark, Switzerland)
Fifth Stage (Declining)	**Lower than death rate**	**Higher than birth rate**	Declining (East European countries, e.g., Germany, Hungary)

Fertility Related Statistics

Table 21: Fertility related indicators

Indicators	Definitions and formulae
Birth rate	Number of birth per 1000 estimated mid-year population in a given year. $\frac{\text{Number of live births during the year}}{\text{Estimated mid-year population}} \times 1000$

Contd...

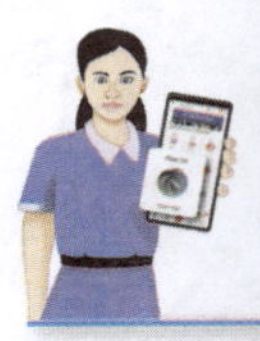

Indicators	Definitions and formulae
General fertility rate (GFR)	The number of live birth per 1000 women in the reproductive age group (15–44 or 49 years) in a given year. $$\frac{\text{Number of live births in an area during the year}}{\text{Mid-year population age 15–44 (or 49) in the same area in the same year}} \times 1000$$
General marital fertility rate	Number of live birth per 1000 married women in the reproductive age group (15–44 or 49) in a given year. $$\frac{\text{Number of live births in a year}}{\text{Mid-year married female population in the age group 15–49 years}} \times 1000$$
Age specific fertility rate	A more precise measure of fertility rate. Number of live birth in a year to 1000 women in any age specific group. $$\frac{\text{Number of live births in a particular age group}}{\text{Mid-year female population of same age group}} \times 1000$$
Age specific marital fertility rate	It is the number of live birth in a year to 1000 married women in any specified age group $$\frac{\text{Number of live births in a particular age group}}{\text{Mid-year married female population of the same age group}} \times 1000$$
Net reproduction rate	It is defined as the number of daughters, a new born girl will bear during her life-time, assuming fixed age specific fertility and mortality rate.
Child-women ratio	Ratio of children under 5 years per 1000 women of reproductive age (15–49 years).
Pregnancy rate	Ratio of number of pregnancies in a year to married women in the age of 15-44 (or 49) years. The number of pregnancies includes all live birth, still-birth or abortion or had not yet terminated.
Abortion rate	It is the annual number of all type of abortion, usually per 1000 women of childbearing age (usually defined as age of 15–49 years)
Abortion ratio	It is number of abortions performed during a particular time period by number of live birth over the same period.
Marriage rate	It is the number of adults getting married in a year per 1000 population
Crude marriage rate	$$\frac{\text{Number of marriages in a year}}{\text{Mid-year population}} \times 1000$$
General marriage	$$\frac{\text{Number of marriages within one year}}{\text{Number of unmarried persons of age 15–49}} \times 1000$$
Eligible couple	It refer to currently married couple where the wife is in the reproductive age, which is generally assumed to lie between the age of 15 and 49.
Couple protection rate	It is an indicator of contraceptive practices in the community. It is defined as the percentage of eligible couple effectively protected against child birth by one or the other approved method of family planning.

Vital Statistics

- Vital statistics provide crucial and critical information about the population in a country.

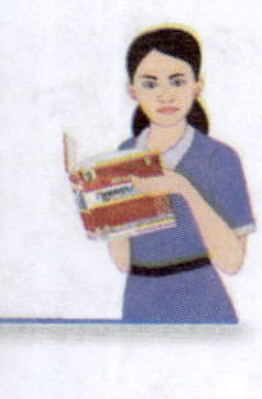

Sources of Vital Statistics in India

- Population Census
  - The population census in India is conducted **once in ten years**.
  - The Census of India 2011 was the **fifteenth census** in the continuous series from 1872.
  - Beginning in 1872 under **British Viceroy Lord Mayo**, the first complete census was taken in 1881
- Civil Registration System (CRS)
  - It is popularly known as birth and death registration system

KEY POINT

The **normal period of 21 days** (from the date of occurrence) has been prescribed for reporting the **birth, death and still birth events**.

- It is the recording of vital events i.e. Birth, Death & Still Birth under the statutory provisions
- CRS falls under the Concurrent list of the Constitution of India

- Sample Registration System (SRS)
  - The Office of Registrar General, India, initiated the sample registration of births and deaths in India popularly known as **Sample Registration System (SRS)** in **1964-65 on a pilot basis** and on **full scale from 1969-70.**
  - The main objective of SRS is to provide reliable estimates of birth rate, death rate and infant mortality rate at the natural division level for major States and at the State level for smaller States.
- Demographic Sample Surveys such as those conducted by the National Sample Surveys Organization (NSSO)
- Health Surveys

Statistics on Mortality Indicators (2020)

Mortality Indicators	Total	Rural	Urban
Crude Death Rate	6	6.4	5.1
Under-five Mortality Rate	32	36	21
Infant Mortality Rate	28	31	19
Neo-natal mortality rate	20	23	12
Peri-natal Mortality Rate	18	21	12
Still Birth Rate	3	4	3

Source: SRS Statistical Report (2020), Govt of India.

Indicator	State	Max./Min. Values	Values
Birth rate	Uttar Pradesh	Maximum	28.5
	Kerala	Minimum	11.4
Death rate	Chattisgarh	Maximum	8.5
	Jammu & Kashmir	Minimum	4.4
Infant mortality rate	Madhya Pradesh	Maximum	48
	Kerala	Minimum	6

Source: SRS Statistical Report (2020), Govt of India.

NATIONAL POPULATION POLICY 2000

- **India** launched family planning program in 1952
- The first **National Population Policy** was formulated and tabled in Parliament in **1976.**
- Population policy generally refers to the policies intended to decrease the birth rate and growth rate.
- **National population policy 2000**: Target free approach in administering family planning services.

CONTRACEPTIVE METHODS/ FAMILY PLANNING METHODS (FERTILITY REGULATION METHOD)

- Contraceptive methods refer to preventive measures which help the women avoid unwanted pregnancies and plan the wanted pregnancy.
- Broadly, contraceptive methods are classified into two types, i.e. Spacing method and Terminal Method.

Spacing Methods

- **Barrier methods**
  - Physical method (condom, diaphragm, female condom, vaginal sponge)
  - Chemical method
  - Combined method
- **Intrauterine devices** (lippes loop, Cu-T)
  - IUD mainly works by changing the intra-uterine environment and makes it spermicidal
  - Non-medicated IUDs cause a sterile inflammatory response to make it spermicidal
  - Copper containing IUDs release free copper that causes alteration in cervical mucus and endometrial secretions.
- **Hormonal methods**
  - Combined methods (MALA-N, MALA-D), **Progestogen** only pills, post-coital contraception, once a month pill, male pill.
  - Levonorgestrel tablets, 0.75 mg is a progestin-only emergency contraceptive pill used for prevention of pregnancy following unprotected intercourse
- **Miscellaneous**
  - Abstinence, coitus interruptus, safe period, natural family planning method).

KEY POINTS

- Sample Registration System (SRS) provides reliable estimates of birth rate, death rate and infant mortality rate.
- State of Uttar Pradesh has the highest birth rate (28.5) in India.
- * Highest infant mortality rate (IMR) is reported in Madhya Pradesh (48 per 1000 live birth)

POINT TO REMEMBER

India is the first country to start Family Planning Program.

KEY POINTS

- The contraceptive method that also offers protection against sexually-transmitted infection is Latex condom.
- Intrauterine devices (IUDs) insertion is scheduled within 7 days from the starting of period.
- **Excessive menstrual bleeding is the most common side effects of IUDs.**
- **The Pearl Index** is the measure of the safety of contraceptives. The smaller the Pearl Index, the safer the method of contraception. For example, Pearl Index 3 refers to 3 contraceptive failures out of 100 women using a specific contraceptive method.

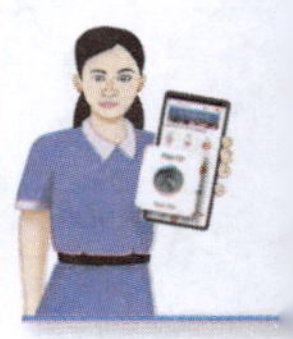

Terminal Methods

- Male sterilization (Vasectomy)
- Female sterilization (Tubectomy)

BARRIER METHODS

- The aim of barrier method is to prevent live sperm from meeting ovum.
- Barrier methods also provide some protection from sexually transmitted disease.

Physical methods: Condom, female condom, diaphragm, vaginal sponge

Condom

- Widely known as barrier technique for males
- In india it is the most popular by the trade name known as nirodh
- Condom will be fitted on erected penis before intercourse.

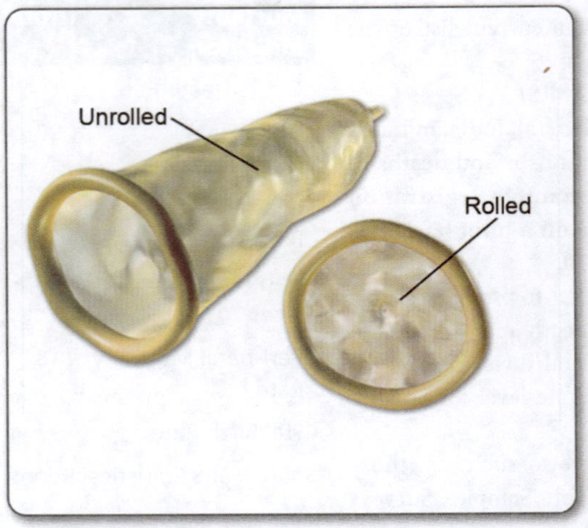

Advantages	Disadvantages
• Easily available • Safe and inexpensive • Easy to use, do not need medical supervision • No side effect • Light, compact and disposable • Provides protection against STD	• May slip off or tear during intercourse due to incorrect use. • Interfere with sex sensation

Female Condom

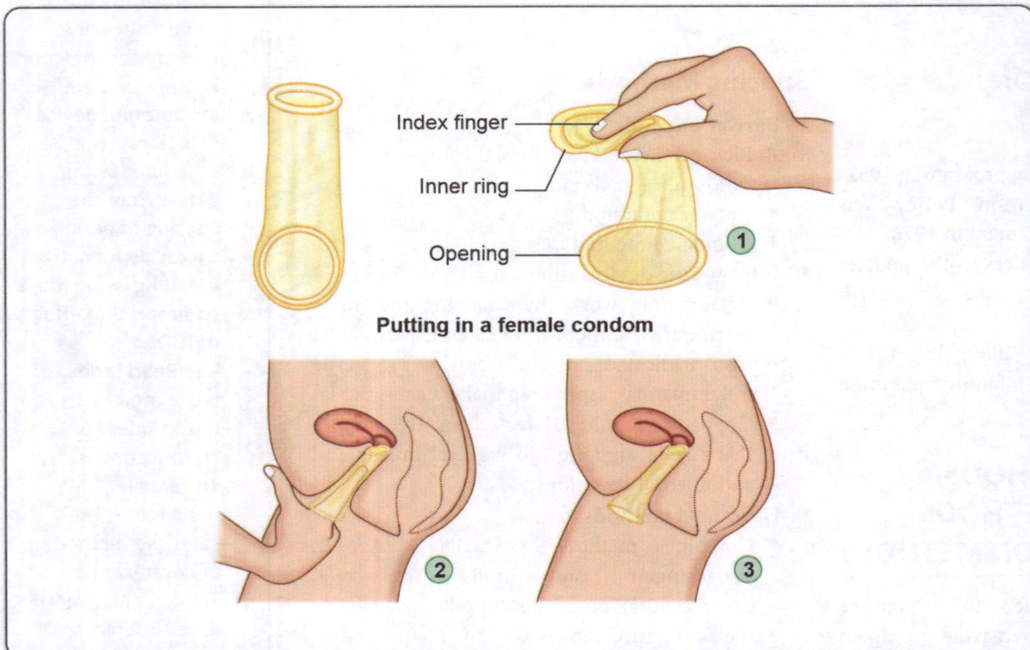

Putting in a female condom

- Female condom is a pouch made up of polyurethane which lines the vagina.
- Internal ring of the closed end covers cervix and external ring remains outside the vagina.
- It is prelubricated with silicon.

KEY POINTS

- Condoms are available in two main types: External condoms, also known as male condoms, which are worn over the penis, and Internal condoms, also known as female condoms, which are inserted into the vagina.
- Female condom is a sheath made of nitrile and is prelubricated with a silicone-based lubrica.

KEY POINTS

- Latex is the material commonly used in the production of most condoms; however, it can pose challenges for individuals with latex allergies or sensitivities.
- As an alternative to latex, polyurethane condoms are available.

Practice Question

20. The effectiveness of population control through birth control programs relies on:

a. Tubectomy
b. Vasectomy method
c. Proper use of contraceptive
d. The acceptance of the above methods by the population.

Ans. (d) The acceptance of the above methods by the population

Diaphragm

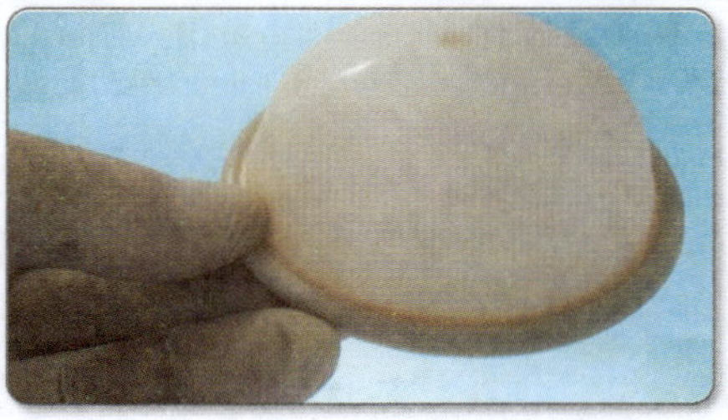

- Diaphragm is a vaginal barrier and is also known as **dutch cap**
- Diaphragm is a shallow cup made up of plastic or synthetic rubber.
- Its diameter ranges from 5 to 10 cm
- It has a flexible rim made up of spiral or metal.
- Diaphragm is held in place because of the spring tension and vaginal muscle tone.
- Diaphragm is inserted before sexual intercourse, and it remains in place for not less than 6 hours.
- Spermicide jelly is used always along with diaphragm.

Advantages	Disadvantages
There is no risk or medical contraindication associated with it	• Trained person is needed initially to demonstrate the technique of insertion. • After delivery it can be used only after involution of uterus is completed • Facilities for washing and storage is needed. • Since the diaphragm is left in vagina for an extended period of time, there is a chance for toxic shock syndrome.

Vaginal Sponge

- Vaginal sponge is marketed in the USA under the trade name of TODAY
- It is a small polyurethane foam sponge measuring 5 × 2.5 cm saturated with the spermicide nonoxynol-9.
- Sponge is less effective than diaphragm with a high failure rate.

Chemical Methods

It is of four categories

- Foam: foam tablets, foam aerosol
- Creams: jellies and pastes
- Suppositories
- Soluble films
  - Spermicide contains a base into which a spermicide is incorporated
  - The modern spermicides are surface active agents, which attach themselves to the spermatozoa and inhibit oxygen intake and kill them.
  - It has **high failure rate** and needs to be used immediately before sex and needs to be repeated after each sex.

Intra Uterine Devices (IUDs)

- IUD is a small device inserted into the uterus to prevent pregnancy.
- Mainly two types are there
  - Non-medicated and medicated
- Both are made up of polyethylene or other polymers.
- Medicated IUDs release either metal ion (copper) or hormone (progesterone).
- Non-medicated IUDs are **first generation**
- IUD which releases copper ion is **second generation**
- IUD which releases hormone is **third generation**
- Earlier in India under National Family Welfare Program, Cu-T-200B was used. From 2002 onward, Cu-T-380A has been added.

KEY POINTS

- Diaphragm must be left in place for six to eight hours after sexual intercourse and should then be removed.
- For women with a history of toxic shock syndrome (TSS), it is generally not recommended to use a diaphragm as a method of contraception.

KEY POINTS

- The cervical cap, known as FemCap made of silicone rubber, is offered in various sizes and is used similarly to a diaphragm.
- It is inserted over the cervix and contains spermicide. It can be left in place for up to 48 hours.
- Cervical cap may not be most suitable for women who have previously given birth because the shape of cervix may not offer secure fit for the cap.

First generation	Second generation	Third generation
Inert and non-medicated devices	IUD with copper.	Hormone releasing IUD
Lippes loop, spirals, coils, rings and bows	• Earlier devices ▪ Copper-7 ▪ Copper T-200 • Newer device ▪ Variants of T devices (Cu-T-220 C, Cu-T-380-A or Ag) ▪ Nova T ▪ Multiload devices (ML-Cu-250, ML-Cu-375)	• Progestasert is the widely using hormonal device. • It is T shaped and is filled with **38 mg of progesterone.** • This hormone is released at a rate of **65 mEg/day.** • It acts on uterine lining, cervical mucosa and sperms and prevent fertilization • Hormonal supply diminished over a period of time so regular replacement is needed.

Contd...

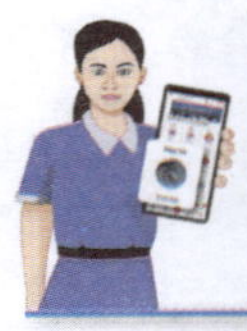

First generation	Second generation	Third generation
• Lippes loop contain small amount of barium sulfate to detect it in X-ray. • After insertion tail of Lippes loop made up of nylon projected outside vagina help us to ensure it in place. • It has 4 sizes. A, B, C and D, in which A is smallest and D is largest. • Larger Lippes loop has more anti-fertility effect and lower expulsion rate, but it has more side effect • Larger size suits multiparous women.	• The number in the name of each device indicated the surface area of copper in sq. mm on each device.	• LNG-20 or Mirena is an another third generation IUD which releases 20 mcg **levonorgestrel**. • Advantages of this type includes low menstrual blood flow and fewer days of bleeding.

Duration of use of IUD

Name of IUD	Duration
Lippes loop	As long as required
Cu-T-380-A or Ag	10 years
Cu-T-200	3 years
Nova T	3 years
ML-Cu-375	5 years
ML-Cu-250	3 years
Progesterone releasing IUD	Every year
Levonorgestrel IUD	7 years

KEY POINTS

Parts of IUCDs

1. T shaped (horizontal arm)
2. Progesterone or copper
3. Vertical stem
4. Suture or string or thread

Advantages and Disadvantages of IUDs

Advantages	Disadvantages
• Simplicity, easy to insert and no hospitalization required • Insertion takes only few minutes • Once inserted can be used for long duration • Inexpensive • Contraception is reversible by removing it	**Absolute contraindications** • Suspected pregnancy, pelvic inflammatory device, vaginal bleeding of undiagnosed etiology, cancer of genital organs, previous ectopic pregnancy **Relative contraindications** • Anemia, menorrhagia, history of pelvic inflammatory disease, purulent cervical discharge, distortion of uterine cavity due to congenital anomalies, fibroids and unmotivated person.

Recent Questions (NORCET 2021)

5. Cu-T is not inserted in:

a. Unexplained vaginal bleeding
b. Multiparous female
c. After delivery
d. Anemia

Ans. (a) Unexplained vaginal bleeding

6. The protection period provided by Cu-T 380 A is:

a. 10 years
b. 20 years
c. 15 years
d. 5 years

Ans. (a) 10 years

Timing of Insertion

- Best time for insertion is during menstruation or within 10 days of the beginning of menstrual period.
- Immediate postpartum insertion occurs within the first week of delivery before the woman leaves the hospital. It can be inserted within 48 hours following delivery.
- Post-puerperal insertion occurs 6-8 weeks following delivery.
- Post-placental insertion is done within 10 min after the expulsion of placenta.
- In LSCS deliveries, IUD can be inserted after removing the placenta.

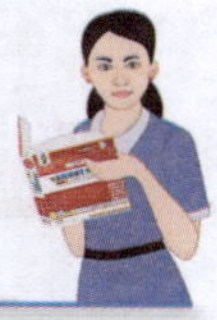

HORMONAL METHODS

- **Synthetic estrogen**: two synthetic estrogen are used in oral contraceptive.
  - Ethinyl-oestradiol
  - Mestranol.
- Mestranol is inactive until converted into ethinyl oestradiol in the liver.

KEY POINTS

- The most common complication associated with IUD is bleeding
- Second most common complication is pain and is the most common reason for removal of IUD before completing shelf life.

- **Synthetic progesterone** : they are of three types
  - **Pregnanes**
  - **Oestranes**
  - **Gonanes**

Classifications

Oral pills	Depot formulations
• Combined pill • Progesterone only pill • Post-coital pill • Once a month pill • Male pill	• Injectables • Subcutaneous implant • Vaginal ring

Combined Pills

- Combined Oral Contraceptive pills (COCs) contain low doses of two synthetic hormones progestin and an oestrogen.
- Combined pills are safe and effective.
- Non-contraceptive benefits- protection against endometrial and ovarian cancer, iron deficiency anemia, polycystic ovarian syndrome and endometriosis.
- It should not be given to breastfeeding women till 6 months postpartum.
- One pill is to be taken every day. For best results, a woman must take pills daily without any break (28 pills packet- 21 oral contraceptive pills and 7 iron tablets).
- Missing pills increases the risk of unwanted pregnancy.

Types of Pills

- Govt of India has made available two types of pills known as mala N and mala D.
- Mala -D is available to the consumer under social marketing at a price of Rs. 3 per packet. Mala-D was developed by CDRI, Dehradun.
- **Mala-N** is supplied through all PHCs, urban family welfare centers free of cost.
- These pills contain Levonorgestrel (0.15 mg) + Ethinyl estradiol (30 micrograms).

How to Use Combined pills?

- Start the combined pill on the first day of the menstrual period.
- One pill should be taken every day, even if there is no intercourse, until the pack is empty.
- 28-pill packs: When she finishes one pack, first pill from the next pack should be taken on the very next day.
- If she vomits within 2 hours of taking a pill, another pill from the pack should be taken as soon as possible and rest of the pills should be continued as scheduled.

KEY POINTS

- Pill should be taken everyday at a fixed time preferably before going to the bed.
- Pill should be started on 5th day of menstrual cycle
- If a woman forgets to take a pill, she should take it as soon as she remembers and continue the remaining pills at usual time.

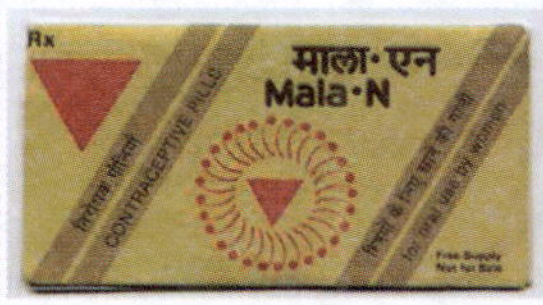

Male N

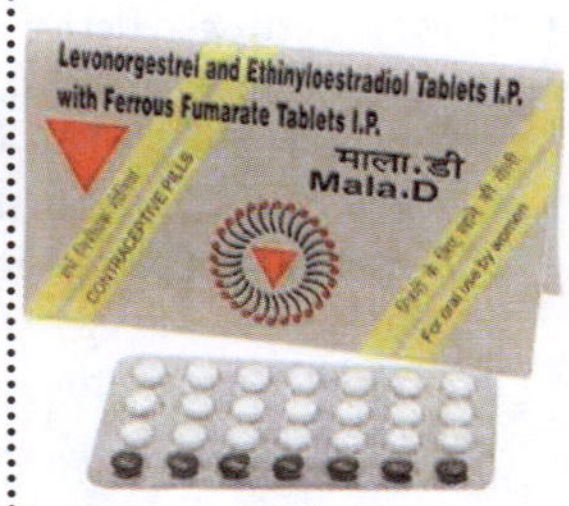

Male D

Problems Associated with Missing Pills

Missed pills	Management
Missed 1 or 2 pills/ started new pack 1 or 2 days late?	• Take one hormonal pill as soon as possible or two pills at scheduled time. • There is little or no risk of pregnancy.
Missed 3 or more pills in the first or second week/started new pack 3 or more days late?	• Take one hormonal pill as soon as possible and continue the scheduled pill. • Use a backup method for the next 7 days. • Also can consider taking ECPs, if she had sex in the past 72 hours.
Missed 3 or more pills in the third week?	• Take one hormonal pill as soon as possible and finish all hormonal pills in the pack as scheduled. Throw away the 7 non-hormonal pills in a 28-pill pack. • Start a new pack the next day. • Use a backup method for the next 7 days. • Also can consider taking ECPs, if she had sex in the past 72 hours.
Missed any nonhormonal pills? (last 7 pills in 28-pill pack)	• Discard the missed non-hormonal pill(s). • Keep taking Combined Oral Contraceptives, one each day. • Start the new pack as usual.
Severe vomiting or diarrhea	• If she vomits within 2 hours after taking a pill, she should take another pill from pack as soon as possible and continue taking the scheduled pills. • If she has vomiting or diarrhea for more than 2 days, follow instructions for 1 or 2 missed pills above.

KEY POINT

Oral contraceptives are the safest and reliable method for newly married couple

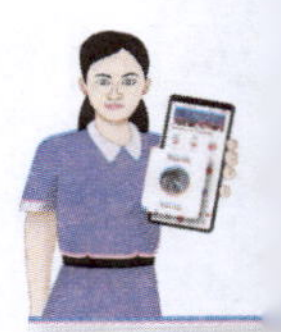

Progesterone Only Pills (POP)

- Also known as Progestin only pills contain very low doses of a synthetic hormone known as progestin which is like the natural hormone progesterone in a woman's body.
- POPs are also called Minipills or micropills.
- The available products are Levonorgestrol (LNG) and Desogestrel.
- POPs are safe and effective.
- In a women with regular period, it should be started in the first day of menstrual period.
- POPs are safe for breastfeeding women as they do not affect quality and quantity of milk.
- POPs can be started in breastfeeding women earlier than 6 weeks.
- One pill is to be taken every day at the same time without any break.
- One pill should be taken every day and at the same time until the pack is empty.
- It is very important to start the new pack on the next day at the same time.

Chhaya and Saheli

- Saheli is a non-steroid non-hormonal contraceptive composed with Ormeloxifene 30 mg.
- Saheli was developed by CDRI, Lucknow.
- It is available with the market name Centchroman-30
- These are estrogen derivative contraceptives
- For the first three months, tablet needs to be taken twice weekly followed by once per week.
- First pill taken on the first day of period. Second pill on 4th day of period and pattern of taking will continue.
- It acts by preventing the implantation of fertilized ovum.

Postcoital Contraception (Emergency Contraceptive Pills)

- It is also known as morning after pills
- These pills are usually indicated within 72 hours of unprotected sex.
- In India, levonorgestrel 0.75 mg tablet is approved for emergency contraception.
- Levonorgestrel 0.75 mg (two tablets): the first tablet should be taken as soon as possible within 72 hours of intercourse. The second tablet should be taken 12 hours later.
- Levonorgestrel 1.5 mg (one tablet): It should be taken as soon as possible within 72 hours after the unprotected sexual intercourse.
- Another method is mifepristone 10mg once within 72 hours.

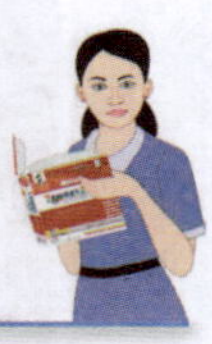

Once a Month Pill

- It is a long acting pill
- In this pill, a long acting estrogen known as quinestrol and a short acting progesterone are present.
- Disadvantages: High failure rate and irregular bleeding method.

Male Pill

- A male pill made up of gossypol—a derivative of cotton seed oil is effective in producing azoospermia or oligospemia.
- But 10% men after taking it for 6 months become permanently azoospermic.

DEPOT FORMULATIONS

Injectable Contraceptives

The injectable contraceptives contain synthetic hormones resembling the natural female hormones.

When administered (IM/SC) there is a slow release of hormone into the blood stream and it provides protection from pregnancy for a long time to the client.

There are two main types of injectable contraceptives:

1. Progestogen-only Injectables (POI) containing only synthetic progesterone. They are of two types:
   - **Depot Medroxy Progesterone Acetate (DMPA-IM)**
     - Dosage is 150 mg IM every 3 months.
     - Acts by suppressing ovulation, thickening of cervical mucosa and thinning of endometrial lining.
     - Initial dose should be given within the first 5 days of menstrual cycle.
     - Safe during breastfeeding
     - **DMPA-SC** – 3 monthly injection
       - Newer formulation injected Subcutaneously
       - Dosage is 104 mg every 3 months
   - **Norethisterone enanthate (NET-EN)**
     - Dosage is 200 mg IM every 2 months
     - Act by inhibiting ovulation and progestogenic effect of cervical mucosa
     - Initial dose within the first 5 days of menstrual cycle.
2. **Combined Injectables Contraceptive (CIC):**
   - These injectables contain a progesterone and an estrogen.
   - It is given at monthly interval plus or minus three days
   - It acts mainly by suppressing ovulation, thickening the cervical mucosa and makes endometrium unfavourable for implantation.
   - Not suitable for breastfeeding women until 6 months
   - Contraindications: confirmed or suspected pregnancy, thromboembolic disorders, cerebrovascular or coronary vascular diseases, focal migraine, malignancy of breast, diabetes with vascular complications

KEY POINTS

Chhaya/Saheli

CSIR-Central Drug Research Institute's (CSIR-CDRI) developed centchroman (ormeloxifene), which is nonhormonal (non-steroid based) in nature and is consumed once a week.

- This product is branded as Chhaya/ Saheli.
- CSIR claims that it is World's first non-steroidal birth control pill.
- It is free of cost.
- It is part of ASHA kit
- Each Chhaya packet contains 8 tablets.
- Tablet has to be taken twice in a week for first three months and then once in a week.

SUBDERMAL IMPLANTS

- Subdermal implants are inserted under the skin of the forearm or upper arm.
- Norplant is one of the subdermal implants.
- It has 6 silastic capsules. Each contains 35 mg of levonorgestrel.
- Another subdermal implant is norplant -2, it has 2 small rods with levonorgestrel
- These will provide contraception for 5 years.
- Insertion and removal require surgical procedure.
- Major disadvantage: irregularities with menstrual cycle.

VAGINAL RINGS

- Vaginal rings contain levonorgestrel.
- Hormone is slowly absorbed through the vaginal mucosa.
- The ring is worn in the vagina for 3 weeks and removed in the fourth week.

POST-CONCEPTIONAL METHODS

Menstrual Regulation

- It consists of aspiration of uterine content following 6-14 days of a missed period.
- Immediate complications are uterine perforation and trauma.
- Late complications are chance for abortion in future, premature labor, infertility, menstrual disorders, increased ectopic pregnancies, Rh isoimmunization.

How it differs from abortion

- It is performed in early weeks and certainty of pregnancy is not known.
- Lack of legal restrictions.
- Increased safety.

Menstrual induction

- This method is accompanied by the intrauterine application of prostaglandin solution.
- This will lead to contraction of uterus and bleeding which will last for 7–8 days.

Oral abortifacient

- Combination of mifepristone and misoprostol is used for this. Following are the regimen used for this:-
  - Mifepristone 200 mg given orally on day 1 followed by misoprostol 800 mcg given vaginally or orally. OR
  - Mifepristone 600 mg on day 1 followed by misoprostol 400 mcg on day 3.

Contraindications

- Allergy to prostaglandin
- Ectopic pregnancy
- IUD in place
- Hemorrhagic disorders
- Inherited porphyria
- Lack of access to medical care

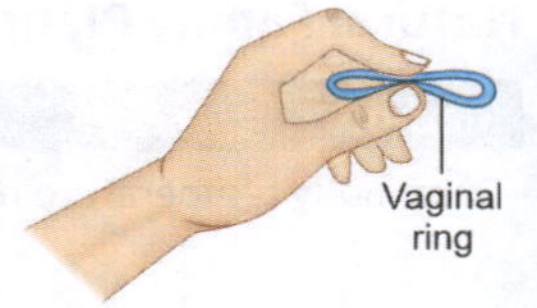

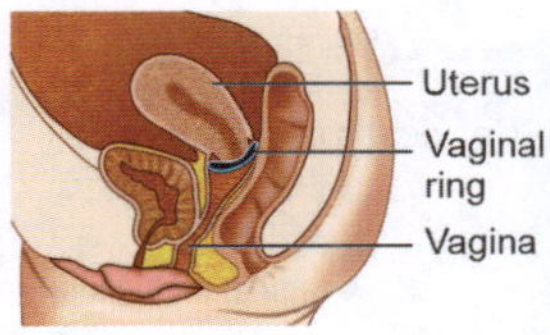

Chapter 4 Community Health Nursing

Practice Question

21. Which birth control method is based on calculating the ovulation period and avoiding sexual intercourse during the fertile window?

a. Coitus interruptus
b. Safe period (rhythm method)
c. Tubectomy
d. Vasectomy

Ans. (b) Safe period (rhythm method)

Other miscellaneous methods

Method	Description
Abstinence	• It means complete sexual abstinence for birth control.
Coitus interruptus	• In this method, the male withdraws before ejaculation and therefore, avoid deposition of semen into the vagina. • Main drawback of this method is precoital secretion of male that may contain sperm. • Slightest delay in withdrawal time may also lead to failure of this method.
Safe period (rhythm method)	• It is also known as calendar method. • First described in 1930 by Ogino. • This method is based upon ovulation. • Ovulation happens 12-16 days before next menstruation. • This method advises to NOT have sex during fertile period. • For a woman whose cycle length is between 28 and 35 days, fertile period can be calculated as follows. • Shortest length of cycle minus 18 (28–18 = 10 day) and longest length minus 10 (35–10 = 25). This means a woman should avoid sex between 10th to 25th day of her cycle, where the first day is the starting day of menstruation. • If the calculation is not possible, couple is advised to not have sex from 8th to 22nd day of menstruation. **Disadvantages** • Not possible for women with irregular menstrual cycle • Only possible for educated and responsible couple • High failure rate

KEY POINTS

- Mifepristone and Misoprostol are medications used together as a combination for medical abortion (nonsurgical abortion).
- They are used as oral abortifacients to terminate a pregnancy during its early stages.
- It is typically used within the first 10 weeks of gestation under medical supervision.

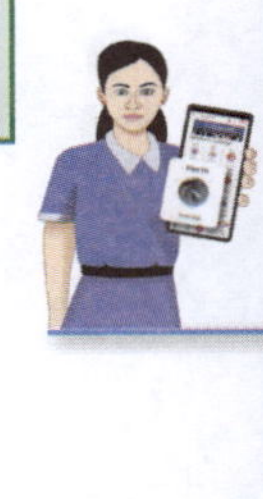

Natural Family Planning Methods

Method	Description
Basal body temperature method	• This is based upon the elevation of body temperature during ovulation. • This elevation of temperature occurs due to hormone progesterone • Elevation is very minimal and is about 0.3°–0.5°C
Cervical mucus method	• It is also known as billing method or ovulation method. • This is based upon the changes happening to cervical mucosa at the time of ovulation. • During ovulation time, cervical mucosa becomes watery clear, resembling egg white, smooth, slippery and profuse. • Due to the effect of increased progesterone after ovulation mucosa becomes thick. • Women should have adequate knowledge regarding different types of cervical mucosa to practice this method.
Symptothermal method	• This method is a combination of temperature, cervical mucosa and calendar technique to identify the fertile period.
Breast feeding	• Lactation prolongs postpartum amenorrhea and provides some degree of protection.
Birth control vaccine	• Immunization with human chorionic gonadotropin prevents pregnancy.

Terminal Methods

- It is also known as sterilization
- It is provided free of cost in government institutions in India

Guidelines

- Age of husband should be between 25 to 50 years
- Age of wife should be between 20 and 45 years
- Motivated couple should have 2 children at the time of sterilization procedure.
- If couple has 3 or more living children, then the lower age limit for husband and wife may be relaxed by the operating surgeon.
- Spouse should give consent

Male Sterilization

- Male sterilization is known as vasectomy.
- It is performed by any trained doctor under local anesthesia, it can be even done at PHC
- A piece of vas deference is removed, and end is folded back and stitched in such a way that cut ends face away from each other. (To reduce the risk of recanalization).
- Following surgery, sperm and hormone production are not going to be affected.
- The sperm produced are destroyed after the surgery through phagocytosis

No-Scalpel Vasectomy

- No-scalpel vasectomy is also known as key-hole vasectomy.
- In this male sterilization procedure, no incisions will be made on the skin. Hemostatic clamp will be used to puncture the scrotal sac and then vas will be clamped.
- This program is funded by UNFPA.

Conventional Vasectomy: an incision is made on each side of the scrotum to access the vas deferens, and then the tubes are cut and sealed to achieve male sterilization.

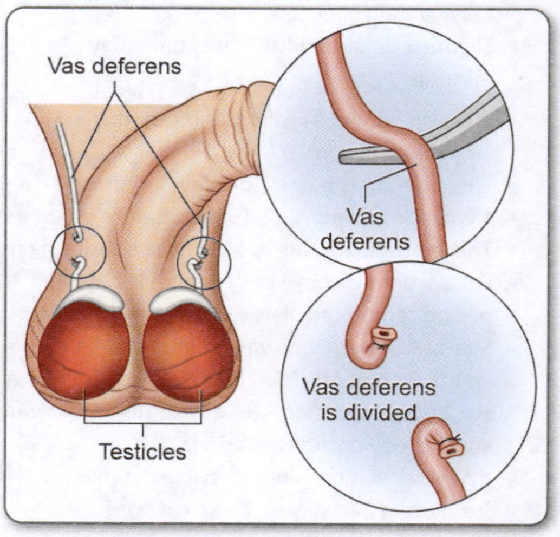

Figure 13: Vasectomy

Recent Question

7. What is the fertile period in the rhythm method (calendar method) of contraception for a woman with a menstrual cycle between 26 to 33 days?

a. 10th to 25th day of her cycle
b. 8th to 23rd day of her cycle
c. 12th to 23rd day of her cycle
d. 14th to 24th day of her cycle

Ans. (b) 8th to 23rd day...

The fertile period in the rhythm method (calendar method) is determined based on the estimated ovulation time. For a woman with a menstrual cycle length between 26 to 33 days, the shortest length of the cycle is subtracted by 18, and the longest length is subtracted by 10 to calculate the fertile period. In this case, the calculation would be 26 - 18 = 8 and 33 - 10 = 23. Therefore, the couple is advised to avoid sexual intercourse between the 8th and 23rd day of the woman's menstrual cycle. This is considered the fertile period in the rhythm method for this specific cycle length range.

KEY POINTS

- **Spontaneous recanalization:** vas deferens may join together and form re-canal after the surgery.
- Client does not become sterile immediately after surgery. It takes 30 more ejaculations to become sterile. Additional contraceptive method is advised for 3 months.
- Avoid cycling and heavy lifting for 2 weeks after surgery, complete bed rest is not needed
- Stiches will be removed on 5th post operative day.

Female Sterilization

- In female sterilization, fallopian tubes are occluded.
- Mainly two types are there
    - Laparoscopy
    - Minilap operation

Laparoscopy

- Female sterilization is done through abdominal approach using laparoscope.
- Falope rings are applied to occlude the tube.

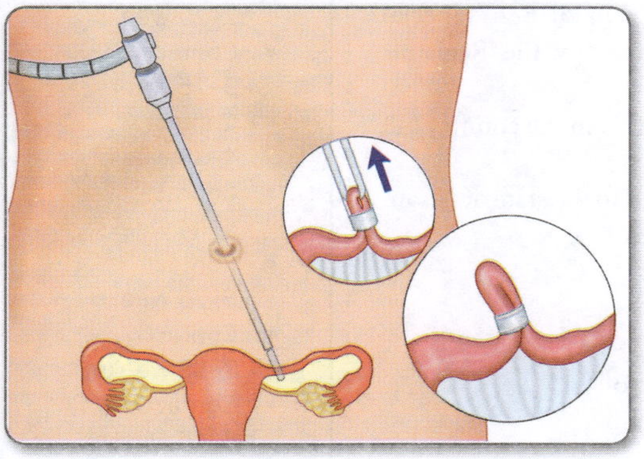

Figure 14: Laparoscopic tubectomy (Falope rings inside)

Minilap Operation

Minilap operation is done under local anesthesia and by creating small incision on the abdomen. In this also, fallopian tube will be clamped.

Pearl index

- Pearl index is a method used to calculate the effectiveness of contraceptive method.
- When the Pearl index is below 10, the effectiveness of particular method is high and when it is more than 20, the effectiveness of method is low.

PRENATAL ADVICE

- **Diet:** On an average normal healthy women gain weight of 10–12 kg during pregnancy
    - Calorie requirement
        - Pregnant women require an additional 300 kcal/day
        - 1800 calories per day during the first trimester
        - 2200 calories per day during second trimester
        - 2400 calories per day during third trimester
    - Iron and folic acid (for 100 days starting from 14-16 weeks of pregnancy)
        - Iron – 100 mg/day
        - Folic acid – 500 mcg/day
- **Personal hygiene:** Personal cleanliness, sleep (8 hours/day at least 2 hours after meal) quit smoking and alcohol, good oral care, sexual intercourse should be restricted especially during the last **trimester.**
- **Drugs:** Without any prescription from doctor, medication intake should be restricted to all pregnant women.
- **Radiation:** Exposure to radiation is dangerous for fetus. Exposure to radiation should be avoided during the pregnancy.
- **Warning signs:** Swelling of the feet, fits, headache, blurring of vision, bleeding or discharge from vagina.
- **Child care:** Advice regarding care of child, nutritional mainte-nance, etc.

Calculation of number of expected pregnancies per year

Expected no of live birth/year (Y) =

$$\frac{\text{Birth rate per 1000 population} \times \text{Population (size) of the area}}{1000}$$

The total number of expected pregnancies (Z) = Y + 10% of Y

Calculation of expected date of delivery (EDD)

Naegele's rule: It is a standard way of calculating EDD for a pregnancy.

EDD: First day of last menstrual cycle + 9 months + 7 days.

INTRANATAL CARE

5Cs

- Clean surface
- Clean hands
- Clean cord cut (blade)
- Clean cord tie
- Clean cord stump

MOTHER AND CHILD HEALTH (MCH)

The main aim is to provide care to vulnerable population (children <5 years and women in the reproductive age group 15–44) in order to decrease the disability and death.

- Components of MCH include:
    - Maternal health
    - Family planning
    - Child health
    - School health
    - Handicapped children.
    - Care of children in special setting such as day care centers.

Recent Question

8. An incision made on each side of the scrotum to reach the vas deferens in vasectomy procedure is called

a. No-scalpel vasectomy
b. Scalpel vasectomy
c. Conventional vasectomy
d. Non-conventional vasectomy

Ans. (c) Conventional vasectomy

POINT TO REMEMBER

Emergency contraception: Two dose regimen - Levonorgestrel tablets, 0.75 mg is taken as soon as possible within 72 hours of unprotected intercourse, with a second 0.75 mg dose taken 12 hours later.
Single dose regimen - 1.5 mg of levonorgesterol within 24 hours to 72 hours of unprotected intercourse.

KEY POINT

Current infant mortality rate (NFHS-5 2019-2021) is 35.2 per 1000 live birth

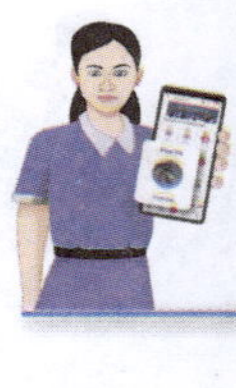

Chapter 4 Community Health Nursing

Recent Trends in MCH Services

- Integration of care
- Risk approach
- Manpower changes
- Primary healthcare

Indicators of MCH Services

- Maternal mortality rate
- Mortality in infancy and childhood
  - Perinatal mortality
  - Neonatal mortality
  - Post neonatal mortality
  - Infant mortality
  - 1-4 year mortality rate
  - Under 5 mortality rate
  - Child survival rate

Infant Mortality Rate (as per NFHS-5 2019-2021)

- Infant Mortality Rate (IMR) in India is 35.2 per 1000 live births.
- The maximum IMR has been reported for Madhya Pradesh (48) and the minimum for Nagaland (4).

Source: Sample Registration System Bulletin, 2020.

Maternal Mortality Rate (MMR) (as per 2018 Sample Registration System)

- Maternal Mortality Rate (MMR) in India
  - 130 per 100,000 live births in 2014-16.
  - 113 per 100,000 live births in 2016-18 (SRS, Govt of India)
  - 97 per 100,000 live births in 2018-20 (Special Bulletin on MMR released by the Registrar General of India)
- Kerala Registered lowest MMR in the country (43 per 1,00,000 live births)
- Highest MMR was registered in the state of Assam (215 per 1,00,000 live births)

$$\textbf{Maternal mortality rate} = \frac{\text{Total number of female deaths due to complications of pregnancy/childbirth within 42 days of delivery from puerperal causes in an area during a given year}}{\text{Total number of live birth in the same area and year}} \times 1{,}00{,}000$$

Universal Children's Day

November 14 is observed as universal children's day. It was started by UNICEF and international Union for Child Welfare. In 1954, the UN Assembly passed the formal declaration.

Table 22: Some important policies related to children and year of implementation

Year	Policy
1974	National Policy for Children
1986	National Policy on Education
1979	The National Children's Fund
2002	National Health Policy
2003	National Charter for Children
2005	Commission for the Protection of Child Right Act
2005	National Plan of Action for Children

REPRODUCTIVE CHILD HEALTH PROGRAM (RCH)

Historical Background

- 1952: National Family Planning Program
- 1977: National Family Welfare Program
- 1985: Universal Immunization Program
- 1992: Child Survival and Safe Motherhood Program
- 1997: RCH–Phase I
- 2005: RCH–Phase II

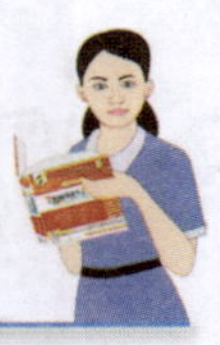

KEY POINTS

- WHO Antental Care Models (ANC) recommends minimum of 8 antenatal contacts to reduce perinatal mortality.
  - Contact 1- up to 12 weeks
  - Contact 2–20 weeks
  - Contact 3–26 weeks
  - Contact 4–30 weeks
  - Contact 5–34 weeks
  - Contact 6–36 weeks
  - Contact 7–38 weeks
  - Contact 8–40 weeks
- SDG set by United Nations aims at reducing the global maternal mortality ratio to less than 70 per 100,000 live births.
- Five states [Kerala (43), Maharashtra (46), Tamil Nadu (60), Telangana (63) and Andhra Pradesh (65)] have already achieved the target of SDG on MMR.
- The **Ujjawala Scheme** was launched in 2007 to prevent trafficking of children and women.
- The objective of the Ujjawala scheme is to prevent, rescue, rehabilitate, reintegrate, and repatriate victims trafficked for commercial sexual exploitation.

Components of RCH

There are 4 components of RCH Phase I as follows:

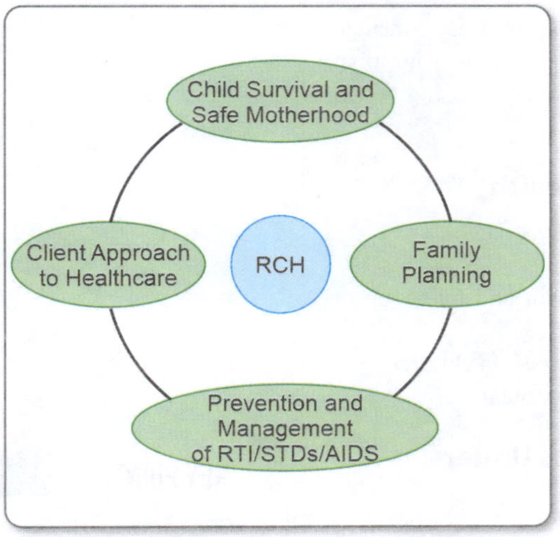

Figure 15: Components of RCH

- **RCH–Phase I**
  - Year of establishment: 15.10.1997
  - Focused on 4 components
- **RCH–Phase II**
  - Started in 1st April 2005
  - Focus on reducing neonatal and child mortality and morbidity
  - Emphasis on rural healthcare
- **Components (3 Es)**
  - Essential obstetric care
  - Emergency obstetric care (EmOC)
  - Emphasis on strengthening of referral system

New Initiatives Under RCH

1. Training of MBBS doctors in life saving anesthetic skills for emergency obstetric care
2. Setting up of blood storage centers at FRUs
3. **Janani Suraksha Yojana (JSY):** Free of cost institutional delivery
4. **Vandemataram Scheme:** Provision of safe motherhood service free of cost
5. Safe abortion services
6. Integrated Management of Neonatal and Childhood Illness (IMNCI)
7. Janani Shishu Suraksha Karyakaram (JSSK) (2011)
8. Child health components–newborn care is given in table as follows:

Table 23: Newborn care

Health facility	All newborns at birth	Sick newborn
PHC/SC	Newborn Care Corner (NBCC) in labor room	Prompt referral
CHC/FRU	Newborn Care Corner CR labor room and in OT	Newborn stabilization Unit (NBSU)
District hospital	Newborn Care Corner CR labor room and in OT	Special newborn care unit (SNCU)

9. Navjat Shishu Suraksha Karyakram (NSSK, 2009): Training of health personnel in basic newborn care and resuscitation.
10. Rashtriya Bal Swasthya Karyakram (RBSK 2013): Focus on early detection of 4 D and its management
    - Defects at birth
    - Diseases in children
    - Deficiency conditions
    - Development delays
11. **RMNCH + A:** Reproductive, Maternal, Newborn Child and Adolescent health (2013). 12th Five Year Plan Initiative.
12. **India Newborn Action Plan (INAP, 2004):** Focus on single digit neonatal mortality

RCH Package

- For mother
  - Early registration, vaccination, Iron and folic acid, institutional delivery, emergency management, referral and transport
- For Children
  - Essential newborn care, exclusive breast feeding, growth monitoring, immunization, vitamin A prophylaxis, Oral Rehydration Therapy, Treatment of anemia, Management of diarrhea and Respiratory Tract infections
- For eligible couples
  - Availability of contraceptive methods, safe MTP services
- Other services
  - Management of RTIs and STIs, Adolescent health, women empowerment gender equity, male participation

UNDER 5 CLINIC

Under 5 clinic is a center, where preventive, promotive curative, referral and educational service are provided to under 5 children under one roof.

Practice Question

22. All of the following are the essential components of RCH Program in India, except:

a. Reduce the under-five mortality to half
b. Maternal care including antenatal delivery & post-natal services
c. Safe abortion service
d. Management of STDs

Ans. (a) Reduce the under-five mortality to half

KEY POINTS

- Janani Suraksha Yojana is a centrally funded scheme launched in 2005.
- JSY aims at lowering maternal mortality and infant mortality by **encouraging institutional deliveries.**
- Janani Shishu Suraksha Karyakaram (JSSK) is an initiative to provide completely **free and cashless services** to pregnant women including normal deliveries and cesarean operations and sick new born (up to 30 days after birth) in Government health institutions in both rural & urban areas.

POINT TO REMEMBER

Under Five Clinics are also known as Growth and Development Clinics

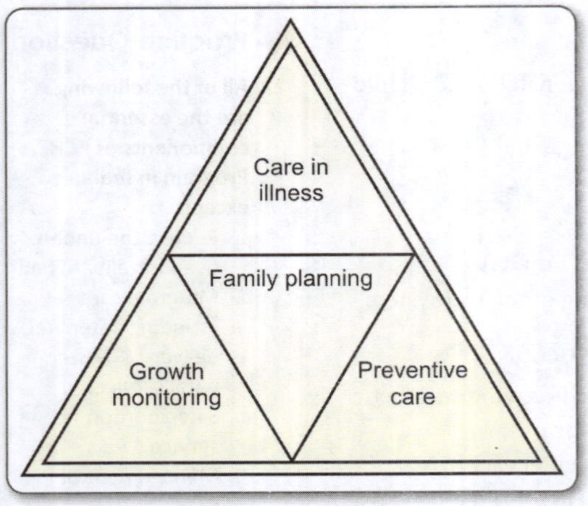

Figure 16: Component of under 5 Clinic

Functions/Components

- Care in illness
- Growth monitoring
- Preventive care
- Family planning
- Health education

UNICEF's GOBI – FFF Programs

G – Growth monitoring
O – Oral rehydration
B – Breastfeeding
I – Immunization
F – Family planning
F – Female education
F – Food supplements

SCHOOL HEALTH SERVICES

- School health services refer to the need based comprehensive services rendered to pupil, teachers and other personnel in the school to promote, protect their health, prevent and control diseases and maintain their health.
- Main school health problems include malnutrition, infectious diseases, intestinal parasite, diseases of skin, eye and ear and dental caries.

Objectives of School Health

- Promotion of positive health
- Prevention of disease
- Early diagnosis and treatment and follow-up of defects
- Awakening health consciousness in children
- Provision of healthful environment

School Health Programs Under Ayushman Bharat

Weekly

- Classroom transaction by health and wellness ambassadors
- Administration of IFA tablets

Fortnightly/Monthly

- Thematic school assembly
- Question box response

Quarterly

- Thematic AHD
- Parent teacher meeting

Bi-annual

- Administration of albendazole tablets (national deworming day).

Age-Appropriate Health Promotion

Primary school	Middle school	High school
• Health, growth, and development • Personal safety • Nutrition and physical activity • Hygiene practices • Prevention of diseases like malaria, dengue, TB, worm infestation, diarrhea, and vaccine preventable diseases.	• Puberty and related changes • Eye care and oral hygiene • Nutrition • Bullying prevention • Meditation and yoga • Internet safety and media literacy • Prevention of substance abuse • HIV/AIDS • Mental health	• Prevention of substance abuse • Sexual and reproductive health • Violence prevention • Unintentional injury • Road safety • Nutrition • Meditation and yoga

NUTRITION AND HEALTH

Nutritional Assessment (ABCDE)

A – Anthropometric measurements (Assessment)
B – Biochemical assay
C – Clinical examination
D – Diet survey
E – Ecological assessment

KEY POINTS

- ICDS comes under Ministry of Women and Child Development.
- Anganwadi is the heart of ICDS Scheme.
- According to the WHO report, malnutrition contributes to 45 percent of deaths of children aged under 5 years (worldwide).
- Anthropometry is the index for nutritional status in children.
- According to WHO childhood Severe Acute Malnutrition (SAM) is diagnosed when the weight-for-height.
- Wasting (low weight for height) indicates acute malnutrition.
- Chronic malnutrition is measured by height for age.
- Stunting (low height for age) indicates chronic malnutrition.

Protein Energy Malnutrition (Weight As % of the Standard - Grade of Malnutrition)

Table 24: Classification of protein energy malnutrition

ICMR classification	Gomez classification
• Normal – 80% and above • Grade I → 70–80% • Grade II → 60–70% • Grade III → 50–60% • Grade IV → Below 50%	• >90% → Normal • 75–89% → 1st degree • 60–74% → 2nd degree • Below 60% → 3rd degree

Age-Independent Anthropometric Indicators

- **Bangle Test:** If a bangle of 4 cm internal diameter crosses elbow
- **Shakir's tape:** Plastic tape with color zones (see figure below)
- **Quac Stick:** Rod with markings for Height and Arm circumference
- **Nabarrow's thinness chart:** Graphic chart for Wt/Ht
- **MAC: Height Ratio:** Normal if >0.32; severe malnutrition if < 0.29
- **Ponderal Index:** Weight (g)/(Height in cm)^3 × 100
- **Dughadale ratio:** Weight (kg)/(height in cm)$^{1.6}$; normal if > 0.79

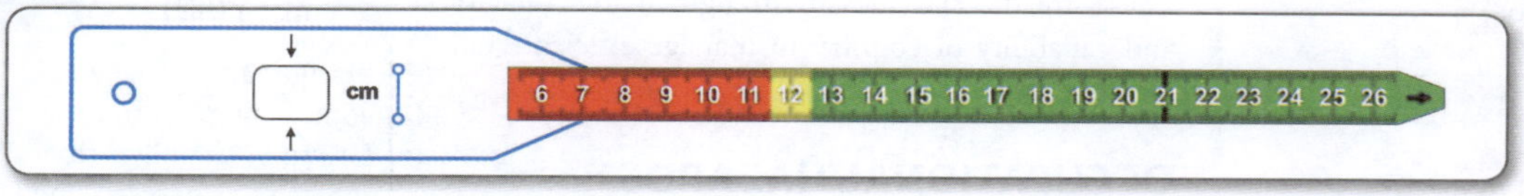

Figure 17: Mid-upper arm circumference (MUAC) measuring tape: Shakir's tape

Interpretation of Color Coding (Shakir's Tape Measurement)

Red	<12.5 cm	Wasted	Severe Protein Energy Malnutrition (PEM)
Yellow	12.5 – 13.5 cm	Borderline	Mild-moderate PEM
Green	>13.5	Normal	Normal

Vitamins

These are organic compounds classified as essential nutrients. They fall in the category of micronutrients. They are chiefly classified as:

- Fat soluble vitamins (vitamins A, D, E, K).
- Water soluble vitamins (vitamin B group and vitamin C).

Vitamins, functions, sources and deficiency diseases: Please refer Appendices

Community Nutrition Program

Table 25: Community nutrition program has been given in tabular form as follows:

Program	Explanation
Vitamin A Prophylaxis Program	Control of blindness through administration of vitamin A preparations
Prophylaxis against Nutritional Anemia	Distribution of iron and folic acid to pregnant women and children (1–12 years). ICDS, MCH, PHC are engaged in the implementation of this program
Control of Iodine Deficiency Disorders	Identification of goiter endemic region and supply of iodized salt and to assess the impact of goiter control measures
Special Nutritional Program	Launched in 1970 for the nutritional benefit of children below 6 years of age, pregnant and nursing mothers. Supplementary food supply having about 300 kcal and 10–12 g of protein per children per day
Balwadi Nutrition Program	Started in 1970 for the benefit of children in the age group of 3–6 years
ICDS Program	Started in 1975, there is strong nutritional component in this program in the form of supplementary nutrition, vitamin A prophylaxis, iron and folic acid distribution. Beneficiaries are children below 6 years of age and adolescent girls 11–18 years, pregnant and lactating mothers

Contd...

KEY POINTS

Leading causes of Under five Mortality (2017):

- Lower Respiratory tract infection—17.9%
- Preterm birth—15.6%
- Diarrheal disease—9.9%

KEY POINTS

Leading causes of Neonatal death (2017):

- Preterm birth—27.7%
- Birth asphyxia and trauma—14.5%
- Lower Respiratory tract infection—11.0%

KEY POINTS

- Green leafy vegetables and other plant foods are rich sources of **carotenoids.**
- National nutritional anemia prophylaxis program launched in the year 1970 as the part of 4th five year plan.
- In August, 1992 the National Goitre Control Programme (NGCP) was renamed as National Iodine Deficiency Disorders Control Programme (NIDDCP)
- In balwadi nutritional programme food supplements provides 300 Kcal and 10 gm protein per child per day.

Recent Question (NORCET 2023)

9. What is the weight-for-height z-score or SD of MUAC for acute malnutrition according to the growth chart?

a. <-2 SD
b. <-3 SD
c. >2SD
d. Equal to 2 SD

Ans. (d) Equal to 2 SD

Program	Explanation
Mid-day Meal Program	Launched in 1961. The major objective of this program is to attract more children for admission to school and retain them so that literacy improvement of children could be brought about.
Mid-day Meal Scheme	It is also known as National Program of Nutritional Support to Primary Education. Launched in 1995 and revised in 2004. The main objective is being universalization of primary education by increasing enrolment, retention and attendance and simultaneously impacting on nutrition of students up to middle level classes

DISASTER MANAGEMENT

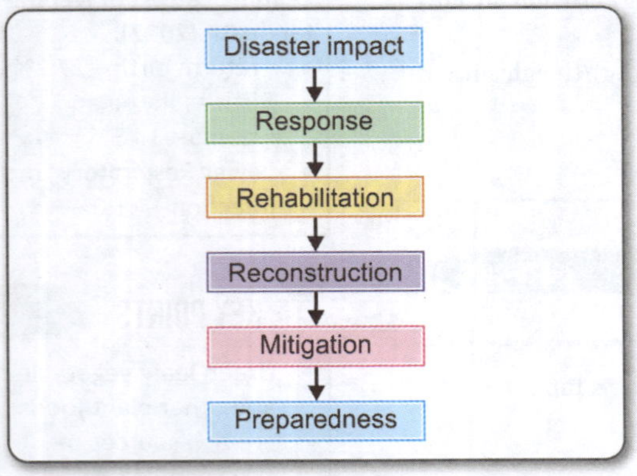

Figure 18: Management sequence of a sudden onset disaster

Disaster Impact and Response

- Search, rescue and first aid
- Field care
- **Triage:** Classify the victims according to the seriousness of injury.
- **Tagging:** All the patients should be provided with a tag which contains their name, age, etc.
- Identification of dead

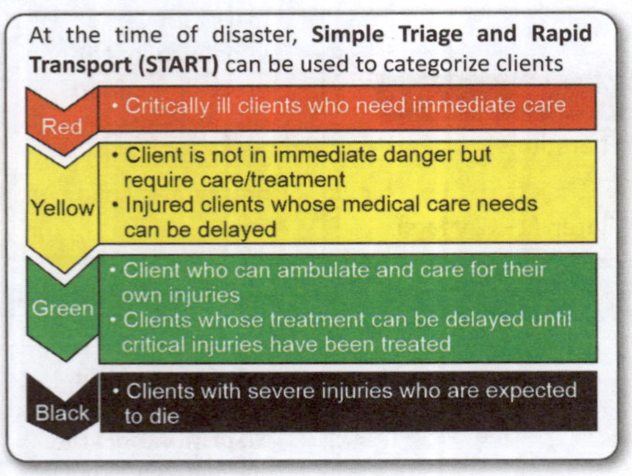

Figure 19: Triage categories

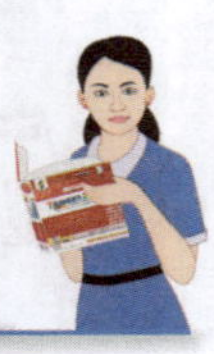

Rehabilitation

- Restoration of predisaster conditions. It starts from the time of disaster.

Disaster Mitigation

It involves the measures, which are adapted to prevent hazard from causing emergency or to lessen the likely effect of emergencies.

Disaster Preparedness

These are the activities to strengthen the capacity and capability of country to manage efficiently all type of emergencies.

OCCUPATIONAL HAZARDS

- **Physical hazards:** Heat and cold; light; noise; vibration; UV radiation; ionizing radiation.
- **Chemical hazards:** Exposure to chemicals such as acids, base, corrosive materials and other toxic compounds.
- **Biological hazards:** Infective and parasitic agents in the place of work
- **Mechanical hazards:** Hazards in the industry because of machinery and other moving parts
- **Psychosocial hazard:** It occurs because of the failure of workers to adapt with an external environment. Frustration, lack of job satisfaction, insecurity and poor human relationship are some of the examples.

Diseases Due to Physical Agent

Table 26: Physical agents and its associated diseases

Physical agent	Disease
Heat	Hyperpyrexia, heat exhaustion, heat syncope, heat cramp, burns
Cold	Trench foot, frost bite, chilblains
Light	Occupational cataract, miner's nystagmus
Noise	Occupational deafness
Radiation	Cancer, leukemia, aplastic anemia, pancytopenia
Mechanical factors	Injuries, accidents
Electricity	Burns

POINT TO REMEMBER

Nodal Center in case of a disaster management is District.

KEY POINT

Pradhan Mantri Ujjwala Yojna scheme is to provide LPG to BPL families (to replace unclean cooking fuels)

Practice Question

23. Nurse Ramya is working as a triage nurse during a disaster situation in an earthquake affected area. Tags placed on injured victims are on the triage color code. Which of the following color tag represents the victim who needs to be treated on priority?

a. Green
b. Yellow
c. Red
d. Black

Ans. (c) Red

Explanation:
Red tag indicates that the victim is critically ill and need immediate care. Black-tagged victims are with severe injuries who are expected to die. Medical care for victim with yellow and green tag can be delayed.

Diseases Due to Chemical Agents

Table 27: Chemical agents and its associated diseases

Agent	Disease	Key points
Coal dust	Anthracosis	• Risk of death in coal miner is twice as general population • Notifiable disease in the Indian Mines Act of 1952 • Progressive massive fibrosis (PMF) • Causes severe respiratory disability and frequently results in premature death
Silica	Silicosis	• Notifiable disease under the Factories Act 1948 and the Mines Act 1952 • First reported in India from Kolar Gold Field (KGF) in 1947 • Common industries — Mining industry, pottery and ceramic industry, sand blasting, metal grinding, building and construction work, rock mining, iron and steel industry • Incubation (exposure) period — 6 months to 6 years • Silicosis is characterized by a dense "nodular" fibrosis • Chest X-ray shows **"snow-storm" appearance** in the lung fields
Asbestos	Asbestosis, cancer lung	• Asbestos are silicates of varying composition; insoluble fibers • Deposited dust causes fibrosis leading to respiratory insufficiency and death; carcinoma of the bronchus, mesothelioma of the pleura or peritoneum and cancer of GI tract • **X-ray shows a ground-glass appearance** in the lower 2/3rd of the lung fields • Clubbing of fingers, cardiac distress and cyanosis are seen in advanced cases
Iron	Siderosis	
Cane fiber	Bagassosis	• First reported in India in 1955 • **Thermoactinomyces sacchari** is a thermophilic actinomycete found predominantly in bagasse • Bagasse control -2% propionic acid and 20% moisture control in the bagasse prevents actinomycete growth. • Skiagram may show mottling in lungs or shadow
Cotton dust	Byssinosis	• Symptoms: Chronic cough and progressive dyspnea, ending in chronic bronchitis and emphysema • 7 to 8% incidence
Hay or grain dust	Farmer's lung	• Growth of thermophilic actinomycetes (Micropolyspora faeni) in the grain dust is a major cause • Characterized by Respiratory symptoms and physical signs • Repeated attacks cause Pulmonary fibrosis and inevitable pulmonary damage and corpulmonale
Tobacco	Tobaccosis	
Gases	CO_2, CO, HCN, CS_2, NH_3, N_2, H_2S, HCl, SO_2, these gases cause poisoning	

KEY POINTS

- Silicosis is the most prevalent occupational disease in the world.
- In Silicosis, Chest X-ray shows **"snow-storm" appearance** in the lung fields.
- In Asbestosis, **X-ray shows a ground-glass appearance** in the lower 2/3rd of the lung fields.
- **Mesothelioma** is caused by crocidolite variety of amphibole asbestos.
- Growth of thermophilic actinomycetes (Micropolyspora faeni) in the grain dust is a major cause of Farmer's lung.
- **Thermoactinomyces sacchari** is a thermophilic actinomycete found predominantly in bagasse (Bagassosis)
- Progressive massive fibrosis is the feature of Anthracosis.
- 75% of all occupational cancer is skin cancer.
- Bladder cancer is associated with Aniline and dyeing industries.
- Hematuria is the most common symptom of bladder cancer.
- Employment of any person <14 years is prohibited as per Factories Act, 1948.
- ESI Act, 1948: Employer contributes 4.75% of total wage bill while employee contributes 1.75%.

Lead Poisoning

- More industrial workers are exposed to lead than to any other toxic metal
- Non-occupational sources: Gasoline; drinking water from lead pipe; chewing paint, toys
- Normal adults ingest about 0.2 to 0.3 mg of lead per day
- Blood levels: 25 mcg/100 mL >70 mcg/100 mL is associated with clinical symptoms
- Management: Chelating agent - D-penicillamine

Occupational Cancer

- Appear after prolonged exposure — 10 to 25 years
- Skin cancer is a most common (75%) type of occupational cancer. It is common among gas workers, tar distillers, oil refiners, dye-stuff workers, road makers
- Cancer bladder first noted in Aniline industry in 1895
- Leukemia is associated with exposure to benzol, roentgen rays and radioactive substances

Measures for Health Protection of Workers

- At least one sanitary convenience for every 25 employees for first 100; and then 1 per 50
- Space required: 500 cu.ft/worker; space more than 14 ft above the floor is not considered
- Recommended lighting
  - Precision work for a high degree of accuracy: 50-75 foot candles
  - Regular work: 6–12 foot candles
  - Illumination in corridor and passages: at least 0.5 foot candles

Protection Available for Women Workers in India

- Maternity leave for 12 weeks of which 6 weeks precede the EDD (ESI Act, 1948)
- The Factories Act (Sec 66) prohibits night work between 7 pm and 6 am
- The Indian Mines Act (1923) prohibits women from working underground
- The Factories Act, 1976 provides for creches in factories where more than 30 women workers are employed
- No child below the age of 14 shall be employed

The Employees State Insurance Act, 1948

- The ESI Act passed in 1948
- Amended in 1975, 1984, 1989, 2010
- It is for Social security and health insurance for employees in India
- ESI Corporation is an autonomous body. Head office is in New Delhi
- Union Minister for Labor is the chairman
- It has 23 regional offices, 37 sub-regional offices, 1418 ESI dispensaries, 2100 panel clinics, 307 diagnostic centers, besides 151 ESI hospitals and 42 hospital annexes with over 27000 beds
- ESI gives coverage to about 343 lakh persons/ family units as on 31.3.2018
- 12.4 crore beneficiaries in total
- The rate of contribution is fixed at 6.5% of the wages (Employers' share = 4.75% & employees' share = 1.75%)
- Benefits: Medical benefit, sickness benefit, Maternity benefit, Disablement benefit, Dependent's benefit, funeral expenses, rehabilitation allowances.

Rajiv Gandhi Shramik Kalyan Yojana

- Unemployment allowance for the employees covered under ESI Scheme due to factory closure
- Came into effect from 1st April, 2005

Prevention of Occupational Hazards

- Preplacement examination
- Periodical examination
- Medical and health services
- Notification
- Supervision of working environment
- Maintenance and analysis of record
- Health education and counseling

Besides these above mentioned points, few acts are present which protect the employees.

The Factories Act (1948)

- The Act defines factory as an establishment where 10 or more employees are there and electricity power is used and 20 or more workers where electricity power is not used.
- This Act covers the areas like health, safety and welfare, employment of young persons, hours of work, leave and wages, occupational disease and employment in hazardous processes.

The Employee State Insurance Act (ESI) 1948

- It is an important Act for the measurement of social security and health insurance.
- It provides certain cash and medical benefits to industrial employees in case of sickness, maternity and employment injury.

Benefits to Employee

- Medical benefit
- Sickness benefit
- Maternity benefit
- Disablement benefit
- Dependents benefit
- Funeral expenses
- Rehabilitation allowance

KEY POINTS

Logo of Employees State Insurance Corporation (ESIC)

- Narayan Meghaji Lokhande (N. M. Lokhande) organized the first labor union in India known as the "Bombay Mill Hand Society" in 1880.
- The Employees State Insurance Act, 1948 (ESI Act) was in 1948.
- The rate of contribution for ESI is fixed at 6.5% of the wages (Employers' share = 4.75% & employees' share = 1.75%)

KEY POINTS

- Recommended lighting for workers:
- Precision work - 50–75 foot candles
- Regular work: 6–12 foot candles.
- Light in corridor: at least 0.5 foot candles.

Recent Question (NORCET 2022)

10. A hospital caught fire. What will be the priority nursing intervention in this case?

a. Evacuate the patient
b. Use the fire extinguisher
c. Shut off the oxygen supply
d. Call fire department

Ans. (d) Call fire ...

Explanation: Shut off the oxygen supply will be the priority in order to limit the rapid spread of fire. Later follow the RACE protocol.

HEALTH POLICY AND PLANNING

National Health Policy 2017

- The National Health Policy 2017 is a comprehensive health policy document for India that was approved by the Union Cabinet on 15 March 2017.
- The National Health Policy 2017 (NHP 2017) is the overarching policy framework for the health sector in India.
- It serves as a roadmap for the government to plan and implement health programs and initiatives over the long term.
- **Key highlights and objectives of the National Health Policy 2017 include:** Attaining the highest possible level of health and well-being for all at all ages. This would be achieved through a preventive and promotive health care orientation in all developmental policies, and universal access to good quality health care services without anyone having to face financial hardship as a consequence.
- **Increase health expenditure by Government** as a percentage of GDP from the existing 1.15% to 2.5 % by 2025.
- **Increasing life expectancy** at birth from 67.5 years to 70 years by 2025.
- **Reduce infant mortality rate** to 28 by 2019
- **Reduce neonatal mortality** to 16 and still birth rate to "single digit" by 2025.
- **Reducing under-five mortality rate** to 23 per 1,000 live births by 2025.
- **Reducing maternal mortality ratio** to 100 per 100,000 live births by 2020.
- **Reduction of Total Fertility Rate (TFR)** to 2.1 at national and sub-national level by 2025.

Achieving universal health coverage by 2030.

- **Increase utilization of public health facilities** by 50% from current levels by 2025.
- **Investing in human resources for health:** This includes increasing the number of doctors, nurses, and other health professionals, and improving their skills and training.
- **Promoting innovation and research in health:** This includes supporting the development of new drugs, vaccines, and diagnostic tools, and promoting research on the prevention and treatment of diseases.
- **Enhancing the financial protection of people against health risks:** This includes expanding health insurance coverage, and providing financial assistance to the poor and vulnerable.

Health Planning in India

Please refer Appendices

Five-Year Plans

Planning Commission was established on March 15, 1950 as an advisory institution to form five plans. The broad objective for the health programs during the five year plans have been given below:

1. Control and eradication of major communicable disease
2. Strengthening of the basic health service through the establishment of PHC and SC
3. Population control
4. Development of health manpower resources.

Table 28: Five-year plans

Sl. no.	Plan	Time period
1.	First-five year plan	1951–1956
2.	Second five-year plan	1956–1961
3.	Third five-year plan	1961–1966
4.	Annual plan	1966–1969
5.	Forth five-year plan	1969–1974
6.	Fifth five-year plan	1974–1979
7.	Outlay	1979–1980
8.	Sixth five-year plan	1980–1985
9.	Seventh five-year plan	1985– 1990
10.	Annual plan	1990–1991
11.	Annual plan	1991–1992
12.	Eighth five-year plan	1992–1997
13.	Ninth five-year plan	1997–2002
14.	Tenth five-year plan	2002–2007
15.	Eleventh five-year plan	2007–2012
16.	Twelfth five-year plan	2012–2017

Recent Question (NORCET 2022)

11. Anthracosis occurs due to:

a. Coal dust
b. Silicon
c. Cotton
d. Sugarcane

Ans. (a) Coal dust

KEY POINTS

Specific Quantitative Goals of NHP 2017

- Reduce neonatal mortality to 16 and still birth rate to "single digit" by 2025
- Achieve and maintain elimination status of Leprosy by 2018, Kala-Azar by 2017 and Lymphatic Filariasis in endemic pockets by 2017.
- To achieve and maintain a cure rate of >85% in new sputum positive patients for TB
- To reduce the prevalence of blindness to 0.25/1000 by 2025 and disease burden by one third from current levels.
- To reduce premature mortality from cardiovascular diseases, cancer, diabetes or chronic respiratory diseases by 25% by 2025.
- Antenatal care coverage to be sustained above 90% and skilled attendance at birth above 90% by 2025.
- More than 90% of the newborn are fully immunized by one year of age by 2025.

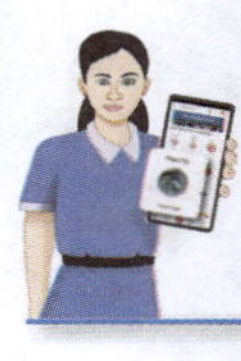

HEALTHCARE OF THE COMMUNITY

Levels of Healthcare

- **Primary care level (essential healthcare)**
  - First level of contact of individual, family and community with national health system.
  - At this level healthcare is most effective.
  - In India, primary healthcare is provided by PHC and SC with the help of multipurpose health workers, village, health guide and trained dais.
- **Secondary care level (intermediate)**
  - This level deals with more complex problems
  - In India this kind of care is provided by CHC and district hospital
  - This level at last is the first referral level
- **Tertiary care level**
  - It is more specialized level of care which provides specific facilities and attention of highly specialized health workers
  - In India, this kind of care is provided by regional or central level institution.

PRIMARY HEALTHCARE

- Following an international conference at **Alma-Ata (1978)**, a new approach to healthcare came into action and this was called primary healthcare.
- Alma-Ata conference defines primary healthcare as an essential healthcare; made universally accessible to individuals and acceptable to them through their full participation and at a cost that the community and country can afford.
- In 1977, Government of India developed rural health scheme based upon the recommendation of Shrivastav committee.
- It is a three-tier system based on the principle of placing people's health in people's hand.

Principles of Primary Healthcare

- **Equitable distribution**: Health services must be shared equally by all people in perspective of their ability to pay and all must have access to health services.
- **Community participation:** The involvement of individuals, families and communities in promotion of their own health and welfare.
- **Intersectoral coordination: Coordination between** related sectors and aspects of national and community development, in particularly agriculture, animal husbandry, food industry, education housing, public works, communication and other sectors.
- **Appropriate technology:** Technology with resources that a community and country can afford
- **Focus on prevention**: Promote health and healthy lifestyles with emphasis on prevention.

Eight Essential Elements of Primary Healthcare

E	Education about health problems and methods of identifying, prevention and control
L	Locally endemic disease prevention and treatment
E	Expanded program of immunization against major infectious disease
M	Maternal and Child Health including family planning
E	Essential drug arrangement
N	Nutritional and Food Supply
T	Treatment of common infections
S	Safe water supply and sanitation control

HEALTHCARE DELIVERY SYSTEM

Village Level

- One of the main features of primary healthcare is equitable distribution and universal coverage.
- To achieve the aim at village level, the following schemes are functional
  - ASHA scheme
  - ICDS scheme
  - Training of local dais

Subcenter

- First contact point between primary healthcare system and community.
- Plain area- one subcenter for 5000 population
- Hilly, tribal or desert areas - one subcenter for 3000 population
- **Type A subcenter** provides basic services
- **Type B subcenter** provides MCH services + Basic services.
- **Type B subcenters** are also known as MCH subcenters
- Ministry of Health and Family Welfare, GOI provides assistance to all the sub centers in the country since April 2002 in the form of salary of ANMs and LHVs, rent (if located in rented building), contingency, drugs and equipment kit.
- The salary of male health worker is borne by state government.

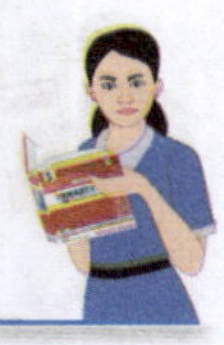

KEY POINTS

- India had a total of 12 Five-Year Plans, the last one being from 2012-2017.
- In 2015, The Planning Commission was dissolved and replaced with NITI Aayog.
- Govt. of India established NITI Aayog (National Institution for Transforming India) on **January 1, 2015,** as replacement for the Planning Commission.

KEY POINTS

- **Type A sub-center** provides basic services
- **Type B sub-center** provides MCH services + Basic services. So it is known as MCH subcenters

KEY POINTS

- The healthcare infrastructure in rural areas has been developed as a **Three tier system** (Subcenter, PHC, CHC).
- Primary healthcare concept was finally accepted at the Alma-Ata Conference, 1978.
- Primary healthcare must be acceptable, Accessible, Available and Affordable.
- Primary healthcare accounts for 52.1 per cent of India's current public expenditure on health as per the National Health Estimates, 2016-17.

Staffing at Subcenter

Type of subcenter	Subcenter A		Subcenter B (MCH Subcenter)	
Staff	Essential	Desirable	Essential	Desirable
ANM/Health worker (Female)	1	+1	2	
Health worker (Male)	1		1	
Staff nurse (or ANM, if staff nurse is not available)				1**
Safai-Karamchari*	1(Part-time)		1 (Full-time)	

*To be outsourced
**If number of deliveries at the Subcenter is 20 or more in a month

Drugs and equipment kit at subcenter level
- Drug kit A for ANM
- Drug kit B
- Kit C (Midwifery Kit) contains subcenter equipment and midwifery kit

Primary Health Center

- First contact point between village community and the medical officer is Primary Health Center.
- One PHC for 3000 population in rural plain areas and one PHC for 2000 population in hilly backward and tribal areas.
- From the delivery case load point of view, PHCs are classified into A and B type.
- **Type A PHC** means less than 20 deliveries per month
- **Type B PHC (Upgraded PHC)** means more than 20 deliveries per month

Staffing Pattern (Essential & Desirable)

Staff	Type A (PHC)		Type B (UPHC)	
	Essential	Desirable	Essential	Desirable
Medical officer (MBBS)	1	1	2	—
MO AYUSH	—	1	—	—
MO Dental	—	1	—	1
Staff Nurses	2	1	1	1
Pharmacist	1	—	1	—
Accountant cum data entry operator	1			1
Lab Technician	1	—	1	—
Optometrist/Ophthalmic Assistant/ Vision Technician	—	1	—	1
Health worker (female)/ANM	1	—	5	—
Health worker/Health assistant (male)	1	—	—	—
Health assistant female/lady health visitor	1	—	1	—
Health Educator/Counselor	—	1	—	1
Dental Assistant*	—	1	—	1
Cold chain/Vaccine logistic Assistant	—	1	—	1
Public Health Manager	—	—	1	—
Dresser	1	—	1	—
LDC-1/Accountant	1	—	1	—
Data Entry Operator	1	—	1	—
Sanitary staff	1	—	1	—

Source: Indian Public Health Standards by NHM, Ministry of Health and Family Welfare (Volume III, 2022)

KEY POINTS

- Subcenter A is managed by one Male and one female Health Worker (ANM) + 1 part time safai-karamchari (oursourced)
- MCH subcenter (Subcenter B) is managed by 2 female health workers and one male health worker + 1 full time safari karamchari (outsourced).

Kit A
Oral rehydration salt
Tab. IFA (large)
Tab. IFA (small)
Vitamin A solution
Tab. Cotrimoxazole (pediatric)

Kit B
T. Methylergometrine Maleate
T. Paracetamol
Inj. Methylergometrine Maleate
T. Mebendazole
T. Dicyclomine HCl
Ointment Povidone iodine 5%
Cetrimide Powder
Cotton bandage
Absorbent cotton

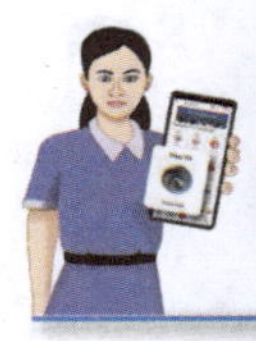

Drug and Equipment Kit at PHC

- Equipment Kit D

Kit-D (PHC Equipment Kit)

- Normal delivery kit
- Equipment for assisted vacuum delivery
- Equipment for assisted forceps delivery
- Standard surgical set for minor procedure
- Equipment for manual vacuum aspiration
- Equipment for newborn care and neonatal resuscitation
- IUCD insertion kit
- Equipment/reagent for essential laboratory investigation

Community Health Center (CHC)

- It has 30 indoor beds with one OT, X-ray, Labor room and Laboratory facilities.
- **Plain areas-** One CHC covers 1,20,000 population
- Hilly and Tribal areas- One CHC covers 80000 population.

Staffing at CHC

Personnel	Strength
Medical Officer (Surgeon, Obstetrician, Physician, Pediatrician, anesthetist – 1 each)	5
Eye surgeon	1
Dental Surgeon	1
Public health manager	1
General duty medical officer	6 (at least 2 females)
Specialist of AYUSH	1
General duty medical officer AYUSH	1
Supporting staff	
Staff nurse	**19**
Public health nurse	1
ANM	1
Pharmacist/compounder	3
Pharmacist AYUSH	1
Lab technician	3
Radiographer	2
Ophthalmic assistant	1
Dresser (certified by Red Cross/St John Ambulance)	2
Ward boy/nursing orderly	5
Sweepers	5
Chowkidar	5
Dhobi	1
Mali	1
Aya	5
Peon	2
OPD attendant	1
Registration clerk	2
Statistical assistant/data entry operator	2
Accountant/admin. assistant	1
OT technician	1

KEY POINTS

- Four PHCs are covered by one CHC.
- One CHC covers 80,000 (hill) to 1,20,000 (plain) population.
- One PHC covers 20,000 (hill) to 30,000 (plain) population
- One Subcenter covers about 3000 (hill) to 5000 (plain) population.

KEY POINTS

- The main aim of PHC is to provide accessible, affordable and available primary care to people.
- PHC is the first contact point between community and Doctors.
- PHC is referral center for 6 subcenters.

Drug and equipment kit at CHC/FRU

Kit-E - Laparotomy set
Kit-F - Mini-Laparotomy set
Kit-G - IUD insertion set
Kit-H - Vasectomy set
Kit-I - Normal delivery set
Kit-J - Vacuum extraction set
Kit-K - Embryotomy set
Kit-L - Uterine evacuation set
Kit-M - Equipment for anesthesia
Kit-N - Neonatal resuscitation set
Kit-O - Equipment and reagent for blood test
Kit-P - Donor blood transfusion set

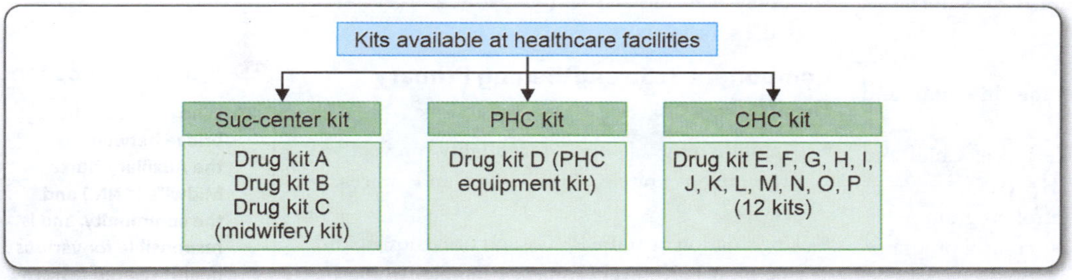

Table 29: Distribution of subcenter, PHC and CHC according to population

Name of the center	Hill/tribal area	Plain's area
One Subcenter	3,000 population	5,000 population
One Primary Health Center	20,000 population	30,000 population
One Community Health Center	80,000 population	1,20,000 population

Average Number of Villages Covered

- Subcenter – 4 villages
- PHC – 27 villages
- CHC – 133 villages

Grass Root Level Workers

- Village health guide
- Local dais
- Anganwadi workers
- ASHA (Accredited Social Health Activist)
- USHA (Urban Social Health Activist)

Table 30: Following table contains summarized information about gross root level workers

Village health guide (VHG)	Local dais
• **Training:** 200 hours • **Stipend:** 200/month • **Work:** 2–3 hours per day • **Salary:** 50/month • **For drugs:** 600/annum	• **Training:** 1 month/30 days • **Stipend:** 300/month • **1 week:** 4 days in field and 2 days in PHC/SC • ₹10/delivery • ₹3/registration
Anganwadi workers (AWW)	**ASHA–Rural areas**
• **1 AWW:** for 1000 population • **100 workers:** 1 project • **Training:** 4 months **Honorarium:** • AWW at main-Anganwadi centers: ₹4,500/month • AWW at mini-Anganwadi centers: ₹2,250/month • There is one Mukhya Sevika (Supervisor) for every 20-25 AWW.	• Covers 1000 population in rural and 1000-2500 in urban • She should be from local area • She should have formal education up to 8th Std. • Major role: Accompanying pregnant women to healthcare center for Institutional delivery. • She is DOTS provider in RNTCP • Monthly incentives: ₹2000.

KEY POINTS

- ASHA must primarily be a woman resident of the village married/ widowed/ divorced, preferably in the age group of 25 to 45 years.
- The ASHAs will receive performance-based incentives for promoting universal immunization, referral and escort services for RCH.

KEY POINTS

WHO norm for health workers:

- 1 Doctor per 1000 population (currently, 1: 1456 in India)
- 3 nurses per 1000 population (currently, 1: 1777 in India)
- 1 Pharmacist per 10,000 population
- 2 ASHA per 1000 population
- 1 Lab technician per 10,000 population
- 1 trained dais per village (1000 population)

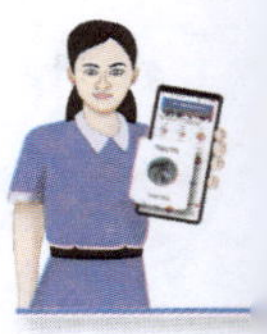

NATIONAL HEALTH MISSION (NHM)

- National Health Mission was approved in May 2013.
- The National Health Mission (NHM) encompasses its two Sub-Missions:
  - The National Rural Health Mission (NRHM) and
  - The newly launched National Urban Health Mission (NUHM).
- Main Program components
  - Health System Strengthening in rural and urban areas
  - Reproductive, Maternal, Newborn, Child and Adolescent Health (RMNCH+A)
  - Communicable Disease control program
  - Non-Communicable Disease control program

National Rural Health Mission (NRHM)

Figure 20: Logo of NRHM

- It was launched on 12th April 2005.
- Its objective is to provide accessible, affordable, and accountable quality health services to the poorest households in the remotest rural regions.
- Under the NRHM, difficult areas with unsatisfactory health indicators were classified as special focus states to ensure greatest attention where needed.
- Plan of action consists of 10 components

Component 1: ASHA (Accredited Social Health Activists)

- **Selection**: every village/large habitat (1000 population) will have a female community health activist
- ASHA must be primarily a woman resident of the village- preferably in the age group of 25-45 years
- She should be a literate woman with formal education up to the 8th class.
- ASHA would act as a bridge between the ANM and the village and be accountable to the panchayat.
- ASHA will be honorary volunteer.

Responsibilities of ASHA Worker

- Awareness campaign, counseling, mobilization of community resources, Escort pregnant women and children requiring treatment to treatment facilities, medical care of minor ailments, depot holder of essential drugs, birth and death registration.

Component 2: Strengthening Subcenters

- Each subcenter will have an untied fund for local action ₹10,000 per annum.
- Supply of essential drugs (allopathic and AYUSH) to the subcenters.

Component 3: Strengthening Primary Health Centers

- Strengthening of PHC for quality preventive, promotive, curative, supervisory and outreach services.
- Upgradation of 100% PHCs, and provision of 2nd doctor at PHC level (1 male, 1 female) would be undertaken on the basis of felt need.

Component 4: Strengthening of CHC for First Referral Care

Operationalizing existing community Health centers (30-50 beds) as 24 hours First Referral Units, including posting of anesthetists.

Component 5: District Health Plan

All Vertical Health and Family Welfare Programs at district and state level merge into one common "District Health Mission" at the district level and the "State Health Mission" at the state level

Component 6: Converging Sanitation And Hygiene Under NRHM

- Total Sanitation Campaign (TSC) is presently implemented in 350 districts, and is proposed to cover all districts in 10th Plan.
- The District Health Mission would guide activities of sanitation at district level
- ASHA would be incentivized for promoting household toilets by the Mission.

Component 7: Strengthening Disease Control Programs

- National Disease Control Programs for Malaria, TB, Kala Azar, Filaria, Blindness and Iodine Deficiency and Integrated Disease Surveillance Program shall be integrated under the Mission, for improved program delivery.

Component 8: Public-Private Partnership for Public Health Goals, Including Regulation of Private Sector

- Management plan for PPP initiatives: at District/ State and National levels

RECENT UPDATE:
National Health Mission (NHM) renamed as Pradhan Mantri-Samagra Swasthya Mission (PM-SSM) in July 2023.

Practice Question

24. Who serves as the bridge between the Auxiliary Nurse Midwife (ANM) and the community, and is responsible for various health-related tasks, including awareness campaigns and birth and death registration, under the NRHM?

a. The Village Headman
b. The District Health Officer
c. Accredited Social Health Activist (ASHA)
d. Female Health Worker

Ans. (c) Accredited Social Health Activist (ASHA)

KEY POINTS

- ASHA collects data about Births and deaths in a village.
- ASHA provides medical care for minor ailments like diarrhea, fever & first aid for minor injuries.
- NUHM would cover all State capitals, district headquarters and cities/towns with a population of more than 50,000.

Component 9: New Health Financing Mechanisms

- A Task Group to examine new health financing mechanism

Component 10: Reorienting Health/ Medical Education To Support Rural Health Issues

- Medical and Para-medical education facilities need to be created in states, based on need assessment.

The National Urban Health Mission (NUHM)

- It is a sub-mission of National Health Mission (NHM).
- It has been approved by the Cabinet on 1st May 2013.
- NUHM envisages to meet healthcare needs of the urban population with the focus on urban poor, by making available to them essential primary healthcare services and reducing their out-of-pocket expenses for treatment.
- Goal: Strengthening the existing healthcare service delivery system and targeting the people living in slums.

Urban Healthcare Delivery Model

The urban health delivery model would basically comprise an Urban Primary Health Center for provision of primary healthcare with outreach and referral linkages.

Urban Primary Health Center (U-PHC)

- Functional for a population of around approximately 50,000–60,000
- It may be located preferably within a slum or near a slum within half a kilometer radius catering to a slum population of approximately 25,000-30,000, with provision for OPD from 12 noon to 8 pm in the evening.
- The cities based upon the local situation may establish a U-PHC for 75,000 for areas with very high density.
- OPD services with basic lab diagnosis, drug/ contraceptive dispensing, and health education services.

Support Staff

- Two doctors (one regular and one on a part time basis)
- There will be 2 multiskilled paramedics (lab technician and pharmacist)
- 2 multi-skilled nurses
- 1 LHV
- 4-5 ANMs (depending upon the population covered)
- Clerical and support staff and one Program Manager

Urban- Community Health Centers (U-CHC)

- May act as a satellite hospital for every 4-5 U-PHCs
- The U-CHC would cater to a population of 2,50,000

Services

- It would provide inpatient services and would be a 30-50 bedded facility.
- It would provide medical care, minor surgical facilities, and facilities for institutional delivery.

Support Staff

- Two doctors (one regular and one on a part time basis)
- There will be 2 multi skilled paramedics (lab technician and pharmacist)
- 2 multi-skilled nurses, 1 LHV, 4–5 ANMs (depending upon the population covered)
- Clerical and support staff and one Program Manager

Urban Social Health Activist (USHA)

- A Frontline community worker for each slum/ community similar to USHA under NRHM
- The USHA would be a woman resident of the slum, preferably in the age group of 25–45 years
- She would be covering about 1000–2500 community level beneficiaries.
- She would be covering between 200–500 households.
- She would serve as an effective demand-generating link between the health facility (Urban Primary Health Center) and the urban slum populations

KEY POINTS

- **Urban Primary Health Center (U-PHC)** is functional for a population of around approximately 50,000–60,000.
- **Urban Community Health Centers (U-CHC)** act as a satellite hospital for every 4-5 U-PHCs (2,50,000 population)

KEY POINTS

- USHA would help the ANM in delivering outreach services
- USHA will be responsible to the Mahila Arogya Samitis (community groups) for which they are designated.

DIFFERENCES BETWEEN NRHM AND NUHM

NRHM	NUHM
National Rural Health Mission	National Urban Health Mission
Improves rural health delivery system	Separate mission for urban areas and focus on slums and other urban poor families.
Launched on 12th April, 2005	Approved on 1st May 2013

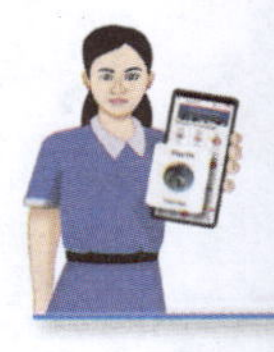

Contd...

NRHM	NUHM
Creation of ASHA (Accredited Social Health Activist)	Creation of USHA (Urban Social Health Activist)
1 ASHA = 1000 population	1 USHA = 1000–2500 beneficiaries, 200-500 households
PHC and CHC present to provide health services	PUHC and CUHC are there to provide health services.
Programs under NRHM are • Janani Suraksha Yojana • Rogi Kalyaan Samiti, • *Rashtriya Swasthya Bima Yojana*	Programs under NUHM are • Nehru Rojgar Yojana • Mahila Arogya Samiti • Urban basic services for the poor • Swarna Jayanti Shahari Yojana.

PROGRAMS UNDER NRHM

Janani Suraksha Yojana (JSY)

- JSY was launched on 12 April 2005 by the Hon'ble Prime Minister
- National maternity benefit scheme has been modified into new scheme called Janani suraksha yojana.
- Janani Suraksha Yojana (JSY) is a safe motherhood intervention under the National Rural Health Mission (NRHM).
- The objective is to reduce maternal and neo-natal mortality by promoting institutional delivery among the poor pregnant women.
- JSY is a centrally sponsored scheme, this scheme integrates cash assistance with delivery and post-delivery care.
- The Yojana has identified **Accredited Social Health Activist (ASHA)** as an effective link between the government and pregnant women
- The success of the scheme would be determined by the increase in institutional delivery among the poor families.
- This program gives special focus to 10 low performing states (LPS) such as Uttar Pradesh, Uttarakhand, Madhya Pradesh, Jharkhand, Bihar, Rajasthan, Chhattisgarh, Odisha, Assam and Jammu and Kashmir.
- In LPS, this JSY extends up to third child if mother chooses to undergo sterilization at health facility immediately after delivery.

Rogi Kalyan Samities (RKSs)/Hospital Management Committees

॥ सर्वे सन्तु निरामयाः॥

ROGI KALYAN SAMITI

- RKS was introduced in 2005 under the National Rural Health Mission (NRHM) as a forum to improve the functioning and service provision in public health facilities, increase participation and enhance accountability.
- RKS/HMC would be a registered society set up in all District Hospitals/Sub District Hospitals/ CHCs/FRUs.
- Objective is to ensure compliance to minimal standard for facility and hospital care and protocols of treatment as issued by the Government.

Rashtriya Swasthya Bima Yojana

राष्ट्रीय स्वास्थ्य बीमा योजना

Rashtriya Swasthya Bima Yojana (RSBY)

- RSBY has been launched by Ministry of Labor and Employment, GoI to provide health insurance coverage for Below Poverty Line (BPL) families.
- The objective of RSBY is to provide protection to BPL households from financial liabilities arising out of health shocks that involve hospitalization.
- Eligibility: Unorganized sector workers belonging to BPL category and their family members (a family unit of five) shall be the beneficiaries under the scheme.
- Benefits: Total sum insured would be ₹30,000/- per family per annum on a family floater basis. Cashless attendance to all covered ailments. Transportation cost-₹100 per visit (over limit of ₹1000).

Mahila Arogya Samiti (MAS)

- MAS is one of the key interventions under National Health Mission aimed at promoting community participation in health at all levels, including planning, implementing and monitoring of health programs.

- MAS is expected to take collective action on issues related to Health, Nutrition, Water, Sanitation and social determinants at the slum level.

Features

- Local women's collective/group with an elected Chairperson and a Secretary
- Covers approximately 50-100 households in slum and slum-like settlements
- Addresses local issues related to Health, Nutrition, Water, Sanitation and social determinants of health at slum level
- Facilitated by the ASHA who acts as the Member Secretary

URBAN POVERTY ALLEVIATION

The Urban Poverty Alleviation Programs (UPAPs) which were in operation during eighth plan are as follows

- Nehru Rozgar Yojana (NRY) – launched in 1989
- Urban Basic Services for the Poor (UBSP) -
- Prime Minister's Integrated Urban Poverty Eradication Program (PM IUPEP) – launched in November 1995.

The Swarna Jayanti Shahari Rozgar Yojana (SJSRY)

- In Ninth five-year plan, it was proposed to launch the Swarna Jayanti Shahari Rozgar Yojana (SJSRY) and phase out NRY, PMIUPEP and UBSP
- The SJSRY is a Centrally Sponsored Scheme applicable to all the urban areas with expenditure to be shared in ratio 75:25 between the Center and States/UTs.
- The program became operational on **December 1, 1997**.
- This program would have two sub-schemes, namely, (i) Urban Self-Employment Program and (ii) Urban Wage Employment Program.
- The SJSRY seeks to provide gainful employment to the urban unemployed or underemployed poor by encouraging the setting up of self-employment ventures or provision of wage employment.

NATIONAL HEALTH PROGRAMS

Ayushman Bharat Yojana

- Ayushman Bharat, a flagship scheme of Government of India, was launched as recommended by the National Health Policy 2017, to achieve the vision of Universal Health Coverage (UHC).
- Ayushman Bharat adopts a continuum of care approach, comprising two interrelated components, which are:
  - Health and Wellness Centers (HWCs)
  - Pradhan Mantri Jan Arogya Yojana (PM-JAY)
- **Cashless and paperless** access to quality healthcare services.
- Government provides health insurance cover of up to **₹5,00,000 per family per year.**
- Free treatment available at all public and empaneled private hospitals in times of need.
- This initiative has been designed to meet Sustainable Development Goals (SDGs) and its underlining commitment, which is to "leave no one behind."
- Covers secondary and tertiary care hospitalization.
- It provides provision of financial protection for access of curative care at the secondary and tertiary levels through engagement with both public and private sector.

Rashtriya Bal Swasthya Karyakram (RBSK)

- It is an important initiative aiming at early identification and early intervention for children from birth to 18 years to cover 4 'D's viz. Defects at birth, Deficiencies, Diseases, Development delays including disability.
- Launched in February 2013.

Mother and Child Tracking System

- Mother and Child Tracking System (MCTS) is an initiative of Ministry of Health & Family Welfare to leverage information technology for ensuring delivery of full spectrum of healthcare and immunization services to pregnant women and children up to 5 years of age.
- It facilitates and monitors service delivery and also establishes a two-way communication between the service providers and beneficiaries.

Integrated Disease Surveillance Project (IDSP)

- It is a decentralized, state-based surveillance program in the country.
- It is intended to detect early warning signals of impending out breaks and help initiate an effective response in a timely manner.
- It is also expected to provide essential data to monitor progress of on-going disease control programs and help allocate health resources more efficiently.

Recent Question (NORCET 2023)

12. Which committee recommended three-tier system of healthcare delivery in India?

a. Shrivastav comittee
b. Bhore comittee
c. Kartarsingh comittee
d. Mudaliar committee

Ans. (a) Shrivastav comittee

Recent Question (NORCET 2021)

13. Which of the following is NOT included in Mission Indradhanush?

a. Measles
b. DPT
c. PCV
d. Hepatitis B

Ans. (c) PCV

Explanation: The diseases covered by Mission Indradhanush are:

- Diphtheria
- Pertussis
- Tetanus
- Polio
- Measles
- Rubella
- Tuberculosis
- Hepatitis B

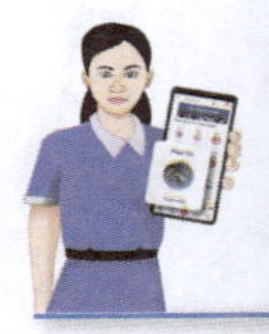

INTERNATIONAL HEALTH AGENCIES

Agency	Description	Objective
World Health Organization (WHO)	Established in 1946 Headquarters: Geneva Constitution came into force: 7th April 1948	**Attainment of highest level of health to all people** **Work** • Prevention and control of specific diseases • Development of Comprehensive services • Family health Biomedical Research • Health Statistics Environmental Health, Health literature and information • Cooperation with other organization
UNICEF (The United Nations Children's Fund)	The United Nations Children's Fund (UNICEF), originally known as the United Nations International Children's Emergency Fund. Established in 1946 Headquarter: New York	• It is created by the United Nations General Assembly on 11 December 1946, to Provide emergency food and healthcare to children and mothers in countries that had been devastated by World War II. • In 1950, UNICEF's mandate was extended to address the long-term needs of children and women in developing countries everywhere. • In 1953 it became a permanent part of the United Nations System, and the words "international" and "emergency" were dropped from the organization's name, though it retained the original acronym, "UNICEF". • Services include child health, child nutrition, family health and child welfare, education (formal and informal) • It derives funds from voluntary governmental and nongovernmental organization.
United Nations Development Program (UNDP)	Established in 1966 Headquarter: New York	• To help poor nations to develop their human and natural sources more fully.
Food and Agricultural Organization (FAO)	Established in 1945 Head quarter: Rome	• It is the specialized agency of the United Nations that leads international efforts to defeat hunger and improve nutrition and food security.
International Labor Organization (ILO)	Established in the year 1919 Headquarters: Geneva, Switzerland	• It deals with labor issues, particularly international labor standards and decent work for all. • 185 of the 193 UN member states are members of the ILO. • In 1969, the organization received the Nobel Peace Prize for improving peace among classes, pursuing justice for workers, and providing technical assistance to other developing nations.
United States Agency for International Development (USAID)	Established: 3rd November 1961 Headquarters : Ronald Reagan Building Washington, DC	• The United States Agency for International Development (USAID) is an independent agency of the United States federal government that is primarily responsible for administering civilian foreign aid and development assistance. • Activities include: (1) Malaria eradication, (2) Medical education, (3) Nursing education, (4) Health education, (5) Water supply and sanitation, (6) Control of communicable diseases, (7) Nutrition, (8) Family planning
Cooperative for Assistance and Relief Everywhere (CARE)	Founded in the year: 1945	• It is one of the world's largest independent, non-profit, non-sectarian international relief and development organization. CARE provides emergency aid and long-term development assistance. Operation in India from 1950.

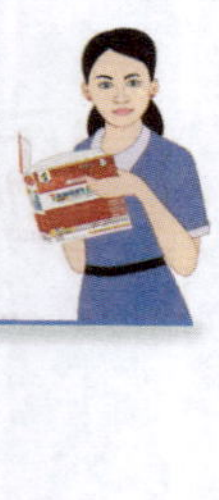

Golden Points to Remember

- The world health day is celebrated on **April 7th.**
- World Tuberculosis day is celebrated on **March 24th**.
- World AIDS day is celebrated on **1st December**.
- Prevention of risk factors refers to primordial prevention. Example: Lifestyle modification.
- **Immunization and fortification of food** with specific nutrients are an example of **primary prevention.**
- Wearing seat belts, safety helmets and other safety equipment are the examples of **primary health promotion behavior.**
- Early diagnosis (screening) and primary treatment (basic treatment) of the disease are known as **secondary prevention.**
- Medical therapy (hospital care), surgical treatment and rehabilitation are the examples of **tertiary level prevention.**
- The ideal **weight** of an adult person is calculated on the basis of **height.**
- **Incidence** is defined as the number of new cases that occur over a given period of time.
- **Prevalence** is the number of cases (old + new cases) in a population in a given period of time.
- **Point prevalence** is defined as proportion of population which has condition in specific point in time.
- **Period prevalence** is defined as proportion of a population which has the condition at some point of time during the given period.
- A sudden outbreak of disease in the community in excess than the normal expectation is known as **epidemic.**
- **Pandemic:** When an epidemic spreads out throughout the world (worldwide).
- **Endemic**: A disease that exists permanently **in a** particular geographical region or population.
- **Entomology** is a scientific study of insects, a branch of zoology.
- The WHO initiative 'Right to Sight' is named as **Vision 2020.** It is a global initiative for the elimination of avoidable blindness.
- India is currently in late expanding stage (third stage) of demographic cycle. In this stage, birth rate begins to decline and death rate further decreases (from 2nd stage).
- **Sex ratio** is defined as the number of female individuals for every 1000 male individuals.
- **General fertility rate** refers to number of live births per 1000 females in reproductive age group.
- **Mass drug administration** is given to control filaria and malaria in many countries but in India it is done in case of lymphatic filaria only.
- The content of Drug Kit A provided at subcenter includes ORS, tablet iron and folic acid, vitamin A solution and tablet cotrimoxazole.
- The population covered by the primary health center is 30,000 in plain areas and 20,000 in tribal area.
- **Bhore Committee** (1946) is known as **Health Survey & Development Committee.**
- **Mudaliar Committee** (1962) is known as **Health Survey & Planning Committee.**
- One **basic health worker** for 10,000 population was recommended by **Chadha Committee (1963).**
- **Kartar Singh Committee (1973)** recommended that ANMs were to be converted to MPW (F).
- The **Rural Health Scheme** was based on the recommendation of **Srivastava Committee.**
- MPWs (multipurpose worker) team include one male health worker and one female health worker which cover 5,000 population in rural areas.
- The new-born birth to be registered in India within 21 days of birth.
- **UNICEF (United Nation International Emergency fund)** was established in 1946.
- **Telemedicine hub** refers to the primary clinical site from where the health provider renders health services to the remote places.
- Antiviral agents used for prevention and treatment of **swine flu** are Oseltamivir (Tamiflu) and Zanamivir (Relenza).
- A **characteristic** feature of the rash in **chicken pox** is its **pleomorphism** (all stages of rash may be seen simultaneously).
- India was free from smallpox in April 1977 but it was officially declared in December 1979.
- Smallpox was officially declared eradicated by the World Health Organization (WHO) on 8th May, 1980.
- **BCG, Hepatitis B, OPV** vaccines are recommended at birth according to National Immunization Schedule.
- The system of storing and transporting vaccines is termed as Cold chain.
- The vaccination can be used if the center square is white in the Vaccination Vial Monitor (VVM).

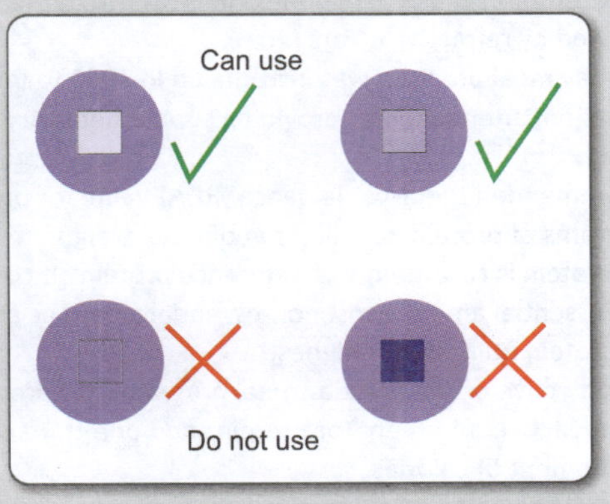

- **Oral Polio Vaccine** (OPV) is live vaccine (Sabin) and **Inactivated Polio Vaccine** (IPV) is a killed vaccine (Salk).
- The diluent used for reconstitution of BCG vaccine is normal saline.

Contd...

- **Pulse Polio Immunization** was introduced in 1995.
- **Hepatitis A** and **Hepatitis E** viruses are mainly transmitted through feco-oral route.
- **Hepatitis B** and **C** are transmitted through blood-to-blood contact.
- **Hepatitis D** only occurs in people who are infected with the **hepatitis B** virus because HDV require help of HBV to replicate.
- The time interval between the invasion by an infectious agent and the appearance of first sign of disease is called **incubation period.**
- **DOTS (Directly Observed Treatment for Short course)** is a strategy used by World Health Organization (WHO) to decrease the number of tuberculosis (TB) patients.
- **Dengue** is spread through the bite of the female *Aedes aegypti* mosquito. This mosquito is a daytime feeder. Biting period is early in the morning.
- ***Culex vishnui*** mosquito from the Culicidae family is the most common vector causing the **Japanese encephalitis virus (JEV)** in India, Sri Lanka.
- **Schick test** is intradermal test used to confirm the diagnosis of **diphtheria.**
- **Trachoma** is contagious and affects the conjunctiva of the eye, cornea and eyelids. It is caused by the Chlamydia trachomatis bacteria.
- **Gonorrhea** is a sexually transmitted infection caused by bacteria ***Neisseria gonorrhoeae.***
- **Measles** is caused by Rubeola virus.
- Amoebiasis is caused by ***Entamoeba histolytica.***
- Glucose is added in ORS solution because it increases the sodium absorption.
- A freshly prepared **ORS solution (Oral rehydration solution)** should be used within 24 hours.
- During cholera outbreak, the best emergency sanitation measures to be adopted will be provision of chlorinated water.
- Most common cause of blindness in India is Cataract (62%) followed by refractive errors (20%).
- Mid-day meal program was **introduced in 1961** to improve the school attendance by providing supplementary food from school.
- Recommended Dietary Allowance (RDA) Value for protein is 0.8 grams of protein per kilogram of body weight.
- Egg protein is considered as 'reference protein'. It contains all nine essential amino acids, non-essential amino acids and its net protein utilization is highest.
- The objective of the mid-day meal program is to provide half of the daily requirement for proteins and one-third of daily requirement of calories.
- The method of waste disposal in which waste is disposed along with night soil is known as **Composting.**
- The Asian 'Tiger Mosquito' (***Aedes albopictus***) is a small black and white mosquito.
- Zinc phosphide is an efficient rodenticide. Rodents include rats, mice, squirrels, beavers, etc.
- Eating maize alone leading to pellagra because maize is a poor source of niacin and tryptophan.
- Integrative approach is a family therapy approach that focuses on both the biological and the psychosocial components of a problem.
- Inhalation of cotton fiber dust over the long period of time results in **Byssinosis.**
- Monday fever is the other name for byssinosis.
- The most satisfactory method of waste disposal where suitable land is available is controlled tipping.
- A method used for individual health education in the community is Counselling and Interview.
- INSPIRE is a technical package for everyone committed to preventing and responding to violence against children and adolescents. Seven strategies for ending violence to children:
    i. I – Implementation and enforcement of laws
    ii. N – Norms and values
    iii. S – Safe environment
    iv. P – Parent and caregiver support
    v. I – Income and economic strengthening
    vi. R – Response and support services
    vii. E – Education and life skills
- Dolutegravir is a new drug added in ARV regimens for post exposure prophylaxis for HIV infection. The dosage of the drug is 50 mg.
- Horrock's apparatus is used to detect the estimation of chlorine demand in water.
- Father of Homeopathy: Samuel Hahnemann
- Koch's phenomenon is seen in Tuberculosis.
- Secondary Attack Rate is number of exposed persons developing the disease within range of incubation period following exposure to the primary case.
- The strain which is used in BCG is Danish – 1331 strain.
- OPV (Sabin) vaccine is associated with a **rare side effect** of vaccine-associated paralytic polio or vaccine-derived poliovirus.
- Cholera vaccine and the yellow fever vaccine should not be given together.
- Most widely used test for diagnosis of Rubella (German measles) is Heme-agglutination Inhibition test.
- TB Mission 2020 was launched at 28th October 2014 by Ministry of health and family welfare. The main objective of this mission is to eliminate TB from India by 2020.
- National Deworming day – 10th February.
- Classical dengue fever is also called breakbone fever.
- Bubonic plague is the most common type of plague.
- The causative agent of scrub typhus is **Rickettsia tsutsugamushi**.
- WHO and UNICEF recommend the use of a cut-off for weight-for-height of below -3 standard deviations (SD) of the WHO standards to identify infants and children as having Severe Acute Malnutrition (SAM) (Red/Pink zone).
- **Underweight**: **Weight for age** is less than –2 standard deviations (SD) of the WHO Child Growth Standards median.

Contd...

- **Stunting**: **Height for age** is less than –2 SD of the WHO Child Growth Standards median.
- **Wasting**: **Weight for height** is less than –2 SD of the WHO Child Growth Standards median.
- **Overweight**: **Weight for height** is more than +2 SD of the WHO Child Growth Standards median.
- Ziehl & Neelsen staining is the staining technique used for tuberculosis.
- The blood pressure is the single most useful test for identifying individuals at a high risk of developing Coronary Heart Disease (CHD).
- **Framingham Study**, has played a major role in establishing the nature of CHD risk factors and their relative importance.
- Essential hypertension is the most prevalent form of hypertension accounting for 90 percent of all cases of hypertension.
- **Reduviidae bugs**, also known as cone-nose bugs, are vectors of **Chagas disease.**
- Trypanosoma cruzi is the causative agent of **chagas disease.**
- Occupational diseases are usually defined as diseases arising out of or in the course of employment.
- “Snow-storm” appearance in the lung fields of a chest X-ray is a characteristic feature of silicosis.
- Pathologically, silicosis is characterized by a dense “nodular” fibrosis, the nodules ranging from 3 mm to 4 mm in diameter.
- The recommended dietary allowance of vitamin E is placed at 10 mg of alpha tocopherol equivalents for adult males and 8 mg for adult females.
- The requirements of thiamine, riboflavin and niacin are closely related to energy intake and utilization, and are stated in terms of 1000 kcal intake of energy as:
  - Thiamine 0.5 mg/1000 kcal
  - Riboflavin 0.6 mg/1000 kcal
  - Niacin 6.0 mg/1000 kcal
- Keratomalacia or liquefaction of the cornea is a grave medical emergency. The cornea may become soft and may burst open rapidly. If the eye collapses, vision is lost.
- Conjunctival xerosis is the first clinical sign of vitamin A deficiency.
- Pleomorphism is a characteristic feature of the rash in chicken pox. All stages of the rash (papules, vesicles and crusts) may be seen simultaneously at one time, in the same area.
- Mumps infection in the first trimester of pregnancy is associated with a 25% incidence of spontaneous abortion.
- The laboratory confirmation of mumps is by positive mumps IgM antibody.
- Avian influenza refers to a large group of different influenza viruses that primarily affect birds.
- **Paroxysmal cough** is the characteristic clinical feature of **Bordetella pertussis.**
- A severely malnourished child is at high risk of developing and dying from pneumonia.
- If a client had burn injury, avoid prolonged cooling with water because it may lead to hypothermia.
- If a client had a snake bite, do not give alcoholic beverages or stimulants. They are known vasodilators and they speed up the absorption of venom.
- Do not incise or manipulate the snake bitten site. Do not apply ice.
- Bitot’s spots in young children usually indicate vitamin A deficiency.
- An excess intake of retinol causes nausea, vomiting, anorexia and sleep disorders followed by skin desquamation and then an enlarged liver and papillary edema.
- Niacin or nicotinic acid is essential for the metabolism of carbohydrate, fat and protein.
- Iron is necessary for many functions in the body including formation of hemoglobin, brain development and function, regulation of body temperature, muscle activity, and catecholamine metabolism.
- Iodine is an essential micronutrient. It is required for the synthesis of the thyroid hormones, thyroxine (T4) and triiodothyronine (T3).
- “Goitrogens”, are chemical substances leading to the development of goiter.
- The daily requirement of iodine for adults is placed at 150 micrograms. The recommendation by WHO is 250 mcg/day for iodine during pregnancy.

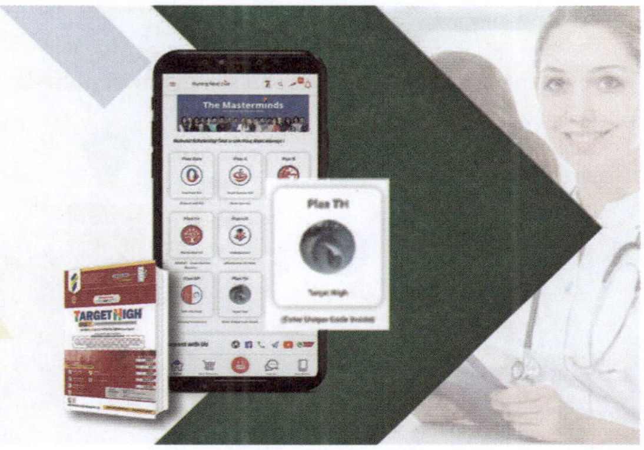

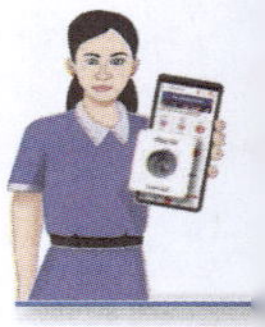

Image-Based Questions

1. Identify the statistical diagram shown

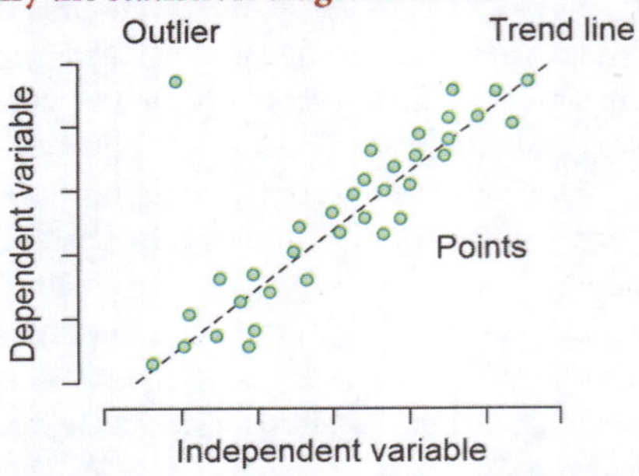

a. Ogive chart
b. Scatter plot
c. Dot matrix
d. Histogram

2. Identify the medication in the strip.

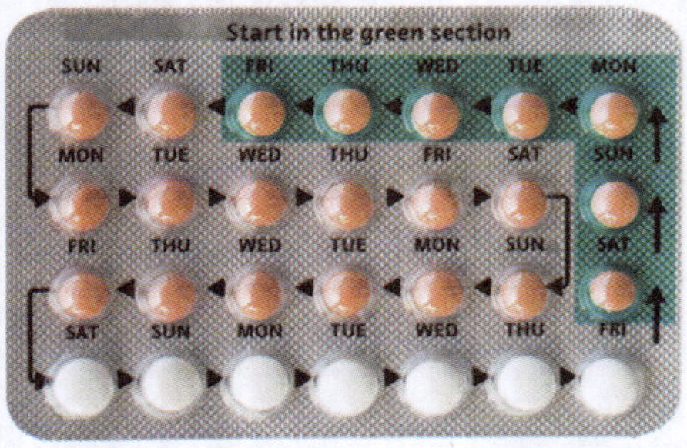

a. DOTS Category I
b. DOTS Category II
c. MDT Kit for Leprosy
d. Combined OCP

3. The type of Copper-T shown in the image is:

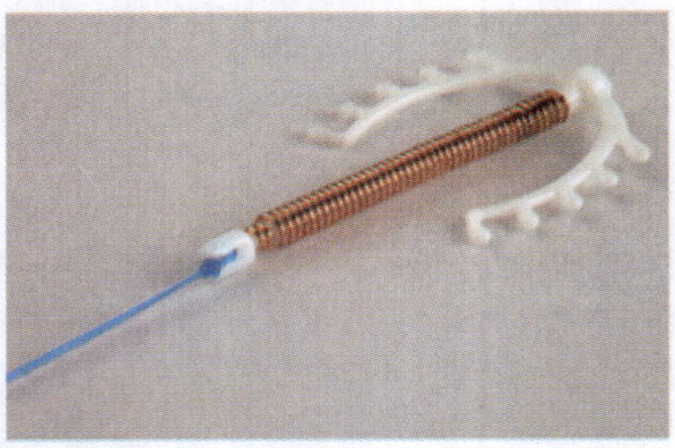

a. Cu T 200
b. Cu T 375
c. Cu T 380 A
d. Nova-T

4. Identify the national health program depicted.

a. Rashtriya Swasthya Suraksha Karyakram
b. Rashtriya Bal Swasthya Karyakram
c. Rashtriya Kishor Swasthya Karyakram
d. Navjat Shishu Suraksha Karyakrama

5. Identify the disease for which program is depicted in symbol.

a. Iodine deficiency
b. Non-communicable diseases, cancer, diabetes
c. Deafness
d. Road traffic accidents

6. Services provided at facility shown in symbol:

[Recent Question 2014]

a. DOTS services
b. HIV Counselling
c. RTI/STI services
d. First aid services

7. The logo shown in the picture belongs to:

a. Ayushman Bharat
b. National Green Tribunal
c. Jan Dhan Yojana
d. Atal Pension Yojana

8. The logo shown in the picture indicates:

a. Ayushman Bharat
b. NRHM
c. Jan Dhan Yojana
d. Atal Pension Yojana

Ans.

1. b
2. d
3. b
4. c
5. c
6. c
7. a
8. c

[*Courtesy*: PHOTON-20® 3th ed. by Vivek Jain, CBS Publishers and Distributors Pvt Ltd]

9. The logo shown in the picture is associated with:

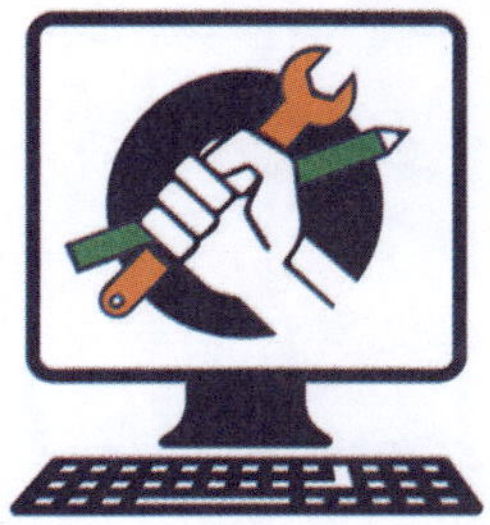

a. Make in India project
b. Skill India Mission
c. Industrial revolution
d. Old age pension scheme

10. The logo image shown in the picture is associated with:

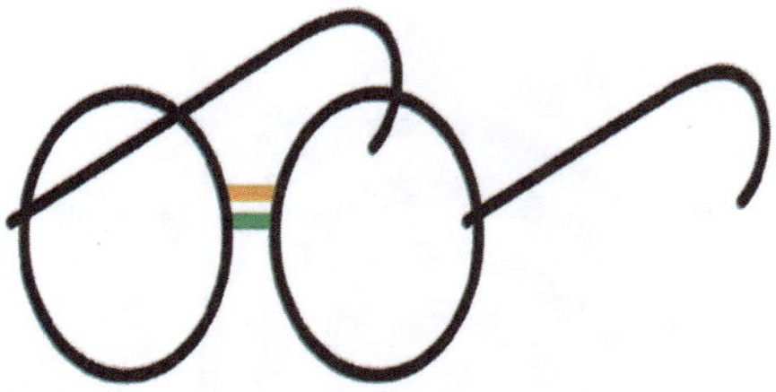

a. Sansad Adarsh Gram Yojana
b. Swachh Bharat Mission
c. Shramew Jayate Yojana
d. Atal Pension Yojana

11. The logo shown in the image is associated with ________ scheme.

a. Skill India Mission
b. Hridaya Plan
c. Beti Bachao Beti Padhao
d. Shramew Jayate Yojana

12. Identify vector shown in photograph:

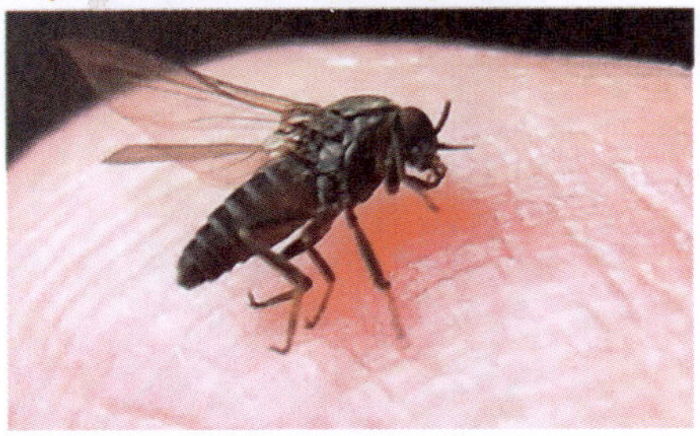

a. Culex
b. Mansonia
c. Sandfly
d. House fly

13. Identify the strip shown in photograph.

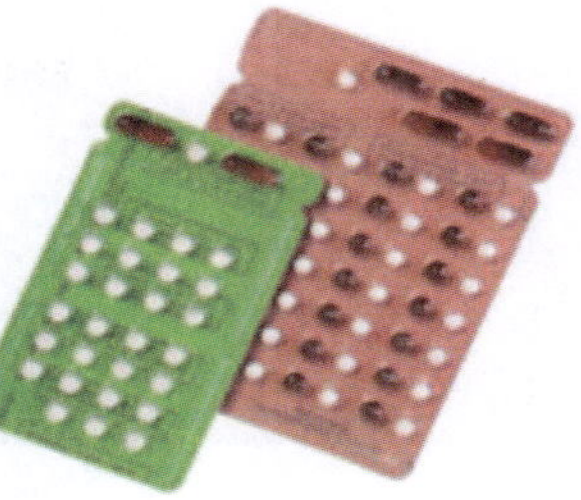

a. Combined OCP
b. Iron Folic acid tablets
c. DOTS
d. MDT

14. Vector shown in photograph can transmit .... disease:

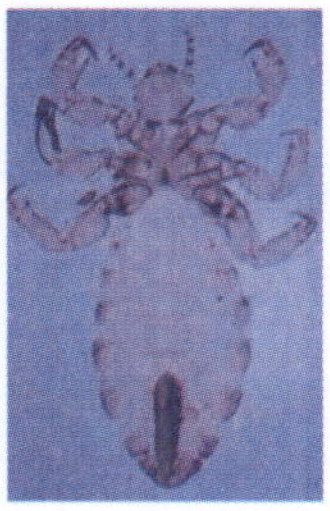

a. Trench fever
b. RMSF
c. Endemic typhus
d. Scrub typhus

15. Animal shown in photograph is reservoir host of:

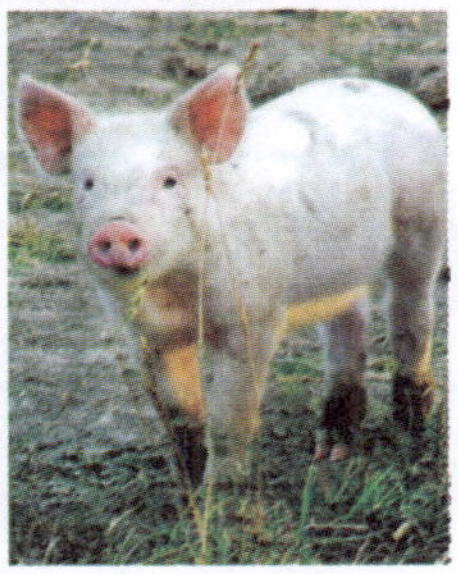

a. Rabies
b. Japanese encephalitis
c. Yellow fever
d. Chikungunya fever

16. The lesion on the skin is most likely a:

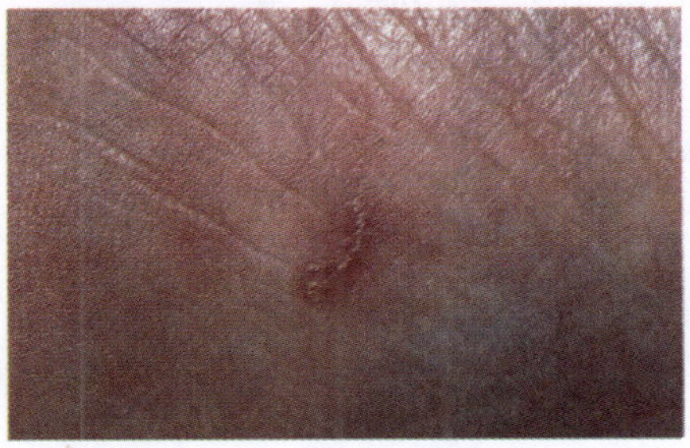

a. Folliculitis
b. Scabies skin lesion
c. Erythema
d. Cellulitis

Ans.

9.	b
10.	b
11.	c
12.	c
13.	d
14.	a
15.	b
16.	b

17. Identify the national health program depicted by the symbol:

a. IDSP
b. NPCDCS
c. RCH
d. National Deworming Program

18. Identify the legislation/scheme shown in symbol:

a. RTI Act 2005
b. RSBY 2008
c. NREGA 2005
d. Factory Act 1948

19. Statutory body (shown in symbol) has been established under the act passed in:

a. 2000
b. 2002
c. 2006
d. 2013

20. Identify the parasitic insect:

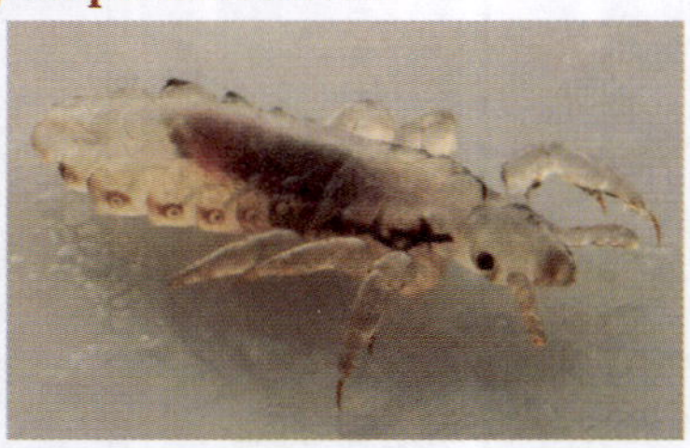

a. Scabies mite
b. Bed bug
c. Mansonia
d. Head lice (Pediculus capitis)

21. Identify the symbol:

a. Vitamin A in Immunization
b. Defluoridation of water
c. Iodization of salt
d. Iron fortification of salt

22. Identify the organization depicted by symbol:

a. National Planning Commission (NPC)
b. National Disaster Management Authority (NDMA)
c. Unique Identification Authority (UIDAI)
d. ESI Corporation

23. Content composition of Pills shown in photograph:

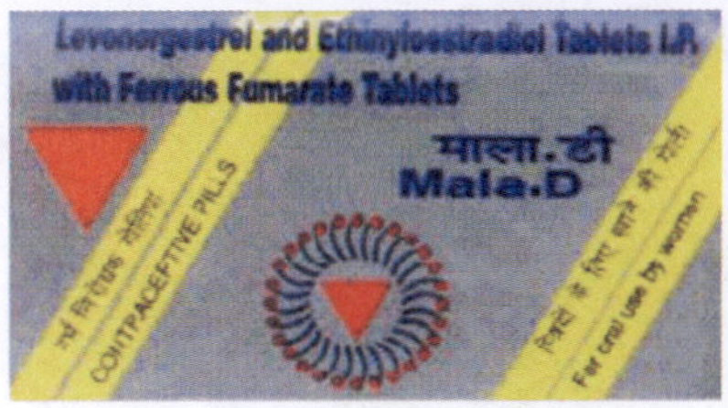

a. 15 mcg Estrogen, 300 mcg Progesterone
b. 150 mcg Estrogen, 30 mcg Progesterone
c. 30 mcg Estrogen, 150 mcg Progesterone
d. 300 mcg Estrogen, 15 mcg Progesterone

24. Identify the contraceptive device shown in the image:

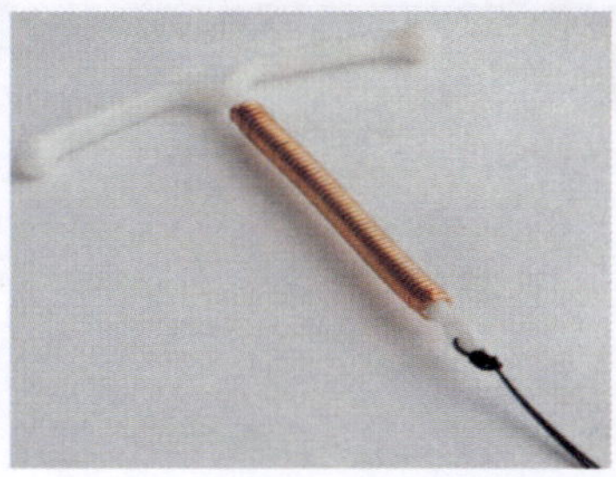

a. CuT 7
b. CuT 220 B
c. CuT 380 A
d. Progestasert

Ans.

17. b
18. b
19. c
20. d
21. c
22. c
23. c
24. c

25. Duration for usage of Barrier methods is recommended after a client underwent the procedure shown in the image:

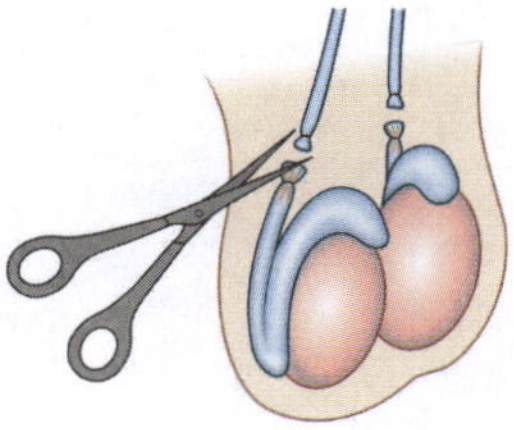

a. 30 days
b. 60 days
c. 90 days
d. 12 months

26. Identify the symbol shown in photograph:

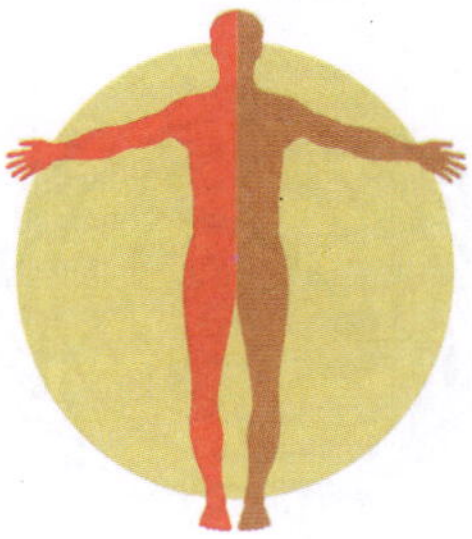

a. MDT
b. DOTS
c. ART
d. Anti-malaria therapy

27. Identify the national health Program depicted by the symbol:

a. RNTCP
b. NIDDCP
c. NRHM
d. NVBDCP

28. Identify the national health program depicted by the symbol:

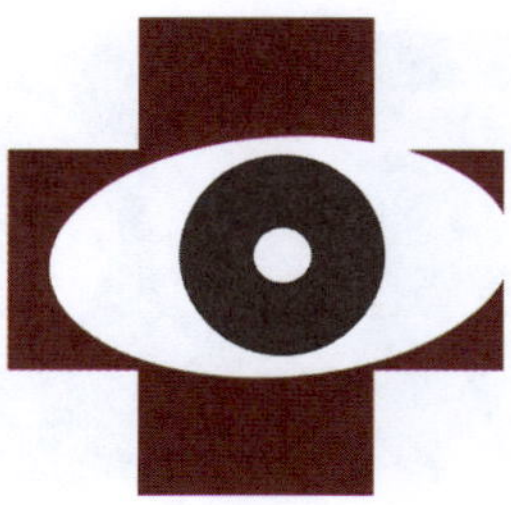

a. IDSP
b. RCH
c. NPCB
d. NVBDCP

29. Identify the scheme program plan launched by government of India:

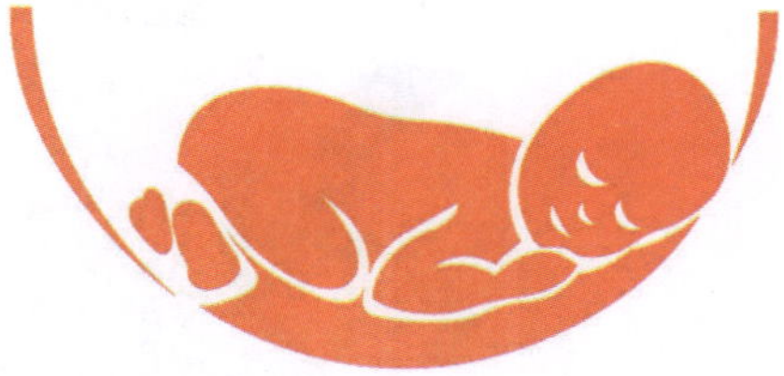

a. Mission Indradhanush
b. Kangaroo Mother Care
c. Reproductive and Child Health
d. India Newborn Action Plan

30. Identify the program associated with the symbol shown:

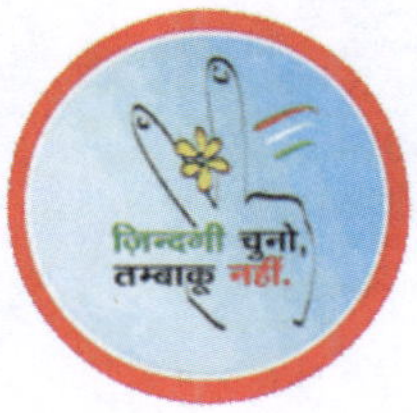

a. NPCDCS
b. NIDDCP
c. National Tobacco Control Program
d. JSY Scheme

31. Identify the campaign depicted by the symbol:

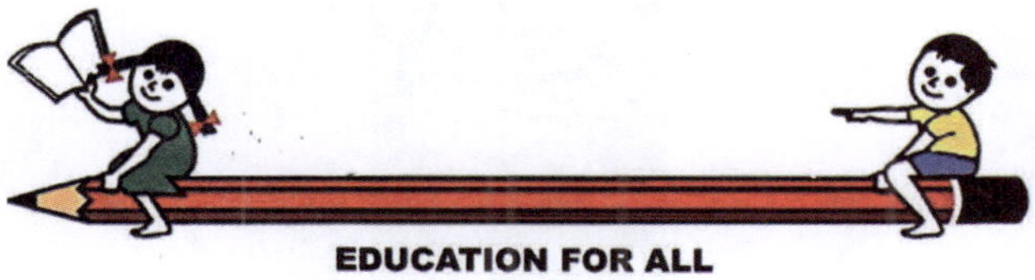

a. Beti Bachao Beti Padhao Andolan
b. Sarva Shiksha Abhiyan
c. Kishori Shakti Yojana
d. Save the girl child

32. Location of organization depicted by symbol in photograph is:

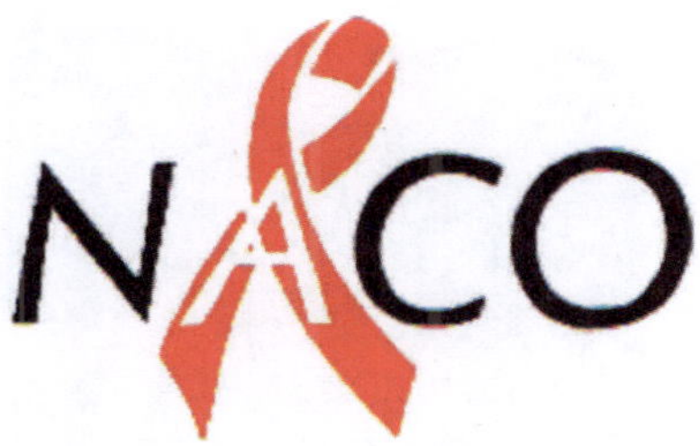

a. New Delhi
b. Kolkata
c. Mumbai
d. Chennai

Ans.

25. c
26. b
27. c
28. c
29. d
30. c
31. b
32. a

33. Number of vaccine vials that can be kept in the equipment shown in photograph:

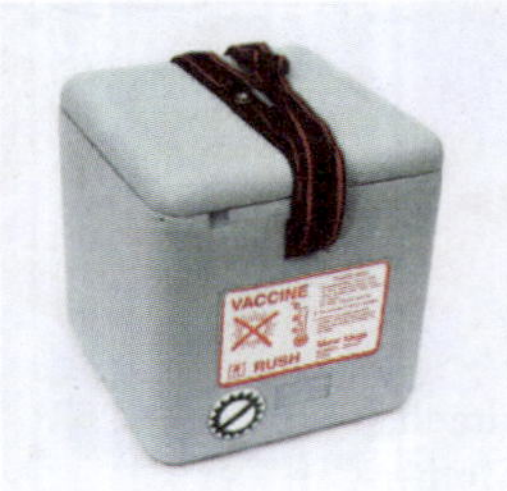

a. 1–2 b. 2–4
c. 6–8 d. 16–20

34. Identify the contraceptive device shown in photograph:

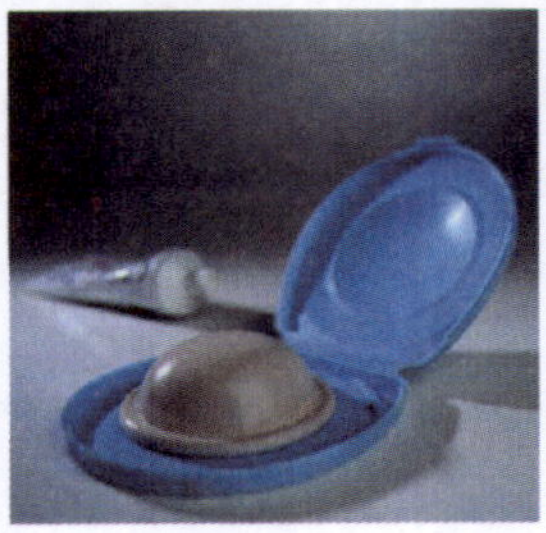

a. Female condom b. Diaphragm
c. Vaginal sponge d. Vaginal ring

35. Identify the contraceptive device shown:

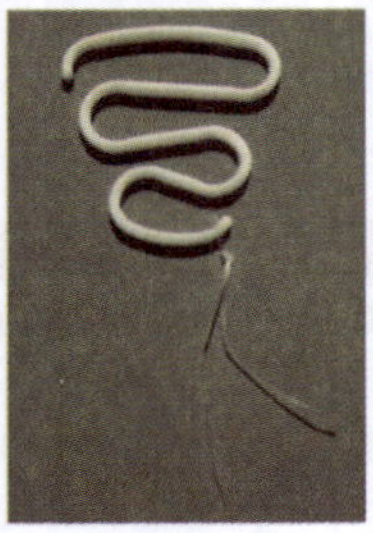

a. Progestasert b. Mirena
c. Lippes loop d. Vaginal ring

36. Content composition of contraceptive shown in photograph is: (Estrogen, progesterone):

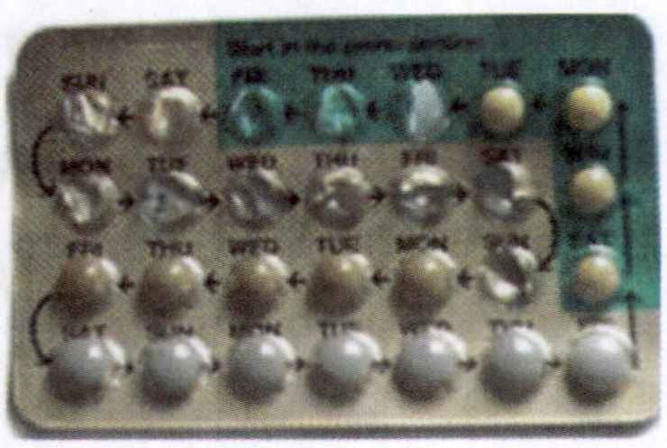

a. 15 mcg, 30 mcg b. 30 mcg, 150 mcg
c. 150 mcg, 30 mcg d. 30 mcg, 15 mcg

37. Identify vector shown in photograph:

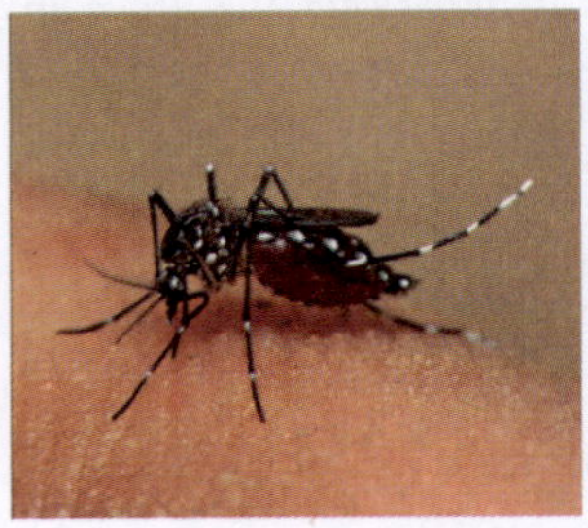

a. Anopheles b. Culex
c. Aedes d. Mansonia

38. Identify the International Health Agency shown in photograph:

a. WHO b. UNICEF
c. ILO d. FAO

39. Location of headquarters of International Health Agency shown in photograph:

a. Geneva b. Rome
c. New York d. New Delhi

40. Location of headquarters of International Health Agency shown in photograph:

CDC

a. Geneva b. Rome
c. New York d. Atlanta

Ans.

33. d
34. b
35. c
36. b
37. c
38. a
39. c
40. d

41. Identify the substance deposited in ring shown in photograph:

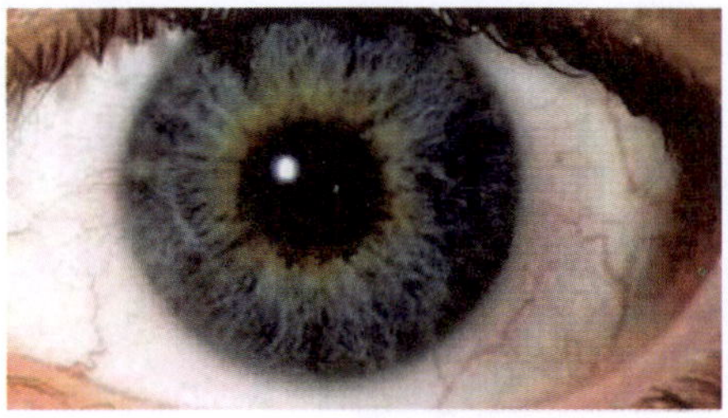

a. Lead b. Mercury
c. Iron d. Copper

42. Identify the type of contraceptive shown in photograph:

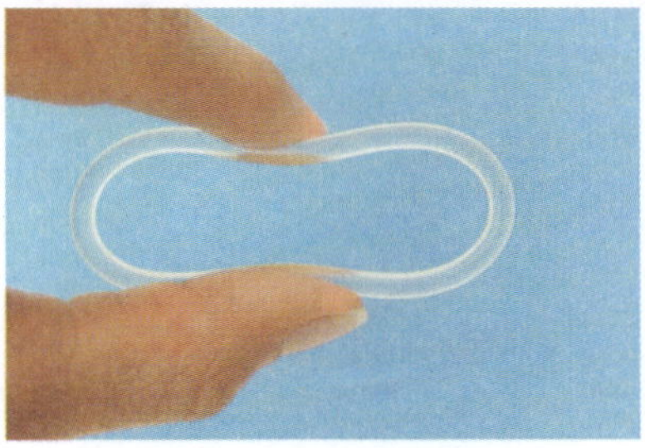

a. Diaphragm b. Cervical cap
c. Vaginal ring d. Contraceptive patch

43. How can the efficacy of the contraceptive in figure be improved?

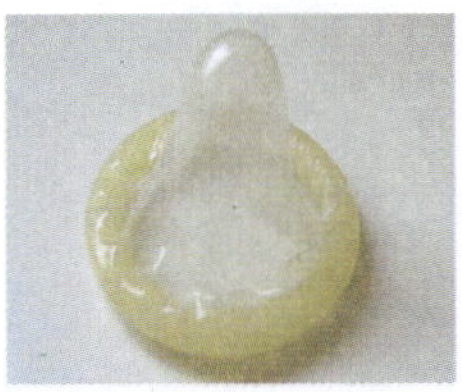

a. By using water based lubricant
b. By using oil based lubricant
c. By using spermicidal jelly
d. By making small hole near teat

44. Identify the contraceptive shown in figure.

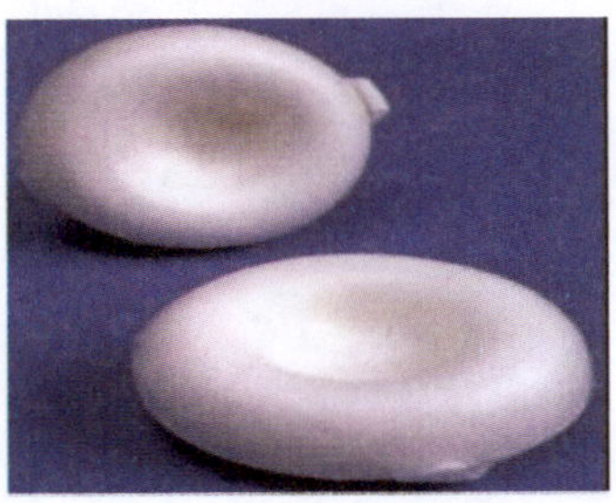

a. Dutch Cap b. Cervical Cap
c. Diaphragm d. Vaginal sponge

45. The symbol shown in figure is related to:

a. National Human Rights Commission
b. Sarva Siksha Abhiyan
c. National Literacy Mission
d. International Yoga Day

46. The diagram shown in figure represents:

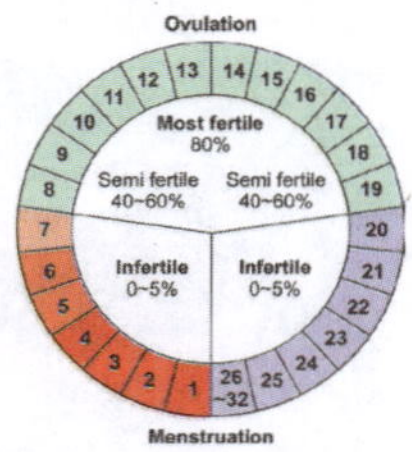

a. Ideal Tubectomy time estimation
b. BBT Method
c. Cervical mucus method
d. Rhythm method

47. The symbol shown in figure is related to:

a. NUHM b. Smart city
c. NHAI d. Swachh Bharat

48. Identify the scheme/program/plan launched by Government of India. ***(Refer explanation at the end)***

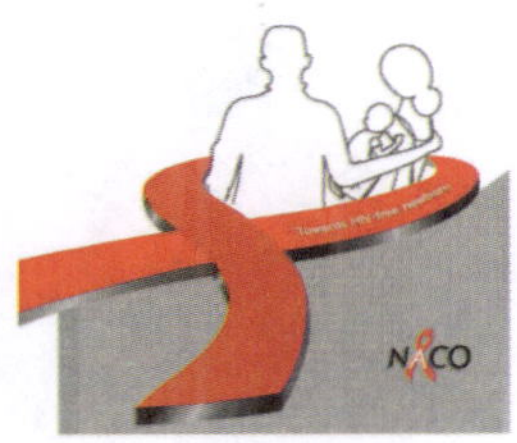

a. HIV/AIDS b. ICTC
c. ART d. PPTCT

Ans.

41.	d
42.	c
43.	c
44.	d
45.	c
46.	d
47.	b
48.	d

49. Identify the scheme shown in symbol:
(Refer explanation at the end)

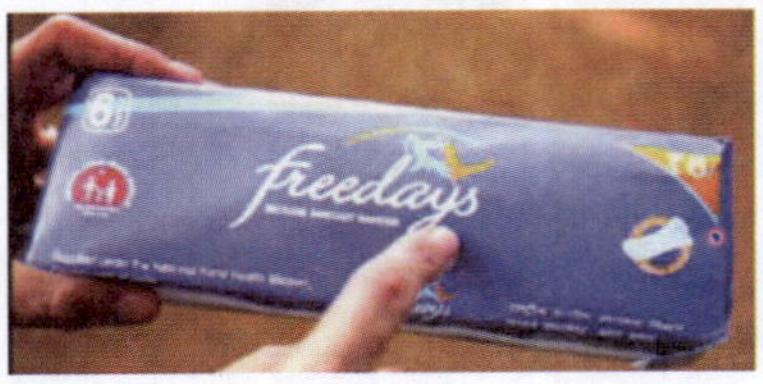

a. SABLA Scheme
b. Kishori Shakti Yojana
c. Janani Suraksha Yojana
d. Menstrual Hygiene Scheme

50. Following Viral diseases are transmitted by Vector shown in Photograph except:

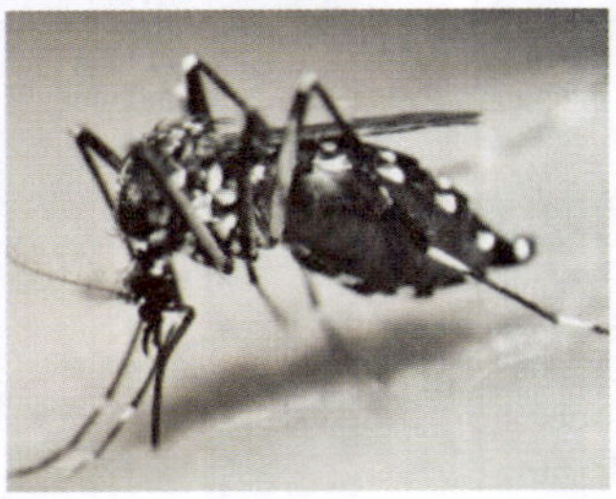

a. Dengue
b. Chikungunya
c. Japanese encephalitis
d. Yellow fever

51. Disease transmitted by Vector shown in photograph is:

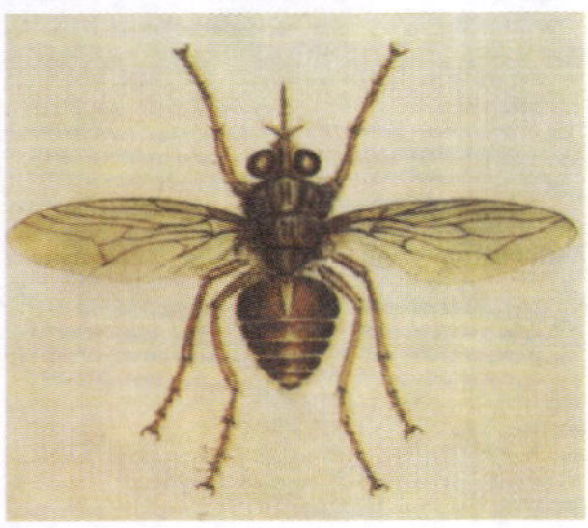

a. Malaria
b. Trypanosomiasis
c. Onchocerciasis
d. Poliomyelitis

52. Which Biomedical waste is disposed in BMW colour coded bag shown in photograph? *[AIIMS May 2017]*

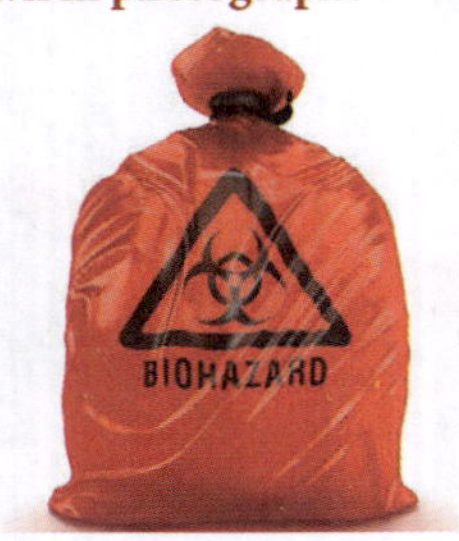

a. Soiled waste
b. Sharp waste
c. Urine bags
d. Anatomical waste

53. Identify the National Health Program depicted by the symbol: *[Recent Question 2013, 2016]*

a. RNTCP
b. NACP
c. NRHM
d. NLEP

54. Identify the National Health Program depicted by the symbol: *[Recent Question 2014]*

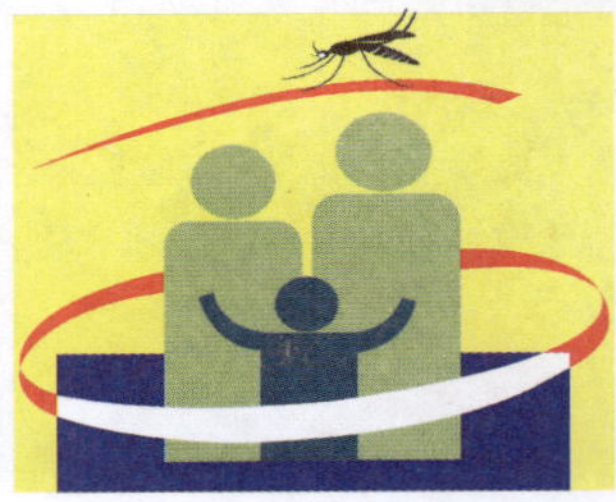

a. IDSP
b. RCH
c. NRHM
d. NVBDCP

55. True about instrument, shown in photograph, is all; except:

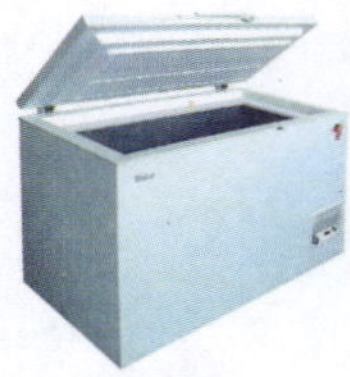

a. Used to store vaccines at PHC
b. Requires 8 hours electricity per day minimum
c. Without electricity, maintain up to 24 hours
d. Should not be used to freeze ice packs

56. Identify Vector shown in photograph: *[Recent Question 2013]*

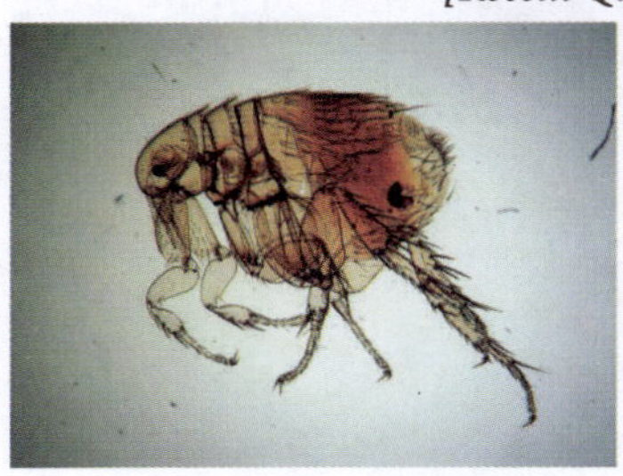

a. Rat flea
b. Louse
c. Soft tick
d. Itch mite

Ans.

49. d
50. c
51. b
52. c
53. d
54. d
55. c
56. a

57. Vector shown in photograph can transmit:

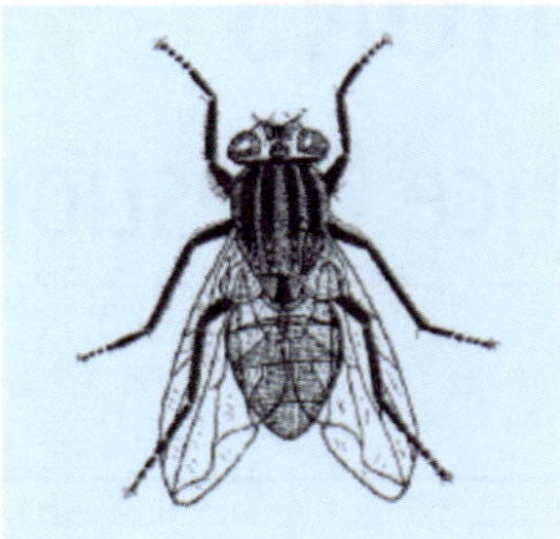

a. Poliomyelitis b. Trachoma
c. Anthrax d. All of these

58. Drug of choice for disease caused by Mite shown in photograph is:

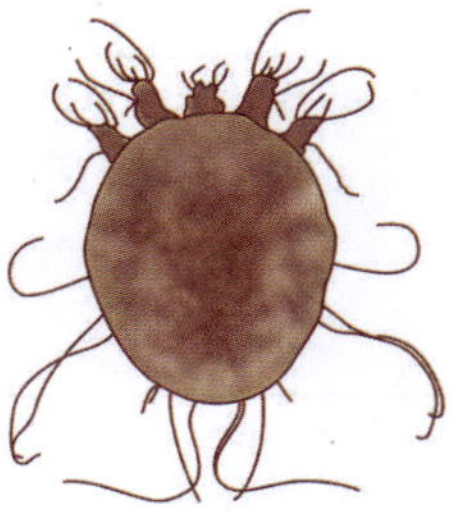

a. Ivermectin b. 1% Permethrin
c. 5% Permethrin d. Azithromycin

59. Disposal mechanism of waste shown in photograph is:

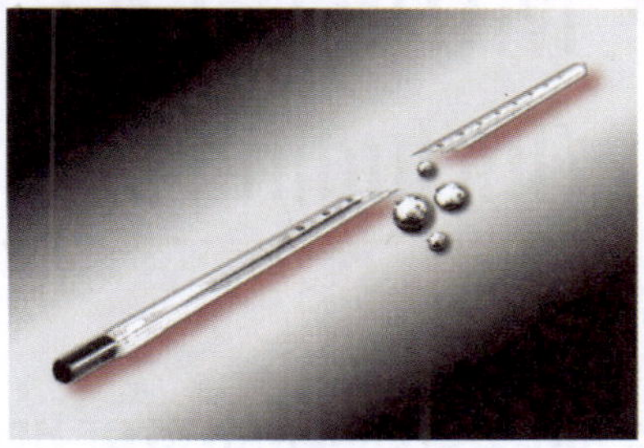

a. Autoclaving b. Incineration
c. Recycling d. Microwaving

60. Identify the diagram used in demography:

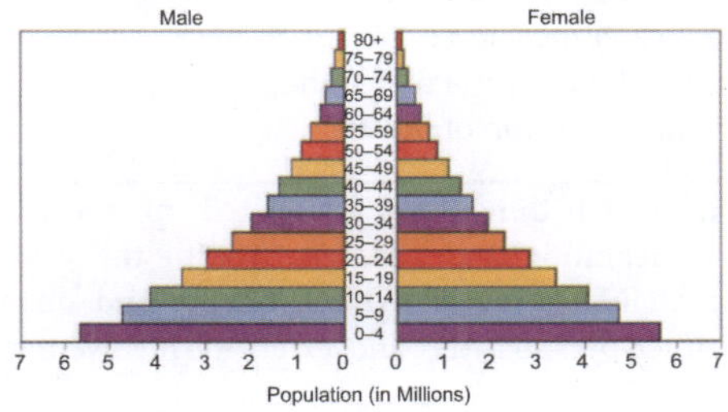

a. Sex ratio pyramid b. Age-sex pyramid
c. Malthusian growth model d. Dependency ratio

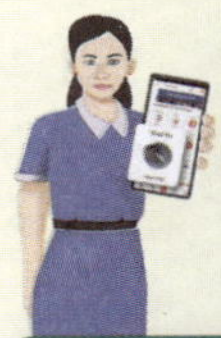

Ans.

57. d
58. c
59. c
60. b

Explanations of Image-Based Questions

48. Ans. (d) PPTCT

[Ref. Obstetrics & Gynecology For PGs by Gopalan, 3e p172]

Prevention of Parent to Child Transmission of HIV India (Photograph)

Modality	Description	Efficacy
Zidovudine	Mother: 300 mg BD from 36 weeks POG + 300 mg 3 h during delivery Child: 2 mg/kg 6 h × 6 weeks	66%
Nevirapine	Single oral dose Mother: 200 mg at labor onset Child: 2 mg/kg within 72 h of birth	50%
Cesarean section	Elective CS	50%
Triple ARV	Tenofovir 300 mg OD Lamivudine 300 mg OD Efavirenz 600 mg OD	90%

49. Ans. (d) Menstrual Hygiene Scheme

[Ref. Adolescence Education by Choudhary, 1/e p186]

Scheme for Promotion of Menstrual Hygiene (Photograph)

- The scheme aims at ensuring that adolescent girls in the target group have adequate knowledge and information about menstrual hygiene and the use of sanitary napkins, that high quality, safe products are made available to them, and that environmentally safe disposal mechanisms are readily accessible
- The scheme has been launched as part of the Adolescent Reproductive and Sexual Health (ARSH) component under RCH II
- The sanitary napkins are provided under NHM's brand, 'Freedays'
- These napkins are being sold to adolescent girls at the rate of ₹6 per pack of six napkins by Accredited Social Health Activists (ASHAs)

"Man needs difficulties; they are necessary for health."
—Carl Jung

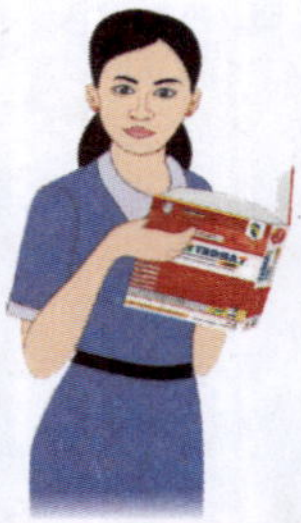

MULTIPLE CHOICE QUESTIONS
(Including Explained and Practice Questions)

CONCEPTS AND DETERMINANTS OF HEALTH & WELL-BEING

1. Quality and quantity of an individual's inter-personal ties and extent of involvement with the community is known as: *(AIIMS BPL NO 2018)*

a. Mental dimension of health
b. Physical dimension of health
c. Spiritual dimension of health
d. Social dimension of health

Explanation: Social dimension is related to social well-being that creates integration and adjustment with the individual and community. Mainly it is defined the quality and quantity of an individual's inter-personal ties and extent of involvement with the community.

2. The functions of community are: *(AIIMS Raipur Grade II 2017)*

a. It provides space for socializing and recreation
b. It provides safety and security
c. Socialization and Education for its members
d. Provides opportunity for interaction among members

a. a, b, c   b. b, c, d
c. a, c, d   d. a, b, c, d

Explanation: The functions of community include socialization, social control, social participation and mutual support

3. Ageism is characterized by:

a. Denial of negative stereotypes regarding aging
b. Positive attitude towards the elderly based on age
c. Negative attitude towards the elderly based on age
d. Negative attitude towards the elderly based on physical disability

4. Entomology is the science that studies: *(RRB SSNE 2015)*

a. Behavior of human beings
b. Insects
c. Behavior of ants
d. Formation of rocks

5. Head Quarters of World Health Organization (WHO) is situated at:

a. New York, United States of America
b. London, England
c. Geneva, Switzerland
d. Paris, France

6. The concept of health which emphasizes that health is a 'sound mind in a sound body in a sound family in a sound environment' is: *(AIIMS Bhopal Grade-I 2018)*

a. Ecological concept   b. Physical concept
c. Psychological concept   d. Holistic concept

Explanation: The health has been described by various scientists according to their concept of viewing the health. The ecologist viewed health as a harmonious equilibrium between man and environment. The physical concept of health describes health as a state of well-functioning of the body and psychological concept describes health as absence of mental illness. The Holistic concept of health is viewed as a multidimensional process involving well-being of the whole person in the context of his environment

7. The World Health Day is observed on:

a. 7th April
b. 4th May
c. 17th August
d. 1st December

Explanation: The World Health Organization observes World Health Day on 7th of April every year.

8. The subjective component of well-being is referred to as:

a. Physical quality of life
b. Quality of work
c. Quality of life
d. Standard of living

Explanation: Subjective well-being is called as quality of life.

9. Health means absence of disease is the concept of:

a. Biomedical
b. Ecology
c. Holistic
d. Psychosocial

Explanation: Health means absence of disease is the biomedical concept.

10. What is the theme for 2016 world health day?

a. Halt the rise: Beat diabetes
b. Food safety
c. Vector-borne diseases: Small bite, big threat
d. Healthy heart beat, Healthy blood pressure

Explanation:

- **2016:** Halt the rise: Beat diabetes
- **2015:** Food safety
- **2014:** Vector-borne diseases: Small bite, big threat
- **2013:** Healthy heart beat, Healthy blood pressure

11. Forerunner of modern public health is: *(JIPMER 2012)*

a. Phoebe
b. John Snow
c. Serelette
d. Louis Pasteur

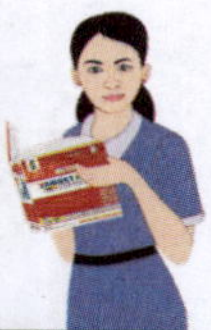

Ans.

1.	d
2.	d
3.	c
4.	b
5.	c
6.	d
7.	a
8.	c
9.	a
10.	a
11.	d

12. Which of the following is not a method of health promotion; EXCEPT:
a. Behavioral modification b. Lifestyle modification
c. Immunization d. Nutritional education

13. One characteristic of the integrative model of health care is:
a. Increased cost
b. A focus on physical disease states
c. An integration of mind-body-spirit
d. The plan of care is directed by the health care provider

14. WHO definition of health is:
a. Complete absence of disease
b. Physical and mental well-being
c. Complete physical, mental and social well-being not merely the absence of disease or infirmity
d. Complete physical, mental, psychological and social well-being

INDICATORS OF HEALTH

15. All of the following components are used in Kuppuswamy classification of socio-economic status; EXCEPT:
a. Family income b. Education
c. Occupation d. Number of children

Explanation: Component of Kuppuswamy scale includes education, occupation and income. Kuppuswamy classification is used in urban and periurban areas which consider the education of the head of family, occupation of head of the family and per capita monthly income.

16. The process of continuous progressive improvement of the health status of a population is:
a. Block development
b. Community development
c. Health development
d. Society development

Explanation: Health development is the progressive improvement of health status of a population.

17. Ongoing measurement of performance of a health service refers to:
a. Evaluation b. Monitoring
c. Scrutinization d. Surveillance

Explanation: Ongoing measurement of performance of health services is known as surveillance.

18. Human Development Index (HDI) does not include:
a. Mean Years of schooling b. Life expectancy at birth
c. Real GDP per capita d. Adult literacy rate

19. The value of Human Developmental Index in India is:
a. 0.500 b. 0.586
c. 0.505 d. 0.540

20. Nursing interventions directed at health promotion in the older adult are primarily focused on:
a. Disease management
b. Controlling symptoms of illness.
c. Teaching positive health behaviors
d. Teaching regarding nutrition to enhance longevity

Explanation: Nursing interventions directed at health promotion in the older adult are primarily focused on teaching positive health behaviors. These interventions aim to empower older adults to take control of their health and make choices that promote well-being and prevent illness. By providing education and guidance on topics such as exercise, healthy eating, stress management, and preventive screenings, nurses can help older adults adopt and maintain healthy habits that enhance their overall health and quality of life.

21. Most important health status indicator of a country:
a. Life expectancy at birth
b. Maternal mortality rate
c. Total fertility rate
d. Infant mortality rate

Explanation: Life expectancy at birth is considered the most important health status indicator of a country. It provides an overall measure of the average number of years a person is expected to live from birth, taking into account factors such as healthcare, living conditions, and socioeconomic factors.

22. Which one of the following is not a socio-economic indicator?
a. Literacy rate
b. Family size
c. Housing
d. Life expectancy at birth

LEVELS OF HEALTHCARE & HEALTH FOR ALL

23. Philosophy of Primary Health Care are as follows; EXCEPT:
(ESIC 2019)
a. Equity and justice
b. Intersectoral approach
c. Primary prevention
d. Inter-relationship of health and development

Explanation: Philosophy of Primary Health Care is based on the values of equity, social justice, solidarity, Intersectoral approach and inter-relationship of health and development, Further, at its core is a focus on population health, illness prevention, and health promotion.

24. The principles of primary health care include:
(AIIMS Raipur Grade II 2017)
a. Equitable distribution
b. Community participation
c. Coverage and accessibility
d. Appropriateness and continuity
a. a, b, c b. b, c, d
c. a, c, d c. a, b, c, d

Explanation: The principles of primary health care include intersectoral coordination, appropriate technology, equitable distribution and community participation.

25. The following are the functions of male health Workers as a Health Team member; EXCEPT:
(AIIMS Raipur Grade II 2017)
a. Conduct survey of the Sub center and maintain record of all families
b. Provide nutrition advice and Immunization to mothers and Children
c. Maintain information of all vital events
d. Promote health education activities

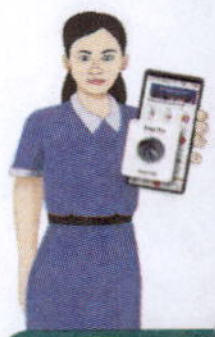

Ans.
12. c
13. c
14. c
15. d
16. c
17. d
18. d
19. b
20. c
21. a
22. d
23. c
24. a
25. b

Explanation: The functions of health worker include community service provider, facilitator, health counselor, co-researcher, member of a team and health educator.

26. Which level of healthcare primarily focuses on providing comprehensive healthcare services to individuals and families within their community? *New Q*

a. Primary healthcare b. Secondary healthcare
c. Tertiary healthcare d. Quaternary healthcare

Explanation: Primary healthcare is the first point of contact for individuals seeking healthcare and is delivered by healthcare professionals such as community health nurses in community settings. It focuses on providing essential healthcare services, promoting health, preventing diseases, and managing common health problems.

27. The focus of secondary health care is:

a. Early detection
b. Early diagnosis and treatment
c. Prevention of risk factors
d. Immunization for preventable diseases

28. The characteristic of primary health care as compared to secondary and tertiary health care is:

a. Less costly b. More costly
c. Less efficient
d. Lack of resources

29. All among the following are the characteristic of secondary health care; EXCEPT:

a. Procedures for diagnosis and treatment available
b. It acts as first referral center.
c. Some degree of specialization
d. Complex surgical procedures

30. Which among the following is not a component of primary health care?

a. Immunization
b. Family planning
c. Essential drug supply
d. Specialized services

31. Eligible couple register is maintained at:

a. Sub center b. PHC
c. CHC d. District hospital

32. Which among the following committee recommended three tier health care delivery system in rural India?

a. Bhore Committee
b. Jungalwalla Committee
c. Srivastava Committee
d. Kartar Singh Committee

33. All among the following are job responsibility of health worker male; EXCEPT:

a. Sputum collection
b. ORS distribution
c. DOTS supervision
d. Growth monitoring

MILLENNIUM DEVELOPMENT GOAL AND SUSTAINABLE DEVELOPMENT GOAL

34. How many millennium development goals are there?

a. 7 b. 8
c. 9 d. 10

35. Which MDG is represented by the following graphics?

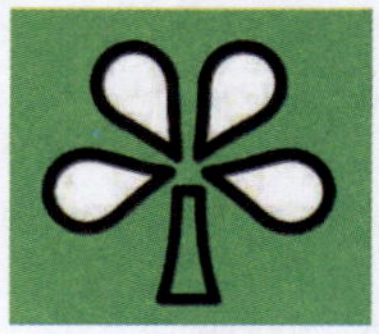

a. Eradicate extreme poverty and hunger.
b. Achieve universal primary education.
c. Ensure environmental sustainability.
d. Improve maternal health

36. MDG3 is to promote gender equality. Which of the following is not a target or indicator?

a. Increase the number of female political representatives
b. End gender-based violence
c. Eliminate gender disparity in primary and secondary education
d. Increase the share of women in waged employment

37. Which country was the first to achieve the goal of halving extreme poverty?

a. Zimbabwe b. Thailand
c. Bolivia d. Ghana

LEVELS OF PREVENTION

38. Secondary prevention is: *(ESIC 2019)*

a. Safe water supply, Vector and animal reservoir control
b. Early detection (diagnosis) of disease and Prompt treatment
c. Good living and working condition
d. Nutritional counseling

Explanation: Secondary prevention aims to reduce the impact of a disease or injury that has already occurred. This is done by detecting (early diagnosis) and promptly treating disease or injury as soon as possible to halt or slow its progress.

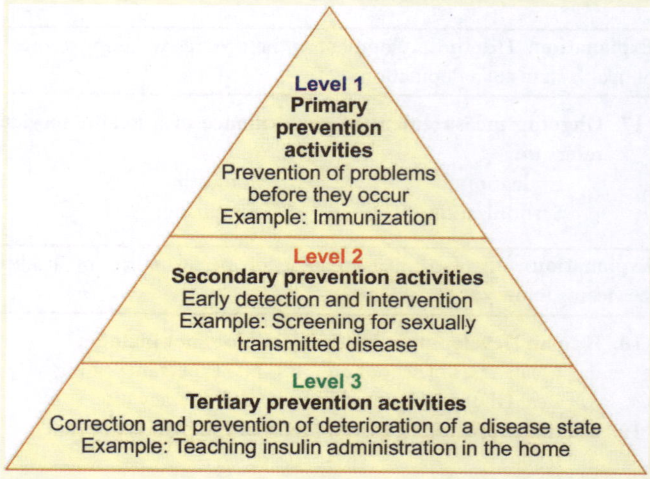

Figure: The 3 levels of prevention

39. Prevention of risk factors related to a disease condition is known as:

a. Primordial prevention b. Primary prevention
c. Secondary prevention d. Tertiary prevention

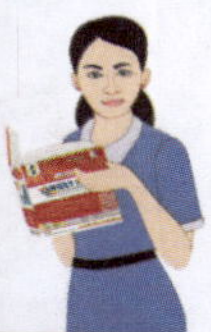

Ans.

26.	a
27.	b
28.	a
29.	d
30.	d
31.	a
32.	c
33.	d
34.	b
35.	c
36.	b
37.	d
38.	b
39.	a

Explanation: Primordial prevention is defined as prevention of risk factors themselves, beginning with change in social and environmental conditions in which these factors are observed to develop, and continuing for high risk children, adolescents and young adults.

40. Which of the following is NOT considered the secondary prevention strategy? *New Q*
- a. Health screening for hypertension
- b. Contact tracing for STI
- c. Case finding for Cholera
- d. Reconstructive surgery for burn patient

Explanation: Reconstructive surgery for burn patients is not considered a Tertiary prevention. It is a form of treatment and rehabilitation aimed at restoring function and appearance after a burn injury has occurred.

Secondary prevention strategies focus on early detection, diagnosis, and treatment of a disease or condition to prevent its progression and minimize its impact.

41. Main intervention in primordial prevention is:
- a. Health education
- b. Immunization
- c. Early diagnosis
- d. Early screening

42. Pap smear screening is an example of:
- a. Primordial prevention
- b. Primary prevention
- c. Secondary prevention
- d. Tertiary prevention

43. An example of Primary Prevention strategies is:
- a. Early diagnosis
- b. Hospitalization and treatment
- c. Rehabilitation
- d. Health Education

44. Prevention of risk factors is known as:
- a. Primordial prevention
- b. Primary prevention
- c. Secondary prevention
- d. Tertiary prevention

45. Which of the following is not an example of primary prevention?
- a. Breast self-examination
- b. Smoking cessation
- c. BCG vaccination
- d. Vitamin A supplementation

46. Which of the following is considered as secondary prevention strategies?
- a. Physiotherapy for arthralgia
- b. Surgery for cataract
- c. DOTS therapy for a tuberculosis patient
- d. All of the above

47. Early diagnosis of disease is known as ________ strategy.
- a. Primary prevention
- b. Secondary prevention
- c. Tertiary prevention
- d. Rehabilitation prevention

48. Example of primary prevention strategies includes:
- a. Colonoscopy at age 50
- b. Avoidance of tobacco products
- c. Intake of a diet low in saturated fat in a patient with high cholesterol
- d. Teaching the importance of exercise to a patient with hypertension

49. Immunization is:
- a. Primary prevention
- b. Secondary prevention
- c. Tertiary prevention
- d. Disability limitation

50. Iodized salt in iodine deficiency control programme is:
- a. Primordial prevention
- b. Primary prevention
- c. Secondary prevention
- d. Tertiary prevention

51. Level of prevention that includes specific protection is:
- a. Primordial
- b. Primary
- c. Secondary
- d. Tertiary

52. When you immunize a child for measles what type of prevention are you doing?
- a. Primordial prevention
- b. Health promotion
- c. Specific protection
- d. Secondary Prevention

53. Monitoring of blood pressure is which level of prevention?
- a. Primordial
- b. Primary
- c. Secondary
- d. Tertiary

54. Patient is on psychotherapy, what is the level of prevention?
- a. Primordial
- b. Primary
- c. Secondary
- d. Tertiary

55. Screening of the disease is which type of prevention?
- a. Primordial prevention
- b. Primary prevention
- c. Secondary prevention
- d. Tertiary prevention

56. Target group in secondary prevention:
- a. Healthy individuals
- b. Healthy-appearing individuals
- c. Patients with advanced stage of disease
- d. Patient recovering from chronic illness

Explanation: Secondary prevention emphasizes early disease detection and its target is healthy-appearing individuals with subclinical forms of the disease. Secondary prevention often occurs in the form of screenings.

Ref: Kisling L.A., Das J.M. Prevention strategies. (https://www.ncbi.nlm.nih.gov/books/NBK537222/)

57. Disability limitation is which mode of prevention?
- a. Primordial prevention
- b. Primary prevention
- c. Secondary prevention
- d. Tertiary prevention

58. Primordial prevention is done in population:
- a. With risk factors
- b. Without risk factors
- c. Whole population with low prevalence of disease
- d. Population with disease

59. A 19-year-old female presents to the gynecology clinic for her annual check-up. During the assessment, the nurse discusses the importance of obtaining a Pap smear test for the detection of cervical carcinoma. This is an example of which level of prevention? *New Q*
- a. Primordial prevention
- b. Primary prevention
- c. Secondary prevention
- d. Tertiary prevention

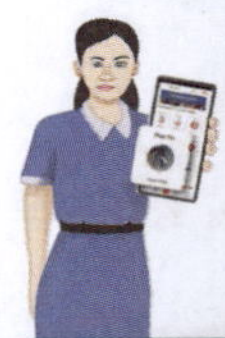

Ans.

40. d
41. a
42. c
43. d
44. a
45. a
46. d
47. b
48. b
49. a
50. b
51. b
52. c
53. c
54. c
55. c
56. b
57. d
58. b
59. c

Explanation: Secondary prevention involves early detection and intervention to identify and treat a disease or condition in its early stages to prevent its progression and reduce its impact. The Pap smear test is a screening tool used to detect abnormal cells in the cervix, which may indicate the presence of cervical carcinoma or precancerous changes.

60. Chemoprophylaxis is _______ level of prevention.
a. Primary b. Secondary
c. Tertiary d. Quaternary

61. Primordial prevention means:
a. Prevention of complications
b. Prevention of infections
c. Preventions of emergence of risk factors
d. None of the above

62. Sputum examination for AFB is an example of:
a. Primordial prevention b. Primary prevention
c. Secondary prevention d. Tertiary prevention

63. A Community Health Nursing is providing health education to a diabetic patient regarding how to self-monitor blood glucose level. Which of the following level of prevention is practiced here?
a. Primordial prevention b. Primary prevention
c. Secondary prevention d. Tertiary prevention

Explanation: Tertiary prevention aims to soften the impact of an ongoing illness or injury that has lasting effects. This can be achieved by helping people to manage long-term illness and complex health problems in order to improve their functionality. In this case scenario, the patient is already diagnosed to have diabetes which is chronic disease. Health education is provided to improve the patient's quality of life and reduce the symptoms of diabetes. So, this is considered to be tertiary prevention.

64. Which of the following is considered as primary prevention strategy?
a. Early identification
b. Reduction of disability
c. Control of spread of disease
d. Early treatment of disease

65. Primary prevention of communicable diseases can be attained by:
a. Quarantine b. Strict isolation
c. Immunization d. Antibiotics

INTRODUCTION TO EPIDEMIOLOGY

66. Father of Indian Surgery is:
a. Dhanvantari b. Charaka
c. Sushruta d. Atreya

67. Outbreak of disease in the community in excess the normal expectation is: *(RAK MSc 2018)*
a. Epidemic b. Pandemic
c. Sporadic d. Endemic

Explanation:
- **Epidemic**- Epidemic is the outbreak of particular diseases in the community in excess form from the normal expectation.
- **Pandemic**- Pandemic is the outbreak of the disease from one country to another country means all over the world.
- **Sporadic**- Sporadic is the prevalence at intervals of a single particular disperses case of a disease.
- **Endemic**- A continuous presence of a particular disease with in a particular geographical area is called as endemic.

68. The constant presence of infection in a given geographical area without any external input is known as:
a. Epidemic
b. Endemic
c. Pandemic
d. Sporadic

Explanation: An infection is said to be endemic in a population when that infection is maintained in the population without the need for external inputs. Epidemic is the rapid spread of infectious disease to a large number of people in a given population within a short period of time.
- A pandemic is an epidemic of world-wide proportions.
- Sporadic refers to diseases that is occurring at irregular intervals or only in a few places

69. A community health nurse is providing education on the different patterns of disease occurrence to a group of nursing students. The nurse asks the students to identify the term that best describes a disease that occurs at irregular intervals or only in few places, scattered in an isolated manner. Which of the following options correctly represents this term? *New Q*
a. Pandemic b. Epidemic
c. Sporadic d. Endemic

70. Outbreak of disease in bird population is:
a. Epidemic b. Endemic
c. Zoonoses d. Epornithic

Explanation: Outbreak of disease in bird's population is epornithic. Zoonoses means a disease which transmits from animal to human being. Epidemic is the sudden outbreak of disease. Endemic means constant presence of infection in a geographical area without external input.

71. Quarantine stands for:
a. Time period between infection and confirmatory diagnosis
b. Time period between diagnosis and initiation of treatment
c. Time period between infection and multiplication of organism
d. Longest incubation period

Explanation: A period of time during which a vehicle, person, or material suspected of carrying a contagious disease is detained at a port of entry under enforced isolation to prevent disease from entering a country. There is restriction on healthy contacts. Time of restriction is a longest incubation period.

72. Father of epidemiology is:
a. John Snow b. Joseph Lister
c. Karl Landsteiner d. Robert Hook

Explanation: John Snow is the father of epidemiology.

73. The initial role of the field forensic epidemiology was investigation related to: *New Q* *(AIIMS MG Tutor 2023):*
a. Medical misadventures
b. Bioterrorism
c. Industrial accidents
d. Drug prevention

Ans.
60. a
61. c
62. c
63. d
64. c
65. c
66. c
67. a
68. b
69. c
70. d
71. d
72. a
73. b

Explanation: Bioterrorism is a serious threat to public health. It can cause widespread illness and death, and it can disrupt society. However, it is a threat that can be prevented. Field forensic epidemiology plays a crucial role in responding to bioterrorism events.

In case of medical misadventures, the response typically involves a collaborative effort from healthcare institutions, regulatory bodies, and legal authorities.

74. Tear out by roots is the literal meaning of:
a. Elimination b. Eradication
c. Isolation d. Transmission

Explanation: Tear out by roots means eradication of the disease.

75. A person with no sign of disease but may transmit, it is called: *(ESIC Chennai May 2012)*
a. An allergic person b. Immune person
c. A resistant person d. A carrier person

76. Decrease in the incidence of a disease to a level where it ceases to be a public health problem is: *(RRB Feb 2012)*
a. Elimination b. Control
c. Surveillance d. Eradication

77. Basic unit of the society: *(RRB Feb 2012)*
a. Individual b. Family
c. PHC d. County

78. All are true about incidence; EXCEPT: New Q
a. Denominator includes population at risk
b. Numerator includes number of new cases
c. Does not include unit of time
d. It is a rate

Explanation: The numerator of an incidence proportion or **rate** consists only of persons whose illness began during the specified interval (time frame).
Formula to calculate incidence:
Incidence =

$$\frac{\text{(Number of new cases of a disease within a specified time period)}}{\text{(Population at risk during the same time period) x K.}} \times K.$$

K denotes 1000 or 10000, used to express the incidence rate per unit of population..

79. Time interval between primary and secondary case is known as:
a. Extrinsic incubation period b. Intrinsic incubation period
c. Serial interval d. Window period

80. 'Silent epidemic' of the century is:
a. Coronary artery disease
b. Chronic liver disease
c. Chronic obstructive lung disease
d. Alzheimer's disease

81. Time between infection and maximum infectivity is known as:
a. Incubation period b. Serial interval
c. Generation time d. Communicable period

82. The obligate refers to the:
a. Host in which the parasite remains asexual
b. Temporary host
c. Only host
d. Multiple hosts

Explanation: An obligate host means the single host in which complete life cycle of infecting agent completes. Without this host life cycle of the parasite will not complete.

83. Transport host is one in which:
a. Parasite passes its sexual stage
b. Parasite remains asexual
c. Organism remains alive but does not undergo development
d. Life cycle is not complete.

Explanation: Transport host is also known as paratenic host. In this the parasite will infect the host but not undergo any development. One that is used until the appropriate definitive host is reached, but is not necessary to completion of the life cycle of the parasite.

84. A community health nurse is teaching a group of nursing students about different types of carriers in relation to infectious diseases. The nurse asks the students to identify the term that best describes a person who is capable of transmitting an infectious agent to others during the incubation period of the disease. Which of the following options correctly represents this term? New Q
a. Incubatory carrier b. Convalescent carrier
c. Asymptomatic carrier d. Carrier

Explanation:
- An incubatory carrier is a person who is capable of transmitting an infectious agent to others during the incubation period of the disease.
- On the other hand, an asymptomatic carrier is a person or organism that has contracted an infectious disease but displays no symptoms. They are unaffected by the disease themselves but can transmit it to others. Unlike incubatory carriers, asymptomatic carriers have passed the incubation period and may have entered the convalescent stage or have a chronic infection.
- Convalescent carriers are those who have recovered from their illness but remain capable of transmitting to others.
- Carrier (option d) is not specific.

85. An infection which is present in an individual but, not sufficient to result in a disease is called as:
a. Latent infection b. Clinical infection
c. Subclinical infection d. Secondary infection

Explanation: Infection means a successful entry, development and or multiplication of organism in the body of living being, but if the organism fails to cause signs and symptoms of disease in the individual, it is called as sub clinical infection.

86. Spread of communicable disease across a large region, country to country is referred to:
a. Endemic b. Epidemic
c. Episodic d. Pandemic

Explanation: Spread of disease among larger population is known as pandemic. Endemic refers to disease or condition that is regularly found among particular people or in a certain area.

Epidemic refers to a widespread occurrence of an infectious disease in a community at a particular time.
Episodic refers to occasional.

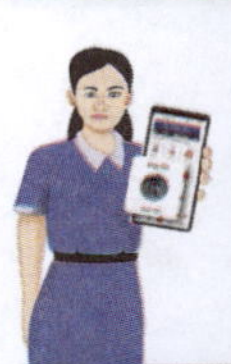

Ans.
74. b
75. d
76. b
77. b
78. c
79. c
80. d
81. c
82. c
83. c
84. a
85. c
86. d

87. Window period means:

a. Time period between infection and detection of antibodies
b. Time period between infection and first sign and symptom
c. Time period between diagnosis and treatment
d. None of the above

Explanation: The window period is time between potential exposure to HIV infection and the point when the test will give an accurate result. During the window period a person can be infected with HIV and infectious but have a negative HIV test. The window period for a 4th generation antigen/antibody test is four weeks.

88. Time period between infection and detection of antibodies against HIV is known as:

a. Acute Infection
b. Chronic Infection
c. Active HIV
d. Window Period

Explanation: The window period is time between potential exposure to HIV infection and the point when the test will give an accurate result. During the window period a person can be infected with HIV and infectious but have a negative HIV test. The window period for a 4th generation antigen/antibody test is four weeks.

89. Quarantine period should be:

a. Minimum incubation period
b. Maximum incubation period
c. Period of communicability
d. Median incubation period

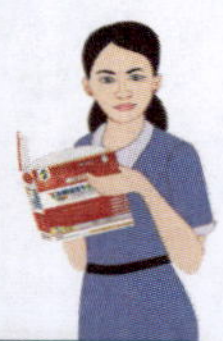

MORTALITY RATES & RATIOS

90. Denominator while calculating maternal mortality rate is:

a. Total number of deliveries
b. Total number of live birth
c. Total number of maternal death
d. Midyear population

Explanation: MMR = Total number of female death due to complications of pregnancy, child birth or within 42 days of delivery from puerperal causes in an area during a given year/total number of live birth.

91. Commonest cause of neonatal morbidity in India is: *(RRB SSNE 2015)*

a. Diarrheal diseases
b. Birth injuries
c. Congenital anomalies
d. Prematurity and low birth weight

92. The most common cause of maternal morbidity in India is: *(RRB SSNE 2015)*

a. Anemia
b. Hemorrhage
c. Abortion
d. Sepsis

93. The major cause of infant mortality rate in India is: *(LNJP H D 2012)*

a. Diarrhea
b. Respiratory infection
c. Congenital anomalies
d. Low birth weight and prematurity

Ref: K. Part. Social and Preventive Medicine. 24th Ed. Pg. 605.

Explanation: The most common cause of Infant Mortality Rate in INDIA is in following order:

- Low Birth Weight - 57%
- Respiratory infection - 17%
- Congenital malformation - 5%
- Diarrheal diseases - 4%.

94. Sex ratio is defined as: *(AIIMS-BBS SNO 2019)*

a. The number of female individuals for every 1000 male individuals
b. The number of male individuals for every 1000 female individuals
c. The number of female individuals for every 100 male individuals
d. The number of male individuals for every 100 female individuals.

95. For calculation of incidence denominator is taken as:

a. Midyear population
b. Population at risk
c. Total number of cases
d. Total number of deaths

96. Denominator in Crude Birth Rate:

a. Mid-year population
b. Total number of birth
c. 1000 live birth.
d. Total number of live birth in a year

97. True about general fertility rate is:

a. Indicator complete family size
b. Measure of fertility
c. Not better than crude birth rate
d. All of the above

98. General fertility rate (GFR) is:

a. Number of live birth in women in the reproductive age group 15-44 years
b. Number of live birth in unmarried women in the age group 15-44 years
c. Number of children a woman would have if she were to pass through her reproductive years
d. Number of abortions, usually per 1000 women of child bearing age

99. Which of the following fertility rates include mortality in it?

a. TFR
b. GFR
c. NRR
d. GRR

100. Dependency ratio numerator is:

a. Less than 15 years and more than 65 years
b. Mid-year population
c. Less than 15 years
d. More than 65 years

101. The denominator used to calculate literacy rate of Indian population is:

a. Population aged 18 year or more
b. Population aged 7 year or more
c. School going population
d. Total midyear population

102. Maternal mortality rate definition includes all except:

a. Death in pregnancy
b. Death during pregnancy
c. Death within 6 weeks post delivery
d. Death within 6 months post delivery

Ans.

87.	a
88.	d
89.	b
90.	b
91.	d
92.	b
93.	d
94.	a
95.	b
96.	a
97.	b
98.	a
99.	c
100.	a
101.	b
102.	d

103. Maternal Mortality Ratio is calculated by:
a. Maternal deaths/live birth
b. Maternal deaths/1000 live births
c. Maternal deaths/100000 live births
d. Maternal deaths/100000 populations

104. Maternal Mortality Ratio (MMR) is expressed as:
a. Per 100,000 live births
b. Per 1000 live births
c. Per 100,000 births
d. Per 1000 population

105. About Maternal Mortality Rate which of the following is true?
a. It is a rate not ratio
b. Numerator includes complications related death up to 42 days after pregnancy
c. Denominator includes stillbirth and abortions
d. Expressed as rate per 1000 live birth

106. Neonatal death is defined as death of a live born neonate –:
a. In the first 28 days after birth
b. In the first 3 months of life
c. In the first 6 months of life
d. In the first year of life

107. Most common cause of infant mortality in India is:
a. Low birth weight
b. Respiratory disease
c. Diarrheal disease
d. Congenital anomalies

Ref: K. Part. Social and Preventive Medicine. 24th Ed. Pg. 605.

Explanation: The most common cause of Infant Mortality Rate in INDIA is in following order:
- Low Birth Weight - 57%
- Respiratory infection - 17%
- Congenital malformation - 5%
- Diarrheal diseases - 4%

108. All the following are the parts of Infant mortality; EXCEPT:
a. Early neonatal mortality
b. Perinatal mortality
c. Post neonatal mortality
d. Late neonatal mortality

109. In a population of 5000, with birth rate of 30/1000 population, 15 children died during first year life in a year: of these 9 died during first month of life. What is the infant mortality rate in this population?
a. 100 b. 60
c. 150 d. 45

Explanation:

Birth rate = 30/1000
In 5000 population, no. of live birth= (30/1000) × 5000 = 150
No. of death before 1 year of age = 15
IMR = (No. of death of children less than one year of age/No. of live birth in the same year) × 1000
IMR = (15/150) × 1000 = 100

110. Infant mortality rate (IMR) is defined as number or deaths of infants under age one per:
a. 1000 births
b. 1000 live births
c. 1000 midyear population
d. 1000 women of reproductive age group

111. To achieve net reproduction rate of 1, the couple protection rate should be: *(RRB Feb 2012)*
a. 50% b. 65%
c. 55% d. 60%

112. Annual Under five deaths globally reported are:
a. 6 million b. 8 million
c. 10 million d. 12 million

113. Physical quality of life is a consolidated index of:
a. MMR, IMR and life expectancy at age 5 years
b. Infant mortality, life expectancy at age one and literacy
c. IMR, MMR and life expectancy at age 14 years
d. MMR, NRR and life expectancy at age of 60 years

114. Perinatal mortality rate includes:
a. 37 weeks to 1st week after birth
b. 28 weeks to 1st week after birth
c. 20 weeks to 1st week after birth
d. Before preterm labor

115. All of the following are common cause of postneonatal infant mortality in India; EXCEPT:
a. Tetanus b. Malnutrition
c. Diarrheal diseases d. Acute respiratory infection

116. Present IMR in India as per the latest data is:
a. 34 per 1000 live births
b. 36 per 1000 live births
c. 39 per 1000 live births
d. 40 per 1000 live births

117. Incidence of chromosomal abnormalities in India is:
a. 1- 2 per 1000 live births
b. 2-3 per 1000 live births
c. 5-6 per 1000 live births
d. 8-9 per 1000 live births

118. Major cause of perinatal mortality is:
a. Malnutrition b. Congenital anomalies
c. Birth asphyxia d. Both a and b

119. Leading cause of neonatal mortality in India is:
a. Infections
b. Birth asphyxia/trauma
c. Diarrhea
d. Prematurity and congenital malformation

120. The highest rate of infant mortality in India is reported from:
a. Madhya Pradesh b. Bihar
c. Uttar Pradesh d. Orissa

121. All are direct causes of maternal mortality in India; EXCEPT:
a. Cardiac disease b. Eclampsia
c. Hemorrhage d. Abortion

122. Mainly included in child survival index:
a. MMR
b. IMR
c. Mortality between 1 and 4 years of age
d. Under 5 mortality

123. Perinatal death includes:
a. After 28 weeks of pregnancy
b. Within seven days after birth
c. Both a and b
d. None of the above

124. Most common cause of perinatal mortality is:
a. Prematurity b. Birth injury
c. Metabolic d. Congenital

125. Most common cause of death in children <5 years age:
a. Respiratory infection b. Diarrhea
c. Prematurity d. Accidents

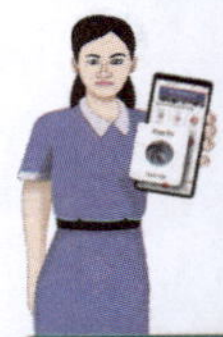

Ans.

103. c
104. a
105. a
106. a
107. a
108. b
109. a
110. b
111. d
112. a
113. b
114. b
115. a
116. a
117. c
118. c
119. d
120. a
121. a
122. d
123. c
124. a
125. a

INCIDENCE AND PREVALENCE OF DISEASE

126. Kaplan Meier method is for:

a. Survival b. Incidence
c. Prevalence d. Frequency

127. Prevalence is a:

a. Rate b. Ratio
c. Proportion d. Mean

128. Other name for Vitamin B12 is:

a. Ascorbic acid b. Cyanocobalamin
c. Thiamine d. Riboflavin

129. Number of current cases (new and preexisting) at a specified point in time divided by population at the same specified point in time is referred as:

a. Point prevalence b. Period prevalence
c. Lifetime prevalence d. Prevalence estimate

Explanation: Point prevalence refers to the number of current cases (both new and preexisting) of a specific condition or disease at a particular point in time divided by the population at the same specified point in time. It provides a snapshot of the proportion of individuals in a population who have the condition at a specific moment.

Period prevalence refers to the number of individuals with a specific condition over a defined period of time.

130. Number of current cases (new and preexisting) over a specified period of time divided by average or mid-interval population:

a. Point prevalence
b. Period prevalence
c. Lifetime prevalence
d. Total prevalence

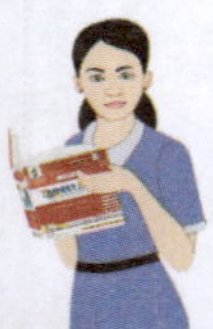

131. The number of new cases occurring in a defined population during a specified period of time is known as:

a. Incidence
b. Point prevalence
c. Period prevalence
d. Current prevalence

EPIDEMIOLOGICAL METHODS

132. A village is divided into five subgroups, for a survey. The sample is proportionately drawn by selecting people randomly from each of these subgroups. What type of sampling has been done? *New Q*

a. Simple random sampling
b. Stratified random sampling
c. Cluster sampling
d. Systematic random sampling

Explanation: In stratified random sampling, the population is divided into distinct subgroups or strata based on certain characteristics. The sample is then selected from each stratum in proportion to its representation in the population.

133. In a research study, first schools are sampled, then sections and finally student. This type of sampling is known as:

a. Stratified sampling
b. Simple random sampling
c. Cluster sampling
d. Multi stage sampling

134. Stratified sampling is ideal for:

a. Hetrogeneous data b. Homogenous data
c. Both a and b d. None of these

135. Simple random sampling is ideal for:

a. Vaccinated people
b. Heterogeneous population
c. Homogenous population
d. All of the above

136. Degree of freedom for 2 × 2 contingency table is:

a. 1 b. 0
c. 2 d. 4

137. Chi square test is for:

a. Standard error of mean
b. Standard error of proportion
c. Difference between population means
d. Difference between population proportion

138. Not required for Chi square test:

a. Null hypothesis
b. Degree of freedom
c. Means in different groups
d. Proportion in different groups

139. Degree of freedom of contingency table with 3 rows and 6 columns is:

a. 2 b. 3
c. 10 d. 18

140. Chi square test 5 rows/4 columns, degree of freedom is:

a. 9 b. 12
c. 16 d. 20

141. If the distribution of Intra-ocular pressure (IOP) seen in 100 glaucoma patients has an average 30 mm with a SD of 1.0, what is the lower limit of the average IOP that can be expected 95% of times?

a. 29 b. 26
c. 32 d. 259

Explanation:

To calculate the lower limit of the average IOP that can be expected 95% of the time, we need to determine the confidence interval (CI).

The formula for the confidence interval is:

Lower limit = Mean – (1.96 × Standard Error)

Standard Error = Standard Deviation / √(Sample Size)

In this case, the sample size is 100, the mean is 30 mm, and the standard deviation is 1.0.

Standard Error = 1.0 / √100 = 1.0 / 10 = 0.1

Lower limit = 30 – (1.96 × 0.1) = 30 – 0.196 = 29.804

Rounded to the nearest whole number, the lower limit of the average IOP that can be expected 95% of the time is 29.

Therefore, the correct answer is: a. 29.

Similarly, the upper limit IOP at 95% CI can be calculated using the formula

Upper limit = Mean + (1.96 × Standard Error)

142. Which is the best distribution to study the daily admission of head injury patients in a trauma care center?

a. Normal distribution b. Binomial distribution
c. Uniform distribution d. Poisson distribution

143. In the left skewed curve, true statement is:

a. Mean = Median b. Mean < Mode
c. Mean > Mode d. Mean = Mode

Ans.

126. a
127. c
128. b
129. a
130. b
131. a
132. b
133. d
134. a
135. c
136. a
137. d
138. c
139. c
140. b
141. a
142. d
143. b

144. For a negatively skewed data mean will be:
a. Less than median b. More than median
c. Equal to median d. One

145. Confidence limit is calculated by using:
a. Mean and standard error
b. Mean and standard deviation
c. Median and standard deviation
d. Median

146. A child's weight for height is more than 2SD of mean, and his height for age is less than 2SD of mean. He is classified as:
a. Normal b. Stunted
c. Wasted d. Wasted and stunted

147. In WHO "Road to Health" chart, upper and lower limit of represents:
a. 30 percentile for boys and 3 percentile for girls
b. 50 percentile for boys and 3 percentile for girls
c. 30 percentile for boys and 5 percentile for girls
d. 50 percentile for boys and 5 percentile for girls

148. If the birth weight of each of the 10 babies born in a hospital in a day is found to be 2.8 kg, then the standard deviation of this sample will be:
a. 2.8 b. 0
c. 1 d. 0.28

149. Most reliable measures of central tendency in a normally contributed data is:
a. Mean b. Median
c. Mode d. Standard deviation

150. Mean, Median and Mode are:
a. Measures of dispersion
b. Measures of association between two variables
c. Test of significance
d. Measures of central tendency

151. Most frequently occurring value in a group of data: *(TNPSC 2015)*
a. Mean b. Mode
c. Median d. Standard deviation

152. Which type of variable "Social Class" is, if it has four categories-I to V and Class I is the highest social class and Class V is the lowest?
a. Dichotomous b. Nominal
c. Ordinal d. Interval

153. A physician, after examining a group of patients of a certain disease, classifies the condition of each one as 'Normal', 'Mild', 'Moderate' or 'Severe'. Which one of the following is the scale of measurement that is being adopted for classification of the disease condition?
a. Normal b. Interval
c. Ratio d. Ordinal

154. In a study following interpretation are obtained: Satisfied, Very satisfied, Dissatisfied. Which type of scale is this?
a. Nominal b. Ordinal
c. Interval d. Ratio

155. All of the following are example of nominal scale; EXCEPT:
a. Race b. Sex
c. Body weight d. Occupation

156. Histogram is used to present which kind of the data:
a. Nominal
b. Continuous
c. Discrete
d. None of the above

157. The best graphic representation of frequency distribution of data gathered of a continuous variable is:
a. Simple bar b. Histogram
c. Line diagram d. Multiple bar

158. Trends can be represented by:
a. Scatter diagram b. Bar diagram
c. Line diagram d. Pie chart

EPIDEMIOLOGICAL TRIAD

159. The agent factor responsible for the occurrence of a disease includes: *(AIIMS Raipur Grade II 2017)*
a. Biological and physical agents
b. Mechanical and chemical agents
c. Vertical and inoculation agents
d. Nutrient and living agents
a. a, b, c b. b, c, d
c. a, b, d d. a, c, d

Explanation: According to being theory factors responsible for occurrence of disease are biological factors, behavioural factors, environmental factors as physical, chemical and biological aspects of environment, immunological factors, nutritional factors, genetic factors, social factors, spiritual factors, service factors related to various aspects of health services.

160. Epidemiological triad comprises all; EXPECT:
A Host b. Environmental factor
c. Agent d. Investigator

161. Which of the following is the most logical sequence?
a. Impairment – Disease – Disability – Handicap
b. Disease –Impairment – Disability – Handicap
c. Disease –Impairment – Handicap – Disability
d. Disease– Handicap –Impairment – Disability

162. Man is an intermediate host of all of the following; EXCEPT:
a. Malaria b. Toxoplasmosis
c. Hydatid disease d. Kala-azar

163. Which of the following chain of infection is in the correct order?
a. Mode of transmission-Source/reservoir-Host
b. Mode of transmission → Host → Source/reservoir
c. Host → source/reservoir → Mode of Transmission
d. Source/reservoir → Mode of Transmission → Host

SURVEILLANCE AND MONITORING FOR DISEASE

164. The continuous, systematic collection, analysis and interpretation of health-related data needed for the planning, implementation, and evaluation of public health practice is known as:
a. Incidence b. Monitoring
c. Surveillance d. Community assessment

Explanation:
- The given sentence is the definition of surveillance. Incidence is the measure of the probability of occurrence of a given medical condition in a population within a specified period of time.
- Community based monitoring is a form of public oversight driven by local information needs and is not systematic. A community assessment is basically a description of a community and its people.

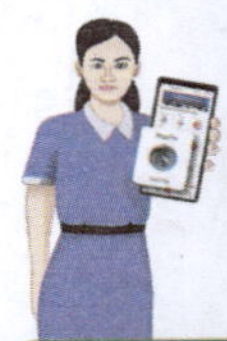

Ans.
144. a
145. d
146. b
147. b
148. b
149. a
150. d
151. b
152. c
153. d
154. b
155. c
156. b
157. b
158. c
159. c
160. d
161. b
162. d
163. d
164. c

165. Sentinel surveillance is used to:
a. Know the total number of affected people
b. Know the hidden cases in the community
c. Compare the incidence
d. Measure incidence and prevalence

Explanation: Public health surveillance is the continuous, systematic collection, analysis and interpretation of health-related data needed for the planning, implementation, and evaluation of public health practice.

There are 3 types of surveillance:
1. Sentinel Surveillance.
2. Accelerated Disease Control - National Active.
3. National Passive.

A sentinel surveillance system is used when high-quality data are needed about a particular disease that cannot be obtained through a passive system.

Active surveillance involves visiting health facilities, talking to health-care providers and reviewing medical records to identify suspected cases of disease under surveillance.

Regular reporting of disease data by all institutions that see patients (or test specimens) and are part of a reporting network is called passive surveillance.

166. The screening of the immigrants for infectious disease is:
a. Mass screening
b. Prescriptive screening
c. Prospective screening
d. Selective screening

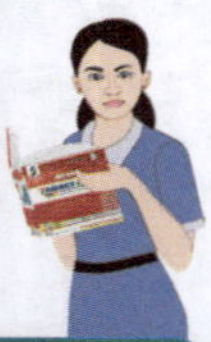

Explanation: Screening of immigrants for infection is known as prospective screening.

167. HIV prevalence can be assessed by:
a. Sentinel surveillance
b. Active surveillance
c. Central register
d. State register

168. Missed cases are identified by: *(AIIMS 1999)*
a. Active surveillance
b. Passive surveillance
c. Sentinel surveillance
d. Prevalence rate

169. Which of the following used to estimate the morbidity in a community?
a. Prevalence rate
b. Active surveillance
c. Passive surveillance
d. Sentinel surveillance

170. Screening of the immigrants for infectious disease is referred as:
a. Primordial screening
b. Prospective screening
c. Prescriptive screening
d. Quarantine screening

171. In India, goiter is found commonly in:
a. Southern region
b. Himalayan region
c. Western region
d. Coastal region

172. Most common cause of stroke in India is:
a. Cerebral thrombosis b. Cerebral embolism
c. Cerebral hemorrhage d. Subarachnoid hemorrhage

Explanation:
- Ischemic strokes are the most common type of stroke, accounting for about 80% of all strokes. There are two main types of ischemic strokes:
  1. Thrombotic stroke: This type of stroke occurs when a blood clot forms in an artery in the brain. It accounts for about 80% of ischemic strokes.
  2. Embolic stroke: Stroke occurs when a blood clot or other foreign object travels to the brain from another part of the body and blocks an artery.

173. National family health survey done in every:
a. 6 months b. 1 year
c. 5 years d. 10 years

ICEBERG PHENOMENON

174. The floating tip of the iceberg represents:
a. Latent cases b. Clinical cases
c. Undiagnosed cases d. None of the above

175. Submerged portion of the iceberg represents:
a. Undiagnosed cases b. Clinical cases
c. Dead cases d. Treated cases

Explanation: The submerged portion of the iceberg represents the hidden mass of the disease (e.g., subclinical cases, carriers, undiagnosed cases). The floating tip represents what the physician sees in his practice/chamber/hospital, etc.

176. Iceberg phenomenon differentiate between:
a. Cases and carriers
b. Diagnosed and undiagnosed
c. Apparent and inapparent
d. Symptomatic and asymptomatic

177. Tip of iceberg phenomenon is most apparently seen in:
a. PEM b. Tetanus
c. Rubella d. Dysentery

178. The tip of iceberg represents:
a. Visible cases
b. Invisible cases
c. Clinical illness
d. Death occurred due to disease

IMMUNITY

179. Immunity acquired through natural infection is:
a. Artificial active immunity
b. Herd immunity
c. Natural Active immunity
d. Specific human immunity

Explanation: Immunity that occurs after the person is exposed to a specific disease is called as natural active immunity, e.g., chicken pox. If immunity developed after immunization then it is known as artificial active immunity.

Ans.
165. b
166. c
167. a
168. c
169. b
170. b
171. b
172. a
173. c
174. b
175. a
176. c
177. a
178. a
179. c

180. Herd immunity is not useful in prevention of:

a. Polio b. Rubella
c. Tetanus d. Measles

Explanation: Herd immunity is a form of indirect protection from infectious disease that occurs when a large percentage of a population has become immune to an infection, thereby providing measure of protection for individual who are not immunized. Herd immunity does not apply to all diseases, just those that are contagious meaning that they can be transmitted from one individual to another. Tetanus for example, is infectious but not contagious, so herd immunity does not apply.

181. Administration of readymade antibody creates: *(AIIMS 2010)*

a. Active acquired immunity b. Passive acquired immunity
c. Active natural immunity d. Passive natural immunity

Explanation: Artificially acquired passive immunity is a short-term immunization by the injection of antibodies, such as gamma globulin, that are not produced by the recipient's cells.

182. Viral proteins called interferons helping innate immunity are classified under: *(Kerala PSC, Nov 2014)*

a. Physical barriers b. Physiological barriers
c. Cytokine barriers d. Cellular barriers

183. Test used to identify the immunity status against diphtheria is:

a. Schick test b. Widal test
c. Mantoux test d. Allen's test

184. All of the following are true about Herd immunity for infectious diseases; EXCEPT:

a. Herd immunity is constant
b. Depends on clinical and sub clinical infections
c. Influenced by immunization
d. Depends on presence of alternative host

IMMUNIZING AGENTS/VACCINES

185. A clinic nurse prepares to administer an MMR (Measles, Mumps, Rubella) vaccine to a five-year-old. The nurse administers this vaccine: *(RAK MSc 2018)*

a. Intramuscularly in the anterolateral aspect of the thigh
b. Intramuscularly in deltoid muscle
c. Subcutaneously in the outer aspect of the upper arm
d. Subcutaneously in the gluteal muscle

Explanation: Measles, mumps, and rubella virus vaccine is a live vaccine to prevent infection of measles, mumps, and rubella viruses.

- The dosage for MMR is 0.5 mL. Vaccine is administered by the subcutaneous route.
- The minimum age for MMR is in 12 months of age.
- The second dose of vaccine is given at 4 to 6 years of age.
- The minimum gap between MMR doses is 4 weeks.
- The recommended injection site in small children is the anterolateral aspect of the thigh and for older children it is in the posterior (outer) triceps of the upper arm.

186. BCG is:

a. Live attenuated vaccine b. Inactivated vaccine
c. Killed vaccines d. Toxoids

Explanation: BCG vaccine is live attenuated vaccine, which provides protection against Tuberculosis.

187. The vaccine that leaves permanent scar in babies is:

a. Measles b. Pentavalent
c. DPT d. BCG

Explanation: Administering BCG vaccine produces a permanent scar. BCG immunization forms a superficial abscess, which begins 2 weeks after immunization. The abscess heals without treatment, but with the formation of a permanent scar.

188. Influenza – A (H1N1) vaccine was approved in the year:

a. 2009 b. 2010
c. 2012 d. 2004

Explanation: Vaccine against H1N1 influenza was approved in the year of 2009.

189. Smallpox was eradicated from the world in the year:

a. 1980 b. 1981
c. 1982 d. 1983

Explanation: In 1980 smallpox was eradicated from the world.

190. Polyvalent vaccine means:

a. Single strain of single microorganism
b. Two or more strains of same microorganism
c. Antibody of single microorganism
d. None of the above

Explanation:

- Mixed viruses are also called as 'Polyvalent vaccines'. If vaccine is prepared from more than two strain of same species then it is known as polyvalent.
- A **monovalent** vaccine is designed to immunize against a single antigen or single microorganism. A **multivalent** or **polyvalent** vaccine is designed to immunize against two or more strains of the same microorganism, or against two or more microorganisms.

191. Anti-rabies vaccine is made from:

a. Wild viruses
b. Live attenuated viruses
c. Mixed viruses
d. Killed viruses

Explanation: Anti-rabies vaccine is an active immunizing agent used to prevent infection caused by the rabies virus. Anti-rabies vaccine is a type of killed/inactivated vaccine.

192. Which of the following vaccines is most sensitive to heat?

a. Pertussis vaccine b. Typhoid vaccine
c. Polio vaccine d. BCG vaccine

Explanation: OPV is the most heat sensitive vaccine and has temperature sensitive label called vaccine vial monitor (VVM). Since this vaccine is heat sensitive it is stored in freezer compartment.

193. Expansion of BCG vaccine is:

a. Bacillus Calmette-Guérin
b. Bacillus Calmette-Guereo
c. Bacilli Calmette-Guerreror
d. Bacilli Calmette-Gurein

Explanation: Camille Guerin and Albert Calmette produced BCG vaccine at Pasteur Institute in Paris.

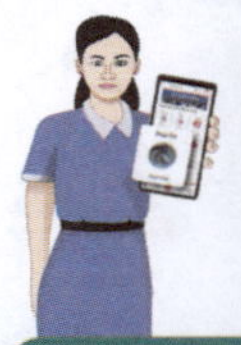

Ans.

180. c
181. b
182. c
183. a
184. a
185. c
186. a
187. d
188. a
189. a
190. b
191. d
192. c
193. a

194. BCG vaccine is available in powder form. It is reconstituted with:

a. Distilled water b. Normal saline
c. 5% Dextrose solution d. Ringer lactate solution

Explanation: Normal saline 1 mL is used to dilute BCG vaccine, it is available along with the vaccine

195. Adjuvant used in DPT vaccine is:

a. Zinc phosphate
b. Aluminium phosphate
c. Aluminium hydroxide
d. Both b and c

Explanation: Aluminium phosphate and aluminium hydroxide both are used as adjuvant in vaccine

196. Which of the following vaccine is contraindicated during pregnancy?

a. MMR b. Hepatitis B
c. DPT d. DT

Explanation: MMR is a live vaccine, if it is given during pregnancy it can affect the fetus. So, it is contraindicated during pregnancy.

197. Measles vaccine is: *(ESI 2009)*

a. Live viral vaccine b. Live bacterial vaccine
c. Killed vaccine d. Toxoid

Explanation: Measles is a live viral vaccine. Measles mumps rubella vaccine (MMR) vaccine is a live attenuated viral vaccine used to induce immunity against measles, mumps and rubella.

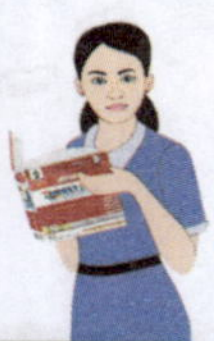

198. Live vaccine is: *(Karnataka PSC)*

a. DPT b. Hepatitis-B
c. TT d. BCG

Explanation: BCG is a live attenuated vaccine. Other live vaccines includes polio (sabin), MMR, measles vaccine. Live attenuated vaccines contain a version of the living microbe that has been weakened in the lab so that it cannot cause disease.

199. Which of the following vaccines are contraindicated in pregnancy?

a. Rubella b. Measles
c. Varicella d. All of these

Explanation: Live vaccines are contraindicated in pregnancy. Above mentioned vaccines are live vaccines and all are contraindicated in pregnancy.

200. A killed vaccine is: *(Safdarjung NO 2018)*

a. OPV b. BCG
c. MMR d. Rabies

201. Which of the following diseases are known as six killer diseases in children?

a. Whooping cough, Yellow fever, Hepatitis, TB, Smallpox, Tetanus
b. Diphtheria, Whooping cough, Measles, Polio, TB, Tetanus
c. Diphtheria, Yellow fever, TB, Leprosy, Malaria, Cholera
d. Whooping cough, Diphtheria, Malaria, Smallpox, TB, Chicken pox

Explanation: These six diseases are killer diseases. National Immunization Program also aims at reducing the incidences of these diseases.

202. Which is the recommended site of administration of DPT in infants?

a. Gluteal muscles
b. Deltoid muscles
c. Lateral aspect of mid-thigh
d. Forearm

Explanation: Lateral aspect of mid-thigh in infant is the safest area for administering vaccine. It will promote vaccine absorption as well as minimize the chances of nerve injury.

203. Salk vaccine is given for the prevention of: *(Kerala PSC, Nov 2014)*

a. Measles b. Mumps
c. Polio d. Rabies

204. Immunization of DPT should be administered by: *(Kerala PSC, Nov 2014)*

a. Intradermal b. Intramuscular
c. Subcutaneous d. Intravenous

205. The age of administration of measles vaccine is: *(Staff Nurse G II 2014, LNJP H D 2012)*

a. 18 months b. 6 months
c. 3 months d. 9 months

206. Dose of BCG vaccination is: *(JIPMER 2012)*

a. 0.5 mL s/c b. 0.5 mL I/D
c. 0.1 mL I/D d. 1 mL I/M

207. B.C.G. vaccine is given to protect the child against: *(ESIC Chennai May 2012)*

a. Diphtheria b. Tuberculosis
c. Tetanus d. Typhoid

208. Example of a live vaccine are: *(LNJP H D 2012)*

a. Hepatitis B b. Rabies
c. Measles d. Typhoid vaccine

209. Varicella vaccine is:

a. Killed vaccine b. Live attenuated vaccine
c. Immunoglobulin d. None of these

210. Smallpox vaccine was invented by:

a. Louis Pasteur b. Edward Jenner
c. Paul Eugene d. John Snow

211. Which of the following is a diarrheal preventive vaccine?

a. DPT vaccine b. Rotavirus vaccine
c. MMR vaccine d. Hepatitis B

212. Salk vaccine is a:

a. Live vaccine b. Live attenuated vaccine
c. Killed vaccine d. Toxoid

213. OPV is a:

a. Live vaccine b. Live attenuated vaccine
c. Killed vaccine d. Toxoid

214. Which of the following is a live attenuated vaccine?

a. BCG b. DPT
c. Hepatitis B d. Tetanus Toxoid

215. The route of administration of live attenuated polio vaccine is:

a. Intradermal route b. Intramuscular
c. Oral route d. Subcutaneous route

Ans.

194. b
195. d
196. a
197. a
198. d
199. d
200. d
201. b
202. c
203. c
204. b
205. d
206. c
207. b
208. c
209. b
210. b
211. b
212. c
213. b
214. a
215. c

216. World immunization week is celebrated in *New Q*

a. April first week
b. April last week
c. June first week
d. June last week

217. HPV vaccine is used to prevent which among the following cancer? *New Q (NORCET 2021)*

a. Cervical cancer
b. Breast cancer
c. Stomach cancer
d. Lung cancer

Explanation: HPV vaccine is a vaccine that protects against the human papillomavirus (HPV), which is a sexually transmitted infection (STI). HPV can cause cervical and other cancers, including cancer of the vulva, vagina, penis, or anus (Ref: CDC)

218. India's first indigenous COVID vaccine is: *(NORCET 2021)* *New Q*

a. Covaxin
b. Covishield
c. Moderna
d. Sputnik

Explanation: Covaxin was approved for emergency use in India in January 2021. Covaxin is an Indian COVID-19 vaccine developed by Bharat Biotech. It is a whole-virion inactivated vaccine, which means that it is made from a virus that has been killed.

219. The first dose of MMR vaccine is given at the age of:

a. At birth
b. 6 month
c. 12-15 months
d. 9 months

Explanation: As per the Indian Academy of Pediatrics (IAP) Recommended Immunization Schedule (2014), the first dose of MMR is given at the age of 9 months. MMR vaccine is not a part of the national immunization schedule of India. As per National Immunization Schedule in India, Measles /MR 1st Dose is given at 9-12 months (can be given till 5 years of age).

220. MMR vaccine provide protection against all; EXCEPT: *(RPSC NG-II-2007)*

a. Mumps
b. Meningitis
c. Rubella
d. Rubeola

221. Zero dose of polio vaccine is given:

a. Before giving DPT
b. At birth
c. When child is having diarrhea
d. When child is having polio

222. Which of the following statements regarding live vaccines is false?

a. Two live vaccines cannot be administered simultaneously
b. Booster doses are not required when live vaccines are administered
c. Single dose gives lifelong immunity
d. Live vaccine contains both major and minor antigens

223. Which of the following is true about BCG vaccination?

a. Distilled water is used as diluent
b. The site of injection should be cleaned with spirit
c. Mantoux test becomes positive after 48 hours of vaccination
d. WHO recommends Danish 1331 strain for vaccine production

224. Adjuvant used in DPT vaccine is:

a. Zinc
b. Aluminium
c. Copper
d. Magnesium

225. True about polio vaccination is all; EXCEPT:

a. Follow up of AFP every 30 days
b. Salk contains three types of polio virus
c. Pulse polio virus are extra and supplemental
d. Oral polio vaccine provides intestinal immunity also

226. Which of the following is not true about Oral Polio Vaccine?

a. Induces both local and systemic immunity
b. Maternal antibody is completely protective
c. Live attenuated vaccine
d. Requires subzero temperature for long term shortage

227. All are true about SALK vaccine; EXCEPT:

a. OPV can be given as booster dose
b. Injections during epidemic prevents paralysis
c. Can be given to immunocompromised
d. Easily transported

228. Following is a live attenuated vaccine:

a. BCG
b. Hepatitis B
c. Japanese encephalitis
d. Salk

229. Vaccine preventable neonatal disease is:

a. Tuberculosis
b. Measles
c. Pertussis
d. Tetanus

230. BCG vaccine is:

a. Killed
b. Live attenuated
c. Toxoid
d. Cellular fraction

231. BCG is given:

a. Intramuscular
b. Intradermal
c. Subcutaneous
d. Intravenous

232. Dose of OPV given at birth in case of institutional deliveries is:

a. Primary dose
b. Initial dose
c. Zero dose
d. First dose

233. Killed vaccine of polio is:

a. Salk
b. Sabin
c. Both a and b
d. None of these

234. Most heat sensitive vaccine is:

a. Measles
b. DPT
c. OPV
d. Hepatitis B

235. Reconstituted measles vaccine should be used within:

a. 1 hour
b. 3 hours
c. 6 hours
d. 12 hours

236. All are true about measles vaccine; EXCEPT:

a. Freeze dried live attenuated vaccine
b. Single in dose 0.5 mL
c. Occasionally associated with TSS
d. Contraindicated in pregnancy

237. Active immunization following exposure is given most commonly for:

a. Rabies
b. Polio
c. Plague
d. Measles

COLD CHAIN

238. Frozen DPT vaccine should be:

a. Discarded
b. Rolled between palms until it reaches room temperature
c. Immersed in hot water
d. Kept out until it reaches room temperature

Explanation: Frozen DPT vaccine should be discarded.

239. In cold chain process the walk-in cold rooms, stores vaccine up to ....months.

a. 4 months
b. 6 months
c. 3 months
d. 1 month

Explanation: In walk-in cold room, vaccines can be stored up to 3 months.

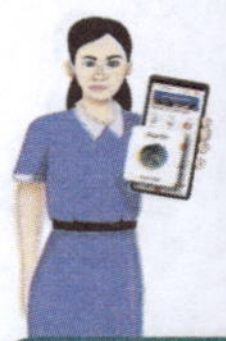

Ans.

216. b
217. a
218. a
219. d
220. b
221. b
222. a
223. d
224. b
225. a
226. b
227. b
228. a
229. d
230. b
231. b
232. c
233. a
234. c
235. b
236. b
237. a
238. a
239. c

240. Measles vaccine are stored in ....part of refrigerator.:
a. Chilled tray
b. Deep freezer
c. Tray below the freezer
d. Shelves in the door

Explanation: Measles and Polio vaccines are very sensitive to heat and maintain their potency at 2-8 degree Celsius. Hence, it is stored in deep freezer.

241. Cold Chain System is the process of preserving:
a. Blood specimen for malarial parasite
b. Chemotherapeutic agents
c. Sputum specimens
d. Vaccines

Explanation: Cold chain transport system is used to store and transport vaccine from site of manufacture to site of administration without losing potency of the vaccine.

242. System of storage and transport of vaccines at low temperature from the manufacturer to the vaccination site is called:
(Safdarjung NO 2018; LNJP H D 2012; DSSSB PHN, 2015)
a. Deep small freezers b. Cold room
c. Cold chain d. Deep freezers

243. The Inactivated Polio Vaccine (IPV) should be preserved at: *(LNJP H D 2012)*
a. 2 to 8°C b. Below 0°C
c. −2 to −8°C d. 0 to 4°C

244. Cold Chain System is the process of:
a. Storing blood specimen for MP and MF
b. Refrigerating chemotherapeutic agents
c. Storing sputum specimens
d. Preserving vaccines

245. ILR is designed for:
a. Storing vaccines
b. Incubating culture medias
c. Sterilization of rubber gloves
d. Disinfection of sharp materials

246. ILR is a part of:
a. Sterilization procedure
b. Disinfection procedure
c. Cold chain
d. Drug transport

247. At what temperature should polio vaccine be stored?
a. 0 degree Celsius
b. 2-5 degree Celsius
c. 15 degree Celsius
d. -20 degree Celsius

248. Which vaccine must be stored in the freezer compartment?
a. DPT b. Polio
c. BCG d. TT

249. Which of the following vaccine should be stored in the freezer compartment?
a. Polio b. Measles
c. DPT d. Both a and b

250. At the Primary Health Center (PHC) level, vaccines are stored in the:
a. Cold box
b. Deep freezer
c. Ice lined refrigerator
d. Walk-in cold room

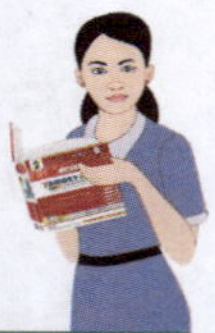

Ans.
240. b
241. d
242. c
243. a
244. d
245. a
246. c
247. d
248. b
249. d
250. c
251. b
252. a
253. a
254. a
255. d
256. c
257. c
258. c

ADVERSE EVENTS FOLLOWING IMMUNIZATION

251. What reaction might occur due to Tetanus vaccine?
a. Febrile seizures b. Brachial neuritis
c. Hypotonic d. Encephalopathy

Explanation: Brachial neuritis is the reaction occurring towards tetanus vaccine.

252. Which of the following vaccines can result in Thrombocytopenia?
a. MMR vaccine b. Typhoid vaccine
c. Influenza vaccine d. HiB vaccine

253. The following vaccine if contaminated can cause Toxic Shock Syndrome:
a. Measles Vaccine b. DPT
c. Hepatitis d. Typhoral

254. The neurological complication of DPT are due to:
a. Pertussis b. Diphtheria
c. Tetanus d. All of these

255. One of the reported side effects of Rotavirus vaccination is:
a. Pain b. Aphthous ulcers
c. Gastritis d. Intususception

"NATIONAL IMMUNIZATION SCHEDULE/ UNIVERSAL IMMUNIZATION PROGRAMME"

256. Route of administration of Hepatitis B Vaccine is:
a. Intradermal b. Subcutaneous
c. Intramuscular d. Intravenous

Explanation: Hepatitis B vaccine is administered via intramuscular route in the deltoid region of arm. BCG vaccine is administered through intradermal route. MMR vaccine is administered through Subcutaneous route. Vaccines should not be administered Intravenously.

257. All the vaccines are in national immunization schedule; EXCEPT:
a. BCG b. Pentavalent
c. Typhoid vaccine d. OPV

Explanation: According to the National immunization schedule BCG is given at birth.

- **OPV:** Birth dose for institutional deliveries, Primary three doses at 6, 10 and 14 weeks and one booster dose at 16-24 months of age. Given orally. Pentavalent (containing Hib+DPT+Hep B) is given at 6, 10 and 14 weeks of age. **(Pentavalent vaccine** introduced in 8 states, i.e., Tamil Nadu, Kerala, Haryana, J & K, Gujarat, Karnataka, Goa and Puducherry.)

Typhoid vaccine is not included in national immunization schedule.

258. Universal immunization program (UIP) was launched in the year of:
a. 1974 b. 1978
c. 1985 d. 1992

Explanation: Expanded program of immunization was launched by WHO in May 1974. It is launched in India in January 1978. EPI emphasizes on children <5 yr and pregnant women. UIP was launched on November 19, 1985. UIP emphasizes on children <1 yr of age.

259. Pulse Polio Immunization was introduced in: *(Safdarjung NO 2018)*

a. 1995 b. 1999
c. 2000 d. 2001

260. Under UIP programme which of the following vaccines is administered at 9 months of age?

a. DPT-1 b. BCG
c. Measles d. Hepatitis B-1

261. Target group for pulse polio immunization is:

a. 0-1 years
b. 0-3 years
c. 0-5 years
d. 0-10 years

262. When should a child receive the first dose of the Hepatitis B vaccine?

a. At birth
b. 6 weeks
c. 10 weeks
d. 14 weeks

263. A person received complete immunization against tetanus 10 years ago; now he presents with a clean wound without any lacerations from an injury sustained 2.5 hours ago. He should be given:

a. Full course of TT
b. Single dose of TT
c. Human Tetanus globulin.
d. Human Tetanus globulin and Single dose of TT

COMMUNICABLE DISEASES

264. The Germ Theory of Disease was propounded by:

a. Robert Koch
b. Hippocrates
c. Louis Pasteur
d. August Weismann

265. Which of the following is not a complete sterilization agent?

a. Glutaraldehyde
b. Hydrogen peroxide
c. Absolute alcohol
d. Sodium hypochlorite

266. During cholera outbreak, the best emergency sanitation measures to be adopted is: *(RAK MSc 2018)*

a. Chemoprophylaxis
b. Mass vaccination
c. Disinfection of stool
d. Provision of chlorinated water

Explanation:

- Cholera is an acute diarrheal disease caused by Vibrio cholera, and it is transmitted from men to men by contaminated water, food and drinks and direct contacts with infected person.
- If the cholera disease is endemic in nature, the best emergency management is boiling or chlorination.
- Mass vaccination and disinfection of stool are also effective measures, but they are all long-term measures it takes time to see the effect of these measures on population.

267. Mass drug administration is related to which disease? *(AIIMS Raipur NO 2019)*

a. Malaria b. Filaria
c. Polio d. Chicken pox

Explanation:

- Mass drug administration (MDA) is the administration of treatment to every member of a defined population living in a defined geographical area (except those for whom the medicine is contraindicated) at approximately the same time and often at repeated intervals.
- Mass drug administration is also given in malaria in many countries **but in India it is given only in case of lymphatic filaria.**

268. Scabies is a/an:

a. Non-communicable disease
b. Contagious disease
c. Bacterial infection
d. Fungal infection

Explanation: Scabies is a contagious (communicable) disease caused by itch mite. It is capable of spreading rapidly from one person to another by contact or close proximity.

269. The other name of pertussis is:

a. Rubella
b. Whooping cough
c. Rubeola
d. Diphtheria

Explanation: Whooping cough is also known as pertussis, which is caused by Bordetella pertussis. Whooping cough (pertussis) is a highly contagious respiratory tract infection. In many people, it is marked by a severe hacking cough followed by a high-pitched intake of breath that sounds like "whoop."

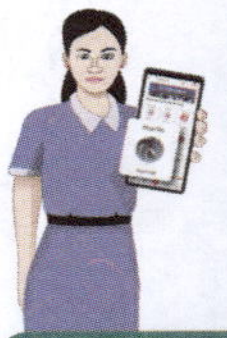

270. Symmetrical unilocular rashes firstly appearing from trunk and then on face, arms and legs are characteristics of ------------disease.

a. Smallpox b. Measles
c. Chicken pox d. Rubella

Explanation: Chicken pox caused by varicella zoster virus presents with clinical feature of dew drops kind of rashes that firstly appear on trunk and then come on face, arms and legs

271. Boiling water helps in killing all organisms; EXCEPT:

a. Fungi b. Bacteria
c. Protozoa d. Spores

Explanation: Spores serve as a resting stage in life cycle of bacteria during unfavorable environmental conditions.

272. The last known natural case of smallpox was reported in the world in: *(MSc RAK 2010)*

a. 1977 b. 1978
c. 1979 d. 1980

Explanation: Smallpox is an acute contagious disease caused by the variola virus, a member of the orthopoxvirus family. It was one of the world's most devastating diseases known to humanity. It was declared eradicated in 1980 following a global immunization campaign led by the World Health Organization. The last known natural case was in Somalia in 1977. Since then, the only known cases were caused by a laboratory accident in 1978 in Birmingham, England, which killed one person and caused a limited outbreak.

Ans.

259. a
260. c
261. c
262. a
263. b
264. c
265. c
266. d
267. b
268. b
269. b
270. c
271. d
272. a

273. Mumps presents with a clinical feature of:

a. Fever with enlargement of thyroid glands
b. Fever with non-supportive enlargement of one or both parotid glands
c. Fever with supportive enlargement of parotid glands
d. Fever, cough and enlargement of submandibular glands

Explanation: Mumps is caused by RNA virus belonging to Myxovirus group, it is a self-limiting infectious disease that spreads through droplet infection. It is associated with sudden onset of fever with non-supportive enlargement of one or both parotid glands.

274. Koplik's spots are seen in: *(AIIMS 1996)*

a. Rubella b. Measles
c. Chikungunya d. Chicken pox

Explanation: Measles is also known as Rubeola. Koplik spots (also Koplik's sign) are characteristic feature of measles manifesting two to three days before the measles rash itself. They are characterized as clustered, white lesions on the buccal mucosa (opposite the lower 1st and 2nd molars) and are pathognomonic for measles.

275. Rabies free zone in India is:

a. Goa
b. Lakshadweep
c. Arunachal Pradesh
d. Tamil Nadu

Explanation: Lakshadweep is the rabies free zone. In India, union territory of Lakshadweep and Andaman and Nicobar islands are free of rabies disease. A "RABIES FREE AREA" has been defined as one in which no case of indigenously acquired rabies has occurred in man or any animal species for 2 years.

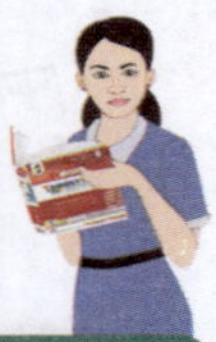

276. Among the following identify the most common complication associated with mumps?

a. Aseptic meningitis b. Mastitis
c. Orchidites d. Oophoritis

Explanation: Aseptic meningitis is one of the most common complications caused by mumps.

277. International Health Regulation is subjected to:

a. Plague b. Yellow fever
c. Cholera d. All of these

Explanation: All of the mentioned diseases are subjected to International Health Regulation.

278. Schick's test is used to diagnose:

a. Diphtheria b. Pertussis
c. Measles d. Mumps

Explanation: Schick test, method for determining susceptibility to diphtheria; it laid the basis for inoculation against the disease. A minute amount of diphtheria toxin is injected into the skin of the forearm. Redness at the site of injection after three days indicates a positive reaction (absence of circulating antibody) or a false positive reaction (hypersensitivity to the toxin). A positive reaction can be distinguished by use of a control injection of the same amount of heated toxin (toxoid) into the other forearm. The Schick test was introduced in 1913 by Béla Schick (1877–1967), an Austrian pediatrician.

279. Most common complication associated with chicken pox in children is:

a. Secondary bacterial infection
b. Meningitis
c. Orchitis
d. Otitis media

Explanation: Secondary bacterial infection is the most common complication associated with chicken pox in children.

280. Complications of chicken pox include:

a. Rey's syndrome
b. Pneumonia
c. Cerebellar ataxia
d. All of the above

Explanation: Pneumonic used for complication associated with chicken pox include RAPE

R = Rey's syndrome
A = Acute cerebellar ataxia
P = Pneumonia
E = Encephalitis

281. Drug of choice for cholera is:

a. Tetracycline b. Penicillin
c. Chloramphenicol d. Co-trimoxazole

Explanation: Tetracycline is the drug of choice for cholera. Adult dose is 500 mg BD. Children between 4-13 years the dose is 125 mg, for children younger than 4 years dose is 50 mg.

282. Congenital rubella is diagnosed in infant with the help of .... antibodies in infant.

a. IgM b. IgG
c. IgE d. IgA

Explanation: This condition is diagnosed when the infant is having IgM antibodies at the time of birth.

283. Chemoprophylaxis of choice in case of meningococcal meningitis is:

a. Chloroquine b. Tetracycline
c. Rifampicin d. Penicillin

Explanation: Chemoprophylaxis is recommended for close contacts of persons with meningococcal disease. Rifampicin is the drug of choice. 600 mg BD for 2 days.

284. People with pertussis are most contagious of whooping cough during: *New Q*

a. One week after cough begins
b. 10 days after cough begins
c. Three weeks after the cough begins
d. Two months after cough begins

Explanation: Pertussis, also known as whooping cough, is a highly contagious respiratory infection caused by the bacterium *Bordetella pertussis*.

The first symptoms generally appear 7 to 10 days after infection. People with pertussis are most contagious up to about 3 weeks after the cough begins, and many children who contract the infection have coughing spells that last 4 to 8 weeks. (Ref: WHO)

Ans.

273.	b
274.	b
275.	b
276.	a
277.	d
278.	a
279.	a
280.	d
281.	a
282.	a
283.	c
284.	c

285. Diphtheria carrier is identified through:
a. Throat swab culture
b. Ziehl-Neelsen stain
c. Gram stain
d. Albert stain

Explanation: Swab taken from nose and throat is subjected to culture and then identify the carrier in diphtheria.

286. WHO declared global eradication of Smallpox on: *(Safdarjung NO 2018)*
a. 26th October 1977
b. 5th July 1975
c. 17th May 1975
d. 8th May 1980

287. Incubation period of chicken pox ranges from: *(Staff Nurse G II 2014)*
a. 20–25 days b. 30–40 days
c. 6–10 days d. 14–16 days

288. Causative agent of mumps is: *(JIPMER 2012)*
a. Bordetella b. Paramyxovirus
c. Toga virus d. H. influenza

289. Most common cause of post measle death: *(RRB Feb 2012)*
a. SSPE b. RTI
c. Weakness d. Diarrhea

290. Congenital varicella is related with which disease? *(RRB Feb 2012)*
a. Mumps b. Germen measles
c. Measles d. Chicken pox

291. The procedure of 'Quarantine' was introduced to protect against importation of: *(RRB Feb 2012)*
a. Yellow fever b. Cholera
c. Leprosy d. Plague

292. Scarlet fever is caused by:
a. S. pyogenes b. Gonococci
c. Meningococci d. S. typhi

293. Which of the following communicable disease has been eradicated from the world?
a. Chicken pox b. Smallpox
c. German measles d. Poliomyelitis

294. Which of the following is also called epidemic parotitis?
a. Measles b. Chicken pox
c. Mumps d. Pertussis

295. Which among the following is an airborne disease?
a. Typhoid b. Kala-azar
c. Tuberculosis d. Malaria

296. Chemoprophylaxis can be done for the following; EXCEPT:
a. Meningitis b. Typhoid
c. Cholera d. Diphtheria

297. Which is the causative organism of Diphtheria?
a. Mycobacterium tuberculosis
b. Treponema pallidum
c. Corynebacterium Diphtheriae
d. Myxovirus parotitis

298. Which of the following is the mode of transmission of Hepatitis A?
a. Sexual contact
b. Use of contaminated needles and syringes
c. Vertical transmission
d. Contaminated food and water

299. Why it was difficult to eradicate small pox?
a. Highly effective vaccine
b. Cross-immunity with animal pox virus
c. Subclinical infection does not transmit the disease
d. Lifelong immunity

300. Characteristic rashes present in measles are known as:
a. Koplik spot
b. Pleomorphic
c. Vesicular rashes
d. Flushing

301. Most serious complication of measles is:
a. Koplik spots b. Parotitis
c. Meningoencephalitis d. Nephritis

302. In measles Koplik spots are seen in:
a. Prodromal stage b. Post measles stage
c. Eruptive Stage d. None of these

303. An example of epidemic disease is:
a. Plague
b. Fracture
c. AIDS
d. Hypertension

304. Which of the following communicable diseases is treated by the drug Dapsone?
a. Tuberculosis b. Hepatitis B
c. Leprosy d. Syphilis

305. Window period for HIV infection is:
a. 3-12 weeks b. 8-20 weeks
c. 6-24 weeks d. None of these

306. Which of the following diseases was declared eradicated from world?
a. Smallpox
b. Guinea worm
c. Polio
d. Diphtheria

307. True about measles is/are:
a. Incubation period is 10 days
b. Infectious 4 days before the rash
c. Kopliks spots are seen
d. All of the above

308. Chicken pox rashes first appear in which body part?
a. Trunk and face
b. Trunk and legs
c. Trunk and arms
d. Arms and legs

309. Measles (rubeola) rashes first appear in which body part?
a. Trunk b. Face
c. Hands d. Legs

310. Rubella (German measles) rashes first appear in which body part?
a. Trunk b. Face
c. Hands d. Legs

311. Keratomalacia is associated with:
a. Diarrhea b. Measles
c. Chicken pox d. a and b

Explanation: Keratomalacia is an eye disorder caused by Vitamin A deficiency. Cornea gets cloudy and softens.

Measles and Diarrhea are associated with Vitamin A deficiency that leads to Keratomalacia.

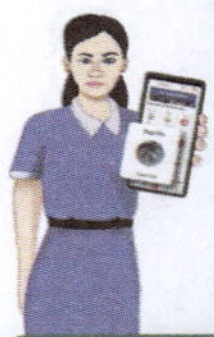

Ans.
285. a
286. d
287. d
288. b
289. b
290. d
291. d
292. a
293. b
294. c
295. c
296. b
297. c
298. d
299. b
300. a
301. c
302. a
303. a
304. c
305. a
306. a
307. d
308. a
309. b
310. b
311. d

312. Commonest complication of Mumps is:

a. Pneumonia b. Encephalitis
c. Aseptic meningitis d. Pancreatitis

313. Multi drug therapy (MDT) is treatment for:

a. T b. Leprosy
c. HIV d. All of these

314. Which type of sample is used to isolate polio virus earliest?

a. Stool b. Blood
c. CSF d. Throat swab

315. Which of the following viruses is excreted through feces?

a. Hepatitis b. HIV
c. Poliomyelitis d. Hepatitis C

316. Incubation period of Plasmodium vivax is:

a. 5-7 days b. 7-10 days
c. 10-14 days d. 15-30 days

317. The most effective way of preventing tetanus is:

a. Surgical debridement and toilet
b. Hyperbaric oxygen
c. Antibiotics
d. TT

318. 'Five clean practices' under strategies for elimination of neonatal tetanus include all; EXCEPT:

a. Clean surface for delivery
b. Clean hand of attendant
c. New blade for cutting the cord
d. Clean airway

319. Which of the following is the major risk factor of candidiasis of oral cavity?

a. Poor personal hygiene b. Alcoholism
c. Thiamine deficiency d. Smoking

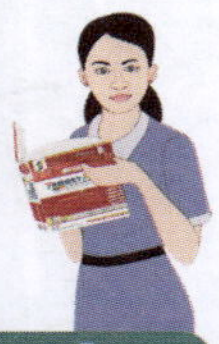

320. Which of the following terms refers to a fungal infection of foot?

a. Tinea corporis b. Tinea pedis
c. Tinea capitis d. Tinea cruris

MODES OF TRANSMISSION OF DISEASES

321. Mode of spread of whooping cough is:

a. Direct contact b. Droplet infection
c. Fomite d. Water borne

Explanation: Whooping cough is transmitted from one person to another by droplets of moisture expelled from the upper respiratory tract through coughing and sneezing.

322. The maximum size of droplet nuclei that can be inhaled into alveoli of lungs is:

a. 1-2 microns b. 1-5 microns
c. 5-7 microns d. 7-10 microns

Explanation: Vehicle of airborne respiratory disease transmission is droplet. 1-5 micron is the size of nuclei that can be inhaled into alveoli of lung easily.

323. Amebiasis is transmitted through ______ route.

a. Feco-oral b. Parenteral
c. Vector borne d. Air borne

Explanation: Amebiasis is a parasitic infection of the intestines caused by the protozoan *E. histolytica*. It is usually transmitted by the fecal-oral route, but it can also be transmitted indirectly through contact with contaminated hands.

324. Diseases which are transmitted by water and food are called as:

a. Vector- borne b. Air -borne
c. Fomite- borne d. Vehicle-borne

Explanation: Disease transmitted via food and water is called as vehicle borne.

325. Which one of the following diseases is not transmitted mainly by Fecal-Oral route? *(Safdarjung NO 2018)*

a. Enteric fever b. Measles
c. Cholera d. Hepatitis - A

326. Mode of spread of polio infection is: *(Staff Nurse G II 2014)*

a. Through vectors b. Droplet infection
c. Fecal-oral route d. Through blood

327. Plague is transmitted by:

a. Hard tick b. Soft tick
c. Rat flea d. Louse

328. Commonest mode of transmission of AIDS in India is:

a. Transplacental/mother to child
b. Use of unsterile syringes and needles
c. Sexual
d. Blood transfusion

329. Chikungunya virus is transmitted through:

a. Aedes mosquito b. Chikungunya mosquito
c. Culex mosquito d. Marsh mosquito

330. Japanese encephalitis is transmitted by:

a. Mosquito b. Tick
c. Mite d. Rat flea

331. Which pathogen is responsible for causing ringworm, and what is the primary mode of transmission for this infection? *New Q*

a. Parasite, direct contact
b. Parasite, waterborne
c. Fungus, direct contact
d. Bacteria, direct contact

Explanation: Ringworm, also known as dermatophytosis, is a fungal infection of the skin. It is caused by various species of dermatophytes, which are fungi that can infect the skin, hair, and nails. The primary mode of transmission for ringworm is through direct contact with an infected person, animal, or object.

332. Transovarian transmission is seen in:

a. Rickettsial disease b. Malaria
c. Filariasis d. None

333. Mosquito is not associated with transmission of:

a. Malaria b. Typhus
c. Dengue fever d. Japanese encephalitis

334. The most common cause of Urinary Tract Infection (UTI) in community is: *(DSSSB PHN, 2015)*

a. E. coli b. Klebsiella
c. Citrobacter d. Proteus Vulgaris

DIARRHEAL DISEASE & MANAGEMENT

335. During home visit, Nurse Mala found no signs of dehydration in 7 weeks old child who had diarrhea for last 2 weeks. The child is having:

a. Persistent diarrhea
b. Acute diarrhea
c. Dysentery
d. Severe dysenter

Ans.

312. c
313. d
314. a
315. c
316. c
317. d
318. d
319. a
320. b
321. b
322. b
323. a
324. d
325. b
326. c
327. c
328. c
329. a
330. a
331. c
332. a
333. b
334. a
335. a

336. Glucose is added to antidiarrheal solution because: *(RAK MSc 2018)*

a. It tastes sweet
b. Increases absorption of amino acids
c. Increases absorption of sodium
d. All of the above

Explanation: Oral rehydration therapy is depending on the glucose observation given orally for the purpose to increase the intestinal absorption of salt and water and it is efficient for managing the fluid and electrolyte imbalance.

337. Oral rehydration solution does not contain: *(DSSSB 1992)*

a. Sodium chloride
b. Calcium lactate
c. Bicarbonate
d. Glucose

Explanation: Calcium lactate is not a component of ORS solution.

338. Dehydration in a child with diarrhea, thirst present, tears absent is:

a. Mild
b. Moderate
c. Severe
d. None

339. During a home visit, a community health nurse found a child who is suffering from diarrhea and vomiting. What would be the nurse teach the mother to prepare first?

a. Oral dextrose solution
b. Oral rehydration solution
c. Oral saline solution
d. Semi solid food

340. New WHO ORS osmolarity is:

a. 270
b. 245
c. 290
d. 310

341. Which of the following is not present in ORS?

a. Glucose
b. Calcium gluconate
c. Potassium chloride
d. Sodium chloride

342. ORS should be discarded after ________ of preparation.

a. 54 hours
b. 6 hours
c. 12 hours
d. 24 hours

FOOD POISONING/FOOD-BORNE DISEASES

343. Which among the following organisms commonly causes food poisoning?

a. Bacteria and virus
b. Fungus
c. Protozoa
d. Yeast

344. Which among the following organisms is most commonly responsible for food-borne disease from undercooked poultry and eggs?

a. Clostridium
b. Salmonella
c. Botulism
d. Alga

345. All statements are true regarding botulinal toxin; EXCEPT:

a. Produced by clostridium botulinum
b. Produced by gram positive anaerobic bacteria.
c. It is neurotoxic.
d. It is a water-soluble endotoxin.

346. Clostridium perfingens poison is associated with:

a. Meat
b. Egg
c. Vegetables
d. Fruits

347. At which of the following temperatures food poisoning bacteria multiply rapidly?

a. 30°C
b. 37°C
c. 40°C
d. 45°C

348. Food poisoning is caused by all; EXCEPT:

a. Clostridium difficile
b. Bacillus cereus
c. Vibrio parahaemolyticus
d. Staph aureus

349. A community health nurse is assessing a neighborhood for potential health risks. The nurse observes that many households have improper waste disposal practices, leading to the storage of water in open areas, accumulation of garbage, and the presence of rodents and insects. Based on this observation, the nurse identifies a high risk of which of the following diseases related to poor sanitation and waste management in the community? *New Q*

a. Dengue fever
b. Measles
c. Tuberculosis
d. Chicken pox

Explanation: Improper waste disposal practices and the storage of water in open areas create breeding grounds for mosquitoes, which are the primary vectors for dengue fever transmission. Mosquitoes breed in stagnant water, and the accumulation of water in open containers provides an ideal environment for their proliferation.

PARASITIC INFECTIONS

350. The drug of choice for chemoprophylaxis in contact of a patient of plague is:

a. Penicillin
b. Rifampicin
c. Erythromycin
d. Tetracycline

351. Kala-azar is transmitted by:

a. Phlebotomus sergenti
b. Phlebotomus argentipes
c. Phlebotomus papatassi
d. All of the above

352. Which of the following is the carrier of Plague virus?

a. Dogs and carnivores
b. Rats and rodents
c. Snakes and Reptiles
d. Frogs and amphibians

353. Management of area with Annual Parasite Index (API) less than 2 include; EXCEPT:

a. Regular insecticidal spray
b. Passive surveillance
c. Detected cases get radical treatment
d. Follow -up blood smears are to be collected

Explanation: Areas are categorized under API to control the malaria cases. API is more than 2 indicates that cases of malaria are more and need more attention, while area with API less than 2 receives less attention. So, management in area with API <2 includes no regular spraying, passive surveillance, radical treatment of detected cases and follow up of blood smears.

354. Which of the following is observed as anti-malaria month? *(Staff Nurse G II 2014)*

a. December
b. May
c. June
d. January

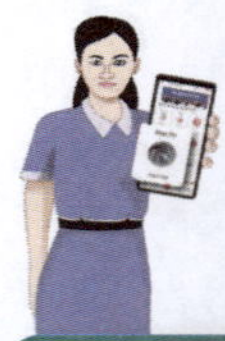

Ans.

336. c
337. b
338. b
339. b
340. b
341. b
342. d
343. a
344. b
345. d
346. a
347. b
348. c
349. a
350. d
351. b
352. b
353. a
354. c

HELMINTH INFESTATIONS

355. Causative organism of Enterobiasis is:
a. Hookworm b. Tapeworm
c. Pinworm d. Roundworm

356. Filarial larva can be collected from man's:
a. Anus at midnight
b. Peripheral blood at midnight
c. Nails after itching
d. Smear of intestinal content

357. Which among the following diseases is caused by nematodes?
a. Filariasis b. Amebiasis
c. Dysentery d. Polio

358. What is the difference between female and male ascariasis?
a. Females are shorter than male with straight posterior tail
b. Males are shorter than females with straight posterior tail
c. Males are shorter than females and have a curved posterior tail.
d. Males are longer than females and have a curved posterior tail.

359. The helminth which enters the body of a person through feet, if he walks bare foot in the contaminated soil is:
a. Hookworm b. Roundworm
c. Tapeworm d. Pinworm

360. Which of the following diseases has been eradicated from India?
a. Measles b. Mumps
c. Guinea worm disease d. Leprosy

361. Scotch tape swab is used to identify:
a. Tapeworm b. Pinworm
c. Angiostoma d. Cryptosporidium

Explanation: Pinworm ova are deposited around the anal orifice. Scotch tape test is done to check for pinworm infestation. The pinworm, also known as threadworm or seatworm, is a parasitic worm. It is a nematode and a common intestinal parasite or helminth, especially in humans.

362. Hookworm penetrates into the body by penetrating the skin of: *(DSSSB PHN, 2015)*
a. Hand b. Foot
c. Ear d. Head

ARTHROPOD-BORNE INFECTIONS/VECTOR-BORNE DISEASES

363. 'Chikungunya' species belongs to which family? *(AIIMS Bhopal Nursing Officer, 2018)*
a. Flaviviridae b. Togaviridae
c. Bunyaviridae d. Reoviridae

Explanation: 'Chikungunya' species belongs to Togaviridae family. Dengue and yellow fever species belongs to Flaviviridae family.

364. Chain of spread of malaria is:
a. Man—arthropod—man b. Man—pig—man
c. Mammal—bird—man d. Bird—arthropod—man

Explanation: Malaria completes its life in mosquito (asexual life cycle) and human being (sexual cycle). So option A is the correct answer.

365. Which of the following is the method of transmission of infection by vector?
a. Biting
b. Regurgitation
c. Scratching in-of infective feces
d. All of the above

Explanation: Biting, regurgitation, scratching-in of infective feces and contamination of host with body fluids of vectors are the methods of transmission of infection by vector.

366. A community health nurse is conducting a health education session on vector-borne diseases for a group of individuals living in a rural area. All of the following preventive measures are advised to reduce the risk of Kyasanur Forest Disease (KFD) disease in the community; EXCEPT: *New Q*
a. Vector control by dusting by Malathion or Pyrethroids
b. Application of insecticide on cattle
c. Advising individuals to wear long-sleeved clothing and pants when outdoors
d. Apply musquito repellent on exposed parts before entering forest.

Explanation:
- Kyasanur Forest Disease (KFD) is a tick-borne disease caused by the Kyasanur Forest Disease virus (KFDV). The virus is transmitted to humans through the bite of an infected tick. Ticks are small, parasitic insects that feed on the blood of animals and humans. They are most active during the spring and summer months. It is also known as **"monkey disease/monkey fever"** because of its association with monkey deaths.
- Vector control by dusting by Malathion or Pyrethroids can kill ticks and mosquitoes. Application of insecticide on cattle can also kill ticks that may be feeding on the cattle. Advising individuals to wear long-sleeved clothing and pants when outdoors can help to protect them from tick bites.
- **However, applying mosquito repellent on exposed parts before entering the forest is not an effective preventive measure for KFD.**
- Application of repellants such as
  - Dimethylphthalate (DMP), NN-Diethylm-Tolumaide (DEET) and certain other proprietary preparations having these or similar chemicals, e.g. Mylol on the exposed parts is effective from one to a few hours.

367. Which of the following viral infections is transmitted by tick? *(DSSSB 2008)*
a. Japanese encephalitis b. Dengue fever
c. Kyasanur forest disease d. Yellow fever

Explanation: Kyasanur Forest disease (KFD) is a tick-borne viral hemorrhagic fever endemic to South Asia The disease is caused by a virus belonging to the family Flaviviridae, which also includes yellow fever and dengue fever.

368. Kala-azar is transmitted by:
a. Aedes mosquito b. Tsetse fly
c. Sandfly d. Mice

Explanation: Sandfly causes kala-azar. Visceral leishmaniasis is spread by sandfly bites. This type of leishmaniasis affects the internal organs, usually the spleen, liver, and bone marrow.

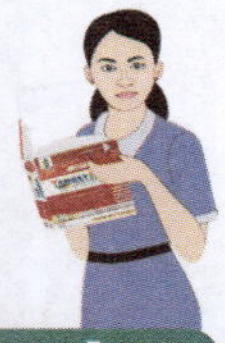

Ans.
355. c
356. b
357. a
358. c
359. a
360. c
361. b
362. b
363. b
364. a
365. d
366. d
367. c
368. c

369. Which disease condition is transmitted by Aedes mosquito?

a. Dengue fever
b. Chikungunya
c. Yellow fever
d. All of these

Explanation: Dengue fever, yellow fever, West Nile fever, chikungunya, eastern equine encephalitis, and Zika virus.

370. The mosquito that lays eggs singly:

a. Aedes
b. Anopheles
c. Culex
d. Mansonia

Explanation: Mosquito that lays egg singly is known as anopheles.

371. The drug of choice for falciparum malaria is:

a. Chloroquine
b. Quinine
c. Vancomycin
d. Amphotericin B

Explanation: Chloroquine is a medication used to prevent and to treat malaria in areas where malaria is known to be sensitive to its effects. Certain types of malaria, resistant strains, and complicated cases typically require different or additional medication.

372. Dengue fever is transmitted by: *(Safdarjung NO 2018)*

a. Culex fatigans
b. Culex vishnui
c. Aedes aegypti
d. Glossina palpalis

373. Malaria infection can be transmitted by: *(DSSSB PHN, 2015)*

a. Blood transfusion
b. Bite of infected female anopheles mosquito
c. Vertical transmission through placental defect
d. All of the above

374. Malarial transmission occurs by: *(Banaras HU 2015)*

a. Vector
b. Food and water
c. Air borne
d. Fomite (inanimate object)

375. Which among the following diseases is not due to Aedes mosquitoes? *(Kerala PSC, Nov 2014)*

a. Filariasis
b. Yellow fever
c. Dengue fever
d. Chikungunya fever

376. Which among the malarial parasites is responsible for cerebral malaria? *(Kerala PSC, Nov 2014)*

a. P. vivax
b. P. ovale
c. P. falciparum
d. P. quartan

377. Incubation period of Chikungunya fever is: *(Kerala PSC, Nov 2014)*

a. 10-13 days
b. 1-2 days
c. 14-16 days
d. 4-7 days

378. Causative organism of yellow fever is: *(Staff Nurse G II 2014)*

a. Myxovirus
b. Rhabdovirus
c. Enterovirus
d. Arbovirus

379. Malaria is caused by a: *(ESIC Chennai May 2012)*

a. Protozoa
b. Virus
c. Bacteria
d. Fungi

380. Vector responsible for Japanese encephalitis is:

a. Anopheles
b. Culex
c. Aedes
d. Mansonoides

381. Life cycle from egg to a complete adult mosquito takes:

a. 2-6 days
b. 7-10 days
c. 10-15 days
d. 14-21 days

382. Insecticide used for ultra-low volume fogging is:

a. Pyrethrum
b. DDT
c. Fenthion
d. Malathion

383. Which among the following is the most important treatment of patients with Dengue H-fever?

a. Aspirin for fever
b. Apply ice cap over abdomen to prevent melena
c. Replace body fluids
d. Use NSAIDs to control fever

384. Malaria parasite was discovered by:

a. Robert Koch
b. Louis Pasteur
c. Laveran
d. Ronald Ross

385. Malaria is transmitted by:

a. Female anopheles
b. Male anopheles
c. Culex
d. Aedes

386. A community health nurse is providing education on the prevention of leishmaniasis for a group of individuals living in an endemic area. The nurse emphasizes the importance of taking preventive measures against sandfly bites. The nurse should include all of the following advises to reduce the risk of leishmaniasis transmission, EXCEPT: *New Q*

a. Using bed nets treated with insecticide
b. Applying insect repellent on exposed skin
c. Clearing vegetation around homes to reduce sandfly breeding sites
d. Administering antiparasitic medications to the community

Explanation: Leishmaniasis is transmitted by the bite of infected sandflies. Preventive measures focus on avoiding sandfly bites and reducing breeding sites. Options a, b, and c are effective strategies to reduce the risk of bites and subsequent transmission of leishmaniasis. However, administering antiparasitic medications to the community is not a preventive measure but a treatment option for individuals who have already contacted the disease.

387. Scabies is caused by:

a. Trichophyton
b. Dermatophyton
c. Mycobacterium
d. Sarcoptes scabiei

388. Drug of choice for Scabies is:

a. 25% Benzyl benzoate
b. 5% Permethrin
c. 1% H
d. 5% Sulfur ointment

389. Q fever is transmitted by:

a. Mosquitoes
b. Mites
c. Ticks
d. Flea

390. Which of the following diseases is transmitted by mosquitoes?

a. Dengue
b. Kala-azar
c. Trypanosomiasis
d. Listeriosis

391. Which of the following vectors causes scabies?

a. Mosquito
b. Itch mite
c. Louse
d. Sandfly

392. Which of the following is not true about Zika Disease?

a. Causes Microcephaly in newborn
b. Caused by a virus and spreads sexually
c. Caused by bacteria and spreads by contamination
d. Mosquitoes are the vectors

393. The following infection is transmitted by Tick:

a. Japanese encephalitis
b. Dengue Fever
c. Kyasanur Forest Disease
d. Yellow Fever

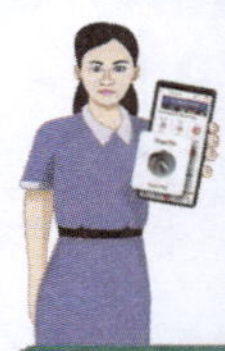

Ans.

369. d
370. b
371. a
372. c
373. d
374. a
375. a
376. c
377. d
378. d
379. a
380. b
381. b
382. d
383. c
384. c
385. a
386. d
387. d
388. a
389. c
390. a
391. b
392. c
393. c

394. Filaria is caused by: *(Banaras HU 2015)*

a. Bacteria b. Protozoa
c. Fungus d. Virus

395. Vector of dengue fever is: *(BHU 2001)*

a. Aedes b. Anopheles
c. Culex d. None

Explanation: Dengue is spread through the bite of the female mosquito (Aedes aegypti). This also can spread dengue fever, chikungunya, Zika fever, Mayaro and yellow fever viruses, and other diseases.

WATER-BORNE DISEASES

396. The following diseases can be transmitted by water and food; EXCEPT: *(AIIMS Bhopal Grade-I 2018)*

a. Hepatitis C b. Hepatitis A
c. Cholera d. Poliomyelitis

Explanation: Cholera is a bacterial infection that causes diarrhea. The cholera bacterium (vibrio Cholerae) is usually found in water or food that has been contaminated with feces. Polio virus and hepatitis-A virus are also transmitted through water and food via feco-oral route. Hepatitis-C is transmitted through blood and blood products.

397. Isolation is required in salmonellosis until:

a. 3 days after initiating antibiotic therapy
b. 3 consecutive stool sample become negative
c. 3 consecutive blood culture become negative
d. Rashes disappear

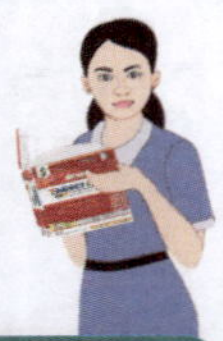

Explanation: In salmonellosis and shigellosis infection, isolation is recommended until three consecutive stool sample become negative for the organism.

398. Widal test is used for the diagnosis of: *(Banaras HU 2015)*

a. Enteric fever b. Malaria
c. Cholera d. Plague

399. The characteristic fever found in typhoid is: *(Staff Nurse G II 2014)*

a. Relapsing fever b. Step ladder fever
c. Intermittent fever d. Continuous fever

400. Which part of body is affected in typhoid? *(ESIC Chennai May 2012)*

a. Lungs b. Intestines
c. Liver d. Pancreas

401. Maximum permissible chloride level in a liter of water is:

a. 200 mg b. 400 mg
c. 600 mg d. 800 mg

402. Who found the link between cholera and contaminated water:

a. Louis Pasteur b. Ronald Ross
c. Edward Jenner d. John Snow

403. Example of a water borne disease is:

a. Malaria b. Cholera
c. Tuberculosis d. Rabies

404. Which of these diseases is not a water borne disease?

a. Typhoid fever b. Cholera
c. Hepatitis A d. Tuberculosis

405. Which of the following disease can be diagnosed by Mantoux test?

a. Diphtheria b. Tuberculosis
c. Pertussis d. Mumps

406. Which is the main agent of Typhoid fever?

a. Salmonella Typhi
b. Salmonella paratyphi A
c. Salmonella paratyphi B
d. Shigella

407. Drug of choice for cholera chemoprophylaxis is:

a. Erythromycin b. Ampicillin
c. Ciprofloxacin d. Tetracycline

408. All are "Water-Washed Diseases"; EXCEPT:

a. Trachoma b. Scabies
c. Conjunctivitis d. Yellow fever

409. Scabies, an infection of the skin caused by Sarcoptes scabiei, is an example of:

a. Water borne disease b. Water washed disease
c. Water based disease d. Water related disease

ZOONOSES

410. Which of the following is Zoonotic disease? *(RAK MSc 2018)*

a. Chikungunya b. Malaria
c. Rabies d. AIDS

Explanation: Rabies is zoonotic disease mainly transmitted to human from vertebrate animals like dogs, cats or wolves. It is also known as Hydrophobia. It is viral infection of central nervous system. Main causative agent is by Lyssavirus type 1 (RNA virus having bullet shaped neurotropic virus). It is transmitted through the deep bite or scratch and saliva by the infected animals.

411. Characteristic feature of a zoonotic infection is: *(AIIMS BBS NO 2018)*

a. Swimming pool granuloma
b. Carbuncle
c. Malignant pustule
d. Vincent's angina

Explanation: Malignant pustule is a form of Anthrax infection developed by papule and became vesicles. It is a very contagious disease caused by bacterium Bacillus anthracis (Zoonotic disease).

- Aquarium (swimming pool) granuloma - caused by Mycobacterium marinum.
- Carbuncle – caused by Staphylococcus aureus
- Vincent angina or trench mouth - caused by Bacillus fusiformis and Borrelia vincentii.

412. Zinc phosphide is an efficient: *(NCFL 2019)*

a. Rodenticide
b. Insecticide
c. Bactericide
d. Disinfectant

Explanation:

- Zinc phosphide is an efficient rodenticide. Rodents include rats, mice, squirrels, chipmunks, woodchucks, nutria, porcupines and beavers.
- Zinc phosphide will not kill insects, bacteria and microbes.

Ans.

394. b
395. a
396. a
397. b
398. a
399. b
400. b
401. c
402. d
403. b
404. d
405. b
406. a
407. d
408. d
409. b
410. c
411. c
412. a

413. **Negri bodies are found in which disease condition?**
   a. Rabies b. Measles
   c. Mumps d. Pertussis

Explanation: Most characteristic pathological finding in rabies is in the Central Nervous System, i.e., Negri body. Negri bodies are eosinophilic, sharply outlined, pathognomonic inclusion bodies (2–10 µm in diameter) found in the cytoplasm of certain nerve cells containing the virus of rabies, especially in Ammon's horn of the hippocampus.

414. **Rabies is caused by a virus called:**
   a. Filarial b. Lyssavirus type 1
   c. Myxovirus d. Adenovirus

Explanation: Rabies is caused by RNA virus called Lyssavirus type 1, it belongs to family rhabdoviridae-serotype 1.

415. **The infection which is acquired from animals to human is:** *(DSSSB PHN, 2015)*
   a. Plague b. Polio
   c. Pertussis d. Malaria

416. **Which of the following disease is transmitted through dog bite?** *(Banaras HU 2015)*
   a. Influenza b. Yellow fever
   c. Herpes d. Rabies

417. **Hydrophobia is the clinical feature of:**
   a. Mumps b. Pertussis
   c. Rabies d. Tetanus

418. **Which of the following is a zoonotic disease?**
   a. Hydatid cyst b. Malaria
   c. Filariasis d. Dengue fever

419. **All are anthropozoonotic disease; EXCEPT:**
   a. Plague
   b. Hydatid disease
   c. Dracunculiasis
   d. Rabies

420. **Zoonotic disease transmitted by arthropods is/ are:**
   a. Plague
   b. Melioidioses
   c. Rabies
   d. Leishmaniasis

421. **Rabies free country is:**
   a. China b. Russia
   c. Australia d. France

422. **High prevalence of Tuberculosis found in which of the following group of people?**
   a. Smokers b. Diabetics
   c. Asthmatics d. HIV positive

LEPROSY (HANSEN'S DISEASE)

423. **......disease has received maximum social stigma in India.**
   a. Tuberculosis b. Leprosy
   c. Polio d. Cholera

Explanation: Leprosy has very negative image among Indians, it is one of the oldest known diseases in human history, people considered it occurred due to past sins and people suffered from it were called 'lepers' and were isolated from the families, societies and communities.

424. **The another name for leprosy is:**
   a. Hansen's disease
   b. Anderson's diseases
   c. Chagas disease
   d. Slim of disease

Explanation: Leprosy gets its name from Latin word leprae means 'Scaly', it is also called as Hansen's disease, named after a Norway physician Gerhard Armauer Hansen who discovered that leprosy was not hereditary but by microorganism.

425. **Strategies of leprosy eradication program includes all of the following; EXCEPT:**
   a. Early detection and complete treatment of new leprosy cases
   b. Early diagnosis and prompt MDT, through routine and special efforts
   c. Strengthening of Disability Prevention and Medical Rehabilitation (DPMR) services
   d. Centralized leprosy services through dedicated hospitals for leprosy treatments

Explanation: Leprosy Elimination in India strategies include :
- Decentralized integrated leprosy services through General Health Care system.
- Early detection and complete treatment of new leprosy cases.
- Carrying out household contact survey in detection of Multibacillary (MB) and child cases.
- Early diagnosis and prompt MDT, through routine and special efforts
- Involvement of Accredited Social Health Activists (ASHAs) in the detection and complete treatment of Leprosy cases for leprosy work
- Strengthening of Disability Prevention and Medical Rehabilitation (DPMR) services.
- Information, Education and Communication (IEC) activities in the community to improve self-reporting to Primary Health Center (PHC) and reduction of stigma.
- Intensive monitoring and supervision at primary health center/ community health center.

426. **Mode of transmission of leprosy is:**
   a. Breast milk b. Insect bite
   c. Droplet infection d. Both b and c

Explanation: Until recently, the most widely held belief was that the disease was transmitted by direct contact between cases of leprosy and healthy persons. More recently the possibility of transmission by the respiratory route is gaining ground. There are also other possibilities such as transmission through insects which cannot be completely ruled out. (As per WHO)

427. **Which of the following is the early sign of leprosy?**
   a. Loss of sensation
   b. Lesions over the skin
   c. Thickened painful nerves
   d. Sinking of the nose bridge

Explanation: Thickened painful nerves is an early sign of Leprosy. Leprosy is caused by infection with the bacterium mycobacterium leprae. It mainly affects the skin and peripheral nerves. Symptoms include pale or red skin lesions, reduced sensation and numbness.

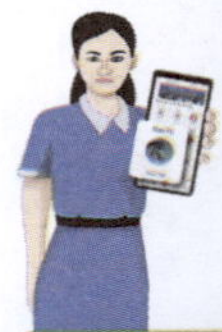

Ans.
413. a
414. b
415. a
416. d
417. c
418. a
419. c
420. a
421. c
422. d
423. b
424. a
425. d
426. d
427. c

428. Lepromin test is used to diagnose:

a. Leprosy b. Malaria
c. TB d. HIV/AIDS

Explanation: The lepromin skin test is used to determine what type of leprosy a person has. A sample of inactivated (unable to cause infection) leprosy-causing bacteria is injected just under the skin, usually on the forearm, so that a small lump pushes the skin up. The lump indicates that the antigen has been injected at the correct depth. The injection site is labeled and examined 3 days, and again 28 days, later to see if there is a reaction.

429. Lepromin test is usually read after:

a. 1 week b. 2 weeks
c. 3 weeks d. 4 weeks

Explanation: A sample of inactivated (unable to cause infection) leprosy-causing bacteria is injected just under the skin, usually on the forearm, so that a small lump pushes the skin up. The lump indicates that the antigen has been injected at the correct depth. The injection site is labeled and examined 3 days, and again 28 days, later to see if there is a reaction.

430. Classification of leprosy is based upon:

a. Bacteriological status
b. Immunological status
c. Histological status
d. All of the above

Explanation: Leprosy classification is based upon clinical, bacteriological, immunological and histological status of the patients.

431. Drug of choice for leprosy: *(RRB Feb 2012)*

a. DEC b. Dapsone
c. Streptomycin d. Ivermectin

432. Lepromin test is used for all of the following; EXCEPT:

a. Classify the lesions of leprosy patients
b. Determine the prognosis of disease
c. Assess the resistance of individuals to leprosy
d. Diagnosis of leprosy

TUBERCULOSIS

433. Who discovered tuberculin skin test?

a. Von Pirquet b. Louis Pasteur
c. Ronald Ross d. Edward Jenner

434. Robert Koch discovered the etiologic agent of: *(Banaras HU 2015)*

a. Typhoid b. Smallpox
c. Tuberculosis d. Polio

435. Among the following which is NOT a contagious disease? *New Q*

a. Chicken pox
b. Measles
c. Influenza
d. Hookworm infestation

Explanation: All contagious diseases are also infectious, but not all infectious diseases are contagious.

A communicable disease that can spread rapidly from person to person through direct contact (touching a person who has the infection), indirect contact (touching a contaminated object), or droplet contact (inhaling droplets made when a person who has the infection coughs, sneezes, or talks) is known as contagious.

436. Which of the following infection of animals primarily can be transmitted through milk? *(AIIMS Raipur Staff Nurse Grade I-2018)*

a. Tuberculosis b. Dengue
c. Plague d. Leptospirosis

Explanation: The infection which transmitted via animal milk is tuberculosis. Dengue fever is spread by Aedes aegypti mosquito which is caused by virus. Plague is a bacterial infection caused by Yersinia pestis transmitted by fleas. Leptospirosis is a bacterial infection spread via urine of the infected animal.

437. Tuberculin test denotes: *(JIPMER 1994)*

a. Previous or present sensitivity to tubercle proteins
b. Patient is resistant to tuberculosis
c. Patient is susceptible to tuberculosis
d. Protective immune status of individual against tuberculosis.

Explanation: A purified protein derivative (PPD) skin test is a test that determines if you suffer from tuberculosis (TB). Tuberculosis is a serious infection, usually of the lungs, caused by the bacteria Mycobacterium tuberculosis.

438. The size of respirable dust is:

a. 20 microns b. 15 microns
c. 10 microns d. 5 microns

Explanation: Solid dust particles produced during grinding, crushing are suspended in the air. Dust particles larger than 10 microns settle down easily, but dust particles of 5 micron and below can be easily inhaled directly into lungs.

439. DOTS is for……………….condition of. *(MSc AIIMS 2005)*

a. Tuberculosis b. Leprosy
c. Malaria d. HIV

Explanation: DOTS (directly observed treatment, short-course) is the name given to the tuberculosis control strategy recommended by the World Health Organization.

440. Among the following secondary prevention of TB is:

a. BCG vaccination b. DOTS treatment
c. Health education d. Sputum testing

Explanation: Primary prevention addresses the root cause of a disease or injury whereas secondary prevention aims to detect and treat a disease early.

441. Staining technique used to diagnose TB is known as:

a. Ziehl-Neelsen stain b. Gram stain
c. Giemsa stain d. PAS

Explanation: Ziehl-Neelsen stain, also known as the acid–fast stain, is a special bacteriological stain used to identify acid-fast organisms, mainly mycobacterium.

442. Which is the full form of DOTS chemotherapy?

a. Directly Observed Treatment- Short-course
b. Digitally Operated Treatment Service
c. De-oxygenated Tetracycline – Streptomycin
d. Doxycyclin–Omaprazole–Tetracycline-Short-course

Explanation: DOTS stands for directly observed treatment short course used to treat tuberculosis.

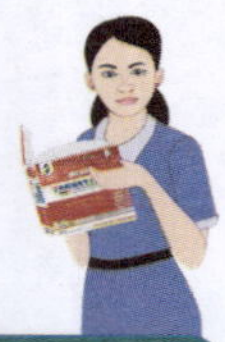

Ans.

428. a
429. d
430. d
431. b
432. d
433. a
434. c
435. d
436. a
437. a
438. d
439. a
440. b
441. a
442. a

443. DOTS is a comprehensive strategy to cure TB. The Primary element of DOTS is: *(AIIMS Raipur Grade II 2017)*
   a. Sputum microscopy services
   b. Regular drug supply to the patients
   c. Health workers counsel and observe their patients swallow each anti-TB medications and monitor progress until cured
   d. Political will in terms of manpower

Explanation: The five elements of DOTS are political commitment with increased and sustained financing, case detection through quality assured bacteriology, standardized treatment with supervision, effective drug supply and monitoring/evaluation system and impact measurement.

444. Disease which is also known as barometer of social welfare is:
   a. TB
   b. Typhoid
   c. Cholera
   d. HIV/AIDS

Explanation: It is the term used for TB.

445. Which of the following diseases is known as "Barometer of social welfare"? *(RRB Feb 2012)*
   a. Leprosy
   b. Tuberculosis
   c. Cholera
   d. Malaria

446. The most appropriate test to assess the prevalence of tuberculosis infection in a community is:
   a. Mass miniature Radiography
   b. Sputum examination
   c. Tuberculin test
   d. Clinical examination

447. Incidence of TB in a community is measured by:
   a. Sputum smear positivity
   b. Positive Tuberculin test
   c. Sputum culture
   d. Mantoux test positive

448. Full form of DOTS chemotherapy is:
   a. Directly Observed Treatment- Short-course
   b. Digitally Operated Treatment Service
   c. Directly Observed Therapy Supervised
   d. Directly Observed Treatment Supervised

449. Which of the following drugs in DOTS therapy can cause deafness?
   a. Ethambutol
   b. Isoniazid
   c. Rifampicin
   d. Streptomycin

450. Which of the following tests is done to test the efficiency of pasteurization of milk?
   a. Coliform count
   b. Methylene blue
   c. Reduction test
   d. Indicator test

451. Which of the following tests is done to check the presence of tuberculosis in human being?
   a. Weston Blot
   b. Widal test
   c. Mantoux test
   d. ELISA test

452. Case finding in RNTCP is based on:
   a. Sputum culture
   b. Sputum microscopy
   c. X-ray chest
   d. Mantoux test/ PCR

453. All among the following are bactericidal ATT drugs; EXCEPT:
   a. Rifampicin
   b. Ethambutol
   c. Streptomycin
   d. Pyrazinamide

454. In Tuberculosis combination of antimicrobials is used:
   a. To delay development of resistance
   b. To reduce toxicity
   c. To broaden antibacterial spectrum
   d. To prevent liberation of toxins from organism.

455. Anti-tubercular drug contraindicated in pregnancy is:
   a. Isoniazid
   b. Rifampicin
   c. Streptomycin
   d. Ethambutol

456. Why a TB patient is recommended a regimen of 4 drugs on 1st visit?
   a. To avoid emergence of resistance
   b. To avoid side effects
   c. To cure disease early
   d. None of the above

457. True about DOTS is:
   a. Drugs are given under supervision
   b. Streptomycin is always given in first 2 months
   c. Intermittent regimen is followed
   d. Same regimen is given in all patient

458. Multidrug resistance in TB is defined as resistance to:
   a. Streptomycin, Rifampicin and Isoniazid
   b. Streptomycin and Rifampicin
   c. Isoniazid and Rifampicin
   d. Streptomycin and Isoniazid

459. Anti-tubercular drug not given in children < 6 years of age is:
   a. Isoniazid
   b. Rifampicin
   c. Streptomycin
   d. Ethambutol

TETANUS

460. What type of toxin is produced by Clostridium tetani?
   a. Exotoxin
   b. Endotoxin
   c. Organic toxin
   d. Inorganic toxin

Explanation: Clostridium tetani produces exotoxins. These are the toxoids that are secreted from the bacterial cells whereas, endotoxins are present within the cells.

461. Strategy for prevention of neonatal tetanus include all; EXCEPT:
   a. TT to all females in reproductive age group
   b. Giving penicillin to all neonates
   c. 2 doses of TT to all unimmunized pregnant women
   d. Three clean's

462. In Tetanus communicable period is:
   a. 7 days
   b. 10 days
   c. 14 days
   d. None of these

463. What reaction might occur due to tetanus vaccine?
   a. Febrile seizures
   b. Brachial neuritis
   c. Hypotonic muscles
   d. Encephalopathy

464. The true statement regarding tetanus is:
   a. 5 dose immunization provides lifelong immunity.
   b. TT affords no protection in the present injury.
   c. TT serves no use once 12 hours have elapsed following injury.
   d. TT and Ig may both be given in suspected tetanus.

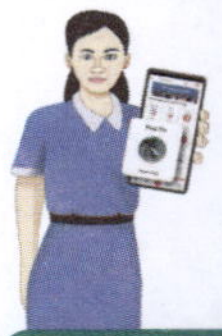

Ans.

443. c
444. a
445. b
446. c
447. a
448. a
449. d
450. a
451. c
452. b
453. b
454. a
455. c
456. a
457. a
458. c
459. d
460. a
461. b
462. d
463. b
464. d

SEXUALLY TRANSMITTED DISEASE

465. The effective preventive measures for AIDS are use of condom, which provides protection against: *(RAK MSc 2018)*

a. Inhibition of sperm action
b. Spermicidal action
c. Agglutination of spermatozoa
d. All of the above

Explanation: Preventive measures are used for AIDS in the use of male and female condoms which reduce the risk for spreading the disease by inhibiting the contact of sperm on vaginal wall. Condom is acting as a barrier between sperm and vaginal mucosal wall.

466. Intervention used under prevention of spreading of AIDS include:

a. Treating STD
b. Providing condoms
c. Behavior change communication
d. All of the above

Explanation: All of the above components are used for preventing spread of HIV.

467. Causative organism of AIDS: *(ESI 2009)*

a. Rabies virus
b. CMV
c. Retro virus
d. Adenovirus

Explanation: AIDS is caused by HIV (Human immunodeficiency virus). This virus belongs to lenti family and it affects the CD4 T cell.

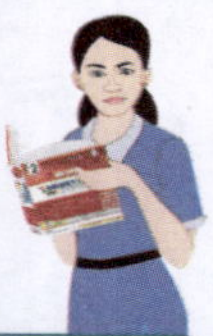

468. Identify the sexually transmitted disease among the following:

a. HIV/AIDS
b. Herpes simplex-2
c. Human papillomavirus infection
d. All of the above

Explanation: All of the above mentioned conditions are sexually transmitting diseases.

469. Fifth disease is also known as:

a. Erythema infectiosum
b. Mumps
c. Measles
d. Rubella

Explanation: Erythema infectiosum (also known as fifth disease) is usually a benign childhood condition characterized by a classic slapped-cheek appearance and lacy exanthem. It results from infection with human parvovirus (PV) B19, an erythrovirus.

470. Refrigerated blood for more than 48 hours cannot transmit:

a. HIV
b. Hepatitis B
c. Syphilis
d. Gonorrhea

Explanation: Syphilis is transmitted in fresh blood. Storage of blood will kill the microorganism.

471. Syphilis is caused by: *(DSSSB PHN, 2015)*

a. HIV
b. Papilloma
c. Neisseria
d. Treponema

472. World AIDS day is celebrated every year on: *(Kerala PSC, Nov 2014)*

a. July 11th
b. December 25th
c. December 1st
d. June 5th

473. First AIDS case in India was reported in the year: *(JIPMER 2012)*

a. 1987
b. 1982
c. 1992
d. 2002

474. HIV virus was discovered in the year:

a. 1981
b. 1983
c. 1986
d. 1996

475. HIV postexposure prophylaxis should be started in:

a. 24 hours
b. 48 hours
c. 72 hours
d. 6 hours

476. The chance of HIV transmission from mother to child can be reduced by all; EXCEPT:

a. Cesarean section
b. Vitamin A supplementation
c. Stopping breastfeeding
d. Nevirapine mother antenatal and newborn after delivery

477. First country in South East Asia to report AIDS was:

a. Sri Lanka
b. India
c. Thailand
d. Bangladesh

478. HIV is not transmitted by:

a. Eating with a person having HIV
b. Unprotected sex
c. Use of unsterile syringes
d. Transfusion of HIV infected blood

479. Which of the following is a sexually transmitted disease?

a. Fibroid uterus
b. Gonorrhea
c. Ovarian cancer
d. SLE

480. Drug used to prevent vertical transmission of HIV infection in a child of HIV positive pregnant mother is:

a. Single dose of Nevirapine to newborn
b. Nevirapine for 6 weeks to 3 months to newborn
c. Single dose of Zidovudine to newborn
d. Zidovudine for 3 months to newborn

481. Which of the following would be the right method of choice of discarding the blood soaked-dressing removed from a HIV patient?

a. Pour 1 % hypochlorite on the dressing material and send it for incineration in an appropriate bag.
b. Pour 5 % hypochlorite on the dressing material and send it for incineration in an appropriate bag.
c. Pour 5% Lysol on the dressing material and send it for incineration in an appropriate bag
d. Pour 1% Lysol on the dressing material and send it for incineration in an appropriate bag.

482. Person with which of the following characteristics has highest chance to become infected with STD?

a. Intravenous drug use
b. Unprotected sex with multiple partners
c. Sex with people they don't know
d. Homosexual

483. Syphilis infection is caused by a:

a. Virus
b. Fungus
c. Spirochete
d. Protozoa

ENVIRONMENTAL POLLUTION

484. Which of the following is true about Global Warming?

a. CO_2 is a major greenhouse gas
b. Stratosphere ozone layer is harmful
c. CFC increases Stratosphere ozone layer
d. Kyoto protocol called for 20% reduction in Greenhouse emissions

Ans.

465. a
466. d
467. c
468. d
469. a
470. c
471. d
472. c
473. a
474. b
475. c
476. b
477. c
478. a
479. b
480. b
481. a
482. b
483. c
484. a

485. Air velocity is measured by:
- a. Hygrometer
- b. Psychrometer
- c. Anemometer
- d. Wet bulb thermometer

486. Which of the following is non natural gas causing greenhouse effect?
- a. Carbon Dioxide
- b. Methane
- c. Ozone
- d. CFCs

487. Exposure to noise above .... causes permanent loss of hearing.
- a. 85 d
- b. 90 dB
- c. 100 db
- d. 160 dB

488. The level of noise that can be tolerated without damage to hearing is:
- a. Up to 60 dB
- b. Up to 85 dB
- c. Up to 95 dB
- d. Up to 120 dB

489. The 'acceptable' noise level is:
- a. 85 dB
- b. 90 dB
- c. 95 dB
- d. 100 dB

490. Unit of absorbed radiation is:
- a. Roentgen
- b. Rad
- c. Rem
- d. Sievert

491. Which of the following day is celebrated as World Environment Day? *(Kerala PSC, Nov 2014)*
- a. May 1
- b. September 5
- c. December 1
- d. June 5

492. Not seen in fecal pollution is:
- a. E. coli
- b. Staphylococcus
- c. Streptococcus
- d. Clostridium perfringens

493. Which among the following is regarded as the most widely and commonly distributed air pollutant?
- a. Carbon monoxide
- b. Carbon dioxide
- c. Hydrocarbons
- d. Ozone

494. Best indication of air pollution is:
- a. SO_2
- b. CO_2
- c. Smoke index
- d. Suspended particle

WATER PURIFICATION PROCESSES

495. Temporary hardness of water is removed by: *(Banaras HU 2015)*
- a. Boiling
- b. Filtration
- c. SODIS method
- d. Addition of chlorine

496. Optimum level of fluoride in drinking water per liter is: *(JIPMER 2012)*
- a. 1-2 mg
- b. 0.05 – 0.08 mg
- c. 0.7 – 1.2 mg/L
- d. 0.5 – 0.8 rl

497. The most effective method of well disinfection is done by: *(RRB Feb 2012)*
- a. Chlorine tablets
- b. $KMnO_4$
- c. Per chlorine
- d. $CaOCl_2$

498. True about slow sand filter is:
- a. Occupies less space
- b. More expensive
- c. Requires longer duration
- d. Sand size 0.4 - 0.7mm

499. Slow sand filter is differentiated from rapid sand filter by:
- a. Bacteria are removed more effectively
- b. Skilled person is needed
- c. Cost construction is cheaper.
- d. Sand particles are of smaller size

500. Purest water in nature is:
- a. River water
- b. Rain water
- c. Deep well
- d. Impounding reservoirs

501. Residual Chlorine after chlorination of water should be: *(Safdarjung NO 2018)*
- a. 1 mg/L after 1 hour
- b. 1 mg/L after ½ hour
- c. 0.5 mg/L after 1 hour
- d. 0.5 mg/L after ½ hour

Explanation: Chlorination is the last step of the purification of water that mainly kills bacteria and safe for drinking. The small excess of chlorine is called free residual chlorine. 0.5 mg chlorine per liter at the end of 1 hour is required for continuous control of bacterial contamination.

502. The minimum recommended level of residual chlorine in the drinking water for one hour is:
- a. 0.25 mg/L
- b. 0.5 mg/L
- c. 1.0 mg/L
- d. 2.0 mg/L

503. Hardness of water is expressed as: *(JIPMER 2012)*
- a. OZ/L
- b. mg/L
- c. mg%
- d. mEq/L

504. How much gram of chlorine tablet is required to disinfect 20 liters of water?
- a. 0.2 g
- b. 0.3 g
- c. 0.5 g
- d. 1.0 g

505. Hardness of water can be removed by:
- a. Adding sodium carbonate into water
- b. Base exchange process
- c. Chlorination
- d. All of the above

506. Contact time for chlorination is:
- a. 4 hours
- b. 1 hour
- c. 1½ hours
- d. 2 hours

507. Disinfecting action of chlorine on water is mainly due to:
- a. Hydrogen Chlorine
- b. Hypochlorous acid
- c. Hypochlorite ions
- d. Hydrogen ions

508. True statement regarding chlorination is:
- a. Orthotolidine test measures free chlorine separately
- b. Chlorine acts best when pH is around 7
- c. It kills bacteria, viruses and spores
- d. Hypochlorite ions are mainly responsible for disinfecting activity

509. Orthotolidine test is used to detect:
- a. Free residual chlorine
- b. Bound chlorine
- c. Free and combined chlorine
- d. Chlorine demand

510. Fresh Bleaching powder contains:
- a. 33% chlorine
- b. 3.3% chlorine
- c. 0.33% chlorine
- d. 0.033% chlorine

511. Temporary hardness of water is primarily due to the presence of:
- a. Calcium and magnesium sulfates
- b. Calcium and magnesium chlorides
- c. Calcium and magnesium bicarbonates
- d. Calcium and magnesium nitrates

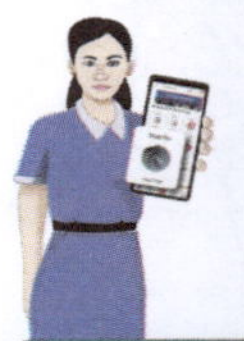

Ans.

485. c
486. d
487. c
488. b
489. a
490. b
491. d
492. b
493. a
494. a
495. a
496. c
497. d
498. c
499. a
500. b
501. c
502. b
503. b
504. c
505. d
506. b
507. b
508. b
509. c
510. a
511. c

512. Not a feature of hard water is:
a. Increased fuel consumption
b. Erosion of lead pipe
c. Scaling of boiler
d. Decreased soap consumption

513. Coliform test is for:
a. Air pollution
b. Water contamination
c. Sound pollution
d. None

514. The best bacterial indicator of water contamination is:
a. Streptococci Fecalis
b. E. coli
c. Clostridium perfringens
d. Klebsiella

515. Fecal contamination of drinking water is indicated by the presence of:
a. Klebsiella
b. E. coli
c. Proteus
d. Coagulase negative staphylococci

516. Which of the following is used as an indicator for recent fecal contamination of water?
a. E. coli
b. Corynebacterium diphtheriae
c. Pseudomonas
d. Streptococci

517. Which of the following is not true about water quality estimation?
a. Clostridium spores indicate recent contamination
b. Not more than 5% samples should have any coliforms
c. Sodium thiosulfate is added to neutralize chlorine
d. Coliforms must not be detectable in any 100 mL sample

518. Maximum permissible chloride level is:
a. 200 mg/L b. 300 mg/L
c. 500 mg/L d. 600 mg/L

519. Vital layer in slow sand filter is seen:
a. Top of water b. On the sand bed
c. Near filter valves d. None

520. Aeration of water is done to remove:
a. Odor b. Color
c. Sledge d. Turbidity

Explanation: Aeration helps in the removal of unpleasant odors present in water. It allows volatile compounds that contribute to odor to escape from the water, improving its smell and taste.

Note: While aeration can have some impact on reducing color and bacteria, it is not primarily used for their removal. Aeration does not remove sledge.

521. Venturi meter is used for measuring:
a. Bed strength in slow sand filter
b. Amount required for chlorination
c. Airflow direction
d. Airflow velocity

522. The heart of the activated sludge process is: *(RRB Feb 2012)*
a. Sludge digester
b. Primary sedimentation tank
c. Aeration tank
d. Final setting tank

WASTE MANAGEMENT

523. All of the following wastewater contains human excreta; EXCEPT:
a. Sewage b. Sullage
c. Feces d. None

524. Best method for disposal of refuse where land is available is:
a. Burial b. Dumping
c. Manure pit d. Controlled tipping

525. Waste water without human excreta is called:
a. Sewage b. Humus
c. Sullage d. Effluent

526. What is the first step in sewage treatment?
a. Aeration b. Chlorination
c. Precipitation d. Sedimentation

527. Most hazardous pesticide color coding is:
a. Red b. Green
c. Yellow d. Black

528. Sputum can be disinfected by all of the following; EXCEPT:
a. Autoclaving b. Boiling
c. Chlorhexidine d. Cresol

529. Best disinfectant of cholera stool is:
a. Bleaching powder b. Lime
c. Cresol d. Phenol

530. Which of the following methods is safe for disposal of mercury? *(PGIMER Chandigarh)*
a. Burry under earth
b. Collect carefully and reuse
c. Autoclaving and discard
d. Treat with chemical

Explanation: Mercury is highly poisonous and mercury containing products are properly and safely recycled or disposed of is one step that can be taken to protect environment and human health. Mercury is a virulent poison. Short-term or long-term exposures to mercury can lead to serious health problems, including death. Human exposure to mercury occurs primarily from breathing contaminated air. Mercury is also readily absorbed though the gastrointestinal tract and through the skin.

531. Universal precautions are applied to:
a. Blood b. Semen
c. Amniotic fluid d. All of these

Explanation: Universal precaution applies to blood, semen, vaginal secretion, amniotic, cerebrospinal, pericardial, peritoneal, pleural and synovial fluid and to other body fluid contaminated blood. This is given by Center for disease control and prevention (CDCP).

532. Color coded bag not to be incinerated as it contains Cadmium is:
a. Black bag b. Yellow bag
c. Blue bag d. Red bag

533. Waste sharps are disposed in:
a. Black container b. Yellow container
c. White container d. Red container

534. Most satisfactory method of Refuse disposal is:
a. Dumping b. Controlled tipping
c. Incineration d. Manure pits

535. If land is available the ideal method of disposal is:
a. Composting b. Incineration
c. Controlled tipping d. None

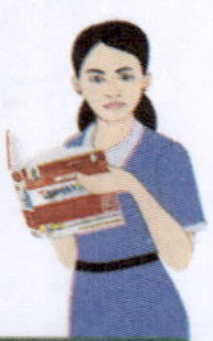

Ans.

512. d
513. b
514. b
515. b
516. d
517. a
518. d
519. b
520. a
521. a
522. c
523. b
524. d
525. c
526. d
527. a
528. c
529. d
530. b
531. d
532. d
533. c
534. b
535. c

536. Discarded and expired medicines are to be thrown into:
a. Blue bag b. Black bag
c. Yellow bag d. Red bag

537. Not true about screw feed technique is:
a. 80% volume reduction
b. Pathological wastes are removed
c. Weight is decreased by 20–30%
d. Based on non burn thermal treatment

538. Good for soil building is:
a. Incineration b. Controlled tipping
c. Composting d. Dumping

539. Which of the following wastes is disposed through incineration?
a. Anatomical waste b. Sharp waste
c. Cytotoxic waste d. Radioactive waste

540. True about incinerator is/are:
a. Red bag can be incinerated
b. No pretreatment required
c. Yellow bag must be incinerated
d. Sharps must not be incinerated

541. Animal waste is disposed of by:
a. Autoclaving b. Incineration
c. Chemical treatment d. Microwave

542. Incineration is done for:
a. Waste sharps b. Human anatomical waste
c. Radiographic waste d. Used batteries

543. What is the best method to dispose hospital waste? *(Banaras HU 2015)*
a. Composting b. Dumping
c. Chemical treatment d. Incineration

544. Incineration is not done for:
a. Cytotoxic drugs b. Waste Sharp
c. Human Anatomical Waste
d. Both a and b

545. Incineration is:
a. High temperature reduction process
b. High temperature oxidation process
c. Low temperature reduction process
d. Low temperature oxidation process

546. Sharp waste should be disposed in:
a. Black b. Blue/White translucent
c. Yellow d. Red

547. "3-D" in hospital waste management is:
a. Disinfection, Disposal, Drainage
b. Discard, Disinfection, Drainage
c. Destruction, Deep burial, Drainage
d. Destruction, Deep burial, Disposal

548. A community health nurse is providing education on biomedical waste management to a group of healthcare workers. The nurse explains the different categories of biomedical waste and their appropriate disposal methods. Which of the following statements by a healthcare worker indicates a correct understanding of the topic? *New Q*
a. "Sharps waste, such as needles and syringes, should be carefully disposed of in regular trash bins."
b. "Unused medications can be discarded in the sink for safe and convenient disposal."
c. "Anatomical wastes should be disposed in yellow container."
d. "Incineration is the preferred method of disposal for all types of biomedical waste."

549. Safe disposal of mercury is:
a. Collect carefully and recycle
b. Controlled combustion
c. Chemical treatment
d. Deep burial

550. Outdated cytotoxic drugs are disposed of by:
a. Disposal in municipal waste
b. Destruction and dumping in secured landfill
c. Store for months and then burial
d. Autoclave

551. Method for waste disposal in small camps is:
a. Burial b. Land filling
c. Incineration d. Dumping

CLIMATE CHANGE AND GLOBAL WARMING

552. Ozonosphere is mainly depleted by:
a. Ozone b. Excess Carbon monoxide
c. Excess Carbon dioxide d. CFCs

553. All of the following are the possible adverse effects of global warming; EXCEPT:
a. Melting glaciers
b. Extraordinary weather patterns
c. Increase in UVB radiation
d. Rise in sea level

554. Which of the following is not a major greenhouse gas?
a. Ozone b. Nitrous oxide
c. Methane d. Carbon dioxide

555. Global warming also refers to as:
a. Ecological change b. Atmosphere change
c. Climate change d. None of the above

556. UNFCCC stands for:
a. United Nations Framework Convention on Climate Change
b. United Nations Feedback Convention on Climate Change
c. United Nations Framework Council on Climate Change
d. United Nations Focus Council on Climate Change

557. All of the following types of sources of energy do not produce carbon dioxide; EXCEPT:
a. Wind energy b. Geothermal energy
c. Hydroelectric energy d. Coal thermal energy

CARDIOVASCULAR DISEASES/HYPERTENSION

558. Which of the following diseases causes most death worldwide? *(NCFL 2019)*
a. Cardiovascular disease b. HIV/AIDS
c. Malaria d. Tuberculosis

Explanation: According to WHO (2015), the top 5 diseases causing the most deaths worldwide are:
1. Ischemic heart disease or coronary artery disease – 8.8 Million deaths
2. Stroke – 6.2 Million deaths
3. Lower respiratory infections – 3.2 Million deaths
4. Chronic obstructive pulmonary disease – 3.1 Million
5. Trachea, bronchus and lung cancers– 1.7 Million deaths

559. Following are major criteria of Jones in Rheumatic Fever; EXCEPT:
a. Carditis b. Polyarthritis
c. Chorea d. Elevated ESR

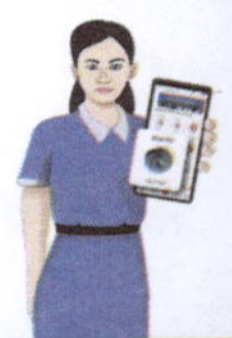

Ans.
536. c
537. b
538. c
539. a
540. b
541. b
542. b
543. d
544. d
545. b
546. b
547. a
548. c
549. a
550. b
551. a
552. d
553. c
554. a
555. c
556. a
557. d
558. a
559. d

560. While teaching a patient with COPD regarding exercise, the community health nurse should emphasize:
a. Rest in between exercise
b. Avoid exercise
c. Exercise strenuously
d. Take medication in between exercise

561. Modifiable risk factor for hypertension is:
a. Ethnicity b. Age
c. Sex d. Obesity

562. Not included among major criteria in acute rheumatic fever is:
a. Erythema marginatum b. Polyarthralgia
c. Chorea d. Pancarditis

563. Not a dietary modification in high risk Cardiovascular Disease group is:
a. LDL Cholesterol less than 100 mg/dl
b. Avoidance of alcohol
c. Saturated fat intake limited to 7% of total calories
d. Salt intake less than 5 gm/day

564. Modifiable risk factors in CHD are all; EXCEPT:
a. Smoking b. Obesity
c. Personality d. Hypertension

565. Ideal cholesterol level should be less than:
a. 200 b. 220
c. 300 d. 350

566. The most common early manifestation of chronic bronchitis:
a. Frequent productive cough
b. Dyspnea on exertion
c. Cyanosis at feet
d. Blood in sputum

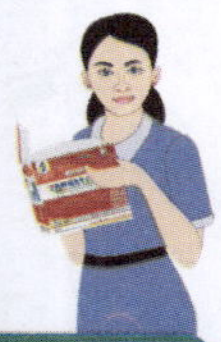

CANCER

567. The most common cancer, affecting both males and females worldwide is:
a. Cancer of the pancreas b. Buccal mucosa cancer
c. Lung cancer d. Colorectal cancer

568. Most common cancer affecting Indian females is:
a. Cervical cancer b. Ovarian cancer
c. Breast cancer d. Colonic cancer

569. Most common cancer among women worldwide is:
a. Lung cancer b. Oral cancer
c. Breast cancer d. Gastric cancer

570. Best method of screening for early detection of carcinoma breast in women aged above 40 years is:
a. Regular X-rays b. Self-examination
c. Mammography d. Regular biopsies

Ref: www.cancer.org

Explanation: Mammography is advised after a woman crosses 40 years of age. If mammography is normal, screening continues every year.

According to American Cancer Society, breast self-exam is also no longer recommended as an option for women of any age.

571. Which is not a predisposing factor for Carcinoma cervix?
a. Early marriage b. Early coitus
c. Early child bearing d. Single childbirth

572. Benzene is associated with cancer of:
a. Skin cancer b. Lung cancer
c. Bladder cancer d. Leukemia

DIABETES MELLITUS

573. While teaching "survival skills" to newly diagnosed type-I diabetic patient, the community nurse should include information about:
a. Foot care
b. Eliminating sugar from diet
c. Prevention of hypoglycemia
d. Need to increase rest

574. Glycosylated hemoglobin reflects the mean blood glucose level of previous:
a. 15 days b. 1 month
c. 3 months d. 6 months

575. Following is not a risk factor for development of diabetes mellitus:
a. Sedentary lifestyle
b. Protein energy malnutrition in infancy
c. Excessive intake of alcohol
d. High intake of vitamin-A

576. A community health nurse is organizing a diabetes screening program for a local community. Which of the following individuals should the nurse prioritize for diabetes screening? ***New Q***
a. A 30-year-old with a BMI of 22 and no family history of diabetes
b. A 45-year-old with a BMI of 30 and a family history of diabetes
c. A 50-year-old with a BMI of 25 and a history of hypertension
d. A 25-year-old with a BMI of 27 with a history of smoking

Explanation: The 45-year-old with a BMI of 30 and a family history of diabetes should be prioritized for diabetes screening. Family history of diabetes and obesity (high BMI) are known risk factors for developing diabetes. The combination of these risk factors increases the likelihood of developing diabetes and warrants screening to identify any potential early signs or symptoms.

577. Most common neonatal disorder screened is:
a. Neonatal hypothyroidism
b. Phenylketonuria
c. Hemoglobinopathies
d. Congenital dislocation of hip

OBESITY

578. Which of the following would the nurse reinforce after a teaching session as the most important lifestyle modification for the patient whose age is 59, height 5'11", weigh 280 pounds, and is hypertensive? *(RAK MSc 2018)*
a. Reduce weight b. Restrict salt intake
c. Increase potassium intake d. Decrease alcohol intake

Explanation: Patient's weight is 280 pounds (127 kg). So the first lifestyle modification needed is to reduce the weight. Though other options are also recommended for a patient with hypertension, the immediate concern is the patient's weight.

579. Childhood obesity prevention is a type of:
a. Primordial prevention
b. Primary prevention
c. Secondary prevention
d. Tertiary prevention

Ans.
560. a
561. d
562. b
563. a
564. c
565. a
566. a
567. c
568. c
569. c
570. c
571. d
572. d
573. c
574. c
575. d
576. b
577. b
578. a
579. a

580. A patient is called obese if BMI is:
- a. 20-30
- b. >25
- c. >30
- d. >40

581. BMI for normal weight:
- a. 18.5-27.99
- b. 18.5-24.99
- c. 23.0-24.99
- d. >30

582. BMI is also known as:
- a. Quetelet Index
- b. Lorentz Index
- c. Broca Index
- d. Corpulence Index

583. BMI (body mass index) is defined as:
- a. Weight (kg) /(Height)2 [meters]
- b. Weight (kg) /(Height)1.6 (cm)
- c. Midarm circumference (cm)/Head circumference (cm)
- d. Midarm circumference (cm) between ages of 1 -5 yrs

584. A community health nurse is providing education to a group of parents on preventing obesity in children. Which of the following strategies should the nurse recommend as an effective approach? *New Q*
- a. Encouraging watching fitness-related videos
- b. Promoting portion control and mindful eating
- c. Providing meal replacement shakes as a dietary option
- d. Implementing strict calorie counting and tracking

Explanation: Promoting portion control and mindful eating is an effective approach to prevent obesity. It focuses on developing healthy eating habits, being aware of portion sizes, and listening to one's body's hunger and fullness cues. Watching fitness-related videos (option a) can be a part of promoting physical activity but may not directly address the prevention of obesity. Meal replacement shakes (option c) may not provide a balanced and sustainable approach to nutrition. Implementing strict calorie counting and tracking (option d) may potentially contribute to disordered eating patterns.

BLINDNESS

585. SAFE strategy is recommended for the control of Trachoma. It contains all the following components; EXCEPT:
- a. Surgery
- b. Annual eye check up
- c. Facial cleanliness
- d. Environmental hygiene

Explanation: SAFE strategy means S–surgery A–antibiotics F–facial cleanliness E–environmental improvements. The SAFE strategy is an innovative public health approach designed to treat and prevent trachoma. Endorsed by the World Health Organization.

586. Leading cause of blindness in India is:
- a. Cataract
- b. Trachoma
- c. Glaucoma
- d. Vitamin A deficiency

Explanation: As per the survey conducted under National Program for Control of Blindness, it was found that the main causes of blindness were as follows. Cataract (62.6%) Refractive Error (19.70%) Corneal Blindness (0.90%), Glaucoma (5.80%), Surgical Complication (1.20%) Posterior Capsular Opacification (0.90%) Posterior Segment Disorder (4.70%), Others (4.19%) Estimated National Prevalence of Childhood Blindness/Low Vision is 0.80 per thousand.

587. Chronic exposure to poor lighting causes:
- a. Miner's nystagmus
- b. White finger
- c. Cataract
- d. Blurring of vision

Explanation: Poor lighting in working area causes eyestrain and on chronic exposure person develops shaking of eyeballs which is called Miner's nystagmus.

588. National Program for Control of Blindness and Visual Impairment (NPCBVI) was launched in the year *New Q*
- a. 1965
- b. 1976
- c. 1984
- d. 1991

Explanation: National Program for Control of Blindness and Visual Impairment (NPCBVI) was launched in the year 1976 as a 100% Centrally Sponsored scheme with the goal to reduce the prevalence of blindness from 1.4% to 0.3%..

Various activities/initiatives undertaken during the Five Year Plans under NPCBVI are targeted towards achieving the goal of reducing the prevalence of blindness to 0.3% by the year 2020.

589. In India the target disease included in vision 2020 is:
- a. Cataract
- b. Refractive errors
- c. Childhood blindness
- d. All of these

Explanation: Target disease areas for Vision 2020 includes Cataract, Refractive error, Trachoma, Childhood blindness, Low vision, Onchocerciasis/river blindness, Glaucoma, Diabetic retinopathy, Age-related macular degeneration, Gender and blindness and Vitamin A deficiency.

590. Which of the following conditions is not included as a component of five key areas for action in vision 2020?
- a. Cataract
- b. Refractory error
- c. Childhood blindness
- d. Viral conjuctivitis

591. Which of the following diseases is not included in "Vision 2020- Right to sight" immediate goals?
- a. Cataract
- b. Onchocerciasis
- c. Trachoma
- d. Epidemic conjunctivitis

592. Social stigma is felt or assumed in case of disability by community brings: *(Safdarjung NO 2018)*
- a. Isolation
- b. Serious problems
- c. Bitterness
- d. All of these

Explanation: The individual perceives his/her disability as a limitation which is associated with social stigma and it brings isolation from the surrounding community. It is a serious social problem, as it decreases the ability of the otherwise healthy individual.

HEALTH PROGRAMS IN INDIA

593. UNICEF was established in the year:
- a. 1946
- b. 1948
- c. 1952
- d. 1955

594. WHO was established in the year of:
- a. 1920
- b. 1948
- c. 1954
- d. 1960

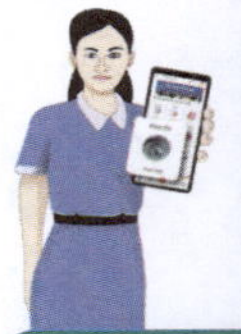

Ans.

580.	c
581.	b
582.	a
583.	a
584.	b
585.	b
586.	a
587.	a
588.	b
589.	d
590.	d
591.	d
592.	a
593.	a
594.	b

595. All of the following are the roles of community nurse in school Health program; EXCEPT: *(ESIC 2019)*

a. Assist in school medical examination and follow up
b. Assist in screening physical, mental and other special examinations of children in school
c. Assist in communicable disease control
d. To provide immunization to the children

Explanation: To provide immunization to the children is not the responsibility of the school health nurse in school health program. The immunization is covered in the Anganwadi program, a day in the week is fixed for immunization.

596. All are true of midday school meal programme; EXCEPT: *(Safdarjung NO 2018)*

a. Should supply one-third daily calories and half of daily protein
b. Substitute for regular food
c. Locally available foods are used
d. Cheap and easy to prepare

597. As per the Mid-day Meal Programme the meals served should supply at least.........of the total energy requirement. *(NCFL 2019)*

a. 1/3rd b. 1/4th
c. 1/6th d. 3/4th

Explanation: As per the set norms, the midday meal is required to meet one-third of energy and one-half of protein requirement (RDA) of school children.

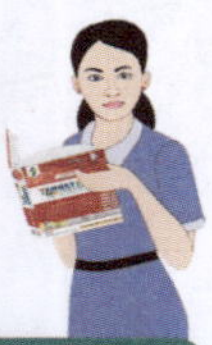

598. The diseases that come under National vector borne disease control program are; EXCEPT:

a. Filariasis b. Japanese encephalitis
c. Malaria d. Swine flu

Explanation: National vector borne disease control program is implemented for prevention and control of vector borne diseases like malaria, filariasis, Japanese encephalitis, Kala-Azar, dengue and chikungunya.

599. National malaria eradication program was launched in the year:

a. 1953 b. 1958
c. 1970 d. 2002

Explanation: National malaria control program was launched in 1953, but after spectacular results in 5 year period, the program was renamed as malaria eradication program in the year 1958. But there was resurgence of malarial cases in the early 1970. In 1999, the whole program was renamed as National Anti-malaria program. Recently in 2002, the program was renamed as National vector borne disease control program.

600. Beti bachao beti padhao programme was first launched in which state?

a. Haryana b. Bihar
c. Uttar Pradesh d. Delhi

Explanation: Launched in Haryana. "Beti bachao beti Padhao" (BBBP) Yojana (save daughter, educate daughter), to save and empower the girl child, making waves all over the nation.

601. Midday meal program started in the year: *New Q*

a. 1960 b. 1961
c. 1995 d. 2001

Explanation:

- Mid-day Meal Scheme was started in 1995 throughout India.
- Tamil Nadu government was the first in India to start the Mid Day Meal Scheme in India.
- **Update:** In September 2021, the Mid-Day Meal Scheme was renamed 'PM POSHAN' or Pradhan Mantri Poshan Shakti Nirman. PM POSHAN will extend the hot cooked meals to students studying in pre-primary levels or Bal Vatikas of government and government-aided primary schools, in addition to those already covered under the mid-day scheme.

602. National tuberculosis control program was adopted in India in the year: *(Staff Nurse G II 2014)*

a. 1960 b. 1966
c. 1962 d. 1964

603. Which of the following is the prime objective of Beti Bachao Beti Padhao Scheme?

a. Financial help for girl child until her 14 years of age
b. Celebrate girl child and enable her education
c. Government of employment for girl children
d. All of the above

604. How many districts are selected throughout the country for Beti Bachao Beti Padhao scheme?

a. 50 districts b. 100 districts
c. 200 districts d. 300 districts

605. Name the special deposit account under Beti Bachao Beti Padhao scheme.

a. Suraksha Samriddhi Account
b. Sukanya Samriddhi Account
c. Beti Samriddhi Account
d. Janani Samriddhi Account

606. Pradhan Mantri Suraksha Bima Yojana will cover:

a. Death due to accident
b. Disablement due to accident
c. Both disablement and death due to accident
d. Death due to communicable diseases

607. What is the cover amount for full disability in Pradhan Mantri Suraksha Bima Yojana?

a. 1 lakh b. 2 lakhs
c. 4 lakhs d. 5 lakhs

608. Vande Mataram scheme is included in:

a. RCH program b. JSY program
c. IMNCI program d. ICDS program

609. Urban malaria scheme is based on:

a. Epidemiological survey
b. Anti-adult mosquito measure
c. Anti-larval measures
d. Chemoprophylaxis

610. Recent Mental Health Act in India is designated as:

a. Mental Health Act (2011)
b. Mental Healthcare Act 2017
c. Mental Health and Lunatics Act (2011)
d. Mental Health and Illness Act (2011)

611. National tuberculosis control programme was launched in the year of:

a. 1962 b. 1992
c. 1995 d. 1997

Ans.

595.	d
596.	b
597.	a
598.	d
599.	b
600.	a
601.	c
602.	c
603.	b
604.	b
605.	b
606.	c
607.	b
608.	a
609.	c
610.	b
611.	a

612. Revised national tuberculosis control programme was launched in the year of:

a. 1962 b. 1992
c. 1995 d. 1997

613. First round of pulse polio immunization programme was launched in the year of:

a. 1962 b. 1993
c. 1995 d. 1997

614. What is the aim of swajal dhara?

a. Providing safe drinking water
b. Promotion of institutional delivery
c. Providing irrigation facilities for barren lands
d. Interlinking of river project

615. Kishori Shakti Yojana has been designed to improve nutritional status of:

a. Adult men
b. Adolescent girls
c. Under five children
d. Senior citizens

616. Kishori Shakti Yojana (KSY) is:

a. Empowerment of females under Maternity Benefit Scheme
b. Adolescent girl's scheme under ICDS
c. Free and compulsory education for girl child
d. Child care home scheme for female juvenile delinquents

617. RNTCP, Category II treatment comprises:

a. 2H3R3Z3E3 + 4H3R3
b. 2H3R3Z3E3S3 + 1H3R3Z3E3+ 5H3R3E3
c. 2H3R3Z3E3 + 5H3R3Z
d. None

618. True statement regarding RNTCP includes all; EXCEPT:

a. Sputum microscopy
b. Exclusion of private practitioners
c. Participation of all health workers
d. Provide latest equipment

619. National malaria control programme was launched in the year of:

a. 1921 b. 1953
c. 1954 d. 1960

620. Red cross society established in the year:

a. 1920 b. 1953
c. 1954 d. 1960

621. Red cross society was founded by: *(RPSC NG-II)*

a. Alfred
b. Henry Dunant
c. Emyllin
d. William James

622. Millennium development goals were declared by WHO in the year of:

a. 2000 b. 2004
c. 2005 d. 2010

623. Which of following health services provide mid-day meal programme?

a. M b. PHC
c. R d. School Health Services

624. In ICDS all of the following are included; EXCEPT:

a. Immunization
b. Health Education
c. Prevention of iodine deficiency disorders
d. Supplementary nutrition

625. In which year, a nationwide family planning programme was launched in India?

a. 1948 b. 1950
c. 1952 d. 1955

626. The main amendments to the Medical Termination of Pregnancy Act, 2021 include all; EXCEPT: *New Q*

a. Increasing the upper gestation limit for abortion from 20 to 24 weeks
b. Consent of the spouse is mandatory in case of married women
c. Establishing Medical Boards to review abortion cases
d. Confidentiality of abortion procedures

Explanation:

The main amendments to the MTP Act, 2021 include:

- Termination of Pregnancy for "special category of woman" (may include rape survivors etc.) till 24 weeks. For substantial fetal anomalies, subject to the permission of the medical board, termination can be done even after 24 weeks.
- Allowing abortion without the consent of the spouse.
- The new amendment establishes Medical Boards to review abortion cases. These Boards will be responsible for reviewing cases where there is a disagreement between the woman and her doctor about whether or not the abortion is justified.
- The new amendment also provides for the confidentiality of abortion procedures.

627. MTP Act of 1971 provides the following indications; EXCEPT:

a. Where continuation of pregnancy endangers mother's life
b. Where pregnancy is a result of rape
c. When acceptors require incentives
d. Failure of contraceptive devices

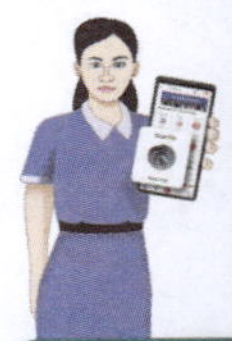

DEMOGRAPHIC TRENDS IN INDIA & NATIONAL POPULATION POLICY 2020

628. In which stage of the demographic cycle is in India currently?

a. High stationary b. Late expanding
c. Early stationary d. Low stationary

629. Magnitude of unemployment is aggravated by: *(Safdarjung NO 2018)*

a. Population control
b. Quality healthcare services
c. Population explosion
d. None of the above

Explanation: Unemployment is aggravated by population explosion. A sudden increase in the size of population is called population explosion.

FERTILITY-RELATED STATISTICS

630. In demographic stages "when birth rate begins to decline and death rate further decreases" is said to be: *(RAK MSc 2018)*

a. High stationary stage b. Early expansion stage
c. Late expansion stage d. Low stationary stage

Ans.

612. d
613. c
614. a
615. b
616. b
617. b
618. b
619. b
620. a
621. b
622. a
623. d
624. c
625. c
626. b
627. c
628. b
629. c
630. c

Explanation: The History of world's population since 1650 suggests the 5 stages of demographic cycle:

- First stage is called as High stationary stage. In this birth rate is high and death rate is also high that will cancel each other, and the population remains stationary.
- Second stage is also called as Early expanding stage. In this the death rate begins to decline and birth rate remains same.
- Third stage is also called as Late expanding stage. In this the death rate decreases still further and birth rate display as fall.
- Fourth stage is also called as Low stationary stage. In this the birth rate is low and death rate is also low this results population becomes stationary.
- Fifth stage is also called as declining stage. In this birth rate is decreasing than the death rate and population is declining.

631. As per WHO 2000 report, India's health expenditure was:

a. 3.2% of GDP b. 4.3% of GDP
c. 6.7% of GDP d. 7.2% of GDP

632. Limit for registration of birth is:

a. 7 days b. 14 days
c. 21 days d. Any of the above

633. Census population count is in reference to:

a. 1st March b. 1st July
c. 30th June d. 1st January

634. Census is conducted in every________ years in India.

a. 10 b. 25
c. 15 d. 20

635. First census in India was done in:

a. 1861 b. 1871
c. 1881 d. 1891

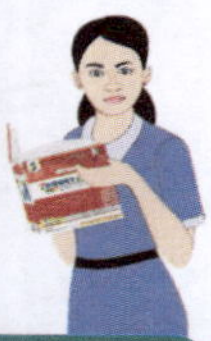

636. In which Century the Vital Statistics was originated? *(Safdarjung NO 2018)*

a. Eighteenth Century b. Seventeenth Century
c. Nineteenth Century d. Sixteenth Century

Explanation: The origin of vital statistics begins at early stage from 1854 with named James Stark for Register House in Edinburgh city associated with the Scottish Registration Act. He created the concept of vital statistics in 1854.

637. Vital statistics include the following; EXCEPT: *(ESIC 2019)*

a. Life expectancy
b. Birth rate
c. Education rate
d. Morbidity and mortality statistics

Explanation: **Vital statistics** include life expectancy, birth rate, death rate and other morbidity and mortality statistics. Education rate or literacy rate are considered as demographic data.

638. The newborn birth to be registered in India within: *(RAK MSc 2018)*

a. 7 days b. 21 days
c. 30 days d. 45 days

639. Eligible couple represents which age group of women?

a. 12-45 years b. 15-49 years
c. 14-45 years d. 18-45 years

Explanation:

- **Eligible couple:** A currently married couple wherein the wife (woman) is in the reproductive age (i.e., 15–49 yr. of age).
- **Target couple:** Eligible couples who have 2–3 living children

640. Eligible couple register is maintained at: *(RRB Feb 2012)*

a. Sub center b. CHC
c. PHC d. District headquarters

641. Best indicator of fertility: *(RRB Feb 2012)*

a. GFR (General fertility rate)
b. TFR (Total fertility rate)
c. CBR (Crude birth rate)
d. NRR (Net reproductive rate)

642. *Eligible couples* are those couples whose wife is in the age group of:

a. 18-35 years b. 18-40 years
c. 15-45 years d. 20-45 years

643. In Duvall's eight developmental stages of a family life cycle, couples come under: *(AIIMS-BBS SNO 2019)*

a. Stage 1 b. Stage 7
c. Stage 8 d. Stage 5

Explanation: Duvall's eight developmental stages of a family life cycle.

- Stage 1. Married couples without children
- Stage 2. Childbearing families with the oldest child between birth and 30 months
- Stage 3. Families with preschool children
- Stage 4. Families with school age children
- Stage 5. Families with adolescent children
- Stage 6. Launching families (First to last child is leaving home)
- Stage 7. Middle age families (Empty nest to retirement)
- Stage 8. Aging families (Retirement to death of both spouses)

CONTRACEPTIVE METHODS

644. A newly married healthy couple is asking for the best method of contraception and which of the following methods a nurse will advise? *(NCFL 2019)*

a. Barrier method
b. Rhythm method
c. Intrauterine devices
d. Combined Oral Pills

Explanation:

- Combined Oral pills have very low failure rate and a lot of non-contraceptive benefits. So it is a preferred option for a newly married healthy couple.
- Barrier method (condom) has high failure rate. Rhythm method is unreliable. IUD is not a first choice for young and never pregnant women.

645. The best time for insertion of I.U.C.D in women is: *(RAK MSc 2018)*

a. Within first week of cessation of menstrual period
b. Fourteen days after menstrual period
c. One week before menstrual period
d. During menstrual period

Explanation: Intrauterine devices made up of polyethylene or polymers with copper metal or progestogens. The IUD insertion is scheduled within 7-10 days of starting period. Because internal os is slightly open during the first 7 days of periods thereafter the os closes and makes the copper T insertion difficult.

Ans.

631. b
632. c
633. a
634. a
635. c
636. c
637. c
638. b
639. b
640. a
641. d
642. c
643. a
644. d
645. a

646. Commonest side effect of copper – T is: *(PGI 2006)*

a. Pain b. Bleeding
c. Vaginal discharge d. Pelvic inflammation

Explanation: Most common side effect associated with CU-T is bleeding.

647. Best response from a nurse to the woman who missed single dose of oral contraceptive pill?

a. Take the missed pill now and continue the course
b. Take 2 pills the next day and continue with the course
c. Discontinue the course because OCP has no more effect
d. Use barrier technique

Explanation: A woman who misses single dose of OCP should take 2 pills on next day and continue with the same cycle.

648. Absolute contraindication to the OCP includes:

a. Thromboembolism b. Liver disease
c. Ca breast d. All of these

Explanation: As per WHO

Absolute contraindication to OCP includes the following:

- Less than 6 weeks postpartum
- Smoker over the age of 35 (>15 cigarettes per day)
- Hypertension (systolic >160 mm Hg or diastolic >100 mm Hg)
- **Current or past history of venous thromboembolism (VTE)**
- Ischemic heart disease
- History of cerebrovascular accident
- Complicated valvular heart disease (pulmonary hypertension, atrial fibrillation, history of subacute bacterial endocarditis)
- Migraine headache with focal neurological symptoms
- **Breast cancer (current)**
- Diabetes with retinopathy/nephropathy/neuropathy
- **Severe cirrhosis (Liver disease)**
- Liver tumor (adenoma or hepatoma)

Relative contraindications include the following:

- Smoker over the age of 35 (<15 cigarettes per day)
- Adequately controlled hypertension
- Hypertension (systolic 140–159 mm Hg or diastolic 90–99 mm Hg)
- Migrai headache over the age of 35
- Currently symptomatic gallbladder disease
- Mild cirrhosis
- History of combined OCP-related cholestasis
- Users of medications that may interfere with OCP metabolism

649. On prescription of oral pills to the user, the health worker will ask about the following; EXCEPT: *(DSSSB 2010)*

a. Number of live children b. Calf tenderness
c. Headache d. Swelling of feet

Explanation: Number of live children is not taken into account while prescribing OCP.

650. Chemical components of Mala-D are:

a. D–norgestrel and ethinylestradiol
b. D–norgestrel and progestogen
c. Progestogen
d. Norethisterone Acetate

Explanation: MALA-D contains combination of D–norgestrel and Ethynyloestradiol.

651. Which of the following is the terminal method of contraceptive in male?

a. IUD
b. Chemical methods
c. Vasectomy
d. Condom

Explanation: Terminal method of contraception is vasectomy. Others are temporary method which are all reversible.

652. The metal which is commonly used for family planning is: *(DSSSB PHN, 2015)*

a. Copper b. Aluminum
c. Iron d. Silver

653. Which of the following is a common side effect of an Intrauterine device? *(RRB SSNE 2015)*

a. Vaginal Bleeding
b. Pelvic Inflammatory disease
c. Uterine perforation
d. Ectopic pregnancy

Ref: K.Park. Preventive Social Medicine. 24th Ed. Pg. 532-533.

Explanation: The commonest side effect of IUD - Increased vaginal bleeding.

- 10–20% of IUD removal are due to complaints of increased bleeding.
- Pain is second major side effect of IUD.
- Pelvic inflammatory disease, uterine perforation and Ectopic pregnancy are more serious side effects but less common compare to vaginal bleeding and pain.

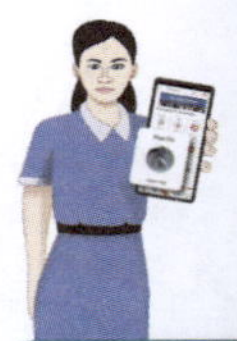

654. Which of the following methods of contraception can prevent sexually transmitted disease? *(Banaras HU 2015)*

a. Oral pills b. Condom
c. Copper–T d. Cervical cap

655. Which of the following neoplasm has been associated with the use of oral contraceptives? *(Banaras HU 2015)*

a. Breast cancer
b. Ovarian cancer
c. Endometrial cancer
d. Hepatic adenoma

656. Which one of the following is not an oral contraceptive pill? *(Banaras HU 2015)*

a. Estrogen only, mini pill
b. Estrogen and progesterone, combined pill
c. Estrogen followed by progesterone, sequential pill
d. Cortisol only pill

657. Natural method of contraception is:

a. Coitus interruptus
b. Breastfeeding
c. Both a and b
d. Condom

658. The emergency contraceptive for woman is:

a. Mala-D
b. Mala-N
c. Levonorgestrel
d. Progesterone

659. Which of the following is a natural contraceptive method?

a. Breastfeeding b. Condom
c. Copper-T d. IUD

Ans.

646. b
647. b
648. d
649. a
650. a
651. c
652. a
653. a
654. b
655. a
656. d
657. c
658. c
659. a

660. Which of the following is a traditional contraceptive method? *New Q*

a. Coitus interruptus b. Condom
c. IUD d. Diaphragm

Explanation:

Contraceptive methods are often classified as either:

Modern: Barrier methods such as male and female condoms, diaphragm, cervical cap and sponge; hormonal contraceptives that include oral, injectable, transdermal, vaginal ring, and implants; intrauterine device (IUD)]

OR

Traditional: Rhythm method (periodic abstinence), withdrawal (coitus interruptus), fertility awareness-based methods, the lactational amenorrhea method and folk methods. (Ref. WHO)

661. Spermicide used in Contraceptive TODAY is:

a. Norethisterone b. 9-Nanoxynol
c. Prostaglandin F2 d. MPA

662. Barrier methods are all; EXCEPT:

a. Diaphragm b. Foam tablets
c. Vaginal-sponge d. Lippes loop

663. Non medicated Intra Uterine Devices (IUDs) are called:

a. 3rd generation IUDs
b. 2nd generation IUDs
c. 1st generation IUDs
d. Multi – load devices

664. Cu T 380A IUD should be replaced once in:

a. 4 years b. 6 years
c. 8 years d. 10 years

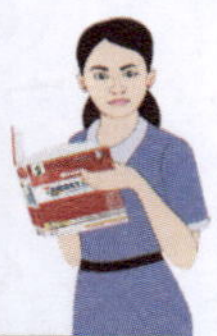

665. IUCD of choice in a woman with menorrhagia is:

a. Lippes loop
b. Cu T 200
c. Cu T 380A
d. Progesterone containing IUCD

666. Multiload device refers to:

a. 1st generation IUCD
b. 2st generation IUCD
c. Oc.
d. Barrier contraceptive

667. Most effective Cu T is:

a. Cu T 380 b. Cu T 220
c. Cu T 200 d. ML-Cu-250

668. In Cu T 200, the number denotes:

a. Weight in microgram b. Weight in milligram
c. Surface area d. Volume of device

669. The following statements are true about IUD; EXCEPT:

a. Multiload Cu-375 is a 3rd generation IUD
b. The pregnancy rate of Lippes loop and Cu-T 200 are similar
c. IUD can be used for Emergency Contraception within 5 days
d. Levonorgestrel releasing IUD has an effective life of 5 years.

670. Which IUCD acts for 10 years?

a. Cu-T 200 b. Nova T
c. Cu-T380 d. Multi load 250

671. Characteristics of an ideal candidate for copper -T insertion include all of the following; EXCEPT:

a. Has borne at least one child
b. Is willing to check IUD tail
c. Has a history of ectopic pregnancy
d. Has normal menstrual periods

672. IUD associated most commonly with expulsion is:

a. Lippes loop b. Cu-T 200
c. Cu –T 380 d. LNG IUD

673. Radiopaque material in copper T is:

a. Silicon b. $BaSO_4$
c. Carbon d. None

674. CuT is preferably inserted postnatal after:

a. 2 weeks b. 4 weeks
c. 5 weeks d. 8 weeks

675. Best contraceptive for a newly married healthy couple:

a. Barrier method b. IUCD
c. Oral contraceptive pills d. Natural methods

676. Packet of oral contraceptive pills consists of ----------- number of pills.

a. 21 contraceptive and 7 iron pills
b. 28 contraceptive pills and 5 iron pills
c. 23 contraceptive pills and 5 iron pills
d. 14 contraceptive and 14 iron pills

677. Which of the following is not an absolute contraindication for OCP?

a. Nursing mother b. Breast cancer
c. Cardiac abnormality d. H/O Thromboembolism

678. Serious complication of oral contraceptive is:

a. Leg vein thrombosis b. Headache
c. Break through bleeding d. Breast tenderness

679. The dose of ethinyl estradiol in Mala-N is:

a. 20 ugm b. 30 ugm
c. 50 ugmq d. 100 ugm

680. Mala-N oral contraceptive pill differs from Mala D, in terms of:

a. Norgestrel dosage
b. Estradiol dosage
c. Sold under social marketing scheme
d. Supplied free of cost

681. Hormonal contraceptive of choice in lactating woman is:

a. Combined pill b. Multiphasic pill
c. Mini pill d. Centchroman

682. Minipill is contraceptive of choices for:

a. Elderly females b. Lactating females
c. Obese women d. Menstruating women

683. Schedule of administration of mini pill containing 75 microgram of desogestrel for contraception is:

a. Once a day pill for 3 months + 7 day pill free interval
b. Once a day pill for 2 months + 7 day pill free interval
c. Taken for 21 days with 7 days pill free interval
d. Taken for 28 days with no pill free interval

684. Minipills contain:

a. Only progesterone in small quantity
b. Progesterone and estrogen in small quantity
c. Estrogen in small quantity and progesterone in large
d. None of the above

685. DMPA is an injectable contraceptive given every:

a. 2 weeks b. 2 months
c. 2 years d. 3 months

686. Safe period is calculated by:

a. Length of menstrual period
b. Duration and date of ovulation
c. Length of ovulation
d. Length of luteal phase

Ans.

660. a
661. b
662. d
663. c
664. d
665. d
666. b
667. a
668. c
669. c
670. c
671. c
672. a
673. b
674. d
675. c
676. a
677. a
678. a
679. b
680. d
681. c
682. b
683. d
684. a
685. d
686. a

687. Which of the following Natural methods of contraception is least effective?
a. Symptothermic method b. Creighton Model
c. Calendar method d. BBT method

Explanation: Among natural method of contraception, Calender method has 5% failure rate when it is perfectly used. Whereas symptothermal method and BBT has 0.4% of failure rate. Symptothermal method is combination of BBT and cervical mucous method. Failure rate in Creighton method is 1% when it is perfectly used.

688. "Persona" is a method of:
a. Natural contraceptive b. Hormonal contraceptive
c. Barrier contraceptive d. IUCD

689. Most common method of sterilization practised in India:
a. Female sterilization b. Male sterilization
c. Both equally common d. None

690. Most cost effective family planning method is:
a. Vasectomy b. Tubectomy
c. Copper T d. Oral pills

691. Which of the following methods is most suitable for the couple who is already having two children?
a. Condom and Contraceptive pills
b. Tubectomy
c. Contraceptive pills and IUDs
d. Condom and Diaphragm

692. Following vasectomy for family planning, a patient should be advised to use some other method of contraception, till:
a. Removal of all sutures b. Pain completely subsides
c. Two weeks d. Eight weeks

693. In emergency contraception which progesterone is used?
a. Norethisterone b. Medroxyprogesterone
c. Desogestrel d. Levonorgestrel

ANTENATAL CARE

694. The diagram that is used to predict possible genotypes in an offspring is known as:
a. Genogram
b. Punnett square
c. Pedigree chart
d. All of the above

695. Detection of high levels of alpha fetoprotein in mother's blood indicates that developing baby has:
a. Coarctation of aorta
b. Delayed skeletal development
c. Neural tube defect
d. Development of tumor

Explanation: Alpha fetoprotein is a type of protein produced from fetal yolk sac and then later in liver and gastrointestinal sac. It is found in both fetal serum and also in amniotic fluid. If its level is above normal it indicates that developing baby has neural tube defect.

696. Kegel exercises during pregnancy help in strengthening of:
a. Pelvic floor muscle b. Psoas muscle
c. Rectus abdominis d. Quadratus lumborum

Explanation: Kegel exercises are named after Arnold Kegel, who recommended these exercises in 1940's. These exercises help in strengthening pelvic floor muscles and improve blood circulation to rectum and vagina.

697. Punnett square is useful for:
a. To determine the probability of an offspring having a particular genotype
b. To determine the incidence of disease condition
c. To determine the surveillance of the disease condition
d. To determine the outcome of a disease condition

Explanation: The Punnett square is a diagram that is used to predict an outcome of a particular cross or breeding experiment. It is named after Reginald C. Punnett, who devised the approach. The diagram is used by biologists to determine the probability of an offspring having a particular genotype.

698. Which of the following ATT drugs is absolutely contra-indicated in pregnancy?
a. Pyrazinamide b. Rifampicin
c. Streptomycin d. Ethambutol

Explanation: Streptomycin is absolutely contraindicated in pregnancy. Streptomycin is a bactericidal antibiotic. Adverse effects of this medicine are ototoxicity, nephrotoxicity, fetal auditory toxicity, and neuromuscular paralysis.

699. Medical methods of abortion using a combination of mifepristone and misoprostol are found to be most effective and safe upto ________ of pregnancy.
a. 18-22 weeks b. 13-20 weeks
c. 13-18 weeks d. 8-12 weeks

700. Medical termination of pregnancy can be done by a registered medical practitioner if the gestation period is less than:
a. 8 weeks b. 12 weeks
c. 20 weeks d. 24 weeks

701. What are the amounts of calories and proteins received by a pregnant woman from the anganwadi worker?
a. 300 cals, 15 gm protein b. 500 cals, 15 gm protein
c. 300 cals, 25 gm protein d. 500 cals, 25 gm protein

702. Which one of the following is categorized as a high risk pregnancy?
a. Birth order 3 b. Maternal height 150 cm
c. Twins pregnancy d. Blood group AB+ve

703. Preterm babies:
a. Born before 37 weeks
b. Born before 40 weeks
c. Born before 42 weeks
d. Born before 47 weeks

704. Most common cause of low birth weight baby is:
a. Prematurity b. Infection
c. Anemia d. Diabetes

INTRANATAL CARE

705. Neural tube defect occurs due to lack of:
a. Folic acid b. Calcium
c. Niacin d. Riboflavin

Explanation: Neural tube defects are birth defects of the brain, spine, or spinal cord. They happen in the first month of pregnancy, often before a woman even knows that she is pregnant. The two most common neural tube defects are spina bifida and anencephaly. In spina bifida, the fetal spinal column does not close completely. Taking a prenatal vitamin with the recommended 400 micrograms (mcg) of folic acid before and during pregnancy can help prevent NTD.

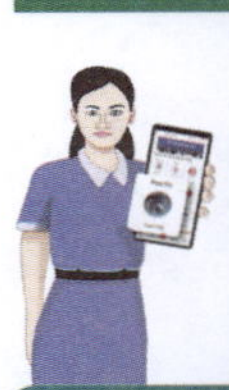

Ans.
687. c
688. a
689. a
690. a
691. b
692. d
693. d
694. b
695. c
696. a
697. a
698. c
699. d
700. c
701. d
702. c
703. a
704. a
705. a

706. Which of the following is not included in '5 cleans' in conduct of delivery?
- a. Clean hands
- b. Clean perineum
- c. Clean cutting and care of cord
- d. Clean surface for delivery

POSTNATAL CARE

707. In which of the following conditions breastfeeding is contraindicated?
- a. Maternal Ebola virus disease
- b. Leprosy
- c. Tuberculosis
- d. Typhoid

708. Rooming in practice means keeping mother and infant together:
- a. For 24 hours a day
- b. For 8 hours
- c. Whenever baby demands for feeding
- d. Whenever infant becomes hypothermic

Explanation: Rooming in is a step taken under baby friendly hospital initiative, in which mother and infant are kept together for 24 hours. This increases neuromotor development, prevents hypothermia and infection. This arrangement gives an opportunity for the mother and father to know their baby. The bond between the parent and the child is well established in roomed-in babies.

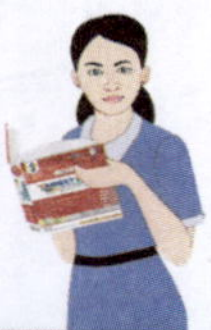

709. Exclusive breastfeeding helps mother in; EXCEPT:
- a. Prevention of cervical cancer
- b. Prevention of breast cancer
- c. Act as a contraceptive method
- d. Helps in quick and early involution of uterus

Explanation: Exclusive breastfeeding helps mother in preventing breast cancer. Breastfeeding acts as a natural contraceptive, prevents conception and it helps in quick involution of uterus and reduces post-partum bleeding. Cervical cancer is not related with breastfeeding.

710. Prolactin reflex in mother causes:
- a. Ejection of milk
- b. Production of milk
- c. Suppression of milk production
- d. Storage of milk

Explanation: As the baby sucks, nerve ending in the nipple stimulates anterior pituitary gland resulting in release of prolactin hormone which stimulates alveolar cells to produce milk. Thus, more the baby sucks more milk will be produced.

711. Baby with birth weight of 1000-2000 g are termed:
- a. Low birth weight babies
- b. Very low birth weight babies
- c. Small for date baby
- d. Extremely low birth weight babies

Explanation: Very low birth weight is very fragile and needs intensive neonatal care in hospital.

Birth weight	Grade
>3500 g	Obese
3500–2500 g	Normal birth weight babies
2500–2000 g	Low birth weight baby
2000–1000 g	Very low birth weight baby
<1000 g	Extremely low birth weight babies

712. Warm chain means:
- a. Drying the baby
- b. Establishing skin to skin contact with mother and immediate initiation of breastfeeding
- c. Warm resuscitation and warm transportation
- d. All of the above

Explanation: Warm chain is a set of 10 interlinked procedures carried at birth and later to prevent hypothermia among newborns, it includes:
- Warm delivery room (>25°C)
- Warm resuscitation
- Immediate drying
- Skin-to-skin contact between baby and the mother
- Breastfeeding
- Bathing and weighing postponed
- Appropriate clothing and bedding
- Mother and baby together
- Warm transportation
- Training/awareness of healthcare providers

713. Apgar score helps to assess depression of:
- a. Cardiopulmonary functions
- b. Psychomotor functions
- c. Integumentary functions
- d. Cardiopulmonary and neurologic function

Explanation: Apgar Scoring system is used to assess the depression of cardiopulmonary and neurologic functions. It considers signs such as color, heart rate, respiratory rate, muscle tone and reflexes.

714. Apgar score of 4-6 of newborn indicates:
- a. Severe depression
- b. Mild depression
- c. Moderate depression
- d. No depression

Explanation: Apgar scoring is done by summing of scores obtained under all 5 parameters. Minimum score is 0 and maximum score is 10.

Apgar Score	Level of depression	Level of attention
0–3	Severe	Intensive neonatal care
4–6	Mild	Needs immediate attention, if Apgar score has not changed after 5 minutes should be treated in intensive care
7–10	No depression	No special attention needed

Ans.

706.	b
707.	a
708.	a
709.	a
710.	b
711.	b
712.	d
713.	d
714.	b

715. Normal umbilical cord contains:

a. 1 artery and 2 veins b. 2 artery and 1 vein
c. 1 artery and 1 vein d. 2 artery and 2 veins

Explanation: Normal newborn gets 2 arteries and 1 vein, abnormality in umbilical artery can be detected during early pregnancy, it is an indication for chromosomal abnormalities, congenital anomalies and potential complication during pregnancy.

716. Primary postpartum hemorrhage occurs within ……… hours of delivery.

a. 6 hours b. 8 hours
c. 12 hours d. 24 hours

Explanation: Bleeding more than 500 mL of blood from vagina after delivery is called Post-partum hemorrhage (PPH). If hemorrhage occurs within 24 hours of delivery it is called primary PPH. Secondary is defined as excessive vaginal bleeding from 24 hours after delivery up to 6 weeks postpartum.

717. The management of postpartum hemorrhage includes all; EXCEPT:

a. Bimanual uterine compression
b. Administration of oxytocin
c. Controlled cord traction
d. Administration of progesterone

Explanation: Post-partum hemorrhage is caused by atonic uterus, retained blood clots or placental products, delay in third stage of labor. In such cases, administering 10 IU of oxytocin, giving bimanual compression or using controlled cord traction can help prevent PPH.

718. Human milk is rich in all; EXCEPT: *(LNJP)*

a. Fat b. Protein
c. Iron d. Carbohydrate

Explanation: Milk is rich in all except Iron. Mature human milk contains 3%–5% fat, 0.8%–0.9% protein, 6.9%–7.2% carbohydrate calculated as lactose, and 0.2% mineral constituents expressed as ash. Its energy content is 60–75 kcal/100 mL. Protein content is markedly higher and carbohydrate content lower in colostrum than in mature milk. Iron is deficient in human milk.

719. Exclusive breastfeeding refers to feeding of infant only with breast milk for the period of:

a. 3 months b. 6 months
c. 8 months d. 12 months

Explanation: As per World Health Organization (WHO) "Exclusive breastfeeding" is defined as no other food or drink, not even water, except breast milk (including milk expressed or from a wet nurse) for 6 months of life, but allows the infant to receive ORS, drops and syrups (vitamins, minerals and medicines).

720. Neonatal tetanus can be prevented through:

a. Clean surface of delivery
b. Clean hand of the attendant
c. Clean cord tie
d. All of the above

Explanation: Neonatal tetanus prevented by 5 cleans: Clean hand, clean delivery surface and clean cord care (it includes clean tie for cord and no application on cord stump, clean blade for cutting cord)

721. Mean birth weight in India is:

a. 2.0 – 2.3 kg b. 2.3 – 2.5 kg
c. 2.5 - 2.9 kg d. 3.0 – 3.5 kg

722. Road-to-Health chart was given by:

a. David Morley b. John Snow
c. Koch Darwin d. Dukes

723. Small for gestational age newborns are at risk for difficulty maintaining body temperature because:

a. They have less fat storage than other infants
b. They are relatively small in size which reduces the body surface area
c. They are more active
d. Their skin is more susceptible to cold

724. A community health nurse is providing postnatal care to a new mother. Which of the following interventions should the nurse prioritize to promote successful breastfeeding? *New Q*

a. Encouraging the mother to supplement with formula milk for adequate nutrition.
b. Assisting the mother in establishing proper latch and positioning for breastfeeding.
c. Providing the mother with a variety of pacifiers to soothe the baby.
d. Advising the mother to avoid breastfeeding in the first 24 hours after birth.

Explanation: Proper latch and positioning are essential for successful breastfeeding. The nurse should provide guidance and support to the mother in achieving a comfortable and effective latch, which promotes optimal milk transfer and prevents nipple soreness and other breastfeeding difficulties.

725. Among causes of maternal mortality, which one of the following is the correct descending order due to which the maternal death occur in India?

a. Hemorrhage, obstructed labor, abortion, sepsis
b. Obstructed labor, hemorrhage, abortion, sepsis
c. Hemorrhage, sepsis, abortion, obstructed labor
d. Sepsis, obstructed labor, abortion, hemorrhage

726. Most common cause of maternal death in India:

a. Unsafe abortion b. Obstructed labor
c. Puerperal sepsis d. Obstetric hemorrhage

727. Which among the following is the most important immediate care of newborn?

a. Resuscitation b. Rooming-in
c. Breastfeeding d. Health assessment

728. Which is the indicator of immediate estimate of the physical condition of the baby?

a. GCS score
b. APGAR Score
c. Complete physical examination
d. Neurological assessment

729. All are included in Kangaroo Mother Care; EXCEPT:

a. Skin to skin contact
b. Early discharge and follow-up
c. Free nutritional supplements
d. Exclusive breastfeeding

730. Kangaroo Mother Care is the management of which of the following conditions?

a. Hypothermia b. Hyperthermia
c. Respiratory Distress d. Jaundice

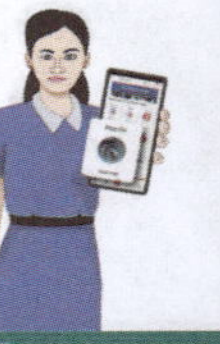

Ans.

715.	b
716.	d
717.	d
718.	c
719.	b
720.	d
721.	c
722.	a
723.	a
724.	b
725.	c
726.	d
727.	a
728.	b
729.	c
730.	a

731. The extra calorie requirement for a lactating mother is:
a. 250 kcal/day b. 400 kcal/day
c. 550 kcal/day d. 650 kcal/day

732. The term used for babies born as a result of retarded intrauterine fetal growth is:
a. Pre-term babies b. Low birth weight babies
c. Small for date babies d. Retarded babies

733. By international agreement, low birth weight has been defined as a birth weight when measured within the first hour of life is:
a. Less than 2000 grams b. Less than 2500 grams
c. Less than 2800 grams d. Less than 3000 grams

734. As per WHO low birth weight is defined as:
a. Birth weight less than 2.5 kg
b. Birth weight <10th percentile
c. Gestational age <34 weeks
d. Gestational age <28 weeks

735. Still birth rate includes fetal death after: *(RRB SSNE 2015)*
a. 20 weeks b. 24 weeks
c. 28 weeks d. 32 weeks

MOTHER AND CHILD HEALTH (MCH)

736. Dehydrated child will have:
a. Skin pinch goes back slowly
b. Depressed fontanels
c. Sunken eyes
d. All of the above

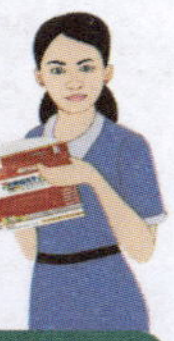

Explanation: In dehydrated child, skin pinch goes back slowly, and has sunken eyes, depressed fontanels, decreased tears, thirst or is unable to drink.

737. IMNCI target group is:
a. Up to 5 yrs b. Up to 10 yrs
c. Up to 15 yrs d. Up to 20 yrs

738. Under MCH programme, IFA tablets to be given daily to mother has:
a. 60 mg iron + 500 mcg folic acid
b. 100 mg iron + 500 mcg folic acid
c. 60 mg iron +100 mcg folic acid
d. 100 mg iron +100 mcg folic acid

739. All are criteria for identifying 'at risk' infants; EXCEPT:
a. Artificial feeding b. Birth order 4 and more
c. Grade II malnutrition d. Working mother

740. Breastfeeding week is celebrated in:
a. 1st week of March b. 1st week of July
c. 1st week of August d. 1st December

741. At which age weaning should start?
a. 5–6 months
b. 7–8 months
c. 8–12 months
d. Above one year

REPRODUCTIVE CHILD HEALTH PROGRAM (RCH)

742. According to WHO, a child with IQ level between 35-50 falls under which of the following category of mental retardation?
a. Mild b. Moderate
c. Severe d. Profound

743. Child Survival and Safe Motherhood (CSSM) programme was replaced by which program in India?
a. MCH b. NRHM
c. RCH d. ICDS

Explanation: CSSM is replaced by RCH.

744. Components of RCH 1 include all of the following; EXCEPT:
a. Family planning b. CSSM
c. Prevention of STD d. Emergency obstetric care

745. Component of RCH II include all; EXCEPT:
a. Emergency obstetric care
b. Essential obstetric care
c. Family planning
d. Strengthening of referral system

746. As per RCH, the community health center is:
a. First referral unit b. Secondary referral unit
c. Tertiary referral unit d. None of the above

747. RCH phase 2 does not include:
a. Immunization of pregnant women
b. Treatment of STD/RTI
c. Feed to malnourished children
d. Early registration of pregnancy up to 12–16 weeks

UNDER-FIVE CLINIC

748. Which of the following is an international agency which assists in Programme that benefits child health most? *(RAK MSc 2018)*
a. UNO b. WHO
c. UNICEF d. Red Cross

Explanation: UNICEF- United Nation International Child Emergency Fund is specialized for the United Nation established in 1946. Main works are maintaining child health, nutrition, maintain family and child welfare and provide formal and nonformal education.

749. Which of the following is an activity of under-five clinics? *(Staff Nurse G II 2014)*
a. Mid-day meal program b. Child education
c. Growth monitoring d. School health services

750. IMNCI refers to:
a. Integrated mother and neonatal critical illness
b. Integrated mother and newborn clinical interventions
c. Integrated management of neonatal and childhood illness
d. Integrated management of neonatal and clinical illness

751. A patient treated at home is allotted which color code according to IMNCI coding:
a. Pink b. Red
c. Green d. Yellow

752. IMNCI includes management of all of the following conditions; EXCEPT:
a. Diarrhea
b. Measles
c. Acute respiratory infections
d. Vitamin A deficiency

753. According to IMNCI, fast breathing in 5 months old child is defined as:
a. >30/min b. >40/min
c. >50/min d. >60/min

Ans.
731. c
732. c
733. b
734. a
735. c
736. d
737. a
738. b
739. b
740. c
741. a
742. b
743. c
744. d
745. c
746. a
747. c
748. c
749. c
750. c
751. c
752. d
753. c

754. IMNCI differs from IMCI in all; EXCEPT:

a. Malaria and Anemia are included
b. 0-7 days infants are included
c. Sick neonates are preferred over sick older children
d. Treatment is aimed at more than one disease (condition) at a time

755. Integrated Management of Neonatal and Childhood Illnesses (IMNCI) includes the following; EXCEPT:

a. Malaria
b. Respiratory infections
c. Diarrhea
d. Tuberculosis

756. Integrated Management of Childhood Illness (IMCI) initiative was taken to prevent morbidity and mortality from all of the following; EXCEPT:

a. Malaria b. Malnutrition
c. Otitis Media d. Neonatal tetanus

757. IMNCI includes all; EXCEPT:

a. Tetanus
b. Acute respiratory tract infection
c. Measles
d. Malaria

758. Guidelines for Baby friendly hospital initiative includes following; EXCEPT:

a. Mother and infant to be together for 24 hours a day
b. Mother to initiate breastfeeding in 4 hours of normal delivery
c. Giving newborn infants no food or drink other than breast milk
d. Encouraging breastfeeding on demand

759. Which of the following would contribute to growth monitoring of under-five children?

a. Health education
b. Road to health chart
c. Apgar Score
d. Weight Monitoring

760. The Children's Act was passed in:

a. 1960 b. 1969
c. 1971 d. 1986

761. Baby friendly hospital initiative was started in India in the year:

a. 1993 b. 1991
c. 1996 d. 1990

Explanation: Baby friendly hospital initiative is a global movement, developed jointly by WHO and UNICEF in the year 1990, later it was launched by WHO in 1991. India adopted the same initiative in the year1993 with an objective to reduce infant mortality and morbidity due to improper breastfeeding techniques.

762. Most reliable indicator to identify the nutritional status in under 2 year's children in community setting is:

a. Mid arm circumference
b. Weight for age
c. Weight for height
d. BMI

Explanation: MUAC is the circumference of the left upper arm, measured at the mid-point between the shoulder and the elbow (olecranon process and the acromion process). In children, MUAC is useful for the assessment of nutritional status.

NUTRITIONAL ASSESSMENT

763. Best indicator for growth measurement is:

a. Height b. Weight
c. Arm circumference d. None

764. Road to health card or the growth chart was first designed by:

a. Edwin Chadwick
b. David Morley
c. Gopalan
d. CE Winslow

765. All are true about growth chart; EXCEPT:

a. It is a tool for educating mothers
b. The position of dots is more important than direction
c. Between top 2 lines, it shows 'Road-to -Health' or 'zone of normality'
d. Lowermost line corresponds to children below 3 percentile

766. Deficiency in Weight for Height in a 3-year-old child indicates:

a. Acute malnutrition
b. Chronic malnutrition
c. Concomitant acute and chronic malnutrition
d. Under weight

767. WHO growth chart is:

a. International based b. National Based
c. Home based d. Community based

768. Mid-arm Circumference is constant during:

a. 0-6 months b. 1-5 years
c. 5-10 years d. 10 years

769. Growth chart used in India has curves:

a. 2 b. 3
c. 4 d. 5

770. At birth head circumference is about:

a. 32 cm b. 34 cm
c. 36 cm d. 38 cm

771. WHO Growth Chart has got information for all except:

a. Immunization procedures
b. Child spacing
c. History of sibling health
d. History of maternal health

772. Which is the best test to detect iron deficiency in a client? *(Karnataka PSC96)*

a. Ferrous sulfate b. Serum Ferritin
c. Serum Iron d. Hemoglobin

Explanation: The amount of ferritin in the blood (serum ferritin level) is directly related to the amount of iron stored in human body. Iron is important for red blood cell production. Doctor may order this test if a client have signs or symptoms of anemia due to low iron.

773. Name the classification developed by WHO for disability:

a. International classification of functioning, disability and health
b. Kuppuswamy classification
c. NYHA classification
d. FAB classification

Explanation: International Classification of Functioning, Disability, and Health (ICF). The ICF is a classification of health and health-related conditions for children and adults that was developed by World Health Organization (WHO) and published in 2001.

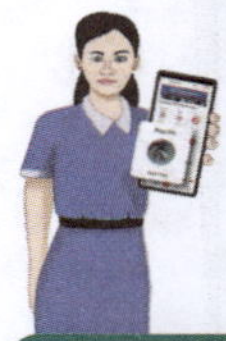

Ans.

754. c
755. d
756. d
757. a
758. b
759. b
760. a
761. a
762. a
763. b
764. b
765. b
766. a
767. c
768. b
769. b
770. b
771. d
772. b
773. a

774. As per WHO blindness is if visual acuity less than:

a. 6/18 b. 6/24
c. 3/60 d. 6/60

Explanation: WHO has defined blindness as "visual acuity of less than 3/60 (Snellen) or its equivalent".

775. The most common congenital lesion in North India is:

a. Cleft lips and cleft palate
b. Club foot
c. Neural tube defect
d. Congenital heart diseases

776. RDA of iodine for an adult is:

a. 50 μg/day b. 75 μg/day
c. 100 μg/day d. 150 μg/day

777. Health survey and development committee is also known as: *(RUHS 2007)*

a. Bhore committee
b. Chadah committee
c. Shrivastav committee
d. Mukherji committee.

778. Bhore Committee was appointed by the Govt. of India in the year: *(Safdarjung NO 2018)*

a. 1933 b. 1953
c. 1943 d. 1963

Explanation: This committee, known as the Health Survey and Development Committee, was appointed in 1943 with Sir Joseph Bhore as its Chairman. It laid emphasis on integration of curative and preventive medicine at all levels. It made comprehensive recommendations for remodeling of health services in India. The report, submitted in 1946, had some important recommendations like:

- Integration of preventive and curative services of all administrative levels
- Development of primary health centers in 2 stages

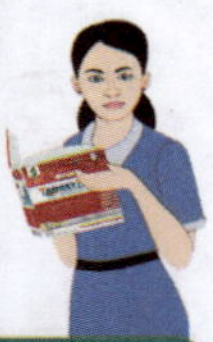

779. Gray baby syndrome is caused by: *(ESI-2009)*

a. Chloramphenicol b. Amphotericin B
c. Vancomycin d. Tetracycline

Explanation: Gray baby syndrome is a serious side effect that occurs in newborn infants following intravenous administration of antimicrobial chloramphenicol because they lack the necessary liver enzymes to metabolize this drug. Chloramphenicol accumulates in the baby, causing hypotension, cyanosis (blue coloring of lips, nail beds, and skin due to lack of oxygen in the blood), and often death. Chloramphenicol is, therefore, usually not given to newborns or premature babies.

780. The best parameter for assessment of chronic malnutrition is:

a. Weight for age
b. Weight for height
c. Height for age
d. Mid upper arm circumference

781. Which of the following parameter is the best indicator for nutritional status of child?

a. Head circumference
b. Mid-arm circumference
c. Chest circumference
d. Rate of increase of height and weight

782. Which of the following foods is accepted as a reference protein?

a. Cow's milk b. Hen's egg
c. Human milk d. Soybean

Explanation: Hen's egg is considered as reference protein.

783. In Simmering, the food is prepared:

a. At Boiling point b. Above Boiling point
c. Below Boiling point d. In normal water

Explanation: Food cooked below the boiling point is known as simmering.

784. Mixing of brick powder with Chili powder is called as:

a. Food intoxication b. Food Additives
c. Food Fortification d. Food Adulteration

Explanation: Adding of non-nutritive substance to nutritive substance is called food adulteration.

785. One gram of protein contains:

a. 4 kcal b. 5 kcal
c. 8 kcal d. 9 kcal

786. One gram of fat contains:

a. 4 kcal b. 5 kcal
c. 8 kcal d. 9 kcal

787. 100 mL of human milk provides:

a. 40 kcal b. 60 kcal
c. 70 kcal d. 400 kcal

788. One gram of carbohydrate contains:

a. 4 kcal b. 5 kcal
c. 8 kcal d. 9 kcal

789. Which of the following is an example of biologically incomplete protein?

a. Egg b. Meat
c. Milk d. Nuts

790. An example of unsaturated fatty acid is:

a. Oleic acid b. Capric acid
c. Myristic acid d. Stearic acid

791. An example of saturated fatty acid is:

a. Oleic acid b. Linoleic acid
c. Palmitoleic acid d. Lauric acid

792. Which of the following is not an essential amino acids:

a. Histidine b. Leucine
c. Lysine d. Arginine

793. Which of the following is not a sulfur containing amino acids? *(AIIMS Jodhpur Lecturer-Nursing screening exam)*

a. Methionine b. Histidine
c. Cysteine d. Homocysteine

794. Which of the following constituents of food is also called Body Building Food?

a. Minerals b. Carbohydrates
c. Proteins d. Fats

795. Mixing of papaya seeds with peppercorns is a case of:

a. Food intoxication b. Food Adulteration
c. Food Additives d. Food Fortification

796. Age independent anthropometric measure of malnutrition is:

a. Weight for age b. Mid arm circumference
c. Head circumference d. Chest circumference

Ans.

774. c
775. c
776. d
777. a
778. c
779. a
780. c
781. d
782. b
783. c
784. d
785. a
786. d
787. c
788. a
789. d
790. a
791. d
792. d
793. b
794. c
795. b
796. b

797. Compared with unprocessed cow's milk, human breast milk contains more of:

a. Lipids b. Proteins
c. Minerals d. Carbohydrates

798. Which of the following diets promote wound healing?

a. Low carbohydrate, high protein and high Vitamin C diet
b. High carbohydrate, high protein and high vitamin C diet
c. High protein, high vitamin A and high vitamin C diet
d. Adequate calorie, Protein, Vitamin D and vitamin E diet

799. Tryptophan is present in all; EXCEPT:

a. Maize b. Cheese
c. Chicken d. Fish

Explanation: Tryptophan is an amino acid needed for normal growth in infants and for nitrogen balance in adults. It is an essential amino acid, which means your body cannot produce it. Except in maize all other given food items contain Tryptophan.

800. Calorie intake of 1 year child per kg is: *(AIIMS 1991)*

a. 100 b. 200
c. 300 d. 400

Explanation: Calculated energy requirement for 1 year child is 100 kcal/Kg. so total calorie intake will be approximately 1000 kcal/day.

801. Phosphatase test is used:

a. To test the presence of nitric acid
b. To determine the type of methemoglobinemia, a blood disorder
c. To test for efficacy of pasteurization of milk
d. None of the above

Explanation: Alkaline Phosphatase is an enzyme which is naturally present in milk, but is destroyed at a temperature just near to the pasteurization temperature. Alkaline Phosphatase test is used to indicate whether milk has been adequately pasteurized or whether it has been contaminated with raw milk after pasteurization.

802. Amino acid deficient in wheat is: *(DSSSB)*

a. Leucine b. Methionine
c. Lysine d. Cystine

Explanation: Wheat is deficient in lysine. Lysine is an amino acid found in the protein of foods such as beans, cheese, yogurt, meat, milk, brewer's yeast, wheat germ, and other animal proteins. Proteins derived from grains such as wheat and corn tend to be low in lysine content. The bioavailability of lysine is reduced with food preparation methods, such as heating.

803. Orthotolidine test is used for detecting:

a. Chlorine
b. Silver
c. Oxygen
d. Ammonia

Explanation: In this test, 10 mL of chlorinated sample of water is taken after the required contact period, in a glass tube. To this 0.1 mL of orthotolidine solution is added. The color formed is observed after 5 minutes. The formation of yellow color normally indicates the presence of chlorine (either combined or free) in the water. The more yellow the color, the greater, is the chlorine residual.

804. Guthrie Test is useful for screening: *(AIPGME 1999)*

a. Pomp's disease b. Phenylketonuria
c. Thalassemia d. Hemophilia

Explanation: Guthrie test: A simple screening blood test for phenylketonuria (PKU). The Guthrie test was the original impetus to newborn metabolic screening. A small drop of blood is taken from the heel of a newborn and applied to a card. In the original form of the test, a punch-out of the dried disc was incubated on a petri dish plated with bacteria (Bacillus subtilis) in the presence of a growth inhibitor, B-2-thienyl-alanine. High levels of Phe in the blood sample overcome the inhibition, and allow the bacteria to grow. If an elevated level of Phe is detected, the child is placed on a phenylalanine-restricted diet for the first several years.

805. Pasteurization of milk is considered better without boiling because:

a. Can be stored for longer period than that of boiled milk
b. Bacterial spores are destroyed
c. Vitamin C reduced only by 20%
d. Calcium forms complex when boiled

Explanation: When boiling the pasteurized milk the amount of Vitamin C present in the milk will reduce. So pasteurized milk is considered as best without boiling.

VITAMINS

806. Vitamin D resistant rickets is a (an):

a. X-linked recessive disorder
b. X-linked dominant disorder
c. Autosomal recessive disorder
d. Autosomal dominant disorder

807. The most characteristic and specific signs of Vitamin-A deficiency is/are:

a. Eye lesions b. Color blindness
c. Blurring of vision d. Double vision

808. Vitamin A prophylaxis is an example of:

a. Primordial prevention
b. Health protection
c. Specific protection
d. Disability limitation

809. Highest source of vitamin A is seen in:

a. Cod liver oil b. Green leafy vegetable
c. Amla d. Guava

810. Which of the following disease is caused by deficiency of Thiamine?

a. Wernicke's encephalopathy
b. Cheilosis
c. Pellagra
d. All of the above

811. Deficiency of _________ causes Wernicke's encephalopathy?

a. Niacin b. Phosphorus
c. B12 d. Thiamine

812. Deficiency of which of the following vitamins causes beriberi?

a. Vitamin B1 b. Vitamin B2
c. Vitamin B6 d. Vitamin B12

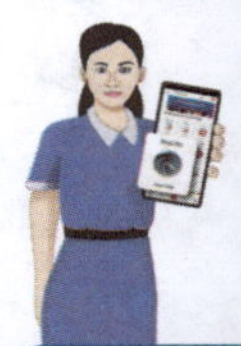

Ans.

797. d
798. b
799. a
800. a
801. c
802. c
803. a
804. b
805. c
806. b
807. a
808. c
809. a
810. a
811. d
812. a

813. Which vitamin deficiency causes night blindness?

a. Vitamin A b. Vitamin B
c. Vitamin C d. Vitamin D

814. Vitamin A is also known as:

a. Thiamine b. Cholecalciferol
c. Tocopherol d. Retinol

815. Vitamin K at birth is administered to .... among newborns.

a. Prevent excessive bleeding
b. Increase immunity
c. Prevent infection
d. Correct malnutrition

Explanation: Vitamin K is one of the clotting factors that helps in clotting the blood. Newborns at birth are unable to produce adequate amount of Vitamin K because baby's bowel is 'sterile' when inside the uterus (meaning no bacteria) and does not start producing vitamin K until after they are born. Most of the Vitamin K needed by the baby is obtained through a slow buildup of their gut bacteria in the weeks, or months, after the birth.

816. Which vitamin is lost during polishing of rice?

a. B12 b. Thiamine
c. Vitamin A d. Vitamin K

Explanation: Polishing of rice can lead to loss of vitamin called thiamine.

817. Vitamin C deficiency causes:

a. Megaloblastic anemia b. Glossitis
c. Scurvy d. Bitot's spots

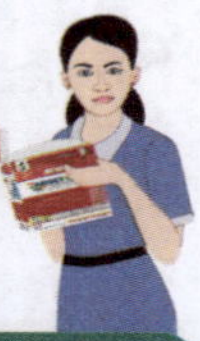

818. Which of the following vitamins is not present in Egg?

a. Folic acid
b. Vitamin C
c. Vitamin
b. Vitamin E

819. Which of the following vegetables is the rich source of Vitamin C?

a. Amla
b. Potatoes
c. Brinjal
d. Black gram

820. Angular stomatitis is usually caused by the deficiency of:

a. Riboflavin b. Thiamine
c. Folic acid d. Pantothenic acid

821. Maximum amount of Vitamin D is present in:

a. Liver b. Egg yolk
c. Cheese d. Cod liver oil

Explanation: The flesh of fatty fish (such as salmon, tuna, and mackerel) and fish liver oils are among the best sources. Small amounts of vitamin D are found in beef liver, cheese, and egg yolks. Dietary sources of vitamin D is habitual liver oil: 500-10000 μg/100 gm.

822. 3D's (diarrhea, dementia, dermatitis) are the characteristics of ....deficiency disorder.

a. Niacin b. Thiamine
c. Riboflavin d. Biotin

Explanation: Niacin deficiency results in pellagra. It is characterized by 3D's Diarrhea, Dermatitis, and Dementia.

COMMUNITY NUTRITION PROGRAM

823. Mass prophylaxis is used in all; EXCEPT:

a. Rabies b. Lymphatic filariasis
c. Trachoma d. Malaria

Explanation: Mass Prophylaxis is the capability to protect the health of the population through the administration of critical interventions in response to a public health emergency in order to prevent the development of disease among those who are exposed or are potentially exposed to public health threats.

824. Which of the following is the macronutrient?

a. Vitamins b. Zinc
c. Proteins d. Calcium

825. Pellagra is characterized by 3Ds. Which of the following describes 3Ds of pellagra?

a. Diarrhea, Dermatitis, Dementia
b. Delusion, Diarrhea, Dementia
c. Deformity, Delusion, Deviated septum
d. Dementia, Delusion, Disarticulation

826. ICDS was launched in:

a. 1955 b. 1968
c. 1975 d. 2005

827. Administrative unit of the ICDS project in rural areas is:

a. PHC
b. Community development block
c. Zila parishad
d. Gram panchayat

828. ICDS does not cover:

a. Nutritional supplementation
b. Formal education
c. Health education
d. Immunization

829. According to ICDS programme, children of age 6 months to 36 months should be supplemented with which of the following?

a. 500 cal + 12-15 g proteins b. 300 cal + 10-15 g proteins
c. 600 cal + 18-20 g proteins d. 500 cal + 18-20 g proteins

830. Which of the following is known as 'Heart of ICDS system'?

a. Mother and Children b. CDPO
c. Primary Health Center d. Anganwadi

DISASTER MANAGEMENT

831. Most potential agent that can be used in bioterrorism:

a. Viral encephalitis b. Brucellosis
c. TB d. Clostridium botulinum

Explanation: The Clostridium botulinum produces an extremely toxic neurotoxin that can cause serious muscle paralyzing in the individual and the ease of production, transport and delivery make this a potential bioterrorism agent. The toxin may be used as an aerosol for people to breathe in or may be put into food supplies.

832. Which of the following disinfectant is used for blood spill?

a. Glutaraldehyde b. Phenol
c. Ethanol d. Sodium hypochlorite

833. 'Monday morning fever' is a common name for:

(RRB Feb 2012)

a. Asbestosis b. Bagassosis
c. Byssinosis d. Mad Hatter's disease

Ans.

813. a
814. d
815. a
816. b
817. c
818. b
819. a
820. a
821. d
822. a
823. a
824. c
825. a
826. c
827. b
828. b
829. a
830. a
831. d
832. d
833. c

OCCUPATIONAL HAZARDS & INDUSTRIAL HEALTH

834. Occupational health practice mainly refers to:
- a. Pre-employment examination
- b. Periodical examinations
- c. Maintenance and analysis of health records
- d. All of the above

835. In acute silicosis clinical manifestation is:
- a. Hypersensitivity pneumonitis
- b. Hypersensitivity pneumonia
- c. Pulmonary alveolar proteinosis
- d. Forms nodules and causes pneumoconiosis

836. Nosocomial infection occurs in:
- a. Agricultural fields
- b. Crowded places
- c. Hospital
- d. Working place

837. Nosocomial infections are those which develop:
- a. Within 24 hours after hospitalization
- b. Within 48 hours of hospitalization
- c. After 48 hours of hospitalization
- d. After 7 days of hospitalization

838. Ergonomics is a science of:
- a. Designing the job to fit to the worker
- b. Training the worker to fit to the job
- c. Prevention of occupational diseases
- d. Recruiting the employee to fit for the job

Explanation: Ergonomics is derived from Greek word Ergon meaning work and Nomo's meaning law, so ergonomics is described as science of "designing the job to fit to the worker, and not forcing the worker to fit to the job".

839. Cutaneous vasoconstriction on exposure to hypothermia results in:
- a. Immersion foot
- b. Frost bite
- c. Erythrocyanosis
- d. All of these

Explanation: Working in cold areas causes the person to experience cutaneous vasoconstriction where the blood supply to the lower limbs reduces leading to development of Immersion foot, frostbite, erythrocyanosis and chilblains.

840. Lead is widely used in variety of industries because of its properties; EXCEPT:
- a. Low boiling point
- b. Anti-corrosive
- c. Non-oxidizing
- d. Mixes with other metals easily

Explanation: Lead is widely used because of its four properties like:
- i. Low boiling point
- ii. Mixes with other metals easily to form alloys
- iii. Easily oxidized
- iv. Anticorrosive

841. Appearance of Burton's line in lead poisoning:
- a. Bluish purple line on gums
- b. Greenish coating on gums
- c. Brown stains on teeth
- d. Pale pinkish gums

Explanation: During inorganic lead poisoning, the gums appear in bluish purple in color.

842. Role of occupational health nurse includes the following; EXCEPT:
- a. Prevention of workplace accidents and injuries
- b. Promotion of health and work ability
- c. Improving environment health for occupational health workers
- d. Improve the productivity outcome of workers

Explanation: As per the recommendation by the WHO, the occupational health nurse role is for:
- Prevention of occupational injury and disease through a comprehensive pro-active occupational health and safety strategy.
- The promotion of health and work ability, by focusing on non-occupational workplace preventable conditions that whilst not caused directly by work, may affect the employee's ability to maintain attendance or performance at work, through a comprehensive workplace health promotion strategy.
- Improving environmental health management, by reducing risk to the working population and the wider community, which contributes to the wider public health agenda.

843. Most common heavy metal poisoning in the world:
- a. Lead
- b. Arsenic
- c. Mercury
- d. Cadmium

844. DDT is a: *(DSSSB)*
- a. Contact poison
- b. CNS poison
- c. Stomach poison
- d. None of these

Explanation: DDT (Dichlorodiphenyltrichloroethane) is a colorless, crystalline, tasteless and almost odorless organochloride known for its insecticidal properties and environmental impacts. DDT has been formulated in multiple forms, including solutions in xylene or petroleum distillates, emulsifiable concentrates, water-wettable powders, granules, aerosols, smoke candles and charges for vaporizers and lotions. Because of the high efficiency, DDT acts as a contact poison against several arthropods.

845. Arc welders are more prone to suffer from.............. occupation hazard.
- a. Glaucoma
- b. Welder' flash
- c. Welder's cataract
- d. Temporary blindness

Explanation: Arc welder gets exposure to ultraviolet radiation which mainly affects eyes causing conjunctivitis and keratitis.

846. Following are the diseases that comes under pneumoconiosis: EXCEPT:
- a. Silicosis
- b. Asbestosis
- c. Siderosis
- d. Psittacosis

Explanation: Psittacosis is caused by bacteria called as Chlamydophila psittaci found in the dropping of bird and on the other hand pneumoconiosis is a group of lung diseases that are caused by inhalation of dust particles with size ranging from 0.5 microns–3 microns.

847. Anthracosis is caused due to inhalation of:
- a. Coal particles
- b. Sugarcane dust
- c. Cotton dust
- d. Silicon dust particles

Explanation: Inhalation of coal dust particles causes anthracosis. Inhalation of sugarcane dust causes bagossis, cotton dust causes Byssinosis, silicon dust causes silicosis.

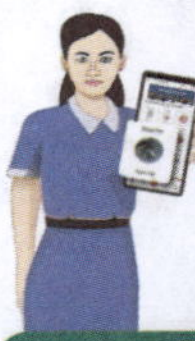

Ans.

834. d
835. c
836. c
837. c
838. a
839. d
840. c
841. a
842. d
843. a
844. a
845. c
846. d
847. a

848. Strategies to prevent occupational dermatitis includes:

a. Pre selection examination
b. Application of barrier creams
c. Use of protective equipment and periodic health checkups
d. All of the above

Explanation: Occupational dermatitis is a big health problem in many industries due to causes like heat, cold, chemical agents, and biological agents. It can be prevented by using suitable preventive measures like pre selection screening, application of barrier creams, use of protective equipment and periodic health checkups.

849. Monday fever is also known as:

a. Bagassosis b. Byssinosis
c. Asbestosis d. COPD

Explanation: Byssinosis is a disease of the lungs brought on by breathing in cotton dust or dusts from other vegetable fibers such as flax, hemp, or sisal while at work.

850. Which of the following agents is responsible for Bagassosis?

a. Smoke b. Silica
c. Sugarcane dust d. Coal

Explanation: Bagassosis is a form of Hypersensitivity pneumonitis caused due to inhalation of sugarcane fiber waste. This disease was first found in India in 1955. This disease basically causes symptoms like shortness of breath and fever.

851. Occupational exposure that may cause sterility in females:

a. Aniline b. Lead
c. Radon d. Nickel

852. All are disease manifestation associated with low temperature; EXCEPT:

a. Frost bite b. Trench foot
c. Prickles d. Chill blains

853. Following are chemical agents, that cause occupational dermatitis by local irritation; EXCEPT:

a. Rubber b. X-ray
c. Lime d. Ether

854. Occupational cancer involves following organs; EXCEPT:

a. Lung b. Breast
c. Bladder d. Liver

855. Most common mode of lead poisoning is:

a. Ingestion b. Skin
c. Inhalation d. Feco-oral

856. Asbestosis is:

a. A water borne disease b. An occupational disease
c. An airborne disease d. A food borne disease

857. Which occupational diseases is caused by extreme cold climate?

a. Occupational cataract b. Miner's nystagmus
c. Pancytopenia d. Frost bite

858. Which of the following disease is caused by inhalation of sugarcane dust?

a. Asbestosis b. Bagassosis
c. Byssinosis d. Silicosis

859. A lung disease caused by prolonged inhalation of cotton fiber dust is:

a. Bagassosis b. Byssinosis
c. Farmers lung d. Pneumonia

860. 'Snow storm appearance' in X-ray of an adult male suggests:

a. Asbestosis b. Siderosis
c. Anthracosis d. Silicosis

861. Diffuse Mesothelioma is seen with:

a. Asbestos b. Tobacco
c. Arsenic d. TB
e. Histoplasmosis

862. "Farmers lung" is due to inhalation of:

a. Cotton fiber b. Sugarcane dust
c. Hay dust d. Coal dust

863. Main cause of Farmer's lung is:

a. Pneumococcus
b. Mycobacterium tuberculosis
c. Micropolyspora faeni
d. Staphylococcus aureus

864. International labor organization is situated in:

a. Geneva
b. Denmark
c. Scotland
d. United States of America

Explanation: International Labor Organization is a United Nation's agency. It founded in 1919. Its headquarters is in Geneva, Switzerland. It mainly focuses on labor related issues. In 1969, the organization received Nobel Peace Prize.

865. Which day is celebrated as Labor Day?

(ESIC Chennai May 2012)

a. 1st June b. 30th May
c. 1st May d. None of these

HEALTH POLICY AND PLANNING

866. Other name of multipurpose worker's committee is:

a. Bhore Committee b. Kartar Singh Committee
c. Mudaliar Committee d. Mukherji Committee

867. Other name of 'health survey and development committee' is:

a. Bhore Committee
b. Kartar Singh Committee
c. Mudaliar Committee
d. Mukherji Committee

868. Health survey and planning committee is also known as:

a. Bhore Committee
b. Kartar Singh Committee
c. Mudhaliar Committee
d. Mukherji Committee

869. Chadha committee was appointed in the year:

a. 1960 b. 1963
c. 1965 d. 1968

870. One basic health worker (multipurpose worker) for 10,000 populations was recommended by: *(AIIMS Nagpur NO 2018)*

a. Chadha committee
b. Mukherjee committee
c. Bhore committee
d. Mudaliar committee

Explanation: Chadha committee in 1963 recommended one basic health worker (multipurpose worker) per 10,000 populations. Multipurpose workers to look after additional duties of collection of vital statistics and family planning in addition to malaria vigilance.

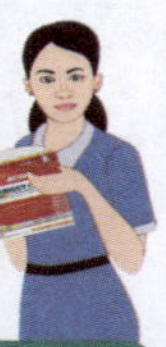

Ans.

848.	d
849.	b
850.	c
851.	c
852.	c
853.	a
854.	b
855.	c
856.	b
857.	d
858.	b
859.	b
860.	d
861.	a
862.	c
863.	c
864.	a
865.	c
866.	b
867.	a
868.	c
869.	b
870.	a

871. The WHO initiative 'Right to Sight' is named as: *(AIIMS-BBS SNO 2019)*

a. Vision 2015 b. Vision 2020
c. Vision 2030 d. Vision 2025

Explanation: The WHO initiative 'Right to Sight' is named as **Vision 2020.** It is a global initiative for the elimination of avoidable blindness, which is a joint Programme of the WHO and the international agency for prevention of blindness. (IAPB)

872. The Act that is recommended for provision of crèches for women in factory:

a. ESI Act 1948
b. The Indian Mines Act 1923
c. The Factories Act 1976
d. CGHS

Explanation: The Factories Act, 1976 made recommendation to provide crèches in factories where more than 30 women workers are employed.

873. ESI Act, 1948 was last amended in the year:

a. 2008 b. 1998
c. 1989 d. 2010

Explanation: ESI Act was passed in the year 1948 later it was amended in 1975, 1984 and 1989. Recently on 1/5/ 2010 the ESI Act was again revised to increase the benefit for wider group employees.

874. An employer contributes ....percentage of wages for the benefit of employee in every wage period under ESI Act.

a. 1.75% b. 4.75%
c. 2.35% d. 3.75%

Explanation: Under ESI Act an employee contributes 1.75% of wages paid and employer contributes 4.75% of wages paid in respect of the employees in every wage period.

875. The goal of "Health for all by 2000 AD" was mooted in world health assembly in the year: *(Staff Nurse G II 2014)*

a. 1966 b. 1948
c. 1957 d. 1978

876. Alma Ata Declaration was made in: *(JIPMER 2012)*

a. 1948 b. 1978
c. 1967 d. 2002

877. MTP Act (1971) in India specifies all of the following; EXCEPT: *(RRB Feb 2012)*

a. Persons who should perform abortion
b. Conditions for abortion
c. Techniques of abortions
d. Place for conducting abortions

878. Rashtriya Swasthya Bima Yojana is a Government run insurance scheme for:

a. Poor people b. Older persons
c. Girl children d. All women

879. In India the ESI Act was enacted in the year:

a. 1947 b. 1948
c. 1950 d. 1952

880. Active strategies of health promotion include:

a. Weight reduction
b. Quit alcohol consumption
c. Smoking cessation
d. All of the above

Explanation: Active strategies for health promotion of individual are promoted to adopt a particular lifestyle or pattern, they are actively involved in the activity.

881. Which of the following is NOT among the three key focus areas outlined in UNDP's HIV and Health Strategy 2022-2025? *New Q*

a. Reducing the inequalities and social exclusion that affect health and drive epidemics
b. Advocating for human rights and strengthening healthcare infrastructure.
c. Promoting effective and inclusive governance for health
d. Building resilient and sustainable systems for health.

882. The headquarters of WHO is situated in:

a. New York b. Geneva
c. London d. Toronto

PRIMARY HEALTHCARE

883. Following are the elements of primary health care; EXCEPT: *(DSSSB 2006)*

a. Health education b. Intersectoral coordination
c. Cost-effectiveness d. Provision of essential drugs

Explanation: Cost-effective care is judged to provide good health value for expenditure. Health value refers to the benefits of a particular medical intervention, which might include longer life, better quality of life, or both. Expenditures should include not only the costs of a test or treatment itself, but the subsequent costs it might cause, including additional medical interventions, work disability, costs of long-term care, and so forth.

884. Primary health care is: *(DSSSB 2004)*

a. Health for all
b. Health for those who are in need
c. Health for an area of 30,000 population
d. Health for children attending primary school

Explanation: In 1978, 134 health ministries signed the Alma Ata Declaration. The Declaration set a deadline of the year 2000 for achieving a level of health that would enable all of the world's people to lead a socially and economically productive life. The strategy to achieve this goal was focused on primary healthcare with the emphasis on community participation and tackling the underlying causes of disease such as poverty, illiteracy and poor sanitation. Many now argue that globalization has become an additional threat to the achievement of the health-for-all principle contained in the declaration, with an estimated 800 million people still lacking access to even the most basic health services. However, those who see greater benefits from globalization feel that it can, in fact, make the health-for-all principle a reality.

885. Primary health care includes all except: *(RAK MSc 2018)*

a. Low cost
b. Equitable distribution
c. Community participation
d. Latest technology

886. All of the following are the essential elements of primary health care; EXCEPT:

a. Multi-sectoral Approach
b. Qualification of health providers
c. Community participation
d. Appropriate technology

Ans.

871. b
872. c
873. d
874. b
875. d
876. b
877. c
878. a
879. b
880. d
881. b
882. b
883. c
884. a
885. a
886. b

887. Community mental health services does not involve:
a. Early diagnosis
b. Treatment with modern psychoactive drugs
c. Psychosurgery
d. Referral services

888. Blood banks get permission to operate from:
a. NACO
b. ICMR
c. DGHS, Ministry of health
d. Drug controller general of India

HEALTHCARE DELIVERY SYSTEM

889. Which of the following functions of community health nurse enables community empowerment?
a. Helping people in achieving personal hygiene
b. Forming partnerships with people
c. Decision making for people in the community.
d. Accepting responsibility for people's action

890. Population covered by a sub-center in hilly area: *(RAK MSc 2018)*
a. 5000 population b. 3000 population
c. 10,000 population d. 30,000 population

Explanation: Sub center is a peripheral area of the village having health care delivery system. One sub center covers 5000 in plain area and 3000 population in hilly and tribal area. It works at the grass-root level and main function is to provide primary health care services and some preventive, promotive and curative services. One PHC contains six Sub centers.

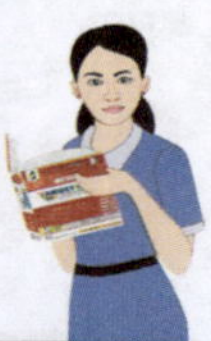

891. Which of the following is not a content of Drug Kit A provided at subcenter? *(AIIMS BPL NO 2018)*
a. Oral rehydration salt b. Tab Co-trimoxazole
c. Tablet paracetamol d. Vitamin A Solution

Explanation:

Contents of Kit-A

Contents	Quantity
Oral rehydration salt	150 packets
Tablet IFA	15000 tablets
Tablet IFA	13000 tablets
Vitamin A solution	6 bottles of 100 mL each
Tab co-trimoxazole for pediatric use	1000 tablets

892. One PHC covers a population of: *(Safdarjung NO 2018; DSSSB PHN, 2015; RRB Feb 2012)*
a. 50,000 b. 30,000
c. 10,000 d. One lakh

Explanation: As a basic unit of health care, PHC covers 20,000 population in hilly and tribal areas and 30,000 for plain areas.

893. In India, which one of the following is the first referral unit? *(AIIMS Raipur Staff-Nurse Grade I-2018)*
a. Sub center
b. Primary health center
c. Community health center
d. Regional hospital

Explanation: As per RCH, first referral unit is a community health center which has the facilities for obstetric surgery, blood transfusion, anesthesia, specialist pediatric care, operation theater and required equipment. This center also has the facilities for MTP, tubectomy, vasectomy and pediatric care for high risk neonates and other severe problems of early childhood.

894. The human resource available in subcenter is:
a. Multipurpose health worker
b. Physician
c. Anganwadi worker
d. Medical officer

Explanation: Multipurpose health worker (Female), Multipurpose health worker (Male) and voluntary worker consist the human resource available in the sub center

895. In health care delivery system grass root level workers include:
a. Anganwadi workers b. ASHA
c. Village health guide d. All of these

896. The Multipurpose Worker in general serves a rural population of: *(DSSSB PHN, 2015)*
a. <500 b. 1000
c. 3000 d. 5000

897. Which one of the health services is not available in rural health unit? *(Banaras HU 2015)*
a. Maternal and child health work
b. Communicational disease control work
c. Environmental sanitation work
d. Cancer treatment facility

898. Population covered by an Anganwadi worker is: *(Kerala PSC, Nov 2014)*
a. 2000 b. 3000
c. 1500 d. 1000

899. The three tier system of local self-government at block level is: *(Staff Nurse G II 2014; JIPMER 2012)*
a. Panchayat Samiti b. Gram Sabha
c. Nyaya Panchayat d. Zilla Parishad

900. The backbone of public health nursing is: *(JIPMER 2012; Staff Nurse G II 2014)*
a. Home visit b. Recording
c. Health education d. Immunization

901. Which of the following actions by a public health nurse is likely to encourage community participation?
a. Invite people from NGOs
b. Refer to the physician for prescription
c. Listen to people when they relate their problems
d. Encourage sponsorship for participation

902. How much population is covered by one Anganwadi Unit?
a. 500 b. 800
c. 1000 d. 1200

903. Population covered in sub-center is:
a. 3000-5000 b. 20,000-30,000
c. 80,000-1,20,000 d. >1,20,00

904. Population covered by primary health center in plain area is:
a. 3000-5000 b. 30,000
c. 80,000- 1,20, 000 d. >1,20,000

905. How much population is covered by one PHC in hilly and tribal area?
a. 5000–15000 b. 20000
c. 25000–30000 d. 30000–40000

Ans.
887. c
888. d
889. b
890. b
891. c
892. b
893. c
894. a
895. d
896. d
897. d
898. d
899. a
900. a
901. c
902. c
903. a
904. b
905. b

906. Population covered in community health center is:

a. 5000–6000 b. 20,000–30,0000
c. 80,000–1,20,000 d. >1,20,000

907. Drug-kit B is given at:

a. PH b. Subcenter
c. CH d. FRU level

908. All of the following are the functions of PHC; EXCEPT:

a. Providing medical care b. Performing surgeries
c. Health education d. Referral services

909. The following are the data collection techniques used in the community assessment; EXCEPT: *(AIIMS Raipur Grade II 2017)*

a. Making appropriate judgments
b. Organization and comparisons of problem
c. Effective communication
d. Investigation and measurements

Explanation: There are various techniques used in community assessment for collection of data that include questionnaires, focus group, interviews, case studies, observations. Organization and comparisons of problems is not a data collection technique but a method of analysis.

910. Providing health education about the environmental hygiene to the community people is an example of: *(AIIMS Raipur Grade II 2017)*

a. Social communication
b. Structural communication
c. Therapeutic communication
d. Formal communication

Explanation: Social communication or pragmatics is the way in which children use language with social situations. Structural communication is an instructional approach which provides a stimulated dialogue between author of instructional materials and students. Therapeutic communication is the face to face process of interacting that focuses on advancing physical and emotional well-being of patient. Formal communication is exchange of official information vertically or horizontally.

911. The female health worker (MPW) does not do: *(RAK MSc 2018)*

a. Distribution of condom
b. Birth and death registration
c. Malaria surveillance
d. Supervision of health volunteer

912. A 14-year-old child lost his father a year ago, and got caught shoplifting. The boy will be sent to:

a. Orphanage b. Remand Home
c. Prison d. Aanganwadi

913. All are true about Anganwadi worker; EXCEPT: *(Safdarjung NO 2018)*

a. Part time worker
b. Covers population of 5000
c. Supply Nutrition and educate about vaccination
d. Under controls ICDS

Explanation: All points are true about Anganwadi worker except they covers 5000 population. Under the ICDS scheme anganwadi worker covers that 1000 population and services are given like health check-up, immunization, supplementary nutrition, health education, referral services, preschool nonformal education.

914. Vitamin A supplement administered under 'National Programme for Prevention of Nutritional Blindness', contains:

a. 25,000 IU/ mL b. 1 Lakh IU/mL
c. 3 Lakh IU/mL d. 5 Lakh IU/mL

915. Disposal of placenta at PHC is done by:

a. Dry burning
b. Deep burial
c. Boiling
d. Treat with bleaching powder and burial

NATIONAL HEALTH MISSION (NHM)

916. JSY stands for: *(Kerala PSC 2002)*

a. Janani Swetchath Yojana b. Jan Suraksha Yojana
c. Janani Suraksha Yojana d. Jan Sulabh-sauchalay Yojana

Explanation: Janani Suraksha Yojana (JSY) is a safe motherhood intervention under the National Rural Health Mission (NRHM). It is being implemented with the objective of reducing maternal and neonatal mortality by promoting institutional delivery among poor pregnant women.

917. The main objective of Janani Suraksha Yojana is:

a. Tetanus immunization
b. Institutional deliveries
c. Iron supplementation
d. Nutritional supplementation

NATIONAL RURAL HEALTH MISSION (NRHM)

918. NRHM was started in:

a. 2005 b. 2006
c. 2007 d. 2009

919. All are included in National Rural Health Mission (NRHM); EXCEPT:

a. Strengthening of JSY (Janani Suraksha Yojana)
b. Formation of family health and social welfare societies
c. State and district health mission
d. Recruitment and training of ASHA

920. Under NRHM, lowest level at which Health Action Plan is prepared is:

a. State level b. District level
c. Village level d. Sub center level

921. Under National Rural Health mission who will be the link person between community and health care services?

a. Anganwadi worker b. TBA
c. ASHA d. ANM

922. The Panchayati Raj consists of 3 tier structure:

a. Panchayat, Panchayat Samiti, Municipal area committee
b. Panchayat, Panchayat Samiti and Zila Parishad
c. Panchayat, Tehsil and Blocks
d. Panchayat, Tehsil Blocks and municipal Board

923. Social stratification implies: *(AIIMS Nagpur NO 2018)*

a. Social injustice b. Social equality
c. Social inequality d. Social justice

Explanation: Social stratification refers to a system by which a society ranks categories of people in a hierarchy. It is perfectly clear that some groups have greater status, power, and wealth than other groups. These differences led to **social inequality** in society.

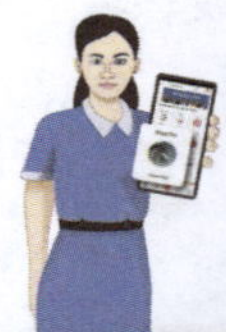

Ans.

906. c
907. b
908. b
909. b
910. b
911. b
912. b
913. b
914. b
915. d
916. c
917. b
918. a
919. b
920. c
921. c
922. b
923. c

924. ASHA (Accredited social health activist) workers are functioning at:

a. Community level b. Village level
c. PHC level d. District level

Explanation: Accredited Social Health Activists (ASHAs) are community health workers instituted by the government of India's Ministry of Health and Family Welfare (MoHFW) as part of the National Rural Health Mission (NRHM).

925. ASHA workers performance is monitored through:

a. Number of deliveries attended
b. Number of home visits done
c. Reduction in IMR
d. Number of training hours attended

Explanation: ASHA workers performance is monitored through reduction in IMR.

926. ASHA is located at:

a. Subcenter b. PHC
c. CHC d. Village

927. ASHA worker works for .... population.

a. 3000 b. 1000
c. 5000 d. 400

928. In which five year plan programme ASHA was introduced?

a. 8th five-year plan b. 9th five-year plan
c. 10th five-year plan d. 11th five-year plan

929. Full form of ASHA is:

a. Accredited Social Health Activist
b. Accredited School Health Act
c. A specific health agent
d. Association of School Health Activist

930. All are correct statement about ASHA; EXCEPT:

a. Female trained village guide
b. One per village
c. One per 1000 population
d. Female untrained guide

931. ASHA scheme is associated with:

a. ICD b. Rural Health Mission
c. 20 Points Programme d. Minimum Needs Programme

NATIONAL URBAN HEALTH MISSION (NUHM)

932. Population covered under Urban Primary Health Center is:

a. 20,000–30,000 b. 30,000–40,000
c. 40,000–50,000 d. 50,000–60,000

933. Population covered under urban CHC is:

a. 200,000 b. 250,000
c. 300,000 d. 350,000

934. NUHM was launched on:

a. 1st May 2013 b. 12th April 2015
c. 1st May 2015 d. 12th April 2013

935. What is the population strength of state capitals, district headquarters and other cities/towns which comes under NUHM?

a. 30,000 and above
b. 50,000 and above
c. 70,000 and above
d. 80,000 and above

936. Front line community worker under NUHM is:

a. ASHA b. USHA
c. MPW d. LHV

937. What is the preferred age group of USHA?

a. 18-25 years b. 20-30 years
c. 25-45 years d. 35-45 years

938. One USHA would be covering .... population.

a. Less than 1000
b. 1000–2500
c. 2000–3000
d. 2500–3500

AYUSHMAN BHARAT

939. Pradhan Mantri Jan Arogya Yojana (PM-JAY) was launched on:

a. 1st May 2012 b. 23rd September 2018
c. 12th April 2016 d. 27th August 2014

940. How much amount is covered under Pradhan Mantri Jan Arogya Yojana (PM-JAY)?

a. 3 lakhs per family per year
b. 5 lakhs per family per year
c. 8 lakhs per family per year
d. 10 lakhs per family per year

941. What type of scheme is Ayushman Bharat PM-JAY?

a. Cashless b. Paperless
c. Both a and b d. None of these

Explanation: Ayushman Bharat, a flagship scheme of Government of India, was launched as recommended by the National Health Policy 2017, to achieve the vision of Universal Health Coverage (UHC). Ayushman Bharat adopts a continuum of care approach, comprising of two inter-related components, which are:

- Health and Wellness Centers (HWCs)
- Pradhan Mantri Jan Arogya Yojana (PM-JAY)

Pradhan Mantri Jan Arogya **Yojana** (PM-JAY) was launched on 23rd September, 2018 in Ranchi, Jharkhand by PM of India. It is a **cashless and paperless** access to services for the beneficiary at the point of service.

942. All of the following statements regarding PM-JAY are true; EXCEPT:

a. PM-JAY is the world's largest health insurance/ assurance scheme fully financed by the government.
b. PM-JAY provides cashless access to health care services
c. There is no restriction on the family size, age or gender.
d. Pre-existing disease conditions during enrolment into the scheme are not covered

Explanation: Key features of PM-Jay:

- PM-JAY is the world's largest health insurance/ assurance scheme fully financed by the government.
- It provides a cover of ₹5 lakhs per family per year for secondary and tertiary care hospitalization across public and private empanelled hospitals in India.
- Cashless access to health care services for the beneficiary at the point of service, that is, the hospital.
- There is no restriction on the family size, age or gender.
- All pre-existing conditions are covered from day one
- Benefits of the scheme are portable across the country
- Public hospitals are reimbursed for the healthcare services at par with the private hospitals

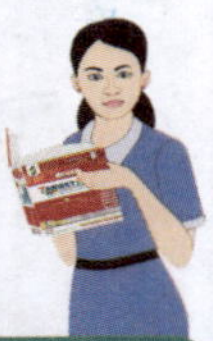

Ans.

924. b
925. c
926. d
927. b
928. c
929. a
930. d
931. b
932. d
933. b
934. a
935. b
936. b
937. c
938. b
939. b
940. b
941. c
942. d

943. In which type of hospitals free treatment is available to the beneficiary under Ayushman Bharat Scheme?
a. Government
b. Private
c. Government and empanelled private hospitals/PM-JAY
d. Any hospital

UPDATED QUESTIONS ON COVID-19

944. Which of the following virus causes the disease COVID-19?
a. NIPAH
b. SARS
c. MERS
d. SARS-CoV-2

945. The outbreak of Novel coronavirus disease (COVID-19) was initially reported from:
a. Madrid city, Spain
b. Wuhan city, China
c. Rome, Italy
d. New York, USA

946. The outbreak of COVID-19 was declared a "Public Health Emergency of International Concern" by WHO on:
a. 31 December, 2019
b. 30 January, 2020
c. 11 March, 2020
d. 19 March, 2020

947. WHO declared COVID-19 as global pandemic on:
a. 31 December, 2019
b. 30 January, 2020
c. 11 March, 2020
d. 19 March, 2020

948. Coronavirus is a:
a. Enveloped RNA virus
b. Enveloped DNA virus
c. Nonenveloped DNA virus
d. Single stranded DNA virus

949. Which of the following diseases is related to coronavirus?
a. Severe Acute Respiratory Syndrome (SARS)
b. Middle East Respiratory Syndrome (MERS)
c. Both a and b
d. None of the above

950. Mode of transmission of COVID-19 is:
a. Direct contact
b. Respiratory droplets
c. Fomites
d. All of these

951. Which of the following patient is at lowest risk of developing complications due to COVID-19?
a. Patient aged > 60 years
b. Under five children
c. Patient with comorbidities
d. Patient with immunosuppression

952. Which of the following sign/symptom is most commonly reported among COVID-19 infected patients?
a. Fever
b. Sore throat
c. Weakness
d. Running nose

953. Some of the common symptoms of COVID-19 are similar to:
a. Scabies
b. Influenza
c. Asthma
d. Cholera

954. Dedicated COVID-19 treatment Unit should have preferably negative pressure rooms with a minimum of:
a. 5 air exchanges per hour
b. 8 air exchanges per hour
c. 12 air exchanges per hour
d. 15 air exchanges per hour

955. In COVID treatment unit, high touch surfaces should be disinfected every:
a. 1-2 hourly
b. 3-4 hourly
c. 2-4 hourly
d. 6-8 hourly

956. An adult patient with which of the following symptoms is considered to be a moderate case of COVID-19:
a. Patients with uncomplicated upper respiratory tract infection
b. Patients with pneumonia, presence of dyspnea or hypoxia and RR ≥24 breaths/min
c. Patients with pneumonia, presence of dyspnea or hypoxia and RR ≥24 breaths/min
d. Patients with severe pneumonia, ARDS, and septic shock

957. An adult patient with which of the following symptom is considered to be a severe case of COVID-19?
a. Patients with uncomplicated upper respiratory tract infection
b. Patients with pneumonia, presence of dyspnea or hypoxia and RR ≥24 breaths/min
c. Patients with pneumonia, presence of dyspnea or hypoxia and RR ≥24 breaths/min
d. Patients with severe pneumonia, ARDS, and septic shock

958. Which of the following is the viral test for COVID-19 case findings recommended by ICMR?
a. Real time or Conventional RT-PCR test
b. SARS-CoV-2 antibody tests
c. Both a and b
d. None of the above

959. Which of the following is the most preferred sample for laboratory diagnosis of COVID-19?
a. Venous blood sample in a heparinized vial
b. Throat and nasal swab in viral transport media (VTM)
c. Mid-stream urine specimen
d. All of the above

960. Which of the following drug is recommended by ICMR for prophylactic use in asymptomatic healthcare workers involved in containment and treatment of COVID-19?
a. Hydroxychloroquine
b. Remdesivir
c. Tocilizumab
d. Methylprednisolone

961. Which of the following solution is used to disinfect the surfaces in COVID treatment units?
a. 1% Hypochlorite solution
b. Dettol
c. Savlon
d. Sterillium

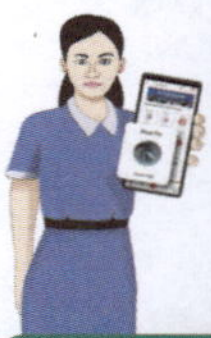

Ans.

943. c
944. d
945. b
946. b
947. c
948. a
949. c
950. d
951. b
952. a
953. b
954. c
955. a
956. b
957. d
958. a
959. b
960. a
961. a

"**Keep your vitality. A life without health is like a river without water.**"

—Maxime Lagacé

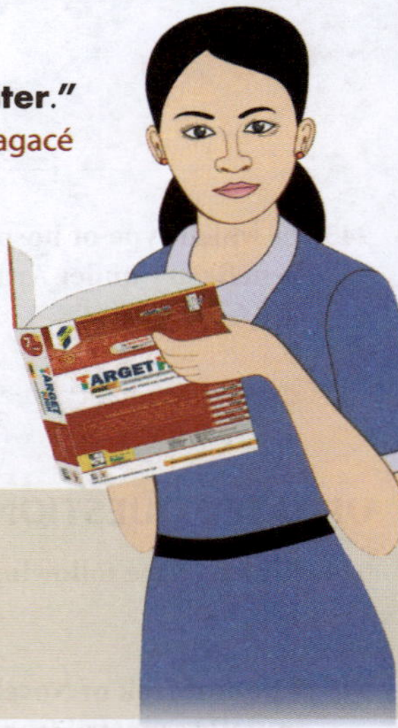

CHAPTER 5

PSYCHIATRIC NURSING

SYNOPSIS

INTRODUCTION

- **Mental health nursing** is a specialized area of nursing practice that deals with promotion of mental health, prevention of mental illness, care and rehabilitation of mentally ill individuals both in hospital and community.
- In**1943,** mental health nursing course was first started for male nurses.
- In **1965, Indian Nursing Council** included psychiatric nursing as a compulsory course in the BSc Nursing program.
- In **1967 TNAI,** formed a separate committee for mental health nursing to improve the perception of mental health nursing as well as to set guidelines for nursing teachers to conduct theory classes and clinical training in psychiatric nursing.
- **In 1976, Masters in Psychiatric Nursing was first started at RAK College of Nursing, New Delhi.**

MENTAL HEALTH

- Mental health is an adjustment of human beings to the world and to each other with maximum effectiveness and happiness.
- Mental health is an equilibrium of body, mind and spirit with the environment.

MENTAL ILLNESS

- Mental illness is maladjustment in living. It produces a disharmony in the person's ability to meet human needs comfortably or effectively and to function within a culture.
- Mental illness is health condition involving changes in emotion, thinking and behavior (or a combination of these).

Mental Healthcare Act 2017

- The Indian **Mental Healthcare Act 2017** replaced the Mental Health Act 1987.
- Mental Healthcare Act 2017 (MHA 2017) received presidential consent on April 7th, **2017** and **replaced** the **1987 Act.**

Salient Features of MHA 2017

- **Decriminalization of suicide attempt:** This Act has overturned **309 Indian Penal Code.** The MHA 2017 decriminalizes suicide attempt by mentally ill person.
- **Rights of persons with mental illness**
  - Every person will have the right to access mental healthcare services.
  - Protect person with mentally ill from inhuman treatment.
  - Mentally ill patients to have access to free legal services and right to complain about shortcoming of provision of treatment.
  - **Advance directive:** Empowers a mentally ill person to have the right to make an advance directive toward the way he/she wants to be treated.
- The government has to set up Central Mental Health Authority at national level and State Mental Health Authority at state level.
- The Act outlines the process of admission, treatment and discharge of patients.
- **No ECT** therapy without use of muscle relaxants.
- **No ECT** therapy for minors.
- **Financial Punishment:** Up to 6 months of imprisonment or ₹10,000 or both for violating of provisions of MHA 2017. Repeat offenders may face up to 2 years imprisonment or fine of ₹50,000 – 5,00,000 or both.
- **Reception order:** Refers to an order for admission and detention of a mentally ill person in a psychiatric hospital.

KEY POINTS

- The term 'Psychiatry' was coined by Christian Reil.
- Linda Richards is considered First Psychiatric Nurse.
- Sigmund Freud is the father of Modern Psychiatry.
- Freud's model of development which comprises 'id, ego and superego' is called Structural Model.
- World Mental Health Day is observed on 10th October.
- The Indian Lunacy Act was passed in the year 1912.
- The Indian Mental Health Act was passed in the year 1987.
- Mental Health Act 2017 decriminalizes suicide attempt by mentally ill person.

DEVELOPMENT OF PERSONALITY

Factors Influencing Personality Development

Biological Factors

- **Heredity:** Genetic characteristics such as height, color of the skin and appearance influence personality of a person.
- **Endocrine glands:** Secretions of endocrine glands heavily influences one's behavior, e.g. Male hormone, testosterone is associated with aggression.
- **Physique:** An individual's physical characters such as height, weight and general appearances determine the behavior toward others.
- **Nervous system:** Nervous systems work in close coordination with endocrine system. The behavior of an individual is managed and controlled by the nervous system.

Environmental/Social Factors

- **Family:** Most important factor in molding personality among environmental factors is family.
- **School:** Schools play a significant role in building personality of a growing child.
- **Teacher:** Desirable personalities of a teacher are often inculcated in student's behavior. Undesirable and prejudicial treatment by teachers often negatively affects student's personality.
- **Peer group:** Peer group plays a vital role in shaping the personalities of the children.
- **Sibling relationship:** The number of siblings, their gender and the age gap influence the children's personality traits, like sharing, cooperativeness, jealousness and aggressiveness.
- **Mass media:** Nowadays, mass media has a major impact on children's behavior as the access and time to these media has increased recently. Use of smart phones and technologies impact the personality of the children as face to face interaction has become less significant at very young age.
- **Culture:** Every culture has its own value system, moral system, beliefs, and norms which shape the behavior of the children. What is considered to be an acceptable behavior in one culture may not be the same in an another culture of the country.

Practice Questions

1. Personality of an individual is developed as a result of

a. Genetic inheritance
b. Environmental factors
c. Both a & b
d. None of the above

Ans. (c) Both a & b

2. Which of the following factors can have an effect on development of an individual's personality?

a. General appearance
b. Peer group influence
c. Cultural beliefs
d. All of the above

Ans. (d) All of the above

THEORIES OF PERSONALITY DEVELOPMENT

Freud's Stages of Psychosexual Development

Table 1: Stages of psychosexual development

Stages of development	Main characteristics	Examples of unsuccessful task completion
Oral (Birth to 18 months)	Focus of libido is on Mouth, Tongue and Lips. Pleasure centers on mouth – sucking, biting, chewing	Smoking, overeating, obesity, alcoholism, nail biting, drug addiction, difficulty in trusting others
Anal (18 months to 3 years)	Pleasure focuses on bowel and bladder. Elimination and toilet training are central focus.	Perfectionism or messiness, obsessive compulsive disorder.
Phallic (3–6 years)	Awareness of genital area as source of pleasure. Child learns sexual identity. Conflicts end as child represses urge and identifies with same sex parent. The development of Electra complex *(female)* and Oedipus complex *(male)* occurs during this stage of development. Freud described this as the child's unconscious desire to eliminate the parent of the same sex and to possess the parent of the opposite sex.	Sexual dysfunction (transexuality, homosexuality, sexual identity problem) difficulty in accepting authority
Latency (6–12 Years)	Quite stage in sexual development. Child learns to socialize.	Inability to conceptualize; lack of motivation in school or job.
Genital (12 years to adulthood)	The genitals are again the focus of stimulation. Sexual maturity and satisfactory relationships with opposite sex is the central focus	Unsatisfactory relationship, impotence, premature ejaculation.

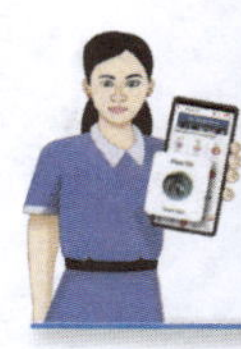

Erikson's Stages of Personality Development

Table 2: Stages of personality development

Stage and approximate ages	Important events	Virtue	Tasks	Consequences of unsuccessful task completion
Infants Trust Vs mistrust Birth to 18 months	Feeding	Hope	Viewing the world as safe and reliable, relationships as nurturing, stable and dependable	Suspiciousness, trouble with personal relationship
Toddler Autonomy Vs shame and doubt 1.5–3 years	Toilet training	Will	Achieving a sense of control and free will	Low self-esteem, dependency
Pre-school Initiative Vs guilt 3–6 years	Explorative	Purpose	Beginning development of conscious learning to manage conflict and anxiety	Passive personality, strong feeling of guilt
School age Industry Vs inferiority 6–12 years	Schooling	Competence	Emerging confidence in child's own ability, taking pleasure in accomplishments	Unmotivated, unreliable
Adolescence Identity Vs role confusion 12–19 years	Social relationship	Fidelity	Formulate a sense of self and belongingness	Substance abuse, difficulty in keeping personal relationship
Young adult Intimacy Vs isolation 20–40 years	Relationship	Love	Formulating adult, loving relationship and meaningful attachment to others	Emotional immaturity, may deny need for personal relationship
Middle adult Generativity Vs stagnation 41–65 years	Risk and parenthood	Care	Being creative and productive, focus is on establishment of family and guiding to the next generation	Inability to show concern for anyone but self
Maturity Ego integrity Vs despair 65 years to death	Reflection of life	Wisdom	Accepting the responsibility for one's self and life	Has difficulty dealing with issues of aging and death, may have feeling of hopelessness

Sigmund Freud Theory

- **Sigmund Freud (1856-1939)** an Austrian neurologist is considered as the **Father of Psychoanalytical Theory**. He emphasized the unconscious processes or psychodynamic factors as the basis for motivation and behavior. He categorized his personality theory according to structure, dynamics and development.
- He organized the structure of the personality into three major components: **id**, **ego** and **superego**.
- The ***id*** contains all our biologically based drives (hunger, sex), etc. It operates according to the "pleasure principle". Id-driven behaviors are impulsive and may be irrational.
- The ***ego*** functions on the basis of "reality principle". It maintains harmony between the external world, the id and the super ego.
- The ***superego*** is referred to as the "perfection principle". It is important in the socialization of the individual as it assists the ego in the control of id impulses. **It works on *ideal principle* and is also called *conscience*.**
- A strong and mature ego will help to shape an ideal personality of an individual.

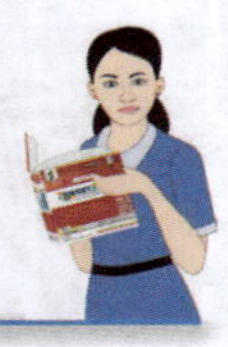

Maslow's Hierarchy of Needs

- **Abraham Maslow (1921–1970)** was an American psychologist who studied the needs or motivation of an individual.
- Maslow's hierarchy of needs model explains individual's differences in terms of one's motivation, which are not necessarily stable throughout the life.
- ***Before moving to next stage, it is necessary to fulfill the needs at lower levels.***
- This theory helps nurses understand patient's behavioral change during life crisis.

KEY POINTS

- Pavlov's experiment is an example of Classical Conditioning.
- Cognitive model suggests that psychological disorders result from acquiring dysfunctional ways of Thinking and Acting.
- Psychoanalytic therapy was developed by Sigmund Freud.
- Id - Pleasure principle
- Ego - Reality principle
- Superego - Perfection principle

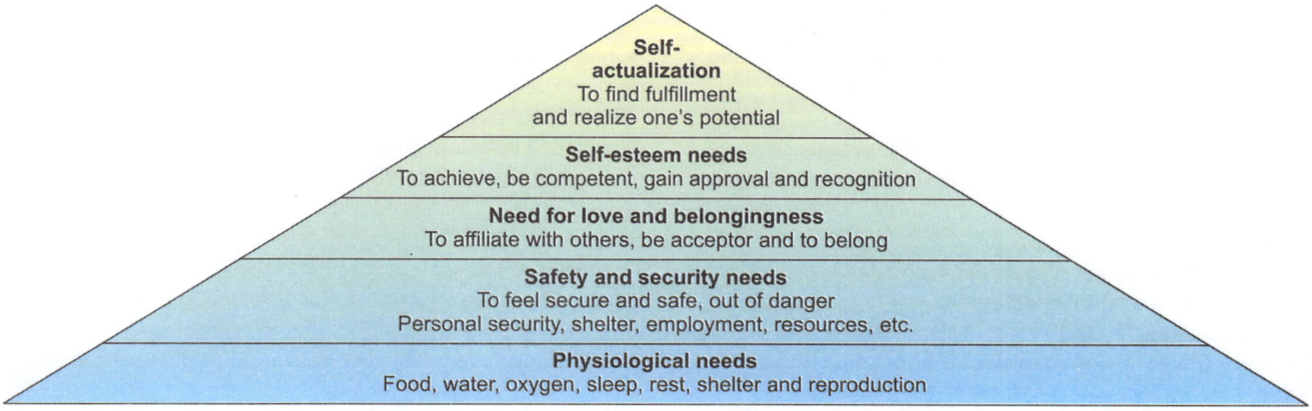

Figure 1: Pyramid of Maslow's hierarchy of needs

Table 3: Levels of **consciousness**

Clouding of consciousness →	Drowsiness →	Stupor →	Coma →
Earliest stage of impaired consciousness Decreased awareness and alertness	Next level of Impaired consciousness Decreased awareness and Alertness If not stimulated constantly, can go into sleep	Non-responsiveness Patient can be aroused by repeated stimulation	Unconscious patient Eyes closed and no mental responses

Ref: Gajandra H. and Singh P. My PGMEE Notes. CBS Publishers and Distributors Pvt ltd.

DEFENSE MECHANISM

Defense mechanism is method of attempting to promote self-esteem and in coping with basic drives or emotionally painful thoughts, feelings or events.

Table 4: Defense mechanism and their descriptions

Defense mechanisms	Examples
Repression It is an unconscious mechanism that keeps the painful ideas and disturbing thoughts away from consciousness. Unconsciously deny impulse.	A child who is abused by a parent, later has no recollection of events, but has trouble in forming relationships.
Suppression A deliberate or conscious attempt to push away unwanted or disturbing thoughts. Consciously suppress impulse.	A voluntary decision not to think about his argument with his girlfriend while going for an interview.
Denial It is the refusal to accept the reality or fact that causes anxiety to a person.	Smokers may refuse to accept that smoking is injurious to health. A patient who is newly diagnosed with lung cancer may not admit even though there is a confirmatory laboratory findings.
Displacement Unwanted feelings and frustrations are discharged on a less threatening object or person.	A husband comes home after a bad day at work and shouts at her wife or children.
Reaction formation Anxiety producing or unacceptable feelings are replaced with their exact opposite feelings and emotions.	A jealous boy who hates his elder brother may show exaggerated respect and affection toward him.
Rationalization Justification of one's unacceptable behavior or failure in a logical manner by giving socially-approved reasons.	A student who comes late to the class may complain that the hostel mess served the food late.

Contd...

Defense mechanisms	Examples
Sublimation It is a practice of acting out socially unacceptable impulses and urges into socially acceptable activities.	Aggressiveness might be transformed into competitiveness in studies and sports.
Compensation People try to over achieve in one area to compensate shortcomings or failure in another area. It is an act of covering up for a weakness by making up a desirable trait.	A student who fails in his studies may compensate by becoming the college champion in sports.
Projection The individual, either consciously or unconsciously, blames another person for his own failure or difficulties.	A surgeon, whose patient does not recover as he anticipated, may tend to blame the scrub nurse who helped at the time of surgery.
Intellectualization Reasoning (thinking) is used to block confrontation with an unconscious conflict and its associated emotional stress. Intellectualization may accompany rationalization but is different from rationalization.	Person shows no emotional expression when discussing serious car accident, he just goes through.
Undoing A person tries to 'undo' an unhealthy, destructive or threatening thought or action by engaging in contrary behavior.	Giving a treat to a child who is being punished for wrong doing.
Regression Unconscious return to an earlier and more comfortable developmental stage. It is an attempt to bring back a time when the person feels safe and taken care of.	An adult throws a temper tantrum when he does not get his own way.
Dissociation The unconscious detachment from immediate surroundings or physical and emotional experiences that cause anxiety.	Amnesia that prevents recall of previous day's car accident.
Conversion Psychological or interpersonal conflicts manifest themselves in physical symptoms	A student awakens with the migraine headache in the morning of a final examination and feels too ill to take the test.
Retroflexion Retroflexion is the turning back of something onto the self. This could be any emotion such as anger, blame, guilt, etc.	Blaming oneself for the death of a friend.
Substitution The replacement of highly-valued unacceptable object with an object that is more acceptable to the ego.	A person who could not get admission to MBBS chose BDS (Dentist).

THERAPEUTIC COMMUNICATION

It is an interpersonal interaction between the nurse and the patient that focuses on the patient's specific needs for promoting an effective exchange of information.

- **Process:** Sender, Message, Channel, Receiver, Feedback.
- **Techniques:** Listening, broad opening, restating, clarification, reflection, humor, informing, focusing, sharing perception, theme identification, silence, suggesting, validating, paraphrasing, pinpointing, linking, questioning and summarizing.

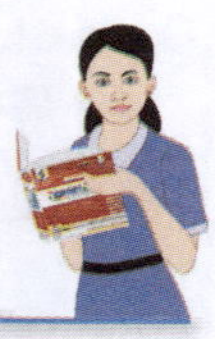

Types

Verbal and Nonverbal

Phases of therapeutic communication techniques include

- Preorientation phase (pre-interaction phase)
- Orientation phase (Interaction phase)
- Working phase
- Termination phase

Pre-interaction phase: This phase comes before the actual interaction with the client. This phase begins after assigning a client to the nurse. A nurse deals with her own anxiety of dealing a psychiatric patient

Clinical Corner

CASE SCENARIO 1:

Nurse Linda is collecting history from a patient who is getting admitted into psychiatric ward. She found that the patient is using rationalization as a defence mechanism. She is aware that the purpose of using defence mechanism is

a. To help an individual to physically defend himself in a threatening situation
b. To protect the ego from anxiousness and feeling of guilt
c. To protect the impulsive desires of the id
d. To release the bottled-up mental pressures

Ans. (b) To protect the ego...

Orientation phase (interaction phase): This is the phase in which client and nurse will come face to face for interaction. In this phase itself termination of the therapeutic relationship will also begin. Goals of the therapeutic relationship will also be discussed during this phase.

Working phase: In this phase, the client and the nurse will work together to meet the goals established in the orientation phase. **Transference** (Patient develops emotional dependency on nurse) and **counter transference** (Nurse develops emotional dependency on patient) occur in this phase.

Termination phase: In this phase, actual termination of the therapeutic relationship will take place.

KEY POINTS

- Process recording is the recording of conversation between the nurse and patient in a psychiatric set up.
- The best approach in helping a severely withdrawn patient is to provide a trusting relationship.
- Giving advice to the patient is one of the barriers of therapeutic nurse-patient communication.
- Open-ended questions are used during psychiatric history collection.

Techniques used in Therapeutic Communication

Table 5: Techniques and their explanations in therapeutic communication

Technique	Explanation
Using open ended question (broad opening)	Using open ended questions will allow the client to express himself/herself.
Using general leads	It will help the client to continue with the conversation.
Restating	It is stating back the sentence said by the client. It will also encourage the client to continue with the communication.
Reflection	Turn back the meaning or the feeling of what has been said by the client. It is to let the client make sense of the conversation.
Using silence	It helps the nurse to observe the non-verbal clues of the client as well as encourage the client to express his/her emotions.
Giving information	During the communication process providing appropriate information to the client will also help the client to make appropriate decision.
Clarifying	If the nurse is not clear about what was said by the client ask the client to clarify what the client said.
Exploring	It means ask the client to explain more about the specific part of the conversation in order to identify further ideas or experiences.
Non-judgmental	Refraining from judgment based on personal ethical standards. A core attitude that psychiatric nurses need to develop to be effective in their work is being non-judgmental.

NEUROTRANSMITTERS

Table 6: Imbalance in neurotransmitters

Neuro-transmitter	Imbalance
Acetylcholine	Decreased level — Alzheimer's disease Increased level — depression
Norepinephrine	Decreased level — depression Increased level – Mania, Anxiety states, Schizophrenia
Dopamine	Decreased level — Parkinson's disease and depression Increased level — Mania and schizophrenia
Serotonin	Decreased level — Depression Increased level — Anxiety state
Histamine	Decreased level — Depression
Gamma amino butyric acid (GABA)	Decreased level — Anxiety disorders, schizophrenia and various forms of epilepsy
Somatostatin	Decreased level — Alzheimer's disease Increased level — Causes Huntington's disease

KEY POINTS

- Biochemical etiology of Alzheimer's disease relates to Acetylcholine.
- Parkinson's disease - low and falling dopamine levels.
- Depression - Deficiency of Serotonin or 5 HT (5-hydroxytryptamine).
- Schizophrenia & Mania - Increased dopamine level

Clinical Corner

CASE SCENARIO 2:
The psychiatric ward in-charge nurse observes inconsistency in the nurse's behavior toward a patient. The nurse is overly concerned and kind toward the patient. This is an act of

a. Transference.
b. Countertransference
c. Empathetic resonance
d. Sympathetic resonance

Ans. (b) Countertransference

CASE SCENARIO 3:
While working in a psychiatric ward, a nurse is expected to use all of the following therapeutic communication techniques in her communication, except

a. Restating
b. Asking the client "why?"
c. Maintain neutral responses
d. Active listening

Ans. (b) Asking the client "why?"

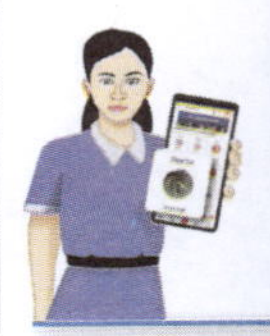

PSYCHOSOCIAL THERAPIES

Various therapies are used to relieve patient's symptoms and help him/her to understand and modify conduct and to lead a well-adjusted life.

Psychoanalytical Therapy

In this, focus is on the cause of the problem, which is buried somewhere in the unconscious. The therapist tries to take the patient into the past in an effort to determine where the problem began. Techniques used are free association, dream analysis, hypnosis, catharsis and abreaction therapy.

Individual Psychotherapy

It is a method of bringing about change in a person by exploring his or her feelings, attitudes, thinking and behavior. It is one to one relationship of therapist with patient.

Indications

- Stress-related disorder
- Alcohol and drug dependence
- Sexual disorders
- Marital disharmony

Behavioral Therapies

Behavioral therapy assumes that the maladaptive behavior can be corrected through provision of learning experiences.

Goal

To modify maladaptive behavior by reinforcing adaptive behaviors

Principles

- **Theory of Classical Conditioning**: Learning by association. (remember dog-saliva experiment)
- **Theory of Operant Conditioning**: Learning by reinforcement (rewards) and punishment. [Remember Rat – lever – food experiment]
- Social learning theory
- Cognitive Behavioral Therapy

Indications

- Social phobia
- Obsessive Compulsive Disorder (OCD)
- Post-Traumatic Stress Disorder (PTSD)
- Eating disorder
- Substance use
- Depression, BPAD, Schizophrenia, Autism

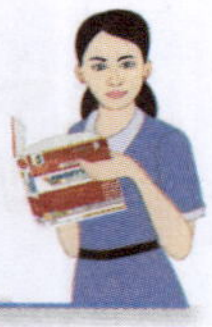

Behavior Therapy Techniques

Systemic Desensitization

- Developed by **Joseph Wolpe**
- **Steps**
  - Relaxation Training → Hierarchy Construction of anxiety provoking situation→ Desensitization of Stimulus
- **Appropriate technique for**
  - Phobic anxiety disorder
  - Anxiety disorder
  - Obsessive compulsive disorder (OCD)
  - Certain sexual disorder

Flooding or Implosion

- A person is exposed directly to the stimulus (fearing object) in the most immediate and unavoidable way.
- No grading or relaxation
- Suitable to treat phobia
- Not suitable for client with heart disease

Shaping

- Based on operant conditioning principle
- Client's behavior leading to the desired behavior is rewarded
- Suitable for speech therapy in Autistic Child

Extinction

Reinforcement that is provided for problem behavior is discontinued in order to eliminate occurrences of these types of problem behaviors.
E.g.: Extinction in temper tantrum

Token Economy

- It is an operant conditioning technique
- 'Token' is distributed to appreciate desired (target) behavior
- The token can be later exchanged for privileges such as food, etc.

Restitution/Over-Correction

- Used to treat disruptive behavior
- A person engaged in disruptive behavior is asked to restore the situation much better than before.
  E.g.: A patient who urinated in the ward will be asked to clean the dirty area and also asked to mop the entire ward.

Time Out

- It is an aversive stimulus/punishment in which the client is isolated from the environment where he/she exhibited unacceptable behavior.
- This is to prevent reinforcement from attention of others.

Exposure and Response Prevention (ERP)

- Most important type of Cognitive Behavior Therapy (CBT) for OCD
- **Exposure:** Encourage client to expose himself/herself to the images, thoughts, objects or situations that make obsessions.

KEY POINTS

- Systemic desensitization is developed by Joseph Wolpe.
- Systemic desensitization is useful for phobic anxiety disorder, OCD and certain sexual disorder.
- Flooding or implosion is useful therapy for phobia.
- Shaping is suitable for speech therapy in autistic child.
- Extinction technique is useful in temper tantrum.
- Exposure and response prevention (ERP) is the most important type of Cognitive Behavior Therapy (CBT) for OCD.
- Brief Cognitive Behavioral Therapy (CBT) focuses on solving current problems. It focuses on 'here and now' approach.
- Aversion therapy is useful alcoholism, impulsive behavior, and paraphilias.

Practice Question

3. A 30-year-old male patient complains of an intense, overwhelming fear of driving a bike. The patient does not go for shopping or job unless someone transports him. The fear has disrupted all elements of the patient's life. He has few social contacts. Which of the following is the most appropriate treatment plan for this patient?

a. Flooding.
b. Assertiveness training.
c. Systematic desensitization
d. Reminiscence therapy

Ans. (c) Systematic...

- **Response prevention:** Encourage client not to do compulsive act after the obsession and anxiety triggered by the exposure.

Aversion Therapy

- Punishment (noxious stimuli) is presented immediately after exhibiting undesired behavior.
- Noxious stimuli can be Electric shock, substance that induce vomiting, social disapproval, corporeal punishment.
- Useful for Alcoholism, impulsive behavior, and paraphilias.

Social Skill Training

Teach the client with verbal and nonverbal behaviors to improve social interactions

Assertiveness Training

- Assertive responses promote positive sense of respect for self and others
- Assertive training helps empowering the client in terms of human interactions

Cognitive Therapy

It focuses on how patients think about themselves and their world, make change in current ways of thinking and behavior. It helps to modify the thinking pattern and develop right thinking.

Indications

- Anxiety, eating disorders
- Personality disorders
- Suicidal thoughts or attempts
- Sexual disorders

Family Therapy

It is used when individual's psychiatric symptoms are inseparably related with the family in which he lives. Thus the focus of the treatment is not the treatment alone but also the family.

Indications

Family problems or marital maladjustment

Behavior Therapy

A trained professional helps a patient to correct the existing maladaptive behavior pattern by application of principles of learning.

Indications

- Specific phobias
- Alcohol abuse
- Paraphilias
- Homosexuality
- Transvestism
- Obsessions
- Compulsions

Milieu Therapy

- **Bettleheim'** coined the term Milieu therapy
- The word "milieu" is French word means "middle". English translation of the word is surroundings or environment.
- Therapy involving the milieu or the environment may be called milieu therapy, therapeutic community or therapeutic environment.
- The goal of milieu therapy is **to manipulate the environment** so that all aspects of the client's hospital experience are considered therapeutic.
- Within this milieu, the client is expected to learn adaptive coping, interaction and relationship skills
- Key concepts of milieu therapy
  - **Containment:** Process of providing safety and security
  - **Validation:** Process that affirms patient individuality.
  - **Structured interaction:** Staff members approach the client in a consistent manner.
  - **Open communication:** Staff and patient willingly share information.
- **Programs within milieu**
  - Client government
  - Work related activities
- Some of the scales for evaluation of therapeutic environment includes Behavioral mapping by **Ittleson**, **Rivlin,** and **Proshansky,** Ward atmosphere scale by Moos.
- **Advantages**
  - The patient learns to adopt an acceptable behavior, decision making and leadership skills.
  - Client becomes socio centric
- **Disadvantages**
  - Role blurring between staff and patient
  - Patient may find transition to community difficult
  - Conflict resolution is needed as part of the staff's skills

ICD 10 CLASSIFICATION OF PSYCHIATRIC DISORDERS

Introduction

- ICD-10 is the 10th revision of the International Statistical Classification of Diseases and Related Health Problems (ICD), a medical classification list by the World Health Organization (WHO).
- Chapter V of the ICD 10 Classifies of Mental and Behavioral Disorders

KEY POINTS

- The goal of milieu therapy is to manipulate the environment so that all aspects of the client's hospital experience are considered therapeutic.
- Concepts of milieu therapy include containment, **validation, structured interaction,** and **open communication.**
- Cognitive Behavior Therapy (CBT) is the treatment of choice for bulimia nervosa and for binge-eating disorder
- CBT is found to be effective in the treatment of PTSD.
- Release of feelings that takes place by talking about an emotionally charged areas is known as abreaction.

Practice Question

4. All of the following are true about psychoanalytic therapy, except

a. Insight-oriented therapy
b. Emphasize operant conditioning and modeling
c. Focused on past
d. Consider disorders as arising from unresolved conflicts

Ans. (b) Emphasize operant conditioning and modeling

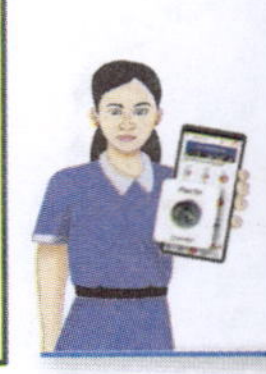

List of Categories

- **F00-F09:** Organic, including symptomatic, mental disorders
- **F10-F19:** Mental and behavioral disorders due to psychoactive substance use
- **F20-F29:** Schizophrenia, schizotypal and delusional disorders
- **F30-F39:** Mood [affective] disorders
- **F40-F48:** Neurotic, stress-related and somatoform disorders
- **F50-F59:** Behavioral syndromes associated with physiological disturbances and physical factors
- **F60-F69:** Disorders of adult personality and behavior
- **F70-F79:** Mental retardation
- **F80-F89:** Disorders of psychological development
- **F90-F98:** Behavioral and emotional disorders with onset usually occurring in childhood and adolescence
- **F99-F99:** Unspecified mental disorder

Important Psychiatric Disorders and its Classification Codes

- **F10:** Mental and behavioral disorders due to use of **alcohol**
- **F11:** Mental and behavioral disorders due to use of **opioid**
- **F20:** Schizophrenia
- **F30:** Manic episode
- **F31:** Bipolar Affective Disorder (BPAD)
- **F32:** Depressive Episode
- **F40:** Phobic Anxiety Disorder
- **F42:** Obsessive Compulsive Disorder
- **F44:** Dissociative Disorder
- **F50:** Eating disorders
- **F52:** Sexual dysfunction
- **F60:** Specific Personality disorders
- **F70:** Mild Mental retardation
- **F71:** Moderate Mental retardation
- **F72:** Severe Mental retardation
- **F73:** Profound Mental retardation
- **F80:** Specific developmental disorders of speech and language
- **F90:** Hyperkinetic disorder
- **F95:** Tic disorders

GENERAL PSYCHOPATHOLOGY

Disorders of Consciousness

- **Consciousness** is awareness of the self and the environment
- **Quantitative changes of consciousness** mean reduced vigility (alertness):
  - **Somnolence**: State of strong desire for sleep, or sleeping for unusually long periods
  - **Stupor**: A state of near-unconsciousness or insensibility
  - **Coma**: A deep state of prolonged unconsciousness in which a person cannot be awakened
- **Qualitative changes of consciousness** mean disturbed per-ception, thinking, affectivity, memory and consequent motor disorders:
  - **Delirium (confusional state):** Characterized by disorien-tation, distorted perception, enhanced suggestibility, misinterpretations and mood disorders
  - **Obnubilation** (twilight state): Starts and ends abruptly, amnesia is complete; the patient is disordered, his acting is aimless, sometimes aggressive, hard to understand. The person may be Stuporous or Delirious
- **Hypnosis:** Artificially incited change of consciousness
- **Syncope:** Short-term unconsciousness

Disorders of Perception

- **Illusions**: Refers to an instance of a wrong or misinterpreted perception of a sensory experience (sensory stimuli).
- **Pseudoillusions**: Distorted perception of objects which may occur when the general level of sensory stimulation is reduced
- **Hallucination:** Perception without any obvious stimulus

KEY POINTS

- ICD-11 has been adopted by the Seventy-second World Health Assembly in May 2019 and comes into effect on 1 January 2022
- International Classification of Diseases is published by World Health Organization (WHO).
- Diagnostic and Statistical Manual (DSM) classification of mental disorders is published by American Psychiatric Association.

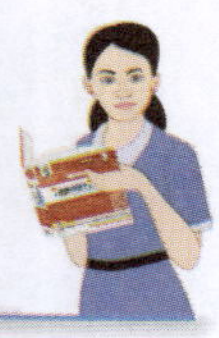

KEY POINT

The traditional division between neurosis and psychosis that was evident in ICD-9 (deliberately left without any attempt to define these concepts) has not been used in ICD-10.

Practice Question

5. A 45-year-old male client with 8 years history of alcohol abuse is admitted for deaddiction treatment. The nurse in the unit is aware the following symptoms are associated alcohol withdrawal delirium, except

a. Hallucinations, disorientation, hypertension, anxiety
b. Ataxia, lethargy, hypotension, hunger
c. Hypotension, lethargy, Stupor, dystonia
d. Muscle rigidity, alertness, Coarse hand tremors, hypothermia

Ans. (a) Hallucinations, disorientation, hypertension, anxiety

Table 7: Types of hallucination with their key features

Types of hallucination	Key points
Auditory hallucination (acousma)	Person hears non-existent sounds. Most common type of hallucination. Common in schizophrenic patient.
Visual hallucination	Person sees something that does not exist Common in acute organic brain stem conditions
Olfactory hallucination (Phantosmia)	Person smells odors that do not exist. Odors are usually unpleasant. Can occur in schizophrenia and organic states. It can also be caused by Epilepsy
Gustatory hallucination	Person tastes something that is not present Seen in depression
Tactile hallucination (or deep somatic)	Person senses that they are being touched when they are not. Commonly associated with substance use such as cocaine or amphetamine
Kinetic hallucination	Sensation of flying or moving the body or a part of body. Also known as motor hallucination.
Delusional zoopathy	Delusional belief + feeling of animals/insects crawling in the body
Pseudohallucinations	Patient can distinguish them from reality

Disorders of Thinking/Thought

Quantitative (Formal) Disorders of Thinking

- **Pressure of thought:** Ideas arise very rapidly and in great variety, passing through the mind quickly. It may be experienced in mania or schizophrenia.
- **Poverty of thought:** The mental state of being devoid of **thought** and having a feeling of emptiness.
- **Thought blocking:** A person stops speaking suddenly and without explanation in the middle of a sentence. Common in Schizophrenia.
- **Flight of ideas:** Rapid speech with frequent shifts in topic with no association between topics.
- **Perseveration:** Repetition of a particular response (such as a word, phrase, or gesture) regardless of the absence or cessation of a stimulus
- **Verbigeration:** Obsessive repetition of random words. It is similar to perseveration, in which a person repeats words in response to a stimulus.
- **Loosening of associations:** Series of ideas are presented with loosely apparent or completely in apparent logical connections.
- **Word salad:** Confused or unintelligible mixture of seemingly random Words and phrases
- **Neologisms:** A newly-created word whose meaning is unknown to others

Qualitative Disorders of Thought (Content Thought Disorders)

Delusion is defined as fixed, false belief that does not change even when a person is presented with conflicting evidence.

Table 8: Types of delusion

Types of delusion	Explanation
Delusion of persecution	Patient thinks that people are planning to kill or harm him/her
Delusion of grandiosity	Patient feels more superior and powerful than he really is
Delusion of infidelity	Patient thinks that his/her spouse is unfaithful on him/her. Feeling of being cheated by spouse.
Delusion of Nihilism	Patient feels that things do not exist (everything including self) and a sense that everything is unreal.

Concerning the Possession of Thoughts

- Thought insertion
- Thought withdrawal
- Thought broadcasting

KEY POINTS

- Auditory hallucination is the most common form of hallucination in schizophrenics.
- Olfactory hallucination occurs due to neurological damage to olfactory system. **It can also be caused by Epilepsy**.
- Visual hallucination is common in acute organic brain stem conditions.
- Tactile hallucination is commonly associated with substance use such as cocaine or amphetamine.
- Circumstantiality is a disorder of thought in which thinking proceeds slowly with many unnecessary trivial details, but finally the point is reached.
- Persecutory delusion and/or suspiciousness is common in paranoid schizophrenia.
- Delusion of grandiosity is common in Mania

Recent Question (NORCET 2022)

1. **Wernicke-Korsakoff syndrome in alcoholic patient occurs due to the deficiency of:**
   a. Thiamine deficiency
   b. Vitamin C
   c. Vitamin D
   d. Vitamin A

Ans. (a) Thiamine deficiency

Obsessions (Obsessive Thought)

Obsessions (obsessive thought) are recurrent persistent thoughts, impulses or images entering the mind despite the person's efforts to exclude them. Obsessive phenomena in acting (usual as senseless rituals – cleaning, counting, dressing) are called **compulsions.**

Disorders of Memory

Types of Memory

- **Short-term memory (working memory)**: For verbal and visual information, retained for 15–20 sec., low capacity, e.g. retaining phone number while dialing.
- **Long-term memory**: Wide capacity and more permanent storage, e.g. childhood memories, language vocabulary

Various disorders of memory are:

- **Amnesia:** Severe memory loss.
  - **Retrograde amnesia:** Cannot recall events that occurred prior to the brain trauma.
  - **Anterograde amnesia:** Cannot recall events that occurred after the brain trauma. Occurs due to failure to make permanent traces.

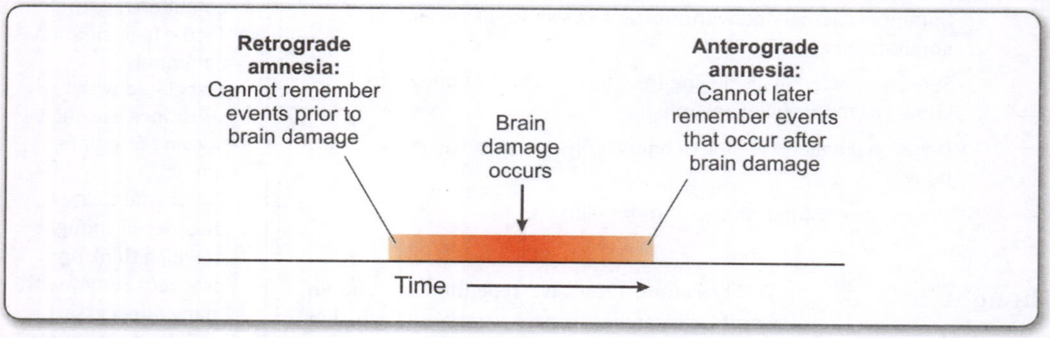

Figure 2: Types of amnesia

- **déja vu:** It comprises the feeling of having experienced a current event in the past, although it has no basis in fact.
- **Jamais vu:** It is opposite to déja vu. The phenomenon of experiencing a situation that one recognizes in some fashion, but that nonetheless seems very unfamiliar.
- **Confabulation:** Gaps in memory are unconsciously filled with fabricated, misinterpreted, or distorted information.
- **Amnesic disorientation:** Characterized by disorientation particularly in time, impairment of immediate recall, loss of recent memory, retroactive loss of remote memory of varying extent and a tendency to confabulation.
- **Hypomnesia:** Abnormally poor memory of the past.
- **Hypermnesia:** Unusual power or enhancement of memory, typically under abnormal conditions such as trauma, hypnosis, or narcosis.
- **Korsakoff's syndrome:** Occurs due to vitamin B1 (thiamin) deficiency. Memory problems are often preceded by ataxia.
- **Transient global amnesia:** It is characterized by a patient's inability to learn new material. Perception and personal identity are normal.

Motor Disorders

Motor disorders occur frequently in all kinds of mental disorders, especially in catatonic schizophrenia.

Quantitative

- **Hypoagility:** An overall lowering or deprivation of activities
- **Hyperagility:** Excessive activity.
- Agitated behavior

Qualitative

- **Mannerisms**: A habitual gesture or way of speaking or behaving
- **Stereotypies**: A motor disorder with onset in childhood involving repetitive, nonfunctional motor behavior (e.g., hand waving or head banging)
- **Posturing**: An abnormal involuntary flexion or extension of the arms, legs and or body parts.
- **Waxy flexibility:** The person is nearly or completely unresponsive to stimuli and remains immobile for long periods of time
- **Echopraxia:** Meaningless repetition or imitation of the movements of others

KEY POINTS

- Confabulation is a symptom of various memory disorders in which made up stories fill in any gaps in memory.
- Unfamiliarity of familiar things is seen in Jamais vu.
- Déjà vu is a feeling of having already experienced the present situation.
- Recent memory loss is a feature of Alzheimer's disease.
- Separation of a thought or memory from its associated feeling or emotion is known as Isolation.
- **Amnesia**: Loss of memory
- **Agnosia**: Unable to recognize inanimate objects
- **Apraxia**: No recognition of object function
- **Aphasia**: Unable to speak

- **Negativism:** Seen in patients with catatonia. opposition or no response to instructions or external stimuli
- **Automatism:** Automatism is more or less coordinated, involuntary motor activity occurring during a state of impaired consciousness either in the course of or after an epileptic seizure and usually followed by amnesia.
- **Agitation:** A state of anxiety or nervous excitement
- **Tics:** Condition that involves brief, uncontrollable, spasm-like movements
- **Compulsions:** Compulsive acts can be defined as repetitious, purposeful physical or mental actions that the individual feels compelled to engage in a stereotyped manner.

ORGANIC MENTAL DISORDERS

These are behavioral or psychological disorders associated with transient or permanent brain dysfunction.

Dementia

It is an acquired global impairment of intellect, memory and personality without impairment at consciousness level. Sundown phenomena is also common in dementia.

Sundown phenomena is characterized by drowsiness, confusion and ataxia. Accidental falls may also occur at night when external stimuli such as light and interpersonal orienting cues are diminished.

Causes of Dementia

- Alzheimer's disease
- Vascular dementia
- Frontotemporal dementia (Pick's disease)
- Head trauma
- Parkinson's disease
- Huntington's disease

Symptoms According to Stages

Stage I: Early Stage (2 to 4 Years)

- Forgetfulness
- Declining interest in the environment
- Hesitancy in initiating actions
- Poor performance at work.

Stage II: Middle Stage (2 to 12 Years)

- Progressive memory loss
- Hesitates in response to questions
- Has difficulty in following simple instructions
- Irritable, anxious
- Wandering
- Neglects personal hygiene
- Social isolation.

Stage III: Final Stage (Several Weeks to Several Years)

- Marked loss of weight because of inadequate intake of food
- Unable to communicate
- Does not recognize family
- Incontinence of urine and feces
- Losses the ability to stand and walk
- Death is unusually caused by aspiration pneumonia.

Treatment

- Psychosocial therapy
- Symptomatic treatment
- Pharmacological treatment
  - Memantine is the drug of choice nowadays.
  - Tacrine hydrochloride (Cognex); rarely used due to potential side effect of hepatotoxicity
  - Donepezil hydrochloride (Aricept)
  - Antipsychotics such as risperidone and haloperidol
  - Benzodiazepines for insomnia and anxiety
  - Antidepressants for depression
  - Anticonvulsants to control seizures.

KEY POINTS

- Presenile dementia occurs in younger person (<65 years). **Causes:** Alzheimer's disease, Pick's disease, Parkinson's disease.
- Senile dementia occurs after 65 years of age. **Cause:** Degenerative brain changes.
- In dementia, symptoms seem to worsen in the late afternoon and evening—a phenomenon termed sundowning.
- For a client with dementia, a complex task will be easier if it is broken down into series.

KEY POINTS

- Mini mental status examination is used to assess cognitive impairment
- Minimize the sensory stimulation. The rooms should be free from distractions, quiet and away from the noise of any activity.
- Speak directly to the client in a low frequency range and enunciate clearly.
- Confusion and disorientation may increase at night.
- If the client is verbally upset, listen briefly give support, then change the topic.
- Provide simple group activities. Encourage the client for group activities that are familiar and simple to perform.
- Assist the client as needed to maintain the daily functions and adequate personal hygiene.
- A complex task will be easier for the client if it is broken down into series.
- Sundowning: Nocturnal episodes of confusion with agitation, restlessness.

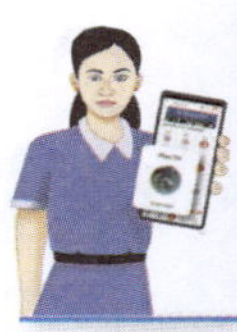

Delirium

It is an acute organic mental disorder characterized by impairment of consciousness (hallmark sign), disorientation and disturbances in perception and restlessness. Dementia can be differentiated from delirium by acute onset and lack of orientation.

Signs and Symptoms

- Impairment of consciousness
- Impairment of attention
- Perceptual disturbances (illusion, hallucination)
- Disturbance of cognition
- Psychomotor disturbances (Asterixis, tremor, unsteady gait)
- Disturbance of sleep wake cycle
- Insomnia at night and Drowsiness during day.
- Emotional disturbances—depression, anxiety, fear, irritability, euphoria and apathy

Treatment

- Identification of cause and its immediate correction
- Symptomatic measures—benzodiazepines or antipsychotics may be given.

Alzheimer's Disease

- Alzheimer's disease is the **most common cause of dementia**, a group of disorders that impairs mental functioning.
- More commonly seen in women than in men.
- Alzheimer's is progressive and irreversible disease.
- Memory loss is one of the earliest symptoms, along with a gradual decline of other intellectual and thinking abilities.

Symptoms of Alzheimer's Disease

- Difficulty in performing otherwise familiar tasks
- Memory loss that affects job skills
- Problems using language
- Disorientation to time and place
- Loss of good judgment
- Problems with abstract thinking
- Misplacing things
- Rapid mood swings
- Personality changes
- Loss of initiative, sleeping longer than usual, and loss of interest in the usual activities

Stages of Alzheimer's Disease

- **Stage 1:** Normal; mentally healthy person
- **Stage 2:** Normal and aged forgetfulness
- **Stage 3:** Mild cognitive impairment
- **Stage 4:** Mild Alzheimer's disease
- **Stage 5:** Moderate Alzheimer's disease
- **Stage 6:** Moderately severe Alzheimer's disease
- **Stage 7:** Severe Alzheimer's disease

Treatment

Memantine, galantamine, rivastigmine, donepezil, tacrine

SUBSTANCE USE DISORDERS

Disorders due to psychoactive substance use and refer to conditions arising from the abuse of alcohol, psychoactive drugs and other chemicals such as volatile solvents.

Types of Substance use are:

- Alcohol
- Opioids
- Cannabis
- Cocaine
- Amphetamines and other sympathomimetic
- Hallucinogens, for example, LSD, phencyclidine
- Sedatives and hypnotics for example barbiturates
- Inhalants, for example, volatile solvents
- Nicotine
- Other stimulants, for example, caffeine

Alcohol-Dependence Syndrome (ADS)

It refers to the use of alcoholic beverages to the point of causing damage to the individual, society or both.

Symptoms

- **Minor complaints:** Malaise, dyspepsia, mood swings or depression, increased incidence of infection.
- Secretive behavior (may attempt to hide disorder or alcohol supply)
- Tendency to blame others and rationalize problems
- Poor personal hygiene, untreated injuries
- Denial of problem
- Usually high tolerance for sedatives and opioids
- Consumption of alcohol containing products
- Nutritional deficiency (vitamin B1)

Phases of Alcoholism

- Pre-alcoholic symptomatic phase
- Prodromal phase
- Crucial phase
- Chronic phase.

Withdrawal Symptoms of Alcoholism

In persons who have been drinking over a prolonged period of time, any rapid decrease in the amount of alcohol in the body is likely to produce withdrawal symptoms. These are:

- Simple withdrawal syndrome
- Delirium tremens

Wernicke's Korsakoff's syndrome occurs due to **thiamine (vitamin B1)** deficiency that is caused by chronic alcohol abuse.

KEY POINTS

- ***Abuse:*** Maladaptive pattern of substance use that impairs health in a broad sense.
- ***Dependence:*** It refers to certain physiological and psychological phenomena induced by the repeated consumption of a substance.
- ***Tolerance:*** It is a state in which after repeated administration, a drug produces a decreased effect, or increasing doses are required to produce the same effect.
- ***Withdrawal state:*** A group of signs and symptoms recurring when a drug is reduced in amount or withdrawn, which last for a limited time.

Clinical Corner

CASE SCENARIO 4:

A 34-year-old male patient admitted into deaddiction unit begins to experience alcoholic hallucinosis. Which of the following is the best intervention at this time?

a. Restrain the patient in bed
b. Restrain the patient in bed and assess vital signs every 30 minutes
c. Discuss with the patient the content of hallucination
d. Provide quite environment and administer medications as prescribed

Ans. (d) Provide quite...

CASE SCENARIO 5:

A 32-yeard-old male patient has been admitted in the deaddiction unit for treatment of alcohol dependency. Which of the following client's possession need to be placed in a locked area?

a. Toothpaste
b. Medicated Shampoo
c. Aftershave lotion
d. Moisturizer lotion

Ans. (c) Aftershave lotion

Wernicke's syndrome: This is characterized by prominent cerebellar ataxia, **palsy of the 6th cranial nerve,** peripheral neuropathy, and mental confusion.

Korsakoff's syndrome: Gross memory disturbance (Irreversible in nature)

- Disorientation
- Confusion
- Confabulation (memory problem)
- Poor attention span and distractibility
- Impairment of insight

Management of Withdrawal Symptoms

- **Detoxification:** It is the treatment for alcohol withdrawal symptoms. The drugs of choice are benzodiazepines, for example,
  Chlordiazepoxide (80–200 mg/day in divided dose), Diazepam (40-80 mg/day)
- **Others:** For **vitamin B1 deficiency a preparation of vitamin B1** containing 100 mg of thiamine should be administered parenterally, twice daily for 3 to 5 days. This should be followed by oral administration of vitamin B1 for at least 6 months.
  - Administration of anticonvulsants is necessary, maintaining fluid and electrolyte balance, strict monitoring of vitals, level of consciousness and orientation.

Maintenance Therapy

Deterrent Agent (Disulfiram)

It is used to ensure abstinence in the treatment of alcohol dependence. It works on classical conditioning theory given by **Ivan Pavlov** (1936) and Operant conditioning theory of **BF Skinner** (1953).

- **Dose:** Initial dose is 500 mg/day orally for the first two weeks, followed by a maintenance dosage of 250 mg/day. It should not exceed 500 mg/day.
- **Indications:** It is used as an aversive conditioning treatment for alcohol dependence.

It is used mainly in patients who are highly motivated in quitting alcohol.

Informed consent is necessary before initiation of disulfiram therapy.

Disulfiram Ethanol Reaction (DER)

Disulfiram ethanol reaction is caused due to accumulation of acetaldehyde, as Disulfiram is an aldehyde dehydrogenase inhibitor that interferes with the metabolism of alcohol and produces acetaldehyde in blood. DER is characterized by nausea, throbbing headache, vomiting, hypotension, flushing, sweating, thirst, dyspnea, tachycardia, chest pain, vertigo, blurred vision and a sense of impending doom associated with severe anxiety.

Role of Nurse

- An informed consent should be taken before starting treatment.
- Ensure that at least 12 hours have elapsed since the last ingestion of alcohol before administering the drug.
- Patient must be instructed that ingestion of even the smallest amount of alcohol brings on a Disulfiram-Ethanol Reaction with all its unpleasant effects.
- Patient should also be warned against ingestion of any alcohol containing preparations such as cough syrups, drops of any kind, and alcohol containing foods and sauces.
- Caution patient against taking CNS depressants or any OTC drugs.
- Instruct patient to avoid driving or other activities requiring alertness until response to drug is known.
- Emphasize the importance of follow-up visits to the physician to monitor the progress in long-term therapy.
- Anticraving Agent: Acamprosate (333 mg) Enteric-coated capsule - two capsules, 3 times a day to maintain abstinence. It reduces craving for alcohol.

Psychosocial therapies

- Behavior therapy
- Group therapy (E.g. Alcoholic Anonymous)
- Motivational therapy

Opioid Dependence

Commonly used opioids are heroin (brown sugar and smack) and synthetic preparations like pethidine, fortwin and tidigesic.

Symptoms of Acute Intoxication

- Apathy
- Bradycardia
- Hypotension
- Respiratory depression
- Subnormal temperature
- Pinpoint pupils

Withdrawal Symptoms

- **Constricted pupil** (acute intoxication) and **dilated pupil** (in chronic use)
  - Watery eyes
  - Running nose
  - Yawning
  - Anorexia
  - Irritability
  - Tremors

Recent Question (NORCET 2023)

2. Opioid tolerance develops rapidly to all of the following, except:
a. Euphoria
b. Respiratory depression
c. Sedation
d. Constricted pupils

Ans. (d) Constricted pupils

Clinical Corner

CASE SCENARIO 6:
Nurse Linda is educating undergraduate college students regarding alcohol dependence. She is aware that sneaking drinks, rapidly gulping drinks, and preoccupation with alcohol are characteristics features at the stage of
a. Prealcoholic phase alcoholism
b. Early alcoholic phase alcoholism
c. Crucial phase of alcoholism
d. Chronic phase of alcoholism

Ans. (b) Early alcoholic phase alcoholism

CASE SCENARIO 7:
Nurse Linda is caring for a patient undergoing opiate withdrawal treatment. Which of the following drug is used during the withdrawal phase to minimize withdrawal effects of opiates
a. Flumazenil
b. Amphetamines
c. Methadone
d. Benzodiazepines

Ans. (c) Methadone

KEY POINT

World's "No Tobacco Day" is observed on 31st May.

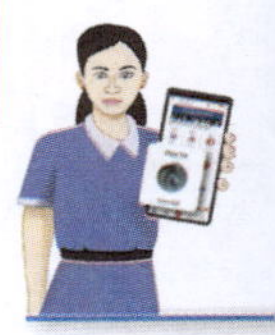

- Sweating
- Muscle cramps
- Nausea
- Diarrhea
- Insomnia
- Raised body temperature
- Piloerection
- Anorexia
- Constipation

Treatment

- **Overdose:** Narcotic antagonist, for example naloxone, naltrexone.
- **Detoxification:** Methadone, clonidine, naltrexone
- **Maintenance therapy**: Methadone, opioid antagonists (naltrexone and naloxone), psychotherapies.

SCHIZOPHRENIA

It is psychotic condition characterized by a disturbance in thinking, emotions, volitions and faculties in the presence of clear consciousness, which usually leads to social withdrawal.

Box 1: Schneider's first rank symptoms of schizophrenia (SFRS)

- Hearing one's thoughts spoken aloud
- Hallucinatory voices in the form of statement and reply
- Hallucinatory voices in the form of a running commentary
- Thought withdrawal
- Thought Insertion
- Thought Broadcasting
- Delusion Perception
- Somatic Passivity
- Made volition or acts
- Made impulses
- Made feelings or affect

Box 2: Nursing assessment criteria

- Collect history of organic brain syndrome.
- Collect history of psychoactive substance use disorder.
- Ensure comorbid psychiatric conditions, like Depression, Anxiety, Substance abuse, Aggression and Suicidal ideation.
- Collect treatment history.
- Assess for Auditory Voice heard. If yes, then record in detail about the voice content, reality, reactions and coping skills.
- Assess for Delusional behavior (false belief). If present, then ask in detail about the content, intentions to harm someone, plans to do so and the means to carry out the plans.
- Assess for insight into illness.
- Assess the patients current and premorbid level of functioning.

Table 9: Objective signs and symptoms of schizophrenia

Objective signs	Subjective symptoms
• **Withdrawal behavior** • **Hostility** • **Inappropriate communications** • **Psychomotor agitation** • **Catatonic rigidity** • **Stereotype behavior** • **Apathy** • **Ambivalence** • **Mutism** • **Inability to trust others**	• Hallucination • Illusions • Paranoid thinking • Anhedonia • Confusion • Ideas of reference • Thought blocking • Retarded thinking • Insomnia

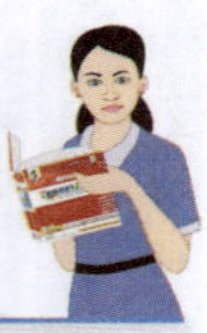

KEY POINT

World Schizophrenia Day is commemorated on **24 May** to increase awareness about the disorder and educate people about the challenges faced by the patients.

Clinical Corner

CASE SCENARIO 8:

A patient is admitted into psychiatric ward with a diagnosis of catatonic stupor. The nurse found the patient lying in a fetal position on the bed. Which of the following is the most appropriate intervention in this situation?

a. Take the client into recreation room to engage with other patients
b. Sit near the client in silence with occasional open-ended questions
c. Minimize the external stimuli and leave the client alone in the room
d. Encourage talking by asking direct close-ended questions

Ans. (b) Sit near the client...

CASE SCENARIO 9:

A 36-year-old male patient admitted into psychiatric ward has become overly aggressive. Which of the following nursing intervention is most appropriate when trying to diffuse a patient's impending violent behavior?

a. Put the patient into seclusion room
b. Help the patient to identify and express feelings of anxiety and anger
c. Involve the patient in a play activity to divert attention
d. Lock the client in isolation room

Ans. (b) Help the patient to...

Table 10: Nursing diagnosis framing

Symptoms	Nursing Diagnosis
Auditory Hallucinations	• Disturb sensory perception • Risk for violence to self or others
Delusions	• Disturb thought process • Ineffective health maintenance • Defensive coping
Alogia **Asociality** **Apathy** **Anergia** **Avolition**	• Impaired social interaction • Social isolation • Risk for loneliness • Ineffective coping • Self-care deficit (Hygiene, dressing, grooming, eating etc.)
Depression/Dysphoria **Ideas of worthlessness** **Poor drug Compliance**	• Low self esteem • Risk for self-directed violence • Non-adherence
Family Members – ignorant of illness, feel stressed or burdened	• Deficient knowledge • Compromised or ineffective family coping • Impaired family coping

Table 11: Nursing outcome criteria

Short-term goals	Long-term goals
Identify the presence of delusions and hallucinations. **Demonstrate decrease hallucinations.**	Identify the emotions and their origin. Eliminate pattern of delusional thinking. Verbalize plans to deal with hallucinations, if occur.
Identify the feelings (fear and anxiety) due to delusions and hallucinations.	Recognize and interprets feelings accurately.
Demonstrate trust in others. **Demonstrate decrease anxiety level.** **Demonstrate increased interest in self-care.**	Demonstrate improve reality orientation. Complete daily activity with minimum assistance.

Types

Table 12: Types of schizophrenia with their key features

Types of schizophrenia	Key points
Paranoid schizophrenia	Most common type of schizophrenia Presence of delusion, hallucination and false belief of grandeur Good prognosis No noticeable change in affect
Hebephrenic schizophrenia (Disorganized Schizophrenia)	Worst prognosis Disorganized thinking, flat affect, inappropriate emotions or behavior
Catatonic schizophrenia	Best prognosis Marked disturbance in motor behavior Rigid posture and waxy flexibility ECT and IV Lorazepam is the treatment of choice
Simple Schizophrenia	Worst prognosis after hebephrenic schizophrenia Predominantly negative symptoms Symptoms are mild and do not exhibit psychotic trait
Undifferentiated schizophrenia	When the patient cannot be categorized into other types
Residual Schizophrenia	It is characterized by past history of at least one episode of schizophrenia but person currently having no positive symptoms
Pfropf schizophrenia	Schizophrenia associated with mental retardation. Also known as grafted schizophrenia

Ref: Gajandra H. and Singh P. My PGMEE Notes. CBS Publishers and Distributors Pvt ltd.

KEY POINTS

- The term schizophrenia is coined by **Eugene Bleuler.**
- In schizophrenia, gradual subtle behavioral changes occur in the prodromal phase.
- Inability to maintain adequate boundaries is the feature of schizophrenic patients.
- Impaired insight is a common feature in Schizophrenia.
- The affect that is most commonly seen in patients with schizophrenia is apathy and flatness.
- Risperidone is the treatment of choice for patients with schizophrenia, who refuses to take treatment.
- Gradual onset is one of the poor prognostic factors in schizophrenia.
- Schizophrenia is more prevalent in lower socioeconomic status group
- Catatonic schizophrenia is the best prognosis
- Hebephrenic schizophrenia has got the worst prognosis
- Paranoid schizophrenia is the most common type of schizophrenia.

Recent Question (NORCET 2022)

3. According to Schneider, All of the following symptoms in schizophrenia patient are known as first rank symptoms, EXCEPT
a. Auditory hallucination
b. Visual hallucination
c. Thought echo
d. Thought broadcast

Ans. (b) Visual hallucination

Thought and Speech Disorders

- Autistic thinking
- Loosening of association
- Thought blocking
- Neologism
- Poverty of speech
- Poverty of ideation
- Echolalia
- Perseveration
- Verbigeration
- Delusions of various kinds

Disorders of Perception

- Auditory hallucination
- Visual hallucination

Disorders of Affect

- Apathy
- Emotional blunting
- Emotional shallowness
- Anhedonia
- In appropriate emotional response

Symptoms

- **Bleuler's four A's-**
    - **Affective disturbance:** Inability to show appropriate emotional responses (inappropriate), blunted or flattened affect.
    - **Autistic thinking:** The individual is unable to relate to others or to the environment. Preoccupation with the self, with little concern for external reality.
    - **Ambivalence:** It refers to contradictory or opposing emotions, attitude, ideas or desires for the same person, thing or situation simultaneous opposite feelings.
    - **Associative looseness:** Inability to think logically. The stringing together of unrelated topics.

Table 13: Positive and negative signs of schizophrenia

Positive signs	Negative signs (5 A's)
Delusions	**A**ffective flattening or blunting
Hallucinations	**A**volition—apathy
Excitement or agitation	**A**ttentional impairment
Hostility or aggressive behavior	**A**nhedonia
Suspiciousness, ideas of reference	**A**logia
Possible suicidal tendencies	

Treatment

- **Pharmacotherapy** includes antipsychotics such as clozapine, risperidone, olanzapine, quetiapine; other drugs are antidepressants, mood stabilizers, and benzodiazepines.
- ECT
- **Psychosocial therapies:** Group therapy, behavior therapy, social skills training, cognitive therapy, family therapy.

PERSONALITY DISORDERS

Personality disorders result when personality traits become abnormal, i.e. become inflexible and maladaptive, and cause significant social or occupational impairment or significant subjective distress.

Table 14: Prognosis factors of schizophrenia

Good Prognosis	Poor Prognosis
Female	Male
Old age of onset	Young age of onset
Positive symptoms	Negative symptoms
No family history of schizophrenia	Family history of Schizophrenia
Married	Unmarried
Good premorbid personality	Personality problems
Treatment compliance	Poor compliance with treatment
Rapid onset	Insidious onset
High IQ	Low IQ

Recent Question (NORCET 2022)

4. Schizophrenia life expectancy is_______ years less than the general population?

a. 1–2 years
b. 2–5 years
c. 8–10 years
d. 11–20 years

Ans. (c) 8–10 years

KEY POINTS

- **Schizophrenia** is the most severe of all psychiatric disorders.
- **Positive symptoms** are typical (hallucinations and delusions) and respond well to antipsychotics.
- **Negative symptoms** of schizophrenia (poor social adjustment, lack of motivation and withdrawal) are more disabling and respond poorly to antipsychotics.

Clinical Corner

CASE SCENARIO 10:

A 25-year-old male patient is diagnosed with dependent personality disorder. Which of the following behavior is most likely to be evidence of ineffective individual coping?

a. Deliberately avoiding relationships
b. Showing interest only in solitary activities
c. Inability to make choices and decisions on his own
d. Self-harming behavior

Ans. (c) Inability to make choices and decisions on his own

CASE SCENARIO 11:

A female client is diagnosed with schizotypal personality disorder is expected to exhibit which of the following signs during social situation?

a. Aggressive behavior
b. Emotional affect
c. Paranoid thoughts
d. Dependence

Ans. (c) Paranoid thoughts

Nursing interventions and responsibilities

- When patients are suspicious (paranoid), they may be afraid of everyone and every interaction around them. The nurse must communicate clearly, directly with simple statements.
- Distract the patients from delusional thoughts.
- Careful monitoring is important in delusional patients, to not harm to self and others.
- Discourage long discussions about irrational thinking.
- Use same staff as far as possible.
- Avoid physical contact in the form of touching the patient.
- Avoid laughing, whispering, or talking quietly where the patient can see but cannot hear what is being said.
- Encourage patient to express feelings as much as possible.
- Provide packed food and fruits if the patient is suspicious about food.
- Maintain structured schedule or routine for patients.
- Encourage patients for independent activities as far as possible.
- Maintain low level stimulation in the patient's environment.
- Remove all dangerous objects from the patients surrounding.
- Be alert for signs of increasing anxiety, fear, agitation so that intervention can be planned as early as possible, and harm can be prevented to self and others.
- Show acceptance attitude and unconditional positive regard.
- Provide positive reinforcement and recognition.
- Provide information to family about the patient's illness, treatment, and long-term prognosis.

Clinical Corner

CASE SCENARIO 12:

A 40-year-old female patient with borderline personality disorder requests the nurse to keep it confidential and then showed self-inflicted, superficial injuries on both forearms. Which of the following would be the best response by the nurse?

a. This is enough. I am putting you on suicide precautions.
b. I am going to inform your treating Doctor right now
c. The treating team should know when something like this occurs in treatment. I need to inform the treating team, but let's talk about it first.
d. Tell me what type of materials used to inflict injuries.

Ans. (c) The treating team should know when...

Types

Table 15: Types of personality disorders with characteristics features

Cluster	Personality disorder	Characteristics
Cluster A	Paranoid personality	Long-standing suspicious, hypersensitive, secretive, hostile and irritable
	Schizoid personality	Passive, seclusive, indifferent, cold and aloof
	Schizotypal personality	Odd thinking, peculiar language, bizarre thinking, idea of reference
Cluster B	Histrionic personality	Attention seeking, provocative, flamboyant, dramatic
	Narcissistic personality	Excessive self-admiration, self-importance, sense of grandiose, egocentric
	Borderline personality	Impulsive, manipulative, self-mutilative
	Antisocial personality	Aggressive, rule breaker, abusive, lying, theft
Cluster C	Avoidant personality	Overly serious, fears criticism, withdrawn, sensitive to rejection, inflexibility
	Dependent personality	Indecisive, submissive, clingy
	Obsessive compulsive personality	Perfectionist, rigid, passive-aggressive

Psychological Test for Assessment of Personality

Table 16: Objective and projective tests

Objective personality tests *(To determine the personality traits of a person)*	**Projective personality tests** *(Test reveals hidden emotions and internal conflicts projected by the person into the test)*
• Minnesota Multiphasic Personality Inventory [MMPI] • 16 Personality factor • Millon clinical multiaxial inventory [MCMI] • Eysenck personality questionnaire	• Draw a Person Test [DAPT] • Thematic Apperception Test [TAT] • Rorschach Inkblot Test • Sentence Completion Test [SCT]

Ref: Pg. No. 807 Table from My PGMEE NOTES (Hemant Gajendra)

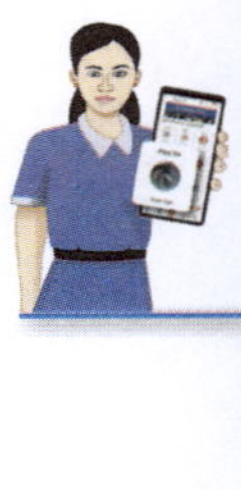

Treatment for Personality Disorders

Group therapy, occupational therapy, recreation therapy, interaction and guidance by therapist.

MOOD DISORDERS

- Mood disorder is a group of conditions where a disturbance in the person's mood is the main underlying feature.
- Common mood disorders are:
  - Depression
  - Hypomania and Mania
  - Bipolar Affective Disorder (BPAD)

Depression

An alteration in mood that is expressed by feelings of sadness, despair and pessimism. There is a loss of interest in usual activities and somatic symptoms may be evident. Change in appetite and sleep patterns are common.

Clinical Features

- Depressed mood
- Depressive cognitions
- Suicidal thoughts
- Psychomotor activity
- Psychotic features—Delusion and hallucinations
- Somatic symptoms—Decrease in appetite or weight, early morning awakening, diurnal variation, psychomotor agitation

Depression Classical Triad Includes

- Hoplessness
- Helplessness
- Worthlessness

Table 17: Common and other symptoms of depression

Common symptoms	Other symptoms
Apathy	Fatigue
Sadness	Thoughts of death
Sleep disturbances	Decreased libido
Hopelessness	Dependency
Helplessness	Spontaneous crying
Worthlessness	Passiveness

Treatment

- It includes use of antidepressants and various therapies such as cognitive behavioral therapy, interpersonal therapy and problem-solving therapy.
  ECT is the choice of treatment in severe depression or when patient does not respond to any other treatment.
- Antidepressant drugs of choice include selective serotonin reuptake inhibitors (SSRIs), Serotonin and norepinephrine reuptake inhibitors (SNRIs), Tricyclic antidepressants (TCAs), Tetracyclic antidepressants (TeCAs), Monoamine Oxidase inhibitors (MAOIs).

Mania and Hypomania

Mania refers to a syndrome in which the central features are over-activity, mood change and self-important ideas. ***It is characterized by pressure of speech, increased psychomotor activity and elevated mood.***

Hypomania is a lesser degree of mania. There is a persistent mild elevation of mood and increased sense of psychological well-being and happiness not in keeping with ongoing events.

Clinical Features

Elevated, Expansive or Irritable Mood

- **Euphoria (Stage I):** Mild elevation of mood; feeling of elevated mood and optimism; Usually present in hypomania.
- **Elation (stage II):** Moderate elevation of mood-feeling of confidence and enjoyment– seen in manic illness.
- **Exaltation (stage III):** Intense (severe) elevation of mood with delusions of grandiosity; usually seen in severe mania.
- **Ecstasy (Stage IV):** Very severe elevation of mood; a sense of extreme well-being. Usually seen in delirious and stuporous mania.

Psychomotor Activity

- Increased psychomotor activity ranging from activeness and restlessness to manic excitement.

Speech and Thought

- Flight of ideas
- Pressure of speech
- Delusion of grandeur
- Delusions of persecution
- Distractibility
- Poverty of thought

Clinical Corner

CASE SCENARIO 13:

A 30-year-old male patient diagnosed with major depression is admitted in the psychiatric unit. He spends majority of the day lying in bed with the sheet covering his head. Which of the following approaches by the nurse would be the most therapeutic for this patient?

a. Sit outside the client's room and wait for the client to get up
b. Initiate contact with the client frequently
c. Keep questioning the client until he responds
d. Wait until the client begins conversation on his own

Ans. (b) Initiate contact with the client frequently

CASE SCENARIO 14:

A 30-year-old male patient is admitted into the psychiatric ward. All of the following biological symptoms are associated with depression, except

a. Loss of appetite
b. Diurnal variation
c. Increased libido
d. Sleep disturbance

Ans. (c) Increased libido

KEY POINT

Omega sign

Ω

Omega sign is the characteristic feature of depression

Recent Question (NORCET 2021)

5. Which among the following causes the occurrence of symptoms of bipolar disorder?

a. Physical activity
b. Return on previous performance level of work
c. Reduced sleep
d. None of the above

Ans. (b) Return on previous performance level of work

Other Features

- Increased sociability
- Impulsive behavior
- Disinhibition
- Hypersexual and promiscuous behavior
- Poor judgment
- High risk activities
- Decreased need for sleep
- Decreased food intake
- Absence of insight (psychosis)
- The **characteristic triad** of symptoms include:
  - Elevated mood
  - Increased psychomotor activity
  - Flight of ideas.

Treatment

- Pharmacotherapy includes lithium carbonate 900–2100 mg/day), carbamazepine (600–1800 mg/day), sodium valproate (15–60 mg/kg/day).
- ECT
- Psychotherapies—Family and marital therapy.

Bipolar Affective Disorder (BPAD)

- Bipolar affective disorders (BPAD) is characterized by mood swings from episodes of profound depression to extreme euphoria (mania), with period of normalcy between episodes.
- The life-long prevalence rate of bipolar disorder is 0.3 to 1.5% (worldwide)
- Types of Bipolar disorders
  - **Bipolar I disorder:** Manic episodes that last at least 7 days, or by manic symptoms that are severe. Usually, depressive episodes occur as well, typically lasting at least 2 weeks.
  - **Bipolar II disorder**: pattern of depressive episodes and hypomanic episodes, but not the full-blown manic episodes that are typical of Bipolar I Disorder
- **Cyclothymic disorder**: chronic mood disturbance characterized by periods of hypomanic symptoms as well as periods of depressive symptoms lasting for at least 2 years' duration. However, the symptoms do not meet the diagnostic criteria for either depressive episode or hypomanic episode.
- **Causes:**
  - Biological
  - Biochemical (depression- decreased levels of norepinephrine and dopamine; Mania – increased levels of norepinephrine and dopamine)
  - Physiological (right-sided lesions in the limbic system)
  - Side effects of medication

Table 18: Signs and symptoms

Manic episode	Depressive episode
Heightened and grandiose mood	Feeling sad, hopeless and down
Exaggerated self esteem	Diminished self-esteem. Social inhibitions
Decreased need for sleep	Trouble falling asleep Wake up too early or sleep too much
Loss of appetite	Increased appetite and weight gain
Feeling of having superpower (delusion of grandiosity)	Feeling of helplessness and worthlessness
Pressured speech and flight of idea	Less social interaction
Risk taking behavior	Little interest in activities
Elated sexual interest	Loss of libido or sexual interest

- **Medical Management**
  - Psychotherapy: helps in decreased relapse rate and improved quality of life
  - Electroconvulsive therapy (ECT)
  - Activity – Regular exercise and develop regular schedule of major activities
- **Pharmacological management**
  - Mood stabilizers (Lithium is commonly used for both prophylaxis and treatment) - (discussed in detail under "psychopharmacology")
  - Anxiolytics
  - Antipsychotics
- **Nursing Management**
  - Provide a safe environment for client and others
  - Decrease environmental stimuli
  - Provide therapeutic communication
  - Promote socially acceptable, large motor activities such as arranging chairs in the ward/ hall
  - Monitor periodic serum lithium level
  - Adequate water and sodium intake to be maintained

Clinical Corner

CASE SCENARIO 15:

A 24-year-old male patient is admitted into psychiatry ward with a diagnosis of Mania. He has symptoms of delusions of grandiosity. This delusion reflects a belief that one is

a. Connected to whatever is happening around him
b. Cheating on him
c. Being killed or plotted to kill others
d. Highly powerful and famous

Ans. (d) Highly powerful and famous

CASE SCENARIO 16:

A 30-year-old female patient is admitted into a psychiatric ward with a diagnosis of bipolar disorder with aggressive social behavior. Nurse Linda is planning activities for this patient. All of the following activities can be included in the plan, Except

a. Writing
b. Chess
c. Finger painting
d. Walks with staff

Ans. (b) Chess

Explanation:

It can be difficult and challenging to try chess game with a patient with BPAD due to lack of attention span and concentration.

KEY POINTS

- Hyponatremia causes lithium toxicity
- The drug of choice for treatment and management of bipolar mania is lithium carbonate.
- Exposure to lithium early in pregnancy is associated with high risk of Ebstein anomaly in the baby.

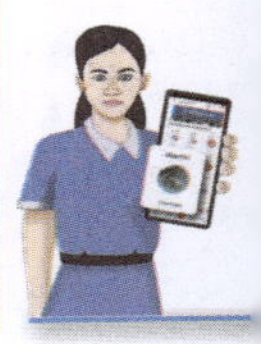

SOMATOFORM DISORDERS

It is characterized by repeated presentation with physical symptoms which do not have any physical basis and persistent request for investigation and treatment.

- **Somatization disorder:** Chronic multiple somatic complaints, unexplained by medical findings.
- **Hypochondriasis:** A persistent preoccupation with a fear or belief of having a serious disease.
- **Somatoform autonomic dysfunction:** In this disorder the symptoms are predominantly under autonomic control, as they were due to a physical disorder.
- **Persistent somatoform pain disorder:** The main feature of this disorder is persistent and severe pain without any physical basis. It may be of sufficient severity so as to cause social or occupational impairment.

STRESS AND ADAPTATION

Stress

- Stress is an adaptive response to a real or perceived threat to physical or psychological integrity of an individual.
- The term "stress" was first used by the endocrinologist ***Hans Selye (1930s)***
- Process which shows on-body responds to stress.

General Adaptation Syndrome (GAS)

- Hans Seyle (1936) termed the body's response to stressors as GAS –general adaptation syndrome.
- There are three stages of GAS:
  (i) Alarm stage
  (ii) Resistance stage
  (iii) Exhaustion stage

Alarm Stage

- It is the emergency response of the body in response to the stressor
- There is a **Flight or fight response**
- Mainly mediated by **sympathetic nervous system**

Resistance Stage

- If continuous stressor is present, body tries to resist the effects
- Hormonal responses of the body come to play (adreno-corticotropic-ACTH- axis) - Cortisol
- High level of Cortisol causes immune suppression, high BP

Exhaustion Stage

- Inability to defend against stressors
- Person may become ill or can even die (due to the high Cortisol) end of relationships

Acute Stress Disorder (ASD)

- Acute stress disorder develops within one month after an individual experiences or sees an event involving a threat or actual death, serious injury, or physical violation to the individual or others, and responds to this event with strong feelings of fear, helplessness or horror.
- Pharmacological treatment includes Anxiolytics, selective serotonin reuptake inhibitors (SSRI) and antidepressants.
- Cognitive behavior therapy may speed up recovery and may prevent ASD from turning into PTSD.

Post-Traumatic Stress Disorder (PTSD)

- Hyperarousal, re-experiencing image of the stressful events and avoidance of reminders.
- It is a reaction to extreme stressor such as floods, earthquakes, war, and rape.
- The symptoms develop after the latency period, within 6 months after the stress or may be delayed.
- Anxiolytics, SSRIs and antidepressants to relieve secondary symptoms.
- Psychotherapy includes cognitive therapy, exposure therapy and Eye Movement Desensitization and Reprocessing (EMDR).

PHOBIA

Phobia refers to a marked, intense and irrational fear or aversion toward something.

Classification of Phobic Disorder

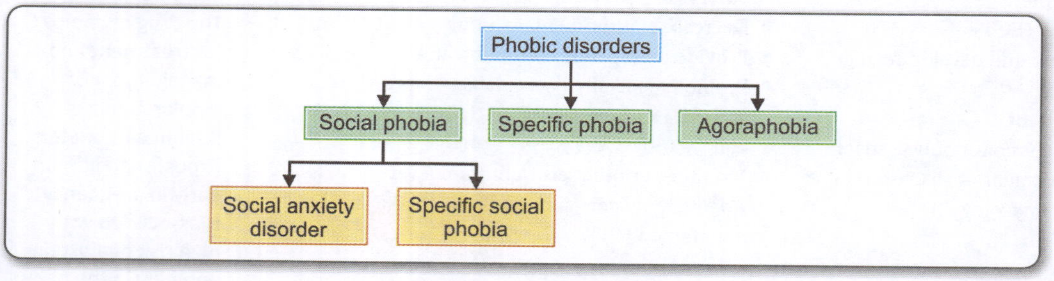

Figure 3: Types of phobic disorders

KEY POINTS

- **Alarm reaction, Resistance and Exhaustion** (in same sequence) are the three stages of General Adaptation Syndrome (GAS) of stress.
- Sympathetic nervous system is responsible for **Fight or Flight response.**
- The ability of a person to readily recover from stressful situations is called Resilience.
- **Nursing Intervention for PTSD:** Encourage the patient to verbalize thoughts and feelings about the trauma.
- Avoidance of stress is not possible but control over one's response to stress is possible.

Recent Question (NORCET 2022)

6. Post-traumatic stress syndrome (PTSD) may be experienced after
a. Divorce
b. Gunshot
c. Financial loss
d. All of above

Ans. (b) Gunshot

Clinical Corner

CASE SCENARIO 17:
Nurse Linda is caring a patient who is experiencing anxiety attack. Which of the following is the most appropriate nursing intervention in this scenario?
a. Turn on the television of music system
b. Stay with the patient and speak in short sentences
c. Ask the patient to engage in play activity with other patients
d. Leave the client alone until his anxiety diminishes

Ans. (b) Stay with the patient and speak...

Agoraphobia

- Fear of the marketplace
- Person experiences fear of being alone in places or situations from where escape may be difficult or immediate help may not be available.

Social Phobia (Social Anxiety Disorder)

- A person with social phobia has persistent, intense fear or anxiety about specific social situations because he/she believes that he/she may be judged, embarrassed or humiliated

Specific phobia: Irrational fear about a specific objects or situation

Classification of Specific Phobias

Table 19: List of specific phobias and their definition

Types of phobia	Definitions
Achluophobia	Fear of darkness
Acrophobia	Fear of heights
Agliophobia	Fear of pain
Aichmophobia	Fear of needles or pointed objects
Androphobia	Fear of men
Anginophobia	Fear of angina or choking
Anthophobia	Fear of flowers
Anthrophobia	Fear of people or society
Aphenphosmphobia	Fear of being touched
Arachnophobia	Fear of spiders
Arithmophobia	Fear of numbers
Astraphobia	Fear of thunder and lightening
Atychiphobia	Fear of failure
Monophobia	Fear of being alone
Bacteriophobia	Fear of bacteria
Belonephobia	Fear of needles
Bibliophobia	Fear of books
Botanophobia	Fear of plants
Cacophobia	Fear of ugliness
Chromophobia	Fear of colors
Claustrophobia	Fear of confined spaces
Cyberphobia	Fear of computers
Cynophobia	Fear of dogs
Domatophobia	Fear of houses
Ecophobia	Fear of the one's home
Ailurophobia	Fear of cats
Entomophobia	Fear of insects
Gamophobia	Fear of marriage
Glossophobia	Fear of speaking in public
Gynophobia	Fear of women
Heliophobia	Fear of the sun
Hemophobia	Fear of blood
Herpetophobia	Fear of reptiles
Homophobia	Fear of homosexuality

Contd...

KEY POINTS

- Systematic desensitization therapy is useful in the treatment of Phobias.
- Clients with a specific phobia typically use avoidance as a coping mechanism to deal with fear.

Clinical Corner

CASE SCENARIO 18:

Mr. Ramu has extreme fear of entering an elevator. He is being treated for claustrophobia with systematic desensitization. The nurse would consider the treatment successful if:

a. Ramu agrees to nurse that he will enter the elevator
b. Ramu verbalizes decreased fear of entering the elevator
c. Ramu enters the elevator for a brief period
d. Ramu recognizes that the fear is irrational

Ans. (c) Ramu enters the elevator for a brief period

Recent Question (NORCET 2022)

7. A 16-year-old client with anorexia nervosa is on an inpatient psychiatric unit. She has a fear of gaining weight and is refusing to eat sufficient amounts to maintain body weight for her age, height, and stature. To assist with the problem of powerlessness and plan for the client to no longer need to withhold food to feel in control, the nurse uses the following strategy:

a. Establish a structured environment with routine tasks and activities. Also, serve meals at the same time each day.

Contd...

Types of phobia	Definitions
Hydrophobia	Fear of water
Iatrophobia	Fear of doctors
Insectophobia	Fear of insects
Lockiophobia	Fear of childbirth
Mageirocophobia	Fear of cooking
Mysophobia	Fear of dirt and germs
Necrophobia	Fear of death or dead things
Noctiphobia	Fear of the night
Nosocomephobia	Fear of hospitals
Obesophobia	Fear of gaining weight
Ophidiophobia	Fear of snakes
Ornithophobia	Fear of birds
Pathophobia	Fear of disease
Pedophobia	Fear of children
Philophobia	Fear of love
Pyrophobia	Fear of fire
Somniphobia	Fear of sleep
Taphophobia	Fear of being buried alive
Thanatophobia	Fear of death
Trichophobia	Fear of hair
Venustraphobia	Fear of beautiful women
Verminophobia	Fear of germs
Wiccaphobia	Fear of witches and witchcraft
Xenophobia	Fear of strangers or foreigners
Zoophobia	Fear of animals.

Management

Pharmacological Management

- Anxiolytics. e.g. Benzodiazepines such as Alprazolam and Clonazepam
- **Antidepressants:** SSRI is the first-line treatment choice
- Antihypertensive agents (for symptom control), e.g. Propranolol and atenolol

Psychosocial Interventions

- Systematic desensitization (introduced by Joseph Wolpe in 1958): Patient is gradually exposed to anxiety-causing situation.
- **Flooding (implosion therapy):** Floods the client with triggering situation/stimuli.

OBSESSIVE COMPULSIVE DISORDER (OCD)

- **OCD** is repetitive, irresistative with unwanted thoughts and ritualistic action
- It is characterized by intrusive thoughts that produce uneasiness, apprehension, fear or worry (obsessions), repetitive behaviors aimed at reducing the associated anxiety (compulsions), or a combination of such obsessions and compulsions.
- Various types of obsessions include obsessional thoughts, obsessional images, obsessional rumination, obsessional doubts, obsessional impulses, obsessional rituals, obsessional slowness.
  Various types of compulsive acts such as washing, checking, knocking are common.
- Pharmacological treatment includes antidepressants including SSRIs. (Clomipramine, Fluvoxamine, Fluoxetine, Sertraline).
- ***Exposure and Response Prevention (ERP) and thought stopping is the most effective treatment.***

ADJUSTMENT DISORDER

- **Adjustment disorder** is a short-term condition that occurs when a person has great difficulty in

b. Distract the client during meals to get her to eat because she must take in sufficient amounts to keep from starving.
c. Do frequent room checks to be sure that the client is not hiding food or throwing it away.
d. Listen attentively and participate in in-depth discussions about food.

Ans. (a) Establish a structured environment...

Recent Question (NORCET 2022)

8. Most common area affected in trichotillomania is:
a. Scalp
b. Face
c. Arms
d. Eyelashes

Ans. (a) Scalp

Practice Question

6. A 28-year-old female patient is admitted into the psychiatric unit with a diagnosis of OCD. She spends most of the time during the day and night washing her hands. After a couple of days, she reported she feels better and more comfortable with the staff and other patients. The most appropriate nursing intervention for this patient is
a. Ignore the ritualistic behavior
b. Allow her to carry out the ritualistic behavior
c. Acknowledge the ritualistic behavior each time and reassure that it is inappropriate.
d. Collaborate with the patient to minimize the amount of time she engages in ritualistic behavior.

Ans. (d) Collaborate with the patient to minimize the amount of time she engages in ritualistic behavior.

coping with, or adjusting to, a particular source of stress. This conduct disorder usually occurs within one month of significant life change.
- Duration of the disorder is usually less than one month.
- It is characterized by predominant disturbance of emotions.
- **Treatment:** Anxiolytics and antidepressants.

EATING DISORDERS

Eating disorders are psychological disorders characterized by abnormal or disturbed eating habits and severe distress or concern about body weight and shape. Eating disorders includes
- Anorexia nervosa
- Bulimia nervosa
- Binge eating disorder

Anorexia Nervosa

- Inadequate food intake leading to visible weight loss.
- Intense fear of weight gain, obsession with weight and persistent behavior to prevent weight gain.

Signs and Symptoms

- Amenorrhea, excessive weight loss, lanugo (fine body hair), abdominal distention, dry hair, and electrolyte disturbances. Nail biting is common.
- Poor self-esteem related to body image.
- Inability to appreciate the severity of the situation.

Treatment

- Neuroleptics, appetite stimulants, antidepressants.
- Individual psychotherapy, behavioral therapy, cognitive behavioral therapy, family therapy.

Bulimia Nervosa

- Frequent episodes of consuming very large amount of food followed by behaviors to prevent weight gain, such as self- induced vomiting.
- A feeling of being out of control during the binge-eating episodes.
- Self-esteem overly related to body image.

Treatment

Psychotherapy, SSRI and Self-help group.

Binge Eating Disorder

- Frequent episodes of consuming very large amounts of food but without behaviors to prevent weight gain, such as self- induced vomiting.
- A feeling of being out of control during the binge eating episodes.
- Feelings of strong shame or guilt regarding the binge eating.

Treatment

Cognitive therapy, interpersonal therapy, anti-depressants, and self-help group.

Nursing Intervention

- Monitor the patient during mealtimes and for a period of one hour after meals
- Identify the patient's elimination pattern to prevent self-induced vomiting
- Establish a minimum weight goal and daily nutritional requirements
- Maintain intake output chart and electrolyte balance
- Encourage patient to verbalize his feelings
- Avoid discussions that focuses on food
- Engage patient in therapeutic alliance to obtain commitment to treatment
- Set a time limit for food
- Explain the complication
- Provide assertiveness training
- Assess the suicide potential.

SLEEP DISORDERS

Physiology of Sleep

Sleep is a state of unconsciousness in which the brain is relatively more responsive to internal than external stimuli. Major sleep center in the body is hypothalamus.

Stages of Sleep

- Stages of sleep are defined based on the patterns of EEG (Electroencephalogram)

Stage 1

- Non-Rapid Eye Movement (NREM) Sleep (Orthodox sleep or Synchronized or 'S' sleep)
  - Further divided into Stage 1, Stage 2, Stage 3, and Stage 4 sleep
  - EEG
    - **Stage 1:** Theta waves (Hypnogogic state)
    - **Stage 2:** Theta waves (Sleep Spindles)
    - **Stage 3:** Delta waves
    - **Stage 4:** Delta waves (**Bed wetting, Night terrors, sleep walk/talk**)

Stage 2

- **Rapid Eye Movement (REM) sleep** (Paradoxical sleep or Desynchronized or 'D' sleep)
  - After 90 minutes of sleep onset → 1st REM episode
  - **EEG: Mimic beta waves**
  - **Associated with dreaming**
  - Difficult to arise
  - Increased/Irregular HR, RR and BP
  - Penile erection or clitoris engorgement
  - Muscle twitches

KEY POINTS

- Neurotransmitter serotonin plays a role in the psycho-pathology of OCD
- **Obsessive thoughts:** Most common obsessive thought is fear of being contami-nated by germs or dirt.
- **Compulsive behaviors:** E.g. spending a lot of time on washing and cleaning. Excessive double-checking of things, such as locks and appliances. Ordering or arranging things.
- Medication with a serotonin reuptake inhibitor is helpful for many OCD patients

Clinical Corner

CASE SCENARIO 19:
Nurse Linda is assessing a 16-year-old adolescent female who reports weight loss, amenorrhea, and depression. Which of the following additional information reported by the client suggests that she has an eating disorder?

a. Wearing tight-fitting clothing
b. Excessive and ritualized exercise
c. Skin appears oily
d. Elevated blood pressure

Ans. (b) Excessive and...

CASE SCENARIO 20:
A 15-year-old adolescent girl with anorexia nervosa has been admitted to the psychi-atric unit. She refuses to eat. Which of the following is the most appropriate response by the nurse?

a. Why do you think you're fat? You are extremely underweight.
b. You can choose whether to eat or not.
c. I hope you will eat your food by mouth. Tube feedings and I.V. lines can be uncomfortable.
d. You don't have to eat if you don't like to eat.

Ans. (c) I hope you will eat...

Circadian Rhythm

- Sleep/wake cycle of body that goes through 24-hour cycle
- It is a natural cycle of physical, mental and behavioral changes in a body.
- **Polysomnography**, also called a sleep study, is a test used to diagnose sleep disorders.

Sleep Disorders

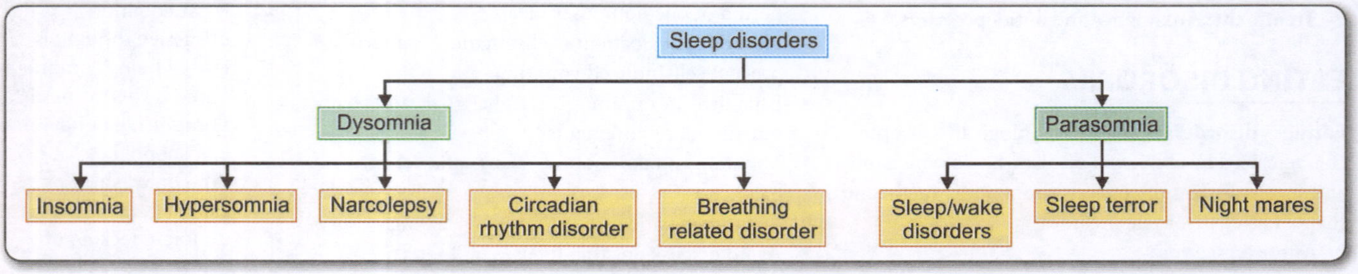

Figure 4: Types of sleep disorders

Dysomnia

Insomnia

- Difficulty in initiating or maintaining sleep.
- Insomnia is the **most common sleep disorders**.
- **Management**: Melatonin, L-Tryptophan, Short acting benzo-diazepines, Zolpidem, etc.

Hypersomnia

- Excessive amount of sleep, excessive day time sleepiness or both.
- **Management**: Non-Sedating SSRI, Stimulant drugs.

Narcolepsy

- It is a chronic sleep disorder characterized by excessive daytime drowsiness and sudden attacks of sleep.
- Uncontrollable sleepiness leading to 10-20 mins of sleep at inappropriate times.
- **Management**: Dexamphetamine, Modafinil, Methylphenidate.

Obstructive Sleep Apnea Syndrome

- Insomnia caused by sleep-related breathing disturbances such as apnea, hypopnea, etc.
- **Management**: encourage weight loss, **CPAP**, treat the cause of respiratory obstruction.

Circadian Rhythm Sleep Disorder

- **Jet lag type:** Difficulty in initiating or maintain sleep. Resolves in 2–7 days without treatment
- **Delayed sleep phase:** Late onset of sleep. (2 am)
- **Shift work type:** excessive sleepiness, symptoms of insomnia
- **Management:** Chronotherapy – Adopt regular waking time. Melatonin and short-acting Benzodiazepines.

Restless Leg Syndrome (Ekbom's Syndrome)

- Painful condition leads to severe insomnia and periodic limb movement during sleep
- **Causes:** Vit B12 deficiency, Anemia
- Aggravated by caffeine, stress or fatigue
- **Management**: Ropinirole, Clonazepam, L-Dopa, Carbidopa, Bromocriptine, Vit B12 supplement.

Kleine-Levin Syndrome

Characterized by Megaphagia, Hypersomnolence, and sexual disinhibition.

Parasominias

- Abnormal behavior associated with sleep/wake cycle or stages
- Includes night mares, sleep walk/talk, or night terror
- **Causes:** PTSD, fever, psychotropic drugs, alcohol intoxication
- **Management**: Sleep hygiene measures, Benzodiazepines or antidepressants

SEASONAL AFFECTIVE DISORDER

Seasonal Affective Disorder (SAD), also known as **winter depression,** winter blues, summer depression, summer blues, or seasonal depression, are mood disorders in which people who have normal mental health throughout the year experience depressive symptoms in the winter or summer. Seasonal depression is because of stop breakdown of melatonin. Sunlight therapy is helpful to treat seasonal depression.

KEY POINTS

- Non-REM sleep has 4 stages
- REM sleep is associated with sleep paralysis and nightmares
- REM sleep normally cycles every 90 minutes during a night of sleep and may last 20 to 25 minutes
- Most vivid dreams occur during REM sleep.
- Restless leg syndrome can be caused by Vitamin B12 deficiency and renal disease.
- Ropinirole is the drug of choice for Restless Leg Syndrome.
- Excessive day time sleepiness is known as narcolepsy.

KEY POINT

Dreams occur in both NREM and REM. but dreams of REM are vivid and more elaborative.

SEXUAL DISORDERS

Disorder of Preference

- **Transvestism**: Sexual arousal occurs by wearing clothes of the opposite sex.
- **Sexual sadism**: The person is sexually aroused by physical and psychological humiliation, suffering, or injury of the sexual partner.
- **Sexual masochism**: Here the person is sexually aroused by physical or psychological humiliation or injury inflicted to self by other.
- **Exhibitionism**: In this the person is sexually aroused by the exposure of one's genitalia to an unsuspecting stranger.
- **Voyeurism**: This is a persistent or recurrent tendency to observe unsuspecting person naked (usually of the other sex) and engaged in sexual activity.
- **Pedophilia:** It is characterized by persistent or recurrent involvement of an adult in sexual activity with prepubertal children.
- **Zoophilia**: Involving in sexual activity with animals.

Sexual Dysfunction

- **Frigidity**: Absence of desire for sexual activity.
- **Impotence**: This disorder is characterized by an inability to have or sustain penile erection till the completion of satisfactory sexual activity.
- **Premature ejaculation:** Ejaculation before the completion of satisfactory sexual activity of both partners.
- **Nonorganic vaginismus:** An involuntary spasm of lower 1/3rd of vagina, interfering with coitus.
- **Nonorganic dyspareunia:** Pain in the genital area of either male or female during coitus which is not having any ruled out organic cause.

ELECTROCONVULSIVE THERAPY (ECT)

Electroconvulsive therapy was first introduced by **Bini** and **Cerletti** in April 1938. From 1980 onwards ECT is being considered as a unique psychiatric treatment. ECT also known as electroshock therapy or shock therapy. It is a form of somatic treatment/ physical therapy.

Voltage: 70–120 volts
Duration: 0.7–1.5 seconds
Frequency: 3 times per week or as indicated
Total number: 6–10 up to 25 may be preferred as indicated
Indications: Major depression, severe catatonia, severe psychosis, organic mental disorder
Contraindication: Raised ICP (absolute contraindication), congestive heart failure, cerebral hemorrhage, retinal detachment, pneumonia, acute myocardial infarction, brain tumor, cerebral aneurysm.

- **Drugs used**
  - Inj. Succinyl choline 0.5 mg/kg (Muscle relaxant)
  - Inj. Thiopentone sodium 3 mg/kg (Anesthetic).
  - Inj. Atropine 0.4–1.0 mg IV or 0.3 mg - 0.6 mg IM (To reduce respiratory secretions and prevent aspiration).

Nursing responsibilities: Informed consent, empty stomach before for 4–6 hours prior to ECT, hold the medication that can increase the threshold of seizure, head shampoo, environment preparation oxygen, suction, medication, monitors. Side lying position after ECT is advised to prevent aspiration.

- **Side effects**
  - Headache and short-term memory loss

Practice Question

7. The phosphodiesterase type 5 inhibitors (PDE-5i) are useful in treatment of which of the following sexual disorders?

a. Paraphilias
b. Gender Identity Disorders
c. Transvestism
d. Male erectile disorder

Ans. (d) Male erectile disorder

Clinical Corner

CASE SCENARIO 21:
A 35-year-old female patient is scheduled for an Electroconvulsive Therapy (ECT). Presence of which of the following condition is absolutely contraindicated for ECT?

a. Hemophilia
b. History of seizures
c. Space occupying lesions in brain
d. Second semester pregnancy

Ans. (c) Space occupying lesions in brain

CHILDHOOD PSYCHIATRIC DISORDERS

Table 20: The childhood psychiatric disorders

Autistic disorder	Rett's disorder	Childhood disintegrative disorder	Asperger's disorder
• Also called **EARLY INFANTILE AUTISM/ KANNER'SAUTISM** • Biological causation onset prior to 3 years of age	• Mutation of Mecp2 gene is involved in maximum cases • It is a genetic brain disorder/ neurodevelopmental disorder	• Also called **Heller's Syndrome/Disintegrative Psychosis** • Shows at least 2 years of normal development	• There is qualitative impairment in social interactions with stereotyped and repetitive behavior
• Mental retardation seen in 2/3rd of patients • Absent social smile • Psychological intervention is the mainstay of treatment	• It most commonly affects girls after 6 - 18 months of age • Normal prenatal and perinatal development with normal motor development in first 5 months after birth	• Significant loss of previously acquired skills • Associated with tuberous sclerosis and epilepsy	• As per DSM-V, it is a part of Autism Spectrum Disorder (ASD) • Also known as "High Functioning" type of ASD

Contd...

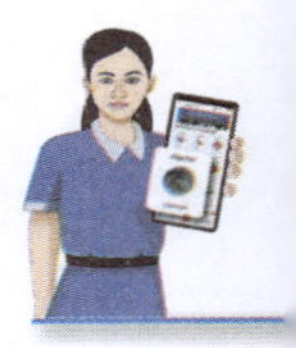

Autistic disorder	Rett's disorder	Childhood disintegrative disorder	Asperger's disorder
	• Normal head circumference at birth and more common in females • There is deceleration of head growth • Development of stereotyped hand movements and poorly coordinated gait and drunk moments • Treatment is physiotherapy for muscular dysfunction anticonvulsants for seizures and behavior therapy+ medications to control self-injurious behavior		

Ref: My PGMEE Notes (Hemant Gajendra) page no. 810

ATTENTION DEFICIT HYPERACTIVE DISORDER (ADHD)

Also known as **hyperkinetic disorder** is persistent pattern of in attention and or hyperactivity. Characterized by neurological disorder, developmentally inappropriate inattention, impulsiveness and in some cases, hyperactivity.

Treatment

- **Drugs**
  - Stimulants, e.g., Methylphenidate (Ritalin), Amphetamine. **Ritalin** is the drug of choice in ADHD
- Behavioral modification technique.
- Cognitive behavior therapy.
- Social skills training.
- Family education.

MENTAL RETARDATION (INTELLECTUAL DISABILITY)

Intellectual disability (ID), also known as general learning disability and mental retardation (MR), is a generalized neurodevelopmental disorder characterized by significantly impaired intellectual and adaptive functioning.

Etiology

- **Down's Syndrome:** Caused due to trisomy 21 (extra chromosome 21)
- **Phenylketonuria (P.K.U)**
- **Maple syrup urine disease**
- **Cat cry syndrome:** Absence of 5 chromosomes
- **Lead poisoning**
- **Maternal age:** >35 yrs has more chances of abnormalities
- **Problems during pregnancy**
- Birth trauma, hypoxia, cord around neck, very low birth weight, brain infections, head injury, cerebral palsy

Levels of Mental Retardation

Table 21: Levels of mental retardation with their characteristics

Types	IQ level	Characteristics
Mild MR	50–70	• Includes 85% of MR population • Many adults with mild MR can live independently with appropriate support
Moderate MR	35–50	• Includes 10% MR population • They are challenged academically • Often are unable to achieve above second to third grade level in academics • Can lead relatively normal lives with supervision
Severe MR	20–35	• Includes about 3–4% of MR population • Often learns to count as well as recognize words that are critical to functioning • Often master the most basic skills of living, e.g. cleaning and dressing themselves • They live in groups
Profound MR	Less than 20	• Includes 1-2% of MR population. • Most individuals may be taught some self-care skills and learn to communicate their needs given the appropriate training.

Clinical Corner

CASE SCENARIO 22:
A child diagnosed with ADHD is displaying disruptive behaviors at home. The most appropriate advice to the parents regarding the treatment plan for the social domain is

a. Instruct the child to complete homeworks assignment at a time.
b. Establish eye contact before giving directions.
c. Initiate a token system, to reward the child for appropriate behavior.
d. Maintain a predictable environment in the home.

Ans. (c) Initiate a token...

CASE SCENARIO 23:
Which of the following intervention would be most effective in changing the behavior of a child with attention deficit hyperactivity disorder (ADHD)?

a. Use punishment to control unwanted behavior
b. Use sedatives to control acting out behavior
c. Reward appropriate behavior of the child
d. Use lengthy time-out session

Ans. (c) Reward appropriate behavior of the child

Assessment of IQ

- A normal individual has IQ between 90 and 110.

Calculating IQ

$$= \frac{\text{Mental Age}}{\text{Chronological Age}} \times 100 = \text{IQ}$$

For example, a 10-year-old that tested at a 12 year old mental age would have an IQ of 120

$$= \frac{12}{10} \times 100 = 120$$

- An intelligence quotient (IQ) is a total score derived from several standardized tests designed to assess human intelligence.
- Standard IQ Tests
  - Stanford-Binet test
  - Wechsler Adult Intelligence Scale (WAIS)
  - Raven color progressive matrices
  - Vineland social maturity scale (for blind deaf and dumb)
  - Seguin form board test (for illiterate patients)

Signs and Symptoms

- Delays in oral language development and memory skills
- Difficulty in learning social rules and problem solving skills
- Lack of social interests
- Delays in the development of adaptive behavior such as self-help or self care skills
- Behavioral problems associated with MR are restlessness, poor concentration, impulsiveness, temper-tantrum, irritability, crying and self injurious behavior (head banging).

Prevention

- Antenatal counselling and screening

MANAGEMENT

- Training on self-care and life skills
- Training in vocation
- Family support and parental teaching.

LEARNING DISABILITIES AND DISORDERS (SPECIFIC LEARNING DISORDER)

- As per DSM-5, Children with learning disability have difficulties in at least one of the following:
  - Difficulty in reading, spelling, understanding the meaning, written expression, number concepts, mathematical reasoning.
- Specific learning disorder (learning disorder or learning disability) is a neurodevelopmental disorder that begins during school-age.
- Approximately 5 to 15 percent of school-age children struggle with a learning disability
- One third of people with learning disabilities also have ADHD

Types of Learning Disorders

- **Dyslexia**: refers to the difficulty with reading. Reading becomes slow and effortful.
- **Dysgraphia**: Difficulties in writing one's thought on paper. It interferes with spelling, word spacing, grammar and punctuations.
- **Dyscalculia**: Difficulties in arithmetic (maths) calculations.

Management

- Strengthening the skills
- Developing a learning strategy tailored to take advantage of a child's strengths.

PSYCHOPHARMACOLOGY

Antipsychotics

These are used to treat psychotic symptoms. Also known as **neuroleptic drugs** as they produce neurological side effect, major tranquilizer, D_2 receptor blockers and anti-schizophrenia drugs. Chlorpromazine is the first and oldest antipsychotics.

Typical Antipsychotic (First Generation)

Drug	Dose
• **Phenothiazines**	
▪ Chlorpromazine	40–800 mg
▪ Perphenazine	12–64 mg
▪ Fluphenazine	1–40 mg
▪ Thioridazine	150–800 mg
• **Thioxanthenes**	
▪ Thiothixene:	6–30 mg
• **Butyrophenones**	
▪ Haloperidol	1–100mg
• **Dibenzothiazepine**	

Atypical Antipsychotics (Second Generation)

Drug	Dose
• Clozapine	300–900 mg
• Risperidone	4–16 mg
• Olanzapine	5–20 mg
• Quetiapine	150–750 mg

Newer drugs: Aripiprazole and blonanserine

Side Effects

- **Anticholinergic effects**
  - Dry mouth, blurred vision, constipation, urinary retention
- Nausea, skin rash, sedation
- Orthostatic hypotension
- Photosensitivity

Clinical Corner

CASE SCENARIO 24:
Nurse Linda is assessing an infant in a genetic clinic. She knows that flattened nasal bridge, short neck, upward slanting eyes, epicanthal folds and transverse palmar creases are the features of a child with ....

a. Angelman syndrome
b. Prader–Willi syndrome
c. Down syndrome
d. Edward's syndrome

Ans. (c) Down syndrome

CASE SCENARIO 25:
A 10-year-old child is admitted into psychiatric ward with Tourette's syndrome. Which of the following conditions is least likely to be associated with Tourette's syndrome?

a. OCD
b. Learning Difficulties
c. Mental retardation
d. ADHD

Ans. (c) Mental retardation

Practice Question

8. Atypical antipsychotics are likely to cause less extrapyramidal side effects in comparison to typical antipsychotics. All of the following drugs are atypical antipsychotics, except

a. Risperidone
b. Quetiapine
c. Fluphenazine
d. Olanzapine

Ans. (c) Fluphenazine

Clinical Corner

CASE SCENARIO 26:
A patient with schizophrenia is on Clozapine. Due to the potential side effect of this drug, the nurse should observe for which of the following symptoms in this patient?

a. Obesity
b. Mood swings
c. Fever and sore throat
d. Renal impairment

Ans. (c) Fever and sore...

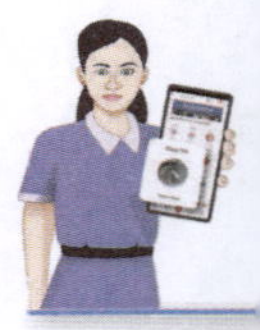

- **Hormonal effects**
  - Decreased libido, retrograde ejaculation, gynecomastia, amenorrhea, weight gain.
- **ECG changes:** Prolongation of the QT interval are possible with most of the antipsychotics.
- Reduction of seizure threshold.
- **Agranulocytosis and hypersalivation**
  - **Clozapine:** Weekly/biweekly blood investigation but more effective in treating treatment-resistant schizophrenia
- **Extrapyramidal symptoms (EPS)**
  - Pseudoparkinsonism
    - Tremor, shuffling gait, drooling, rigidity
    - 1–5 days after initiation of antipsychotics
  - Akinesia
  - Akathisia: Restlessness characterized by inability to sit still (50–60 days after initiation of therapy)
  - Dystonia: Men; older than 25 years of age
    - **Acute Dystonia:** Sustained muscle contraction frequently causing twisting, repetitive movement or abnormal posture
  - Oculogyric crisis
    - Treated as emergency
    - Physician should be contacted immediately
    - **Management:** IV benztropine mesylate
  - **Tardive dyskinesia:** Continuous movement of mouth, tongue and jaw.
- **Neuroleptic malignant syndrome (NMS)**
  - Severe Parkinsonian muscle rigidity
  - Body temperature up to107° F, tachycardia, tachypnea
  - Fluctuations in blood pressure, diaphoresis, and rapid dete-rioration of mental status to stupor and coma
  - This is rare but potentially fatal complication of treatment with neuroleptic drugs
  - It may precipitate within hours – years after drug initiation
    - Discontinue neuroleptic immediately.
    - **Management:** Bromocriptine or dantrolene.

Antiparkinsonian Drugs for Drug Induced Extrapyramidal Symptoms (EPS)

- **Anticholinergics**
  - **Benztropine:** 0.5–9 mg
  - **Biperiden:** 2–8 mg
  - **Procyclidine:** 5–20 mg
  - **Trihexyphenidyl:** 1–15 mg
- **Antihistamines**
  - **Diphenhydramine:** 10–400 mg
- **Dopaminergic agents**
  - **Amantadine:** 200–400 mg
  - **Bromocriptine:** 10–40 mg

Antidepressants

These are the drugs, which are used for the treatment of the depressive illness. Also known as **mood elevators** or thymoleptics.

Monoamine Oxidase Inhibitors (MAOI)

For example, Phenelzine, Tranylcypromine, Selegiline

Side Effects

Nausea, Headache, stiff neck and dry mouth.

Caution

Avoid tyramine containing food items (i.e. red meat, wine, liver, dried fish, chicken, chocolate, beer and coffee) in a patient who is getting MAOI to prevent hypertensive crisis.

Tricyclic Antidepressants (TCAs)

- NA + 5-HT reuptake inhibitors
  - Imipramine, Amitriptyline, Trimeprazine,
- Doxepin, Dothiepin, Clomipramine
  - Predominantly NA reuptake inhibitors
    - Desipramine, Nortriptyline, Amoxapine

Side Effects

- Dry mouth, bad taste, constipation, epigastric distress, urinary retention, blurred vision, palpitation, sedation, mental confusion, and weight gain.
- Some patients may switch to hypomania or mania
- Sweating and fine tremors are relatively common
- Seizure threshold is lowered fits may be precipitated
- Postural hypotension, especially in older patients

Selective Serotonin Reuptake Inhibitors (SSRI)

- Fluoxetine, Fluvoxamine, Paroxetine, Sertraline, Citalopram.

Clinical Corner

CASE SCENARIO 27:

The severe feeling of restlessness and an urge to move produced by some psychotropic medications, which is often misinterpreted by patients as anxiety or a recurrence of psychiatric symptoms, is known as

a. Myoclonus
b. Akinesia
c. Akathisia
d. Neuroleptic malignant syndrome.

Ans. (c) Akathisia

CASE SCENARIO 28:

Which of the following food and drug combination may lead to hypertensive crisis?

a. Cheese and Ergotamine
b. Beer and Reserpine
c. Coffee and Dopamine
d. Smoked fish and Phenelzine

Ans. (d) Smoked fish and Phenelzine

Explanation:

Phenelzine is a non-selective and irreversible monoamine oxidase inhibitor (MAOI). Ingestion tyramine containing food such as smoked meat or fish with phenelzine can precipitate hypertensive crisis.

KEY POINT

It is recommended to take Sertraline at the same time of each day preferably in the evening.

KEY POINTS

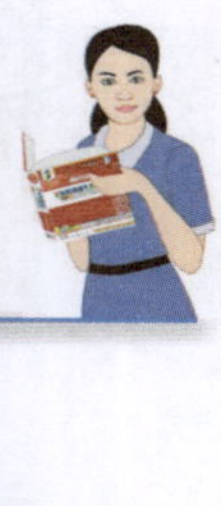

- First generation antipsychotics known as Typical Antipsychotic was discovered in 1950
- Chlorpromazine (typical antipsychotic) was discovered in 1950 and was the first antipsychotic drug
- Second generation antipsychotics known as Atypical Antipsychotic in which Clozapine was discovered in 1950 and introduced clinically in 1970.
- Anticholinergics (e.g. Benztropine) are used to treat Extra-pyramidal symptoms (EPS)
- The major side effect of Clozapine is agranulocytosis. So periodical Complete Blood Count is suggested.
- EPS is most common with Fluphenazine and Haloperidol
- Orthostatic hypotension is most common with Chlorpromazine, Thioridazine, and Clozapine.

Side Effects

Dry mouth, insomnia, restlessness, agitation, difficulty reaching orgasm, erectile dysfunction.

Atypical Antidepressants

Trazodone, Mianserin, Mirtazapine, Venlafaxine, Tianeptine, Amineptine, Bupropion.

Side Effect

Dry mouth, nervousness and seizure at high dose.

Anxiolytics

- Anxiolytics are mostly mild CNS depressants which are aimed to control the symptoms of anxiety
- The anxiolytic-sedative drugs are more closely resemble sedative-hypnotics
- They do not produce extrapyramidal side effects

Classification

Benzodiazepines

- Diazepam (5–30 mg/day; Valium, calmpose)
- Chlordiazepoxide (20–100 mg/day; Librium, equilibrium)
- Oxazepam (30–60 mg/day in 2–3 divided portions; Serepax)
- Lorazepam (1–6 mg/day; Larpose, ativan, Calmese)
- Alprazolam (0.25–1.0mg tds up to 6 mg/day in panic disorder; Alprax, alzolam)

Mechanism of Action

Benzodiazepines act preferentially on midbrain ascending reticular formation and on limbic system

Indications

- Generalized anxiety disorders
- Panic anxiety disorders
- Anxiety disorders with or without depressive symptoms

Side Effects

- Drowsiness
- Sedation
- Confusion
- Dependence and withdrawal symptoms
- Sexual dysfunction

Azapirones

- **Buspirone (5–15 mg OD-TDS; Anxipar, Buspin), Gepirone**
- Ispapirone

Sedative Antihistaminic

Hydroxyzine (100-200 mg/day; Atarax 10, 25 mg tab)

Beta Blocker

Propranolol

Mood Stabilizers

Mood stabilizers are used for the treatment of bipolar affective disorders, more commonly used mood stabilizers are: lithium carbonate, carbamazepine and sodium valproate.

Lithium Carbonate

- **Dose:** In acute mania—900–2100 mg/day in 2-3 divided dose
- Serum Therapeutic level: 0.8–1.2 mEq/L
- Prophylactic level: 0.6–1.2 mEq/L
- Toxic lithium level: >2.0 mEq/L

Side Effect

- **Adverse reactions:** below 1.5 mEq/L.
- **Mild to moderate adverse reactions:** 1.5–2.5 mEq/L
- **Severe reactions:** 2.5 mEq/L and above.
- Fine hand tremor, polyuria, and mild thirst
- **EEG Changes:** Diffuse slowing, widening of the frequency spectrum
- **ECG Changes:** Reversible flattening, isoelectricity or inversion of T-waves.

Lithium Toxicity

Symptoms of lithium toxicity begin to appear at blood levels greater than 1.5 mEq/L and are dosage determinate.

Table 22: Serum level of lithium and toxicity symptoms

Serum level of lithium	Toxicity symptoms
1.5–2.0 mEq/L	• Blurred vision, ataxia, tinnitus, persistent nausea and vomiting, severe diarrhea.
2.0–3.5 mEq./L	• Excessive output of dilute urine, increasing tremors, muscular irritability, psychomotor retardation, mental confusion, giddiness.
Above 3.5 mEq/L	• Impaired consciousness, nystagmus, seizures, coma, oligurea/anuria, arrhythmias, myocardial infarction, cardio vascular collapse.

Recent Question (NORCET 2022)

9. Patients taking MAO are not allowed to consume tyramine-rich food as it causes:
a. Diarrhea
b. Hypertensive crisis
c. Delayed drug effect
d. Apnea

Ans. (b) Hypertensive crisis

POINT TO REMEMBER

Dangerous hypertensive crisis with excitement and hallucinations occurs when **TCAs are given with SSRI.**

POINT TO REMEMBER

Antidepressants, especially the SSRIs are effective in OCD, phobias, panic and many types of severe generalized anxiety disorders

Clinical Corner

CASE SCENARIO 29:

A 39-year-old male patient was discharged on bupropion for the treatment of depression. Nurse Linda is assessing the patient on his follow-up visit. Which of the following adverse effect, if found, is an indication of overdose of this drug?
a. Increased weight
b. Orthostatic hypotension
c. Seizure activity
d. Constipation

Ans. (c) Seizure activity

CASE SCENARIO 30:

Which of the following sign or symptom has to be closely observed from a patient who was taking escitalopram daily for the 15 days?
a. Increased appetite
b. Increased energy level
c. Suicidal ideation
d. Sleep disturbance

Ans. (c) Suicidal ideation

Client/Family Education

- **Not drive or operate dangerous machinery** until lithium levels are stabilized
- The client should drink **6 to 8 large glasses of water** each day and avoid excessive use of beverages containing caffeine
- Notify the physician if vomiting or diarrhea occur. These symptoms can result in sodium loss and an increased risk of toxicity.
- Include **adequate sodium** in the diet (in case or heavy sweating in labor work, add more sodium in the diet or else maintain normal intake)
- **Avoid pregnancy** while receiving lithium therapy. Lithium is teratogenic agent which is likely to cause Ebstein's Anomaly.

Nurses Responsibilities

- Lithium should be taken along with food
- In a patient who is stabilized on lithium therapy, blood lithium levels should be checked
  - 8–12 hours after the first dose
  - 2 or 3 times weekly during the first month
  - Weekly to monthly during maintenance therapy.
- Discontinue medication in case of sign of lithium toxicity (excessive vomiting, extreme hand tremors, sedation, muscles weakness and vertigo) and report physician immediately.
- Increase water intake with salt to prevent lithium toxicity
- A patient who is taking lithium for bipolar affective disorder must maintain a balanced diet with adequate salt intake.
- Low calorie diet to prevent weight gain.
- Explain the patient about dehydration and lithium toxicity.

NATIONAL MENTAL HEALTH PROGRAM (NMHP)

- The National Mental Health Program (NMHP, 1982) was **launched in 1982,** by the government of India
- The NMHP was re-strategized in 2003 to include two schemes, viz.
  - Modernization of State Mental Hospitals and
  - Up-gradation of Psychiatric Wings of Medical Colleges/General Hospitals.
- The Manpower Development Scheme (Scheme-A and B) became part of the Program in 2009.

Components of NMHP

Three main components of NMHP are as follows:

1. Treatment of Mentally ill
2. Rehabilitation
3. Prevention and promotion of positive mental health.

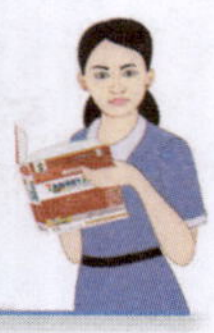

Objectives of NMHP

- To ensure the availability and accessibility of minimum mental healthcare for all in the foreseeable future
- To encourage the application of mental health knowledge in general healthcare and in social development
- To promote community participation in the mental health service development
- To enhance human resources in mental health sub-specialties

Strategies

- Integration of mental health with primary healthcare through the NMHP
- Provision of tertiary care institutions for treatment of mental disorders
- Eradicating stigmatization of mentally ill patients and protecting their rights

OBJECTIVES OF DISTRICT MENTAL HEALTH PROGRAM (DMHP)

- To provide sustainable basic mental health services to the community and to integrate these services with other health services
- Early detection and treatment in community itself
- To reduce stigma of mental illness through public awareness
- To treat and rehabilitate mental patients within the community.

Components of DMHP

- Training of medical, paramedical personnel and community leaders
- Community Mental Health care through existing infrastructure of the health services
- Information, Education and Communication (IEC) activities

DEADDICTION DRUGS/ANTABUSE DRUGS

These drugs are used for the treatment of substance use disorders.

Criteria for Treatment on Out Patient Department (OPD) Basis

- Mild to moderate dependence, Medically stable, Good social support, High motivation,
- Willing to give body fluids for exam.

Criteria for Inpatient Treatment

- Having severe withdrawals (current or past history), with medical complications, co-morbid psychiatric/mental illness, poor social support, Patient in crisis

KEY POINTS

- For determining the serum lithium, the blood specimen is to be obtained before breakfast. It is advisable to take the blood sample after 12 hours of last dose.
- Therapeutic serum level of lithium is 0.8-1.2 mEq/L.
- Acetazolamide, theophylline, and sodium bicarbonate may increase renal excretion of lithium, reducing its effectiveness.
- Diuretics should be avoided in clients taking lithium.
- Three main components of NMHP include treatment of mentally ill, rehabilitation and prevention and promotion of positive mental health.
- The Manpower Development Scheme Scheme-A & B became part of NMHP in 2009.

Recent Question (NORCET 2022)

10. All of the following results in delirium, except:

a. Benzodiazepines withdrawal
b. Opioid withdrawal
c. Hyponatremia
d. Depression

Ans. (d) Depression

Phases of Treatment

- Withdrawal phase (detoxification)
- Maintenance phase

Table 23: Drugs used in withdrawal and maintenance phase of deaddiction treatment

Substance	Treatment	
	Withdrawal phase	Maintenance phase
Opioid	• Opioid detoxification requires 2 weeks • Buprenorphine, dextropropoxyphene, and clonidine are used • Starting dose of depends on amount of opioids consumed. • Divided doses of 1.2-4 mg of buprenorphine/ 6-12 capsules of dextropropoxyphene is preferred	• **Opioid agonist:** Methadone, Buprenorphine, Morphine • **Antagonist**: Naltrexone
Alcohol	• Long acting benzodiazepines (chlordiazepoxide/ diazepam) are used • Usually daily divided doses of 20-40 mg of diazepam/ 40-80 mg of chlordiazepoxide • Taper off the dose of benzodiazepines gradually over next 7–10 days. • Oral administration of thiamine to treat Wernicke-Korsakoff syndrome • **Loading dose**: 20 mg diazepam every 2 hourly till sedated on the first day of withdrawal.	• Deterrent agents: Disulfiram (**dose:** 250 mg tab.; 1-2 tab per day), calcium carbimide • **Anticraving agents:** Acamprosate (333 mg, 2-3tabs TDS, commonly used), naltrexone (50mg, 1tab OD), fluxetine (20/40mg).
Benzodiazepine	• Shift to long acting benzodiazepines, e.g. Diazepam	Taper off Long acting benzodiazines.
Nicotine	• Nicotine gum, Nicotine transdermal patch	• Nicotine chewette • 2/4 mg, every 2-3 hourly. • Gradual tapering over few weeks. • Nicotine transdermal patch • Bupropion – 300-600 mg/day. Onset of action takes 2 week time.

CRISIS AND CRISIS INTERVENTION

- Crisis is an acute time limiting state of physiological disequilibrium resulting from situational, developmental or societal source of stress
- Crisis is acute, will be solved by one or another means within a brief period

Stages of Crisis

Exposure to Hazardous event (stressor) → The vulnerable state → The precipitating factor → Active crisis state → Reintegration/restoration of equilibrium

Types of Crisis

- **Developmental Crisis/Maturational crisis:** It is the result of a normal life event, e.g. Pregnancy, graduation
- **Situational Crisis:** Most common type of crisis. An event that is so overwhelming and sudden that it overwhelms normal coping, e.g. sexual assault, Road traffic accident or sudden loss or grief.
- **Existential Crisis:** These are related to situations of regret or belief that one will not reach goals they had set for themselves at a certain age. Existential crises are particularly common at life transition points like 30, 40, and 50 when people "take stock" of their life.
- **Adventitious Crisis/ social crisis:** Adventitious crises have been called events of disaster. Social crisis is accidental, uncommon, unplanned and unanticipated and results in multiple losses and environment changes.
- Examples are: Natural disasters, hurricanes, flood, fire, earthquake, war, riots, Crime of violence, bombing in crowded areas, etc.

Crisis Intervention

Goals: Relieving the client's symptoms and restoration of client's previous level of functioning

Stages of Crisis Intervention

- **Assessment**
  - Identify the precipitating factor
  - Determine client's subjective reaction to the precipitating event
  - Define the context of the crisis situation
  - Assess previously used coping mechanisms
- **Planning and implementation**
  - Obtain relevant background information
  - Set immediate goals based on available resources and support system
  - Identify tasks that allow the client to achieve those goals

Clinical Corner

CASE SCENARIO 31:

A patient comes to the psychiatric OPD with sleeping problems, irritability, anxiety, and headaches. The symptoms started a week before when he was terminated from his current work. The patient is worried that he is without work and it will affect the entire family. The patient is most likely experiencing:

a. A developmental crisis.
b. A situational crisis.
c. A maturational crisis.
d. An existential crisis

Ans. (a) A situational crisis

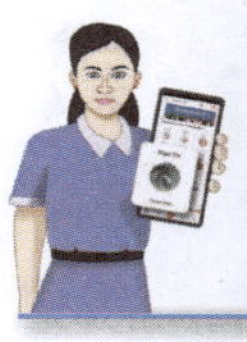

- **Termination**
  - The client and therapist review the client's progress in terms of the goals of the intervention
  - Make a decision on termination
  - Discuss the client's plan for future
- **Crisis intervention technique**
  - **Sustainment:** During initial stages of crisis intervention
  - **Direct influence:** Involves contact with other agencies to mobilize support system
  - **Person-situation reflection:** Help the client to understand the crisis situation
  - **Dynamic and developmental understating:** Used to explore deeply the client's role in the crisis situation.
- **Catharsis:** Expressions and release of feelings that take place as the patient talks emotionally charged areas
- **Clarification:** Encouraging the patient to express more clearly the relationship between certain events.
- **Manipulation:** Using the patient's emotions, wishes or values to benefit the patient in the therapeutic process.
- **Reinforcement of behavior:** giving the patient positive reinforcement to adaptive behavior.
- **Support of defences**: encouraging the use of healthy, adaptive defences and discouraging those that are unhealthy or maladaptive.
- **Increasing self- esteem:** helping the patient to regain feelings of self-worth.
- **Exploration of solution:** examining alternative ways of solving the immediate problem.

PSYCHIATRIC EMERGENCIES

- Psychiatric emergency is a condition wherein the patient has disturbances of thought, affect and psychomotor activity leading to a threat to self (suicide), or threat to others.
- Psychiatric emergencies require action without delay to save the patient and other persons from mortal danger or other serious consequences.

Examples of psychiatric emergencies

- Suicidal threat
- Violent or aggressive behavior or excitement
- Panic attacks
- Catatonic stupor
- Hysterical attacks
- Transient situational disturbances
- Intoxication

Suicide

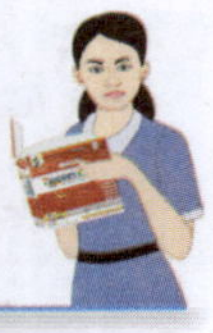

- Suicide is the intentional taking of one's own life in a culturally non-endorsed manner. Attempted suicide is any act of self-damage carried out with the apparent intention of self-destruction however half-hearted, vague and ineffective.

Management

- Assessment (ask directly about suicidal thoughts)
- Brief psychotherapy
- Medication
  - Mild tranquillizers 5–10 mg
  - Diazepam/lorazepam—1–2 mg
  - Antidepressants
- Counseling–support/encouragement, instilling hope, be always with patient.
- ECT—in case of depression with suicidal ideation

Precautions

- Continuous observation of the patient
- Place in hospital gown without ties, shoelaces, sharp instruments, stockings
- Sedate the agitated and restrain if necessary
- Evaluate the precautions regularly

Nursing Management

- Assess suicidal risk daily. Ask the suicide plan
- Have staff member with the patient all the time
- Explain suicide precautions
- Remove all sharp objects and potentially dangerous items from patient's possession
- Keep the window locked so that the patient cannot open
- Be alert to the possibility of the patient saving up his medications
- Talk about his feelings, relationships, or life situations. Encourage and support the client's expression of anger/emotions
- Be alert about decreased communication, conversation about death, low frustration tolerance and dissatisfaction with dependency
- Do not joke about death
- Refer to spiritual source
- Involve the patient for his own treatment
- Teach problem solving approach, social skills and self-care activities

Violent or Aggressive Behavior or Excitement

- **Violence** is physical aggression by one person on other. Violence is associated with psychotic disorders, personality disorders, delirium, drug intoxication, or withdrawal, mental retardation, CNS disorders and domestic quarrel.

Management

- **Medication (chemical restraints)**
  - Chlorpromazine 50–150 mg IM
  - Haloperidol 5–10 mg IM/IV repeat every 20 minutes to a maximum of 120 mg per day.
  - Trifluoperazine 10–30 mg IM 8 hourly.
  - Diazepam 10–40 mg IV preferably when violent behavior is associated with epilepsy
  - **NOTE**: Give medication in juice or water. Avoid giving tablet or capsule

Clinical Corner

CASE SCENARIO 32:

Nurse Linda is developing a plan for care for a 24-year-old male patient who is admitted into psychiatric ward with severe depression and suicidal ideation. Which of the following issue is of highest priority for the nurse?

a. Stress
b. Safety
c. Sleep
d. Self-esteem

Ans. (b) Safety

KEY POINTS

- Incidence of suicide in India is 10-11/1,00,000 population.
- Hanging is the most common method of suicide in India according to National Crime Records Bureau 2014.
- The behavioral clues for impending suicide include giving away valuable possessions, becoming energetic after a period of server depression, withdrawals from social activities, farewell quotes and letters, and avoiding serious decision making.

- **Therapeutic communication (verbal de-escalation)**
  - Softly even if he is talking loudly
  - Avoid closed-ended questions
  - Question should be concise and direct and assist him in defining problem and focusing on the issue
  - Ask the patient direct and firm manner 'how can we help you?' most patients appreciate that someone bothers to ask what is going on.
- **Food**
  - Offer patient something to eat and drink; food may have a calming effect on the patient's anxiety.
- **Physical restraints**
  - The nurse should make sure that there is a physician order to restrain (except emergency situations)
  - Approach the patient from front. Never see potentially violent patient alone.
  - Have four members team to hold the extremities to tie up.
  - Use leather belts, padded bandages to restrain. After restraining do not leave him unattended.
  - Keep a comfortable distance away from the patient.
  - Maintain a clear exit route for both the staff and the patient.
  - Be supportive to the patient and intervene to increase his self-esteem.
  - Avoid excessive stimulation.
  - Remove all the sharp weapons, open electric circuit, ropes, etc. in his room.
  - Frequent circulations checks (distal to the knot) should be performed when extremities are restrained.
  - Offer bedpan or bathroom every 2 hours
  - Review the incident to the patient after he achieves control.
- ECT may be given to help him control aggression.
- Teach him alternative coping methods.

GLOSSARY OF COMMON TERMINOLOGIES

- **Akathisia**: Motor restlessness, inability to sit still.
- **Anhedonia:** Inability to experience pleasure in any activity.
- **Amnesia:** Partial or total inability to recall fast experience may be organic or emotional.
- **Apathy:** Lack of emotional feeling.
- **Anorexia nervosa**: Characterized by extreme concern with body weight, an intense fear of becoming fat, and maintenance of body weight below expected level.
- **Blunt affect**: A reduction in emotional experience.
- **Circumstantiality**: A pattern of communication that includes many irrelevant and unnecessary trivial detailed in his speech before he is able to come to the point.
- **Idea of reference:** It is an incorrect belief that the statements or actions of others are related to oneself.
- **Déjà vu**: A subjective feeling that an event which is occurring for the first time has been experienced before.
- **Delusion**: A false, fixed and unshakeable belief which is not amenable to reasoning and is not in keeping with the patient's sociocultural and educational background.
- **Dystonia**: Muscle rigidity that affects posture, gait, and eye movement.
- **Echolalia**: Pathological repetition by imitation of the speech of another.
- **Echopraxia**: Pathological repetition by imitation of the behavior or act of another.
- **Encopresis**: Involuntary passage of feces in inappropriate place after age of voluntary control has been established.
- **Euphoria**: Excessive feeling of happiness.
- **Grandiose**: Unrealistic or exaggerated sense of self-worth importance wealth or ability.
- **Hallucination:** A false sensory perception in the absence of an actual external stimulus.
- **Illusion:** The misinterpretation of real external sensory experience. It is mental misperception of actual sensory stimuli.
- **Insight:** Awareness of one's own mental illness.
- **Jamais vu**: Failure to recognize events that have been encountered before.
- **Palilalia:** Compulsive repetition of one word (usually last one) phrase.
- **Stupor**: A state in which the individual does not reach to his surroundings and appears to be unaware of them.
- **Tangentiality:** A form of thinking/speech in which the client tends to wander away from the intended point, and never returning to the original idea.
- **Thought block**: A sudden interruption in the thought process before the thought is completed. After a pause, the subject cannot recall what he had meant to say.
- **Tic**: Sudden, repetitive, stereotyped motor movement or verbal speech.
- **Waxy flexibility**: A condition by which the individual with schizophrenia passively yields all movable parts of the body to any efforts made at placing them in certain position.

Practice Question

9. Tourette syndrome is a disorder that involves repetitive movements (motor tics) or unwanted sounds (vocal tics). A vocal tic that involves repeating one's own sounds or words termed

a. Echolalia
b. Echopraxia
c. Palilalia
d. Verbigeration

Ans. (c) Palilalia

Recent Questions (NORCET 2022)

11. A schizophrenic client who is experiencing thoughts of having special powers states that "I am a messenger from another planet and can rule the earth." The nurse assesses this behavior as:

a. Ideas of reference
b. Delusions of persecution
c. Thought broadcasting
d. Delusions of grandeur

Ans. (d) Delusions of...

12. A 56-year-old client is admitted to the psychiatric unit in a state of total despair. She feels hopeless and worthless, has a flat affect and very sad appearance, and is unable to feel pleasure from anything. Her husband has been assisting her at home with the housework and cooking: however, she has not been eating much, lies around or sits in a chair most of the day, and is becoming confused and thinks her family does not want her around anymore. In assessing the client, the nurse determines that her behavior is consistent with:

a. Transient depression
b. Mild depression
c. Moderate depression
d. Severe depression

Ans. (d) Severe depression

Golden Points to Remember

- The Nobel Prize for experiments on split brain was given to Roger Sperry.
- The theory of operant conditioning was experimented by B F Skinner.
- Mental Healthcare Act 2017 (MHA 2017) received presidential assent on April 7th, 2017 and replaced the 1987 Act.
- Mental Health Act 2017 decriminalizes suicide attempt by mentally ill person.
- As per MHA 2017, No ECT therapy without use of muscle relaxants and No ECT therapy for Minors.
- Mental Health Act (MHA 2017) empowers a mentally ill person to have the right to make an advance directive toward the way he/she wants to be treated.
- Reception order refers to an order for admission and detention of a mentally ill person in a psychiatric hospital.
- Temporary discharge of the patient from the psychiatric hospital is referred to as Parole.
- Trust is the most important factor in a therapeutic relationship.
- Termination of interpersonal relationship starts in orientation phase.
- Transference is a phenomenon in which the person in treatment redirects feelings for others onto the therapist.
- Countertransference occurs when a therapist transfers emotion to a person in therapy.
- ICD stands for International Classification of Diseases.
- The National Mental Health Program (NMHP, 1982) was launched in 1982 by the Government of India.
- National Mental Health Program (NMHP) was re-strategized in 2003 to include two schemes, viz. Modernization of State Mental Hospitals and Up-gradation of Psychiatric Wings of Medical Colleges/General Hospitals.
- Parkinson's disease is caused by a loss of nerve cells in the part of the brain called the substantia nigra (low dopamine levels).
- Part of the brain that is responsible for emotional aspects of behavior is limbic system.
- The part of the brain that regulates cognitive function is cerebrum.
- Mini mental status examination is used to assess cognitive impairment.
- Total score of Mini Mental Status Examination (MMSE) is 30. A score of 24 or more indicates a normal cognition.
- Mini Mental Status Examination (MMSE) score of 19 to 23 indicates mild cognitive impairment; scores of 10 to 18 indicate moderate cognitive impairment. Scores below 10 indicate severe cognitive impairment.
- The most significant characteristics experienced by a patient with depression is depressed mood and loss of pleasure or interest.
- 'Omega sign' is seen in depressed patient.
- Depressed mood and loss of pleasure or interest are the most significant characteristics experienced by a patient with depression.
- Common risk factor in patient with severe depression is suicidal tendency.
- For a patient with severe depression, the setting where there are simple daily routines will be least stressful.
- Aphonia is the inability to produce voiced sound.
- Apathy is a state of indifference, or the suppression of emotions such as concern, excitement, motivation, and passion.
- Kleptomania means irresistible desire to steal things.
- Tardive dyskinesia is the adverse effect resulting from the chronic use of antipsychotics.
- The term schizophrenia is coined by Eugene Bleuler.
- Meaning of term 'Schizophrenia' is split mind.
- Negative symptoms of Schizophrenia include Affective flattening, Alogia, Avolition, and Apathy.
- First rank symptoms of schizophrenia (FRSS) was described by Schneider.
- Four A_s of Schizophrenia (According to Eugen Bleuler) are: Associative looseness, ambivalence, autistic thinking, and affective changes.
- Waxy flexibility, mutism, bizarre posture and stupor are characteristics of catatonic schizophrenia.
- Persecutory delusion and/or suspiciousness is common in paranoid schizophrenia.
- Late adolescence to early adulthood is the most common period of onset of schizophrenia.
- Flight of ideas is typical feature of mania.
- Type of diet is recommended for a patient with manic episode is finger foods.
- Most appropriate intervention to manage manipulative behavior of a manic patient is to set limits on patient behavior.
- Calling hospital security should be the first step by the nurse following a violent episode on a psychiatric unit.
- False sensory perceptions with no basis in reality (no external stimuli) is known as hallucination.
- Illusion is a distortion of senses characterized by misinterpretation of stimuli.
- Formed visual hallucinations are usually from lesion of temporal region.
- Unformed hallucinations are common with disorders of the occipital lobe.
- Auditory hallucination is the most common type of hallucination experienced by patients with mental illness.
- Mood congruent hallucination refers to hallucination whose content represents or reflects the mood state of the individual.

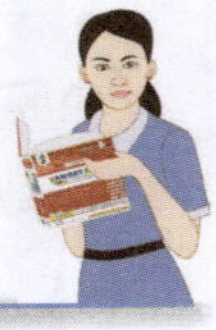

Contd...

- Fixed false belief of a person which cannot be changed by logical reasoning is known as delusion.
- The belief that oneself, a part of one's body, or the real world does not exist is known as nihilistic delusion.
- Schizophrenia is treated by antipsychotics.
- Presenting the patient with a 'hypothetical situation' helps in the assessment of judgement.
- Catharsis is the process of releasing strong emotions through a particular activity or experience.
- Catatonia is a state of psychomotor immobility and behavioral abnormality manifested by stupor.
- Cataplexy is a sudden and transient episode of muscle weakness accompanied by full conscious awareness which is precipitated or triggered by emotions as laughing, crying, etc.
- A state of diminished consciousness in which the patient remains mute and still with the eyes open is called stupor.
- Systematized delusions occur in the dementia only. It does not occur in delirium.
- Delirium is an acute state of confusion but dementia develops over time with slow progression of cognitive decline.
- Hypothyroidism is one of the most important causes of potentially reversible dementia.
- Best test for diagnosis of organic mental disorder is Bender gestalt test.
- Rorschach Test (RT) and Thematic Apperception Test (TAT) are projective tests to assess personality structure, pattern of thoughts, emotional problems and mental disorders.
- Rorschach's projective test is designed to measure unconscious intentions.
- The extreme feeling of happiness is known as Euphoria.
- When a patient is not aware of his/her mental disorder, it is called lack of insight.
- A person who is aloof, isolated and does not socialize, is considered to be withdrawn.
- Verbal utterance that are often obscene is known as Coprolalia.
- Echolalia is the repetition of the words spoken by others.
- Echopraxia is the repetition of movements performed by others.
- Neologism is the coining of new words without any meaning.
- Persistent and inappropriate repetition of the same thoughts is known as Perseveration.
- An unwanted thought that a person finds intrusive and distressing is called obsession.
- A behavior that a person feels compelled to perform is defined as compulsion.
- Polysomnography, also called a sleep study, is a test used to diagnose sleep disorders.
- Most vivid dreams occur during REM sleep.
- Penile erection or clitoris engorgement occurs during REM sleep.
- Non-Rapid Eye Movement (NREM) sleep is also known as Orthodox sleep or Synchronized or 'S' sleep.
- Restless leg syndrome (Ekbom's Syndrome) - Painful condition leads to severe insomnia and periodic limb movement during sleep.
- Sleep walking is otherwise called somnambulism.
- Repetitive, uncontrollable thoughts and acts are termed as Obsessive-compulsive disorders (OCDs).
- Exposure and response prevention (ERP) is the most important type of Cognitive Behavior Therapy (CBT) for OCD.
- Chlorpromazine (typical antipsychotic) was discovered in 1950 and was the first antipsychotic.
- Extra pyramidal symptoms are most common with Fluphenazine and Haloperidol.
- Orthostatic hypotension is most common with Chlorpromazine, Thioridazine, Clozapine.
- Agranulocytosis is more common with typical than atypical antipsychotics (except Clozapine).
- The major side effect of Clozapine is agranulocytosis. So periodical complete blood count is suggested.
- Bromocryptine or dantrolene is the treatment of choice for Neuroleptic Malignant syndrome (NMS).
- Anticholinergics (e.g. Benztropine) are used to treat extrapyramidal symptoms (EPS).
- The drug of choice for treatment and management of bipolar mania is lithium carbonate.
- Daily adult dosage of lithium for acute mania is 1800-2400 mg. For maintenance—900–1200 mg.
- Therapeutic Plasma Range for acute mania—1.0–1.5 mEq/L; For maintenance - 0.6–1.2 mEq/L.
- Patient who is on lithium therapy should drink 6 to 8 large glasses of water each day and avoid excessive use of beverages containing caffeine (coffee, tea, colas), which promote increased urine output. The client must consume a diet adequate in sodium.
- Neurotransmitter serotonin plays a role in the psychopathology of OCD.
- Medication with a serotonin reuptake inhibitor is helpful for many OCD patients.
- The type of loss in which the client is aware that a loss will occur is known as anticipatory loss.
- Willis Ekbom Syndrome is also known as Restless legs syndrome.
- Excessive sleep is termed as Hypersomnia.
- Dhat syndrome: It is considered as a culture-bound syndrome (CBS) specific to the Indian subcontinent.
- Kleine–Levin syndrome is a rare sleep disorder mainly affecting teenage boys in which the main features are intermittent hypersomnolence.
- Ganser syndrome is a type of factitious disorder, in which a person deliberately and consciously acts as if he or she has a physical or mental illness when he or she is not really sick.
- The immediate nursing intervention for the patient who has just awakened from an electroconvulsive therapy (ECT) treatment is to orient the patient.

Contd...

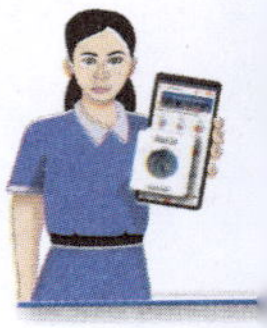

- The most common indication of ECT is Major depression.
- Type of schizophrenia best responds to ECT is Catatonic Schizophrenia.
- The voltage needed to produce seizures while giving ECT is 70 to 130 volts.
- Succinylcholine (smooth muscle relaxant) is administered during ECT to prevent injuries to patient during seizure.
- Atropine is given to patient before Electroconvulsive Therapy (ECT) is to minimize secretions and to prevent transient postictal brady arrhythmia due to excessive vagal tone.
- Most common side effect of ECT is temporary memory loss.
- Agoraphobia is fear of open spaces. It is the most common type of phobia seen in clinical practice.
- Irrational fear related to closed spaces is referred to as claustrophobia.
- Fear of high places is called acrophobia.
- Preoccupation with a fear of having a serious physical illness, not based on real or organic pathology is hypochondriasis.
- The part of mind that distinguishes right from wrong and acts as censor of behavior is known as superego.
- An attempt to integrate values learned from parents and society is referred to as superego.
- Another term for superego is conscience.
- As per psychoanalytic theory the ability to tolerate frustration is seen in Ego.
- As per Freud, the development of Oedipus Complex (male) and Electra Complex (female) occurs during the phallic (3-6 years) stage of development.
- A male child's unconscious sexual desire for the parent of the opposite sex is termed as Oedipus Complex.
- A female child's unconscious sexual desire for the parent of the opposite sex is termed as Electra complex.
- Topographical model of mind by Freud is Conscious - Preconscious – Unconscious.
- Father of Intelligence Test is Alfred Binet (Early 1900s).
- Milieu theory insists on community participation by abiding unit rules.
- In psychoanalytic terms, obsessive compulsive disorder is fixed at Anal Stage.
- Ego defense mechanism is a mechanism designed to reduce stress and conflict caused by specific experiences.
- Rechanneling of socially unacceptable drives into activities that are more tolerable and constructive is known as Sublimation.
- A young man who is dealing with aggression by playing football is an example of Sublimation (Defense Mechanism).
- Attributing unacceptable feeling to others is the mechanism known as Projection.
- Rationalization is an **adaptive mechanism of giving excuses when a person cannot solve a problem.**
- Repression involves placing uncomfortable thoughts in relatively inaccessible areas of the subconscious mind.
- Intellectualization is an attempt to avoid expressing actual emotions associated with a stressful situation by using the intellectual process of logic, reasoning and analysis.
- Most commonly using defensive mechanism by a physically abusive individual is Displacement.
- Situational crisis is term given to a person whose coping mechanisms are affected due to their circumstances, e.g. job loss, financial crisis, etc.
- In conversion disorder, anxiety is expressed through physical symptoms.
- Integrative approach is a combined approach to psychotherapy that brings different elements of specific therapies.
- Eradication of unwanted habits by associating unpleasant condition with it is called Aversive Conditioning.
- Flooding is a behavioral therapy in which the patient is suddenly exposed to a direct and maximum fear producing stimulus.
- Supportive confrontation can be used in a patient with narcissistic personality disorder to point out discrepancies between what the client states and what actually exists.
- The ideal size for group therapy is 8 to 10 members.
- Most common symptom of alcohol withdrawal is tremor.
- The health education to a group of alcoholic people should be able to change their behaviors.
- Korsakoff's Psychosis is a long-term effect of 'Medical Complication of Alcoholism'. It occurs due to deficiency of the Vitamin Thiamine.
- Chronic alcoholic patients are treated initially by IM injection of thiamine 100 mg.
- Heroin (like opium and morphine) is made from the resin of poppy plants.
- Total abstinence is the only effective treatment for alcoholism, particularly in short-term alcoholic addicts.
- Regular coffee is contraindicated in a patient who is on alcohol withdrawal phase.
- Alcohol anonymous group is a self-help group, who meets together to maintain sobriety.
- Most severe alcohol withdrawal syndrome is Delirium tremens.
- Chlordiazepoxide is used to treat withdrawal symptoms of alcoholism.
- Acamprosate is an anti-craving agent used in maintenance phase of treatment of alcohol dependence.
- Disulfiram is the deterrent agent used in the maintenance phase of treatment of alcohol dependence syndrome.
- Combination of alcohol and Disulfiram results in nausea and hypertension as a result of accumulation of Acetaldehyde.
- Flumazenil is an antidote of benzodiazepines.
- Naloxone is an antidote of opioids.
- Naltrexone is an opioid antagonist.
- Suspiciousness and mistrust of others (paranoia) is a characteristic feature of schizotypal personality disorder.
- Patient with schizotypal personality has great difficulty in establishing and maintaining close relationships with others.
- Characteristic of schizoid personality disorder is introverted and emotionally withdrawn.

  Dependent personality disorder is characterized by intense lack of self-confidence, low self-esteem, and inability to make decisions.
- Clients with borderline personality disorder are likely to develop dysfunctional coping and act out in self-destructive ways such as binge eating.

Contd...

- Dissociative fugue or psychogenic fugue is a dissociative disorder characterized by reversible amnesia for personal identity.
- A nurse who is caring for a client with antisocial behavior should stress on setting clear rules and expectations about the client's behavior.
- Sheldon's classification of personality includes Ectomorphs, Endomorphs, and Mesomorphs.
- Characteristic of histrionic personality is dramatic, theatrical and attention seeking.
- People with anti-social behavior lack ego and super-ego that controls behavior. They have little or no concern for others.
- A naive, inappropriate lack of emotion or concern for the perceptions by others of one's disability is known as La belle indifference.
- Derealization and depersonalization are seen in Dissociative disorder.
- A person who is kind, quiet, submissive, sympathetic and gloomy has Melancholic personality.
- Loss of personal identity and wandering away from psychiatric hospital is referred to as Dissociative Fugue.
- Uncertainty and excessive sense of responsibility is seen in generalized anxiety disorder.
- Diagnostic interview with sodium amytal or hypnosis is a special feature of Post-traumatic neurosis.
- Grief is a reaction of an individual to a significant loss. The loss may be real or anticipated one.
- The basis of ritualistic behavior seen in Obsessive Compulsive disorder (OCD) is aimed at controlling guilt and inadequacy by maintaining an absolute set pattern of behavior.
- The most common psychotherapy used to help a person with Obsessive Compulsive Disorder is behavior modification.
- In a client with OCD, the rituals performed by the client will help to control the anxiety.
- Drug most useful in treatment of obsessive compulsive disorder is Fluoxetine (SSRI).
- Lateral hypothalamus (to start) and Ventromedial Nuclei (to stop) of hypothalamus controls hunger and eating.
- Establishing a consistent eating plan and monitoring the client's weight are important in developing care plan for a client with anorexia nervosa.
- Bulimic behavior is generally a maladaptive coping response to stress and underlying issues.
- The most appropriate goal for a client with bulimia nervosa is that the patient must identify anxiety-causing events or situations that stimulate the bulimic behavior.
- Trichotellomania is a disorder that involves recurrent irresistible urge to pull out hair.
- Juvenile delinquency is a legal classification of children's behavior that violates the law.
- Methylphenidate is the first line drug of choice for the treatment of ADHD.
- Autistic child turns inward to his/her own self stimulating acts and responds less to environmental stimuli.
- Language development of an autistic child resembles Echolalia.
- Dyslexia is a learning disorder that involves difficulty reading.
- Dyscalculia refers to severe difficulty in making arithmetical calculations.
- Tic is an abnormal involuntary movement which occurs suddenly, repetitively and purposelessly.
- Tourette syndrome is a disorder of Tic.
- Magical thinking is commonly seen in Toddlers and Preschoolers.
- Haloperidol is the drug of choice to treat Tourette's disorder.
- Patients who are taking monoamine oxidase inhibitor should avoid taking food rich in tyramine.
- Examples of tyramine rich foods are aged cheeses, alcohol beverages, cured meats, etc.
- Antipsychotic drugs are also known as neuroleptic drugs or tranquilizers.
- Tardive dyskinesia is a side effect of long-term use of certain antipsychotics.
- Neuroleptic malignant syndrome (NMS) is a life-threatening, neurological disorder most often caused by an adverse reaction to antipsychotic drugs.
- Neuroleptic malignant syndrome (NMS), an adverse effect of antipsychotics, can occur within hours after drug initiation.
- Chlorpromazine depresses hypothalamic thermoregulatory mechanism, exposure to extreme temperature may cause hyperthermia.
- Patients who are on haloperidol are advised not to drive or operating machines due to the side effect of dizziness and drowsiness.
- Abrupt withdrawal of barbiturate could cause withdrawal symptoms such as seizure, restlessness, insomnia, sweating and anxiety.
- Drug of choice to reverse a dystonic reaction is Diphenhydramine (Benadryl), 25 to 50 mg IM or IV.
- Disulfiram therapy is an overt sensitization, a type of aversion therapy which produces unpleasant consequence for undesirable behavior.
- Antidote for methanol is Ethanol.
- Atypical antipsychotics has a lower incidence of extra pyramidal effects than the typical antipsychotics.
- Agranulocytosis is the side effect of Clozapine (atypical antipsychotics). So periodical Blood screening for CBC is required.
- Psychology is a Natural science.
- Psychology as a 'Science of Mind', is defined by Psychoanalysts.
- E.B. Titchener (1867-1927) defined 'Psychology' as the science of mind.
- Abnormal Psychology is mainly the study of Abnormality of mind.
- Grimacing and mirror gazing is seen in hebephrenic schizophrenia.
- The frequency of alpha rhythm in EEG is 8–12 HZ
- The frequency of beta rhythm in EEG is >12 HZ
- Sleeping beauty syndrome (Kliene – Levine syndrome): Hypersomnia, hypergraphia, hypersexuality with mood changes.
- Dramatic self-mutilation occurring in schizophrenia is called Capgras syndrome

Contd...

- Carphologia is defined as picking movements on clothes and bedsheets
- Legal limit of blood alcohol concentration for driving in India is 30 mg/100 ml
- Minnesota Multiphasic Personality Inventory (MMPI) is a used for the assessment of Personality disorder.
- The commonest type of post-partum psychiatric disturbance is postpartum blues.
- Abnormal and excessive fear of cats is called ailurophobia
- Fear of beautiful women is called venustraphobia.
- Monophobia is fear of being alone.
- Psuedologia fantastica is also called pathological lying.
- A woman believes that man of higher status is in love with her is called declerembault's syndrome.
- To diagnose pica, child has to be consuming non-nutritive substance for at least one month.
- La belle indifference is seen in conversion/Dissociative disorder.
- A patient who has a phobic disorder uses self-protective avoidance as an ego defense mechanism.
- Disulfiram should not be taken concurrently with metronidazole because they may interact and cause psychotic reaction.
- Al-Anon is a self-help group for families of alcoholics.
- Amphetamines are powerful CNS stimulants with peripheral sympathomimetic effects.
- Recreation is a form of activity therapy that enables people with limitations to engage in recreational experiences.
- Client information should be released only with the client's informed consent except in the emergency situation.
- The immediate nursing action for a client with anxiety is to decrease the environmental stimuli and provide a calm and quite environment.
- The most common conversion symptoms are blindness, deafness, paralysis and the inability to talk.
- If a client had a risk for harm, do not leave the client alone for extended periods.
- Monitor closely if a client with a history of depression presents with increased energy because it could mean that the client has the energy to perform the suicide act.
- Safety is the first priority for a client with hallucination.
- Do not whisper or laugh in front of a client with paranoid personality disorder because the client will think that you are talking about or laughing him/her, this will increase the paranoia.
- Histrionic personality disorder is characterized by overly dramatic and intensely expressive behavior.
- MAST – Michigan alcohol screening test, DAST – Drug abuse screening test and CAGE screening questionnaire helps to assess a substance abuse disorder.
- The client must avoid drinking alcohol for 14 days after the last dose of disulfiram because there is a risk for a disulfiram – alcohol reaction.
- Mourning is the outward and social expression of loss.
- Dysfunctional grief occurs with prolonged emotional instability and lack of progression to successful coping with the loss.
- The SSRI should be withheld if the client develops priapism.
- If a client having long-term SSRI therapy monitor liver and renal function test.
- Cardiac toxicity can occur for a client having tricyclic antidepressants, so before treatment the client should receive electrocardiogram.
- When discontinuing antipsychotics, the medication dosage should be reduced gradually to avoid sudden recurrence of psychotic symptoms.
- Acetylcholinesterase inhibitors may be used in clients with Alzheimer's disease to improve cognitive functions in early stages.
- **Sleep apnea:** It is a sleep disorder characterized by repetitive pauses in breathing or shallow breaths during sleep. These pauses can last for a few seconds to minutes and can occur numerous times throughout the night. Sleep apnea can be of three primary types:
  - Obstructive Sleep Apnea (OSA): This is the most common form of sleep apnea. It occurs when the muscles at the back of the throat fail to keep the airway open, leading to blockage or partial blockage, resulting in breathing difficulties during sleep.
  - Central Sleep Apnea (CSA): In this type, the brain fails to transmit the appropriate signals to the muscles that control breathing, leading to disruptions in the breathing pattern during sleep.
  - Complex Sleep Apnea Syndrome (Mixed Sleep Apnea): Also known as treatment-emergent central sleep apnea, this type is a combination of both obstructive and central sleep apnea.
- **Excessive daytime sleepiness (EDS):** It is a condition characterized by an overwhelming and persistent desire to sleep during the daytime, even in situations that require alertness and attention.
- **Sleep deprivation:** It refers to the condition of not getting enough sleep, either in terms of quantity or quality, to meet the body's physiological and cognitive needs. It can result from a variety of factors, including voluntary choices, lifestyle, work or school demands, medical conditions, or sleep disorders.
- **Fetishism:** It is a type of sexual preference or arousal pattern in which an individual becomes sexually fixated on a particular object, body part, or non-genital body feature. The object of fetishism, known as a fetish, may be something non-human, such as clothing (e.g., high heels, latex), specific body parts (e.g., feet, hair), or even particular materials or textures.
- **Frotteurism:** It is a paraphilic disorder characterized by a recurrent and intense sexual arousal from touching or rubbing one's genitals against a non-consenting person, usually in a crowded public place.

"He who has health has hope; and he who has hope has everything."
—Arabian proverb

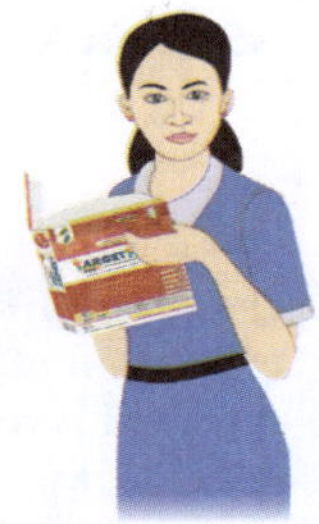

CLINICAL CASE-BASED QUESTIONS

1

A 32-year-old woman complains of intense depressed mood for last 6 to 8 months. She also reports inability to enjoy previously pleasurable activities. The nurse recognizes this symptom as:

a. Avolition
b. Ambivalence
c. Anhedonia
d. Apathy

Ans. (c) Anhedonia

Explanation: Anhedonia is the inability to experience pleasure or lack of interest in previously enjoyable activities. Avolition is the inability to initiate or persist in goal-directed activities. Ambivalence is the state of having mixed feelings about something. Apathy is a lack of interest or concern in the world around oneself.

2

A patient was standing still near his bed and the examiner tried to move his hand as given in the picture below. The catatonic feature demonstrated is:

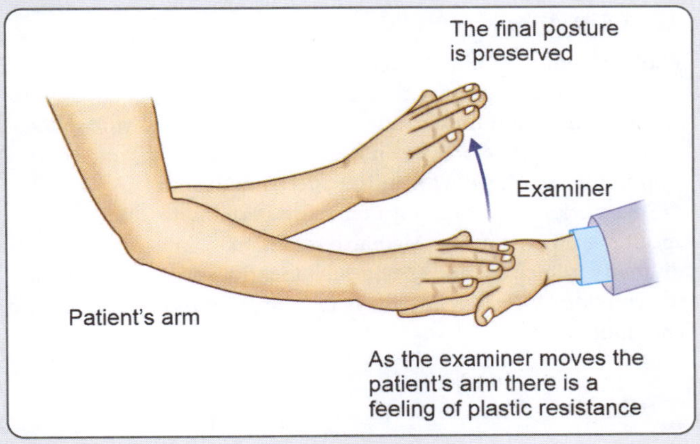

a. Negativism
b. Posturing
c. Waxy Flexibility
d. Echopraxia

Ans, (c) Waxy Flexibility

Explanation: Waxy flexibility is a condition in which a person's limbs can be moved into and held in any position, even a bizarre or uncomfortable one, without any resistance. The main difference between waxy flexibility and posturing is that waxy flexibility refers to the maintenance of a rigid or fixed posture when someone else moves or positions the individual's body, as if it were made of wax. On the other hand, posturing involves assuming unusual or rigid body positions voluntarily, often adopting bizarre or unnatural postures for an extended period of time without external manipulation.

3

A patient says she loves her child and wants to hug him but also hates him and wants to hurt him. She is unable to decide what to express. This is known as:

a. Abulia
b. Ambivalence
c. Anhedonia
d. Apathy

Ans. (b) Ambivalence

Explanation: Ambivalence refers to having conflicting feelings or emotions toward someone or something. In the given case, the patient expresses both love and hate toward her child, indicating conflicting emotions. She wants to hug him but also wants to hurt him, demonstrating ambivalence.

4

Mr. X is diagnosed with major depression and is admitted into an acute care psychiatric ward. He has recently attempted to commit suicide. While having a conversation with the nurse, he says to the nurse, "I wish I were dead! I've always been a failure. Things never go well for me." Which of the following statement by the nurse suggests that she has used appropriate therapeutic communication technique?

a. "You have many reasons to continue to live for"
b. "What makes you to feel that you are a failure"
c. "Experiencing these emotions are a part of being depressed"
d. "You've been feeling like a failure for a while"

Ans. (d) "You've been feeling like a failure for a while"

Explanation: The therapeutic technique used in this statement is reflection or paraphrasing. The nurse restates or reflects the patient's expressed feelings of being a failure by saying, "You've been feeling like a failure for a while" This technique demonstrates active listening and understanding, allowing the nurse to confirm and acknowledge the patient's emotions.

The other options are not therapeutic communication techniques. Option (a), " You have many reasons to continue to live for " is a form of positive reinforcement, which is not appropriate for a patient who is feeling suicidal. Option (b), " What makes you to feel that you are a failure?", is a form of probing, which can be counterproductive in a therapeutic setting. Option (c), " Experiencing these emotions are a part of being depressed," is a form of labeling, which can be invalidating for the patient.

5

The junior trainee nurse is helping the assigned nurse in the application of restraint to the patient as per the doctor orders as patient is very agitated and try to remove its intravenous line and nasogastric tube. While preparing for this, the trainee nurse wants to know about which different method of restraints?

a. Physical restraint
b. Chemical restraint
c. Environmental restraint
d. All of the above

Ans. (d) All of the above

Explanation: The patient may be restrained physically using restraint devices, chemically using medications, or environmentally by confining to a seclusion room.

6

A patient was caught by police for fighting with classmates because he thought they were planning to kill him. He states that his dead grandfather talks to him every now and then for last one month. He is delusional from past few weeks also. What will be the most likely diagnosis?

a. Delusional disorder
b. Mania
c. Post-traumatic stress disorder
d. Schizophrenia

Ans. (d) Schizophrenia

Explanation: Schizophrenia is a mental disorder characterized by delusions, hallucinations, disorganized thinking, and abnormal behavior. The patient's belief that classmates were planning to kill him, along with the hallucination of his deceased grandfather talking to him, are consistent with symptoms of schizophrenia. Additionally, the presence of delusions and the duration of symptoms for several weeks suggest a psychotic disorder like schizophrenia.

7

A 29-year-old female was brought to psychiatry OPD. She appeared agitated and claimed that her husband has stolen baby from her womb. Patient was also muttering to herself and has not slept for last 4 days. She had delivered a healthy female child three weeks back, however, was not taking care of the baby. The symptoms started in second week postpartum. The likely diagnosis is:

a. Postpartum blues
b. Postpartum depression
c. Postpartum psychosis
d. Schizophrenia

Ans. (c) Postpartum psychosis

Explanation: Postpartum psychosis is a severe psychiatric disorder that can occur in some women following childbirth. It is characterized by symptoms such as agitation, delusions (e.g., believing the baby has been stolen from the womb), muttering to oneself, and sleep disturbances. The onset of symptoms in the second week postpartum, along with the patient's lack of care for the baby, further supports the diagnosis of postpartum psychosis.

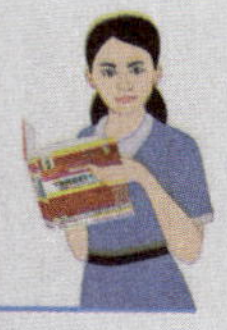

8

A 65-year-old lady is brought to the psychiatrist by her son. Son reported that she has gone absent minded six months after her husband's death. She has become more spiritual and gives lots of donations. She strongly believes that she has special powers to change society. She is occupied in too many activities and sleeps very less. She does not like being brought to the hospital and is argumentative on being questioned on her doings. The probable diagnosis is:

a. Delusional disorder
b. Impulse control disorder
c. Schizophrenia
d. Mania

Ans. (d) Mania

Explanation: The lady's symptoms are consistent with mania. The presence of absent-mindedness, increased spirituality, excessive donations, grandiose beliefs about having special powers to change society, high levels of activity, decreased sleep, resistance to hospitalization, and argumentative behavior are indicative of manic episodes.

9

A 3-year-old male child has normal developmental milestones, except delayed language development and poor speech development. He doesn't respond to name. He has difficulty in concentration, communication, and making friends. He prefers playing alone and avoids eye contact with others. The most probable diagnosis is:

a. Mental retardation
b. Specific learning disability
c. Autism
d. ADHD

Ans. (c) Autism

Explanation: The child's delayed language development, poor speech development, lack of response to name, difficulty in concentration, communication challenges, preference for solitary play, and avoidance of eye contact are indicative of characteristics commonly associated with autism spectrum disorder (ASD).

Specific learning disability typically pertains to difficulties in specific academic areas. Mental retardation refers to intellectual disability, which is not specifically mentioned in the provided information. ADHD primarily involves symptoms of hyperactivity and impulsivity.

10

A 45-year-old woman is complaining of weakness, sleep disturbances, loss of appetite, reduced interest in work, and avoidance of social interactions with friends and relatives for the past two years. The most likely diagnosis for her is:

a. Somatoform pain disorder
b. Major depression
c. Somatization disorder
d. Dissociative disorder

Ans. (b) Major depression

Explanation: Major depression is a mood disorder characterized by persistent depressive symptoms, including changes in sleep patterns, appetite, energy levels, and interest in activities. The woman's symptoms of weakness, sleep disturbances, loss of appetite, reduced interest in work, and avoidance of social interactions are consistent with the criteria for major depression.

11

A patient who is on lithium therapy for his BPAD is brought to the casualty in a state of altered sensorium. He had an episode of vomiting. On examination, he has coarse tremor, unsteady gait and muscle fasciculations. The serum lithium was found to be 1.95 mEq/L. The adverse effects of lithium is graded as:

a. Mild lithium toxicity
b. Moderate lithium toxicity
c. Severe lithium toxicity
d. Life threatening lithium toxicity

Ans. (b) Moderate lithium toxicity

Explanation: The given laboratory value and presenting symptoms suggest moderate level of lithium toxicity in patient.

Level of lithium toxicity	Plasma Lithium Level (mEq/L)	Symptoms
Mild	1.2–1.5	Nausea, vomiting, lethargy, fine tremor, fatigue
Moderate	1.5–2.5	Tachycardia, ataxia, agitation, confusion, delirium, hypertonia
Severe	2.5–3.5	Hyperthermia, hypotension, seizures, renal failure, coma to death
Life-threatening	>3.5	Coma to death

12

A 60-year-old patient with pneumonia has been hospitalized for six days but is now experiencing a change in mental status. He suddenly fails to recognize the medical staff and believes he is imprisoned, reporting of snake attacks. The likely diagnosis for this patient is:

a. Acute dementia
b. Acute delirium
c. Delusional disorder
d. Acute paranoia

Ans. (b) Acute delirium

Explanation: Delirium is characterized by a decreased level of consciousness, confusion, disorientation, and often hallucinations or delusions. The symptoms of acute delirium can fluctuate over time, and they can be caused by a variety of factors, including infections, medications, and metabolic imbalances. The given symptoms are consistent with acute delirium.

13

A 55-year-old male with chronic alcoholism presented with irrelevant talks, tremor and sweating. He had his last drink 3 days back. What will be the probable diagnosis?

a. Delirium tremens
b. Korsakoff psychosis
c. Post-Acute withdrawal syndrome
d. Discontinuation syndrome

Ans. (a) Delirium tremens

Explanation: Delirium tremens (DT) is a severe and potentially life-threatening form of alcohol withdrawal that typically occurs within 2-3 days after the last drink. It is characterized by symptoms such as confusion, disorientation, agitation, tremors, sweating, hallucinations (usually visual), and autonomic hyperactivity. The presentation of irrelevant talks, tremor, and sweating aligns with the symptoms commonly seen in delirium tremens.

14

A patient with post-traumatic stress disorder (PTSD) appears to be having a flashback. Which of the following nursing interventions is most appropriate for this patient?

a. Firmly inform the patient that what the patient experiencing is unreal.
b. Persuade the patient to express the current emotions to the nurse
c. Calmly reorient the patient to the current situation.
d. Help the patient in acting out the event.

Ans. (c) Calmly reorient the patient to the current situation.

Explanation: Flashbacks are distressing and vivid recollections of past traumatic events that can be experienced by individuals with PTSD. When a patient is having a flashback, it is important for the nurse to provide a calm and supportive environment. Calmly reorienting the patient to the present situation can help ground them and reduce the intensity of the flashback.

15

A patient was brought to the emergency room with nonstop talking, singing, agitation, uncontrollable behavior and apparent loss of contact with reality. It is diagnosed as a case of acute mania. Which of the following drugs is most suitable for rapid control of his symptoms?

a. Lithium
b. Haloperidol
c. Valproate
d. Diazepam

Ans. (b) Haloperidol

Explanation: Haloperidol used alone is recommended to help calm situations of aggression or agitation for people with psychosis. IV haloperidol can be used effectively to treat acute psychotic agitation in a low dosage of 1-2 mg every 8 hours for 2–3 days, and the drug can be continued orally for the next several days until symptoms completely subside.

16

During assessment of a patient, the nurse asked the meaning of "Strike when the rod is hot" and the patient replied, "It means that you should strike when the iron rod is hot to melt it because it is the most malleable then." What aspect of the patient thinking is demonstrated?

a. Abstract thinking
b. Concrete thinking
c. Content of thought
d. Form of thought

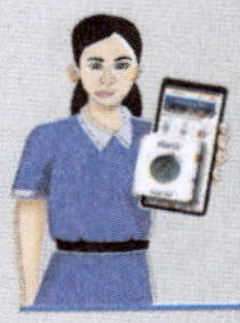

Ans. (b) Concrete thinking

Explanation: Concrete thinking refers to understanding of literal meaning of a sentence/proverb. In this case, the patient's reply demonstrates the direct and literal meaning of the proverb. Abstract thinking refers to the deeper meaning of a sentence/proverb. For example, a person capable of abstract thinking would have answered the metaphorical meaning of the proverb given in the question (strike when the iron is hot), which is to take action when the opportunities are favorable.

17

The maternity nurse is educating a new mother about the psychosocial development of her newborn using Erikson's psychosocial development theory. The nurse would advise the mother to:

a. Be proactive in anticipating the needs of the newborn infant
b. Allow the newborn to signal a need
c. Allow the infant to cry initially and then provide attention once crying subsides
d. Let the infant cry for first 10 minutes and then attend

Ans. (b) Allow the newborn to signal a need

Explanation: According to Erikson's psychosocial development theory, infants develop a sense of trust in their caregivers when their needs are consistently met. By allowing the newborn to signal their needs, the mother can respond appropriately and establish a trusting relationship with the infant. This approach supports the development of a secure attachment between the mother and the infant.

18

The nurse is caring a 60-year-old man with dementia. The nurse knows that which of the following should be the priority in caring for this client?

a. Provide the client with emotional support
b. Institute various fall prevention measures
c. Give clear written instructions
d. Encourage daytime sleep for extended periods

Ans. (b) Institute various fall prevention measures

Explanation: Falls are a significant concern for individuals with dementia, as they may experience difficulties with balance, coordination, and judgment. Implementing fall prevention measures is crucial to ensure the safety and well-being of the client.

19

A 65-year-old patient with dementia is admitted into the ward. Which among the following should be the priority in caring for this client?

a. Provide emotional support to the patient and his family
b. Establish an effective communication system with the patient and his family
c. Provide rest periods between activities
d. Encourage the patient to exercise as ordered to help maintain mobility

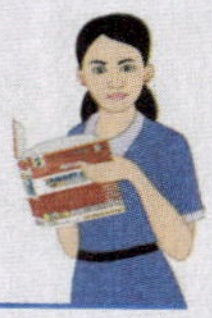

Ans. (b) Establish an effective communication system with the patient and his family

Explanation: Although all of the given options are important in caring of patient with dementia, ensuring effective communication takes priority as it facilitates overall care and understanding. Establishing an effective communication system with the patient and their family is crucial in providing comprehensive care for individuals with dementia. Communication difficulties are common in dementia, and establishing effective communication strategies helps to enhance understanding, address needs, and reduce frustration for both the patient and their family.

20

An agitated patient throws a chair across the OPD waiting room on the psychiatry floor and threatens the other patients with physical harm. Which of the following action should be taken first by the nurse?

a. Remove the other patients from the waiting room
b. Tell patient that a family member will be called to the hospital
c. Call security staff to help put the patient in preventive seclusion
d. Ask the patient to explain the cause of anger

Ans. (c) Call security staff to help put the patient in preventive seclusion

Explanation: Ensuring the immediate safety of all individuals involved is the priority in such a situation. Calling security staff is crucial to handle the aggressive behavior and protect the safety of the other patients and staff members. The patient's behavior poses a risk to others, and preventive seclusion, with the assistance of security staff, may be necessary to manage the situation.

21

A psychiatrist has prescribed Escitalopram Oxalate 10 mg PO daily for an 18-year-old male diagnosed with depression. After an initial assessment of the patient and review of the prescription, the nurse calls the psychiatrist to verify the prescription. Which of the following should be the concern for the nurse in relation to the safety of the prescription?

a. Prescribed dose is higher than the recommended dose
b. Prescribed dose is lower than the effective dose
c. Patient has a history of facial swelling and difficulty breathing with citalopram therapy
d. Medication is not recommended for use in an 18-year-old

Ans. (c) Patient has a history of facial swelling and difficulty breathing with citalopram therapy

Explanation: The nurse's concern lies in the patient's history of allergic reactions, specifically facial swelling and difficulty breathing, in response to citalopram therapy. Since escitalopram is closely related to citalopram in chemical structure, there is a potential for cross-reactivity and an increased risk of allergic reactions. Therefore, verifying the prescription with the psychiatrist is necessary to ensure patient safety.

22

A young woman who appears depressed is brought to the emergency room. On initial assessment, the nurse ascertains that her child passed away a year ago as a result of an accident. The initial nursing diagnosis is dysfunctional grieving. Which of the following statement by the women supports this nursing diagnosis?

a. "I feel envious of mothers who have toddlers."
b. "I haven't been able to open the door and enter my child's room."
c. "I observe other toddlers playing and it brings me to tears."
d. "I frequently contemplate how I could have prevented the death."

Ans. (b) "I haven't been able to open the door and enter my child's room."

Explanation: Dysfunctional grieving is characterized by difficulty in accepting the loss and engaging in behaviors that hinder the grieving process. The woman's statement indicates that she is unable to enter her child's room, suggesting that she is struggling with the process of accepting the loss and coping with her grief. This statement aligns with the diagnosis of dysfunctional grieving.

23

A patient with end-stage cancer tells the nurse, "If I can just survive to see my first grandson who is expected in 6 months, then I can die happy." The nurse understands that the patient is demonstrating which of the following stages of grieving?

a. Prolonged grief disorder
b. Kübler-Ross's stage of acceptance
c. Kübler-Ross's stage of bargaining
d. Kübler-Ross's stage of depression

Ans. (c) Kübler-Ross's stage of bargaining

Explanation: In Kübler-Ross's stages of grief, bargaining is one of the stages that individuals may go through when facing a terminal illness or impending death. During this stage, individuals may make deals or negotiate with a higher power (e.g., God), hoping to delay or alter the outcome. The patient's statement reflects a form of bargaining, as they express a desire to survive long enough to witness the birth of their first grandson.

24

The nurse is caring for a patient who is experiencing depressed mood, poor concentration, decreased sleep and poor appetite for the past five months. The nurse anticipates administering which of the following medications to the patient?

a. Haloperidol
b. Clonazepam
c. Quetiapine
d. Mirtazapine

Ans. (d) Mirtazapine

Explanation: The symptoms described are consistent with major depressive disorder. Mirtazapine is an antidepressant medication commonly used to treat depression. Haloperidol and Quetiapine are antipsychotics used to manage psychosis. Clonazepam is a benzodiazepine, used as an antianxiety agent and sedative.

25

An 82-year-old patient accompanied by his daughter presents at the hospital seeking diagnostic confirmation and management for suspected delirium. Which statement made by the patient's daughter provides the best support for the diagnosis?

a. "Perhaps it's just a result of aging. It's common at his age, right?"
b. "Dad has always been very self-sufficient. He has lived alone since mom passed away."
c. "His behavioral changes occurred so rapidly! I wasn't sure what was going on."
d. "Dad didn't seem to know what he was doing. He couldn't recall what he had for breakfast."

Ans. (c) "His behavioral changes occurred so rapidly! I wasn't sure what was going on."

Explanation: Delirium is characterized by a rapid onset of cognitive changes, including disturbances in attention, awareness, and perception. The daughter's statement about the sudden onset of behavioral changes aligns with this characteristic of delirium, providing support for the diagnosis.

26

The nurse is preparing to administer electroconvulsive therapy (ECT) to a patient and explains to the student nurses the primary reason for administering atropine before the treatment. Which of the following is the main purpose of administering atropine before ECT?

a. To minimize gastrointestinal contractions and promote digestion.
b. To reduce anxiety and help the patient relax before the procedure.
c. To prevent aspiration and protect the patient's airway.
d. To increase body secretions and improve overall hydration.

Ans. (c) To prevent aspiration and protect the patient's airway.

Explanation: The main purpose of administering atropine before ECT is to prevent aspiration and protect the patient's airway. ECT can sometimes cause excessive salivation, and atropine, as an anticholinergic medication, helps to dry up secretions, reducing the risk of saliva entering the lungs and causing aspiration pneumonia.

27

The nurse is providing care for a patient experiencing a manic episode. Which intervention would be most appropriate for the nurse to perform in this situation?

a. Encourage the patient to attend a group focused on managing emotions.
b. Provide the patient with art materials to engage in a creative activity.
c. Facilitate a board game session with other patients.
d. Encourage the patient to engage in physical activity using an exercise bike.

Ans. (d) Encourage the patient to engage in physical activity using an exercise bike.

Explanation: During a manic episode, individuals often have excess energy and restlessness. Engaging in physical activity can

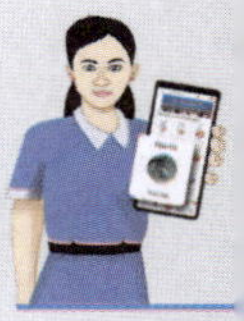

help channel and release this energy in a productive and healthy way. Exercise can also help promote relaxation, reduce agitation, and improve overall mood. Encouraging the patient to use an exercise bike provides a structured and safe means of physical activity.

28

A 17-year-old girl who has experienced sexual abuse has no memory of the event and is unable to recall any details despite her best efforts. What is the likely diagnosis for this girl?

a. Dementia
b. Dissociative amnesia
c. Delirium
d. Malingering

Ans. (b) Dissociative amnesia

Explanation: Dissociative amnesia is a type of dissociative disorder characterized by the inability to recall important personal information, typically associated with traumatic or stressful events. In cases of traumatic experiences such as sexual abuse, the mind may use dissociation as a defense mechanism to protect the individual from the overwhelming emotions and memories associated with the event.

29

A 50-year-old male presents with a three-year history of irritability, low mood, lack of interest in his surroundings, and a general sense of dissatisfaction. There are no significant disturbances in sleep and appetite. What is the likely diagnosis for this patient?

a. Major depression
b. No psychiatric disorder
c. Dysthymia
d. Somatoform disorder

Ans. (c) Dysthymia

Explanation: Dysthymia, also known as persistent depressive disorder, is characterized by chronic depressive symptoms that last for at least two years in adults (one year in children/adolescents). The symptoms may not be as severe as those seen in major depression but persist for an extended duration and significantly impact daily functioning.

30

A 40-year-old male was brought to the psychiatry OPD by the family members and the following clinical features are noted which are seen for about three weeks in the last one month. He speaks to himself, complains of hearing two people talking about him, reduced affect and impaired judgment. What is the probable diagnosis?

a. Brief psychotic episode
b. Dementia
c. Manic episode
d. Fugue state

Ans. (a) Brief psychotic episode

Explanation: Based on the given information, the most probable diagnosis is a brief psychotic episode. A brief psychotic episode is characterized by the presence of psychotic symptoms, such as hallucinations (e.g., hearing voices) and impaired judgment, which last for a brief duration, typically less than one month. The symptoms described in the scenario align with the criteria for a brief psychotic episode.

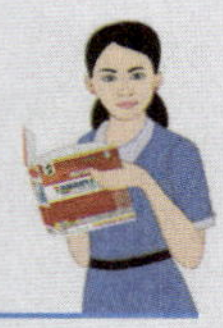

31

A 46-year-old male presented to the psychiatry OPD with the clinical features of speaking to himself, hearing two people talk about him, reduced affect and impaired judgment which were present for more than 6 months. What is the diagnosis?

a. Brief Psychotic disorder
b. Major depression with psychosis
c. Schizophrenia
d. Schizophreniform disorder

Ans. (c) Schizophrenia

Explanation: Schizophrenia is a psychiatric disorder characterized by symptoms such as hallucinations (such as hearing voices), delusions (such as believing others are talking about oneself), reduced affect (emotional expression), and impaired judgment. To make a diagnosis of schizophrenia, symptoms must be present for a significant portion of time over a 1-month period and continue for at least 6 months, including active-phase symptoms (such as hallucinations or delusions).

32

Patient A and B are on different antipsychotics. A has gained a lot of weight and has been feeling dizzy when she stands. B has not gained weight, but is very restless and keeps pacing around the room. The drug they are taking most likely are:

a. A-Haloperidol, B- Chlorpromazine
b. A- Haloperidol, B- Risperidone
c. A- Clozapine, B- Quetiapine
d. A- Olanzapine, B- Haloperidol

Ans. (d) A- Olanzapine, B- Haloperidol

Explanation: Olanzapine is an atypical antipsychotic that is known to cause weight gain and dizziness. Haloperidol is a typical antipsychotic that is not known to cause weight gain, but can cause restlessness.

33

A 50-year-old individual with a history of chronic alcoholism is admitted to the hospital in a confused state, exhibiting loss of muscle coordination and double vision. During evaluation, the clinician asks the patient if he remembers what he had for breakfast, to which the patient confidently responds that they had Dosa. However, the attendant disputes this claim, stating that the patient did not have any breakfast that day. The patient then insists that he had Dosa for breakfast with his wife. The attendant confirmed that the patient did not meet his wife that day. What is this phenomenon referred to as?

a. Dementia and Lewy bodies
b. Confabulation
c. Delusion
d. Preservation

Ans. (b) Confabulation

Explanation: Confabulation is a cognitive phenomenon where an individual produces false or fabricated memories or information without the intention to deceive. In this case, the patient confidently states that he had Dosa for breakfast with his wife, despite the attendant confirming that the patient did not have breakfast or meet his wife that day.

34

A patient says that he feels that there is something wrong with him mentally and it is because of the winter season. How much would he score on the insight scale?

a. 2/6 b. 3/6
c. 4/6 d. 5/6

Ans. (b) 3/6

Explanation:

Grade 1	Complete denial of illness
Grade 2	Slight awareness of being sick and needing help but denying at the same time
Grade 3	Awareness of being sick but blaming it on others, external factors, organic factors (**as applicable in the given case scenario**)
Grade 4	Awareness that illness is due to something unknown in patient
Grade 5	Intellectual insight: admission that the patient is ill without applying that knowledge for future experience
Grade 6	True emotional insight: emotional awareness of the motives and feelings within patient and the important people in his / her life.

35

A 30-year-old married man strongly believes that his wife is unfaithful to him. He remains firm on his belief despite reassurances from his wife and his family members that his belief is untrue and baseless. This is referred to as:

a. De Clerembault syndrome b. Ekbom syndrome
c. Fregoli syndrome d. Morbid jealousy

Ans. (d) Morbid jealousy

Explanation: Morbid jealousy, often referred to as pathological jealousy or Othello syndrome, is a condition which occurs when a person feels an irrational fear of their partner being unfaithful toward them. Individuals with morbid jealousy may engage in behaviors such as stalking, persistent accusations of infidelity, and, in severe cases, domestic abuse.

36

Which of the following is the nurses' correct interpretation when the patient has serum lithium level 2.0 mEq/L?

a. The levels are below therapeutic range; inform the physician
b. The levels are within therapeutic range; do nothing
c. The levels are elevated; patient should be assessed for lithium toxicity manifestation.
d. The levels are slightly elevated; do nothing.

Ans. (c) The levels are elevated; patient should be assessed for lithium toxicity manifestation.

Explanation: The therapeutic level of lithium is 0.8–1.2 mEq/L, Prophylactic level is 0.6–1.2 mEq/L. Here the patient had the level of >2.0 mEq/L, more than 2.0 mEq/L indicates lithium toxicity.

37

A patient is taking chlorpromazine drug. On evaluation, the patient demonstrates a shuffling gait, curved posture, drooling, and exhibits ataxia. The patient has developed:

a. Tardive dyskinesia b. Drug-induced parkinsonism
c. Dystonia d. Akathisia

Ans. (b) Drug-induced parkinsonism

Rationale: Chlorpromazine is an antipsychotic drug. Drug-induced parkinsonism is one of the adverse effects of antipsychotic drugs. The symptoms of drug-induced parkinsonism are muscular rigidity, tremors, ataxia, drooling, inability to sit still and bradykinesia. The other side effects of antipsychotics include akathisia, Tardive dyskinesia, acute dystonia and neuroleptic malignant syndrome.

38

A patient is receiving clozapine. Which of following blood investigation the patient should routinely undergo?

a. TLC, DLC. b. Thyroid Profile.
c. Lipid Profile. d. Liver Function Test

Ans. (a) TLC, DLC

Explanation: If a patient is receiving clozapine, he/she is at risk of developing agranulocytosis (deficiency of a granulocytes in the blood). So the monitoring of total leukocyte count and differential leukocyte count is essential. If the WBC level is below 3000/mm^3, the drug should be stopped immediately.

39

Few days after regularly taking antipsychotic drugs, the patient develops feeling of muscle discomfort that is making the patient agitated, restless, generally dysphoric. Which side effect the patient is experiencing?

a. Neuroleptic malignant syndrome
b. Tardive dyskinesia.
c. Dystonia
d. Akathisia

Ans. (d) Akathisia

Explanation: Akathisia means inability to sit still. It is a feeling of muscular discomfort that will cause restlessness, agitation and uneasiness/dissatisfaction. Akathisia is one of the adverse effects of antipsychotic drugs.

40

What is the other name of antidepressant drugs?

a. Neuroleptics b. Thymoleptics
c. Mood stabilizers d. Major tranquilizers

Ans. (b) Thymoleptics

Explanation: Thymoleptics are the drugs which can change the person's mood and are also called antidepressant drugs. Neuroleptic drugs/major tranquilizers are also known as

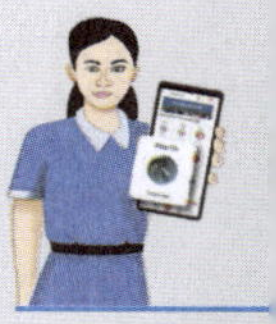

antipsychotic drugs. They are is used to treat various psychiatric conditions. Mood stabilizers are also known as antiepileptic medication/anticonvulsant medication which are used to treat mania and seizures.

41

After taking antipsychotic drugs, the patient experiences sedation because antipsychotic drugs:

a. Block D2 receptors in mesolimbic systems.
b. Block D2 receptors basal ganglia.
c. Cause alpha-adrenergic blockage.
d. Block D2 receptors mesofrontal system.

Ans. (c) Cause alpha-adrenergic blockage

Explanation: The blockage of D2 receptors in mesolimbic and mesofrontal system may result in emotional reactions. Sedation is caused due to the blockage of alpha-adrenergic receptor. The extra pyramidal symptoms are due to the anti-dopaminergic actions in the basal ganglia.

42

After 5 days of taking Haloperidol, the patient develops abnormal, irregular, choreoathetoid movement of muscles of head, limbs and trunk. Which of the following symptom is the patient experiencing?

a. Tardive dyskinesia
b. Akathisia
c. Drug-induced parkinsonism
d. Acute dystonia

Ans. (a) Tardive dyskinesia

Explanation: Tardive dyskinesia is a movement disorder, in which the clients experience involuntary and repetitive choreoathetoid movements of the limbs, trunk and head. It is the late adverse effect of antipyschotics.

43

The mental health care bill was introduced in Rajya Sabha on the following date:

a. 19th April 2011
b. 25th July 2016
c. 18th January 2013
d. 19th August 2013

Ans. (d) 19th August 2013

44

A patient experiences that he is hearing voices of people who are talking several kilometers away. What type of hallucination it is?

a. Visual hallucination
b. Auditory hallucination
c. Extracampine hallucination
d. Reflex hallucination

Ans. (c) Extracampine hallucination

Explanation: Extracampine hallucination is a type of hallucination which is outside the limits of one's sensory field that is either outside the visual field or not within the range of audibility.

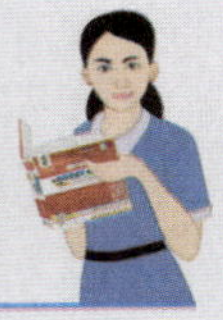

45

A jealous employee who hates his/her senior may show exaggerated respect and affection toward him. Which type of defense mechanism is it?

a. Displacement
b. Reaction formation
c. Denial
d. Projection

Ans. (b) Reaction formation

Explanation: Reaction formation is replacing unacceptable feelings with their exact opposites. Displacement means unconsciously discharging pent-up feelings to a less threatening objects. Projection means unconsciously or consciously blaming someone else for one's difficulty. Denial is defined as unconscious refusal to admit an unacceptable idea or behavior, usually the first defense is learned and used.

46

After completing the viva of psychiatric nursing successfully, Mr X felt calm and relaxed. He stopped sweating and felt hungry. Which part of his nervous system is activated?

a. Somatic
b. Cerebellum
c. Parasympathetic
d. Sympathetic

Ans. (c) Parasympathetic

Explanation: The primary process in sympathetic nervous system is mainly responsible to stimulate the body's 'fight or flight response'. The parasympathetic nervous system is responsible for stimulation of 'rest and digest' response of our body. The sympathetic nervous system will prepare the body for any potential danger. The parasympathetic nervous system will inhibit the body from a stressful situation and restores the body to a calm state.

47

During mental status examination, a nurse asks a patient about similarity between paired objects. Which component of the cognitive functioning the nurse is testing?

a. Abstract thinking
b. Intelligence
c. Memory
d. Orientation

Ans. (a) Abstract thinking

Explanation: Abstract thinking is defined as the ability to use concepts and to use metaphors and hypotheses appropriately. Abstract thinker can conceptualize, generalize and understand that each concept can have multiple meaning.

48

Which of the following is an appropriate statement for the principle "use self understanding as a therapeutic tool"?

a. Being nonjudgmental and nonpunitive
b. Routine pattern that does not change from one day to the other
c. Analysis and study of symptoms.
d. Keep reflecting on why you feel or act the way you do

Ans. (d) Keep reflecting on why you feel or act the way you do.

Explanation: A psychiatric nurse should have a realistic self-concept and should be able to recognize one's own feelings, attitudes and responses. It will help her to care the patients effectively.

49

A nurse is performing intelligence testing of the patient. Which of the following instrument she should use?

a. Bhatia battery test
b. Rorschach inkblot test
c. Thematic apperception test
d. Mini mental status examination

Ans. (a) Bhatia battery test

Explanation: Bhatia battery test is used to assess the intelligence of a patient. There are five sub tests in this test which include, Kohs block design – discrimination of patterns, Alexander's pass along test- Discrimination of movement of concrete material, Pattern drawing test – analysis in terms of line, Immediate memory – Verbal memory, Picture Construction – Discrimination of picture parts.

Rorschach inkblot test is used as a projective psychological test. It is used to identify the emotional functioning and personality. Thematic apperception test is projective personality test. Mini mental status examination is used to assess the cognitive functions.

50

While performing a deep tendon reflex test, the nurse gently scraps the sole of the foot with a blunt object. She observes dorsiflexion of the great toe and often fanning of the other toe. Which reflex she is testing for?

a. Glabella reflex
b. Babinski reflex
c. Snout reflex
d. Rooting reflex

Ans. (b) Babinski reflex

Explanation: Babinski reflex is normal in infants. In adults with a positive Babinski reflex, the greater toe dorsiflex and the other toes fan outward. The positive Babinski reflex indicates there is an underlying nervous system or any brain condition that will cause the reflexes to react abnormally. A negative Babinski reflex (normal) elicits flexion of all toes.

51

Which component of nursing process requires three part statement, i.e., the health problem, contributing factor and the defining characteristic?

a. Assessment
b. Nursing intervention
c. Nursing diagnosis
d. Expected outcome

Ans. (c) Nursing diagnosis

Explanation: Nursing diagnosis statement includes three main components, actual or potential problem, etiology or risk factors of the problem and the defining characteristic of problem. These three components are needed for a nursing diagnosis statement. In assessment, two types of data are collected—one is subjective data and the other is objective data.

52

While performing neurological examination, the nurse asks the patient to place his index finger on the nurse's index finger. He is asked to repeat this for several times. Which component of neurological examination the nurse is assessing?

a. Cerebellar function
b. Motor function
c. Cranial nerve examination
d. Cerebral function

Ans. (a) Cerebellar function

Explanation: The purpose of cerebellar functioning assessment is for the evaluation of balance and coordination. In this the nurse asked the client to perform finger to finger test. The other tests like finger to nose test, Romberg test and tandem walking test are used to assess cerebellar function.

53

A patient with schizophrenia exhibits preoccupation with the self, with little concern to external environment and inability to relate with others. The nurse documents this finding as :

a. Ambivalence
b. Anhedonia
c. Alogia
d. Autistic Thinking

Ans. (d) Autistic Thinking

Explanation: Autistic thinking is defined as preoccupations that totally remove a person from the reality. In this the client experiences narcissistic, ego centric, fantasizing and day dreaming. Anhedonia means inability to experience pleasure in any activity. Ambivalence is defined as the coexistence of two opposite feelings or emotions for the same person. Alogia means poverty of speech.

54

A patient exhibits delusional belief that other people in the environment is not their actual selves but are their own doubles. The nurse concludes this finding as:

a. Somatic delusion
b. Visual hallucination
c. Capgras syndrome
d. Acute and transient psychotic disorder

Ans. (c) Capgras syndrome

Explanation: Capgras syndrome is one of the delusional misidentification syndromes. The person with this syndrome cannot be able to identify the persons in the environment. Person having delusion that a well known person has been replaced by an identical looking imposter. It is also known as Imposter syndrome.

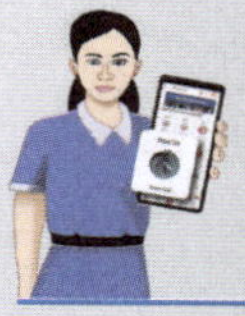

55

During mental status examination, a schizophrenic patient tells the nurse, "my family members are setting conspiracy to kill me, they have even poisoned my food." The nurse documents that the patient is experiencing:

a. Delusion of grandiosity
b. Delusion of persecution
c. Delusion of control
d. Delusion of jealousy

Ans. (b) Delusion of persecution

Explanation: Delusion of persecution is defined as the person believes that he/she is being cheated, tracked, slandered or harmed by some other persons. Delusion of grandiosity is defined as the person develops false belief that he or she is having super powers or he/she is the supreme member in the world. Delusion of jealousy centers around that the person's partner is not faithful.

56

A patient with schizophrenia has potential to harm self as well as others in the ward. Which of the following is the most appropriate nursing intervention?

a. Maintain low level of stimulation; be alert for signs of increasing anxiety and agitation
b. Assess the nature of severity
c. Apply mechanical restraints if necessary
d. Ask the patient directly "have you thought about harming yourself or others"

Ans. (a) Maintain low level of stimulation; be alert for signs of increasing anxiety and agitation

Explanation: Always assess the schizophrenia patients for any suicidal attempts or to harm other persons in the ward. Create a safe environment for the patients, remove the sharp and harmful objects from the patient's sight. Assess the nature and severity of hallucinations periodically.

57

A person who was wandering purposelessly around the roads, untidy, on examination he is found muttering to self and irritable sometimes. Which of the following disorder the patient may be suffering from?

a. Major depressive disorder
b. Schizotypal personality disorder
c. Obsessive compulsive disorder
d. Chronic schizophrenia

Ans. (d) Chronic schizophrenia

Explanation: Chronic schizophrenia is defined as a severe mental disorder that affects how a person thinks, feels and behaves. Client with schizophrenia has lost touch with the reality. The symptoms of chronic schizophrenia include affective flattening, alogia, anhedonia, avolition and poor attention. These are the negative symptoms of schizophrenia having poorest prognosis.

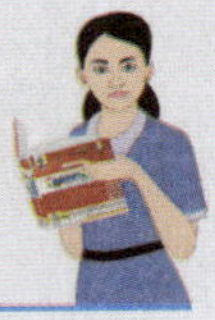

58

On family assessment, patient's family members show; critical, hostile and overinvolvement behavior toward patient. Document the attitude that the family is showing:

a. Adequate support system
b. Expressed emotions
c. Care and concern toward patient
d. Judgmental attitude toward patient

Ans. (b) Expressed emotions

Explanation: Expressed emotion is the critical and emotionally overinvolved attitude that the family members show toward the client. This negative family atmosphere will lead to relapse of the symptoms and rehospitalization and will also put significant effect on the course of illness.

59

A patient with excited catatonia shows extreme excitement with rigidity, appears hyperthermic and dehydrated. The nurse documents this finding as:

a. Pernicious catatonia
b. Catatonic stupor
c. Ecstasy
d. Extremely excited catatonia

Ans. (a) Pernicious catatonia

Explanation: The clinical features of catatonic schizophrenia include loosening of associations, increase in speech production, increase in excitement, aggressiveness, restlessness, agitation, loosening of association. If the excitement becomes very severe and is accompanied by hyperthermia, dehydration, rigidity and can lead to death, it is called pernicious catatonia or acute lethal catatonia.

60

Mr Suresh and Mr Mohan have close emotional bond. Mr Suresh experiences delusion of grandiosity (in actuality), after some time Mr Mohan also experiences the same symptoms as Mr Suresh. Which type of disorder the two are experiencing?

a. Persistent delusional disorder
b. Capgras syndrome
c. Induced delusional disorder
d. Acute and transient psychotic disorder

Ans. (c) Induced delusional disorder

Explanation: A delusional disorder shared by two closely related persons in which only one person is having genuine psychotic disorder, the other person is induced and mutually share the same delusion. It is popularly called folieadeux.

MOOD DISORDERS

61

According to Sigmund Freud, loss of loved object and fixation in the oral sadistic phase of development leads to development of which disorder?

a. Mania
b. Schizophrenia
c. Depression
d. Phobia

Ans. (d) Depression

Explanation: According to Sigmund Freud, the oral stage is divided into two sub-phases. The first is oral incorporative phase (0 – 6 months). The oral incorporative behavior occurs first and involves the pleasurable stimulation of the mouth by other people and by food. Adults fixated at the oral incorporative stage are excessively concerned with oral activities such as smoking, drinking and kissing. The second oral behavior is oral sadistic phase which occurs during the painful, frustrating eruption of teeth. Persons fixated at this level are prone to excessive pessimism, hostility and aggressiveness.

62

A patient is taking selective serotonin reuptake inhibitor for the treatment of depression and asks the nurse about the time lag for the maximum therapeutic affect to occur. The best response of the nurse is:

a. Two days
b. One week
c. Four weeks
d. Three weeks

Ans. (d) Three weeks

Explanation: SSRI will slow down the reabsorption of serotonin which helps to regulate the mood and anxiety. The maximum therapeutic response of the drug SSRI will take up to three weeks. So the nurse should educate the client that it will take three weeks for the maximum therapeutic response.

63

A patient with mania states " Rock, clock, lock, mock". The nurse documents this verbal expression as:

a. Flight of ideas
b. Word salad
c. Clang association
d. Euphoria

Ans. (c) Clang Association

Explanation: Clang association is the disorder of stream of thought. It refers to the sequence of thought stimulated by the sound of previous word rather than by the meaning. It is mostly based on the rhyming of the word without the proper meaning of the word.

64

A patient with suicidal ideation gives a written agreement to the health care team regarding not to harm himself and herself. Such type of contract is known as:

a. No harm contract
b. No suicide pledge
c. No injury contract
d. No suicide contract

Ans. (d) No suicide contract

Explanation: No suicide contract is a written agreement between the patient and the nurse that the patient will not act on any suicidal impulses. It is considered one of the forms of management for suicide.

65

Although there is a risk of suicide in all patients with depression. The risk is higher in which of the following situation?

a. Recovery from depression
b. At peak of depression
c. Being married women
d. Female gender

Ans. (a) Recovery from depression

Explanation: The risk of suicide is more after the recovery from depression because the characteristic psychomotor retardation has improved and the patient has more energy to carry out the suicidal plans.

66

A patient with mood disorder is getting discharged from hospital. The nurse educates the patient and family members about inclusion of good bowel regimen and high fiber diet, and increase fluid intake in lifestyle as medicines may cause constipation. Which medicine the patient is on?

a. Lithium
b. Carbamazepine
c. Antidepressants
d. Atypical antipsychotics

Ans. (c) Antidepressants

Explanation: One of the side effects of antidepressants is constipation. So in order to avoid constipation, the nurse should educate the client to follow good bowel regimen and high-fiber diet. The other autonomic side effects are dry mouth, mydriasis, urinary retention, orthostatic hypotension, impotence, delirium and aggravation of glaucoma.

67

A nurse accepts free gifts from patient and develops personal or social relationship with the patient. Such act from the nurse will be called:

a. Resistance
b. Boundary violation
c. Transference
d. Countertransference

Ans. (b) Boundary violation

Explanation: Boundary violation is defined as the nurse goes outside the boundaries of the therapeutic relationship and establishes a personal relationship with the patient, like she accepts gifts from the patient, hugs or has physical contact with patient, reveals personal information to the patient, etc.

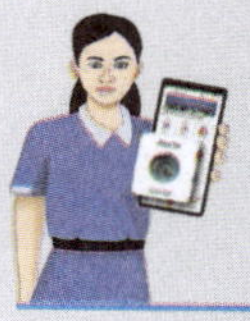

68

While conducting interview of a patient and after the patient's response, the nurse replies, "I am Not sure what you mean". Could you please tell me about that again? Which technique of therapeutic communication the nurse is using?

a. Seeking clarification
b. Focusing
c. Reflection
d. Sharing perception

Ans. (a) Seeking clarification

Explanation: Seeking clarification is a technique of therapeutic communication in which the nurse attempts to put vague ideas into words.

69

A patient with a paranoid personality disorder mistrusts people and doesn't work together with others as a way to handle the problems. Which one is the most appropriate nursing intervention?

a. Directly confronting the patient
b. Diverting patient's mind into the recreational activities
c. Taking feedback about the patient from his family
d. Clarifying thoughts and belief regarding an incident

Ans. (d) Clarifying thoughts and belief regarding an incident

Explanation: The paranoid personality disorder is marked by unrelenting mistrust and suspicion of others, even when there is no reason to be suspicious. Person with paranoid personality disorder searches for hidden meaning and hostile intentions in everything others say. So the most appropriate nursing intervention is to clarify thoughts and belief regarding an incident.

70

A patient demonstrates persistent social inhibition, agoraphobia, fear of criticism, thoughts of inferiority to others, and feelings of being totally unattractive to others.The nurse interprets these actions as features of which disorder?

a. Schizoid personality disorder
b. Schizotypal personality disorder
c. Avoidant personality disorder
d. Borderline personality disorder

Ans. (c) Avoidant personality disorder

Explanation: Avoidant personality disorder is characterized by social inhibition, feelings of inadequacy, and sensitivity to rejection and criticism that cause problems in work situations and relationships. The disorder is characterized by extreme shyness and sensitivity to criticism from others and is known as a Cluster C personality disorder or one that involves anxious and fearful personality disorders.

71

A newly-admitted patient had an argument with another patient of his room. After the argument, the patient requests the nurse to change his room because he believes that all patients in the room are same and have a tendency to argue all the time with one another. The most appropriate interpretation of patient's belief is:

a. Overgeneralization
b. Free association
c. Unrealistic assumption
d. Faulty inference

Ans. (a) Overgeneralization

Explanation: Over-generalization mainly affects the clients with anxiety and depression. It is a cognitive distortion in which an individual views a single event as an invariable rule. The way of thinking an individual had one experience expecting the same to all experiences, including those in the future.

72

A patient has thrown his food into the ward. The nurse makes him to clean the dirty area and mop the entire ward. Which behavior therapy technique the nurse has used?

a. Punishment
b. Time out
c. Channing
d. Restitution

Ans. (d) Restitution

Explanation: Restitution is defined as restoring the disturbed situation to a state that is better than before the occurrence of problematic behavior. It is a procedure that requires an individual returns the environment to its state prior to the behavior which changes the environment.

73

While caring for a patient with panic anxiety, the nurse maintains calm, nonthreatening matter-of-fact approach. What is the rationale behind this intervention?

a. Anxiety is contagious
b. To make the patient relax
c. It may provide feeling of security
d. It will decrease the patient's anxiety

Ans. (a) Anxiety is contagious

Explanation: A person with anxiety always faces trouble-relaxing so the relaxation technique is essential for the anxiety patients. While maintaining calm and nonthreatening environment, client can slowly get relief from the anxiety behavior. Cognitive therapy focuses on changing patterns of thinking and beliefs that are associated with trigger and anxiety.

74

A patient with OCD was made to sit comfortably in a chair. Patient was made to recall the unwanted thoughts and as soon as the thoughts appear the patient was instructed to stop followed by a relaxation. The therapist is using which technique?

a. Exposure and response prevention.
b. Systemic desensitization.
c. Thought stoppage
d. Thought balancing

Ans. (c) Thought stoppage

Explanation: Thought stoppage in OCD is a cognitive intervention technique in which the process of suppressing or pushing away the unwanted repeated thoughts takes place. Whenever the unwanted thoughts reoccur, a command like 'stop' or using rubber band on the wrist of the patient is given to punish himself/herself in the intention of stopping the negative behavior.

75

A patient complains that he is experiencing urges to perform unusual acts like beating a child, or giving threats to a child. The nurse documents that the patient is experiencing:

a. Obsessional doubts
b. Obsessional impulses
c. Obsessional rituals
d. Obsessional images

Ans. (b) Obsessional impulses

Explanation: Obsessional impulses are the ideas, thoughts and beliefs that force the client's mind to execute the obsessional impulse like behaving violently, shouting in the calm environment, hurting a child. Obsessional images mean repeated images or pictures about abnormal sexual activity. Obsessional doubts mean lack of confidence in one's own memory, attention and perception. Obsessional rituals mean repeating a certain form of words or senseless behavior.

76

A person fears that something bad will happen if he throws anything away. He compulsively accumulates things that he doesn't need or use. The patient falls in which category of OCD?

a. Arrangers
b. Doubters
c. Counters
d. Hoarders

Ans. (d) Hoarders

Explanation: A person with hoarding disorder had excessive acquiring tendency and difficulty in discarding the items. In hoarding disorder, excessive accumulation of items rather than their use or there is no space for keeping the items, always had the feeling of need to save the items. The patients believe that the saved items are unique and will be needed in some point of time.

77

A patient complains of persisting and distressing increase in fatigue after any mental and physical effort. The nurse documents this as:

a. Neurasthenia
b. Derealization
c. Pathological fatigue
d. Patient is lazy

Ans. (a) Neurasthenia

Explanation: It is a medical condition in which the client is having the symptoms of dizziness, dyspepsia, muscle aches, irritability and physical fatigue. Fatigue is predominant in the neurasthenia. It is caused by a physical, neurological disease that affected the entire body, causing intense, long-term fatigue.

78

A person has preoccupation with an imagined defect in appearance. If a slight physical anomaly is present, the person's concern is markedly excessive. He is likely to be suffering from:

a. Somatization
b. Hypochondriasis
c. Body dysmorphic disorder
d. Generalized anxiety disorder

Ans. (c) Body dysmorphic disorder

Explanation: Body dysmorphic disorder means person preoccupied with an imagined physical defect or minor defect that the other person cannot see. These people see themselves as ugly and avoid public exposure and try to improve their appearance by involving in plastic surgery. It affects both men and women equally and usually begins at the age group of early adulthood.

79

In which disorder the most appropriate nursing intervention is to "encourage a patient to express her grief, complete the mourning process and use crisis intervention techniques as needed."

a. Depression
b. Dysthymia
c. Anxiety disorder
d. Post-traumatic stress disorder

Ans. (d) Post-traumatic stress disorder

Explanation: Post-traumatic stress disorder is an anxiety disorder caused by very stressful, frightening or distressing events. The symptoms of PTSD are disturbed sleep, difficulty in concentration, irritability and guilt. Encouraging the clients to express their grief, will help to relieve the client from distress.

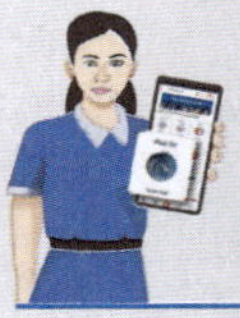

Image-Based Questions

1. Identify the behavioral syndrome as shown in photograph: *[Recent Question 2013]*

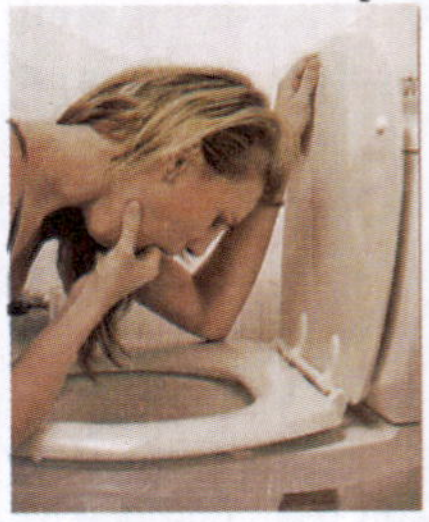

a. Anorexia nervosa b. Bulimia nervosa
c. Obesity d. Binge-eating disorder

2. Fear of situation shown in the photograph is known as:

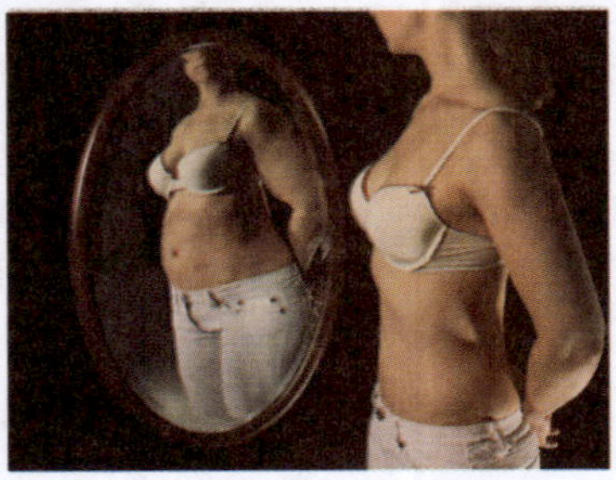

a. Xenophobia b. Sitophobia
c. Algophobia d. Ichthyophobia

3. Disorder in which a person develops sexual arousal with object shown in photograph:

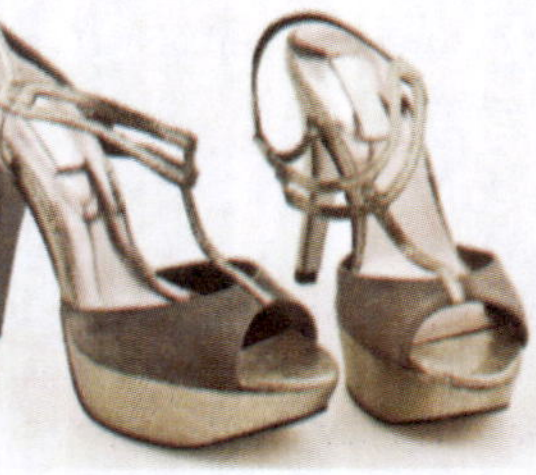

a. Sexual masochism b. Voyeurism
c. Frotteurism d. Fetischism

4. Identify paraphilia shown in photograph:

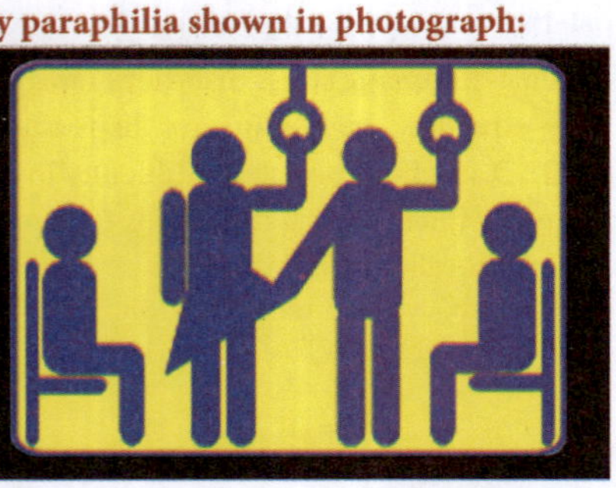

a. Sadism b. Exhibitionism
c. Sexual masochism d. Frotteurism

5. Method of substance use shown in figure is mainly used for:

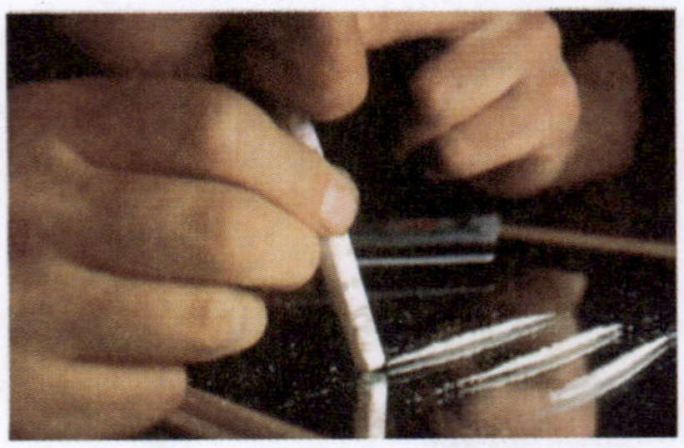

a. Ganja b. Bhang
c. Charas d. Cocaine

6. Plant shown in photograph is NOT a source of:

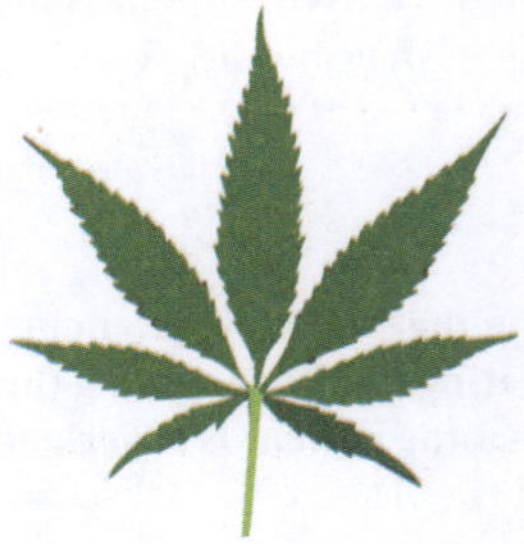

a. Bhang b. Charas
c. Cocaine d. Ganja

7. Plant shown in the photograph can lead to .... poisoning: *[Recent Question 2017]*

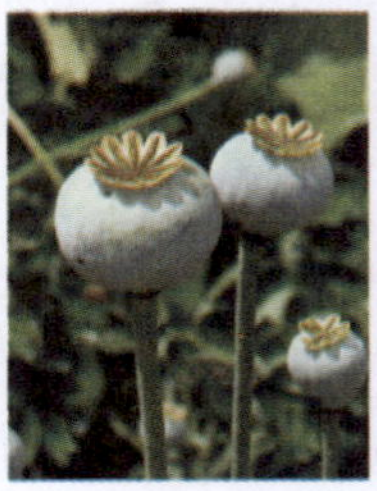

a. Cocaine b. Opioid
c. Cannabis d. None of these

8. Maximum score of test shown in photograph is:

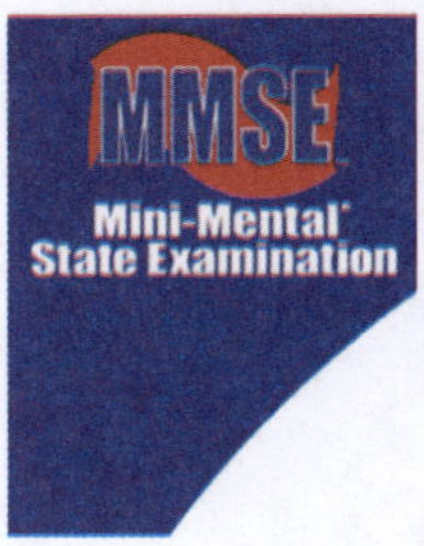

a. 13 b. 30
c. 47 d. 55

Ans.

1.	b
2.	b
3.	d
4.	d
5.	d
6.	c
7.	b
8.	b

[*Courtesy*: PHOTON-20® 3th ed. by Vivek Jain, CBS Publishers and Distributors Pvt Ltd]

9. Psychiatric test shown in photograph is a type of:

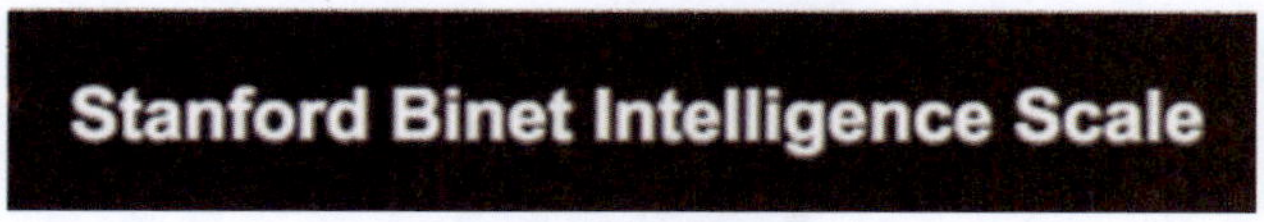

a. Objective test
b. Projective test
c. Neuropsychological test
d. Rating scale

10. Fear of situation shown in the photograph is known as:

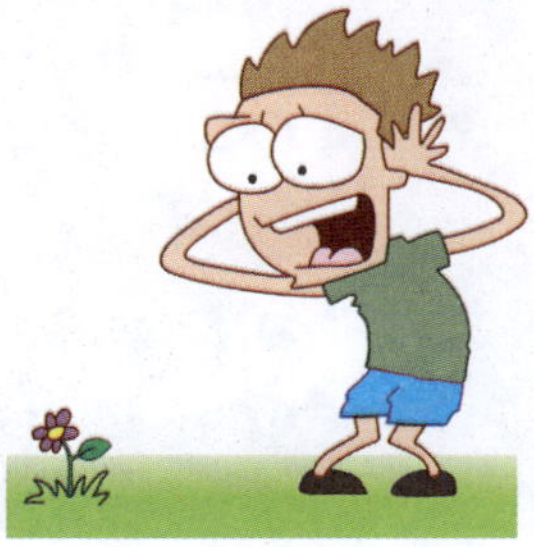

a. Xenophobia
b. Algophobia
c. Antlophobia
d. Claustrophobia

11. Identify the child psychiatric disorder as shown in photograph:

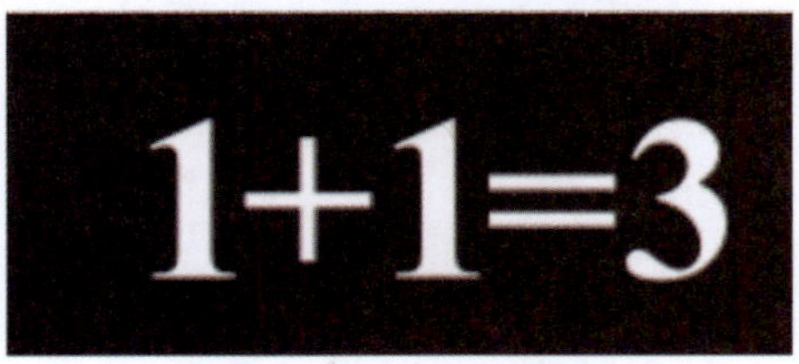

a. Dyscalculia
b. Dysphasia
c. Dyspraxia
d. Echolalia

12. Identify fear shown in photograph:

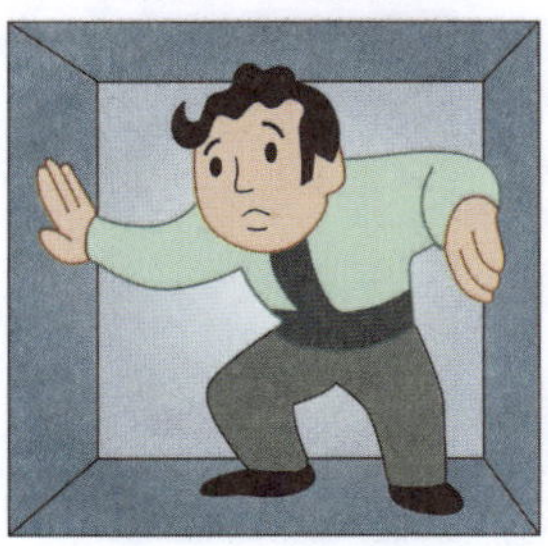

a. Agoraphobia
b. Acrophobia
c. Claustrophobia
d. Xenophobia

13. Impulse disorder associated with photograph is:

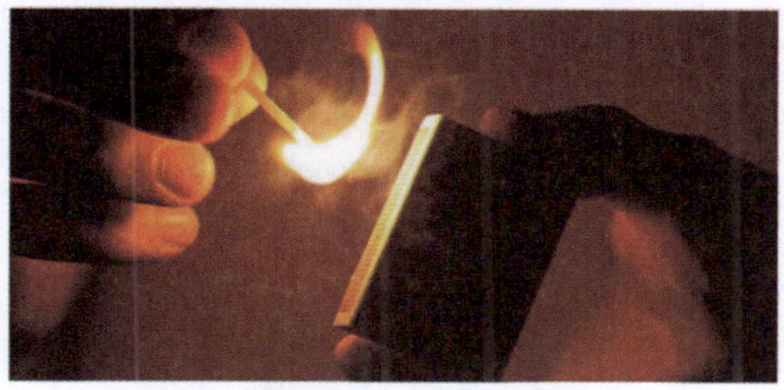

a. Kleptomania
b. Trichotitillomania
c. Onychophagia
d. Pyromania

14. Sexual perversion shown in the Photograph is:

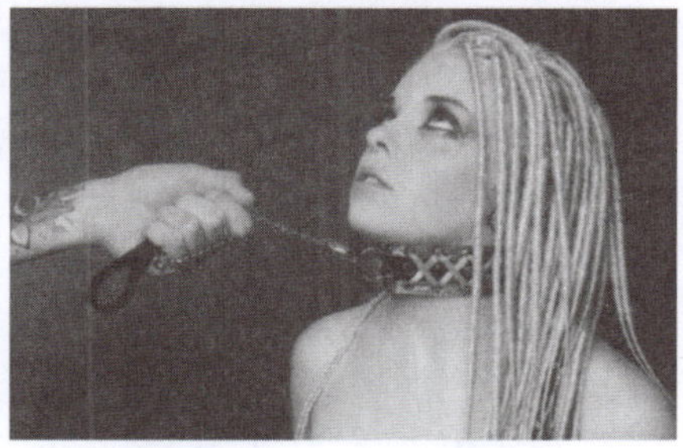

a. Incest
b. Sadism
c. Scotophilia
d. Eonism

15. Sexual perversion shown in the photograph is:

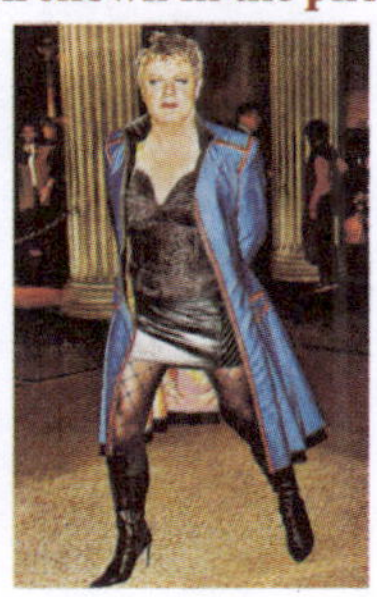

a. Fetichism
b. Masochism
c. Transvestism
d. Sadism

16. Sexual perversion shown in the photograph is:

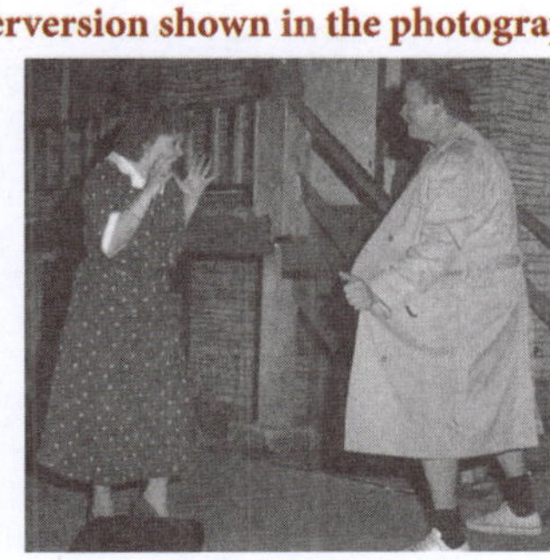

a. Undism
b. Scotophilia
c. Eonism
d. Exhibitionism

Ans.

9.	a
10.	c
11.	a
12.	c
13.	d
14.	b
15.	c
16.	d

17. Opium is derived from ……… part of plant shown in photograph. *[Recent Question 2013]*

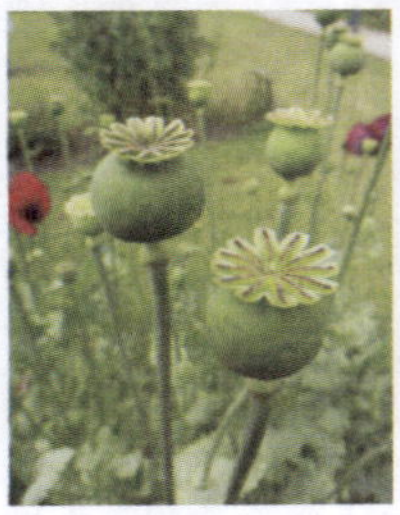

a. Leaf b. Root
c. Seed d. Unripe capsule

18. Identify the Neurologist shown in photograph:

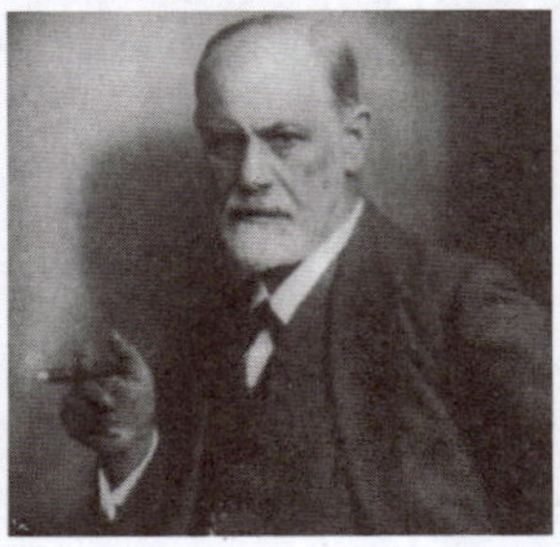

a. Eugene Bleuer b. Cloninger
c. Sigmund Freud d. Jellinek

19. Symbol shown in photograph is related to ……… disorder

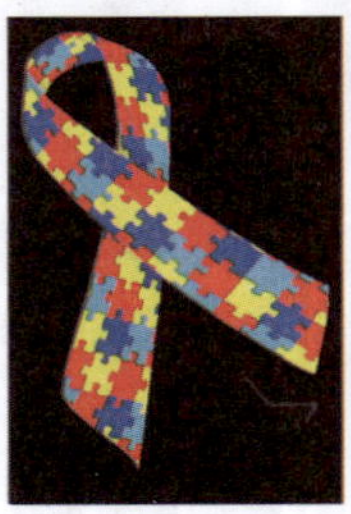

a. Alcoholism b. Depression
c. Substance use disorders d. Autism

20. Identify psychiatrist shown in photograph: *[Recent Question 2014]*

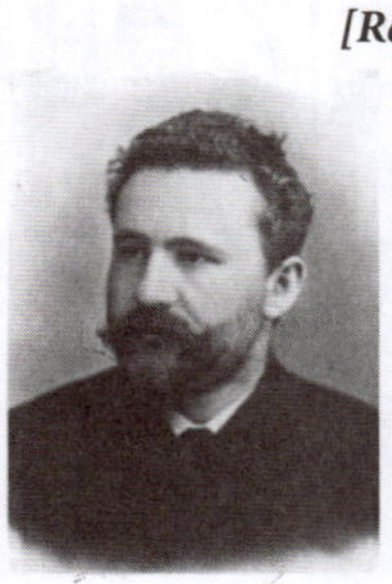

a. Eugene Bleuer b. Emil Kraepelin
c. Freud d. Cloninger

21. Identify the Psychiatrist shown in photograph: *[Recent Question 2014]*

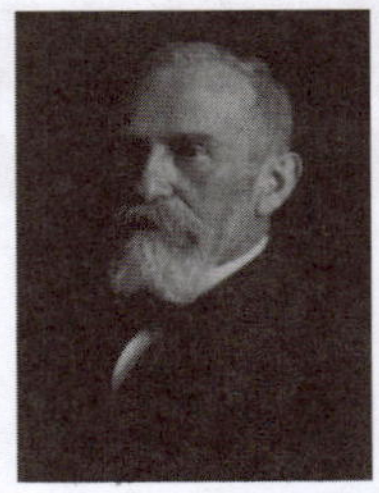

a. Cloninger b. Jellinek
c. Eugene Bleuer d. Sigmund Freud

22. Fear of Situation shown in the photograph is known as:

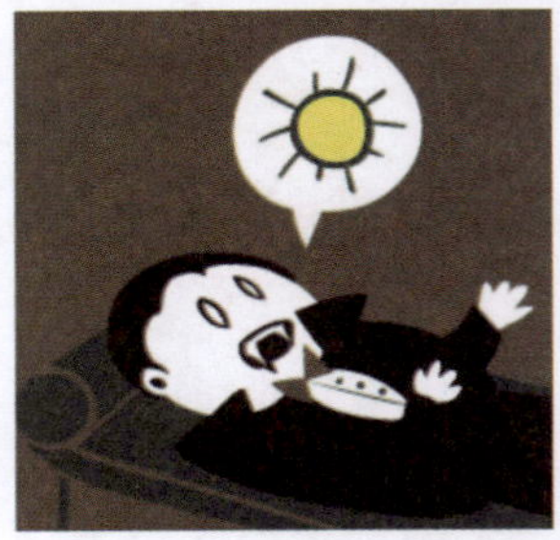

a. Xenophobia b. Heliophobia
c. Iatrophobia d. Hypnophobia

23. Identify Obsession seen in a Patient shown in photograph:

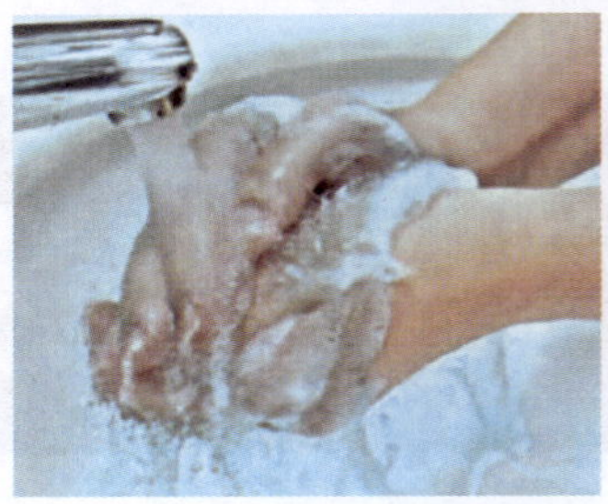

a. Checkers b. Washers
c. Cleaners d. None

24. Identify disorder of childhood shown in photograph:

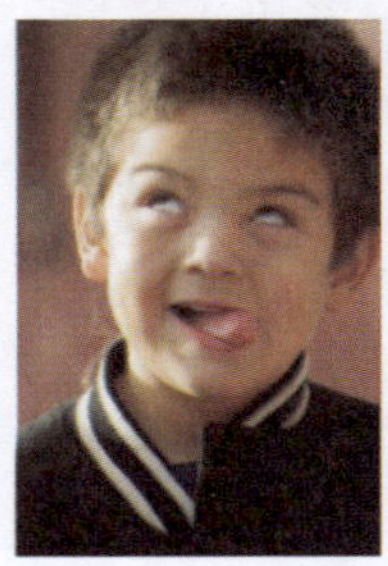

a. Tourette syndrome b. ADHD
c. Dyslexia d. Autism

Ans.

17.	d
18.	c
19.	d
20.	b
21.	c
22.	b
23.	b
24.	c

25. Identify Bleuler's symptom of Schizophrenia shown in photograph:

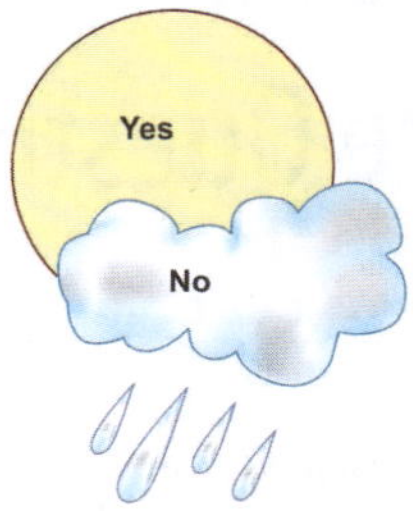

a. Autism b. Affect disturbance
c. Association disorder d. Ambivalence

26. Identify Defence mechanism shown in photograph: ***[Recent Question 2012]***

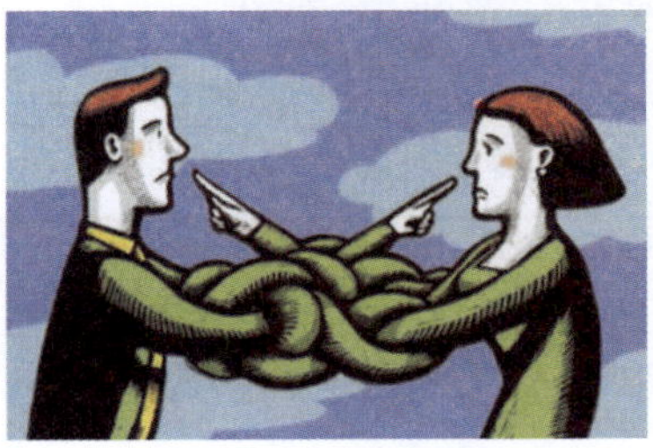

a. Repression b. Projection
c. Denial d. Distortion

27. Identify delusion shown in photograph:

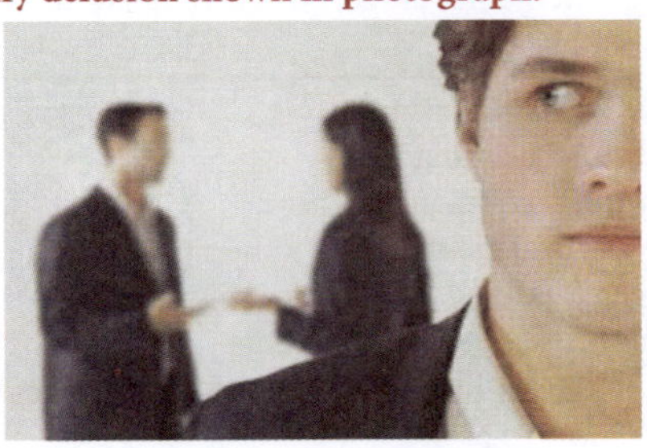

a. Nihilistic b. Doubles
c. Persecution d. Religious

28. Identify specific Paraphilia shown in photograph:

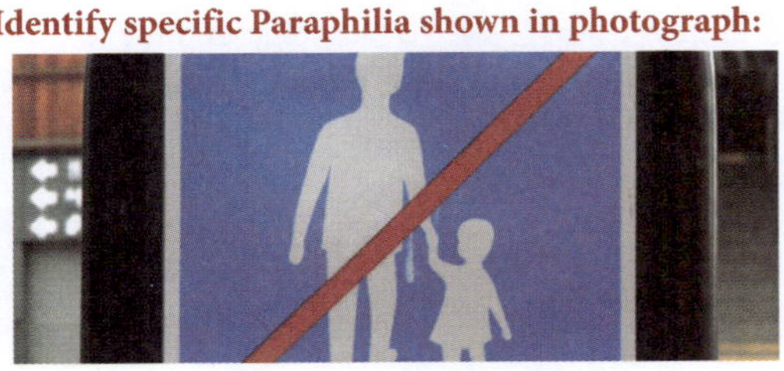

a. Sadism
b. Voyeurism
c. Pedophilia
d. Frotteurism

29. Personality disorder shown in photograph:

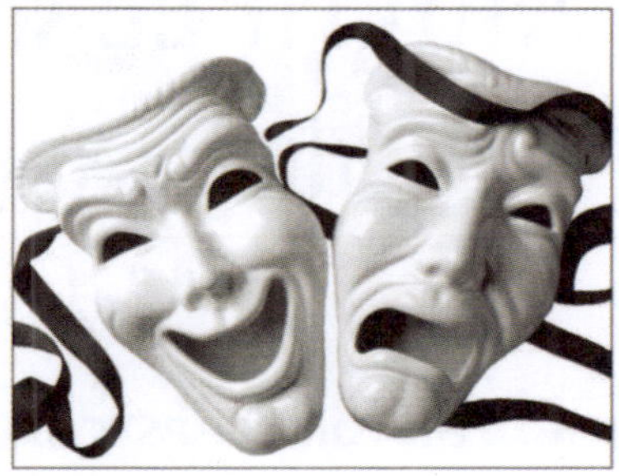

a. Histrionic b. Anxious
c. Narcissistic d. Avoidant

30. Most Severe Withdrawal syndrome of Dependence shown in photograph is:

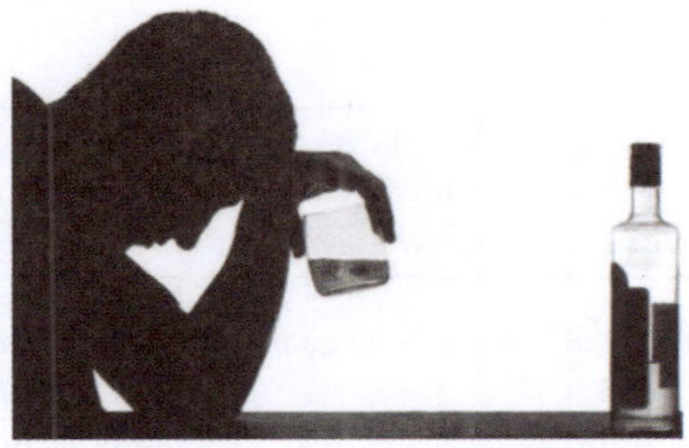

a. Delirium tremens b. Alcoholic seizures
c. Alcoholic hallucinosis d. Vomiting

31. Plant shown in photograph is used for production of which recreational drug?

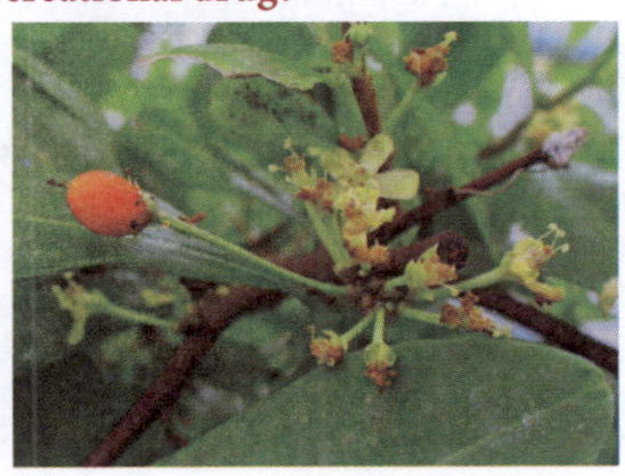

a. Cocaine b. Cannabis
c. LSD d. Heroin

Ans.

25. d
26. b
27. c
28. c
29. a
30. a
31. a

"To keep the body in good health is a duty... otherwise we shall not be able to keep our mind strong and clear."

—Buddha

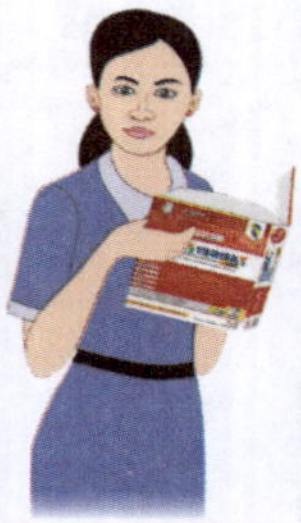

MULTIPLE CHOICE QUESTIONS
(Including Explained and Practice Questions)

DEFINITION AND HISTORY OF PSYCHIATRIC NURSING

1. A psychiatric illness may be manifested by all of the following; EXCEPT:

a. Impairment in pre-existing functioning
b. Impoverishment of feelings
c. Disturbance in behavior
d. Unpopular beliefs

Explanation: Unpopular beliefs or opinion by an individual is not considered as psychiatric illness. Fixed false belief that is not changed by rational explanation is known as delusion.

2. Which of the following is not a medicopsychiatric condition? *(AIIMS BPL NO 2018)*

a. Insulinoma b. Agitated depression
c. Hyperthyroidism d. Angina

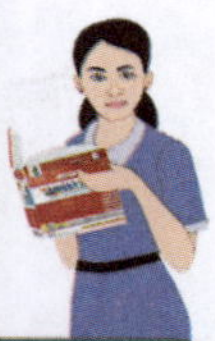

Explanation:

- Agitated depression is a psychiatric condition without organic involvement (medical condition). Agitated depression is also known as "melancholia agitation." It is known as "mixed mania" or "mixed features." Other conditions are medico-psychiatric condition.
- **Strategy**: Use the rule of elimination to solve this question. Find out three medical condition which are associated with psychiatric condition (medicopsychiatric condition) and eliminate them. Among given options, the medical conditions that are associated with psychiatric conditions are Insulinoma, Hyperthyroidism and Angina.

3. The state of complete disorganization and confusion which leads to loss of identity and direction. It is known as: *(Safdarjung NO 2018)*

a. Equilibrium
b. Bargaining
c. Chaos or disruption
d. Resistance

Explanation:

- The state of complete disorganization and confusion which leads to loss of identity and direction is chaos and disruption. When a person is not able to cope up with the existing problems and become disorganized externally or internally is called Chaos and disruption. It hugely affects the harmony and performance of the person.
- Equilibrium is a state of balance. Bargaining is a process of negotiation. Resistance is an action or inaction towards the change.

4. Assuming the all members of a group are alike is called: *(AIIMS BBS NO 2018)*

a. Cultural imposition b. Cultural competency
c. Clustering d. Stereotyping

Explanation: A stereotype is a belief that all members of a certain group act and think in the same fashion.

5. Who is the first psychiatric nurse? *(AIIMS Raipur Staff Nurse Grade I-2018)*

a. Hildegard Peplau b. Linda Richards
c. Sigmund Freud d. Jean Watson

Explanation: Linda Richards is considered as the first psychiatric nurse.

6. Who is the father of modern psychiatry?

a. Benjamin Rush
b. Philippe Pinel
c. Emil Kraepelin
d. William Tuke

Explanation: Philippe Pinel is considered as the father of modern psychiatry and Benjamin Rush is considered as the father of American psychiatry.

7. Which of the following is one of the general principles of mental health nursing?

a. Judgment of patient symptoms
b. Use self-understanding as a therapeutic tool
c. Repeated talking
d. Focus on symptoms of patients

8. Which of the following statement about mental illness is true?

a. Marriage can cure mental illness
b. Metal illness is connected to committing sin in the past
c. Mental illness is curable
d. Mentally ill patients are dangerous for the society

9. Term 'Psychiatry' was coined by:

a. Skinner b. Sigmund Freud
c. Christian Reil d. Eugene Blueur

10. Nobel Prize for experiments on Split brain was given to:

a. M. Morgia b. Penfield
c. M. Gazzaniga d. Roger Sperry

11. Name the author who propounded psychoanalysis:

a. Sigmund Freud
b. Carl Jung
c. Jean Piaget
d. Wilhelm Wundt

12. Father of Intelligence test is: *(DSSSB PHN, 2015)*

a. Alfred Binet b. Erick Erickson
c. Alfred Adler d. Carl Jung

Ans.

1.	d
2.	b
3.	c
4.	d
5.	b
6.	b
7.	b
8.	c
9.	c
10.	d
11.	a
12.	a

Explanation:

- **Alfred Binet (early 1900s)** is known as the man who created the first ‹intelligence test› in the form as we know them today. He is commonly known as the father of IQ testing.

Theorists	Theory
Alfred Binet	Father of intelligence test
Erikson's	Psychosocial development
Alfred Adler	School of individual psychology.
Carl Jung	Theory of the Collective Unconscious, Meyers-Briggs personality tests

13. Psychoanalytic therapy was developed by: *(RRB SSNE 2015)*
a. Sigmund Freud b. Jacobson
c. Franklin d. Aristotle

14. Cognitive model of depression was given by:
a. Beck b. Skinner
c. Cerletti d. Freud

THEORIES OF PERSONALITY DEVELOPMENT

15. In Erickson's theory, adolescent develops a sense of_______ *(ESIC 2019)*
a. Initiative b. Intellect
c. Identity d. Industry

Explanation: In Erickson's theory, adolescent develops a sense of identity, preschooler child develops sense of initiative, and school age child develops sense of industry. Intellect is a distractor that is not associated with Erickson's stages of development. [*Refer to Erickson's stage of personality development in Synopsis (Page no. 562)*]

16. Freud's model of development which comprises 'id, ego and superego' is called:
a. Genetic model
b. Unconscious model
c. Constructive model
d. Structural model

Explanation: Structural model: Freud developed the psychoanalytic theory of personality development, which argued that personality is formed through conflicts among three fundamental structures of the human mind: the id, ego, and superego.

17. According to Kubler-Ross theory of grief, which among the following behavior is observed in stage II? *(AIIMS Bhopal Grade-I 2018)*
a. Depression b. Anger
c. Bargaining d. Denial

Explanation: The 5 stages of grief according to Kubler-Ross are as follows:
1. **Denial: E.g.** "This can't be happening to me"
2. **Anger: E.g.** "Why is this happening to me?" "Who is to blame for this?"
3. **Bargaining:** Stage of false hope. E.g. "Make the loss less significant"
4. **Depression:** E.g. "I am too sad to do anything"
5. **Acceptance:** E.g. "I am able to exist and adjust what happened to me"

18. The techniques of psychoanalysis include the following; EXCEPT: *(AIIMS Raipur Grade II 2017)*
a. Exploration
b. Free association
c. Clay association
d. Transference

Explanation: Transference is psychological phenomenon in which an individual redirects emotions and feelings, often unconsciously, from one person to another. Free association refers to process of discovering thoughts, memories and feelings by freely sharing all the seemingly random thoughts that pass through the mind. Exploration refers to action of exploring an unfamiliar area though examination of a subject.

19. Which of the following behavior by a 35-year-old male client indicates cognitive development?
a. Acquire object permanence
b. Generates new levels of awareness
c. Intelligence is demonstrated through logical and systematic manipulation
d. Egocentric thought diminishes

Explanation: An adult of age 31 to 45 years generates new level of awareness. As per Piaget's theory of cognitive development object permanence is developed during infancy. Intelligence is demonstrated through logical and systematic manipulation and egocentric thought diminishes are seen among elementary and early adolescence period.

20. The part of mind that distinguishes right from wrong and acts as censor of behavior is known: *(RPSC Nursing Tutor 2009)*
a. Id b. Ego
c. Superego d. Libido

Explanation: The id, ego, and superego are names for the three parts of the human personality which are part of Sigmund Freud's psychoanalytic personality theory. The superego is the ethical component of the personality and provides the moral standards by which the ego operates. The superego develops last, and is based on morals and judgments about right and wrong.

21. Identity v/s role confusion is the task of which stage of development according to Erik Erikson:
a. Toddler
b. Preschool
c. Adolescent
d. Adult

Explanation:

Age	Psychosocial Crisis
Infancy (0–2 years)	Trust Vs Mistrust
Early childhood (2–4 years)	Autonomy Vs Shame doubt
Preschool (4– 5 years)	Initiative Vs Guilt
School age (5–12 years)	Industry Vs Inferiority
Adolescence (13–19 years)	Identity Vs role confusion
Early adulthood (20–39 years)	Intimacy Vs Isolation
Adulthood (40– 64 years)	Generativity Vs Stagnation
Maturity (65–Death)	Ego integrity Vs despair

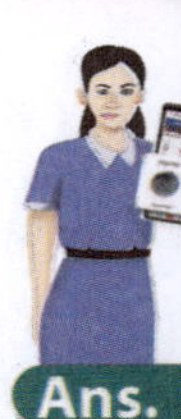

Ans.
13. a
14. a
15. c
16. d
17. b
18. c
19. b
20. c
21. c

22. As per Freudian theory, a male child's unconscious sexual desire for the parent of the opposite sex and wish to exclude the parent of the same sex is known as:

a. Oedipus complex b. Electra complex
c. Phallic complex d. Latency complex

Explanation: As per Freud, the development of Oedipus complex (male) and Electra complex (female) occurs during the phallic (3-6 years) stage of development. Freud described this as the child's unconscious desire to eliminate the parent of the same sex and to possess the parent of the opposite sex.

23. As per psychoanalytic theory the ability to tolerate frustration is seen in:

a. Id b. Ego
c. Superego d. Unconscious

Explanation: Mediating frustration within the real world is an ego function.

24. You need to abide by the unit rules and attend the community meeting. This statement by the nurse is indicative of ------------------- theory.

a. Crisis theory
b. Milieu theory
c. Family system theory
d. Biological theory

Explanation: Milieu theory insists community participation by abiding unit rules. Crisis communication theory is designed to protect and defend an individual facing a challenge to his reputation/existence.

25. Topographical model of mind by Freud is:

a. Id - ego - superego
b. Conscious - preconscious - unconscious
c. Regression - repression - suppression
d. Denial - rationalization - projection

Explanation: Freud topographical model represents his configuration of the mind. According to Freud, there are three levels of consciousness:

- **Conscious (small)** This is the part of the mind that holds what the person is aware of.
- **Preconscious (small-medium)** This is ordinary memory. So although things stored here are not in the conscious, they can be readily brought into conscious.
- **Unconscious (enormous)** Freud felt that this part of the mind was not directly accessible to awareness. In part, he saw it as a dump box for urges, feelings and ideas that are tied to anxiety, conflict and pain.

26. Another term for superego is: *(JIPMER 2012)*

a. Self b. Ideal self
c. Conscience d. Sub conscious

27. An attempt to integrate values learned from parents and society is referred to as:

a. The id b. Superego
c. Sublimation d. Projection

28. According to Erikson's stages of psychosocial development, which of the following developmental task is associated with Infancy?

a. Trust vs Mistrust b. Autonomy vs Shame
c. Initiative vs Guilt d. Intimacy vs Isolation

29. According to Erikson's stages of psychosocial development, which of the following developmental task is associated with adolescence?

a. Trust vs Mistrust
b. Identity vs Role confusion
c. Industry vs Inferiority
d. Intimacy vs Isolation

30. Interpersonal theory of nursing was proposed by:

a. Betty Neuman b. Dorothy Orem
c. Hildegard Peplau d. Jean Watson

31. A 5-year-old girl is struggling with whether to take chocolates cookies out of the jar without her mother's permission. Which of Freud's personality structures is activated in this scenario?

a. Suppression b. Id
c. Ego d. Superego

32. The contributions of Sigmund Freud are all; EXCEPT:

a. Effects of cocaine *(JIPMER 1996)*
b. Interpretation of dream
c. Psychosexual stages of development
d. Superiority inferiority complex

33. The term 'id' was coined by:

a. Freud b. Skinner
c. Wayker d. Bleuler

34. Pavlov's experiment is an example of:

a. Operant conditioning
b. Classical conditioning
c. Learned helplessness
d. Modeling

35. Which of the following model suggests that psychological disorders result from acquiring dysfunctional ways of thinking and acting?

a. Social model b. Somatic model
c. Behavioral mode d. Cognitive model

36. According to Freud's psychoanalytic view, pleasure principle is the driving force of:

a. Id b. Ego
c. Superego d. All of the above

37. According to Freud's psychoanalytic view, social component of personality consists:

a. Id b. Ego
c. Superego d. All of the above

38. According to Freud's psychoanalytic view, psychological component of personality consists:

a. Id b. Ego
c. Superego d. All of the above

39. Oedipal stage of mental development occurs at the age of:

a. 2 years b. 3–5 years
c. 5–6 years d. 6–8 years

40. That part of mind which is working on reality principle is:

a. ID b. Ego
c. Super ego d. Ego-ideal

41. Fixation of Hysteria is:

a. Genital b. Anal
c. Oral d. Phallic

42. Oedipus complex (given by Sigmund Freud) is seen in: *(JIPMER 1998, 2004)*

a. Boys of 1–3 years of age
b. Girls of 1–3 years of age
c. Boys of 3–5 years of age
d. Girls of 3–5 years of age

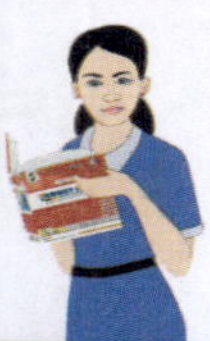

Ans.

22. a
23. b
24. b
25. b
26. c
27. b
28. a
29. b
30. c
31. c
32. d
33. a
34. b
35. d
36. a
37. c
38. d
39. b
40. b
41. d
42. c

43. In psychoanalytic terms, obsessive compulsive disorder is fixed at:

a. Oedipal stage b. Genital stage
c. Oral stage d. Anal stage

44. Which of the following is an example of classical conditioning?

a. Dog learns to salivate on hearing bell
b. Rat presses lever to get food delivered
c. Crow pecks at key for food delivery
d. All of the above

45. Which of the following is an example of operant conditioning?

a. Dog learns to salivate on hearing bell
b. Rat presses lever to get food delivered
c. Crow pecks at key for food delivery
d. All of the above

46. The theory of operant conditioning was experimented by:

a. William James b. Ivan Pavlov
c. Harry Stock Sullivan d. B F Skinner

47. Which of the following therapy is based on learning theory?

a. Cognitive therapy b. Psychoanalysis
c. Behavior therapy d. Milieu therapy

48. 'Reinforcement' is used in:

a. Psychoanalysis
b. Hypno-analysis
c. Abreaction
d. Conditioned learning

49. According to Freud, Child adopts parental standards, traits and habits through:

a. Regression b. Imitation
c. Introjection d. Identification

DEFENCE MECHANISM

50. Which of the following is an example of sublimation? *(AIIMS BPL NO 2018)*

a. Blaming the teacher for failing in exams
b. A woman has no memory of being sexually assaulted as a child
c. Child starts bedwetting after the birth of sibling
d. A young man who is dealing with aggression by playing football

Explanation: Rechanneling of drives or impulses (**aggression**) that are personally or socially unacceptable into activities that are constructive (**playing football**) is known as sublimation.

51. Adaptive mechanism of giving excuses when a person cannot solve a problem: *(AIIMS Nagpur NO 2018)*

a. Projection b. Substitution
c. Rationalization d. Compensation

Explanation: Rationalization is a process in which an individual justifies his failure and socially unacceptable behavior by giving socially approved reasons. **Example:** A student who fails in the examination may complain that the hostel atmosphere is not favorable and resulted in his failure.

52. In which defense mechanism anxiety is expressed through physical symptoms? *(AIIMS Raipur Staff Nurse Grade I-2018)*

a. Projection b. Regression
c. Conversion d. Hypochondriasis

Explanation:

- Conversion as a defense mechanism occurs where cognitive tensions manifest themselves in physical symptoms. The symptom may well be symbolic and dramatic and it often acts as a communication about the situation. Extreme symptoms may include paralysis, blindness, deafness, becoming mute or having a seizure.
- Regression is an ego defense mechanism in which person goes back to the earlier stage of development. Hypochondriasis means person believe that he/she may having serious but undiagnosed medical condition. Projection is blaming someone else for one's own difficulty.

53. Which of the following describes "ego defense mechanism"? *(DSSSB)*

a. A mechanism designed to reduce stress and conflict caused by specific experiences.
b. A mechanism designed to remove psychological barriers
c. Any form of martial arts
d. A method for negotiating a stage of development

Explanation: Defense mechanisms operate at an unconscious level and help ward off unpleasant feelings, (i.e., anxiety) or make good things feel better for the individual.

54. Rechanneling of socially unacceptable drives into activities that are more tolerable and constructive is known as:

a. Displacement b. Sublimation
c. Intellectualization d. Projection

Explanation: It is the definition of sublimation. Displacement means transfer of feeling from one target to another. Intellectualization means avoidances of expression of actual emotion associated with stressful situation. Projection is attributing feelings or impulses unacceptable to one's self to another person.

55. Which of the following client behavior indicates displacement?

a. Ignoring unpleasant aspects of reality
b. Resisting any demand made by others
c. Using imaginary activity to escape reality
d. Directing pent-up emotions to other than the primary source.

Explanation: Acting out angry or express feeling on a weaker or safer object indicates displacement.

56. A client stated that "people get angry and take it out on me". This sentence indicates which of the following defense mechanism.

a. Denial b. Projection
c. Displacement d. Intellectualization

Explanation: Attributing unacceptable feeling to others is the mechanism known as projection.

57. Imposing one's own weaknesses to others is a defense mechanism, known as:

a. Projection b. Intellectualization
c. Suppression d. Displacement

Explanation: Projection is a defense mechanism that involves taking our own unacceptable qualities or feelings and imposing them to other people.

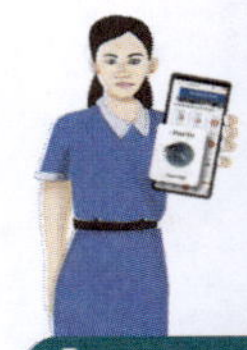

Ans.

43.	d
44.	a
45.	b
46.	d
47.	c
48.	d
49.	d
50.	d
51.	c
52.	c
53.	a
54.	b
55.	d
56.	b
57.	a

58. Finding a logical reason for the things that one wants to do 'sour grapes' mechanism is:

a. Projection b. Rationalization
c. Identification d. Sublimation

Explanation: In psychology, rationalization (also known as making excuses) is a defense mechanism in which controversial behaviors or feelings are justified and explained in a seemingly rational or logical manner to avoid the true explanation, and are made consciously tolerable – or even admirable and superior – by plausible means. It is also an informal fallacy of reasoning.

59. The involuntary blocking of unpleasant feeling and experiences from one's awareness is known as: *(RPSC Nursing Tutor 2009)*

a. Displacement b. Repression
c. Regression d. Suppression

Explanation: Repression involves placing uncomfortable thoughts in relatively inaccessible areas of the subconscious mind.

60. An attempt to avoid expressing actual emotions associated with a stressful situation by using the intellectual process of logic, reasoning and analysis is: *(AIIMS)*

a. Suppression b. Regression
c. Intellectualization d. Displacement

Explanation: Intellectualization is a defense mechanism where reasoning is used to block confrontation with an unconscious conflict and is associated with emotional stress where thinking is used to avoid feeling. The given situation refers to an intellectualization.

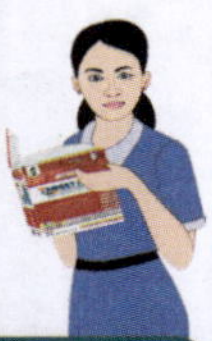

61. Most commonly using defensive mechanism by a physically abusive individual is:

a. Transference b. Manipulation
c. Displacement d. Reaction formation

Explanation: In displacement one's pent up feelings are discharged from threatening person to less threatening individuals.

62. "Doctor shopping" is the characteristic of hypochondriac disease, which defense mechanism is the root of this behavior?

a. Denial b. Compensation
c. Displacement d. Identification

Explanation: Patient with hypochondriasis believe that their physical symptoms are having some underlying pathology, but whenever the doctor says everything is normal and there is no underlying pathology, and the cause may be psychological they deny the words of doctor and go to another doctor.

63. The defense mechanism which returns to the earlier developmental stage is:

a. Regression b. Repression
c. Projection d. Rationalization

Explanation: Going back to the earlier stages of development is the characteristic of regression. Involuntary blocking of unpleasant feelings is repression. Projection means attributing to another person feeling or impulses.

64. A defense mechanism that allows to convert our unacceptable behavior into acceptable form is: *(JIPMER 2015)*

a. Introjection b. Sublimation
c. Projection d. Displacement

65. An unconscious exclusion (forgetting) of distressing memories, thoughts, or feelings from the conscious mind is known as:

a. Repression b. Fantasy
c. Displacement d. Identification

66. A conscious exclusion (forgetting) of distressing memories, thoughts, or feelings is known as:

a. Repression b. Suppression
c. Displacement d. Identification

67. A surgeon, whose patient did not respond as he anticipated, blamed the theatre nurse who helped him at the time of surgery. Which of the following defense mechanism was used by the surgeon?

a. Intellectualization b. Rationalization
c. Suppression d. Projection

68. Mr Prakash says, "I don't cry because my wife can't bear it". This is an example of:

a. Suppression b. Undoing
c. Rationalization d. Reaction formation

69. Defense against feelings of inferiority and inadequacy is known as:

a. Repression b. Sublimation
c. Regression d. Compensation

70. The defense mechanism in which the controversial behaviors or feelings are justified and explained in a seemingly rational or logical manner is known as:

a. Intellectualization b. Rationalization
c. Identification d. Regression

71. Individuals attributing their own thoughts, feeling and motives to another person is known as:

a. Rationalization b. Projection
c. Reaction formation d. Displacement

72. Patient who is newly-diagnosed with cancer frequently use the defense mechanism of:

a. Displacement b. Reaction formation
c. Denial d. Projection

73. A mechanism designed to reduce stress and conflict caused by specific experiences is known as:

a. Immune mechanism b. Defense mechanism
c. Catharsis mechanism d. Coping mechanism

74. A client with substance use disorder joins a self-help group and preaches against substance abuse. He is likely demonstrating the use of defense mechanism:

a. Displacement b. Suppression
c. Reaction formation d. Projection

75. A dishonest person thinks other persons are also dishonest. Defense mechanism used by him is:

a. Projection b. Introjection
c. Suppression d. Rationalization

76. Which of the following defense mechanism is often used by drug dependents to forget shame and pain?

a. Sublimation b. Compensation
c. Repression d. Displacement

Ans.

58. b
59. b
60. c
61. c
62. a
63. a
64. b
65. a
66. b
67. d
68. c
69. d
70. b
71. b
72. c
73. b
74. c
75. a
76. c

THERAPEUTIC COMMUNICATION

77. How many quadrants are there in the Johari Window?

a. 2 b. 6
c. 4 d. 8

Explanation: The Johari Window model is a simple and useful tool for illustrating and improving self-awareness, and mutual understanding between individuals within a group. The Johari Window model can also be used to assess and improve a group's relationship with other groups.

78. Presenting the patient with a 'hypothetical situation' helps in the assessment of: *(AIIMS Bhopal Grade-I 2018)*

a. Abstractability b. Insight
c. Comprehension d. Judgment

Explanation: Judgment involves ability to understand the facts and draw conclusions. Judgment can be evaluated by exploring the patient's involvement in hypothetical situations, relationships and vocational choices by the use of situational judgment test

79. Emotion can be best expressed through: *(Nursing Grade- II 2007)*

a. Gesture b. Language
c. Posture d. All of the above

Explanation: Emotional expressions are observable through verbal and nonverbal behaviors. Language is verbal communication and gesture and posture are the non-verbal communication.

80. When a clients's behavior is considered abnormal the nurse first need to:

a. Ignore the client's behavior
b. Point out the client's disturbed behavior
c. Focus on the emotions
d. Focus on the positive behavior

81. Which is not a therapeutic communication technique?

a. Informing b. Reflection
c. Humor d. Automatic response

82. Responses to avoid in therapeutic communications are as follows; EXCEPT: *(ESIC 2019)*

a. Advice giving
b. Closed-ended questions.
c. Reflecting and clarifying
d. Arguing and judgmental responses

Explanation: **Reflecting and clarifying** are therapeutic communication techniques. Advise giving, closed-ended questions and arguing and judgmental responses are antitherapeutic communication techniques, so it should be avoided.
notE: There are double negatives in the stem. "Avoid" and "EXCEPT". So carefully read the question twice before answering.

83. An example of non-therapeutic communication techniques:

a. Validating b. Reflecting
c. Belittling d. Listening

Explanation: Belittling means putting down or making another person feel as less important than you.

84. The most important factor in a therapeutic relationship is:

a. Trust b. Knowledge
c. Professionalism d. Motivation

Explanation: Without trust in a relationship, there is no relationship. Trust is one of the most important aspects of a relationship.

85. Most difficult part of a nurse-client relationship in therapeutic relationship for the nurse is:

a. Remain as therapeutic and professional
b. Being able to understand and accept client's behavior
c. Developing an awareness of self and professional role relationship
d. Accepting responsibility in identifying and evaluating the real need of the client

Explanation: Psychiatric nurse identify their own feeling and understand how they affect the situation.

86. Termination of interpersonal relationship starts in ....phase.

a. Preinteraction b. Orientation
c. Working d. Termination

Explanation: Terminating phase starts during the orientation phase when the therapeutic nurse-patient relationship is established. The length of this therapeutic relationship in terms of termination should be discussed when the nurse and patient initially agree to work together.

87. In a mental health unit nurse is showing undue concern and kindness towards a patient, this can be identified as:

a. Transference
b. Counter transference
c. Emotional attachment
d. Sympathy

Explanation: Countertransference, which occurs when a therapist transfers emotion to a person in therapy, is often a reaction to transference, a phenomenon in which the person in treatment redirects feelings for others onto the therapist.

88. While communicating to a client nurse ask, what time it is, place where they admitted and person with them, these questions help the nurse to assess:

a. Memory b. Orientation
c. Thought process d. For good rapport

Explanation: Questions related to time, place and person will give information regarding the orientation of the patient.

89. The patient states "Give me five minutes to recall the name of the college lecturer who failed most of us in pediatric nursing exam". The patient is operating his:

a. Conscious self b. Subconscious
c. Unconscious d. Superego

90. The recording of conversation between the nurse and patient in a psychiatric set up is termed as: *(JIPMER 2015)*

a. Therapeutic communication
b. Interview technique
c. Process recording
d. Case study

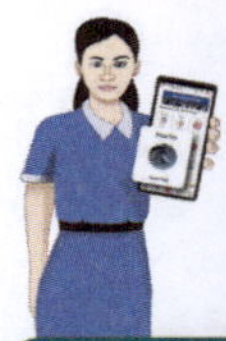

Ans.

77. c
78. d
79. d
80. b
81. d
82. c
83. c
84. a
85. c
86. b
87. b
88. b
89. b
90. c

91. The best approach in helping a severely withdrawn patient is:
a. Engage in group activities
b. Establish a specific routine
c. To provide a trusting relationship
d. Engage in ward activities

92. The process of encouraging or establishing a belief or pattern of behavior is known as:
a. Exploration b. Reinforcement
c. Sensitization d. Enforcement

93. A nurse is caring for a patient who recently experienced the loss of a loved one. The patient is displaying signs of sadness, withdrawal, and tearfulness. The nurse engages in therapeutic communication to support the patient. Which therapeutic communication technique is the nurse demonstrating in this scenario? *New Q*
a. Providing reassurance
b. Offering advice
c. Reflecting feelings
d. Interpreting the patient's emotions

Explanation: In this scenario, the nurse is demonstrating the therapeutic communication technique of reflecting feelings. Reflecting feelings involves acknowledging and verbalizing the patient's emotions to show understanding and empathy. By reflecting the patient's feelings, the nurse validates the patient's experience and creates a supportive environment for emotional expression.

94. Communication technique of confrontation is used during which phase of nurse-patient relationship?
a. Pre-orientation b. Orientation
c. Working d. Termination

95. Cultural barrier of communication is:
a. Intelligence b. Sound
c. Fear d. Language

96. Which of the following is one of the barriers of therapeutic nurse-patient communication?
a. Reflection b. Restating
c. Giving advice d. Silence

97. One of the barriers in nurse-patient therapeutic relationship is:
a. Reflection b. Transference
c. Listening d. Nodding

98. A prerequisite for a nurse to develop an effective communication with patient is:
a. A good understanding the pathophysiology of mental disorders
b. To use transference and counter transference
c. To use self-awareness as a tool to understand the patient
d. To have good knowledge of various treatment modalities

99. Which of the following is an example of non-therapeutic communication techniques?
a. Non-judgmental attitude b. Silence
c. Reflection d. Informing

100. A nurse, during the course of treatment, develops positive or negative feelings toward the patient. This is termed as:
a. Empathy
b. Counter-transference
c. Sympathy
d. Transference

101. The attitude of nurse who is taking care of a patient with mania should be:
a. Active friendliness
b. Jovial
c. Passive friendliness and firm
d. Threatening

102. Repeating the main thoughts expressed by the patient is called as:
a. Restating b. Clarification
c. Reflection d. Validation

103. Which of the following type of questions are used during psychiatric history collection?
a. Forced choice questions
b. Objective type questions
c. Open ended questions
d. Closed ended questions

104. First step in counseling process is:
a. Relationship building
b. Goal setting
c. Problem assessment
d. Interventions

105. A written documentation of verbal interaction between a client and nurse is known as?
a. Mental status examination
b. Process recording
c. Mini mental status examination
d. Anecdotal record

106. A client is very affectionate toward one of the staff members in the ward. The client is manifesting:
a. Empathy
b. Resistance
c. Transference
d. Counter transference

107. All of the following are the elements of therapeutic community; EXCEPT:
a. Validation
b. Restricted communication
c. Structured interaction
d. Active participation

108. A mental health nurse performs a process recording with a 30-year-old male patient with BPAD. Which of the following is not a component of a process recording?
a. Verbal narrative account
b. Nonverbal narrative account
c. Audio-visual recording
d. Audio and interpretation

ROLE OF NEUROTRANSMITTERS IN PSYCHIATRIC DISORDERS

109. The junction at which impulses are being transmitted from one neuron to another is: *(Nursing Grade- II 2007)*
a. Schwan cell b. Axon
c. Synapse d. Dendron

Explanation: Synapse is a junction between two nerve cells, consisting of a minute gap across which impulses pass by diffusion of a neurotransmitter.

Ans.

91. c
92. b
93. c
94. c
95. d
96. c
97. b
98. c
99. d
100. b
101. c
102. a
103. c
104. a
105. b
106. c
107. b
108. c
109. c

110. Increased dopamine level will cause:
a. Schizophrenia b. Depression
c. OCD d. BPAD

Explanation: Increased dopamine level can cause schizophrenia in the person.

111. The major neurotransmitter involved in causation of schizophrenia is:
a. GABA
b. Acetylcholine
c. Dopamine
d. Epinephrine

112. Typical antipsychotics act predominantly on _____ receptors.
a. GABA b. D1
c. D2 d. D3

113. Which of the following neurotransmitter is deficient in depression? *(AIIMS)*
a. Serotonin b. 5 HT
c. Both A and B d. GABA

Explanation: Serotonin or 5 HT (5-hydroxytryptamine) is a excitatory neurotransmitter. Deficiency of these neurotransmitter found to cause depression.

114. The neurotransmitter believed to be associated with Bipolar Disorder is:
a. GABA b. Norepinephrine
c. Serotonin d. Acetylcholine

115. Neurotransmitters elevated in manic episode are:
a. Acetylcholine and serotonin
b. Norepinephrine and dopamine
c. GABA and dopamine
d. Serotonin and GABA

116. Read the Assertion (A) and Reason (R) given below and choose the appropriate option. ***New Q***
Assertion (A): Imbalances in the neurotransmitter dopamine can contribute to symptoms of Parkinson's disease.
Reason (R): In Parkinson's disease, there is a loss of dopamine-producing cells in the brain, leading to motor symptoms such as tremors, rigidity, and difficulty with movement.
a. Both assertion (A) and reason (R) are true, and the reason (R) is the correct explanation of the assertion (A).
b. Both assertion (A) and reason (R) are true, but the reason (R) is not the correct explanation of the assertion (A).
c. Assertion (A) is true, but the reason (R) is false.
d. Assertion (A) is false, but the reason (R) is true.

Explanation: Parkinson's disease is characterized by the degeneration of dopamine-producing cells in the brain, particularly in an area called the substantia nigra. This loss of dopamine leads to a dopamine imbalance, resulting in the motor symptoms associated with the disease. The reason provided accurately explains how the imbalance in dopamine contributes to the development of Parkinson's disease.

117. The neurotransmitter associated with anxiety is:
a. GABA
b. Acetylcholine
c. Dopamine
d. Serotonin

118. The major neurotransmitter involved in the occurrence of Obsessive compulsive disorder is: *(AIIMS Bhopal Grade-I 2018)*
a. Dopamine b. Acetylcholine
c. Epinephrine d. Serotonin

Explanation: Serotonin neurotransmitter involved in core physical processes such as regulation of sleep, aggression, anxiety, mood, fear etc. Low level of serotonin is linked to the repetitive thoughts or obsessions and initiating the disorder. So, serotonin is the primary neurotransmitter associated with the symptoms of OCD.

119. Benzodiazepines reduce anxiety by acting on which neurotransmitter? *(Banaras HU 2015)*
a. GABA b. Serotonin
c. Noradrenaline d. Dopamine

PSYCHOSOCIAL THERAPIES

120. Among the following identify the overall priority goal of in-patient psychiatric treatment?
a. Prevention of violence
b. Monitor and minimize self-harm behavior
c. Stabilization and return to the community
d. Encourage to come for regular follow up

Explanation: The goals of in-patient psychiatric treatment are to reduce stress on the patient and prepare the patient to lead a normal life in the community setting. It also focuses upon to prevent the relapses and also enhance the patient adaptation and coping skill with new life situation in the community.

121. The act of purging or purification or elimination of complex emotions by bringing it to consciousness and affording to expression is:
a. Abreaction therapy b. Hypnosis
c. Catharsis d. Biofeedback

Explanation: Catharsis (from the Greek katharsis meaning "purification" or "cleansing") is the purification and purgation of emotions—especially pity and fear—through art or any extreme change in emotion that results in renewal and restoration.

122. A form of psychotherapy that involves the use of therapeutic communities is known as:
a. Group therapy
b. Cognitive behavior therapy
c. Milieu therapy
d. Interpersonal psychotherapy

123. Which of the following is not true regarding Brief Cognitive Therapy? *(AIIMS-BBS SNO 2019)*
a. It puts greater emphasis on the cause of the problem
b. It uses here-and now approach
c. It uses goal-oriented approach
d. It uses time-limited approach

Explanation: Brief Cognitive Therapy has gained widespread application in treatment of substance abuse. The aim is to help the client address specific, identifiable problems in such a way that the client is able to apply basic techniques and skills learned, without assistance of therapist. It focuses on **'here and now' approach**. Instead of focusing on cause.

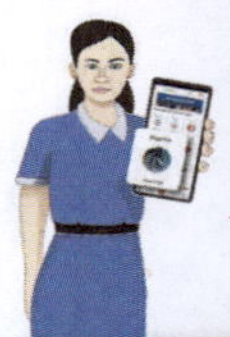

Ans.
110. a
111. c
112. c
113. c
114. b
115. b
116. a
117. a
118. d
119. a
120. c
121. c
122. c
123. a

124. ___________is a family therapy approach that focuses on both the biological and the psychosocial components of a problem. *(AIIMS-BBS SNO 2019)*

a. Integrative approach
b. Bowen approach
c. Psychoanalytic approach
d. Structural approach

Explanation: Integrative approach is a combined approach to psychotherapy that brings different elements of specific therapies. It also refers to the infusion of a person's personality and needs-integrating the affective, behavioral, cognitive, and physiological systems within one person, as well as addressing social and spiritual aspects.

125. Eradication of unwanted habits by associating unpleasant condition with it is called: *(AIIMS BPL NO 2018)*

a. Biofeedback
b. Desensitization
c. Aversive conditioning
d. Classical conditioning

Explanation: Aversion therapy is a form of behavior therapy in which an aversive (causing a strong feeling of dislike or disgust) stimulus is paired with an undesirable behavior in order to reduce or eliminate that behavior. The aim of aversion therapy is to decrease or eliminate unwanted behaviors.

126. Which of the following therapy is based on learning theory?

a. Logo therapy
b. Psychoanalysis
c. Behavior therapy
d. Interpersonal therapy

Explanation: Behavior therapy is a broad term referring to psychotherapy, behavior analytical, or a combination of the two therapies. In its broadest sense, the methods focus on either just behaviors or in combination with thoughts and feelings that might be causing them.

127. The purpose of self-help group is to provide:

a. Support
b. Confrontation
c. Psychotherapy
d. Self-awareness

Explanation: Self-help group members share similar experiences and can provide support to each other

128. Identify the correct statement regarding Milieu therapy (therapeutic community)

a. Manipulate the environment to bring about positive changes in behavior
b. The client owns his or her own environment
c. Each client owns his or her own behavior
d. All of the above

Explanation: Milieu therapy manipulates the environment so that all aspects of the client's hospital experience become therapeutic. All the above-mentioned statements are correct in relation to Milieu therapy.

129. Desensitization is a type of:

a. Psychotherapy
b. Psychoanalysis
c. Behavioral therapy
d. None

130. Behavior therapy is useful in all of the following conditions; EXCEPT:

a. OCD
b. Phobia
c. Mania
d. Hysterical conversion reaction

131. A specialized type of group therapy that uses role-playing to help people explore their thoughts

a. Psychodrama
b. Psychotherapy
c. Cognitive behavioral therapy
d. Reminiscence therapy

132. Group therapy can most useful for those who are:

a. Dependent on others
b. Distressed
c. Emotionally ill
d. Isolated

133. The most effective psychotherapy for a 9-year-old child diagnosed with attention deficit hyperactivity disorder (ADHD) is: *(Banaras HU 2015)*

a. Play therapy
b. Milieu therapy
c. Behavior therapy
d. Family therapy

134. Read the (A) and (R) given below and choose the appropriate option.

Assertion (A): Clients in a milieu therapy setting are encouraged to participate in activities that promote their physical and mental health.

Reason (R): Milieu therapy typically takes place in a residential setting, such as a psychiatric hospital or a halfway house. *New Q*

a. Both assertion (A) and reason (R) are true, and the reason (R) is the correct explanation of the assertion (A).
b. Both assertion (A) and reason (R) are true, but the reason (R) is not the correct explanation of the assertion (A).
c. Assertion (A) is true, but the reason (R) is false.
d. Assertion (A) is false, but the reason (R) is true.

Explanation: While both statements (A) and (R) are true about milieu therapy. However, the reason (R) is not the correct explanation of the assertion (A). The reason (R) only states that milieu therapy typically takes place in a residential setting. It does not explain why clients in a milieu therapy setting are encouraged to participate in activities that promote their physical and mental health.

The correct explanation of the assertion (A) is that these activities can help to improve mood, reduce stress, and increase energy levels.

135. Psychoanalysis is an attempt to explain:

a. Normal psychological functioning
b. Abnormal psychological functioning
c. Normal and abnormal psychological functioning
d. Cognitive thinking

136. Which of the following action can minimize agitation in a disturbed client?

a. Increasing environmental stimuli
b. Limiting unnecessary interaction with patient
c. Discussing the reasons for suspicious belief
d. All of the above

137. Characteristics of milieu therapy include:

a. Distribution of power
b. Structured interactions
c. Work-related activities
d. All of the above

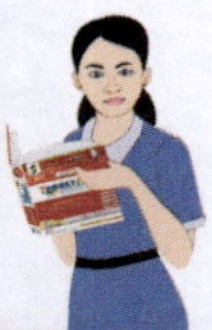

Ans.

124. a
125. c
126. c
127. a
128. d
129. c
130. c
131. a
132. c
133. c
134. b
135. c
136. b
137. d

138. All of the following behavioral techniques are used to treat OCD; EXCEPT:
- a. Exposure and response prevention
- b. Aversive conditioning
- c. Flooding
- d. Thought stoppage

139. Steps of systematic desensitization include following steps; EXCEPT:
- a. Hierarchy construction
- b. Testing anxiety level
- c. Learning of relaxation techniques
- d. Desensitization of stimulus

140. Which of the following is a type of relaxation therapy?
- a. Reiki therapy
- b. Acupuncture
- c. Catharsis
- d. Deep breathing exercise

141. A treatment for phobias in which the patient is exposed to progressively more anxiety-provoking stimuli and taught relaxation techniques is known as:
- a. Aversive therapy
- b. Flooding
- c. Deterrent therapy
- d. Systematic desensitization

142. Which of the following behavior modification technique is useful in the treatment of phobias?
- a. Positive reinforcement
- b. Modeling
- c. Desensitization therapy
- d. Token economy

143. The technique used in hypnosis is:
- a. Exploration
- b. Questioning
- c. Suggestion
- d. Sensitization

144. The induction of a state of altered consciousness in which a person apparently loses the power of voluntary action and is highly responsive to suggestion is known as:
- a. Psychotherapy
- b. Rehabilitation
- c. Hypnosis
- d. Cognitive therapy

145. The most effective form of somatic therapy for patient with schizophrenia is:
- a. Minor tranquilizers
- b. Electroconvulsive Therapy
- c. Major tranquilizers
- d. Biofeedback

146. Useful intervention for a patient with adjustment disorder is:
- a. Extended follow-up
- b. Individual Psychotherapy
- c. Group therapy
- d. CBT

147. The ideal size for group therapy is:
- a. 8-12 members
- b. 10-55 members
- c. 15-20 members
- d. 15-25 members

148. Pre-sleep rituals that help to initiate relaxation each night before sleep include all of the following EXCEPT:
- a. Warm bath before bedtime
- b. Eating heavy meals near bedtime
- c. Eating light snacks
- d. Reading or listing to music

149. Behavioral therapy is helpful in:
- a. Schizophrenia
- b. Agoraphobia
- c. Personality disorder
- d. Neurotic depression

150. Cognitive behavior therapy deals with:
- a. Unconscious motive
- b. Maladaptive assumptions
- c. Pseudo-dynamic conflict
- d. Emotional consciousness of automatic thoughts

151. It is an aspect of treatment that focuses on helping the person return to an optimal level of functioning and to achieve maximum range of interest and activity.
- a. Primary Prevention
- b. Secondary Prevention
- c. Psychiatric Intervention
- d. Psychiatric Rehabilitation

152. PLISSIT model is for:
- a. Sex therapy
- b. Spiritual therapy
- c. Family therapy
- d. Behavioral therapy

Explanation:

PLISSIT Model of addressing sexual functioning (Annon, 1976)

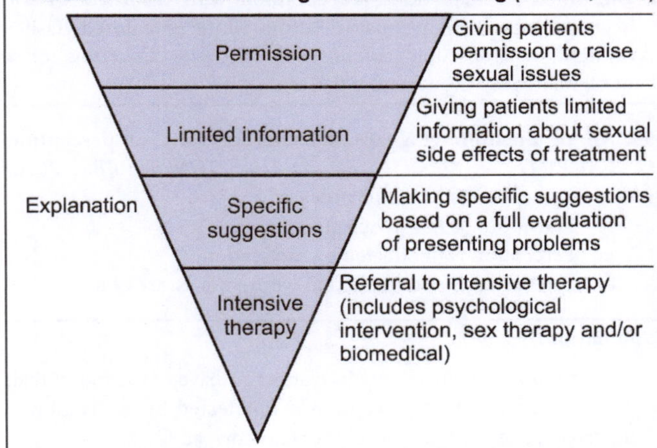

ICD-10 CLASSIFICATION OF PSYCHIATRIC DISORDERS

153. With regard to diagnosis of mental disorders, the term DSM stands for:
- a. Disease System Manual
- b. Diagnostic System Manual
- c. Diagnostic and Statistical Manual
- d. Diagnostic System for Mental disorders

154. DSM classification of mental disorders is published by:
- a. World Health Organization
- b. American Psychiatric Association
- c. International Psychiatric Association
- d. American Psychological Association

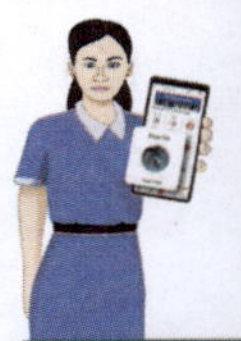

Ans.

138. c
139. b
140. d
141. d
142. c
143. c
144. c
145. b
146. b
147. a
148. b
149. b
150. b
151. d
152. a
153. c
154. b

155. With regard to diagnosis of Mental disorders, the term ICD stands for:

a. International Classification of Diseases
b. Indian Classification of Diseases
c. International Criteria for Diagnoses
d. Indian Criteria for Diagnoses

156. The ICD classification of diseases is published by:

a. American Psychiatric Association (APA)
b. Indian Society of Psychiatric Nurses (ISPN)
c. International Psychiatric Association
d. World Health Organization

157. Which of the following statement is most appropriate for Psychosis?

a. The person has suffered memory loss
b. The person suffers from extreme sleeplessness
c. Viral infection of the brain
d. The person has not distinguished imagination from reality

158. Formed visual hallucinations are seen in the lesion of: *(AIIMS BBS NO 2018)*

a. Occipital b. Temporal
c. Parietal d. Frontal

Explanation:

- Formed visual hallucinations are usually from lesion of temporal region. The content are vivid objects, flowers, animals and persons
- Unformed hallucinations are common with disorders of the occipital lobe. Patients may describe white or colored flashes of light, kaleidoscopic colors, moving discs, flickering, or a hexagonal array (honeycomb pattern).

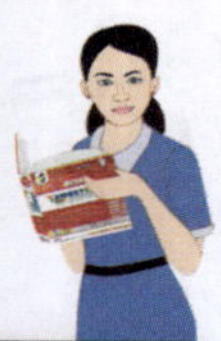

159. All of the following are the characteristic of perception EXCEPT: *(IGNOU PBBSC 2016)*

a. Perception is an active process.
b. Perception is highly selective.
c. Perception is unaffected by motivation.
d. Perception is automatic that we are not aware of it.

Explanation:

- Perception is influenced by motivation or drive of the individual. So the statement that perception is unaffected by motivation is incorrect statement. So the answer C is correct.
- All other statements are characteristics of perception.

160. A 52-year-old man has an altercation with his neighbor. The next day he feels that his neighbors are following him and recording his movements and he fears that they are planning to kill him. What do his symptoms represent? New Q

a. Thought insertion
b. Delusion of control
c. Delusion of persecution
d. Delusion of reference

Explanation: Delusion of persecution is a type of delusion where an individual falsely believes that others are out to harm, threaten, or persecute them. In this case, the man's belief that his neighbors are following him, recording his movements, and planning to kill him indicates a paranoid and persecutory delusion.

161. Rorschach inkblot test is: *(Rohtak PGMEE 2003)*

a. Projective b. Subjective
c. Both d. None

162. Rema is admitted in psychiatric ward, refused to eat breakfast by stating that the food is poisoned. This kind of response is an example of:

a. Hallucination b. Illusion
c. Delusion d. Empathy

Explanation: An erroneous belief that is held without evidence and irrational is known as delusion.

163. Unshakable and persistent ideas or false fixed belief are called:

a. Delusion
b. Obsession
c. Compulsion
d. Illusion

Explanation: Delusion refers to a fixed, false belief that persists despite evidence to the contrary. It is a symptom commonly associated with psychotic disorders such as schizophrenia, but can also occur in other mental health conditions.

Example: A person believes that they have been implanted with a microchip by the government that is controlling their thoughts and actions. Despite the lack of evidence and the implausibility of such a scenario, the individual firmly holds onto this belief.

164. False sensory perceptions with no basis in reality is known as: *(DSSSB 2013; Safdarjung NO 2018)*

a. Hallucinations b. Delusions
c. Illusions d. Thought insertion

Explanation: Hallucination is an experience involving the apparent perception of something not present. It is a perception without a presence of sensory stimuli. Types of hallucination includes Auditory (sound), visual (vision), olfactory (smell), tactile (touch) and gustatory (taste). Auditory hallucination is the most common type of hallucination experienced by patients with mental illness.

165. Persecutory delusion is common in: *(RPSC Nursing Tutor 2009)*

a. Schizophrenia b. Paranoid Schizophrenia
c. BPAD d. OCD

Explanation: Individual with persecutory delusion believes that they are being malevolently (vindictively) treated in some way. Persecutory delusion is common in Paranoid Schizophrenia.

166. Gustatory hallucination affects the: *(RPSC Nursing Tutor 2009)*

a. Ears b. Taste buds
c. Nose d. Eyes

Explanation: A hallucination is a perception in the absence of a stimulus. A gustatory hallucination is a perception of taste without a stimulus. These hallucinations, which are typically strange or unpleasant, are relatively common among individuals who have certain types of focal epilepsy, especially temporal lobe epilepsy.

167. Client with schizophrenia experiencing voice which stated that "you are bad and should die". This is called:

a. A delusion b. Illusion
c. Grandiosity d. Hallucination

Explanation: A hallucination is a sensory perception without a real stimulus. Hearing voice without a stimulus is known as auditory stimulus.

Ans.

155. a
156. d
157. d
158. b
159. c
160. c
161. a
162. c
163. a
164. a
165. b
166. b
167. d

168. Nihilistic delusion is:

a. A false belief about the functioning of the body
b. False idea that others are talking about the person
c. Part of self, other or world is nonexistent
d. The inability to carry out somatic functioning

Explanation: Nihilistic delusions are false ideas about the self, others, or the world. A false belief about the functioning of the body is somatic delusion.

169. Most common type of hallucination seen in schizophrenia patient is:

a. Auditory b. Visual
c. Tactile d. Olfactory

Explanation: The most commonly seen hallucination among schizophrenia patient is auditory hallucination.

170. Among the following all are positive symptoms of schizophrenia; EXCEPT:

a. Apathy b. Agitation
c. Hallucination d. Aggression

Explanation: Apathy is considered as one of the negative symptoms of schizophrenia.

171. Condition indicating abnormality in perception is:

a. Illusion b. Obsession
c. Persecution d. Compulsion

Explanation: Illusion is a distortion of senses characterized by misinterpretation of stimuli. For example, a rope could be misinterpreted as snake.

172. Perception of an object in the absence of a stimuli is called:

a. Illusion b. Hallucination
c. Delusion d. Confabulation

173. Misinterpretation or misperception of real external stimuli is known as:

a. Illusion b. Hallucination
c. Delusion d. Confabulation

174. Which of the following is the disorder of perception?

a. Delusion b. Hallucination
c. Amnesia d. Delirium

175. An 8-year-old child after a tonsillectomy sees a bear in her room. She screams in fright. A nurse who rushes in switches on the light, finds a rug wrapped on an arm chair. She pacifies the child. What the child experienced was:

a. Delusion
b. Illusion
c. Hallucination
d. None of the above

176. Hallucinations are seen in All; EXCEPT:

a. Schizophrenia
b. Seizure due to intracerebral space occupying lesions
c. LSD
d. Anxiety

177. Auditory hallucinations not seen in:

a. Schizophrenia
b. Mania
c. Hysteria
d. Amphetamine toxicity

178. A patient was caught by police for fighting with classmates because he thought they were planning to kill him. He states that his dead grandfather talks to him every now and then for last one month. He is delusional from past few weeks also. What will be the most likely diagnosis? *New Q*

a. Delusional disorder
b. Mania
c. Post-traumatic stress disorder
d. Schizophrenia

Explanation: Schizophrenia is a mental disorder that is characterized by delusions, hallucinations, disorganized thinking, and impaired social functioning. Delusions are false beliefs that are held with conviction despite evidence to the contrary. Hallucinations are sensory experiences that occur in the absence of external stimuli.

The patient in this case is experiencing delusions, hallucinations, and disorganized thinking. So the most likely diagnosis is Schizophrenia.

179. Altered perception of real objects is:

a. Illusion b. Delusion
c. Hallucination d. Delirium

180. Lack of insight is not a feature of: *(JIPMER 2003)*

a. Panic disorder
b. Schizophrenia
c. Mania
d. Reactive Psychosis

181. Hallucination is caused by:

a. Gastrointestinal disorder
b. Mental illness
c. Disorder of reproductive organs
d. Infectious disease

182. A person seeing a design on the floor thought it was a fossil. It is an example of: *(Banaras HU 2015)*

a. Illusion
b. Delusion
c. Hallucination
d. Idea of reference

183. What is the diagnosis code of dual-role transvestism in ICD-10? *New Q (AIIMS Bibinagar, Fac 2023)*

a. F 64.0 b. F 64.1
c. F 64.2 d. F 64.3

Explanation:

- The ICD-10 code for dual-role transvestism is F64.1
- F64.0 is the diagnosis code for trans-sexualism.
- F64.2 is the diagnosis code for gender identity disorder in children.
- F64.8 is the diagnosis code for Other gender identity disorders.
- F64.9 is the diagnosis code for Gender identity disorder, unspecified

184. The most common type of hallucination seen in patients with mental illness is: *(JIPMER Nursing Tutor Entrance 2011)*

a. Gustatory hallucination
b. Auditory hallucination
c. Olfactory hallucination
d. Visual hallucination

Ans.

168. c
169. a
170. a
171. a
172. b
173. a
174. b
175. b
176. d
177. c
178. d
179. a
180. a
181. b
182. a
183. b
184. b

185. Patient tells the nurse that the news announcer on TV is talking about me. The nurse documents this as:

a. Delusion of reference
b. Delusion of grandiosity
c. Delusion of persecution
d. Delusion of infidelity

186. Mrs. Anita refuses to eat her breakfast in the hospital, stating that the food is poisoned. This is an example of:

a. Delusion of nihilism
b. Delusion of grandiosity
c. Delusion of persecution
d. Delusion of reference

187. According to the ICD-10 classification, which code represents "Mania with psychotic symptoms"? ***New Q***

a. F 30.0 b. F 30.1
c. F 30.2 d. F 30.3

Explanation:

- F 30-F39 describes Mood (affective) Disorders.
- F30.2- Mania with psychotic symptoms
- F30 - Manic episode
- F 30.0 - Hypomania
- F 30.1 - Mania without psychotic symptoms

188. A patient expresses the belief that the Army is out to shoot him. This is an example of:

a. Delusion of grandiosity
b. Idea of reference
c. Delusion of persecution
d. Delusion of nihilism

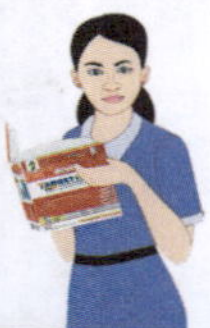

189. Delusion is a disorder of:

a. Thought b. Perception
c. Insight d. Cognition

190. According to the ICD-10 classification, which code represents "Bulimia Nervosa"? ***New Q***

a. F 50.1 b. F 50.2
c. F 60.1 d. F 60.2

Explanation:

- F50-F59: Behavioral syndromes are associated with physiological disturbances and physical factors. Under this classification, the code for bulimia nervosa is F 50.2.
- F 50.0 is for Anorexia nervosa and F50.1 is for Atypical anorexia nervosa.
- F 60 - F69 describes Disorders of adult personality and behavior

191. A man hits his neighbor. Next day he feels that police is behind him and his brain is being controlled by radio waves by his neighbor. The probable diagnosis is: *(JIPMER 1999)*

a. Thought insertion
b. Passivity feeling
c. Delusion of persecution
d. Obsessive Compulsive Disorder

192. Persecutory delusion is a feature of:

a. OCD
b. Paranoid Schizophrenia
c. Catatonic Schizophrenia
d. BPAD

193. Loss of insight and judgement is seen in patients with:

a. Phobic disorder b. Psychosis
c. Alcoholism d. Dissociative disorder

194. A person is saying his family members are dying. He is also decaying, nothing exists in the world? ***New Q*** *(NORCET 2022)*

a. Delusion of persecution
b. Paranoid delusion
c. Nihilistic delusion
d. Delusion of reference

Explanation: Nihilistic delusion, also known as Cotard's syndrome, is characterized by the belief that oneself, others, or the world do not exist, are decaying, or are dead. In this case, the person is expressing the delusional belief that their family members are dying and that nothing exists in the world.

195. Olfactory and gustatory hallucinations are seen in:

a. Depression
b. Paranoia
c. Temporal lobe epilepsy
d. Alzheimer's disease

196. The hallucination in which the content is consistent with either a depressed or manic mood is called: *(AIIMS Raipur Grade II 2017)*

a. Somatic hallucination
b. Mood - congruent hallucination
c. Mood - incongruent hallucination
d. Haptic hallucination

Explanation: Mood congruent hallucination refers to hallucination whose content represents or reflects the mood state of the individual. Mood congruence is a psychotic symptom of bipolar disorder. Mood incongruence is a psychotic feature of the disease wherein the person's belief or action, whether by hallucination or delusion, does not match with his or her mood. Haptic hallucination is the sensation of touch mostly seen in alcoholic delirium tremens. Somatic hallucination is the perception of a physical experience occurring within the body.

197. Type of delusion in which an individual feels extreme power, intelligence or fame is called, delusion of:

a. Persecution
b. Nihilism
c. Control
d. Grandiosity

DISORDERS OF THINKING/THOUGHT

198. Rorschach's projective test designed to measure? *(VIHMANS 1996)*

a. Unconscious intentions
b. Dreams
c. Conscious desires
d. Brain size

Explanation: Rorschach's Inkblot Test: The inkblot test (also called the "Rorschach's test") is a method of psychological evaluation. Psychologists use this test in an attempt to examine the personality characteristics and emotional functioning of their patients. This test is often employed in diagnosing underlying thought disorders and differentiating psychotic from nonpsychotic thinking in cases where the patient is reluctant to openly admit to psychotic thinking.

Ans.

185. a
186. c
187. c
188. c
189. a
190. b
191. c
192. b
193. b
194. c
195. c
196. b
197. d
198. a

199. Part of the brain that is responsible for emotional aspects of behavior is:
a. Cerebellum
b. Limbic system
c. Gyri and Sulcus
d. Cerebrum

200. The part of the brain that regulates cognitive function is.:
a. Cerebrum
b. Cerebellum
c. Limbic system
d. Pons

201. Loosening of association is an example of:
a. Formal thought disorder
b. Schneider's first symptoms
c. Preservation
d. Concrete thinking

202. Which of the following assessment method is used to assess cognitive impairment?
a. Mini mental status examination
b. Ishihara polychromatic plates
c. Ink blot test
d. Projective technique

203. A 60-year-old man had undergone cardiac bypass surgery two days back, now he started forgetting things and was not able to recall names and phone numbers of his relatives. What is the probable diagnosis? *New Q*
a. Depression
b. Post-traumatic psychosis
c. Cognitive dysfunction
d. Alzheimer's disease

Explanation: Cognitive dysfunction is a decline in cognitive functions, such as memory, attention, and thinking skills. It can be caused by a number of factors, including surgery, medications, and medical conditions.

In this case, the 60-year-old man had undergone cardiac bypass surgery two days back and started forgetting things and was not able to recall names and phone numbers of his relatives. This suggests that he is experiencing cognitive dysfunction.

204. Separation of a thought or memory from its associated feeling or emotion is known as: *(AIIMS BPL NO 2018)*
a. Idealization
b. Projection
c. Intellectualization
d. Isolation

Explanation: Isolation is a defense against harmful thoughts. Isolation prevents the self from allowing these cognitions of harmful thoughts or memory to become recurrent and possibly damaging to the self-concept.

205. The belief that oneself, a part of one's body, or the real world does not exist or has been destroyed is termed as:
a. Persecutory delusion
b. Somatic delusion
c. Nihilistic delusion
d. Secondary delusion

206. The commonest form of puerperal psychosis:
a. Organic
b. Schizophreniform
c. Affective
d. Anxiety neurosis

207. Presence of which of the following feature is seen in patients with neurosis?
a. Hallucination
b. Insight
c. Delusion
d. Disorganized speech

208. Visual hallucinations without auditory hallucinations are seen in:
a. Organic brain damage
b. Obsessive compulsive neurosis
c. Agoraphobia
d. Schizophrenia

209. An individual with broadcasting will have, a feeling of:
a. Being persecuted or harassed
b. Being spiritual and having superpower
c. Being responsible for every activity happening in the world
d. Being in a state of their thoughts escaping their mind.

210. A person quarrels and hits his neighbor, as he feels that he had conspired with the police to arrest him and beat him. This symptom is:
a. Auditory hallucination
b. Social withdrawal
c. Avolition
d. Persecutory delusion

DISORDERS OF MEMORY

211. Confabulation is a disorder of:
a. Perception
b. Thought
c. Memory
d. Mood

212. All are true about Ganser syndrome except: *(JIPMER 1999, 2000, 2000)*
a. Approximate answer
b. Apparent clouding of consciousness
c. Only found in prisoners
d. Hallucinations

213. Psychogenic amnesia is characterized by:
a. Antegrade Amnesia
b. Retrograde Amnesia
c. Both with confabulation
d. Patchy impairment of Personal memories

214. 60-year-old man had undergone cardiac bypass surgery 2 days back. Now he started forgetting things and was not able to recall names and phone numbers of his relatives. What is the probable diagnosis? *(JIPMER 2010)*
a. Depression
b. Post traumatic psychosis
c. Cognitive dysfunction
d. Alzheimer's disease

215. Deja vu is seen in: *(JIPMER 1994)*
a. Temporal lobe epilepsy
b. Normal person
c. Psychosis
d. All of the above

216. Disturbances of orientation memory and intelligence is present in which of the following condition?
a. Organic Psychosis
b. Functional Psychosis
c. Hallucination
d. Phobia

Explanation: Psychosis may be divided into two categories: organic and functional. Organic psychosis is characterized by abnormal brain function that is caused by a known physical abnormality, which in most cases is some organic disease of the brain.

MOTOR DISORDERS

217. Which among the following activity need to be restricted in a client with Parkinson's disease?
a. Taking cold water bath
b. Walking on the yard on a cold winter day
c. Taking food item which is high in water content
d. Sitting on the beach in the sun on a summer day

Explanation: The patient with Parkinson's should be advised to avoid exposure to sun during summer. The patient may be oversensitive to heat and increases the risk of hyperthermia.

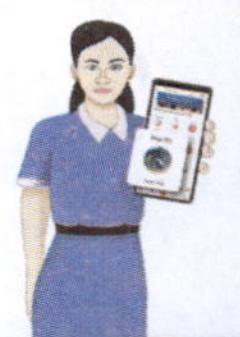

Ans.

199. b
200. a
201. a
202. a
203. c
204. d
205. c
206. c
207. b
208. a
209. d
210. d
211. c
212. c
213. b
214. c
215. d
216. a
217. d

218. Parkinson stuporous disease is caused by: *(DSSSB 2013)*
- a. Death of brain cells due to old age
- b. Hereditary factors
- c. Impairment of dopamine producing cells in the brain
- d. Demyelination of the nerve cells

Explanation: Parkinson's disease is primarily caused by low and falling dopamine levels. Parkinson's disease is caused by a loss of nerve cells in the part of the brain called the substantia nigra.

219. All of the following are features of Parkinsonism; EXCEPT: *(JIPMER 2011)*
- a. Rest-tremors
- b. Mask-like face
- c. Rigidity
- d. Preserved postural reflexes

220. Parkinson's disease is characterized by all of the following clinical features; EXCEPT:
- a. Hyperactivity
- b. Tremor
- c. Bradykinesia
- d. Rigidity

221. Sudden involuntary movement which is purposeless in nature is termed as:
- a. Mannerisms
- b. Tic disorder
- c. Catatonia
- d. Waxy flexibility

DEMENTIA

222. Which of the following features is present only in dementia when compared with Delirium? *(AIIMS BPL NO 2018)*
- a. Misperception
- b. Vivid illusions
- c. Hallucination
- d. Systematized delusions occur early

Explanation:
- Systematized delusions occur in the dementia only. It does not occur in delirium.
- Misperception, vivid illusions and Misperception are the symptoms of delirium.

223. Best test for diagnosis of organic mental disorder is: *(AIIMS BBS NO 2018)*
- a. Bender gestalt test
- b. Sentence completion test
- c. Rorschach test
- d. Thematic appreciation test

Explanation:
- The Bender-Gestalt test is a psychological test used by mental health professionals that assesses visual-motor functioning, developmental disorders, and neurological impairments in children ages 3 and older and adults.
- Sentence completion test – diagnosis of personality.
- Rorschach test and Thematic Apperception Test (TAT) - projective test to assess personality structure, pattern of thoughts, emotional problems and mental disorders.

224. Reversible dementia is seen in:
- a. Wilson
- b. Myxedema
- c. Alzheimer's
- d. Huntington disease

Explanation: Hypothyroidism is one of the most important causes of potentially reversible dementia. Myxedema is caused by hypothyroidism.

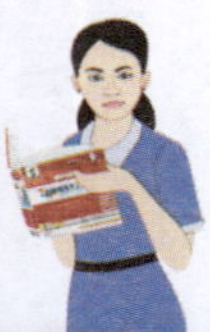

Ans.

218. c
219. d
220. a
221. b
222. d
223. a
224. b
225. b
226. b
227. b
228. c
229. a
230. b
231. a
232. c
233. c

225. All are true about Dementia; EXCEPT:
- a. Loss of short term memory
- b. Loss of long term memory
- c. Deterioration of personality
- d. Impaired learning

226. The most common cause of dementia is:
- a. Stroke
- b. Alzheimer's disease
- c. Thyroid abnormalities
- d. Trauma

227. An acquired global impairment of intellect, memory and personality without impairment of consciousness is referred to as:
- a. Amnesia
- b. Dementia
- c. Delirium
- d. Parkinsonism

228. In dementia patients, mood changes can be eased by:
- a. Use of mood stabilizers such as lithium
- b. Keeping the client busy with activities
- c. Keeping a calm environment with fixed daily routine
- d. Engaging the client in group activities

229. Disorientation is most evident in:
- a. Organic brain damage
- b. Paranoid schizophrenia
- c. BPAD
- d. OCD

Explanation: A person with dementia (organic brain syndrome) is usually disoriented in terms of time and space, and has incoherent thoughts and speech.

230. A sudden unexpected travel away from home/work place with inability to recall one's past is called:
- a. Possession disorder
- b. Dissociative fugue
- c. Selective amnesia
- d. Multiple personality disorder

231. Dissociative fugue is characterized by: *(JIPMER 2012)*
- a. Wandering away from home
- b. Irreversible amnesia
- c. Gradual recovery
- d. Normal recall

DELIRIUM

232. Which of the following is considered under acute neuro-psychiatric complications of AIDS? *(AIIMS Bhopal Nursing officer, 2018)*
- a. Organic hallucinosis
- b. Organic personality disorder
- c. Delirium
- d. AIDS dementia

Explanation: Delirium is considered under acute neuropsychiatric complications of AIDS

233. All of the following are true about nursing care for a patient with delirium; EXCEPT: *(Banaras HU 2015)*
- a. Allow the client to wear his/her own clothes
- b. Avoid room changes, especially at night
- c. Refrain family members to stay with the patient
- d. Avoid physical restraint whenever possible

234. Clouding of consciousness is a feature of:

a. Selective amnesia b. Dementia
c. Delirium d. Alzheimer's disease

235. Delirium is seen mainly in disorders associated with: *(JIPMER 2012)*

a. Alcohol b. Barbiturate
c. Opium d. Cocaine

236. Signs and symptoms of delirium tremens include all of the following; EXCEPT: *(JIPMER 2011)*

a. Clouding of consciousness b. Tremors
c. Hypothermia d. Disorientation

237. Delirium and amnestic reaction are seen with:

a. Alcohol b. Opiates
c. Cannabis d. Amphetamines

ALZHEIMER'S DISEASE

238. Biochemical etiology of Alzheimer's disease relates to: *(AIIMS BBS NO 2018)*

a. Epinephrine b. Acetylcholine
c. Serotonin d. Dopamine

Explanation: The decrease in production of acetylcholine reduces the amount of the neurotransmitter that is released to cells in the cortex and hippocampus, resulting in a disruption of the cognitive processes.

239. A 73-year-old client is admitted to the hospital with the diagnosis of dementia of the Alzheimer's type and depression. The symptom that is unrelated to depression would be: *(Safdarjung NO 2018)*

a. Apathetic response to the environment
b. "I don't know" answer to questions
c. Shallow of labile effect
d. Neglect of personal hygiene

Explanation:

- Apathetic response to the environment, neglect of personal hygiene, and "I Don't Know" answer to questions are signs of depression.
- Labile affect is also known as pseudobulbar affect, emotional incontinence, or involuntary emotional expression disorder (IEED). Shallow effect refers to little or no emotions of a person. It is referred to as marked fluctuation of mood; can be a symptom of a disorder such as schizophrenia.

240. A 65-year-old man with Alzheimer's disease exhibits frequent episodes of emotional liability. Which of the following intervention is most appropriate for this patient?

a. Logically explains the reality
b. Reduce environmental stimuli to redirect attention
c. Try humor to alter the patient's mood
d. Explore the cause of altered mood

241. Which of the following is a short-term goal for a patient with Alzheimer's disease?

a. Optimum functioning in the least restrictive environment
b. Improved self-esteem
c. Improved self-confidence
d. Regain of sensory and cognitive function

242. All of the following are an example of organic brain disorders; EXCEPT:

a. Alzheimer's disease
b. Delirium
c. Dementia
d. PTSD

243. Which of the following is feature of Alzheimer's disease? *(JIPMER 2007)*

a. Early memory loss
b. Recent memory loss
c. Recent and past memory loss
d. Global memory loss

244. Alzheimer's disease is associated with: *(JIPMER 2008)*

a. Delusion
b. Dementia
c. Delirium
d. Depression

ALCOHOL DEPENDENCE SYNDROME (ADS)

245. A chronic alcoholic developed ataxia, nausea, vomiting, and ophthalmoplegia. The possible diagnosis is:

a. Korsakoff psychosis
b. Wernicke's encephalopathy
c. Cerebellar infarction
d. Alcohol Intoxication

246. Which of the following medications are the safest to administer to adults needing assistance in falling asleep?

a. Barbiturates
b. SSRIs
c. Minor tranquilizers
d. Benzodiazepines

247. A patient approached nurse asking for advice on how to deal with his alcohol addiction. Nurse should tell the client that the only effective treatment for alcoholism is: *(Safdarjung NO 2018)*

a. Psychotherapy
b. Alcoholics anonymous (AA)
c. Total abstinence
d. Aversion Therapy

Explanation: For alcoholism total abstinence is the only effective treatment. Psychotherapy, attendance at alcoholics anonymous (AA) meeting, and aversion therapy are all adjunctive therapies that can support the client in efforts to abstain.

248. Most common symptom of alcohol withdrawal is: *(AIIMS BBS NO 2018)*

a. Body ache b. Tremor
c. Rhinorrhea d. Diarrhea

Explanation:

- Within 4–12 hours of cessation of or reduction in heavy or prolonged alcohol use, the following symptoms may appear—coarse tremor of hands, tongue, or eyelids, nausea or vomiting, weakness, tachycardia, sweating, elevated BP, anxiety, depressed mood or irritability, and insomnia.
- Body ache, Rhinorrhea and diarrhea are more common in Opioid withdrawal.

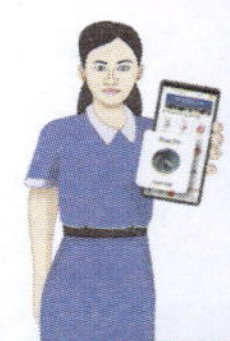

Ans.

234. c
235. a
236. c
237. a
238. b
239. c
240. b
241. a
242. d
243. c
244. b
245. b
246. d
247. c
248. b

249. The health education to a group of alcoholic people should be able to: *(RAK MSc 2018)*

a. Teach the bad effects of alcoholism
b. Change their behavior
c. Inform about constituents of alcohol
d. Create awareness among them about family crisis

Explanation: In alcohol and drug education, the goal is to alter several negative behaviors. Other options are the way of approach to achieve the goal of behavioral change. The goal of health education is to bring behavioral change in an alcoholic.

250. Which of the following foods would the nurse eliminate from the diet of a client in alcohol withdrawal: *(Safdarjung NO 2018)*

a. Milk b. Orange juice
c. Tea d. Regular coffee

Explanation: Caffeine is present in regular coffee, which stimulates psychomotor activity and results in feelings of anxiety and agitation. Serving coffee to the client may add to tremors and wakefulness. Orange juice, milk and tea are part of balanced diet needed for the client who is on alcohol withdrawal.

251. Which of the following is a long-term effect of 'Medical complication of Alcoholism'? *(AIIMS Bhopal Nursing officer, 2018)*

a. Korsakoff's Psychosis
b. Depression
c. Delirium Tremens
d. Paranoia

Explanation: In alcohol misuse a chronic memory disorder can occur due to the deficiency of thiamine (vit B1). It is called Korsakoff's Psychosis.

252. Chronic alcoholic patients are treated initially by:

a. Use of paraldehyde
b. Use of tranquilizers
c. Providing high protein diet
d. IM injection of thiamine

Explanation: Parenteral administration of thiamine is unanimously considered the route of choice to replenish thiamine stores as rapidly as possible.

253. The most effective treatment for alcoholism is:

a. Group therapy b. Disulfiram therapy
c. Total abstinence d. Chlorpromazine

Explanation: Abstinence is the total avoidance of an activity. Total abstinence is the marker of success of deaddiction treatment. Abstinence is the only effective treatment for alcoholism, particularly in short-term alcoholic addicts.

254. An alcoholic client is showing confabulation, which complication of alcoholism did the nurse need to suspect?

a. Seizure
b. Wernicke's encephalopathy
c. Korsakoff's psychosis
d. Dementia

Explanation: It is a syndrome of confusion, loss of recent memory, and confabulation in alcoholic client caused by deficiency of thiamine (vitamin B1).

255. Drug of choice to treat alcohol withdrawal symptoms such as tremors, and high BP include:

a. Disulfiram b. Lorazepam
c. Cloxacillin d. Benztropine

Explanation: The drug of choice to treat the alcohol withdrawal symptoms include lorazepam, its onset of action is also fast.

256. Alcohol anonymous group is classified as:

a. Social group
b. Self-help group
c. Resocialization group
d. Psychotherapeutic group

Explanation: It is a self-help group, who meet together to maintain sobriety.

257. An alcoholic client experiencing burning and tingling sensations of the feet. It is suggestive of:

a. Peripheral neuropathy b. Wernicke's encephalopathy
c. Korsakoff psychosis d. Seizure

Explanation: Peripheral neuropathy, characterized by peripheral nerve damage, results in pain, burning, tingling, or prickly sensations of the extremities.

258. Most severe alcohol withdrawal syndrome is: *(Staff Nurse G II 2014)*

a. Alcoholic hallucinosis b. Hangover
c. Alcoholic seizures d. Delirium tremens

259. Thiamine therapy in alcoholic patient is to prevent: *(ISRO)*

a. Alcoholic Dementia
b. Wernicke-Korsakoff syndrome
c. Huntington's disease
d. All of the above

260. The most common deficiency seen in patient with chronic alcoholism is: *(ISRO)*

a. Thiamine b. Cyanocobalamin
c. Niacin d. Vitamin C

261. Which of the following drug is used to treat withdrawal symptoms of alcoholism?

a. Naloxone b. Naltrexone
c. Chlordiazepoxide d. Bupropion

262. A 35-year-old male patient is discharged on Disulfiram as maintenance therapy for alcohol dependence syndrome. The nurse should educate patient to avoid which of the following product?

a. Carbonated beverages b. Cheese
c. Red meat d. After shave lotion

263. Amount of alcohol an average healthy adult person can metabolize in 24 hours is:

a. Two ounces (60 mL)
b. Four ounces (120 mL)
c. Five ounces (150 mL)
d. Six ounces (180 mL)

264. A 35-year-old male client was admitted to emergency room with alcohol intoxication. Which of the following intervention by the nurse is most appropriate for this client?

a. Counsel the patient on harmful effects of alcoholism
b. Motivate the client to stop alcoholism
c. Decrease in environmental stimuli
d. Use harm minimization principles to counsel the patient

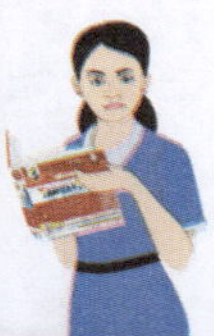

Ans.

249. b
250. d
251. a
252. d
253. c
254. c
255. b
256. b
257. a
258. d
259. b
260. a
261. c
262. d
263. a
264. c

265. A nurse is observing a patient for alcohol withdrawal symptoms. Which of the following finding indicates a potential risk for delirium tremens?
a. Muscular rigidity and stupor
b. Hypertension, hallucinations and changes in LOC
c. Agitation and hypotension
d. Hypotension and ataxia

266. Treatment for withdrawal symptoms of substance abuse is otherwise known as:
a. Detoxification phase
b. Maintenance phase
c. Harm reduction
d. Harm minimization

267. Wernicke-Korsakoff syndrome in chronic alcoholic patients is caused by a deficiency of:
a. Riboflavin
b. Thiamine
c. Pyridoxine
c. Niacin

268. A 40-year-old man presents with a 20 years history of alcohol intake with a 10 years' history of a dependence pattern. He presents with a 2-day history of altered behavior, restlessness, tremors, sleep disturbance, irritability and difficulty in walking. On examination he has gaze palsy and is disoriented. What is the most likely diagnosis?
a. Delirium tremens
b. Wernicke's encephalopathy
c. Korsakoff s psychosis
d. Alcohol induced psychosis

269. Wernicke's encephalopathy features are all; EXCEPT: *(JIPMER 2012)*
a. Confusion
b. Ataxia
c. Aphasia
d. Nystagmus

270. Heavy users of alcohol are from:
a. Upper social class
b. Middle class
c. Lower class
d. None of social class predominance

271. Direct evidence of alcohol addiction is: *(JIPMER 1995)*
a. Memory disturbance
b. Confabulation
c. Cirrhosis
d. Withdrawal symptoms

272. Alcohol hallucinations occur within: *(JIPMER 2005)*
a. 24 hours
b. 36 hours
c. 72 hours
d. 96 hours

273. Recommended treatment for extremely agitated behavior by a person who is grossly intoxicated with alcohol is:
a. Diazepam
b. Phenobarbital
c. Chlorpromazine
d. Haloperidol

274. All of the following drugs may be used for the treatment of alcohol dependence; EXCEPT: *(JIPMER 2012)*
a. Naltrexone
b. Disulfiram
c. Flumazenil
d. Acamprosate

275. Visual hallucination is seen in:
a. Alcoholism
b. Mania
c. Depression
d. Phobia

OPOID DEPENDENCE

276. Heroin is a form of:
a. Tobacco
b. Poppy
c. Datura
d. Cannabis

Explanation: Heroin is a highly addictive, illegal drug. Heroin (like opium and morphine) is made from the resin of poppy plants. Milky, sap-like opium is first removed from the pod of the poppy flower.

277. Among the following identify the late sign of heroine withdrawal:
a. Dysphoric mood
b. lacrimation
c. Vomiting and Diarrhea
d. Muscle cramps

Explanation: Vomiting, diarrhea, muscle spasm, fever, nausea, abdominal cramps and backache are the common late signs of heroin withdrawal.

278. LSD is also known as: *(JIPMER 1992)*
a. Brown sugar
b. Mind blocker
c. Mind expander
d. Glue

279. Which of the priority concern in a nurse while caring for a client with opioid addiction is:
a. Difficulty arousing the patient
b. Oxygen saturation of 95%
c. Respiratory rate 12 breaths/min
d. Pain score 50 on scale of 0 to 100

OTHER SUBSTANCE USE DISORDERS

280. In a client with substance abuse, which is the best indicator to assess the client's progress in rehabilitation?
a. Perform all the activities of daily living independently
b. The number of drug-free days he has
c. Taking all the prescribed drugs on time
d. Willing to come for follow up

Explanation: Number of drug-free days is the best indicator to determine the progress of rehabilitation of patient with substance use disorder. Maintenance of abstinence from the substance is the ultimate goal of the deaddiction treatment.

281. Substance abuse refers to:
a. Developing tolerance for substance
b. Maladaptive pattern of substance use
c. Experiencing withdrawal symptoms on stopping the substance
d. Psychological dependence on drugs

282. ICD-10 diagnostic criteria for drug dependence syndrome include all; EXCEPT:
a. Development of tolerance
b. Episodic use of substances
c. Appearance of withdrawal symptoms on stopping the substance
d. A strong craving for the substance

283. Drug dependence refers to:
a. Harmful pattern of substance use
b. Physiological and psychological dependence on substances
c. Habitual use of substances
d. Experiencing psychotic symptoms due to substance use

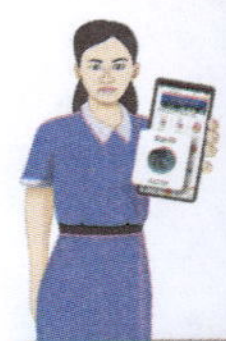

Ans.
265. b
266. a
267. b
268. b
269. c
270. d
271. d
272. a
273. a
274. c
275. a
276. b
277. c
278. c
279. a
280. b
281. b
282. b
283. b

SCHIZOPHRENIA

284. Who coined the term schizophrenia?

a. Eugene Bleuler b. William Tuke
c. Karl Menninger d. John Weber

Explanation: The term schizophrenia is coined by Eugene Bleuler

285. In schizophrenia, gradual subtle behavioral changes occur in: *(AIIMS-BBS SNO 2019)*

a. The premorbid phase
b. The prodromal phase
c. The onset phases
d. The progressive phase

Explanation: Features of prodromal phase include Functional impairment, nonspecific symptoms, and gradual subtle behavioral changes (disorientation in role functioning, social withdrawal, and positive symptoms appear).

286. The following are presenting symptoms of patient with catatonic schizophrenia; EXCEPT: *(ESIC 2019)*

a. Sudden onset of mutism
b. Have dangerous periods of agitation and explosive behavior
c. Disorganized behavior and speech
d. Stereotyped position with waxy flexibility.

Explanation: **Catatonic schizophrenia** is a type of schizophrenia that is characterized by disruptions in a person's movement. The features may include:

- Catatonic excitement (periods of agitation and explosive behavior) or
- Catatonic stupor (mutism or Stereotyped position with waxy flexibility)

Disorganized behavior and speech are not the presenting symptoms of patient with catatonic schizophrenia.

287. Which of the following is not a part of Bleuler's 4 A's? *(AIIMS Bhopal Grade-I 2018)*

a. Ambivalence b. Avolition
c. Associative loosening d. Autistic thinking

Explanation: Eugen Bleuler's gave the famous 4 A's that he presumed lied at the core of the schizophrenia and were fundamental aspects of the disorder. These 4 A's are: Affect, Autism, Ambivalence and Associative loosening.

288. According to DSM IV, the positive symptoms of Schizophrenia include: *(AIIMS Raipur Grade II 2017)*

a. Hallucinations b. Delusions
a. Flat affect d Bizarre behavior
a. a, b, c b. b, c, d
c. a, c, d d. a, b, d

Explanation: The positive symptoms of schizophrenia include delusions, thought disorder, disorganized behavior and movement disorder (agitated or repeated movements). The negative symptoms include lack of emotion or small emotional range, reduced ability to plan and follow through the activities, neglect of personal hygiene, social withdrawal and decrease in talkativeness and loss of motivations.

289. Mr. Raju says that he is the first lead of the world and he is born with a special mission in life. These are the symptoms of: *(AIIMS Raipur Grade II 2017)*

a. Autochthonous delusion b. Delusion of grandeur
c. Delusion of persecution d. Delusion of reference

Explanation: A primary delusion is a delusion which arises "out of the blue" with no morbid antecedents is called autochthonous delusion. Persecutory delusions are a set of delusional conditions in which the affected persons believe they are being persecuted. A delusion of reference is a type of delusion wherein the individual perceives unrelated events or objects in his/her surroundings to be of significance for himself/herself. Delusion of grandeur refers to feeling superior.

290. Mrs. Gowri, on assessment, shows the following behavior. *(AIIMS Raipur Grade II 2017)*

a. Maintaining rigid posture
b. Being mute
c. Hears "God's voice"
d. Repeating the phrases.

These are the characteristics of:

a. Paranoid Schizophrenia
b. Undifferentiated schizophrenia
c. Catatonic schizophrenia
d. Residual Schizophrenia

Explanation: Catatonia includes extremes of behavior such as excessive and peculiar motor behaviors and decreased motor activity and engagement. In paranoid schizophrenia people may have false beliefs or delusions that an individual or group of people are conspiring to harm them or members of their family. When a person has a past history of at least one episode of schizophrenia but currently has no symptoms, are called residual schizophrenia. Undifferentiated schizophrenia is categorized when features of no other subtypes of schizophrenia are fully present of features of more than one type of subtype are exhibited.

291. A client with schizophrenia unlikely to demonstrate:

a. Low self-esteem
b. Ambivalence
c. Effective self-boundaries
d. Weak ego

Explanation: Inability to maintain adequate boundaries is the feature of schizophrenic patients.

292. The most frequent period of onset of schizophrenia is:

a. Late adolescence to early adulthood
b. Childhood
c. Middle age
d. Old age

Explanation: Schizophrenia is a disease that typically begins in early adulthood; between the ages of 15 and 25. Men tend to develop schizophrenia slightly earlier than women; whereas most males become ill between 16 and 25 years old, most females develop symptoms several years later, and the incidence in women is noticeably higher in women after age 30. The average age of onset is 18 in men and 25 in women.

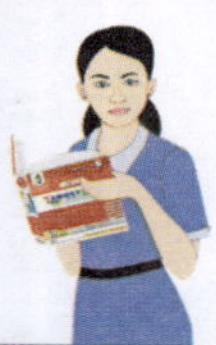

Ans.

284. a
285. b
286. c
287. b
288. d
289. b
290. c
291. c
292. a

293. The priority nursing intervention for a client who is admitted with paranoid schizophrenia is:
a. Establish a structured daily routine
b. Plan a programme of self-fulfillment.
c. Provide patient and others with safe environment
d. Do mini mental status examination

Explanation: Patient is suffering from paranoid schizophrenia, so the priority nursing intervention is to provide a safe environment for patient and others.

294. Characteristics of Paranoid personality disorder include:
a. Constantly on guard and hypervigilant
b. Appear tense and irritable
c. Avoid interaction with other people
d. All of the above

Explanation: Characteristics of paranoid personality disorder include doubt the commitment, loyalty, or trustworthiness of others, believing others are using or deceiving them, reluctant to confide in others or reveal personal information due to a fear that the information will be used against them, unforgiving and hold grudges, hypersensitive and take criticism poorly, read hidden meanings in the innocent remarks or casual looks of others, perceive attacks on their character that are not apparent to others; they generally react with anger and are quick to retaliate, have recurrent suspicions, without reason, that their spouses or lovers are being unfaithful, generally cold and distant in their relationships with others, and might become controlling and jealous. They cannot see their role in problems or conflicts and believe they are always right. Have difficulty in relaxing, hostile, stubborn, and argumentative.

295. Delusions of grandeur means: *(IHBAS, Delhi)*
a. Someone usually in higher status is in love with them
b. Irrational ideas regarding their own worth, talent, knowledge or power
c. Sexual partner is unfaithful.
d. They are being malevolently treated in some way

Explanation: Option b is the correct answer. Option a is delusion of erotomanic type. Option c is jealous type delusion. Option d is persecutory type delusion.

296. The prominent symptom thats lasts at least for 1 month and helpful to diagnose paranoid schizophrenia is:
a. Delusions and hallucination
b. Poverty of speech with apathy
c. Bizarre behavior associated with drug use
d. Disturbed relationship and poor grooming

Explanation: Diagnostic criteria for paranoid schizophrenia include persistence of two or more symptoms such as delusion or hallucination for more than 1 month.

297. When the person feels both positive and negative toward same object it is known as:
a. Ambivalent
b. Occasionally appropriate
c. Positive affect
d. Inappropriate

Explanation: Ambivalence is a state of having simultaneous conflicting reactions, beliefs, or feelings toward some object. Stated another way, ambivalence is the experience of having an attitude toward someone or something that contains both positively and negatively balanced components.

298. Impaired insight is evident in: *(JIPMER 1992, 2009)*
a. Psychosomatic disorder
b. Anxiety neurosis
c. Post-traumatic Stress Disorder
d. Schizophrenia

299. Which of the following is not true about hallucinations?
a. It is a disorder of perception
b. It is always pathological
c. It is different from imagery
d. It occurs on objective space

300. Catatonic behavior in schizophrenia is characterized by which of the following: *(LNJP H D 2012)*
a. Resisting attempts to be moved
b. Maintaining rigid, immobile postures
c. Decrease in reactivity to the environment
d. All of the above

301. The parents of a 20-year-old male patient with schizophrenia express feelings of guilt for their son's problems. Which of the following should be a part of family education?
a. Teach the parents that they must change
b. Acknowledge the parent's responsibility and commitment
c. Explain the biological process of schizophrenia
d. Refer the family to a support group

302. The characteristic feature of catatonic schizophrenia is:
a. Paranoid thoughts
b. Motor disturbances
c. Delusion of persecution
d. Thought broadcasting

303. The four A's of schizophrenia include all the following EXCEPT:
a. Auditory hallucinations
b. Ambivalence
c. Associative looseness
d. Autistic thinking

304. First rank symptoms of schizophrenia (FRSS) were described by:
a. William Wundt
b. Eugen Bleuler
c. Schneider
d. Evan Pavlov

305. Schizophrenia is a disorder of:
a. Perception
b. Thinking
c. Speech
d. Mood

306. A patient in acute care psychiatric ward assessed to have hallucination and intense delusions. The nurse understands that this patient should be closely monitored for:
a. Negligence of personal hygiene
b. Grandiosity
c. Suicidal behavior
d. Injury to others

307. Example of nonaffective psychosis is:
a. Schizophrenia
b. Mental Retardation
c. Anxiety Neurosis
d. Hysteria

308. The effect that is most commonly seen in patients with schizophrenia is:
a. Elation and Euphoria
b. Sadness and depression
c. Apathy and flatness
d. Anger and Aggression

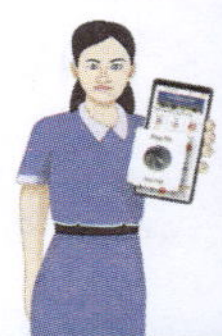

Ans.

293. c
294. d
295. b
296. a
297. a
298. d
299. b
300. d
301. c
302. b
303. a
304. c
305. b
306. d
307. a
308. c

309. A 32-year-old woman who is admitted to acute care psychiatric ward with a diagnosis of paranoid schizophrenia refuses to take food saying that the food is poisoned. The appropriate nursing intervention for this client is to:
a. Reassure the patient by tasting the food before patient
b. Assure the patient that the food is safe to take
c. Allow the patient to take packed/canned foods
d. Warn the patient of the consequences if she refuses to take food

310. Waxy flexibility, mutism, bizarre posture and stupor are characteristics of:
a. Undifferentiated schizophrenia
b. Catatonic schizophrenia
c. Paranoid schizophrenia
d. BPAD with depressive episode

311. Suspiciousness is a typical feature of:
a. BPAD with Mania
b. Paranoid schizophrenia
c. Undifferentiated schizophrenia
d. Hebephrenic schizophrenia

312. A schizophrenic patient is suspecting his faithful partner of infidelity (extramarital affair). The nurse understands that the patient is experiencing:
a. Delusion of nihilism b. Delusion of grandiosity
c. Delusion of persecution d. Delusion of infidelity

313. Which of following is a negative symptom of schizophrenia?
a. Delusions b. Aggression
c. Hallucinations d. Affective flattening

314. In Schizophrenia, all are considered negative symptoms; EXCEPT: *(JIPMER 2011)*
a. Anhedonia
b. Decreased emotional expression
c. Impaired concentration
d. Hallucinations

315. Schizophrenia is treated by: *(JIPMER 2011)*
a. Antidepressants b. Antipsychotics
c. Antiepileptics d. Mood stabilizers

316. Wax-molding posture is seen in: *(JIPMER 2001)*
a. Schizoaffective disorder
b. Manic depressive psychosis
c. Bipolar-II disorder
d. Catatonic schizophrenia

317. Prognosis in Schizophrenia is less favorable if: *(JIPMER 2003)*
a. Occurs in women
b. Anxiety is prominent
c. Emotional blunting occurs
d. Rapid onset of psychosis occurs

318. First rank symptoms of schizophrenia are all; EXCEPT: *(JIPMER 2012)*
a. Ambivalence b. Running commentary
c. Primary delusion d. Somatic passivity

319. First rank symptoms of schizophrenia are all; EXCEPT:
a. Depersonalization b. Running commentary
c. Primary delusion d. Somatic passivity

320. Poor prognostic factor in schizophrenia is:
a. Acute onset
b. Middle age
c. Family history of affective disorder
d. Gradual onset

321. Which of the following is the treatment of choice for patients with schizophrenia, who refuse to take treatment? *(JIPMER 2012)*
a. Clozapine b. Risperidone
c. Olanzapine d. Fluphenazine

322. Schizophrenia drugs mainly act on: *(JIPMER 2014)*
a. D1 Dopamine receptors
b. D2 Dopamine receptors
c. D3 Dopamine receptors
d. Ach receptors

323. Meaning of term 'Schizophrenia' is: *(JIPMER 2014)*
a. Free mind b. Euphoric mind
c. Split mind d. Confused mind

324. Cause of premature deaths in Schizophrenia is: *(JIPMER 2011)*
a. Hospital acquired infections
b. Homicide
c. Suicide
d. Toxicity of anti-psychotic drugs

325. Schizophrenia is characterized by all; EXCEPT:
a. Delusion b. Auditory Hallucination
c. Elation d. Catatonia

326. Characteristic clinical manifestation of Schizophrenia is: *(JIPMER 1998)*
a. Confusion b. Anxiety
c. Auditory hallucinations d. Visual hallucinations

327. Most common hallucination in Schizophrenia is: *(JIPMER 1995, 1999)*
a. Auditory b. Visual
c. Olfactory d. Tactile

328. All of the following factors are associated with poor prognosis in schizophrenia; EXCEPT:
a. Rapid onset of symptoms
b. Family history of schizophrenia
c. Prodominantly negative symptoms
d. Onset of illness in early age

329. Most common types of schizophrenia:
a. Simple b. Hebephrenic
c. Catatonic d. Paranoid

330. Waxy flexibility characteristic of schizophrenia is: *(JIPMER 2006)*
a. Excitatory catatonia
b. Stuporous catatonia
c. OCD
d. All of these

331. Which is not classical 4 A's of Schizophrenia?
a. Ambivalence b. Autism
c. Affective flattening d. Automatism

332. Ambivalence is most commonly associated with: *(MP PGMEE 2002)*
a. Depression
b. Generalized anxiety disorder
c. Schizophrenia
d. OCD

333. Schizophrenia with early onset and poor prognosis is:
a. Catatonic
b. Hebephrenic
c. Paranoid
d. Schizoaffective

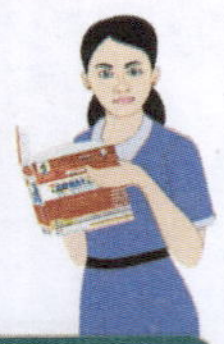

Ans.

309.	c
310.	b
311.	b
312.	d
313.	d
314.	d
315.	b
316.	d
317.	c
318.	a
319.	a
320.	d
321.	b
322.	b
323.	c
324.	c
325.	c
326.	c
327.	a
328.	a
329.	d
330.	b
331.	d
332.	c
333.	b

334. Grimacing and Mannerism is: *(JIPMER 1992)*
   a. Simple Schizophrenia
   b. Catatonic Schizophrenia
   c. Hebephrenic Schizophrenia
   d. Phobia

335. ____________ is a functional psychosis:
   a. Schizophrenia   b. Conversion disorder
   c. Panic anxiety   d. Phobia

336. The neurotransmitter theory of schizophrenia known as dopamine hypothesis refers to:
   a. Insufficient dopamine activity
   b. Mixture of dopamine
   c. Excess of dopamine
   d. Hypersensitivity to dopamine

337. In the context of schizophrenia, "expressed emotions" refer to:
   a. An individual who has difficulty in expressing his feelings
   b. An adverse family environment with the decreased quality of interaction patterns
   c. A family which is overemphasized with positive comments
   d. A family with complete lack of expressing emotions.

338. Which among the following drugs has therapeutic benefit in the treatment of schizophrenia?
   a. Lithium   b. Imipramine
   c. Haloperidol   d. Alprazolam

PERSONALITY DISORDERS

339. In psychosomatic disorders, which are of the following factors causes physical symptoms? *(Nursing Grade- II 2007)*
   a. Genetic factors
   b. Emotional factors
   c. Social factors
   d. Physical factors

Explanation: A psychosomatic disorder is a disease which involves both mind and body. Some physical symptoms are thought to be particularly prone to be made worse by emotional factors such as stress and anxiety.

340. Behavior of pretending to be ill is:
   a. Psychotic
   b. Malingering
   c. Out of contact with reality
   d. Using conversion defenses

Explanation: Pretending to be ill without any physical cause is called Malingering.

341. Disturbances of orientation, memory and intelligence is seen in:
   a. Functional Psychosis   b. Organic Psychosis
   c. Delusion   d. Anxiety disorder

342. Which of the following approaches would be most appropriate to use with a client suffering from narcissistic personality disorder when discrepancies exist between what the client states and what actually exist: *(Safdarjung NO 2018)*
   a. Rationalization
   b. Supportive confrontation
   c. Limit setting
   d. Consistency

Explanation: Supportive confrontation can be used to point out discrepancies between what the client states and what actually exists. This will increase the client's responsibility for self. Limit setting may help the client control unacceptable behavior but do not point out discrepancies. Rationalization usually used by the client as defense mechanism, not the nurse. Consistency helps gain control but does not point out discrepancies.

343. A patient with antisocial personality disorder belches loudly. A staff member asks "Do you know why people find you repulsive?" this statement most likely would elicit which of the following client reaction: *(Safdarjung NO 2018)*
   a. Defensiveness   b. Embarrassment
   c. Shame   d. Remorseful

Explanation: Since the question from the nurse is demeaning (belittling) the client, the client may likely feel defensive because the question may attack the self-image of the client. It is the natural tendency of the client to counterattack the threat to self-image.

344. A male client is diagnosed with schizotypal personality disorder. Which signs would this client exhibit during social situation: *(Safdarjung NO 2018)*
   a. Paranoid thoughts
   b. Emotional affect
   c. Independence need
   d. Aggressive behavior

Ref: Mary C Townsend. Essentials of Mental Health Nursing. 6th edition. pp. 608-14.

Explanation:
- Suspiciousness and mistrust of others (paranoia) is a characteristic feature of schizotypal personality disorder.
- Emotional affect and independence needs are not related to schizotypal personality disorder. Aggressive behavior is not seen in person with schizotypal personality.

345. A 20-year-old client was diagnosed with dependent personality disorder. Which behavior is most likely to be evidence of ineffective individual coping? *(Safdarjung NO 2018)*
   a. Recurrent self-destructive behavior
   b. Avoiding relationship
   c. Showing interest in solitary activities
   d. Inability to make choices and decision without advice

Explanation: Dependent personality disorder is characterized by intense lack of self-confidence, low self-esteem, and inability to make decisions.

346. A patient with borderline personality disorder who is to be discharged soon threatens to "do something" to herself if discharged. Which of the following actions by the nurse would be most important? *(Safdarjung NO 2018)*
   a. Ask a family member to stay with the client at home temporarily
   b. Discuss the meaning of the client's statement with her
   c. Request an immediate extension for the client
   d. Ignore the client's statement because it's a sign of manipulation

Ans.
334. b
335. a
336. c
337. b
338. c
339. b
340. b
341. b
342. b
343. a
344. a
345. d
346. b

Explanation:

- The nurse should assess for suicidal risk. The nurse should attempt to assess any suicidal statement and determine its meaning in terms of suicide. It is common among clients with borderline personality disorder to make threatening comments before discharge.
- Asking family members to stay with a client will transfer the responsibility to the family instead of client. Granting extension will encourage dependency of client. Ignoring client's statement may lead to error in judgment.

347. A hospitalized client, diagnosed with a borderline personality disorder, consistently breaks the unit rules. This behavior should be confronted because it will help the client:

(RAK MSc 2018)

a. Control anger
b. Become more self-aware
c. Reduce anxiety
d. Set realistic goals

Explanation:

- Clients with borderline personality disorder are likely to develop dysfunctional coping and act out in self-destructive ways such as binge eating. Clients must first become aware of their behavior before they can change it. So, confrontation of their rules breaking behavior will help the client to become more self-aware.
- After the client is aware of the behavior and has a desire to change the behavior, then other options like setting the realistic goal reducing anxiety and controlling anger should be done.

348. A person has run away from home adopting a new identity with complete amnesia about his earlier life. This disorder is known as: *(AIIMS Bhopal Grade-I 2018)*

a. Dissociative fugue
b. Multiple personality disorder
c. Dissociative amnesia
d. Conversion disorder

Explanation: Dissociative fugue or psychogenic fugue is a dissociative disorder characterized by reversible amnesia for personal identity. The state can last for days, months or longer and is sometimes accompanied by the establishment of new identity.

349. A person who is aloof, isolated and does not socialize, falls into which of the following category?

(AIIMS Raipur Staff Nurse Grade I-2018)

a. Withdrawn
b. Anxious
c. Aggressive
d. Obsessive

Explanation: Above given description indicates withdrawn person. In anxious personality, worry and fear become overwhelming and can interfere with activity of daily living. In aggressive personality persistent maladaptive aggression is expressed in different ways. In obsessive personality, preoccupation with orderliness and perfectionism can be seen.

350. A nurse who is caring for a client with antisocial behavior should stress on:

a. Close supervision of the client
b. Educate the family members that someone should be with the client all time
c. Setting clear rules and expectations about the client's behavior
d. Provide stimuli free environment to the client

Explanation: The nursing care plan for the antisocial client should stress on setting the clear rules and expectation about the client's behavior.

351. Which is the most appropriate nursing intervention for a schizotypal personality disorder client with a nursing diagnosis of impaired verbal communication?

a. Helping the client to participate in social interactions
b. Establishing a one-on-one relationship with the client
c. Establishing alternative forms of communication
d. Allowing the client to decide when he wants to participate in verbal communication with the nurse.

Explanation: Patient with schizotypal personality has great difficulty in establishing and maintaining close relationships with others. By establishing a one-to-one relationship, the nurse can help the client to learn how to interact with other people in different environment.

352. The main treatment for Dissociative Identity Disorder is:

a. Hypnosis
b. Individual psychodynamic psychotherapy
c. Family therapy
d. Group psychotherapy focusing on family issues

Explanation: Individual psychotherapy is the most widely used modality as opposed to family, group or couple's therapy. The main goal for treatment is the integration of the separate personality states into one cohesive, unified personality, unless the person with DID is not ready or motivated to work with trauma.

353. Which of the following sign would be exhibited by a client with schizotypal personality in a social situation?

a. Blunt emotional affect
b. Violent behavior
c. Paranoid thoughts
d. Anhedonia

Explanation: Patients with schizotypal personality disorder develop excessive social anxiety in a social situation. This may lead to paranoid thoughts.

354. Which among the following activity is best suited for a client with histrionic personality disorder who is responding to situations in an exaggerated manner?

a. Behavioral therapy
b. Role playing
c. Isolate the client
d. Therapeutic community

Explanation: Use of role-playing can be used to teach the client appropriate responses to others and in different situations.

355. Splitting is the trait of .... Disorder.

a. Borderline personality disorder
b. Passive aggressive personality
c. Dependent personality disorder
d. Narcissistic personality disorder

Explanation: It is the characteristic of borderline personality disorder. It arises from their lack of achievement of object constancy and is manifested by an inability to integrate and accept both positive and negative feeling.

356. Schizotypal personality disorder exhibits:

a. Paranoid thoughts
b. Inappropriate/constricted affect
c. Odd thinking and speech
d. All of the above

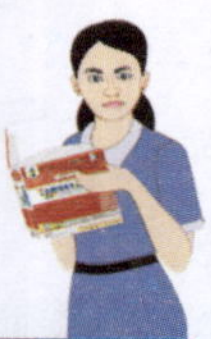

Ans.

347. b
348. a
349. a
350. c
351. b
352. b
353. c
354. b
355. a
356. d

Explanation: Schizotypal personality disorder (STPD) is a personality disorder characterized by all the above-mentioned signs and symptoms.

357. Sheldon's classification of personality includes:

a. Ectomorphs b. Endomorphs
c. Mesomorphs d. All of the above

Explanation: All the above-mentioned components are the part of Sheldon's classification of personality.

358. Narcissistic personality disorder is characterized by:

a. Callous unconcern for feelings of others
b. Self-dramatization, theatrically
c. Ideas of grandiosity and inflated sense of self-importance
d. Significant and persistent disturbances of identity of self

Explanation: Ideas of grandiosity and inflated sense of self-importance are the characteristic of narcissistic personality.

359. Characteristic of schizoid personality disorder is:

a. Rigid and controlling
b. Submissive and immature
c. Arrogant and attention seeking
d. Introverted and emotionally withdrawn

Explanation: These clients show social inadequacy and lack of emotional contact with others.

360. Characteristic of histrionic personality is:

a. Dramatic and theatrical b. Boastful and egocentric
c. Rigid and perfectionistic d. Aggressive and manipulative

Explanation: Client with histrionic personality draws attention to themselves and demonstrates emotionally and attention-seeking behavior

361. People with anti-social personality have difficulty in relating to others because:

a. Will not count on others
b. Cannot empathize with others
c. Never learned to be dependent on others
d. Have difficulty in communicating socially with others

Explanation: People with anti-social behavior lack ego and super-ego that control behavior. These people have little or no concern for others.

362. Which of the following intervention is appropriate for handling a patient with an antisocial personality?

a. Ignore the patient
b. Agree with the patient's demands
c. Set limits with patient
d. Be friendly with patient

363. Lack of self-esteem, strong dependency needs and impulsive behavior are characteristics of:

a. Schizoid personality disorder
b. Paranoid personality disorder
c. Borderline personality disorder
d. Narcissistic personality disorder

364. The primary treatment for dissociative identity disorder is:

a. Individual psychodynamic psychotherapy
b. Narcoanalysis
c. Cognitive therapy
d. Group psychotherapy

365. Which of the following is a type of dissociative disorder?

a. Panic anxiety disorder
b. Trans and possession disorder
c. Acute stress disorder
d. Obsessive compulsive disorder

366. In which of the following disorders the "La belle indifference" is a typical feature?

a. Post-traumatic stress disorder
b. Dissociative disorders
c. Phobic disorders
d. Mood disorders

367. Insensitive to others, no sense of remorse and abusive behaviors toward others are characteristics of:

a. Antisocial personality
b. Paranoid personality
c. Schizoid personality
d. Narcissistic personality

368. Derealization and Depersonalization are seen in which type of disorder? *(JIPMER 2012)*

a. Dissociative disorder
b. Personality disorder
c. Mania
d. None

369. Person who is kind, quiet, submissive, sympathetic and gloomy has: *(Kerala PSC, Nov 2014)*

a. Melancholic personality
b. Narcissistic personality
c. Cyclothymic personality
d. Histrionic personality

370. While providing care to a patient with antisocial personality, which of the following intervention is appropriate?

a. Focus on group, not individual therapy
b. Provide an organized and structured environment
c. Withdraw basic privileges until showing positive response to treatment
d. Recognize that the disorder is a form of social withdrawal

371. Which of the following assessment information is most important for a nurse to collect while assessing a patient with a personality disorder?

a. A family history of sexual abuse
b. Number of close friends
c. Ability to form close relationship
d. History of substance abuse

372. Narcissistic personality disorder is characterized by:

a. Unconcern for feelings of others
b. Ideas of grandiosity and inflated sense of self-importance
c. Self- dramatization
d. Disassociation

373. The characteristics of schizoid personality disorder include:

a. Dramatic, emotional, and suspicious behavior
b. Shy, quiet, passive, daydreaming, and introverted
c. Self-centric and maladjustment
d. Suspicious ideas and mistrust

374. The most prominent characteristics of a person with border-line personality disorder is:

a. Paranoid thinking
b. Instability in personal relationships
c. Mistrust
d. Antisocial activity

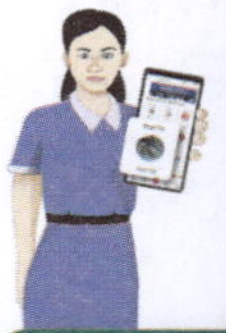

Ans.

357. d
358. c
359. d
360. a
361. b
362. c
363. c
364. a
365. b
366. b
367. a
368. a
369. a
370. b
371. d
372. b
373. b
374. b

375. All of the following are Cluster-A personality disorders; EXCEPT: *(JIPMER 2005)*

a. Paranoid b. Schizoid
c. Schizotypal d. Histrionic

376. Most effective treatment in borderline personality disorders is: *(JIPMER 2012)*

a. Pharmacotherapy
b. Behavior therapy
c. Combination of both pharmacotherapy and behavioral therapy
d. None

377. In schizoid personality disorder all are seen; EXCEPT: *(JIPMER 2013)*

a. Aloof and detached b. Prone to fantasy
c. Suspicious d. Introspective

378. Lifelong theatricality of behavior is seen in: *(JIPMER 1992)*

a. Obsessive personality b. Schizoid personality
c. Hysterical personalities d. Avoidant personalities

379. Which of the following is a Cluster C personality disorder? *(JIPMER 2012, 2013)*

a. Avoidant personality disorder
b. Histrionic personality disorder
c. Paranoid personality disorder
d. Narcissistic personality disorder

380. Anti-social personality disorder is characterized by: *(JIPMER 2014)*

a. Excessive sensitivity and suspiciousness
b. Emotional coldness, lack of pleasure
c. Unconcern for feeling of others, disregard for social norms
d. Self-dramatization, exaggerated expression of emotions

381. All are cluster B disorders of personality; EXCEPT: *(JIPMER 1999)*

a. Antisocial b. Narcissistic
c. Avoidant d. Borderline

382. Characteristic feature of Schizoid personality is: *(JIPMER 1999)*

a. Conversion reaction
b. Not concerned with disease
c. Checks details of all things
d. Emotional coldness

383. Antisocial personality is seen with: *(JIPMER 1999)*

a. Drug abuse
b. Paranoid schizophrenia
c. OCN
d. None

384. Loss of personal identity and wandering away from psychiatric hospital is referred to as: *(JIPMER 2015)*

a. Fugue b. Split personality
c. Possession state d. Trance state

385. All of the following are the core features of personality disorder; EXCEPT:

a. Emotionally Cold b. Argumentative
c. Suspicious d. Trustworthy

386. Suspicious, sensitive, mistrustful, stubborn, and argumentative are the main features of which of the following personality disorder?

a. Paranoid Personality Disorder
b. Antisocial Personality Disorder
c. Schizotypal Personality Disorder
d. Histrionic Personality Disorder

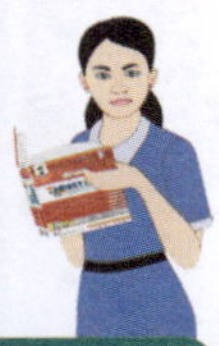

Ans.

375. d
376. b
377. c
378. c
379. a
380. c
381. c
382. d
383. a
384. a
385. d
386. a
387. c
388. c
389. c
390. c
391. b

387. A nursing officer working in psychiatric unit is assessing a patient with histrionic personality disorder. The nursing officer might identify which of the following characteristic behavior?

a. Impulsive Actions & aggressiveness
b. Odd Eccentric & Magical Thinking
c. Excessive Emotionally & Attention Seeking Behavior
d. Preoccupation with Orderliness & Cleanliness

388. All of the following features are characteristic of an antisocial personality; EXCEPT:

a. Disregard for other's feelings and emotions
b. Impulsive and aggressive actions
c. Exaggerate achievement and talents
d. Low tolerance to Frustration

389. The following features are characteristics of antisocial personality; EXCEPT:

a. Pleasure seeking
b. Inability to work under supervision
c. Deep emotional relationship
d. Drug abuse and alcohol dependence

Explanation: People with antisocial personality are likely to have Poor or abusive relationships. All other given characteristics are the features of antisocial personality disorder.

390. Unstable relationships, impulsive behavior, variable moods, lack of control on anger recurrent suicidal threats are the main clinical features of which type of personality disorder?

a. Narcissistic Personality
b. Histrionic Personality
c. Borderline Personality
d. Schizoid Personality

391. The most recent 5th edition of the Diagnostic and Statistical Manual (DSM V) of Mental Disorders grouped personality disorders into clusters. Which of the following cluster is correctly matched with its characteristics?

a. Cluster A (anxious or fearful disorders)
b. Cluster B (dramatic, emotional or erratic disorders)
c. Cluster C (Odd, eccentric disorders)
d. Cluster D (Unpredictable cluster)

Explanation: DSM V of Mental Disorders grouped personality disorders into three clusters (A, B, C) only

The three personality disorder clusters

Cluster A	Cluster B	Cluster C
The odd, eccentric cluster	The dramatic, unpredictable cluster	The anxious, fearfull cluster
Includes: • Paranoid personality disorder • Schizoid personality disorder • Schizotypal personality disorder	Includes: • Antisocial personality disorder • Borderline personality disorder • Histrionic personality disorder • Narcissistic personality disorder	Includes: • Avoidant personality disorder • Dependent personality disorder • Obsessive-compulsive personality disorder

DEPRESSIVE DISORDERS

392. The ability of a person to readily recover from stressful situations is called: *(AIIMS BPL NO 2018)*

a. Mental freedom b. Androgyny
c. Hardiness d. Resilience

Explanation: Psychological resilience is the ability to successfully cope with a crisis and to return to pre-crisis status quickly. Resilience exists when the person uses "mental processes and behaviors in promoting personal assets and protecting self from the potential negative effects of stressors".

393. 'Omega sign' is seen in which of the following? *(AIIMS BPL NO 2018)*

a. Anxious patient
b. Depressed patient
c. Deluded patients
d. Negativistic patient

Explanation: Omega sign is a sign in melancholia (depression) in which the patients have a furrowed brow due to sustained contraction of the corrugator muscle, often accompanied by Veraguth's folds, a finding likened to the Greek letter omega.

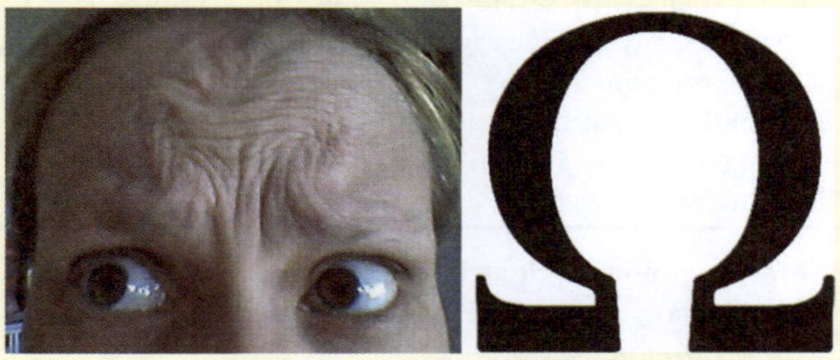

Figure: Omega sign seen in depressed patients

394. Behavioral clues of impending suicide are as follows; EXCEPT: *(ESIC 2019)*

a. Gives away valuable possessions
b. Becomes energetic after a period of severe depression
c. Withdraws from social activities and plans
d. Hypervigilance and exaggerated startle response

Explanation: The behavioral clues for impending suicide include:

- **Gives away valuable possessions.**
- **Becomes energetic after a period of severe depression**
- **Withdraws from social activities and plans**
- Farewell quotes and letters
- Avoid taking serious decisions

395. The most significant characteristics experienced by a patient with depression is: *(ESIC 2019)*

a. Aggressive, abusive or violent behavior
b. Hypervigilance and nightmares.
c. Lack of impulse control
d. Depressed mood and loss of pleasure or interest

Explanation:

- **Aggressive, abusive, violent behavior and lack of impulse control** are feature of mania. **Hypervigilance and nightmares** are the feature of anxiety disorders and/or paranoid schizophrenia. **Lack of impulse control:** Is common among manic patients.
- **Strategy**: Use the key word 'depression' to find out the answer. Depression is the key term which is common in stem and in option 'D'.

396. Which of the following is exhibited by a mother with postpartum depression? *(Daman and Diu NO 2018)*

a. Hallucinations b. Delusions
c. Uncontrolled crying d. Confusion

Explanation:

- Postpartum depression (PPD), also called postnatal depression, is a type of mood disorder associated with childbirth. Symptoms may include extreme sadness, low energy, anxiety, crying episodes, irritability, and changes in sleeping or eating patterns.
- Hallucinations, delusion and confusion are seen in postpartum psychosis.

397. A clinical feature of patient with major depression includes: *(AIIMS Raipur Grade II 2017)*

a. Psychomotor agitation b. Insomnia
c. Feelings of worthlessness d. Increased libido

a. a, b, c b. b, c, d
c. a, b, d d. a, c, d

Explanation: As per DSM IV criteria for major depressive disorder are 5 more of the following symptoms present during the same 2-week period and represent a change from previous functioning.

1. Depressed mood most of the day
2. Markedly diminished interest or pleasure in all activities
3. Significant weight loss when not dieting or weight gain
4. Insomnia or hypersomnia every day
5. Psychomotor agitation or retardation
6. Fatigue or loss of energy every day
7. Feelings of worthlessness or inappropriate guilt
8. Diminished ability to think and concentrate
9. Recurrent thoughts of death

398. The most significant causative factor of depression is:

a. Family environment
b. Chemical imbalance
c. Social environment
d. Hereditary

Explanation: Mental disorders, such as depression and anxiety, are caused by a chemical imbalance in the brain. The hypothesis is sometimes called the chemical imbalance hypothesis or chemical imbalance theory. Imbalances in serotonin, particularly relative to norepinephrine and dopamine, are common causes of certain types of depression.

399. Which of the following is not a characteristic of Endogenous Depression? *(AIIMS Bhopal Nursing officer, 2018)*

a. Feeling of more sadness during morning
b. Having suicidal tendency
c. A better feeling when in solitude
d. Feeling of more sadness during evening

Ans.

392. d
393. b
394. d
395. d
396. c
397. a
398. b
399. d

Explanation: Feeling of more sadness during evening is not the characteristic of endogenous depression. Feeling of sadness in the morning is the characteristic of endogenous depression.

400. Which of the following is the most lethal method of suicide?

a. Wrist cutting   b. Taking poison
c. Use of gun   d. Drowning

Explanation: Lethality method of suicide is determined based on the amount of time that occurs between initiating the attempt and the lethal impact of the method. Out of the given options above, use of gun is most lethal.

401. Common risk factor in patient with severe depression is: *(DSSSB 2013)*

a. Fatigability   b. Hallucinations
c. Agitation   d. Suicidal tendency

Explanation: Suicidal ideation is generally associated with mood disorders such as depression. Depression alone can cause suicidal thoughts and behavior. Suicidal risk assessment of patients diagnosed with depression is an important nursing intervention.

402. Which of the following comments, if made by a patient who has major depression would indicate an increased risk of suicide? *(RAK MSc Entrance 2010)*

a. I don't want to share my problem with any one
b. I won't be a problem much longer
c. my family members are not giving me the medication daily
d. I don't have any plan to kill my self

Explanation: Option b indicated the patient is having suicidal ideas and nurse has to intervene immediately.

403. The type of delusion commonly seen in depression is/are:

a. Delusion of Nihilism
b. Delusion of poverty
c. Delusion of persecution
d. All of the above

Explanation: All the above-mentioned delusions are apparent in depression.

404. Identify the correct statement regarding suicide:

a. Suicidal people have definitive clues and warning about their plan
b. Suicidal people are ambivalent about their feelings
c. Suicidal thoughts are only for limited period of time
d. All of the above

Explanation: All of the above statements are true regarding suicidal thought in an individual.

405. Most appropriate nursing intervention for a client who has a history of suicidal attempt and currently on suicidal tendency is:

a. Give him privacy
b. Allow him to urinate
c. Open the window and allow him to get some fresh air
d. Observe him continuously

Explanation: Continuous nursing observation is regularly involved for patient at risk of suicide. Providing privacy will affect observation. Other interventions are not appropriate for suicidal client.

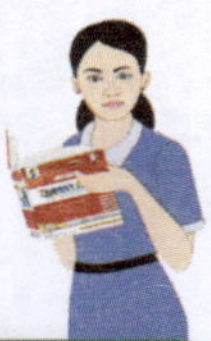

Ans.

400. c
401. d
402. b
403. d
404. d
405. d
406. d
407. b
408. b
409. c
410. c
411. d

406. Go through the following statement and identify the most appropriate one for depression:

a. Causes may include chemical imbalance in the brain and stressful life events
b. Dysthymia is also a type of depressive disorder.
c. Includes symptoms such as loss of interest, sadness, weight loss and worthless feelings
d. All of the above

Explanation: As per WHO, depression is a common mental disorder, characterized by sadness, loss of interest or pleasure, feelings of guilt or low self-worth, disturbed sleep or appetite, feelings of tiredness and poor concentration. Dysthymia is known as persistent mild depression. Causes include imbalance in neurotransmitters (serotonin) and stressful life events.

407. Extremely depressed clients are anticipated to perform well in settings where they:

a. Have support from someone
b. Do routine activities
c. Have somebody to assist
d. Have varied daily activities

Explanation:

- For a patient with severe depression, the setting where there are simple daily routines are followed will be least stressful and anxiety producing.
- **Elimination Tips:** Eliminate Option A and C because both are seeming to be very similar. None of the two similar options may be right answer.

408. Most common psychiatric illness seen in majority in India is:

a. Mania   b. Depression
c. Schizophrenia   d. OCD's

409. A 50-year-old male presents with a three year history of irritability, low mood, lack of interest in surrounding and general dissatisfaction with everything. There is no significant disruption in sleep and appetite. He is likely to be suffering from: *New Q*

a. Major depression
b. No psychiatric disorder
c. Dysthymia
d. Chronic fatigue syndrome

Explanation: Dysthymia is a chronic form of depression that is characterized by low mood, loss of interest or pleasure, and low energy. Symptoms of dysthymia are typically less severe than those of major depression, but they can last for years.

410. Which of the following would be the most appropriate cognitive intervention for a client with major depressive disorder?

a. Promote active socialization with other patients
b. Role play to increase assertiveness skills
c. Focus on identifying strengths and accomplishments
d. Encourage journaling of underlying feelings

411. Which of the following symptoms is not a sign of depression?

a. Disrupted sleep
b. Lethargy
c. Worthlessness
d. Uninhibited socialization

412. Which of the following is not a symptom of depression? *(JIPMER 2015)*

a. Loss of interest in daily activities
b. Delusion of guilt
c. Suicidal ideas
d. Delusion of grandiosity

413. Structural and functional abnormalities in which of the following part of brain is associated with Major Depression?

a. Amygdala
b. Brain stem
c. Pituitary gland
d. Cerebrum

414. Helplessness, hopelessness and worthlessness are the characteristic features of:

a. BPAD with mania
b. Paranoid schizophrenia
c. Depression
d. Acute stress disorder

415. Risk of suicide is high in patients with:

a. Mania
b. Major depression
c. Paranoid schizophrenia
d. Substance abuse

416. Prevalence of suicide is high among patients with: *(JIPMER 2008)*

a. Schizophrenic disorders
b. Neurotic stress related disorders
c. Personality disorders
d. Mood disorders

417. A mood disorder that consists of the same cognitive and physical problems as in depression, with less severe but longer-lasting symptoms is known as:

a. Melancholia
b. Dysthymic Disorder
c. Cyclothymic disorder
d. Bipolar affective disorder with depression

418. In Bipolar II Disorder, hypomanic episodes alternate with periods of:

a. Hyperventilation.
b. Major depressive disorders
c. Elation and euphoria
d. Obsession and compulsion

419. Which of the following is not true about major depressive disorder? *(JIPMER 2003)*

a. Commonly seen in females
b. Recovery is complete after treatment
c. Associated with hypothyroidism
d. Family history of major depression

420. A 25-year-old woman complains of intense depressed mood for 6 months with inability to enjoy previously pleasurable activities. This symptom is known as: *(JIPMER 2005)*

a. Anhedonia
b. Avolition
c. Apathy
d. Amotivation

421. An example of hybrid disorder is:

a. Borderline personality disorder
b. Eating disorder
c. Paranoid personality disorder
d. Mixed-anxiety depressive disorder

422. The best way to assess suicidal risk of a patient is by:

a. Indirectly asking for the clues
b. Directly question the patient on suicidal thoughts
c. Observe for cues
d. None of the above

423. Which of the following takes priority while planning care plan for a patient with suicidal risk?

a. Safety
b. Sleep
c. Self-esteem
d. Elimination

424. Recurrent suicidal tendencies are seen in: *(JIPMER 2009)*

a. Schizophrenia
b. Severe depression
c. Borderline personality disorders
d. All of the above

425. Suicidal tendencies are least common with: *(JIPMER 2013)*

a. Alone
b. Depression
c. Male
d. Married person

426. Incidence of suicide in India is:

a. 10-11/1000 population
b. 10-11/10000 population
c. 10-11/100000 population
d. 10-11/1000000 population

427. Most common mental disorder as a cause of suicide: *(JIPMER 2002; 2003)*

a. Mania
b. Depression
c. Alcohol dependence
d. Schizophrenia

428. What is most common method of suicide in India according to National Crime Records Bureau 2021?

a. Hanging
b. Drowning
c. Poisoning
d. Fall from height

429. Which of the following intervention is appropriate for a patient with depression?

a. Limiting interpersonal interaction
b. Protecting the client against harm to others
c. Providing motor outlets for feelings
d. All of the above

430. The Psychological disorder most commonly associated with myxoedema:

a. Mania
b. Depression
c. Phobia
d. Paranoia

431. "Learned helplessness" is typically seen in:

a. Delirium
b. Dementia
c. Schizophrenia
d. Depression

MANIA AND HYPOMANIA

432. Intense elation of mood with delusions of grandeur is known as:

a. Euphoria
b. Elation
c. Exaltation
d. Euthymia

Explanation: Exaltation is a severe elevation of mood. There is intense elation with delusions of grandeur; seen in severe mood mania.

433. A term used to explain a disorder of thought in which thinking proceeds slowly with many unnecessary trivial details, but finally the point is reached known as:

a. Flight of ideas
b. Prolixity
c. Tangentiality
d. Circumstantiality

Explanation: In circumstantiality, client will talk too much details and finally comes to the original topic.

434. Verbal utterance that are often obscene is known as:

a. Palilalia
b. Coprolalia
c. Echokinesis
d. Agoraphobia

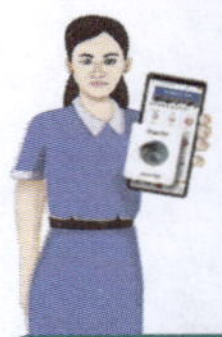

Ans.

412. d
413. a
414. c
415. b
416. d
417. b
418. b
419. b
420. a
421. d
422. b
423. a
424. d
425. d
426. c
427. b
428. a
429. c
430. b
431. d
432. c
433. d
434. b

Explanation: Use of involuntary vocalizations that are often obscene is termed coprolalia.
- Palilalia is repeating one's own sound or words.
- Echokinesis means imitating someone else movement.
- Agoraphobia means fear of being alone in public place.

435. Flight of ideas is typical feature of:
a. Schizophreni b. Mania
c. Conduct disorder d. Tic

436. A patient with mania says, "we can slam, glam, plam and flam". The nurse documents this as:
a. Verbigeration b. World salad
c. Clang association d. Neologism

437. All of the following are neurotic disorders; EXCEPT:
a. Panic anxiety b. Delirious mania
c. Conversion reaction d. Depersonalization

Explanation: Delirious mania is a severe but under-recognized neuropsychiatric syndrome characterized by the rapid onset of delirium, mania, and psychosis, not associated with a prior toxicity, physical illness, or mental disorder.

438. Mania is a type of: *(DSSSB 2013)*
a. Thought disorder b. Dissociative disorder
c. Mood disorder d. Neurotic disorder

Explanation: Mania is an abnormally elated mental state, typically characterized by feelings of euphoria, lack of inhibitions, racing thoughts, diminished need for sleep, talkativeness, risk taking, and irritability. In extreme cases, mania can induce hallucinations and other psychotic symptoms.

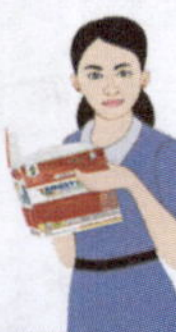

439. How can agitation in a disturbed client be minimized? *(JIPMER)*
a. Communicate to the client regarding his problem
b. Keep control on unnecessary interaction
c. Involve the client in psychotherapies
d. Encourage the family members to interact with the client

Explanation: Agitation can be minimized by reducing the environmental stimuli and with limited interaction to the client.

440. A client with manic phase of BPAD exhibits:
a. Passivity b. Dysphonia
c. Anhedonia d. Grandiosity

Explanation: Grandiosity is the most commonly seen behavior in the manic phase of BPAD.

441. Pyromania is a type of: *(JIPMER 2005; 2003)*
a. Phobia b. Impulse
c. Delusion d. Obsession

442. Elevated mood with increased psychomotor activity is a characteristic feature of: *(JIPMER 2015)*
a. Mania b. Euphoria
c. Bipolar Disorder d. Dysthymia

443. Which of the following type of diet is recommended for a patient with manic episode?
a. High-fiber diet
b. Liquid diet
c. Finger foods
d. High Calorie diet

444. Most appropriate intervention to manage manipulative behavior of a manic patient is to:
a. Set limits on patient behavior
b. Reduce environmental stimuli
c. Punish the patient for inappropriate behaviors
d. Engage patient in physical activities

445. Grandiose delusions are associated with:
a. Manic disorder
b. Obsessive compulsive disorder
c. Schizophrenia d. PTSD

446. Hyperactive behavior of a manic patient can be best channelized by:
a. Engaging in a writing activities
b. Engage patient in aerobic exercise
c. Engaging in craft activities
d. Engaging in activities which requires intellectuality

447. Which of the following disorder is classified under mood disorders?
a. Neurosis b. OCD
c. Schizophrenia d. Mania

448. All of the following symptoms are characteristics of mania; EXCEPT:
a. Grandiosity b. Suicidal ideas
c. Hyperactivity d. Flight of ideas

449. Which of the following activities can be suggested by a nurse for a patient with manic behavior?
a. Playing chess
b. Playing carom
c. Solitary activity (writing)
d. Hammering on metal (Jewelry making)

450. Stimulation of which of the nerve leads to elevated mood? *(JIPMER 2009)*
a. Optic b. Olfactory
c. Trochlear d. Vagus

451. The appropriate nursing intervention for a patient acting out aggression is:
a. Maintain low level of stimuli in the environment
b. Verbal de-escalation
c. Remove all dangerous objects from the patient environment
d. All of the above

BIPOLAR AFFECTIVE DISORDER (BPAD)

452. Clients with the diagnosis of bipolar disorders, manic episode, most likely will exhibit signs of: *(RAK MSc 2018)*
a. Passivity b. Dysphoria
c. Anhedonia d. Grandiosity

Explanation:
- As per ICD-10 diagnostic criteria, mania is the episode which should last for at least 1 week and should be severe enough to disrupt ordinary work and social activities more or less completely. The mood change is usually accompanied by increased energy, pressure of speech, decreased need for sleep, **grandiosity**, and excessive optimism (opposite to passivity).
- All other given symptoms are characteristics of patient with depression.

Ans.
435. b
436. c
437. b
438. c
439. b
440. d
441. b
442. a
443. c
444. a
445. a
446. b
447. d
448. b
449. d
450. d
451. d
452. d

453. Which of the following is the priority nursing diagnosis for the patient with BPAD who exhibits extreme excitement, delusion and command hallucinations?
- a. Impaired social interaction
- b. Altered sensory perception
- c. Risk for other-directed violence
- d. Altered thought process

454. The most common psychiatric disorder seen in Indian population?
- a. Schizophrenia
- b. Personality Disorder
- c. Endogenous depression
- d. BPAD

455. A mild form of bipolar disorder, in which a person has mood swings over a period of years that go from mild depression to mild elation is known as:
- a. Dysthymic Disorder
- b. Cyclothymic Disorder
- c. Conversion disorder
- d. Multiple personality disorder

456. OCD is best managed with which of the following psychotherapy?
- a. Psychodynamic psychotherapy
- b. Interpersonal psychotherapy
- c. Cognitive behavior therapy
- d. Supportive psychotherapy

Explanation: Cognitive behavioral therapy (CBT) can help you manage your problems by changing the way you think and behave. It is most commonly used to treat anxiety and depression, but can be useful for other mental and physical health problems.

SEASONAL AFFECTIVE DISORDER

457. Phototherapy is used in which Psychiatric illness?
- a. Involutional melancholia
- b. Seasonal mood disorder
- c. Masked depression
- d. Bipolar depression

SOMATOFORM DISORDERS

458. All of the following conditions are included in somatoform disorder; EXCEPT:
- a. Conversion disorder
- b. Body dysmorphic disorder
- c. Pain disorder
- d. Anorexia Nervosa

Explanation: Somatoform disorders are characterized by recurrent multiple somatic complaints which are not accounted for by any underlying physical illness. Somatoform disorders include conversion disorder, somatization disorder, hypochondriasis, body dysmorphic disorder and pain disorder. Anorexia nervosa is a type of eating disorder.

459. Identify common motor symptoms in conversion disorder:
- a. Paralysis
- b. Impaired balance
- c. Double vision
- d. All of the above

Explanation: Conversion disorder involves symptoms or deficits affecting voluntary motor or sensory function. Common examples of conversion symptoms include blindness, diplopia, paralysis, dystonia, psychogenic nonepileptic seizures (PNES), anesthesia, aphonia, amnesia, dementia, unresponsiveness, swallowing difficulties, motor tics, hallucinations, pseudocyesis and difficulty in walking.

460. A condition wherein the individuals have overwhelming fear that they are suffering from a physical illness despite no medical evidence of illness, is known as:
- a. Generalized anxiety disorder
- b. Conduct disorder
- c. Hypochondriasis
- d. Dissociative disorder

461. The symptoms of conversion disorder include all of the following; EXCEPT:
- a. Neurological symptoms
- b. Altered motor and sensory function
- c. Stress exacerbated symptoms
- d. Lack of insight

462. When psychological distress causes physical symptoms, the condition is known as:
- a. Hypochondiasis
- b. Hysteria
- c. Somatization disorder
- d. Dissociative disorder

463. Most common form of dissociation hysteria is: *(JIPMER 1998)*
- a. Fugue
- b. Amnesia
- c. Multiple personality
- d. Somnambulism

464. Hypochondriasis is: *(JIPMER 1994)*
- a. Fear of fatal disease
- b. Too much concern of own health and misinterpretation of normal body function
- c. Marked mental and physical fatigue
- d. Repeated hospitalization

465. A 45-year-old male presents with history of headache, and vague body pains, off and on diarrhea and constipation, Impotence and tingling and paresthesia in glove stocking pattern. The probable diagnosis is: *(JIPMER 2000; 2002)*
- a. Hypochondriasis
- b. Somatization disorder
- c. Conversion disorder
- d. Factitious disorder

STRESS AND ADAPTATION

466. A client is experiencing anxiety attack. The most appropriate nursing intervention should include: *(Safdarjung NO 2018)*
- a. Turning on the television
- b. Leaving the client alone
- c. Staying with the client and speaking in short sentences
- d. Ask the client to play with other clients

Explanation:
- Nursing interventions during anxiety include using short sentence, staying with the client, decreasing stimuli, remaining calm, and medication administration.
- Leaving client alone, turning on television and playing with other may exaggerate the anxiety of the client.

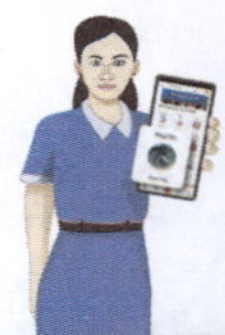

Ans.

453. c
454. c
455. b
456. c
457. b
458. d
459. d
460. c
461. d
462. c
463. b
464. b
465. b
466. c

467. The level of anxiety that enhances the individual's power of perception is known as:

a. Mild b. Panic
c. Moderate d. Severe

Explanation: Mild anxiety enhances the perception while higher level of anxiety interferes with one's functioning.

468. Which physiological response is typically observed during the exhaustion stage of the general adaptation syndrome? *New Q*

a. Increased mental alertness
b. Vasoconstriction
c. Initiation of neuroendocrine activity
d. Decreased blood pressure

Explanation: The general adaptation syndrome (GAS) is a theoretical model that describes the body's response to stress. It consists of three stages: alarm, resistance, and exhaustion.

During the exhaustion stage, the body's resources become depleted due to prolonged exposure to stress. As a result, various physiological systems start to dysfunction and may lead to a decline in overall health. One of the common physiological responses during this stage is a decrease in blood pressure.

469. While assessing a client with generalized anxiety disorder, which among the following is the best indicator of client's present situation?

a. Memory b. Behavior
c. Judgment d. Responsiveness

Explanation: Client's current behavior is the best indicator of client's present situation.

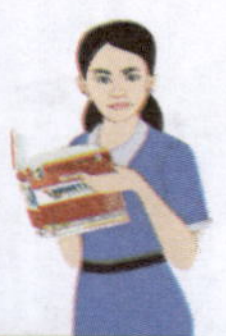

470. Physical symptom which is present in panic attack is:

a. Sweating and palpitation b. Seizure
c. Vomiting d. Restlessness

Explanation: Sweating and palpitations are the signs and symptoms associated with panic attack.

471. The stage which keeps an individual physically alert to face the danger arising out of stress is termed: *(DSSSB PHN, 2015)*

a. Adjustment reaction b. Stage of resistance
c. Exhaustion stage d. Alarm reaction

Explanation: There are three stages in General Adaptation Syndrome:

i. **Alarm reaction stage:** The alarm stage is also known as the fight or flight stage. The person is physically alert and the sympathetic nervous system is stimulated. There is increased heart rate and blood supply to arms and legs.
ii. **Resistance stage:** After initial shock of stressful event, the body begins to resist. The parasympathetic system attempts to bring physiological functions to normal level.
iii. **Exhaustion stage:** If the stressor continues beyond the body's capacity, the resources get exhausted and the body is susceptible for disease and eventual death.

472. Anxiety expressed through physical symptoms is: *(JIPMER 2012)*

a. Depersonalization b. Sublimation
c. Regression d. Hypochondriasis

473. Stress is always .... of the client.

a. Adaptation b. Life style
c. Perception d. Tolerance

474. State of apprehension arising out of anticipation of danger is referred to as:

a. Phobia b. Amnesia
c. Anxiety d. Obsession

475. Which of the following is a characteristic feature of hysterical fits?

a. Tongue bite is absent
b. It usually occurs in unsafe places
c. It usually occurs in the absence of people
d. Incontinence of urine occurs

476. Which of the following is not an anxiety reduction technique? *(JIPMER 2010)*

a. Using anxiolytics
b. Biofeedback techniques
c. Implosion of flooding techniques
d. Jacobson progressive muscle relaxation

477. Features of anxiety neurosis are the following; EXCEPT: *(JIPMER 1998, 2007)*

a. Excessive sweating
b. Palpitations
c. Loss of consciousness
d. Tremors

478. Thyrotoxicosis is most commonly associated with: *(JIPMER 1993)*

a. Anxiety b. Paranoid states
c. Mania d. Delirium

479. Anxiety is: *(JIPMER 2012)*

a. Neurosis b. Psychosis
c. Personality disorder d. None

480. Differentiation of hysterical fits from epileptic fit: *(JIPMER 1995, 1999, 2001, 2004, 2006)*

a. Occurs in sleep
b. Injuries to person
c. Incontinence
d. Occurs when people are watching

481. Uncertainty and excessive sense of responsibility is seen in: *(JIPMER 2015)*

a. OCD
b. Depression
c. Personality disorder
d. Generalized anxiety disorder

482. Diagnostic interview with sodium amytal or hypnosis is a special feature of: *(AIIMS BPL SNO, NO 2018)*

a. Post-traumatic neurosis
b. Mania
c. Hyperventilation syndrome
d. Phobia

Explanation: Therapeutic indications of amytal interviews include the abreaction of traumatic neurosis, recovery of memory in amnesic and fugue states, and recovery of function in conversion disorders. Amytal interviews have a valid role in the assessment and initial management of catatonia, hysterical stupor, and unexplained muteness as well as in distinguishing between depressive, schizophrenic, and organic stuporous states.

Ans.

467. a
468. d
469. b
470. a
471. d
472. d
473. c
474. c
475. a
476. c
477. c
478. a
479. a
480. d
481. d
482. a

483. Cognitive manifestation of stress includes:

a. Inability to concentrate
b. Higher level of anxiety
c. Obsessive thoughts
d. All of the above

Explanation: Cognitive manifestation of stress includes:

- Constant worrying
- Racing thoughts
- Forgetfulness and disorganization
- Inability to focus/concentrate
- Poor judgment
- Being pessimistic or seeing only the negative side
- Obsessive thoughts and
- Higher level of anxiety

484. The symptom that differentiate PTSD from other anxiety disorder is:

a. Avoding similar situation that causes stress
b. Depression and a blunted affect when discussing the traumatic situation
c. Lack of interest in family and others
d. Bring back memories of the trauma accompanied by intense emotional and physical reactions

Explanation: Post-traumatic Stress Disorder (PTSD) is a mental health condition that's triggered by a terrifying event — either experiencing it or witnessing it. Symptoms may include flashbacks, nightmares and severe anxiety, as well as uncontrollable thoughts about the event.

485. Screening family members for PTSD after a major disaster comes in .... level of prevention.

a. Primordial
b. Primary
c. Secondary
d. Tertiary

Explanation: Early identification and treatment come under secondary prevention. So, screening after PTSD will be secondary prevention.

486. Which of the following is the correct sequence of stages of General Adaptation Syndrome?

a. Alarm – Exhaustion - Resistance
b. Alarm – Resistance – Exhaustion
c. Resistance - Alarm – exhaustion
d. Exhaustion – alarm – resistance

487. The emotional state an individual experiences to the loss of loved object is:

a. Grief
b. Mourning
c. Bereavement
d. Agony

488. Release of feelings that takes place by talking about an emotionally charged areas is:

a. Clarification
b. Abreaction
c. Suggestion
d. Exploration

489. True for PTSD are all; EXCEPT:

a. Past h/o psychiatric illness
b. Women are more predisposed
c. Occurs in intellectuals
d. Numbness

490. Drug of choice for Panic Disorder is: *(JIPMER 1994)*

a. Fluoxetine
b. Lithium
c. Diazepam
d. Chlorpromazine

491. Post-traumatic stress disorder, treatment of choice is:

a. Cognitive behavior therapy *(JIPMER 2014)*
b. Hypnosis
c. Rational emotive therapy
d. Eye movement desensitization and reprocessing

492. Which of the following is the priority nursing action for a patient who is experiencing acute panic attack?

a. Remain with the client all the time
b. Teach signs and symptoms of escalating anxiety
c. Reduce external stimuli
d. Teach coping measures

493. How long can the low-level depressive feelings in persistent depressive disorder typically persist for? *New Q*

a. Less than one year
b. More than 5 years
c. At least 1 year in children/adolescents and 2 years in adults
b. At least 2 years in children/adolescents and 3 years in adults

494. In patient with Post-Traumatic Stress Disorder (PTSD), the most common factor associated with disturbed sleep pattern is:

a. Drinking alcohol at bed time
b. Persistent dreams of the traumatic event
c. Apprehension of being harmed while asleep
d. None of the above

495. Four months after a traumatic incident, Mr X is re-experiencing flashbacks of incident, insomnia and depression. He is most likely to be suffering with:

a. Conversion disorder
b. Acute stress disorder
c. Post-traumatic stress disorder
d. Hysteria

496. Sudden attacks of anxiety accompanied by a fear of serious consequence such as a heart attack is a characteristic feature of:

a. Acute stress disorder
b. Phobic disorder
c. Panic disorder
d. PTSD

497. Post-Traumatic stress syndrome is due to: *(JIPMER 1998)*

a. Head Injury
b. CVD
c. Minor Stress
d. Major life-threatening events

498. A 20-year-old female complains of sudden onset palpitation and apprehension. She is sweating for last 10 minutes and fears of impending death. Diagnosis is: *(JIPMER 2001)*

a. Hysteria
b. Generalized Anxiety Disorder
c. Cystic fibrosis
d. Panic attack

499. What is the most important information the nurse should teach to prevent relapse in a client with a psychiatric illness? *(RAK MSc 2018)*

a. Develop a close support system
b. Create stress-free environment
c. Refrain from activities that cause anxiety
d. Follow the prescribed medication regimen

Explanation: Compliance with the medications is important because side effects and denial of illness may cause clients to stop taking their medications; Research studies highlighted that chance of relapse is very high when medication are discontinued.

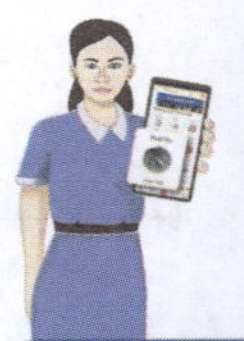

Ans.

483. d
484. d
485. c
486. b
487. a
488. b
489. c
490. c
491. a
492. a
493. c
494. b
495. c
496. c
497. d
498. d
499. d

PHOBIA

500. Kleptomania means: *(JIPMER 1999)*

a. Irresistible desire to set fire
b. Irresistible desire to steal things
c. Compulsive hair pulling
d. Pathological gambling

501. Commonest type of phobia seen in clinical practice: *(JIPMER 1992, 2004)*

a. Social phobia b. Simple phobia
c. Agoraphobia d. Claustrophobia

502. Mental illnesses that cause bodily symptoms, including pain and the symptoms can't be traced back to any physical cause is known as:

a. PTSD
b. Obsessive- compulsive disorder
c. Somatoform disorder
d. Dissociative disorder

Explanation: Somatoform disorders are mental illnesses that cause bodily symptoms, including pain. The symptoms cannot be traced back to any physical cause and they are not the result of substance abuse or another mental illness. People with somatoform disorders are not faking their symptoms. The pain and other problems they experience, are real. The symptoms can significantly affect daily functioning.

503. The sleep stage at which majority of the dreams appears is: *(ISRO)*

a. Stage 1 NREM sleep b. Stage 2 NREM sleep
c. Stage 4 NREM sleep d. REM sleep

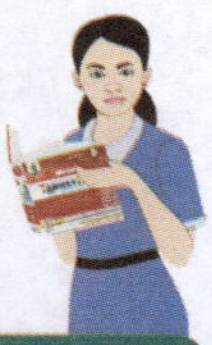

504. Gamophobia means:

a. Fear of sound b. Fear of marriage
c. Fear of social isolation d. Fear of speed

Explanation: Fear of marriage is known as gamophobia.

505. The acquisition of phobia can best be explained by which of the following model?

a. Behavioral model b. Tetrad model
c. Interpersonal model d. Environmental model

Explanation: Phobias can be acquired by classical conditioning (behavioral model) by simply pairing the neutral stimulus with the potent stimulus.

506. Which of the following modality has highest success rate in client with phobia?

a. Systematic desensitization with relaxation technique
b. Insight therapy to determine the origin of anxiety and fear
c. Psychotherapy aimed at rearranging psychotic thought process
d. Psychoanalytic exploration of repressed conflict of an earlier developmental phase

Explanation: Highest success rate is present in systematic desensitization with relaxation therapy.

507. Which of the following condition is not a psychotic illness?

a. BPAD b. Phobia
c. Depression d. Schizophrenia

508. Agoraphobia is fear of: *(JIPMER 2007; 2003; ESI IMO 2014)*

a. Agar b. Strangers
c. Open spaces d. Closed spaces

509. Patient of contamination phobia was asked by therapist to follow behind and touch everything he touches in patient's house. Therapist kept talking quietly and calmly all the time and the patient was asked to repeat the procedure twice daily. The procedure is:

a. Flooding b. Modeling
c. Positive reinforcement d. Aversion therapy

510. Definitive treatment of all types of phobia is: *(JIPMER 2008)*

a. Behavior therapy b. Social therapy
c. Avoidance d. Drug therapy

511. Irrational fear related to closed spaces is referred to as: *(JIPMER 2015)*

a. Acrophobia b. Agoraphobia
c. Claustrophobia d. Nosophobia

512. A behavioral therapy of sudden, direct and maximum exposure to the fear producing stimulus: *(JIPMER 2015)*

a. Biofeedback b. Flooding
c. Desensitization d. Response prevention

513. Fear of high places is called: *(JIPMER 2014; Staff Nurse G II 2014)*

a. Agoraphobia b. Algophobia
c. Acrophobia d. Claustrophobia

514. A mental health nurse conducted a session on conversion disorders for nursing students. During the evaluation, she asked the students to identify a symptom that is not typically associated with conversion disorders. Which option identified by the student would indicate that the session was effective? *New Q*

a. Neurological manifestations
b. La belle indifference
c. Lack of insight
d. Weakness on one side of body

515. Mr. X, who has recently been prescribed T. Fluoxetine, approaches the nurse on duty to inquire about when he can expect to observe the effects of the medication and experience improvements in his condition. The nurse's appropriate response would be: *New Q*

a. Significant improvement may become evident after a couple of days of taking the prescribed regimen.
b. You should start noticing improvement within the first week of therapy.
c. You might see improvements after approximately 30 days of therapy.
d. It typically takes about 2 to 3 weeks to observe noticeable improvements.

516. Irrational fear of being in places away from home setting is referred to as:

a. Agoraphobia
b. Claustrophobia
c. Acrophobia
d. Homophobia

517. Predominant evolutionary theory of phobias is:

a. Hypersensitivity
b. Biological preparedness
c. Learned responses
d. Fight or flight response

518. Social phobia can be treated with:

a. Serotonin reuptake inhibitors
b. Mood stabilizers
c. Antipsychotic drugs
d. NSAIDs

Ans.

500.	b
501.	c
502.	c
503.	d
504.	b
505.	a
506.	a
507.	b
508.	c
509.	b
510.	a
511.	c
512.	b
513.	c
514.	c
515.	d
516.	a
517.	b
518.	a

519. A person has poor performance in front of his seniors in public place, has tachycardia when he has to deliver a lecture, avoids going to parties. The diagnosis is: *(JIPMER 1999)*

a. Panic disorder
b. Schizophrenia
c. Social Phobia
d. Avoidant Personality

OBSESSIVE COMPULSIVE DISORDER (OCD)

520. Which is the best nursing intervention to meet the needs of individuals who demonstrate obsessive compulsive behavior? *(RAK MSc 2018)*

a. Restricting their movements
b. Calling attention to their behavior
c. Keeping them busy to distract them
d. Supporting but limiting their behavior

Explanation:

- Accepting these clients and their symptomatic behavior sets the foundation for the nurse-patient relationship. Setting limit provide external control and helps lower anxiety.
- Calling attention and restricting their movement will increase the anxiety. Distraction is unrealistic.

521. A 39-year-old mother with obsessive-compulsive disorder has become immobilized by her elaborate hand washing and walking rituals. Nurse recognizes that the basis of Obsessive-compulsive disorder is often: *(Safdarjung NO 2018)*

a. Problems with being too conscientious
b. Problems with anger and remorse
c. Feelings of guilt and inadequacy
d. Feeling of unworthiness and hopelessness

Explanation:

- The basis of ritualistic behavior seen in Obsessive Compulsive Disorder (OCD) is aimed at controlling guilt and inadequacy by maintaining an absolute set pattern of behavior.
- Being too conscientious is a healthy perfectionism (adaptive perfectionism).

522. The most common psychotherapy used to help a person with Obsessive Compulsive Disorder is:

a. Behavior modification
b. Transaction therapy
c. Abreaction
d. Flooding

Explanation: Behavior modification is a treatment approach, based on the principles of operant conditioning that replaces undesirable behaviors with more desirable ones through positive or negative reinforcement.

523. In a client with OCD, the rituals performed by the client will help to:

a. Maintain hygiene
b. Control the anxiety
c. Provide safe environment
d. Attain primarily for secondary gains

Explanation: Obsessive-compulsive disorder is characterized by unreasonable thoughts and fears (obsessions) that lead to compulsive behaviors. OCD often centers on themes such as a fear of germs or the need to arrange objects in a specific manner. Symptoms usually begin gradually and vary throughout life. It is an anxiety disorder characterized by unwanted thoughts and repetitive, ritualized behaviors.

524. A condition in which thoughts enter into the mind of the person though he/she does not want to think about them, is known as:

a. Obsession
b. Delusion
c. Regression
d. Suppression

Explanation: Compulsive pre-occupation with a fixed idea or an unwanted feeling or emotion, often accompanied by symptoms of anxiety, is known as obsession.

525. The compulsive act seen in OCD is:

a. Has a purpose but useless
b. Is performed after long urging
c. Appear to be performed willingly
d. Seems absurd but necessary to that person

Explanation: Carrying out of this kind of compulsive activity is a way for the client to relive anxiety. These activities are important for the client.

526. A client with OCD is on her way to the clinic for an appointment. While driving, she suddenly becomes anxious and starts thinking, "Did I remember to turn off the stove?" This thought keeps bothering her, and she feels the need to return home to check. ***New Q***
Which subtype of OCD is most likely affecting this client?

a. Contamination
b. Checking
c. Hoarding
d. Symmetry and ordering

Explanation: In the given scenario, the client experiences intrusive thoughts about whether she remembered to turn off the stove and feels compelled to check. This indicates a checking subtype of OCD. Individuals with checking OCD have persistent doubts and fears that something negative will happen if they don't repeat or verify specific actions multiple times.

527. Drug most useful in treatment of obsessive compulsive disorder is:*(JIPMER 1997, 2000, 2001, 2003, 2005, 2006, 2007)*

a. Amoxapine
b. Fluoxetine
c. Doxepin
d. Dothiepin

528. Treatment of choice for OCD is: *(JIPMER 2006)*

a. Behavior therapy
b. Drug therapy
c. Psychosurgery
d. Combination of behavior and drug therapy

529. Which of the following drugs is not effective in the treatment of Obsessive-Compulsive symptoms?

a. Fluvoxamine
b. Imipramine
c. Fluoxetine
d. Sertraline

530. The ego defense mechanism commonly used by patients with OCD is:

a. Displacement
b. Reaction formation
c. Undoing
d. Projection

531. "Raghu feels that his hands become contaminated and dirty after touching a water tap handle and wash his hands repeatedly." ***New Q***
Which part of the above statement indicate 'obsession'?

a. Feels that his hands become contaminated and dirty.
b. Touching a water tap handle.
c. Washing hands repeatedly.
d. Feels that he should never touch the tap handle.

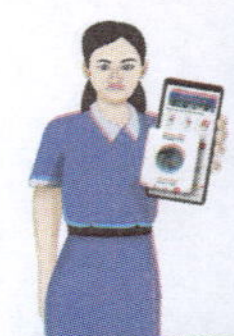

Ans.

519. c
520. d
521. c
522. a
523. b
524. a
525. d
526. b
527. b
528. d
529. b
530. c
531. a

Explanation: Obsessions are intrusive and persistent thoughts, urges, or images that cause distress or anxiety. In this case, the individual's belief that their hands become contaminated and dirty after touching a water tap handle represents an obsession. The focus on hand contamination is a recurring and distressing thought that drives the individual's behavior.

532. Characteristics of obsessional thoughts include all of the following; EXCEPT:
a. Unwanted thoughts
b. Subjective distress
c. Feeling of subjective compulsions
d. Feeling of worthlessness

533. An appropriate nursing intervention for a client with OCD is:
a. Recognize that the compulsive act is a part of OCD
b. Provide positive reinforcement for non-ritualistic behavior
c. Ignore patient behavior completely
d. Restrict the client's compulsive acts

534. Which of the following is the most appropriate nursing diagnosis for a patient exhibit obsessive compulsive behavior?
a. Altered nutritional status
b. Ineffective individual coping
c. Impaired socialization
d. Risk for injury to self and others

535. Which of the following statement about OCD is incorrect?
a. Anxiety is the key reason for OCD
b. Compulsions relive anxiety
c. Obsessive thoughts are not associated with level of neurochemicals
d. Antidepressant medications increase serotonin levels

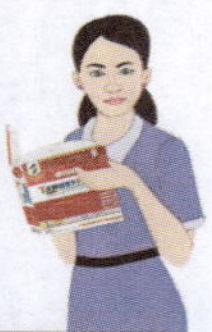

536. Signs and symptoms of Obsessive Compulsive Disorder (OCD) include all; EXCEPT:
a. Thought broadcasting
b. Feeling of guilt
c. Obsessive thoughts
d. Ritualistic behavior

537. Obsessional personality is also known as:
a. Schizoid personality
b. Histrionic personality
c. Anankastic personality
d. Borderline personality

538. A psychotherapy technique that is most effective in obsessive ruminations is:
a. Thought stopping
b. Desensitization
c. Flooding
d. Sensitization

ADJUSTMENT DISORDERS

539. In community mental health nursing, primary prevention refers to:
a. Identification and specific protection of vulnerable population
b. Early diagnosis and prompt treatment
c. Reduce the severity associated with mental disorders
d. Rehabilitation of mentally ill patients

540. Following are correctly matched; EXCEPT:
a. Schizophrenia-Auditory hallucination
b. OCD-infidelity
c. Alcoholism-auditory hallucination
d. Depression-guilt feeling

EATING DISORDERS

541. Which of the following is a characteristics of an adolescent with bulimia nervosa?
a. A positive body image
b. A positive self-concept
c. Excessive stained teeth
d. Previous history of gastritis

542. Nurse is caring for a client diagnosed with bulimia nervosa. The most appropriate initial goal for a client diagnosed with bulimia nervosa is: *(Safdarjung NO 2018)*
a. Encourage to avoid foods
b. Identify anxiety causing situations
c. Eat only three meals a day
d. Avoid shopping plenty of groceries

Explanation: Bulimic behavior is generally a maladaptive coping response to stress and underlying issues. The most appropriate goal for the client is that the patient must identify anxiety-causing events or situations that stimulate the bulimic behavior. This is followed by learning new ways or methods to cope with the anxiety.

543. Intractable anorexia nervosa is associated with: *(Safdarjung NO 2018)*
a. Cardiac dysrhythmia resulting to cardiac arrest
b. Glucose intolerance resulting in protracted hypoglycemia
c. Endocrine imbalance causing cold amenorrhea
d. Decreased metabolism causing cold intolerance

Explanation: Patients with intractable anorexia nervosa often have severe electrolyte imbalance such as decreased levels of sodium and potassium because of their starvation diet and energy expenditure, these electrolytes are very essential for cardiac functioning. Anemia, constipation, dehydration, electrolyte imbalances and orthostatic hypotension are the potential medical complications of anorexia nervosa. So cardiac dysrhythmias due to electrolyte imbalance is one of the major complications among the given options.

544. Nurse is developing a plan of care for a female client with anorexia nervosa. Which action should the nurse include in the plan? *(Safdarjung NO 2018)*
a. Provide privacy during meals
b. Set-up a strict eating plan for the client
c. Encourage client to exercise to reduce anxiety
d. Restrict visits with the family

Explanation:

- Establishing a consistent eating plan and monitoring the client's weight are important in developing care plan for a client with anorexia nervosa.
- Inclusion of family members in plan of care is important. Client should be monitored during meals, so client privacy is not necessary. Only limited and supervised exercise is recommended.

545. The morbid fear of becoming obese with a persistent lack of appetite and severe weight loss is:
a. Anorexia nervosa
b. Bulimia nervosa
c. Binge eating disorder
d. Pica

Explanation: Option a is the correct answer. Bulimia nervosa is excessive insatiable appetite.

Ans.

532. d
533. b
534. b
535. c
536. a
537. c
538. a
539. a
540. b
541. c
542. b
543. a
544. b
545. a

546. Among the following groups of sign and symptoms identify the most specific signs and symptoms that would be used for diagnosis of anorexia nervosa?

a. Binge eating behavior is present
b. Excessive weight loss, amenorrhea and abdominal distension
c. Eating only homemade food and avoiding fast food
d. Lazy and not doing any activity

Explanation: Anorexia nervosa is a serious eating disorder primarily of young women in their teens and early twenties that is characterized especially by a pathological fear of weight gain leading to faulty eating patterns, malnutrition, and usually excessive weight loss. Common signs and symptoms include excessive weight loss, amenorrhea and abdominal distension.

547. While communicating to a client who is admitted in psychiatry ward because of the disordered thinking process about food being poisoned, which of the following technique need to be adopted by the nurse to encourage the client to have dinner?

a. Have dinner with client
b. Using open-ended question and silence
c. Explain the client that food is not poisoned
d. Allow the client to express his thoughts

Explanation: Open-ended questions are exploratory in nature. Open-ended questions along with silence encourage the patient to discuss his/her problem in a friendly manner.

548. Which of the following part controls eating behavior?
(Nursing Grade- II 2007)

a. Hypothalamus b. Pituitary gland
c. Pineal gland d. Pancreas

Explanation: There are two places in the hypothalamus (part of the brain) that controls hunger and eating. The Ventromedial Nuclei gives a signal when to stop eating, and the Lateral hypothalamus gives a signal to start eating.

549. Which is the characteristic of anorexia nervosa?

a. Obsessed with weight loss
b. Body image disturbance
c. Healthy family relation ship
d. Both a and b

Explanation: Anorexia is characterized by a distorted body image, with an unwarranted fear of being overweight. Symptoms include trying to maintain a below-normal weight through starvation or too much exercises.

550. An adolescent with a diagnosis of bulimia nervosa is likely to exhibit:

a. Affective instability
b. Anhedonia
c. Repetitive motor mechanism such as tics
d. Unkempt appearance

Explanation: Affective instability, impulsivity, and anger are associated with Bulimia Nervosa and Anorexia Nervosa. These symptoms are observed more in bulimia nervosa than in anorexia nervosa. Identity disturbance is strongly associated with anorexia nervosa than bulimia nervosa.

551. A patient with anorexia nervosa shows signs of malnutrition. During initial re-feeding, the nurse carefully assesses the patient for:

a. Hyperkalemia b. Hypoglycemia
c. Hypercalcemia d. Hypophosphatemia

552. Anorexia nervosa is characterized by all; EXCEPT:

a. Amenorrhea b. Weight loss
c. Hypothermia d. Alopecia

553. A young lady is present with H/O repeated episode of over eating (binge) followed by purging using laxatives she probably suffering from
(JIPMER 2010; 2007; 2004; 2001)

a. Bulimia nervosa b. Schizophrenia
c. Anorexia nervosa d. Benign eating disorders

554. All of the following are signs of anorexia nervosa; EXCEPT:
(Banaras HU 2015)

a. Frequent eating habits b. Dry hair and skin
c. Fatigue d. Anxious and hopeless look

555. The most appropriate initial goal for an adolescent patient with bulimia is to:

a. Control eating bouts
b. Identify anxiety-causing situations
c. Control shopping for large amounts of food
d. Eat only limited meals

556. Which of the following is the highest priority for a 18-year-old female patient diagnosed with anorexia nervosa?

a. The patient will develop insight about body size
b. The patient will understand the physical consequences of fasting
c. The patient will establish adequate nutritional intake
d. The patient will set a target weight in consultation with nurse

557. An 18-year-old female patient diagnosed with anorexia nervosa tells the nurse, "I have what I see at mirror. I look so ugly and fat." Which of the following strategy by a nurse is appropriate to deal with distorted perceptions of the patient?

a. Focus discussions on food and weight
b. Provide objective data feedback about patient's weight
c. Avoid discussing the patient's perceptions about weight
d. All of the above

558. Which of the following is a type of eating disorder?

a. Anorexia nervosa b. Phobic anxiety disorder
c. Conversion disorder d. Fetishism

559. Characteristics of a client with anorexia nervosa include all of the following; EXCEPT:

a. Fear of gaining weight
b. Distorted body image
c. Fasting and dieting
d. Binge eating followed by purging

560. Bulimia nervosa is a type of:

a. Anxiety disorder b. Eating disorder
c. Stress disorder d. Organic disorder

561. Characteristics of a client with bulimia nervosa include all of the following; EXCEPT:

a. Binge eating b. Feeling of thinness
c. Use of laxatives d. Induce vomiting

562. Craving and eating of non-edible substances such as chalk and mud is known as:

a. Bulimia b. Pica
c. Paraphagia d. Verbigeration

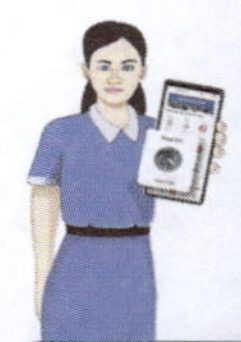

Ans.

546. b
547. b
548. a
549. d
550. a
551. d
552. d
553. a
554. a
555. b
556. c
557. b
558. a
559. d
560. b
561. b
562. b

563. Anorexia nervosa is an eating disorder characterized by all; EXCEPT: *(JIPMER 2012)*

a. Menorrhagia
b. Salivary gland enlargement
c. Acrocyanosis
d. Bradycardia

564. Ms. Kavita, a female patient, got admitted to psychiatric ward with the complaints of intense fear of becoming obese. This fear does not decrease even if the person loses weight grossly and becomes very thin. The body weight is 15 percent below the standard weight. identify the diagnosis of the patient.

a. Anorexia Nervosa
b. Bulimia Nervosa
c. Binge eating disorder
d. Increased BMR

565. Which of the following is one of the clinical manifestations of Bulimia Nervosa?

a. Set themselves daily calorie limits
b. Pursuit of thinness
c. Repeated bouts of overeating & self-induced vomiting
d. Body weight is 15 percent below the standard weight

566. A patient with eating disorder is being admitted in a psychiatric unit. Patient has been diagnosed as anorexia nervosa and is on treatment. The psychiatric nurse is aware that the short-term management for this condition is to:

a. Help the client to develop compensatory behaviors
b. Achieve a weight gain of 0.5 to 1 kg per week
c. Listen to patient & give full freedom not to eat
d. None of the above

567. A patient is brought by relatives to psychiatric OPD. After detailed investigation, patient is diagnosed as anorexia nervosa. Which of the following manifestation requires hospitalization of this patient?

a. Pulse Rate 88–98 per minute
b. Hyperthermia
c. Blood Pressure of 84/55 mm Hg
d. Amenorrhea

568. Ms. Madhu is a postgraduate history student, highly concerned for her overweight. Assessment revealed that her BMI is normal. She is presently having weight phobia, feature of dread of fatness, and a drive for thinness. Which of the following is the probable diagnosis?

a. Hallucination
b. Misinterpretation
c. Sexual Disorder
d. Eating Disorder

SLEEP DISORDERS

569. Abnormal drowsiness or excessive sleep in the day time is known as:

a. Narcolepsy | b. Somnolence
c. Somnambulism | d. Sleep ataxia

Explanation: One of the most prominent symptoms of narcolepsy is excessive daytime sleepiness. People with narcolepsy feel moderately or severely tired during the day.

570. Number of sleep stages are:

a. 2 | b. 4
c. 5 | d. 6

571. Narcolepsy is due to abnormality in:

a. Hypothalamus | b. Neocortex
c. Cerebellum | d. Medulla oblongata

572. Excessive sleep is termed: *(LNJP H D 2012)*

a. Insomnia | b. Asomnia
c. Somnambulism | d. Hypersomnia

573. Sleep walking is otherwise called:

a. Somnambulism
b. Somnokinesis
c. Insomnia
d. Enuresis

574. Which of the following is not true about sleep? *(AIIMS-BBS SNO 2019, Daman and Diu NO 2018)*

a. It consists of REM and non-REM sleep.
b. Sleep cycles are controlled by the suprachiasmatic nucleus.
c. Most growth hormones are produced during stages 3 and 4 of sleep
d. Dreams occur during non-REM sleep

Explanation: REM means Rapid eye movements and non-REM means non-rapid eye movements. REM sleep first occurs about 90 minutes after falling asleep. Most of the dreams occur during REM sleep.

575. All are true regarding REM sleep; EXCEPT:

a. Frequent and rapid movement of the eyes
b. Difficult to open eyes/arise
c. It is also known as Synchronized or 'S' sleep
d. It is associated with dream

Explanation:

Stages of sleep

- Stages of sleep are defined based on the patterns of EEG (Electroencephalogram)
- Non-rapid Eye Movement (NREM) sleep (Orthodox sleep or Synchronized or 'S' sleep)
- Rapid Eye Movement (REM) sleep (paradoxical sleep or Desynchronized or 'D' sleep)

Non-rapid Movement (NREM) Sleep

- Further divided into Stage 1, Stage 2, Stage 3, and Stage 4 sleep

EEG

- Stage 1: Theta waves (hypnogogic state)
- Stage 2: Theta waves (Sleep Spindles)
- Stage 3: Delta waves
- Stage 4: Delta waves **(bed wetting, Night terrors, sleep walk/talk)**

Rapid Eye Movement (REM) sleep

- After 90 minutes after sleep onset → 1st REM episode

EEG: Mimic beta waves

Associated with dreaming

- Difficult to arise
- Increased/Irregular HR, RR and BP
- Penile erection or clitoris engorgement
- Muscle twitches

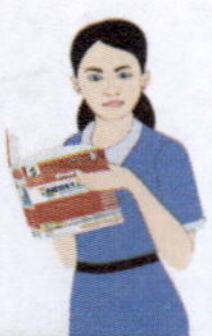

Ans.

563. a
564. a
565. c
566. b
567. c
568. d
569. a
570. c
571. a
572. d
573. a
574. d
575. c

576. During a health teaching session regarding sleep hygiene among insomnia client nurse need to focus upon:

a. Encourage day time nap
b. Exercise before going to bed
c. Use hypnotics
d. Avoiding caffeine-containing beverages

577. Disruptive sleep disorders that can occur during arousals from REM sleep or partial arousals from non-REM sleep is known as:

a. Somnabulism b. Parasomnia
c. Narcolepsy d. Somnambulism

578. How long does the first period of Rapid Eye Movement-REM sleep last? *New Q*

a. 10 minutes
b. 15 minutes
c. 20 minutes
d. 5 minutes

Explanation: REM sleep stage usually starts 90 minutes after one fall asleep, with each of the REM cycles getting longer throughout the night. The first period typically lasts 10 minutes, with the final one lasting up to an hour.

579. True about NREM sleep is:

a. Teeth grinding b. Narcolepsy
c. Nightmares d. Sleep paralysis

580. The disorder in which the child suffers from incontinence of urine during sleep:

a. Incontinence b. Somnambulism
c. Enuresis d. Uropsychogenesis

581. Among the following condition which one is treated with hypnotic drugs?

a. Psychosis b. Sleep disorders
c. Delusion d. Hallucination

Explanation: Hypnotic drugs are used to treat sleep disorders.

582. Vivid dreaming most commonly occurs during:

a. Stage 2 NREM sleep
b. Stage 4 NREM sleep
c. REM sleep
d. Transition period from NREM to REM sleep

SEXUAL DISORDERS

583. All of the following psychiatric disorders are more prevalent in women than in men; EXCEPT:

a. Social Phobia b. Anorexia Nervosa
c. Depression d. Transvestism

584. Voyeurism means:

a. Person receives sexual gratification from seeing the genitalia of others or witnessing others' sexual behavior
b. Sexual urges or fantasies involving unusual sources of gratification problems
c. An individual is dissatisfied with his/her own biological sex and has a strong desire to be a member of the opposite sex
d. Using opposite sex undergarments to satisfy sexual drive

Explanation: Option a is the correct definition of voyeurism.

585. Excessive sexual desire in males is known as: *(JIPMER 2008)*

a. Nymphomania b. Satyriasis
c. Tribadism d. Sadism

586. Squeeze Technique is used for: *(JIPMER 2000)*

a. Impotence b. Premature ejaculation
c. Infertility d. Priapism

587. The force by which the sexual instinct represented in the mind is known as:

a. Propositions b. Fetishism
c. Condensation d. Libido

588. A paraphilic interest in which the person gets sexual gratification by rubbing against an unsuspecting, non-consenting person. This is termed:

a. Frotteurism
b. Sadism
c. Voyeurism
d. Exhibitionism

589. Practice of dressing and acting in a style or manner traditionally associated with the opposite sex is known as:

a. Voyeurism b. Exhibitionism
c. Fetishism d. Transvestism

590. The practice of obtaining sexual gratification by looking at sexual objects or acts, especially secretively, is known as:

a. Fetishism b. Voyeurism
c. Sexual sadism d. Frotteurism

591. A feeling of sexual excitement resulting from administering pain, suffering, or humiliation to the partner is known as:

a. Fetishism b. Masochism
c. Voyeurism d. Sadism

592. Bestiality is also known as:

a. Social phobia b. Zoophilia
c. Pedophilia d. Zoophobia

593. A male patient is admitted by relatives to psychiatric hospital with the complaints of persistent involvement in the act of touching and rubbing against an unsuspecting person. Which of the following is the most probable diagnosis for this client?

a. Sexual Masochism b. Frotteurism
c. Frigidity d. Voyeurism

594. In these disorders, the sense of one's masculinity or femininity is disturbed. Identify the name of the disorder from the options:

a. Gender identity disorders
b. Sexual development and maturation disorder
c. Disorders of sexual preference (paraphilia)
d. Sexual dysfunction

595. Mr. Vishal's family members explain that he is having some abnormal behavior which includes tendency to observe unsuspecting persons of opposite sex naked and engaged in sexual activity. This behavior suggests that Mr. Vishal is suffering from:

a. Exhibitionism
b. Voyeurism
c. Transvestism
d. Sexual sadism

596. All of the following nursing Interventions are planned for a patient with sexual disorder admitted in a psychiatric ward; EXCEPT:

a. Provide information regarding sexuality and sexual functioning
b. Refer for additional counselling
c. Decrease variant behavior
d. Express a non-accepting attitude as a coercive and limit setting measure

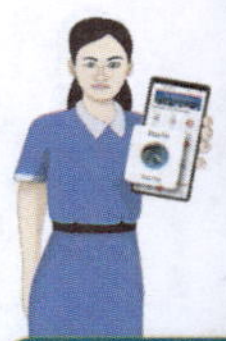

Ans.

576. d
577. b
578. a
579. a
580. c
581. b
582. c
583. d
584. a
585. b
586. b
587. d
588. a
589. d
590. b
591. d
592. b
593. b
594. a
595. b
596. d

597. It is a persistent and significant sense of discomfort regarding one's anatomic sex and a desire to live and be accepted as a member of the opposite sex is known as:

a. Transsexualism
b. Intersexuality
c. Dual-role transvestism
d. Exhibitionism

ELECTROCONVULSIVE THERAPY (ECT)

598. A neuromuscular blocking agent is administered to a client before ECT therapy. The Nurse should carefully observe the client for: *(Safdarjung NO 2018)*

a. Respiratory difficulties
b. Nausea and vomiting
c. Dizziness
d. Seizures

Explanation: Neuromuscular blocking agents (NMBA) reduce muscular convulsions and decrease the risk of serious injury during ECT procedure. Succinylcholine (0.5 mg kg^{-1}) is most commonly used NMBA in ECT. NMBA induces reversible muscle paralysis that leads to respiratory difficulties. So, the nurse should carefully observe the client for respiratory difficulties.

599. A nurse was discussing with the psychiatrist about the possibility of electroconvulsive therapy for a 45-year-old patient who was recently admitted into a psychiatric ward. Which of the following diagnosis of the patient indicates a situation where ECT is not typically considered a first-line treatment? *New Q*

a. Acute Schizophrenia.
b. Major depressive disorder
c. Chronic schizophrenia
d. Catatonic schizophrenia

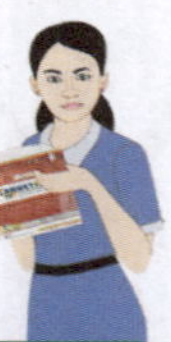

Explanation: ECT (Electroconvulsive Therapy) is generally not considered a first-line treatment for chronic schizophrenia. For chronic schizophrenia, antipsychotic medications are typically the primary treatment approach.

600. Following ECT a client is receiving oxygen via positive pressure ventilation method. The nurse should understand that positive pressure ventilation is necessary because:

a. Seizure activity can depress respirations
b. Decreased oxygen to the brain leads to confusion and disorientation
c. Anesthesia is administered during the procedure
d. Succinylcholine administered during procedure can cause respiratory depression

Explanation: Succinylcholine (smooth muscle relaxant) is administered during ECT to prevent injuries to patient during seizure. The effect of this drug can cause respiratory depression.

601. Prior to ECT therapy client is given with atropine to:

a. Induce sleep
b. Minimize the secretions
c. To decrease pain
d. Relax smooth muscles

Explanation: Atropine is given to patient before Electroconvulsive Therapy (ECT) is for two reasons:

i. To prevent transient postictal bradyarrhythmia due to excessive vagal tone
ii. To minimize secretions within the respiratory tract. No option related to postictalbrady arrhythmia was given which leads you to select the option (B).

602. The most common side effect of ECT is:

a. Permanent memory loss
b. Temporary memory loss
c. Fracture of cranial bone
d. MI and cardiac arrest

Explanation: Most common side effect of ECT is temporary memory loss.

603. Among the following what is the important nursing intervention to maintain safety of a client who is receiving ECT?

a. Tyramine free meals
b. Avoidance of exposure to sun
c. Maintenance of a safety sodium intake
d. Elimination of benzodiazepine for night time sedation

Explanation: The use of these drugs can raise the seizure threshold, which is counterproductive.

604. The sequence of administration of medications in anesthesia for ECT is:

a. Atropine--- thiopentone/methohexitol --- succinylcholine
b. Succinylcholine--- atropine --- thiopentone/methohexitol
c. Atracurium --- succinylcholine --- atropine
d. Atropine---succinylcholine --- thiopentone/methohexitol

Explanation: Atropine is to decrease secretions, thiopentone is for anesthesia effect and succinylcholine is for muscle relaxation.

605. The drugs need to be administer to a client immediately before ECT include:

a. Thiopental sodium
b. Succinylcholine
c. Methohexital sodium
d. All of the above

Explanation: All the above-mentioned drugs need to administer immediately before the procedure, anti-cholinergic drug such as atropine will administer 30 min prior to the procedure. Option A and C are short acting anesthetic drugs, while option B is a muscle relaxant.

606. When explaining the procedure about ECT, nurse should emphasize that:

a. Answer to all questions will be provided
b. Periods of amnesia will be there following treatment
c. Treatment will make the client feel better
d. Client will not be alone during the treatment

Explanation: Staff present in the unit will provide continuous support to the client.

Ans.

597. a
598. a
599. c
600. d
601. b
602. b
603. d
604. a
605. d
606. d

607. Nurse attending to a patient receiving electroconvulsive therapy (ECT) in a psychiatry department should ensure the compliance of all of the following; EXCEPT: *(Banaras HU 2015)*
- a. Emptying of bladder and bowel is not necessary
- b. Patient's hair should be kept clean and dry
- c. Hairpins, bracelets, body piercing should be removed
- d. Take the informed consent from a patient/legal heir

608. ECT is not the first-line treatment for:
- a. Hypomania
- b. Severe depression with psychosis
- c. Depressive stupor
- d. Catatonia

609. The first therapeutic use of electrically induced seizures in the treatment of mental disorders was by: *New Q*
- a. Eugen Blueler
- b. Luigi Bini and Ugo Cerletti
- c. D. Goldman
- d. G. Holmberg and S. Thesieff

610. In Direct ECT, the intraocular tension is: *(JIPMER 1991)*
- a. Increased
- b. Decreased
- c. No change
- d. Variable

611. The voltage needed to produce seizures while giving ECT is: *(JIPMER 2015; 2012)*
- a. 180 to 220 volts
- b. 40 to 70 volts
- c. 150 to 180 volts
- d. 70 to 130 volts

612. Nursing care in electroconvulsive therapy includes: *(ESIC Chennai May 2012)*
- a. Preparing and monitoring the patient during the actual procedure
- b. Providing educational and emotional support
- c. Pretreatment planning and assessment
- d. All the above

613. As per the Mental Healthcare Act 2017, which of the following statement is not TRUE regarding ECT therapy?
- a. ECT should not be used without muscle relaxant
- b. ECT should not be used without anesthesia
- c. ECT therapy will not be performed for minors
- d. Direct ECT can be given with the consent of the patient

614. The immediate nursing intervention for the patient who has just awakened from an electroconvulsive therapy treatment is to:
- a. Orient the patient
- b. Assess for suicidal behavior
- c. Serve the food
- d. Assess for auditory hallucination

615. Which of the following is an absolute contraindication for ECT treatment?
- a. Recent stroke
- b. Recent myocardial ischemia
- c. Aortic aneurysms
- d. Pheochromocytoma

616. ECT procedure was first used for the treatment of psychosis in the year:
- a. 1930
- b. 1938
- c. 1940
- d. 1942

617. The normal range of duration of electricity delivery during ECT is:
- a. 0.1–0.2 seconds
- b. 0.7–1.5 seconds
- c. 0.5–2.5 seconds
- d. 1.0–2.5 seconds

618. The most common indication of ECT is:
- a. Schizophrenia
- b. Phobia
- c. Mania
- d. Major depression

619. Which of the following type of schizophrenia best responds to ECT?
- a. Catatonic schizophrenia
- b. Simple schizophrenia
- c. Paranoid schizophrenia
- d. Hebephrenic schizophrenia

620. The commonest side effect of ECT is:
- a. Dislocation of mandible
- b. Fracture of a long bone
- c. Nausea and vomiting
- d. Body pain particularly in lower extremities

621. Electroconvulsive therapy (ECT) is primarily used to treat patients with:
- a. Conversion disorder
- b. Organic brain Syndrome
- c. Depression
- d. OCD

622. A mental disturbance characterized by confusion, disordered speech, clouding of consciousness and hallucinations is known as:
- a. Dementia
- b. Delirium
- c. Hallucination
- d. Psychosis

CHILDHOOD PSYCHIATRIC DISORDERS-INTRODUCTION

623. Thinking containing erroneous conclusions and internal contradiction is called: *(AIIMS Raipur Grade II 2017)*
- a. Autistic thinking
- b. Critical thinking
- c. Illogical thinking
- d. Logical thinking

Explanation: Autistic thinking comprises inner thoughts and individual reality. Day dreaming and fantasies are elements of autistic thinking. Critical thinking means making reasoned judgements that are logical and well thought out. Logical thinking is the process in which one uses reasoning consistently to come to a conclusion.

624. What is the condition in which children is pulling out hair? *(AIIMS Raipur Staff Nurse Grade I-2018); (AIIMS Bhopal Nursing officer, 2018)*
- a. Trichotillomania
- b. Acrophobia
- c. Imipramine
- d. Olanzapine

Explanation: **Trichotillomania:** a disorder that involves recurrent irresistible urge to pull out hair
- **Acrophobia:** Irrational fear of height
- **Imipramine:** It is a tricyclic antidepressant drug
- **Olanzapine:** It is an antipsychotic drug

625. A legal classification of children's behavior that violates the law:
- a. Juvenile delinquency
- b. Enuresis
- c. Pica
- d. ADHD

Explanation: Juvenile delinquency, also known as "juvenile offending", is participation in illegal behavior by minors (juveniles, i.e. individuals younger than the statutory age of majority).

626. Autistic child gives best response to:
- a. Large group activity
- b. Loud cheerful music
- c. Small group activities
- d. Their own self stimulating acts

Explanation: Autistic child turns inward and responds less to environmental stimuli.

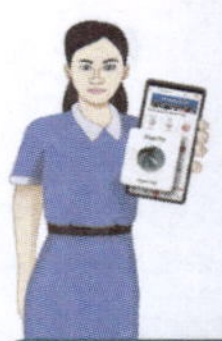

Ans.

607.	a
608.	a
609.	b
610.	b
611.	d
612.	d
613.	d
614.	a
615.	d
616.	b
617.	b
618.	d
619.	a
620.	a
621.	c
622.	b
623.	c
624.	a
625.	a
626.	d

627. Autistic child's language resembles:

a. Stuttering
b. Confabulation
c. Neologism
d. Echolalia

Explanation: Language development of an autistic child resembles Echolalia, i.e., the uncontrollable and immediate repetition of words spoken by another person.

628. Which of the following are risk factors for childhood psychiatric disorders? *(LNJP H D 2012)*

a. Parental psychopathology
b. Repeated early separation from parents
c. Harsh parents
d. All of the above

629. Autism is: New Q *(LNJP H D 2012)*

a. Metabolic disease
b. Neuromuscular disorders
c. Social and language communication problems
d. Mainly due to hypothalamic damage

630. Which of the following should be a primary focus of a nurse in terms of primary prevention of psychiatric disorder in children?

a. Lack of friends
b. Culture of the family
c. Family history of mental illness
d. Single parent

631. Which of the following is NOT a physical cause often associated with Phonological disorder? New Q

a. A hearing impairment
b. Cleft palate
c. Small frontal lobes
d. Cerebral palsy

Explanation: Phonological disorder, also known as speech sound disorder, is a communication disorder characterized by difficulties in producing or using speech sounds correctly. Hearing impairment, cleft palate and cerebral palsy are considered to be physical causes for phonological disorder. However, small frontal lobes are not a commonly recognized physical cause associated with phonological disorder. Frontal lobes are primarily involved in higher cognitive functions, decision-making, and motor control, rather than specific speech sound production.

632. The major cause of enuresis in children is:

a. Overprotection by parents
b. Emotional insecurity in a child
c. Drinking too much fluid at bedtime
d. Dehydration

633. Example of a specific learning disability is:

a. Mental Retardation
b. Dyslexia
c. Hyperkinetic disorder
d. Childhood autism

634. Children with hyperkinetic disorder are likely to have deficits in which of the following brain areas?

a. Motor functioning
b. Executive functioning
c. Limbic system
d. Perception

635. Tourette is a disorder of: *(JIPMER 2015)*

a. Attention deficit
b. Tics
c. Autism
d. Mental retardation

ATTENTION DEFICIT HYPERACTIVE DISORDER (ADHD)

636. Treatment of ADHD involves the following drugs; EXCEPT: *(Kerala PSC 2004)*

a. Amphetamine
b. Antidepressants
c. Benzodiazepine
d. Methylphenidate

Explanation: Drugs of choice for the management of ADHD includes amphetamines, methylphenidate, dexmethylphenidate, antidepressants and lithium carbonate. Benzodiazepine is not the drug of choice.

637. Major behavioral characteristic of child with ADHD is:

a. Overreaction to stimuli
b. Continued use of rituals
c. Delayed speech development
d. Inability to use abstract thought

Explanation: ADHD children are highly reactive to external stimuli.

638. ADHD is usually treated with:

a. Lorazepam
b. Haloperidol
c. Methylphenidate
d. Methocarbamol

Explanation: Methylphenidate acts by stimulating the release of norepinephrine.

639. Most effective nursing action to change child's behavior in a child with Attention Deficit Hyperactivity Disorder (ADHD) is:

a. Sedate child for hyperactivity
b. Reward appropriate behavior
c. Use of seclusions and restraints
d. Aggressive punishments

640. Characteristics of children with ADHD is:

a. More attentive, hyperactive, and impulsive
b. Less attentive, hyperactive, and impulsive
c. More attentive, impulsive and focused
d. Less attentive, focused and calm

641. The first-line treatment approach for ADHD often includes: New Q

a. Cognitive-behavioral therapy (CBT)
b. Antidepressant medications
c. Stimulant medications
d. Antipsychotic medications

642. Stimulant drug is given to child for: *(JIPMER 2012)*

a. Conduct disorder
b. Speech developmental disorder
c. Pervasive disorder
d. ADHD

643. Which group of drug is the choice for ADHD?

a. Benzodiazepine
b. CNS stimulant
c. Anti-psychotics
d. Anticonvulsant

Explanation: CNS stimulant is the drug of choice to treat ADHD. Methylphenidate, a CNS stimulant, is the drug of choice for the treatment of ADHD.

Ans.

627. d
628. d
629. c
630. c
631. c
632. b
633. b
634. b
635. b
636. c
637. a
638. c
639. b
640. b
641. c
642. d
643. b

MENTAL RETARDATION/INTELLECTUAL DISABILITY

644. X-linked disease leading to mental retardation is:
- a. Myotonic dystrophy
- b. Fragile-X syndrome
- c. Tuberous sclerosis
- d. Phenylketonuria

645. Person included in Disability Act 1999:
- a. Mental retardation
- b. Phobia disorder
- c. Alcohol dependence
- d. Personality disorder

646. IQ level of 45 is called: *(JIPMER 2005)*
- a. Mild mental retardation
- b. Moderate mental retardation
- c. Severe mental retardation
- d. Profound mental retardation

647. Patient with IQ of 65 has:
- a. Mild Mental Retardation
- b. Moderate M.R.
- c. Severe M.R.
- d. Profound M.R.

648. Person with I.Q below _______ is considered to be mentally retarded.
- a. 60
- b. 70
- c. 80
- d. 100

649. Which of the following is an example of intellectual disability?
- a. Dyscalculia
- b. Mental Retardation
- c. Hyperkinetic disorder
- d. Childhood autism

650. Profound Mental Retardation is:
- a. IQ below 20
- b. IQ 20-35
- c. IQ 50-70
- d. IQ 35-50

651. Which of the following intervention is most appropriate to develop language skills among autistic children?
- a. Provide child with his/her favorite toys
- b. Restrict number of care givers to autistic child
- c. Teach the names of the objects by linking them with the actual object
- d. Encourage child to interact

652. A characteristic feature of autism is:
- a. Over activity
- b. Inattention
- c. Poor communication
- d. Poor intelligence

653. A child with moderate mental retardation is capable of:
- a. Performing an intellectual job
- b. Performing ADL independently
- c. Performing certain self-care activities
- d. Performing complex task which requires intellectuality

ANTIPSYCHOTICS

654. When administering an oral medication to a patient with psychiatric disorder, it is important to:
- a. Give the medication to the patient's attendant
- b. Keep the medication on the bedside table
- c. Give to the patient and observe that it is swallowed
- d. Tell the patient to take the medication

Explanation: There are chances that they may not take the medicines or even throw them away. So it is important to give the medicine to patient and observe that is swallowed.

655. Blocking of acetylcholine receptor by a psychotropic drug resulting in:
- a. Diarrhea
- b. Dry mouth
- c. Dementia
- d. Vomiting

Explanation: Blocking of acetylcholine receptor will result in dry mouth, blurred vision, constipation, and urinary incontinence.

656. The nurse understands that neuroleptics are the drugs of choice to relieve symptoms of: *(RAK MSc 2018)*
- a. Psychosis
- b. Depression
- c. Excessive activity
- d. Narcotic withdrawal

Explanation: Antipsychotic drugs are also known as neuroleptic drugs or tranquilizers which are used to treat or manage psychosis basically in bipolar disorder or schizophrenia.

657. Which one of the following is the adverse effects resulting from the chronic use of antipsychotics? *(AIIMS Raipur NO 2019)*
- a. Parkinson's tremor
- b. Akathisia
- c. Neurologic malignant syndrome
- d. Tardive dyskinesia

Explanation:
- All the given symptoms are extrapyramidal symptoms of antipsychotics.
- **Tardive dyskinesia:** Bizarre facial and tongue movements, stiff neck, difficulty swallowing. It can be a side effect of **long-term use of certain antipsychotics.**
- **Parkinson's tremors:** The symptoms may appear within 1–5 days after the initiation of antipsychotic medications.
- **Akathisia** may occur 50–60 days after initiation of therapy.
- **Neuroleptic malignant syndrome (NMS)** - onset occurs within hours after drug initiation.

658. A client with schizophrenia is receiving chlorpromazine (Thorazine) 400 mg twice a day. An adverse side effect of the medication is: *(AIIMS Raipur NO 2019)*
- a. Photosensitivity
- b. Elevated temperature
- c. Weight gain
- d. Elevated blood pressure

Explanation: **Chlorpromazine** depresses hypothalamic thermo-regulatory mechanism, exposure to extreme temperature may cause hyperthermia. Other adverse effects are EPS, sedation and hypotension (IM use), etc.

659. A client is to be discharged from a psychiatric unit with suggested haloperidol therapy. As a part of the teaching plan concerning this medication, the nurse should teach the client to avoid: *(RAK MSc 2018)*
- a. Driving at night
- b. Staying in the sun
- c. Ingesting aged cheese
- d. Taking medications containing aspirin

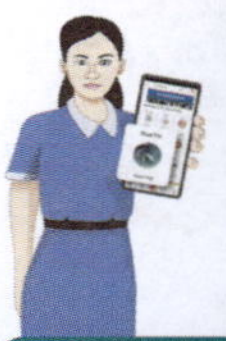

Ans.

644. b
645. a
646. b
647. a
648. b
649. b
650. a
651. c
652. c
653. c
654. c
655. b
656. a
657. d
658. b
659. a

Explanation:

- Patients who are on haloperidol are advised not to drive or operating machines due to the side effect of dizziness and drowsiness.
- Photosensitivity is an uncommon (0.1% to 1%) side effect of haloperidol. Ingesting aged cheese should be avoided in case of MAO inhibitors. Aspirin is not contraindicated with haloperidol therapy.

660. Which among the following is the most appropriate nursing action if the client is experiencing muscle rigidity following haloperidol administration?

a. Administer one more dose of haloperidol per orally as the dose is less for the client.
b. Administer a dose of benztropine IM as ordered.
c. Withhold the next dose of haloperidol as it occurs because of toxicity
d. Inform the physician immediately

Explanation: Haloperidol can trigger oculogyric crisis (OGC) which is characterized by muscle rigidity. Immediate treatment of drug-induced OGC can be achieved with benztropine.

661. What is the advantage of liquid chlorpromazine over its tablet forms?

a. Has a more predictable onset of action
b. Easy to swallow and early absorption in GI tract
c. It is more palatable than the tablet form
d. Has few drug interactions

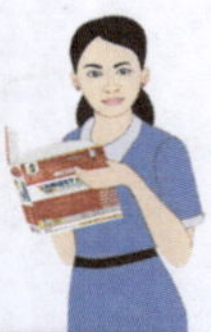

Explanation: The onset of liquid chlorpromazine is rapid and predictable compared to tablet because the liquid form produces therapeutic effects within 2–4 hours time.

662. Drug of choice to reverse a dystonic reaction is: *(Karnataka PSC)*

a. Prochlorperazine (Compazine)
b. Diphenhydramine (Benadryl)
c. Chlorpromazine (Thorazine)
d. Fentanyl

Explanation: Diphenhydramine (Benadryl), 25–50 mg IM or IV, is an antihistamine. Diphenhydramine blocks the effects of the naturally occurring chemical histamine in the body. Benadryl is used to treat sneezing; runny nose; itching, watery eyes; hives; rashes; itching; and other symptoms of allergies and the common cold.

663. Which among the following indicates that client is experiencing pseudo-parkinsonism induced by chlorpromazine? *(CMC Vellore)*

a. Restlessness and showing tics
b. Continuous muscle twitching
c. Tremors, shuffling gait, and mask like face
d. Extremity spasm and difficulty to walk

Explanation: Drug induced parkinsonism (pseudoparkinsonism) may develop 1 to 5 days after starting an antipsychotic medication. Symptoms mimic Parkinson disease such as tremor, shuffling gait, drooling, mask like face and rigidity.

664. Important teaching for women in their childbearing years who are receiving antipsychotic medications includes *(DSSSB)*

a. Instruction that amenorrhea is irreversible
b. Increased incidence of dysmenorrhea while taking the drug
c. Continuing previous use of contraception during periods of amenorrhea
d. Occurrence of increased libido due to medication adverse effects

Explanation: Antipsychotics may cause amenorrhea, which is reversible. The client must be instructed to continue her previous use of contraception despite amenorrhea present.

665. A client on antipsychotic therapy developed muscle rigidity, higher fever, tachycardia, fluctuations in BP, diaphoresis, and rapid deterioration of mental status to stupor and coma. These signs and symptoms indicative of:

a. Extra pyramidal symptoms
b. Oculogyric crisis
c. Tardive dyskinesia
d. Neuroleptic malignant syndrome

Explanation: Neuroleptic malignant syndrome (NMS) is a life-threatening, neurological disorder most often caused by an adverse reaction to antipsychotic drugs. Symptoms include high fever, sweating, unstable blood pressure, stupor, muscular rigidity, and autonomic dysfunction.

666. Drug of choice for Tourette's disorder?

a. Chloramphenicol
b. Methylphenidate
c. Haloperidol
d. Faith in his wife

Explanation: Haloperidol is the drug of choice to treat Tourette's disorder.

667. Neuroleptic drugs are the drugs of choice to relieve:

a. Psychosis
b. Depression
c. Excessive activity
d. Narcotic withdrawal

Explanation: Neuroleptic drugs modify the behavior of psychotic client.

668. Common manageable side effect of neuroleptic drug is:

a. Jaundice
b. Melanocytosis
c. Drooping eyelids
d. Unintentional tremors

Explanation: Unintentional tremors are the common and manageable side effect of neuroleptic drugs.

669. A patient with schizophrenia is not taking medication as advised, for this client a medication that is to be administered I/M by the nurse every 2–3 weeks is:

a. Haloperidol
b. Valium
c. Lithium carbonate
d. Prolixin decanoate

Explanation: Prolixin decanoate (Fluphenazine decanoate injection) is a long-acting parenteral antipsychotic drug. It is administered 2–3 times weekly to the client to control the sign and symptoms.

Ans.

660. b
661. a
662. b
663. c
664. c
665. d
666. c
667. a
668. d
669. d

670. What is the important nursing action while administering imipramine?
- a. Avoid administration of barbiturates or steroids with this drug
- b. Warn the client not to eat cheese, fermented products and chicken liver
- c. Observe client for increased tolerance so that dosage is maintained
- d. Have the client checked the intraocular pressure and provide instruction to be alert for symptoms of glaucoma.

Explanation: Development of glaucoma is the side effect of imipramine. It belongs to tricyclic group of antidepressants. Option b is applicable to MAOI group of antidepressants.

671. Identify the classic manifestations of Parkinson's disease:
- a. Bradykinesia, ataxia and dysarthria
- b. Tremor, ataxia and drowsiness
- c. Dysarthria, rigidity and bradykinesia
- d. Tremor, rigidity and bradykinesia

672. A diabetic client taking insulin is psychotic and started with olanzapine, this combination can cause:
- a. Depress respiration
- b. Decreased control of diabetes
- c. Intensify the action of both drugs
- d. Increase chances for extra pyramidal symptoms

Explanation: Olanzapine alter the effect of exogenous insulin and the combination must be used with caution.

673. Photosensitivity is a side effect of:
- a. Sertraline
- b. Lithium carbonate
- c. Methylphenidate hydrochloride
- d. Chlorpromazine hydrochloride

Explanation: Acute phototoxic dermatitis on sun exposure is a well-known side-effect of chlorpromazine.

674. Antidote for methanol is:
- a. Ethanol
- b. Fomepizole
- c. Both a and b
- d. Flumazenil

Explanation: The mainstay of treatment for both Methanol and Ethylene glycol ingestion is the administration of an antidote which blocks the function of Alcohol Dehydrogenase (ADH). Currently there are two antidotes used to block ADH metabolism: ethanol, a competitive ADH substrate, and fomepizole, an ADH inhibitor.

675. Drug of choice to treat extra pyramidal symptom includes:
- a. Noradrenaline
- b. Benztropine
- c. Carbamazepine
- d. Haloperidol

Explanation: Benztropine is an anticholinergic drug which is used to treat the extrapyramidal symptoms associated with anti-psychotic drugs.

676. A client who was started on antipsychotics a week back developed parkinsonism. Which of the following drugs is used for the treatment of parkinsonism in this patient?
- a. Anticholinergics
- b. Anti-depressants
- c. Atypical antipsychotics
- d. Mood stabilizer

Explanation: Anticholinergics (i.e. Benztropine) are used in the treatment of antipsychotic drug-induced Parkinsonism (peudoparkinsonism).

677. Extrapyramidal symptoms are the side effect of:
- a. Antipsychotic
- b. Antianxiety drugs
- c. Antidepressants
- d. Antimalarial drugs

Explanation: Complication of using antipsychotic drug includes extrapyramidal symptoms (EPS).

678. Advantage of risperidone is:
- a. Cholinergic effects are more
- b. A lower incidence of extrapyramidal effects
- c. It causes sedation and sleep in the patient
- d. No incidence of neuroleptic malignant syndrome

Explanation: Risperidone is an atypical antipsychotic which has a lower incidence of extrapyramidal effects than the typical antipsychotic.

679. Health education regarding imipramine should includes:
- a. It causes dry mouth
- b. It causes urinary retention
- c. Should not stop abruptly
- d. All of the above

Explanation: All the above-mentioned statements are correct regarding imipramine, which is an anti-depressant drug. It can cause photosensitivity and nausea among the individual.

680. Drug which causes hallucinations is: *(JIPMER March 2008)*
- a. Ketamine
- b. Gallamine
- c. D-tubocurare
- d. Pancuronium

681. A 30-year-old manic patient was prescribed Haloperidol one week back. For the last two days he has become restless and kept pacing in the room for a day. On examination he was found to have tremors of hand. He is most likely suffering from: *(JIPMER 2003)*
- a. Anhedonia
- b. Dystonia
- c. Restless leg syndrome
- d. Akathisia

682. Risperidone is an example of:
- a. Antipsychotics
- b. Anxiolytics
- c. Anticonvulsants
- d. Antidepressants

683. All of the following drugs belong to antipsychotics; EXCEPT:
- a. Haloperidol
- b. Clozapine
- c. Chlorpromazine
- d. Imipramine

684. Haloperidol is an example of:
- a. Anxiolytic
- b. Antipsychotic
- c. Antidepressant
- d. Sedative

685. Atypical antipsychotics include:
- a. Haloperidol and Olanzapine
- b. Chlorpromazine and Trifluoperazine
- c. Olanzapine and Quetiapine
- d. Chlorpromazine and Haloperidol

686. Which of the following drug needs a blood screening for CBC periodically?
- a. Clozapine
- b. Lithium
- c. Alprazolam
- d. Haloperidol

687. Chlorpromazine belongs to:
- a. Antipsychotic group
- b. Antianxiety group
- c. Anticonvulsive group
- d. Antibiotic group

688. One of the potential adverse effects of Mellaril (thioridazine) is:
- a. Weight loss
- b. Photosensitivity
- c. Diarrhea
- d. Color blindness

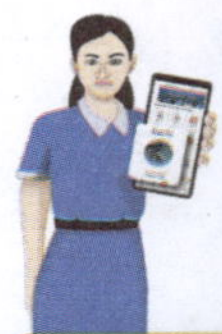

Ans.

670. d
671. d
672. b
673. d
674. c
675. b
676. a
677. a
678. b
679. d
680. a
681. d
682. a
683. d
684. b
685. c
686. a
687. a
688. b

689. Drug induced extra pyramidal symptoms (EPS) such as tardive dyskinesia is treated with:

a. Anxiolytics
b. Anticholinergic drugs
c. Tranquilizers
d. Sedatives and hypnotics

690. One of the side effects of an antipsychotic drug that is characterized by involuntary movements of the face and jaw is known as:

a. Tardive dyskinesia
b. Facial palsy
c. Akathisia
d. Neuroleptic malignant syndrome

691. Antipsychotic drugs mainly work by their action on receptors of:

a. Dopamine
b. Acetylcholine
c. Epinephrine
d. GABA

692. Atypical antipsychotics are all; EXCEPT:

a. Olanzapine
b. Clozapine
c. Risperidone
d. Thioridazine

693. Least Extrapyramidal side-effects are seen in:

a. Haloperidol
b. Thioridazine
c. Clozapine
d. Chlorpromazine

694. Adverse effect of clozapine is:

a. Hypertension
b. Sialorrhea
c. Extrapyramidal side effects
d. Neuroleptic malignant syndrome

695. Tardive dyskinesia is produced by the following; EXCEPT:

a. Fluphenazine
b. Haloperidol
c. Chlorpromazine
d. Clozapine

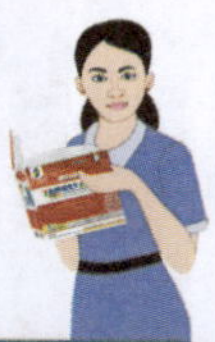

ANTIDEPRESSANTS

696. What will be the side effect if a client on monoamine oxidase fail to follow the diet restriction? *(RAK MSc 2018)*

a. Occipital headache
b. Generalized urticaria
c. Severe muscle spasm
d. Sudden drop in blood pressure

Explanation: Patients who are taking monoamine oxidase inhibitor should avoid taking food rich in tyramine. Tyramine is an amino acid found in fermented, aged or overripe food. This may cause sudden rise in blood pressure due to release of norepinephrine directly into the blood stream, causing occipital headache.

697. A monoamine oxidase inhibitor (MAOI) is prescribed. What should the nurse teach the client to avoid? *(RAK MSc 2018; AIIMS Bhopal Grade-I 2018)*

a. Prolonged exposure to the sun
b. Ingesting wines and aged cheese
c. Engaging inactive physical exercise
d. Over the counter NSAID medications

Explanation: Nurse suggest the patient to avoid ingesting wines and aged cheese as it contains tyramine which will otherwise cause sudden rise in blood pressure by releasing norepinephrine directly into the blood stream. Sudden rise in blood pressure causes hypertension crises which require immediate treatment. Tyramine rich foods (aged cheeses, alcohol beverages, cured meats etc.) must be avoided or used cautiously.

698. Important nursing intervention for a client who is on lithium therapy is: *(RAK MSc 2018)*

a. Restrict daily sodium intake
b. Test client's urine specific gravity
c. Monitor drug level in blood
d. Withhold all other medication

Explanation: It is very important to monitor blood levels of drug when patient is on lithium carbonate therapy since the plasma concentrations (>2 mmol/L) can be fatal, and causes lithium toxicity producing symptoms, like vomiting, severe diarrhea, albuminuria, hypotension and cardiac arrhythmias.

699. For determining the serum lithium, the blood specimen to be obtained: *(AIIMS Raipur NO 2019)*

a. Afternoon
b. Before lunch
c. Before breakfast
d. Before bedtime

Explanation: It is advisable to take the blood sample after 12 hours of last dose. If the last dose is administered at bedtime, it is convenient for the patient to provide a blood sample before next morning dose. So, the sample should be drawn before breakfast.

700. The side effects of antidepressant include: *(AIIMS Raipur Grade II 2017)*

a. Dry mouth, difficult in micturition and constipation
b. Epileptic seizures, tremors and muscle twitching
c. Skin rashes and jaundice
d. Somnolence and orthostatic hypotension

a. a, b, c
b. b, c, d
c. a, b, d
d. a, b, c, d

Explanation: The side effects of antidepressants include nausea, increased appetite and weight gain, loss of sexual desire and sexual problems such as erectile dysfunction and decreased orgasm, fatigue and drowsiness, insomnia, dry mouth, blurred vision and constipation.

701. After initiating lithium therapy, the therapeutic effective serum lithium concentration level is monitored: *(RPSC Nursing tutor 2009)*

a. <12 hours
b. 12–24 hours
c. 1–2 days
d. After 1 week

Explanation: The therapeutic effective serum lithium concentration level is monitored within 12-24 hours of Lithium administration.

702. Abrupt withdrawal of barbiturate causes: *(RPSC 2010)*

a. Sleepiness
b. Itching
c. Erythema
d. Seizures

Explanation: Abrupt withdrawal of barbiturate could cause withdrawal symptoms. These includes seizure, restlessness, insomnia, weakness, dizziness, nausea, sweating and anxiety.

703. All are anti-depressant drug; EXCEPT:

a. Tricyclic antidepressants
b. Monoamine oxidase inhibitors (MAOIs)
c. Selective serotonin reuptake inhibitors (SSRIs)
d. Thiazides

Explanation: Thiazide is a diuretic. All other drugs given above are antidepressants.

Ans.

689.	b
690.	a
691.	a
692.	d
693.	c
694.	b
695.	d
696.	a
697.	b
698.	c
699.	c
700.	a
701.	b
702.	d
703.	d

704. Antenatal use of lithium by mother can lead to .... malformation in fetus.

a. Neural tube defects
b. Cardiac malformations
c. Esophageal atresia
d. Cleft lip

Explanation: Lithium use during pregnancy (antenatal period) can cause Ebstein's anomaly in the fetus. Ebstein's anomaly is a congenital heart defect in which the septal and posterior leaflets of the tricuspid valve are displaced towards the apex of the right ventricle of the heart.

705. Antidote of benzodiazepine:

a. Lithium
b. Methadone
c. Flumazenil
d. Chlorpromazine

Explanation: Flumazenil competitively inhibits activity at benzodiazepine recognition site on GABA/benzodiazepine receptor complexes.

706. Which of the following food item is contraindicated to a client who is on MAOI therapy?

a. Banana
b. Red wine
c. Milk
d. Legumes

Explanation: A hypertensive crisis can result from ingestion of tyramine-rich foods in conjunction with monoamine oxidase inhibitors (MAOIs). So, the tyramine-rich foods should be strictly avoided for the clients on MAOI therapy. For tyramine rich food aged cheeses, red wine, yeast extract, pickles and canned sardines and liver.

707. Therapeutic serum level of lithium is:

a. 0.5-1.2 mEq/l
b. 0.8-1.2 mEq/l
c. 0.9-1.2 mEq/l
d. 1-1.2 mEq/l

Explanation: Normal therapeutic serum level of lithium is 0.8 to 1.2 mEq/L. Lithium is an antimanic drug with very low therapeutic index (low safety margin). So therapeutic serum level of the drug should be strictly monitored to prevent adverse effect of the drug.

708. A common anti-obsessional medication usually prescribed by practitioner are:

a. Fluvoxamine
b. Benztropine
c. Amantadine
d. Diphenhydramine

Explanation: Fluvoxamine blocks the uptake of serotonin and decreases the obsessive-compulsive behavior.

709. Anticholinergic side effect of TCA therapy includes:

a. Urine retention and blurred vision
b. Kussmaul breathing
c. Sleeplessness
d. Tremors and cardiac arrhythmia

Explanation: Anticholinergic effects of tricyclic antidepressants (TCA) include dry mouth, blurred vision, constipation, urinary retention, drowsiness, orthostatic hypotension, and perspiration.

710. Which of the following lab test will be prescribed for a client who is getting sodium Valproate for BPAD?

a. Platelet count and bleeding time
b. Liver function test
c. Both a and b
d. Blood sugar

Explanation: It is an anticonvulsant and used as a mood stabilizer. It will cause blood dyscrasias, so platelet count and bleeding time need to monitor, it has liver toxicity as side effect, so monitor aminotransferase level.

711. The function of gland which is affected in lithium toxicity is: *(JIPMER 2015)*

a. Parathyroid
b. Pituitary
c. Adrenal
d. Thyroid

712. A 35-year-old patient diagnosed with depression visits a health care provider. The provider decides to prescribe trazodone to help improve sleep quality. During the assessment, the patient mentions that he recently started taking a new medication. The provider reviews the patient's medication list and identifies a potential contraindication. Which medication, if already being taken by the patient, would be a contraindication for prescribing trazodone?

a. Selective serotonin reuptake inhibitors (SSRIs) *New Q*
b. Benzodiazepines
c. Monoamine oxidase inhibitors (MAOIs)
d. Atypical antipsychotics

Explanation: Trazodone, an antidepressant medication, is contraindicated when a patient is already taking monoamine oxidase inhibitors (MAOIs). MAOIs inhibit the activity of the enzyme monoamine oxidase, which play a role in the breakdown of certain neurotransmitters, including serotonin. Combining trazodone with MAOIs can lead to an excessive accumulation of serotonin in the brain, potentially resulting in serotonin syndrome.

713. The following drugs cause CNS depression; EXCEPT: *(JIPMER 1998)*

a. Amphetamine
b. Alcohol
c. Barbiturates
d. Diazepam

714. Lithium toxicity affects all of the following organs; EXCEPT: *(JIPMER 2006)*

a. Liver
b. Brain
c. Heart
d. Kidney

715. Absolute contraindication to Lithium therapy: *(JIPMER 2004)*

a. Renal failure
b. Angina
c. Glaucoma
d. Epilepsy

716. Drugs used for recurrent depressive episode is: *(JIPMER 2009)*

a. Imipramine
b. Carbamazepine
c. Fluoxetine
d. Sodium valproate

717. Non-sedating Antidepressant is: *(JIPMER 1993)*

a. Fluoxetine
b. Mianserin
c. Amoxaprine
d. Imipramine

718. Serum Lithium level should be checked earliest after how many days of constant dosing? *(JIPMER 2015)*

a. 3
b. 5
c. 14
d. 20

719. Which of the following class of drugs used to treat enuresis in children?

a. Benzodiazepines
b. MAOI
c. Tricyclic antidepressants
d. Sedative and hypnotics

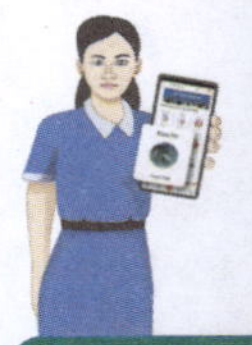

Ans.

704. b
705. c
706. b
707. b
708. a
709. a
710. c
711. d
712. c
713. a
714. a
715. a
716. a
717. a
718. b
719. c

720. Fluoxetine is used in which of the following childhood condition? *(JIPMER 2002)*
a. Depression b. Autism
c. Enuresis d. None of these

721. Consumption of tyramine-rich food by a patient who is on MAOI therapy may lead to:
a. Hypertensive crisis
b. Extrapyramidal symptoms
c. Neuroleptic Malignant syndrome
d. Severe vomiting

722. Serene is an example of: *(JIPMER 2015)*
a. Antipsychotic b. Antidepressant
c. Mood stabilizer d. Anxiolytic

723. The most common serious adverse effect of using flumazenil to reverse benzodiazepine overdose is:
a. Shivering b. Chest pain
c. Anorexia d. Seizures

724. Which of the following part of the brain is the target of Selective serotonin reuptake inhibitors (SSRI)?
a. Limbic system b. Basal ganglia
c. Frontal cortex d. Hippocampus

725. Which of the following drug is an antidepressant?
a. Clozapine b. Fluoxetine
c. Haloperidol d. Risperidone

726. All of the following are antidepressants; EXCEPT:
a. Sertraline b. Imipramine
c. Valproate d. Trazodone

727. Which of the following drug is not an example of SSRI?
a. Phenelzine b. Citalopram
c. Fluoxetine d. Sertraline

728. Which of the following antidepressant drug is not an MAOI?
a. Selegiline b. Phenelzine
c. Trazodone d. Isocarboxazid

729. Patients on MAOI's should not consume foods rich in:
a. Thiamine b. Tyramine
c. Vitamin C d. Iron

730. Which of the following receptors is blocked by tricyclic antidepressants (TCA)?
a. Acetylcholine receptor b. Norepinephrine transporter
c. GABA receptor d. D2 receptor

731. Time lag for maximum therapeutic response after initiation of fluoxetine hydrochloride is:
a. One week b. Two weeks
c. Three weeks d. Four weeks

732. Side effects of Fluoxetine are all; EXCEPT: *(AP PGMEE 1994)*
a. Weight gain b. Sweating
c. Urinary retention d. Diarrhea

733. Mode of action of fluoxetine:
a. GABA agonist b. GABA antagonist
c. Inhibit uptake of 5-HT d. Increase uptake of 5-HT

MOOD STABILIZERS

734. The parrot-like repetition of words spoken by others is known as: *(RPSC Nursing Tutor 2009)*
a. Enmeshment b. Echopraxia
c. Echolalia d. Neologism

Explanation: Echolalia is a meaningless repetition of another person's spoken words, i.e., patient keeps repeating the last few words of what he/she hears. Echopraxia is imitating the movement of others. Enmeshment is a psychological state that describes blurring of boundaries between individuals, especially family members. This occurs when a parent tries to get his/her needs met through the child. Neologism refers to the coining or use of new words which has no meaning.

735. Adverse effect due to Sodium valproate seen only in children is: *(JIPMER 2007)*
a. Tremor b. Hepatitis
c. Anorexia d. Loss of hair

736. Best prophylactic drug for febrile seizure is:
a. Acetaminophen b. Phenytoin
c. Diazepam d. Phenobarbitone

Explanation: Phenobarbitone is effective in preventing the recurrence of simple febrile seizures.

737. All of the following are used in treatment of Bipolar disorders; EXCEPT: *(JIPMER 2012)*
a. Lithium b. Antipsychotics
c. Phenytoin d. Sodium valproate

738. Treatment of choice of bipolar mood disorder: *(JIPMER 2012)*
a. Fluoxetine b. Imipramine
c. Lithium d. Chlorpromazine

739. Drug of choice for prophylaxis of Mania is: *(JIPMER 1994)*
a. Diazepam b. Lithium
c. Haloperidol d. Fluoxetine

740. All are side-effects of prolonged Phenytoin therapy; EXCEPT: *(JIPMER 2008)*
a. Osteomalacia
b. Gum hyperplasia
c. Gynaecomastia
d. Megaloblastic anaemia

741. Which of the following anti-epileptic drugs act by affecting levels of GABA? *(JIPMER 2008)*
a. Phenytoin sodium
b. Ethosuximide
c. Sodium valproate
d. Carbamazepine

742. A patient suffering from mixed seizure syndrome has not responded to other oral anticonvulsant drug therapy. Which drug would the nurse expect to be prescribed for this patient? *New Q*
a. Carbamazepine
b. Diazepam
c. Ethosuximide
d. Valproic acid

Explanation: Valproic acid is a broad-spectrum anticonvulsant medication that is commonly used in the treatment of various seizure disorders, including mixed seizure syndrome.

When a patient with mixed seizure syndrome has not responded to other oral anticonvulsant drug therapy, valproic acid is a medication that the nurse would typically expect to be prescribed.

743. Use of Carbamazepine in psychiatry is as a: *(JIPMER 2012)*
a. Mood stabilizer b. Antidote
c. Anticonvulsant d. Neuroleptic

744. Which of the following is a first generation antipsychotic? *New Q*
a. Clozapine b. Chlorpromazine
c. Quetiapine d. Risperidone

Ans.
720. a
721. a
722. b
723. d
724. c
725. b
726. c
727. a
728. c
729. b
730. b
731. c
732. c
733. c
734. c
735. b
736. d
737. c
738. c
739. b
740. c
741. c
742. d
743. a
744. d

745. Normal dose of lithium in the treatment of mania is:
a. 900-3000 mg b. 600-900 mg
c. 500-750 mg d. 900-2100 mg

746. A 32-year-old patient with schizophrenia has a history of poor medication adherence and frequent relapses. The nurse advises a different treatment approach to enhance treatment compliance. Which of the following options would be most suitable for this patient? *New Q*
a. Prescribing a daily oral antipsychotic medication
b. Recommending depot formulation of an antipsychotic
c. Initiating psychotherapy alone
d. Suggesting non-pharmacological interventions

747. Which of the following drug is an anxiolytic?
a. Risperidone b. Chlorpromazine
c. Alprazolam d. Haloperidol

748. Contraindications of lithium includes:
a. Renal diseases b. Cardiovascular disease
c. Sodium depletion d. All of these

749. Which of the following electrolyte should be consumed in adequate amount by a patient who is on lithium therapy?
a. Sodium b. Calcium
c. Potassium d. Zinc

750. Gender specific side effect of Valproate?
a. Alopecia b. Weight loss
c. Tremor d. PCOD

DEADDICTION/ANTABUSE DRUGS

751. Disulfiram therapy is indicated in:
a. Acute alcohol intoxication
b. Nicotine dependence
c. Acute opium intoxication
d. Alcohol dependence

752. Which of the following is an anticraving agent used during the maintenance phase of treatment of alcoholism?
a. Naltrexone b. Calcium carbonate
c. Disulfiram d. Acamprosate

753. Which of the following is the deterrent agent used in the maintenance phase of treatment of alcohol dependence syndrome?
a. Naloxone b. Disulfiram
c. Acamprosate d. Naltrexone

754. What is a relapse?
a. Worsening of symptoms after temporary improvement
b. It is a stage of diminution in symptom
c. Deterioration of symptoms
d. Recurrence of symptoms

755. The primary function of Alcoholic Anonymous (AA) is:
a. To teach harmful effects of alcoholism to public
b. To help members to maintain sobriety
c. To provide financial assistance for treatment
d. To provide detoxification and maintenance treatment

756. Disulfiram-like reaction is not seen with:
a. Disulfiram b. Amoxycillin
c. Metronidazole d. Cefoperazone

757. Combination of alcohol and Disulfiram results in nausea and hypertension as a result of accumulation of:
a. NADH b. Methanol
c. Acetate d. Acetaldehyde

758. The drug which is used to create aversion of the Alcohol Dependence: *(JIPMER 2015)*
a. Apomorphine b. Propranolol
c. Diazepam d. Disulfiram

759. Chronic Alcoholic patients are treated initially with ________ to prevent Wernicke-Korsakoff Syndrome.
a. Disulfiram
b. I/M injection of thiamine
c. I/V Diazepam
d. Acamprosate

760. Disulfiram therapy is .... type of behavioral therapy.
a. Systematic desensitization b. Overt sensitization
c. Token economy d. Flooding

Explanation: Disulfiram therapy is an overt sensitization, a type of aversion therapy which produces unpleasant consequence for undesirable behavior.

761. Higher dose of thioridazine (Mellaril) results in:
a. Widened or narrowed pupils
b. Stuffed nose
c. Retinal pigmentation
d. All of the above

Explanation: All the above-mentioned signs and symptoms are the side effect of overdose with thioridazine (Mellaril).

762. Which of the following is a potential complication of disulfiram therapy? *New Q*
a. Hypotension b. Hypokalemia
c. Hypothyroidism d. Hepatotoxicity

763. Which of the following is an example of a universal prevention strategy for substance use? *New Q*
a. Providing substance use treatment to people with addiction
b. Targeting at-risk individuals with individualized interventions
c. Implementing community-wide education campaigns
d. Increasing law enforcement efforts to reduce drug availability

Explanation: Community-wide education campaigns are an example of a universal prevention strategy for substance use. Universal prevention strategies aim to reach and provide information, resources, and support to the entire population, regardless of their individual risk factors.

NATIONAL MENTAL HEALTH PROGRAM (NMHP)

764. National mental health programme was launched in the year of:
a. 1982 b. 1981
c. 1980 d. 1979

Explanation: The Government of India launched the National Mental Health Programme (NMHP) in 1982, keeping in view the heavy burden of mental illness in the community, and the absolute inadequacy of mental health care infrastructure in the country to deal with it.

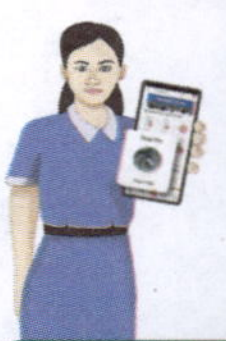

Ans.
745. d
746. b
747. c
748. d
749. a
750. d
751. d
752. d
753. b
754. a
755. b
756. b
757. d
758. d
759. b
760. b
761. d
762. d
763. c
764. a

765. All are the specific approaches suggested for implementation of the NMHP; EXCEPT:

a. Diffusion of mental health skills to the periphery of the health service system.
b. Appropriate appointment of tasks in mental health care
c. Integration of basic mental health care into general health services
d. Centralization in distribution of resources

766. District Mental Health Program (DMHP) was launched under NMHP in the year 1996. All of the following are the components of DMHP; EXCEPT:

a. Public education in the mental health to increase awareness
b. Outpatient services for early detection & treatment
c. Providing food and thiamine supplements to all
d. Imparting short term general physician for diagnosis and treatment

767. National Institute of Mental Health and Neuro Sciences (NIMHANS), Bengaluru, had developed District Mental Health Programme (DMHP), to achieve the objectives of National Mental Health Programme (NHMP). DMHP started based on which of the following model?

a. Nagori Model
b. Belgam Model
c. Chakkalwara model
d. Bellary Model

CRISIS INTERVENTION

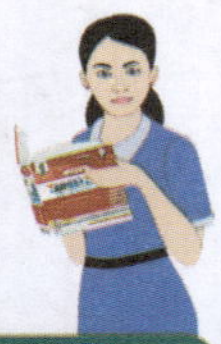

768. The crisis that is precipitated by an unanticipated stressful event that creates disequilibrium by threatening one's sense of biological, social or psychological integrity is called:

(AIIMS Bhopal Grade-I 2018)

a. Situational crisis
b. Adventitious crisis
c. Maturational crisis
d. Social crisis

Explanation: Situational crisis is term given to a person whose coping mechanisms are affected due to their circumstances (situations). Circumstances include loss of a job, financial situation, death of loved one, divorces, abortion or physical illness. It differs from adventitious crisis (unplanned or accidental) which includes rape, flood, fire, earthquake, terrorist attack, murder, child abuse, etc. Maturational crisis includes puberty, marriage, etc.

769. Following the death of spouse the person is experiencing Crisis. This type of crisis is known as:

a. Dispositional crisis
b. Crisis resulting from traumatic life experiences
c. Developmental crisis
d. Crisis reflecting psychopathology

Explanation: Crisis precipitated by unexpected external stress over which the individual has little or no control and as a result of which he/she feels emotionally overwhelmed and defeated.

770. Identify the characteristic of crisis among the following:

a. Crisis occurs in all individual and is not equated with psychopathology
b. Crisis is precipitated by specific identifiable event
c. Crisis is personal in nature and can vary from one person to another
d. All of the above

Explanation: A crisis is any event that is going to lead to an unstable and dangerous situation affecting an individual:

The following are the characteristics of crisis:

- The event is unexpected
- It creates uncertainty
- Crisis is seen as a threat to important goals
- Crisis is precipitated by specific events
- Crisis is personal in nature and can vary from person to person
- Crisis occurs in all individual and is not equated with psychopathology.

771. The crisis experienced by middle-aged adult during midlife is most commonly due to:

a. Many role changes experienced by the person
b. Individual's perception about his or her own life
c. Anticipation of negative changes associated with old age
d. Lack of support from family

Explanation: Most significant factor in avoiding or precipitating crisis is how individual perceive them.

772. The main goal in planning care for a client in crisis is:

a. Schedule follow up counselling for the client
b. Restore the client's psychological equilibrium
c. Have the client gain insight into the problems
d. Refer the client for occupational and physiotherapy

Explanation: Crisis intervention always focused on restoring the psychologic equilibrium.

773. During crisis intervention nurse should adopt:

a. Passive and reflective approach
b. Active and goal directed
c. Future oriented and passive
d. Interpretive and analytical

Explanation: Nurse should be active and goal-directed in crisis intervention. Other approaches are not appropriate for crisis management.

774. Which of the following information is the most important assessment data for the nurse to collect from a patient in crisis?

a. Socio-economical background
b. Strength and weaknesses
c. Food habits
d. Occupational history

775. An example of maturational crisis is:

a. Retirement
b. Earthquake
c. Road traffic accident
d. Financial loss

776. Rape is an example of:

a. Adventitious crisis
b. Social crisis
c. Maturational crisis
d. Cultural crisis

777. The primary goal of crisis intervention is to:

a. Help the patient return to pre-crisis level of functioning
b. Identify predisposing factors
c. Help the patient to ventilate his/her feelings
d. Support the family members to cope with the crisis

Ans.

765. d
766. c
767. d
768. a
769. b
770. d
771. b
772. b
773. b
774. b
775. a
776. a
777. a

778. Which among the following information is required by the nurse to make the client return to pre-crisis level of functioning?
   a. Full knowledge regarding the event
   b. Family support system
   c. Social support system
   d. Personal strength of the client

Explanation: Information regarding the personal strength and weakness is necessary to make the client return to pre-crisis phase of functioning.

779. These types of groups are composed of people who are trying to cope with a specific problem or life crisis and share their experience good or bad, successful or unsuccessful, with one another.
   a. Primary group   b. Secondary group
   c. Tertiary group   d. Self-help group

PSYCHIATRIC EMERGENCIES

780. Most common psychiatric emergency: *(JIPMER 2005)*
   a. Rape   b. Violence
   c. Panic attack   d. Suicide

781. Psychiatric emergencies include all; EXCEPT: *(JIPMER 2014)*
   a. Suicide   b. Panic disorder
   c. Drug use disorder   d. Insomnia

782. Which of the following actions should the nurse take first following a violent episode in a psychiatric unit? *(RAK MSc Entrance 2010)*
   a. Restrain the client
   b. Administer sedatives
   c. Call physician
   d. Call hospital security

Explanation: During a violent behavior in psychiatric unit, first nursing responsibility is to call the hospital security.

783. A patient presents to the emergency department with self-harm and indicates suicidal intent. Which of the following conditions does not warrant an immediate specialist assessment? *New Q*
   a. Formal thought disorder
   b. Acute alcohol intoxication
   c. Chronic severe physical illness
   d. Social isolation

Explanation: Acute alcohol intoxication is a medical emergency, but it does not warrant an immediate specialist assessment. This is because the patient's condition is usually stabilized by medical staff in the emergency department. Once the patient is stabilized, he can be transferred to a psychiatric ward for further evaluation and treatment.

Other conditions require an immediate specialist (psychiatrist) assessment.

Social isolation can also increase the risk of suicide. This is because people who are socially isolated may feel lonely and disconnected.

People with chronic severe physical illness may feel hopeless and helpless. They may also feel like they are a burden to their loved ones. This can lead to suicidal thoughts and behaviors.

Formal thought disorder is a symptom of schizophrenia and other psychotic disorders, so the client needs help from specialist.

784. Panic attack is characterized by all; EXCEPT: *(JIPMER 2001)*
   a. Fear of dying
   b. Visual hallucinations
   c. Choking sensation
   d. Fear of losing control

LEGAL ASPECTS OF PSYCHIATRIC NURSING

785. Relative of Mrs. X brought her to psychiatry hospital with an application made out to the magistrate and got her admitted in the hospital. The nurse knows that this type of admission is:
   a. Admission on voluntary basis
   b. Admission on involuntary basis
   c. Admission under special circumstances
   d. Admission under reception order

786. All among the following are the role of community psychiatric nurse; EXCEPT:
   a. Counsellor   b. Client Advocate
   c. Prescribe drugs   d. Crisis worker

787. Which of the following is not one of the revisions made in the Mental Healthcare Act 2017 which repealed the Mental Health Act, 1987?
   a. Decriminalizing the attempt to commit suicide
   b. Provisions for the registration of mental health related institutions and for the regulation of the sector
   c. Restriction of usage of electroconvulsive therapy (ECT) in children
   d. Electroconvulsive therapy to be used without muscle relaxants and anesthesia

Explanation: Following procedures are prohibited in Mental Healthcare Act 2017 (S.no 95a-d)-
- Electro-convulsive therapy without the use of muscle relaxants and anesthesia
- Electro-convulsive therapy for minors
- Sterilization of men or women, when such sterilization is intended as a treatment for mental illness
- Chained in any manner or form whatsoever.

788. A patient is brought by family members to psychiatric OPD. The psychiatric nurse understands that an assessment tools is needed to assess personality disorder. Which of the following instrument is related to assessment of personality traits?
   a. BPRS   b. PANSS
   c. MMSE   d. MMPI

MENTAL HEALTHCARE ACT 2017

789. Mental Healthcare Act 2017 bill received president assent on:
   a. April 7, 2017
   b. April 15, 2017
   c. July 7, 2017
   d. July 15, 2017

790. The Indian Lunacy Act was passed in the year:
   a. 1898   b. 1912
   c. 1982   d. 1987

791. The Indian Mental Health Act was passed in the year:
   a. 1912   b. 1947
   c. 1982   d. 1987

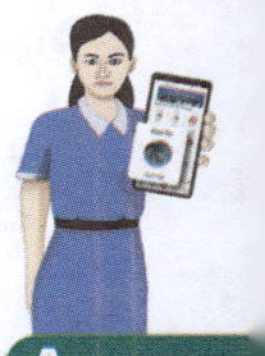

Ans.
778. d
779. d
780. d
781. d
782. d
783. b
784. b
785. d
786. c
787. d
788. d
789. a
790. b
791. d

792. According to Mental Health Act 1987, leave of absence refers to:

a. Mentally ill patient is forcefully removed from the hospital
b. Mentally ill patient is denied entry into the hospital
c. Mentally ill patient is given time limited leave
d. Mentally ill patient is leaving the hospital without permission

793. Which of the following is not a feature of Mental Healthcare Act 2017:

a. Every person except minor has right to take advance directive in writing
b. It does not allow the patient to appoint a representative to take decision on behalf of patient
c. This Act abolished the ECT for children and made provisions for Modified ECT
d. Decriminalization of suicide

794. According to Mental Health Act 1987, admission under special circumstances refers to:

a. Application for admission is made by the patient voluntarily
b. Application for admission is made by relatives or friends of the patient
c. Application for admission is made by a relative or friends of the patient through a magistrate
d. Application for admission is made by Police through a Magistrate

COMMON TERMINOLOGY IN PSYCHIATRY

795. Temporary loss of muscle tone and weakness precipitated by a variety of emotional states is called:

(AIIMS Raipur Grade II 2017)

a. Cataplexy　　b. Catharsis
c. Compulsion　　d. Confabulation

Explanation: Cataplexy is a sudden and transient episode of muscle weakness accompanied by full conscious awareness which is precipitated or triggered by emotions as laughing, crying, etc. Catharsis is the process of releasing strong emotions through a particular activity or experience. Compulsive behavior is a psychological condition in which a person does behavior compulsively having an overwhelming feeling that they must do so. Confabulation is a symptom of various memory disorders in which made up stories fill in any gaps in memory.

796. A state of diminished consciousness in which the patient remains mute and still with the eyes open is called:

(AIIMS Raipur Grade II 2017)

a. Catatonia　　b. Stupor
c. Panic　　d. Hysteria

Explanation: Catatonia is a state of psychomotor immobility and behavioral abnormality manifested by stupor. Panic is a sudden, strong feeling of anxiety or fear that prevents reasonable thought and actions and may spread to influence many people. Hysteria is exaggerated or uncontrollable emotion or excitement.

797. When a patient is not aware of his/her mental illness, it is called?

(AIIMS Raipur Staff Nurse Grade I-2018)

a. Disorientation　　b. Lack of insight
c. Unconsciousness　　d. Lack of concentration

Explanation:

- **Disorientation:** Cognitive disability in which person is not aware about time place and person.
- **Lack of insight:** Also known as anosognosia in which person is not aware about his or her own mental illness.

798. The person is able to speak only in whisper:

a. Aphonia　　b. Mutism
c. Aphasia　　d. Stuporness

Explanation: Aphonia is the inability to produce voiced sound.

799. Creating imaginary events to fill up the memory gap is known as:

a. Circumstantiality　　b. Neologism
c. Confabulation　　d. Compulsion

Explanation: Confabulation is the falsification of memory in which gaps in recall are filled by fabrications that the generating individual accepts as fact.

800. While talking to a psychiatric client, nurse came to know that the client moves from one idea to other which are not related. This phenomenon is called:

a. Echopraxia　　b. Echolalia
c. Circumstantiality　　d. Loosening of association

Explanation: Loosening of association is a thought disorder characterized by discourse consisting of a sequence of unrelated or only remotely related ideas. The frame of reference often changes from one sentence to the next.

801. In a group therapy members express both positive and negative feeling in a non-threatening atmosphere is called:

a. Catharsis　　b. Echopraxia
c. Cognition　　d. Apraxia

Explanation: The given statement indicates catharsis, which is identified by Yalom.

802. The patient may not talk at all. This term is known as:

a. Mutism　　b. Aphonia
c. Stupor　　d. Thought block

Explanation: This condition is mutism, Aphonia is inability to talk.

803. Clang association means:

a. Impaired verbal communication
b. Risk for violence
c. Ineffective health maintenance
d. Disturbed sensory perception

Explanation: In psychiatry, clanging refers to a mode of speech characterized by association of words based upon sound rather than concepts. It usually includes compulsive rhyming. As speech is verbal form, it is under impaired verbal communication.

804. Temporary discharge of the patient from the psychiatric hospital is referred to as: *(DSSSB PHN, 2015)*

a. Parole　　b. Abscond
c. Termination　　d. Escape

805. Unfamiliarity of familiar things is seen in:

a. Déjà Vu　　b. Jamais Vu
c. Deja Entend　　d. Deja pence

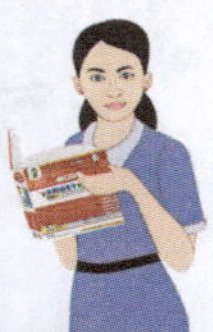

Ans.

792.	c
793.	b
794.	b
795.	a
796.	b
797.	b
798.	a
799.	c
800.	d
801.	a
802.	a
803.	a
804.	a
805.	b

806. Preservation is:
- a. Persistent and inappropriate repetition of the same thoughts
- b. When a patient feels very distressed about it
- c. Characteristic of schizophrenia
- d. Characteristic of obsessive compulsive disorder (OSD)

807. If the activities done by the people are repeated by a patient, it is called: *(Kerala PSC, Nov 2014)*
- a. Echolalia
- b. Hyperactivity
- c. Compulsion
- d. Echopraxia

808. A false memory that the patient believes to be true is: *(Staff Nurse G II 2014)*
- a. Confabulation
- b. Fugue
- c. Cataplexy
- d. Anergia

809. A condition in which person maintaining the body posture into which it is placed is: *(Staff Nurse G II 2014)*
- a. Anergia
- b. Echopraxia
- c. Cataplexy
- d. Catalepsy

Explanation: Catatonia is a motor inactivity manifested by waxy flexibility or catalepsy, mutism, and increased muscle tone. Catalepsy is a condition characterized by a trance or sudden loss of sensation and consciousness along with rigidity of the body. Cataplexy is sudden loss of muscle tone leading to fall precipitated by laughter or excessive emotions.

810. Abnormal involuntary movement which occurs suddenly, repetitively and purposeless is: *(Staff Nurse G II 2014)*
- a. Mannerism
- b. Compulsion
- c. Cataplexy
- d. Tic

811. When Ramya first saw violent movie, she was scared and disgusted. But now she has seen several such movies, she is barely affected by them. Ramya has experienced: ***New Q***
- a. Habituation
- b. Displacement
- c. Cultivation
- d. Catharsis

Explanation: Habituation is the process of becoming less sensitive to a stimulus over time. In this case, Ramya has become less sensitive to violence in movies over time. This is because her brain has learned to expect violence in movies, and it no longer responds to it in the same way.

812. Persistent mechanical repetition of speech or movement is known as:
- a. Echolalia
- b. Stereotype
- c. Tangentiality
- d. Circumstantiality

Explanation:
- Stereotype of stereotyped behavior is characterized by repetition of speech or movement.
- **Echolalia is meaningless repetition of another person's words. Echopraxia refers to involuntary repetition or imitation of another person's actions.**

813. A state of indifference, or the suppression of emotions such as concern, excitement, motivation, and passion is known as:
- a. Apathy
- b. Ambivalence
- c. Catatonia
- d. Mutism

814. Having the strong sensation that an event or experience currently being experienced has already been experienced in the past is known as:
- a. Déjà Vu
- b. Jamais vu
- c. Selective amnesia
- d. Dissociative amnesia

815. The process of rapidly releasing negative emotions is known as:
- a. Reminiscence therapy
- b. Hypnosis
- c. Biofeedback
- d. Catharsis

816. Flattening of emotions is otherwise known as:
- a. Loose association
- b. Ambiguity
- c. Blunted affect
- d. Suppression

817. A person who laughs one minute and cries the next without any clear stimulus is said to have:
- a. Incongruent affect
- b. Euphoria
- c. Labile affect
- d. Split personality

818. Abnormal sensitivity to light is known as: *(JIPMER 2012)*
- a. Aphasia
- b. Photophobia
- c. Hydrophobia
- d. Diplopia

819. A form of speech in which the client tends to wander away from the intended point and never returning to the original idea is called: *(AIIMS Raipur Grade II 2017)*
- a. Verbigeration
- b. Thought insertion
- c. Tangentiality
- d. Thought block

Explanation: Verbigeration is the obsessive repetition of random words. Thought insertion is associated with schizophrenia. Thought insertion along with thought broadcasting, thought blocking and thought withdrawal are primary first rank symptoms of schizophrenia.

820. Pattern of speech that is very indirect and delayed in reaching the central point (goal) is known as:
- a. Word salad
- b. Clang association
- c. Circumstantiality
- d. Tangentiality

821. A naive, inappropriate lack of emotion or concern for the perceptions by others of one's disability is known as:
- a. Apathy
- b. La belle indifference
- c. Déjà vu
- d. Jamme vu

822. Feeling of sadness and irritability is referred to as:
- a. Dysphoria
- b. Anhedonia
- c. Cyclothymia
- d. Dysthymia

823. La Bella indifference is related to: *(RPSC Nursing tutor 2009)*
- a. Body dysmorphic disorder
- b. Pain disorder
- c. Somatization disorder
- d. Conversion disorder

Explanation: La Bella indifference is related to conversion disorder. It is a symptom of conversion disorder in which there is a relative lack of concern that is out of keeping with the severity of impairment.

824. Psychiatrist orders "restraints PRN", the nurse should understand that:
- a. Use restraints if client begin to act out
- b. Ask to the doctor regarding the type of restraints
- c. Ensure that all staffs are aware about restraints
- d. Identify that PRN orders are not valid for restraints

Explanation: Order for restraints should be prescribed each time when it is required. PRN orders are not acceptable for restraints.

MISCELLANEOUS

825. According to Marie Jahoda, all of the following statements are correct regarding ideal mental health, EXCEPT: ***New Q*** *(AIIMS MG Faculty 2023)*
- a. Capability for growth and development
- b. Accurate perception of reality
- c. Dependence on each other
- d. Positive view of self

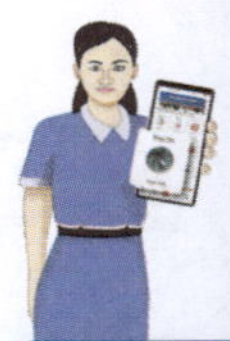

Ans.

806.	a
807.	d
808.	a
809.	d
810.	d
811.	a
812.	b
813.	a
814.	a
815.	d
816.	c
817.	c
818.	b
819.	c
820.	c
821.	b
822.	a
823.	d
824.	d
825.	c

826. Which of the following disorders is NOT a category of psychosis? *New Q*

a. Hallucination b. Disorganized behavior
c. Phobia d. Delusion

827. Which of the following is a symptom of alcohol withdrawal syndrome? *New Q*

a. Anxiety and agitation b. Increased appetite
c. Bradycardia d. Dry mouth

828. Disorders of adult personality and behavior is classified under which of the following classification of ICD 10? *New Q*

a. F40-49 b. F50-59
c. F60-69 d. F70-79

829. What is the Intelligence Quotient (IQ) of an individual with the mental age of 30 and chronological age of 25? *New Q*

(AIIMS MG Tutor 2023)

a. 100 b. 123
c. 83 d. 120

Explanation: To determine the Intelligence Quotient (IQ) of an individual, we use the formula:
IQ = (Mental Age / Chronological Age) * 100
In this case, the individual has a mental age of 30 and a chronological age of 25. Applying these values into the formula, we get:
IQ = (30 / 25) * 100 = 120
Therefore, the correct answer is:
d. 120

830. Immunization against which of the following maternal infections is a primary prevention measure for mental retardation? *New Q*

a. Mumps b. Rubella
c. Tetanus d. Measles

Explanation: Immunization against rubella is a primary prevention measure for preventing mental retardation. If a pregnant woman contracts rubella during early pregnancy, it can result in congenital rubella syndrome (CRS) in the developing fetus. CRS can lead to various complications, including mental retardation, hearing impairment, vision problems, and other developmental disabilities.

831. All of the following result in delirium; EXCEPT: *New Q*

(NORCET 2022)

a. Benzodiazepines withdrawal
b. Opioid withdrawal
c. Hyponatremia
d. Depression

832. A schizophrenic client who is experiencing thoughts of having special powers states that, "I am a messenger from another planet and can rule the earth." The nurse assesses this behavior as: *New Q* *(NORCET 2022)*

a. Ideas of reference b. Delusions of persecution
c. Thought broadcasting d. Delusions of grandeur

833. A person, suffering from severe anxiety disorder, is able to speak freely with certain people only and is not able to speak with others, especially with certain social groups such as classmates at school: *New Q*

a. Aphasia b. Mutism
c. Epilepsy d. Selective mutism

Explanation: Selective mutism is a childhood anxiety disorder characterized by the consistent failure to speak in specific social situations, despite having the ability to speak in other settings. Individuals with selective mutism may be able to speak freely and comfortably with certain people or in familiar environments but experience extreme difficulty speaking or communicating effectively in other situations, such as at school or in public.

834. A patient comes in stuporous condition. Patient's parents give history of patient being continually sad and suicidal attempts and not eating and sleeping for most of the time. The preferred treatment is: *New Q*

a. ECT b. Antidepressant
c. Antipsychotic d. Sedative

835. Thought process characterized by a series of ideas without apparent logical connections is referred to as: *New Q*

a. Loosening of association
b. Flight of ideas
c. Tangentiality
d. Preservation

836. First discovered tricyclic antidepressant is: *New Q*

a. Sertraline b. Clomipramine
c. Imipramine d. Trazadone

Explanation: Imipramine was approved in 1959 by the Food and Drug Administration (FDA) for the treatment of Major depressive Disorder, which established the class of drugs called tricyclic antidepressants (TCA).

837. Services aimed at reducing the prevalence of psychiatric illness by shortening the course of the illness is called:

(AIIMS Bhopal Grade-I 2018)

a. Secondary prevention
b. Primary prevention
c. Tertiary prevention
d. Primordial prevention

Explanation: Disease prevention includes measures not only to prevent the occurrence of disease (primary level prevention-reduce risk, immunization) but also to arrest its progress (secondary level prevention- early diagnosis and prompt treatment) and reduce its consequences once established (tertiary level prevention-rehabilitations).

838. What is total score in Mini Mental Status Examination (MMSE)? *(AIIMS Raipur Staff Nurse Grade I-2018)*

a. 25 b. 30
c. 32 d. 35

Explanation: Total score of mini mental status examination is 30 and is divided among the following categories such as orientation, registration, attention and calculation, recall and language.

839. Full form of MMSE is:

a. Multi memory state status examination
b. Multiple mental strata evaluation
c. Mini mental status examination
d. Meta mental structural evaluation

Explanation: MMSE stands for Mini Mental Status Examination. It is otherwise called Folstein test. The maximum score is 30.

840. Touching one's body without consent is known as:

a. Battery
b. Fraud
c. Breach of confidentiality
d. Harassment

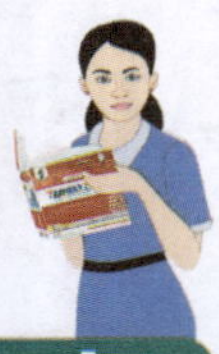

Ans.

826. c
827. a
828. c
829. d
830. b
831. d
832. d
833. d
834. a
835. b
836. c
837. a
838. b
839. c
840. a

Explanation: A battery is an intentional and wrongful physical contact with another person without that person's consent that includes some injury or offensive touching.

841. Co-occurrence of how many psychiatric disorders in a single patient can be termed comorbidity?

a. 2 b. ≥2
c. ≥3 d. 3

842. Which of the following component is not a part of mental status examination (MSE)?

a. Insight b. Judgment
c. Mood and affect d. Language

843. Mini mental status examination is: *(JIPMER 2002, 2007)*

a. Method to investigate common psychiatric problem
b. 30-point programme to evaluate cognitive function
c. To evaluate schizophrenia
d. Instrument to measure delirium

844. What cut-off score of Mini-Mental State Examination (MMSE) is used to detect dementia?

a. Less than 20
b. Less than 24
c. Less than 27
d. Less than 29

845. Paroxysmal cerebral dysfunction is otherwise called:

a. Depression b. Epilepsy
c. Coma d. Brain death

846. The major cause of neurotic disorders is:

a. Physical factor b. Genetic disorder
c. Stress factor d. Biological factor

847. Which of the following is not a neurotic disorder?

a. Panic anxiety b. Conversion reaction
c. Delirious mania d. Dissociative fugue

848. Which of the following is not a characteristic feature of neurotic disorders?

a. Intact insight b. Subjective distress
c. Anxiety d. Delusions

849. Insight is present in all; EXCEPT:

a. Neurosis
b. Obsessive compulsive disorders
c. Phobias
d. Psychosis

ANTIPSYCHOTICS AS LONG ACTING INJECTABLES (LAI) OR DEPOTS

850. Which of the following statements about long-acting injectable (LAI) antipsychotics is true?

a. LAIs were introduced in the 1970s as the first-line treatment for schizophrenia.
b. LAIs were initially met with resistance from the medical profession due to fears of increased side effects.
c. LAIs are associated with daily peaks and troughs of medication levels in the plasma.
d. LAIs have shown no improvement in the morbidity of schizophrenia compared to oral formulations.

851. Second-generation antipsychotics available as long-acting injectable are all, except:

a. Olanzapine pamoate
b. Risperidone microspheres
c. Fluphenazine decanoate
d. Paliperidone palmitate

Explanation: Fluphenazine decanoate is a first generation long acting injectable (LAI). All other given formula are second generation antipsychotics which is available in LAI form.

852. Before the first injection of RLAI, the patient is recommended to be on oral risperidone for not less than:

a. One week
b. Two weeks
c. Three weeks
d. Four weeks

Explanation: Before the first injection of RLAI, the patient is recommended to be on oral risperidone no shorter than 2 weeks. RLAI doses are available as: 25, 37.5, and 50 mg. RLAI should be used in the lowest effective dose, usually given every 2 weeks. The administration of RLAI less frequently than every four weeks is not recommended.

In the event of discontinuation, it needs to be taken into account that the risperidone level will maintain for at least 3 weeks after the last injection.

853. When the patient had already been stabilized on oral olanzapine, the Olanzapine Long Acting Injectables (OLAI) should be given at the:

a. Lowest possible dosage, usually at the intervals of 2 weeks
b. Lowest possible dosage, usually at the intervals of 4 weeks
c. Highest possible dosage, usually at the intervals of 2 weeks
d. Highest possible dosage, usually at the intervals of 4 weeks

Explanation: OLAI is available in three doses: 210, 300 and 405 mg of olanzapine pamoate monohydrate powder and solvent for prolonged-release suspension for injections. The half-life of OLAI is 30 days. When the patient had already been stabilized on oral olanzapine, the OLAI should be given at the lowest possible dosage, usually at the intervals of 4 weeks.

The drug should be administered deeply into the gluteal muscle.

854. Aripiprazole long-acting injectables is indicated for the maintenance treatment of:

a. Patients with schizophrenia who have been stabilized by oral antipsychotics
b. Elderly patients with schizophrenia
c. Schizophrenic patients with dementia
d. Children less than 18 years of age

Explanation: Aripiprazole long-acting injection (ALAI) is indicated for maintenance treatment of patients with schizophrenia who have been stabilized by oral antipsychotic treatment. ALAI is not indicated for elderly and dementia patients. It is not indicated for patients less than 18 years.

855. Advantages of DEPOT preparations includes all; except: *New Q*

a. Eliminates bioavailability problems
b. Reduces risk of an overdose
c. Flexibility of dose adjustment
d. Reduced relapse frequency

Explanation: Depot preparations may have limited flexibility for dose adjustment compared to oral medications. Once the depot preparation is administered, the medication is slowly released into the bloodstream over an extended period. This sustained release limits the ability to adjust the dose on a daily or immediate basis.

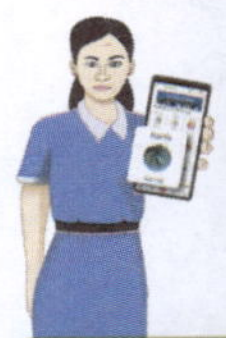

Ans.

841. b
842. d
843. b
844. b
845. b
846. c
847. c
848. d
849. d
850. b
851. c
852. b
853. b
854. a
855. c

"One day in perfect health is much."
—Arabic

CHAPTER 6

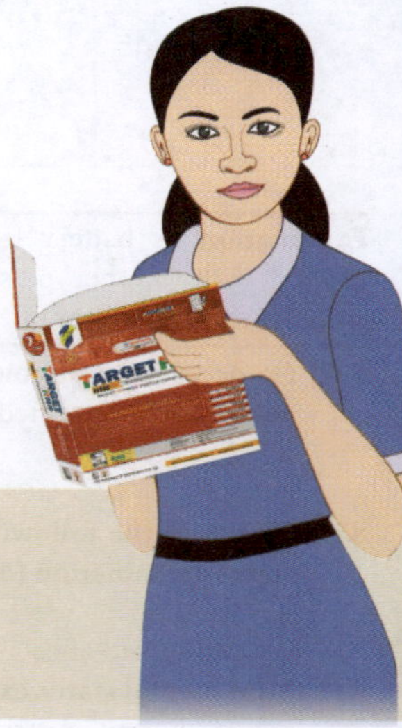

PEDIATRIC NURSING

SYNOPSIS

GROWTH AND DEVELOPMENT

Growth

Growth denotes the net increase in size or mass of tissue. It is a quantitative measurement.

Development

Development specifies the maturation of function. It is a qualitative measurement.

Stages of Growth and Development

Prenatal Period

Ovum	0–14 days after conception
Embryo	14 days to 8 weeks
Fetus	8 weeks to birth (8–40 weeks)

Postnatal Period

Neonate/newborn	0–28 days
Infancy	29 days – 1 year
Toddler	1–3 years
Pre-school child	3–6 years
School going child	6–10 years (girls) 6–12 years (boys)
Adolescent	puberty–adulthood
Early adolescent	12–14 years
Middle adolescent	14–16 years
Late adolescent	16–20 years

Factors Affecting Growth and Development

- Age
- Race
- Genetic factors
- Antenatal factors
- Natal factors
- Nutritional factors
- Hormonal factors
- Sex
- Biorhythm
- Seasonal variation
- Environmental factors (Infections, illness, trauma to growing parts of bones)
- Social factors (Socioeconomic class, cultural habits, education of parents, education of child, psychological factors and psychosocial factors)

Principles of Growth and Development

- Growth and development in children is a continuous orderly process.
- Growth pattern of every individual is unique.
- Different body tissues grow at different rates.
- Development is a continuous process.
- Development depends upon the maturation of nervous system.
- The sequence of attainment of milestone is same in all children.
- The process of development progresses is in cephalocaudal direction and proximodistal direction.
- Certain primitive reflexes have to be lost before attainment of relevant milestone.
- The initial disorganized mass activity is gradually replaced by specific and willful actions.
- Development depends on maturation and learning.

Weight

The average weight of a neonate is 3 kg. In Indian children, 2.5–3.5 kg weight of a neonate is considered as normal.

In the first few days after birth, newborn loses extracellular fluid equivalent to 10% of the body weight. So, there will be slight decline in the birth weight of the baby. The usual pattern of gaining weight is shown in the table.

KEY POINTS

- Growth and development in children are the continuous orderly processes.
- The sequence of attainment of milestone is same in all children.
- The process of development progresses in cephalocaudal direction and proximodistal direction.
- The baby attains three times of its birth weight by one year of age.
- The baby attains four times of its birth weight by two years and 5 times by three years of age.

Recent Question
(NORCET 2023)

1. **A baby at 3 year will be considered as for having developmental delay if he or she**
   a. Cannot hop on one foot
   b. Cannot catch ball reliably
   c. Cannot hold spoon effectively
   d. Cannot copy a square

Ans. (c) Cannot hold ...

Table 1: Average weight chart for children

Age of the baby*	Weight of the baby*
Birth	X
5–6 months	2x
1 year	3x
2 years	4x
3 years	5x
5 years	6x
7 years	7x
10 years	10x

*(*approximate values are given in the table)*
'x' denotes birth weight of the baby.

Weight between ages of 3 months and 12 years can be calculated by using Weech's formula;

3–12 months: Expected weight (kg) = $\frac{\text{Age in months} + 9}{2}$

1–6 years: Expected weight = (Age in years × 2) + 8

7–12 years: Expected weight (kg) = $\frac{(\text{Age in years} \times 7) - 5}{2}$

An easy formula to calculate weight in children between 2 and 12 years is

Weight (kg) = Age $\frac{(\text{Age in years} + 3) \times 5}{2}$

Length/Height

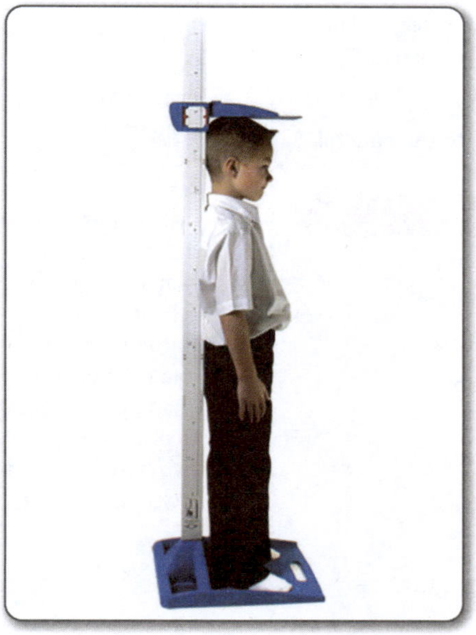

Figure 1: Stadiometer

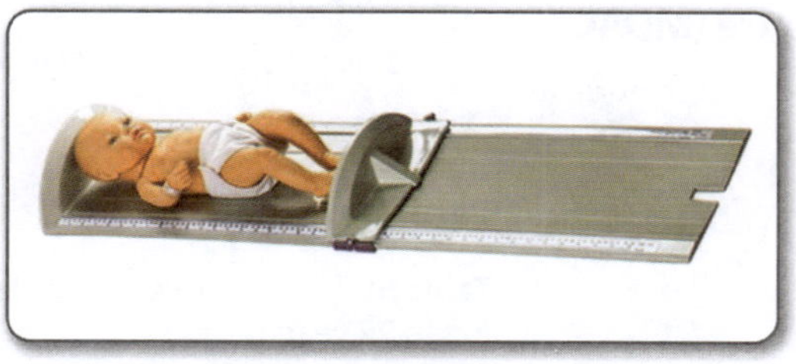

Figure 2: Infantometer

Table 2: Length/Height of children

Age of the baby*	Length/height of the baby*
Birth	50 cm
3 months	60 cm
6 months	65 cm
9 months	70 cm

Contd...

Recent Questions (CNCI 2021)

2. A baby whose birth weight is 3 kg, what will be his required weight at the age of 4 years?
a. 6 kg
b. 12 kg
c. 14 kg
d. 16 kg
Ans. (d) 16 kg

3. The expected height of a normal child at 12 months is:
a. 45 cm
b. 50 cm
c. 75 cm
d. 100 cm
Ans. (c) 75 cm

Recent Question (NORCET 2023)

4. Up to which age height of the child is measured in lying down posture?
a. 12 months
b. 18 months
c. 24 months
d. 36 months
Ans. (c) 24 months

KEY POINTS

- Head circumference is a measurement of a child's head around its largest area.
- Head circumference is measured over the most prominent part on the back of the head (occiput) and just above the eye-brows (supraorbital ridges).
- Microcephaly is defined as a head circumference 2 standard deviations (SDs) below the mean for age and sex or roughly less than the 3rd per-centile.

(NORCET 2021)

Length of baby doubles by 4 years of age

Age of the baby*	Length/height of the baby*
1 year	75 cm
2 years	90 cm
4 years	100 cm

*(*approximate values are given in the table)*

After 4 years, a child gains approximately 6 cm height every year until 12 years of age.

- >5 years age—height measured in standing position using stadiometer.
- 5 years or below—height measured in lying position using infantometer.

Head Circumference (HC)

Table 3: Head circumference for various ages

Age	Head circumference (cm)
At birth	34–35
2 months	38
3 months	40
4 months	41
6 months	42–43
1 years	45–46
2 years	47–48

- Head circumference is measured by placing tape over occipital protuberance at the back and just over the supraorbital ridge and glabella in front.
- Increased head circumference: Hydrocephalous, Macrocephaly
- Decreased head circumference: Microcephaly

Chest Circumference (CC)

- The CC is about 3 cm less than the HC at the time of birth (31 cm approx.)
- HC and CC become almost equal by 1 year of age and after that CC exceeds the HC.
- CC is measured at the level of nipples in mid inspiration.

Mid Upper Arm Circumference (MUAC)

At birth, average MUAC is about 9–11 cm in normal newborn baby

- At 1 year it is 12–16 cm
- At 1–5 year it is 16–17 cm
- At 12 years it is 17–18 cm
- At 15 years it is 20–21 cm

Arm Span (Wing Span)

- Arm span is the distance between the tips of the middle finger of both arms when they are outstretched at right angles to the body. The arm span is 1–2 cm less than the height of children below 5 years and by 10–12 years both will be equal.
- Arm span is greater than height in:
  - Marfan syndrome, Klinefelter syndrome, Homocystinuria

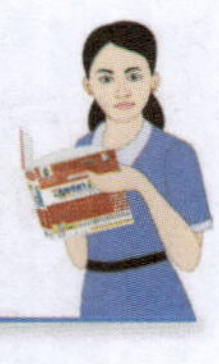

- Arm span is less than height in:
  - Achondroplasia, cretinism

Skin Fold Thickness (SFT)

- Instrument used for measurement is Lange's or Harpenden's skin-fold calipers.
  - It holds a fold of skin over triceps area on the left side
  - Measure the area between thumb and index finger
  - Triceps skin fold are most popular
  - Ratio of total body water and body weight is a more accurate index of body fat.

Eruption of Teeth

Primary Teeth

The primary dentition consists of 20 teeth. There are four incisors (two central and two lateral), two canines and four molars in each jaw.

Table 4: Teeth eruption according to the age (till 33 months)

Age	Eruption
Birth	Nil
8–12 months	Central incisors
9–13 months	Lateral incisors
13–19 months	First molar
16–22 months	Canines
25–33 months	Second molars

Permanent Teeth

Table 5: Teeth eruption according to the age (up to 22 years)

Age (Years)	Eruption
6 years	First molars
7–8 years	Central and lateral incisors
9 years	First premolar
10–11 years	Second premolar
11–12 years	Canines
12-13 years	Second molars
17–22 years	Third molars (wisdom teeth)

KEY POINTS

- The Chest Circumference (31 cm approx) is about 3 cm less than the Head Circumference at the time of birth.
- Head Circumference (HC) and Chest Circumference (CC) are almost equal by 1 year of age and after that CC exceeds the HC.
- The arm span is 1-2 cm less than height of children below 5 years and by 10-12 years both will be equal. Then arm span exceeds the height.
- In children, arm span is greater than height in Marfan's syndrome, Klinefelter's syndrome and Homocystinuria.
- Arm span is less than height in Achondroplasia, cretinism.
- Instrument used for measurement of skin fold thickness is Lange's or Harpenden's skin fold callipers.
- The first two teeth to erupt are the two bottom central incisors.

Recent Question (NORCET 2023)

5. Identify an example of age-independent anthropometry?

a. MUAC
b. Weight
c. Head circumference
d. Chest circumference

Ans. (a) MUAC

GROWTH CHART

If the growth measurements are recorded in a child over a period of time and are plotted on a graph, the deviation in the growth profile can be easily interpreted. This is a good tool to diagnose deviation of growth from normal. Growth chart is also known as "road to health chart."

Uses of Growth Charts

- Growth monitoring
- Diagnostic tool
- Tool for action
- Tool for evaluation
- Tool for teaching.

Recent Question (NORCET 2023)

6. Which of the following is the correct height velocity in children aged 2–10 years:
a. 8–18 cm/year
b. 4–6 cm/year
c. 2–4 cm/year
d. 6–8 cm/year

Ans. (b) 4–6 cm/year

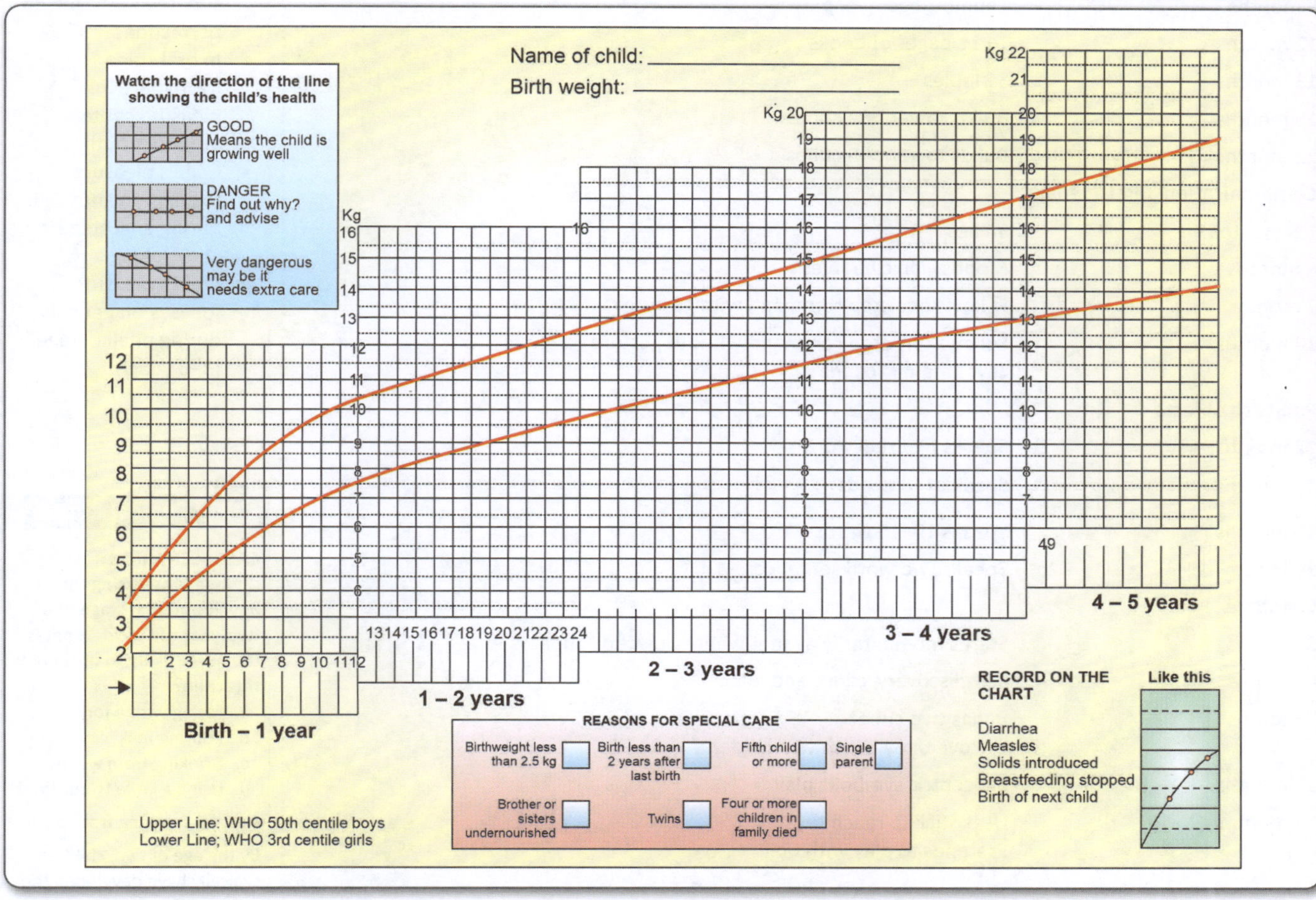

Figure 3: Growth chart

MILESTONES

Table 6: Milestones according to the age

Age in months	Milestones
Gross motor	
2 months	Holds Head steady while sitting
3 months	No head lag Self-discovery of hands
4 months	Asymmetric tonic neck reflex disappears
6 months	Sits without support
6.5 months	Roll back to stomach

Contd...

KEY POINT

Growth charts consist of a series of percentile curves that illustrate the distribution of selected body measurements in children.

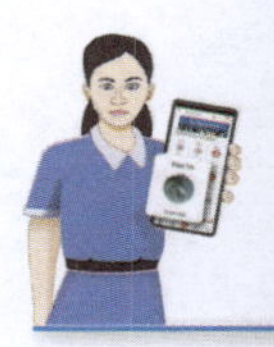

Age in months	Milestones
12 months	Walks alone
16 months	Runs
Fine motor	
3.5 months	Grasps rattle
4 months	Palmer grasps disappears Reaches for objects
5.5 months	Objects are transferred from hand to hand
8 months	Thumb-finger grasp
12 months	Turns pages of books
13 months	Scribbles
15 months	Builds tower of 2 cubes
22 months	Builds tower of 6 cubes
Communication and Language	
1.5 months	Smiles
6 months	Monosyllabic babbles
7 months	Follows one step command with gesture
10 months	Follows one step command without gesture Says "mama" or "dada"
Points to objects	
12 months	Speaks first real word
15 months	Speaks 4–6 words
18 months	Speaks 10–15 words
19 months	Speaks two word sentences
Cognitive	
2 months	Stares momentarily at spot where object disappears
4 months	Self-discovery, cause and effect
8 months	Bangs two cubes Uncovers toy which was hidden
12 months	Egocentric symbolic play
17 months	Uses stick to reach toy Pretends to play with doll

THEORIES OF GROWTH AND DEVELOPMENT

Psychosexual Development (Sigmund Freud)

- Defined the terms Id, Ego and Superego
- Id is pleasure principle, ego is based on reality and superego is based on perfection.
- Freud considered sexual instinct to be significant in personality development.
- During childhood certain regions of the body assume a prominent psychological significance as the source of pleasure and new conflicts gradually shift from one part of the body to another at particular stage of development
- Birth to 1 year (Oral stage): Infant's pleasure centers on mouth
- 1-3 years (Anal stage): Child's pleasure focuses on anus
- 3–6 years (Phallic stage): Child's pleasure focuses on genitals
- 6 years to puberty (Latency stage): Child represses sexual interest and develops social and intellectual skills
- Puberty to death (Genital stage): A time of sexual re-awakening; source of sexual pleasure becomes someone outside of the family.

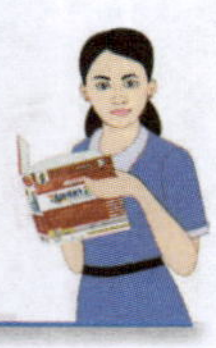

KEY POINTS

- Sigmund Freud's psychosexual development defined the terms Id, Ego and Superego.
- Id is pleasure principle; ego is based on reality and superego is based on perfection.
- In oral stage (0–1 year), infant's pleasure centers around mouth.
- Child's pleasure focuses on anus during anal stage (1–3 years).
- Child's pleasure focuses on genitals during phallic stage (3–6 years).

Clinical Corner

CASE SCENARIO 1:

A nurse is assessing the developmental stage of a two-year-old child. What is the nurse likely to observe in this child?

a. Eating with a fork
b. Pouring milk into a cup
c. Drinking from a cup
d. Using a knife to cut food

Ans. (c) Drinking from a cup

By the age of two, children typically have developed the motor skills necessary to hold and use a cup for drinking. They can usually handle a sippy cup or a regular cup with some assistance. This milestone represents an important step in their self-feeding and self-care abilities.

Using a fork to eat and using a knife for cutting food are skills that typically develop later.

Psychosocial Development [Erikson]

- Erikson described eight stages of development
- Each stage is characterized by a psychosocial crisis, representing a conflict between the individual and society
- The progression to the next stage depends on the resolution of these conflicts
- Out of eight stages only five are related to the childhood.

Erikson's Stages of Personality Development

For details of Erikson's stages of personality development please "Refer Synopsis of Psychiatric Nursing"

Moral Development (Lawrence Kohlberg)

- Moral development is based on cognitive development theory.
- It consists of three major levels (preconventional, conventional and postconventional) each with two distinct stages.
- Kohlberg's theory allows for prediction of behavior, but pays little attention to individual differences.

Spiritual Development (James W Fowler)

- Related to the moral and ethical portion of children's self–concepts.
- Fowler (1974) has identified 7 stages in development of faith, five of which are parallel and closely associated with cognitive and psychosocial development in childhood.

Stages

- **Stage 0:** Undifferentiated
- **Stage 1:** Intuitive—projective faith
- **Stage 2:** Mythical—literal faith
- **Stage 3:** Synthetic—convention
- **Stage 4:** Individuating—reflective
- **Stage 5:** Conjunctive
- **Stage 6:** Universalizing

Development of Logical Thinking (Jean Piaget)

Piaget believed that there are four stages in the development of logical thinking.

- **Birth to 2 years of age (Sensorimotor stage):** The infant constructs an understanding of the world by coordinating sensory experiences with physical actions: progressing from reflexive, instinctual action at birth to the beginning of symbolic thought towards end of the stage.
- **2–7 years of age (Preoperational stage):** The child begins to represent the world with words and images. These words and images reflect increased symbolic thinking and go beyond the connection of sensory information and physical action.
- **7–11 years of age (Concrete operational stage):** The child can now reason logically about concrete events and classify objects into different sets.
- **11–15 years of age through adulthood (Formal operational stage):** The adolescent reasons in more abstract idealistic and logical ways.

ESSENTIAL NEWBORN CARE

Neonates

Neonates are babies who all are less than 28 days after birth. In India, current neonatal mortality rate is 23 per 1000 live births. (2018, SRS report)

Early neonatal period: first 7 days of life

Late neonatal period: 7th to 28 days of life

Term normal neonate: Baby born between 37–42 weeks of gestation and weighing more than 2500 g.

Preterm neonate: Baby born before 37 completed weeks irrespective of birth weight.

Post term neonate: Baby born after 42 weeks of gestation irrespective of birth weight.

Low birth weight: Baby weighing less than 2500 g irrespective of gestational age.

Very low birth weight: Baby weighing less than 1500 g at birth.

Extremely low birth weight: Baby weighing less than 1000 g at birth.

Small for gestational age: Neonate weighing less than 10th centile.

APGAR Scoring

- A quantitative method to assess newborn's respiratory, circulatory and neurological status.
- Introduced by Dr Virginia Apgar (1952).
- The score is taken at one minute and five minutes after neonate birth.

KEY POINT

Injection vitamin K is routinely administered to a newborn to prevent bleeding.

Recent Questions (AIIMS 2020)

7. According to psychosocial theory of Erikson, which behavior is seen in toddler age group?
a. Autonomy vs. shame
b. Generativity vs. stagnation
c. Ego integrity vs. despair
d. Trust vs. mistrust
Ans. (a) Autonomy...

8. When does the posterior fontanel close in the baby?
a. 2 to 3 months
b. 2 to 3 years
c. 2 to 3 weeks
d. 2 to 3 days
Ans. (a) 2 to 3 months

Recent Questions (NORCET 2020)

9. After 2 hours of birth, baby has acrocyanosis. What should the nurse do?
a. Inform to physician
b. Intubate the infant
c. Document the finding
d. Give oxygen
Ans. (c) Document the...

10. What is the normal neonatal heart rate?
a. 120-160 BPM
b. 100-120 BPM
c. 160-200 BPM
d. 80-100 BPM
Ans. (a) 120-160 BPM

11. A nurse was giving instruction to a postpartum mother of a newborn with hyperbilirubinemia. Which of the following is an appropriate instruction?
a. Withhold breastfeeding if phototherapy is continued
b. Substitute breastfeeding with formula feeding
c. Continuous breastfeeding every second hourly
d. Routine supplementary feeds are recommended
Ans. (c) Continuous...

APGAR Scoring System

Table 7: APGAR system of scoring

	0 Points	1 Point	2 Points	Total points
Activity (muscle tone)	Absent	Arms and legs flexed	Active movement	
Pulse	Absent	Below 100 bpm	Over 100 bpm	
Grimace (reflex irritability)	Flaccid	Some flexion of Extremities	Active motion (sneeze, cough, pull away)	
Appearance (skin color)	Blue, pale	Body pink, Extremities blue	Completely pink	
Respiration	Absent	Slow, irregular	Vigorous cry	

Severely depressed	0–3
Moderately depressed	4–6
Excellent condition	7–10

Recent Question (CNCI 2021)

12. Cord clamping is delayed by 1-3 minutes in neonates because:
a. Prevents anemia in women
b. Placenta separates easily
c. Prevents jaundice in neonate
d. Neonate gets cord blood

Ans. (d) Neonate gets...

KEY POINTS

- APGAR score is considered excellent if the score is 7-10.
- While assessing APGAR, pulse or heart rate has to be assessed first and then the respirations.

Assessment of Gestational Age

- The **Ballard maturational assessment/Ballard score/Ballard scale** is a commonly used technique of gestational assessment.
- Developed in 1979.
- Criteria used for the assessment of gestational age is divided into two categories, **physical and neurological criteria.**
- Scoring provides the estimation of gestational age ranging from 20 to 44 weeks.
- It can be used up to 4 days after birth (in practice, the **Ballard score** is usually used in the first 24 hours).

Recent Question (INC PhD 2020)

13. APGAR score 8 means
a. Severely depressed
b. Moderately depressed
c. Thermoregulation is not good
d. Adapted with extrauterine life

Ans. (d) Adapted with...

Table 8: Components of physical and neuromuscular maturity in Ballard scale

Physical Maturity	Neuromuscular maturity
Skin	Posture
Lanugo	Square window (wrist)
Plantar surface	Arm recoil
Breast	Popliteal angle
Eye/ear	Scarf sign
Genitals	Heel to ear

Neonatal Reflexes

Table 9: Reflexes of a normal neonate

Reflexes	Stimulation	Response	Duration
Blinking	Flash of light or puff of air	Closes eyes	Permanent
Rooting	Cheek stroked or side of mouth touched	Turns toward source, opens mouth and sucks	Disappears at 3–4 months
Sucking	Mouth touched by object	Sucks on object	Disappears at three to four months
Grasping	Palms touched	Grasps tightly	Fully developed at 32-week POG. Disappears at 6 months of age.
Tonic neck	Placed on back	Makes fists and turns head to the right	Fully developed at 1 month and disappears during 4-6 months
Stepping	Infant held upright with feet touching ground	Moves feet as if to walk	Disappears at 3–4 months
Swimming	Placed face down in water	Makes coordinated swimming movements	Disappears at 6–7 months

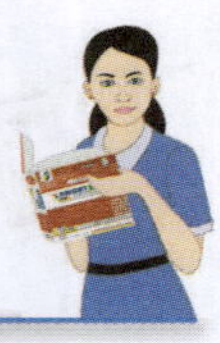

Contd...

Reflexes	Stimulation	Response	Duration
Babinski	Sole of foot stroked	Fans out toes and twists foot and is known as positive Babinski which is considered as normal in children and abnormal in adult	Disappears at 9 months to 1 year
Moro	Sudden move; loud noise	Startles; throws out arms and legs and then pulls them toward body	Disappears at 6 months
Startle	Sudden loud noise or trapping the sternum	Elbow flexed, hand remains closed	Disappears at 4-6 months
Magnet	Child is supine examiner's finger pushed against sole of foot, and the knee and hip flex and finger is withdrawn	Follows the finger	
Parachute	While on ventral suspension with sudden change of equilibrium	Causes extension of hands and legs	Never disappear
Landau	While in prone position, trunk is being supported	Baby exhibit some muscle tone	Disappears by 6-9 months
Trunk incurvation (Galant reflex)	In prone position and the paravertebral area is stimulated	It causes flexion of the trunk and swings his pelvis toward the touch	Disappears by 4 months

Neonatal Seizure

- Most common type: Subtle seizure
- Least common type and worst prognostic seizure: Myoclonic seizure
- Best prognostic seizure: Focal clonic
- Most common cause of seizure is hypoxia
- Drug of choice for neonatal seizure is phenobarbitone
- Most common cause of seizure among preterm babies: intraventricular hemorrhage.
- Vitamin deficiency of vitamin B6 (pyridoxine) is responsible for neonatal seizure.

THERMOREGULATION IN NEWBORN

Warm Chain

Set of interlinked procedures carried out during birth and following days to prevent heat loss.

Components of Warm Chain

- Warm delivery room
- Warm resuscitation
- Immediate drying
- Skin to skin contact
- Breastfeeding
- Bath postponed
- Appropriate clothing
- Mother and baby together
- Professional alertness
- Warm transportation

Hypothermia

Axillary temperature is less than 36.5°C .

Mild Hypothermia

- Temperature: 36°C–36.4°C
- Baby has warm trunk and cold extremities
- Extremities are cold and bluish in color
- Lethargy and poor weight gain

Management

- Skin-to-skin contact with caregiver if possible
- Keep the baby in close contact with caregiver
- Cover the baby adequately
- Ensure room is warm
- Provide warmth
- Encourage breastfeeding

Moderate Hypothermia

- Temperature: 32°C–35.9°C
- Baby has cold trunk and cold extremities
- Poor sucking and feeding, lethargy, weak cry, fast breathing

Management

- Cover mother and baby together using prewarmed clothes
- Provide warmth
- Vitamin K injection for newborn babies if not given earlier
- Reassess after 15 minutes, if temperature does not improve provide additional heat
- Encourage breastfeeding

Severe Hypothermia

- Temperature <32°C
- Baby has cold trunk and cold extremities
- Lethargic baby, poor perfusion and mottling, slow heart rate, hardening of skin with redness and edema, bleeding, low blood sugar

KEY POINTS

- Plantar grasp disappears in infant around 9–12 months of age. It is the last neonatal reflex to disappear.
- The last neonatal reflex to emerge is rooting reflex. It develops at around 28–30 weeks of gestational age.
- Rooting reflex in infant disappears at 3–4 months.
- Asymmetric Moro's reflex at birth is indicative of Kernicterus.

KEY POINTS

The sequence of vital signs assessment in newborn is Respiratory Rate, Pulse and Temperature.

- A newborn's temperature on an average ranges from 36.5°–37.5°C.
- Immediately after the delivery baby should be placed on mother's chest.

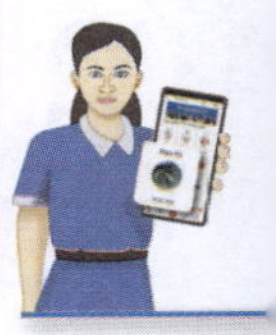

Management

- Rapid rewarming till baby is 34°C and then slow rewarming
- Oxygen administration
- IV fluids (warm dextrose)
- Injection of vitamin K
- Reassess after 15 minutes

How newborns keep themselves warm?

- Universal flexion
- Vasoconstriction caused by sympathetic surge
- Increased heart rate which supplies more oxygen
- Brown fat in the body which helps in non-shivering thermogenesis.

Mechanisms of Heat Loss

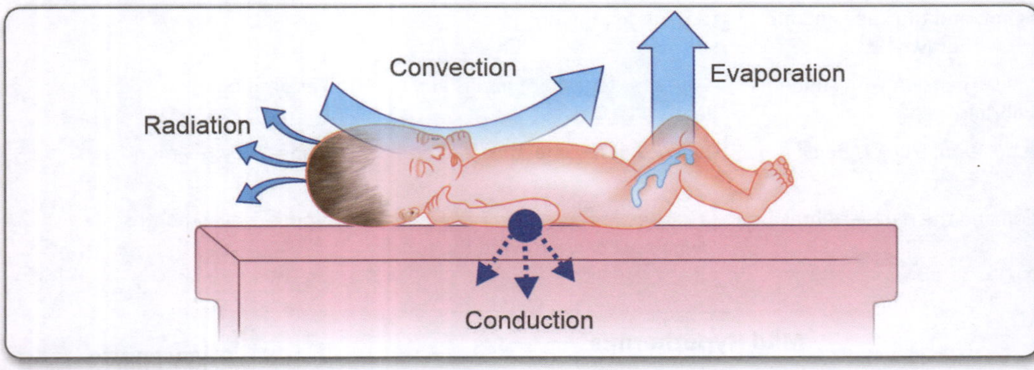

Figure 4: Mechanisms of heat loss

Table 10: Heat loss mechanism along with their description and nursing implications

Heat loss mechanism	Description	Nursing implications
Conduction	Heat loss occurs when body comes in direct contact with cooler objects.	• Put the child always on a prewarmed sheet • Cover the weighing scale and X-ray cassettes with sheet before coming in contact with the baby
Convection	Transfer of heat from body surface to cooler surrounding air.	• Avoid air current. • Manage high risk newborn babies inside incubator • Provide warm humidified oxygen.
Radiation	Heat loss occurs when the body emits infrared radiation. Heat transfer takes place without physical contact.	• Keep the baby's cot away from solid objects such as wall, almirah, etc. • Cover the baby.
Evaporation	Heat loss occurs when water evaporates from the skin.	• Keep baby dry • Dry the baby immediately after birth • Remove wet nappies

KANGAROO MOTHER CARE (KMC)

Special way of care for low-birth-weight babies by placing them on caregiver's chest between breast, which establishes skin to skin contact and promotes breastfeeding.

Components: Skin to skin contact and exclusive breastfeeding.

Kangaroo Mother Care (KMC) Procedure

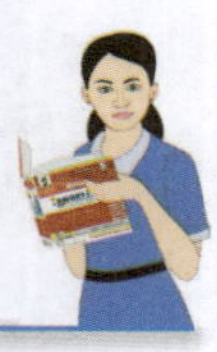

Positioning

- Place the baby between mother's breast in upright position
- Head turned to one side and slightly extended
- Hip flexed and abducted in frog position
- Baby's abdomen in mother's epigastrium
- Support baby's bottom
- KMC provider will be in semi-reclining position to prevent GERD in the infant.

Purposes

- It is very useful for low birth weight babies.
- It helps them to gain weight, increase feeding, reduce incidence of infection and respiratory complications.
- It promotes breastfeeding and mother-baby bonding.

Recent Question (NORCET 2023)

14. The expected SPO2 level in new-born in first 5 min is
a. 60–65
b. 70–75
c. 80–85
d. 90–95
Ans. (c) 80–85

Recent Question (NORCET 2021)

15. Premature babies have more chances of hypothermia because of all of the following, EXCEPT:
a. Cold environment
b. Less developed epidermis
c. Less brown fat
d. Small body surface area in comparison of weight
Ans. (d) Small body surface area in comparison of weight

Recent Question (NORCET 2023)

16. Which of the following is true about Kangaroo Mother care?
a. Exclusive breastfeeding, Early discharge, Belongingness
b. Exclusive breastfeeding, Early discharge, Prevention of Infection
c. Exclusive breastfeeding, Early discharge, Prevention of hypothermia
d. Exclusive breastfeeding, Early discharge, Supplementary nutrition
Ans. (c) Exclusive breastfeeding, Early discharge, Prevention of hypothermia

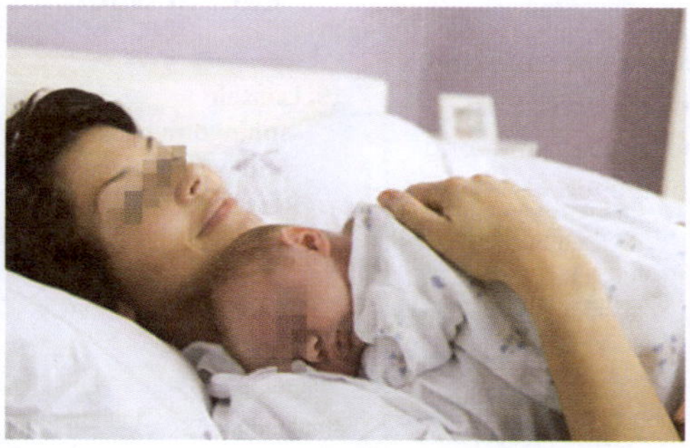

Figure 5: Kangaroo mother care

HIGH RISK NEWBORN

Low Birth Weight

Birth weight less than 2500 g is known as low birth weight.

Table 11: Classification of birth weight

Classification	Birth Weight
Low birth weight	<2500 g
Very low birth weight	<1500 g
Extremely low birth weight	<1000 g

Prematurity

A neonate born before 37 weeks of complete gestation is known as premature neonate.

Table 12: Differences between term and preterm baby

Characteristic	Term baby	Preterm baby
Posture	Fully flexed	Lies in relaxed attitude with limbs extended.
Size of head	Head and body are proportionate in size	Head is larger than body
Skin	More subcutaneous fat, less lanugo and covered with vernix caseosa	Less subcutaneous fat, abundant lanugo, and little amount of vernix caseosa
Ear	Well-developed and good recoil capacity	Not well-developed and recoil is poor
Sole	Deep sole creases are present	Sole is more turgid and has fine creases only.
Genitalia	Male: well-developed scrotum with descended testis. Female: well-developed labia majora which covers labia minora and clitoris.	Male: underdeveloped scrotum and is not pendulous and testis may be undescended. Female: poorly developed labia majora with labia minora and clitoris exposed.
Reflex	Well-developed reflexes	Sluggish reflexes.
Scarf sign	Elbow may be brought to the midline of the chest with resistance beyond midline	Elbow may be easily brought across the chest with less or no assistance
Heel to ear	Not possible to bring heel to ear	Heel can be easily brought to ear without any resistance.

Intra-uterine Growth Retardation

Table 13: Comparison between symmetrical IUGR and asymmetrical IUGR

Factor	Symmetrical IUGR	Asymmetrical IUGR
Time of insult	In the first trimester and in the early weeks of second trimester	In the 2nd and 3rd trimester
Etiology	TORCH infection Chromosomal abnormality Genetic issues	Medical and obstetrical issues of mother in the late trimester of pregnancy such as poor maternal nutrition, placental insufficiency, maternal hypertension.
Effect on cells	Fetal cell number decreased	Rather than number of cells, size of the cells is more affected.
Anthropometric parameters	All parameters such as head circumference, height and weight are equally affected	Head circumference affected
Ponderal index	≥2	<2
Brain: liver size	<5	>5
Prognosis	Poor	Better outcome

KEY POINTS

- KMC can be done by any family member who is free from infection.
- Each session should last for at least one hour.
- Newborns lose 10% of their birth weight by 3-4 days of age. Newborns gain the lost birth weight by 10th day of life.
- Normal birth weight of an Indian child is 2.5-3.5 kg.
- Baby's birth weight doubles at 5-6 months of age.
- Baby's birth weight triples at 1 year of age.
- LBW babies showing rapid catch up growth in infancy are at increased risk for developing coronary heart disease and hypertension in adult life and is known as **adult metabolic syndrome**.

Recent Questions (NORCET 2022)

17. A low birth weight baby is:
a. <1500 g
b. <500 g
c. <2500 g
d. <1000 g
Ans. (c) <2500 g

18. When does the child identify gender?
a. 3 years
b. 6 years
c. 7–8 years
d. At puberty
Ans. (a) 3 years

NEWBORN RESUSCITATION

Technique of Chest Compression

- **Thumb technique**: Two thumbs depress the sternum while hands encircle the torso.
- **Two finger techniques**: Tips of middle finger and index finger of one hand are used to compress the sternum while the other hand is used to support the baby's back.
- Thumb technique is preferred because it is less tiring and generates high peak systolic pressure and coronary perfusion pressure.
- Two finger technique is preferred to provide access to umbilicus for medication administration.

Site and Depth of Compression

- Compression provided at lower third of the sternum to a depth of one third of the anterio-posterior diameter.
- The site lies between the xiphoid and a line drawn between the nipples.

Rate of Compression

- 3:1 is the ratio between chest compression and breaths irrespective of the number of rescuers.
- One cycle consists of 3 compressions and one breath will take 2 seconds to complete.
- Total of 120 events (90 compressions and 30 breaths per minute) should be given.

Epinephrine

- Available concentration is 1:1000
- Dilute 1 mL of epinephrine with 9 mL of water for injection then volume is 10 mL and concentration is 1:10,000.
- Dilute 0.1 mL of epinephrine with 0.9 mL of water for injection then volume is 1 mL and concentration is 1:10,000.

Note: While providing PPV appropriate squeezing of bag will provide 40-60 breaths per minute.

Recent Questions (INC PhD 2020)

19. Lecithin -sphingomyelin ratio which suggests Respiratory Distress Syndrome is
a. <2
b. 2
c. >2
d. 2.5
Ans. (a) <2

20. Preterm babies are more prone to develop alveolar collapse because of
a. Low lung compliance
b. Lack of surfactant
c. Body surface area is more
d. Poor breathing capacity
Ans. (b) Lack of surfactant

21. Dosage of 1:10,000 adrenaline during pediatric resuscitation is:
a. 0.1–0.3 mL/kg
b. 0.2–0.5 mL/kg
c. 0.3–0.5 mL/kg
d. 0.4–0.6 mL/kg
Ans. (a) 0.1–0.3 mL/kg

KEY POINTS

- Immediate action by the nurse after the birth of a baby is to clear the mucus in nose and mouth that will help the baby to breathe.
- Lack of stridor and adventitious breath sounds are the signs of shaken baby syndrome.
- Total lung capacity in full term newborn is **150 mL**.

COMMON RESPIRATORY CONDITIONS IN NEWBORNS

Table 14: Respiratory conditions in newborns

Condition	Descriptions
Respiratory distress syndrome (RDS)	• Seen primarily in preterm infants due to a deficiency of surfactant in the lungs. • Often also called hyaline membrane disease • Typical appearance on the X-ray is termed as ground glass appearance. • Antenatal maternal administration of corticosteroids and exogenous surfactant therapy have revolutionized the management of RDS.
Chronic lung disease (CLD)	• Often called broncho-pulmonary dysplasia (BPD), it is the most common long-term respiratory consequence of prematurity. • CLD is defined as supplemental oxygen dependency for at least 28 days from birth, and at 36 weeks corrected gestational age
Transient tachypnea of newborn (TTN)	• TTN is a benign, self-limited condition that can present in infants of any gestational age, shortly after birth. • It is caused due to delay in the clearance of fetal lung fluid after birth which leads to ineffective gas exchange, respiratory distress, and tachypnea.
Persistent pulmonary hypertension of newborn (PPHN)	• PPHN is often secondary to parenchymal lung disease or lung hypoplasia but can also be idiopathic. • It is characterized by elevated pulmonary vascular resistance, resulting in right-to-left shunting of blood and hypoxemia.
Meconium aspiration syndrome (MAS)	• The healthy fetus does not normally pass meconium in utero. • Fetal distress, usually during labor, can cause the fetus to pass meconium into the amniotic fluid before delivery. • As a physiological response to worsening fetal distress, the fetus attempts gasping respiratory effort. During such gasps, the fetus may inhale meconium-stained liquor into the lungs. • The inhaled meconium adversely affects the lung.

Contd...

Recent Question (NORCET 2023)

22. Ratio of chest compression to ventilation/Minute in neonates?
a. 90:30
b. 3:1
c. 15:2
d. 30:2
Ans. (a) 90:30

Condition	Descriptions
Pneumothorax	• Leak of air from the lungs into the pleural cavity. • Underlying respiratory disease (RDS) and positive pressure ventilation, are associated with increased risk of developing a pneumothorax in a newborn.
Congenital diaphragmatic hernia (CDH)	• A developmental failure of the diaphragm during its embryological formation allows herniation of abdominal organs into the chest affecting lung growth and alveolar development.

Silverman-Andersen Retraction Scoring

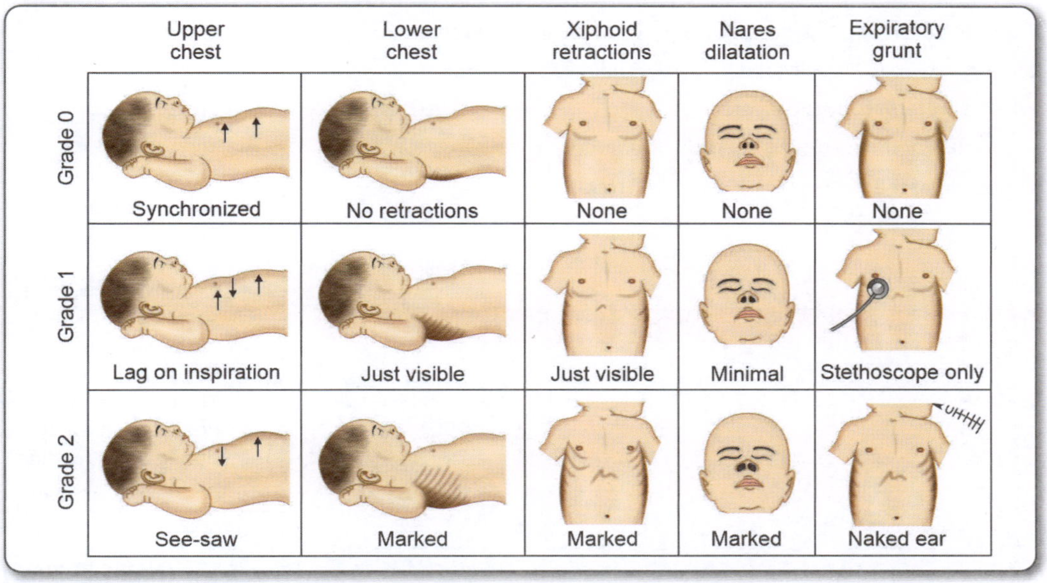

Interpretation

Table 15: Silverman-Andersen score and interpretation

Score	Interpretation
0-3	Mild respiratory distress
4-6	Moderate respiratory distress
>6	Impending respiratory distress
10	Severe respiratory distress

Gastric Shake Test

- 0.5 mL of gastric fluid is mixed with equal volume of NS and then with 95% ethanol and the mixture is agitated for 15 sec.
- After standing for 15 min, the air-liquid interface was examined for bubbles.
- If no bubbles are present, then the test is NEGATIVE (very little surfactant is present).
- If bubbles are present right across the surface of the fluid, then the test is POSITIVE (adequate amounts of surfactant).

FEEDING IN CHILDREN

Nutritional management influences immediate survival of as well as subsequent growth and development of low birth weight (LBW) infants.

Table 16: Feeding in children according to birth weight

Birth weight	Preferred method of feeding
<1250 g	Baby may need I/V fluids initially, then initiate orogastric feeding gradually
1250–1500 g	Most would need spoon/paladai while some need orogastric feeding
1501–2000 g	Most babies would accept breastfeeding while some might need paladai feeding
>2000 g	Breastfeed in normal birth weight baby, but with monitoring

KEY POINTS

- Silverman score is used to assess respiratory distress in preterm neonate.
- The maximum score in Silverman score is 10.
- Human milk contains little iron, so infants who are exclusively breastfed are at increased risk of iron deficiency after four months of age. This is more common among preterm infants as they are born with lower iron stores.
- A newborn who is adequately breastfed will sleep at least 2 hours, pass urine 8 to 10 times a day and will gain weight.
- Expressed breast milk can be stored at room temperature for up to 4 hours.
- Cow's milk is deficient of iron.
- Bottle-fed babies are more prone to develop diarrhea.

KEY POINTS

Signs of good attachment while breastfeeding

- Babies mouth should be wide open.
- Baby's chin touching mother's breast.
- Lower lip turned outward.
- More areola visible above than below.

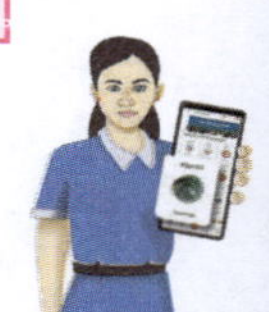

Breastfeeding

Frequency of Feeds

- First few weeks: 8–12 times a day during first few weeks
- Demand feeding: 1–4 hours as per demand
- By 9–12 months: 3–5 meals

Composition of Breast Milk

Table 17: Composition of breast milk

Types of breast milk	Time	Appearance
Colostrum	3-4 days after birth	Yellowish and thick
Transitional milk	4 days to 10–14 days	Thinner, lighter in color
Mature milk	2 weeks after baby is delivered	Thinner
Preterm milk	When a preterm baby is delivered	
Foremilk	At the start of the feed	Watery
Hind milk	At the end of the feed	Thick

Nutrients in Breast Milk

Table 18: Nutrients content in breast milk

Component	Content/100 mL
Calories	71 kcal
Carbohydrates	7 g
Proteins	1.1 g
Fat	3.8–4.2 g
Lactose	7.0 g
Sodium	0.9 mEq/L
Potassium	1.4 mEq/L
Calcium	34 mg
Phosphorous	15 mg
Iron	0.05–0.1 mg/L
Zinc	120 microgram
Vitamin A	170–670 IU
Vitamin C	5.2–10 mg
Vitamin D	0.5–10 IU
Vitamin E	0.56 microgram
Vitamin K	1.5 microgram
Water	88%
Protective factors	IgA, IgG, IgM, Bifidus factor, Lactoferrin, Lysozyme, Para-aminobenzoic acid

IMMUNIZATION

Active immunity: Protective response occurs following exposure to infectious agent or administration of live or killed vaccine or toxoid.

Passive immunity: Providing immunity by direct administration of antibodies in the form of immunoglobulin.

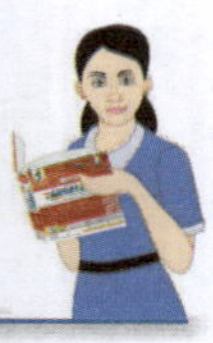

KEY POINTS

- The first milk produced after delivery is known as Colostrum. It appears thick and yellow colored.
- Milk secreted following colostrum is transition milk.
- Foremilk (milk secreted at the start of feed) is rich in proteins, sugar and minerals whereas hindmilk is rich in fat and provides more energy.
- Immunoglobulin present in breast milk is IgA.
- Exclusive breastfeed should be provided to the baby up to 6 months.
- The extra calories needed by mother during breastfeeding is 500 calories.

(NORCET 2023)

Vastus lateralis is the best choice for IM injection in infants and younger children.

Recent Question (NORCET 2020)

23. Which of the following is the first discovered vaccine?
a. Chicken Pox
b. Rabies
c. Small pox
d. H1NI Flu

Ans. (c) Small pox

Recent Question (NORCET 2023)

24. The preferred muscle site of IM injection in case of pediatrics immunization is:
a. Vastus lateralis
b. Deltoid
c. Dorsogluteal
d. Ventro gluteal

Ans. (a) Vastus lateralis

Types of Vaccines

Table 19: Vaccines and their types

Types of vaccines	Description
Live attenuated vaccine	Prepared from live organism to produce immune response mimicking natural infection. **E.g.:** BCG, oral typhoid, MMR, measles, mumps, rotavirus, varicella, yellow fever
Killed vaccine	Organism is inactivated and able to produce immune response without causing infection. **E.g.:** DPT, IPV, Rabies, Hepatitis A
Toxoids	Toxins produced by certain organisms are detoxified and used as vaccine. **E.g.:** Diphtheria, tetanus
Subunit vaccine	They are made by isolating a specific protein or antigen from the pathogen and using it to stimulate an immune response. These vaccines contain only those parts of the pathogen which are necessary to elicit an immune response, and do not contain any live or inactivated virus or bacteria. **E.g.: Hep b vaccine, HPV vaccine**
Recombinant vaccines	They are made by using genetic engineering techniques to produce a protein or antigen that is identical or similar to the one found in the pathogen. **E.g.: Human Papillomavirus Vaccine (HPV), Shingles Vaccine**
Polysaccharide vaccines	Polysaccharide vaccines are a type of vaccine that contains sugars (polysaccharides) that are found on the surface of certain bacteria. These sugars can trigger an immune response in the body, leading to the production of antibodies. **E.g.: Pneumococcal conjugate vaccine (PCV)**

Recent Question (AIIMS 2020)

25. With which of the following, the "Indradhanush scheme" is associated with?
a. Immunization
b. Sanitation
c. Mid-day meal program
d. All of the above

Ans. (a) Immunization

Clinical Corner

CASE SCENARIO 2:
An infant developed redness and swelling at the injection site after receiving a diphtheria, tetanus, and acellular pertussis (DTaP) vaccine at PHC. The patient contacted the community health nurse and reported the problem. Which intervention should the nurse suggest to the parent?
a. Advise the patient to monitor the infant for a fever
b. Instruct the parent to bring the infant back to the clinic
c. Advise the parent to apply a hot pack to the injection site
d. Advise the parent to apply a cold pack to the injection site

Ans. (d) Advise the parent to apply a cold pack to the injection site

Immunization Schedule

Table 20: Immunization schedule

Vaccine	Age	Dose	Route	Site
For pregnant women				
Tetanus and adult Diphtheria (Td) -1	Early in pregnancy	0.5 mL	Intramuscular	Upper arm
Td-2	4 weeks after Td-1*	0.5 mL	Intramuscular	Upper arm
Td- Booster	If received 2 TT/Td doses in a pregnancy within the last 3 years	0.5 mL	Intramuscular	Upper arm
For Infants				
BCG	At birth or as early as possible till one year of age	0.1 mL (0.05 mL until 1 month age)	Intradermal	Left upper arm
Hepatitis B - Birth	At birth or as early as possible within 24 hours	0.5 mL	Intramuscular	Anterolateral side of mid-thigh
OPV-0	At birth or as early as possible within the first 15 days	2 drops	Oral	Oral
OPV 1, 2 and 3	At 6 weeks, 10 weeks and 14 weeks (OPV can be given till 5 years of age)	2 drops	Oral	Oral

Vaccine	Age	Dose	Route	Site
Pentavalent 1, 2 and 3[‡]	At 6 weeks, 10 weeks and 14 weeks (can be given till one year of age)	0.5 mL	Intramuscular	Anterolateral side of mid-thigh
Pneumococcal Conjugate Vaccine(PCV)	Two primary doses at 6 and 14 weeks followed by booster dose at 9-12 months	0.5 mL	Intra-muscular	Anterolateral side of mid-thigh
Rotavirus[#]	At 6 weeks, 10 weeks and 14 weeks (can be given till one year of age)	5 drops	Oral	Oral
IPV	Two fractional dose at 6 and 14 weeks of age	0.1 mL	Intradermal two fractional dose	Intradermal right upper arm
Measles /MR 1st Dose	9 completed months-12 months. (can be given till 5 years of age)	0.5 mL	Subcutaneous	Right upper arm
JE - 1**	9 completed months-12 months.	0.5 mL	Subcutaneous (Live attenuated vaccine) Intramuscular (Killed vaccine) aspect of mid thigh (Killed vaccine)	Left upper arm (Live attenuated vaccine) Anterolateral aspect of mid thigh (Killed vaccine)
Vitamin A (1st dose)	At 9 completed months with measles-Rubella	1 mL (1 lakh IU)	Oral	Oral
For Children				
DPT booster-1	16–24 months	0.5 mL	Intramuscular	Anterolateral side of mid-thigh
Measles/MR 2nd dose[†]	16–24 months	0.5 mL	Subcutaneous	Right upper arm
OPV Booster	16–24 months	2 drops	Oral	Oral
JE-2	16–24 months	0.5 mL	Subcutaneous (Live attenuated vaccine) Intramuscular (Killed vaccine) aspect of mid thigh (Killed vaccine)	Left upper arm (Live attenuated vaccine) Anterolateral aspect of mid thigh (Killed vaccine)
Vitamin A*** (2nd to 9th dose)	16–18 months. Then one dose every 6 months up to the age of 5 years.	2 mL (2 lakh IU)	Oral	Oral
DPT Booster-2nd	5–6 years	0.5 mL	Intramuscular	Upper arm
Td	10 years and 16 years	0.5 mL	Intramuscular	Upper arm

*Give TT-2 Booster doses before 36 weeks of pregnancy. However, give these even if more than 36 weeks have passed. Give TT to a woman in labor, if she has not previously received TT

**JE Vaccine is introduced in select endemic districts after the campaign.

***The 2nd to 9th doses of Vitamin A can be administered to children 1–5 years old during biannual rounds, in collaboration with ICDS.

[#]Phased introduction, at present in Andhra Pradesh, Haryana, Himachal Pradesh and Odisha from 2016 and expanded in Madhya Pradesh, Assam, Rajasthan, and Tripura in February 2017 and planned in Tamil Nadu and Uttar Pradesh in 2017.

[†]Phased introduction, at present in five states namely Karnataka, Tamil Nadu, Goa, Lakshadweep and Puducherry (As of Feb' 2017)

[‡]Pentavalent vaccine: Provides protection against Diphtheria, Pertussis, Tetanus, Hepatitis B and Hemophilus influenza type B.

Recent Question (NORCET 2022)

26. Vaccine given at birth, except:

a. BCG
b. OPV
c. Hepatitis B
d. IPV

Ans. (d) IPV

Recent Question (NORCET 2023)

27. If child has done routine immunization of DPT and after giving injection it develops fever, swelling over the vaccine site then what should be the nurse's advice to parents

a. It is normal reaction nothing to do
b. It is mild reaction tell them to bring to the clinic
c. Tell to withhold next dose of DPT
d. Refer child to emergency

Ans. (a) it is normal reaction nothing to do

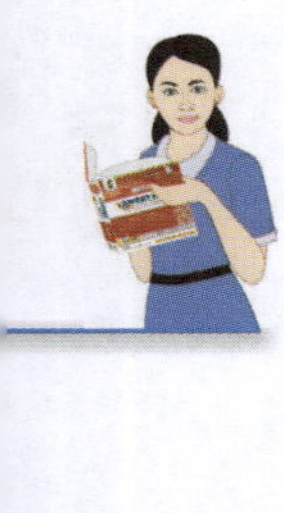

Catch up Vaccinations

- Catch-up vaccination refers to a vaccination schedule that is designed to help individuals who may have missed one or more doses of a vaccine "catch up" and receive the full recommended course of immunization.
  E.g.: BCG vaccination up to 1 year of age (according to NIS) and up to 5 years of age (according to IAP).

Table 21: Side effect and contraindications of vaccines

Vaccine	Side effects	Contraindications
Oral Polio Vaccine (OPV)	Paralytic polio, vaccine derived polio virus	Immunocompromised
BCG	Axillary lymphadenitis, cervical lymphadenopathy (if given vis S/C route), ulceration, infection.	Immunocompromised
Rota virus (oral)	Intussusception, irritability, diarrhea, vomiting	Egg allergy, GBS
Measles	Toxic shock syndrome	Immunocompromised
DPT	Persistent cry, hyperpyrexia, seizure, encephalopathy.	Progressive neurological disorder, encephalopathy, anaphylaxisis.

Cold Chain

Cold chain is the system of transporting and storing vaccines at recommended temperature from the point of manufacture to the point of use.

Cold Chain Equipment

Table 22: Cold chain equipment

Equipment	Description
Walk-in coolers	• Used for bulk storage of vaccine at state and regional levels. • Maintain temperature between 2 and 8° C.
Deep freezer	• It has a top opening lid which maintains temperature between –15 and –25°C. • Utilized for storing OPV (district level and above) and for freezing ice packs at PHC level.
Ice lined refrigerator	• These are top opening refrigerators because they can hold cold air better than front open refrigerators. • It has bottom and top sections. Bottom or section A is the coolest part. • Top or section B maintains temperature between 2°C and 8°C. • All vaccines are kept in the basket inside the ILR. • OPV and measles can be kept in the bottom of the basket while BCG, DPT, DT, TT are kept in the upper part of the basket.
Cold boxes	• These insulated boxes are used for transportation of vaccine and to store vaccine and ice packs in emergency. • Before placing vaccine in the cold box, conditioned ice pack should be placed at bottom and side of the cold box. • Vaccine should be placed in a carton or polythene bag and then placed inside the cold box. • Vials of DPT, DT, TT and Hep B should not be placed in the direct contact with ice packs. These vaccines should be surrounded by OPV/BCG/Measles vaccine.
Vaccine carriers	• Used for carrying small quantities of vaccine (16-20 vials) to the subcenters or to session site. • Four ice packs are laid in the vaccine carrier.

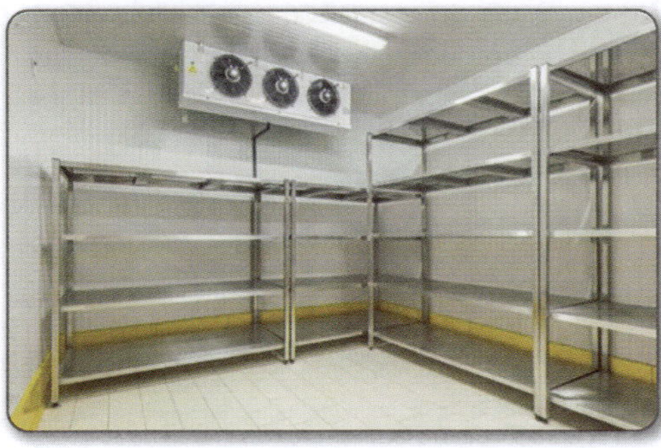
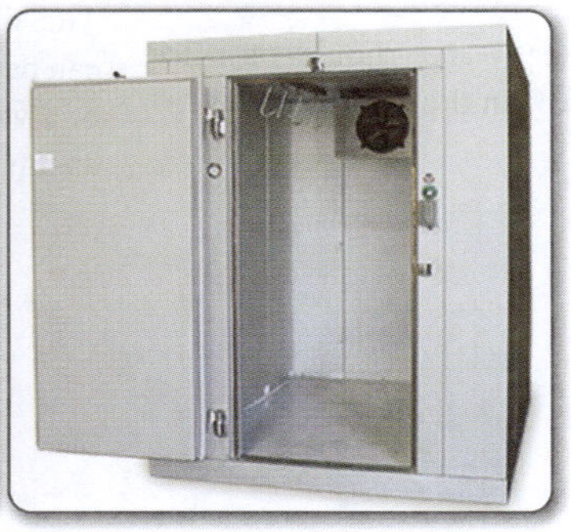

Walk-in cooler

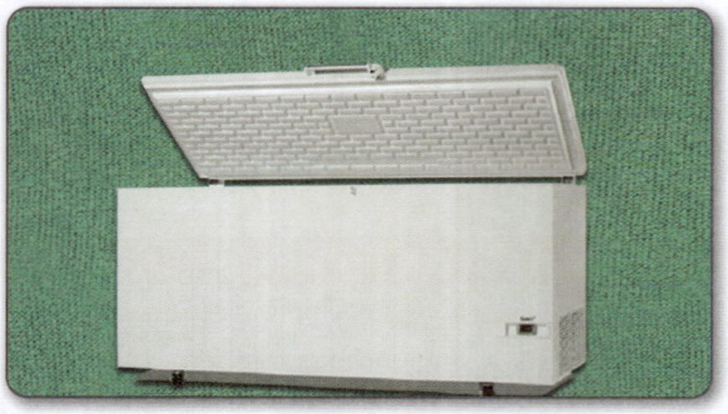

Deep freezer

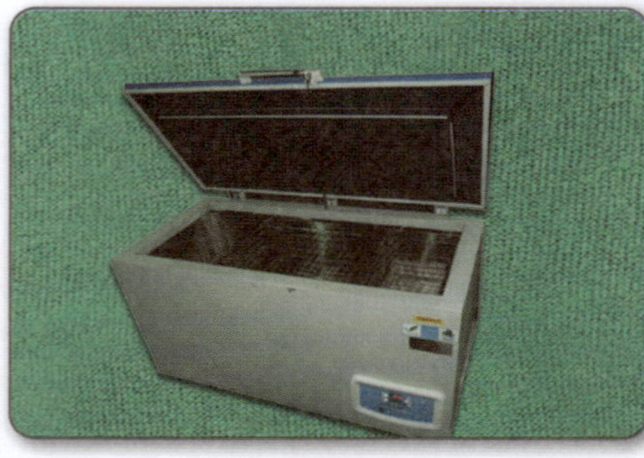

Ice-lined refrigerator

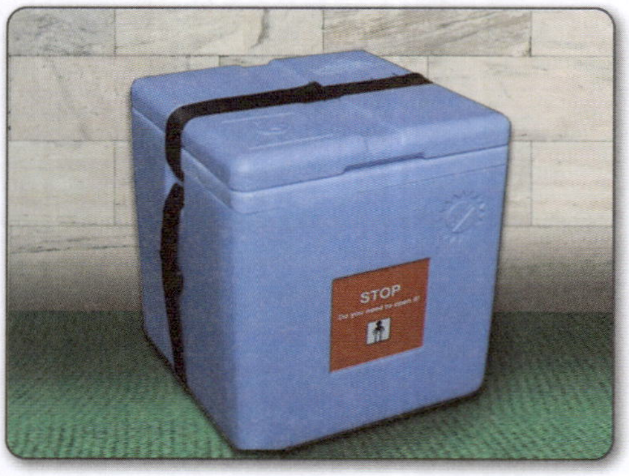

Cold boxes

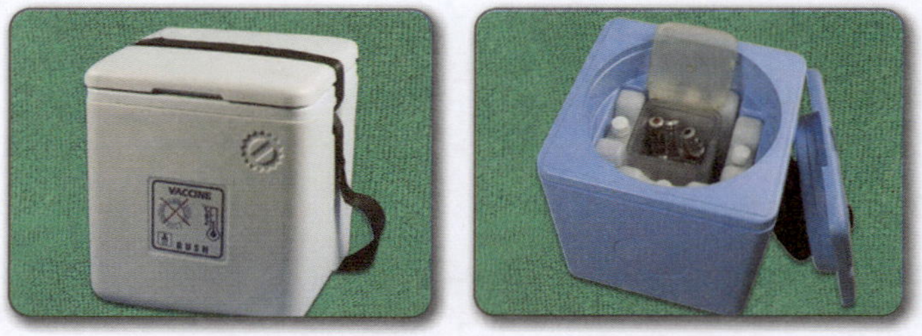

Vaccine carriers

Ice Packs

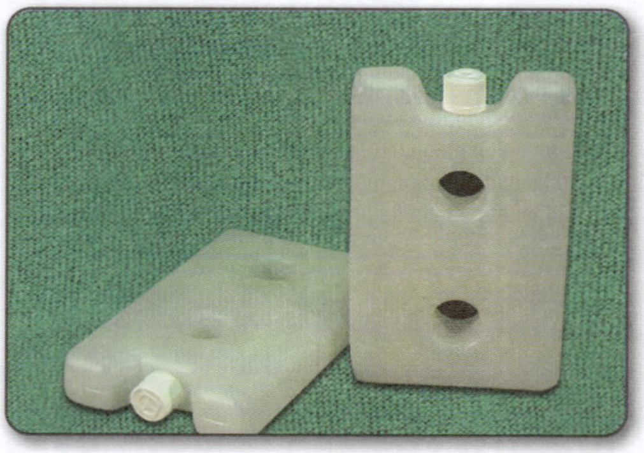

- These are frozen inside the deep freezer under the temperature range of -15 to -25°C.
- Ice packs contain water. Water should be filled only up to the level mark on the side.
- **Salt should not be added** to the water as it lowers the temperature to sub-zero level.

Vaccine Vial Monitoring (VVM)

A vaccine vial monitor (VVM) is a label containing a heat sensitive material which is placed on a vaccine vial to register cumulative heat exposure over time. The combined effects of time and temperature cause the inner square of the VVM to darken, gradually and irreversibly. A direct relationship exists between the rate of color change and temperature:

- The lower the temperature, the slower the color change.
- The higher the temperature, the faster the color change.

The VVM is a circle with a small square inside it. It can be printed on a product label, attached to the cap of a vaccine vial or tube, or attached to the neck of an ampoule.

Recent Questions (NORCET 2020)

28. In which of the following vaccine cold chain must be maintained

a. Killed Vaccine
b. Live vaccine
c. Toxoids
d. Serums

Ans. (b) Live vaccine

29. Which of the following vaccine should not be frozen and it should be discarded if frozen?

a. OPV
b. Measles
c. DPT
d. MMR

Ans. (c) DPT

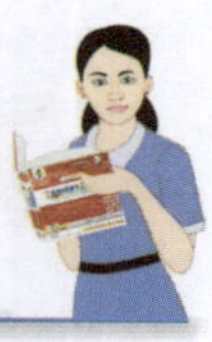

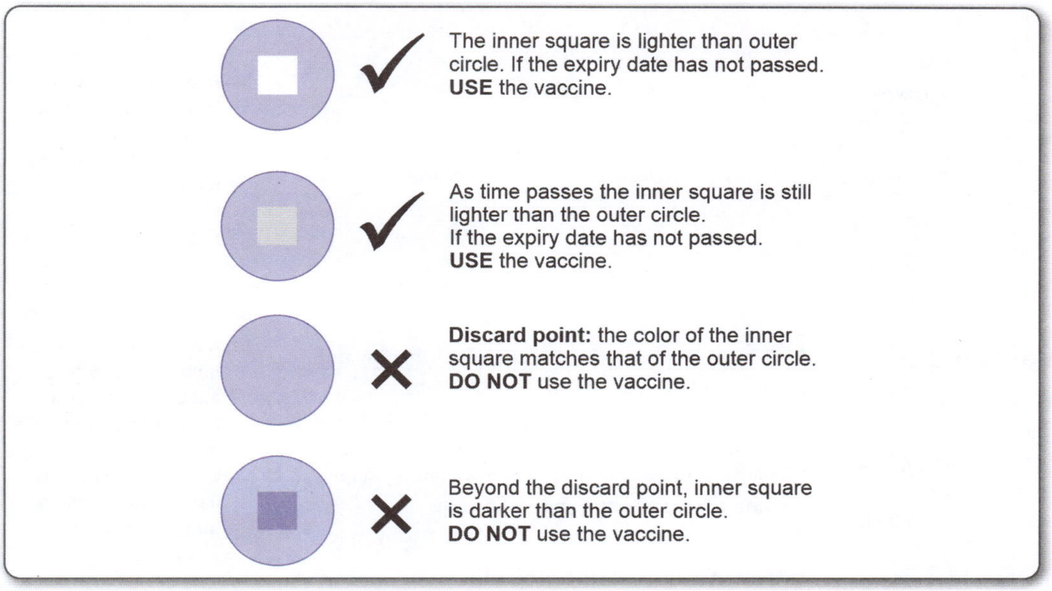

KEY POINTS

- Oral Poliovirus (OPV) and measles are sensitive to heat and can be frozen without harm.
- DTP vaccine should be stored at **4°-8°C**.

UNDER-FIVE CLINICS

- It is a center where preventive, promotive, curative, referral and educational services are provided in a package manner to under five age group children.
- Its functions include care of illness, growth monitoring, preventive care, family planning and health education.

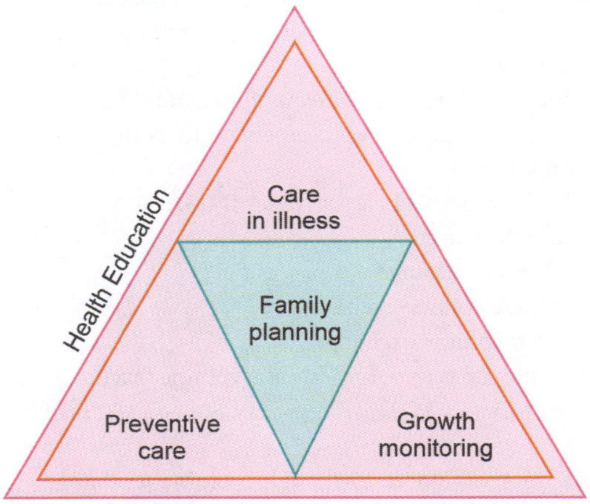

Figure 6: Functions of under-five clinics

KEY POINTS

- The symbol of under-five clinic is triangular in shape.
- The apex of the large triangle represents care in illness.
- The left and right triangle consecutively indicates nutrition and immunization.
- The central triangle represents family planning.
- The outer line indicates health education.
- Neonatal physiological jaundice appears after 24 hours of life due to breakdown of Red Blood Cells.
- Neonatal pathological jaundice appears within first 24 hours after birth.
- Drug used in the treatment of neonatal jaundice is phenobarbitone.
- Eyes and genitalia need to be covered during phototherapy.

JAUNDICE

Physiological and Pathological Jaundice

Table 23: Comparison of physiological and pathological jaundice

Characteristics	Pathological jaundice	Physiological jaundice
Onset	Within 24 hours	Appears between 24 and 72 hours
Duration	Term: >2 weeks Preterm: >3 weeks	Term: <2 weeks Preterm: <3 weeks
Raise in serum bilirubin	>0.2 mg/dL/hr or >5 mg/dL/day	<0.2 mg/dL/hr or <5 mg/dL/day

Contd...

Characteristics	Pathological jaundice	Physiological jaundice
Total Serum bilirubin	>15 mg/dL	<15 mg/dL
Direct bilirubin	>2 mg/dL	<2 mg/dL
Involvement of sole and palm	Yes	No
Urine	Dark stain of nappies and clay color stool	Urine does not stain diaper.
Signs of Acute Bilirubin encephalopathy	Yes	No

Management of Neonatal Jaundice

- Neonatal jaundice causes elevated level of total serum bilirubin level in the blood.
- It can happen either because of elevated conjugated hyperbilirubinemia/ direct hyperbilirubinemia (CHB) or due to elevated unconjugated hyperbilirubinemia (UHB).
- UHB is the most common clinical type among neonates.
- CHB always indicates certain underlying medical pathology and is always pathological jaundice.
- Most common cause of CHB among infants is biliary atresia.
- Uridine diphosphate glucuronosyltransferase (UGT) is the enzyme that is responsible for conjugating bilirubin in the liver, which is necessary for its excretion from the body. E.g., Gilbert's syndrome or Crigler-Najjar
- In neonatal jaundice, the activity of UGT is not necessarily impaired, but the enzyme may not be fully developed in the liver of a newborn.
- Barbiturate group of drugs can increase the level of UGT.

Phototherapy

- Phototherapy works through the mechanism mainly as photoisomerization, structural isomerization and photo-oxidation.
- Photoisomerization: It converts the toxic bilirubin to non-toxic one.
- Structural isomerization: Bilirubin is converted as lumirubin which can be easily excreted.
- The aim of phototherapy is to decrease the level of unconjugated bilirubin in order to prevent acute bilirubin encephalopathy, hearing loss and kernicterus.
- The required wavelength of the light is 425–475 nm.
- The distance between the baby and light should be **30–45 cm** or as per the manufacturer recommendation.
- The ambient room temperature is optimum 25 to 28° Celsius to prevent hypothermia or hyperthermia in the baby.
- While placing the baby under phototherapy unit, cover eyes and genital areas of the baby.
- Monitor hydration status of the baby and breastfeed needs to be encouraged.
- Monitor urination of baby and weigh the diaper.
- Monitor temperature every 2 hourly.
- Regularly check bilirubin level in the baby.

Intravenous immunoglobulin

- IVIg in infants with Rh or ABO isoimmunization can significantly reduce the need for exchange transfusions. It is mainly used when there is an immune mediated hemolysis.

Exchange Transfusion

- It provides rapid reduction of circulating bilirubin, so it could represent appropriate treatment in many cases of severe **hyperbilirubinemia** in the **neonatal** period.
- Treatment involves removal of the **infant's** blood and simultaneous replacement with compatible donor blood.
- Three types of exchange transfusions are commonly used:
  1. Partial exchange
  2. Single volume exchange
  3. Two volume exchange
- Volume of blood for double volume exchange transfusion = Weight (kg) × 2 × 80, i.e., 160 mL/kg
- Volume of blood for Single volume exchange transfusion = Weight (kg) × 80, i.e., 80 mL/kg

NEONATAL CARE

Neonatal Hypoglycemia

- Neonatal hypoglycemia is defined as a plasma glucose level of less than 30 mg/dL in the first 24 hours of life and less than 45 mg/dL thereafter.
- Neonatal hypoglycemia is the most common metabolic problem in newborns.
- Neonates at risk of hypoglycemia: Preterm babies, babies <2 kg weight, infants of diabetic mother, large for gestational age.

Recent Questions (NORCET 2023)

30. Phototherapy for an infant of age 90 hours should be instituted when the total serum bilirubin level is?

a. 10 g
b. 12.5 g
c. 15 g
d. 20 g

Ans. (c) 15 g

31. A new-born nursery notes that a 36-hour-old baby is jaundiced. Phototherapy has initiated. Which of the following nursing interventions will be most therapeutic?

a. Maintain a warm ambient environment
b. Have the mother feed the baby frequently
c. Have the mother hold the baby skin to skin
d. Place the baby naked by a closed sunlight window

Ans. (b) Have the mother feed the baby frequently

KEY POINTS

- Exchange transfusion is needed in a neonate with erythroblastosis fetalis to prevent kernicterus that is caused by the deposition of bilirubin in brain cells.
- Single volume exchange transfusion = 80 mL/kg
- Double volume exchange transfusions = 160 mL/kg
- Nevirapine is more potent than zidovudine in inhibiting HIV-1, but do not inhibit HIV-2.

- Symptoms: Lethargic, weak cry, poor feeding, poor respiratory effort, excessive jitteriness, convulsions and hypotonia.
- **Treatment:**
  - 200 mg/kg of dextrose (2 mL/kg of 10% dextrose as bolus, slowly over 3–5 minutes and start maintenance dose)
  - Resistant or persistent hypoglycemia: Hydrocortisone, Glucagon, Diazoxide, Octreotide.

Care of Neonate Born to Diabetic Mother

- Babies born to diabetic mother are more prone to develop cardiac abnormalities like Ventricular Septal Defect (VSD) and transposition of great arteries.
- Mothers develop polyhydramnios and babies are having macrosomia.
- Babies born to diabetic mothers are prone to develop hypoglycemia.

Care of Neonate Born to HIV Positive Mother

- Maintain universal precaution.
- Wipe baby's mouth and nose as soon as head delivered.
- Clamp the cord early and avoid milking.
- Exclusive breastfeeding is recommended for first six months of age unless replacement feeding is acceptable, feasible, affordable, sustainable and safe (AFASS).

WHO 2009 Recommendations

Infant Born to HIV Infected Mother Receiving ART

- Breastfeeding infant: Daily Nevirapine (NVP) from birth until 6 weeks of age[NORCET 2023]
- Non-breastfeeding infant: Daily Azidothymidine (AZT)/Nevirapine (NVP) from birth until 6 weeks of age.

Infant Born to HIV Infected Mother who did not Receive ART

- **Mother:** AZT
- **Breastfeeding infant:** Daily NVP from birth until one week after all exposure to breast milk has ended.
- **Non-breastfeeding infant:** AZT/NVP for 6 weeks.

Diagnosis of HIV Infection in Infants

- First HIV DNA PCR should be tested within 4 to 6 weeks. If positive repeat test immediately.
- If first PCR is negative in non-breastfed infant second PCR at 6 months.
- If breastfed with first PCR negative repeat PCR at 6–8 weeks of cessation of breastfeeding.
- The infant is considered to be HIV positive if two PCR reports are positive.
- Infant is considered negative for HIV if two PCR reports are negative.

Recent Question (NORCET 2023)

32. An image of the baby is shown with different zones of bilirubin level. How much bilirubin level in baby is likely to have up to 3rd zone?

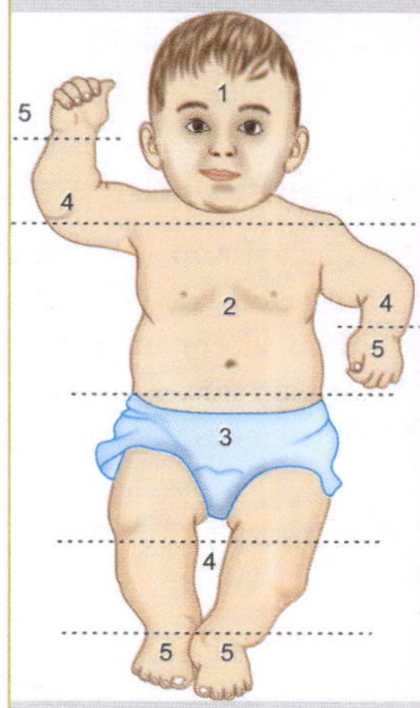

a. 4–6 mg/dL
b. 9–12 mg/dL
c. 13–16 mg/dL
d. 15–20mg/dL

Ans. (b) 9–12 mg/dL

BIRTH INJURIES

Caput Succedaneum versus Cephalohematoma

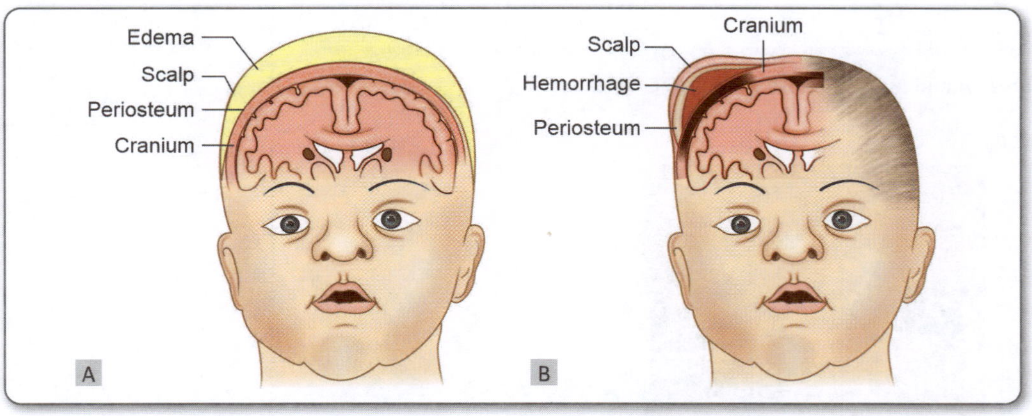

Figures 7A and B: **A.** Caput succedaneum; **B.** Cephalohematoma

Recent Question (NORCET 2023)

33. What is the management for a baby born to a mother who was on ART during the antenatal period?

a. Exclusive breast feeding, nevirapine for 6 weeks
b. Exclusive replacement feeding, nevirapine for 6 weeks
c. Exclusive breastfeeding, nevirapine for 12 weeks
d. Exclusive replacement feeding, nevirapine for 12 weeks

Ans. (a) Exclusive breast feeding, nevirapine for 6 weeks

Table 24: Differences between caput succedaneum and cephalohematoma

Caput succedaneum	Cephalohematoma
Present at birth	Develops hours or days after birth
Diffuse tissue edema overlying more than one bone	Localized hematoma to one bone limited by sutures at its edges.
Ill-defined edges	Well-defined edges.
Soft, pits on pressure	Elastic does not pit on pressure
Disappears within 1-2 days	Disappears within few weeks
It is common at birth	It is less common at birth and is associated with linear skull fracture, hyperbilirubinemia.

Duchenne-Erb Paralysis (C5-C6)

- Affected arm is adducted and internally rotated with elbow extended (waiter's tip position)
- Moro, biceps and radial reflexes are absent on the affected side.
- Grasp reflex intact

Klumpke's Paralysis (C7, C8 and T1)

- Intrinsic muscles of the hand are affected and grasp is absent (claw hand).
- Biceps and radial reflexes are absent.
- Complication is contracture.

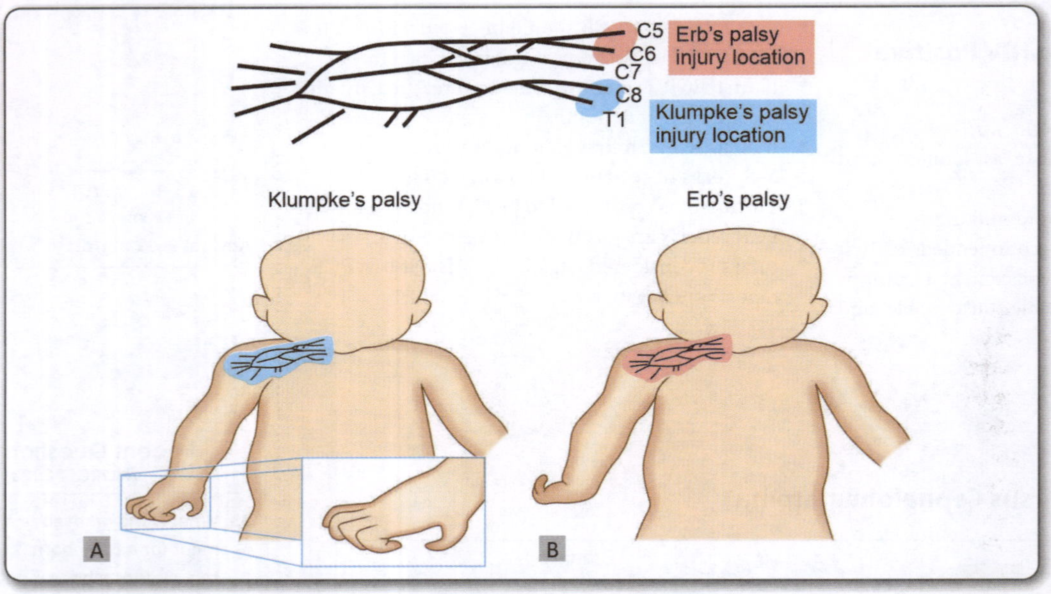

Figures 8A and B: **A.** Klumpke's palsy; **B.** Erb's palsy

Erythema Toxicum

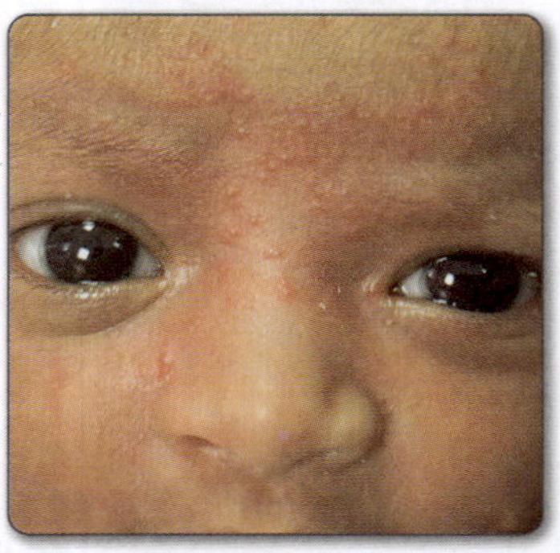

- Erythematous papular pustular lesions occur in newborn after 1-3 days of birth.
- Exact cause is unknown but it is thought to be a normal response of a baby's skin to the new environment outside the womb.

KEY POINTS

- The formation of swelling due to stagnation of fluid in the layers of the scalp is called **caput succedaneum.**
- Caput succedaneum presents as a scalp swelling that extends **across the midline** and over suture line and is associated with head molding.
- Cephalohematoma - increases size for 12–24 hours then becomes stable. It does not cross the suture line.
- **Erb's palsy** is one of the complications of breech delivery. It is characterized by flaccid arms with elbows extended.
- Police man tip hand condition is known as Erb's palsy.
- Erb's palsy is a paralysis of the arm caused by injury to the upper group of the arm's main nerves (C5–C6)
- Klumpke's paralysis (or Déjerine-Klumpke palsy) is a variety of partial palsy of the lower roots of the brachial plexus (C7, C8 and T1)

INTEGRATED MANAGEMENT OF NEONATAL AND CHILDHOOD ILLNESS (1995)

- WHO, UNICEF and other international partners introduced new strategy known as integrated management of childhood illness (IMCI) in 1995.
- This strategy expanded in India with a view to include neonate as well and the program is renamed as integrated management of neonatal and childhood illness (IMNCI).
- IMNCI beneficiaries include newborn and young infants less than 2 months of age and children between 2 months to 5 years of age.
- IMNCI classifies the children into various categories and the classifications are color coded.
  - Pink: Urgent referral after treatment at OPD (for stabilization)
  - Yellow: Treatment at outpatient department (OPD)
  - Green: Home care
- Diarrhea, acute respiratory infection (pneumonia), malaria, acute ear infection, measles, malaria, malnutrition and anemia are the conditions managed for children between 2 months to 5 years under IMNCI.
- Children up to 2 months of age are assessed for serious bacterial infection or other severe disease, jaundice, eye infection, diarrhea and dehydration, feeding problem and nutrition.

BABY FRIENDLY HOSPITAL INITIATIVE

Baby friendly hospital initiative (BFHI) was launched by WHO and UNICEF in 1991, following Innocenti Declaration of 1990.

Ten steps to successful breastfeeding:

1. Have a written breastfeeding policy that is routinely communicated to all health care staff
2. Train all health care staff in skills necessary to implement this policy
3. Inform all pregnant women about benefits and management of breastfeeding
4. Help mothers initiate breastfeeding within one and half hours of birth
5. Show mothers how to breastfeed and maintain lactation, even if they should be separated from their infants
6. Give newborn no food or drink other than breast milk unless medically indicated
7. Practice rooming in that allows mothers and infants to remain together 24 hours a day
8. Encourage breastfeeding on demand
9. Giving no artificial teats or pacifiers to breastfeeding infants
10. Foster establishment of breastfeeding support groups and refer mothers to them on a discharge from hospital or clinic.

Recent Question
(AIIMS 2020)

34. According to hospital's protocol during emergency situation "code pink" is used for which condition?
a. Infant and child abduction
b. Disastrous situation
c. Bomb threat nearby
d. Fire in hospital
Ans. (a) Infant and child...

KEY POINTS

Color-coded treatment under IMNCI:
Green: Home care
Yellow: Treatment at Outpatient Department (OPD)
Pink: Urgent referral after treatment at OPD

(NORCET 2021)

Complementary feeding starts at 6 months of age.

CHILD WELFARE PROGRAMS

Table 25: Common Child Welfare Programs

Program	Highlights
Universal Immunization Program (UIP)	• In India, UIP was introduced in 1978 as 'Expanded Program of Immunization' (EPI) by the Ministry of Health and Family Welfare, Government of India. • In 1985, the programme was modified as 'Universal Immunization Program' (UIP) to be implemented in phased manner to cover all districts in the country by 1989-90 with one of the largest health programs in the world.
Child survival and safe motherhood program (CSSM)	• Integrated approach of maternal and child health and immunization program started during 1992-93 and was called CSSM. • Main objective: **To improve the health status of infant** and **to reduce maternal morbidity and mortality**.
Reproductive and child health program -I (RCH-I)	• Program launched in October 1997 • Main aim of the program was to reduce infant, child and maternal morbidity and mortality rate.
Reproductive and child health program-II (RCH- II)	• It was launched in April 2005 under NRHM. • Components: Maternal health, neonatal and child health, family planning, adolescent health and control of RTI and STD.
Integrated child development service scheme (ICDS):	• Beneficiaries of this program include children below 6 years of age, pregnant and lactating women, adolescent girls, women of age group 15–45.
School health program	• It is under NRHM to address the health needs of the school going children and adolescents in 6–18 years of age. • Components: Screening, health care and referral, immunization, micronutrient (vitamin A and IFA) management, de-worming, health promoting services.

Program	Highlights
National nutritional program	• Some of the programs which come under this are • Mid-day meal program (1961) • Applied nutrition program (1963) • Balawadi nutrition program (1970) • Vit A prophylaxis program (1970), etc.
National rural health mission (NRHM)	• Launched by government of India on 13th April 2005 for a duration of 7 years (2005-2012).
RMNCH + A strategy	• This strategic approach to reproductive, maternal, neonatal, child health plus adolescent health to ensure continuum of care throughout the various phases of lifecycle was launched by government of India in 2013 under 12th five-year plan.
LaQshya	• Labor room and Quality improvement initiative is a program of ministry of health and family welfare launched on 11th December 2017 to reduce maternal and neonatal mortality and provide a safe and respectful maternity care.
Mission Indradhanush	• Launched by ministry of health and family welfare in December 2014 to ensure full immunization. • It depicts 7 colors of rainbow targeting 7 vaccine preventable diseases.
Mother's Absolute Affection (MAA)	• Nationwide program of ministry of health and family welfare to revitalize efforts towards promotion, protection and support of breastfeeding practice through health system to achieve higher breastfeeding rates.

CHILD WELFARE MILESTONES

- UN Convention on the Rights of the Child—11th December 1992.
- National Policy for Children—August 22nd 1974.
- National Policy on Education—1986.
- National Policy on Child Labor—August 1987 (child labor prohibition and regulation act on 1986).
- National Nutrition Policy—1993
- National Plan for SAARC—decade for girl child—1990–2000
- UN Millennium Summit-MDG September 30, 2000
- National Health Policy—2002.
- National Plan of Action for Children—2005
- The Commissions for Protecting of the Child Right Act—2005.
- National Policy for Children—2013.

KEY POINTS

- The type of play commonly exhibited by toddlers where they play by themselves in the presence of other children is called parallel play.
- The child plays intently with available materials but remains totally alone is known as solitary play.

TYPES OF PLAY AMONG CHILDREN

Table 26: Types of play

Types of play	Description
Unoccupied play	• Seen from birth to months. • Child makes random movements without any purpose.
Solitary play	• Seen from 3 to 18 months. • Babies play on their own. • During this play, child is engaged in playing with own toys and may not seem to notice other children sitting or playing nearby.
Onlooker play	• It happens most during toddlerhood. • Child watches other children play. • Child learns how to relate to others and learning languages. Child may ask question but there is no effort to join the play
Parallel play	• Seen in the age group of 18 months to 2 years. • Child begins to play alongside other children without any interaction. • Child observes others and may copy how others are playing but seldom interact.
Associative play	• Preschool children demonstrate this type of play. • They are interested in playing and socializing with other children. • This type of play is loosely organized play.
Cooperative play	• Common among preschool and school age children. Children play cooperatively with others.

Recent Question (INC PhD 2020)

35. Characteristic of play seen in autistic child:
a. Self-centric play
b. Cooperative play
c. Associative play
d. Exploratory play

Ans. (a) Self-centric play

PROTEIN ENERGY UNDERNUTRITION

Protein energy undernutrition was previously known as protein energy malnutrition (PEM). It is an energy deficit due to deficiency of all macronutrients and commonly includes deficiencies of many micronutrients.

Kwashiorkor

- It is a form of PEM which is also called as wet -PEM (because its main characteristic is the presence of edema).
- It occurs primarily by protein deficiency.
- Main symptoms include edema, lethargy and growth failure, mental changes and fatty liver.

Recent Question
(NORCET 2020)

36. The assessment of acute malnutrition in children is done by
a. Height
b. Weight
c. BMI
d. Weight for Height
Ans. (d) Weight for Height

Clinical Features

Skin	Dry, scaly skin with mosaic pattern. Flaky paint dermatosis (hyperpigmented area alternate with hypopigmented area).
Hair	Scanty and easily pluckable. Flag sign is present (segmental discoloration)
Face	Moon face with baggy cheeks
Psychomotor	Apathy, irritability, mental retardation

Marasmus

It is a form of severe protein-energy malnutrition characterized by energy deficiency and emaciation.

Clinical Features

Gross wasting of muscles, poor muscle tone, complete loss of subcutaneous fat, prominent bone uncovered by fat and muscles, aged look, hollow cheeks (monkey face appearance).
Skin is loose and wrinkled with loss of elasticity, marasmic purpura.

Table 27: Comparison between kwashiorkor and marasmus

Features	Marasmus	Kwashiorkor
Deficiency	Mainly energy	Protein deficiency
Muscle wasting	Obvious	Sometimes hidden by edema and fat
Edema	None	Present in lower legs, face and lower arms
Face	Monkey face	Moon face
Weight for height	Very low	Masked by edema
Skin changes	Usually not seen	Diffuse pigmentation, flaky paint dermatitis
Hair changes	Seldom	Sparse, silky, easy to pluck out

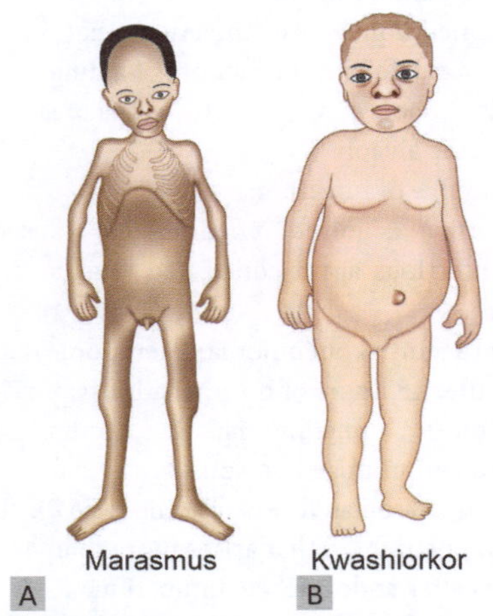

Figures 9A and B: **A.** Marasmus; **B.** Kwashiorkor

KEY POINTS

- **Marasmus** is a condition primarily caused by a deficiency in calories and energy **(theory of dysadaptation/ adaptation failure)**, whereas **kwashiorkor** indicates an associated protein deficiency **(theory of adaptation/good adaptation)**
- Children with marasmus have Good appetite whereas Kwashiorkor child exhibits poor appetite and apathy.
- **Marasmus** is characterized by failure to gain weight and irritability, followed by weight loss and listlessness until emaciation results
- **Kwashiorkor** is characterized by development of pedal edema which can mask weight loss
- Triad of complications seen in severe acute malnutrition includes hypoglycemia, hypothermia and infection.

DISORDERS OF RESPIRATORY SYSTEM

Table 28: Respiratory tract infections

Upper respiratory tract	Lower respiratory tract
Common cold Rhinitis Nasopharyngitis Pharyngitis Otitis media	Epiglottitis Laryngitis Bronchitis Bronchiolitis Pneumonia

Table 29: Microorganisms responsible for respiratory infections

Disease	Microorganism
Common cold	Rhinovirus
Pharyngitis	Adenovirus, *Streptococcus pyogenes*
Croup	Parainfluenza virus
Whooping cough	*Bordetella pertussis*
Bronchiolitis	Respiratory syncytial virus
Epiglottitis	*Streptococcus pyogenes*

Bronchiectasis

- It is the abnormal and irreversible dilatation of one or more bronchi due to inflammatory destruction of bronchial and peri bronchial tissue.
- Persistent and recurrent cough, increased production of copious, foul smelling sputum and sputum color alteration from yellow to green, and hemoptysis are the manifestations.
- Chest X-ray shows honeycomb appearance in the affected area.

Epiglottitis

Microorganism: *Streptococcus pyogenes*

Clinical manifestations: Fever, sore throat, tripod sitting and 4Ds (dysphagia, dysphonia, drooling, and distress)

Cherry red epiglottis: The epiglottis may turn a cherry red color due to the increased blood flow and inflammation in the area.

Thumb sign: It is created by the swollen and inflamed epiglottis, which can cause the trachea to be pushed backward and appear widened on X-ray.

Treatment: Ceftriaxone

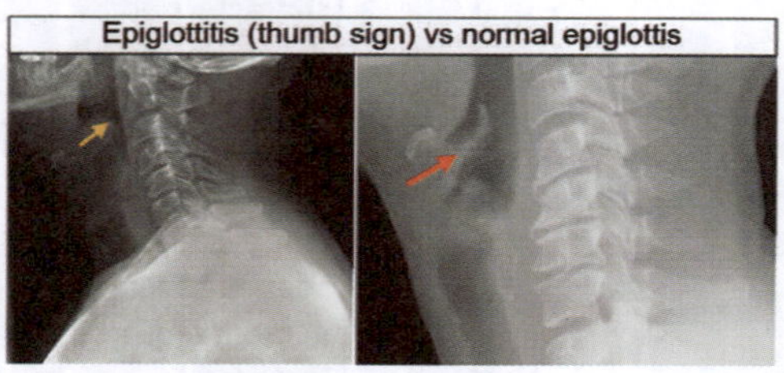

Figure 10: Epiglottitis (thumb sign) vs normal epiglottis

Pneumonia

- It is the inflammation and consolidation of lung tissue due to an infectious agent.
- Pathophysiology of pneumonia include congestion, red hepatization (Presence of erythrocytes in the cellular intraalveolar exudate), grey hepatization (No new erythrocytes are extravasating, and those already present have been lysed and degraded, neutrophil is the predominant cell, fibrin deposition is abundant) resolution (Macrophage is the dominant cell type in the alveolar space, Debris of neutrophils, bacteria, and fibrin has been cleared).

Types of Pneumonia

- Anatomical classification:
  - Bronchopneumonia: It affects the lungs in patches around bronchi.
  - Lobar pneumonia: An infection that only involves a single lobe, or section, of a lung.
  - Interstitial pneumonia: It involves the areas in between the alveoli.
- Based on source of infection:
  - Community acquired pneumonia: Caused by an infectious agent contracted outside the hospital.
  - Hospital acquired pneumonia: Pneumonia that occurs after 48 hours of hospital admission.
  - Opportunistic pneumonia: It occurs in immunocompromised persons.
  - Ventilator Associated Pneumonia (VAP): It refers to pneumonia that arises more than 48–72 hours after endotracheal intubation.

KEY POINTS

- Bronchiectasis is characterized by destruction of bronchial and peribronchial tissues
- Treatment of Choice in Bronchiectasis is postural drainage
- Confirmatory test for pneumonia to determine the extent and location of the infection is X-ray
- β-lactam or macrolide antibiotics are the Drug of Choice for Pneumococcal Pneumonia.
- An acute, severe prolonged asthma attack and is unresponsive to usual treatment is known as Status Asthmaticus
- Highest nursing priority for a client with status asthmatics is avoiding intubation

Recent Question (NORCET 2023)

37. An 8-year-old child comes to the physician's office complaining of swelling and pain in the knees. His mother says, the swelling occurred for no reason, and it keeps getting worse." The initial diagnosis is Lyme disease. When talking to the mother and child, questions related to which of the following would be important to include in the initial history?

a. A decreased urinary output and flank pain
b. A fever of over 103F occurring over the last 23 weeks
c. Rashes covering the palms of the hands and the soles of the feet
d. Headaches, malaise, or sore throat

Ans. (d) Headaches, malaise, or sore throat

Bronchial Asthma

- Asthma is a chronic inflammatory disease of the airways that causes airway hyper responsiveness, mucosal edema, and mucus production. This inflammation ultimately leads to recurrent episodes of asthma symptoms: cough, chest tightness, wheezing, and dyspnea.
- Risk factors for asthma: Positive family history, allergy (strongest risk factor), chronic exposure to airway irritants or allergens.
- The three most common symptoms of asthma are cough (especially at night), dyspnea, and wheezing.
- Two general class of medications to treat asthma include quick relief medication and long-acting medication.
- Quick-relief medications: Short-acting beta-adrenergic agonists for relieving acute symptoms and preventing exercise-induced asthma.
  - E.g.: salbutamol, terbutaline, ipratropium.
- Long-acting control medications: Corticosteroids are the most potent and effective anti-inflammatory medications currently available. They are broadly effective in alleviating symptoms, improving airway function, and decreasing peak flow variability.
  - E.g.: budesonide, beclomethasone.

Status Asthmaticus

- A prolonged severe attack of asthma that is unresponsive to initial standard therapy, is characterized especially by dyspnea, dry cough, wheezing, and hypoxemia, and that may lead to respiratory failure.
- In the emergency setting, the patient is treated initially with a short-acting beta-adrenergic agonist and corticosteroids.
- The patient usually requires supplemental oxygen and intravenous fluids for hydration.

Drug delivery devices

- Metered dose inhaler (MDI)
- Children <4 years: MDI + spacer + face mask
- Children 4–12 years: MDI + spacer
- Children > 12 years: MDI directly
- Dry powder inhaler
- Nebulizer

Chronic Obstructive Pulmonary Disease (COPD)

- Chronic obstructive pulmonary disease (COPD) is a disease state characterized by airflow limitation that is not fully reversible.
- COPD may include diseases that cause airflow obstruction (e.g., emphysema, chronic bronchitis)
- Chronic bronchitis: It is a chronic inflammation of the lower respiratory tract characterized by excessive mucous secretion, cough, and dyspnea associated with recurrent infections of the lower respiratory tract.
- Emphysema: Pathological condition of the lung characterized by abnormal dilatation of alveoli and its rupture eventually causes decreased lung function.
- COPD is characterized by three primary symptoms:
  1. Cough
  2. Sputum production and
  3. Dyspnea on exertion (DOE)—Weight loss is common because dyspnea interferes with eating.
- **Barrel chest** is seen in emphysema.
- Treatment concept of COPD:
  - Risk reduction (smoking cessation)
  - Bronchodilators
  - Inhaled corticosteroids
  - Pulmonary rehabilitation and surgery (bullectomy, lung volume reduction surgery and lung transplantation).

(NORCET 2022)

Correct placement of simple oxygen mask in pediatric patients

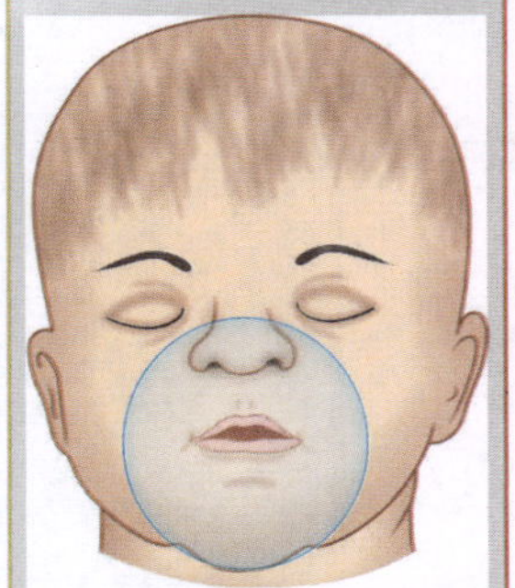

POINT TO REMEMBER

Oxygen needs to be administered judiciously in COPD patient because hypercapnia (increased CO_2) cause respiratory stimuli in this patient, increased oxygen may lead to poor respiratory efforts in these clients.

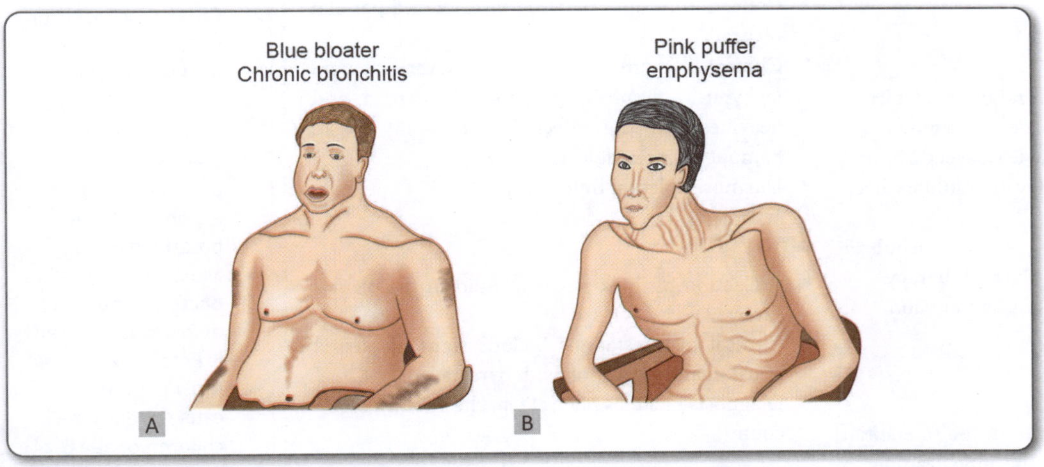

Figures 11A and B: **A.** Chronic bronchitis; **B.** Emphysema

Table 30: Differences between chronic bronchitis and emphysema

Chronic bronchitis (blue bloaters)	Emphysema (pink puffers)
Patients may be obese	Patients may be very thin with a barrel chest
Frequent cough and expectoration are typical	They typically have little or no cough or expectoration.
Use of accessory muscles of respiration is common	Breathing may be assisted by pursed lips and use of accessory respiratory muscles; they may adopt the tripod sitting position.
Coarse rhonchi and wheezing may be heard on auscultation. Patients may have signs of right heart failure (cor pulmonale), such as edema and cyanosis	The chest may be hyper resonant, and wheezing may be heard; heart sounds are very distant.

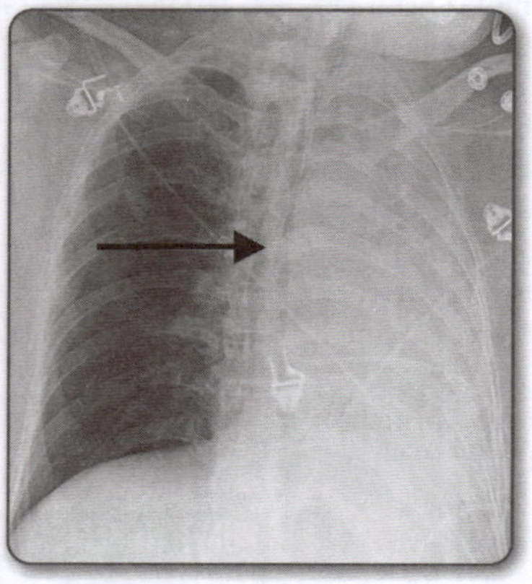

Figure 12: Atelectasis

Atelectasis

- Collapse of the part of lung or entire lung is known as atelectasis.
- It occurs due to foreign body on the airway or due to diminished distention of alveoli
- X-ray shows patchy infiltrates or consolidated area.
- SPO_2 <90%
- Physical examination shows decreased breath sounds and crackles are heard over the affected area.

Management

- Frequent turning, early mobilization, strategies to expand the lungs and to manage secretions.
- Deep-breathing maneuvers (at least every 2 hours)
- The use of incentive spirometry or voluntary deep breathing
- Directed cough, suctioning, aerosol nebulizer treatments followed by chest physical therapy.
- Postural drainage and chest percussion, or bronchoscopy

Pulmonary Edema

- Excessive accumulation of fluid in the interstitial space and alveolar space of the lung leading to oxygen desaturation and respiratory distress.
- **Manifestations**: Dyspnea, tachypnea, fine crackles, wheezing cough and expectoration of frothy edema fluid.
- One of the classical signs of pulmonary edema is coughing up blood (classically seen as **pink, frothy sputum**).

Pulmonary Embolism

- It is an obstruction in one of the major blood vessels in the lung usually due to blood clot.
- Causes: Deep vein thrombosis, fatty material from the marrow of a broken bone, foreign material from an impure injection, a large air bubble in the vein, small piece of neoplastic material that has broken off from a large tumor body.
- Clinical features: Severe breathlessness, hemoptysis, chest pain (felt in the center of chest behind breast bone)
- Diagnosis: Chest X-ray, echocardiography, pulmonary angiography
- Management: Anticoagulant therapy, clot dissolving injection (alteplase, streptokinase, urokinase).
- **Surgery:** Embolectomy

Pleural Effusion

- Collection of fluid between visceral and parietal pleura.
- Clinical features: Persistent fever, cough, tachypnea, dyspnea, pleuritic chest pain and heaviness on the affected side, night sweat, hemoptysis, weight loss.
- Diagnosis: pleural fluid analysis.

Empyema

- Collection of thick purulent fluid in the pleural cavity
- Clinical manifestations include signs of pleural effusion and toxic look with pyrexia
- Diagnosis includes pleural tap, chest X-ray, blood count

KEY POINTS

- Pus in the pleural cavity is known as Empyema.
- Absence of breaths sound during auscultation in the right thorax suggests a right pneumothorax. Similarly, absent breath sound in left thorax suggests left pneumothorax.
- Confirmatory diagnostic test for pneumothorax is chest X-ray.
- Feeding a child with choanal atresia can cause chokes on feeding.
- Chest tube insertion is the management for Pleural effusion.
- A chest tube helps remove the excess fluid or air and allows the lung to expand, making breathing easier.
- Most common **bacterial cause** of diarrhea in children is *Enterotoxic E. coli*.
- Most common cause of diarrhea in children of age 6-24 months: **Rotavirus**

Pneumothorax

- Presence of air between visceral pleura and parietal pleura leads to lung collapse.
- When air enters the pleural space, positive pressure leads to collapse of the affected lung and mediastinum to shift to the opposite side which leads to decline in cardiac output.

Choanal Atresia

- Congenital disorder in which back of the nasal passage is obstructed.
- It can be unilateral or bilateral. In bilateral choanal atresia, symptoms appear immediately after birth with severe respiratory distress and cyanosis. Unilateral choanal atresia is less life threatening and symptoms may appear later in childhood.

Croup

- Croup is a respiratory illness characterized by inspiratory stridor, cough, and hoarseness.
- These symptoms result from inflammation in the larynx and subglottic airway.
- A barking cough is the hallmark of croup among infants and young children, whereas hoarseness predominates in older children and adults.
- The term croup has been used to describe a variety of upper respiratory conditions in children including laryngitis, laryngotracheitis, laryngotracheobronchitis, bacterial tracheitis or spasmodic croup.
- Clinical manifestations include hoarse or barking cough, nasal drainage, sore throat, low grade fever, tachycardia, tachypnea, inspiratory stridor.

DISORDERS OF GASTROINTESTINAL SYSTEM

Diarrhea

It is the **second most leading cause of death** among the age group of under five children after pneumonia (WHO, UNICEF). **Diarrhea** is the passage of watery stool at least three times in 24-hour period. Consistency is more important than frequency.

Acute watery diarrhea: Change in frequency and consistency of stool

Dysentery or bloody diarrhea: Visible blood in the stool

Persistent diarrhea: Episodes of diarrhea with or without blood that lasts for at least 14 days are associated with HIV infection or malnutrition.

Traveller's diarrhea: It is a common condition that affects many people who travel to developing countries or areas with poor sanitation. Most common organism responsible for this is ***E. coli.***

Etiology

Bacteria	*E. coli*, Campylobacter jejuni, Vibrio cholerae, Shigella, Salmonella, Yersinia enterocolitica
Virus	Rotavirus, norovirus, adenovirus, cytomegalovirus, astrovirus
Protozoa	Cryptosporidium parvum, Giardia intestinalis, Entameba histolytica
Helminths	Strongyloides stercoralis, Angiostrongylus costaricensis

Clinical Features

- Frequent watery stool
- Irritability
- Dehydration
- Weak and thready pulse
- Hypotension
- ECG changes ST depression and flat T wave
- Kussmaul breathing in acidosis

Table 31: Degrees of dehydration

Assessment	No dehydration	Some dehydration (two or more signs are present)	Severe dehydration (two or more signs are present)
Look at general condition	Well alert	Restless, irritable	Lethargic or unconscious or floppy
Eyes	Normal	Sunken	Sunken
Tears	Present	Absent	Absent
Mouth and tongue	Moist	Dry	Very dry
Thirst	Drinks normally, no thirst	Drinks eagerly, thirsty	Unable to drink or drinking poorly
Feel : skin pinch	Goes back quickly	Goes back slowly	Goes back very slowly

Recent Question (NORCET 2023)

38. Which of the following has low risk of Sudden infant death syndrome?

a. Baby who sleeps on his back
b. Has family history of sudden infant death syndrome.
c. Baby with prenatal drug exposure
d. Baby who is premature

Ans. (a) Baby who sleeps on his back

Sudden infant death syndrome (SIDS) is the sudden and unexplained death of an infant under the age of 1 year. There is no single cause of SIDS, but there are some risk factors that have been identified.

One of the most important risk factors for SIDS is sleeping on the stomach. Babies who sleep on their stomachs are more likely to have their faces pressed against the mattress, which can block their airways which leads to suffocation.

POINT TO REMEMBER

Rotavirus is the most common cause of infective diarrhea in children.

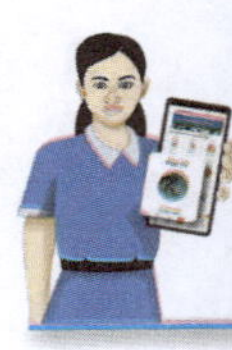

Management

Plan A: No dehydration: Child with no signs of dehydration needs home treatment

- Breastfeed child frequently and for longer duration.
- If the child is exclusively breastfed, give ORS or clean water along with breastfeed.
- If the child is not exclusively breastfed, provide one or more of the solutions like ORS, food-based fluids (soup, rice water, yoghurt) or clean water.
- Up to two years of age — give 50–100 mL of fluids with each loose stool.
- Child more than two years of age - give 100-200 mL after each loose stool.
- If child vomits, wait for 10 minutes and feed again more slowly.
- Zinc supplement: Up to 6 months half tablet per day for 14 days and more than 6 months 1 tablet per day for 14 days.
- Return to health care facility: If the child is not getting better in 3 days or continue to have symptoms.

Plan B: Child with some dehydration

Give ORS in the health care facility until the skin pinch is normal, the thirst is over, the child is calm.

Table 32: Requirement of ORS

Age	Weight	Amount (mL)
Up to 4 months	<6 kg	200–400
4–12 months	6 to <10 kg	400–700
12 months to 2 years	10 to <12 kg	700–900
2–5 years	12-19 kg	900–1400

If child wants more than the recommended, give more.

- Infants below 6 months of age who all are not breastfed, give additional 100-200 mL clean water during this period.
- Continue breastfeeding whenever the child wants.
- Reassess after 4 hours. If there is no dehydration switch to plan A, if some dehydration is still present continue plan B and if signs indicate severe dehydration switch to plan C.

Plan C: Child with severe dehydration

- Children need to be treated with IV fluids at hospital.
- Give 100 mL/kg RL solution (if RL not available then NS)
- Infants (under 12 months): 30 mL/kg for 1 hour then 70 mL/kg for 5 hours.
- Children 12 months to 5 years: 30 mL/kg for 30 minutes followed by 70 mL/kg for 2 and half hours.
- If IV fluid therapy is not available, then insert NG or OG and give ORS
    - 20 mL/kg/hr for 6 hours, reassess every 1–2 hours
    - If not improving after 3 hours refer the child to a hospital urgently for IV
    - After 6 hours reassess the child and reclassify for plan A, B, C

ORS

The most widely used ORS is designed by WHO. In 2004, WHO and UNICEF recommended a new ORS formula known as low osmolarity ORS to treat dehydration among all age groups.

Table 33: Differences between traditional and low osmolarity formula of ORS

Traditional formula		Low osmolarity formula	
Composition	g/L	Ions/osmole	Mmol/L
Sodium chloride	2.6	Sodium	75
Glucose, anhydrase	13.5	Chloride	65
Potassium chloride	1.5	Glucose, anhydrase	75
Trisodium citrate	2.9	Potassium	20
		Trisodium citrate	10
		Osmolarity = 245	

Gastroesophageal Reflux Disease (GERD)

The cardiac sphincter and lower portion of the esophagus are weak allowing regurgitation of gastric content back into the esophagus.

Recent Question (NORCET 2020)

39. Which among the following is added with ORS to control diarrhea?
a. Copper
b. Calcium
c. Zinc
d. Potassium
Ans. (c) Zinc

KEY POINTS

- Glucose is added in ORS solution because it increases the sodium absorption.
- A freshly prepared **ORS solution (Oral rehydration solution)** should be used within 24 hours.

Recent Question (INC PhD 2020)

40. Identify the potassium-rich food among the following.
a. Lemon
b. Amla
c. Green leafy vegetables
d. Mango
Ans. (c) Green leafy...

Recent Question (NORCET 2023)

41. Which of the following is not a sign of dehydration in an infant:
a. Perianal excoriation
b. Delayed skin pinch
c. Dry mouth
d. Drying of tears
Ans. (a) Perianal excoriation

- **Interventions:**
  - Feeding changes including restricting milk and egg intake in maternal diet of breastfeeding mothers.
  - Thicken the formula and reducing the volume and increasing the frequency.
  - Sitting and supine position while feeding is avoided. Left lateral position with head end elevated at 30 degrees can be used for feeding children.
  - Lifestyle modifications: Weight loss in overweight patients, cessation of smoking, avoiding alcohol, caffeine, chocolate and spicy foods from the diet.
- **Medical management**
  - Antacid, histamine 2 receptor antagonist and protein pump inhibitors
  - Prokinetic agents like metoclopramide may be used
  - Surgery: Fundoplication may reduce the reflex

Malabsorption Syndrome

- It is a condition in which intestine's ability to absorb certain nutrients into the blood stream is negatively affected resulting in chronic diarrhea, abdominal distention and failure to thrive.
- **Clinical manifestations**
  - Carbohydrate malabsorption: Bloating, flatulence, explosive diarrhea, anorexia, fatigue, weight loss
  - Protein malabsorption: Fluid retention, dry hair and hair loss
  - Fat malabsorption: Light colored foul smelling and soft and bulky stool
  - Vitamin malabsorption: Anemia, malnutrition, low BP, weight loss, wasting

Lactose Intolerance

- It is the inability to digest lactose found in dairy products due to the deficiency of lactase enzyme.
- Manifestations: Abdominal pain, watery diarrhea, nausea, flatulence, bloating.
- Diagnosis: 2-week trial of strict lactose free diet, hydrogen breath test, clinical examination of stool.
- Management: Lactose free diet, breastfeeding mothers are advised to eliminate lactose from diet, mineral and vitamin supplements, and lactase enzyme as medication.

Celiac Disease

- It is an autoimmune disease
- Inability to fully digest gliadin, which is a by-product of the protein gluten. Also called as gluten induced enteropathy, gluten-sensitive enteropathy, celiac sprue.

Treatment

- Lifelong gluten free diet is advised
- Rice can be used instead of wheat, barley and rye

Cystic Fibrosis

- It is an autosomal recessive inheritance affecting exocrine glands.
- It is caused by mutation in cystic fibrosis transmembrane regulator (CFTR) located in chromosome 7.
- Abnormality in CFTR blocks chloride transport leading to dehydration, thus affecting organs and causing thick secretion of exocrine gland.
- Abnormally thick secretions affect respiratory, GI, exocrine and reproductive system.
- Diagnosis: sweat chloride test (>60 mEq) on at least two occasions. Sodium and chloride levels are elevated.
- Sweat glands normally absorb sodium back and in this condition salty sweat will be there.
- Clinical manifestations: Salty taste skin, respiratory tract infection (upper and lower), poor growth, meconium ileus.

Management

- Prevention and management of pulmonary infection with antibiotics
- Chest physiotherapy for sputum expectoration
- Management of dietary supplements (enzyme with meals and snacks)

Inflammatory Bowel Disease

It refers to two forms of chronic intestinal inflammation: Ulcerative colitis and Crohn's disease.

KEY POINTS

- In gastroesophageal reflux disease (GERD), the purpose of esophageal pH monitoring is to assess the frequency of reflex.
- Preferred position for nursing babies with GERD is left lateral.
- Effectiveness of use of thickened formula feed in a client with GERD is evaluated with decrease in regurgitation and vomiting.
- Lactose intolerance is an inability to tolerate the lactose found in dairy products as a result of an absence or deficiency of lactase.
- Child with celiac disease needs to avoid food items containing gluten protein.

Recent Question
(INC PhD 2020)

42. Which among the following is the manifestation of cystic fibrosis at birth?
a. Meconium ileus
b. Drooling of saliva
c. Scaphoid abdomen
d. Currant jelly like stool

Ans. (a) Meconium ileus

POINT TO REMEMBER

During postoperative care of an infant with a cleft palate repair, the nurse should position the baby in prone position.

Table 34: Features of ulcerative colitis and crohn's disease

Features	Ulcerative colitis	Crohn's disease
Location	Limited to large intestine	Entire GI tract most commonly affects terminal ileum
Pattern of inflammation	Inflamed areas are continuous with no patchy area. Ulcers penetrate only inner lining of the intestine	Patches of inflammations are seen between affected areas. Involves entire thickness of the intestinal lining
Location of pain	Commonly on left lower abdomen	Commonly on right lower abdomen
Bleeding	During bowel movement	Less common
Growth failure	Less common	Common

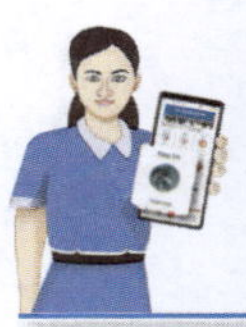

CLEFT LIP AND CLEFT PALATE

Cleft lip (cheiloschisis): It is a gap or split continued up to the nostril due to failure of fusion of the maxillary and medial nasal process.

Cleft palate (palatoschisis): It is a condition in which two plates of the skull that forms hard palate are not completely joined due to the failure of the fusion of the lateral palatine processes, nasal septum, and medial palatine processes.

Risk Factors

- Smoking during pregnancy—increased risk to have baby with an orofacial cleft.
- Maternal Diabetes—increased risk of having a child with a cleft lip with or without cleft palate.
- Use of certain medicines—Antiepileptics such as **topiramate, valproic acid, phenytoin, retinoic acid** during the first trimester of pregnancy have an increased risk of having a baby with cleft lip with or without cleft palate.

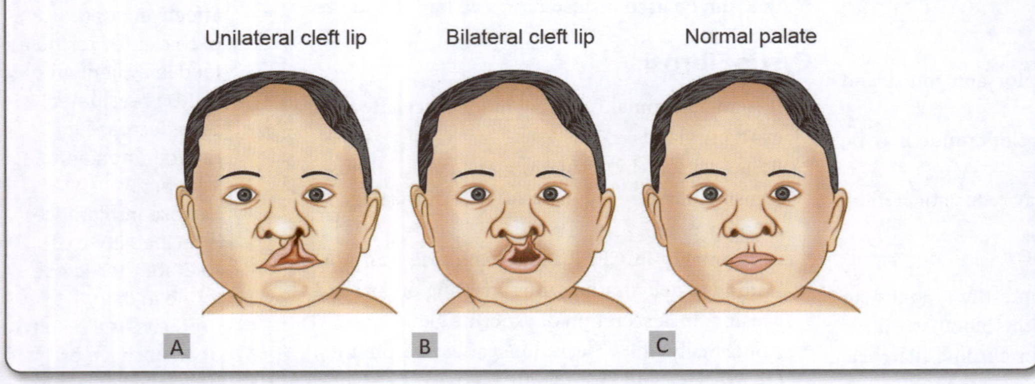

Figures 13A to C: A. Unilateral cleft lip; **B.** Bilateral cleft lip; **C.** Normal palate

Problems with Cleft Lip and Cleft Palate

- **Feeding difficulty:** Difficulty in creating enough suction.
- **Breathing**: Increased chance for aspiration due to air entry during feeding through the gap.
- Recurrent ear infection and hearing loss
- **Speech difficulty:** Due to palatal deformity air escapes into nose and causes an excessively nasal sounding voice.
- **Malocclusion of teeth**: Missing teeth particularly in the line of cleft. They may have extra teeth or malformed teeth. Because of this their teeth can be crowded, tilted, or rotated.

Management

- Hold the baby in upright position while feeding and make the baby burp frequently in between feeding to prevent air trapping and choking.
- For bottle feeding, large hole especially designed for cleft lip and palate should be used.
- **Haberman feeder** is a specially designed bottle with a valve to control the air entry and prevent back flow.

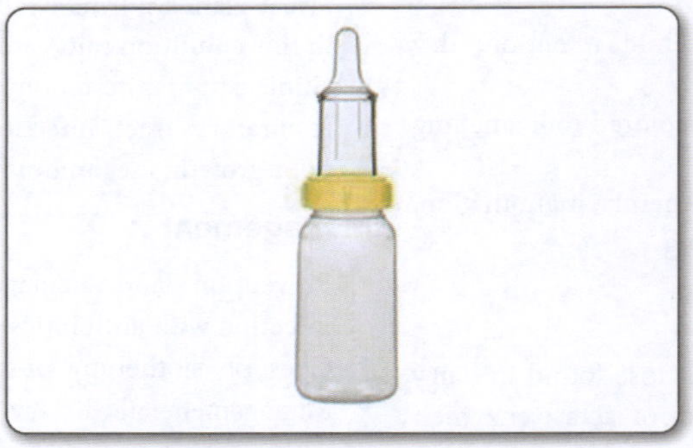

Figure 14: Haberman feeder

- NUK nipple, which can be adjusted with size of the hole by making crisscross cut in midline can be used with regular bottle.

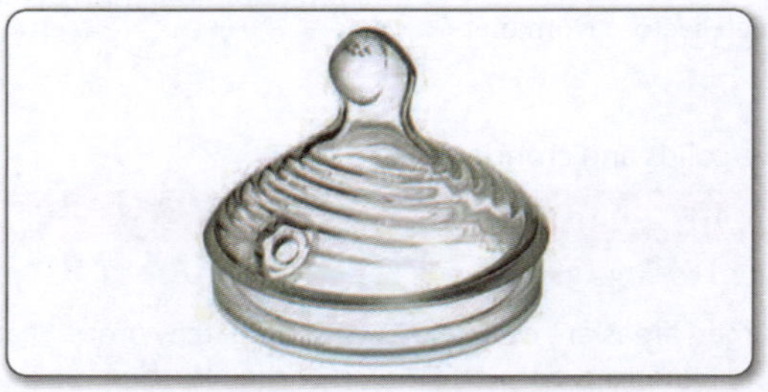

Figure 15: NUK nipple

Recent Questions (INC PhD 2020)

43. Child with cleft lip has problem with
a. Sucking
b. Swallowing
c. Breathing
d. Smiling
Ans. (a) Sucking

44. Nutrient deficient in phenytoin therapy.
a. Vitamin C
b. Vitamin A
c. Calcium
d. Potassium
Ans. (c) Calcium

Recent Question (NORCET 2020)

45. During postoperative care of an infant with a cleft palate repair, the nurse should position the baby in which of the following positions?
a. On side lying position
b. In an infant seat
c. Prone
d. Supine
Ans. (c) Prone

Clinical Corner

CASE SCENARIO 3:
Mother of a child with cleft lip asked the nurse that why her infant is more prone to developing infections as compared to other children of same age group. The best response from nurse is:
a. Imbalanced nutrition
b. Poor sucking
c. Mouth breathing
d. Inadequate circulation in the affected area

Ans. (c) Mouth breathing
Infant with cleft lip breathes through mouth and by passing natural humidification, which leads to dryness of oral mucosa and makes it crack and is easily gets infected.

- In case of katori spoon feeding, long straight handled spoon is used.
- A **cleft lip** is **usually repaired between 3 and 6 months** of age and the surgery is known as cheiloplasty.
- A **cleft palate is commonly fixed between 9 and 14 months** of age and the surgery is known as palatoplasty.

Table 35: Feeding considerations for a baby with cleft lip and cleft palate.

Criteria	Description
Position	Baby in an upright position with the head slightly elevated during feeding. This position helps prevent choking, facilitates swallowing, and minimizes the risk of aspiration.
Special feeding devices	Utilize specialized cleft palate bottles or nipples that are designed to accommodate the cleft and facilitate feeding. These devices can help control the flow of milk and make feeding easier for the baby.
Burping	Burp the baby frequently during feeding to release any swallowed air. Gently pat or rub the baby's back in an upright position to facilitate burping.
Feeding technique	Tilt the bottle to allow the milk to flow more slowly, helps the baby to swallow comfortably. Avoid forcing the baby to drink quickly or gulp down large amount of milk.
Adequate time for feeding	Allow ample time for feeding and be patient. It is essential not to rush or force-feed the baby.
Feeding cues	Look for cues such as rooting, lip smacking, or turning away when full. Recognize when the baby is no longer interested in feeding and avoid overfeeding.

TRACHEOESOPHAGEAL FISTULA AND ESOPHAGEAL ATRESIA

- Esophageal atresia (EA): Congenital discontinuity of esophageal lumen is known as esophageal atresia.
- Tracheoesophageal fistula (TEF): It is the abnormal communication between trachea and esophagus.
- Two syndromes associated with EA
  - VACTERAL — vertebral anomalies, anal atresia, cardiac malformation, tracheoesophageal fistula, renal abnormalities and radial aplasia and limb abnormalities
  - CHARGE — coloboma, heart defect, atresia of choanae, retardation of physical and mental development, genital hypoplasia, ear abnormalities.

Classification

- Most common type is Type C esophageal atresia with distal TEF.
- Cardinal signs: Drooling of saliva, 3C's (coughing, choking, cyanosis)
- Other signs and symptoms: Respiratory distress, abdominal distention, regurgitation, aspiration pneumonia.
- Diagnosis: Antenatal USG, inability to pass stiff red rubber catheter to stomach, chest X-ray. If distal TEF is present, air in the stomach will be seen on X-ray film with abdominal distention.
- Tracheobronchoscopy

KEY POINTS

- Cheiloplasty is the surgical management of Cleft lip.
- Cleft lip is usually repaired at four to six months of age and a cleft palate is usually repaired around 12 months of age.
- Double bubble sign in the X-ray is suggestive of **duodenal atresia.**
- Continuous drooling immediately after birth indicates tracheoesophageal fistula.
- Esophageal atresia with or without tracheoesophageal fistula is the most common congenital anomaly of the esophagus.

Recent Question (NORCET 2023)

46. In Tracheoesophageal fistula, which position is preferred for the child?
a. Prone
b. Head of bed elevated at 30 degree
c. Supine
d. Lateral

Ans. (b) Head of bed elevated at 30 degree

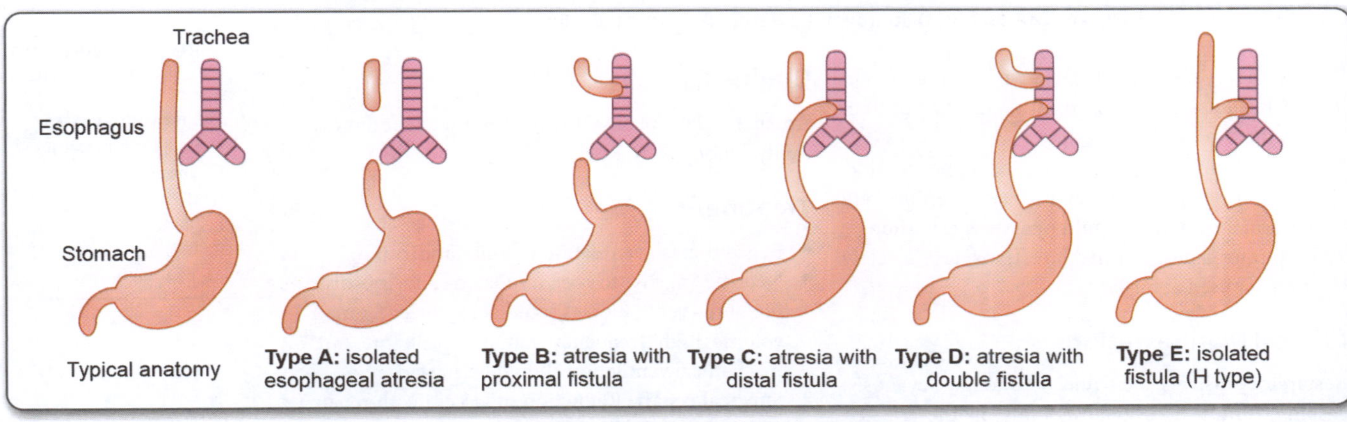

Figure 16: Types of esophageal atresia

Management

- Supine position with head end elevated to reduce the risk of gastric secretions entering in the lung.
- Primary repair is done by ligation of the fistula and end to end anastomosis.

Complications

Anastomotic leak, dysphagia, esophageal stricture, GERD, recurrent pneumonia, tracheomalacia and chest wall deformity.

HYPERTROPHIC PYLORIC STENOSIS

Characterized by hypertrophy of two muscle layers of pylorus resulting in obstruction of gastric outlet.

Clinical Manifestations

- Non-bilious projectile vomiting
- Persistently hungry
- **Olive like mass** on the right upper quadrant of the abdomen
- Visible peristaltic movement from left hypochondrium to umbilicus
- Dehydration and alkalosis

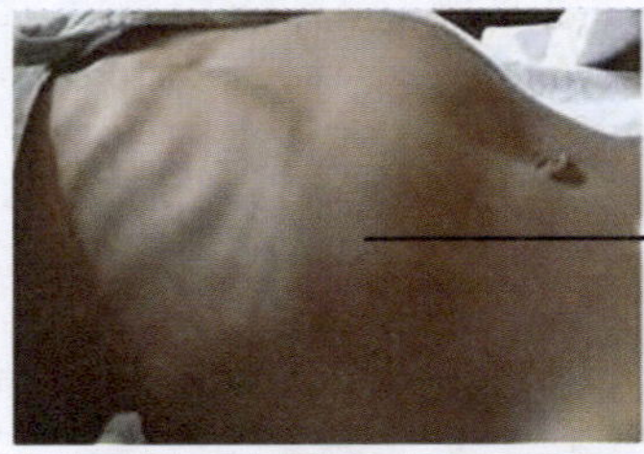

Figure 17: Hypertrophic pyloric stenosis (olive shaped)

Diagnosis

- Ultrasound abdomen shows thickened pyloric mass
- Upper GI barium study shows elongated pyloric canal (string sign) or thickened pyloric mucosa (double track sign).
- Upper GI endoscopy

Surgery

- Ramstedt pyloromyotomy: Longitudinal incision on the pylorus thus relieves gastric outlet obstruction
- Laparoscopic pyloromyotomy
- Endoscopic balloon dilatation

Recent Question (AIIMS 2020)

47. Which of the following is the cardinal sign of pyloric stenosis?
a. Projectile Vomiting
b. Fever
c. Diarrhea
d. Constipation
Ans. (a) Projectile...

KEY POINTS

- **Hypokalemic metabolic alkalosis** is the classic electrolyte and acid-base imbalance of **pyloric stenosis.**
- Olive-like mass, Projectile vomiting and String sign in the X-ray are the characteristic features of pyloric stenosis.

KEY POINT

4 Ps of Pyloric stenosis
Punny infant
Projectile vomiting
Palpable olive shaped mass
Peristaltic movement highly invisible.

CONGENITAL DIAPHRAGMATIC HERNIA (CDH)

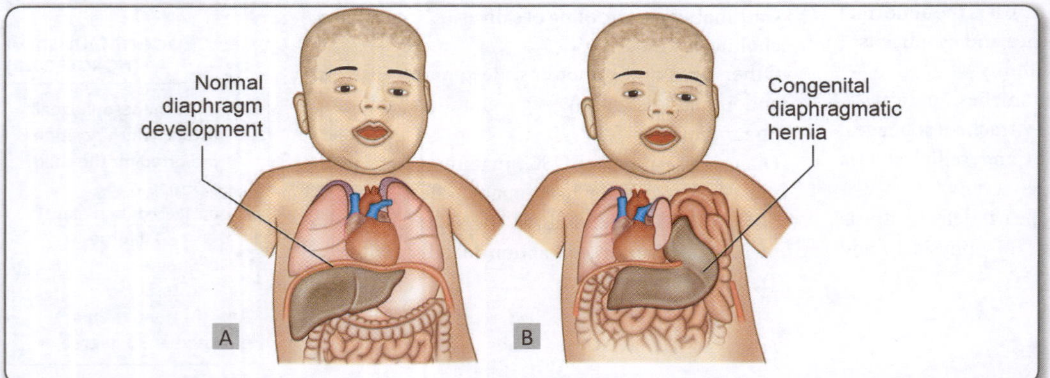

Figures 18A and B: Diaphragmatic Hernia **A.** Normal; **B.** Hernia

- It is the posterolateral defect in the diaphragm which allows the passage of abdominal content into the thorax.
- Mediastinum is displaced to the opposite side, lungs are hypoplastic and their arterioles are abnormal resulting in pulmonary hypertension.
- Respiratory and cardiac functions are severely compromised at birth.

Clinical Manifestations

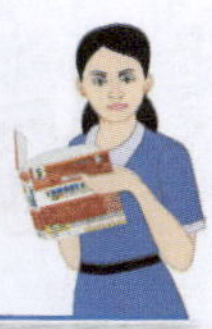

Respiratory distress, tachypnea, retractions, cyanosis, gasping, diminished breath sounds on the affected side, evacuated abdomen with sternal protrusion, displacement of heart sound to the contralateral side, bowel sounds heard over the chest, scaphoid abdomen.

Diagnosis

Antenatal USG, plain X-ray of thorax and abdominal cavity, blood gas and pH

Treatment

- Bag and mask ventilation is **contraindicated**.
- Neonate needs to be intubated and positive pressure ventilation should be started. Small volume high frequency reduced peak pressure mechanical ventilation should be started.
- **Surgical repair:** Reduction of viscera with repair of diaphragm is done after 6-18 hours of birth or when the baby is physiologically stable.

Recent Question (NORCET 2022)

48. The newborn passes the meconium within:
a. 6 hours
b. 12 hours
c. 24–48 hours
d. 96 hours
Ans. (c) 24–48 hours

Intestinal Obstruction

Condition in which normal passage bowel content is obstructed through the lumen. It can affect both small intestine and large intestine.

Clinical Manifestations

- Nonbilious vomiting implies that the obstruction is proximal to the ampulla of Vater.
- Proximal intestinal obstruction leads to bilious vomiting with minimal abdominal distention.
- In case of distal obstruction, bilious vomiting with abdominal distention, abdominal pain, fever, tenderness, decreased bowel sounds, dehydration, constipation occur.

Diagnosis

History, physical examination, barium enema, plain X-ray.

Intussusception

Telescopic movement of proximal part of intestine into the distal part of the intestine leading to disruption in blood supply and necrosis.

Clinical Manifestations

- Non-bilious vomiting progressing to bilious vomiting
- Passage of **currant jelly-like stool**
- Sausage-shaped mass in the abdomen
- Empty right lower quadrant (Dance's sign)

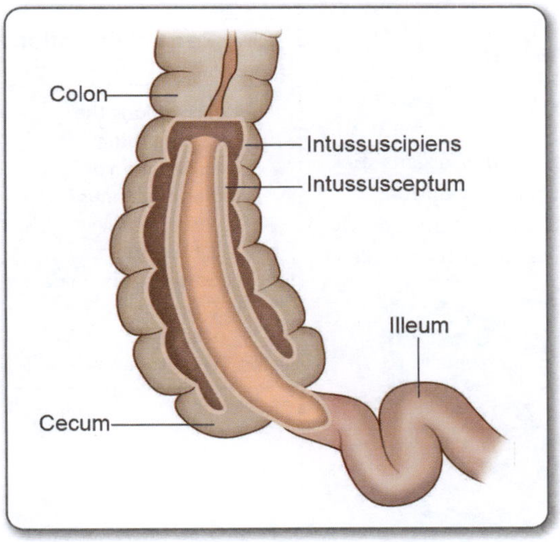

Figure 19: Intestinal obstruction

Diagnosis

- Plain X-ray of abdomen:- Crescent sign showing soft tissue density projecting into the gas of the large bowel and target sign
- Ultrasound: Bull's eye or coiled spring lesion representing layers of intestine within intestine.
- Barium enema: Inverted cup or claw sign showing intussusception.

Management

- Nonsurgical hydrostatic reduction: With the help of barium enema, water soluble contrast or air try to push the invaginated portion of the bowel back into the normal position.
- Surgical management: Resection and primary anastomosis

Hirschsprung's Disease

Absence of ganglionic cells in all or part of the colon leading to functional colonic obstruction. It is also known as **congenital megacolon or aganglionosis.**

Clinical Manifestations

- Failure to pass meconium in 24 hours of life, bilious vomiting, difficult bowel movements, abdominal distension, tight anal sphincter with empty rectum.
- **Ribbon like stools are common symptom of Hirschsprung's disease.**

Red Flag Signs

- Delayed meconium (>24 hrs)
- Neonatal constipation
- Family history
- Poor growth
- Abdominal distention
- Down syndrome and other chromosomal abnormalities

Diagnosis

- Rectal suction biopsy: Shows absence of **Meissner and Auerbach's plexuses**.
- Anal manometry
- Abdominal X-ray

Surgery

- Primary aim of the surgery is to remove the affected colon. Most of the time surgeries are performed in stages.
- **Colostomy:** Creation of an opening for the colon to excrete the stool content
- **Pull through procedure**: Aganglionic portion is removed and healthy portion is pulled down into the rectum after 4-6 months of colostomy. Common pull through procedures are **Soave, Duhamel and Swenson.**
- **Closure of colostomy:** Colostomy will be closed and gradual return to normal bowel functions.

Meckel's Diverticulum

- It is a congenital diverticulum arising from the antimesenteric border of terminal ileum.
- During the eighth week of gestation, incomplete obliteration of vitelline duct results in some congenital abnormalities, the **most common of which is Meckel's Diverticulum.**

Recent Question
(INC PhD 2020)

49. Which part of the colon is most affected in Hirschsprung's disease?
a. Ascending colon
b. Transverse colon
c. Descending colon
d. Rectosigmoid colon

Ans. (d) Rectosigmoid...

KEY POINTS

- Currant jelly-like stools is the characteristic feature of intussusception.
- Ribbon-like stool is the feature of Hirschsprung's disease.
- Suction biopsy is the confirmatory diagnostic test for Hirschsprung's disease.
- Meckel's diverticulum is an outpouching or bulge in the lower part of the small intestine. The bulge is congenital (present at birth) and is a leftover of the umbilical cord.

Clinical Corner

CASE SCENARIO 4:
Child admitted with Hirschsprung's disease developed fever and explosive diarrhea. Assigned nurse immediately informs this event to the physician. What complication she would have anticipated?
a. Intussusception
b. Enterocolitis
c. Volvulus
d. Perforation

Ans. (b) Enterocolitis
One of the complications associated with Hirschsprung's disease is enterocolitis. Hirschsprung-associated enterocolitis often presents with fever, explosive diarrhea, abdominal swelling, lethargy, and vomiting.

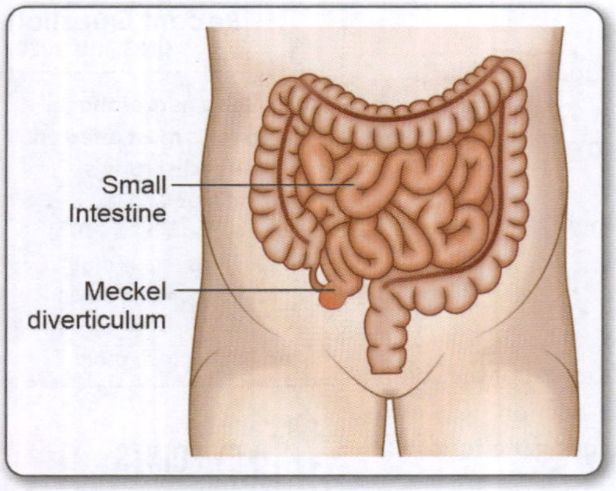

Figure 20: Meckel's diverticulum

Clinical Manifestations

Mostly asymptomatic, painless rectal bleeding, nausea and vomiting, anemia.

Diagnosis

Barium enema, Meckel scan, rectosigmoidoscopy

Treatment

Diverticulum is removed under general anesthesia.

Appendicitis

Inflammation of vermiform appendix located at the end of cecum.

Clinical Manifestations

- Rebound tenderness.
- **Positive Rovsing's sign**: Palpation of left lower quadrant of the abdomen increases pain in the right lower quadrant.
- **Pain at McBurney's point**: Finger pressure at Mc Burney's point (midway between superior iliac spine and umbilicus on right side) elicits a major pain response.

Management

- Appendectomy is the surgery of choice.
- Enema is contraindicated in this condition.

UMBILICAL CORD ANOMALIES

Umbilical Granuloma

- It is a small round, wet, often pink, pedunculated lesion measuring up to 1 cm arising from the base of umbilicus.
- Treatment includes cauterization with silver nitrate, ligation, use of alcoholic wipes and rarely surgical excision.

Omphalitis

- Inflammation of cord stump or its surrounding tissue.
- It needs to be treated with antibiotics otherwise it may lead to umbilical phlebitis, portal vein thrombosis, liver abscesses, peritonitis.

Umbilical Hernia

An umbilical hernia occurs when part of intestine bulges through the opening in abdominal muscles near umbilicus.

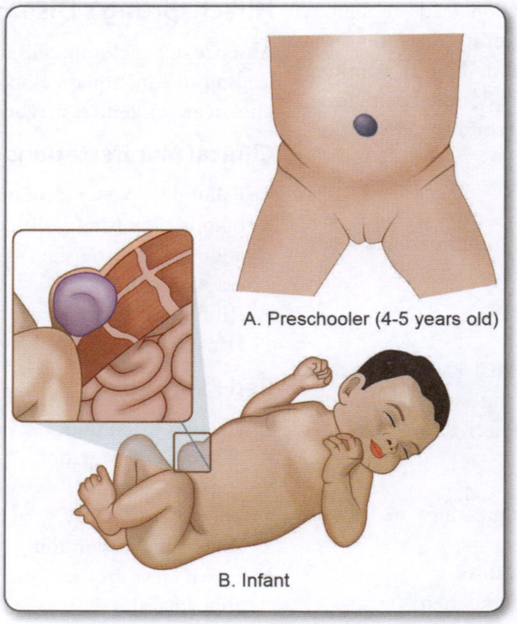

Figure 21: Umbilical Hernia

Omphalocele (Exomphalos)

- Omphalocele is a birth defect of the abdominal wall.
- The infant's intestines, liver, or other organs stick outside of the belly through the belly button.
- The organs are covered in a thin, nearly transparent sac that hardly ever is open or broken.

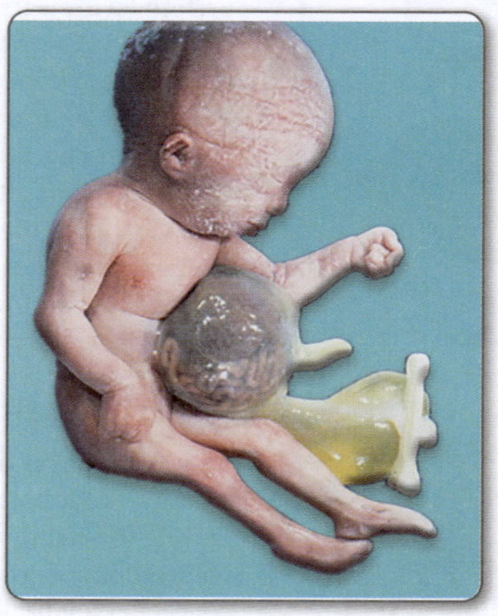

Figure 22: Omphalocele

KEY POINT

Enema is contraindicated in appendicitis.

KEY POINT

In appendicitis, pain is located in the right lower quadrant of the abdomen (McBurney's point)

Recent Question (INC PhD 2020)

50. Which among the following is the manifestation of imperforate anus?

a. Meconium ileus
b. Ribbon-like stool
c. Scaphoid abdomen
d. Currant jelly-like stool

Ans. (a) Meconium ileus

KEY POINT

Sponge bath the baby until stump falls off because moisture will delay the stump to fall off.

Gastroschisis

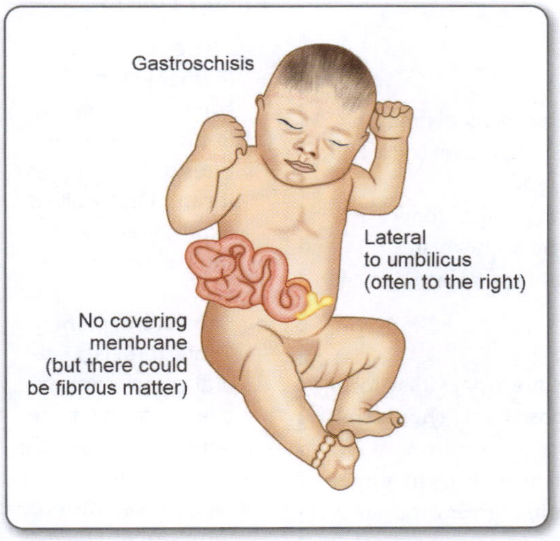

Figure 23: Gastroschisis

- It is a birth defect of the abdominal (belly) wall.
- The baby's intestines are found outside of the baby's body, exiting through a hole beside the belly button.
- A hole occurs which allows the intestines and other organs to extend outside of the body, usually to the right side of belly button.

DISORDERS OF HEPATIC SYSTEM

Hepatitis

- Acute viral hepatitis is a systemic infection and inflammation predominantly affecting the liver.
- Hepatitis A is caused by RNA virus and spreads through fecal-oral route.
- Hepatitis B is caused by DNA virus and spreads via blood and body fluids.
- Hepatitis C is caused by RNA virus and is transmitted through blood and body fluids.
- Hepatitis D virus is also an RNA virus which is also called as delta virus and is transmitted by blood and body fluids.
- Hepatitis E virus is RNA virus and its mode of transmission is fecal-oral route.

Clinical Manifestations

Jaundice, fever, fatigue, nausea, anorexia, abdominal pain, dark urine

Diagnosis

- Liver enzyme like AST and ALT
- Serum bilirubin
- ESR
- HAV infection by anti-HAV immunoglobulin M
- HBV infection by detection of HBsAg antigen and IgM antibodies to HBcAg.
- HCV is diagnosed by anti HCV, HCV core Ag

Management

- Hand hygiene and low-fat balanced diet
- Adequate rest and avoid vigorous physical activities
- Safe water and sanitation
- Vaccination

Liver Cirrhosis

It is a chronic degenerative state of liver which leads to development of bands of fibrous tissues.

Clinical Manifestations

Irritability, chalky, pasty stool, abdominal distention, fever, jaundice, hepatomegaly, splenomegaly, ascites, esophageal varices, hemoptysis, anemia, muscle weakness, lethargy and GI bleeding.

Diagnosis

History collection and physical examination, liver function test (ALT, GGT), prothrombin time, clotting time and bleeding time, liver biopsy, cupriuresis.

Management

- There is no specific treatment
- Adequate diet with good quality of protein, vitamins, and minerals
- Antibiotics to treat infections
- D-penicillamine to chelate copper
- Immunomodulators
- Corticosteroids and gamma globulins
- IV fluids to treat dehydration

Extrahepatic Biliary Atresia

- Characterized by destruction or absence of all or a portion of the bile duct that lies outside the liver.
- Absence or destruction of the bile ducts results in the abnormal accumulation of bile in the liver.
- Affected infants have **yellowing of the skin and sclera (jaundice)** and scarring of the liver (fibrosis).

Clinical Manifestations

- Symptoms appear by the age of two to six weeks.
- Jaundice, abnormally pale stools, and dark urine, abdominal distention, hepatomegaly, poor weight gain, portal hypertension

Diagnosis

- Deranged LFT including bilirubin and liver enzyme.
- Elevated prothrombin time, partial thromboplastin time.
- USG, Viral serology and Liver biopsy
- Endoscopic retrograde cholangiopancreatography (ERCP)

KEY POINTS

- Hepatitis-B vaccine to a newborn is administered intramuscularly in Vastus lateralis.
- Serum hepatitis is also known as Hepatitis B
- The primary cause of abdominal ascites in a patient with cirrhosis of the liver is a decreased serum albumin level.
- Most common cause of obstructive jaundice in children is biliary atresia.
- Magnetic resonance cholangiopancreatography (MRCP) is investigation of choice to diagnose biliary atresia in infants.

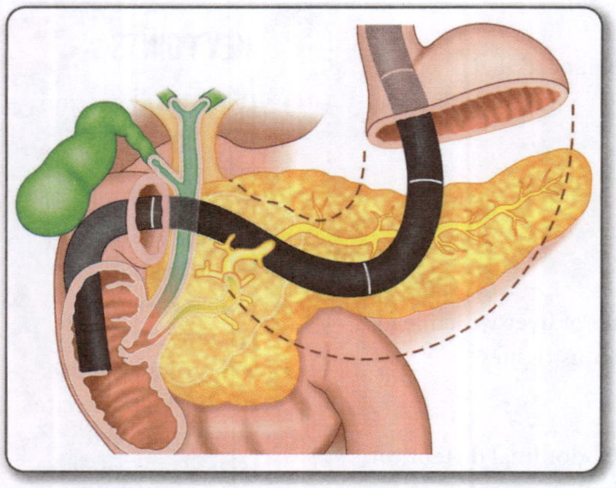

Figure 24: Endoscopic retrograde cholangiopancreatography

Management

- If correctable lesion, then choledochojejunostomy (surgical anastomosis of common bile duct and jejunum).
- If any correctable lesion is found, then hepatic portoenterostomy or **kasai** procedure (in this, extra hepatic duct is removed and jejunum is anastomosed with the hilus of liver) is done.
- Liver transplantation is the definitive treatment for atresia.

Wilson's Disease

- It is also called as hepatolenticular degeneration and lenticular degeneration.
- It is a rare autosomal recessive disorder of copper metabolism characterized by the multiple mutations in the ATP-ase 7B gene on chromosome 13q.

Clinical Manifestations

- **Kayser-Fleischer ring:** Color of the ring may be golden to brown or green seen in cornea.
- **Sunflower cataract**: Copper deposition in the lens gives sunflower appearance.
- Jaundice, Fatigue, nausea, vomiting, weight loss, and pain in abdomen
- **Spider angiomas**, muscle cramps and edema
- Hepatosplenomegaly and elevated liver enzyme
- Seizures, gait abnormalities, olfactory impairment
- Personality changes, cognitive impairment and depression
- Bone and joint involvement
- Hemolytic anemia, thrombocytopenia
- Hypercalciuria, hyperphosphaturia and hypokalemia
- Hypopigmentation of lower legs

Diagnosis

- Liver biopsy (hepatic copper determination)
- Slit lamp examination (for Kayser-Fleischer ring)
- Serum ceruloplasmin
- 24-hour urinary copper excretion
- Serum copper and serum free copper
- MRI
- Genetic testing

Management

- Chelating agents like trientine, penicillamine
- Zinc acetate: It blocks the digestive tract and absorption of copper from food
- Diet: Avoid foods containing high copper like shellfish, liver, mushroom, nuts, chocolate
- Liver transplantation in case of severe liver damage

Cholelithiasis

- Gallstones or cholelithiasis are stones that form in the gallbladder composed of cholesterol, bilirubin, and bile.
- Symptomatic patients present with **right upper abdominal pain** after eating greasy or spicy food, nausea, vomiting, pain in epigastrium that radiates to the right scapula or mid-back.

Diagnosis

USG, MRCP, ERCP, cholescintigraphy

Treatment

- Asymptomatic cases can be observed for spontaneous passage of stool
- Laparoscopic cholecystectomy
- Extracorporeal shock wave lithotripsy
- Cholecystectomy with splenectomy

Choledochal Cyst

- These are cystic dilation of extrahepatic duct, intrahepatic duct, or both that may result in progressive biliary obstruction and biliary cirrhosis.

Clinical Manifestations

- Triad of symptoms include pain in abdomen, palpable abdominal mass, jaundice
- Liver dysfunction, hepatomegaly

Diagnosis

- LFT
- USG, CT, HIDA scan, MRCP, ERCP

Management

- Laparoscopic excision of cyst
- Roux-en-Y hepaticojejunostomy

DISORDERS OF CARDIOVASCULAR SYSTEM

Congenital Heart Disease

- These are cardiac anomalies arising because of a defect in the structure or function of the heart and great vessels which are present at birth.
- Two types: Acyanotic heart disease and cyanotic heart disease.

KEY POINTS

Two types of gallstones:

- **Pigment stone:** Unconjugated pigment in the bile precipitates to form stones. It can't be dissolved. Surgical removal is the treatment of choice.
- **Cholesterol stone:** Cholesterol is a natural component of bile. Its solubility depends upon bile acid and lecithin. Cholesterol precipitates to form stones when bile acid synthesis is less than cholesterol synthesis.

KEY POINTS

- Kayser-Fleischer (golden brown) ring at the limbus of cornea seen with a hand lens is observed in Wilson's disease.
- Sunflower cataract in Wilson's disease is due to copper deposition in lens.

Acyanotic Heart Disease

The shunt is from left to right side of the heart.

Table 36: Classification of acyanotic heart disease

Increased pulmonary blood flow	Obstruction to blood flow from ventricles
ASD VSD PDA	Coarctation of aorta Aortic stenosis Pulmonic stenosis Mitral stenosis

Atrial Septal Defect (ASD)

- An abnormal opening in the atrial septum which allows oxygenated blood from the left atrium to mix with deoxygenated blood in the right atrium at a minor pressure difference.
- When blood passes through the ASD from the left atrium to the right atrium, a larger volume of blood than normal must be handled by the right side of the heart. Extra blood then passes through the pulmonary artery into the lungs leading to pulmonary hypertension and pulmonary congestion.
- If the ASD is left uncorrected, then pulmonary hypertension progresses and pressure in the right side of the heart will become greater than the left side of the heart. This reversal of the pressure gradient across the ASD causes the shunt to reverse from right to left. This phenomenon is known as **Eisenmenger's syndrome**.
- Once right-to-left shunting occurs, a portion of the oxygen-poor blood will get shunted to the left side of the heart and ejected to the peripheral vascular system. This will cause signs of cyanosis.

Types of Atrial Septal Defect

Table 37: Types of ASD

Type	Description
Ostium primum	Opening at the lower end of the septum.
Ostium secundum	Most common type of ASD. Opening at the center of the septum.
Sinus venosus	Opening near the junction between superior vena cava and right atrium.

Clinical Manifestation

- Most infants and children are asymptomatic but over years to decades may experience the symptoms depending on type and severity of ASD
- Infant gets tired during feeding
- Child gets tired with playing/eating
- Shortness of breath
- Fatigue, Sweating, Palpitations
- Stunted growth

Management

- **20% of atrial septal defects will close spontaneously** in the first year of life or as the child grows
- **For defects of 3–8 mm** or smaller: Supportive medical management like digoxin, diuretics and prophylactic antibiotics up till spontaneous closure.
- **If defect is >8 mm:** Surgical repair may be required.
- If spontaneous closure does not occur by school-going age, surgical repair becomes essential.
- **Surgical repair:**
  - Defect may be closed with **stitches or a special patch.**
  - **The material used for patch closure** - Patient's own pericardium or commercially available bovine pericardium, or synthetic material (Gore-Tex, Dacron).

KEY POINTS

- **Foramen ovale is** a structure with functional closure immediately after birth.
- Failure of the foramen ovale closure will lead to atrial septal defect.
- Patent ductus venosus results in irregular transmission of blood between **left umbilical vein and inferior vena cava.**
- After the closure, ductus venosus is known as **ligamentum venosum.**
- After the closure, ductus arteriosus is known as **ligamentum arteriosum.**
- After the closure, foramen ovale is known as **fossa ovalis.**

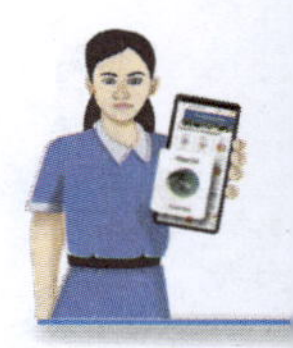

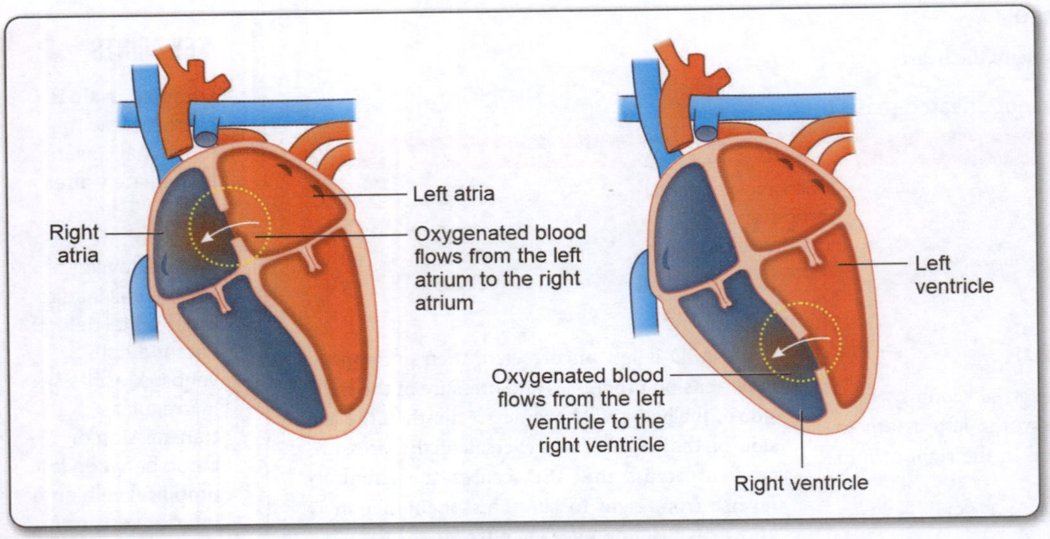

Figure 25: Atrial septal defect

Ventricular Septal Defect (VSD)

- An opening in the ventricular septum which allows oxygenated blood to pass from the left ventricle, through the opening in the septum, and then mix with unoxygenated blood in the right ventricle.
- **VSDs are the most commonly occurring type of congenital heart defect,**[NORCET 2022] occurring in 14–17% of babies born each year.

Clinical Manifestation

- Small VSD: Usually asymptomatic
- Moderate to large VSD: Dyspnea, tachypnea, exercise intolerance, delayed growth, feeding difficulty, recurrent respiratory tract infection, features of cardiac failure, cardiomyopathy
- Large VSD with shunt reversal: Cyanosis, clubbing, right ventricular hypertrophy

Diagnosis

Cardiac auscultation of murmur, ECG, chest X-ray, echo, cardiac catheterization, Doppler study.

Management

- Closure of VSD using Dacron patches.
- Pulmonary artery banding is done for large or multiple VSD.

Patent Ductus Arteriosus

- It is the persistent communication between pulmonary artery and aorta that results from failure of normal physiologic closure of the fetal ductus after birth.

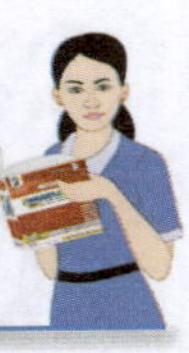

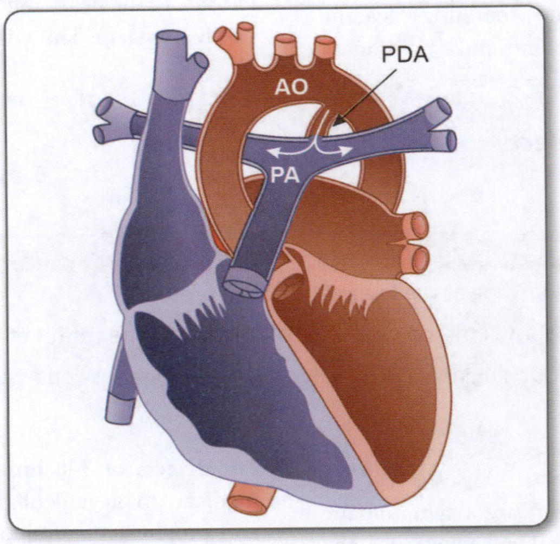

Figure 26: Patent ductus arteriosus (PDA)

Clinical Manifestation

Dyspnea on exertion, fatigue, poor growth, respiratory infection, continuous machinery murmur, increased heart rate, gallop rhythm, bounding pulse, widened pulse pressure.

Diagnosis

ECG, chest X-ray, echo, Doppler study, cardiac catheterization.

Management

- Small PDA: Spontaneous closure
- Moderate PDA: Wait up to 2 years or 10 kg weight
- PDA with CCF: Surgical closure
- **Indomethacin** 0.2 mg/kg/dose helps in closure of PDA
- **Ibuprofen** can be given where indomethacin is contraindicated

KEY POINTS

- Most common heart abnormality in children is **Ventricular Septal Defect.**
- Patent ductus arteriosus results in irregular transmission of blood between pulmonary artery and aorta.
- Sternum is the best site to demonstrate capillary refilling in infants.

Recent Question (NORCET 2023)

51. Most common congenital malformation in overt diabetes in pregnancy:
a. Ventricular septal defect
b. Sacral agenesis
c. Tetralogy of fallot
d. Atrial septal defect

Ans. (a) Ventricular septal defect

POINTS TO REMEMBER

- ***Prostaglandin infusion helps to keep the PDA patent.***
- Indomethacin/ ibuprofen helps to close the PDA.

Coarctation of Aorta

Narrowing of the aorta can occur anywhere, but is most likely to happen in the segment just after the aortic arch.

Clinical Manifestation

- High blood pressure in the arms and low blood pressure in the legs.
- Delayed and weak femoral pulse and strong brachial pulse.
- Intermittent claudication, pain and weakness in legs.
- Leg may be cooler than arms.

Diagnosis

- ECG: Ventricular hypertrophy
- Chest X-ray: Prominent ascending aorta
- Barium swallow: Confirm the site of coarctation
- Echo: Shell like constriction in descending aorta
- Color Doppler: Acceleration of blood flow in the site of narrowing

Treatment

- Balloon dilation
- Resection of narrowing segment and end to end anastomosis.

Aortic Stenosis

Narrowing or stricture of the aortic valve.

Management

- Percutaneous balloon valvuloplasty
- Aortic valve commissurotomy
- Aortic valve replacement

Pulmonic Stenosis

Narrowing at the entrance of pulmonary artery.

Mitral Stenosis

Narrowing of the heart's mitral valve.

Cyanotic Heart Disease

The shunt present is predominantly from Right to Left leading to shunting of venous blood without passing through the lungs to be oxygenated. Unoxygenated blood circulates in arteries.

Recent Question (NORCET 2020)

52. Cyanotic spell is seen in which of the following conditions?
a. Atrial septal defect
b. Ventricular septal defect
c. Tetralogy of Fallot
d. Transposition of arteries

Ans. (c) Tetralogy of...

KEY POINTS

- A child who is suffering from cyanotic heart diseases is more comfortable in knee-chest position.
- In X-ray, the heart of a child with tetralogy of Fallot appears boot-shaped.

Table 38: Manifestations, diagnosis and management of various conditions

Condition	Manifestations	Diagnosis	Management
Tetralogy of Fallot: Consists of four problems 1. VSD 2. Pulmonic stenosis (right ventricular outflow tract obstruction) 3. Overriding of aorta 4. Right ventricular hypertrophy	• Cyanosis • Shortness of breath (SOB) on exertion/ feeding • Hypercyanotic spells • Clubbing of fingers • Tachypnea • Systolic thrill	Chest X-ray: boot-shaped heart 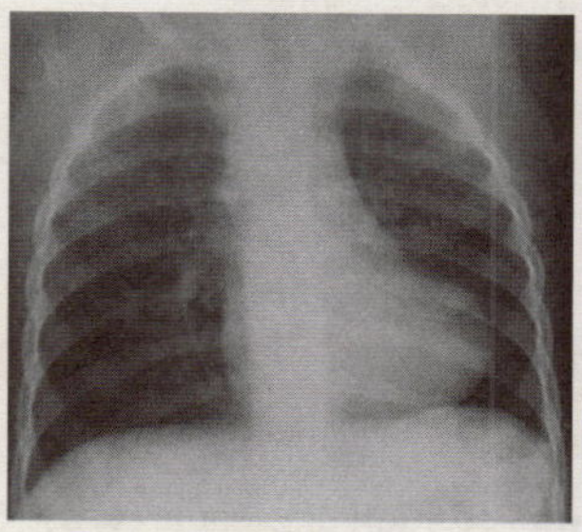 ECG: Right ventricular hypertrophy	**Hypoxic spell management:** • Oxygen administration. • Knee-chest position. • Morphine: to abolish hyperpnea. **Surgical Management:** **Pott's procedure:** Anastomosis of the upper descending aorta with left pulmonary artery. **Waterston shunt:** Side to side anastomosis of ascending aorta with right pulmonary artery. **Brock's procedure:** Pulmonary valvotomy done to correct pulmonary stenosis. **Classic Blalock-Taussig shunt:** Subclavian artery and the ipsilateral pulmonary artery are anastomosed.
Transposition of great arteries (TGA): Aorta arises from right ventricle and pulmonary artery arises from left ventricle. So deoxygenated blood is carried by aorta to systemic circulation and oxygenated blood returns to lung by pulmonary artery.	• Cyanosis • Rapid breathing • Indrawing beneath the rib cage • Congestive heart failure • Ejection systolic murmur	• ECG • Chest X-ray (egg on string appearance) • Cardiac catheterization	**Palliative** Non-surgical procedures to enlarge foramen ovale or balloon atrial septostomy. Prostaglandin infusion to keep PDA open. **Total correction** Arterial switch operation: Distal aorta is connected to pulmonary stump and pulmonary artery is connected to proximal aortic stump.
Truncus arteriosus: The aorta and pulmonary artery start as a single blood vessel, which eventually divides and becomes two separate arteries.	• Cyanosis after birth • Signs of CHF • Dyspnea with feeding • Failure to thrive • Frequent respiratory infections	ECG Echo X-ray	**Surgery** • Closing the VSD • Excising the pulmonary arteries from aorta and attaching them to the RV by means of homograft

Contd...

Condition	Manifestations	Diagnosis	Management
Tricuspid atresia: There is no tricuspid valve in this condition, so there is no blood flow from right atrium to right ventricle.	• Cyanosis • Tachypnea • Poor feeding • A small right ventricle, a large left ventricle, small VSD and PDA.	ECG X-ray Echo	**Palliative procedure** • PGE1 should be started in neonates with severe cyanosis to maintain the patency of the ductus arteriosus. • The **Rashkind procedure** (balloon atrial septostomy) may be performed to improve the RA-to-LA shunt. **Surgery** • Modified blalock-taussig shunt.
Total anomalous pulmonary venous return (TAPVR): Oxygen-rich blood does not return from the lungs through pulmonary vein to the left atrium, instead the oxygen-rich blood returns to the right side of the heart.	• Cyanosis • Rapid breathing, grunting and retractions • Chest infections	• ECG • Chest X-ray: Enlargement of the right side and pulmonary edema. • Echo • Cardiac catheterization	In surgery, the pulmonary veins are connected to the left atrium and the defect between the right and left atrium is closed.
Hypoplastic left heart syndrome: Underdevelopment of the left side of the heart resulting in a hypoplastic left ventricle and aortic atresia.	• Neonate becomes critically ill within the first few hours to the first few days of life. • Tachycardia • Dyspnea • Pulmonary crackles • Weak peripheral pulses • Vasoconstricted extremities • Cyanosis • S2 is loud and single.	ECG shows RVH. Chest X-ray films characteristically show pulmonary venous congestion or pulmonary edema. Arterial blood gas levels reveal a slightly decreased PO_2 and a normal PCO_2.	**Therapeutic Mx** PGE1 infusion to maintain ductal patency. **Surgical Mx** 1st stage: Norwood procedure 2nd stage-Bidirectional Glenn Shunt

Table 39: X-ray appearance in various congenital heart diseases

X-ray characteristics	Congenital heart disease
Boot shaped heart	Tetralogy of Fallot
Egg on string appearance	Transposition of great arteries
Snow man or figure of 8 appearance	Supra-cardiac total anomalous pulmonary venous return
Box shaped heart	Ebstein's anomaly

Acute Rheumatic Fever

Immune-mediated delayed response to infection with specific strains of group A beta hemolytic streptococcus—Antigens that may cross-react with cardiac myosin and sarcolemmal membrane protein.

Child with history of streptococcal pharyngitis with fever is at risk for developing this.

Revised Jones Criteria

Major Manifestation

- Carditis
- Polyarthritis
- Chorea
- Erythema marginatum
- Subcutaneous nodule

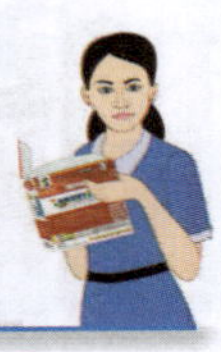

Minor Manifestation

- Hyperpyrexia
- Arthralgia, without other signs of inflammation
- **Lab:** Elevated ESR, CRP
- Prolonged PR interval in ECG
- And evidence of antecedent streptococcal infection
  - Throat swab culture or rapid antigen test
  - Elevated/increasing anti-streptococcal antibody titer in serum

Diagnosis of initial episode:

Primary episode of rheumatic fever: 2 major or 1 major + 2 minor manifestation plus evidence of preceding group A streptococcal infection.

Management

- Single dose of benzyl penicillin 1.2 million U IM

KEY POINTS

- The Fontan procedure is used to correct tricuspid atresia.
- **Group A β-hemolytic streptococcus is the** causative organism for rheumatic fever.
- Drug of choice for rheumatic fever prophylaxis in penicillin allergic patient is Erythromycin.
- Most common cyanotic congenital heart disease on day 1 of life is transposition of great arteries.
- Intake of lithium during pregnancy can cause Ebstein anomaly.

- Oral phenoxymethylpenicillin 250 mg 6-hourly for 10 days
- Penicillin-allergic patients: Erythromycin or a cephalosporin
- Analgesia: Optimally achieved with high doses of salicylates
- Treatment is then directed towards limiting cardiac damage and relieving symptoms

Rheumatic Heart Disease

Rheumatic heart disease is a condition in which the heart valves have been permanently damaged by rheumatic fever.

The order of affecting valve is mitral > aortic > tricuspid.

Diagnosis

- ECG
- Echo: Echo can show damage to the valve flaps, backflow of blood through a leaky valve, fluid around the heart, and heart enlargement.
- Chest X-ray
- Cardiac MRI
- Blood test like CRP, ESR

Rheumatic heart disease most commonly affects valves in the following order: Mitral, Aortic, tricuspid and pulmonic.

Infective Endocarditis

Infective endocarditis (IE) is a microbial infection of the endocardial (endothelial) surface of the heart.

Diagnosis

Duke criteria are used to diagnose infective endocarditis.

Major Criteria

- Positive blood cultures for infective endocarditis
- Echocardiogram: Vegetation, dehiscence, abscess, new valvular regurgitation murmur
- Positive Coxiella burnetii or anti-phase IgG antibody titer >1:800

Minor Criteria

- Predisposing heart condition or IV drug use
- Fever >38°C
- Vascular phenomena: Emboli to organs/brain, hemorrhages
- Immunologic phenomena: Glomerulonephritis, Osler nodes, Roth spots, rheumatoid factor
- Positive blood culture with organism is consistent with infective endocarditis.
- Echocardiography findings are consistent with infective endocarditis but not meeting major criterion as noted previously.

To Diagnose the Condition

- 2 major criteria
- 1 major criterion and any 3 minor criteria
- 0 major criterion and any 5 minor criteria

Management

- Antibiotic: Penicillin or ampicillin (vancomycin if allergic to penicillin) plus gentamycin for 4-6 weeks.
- Surgery is indicated if there is continued bacteremia after 2 weeks of appropriate therapy.

Kawasaki Disease

- Kawasaki disease (KD), formerly known as Mucocutaneous lymph node syndrome and Infantile polyarteritis nodosa, is an acute febrile illness characterized by inflammation of blood vessels throughout the body that primarily affects young children and infants.
- It is now the **most common cause of acquired heart disease** in children.

Phases of Disease

- **Acute febrile phase (0–10 days)** — Fever and the other acute signs of illness.
- **Subacute phase (10–28 days)** — Associated with desquamation, thrombocytosis and the highest risk of sudden death in patients in whom aneurysms have developed.
- **Convalescent phase:** 6-8 weeks after the onset of illness.

Manifestation

- Fever that is often higher than 102.2°F
- Change in extremities
  - Acute: Erythema and edema of hands and feet
  - Convalescent: Membranous desquamation of fingertips
- Polymorphous exanthema
- Bilateral painless bulbar conjunctival infection without exudate
- Erythema and cracking of lips, **strawberry tongue**, diffuse infection of oral and pharyngeal mucosa
- Cervical lymphadenopathy, usually unilateral

Management

- Intravenous immunoglobulin in a single dose of 2 g/kg in the first 10 days of illness along with aspirin 70–80 mg/kg/day given every 6 hours.
- Antiplatelet drugs and heparin may be required for patients with more severe diseases.
- Corticosteroids may be given in unresponsive patients.

Clinical Corner

CASE SCENARIO 5:
Rashmi, a 4-year-old girl, has been diagnosed with Kawasaki disease. In addition to the recognized symptoms of the disease, the nurse is aware that she may also be at risk of developing which of the following conditions?

a. Sepsis
b. Meningitis
c. Mitral valve disease
d. Aneurysm formation

Ans. (d) Aneurysm formation

Clinical Corner

CASE SCENARIO 6:
A 4-year-old girl presents with fever for the past five days, strawberry tongue, generalized erythematous rash, and cervical lymphadenopathy. Echo suggested coronary artery abnormalities. The most likely diagnosis is?

a. Rosie-Dorfaman disease
b. Scrub Typhus
c. Kawasaki disease
d. Scarlet fever

Ans. (c) Kawasaki disease

POINTS TO REMEMBER

Administration of parenteral vaccine (measles, mumps, rubella, varicella) should be delayed for at least 3 months after IV immunoglobulin for Kawasaki Disease.

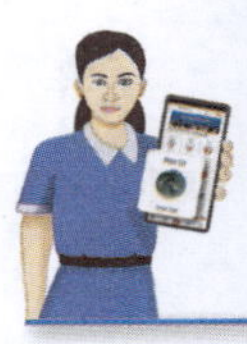

DISORDERS OF GENITOURINARY SYSTEM

Nephrotic Syndrome

It is a disorder characterized by alteration in permeability of glomerular capillaries which leads to massive **proteinuria, hypoalbuminemia, edema and hyperlipidemia**.

Clinical Manifestation

- **Edema:** Starting at face around the eyes and subsequently pedal edema progressing to presacral and genital area to generalized subcutaneous edema. **Generally, edema increases in the morning and subsides in the evening.**
- Decreased urine volume
- Massive proteinuria
- GI symptoms: Pain in abdomen and diarrhea
- Respiratory symptoms: Pulmonary edema, hydrothorax

Diagnosis

- Urine examination for proteinuria and cast
- Serum biochemistry: WBCs, hemoglobin, protein, albumin, cholesterol,
- Chest X-ray
- C3 and ASO titer
- Renal biopsy in some conditions

Management

- **For initial episode**: Prednisolone 2 mg/kg/day (max 60 mg) for 6 weeks followed by 1.5 mg/kg/day (max. 40 mg) as a single morning dose every alternative day for 6 weeks.
- **For relapse**: Prednisolone 2 mg/kg/day until urine albumin trace is nil or trace for 3 consecutive days followed by 1.5 mg/kg/day as a single morning dose every alternative day for 4 weeks and then stopped.
- **Frequent relapse or steroid dependent**: Alternative day single morning dose of prednisolone 0.5 to 0.7 mg/kg for 9-18 months.
- **Steroid resistant case:** Prednisolone and cyclophosphamide and high dose methylprednisolone and cyclophosphamide.
- **For edema:** Diuretics — oral furosemide 1-3 mg/kg/day. For refractory edema, albumin infusion is given on alternative days followed by IV furosemide.
- **Diet:** Protein intake should be 2-2.5 g/kg/day daily.
- Immunization: Children under steroid therapy are immunocompromised. Hence **live vaccines cannot be given during treatment**. These can be given after 6 weeks of discontinuation of steroid therapy.

All killed vaccines can be given. Pneumococcal vaccine should be given to prevent Streptococcus pneumonia infection. Varicella vaccine should be given during remission.

Acute Glomerulonephritis

- It is an inflammatory process primarily affecting the glomerulus characterized by sudden onset of **hematuria, oliguria, edema and hypertension.**
- Acute post streptococcal glomerulonephritis is the commonest type affecting children.

Clinical Manifestation

- Edema: Puffiness of face, periorbital edema and pedal edema.
- Mild proteinuria
- Hematuria: Cola-colored urine and smoky urine
- Oliguria
- Hypertension
- Fever, malaise
- History of sore throat or pyoderma
- **Classic triad of symptoms** in post streptococcal acute glomerulonephritis are **edema, hematuria, hypertension.**

Diagnosis

- Urine: RBC, cast, neutrophils, and albumin
- Blood: Raised urea creatinine, low serum C3 level, raised ASO titer, low sodium and high potassium.
- Chest X-ray and Renal biopsy

Management

- **Diuretics:** Edema is treated with oral furosemide 1-3 mg/kg.
- **Hypertension**: Mild hypertension is treated with fluid and water restriction. Commonly used anti-hypertensives are amlodipine, nifedipine or diuretics. Hypertensive emergency is managed with IV nitroprusside or labetalol.

Wilm's Tumor

It is also known as nephroblastoma. It is a highly malignant neoplasm affecting one or both kidneys.

Clinical Manifestation

- Large abdominal mass
- Hematuria
- Hypertension
- Abdominal pain
- Fever
- Anorexia and vomiting
- Polycythemia

Diagnosis

- Abdominal X-ray
- USG and Doppler
- CT scan
- Intravenous pyelography

POINTS TO REMEMBER

- Other name of mucocutaneous lymph node syndrome is **Kawasaki Disease**.
- The most serious complication of Kawasaki disease is cardiac involvement.

KEY POINTS

- Wilms' tumor is the most common primary malignant renal tumor of childhood
- 80% of patients with Wilms' tumor are aged below 5 years
- **Classic triad of symptoms** in post streptococcal acute glomerulonephritis are **edema, hematuria, hypertension**
- Acute glomerulonephritis most often occurs due to streptococci infection
- Type of anemia present in Hemolytic- uremic syndrome is Microangiopathic anemia

Management

Surgery: Radical nephrectomy
Chemotherapy:

- Most used drug is **actinomycin-d and vincristine**
- Doxorubicin and cyclophosphamide also used in some cases

Note: Abdominal palpation is contraindicated

Hemolytic Uremic Syndrome

- It is a condition characterized by triad of symptoms like microangiopathic hemolytic anemia, thrombocytopenia and renal failure.
- It is of two types. Typical or diarrhea associated HUS and atypical or diarrhea negative HUS.

Diagnosis

- Peripheral blood smear reveals fragmented RBC
- Low platelet and high reticulocyte count
- Unconjugated hyperbilirubinemia
- Normal PT and APTT
- Positive direct Coombs test
- Renal biopsy

Treatment

- Fluid restriction and diuretics
- Antihypertensive
- Salt and potassium limitation
- Plasma exchange therapy
- Hemodialysis and peritoneal dialysis

Hypospadias and Epispadias

Hypospadias: Urethra opens on the ventral (underside) part of the penis.

Epispadias: Urethra opens in the dorsal (upper surface) aspects of the penis.

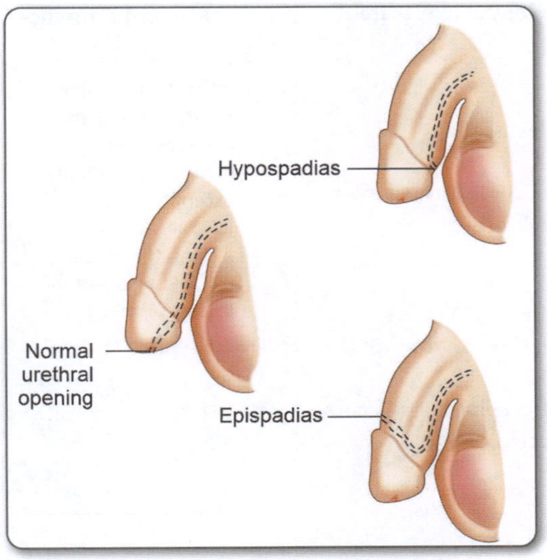

Figure 27: Hypospadias and epispadias

Exstrophy of Bladder

Bladder and urethra abnormality in which bladder is turned inside out.

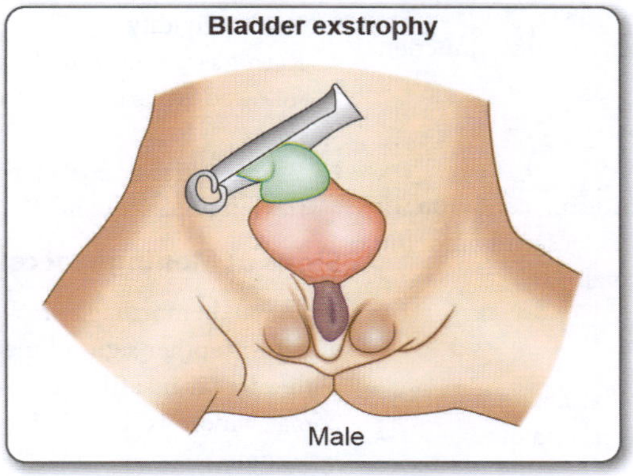

Figure 28: Exstrophy of bladder

Clinical Features

- Absent anterior bladder wall and exposed bright red posterior bladder
- Seepage of urine into posterior bladder
- Constant urine odor and skin excoriation
- Flattened puborectal sling
- Separation of pubic symphysis
- External rotation of pelvis
- Female frequently have displaced and narrowed vaginal orifice

Management

- **Modern staged repair of exstrophy (MRSE):** Initial step is the closure of abdominal wall at 6 months of age. The patient then undergoes repair of the epispadias after testosterone stimulation. Finally, bladder neck repair usually occurs around the age of 4–5 years.
- **Complete primary repair of exstrophy:** The bladder closure is combined with an epispadias repair, to minimize costs and morbidity.

Hydronephrosis

It happens when there is either blockage of urine outflow or reverse flow of urine already in the bladder that can cause the renal pelvis to become enlarged.

Clinical Features

- Pain in the abdomen or flank
- Painful urination
- Frequency and urgency of urine
- Urinary tract infection

Diagnosis

USG, Voiding cystourethrogram, renal scan with Lasix, X-ray, CT, MRI

KEY POINTS

- Preoperatively cover the bladder exstrophy with a thin dressing or clear plastic wrap.
- Avoid petroleum jelly to prevent damage to the mucous.
- Pyeloplasty is the treatment of choice in bilateral hydronephrosis.
- Measuring the child's weight daily on the same scale is most accurate method to determine fluid balance in child. This method is more accurate than intake-output chart.
- Most common cause of neonatal meningitis: Group B streptococci is followed by *E. coli.*
- *Streptococcus pneumoniae* is the most common cause of bacterial meningitis in infants, children and adults.

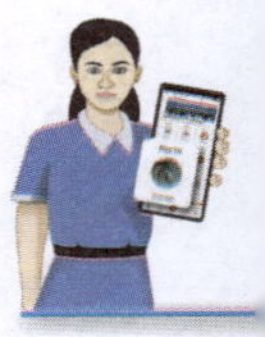

Treatment

- Antibiotic to prevent infection.
- Pyeloplasty: Surgery to correct UPJ obstruction.
- Ureteral re-implantation: Surgery to correct vesicoureteral reflux or ureterovesical junction obstruction.

Undescended Testis

It is also known as cryptorchidism, condition in which one or both testis fail to descend into the scrotum through the inguinal canal.

Ambiguous Genitalia

It is a birth defect of sex organ that makes it unclear whether an affected newborn is girl or a boy.

DISORDERS OF CENTRAL NERVOUS SYSTEM

Meningitis

Defined as an inflammation of meninges.

Classification

- **Bacterial or pyogenic meningitis or septic meningitis:** Caused by bacterial organisms
- **Aseptic meningitis:** Caused by virus, fungal and protozoal agents

Signs of Meningeal Irritation

- Nuchal rigidity
- Kernig's sign: Flexing the patient's hip at 90 degree followed by extending the patient's knee causes pain.
- Brudzinski's sign: Flexing patient's neck causes flexion of patient's hip and knees.

Signs of Meningococcal Meningitis

Petechial hemorrhagic rash on skin and mucosa along with other signs of meningitis. It may proceed with adrenal insufficiency, hypotension, shock and coma which is called **Waterhouse–Friderichsen** syndrome.

Diagnosis

- CSF study
- CT scan
- Rapid diagnostic test: Latex agglutination, PCR, loop mediated amplification method, microarray or biochip, immunochromatography

KEY POINTS

- Positive Kernig's sign, Brudzinski's sign and nuchal rigidity are signs of meningitis.
- **Brudzinski's sign:** Hips and knees to flex when the neck is flexed.
- **Kernig's sign:** Inability to straighten the leg when the hip is flexed to 90°.

Table 40: Types of meningitis

Type of meningitis	Appearance	Leukocyte count (cells/mm³)	Glucose (mg/dL)	Protein (mg/dL)	Opening pressure (mmHg)
Normal	Clear	<8	50-80	15-45	90-180
Bacterial meningitis	Turbid	>1000-2000	<40	>200	Elevated
Viral meningitis	Clear	<300	Normal	<200	Normal
Fungal meningitis	Turbid	<500	Normal to low	>200	Normal to elevated

Treatment

- Antibiotic therapy
- Steroid therapy as an adjuvant method
- Supportive therapy: Osmotic diuretic

Hydrocephalus

Hydrocephalus is the abnormal accumulation of cerebrospinal fluid in the intracranial spaces.

Cerebrospinal Fluid

- The normal amount of CSF is about 150 mL
- CSF is formed by choroid plexuses
- Absorbed by arachnoids villi
- Normally about 500 mL of CSF is formed every day and an equal amount is absorbed

Types of Hydrocephalus

- Communicating hydrocephalus: Occurs due to the over production of CSF or due to the inadequate absorption of CSF.
- Non-communicating hydrocephalus: Occurs when the CSF flow is obstructed.

Recent Question (INC PhD 2020)

53. A Six-months-old child is brought to emergency with hydrocephalus. Which among the following needs to be assessed by the nurse?

a. Level of consciousness
b. Fever and vomiting
c. Anterior fontanelle
d. Posterior fontanelle

Ans. (c) Anterior...

Recent Question (NORCET 2023)

54. All of the following are the early signs and symptoms of meningitis in infant, except

a. Poor feeding
b. Tensed fontanel
c. Vomiting & Irritability
d. High pitched cry

Ans. (b) Tensed fontanel

A tense or bulging fontanel is a late sign of meningitis. All other given options are associated with early sign of meningitis in infants.

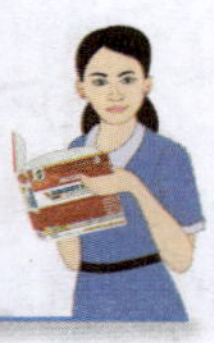

Clinical Manifestation

Table 41: Differences between manifestation of infant and children

Infant (0–2 years)	Children
• Increased head circumference • Bulging fontanelle and bulging scalpel vein • Occipital prominence • Irritability, lethargy, fever and vomiting • Sunsetting eyes • Macewen sign • Impaired vision due to compression of optic chiasma • Increased deep tendon reflex and muscle tone in the lower extremities • Seizure	• Headache, feeling sleepy and lethargy • Sunsetting eyes • Papilledema and strabismus • Convulsion • Delayed milestones • Poor coordination and decreased bladder control

Diagnosis

- Serial recording of head circumference
- Serial USG
- CT/MRI

Management

- Medical management: Acetazolamide to reduce CSF production
- Surgical management: A shunt is made up of radio plastic and has ventricular catheter, pressure valve, pumping chamber, and distal catheter that directs the flow of CSF from the ventricles to other areas of body from where it is absorbed

E.g., ventriculoperitoneal shunt, ventriculoatrial shunt and ventriculopleural shunt

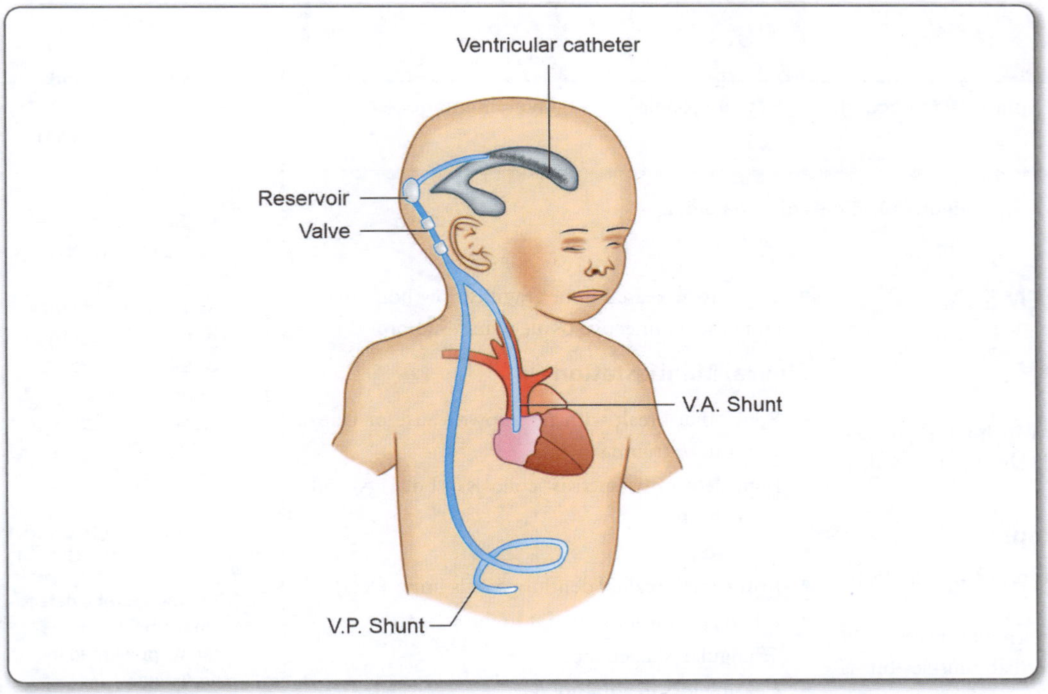

Figure 29: Hydrocephalus

Neural Tube Defect

A neural tube defect (NTD) is a type of birth defect that affects the development of the brain, spinal cord, or their protective coverings.

Types of NTD: Spina bifida, encephalocele, meningomyelocele, iniencephaly, anencephaly, caudal regression syndrome, dermal sinus (tethered cord and syringomyelia).

KEY POINTS

- Sunset sign is seen in Hydrocephalus. In this, eyes are often rolled downward so that the white part of the eyes (sclera) is visible below the upper eyelid.
- Most common seizure disorder during childhood: Febrile seizure.
- Most common cause of neonatal seizure: Hypoxia.
- Most common presentation of neonatal seizure: subtle type.

Recent Question (NORCET 2023)

55. A newborn baby had lumbosacral meningocele. Till the period of surgery, the sac should be well protected by covering it with a sterile gauze piece soaked in

a. Spirit
b. Normal Saline
c. Methylene Blue
d. Betadine

Ans. (b) Normal Saline

Spina Bifida

It is a congenital disorder in which the vertebral arch of the spinal column is either incompletely formed or absent.

Classification

- Spina bifida occulta
- Spina bifida cystica
    - Meningocele
    - Meningomyelocele

Spina bifida occulta: Mildest form of the disease. Overlying skin covering the defect or it may have some hair growing from it; there may be a dimple in the skin, or a birthmark.

Spina bifida cystica: Vertebral defect that is not covered and is exposed to outside environment. It is of two types.

Meningocele: The sac is composed of CSF and meningeal sac there are no nerve roots. Most common location is lumbosacral.

Meningomyelocele: The sac contains both CSF and nerve roots.

Management

Provision of folic acid during pregnancy helps to prevent this condition.

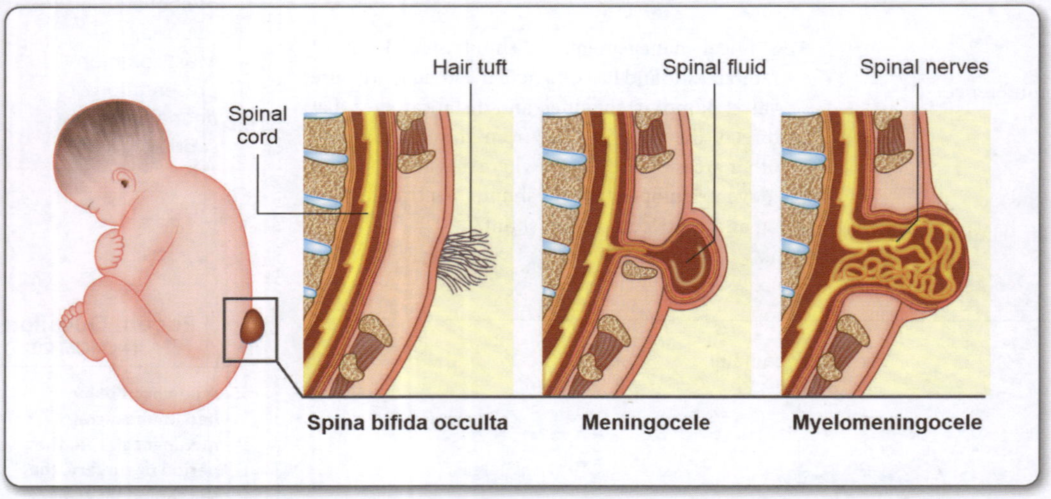

Figure 30: Types of spina bifida

ORTHOPEDIC PROBLEMS IN CHILDREN

Muscular Dystrophies

Group of inherited disorders in which face, arm, leg, spine or heart muscles gradually shrink and weaken over time.

Duchenne Muscular Dystrophy

- It is an X-linked recessive disorder which affects males, while girls are carriers.
- Dystrophin is a protein normally present in skeletal muscle, brain and cardiac muscles but is deficient in this condition.
- Deficiency of dystrophin leads to sarcolemma membrane weakness that results in calcium influx and necrosis of membrane.

Osteogenesis Imperfecta

- It may be autosomal dominant or recessive disorder. It is also known as **brittle bone disease**.
- There is increased bone fragility, low bone mass and other connective tissue manifestation.

Clinical Manifestation

- Bones that break with no known cause or from very minor trauma
- Bone deformity (such as scoliosis or bowlegs) and loose joints
- Short stature
- Brittle teeth (called dentinogenesis imperfecta)
- A blue, purple, or gray tint to the sclera
- Triangular-shaped face
- Hearing loss in adulthood

Diagnosis

- Physical examination
- Bone biopsy
- Bone density measurement
- Serum phosphate and calcium
- Genetic counseling

KEY POINTS

- Since there is chance of shunt malfunction, the nurse needs to measure head and abdominal circumference of the infant in order to monitor the early signs of intracranial pressure and abdominal distension.
- Most common site of Neural Tube Defect: Lumbosacral region.
- In Neural Tube Defect, the following markers increase in the amniotic fluid:
    - Alpha fetoprotein
    - ACh esterase
- Peri-conceptional use of folic acid decreases the incidence of Neural Tube Defect by: 50-70%.
- **Dose of folic acid for:**
    - Primary prevention of NTD: 0.4 mg/day.
    - Secondary prevention of NTD: 5 mg/day.
- Spina bifida occulta is a malformation of one or more vertebrae, it is also called closed or hidden spina bifida.

Recent Question (CNCI 2021)

56. The neural tube defect among newborns can be prevented by providing?

a. Iron to the mother in third trimester
b. Folic acid to mother in first trimester
c. Iron & folic acid throughout pregnancy
d. Vitamin K to the mother in first trimester

Ans. (b) Folic acid to...

Treatment

- Bisphosphonate treatment: Oral pamidronate
- Vitamin D and calcium supplement
- Analgesics
- Traction, casting and fixation
- Genetic counseling

Developmental Dysplasia of Hip

It is also known as congenital dysplasia of hip.

Clinical Manifestation

- Newborns present with hip instability: Infants have limited hip abduction until they begin walking
- Asymmetric skin fold on medial aspect of thigh and gluteal region
- Shortening of limb on the affected side

Physical Examination

Barlow test: The examiner grasps the infant's thigh near the hip and with gentle posterior/lateral pressure, attempts to dislocate the femoral head from the acetabulum. If the hip is dislocatable, a distinct "clunk" may be felt as the femoral head pops out of joint.

Ortolani test: Hip is abducted, and gentle pressure is applied to the proximal thigh from behind. Here, the examiner attempts to relocate an already dislocated femoral head back into the acetabulum. If the joint is dislocated, a palpable "clunk" is noticed as the head slides back into place.

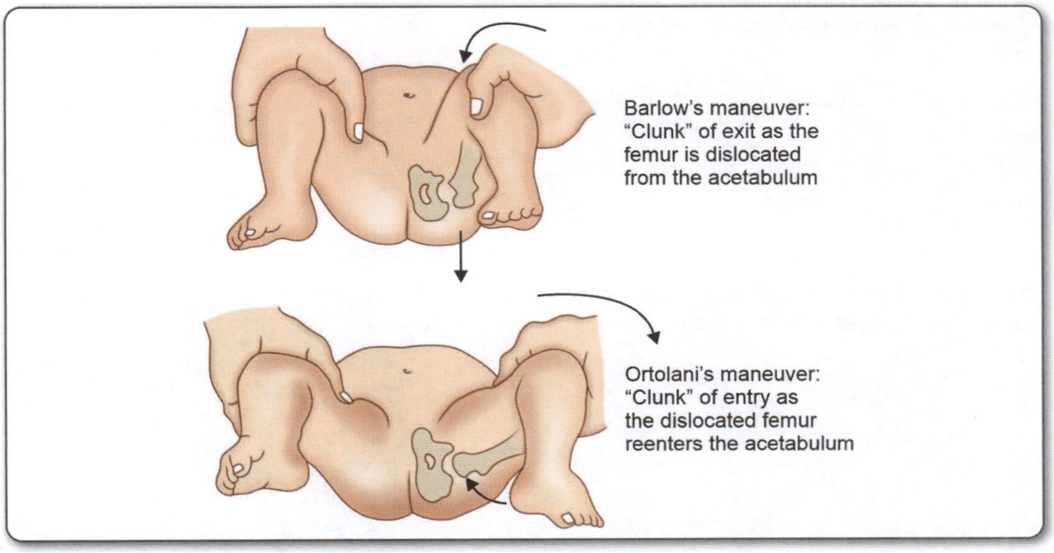

Figure 31: Dysplasia of hip

Galeazzi sign: Child is placed in supine position with both hip and knees flexed. An inequality in the height of the knees is the positive Galeazzi sign.

Trendelenburg's test: A limp on the affected side when the child is walking.

Duck waddle gait: Marked lordosis in bilateral dysplasia.

Treatment

For a newborn up to 6 months, closed reduction and immobilization in a Pavlik harness.

For children older than 6 months, closed reduction under general anesthesia and hip spica casting is done.

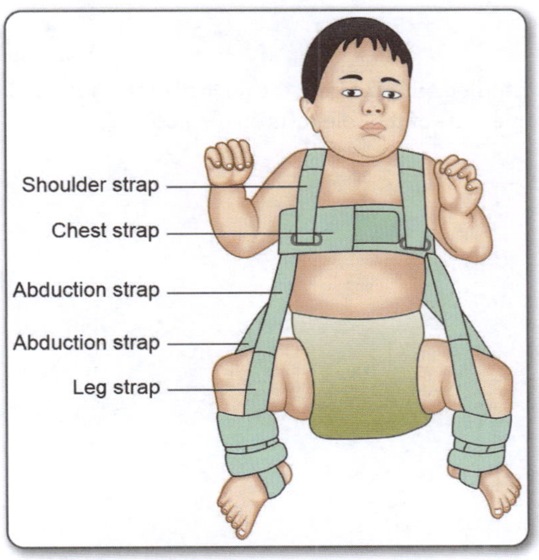

Figure 32: Pavlik harness

Recent Question
(INC PhD 2020)

57. Baby with no legs at birth. Prosthesis can be fitted:
a. Once the body is strong
b. After attaining head control
c. After sitting independently
d. After standing independently

Ans. (c) After sitting...

KEY POINT

- Osteogenesis imperfecta is also known as **brittle bone disease.**

The ninety – ninety traction is used for the fracture of a child's femur or tibia.

Clinical Corner

CASE SCENARIO 7:
One-year-old child diagnosed with congenital dysplasia of hip is waiting for traction. As an experienced nurse you should know that the child will be on:
a. Buck's traction
b. Bryant's traction
c. Tulloch Brown traction
d. Perkin's traction

Ans. (b) Bryant's traction

Bryant's traction is used to treat femoral fracture and congenital dislocation of lip. Buck's traction is used to treat femoral neck fractures and femoral shaft fractures in older and larger children. Perkin's traction used in case of fracture tibia, fracture of femur from subtrochanteric region distally in all ages and fracture trochanter in <50 years.

Club Foot

It is a congenital defect which is also known as congenital talipes equinovarus (TEV).

Classification

Table 42: Classification of clubfoot

Type of clubfoot	Description	Image
Talipes equinovarus	This is the most common type of clubfoot accounting for almost 95% of these. This is characterized by planter flexion of the foot deviating medially and elevated heel than toes.	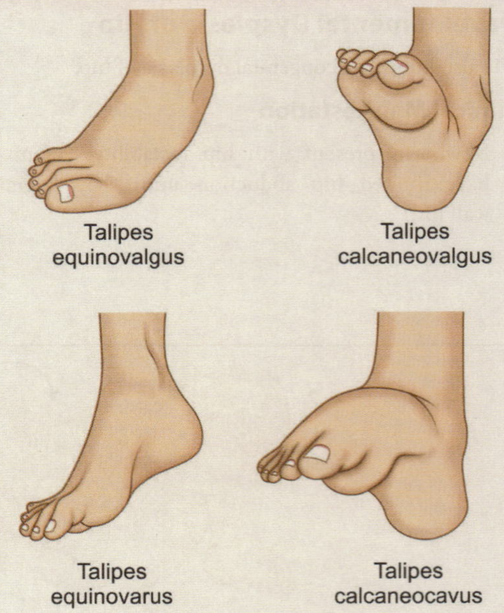
Talipes equinovalgus	The heel is elevated and turned outwards from the midline of the body.	
Talipes calcenovalgus	This is characterized by dorsiflexed and laterally deviated foot. This means the heel is turned outward from midline of the body and anterior part of the foot is elevated on the outer border.	
Talipes calcenovarus	The heel is turned toward of the midline of the body and anterior part of the foot is elevated with heel resting on the floor.	
Talipes varus	Heel is turned inward from the midline of the body and only outer portion of the sole rests on the floor.	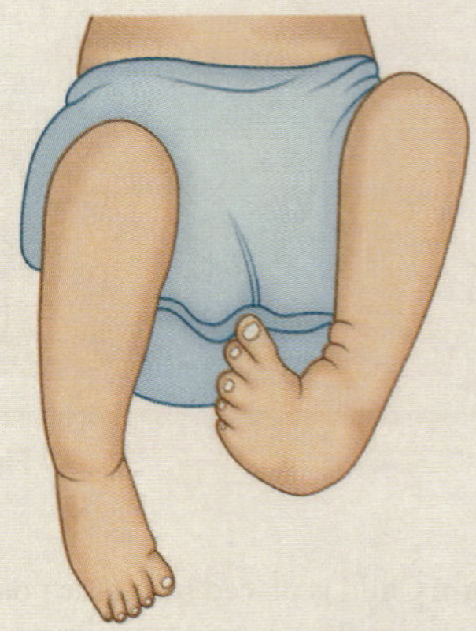
Talipes valgus	Heel is turned outward from the midline of the body and only inner side of the sole rests on the floor	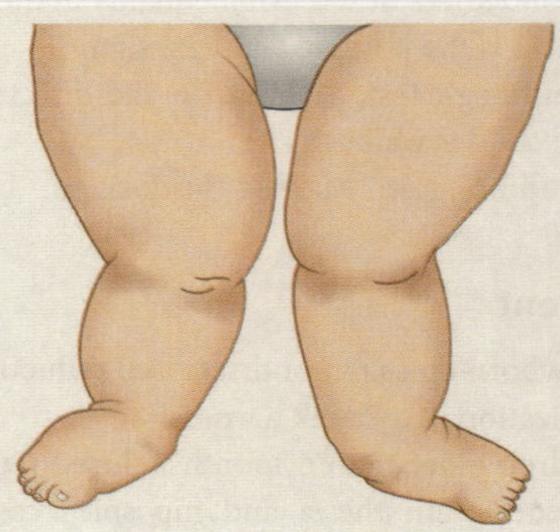

Contd...

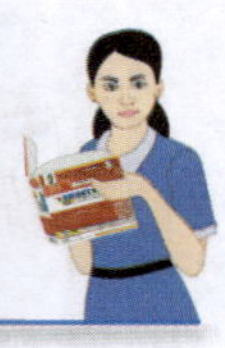

Type of clubfoot	Description	Image
Talipes calcaneus	The foot is fully dorsiflexed, almost touching the anterior part of the leg, and the strongly marked heel seems to be the direct extension of the leg.	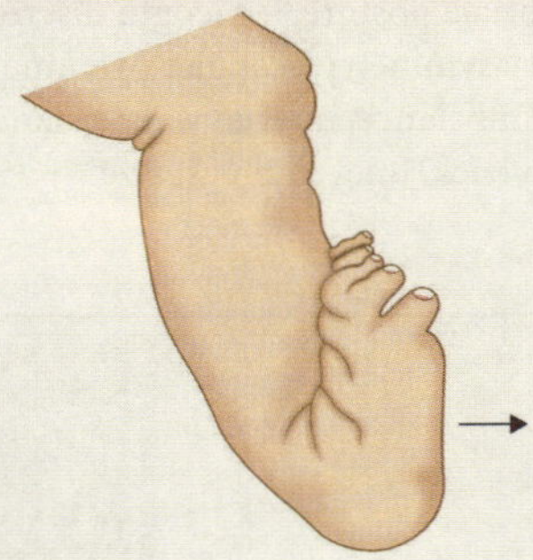
Convex pes valgus	Rare deformity associated with equinus of the rearfoot and dorsiflexion of the forefoot. This results in the break between the forefoot and the rearfoot.	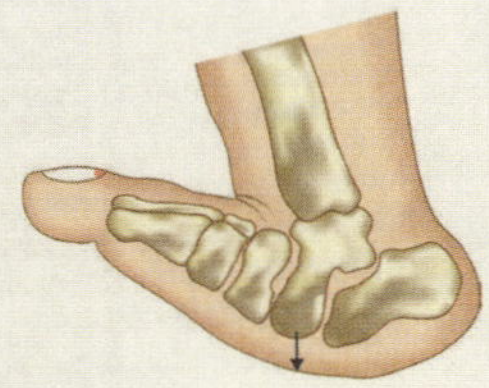
Pes supinatus	The sole of the foot faces inward and the dorsal part of the foot is oriented externally. This abnormal position can be reduced manually and the rearfoot shows no equinus deformity.	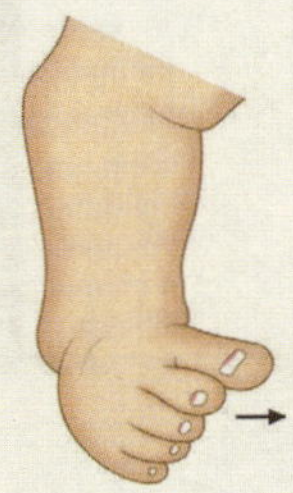
Metatarsus adductus	Inward bending of the metatarsal bones and toes. When looking at the sole of the foot, the forefoot forms an open angle with the rearfoot. The external edge of the foot has a convex shape, while the internal edge is curved inward. The big toe looks longer and has a more distal position compared with the other toes.	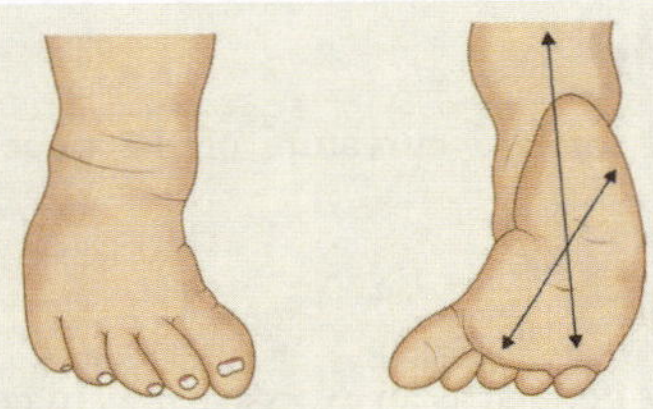

Management

- Manipulation and casting
- Achilles tenotomy
- Bracing

Juvenile Rheumatoid Arthritis

It is an autoimmune disease, characterized by inflammation and stiffness of joint for more than 6 weeks in a child aged 16 years or less.

Diagnosis

- Positive rheumatoid factor, Antinuclear antibody (ANA)
- Elevated ESR and C-reactive protein
- Leukocytosis, anemia, etc.
- X-ray

Management

- NSAIDs: Ibuprofen, naproxen, indomethacin
- Intra articular corticosteroid injections: Triamcinolone hexacetonide
- Oral or intravenous corticosteroids: Prednisolone, high dose Solumedrol or pulse therapy
- Disease modifying antirheumatic drugs: Sulfasalazine, azathioprine, hydroxychloroquine, leflunomide, cyclosporine, methotrexate

Osteomyelitis

Infection of the bone due to hematogenous seeding of bacteria to the metaphyseal region of the bone.

Clinical Features

Limb pain, refusal to wear weight or limping, restricted motion of joints, fever, tenderness.

Treatment

Antibiotic therapy, surgical drainage, debridement.

Scoliosis

Sideways curvature of spine.

Clinical Manifestation

- Inappropriate posture, leg length discrepancy
- Shoulder asymmetry, scapular prominence
- Truncal imbalance, uneven waist balance
- Lump on back, uneven breast size

Management

Scoliosis brace: Most common type of brace is made up of plastic and is contoured to conform to the body. This brace is invisible under the clothes.

Surgery: Spinal fusion is indicated when surgery is unsuccessful.

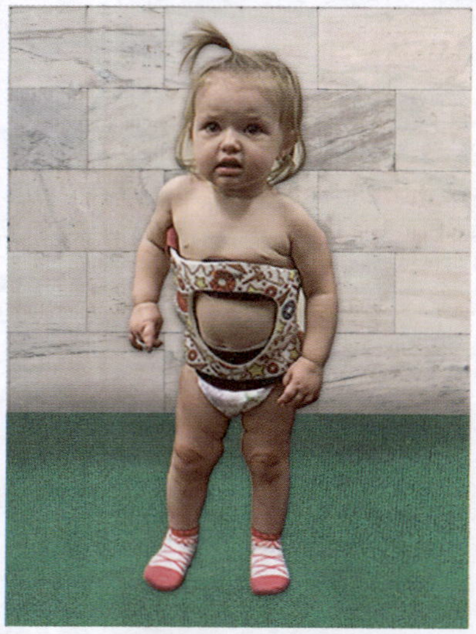

Figure 33: Scoliosis brace

Kyphosis

Abnormal forward curvature of the upper bone. Children with kyphosis have a round or hunchback appearance.

Lordosis

Lordosis is defined as an excessive inward curve of the spine at lower back.

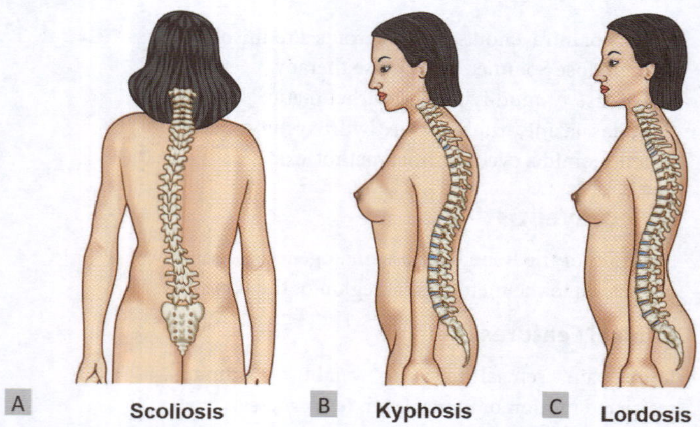

Figures 34A and B: **A.** Scoliosis; **B.** Kyphosis; **C.** Lordosis

KEY POINTS

- Volkmann contracture is a **deformity of the hand, fingers, and wrist caused by injury to the muscles of the forearm. Sometimes it occurs** due to the improper use of the tourniquet or cast.
- Dupuytren's contraction is a flexion deformity of the fingers or toes caused by the shortening, thickening and fibrosis of the palmar or plantar fascia.
- The Milwaukee brace is commonly used in the treatment of scoliosis.

DISORDERS OF SKIN

Atopic Dermatitis

It is chronic, pruritic inflammatory skin disease characterized by intense itching with episodes of exacerbation and remission.

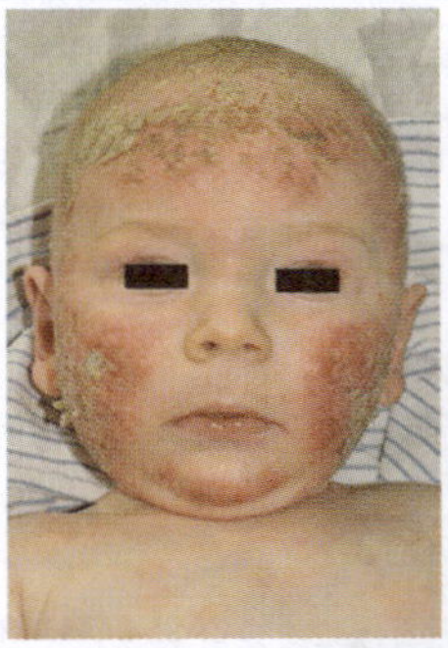

Figure 35: Child with Atopic dermatitis

Clinical Manifestation

- Pruritis
- Lesion may appear as xerosis
- Ill-defined erythema

Treatment

- Tepid bath without washcloths, mild soap, pat dry
- Gentle skincare (emollients), i.e., use of ointments or thick cream
- Wet dressing
- Identification and avoidance of triggers and irritants
- Topical corticosteroids to treat acute inflammation
- Antihistamine for pruritis
- Antibiotics to treat co-existing inflammation

Seborrheic Dermatitis (Cradle Cap)

It is a chronic inflammatory reaction of the skin, most commonly in the scalp but may involve eyelids, external ear canal, nasolabial fold and inguinal region.

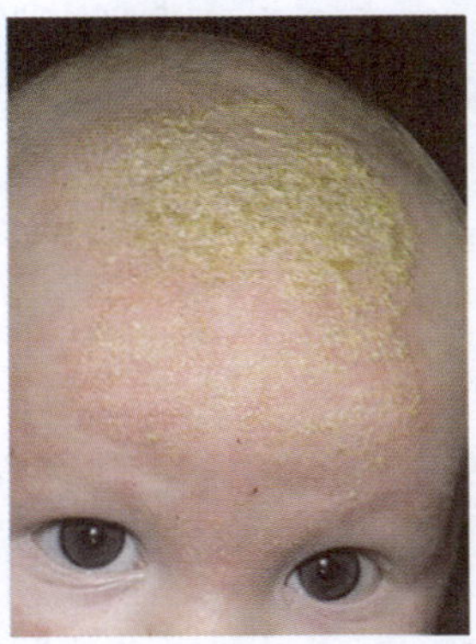

Figure 36: Seborrheic dermatitis (cradle cap)

Clinical Manifestation

- Greasy yellow scale on erythematous base
- Reddish, somewhat swollen patches of skin
- Itching and burning

Treatment

- Crusts should be removed by pretreatment with oil
- 2% ketoconazole shampoo, mild topical steroids
- Wet compression over the fissured lesion before application of ointments

Diaper Dermatitis

- It is an example of irritant contact dermatitis caused by over hydration of the skin, maceration, prolonged contact with urine and feces.
- Candida albicans has been identified as another contributing factor.

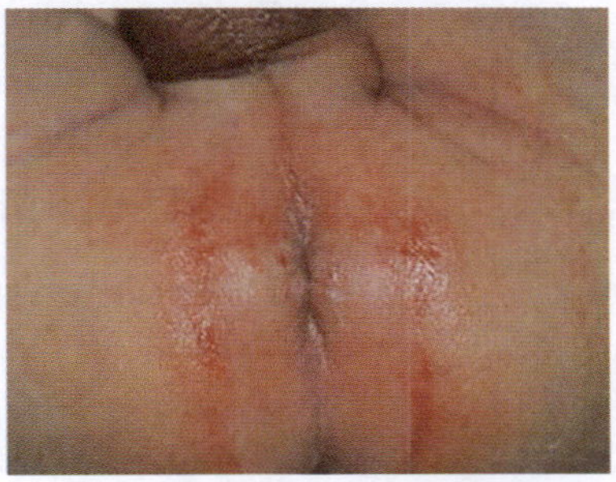

Figure 37: Diaper dermatitis

Clinical Manifestation

Deep red shiny rashes

Treatment

- Zinc oxide ointment
- Emollient like pure petroleum jelly
- If candidiasis proved, then antifungal like **nystatin or econazole nitrate cream**
- Diaper area should be left open to air

DISORDERS OF ENT

Mastoiditis

Inflammation of the mastoid air cells in the temporal bone.

Clinical Manifestation

- Pain behind the ear
- Fever, irritability, and lethargy
- Swollen ear lobe
- Redness and tenderness behind the ear
- Drainage from the ear
- Bulging and drooping of ear

Complications: Meningitis, brain abscess, hearing loss.

KEY POINTS

- Diaper rashes most commonly are caused by *Staphylococcus aureus*.
- A common site for the lesions associated with atopic dermatitis is antecubital space.
- A seborrheic crusting over the scalp of a newborn is known as cradle cap.
- Most common complication of Chronic Suppurative Otitis Media (CSOM) is **Mastoiditis**.

Management: Parenteral antibiotics, myringotomy, mastoidectomy.

Hearing Impairment

Impairment in hearing leads to difficulty in perceiving or identifying sounds clearly.

Types

- Conductive hearing loss: Dysfunction of the conduction pathway for sound to reach the inner ear caused by disease or obstruction in the outer or middle ear.
- Sensorineural hearing loss: Damage to delicate hair cells of the inner ear or nerve.
- Mixed hearing loss: Combination of conductive and sensory neural hearing loss, indicating problem with outer, middle, and inner ear.
- Central hearing loss: Injury or impairment to the nerve or nuclei of the CNS.

DISORDERS OF EYE

Retinopathy of Prematurity

Vaso proliferative disorder of retina among premature babies which was previously termed retrolental fibroplasia.

Risk Factors

- Premature birth
- Unconditional oxygen therapy
- Systemic problem associated with prematurity such as anemia, sepsis

Treatment

Peripheral retinal ablation of avascular retina.

Amblyopia

- Subnormal vision in one or both eyes despite correction of refractive error.
- It is the disease of the visual cortex that develops in children younger than 6–8-year-old.

Strabismus

- Crossed eyes, or strabismus, is a condition in which both eyes do not look at the same place at the same time.
- It usually occurs in people who have poor eye muscle control or are very farsighted.

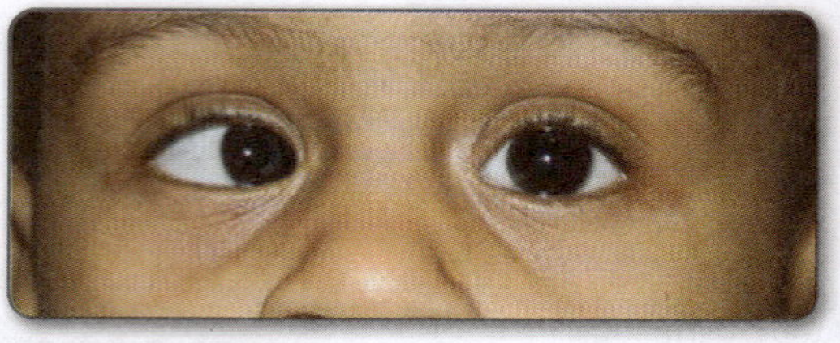

Figure 38: Strabismus

PEDIATRIC EMERGENCY

Cardiopulmonary Resuscitation in Children

- Pediatric Basic Life Support (PBLS) is a rescue procedure which has purpose of preventing the anoxic brain damage by promoting the return of spontaneous circulation and breathing. (AHA)
- Compression, airway and breathing (CAB) is the pattern used for CPR.

NATIONAL IMMUNIZATION SCHEDULE

Age	Vaccines given
Birth	Bacillus Calmette Guerin (BCG), Oral Polio Vaccine (OPV)-0 dose, Hepatitis B birth dose
6 Weeks	OPV-1, Pentavalent-1, Rotavirus Vaccine (RVV)-1, Fractional dose of Inactivated Polio Vaccine (fIPV)-1, **Pneumococcal Conjugate Vaccine (PCV) -1***
10 weeks	OPV-2, Pentavalent-2, RVV-2
14 weeks	OPV-3, Pentavalent-3, fIPV-2, RVV-3, **PCV-2***
9-12 months	Measles & Rubella (MR)-1, **JE-1****, **PCV-Booster***
16-24 months	MR-2, **JE-2****, Diphtheria, Pertussis & Tetanus (DPT)-Booster-1, OPV – Booster
5-6 years	DPT-Booster-2
10 years	Tetanus & adult Diphtheria (Td)
16 years	Td
Pregnant Mother	Td-1, Td-2 or Td-Booster***

* **PCV** in selected states/districts: Bihar, Himachal Pradesh, Madhya Pradesh, Uttar Pradesh (selected districts) and Rajasthan; in Haryana as state initiative

** JE in endemic districts only

*** One dose if previously vaccinated within 3 years

KEY POINTS

- Untreated strabismus can lead to loss of vision in the affected eye.
- Oxygen toxicity in premature infants is known as retinopathy of prematurity.
- Vitamin E is used to treat retinopathy of prematurity.

Clinical Corner

CASE SCENARIO 8:
Nurse Amli responds to a call bell and finds a distressed mother with her child. The child is having a seizure. Which of the following is the priority nursing action in this situation?

a. Restrain the child to prevent any injury to the child
b. Insert a padded tongue blade in the patient's mouth to prevent the child from swallowing or choking on his tongue
c. Contact the operator to request for seizure assistance
d. Ensure that the area is clear and position the child safely

Ans. (d) Ensure that the...

Recent Questions (NORCET 2023)

58. What is the targeted oxygen saturation in both preterm and term neonates receiving oxygen therapy?
a. 81–85%
b. 85–90%
c. 91–95%
d. 95–100%

Ans. (c) 91–95%

59. What is the dose of adrenaline in neonates in CPR?
a. 0.5 mg/kg (1:10,000 dilution)
b. 0.05 mg/kg. (1 ml of 1:10,000 dilution)
c. 0.1 mg/kg (1:1000)
d. 0.1 mg/kg (1:10,000)

Ans. (b) 0.05 mg/kg...

Pediatric basic life support algorithm for healthcare providers—Single rescuer

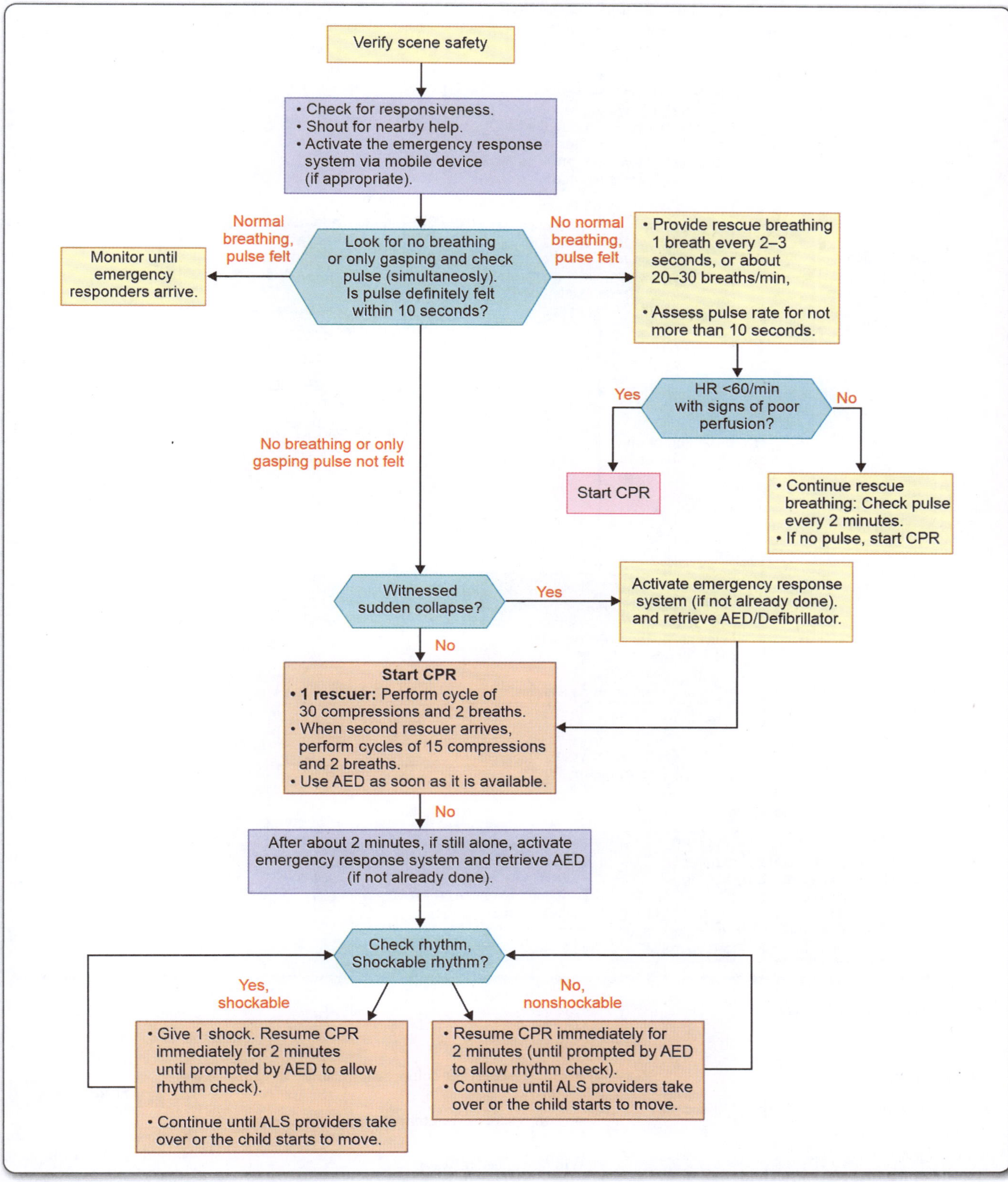

Source: American Heart Association

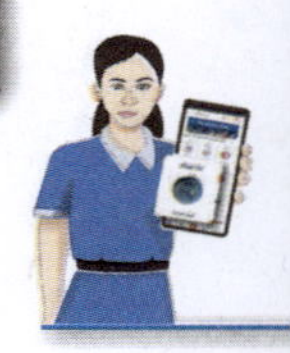

Pediatric basic life support algorithm for healthcare providers—2 or More Rescuers

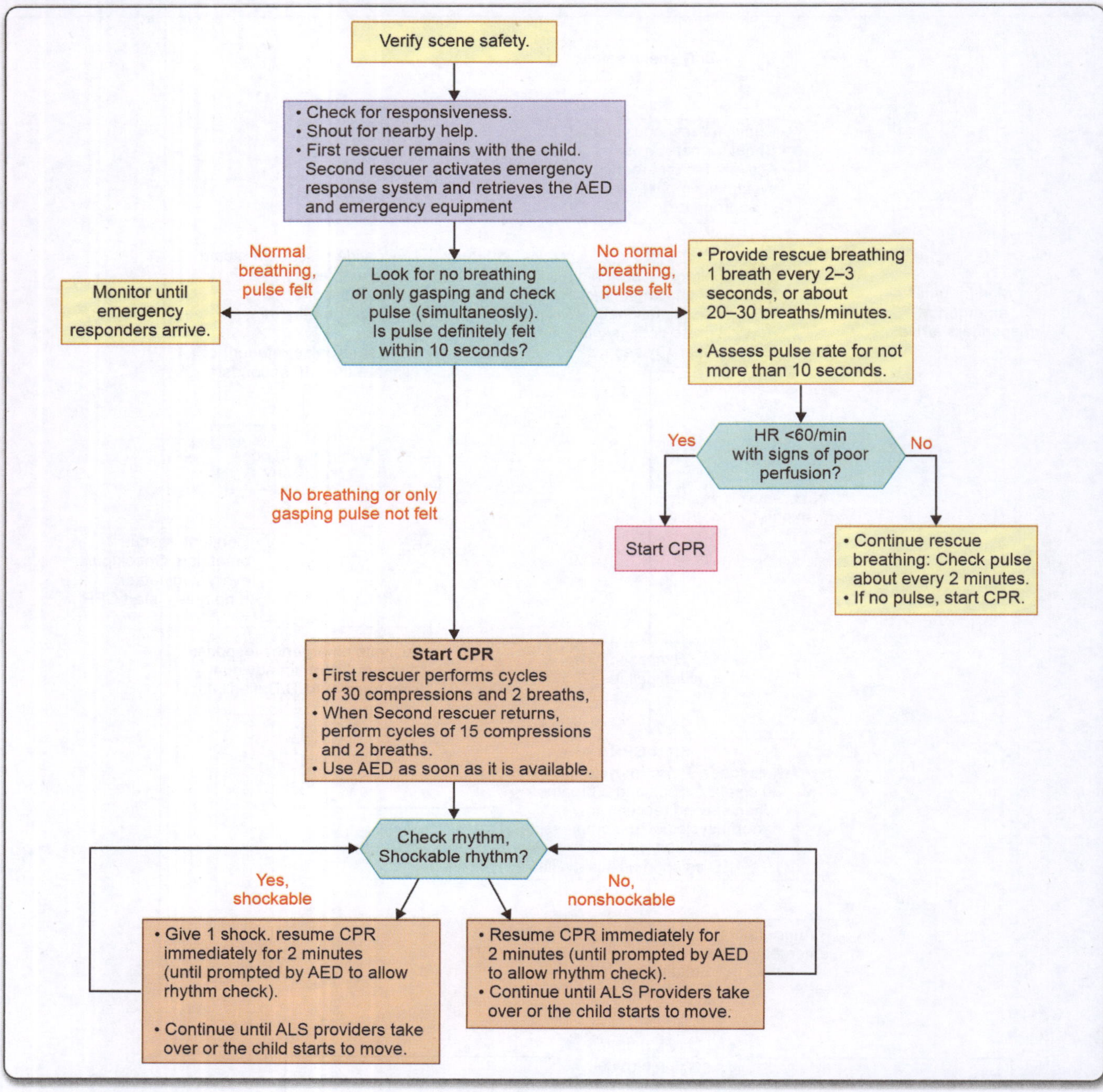

Source: American Heart Association

Pulse Checking

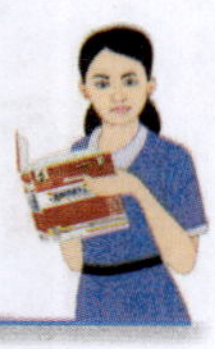

Healthcare providers may take up to 10 seconds to attempt to feel for a pulse:

- Brachial pulse in an infant
- Carotid or femoral pulse in a child

Chest Compression

- Without advanced airway:
  - One rescuer: 30 compressions and 2 breaths (30:2)
  - Two rescuers: 15 compressions and 2 breaths (15:2)
- With advanced airway:
  - Continuous compressions at a rate of 100-120/min
  - Give 1 breath every 6 seconds (10 breaths/min)

KEY POINT

In infants, brachial pulse is used to detect the presence or absence of pulse rate during cardiac arrest.

Chest Compression Techniques

- 2 hands or 1 hand (optional for very small child) on the lower half of the breastbone (sternum)
- Infant:
  - 1 rescuer: 2 fingers in the center of the chest, just below the nipple line
  - 2 or more rescuers: 2 thumb–encircling hands in the center of the chest, just below the nipple line

Depth of Chest Compression

- Compression that depresses the chest at least **one third** of the anteroposterior diameter.
- Approximately 1.5 inches (4 cm) in infants to 2 inches (5 cm) in children.
- Once children have reached puberty (i.e., adolescents), the recommended adult compression depth of at least 2 inches (5 cm) but not greater than 2.4 inches (6 cm) is used.

Chest Compression Rate

Compression rate of 100–120/min for infants and children

Opening the Airway

- Head tilt-chin lift method
- Jaw thrust method (if cervical spine injury is suspected)

High Quality CPR

- Compression of adequate rate and depth
- Allowing complete chest recoil between compressions
- Minimizing interruptions in compression
- Avoiding excessive ventilation

Defibrillation

- Ventricular fibrillation (VF) and pulseless Ventricular Tachycardia (VT) are referred to as "shockable rhythms" because they respond to electric shocks (defibrillation).
- Infant: Prefer manual defibrillation/Pediatric dose attenuator
- Age 1–8 years: AED with a pediatric attenuator
- Age >8 years: AED for adult is used

Paddle Size

Adult size (>10 kgs) and Pediatric size (<10 kg)

Energy

Acceptable to use an initial dose of 2–4 J/kg not to exceed 10 J/kg or the adult maximum dose.

GENETIC DISORDERS

Down Syndrome

Down syndrome has an extra copy of chromosome 21 known as Trisomy of 21st chromosome.

KEY POINTS

- X-linked recessive disorders are more common among males as compared to females.
- Trisomy 13 is identified as **Patau's syndrome.**
- **Trisomy 18** is identified as Edward's syndrome.
- **Trisomy 21** is identified as Down's syndrome.
- A chromosomal disorder in which a female is born with only one X chromosome is known as Turner's syndrome.
- Triple marker screen test involves Alpha-fetoprotein, Human chorionic gonadotropin, and Estriol. It is performed during second trimester of pregnancy to diagnose the risk for chromosomal abnormalities in fetus.

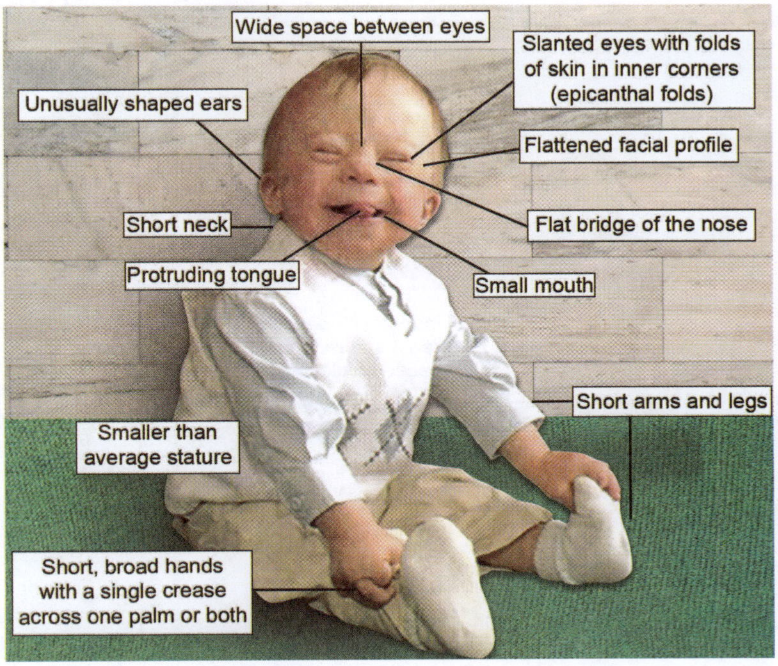

Figure 39: Features of down syndrome

Clinical Manifestation

- A flattened face, especially the bridge of the nose
- Almond-shaped eyes that slant up
- A short neck, small ears
- A tongue that tends to stick out of the mouth
- Tiny white spots on the iris (colored part) of the eye
- Small hands and feet
- A single line across the palm of the hand (palmar crease)
- Small pink fingers that sometimes curve towards the thumb
- Poor muscle tone or loose joints
- Shorter in height

Turner Syndrome

- It is a condition affecting only females. These females have only single copy of X chromosome (45 X) instead of two.
- The most common feature of Turner syndrome is short stature.

Clinical Features

- Short neck with a webbed appearance
- A low hairline at the back of the head
- Low-set ears
- Narrow fingernails and toenails that are turned upward
- A broad chest with widely spaced nipples may occur (shield chest)
- Some individuals may have swollen, puffy hands and feet.

Management

- Growth promoting therapy: GH increases childhood growth and final adult height.
- Estrogen replacement therapy: It is for sexual development and preservation of bone mineral density.

Klinefelter Syndrome

Klinefelter Syndrome is a chromosomal variation in males in which one extra X chromosome is present, resulting in a 47, XXY karyotype.

Clinical Manifestation

- Small, firm testicles
- Cryptorchidism
- Delayed or incomplete puberty with lack of secondary sexual characteristics
- Breast growth (gynecomastia)
- Reduced facial and body hair
- Infertility
- Tall stature
- Abnormal body proportions (long legs, short trunk, shoulder equal to hip size)
- Learning disability, speech delay
- Hypospadias
- Social, psychologic and behavioral problems

Treatment

- Testosterone replacement therapy
- Infertility treatment

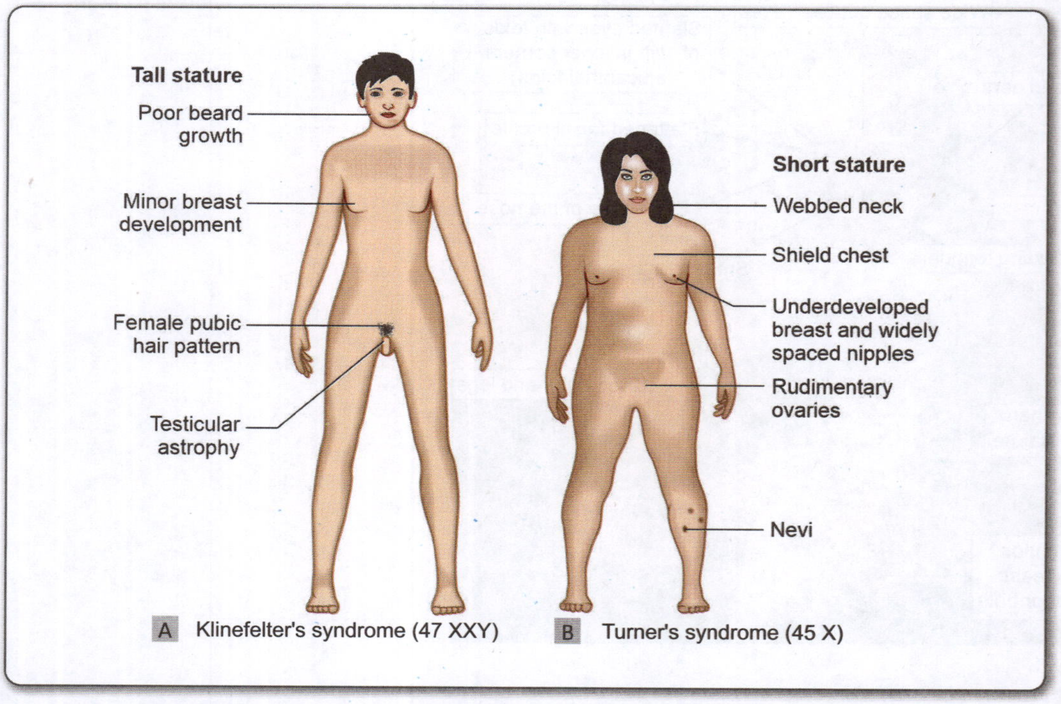

Figures 40A and B: Clinical features of Klinefelter's syndrome and Turner's syndrome

Recent Question (CNCI 2021)

60. In which of the following genetic condition, Karyotype 47, XXY is seen?

a. Down's syndrome
b. Klinefelter's syndrome
c. Edward's syndrome
d. Patau's syndrome

Ans. (b) Klinefelter's...

KEY POINTS

- Turner syndrome is not an inherited abnormality. Because women with Turner syndrome are sterile and cannot have children.
- Klinefelter syndrome is the most common cause of primary hypogonadism and infertility in males.
- "Jerky ataxic movement (Happy Puppet)" is seen in Angelman syndrome, a genetic disorder.
- Anti–mongoloid slant is seen in Treacher Collins syndrome and Cri du chat syndrome
- Rocker bottom foot is seen in Edward syndrome

BEHAVIORAL DISORDERS IN CHILDREN

Refer to Mental Health Nursing synopsis

CHALLENGED CHILDREN

Refer to Mental Health Nursing synopsis

DRUGS IN PEDIATRICS

Instillation

Eye drop/ointment:

- Instill eye drop in the lower conjunctival sac.
- Ointment is applied from inner canthus to outer canthus.
- If using both drop and ointment, then instill drop first then after few minutes apply ointment.

Nasal Drops

Instill with head tilted upward and maintain position for 1 minute.

Ear Drops

- Pull pinna downward and backward if child is less than 3 years and pull pinna upward and backward if child is more than 3 years old.
- Massage the area in front of ear. Maintain position with affected ear up to 5 minutes.

Rectal Medication

- Use side lying position.
- Insert lubricated suppository up to first knuckle.
- Hold buttocks together for 1-2 minutes.

Guidelines for Calculating Pediatric Drug Dosage

- **Formula:**
  - Young's rule (For children 2 years and above):
    $$\frac{[\text{Age (yr)}]}{\text{Age (yr)} + 12} \times \text{adult dose}$$
  - Clark's rule:
    $$\frac{[\text{Weight (lb)}]}{50}$$
  - Fried's rule (For infants up to 2 years old):
    $$\frac{[\text{Age (month)}]}{150} \times \text{adult dose}$$
  - Square meter surface area OR Mosteller's equation SA in $m^2 = \frac{(\text{height} \times \text{weight})}{60}$ 1/2

Commonly used Drugs

Atropine

- Treatment of sinus pulseless electrical activity, bradycardia, or asystole
- Neonates and children: 0.02 mg/kg intratracheal (max. 0.5 mg); may repeat 5 min later, one time
- As a preoperative medication to inhibit secretions and salivation
- Antidote to organophosphate poisoning: 0.02–0.05 mg/kg every 10–20 min until atropine effect is seen, then 1–4 hours for at least 24 hrs.
- Cautions: Gastrointestinal obstruction, thyrotoxicosis, and tachycardia.
- Adverse events: Tachycardia, palpitations, delirium, ataxia, dry hot skin, tremor, urinary retention

Epinephrine

- **Indications:** Treatment of cardiac arrest, bronchospasm, anaphylactic reaction.
- For asystole or for heart failure- Epinephrine (0.1–0.3 mL/kg of a 1: 10,000 solution, intravenously or intratracheally) is given.
- The dose may be repeated every 5 min
- Routes- IV, intratracheal, continuous infusion and nebulization
- Adverse events: Tachycardia, hypertension, tremor, weakness, acute urinary retention, peripheral soft tissue damage if they extravasate from peripheral lines into the local tissues

Hydrocortisone

- **Indications**: Status asthmaticus, shock [50 mg/kg/dose], treatment of adrenal insufficiency, congenital adrenal hyperplasia
- **Caution**: Abrupt withdrawal-acute adrenal insufficiency
- **Adverse events**: Hypertension, hyperglycemia, hypokalemia, euphoria, insomnia, headache, Cushing syndrome, peptic ulcer, cataract, immunosuppression, skin and muscle atrophy, acne, edema.

Furosemide

- **Indications**: Pulmonary edema, cardiac failure, SIADH, reduction of ICP in combination with mannitol, broncho-pulmonary dysplasia.
- **Adverse events:** Dehydration, electrolyte loss, hyperuricemia, photosensitivity, ischemic hepatitis, hypercalciuria, renal stones, ototoxicity (IV infusion rate >4 mL/min), gastrointestinal intolerance
- Careful monitoring of electrolytes is necessary with long-term furosemide therapy because of the **potential for significant loss of potassium.**
- Potassium chloride supplementation is usually required unless the potassium-sparing diuretic spironolactone is given concomitantly.
- When furosemide is administered every other day, dietary potassium supplementation may be adequate to maintain normal serum potassium levels.

KEY POINTS

Behavioral disorders:

- Passage of feces in inappropriate places after bowel control would be expected is known as **Encopresis.**
- To diagnose pica, child has to be consuming non-nutritive substance for at least one month.
- Intelligence quotient (IQ) is the index of intellectual brightness of the child and is calculated as: **IQ = Mental age/ Chronological age × 100**
- The new terminology for mental retardation is **intellectual disability.**

Recent Question (NORCET 2020)

61. A 7-year-old child intermittently bedwetting at least 2 times a week. The nurse anticipates which of the following drugs to be prescribed by the physician?

a. Desmopressin
b. Diazepam
c. Methylphenidate
d. Fluoxetine

Ans. (a) Desmopressin

Recent Question (CNCI 2021)

62. The nurse administers ear drop to a 7-year-old child. How does the nurse pull the patient's ear?

a. Outward
b. Backward
c. Upward and Backward
d. Backward and Downward

Ans. (c) Upward and...

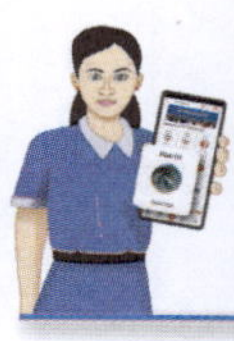

Digoxin

- **Indications**: Treatment of systolic heart failure and supraventricular tachyarrhythmias.
- **Cautions**: Contraindicated in AV block, idiopathic hypertrophic subaortic stenosis, or constrictive pericarditis.
- The drug crosses the placenta, and therefore a fetus with heart failure (secondary to arrhythmia) can be treated by administering digoxin to the mother.
- The kidney eliminates digoxin, so dosing must be adjusted according to the patient's renal function.
- Check post-distribution digoxin levels (drawn at least 6–8 hrs post dose) at steady-state (2–4 weeks) or if ECG or clinical signs of toxicity. Check ECG, serum electrolytes, calcium, and magnesium.
- **Digoxin Immune Fab:** Treatment of digitalis intoxication from digoxin.
- **Adverse events:** Worsening of heart failure or atrial fibrillation, hypokalemia, anorexia, **yellow or green vision, blurred vision, diplopia**, photophobia, facial swelling, and redness.

Conversions you need to remember

- 1 teaspoon = 5 mL/cc
- 1 tablespoon = 15 mL/cc
- 1 ounce = 30 mL/cc
- 1 gram (g) = 1000 milligrams (mg)
- 1 milligram (mg) = 1000 micrograms (mcg)
- 1 liter (L) = 1000 milliliters (mL)

Dosage Calculation

$$\frac{\text{Desired amount or prescribed amount } (\mathbf{D})}{\text{Available dosage (what's on hand) } (\mathbf{A})} \times \text{Quantity (e.g., 1 pill or 1 tablet or 5 mL} = X)$$

$$\frac{\text{Desired amount}}{\text{Available dosage}} \times \text{Quantity amount to give}$$

COMMON PEDIATRIC NURSING PROCEDURES

Peak Flow Meter

Peak Flow Meter Parts:

- Mouthpiece
- Indicator/cursor
- Measuring scale

Uses

- To classify severity of asthma.
- To see whether the management plan is working or not.
- To decide when to add or stop medicine.
- Peak flow meter is **not usually applicable for less than 5 years of age.**

Procedure

- Place the indicator at the base of numbered scale.
- **Position:** Stand up or sit in the upright posture.
- Take a deep breath.
- Place the meter in mouth and close lips around the mouthpiece.
- Do not put tongue inside the hole and do not put finger over measuring scale.
- Blow out as hard and as fast as can.
- Write down the number you get.
- Repeat the steps two more times.
- Note the highest reading.

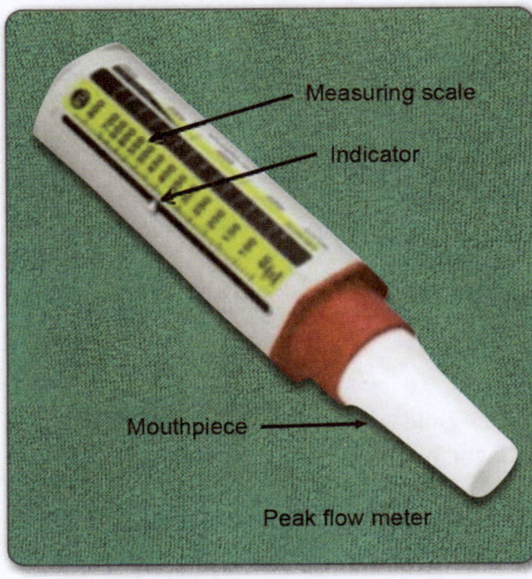

Figure 41: Peak flow meter

Nebulization

Purpose of Nebulization

- To administer various drugs to the airways like- – Bronchodilator (mostly used) – Steroids, etc.
- To hydrate thick sputum and prevent mucus plugging.

Procedure

- Clean all parts before use.
- At first, attach the air tube to the outlet of the machine.
- Fit the air tube with mixing chamber and mask.
- Take measured amount of drugs into the mixing chamber by syringe or dropper and mix with normal saline.
- Connect the electrical line and turn on the switch.
- Look whether fine mist is coming out through the mask adequately.
- Place the child in comfortable position **(head upright).**
- Put the mask to the face of the child covering nose and mouth adequately (but not so tight).
- In case of mouthpiece, place it between patient's lips into oral cavity.

Recent Questions (INC PhD 2020)

63. Dosage of 1:10,000 adrenaline required during resuscitation of a 5kg child is:
a. 0.1 mL b. 0.3 mL
c. 0.5 mL d. 1 mL
Ans. (c) 0.5 mL

64. Drug of choice in bee sting anaphylaxis is:
a. Adrenaline
b. Dopamine
c. Dobutamine
d. Dexamethason
Ans. (a) Adrenaline

KEY POINTS

- BROSELOW TAPE: Tape is used for quick categorization of a child into a certain weight range based on the child's length.
- The Broselow Tape is a color coded tape used to simplify the treatment of children in pediatric medical emergencies.
- The earliest and most frequent manifestation of digoxin toxicity in infants and children is the appearance of cardiac arrhythmias, including sinus bradycardia.
- Working principle of a nebulizer is Bernoulli's principle.
- There are two main types of nebulizers: Compressed-air nebulizers and Ultrasonic nebulizers.
- **Compressed-air nebulizer:** Uses compressed air to transport medicine to the lungs. Also called jet nebulizer or atomizer. The disadvantage of a jet nebulizer is its noise and weight.
- **An ultrasonic nebulizer:** It has a transducer which produces ultrasonic sound waves that convert the medicated liquid into vapors.

- Continue nebulization until fine mist is no longer present.

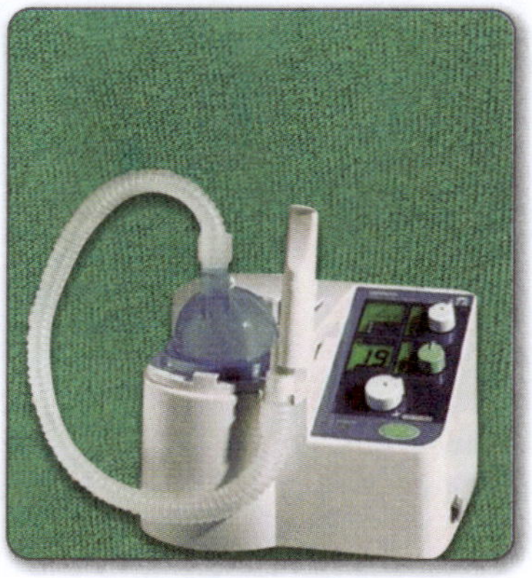

Figure 42: Ultrasonic nebulizer

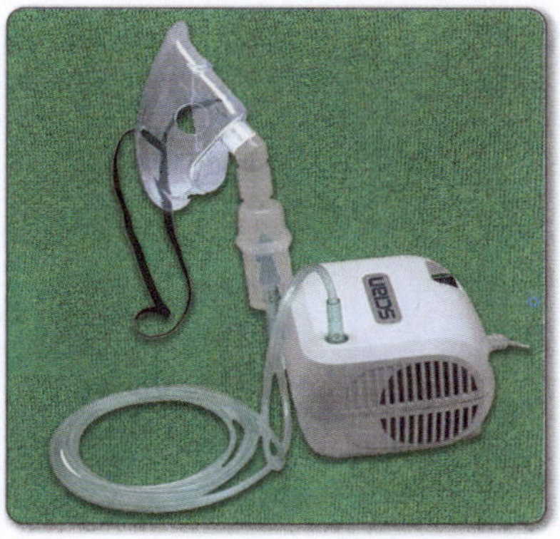

Figure 43: Compressor nebulizer (atomizer jet)

Pulse Oximeter

- It is a device used to determine the percentage of hemoglobin (Hb) that is saturated with oxygen.

The oxygen saturation (SpO_2) is a measure of how much oxygen the blood is carrying as a percentage of the maximum it could carry.

- Types of pulse oximeter: 1) Desktop 2) Finger/ Mobile

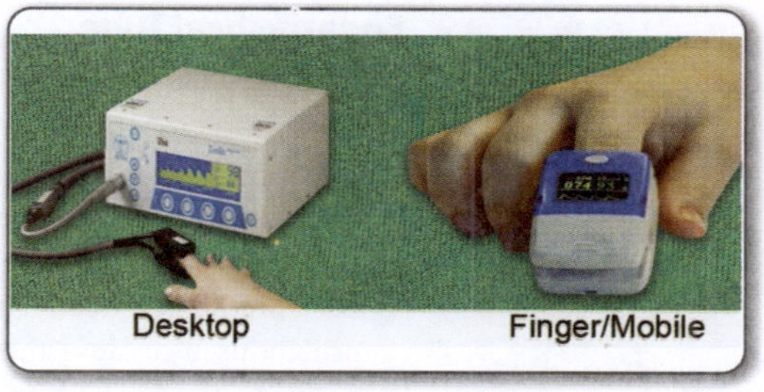

Figure 44: Types of oximeter

How it Works

The measurements are obtained by simply shining two wavelengths of light. One is a visible red beam, the other an invisible infrared beam. By measuring how much light has been absorbed by the oxygen in the blood, an oxygen saturation reading is established and displayed as a percentage of the maximum amount of oxygen the blood could carry.

Benefits of Pulse Oximeter

- A pulse oximeter can detect before a patient shows signs of becoming cyanotic.
- In the ICU, pulse oximeter is used extensively on mechanically ventilated patients, as it can frequently detect problems with oxygenation before they are noticed clinically, as well as a valuable guide for weaning patients off ventilation and helping to assess the adequacy of a patient's oxygen therapy.

KEY POINTS

- Pulse oximetry is based on Beer-Lambert law
- Oxyhemoglobin absorbs more infrared light and deoxyhemoglobin absorbs more red light.

AMBU (Artificial Manual Breathing Unit)

AMBU Parts

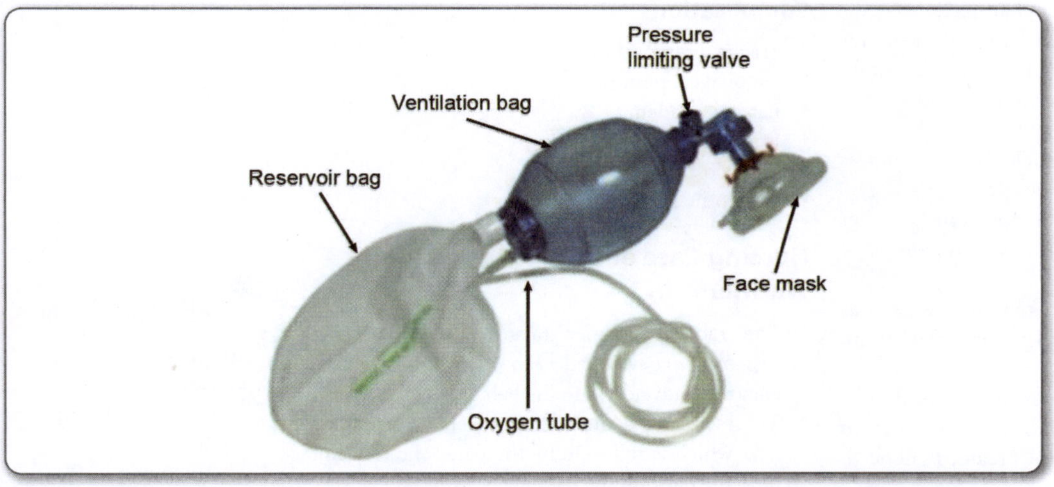

Figure 45: Parts of AMBU

Indications of Use

- Neonatal resuscitation in case of perinatal asphyxia
- Respiratory distress syndrome
- Respiratory failure due to any cause (any age) like pneumonia, severe acute asthma, poisoning, GBS, etc.

Contraindications

- Diaphragmatic hernia
- Tracheoesophageal fistula

Prerequisites

- Sniffing position
- Thumb + index finger to maintain face seal
- Middle finger under mandibular symphysis
- Ring and little finger under the angle of mandible

Endotracheal Intubation

Indications

- To provide mechanical respiratory support
- Obtain aspirates for culture
- Assist in bronchopulmonary hygiene
- Alleviate subglottic stenosis
- Endotracheal medications (e.g., epinephrine, lidocaine, atropine, etc.)

Endotracheal Tube

- ET tubes can be cuffed or uncuffed.
- Cuffed ET tubes are usually used in children >8 years. The cuff when inflated maintains the ET tube in proper position and prevents aspiration of contents from GI tract into respiratory tract.
- In children <8 years, uncuffed ET tubes are usually used because the narrow subglottic area performs the function of a cuff and prevents the ET tube from slipping.

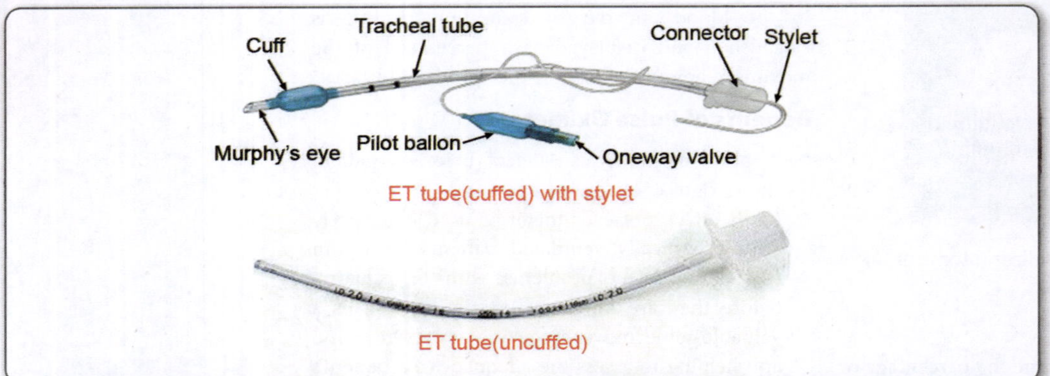

Figure 46: Endotracheal tube

Procedure

- Position: Sniff position (rolled towel under shoulder) or Supine (do not hyperextend)
- Suction oropharynx and nasopharynx as needed
- Pre-oxygenation with high flow oxygen for 1 minute if possible (do not bag if meconium aspiration, diaphragmatic hernia)
- Monitoring vital signs and SpO_2
- Drugs: Following drugs should be used unless patient is flaccid and unresponsive:
  - Initially hypnotic such as thiopentone (3–5 mg/kg), midazolam (0.5 mg/kg) or propofol (2–4 mg/kg)
  - Followed by muscle relaxant such as suxamethonium (1 mg/kg) or rocuronium (1 mg/kg).
- Then intubate the trachea as soon as relaxed
- Auscultation of the chest on both sides (and also of stomach) with mechanical breath, is done to confirm proper ET tube position
- Secure the tube in place using tape
- Cut the tube at about 0.5 cm from where it is taped (to reduce dead space)

Complications

- Tracheal perforation
- Esophageal perforation
- Laryngeal edema
- Improper tube positioning
- Tube obstruction or kinking
- Subglottic stenosis

Nursing Care of Baby Under Radiant Warmer

- The radiant warmer (also called open care system) was developed as an 'open incubator' that ensures ready access to the baby.
- The overhead quartz heating element produces heat which is reflected by the parabolic reflector onto the baby on the bassinet.

Recent Question (NORCET 2020)

65. The ET Tube size 5.5 is used for:
a. Infants
b. Adults
c. Children
d. Geriatric patients
Ans. (c) Children

KEY POINTS

Articles to be arranged for intubation SOAP-ME

S – Suction
O – Oxygen
A – Airway (appropriate size ET tube, oral and nasal airway)
P – Personnel
M – Medications
E – Equipment (AMBU bag and mask, syringe, ET-securing tape, stethoscope, etc.)

KEY POINTS

Two types of laryngoscope blades are available.

- Miller & Macintosh

Miller blade

- Thin and straight one
- Preferred for infants and young children
- Facilitate lifting of epiglottis and expose glottis
- Possibly better control of tongue

Macintosh

- Wide and curved blade
- Used in older children and adult
- Curves around tongue

KEY POINTS

Size of ET tube:

- **Uncuffed:** **4 + (Age (yrs)/4)**
- **Cuffed:** **3 + (Age (yrs)/4)**

Modes Used

- Servo mode
- Manual mode

Servo Mode

- Set temperature at 36.5°C, heater output will adjust automatically to keep baby at set temperature.
- If the baby temperature is below the set temperature, the heater output will increase.
- If the baby is at set temperature or higher, the heater output will become zero.

Manual Mode

The heat output from the quartz heating rod could also be increased or decreased manually.

Disinfecting Radiant Warmer

- When the equipment is in use, all approachable external surfaces should be cleaned daily with an antiseptic solution like 2% bacillocid or glutaraldehyde.
- Spirit or other organic solvents **must not be used** to clean the glass side panels or display panels.
- For disinfection of reusable probe, isopropyl alcohol swab should be used.
- Every seventh day, after shifting the baby to another cot, the used equipment should be cleaned thoroughly, first by light detergent solution and then by antiseptic solution.
- All detachable assemblies are to be treated similarly.

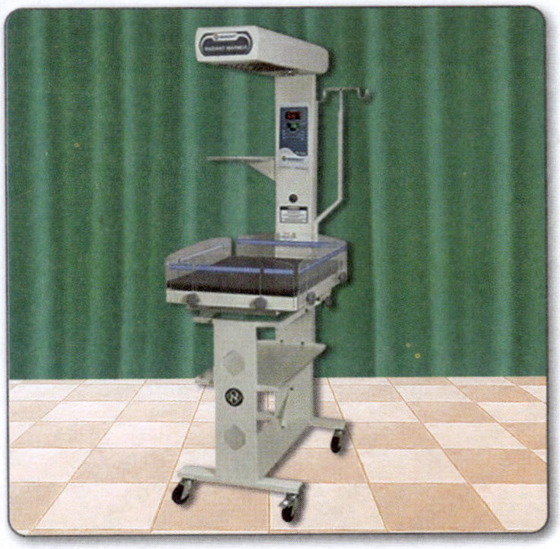

Figure 47: Radiant warmer

Nursing Care of Child in Incubator

- Maintain axillary temperature between 36.5°C and 37.5°C.
- Access baby by using the portholes, limit opening of the large door as this interferes with air temperature.
- Ensure baby is nursed naked apart from a nappy.
- Position baby using rolled towels/cloth nappies to provide boundaries that support 'nesting' and flexion of limbs but keeping face clear.
- Should not tap on the canopy.
- No equipment is placed on top of the canopy.
- Axillary temperature is taken on admission into the incubator and rechecked in the first hour. Temperature is documented 4–6 hourly as per the condition.
- Humidification is utilized for incubator care of preterm babies only — NOT required for babies >32 weeks.
- Cleaning and sterilization: When the incubator is occupied, it should be cleaned daily with mild detergent. Humidifier chamber must be emptied and cleaned daily.
- After seven days, the neonate should be shifted to another incubator and used incubator should be cleaned with antiseptic solution.
- Sensory stimuli like light and pain should be kept to the minimal.
- When the neonate develops fever, the incubator modes have to be changed in normal modes.
- When the neonate is nursed in prone position, skin sensor is placed over the flank and it should not touch the bed.

Incubator

- Incubator is an apparatus for maintaining an infant, especially a premature infant, in an environment of controlled temperature, humidity, and oxygen concentration
- **Purposes of incubator:**
  - Maintenance of thermoneutral ambient temperature
  - Provision of desired humidity and oxygenation
  - Observation of very sick neonates
  - Isolate newborn babies from infections, unfavorable external environment
- **Modes used:**
  - Air mode (which is similar to the manual mode of radiant warmer)
  - Skin mode or servo mode

FETAL CIRCULATION

Refer to Obstetrics and Gynecological Nursing synopsis

KEY POINTS

- While caring for a baby in servo mode, make sure that skin probe is attached to the baby.
- In supine position, temperature probes need to be attached to the right hypochondriac region and in the prone position, probe attached to the flank region.
- Manual mode is used for prewarming purposes, rapid rewarming of a hypothermic baby and caring for a baby with fever to prevent repeated skin temperature alarm due to temperature fluctuations.

Recent Question (INC PhD 2020)

66. Child with burn injury develops edema. What is the mechanism behind this?
a. Loss of fluid from body
b. Increased capillary permeability
c. Decreased urine output
d. Excessive tissue damage

Ans. (b) Increased...

Recent Question (CNCI 2021)

67. What is the name of the opening that connects two atria of fetal heart?
a. Ductus arteriosus
b. Ductus venosus
c. Foremen ovale
d. Ligamentum teres

Ans. (c) Foremen ovale

KEY POINT

1–2 mL of Glacial acetic acid or vinegar can be added to water in the humidifier to prevent bacterial growth.

Golden Points to Remember

- New Ballard Scale is frequently used scale for assessment of the gestational age. It assesses six external physical and six neuromuscular characteristics.
- Loving, consistent care, including playing by parents help in infant's cognitive and psychosocial development.
- Negativism is commonly seen in young children (Toddlers). It is a behavior characterized by the tendency to resist direction from others, and refusal to comply with requests.
- The normal newborn hemoglobin level is 17-20 g/dL.
- Drug of choice for neonatal seizure: Phenobarbitone.
- Vitamin deficiency responsible for neonatal seizure: Pyridoxine (Vitamin B_6).
- Descending motor paralysis is seen in:
  - Botulinum
  - Polio
  - Diphtheria
- If a newborn's head and trunk are allowed to fall backward it elicits moro reflex.
- Neonatal reflex elicited by touching the cheeks of the baby is rooting reflex.
- Most common cause of meningitis in the age group of 3 months-3 years: H. influenza.
- The most common form of childhood brain tumor is Medulloblastoma.
- Phototherapy is indicated for children with hyperbilirubinemia.
- Artificially acquired immunity is obtained by immunization with antibody response. Antibodies are administered, not produced by the body.
- Breastfeeding is natural passive immunity which is obtained by immunoglobins in mother's breast milk.
- BCG vaccine is given Intradermally. In intradermal injection, needle is placed almost flat against patient's skin (15°).
- Tetralogy of Fallot (TOF) is a combination of four heart defects present at the time of birth. It includes Ventricular Septal Defect (VSD), Pulmonary Valve Stenosis (PVS), overriding of aorta, Right Ventricular Hypertrophy (RVH).
- A complication of erythroblastosis fetalis is kernicterus, which is caused by deposition of bilirubin in the brain. Exchange transfusion is needed to prevent the complication.
- Drug used to keep Patent Ductus Arteriosus (PDA) open is **PGE1 (Misoprostol].**
- Drug used to treat PDA is Indomethacin.
- Bulging sack-like lesion filled with spinal fluid and spinal cord element is known as myelomeningocele.
- Reye's syndrome is associated with the use of aspirin with viral illness. Reye's syndrome most often affects children. It causes swelling in the liver and brain.
- The ratio of lung inflation to chest compression in cardiopulmonary resuscitation is 1:3.
- Both Indomethacin and Ibuprofen are equally effective in closing Patent Ductus Arteriosus.
- Commonly occurring accident among newborn babies is falling from bed.
- **Myoclonic seizure is the most common type of seizure occurring in newborn.**
- Baby-Friendly Hospital Initiative (BFHI) was launched by WHO in the year of 1991.
- Most abundant immunoglobulin of human body is IgG.
- Only class of immunoglobulin which is transported across the placenta is IgG.
- Vaccine of Diphtheria, Tetanus Toxoids and Pertussis (DTP) is contraindicated in **progressive neurological illness.**
- Method used for the transportation of vaccine from the site of production to the vaccination site is Cold Chain.
- Bacillus Calmette–Guérin (BCG) vaccine is administered through intradermal route.
- Measles, Mumps, and Rubella (MMR) are live vaccines and route of administration is subcutaneous.
- Varicella vaccine provides protection against chicken pox.
- Subacute sclerosing panencephalitis may occur years after measles vaccination as a complication.
- Diaper rashes most commonly caused by *Staphylococcus aureus*.
- Site of lesion in polio is **ventral horn of spinal cord.**
- Parenteral polio vaccine is also known as Salk.
- Oral Polio Vaccine is also known as Sabin.
- Burns are the most common documented cause of accidents in toddlers followed by choking, toxic ingestions and drowning.
- Child's participation in decision-making process about health care is termed as Assent.
- Normal adult hemoglobin contains two alpha chains and two beta chains.
- Neonatal anemia is defined as hemoglobin less than 13 g/dL.
- Anemia in children is defined as hemoglobin less than 11 g/dL.
- Treatment of choice for thalassemia major is **blood transfusion and desferrioxamine.**
- Hemophilia affects only male.
- A female who inherits one affected X chromosome becomes a 'carrier' of hemophilia.
- Vitamin 'A' deficiency leads to diarrhea and hyperkeratosis in children.
- Cleft palate is usually repaired around 12 months of age.
- Cleft lip is usually repaired at four to six months of age.
- Congenital absence of ganglion cells in the submucosal and myenteric plexus of the distal intestine is known as **Hirschsprung's disease.**
- Projective vomiting is a feature of **hypertrophic pyloric stenosis.**
- Drug of choice to treat scabies in younger children is 5% permethrin cream.
- Frequent swallowing is a sign of hemorrhage in child who underwent tonsillectomy.
- Drug of choice in trachoma for children is oral tetracycline.
- Tetracycline is contraindicated in infants and young children.
- To administer eardrop in children below age 3, pull the pinna downward and backward. In adult the pinna will be hold upward and backward.
- Toddler and preschooler are more prone to accidental poisoning due to their curiosity and desire to explore the world.
- Damage caused by lead poisoning is irreversible in CNS, but in all other body system the damage is reversible.

Contd...

- Folic acid helps in prevention of neural tube defect in fetus.
- Meningomyelocele is a sac-like protrusion containing meninges, *Cerebrospinal Fluid* (CSF) and neural elements.
- Excess or deficiency of vitamin pyridoxine leads to peripheral neuropathy.
- Tetralogy of Fallot is a cyanotic heart disease.
- Tetralogy of Fallot is congenital heart disease which includes four heart defects, namely:
  - Overriding aorta
  - Pulmonic stenosis
  - Ventricular septal defect
  - Right ventricular hypertrophy
- The heart disease most commonly associated with rubella infection is Patent Ductus Arteriosus.
- Common symptom of TOF is **clubbing of fingers.**
- Deficiency of growth hormone leads to **proportionate dwarfism.**
- Hyper secretion of growth hormone before the closure of epiphyseal plates can cause **Gigantism.**
- Hyper secretion of growth hormone after the closure of epiphyseal plates can cause **Acromegaly.**
- Adrenocorticotropic hormone (ACTH) secretion is highest in **morning.**
- Term used for undescended testis is **Cryptorchidism.**
- Unilateral renal agenesis is associated with **single umbilical artery.**
- Wilm's Tumor is commonly present as **abdominal mass.**
- In Acute Renal Failure (ARF), hyperkalemia is treated with **calcium gluconate.**
- Red urine without RBC is seen in **Rhabdomyolysis.**
- Color codes used in IMNCI are **Pink, Green** and **Yellow.**
- Most common form of childhood cancer is Leukemia.
- The Human Genome Project was completed in 2003.
- The first human gene therapy was instituted in 1990.
- The science of betterment of human race by application of the law of inheritance is called Eugenics.
- Deficiency of vitamin-D in children may cause Rickets.
- Chvostek sign and trousseau signs are seen in **Hypocalcemia.**
- Restraints used during upper chest/abdominal procedure which immobilize all the extremities is **Mummy restraints.**
- An axillary temperature should be taken for 3 minutes.
- The rectal temperature should be taken in 1 minute.
- Late neurological complication of measles is SSPE (Subacute sclerosing Panencephalitis).
- Most common complication of measles – Otitis media.
- Most common death in measles is due to Pneumonia.
- Roseola infantum (Nagayama spots) is also known as **exanthema subitum** or **sixth disease** typically presents in children between six and 12 months of age; ninety percent of cases occur in children younger than two years.
- Erythema infectiosum (also known as fifth disease) is usually a benign childhood condition characterized by a classic slapped-cheek appearance.
- Iron should not be administered fast because unbound iron may cause free radical formation.
- Expected hematocrit level of one-year-old infant is 29–41%
- 'Puff of smoke' appearance in cerebral angiography is seen in moyamoya disease.
- Pediatric assessment triangle includes appearance of skin, work of breathing and circulation to skin. It is used to determine whether the child is in respiratory distress or shock.
- Prader Willi syndrome is the most common syndromic form of obesity.
- Spiramycin is given during pregnancy to prevent vertical transmission of toxoplasma.
- The Sabin-Feldman dye test is a sensitive and specific neutralization test for toxoplasmosis. It is used to measure primarily IgG antibody and is the standard reference test for toxoplasmosis.
- Hutchinson's triad is seen in late congenital syphilis consists of interstitial keratitis, notched incisors and deafness.
- Iron is absorbed from proximal small intestine mainly from duodenum.
- Hair-on-end appearance of the skull is a characteristic feature of chronic hemolysis usually seen in patients with thalassemia and sickle cell anemia.
- Bartter syndrome is a group of rare genetic disorder in which there are specific defects in the kidney function. These defects impair the kidney's ability to reabsorb the salt and causes various electrolyte imbalances in the body.
- In an infant, a bulging fontanel is the most significant sign of increasing intracranial pressure.
- The arterial switch procedure is also known as Jatene switch procedure. This procedure is used to repair the D-transposition of the greater arteries (D-TGA).
- The main advantage of delayed cord clamping is lesser chance of anemia.
- Triad of celiac disease: Failure to thrive, Chronic diarrhea and iron deficiency anemia.
- Scabies is transmitted by close personal contacts.
- To determine the adequacy of fluid resuscitation, vital signs, urine output, adequacy of capillary filling and sensorium status are assessed.
- Pearl-gray tympanic membrane is a normal finding.
- Hemolytic uremic syndrome is characterized by the triad of: Anemia, renal failure and thrombocytopenia.
- Henoch-schonlein purpura is the vasculitis of small vessels and characterized by the deposition of IgA in the wall of involved vessels.
- Ramstedt procedure and pyloromyotomy is the surgical procedure of choice for pyloric stenosis.
- Ventricular Septal Defect (VSD) is the most common congenital heart disease involved in infective endocarditis.
- Common signs and symptoms of viral meningitis include fever, nuchal rigidity, irritability and photophobia.
- Nada's criteria are used for the assessment of congenital heart disease.
- **Wimburger sign** is the radiological feature seen in scurvy.
- Applying petroleum jelly to exstrophy bladder is avoided because it tends to dry out, adhere to the bladder mucosa and damage the delicate tissues when the dressing is removed.
- The vaccine that forms blister and leaves permanent scar in babies is BCG.

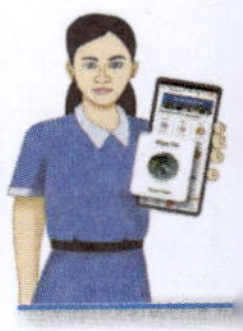

"He who has health has hope; and he who has hope has everything."
—Arabian proverb

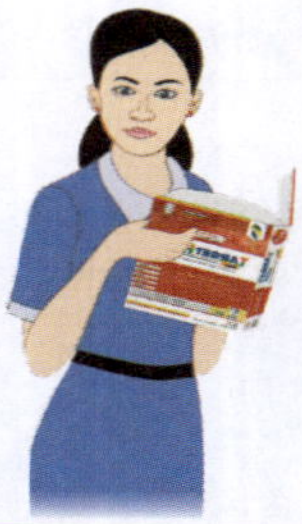

CLINICAL CASE-BASED QUESTIONS

1

What is the possible diagnosis for a one-year-old baby brought by the mother with a cystic mass on the lumbosacral area and the inability to move both legs since birth?

a. Pilonidal cyst
b. Meningocele
c. Meningomyelocele
d. Sacrococcygeal teratoma

Ans. (c) Meningomyelocele

Explanation: Meningomyelocele is a type of neural tube defect where the spinal cord and its protective covering, the meninges, protrude through an opening in the spine. It usually presents as a cystic mass on the back, commonly in the lumbosacral area. This condition can cause paralysis or weakness in the lower limbs, as well as other neurological complications.

Pilonidal cyst: Cyst or abscess in the cleft of the buttocks near the tailbone. Unrelated to the presented symptoms.

Meningocoele: Protrusion of the meninges through a defect in the skull. Unrelated to the cystic mass on the back.

Sacrococcygeal teratoma: Tumor at the base of the tailbone. Not present at lumbosacral area.

2

A mother of a newborn calls the health and wellness clinic to express her concern about the umbilical cord care, as she noticed the cord was wet and had some discharge when she was cleaning it. What would be the most suitable instruction for the nurse to give to the mother?

a. Bring the infant to the health and wellness clinic for further assessment
b. Continue monitoring as this is a normal occurrence and no further action is needed
c. Increase the number of times that the cord is cleaned per day
d. Monitor the cord for another 24–48 hours and call the clinic if the discharge continues

Ans. (a) Bring the infant to the health and wellness clinic for further assessment

Explanation: If the mother notices any signs such as the umbilical cord being wet, discharging, oozing, or redness around its base, it may be sign of infection. The mother should be advised to visit the clinic for further evaluation and appropriate treatment.

3

In the emergency department, a mother presents with her 5-year-old child who fell off a bunk bed, and a head injury is suspected. The nurse evaluates the child's airway and monitors for both early and late indicators of increased intracranial pressure (ICP). Which of the following is a late sign of increased ICP?

a. Nausea
b. Irritability
c. Headache
d. Bradycardia

Ans. (d) Bradycardia

Explanation: Increased intracranial pressure refers to a condition where there is an abnormal increase in pressure within the skull. As ICP rises, it can cause compression and compromise of brain tissue, leading to various signs and symptoms. The options provided include both early and late signs of increased ICP. Early signs of increased ICP include headache, nausea, vomiting, and irritability. Late signs of increased ICP include bradycardia, hypertension, and abnormal breathing patterns.

4

A 5-year-old child is brought to the emergency department after a fall from a bicycle. Nurse in the emergency department is assessing for signs of increased intracranial pressure, resulting in head trauma. Which of the following signs or symptoms would be cause for concern?

a. Bulging anterior fontanel
b. Repeated vomiting
c. Signs of sleepiness at 10 p.m.
d. Inability to read short words from a distance of 18 inches

Ans. (b) Repeated vomiting

Explanation: Early signs of increased ICP include headache, nausea, vomiting, and irritability. Late signs of increased ICP include bradycardia, hypertension, and abnormal breathing patterns. So, repeated vomiting (option b) is the correct answer. The fontanel of a 4-year-old child would be closed already, so option a is wrong. Other options are nonspecific to increased ICP.

5

An 8-year-old baby presents with fever, cough and confluent rash on hairlines, face, neck and body. The most likely causative agent is:

a. Rubella
b. Varicella
c. Rubeola
d. Variola

Ans. (c) Rubeola

Explanation: Rubeola, also known as measles, commonly presents with symptoms such as fever, cough, and a rash that starts on the face and spreads downward to the rest of the body.

Rubella (German measles) typically causes a milder rash and is less likely to present with a cough. Varicella (chickenpox) causes a characteristic vesicular rash, and variola refers to smallpox, which is an eradicated disease.

6

During the discharge process of a 12-year-old child with hemophilia, the nurse advises the parents regarding the most appropriate sport activity for the child. What sport activity does the nurse recommend?

a. Swimming
b. Football
c. Field hockey
d. Basketball

Ans. (a) Swimming

Explanation: When providing instructions to the parents of a 12-year-old child with hemophilia regarding sport activities, the nurse should consider the safety and potential risks associated with the child's condition. Hemophilia is a bleeding disorder characterized by a deficiency or dysfunction of clotting factors in the blood. Therefore, high-impact or contact sports should generally be avoided to minimize the risk of bleeding and injury. With that in mind, the nurse should recommend low-impact and noncontact sports. So among the given options most appropriate sport activity for the child is swimming.

7

A 1-month-old infant with hydrocele visits the clinic for a follow-up appointment. The scrotum has reduced in size since birth, but fluid is still visible upon illumination. What recommendation is the physician likely to provide?

a. Advise massaging the groin area few times a day until the fluid is absorbed
b. Referral to a surgeon for repair
c. No treatment is necessary; the fluid is reabsorbing normally
d. Advise to keep the infant in a flat, supine position to promote absorption of fluid.

Ans. (c) No treatment is necessary; the fluid is reabsorbing normally

Explanation: A hydrocele is a collection of fluid in the scrotum. In infants, hydroceles often resolve spontaneously without any intervention. It is normal for the fluid to gradually reabsorb over time. Therefore, in this case, since the scrotum has become smaller, the physician is likely to reassure the parents that no treatment is necessary at this time and it will resolve with time.

8

In a 5-year-old child with microcytic, hypochromic anemia, iron therapy was initiated. Despite the child's adherence to the treatment, there was no improvement in hemoglobin levels. On examination, the following finding is noted. What could be the probable etiology?

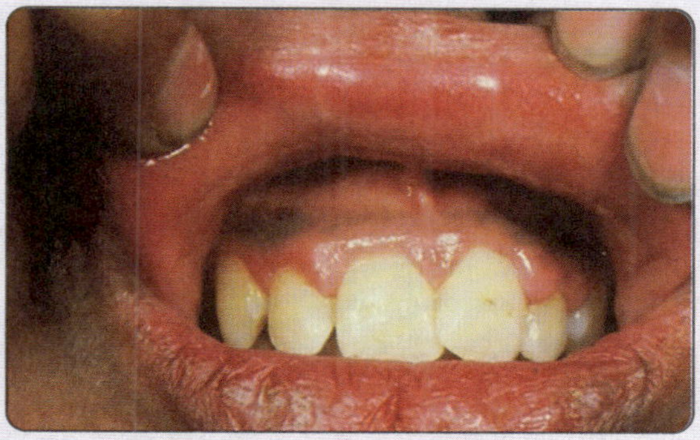

a. Liver dysfunction
b. Celiac disease
c. Plumbism
d. Vitamin C deficiency

Ans. (c) Plumbism

Explanation: The thin black-blue visible along the margins of gum is known as Burton's line. It is found in patients with significantly higher blood levels of lead. This is caused by the reaction between lead and sulfur ions released by oral bacteria, which deposits lead sulfide at the junction of the teeth and gums.

Lead poisoning is also known as **Plumbism**. The anemia of **lead intoxication** is hypochromic and normo -or microcytic with associated reticulocytosis.

9

A mother brings her male infant to the clinic because she has observed that the infant holds his head in an abnormal position and consistently faces one side. Which of the following is a most likely cause?

a. Torticollis, characterized by shortening of the sternocleidomastoid muscle
b. Craniosynostosis, involving premature closure of the cranial sutures
c. Plagiocephaly, resulting in flattening of one side of the head
d. Hydrocephalus, leading to increased head size

Ans. (a) Torticollis, with shortening of the sternocleidomastoid muscle

Explanation: Torticollis is a condition characterized by the shortening or tightness of the sternocleidomastoid muscle, which runs along the side of the neck. This muscle helps to control the movement and position of the head. When the sternocleidomastoid muscle is shortened or tight on one side, it can cause the infant to hold their head tilted to one side and have difficulty turning it in the opposite direction.

10

A 3-year-old child had a fall from tricycle and sustained an injury to the leg. The child refuses to walk. The nurse in the emergency department observed swelling of the affected lower leg. Which of the following does the nurse suspect as the possible cause of the child's symptoms?

a. Fracture of the tibia
b. Bruising of the gastrocnemius muscle
c. Fracture of the radius
d. No anatomic injury, the child wants attention from mother

Ans. (a) Possible fracture of the tibia

Explanation: Swelling, along with the refusal to bear weight on the leg, is a common presentation in the case of a possible fracture. The tibia, which is one of the long bones in the lower leg, is susceptible to fractures, particularly in young children who engage in active play and may experience falls or other accidents. Radius is situated in the arm (upper limb), so it is not appropriate.

11

In the clinic, a baby is brought in with multiple physical abnormalities including cleft lip, cleft palate, microcephaly, small eyes, scalp defect, and polydactyly. These features collectively suggest a specific syndrome. What is the likely syndrome underlying these clinical findings?

a. Trisomy 13
b. Trisomy 18
c. Trisomy 21
d. Trisomy 23

Ans. (a) Trisomy 13

Explanation: Trisomy 13, also known as patau syndrome, is a genetic disorder caused by the presence of an extra copy of chromosome 13. The symptoms of Trisomy 13 can vary from mild to severe. Common features include: Cleft lip and palate, Microcephaly, Small eyes, Scalp defect, Polydactyly (born with one or more extra fingers), Heart defects, Brain defects, and Mental retardation.

12

A child is hospitalized a few days after sustaining a puncture wound on her foot from stepping on a sharp object. The physician suspects osteomyelitis and prescribes parenteral antibiotics. What is the immediate action taken before initiating antibiotic therapy?

a. Prepare admission orders
b. A complete blood count (CBC) with differential is drawn
c. A sample for blood culture is drawn
d. Wait until the parents arrive

Ans. (a) A sample for blood culture is drawn

Explanation: Before starting antibiotics, it is important to identify the bacteria that are causing the infection. This is done by drawing a blood culture, which is a test that cultures the blood to see what bacteria are growing. The blood culture is drawn immediately before the antibiotic is started so that the bacteria that are causing the infection can be identified and treated appropriately. Inappropriate antibiotic usage can lead to extended hospitalization, higher expenses, and negatively impact the patient's overall prognosis.

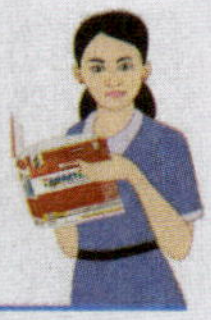

13

A 21-year-old patient arrives at the emergency department (ED) with a sudden onset of asthma symptoms. The patient's respiratory rate is 42 breaths per minute, indicating acute respiratory distress. What should be your immediate course of action?

a. Obtain a comprehensive medical history
b. Attach a cardiac monitor to the patient
c. Administer a bronchodilator by nebulizer
d. Provide emotional support for the patient

Ans. (c) Give a bronchodilator by nebulizer

Explanation: The patient is in acute respiratory distress, so the first priority is to improve his breathing. A bronchodilator is a medication that opens up the airways, so it will help to relieve the airway obstruction that is causing the respiratory distress.

The other options are important, but they are not as urgent as giving the bronchodilator.

14

You are called to assess a 1-day-old female infant with unusual physical findings. Upon examination, you observed that the neonate's hands are clenched with overlapping digits and her lower extremities are extended and crossed. Additionally, you observe the presence of feet with a rocker bottom appearance and delicate, small facial features. What chromosomal abnormality is the most probable explanation for the observed features in the patient?

a. Trisomy 13
b. Trisomy 18
c. Trisomy 21
d. Absence of chromosome 15

Ans. (b) Trisomy 18

Explanation: The described physical findings are the characteristics of a condition called Edward syndrome, also known as Trisomy 18. Trisomy 18 is a chromosomal abnormality caused by the presence of an extra copy of chromosome 18. The specific physical findings mentioned, such as clenched hands with overlapping digits (known as "rocker bottom" feet), extended and crossed lower extremities, and delicate small facial features, are commonly seen in infants with Trisomy 18. Therefore, the most likely cause of the patient's features in this scenario is b. Trisomy 18.

15

A child who has undergone spinal fusion surgery for scoliosis reports abdominal discomfort and experiences episodes of vomiting. The nurse observes abdominal distention during assessment. In view of these findings, what action should the nurse take?

a. Position the child in a Sims' position
b. Administer an antiemetic to control nausea and vomiting
c. Adjust the IV fluid flow rate.
d. Notify the physician

Ans. (d) Notify the physician

Explanation: Scoliosis is a spinal deformity that can cause lateral curvature, spinal rotation, and hypokyphosis of the thorax.

Superior mesenteric artery syndrome is a potential complication following surgical treatment for scoliosis. It occurs due to mechanical changes in the abdominal contents caused by the lengthening of the body. This can lead to symptoms such as vomiting and abdominal distention, resembling intestinal obstruction or paralytic ileus. Postoperative vomiting in children with body casts or those who have undergone spinal fusion should be monitored closely for signs of superior mesenteric artery syndrome. So, the physician need to be informed immediately.

16

A 12-year-old boy came to the emergency department with her mother. While taking the history the mother of the child said that he was playing with the coins and accidently ingested one coin. The doctor assessed the airway and concluded that the airway is partially obstructed. The doctor asked you to pass him the instrument used to remove the foreign body. Select which among the following instrument you will provide to the doctor?

a. 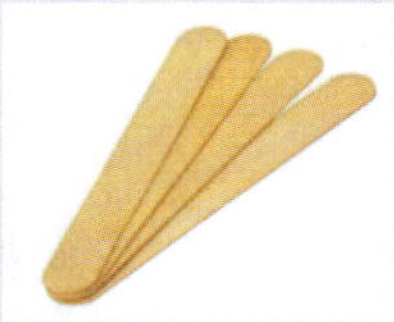

b. 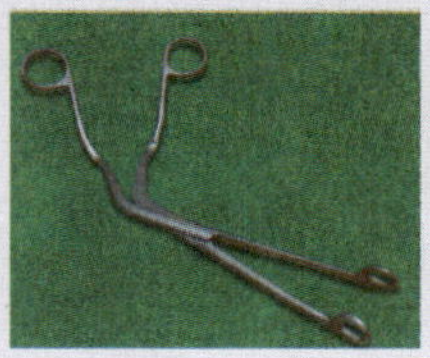

c. 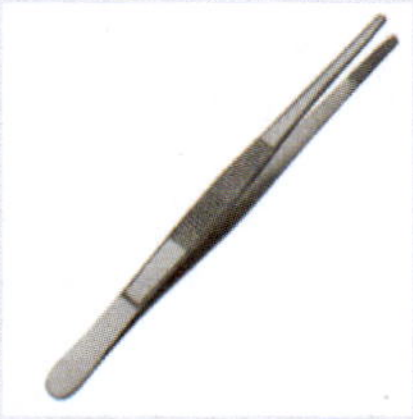

d. 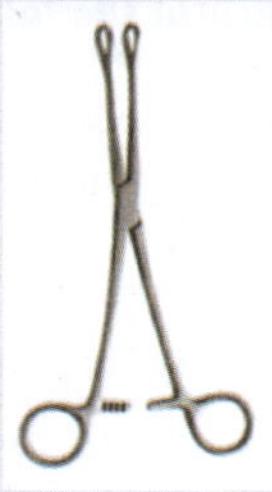

Ans. (b)

Explanation: In this scenario, the most appropriate instrument to provide to the doctor for the removal of a partially obstructing coin in the airway of a 12-year-old boy is Magill forceps. Magill forceps are specially designed curved forceps commonly used for the removal of foreign bodies from the upper airway. They have a curved tip that allows for better maneuverability and grasping of objects, such as coins, lodged in the airway.

17

The nurse is about to administer a phytonadione (vitamin K) injection to a newborn. The mother asks the nurse why her infant needs the injection. How should the nurse best respond?

a. "Your newborn requires the injection to develop immunity."
b. "Newborns have sterile bowels, and the injection stimulates the growth of bowel bacteria."
c. "Newborns have a vitamin K deficiency, and this injection prevents bleeding in your newborn."
d. "The injection will prevent jaundice in your newborn."

Ans. (c) "Newborns have a vitamin K deficiency, and this injection prevents bleeding in your newborn."

Explanation: Vitamin K plays a crucial role in the clotting of blood. Newborns are born with low levels of vitamin K and have an immature liver that is not yet capable of producing adequate amounts of this vitamin. As a result, they are at risk of developing a condition called vitamin K deficiency bleeding (VKDB), which can lead to severe bleeding, including bleeding in the brain.

Administering a vitamin K injection to newborns shortly after birth helps prevent this deficiency and reduces the risk of bleeding complications. It is a standard practice recommended by healthcare professionals to ensure the newborn's well-being and safety.

18

Nurse Ramya is assessing a male newborn following circumcision and observes that the circumcised area appears red with a slight amount of bloody drainage. What would be the most appropriate nursing action in this situation?

a. Apply gentle pressure to the area
b. Reinforce the dressing
c. Document the findings
d. Notify the Physician

Ans. (c) Document the findings

Explanation: After circumcision, it is normal for the circumcised area to appear red and have a small amount of bloody drainage. This is a common and expected finding in the immediate postcircumcision period. By documenting these findings, the nurse is maintaining an accurate record of the newborn's condition, which is important for ongoing assessment and communication among healthcare providers.

19

The pediatrician prescribed an IV solution of 5% dextrose and half-normal saline with 40 mEq of potassium chloride at the rate of 1000 mL over 8 hours for a child with hypotonic dehydration. Which of the following assessments is carried out by the nurse before administering this IV prescription?

a. Obtains the child's weight
b. Checks the amount of urine output
c. Measures the temperature
d. Measures the blood pressure

Ans. (b) Checks the amount of urine output

Explanation: Hypotonic dehydration is a condition in which the body loses too much water and electrolytes. This can lead to low blood pressure, decreased urine output, and other problems. Therefore, the priority assessment before administering the IV solution is to check the amount of urine output. This will help to determine how dehydrated the child is and how much fluid they need to replace.

The pediatrician prescribes the fluid volume for replacement based on the child's body weight. Therefore, the nurse would have already obtained the child's body weight as part of the initial assessment.

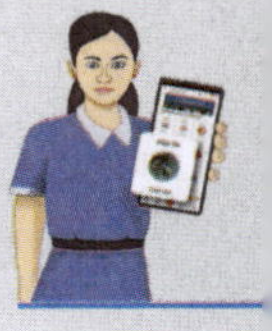

20

After exploring home remedies and alternative treatments for a 10-year-old child with enuresis, the nurse is aware that a specific medication may be prescribed to address this condition. Which of the following medications is likely to be prescribed in this condition?

a. Citalopram
b. Sertraline
c. Fluvoxamine
d. Imipramine

Ans. (d) Imipramine

Explanation: Imipramine is a tricyclic antidepressant which has shown effectiveness in the treatment of enuresis (bedwetting) in children. It works by increasing the bladder's capacity and reducing night-time urine production. Imipramine is often prescribed as a second-line treatment option when other interventions and behavioral modifications have been explored but proved ineffective. Desmopressin is often the first choice of medicine for bedwetting.

21

In the delivery room, a nurse assists with the delivery of a newborn infant. Following the delivery, the nurse prepares to prevent heat loss in the newborn due to evaporation effect by:

a. Heating the surface of the crib mattress
b. Turning on the radiant warmer
c. Shutting the room doors
d. Drying the infant in a warm blanket

Ans. (d) Drying the infant in a warm blanket

Explanation: Evaporation occurs when moisture on the newborn's skin evaporates and cools the body. To prevent this, the nurse should dry the infant thoroughly with a warm blanket or towel. This helps in removing any wetness on the skin, reducing heat loss through evaporation.

Warming the crib pad, turning on the overhead radiant warmer, and closing the doors to the room primarily address other modes of heat loss, not evaporation.

22

While monitoring a preterm newborn infant, a nurse in the newborn nursery is looking for specific assessment signs that may indicate the presence of respiratory distress syndrome. Presence of which of the following signs would alert the nurse for the possibility of this syndrome?

a. The presence of a barrel chest with grunting
b. Bradycardia and decreased BP
c. Tachypnea and retractions
d. Grunting and acrocyanosis

Ans. (c) Tachypnea and retractions

Explanation: Respiratory distress syndrome (RDS) is a common condition in preterm newborn infants, also known as hyaline membrane disease. It occurs due to the inadequate production of surfactant in the immature lungs, leading to difficulty in breathing. The following signs and symptoms are commonly seen in newborns with RDS: Tachypnea (>60 breaths per minute), a hallmark sign of RDS. Retractions: Muscles between the ribs and in the neck pull inward during inspiration, indicating increased effort to breathe.

Other given symptoms also present in RDS, however, they are nonspecific. Therefore, the most specific assessment signs for identifying respiratory distress syndrome in a preterm newborn infant are tachypnea and retractions (choice b).

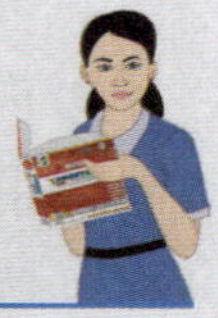

23

Which of the following is most likely associated with a cerebrovascular accident (CVA) resulting from congenital heart disease?

a. Polycythemia
b. Cardiomyopathy
c. Endocarditis
d. Low blood pressure

Ans. (a) Polycythemia

Explanation: Congenital heart defects can cause chronic hypoxemia, leading to compensatory polycythemia. The increased viscosity of the blood in polycythemia increases the risk of clot formation and subsequent cerebrovascular accidents.

24

The nurse is preparing to provide care for a five-year-old child who is in traction after fracturing their femur. The nurse is aware that which of the following activities would be the most suitable for this child?

a. Reading large picture books
b. Using crayons and coloring book
c. Listening to a radio
d. Watching a sports video

Ans. (b) Using crayons and coloring book

Explanation: Providing crayons and a coloring book would be the most appropriate activity as this activity promotes creativity, engagement, and cognitive development while keeping the child occupied during their recovery period.

25

A 15-year-old boy is hospitalized for acute appendicitis and undergoes an appendectomy. Which nursing intervention would best support the client's normal growth and development?

a. Permit the family to bring the child's favorite computer games
b. Allow the child to participate in activities with peer group when condition permits
c. Encourage the parents to stay with the child in room
d. Encourage the child to rest and read

Ans. (b) Allow the child to participate in activities with peer group when condition permits

Explanation: Allowing the 15-year-old boy to participate in activities with his peer group is particularly important because it aligns with the developmental stage of identity versus role confusion. Adolescence strive to form their own identity and establish a sense of self. Interacting with peers allows them to explore different roles, develop social skills, and gain a sense of belonging and acceptance within their peer group.

26

When providing care for a child with iron deficiency anemia, which of the following blood study findings would the nurse anticipate as the most probable?

a. Hemoglobin level above the reference range
b. Normal hematocrit level
c. Normal total iron-binding capacity (TIBC)
d. Decreased mean corpuscular volume (MCV)

Ans. (d) Decreased mean corpuscular volume (MCV)

Explanation: Iron deficiency anemia is a condition in which there is not enough iron in the body to produce healthy red blood cells. This can lead to a decrease in the size of the red blood cells, which is known as microcytosis. Microcytosis is reflected in a decreased mean corpuscular volume (MCV).

27

Nurse Ramya is caring for a neonate. During assessment, Ramya observes that the infant is exhibiting signs of rapid breathing, cyanosis, nasal flaring, and grunting. The diagnosis of respiratory distress syndrome is made, and the physician orders surfactant replacement therapy. How should the nurse prepare to administer this therapy?

a. Instillation into the lungs through an Endotracheal Tube
b. Subcutaneous injection
c. Intravenous injection
d. Intramuscular injection

Ans. (a) Instillation into the lungs through an Endotracheal Tube

Explanation: Surfactant replacement therapy is a treatment used to manage respiratory distress syndrome (RDS) in premature infants. RDS is a condition caused by the insufficient production of surfactant, a substance that helps keep the air sacs open in the lungs. To administer surfactant replacement therapy, the surfactant preparation is delivered directly into the baby's lungs through an endotracheal tube (ET).

28

Rohini, a 13-year-old girl, has undergone a lumbar puncture to assess the cerebrospinal fluid (CSF) for possible bacterial infection. Which position is most suitable for her to maintain after the procedure?

a. Prone for two hours to prevent the risk of aspiration in case of vomiting
b. Sitting in semi-upright position for 6 hours
c. Supine for several hours, to prevent headache
d. Left lateral position to facilitate return of CSF

Ans. (b) Supine for several hours, to prevent headache

Explanation: After a lumbar puncture, it is common for some patients, including adolescents like Rohini, to experience a postlumbar puncture headache. This headache is caused by a temporary decrease in cerebrospinal fluid (CSF) pressure around the brain and spinal cord. Keeping the patient in a supine position for several hours after the procedure can help prevent or minimize the development of this headache.

29

Nurse Ramya is closely monitoring the intake and output of an infant with heart failure who is on diuretic therapy. Which of the following method is most appropriate to assess the urine output in this case?

a. Measuring the quantity of water added to formula
b. Comparing intake to the output
c. Weighing the diapers
d. Using a urinary catheter

Ans. (c) Weighing the diapers

Explanation: When an infant is receiving diuretic therapy, it is important to closely monitor their urine output. The most accurate way to do this is to weigh the diapers. The weight of the diaper before and after the infant urinates will an accurate measure of the urine output.

30

The 14-year-old boy has fractured his arm because of a fall from the stairs. Following the application of a cast to the injury, the nurse recognizes the significance of conducting several assessments on the region distal to cast. Which of the following assessment is least important?

a. Capillary refill
b. Radial and ulnar pulse
c. Finger movement
d. Skin integrity

Ans. (d) Skin integrity

Explanation: Assessments such as capillary refill, pulses, skin temperature, and color are important for evaluating circulation and ruling out compartment syndrome in a patient with a cast. Assessment of skin integrity at this point is least important.

31

Nurse Ramya is preparing to care for a child diagnosed with intussusception. Which specific sign is the nurse likely to find documented in the child's medical record?

a. Profuse projectile vomiting
b. Watery diarrhea
c. Ribbon-like stools
d. Rectal bleeding, often with "red currant jelly" stool

Ans. (d) Rectal bleeding, often with "red currant jelly" stool

Explanation: Intussusception is a medical emergency that occurs when a portion of the intestine telescopes into another part of the intestine, causing a blockage. It is most seen in infants and young children.

One of the hallmark signs of intussusception is the presence of bright red, "currant jelly"—like stools, which contain blood and mucus. As the intestine telescopes into itself, it can cause irritation, inflammation, and bleeding, leading to the appearance of blood and mucus in the stool.

Ribbon like stool is seen in Hirschsprung disease.

Projectile vomiting is seen in hyper pyloric stenosis. watery diarrhea is nonspecific.

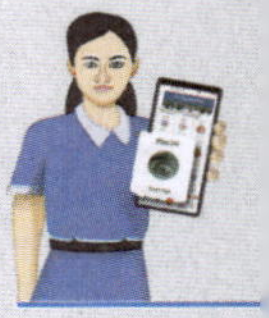

32

The adolescent patient is exhibiting symptoms of meningitis such as nuchal rigidity, vomiting, fever, and lethargy. The nurse is aware that it is necessary to prepare for which of the following specific test?

a. Blood and throat culture b. Lumbar puncture
c. MRI scan d. CAT scan

Ans. (b) Lumbar puncture

Explanation: Meningitis is an inflammation of the meninges, the membranes that surround the brain and spinal cord. The most definitive test for meningitis is a lumbar puncture. A lumbar puncture is a procedure in which a needle is inserted into the spinal canal to collect cerebrospinal fluid (CSF). Lumbar puncture is the most definitive test for meningitis because it allows the doctor to collect CSF and test it for bacteria, viruses, or fungi

33

A child, born two days ago, presents with bilious vomiting and the mother reported history of polyhydramnios. The radiological imaging is shown. Which of the following is the probable diagnosis?

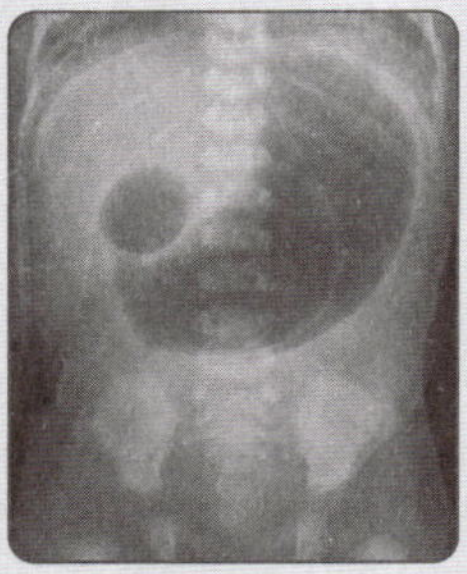

a. Duodenal atresia b. Hypertrophic pyloric stenosis
c. Ileal atresia d. Congenital megacolon

Ans. (a) Duodenal atresia

Explanation: The "double bubble sign" seen on the radiograph indicates the presence of two dilated loops of bowel, one in the stomach (gastric bubble) and another in the first part of the duodenum (duodenal bubble). Duodenal atresia is a congenital condition where there is a blockage or complete absence of the lumen in the duodenum, which is the first part of the small intestine.

34

Mother brought her 18-month-old infant to well-baby clinic with the complaining of consumption of clay, crayons, and paper by her baby. As an experienced pediatric nurse, which among the following you will assess first?

a. Nutritional intake of the baby
b. Parental attention to the baby
c. Recent change in home environment
d. New tooth eruptions

Ans. (c) Recent change in home environment

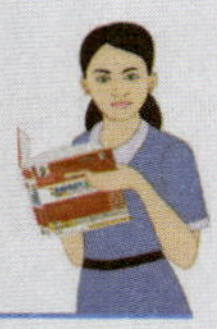

Explanation: Oral gratification is a method to cope up with anxiety among toddlers. Therefore, any recent change in the home environment is needed to assess first.

35

Mother brought her 9-month-old baby to under five clinics stating that her baby's development is slow. While assessing the infants development absence of which among the following indicates a need for further development screening?

a. Creeping b. Stand holding onto the object
c. Drinking from cup with spoon
d. Single syllables

Ans. (d) Single syllables

Explanation: Creeping and standing holding onto the object is expected at 9 months. Drinking from cup with a spoon is seen by the age of 15 months of age. Single syllables are seen in 6 months old baby. Absence of single syllables in a 9 month old baby needs further evaluation.

36

Baby Hima diagnosed with truncus arteriosus. Her parents ask nurse Lina regarding the condition. Nurse explained this condition as:

a. Single blood vessel arising from both ventricles
b. Obstruction to the blood from left ventricle
c. Obstruction of blood from right ventricle
d. Abnormal connection between left and right atrium

Ans. (a) Single blood vessel arising from both ventricles

Explanation: Single blood vessel is coming out from both right and left ventricles is known as truncus arteriosus. Obstruction of blood from right ventricle is known as pulmonic stenosis. Abnormal connection between left and right atrium is known as atrial septal defect.

37

Nurse was instructing a group of mothers how to encourage autonomy among their 4-year-old child. Which among the following statements identified by mothers indicates that session was effective?

a. Help them to button the dress and tie the shoelace.
b. Let them select the dress they need to wear.
c. Tell the child whenever they did not dress well.
d. Give instruction to them regarding cloth selection.

Ans. (b) Let them select the dress they need to wear.

Explanation: If child is allowed to select dress for self, it will boost autonomy and self-esteem. Other options are discouraging autonomy and self-esteem.

38

After a class on growth and development, students identified which age group's primary psychosocial task as "Identity development"?

a. Infancy b. Toddler
c. School-going d. Adolescence

Ans. (d) Adolescence

Explanation: As per the Erikson's psychosocial development identity v/s role confusion is seen in adolescence.

39

Mother complained about the temper tantrum behavior of her 3-year-old child to a nurse. Most appropriate response from nurse is:

a. Punish the child whenever the unwanted behavior occurs.
b. It is normal as per her age group.
c. Set limit on her behavior.
d. Ignore the child completely whenever the unwanted behavior occurs.

Ans. (c) Set limit on her behavior.

Explanation: Being consistent and setting limits on the child's behavior are necessary to control behavior of toddlers. Ignoring and punishing a child may not be helpful to control behavior as they have some unseen effect on their later behaviors.

40

Nurse is teaching to a group of mothers whose children are affected with Cystic fibrosis. Nurse could understand, teaching was effective if parents correctly identified the INCORRECT statement about Cystic fibrosis as:

a. It affects body's mucous secreting glands.
b. Intake of high calorie, high protein and moderate fat is required.
c. Postural drainage is required and to be done before meals.
d. When disease is under control, large quantities of foul-smelling stool occur.

Ans. (d) When disease is under control, large quantities of foul-smelling stool occur.

Explanation: Cystic fibrosis is a condition which affects exocrine glands in the body and produce thick secretions. Because of difficulty with absorption and digestion high calorie, high protein moderate fat is needed. Postural drainage helps to remove secretions and to be done before meals to avoid the possibility of vomiting and regurgitation. If the disease is under control, stool will be soft and with little odor.

41

Nurse is collecting history of a child admitted with rheumatic fever. While collecting history, which among the following informations is most important?

a. Recent travel history to restricted countries
b. Recent history of viral infection
c. Recent episode of pharyngitis
d. Lack of interest in food

Ans. (c) Recent episode of pharyngitis

Explanation: There is an antigen antibody reaction usually following streptococcal sore throat which predisposes a client to sore throat.

42

Client came to emergency department with cardiac failure from his relative, nurse came to know that he was on digoxin therapy. Which among the following signs indicates digoxin toxicity as a cause of cardiac failure?

a. Extreme bradycardia
b. Profuse diarrhea
c. Headache
d. Chest pain

Ans. (a) Extreme bradycardia

Explanation: Digoxin decreases the heart rate; extreme bradycardia is a cardinal sign of heart failure associated with digoxin toxicity.

43

Labor room nurse was assessing a baby following term delivery. Which among the following characteristics will be present in the baby?

a. Baby is in extended posture.
b. Lanugo is covering most of the body part.
c. Ear cartilage has poor recoiling capacity.
d. Sole creases covering the entire foot.

Ans. (d) Sole creases covering the entire foot.

Explanation: Sole creases covering the entire foot is the characteristic of term delivery. All other options are the characteristics of preterm babies.

44

Pediatric ICU nurse was performing suction on a child. Following suction, which among the following findings needs to be observed in the child?

a. Bradycardia
b. Tachypnea
c. Hypertension
d. Jerking movement

Ans. (a) Bradycardia

Explanation: Bradycardia following suction is an expected finding because of the vagal stimulation. Other given options are not a normal observation following suction.

45

Nurse was assessing a male neonate and observed urinary meatus was opening on the dorsal side of the penis. This condition is known as:

a. Phimosis
b. Epispadias
c. Hypospadias
d. Cryptorchidism

Ans. (b) Epispadias

Explanation: Urinary meatus on the dorsal side is known as epispadias and on the ventral side is known as hypospadias. Phimosis is a condition in which foreskin is too tight to be pulled back over the head of the penis. Cryptorchidism is a condition in which one or both of the testes fail to descend from the abdomen into the scrotum.

46

CPR was going on in NICU. After 30 seconds of chest compression heart rate was 52 bpm. Adrenaline injection given to the baby. What is the normal expected finding following the injection?

a. Increase in heart rate
b. Hypotension
c. Polyurea
d. Sedation

Ans. (a) Increase in heart rate

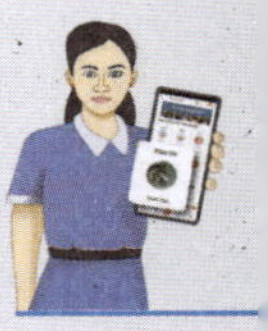

Explanation: Adrenaline or Epinephrine injection is given to treat severe bradycardia or hypotension. Following injection, normal expected finding is rise in BP and heart rate. Adrenaline decreases renal blood flow and causes decrease in urine output. It stimulates alpha- and beta-adrenergic receptors so sedation cannot be expected.

47

A mother with her 15-month-old child came to developmental clinic with the concern that her child is not yet walking. The nurse working in the clinic understood that according to the Denver Developmental Screen, the median age for walking is:

a. 12 months b. 15 months
c. 18 months d. 24 months

Ans. (a) 12 months

Explanation: According to the Denver Developmental Screen, the median age for walking is 12 months and the concern of mother is genuine and baby needs further assessment.

48

Nurse received baby following lumbar puncture procedure. Which position needs to be given to the baby in post procedural period?

a. Supine b. Prone
c. Fowlers d. Knee chest

Ans. (a) Supine

Explanation: Following lumbar puncture, baby has to be placed in supine position to prevent post lumbar puncture headache. Increasing fluid intake will replenish the lost fluid during this time.

49

Nurse educator was explaining to a junior nurse about iron deficiency anemia. Nurse educator can identify her class was effective if junior nurse identifies INCORRECT statement regarding iron deficiency anemia as:

a. Microcytic anemia
b. Decreased total iron binding capacity
c. Decreased MCV
d. Decreased hemoglobin

Ans. (b) Decreased total iron binding capacity

Explanation: In a child with iron deficiency anemia, the blood study results most likely would reveal decreased mean corpuscular volume (MCV) which demonstrates microcytic anemia, decreased hemoglobin, decreased hematocrit and elevated total iron binding capacity.

50

An undergraduate nursing student was performing physical examination on a toddler, her educator asked her about the best method to perform physical examination on a toddler. She correctly responds as:

a. Cephalocaudal direction b. System wise assessment
c. Least to most intrusive d. Proximal to distal

Ans. (c) Least to most intrusive

Explanation: Best method to perform physical examination on a toddler is least intrusive to most intrusive. All other given options are inappropriate.

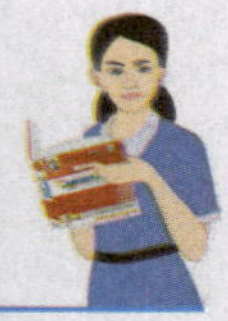

51

Baby Riya underwent for ventriculoperitoneal shunt last week, which among the following signs indicates early shunt malfunction?

a. High pitched cry, changes in pulse and respiration
b. Pupillary changes and high-pitched cry
c. Tense fontanelle, vomiting and irritability
d. Headache, anorexia and irritability

Ans. (c) Tense fontanelle, vomiting and irritability

Explanation: Early signs of shunt malfunction include irritability, vomiting and tensed fontanelle. Change in pulse and respiration is a late sign.

52

During the visit to well-baby clinic, mother asked the clinic nurse regarding weaning and introduction of home food. Which among the following food items needs to be introduced by the mother first?

a. Smashed potato b. Mashed fruit
c. Hen's egg d. Rice cereals

Ans. (d) Rice cereals

Explanation: Rice cereals are the best food to introduce after weaning as they are easily digestible and associated with less allergic reaction. Following cereals, mashed vegetables and fruits can be given. Introduction of egg should be delayed as it causes allergic reaction in most of the babies.

53

While going through the case file of a patient, nurse saw diagnosis as Wilson disease. What all characteristics she needs to expect in the file; except:

a. Kayser-Fleischer rings in the eyes
b. It is inherited as an autosomal recessive trait
c. Excess copper stored in various body tissues
d. Sweat chloride test is the diagnostic method

Ans. (d) Sweat chloride test is the diagnostic method

Explanation: Except option d all are the characteristics of Wilson disease. Sweat chloride test is the diagnostic method for cystic fibrosis. Wilson disease is diagnosed with blood levels.

54

Newborn child diagnosed with developmental dysplasia of the hip (DDH). As an experienced nurse you should understand that most common type of DDH is:

a. Subluxable b. Dislocatable
c. Teratologic hip d. Late dysplasia

Ans. (a) Subluxable

Explanation: Developmental Dysplasia of the Hip is a disorder of abnormal development resulting in dysplasia, subluxation, and possible dislocation of the hip secondary to capsular laxity and mechanical instability. Most common type of DDH is subluxable.

55

Nurse was educating a mother about iron deficiency anemia. On identifying, which among the following items is not the best source for iron?

a. Spinach
b. Liver and organ meat
c. Legume
d. Yellow vegetables

Ans. (d) Yellow vegetables

Explanation: Shellfish, spinach, liver and other organ meats, legumes, red meat, pumpkin seeds, etc. are good source of iron. Yellow vegetables are poor source of iron.

56

Nurse was educating parents of a child with newly diagnosed attention deficit hyperactivity disorder (ADHD). All among the following are features of ADHD; except:

a. Difficulty paying attention
b. Being overactive
c. Acting without thinking
d. Excessive fatigue

Ans. (d) Excessive fatigue

Explanation: ADHD is a mental condition in which child has differences in brain development and brain activity that affect attention, the ability to sit still, and self-control. Except option d all other options are the characteristics of ADHD.

57

Lucy, an 8-year-old child known case of diabetes, came to emergency complaining of nausea, vomiting, fruity-scented breath. Diagnosis of diabetes ketoacidosis was made. Which among the following is not the expected management for this child?

a. Isotonic fluid infusion
b. Potassium supplementation
c. Sodium supplementation
d. Insulin infusion

Ans. (c) Sodium supplementation

Explanation: Diabetes ketoacidosis is a complication of diabetes in which excessive fat destruction leads to the production of ketone bodies. Insulin deficiency, increased insulin counter-regulatory hormones and peripheral insulin resistance leading to hyperglycemia, dehydration, ketosis, and electrolyte imbalance, which underlie the pathophysiology of DKA. Except option d all other options are the treatment guideline for DKA.

58

Senior nurse was orienting junior nurse to a neurosurgical ICU. After the orientation, senior nurse asked the junior nurse why the head end is elevated 10-20 degree for patients with increased ICP. All among the following are correct response by the junior nurse; except:

a. Helps to reduce headache
b. Maintain neutral position
c. Decreases intra-abdominal and intrathoracic pressure
d. Helps to relieve neck stiffness

Ans. (d) Helps to relieve neck stiffness

Explanation: Except option d all are the advantages of elevating head end 10–20 degree angle for a patient with increased ICP.

59

Nurse was collecting history from a child's parents who is scheduled for IPV vaccination. Which among the following informations nurse should brought into the attention of doctor?

a. Recent history of upper respiratory tract
b. Anaphylaxis reaction to neomycin
c. Redness and itching at previous injection site
d. Child is having diarrhea

Ans. (b) Anaphylaxis reaction to neomycin

Explanation: Anaphylaxis reaction to neomycin should brought into the attention of doctor as IPV contains trace amount of streptomycin, neomycin, and polymyxin.

60

Nurse Liza is caring for a school going child diagnosed with asthma. Which among the following observations would be more concerning?

a. Child is getting O_2 via nasal prongs and SpO_2 is 97%
b. Child is having intercostal and subcostal retraction
c. Child is unable to speak one complete sentence
d. Child is using MDI without spacer

Ans. (c) Child is unable to speak one complete sentence

Explanation: Option a and d are normal findings in a preschool child with asthma. Intercostal and subcostal retraction can be seen in a child with mild respiratory distress. If child is unable to speak one complete sentence it is because of their increased work for breathing and risk for airway obstruction. Among options b and c most appropriate option is c.

61

OPD nurse notices one of the childs with a crusty yellow honey-colored scab forms over the sore on the face of the child. She should understand that the condition is:

a. Scabies
b. Impetigo
c. Psoriasis
d. Dermatitis

Ans. (b) Impetigo

Explanation: Impetigo is a skin infection caused by group A *Streptococcus or Staphylococcus aureus*. Crusty yellow or "honey-colored" scab forms over the sore, which then heals without leaving a scar is the characteristic lesion of impetigo.

Scabies is a skin condition caused by a tiny burrowing mite called Sarcoptes scabiei and the condition is characterized by intense itching and the urge to scratch may be especially strong at night.

Psoriasis is a noncontagious, chronic skin disease that produces plaques of thickened, scaly skin. The dry flakes of silvery-white skin scales result from the excessively rapid proliferation of skin cells.

Dermatitis (eczema) is inflammation of the skin, typically characterized by itchiness, redness and a rash.

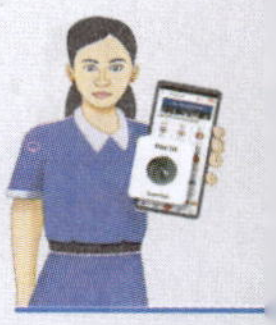

62

Nurse was educating parents about febrile seizures. Nurse understands further teaching is needed. Which among the following is not the characteristic of febrile seizure?

a. It can be prevented by giving paracetamol syrup when child falls sick with fever
b. It does not cause brain damage
c. Antiseizure medications may need to continue for couple of years
d. Children usually outgrow this kind of seizure around six years

Ans. (c) Antiseizure medications may need to continue for couple of years

Explanation: All options except c are correct about febrile seizures. Usually antiseizure medications are not needed to manage febrile seizures as they tend to last less than 5 minutes.

63

Mother of a child diagnosed with phenylketonuria asked the nurse regarding her diet. What type of diet nurse should advise the mother?

a. Low protein
b. Low fat
c. Low calorie
d. High fiber

Ans. (a) Low protein

Explanation: Phenylketonuria (PKU) is caused by deficient activity of the enzyme phenylalanine hydroxylase, needed to convert the essential amino acid (AA) phenylalanine (Phe) to tyrosine. Phenylalanine is an amino acid found in protein, so the child should be encouraged to have low protein diet.

64

Nurse Julie was attending a 1-year-old child on the first post-operative day of cheiloplasty. Which among the following restrains she should prepare for the child?

a. Mummy restrain
b. Jacket restrain
c. Elbow restrain
d. Hand restrain

Ans. (c) Elbow restrain

Explanation: Elbow restrain is used around the elbow to prevent from bending the arm. In this situation we need to prevent the child from bending arm, so that he can't access the repaired lip. All the other given restrains are not suiting with the given situation.

65

Labor room nurse was assessing a new born baby after delivery and she noticed umbilical hernia in the baby. Which among the following conditions is most susceptible to the baby?

a. Tracheoesophageal fistula
b. Renal agenesis
c. Congenital cardiac disease
d. Down syndrome

Ans. (d) Down syndrome

Explanation: Umbilical hernia is most associated with down syndrome. All other given options are not associated with umbilical hernia.

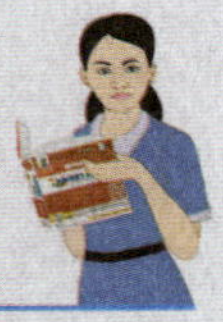

66

Nursing instructor was performing physical examination on a child diagnosed with appendicitis. Instructor made the patient to lie on his left side and asked him to flex the right thigh. Upon doing this, patient complains of pain. Instructor explained to the student this sign as:

a. Rovsing's sign
b. Dunphy's sign
c. Psoas sign
d. Obturator sign

Ans. (c) Psoas sign

Explanation: Here the mentioned sign is psoas sign. Rovsing's sign is palpation of left lower quadrant and elicit pain in the right lower quadrant. Dunphy's sign is coughing, causing increased pain in abdomen with appendicitis. Obturator sign is pain on passive internal rotation of the hip when the right knee is flexed. It is present when the inflamed appendix is in contact with the obturator internus muscle.

67

An infant came to emergency with gastroenteritis and dehydration. ABG analysis reveals that the child is having metabolic acidosis. Which among the following clinical manifestations will be present in the child?

a. Tachypnea
b. Shallow respiration
c. Polycythemia
d. Anemia

Ans. (a) Tachypnea

Explanation: Tachypnea will be present in the infant. Body tries to eliminate buffered acids via respiratory system and there will be increase in ventilation which manifest as tachypnea.

68

Nurse working in ICU was preparing TPN for her assigned child. The child has peripheral line. While preparing TPN, she should keep in mind that the maximum safest amount of glucose that can be administered via peripheral line is:

a. 5% glucose
b. 10% glucose
c. 25% glucose
d. 50% glucose

Ans. (b) 10 % glucose

Explanation: Safest amount of glucose that can be given via peripheral line is 10% glucose. Any concentration above that is to be administered via central line.

69

Nurse received a call from emergency that a new admission of child with meningococcal meningitis is going to be there in her ward. What all preadmission requisites she needs to do?

a. Arrange O_2 supply.
b. Ready with the emergency medicine and intubation system.
c. Arrange isolation with droplet precaution.
d. Get ready with ICP lowering agents.

Ans. (c) Arrange isolation with droplet precaution.

Explanation: A child with meningococcal meningitis should be placed on droplet precautions until they have completed 24 hours of appropriate antibiotic therapy. Oxygen supply and intubation arrangements are based on sickness level of child. There was no communication from emergency department regarding any special arrangements.

70

A child diagnosed with asthma receiving inhaler with bronchodilator and steroid. Parents asked the nurse which inhaler needs to be used first. Correct response from the nurse is:

a. Bronchodilator inhaler first then steroid inhaler
b. Steroid inhaler first then bronchodilator inhaler
c. Any inhaler can be used first
d. There is no specific order

Ans. (a) Bronchodilator inhaler first then steroid inhaler

Explanation: When using two inhalers, one must use bronchodilator inhaler first followed by steroid inhaler.

71

A child with sickle cell disease started on oral deferoxamine therapy. While initiating this therapy, what sign/symptom should the client report immediately?

a. Red color urine
b. Itching
c. Diarrhea
d. Hearing changes

Ans. (d) Hearing changes

Explanation: All above the following are the side effects of deferoxamine. But the serious side effect which needs immediate attention from the medical practitioner is vision changes (such as vision loss, loss of color vision, cataracts) eye pain, or hearing changes (decreased hearing/loss).

72

Child brought to the emergency by parents by complaining that child has ingested some unknown drug in unknown amount. Upon assessment nurse found that GCS 4, HR 80 bpm and regular respiratory rate is 20 bpm, BP: 70/50 and RBS is 36 mg/dL. Based upon the findings, which among the following drugs is suspected as the cause of poisoning?

a. Beta blocker
b. Calcium channel blocker
c. ACE inhibitors
d. Cholinesterase

Ans. (a) Beta blocker

Explanation: Beta blockers not only affect heart and lungs but also affect the beta site in the liver and cause hypoglycemia.

73

18-month-old toddler with the diagnosis of spina bifida meningomyelocele is posted for cardiac catheterization. Mother expresses concern about the use of dye in the procedure. The child does not have any known allergies. In addition to the iodine allergy, what allergy should the surgical team anticipate?

a. Antibiotic penicillin
b. Betadine
c. Shelly fish
d. Latex

Ans. (d) Latex

Explanation: Often the patient with meningomyelocele develops allergy to latex. In the catheterization procedure the catheter is made up of latex and the personnel doing the procedure is also wearing rubber gloves. Child who is sensitive to latex may also develop allergy to kiwi fruits and bananas.

74

Nurse Julie is assessing a child with chickenpox, and she noticed papules, vesicles, and crusts in her body. How will she document this finding?

a. Pleomorphism
b. Kolpik spot
c. Blotchy rash
d. Sandpaper rash

Ans. (a) Pleomorphism

Explanation: A characteristic feature of the rash in chickenpox is pleomorphism, which means all stages of the rash (papules, vesicles and crusts) may be seen simultaneously at one time, in the same area. This is due to the rash appearing in successive crops for 4–5 days in the same area.

Koplik spots are the peculiar spots present on the buccal mucosa and are considered a diagnostic/pathognomic feature of measles/rubeola in the pre-eruptive stage.

A rash is the most common sign of scarlet fever in both adults and children. It usually begins as a red blotchy rash and becomes fine and rough like sandpaper.

75

Doctor ordered visual acuity test for 1-year-old child, which among the following nurse needs to prepare for visual acuity check?

a. Any object which child needs to look and follow
b. Snellen's chart
c. Symbol chart
d. All of these

Ans. (a) Any object which child need to look and follow

Explanation: 1-year-old child is not able to understand symbol chart or Snellen's chart. In order to assess visual acuity in them, nurse needs to hold any object in child's visual feed and needs to check whether the child is able to follow the object or not.

76

Which among the following describes the play seen among school going children?

a. Child observes others and play alone.
b. Child is playing independently among other children.
c. Children are playing together without any organization.
d. Children are playing together with organization.

Ans. (d) Children are playing together with organization.

Explanation: Child is observing other children and does not join to play with them is the characteristic of solitary play. Child is playing alone is solitary play. Child is playing independently among group of children is the characteristic of parallel play and is seen among toddlers. Children are playing together without organization is associative play and is seen among preschool children. Children are playing together with organization is seen among school going children.

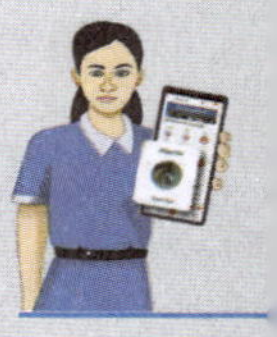

77

Nisha, friend of nurse Julie asked her which type of toy is appropriate for 5-month-old baby as she is going to visit one of her friend's family. Which among the following is the most appropriate response from Julie?

a. Light and sound producing toys
b. Noise-making objects and soft toys
c. Teething toys and social interaction
d. Large blocks, toys that pop apart, and push and pull toys

Ans. (b) Noise-making objects and soft toys

Explanation: Appropriate toys as per the age group is birth to 3 months: visual and auditory stimuli toys, 3 to 6 months: noise-making objects and soft toys, from 6 to 9 months: teething toys and social interaction and from 9 to 12 months: large blocks, toys that pop apart, and push and pull toys.

78

Mother of a preterm newborn admitted in NICU was expressing breastmilk. She asked the nurse that there was some leftover milk from previous feeding, can I use the milk to feed the newborn. What is the correct response from nurse?

a. Leftover feed can be used within 2 hours.
b. Leftover feed can be used within 5 hours.
c. Leftover feed can be used within 6 hours.
d. Leftover feed can be used within 8 hours.

Type of breast milk	Storage location and temperatures		
	Countertop 77°F (25°C) or colder (room temperature)	Refrigerator 40°F (4°C)	Freezer 0°F (–18°C) or colder
Freshly expressed or pumped	Up to 4 hours	Up to 4 days	Within 6 months is best. Up to 12 months is acceptable
Thawed, previously frozen	1–2 hours	Up to 1 day (24 hours)	Never refreeze human milk after it has been thawed
Leftover from a feeding (baby did not finish the bottle)	Use within 2 hours after the baby is finished feeding		

Ans. (a) Leftover feed can be used within 2 hours.

Explanation: Leftover from a feeding (baby did not finish the bottle) has to be used within 2 hours after the baby is finished feeding (from CDC).

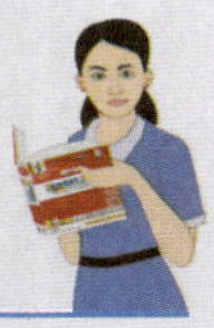

79

Mother brought her 18-month-old child with the complaining of falling unconsciously and becoming blue-colored after the episode of excessive cry. From the description, nurse understood that the child is having:

a. Seizure attack
b. Breath holding spells
c. Temper tantrum
d. Anoxia

Ans. (b) Breath holding spells

Explanation: A breath holding spell is a benign paroxysmal nonepileptic disorder occurring in healthy children 6 to 48 months of age. The episodes start with a provocation such as emotional upset or minor injury, and might progress to breath holding, cyanosis, and syncope.

80

Nurse was feeding a baby with the diagnosis of choanal atresia. Which among the following she needs to monitor while feeding the baby?

a. Sucking and swallowing ability
b. Cough and choke on feeding
c. Regurgitation and vomiting
d. Amount of milk and time taken to consume it

Ans. (b) Cough and choke on feeding

Explanation: Infant with choanal atresia has no opening between nose and nasopharynx. As they are taking breaths through mouth, there is a chance for choking and coughing while giving feeds.

81

Nurse Julie is assigned with a child suffering from Croup. While caring for the child, which among the following is the most important nursing responsibility?

a. Provide humidified environment.
b. Keep emergency tray nearby.
c. Assess respiratory status.
d. Provide bronchodilators.

Ans. (c) Assess respiratory status.

Explanation: Croup refers to an infection of the upper airway, which obstructs breathing and causes a characteristic barking cough. Laryngeal spasm can occur at any time in these patients, so continuous monitoring of respiratory status is necessary.

82

A child with AML started on chemotherapy and prednisolone. What is the expected side effects of prednisolone in the patient?

a. Euphoria
b. Increased appetite
c. Weight gain
d. All of these

Ans. (d) All of these

Explanation: Prednisolone is a steroid medication used to treat certain types of allergies, inflammatory conditions, autoimmune disorders, and cancers. All the given options are expected side effects of prednisolone.

83

Nurse was doing physical examination of a child with the diagnosis of asthma. While doing physical examination, at what point she should assess the child for retraction?

a. Inspiration
b. Expiration
c. Wheezing
d. Ask them to hold the breath

Ans. (a) Inspiration

Explanation: Indrawing of skin between ribs when a patient tries to inhale. It indicates respiratory difficulty. In an asthmatic patient, we can observe it during inspiration.

84

Parents of a 4-month-old child with eczema asked the nurse which toy is appropriate for their child. Which among the following will be the response from nurse?

a. Plush toys
b. Snake and ladder game
c. Soft washable toys
d. Toy train

Ans. (c) Soft washable toys

Explanation: Eczema which is also known as dermatitis is an itchy inflammatory condition of the skin. So, while selecting toys for these kids, keep in mind that it should not stimulate itching. Plush toy which is also known as stuffed toy will accumulate dirt and dust and aggravate their skin condition. Snake and ladder game is not an age-appropriate toy for 4-month-old child. Toy train has sharp edges and child may use them for itching and scraping over the body lesions. So soft washable toys are age-appropriate toys for these group of kids.

85

3-year-old child admitted in the hospital. Child's parents are leaving the hospital. Which among the following reactions is normal and expected in the child?

a. Crying and clinging to the parents
b. Saying bye to them
c. Going and playing with peer groups
d. Stay silent without any reaction

Ans. (a) Crying and clinging to the parents

Explanation: Separation anxiety is one of the most common problems among this age group, and these age groups show it as crying and clinging to the parents, throwing tantrum, etc.

86

7-year-old child admitted for adenoidectomy. While doing pre-anesthetic physical examination for the child, which among the following needs to be assessed?

a. Characteristic of tongue, gum, and adenoid
b. Existing other medical conditions
c. Number of milk teeth
d. Any loose teeth and its location

Ans. (d) Any loose teeth and its location

Explanation: From the age of six children will lose their milk teeth. In a 7-year-old child, there is a chance for loose teeth. So, while doing physical examination, this is the most important thing to notice. Existing other medical conditions' information could have been obtained through history collection.

87

Mother came with her 3-year-old child to under-five clinics. Mother told the clinic nurse that, child needs the same plate and glass even if they go the restaurant. Which among the following is the best response from the nurse?

a. It is an excuse for not having food
b. It is because of their negativism behavior
c. It is because of their ritualistic behavior
d. It is because of their separation anxiety from home

Ans. (c) It is because of their ritualistic behavior

Explanation: Toddlers have typical ritualistic behaviors. The above situation is an example of displaying ritualistic behaviors.

88

What is the rationale for saying by the nurse that peanuts are not good food for toddlers?

a. Low nutritional value
b. Easily spilled by toddlers
c. Can cause fatty liver disease
d. Can be easily aspirated

Ans. (d) Can be easily aspirated

Explanation: Toddlers may easily aspirate peanut. Due to the risk for aspiration, nurse stated that peanuts are not a good food choice for toddlers.

89

Child came to school health nurse with the complaining of itchy skin. On further evaluation, she found out it as impetigo. What should be the next step?

a. Educate the child and family not to use soap.
b. Apply thick layer of moisturizer over the itchy skin and send the child back to class.
c. Cover the itchy skin with thin layer of gauze piece.
d. Send the child back to home with parents and advise them to visit medical practitioner.

Ans. (d) Send the child back to home with parents and advise them to visit medical practitioner.

Explanation: Impetigo is a contagious skin infection. To prevent it spreading, child should be sent back to home along with parents with the advise to consult medical practitioner.

90

Nurse Lucy working in postoperative unit is caring for a child with appendectomy, postoperative day one. Nurse noticed NG tube in situ for a client. What is the purpose of NG tube for this client?

a. To promote wound drainage
b. To maintain water electrolyte balance
c. To prevent abdominal distention
d. To prevent wound dehiscence

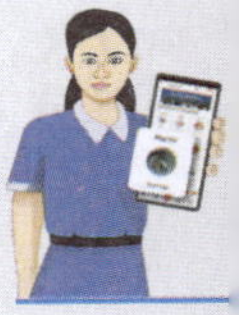

Ans. (c) To prevent abdominal distention

Explanation: After abdominal surgery, NG tube is inserted to prevent abdominal distention.

91

A 6-month-old infant admitted in postanesthesia care unit with elbow restrain in place. Child is intubated and about to be extubated. Which among the following is correct intervention for this child?

a. Remove both restrain as child is about to be extubated.
b. Do not remove restrain until the child is extubated.
c. Remove one restrain at a time and provide range of motion exercises.
d. Remove both restrains simultaneously and provide range of motion exercise.

Ans. (c) Remove one restrain at a time and provide range of motion exercises.

Explanation: Removing one restrain and providing range of motion exercises will improve extremities functional ability. Removing both restrain at a time may cause accidental extubation.

92

Parents bring their child to pediatric emergency with severe diarrhea following rotavirus infection. Which among the following is the most important nursing intervention?

a. Insert indwelling urinary catheter
b. Inset IV line and start IV fluid
c. Check weight of the child
d. Start to give ORS

Ans. (b) Inset IV line and start IV fluid

Explanation: Child is having severe diarrhea. Rehydration is the most important nursing intervention in this situation. Starting IV fluid is the most important thing to do. Giving ORS is not recommended in severe diarrhea. First and important management in a child with severe diarrhea is initiation of IV fluids.

93

A 9-year-old child diagnosed with sickle cell anemia came to emergency with the complaining of severe headache and vaso-occulsive diagnosis is made for the child. Which among the following will be the first intervention?

a. Administer oxygen via mask
b. Assess the pain intensity and give fentanyl
c. Assess the neurological status of the child
d. Administer IV fluids

Ans. (c) Assess the neurological status of the child

Explanation: Child is diagnosed with vaso-occulsive crisis and complaining of severe headache. So, first thing to be done is rule out stroke, for that neurological assessment needs to be done. Following that hydration status to be ensured.

94

Nurse was assessing children admitted in pediatric ward. Which among the following cases needs to notify the physician?

a. Proteinuria in a child with nephrotic syndrome
b. Breathing difficulty in a child with rheumatic fever
c. Crying and irritable infant with the diagnosis of rheumatic fever
d. Dark cola-colored urine in a child with glomerulonephritis

Ans. (b) Breathing difficulty in a child with rheumatic fever

Explanation: While doing assessment, priority is always ABC. So, a child with breathing difficulty needs to be informed to the physician first. All other options are expected findings in a child with that diagnosis.

95

While interviewing an adolescent client, which among the following strategies is the most appropriate to establish trust?

a. Ask open ended questions
b. Ask personal questions
c. Record or note down everything they are saying
d. Allow them to accompany their friends with them

Ans. (a) Ask open ended questions

Explanation: Asking open ended questions allow them to share their feelings. All other options are not helpful to establish trustworthy relationship with adolescent.

96

During the stages of growth and development, infant develops arm movement then fine motor skills. How can this characteristic be explained?

a. Cephalocaudal
b. Less to more intrusive
c. Proximodistal
d. General to specific

Ans. (c) Proximodistal

Explanation: Proximodistal means child acquire developmental progress from center of the body to the extremities, such as from arm to fingers. The above given situation is an example of proximodistal development.

97

Nurse was assessing a 4-year-old child admitted in the emergency. Which among the following suggests parental neglect?

a. Child shows temper tantrum and kicking parents.
b. Do not cooperate with medical staff.
c. Weight loss and poor hygiene.
d. Pulling hair and eating non-nutritious material.

Ans. (c) Weight loss and poor hygiene

Explanation: Poor hygiene and weight loss suggestive of parental neglect. Temper tantrum, kicking parents, noncooperation with medical staff are the normal behavior for the age group.

98

Mother brought her 4-year-old child to the emergency with severe dehydration and history of vomiting and diarrhea for the last 3 days. Mother told the nurse that child's illness is her mistake, and she is responsible for the present situation. Which among the following is the most appropriate response from the nurse?

a. Tell me why you think so.
b. Don't think like that everything is going to be alright.
c. You could have brought the child earlier.
d. If you cry in front of the child, it will make her upset more.

Ans. (a) Tell me why you think so

Explanation: Option a will help the mother to express her feelings and concern and also feel somebody is there to listen and understand her. All other options are not appropriate for mother to express her feelings.

99

A 2-year-old child is recently diagnosed to have cystic fibrosis. The pediatric nurse is educating the parents on care of child. The nurse is aware that the child is at risk of which of the following vitamins deficiency?

a. Folic acid
b. Vitamin C
c. Thiamin and Niacin
d. Vitamins A, D and K

Ans. (d) Vitamins A, D and K

Explanation: Cystic fibrosis patients have problem absorbing fats, making them at risk of developing deficiencies in fat-soluble vitamins (vitamins A, D, E, and K).
B-complex, C, folic acid, biotin, and pantothenic acid are water soluble and easily absorbed.

100

An infant whose mother is HIV positive is admitted in the ward, and they planned to start zidovudine. Before administering the medication, which lab test results should the nurse analyze?

a. Plasma viral load
b. CBC with creatinine
c. CBC and ALT
d. CBC with APTT

Ans. (c) CBC and ALT

Explanation: Laboratory parameters for HIV-infected infants and children at baseline during ART include Hb, CBC, LFT, ALT, Urinalysis, CD4, and X-ray chest. Creatinine should be done if planning for Tenofovir Disoproxil Fumarate (TDF). Lipid profile should be done if planning for Efavirenz (EFV) or Protease Inhibitor (PI).

101

An 8-year-old male child with leukemia is admitted into a long term care facility and developed a stage 2 pressure ulcer. Which of the following method of wound debridement should the nurse prefer to use for this patient?

a. Autolytic debridement
b. Enzymatic debridement
c. Mechanical debridement
d. Sharp debridement

Ans. (a) Autolytic debridement

Explanation: Autolytic Debridement - This type of debridement is a natural process by which endogenous phagocytic cells and proteolytic enzymes break down necrotic tissue. Consider autolytic debridement with appropriate dressings for dead tissue in neonates, infants, children and young people. Consider sharp and surgical debridement by trained staff only if autolytic debridement is unsuccessful. (Ref: https://www.ncbi.nlm.nih.gov/books/NBK333114/)

102

A patient with pressure ulcer is being treated with autolytic debridement. The patient reports to the nurse that his wound has a foul odor. Which of the following interventions should the nurse implement?

a. Assess the wound site immediately
b. Explain the client that it is the expected finding
d. Check the client's vital status
d. Notify the physician

Ans. (b) Explain the client that it is the expected finding

Explanation: The foul odor is produced by the breakdown of cellular debris and does not indicate that the wound is infected. It is an expected finding.

103

A 6-month-old baby is brought to under-five clinic with cough. After the initial assessment, the nurse classifies the child as having severe pneumonia. Which of the following is the best management for this child?

a. Prescribe antibiotic
b. Instruct the mother to increase fluid intake
c. Instruct the mother to continue exclusive breastfeeding
d. Refer the child immediately to the hospital

Ans. (d) Refer the child immediately to the hospital

Explanation: Severe pneumonia requires urgent referral to hospital. Other interventions are appropriate for mild pneumonia.

104

On a home visit, a 3-month-old infant with the chief complaint of diarrhea is classified under the category of 'some dehydration' by the nurse. As per the IMCI guidelines, which of the following is the appropriate intervention?

a. Bring the child to health center and observe for next 24 hours
b. Educate the mother on home management
c. Supervise the mother in giving 200 mL to 400 mL ORS in 4 hours
d. Bring the child immediately to health center and start IV fluids

Ans. (c) Supervise the mother in giving 200 mL to 400 mL ORS in 4 hours

Explanation: In the IMCI management guidelines, 'some dehydration' is treated with the administration of ORS within a period of 4 hours. The amount of ORS solution to be administered is calculated on the basis of the child's weight (75 mL/kg body weight). The amount of ORS is based on child's age if weight is unknown.

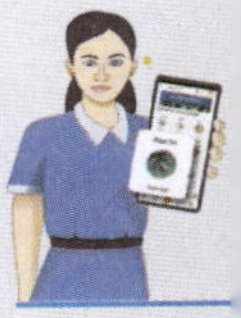

Image-Based Questions

1. Identify the type of conjoined twins

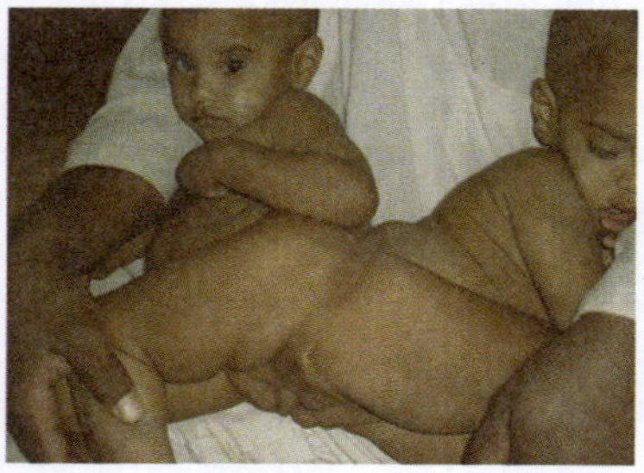

a. Ischiopagus twins b. Pygopagus twins
c. Eluidi twins d. Craniopagus twins

2. Identify the type of conjoined twins

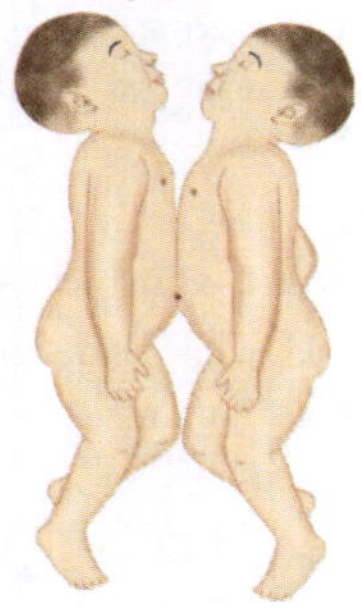

a. Pygopagus b. Thoracophagus
c. Omphalopagus d. Parapagus

3. A child diagnosed with VSD (ventricular septal defect) presents with the findings as show in the image. There is no history of fever. Based on this information, what is the most probable cause of these findings?

(Refer explanation at the end)

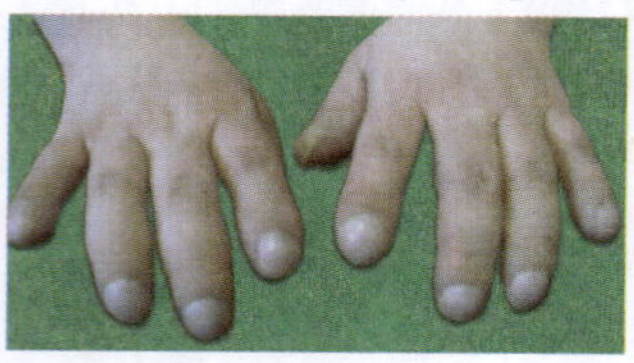

a. Infective endocarditis b. Eissenmenger syndrome
c. Patent Ductus Arteriosus d. Mitral valve prolapse

4. A pregnant mother experienced a fever and rash during the antenatal period. After delivery, the newborn is found to have Patent Ductus Arteriosus (PDA) and deafness. Further examination with an ophthalmoscope revealed the following findings. what is the most likely cause of these clinical manifestations?

(Refer explanation at the end)

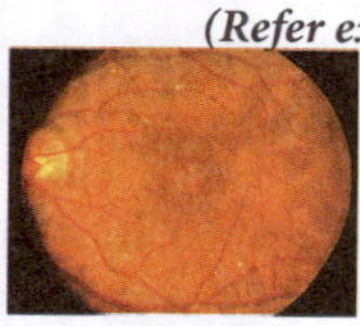

a. Congenital toxoplasmosis b. Congenital rubella
c. Congenital syphilis d. Congenital Tuberculosis

5. Identify the instrument shown in the image

(Refer explanation at the end)

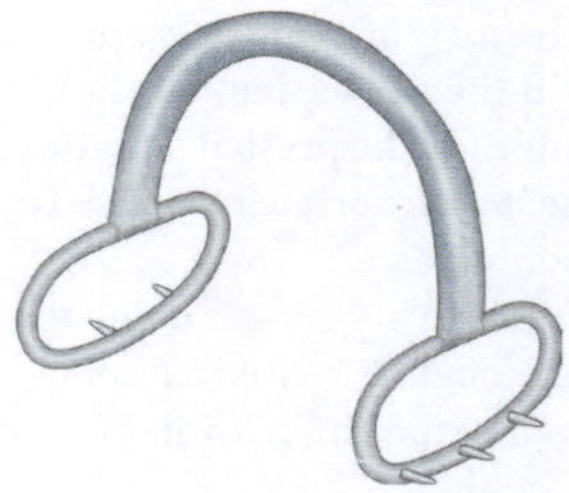

a. Logan bow b. Allen bow
c. Root elevator d. Periosteal elevator

6. The devise/kit used in this procedure is known as

(Refer explanation at the end)

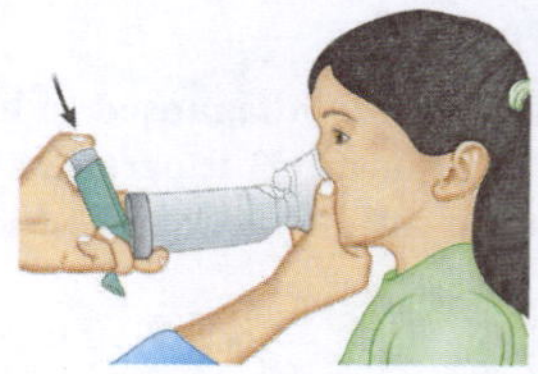

a. Metered dose inhaler
b. Rotahaler
c. Metered dose inhaler with spacer
d. Rotahaler with spacer

7. Identify the device used for the treatment in the neonate show in the picture? ***(Refer explanation at the end)***

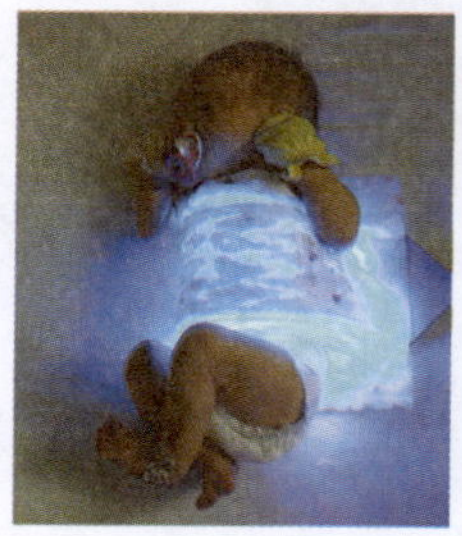

a. Thermal blanket b. Bili blanket
c. Neonate cooler d. None of these

8. Identify the device shown in the image below

(Refer explanation at the end)

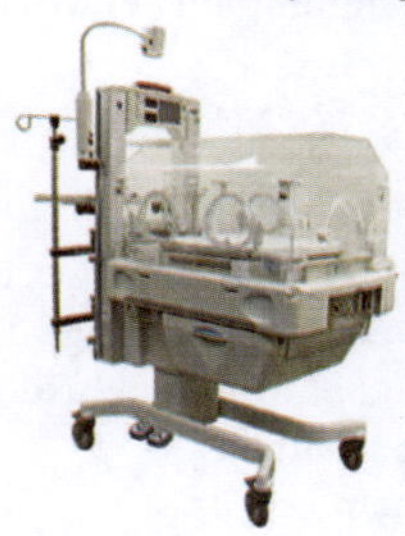

a. Radiant warmer b. Giraffe incubator
c. Portable incubator d. Shaker incubator

Ans.

1. b
2. c
3. b
4. b
5. a
6. c
7. b
8. b

[*Courtesy*: PHOTON-20® 3th ed. by Vivek Jain, CBS Publishers and Distributors Pvt Ltd]

9. Instrument shown in photograph is used in public health for:

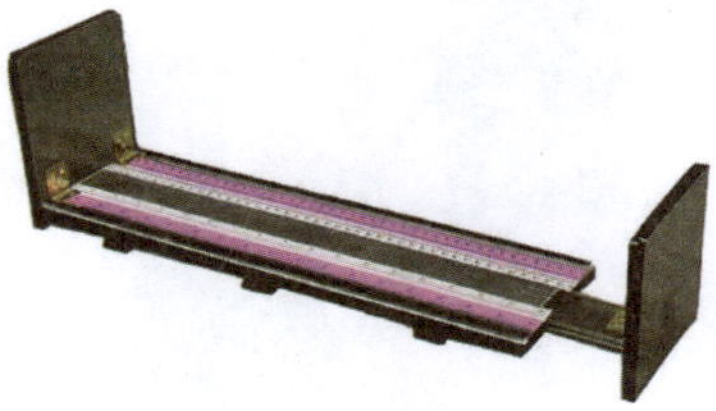

a. Birth weight
b. Birth length
c. Mid arm circumference
d. Abdominal circumference

10. Monitor shown in photograph is a marker of:

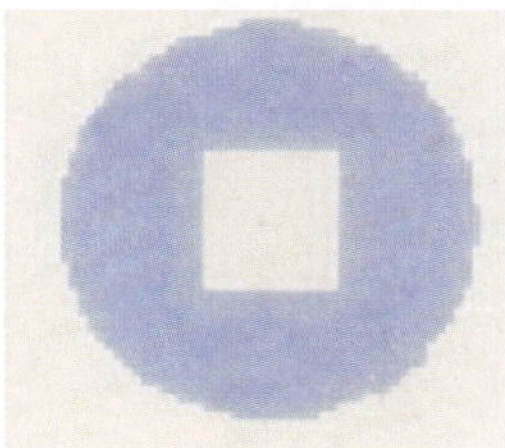

a. Efficacy of vaccine
b. Expiry of vaccine
c. Cold chain maintenance
d. Number of doses in vaccine vial

11. Suture (Arrow) shown in the photograph closes by the age of: ***[Recent Question 2012]***

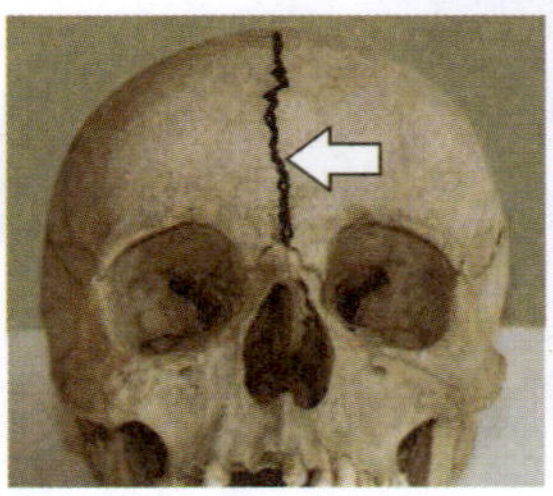

a. 6 months
b. 2 years
c. 3 years
d. 6 years

12. Urine sample collection method shown in photograph is preferred in:

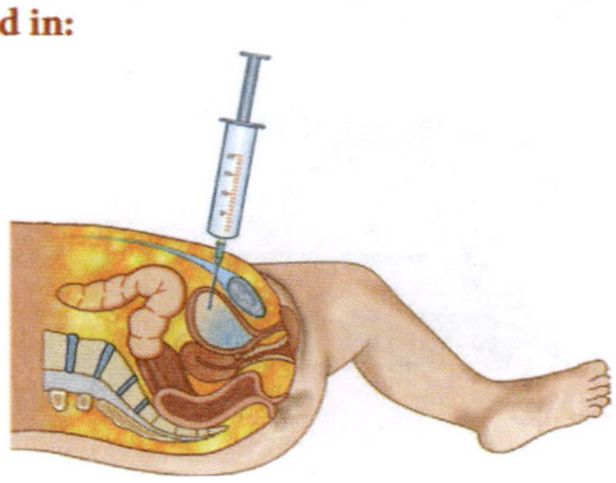

a. Infants
b. Adolescents
c. Adults
d. Older persons

13. Which of the following vaccines is given by route shown in photograph? ***[Recent Question 2012]***

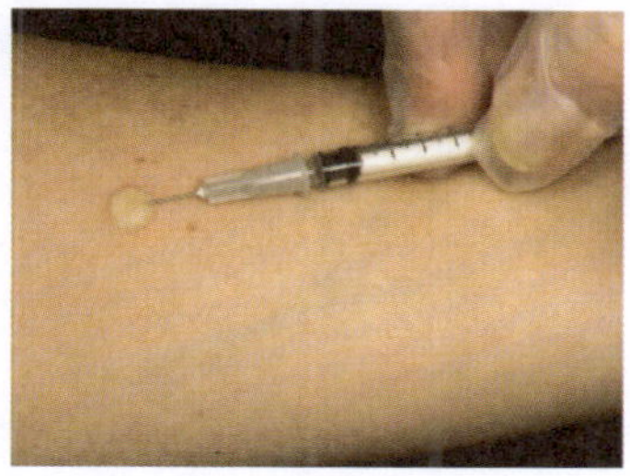

a. DPT
b. Hepatitis B
c. MMR
d. BCG

14. Vaccine administered by following route is:

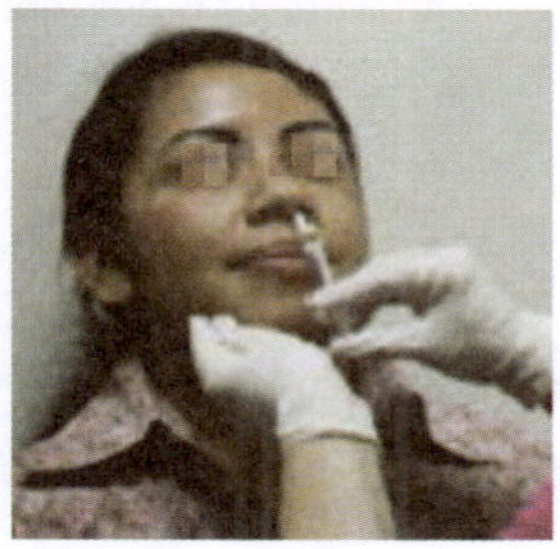

a. Typhoid live
b. H1N1 killed
c. H1N1 live
d. Yellow fever live

15. Identify the Reflex shown (First stage) in the photograph: ***[Recent Question 2014]***

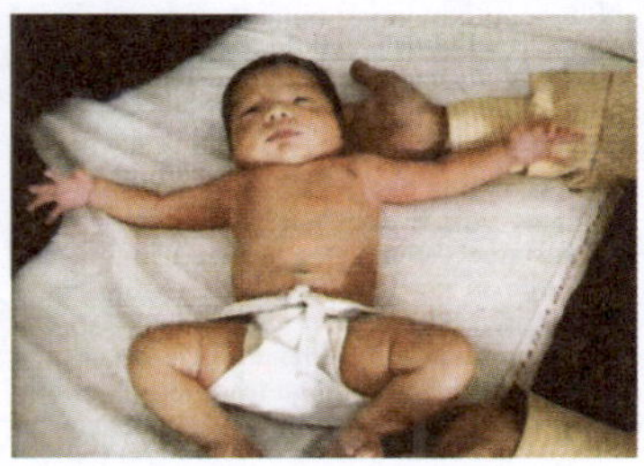

a. Tonic neck reflex
b. Moro's reflex
c. Parachute reflex
d. Rooting reflex

16. Identify the therapy:

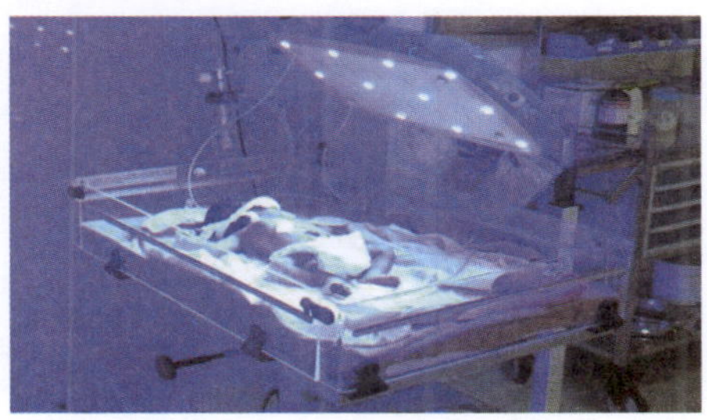

a. Phototherapy
b. Radiant warmer
c. Heater
d. IR therapy

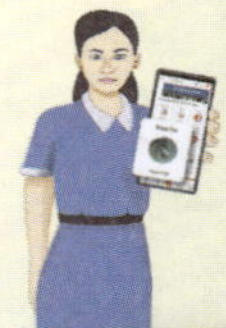

Ans.

9. b
10. c
11. a
12. a
13. d
14. c
15. b
16. a

17. Cut-section of Structure shown in the photograph contains:

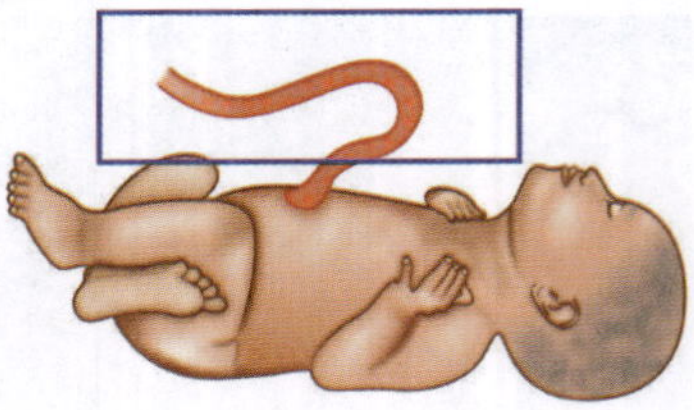

a. 1 artery, 2 veins
b. 2 arteries, 2 veins
c. 2 arteries, 1 vein
d. 1 artery, 1 vein

18. In the given image, which of the following breastfeeding practices for good attachment is not complied?

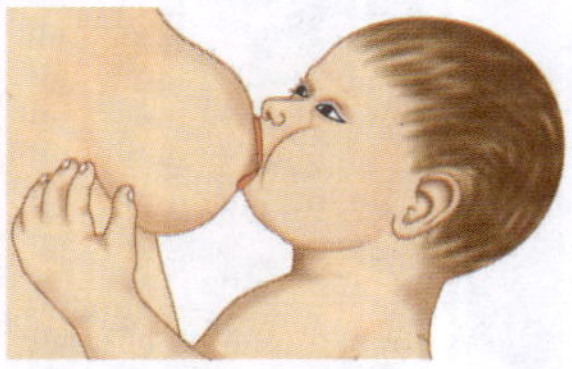

a. Wide open mouth
b. Most nipple and areola in mouth
c. Chin touching breast
d. Lower lip turned outwards

19. Disorder based on line (arrow) shown in photograph:

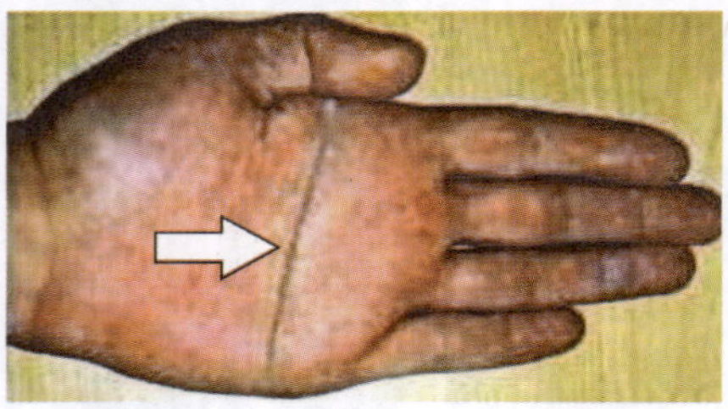

a. Hyperthyroidism
b. Bronchogenic carcinoma
c. PDA
d. Down's syndrome

20. Identify the instrument shown in the photograph:

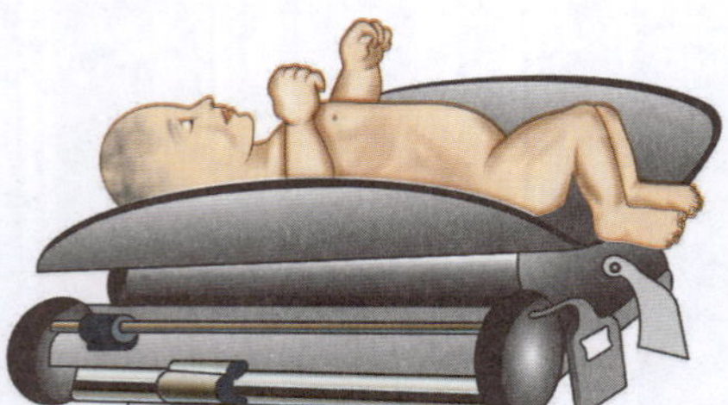

a. Salter scale
b. Spring balance
c. Electronic weighing scale
d. Beam balance

21. Milestone shown in photograph appears at age of:

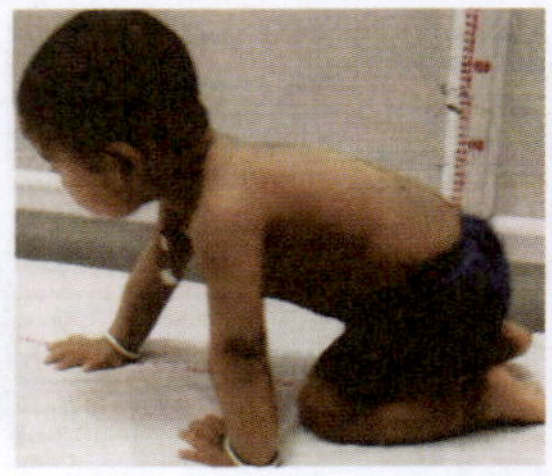

a. 3 months
b. 5 months
c. '7 months
d. 10 months

22. Milestone shown in photograph appears at age of:

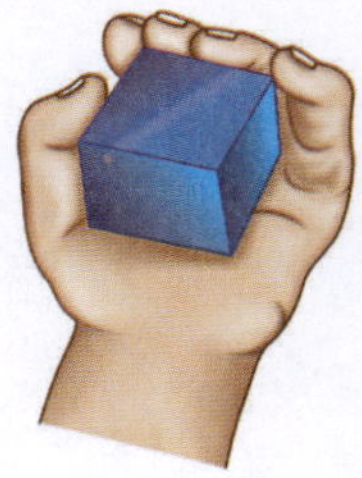

a. 6 months
b. 9 months
c. 12 months
d. 18 months

23. Milestone shown in photograph appears at age of:

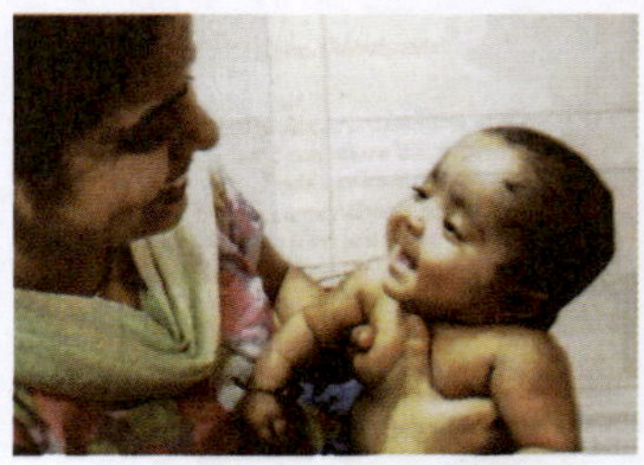

a. 2 months
b. 4 months
c. 6 months
d. 12 months

24. Identify the apparatus used in pediatrics as shown in photograph:

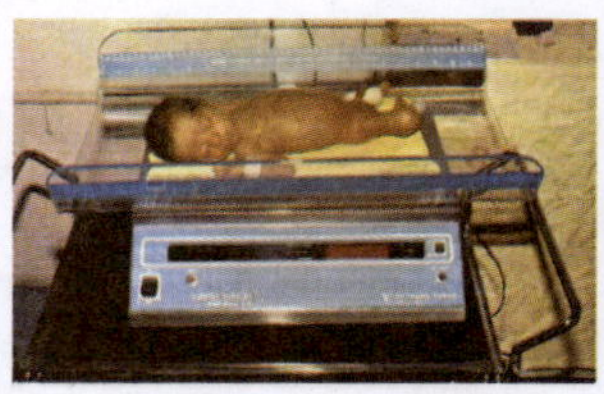

a. Radiant warmer
b. Infantometer
c. Electronic weighing scale
d. Salter weighing scale

Ans.

17. c
18. c
19. d
20. d
21. d
22. a
23. a
24. c

25. The item shown in the figure is:

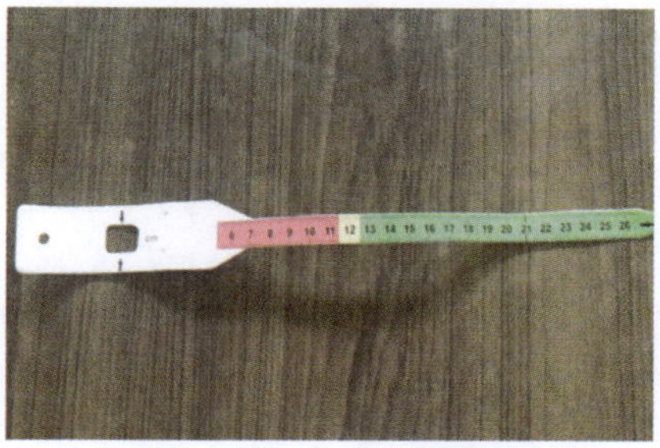

a. Shakir's tape
b. Triage tape
c. Multipurpose tape
d. Wrist tape

26. The condition depicted in figure is:

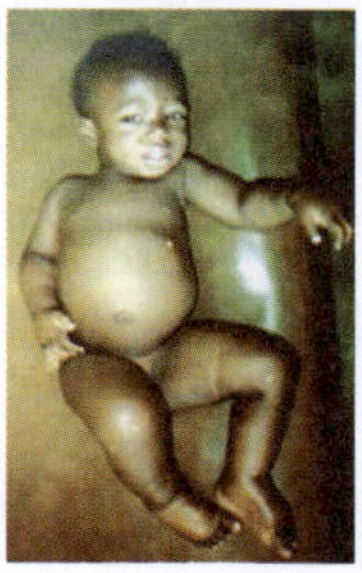

a. Kwashiorkor
b. Marasmus
c. Nephrotic syndrome
d. Epidemic dropsy

27. Injection technique shown in figure is used to administer?

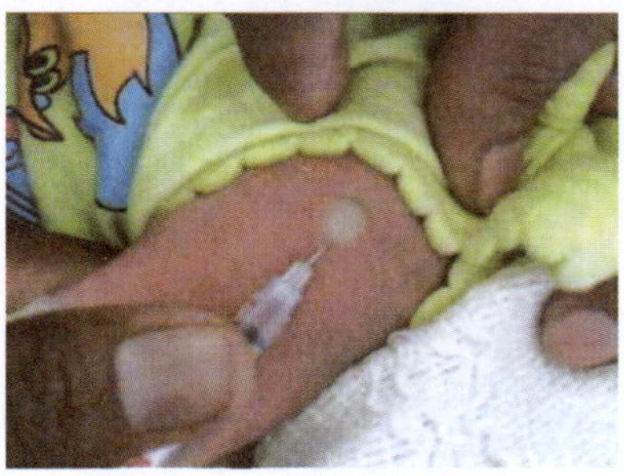

a. BCG
b. Measles
c. Hepatitis B
d. Japanese Encephalitis

28. Identify the scheme/program/plan launched by Government of India: ***(Refer explanation at the end)***

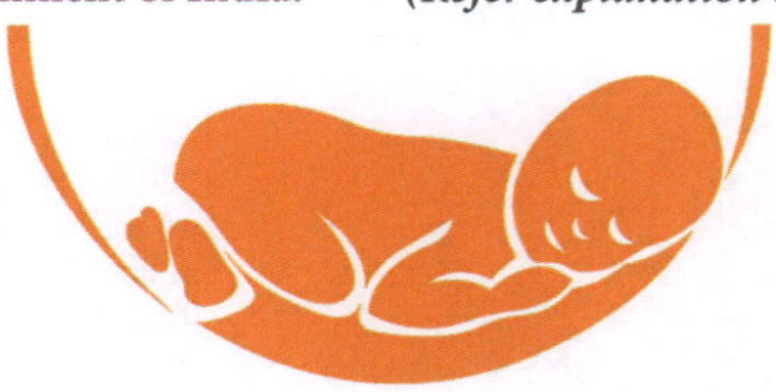

a. Mission Indradhanush
b. Kangaroo Mother Care
c. BFHI
d. India Newborn Action Plan

29. What is the target year for the mission depicted in the symbol? ***(Refer explanation at the end)***

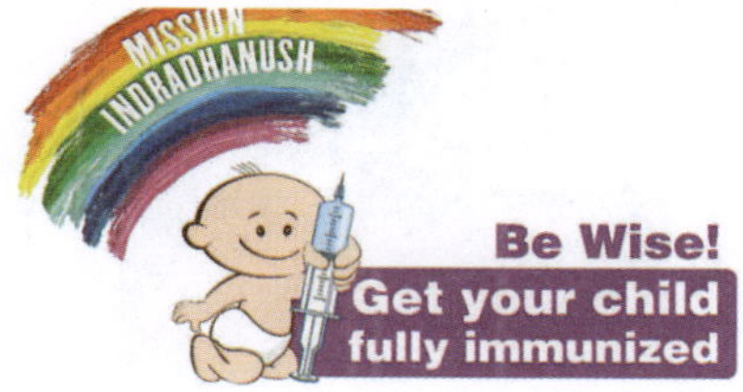

a. 2017
b. 2020
c. 2025
d. 2030

30. Identify the scheme/program/plan launched by WHO/ UNICEF: ***(Refer explanation at the end)***

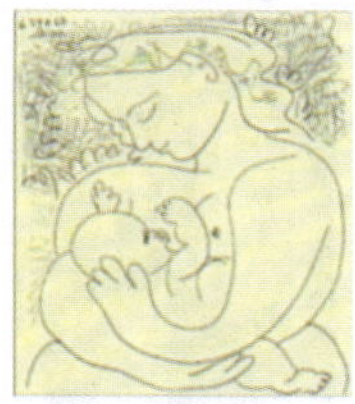

a. Janani Shishu Suraksha Karyakram
b. Kangaroo Mother Care
c. BFHI
d. RCH Program

31. True about instrument shown in photograph is: ***(Refer explanation at the end)***

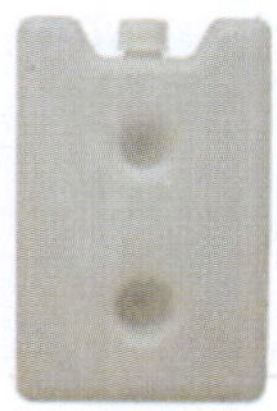

a. Filled with tap water
b. Salt is added
c. Filled up to brim
d. Holes used to hold when taking out of Freezer

32. In the picture which area is being auscultated? ***(Refer explanation at the end)***

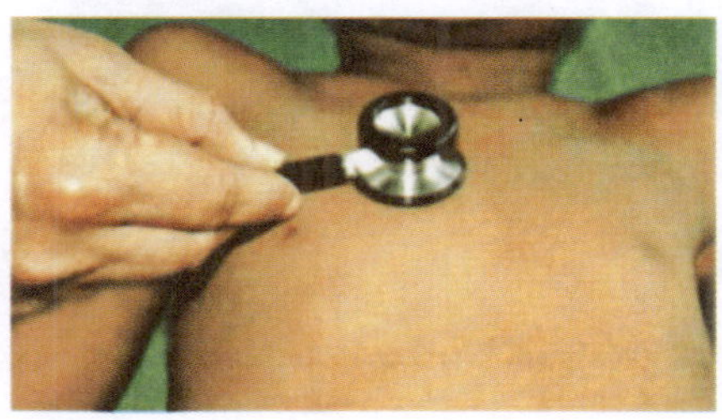

a. Tricuspid area
b. Pulmonic area
c. Aortic area
d. Mitral area

Ans.

25. a
26. a
27. a
28. d
29. b
30. c
31. a
32. c

33. The following auscultation is done for diagnosis of?
(Refer explanation at the end)

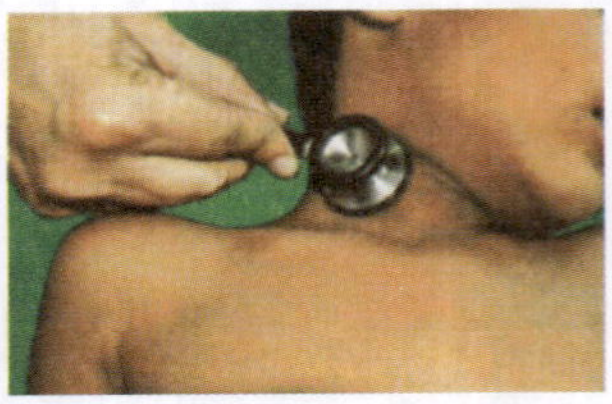

a. Radiation of aortic regurgitation murmur
b. Carotid artery bruit
c. Carotid artery dissection
d. Venous hum

34. The device being used by the child is:
(Refer explanation at the end)

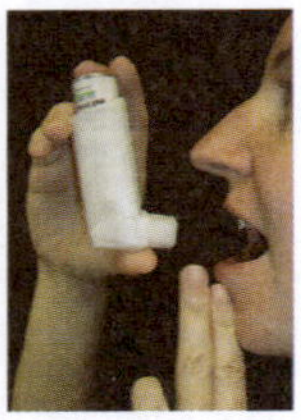

a. Spirometer
b. Metered dose inhaler
c. Peak expiratory flow rate meter
d. Nebuliser

35. Which among the following depicts the correct fitting of face mask used during neonatal resuscitation?
(Refer explanation at the end)

a. 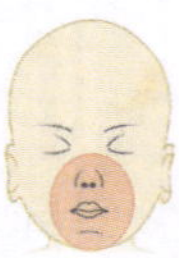

b. 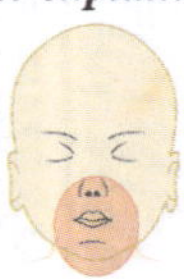

c. 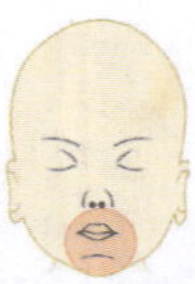

d. 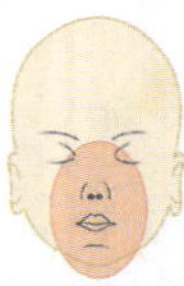

36. Name the condition shown in the image on the right side:

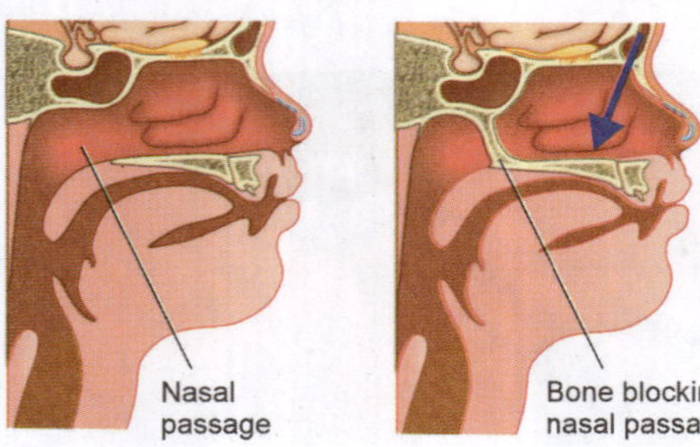

a. Choanal atresia
b. Deviated Nasal septum
c. Nasal polyps
d. Sinusitis

37. Name the condition shown in the picture:

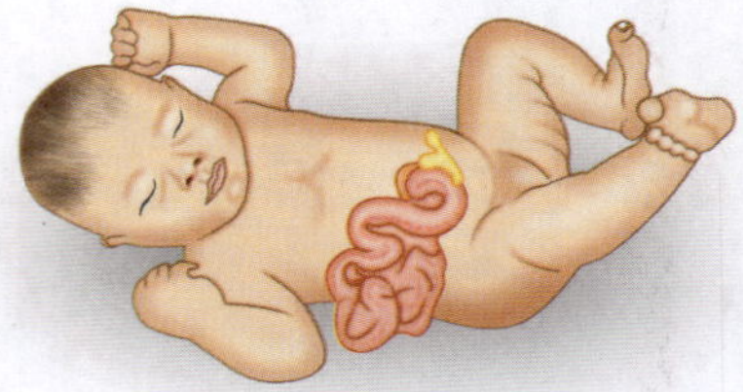

a. Omphalocele
b. Umbilical hernia
c. Gastroschisis
d. Hirschsprung's disease

38. Identify the rare genetic condition shown in this picture:

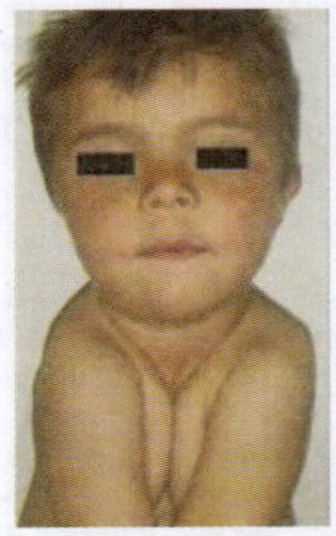

a. Cleidocranial dysplacia
b. Down syndrome
c. Trisomy 13
d. Edward's syndrome

39. Identify the condition shown in the picture:
(Refer explanation at the end)

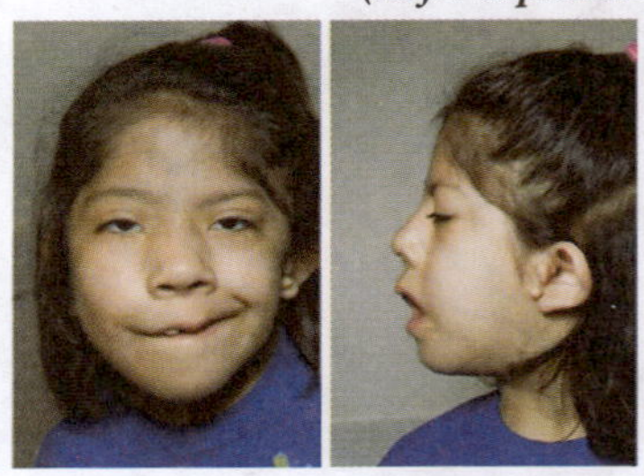

a. Bell's palsy
b. Facial palsy
c. Goldenhar syndrome
d. Myasthenia gravis

40. Name of the assessment being performed to assess hip dislocation:

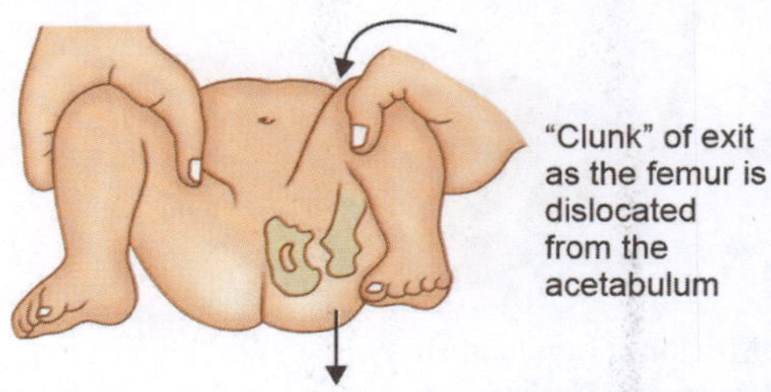

a. Barlow's maneuver
b. Ortolani maneuver
c. Trendelenburg's test
d. Galeazzi test

Ans.

33.	b
34.	b
35.	a
36.	a
37.	c
38.	a
39.	c
40.	a

41. Name of the assessment being performed to assess hip dislocation:

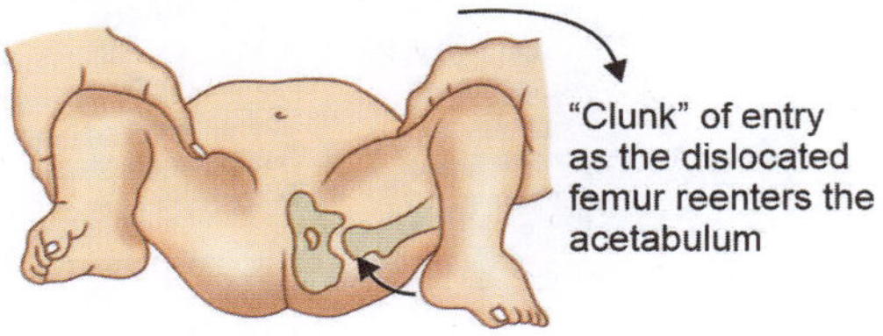

a. Barlow's maneuver
b. Ortolani maneuver
c. Trendelenburg's test
d. Galeazzi test

42. Identify the procedure shown in this picture:

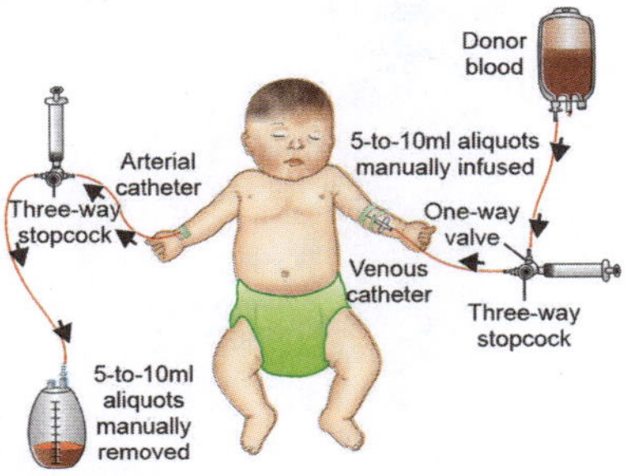

a. Blood transfusion
b. Hemodialysis
c. Exchange transfusion
d. Plasma therapy

43. Identify the device used post-operatively after cheiloplasty to maintain post-operative apposition?

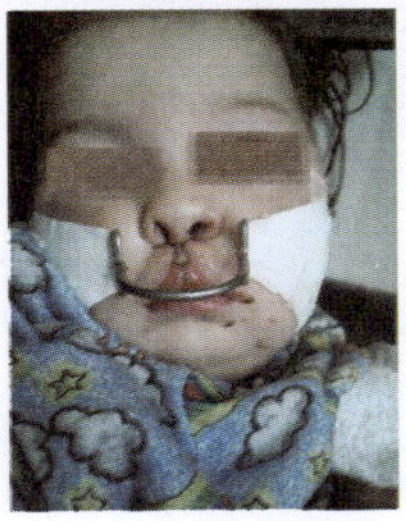

a. Nose splints
b. Nasal dilator
c. Logan bow
d. NAM device

44. Identify the condition shown in the picture:

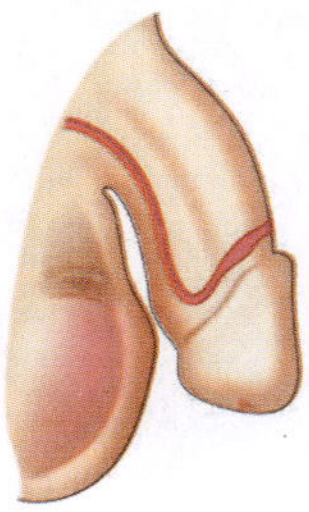

a. Hypospadias
b. Epispadias
c. Cryptorchidism
d. Phimosis

45. Identify the condition shown in the picture:

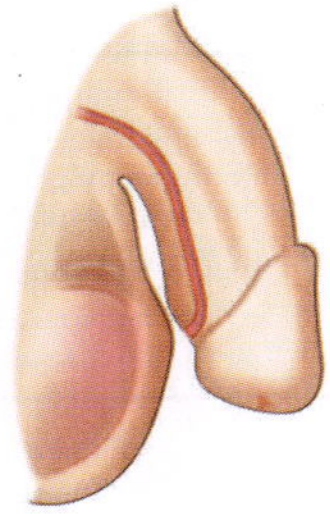

a. Hypospadias
b. Epispadias
c. Cryptorchidism
d. Phimosis

46. Diagnose the Congenital disorder shown in Photograph:

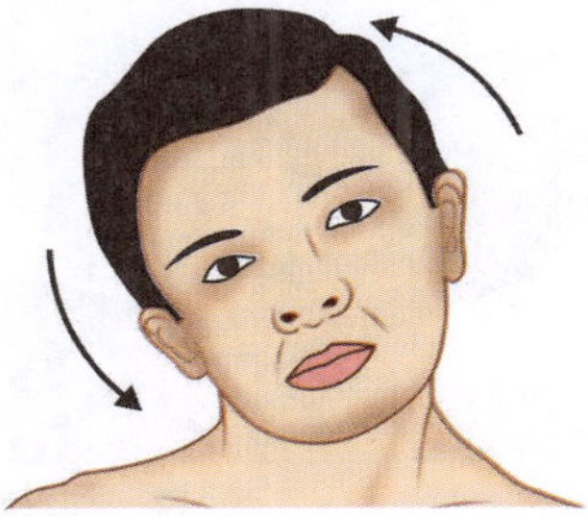

a. Cleidocranial dysostosis
b. Sprengel's shoulder
c. Congenital Torticollis
d. Absence of clavicle

47. Diagnose the Developmental disorder shown in Photograph:

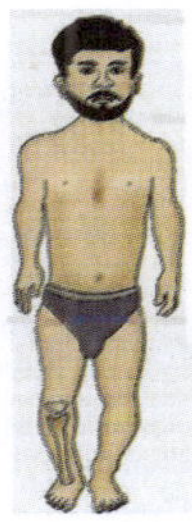

a. Osteogenesis imperfecta
b. Fibrous dysplasia
c. Achondroplasia
d. Paget's disease

48. Diagnose the Underlying Condition as shown in Photograph:

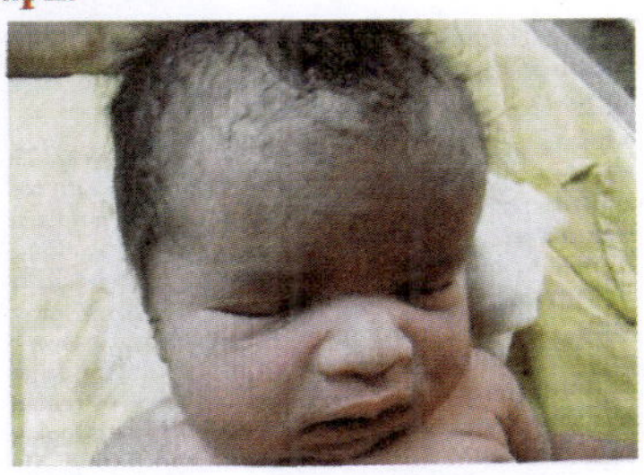

a. Dolichocephaly
b. Macrocephaly
c. Plagiocephaly
d. Scaphocephaly

Ans.

41. b
42. c
43. c
44. b
45. a
46. c
47. c
48. b

49. A child is able to draw figure shown in Photograph at age of: ***[Recent Question 2014]***

a. 2 years b. 3 years
c. 4 years d. 5 years

50. Technique used in Pediatrics as shown in Photograph is known as:

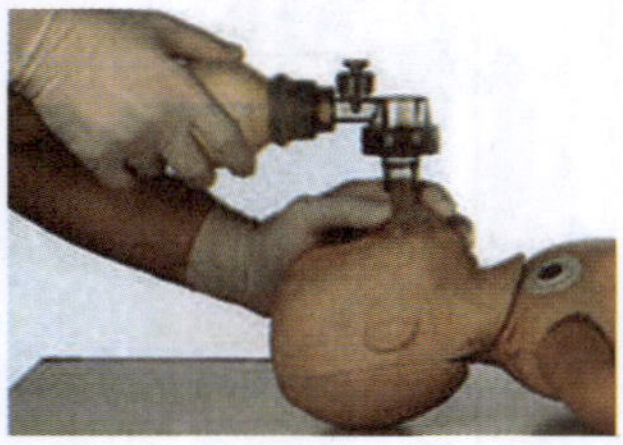

a. Laryngoscopy b. Bag and Mask ventilation
c. Mouth-to-mouth resuscitation
d. Slit lamp examination

51. Instrument shown in Photograph is known as:

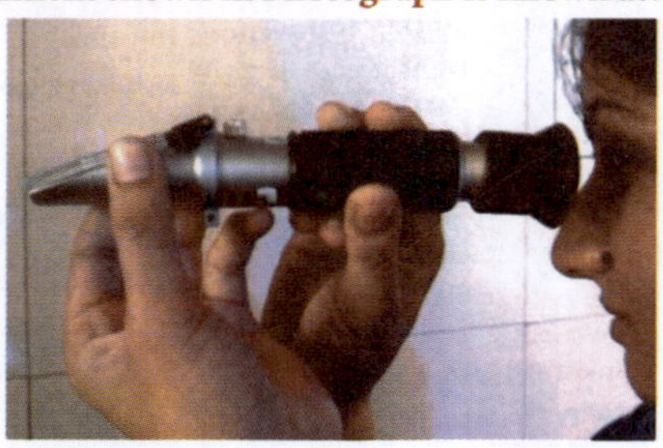

a. Otoscope b. Ophthalmoscope
c. Refractometer d. None of these

52. Physical characteristic shown in Photograph is seen in: ***[Recent Question 2012]***

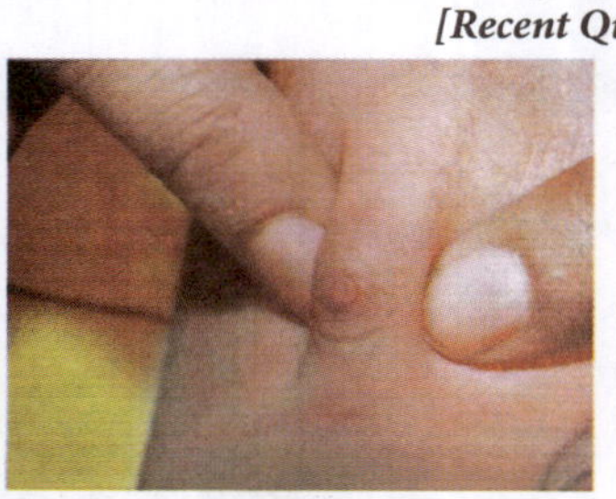

a. Pre-term neonate b. Term neonate
c. Post-term neonate d. Cannot be determined

53. Neonatal reflex shown in the Photograph is:

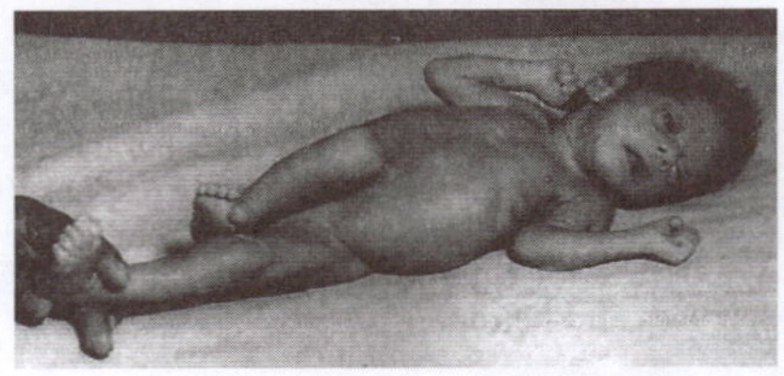

a. Moro's reflex
b. Crossed extension reflex
c. Tonic neck reflex
d. Grasp reflex

54. Pediatric disorder as shown in Photograph is:

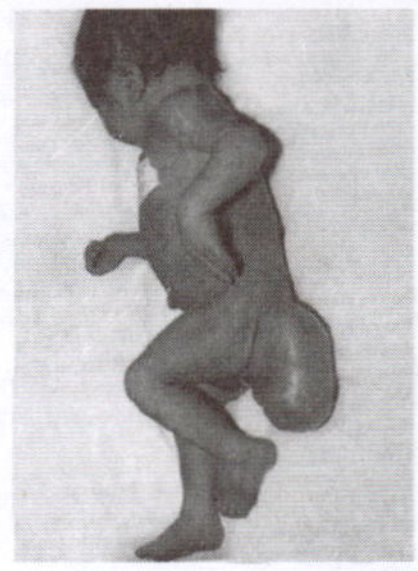

a. Rectal prolapse b. Neuroblastoma
c. Sacrococcygeal teratoma d. Nephroblastoma

55. Neonatal reflex shown in the Photograph is:

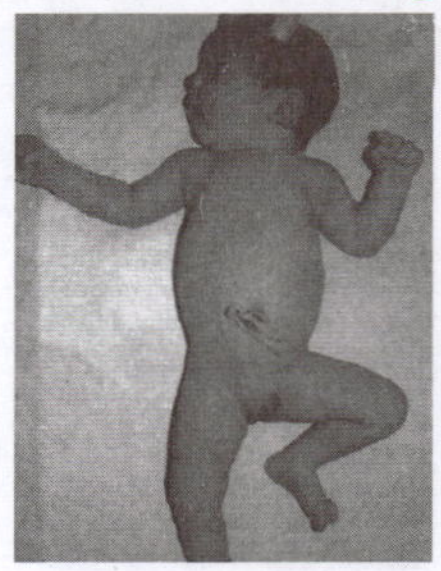

a. Moro's reflex b. Crossed extension reflex
c. Tonic neck reflex d. Grasp reflex

56. Physical characteristic shown in Photograph is seen in:

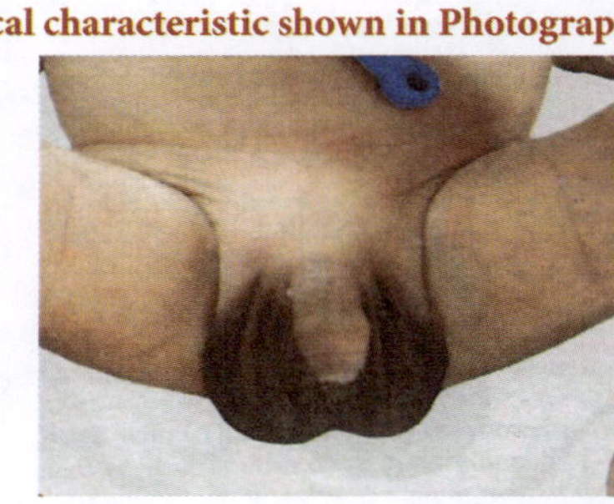

a. Pre-term neonate b. Term neonate
c. Post-term neonate d. Cannot be determined

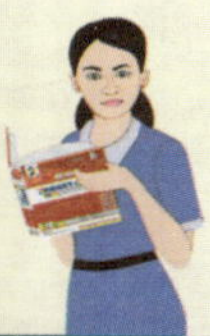

Ans.

49. c
50. b
51. c
52. b
53. b
54. c
55. c
56. b

57. Identify the GIT disorder shown in Photograph: *[Recent Question 2012]*

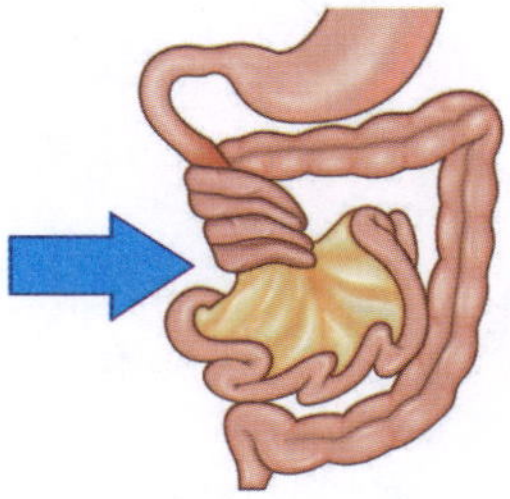

a. Acute appendicitis
b. Intussusception
c. Malrotation
d. Choledochal cyst

58. Diagnose the Vascular birthmark shown in Photograph: *[Recent Question 2013, 2016]*

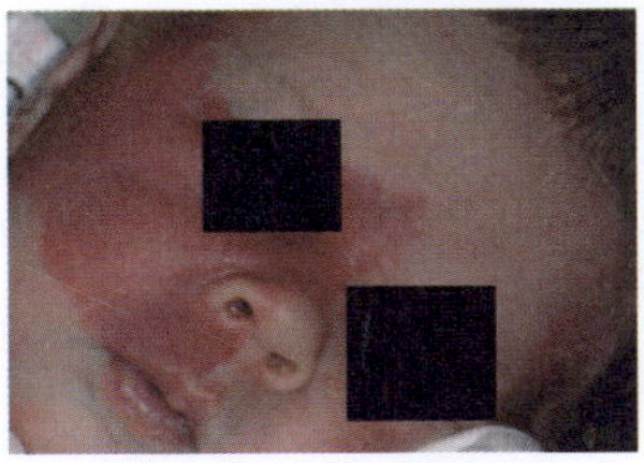

a. Infantile hemangioma
b. Salmon patch
c. Port wine stain
d. Lymphangioma

59. Diagnose the Skin disorder as shown in Photograph: *[Recent Question 2013]*

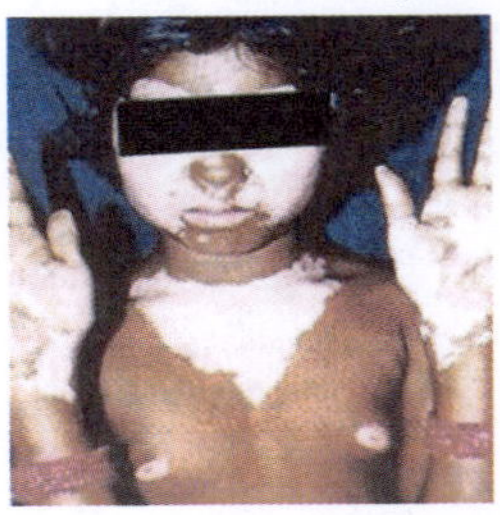

a. Burn injury
b. Seborrheic dermatitis
c. Leprosy
d. Vitiligo

60. Diagnose the Skin disorder as shown in Photograph: *[Recent Question 2017, 2012]*

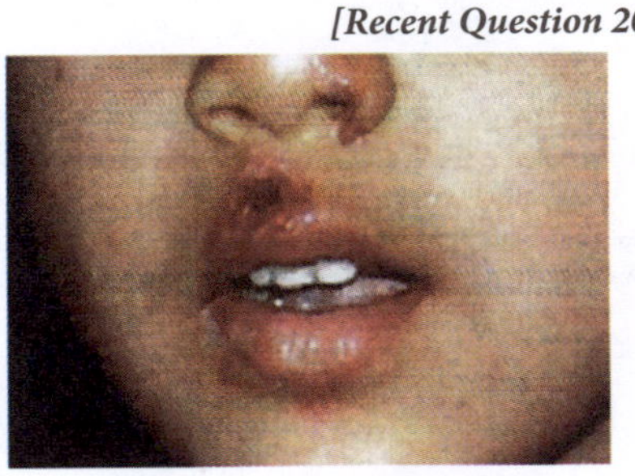

a. Impetigo contagiosa
b. Scrofuloderma
c. Ichthyosis
d. Bullous impetigo

61. Identify the Congenital malformation shown in the Photograph:

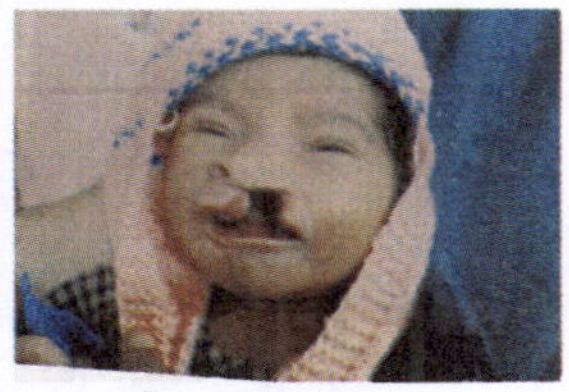

a. Unilateral cleft lip
b. Unilateral cleft lip and palate
c. Bilateral cleft lip
d. Bilateral cleft lip and palate

62. Technique shown in the Photograph is used for:

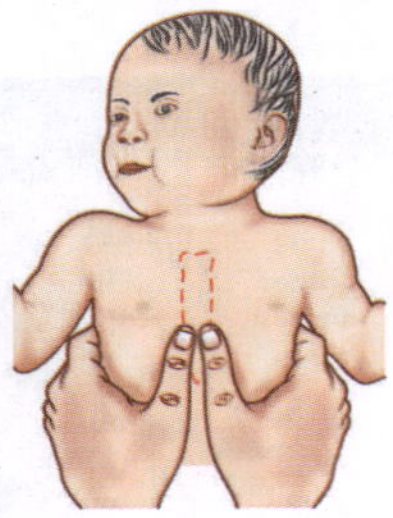

a. Tactile stimulation
b. External cardiac massage
c. Heimlich's maneuver
d. Burping

63. Dermal zones shown in Photograph are used for estimation of: *[Recent Question 2013]*

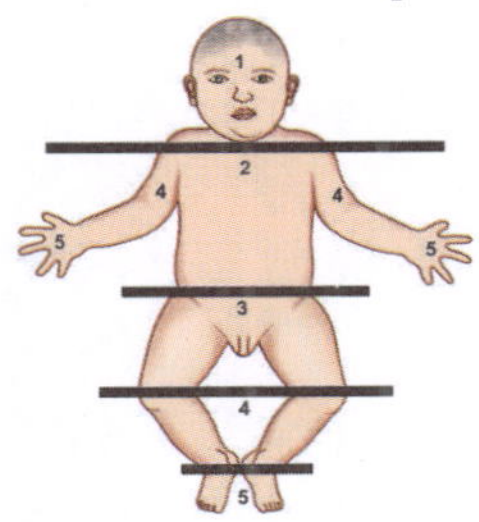

a. Serum hemoglobin levels
b. Serum bilirubin levels
c. Serum glucose levels
d. Serum calcium levels

64. Sign shown in Photograph occurs due to: *[Recent Question 2014, 2012]*

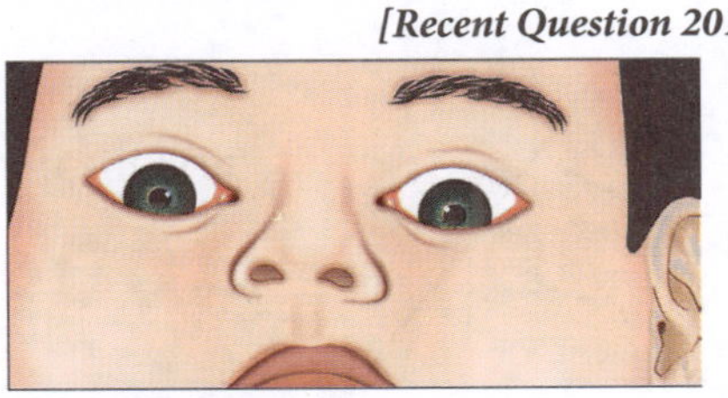

a. Subdural hemorrhage
b. Hydrocephalus
c. Craniotabes
d. Dolichocephaly

Ans.

57. c
58. c
59. d
60. a
61. b
62. b
63. b
64. b

65. Reflex used in Neonate shown in the Photograph is:
[Recent Question 2014]

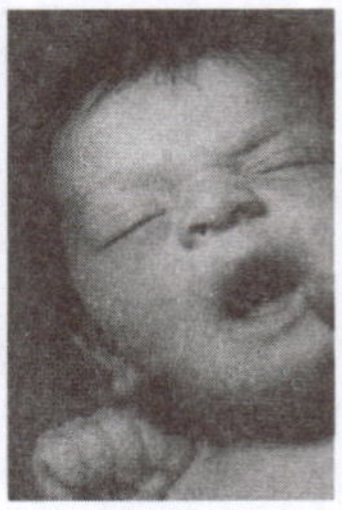

a. Moro's reflex b. Rooting reflex
c. Parachute reflex d. None of these

66. Identify the Childhood Malignancy shown in Photograph based on Sign (Box) shown:

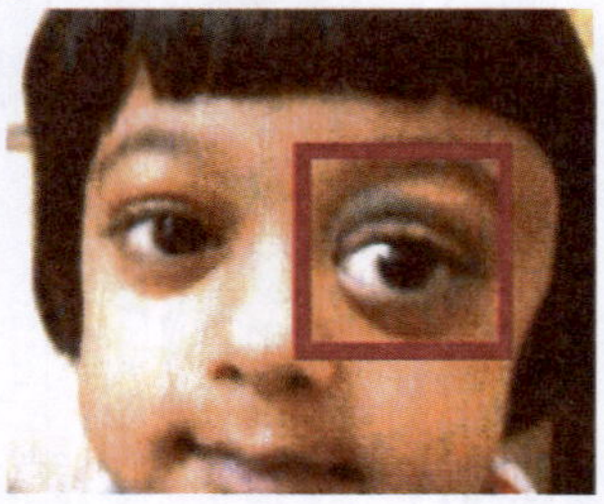

a. Retinoblastoma b. Neuroblastoma
c. Meningioma d. Wilms' tumor

67. CPR Method shown in Photograph is:

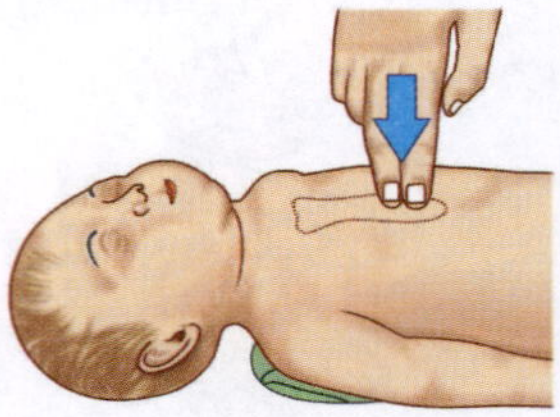

a. Cardiac massage
b. Two finger cardiac compression
c. Two thumb cardiac compression
d. Cardiac thump

68. CPR Method shown in Photograph is:
[Recent Question 2012]

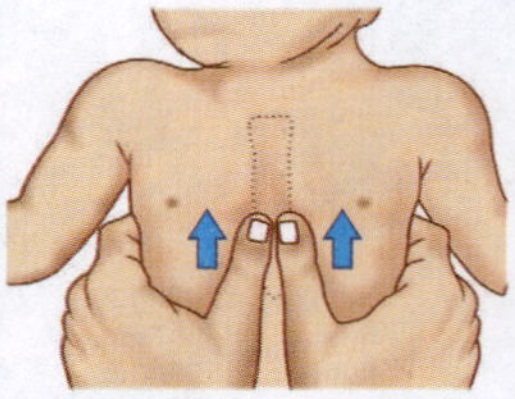

a. Cardiac massage
b. Two finger cardiac compression
c. Two thumb cardiac compression
d. Cardiac thump

69. Identify the foot condition shown in photograph: *[Recent Question 2014]*

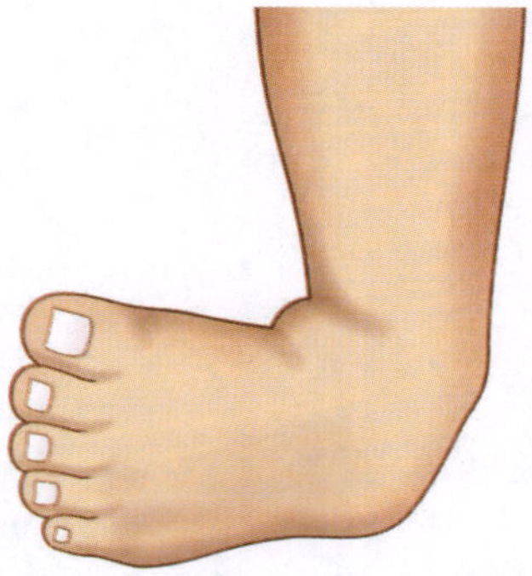

a. Talipes calcaneus b. Talipes varus c. Talipes equinus d. Talipes valgus

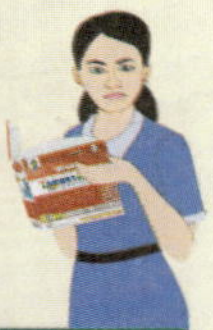

Ans.

65. b
66. b
67. b
68. c
69. b

Explanations of Image-Based Questions

3. Ans. (b) Eissenmenger syndrome

In Eisenmenger syndrome, a large VSD allows the blood to shunt from the left ventricle to the right ventricle, causing increased pressure in the pulmonary arteries. Over time, this elevated pressure in the lungs leads to changes in the blood vessels and the development of pulmonary hypertension. As a consequence, blood flow is redirected from right to left, causing deoxygenated blood to mix with oxygenated blood and result in cyanosis (bluish discoloration of the skin, lips, and nails). Nail clubbing is often associated with chronic hypoxia (low oxygen levels) and is characterized by the thickening and rounding of the fingertips and enlargement of the nail beds. In Eisenmenger syndrome, chronic hypoxia due to the right-to-left shunting of blood can lead to nail clubbing.

4. Ans. (b) Congenital rubella

In Congenital Rubella Syndrome, ophthalmoscope findings often reveal characteristic abnormalities, including cataracts (clouding of the lens), retinopathy (retinal abnormalities), and microphthalmia (smaller-than-normal eye size). Taken together, the clinical manifestations of a fever and rash in the mother, along with the presence of PDA, deafness, and specific ophthalmoscope findings in the newborn, strongly support the diagnosis of Congenital Rubella Syndrome.

5. Ans. (a) Logan bow

The Logan Bow is an external device comprising a curved bow-shaped metal bar, with spikes attached to its cross bars, and is widely used as part of a cleft lip management to maintain postoperative apposition and to avoid excessive strain after cheiloplasty for a cleft lip.

6. Ans. (c) Metered dose inhaler with spacer

A spacer is a device that attaches to the metered-dose inhaler. This allows the child to breathe in the medicine more easily. It helps deliver the medicine to the airways of the lungs instead of the mouth.

7. Ans. (b) Bili blanket

Bili Blanket Led Phototherapy is the next generation fiber optic based technology for treatment of indirect hyperbilirubinemia in newborns. A biliblanket consists of a fiber-optic blanket designed to transfer the light from a lamp unit all around the baby's body.

8. Ans. (b) Giraffe incubator

GE (Giraffe Incubator) is an enclosed neonatal intensive care microenvironment incubator with an innovative design and exceptional thermal performance that creates an unsurpassed healing environment for intensively ill infants. It has a centralized display/control unit providing accessibility from either side of the bed plus excellent viewing of all equipment and patient parameters. It is patented by GE (General Electric) company.

28. Ans. (d) India Newborn Action Plan

[Ref. Park, 23/e p 467]

India Newborn Action Plan (INAP) (Photograph)

- India Newborn Action Plan (INAP) was launched in September 2014 with the aim of ending preventable newborn deaths and stillbirths by 2030
  - **Goal 1:** Ending Preventable Newborn Deaths to achieve "Single Digit NMR" by 2030, with all the states to individually achieve this target by 2035
  - **Goal 2:** Ending Preventable Stillbirths to achieve "Single Digit SBR" by 2030, with all the states to individually achieve this target by 2035

29. Ans. (b) 2020

[Ref. Park, 23/e p442]

Mission Indradhanush 2014 (Photograph)

- **Launch:** 25 December 2014
- **Description:** Indradhanush depicting seven colors of the rainbow, aims to cover all those children by 2020 who are either unvaccinated, or are partially vaccinated against 7 vaccine preventable diseases (7 VPD's)
  - Diphtheria
  - Pertussis
  - Tetanus
  - Childhood Tuberculosis
  - Poliomyelitis
  - Hepatitis B
  - Measles
- **Strategy:**
  - **Focused and systematic immunization drive:** "Catch-up" campaign mode to cover all the children who have been left/ missed out
  - **Four special vaccination campaigns:** January-June 2015 with intensive planning and monitoring

30. Ans. (c) BFHI

[Ref. Park, 23/e p540]

WHO-UNICEF and BFHI 1991 Baby Friendly Hospital Initiative (Photograph)

- Ten Steps to Successful Breastfeeding
- Every facility providing maternity services and care to the newborn infants should,
  - Have a written breastfeeding Policy that is routinely communicated to all healthcare staff
  - Train all healthcare staff in skills necessary to implement this policy
  - Inform all pregnant women about benefits and management of breastfeeding
  - Help mother Initiate breastfeeding 'within half hour of birth'
  - Show mothers how to breastfeed, and how to maintain lactation even if they are separated from their infants

- Give newborn infants no food or drink other than breast milk, unless medically indicated
- Practice Rooming-in: Allow mothers and infants to remain together 24 hours a day
- Encourage 'breastfeeding on Demand'
- Foster Establishment of breastfeeding support groups and refer mothers to them on discharge from the hospital or clinic:
  - Eliminate any support by the manufacturers of infant-formula/infant-food or feeding bottles
  - Prohibit distribution of free and low-cost supplies of breast milk supplies
  - Provide additional lactation assistance to mothers of special cases, i.e., low birth weight, cesarean section
  - Assure a safe and healthy, and positive birthing experience for mother and Infant

31. Ans. (a) Filled with tap water

[Ref. Park, 23/e p109]

ICE-PACK (Photograph)

- Is prepared by keeping in a Deep freezer
- Is used for:
  - Temperature maintenance during vaccine transportation, in a vaccine carrier
  - Temperature maintenance during an immunization session
- Is of total 320 – 340 ml capacity
- Has a 'horizontal mark' – water fill level (as water expands on freezing)
  - NOTHING should be added to water for freezing in an ice-pack
- Has generally 2 holes – MEANT FOR keeping vaccines

32. Ans. (c) Aortic area

- The stethoscope has been put on right second intercostal area just lateral to sternal border and this represents aortic area.
- The auscultation should proceed in a logical manner over 4 general areas on the anterior chest, beginning with the patient in the supine position. The 4 precordial areas are examined with diaphragm, including:
  - Aortic region (between the 2nd and 3rd intercostal spaces at the right sternal border) (RUSB – right upper sternal border).
  - Pulmonic region (between the 2nd and 3rd intercostal spaces at the left sternal border) (LUSB – left upper sternal border).
  - Tricuspid region (between the 3rd, 4th, 5th, and 6th intercostal spaces at the left sternal border) (LLSB – Left Lower Sternal Border).
  - Mitral region (near the apex of the heart between the 5th and 6th intercostal spaces in the mid-clavicular line) (apex of the heart).

33. Ans. (b) Carotid artery bruit

- The stethoscope over the carotid artery indicates attempt to evaluate for carotid artery bruit.

34. Ans. (b) Metered dose inhaler

The image shows a child blowing into the mouthpiece of a peak expiratory flow rate meter. It is shown next:

- PEFR is the maximum flow rate generated during a forceful exhalation, starting from full lung inflation. Peak flow rate primarily reflects large airway flow and depends on the voluntary effort and muscular strength of the patient.
- Maximal airflow occurs during the effort-dependent portion of the expiratory maneuver, so low values may be caused by a less than maximal effort rather than by airway obstruction.
- Nevertheless, the ease of measuring peak flow rate with an inexpensive small portable device has made it popular as a means of following the degree of airway obstruction in patients with asthma and other pulmonary conditions.

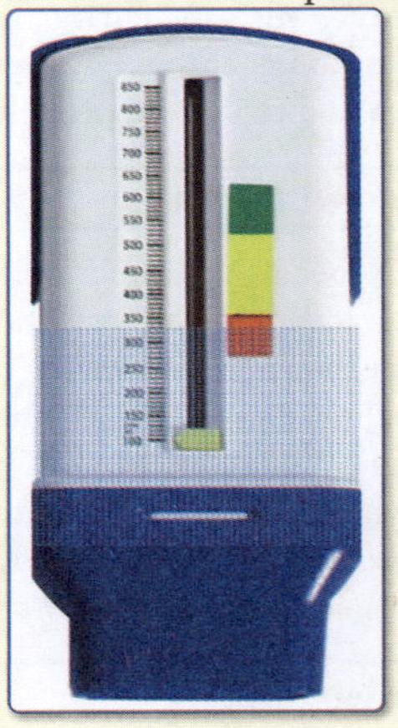

35. Ans. (a)

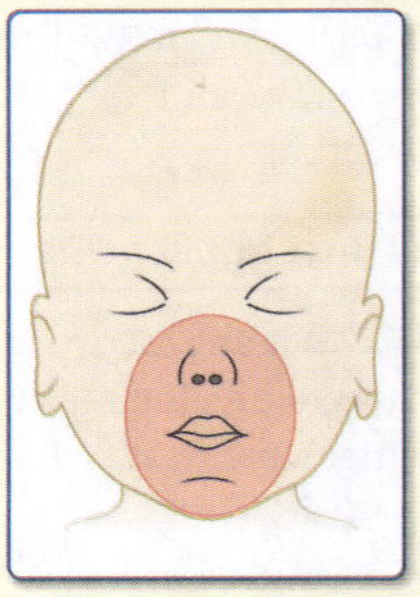

- Using an appropriately sized mask will reduce leakage and is vital for successful effective resuscitation
- The mask or facemask is connected to the bag and covers the mouth and nose of the newborn during resuscitation.
- A correctly sized **mask** should **cover the mouth and nose**, but not the eyes, and should not extend beyond the chin.

39. Ans. (c) Goldenhar syndrome

- **Goldenhar syndrome** is a rare congenital condition characterized by abnormal development of the eye, ear and spine.

"A good laugh and a long sleep are the best cures in the doctor's book."
—Irish Proverb

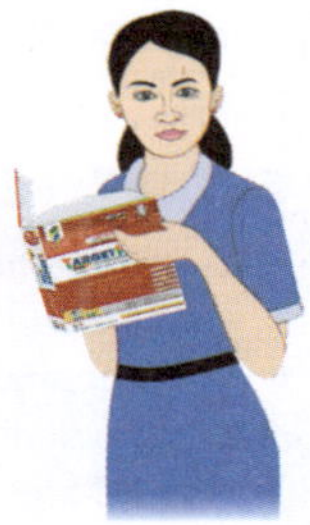

MULTIPLE CHOICE QUESTIONS
(Including Explained and Practice Questions)

INTRODUCTION TO GROWTH & DEVELOPMENT

1. The modern concept of pediatrics means:
(Safdarjung NO 2018)
a. Short term care of the child
b. Basic care of the child
c. Continuous and preventive care of whole child
d. Terminally ill care of the child

Explanation: Pediatrics is defined as the branch of medical science that deals with child development and care during illnesses. As the major causes leading to under five mortality and morbidity are preventable in nature, the modern concept of pediatrics focuses on prevention of illness and promotion of health rather than treatment of illnesses alone.

2. Which part of the brain controls and integrates activities of the autonomic nervous system?
a. Hypothalamus
b. Epithalamus
c. Midbrain
d. Thalamus

3. Child can help in household chores, dresses and undresses at?
a. 2 years
b. 3 years
c. 4 years
d. 5 years

Explanation: Key social milestones achieved at five years of age include Dressing and undressing asking questions about meaning of words; engaging in domestic role-playing

4. In development of language, a child can tell stories by the age of:
a. One year
b. Two years
c. Three years
d. Four years

5. Low recurrence in nocturnal enuresis is seen with which of the following interventions?
a. Desmopressin
b. Oxybutynin
c. Imipramine
d. Bed alarms

Explanation: Best success rate is seen with bed alarms which when goes off, child should get up and go to the toilet. Participation of parents is critical in success of this intervention. However, initial management is behavior modification like limiting fluid intake in evening hours and awakening the child during night to go to bathroom. Parents should avoid shaming of the child.

6. Early strict toileting can result in which of the following condition?
a. Night terror
b. Temper tantrums
c. Encopresis
d. Nocturnal enuresis

Explanation: Night terrors refers to disconcerting, screaming or crying that a toddler or young child may have at night during sleep. When a child is toilet-training, he may feel torn between pleasing his parents and being unable to resist soiling. He wants to assert his independence, but he also has a fear of a lack of control. This anxiety and stress can contribute to a child experiencing night terrors.

7. Which of the following milestone is a red flag sign in child development if not attained?
a. Walking at 12 months
b. Talking single word at 12 months
c. Social smile at 3 months
d. Vocalization at 2 months

8. Which of the following is the most common cause of short stature in child?
a. Hypothyroidism
b. Constitutional developmental delay
c. Growth hormone deficiency
d. Psychosocial disturbances

Explanation: Short stature is said to be present if the height of the child is below the 3rd percentile or less than 2 SD of mean height of the corresponding age. Constitutional developmental delay is a significant cause of short stature in mid childhood period. Short stature can be proportional or disproportional.

9. Aspergers syndrome is a:
a. Metabolic disorder
b. Neuromuscular disorder
c. Degenerative disorder
d. Developmental delay

10. Taste perception of a baby develops at:
a. Birth
b. 3 months
c. 6 months
d. 8 months

Explanation: Newborns are born with odor and taste preferences acquired in the womb from the smell and taste of amniotic fluid which is influenced by what mother eats. At birth, infants can show expressions of pleasure or disgust when presented with pleasant odors such as honey/milk or unpleasant odors and taste.

11. What does it mean when a baby has 25th percentile of head circumference (HC)?
a. 25% of children will have HC more than that
b. The child is having 25% of normal HC
c. 25% of children will have HC less than that
d. 75% of the children will have HC less than that

Explanation: Percentile is a number where a certain percentage of scores fall below that number. If a child has 25th percentile HC means that there are 25% of children who has HC less than that.

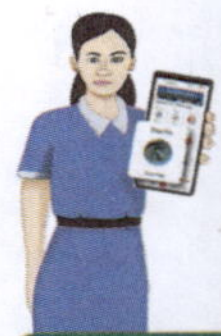

Ans.
1. c
2. a
3. d
4. d
5. d
6. a
7. c
8. b
9. d
10. a
11. c

GROWTH CHART

12. During the first year after birth an infant's birth weight normally:
- a. Quadruples
- b. Doubles
- c. Remain stable
- d. Triples

13. Expected weight of one-year-old child, when the birth weight is 3.5 kg: *(RAK MSc 2018)*
- a. 7 kg
- b. 6 kg
- c. 9.5 kg
- d. 10.5 kg

Explanation: As the child ages the weight increase is as follows:

- X Weight at Birth
- 2x 5 months
- 3x 1 year
- 4x 2 years
- 5x 3 years
- 6x 5 years
- 7x 7 years
- 10x 10 years

So, Birth weight triples (3x) at one year.
Therefore, the correct answer is 3.5 × 3 = 10.5 in a year

14. Which of the following best describes typical annual growth during the school age years?
- a. Few physical differences are noticeable between age mates throughout this period
- b. Fat pads increase in number and add to the normal "chubby" appearance of the child
- c. Child grows an average of 2 inches (5.2 cm) per year
- d. Child gains an average of 3 pounds (1.4 kg) per year

15. Growth chart is used for:
- a. Growth monitoring
- b. Diagnostic tool
- c. Tool for action
- d. All of these

16. Growth chart is also known as:
- a. New Ballard scale
- b. Road to health chart
- c. Apgar Score
- d. GCS score

17. Identify the correct statement among the following related to weight of the child:
- a. Normal birth weight of an Indian child is 2.5–3.5 kg
- b. Baby's birth weight doubles at 5-6 months of age
- c. Baby's birth weight triples at 1 year of age
- d. All of the above

18. Normal chest circumference of a newborn is: New Q
- a. 30-32 cm
- b. 35-37 cm
- c. 31-33 cm
- d. 33-35 cm

19. Which of the following is not true regarding the birth weight of a newborn? *(AIIMS-BBS SNO 2019)*
- a. Birth weight less than 5% of normal on the day of birth requires further investigation
- b. Typical birth weight of newborn is between 2.7 kg and 4.0 kg
- c. Newborns lose 10% of their birth weight by 3-4 days of age
- d. Newborns gain the lost birth weight by 10th day of life

Explanation: Normal birth weight of the baby is between 2.5 kg and 4.5 kg. Newborns often lose around 10% in the first 4 to 5 days after birth but regain it by about 10 to 12 days of age. So, 5% loss on day of birth is considered normal and requires no further investigation.

20. Identify the incorrect statement related to height/length of a child:
- a. Length of the baby at the time of birth is approximately 45-51 cm
- b. Length of the baby doubles at 4 years of age
- c. Height of a child will increase till the closure of epiphyseal plate
- d. Rate of growth in height is highest during toddler

21. Identify the correct statement related to head circumference/chest circumference:
- a. At the time of birth, head circumference is about 33-35 cm
- b. At the time of birth chest circumference is about 30-33 cm
- c. In a healthy child, the head and chest circumference will become equal at around 12 months
- d. All of the above

22. In a healthy child, the head and chest circumference equal each other around the age of:
- a. 3-6 months
- b. 6-9 months
- c. 9-12 months
- d. 15-18 months

Ref: OP Ghai 8th ed. p 13

Explanation: In a healthy child, the circumference of the chest is about 2-3 cm less than head circumference at birth.

The circumference of head and chest are almost equal by the age of 1 year. Thereafter, the chest circumference exceeds the head circumference.

23. What is the relationship between head circumference (HC) and chest circumference (CC) in a newborn baby?
- a. Both are equal at the time of birth
- b. HC more at the time of birth and both become equal by 1 year and then CC exceeds
- c. CC is more at the time of birth and then both become equal by 1 year and then HC exceeds
- d. None of the above

24. Normal head circumference of a newborn is: *(Staff Nurse G II 2014)*
- a. 30-32 cm
- b. 35-37 cm
- c. 31-33 cm
- d. 33-35 cm

25. Normal mid upper arm circumference (MUAC) at birth is about:
- a. 6–8 cm
- b. 9–11 cm
- c. 12–14 cm
- d. 14–16 cm

26. The best method to perform physical examination on a 2-year-old child is:
- a. Proximally to distal
- b. From head to toe
- c. From least to most intrusive
- d. Abdomen to head

27. The nurses assess a six-month-old child during well-baby-clinic. Nurse makes all the following observations. Which of the following assessments made by the nurse is an area of concern indicating a need for further evaluation? *(RAK MSc 2018)*
- a. Absence of Moro reflex
- b. Closed posterior fontanel
- c. Three pounds weight gain in two months
- d. Moderate head lag when pulled to sitting position

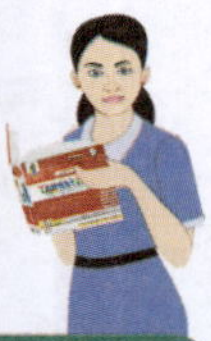

Ans.

12.	d
13.	d
14.	c
15.	d
16.	b
17.	d
18.	c
19.	a
20.	d
21.	d
22.	c
23.	b
24.	d
25.	b
26.	c
27.	d

Explanation: Head control is expected at the age of 3 months in a baby. Starting at 6 weeks head control develops and there is only a slight lag at 12 weeks of age. Infant lifts head from supine position when pulled up at 5 months of age. So, head lagging in 6-month-old infant requires attention.
All other findings are normal for a 6-month-old infant.

28. Maximum absolute growth is seen at: ***(AIIMS 2001)***
a. 0–3 years b. 3–5 years
c. 5–10 years d. 14–16 years

Explanation: Maximum growth can be seen in girls by 10 years (8–13) and in boys by 12 years (10–15). This growth spurt is because of puberty attainment.

29. Identify the high-risk infant among the following:
a. Infant with birth weight 2.5 kg
b. Infant on artificial feeding
c. Infant with birth weight 2 kg
d. Infant with Apgar score 8

30. The premature closure of the sagittal suture is called: *(AIIMS Raipur Grade II 2017)*
a. Scaphocephaly b. Oxycephaly
c. Acrocephaly d. Anencephaly

Explanation: Scaphocephaly is a type of cephalic disorder which occurs when there is a premature fusion of the sagittal suture.
- **Oxycephaly:** Premature closure of coronal suture.
- **Acrocephaly:** Premature closure of the lambdoid and coronal sutures.
- **Plagocephaly:** Asymmetrical distortion (flattening of one side) of the skull.
- **Anencephaly:** Absence of major portion of brain.

31. The average length of a normal newborn baby is:
a. 45 cm b. 43 cm
c. 50 cm d. 35 cm

32. All the following are normal manifestation in a newborn baby; EXCEPT:
a. Uneven head shape
b. Respirations are irregular, abdominal, 30-60 bpm
c. Positive moro reflex
d. Heart rate is 80 bpm

33. Macrosomia means:
a. Baby with large tongue
b. Baby with large head
c. Large size baby
d. Baby whose birthweight is not adequate to the length

34. Correct regarding fontanel is:
a. Anterior fontanel closed at 18 months of age
b. Posterior fontanel closed at 6-8 weeks of age
c. Anterior fontanel known as bregma and posterior is lambda
d. All of the above

35. How much a neonate should gain weight after a successful feeding?
a. 3-8 g/day b. 10-15 g/day
c. 15-20 g/day d. 25-30 g/day

36. Mid upper arm circumference value in a moderately malnourished child is:
a. <11.5 cm b. <12.5 cm
c. <13.5 cm d. <14.5 cm

MILESTONES

37. At what age does a child normally develop 'social smile' milestone? *(AIIMS Bhopal Nursing Officer, 2018)*
a. 12 weeks b. 4 weeks
c. 16 weeks d. 8 weeks

Explanation: By 2 months of age child develops social smile. At this age, the baby also looks at parent, coos, makes gurgling sounds and turns head toward sounds.

38. Brain growth is at its maximum during:
a. 1st trimester of pregnancy b. Infancy
c. Toddler d. School going

Explanation: The last 3 months of pregnancy and first 3 years of post-natal life are most crucial for brain development.

39. Crawling of an Infant occurs at: ***(DSSSB PHN, 2015)***
a. 8 to 9 months b. 2 to 3 months
c. 4 to 5 months d. 6 to 8 months

40. An infant sits alone momentarily by about......month of age.
a. 2 b. 3
c. 4 d. 6

41. A male baby will be having an optimal (50th percentile) head circumference of 45 cm at .... age.
a. 5 months b. 7 months
c. 9 months d. 12 months

Explanation: As per the WHO growth chart for boys, head circumference is 45 cm at 9 months and 46 cm at 12 months (50th percentile).

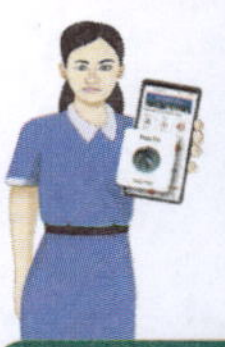

42. Which of the following is a milestone typically achieved by a newborn within the first month of life? ***New Q***
a. Rolling over b. Sitting independently
c. Crawling d. Lifting and turning the head

43. Which of the following is a milestone typically achieved by an infant at around 9 months of age? ***New Q***
a. Walking independently
b. Crawling
c. Saying simple words
d. Rolling over

44. Anterior fontanel is closed at:
a. <3 months b. 12 months
c. 12–18 months d. >3 years

Ref: Nelson 20th ed. p 2972

Explanation: The average time of closure is 18 months but the fontanel may normally close as early as 9 months. The fontanel is normally slightly depressed and pulsatile and is best evaluated when an infant is held upright while asleep or feeding.

45. 1-year-old child comes to well-baby clinic and nurse noticed the child's anterior fontanel is still open. What is the appropriate nursing intervention?
a. Report to doctor
b. Normal findings
c. Measure head circumference
d. Look for sign and symptoms of infection

Explanation: Anterior fontanel close by 18 months of age, so in a 1-year-old child this is a normal finding.

Ans.

28. d
29. c
30. a
31. c
32. d
33. c
34. d
35. d
36. b
37. d
38. b
39. a
40. d
41. c
42. d
43. b
44. c
45. b

46. A child likes to look at self in a mirror at age of _______ months:

a. 1 month
b. 2 months
c. 4 months
d. 6 months

Ref: OP Ghai 8th ed. p 52

Explanation: Milestones achieved at age of 6 months:

Social and Emotional

- Knows familiar faces and begins to know if someone is a stranger
- Likes to play with others, especially parents
- Likes to look at self in a mirror

Language/Communication

- Responds to sounds by making sounds
- Strings vowels together when babbling ("ah," "eh," "oh") and likes taking turns with parent while making sounds
- Responds to own name
- Makes sounds to show joy and displeasure

Cognitive (learning, thinking, problem-solving)

- Looks around at things nearby
- Brings things to mouth
- Shows curiosity about things and tries to get things that are out of reach
- Begins to pass things from one hand to the other

Movement/Physical Development

- Rolls over in both directions (front to back, back to front)
- Begins to sit without support
- When standing, supports weight on legs and might bounce
- Rocks back and forth, sometimes crawling backward before moving forward

47. A 3-year-old child cannot:

a. Draw a square
b. Draw a circle
c. Knows gender
d. Ride a tricycle

Ref: OP Ghai 8th Ed, p 51

Explanation: A child is able to draw a square at approximately 4 ½ years of age.

Important developmental milestones at 3 years of age:

- Rides tricycle
- Draw a circle
- Can dress or undress completely
- Build a tower of 10 cubes
- Knows gender and age
- Counts 3 objects correctly

48. A 3-year-old child is said to have delayed milestone if he fails to:

a. Use spoon
b. Draw a square
c. Skip
d. Climb with alternating foot downwards in the steps

Ref: Nelson 20th ed. p 75

Explanation: A child is expected to use a spoon by 18 months of age, hence not attaining it at 3 years is definitely developmental delay.

All other milestones in the question, namely drawing a square, skipping and climbing with alternating foot downwards are achieved at 4 years of age or afterwards.

49. Popcorn and nuts should not be given to a toddler primarily because they:

a. Will spoil the child's appetite
b. Can cause tooth decay
c. Are easily aspirated
d. Have very little food value

50. First appearing teeth in a child is:

a. Premolar
b. Incisors
c. Canines
d. Third molar

Explanation: The bottom incisors are the first teeth that tend to erupt in children at 6-8 months of age.

51. The child has a complete set of deciduous teeth at the age of ......years.

a. 1 ½ year
b. 2 years
c. 1 year
d. 2 ½ years

52. A 3-year-old male child is likely to perform which of the following act?

a. Tie the shoelaces
b. Pedaling a tricycle
c. Threading beads
d. Write letters

53. Identify the correct statement related to teeth development in children:

a. First erupted teeth in a newborn baby is lower central incisor
b. First teeth erupted in a baby at 4-6 months of age
c. Number of milk teeth in children are 20 in number
d. All of the above

54. At what age do first permanent teeth appear?

a. 5 years
b. 6 years
c. 7 years
d. 8 years

55. Delayed dentition is the most important characteristic of:

a. Mongolism
b. Milia
c. Cretinism
d. Malnutrition

56. A mature Pincer grasp is attained by___________month.

a. 8
b. 10
c. 12
d. 18

Ref: OP Ghai 8th ed. p 50

Explanation: Development of pincer grasp

- 9 months radial digital grasp
- 10 months inferior pincer grasp
- 10–12 months mature pincer grasp

57. Voluntary palmar grasp appears at what age?

a. 28 weeks
b. 20 weeks
c. 12 weeks
d. At birth

Explanation: The **palmar grasp reflex** (known as involuntary palmar grasp) is an involuntary response to a mechanical stimulus that is present in newborns. Palmar grasp usually appears at 16 weeks of gestation and disappears around 3 to 4 months of age. **Voluntary palmar grasp**, on the other hand, is a conscious and intentional act. It is a sign that the infant's brain has developed to the point where they can control their hand movements. Voluntary palmar grasp typically appears between 4 and 6 months of age.

58. Identify the correct statement related to milestones achievement in child:

a. Running seen at the age of 15 months
b. 1-year-old child speaks two words with meaning
c. Recognizing mother is seen at 3 months of age
d. All of the above

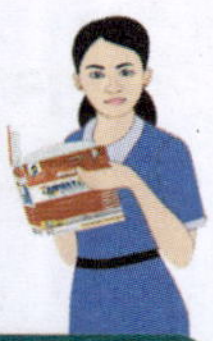

Ans.

46. d
47. a
48. a
49. c
50. b
51. d
52. b
53. d
54. b
55. c
56. c
57. b
58. d

59. When Rajan was 3 months old, he had a toy train; when his view of the train was blocked, he did not search for it. Now that he is 9 months, old, he looks for it, reflecting the presence of:

a. Object permanence
b. Sensorimotor play
c. Schemata
d. Magical thinking

60. A baby with tripod position, bi dextrous approach, recognizes strangers and can spell out mono syllable by what age?

a. 7 months
b. 12 months
c. 9 months
d. 10 months

61. Identify the correct statement related to milestones achievement in child:

a. Sit without support seen at 8 months of age
b. Developmental milestone achieved by a 9-month-old child is creeping
c. Stand without support seen at 12 months of age
d. All of the above

62. At what age child can eat food without spilling, identify her gender, say her full name, can dress self with supervision?

a. 2 yrs
b. 3 yrs
c. 4 yrs
d. 5 yrs

63. When assessing physical development of a five-year-old, you would find it abnormal if he: *(ESIC 2019)*

a. Needed to go up a stairway one step at a time.
a. Could catch a large rubber ball
b. Could stack up pile of six blocks.
c. Could jump on one foot a few times.

Explanation: A 3-year-old child should be able to walk up the stairs using a reciprocal pattern, placing only one foot on each step, without requiring the use of a railing for support. Four-year-old child should be able to go both up and down stairs using a reciprocal pattern and no rail.

Other mentioned milestones are expected in a 5-year-old child.

64. Toilet training need to be initiated at .... of age.

a. 15 months
b. 18 months
c. 20 months
d. 24 months

65. A child can withhold and postpone his bowel movements at age of:

a. 1 year
b. 2 years
c. 3 years
d. 4 years

66. The nurse is aware that preschoolers often display a developmental characteristic that makes them treat dolls or stuffed animals as if they have thoughts and feelings. This is an example of:

a. Logical reasoning
b. Egocentrism
c. Concrete thinking
d. Animism

67. According to Denver Development Screening Test (DDST) an infant normally starts standing with support in:

a. 6 months
b. 9 months
c. 12 months
d. 15 months

68. A mature Pincer grasp is attained by__________months.

a. 8
b. 10
c. 12
d. 18

Ref: OP Ghai 8th ed. p 50

Explanation: Development of pincer grasp

- 9 months radial digital grasp
- 10 months inferior pincer grasp
- 10–12 months mature pincer grasp

THEORIES OF GROWTH AND DEVELOPMENT

69. The prime principles of growth and development include all; EXCEPT:

a. Growth is a continuous process
b. Development occurs in orderly manner and follows a certain sequence
c. Growth and development go hand in hand
d. Development occurs in a Caudocephalad fashion

70. Identify the correct statement related to growth and development among the following:

a. Size and mass of child's body increasing is called as growth
b. Specific maturations of functions in a child is known as development
c. In a child during initial period of growth and development brain growth is faster, then it became almost static
d. All of the above

71. Which age group identifies illness as a punishment for misdeeds?

a. Infant
b. Toddler
c. Preschool
d. School going

72. You are working in a pediatric clinic, during developmental assessment of the toddler, his parents report that their son is able to point to three to five body parts, uses 20–30 words that his parents understand, and is beginning to put together two-word phrases. Assuming his language skills are normal for age, how old is this child? *New Q*

a. 15 months
b. 18 months
c. 24 months
d. 30 months

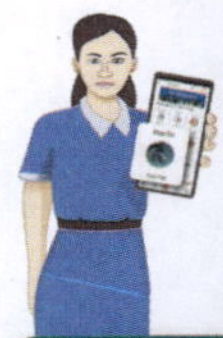

Explanation: By 18 months of age (option b), toddlers generally have a vocabulary of 20–50 words, which aligns with the reported 20-30 words that the child is using. They also begin to combine words into two-word phrases, which is consistent with the reported development in the question.

73. The following are features of premature thelarche:

a. Association with Turner Syndrome
b. Asymmetrical breast enlargement
c. Associated growth spurt
d. Areola pigmentation

74. First sign of puberty in boys is:

a. Testis enlargement
b. Breast enlargement
c. Penis enlargement
d. Scrotum enlargement

75. When considering the principle of growth and development, remember that: *(ESIC 2019)*

a. Although development occurs in an orderly sequence, the rate may vary between individuals.
b. Most children can run before they walk
c. Development occurs evenly, with periods of no growth occurring every third year.
d. All children should grow in the same rate, all four-year-olds should weight within 4 kg of each other.

Explanation: Although development of child follows an orderly sequence, it is not necessary that the rate of growth and development is similar in all individuals. It is subject to individual variations. Statements given in option b, c, d are incorrect as per the principles of Growth and Development.

Ans.

Q	Ans
59.	a
60.	a
61.	d
62.	b
63.	a
64.	b
65.	b
66.	d
67.	b
68.	c
69.	d
70.	d
71.	c
72.	b
73.	b
74.	a
75.	a

76. All among the following indicate principles of normal growth and development; EXCEPT:

a. Proximal to distal b. Cephalocaudal
c. General to specific d. Physical to psychological

Explanation: Physical to psychological is not used to describe normal growth and development. All others are the characteristics of normal growth and development.

77. In the stages of growth and development, the infancy extends from: *(AIIMS Raipur Grade II 2017)*

a. Birth to 4 weeks b. Birth to 1 year
c. 4 weeks to 1 year d. 1 to 3 years

Explanation:
0–28 days - Newborn
1 month-year: Infant
1–3 years: Toddlers
3–6 years: Preschoolers
6–12 years: Schoolers
12–18 years: Adolescents

78. Psychosocial development of children was proposed by:

a. Erikson b. Freud
c. Piaget d. Kohlberg

Explanation: Psychosocial development was proposed by Erikson.
Psychosexual development - Freud
Cognitive development - Piaget's
Moral development - Kohlberg

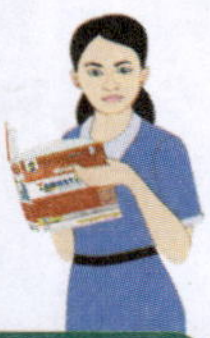

79. According to Piaget's theory, 6-month-old infant will demonstrate:

a. Negativism b. Transductive reasoning
c. Imitation
d. Beginning of object permanence

Explanation: The beginning of object permanence will start by around 6 months of age. Object permanence is the understanding that objects continue to exist even when they cannot be observed (seen, heard, touched, smelled or sensed in any way).

80. As per Erik Erikson's stages of development, child takes decision at the age of: *(Kerala PSE 1991)*

a. 3 years b. 5 years
c. 7 years d. 9 years

Explanation: From 1–3 years, child develops autonomy and reaches peak at 3 years.

81. According to Erikson's psychosocial theory, what is the developmental task of a toddler? *(AIIMS Bhopal Grade-I 2018)*

a. Autonomy/shame and doubt
b. Trust/Mistrust
c. Industry/Inferiority
d. Initiative/Guilt

Explanation: Toddlers are 1–3 years old children. In this age group, the child is developing physically and become more mobile and discovering that he/she has many skills or abilities like putting on clothes and shoes, etc. If children in this stage are supported in their increased independence, they develop a sense of autonomy and if they are criticized or not given opportunity to assert themselves then they feel a sense of shame and doubt in their abilities.

82. Psychosexual development stage of a toddler:

a. Phallic stage b. Anal stage
c. Genital stage d. Oral stage

Explanation: As per the psychosexual development theory proposed by Freud, toddler belongs to anal stage of development.

83. A child's growth is slower than his peers but normal when compared to his father's childhood records. If the child ultimately achieves normal height, what can be the possible diagnosis? *New Q*

a. Delayed puberty b. Constitutional delay
c. Hormonal imbalance d. GH deficiency

Explanation: Constitutional delay refers to a pattern of growth and development that is slower than average but is still within the normal range. In constitutional delay, a child's growth is slower compared to their peers, but they eventually catch up and achieve a normal height.

This condition is often inherited from parents, and it is not a sign of any underlying medical condition.

84. Guidelines for assessing toilet training readiness are:

a. Parental readiness b. Psychological readiness
c. Mental readiness d. All of these

Explanation: Guideline for assessing readiness for toilet training includes parental readiness, psychological readiness, mental readiness and physical readiness.

85. Occurrence of 'Oedipus complex' is commonly seen in:

a. Girls between 1–3 years of age
b. Girls between 3–5 years of age
c. Boys between 1–3 years of age
d. Boys between 3–5 years of age

Ref: Textbook of Developmental Pediatrics by John E. Williams, p 266

Explanation: In Freudian psychoanalytical theory, 'Oedipus complex' is the complex of emotions aroused in a young child, typically around the age of four, by an unconscious sexual desire for the parent of the opposite sex and wish to exclude the parent of the same sex.

- The term was originally applied to ***boys***, the equivalent in girls being called the Electra complex

86. The parents of a child aged 6 years who will begin school ask the nurse for anticipatory guidance. The nurse should explain that a child of this age: *(DSSSB 2010)*

a. Still depends on the parents
b. Rebels against scheduled activities
c. Is highly sensitive to criticism
d. Loves to battle

Explanation: 6-year-old child is independent in most of his activities and highly sensitive to criticism.

87. Eight-year-old Suman has difficult time making friends at school and being chosen to play on the team. He also has trouble completing his homework and, as a result, receives little positive feedback from his parents or teachers. According to Erikson's theory, failure at this stage of development results in:

a. A sense of guilt b. A sense of shame
c. Feelings of inferiority d. A poor sense of self

Ans.

76.	d
77.	c
78.	a
79.	d
80.	a
81.	a
82.	b
83.	b
84.	d
85.	d
86.	c
87.	c

88. To encourage an infant's cognitive and psychosocial development parents and other caregivers should:

(ESIC 2019)

a. Allow the baby to play alone several hours each day
b. Firmly explain the rules of acceptable behavior
c. Give loving consistent care, including playing
d. Keep the baby with them at all times so he or she is safe

Explanation: Giving a loving consistent care, including playing helps in the development of higher mental functions and the behavior related development of the child.

- Allow the baby to play alone several hours each day does not help in behavioral development.
- Firmly explaining the rules increases the discipline in child.
- Keep the baby with them at all times increases the dependency in child.

89. WHO defines adolescent age group between:

a. 10-19 years b. 9-14 years
c. 10-25 years d. 10-14 years

Ref: OP Ghai 8th ed. p 63

Explanation: As per WHO, adolescents are children between the age group of 10 and 19 years.

90. The primary psychosocial task during adolescence is to establish:

a. Identity b. Intimacy
c. Autonomy d. None of these

91. The nurse teaches parents how to have their children learn impulse control and cooperative behaviors. This would be during which of Erikson's stages of development?

a. Trust versus mistrust
b. Initiative versus guilt
c. Industry versus inferiority
d. Autonomy versus sense of shame and doubt

92. During adolescence, psychosocial development focuses on:

a. Becoming independent
b. Establishing an identity
c. Peer group relationship
d. Developing initiative

93. In twin to twin transfusion syndrome, donor twin has all the signs and symptoms; EXCEPT:

a. Oligohydramnios b. Anemia
c. Hypovolemia d. Plethora

Explanation: Donor twin is likely to have oligohydramnios, anemia, and hypovolemia and the recipient twin is likely to have polyhydroamniosis and plethora (abundance or excess) and to be larger than the donor twin

94. Terrible twos is the term used to describe .... age group of children.

a. Infant b. Toddler
c. Pre School d. School going

Explanation: The term terrible twos is used to describe the toddler years, the period ranging from 1 to 3 year of age. It is the challenging time for parents and child as each learn to know the other better. It is an extremely important period for developmental achievement and intellectual growth.

95. Which among the following represents the most common type of accidents found in case of toddlers?

(AIIMS BPL NO 2018)

a. Toxic ingestions b. Choking
c. Drowning d. Burns

Explanation: Burns are the most common documented cause of accidents in toddlers followed by choking, toxic ingestions and drowning. Toddlers use their newly acquired motor skills in an autonomous manner (lack of supervision).

96. Concept regarding death among preschool children is:

a. Not a permanent condition
b. Permanent and irreversible
c. It is because of some bad doing
d. An event that eventually happens to everyone

Explanation: Preschoolers are having no cognitive ability to understand that death is not reversible. So, they think that it is a reversible condition.

ESSENTIAL NEWBORN CARE

97. Follow up care is required for the newborn with:

a. Mongolian spots are present
b. Head circumference 39 cm
c. Milia is present
d. Umbilical cord has 2 arteries and 1 vein

Explanation: Normal head circumference is 33-35 cm in a newborn baby. 39 cm is abnormally large head circumference which is suggestive of hydrocephalus. So, this child require follow up care.

98. All are the characteristics of term baby; EXCEPT:

a. Well curved pinna reaching up to the periphery
b. No deep creases in the soles
c. Pigmented and pendulous scrotal sac
d. Silky hair individual hair strands can be made out

Explanation: In term baby deep creases will be present in the palms and soles of the baby. All others are the characteristic of term baby.

99. The Apgar score should be assessed: *(Safdarjung NO 2018)*

a. Immediately after birth and at 30 minutes after birth
b. At 5 minutes after birth and at 30 minutes after birth
c. At 1 minute after birth and at 5 minutes after birth
d. Immediately after birth and at 5 minutes after birth

Explanation: APGAR scoring is useful for quantitative assessment of newborn for respiratory, circulatory and neurologic status. APGAR is assessed at 1 minute and 5 minutes of birth. Usually newborns have lower score at birth due to depression than the score after 5 minutes of birth. The 1 minute's score determines how well the baby tolerated the process of birth. The 5-minute score determines how well the baby is doing in the outside environment (outside womb).

100. What is nurse's primary critical observation when performing an assessment for determining an Apgar score? *(NCFL 2019)*

a. Heart rate b. Respiratory rate
c. Presence of meconium d. Evaluation of Moro reflex

Explanation: Pulse or heart rate has to be assessed first and then the respirations.

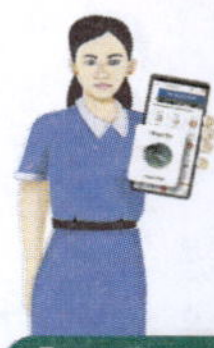

Ans.

88. c
89. a
90. a
91. d
92. b
93. d
94. b
95. d
96. a
97. b
98. b
99. c
100. a

101. Which is the indicator of immediate estimate of the physical condition of the baby?

a. New Ballard scale b. Apgar score
c. Growth chart d. Health assessment

102. In the term APGAR 'G 'stands for:

a. Grunting b. Growth
c. Gross d. Grimace

103. A nurse in a newborn nursery receives a phone call to prepare for the admission of a 43-week-gestation newborn with 1-min and 5-min Apgar scores of 1 and 4. In planning for the admission of this infant, the nurse's highest priority should be to: *New Q*

a. Connect the resuscitation bag to the oxygen outlet
b. Turn on the apnea and cardiorespiratory monitors
c. Set up the intravenous line with 5% dextrose in water
d. Set the radiant warmer control temperature at 36.5° C (97.6°F)

Explanation: The Apgar scores of 1 and 4 indicate that the infant is in severe distress and requires immediate intervention. The nurse's highest priority is to ensure that the infant has a patent airway and is receiving adequate oxygen. This can be done by connecting the resuscitation bag to the oxygen outlet and ventilating the infant.

The other options are important, but they are not as urgent as ensuring that the infant has a patent airway and is receiving adequate oxygen.

104. Which of the following is not a component of Apgar score? *(Recent Question 2015)*

a. Color of the body
b. Muscle tone
c. Heart rate/min
d. Respiratory rate per minute

Ref: OP Ghai 8th ed. p 126

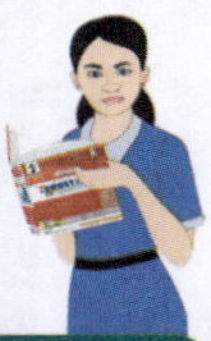

Explanation: It is respiratory effort and not respiratory rate per minute that is taken into consideration in Apgar score.

Apgar scale (evaluate @ 1 and 5 minutes postpartum)

Sign		2	1	0
A	Activity (muscle tone)	Active/fully flexed	Arms and legs flexed	Absent
P	Pulse	>100 bpm	<100 bpm	Absent
G	Grimace (reflex irritability)	Sneezes, coughs, pulls away	Grimaces	Cyanotic or pale all over
A	Appearance (Skin color)	Normal over entire body	Normal except extremities	Cyanotic or pale all over
R	Respirations	Good, crying	Show, irregular	Absent

105. Which of the following are components of Apgar score?

a. Activity, heart rate, grimace, respiratory rate
b. Apnea, heart rate, grimace, tone
c. Activity, color, tone, respiratory effort
d. Appearance, tone, heart rate, respiratory rate

Ref: Nelson 20th Ed, p 798

Explanation: Components of Apgar score:

- Heart rate
- Respiratory effort
- Tone
- Response to catheter in nose
- Color

106. Initial nursing action after the birth of a preterm baby with Apgar score 8 is:

a. Weigh the baby
b. Do suction
c. Inform the family members about the birth and sex of the baby
d. Receive the baby in a pre-warmed towel and dry the baby

Explanation: Preterm babies are more prone to develop hypothermia which causes hypoxia and academia. Because of physiological factors, such as lack of brown fat, the preterm infant is more vulnerable to cool temperatures.

107. A newborn of one minute after vaginal delivery is pink with blue hands and feet has a lusty cry, and heart rate of 140. Prompt response to stimulation with crying and maintains minimal flexion with sluggish movement. The nurse should know that this newborn's Apgar score is:

a. 10 b. 8
c. 9 d. 7

108. Among the following identify the feature that is not expected in a full term newborn baby:

a. Creases cover sole
b. Well pigmented pendulous scrotum
c. Pinna firm, stand erect from head
d. Breast nodule 1-2 mm

Explanation: Breast nodule is small with size less than 5 mm in a preterm child. Average breast diameter at term birth is 8 mm. So breast nodule 1-2 mm is not a feature of full term baby. All other given features are characteristics of a term baby.

109. An infant is born precipitously outside the labor room. What should the nurse do first? *(NCFL 2019)*

a. Tie and cut the umbilical cord
b. Establish an airway for the newborn
c. Ascertain the condition of the uterine fundus
d. Arrange transport for mother and infant to the birthing unit

Explanation: Immediate action by the nurse after the birth of a baby is to establish an airway by clearing the mucus in nose and mouth. This will help the newborn to breathe. Other actions can be followed after that.

110. Which of the following is true about Mongolian Spots?

a. Disappears in about a year
b. It will persist throughout life time
c. Can be treated with emollient
d. Are indicative of parental abuse

111. Identify the incorrect statement related to Mongolian spot in newborn baby:

a. Disappears in about a year
b. Are indicative of parental abuse
c. They are flat, gray-blue in color
d. Any part of the body of dark-skinned babies

Ans.

101. b
102. d
103. a
104. d
105. c
106. d
107. b
108. d
109. b
110. a
111. b

Explanation: Mongolian spots are very common in any part of the body of dark-skinned babies. They are flat, gray-blue in color (almost looking like a bruise), and can be small or large. They are caused by some pigment that did not make it to the top layer when baby's skin was being formed. Most of the time it will disappear by 1 year of age.

112. Sequence of taking vital sign in a newborn infant is:
a. TPR b. PRT
c. RPT d. RTP

Explanation: Respiratory Rate should be assessed first before touching or handling the newborn because the newborn may cry while touching for temperature or pulse assessment that results in increased respiratory rate. So the sequence is respiratory rate, pulse and temperature.

113. Which of the following injections is routinely administered to a newborn to prevent bleeding? *(AIIMS Bhopal Nursing Officer, 2018)*
a. Injection vitamin K b. Soda bicarbonate
c. Calcium gluconate d. Methylergometrine

Explanation: Immediately after the birth of newborn inj. Vit K will be administered to newborn in order to prevent bleeding. Neonate have low plasma concentrations and low levels of vitamin K dependent clotting factors.

114. Gestational age of a newborn baby can be assessed by which one of the following scoring system:
a. Sarnat and Sarnat b. Downeys
c. Silvermans d. New Ballard

115. A newborn baby' skin covered with white sticky material which is known as:
a. Mongolian spot
b. Lanugo
c. Milia
d. Vernix

116. Identify the correct among the following related to umbilical cord care:
a. Apply peroxide to the cord with each diaper change
b. Cover the cord with petroleum jelly after bathing
c. Keep the cord dry and open to air
d. Wash the cord with soap and water each day during a tub bath

117. What all are the advantages of delayed cord clamping?
a. Improved hematologic status
b. Improved iron status
c. Reduced risk of IVH I preterm babies
d. All of the above

Explanation: All the above mentioned are the clinical advantages of delayed cord clamping. It will also decrease the incidence of anemia.

118. While teaching a primi mother about the care of umbilical cord, nurse should teach:
a. Apply lotions over the umbilical cord to keep it as moist
b. Cover the stump tightly
c. Drainage from the umbilical cord is the normal finding
d. Sponge bath the baby until the cord stump fall off

Explanation: Moisture will delay the stump to fall off. So sponge bath the baby until stump fall off. Nothing is supposed to apply in the stump and it should be exposed to air. Cord will fall of itself within a week.

119. Immediately after the delivery baby should be placed:
a. Mother's breast
b. Mother's abdomen
c. Side of the mother
d. Radiant warmer

120. Neonatal period is considered from:
a. Birth to 15 days
b. Birth to 21 days
c. Birth to 28 days
d. Birth to 1 month

121. When should the normal baby take bath?
a. After 1 hour of delivery b. After 24 hours
c. On 3rd day d. On 5th day

Explanation: It is recommended to wait at least 24 hours before bathing the baby. This will give the vernix time to absorb into the skin and protect it. After the initial 24 hours, a full bath can be given using warm water and mild soap specifically formulated for babies.

122. The expected respiratory rate of a neonate within 3 minutes of birth is:
a. 20-40 breaths per minute b. 40-60 breaths per minute
c. 60-80 breaths per minute d. >80 breaths per minute

123. The expected heart rate of a neonate within 3 minutes of birth is:
a. 90–120 b. 100–180
c. 100–130 d. 120–160

124. For accurate measurement of axillary temperature in newborn, thermometer is kept for how many minutes?
a. 1 minutes b. 2 minutes
c. 3 minutes d. 5 minutes

125. Small for gestational age and large for gestational age infants have polycythemia because of: *(AIIMS-BBS SNO 2019)*
a. Hypocalcemia b. Hypoglycemia
c. Hypoxia d. Hypothermia

Explanation: Polycythemia is defined as a venous hematocrit above 65% (too many RBCs in the blood). It can be caused by low oxygen level, chromosomal abnormalities, etc. It affects babies who are small for gestational age or large for gestational age.

126. Signs and symptoms of which of the following would be priority when caring for a newly delivered term neonate diagnosed as small for gestational age? *(RAK MSc 2018)*
a. Iron deficiency anemia
b. Birth asphyxia
c. Persistent pulmonary hypertension
d. Hyperglycemia

Explanation: Birth asphyxia is a major cause of neonatal mortality. Among the given options birth asphyxia in a small for gestational age (SGA) baby needs more concern & priority. Interventions of all other mentioned conditions can be delayed and addressed after managing a newborn for birth asphyxia.

NEONATAL REFLEXES

127. In Babinski's reflex among neonates, the movement of great toe undergoes:
a. Dorsi extension b. Dorsiflexion
c. Plantar flexion d. Plantar adduction

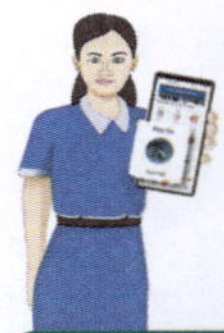

Ans.

112. c
113. a
114. d
115. d
116. c
117. d
118. d
119. a
120. c
121. b
122. b
123. d
124. d
125. c
126. b
127. b

128. Babinski sign is considered as normal in: *(AIIMS Raipur NO 2019)*

a. Newborn b. Adolescents
c. Youth d. Older adults

Explanation: Babinski sign is considered as normal in newborns and infants. Positive Babinski reflex in adults is indicative of abnormalities in the motor control pathways leading from the cerebral cortex.

129. All the following reflexes are present in the newborn baby; EXCEPT:

a. Sucking b. Rooting
c. Mature pincer grasp d. Pupillary reflex

Explanation: Mature pincer grasp will be developing by 9 months of age. All the other reflexes are present in a newborn baby.

130. The last neonatal reflex to emerge is:

a. Rooting reflex b. Grasp reflex
c. Babinski reflex d. Moro's reflex

Ref: Illingworth 10th ed,p 72; Achar Textbook of Pediatrics 4th ed, p 70, Table 6.2

Explanation:

Reflex	Emerges at gestational age
Palmar grasp	11 weeks
Babinski reflex	18 weeks
Moro reflex	8-9 weeks
Rooting reflex	28-30 weeks

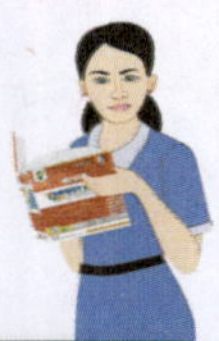

131. If a newborn's head and trunk is allowed to fall backward it elicits:

a. Step in reflex b. Plantar reflex
c. Startled reflex d. Moro reflex

132. Reflex response to a sudden loss of support, when the infant feels as if it is falling is known as:

a. Startle reflex
b. Glabella reflex
c. Moro reflex
d. Tonic neck reflex

133. The last neonatal reflex to disappear is:

a. Rooting reflex b. Grasp reflex
c. Plantar grasp d. Moro's reflex

134. Rooting reflex in infant disappears at:

a. 1 month b. 3 to 4 months
c. 6 to 8 months d. 9 to 12 months

Explanation:

Reflex	Age when reflex appears	Age when reflex disappears
Moro reflex	Birth	2 months
Walking/stepping	Birth	2 months
Rooting	Birth	4 months
Tonic neck reflex	Birth	5-7 months
Palmar grasp	Birth	5-6 months
Plantar grasp	Birth	9-12 months

Source: Caring for Your Baby and Young Child: Birth to Age 5 (Copyright © 2009 American Academy of Pediatrics

135. Newborn reflexes which are present at birth and remain unchanged throughout adulthood: *(Safdarjung NO 2018)*

a. Blinking, coughing, rooting and gag reflex
b. Blinking, coughing, sneezing and gag reflex
c. Rooting, sneezing, swallowing and coughing
d. Stepping, blinking, coughing and sneezing

Explanation: **Blinking, coughing, sneezing and gag** reflexes are mature reflexes and as we grow, they do not disappear as they are needed for normal survival. They are known as protective reflexes.

136. Neonatal reflex elicited by touching the cheeks of the baby is:

a. Moro reflex b. Rooting reflex
c. Startle reflex d. Sucking reflex

137. Asymmetric Moro's reflex at birth is indicative of:

a. Hypoxic ischemic encephalopathy
b. Brain damage
c. Erb's palsy d. Kernicterus

THERMOREGULATION IN NEWBORN

138. The normal axillary temperature of a newborn is between which of the following ranges? ***(AIIMS Bhopal Nursing Officer, 2018)***

a. 40°–42°C b. 30°–32°C
c. 32.5°–34°C d. 36.5°–37.4°C

Explanation: 36.5°–37.4°C is the normal axillary temperature of a newborn baby. If temperature is less than 36.5°C, it is called as hypothermia.

139. Which of the following is not a nursing intervention to maintain the temperature of a newborn? *(AIIMS-BBS SNO 2019)*

a. Dry the newborn immediately after birth
b. Wrap the newborn in warmed blankets
c. Use a warmed cloth for weighing the unclothed newborn
d. Place the newborn near draughts or air vents

Explanation: One of the basic needs of newborn is "warmth". Placing the newborn near air vents will put the newborn at risk of hypothermia due to convection heat loss.

140. Which babies are at higher risk to have hypothermia?

a. Baby with any congenital abnormality
b. Low birth weight babies
c. Healthy baby
d. One year old child.

141. The best method to prevent hypothermia in LBW babies is:

a. Temperature recording b. Hot sponging
c. Warm chain d. Keep baby in cradle

142. While assisting delivery, which of the following intervention by the nurse will prevent heat loss in the newborn due to evaporation?

a. Pre-warming the crib pad
b. Turn on overhead radiant warmer
c. Drying the newborn in a warm blanket
d. Closing the doors of the room

143. Which of the following assessment findings is most suggestive of hypothermia in a neonate?

a. Perspiration b. Tachycardia
c. Bradycardia d. Metabolic alkalosis

Ans.

128.	a
129.	c
130.	a
131.	d
132.	c
133.	c
134.	b
135.	b
136.	b
137.	c
138.	d
139.	d
140.	b
141.	c
142.	c
143.	c

Explanation: Bradycardia proportional to the degree of core temperature is seen in neonates with hypothermia. Perspiration and tachycardia is seen in hyperthermic neonates. Metabolic acidosis is seen in hypoglycemia.

144. Hypothermia is characterized by all; EXCEPT:
- a. Poor feeding
- b. Metabolic acidosis
- c. Increased peripheral perfusion
- d. Respiratory distress

145. All interventions prevent hypothermia in preterm babies; EXCEPT:
- a. Use of polyethylene plastic wraps
- b. Using double layered incubators
- c. Using woolen caps to cover head
- d. Keeping the delivery room temperature at 22°C

146. Moderate hypothermia in neonate is defined as an axillary temperature of:
- a. <32°C
- b. <34°C
- c. 35°–36.9°C
- d. 32°–35.9°C

147. A 1-month-old infant was brought to the casualty with complaints of lethargy and mild increase in temperature and poor feeding. There is no history of cough cold or loose stools. On examination, the infant had sunken eyes and skin pinch was not immediate, temperature was 99°F. What is the most probable diagnosis? *New Q*
- a. Dehydration fever
- b. Sepsis
- c. Normal phenomenon
- d. Post immunization reaction

Explanation: The symptoms of dehydration fever are similar to the symptoms of sepsis, but the absence of loose stools and presence of sunken eyes suggest dehydration fever. No immediate skin pinch is also a sign of dehydration.

148. Hypothermia is stated as a body temperature:
- a. Equal to 35°C
- b. Below 36.5°C
- c. Between 36.5 to 37.5°C
- d. Above 38°C

149. On what basic principle the heat exchange occur in infant incubator? *New Q*
- a. Convection
- b. Evaporation
- c. Conduction
- d. Radiation

150. Severe hypothermia in a neonate is:
- a. When the body temperature is below 30°C.
- b. When the body temperature is below 32°C.
- c. When the body temperature is above 34°C.
- d. When the body temperature is above 36°C.

151. Hypothermia in neonate is characterized by all of the following; EXCEPT: *(PGI Dec 2002)*
- a. Hyperactivity
- b. Respiratory distress
- c. Apnea
- d. Tachypnea

Explanation: Signs and symptoms of hypothermia in neonate include:
- Peripheral vasoconstriction
- Acrocyanosis, cold extremities
- Decreased peripheral perfusion
- CNS depression
- Lethargy, bradycardia, apnea, poor feeding
- Increased pulmonary artery pressure
- Respiratory distress, tachypnea
- Chronic signs
- Weight loss, failure to thrive

152. Signs and symptoms of Hypothermia are all; EXCEPT: *(Recent Question 2015)*
- a. Poor feeding
- b. Apnea
- c. Central cyanosis
- d. Cool extremities

Ref: CPDT 22nd e, p 352

Explanation:
Signs and symptom of hypothermia:
- Acrocyanosis (peripheral cyanosis)
- Cool extremities
- Decreased peripheral perfusion
- Lethargy, bradycardia, apnea, poor feeding
- Hypoglycemia, hypoxia, metabolic acidosis
- Respiratory distress, Tachypnea
- Weight loss

153. What are the causes of hypothermia?
- a. Congenital disorders
- b. Trauma, dehydration and diarrhea
- c. Birth asphyxia, infections and prematurity
- d. Atresia, spina bifida

154. The early symptoms occur in hypothermia:
- a. Weight loss, pale body, hypoglycemia
- b. Edema and central cyanosis, sclerema
- c. Respiratory distress and bradycardia
- d. Feet and hand are cold and body becomes blue, weak suckling, lethargy and weak cry

155. Which of the measures should be chosen to prevent hypothermia after delivery?
- a. Drying, bathing, weighing and vital recording
- b. Wrapping, vital recording, bathing and breastfeeding
- c. Drying, wrapping, weighing, and breastfeeding
- d. Wrapping, bathing, vital recording, bottle feeding

156. Treatment used to provide standard thermal care to prevent neonatal hypothermia in NICU is:
- a. Use of phototherapy
- b. Incubator/radiant warmer
- c. Bathing & weighing
- d. Oxygen support

157. The most prone period of neonatal death due to hypothermia is:
- a. First 24 hours/first week
- b. 2 months
- c. 6 months
- d. 8- 12 months

158. What should be the temperature of delivery room to maintain warmth for neonate?
- a. 21°–24°C
- b. 25°–28°C
- c. 28°–30°C
- d. Above 30°C

KANGAROO MOTHERCARE

159. Kangaroo mother care is necessary till baby attains a weight of: *(J&K PG 2011)*
- a. 1500 g
- b. 2000 g
- c. 2500 g
- d. 3000 g

Ref: OP Ghai 8th ed. p 148

Explanation: WHO recommends that KMC to be continued till baby attains a weight of 2.5 kg or till babies wriggle out, indicating that they do not need kangaroo mother care any further.

160. KMC is mostly applicable to which women:
- a. All pregnant women
- b. Only women who are at high risk of delivering a pre- term/ LBW babies
- c. Only women who are booked to deliver in hospital
- d. Only primigravid women

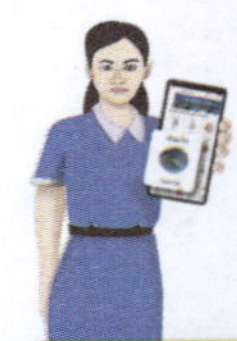

Ans.

144.	c
145.	d
146.	d
147.	a
148.	b
149.	a
150.	b
151.	a
152.	c
153.	c
154.	d
155.	c
156.	b
157.	a
158.	b
159.	c
160.	b

161. The position of the baby during KMC should be:
a. A special garment is needed
b. A blanket is used to keep the infant on the mother's back
c. Keep baby on mother's chest, head turned to one side and support bottom with belt or hand
d. Baby should be kept on mother's lateral side

162. Who should take the infant out of the incubator for KMC?
a. Only the doctor
b. The nurse
c. Either the doctor or the nurse
d. The mother

163. How the baby should be monitored during KMC?
a. With an apnea alarm.
b. A nurse must observe the infant while the mother is giving KMC.
c. Usually no monitoring is needed.
d. The baby vital signs must be recorded every 30 minutes.

164. Which baby should not be given KMC?
a. Babies in incubators.
b. Babies who are having recurrent apnea.
c. Babies who are not breastfeeding yet.
d. Babies whose weight is less than 1200 gram

165. The duration of providing KMC should be:
a. ½ hour b. 1 hour
c. 2 hours d. 3 hours

166. Key features of kangaroo mother care are all the following; EXCEPT: *(AP PG 2014)*
a. Skin to skin contact between mother and baby
b. Exclusive breastfeeding
c. Initiated in a facility and continued at home
d. Done for babies with cyanosis

Ref: OP Ghai 8th ed. p 150

Explanation: Kangaroo care is a technique practiced on newborn, usually preterm, infants wherein the infant is held, skin-to-skin, with an adult.
- The kangaroo position provided ready access to nourishment.
- The parent's stable body temperature helps to regulate the neonate's temperature more smoothly than an incubator, and allows for readily accessible breastfeeding.
- Babies who are eligible for kangaroo care include pre-term infants, weighing less than 1,500 grams, and breathing independently.
- Cardiopulmonary monitoring, oximetry, supplemental oxygen or nasal continuous positive airway pressure ventilation, intravenous infusion, and monitor leads do not prevent kangaroo care.
- Babies who are in kangaroo care tend to be less prone to apnea and bradycardia and have stabilization of oxygen needs.

167. Which of the following is not a component of Kangaroo mother care (KMC)?
a. Skin to skin contact
b. Supplementary nutrition
c. Exclusive breastfeeding
d. Early discharge and follow-up

168. KMC means:
a. Skin to skin contact
b. Back to back contact
c. Hand to hand contact
d. Contact of baby with mother clothes

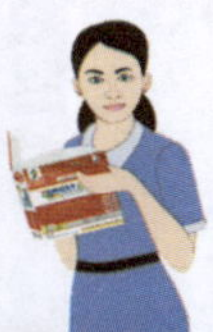

Ans.
161. c
162. c
163. d
164. b
165. b
166. d
167. b
168. a
169. c
170. b
171. a
172. a
173. d
174. c

HIGH RISK NEWBORN (LBW, PREMATURITY)

169. For assessing the gestational age of preterm infant the nurse should use:
a. Palmar creases b. Reflex stability
c. Breast bud size d. Head to toe length

Explanation: The size of breast bud is an indication of gestational age. Small under developed nipple indicate prematurity.

170. In preterm labor, medication given to the mother to establish fetal lung maturity is:
a. Prostaglandin b. Betamethasone
c. Oxytocin d. Adrenaline

171. Lecithin/Sphingomyelin ratio is done to assess the maturity of: *(JIPMER 2014)*
a. Lung b. Fetal circulation
c. Brain d. Gonad

Ref: OP Ghai 8th ed. p 169

Explanation: The Lecithin-Sphingomyelin (L/S) Ratio
- Assessment of fetal lung maturity (FLM) prenatally by testing amniotic fluid obtained by amniocentesis.
- It is performed by thin-layer chromatography.
- The risk of RDS is very low if the L/S ratio is >2.
- Exceptions to L/S ratio >2 are:
- Infants of diabetic mothers (IDMs).
- Intrapartum asphyxia.
- Erythroblastosis fetalis.

172. Most common cause of neonatal death in India: *(AIIMS Nov 2010)*
a. Prematurity b. Infection
c. RDS d. HIE

Ref: Lancet 2010 November 27; 376(9755) 1853-1860

Explanation: The major causes of newborn deaths in India are:
- Prematurity/preterm - 35%
- Neonatal infections - 33%
- Intrapartum related complications/birth asphyxia - 20% and
- Congenital malformations - 9%

Source: UNICEF

173. Which of the following is a major risk factor for having a low birth weight baby? *(RAK MSc 2018)*
a. Heredity
b. Smoking
c. Drugs used during pregnancy
d. Poor nutrition

Explanation:
- **Poor nutrition** is a major risk factor for having a low-birth-weight-baby. Nutritional status of the mother is extremely important for the growth of the fetus.
- Other primary factors associated with low birth weight baby includes genetics, age of the mother, smoking status of mother and prenatal care.

174. According to World Health Organization, "low birth weight" means a weight of less than: *(SSNE 2015)*
a. 2.8 kg b. 2.7 kg
c. 2.5 kg d. 2.3 kg

175. 'Extremely low birth weight' babies have a birth weight of: *(AIIMS Bhopal Nursing Officer, 2018)*

a. 1000 to 1,500 g b. Less than 1000 g
c. 3000 to 2,500 g d. 2,500 to 1,500 g

Explanation:

1500 g - 2500 g	Low birth weight
1000 g to 1500 g	Very low birth weight
Less than 1000 g	Extremely low birth weight

176. Antenatal smoking by the pregnant women may lead to:

a. Coarctation of aorta b. Low birth weight
c. Macrosomia d. Acromegaly

177. The most common complication in low birth weight infant is: *(RAK MSc 2018)*

a. Respiratory distress
b. Mucus damage
c. Brain damage
d. Hemorrhage

Explanation: Low birth weight is most often caused by premature birth. Respiratory distress is the most common complication in preterm babies as their lungs are not mature at the time of delivery. Other complications of LBW babies include hypothermia, perinatal asphyxia, bacterial sepsis, apnea of prematurity, etc.

178. How to keep a LBW baby warm:

a. Keeping the room warm
b. Kangaroo mother care (KMC)
c. Adequate breastfeeding
d. All of the above

179. The LBW baby gets discharged to home:

a. When the baby weight reaches to 1800 grams
b. When the baby weight is 2000 grams
c. When the baby reaches to term period
d. When the baby is feeding well & gaining weight

180. The calories needed in LBW infant is:

a. 50–60 kcal/kg/day
b. 70–110 kcal/kg/day
c. 120–140 kcal/kg/day
d. 150–200 kcal/kg/day

181. All of the following are features of prematurity in a neonate; EXCEPT:

a. No creases on sole
b. Abundant lanugo
c. Thick ear cartilage
d. Empty scrotum

NEWBORN RESUSCITATION

182. The ratio of lung inflation to chest compression in cardio pulmonary resuscitation is: *(UP 2010)*

a. 1:5 b. 2:5
c. 1:3 d. 3:1

Ref: OP Ghai 8th ed. p 131

Explanation: Provider should perform chest compressions while the other maintains the airway and performs Ventilations: Compressions at a ratio of 1:3 with as short a pause in compression as possible.

183. Expanded form of TABC used in neonatal resuscitation is:

a. Thermometer, airway, breathing, circulation
b. Temperature, atmosphere, breathing, compression
c. Temperament, airway, breathing, circulation
d. Temperature, airway, breathing, circulation

184. What is the ideal temperature of the newborn resuscitation room? *(AIIMS Nov 2016)*

a. 37–39°C b. 32–34°C
c. 28–30°C d. 25–27°C

Ref: O.P Ghai 8th Ed, pg 133

Explanation: Immediately after birth the newborn is at high risk for hypothermia. The temperature of delivery room should be 25 degrees Celsius and it should be free from draft of air.

185. Recommended dose of Adrenaline used for neonatal resuscitation is: *New Q*

a. 0.01 mg/kg/body weight (0.1 mL/kg, 1:10000)
b. 1 mg/kg body weight (1 mL, 1:1000)
c. 0.1 mg/kg body weight (0.1 mL, 1:10000)
d. 0.5 mg/kg body weight (0.1 mL/kg, 1:1000)

186. When caring for an infant during cardiac arrest, which pulse must be palpated to determine cardiac function? *(NCFL 2019)*

a. Carotid b. Brachial
c. Pedal d. Radial

187. The first medication that may be required in the resuscitation of baby with prolonged birth asphyxia is:

a. Sodium bicarbonate
b. Adrenalin in 1:10000 dilution
c. Calcium gluconate
d. 25% dextrose

188. Size of suction catheter used in neonate for oral and nasal suction is:

a. 8 Fr b. 12 Fr
c. 14 Fr d. 16 Fr

189. In Neonatal Resuscitation __________ are seldom needed to stimulate the heart, increase tissue perfusion, and restore acid base balance.

a. Medication b. Chest Compression.
c. Bag and mask ventilation d. Tactile stimulation.

190. In Neonatal resuscitation, compressions should be delivered on the:

a. Upper half of sternum
b. Lower half of sternum
c. Upper third of sternum
d. Lower third of sternum

Explanation: Compressions should be delivered on the lower third of the sternum to a depth of approximately one-third of the anterior-posterior diameter of the chest.

Two techniques have been described: compression with 2 thumbs with fingers encircling the chest and supporting the back (the 2 thumb–encircling hands technique) or compression with 2 fingers with a second hand supporting the back. (AHA Guidelines 2010)

191. Bag and mask ventilation is contraindicated in newborn resuscitation with clinical suspicion of all of the following conditions; EXCEPT:

a. Diaphragmatic hernia b. Tracheoesophageal fistula
c. Meconium aspiration d. Lung malformation

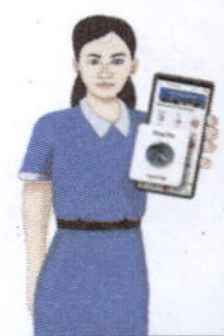

Ans.

175. b
176. b
177. a
178. d
179. d
180. c
181. c
182. c
183. d
184. d
185. a
186. b
187. b
188. a
189. a
190. d
191. d

Explanation: In diaphragmatic hernia, bag and mask ventilation (BMV) leads to further distension of bowel.

Air through Tracheoesophageal fistula can result in increased gastric pressure.

In meconium aspiration, BMV will further increase the risk of aspiration.

192. During resuscitation shoulder roll is placed under baby's shoulder to slightly extent the neck. This is because:

a. It brings posterior pharynx, larynx and trachea in a line
b. Facilitate drainage from the mouth
c. More amount of air will pass
d. It promotes inspiration and expiration

Explanation: Shoulder roll brings posterior pharynx, larynx and trachea in a line and it will facilitate breathing in newborn baby and will also help in easy intubation.

193. During neonatal resuscitation, what is the order of clearance of secretions?

a. Mouth first followed by nasal cavity
b. Nasal cavity followed by mouth
c. Pharynx followed by mouth
d. None of the above

Ref: OP Ghai 8th Ed, p 128

Explanation: During neonatal resuscitation, secretion may be removed from the airway by wiping the nose and mouth with a clean cloth or by suctioning with a bulb syringe or suction catheter.

The mouth is suctioned before nose (*remember, 'M' before 'N'*) to ensure the infant does not aspirate, if she should gasp when the nose is suctioned.

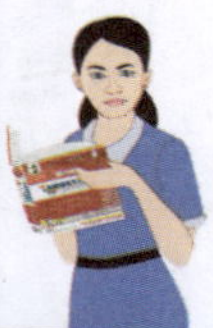

194. Which is the ideal route for administration of drugs during newborn resuscitation? *(AIIMS Nov 2016)*

a. Endotracheal
b. Umbilical artery
c. Umbilical vein
d. Intraosseous

Ref: Cloherty 7th Ed., pg 56

Explanation: The most accessible intravenous (IV) route for neonatal administration of medications is catheterization of the umbilical vein, which can be done rapidly and aseptically.

The most commonly used medication is epinephrine (as 1:10,000 solution). Intravenous fluids and naloxone can also be given.

195. What should be the size of the endotracheal tube for a newborn weighing 2,000 to 3,000 gms? *(AIIMS Bhopal Nursing Officer, 2018)*

a. 4. 0
b. 3. 0
c. 2. 5
d. 3. 5

Explanation:

Tube size	Birth weight	Gestational age
4. 0	>3 kg	Term
3. 5	2–3 kg	34–38 weeks
3. 0	1–2 kg	28–34 weeks
2. 5	<1 kg	≤28 weeks

196. Which one of the following includes the immediate step in resuscitation of the newborn?

a. Squeezing the chest to remove secretions from the airway
b. Routinely giving sodium bicarbonate
c. Clearing the oral and nasal airway
d. Suction of the baby's stomach

RESPIRATORY ISSUES IN NEWBORN

197. All are the characteristics of neonatal asphyxia; EXCEPT:

a. Hypoxia
b. Hypoperfusion
c. Hypocapnia
d. Acidosis

198. The nurse would expect to find in a newborn with birth asphyxia: *(Safdarjung NO 2018)*

a. Hyperoxia
b. Acidosis
c. Hypocapnia
d. Ketosis

Explanation: In birth asphyxia, there is accumulation of carbon dioxide in the blood resulting in respiratory acidosis.

199. In full term newborns, functional closure of ductus arteriosus occurs ______ after birth.

a. Within 3 weeks
b. Within 2 weeks
c. Within 1 week
d. Within 24-72 hours

Explanation: Normally, the ductus arteriosus closes within 24–72 hours after a full-term birth; if after 72 hours the ductus fails to close, a diagnosis of persistent PDA may be made. This is known as functional closure. Permanent or anatomic closure is complete within 2 to 3 weeks.

200. Which drug is used to treat PDA?

a. Oxaceprol
b. Morphine
c. Dopamine
d. Indomethacin

201. Drug used for closure of patent ductus areteriosus:

a. Paracetamol
b. Ibuprofen
c. Indomethacin
d. All of the above

202. Drug of choice to keep ductus arteriosus patent is:

a. Paracetamol
b. Ibuprofen
c. Indomethacin
d. Prostaglandin

Explanation: Prostaglandin [PGE1 (Misoprost)] is the drug of choice to keep PDA open.

FEEDING IN CHILDREN

203. After birth of a baby, breastfeeding should be started:

a. Within first half hour to 2 hours
b. Within 2 hours to 6 hours
c. Within 8 hours to 16 hours
d. After 24 hours

204. Which one of the following is most suggestive of neonatal small bowel obstruction?

a. Generalized abdominal distension
b. Failure to pass meconium in the first 24 hours
c. Bilious vomiting
d. Refusal of feeds

Ans.

192. a
193. a
194. c
195. d
196. c
197. c
198. b
199. d
200. d
201. d
202. d
203. a
204. b

205. Adequate breastfeeding in baby indicates: *(MP PG 2008)*

a. Baby sleeps 2 hour after feeds
b. Does not cry frequently
c. Urine 5-7 times/day
d. Stool 4 times/day

Ref: OP Ghai 8th ed. p 151; 7th e, p 452

Explanation: A newborn who is adequately breastfed will sleep at least 2 hours, pass urine 8 to 10 times a day and will gain weight.

206. The first milk produced after delivery is known as:

a. Colostrum b. Lactose
c. Hindmilk d. Pseudo milk

207. The thick yellow color breast milk secreted initially is:

a. Colostrum b. Foremilk
c. Hindmilk d. Mature milk

208. Milk secreted following colostrum is:

a. Foremilk b. Hindmilk
c. Transition Milk d. Mature milk

209. What is correct about breast milk?

a. Hindmilk is rich in proteins
b. Fat in breast milk is rich in iron
c. Colostrum must be discarded
d. Feeding in supine position increases risk of otitis media

Ref: O.P Ghai 8th Ed., pg 151

Explanation: Fat content in breast milk and cow's milk is similar. However, the amount of PUFA (Polyunsaturated) is significantly higher in breast milk which helps in the myelination of nervous system.

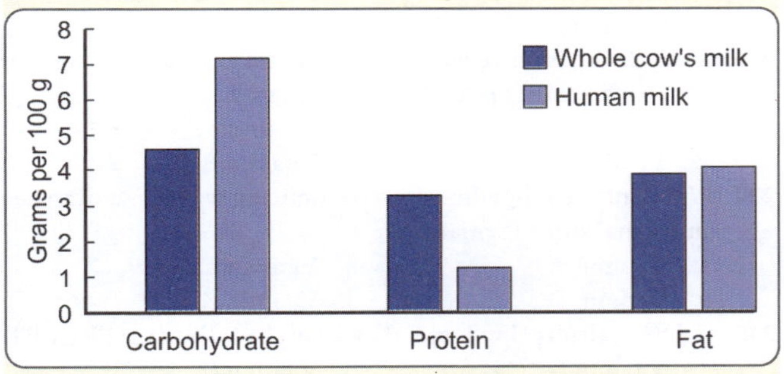

Foremilk (milk secreted at the start of feed) is rich in proteins, sugar and minerals whereas hindmilk is rich in fat and provides more energy.

Colostrum is the milk that is secreted during initial during first 3–4 days after delivery which should not be discarded.

Improper breastfeeding techniques like supine feeding is significantly associated with occurrence of acute otitis media in infants.

210. Exclusive breastfeeding is advised in all; EXCEPT:

a. Diarrhea b. Evening colic
c. Jaundice d. Typhoid

211. Exclusive breastfeed should be provided to the baby:

a. Up to 2 months b. Up to 6 months
c. Up to 1 year d. More than 1 year

212. The extra calories needed by mother during breastfeeding is:

a. 100 calories b. 300 calories
c. 500 calories d. 1000 calories

213. The parents of a 5-day-old term infant notice that he is jaundiced. Your physical examination is remarkable only for scleral icterus and jaundice. The infant's total bilirubin level is 15 mg/dL, with a direct component of 0.4 mg/dL. Which of the following is the most likely diagnosis? *New Q*

a. Pyloric stenosis b. Biliary atresia
c. Breast milk jaundice d. Neonatal hepatitis

Explanation: Breast milk jaundice typically presents within the first two weeks of life in an otherwise healthy infant who is predominantly breastfed.

214. Initially the mother should feed the baby at least:

a. 3 times a day
b. 5-6 times a day
c. 8-12 times a day
d. 10-16 times a day

215. The initial feeding should last for:

a. 1–2 min on each breast
b. 2–4 min on each breast
c. 5–10 min on each breast
d. 10–15 min on each breast

216. Which of the statements is true about breastfeeding?

a. It promotes infections in the baby
b. It reduces risk of developing breast cancer in mother
c. It worsens the baby's digestive system
d. It makes the mother susceptible to infections

217. The benefit of breastfeeding is:

a. To strengthen the bond between the mother and the baby
b. To help the uterus contract after delivery
c. To reduce the risk of breast cancer
d. All of the above

218. Which of these medications should be avoided while breastfeeding?

a. Birth control pills
b. Iodine
c. Antibiotics
d. All of these

219. When the burping should be done?

a. Before each feed
b. Middle and at the end of each feed
c. Only at the end of each feed
d. After 1 hour of feed

220. The symptoms of adequate feeding in baby is:

a. Baby stools are yellow & loose
b. Baby empties his bladder often
c. Baby steadily gains weight
d. All of the above

221. At what interval the mother should feed the baby:

a. 1/2 – 1 hour b. 2-3 hours
c. 3-4 hours d. 4-5 hours

222. Breast milk storage in a refrigerator is up to:

a. 4 hours b. 8 hours
c. 12 hours d. 24 hours

223. Expressed breast milk can be stored at room temperature for how many hours? *(Recent Question 2015)*

a. 4 b. 8
c. 16 d. 24

Ref: OP Ghai 8th ed. p 155

Ans.

205. a
206. a
207. a
208. c
209. d
210. b
211. b
212. c
213. c
214. c
215. c
216. b
217. d
218. d
219. b
220. d
221. b
222. d
223. a

Explanation:

Human Milk Storage Guidelines

Storage Locations and Temperatures

Type of Breast Milk	Countertop 77°F or colder (25°C) (room temperature)	Refrigerator 40°F (4°C)	Freezer 0°F or colder (–18°C)
Freshly Expressed or Pumped	Up to 4 hours	Up to 4 days	Within 6 months is best up to 12 months is acceptable
Thawed, Previously Frozen	1–2 hours	Up to 1 day (24 hours)	Never refreeze human milk after it has been thawed
Left Over from a Feeding (baby did not finish the bottle)	Use within 2 hours after the baby is finished feeding		

Source: Center for Disease Control and Prevention. Revised 2017.

224. Cow's milk is deficient of:
a. Calcium b. Fat
c. Iron d. Lactose

225. What is the sign of good attachment?
a. Baby's chin touches the breast.
b. Baby's mouth is wide open with the lower lip curled out.
c. Baby suckles with slow, deep sucks and pauses sometimes.
d. All of the above.

226. Nipple confusion means: *(AP PG 2014)*
a. Baby fed with a bottle finding it difficult and confusing to suckle at breast
b. Baby not able to suckle with bottle
c. Baby not able to feed with spoon
d. Baby not able to feed with paladai

227. Breastfeeding is contraindicated if the mother is receiving:
a. Aspirin b. Prednisone
c. Amiodarone d. Erythromycin

228. Breastfeeding is contraindicated if mother has: New Q
a. Hepatitis C
b. Cardiomyopathy
c. Active untreated tuberculosis
d. Typhoid

229. Food item need to be introduced following weaning is:
a. Solid diet b. Semi solid diet
c. Liquid diet d. Spicy food

230. Which is the best solid food that can be used during the process of weaning?
a. Fruits b. Vegetables
c. Egg white d. Rice cereals

231. Age at which weaning needs to be initiated is: *(NORCET 2021)*
a. 4 to 6 months b. 6 to 8 months
c. 8 to 10 months d. 10 to 12 months

232. In India, the only true contraindication to breastfeeding is: New Q
a. Maternal HIV
b. Infants with classic galactosemia
c. Infants with G6PD deficiency
d. Maternal typhoid infection

Explanation: Galactosemia in an infant is a contraindication to breastfeeding. This is because galactose, a sugar found in breast milk, can be harmful to babies with classic galactosemia.

There are no medical conditions in the mother that are absolute contraindications, although diagnostic procedures, treatment, or illness can interfere.

In the USA, mothers with HIV are not recommended to breastfeed.

233. Nutritional advice given to the mother of a 5-month-old non-breastfeeding child is:
a. Cow's milk
b. Formula feeds available
c. Skim milk and baby food
d. Iron-rich formula only

Explanation: At the age of 5 months, a child should receive iron-rich formula and that they should not receive solid food even baby food until age of 6 months. Iron rich feed is essential because baby is depending upon the stored iron in the initial months, so depletion of stored iron will be there. So to replenish, the source iron should be supplied to the baby.

234. Identify the management of breast engorgement among the following:
a. Wear a tight-fitting bra or breast binder
b. Apply warm, moist heat to the breasts
c. Contact the nurse midwife for a lactation suppressant
d. Restrict fluid intake to 1000 mL daily

235. In malnourished children the following parameters are reliable indicators of dehydration; EXCEPT?
a. Skin turgor b. Dry buccal mucosa
c. Oliguria d. Thirst

236. A child who is on vegetarian diet only. The pediatric nurse is alert to the child's potential deficiency of:
a. Niacin b. Thiamin
c. Vitamin B6 d. Vitamin B12

237. Which of the following vitamins deficiency leads to diarrhea and, renal stone formation?
a. Vitamin A b. Vitamin C
c. Vitamin D d. Vitamin K

238. Calcium absorption is aided by all of the following; EXCEPT:
a. Vitamin D b. Vitamin C
c. Lactose d. Fat

239. Identify correct statement in relation to vitamin A:
a. Recommended dose of vitamin A at 9 months of age is 1,00,000 IU
b. Vitamin A administered via oral route
c. After the first dose of Vit. A dose need to be repeated every 6 months till 5 years of age
d. All of the above

240. In children, rickets occurs because of the deficiency of:
a. Vitamin A b. Vitamin B
c. Vitamin D d. Vitamin E

241. Anti-infective vitamin is:
a. Vitamin- A b. Vitamin- B
c. Vitamin- C d. Vitamin- D

242. Failure to thrive is:
a. Child is unable to stand
b. Child is unable to sit
c. Child is not gaining weight adequately
d. Child is unable to speak

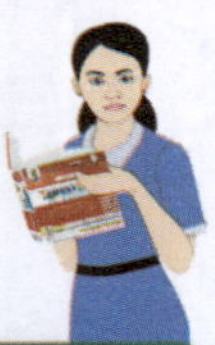

Ans.
224. c
225. d
226. a
227. c
228. c
229. b
230. d
231. a
232. b
233. d
234. b
235. d
236. d
237. c
238. d
239. d
240. c
241. a
242. c

243. Failure to thrive include all among the following; EXCEPT:
a. Growth is lagging behind
b. Infant not gaining weight adequately
c. Infant looks small for age
d. Poor response to social stimuli

IMMUNIZATION SCHEDULE

244. If a mother had measles during pregnancy, her newborn baby would be immunized to this disease for:
a. 4 to 6 months
b. 6 to 12 months
c. 1 to 3 years
d. 3 to 6 years

245. Artificially acquired immunity is obtained by: *(ESIC 2019)*
a. Recovering from a disease
b. Exposure to a disease
c. Being breastfed
d. Immunization with antibody response

Explanation: Recovering from a disease, exposure to a disease (natural active) and breastfeeding (natural passive) are examples of natural immunity. Immunization with antibody response is an artificial immunity. Antibodies are administered from outside, not prepared by body.

246. What are the vaccines recommended at birth as per the universal immunizations program? *(Recent Question 2015)*
a. BCG
b. BCG and Hepatitis B
c. BCG and DPT
d. DT and oral Polio-vaccine

Explanation: OP Ghai 8th ed. p 203

247. DPT is contraindicated in: *(UP 2009)*
a. Family history of convulsions
b. Acute respiratory tract infections
c. Progressive neurological illness
d. Mild diarrhea

Ref: OP Ghai 8th ed. p 193, 194

Explanation: Following are not contraindication for administration of DPT vaccine.
- Mild acute illness
- Low grade fever
- Mild diarrhea
- Current antibiotic therapy
- Prematurity
- Recent exposure to an infectious disease
- History of allergies
- Allergy to penicillin
- Malnutrition

248. An 18-month-old child was brought to the well-baby clinic for booster dose of DPT vaccine. Which among the following muscles is preferred by the nurse to administer vaccine? *(AIIMS Bhopal Grade-I 2018)*
a. Dorsogluteal
b. Ventrogluteal
c. Deltoid
d. Vastus lateralis

Explanation: Vastus lateralis is the best choice for IM injection because in infants or younger children this muscle has an adequate amount of muscle mass. If another muscle is used the delivery of vaccine could be compromised or needle may hit the bone which may cause severe pain.

249. A parent brings her 4-month-old infant to a well-baby clinic for immunizations. The child is up to date with the immunization schedule. The nurse should prepare to administer which immunizations to this infant? *New Q*
a. Varicella, hepatitis B vaccine (HepB)
b. Diphtheria, tetanus, acellular pertussis (DTaP); measles, mumps, rubella (MMR); inactivated poliovirus vaccine (IPV)
c. MMR, Haemophilus influenza type b (Hib), DTaP
d. OPV-3, Pentavalent-3, fIPV, pneumococcal vaccine (PCV), rotavirus vaccine (RV)

250. What is the route of administration of MMR vaccine? *(AIIMS Bhopal Nursing Officer, 2018)*
a. Subcutaneous
b. Oral
c. Nasal
d. Intradermal

Explanation: MMR is a live vaccine and route of administration is subcutaneous. OPV is administered via oral route and BCG is administered via intradermal route.

251. Which of the following is a viral vaccine? *(AIIMS Bhopal Nursing Officer, 2018)*
a. Oral polio vaccine
b. Cholera
c. Bacilli calmette guerin
d. Tetanus toxoid

Explanation: OPV is viral vaccine, cholera is inactivated vaccine, BCG is live bacterial vaccine and tetanus is toxoid.

252. Which of the following vaccines is administered to the newborn within 12 hours of birth?
a. Rubella
b. Hepatitis B
c. Rotavirus
d. Measles

Explanation: The World Health Organization recommends all infants receive the first dose of the hepatitis B vaccine within 24 hours of birth. According to Center for Disease Control (CDC), Hepatitis B vaccination works best when the baby gets it within the first 12 hours of his life. Rubella, Rotavirus vaccine is given at 6 weeks. Measles and Rubella vaccine are given at 9 months.

253. A 13-month-old child who has never been immunized now comes to the hospital. What will your advice regarding immunization according to National immunization schedule?
a. 1 dose BCG, 3 doses OPV, 3 doses DPT
b. 1 dose IPV, 3 doses OPV, 3 doses Pentavalent
c. 3 doses OPV, 3 doses DTP
d. 3 doses Hib, 3 doses Hep B

Explanation: As per the latest immunization schedule, BCG can be given till 1 year of age. Since this child is now 13 months old, BCG need not be given. Also, in the latest schedule, pentavalent vaccines are included in the schedule instead of DPT. Hence this child requires 1 dose IPV, 3 doses OPV, 3 doses of pentavalent vaccine.

254. Which vaccine is contraindicated in child with history of convulsions? *(AIIMS June 2008)*
a. DPT
b. Measles
c. Typhoid
d. BCG

Ref: OP Ghai 8th ed. p 205; IAP Guide Book on Immunization, 3/e p14

Explanation: Pertussis component of DPT vaccine is contraindicated in children with neurological problems such as convulsion.

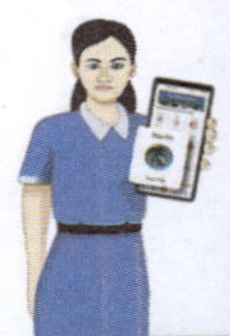

Ans.
243. d
244. a
245. d
246. b
247. c
248. d
249. d
250. a
251. a
252. b
253. b
254. a

255. Varicella vaccine provide protection against:

a. Chicken pox b. Dengue
c. Encephalitis d. Meningitis

Explanation: Varicella vaccine provide protection against chicken pox.

256. What is the Percentage of polio infections that is asymptomatic? *(PGI 2008)*

a. 1% b. 20%
c. 30% d. 90%

Explanation: 90% of polio infection are asymptomatic.

257. All are true about killed vaccine; EXCEPT:

a. Prepared by growing bacteria/virus in a media followed by inactivation with heat/chemical
b. Do not cause infection but elicit immune response
c. Multiple dose is required
d. Between two killed vaccines minimum 4 weeks gap is required.

Explanation: Between two killed vaccines there is no recommended duration. All other statements are true in relation with killed vaccines

258. Identify the incorrect pair among the following:

a. BCG- TB- Intradermal b. DPT - Pertussis - SC
c. MMR- Rubella-S/C d. OPV-Polio- Oral

Explanation: DPT stands for Diphtheria, Pertussis and Tetanus. But the route of administration of DPT vaccine is Intramuscular (IM).

259. Subacute sclerosing panencephalitis is a complication associated with ....vaccine.

a. BCG b. Measles
c. MMR d. OPV

Explanation: Subacute sclerosing panencephalitis may occur years after measles vaccination. In this condition progressive, debilitating, and deadly brain disorder related to measles (Rubeola) infection.

260. A 6-year-old child is scheduled to have measles, mumps, and rubella (MMR) vaccine. Which of the following routes will you expect the nurse to administer the vaccine? New Q

a. Intramuscularly in the vastus lateralis muscle
b. Intramuscularly in the deltoid muscle
c. Subcutaneously in the gluteal area
d. Subcutaneously in the outer aspect of the upper arm

261. The process administering the vaccine/antigen is known as:

a. Immunization b. Seroconversion
c. Herd effect d. Inactivation

262. Polio vaccination in children is an example of:

a. Primary prevention
b. Secondary prevention
c. Tertiary prevention
d. Rehabilitation

263. Site of lesion in polio is:

a. Dorsal horn of spinal cord
b. Ventral horn of spinal cord
c. Spinal canal
d. All muscles

264. Which vaccine is not administered to an HIV-positive child?

a. OPV b. MMR
c. Hepatitis B d. DPT

265. Following DPT immunization a child developed swelling and tenderness at the injection site, a low-grade fever, and malaise. What is the appropriate nursing reaction?

a. Ask the parents to take the child to emergency
b. Educate them that this is occurring because of allergy to the vaccine
c. This is the expected reaction and teach them how to manage
d. In future avoid DPT injections to the child

266. Identify correct statement related to measles vaccine:

a. Measles vaccine is stored at 2–8°C
b. Measles vaccine is a live vaccine
c. Immediately after administration of measles vaccine, immunity develops
d. All of the above

267. Contraindicated vaccine in child with history of convulsions is:

a. Diphtheria b. Pertussis
c. Tetanus d. BCG

268. 4-weeks-old infant who have never been immunized earlier needs to be immunized with the following vaccines:

a. BCG, OPV, Measles
b. BCG, OPV, DPT
c. BCG, DPT, Measles
d. BCG, OPV, Vitamin A

269. True statement about DPT vaccine is:

a. Route of administration of DPT vaccine is IM
b. DPT booster is given at 16-24 months
c. It is a killed vaccine
d. All of the above

270. Identify correct statement related to BCG vaccination:

a. Dose of BCG at birth is 0.05 mL
b. Dose of BCG if not given at birth is 0.1 mL
c. BCG protects against Tuberculosis
d. All of the above

271. Site for BCG vaccination is:

a. Left upper arm
b. Right upper arm
c. Lateral aspect of mid-thigh
d. Anterior aspect of hand

272. A child is vaccinated for MMR at what age?

a. At birth b. 3 months
c. 6 months d. 15 months

273. All are true about BCG; EXCEPT:

a. It is a live vaccine
b. Route of administration is intradermal
c. It is available in powder form and need to dilute before administration
d. It provides protection against MMR

274. Correct regarding polio is:

a. Paralytic polio is caused by Polio virus type - 1
b. Polio is most commonly affecting 6 months to 3 years
c. Flaccid paralysis, tripod sign, fever, nausea and vomiting are the clinical features
d. All of the above

275. Oral polio vaccine is also known as:

a. Sabin b. Salk
c. Pentavalent d. Easy

276. Parenteral polio vaccine is also known as:

a. Sabin b. Salk
c. Pentavalant d. Easy

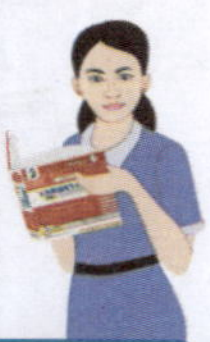

Ans.

255. a
256. d
257. d
258. b
259. b
260. d
261. a
262. a
263. b
264. a
265. c
266. d
267. b
268. b
269. d
270. d
271. a
272. d
273. d
274. d
275. a
276. b

277. Pentavalent vaccine provides protection against:
a. Diphtheria, pertussis, tetanus, hepatitis-B, hemophilus B
b. polio, TB, Measles, Mumps, hemophilus B
c. Measles, mumps, rubella, TB, hemophilus B
d. Measles, mumps, rubella, hepatitis B and hemophilus B

278. What all are the six killer diseases against which immunization provides protection?
a. Polio, diphtheria, pertussis, tetanus, TB, measles
b. Measles, mumps, rubella, TB, polio, hepatitis B
c. Diphtheria, pertussis, tetanus, hepatitis B, hemophilus B, polio
d. Polio, Diphtheria, pertussis, tetanus, Hepatitis B mumps

279. Neonatal tetanus can be prevented through:
a. Conducing deliveries under hygienic conditions
b. Proper cord care practices
c. Maternal immunization with TT in the antenatal period
d. All of the above

Explanation: Maternal and neonatal tetanus (MNT) have been among the most common lethal consequences of unclean deliveries and umbilical cord care practices. When tetanus develops, mortality rates are extremely high, especially when appropriate medical care is not available. Immunizing pregnant mother with TT also help us to prevent neonatal tetanus.

280. All are live vaccine; EXCEPT:
a. OPV
b. BCG
c. Measles
d. TT

281. Expanded Programme of Immunization (EPI) launched in India:
a. 1974
b. 1978
c. 1980
d. 1982

282. WHO launched expanded program of immunization in the year of:
a. 1974 b. 1978
c. 1980 d. 1982

283. Go through the following statements related to vaccination and identify the false statement:
a. Administration of 2 live antigens- a minimum interval of 4 weeks is recommended, if not administered simultaneously.
b. Two or more killed antigens may be administered simultaneously or at any interval between the doses
c. There is no minimum recommended time interval between two types of vaccines
d. If not sure about the immunization status of the child all the vaccine recommended in the immunization schedule need to give from the beginning

284. DPT vaccine should be stored:
a. -20°C
b. 0°C
c. 4-8°C
d. 20°C

285. For children IM injection need to be administered at:
a. Middle aspect of mid-thigh
b. Lateral aspect of mid-thigh
c. Lateral aspect of upper arm
d. Anterior aspect of mid-thigh

COLD CHAIN

286. Which vaccine stored at the Freezer compartment of refrigerator? *(AIIMS Raipur Staff Nurse Grade I-2018)*
a. OPV
b. Hep B vaccine
c. DTwP-hepatitis B-Hib (pentavalent)
d. HPV

Explanation: Vaccines such as OPV, measles, MMR, BCG and Rabies vaccines are most sensitive to heat and can be frozen without harm. Hepatitis B vaccine, Hepatitis A vaccine, DTwP-hepatitis B-Hib (pentavalent), DTaP-hepatitis B-Hib-IPV (hexavalent), DTaP, meningitis C, Pneumoccal vaccine, T, DT, dT and Human papillomavirus (HPV) vaccine are freeze sensitive. Never expose these vaccines to zero or subzero temperatures. *(Ref: WHO).*

287. Method used for the transportation of vaccine from the site of production to the vaccination site by protecting its potential to provide immunity is known as:
a. Cold chain b. Vaccine carrier
c. Transportation d. Cold box storage

288. Which of the following is the most heat sensitive vaccine?
a. Polio b. Measles
c. DPT d. BCG

289. Which among the following vaccine is least sensitive to heat?
a. Polio b. MMR
c. Hepatitis-B d. JE vaccine

290. Which of the following vaccine can be frozen?
a. Hepatitis-B b. DTP
c. Hib Vaccine d. OPV

291. Which of the following is the primary level in the cold chain delivery system?
a. Primary health center b. District level
c. State level d. National level

292. Which of the following test is used to check whether freeze-sensitive vaccines have been damaged by exposure to temperature below zero degree Celsius?
a. Shock test b. Stick test
c. Shake test d. Shick test

Explanation: The "**shake test**" was designed to detect freeze damage in freeze sensitive **vaccines** such as DTP, DT, Td, TT, typhoid, and hepatitis-B. These **vaccines** must never be frozen as this reduces their immunogenicity.

293. What is the name of small digital devices that are placed with freeze-sensitive vaccines during storage or transport?
a. Vaccine vial monitor
b. Digital thermometer
c. Electronic freeze indicators
d. Temperature loggers

UNDER-FIVE CLINIC

294. All of the following information are sought in the well-baby clinic; EXCEPT: *(Banaras HU 2015)*
a. Schooling
b. Breastfeeding
c. Sleep pattern
d. Child growth and development

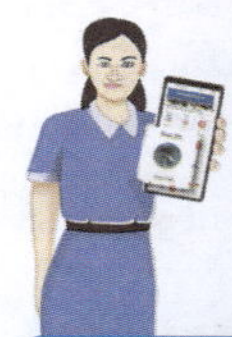

Ans.
277. a
278. a
279. d
280. d
281. b
282. a
283. d
284. c
285. b
286. a
287. a
288. a
289. c
290. d
291. d
292. c
293. c
294. a

295. Outer enveloping triangle that presents around the whole symbol of under 5 clinic represents:

a. Immunization
b. Family planning
c. Treatment of sick children
d. Health teaching

296. The inverted triangle at the center of the under-five clinic logo represents:

a. Immunization
b. Family planning
c. Treatment of sick children
d. Health teaching

297. The apex of the large triangle in the logo of under-five clinic represents:

a. Care in illness
b. Family planning
c. Immunization
d. Nutrition

Explanation:

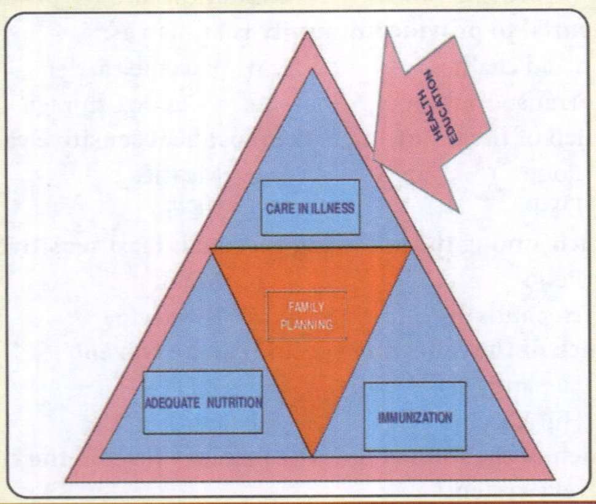

298. Nowadays, well-baby clinics has been replaced by:

a. Child clinics
b. Superspeciality pediatric hospitals
c. Under-five clinics
d. Anganwadis

PHYSIOLOGICAL AND PATHOLOGICAL JAUNDICE

299. All the following are causes of neonatal jaundice; EXCEPT:

a. Hyperthyroidism
b. α-Thalassemia
c. G6PD deficiency
d. Rh incompatibility

300. Which one of the following is considered abnormal in a neonate?

a. Erythema Toxicum
b. Mongolian spot
c. Caput succedaneum
d. Jaundice within the first 24 hours

301. Three days after the birth newborn appears slightly jaundiced. Nurse need to understand that this is due to:

a. Immature liver function
b. Prolonged RBC lifespan
c. Maternal antibody reaction
d. High hemoglobin with low hematocrit value

Explanation: Physiological jaundice occurs because of the short lifespan of RBCs and inability of the immature newborn liver to conjugate them.

302. All are features indicative of physiological jaundice of a newborn; EXCEPT: *(AIIMS BBS NO 2018)*

a. It appears before attaining 24 hours of age
b. It fades by 7th day of life
c. It peaks by 3rd day of life
d. It appears after attaining 24 hours of age

Explanation: Neonatal physiological jaundice appears after 24 hours of life due to breakdown of Red Blood Cells. Jaundice in the first 24 hours after birth is often considered pathologic.

303. Pathological jaundice criteria, all are included; EXCEPT:

a. 24 hours later but within 72 hours
b. >14 days persistence
c. >2 mg/dL conjugated bilirubin
d. Clay colored stool

304. Identify the characteristic of pathological jaundice among the following:

a. It appears in between 24-72 hours of age
b. It occurs because of the physical immaturity of the baby
c. Prematurity, asphyxia and infections may aggravate it
d. It appears within 24 hours

305. All are the characteristics of pathological jaundice; EXCEPT:

a. It appears within 24 hours of birth
b. Total bilirubin level is more than 15 mg/dL
c. Serum bilirubin level does not exceed 15 mg/dL
d. Direct bilirubin level more than 2 mg/dL

306. Kernicterus, which may occur as a complication of jaundice, is a pathological condition of the: *(Safdarjung NO 2018)*

a. Liver
b. Brain
c. Kidney
d. Heart

Explanation: Indirect Bilirubin more than 20 mg/dL can cause a condition called kernicterus in which bilirubin deposition occurs in brain. It can cause athetoid cerebral palsy and hearing loss.

Pathological condition of liver may cause jaundice (hyperbilirubinemia). Here, the question is complication of jaundice. Kernicterus is a complication due to hyperbilirubinemia.

307. Kramer's rule used for:

a. Jaundice
b. Necrotizing enterocolitis
c. Burns
d. Asphyxia

Explanation: Kramer's rule is used for the estimation of bilirubin level in jaundice.

308. Drug used in the treatment of neonatal jaundice is:

a. Phenobarbitone
b. Calcium gluconate
c. Betamethasone
d. Diazepam

Explanation: Phenobarbitone acts in the liver and induces glucuronyl transferase. So, it is the drug of choice in neonatal jaundice.

309. Correct regarding phototherapy:

a. Wavelength of lights used in phototherapy is 500–550 nm
b. 30-45 cm is the distance between light source and baby
c. Biliblanket is used in double surface phototherapy
d. All of the above

Ans.

295. d
296. b
297. a
298. c
299. a
300. d
301. a
302. a
303. a
304. d
305. c
306. b
307. a
308. a
309. d

310. Phototherapy acts by:
- a. Configurational isomerization
- b. Structural isomerization
- c. Photooxidation
- d. All of the above

Explanation: In configurational isomerization, Z isomer is converted to E isomers, in structural isomerization, bilirubin is converted as lumirubin and in photo oxidation, photo products are excreted via urine.

311. In phototherapy unit, what is the importance of using white clothes or aluminum foil around the unit?
- a. To provide privacy to the child
- b. To reflect the light, back on to the baby
- c. To avoid exposure to other lights in the unit
- d. All of the above

Explanation: The purpose is to reflect back the light on to the baby. While using these make sure that air flow is not impede.

312. Eyes need to be covered during phototherapy section because:
- a. To make sure that newborn closed the eyes well
- b. To induce sleep in the baby
- c. To prevent injury to conjunctiva and retina
- d. To minimize repeated blinking of the eyes which causes tiredness to eye muscles

Explanation: Eye patches are applied to prevent dryness of conjunctiva and injury to retina.

313. Pathological jaundice treatment:
- a. Exchange transfusion
- b. Phototherapy
- c. Administration of phenobarbitone
- d. All of the above

314. All are complications of phototherapy; EXCEPT:
- a. Passing loose green stools
- b. Hypercalcemia
- c. Hyperthermia
- d. Bronze discoloration of skin

315. Complication of phototherapy is:
- a. Hyperthermia
- b. Retinal damage
- c. Bronze-baby syndrome
- d. All of these

316. Which all body parts need to be covered of a child getting phototherapy?
- a. Eyes and abdomen
- b. Eyes and genitalia
- c. Eyes and extremities
- d. Genitalia and extremities

317. All of the following are required while caring for a child who is on phototherapy; EXCEPT:
- a. Infant should be fully naked with eyes and genitalia covered
- b. Breastfeeding should be continued unless it is contra-indicated
- c. Frequent monitoring of infant temperature need to be done
- d. Baby should be completely naked

NEONATAL HYPOGLYCEMIA

318. Which of the following babies is at lowest risk of developing hypoglycemia?
- a. Appropriate for gestational age babies
- b. Infant of diabetic mothers
- c. A baby born to mother on beta blockers
- d. IUGR babies

319. In a full term newborn, operational threshold for hypoglycemia is defined as plasma glucose level less than:
- a. 30 mg/dL
- b. 45 mg/dL
- c. 55 mg/dL
- d. 65 mg/dL

Explanation: The operational threshold for hypoglycemia is defined as that concentration of plasma or whole blood glucose at which clinicians should consider intervention, based on the evidence currently available in literature. Operational threshold has been defined as BGL of less than 40 mg/dL (plasma glucose level less than 45 mg/dL).

320. All of the following newborns are at risk of hypoglycemia; EXCEPT:
- a. Newborns born to diabetic mother
- b. Newborns large for their gestational age
- c. Newborns small for their gestational age
- d. Newborns born at term with forceps delivery

321. All of the following are symptoms of hypoglycemia in a newborn baby; EXCEPT:
- a. Hyperthermia
- b. Floppy muscles
- c. Not interested in feeding
- d. Lethargy

322. Seizures in neonates due to hypoglycemia can be treated with a loading dose of:
- a. 2 mL/kg of 50% dextrose
- b. 2 mL/kg of 10 dextrose
- c. 4 mL/kg of 50% dextrose
- d. 4 mL/kg of 10% dextrose

323. All of the following are the possible causes of seizure in first 24 hours of life of a newborn; EXCEPT:
- a. Asphyxia
- b. Intraventricular bleeding
- c. Hypoglycemia
- d. Tetanus

324. All of the following are causes of neonatal hypoglycemia; EXCEPT:
- a. Galactosemia
- b. Congenital adrenal hypoplasia
- c. Glycogen storage disease type-I
- d. Maternal treatment with sodium valporate

CARE OF NEONATE BORN TO DIABETIC MOTHER

325. Which of the following is not a common problem of infants born to diabetic mothers? *(AIIMS-BBS SNO 2019):*
- a. Hyperglycemia
- b. Hypocalcemia
- c. Polycythemia
- d. Macrosomia

Explanation: Gestational diabetes results in neonatal problems like hypoglycemia, polycythemia (venous hematocrit greater than equal to 65), macrosomia (newborn larger than average), and respiratory distress syndrome (breathing disorder).

326. Which of the following complications is expected in a neonate of a diabetic mother?
- a. Thrombocytopenia
- b. Anemia
- c. Hypoglycemia
- d. Oliguria

327. A newborn infant is exhibiting signs of respiratory distress. Which of the following would the nurse recognize as the earliest clinical sign of respiratory distress? *(NORCET 2022)* ***New Q***
- a. Cyanosis
- b. Increased respirations
- c. Sternal and subcostal retractions
- d. Decreased respirations

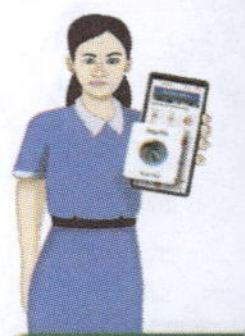

Ans.

310. d
311. b
312. c
313. d
314. b
315. d
316. b
317. d
318. a
319. b
320. d
321. a
322. b
323. d
324. d
325. a
326. c
327. c

Explanation:
- Retractions are a sign that the baby is having to work harder to breathe. They occur when the muscles between the ribs and below the rib cage pull in to help the lungs expand.
- Cyanosis, or bluish skin, is a later sign of respiratory distress.
- Increased respirations are also a sign of respiratory distress, but they are not the earliest sign.
- Decreased respirations are a sign of respiratory failure, which is a more serious condition than respiratory distress.

328. Surfactant deficiency occurs in:
a. Bronchopulmonary dysplasia
b. Infant of diabetic mother
c. Meconium aspiration syndrome
d. Transient tachypnea of neonate

Explanation: Newborns of diabetic mothers are frequently hyperinsulinemic and have an increased incidence of neonatal respiratory distress syndrome, a disease caused by a deficiency in the production of pulmonary surfactant by alveolar type II cells. It has been hypothesized that insulin inhibits fetal lung type II cell differentiation.

CARE OF NEONATE BORN TO HIV POSITIVE MOTHER

329. Which of the following vaccines can be given to HIV positive child?
a. DPT b. Hepatitis B vaccine
c. IPV d. All of these

330. Which of the following immunizations should be given to a client who is HIV positive and immune compromised?
a. MMR b. OPV
c. IPV d. Rotavirus

331. Which drug is given to prevent HIV transmission from mother to child?
a. Nevirapine b. Lamivudine
c. Stavudine d. Abacavir

332. All are the correct nursing interventions while caring for a newborn baby affected with HIV; EXCEPT:
a. Follow standard precautions
b. Educate the family regarding the disease transmission process
c. Educate them that vaccination need to be done after consultation with doctors only
d. If baby is not satisfied with breast milk, then provide formula feed

Explanation: Mixed feeding is never recommended in HIV positive child because it will increase the risk of infection. Vaccination needs to be done after consultation with doctors, because live vaccines need to be avoided in these patients.

BIRTH INJURIES

333. Identify the correct statement regarding caput succedaneum:
a. Maximum size and firmness at birth
b. Occur between skull and periosteum
c. Increases size for 12–24 hours then stable
d. Does not cross the suture line

Explanation: Option a is the correct statement regarding caput succedaneum all other statements are related to cephalohematoma

334. Premature closure of coronal suture is known as:
a. Albert syndrome b. Apert syndrome
c. Neurofibromatosis d. Trachoma

Explanation: Apert syndrome is a genetic disorder characterized by the premature closure of the bones of the skull (craniosynostosis).

335. Craniopagus refers to:
a. Fusion at head and spine b. Fusion at head only
c. Fusion at head and legs d. None of the above

Ref: Cloherty Neonatology manual, 7th Ed, p 129

Explanation: Craniopagus refers to conjoined twins with partially fused skulls; the union may be frontal occipital or parietal.
- They can share scalp, calvarium, dural sinuses and surface of the brain, but the face, foramen magnum and the spine remain separate.
- Conjoined twins result when incomplete embryonic division occurs late, after day 14 postconception.
- **Illustration of a craniopagus twin is shown below.**

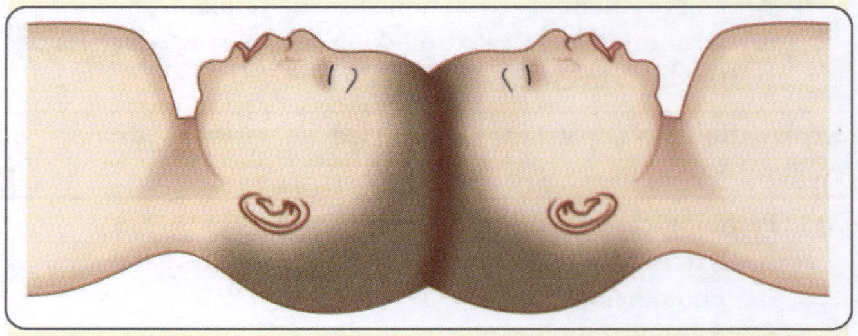

336. Sunset sign is seen in the following condition:
(AIIMS Raipur NO 2019)
a. Pyloric Stenosis
b. Hydrocephalus
c. Tetralogy of Fallot
d. Seizures

Explanation: Sunset sign phenomenon is an ophthalmologic sign seen in children with Hydrocephalus due to increased ICP. In this, eyes are often rolled downward so that the white part of the eyes (sclera) is visible below the upper eyelid.

337. Commonly occurring accident among newborn babies:
a. Road traffic accidents b. Falls
c. Burns d. Poisoning

338. Swelling of tissue over the presenting part of the fetal scalp due to sustained pressure; it resolves in 3-4 days is known as:
a. Caput succedaneum b. Cephalohematoma
c. Mongolian spot d. Anasarca

339. Feeding a child with choanal atresia can cause:
a. Chokes on feeding
b. Lack of swallowing reflexes
c. Does not appear to be hungry
d. Takes about half of the feeding

Explanation: There is no opening between nasal passage and nasopharynx, so infant can breathe only through mouth, it will lead to choking during feeding.

Ans.
328. b
329. d
330. c
331. a
332. d
333. a
334. b
335. b
336. b
337. b
338. a
339. a

IMNCI

340. Correct regarding IMNCI is:
- a. It aims to reduce under five morbidity and mortality
- b. It means integrated management of neonatal and childhood illness
- c. Pink, yellow and green are the color codes used in IMNCI
- d. All of the above

341. According to UNICEF, the most common cause of death among under five children is:
- a. Diarrhea
- b. Malnutrition
- c. Malaria
- d. Pneumonia

Explanation: **Pneumonia** kills **more children** than any other infectious **disease**, claiming the lives of over 800,000 **children under five** every year, or around 2,200 every day. This includes over 153,000 newborns. Almost all of these **deaths** are preventable. (source: UNICEF analysis based on WHO and Maternal and Child Epidemiology Estimation Group)

342. If a child presents with only one of the danger sign stated in the IMCI guideline, this child will be categorized under which of the following color?
- a. Green b. Pink
- c. Red d. Yellow

343. Which of the following vital signs is important in classifying a child with pneumonia from those who do not have?
- a. Blood pressure b. Chest indrawing
- c. Respiratory rate d. Breath sound

344. A five-month-old male baby was brought to the under-five clinic with cough. His respiratory rate is 40/minute. As per the IMCI guidelines of assessment, his respiratory rate is considered to be:
- a. Normal b. Fast
- c. Slow d. Insufficient data to conclude

BABY FRIENDLY HOSPITAL INITIATIVE

345. Ultimate aim of baby friendly hospital initiative was to promote:
- a. Immunization
- b. Hospital deliveries
- c. Breastfeeding
- d. Family planning

346. Baby Friendly Hospital Initiative (BFHI) was launched by WHO in the year of:
- a. 1990 b. 1991
- c. 1992 b. 1993

347. Among the following which is best for a better hospital experience in a 3.5-year-old child?
- a. Tricycle
- b. Clay modeling
- c. Building blocks
- d. Doll and syringe play

Explanation: Therapeutic play allows the child to manipulate unfamiliar equipment and thereby reduces the tension of hospitalization. So, by providing syringe and doll we can make the unfamiliar situation to a familiar one.

CHILD WELFARE PROGRAM AND AGENCIES

348. Supplementary Nursing, Immunization, Health check-up and referral services under Integrated child developmental services are applicable to which of the following age groups?
(AIIMS Bhopal Nursing Officer, 2018)
- a. 12–14 years b. 3–6 years
- c. 8–10 years d. 7–9 years

Explanation: Supplementary Nursing, Immunization, Health check-up and referral services' under Integrated child developmental services are applicable to 3–6 years of age group.

349. Among the following all are the components of GOBI F3; EXCEPT:
- a. Global warming b. Female education
- c. Immunization d. Food supplementation

Explanation: UNICEF'S GOBI F3 contains the following components such as Growth monitoring, oral rehydration, breast-feeding, immunization, female education, family spacing and food supplements.

350. Mission Indradhanush programme is related to:
- a. Immunization
- b. Breastfeeding
- c. Female education
- d. Nutritional supplementation

Explanation: Mission Indradhanush was launched by Ministry of Health and Family Welfare (MoHFW), Government of India on 25th December, 2014. The objective of this mission is to ensure that all children under the age of two years as well as pregnant women are fully immunized with seven vaccine preventable diseases. The diseases are Diphtheria, Pertussis (Whooping Cough), Tetanus, Tuberculosis, Polio, Hepatitis B, Measles.

351. Child Survival and Safe Motherhood programme was replaced by:
- a. MCH b. JSY
- c. RCH d. KSY

352. Midday meal programme is also known as:
- a. Nutrition supplement programme
- b. Beti bachao beti padhao
- c. Iodine deficiency control programme
- d. Sarva Shiksha Abhiyan

PLAY THERAPY

353. When preparing a 4-year-old child for a procedure, which method is developmentally most appropriate for the nurse to use?
- a. Allowing the child to watch another child undergoing the same procedure
- b. Showing the child pictures of what he or she will experience
- c. Talking to the child in simple terms about what will happen
- d. Preparing the child through play with a doll and toy or a medical equipment

354. Importance of play therapy during infancy is:
- a. Physical development
- b. Social development
- c. Psychological development
- d. Emotional development

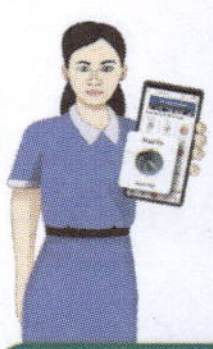

Ans.

340. d
341. d
342. b
343. c
344. a
345. c
346. b
347. d
348. b
349. a
350. a
351. c
352. a
353. d
354. a

Explanation: Play during infancy promotes physical development through the use of different kinds of toys. All others are also the functions of play therapy but during infancy its main importance is physical development of the child.

355. The type of play exhibited by toddlers where they play by themselves in the presence of other children is called: *(AIIMS BPL NO 2018)*

a. Passive play
b. Cooperative play
c. Solitary play
d. Parallel play

Explanation: Parallel play can be defined as children playing side by side from one another. Parallel play is most common among toddlers and can take place at any age. Cooperative play begins in the late preschool period. The play is organized by group goals.

Solitary play - The child plays intently with available materials but remains totally alone.

356. Which among the following statements describes the parallel play between two toddlers?

a. Sharing crayons to color two different pictures
b. Playing a board game with nurse
c. Sitting near to each other and playing with own toys
d. Sharing their toys with two different nurses

357. Typical type of play in a toddler is: *(Staff Nurse G II 2014)*

a. Parallel play b. Cooperative play
c. Associative play d. Onlooker play

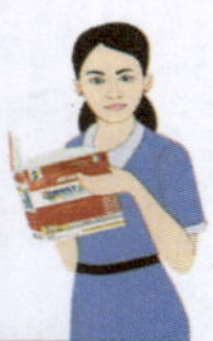

Explanation:
Infant-onlooker play,
Toddler-parallel play,
Preschool – associative play,
School going –cooperative play

Ans.
355. d
356. c
357. a
358. b
359. a
360. a
361. d
362. d
363. a
364. b

358. Which of the following examples represents parallel play? *(Safdarjung NO 2018)*

a. Ajay and Arun share their toys
b. Ajay plays with his car beside Merin, who is playing with her doll
c. Kavin plays a game of Scrabble with Subash and Sathish
d. Kavya plays with a handheld game while sitting in her mother's lap

Explanation: Parallel play can be defined as children play side by side from one another. Parallel play is most common among toddlers and can take place at any age.

PROTEIN ENERGY MALNUTRITION

359. The major cause for childhood illness is: *(AIIMS BPL NO 2018)*

a. Malnutrition b. Accidents
c. Infestation d. Infection

Explanation: According to the World Health Organization (WHO), malnutrition is the gravest single threat to global public health. Globally, it contributes to 45% of deaths of children aged under 5 years.

360. 'Edema' is a sign in which of the following nutritional disorders? *(AIIMS Bhopal Nursing Officer, 2018)*

a. Kwashiorkor
b. Marasmus
c. Underweight
d. Nutritional dwarfism

Explanation: Kwashiorkor is also known as "edematous malnutrition" because of its association with edema (fluid retention). It occurs due to protein deficiency.

361. As per Gomez classification, which of the following 'weight per age' comes under 'IIIrd degree malnutrition' when compared with the Harvard growth standard? *(AIIMS Bhopal Nursing Officer, 2018)*

a. 75–90% of the standard
b. 60–74% of the standard
c. 90–110% of the standard
d. Less than 60% of the standard

Explanation: Gomez classification: One of the earliest systems for classifying protein-energy malnutrition in children, based on percentage of expected weight for age: over 90% is normal, 76–90% is mild (first degree) malnutrition, 61–75% is moderate (second degree) malnutrition and less than 60% is severe (third degree) malnutrition.

362. Which of the following is seen in marasmus, but not in kwashiorkor?

a. Edema
b. Fatty change in liver
c. Hypoalbuminemia
d. Good appetite

Ref: OP Ghai 8th ed. p 99

Explanation: Children with marasmus have voracious appetite versus kwashiorkor child exhibiting poor appetite and apathy.

Clinical finding	Marasmus	Kwashiorkor
Edema	Absent	Present
Activity	Active	Lethargic
Appetite	Voracious (Eager to eat)	Poor
Liver size	Normal	Enlarged (Fatty liver)
Infection	Less prone	More prone
Prognosis	Less than kwashiorkor	-

363. Which is the best parameter for acute severe malnutrition?

a. Weight/height b. Height/age
c. Weight/age d. Mid arm circumference

Ref: Nelson 20th ed. p 297

Explanation: Weight for height is the most reliable long-term indicator regarding the growth status of the child.

364. All are seen in marasmus; EXCEPT: *(Recent Question 2014)*

a. Muscle wasting b. Hepatomegaly
c. Low insulin d. Muscle wasting

Ref: OP Ghai 8th ed. p 99

Explanation:

- **Marasmus:** Is characterized by failure to gain weight and irritability, followed by weight loss and listlessness until emaciation results. The skin loses turgor and becomes wrinkled and loose as subcutaneous fat disappears. Loss of fat from the sucking pads of the cheeks often occurs late in the course of the disease; thus, the infant's face may retain a relatively normal appearance compared with the rest of the body, but this, too, eventually becomes shrunken and wizened.
- *The abdomen may be distended or flat,* with the intestinal pattern readily visible. There is muscle atrophy and resultant hypotonia.
- **Kwashiorkor:** Is characterized by development of pedal edema which can mask weight loss. Dietary protein deficiency leads to brain damage and apathy, and/or irritability. When advanced, there is lack of growth, lack of stamina, loss of muscle tissue, increased susceptibility to infections, vomiting, diarrhea, anorexia, flabby subcutaneous tissues, and edema. It is often present in internal organs before it is recognized in the face and limbs.
- ***Hepatomegaly due to fatty liver is seen with flag sign on hair*** and skin showing ***FLAKY PAINT DERMATOSIS***

365. All are seen in Kwashiorkor; EXCEPT: *(Recent Question 2014)*

a. Increase appetite b. Flag sign on hair
c. Hepatomegaly d. Apathy

Ref: Nelson 20th ed. p 3239-40

Explanation:

- Kwashiorkor is protein and calorie deficiency and hence the serum albumin of the child is very low. This causes the child to develop pedal edema and generalized anasarca later.
- Since the child is not eating proteins, essential amino acids like phenylalanine is deficient and therefore the child forms less of melanin. This results in hair of the child being reddish in color. This color change of hair strand is seen as FLAG sign.
- The children with kwashiorkor have a FATTY liver and thereby a hepatomegaly.
- Apathy means lack of interest in surroundings and therefore this child is not interested in playing with the mother or toys. This occurs due to brain damage secondary to chronic protein deprivation.

Increased appetite can be seen in patients with marasmus.

366. In children which disease occurs due to protein deficiency?

a. Marasmus b. Kwashiorkor
c. Beriberi d. Scurvy

367. "Flag sign" is a characteristic feature of which disease? *(Staff Nurse G II 2014)*

a. Poliomyelitis b. Kwashiorkor
c. Rickets d. Marasmus

368. Essential clinical features of kwashiorkor are:

a. Baggy pants
b. Muscle wasting, and skin and bone appearance
c. Markedly retarded growth, mental changes and edema
d. Low weight and no edema

369. Identify correct statement in relation to marasmus/ kwashiorkor:

a. In kwashiorkor child, edema is present because of Hypoalbuminemia
b. Monkey face, baggy pants, skin and bone appearance are the clinical features of marasmus
c. Marasmus is an energy deficiency disorder
d. All of the above

370. A 4-year-old child was born at term from a low socioeconomic group family, with no congenital anomalies. She is now only 70% of normal body weight. On examination, she shows pitting pedal edema of the lower extremities as well as an enlarged abdomen with palpable fluid wave. Her desquamating skin shows irregular areas of depigmentation, and hyperpigmentation. Which of the following nutritional problems is most likely present in this child? ***New Q***

a. Kwashiorkor b. Marasmus
c. Niacin deficiency d. Vitamin A toxicity

Explanation: Kwashiorkor is a protein-energy malnutrition (PEM) that is characterized by edema, a distended abdomen, and skin changes. It is most common in children who are weaned from breast milk and switched to a diet that is low in protein.

Marasmus is a PEM that is characterized by wasting and emaciation.

371. Following are the clinical manifestations of marasmus; EXCEPT:

a. Sugar baby b. Monkey face
c. Baggy pants d. Skin and bone appearance

372. A 6-month-old infant has developmental delays. His weight falls below the 5th percentile when plotted on a growth chart. A diagnosis of failure to thrive is made. What behaviors might indicate the possibility of maternal deprivation? ***New Q*** *(NORCET 2022)*

a. Responsive to touch, wants to be held
b. Uncomforted by touch, refuses bottle
c. Maintains eye-to-eye contact
d. Finicky eater, easily pacified, cuddly

Explanation:

- Maternal deprivation is a condition in which an infant or child does not receive adequate physical and emotional care from their mother or primary caregiver. This can lead to a number of problems, including failure to thrive, developmental delays, and emotional problems.
- Some of the behaviors that may indicate the possibility of maternal deprivation include:
  - Uncomforted by touch
  - Refuses to be held
  - Does not maintain eye contact
  - Is withdrawn or apathetic
  - Is irritable or aggressive
  - Has developmental delays

373. Best indicator for nutritional status for a child is: *(Recent Question 2014)*

a. Mid arm circumference
b. Head circumference
c. Rate of increase of height and weight
d. Chest circumference

Ref: Nelson 20th ed. p 297, OP Ghai 8th ed. p 18

Explanation: "Rate of increase of anthropomorphic features as shown by growth charts is the most reliable method of assessment": *WHO Handbook*

374. Chronic malnutrition is measured by:

a. Weight/height b. Height/age
c. Weight/age d. Mid arm circumference

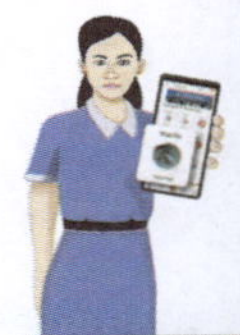

Ans.

365.	a
366.	b
367.	b
368.	c
369.	d
370.	a
371.	a
372.	b
373.	c
374.	b

375. Which of the following is the best indicator of long-term nutritional status? *(UP 2010)*

a. Mid arm circumference
b. Height for age
c. Weight for age
d. Weight for height

Explanation:

Weight for height	Acute undernutrition generally characterized by low weight for height has been termed wasting. Conversely, overnutrition or obesity is characterized by high weight for height.
Height for age	This is a measure of linear growth. Frequent periods of acute food deprivation or infection or prolonged period of inadequate food intake — especially during the rapid growing years (esp. first 2 years of life) may cause measurable growth retardation—the result is a child who is low in height for age—called stunting. This is an indicator of long-term nutritional adequacy.
Weight for age	Does not distinguish between present and long-term malnutrition. Useful in children under 1 year of age in whom length measurement may not be accurate.

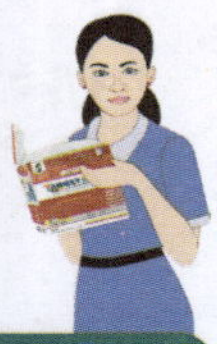

376. According to IAP classification, if weight for age is 61–70% which grade of malnutrition it is?

a. Grade 1
b. Grade 2
c. Grade 3
d. Grade 4

Explanation:

Grade	Weight for age
Grade 1	71–80%
Grade 2	61–70%
Grade 3	51–60%
Grade 4	<50%

377. Identify the age independent indicators of malnutrition among the following:

a. Mid upper arm circumference
b. Shakir tape method
c. Bangle test
d. All of the above

Explanation: All of the above are age independent indicators of malnutrition. Any MUAC below 13.5 is abnormal. In Shakir tape method also mid upper arm circumference which is less than 13.5 is abnormal. In bangle test if 4 cm diameter bangle freely passes the elbow that suggestive of malnutrition. All these parameters, do not require age of the baby to calculate the level of malnutrition so it is called as age independent indicators of malnutrition.

DISORDERS OF RESPIRATORY SYSTEM

378. A nurse is assessing a one-month-old infant. Which of the following findings should be reported by the nurse immediately?

a. Heart rate of 140 beats per minute
b. Respiratory rate of 40 breaths per minute
c. Inspiratory grunt
d. Abdominal respirations

379. What is the most common complication for which a nurse must monitor preterm infant? *(NCFL 2019)*

a. Hemorrhage
b. Brain damage
c. Respiratory distress
d. Aspiration of mucus

Explanation: Respiratory Distress Syndrome (RDS) occurs most often in newborns born preterm, affecting nearly all newborns who are born before 28 weeks of pregnancy. Less often, RDS can affect full term newborns. Since the exact period of preterm (gestational age) is not given, Respiratory distress is the most likely answer.

380. Which assessment data alert the nurse to suspect shaken baby syndrome?

a. Preterm baby
b. Lack of stridor and adventitious breath sounds
c. Previous episode of apnea which lasted for 10–15 seconds
d. Previous episode of seizure

Explanation: Lack of stridor and adventitious breath sounds are the most common signs which occur in shaken baby syndrome following CNS trauma.

381. Which of the following action would the nurse anticipate using while caring for a term neonate diagnosed with transient tachypnea at 2 hours after birth? *(RAK MSc 2018)*

a. Monitoring the neonates color and cry every four hours
b. Feeding the neonate with a bottle every three hours
c. Obtaining extra corporeal membrane oxygenation equipment
d. Providing warm, humidified oxygen in a warm environment

Explanation: Transient Tachypnea of newborn (TTN) is a self-limiting disease that occurs especially among term neonate & due to delayed clearance of lung field. These babies have tachypnea with minimal or no respiratory distress. Oxygen treatment is adequate to treat this condition.

382. Cessation of breathing for 20 seconds is known as:

a. Respiratory arrest
b. Respiratory distress syndrome
c. Apnea
d. Transient tachypnea

383. Surfactant inactivation occurs in:

a. Infant of diabetic mother
b. Meconium aspiration syndrome
c. Transient tachypnea of newborn
d. Bronchopulmonary dysplasia

384. The neonatal feature of cystic fibrosis is:

a. Bronchitis　　b. Bronchiolitis
c. Meconium ileus　　d. Bronchiectasis

Ans.

375. b
376. b
377. d
378. c
379. c
380. b
381. d
382. c
383. b
384. c

385. Which of the following is not true regarding meconium aspiration syndrome? *(AIIMS-BBS SNO 2019)*

a. It is common cause of respiratory distress
b. It occurs when a newborn inhales particulate meconium mixed with amniotic fluid in utero
c. It does not progress to persistent pulmonary hypertension in severe cases
d. Chest X-ray shows fluffy infiltrates with areas of atelectasis.

Explanation: Features of meconium aspiration syndrome include

- Asphyxiated at birth
- Develops progressive respiratory distress soon after birth
- Life threatening persistent pulmonary hypertension
- Chest X-ray shows bilateral coarse irregular densities with patches of obstructive emphysema.

So, the option (c) which states that "it does not progress to persistent pulmonary hypertension" is incorrect.

386. Surfactant production in fetus begins at the age of:

a. 16-20 weeks b. 20-24 weeks
c. 26-30 weeks d. 30-34 weeks

387. Total lung capacity in a newborn is: *(Safdarjung NO 2018)*

a. 100 mL b. 350 mL
c. 500 mL d. 150 mL

Explanation:

- Total lung capacity in a newborn is 150 mL. The estimate of total lung volume of infant is 44±9 mL/kg. An average newborn weighs approximately 3 kg. Therefore, lung capacity is $50 \times 3 = 150$ mL.
- The average total lung capacity of an adult human male is about 6 liters of air.

388. Important sign of cold stress is:

a. Irritability b. Fever
c. Increased Respiratory rate d. Shaking

389. Small baby with intrauterine growth retardation, cataracts, microphthalmia, myocarditis, and a red or purple macular rash ("blueberry muffin" rash) are the characteristics of:

a. Congenital rubella b. Congenital syphilis
c. Congenital varicella d. Congenital herpes

390. A 2-day-old neonate underwent corrective surgery for tracheoesophageal fistula two days back. Which of the following needs to be reported by the nurse? *(AIIMS Bhopal Grade-I 2018)*

a. Diminished bowel sounds
b. Excessive crying, irritability
c. Pulse rate 130 beats/min
d. Dislodgement of orogastric tube

Explanation: Esophageal atresia with or without tracheoesophageal fistula is the most common congenital anomaly of the esophagus. The primary surgical correction is the best option in the absence of severe malformation. But the primary complications during postoperative period are leak and stenosis of the anastomosis, gastroesophageal reflux and respiratory disorders. The dislodgement of the orogastric tube increases the risk for developing the complications. So, this should be reported to the Physician immediately.

391. Immediate postoperative care following tracheoesophageal repair surgery is:

a. Administer pain killers
b. Maintain patent airway
c. Maintain parenteral fluid infusion
d. Do careful oral suction

Explanation: Airway maintenance is the highest priority after surgery. So maintaining a patent airway play an important role in the immediate post-operative period.

392. Which of these signs indicates tracheoesophageal fistula immediately after birth? *(Daman and Diu NO 2018)*

a. Passage of frothy meconium
b. Continuous drooling
c. Slow response to stimuli d. Diaphragmatic breathing

Explanation: Tracheoesophageal fistula is an abnormal connection in one or more places between the esophagus and the trachea. Symptoms may include frothy, white bubbles, drooling in the mouth, coughing or choking when feeding, vomiting, in blue color of the skin especially when the baby is feeding, difficulty in breathing, round and full abdomen.

393. A 10-year-old child with asthma is admitted to the ward. Which of the following observations needs immediate action by the nurse? *(AIIMS Bhopal Grade-I 2018)*

a. Breath rate 20/min
b. Sitting upright and refusing to lie down
c. Refusing to eat food d. Oxygen saturation 96%

Explanation: In children, Asthma Attack Scale is used to determine the disease severity and it has four levels, i.e., Mild (no SOB at rest, mild SOB with walking, can talk normally, can lay down normally, wheezes not heard or mild), Moderate (SOB at rest, speaks in phrases, sitting upright and refusing to lie down, wheezing can be heard), Severe (severe SOB at rest, can talk in single words, wheezing may be loud) and Peak flow rate which tells how well a person can move air out of the lungs. In above scenario, nurses need to take immediate action because the child develops a moderate type of asthma attack.

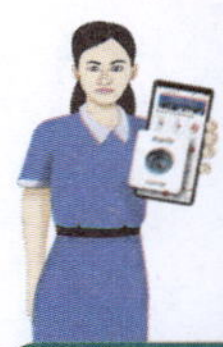

394. A 5-year-old child gets admitted to the hospital with the diagnosis of Bronchopulmonary Dysplasia (BPD). If the child is at the third stage, what would be the clinical symptoms? *(AIIMS Raipur Grade II 2017)*

a. Profuse hyaline membranes and patchy mucosal cilia loss
b. Interstitial fibrosis and epithelial proliferation
c. Edema of the interstitium and necrosis of alveolar cells
d. Alveolar collapse and difficulty in oxygenation

Explanation:

Table

Stage 1 (1–3 days)	Stage 2 (4–10 days)	Stage 3 (11–20 days)	Stage 4 (>1 month)
Presence of hyaline membranes, atelectasis, vascular hyperemia, and lymphatic dilatation	Lung destruction resulting in ischemic necrosis of airways and bronchiolar obstruction	Hypertrophy of the remaining alveoli, bronchial-wall muscle and glands, Airtrapping, pulmonary hyperinflation, tracheomegaly, tracheomalacia, interstitial edema, and ciliary dysfunction	Emphysematous alveoli are seen. Pulmonary hypertension, cor pulmonale. Fibrosis, atelectasis, a cobblestone appearance due to uneven lung aeration, and pleural pseudofissures are seen.

Ans.

385. c
386. b
387. d
388. c
389. a
390. d
391. b
392. b
393. b
394. d

395. What is the priority need that must include in the care of a child who is having pneumonia?

(AIIMS Raipur Staff Nurse Grade I-2018)

a. Rest b. Respiratory exercises
c. Nutrition d. Tricycle riding

Explanation: In a child with pneumonia, rest is the most priority need. The child is having limited energy and nutritional status will be compromised, so unnecessary energy expenditure need to be avoided in order to spend those energy in the airway need of the patient.

396. The most common indication of respiratory illness in infant is:

a. Poor feeding
b. Longer period of sleep
c. Rapid grunting respiration
d. Cough

Explanation: Rapid grunting is the most common sign indicating respiratory distress in an infant. It is a mechanism by which infant tries to keep alveoli open and to increase arterial oxygenation.

397. A newborn is suspected to have respiratory distress if there is:

a. Flaring of nostrils b. Acrocyanosis
c. Breath holding spells d. Irregular respiration

Explanation: According to Silverman-Anderson index for respiratory function, flaring of nostrils indicate respiratory distress.

Table

Feature	Score 0	Score 1	Score 2
Chest movement	Equal	Respiratory lag	Seesaw respiration
Intercostal retraction	None	Minimal	Marked
Xiphoid Retraction	None	Minimal	Marked
Nasal flaring	None	Minimal	Marked
Expiratory grunt	None	Audible with (stethoscope)	Audible

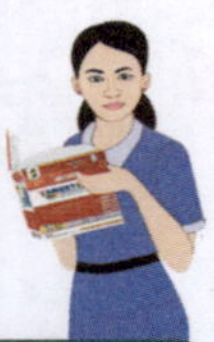

Ans.

395. a
396. c
397. a
398. b
399. a
400. d
401. b
402. d
403. c
404. b
405. a
406. d

398. Choanal atresia affects:

a. Nose b. Nasopharynx
c. Anus d. Sigmoid colon

Explanation: Congenital failure of the nasal cavities to open posteriorly into the nasopharynx (choanae) is called choanal atresia.

399. Which lobe is most commonly affected in children with pulmonary atelectasis?

a. Right middle lobe
b. Right lower lobe
c. Left upper lobe
d. Left lower lobe

Explanation: Right middle lobe is more prone to atelectasis because it is bronchus has a narrow diameter, acute angle of take-off and a relatively long course.

400. What should be the priority nursing intervention in a child with croup?

a. Pad side rails of the ribs
b. Arrange for a quiet, cool environment
c. Obtain a cot so that a parent can stay
d. Place a tracheostomy set at the bedside

Explanation: Priority is the patent airway and necessary equipment must be immediately available.

401. What is the priority nursing intervention for a child who is admitted with respiratory syncytial virus (RSV)?

a. Administering an antiviral agent
b. Clustering care to conserve energy
c. Send daily blood sample
d. Offering oral fluids to promote hydration

Explanation: Often the infant will have decreased pulmonary reserve and the clustering of care is essential to provide for period of rest.

402. When a small child is shaken by the arms or shoulders in a repetitive, violent manner, this condition is called:

a. Marfan syndrome b. Munchausen syndrome
c. De Quervain syndrome d. Shaken baby syndrome

403. What instruction should be included in the nursing care plan of a child with RSV infection?

a. Administering an antiviral agent
b. Allow parents and siblings to visit
c. Maintain standard and contact precautions
d. Administer IV fluids to promote hydration

Explanation: RSV is highly contagious so child needs to be isolated and needs to maintain standard and contact precautions.

404. All are present in a child with croup; EXCEPT:

a. Fever b. Bronchospasm
c. Barking cough d. Inspiratory stridor

Explanation: Fever, barking cough and inspiratory stridor are the manifestation of croup. Croup is a general term applied to conditions characterized by hoarseness of voice and resonant cough it includes acute epiglottitis, laryngitis, laryngotracheobronchitis, spasmodic laryngitis.

405. When assessing a child with chronic hypoxia, nurse has to look for:

a. Clubbing of fingers b. Decreased RBC count
c. $SPO_2 > 90\%$ d. Fluid intake

Explanation: Hypoxia leads to poor peripheral circulation; clubbing occurs as a result of tissue hypertrophy and additional capillary development in fingers. The nail widening that characterizes clubbing occurs because the tissue under the nail plate becomes thicker. This can be caused by a number of conditions that lead to a decrease in the amount of oxygen in the blood, such as lung disease and heart disease.

406. Beclomethasone helps to:

a. Bronchodilation
b. Increases cardiac output
c. Increases surfactant production
d. Decreases inflammatory process

Explanation: This drug reduces the inflammation and inflammatory response of the bronchial wall. Beclomethasone is a steroid. It prevents the release of substances in the body that causes inflammation. Beclomethasone inhalation is used to prevent asthma attacks.

407. A nurse caring for a child with spasmodic croup need to understand that immediate nursing care is required for:
a. Irritability b. Hoarseness
c. Crocking sound d. Rapid respiration

Explanation: Rapid respiration indicates impending airway obstruction.

408. What should the nurse emphasize in discharge teaching of a child with persistent asthma?
a. Indoor plants and pet animals help to increase the activity in asthmatic child
b. Dry dusting of the room need to be done daily
c. Diminishing signs and symptoms helps to taper the drug
d. Medication must be continued even if the child is asymptomatic

Explanation: Children who all are suffering from asthma need to continue the medication even if they are asymptomatic and they always need to carry medications with them.

409. In croup, humidified oxygen is given to:
a. Maintain moist mucosa
b. Provide mode for giving inhaled drugs
c. Decrease tissue inflammation and edema
d. Provide an environment free of pathogenic organisms

Explanation: Cool mist helps to reduce inflammation and tissue edema.

410. A 6-year-old child is admitted to the hospital with pneumonia. An immediate priority in this child's nursing care would include all of the following; EXCEPT: *(Banaras HU 2015)*
a. Provide nutrition to the child
b. Assess respiratory status and signs of cyanosis
c. Give fowler position/semi-fowler position
d. Give oxygen according to the program

411. Which among the following respiratory conditions is always treated as medical emergency?
a. Pneumonia b. Asthma
c. Epiglottitis d. Cystic fibrosis

412. Bronchiolitis is commonly seen in which age group?
a. 6-12 b. <2 years
c. 2-3 years d. All age group

413. In which of the following condition the main presenting symptom is peculiar brassy cough (barking cough)?
a. Acute tonsilopharyngitis b. Croup
c. Pneumonia d. Cystic fibrosis

414. Failure of distension of alveoli due to loss of elasticity of the lung, is known as:
a. Respiratory failure b. Atelectasis
c. Emphysema d. Empyema

415. Which of the following organisms is commonly associated with bacterial tracheitis in children?
a. Hemophilus influenzae b. Staphylococcus aureus
c. Moraxella catarrhalis d. Streptococcus pneumonia

416. Most common cause of Acute Epiglottitis is:
a. S. pneumoniae b. Influenza
c. H. influenza d. Meningococci

417. Most common complication of bronchial asthma is:
a. Hypoxemia b. Atelectasis
c. Hypoxemia d. Respiratory failure

418. Inhaled corticosteroid used in bronchial asthma are all; EXCEPT:
a. Beclomethasone b. Budesonide
c. Fluticasone d. Dexamethasone

419. All the following statements are true related to wheezing; EXCEPT:
a. It is a high pitch whistling sound
b. It can be auscultated by the stethoscope only
c. It occurs due to partial obstruction of lower airway
d. It is predominantly expiratory in nature

420. Identify the lower respiratory tract infection among the following:
a. Coryza b. Common cold
c. Bronchitis d. Rhinitis

421. Which among the following conditions is characterized by destruction of bronchial and peribronchial tissues?
a. Laryngitis b. COPD
c. Bronchiectasis d. Pneumonia

422. Cyanosis in a child can be seen in all the place mentioned below; EXCEPT: *(Banaras HU 2015)*
a. Sclera b. Tongue
c. Nail beds d. Lips

423. Noisy breathing due to airway obstruction is known as:
a. Ronchi b. Stridor
c. Snoring d. Crackles

424. An acute, severe prolonged asthma attack and is unresponsive to usual treatment is known as:
a. Nocturnal asthma b. Intrinsic asthma
c. Extrinsic asthma d. Status asthmaticus

425. Risk factors for persistent asthma in children include all; EXCEPT:
a. Previous episodes of Bronchiolitis in infant
b. Previous episodes of pneumonia
c. Food allergy
d. First born infant to asthmatic parents

426. Best method of oxygen administration to a 2-month-old baby is:
a. Oxyhood b. Nasal cannula
c. Face mask d. Oxygen tent

427. A child is suffering from dyspnea, at first what nursing care you would provide to the child:
a. Start IV infusion
b. Provide supine position
c. Start oxygen therapy
d. Start nebulization

428. When the respiratory rate of a 12-month-old child is 35 breaths/minute, the most appropriate nursing action is:
a. Notify the physician
b. Administer oxygen
c. Reassess respiratory rate in 15 minutes
d. Document the findings

429. Positive Mantoux is seen in:
a. Immunocompromized b. Chicken pox
c. TB d. All of these

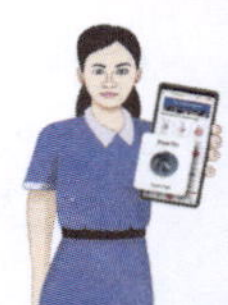

Ans.

407. d
408. d
409. c
410. a
411. c
412. b
413. b
414. c
415. b
416. c
417. b
418. d
419. b
420. c
421. c
422. a
423. b
424. d
425. d
426. a
427. c
428. d
429. d

Explanation: In all of the above-mentioned conditions, mantoux test will be positive. Host related factors such as very young age, malnutrition, immunosuppression by disease or drugs, viral infections also play a role.

DISORDERS OF GI SYSTEM

430. What is main reason for under five morbidity and mortality? *(AIIMS Raipur Staff Nurse Grade I-2018)*

a. Malnutrition
b. Diarrheal disease
c. Asphyxia
d. Leukemia

Explanation: Diarrheal disease is the most common cause of under-five mortality rate in India. Malnutrition is the factor which is making children more vulnerable to other disease condition.

431. Projectile vomiting is a characteristic of which of the following conditions? *(AIIMS Bhopal Grade-I 2018; Safdarjung NO 2018)*

a. Pyloric stenosis
b. Hernia
c. Imperforate anus
d. Appendicitis

Explanation: Pyloric stenosis is a narrowing of the opening from the stomach to the first part of the small intestine characterized by projectile vomiting (Ejection of gastric content up to 3 feet) without the presence of bile. This occurs due to the hypertrophic pylorus muscles which obstructs the gastric pathway.

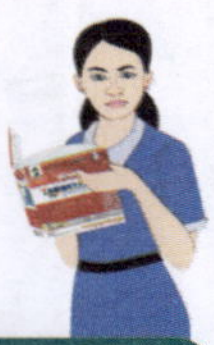

432. Identify the food items need to be avoided in a child with celiac disease: *(AIIMS Raipur Staff Nurse Grade I-2018)*

a. Wheat
b. Rye
c. Oats
d. All of these

Explanation: Celiac disease is an auto immune disease and child with celiac disease need to avoid food items that contain gluten protein. This protein is present in food items such as wheat, barley, oats and rye.

433. A child suffering from acute diarrhea is brought to the emergency room and is diagnosed as having severe dehydration with pH of 7.25- Serum Sodium-126 mEq/L, Serum Potassium-3.0 mEq/L, HCO_3-16. The best IV fluid of choice in this condition is:

a. Half normal saline
b. N/3 Saline+ 5% dextrose
c. Normal Saline
d. N/3 saline + 10% dextrose

434. In a child with lactose intolerance and absent lactase activity, which of the following foods is least likely to cause symptoms?

a. Ice cream
b. Skimmed milk
c. Condensed milk
d. Yogurt

Ref: Nelson 20th Ed, p 289

Explanation: Lactose intolerance is a clinical syndrome of 1 or more of the following; abdominal pain, diarrhea, nausea, flatulence and/ or bloating after the ingestion of lactose or lactose containing food substances

- Avoidance of milk and other dairy product will relieve symptoms in these children.

Among the given options, yogurt is least likely to cause symptoms due to following reasons:

- Yogurt contains inactive lactase enzyme, which is activated by the temperature and pH of the duodenum; this lactase activity in the yogurt substitutes for the lack of endogenous lactase
- Bacteria in yogurt partially digest lactose into glucose and galactose before consumption
- Yogurt's semisolid state slows gastric emptying and gastrointestinal transit resulting in fewer symptoms of lactose intolerance

435. Which of the following vitamins deficiency leads to diarrhea and hyperkeratosis?

a. Vitamin A
b. Vitamin C
c. Vitamin D
d. Vitamin K

Ref: Nelson 20th ed. p 319, 3240, 18th ed. Ch 45

Explanation: The disturbance of the integrity of the intestinal epithelium with an increased risk for bacterial translocation is one of the suggested factors underlying the increased incidence of infections and sepsis during vitamin A deficiency.

- Squamous metaplasia of the renal pelvis, ureters, vaginal epithelium, and the pancreatic and salivary ducts may lead to increased infections in these areas. In the urinary bladder, loss of epithelial integrity may result in pyuria and hematuria.
- Similarly, in the respiratory tract, mucus-secreting epithelium is essential for the disposal of inhaled pathogens and toxicants. Epithelial changes in the respiratory system can result in *bronchial obstruction.*
- Epithelial changes in the skin due to vitamin A deficiency are manifested as dry, scaly, *hyperkeratotic patches,* commonly on the arms, legs, shoulders, and buttocks.

436. Most common bacterial cause of diarrhea in children is: *(Recent Question 2014)*

a. E. coli
b. Salmonella
c. Staphylococcus
d. Shigella

Ref: CPDT 22nd e, p 1353

Explanation: Most common bacterial cause of diarrhea is ETEC (Enterotoxic E. coli).

437. Initial fluid of choice for diarrhea in an infant: *(AIIMS May 2015)*

a. ORS
b. Salt water
c. Sugar water
d. Dextrose

Ref: Nelson 20th ed. p 882t

Explanation: Compared with standard ORS, lower sodium and glucose ORS (containing 75 mEq of sodium and 75 mmol of glucose per liter, with total osmolarity of 245 mOsm per liter) reduces stool output, vomiting, and the need for intravenous fluids without substantially increasing the risk of hyponatremia.

Ans.

430. b
431. a
432. d
433. c
434. d
435. a
436. a
437. a

438. A 4-week-old male infant is brought to the emergency department because of persistent vomiting. Examination shows infant with dry mucus membranes and an olive-shaped mass is palpated in the right upper quadrant of the abdomen. Which of the following acid-base abnormalities is most likely in this patient? *(Recent Question 2015)*

pH, $PaCO_2$ (mm Hg), HCO_3 (mEq/L)

a. 7.10, 80, 24 b. 7.40, 40, 24
c. 7.55, 46, 42 d. 7.62, 21, 21

Ref: Nelson 20th ed. p 1797

Explanation:

- This patient has congenital hypertrophic pyloric stenosis.
- The loss of acidic gastric fluid via vomiting causes a metabolic alkalosis. Additionally, the loss of large volumes of fluid via vomiting leads to contraction alkalosis due to the action of aldosterone.
- In order to compensate for the metabolic alkalosis, the respiratory system responds via hypoventilation to create a secondary respiratory acidosis. The patient described is expected to have a primary metabolic alkalosis with respiratory compensation.
- This is characterized by a plasma pH greater than 7.45, $PaCO_2$ greater than 40 mm Hg and HCO_3^- greater than 24 mEq/L.
- Choice A is ruled out as it has acidosis. Choice B has normal pH and is ruled out. Choice D has alkalosis but HCO_3 is reduced (normal HCO_3= 22-26 mEq) and is hence ruled out.

439. All are true regarding cystic fibrosis; EXCEPT:

a. Secretions to become thick and sticky. Instead of acting as a lubricant
b. It is an inherited disorder
c. Sweat chloride test is used to diagnose the condition
d. Digestion and absorption of nutrients are least likely to be affected

Explanation: Thick mucus can block the tubes that carry digestive enzymes from pancreas to intestines. Without these enzymes, body cannot absorb proteins, fats or fat-soluble vitamins. So there will be nutritional deficiency.

440. All of the following statements about colic in a baby is correct; EXCEPT:

a. Repeated bouts of excessive crying in a baby is observed.
b. Colic is common and can affect up to 3 out of 10 babies.
c. Colic is more common in babies who are born prematurely.
d. All the babies with colic have an intolerance to cow's milk.

Explanation: Colic is a condition where there are repeated bouts of excessive crying in a baby who is otherwise healthy. Colic is common and can affect up to 3 out of 10 babies. It is more common among babies who are prematurely. Some babies with colic have an intolerance to cow's milk but certainly not majority of all the babies with colic have intolerance to cow's milk.

441. Invertogram is used for the diagnosis of ……….. condition.

a. Anorectal malformations b. Tracheoesophageal fistula
c. Cleft lip and palate d. Hirschprungs disease

Explanation: Invertogram is a specific diagnostic test done to find out anorectal malformations. Skiagram is used for the diagnosis of tracheoesophageal fistula.

442. What is persistent diarrhea?

a. Diarrhea last > 1 week
b. Diarrhea last > 2 weeks
c. Diarrhea last > 3 weeks
d. Diarrhea last > 4 weeks

Explanation: Diarrhea lasts more than 2 weeks is persistent diarrhea.

443. In a child with the diagnosis of hyperpyloric stenosis nurse should look for the possible sign of:

a. Dehydration b. Diarrhea
c. Cyanosis d. Malena

Explanation: A child with HPS will develop projectile vomiting and can lead to dehydration. Dehydration occurs as a complication of vomiting. So, nursing responsibility include assessment for dehydration.

444. Confirmatory diagnostic test for Hirschsprung's disease is:

a. Invertogram
b. Suction biopsy
c. Abdominal CT
d. Fiber optic nasoenteric tube

Explanation: Suction biopsy removes some rectal tissues which will be observed under microscope for ganglionic cells.

445. What is the most important nursing intervention while caring an infant with diarrhea?

a. Maintain Intake Output chart
b. Take daily weight at same time and in same scale
c. Teach family how to prepare ORS
d. Promote hand hygiene

Explanation: Weight is the best indicator of fluid loss or gain if measured daily at same time and in same scale. During infancy, mild dehydration is indicated by a loss of weight up to 5%, moderate dehydration by 5-10%, and severe dehydration by more than 10%. The infant's life is threatened if there is greater than 15% weight loss.

446. Nurse was going through the file of a child who is admitted with hypertrophic pyloric stenosis. All among the following except one can be seen in the file:

a. Olive like mass
b. Projectile vomiting
c. String sign in the X-ray
d. Radiating pain towards left shoulder

Explanation: Except d all are the manifestation related to hypertrophic pyloric stenosis. Projectile vomiting leads to dehydration among children. The definitive treatment of pyloric stenosis is with surgical pyloromyotomy known as Ramstedt's procedure (dividing the muscle of the pylorus to open up the gastric outlet).

447. Which among the following indicates parent have adequate knowledge regarding the dietary management of cystic fibrosis?

a. There is no need for any enzyme supply
b. Low salt food needs to be given
c. Provide high calorie food between the meals
d. Eliminate milk and milk products from meal

Explanation: High calorie food needs to be given, because absorption of fats and nutrients are compromised by disease process.

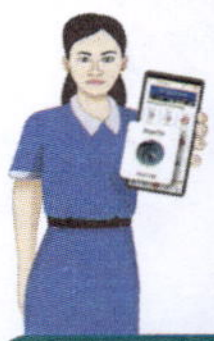

Ans.

438. c
439. d
440. d
441. a
442. b
443. a
444. b
445. b
446. d
447. c

448. Father of a child with cystic fibrosis is concerned about the low weight of his child. The most appropriate nursing education is:

a. Digestive enzymes will be given to help your child digest food
b. Weight gain is not possible for the child
c. In cystic fibrosis, demand for energy is more and intake is less
d. Prepare tasty food and encourage the child to have it

Explanation: In CF, pancreatic ducts are blocked and pancreatic enzymes are not available for digestion process. So supplying pancreatic enzyme will help in digestion process. Enzymatic supplementation helps in proper digestion as well as absorption of nutrient and fat-soluble vitamin.

449. Following Albendazole therapy, nurse needs to educate the parents to observe stool for:

a. Malena   b. Hematochezia
c. Passage of worm   d. Clay colored stool

Explanation: Albendazole is a deworming medication, it's administration leads to killing and passage of worms in the stool.

450. Rice water stools are observed in:

a. Typhoid   b. Cholera
c. Food poisoning   d. Amebic dysentery

451. All are essential requirements of nursing care of a child admitted with severe diarrhea; EXCEPT:

a. Administration of fluids orally/parentally
b. Restrict oral feeding
c. Assess daily weight
d. Maintaining normal body temperature

452. Which vitamin in Excess may lead to necrotizing enterocolitis?

a. Vitamin A   b. Vitamin E
c. Pyridoxine   d. Vitamin C

453. Initial Fluid of choice for diarrhea in an infant?

a. ORS   b. Salt water
c. Sugar water   d. Dextrose

454. Infants who all are recovering from diarrhea often fed with soya-based formula because milk-based formula cause:

a. GI bleeding
b. Soya milk is rich in electrolyte
c. Intestine is unable to digest normal fat
d. Lactase activity is decreased

455. The most important cause of diarrhea in infants and children is: *(Kerala PSC, Nov 2014)*

a. Escherichia coli   b. Rotavirus
c. Salmonella   d. Vibrio cholera

456. Skin turgor in children is assessed at:

a. Dorsum of hand   b. Chest
c. Forehead   d. Abdomen

457. Diarrhea is caused by:

a. E-coli   b. Shigella
c. Salmonella   d. All of these

458. A child had repeated vomiting and developed metabolic alkalosis. The appropriate treatment in this condition is:

a. ORS
b. IV normal saline
c. Ringer lactate
d. IV normal saline and potassium

459. Soy-based formulas are given to a child who is suffering from diarrhea because:

a. Milk-based formulas may cause gastrointestinal irritation and bleeding
b. Supply deficient electrolytes needed for the child
c. Their intestines are unable to digest normal fats
d. Their lactase activity is decreased

460. The common pathogen causing diarrhea in infancy is:

a. Rotavirus   b. E. coli
c. Klebsiella   d. Shigella

461. Bottle fed babies are more prone to develop:

a. Fever   b. Diarrhea
c. Typhoid   d. Malaria

462. A 7-year-old child is brought to the ER at midnight by his mother after symptoms appeared abruptly. The nurse's initial assessment reveals a temperature of 104.5°F (40.3°C), difficulty swallowing, drooling, absence of a spontaneous cough, and agitation. These symptoms are indicative of which one of the following? **New Q** *(NORCET 2022)*

a. Acute tracheitis
b. Acute spasmodic croup
c. Acute epiglottitis
d. Acute laryngotracheobronchitis

Explanation: Acute epiglottitis is a serious condition characterized by a rapid onset of symptoms, usually affecting children between the ages of 2 and 8. The high fever (104.5°F or 40.3°C) is a common feature of epiglottitis. Other hallmark symptoms include difficulty swallowing, drooling, absence of a spontaneous cough, and agitation.

Acute epiglottitis is a medical emergency, as it can rapidly progress to airway obstruction and respiratory distress.

463. Surgery of choice for congenital hypertrophic pyloric stenosis is:

a. Gastrostomy   b. Pyloromyotomy
c. Colostomy   d. Gastrectomy

464. Most common biochemical abnormality in congenital hypertrophic pyloric stenosis:

a. Hypokalemic metabolic alkalosis
b. Hyperkalemic metabolic acidosis
c. Hypokalemic metabolic acidosis
d. Hyperkalemic metabolic alkalosis

465. Congenital absence of ganglion cells in the submucosal and myenteric plexus of the distal intestine is known as:

a. Congenital hypertrophic pyloric stenosis
b. Hirschsprung's disease
c. Intussusception
d. Intestinal obstruction

466. Child is failing to pass meconium and there is protruded abdomen, child is passing ribbon like stool. These are the typical clinical features of:

a. Necrotizing enterocolitis
b. Intestinal obstruction
c. Anorectal malformations
d. Aganglionic megacolon

467. A congenital condition in which abdominal content protrudes through the defect in the abdominal wall and is not covered with sac is called:

a. Gastroschisis   b. Omphalocele
c. Umbilical hernia   d. Abdominal hernia

Ans.

448.	a
449.	c
450.	b
451.	b
452.	b
453.	a
454.	d
455.	b
456.	d
457.	d
458.	c
459.	d
460.	a
461.	b
462.	c
463.	b
464.	a
465.	b
466.	d
467.	a

468. A congenital condition in which abdominal content protrudes through the defect in the abdominal wall and is covered with sac is called:

a. Gastroschisis b. Omphalocele
c. Umbilical hernia d. Abdominal hernia

469. Cleft lip baby diet post-surgery must include: *(NORCET 2022)* **New Q**

a. Fruit pulp b. Crackers
c. Purees d. Cold cereals

Explanation: After cleft lip surgery, babies should be fed a soft diet that is easy to swallow. This includes purees, which are smooth and liquidized foods. Purees are a good way to get the nutrients that babies need after surgery, and they are also easy to digest.

Fruit pulp might be challenging for the baby to consume due to the potential need for suctioning or difficulty creating a seal around a bottle or nipple.

Crackers and cold cereals may be harder to chew and swallow, which could be problematic during the healing phase post-surgery.

470. The important aspect to be included in the discharge plan of a child with cleft lip and palate is: *(Daman & Diu NO 2018)*

a. Adherence to antibiotic therapy
b. Application of sterile dressing over the lip
c. Administration of vitamin supplements
d. Administering oxygen

Explanation: Infection is a potential complication of any surgery. The nurse should inform to give the antibiotic medication to the child on time, as directed. Logan's Bow (U shaped metal bar) or Steri-Strips is left in place after surgery for a week which needs not be changed with any dressing at home.

471. The most common manifestation of ulcerative colitis in children is:

a. Anal fissures b. Abdominal distension
c. Abdominal cramps d. Profuse diarrhea

472. Intense abdominal cramps, anal fissures and abdominal distensions in a child are suggestive of:

a. Ulcerative colitis b. Crohn's disease
c. Diverticulosis d. Diverticulitis

473. Infants with cystic fibrosis (CF) are likely to develop:

a. Meconium ileus b. Loose motions
c. Vomiting d. Constipation

474. All are the manifestation of Crohn's disease; EXCEPT:

a. Intense abdominal cramps b. Profuse diarrhea
c. Anal fissures d. Abdominal distention

475. In gastroesophageal reflux disease (GERD), the purpose of esophageal pH monitoring is:

a. Look for esophagitis
b. Assess the frequency of reflex
c. Assess time taken for gastric emptying
d. Identify possible obstruction

476. A child presents with abdominal colic and hematuria. On ultrasonography, a stone 2.5 cm in diameter is seen in the renal pelvis. The next step in management of this case is:

a. Pyelolithotomy b. Nephroureterostomy
c. Conservative d. ESWL

477. Preferred position for nursing babies with GERD?

a. Right lateral b. Football position
c. Left lateral d. Head down position

478. In a child with Hirschsprung's disease, nurse noticed fever and explosive diarrhea, what is the immediate nursing intervention?

a. Notifying the physician immediately
b. Administer antidiarrheal medication
c. Monitor child every 30 minutes
d. Record the findings

479. Effectiveness of use of thickened formula feed in a client with GERD is evaluated with:

a. Decrease in regurgitation and vomiting
b. Decrease in frequency of stool
c. Increased urine out put
d. All of the above

480. Which is the most common intra-abdominal tumor in children?

a. Wilms' tumor b. Rhabdomyosarcoma
c. Hepatocellular carcinoma d. Osteosarcoma

DISORDERS OF HEPATIC SYSTEM

481. Which of the following statements regarding Wilson's disease are true?

a. Normal hepatic copper level
b. Hemolytic anemia can occur
c. It is an autosomal dominant disease
d. Decreased urinary copper excretion

Explanation: Hemolytic episodes can occur due to increased copper level in the RBC. Wilson's disease is an autosomal recessive disorder. Increased urinary copper level and elevated copper content of liver is seen in Wilson's disease.

482. Which of the following is the most common cause of hepatitis-B in a three-year-old child?

a. Blood transfusion b. Pin prick
c. Saliva exchange d. Perinatal

483. What is the dose of hepatitis B angigen in Hepatitis B vaccine to be given to children?

a. 5 IU b. 10 IU
c. 20 IU d. 50 IU

Explanation: 10 IU dose is administered for children and adolescents below 18 years of age. For adults, the dose is 20 IU.

484. Which of the following is the characteristic feature of congenital Wilson's disease?

a. Decreased urinary copper excretion
b. May present as acute hepatitis
c. KF ring is present at birth
d. Decreased hepatic copper concentration

DISORDERS OF CARDIOVASCULAR SYSTEM

485. Outcome on fetus if the mother is suffering from serious conditions like cyanotic heart disease is:

a. Macrosomia b. Acromegaly
c. VSD d. IUGR

486. The normal resting heart rate for a newborn is?

a. 75 to 115 bpm b. 85 to 125 bpm
c. 110 to 150 bpm d. 140 to 200 bpm

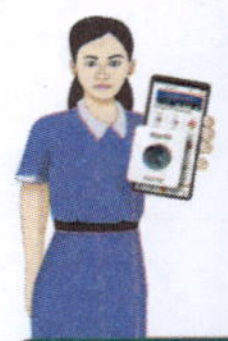

Ans.

468. b
469. c
470. a
471. d
472. b
473. a
474. b
475. b
476. a
477. c
478. a
479. a
480. a
481. b
482. d
483. b
484. b
485. d
486. c

487. The single-most important indicator of cardio-respiratory function in a neonate is: criterion to classify a death as brain death: *(AIIMS BPL NO 2018)*

a. Good cry
b. Good skin color
c. Good muscle tone
d. Good eye contact

Explanation: Good skin color is the most important indicator of cardiopulmonary function in neonate. Adequate oxygenation and good contractility of heart is necessary to have good skin color. Bluish color (cyanosis) of the skin is an indication of defective cardiac function.

488. Most common heart abnormality in child:

a. Tetralogy of Fallot
b. Atrial septal defect
c. Total anomalous pulmonary venous connection
d. Ventricular septal defect

489. What is the normal range of pulse rate of a child of 1 to 2 years? *(AIIMS Bhopal Nursing Officer, 2018)*

a. 60 to 100/min
b. 76 to 120/min
c. 120 to 160/min
d. 80 to 130/min

Explanation: Normal range of pulse rate based upon age of the children is as follows:

Newborns (0–3 months)	:	100–150 BPM
Infants (3–6 months)	:	90–120 BPM
Infants (6–12 months)	:	100–160 BPM
Children (1–10 years)	:	70–130 BPM
Children over age 10 and adults	:	60–100 BPM

In the above given options, 80 to 130 BPM is within the normal range of a child of 1 to 2 years.

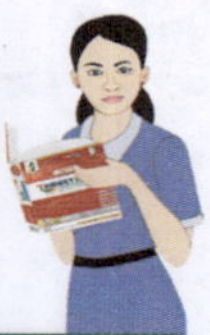

490. All among the following are cyanotic heart diseases; EXCEPT:

a. Tetralogy of Fallot
b. Ebstein's anomaly
c. Transposition of great arteries
d. Patent ductus arteriosus

491. Which of these is a cyanotic heart defect? *(Kerala PSC, Nov 2014; Staff Nurse G II 2014; 2012; AIIMS BPL NO 2018)*

a. Ventricular septal defect
b. Patent ductus arteriosus
c. Tetralogy of Fallot
d. Atrial septal defect

Explanation: Cyanotic heart disease refers to a group of many different heart defects that are present at birth (congenital). They result in a low blood oxygen level. Cyanosis refers to a bluish color of the skin and mucous membranes.

Example of cyanotic heart defect: Tetralogy of Fallot, Tricuspid atresia.

492. Which of the following conditions can present with cyanosis at birth?

a. Tetralogy of Fallot
b. ASD
c. PDA
d. VSD

493. Which of the following is not included in tetralogy of Fallot? *(AIIMS Raipur NO 2019)*

a. Pulmonary stenosis
b. RVH
c. ASD
d. VSD

Explanation: TOF is a combination of four heart defects present at birth. Ventricular septal defect (VSD), pulmonary valve stenosis, overriding of aorta, and right ventricular hypertrophy (RVH).

494. An infant with congestive heart failure (CHF) is admitted to the hospital. Which goal has the highest priority when planning nursing care? *(RAK MSc 2018)*

a. The infant will maintain an adequate fluid balance
b. The infant will have digoxin at the bedside
c. Skin integrity will be assessed
d. Administer medication on time

Explanation: While caring an infant with CHF, the priority is to maintain an adequate fluid balance in the infant. Excessive fluid retention results in symptoms of pulmonary and systemic congestion.

495. In X-ray, the heart of a child with tetralogy of Fallot appears:

a. Cone-shaped
b. Boot-shaped
c. Pea-shaped
d. Apple-shaped

496. Pulmonary blood flow is decreased in?

a. Ventricular septal defect
b. Atrial septal defect
c. Tetralogy of Fallot
d. Truncus arteriosus

497. A child with tetralogy of Fallot and history of severe hypoxic episodes is to be admitted to pediatric unit. Which of the following would be the most important for the nurse to have at the bedside? *(RAK MSc 2018)*

a. Morphine sulfate in a syringe ready to administer
b. Oxygen tubing and gauze plugged in
c. Blood pressure cuff and stethoscope
d. Suction tubing and equipment

Explanation: Tetralogy of Fallot is a complex congenital heart disease. In this disease, cyanosis is the main symptom and the degree of cyanosis depends upon the size of ventricular septal defect and the severity of the obstruction in the right ventricle. The uncontrolled cyanosis leads to respiratory distress. Therefore, oxygen tubing and gauze should be at bed side to meet the emergency signs of respiratory distress.

498. A six-year-old child is admitted to the hospital for heart surgery to repair tetralogy of Fallot, the nurse should anticipate, when the child goes home the parents will most likely have a concern about: *(RAK MSc 2018)*

a. Allowing the child to lead a normal active life
b. Persuading the child to get enough rest
c. Having the child develop post-operative complications
d. Having the child out of the school for a month

Explanation: Last phase of treatment is rehabilitation and principle of rehabilitation is to restore optimal level of health. Rest other options are distractors opposite to leading normal life.

499. Peripheral pulmonic stenosis may be seen in all; EXCEPT: *(Recent Question 2014)*

a. Williams syndrome
b. Alagille syndrome
c. Rubella syndrome
d. CMV

Ref: Nelson 20th ed. p 1551

Ans.

487. b
488. d
489. d
490. d
491. c
492. a
493. c
494. a
495. b
496. c
497. b
498. a
499. d

Explanation:
- A familial tendency has been recognized in some patients with peripheral pulmonic stenosis.
- A high incidence is found in infants with congenital rubella syndrome.
- The combination of supravalvular aortic stenosis with pulmonary arterial branch stenosis, idiopathic hypercalcemia of infancy, elfin facies, and mental retardation is known as Williams syndrome, a condition associated with deletion of the elastin gene in region 7q11.23 on chromosome 7.
- Peripheral pulmonary stenosis is also associated with the Alagille syndrome, which may be associated with a mutation in the Jagged 1 gene.

500. The complications for ventricular septal defect are all of the following; EXCEPT: *(ESIC 2019)*
a. Pulmonary hypertension b. Cerebral palsy
c. Endocarditis d. Heart failure

Explanation: VSD or ventricular septal defect is a cardiac defect in which there is an abnormal communication between two ventricles. Cerebral palsy is neurological disorder that affects balance, movement and muscle tone. All other conditions are complications of VSD.

501. A child who is suffering from cyanotic heart disease is more comfortable in .... position.
a. High Fowler's b. Knee chest
c. Prone d. Supine

Explanation: Assuming the knee-chest position is thought to increase peripheral resistance, decreasing the amount of right-to-left shunting and thus increasing pulmonary blood flow.

502. The most common symptom in children with symptomatic cardiac malformation is:
a. Poor feeding
b. Hypothermia
c. Delayed physical growth
d. Clubbing of the fingertips

Explanation: Children with cardiac malformation often use increased energy in activities of daily living, decreased oxygen utilization and increased energy output in developing child resulting in slow growth rate.

503. In a child with right to left shunt which finding the nurse should; EXPECT?
a. Low BP b. Peripheral edema
c. Elevated hematocrit d. Bounding pulse

Explanation: Polycythemia is a common finding in children with right to left shunt and thereby increased HCT will be present.

504. In pre-operative period of cardiac surgery, prophylactic antibiotics are given to prevent:
a. Pericarditis
b. Myocarditis
c. Sub-acute bacterial endocarditis
d. Upper respiratory tract infection

Explanation: Antibiotics are given to prevent sub-acute bacterial endocarditis which is most commonly present in children with cardiac malformation.

505. While taking vital signs of a child with coarctation of aorta (CoA) nurse should suspect:
a. A weak radial pulse
b. A strong pedal pulse
c. A decreased blood pressure in the arm
d. An elevated blood pressure in the arm

Explanation: CoA is narrowing of aorta usually thoracic segment which causes accumulation of blood above the constriction and increased blood volume and pressure in the arm.

506. Which of the following nursing interventions is a priority after cardiac catheterization?
a. Provide hydration
b. Monitor site for bleeding
c. Check for gag reflex
d. Administer antibiotics as ordered

Explanation: Hemorrhage is a life-threatening complication following catheterization, because catheter is inserted into the artery during the procedure. So, monitor the catheter insertion site for bleeding is the important nursing intervention.

507. In cyanotic heart disease, polycythemia is a compensatory mechanism for:
a. Tissue oxygen need
b. Decreased blood volume
c. More capillary refill time
d. Hypertrophy of cardiac muscles

Explanation: Decreased oxygenation stimulate erythropoiesis, resulting in excessive production of RBCs, so polycythemia will be there.

508. In post-operative period following repair of TOF important nursing intervention is to prevent:
a. Diarrhea b. Sneezing
c. Hard stool d. Unnecessary movement

Explanation: Forceful evacuation resulting in taking deep breath and holding it. This will cause increase in intra-abdominal pressure, which put excessive strain on heart structure.

509. The parents of a 2-day-old girl baby are concerned because her feet and hands are slightly blue. How should the nurse respond? *(AIIMS Raipur NO 2019)*
a. "Your daughter has acrocyanosis; this is causing her blue hands and feet"
b. "Let's watch her carefully to make sure she does not have a circulatory problem"
c. "This is normal; her circulatory system will take a few days to adjust"
d. "This is vasomotor response caused by cooling or warming"

Explanation: In a 2-day-old newborn, slightly blue hands and feet are not an abnormality, but rather a minor immaturity of the circulatory system, which will be resolved after some time. So the reassurance by the nurse is the correct response.

510. In rheumatic fever Sydenham's chorea occurs because of the involvement of:
a. CNS b. Cardiovascular
c. Gastrointestinal d. Genitourinary

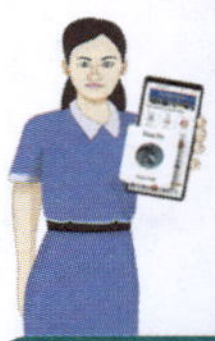

Ans.
500. b
501. b
502. c
503. c
504. c
505. d
506. b
507. a
508. c
509. c
510. a

511. Name the causative organisms responsible for rheumatic fever:
a. Klebsiella
b. Monococcus
c. Group A β-hemolytic streptococcus
d. Staphylococcus aureus

Explanation: Rheumatic fever results as a delayed reaction to inadequately treated group A β-hemolytic streptococcal infection. Poverty, poor hygiene, lack of access to medical care are the risk factors for the development of rheumatic fever. Jones criteria is used to diagnose this condition.

512. A nurse was collecting history from a child who was admitted with suspected rheumatic fever. Which of the following informations is specific to rheumatic fever?
a. A fever that started 2 days back
b. Vomiting for last two days
c. Loss of appetite
d. A recent episode of pharyngitis

513. Drug of choice for Rheumatic fever prophylaxis in penicillin allergic patient:
a. Erythromycin
b. Clindamycin
c. Vancomycin
d. Gentamycin

514. Identify the correct statement(s) related to rheumatic fever:
a. Most common causative organism responsible for rheumatic fever is Group a beta hemolytic streptococci
b. 5-15 years children are most commonly affected with rheumatic fever
c. Jones criteria is the diagnostic criteria used for diagnosing rheumatic fever
d. All of the above

515. Clinical criteria for diagnosing rheumatic fever is developed by:
a. Karl Landsteiner
b. Alexander Fleming
c. Leeuwenhoek
d. T. Duckett Jones

516. All among the following are major criteria for diagnosing rheumatic fever as per Jones criteria; EXCEPT:
a. Erythema marginatum
b. Carditis
c. Arthralgia
d. Polyarthritis

517. All among the following are minor criteria for diagnosing rheumatic fever as per Jones criteria; EXCEPT:
a. Fever
b. Arthralgia
c. Chorea
d. Prolonged PR interval

518. Most commonly affected valve in rheumatic heart disease is:
a. Tricuspid
b. Aortic
c. Mitral
d. Pulmonic

519. As per Jones criteria for diagnosis of rheumatic fever, what is the minimum recommended criterion needs to be presented to diagnose acute rheumatic fever?
a. Presence of one major or two minor signs in the presence of essential criteria
b. Presence of two major signs and no minor signs in the presence of essential criteria
c. Both a and b
d. Presence of one major and one minor sign

520. A classic characteristic of coarctation of aorta includes:
a. Cyanotic episodes
b. Clubbed fingers
c. Absent of diminished femoral pulses
d. Squatting posture of the child

521. In transposition of the great arteries, which of the following procedures is performed to shift the high pressure from the right ventricle to the left ventricle?
a. Rastelli procedure
b. Jatene procedure
c. Nikaidoh procedure
d. Richmond procedure

522. Ductus arteriosus refers to:
a. Communication between pulmonary vein and inferior vena cava
b. A small hole located in the septum between atria
c. Communication between Pulmonary vein and aorta
d. Communication between Pulmonary artery and aorta

523. A child with cyanotic heart disease brought to emergency with cyanotic spell, most important nursing management is:
a. Place the child in high Fowler's position
b. Start IV fluid
c. Decrease hypoxic spells
d. Minimize activity

524. The best position for examination of cardiac murmurs in a child is:
a. Sitting
b. Standing
c. Right lateral
d. Recumbent

525. Common symptom of TOF is:
a. Diarrhea
b. Bradycardia
c. Clubbing of fingers
d. Fever

526. Most sensitive indicator of intravascular volume depletion in infant is:
a. Stroke volume
b. Heart rate
c. Cardiac output
d. Blood pressure

527. Which among the following nursing interventions expects to be performed by the nurse to decrease the joint pain associated with rheumatic fever?
a. Maintaining the joints in a neutral position
b. Do ice compression
c. Apply traction to the joint
d. Use bed cradle to avoid weight of the linen

528. Identify the most frequent complication for a child with congenital cardiac disease?
a. Frequent chest infection
b. Malnutrition
c. Activity intolerance
d. Prolonged bleeding

Explanation: Children with congenital heart disease are more prone to chest infections. Most of the time, these children will be presented with the signs and symptoms related to chest infection.

DISORDERS OF GENITOURINARY SYSTEM

529. A newborn with acquired herpes simplex type 2 infection often exhibits deficit in:
a. GI function
b. Renal function
c. GU function
d. Skeletal function

Explanation: These infants may have renal dysplasia so impaired renal function will be there.

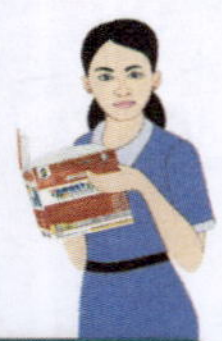

Ans.

511. c
512. d
513. a
514. d
515. d
516. c
517. c
518. c
519. c
520. c
521. b
522. d
523. c
524. b
525. c
526. d
527. d
528. a
529. b

530. If there is delayed passage of meconium stools in newborn and barium enema radiograph shows dilated proximal colon and small obstructed distal colon. What diagnostic test will the nurse anticipate next? *New Q*

a. Abdominal CT-scan
b. Stool studies
c. Rectal suction biopsy
d. Sweat chloride testing

Explanation: The described presentation is suggestive of Hirschsprung's disease, a congenital condition characterized by the absence or insufficient number of ganglion cells in the rectum and/or colon. This results in a functional obstruction of the distal colon and failure to pass meconium in the newborn period.

Rectal suction biopsy is a common diagnostic procedure used to confirm the diagnosis of Hirschsprung's disease. During the procedure, a small suction catheter is inserted into the rectum to obtain a biopsy sample from the affected area.

531. The nurse is planning care for a 2-year-old who has nephrotic syndrome and is in remission. What type of diet would the nurse plan to feed this child? *(RAK MSc 2018)*

a. High protein low caloric
b. High caloric low proteins
c. Low sodium, low fat
d. Regular diet no added sugar

Explanation:

- As child is in remission state, i.e., the protein in the urine disappears and the swelling in the tissues goes away, regular diet with adequate proteins and calories is to be given.
- High protein diet is not given due to compromised kidney function.
- Low calorie diet is not given as the energy requirements of the body are to be met.
- Low sodium and low-fat diets are given only when proteinuria is significantly present.
- High calorie diet is restricted as metabolic functions of the body are altered.

532. The clinical manifestation of nephrotic syndrome includes which of the following: *(RAK MSc 2018)*

a. Hematuria
b. Massive proteinuria
c. Increased serum albumin
d. Weight loss

Explanation: Nephrotic syndrome is a kidney disorder that causes the body to excrete protein (albumin) in the urine more than the normal value due to which urine appears foamy. Nephrotic syndrome is caused by the damage to the glomeruli. Nephrotic syndrome causes edema particularly in the feet and ankles.

Weight gain occurs due to excess fluid retention in the body.

Serum albumin levels are decreased.

Hematuria is also a clinical manifestation of nephrotic syndrome, but it is not always present.

533. A 6-year-old child is admitted with nephrotic syndrome. Which is the significant nursing intervention to be done daily by a nurse? *(AIIMS Bhopal Grade-I 2018)*

a. Checking temperature
b. Measuring mid arm circumference
c. Checking capillary refill
d. Monitoring intake output

Explanation: Nephrotic syndrome is defined as a group of symptoms characterized by number of renal or extra renal features, most prominent of which are proteinuria (>3.5 gm/24 hrs), hypoalbuminemia, edema, hyperlipidemia and hypercoagulability. So, it is very important to maintain intake output chart to maintain fluid and electrolyte balance and prevent dehydration.

534. A child is diagnosed with Wilms' tumor. During assessment, the nurse expects to detect:

a. Gross hematuria
b. Dysuria
c. Oliguria
d. Abdominal mass

Explanation: The most common sign of Wilms' tumor is a painless, palpable abdominal mass, sometimes accompanied by an increase in abdominal girth. Gross hematuria is uncommon, although microscopic hematuria may be present. Usually abdominal palpation is contraindicated in these group of patients.

535. A pediatric nurse is assigned to care for a child with a diagnosis of Wilms' tumor. In planning care for the child, the nurse understands that this tumor is: *(RAK MSC 2018)*

a. An abdominal tumor
b. A renal tumor
c. A brain tumor
d. A bone tumor

Explanation: Wilms' tumor or nephroblastoma is one of the common malignant diseases of children. It is a renal tumor originating from embryonic tissue. Abdominal palpation is contraindicated in this condition.

536. In a child with exstrophy bladder, what covering should the nurse use to protect the exposed area?

a. Loose diaper
b. Moist dressing
c. Dry gauze dressing
d. Petroleum jelly gauze pad

Explanation: Exposed area should be moistened and covered well.

537. Additional defects associated with exstrophy bladder is:

a. Separation of the pubic bones
b. Puborectal slings
c. Abdominal wall defect
d. All of the above

Explanation: All the above-mentioned defects are associated with exstrophy bladder. Bladder exstrophy is a rare genitourinary malformation that, when simply defined, refers to the eversion of the bladder to the outside of the body. It is a rare genitourinary malformation for which the management still challenges the field of pediatric urology.

538. Following circumcision, discharge teaching includes:

a. Apply diaper loosely
b. Clean the site with alcohol and betadine
c. Perform intermittent catheterization
d. Perform Kegel exercises

Explanation: Apply diaper loosely for 2–3 days to lessen the pressure on the penis.

539. Nursing care of a child with acute streptococcal glomerulonephritis is:

a. Monitor I/O chart
b. Monitoring for convulsions
c. Monitor BP
d. All of the above

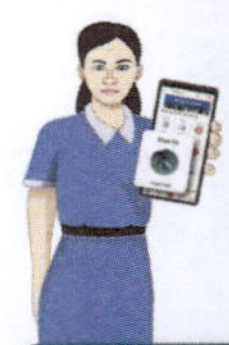

Ans.

530. c
531. d
532. b
533. d
534. d
535. b
536. b
537. d
538. a
539. d

540. All the following are the expected diagnostic tests for Wilms' tumor; EXCEPT:
a. Abdominal CT b. Abdominal MRI
c. Abdominal USG d. Renal biopsy

Explanation: Abdominal palpation and renal biopsy are contra-indicated in a child with Wilms' tumor because it may break the encapsulated tumor and may cause spreading of the disease.

541. Poststreptococcal glomerulonephritis in children is diagnosed by?
a. Heavy proteinuria, high cholesterol, high ASO titre
b. Heavy proteinuria, hematuria, low ASO titre
c. Mild proteinuria, high hematuria, high ASO titre
d. Mild proteinuria, high cholesterol, normal ASO titre

542. Which among the following signs in a child who is suffering from acute poststreptococcal glomerulonephritis indicates early signs of improvement?
a. Weight gain
b. Increased urine output
c. Have good appetite
d. Decreased incidence of fever

543. The child with acute glomerulonephritis is under treatment in a ward. The nurse should look for following as an indicator for acute renal failure: *(Banaras HU 2015)*
a. Polyuria b. Oliguria
c. Hematuria d. Glycosuria

544. Condition in which the foreskin is narrowed and cannot be retracted over the glans is known as:
a. Phimosis b. Cryptorchidism
c. Exstrophy bladder d. Anorectal malformation

545. Circumcision is used for the treatment of:
a. Epispadia b. Hypospadia
c. Cleft palate d. Phimosis

546. Complications of cryptorchidism include:
a. Atrophy of testes b. Strangulated hernia
c. Sterility d. All of these

547. Orchidopexy is the treatment of choice for:
a. Cryptorchidism b. Phimosis
c. Exstrophy bladder d. Anorectal malformation

548. Term used for undescended testis is:
a. Cryptorchidism b. Omphalocele
c. Hypospadiasis d. Epispadiasis

549. Management of cryptorchidism is:
a. Testosterone b. Aldosterone
c. Mineralocorticoids d. Estrogen and progesterone

550. Unilateral renal agenesis is associated with:
a. Polycystic disease of pancreas
b. Hiatus hernia
c. Single umbilical artery
d. Hypogonadism

551. All are the clinical features of Wilms' tumor; EXCEPT:
a. Microscopic hematuria
b. Painless, palpable abdominal mass
c. Increase in abdominal girth
d. Dysuria

552. Wilms' tumor affects:
a. Kidney b. Abdominal muscles
c. Uterus d. Liver

553. Estimation of GFR includes all; EXCEPT:
a. Serum creatinine b. Age of child
c. Weight of child d. Height of child

554. Renal artery stenosis can result in:
a. Persistent hypertension
b. Chronic glomerulonephritis
c. Renal failure
d. Nephrotic syndrome

555. Acute glomerulonephritis most often occurs because of:
a. Streptococci
b. Diphtheria
c. Pneumococci
d. Salmonella

556. Edema is first noticed .... in nephrotic syndrome.
a. On the legs b. Around the eyes
c. All over the body d. On extremities

557. In an edematous child, 1 kg increase in weight indicates approximately how much fluid retention?
a. 100 mL b. 450 mL
c. 750 mL d. 1000 mL

558. The main indication for giving corticosteroids in nephrotic syndrome is to manage:
a. Proteinuria b. Edema
c. Hyperlipidemia d. Hypertension

559. All are the treatment of nephrotic syndrome; EXCEPT:
a. Corticosteroids
b. Daily weight check and urine protein monitoring
c. Low fat diet
d. Extra salt in the diet

560. All serum proteins are reduced in nephrotic syndrome; EXCEPT:
a. Fibrinogen b. Ceruloplasmin
c. Transferrin d. Albumin

561. In ARF, hyperkalemia is treated with:
a. Normal saline
b. Calcium gluconate
c. Corticosteroids
d. 50%dextrose

562. Which nursing care is to be provided pre-operatively to a baby born with exstrophy of bladder?
a. Initially cover the bladder with a thin dressing or clear plastic wrap
b. Cover the bladder with petroleum gauze
c. Immerse the baby in water while bathing
d. Cover with adhesive tape

Explanation: Cover with petroleum jelly causes dryness and damage to mucosa. Thin film dressing without adhesive is preferred.

563. Causes of painless hematuria in children include all; EXCEPT:
a. Acute glomerulonephritis
b. Renal calculus
c. IgA nephropathy
d. Wilms' tumor

564. Red urine without RBC is seen in:
a. Lupus nephritis
b. Pyelonephritis
c. Hemolytic uremic syndrome
d. Rhabdomyolysis

565. Which of the following is the most appropriate method for obtaining a urine specimen for culture in an 8-month-old girl?
a. Suprapubic aspiration b. Indwelling catheter sample
c. Clean catch void d. Urinary bag sample

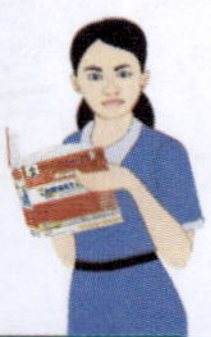

Ans.
540. d
541. c
542. b
543. b
544. a
545. d
546. d
547. a
548. a
549. a
550. c
551. d
552. a
553. d
554. a
555. a
556. b
557. d
558. a
559. d
560. b
561. b
562. a
563. b
564. d
565. c

DISORDERS OF CENTRAL NERVOUS SYSTEM (CNS)

566. Which of the following is not found in cerebral palsy?
- a. Hypotonia
- b. Symmetrical
- c. Ataxia
- d. Flaccid paralysis

567. Which of the following helps in prevention of neural tube defect in fetus? *(RAK MSc 2018)*
- a. Vitamin A
- b. Vitamin C
- c. Vitamin E
- d. Folic Acid

568. An infant born with non-communicating hydrocephalus has just had a ventro peritoneal shunt inserted. In addition to neuromuscular assessments, what measures should the nurse use in child's care plan?:
- a. Reinforce wet dressings every 2 hourly
- b. Position the infant on operative side
- c. Place infant in semi Fowler's position
- d. Measure head and abdominal circumference

Explanation: Nurse needs to measure head and abdominal circumference since there is chance of shunt malfunction and in order to monitor the early signs of intra-cranial pressure and abdominal distension.

569. Isolation period of a child with bacterial meningitis:
- a. 12 hours after starting antibiotics
- b. 24 hours after starting antibiotics
- c. Till antibiotic course completion
- d. Till culture negative

Explanation:
- Isolation is generally required for bacterial meningitis due to meningococci only; it usually spreads by droplet infection.
- The affected children should be placed on droplet precautions (private room, mask for all entering the room) until they have completed 24 hours of appropriate antibiotic therapy.

570. Most common type of meningitis that affects children less than 5 years is: *(AIIMS BPL NO 2018)*
- a. Idiopathic meningitis
- b. Aseptic meningitis
- c. Bacterial meningitis
- d. Tuberculous meningitis

Explanation: Bacterial meningitis: Acute bacterial meningitis is a chief cause of high morbidity and mortality among under five children due to H. influenza type b, S. pneumonia and meningitidis. Bacterial meningitis is also known as septic meningitis.

571. Which of the following informations obtained from the mother of a child with cerebral palsy most likely correlates to the diagnosis? *(Safdarjung NO 2018)*
- a. She was born at 42 weeks gestation
- b. She had meningitis when she was 6 months old
- c. She had physiologic jaundice after delivery
- d. She has frequent sore throats

Explanation: Abnormal brain development, injury or infection to the developing brain can cause Cerebral palsy. Therefore, history of meningitis at the age of 6 months is the correct answer causing cerebral palsy.

572. Meningismus refers to: *(Recent Question 2016-17)*
- a. Meningeal irritation sign without meningitis
- b. Meningitis without meningeal irritation sign
- c. Headache leads to meningitis
- d. It occurs commonly in adults

Ref: Nelson 20th/e/p ch 603

Explanation:
- Meningism, also called meningismus or pseudomeningitis is a set of symptoms similar to those of meningitis but not caused by meningitis.
- Whereas meningitis is inflammation of the meninges, meningism is caused by non-meningitic irritation of the meninges, usually associated with acute febrile illness, especially in children and adolescents.

  Meningism involves the **triad** of nuchal rigidity (neck stiffness), photophobia and headache.

573. Most common diagnostic test performed in a child who is suspected to be suffering from meningitis is:
- a. MRI
- b. X-ray spine
- c. CT scan
- d. Lumbar puncture

Explanation: Inflammation of meninges which is covering brain and spinal cord is known as meningitis. LP is the most commonly performed diagnostic test in a child with meningitis.

574. Cerebrospinal fever is well known as:
- a. Meningococcal meningitis
- b. Pneumococcal meningitis
- c. Staphylococcus meningitis
- d. Hemophilus influenzae type B meningitis

Explanation: Meningococcal meningitis is also known as Cerebrospinal fever caused by Neisseria meningitidis. Meningococcal meningitis is a severe bacterial infection of the bloodstream and meninges which is a thin lining covering the brain and spinal cord. Hence it is also called cerebrospinal fever.

575. All among the following are the characteristics of aseptic meningitis; EXCEPT:
- a. Non-bacterial meningitis
- b. Meningitis with negative bacterial culture
- c. Meningitis with normal CSF glucose, normal to elevated protein
- d. Caused by E. coli

Explanation: Option d is the characteristic of bacterial meningitis. All other are the characteristics of aseptic meningitis caused by viruses.

576. In bacterial meningitis, CSF reveals:
- a. Decreased cell count
- b. Elevated protein level
- c. Increased glucose
- d. Low spinal fluid pressure

Explanation: Blood brain barrier is impaired which allows the passage of protein into the CSF. Cell count will increase and glucose will decrease.

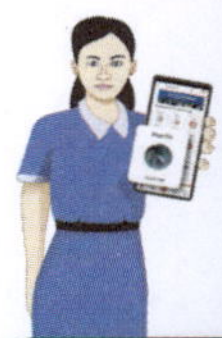

Ans.

566. b
567. d
568. d
569. b
570. c
571. b
572. a
573. d
574. a
575. d
576. b

577. While caring for a child with meningococcal meningitis, the nurse should observe for:

a. Presence of dysphagia
b. Identifying purpuric skin rashes
c. Presence of frontal headache
d. Ataxia

Explanation: Meningococcal meningitis is identified by its epidemic nature and purpuric skin rashes.

578. Clinical features of meningitis:

a. Stiff neck b. Kernig's sign
c. Brudzinski's sign d. All of these

579. The CSF findings in TB meningitis include:

a. High sugar + low protein
b. Low sugar + high protein and Lymphocytosis
c. High sugar + high chloride
d. Low sugar + high protein and Lymphopenia

580. Positive Brudzinski's sign is suggestive of:

a. Craniopharyngioma b. Meningitis
c. Hydrocephalus d. Glioma

581. In a small child diagnosed with H. influenza meningitis, what investigation must be done before discharging him from the hospital?

a. BERA b. MBI
c. CT scan d. X-ray skull

582. Most common cause for communicating hydrocephalus?

a. Bacterial meningitis
b. Intraventricular hemorrhage
c. Aqueductal stenosis
d. Bony malformation of skull

583. While caring for a child with ventriculoperitoneal shunt, what observation might alert the nurse that the child is having infected shunt?

a. Lethargy b. Tachycardia
c. Fever d. Complaining of stiff neck

Explanation: Shunt infection resulting in meningitis and stiff neck is the sign of meningitis.

584. Which among the following anti-seizure medications requires ventilator facility to administer?

a. Phenytoin b. Phenobarbitone
c. Lorazepam d. Calcium gluconate

Explanation: Lorazepam can cause severe respiratory depression, so this drug will be administered only if ventilator facility is available in the unit.

585. Commonly used shunt in hydrocephalus management:
(AIIMS May 2015)

a. Ventriculoatrial b. Ventriculoperitoneal
c. Ventriculo pericardial d. Ventriculo pleural

Ref: Nelson Textbook of Pediatrics 19th e, p 2008-2011; Bailey and Love Textbook of Surgery 25th e, p 627

Explanation: Cerebrospinal fluid shunting is required for the treatment of many children with hydrocephalus.

- The procedure uses a silicone rubber device with a proximal portion inserted into the ventricle, a unidirectional valve, and a distant segment that diverts the CSF from the ventricles to the peritoneal cavity (ventriculoperitoneal shunt).

586. Bulging fontanel indicates:

a. Increased ICP b. Hydrocephalus
c. Both a and b d. Dehydration

Explanation: In hydrocephalus and increased ICP, bulging of fontanel will be there. In dehydration, depressed fontanel will be there.

587. Cracked pot sound on percussion over hydrocephalus baby is called:

a. Chadwick's sign b. Homan's sign
c. Kerning's sign d. Macewen's sign

Explanation: Cracked pot sound in hydrocephalus baby is Macewen sign. Chadwick's sign is a bluish discoloration of the cervix, vagina, and labia resulting from increased blood flow. Homans' sign: Pain in the calf of the leg upon dorsiflexion of the foot with the leg extended that is diagnostic of thrombosis in the deep veins of the area. Kerning's sign: Severe stiffness of the hamstrings causes an inability to straighten the leg when the hip is flexed to 90 degrees. It is suggestive of meningitis.

588. Among the following all are the characteristics of seizure; EXCEPT:

a. Have both fast and slow components
b. Provoked by stimulation
c. Often associated with eye movements
d. Does not stop with restraints

Explanation: Provoked by stimulation is the characteristic of jitteriness, seizure is not provoked by stimulation.

589. Which is the most appropriate diagnostic test to identify phrenic nerve paralysis?

a. Fluoroscopy
b. Bronchoscopy
c. Chest X-ray
d. CT scan

Explanation: An ultrasound or fluoroscopy of the chest would reveal asymmetric diaphragmatic motion in a see-saw manner.

590. Most priority nursing intervention while caring for a child who is suffering from tonic-clonic seizure?

a. Start oxygen by mask
b. Make child sit and provide water
c. Protect child from self-injury
d. Apply restraints

Explanation: Most important nursing intervention during seizure activity is to protect the child from injury.

591. Among the following signs and symptoms, which is not typically seen in increased ICP? *New Q*

a. Vomiting
b. Confusion
c. Blurred vision
d. Dry flushed skin

592. Encephalitis is a complication of:

a. Pertussis b. Varicella
c. Diphtheria d. Rubella

Explanation: Varicella is caused by virus and may be followed by encephalitis.

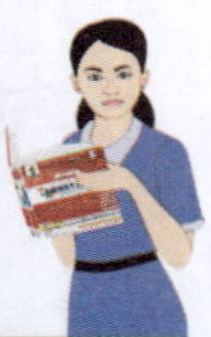

Ans.

577. b
578. d
579. b
580. b
581. a
582. a
583. d
584. c
585. b
586. c
587. d
588. b
589. a
590. c
591. d
592. b

593. Meningomyelocele is:
- a. Herniation of brain, meninges and spinal cord occur through a defect in the base of skull
- b. Protrusion of meninges and spinal fluid but no neural elements
- c. Sac like protrusion through the defect in the vertebra but does not contain CSF
- d. Sac like protrusion contains meninges, CSF and neural elements

Explanation: Meningomyelocele is a condition in which meninges, CSF and neural elements are present in the protruded sac. But in meningocele, meninges and spinal fluid are only involved, but no nerve elements.

594. Immediate nursing care for a child with meningomyelocele is:
- a. Maintain perineal hygiene
- b. Administer antibiotic as ordered to prevent infection
- c. Apply sterile moist non-adherent dressing to the sac
- d. Measure head circumference of the child

Explanation: This is to done to prevent the breakage and dryness of sac and also to prevent the infection which can lead to infection in the CNS. All other options are also the management of a child born with meningomyelocele but the immediate management required is covering of the sac to prevent infection and dehydration.

595. Priority nursing intervention for a child who has meningomyelocele is:
- a. Maintain hydration
- b. Antibiotic therapy
- c. Measurement in head circumference daily
- d. I/O chart maintenance

Explanation: Meningomyelocele predisposes the child to develop hydrocephalus. So, it is important for the nurse to recognize signs and symptoms related to hydrocephalus earlier. Increase in head circumference suggestive of hydrocephalus.

596. The earliest congenital anomaly identified by ultrasound is:
- a. Hydrocephalus
- b. Encephalocele
- c. Renal agenesis
- d. Anencephaly

597. Excess or deficiency of which vitamin leads to peripheral neuropathy?
- a. Pyridoxine
- b. Thiamine
- c. Vitamin B_{12}
- d. Niacin

598. Signs of increased intracranial pressure are all; EXCEPT:
- a. Papilledema
- b. Eighth nerve palsy
- c. Dilated scalp vein
- d. Diplopia

599. A patient is placed in a supine position. The examiner then flexes the patient's neck by bringing the chin toward the chest. If the patient's hips and knees flex involuntarily, the examiner records this observation as: *New Q*
- a. Kernig's sign positive
- b. Kernig's sign negative
- c. Brudzinski's sign positive
- d. Brudzinski's sign negative

Explanation: Brudzinski's sign is a physical exam maneuver used to assess for meningeal irritation (to assess meningitis).

To elicit Brudzinski's sign, the patient is placed in a supine position. The examiner then flexes the patient's neck by bringing the chin towards the chest. If the patient's hips and knees flex involuntarily, Brudzinski's sign is considered positive.

600. Inability or resistance to straighten the leg when the hips and knees are flexed to 90 degrees is known as: *New Q*
- a. Kernig's sign
- b. Brudzinski's sign
- c. Babinski's sign
- d. Battle's sign

Explanation: Kernig's sign is a physical exam maneuver used to assess for meningeal irritation.

To elicit Kernig's sign, the patient is placed in a supine position with the hips and knees flexed to 90 degrees. The examiner then attempts to extend the patient's leg at the knee. If the patient experiences pain or resistance when the leg is extended, Kernig's sign is considered positive.

601. Which neonatal reflex is absent in a child with spastic cerebral palsy?
- a. Moro reflex
- b. Symmetric tonic neck reflex
- c. Asymmetric tonic neck reflex
- d. Grasp reflex

602. Increased accumulation of cerebrospinal fluid in brain is:
- a. NTD
- b. Spinal bifida
- c. Hydrocephalus
- d. None of these

603. A child with Kawasaki disease is likely to develop:
- a. Meningioma
- b. Mitral valve prolapsed
- c. Aneurysm formation
- d. Sepsis

604. Commonest cause of obstructive hydrocephalus in children:
- a. Aqueductal stenosis
- b. Dandy-Walker syndrome
- c. Subarachnoid hemorrhage
- d. Tubercular meningitis

605. Signs and symptoms of increased ICP include:
- a. Bulging fontanel
- b. Headache
- c. Vomiting
- d. All of these

606. Early signs of ventricular shunt malfunction in a child are:
- a. A high-pitched cry, colic, and pupillary changes
- b. A tense fontanel, vomiting, and irritability
- c. Anorexia, and changes in pulse and respiration
- d. Headaches, lethargy, and a loss of appetite

607. Position given after lumbar puncture procedure is:
- a. Fowler's
- b. Supine
- c. Prone
- d. Side lying

608. In an infant the important clinical finding which makes one to suspect increased intracranial tension is:
- a. Fever
- b. Sunken eyes
- c. Tachypnea
- d. Bulged Anterior Fontanel

609. Absent seizures are characterized by:
- a. Infrequent occurrence
- b. Frequent association with vocalization
- c. Aura proceeding the incident
- d. Induction by hyperventilation

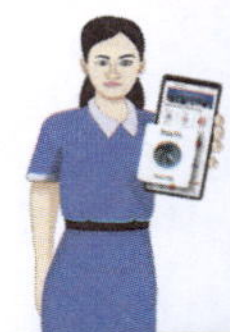

Ans.

593. d
594. c
595. c
596. d
597. a
598. b
599. c
600. a
601. b
602. c
603. c
604. a
605. d
606. b
607. b
608. d
609. d

610. All among the following signs and symptoms are related to increase ICP; EXCEPT:

a. Irritability
b. Bradycardia
c. Decreased alertness
d. Decreased pulse pressure

Explanation: Increased pulse pressure is evident in increased ICP. So option d is not manifested in case of increased ICP. Vomiting, headache, blurring of vision are also often associated with increased ICP.

611. Identify an early symptom of spinal cord tumor from the options:

a. Pain worsens with activity, straining and lying down
b. Position changes leading to complete anesthesia
c. Impaired sensation of temperature, touch pain
d. Clumsiness, weakness, spasticity

612. Which of the following structures is located just inferior to thalamus? *(AIIMS Bhopal Nursing Officer, 2018)*

a. Cerebellum
b. Medulla
c. Epithalamus
d. Hypothalamus

Explanation: The hypothalamus is located below the thalamus and is part of the limbic system. One of the most important functions of the hypothalamus is to link the nervous system to the endocrine system via the pituitary gland.

613. A 3-year-old child was brought to emergency room with hypovolemic shock. The initial fluid bolus should be administered at:

a. 10 mL/kg body weight
b. 20 mL/kg body weight
c. 30 mL/kg body weight
d. 40 mL/kg body weight

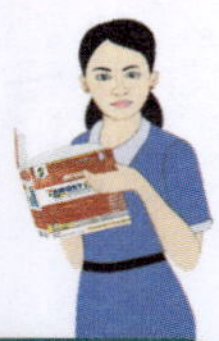

DISORDERS OF HEMATOLOGICAL SYSTEM

614. Rh negative mother delivered a baby. Which among the following tests is more likely to be ordered for the baby?

a. Direct Coombs
b. Indirect Coombs
c. Blood cultured
d. Platelet count

Explanation: Coombs test is the test to determine if RH antibodies are present. Indirect Coombs is done to the mother and Direct Coombs is done to the baby. Blood culture and Platelet count do not help detect Rh antibodies.

Direct Coombs test is used to detect antibodies that are stuck to the surface of red blood cells. Many diseases and drugs can cause this. These antibodies sometimes destroy red blood cells and cause anemia. A normal result means there was no clumping of cells (agglutination). This means there is no antibodies to red blood cells.

615. A newborn with Rh positive group born to a mother with Rh negative blood, during exchange transfusion blood of choice is Rh negative. This is because:

a. To give same blood of mother
b. It is neutral and will not react with baby's blood
c. Can easily obtain from mother
d. To prevent RBC destruction because of maternal anti Rh antibodies

Explanation: Giving Rh positive blood will lead to further hemolysis. Rh negative cells are not attacked by maternal antibodies which are present in infant's blood. So Rh negative blood is the choice.

616. The nurse explains to the mother of a neonate diagnosed with erythroblastosis fetalis, that the exchange transfusion is necessary to prevent damage to: *(NCFL 2019)*

a. Liver
b. Lungs
c. Kidneys
d. Brain

Explanation Erythroblastosis fetalis is a hemolytic anemia caused by transplacental transmission of maternal antibodies to fetal RBCs. The disorder usually results from incompatibility between maternal and fetal blood groups, often RhO(D) antigens.

Exchange transfusion is needed to prevent kernicterus that is caused by the deposition of bilirubin in brain cells.

617. In a child with mild hemophilia A, the factor VIII level is: *(AIIMS Bhopal Grade-I 2018)*

a. 5–50%
b. <1%
c. 50–60%
d. 1–5%

Explanation: The severity of Hemophilia has been defined by a traditional classification into three forms: Mild form in which factor VIII level is more than 5 to 40 % of normal (factor level: >0. 05 to 0. 40 IU/mL), Moderate form in which factor VIII level is 1 to 5% of the normal (factor level: 0.01 to 0.05 IU/mL) and Severe form in which factor VIII level is <1% of the normal (factor level is <0.01 IU/mL).

618. Go through the following statements related to hemophilia and identify the incorrect statement:

a. Hemophilia B is inherited in an X-linked recessive pattern
b. Most of the time females are affected with this condition
c. Fathers cannot pass X-linked traits to their sons
d. In hemophilia B, factor 9 is absent

Explanation: Hemophilia is affecting males and most of the time females are the carrier because it is unlikely that females will have two altered copies of this gene.

619. Normal adult hemoglobin contains: *(Safdarjung NO 2018)*

a. Two alpha chain and one beta chain
b. One alpha chain and two beta chains
c. One beta chain and two alpha chains
d. Two alpha chains and two beta chains

Explanation: Hemoglobin is the protein that makes blood red. It is composed of four protein chains, two alpha chains and two beta chains, each with a ring-like heme group containing an iron atom. Oxygen binds reversibly to these iron atoms and is transported through blood.

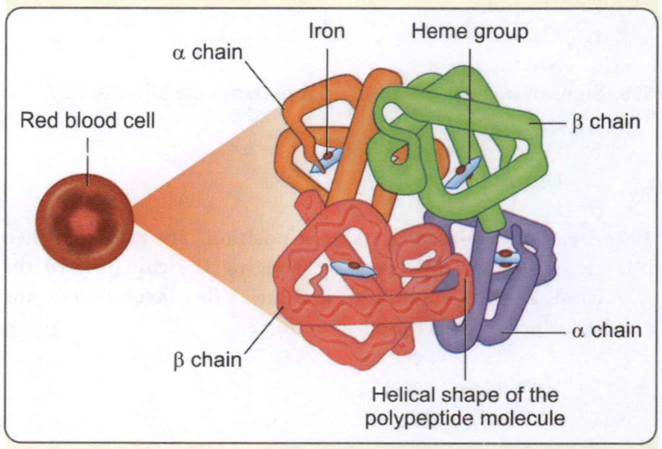

Ans.

610.	d
611.	a
612.	d
613.	b
614.	a
615.	d
616.	d
617.	a
618.	b
619.	d

620. Signs and symptoms of sickle cell anemia most often appear by 4 months of age. This is because:

a. Breastfeeding provides protection against the condition
b. IgG act as a protective factor
c. Fetal hemoglobin act as a protective factor
d. Immunization given at birth provides protection against the condition

Explanation: In newborn baby, fetal hemoglobin acts as a protective factor. Fetal hemoglobin is replaced with adult hemoglobin by the age of 3-4 months, so till that time child remains asymptomatic.

621. A hereditary hemolytic anemia is: *(Safdarjung NO 2018)*

a. Aplastic anemia b. Thalassemia
c. Megaloblastic anemia d. All of these

Explanation: Inherited hemolytic anemia (also known as intrinsic hemolytic anemia) is caused by a defect in the RBC themselves and results when one or more genes that control red blood cell production malfunction. Types of inherited hemolytic anemia include: Thalassemia, Sickle cell anemia, Hereditary Spherocytosis, Pyruvate Kinase Deficiency (PKD), Glucose-6-Phosphate Dehydrogenase (G6PD) Deficiency

622. Inherited pattern of thalassemia is:

a. Autosomal recessive pattern
b. Autosomal dominant
c. X-linked recessive
d. X-linked dominant

Explanation: Autosomal recessive is one of several ways that a trait, disorder, or disease can be passed down through families. An autosomal recessive disorder means two copies of an abnormal gene must be present in order for the disease or trait to develop.

623. Neonatal anemia is defined as hemoglobin:

a. <13 g/dL b. <12 g/dL
c. <11 g/dL d. <10 g/dL

624. According to WHO, cutoff level for hemoglobin in child anemia is:

a. 10 g b. 11 g
c. 12 g d. 13 g

625. Which among the following food items needs to be included in the diet plan of a child with iron deficiency anemia?

a. Rice, cereals and milk
b. Green leafy vegetables and jaggery
c. Bread, jam and cheese
d. Pudding potato and rice

626. In a child with iron deficiency anemia, which among the following activities will be helpful to decrease the oxygen demand?

a. Dancing b. Playing video games
c. Reading a book d. Riding bicycle

627. Most commonly seen anemia in children is:

a. Hemolytic anemia b. Iron deficiency anemia
c. Sickle cell anemia d. Beta thalassemia

628. Vitamin-B12 deficiency anemia also known as:

a. Macrocytic normochromic
b. Microcytic hypochromic anemia
c. Megaloblastic anemia
d. Microcytic normochromic

629. Characteristic of iron deficiency anemia is:

a. Macrocytic normochromic
b. Megaloblastic anemia
c. Microcytic hypochromic anemia
d. Microcytic normochromic

630. Which of the following is a hereditary hemolytic anemia:

a. Aplastic anemia
b. Iron deficiency anemia
c. Vitamin B12 deficiency anemia
d. Thalassemia

Explanation: Aplastic anemia is hereditary but not hemolytic. Thalassemia is a hereditary hemolytic anemia.

631. Bilirubin is the by-product occurred after the metabolism of:

a. Albumin b. Hemoglobin
c. Calcium d. Globulin

632. Hemoglobin level in neonate is:

a. 10–12 g% b. 12–14 g%
c. 14–16 g% d. 16–18 g%

633. In a child with hemophilia, swollen knees occur after falling from bicycle, which among the following is the first nursing intervention?

a. Put an IV cannula and start blood transfusion
b. Monitor client's vital sign
c. Apply ice pack and compressions
d. Provide health education

634. The most common site of bleeding in children with hemophilia is: *(Kerala PSC, Nov 2014)*

a. Joints b. Stomach
c. Gum d. Nose

635. Hemophillia commonly affects:

a. Males
b. Females
c. Transgenders
b. Both males and females equally

636. Which among the following conditions requires repeated blood transfusion?

a. Iron deficiency anemia
b. Pernicious anemia
c. Thalassemia
d. Vitamin B12 deficiency anemia

637. Hemophilia-A is due to deficiency of:

a. Coagulation factor-VIII b. Coagulation factor -IX
c. Coagulation factor -X d. Coagulation factor –XI

638. Hemophilia-B is due to deficiency of:

a. Coagulation factor-VIII b. Coagulation factor -IX
c. Coagulation factor -X d. Coagulation factor -XI

639. Hallmark of the hemophilia is?

a. Epistaxis b. Hemarthrosis
c. Abdominal pain d. Anemia

640. The Best screening test in hemophilia is?

a. Bleeding time b. Clotting time
c. Partial thromboplastin time d. Thrombin time

641. Which of the following would be least likely to result in a prolonged bleeding time?

a. Thrombocytopenia b. Von Willebrand disease
c. Hemophilia A d. Scurvy

642. Treatment of choice for thalassemia major is:

a. Blood transfusion and iron therapy
b. Folic acid and desferrioxamine
c. Blood transfusion and desferrioxamine
d. Iron, blood transfusion and desferrioxamine

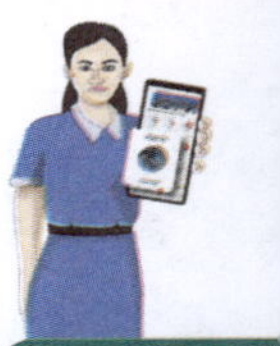

Ans.

620. c
621. b
622. a
623. a
624. b
625. b
626. c
627. b
628. c
629. c
630. d
631. b
632. d
633. c
634. a
635. a
636. c
637. a
638. b
639. b
640. c
641. d
642. c

643. Uncontrolled proliferation of immature WBCs known as:

a. Leukemia b. Anemia
c. Thrombocytopenia d. Leukocytosis

644. All are the diagnostic tests for iron deficiency; anemia; EXCEPT:

a. Total iron-binding capacity
b. Hemoglobin
c. Serum transferrin levels
d. Total protein

645. Laboratory results of a patient who is suffering from disseminated intravascular coagulation (DIC) show:

a. Decreased prothrombin time
b. Decreased partial thromboplastin times
c. Increased platelet counts
d. Prolonged prothrombin and partial thromboplastin times

DISORDERS OF ENDOCRINE SYSTEM

646. A nurse is performing assessment on a 10-year-old suspected of having Hodgkin's disease. The nurse understands that which data are most characteristics of this disease? *(RAK MSc 2018)*

a. Painful, enlarged inguinal lymph nodes
b. Fever and malaise
c. Painless, firm, movable adenopathy in cervical area
d. Anorexia and weight loss

Explanation: Hodgkin's disease is a neoplasm of lymphatic tissue. The presence of Reed-Sternberg cells (giant multinucleated cells) is the hallmark sign of Hodgkin's disease. Specific clinical manifestations associated with Hodgkin's disease include painless, firm, and movable adenopathy in the cervical, supraclavicular, and mediastinal areas. Mediastinal presentation is common in adolescents and young adults. Hepatosplenomegaly is also is seen in this condition.

Other given symptoms are present with many other disorders while painless, firm and movable adenopathy is associated with Hodgkin's disease only.

647. Nelson syndrome is seen after:

a. Hypopituitarism
b. Hyperpituitarism
c. Adrenalectomy
d. Deficiency of growth hormone

648. Which of the following is the most common cause of congenital hypothyroidism?

a. Maternal medications b. Maternal antibiotics
c. Dyshormonogenesis d. Thyroid dysgenesis

Explanation: **Thyroid dysgenesis** is the term used to describe abnormalities in thyroid gland development, includes both the complete absence of **thyroid** tissue (agenesis) and a **thyroid** of decreased size (hypoplasia) with or without associated ectopy. Most cases of congenital hypothyroidism are not hereditary and result from thyroid dysgenesis.

649. An infant has been diagnosed with congenital hypoparathyroidism. All of the following features are associated with congenital hypoparathyroidism; EXCEPT:

a. Esophageal atresia
b. Congenital heart disease
c. Microcephaly
d. Facial abnormalities

Explanation: Congenital hypoparathyroidism refers to defect in development of parathyroid gland due to defect in chromosome 22. Facial abnormalities, esophageal atresia, congenital heart disease and bifid uvula are some of the anomalies associated with congenital hypoparathyroidism.

650. Secretion of ACTH is highest during:

a. Morning b. Noon
c. Evening d. Night

Explanation: In humans, 75% of the daily production of the cortisol occurs between 4 AM and 10 AM. The bursts in secretion is least frequent in the evening.

651. Which of the following conditions leads to delayed fetal lung maturity?

a. Hyperthyroidism b. Diabetes
c. Anemia d. Heart disease

652. All of the following are the possible complications of hypothyroidism; EXCEPT: New Q

a. SIADH b. Muscle weakness
c. Hypokalemia d. Coagulopathy

Explanation: There is impaired renal free water excretion hence hyponatremia due to SIADH. There is not hypokalemia due to hypothyroidism. Muscle dystrophy and muscle weakness can occur as a long term complication of hypothyroidism.

653. Type I diabetes in children is most commonly associated with:

a. Down's syndrome b. Obesity
c. Celiac disease d. Hyperthyroidism

Explanation: **Children** with **celiac disease** were at increased risk of **type 1 diabetes**. The prevalence of **celiac disease** in people with **Type 1 diabetes** is about 6% worldwide. Obesity is associated with Type II diabetes.

ORTHOPEDIC PROBLEMS IN CHILDREN

654. Short stature is a type of __________ disorder.

a. Orthopedic b. Cardiac
c. Metabolic d. Psychiatric

655. Bone dysplasia is because of: *(ILBS, MAHE)*

a. Faulty nutrition b. Faulty development
c. Calcium deficiency d. Fall injury

Explanation: It is an intrinsic disturbance resulting in short stature. Bone or cartilage abnormality that leads to change in size and shape of legs, arms and trunk is known as bone dysplasia.

656. Deformity of...........bone resulting in Sprengel's shoulder.

a. Scapula b. Radius
c. Ulna d. Tibia

Explanation: Sprengel's deformity is a complex anomaly that is associated with malposition and dysplasia of the scapula.

657. The nurse is assessing a child's skeletal traction and notices that the weights are on the floor. Which of the following would the nurse do next? *(RAK MSc 2018)*

a. Raise the weight so that child can move up in bed
b. Notify physician immediately
c. Put the foot of the bed on blocks
d. Move the child up in bed

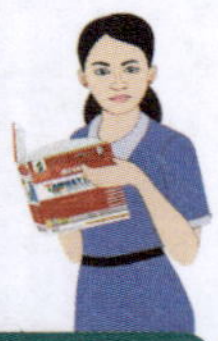

Ans.

643. a
644. d
645. d
646. c
647. c
648. d
649. c
650. a
651. b
652. c
653. c
654. a
655. b
656. a
657. d

Explanation: When a child is in traction the nurse would verify the prescribed amount of traction weight and ensure that the weights hang freely and also ensure that the ropes are on the pulleys. When the child is moved up in the bed the weights lying on the floor will be hanged freely due to counter action of the force and further the fixed alignment of the bone will not be disturbed.

658. Bone age is advanced in:
a. Congenital adrenal hyperplasia
b. Hypothyroidism
c. Hypopituitarism
d. Constitutional delay in growth

659. Deficiency of vitamin-D in children may cause:
a. Osteomalacia
b. Rickets
c. Pellagra
d. Beriberi

660. Break bone fever is commonly known as:
a. Malaria
b. Dengue
c. Kala-azar
d. Q fever

661. Ortolani's test is diagnostic in: *(Staff Nurse G II 2014)*
a. Congenital hip dislocation
b. Induction of labor
c. Respiratory distress
d. Congenital anomalies

662. Which of the following tractions is used to treat femoral fractures of congenital hip dislocation in children under 2 years of age who weigh less than 13.5 kg?
a. Buck's extension traction
b. Bryant's traction
c. Overhead traction
d. Thomas splint traction

663. Ortolani's sign is:
a. Hips and knees to flex when the neck is flexed.
b. Inability to straighten the leg when the hip is flexed to 90 degrees.
c. Palpation of right side of abdomen cause pain and guarding behavior on left side of abdomen
d. The examiner's fingers are extended along the outside of the thighs and a click or a popping sensation may be felt if the joint is unstable

664. A condition in which the sternocleidomastoid muscle is contracted, limiting range of motion of the neck and causing the chin to point to the opposing side is known as:
a. Craniosynostosis
b. Plagiocephaly
c. Torticollis
d. Hydrocephalus

665. Which of the following tractions is used to treat femoral fracture in children over 2 years of age?
a. Buck's extension traction
b. Bryant's traction
c. Thomas splint traction
d. 90-90 traction

666. Which of the following tractions is used for short-term immobilization or to correct bone deformities or contractures?
a. Buck's extension traction
b. Bryant's traction
c. Thomas splint traction
d. 90-90 traction

667. Which of the following tractions is used to treat fractures of the humerus?
a. Bryant's traction
b. Overhead suspension traction
c. Thomas splint traction
d. 90-90 traction

668. In which of the following children the intraosseous drug administration is typically used?
a. Child under 3 years of age
b. Child over 3 years of age
c. Child under 3 years of age and critically ill
d. Child over 3 years of age and critically ill

DISORDERS OF SKIN

669. Drug of choice in treating scabies among younger children is:
a. Gamma benzene hexachloride
b. 5% permethrin cream
c. 0.1% Benzoyl peroxide
d. 0.1% Nicotinamide

Explanation: Gamma benzene hexachloride can cause neurotoxicity through subcutaneous absorption especially in younger children, so drug of choice in younger children is 5% permethrin cream.

670. Drug of choice in trachoma for children is: *(SGPGI 2001)*
a. Oral tetracycline
b. Oral penicillin
c. Aminoglycosides
d. None of these

Explanation: Oral tetracycline (20/mg/kg) is recommended by WHO for the treatment of trachoma in children.

671. Which of the following antibiotics is contraindicated in infants and young children?
a. Amoxicillin
b. Cephalosporins
c. Tetracycline
d. Erythromycin

672. Other name of mucocutaneous lymph node syndrome is:
a. Kawasaki disease
b. Minamata disease
c. Edward syndrome
d. Laughing disease

Explanation: A condition that causes inflammation in the walls of some blood vessels in the body. It is most common in infants and young children. Early stages include a rash and fever. Symptoms include high fever and peeling skin. In late stages, there may be inflammation of medium size blood vessels (vasculitis). It also affects lymph nodes, skin and mucous membranes, such as inside the mouth. Kawasaki disease is usually treatable. Initial treatments include aspirin and IV immunoglobulin therapy are given in a hospital.

673. Child who is on cast is complaining of itching. Action need to taken by the nurse to relieve itching is:
a. Apply cool air under the cast with a blow-dryer
b. Apply lotions on the body
c. Remove the cast
d. Apply mitten to prevent the child from itching

Explanation: Applying cold air under the cast reduces itching.

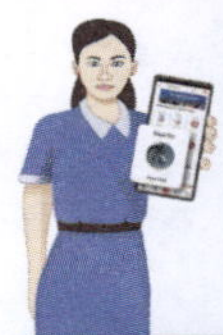

Ans.
658. a
659. b
660. b
661. a
662. b
663. d
664. c
665. d
666. a
667. b
668. c
669. b
670. a
671. c
672. a
673. a

674. Untreated strabismus can lead to:
- a. Cataract
- b. Glaucoma
- c. Amblyopia
- d. Loss of vision in the affected eye

Explanation: By not using affected eye vision in that particular eye will be lost and leads to partial blindness.

DISORDERS OF ENT

675. Neonate with retrolental fibroplasia is associated with:
- a. Hypoxia
- b. Hypocapnea
- c. Hypoxemia
- d. Hyperoxemia

676. Most suitable position for a child who come to OPD with the complaint of epistaxis:
- a. Supine
- b. Prone
- c. Sitting
- d. Lithotomy

Explanation: Sitting is the most appropriate position because keep child's heads elevated but not hyperextended because hyperextension may cause bleeding into the pharynx and possible aspiration.

677. In newborn hearing assessment test done is:
- a. BERA (brain stem evoked response audiometry)
- b. Tuning fork test
- c. Audiometer test
- d. Bone conduction test

Explanation: In newborn baby hearing is assessed with the help of BERA test. Brain stem evoked response auditory (BERA) is a test to measure the brain wave activity that occurs in response to clicks or certain tones.

678. Following tonsillectomy appropriate position in the post-operative period is:
- a. Lithotomy
- b. Side-lying
- c. Fowlers
- d. Prone

Explanation: Side lying position helps in the drainage of secretions from oral cavity and reduces the risk of aspiration.

679. Which of the following would first alert the nurse that a child is hemorrhaging after tonsillectomy? *(RAK MSc 2018)*
- a. Mouth breathing
- b. Frequent swallowing
- c. Requests for drinks
- d. Increased pulse rate

Explanation: Postoperative care for patient with tonsillectomy is to observe for hemorrhage. If hemorrhage occurs patient will show frequent swallowing, pallor, and increase in pulse rate. Hematemesis also can occur.

680. Correct method of holding the pinna in children is:
- a. Upward and backward
- b. Downward and backward
- c. Backward directly
- d. Downward directly

Explanation: By pulling pinna downward and backward, it makes the ear canal straight, and promote visibility and easy administration of medication. In adult the pinna will be held upward and backward.

681. Otitis media in children is caused by:
- a. Streptococcus pneumoniae
- b. Hemophilus influenzae
- c. E-coli
- d. Both a and b

682. Clinical features of "hypothyroidism" in a newborn are all; EXCEPT: *(Recent Question 2014)*
- a. Sluggishness
- b. Large tongue
- c. Large posterior fontanel
- d. Mental retardation

Ref: Nelson 20th ed. p 2668-69

Explanation: Clinical Features of Hypothyroidism in a newborn:
- Birth weight more than average
- Prolongation of physiological jaundice
- Feeding difficulties
- *Respiratory difficulties – large tongue*
- *Sluggishness, poor activities, somnolence*
- Obstinate constipation
- Cold and mottled extremities
- *Umbilical hernia*
- Large posterior fontanel
- Mental Retardation cannot be seen at birth.

683. Identify the correct statement in relation to congenital hypothyroidism:
- a. Oral levothyroxine sodium is used for treatment
- b. Periodic measurement of T3, T4, and TSH is necessary
- c. Monitoring bone age is essential.
- d. All of the above

Explanation: All the above statements are correct in relation to the management of a child with congenital hypothyroidism

684. Hormone responsible for the onset and progression of puberty is:
- a. Estrogen
- b. Testosterone
- c. Progesterone
- d. GnRH

Explanation: GnRH is a hypothalamic gonadotropin-releasing hormone which is responsible for the onset and progression of puberty.

685. Hormone responsible for milk secretion is:
- a. Prolactin
- b. Oxytocin
- c. Estrogen
- d. Progesterone

Explanation: Prolactin stimulates milk production/secretion by inducing the enzyme that synthesizes the constituents of milk, such as lactose, casein, and lipids. The release of the hormone oxytocin leads to the milk ejection or let-down reflex.

686. Prolonged steroid use can cause all; EXCEPT:
- a. Buffalo's hump
- b. Moon faces
- c. Thin extremity
- d. Loss of hair in the body

Explanation: Hirsutism (abnormal hair growth in the body) is the side effect of steroid use.

687. Thelarche is:
- a. It is the onset of secondary breast development, usually occurring at the beginning of puberty in girls.
- b. First menstrual bleeding, in female humans.
- c. The adrenal cortex secretes increased levels of androgens but without increased cortisol levels
- d. The first pregnancy occurs in female human being

Explanation: Option a is the correct answer. Option b indicates menarche. Option c indicates adrenarche.

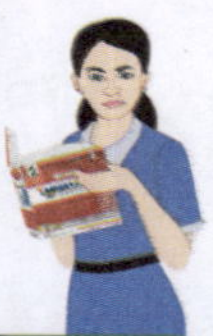

Ans.

674.	d
675.	d
676.	c
677.	a
678.	b
679.	b
680.	b
681.	d
682.	d
683.	d
684.	d
685.	a
686.	d
687.	a

688. Deficiency of Growth Hormone leads to:
a. Delayed union of epiphysis
b. Proportionate dwarfism
c. Acromegaly
d. Mental retardation

689. ACTH secretion is highest during:
a. Noon
b. Evening
c. Morning
d. Night

690. Gigantism is caused by abnormality in the secretion of:
a. Growth hormone
b. Thyroxin
c. Adrenaline
d. Vasopressin

691. Identify the false statement among the following:
a. Acromegaly and gigantism occur due to the problem with growth hormone secretions
b. Gigantism occur in adult and acromegaly occur in children
c. Both are growth defect
d. In gigantism linear growth is more while in acromegaly it occurs after the closure of epiphyseal plate

692. Hypersecretion of growth hormone after the closure of epiphyseal plates can cause:
a. Gigantism b. Acromegaly
c. Myxedema d. Cretinism

693. Hypersecretion of growth hormone before the closure of epiphyseal plates can cause:
a. Gigantism b. Acromegaly
c. Myxedema d. Cretinism

694. Which among the following hormone helps in skeletal maturation of fetus?
a. Testosterone b. Oxytocin
c. Thyroxin d. Prolactin

Explanation: Hormone thyroxin plays an important role in the intrauterine growth and development. This hormone will help in the skeletal maturation of fetus.

695. Thyroxine secretions starts in the fetal life from .... POG onwards.
a. 6th week b. 10th week
c. 12th week d. 14th week

696. In the antenatal period if the mother is suffering from myxedema, then her unborn newborn is at risk for developing:
a. Hyperthyroidism b. Hypothyroidism
c. Both a and b d. Myxedema

697. All are the signs and symptoms of congenital hypothyroidism; EXCEPT:
a. Large fontanels b. Large protruding tongue
c. Umbilical hernia d. Tachycardia

698. Congenital hypothyroidism result in:
a. Myxedema b. Cretinism
c. Gigantism d. Acromegaly

699. Hirsutism is seen in all; EXCEPT:
a. Testicular feminization
b. Polycystic ovary syndrome
c. Cushing's syndrome
d. Congenital adrenal hyperplasia

700. Glycated hemoglobin is a form of hemoglobin that is measured primarily to identify:
a. Oxygen carrying capacity of hemoglobin
b. Glucose absorbing capacity of hemoglobin
c. 3 months average plasma glucose concentration
d. Life span of hemoglobin

701. All are the features of hyperthyroidism; EXCEPT:
a. High amounts of T4, T3
b. High metabolic rate
c. Hand tremors
d. Bradycardia

702. TYPE I Diabetes in children is most commonly associated with:
a. Obesity
b. Celiac disease
c. Downs syndrome
d. Hypothyroidism

703. One of the leading causes of hyperthyroidism is:
a. Graves' disease
b. Exophthalmos
c. Hashimoto's disease
d. Congenital hypothyroidism

704. All are the features of type 1 DM; EXCEPT:
a. Age of onset early
b. Human leukocyte antigen present
c. Can manage with nutritional management
d. Complete absence of insulin

705. All are the features of type 2 DM; EXCEPT:
a. Late onset
b. Family history
c. Tissue resistance is less
d. Manage with diet and exercises

COMMON COMMUNICABLE DISEASES

706. In India, last case of smallpox was reported in the year:
a. 1970 b. 1975
c. 1978 d. 1980

707. India was declared smallpox free in the year:
a. 1970 b. 1977
c. 1980 d. 1982

708. World was declared smallpox free in the year:
a. 1977 b. 1980
c. 1982 d. 1985

709. Thrombocytopenia, increased hematocrit value and positive tourniquet test are seen in:
a. Cholera b. Dengue
c. Mumps d. Measles

710. Important complication of mumps in postpubertal male is:
a. Sterility b. Cryptorchidism
c. Decrease in libido d. Decrease in androgen

Explanation: Mumps causes orchitis in male and can cause sterility.

711. In a 3-year-old child, most common cause of hepatitis B is:
a. Pin prick b. Saliva exchange
c. Perinatal d. Blood transfusion

712. Myxovirus is responsible for:
a. Diphtheria b. Pertussis
c. Mumps d. Tetany

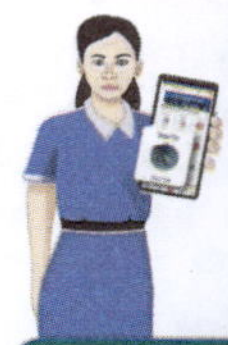

Ans.
688. b
689. c
690. a
691. b
692. b
693. a
694. c
695. c
696. b
697. d
698. b
699. a
700. c
701. d
702. b
703. a
704. c
705. c
706. b
707. b
708. b
709. b
710. a
711. c
712. c

713. Rubeola is:

a. German Measles b. Measles
c. Paratoditis d. Meningitis

714. Commonest complication of Mumps in children is:

a. Orchitis b. Meningitis
c. Myocarditis d. Pancreatitis

715. Mode of transmission of measles is:

a. Droplet b. Transplacental
c. Contaminated food d. Fomite

716. "German measles" is:

a. Mumps b. Rubella
c. Rubeola d. Pertusis

717. Diphtheria is characterized by:

a. Sore throat, dysphasia and low grade fever
b. Sore throat, high grade fever and rash
c. Swelling of parotid gland, earache, fever
d. Sore throat, rash and pain in abdomen

718. Rashes are the clinical manifestation of all the following diseases; EXCEPT:

a. Measles b. Mumps
c. Chickenpox d. Diphtheria

719. The clinical manifestation of Measles which appears last is:

a. Convulsion b. Fever
c. Rash d. Rhinitis

720. Maximum rate of incidence of pertussis is seen in the age group of:

a. < 1 year b. 1-5 years
c. 3-6 years d. 5-10 years

721. Commonly used name for the disease 'hundred-day cough is:

a. Rubella b. Rubeola
c. Cholera d. Pertussis

722. Treatment of choice in community-acquired pneumonia in neonates is?

a. Cefotaxime + Gentamycin
b. Cefotaxime + Amikacin
c. Ampicillin + Amikacin
d. Ampicillin + Gentamycin

723. In the following, which is the first sign of chickenpox in children?

a. Fever b. vesicles
c. Shivering d. Malaise

724. Varicella zoster causes:

a. Chicken pox b. Pertussis
c. Diphtheria d. Polio

725. Most common cause of sore throat in children is:

a. RSV b. Rhinovirus
c. Influenza d. Allergic

726. Which heart disease is most commonly associated with rubella infection?

a. Patent ductus arteriosus
b. Ventricular septal defect
c. Atrial septal defect
d. Eisenmenger's syndrome

727. Infant found to be +ve for HbsAg. The mother was also HbsAg carrier. The mother's hepatitis B serological profile is likely to be: *(AI 2003)*

a. Hbs Ag +ve only
b. Hbs Ag and Hbe Ag +ve
c. Hbs Ag negative and anti HbeAb +ve
d. Hbc Ag positive

Explanation: The hepatitis B blood panel requires only one blood sample but includes three tests:

- HBsAg (hepatitis B surface antigen)
- HBsAb or Anti-HBs (hepatitis B surface antibody)
- HBcAb or anti-HBc (hepatitis B core antibody)

(HBsAg) positive means, this tests for the presence of virus. A "positive" or "reactive" HBsAg test result means that the person is infected with the hepatitis B virus,

A "positive" or "reactive" HBsAb (or anti-HBs) test result indicates that a person has successfully responded to the hepatitis B vaccine or has recovered from an acute hepatitis B infection.

The HBcAb is an antibody that is part of the virus- it does not provide protection. A "positive" or "reactive".

HBcAb (or anti-HBc) test result indicates a past or present infection, but it could also be a false positive.

728. Mother had the onset of varicella zoster before 5 days prior to the onset of delivery. The most appropriate nursing action is:

a. Advise the mother to terminate the pregnancy
b. Varicella-zoster immunoglobulin (VZIG) should be administered to the infant immediately after delivery
c. No need of any action as varicella cannot cross the placental barrier
d. Isolate the baby after the delivery and start formula feed

Explanation: Option b is the correct response; all others are incorrect responses.

729. Which one of the following hepatitis viruses have significant perinatal transmission?

a. Hepatitis E virus b. Hepatitis C virus
c. Hepatitis B virus d. Hepatitis A virus

PEDIATRIC EMERGENCY

730. Sudden infant death syndrome (SIDS) is most likely to occur at what age?

a. 1 to 6 weeks of age, peaking at 3 weeks
b. 1 week to 1 year of age, peaking at 2-4 months
c. 1 week to 1 year of age, peaking at 8-12 months
d. 1 to 3 years of age, peaking at 12-18 months

731. A 2-year-old child is admitted to a burn-unit with partial and full thickness burns over 35% of the body. After admission assessment and review of physician's order, the priority intervention focuses on: *(RAK MSc 2018)*

a. Sedating with morphine sulfate
b. Restricting I/V fluids
c. Inserting nasogastric tube
d. Inserting a Foley catheter

Explanation: Fluid resuscitation is the important treatment for a child with burn injury. Assessment of Urine Output is the best guide regarding fluid resuscitation. Insert a Foley catheter in patients with burns >15% TBSA. Adequate urine output is 0.5 mL/kg/h in adults and 1.5 mL/kg/h in children.

732. Which one of the following is considered a reliable indicator for assessing the adequacy of fluid resuscitation in a 3-year-old child who suffered partial- and full-thickness burns to 25% of her body? **New Q** *(NORCET 2022)*

a. Urine output b. Edema
c. Hypertension d. Bulging fontanelle

Ans.

713.	b
714.	b
715.	a
716.	b
717.	b
718.	b
719.	c
720.	a
721.	d
722.	d
723.	a
724.	a
725.	b
726.	a
727.	b
728.	b
729.	c
730.	b
731.	d
732.	a

Explanation: Urine output is the most reliable indicator of adequate fluid resuscitation in a child who has suffered burns. This is because burns cause a significant loss of fluids, and urine output is a good measure of how well the body is able to replace those fluids.

POISONING

733. Following the poisoning with acetaminophen which among the following sign the nurse needs to expect? *(AIIMS 2004)*

a. Fever
b. Jaundice
c. Right upper quadrant pain
d. Headache

Explanation: Acetaminophen causes hepatic damage because of which child may be complaining of right upper quadrant pain and Jaundice may be a late manifestation.

734. In poisoning, the first action expected from a parent is: *(RML 2000)*

a. Give ample water to the child to drink
b. Call an ambulance immediately
c. Call the poison control center
d. Note down the signs and symptoms developed by the child

Explanation: Before doing any intervention, the parents should call the poison control center for specific directions and help.

735. Assuming that all have achieved normal cognitive and emotional development, which of the following children is at greatest risk for accidental poisoning? *(Safdarjung NO 2018)*

a. A 6-month-old
b. A 4-year-old
c. A 10-year-old
d. A 13-year-old

Explanation: Toddler and preschooler are more prone to accidental poisoning due to their curiosity and desire to explore the world. They learn to eat and drink by their own without knowing, whether it's eatable or not making them vulnerable to eat or drink poisonous substances.

736. Lead poisoning most commonly affects ------------------- body system with it irreversible side effect.

a. Cardiac
b. CNS
c. Gastrointestinal
d. Genitourinary

Explanation: Damage caused by lead is irreversible in CNS, but in all other body system the damage caused by lead is reversible.

737. Oxygen toxicity in pre-term babies causes:

a. Retrolental fibroplasia
b. Respiratory distress syndrome
c. Neonatal sepsis
d. Neonatal hypoglycemia

738. AIDS in children is characterized by:

a. Cryptococcus causing diarrhea
b. Rash on extremities
c. Kaposi's sarcoma
d. Recurrent candidiasis seen

GENETIC DISORDERS

739. All of the following are true about Phenylketonuria; EXCEPT: *(Safdarjung NO 2018)*

a. Deficiency of Phenylalanine Hydroxylase
b. Mental retardation
c. Increased urinary excretion of 4-hydroxy phenyl pyruvic acid
d. Decrease serotonin formation

Explanation: Phenylketonuria is an inborn metabolism error wherein there is absence of phenylalanine metabolism. It results in increased levels of phenylalanine in urine which gives it a musty odor. Hydroxy phenylpyruvic acid is an intermediate product of phenylalanine metabolism. Hence it is found to be a negative statement among the options.

740. All the statement are true about phenylketonuria (PKU); EXCEPT:

a. Inability to properly break down an amino acid called phenylalanine.
b. PKU is an inherited condition
c. Phenylalanine plays a role in the body's production of melanin
d. Diet restriction play least important role in PKU

Explanation: Treatment involves a diet that is very low in phenylalanine, particularly when the child is growing. The diet must be strictly followed. All other statements are true related to PKU.

741. Human has 46 chromosomes was established in the year of:

a. 1954 b. 1955
c. 1956 d. 1957

742. In which year The Human Genome Project was completed?

a. 2001 b. 2003
c. 2005 d. 2008

743. In which year the first human gene therapy was instituted?

a. 1985 b. 1988
c. 1990 d. 1993

744. Commonest DNA variation among the following is:

a. Single nucleotide polymorphism
b. Reciprocal translocation
c. Translocation
d. Mutations

745. One among the following nucleic acid bases is present only in RNA and is:

a. Adenine b. Uracil
c. Guanine d. Thymine

746. The hereditary determinants of humans are received from: *(RRB Feb 2012)*

a. Allele b. Genes
c. Nucleus d. Cytoplasm

747. The science of betterment of human race by application of the law of inheritance is called: *(AIIMS BPL NO 2018)*

a. Genetics b. Eugenics
c. Euphenics d. Euthenics

Explanation: Eugenics is the science of betterment of human race by application of the law of inheritance or *science* of improving the *human species* by selectively mating people with specific desirable hereditary traits.

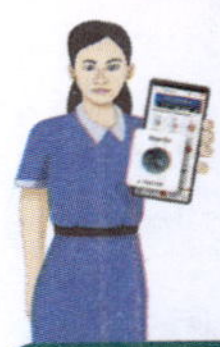

Ans.

733. c
734. c
735. b
736. b
737. a
738. d
739. c
740. d
741. c
742. b
743. c
744. a
745. b
746. b
747. b

748. Cri-du-chat syndrome is:
a. Deletion involving short arm of chromosome 5
b. Addition to the long arm of chromosome 5
c. Deletion of short arm of chromosome 11
d. Addition to the long arm of chromosome 11

749. Webbing of the neck is the characteristic feature of:
a. Edward syndrome b. Neurofibromatosis
c. Turner Syndrome d. Fanconi anemia

750. Karyotype of Klinefelter syndrome is:
a. 47, YYY b. 47, XXY
c. 47, XXX d. 47, XYY

751. Phenylketonuria follows which types of patterns of inheritance? *New Q*
a. Autosomal dominant b. X-linked dominant
c. Autosomal recessive d. X-linked recessive

752. Identify the condition in which Heterozygote (carrier) detection screening can be done:
a. Cystic fibrosis b. Tay-Sachs disease
c. Sickle cell disease d. All of these

753. A normal female, whose father was color blind, marries a normal man. What are the chances of color blindness in their son?
a. 25% b. 50%
c. 75% d. All the male child

754. Among the following autosomal dominant condition is:
a. Albinism b. Sickle cell anemia
c. Thalassemia d. Hereditary spherocytosis

755. In an autosomal dominant couple chances of having an unaffected baby is:
a. 0% b. 25%
c. 50% d. 75%

756. Watson and Crick are associated with:
a. Discovery of helical structure of DNA
b. Find out the bases
c. Explained transcription
d. Explained translocation

757. Identify the X-linked dominant trait among the following?
a. PKU
b. Wilson disease
c. Gaucher disease
d. Vitamin D—resistant rickets

758. X-linked recessive condition is:
a. G6PD deficiency
b. Hemophilia
c. Thalassemia
d. Both a and b

759. Chance of occurrence of an Autosomal Dominant disorder in children if the mother is affected heterozygous and father is normal is:
a. 25% affected b. 50% affected
c. 75% affected d. 100% affected

760. Correct statement regarding X-linked recessive trait is:
a. 50% of boys of carrier mother are affected
b. 50% of girls of diseased fathers are carriers
c. All the children will be affected
d. None of the children will be affected

761. Which type of chromosomal disorders are more common among males as compared to females? *New Q*
a. Autosomal dominant b. Autosomal recessive
c. X-linked dominant d. X-linked recessive

762. Father has an X-linked recessive disorder and mother has a normal genotype. What is the expected outcome?
a. Pass the carrier state to his male children
b. Pass the carrier state to all of his children
c. Pass the carrier state to his female children
d. Not pass on the genetic mutation to any of his children

763. The first son of a couple is affected with hemophilia. Which of the following is the possible outcome of their subsequent pregnancies?
a. Boy will be affected with hemophilia A.
b. Boy will be a carrier of hemophilia A.
c. Girl child will be affected with hemophilia A
d. 50% chance for a girl child to be a carrier of hemophilia A

764. Trisomy 13 is identified as: *(Recent Question 2015)*
a. Edward's syndrome
b. Patau's syndrome
c. Down's syndrome
d. Klinefelter's syndrome

Ref: Nelson 20th ed. p 611t

Explanation: Trisomy 13, also called Patau syndrome, is a chromosomal condition associated with severe intellectual disability and physical abnormalities in many parts of the body. Individuals with trisomy 13 often have heart defects, brain or spinal cord abnormalities, very small or poorly developed eyes (microphthalmia), extra fingers or toes, an opening in the lip (a cleft lip) with or without an opening in the roof of the mouth (a cleft palate), and weak muscle tone (hypotonia).

765. Mapping of genes is possible only if there is a cross between: *(Kerala PSC, Nov 2014)*
a. Dominant heterozygous alleles and dominant heterozygous alleles
b. Dominant heterozygous and dominant homozygous alleles
c. Dominant homozygous and dominant homozygous alleles
d. Dominant heterozygous and recessive homozygous alleles

766. Chromosome pattern in Down's syndrome is:
a. Trisomy 18
b. Trisomy 21
c. Trisomy 22
d. Trisomy 23

767. Most common cardiac lesion in Down's syndrome is?
a. VSD
b. Coarctation of aorta
c. Atrioventricular Septal Defect
d. Transposition of great vessels

768. Chromosome pattern in Edwards syndrome is:
a. Trisomy 18 b. Trisomy 21
c. Trisomy 22 d. Trisomy 23

769. Number of chromosomes in Turner syndrome is:
a. 45 b. 46
c. 47 d. 48

770. In Klinefelter syndrome, no. of chromosomes is: *New Q*
a. 45 b. 46
c. 47 d. 48

771. All are true about Down's syndrome; EXCEPT:
a. Decreased humerus length.
b. Decreased nuchal fold thickness.
c. Mongolian face.
d. Low set ears

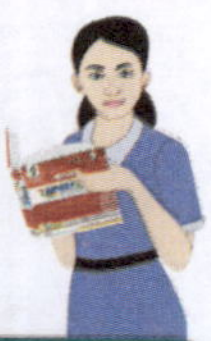

Ans.

748. a
749. c
750. b
751. c
752. d
753. b
754. d
755. b
756. a
757. d
758. d
759. b
760. a
761. d
762. c
763. d
764. b
765. d
766. b
767. c
768. a
769. a
770. c
771. b

Explanation: Increased nuchal fold thickness is a feature of Down's syndrome. So decreased nuchal fold thickness is not true about Down's syndrome.

Decreased humerus length, Mongolian face and low set ears also some of the features of Down's syndrome.

772. All are true about Down syndrome; EXCEPT:
(Recent Question 2014)

a. Mental retardation b. Brushfield spots
c. Microcephaly d. Hypothyroidism

Ref: Nelson 20th ed. p 611

Explanation:

Table: Common characteristics of Down syndrome

Characteristics	Percentage	Characteristics	Percentage
Stunted growth	100%	Short neck	50%
Mental retardation	99.8%	Shortened hands	50%
Atypical fingerprints	90%	Congenital heart disease	45%
Low-set and round ear	60%	Macroglosia (larger tongue)	43%
Flattened nose	60%	Epicanthic fold	42%
Small teeth	60%	Brushfield spots (iris)	35%

- Hematologic malignancies such as leukemia are more common in children with DS.
- ***In particular, acute lymphoblastic leukemia is at least 10 times more common in DS*** and the megakaryoblastic form of acute myelogenous leukemia is at least 50 times more common in DS.
- Hypothyroidism is adults with patients of Down's syndrome.

773. All are seen in Down's syndrome; EXCEPT:
(Recent Question 2014)

a. Low IQ b. Brachycephaly
c. Hypertonia d. Hypothyroidism

Ref: Nelson 20th ed. p 611

Explanation: Brachycepahly implies skull like an American football, due to premature fusion of the coronal suture. Therefore, the brain is not able to grow and it results in mental retardation.

- Overall the most common cause of mental retardation is Down syndrome.
- Thyroid abnormalities in form of either thyroid agenesis or autoimmune thyroiditis are seen in Down syndrome.
- Eye findings of Down syndrome have also been asked and should be remembered as (MEBB)
  - Mongoloid slant of eyes
  - Epicanthal folds
  - Blue dot cataract
  - Brushfield spots in the iris

774. All of the following disorders/diseases are commonly associated with Down's syndrome; EXCEPT:

a. Solid tumors
b. Hirschsprung's disease
c. Congenital Heart Disease
d. Leukemia

Explanation: The conditions associated with Down's syndrome are Heart defects (Congenital Heart Disease), cataracts, hearing loss, infections, hypothyroidism, Leukemia, poor muscle tone, atlantoaxial instability (spinal problem), Epilepsy, celiac disease, Hirschsprung's Disease and mental health problems.

Risk of Hirschsprung's Disease (HD) increases by 50 to 100 fold in children with Down's syndrome (DS) if compared to general population. The incidence of HD in DS patients is 2-3% .

Children with Down's syndrome exhibits a 10 to 20-fold elevated risk of developing acute myeloid leukemia (AML), and acute lymphoblastic leukemia (ALL). The incidence of ALL in Down's syndrome (ALL-DS) is estimated at 1 in 300 (Lange, 2000).

775. Happy Puppet syndrome is also known as:

a. Angelman syndrome b. Prader-Willi
c. Cri du chat syndrome d. Down's syndrome

Explanation: Angelman syndrome is also called "Happy Puppet syndrome" because of the unusual gait and the unprovoked outbursts of laughter. In this condition, interstitial deletion of chromosome 15q1-q13 from maternal side will occur, if it is from the paternal side then it is Prader-Willi syndrome. Trisomy of 21 chromosome is known as Down's syndrome.

776. Short stature, neck webbing, sexual infantilism, and a shield like chest with widely spaced nipples are signs of:

a. Turner's syndrome b. Klinefelter's syndrome
c. Down's syndrome d. Edward's syndrome

Explanation: Mentioned signs and symptoms are the typical features of Turner's syndrome. It occurs because of missing or incomplete sex chromosome.

777. Which of the following would the nurse identify as an appropriate goal for caring a child with Down's syndrome?
(Karnataka PSC 1996)

a. Encouraging self-care skills in the child
b. Adhering to medication regimen
c. Counseling of the family members
d. Allowing them to participate is sports activities

Explanation: Goal of caring mentally-challenged children includes making them independent as much as possible. So teaching them self-care activities will be more effective.

778. Dietary treatment of a child with PKU includes:

a. Protein free diet
b. Protein enriched diet
c. Phenylalanine free diet
d. Low phenylalanine diet

Explanation: Phenylalanine is an essential amino acid, it must be provided in quantities sufficient for promoting growth while maintaining safe blood level.

779. Which is the common nutritional problem associated with Down's syndrome?

a. Obesity b. Kwashiorkor
c. Marasmus d. Vitamin A deficiency

Explanation: Obesity is the most common nutritional problem associated with Down's syndrome, it is associated with impaired growth and excessive calorie intake.

Ans.

772. c
773. c
774. a
775. a
776. a
777. a
778. d
779. a

780. The enzyme deficient in Galactosemia is:
a. Galactose-1 phosphate uridyl transferase
b. Galactose kinase
c. Galactose-6-phosphate epimerase
d. All of the above

Explanation: Above-mentioned enzymes are responsible for galactosemia. Galactose-1 phosphate uridyl transferase causes most serious and classic galactosemia.

781. An inborn error of metabolism that causes premature destruction of RBC:
a. G6PD b. Homocystinuria
c. Phenylketonuria d. Pomps disease

782. A child with low blood glucose is not able to do glycogenolysis or gluconeogenesis. Which of the following enzyme is missing in the child?
a. Fructokinase b. Glucokinase
c. Glucose 6 phosphatase d. Transketolase

783. Darkening of urine on standing is associated with: ***(AI 2007)***
a. Alkaptonuria b. Cystinuria
c. Fabry's disease d. Tyrosinemia

784. Which of the following is true about Asperger syndrome?
a. More common in girls
b. Repetitive activity pattern
c. Subnormal intelligence is consistent feature
d. Severe language impairment is characteristic

Explanation: Severe and sustained impairment in social interaction, and the development of restricted, repetitive patterns of behavior are the features of Asperger's syndrome.

It is more common in boys than girls (4:1). Normal language development as well as normal intelligence is seen in children with Asperger's syndrome.

785. Which among the following finding suggestive of Down's syndrome?
a. Drooling of saliva b. Transverse palmar crease
c. Protruded mass at the back
d. Restricted joint movement

786. Which type of chromosomal disorder is more common among males as compared to females?
a. Autosomal dominant b. Autosomal recessive
c. X-linked dominant d. X-linked recessive

787. Most commonly seen subtype of Down's syndrome in children is:
a. Atopy b. Mosaicism
c. Replication d. Monosomy

788. In Klinefelter syndrome, no. of chromosomes is:
a. 45 b. 46
c. 47 d. 48

Explanation: Klinefelter syndrome is a chromosomal disorder that occurs in males. It is characterized by the presence of an extra X chromosome, resulting in a total of 47 chromosomes instead of the typical 46. The most common karyotype in Klinefelter syndrome is 47,XXY, where there is an additional X chromosome in addition to the usual pair of sex chromosomes (XY).

789. A chromosomal disorder in which a female is born with only one X chromosome is known as:
a. Patau syndrome b. Edward's syndrome
c. Down's syndrome d. Turner's syndrome

Ans.

780.	d
781.	a
782.	c
783.	a
784.	b
785.	b
786.	d
787.	b
788.	c
789.	d
790.	d
791.	a
792.	c
793.	c
794.	b

790. Inborn errors of metabolism are the following; EXCEPT: ***(ESIC 2019)***
a. Cystic fibrosis b. Phenylketonuria.
c. Tay-Sachs disease. d. Turner's syndrome

Explanation: Inborn errors of metabolism are rare genetic (inherited) disorders in which the body cannot properly turn food into energy. The disorders are usually caused by defects in specific proteins (enzymes) that help break down (metabolize) parts of food. Example - Maple sugar urine disease (MSUD), Phenylketonuria (PKU), Cystic fibrosis, Tay-Sachs disease, Glucose-6-phosphate dehydrogenase deficiency (G6PDD).

Turner's syndrome is a chromosomal condition that affects development in females. One of the X chromosomes (sex chromosomes) is missing or partially missing. Short stature is the most common feature of Turner's syndrome.

791. A 10-year-old child is discharged from hospital after, who is suffering from hemophilia. Which of the following sports activity would be recommended by the nurse to this child?
a. Swimming ***New Q***
b. Soccer
c. Field hockey
d. Basketball

Explanation: Swimming is a good sport for children with hemophilia because it is a low-impact activity that does not put stress on the joints. Soccer, field hockey, and basketball are all high-impact sports that can increase the risk of bleeding.

792. All are seen in Down's syndrome; EXCEPT:
a. Low IQ b. Brachycephaly
c. Umbilical hernia d. Hypothyroidism

BEHAVIORAL DISORDERS IN CHILDREN

793. Formula to calculate intelligence quotient (IQ):
a. Chronological age/Mental age*100
b. Mental age-Chronological age *100
c. Mental age/Chronological age*100
d. Mental age + Chronological Age *100

Ref: Achar's Textbook of Pediatrics, 3rd ed, p 31

Explanation: Intelligence quotient (IQ) is the index of intellectual brightness of the child and is calculated as:

IQ = Mental age/Chronological age × 100

- The new terminology for mental retardation is intellectual disability

IQ classification	Level of intellectual disability
50–70	Mild intellectual disability
35–49	Moderate intellectual disability
20–34	Severe intellectual disability
0–19	Profound intellectual disability

794. A mother asks her two-year child, "Do you want to eat now?" The child responds "No". Which of the following behavioral characteristics does the child elicit? ***(AIIMS Bhopal Grade-I 2018)***
a. Egocentrism b. Negativism
c. Egomania d. Ritualism

Explanation: Negativism is a behavior characterized by the tendency to resist direction from others, and refusal to comply with requests. This behavior is commonly encountered with young children (toddlers).

795. Toddler have a tendency to say NO to everything. This feature is known as:

a. Imitation
b. Ritualism
c. Negativism
d. Autonomy

Explanation: A tendency to say no to everything is known as negativism. Imitation means mimicking someone else's behavior. Ritualism means toddlers try to adhere to a specific type of behavior.

796. Which of the following best describes the language of a 24-month-old? *(Safdarjung NO 2018)*

a. Doesn't understand 'yes' and 'no'
b. Understands the meaning of words
c. Able to verbalize needs
d. Continuously asks "Why?" to most of the topics

Explanation: By 2 years of age, a child will be able to understand the meaning of words. Between 8 to 12 months babies start to understand simple requests such as 'yes' or 'no'. At the age of one year, babies begin to communicate beyond crying and are able to verbalize needs in one word. At the age 2 to 3 years, a child will ask 'why' to most of the topic.

797. Passage of feces in inappropriate places after bowel control would be expected, is known as:

a. Encopresis
b. Enuresis
c. Pica
d. Dyslexia

Explanation: Passage of fecal matter in inappropriate locations after bowel control would be expected, is known as encopresis or paradoxical diarrhea. It is voluntary or involuntary faecal soiling in children who have already been toilet-trained.

Enuresis: Refers to a repeated inability to control urination

Pica: eating non-nutritive substances

Dyslexia: Dyslexia, also known as reading disorder, is characterized by trouble with reading

798. A person has not yet fully realized his social identity or defined his personality traits - and he is not actively seeking to, is known as:

a. Role identification
b. Delinquency
c. Negativism
d. Role diffusion

Explanation: According to Erikson, role diffusion develops when the adolescent does not develop a sense of identity and a sense or where he fits in.

799. An 18-month-old child is noted by the parents to be 'anger' about any change in routine. This child's temperament is most likely to be described as:

a. Slow to warm up
b. Difficult
c. Hyperactive
d. Easy

800. Long-term thumb sucking may cause........in the child.

a. Dental problems
b. Worm infestation
c. Decreased nutritional intake
d. All of the above

801. Bedwetting is considered normal in girls and boys till the age of?

a. 3 and 4 years respectively
b. 4 and 5 years respectively
c. 5 and 4 years respectively
d. 4 and 3 years respectively

802. Which is true concerning attention deficit hyperactivity disorder?

a. Impulsive behavior is a feature
b. Higher incidence in tic disorders
c. May respond to treatment with stimulants such as amphetamine
d. All of the above

803. What is the condition in which children is pulling out hair?

a. Trichotellomania
b. Acrophobia
c. Enuresis
d. Encopresis

804. Nocturnal Enuresis is occurrence of involuntary voiding at night in a child more than?

a. 2 ½ yrs
b. 3 ½ yrs
c. 4 yrs
d. 5 yrs

805. Drug of choice to treat Enuresis:

a. Clozapine
b. Diazepam
c. Imipramine
d. Olanzapine

806. Identify the effective nasal spray to control enuresis:

a. Pitressin
b. Desmopressin
c. Lypressin
d. Oxytocin

807. All of the following are common problems of pre-school children; EXCEPT:

a. Temper tantrums
b. Sleep problems
c. Truancy
d. Pica

808. What is the term used for sudden abnormal involuntary repetitive purposeless movement?

a. Obsession
b. Tic
c. Compulsion
d. ADHD

809. Management of attention deficit hyperactivity disorders (ADHD) child is:

a. Calm approach
b. Use simple instructions with the child
c. Reward the child for acceptable behavior
d. All of the above

810. Temper Tantrum is the normal behavior of .... group.

a. Infancy
b. Toddlers
c. Preschool age
d. School age

811. Child's participation in decision making process about health care is termed: *(AIIMS BBS NO 2018)*

a. Assent
b. Collegiality
c. Ethics
d. Advocacy

Explanation: For child less than 18 year of age, assent is taken, procedure is explained to the child in the simpler form while informed written consent is taken from adult (age more than 18 years). This is known as Assent.

812. Repeated urination while sleeping, even after five years of age is called:

a. Enuresis
b. Tic
c. Stuttering
d. Encopresis

813. Which among the following statement indicates that adolescent is having anorexia nervosa?

a. I have my mensuration every month
b. I often go out and eat with my friends
c. I used to exercise three times in a day for total of five hours
d. I always try to maintain my weight around 55-60 kg.

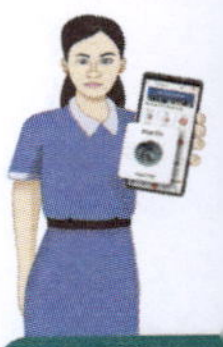

Ans.

795. c
796. b
797. a
798. d
799. c
800. a
801. b
802. d
803. a
804. d
805. c
806. b
807. c
808. b
809. d
810. b
811. a
812. a
813. c

CHALLENGED CHILDREN

814. The term 'educable' is used for which category of mental retardation?
- a. Mild mental retardation
- b. Moderate mental retardation
- c. Severe mental retardation
- d. Profound mental retardation

815. The term 'trainable' is used for which category of mental retardation?
- a. Mild mental retardation
- b. Moderate mental retardation
- c. Severe mental retardation
- d. Profound mental retardation

816. The term custodian is used for which category of mental retardation?
- a. Moderate mental retardation
- b. Severe mental retardation
- c. Profound mental retardation
- d. Both b and c

817. Identify the correct statement related to mental retardation:
- a. In mild MR IQ range is 51–70
- b. In moderate MR IQ range is 36–50
- c. In sever MR IQ range is 20–35
- d. All of the above

818. In a pregnant woman with raised phenylalanine in blood, offspring is most likely to have:
- a. Mental retardation
- b. Lighter complexion
- c. Microcephaly
- d. Reduction of limb growth

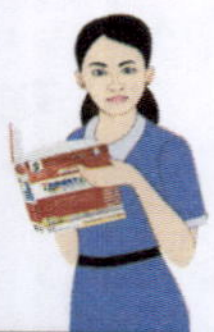

DRUGS IN PEDIATRICS

819. What is the best and most accurate method of measuring the medication dosage for infants and children? *(Safdarjung NO 2018)*
- a. Weight
- b. Height
- c. Nomogram
- d. Weight and Height

Explanation:
- Most drugs in children are dosed according to body weight (mg/kg). Doses are often expressed as mg/kg/day or mg/kg/dose. Chemotherapeutic drugs are commonly dosed according to body surface area:
  - Clarke's Formula = $\frac{\text{Weight (Pounds)}}{150} \times \text{Adult dose}$
  - Fried Formula = $\frac{\text{Age (month)}}{150} \times \text{Adult dose}$
  - Young's Formula = $\text{Adult dose} \times \frac{\text{Age (Years)}}{\text{Age} + 12}$
- Nomogram is a graphical calculating device used to calculate Body surface area.

820. In the antenatal period, there is a history of exposure to morphine in pregnant mother. After the delivery, which among the following drug is most likely ordered by the doctor?
- a. Naloxone
- b. N-acetyl cysteine
- c. Acetazolamide
- d. Sodium bicarbonate

Explanation: Morphine is narcotics and its antidote is naloxone which is essential to prevent respiratory depression in newborn child.

821. Clinical manifestation of fetal alcohol syndrome includes:
- a. Anencephaly, hydrocephalus and microglossia
- b. Hepatomegaly, hypotonia, and microphthalmia
- c. Hyperbilirubinemia, jaundice, and failure to thrive
- d. Microcephaly, short philtrum, and prenatal growth retardation

822. All are seen in fetal alcohol syndrome; EXCEPT:
- a. Microcephaly
- b. Poor coordination
- c. Overgrowth of body
- d. Flat face

823. The fluid requirements for a full-term newborn on day 1 is:
- a. 60-80 mL/kg/day
- b. 80-100 mL/kg/day
- c. 100-140 mL/kg/day
- d. 120-150 mL/kg/day

824. The purpose of Vitamin K injection in newborn is:
- a. For thermogenesis
- b. To establish intestinal flora
- c. To stimulate vitamin K production in the body
- d. To provide protection against bleeding until intestinal flora is established

Explanation: In the newborn baby, gut is sterile, so until intestinal flora is established to provide protection against bleeding, Vitamin K is given to newborn baby. It helps to prevent bleeding problems in the newborn baby. A baby who is less than 1 kg 0. 5 mg I/M is the dose, a baby who is more than 1 kg 1 mg I/M is the dose.

825. Dose of Vitamin K in pre-term baby is:
- a. 0.5 mg
- b. 1 mg
- c. 1.5 mg
- d. 2 mg

826. Dose of Vitamin K in term baby is:
- a. 0.5 mg
- b. 1 mg
- c. 1.5 mg
- d. 2 mg

827. Route of administering Vitamin K in newborn baby is:
- a. IV
- b. IM
- c. SC
- d. ID

828. Iron supplementation in a healthy term breastfed baby should be started at the age of:
- a. 2 months
- b. 4 months
- c. 8 months
- d. 6 months

829. A nurse is assigned to the pediatric rheumatology clinic and is assessing a child who has just been diagnosed with juvenile idiopathic arthritis. Which of the following statements about the disease is most accurate? *New Q*
- a. The child has a poor chance of recovery without joint deformity
- b. Most children progress to adult rheumatoid arthritis
- c. Nonsteroidal anti-inflammatory drugs are the first choice in treatment
- d. Physical activity should be minimized

830. Correct regarding Rh isoimmunization is:
- a. It is also known as Erythroblastosis fetalis
- b. Anti-D gammaglobulin is given to mother to prevent Rh isoimmunization
- c. It is a cause for pathological jaundice
- d. All of the above

831. Cleaning of eyes need to be done in .... direction.
- a. Middle to outer side
- b. Middle to inner side
- c. Inner canthus to outer canthus
- d. Outer canthus to inner canthus

Ans.

814.	a
815.	b
816.	d
817.	d
818.	a
819.	a
820.	a
821.	d
822.	c
823.	a
824.	d
825.	a
826.	b
827.	b
828.	b
829.	c
830.	d
831.	c

832. Excess Vitamin A cause all among the following sign; EXCEPT:

a. Increased appetite b. Blurred vision
c. Bone pain or swelling d. Dryness in the skin

Explanation: Signs and symptoms of Hypervitaminosis A include decreased appetite. Blurred vision, bone pain or swelling, dryness in the skin, bulging fontanel, changes in consciousness, dizziness, drowsiness, double vision, hypercalcemia, heart valve calcification and hair loss are some of the side effects of excessive intake of vitamin A.

833. Agent used for iron chelation is:

a. Deferoxamine b. Iron sulphate
c. Calcium gluconate d. Calcium sulphate

834. The most important toxic side effect of NSAIDs is:

a. Constipation b. Hyperthermia
c. Hematuria d. Feed intolerance

Explanation: Long-term use of NSAIDs can lead to hematuria because of nephrotoxicity.

835. A child weighing 30 kg arrives at the clinic with diffuse itching as the result of an allergic reaction to an insect bite. Diphenhydramine (Benadryl) 25 mg 3 times a day is prescribed. The correct pediatric dose is 5 mg/kg/day. Which of the following best describes the prescribed drug dose?

New Q

a. It is the correct dose
b. The dose is too low
c. The dose is too high
d. The dose should be increased or decreased, depending on the symptoms

Explanation: The recommended pediatric dose for diphenhydramine is 5 mg/kg/day. To calculate the appropriate dose for this child, we can multiply their weight (30 kg) by the recommended dose (5 mg/kg/day).

30 kg × 5 mg/kg/day = 150 mg/day

Since the prescribed dose is 25 mg three times a day, the total daily dose is 75 mg (25 mg × 3 times). Therefore, the prescribed dose of 75 mg is lower than the calculated appropriate dose of 150 mg/day.

836. The primary purpose of administering corticosteroids to a child with nephrotic syndrome is to:

a. Prevent infection b. Control edema
c. Decrease proteinuria d. Increase blood pressure

Explanation: The primary purpose of administering corticosteroids to a child with nephritic syndrome is to achieve complete remission (absence of proteinuria). Corticosteroids have no effect on blood pressure. Steroids may predispose a patient to infection. Diuretics are used to reduce edema.

837. Aspirin overdose in a child can cause:

a. Metabolic alkalosis b. Respiratory alkalosis
c. Metabolic acidosis d. Respiratory acidosis

Explanation: Aspirin is also known as salicylic acid. Overdose with aspirin can lead to metabolic acidosis.

838. For a sick child 500 mL of 5% Isolyte P is to be infused over a period of 48 hrs. The drop factor is 60 gtt/ml. How many drops per minute have to be infused?

a. 10 drops b. 12 drops
c. 15 drops d. 15 drops.

839. Formula used to calculate medication in children is:

a. Young's rule
b. Clark's rule
c. Fried's rule
d. All of the above

840. Intraosseous drug administration is typically used for children:

a. Under age 6 b. Over age 6
c. Critically ill under age 6 d. Critically ill and over age 6

841. Drop factor of pediatric drip set is:

a. 16 b. 20
c. 30 d. 60

842. Priority nursing concern while administering sulfonamide preparation is:

a. Weigh the child daily
b. Maintain I/O chart
c. Administer the drug at prescribed times
d. Monitor drug level in the blood

PEDIATRIC NURSING PROCEDURES

843. Cannula size used in newborn baby is:

a. 24 size b. 22 size
c. 20 size d. 18 size

844. Best site to demonstrate capillary filling in infants:

a. Nail bed b. Sternum
c. Ear lobule d. Great toe

845. Amount of blood used for single volume exchange transfusion in full term newborn is:

a. 50 mL/kg body weight b. 65 mL/kg body weight
c. 80 mL/kg body weight d. 100 mL/kg body weight

Explanation: Estimating the blood volume of newborn as 80 mL/kg, exchange involving replacement of 80 mL/kg has been termed single volume exchange transfusion (SVET) and that involving 160 mL/kg is termed double volume exchange transfusion (DVET).

846. Which one of the following statements is most appropriate to convince a mother for immunization of her child? *(Banaras HU 2015)*

a. Immunization is okay for your baby
b. Vaccines are expensive and you are getting it free
c. Vaccines will prevent the occurrence of that disease in future for which it is meant
d. Government will take care of all post-immunization complications

847. Which of the following symptoms suggest that the child has severe dehydration: *(AIIMS Bhopal Nursing Officer, 2018)*

a. Irritable b. Restless
c. Who drinks water eagerly d. Lethargic or unconscious

Explanation: Lethargic and unconsciousness is the sign of severe dehydration in child. It requires immediate IV fluid replacement. Irritability, restlessness and drinking water eagerly are symptoms of mild to moderate dehydration.

Children with severe dehydration may also have:

- Excessive sleepiness
- Sunken eyes
- Discolored hands and feet
- Persistent wrinkling of the skin
- Faster heart rate
- Extreme thirst

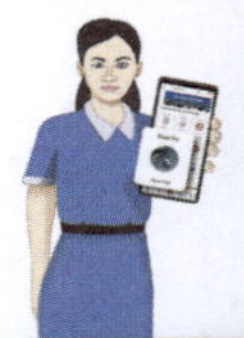

Ans.

832. a
833. a
834. c
835. b
836. c
837. c
838. a
839. d
840. c
841. d
842. c
843. a
844. b
845. c
846. c
847. d

848. A clinic nurse is assessing a child for dehydration. The nurse determines that the child is moderately dehydrated if which symptom is noted on assessment: *(RAK MSc 2018)*

a. Flat fontanels
b. Moist mucous membranes
c. Pale skin color
d. Oliguria

Explanation:

- Oliguria is a sign of dehydration. It is defined as a urine output that is less than 1 mL/kg/hr in infants, less than 0.5 mL/kg/h in children, and less than 400 mL or 500 mL per 24 hours in adults - this equals 17 or 21 mL/hr.
- Sunken or depressed fontanels are seen in dehydration.
- Mucus membrane would be dry in dehydration.
- Skin can be cold or turgor, not pale.

849. While administering IV fluid for the management of dehydration, among the following is the most important nursing intervention?

a. Change the IV set 24 hourly
b. Maintain I/O chart
c. Continuing the prescribed rate of flow
d. Maintaining the fluid at body temperature

Explanation: Prescribed flow rate need to be followed, otherwise it can lead to fluid overload and further problems in children.

850. When administering Total Parenteral Nutrition (TPN) through a peripheral IV line to a school age child, what is the lowest glucose concentration that is considered safe to small veins that will also provide adequate TPN?

a. 5% glucose
b. 10% glucose
c. 15% glucose
d. 20% glucose

Explanation: Any amount above 10% glucose must be administered via central venous access. Glucose 5% is not sufficient concentration to provide sufficient TPN.

851. Parents brought a 4-month-old to OPD with lethargy and poor feeding. Which among the following finding suggestive of fluid volume deficit in child?

a. A sunken fontanel
b. Drinking water
c. Increased blood pressure
d. Enough tears

Explanation: A noticeable sunken fontanel, lethargy, poor feeding and decreased skin turgor suggestive of fluid volume deficit.

852. Which of the following is true about measurement of nasogastric tube in infants?

a. From the tip of head to middle of sternum
b. From the nostril to the end of sternum
c. From the nostril to ear lobe, then to a point midway between the xiphoid process and umbilicus
d. Any of the above measurements can be used

Ref: Primary Care of the Premature Infant by Dara Brodsky, p 111

Explanation: The approximate length of nasogastric tube to be inserted is calculated as "the length from the nostril to the base of the ear lobe, then to a point midway between the xiphoid process and umbilicus".

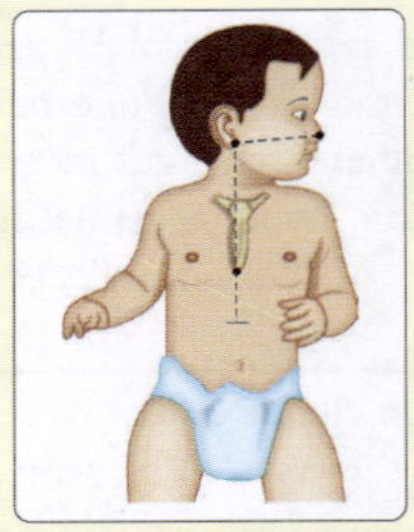

853. Prepared ORS solution is stable for a period of: *(Recent Question 2016-17)*

a. 24 hours
b. 48 hours
c. 72 hours
d. 7 days

Ref: Ghai 8th/e/p 293

Explanation: "Generally, a prepared ORS solution should be covered and not kept for more than 24 hours, due to the risk of bacteriological contamination. Packets of ORS should be stored carefully and not kept in temperatures of over 30 degree C or in conditions of high humidity".

854. Electrolyte is present in ORS is:

a. Calcium carbonate
b. Calcium gluconate
c. Potassium sulfate
d. Sodium chloride

855. All of the following are the signs of fluid volume deficit in an infant; EXCEPT:

a. Low urine specific gravity
b. Increased pulse rate
c. Decreased blood pressure
d. Sunken fontanels

856. Safest position of neonate is on its back or side lying, this is because incidence of .... is very less in these positions.

a. Asphyxia
b. Apnea
c. Sudden infant death syndrome
d. Aspiration

Explanation: Sudden infant death syndrome (SIDS) is the unexplained death, usually during sleep, of a seemingly healthy baby less than a year old. SIDS is sometimes known as crib death because the infants often die in their cribs. Exact cause for this condition is not known. By making them lying down in the back or side lying position will help to reduce the incidence of this condition.

857. Prior to feeding an infant by gastrostomy tube, the nurse should: *(Banaras HU 2015)*

a. Aspirate the tube
b. Slowly instill 5 mL of water
c. Provide the baby with a pacifier
d. Place the baby in Semi-Fowler's position

858. Which measure would be most appropriate for the nurse to do to ensure that a child's ET tube is correctly positioned? *(AIIMS Raipur NO 2019)*

a. Auscultate for abdominal breath sounds
b. Mark the tracheal tube at the child's lip
c. Watch for yellow display on CO_2 monitor
d. Inspect for water vapor in the tracheal tube

Ans.

848. d
849. c
850. b
851. a
852. c
853. a
854. d
855. a
856. c
857. d
858. c

Explanation: Capnography is a noninvasive method for monitoring the level of CO_2 in exhaled breath to assess a patient's ventilatory status. It has become a standard of care. The CO_2 detector should change color from purple to yellow.

Checking for the presence of water vapor is an unreliable method because condensation may be present even if the tube is in esophagus.

859. During child CPR, chest compressions should be given at: *(NORCET 2022)*

a. Upper half of sternum
b. Xiphisternum
c. Lower half of sternum
d. Below sternum

Explanation: The recent CPR guidelines have recommended the lower half of the sternum as the site for proper hand positioning during chest compressions, in order to effectively compress the left ventricle.

860. While performing cardiopulmonary resuscitation (CPR) on a 5-year-old, the nurse palpates for a pulse. Which of the following sites is best for checking the pulse during CPR in a 5-year-old child? *(RAK MSC 2018)*

a. Femoral
b. Carotid
c. Radial
d. Brachial

Explanation: Carotid artery is the best for checking the pulse during CPR in a 5-year-old child. The pulse is located most easily by checking carotid artery on the neck just below the jaw using two fingers. Brachial artery is assessed to locate the pulse in infants.

861. A physician orders I/V potassium for a child with hypertonic dehydration. A nurse performs which of the following highest priority assessment before administering the potassium? *(RAK MSC 2018)*

a. Taking temperature
b. Taking blood pressure
c. Obtaining a weight
d. Checking urine output

Explanation: Before administering potassium to the child, urine output needs to be monitored because main route of excretion of potassium is renal system. If urine output is less than 30ml/hour the patient is at risk for developing hyperkalemia.

862. During the assessment of fluid and electrolyte status in a child, the nurse need to keep in mind that:

a. Kidney is as mature as adult's kidney
b. Intake of fluid will be less
c. Infant body has less percentage of water as compared to an adult
d. Children are having large body surface area

863. Intraosseous drug administration is typically used when a child is:

a. Acutely ill under age 3
b. Acutely ill over age 3
c. Critically ill and under age 3
d. Critically ill and over age 3

Explanation: In critically ill children if other routes are not possible then in emergency situation intraosseous is the route of choice. It is the process of injecting directly into the marrow of a bone.

864. The primary role of the pediatric nurse is to provide nursing care as: *(AIIMS Raipur Grade II 2017)*

a. A collaborator, Care coordinator and consultant
b. An advocate, educator and manager
c. An independent and autonomous practitioner
d. Clinical specialist and case manager

Explanation: The roles of pediatric nurse are primary caregiver, coordinator, collaborator, advocate, health educator, consultant. counsellor, case manager, recreationist, social worker and researcher.

865. Which of the following is the preferred site of intramuscular injections in infants? *(AIIMS BPL NO 2018)*

a. Triceps muscle
b. Vastus lateralis muscle
c. Deltoid muscle
d. Gluteal muscle

Explanation: **Vastus lateralis muscle** is the preferred site of intramuscular injections. The anterolateral thigh is the preferred site for IM injection in infants under 12 months of age.

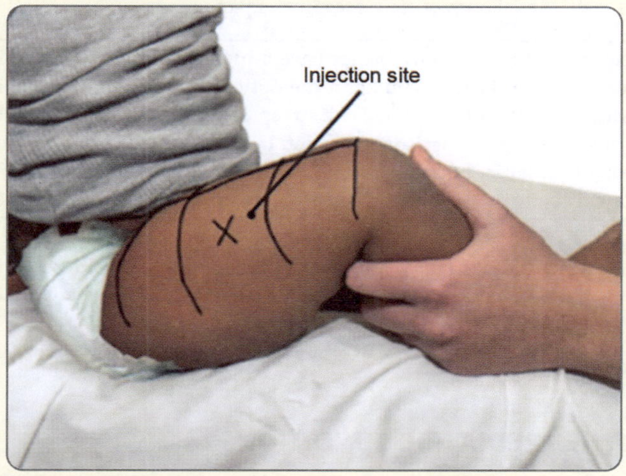

866. Most common congenital malformation in overt diabetes in pregnancy: New Q *(NORCET 2022)*

a. Ventricular septal defect
b. Sacral agenesis
c. Tetralogy of Fallot
d. Atrial septal defect

Explanation: Ventricular septal defect (VSD) is the most common congenital malformation in overt diabetes in pregnancy. The other options are also congenital malformations that can occur in infants of diabetic mothers, but they are not as common as VSDs. Sacral agenesis is rare but specific to overt diabetes in pregnancy.

867. All are true regarding restraints; EXCEPT:

a. Restraints should be used only when it is required
b. It should not be used in SOS basis
c. It should be very tight so that complete immobilization can be achieved
d. Sufficient padding must be used for extremity restraints

868. Restraints used during upper chest/abdominal procedure which immobilize all the extremities is:

a. Clove hitch restraint
b. Crib-net restraint
c. Mummy restraint
d. All of these

Ans.

859. c
860. b
861. d
862. d
863. c
864. b
865. b
866. a
867. c
868. a

869. Main reason for under five morbidity and mortality is:
a. Malnutrition b. Diarrheal Disease
c. Asphyxia d. Leukemia

870. An axillary temperature should be taken for how much period?
a. 15 second b. 30 second
c. 1 minute d. 3 minutes

871. The rectal temperature should be taken in:
a. 30 min b. 1 min
c. 2 min d. 3 min

872. Length of thermometer need to be inserted while taking rectal temperature is:
a. 1 inch
b. 2 inch
c. 2 ½ inch
d. 3 inch

873. Premature babies have more chances of hypothermia because of all of the following; except: **New Q** *(NORCET 2021)*
a. Cold environment
b. Less developed epidermis
c. Less brown fat
d. Small body surface area in comparison of weight

Explanation: Premature babies have a higher risk of hypothermia due to several factors, and all of the options mentioned are usually associated with this increased risk, except for the option d. Small body surface area in comparison to weight. In fact, premature babies have a relatively larger body surface area compared to their weight, which actually contributes to their increased susceptibility to hypothermia.

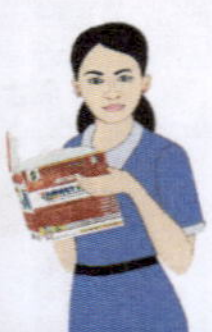

874. What's the smallest amount of glucose that's considered safe and not caustic to small veins, while also providing adequate TPN?
a. 5% glucose b. 10% glucose
c. 25% glucose d. 50% glucose

OTHER PEDIATRIC CONDITIONS

875. Numerator for neonatal mortality rate is calculated by newborn death within:
a. 28 days b. One year
c. 24 hours d. One week

876. Commonest type of seizure in newborn:
a. Atonic b. Tonic
c. Subtle d. Myoclonic

877. Newborn with neonatal tetanus shows:
a. Risus Sardonicus b. Opisthotonus
c. Poor feeding and rigidity d. Trismus and lockjaw

878. Bronze-baby syndrome is characterized by:
a. Decreased urine output and macroglossia
b. Bow-like legs and curved legs
c. Brownish black color of skin, serum and urine
d. Yellowish discoloration of skin

879. Which amongst the following is the most common cause of neonatal death?
a. Mother's lack of knowledge
b. Improper care or due to infections
c. Low family income
d. Any congenital disease

880. In following which is not a preventive measure for tetanus neonatorum?
a. T.T. vaccination
b. Follow five clean rule
c. T.T. immunization during reproductive age
d. Penicillin antibiotic

881. Diaper rashes most commonly are caused by:
a. Streptococci
b. Staphylococcus aureus
c. E-coli
d. Diphtheria

Explanation: Culture of rashes at diaper area will show the growth of **Staphylococcus aureus**

882. Identify the correct statement related to late onset neonatal sepsis?
a. Organisms responsible are present in maternal genital tract
b. Foul smelling liquor and multiple vaginal examination are the risk factors
c. Most commonly manifests as pneumonia
d. Infection is transmitted through the hands of care providers

Explanation: Option d is the correct statement related to late onset neonatal sepsis which occurs after 72 hours, all other statements indicate early onset neonatal sepsis.

883. As per the recent WHO classification of dehydration in children, all of the following are type of dehydration; EXCEPT:
a. No dehydration
b. Moderate dehydration
c. Severe dehydration
d. Some dehydration

Explanation:

Table: WHO guideline for the classification of dehydration

Parameters	No dehydration	Some dehydration	Severe dehydration
Appearance	Well, alert	Restless, irritable	Lethargic or unconscious; floppy
Eyes	Normal	Sunken	Very sunken
Thirst	Drinks nomally, not thirsty	Thirsty, drinks eagerly	Drinks poorly or not able to drink
Skin pinch	Goes back quickly (< 1 second)	Goes back slowly (1 second)	Goes back very slowly (≥2 second)

884. Reye's syndrome is associated with: *(ESIC 2019)*
a. Hemolytic transfusion reactions
b. Biliary colic
c. Sickle cell crisis
d. Use of aspirin with viral illness

Explanation: Reye's syndrome is associated with the use of aspirin with viral illness. It is a rare but serious condition that causes swelling in the liver and brain. Reye's syndrome most often affects children.

Ans.
869. b
870. d
871. b
872. a
873. d
874. b
875. a
876. c
877. d
878. c
879. b
880. d
881. b
882. d
883. b
884. d

885. Child who is affected with Bell's palsy, moistening of the affected eye has to be done to prevent:
a. Keratitis
b. Damage to retina due to light
c. Conjunctivitis
d. Drooping of the eye lid

Explanation: Maintaining moisture to the affected eye (especially at night) to prevent keratitis is required in a child who is affected with Bell's palsy.

886. The nurse is caring for a 6-year-old client with conjunctivitis. Before administering eye drops, the nurse should recognize that it is essential to consider: *(Safdarjung NO 2018):*
a. The eye should be cleansed with warm water, removing any exudate, before instilling the eye drops
b. The child should be allowed to instill his own eye drops
c. The mother should be allowed to instill the eye drops
d. If the eye is clear of any redness or edema, the eye drops should be withheld

Explanation: Conjunctivitis can be manifested as exudates, redness, or edema. Before instilling eye drops, cleansing of eye is done with sterile cotton swab soaked in warm saline using strict aseptic technique.

887. What is the most common form of childhood cancer?
a. Lymphoma
b. Leukemia
c. Brain tumor
d. Osteosarcoma

888. A 6-year-old is newly diagnosed with acute lymphoid leukemia (ALL). During assessment, which of the following signs and symptoms would you expect? *(RAK MSc 2018)*
a. Fever, pallor, bone and joint pain
b. Fever, ruddy complexion, petechiae
c. Abdominal pain, cystitis, swollen joint
d. Enlarged lymph nodes, low-grade fever, night sweat

Explanation: Acute lymphoid leukemia is also known as acute lymphocytic leukemia (ALL). It is a type of blood and bone marrow cancer, in which immature lymphocytes (WBC) are formed. Patients commonly present with pallor caused by anemia and petechiae and bruising secondary to thrombocytopenia. Other signs and symptoms include bleeding gums, bone pain, fever, frequent infections, frequent or severe nosebleeds, lumps caused by swollen lymph nodes in and around the neck, underarm, abdomen or groin, pale skin and shortness of breath.

889. A malignant tumor of childhood, which metastasizes to bones most often, is:
a. Wilms' tumor
b. Neuroblastoma
c. Adrenal gland tumors
d. Granulose cell tumor of ovary

890. What is the most common malignancy of childhood?
a. Medulloblastoma b. Wilms' tumor
c. Leukemia d. Neuroblastoma

891. Chvostek sign and trousseau signs are seen in:
a. Hypokalemia b. Hyperkalemia
c. Hypocalcemia d. Hypercalcemia

Explanation: Chvostek sign means twitching of the orbicularis oculi and mouth elicited by tapping the facial nerve anterior to the external auditory meatus. Trousseau signs mean carpopedal spasm elicited by inflating a BP cuff on the arm to a pressure above the systolic. Both these signs are the characteristic signs of hypocalcemia.

892. ABO incompatibility common in:
a. Mother O+ve baby A+ve
b. Mother O+ve baby B+ve
c. Mother A and baby AB
d. Mother O and baby AB

Explanation: Anti-A and anti-B antibodies are usually IgM and do not pass through the placenta, but some mothers "naturally" have IgG anti-A or IgG anti-B antibodies, which can pass through the placenta. Exposure to A-antigens and B-antigens, which are both widespread in nature, usually leads to the production of IgM anti-A and IgM anti-B antibodies but occasionally IgG antibodies are produced.

893. Most abundant immunoglobulin of human body is:
a. IgG b. IgM
c. IgA d. IgD

894. A child is admitted to the hospital several days after stepping on a sharp object that punctured her athletic shoe and entered the flesh of her foot. The physician is concerned about osteomyelitis and has ordered parenteral antibiotics. Which of the following actions is done immediately before the antibiotic is started? *New Q*
a. The admission orders are written
b. A blood culture is drawn
c. A complete blood count with differential is drawn
d. Written informed consent is obtained

Explanation: Before starting parenteral antibiotics in a child with a suspected case of osteomyelitis, it is crucial to obtain a blood culture. A blood culture helps identify the causative organism responsible for the infection, allowing for targeted antibiotic treatment.

CONGENITAL DISORDERS

895. Cleft-palate is ideally repaired at:
a. Between 6 months and 18 months
b. Between 6 weeks and 8 weeks
c. Between 6 years and 8 years
d. 1st week of birth

896. Double bubble sign in the X-ray is suggestive of:
a. Duodenal atresia
b. Intestinal obstruction
c. Aganglionic megacolon
d. Trachea esophageal fistula

897. Which among the following activity is compromised in a newborn baby with cleft lip? *(AIIMS Raipur Staff Nurse Grade I-2018)*
a. Sucking
b. Swallowing
c. Respiration
d. Facial expression

Explanation: Sucking is the activity compromised in baby with cleft lip and swallowing will be compromised in baby with cleft palate.

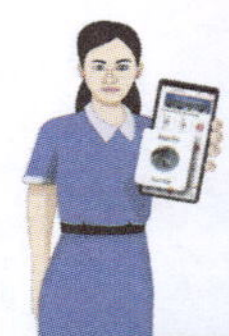

Ans.
885. a
886. a
887. b
888. a
889. a
890. c
891. c
892. d
893. a
894. b
895. a
896. a
897. a

898. Important health teaching regarding feeding practices for a child who is suffering from cleft lip and palate includes:

a. Make the patient lie down and provide feed
b. He should be held in a horizontal position and fed slowly to avoid aspiration
c. Try soft nipple with enlarged opening so he can get the milk through chewing motion
d. Brief rest period and frequent burping during feeding to get rid of swallowed air

Explanation: Providing nutrition and preventing aspiration are the two important nursing responsibilities while caring a child with cleft lip and cleft palate. Child should is be held in upright position during feeding.

899. The cleft palate usually gets repaired during: *(ESIC 2019)*

a. 6 months b 3 months
c. 12-18 months d. 2-3 years

Explanation: Cleft palate is usually repaired around 12 months of age. Cleft lip is usually repaired at four to six months of age.

900. Position used post-operatively while caring for a child with cleft palate is:

a. Supine b. Prone
c. Sitting d. Left lateral

901. Police man tip hand condition is:

a. Erb's palsy
b. Klumpke's paralysis
c. Median never injury
d. Peroneal nerve injury

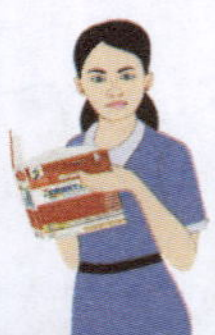

Explanation: Erb's palsy or Erb–Duchenne palsy is a paralysis of the arm caused by injury to the upper group of the arm's main nerves, specifically the severing of the upper trunk C5–C6 nerves. These form part of the brachial plexus, comprising the ventral rami of spinal nerves C5–C8 and thoracic nerve T1

Klumpke's paralysis (or Klumpke's palsy or Dejerine-Klumpke palsy) is a variety of partial palsy of the lower roots of the brachial plexus.

902. As a management of congenital heart disorders one child is posted for the anastomosis of the subclavian artery to the pulmonary artery. This procedure is known as:

a. Glenn shunt
b. Raskkind Procedure
c. Ross procedure
d. Blalock-Taussig

903. Most common acyanotic congenital heart disease:

a. Pulmonic stenosis
b. Atrial septal defect
c. Patent ducts arteriosus
d. Tricuspid atresia

904. The mother of a 2-month-old infant brings the child to the clinic for a well-baby check. She is concerned because she feels only one testis in the scrotal sac. Which of the following statements about the undescended testis is the most accurate?

New Q

a. Normally, the testes are descended by birth
b. The infant will likely require surgical intervention
c. The infant probably has with only one testis
d. Normally, the testes descend by 1 year of age

Explanation: In most cases, the testicles descend into the scrotum by birth. However, in about 1-3% of boys, one or both testicles do not descend. This is called undescended testicles, or cryptorchidism.

In most cases, undescended testicles will descend on their own within the first 6 months of life. However, if the testicle has not descended by 1 year of age, it is likely to require surgical intervention.

905. The clinic nurse asks a 13-year-old female to bend forward at the waist with arms hanging freely. Which of the following assessments is the nurse most likely conducting? New Q

a. Spinal flexibility b. Leg length disparity
c. Hypostatic blood pressure d. Scoliosis

Explanation: Scoliosis refers to an abnormal sideways curvature of the spine. The forward bending test, also known as the Adams forward bend test, is a common screening method used to assess for scoliosis. During this test, the individual is asked to bend forward at the waist while keeping their knees extended and arms hanging freely. The nurse closely observes the curvature of the spine and checks for any asymmetry or abnormal protrusion of the ribs, shoulder blades, or other bony prominences.

906. Low-set ears and wide-set eyes in a child is suggestive of:

a. Exstrophy bladder b. Tracheoesophageal fistula
c. Renal agenesis d. Congenital heart defects

Explanation: Bilateral renal agenesis is characterized by the absence of kidneys and of urine in a baby. The face usually consists of wide-set eyes; a "parrot beak" nose; a receding chin, and large low set ears deficient in cartilage.

907. Polyhydramnios is seen in all the following conditions; except:

a. Duodenal atresia
b. Tracheoesophageal fistula
c. Anencephaly
d. Congenital abnormalities of the fetal kidney

Explanation: Congenital abnormalities of the fetal kidney lead to oligohydramnios. In all other conditions polyhydramnios is there because of the interference with reabsorption of swallowed amniotic fluid.

908. What is the main cause of perinatal mortality?

a. LBW b. Congenital anomalies
c. Birth asphyxia d. Respiratory infection

Ans.

898. d
899. c
900. b
901. a
902. d
903. c
904. d
905. d
906. c
907. d
908. c

"One day in perfect health is much."
—Arabic

CHAPTER 7

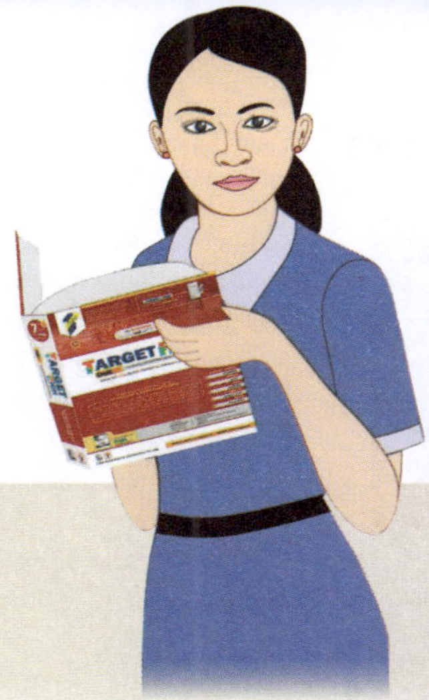

OBSTETRIC AND GYNECOLOGICAL NURSING

SYNOPSIS

ANATOMY OF FEMALE REPRODUCTIVE SYSTEM-OVERVIEW

The female reproductive system refers to the organs and structures involved in the production, transport, and nurturing of the female gamete (egg) and the development and birth of offspring.

It is broadly divided into three categories.

1. External genitalia
2. Internal genitalia
3. Accessory reproductive organs

1. External Genitalia

- It is also known as **vulva** or pudendum.
- It refers to the external structures of the female reproductive system.
- It plays an important role in sexual function.
- It provides a protective barrier for the internal reproductive organs.

External Genitalia (Vulva) Includes

- **Mons pubis:** It is the fatty tissue above the pubic bone that is covered with pubic hair. The hair pattern is triangular among most of the women with base directed upward.
- **Labia majora:** Two folds of skin that extend down from the mons pubis and enclose the labia minora and other vulvar structures. It is **homologous to scrotum in male.** It has own sweat gland and apocrine gland.

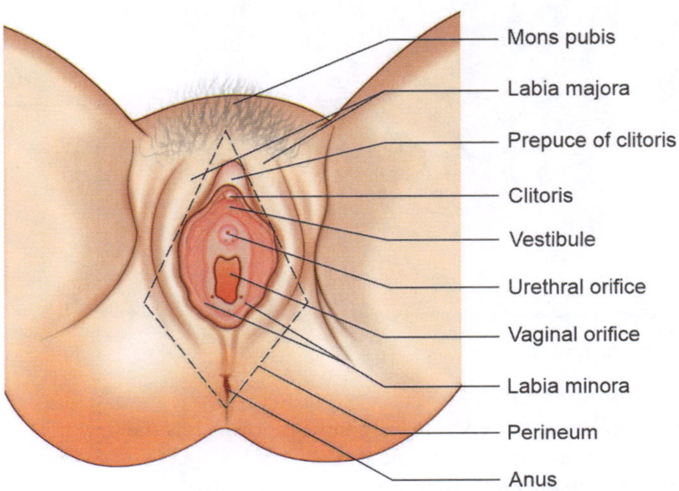

Figure 1: External genitalia

Practice Question

1. While doing pelvic assessment of a pregnant woman nurse noticed red swollen area on the right side of the vaginal orifice. Nurse documented this finding as:

a. Hematoma
b. Montgomery's tubercles
c. Bartholin's gland
d. Bulbourethral glands

Ans. (c) Bartholin's gland

Explanation: Bartholin's glands are homologous to bulbourethral glands in males. Bartholin's glands are located on either side of the vaginal opening and can become swollen and inflamed due to blockage or infection, leading to the formation of a Bartholin's gland cyst or abscess. Montgomery's tubercles are sebaceous (oil) glands that appear as small bumps around the dark area of the nipple.

- **Labia minora:** Two thin folds of skin located inside the labia majora that enclose the vestibule. It is **homologous to penile urethra among males.**
- **Vestibule:** The area between the labia minora. It has total six openings. They are: vaginal opening (1), urethral opening (1), Bartholin's duct opening (2) and Skene's gland opening (2).
- **Clitoris:** A small, highly sensitive organ located at the front of the vulva, involved in sexual arousal and orgasm. It is **homologous to penis in the male**.
- **Hymen:** The hymen is a thin membrane that partially covers the vaginal opening in some females. It is typically located about 1–2 centimetres inside the vaginal opening.
- **Urethra:** It is the opening of the bladder and is located between the clitoris and the vaginal opening.
    - **Bartholin's glands:** Two small glands located on either side of the vaginal opening that secrete alkaline mucus to lubricate the vestibule during sexual arousal. It is **homologous to bulbourethral gland** (Cowper gland) among male. A Bartholin's cyst is a fluid-filled sac that forms in one of the Bartholin's glands, which are located on either side of the vaginal opening. These glands secrete fluid that helps lubricate the vagina.
- **Skene's gland:** It is also known as paraurethral glands. It is composed of two smaller glands, located on either side of the urethral opening. The gland produces a fluid that is similar in composition to male prostate fluid. It is also known as female prostate.

2. Internal Genitalia

It consists of organs named vagina, uterus, fallopian tube, and ovary.

Vagina

- The vagina is a muscular tube that connects the cervix (the opening of the uterus) to the outside of the body. The vagina can expand during sexual arousal and childbirth.
- **It measures** about **2.5 cm in diameter**, it is widest in upper part and narrowest at introitus.
- From puberty, vaginal pH is acidic (4–5 pH) because of lactic acid produced by Doderlein's bacilli.
- Layers of vagina are mucosa, submucosa, muscular and fibrous layer.

Uterus

- The uterus is a pear-shaped muscular organ that is responsible for housing and nourishing a developing fetus during pregnancy. It is in the pelvis and is held in place by ligaments.

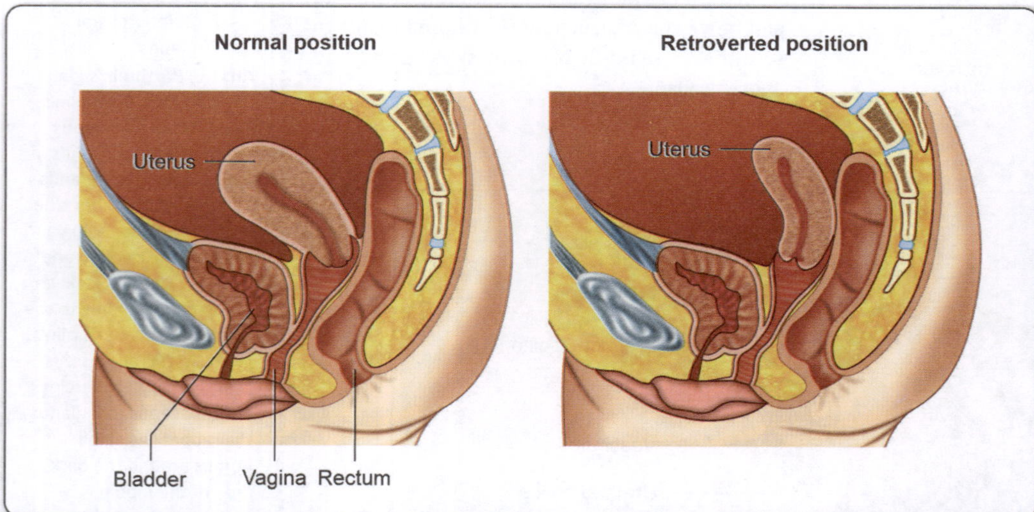

Figure 2: Uterus position

- It is situated between bladder (anterior) and rectum (posterior).
- Normal position of uterus is anteversion and anteflexion and dextrorotation.
- Measurement: It measures 8 cm long, 5 cm across, and 1.35 cm thick and weighs 50–80 g.
- Uterine artery primarily supplies it which is the branch of internal iliac artery.
- **Ligaments supporting uterus (primary support):** Round ligament, uterosacral, transverse cervical, pubocervical.
- Uterus is developed from **Mullerian ducts**.

KEY POINTS

- External genitalia of a female are also known as vulva or pudendum
- Clitoris in female is homologus to penis in male.
- **Blood supply** to the vulva- pudendal artery
- Nerve supply to vulva - pudendal nerve
- From puberty, vaginal pH is acidic (4–5 pH) because of lactic acid produced by Doderlein's bacilli.

Practice Question

2. Which female genital structure is homologous to the scrotum in males?

a. Mons pubis
b. Labia majora
c. Labia minora
d. Clitoris

Ans. (b) Labia majora

KEY POINTS

- Uterus is developed from **Mullerian ducts**.
- Primary blood supply to Uterus: Uterine artery
- Uterine artery is the branch of internal iliac artery

- Uterine wall is composed of three layers:
  i. **Perimetrium:** Outermost serous layer
  ii. **Myometrium:** Middle layer
  iii. **Endometrium:** Innermost mucosal lining of uterine cavity. Thickness changes during menstrual cycle. It changed to decidua during pregnancy.

Parts of the uterus
- Fundus
- Body or corpus
- Isthmus
- Cervix

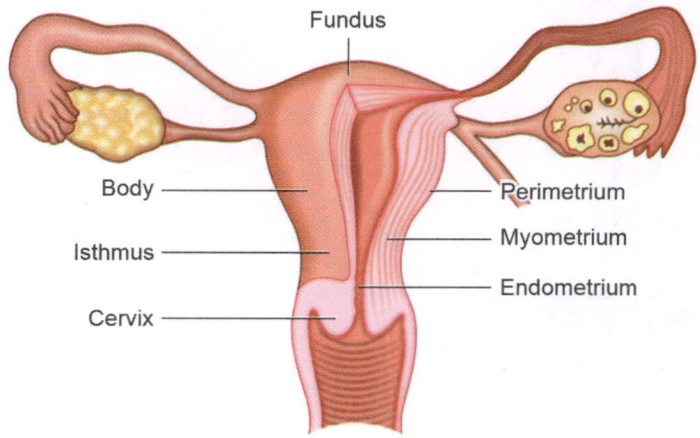

Figure 3: Uterus and its parts

Fundus: The fundus is the upper portion of the uterus, which is located above the level of the fallopian tubes.

Body

- The body is the central portion of the uterus. It is muscular and can stretch to accommodate a developing fetus.
- The uterine tubes are attached to the upper part of the body.
- The point of fusion between the uterine tube and body is called **cornua of the uterus.**
- **Cornua of uterus** is known as **pacemaker of contraction** as uterine contractions begins from this point during labor.

Isthmus: It is the junction between the body and cervix is called isthmus. It is the constricted part.

Cervix:

It connects the vagina with the main body of the uterus

The cervix is composed of two regions:
1. The endocervix is the proximal and inner part of the cervix. It is **lined by simple columnar epithelium** (mucus secreting).
2. The **ectocervix portion** of the cervix projects in the vagina. It is lined **stratified squamous non-keratinized epithelium.**

- **Functions:**
  - Facilitates passage of sperm into the uterine cavity.
  - Prevents uterine cavity from bacterial invasion by frequent shedding of the endometrium, thick cervical mucous and a narrow external os.
- **Blood supply:** Descending branches of the uterine arteries supply cervix and vagina.
- **Nerve supply:** Sympathetic nerves from the **inferior hypogastric plexus (T10–L1)** supply the uterus and cervix. The **pudendal nerve (S2,3,4)** supplies the vagina and pelvic outlet.

Recent Question
(NORCET 2022)

1. **Primary prevention for CA Cervix can be done by:**
   a. HPV vaccine
   b. Pap smear
   c. Drug therapy
   d. Preventing complications

Ans. (a) HPV vaccine

KEY POINTS

- Almost all **cervical cancer** cases (99%) are linked to infection with human papillomaviruses (HPV).
- The combination of **HPV vaccination** and cervical screening can prevent most cervical cancer cases.
- The **inferior hypogastric plexus (T10–L1)** supplies the uterus and cervix.

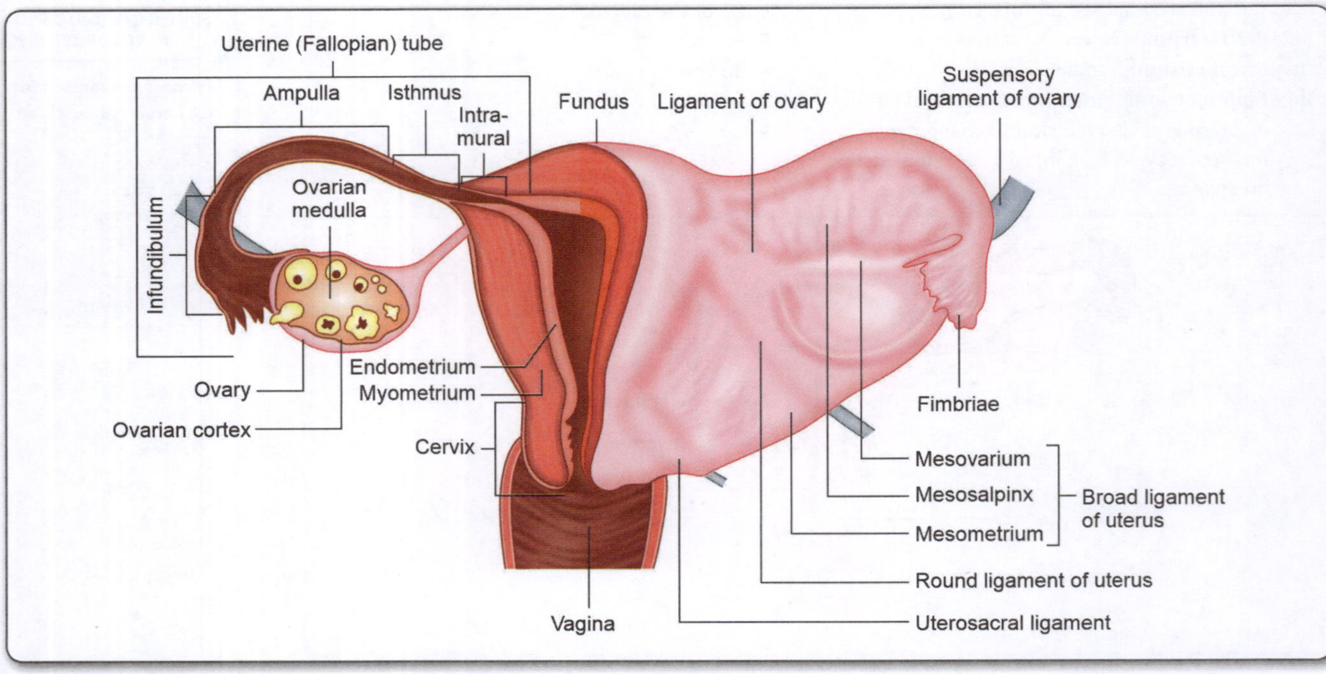

Figure 4: Anatomy of uterus and fallopian tube

Fallopian Tubes (Uterine Tube/ Oviduct/ Salpinx)

- These are paired structures measuring 10 cm.
- They have four parts
  i. Intramural or interstitial (1.25 cm in length 1mm in diameter)–**narrowest part**
  ii. Isthmus (3–4 cm in length and 2 mm in diameter)
  iii. Ampulla: (5 cm in length)–torturous part, **fertilization** occurs in this part. **Longest part** of the fallopian tube.
  iv. Infundibulum: (1.25 cm in length). It has got finger-like projection known as fimbriae.
- **They have the following functions**:
  - Transport gametes
  - Provide suitable environment for fertilization
  - Help in the survival of zygote by its secretions

Ovary

- The ovaries are two small, almond-shaped organs that are located on either side of the uterus.
- It is a retroperitoneal structure.
- Each ovary is approximately 3–5 cm long, 2–3 cm wide and 1–3 cm thick in the menstrual years.
- The ovary is attached to the broad ligament by the **mesovarium.**
- Ovarian ligament connects ovary to the uterus.
- The ovary is composed of a medulla and cortex, covered with germinal epithelium.
- Arterial blood supply is through ovarian artery which is a branch of abdominal aorta.

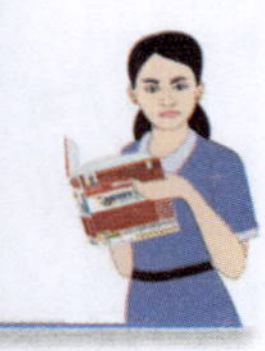

Functions of Ovary

- **Oogenesis:** Formation of mature ovum from the follicle into pelvic cavity.
- **Ovulation:** Expulsion of the matured ovum from Graffian follicle into the fimbriated end of the fallopian tube.
- **Secretion of hormones (steroidogenesis):** Estrogens and progesterone.
  - **Estrogen:** A hormone secreted under the influence of FSH and works to promote the development and maintenance of female reproductive structures, feminine secondary characteristics, and breasts. It also increases protein anabolism and stimulate long bone calcification.
  - **Progesterone:** A hormone secreted under the influence of LH and work with estrogen to prepare endometrium for implantation of fertilized ovum. It inhibits uterine contraction during pregnancy and prepares mammary glands to secrete milk.

Puberty

- Puberty is a natural biological process that marks the onset of sexual maturation and the development of secondary sexual characteristics in humans.
- Main hormone responsible in **female** for the development of secondary sexual characteristic is **estrogen**.

KEY POINTS

- Intramural part of fallopian tube is known as anatomical sphincter.
- Isthmus part of the fallopian tube is known as physiological sphincter.
- In tubal ligation isthmus is the part usually cut.
- Ampulla is the most common site for ectopic pregnancies.

Recent Question
(NORCET 2020)

2. A female came to the gynecologist with chief complaints of irregular vaginal bleeding. The nurse knows well that a decrease in this hormone is responsible for causing bleeding during the menstrual cycle under normal physiological condition:
a. Estrogen
b. Progesterone
c. FSH
d. Thyroxine

Ans. (b) Progesterone

- Main hormone which is responsible for development of secondary sexual characteristic among male is **testosterone**.
- Sequence of puberty among female is thelarche (development of breast buds) → pubarche (appearance of pubic hair) → adrenarche (appearance of axillary hair) → height increases → menarche.
- First sign of puberty among male is **testicular enlargement**.
- **Precocious puberty:** Early onset of puberty <8 years among female and <9 years among males.
- **Delayed puberty:** Late onset of puberty ≥13 years among females and ≥14 years among males.
- **Precocious menstruation:** Early onset of menstruation at <10 years of age.

Anatomical Perinium Vs Obstetrical Perinium

- **Anatomic perineum:** It refers to the region of skin and muscles that is visible on the outside the body. It includes the external genitalia, anus, and the surrounding skin and muscles.
- **Obstetrical perinium (perineal body):** It includes the soft tissues between the vagina and anus. It is the area which stretches during childbirth. Episiotomy is given to this area. This is the area subjected to perineal tear during childbirth. During delivery perineal support is also given to this area.

3. Accessory Reproductive Organs

- The accessory reproductive organs are the organs that support the reproductive function of the gonads.
- It includes pelvic floor muscles, pelvic fascia, pelvic cellular tissue, female urethra, urinary bladder, pelvic ureter, and breast.

Breast

- These are accessory reproductive organs located bilaterally in females and help in lactation following childbirth.
- Mammary glands are the specialized (modified) **apocrine** gland. Apocrine glands are a type of sweat gland that produce a milky fluid that contains proteins, lipids, and other substances.
- It extends from 2nd to 6th ribs in the mid-clavicular line.
- It is made-up of 15–20 lobules of glandular tissue embedded in fat.
- Lobes are separated by fibrous septa.
- Each lobule drains by its **lactiferous duct** on to the **nipple**.
- The pigmented area surrounding nipple is known as **areola**.
- **Montgomery tubercles** are small glands around the nipples on the areola.
- **Blood supply:** Axillary artery, Internal thoracic (Internal Mammary) artery, Intercostal artery.

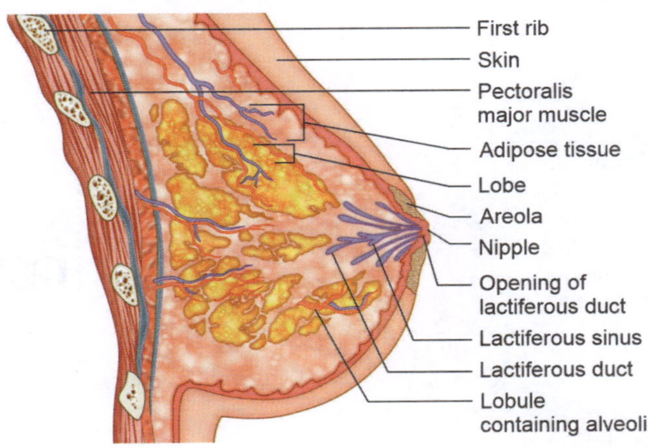

Figure 5: Anatomy of breast

MENSTRUAL CYCLE

- **Menstruation:** Discharge of bloody fluid containing endometrial cells, glandular secretions and blood cells, lasts for 3–5 days.
- **Average length of a menstrual cycle:** 28 days but varies from 21 to 35 days with shorter and longer cycles.
- **Menarche:** A woman's first menstruation; typically occurs around age 12.

Clinical Corner

CASE SCENARIO 1:
Following a class on hormones and pregnancy, teacher asked the students regarding the function of follicle stimulating hormone. The correct answer from the student is:

a. Prepare the endometrium for potential pregnancy
b. Maturation of the Graafian follicle
c. To control the menstrual cycle
d. Regulating the function of the testes

Ans. (b) Maturation of the Graafian follicle

KEY POINTS

- Shape of the nonpregnant uterus is **pyriform**.
- During pregnancy, uterus becomes **globular at 12 weeks**.
- The normal position of the uterus is either **anteversion** or **anteflexion** in the nonpregnant state.
- The uterus **weight** varies from **50 to 80 g**, and **average is 60 g**.
- Uterine measures about 7.5 cm in length, 5 cm wide at its upper part, and nearly 2.5 cm in thickness in adults. **(7.5 x 5 x 2.5)**
- Peritoneal fold present behind the uterus is called **pouch of Douglas.**
- The **length** of each **fallopian tube** is approximately **10 cm**.
- The **diameter** of the fallopian tube is about 1 cm.
- The **length** of each **ampulla** is **5 cm**.

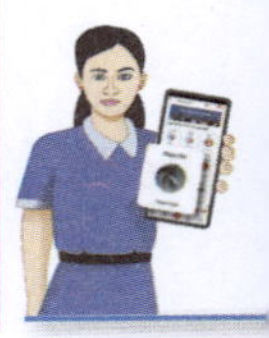

- **Menopause:** End of a woman's reproductive phase, commonly occurs between ages 45 and 55. Age of menopause is largely the result of genetics. To diagnose as menopause, menstruation is absent for 12 months.
- **Precocious menstruation:** If menarche occurs in a girl who is less than 10 years of age.
- **Cryptomenorrhea (hematocolpos):** Menstrual bleeding occurs normally but the blood fails to come out as there is any obstruction in the passage.

Menstrual cycle can be divided into the following phases:

Menstrual Phase (Day 1–5)

- This is the first phase of the menstrual cycle, which starts on the first day of bleeding and lasts till 5 days.
- During this phase, the uterus sheds its lining, which results in menstrual bleeding.
- During this phase, person may experience abdominal cramp due to the contraction of uterine and abdominal muscles to expel menstrual fluid.

Follicular Phase (Day 1–13)

- The follicular phase starts on the first day of bleeding and lasts until ovulation.
- This phase can vary in length from person to person and cycle to cycle.
- During this phase, follicle-stimulating hormone (FSH) stimulates the development of follicles in the ovaries, each containing an egg.
- Eventually, one follicle will become dominant and mature (Graafian follicle), while the others will shrink and disappear.
- Uterus develops endometrium.

Ovulatory Phase (Day 14)

- Pituitary glands secrete **Luteinizing hormone** that causes ovary to release mature egg cell.
- Mature follicle ruptures, and the egg is released from the ovary.
- This usually occurs around day 14 of a 28-day cycle, but it can vary from person to person.
- The released egg then travels through the fallopian tube toward the uterus.

Secretory/Luteal Phase (Progesterone) Phase (15th to 28th day)

- The luteal phase begins after ovulation and lasts until the start of the next menstrual cycle.
- The ruptured Graafian follicle forms a corpus luteum, which produces progesterone to prepare the uterus endometrium for the implantation of the blastocyst.
- If the egg is not fertilized, the corpus luteum will break down, and the levels of estrogen and progesterone will drop, resulting in the start of a new menstrual cycle.

KEY POINTS

- A breast is made-up of three main parts: lobules, ducts, and connective tissue
- **Montgomery's tubercles:** During pregnancy **sebaceous glands in areola** become hypertrophied and called **Montgomery's tubercles.**
- **Thelarche** refers to the onset of female breast development.
- Medicine used to increase the secretion of breast milk is **Metoclopramide (10 mg TDS).**
- Menstruation and ovulation occur around 10 weeks after delivery in lactating mothers and in 4 weeks after delivery in non-lactating mothers.
- **Bilateral oophorectomy** is the term used for surgical menopause.

POINT TO REMEMBER

This diagram shows a 28-day cycle. Some women's cycle may be longer or shorter.

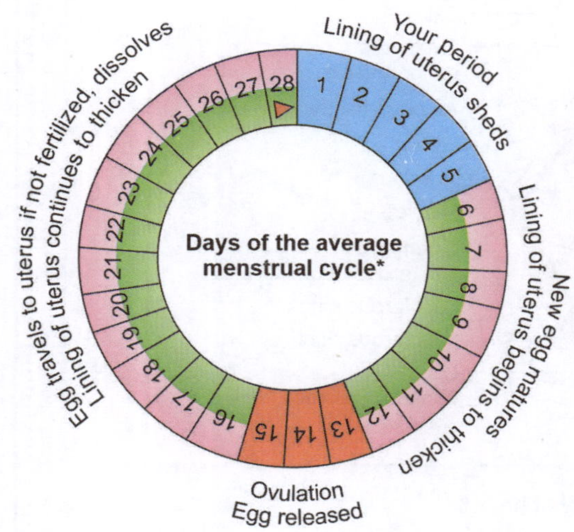

Figure 6: Menstrual cycle

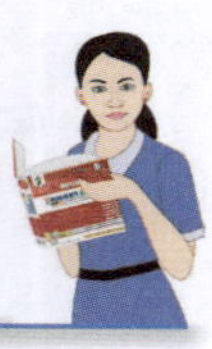

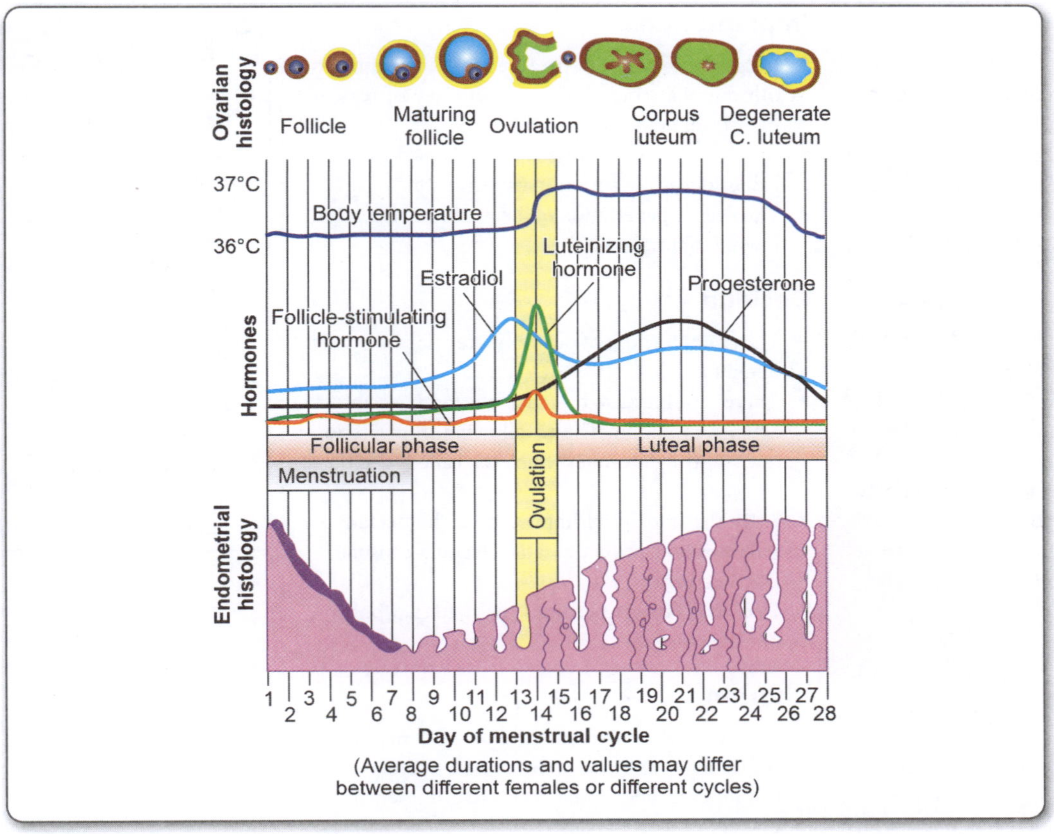

Figure 7: Changes during a normal menstrual cycle

Facts about estrogen

- It is secreted by the follicles/ovary.
- It causes the uterine endometrium to proliferate
- Estrogen decreases FSH and increases LH.
- Maximum estrogen level is present on 12th day of the cycle.

Dysmenorrhea

- Painful menstrual cramps
- Painful menses without evidence of a physical abnormality
- Primary dysmenorrhea does not have pathology
- Believed to be normal body response to uterine contractions.
- **Other symptoms:**
    - Nausea, vomiting, gastrointestinal disturbances and fainting.
    - Prostaglandins cause frequent uterine contractions called cramps.
    - Fibroids, polyps, IUD, PID, or endometriosis.
- **Menorrhagia:** Abnormally heavy (>80 mL) or prolonged (≥8 days) menstrual bleeding. Seen in patient with fibroid uterus.
- **Hypomenorrhea:** Less bleeding (only >5 mL for less than 2 days) during menstruation. Seen in asherman syndrome.
- **Polymenorrhea:** Frequent cycles of <21 days duration.
- **Oligomeorrhea:** Long cycles of >35 days i.e. infrequent menstruation.
- **Metrorrhagia:** Intermenstrual bleeding. Seen in case of uterine polyps.
- **Mittelschmerz syndrome:** Pain at the time of ovulation.

FUNDAMENTALS OF REPRODUCTION

- **Gametogenesis:** Process involved in the maturation of spermatozoa in males and ovum in females.
- **Oogenesis:** The process of development of a mature ovum is called **oogenesis**.
- **Spermatogenesis:** The process of development of spermatids from primordial male germ cells and differentiation into spermatozoa is called spermatogenesis. Time taken for it is 70–75 days.
- **Ovulation:** Release of secondary oocyte from ovary following maturation of Graafian follicles (to become available for conception).

KEY POINTS

- Development of mature ovum is called **oogenesis.**
- Ovulation usually occurs 14th day in a 28-day cycle.
- **Fertilizable life span** of oocyte ranges from 12 to 24 hours.
- **Fertilization** occurs in **ampullary part** of the fallopian tube.
- Penetration of zona pellucida is facilitated by the release of **hyaluronidase** from the **acrosomal** cap.

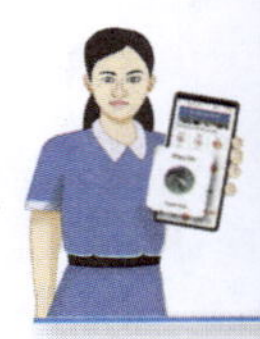

Fertilization

- Fusion of male spermatozoon with mature ovum.
- It usually takes place in the ampulla of uterine tube (fallopian tube).
- The result of fertilization is the production of a zygote, or fertilized egg, initiating prenatal development.
- The life span of oocyte is 12–24 hours and that of the sperm is 48–72 hours.
- After the fusion of sperm with eggs, penetration of other sperms is prevented by Zona reaction (hardening) and oolemma block.
- The spermatozoon determines the sex of the child.

Morula

- After zygote formation nucleus divides into two blastomeres by mitotic division.
- The blastomeres continue to divide until **16 cell stage** occurs called the ***morula***.

Blastocyst

- On day 4th and 5th the morula is covered by mucus and the cells of morula separates to form blastocyst.
- **Outer side** of morula becomes the **trophectoderm** that finally, differentiates into **chorion** while the **inner cells** become inner cell mass which subsequently forms the **embryo.**

Trophoblast

- Before implantation, the trophectoderm differentiates into inner cellular layer called the **cytotrophoblast** and other **syncytiotrophoblast**.
- Placenta and the fetal membranes (chorion) are derived from cytotrophoblast. It also become the umbilical cord in the future.

Implantation

- Implantation occurs in the endometrium on **6th day** that corresponds to 20th day of regular menstrual cycle.
- It involves ***four stages***:- (i) Apposition (ii) Adhesion (iii) Penetration (iv) Invasion.
- The deeper penetration of the blastocyst is termed interstitial implantation.

Decidua

- The endometrium of pregnant uterus is called the **decidua**.
- There is increased structural and secretory activity in endometrium following implantation due to progesterone which is called decidual reaction.
- After the interstitial implantation the decidua is renamed as Decidua basalis, Decidua capsularis, Decidua vera.
- ***Deciduas basalis*** becomes the maternal portion of placenta at term.

Chorion

- Chorion is the outermost layer of fetal membrane consisting of two embryonic layers-outer trophoblast and inner primitive mesenchyme that appears on 9th day.
- The chorion and the amnion together form the **amniotic sac.**

Chorionic Villi

At 3 weeks, the syncytiotrophoblast produces finger-like projections called the primary stem villi which later develop into chorionic villi.

KEY POINTS

- The major sites of **synthesis of prostaglandins** are amnion, chorion, decidual cell and myometrium.
- The **embryo** can be differentiated as human at 8th week of pregnancy.
- Implantation occurs in the form of blastocyst.
- Implantations occur in the human is interstitial implantation.

DEVELOPMENT OF THE INNER MASS CELLS

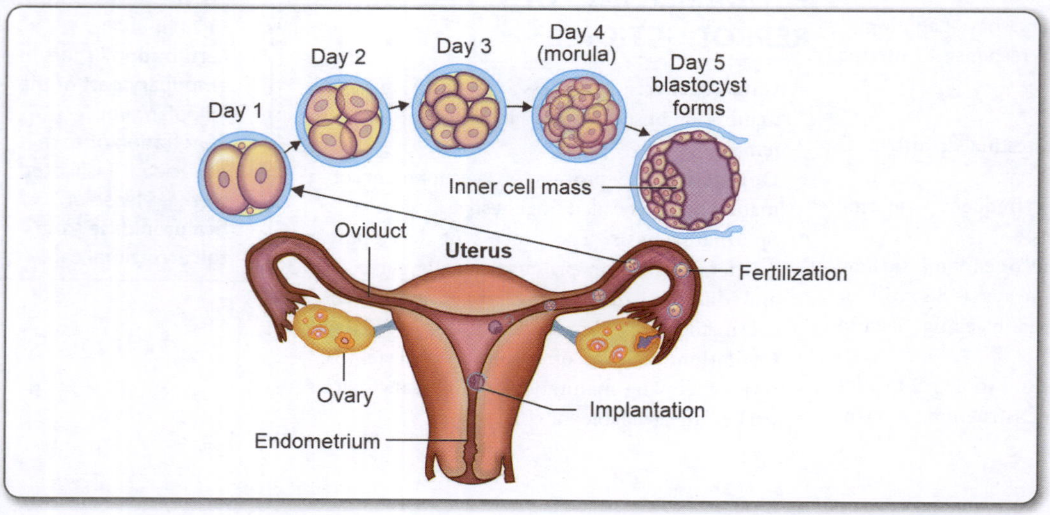

Figure 8: Schematic representation on mitotic division of zygote

Recent Question (NORCET 2020)

3. Which statement among the following is true as far as maturation of Graafian follicle is concerned?

a. Maturation is influenced by both FSH and LH
b. Maturation is only influenced by FSH
c. Maturation is only influenced by LH
d. Maturation is only influenced by progesterone

Ans. (a) Maturation is influenced by both FSH and LH

HUMAN CHORIONIC GONADOTROPIN

- Human chorionic gonadotropin (hCG) is a hormone produced by the placenta during pregnancy
- hCG helps thicken the lining of the uterus to support a growing embryo
- Urinary Pregnancy Test (UPT) works by detecting hCG in the urine.

Increased levels of hCG	Decreased levels of hCG
• Hydatidiform mole • Choriocarcinoma • Down syndrome • Rh incompatibility • Twin pregnancy	• Patau syndrome • Edward syndrome • Ectopic pregnancy • Abortion

KEY POINT

Morning sickness in pregnancy is due to hCG.

PRINCIPAL EVENTS OF EMBRYONIC AND FETAL DEVELOPMENT

Table 1: Stage, gestational age and principal event

Stage	Gestational age	Principal event
Embryonic stage	14–21 days	Notochord develops Ectoderm thickens to form neural plate and neural fold
	21–28 days	Neural fold fuses to form neural tube. Four primitive cardiac chambers, first heart beat on day 21
	4–6 weeks	Optic vesicles appear, complete neural tube closure, limb buds appear, formation of face
	6–8 weeks	All major structures form. Complete ventricular septum
Fetal stage	8–12 weeks	External genitalia develop
	10–12 weeks	Sexual organs differentiate. External genitals can be distinguished
	16 weeks	Fingers and toes develop
	20 weeks	Skin is covered with lanugo, vernix caseosa present Hearing begins
	24–28 weeks	Lungs begin to develop surfactant
	28 weeks	Testis descends into the internal inguinal ring, baby viable Brain grows rapidly
	32 weeks	Bones fully develops
	36 weeks	One testicle descends into the scrotum. Lanugo tend to disappear Muscles fully develop
	40 weeks	Both testicles descend into the scrotum. Nails project beyond finger tip

THE PLACENTA AND FETAL MEMBRANES

Placenta

- Placenta is a circular disc attaches to the uterine wall.
- Human placenta is discoid (disc/circular shape), deciduate (shed after pregnancy), hemochorial (lies in direct contact with maternal blood).
- Measurement: diameter **15–20 cm** and **3 cm thick** at its center.
- Weight: around 500 gms. Its weight proportion to baby's weight is 1:6
- It has two surfaces:
    - **Fetal surface:** It is covered by smooth glistening amnion with umbilical cord attached at or near its center. It develops from chorion frondosum. It forms the 4/5th of the placenta.
    - **Maternal surface:** It is rough and spongy and has a dull red color due to maternal blood. It has 15–20 convex polygons called the lobes or cotyledons. It develops from decidua basalis. It forms 1/5th of the placenta.
- Volume of blood in mature placenta is about **500 mL** (fetal blood 350 mL and maternal blood in the intra-villus space is 150 mL).

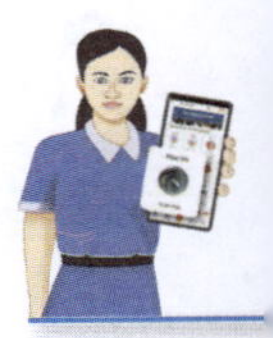

- Placenta attaches to upper part of the body of uterus anterior or posterior with equal frequency.
- After birth placenta separate through decidua spongiosum.
- Section of placenta from inside to outward is amnion, chorionic plate, chorionic villi, intervillous space, decidua (basal plate) and myometrium.

Placental Circulation

It consists of two independent circulations in two system. They are uteroplacental circulation and fetoplacental circulation.

Uteroplacental circulation (maternal circulation)

- Uteroplacental circulation refers to the blood flow between the mother's uterus and the placenta during pregnancy.
- Blood in the intervillous space is replaced 3–4 times per minute.
- Villi received its nutrition from maternal blood.
- 120 spiral (uterine arteries) are opening into intervillous space.

Fetoplacental circulation

- It is the flow of blood between fetus and placenta.
- Fetoplacental circulation is established *via* 2 umbilical artery and 1 umbilical vein.
- Umbilical artery carries impure blood from fetus to placenta.
- Umbilical vein supplies nutrients to fetus.
- Fetal blood flow through the placenta is 400 mL/min.

Functions

- **Nutritive function:** Transfer of nutrients and wastes products between mother and fetus, i.e., respiratory, excretory and nutritive function.
- **Endocrine function:** Produces steroid and peptide hormones to sustain pregnancy.
- **Barrier function:** Protects fetus against noxious agents circulating in maternal blood.
- **Immunological function:** Though fetus and placenta contains antigens foreign to mother, it is not rejected due to immunological protection of placenta.

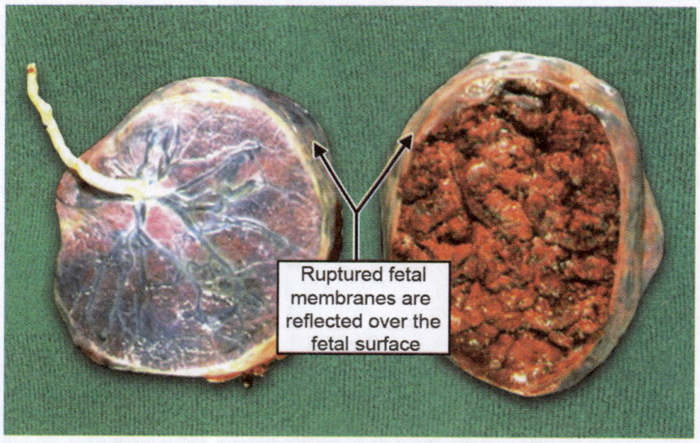

Figure 9: Placenta with ruptured fetal membrane

PLACENTAL ABNORMALITIES

Placental abnormality	Image
Placenta succenturiate Placenta is divided into two or more accessory lobes and are connected to the main body of the placenta by membrane with blood vessels.	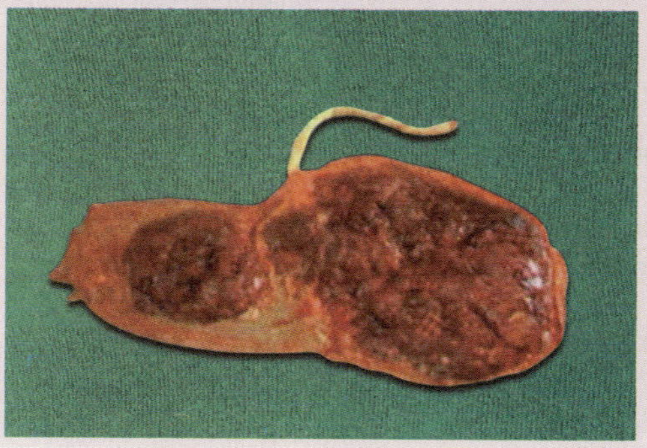

Contd...

Clinical Corner

CASE SCENARIO 2:

A hypertensive pregnant woman at 35 weeks' comes with history of pain in abdomen, bleeding per vaginum and loss of fetal movements. On examination the uterus is contracted with increased uterine tone. Fetal heart sounds are absent.

The most likely diagnosis is:

a. Placenta previa
b. Hydramnios
c. Premature labor
d. Abruptio placenta

Ans. (d) Abruptio placenta

Abruptio placenta, also known as placental abruption, is a condition where the placenta detaches partially or completely from the uterine wall before delivery. It is a medical emergency and can lead to significant maternal and fetal complications.

Pain in the abdomen, bleeding per vaginum, and loss of fetal movements raises suspicion for abruptio placenta. The uterus is contracted with increased uterine tone, which can be a result of uterine irritability caused by the abruption. The absence of fetal heart sounds indicates fetal demise, which is a severe consequence of placental abruption.

Placenta Previa does not typically cause abdominal pain on its own. In palcenta previa, the patient may experience painless vaginal bleeding.

Placental abnormality	Image
Placenta spuria Small part of the placenta is separated from main placenta and is covered by communicating membrane which has no blood vessel to connect it to main placental body.	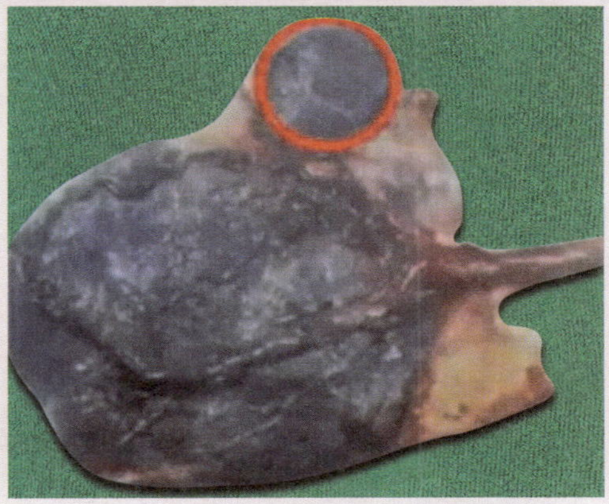
Bilobed placenta/placenta bilobata (bipartite) When placenta divided as roughly two equal parts and both parts are connected to each other by means of blood vessels.	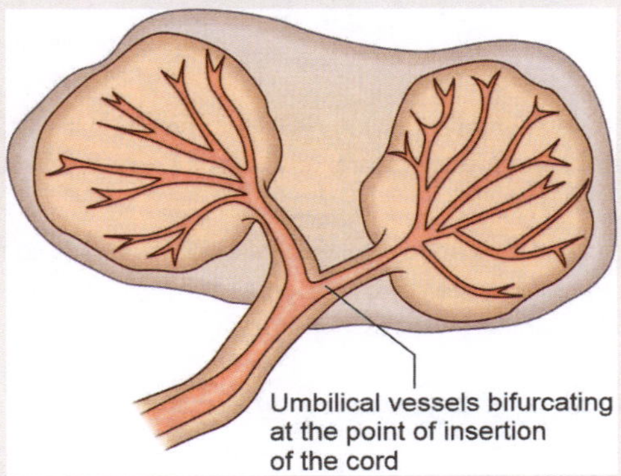
Multilobed placenta Placenta with three or more equal sized lobes. Each lobe is connected by blood vessels to the umbilical cord.	
Extrachorial placenta: It has two variations. **Circumvallate placenta:** In this condition maternal side (basal plate) of the placenta is big and the fetal side (chorionic plate) of the placenta is small. So maternal surface of placenta surrounds the fetal surface like a ring. Misalignment between two plates leads to hematoma retention in the placental margin.	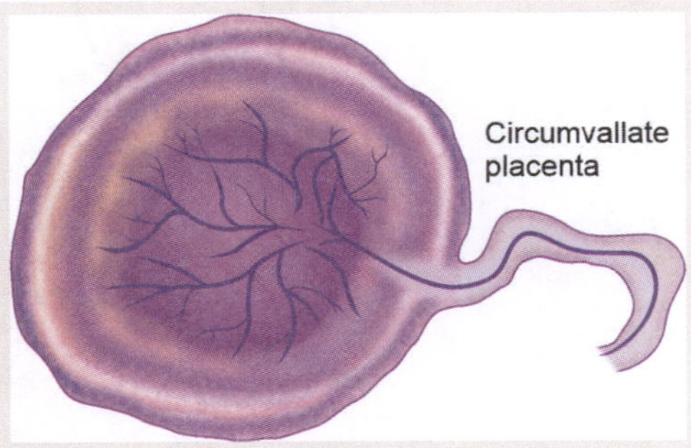
Circummarginate placenta (placenta marginata): In this condition a thin fibrous ring is present at the margin where the fetal blood vessels are terminating.	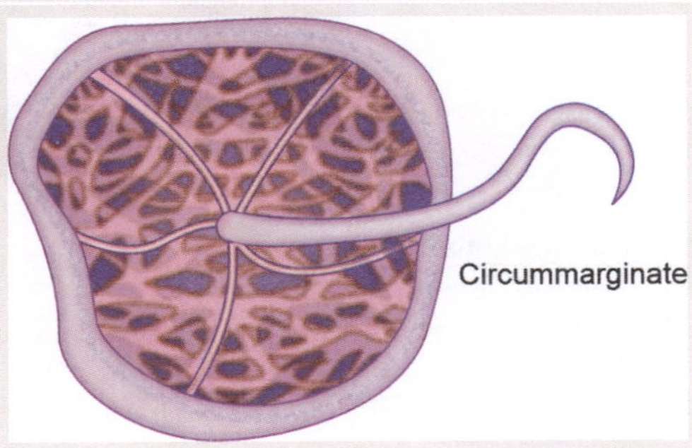

Contd...

Placental abnormality	Image
Placenta membranacea In this condition, placenta is large and thin. Placenta is developed from chorion frondosum and chorion leave. It is characterized by fetal membrane (partially or completely) covered by chorionic villi.	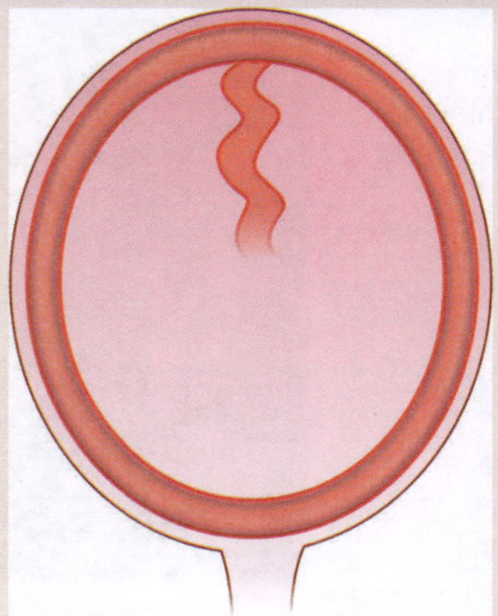 Placenta membranacea
Larger and heavier placenta Placenta weigh up to 1kg or more. It is seen in conditions like gestational DM, multiple gestations (twins, triplets, etc.), fetal growth restriction, and preeclampsia, fetal syphilis, erythroblastosis.	
Smaller and lighter placenta • A smaller and lighter placenta may be indicative of **placental insufficiency**, a condition in which the placenta is unable to provide adequate oxygen and nutrients to the growing fetus. • Placental insufficiency can result in fetal growth restriction, preterm birth, stillbirth, and other complications. • Other possible causes of a smaller and lighter placenta include maternal factors such as malnutrition, smoking, drug use, and certain infections.	
Placenta accreta (adherent placenta) Chorionic villi attached to the surface of myometrium without any intervening decidua basalis.	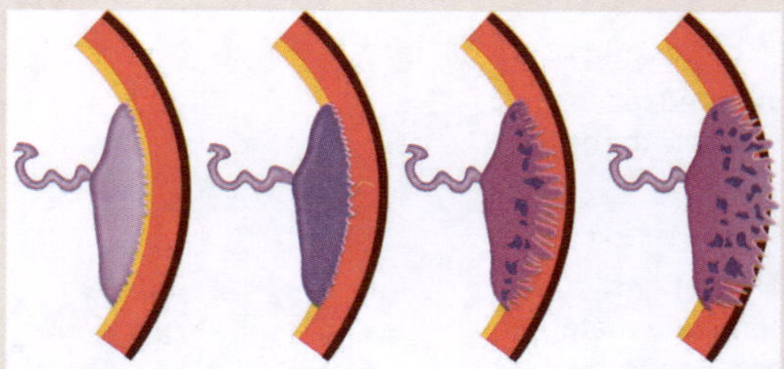
Placenta increta Chorionic villi invade the myometrium (deeply attached).	
Placenta percreta Chorionic villi are attached to the serosa and may invade the nearby organs such as bladder.	
Placenta fenestrate: Placental disc has missing central portion.	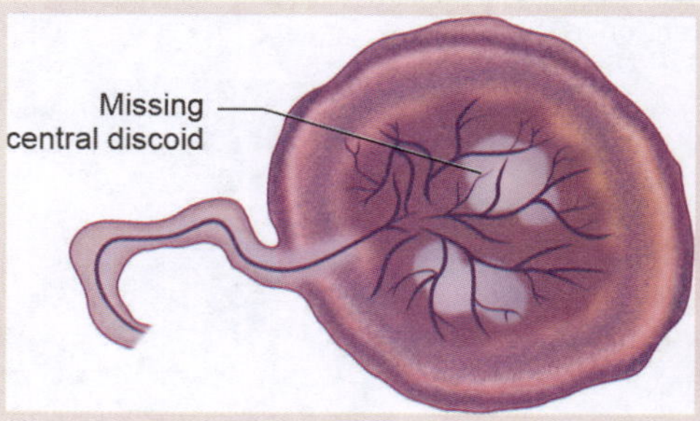

Placentomegaly: When the placental thickness is **more than 4 cm,** it is seen in conditions, like twin pregnancy, diabetes, Rh negative pregnancy.

Small size placenta is seen in patient with pregnancy-induced hypertension and IUGR.

KEY POINTS

- The presence of lambda or twin peak sign indicates dichorionic placenta.
- When the placenta invades the myometrium, it's called placenta accreta.
- Placenta percreta is a **condition where placenta attaches itself and grows through the uterus** and potentially to the nearby organs.
- Vasa previa–Umbilical cord attached to is trapped between the fetus and the opening to the birth canal.
- The **classic presentation of vasa previa** is painless vaginal bleeding, rupture of membranes, and fetal bradycardia.

Recent Question (NORCET 2021)

4. A placenta that is partially or completely attached to myometrium without disbursing the decidua is called:

a. Placenta accreta
b. Increta
c. Percreta
d. Placenta succunturiata

Ans. **(a) Placenta accreta**

Fetal Membranes

- **Chorion:** It is outer layer representing remnants of chorion leave and ends at the margin of placenta.
- **Amnion:** It is inner layer of fetal membrane. Amnion is smooth and shiny and is in contact with liquor amnii. Amnion has no blood and nerve supply and no lymphatic drainage.

Functions

- Formation of liquor amnii
- Prevent ascending uterine infection
- Helps in cervical dilatation during labor
- Regulates enzymatic activity for steroid metabolism.
- Rich source of glycerophospholipid, precursor of prostaglandin.

AMNIOTIC FLUID

Amniotic Fluid

- **Amount**:
  - 50 mL at 12 weeks
  - 400 mL at 20 weeks
  - Reaches its peak of 1 liter at 36–38 weeks and finally starts diminishing afterward and it is about 600–800 mL at term.
  - If pregnancy continues post term, it further reduces to 200 mL at about 43 weeks.
  - **Specific gravity:** 1.010
  - **Osmolarity:** 250 mOsm/L suggests fetal maturity.
  - **Color:** In early pregnancy—colorless, near term pale straw color due to the presence of exfoliated lanugo and epidermal cells, may look turbid due to vernix caseosa.

Table 2: Colors of amniotic fluid and their interpretation

Color of amniotic fluid	Interpretation
Colorless, pale straw color	Normal
Green	Fetal distress/Meconium aspiration
Golden	Rh incompatibility
Greenish yellow of saffron	Post maturity
Dark colored or blood stained	Abruption (concealed accidental hemorrhage)
Dark brown (tobacco juice)	Intrauterine death
Purulent	Chorioamnionitis

Functions

During pregnancy	During labor
• Shock absorber • Maintains even temperature • Allows the growth of fetus and its movement within the amniotic cavity • Adequate water supply with minimal nutritive value • Nutritive value is negligible because of small amount of protein and salt content.	• Helps in dilatation of cervix • Prevents interference with placental circulation during uterine contraction • Prevents umbilical cord compression • Flushes the birth canal to prevent ascending infection into uterine cavity at first stage of labor.

Clinical Importance of Amniotic Fluid

- Amniotic fluid studies help us to find out the fetal maturity and wellbeing.
- Intra amniotic instillation helps in induction of labor.

AMNIOTIC FLUID DISORDERS

Polyhydraminos

- Amniotic fluid exceeds 2000 mL.
- Sonographically seen when Amniotic Fluid Index (AFI) is greater than 25 cm (>95th percentile)
- **Polyhydraminos can be:**
  - **Mild:** DVP >8–11 cm
  - **Moderate:** DVP 12–15 cm
  - **Severe:** DVP ≥16 cm (DVP = deepest vertical pocket)

Etiology

- ***Fetal anomalies***: Anencephaly, open spina bifida, esophageal/duodenal atresia, facial clefts, hydrops fetalis, genetic syndrome, intestinal obstruction.
- **Placental abnormalities:** Chorioangioma of placenta (tumor)
- Multiple pregnancy
- ***Maternal cause***: Commonly associated with diabetes cardiac or renal disease
- ***Idiopathic***: 50–60%

KEY POINTS

- Failure of secretion by the cell of the amnion covering the placenta is called **amnion nodosum**.
- Absence of communicating blood vessels in placenta is **called placenta spuria**.
- There are two surfaces present in the placenta, namely maternal and fetal surface.
- The **maternal surface** of placenta is rough and spongy.
- Fetal membrane consists of **two layers** known as the **outer chorion** and **inner amnion**.
- The umbilical cord is attached to the **chorionic plate**.

KEY POINTS

- Amniocentesis, chorionic villi and alpha-fetoprotein sampling are performed to diagnose any genetic abnormalities in fetus.
- The amniocentesis procedure is not done before the 15th-16th weeks after conception.
- **Amniotic fluid volume** reaches the **peak (1000 mL) at 36–38 weeks**.
- The specific gravity of amniotic fluid is **1.010**.
- Amniotic fluid is **alkaline in nature**.
- Amniotic fluid contains 98-99% water, 1–2% solid.
- **Nitrazine paper test** is used to distinguish amniotic fluid from urine. Paper turns **blue** in case of amniotic fluid and **yellow** in case of urine.
- **Protection of the fetus** is the main function of amniotic fluid.

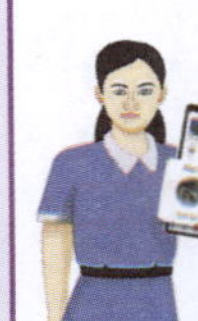

Complications

Pulmonary hypoplasia, cord compression, meconium aspiration syndrome.

Oligohydramnios

- Amniotic fluid is less than 200 mL
- Sonographically, when AFI is less than 5 cm (<5th percentile)

Etiology

- **Fetal conditions:** Chromosomal disorders, renal agenesis, obstructive uropathy, spontaneous rupture of membranes, post maturity, intrauterine infection, drugs-ACE inhibitors and PG inhibitors, amnion nodosum, IUGR.
- **Maternal conditions:** Hypertensive disorders, dehydration, uteroplacental insufficiency, idiopathic.

UMBILICAL CORD

Features of Umbilical Cord

- It connects fetus and placenta though fetal blood flows to and from placenta.
- Average length is 40 cm. It varies from 30 cm to 100 cm.
- Diameter about 1.5 cm (range 1–1.25 cm) with non-uniform thickness having nodes or swelling at places.
- It consists of covering epithelium, Wharton's jelly and blood vessels.
- The umbilical vein carries the oxygenated blood from placenta to fetus.
- There are **two arteries and one vein** present in the umbilical cord singleton pregnancy.
- Umbilical cord usually attached to the fetal surface of placenta somewhere between center and the edge and is known as eccentric insertion.

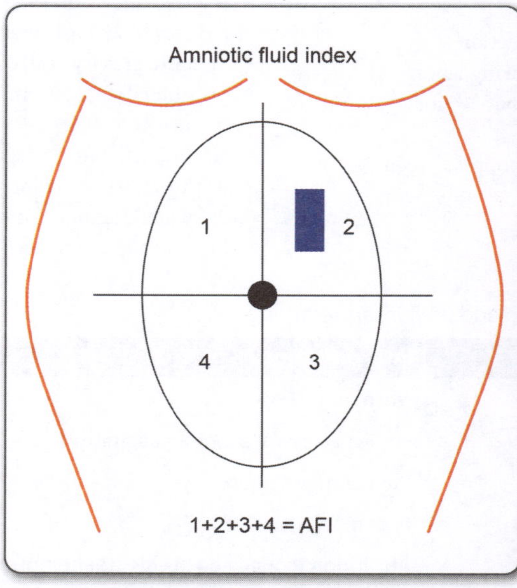

Figure 10: Amniotic fluid index

KEY POINTS

- **Funis** is other name of the **umbilical cord.**
- There are **two arteries** and **one vein** present in the umbilical cord singleton pregnancy.
- Oxygenated blood enters the fetal circulation from umbilical vein *via* ductus venosus.
- Closure of the umbilical arteries takes about 2–3 months after delivery.
- Umbilical artery is not having internal elastic lamina but has got well-developed muscular coat which helps in the effective closure of artery following delivery.

Recent Question (NORCET 2020)

5. **Which of the following position is advised to relieve cord compression during labor?**
   a. Supine
   b. Left lateral
   c. Steep Trendelenburg
   d. Lithotomy

Ans. (b) Left lateral

UMBILICAL CORD ABNORMALITIES

Cord Abnormalities

Cod abnormality	Image
Battledore placenta: Placental cord is attached to the margin. The umbilical cord attaches to the placenta at less than 2 cm from the edge.	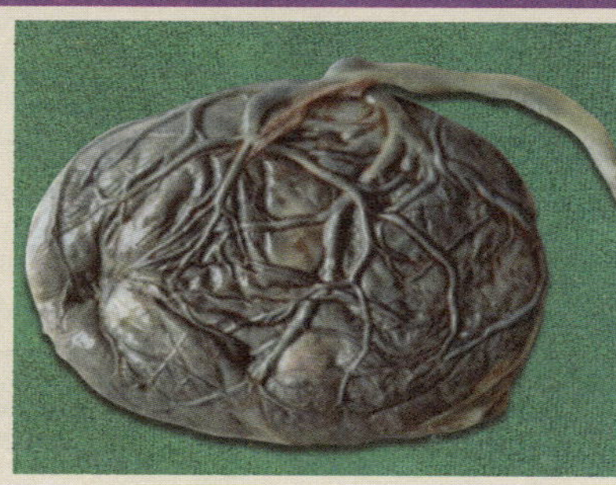 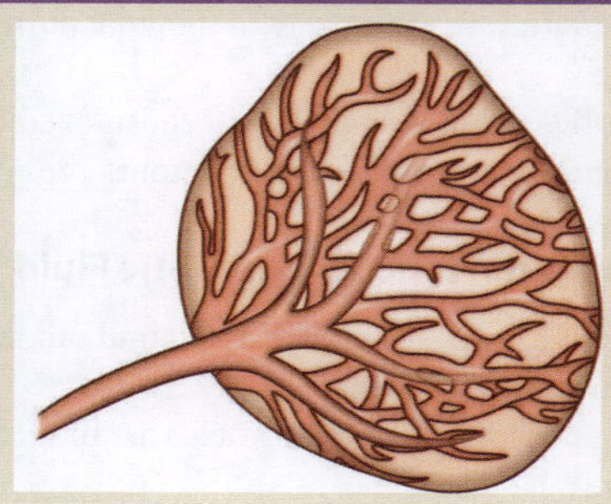
Velamentous placenta: Cord is attached to the membrane instead of placenta. So umbilical vessels are unsupported and may lie below the presenting part and run across the cervical os and known as **vasa previa.**	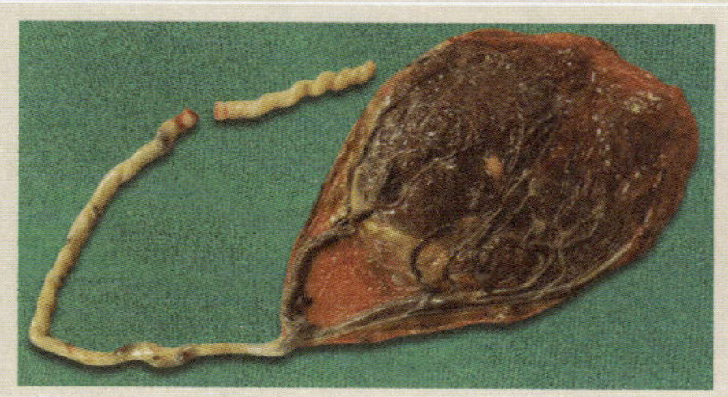 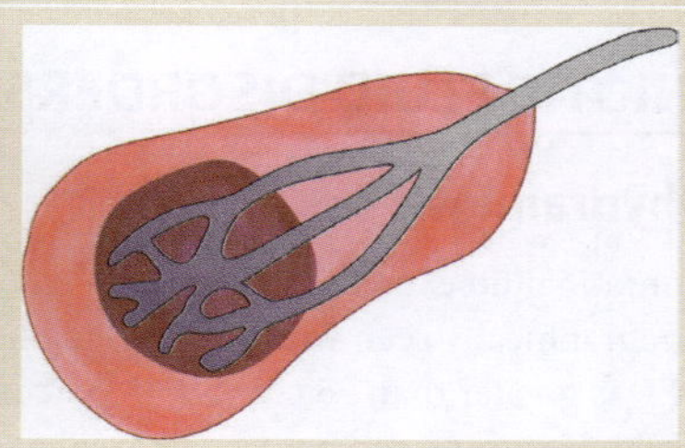

Contd...

Cod abnormality	Image
Long cord: The length of the cord is more than 100 cm. Long cord may loop around the fetal neck and can also cause cord prolapse.	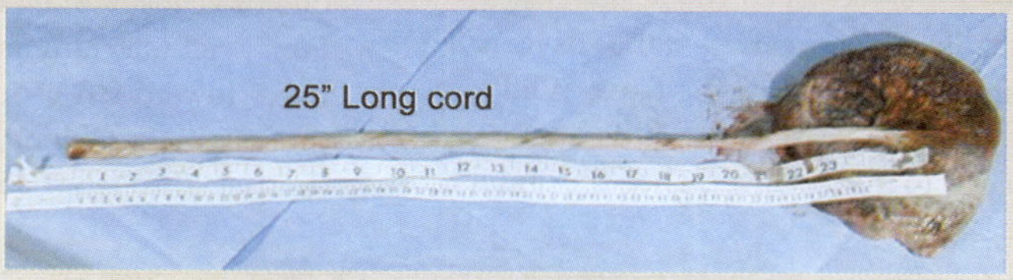
Short cord: True short cord may be less than 20 cm. It may cause failure to the fetus to descend during the delivery. It may brake easily and prevent version.	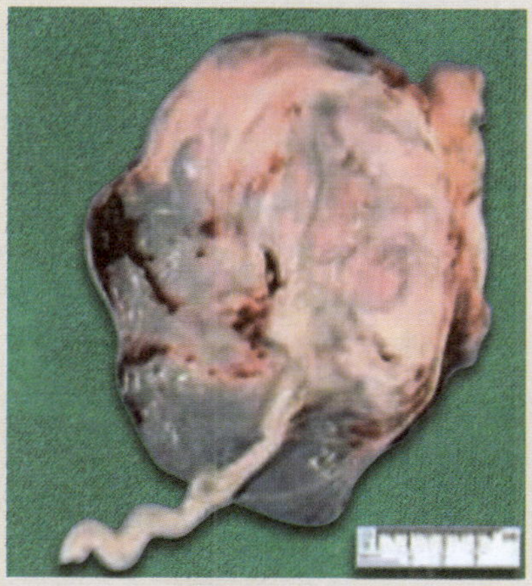
False knot: Knot-like bulge which is seen in umbilical cord due to the accumulation of Wharton's jelly or due to varices.	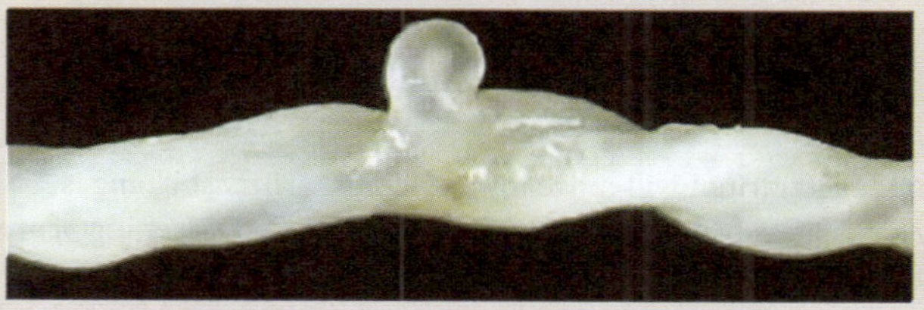
True knot: When real knots are present in the umbilical cord which interfere with the circulation.	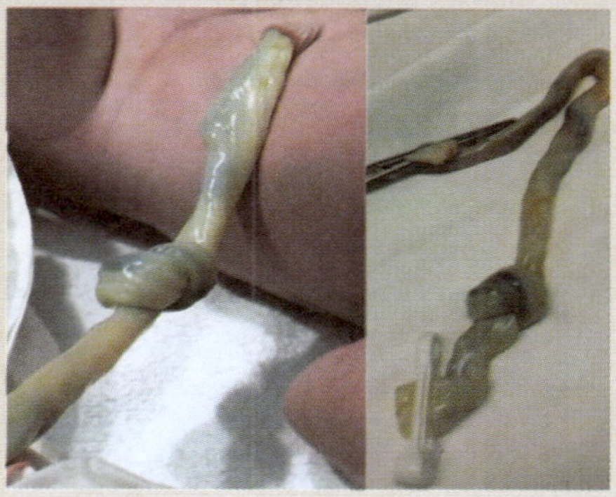
Single umbilical artery: Single umbilical artery may be present due to failure of development or atrophy in later months. It is seen in congenital conditions like renal and genital abnormality, trisomy 18, etc.	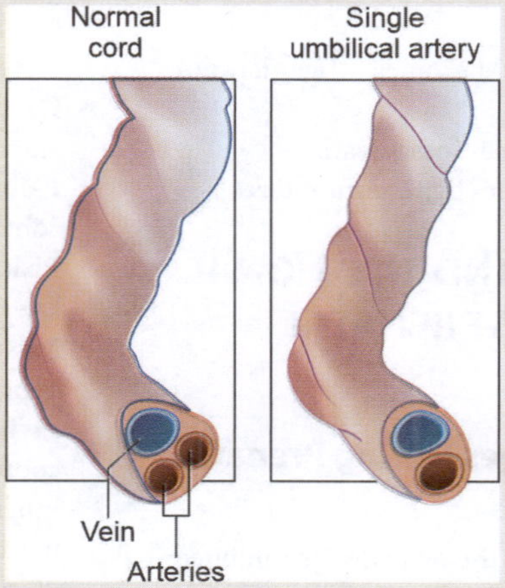
Acordia: Absent cord	

FETAL CIRCULATION

- Single umbilical vein carries 80% oxygenated blood from placenta toward the fetus. While it is moving toward the heart of the fetus one branch will give blood to the fetal liver. Then the umbilical vein enters into the inferior vena cava through ductus venosus and it empties into right atrium.
- From right atrium majority of the blood will move toward left atrium via foramen ovale and the remaining blood will move toward right ventricle through tricuspid valve.

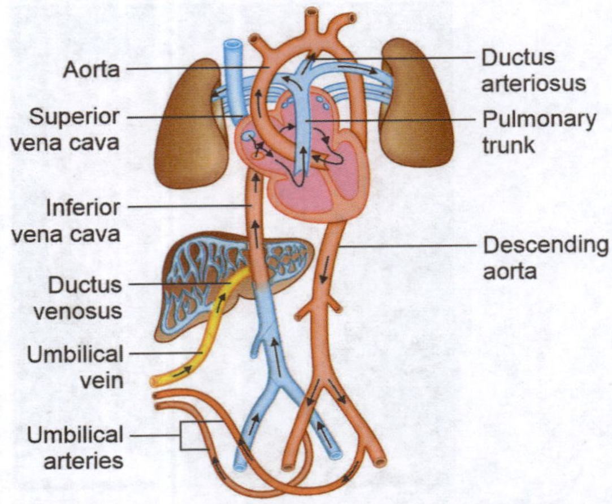

Figure 11: Fetal circulation

- The blood in the left atrium will move toward left ventricle *via* bicuspid valve (mitral valve).
- During systole, the blood in the left ventricle moves toward aorta and it supplies the body parts of fetus.
- The blood in the right ventricle moves toward pulmonary artery. But in the fetal state pulmonary system pressure is higher than the systemic pressure so blood will move from pulmonary artery to aorta via ductus arteriosus.
- Two umbilical arteries carry deoxygenated blood from various parts of the fetal body toward the placenta.
- After the birth of the newborn, all these connections will close and:
  - Ductus venosus becomes **ligamentum venosum**
  - Ductus arteriosus becomes **ligamentum arteriosum**
  - Foramen ovale becomes **fossa ovalis**
  - Umbilical vein becomes **ligamentum teres**

PHYSIOLOGICAL AND EMOTIONAL CHANGES DURING PRENATAL PERIOD

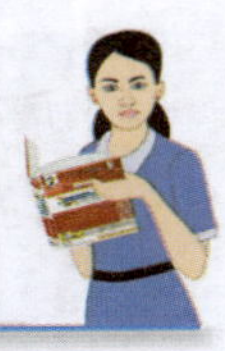

Physiological Changes During Prenatal Period

Amenorrhea occurs when the ovulation is inhibited by the high levels of circulating estrogen and progesterone.

- **Breast changes**
  - Darkening of areola and nipples
  - Montgomery's tubercles: Hypertrophied sebaceous gland termed **fullness, tingling, soreness.**
  - Secretions can be squeezed from breast at 12-week POG which is sticky in nature, thick yellow secretions can be squeezed from milk at 16-week POG.
- **Changes in uterus**
  - **Goodell's sign:** Softening of the cervix as early as 6th week. This sign may occur little earlier in multipara.
  - **Hegar's sign:** Softening of the lower uterine segment.
  - **Chadwick's sign/Jacquemier's sign:** Purplish hue to the cervix and vaginal mucosa due to increased vascularity by 8th week.
  - **Osiander's sign:** Increased pulsation felt at lateral fornices from 8th week onwards.
  - **Palmar sign:** Regular rhythmic uterine contractions. Detected at 4–8 weeks.
  - **Piskacek's sign:** There is asymmetrical
  - **Uterus** enlarges from 70 g to 1000 g at term.
  - Muscles in the uterus undergo hypertrophy, hyperplasia and stretching.
  - **Living ligature:** It is a term used to describe the coordinated action of the outer longitudinal, inner circular, and intermediate muscles of the uterus to prevent excessive bleeding during uterine contractions.

- During pregnancy asymmetrical enlargement of the uterus occur, where the fundus enlarges more than the body.

Shapes of uterus

Time	Shape
Non-pregnant /early weeks of gestation	Pyriform
6th week	Hen's egg
8th week	Cricket ball
12 weeks	Globular/size of fetal head
28 weeks	Pyriform/ovoid
36 weeks and beyond	Spherical

- **Endocrine system**
  - FSH and LH inhibited during pregnancy.
  - Thyroid gland enlarges and basal metabolic rate increases. So untreated maternal hypothyroidism can lead to mental retardation in fetus.
  - Fetus starts producing thyroxine by 11–13 POG. Till then fetus is depends upon materanla thyroxine for brain development.
  - Increased level of ACTH and cortisol.
  - Hyperinsulinism occurs if mother is diabetic.
  - **Human chorionic gonadotrophin (hCG)** is secreted by **syncytiotrophoblast** cells of the placenta during 2nd week of the pregnancy. It maintains corpus luteum during 1st trimester. Responsible for a positive pregnancy test.
  - Estrogen and progesterone level increases and continues to be secreted by placenta during the last 6 months of pregnancy.
  - Thyroid and parathyroid activity is increased
- **Circulatory system**
  - Physiologic anemia occurs due to hemodilution of blood **(in the Second Trimester of the pregnancy)**
  - Reduced haematocrit value.
  - Cardiac output increases 30–50%, peaking at 28–32 weeks.
  - Heart rate increases 10–15 beats/min in second half of pregnancy.
  - **BP may drop** in second trimester of pregnancy.
  - Femoral pressure will increase as gravid uterus compress the common iliac vein and is more on right side due to dextrorotation of the uterus.
  - WBC, fibrinogen, and **clotting factors increase**.
  - Edema of extremities is common in the last 6 weeks of pregnancy.
  - Supine hypotensive syndrome occurs because of compression of inferior vena cava by enlarging uterus during late second and third trimester.
  - Pregnancy is hypercoagulable state with increased fibrinogen level.
- **Respiratory system**
  - Oxygen circulation is increased by about 15% from 16th week of pregnancy.
  - Dyspnea occurs due to the presence of enlarged uterus on diaphragm during 3rd trimester.
  - Dyspnea subsides when lightening occurs at 38 weeks.
- **Gastrointestinal system**
  - Nausea and vomiting (morning sickness) in the first trimester.
  - Constipation is caused by hypoperistalsis, lack of fluids and low fiber intake.
  - Excessive salivation (ptyalism) may occur.
  - Food craving may occur.
  - Increased vitamin C and iron intake is indicated.
- **Skin changes system**
  - Dark patches on the face (**melasma, chloasma gravidarum**)
  - **Linea nigra:** Brownish black pigmented area in the midline stretching from the xiphisternum to the symphysis pubis. It is due to increased melanin.
  - **Striae gravidarum:** Striae on abdomen and thighs caused by skin stretching as pregnancy advances. Initially they are pinkish but after delivery they become glistening white in appearance and are called **striae albicans**
- **Excretory system**
  - Increased urinary frequency.
  - Bladder capacity increases to 1500 mL.
  - Glycosuria and occasional proteinuria occurs.
- **Skeletal system**
  - Softening of ligaments and joints (symphysis pubis and sacroiliac joints) due to hormonal activity.

Psychological (Emotional) Changes

- Pregnancy is identified as a potent stressor that can seriously affect the psychic status of pregnant women and perinatal outcome.
- It is usually associated with ambivalence, frequent mood changes, varying from anxiety, fatigue, exhaustion, sleepiness, depressive reactions to excitement.

DIAGNOSIS OF PREGNANCY

Duration of Pregnancy

- 10 lunar months or 9 calendar months and 7 days or 280 days or 40 weeks
- It is calculated from the first day of last menstrual period (LMP)
- Ovulation and fertilization occur 14 days after the LMP (28 days cycle)
- So gestational period can be calculated by subtracting 14 days from 280 days.

KEY POINTS

- **Aldosterone production** during pregnancy is responsible for stretching of skin in mother.
- **Linea nigra** is visible as early as 20th week of pregnancy.
- **Chloasma** appears at 24 weeks of pregnancy.

KEY POINTS

- **Gravida:** A woman who is or has been pregnant
- **Primigravida:** A woman who is in or who has experienced her first pregnancy (pregnant for first time).
- **Multigravida:** A woman who has been pregnant more than once.
- **Nulligravida:** A woman who has never been pregnant.
- **Parity:** Denotes the state of pregnancy beyond viability. Period of viability can vary from country to country. In India period of viability is 28 weeks while according to WHO it is 24 weeks.
- **Primipara:** A woman who is giving birth for first time.
- **Multipara:** A woman who has given birth two or more times.

Trimesters of Pregnancy

- First trimester: first 12 weeks
- Second trimester: 13–28 weeks
- Third trimester: 29–40 weeks

Presumptive v/s Probable V/S Positive Signs of Pregnancy

Presumptive sign (subjective)	Probable sign (objective)	Positive sign (confirmatory)
Presumptive signs are those that suggest the possibility of pregnancy but do not definitively confirm. These are the maternal physiological changes experienced by the mother. e.g.: • Amenorrhea • Nausea and vomiting • Tingling • Frequency of micturition • Fatigue • Breast tenderness • Presence of colostrum in the nipple • Quickening • Skin pigmentation.	These are more reliable indicators of pregnancy, but still do not provide a definitive diagnosis. These are detected during examination and documented by the examiner. e.g.: • Enlargement of uterus • Presence of hCG in the blood • Urine pregnancy test (UPT) • Vaginal discharge • Hegar's sign • Jacquemier's/Chadwick sign • Osiander's sign • Palmar sign • Goodell's sign • Baxton hick's contraction • Ballottement of fetus	These are those signs that provide definitive evidence of the presence of a fetus: e.g: • Fetal heartbeat • Visualization of the fetus by USG • Palpable fetal movements, • Palpation of the entire fetus.

- **Nullipara:** A woman who has never given birth or who has never had a pregnancy progress beyond 28 weeks.
- **Grand multipara:** Female who has 4 or more viable pregnancies.
- **Term birth:** Birth between 37 and 42 weeks of gestation.
- **Preterm birth:** Birth between 20 and 36 weeks of gestation.
- **Post-term birth:** Birth after 42 weeks of gestation
- **Elderly primigravida:** First pregnancy is at the age of 35 years or more.
- **Parturient:** A women who is in labor.
- **Puerpera:** A women who has just given birth.

Signs of Pregnancy

Table 3: Signs of pregnancy and their explanations

Time	Sign	Explanation
First three months	Hartman sign	Implantation bleeding
4–8 weeks	Palmer's sign	Regular rhythmic contraction during bimanual examination
6 weeks	Goodell's sign	Softening of lower part of cervix
6–10 weeks	Hegar's sign	And by manual examination abdominal and vaginal fingers opposes each other
6–8 weeks	Piskacek sign	Asymmetric enlargement of uterus
8 weeks	Osiander's sign [Octa–8]	Increased pulsation felt through lateral fornix of vagina
8 weeks	Chadwick sign/ Jacquemier's sign	Bluish coloration of vestibule
>20 weeks of pregnancy	Braxton Hicks contractions	Painless irregular spasmodic contraction without any effect on dilation of cervix can also be felt in pedunculated fibroid submucous type and hematometra

Quickening: It is the fetal movement felt by the mother. In primigravida it occurs at 18th week POG while in multigravida it may felt at 16th week POG.

KEY POINTS

- RBC mass increases by 20-30% during pregnancy.
- Blood volume of pregnant women expands by 40-50% above non-pregnant women, i.e., 1500 mL (1000 mL plasma + 500 mL RBC)
- Cardiac output increases by 30–50% during first trimester.

KEY POINTS

- Vaginal hypertrophy during pregnancy occurs due to increase in estrogen levels.
- Pregnancy test using detection of hCG in maternal serum or urine is possible from 8 to 11 days after conception.
- **Urine pregnancy test** is not reliable after 12 weeks of conception.

ESTIMATION OF EDD AND GESTATIONAL AGE

Estimation of Expected Date of Delivery (EDD)

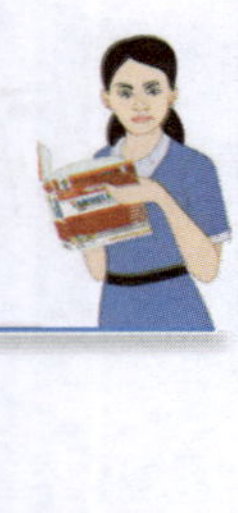

- **Naegele's Rule:** LMP - 3 months + 7 days + 1 year = EDD.
- It can also be calculated by adding 9 months and 7 days to the date of LMP, when the cycle is of 28 days and is also regular.

Estimation of Gestational Age

- **Symphysial fundal height**
  - *At 16 weeks:* Fundus found halfway between symphysis pubis and umbilicus.
  - *At 18–20 weeks:* Fundal height approximately equals the fetus age in weeks ± 2 cm.
  - *At 20–24 weeks:* Fundus is at umbilicus.
  - *At 36 weeks:* Fundus is at xiphoid process.
- **Ultrasonography** establishes gestational age by crown to rump measurement during first 11 weeks.

SCREENING TESTS DURING PREGNANCY

Fetal Well-being

Various tests used for fetal wellbeing during the antenatal period are as follows:

Fetal Movement Count

The count should be performed daily starting at 28 weeks of pregnancy.

Cardiff Count 10 Formulae:

- Mother counts fetal movement starting from 9 a.m. The counting comes to an end as soon as 10 movements felt.
- She is instructed to report if less than 10 movements occur during 12 hours on 2 successive days or no movement felt after 12 hours.

Daily Fetal Movement Count

- Count fetal movements three times a day each of one hour duration.
- Total count multiplied by 4 gives 12-hours fetal movement.
- She is instructed to report if there is diminution of the number of movements to less than 10 in 12 hours.

Non-Stress Test

Continuous FHR monitoring along with the record of fetal movements. There is an observed association of FHR acceleration with fetal movement. It is suggestive of healthy fetus.

Interpretation

- Reactive (reassuring): When two or more acceleration of more than 15 beats/min above the baseline and longer than 15 seconds in duration are present in 20-minute observation.
- Non-reactive: Absence of any fetal activity.

Vibroacoustic Stimulation (VAS)

- Vibroacoustic stimulation is a non-invasive method used during pregnancy to assess fetal well-being.
- This technique involves using a device that produces sound waves and vibrations to stimulate the fetus.
- When the device is applied to the mother's abdomen, the fetus will typically respond by increasing its heart rate.
- This response indicates that the fetus is healthy and responsive to stimuli.
- This test also helps to change the fetal sleep activity from NREM to REM.

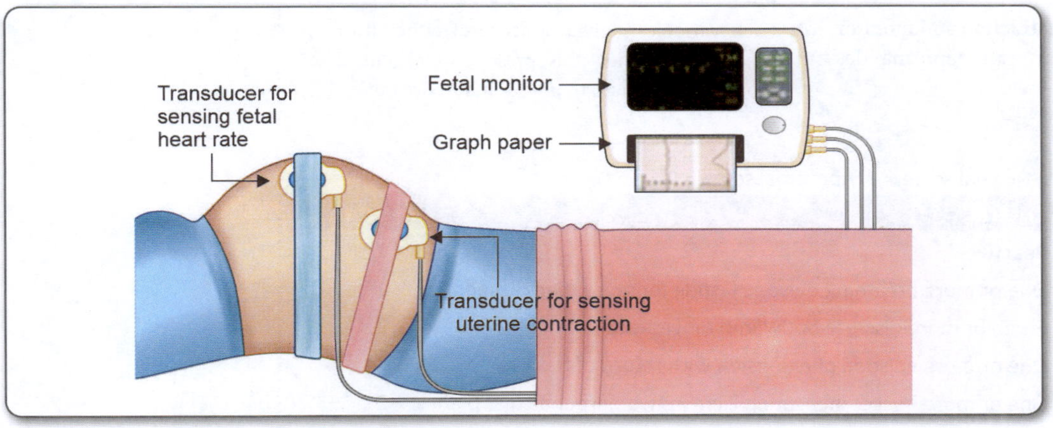

Figure 12: Cardiotocography (CTG)

- It is used to find out the correlation between feal heart rate and uterine contractions.
- A normal baseline FHR range is between 110 and 160 bpm.
- Normal fetal heart rate variability is between 5 and 25 bpm. Reduced variability may indicate fetal distress.
- Normally there should not be any deceleration.
- There should be two or more fetal heart rate acceleration in response to uterine contraction in 20 minutes time.
- If FHR decreased by 15 bpm for 15 seconds with uterine contraction it indicates fetal distress.

KEY POINTS

- Highest level of Alpha-Feto Protein (AFP) in fetal serum and amniotic fluid is reached around 13 weeks.
- **Amniocentesis** is performed between 14 and 16 weeks of pregnancy.
- **Cordocentesis** is also known as percutaneous umbilical blood sampling.
- Fetus length from vertex to the coccyx is known as **Crown-rump length**.
- Fetus length from vertex to the heel is **crown-heel length**.

Recent Question (NORCET 2020)

6. At which week mother feels movement of the baby?
a. 10–12 Weeks
b. 12–14 Weeks
c. 16–20 Weeks
d. 20–25 Weeks

Ans. (c) 16–20 Weeks

Clinical Corner

CASE SCENARIO 3:
Nurse Amli working in antenatal clinic was going through the maternal serum alpha fetoprotein (MSAFP) values of her client. She noticed elevated levels of MSAFP. There is a high chance for all among the following conditions; EXCEPT:
a. Open neural tube defect
b. Intrauterine fetal death
c. Renal abnormalities
d. Gestational trophoblastic disease

Ans. (d) Gestational trophoblastic disease

Ultrasonography

Transvaginal Scanning

Gestational sac visible at 5 weeks

Abdominal Ultrasound

- Gestational sac is seen at 4–5 weeks
- Yolk sac is seen at 5–6 weeks
- Fetal pole is seen at 6–7 weeks
- Cardiac activity is seen at 6–7 weeks

This non-invasive test takes series of measurement from baby such as bi-parietal diameter (BPD), abdominal circumference (AC), head circumference (HC), femoral length (FL) and amniotic fluid index (AFI).

- AC is the parameter which reflect the nutritional status of the fetus.
- If the ratio between HC/AC >1 after 34 weeks IUGR is suspected.

Amniotic Fluid Index (AFI)

- It is calculated by dividing maternal abdomen as **four quadrants** by taking umbilicus, symphysis pubis and fundus as reference point.
- It is assessed with the help of ultrasound.
- The **normal range for AFI** is usually between 5 and 25 centimetres.
- AFI less than 5 cm is considered **oligohydramnios**, and greater than 25 cm is considered **polyhydramnios.**

Contraction Stress Test

- It is performed at the end of pregnancy to identify whether the fetus will cope with the contraction during the labor or not.
- The purpose is to induce contraction and monitor the fetus to check for heart rate abnormalities using a cardiotocograph.

Methods

- **Nipple stimulation:** One nipple is massaged gently through clothing until contraction begins or for a maximum of 2 minutes. This test relies on the endogenous release of oxytocin.
- **Oxytocin challenge test:** Intravenous oxytocin is administered to a pregnant woman with the purpose to achieve three contractions in every 10 minutes.

Interpretation

- **Positive:** Persistent late deceleration of FHR with 50% or more of uterine contraction.
- **Negative:** No late deceleration or significant variable deceleration.

Doppler Ultrasound Velocimetry

- Doppler ultrasound is a non-invasive test that uses sound waves to evaluate blood flow through the fetal vessels.
- It is used during pregnancy to detect abnormalities in blood flow and assess fetal well-being, especially in high-risk pregnancies.
- In normal pregnancy, systolic diastolic ratio, pulsatility index and resistance index decreases as gestational age advances.
- **Increased values** in these parameters indicate **placental vascular resistance.**

Fetal Biophysical Profile (BPP)

- The test evaluates five different fetal biophysical variables.
- It includes NST, fetal breathing movements, gross body movements, fetal muscle tone and amniotic fluid.
- Each variable is given a score of either 0 or 2, based on whether it is present or absent. The scores are added up to give a final score out of 10.

Recent Question (NORCET 2023)

7. **A 34-weeks-pregnant client is undergoing a non-stress test (NST). During the 20-minute examination, the nurse notes three fetal movements accompanied by accelerations of the fetal heart rate, each 15 bpm, lasting 15 seconds. The nurse interprets this test to be:**
   a. Nonreactive
   b. Reactive
   c. Positive
   d. Negative

Ans. (b) Reactive

Explanation: In a reactive NST, the fetal HR shows accelerations of at least 15 beats per minute (bpm) above the baseline, lasting for at least 15 seconds, and occurring at least three times within a 20-minute period. This indicates that the fetus is responding well to its own movements, suggesting a healthy fetal state.

Observation time: 30 minutes, Normal score = 2, Abnormal score = 0

Parameter	Criteria	Score
Non-stress test (NST)	Reactive	2
Fetal breathing movement	One or more breathing episode lasting for more than 30 sec	2
Gross body movement	Three or more discrete body/limb movement	2
Fetal muscle tone	One or more episode of extension with return of flexion	2
Amniotic fluid	One or more pocket measuring 2 cm in two perpendicular planes	2

Interpretation of BPP

Score	Interpretation
8–10	Normal
6	Suspect chronic hypoxia
4	Suspect abnormal chronic asphyxia
0–2	Strongly suspect chronic asphyxia.

Test for Pulmonary Maturity

- Respiratory distress syndrome is caused by the deficiency of lung surfactant.
- It is produced by type II alveolar cells.
- Lung surfactant production begins in the fetus around 24 weeks gestational age.
- Suspect surfactant deficiency in a pre-term newborn.

Lecithin/Sphingomyelin (L/S) Ratio

- The L/S ratio is a test used to assess fetal lung maturity during pregnancy.
- It measures the ratio of two types of lung surfactant phospholipids, lecithin and sphingomyelin, in the amniotic fluid surrounding the fetus.
- Lecithin is a major component of pulmonary surfactant, and its concentration in the amniotic fluid increases as fetal lung maturity progresses.
- Sphingomyelin remains relatively constant in the amniotic fluid throughout pregnancy.
- **A ratio of 2:1 or greater is indicative of fetal lung maturity.**
- Ratio of less than 2:1 may suggests an increased risk of respiratory distress syndrome (RDS) if the fetus is delivered prematurely.
- **Corticosteroids (Betamethasone, dexamethasone)** are the drugs which help in the increased production of surfactant.

Phosphatidylglycerol

The presence of phosphatidylglycerol in the amniotic fluid is suggestive of lung maturity in fetus.

Shake Test (Bubble test)

- It is also called Clements' test.
- A small amount of amniotic fluid is collected and mixed with ethanol or isopropanol.
- The mixture is then agitated or shaken for 15 seconds to create bubbles.
- The number and size of the bubbles is then observed after 15 minutes.
- Presence of complete ring of bubbles at meniscus indicates lung maturity.

Nile Blue Sulphate Test

Amniotic fluid collected is mixed with Nile blue solution. If >50% cells are in orange color it indicates lung maturity.

Maternal Serum Alpha Fetoprotein (MSAFP)

- Alpha-fetoprotein (AFP) is a protein that is produced by the yolk sac and fetal liver and can be detected in the mother's blood.
- AFP level is high in fetal serum by 13 weeks and then it decreases.
- In maternal serum, it reaches its peak around 32 weeks.

KEY POINTS

- **Surfactant** is a lipoprotein that lowers the surface tension in the alveoli and decreases the tendency of the alveoli to collapse
- An L–S (Lecithin-Sphingomyelin) ratio of more than 2:1 in the liquor amnii indicates fetal lung maturity and a relatively low risk of infant respiratory distress syndrome.
- Surfactant production in fetus begins at 24 weeks of gestation.
- **Alveoli of fetus** expands at 24 weeks.
- **Fetal cortisol** is the natural trigger for augmentation **surfactant synthesis.**

AFP increased	AFP decreased
• Wrong gestational age • Open neural tube defects (NTDs) • Multiple pregnancy • Intrauterine Fetal Death (IUFD) • Anterior abdominal wall defects • Renal anomalies • Sacrococcygeal teratoma • Pilonidal sinus	• Trisomy's (Down's syndrome) • Gestational trophoblastic disease • Molar pregnancy • Abortion • Diabetes mother

Triple Marker Test

- It is a combined biochemical test which includes **MSAFP, HCG and UE3 (unconjugated estriol).**
- It is used for detection of **Down's syndrome.**
- In an affected pregnancy, level of **MSAFP and UE3 is low** while that of **hCG is high**.
- It is **ideally performed at 15–18 weeks**.

Dual Test

- Also known as the first-trimester combined test or the screening test.
- **Performed between 10–13 weeks** gestation.
- The test combines two separate screening tests: a blood test and an ultrasound scan.
- The blood test measures the levels of two specific hormones, beta-human chorionic gonadotropin **(beta-hCG)** and **pregnancy-associated plasma protein-A (PAPP-A)**, in the mother's blood.
- The ultrasound scan measures the **nuchal translucency (NT)**, which is the thickness of a fluid-filled space at the back of the fetus' neck.
- The results of these two tests are combined to calculate the risk of the fetus having chromosomal abnormalities, such as Down syndrome.
- **The test is not a definitive diagnosis** of a chromosomal abnormality, but rather a **screening test** that identifies pregnancies that are at a higher risk and may require further testing.

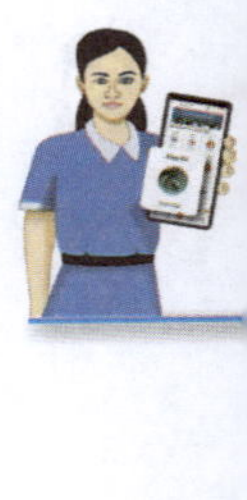

Acetylcholine Esterase (AChE)

- Amniotic fluid AChE level is elevated in most cases of open neural tube defects.
- It has got better diagnostic value than AFP. It is the **best biochemical marker to diagnose Anencephaly**.

Inhibin A

- It is a dimeric glycoprotein produced by the corpus luteum and the placenta.
- Serum level of inhibin A is raised in women carrying a fetus with Down syndrome.

Amniocentesis

- Refers to the aspiration of amniotic fluid from the pregnant uterus for examination.
- It is typically scheduled between the 14th and 16th weeks of pregnancy.
- The **patient** is placed on an examination bed in the **dorsal lithotomy position.**
- An ultrasound is done to determine the position of the fetus and the location of a pocket of amniotic fluid and the placenta.
- Following the procedure patient may experience hyperactive uterus, vaginal discharge and fetal movements.

> **KEY POINT**
> Result of quadruple test in down syndrome is as follows. **AFP and E3 decreses while hCG and Inhibin increases.**

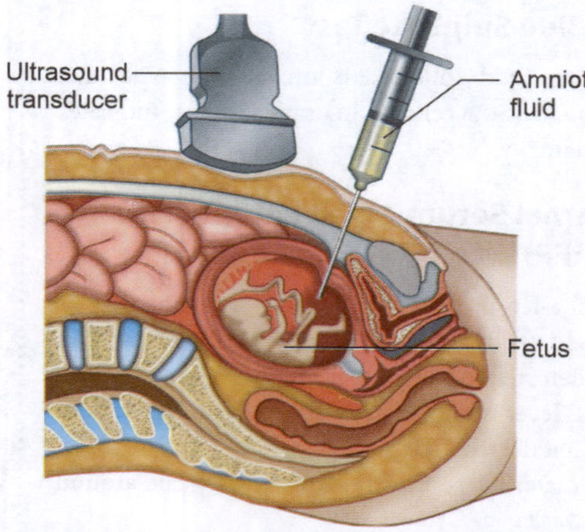

Figure 13: Amniocentesis

Chorionic Villus Sampling (CVS)

- CVS is performed for prenatal diagnosis of genetic disorders.
- It is carried out transcervically between 10 and 12 weeks and transabdominally from 10 weeks to term.
- A few villi are collected from the chorion frondosum under ultrasonic guidance.
- Complications: Fetal loss (1–2%), oromandibular limb deformities or vaginal bleeding are higher.

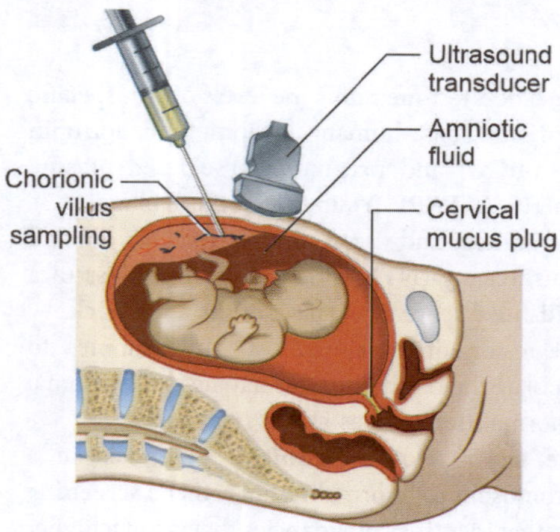

Figure 14: Chorionic villus sampling

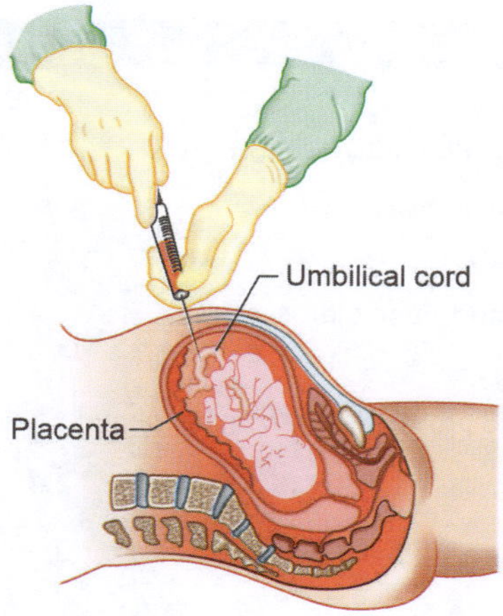

Figure 15: Cordocentesis

Fetal Blood Sampling (cordocentesis)

- This technique is used to take a sample of fetal blood during pregnancy to screen for chromosomal abnormalities, hemoglobinopathies and other disorders affecting blood or cells.
- It is performed under local anesthetic usually after 18 weeks' gestation.

Risks: Abortion, preterm labor and intrauterine fetal death.

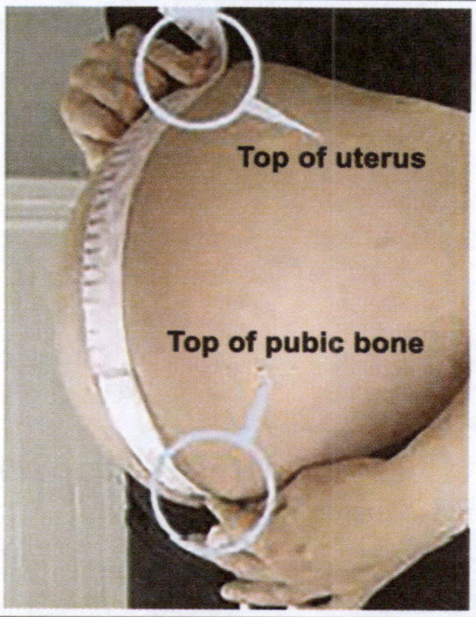

Figure 16: Symphysis-fundus height

ANTENATAL ASSESSMENT OF FETAL WELL-BEING

Antenatal assessment of fetal well-being includes:

- Abdominal examination
- Vaginal examination
- Breast examination

Abdominal Examination

- **Position:** Make the women lay down in supine position with knees flexed after emptying her bladder. Place a pillow under her head and shoulder, keep her arms by her side. Expose her abdomen below the breast to the symphysis pubis.
- **Measure the symphysis-fundus (SF) height:** Measure the distance in centimeters from the symphysis pubis to the top of the fundus. This is the symphysis-fundus height.
- After 24 weeks the SFH is equal to that of period of gestation.

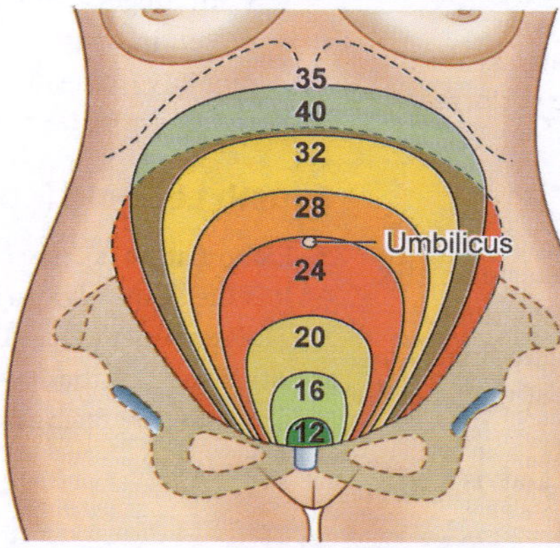

Figure 17: Symphysio-fundal height

KEY POINTS

- Amniocentesis can be performed to reduce the volume of the amniotic fluid.
- Second trimester amniocentesis is safer than early amniocentesis or transcervical CVS
- Transabdominal CVS should be regarded as the procedure of first choice when testing is done before 15 weeks' gestation.
- **Chorionic villus sampling** is more than 99 percent accurate when it comes to diagnosing chromosomal results, such as **Down syndrome**
- Cordocentesis, also known as percutaneous umbilical blood sampling, is a diagnostic prenatal test
- Cordocentesis is usually done after week 18 of pregnancy, can be used to detect certain genetic disorders, blood conditions and infections.

KEY POINTS

- **Contraction Stress Test (CST)** is to observe the response of the fetus at risk for uteroplacental insufficiency in relation to uterine contraction.
- CST is considered positive if late deceleration occurs in 50% or more of contraction.

Fundal Height Location

Period of gestation in weeks	Fundal height location
12	At the level of symphysis pubis
16	Midway between umbilicus and symphysis pubis
20	1–2 finger breadth below the umbilicus.
24	At the level of umbilicus.
32	Halfway between umbilicus and xiphoid process
36	At the level of xiphoid process
40	2–3 fingers below the xiphoid process if lightning happened. Sides of abdomen are full.

Use ulnar border of the hand to assess fundal height.

Abdominal Palpation

Key Terminology

Attitude: The relationship of the fetal head and limbs to its trunk is called attitude.

Presentation: It is the leading anatomical part of the fetus closest to the pelvic inlet of the birth canal. **Example:** Cephalic, breech, or shoulder presentation.

Denominator: The arbitrary bony part of the presenting part is called denominator. **Example:** Occiput in vertex, brow in face, sacrum in breech presentation.

Leopold Maneuvers (Obstetric Grips)

- Leopold in 1984, described four maneuvers. It is used to diagnose fetal presentation in late pregnancy and during labor.
- Ask the client to empty the bladder before procedure.
- Stand on the right side of the patient.
- Client should lie in dorsal position with flexed knees.
- Rub the hand to make it warm before touching the mother's abdomen.
- During Braxton Hicks' contractions or during uterine contractions it should not be performed.

First Maneuver (Fundal Grip)

- Palpation is done facing patient's face.
- The first maneuver aims to determine the gestational age, fetal lie and the presentation.
- The fundus is gently palpated with the fingers of both hands, to discover which pole of the fetus is present.
- The head feels hard and round, and is easily movable and ballotable.
- The breech feels soft, triangular and continuous with the body.

Second Maneuver (Lateral Grip or Umbilical Grip)

- Palpation is done facing patient's face.
- This grip tells us about the position of the fetus.
- Place the hands on both sides of the uterus about midway between symphysis pubis and the fundus.
- The hands are to be placed on the sides of the umbilicus.
- Smooth curve suggests the location of back and comparatively empty and irregular shapes suggests limb side.

Third Leopold Maneuver (Pawlik's Grip)

- The third maneuver was modified by Karel Pawlík (1849–1914)
- Palpation is done facing patient's face.
  - It is done with single hand.
  - With fingers and thumb approximated, the presenting part is grasped distinctly and the mobility from side to side is tested.
  - In transverse lie, Pawlik's grip is empty.

Fourth Leopold Maneuver (Pelvic Grip)

- Examination is done facing patient's feet.
- It is the deep pelvic grip.
- The examiner places the palms of both hands on either side of the lower abdomen, with the tips of the fingers facing downward toward the pelvic inlet.

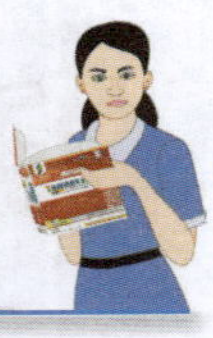

KEY POINT

Recommended antenatal visit schedule according to the 2016 WHO ANC model (8 visits):

1. Contact 1–up to 12 weeks
2. Contact 2–20 weeks
3. Contact 3–24 weeks
4. Contact 4–30 weeks
5. Contact 5–34 weeks
6. Contact 6–36 weeks
7. Contact 7–38 weeks
8. Contact 8–40 weeks

Recent Questions (NORCET 2020)

8. A pregnant woman visiting antenatal clinic complains that she gets frequent leg cramps and pain during night. Which of the following is an appropriate intervention to be suggested for the client?

a. Dorsiflexion with knee extension exercise
b. Complete bed rest is advised
c. Use of compression stockings
d. All of the above

Ans. (a) Dorsiflexion...

9. Extra calories needed during second trimester of pregnancy is:

a. 300 kcal/day
b. 500 kcal/day
c. 600 kcal/day
d. 700 kcal/day

Ans. (a) 300 kcal/day

Leopold Maneuver Consist of Four Grips

Table 4: Four grips of leopold maneuver

Leopold's maneuver	Name of grip	Purpose
First Leopold	Fundal grip	To determine what part of fetus is lying in the fundus
Second Leopold	Lateral or Umbilical grip	To find out the position of back, limbs and the anterior shoulder
Third Leopold	Pawlik's grip	To assess the engagement of presenting part. If the fetal head is ballotable it does not enter the pelvis.
Fourth Leopold	Pelvic grip Deep pelvic grip	To note precise of presenting part, attitude and engagement in vertex presentation. If the fingers are converging below the head of the baby means head has not entered the pelvis.

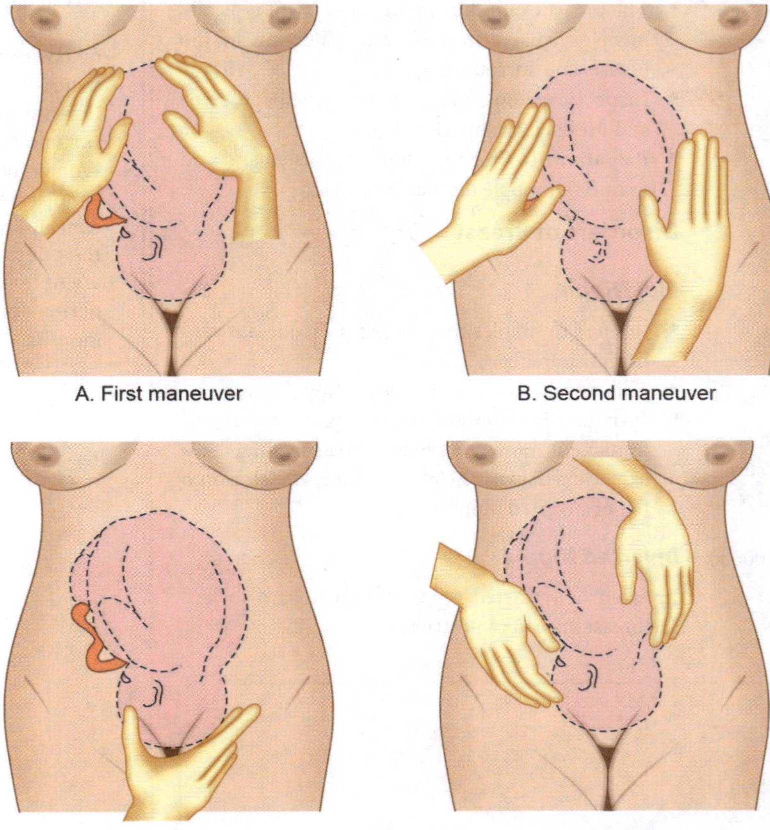

Figures 18A to D: Leopold's maneuver

KEY POINTS

- **Pawlik's grip** is the 3rd obstetric grip on abdominal palpation.
- **Obstetric grip** is also known as **Leopold maneuvers**.
- **Pelvic grip** examination is done facing the patient's feet.
- On examination, divergence of fingers shows engaged head.

Practice Questions

3. **Abdominal examination (Leopold's maneuver) revealed breech presentation. Fetal back is found to be at the right side of the mother. In this scenario, the fetal heart rate can be best heard at:**
   a. Left upper quadrant
   b. Around umbilicus
   c. Team nursing
   d. Right lower quadrant

Ans. (d) Right lower...

4. **While performing step 3 of Leopold's maneuver, the nurse palpated a hard round movable mass at the supra pubic area. She is aware that the mass palpated is:**
   a. Fetal back
   b. Fetal head
   c. Buttocks of the fetus
   d. None of the above

Ans. (b) Fetal head

KEY POINTS

- Ask the client to empty the bladder before abdominal palpation.
- Stand on the right side of the patient during abdominal palpation.
- Client position for abdominal palpation-dorsal position with flexed knees
- The most common normal position of the fetus in utero is vertical position.

Auscultation

- Fetal Heart Sounds are best audible through the back of the fetus in vertex and breech presentation.
- In face presentation, the heart sounds are heard through fetal chest.
- Maximum intensity of FHS is below the umbilicus in cephalic presentation and around the umbilicus in breech position.
- FHR can be heard using doppler at 10 week and with stethoscope at 18–20 weeks.

Table 5: FHR location Location of FHR

Presentation	Location of FHR
Cephalic or vertex	Midway between umbilicus and level of anterior superior iliac spine
Breech	Level with or above the umbilicus
Anterior	Close to the abdominal midline
Occiput transverse	In lateral abdominal area
Occiput posterior	In flank area.

Vaginal Examination

- No internal ballottement is seen
- Often enlarged, tender ovaries
- Gape-like vesicles per vagina
- Cervical os open

Investigations

- Urine pregnancy test is positive in high dilution. 1/200 is highly suggestive, 1/500 is surely diagnostic. In normal pregnancy, it is positive in dilutions up to 1/100.
- Serum β-hCG level is highly elevated (>100000 mIU/mL)
- **USG:** Characteristic intrauterine "**snow storm**" appearance
- No identifiable fetus, bilateral ovarian cysts may be detected, no fetal skeleton.

Complications

- Hemorrhage
- Infection due to absence of the amniotic sac
- Perforation of the uterus
- Pregnancy induced hypertension
- Hyperthyroidism
- Subsequent development of choriocarcinoma.

Treatment

Evacuate the uterus as soon as diagnosis is made.

Breast Examination

- The breast exam during pregnancy will typically involve visual inspection and palpation of the breasts and surrounding tissue.
- **Inspection:** Look for size, symmetry, shape, color and presence of superficial vein.
- **Palpation:** To find out nodules if present and also to find out nipple discharge.

Disorders of Breast

Flat Nipple

- It refers to nipples that do not protrude outward from the areola.
- This condition makes breast feeding difficult.
- Syringing is a method of drawing out the nipple to make it more erect before breastfeeding. This can be particularly helpful for babies to latch onto flat or inverted nipples.

Inverted Nipple

Inverted or retracted nipples point inward toward the breast instead of protruding outward.

KEY POINTS

- A complete molar pregnancy occurs when an egg that contains no genetic information is fertilized by a sperm **(Diploid – 45, XX; rarely 46, XY)**.
- A partial molar pregnancy occurs when a normal egg is fertilized by two sperms **(Triploid – 69, XXY; 69, XXX)**.
- A complete molar pregnancy can be detected by Ultrasound as early as eight or nine weeks of pregnancy. It may show: No embryo or fetus. No amniotic fluid.
- Women who have had a molar pregnancy can conceive again once their Beta HCG levels are normal and remain normal for 6 to 12 months.

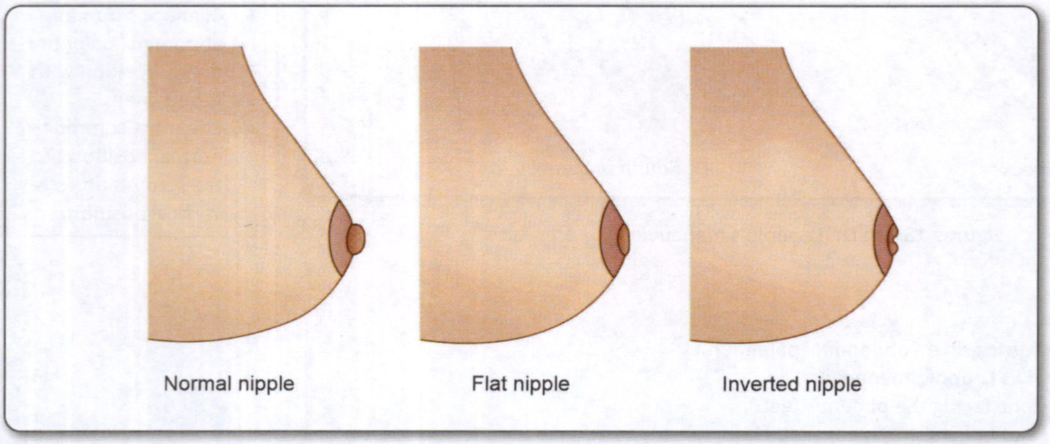

Figure 19: Nipple types

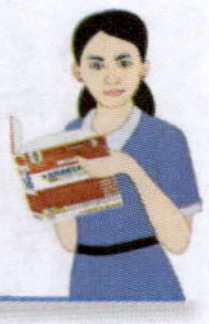

Self-Examination

- The breast self-examination is the best means of early detection of breast cancer combined with routine mammography and regular breast self-examination (BSE).
- **Inspection:** The breast is first examined by inspection, with the patient's arms at her sides and then with her hands pressed against her hips and/or with her arms raised over her head.

Breast Palpation Technique

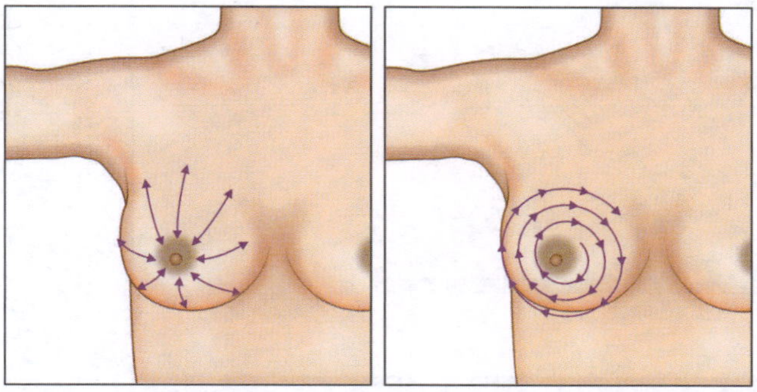

Figure 20: Radial and spiral

- Discoloration or ulcerations of the skin of the breast, areola, or nipple, or edema of the lymphatics are abnormal.
- A clear or milky breast discharge is usually bilateral and associated with stimulation or elevated prolactin levels (galactorrhea).
- Bloody discharge from the breast is abnormal and usually unilateral. It usually does not represent carcinoma, but rather shows inflammation of a breast structure.
- Pus usually indicates infection, although an underlying tumor may be encountered.
- **Palpation** follows inspection, first with the patient's arms at her sides and then with the arms raised over her head.
- This part of the examination is usually done with the patient in the supine position.
- The examiner should cover the entire breast in a spiral or radial pattern, including the axillary tail. If masses are found, their size, shape, consistency (soft, hard, firm, cystic) and mobility, as well as their position, should be determined.
- If fluid is noted on inspection or is expressed, it should be sent for culture and sensitivity and cytopathology.

KEY POINTS

Self-Examination of breast

- BSE is a procedure that a woman can perform physically and visually examine her breasts and underarm areas for changes.
- The best time to do a self-breast exam is a week after menstruation.
- Postmenopausal women should do the examination on **the same day on every month**.
- Any lumps, tenderness or abnormal discharge should be notified to the physician.

Recent Question (NORCET 2020)

10. Which of the following antipsychotic drug causes hyperprolactinemia?
a. Clozapine
b. Risperidone
c. Quetiapine
d. Olanzapine

Ans. (b) Risperidone

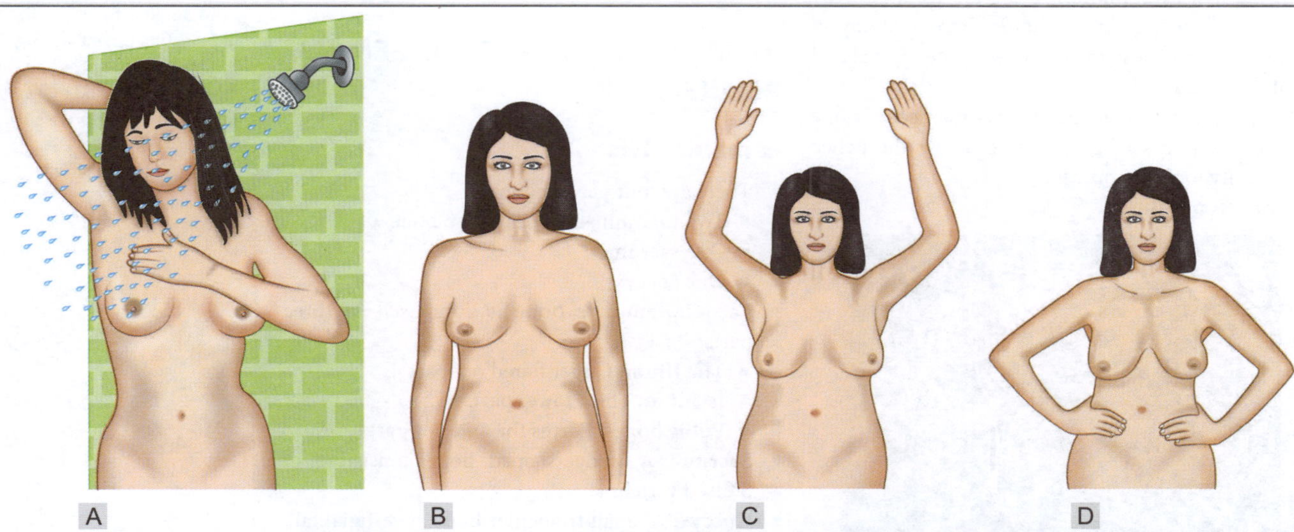

Figures 21A to D:

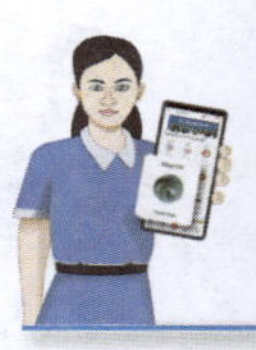

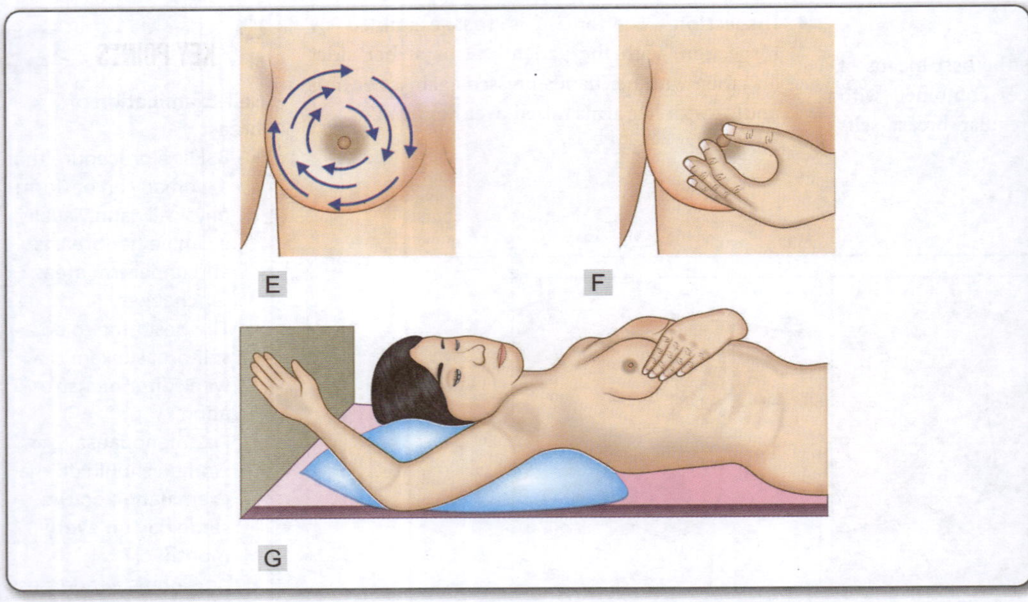

Figures 21A to G: Breast self-examination (From step A to G)

Pelvic Examination

- Patient must empty the bladder before examination.
- Talk before you touch. Avoid anything unexpected.
- Pelvic examinations require relaxation of the muscles. Ask the patient to gently breath in through nose and breath out through mouth.
- **Position:** Lithotomy position.
- **Steps**
  - Inspection and examination of external genitalia
  - Speculum examination: **Pederson speculum** is suitable for nulliparous and postmenopausal women**. Graves speculum** for multiparous women.
- **Bimanual examination** of the uterus is done by lifting the uterus up toward the abdominal fingers so that it may be palpated between the vaginal and abdominal hands.
- In pregnant women pelvic examination is done after 37 weeks of gestation to assess the pelvic capacity for labor process.
- **Graves speculum**

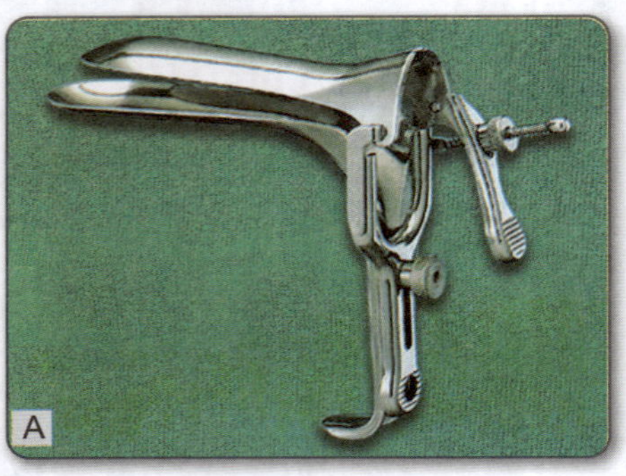

Figures 22A:

- **Pederson speculum**

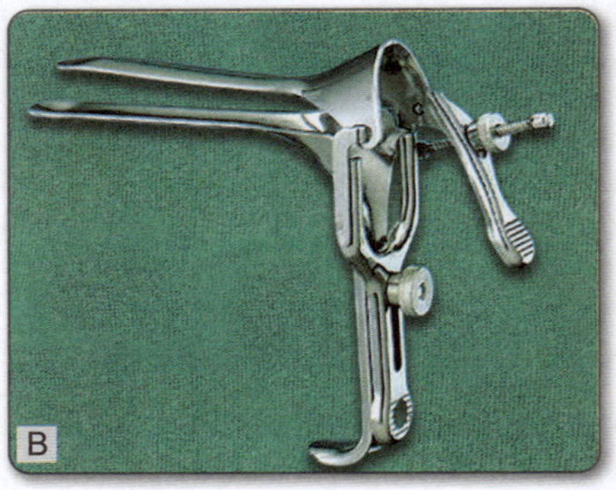

Figures 22A and B: A. Graves speculum B. Pederson speculum

ANATOMY AND TYPES OF FEMALE PELVIS

Female Pelvis

- There are four pelvic bones:
  - Two innominate bones or hip bones
  - One sacrum
  - One coccyx
- Each **innominate bone** is composed of three parts:
  - **The Ilium:** Larger flared out part
  - **Ischium:** Thick lower part
  - **Pubic bones:** Forms the anterior part
- **Sacrum:** A wedge-shaped bone consisting of 5 fused vertebrae.
- **Coccyx:** A small triangular bone, a vestigial tail. Consists of 4 fused vertebrae.

Recent Question (NORCET 2023)

11. During an antenatal visit, a pregnant client, while lying supine on the examining table, tells the Nurse that she is becoming light-headed. The Nurse notices that the client has pallor in her face and is perspiring profusely. The Nurse should initiate to:

a. Place the clent in the Trendelenburg position
b. Assess the client to see if she is having vaginal bleeding
c. Obtain the client's vital signs immediately
d. Help the client to a sitting position

Ans. (d) Help the client to a sitting position

Explanation: The client is experiencing supine hypotension, which is a decrease in blood pressure that occurs when a pregnant woman lies flat on her back. This is caused by the weight of the uterus pressing on the vena cava, a major vein that returns blood to the heart. The symptoms of supine hypotension include lightheadedness, dizziness, pallor, and sweating. The first thing the nurse should do is help the client to a sitting position. This will relieve the pressure on the vena cava and allow blood to flow more freely to the heart.

- There are **four pelvic joints:**
  - **One symphysis pubis:** Form the junction of two pubic bones.
  - **Two sacroiliac joints:** Connects the spine to the pelvis.
  - **One sacro:** Coccygeal joint.

Types of Female Pelvis

- **Gynecoid pelvis (Female pelvis)**
  - It is the most suitable female pelvic shape. Round pelvic inlet and shallow pelvic cavity with short ischial spines.
  - Transverse diameter is more than anteroposterior diameter.
  - It allows normal child birth with ease and is most suitable for child birth.
- **Android pelvis (Male pelvis)**
  - Male type or wedge-shaped pelvis.
  - Has triangular or heart-shaped inlet and is narrower from the front.
- **Anthropoid pelvis**
  - Oval-shaped inlet with large anteriorposterior diameter and comparatively smaller transverse diameter.
  - It has larger outlet. The problem in this pelvis is the inlet.
- **Platypelloid pelvis**
  - Flat type pelvis. It has narrow anterioposterior diameter of pelvic inlet.
  - The pelvic inlet is specifically kidney shaped.

Recent Question (NORCET 2020)

12. The pelvic shape has the poorest prognosis from vaginal delivery is-------------

a. Platypelloid
b. Anthropoid
c. Android
d. Gynecoid

Ans. (c) Android

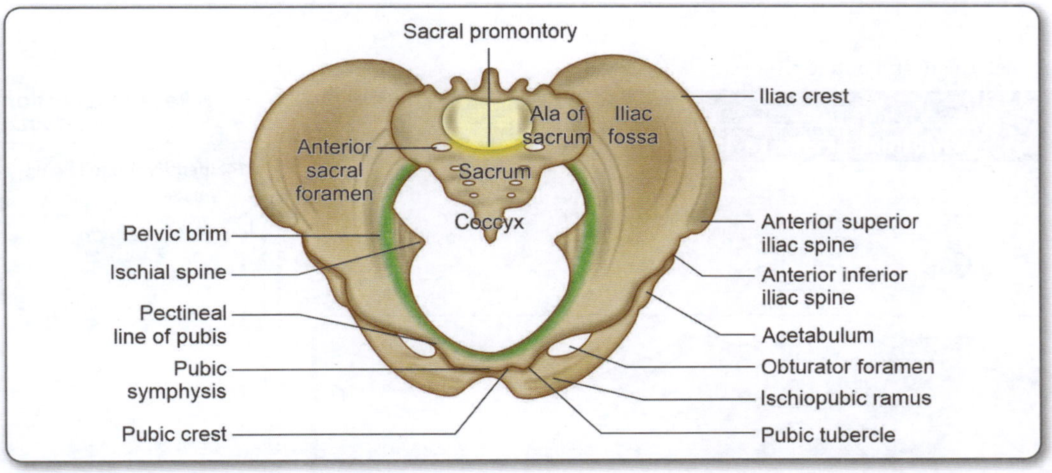

Figure 23: Female pelvis

Types of Pelvis

Characteristic	Gynecoid	Android	Anthropoid	Platypelloid
Shape of inlet	Transverse oval	Heart shaped	Long oval	Flat bowl like
Transverse diameter (TD) and Anterio-Posterior diameter (AP).	TD > AP	TD > AP	AP > TD	TD >>> AP
Side wall	Parallel broad	Converge	Parallel narrow	Divergent
Ischial spine		Prominent		
Subpubic angle	>90°	<90°		

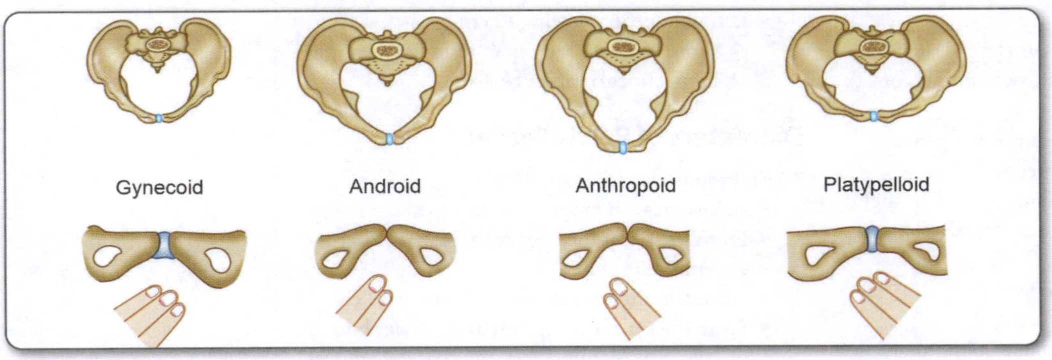

Figure 24: Types of pelvis

KEY POINTS

- Absence of both sacral alae is called **Robert's pelvis.**
- Both naegele's pelvis and Robert's pelvis are **contracted pelvis.**
- **Gynecoid pelvis** is the **most suitable** pelvic shape for **childbirth.**
- The shape of gynecoid is round.
- **Android pelvis** is least suited pelvis type for childbearing.
- Least common variety of pelvis is **platypelloid.**
- An ischial spine is prominent in android pelvic.
- Obstetric conjugate is the shortest anteroposterior diameter.

PELVIC DIAMETER

Diameters of Pelvic Inlet

- **Anteroposterior diameter:**
  - Anatomical anteroposterior diameter (true conjugate) = 11 cm
  - From the mid of the sacral promontory to the inner margin of upper border of the symphysis pubis.
  - Obstetric conjugate = 10 cm

From the tip of the sacral promontory to the most bulging point on the back of symphysis pubis. **It is the shortest anteroposterior diameter.**

- Diagonal conjugate = 12 cm
  - 1.5 cm longer than the true conjugate. From the tip of sacral promontory to the lower border of symphysis pubis.

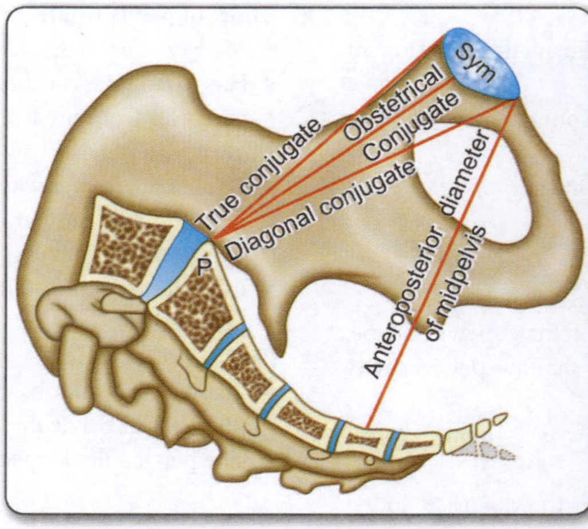

Figure 25: Pelvic diameter

Recent Question (NORCET 2022)

13. Identify the following image.

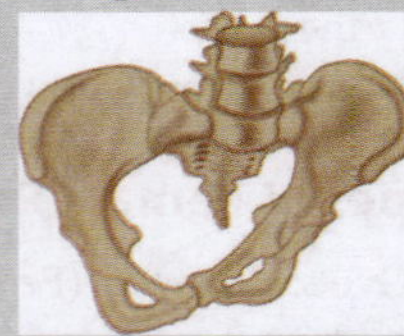

a. Naegele's Pelvis
b. Robert's Pelvis
c. Scoliotic Pelvis
d. Android Pelvis

Ans. (a) Naegele's Pelvis

Table 6: Diameters of pelvis at inlet, cavity and outlet

Diameter of pelvis	Pelvis type		
	Pelvic inlet	**Pelvic cavity**	**Pelvic outlet**
Anteroposterior diameter (cm)	11	12	13
Oblique diameter (cm)	12	12	—
Transverse diameter (cm)	13	12	11

Recent Question (NORCET 2022)

14. Identify the following image.

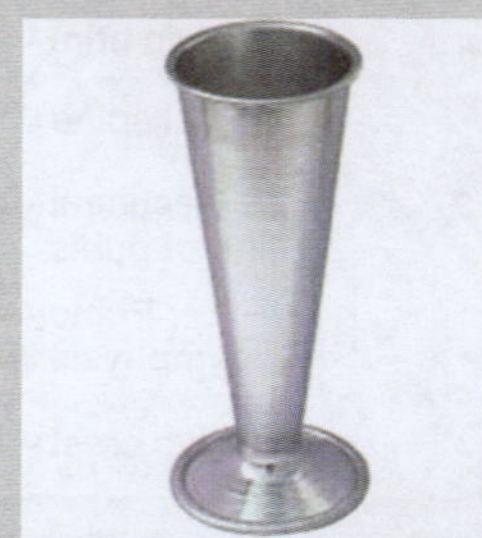

a. Stethescope
b. Pinard fetoscope
c. Endoscope
d. Doppler

Ans. (b) Pinard fetoscope

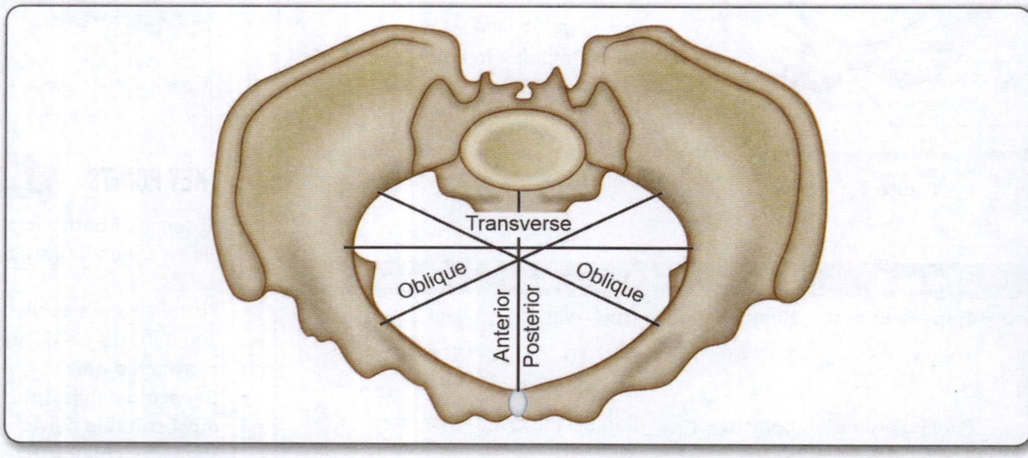

Figure 26: Diameters of pelvis at inlet, cavity and outlet

- **Transverse diameters:**
  - Anatomical transverse diameter = 13 cm
    - Between the farthest two points on the iliopectineal lines.
    - It is the **largest diameter** in the pelvis.
  - Obstetric transverse diameter:
    - It bisects the true conjugate and is slightly shorter than the anatomical transverse diameter.
- **Diagonal/Oblique diameters:**
  - Right oblique diameter = 12 cm
    - From the right sacroiliac joint to the left iliopectineal eminence.
  - Left oblique diameter = 12 cm
    - From the left sacroiliac joint to the right iliopectineal eminence.

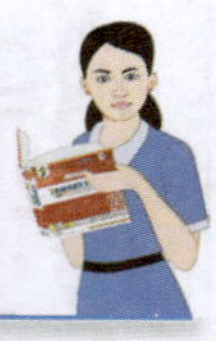

Diameters of Pelvic Outlet

- Anteroposterior diameters:
  - Anatomical anteroposterior diameter = 11 cm
  - From the tip of the coccyx to the lower border of symphysis pubis.
  - Obstetric anteroposterior diameter = 13 cm
  - From the tip of the sacrum to the lower border of symphysis pubis as the coccyx moves backwards during the second stage of labor.

- Transverse diameters:
  - Bituberous diameter = 11 cm
    Between the inner aspects of the ischial tuberosities.
  - Bispinous diameter = 10.5 cm
    Between the tips of ischial spines.

Contracted pelvis: major diameter of the pelvis is decreased by 0.5 cm or more is known as contracted pelvis.

FETAL SKULL

Compared to an adult skull, a fetus's skull is a larger proportion of its body.

Adaptation of this fetal skull with maternal pelvis is one of the important things need to take place during the process of delivery to avoid further complication or adverse events.

Parts of Fetal Skull

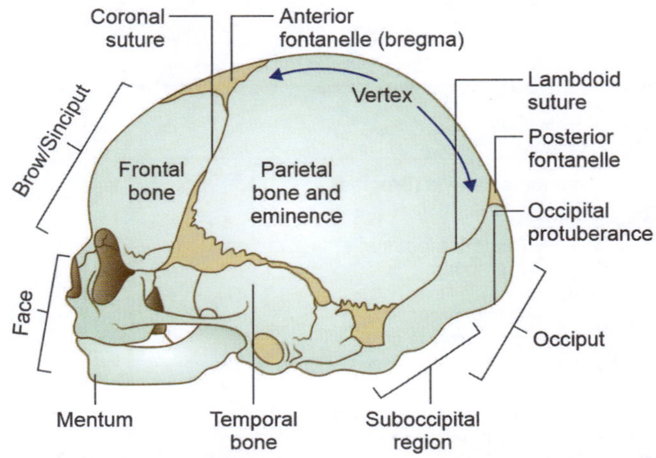

Figure 27: Fetal skull

Bones in Fetal Skull

- 2 Frontal bone
- 2 Parietal bone
- 2 Temporal bone
- 1 Occipital bone

Table 7: Types of sutures and their location on fetal skull

Sutures	Locations
Frontal suture	Between two frontal bones
Coronal suture	Between frontal and parietal bone
Lambdoid suture	Two parietal bone and occipital bone
Sagittal suture	Two parietal bones

Vertex: It is a quadrilateral area bounded by the anterior fontanelle and coronal suture in front, the posterior fontanel and lambdoid suture behind and longitudinal line passing through the parietal eminences laterally.

Brow/sinciput: It is an area bounded by the supraorbital ridges in front, anterior fontanel and coronal suture behind and longitudinal line passing through the frontal eminences laterally.

Face: It is an area between orbital ridges and root of nose to the junction of chin and neck.

Fontanelle

- Two frontal bone forms sinciput of the fetal skull.
- The space between the bones of the skull is suture and the area where the sutures meet is known as fontanelle.
- These sutures and fontanelle help the fetal skull to mold during the process of delivery.
- **Anterior fontanelle (bregma):**
  - Formed at the junction between frontal, coronal and sagittal sutures, since it is at the junction of 4 sutures
  - It is like a **diamond in shape**.
  - It is closed by 18 months of age.
  - It is the largest fontanel. Its length is 2.5 cm and width is 1.5 cm.
- **Posterior fontanelle (lambda):**
  - It is formed at the junction between lambdoid suture on either side and sagittal suture
  - It is like a **triangle in shape**.
  - It is closed by the age of 2–3 months of age. It measures about 1.2 × 1.2 cm.

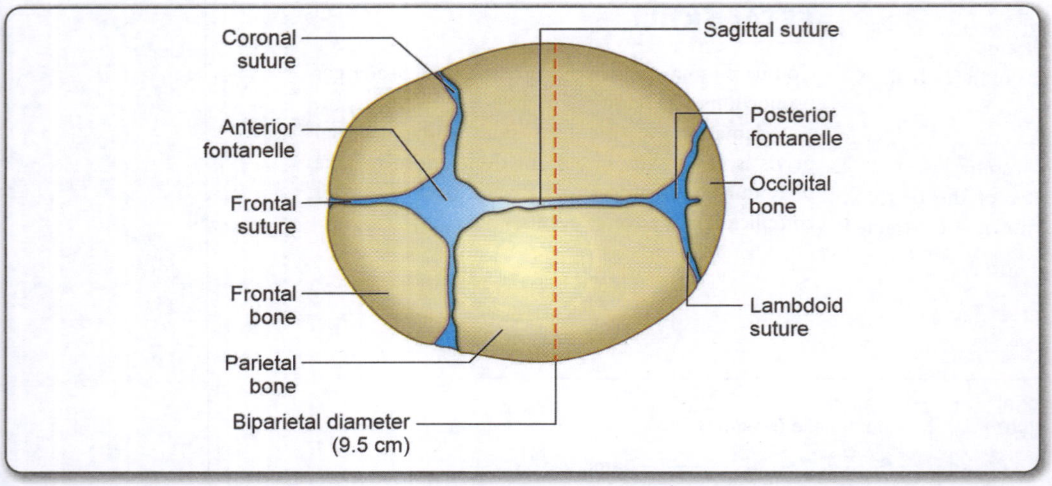

Figure 28: Parts of fetal skull

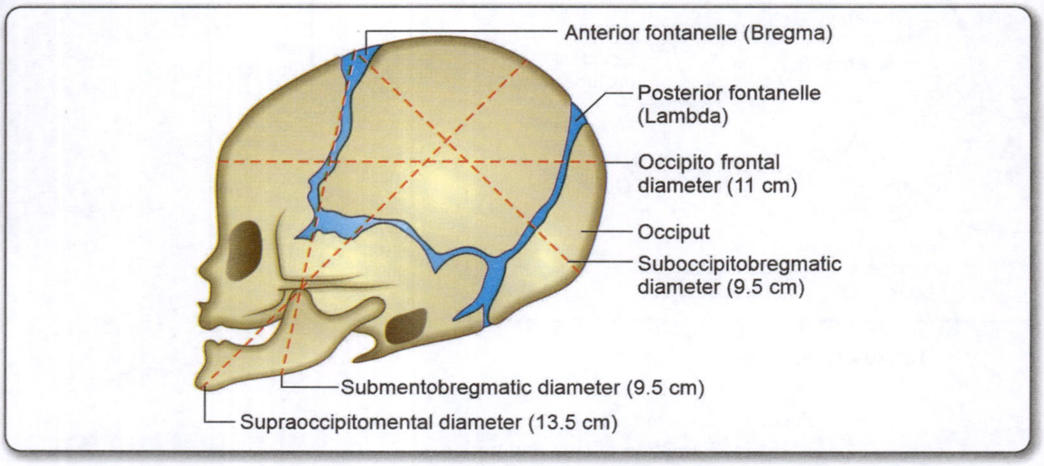

Figure 29: Fetal skull—Diameters

KEY POINTS

- Gap between the suture line is known as fontanelle.
- In an infant, a bulging fontanel is the most significant sign of increasing intracranial pressure.
- **Anterior fontanelle** becomes ossified around 18th month after birth.
- **Posterior fontanelle** becomes ossified around 6 weeks after birth.
- At time of birth there are 6 fontanelles in fetal skull.
- Anterior fontanelle is diamond shaped.
- Posterior fontanelle is triangular shaped.

Diameters of Fetal Skull

Diameter	Length
Bimastoid diameter: Distance between the tip of mastoid process	7.5 cm
Bitemporal diameter: Distance between the anterior inferior end of coronal suture	8 cm
Super subparital diameter: Extends from one point placed below one parietal eminence to a point placed above the other parietal eminence of the opposite side	8.5 cm
Biparietal diameter: Distance between two parietal eminences	9.5 cm
Suboccipito bregmatic: From nape of neck to center of bregma	9.5 cm
Suboccipito frontal: Nape of neck to center of sinciput or anterior end of anterior fontanel	10 cm
Occipito frontal: From occipital eminence to root of nose (glabella)	11.5 cm
Mentovertical: From midpoint of the chin to the highest point in sagittal suture	14 cm
Submentovertical: From junction of floor of mouth and neck to the highest point on sagittal suture.	11.5 cm
Submento-bregmatic: From junction of floor of mouth and neck to the center of the bregma.	9.5 cm

KEY POINTS

- **Coronal sutures** run between parietal and frontal bones on either side.
- Lambdoid sutures separate the occipital bone and the two parietal bones.
- Largest diameter of the fetus skull is **mentovertical (14 cm)**.
- **Biparietal diameter** of fetal head measure about 9.5 cm

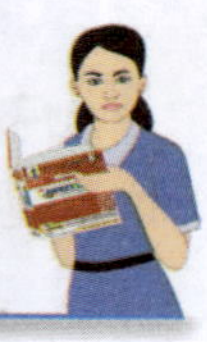

FETUS IN UTERO (LIE, PRESENTATION AND POSITION)

Lie

The lie refers to the relationship of the long axis of the fetus to the long axis of the centralized uterus or maternal spine, the most common lie being longitudinal (99.5%).

Types of Lie

Longitudinal lie	Oblique lie	Transverse lie

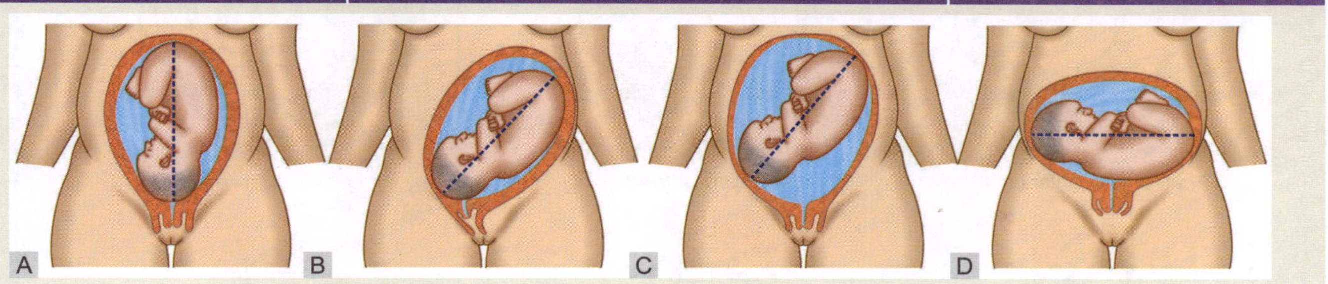

Figures 30A to D: Different types of lies

Attitude: The relationship between fetal limb and head to its trunk. Normal attitude is well flexed.
Denominator: It is the part of presentation that determine the position.

Fetal presentation	Denominator
Vertex presentation	Occiput
Breech presentation	Sacrum
Face presentation	Mentum
Shoulder presentation	Acromion process of the scapula

Presentation

Body parts of the fetus that engage in the true pelvis.

- **Cephalic (head):** Vertex, brow or face.
- **Breech:** Frank, complete, on single or double footling
- **Shoulder:** Fetus cannot travel through birth canal.

Presenting part: Part of the fetus that lies over the cervical OS during labor. It should not be confused with presentation.

Attitude of fetus	Presenting part
Fully flexed	Vertex
Deflexed	Vertex
Partially extended	Brow
Fully extended	Face

Position

Relationship of presenting fetal part to four quadrants of the mother's pelvis.

- (L-left; R-Right; O-Occiput; A-Anterior; P-Posterior; M-Mentum; S-Sacrum).
- **Vertex:** Occiput; LOA, LOP, ROA, ROP
- **Face:** Chin; LMA, LMP, RMA, RMP
- **Breech:** Sacrum; LSA, RSA, LSP, RSP
- **Station:** Relationship of presenting part of the fetus to the ischial spines of mother's pelvis.
- **Floating:** Presenting part movable above the true pelvic inlet.
- **Engaged:** Suboccipitobregmatic diameter fixed into the pelvic inlet.
- **Station 0:** Presenting part at the level of ischial spines; level above spines: –1, –2, –3; level below spins: +1, +2, +3.

Recent Question
(NORCET 2020)

15. The uterine fundal height of a pregnant patient is at the level of the umbilicus, her pregnancy is about_________?
a. 10–12 weeks
b. 14–16 weeks
c. 20–24 weeks
d. 30–32 weeks

Ans. (c) 20–24 weeks

Clinical Corner

CASE SCENARIO 4:
During an internal vaginal examination nurse palpated posterior fontanel on the right side of the mother at the upper quadrant. Nurse interpreted the position of fetus as:
a. LOA
b. ROA
c. LOP
d. ROP

Ans. (b) ROA

POSITIONS AND PRESENTATIONS OF FETUS DURING LABOR

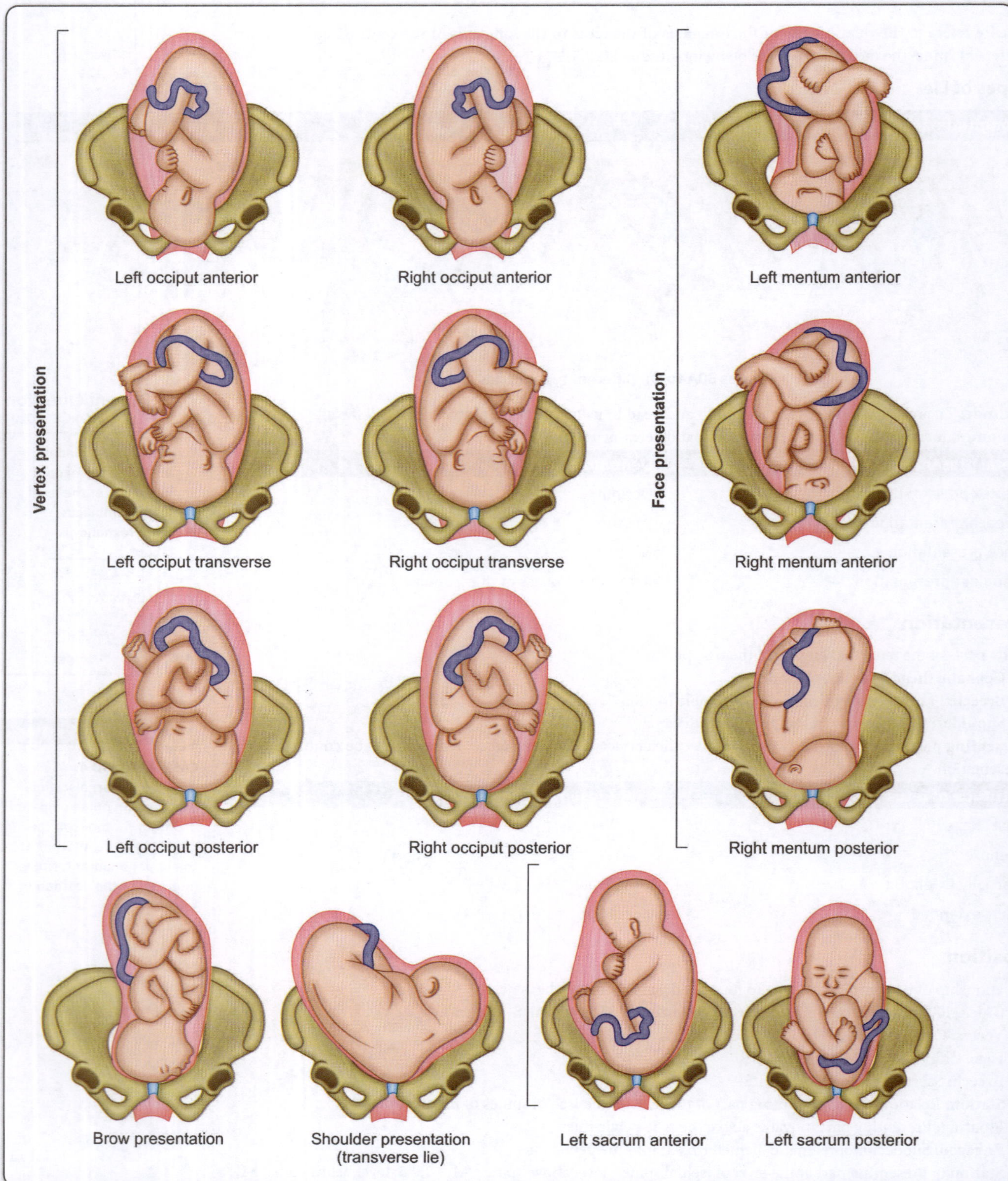

Figure 31: Position and presentation of fetus

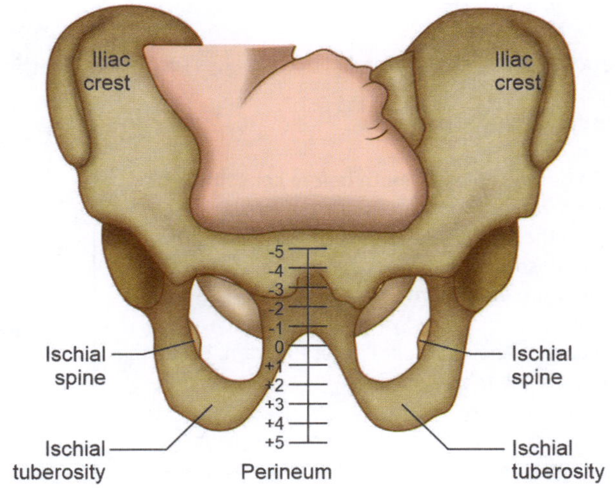

Figure 32: Station of head in relation to ischial spine

Spontaneous rupture of membranes (SROM or SRM): Usually occurs during mid or late labor but can also occur before labor begins.

Artificial rupture of membrane (AROM): Should not be done until presenting part is engaged against cervix.

Nitrazine paper test: Used to confirm the presence of amniotic fluid. Test positive when pH is above 7.

Signs of Previous Childbirth

Breast: Flabbier, nipples are more prominent whoever breastfed their infant. Primary areola pigmentation remains and so the white striae.

Abdomen: Wall is more lax and loose. There may be presence of silvery white striae and linea alba.

Cervix: Nulliparous cervix is conical in shape with a round external os. In parous women, it becomes cylindrical and external os may admit a fingertip.

Vagina: More spacy

Perineum: It is lax and evidence of old scarring from perineal laceration or episiotomy may be present.

POINTS TO REMEMBER

Antenatal Care

- Immunization against tetanus (2 dose) 0.5 mL IM 6 weeks apart. Women who immunized in the past can be given with booster dose.
- Generally, ANC visit should be done every 4 weekly up to 28 weeks, then every 2 weekly up to 36 weeks after that weekly till delivery.
- **According to GOI,** minimum **4 ANC visit** is needed. First visit is in 8–12 weeks for registration, second visit between 24 and 26 weeks, third visit at 32 weeks and fourth visit at 36–38 weeks.
- **According to WHO**, minimum **8 visit is needed**. One in first trimester, 2nd and 3rd in second trimester and 5 visits in third trimester. Earlier it was minimum of three visits.
- Supplementary iron therapy is needed in pregnant women. One ferrous sulphate tablet containing 60 mg elemental iron. Three such tablet provides 45 mg of absorbable iron.
- Air travel is safe up to 36 weeks and is contraindicated in case of placenta previa.
- Backache is common in pregnancy because of hormone like relaxin and estrogen. It is also due to the hyper lordosis during pregnancy, weight gain and anterior tilt of pelvis.
- **Leg cramps** occur in pregnancy due to the **lack of diffusible calcium in serum** and elevation in phosphorus.
- Physiological edema among pregnant women subsided by rest but pathological edema is not subsided and is present above the ankle.
- Constipation occurs in pregnancy due to the pressure exerted by gravid uterus on gut, physical inactivity and atonicity of gut due to progesterone.

Contd...

Recent Question
(NORCET 2020)

16. The leading anatomical part of the fetus closest to the pelvic inlet of the birth canal refers to:
a. Presentation
b. Lie
c. Denominator
d. Position

Ans. (a) Presentation

KEY POINTS

- Most common presentation is cephalic presentation.
- Most common malpresentation is breech.
- Shoulder presentation (transverse lie) with dead baby is called neglected shoulder syndrome
- Maximum chance of cord prolapse is with transverse lie.
- Hand prolapse is seen in transverse lie.

Recent Question
(NORCET 2022–23)

17. A pregnant woman at 27 weeks of gestation visited antenatal clinic at a primary health center for the first time. Her hemoglobin level was found to be 9 gm%. The management will include:
a. Tab iron and folic acid - one tablet (containing 60 mg elemental iron and 500 microgram of Folic acid) daily
b. Tab iron and folic acid - one tablet (containing 50 mg elemental iron and 500 microgram of Folic acid) weekly
c. Blood Transfusion
d. Tab iron and folic acid - two tablet (containing 60 mg elemental iron and 500 microgram of Folic acid) daily

Ans. (d) Tab iron and folic...

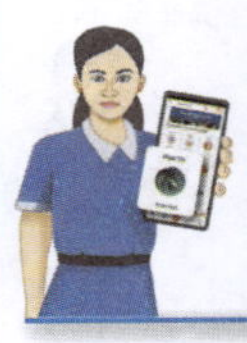

- Crown rump length less than the gestation is associated with increased risk for chromosomal abnormalities such as trisomy.
- Increased nuchal translucency at 10–14 weeks associated with chromosomal abnormalities such as trisomy or monosomy.
- Absence of nasal bone at 10–12 weeks USG suggestive of down syndrome.
- Hemoglobin less than 11 g is considered anemia in pregnancy.
- For all pregnant mothers, folic acid 400 mcg need to be started one month before conception to 3 months after conception. This dose of folic acid is known as prophylactic dose of folic acid.
- Females with previous history of neural tube defect in their baby takes 4 mg folic acid 3 months before conception to 3 months after conception. This dose is called therapeutic dose of folic acid.
- Once folic acid is stopped iron therapy will be started from 4th month onward.
- Total amount of iron needed in pregnancy is 1000 mg.
- GOI supplies iron and folic acid for free of cost as a part of Anemia Mukt Bharat Program. Fe: 60 mg and folic acid 500 mcg. All pregnant women should take one tablet per day.
- This iron therapy should continue till 180 days following delivery.
- As a rule all live vaccines are contraindicated in pregnancy while killed vaccine can be given.
- Absolutely contra-indicated vaccines are Mumps. Measles, Rubella, smallpox, chicken pox, HPV vaccine.
- If any women take live vaccine, then pregnancy is contraindicated for a period of 1 month.
- Absolutely safe vaccines during pregnancy include Hepatitis, Influenza, tetanus, and rabies.
- Tetanus vaccination: nowadays Td (tetanus and diphtheria) is given. First dose in early pregnancy usually at first visit itself and second dose at 4 weeks later.
- Td Booster: If pregnancy occurred within three years after the 2nd dose of Td, then only booster dose is needed in third trimester.
- Td dose is 0.5 mL IM over the upper arm.
- Lying down supine is contraindicated in pregnancy as it causes supine hypotension syndrome. Advise mother to lie down either right or left lateral position.
- Formulas used to calculate fetal weight include Hadlock formula, Shephard formula and Johnson formula.

Recent Question (NORCET 2021)

18. Iron and folic acid dose in pregnant woman is:
a. 60 mg iron, 0.4 mg folic acid
b. 30 mg iron, 0.4 mg folic acid
c. 100 mg iron, 0.3 mg folic acid
d. 60 mg iron, 0.2 mg folic acid

Ans. (a) 60 mg iron, 0.4 mg folic acid

Weight Gain in Pregnancy

- Weight gain expected during pregnancy is 11 kg.
- Normal weight gain is <0.5kg/week or <2kg/month.

More weight gain	Less weight gain	Rapid weight gain
• Diabetic pregnancy in which baby macrosomia and polyhydramnios is present. • Twin pregnancy • Post-term pregnancy	IUGR baby	Weight gain is >0.5kg/week or >2kg/month then pregnancy induced hypertension need to be suspected.

KEY POINTS

- In the **breech delivery** the engaging diameter of the shoulder is bisacromial.
- **Frank breech** is the most common type of breech presentation.
- Burns Marshall Method is used to deliver the fetus in breech presentation.
- The number of positions in the face presentation is **four.**

DIFFERENT POSITIONS AND PRESENTATIONS DURING LABOR

Different Positions and Presentations of Fetus

Figure: Different fetal presentations and positions during labor
(Ref: See Figure in Appendices)

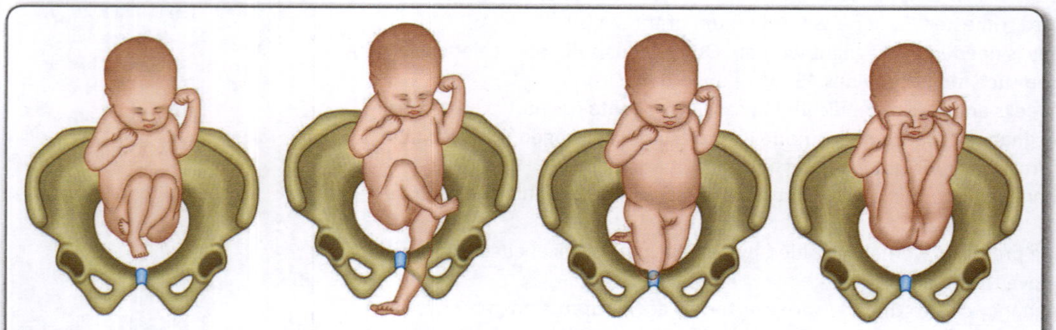

Figure 33: Breech presentation

Recent Question (NORCET 2022)

19. A 26-year-old client is admitted to the labor, delivery, recovery, postpartum unit. The nurse completes her assessment and determines the client is in the first stage of labor. The nurse should instruct her:
a. To hold her breath during contractions
b. To be flat on her back
c. Not to push with her contractions
d. To push before becoming fully dilated

Ans. (c) Not to push with her contractions

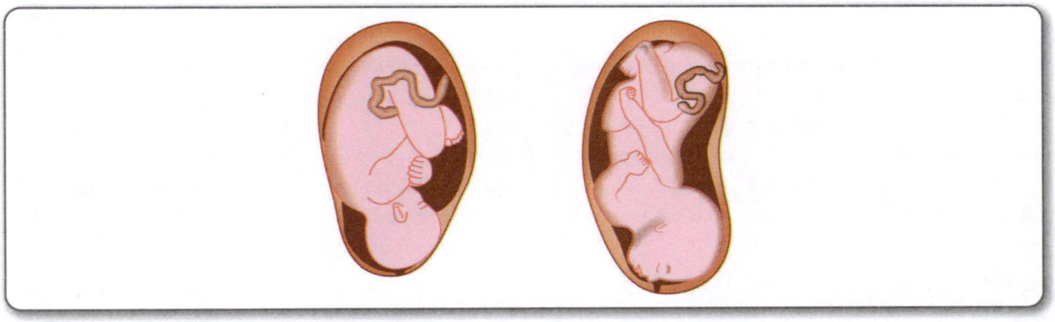

Figure 34: Normal and extended attitude

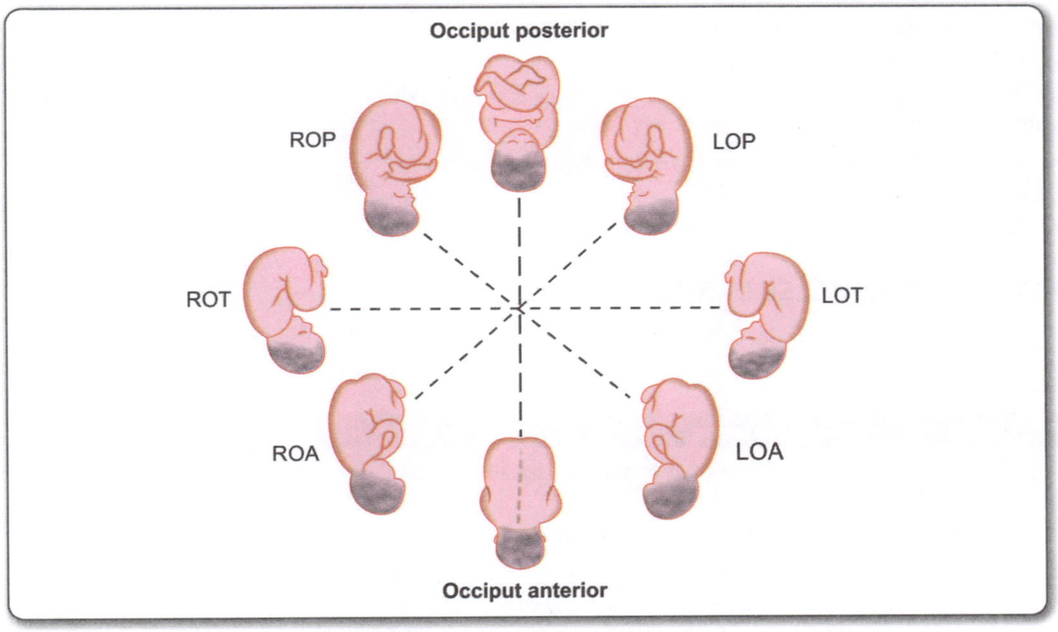

Figure 35: Fetal positions in uterus

Abbreviations: ROT, Right occiput transverse; ROP, right occiput posterior; ROA, right occiput anterior; LOP, left occiput posterior; LOT, left occiput transverse; LOA, left occiput posterior

LABOR AND DELIVERY

Labor: Series of events taking place in the genital organs to expel the viable product of conception from the womb through the vagina into the outer world.

Delivery: Process of extraction/expulsion of viable product of fetus out of the womb. Delivery and labor are not same.

Pre-labor: It is also called pre-monitory stage. It is beginning 2–3 weeks before in primi and 2–3 days before in multi.

Eutocia: It is also known as normal labor. Characteristics of normal labor include the following.

- Occurs spontaneously at term
- Vertex presentation
- Complete in normal time duration
- Natural termination with minimal aids
- No complication to mother and fetus

Dystocia: It is known as abnormal labor. Any changes from the criteria for normal labor is considered abnormal labor.

Preterm labor: If labor occurs before 37 completed weeks.

Term labor: If labor occurs between 37 and 42 weeks.

Post term labor: If labor occurs after 42 completed weeks.

Causes of Labor

Exact cause is unknown. But the following factors are believed to be contributing:

- Uterine distention
- Pressure from the presenting part on the cervical nerve endings
- Myometrial involvement with increased oxytocin receptors
- Oxytocin, estrogen and prostaglandin stimulation
- Progesterone withdrawal
- Fetal cortisol: Increased level of fetal cortisol in late pregnancy increases the estrogen level
- Fetoplacental contribution

Recent Question (NORCET 2023)

20. A pregnant woman is in active labor experienced spontaneous rupture of membrane. What will be the priority nursing intervention?

a. FHR assessment
b. Amniotic fluid color
c. Vital Signs of mother
d. Call the doctor

Ans. (a) FHR assessment

The priority nursing intervention when a pregnant woman in active labor experiences spontaneous rupture of membranes (SROM) is to assess the fetal heart rate (FHR). Spontaneous rupture of membranes means that the amniotic sac surrounding the baby has broken, leading to the release of amniotic fluid. Assessing the FHR is crucial in this situation to ensure the well-being of the baby

Recent Question (NORCET 2022)

21. A client has been admitted to the labor and delivery unit in active labor. After assessing her, the RN notes that the client's fetus position is left occipital posterior. Which of the following statements best describes what this means to the labor process:

a. Decreases the overall time of the labor process
b. Prolongs the client's first stage of labor
c. Decreases the time of the client's first stage of labor
d. Prolongs the client's third stage of labor

Ans. (b) Prolongs the client's first stage of labor

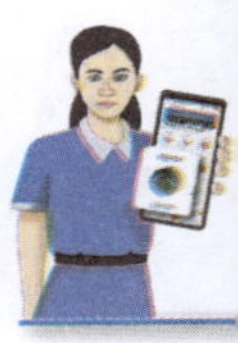

Pre-Labor Signs

Lightening	• Lightening is the process by which the baby's head descends lower into the pelvis in preparation for birth. • It happens days or weeks prior to the labor **(around 37 weeks or later).** • It is considered **welcome sign** and it rules out cephalopelvic disproportion. • After lightening pregnant lady can breathe easier as baby is no longer pressing on her diaphragm, however, frequency of micturition increases as bladder is pressed by the presenting part.
Cervical changes	• The cervix starts to soften, which is known as **ripening**. • The cervix starts to thin out or efface (it becomes shorter and thinner) and it admits one finger and is dilatable.
False labor pain	• Painful uterine contraction which has no effect on cervical dilation. • It may occur 1–2 weeks prior to the onset of labor.
GI upset	In the absence of any contributing factor women may experience diarrhea, indigestion, nausea or vomiting. Women experience either all or any of these signs.
Energy spurt	Women may experience energy spurt approximately 24–48 hours before the onset of labor.
Mood swing	Both high and low mood can occur before the delivery.

DIFFERENCE BETWEEN TRUE AND FALSE LABOR

Refer to Table 8

Table 8: True labor and false labor

True labor	False labor
Regular uterine contractions that increase in frequency, intensity and duration.	Contractions are irregular and dull in nature.
Increases in intensity and duration with walking	Usually stops with walking
Felt in lower back, radiating to lower portion of abdomen and thighs.	Contractions felt in abdomen above umbilicus
Bloody show	No bloody show
Dilation and effacement	No change in cervix
Fetus usually engaged	Fetus is ballotable
Not relieved with enema or sedation	Relieved by enema or sedation
Bag of water will be formed	Bag of water not formed.

Normal Mechanism of Labor (Steps)

The movement that occurs when the fetus passes through the maternal pelvis are called cardinal movements. Earlier 9 cardinal movements were there, including crowning. Nowadays crowning is not considered a cardinal movement.

1. **Engagement:** The b'by's head descends into the pelvis and is engaged in the mother's pelvis.
2. **Descent:** The b'by's head continues to descend through the birth canal with each contraction. It is a continuous process if there is no obstruction in the birth canal.
3. **Flexion:** As the b'by's head reaches the pelvic floor, it flexes to fit through the narrow opening.
4. **Internal rotation:** Head internally rotates to pass through the ischial spines. Internal rotation occurs at the level of ischial spine.
5. **Crowning:** Occiput slips beneath the subpubic arch when the head no longer recedes back.
6. **Extension:** Occiput pivot under symphysis pubis and the head is born with extension.
7. **Restitution:** Visible passive movement occurred in the head due to untwist the neck sustained during internal rotation.
8. **External rotation of head and Internal rotation of the shoulder:** Movement or rotation of head is visible externally due to the internal rotation of shoulder. As the fetus descends through the birth canal, the anterior shoulder rotates approximately $^{1}/8$th of a circle anteriorly, bringing it under the symphysis pubis. At this point, both shoulders are in the anteroposterior diameter of the pelvic outlet, which is the widest diameter of the pelvic outlet.
9. **Expulsion (birth of shoulder and trunk):** Rest of the body is born with lateral flexion.

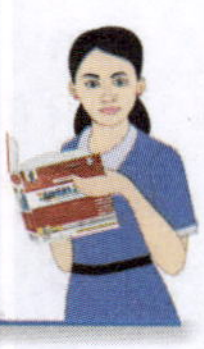

Recent Question (NORCET 2023)

22. A client is admitted in hospital for an induction of labor owing to gestational age of 42 weeks confirm by dates and ultrasound. When she has dilated 3 cm she has contractions of 70 sec. She is receiving IV oxytocin. Nurse priority intervention should be?

a. Stop IV oxytocin Infusion
b. Notify physician.
c. Prepare for delivery.
d. Check FHR

Ans. (a) Stop IV oxytocin Infusion

Contractions that last longer than 60 seconds, if persistent, may indicate that the uterus is contracted for excessive periods of time, contributing to fetal stress. So the nurse should stop the oxytocin infusion and then assess FHR.

Recent Question (NORCET 2023)

23. What is crowning?

a. Rotation at pelvic floor
b. Largest skull diameter fixed that doesn't go back
c. Largest diameter at ischial spines
d. None of the above

Ans. (b) Largest skull diameter fixed that...

Practice Question

5. All of the following are the characteristics of the contractions associated with true labor; Except:

a. Increase in intensity
b. Felt in the back and radiates to lower abdomen
c. Felt in abdomen above umbilicus
d. Consistent

Ans. (c) Felt in abdomen above umbilicus

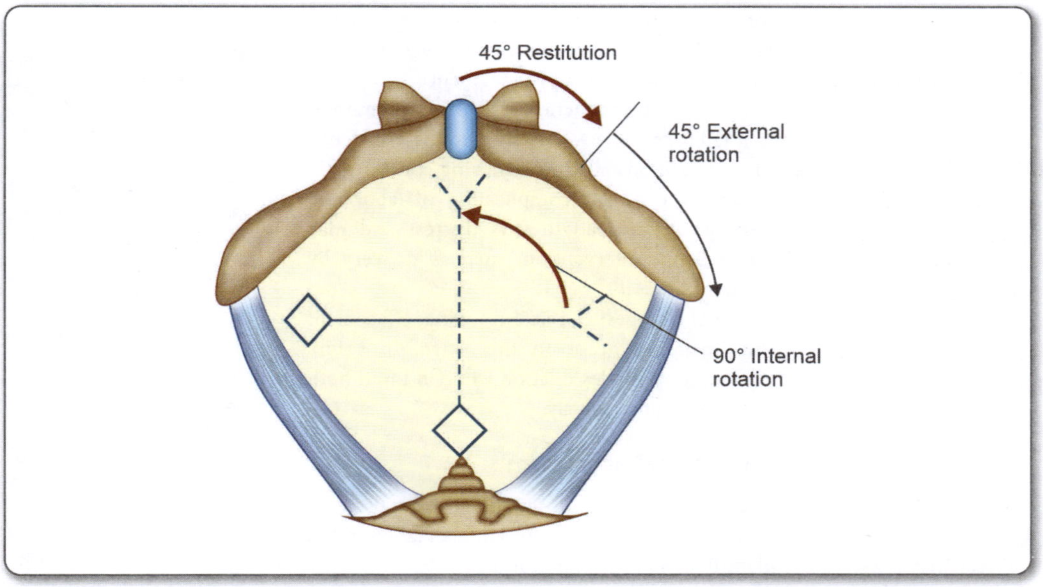

Figure 36: Degree of internal rotation, restitution and external rotation in left occipitolateral position

Stages of Labor

Summary of Stages of labor

Stages	Description	Duration in primi	Duration in multi
First stage	Start with the onset of labor pain and end with full dilation (10 cm) of cervix. It is also known as cervical stage of labor.	12 hours WHO-12 hours	6 hours WHO-10 hours
Second stage	Start with full dilation of cervix and ends with expulsion of fetus. It is divided into two stages---- propulsive stage and expulsive stage. **Propulsive stage:** Full dilation of cervix to the descent of presenting part into the pelvic floor **Expulsive stage:** This stage is with maternal bearing down efforts and ends with the expulsion of fetus from the birth canal.	2 hours WHO-3 hours	30 minutes WHO-2 hours
Third stage	Starts with the expulsion of fetus and ends with the expulsion of placenta from the birth canal.	15 minutes in primi and multi. Duration can be reduced to 5 minutes with active management.	
Fourth stage	It is the observation and monitoring of mother and new-born after the expulsion of placenta for 1 hour	1 hour	

First Stage of Labor (From Onset of True Labor to Full Dilation of Cervix)

- **Latent Phase**
  - Cervix dilates up to 5 cm
  - Mild and short contractions
- **Active Phase**
  - It is the period from 6 cm cervical dilation to 10 cm cervical dilation
  - Moderate to strong contractions (5 minutes apart)
  - Bloody show
  - Membranes may rupture
  - Supportive measures (encouragement, back rubs, rest between contractions)
  - Medications may be necessary for discomfort
- **Transition Phase**
  - This phase marks the transition from the active phase to the pushing stage
  - It typically occurs when the cervix is around 8 cm dilated and continues until the cervix is fully dilated to 10 cm.
  - Strong contractions (1–2 minutes apart).

Clinical Corner

CASE SCENARIO 5:

Labor room nurse noted the findings in one of her primigravida client as follows, cervix dilation 5 cm and fetal station is -1 and 40% effaced. Based upon the findings nurse should understand that her client is in ------------ phase of labor.

a. Latent phase
b. Active phase
c. Transitional phase
d. Expulsive phase

Ans. (b) Active phase

In latent phase, cervical dilation is 0–3 cm, in active phase cervical dilation is 4–7 cm, in transitional phase cervical dilation is 8–10 cm and expulsive phase begins immediately after the birth and ends with separation and expulsion of the placenta.

- Increased bloody show.
- Irritable, restless, agitated, emotional.
- Leg tremors, perspiration, flushed face, sudden nausea and vomiting.

Physiology of First Stage of Labor

- **Fundal dominance:** Contractions begin at the fundus of uterus and then propagate downward toward the cervix.
- **Polarity:** It is the coordination between upper and lower uterine poles throughout the labor.
- **Retraction:** It is the phenomenon in uterine muscles in which muscle fibers are permanently shortened.
- **Formation of upper and lower uterine segment**: Before the onset of labor there is no anatomical and functional division of uterus. As labor progresses, there is an active upper segment (walls are progressively thickened) and relatively passive lower segment (walls are progressively thinning) will emerge.
- **Development of retraction ring (Bandl's ring):** Ring of tissue that forms at the junction between the upper and lower segments of the uterus during labor. This ring is formed because of the differential contraction of the upper and lower segments of the uterus, which causes the lower segment to be pulled up toward the upper segment.

In some cases, the retraction ring may become too tight or fail to relax between contractions, which can lead to a condition called **Bandl's ring constriction**. This can be a serious complication of labor and delivery, as it can lead to fetal distress and may require prompt intervention, such as delivery by cesarean section.

- **Cervical changes:** Cervical ripening, effacement and dilatation occur in this stage. In primi, effacement precedes dilation while in multi both happens simultaneously.

Partograph/Partogram

- The partograph is a graphical tool used in obstetrics to monitor the progress of labor and to identify potential complications.
- Older partograph is known as modified WHO partograph. It was based upon older WHO recommendation.
- New partograph is also known as **labor care guide** or **next generation partograph**. This is based upon modified WHO criteria.

Criteria	Modified partograph	Labor care guide
Latent phase	Up to 3 cm	Up to 5 cm
Active phase	4–10 cm dilation of cervix	6–10 cm dilation of cervix
Plotting on partograph	Begins at 4 cm	Begins at 5 cm
Duration between alert line and action line	4 hours	No alert and action line
Second stage of labor	Not represented	Represented (enhanced monitoring in second stage).
Supportive care	Not represented	Represented such as • Position during delivery • Oral intake • Pain relief • Attendant
Uterine contraction	Represented in terms of duration, frequency, and strength	Represented in terms of duration and frequency only.

Structure of WHO Labor Care Guide

The Labor Care Guide, has 7 sections.

- **Section 1:** Identifying information and labor characteristics at admission
- **Section 2: Supportive care** includes providing various forms of support to women during labor. This ensure respectful maternity care which is considered a fundamental right of a pregnant women.
- **Section 3:** Care of the baby- record of FHR, amniotic fluid, fetal position, caput, etc.
- **Section 4:** Care of the woman – vital parameters of mother
- **Section 5: Labor progress** – records monitoring of labor progression parameters
- **Section 6: Medication** – records the medications including oxytocin and IV fluids administered to the pregnant women.
- **Section 7: Shared decision making** – documents assessment and agreed-upon plans.

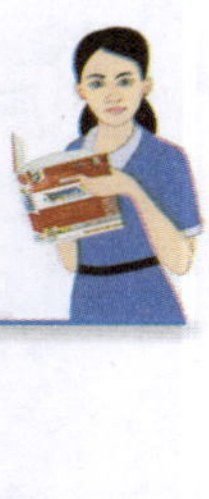

KEY POINT

Change the position of the mother if fetal bradycardia or tachycardia occurs and also assess the mother's vital signs.

Recent Questions (NORCET 2020)

24. How to measure the uterine contraction of the pregnant lady who is on labor pain?

a. Asking question to the lady
b. By using pantograph
c. Assess by placing the hand on abdomen
d. Assess by performing Leopold's maneuver

Ans. (c) Assess by placing the hand on abdomen

25. A female in labor room with cord prolapse should be given which of the following position?

a. Semi-Fowler's position
b. Prone position pantograph
c. Lithotomy position
d. Knee chest position

Ans. (d) Knee chest position

KEY POINTS

- **Steep Trendelenburg** position is advised to relieve cord compression during labor
- Ring of tissue that forms at the junction between the upper and lower segments of the uterus during labor is known as Bandl's ring.

Modified Partograph

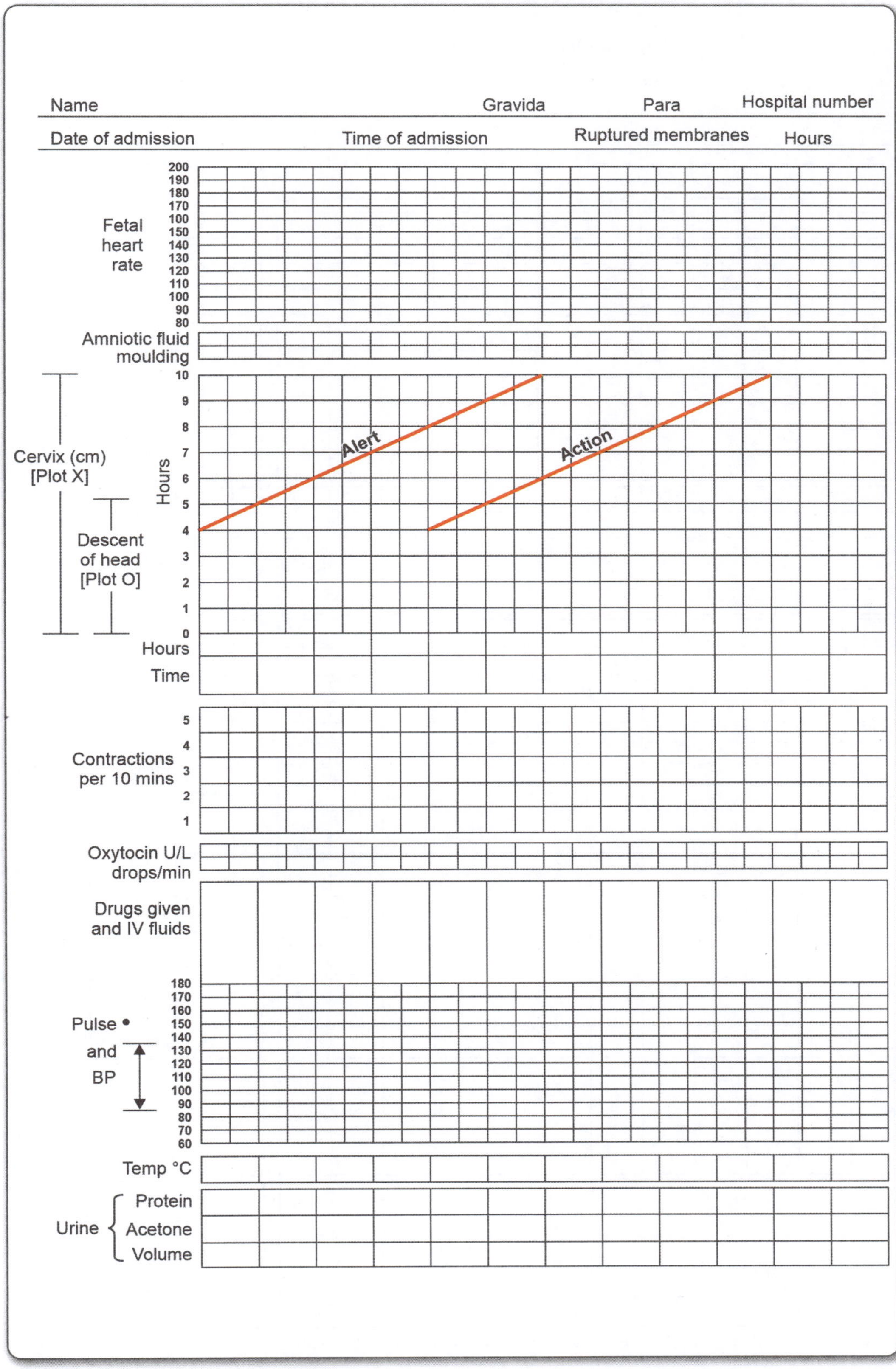

Recent Question
(NORCET 2022)

26. A patient is transferred to labor room and the nurse identifies that the patient is in first stage of labor. When will the nurse document the progress of labor with respect to the cervical dilation on a WHO labor care guide?

a. 4 cm
b. 5 cm
c. 7 cm
d. 10 cm

Ans. (b) 5 cm

WHO Labor care guide is applicable for the active phase of first stage of labor i.e., from cervical dilatation >=5cm to full dilatation of cervix.

In modified WHO Partograph, charting starts from 4 cm of cervical dilation.

Modified Partograph

WHO LABOUR CARE GUIDE

Name Parity Labour onset Active labour diagnosis [Date]

Ruptured membranes [Date Time] Risk factors

Section	Parameter		ALERT	Active first stage (hours 1–12)	Second stage (hours 1–3)
	Time			: : : : : : : : : : : :	: : :
	Hours			1 2 3 4 5 6 7 8 9 10 11 12	1 2 3
			ALERT	← ACTIVE FIRST STAGE →	← SECOND STAGE →
SUPPORTIVE CARE	Companion		N		
SUPPORTIVE CARE	Pain relief		N		
SUPPORTIVE CARE	Oral fluid		N		
SUPPORTIVE CARE	Posture		SP		
BABY	Baseline FHR		< 110, ≥ 160		
BABY	FHR deceleration		L		
BABY	Amniotic fluid		M+++, B		
BABY	Fetal position		P,T		
BABY	Caput		+++		
BABY	Moulding		+++		
WOMAN	Pulse		< 60, ≥ 120		
WOMAN	Systolic BP		< 80, ≥ 140		
WOMAN	Diastolic BP		≥ 90		
WOMAN	Temperature °C		< 35.0, ≥ 37.5		
WOMAN	Urine		P++, A++		
LABOUR PROGRESS	Contraction per 10 min		≤ 2, > 5		
LABOUR PROGRESS	Duration of contractions		< 20, > 60		
LABOUR PROGRESS	Cervix [Plot X]	10			
LABOUR PROGRESS		9	≥ 2h		In active first stage, plot 'X' to record cervical dilatation. Alert triggered when leg time for current cervical dilatation is exceeded with no progress. In second stage, insert 'P' to indicate when pushing begins.
LABOUR PROGRESS		8	≥ 2.5h		
LABOUR PROGRESS		7	≥ 3h		
LABOUR PROGRESS		6	≥ 5h		
LABOUR PROGRESS		5	≥ 6h		
LABOUR PROGRESS	Descent [Plot O]	5			
LABOUR PROGRESS		4			
LABOUR PROGRESS		3			
LABOUR PROGRESS		2			
LABOUR PROGRESS		1			
LABOUR PROGRESS		0			
MEDICATION	Oxytocin (U/L, drops/min)				
MEDICATION	Medicine				
MEDICATION	IV fluids				
SHARED DECISION-MAKING	ASSESSMENT				
SHARED DECISION-MAKING	PLAN				
	INITIALS				

INSTRUCTIONS: CIRCLE ANY OBSERVATION MEETING THE CRITERIA IN THE 'ALERT' COLUMN, ALERT THE SENIOR MIDWIFE OR DOCTOR AND RECORD THE ASSESSMENT AND ACTION TAKEN, IF, LABOUR EXTENDS BEYOND 12 h, PLEASE CONTINUE ON A NEW LABOUR CARE GUIDE.

Abbreviations: **Y** – Yes, **N** – No, **D** – Declined, **U** – Unknown, **SP** – Supine, **MO** – Mobile, **E** – Early, **L** – Late, **V** – Variable, **I** – Intact, **C** – Clear, **M** – Meconium, **B** – Blood, **A** – Anterior, **P** – Posterior, **T** – Transverse, **P+** – Protein, **A+** – Acetone

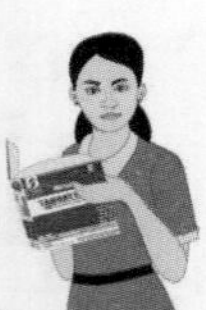

Second Stage of Labor (From Full Dilation of Cervix to Birth of Newborn)

- **Latent Phase**
  - May last up to 1 hour
  - Decrease in frequency and increase in strength of contraction
- **Active Phase**
  - Urge to push
  - Stronger and closer contractions
- **Transition phase**
  - Begins with fetal head on perineum; perineum bulges
  - Leg cramps are common

Episiotomy

It is a planned surgical incision made in the perineum during second stage of labor to enlarge the vaginal opening and to facilitate the delivery.

Purposes

- To enlarge the vaginal opening
- To prevent perineal tear
- To shorten the second stage of labor

Timing for episiotomy: Thinning of the perineum along with uterine contraction and maternal bearing down effect and just before the crowning.

According to WHO it is not a routine practice, it is selective.

Indications for episiotomy: Indications are as follows:

- Shoulder dystocia
- Instrumental delivery
- Macrosomia
- Rigid perineum

When to perform episiotomy: Bulging of the perineum during contraction just before crowning.

Suture: Polyglycolic acid suture (Dexon) or chromic catgut

Types of Episiotomies

Type	Description
Mediolateral	Surgical cut made at an angle, usually about 60°, to the midline of the body, toward the right or left side of the perineum, from the midpoint of the fourchette. This type of episiotomy is typically about 2.5 cm long. It is **the most preferred episiotomy** and it **never involves anal sphincter** no matter how much it is extended.
Median/midline	A surgical cut made in the midline of the perineum, the area between the vaginal opening and the anus. A straight incision made from the posterior vaginal fourchette directly toward the anus.
Lateral	A surgical cut made at an angle to the midline of the perineum about 1 cm away from fourchette, but the direction of the incision is toward either the right or left side of the perineum. Drawback of this is **damage to the Bartholin's gland.**
J-shaped	Starts at the center of the posterior fourchette, extends posteriorly for 1.5 cm, and then curves downward and outward toward either the 5 or 7 o'clock position of the perineum to avoid injury to the anal sphincter.
Radical lateral (Schuchardt) incision)	It is a surgical incision made on one side of the perineum, extending from the vaginal opening to the ischial tuberosity (a bony protrusion on the pelvis), and used to enlarge the vaginal outlet during difficult childbirth. This incision is **less commonly used today,** as other techniques such as forceps, vacuum extraction, or cesarean section are preferred to manage difficult deliveries.

KEY POINTS

Nursing Care during second stage of labor

- Permit mother to choose pushing and position technique (If unmedicated)
- Assist mother in pushing
- Position both legs simultaneously to avoid trauma to uterine ligaments
- Monitor FHR every 5 minutes
- Administer Inj. Methergin after delivery of anterior shoulder contraindicated in cardiac and hypertensive mothers.

KEY POINTS

Nursing care of newborn

- Clear airway mucous
- APGAR scoring: 1 and 5 minutes after birth
- Temperature maintenance; dry infant; skin-to-skin positioning
- Administer antibiotic ophthalmic medication into each eye
- Vitamin K injection to prevent hemorrhagic disorder
- Apply identification bracelets to mother and infant
- Assist with expulsion of placenta

Recent Question (NORCET 2021)

27. Which muscle doesn't play any role in episiotomy?

a. Ischiocavernosus
b. Superior Transverse perineal muscles
c. Deep transverse perineal muscles
d. Bulbospongiosus

Ans. (a) Ischiocavernosus

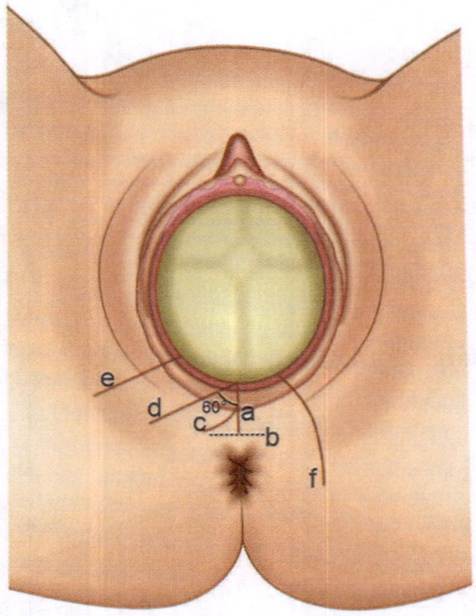

Figure 37: Episiotomies

KEY POINTS

- Mediolateral episiotomy It is **the most preferred episiotomy** and it **never involves anal sphincter** no matter how much it is extended.
- Lateral episiotomy has the **risk of damaging Bartholin's gland.**

Third Stage of Labor (From Birth of Newborn to Delivery of Placenta)

Before the placental separation	After the placental separation
Uterus become discoid, firm and non-ballotable	Uterus becomes globular. Firm and ballotable
Fundal height is slightly below the umbilicus	Fundal height is between symphysis pubis and umbilicus.
Per vagina: Slight trickling of blood and length of umbilical cord is as visible as and remain static	Per vagina: Sudden gush of blood and permanent lengthening of umbilical cord.

POINTS TO REMEMBER

- Constant watch of the mother is recommended during this time.
- In some institution they are following no touch or hands off policy to aid in the separation and delivery of placenta.
- After the delivery of the baby, mother is expected to deliver the placenta within 20 minutes with the aid of gravity.

Management of Third Stage of Labor

Expectant Management (Physiological)

It is allowing the placenta to deliver naturally without intervention.

Issues

- Longer third stage of labor
- Higher risk of postpartum hemorrhage
- Higher likelihood of the need for blood transfusion.

Active Management

This is the most preferred method in which use of interventions to actively assist in the delivery of the placenta, such as:

- Administration of a uterotonic drug (oxytocin)
- Controlled cord traction
- Uterine massage

Purposes

- Shorter third stage of labor
- Reduced risk of blood loss and postpartum hemorrhage
- Reduced risk for maternal anemia
- Reduced need for blood transfusion

Main aim of active management is to excite powerful uterine contraction within 1 min of delivery of baby (WHO).

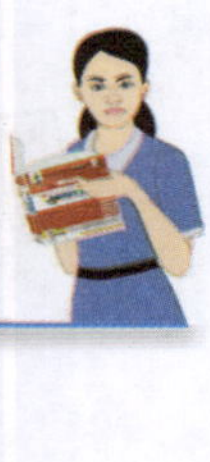

Procedure/steps

- Administer Inj. Oxytocin 10 units I/M (preferred)

  or

  T. Misoprostol 600 mcg PO/PR

  or

  Inj. Methergine 0.2 mg IM to the mother within 1 minute of birth of baby.
- The placenta is expected to deliver soon.
- If not delivered, then use **controlled cord traction** (Brandt-Andrews) during the first uterine contraction.

Assisted Delivery of Placenta

It may be used as part of active management of the third stage of labor or as a standalone intervention if there are concerns about the placenta not delivering on its own.

It includes:

- Controlled cord traction (modified Brandt-Andrews method)
- Fundal pressure

Controlled cord traction (modified Brandt-Andrews method)

After the baby is born, the healthcare provider will apply gentle traction to the umbilical cord while simultaneously applying pressure at the junction of upper and lower uterine segment using palmar

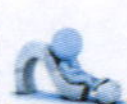

Recent Question (NORCET 2023)

28. After normal vaginal delivery the women is shifted to post-operative ward. What is the first priority?

a. Observe bleeding and color of lochia
b. Start IV fluid
c. Check vital signs
d. Assess mobility

Ans. (c) Check vital signs

The first priority after a normal vaginal delivery is to check vital signs. This includes checking the woman's blood pressure, heart rate, respiratory rate, and temperature. Once the woman's vital signs are stable, the next priority is to observe bleeding and color of lochia.

surface of the fingers of the left hand. The traction applied is controlled, meaning that it is gentle and not forceful.

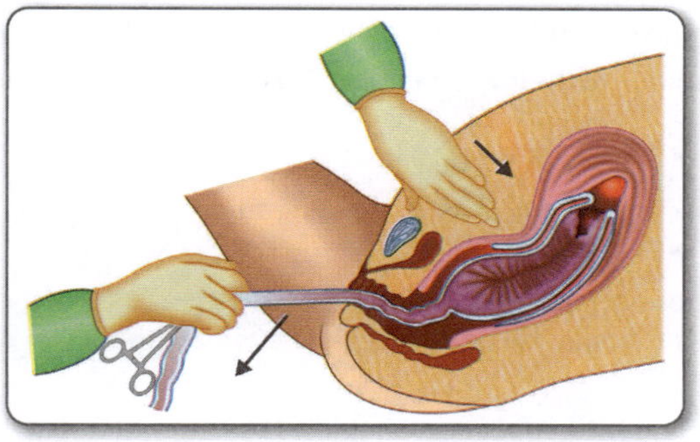

Figure 38: Controlled cord traction

Fundal Pressure

Gentle pressure on the fundus of the uterus can be applied during the second stage of labor by placing four fingers behind the fundus and the thumb in front, using the uterus as a piston, but pressure should only be given when the uterus becomes hard, and this technique should only be used by experienced healthcare providers in specific situations.

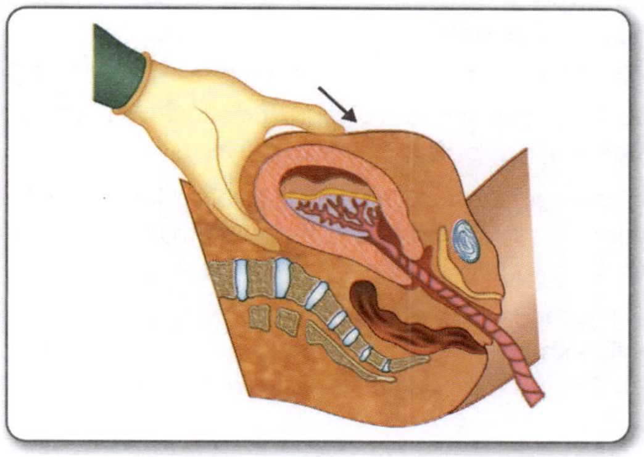

Figure 39: Fundal pressure

Placental Separation

Central separation (Schultze)	Marginal separation (Matthews-Duncan)
During placental separation, the placenta detaches from its attachment to the uterine wall, typically starting in the center and resulting in the accumulation of blood behind the placenta. The detachment is facilitated by uterine contractions, the weight of the placenta, and the accumulated blood, which can lead to the complete detachment of the placenta. 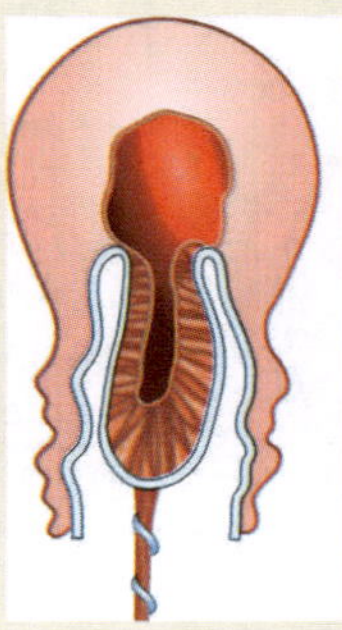	In marginal placental separation, the separation of the placenta from the uterine wall begins at the edges, where it is less supported, and gradually progresses toward the center with increasing uterine contractions. 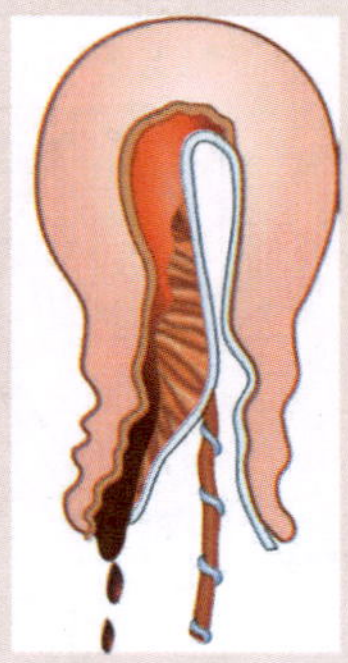

Fourth Stage of Labor

Observe mother and baby for 1 hour following delivery. If the vitals are in normal range, then they can be shifted to ward.

Pain Management during Labor

Sedatives and analgesics: There are several types of sedatives and analgesics that can be used during labor to manage pain, e.g: Pethidine, fentanyl, morphine, meperidine.

Inhalational agents:

- **Entonox:** It is a commonly used inhalational analgesia for pain management during labor. It is a 50:50 mixture of nitrous oxide and oxygen that is delivered through a mask.
- **Isoflurane, desflurane, and sevoflurane:** These are inhalational gases that can be used with or without nitrous oxide for pain management during labor. Sevoflurane is the preferred choice for most women.

Regional Anesthesia

It involves injecting medication to numb specific nerves or nerve groups in the body, thereby blocking pain signals to the brain.

KEY POINTS

Nursing Care

- Palpate fundus every 15 minutes for firmness and height, if relaxed, massage until it becomes firm
- Fundus should be 2 cm below umbilicus immediately after birth.
- It is raised at the level of umbilicus 1 hour after birth.
- Encourage voiding. Check for bladder distention.
- Check perineum for vaginal or suture line bleeding.
- Check for hematoma at episiotomy and laceration site.
- Administer oxytocic medications as ordered.
- Provide food and fluid as tolerated.
- Within first hour of birth, encourage and teach breastfeeding.
- To initiate labor, hormone needed is fetal CRH.
- Adequate uterine contraction is when there is 3 contractions in 10 minutes and each contraction lasts for 45 seconds.
- Tachysystole is excessive uterine contraction. It means there will be 5 or more contractions in 10 minutes.
- Fetal distress associated with tachysystole is called hyper stimulation.

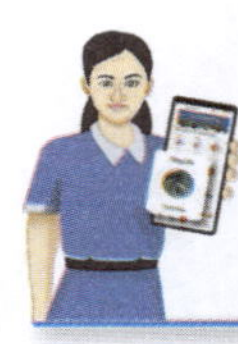

Epidural anesthesia	A catheter is inserted into the epidural space in the lower back, and medication is administered continuously to provide pain relief during labor. 0.5% bupivacaine is injected into the epidural space. It provides complete anesthesia from T10 to S5.
Paracervical block	It involves injecting medication into the cervix to block the pain signals transmitted to the brain during labor.
Pudendal block	Injecting medication into the pudendal nerve, which provides sensation to the lower part of the vagina and perineum. It is given prior to episiotomy suturing and forceps delivery. Site for pudendal nerve block **is ischial spine** and ligament pierced is sacrospinous ligament.
Spinal anesthesia	Medication is injected into the cerebrospinal fluid in the lower back to provide pain relief during labor. **Bupivacaine** 5–10 mg or **lignocaine** 25–50 mg is used.
Combined Spinal Epidural (CSE)	It is a pain management technique that involves injecting a low dose of local anesthetic and opioid (e.g., bupivacaine 2.5 mg + fentanyl 15 – 25 mcg) into the subarachnoid space, followed by an epidural top-up, to provide continuous pain relief during labor or surgery.
Perineal infiltration	It involves injecting a local anesthetic directly into the tissues around the perineum 2–5 minutes before episiotomy. 10 mL 1% lignocaine is the drug of choice. **Note**: Each time prior to the infiltration aspirate and confirm there is no blood.

ASSISTED DELIVERIES/OPERATIVE VAGINAL DELIVERIES

It refers to any delivery process which is assisted by vaginal operation. Delivery by forceps and Ventouse are generally included.

Indications

- Inadequate maternal efforts
- Maternal exhaustion
- Non-reassuring FHR
- After coming head in breech delivery
- Non-progressive labor
- Cervix fully dilated
- Rupture of membranes
- Fetal head engaged (vertex presentation)
- Knowledge of the fetal position
- Fetal weight has been estimated
- Maternal pelvis adequate for vaginal delivery
- Anesthesia administered
- The maternal bladder is empty
- Maternal consent obtained, risks and benefits thoroughly explained
- A back-up plan if the operative delivery method fails.
- Maternal cardiac or neurologic disease when maternal pushing is not feasible.

Absolute Contraindications

For mother	For fetus
• Cervix not fully dilated • Membranes intact • Fetal head not engaged • Unknown fetal position • Cephalopelvic disproportion	• Bleeding disorders (hemophilia, thrombocytopenia, von Willebrand disease) • Bone de-mineralization (osteogenesis imperfecta)

FORCEPS DELIVERIES

Obstetric forceps: It is a pair of instruments, especially designed to assist extraction of the head and thereby accomplishing delivery of the fetus. Traction force needed in primigravida is 20 kg and that of multigravida is 13 kg. Pulling force is directed to the base of the skull.

Types of Forceps

- Long curve forceps with or without axis traction device
- Short curve forceps (Wrigley)
- Kielland's forceps

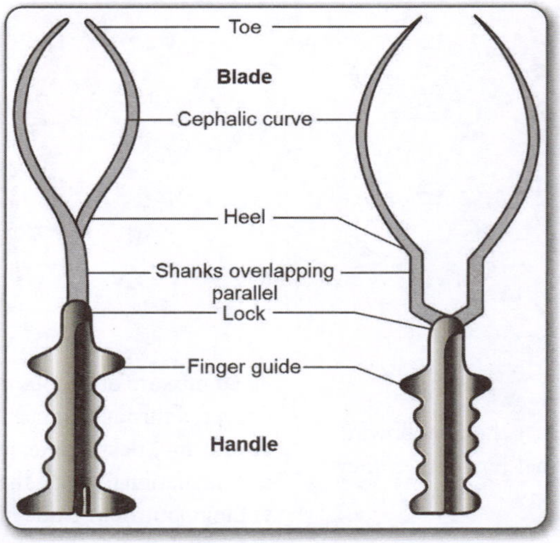

Figure 40: Parts of a forceps

High forceps operation: Application of the forceps on the fetal head where the biparietal diameter has not yet passed the plane of the pelvic inlet (not engaged head).

Mid-forceps operation: Application of the forceps is where the biparietal diameter has passed the plane of the inlet but has not passed the level of ischial spines.

POINTS TO REMEMBER

- For painless labor, epidural anesthesia is the choice.
- The epidural may be placed at the lower thoracic or upper lumbar levels (T10-L1), which can provide analgesia to the lower abdomen and pelvis.
- Preferred anesthesia for c-section is spinal and is at the level of T4 segment.
- For instrumental deliveries pudendal block is the preferred one.

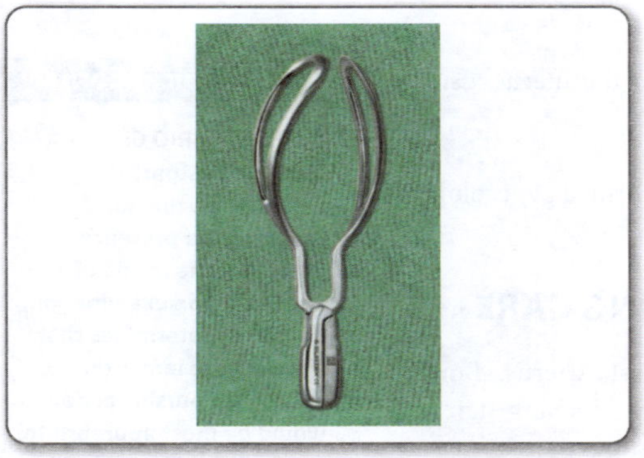

Figure 41: Wrigley forceps

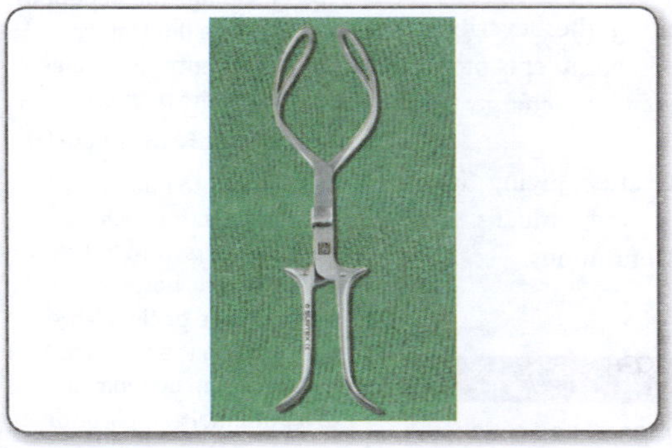

Figure 42: Kielland's forceps

- **Low forceps operation:** Application of the forceps where the biparietal diameter has passed the level of ischial spine.
- **Outlet forceps:** Forceps are applied on the fetal head lying on the perineum and is visible at the introitus in-between contraction. Wrigley's forceps are exclusively for outlet operation.

Table 9: Complications of forceps operation

Maternal	Fetal
Vaginal laceration Cervical tear PPH due to trauma Atonic uterus Low backache Genital prolapse or stress incontinence	Asphyxia due to intracranial stress Intracranial hemorrhage Cephalohematoma Facial palsy Cerebral or spastic palsy

Ventouse

It is a device designed to assist delivery by creating a vacuum between it and the fetal scalp. The pulling force is dragging the cranium.

The scalp, sucked into the cup during ventouse application, forms an elongated portion in the scalp and is known as chignon. It will disappear within few hours.

Practice Questions

6. All of the following are Indications for operative vaginal delivery, except:

a. Maternal exhaustion
b. Maternal heart disease
c. Prolonged first stage of labor
d. Pulmonary compromise

Ans. (c) Prolonged first stage of labor

7. All of the following are maternal complications associated with forceps-assisted delivery, except:

a. Vaginal laceration
b. Atonic uterus
c. Cerebral palsy
d. Genital prolapse

Ans. (c) Cerebral palsy

Explanation:
Cerebral palsy is fetal complication associated with forceps-assisted delivery. All other given options are maternal complications.

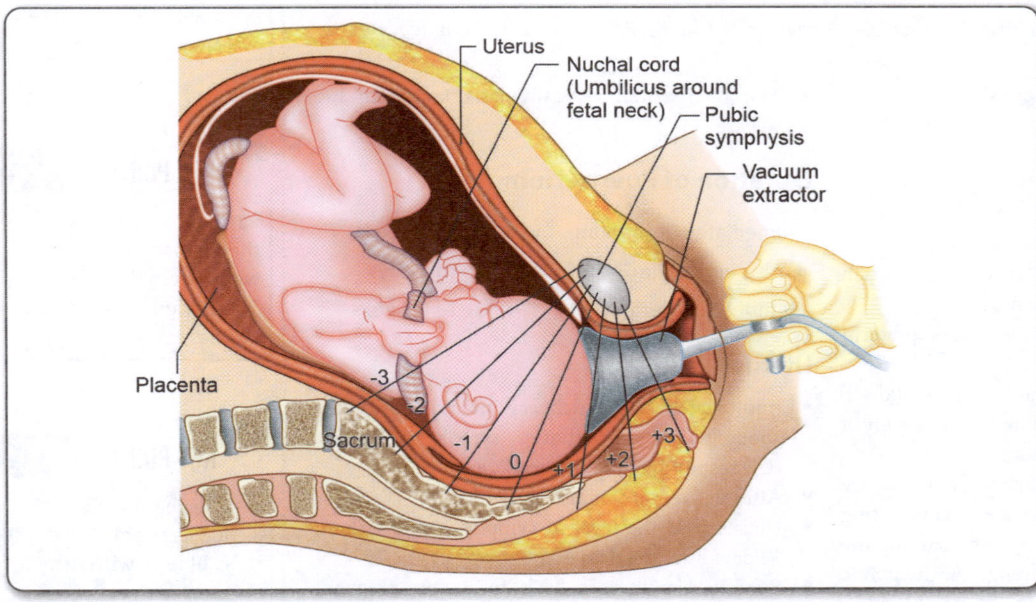

Figure 43: Vacuum extractor (Ventouse) assisted delivery

Practice Question

8. All of the following are the indications for forceps-assisted delivery, except

a. Delay in the second stage of labor
b. Cord prolapsed
c. Maternal distress
d. Cephalopelvic disproportion

Ans. (d) Cephalopelvic disproportion

Complications

- **Fetal:** Sloughing of the scalp, Cephalohematoma, sub–aponeurotic hemorrhage, intracranial hemorrhage (rare).
- **Maternal:** The injury may be due to inclusion of the soft tissue such as the cervix or vaginal wall inside the cup.

Cesarean Delivery

- Cesarean section is a surgical procedure in which one or more incisions are made through a mother's abdomen and uterus to deliver one or more babies.
- Incision can be Vertical Incision or horizontal incision.

- **Vertical incisions:** They are very rare, quickest to make, greater chance of dehiscence.
- **Horizontal incision:** It is placed at the top of pubic hair or just over the hairline. Less chance of dehiscence.

Indications

- Prolonged labor
- Dystocia or failure to progress in labor
- Breech presentation
- Those performed out of concern for fetal well-being
- Failed labor induction
- Failed instrumental delivery (by forceps or ventouse)
- Uterine rupture
- Multiple births
- Previous transverse cesarean section
- Central placenta previa
- Vaginal obstruction

Hysterectomy

- It is the surgical removal of the uterus, usually performed by a gynecologist.
- It can be total or partial.
- It is the most commonly performed gynecological surgical procedure.

POSTPARTUM NURSING CARE

- **Postnatal assessment:** Breast, Uterus, Bowels, Bladder, Lochia, Episiotomy, Homan's sign and Emotional (BUBBLEHE) status.
- **Homans' sign:** To assess for Deep Venous Thrombosis (DVT).
- **REEDA** is a scale for grading the severity of perineal trauma associated with episiotomy. Redness, Edema, Ecchymosis, Discharge and Approximation (REEDA).
- **Lochia:** Vaginal discharge after giving birth (puerperium) containing blood, mucus and uterine tissue. It is typically continuous.

Table 10: Types of lochia and characteristics

Types of Lochia	Color	Postpartum day	Composition
Lochia rubra	Dark red	Lasts 1–4 days	Blood, decidual fragments, and mucus
Lochia serosa	Brownish pink	Lasts 5–9 days	Old blood, serum, invading leucocytes and tissue debris
Lochia alba	White or yellow	Lasts 10–15 days	Mucus, Epithelial cells, old leucocytes

- **Amount (pad in use for <2 hours)**
  - **1 g (pad):** 1 mL of discharge.
  - **Scant:** Less than 1 inch.
  - **Light:** 1–4 inches.
  - **Moderate:** 4–6 inches.
  - **Heavy:** More than 6 inches.
- Amount of lochia is more following cesarian delivery, twin delivery, hydramnios
- Amount of lochia is scanty in case of preterm delivery.
- **Observe vital signs:** Temperature above 100.4°F for 2 consecutive days considered to be a sign of beginning of puerperal infection.
- **Encourage Kegel exercises:** Pelvic floor exercise or **Kegel** exercise consists of repeatedly contracting and relaxing the muscles that form part of the pelvic floor. Kegel exercises strengthen the **pelvic floor** muscles, which support the **uterus**, **bladder**, **small intestine** and **rectum**.
- If Rh- mother, assesses need for administration of RhoGAM.

PUERPERIUM

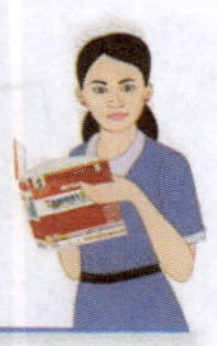

- It is the period after childbirth during which the mother's body undergoes various physiological and psychological changes to return to its pre-pregnancy state.
- The puerperium typically lasts for around 6 weeks.

Duration of Puerperium

Immediate puerperium	First 24 hours
Early puerperium	Up to 7 days
Remote puerperium	Up to 6 weeks

Uterus

- Immediately after delivery uterus positioned about 13 cm above symphysis pubis. (Corresponding to 22-week POG).
- After delivery it weighs about 1 kg
- Uterus is at the level of symphysis pubis about 12 days after the delivery.
- By 6 weeks it goes back to its pre-pregnant position.

Subinvolution

- The uterus does not return to its non-pregnant state as quickly as it should.
- Main two reason for this includes **retained placenta** and **infection.**
- Prolonged or heavy vaginal bleeding, abdominal pain or discomfort, and fever are the major clinical manifestations of subinvolution.

Clinical Corner

CASE SCENARIO 6:

During a postpartum assessment, the nurse observes the presence of clots in the lochia of a patient. Upon examination, the nurse determines that the clots are larger than 1 cm. Which nursing action would be most appropriate?

a. Reassess the patient after 2 hours
b. Encourage the patient to increase fluid intake
c. Document the findings
d. Notify the physician

Ans. (d) Notify the physician

It is normal to find a few small clots in the lochia during the first 1 to 2 days after delivery, however, the presence of clots larger than 1 cm in the lochia after childbirth can be indicative of a potential complication, such as uterine atony or retained placental fragments. This needs to be informed to the physician for further evaluation and intervention.

KEY POINT

Vaginal discharge for the first fortnight (two weeks from delivery) Puerperium is called **Lochia.**

KEY POINTS

- The characteristic of lochia rubra (1–4 days) is **bloody with fishy odor**.
- Adolescents and women age of 40 years and older are at increased risk for molar pregnancies.
- Molar pregnancies are caused by **an imbalance in genetic material (chromosomes)** in the pregnancy.

Afterpains

- It is the spasmodic colicky pain over the abdomen in the immediate post-partum period due to the vigorous contraction of uterus.
- It increases during breastfeeding due to the increased production of oxytocin which in turn further increases the uterine contraction.

Puerperal Pyrexia

Body temperature of more than 38°C or 100.4°F on 2 occasions at 24 hours apart.

It usually manifests within 10 days following delivery.

Most Common about Puerperal Pyrexia

Most common	Site	Endometrium
	Cause	Group A streptococci
	Mode of transmission	Direct spread from cervix to vagina
	Mode of delivery associated with it	Caesarean delivery.

INDUCTION OF LABOR

- Induction of labor is the process of starting labor artificially before it begins spontaneously.
- Status of cervix need to be checked before induction of labor. It can be done through **Bishop Score**.

Bishop Score

Bishop score component	Score value
Cervical dilation (cm)	0 = closed 1 = 1–2 cm 2 = 3–4 cm 3 = 5–6 cm 4 = ≥7 cm
Cervical effacement (%)	0 = 0–30% 1 = 40–50% 2 = 60–70% 3 = ≥80%
Cervical consistency	0 = firm 1 = medium 2 = soft
Cervical position	0 = posterior 1 = mid-position 2 = anterior
Fetal station	0 = -3 or higher 1 = -2 2 = -1 3 = 0 4 = +1 or higher

- The total Bishop score ranges from 0 to 13, with a higher score indicating that the cervix is more favorable for induction of labor.
- A score of 9 or higher is generally considered favorable for induction.
- In modified bishop score, effacement of cervix is replaced by cervical length.
- To measure the length of cervix, USG need to be done. So, Bishop score is done clinically.

Types of Induction of Labor

- Medical
- Mechanical
- Surgical
- Combined

Clinical Corner

CASE SCENARIO 7:

Nurse was palpating the uterus in a primipara mother following vaginal delivery in the immediate post-partum period. One of the nursing students asked the nurse why she is using both hands to palpate. Which among the following responses is correct from the nurse?

a. To prevent PPH
b. To prevent uterine involution
c. To prevent uterine inversion
d. To prevent uterine atony

Ans. (c) To prevent uterine inversion

Using both hands during the post-partum period to palpate the uterus will help to prevent uterine inversion.

Clinical Corner

CASE SCENARIO 8:

After being admitted to the hospital with a diagnosis of inevitable abortion, a client at 16 weeks gestation starts feeling a bearing down sensation and suddenly expels the products of conception while in bed. What is the first action the nurse should take?

a. Inform the physician
b. Assess the firmness of the client's fundus
c. Transfer the client to the OT
d. Administer the sedative as prescribed

Ans. (b) Assess the firmness of the client's fundus

In the given scenario, the nurse's initial priority is to assess the firmness of the client's fundus. Assessing the fundus helps determine if there is uterine atony (lack of uterine muscle tone) or retained products of conception, which can lead to postpartum hemorrhage or other complications. The assessment findings will guide further actions and interventions accordingly.

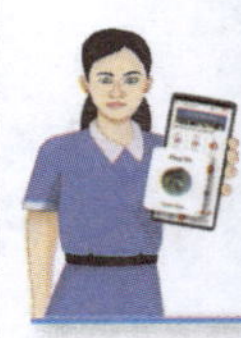

Medical Methods of Induction of Labor

Drug	Description	Points to remember
PGE 1 (misoprostol)	Currently used for induction. Route: Orally or transvaginally. Oral routes are less effective than vaginal route. **Dosage**: 25 mcg PV every 4 hourly. **Side effect** is tachysystole. So, it is contraindicated in women with previous LSCS.	• Ask the mother to empty the bladder before administering the drug. • Remain in lateral position for 30–60 minutes after giving the drug.
PGE2 (dinoprostone or cerviprime gel)	It increases the sensitivity of myometrium to oxytocin. It is considered gold standard for cervical ripening. **Dosage**: 0.5 mg cervically every 6 hourly for 4 doses	
Mifepristone (anti-progesterone)	RU 486 200 mg per vaginally.	
Oxytocin	It is used for both induction and augmentation of labor.	Check maternal vial sign and FHR Check for the signs of water intoxication such as confusion, drowsiness, headache. If fetal distress or uterine hyperstimulation occur, then stop oxytocin and give left lateral position to the client.

Mechanical Methods of Induction of Labor

Method	Description
Foley's induction	Foley's catheter inserted through the cervix and into the uterus, and then inflated with sterile water to put pressure on the cervix and stimulate its dilation.
Laminaria tents	It involves inserting a small, sterile seaweed or synthetic material into the cervix. As the tent absorbs moisture from the cervical tissues, it swells and gradually expands, which can help to dilate and soften the cervix over time.

Surgical Methods of Induction of Labor

Method	Description
Artificial rupture of membrane (ARM)	It involves the intentional breaking of the amniotic sac, which surrounds the fetus in the uterus. This helps to stimulate labor by stretching of cervix, release of PGs and reduction in amniotic fluid volume. **Contraindications** • Free floating head as it can lead to cord prolapse • Intra uterine death • HIV positive mother • Active genital herpes infection
Low rupture of membrane	Membrane below the presenting part covering the internal os are ruptured. Kocher's forceps or amnion hooks are used to rupture the membrane.
Stripping of the membranes (membrane sweeping)	It involves the healthcare provider inserting a gloved finger into the cervical opening and separating the amniotic sac from the uterus by sweeping the finger in a circular motion. This separation releases prostaglandins, which are hormones that can help ripen the cervix and stimulate contractions.

CONTRACEPTIVE METHOD (FERTILITY REGULATION METHOD)

- It is a preventive measure which helps the women to avoid unwanted pregnancies and plan the wanted pregnancy.
- Broadly, contraceptive methods are classified into two types, i.e., Spacing method and Terminal Method.

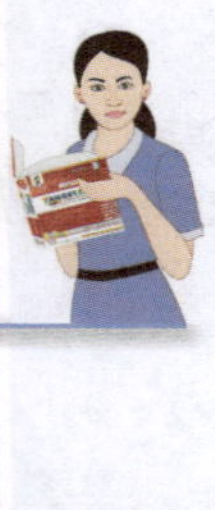

Spacing Method

Barrier Method

- Physical method (condom, diaphragm, female condom, vaginal sponge)
- Chemical method
- Combined method

Recent Question (NORCET 2022)

29. All among the following are the Emergency contraceptives, except:
a. Danazol
b. Levonorgestrel
c. Cu T
d. Mifepristonefor free

Ans. (a) Danazol

Intrauterine Devices

- IUD mainly works by changing the intra-uterine environment and make it spermicidal.
- Non-medicated IUDs cause a sterile inflammatory response to make it spermicidal.
- Copper containing IUDs release free copper that causes alteration in cervical mucous and endometrial secretions.

Hormonal Methods

- Combined methods (MALA-N, MALA-D), **Progestogen** only pills, post-coital contraception, once a month pill, male pill.
- Levonorgestrel tablets, 0.75 mg is a progestin-only emergency contraceptive pill used for prevention of pregnancy following unprotected intercourse.
- Miscellaneous (abstinence, coitus interrupts, safe period, natural family planning method).

Terminal Method

- Male sterilization (Vasectomy)
- Female sterilization (Tubectomy)

ABORTION

- **Abortion:** Loss of fetus before viability (20 weeks)
  - **Spontaneous:** It is the termination of pregnancy before the period of viability because of natural cause. The World Health Organization (WHO) defines spontaneous abortion as the loss of a fetus before the 22nd week of pregnancy or when the fetus weighs less than 500 grams and is not capable of independent survival.
  - **Induced:** Therapeutic or elective reasons for terminating the pregnancy.
  - **Inevitable abortion:** It is a state of abortion in which continuation of pregnancy is not possible.
  - **Complete:** When all the products of conception are expelled.
  - **Incomplete:** When entire products of conception are not expelled, some parts are left in uterine cavity.
  - **Threatened abortion:** Closed cervix, spotting and uterine cramping. Continuation of pregnancy is possible. **Nursing care:** Complete bed rest, check for vaginal bleeding and observe for uterine contractions.
  - **Missed abortion:** The pregnancy is lost and the products of conception is retained inside the uterine cavity for variable period of time. Fetus is dead and is inside the uterus.
  - **Septic abortion:** Abortion with clinical evidence of infection of uterus or its content. Following are the main manifestation of this condition 1. Elevated temperature of at least 100.4°F for 24 hours or more, foul smelling vaginal discharge, other evidences of pelvic infection such as lower abdominal pain and tenderness.
  - **Habitual abortion:** Consecutive abortions
  - **Recurrent abortion:** When a female has two or more episodes of abortion as documented either by sonography or histopathology before 24 weeks POG. (American Society for Reproductive Medicine 2013).

Recent Question (NORCET 2023)

30. The given below statement is true about DMPA (Antara) except?
a. It is injectable
b. It is irreversible
c. Can be used in 15 to 45 years of age group
d. Provided by government of India for free

Ans. (b) It is irreversible

Recent Question (NORCET 2021)

31. According to Govt. of India, the emergency contraceptive is:
a Levonorgestrel 1.5 mcg
b. Levonorgestrel 1.5 mg
c. Levonorgestrel 150 mg
d. Progestogen-only pill (POPs)

Ans. (a) Levonorgestrel 1.5 mcg

Table 11: Types of abortion

Type	Incomplete	Complete	Missed	Threatened	Inevitable
Pain and BPV	Present	Present	Present	Present	Present
External OS	Open	Closed	Closed	Closed	Open
Uterine size	Size is smaller than the period of amenorrhea.	Size is smaller than the period of amenorrhea. (empty uterus)	Size is smaller than the period of amenorrhea.	Corresponds to period of amenorrhoea.	Size is less than 12 weeks.
Cardiac activity	Absent	Absent	Absent	Present	
Other points	Products of conception in cervical canal felt on PV examination. Bleeding profusely	No retained products of conception. Trans vaginal scan reveals uterine cavity is empty.	Fetus dead and is inside uterus	Pain appears usually following haemorrhage. Internal os closed.	The abortion can't be prevented. Dilated internal os through which product of conception can be felt.
Management	Check curettage for retained POCs	Conservative management.	Induce the abortion.	Conservative management + bed rest	Evacuation

BPV= Bleeding Per Vagina;

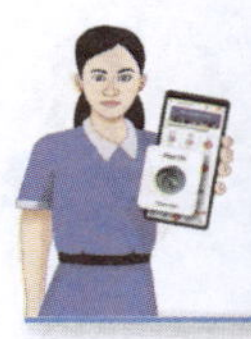

Nursing Care

- Check the vital signs of mother to detect internal bleeding and infection at the earliest
- Psychological care: Sympathizing, understanding and caring
- Assess severity of pain and need for analgesics
- Strict intake-output monitoring and encourage fluid intake
- Maintain strict aseptic technique to prevent cross infection
- Healthy diet to promote recovery
- **Emotional support:** Encourage family support due to pregnancy loss
- Allow grieving and expression of her concern over the loss of pregnancy.

MEDICAL TERMINATION OF PREGNANCY

Medical Termination of Pregnancy

- Medical Termination of Pregnancy (MTP) Act, 1971 provides the legal framework for making Comprehensive Abortion Care (CAC).
- Legal abortion is the deliberate induction of abortion prior to 20 weeks gestation by registered medical practitioner in the interest of mother's health and life.

Provision of MTP under MTP Act, 1971

- Continuation of pregnancy would involve serious risk of life or grave injury to physical and mental health of pregnant women.
- There is substantial risk of the child being born with serious physical and mental abnormalities to be handicapped in life.
- Pregnancy because of rape.
- Pregnancy because of failure of contraceptive methods.
- Where there are actual or reasonably foreseeable environments which could lead to risk of injury to the health of mother.
- Abortion requires the opinion of one doctor if it is done within 12 weeks of conception and two doctors if it is done between 12 and 20 weeks.

Highlights of MTP Act Amendment in 2021

- The amendment (2021) Bill allows abortion to be done on the advice of one doctor up to 20 weeks, and two doctors in the case of certain categories of women between 20 and 24 weeks.
- Increasing the upper gestation limit from 20 to 24 weeks for special categories of women, including survivors of rape, victims of incest and other vulnerable women (differently abled women, minors, among others).
- Upper gestation limit to NOT apply in cases of substantial fetal abnormalities diagnosed by a Medical Board.
- The name and other particulars of a woman whose pregnancy has been terminated cannot be revealed except to a person authorized by law.

Table 12: Methods of termination of pregnancy

First trimester up to 12 weeks	Second trimester 13–20 weeks
Medical • Mifepristone and misoprostol • Misoprostol • Methotrexate and misoprostol • Tamoxifen and misoprostol **Surgical** • Menstrual regulation • Vacuum aspiration • Suction evacuation and curettage • Dilatation and evacuation (rapid method and slow method)	**≤14 weeks** • Mifepristone and misoprostol • Misoprostol alone • Letrozole and misoprostol • Dinoprostone • Concentrated oxytocin **>14 weeks** **Surgical abortion:** Firstly, cervical ripening by medical methods such as Mifepristone and Misoprostol or with osmatic dilators or combination oof both. Then by dilation and evacuation.

Ectopic Pregnancy

- A pregnancy in which the fetus develops outside the uterus.
- Most common site is a fallopian tube (ampulla).
- Second common site for ectopic pregnancy is ovary.
- Risk factors for ectopic pregnancy include pelvic inflammatory disease (PID), tobacco, smoking and the use of assisted reproductive technology.
- **Signs and symptoms** classically include abdominal pain and vaginal bleeding.
- Triad of ectopic pregnancy includes amenorrhea, vaginal bleeding and abdominal pain.
- **Diagnosis:** Urine pregnancy test; ultrasonography; beta-hCG measurement (do not increase appropriately)
- **Treatment:** Methotrexate to terminate the fetal growth and subsequent abortion. Surgical intervention may be necessary.

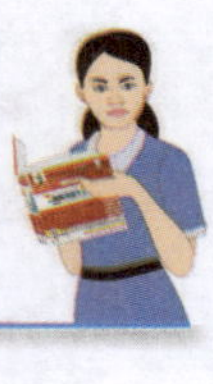

KEY POINTS

- Vaginal misoprostol associated with oxytocin infusion (30 units) is more effective than misoprostol alone in termination of second-trimester pregnancy.
- A client with a missed abortion will have induction of labor. Dinoprostol (Prostin E) is a form of prostaglandin used to soften the cervix.
- Missed abortion is most often associated with septic abortion.
- The most common cause of 1st trimester abortion is **trisomy**.
- Second **trimester abortions** occur mostly due to incompetent cervix.
- In missed abortions, D&C or suction evacuation should be performed by 4–6 weeks if expulsion of the fetal products has not occurred.
- Cervical incompetence is the major cause of abortion in second trimester.

POINTS TO REMEMBER

- In India, the abortion was legalized by Medical Termination of Pregnancy Act (MTP Act) of 1971, and has been **enforced in April 1972**.
- If pregnancy is more than 20 weeks, the opinion of two medical practitioners, is necessary.
- The MTP procedure can be performed only in hospital or places approved by government for MTP.

- Administer RhoGAM to Rh negative mothers.
- Heterotopic pregnancy: in twin pregnancy one is inside the uterus and other is ectopic.

INTRA-UTERINE FETAL DEATH (IUFD)

- All types of fetal loss after 22-week Period of Gestation (POG) and weighing more than 500 g occurring during pregnancy or labor.
- **Signs and symptoms**: fundal height is less than POG. FHR absent.

Signs of Fetal Death in X-Ray

- **Robert sign:** Presence of gas in great vessels of fetus such as aorta and IVC. It occurs within 12 hours of fetal death and is the first IUFD sign seen in X-ray.
- **Spalding sign:** Overlapping of skull bone of fetus. Usually seen after 7 days or more of fetal death.
- **Ball sign:** It is the hyperflexion or hyperextension of the fetal spine. It occurs after the 3 to 4 weeks of IUFD.
- Complication due to the retention of dead fetus in the intra uterine cavity is DIC.

GESTATIONAL TROPHOBLASTIC DISORDERS

- It is the benign neoplasm of the chorionic villi. The uterus is distended by thin walled translucent, grape-like vesicles of different size. These are degenerated chorionic villi filled with fluid.
- There is no vasculature in the chorionic villi which leads to early death and absorption of the embryo.
- **Classification of gestational trophoblastic disorders:** Hydatidiform mole, gestational trophoblastic neoplasia, invasive mole, placental site trophoblastic tumor, choriocarcinoma.

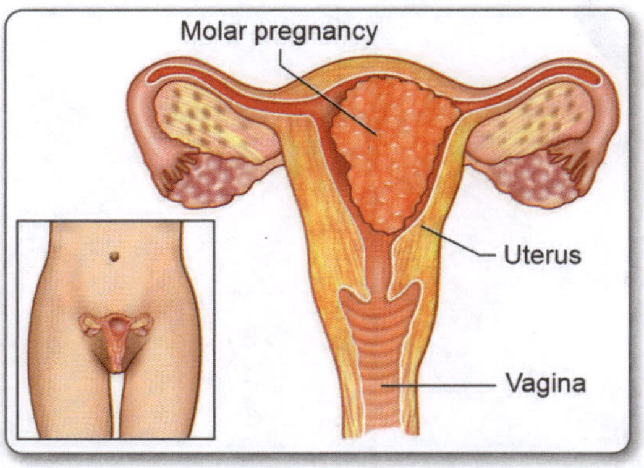

Figure 44: Molar pregnancy

Signs and Symptoms

- Patient shows early signs of pregnancy
- Anemia
- Pregnancy induced hypertension, preeclampsia
- **Uterine bleeding:** Blood mixed with the fluid from the ruptured cyst gives the appearance as **white currant in red currant juice**
- Lower abdominal pain
- Expulsion of grape-like vesicles per vagina
- No quickening even after 20 weeks.

Diagnosis

- Uterus size: Large for dates uterus
- On palpation: Uterus feels doughy or elastic
- Fatal parts not felt
- No fetal movement or fetal heart rate.

MULTIPLE PREGNANCY

- When more than one fetus simultaneously develops in the uterus, then it is called multiple pregnancy.
- Two fetuses (twins) are the commonest.
- Three fetuses (triplets), four fetuses (quadruplets), five fetuses (quintuplets), six fetuses (sextuplets) are also seen.

Classification

- Dizygotic twins (binovular or fraternal) are the commonest (two-third of all twins) and results from the fertilization of two ova. They are non-identical twins.
- Monozygotic twins (uniovular): Fertilization of single ovum. Less common (one-third of all twins)

Twin to Twin Transfusion Syndrome

- Complications are seen in monochorionic twins.
- One twin appears to bleed into other through placental vascular anastomosis.
- Receptor twin becomes larger with hydramnios, polycythemic, hypertensive and hypervolemic.
- Donor twin becomes smaller with oligohydramnios, anemic, hypotensive and hypovolemic.
- Donor may appear stuck due to severe oligohydramnios.

ANTEPARTUM HEMORRHAGE

Any bleeding from the genital tract or in the genital tract after the completion of 28 weeks of pregnancy till delivery.

Causes

Placental cause	Fetal cause	Local cause
• Placenta previa • Abruptio placenta • Circumvallate placenta	Vasa previa	Cervical polyp Trauma to the cervix.

Recent Question (NORCET 2021)

32. Stallworthy sign is seen in:

a. Posterior placenta previa
b. Hydatidiform mole
c. APH
d. PPH

Ans. (a) Posterior...

Recent Question (NORCET 2023)

33. A patient in 28-week gestation is receiving labetalol and magnesium sulfate for her pre-eclampsia treatment. On checking her BP you find that it is 86/56. The most likely cause of this finding is:

a. False BP reading
b. Accidental overdose of labetalol
c. Patient is anxious
d. Magnesium toxicity

Ans. (d) Magnesium...

KEY POINT

Type II Posterior placenta previa is known as dangerous placenta previa.

Clinical Corner

CASE SCENARIO 9:

A client arrives at the hospital at 37 weeks gestation with profuse vaginal bleeding. She states that it occurred suddenly without any noticeable pain. Which condition may the client be experiencing that may require immediate attention?

a. Placenta previa
b. Abruptio placenta
c. Ruptures uterus
d. Concealed abruptio

Ans. (a) Placenta previa

Placenta previa occurs when the placenta partially or completely covers the opening of the cervix. It can cause painless vaginal bleeding, which can be sudden and profuse, especially in the later stages of pregnancy.

Placenta Previa

- Placenta is implanted partially or wholly in the lower uterine segment (near cervical os).
- It is a leading cause of antepartum hemorrhage.
- There are four types of placenta previa:
  - **Type I: Low-lying:** Placenta implanted in the lower segment of uterus but does not reach (covers) the cervical os. Vaginal birth is possible.
  - **Type II: Marginal:** Border of the placenta touches (approaches) the cervical os. Vaginal birth is normally safe.
    - **Type II anterior:** Placenta is located on the front wall (anterior) of the uterus, closest to the mother's abdomen. It does not comprise fetal oxygenation as that of type 2 posterior.
    - **Type II posterior:** Placenta is located on the wall of the uterus closest to the mother's spine (posterior wall). **It is also known as dangerous placenta previa.**
    - **Type 3: Partial:** The placenta only partially obstructs cervical os. Vaginal birth is still possible, mostly CS is preferred for partial type.
    - **Type 4: Complete:** Implantation totally covers the cervical os. Cesarean section is usually recommended.
- **Risk factors:** Advanced maternal age (age greater than 35-year-old), multiparity, smoking, history of curettage, use of cocaine, and history of cesarean section.
- **Signs and symptoms:** Vaginal bleeding, which is painless, sudden onset, causeless and recurrent. bright red bleeding, soft uterus, anemia, uterine contractions.
- **Treatment:** For minimal to no bleeding, bed rest. For Heavy bleeding, C-section may be recommended.
- Vaginal examination should not be done in a suspected or confirmed case of placenta previa.
- **Stall worthy's sign:** Dropping of FHR when the presenting part press down into the pelvis and recovery of FHR once the pressure is released. It is seen mainly in type 1 posterior and Type 2 posterior.

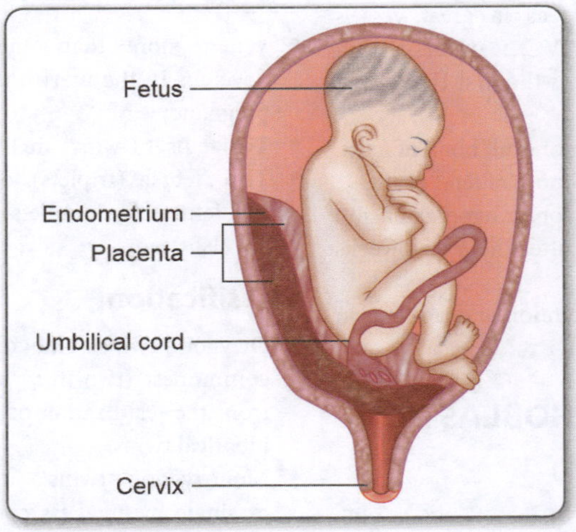

Figure 45: Placenta previa

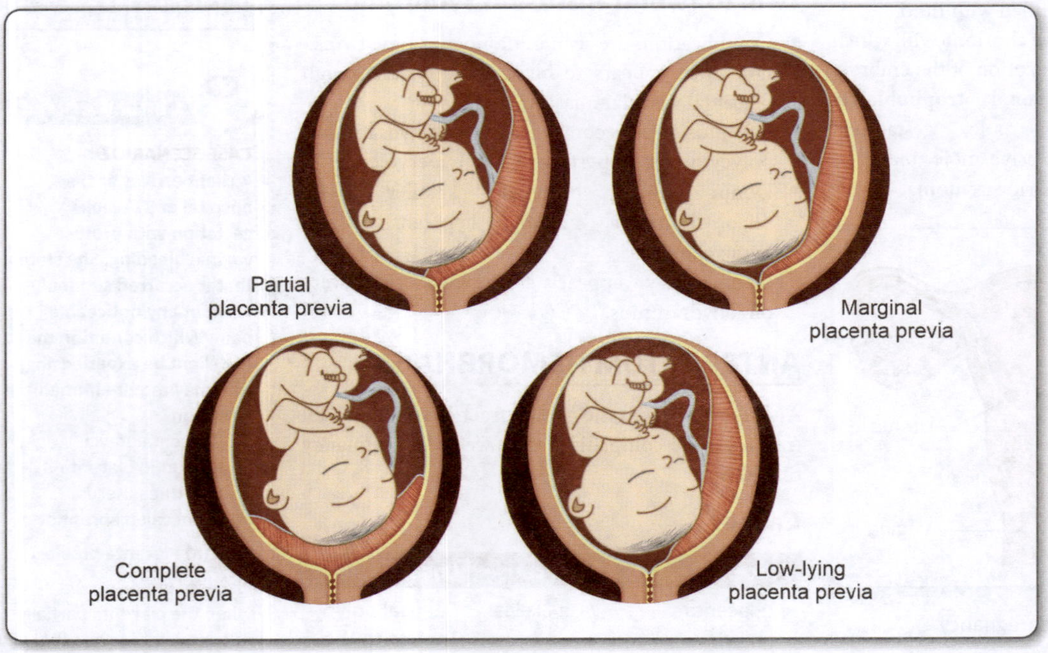

Figure 46: Types of placenta previa

Clinical Corner

CASE SCENARIO 10:

A primigravida mother with 18+ weeks of period of gestation is diagnosed with placenta previa. She asked the nurse what is the management for this condition. The most appropriate response from the nurse is:

a. Heparin therapy
b. Abortion to safeguard mother's life
c. Blood transfusion
d. Activity restriction and bed rest

Ans. (d) Activity restriction and bed rest

Placenta previa is a condition in which placenta covers all or part of the cervix. This condition is one of the causes for antepartum hemorrhage. In the early periods of gestation when the placenta previa diagnosis is made, activity restriction and bed rest are needed as management.

Abruptio Placenta

- The pre-mature separation of the placenta from its normal site of implantation which cause bleeding.
- **Types**
  - **Concealed abruption:** Blood is collected between the membrane and decidua or collected behind the separated placenta.
  - **Revealed abruption:** After the pre-mature separation of placenta blood is visible outside through the cervical canal.
  - **Mixed type:** Some blood is collected inside and some portion of blood is expelled outside the body.
- **Risk factors:** Increased age and parity; vascular diseases, Supine hypotensive syndrome, Smoking, cocaine use, uterine myoma, poor socio-economic status, hypertensive pregnancy, folic acid deficiency.
- **Signs and symptoms:**
  - Vaginal bleeding accompanied with abdominal pain
  - Bright to dark red bleeding
  - Uterine size will increase in case of concealed hemorrhage.
  - Bloody amniotic fluid
  - Pallor skin, hypotension
  - Signs of shock.
- **Treatment:** Depends on gestational age. It ranges from symptomatic management to C-Section or vaginal delivery.

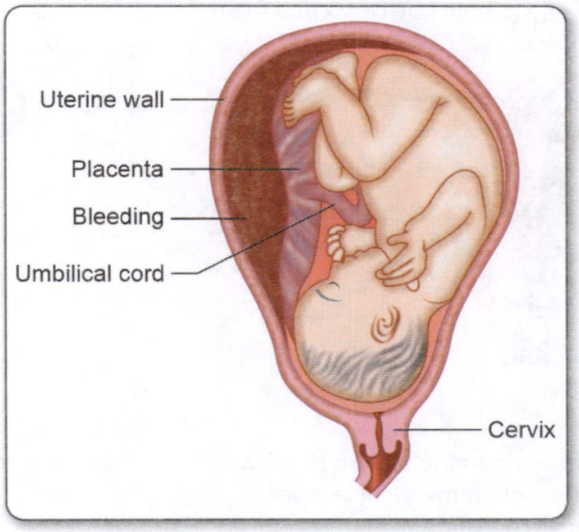

Figure 47: Abruptio placenta

KEY POINTS

- Premature separation of normally situated placenta is called **abruptio placenta**.
- Absence of communicating blood vessels in placenta is **called placenta spuria.**
- Major complication associated with abruptio placenta is Disseminated intravascular coagulopathy (DIC).

Recent Question (NORCET 2020)

34. Which is not a cause of APH?
a. Placenta previa
b. Cord presentation
c. Abruptio placentae
d. Rupture of uterus

Ans. (b) Cord presentation

Comparison of Placenta Previa vs Abruptio Placenta

Characteristic	Placenta previa	Abruptio placenta
Bleeding	Painless, causeless, and recurrent. Bleeding is always revealed type	Painful bleeding. It can be concealed, revealed, or mixed.
Blood type	Bright red	Dark coloured
Condition of patient and anemia	Proportionate to bleeding	Disproportionate
Per abdomen examination	Uterus is soft and height of uterus is equal to POG. FHR present	Uterus is hard and tensed. Size of uterus is more than POG. FHR may not be heard.
PV Examination	Contra indicated	Contra indicated

Uterine Malformations

Malformation

Unicornuate uterus

A condition where the female reproductive system develops with a single-horned shape instead of the usual two-horned structure. It occurs when Mullerian ducts fails to properly fuse during fetal development.

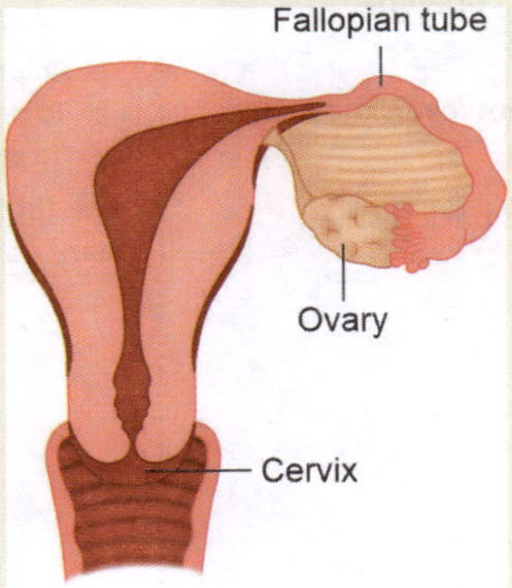

Didelphic uterus

It is also known as a double uterus, is a rare congenital abnormality of the female reproductive system in which the uterus develops as two separate structures instead of one.

Each uterus has its own cervix, and in some cases, each may also have its own vagina.

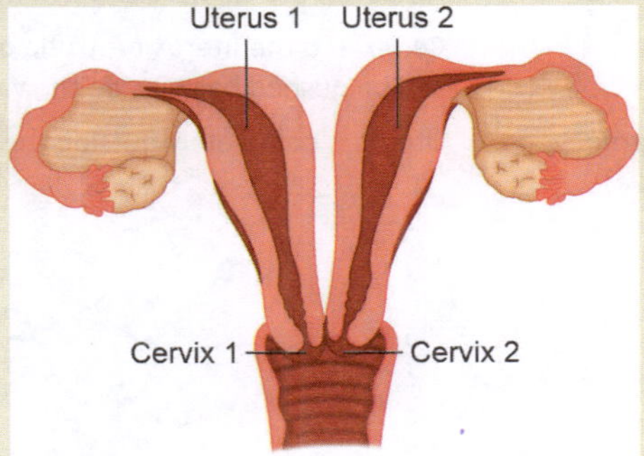

Contd...

Malformation

Bicornuate uterus

It is a type of uterine anomaly where the uterus has a characteristic **heart-like shape**, with a deep indentation at the top.

This is due to incomplete fusion of the two Mullerian ducts, which results in the uterus developing two separate horns instead of fusing into a single organ. Here one cervix and vagina will be present.

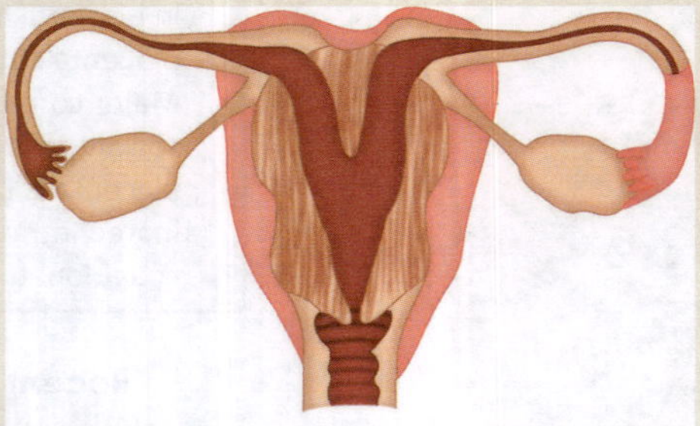

Septate uterus

In this condition uterus is divided into two by a septum which is starting from top of uterus and can extend up to cervix.

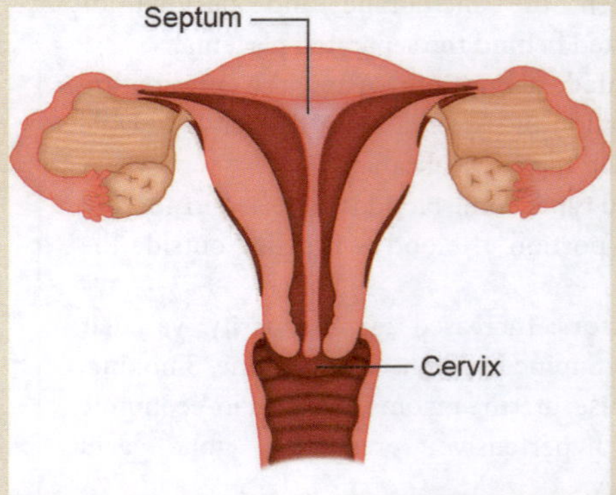

Arcuate uterus

It is the mild indentation of the endometrium at uterine fundus due to the incomplete resorption of uterovaginal septum.

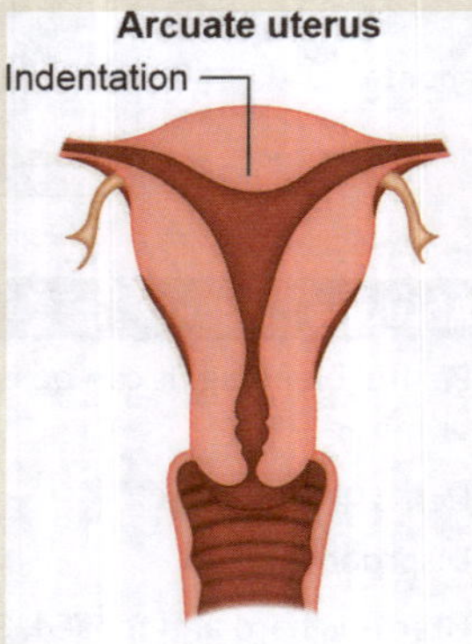

DES uterus (T-shaped)

It is associated with the in-utero exposure to diethylstilbestrol.

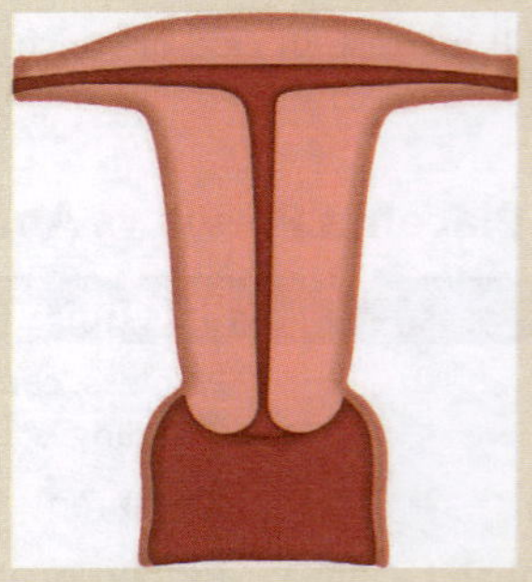

Uterine Prolapse

It is a condition in which pelvic floor muscles are weak and are not strong enough to support uterus. Then uterus is protruding toward or through the vagina.

Classification

Degree of prolapse	Description
First degree	Uterus descends into the lower part of the vagina, but doesn't protrude outside the opening of the vagina
Second degree	The uterus descends further and protrudes outside the vaginal opening. However, the cervix is still within the vagina.
Third degree	Cervix and the uterus protrude outside the vaginal opening. However, they can still be pushed back inside the vagina.
Fourth degree (procidentia)	Uterus is completely outside the vagina and cannot be pushed back inside.

Clinical Corner

CASE SCENARIO 11:

While going through the delivery notes of a mother, nursing student observed it is written as Ritgen's technique. She should understand that this method is used:

a. To expel the placenta
b. To prevent perineal tear
c. To provide episiotomy
d. To prevent PPH

Ans. (b) To prevent perineal tear

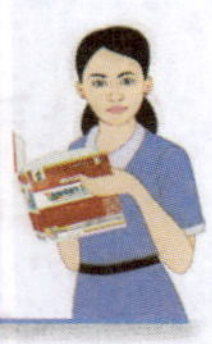

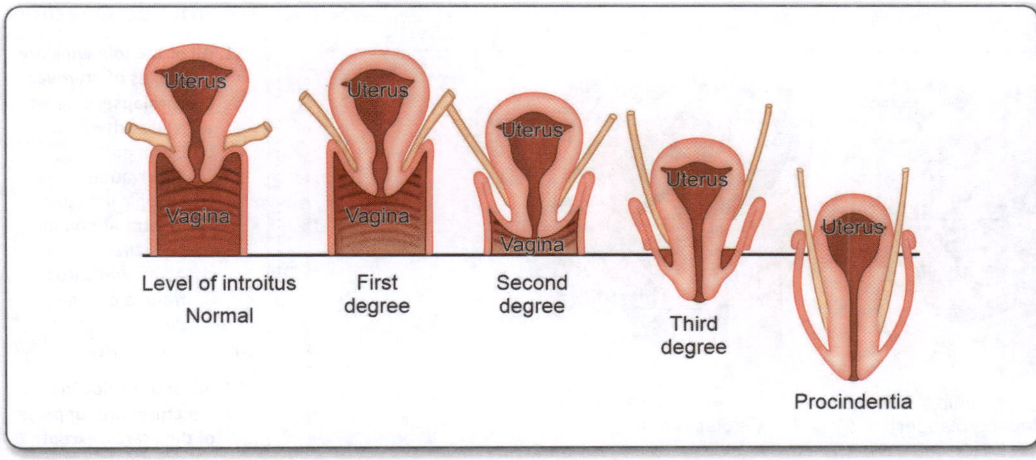

Figure 48: Uterine prolapse

- The three ligaments which primarily support the uterus are cardinal ligament, uterosacral ligament, pubocarvical ligament.
- Secondary support to the uterus is through round ligament.
- The ligament which does not involve in the support of the uterus is broad ligament.

Risk factors: Multipara with many vaginal deliveries, postmenopausal, family history of pelvic organ prolapse.

Major Causes

- Birth injury-perineal tear, excessive stretching of pelvic floor muscles and ligaments
- Peripheral nerve injury- Pudendal nerve injury during childbirth
- Delivery of big baby
- Rapid succession of pregnancy
- Loss of pelvic support
- Post-partum cough or heavy work just after delivery

Symptoms

Feeling of pressure or heaviness in the pelvis, a sensation of something bulging out of the vagina, difficulty emptying the bladder or bowel, urinary or fecal incontinence, or pain during intercourse.

Treatments

- Pelvic floor exercises
- Weight loss
- Avoiding heavy lifting.
- More severe cases may require a pessary (a device inserted into the vagina to support the uterus) or surgery.

Prevention and Management

- **Prevention:**
  - 1st stage of labor: Avoid bearing down. Breech or forceps delivery should not be attempted before full dilatation of cervix.
  - 2nd stage of labor: Avoid prolongation of 2nd stage. Perform episiotomy if overstretching of perineum occurs.
  - 3rd stage of labor: Tears or episiotomy should be carefully sutured.
  - Prevent cough and constipation with appropriate interventions.
  - Kegel exercise to tone up pelvic musculature.
- **Management:**
  - Pessary treatment – A mechanical device for controlling and correcting UV prolapse. Types – Ring pessary and Hodge pessary.

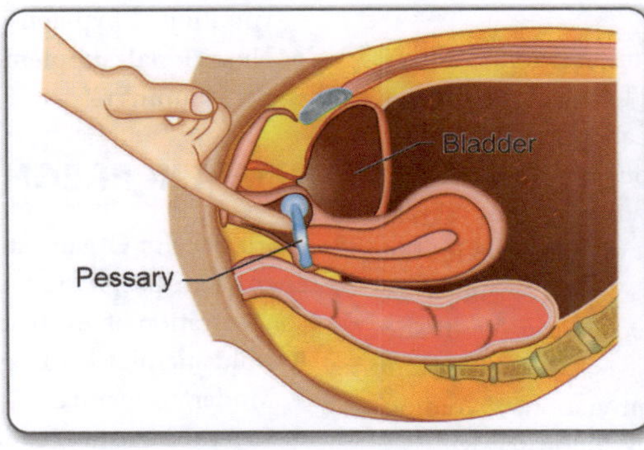

Figure 49: Insertion of ring pessary

  - Surgical treatment: Vaginal hysterectomy, Burch operation, Anterior Colporrhaphy, posterior colporrhaphy, Manchester repair.
- **Nursing management:**
  - Change the pessaries every 3–4 months
  - Teach the client about pelvic floor muscle exercise
  - Provide adequate comfortable devices

KEY POINTS

- Vaginal pessary can be used in elderly patients with prolapse with associated medical complications which contradict surgery
- Sling surgeries are indicated in women desiring to retain reproductive function

Practice Questions

9. Management of 3rd degree uterine prolapse in a 26-year-old woman of P1+0 can be all, except:
a. Sling surgery
b. Ring pessary
c. Hodge pessary
d. Vaginal hysterectomy

Ans. (d) Vaginal hysterectomy

10. Which of the following is NOT a posterior vaginal wall defect:
a. Rectocele
b. Perineal tear
c. Cystocele
d. Perineal body descent

Ans. (c) Cystocele

KEY POINTS

- Prolapse of the uterus with eversion of the entire vagina is termed Procidentia.
- **Cerclage operation** (encircling cervix with suture) is done for patients with incompetent cervix.

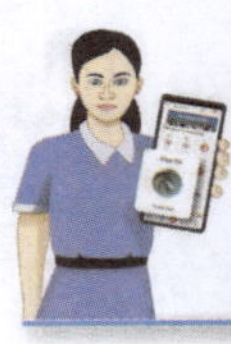

Cystocele and Rectocele

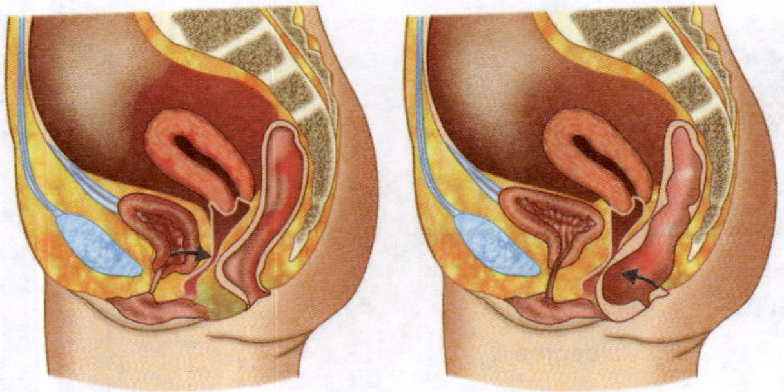

Figure 50: Cystocele and rectocele

- **Cystocele:** A condition in which supportive tissues around the bladder and vaginal wall weaken and stretch, allowing the bladder and vaginal wall to fall into the vaginal canal.
- **Rectocele:** There is a defect in the fascia between the rectum and the vagina. This allows part of the wall of the rectum to bulge into the vagina.
- **Causes:**
  - Difficult vaginal births
  - Forceps assisted delivery
  - Frequent weight-lifting
  - Stress on supportive structure during labor
  - Chronic cough or constipation
  - Obesity
  - Previous pelvic surgery
- **Symptoms:**
  - **Cystocele:** Frequent micturition, Stress incontinence, Frequent UTI, Pain or discomfort in vagina, pelvis, lower abdomen, groin or lower back, Painful intercourse.
  - **Rectocele:** Pain or pressure in the vagina, painful intercourse, pain or pressure in the rectum, difficult to pass stool, feelings of incomplete stool passage, feeling of tissue building out of vagina.
- **Investigation:** Pelvic examination, Voiding cystourethrogram, Cystoscopy, Fluoroscopy
- **Treatment:** Kegel exercises, Estrogen replacement therapy, pessary, surgery
- **Complication:** Urinary retention.

HYPEREMESIS GRAVIDARUM

- Severe vomiting in pregnancy that can deteriorate mother's health and interfere in her daily activities.
- **Incidence:** 1 in 1000 pregnancies
- **Adverse effects:** Dehydration, **metabolic alkalosis**, electrolyte imbalance, weight loss
- **Common measures to be taken:**
  - Small and frequent meals
  - Avoid drinking fluid after meals and take in between meals
  - Do not lie down after having meals
  - Avoid food causing gastric irritation
  - Avoid fatty food or food with odors that can trigger nausea and vomiting.
- **Management:**
  - Admission is required
  - Oral feed is withheld for at least 24 hours or till vomiting persists
  - IV fluids
  - **Antiemetic drugs:** Promethazine (phenergan)-25 mg or prochlorperazine (stemetil) 5 mg, metoclopramide
  - **Hydrocortisone:** 100 mg in case of intractable vomiting or hypotension
  - **Nutritional supplement:** Vitamins B1, B12, B6, vitamins C

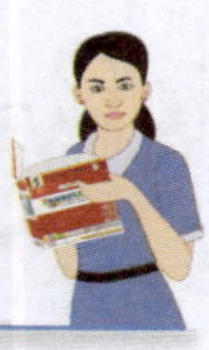

ANEMIA IN PREGNANCY

- World Health Organization (WHO) has **defined anemia in pregnancy** as the hemoglobin (Hb) concentration of less than 11 g/dL.
  - Mild anemia: 9–10.9 g/dL
  - Moderate anemia: 7.8–9 g/dL
  - Severe anemia: <7 g/dL
  - Very severe anemia: <4 g/dL
- The average *pregnant* woman *needs* about 30 mg of elemental *iron* per day.

Causes

- Reduced intake or absorption of iron.
- Excess demand such as multiple pregnancy.
- Blood loss.

Effects of Anemia on the Mother

- Reduced resistance to infection.
- Reduced ability to withstand postpartum hemorrhage.

Practice Questions

11. All of the following are etiologies of uterovaginal prolapse, except:
a. Nulliparity
b. Estrogen deprivation
c. Chronic increase in intra-abdominal pressure
d. Acute and chronic trauma of vaginal delivery

Ans. (a) Nulliparity

12. All of the following structures are supports of the uterus, except:
a. Cardinal ligaments
b. Anterior cruciate ligament
c. Uterosacral ligaments
d. Pubocervical ligaments

Ans. (b) Anterior cruciate...

Recent Questions (NORCET 2020)

35. What mean by posthumous child?
a. Abused child
b. Child who lost the parents after birth
c. Childbirth after death of the biological parents
d. Child who doesn't have mother

Ans. (c) Childbirth after...

36. What is hyperemesis gravidarum?
a. Morning sickness
b. Lethargy
c. Excessive vomiting
d. Excessive loose motion

Ans. (c) Excessive vomiting

KEY POINTS

National iron plus initiative (NIPI) recommends **iron folic acid [IFA]** supplementation of **100 mg elemental iron** and **500 µg of folic acid** every day for at least 100 days starting after the first trimester at **14–16 weeks of gestation** for all non-anemic pregnant women followed by the same dose for 100 days postpartum.

- Strain of even an uncomplicated labor may cause cardiac failure.
- Predisposition to PIH and preterm labor due to associated malnutrition.
- Potential threat to life.

Effects to Fetus/ Baby

- Intrauterine hypoxia and growth retardation
- Prematurity and Low Birth Weight (LBW) baby
- Anemia a few months after birth due to poor stores
- Increased risk of perinatal morbidity and mortality.

Management

- The RDA of iron in third trimester is 30 mg/day
- Supplementary iron therapy (WHO guidelines):
  - Daily oral iron supplementation with 30 mg to 60 mg of elemental iron
  - 60 mg of elemental iron is equal to 300 mg ferrous sulfate heptahydrate, 180 mg ferrous fumarate or 500 mg of ferrous gluconate.
  - If a woman is diagnosed with anemia during pregnancy, her daily elemental iron should be increased to 120 mg until her Hb concentration rises to normal (Hb 110 g/L or higher)
- Iron rich diet
- Adequate treatments to eradicate illnesses likely to cause anemia
- Early detection of falling hemoglobin level.

HIV IN PREGNANCY

- **HIV in pregnancy:** Incidence in asian countries <0.5%
- **Management:**
  - For all pregnant and lactating women, NACO recommends starting Antiretroviral Therapy (ART) irrespective of CD4 count.

Table 13: ART for pregnant women presenting in active labor with no prior ART

Maternal status	Intrapartum	Postpartum
Presenting in active labor, No Prior ARV prophylaxis	Tenofovir (TDF) – 300 mg OD Lamivudine (3TC) – 300 mg OD Efavirenz (EFV) – 600 mg OD	Tenofovir (TDF) – 300 mg OD Lamivudine (3TC) – 300 mg OD Efavirenz (EFV) – 600 mg OD

Intrapartum Care

- Zidovudine infusion to be started at:
  - Onset of labor
  - Four hours before cesarean section
  - Loading dose 2 mg/kg/hr
  - Maintenance dose 1 mg/kg/hr until cord is clamped.
- Women who were on ART:
  - Have vaginal delivery if viral load <50 copies/mL
  - Elective cesarean delivery at 38 weeks if viral load >50 copies/mL
- Broad spectrum antibiotics to be administered as per hospital policy
- Invasive procedures like instrumentation are contraindicated
- Universal precautions to be taken.

Postpartum Care (Neonatal Care)

Antiretroviral therapy (ARV)– To be given within 4 hours of delivery

Table 14: Infant nevirapine (NVP) prophylaxis

Birth weight	NVP daily dose (in mg)	Duration
Less than 2000 g	2 mg/kg once daily	Up to 6 weeks irrespective of whether exclusively breastfed or exclusive replacement fed
2000–2500 g	10 mg, once daily	
More than 2500 g	15 mg once daily	

Source: National Aids Control Organization (NACO), India.

RH INCOMPATIBILITY

- Rh incompatibility is a condition which develops when there is difference in Rh blood type between the Mother (Rh-) and Fetus (Rh+). (Mother-Rh- and fetus Rh+).
- The woman's immune system reacts by producing anti-D antibodies that cause sensitization.
- In subsequent pregnancies, antibodies can cross placenta and destroy fetal erythrocytes.
- **Symptoms:**
  - **Mild to moderate:** Hemolysis, jaundice
  - **Severe:** Hydrops fetalis, severe anemia, fetal heart failure, respiratory distress, kernicterus

KEY POINTS

- In India, mothers known to be HIV-infected (and whose infants are HIV uninfected or of unknown HIV status) should exclusively breastfeed their infants for the first 6 months of life.
- Mothers known to be HIV-infected should be provided with lifelong antiretroviral therapy or antiretroviral prophylaxis interventions to reduce HIV transmission through breastfeeding.
- Elective cesarean reduces the risk of vertical transmission by 50%

Recent Question
(NORCET 2020)

37. Which of the following causative organism is responsible for syphilis?
a. Human immune deficiency virus
b. Sarcoptes scabi
c. Neisseria gonorrhea
d. Treponema pallidum

Ans. (d) Treponema pallidum

KEY POINTS

- **Landsteiner** and **Weiner (1940)** discovered **Rh antigen**.
- Amniotic fluid appears **golden color** in case of Rh incompatibility.
- **Antenatal prophylaxis for Rh incompatibility:** RhoGAM (anti-D immunoglobulin) 1500 IU (300 mcg) IV/IM given at 28–34 weeks of pregnancy in non-sensitized Rh-Negative pregnant women. Another dose within 72 hours of delivery if the baby is Rh+.

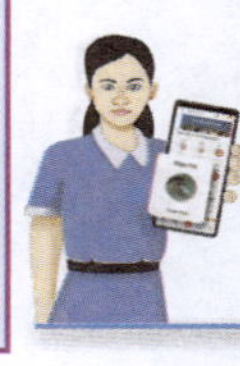

- **Diagnosis**
  - Coomb's test is used to detect Rh incompatibility. It can be direct coombs test or indirect coombs test.
    - **Direct coombs test [direct antiglobulin test (DAT)]:** Presence of antibodies that have coated the surface of fetal red blood cells are detecting. A positive test result indicates that the baby is at risk of developing haemolytic diseases of newborn.
    - **Indirect Coombs test:** Test is often performed during pregnancy to determine if a woman has developed antibodies against her baby's blood. If the mother has developed antibodies against the baby's blood, it can cause hemolytic disease of the newborn (HDN). Test is used to detect unbound antibodies to RBCs, which may be present in the patient's serum.
  - **Prevention:**
    - **Antenatal prophylaxis:** RhoGAM (Anti-D immunoglobulin) 1500 IU (300 mcg) IV/IM at 28–34 weeks of pregnancy is given for non-sensitized Rh-negative pregnant women. (WHO recommendation)
    - Another dose administered within 72 hours after delivery if the baby is Rh+.
    - Rh-negative unsensitized women should receive 1500 IU (**300 mcg**) **RhoGAM (Anti-D immunoglobulin)** within **72 hours** of induced or spontaneous abortion or full-term delivery.
    - Immediate cord ligation is done.

GESTATIONAL DIABETES MELLITUS (GDM)

- Carbohydrate intolerance of variable severity with onset or detection first time during pregnancy.
- Increased insulin resistance is seen among all pregnant women so that developing fetus will get enough glucose from mother.
- Maximum insulin resistance is seen between 24 and 28 weeks POG.

Risk factors for GDM

- Family history, Age >30 years
- Previous overweight baby of 4 kg or more
- Previous stillbirth (pancreatic islet hyperplasia)
- Unexplained perinatal loss
- Obesity
- Persistent glycosuria
- Polyhydramnios or recurrent vaginal candidiasis
- Ethnic group-East Asian, pacific island ancestry
- **Screening for gestational diabetes mellitus:** Glucose Tolerance Test with 75 g. Glucose between 24 and 28 weeks of pregnancy.

Table 15: Glucose tolerance test with 75 g oral glucose (WHO)

Time	Normal tolerance	Impaired glucose tolerance	Diabetes
Fasting	<100	≥100 and <126	≥126
2-hour post glucose	<140	≥140 and <200	≥200

Management

- Diet with 2000–2500 kcal/day for normal weight women
- Diet with 1200–1800 kcal/day for overweight women
- Complex carbohydrates preferred
- Mean plasma glucose level of 105–110 mg/dL gives good fetal outcome
- Exercise like brisk walking and aerobics
- Insulin therapy if fasting blood sugar >90 mg/dL and 2 hours postprandial >120 mg/dL
- Women with good glycemic control may wait for spontaneous induction of labor
- Elective delivery (cesarean/induction) with patients requiring insulin or complications like macrosomia at around 38 weeks
- The two oral hypoglycemic agents used in pregnancy include Metformin and Glyburid.
- Drug of choice for GDM is Insulin.

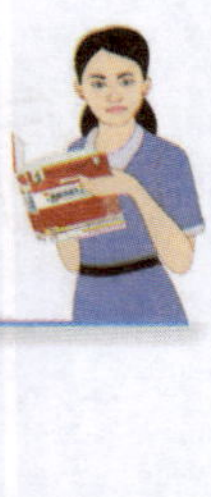

HEART DISEASE IN PREGNANCY

- Most common heart disease during pregnancy is mitral stenosis.
- In certain heart disease such as pulmonary hypertension and Marfan syndrome with aorta involvement, pregnancy is contraindicated.

HYPERTENSION IN PREGNANCY

Clinical types of pregnancy-induced hypertension include:

- Preeclampsia
- Eclampsia
- Gestational hypertension.

Preeclampsia

- A condition in pregnancy characterized by combination of hypertension, proteinuria and pathological edema or pitting edema (fluid retention).

KEY POINT

Rh-negative unsensitized women should receive 1500 IU (**300 mcg**) **RhoGAM (Anti-D immunoglobulin)** within **72 hours** of induced or spontaneous abortion or full-term delivery.

KEY POINTS

- Prematurity and still birth, Congenital anomalies, Macrosomia (large size of the baby) are common in woman with Gestational Diabetes Mellitus.
- Formal Diabetes screening should be done at 24–28 weeks of gestation to identify gestational diabetes mellitus (American Diabetes Association).

Clinical Corner

CASE SCENARIO 12:

Nurse Amli reviews the assessment findings a 32-year-old pregnant woman in her last trimester who has been diagnosed with severe preeclampsia. Amli determines which finding is most closely associated with the complication of this diagnosis?

a. Complaints of feeling hot when the room is cool
b. Breast enlargement
c. Evidence of bleeding, such as in the gums, purpura, and petechiae
d. Periods of fetal movement followed by quiet periods.

Ans. (c) Evidence of bleeding, such as in the gums, purpura, and petechiae

- **Mild preeclampsia:** BP >140/90 mm Hg on 2 or more occasions and proteinuria >300 mg/24 hours or end organ damage.
- **Severe preeclampsia**: BP >160/100 mm Hg on 2 or more occasions and proteinuria >5 g/24 hours.
- **Signs and symptoms:** While waking up in the morning there is edema in the foot and is gradually extending into face, abdominal cavity, vulva and whole body, headache, diminished urine output, blurring of vision, abnormal weight gain.
- Diuretics, antihypertensive drugs such as labetalol, hydralazine, nifedipine, nitroglycerine, sodium nitroprusside are the drugs of choice.

Eclampsia

- Preeclampsia with convulsions.
- **Signs and symptoms:** Flushing, headaches, blurred vision, deep tendon reflex, decreased urinary output.
- Eclamptic fits consist of four stages:
  1. **Premonitory stage:** Patient becomes unconscious. Twitching of muscles in the face, tongue and limbs. Eye balls roll and are turned around and become fixed. Duration of this stage is about 30 seconds.
  2. **Tonic stage:** Whole body goes into spasm. Trunk becomes opisthotonos and respiration ceases and tongue protrude between teeth. Duration of this stage is about 30 seconds.
  3. **Clonic stage:** Whole body goes into contraction and relaxation. Tongue bite occurs. Mouth filled with blood-stained frothy secretions. Patient become cyanosis and this stage lasts for 1–4 minutes.
  4. **Stage of coma:** Following convulsion patient goes into the stage of coma. It may last for a brief period or until another convulsion.
- **Management**
  - Control of hypertension with labetalol, hydralazine.
  - Magnesium sulfate is effective in eclampsia.
  - Magnesium sulfate acts as membrane stabilizer and neuroprotector
  - Repeat this injection only if knee jerk reflexes are present, respiratory rate >12/min and urine output exceeds 30 mL/hr.
  - Therapeutic level of Magnesium is 4–7 mEq/L
  - Recovery/lateral recumbent position to be given
  - Maintain open airway
  - O_2 administration through non-rebreather mask (10 L/min)
  - Fluids administration—colloid/crystalloid ≤125 mL/hr

Magnesium sulfate ($MgSO_4$)

- Loading dose is given as 4 g 20% I/V and 10 g 50% as I/M (5 g in each buttocks).
- Maintenance dose: 5 g 50% $MgSO_4$ as I/M in alternative buttocks every 4 hourly.

Toxicity of $MgSO_4$

- Earliest sign of toxicity is loss of deep tendon reflex. Other than this diaphoresis, respiratory depression and arrest can also be seen.
- **Antidote** for $MgSO_4$ is 10% calcium gluconate.
- Decreased urine output is not a sign of $MgSO_4$ toxicity. In a client on $MgSO_4$ therapy urine output is monitored because it is a drug which is excreted *via* kidney. If urine output is less, then there is a chance that excretion of drug is less and higher chance for toxicity.

POSTPARTUM HEMORRHAGE (PPH)

- Excessive blood loss after delivery is called PPH. In vaginal delivery it is >500 mL and in c-section it is >1000 mL.
- **Types of PPH:**
  - **Primary PPH:** After expulsion of placenta within 24 hours
    - **Third stage hemorrhage:** Before expulsion of placenta
    - **True PPH:** bleeding occur after the expulsion of placenta.
  - **Secondary PPH:** After 24 hours to 6 weeks. It is also known as delayed or puerperal haemorrhage.
- **Causes:** (Four T's)
  - Tone: Atonicity of uterus
  - Traumatic injury
  - Tissues: Retained tissues
  - Thrombin: Blood coagulation disorders
- **Signs and symptoms:** Decreased BP, increased heart rate and uncontrolled bleeding.
- **Management:**
  - Bimanual massage of the uterus
  - Sengstaken Blakemore oesophageal tube or bakri balloon catheter to compress the uterus.
  - Maximum capacity of bakri balloon catheter is 500 mL.
  - Start NS/RL with oxytocin (1 L with 20 units) at 60 drops/min.
  - Administer oxytocin 10 units IM/methergine 0.2 mg IV

Recent Question (NORCET 2022)

38. Which of following is helpful in prevention of pre-eclampsia?

a. Ascorbic acid
b. Vitamin E
c. Calcium
d. Vitamin A

Ans. (c) Calcium

Recent Question (NORCET 2022)

39. Which of the following is needed in the management of the PIH?

a. Vitamin C
b. Vitamin E
c. Folic acid
d. Calcium

Ans. (b) Vitamin E

KEY POINTS

- Hypertension extent of 140/90 mm Hg with proteinuria after the 20th week of pregnancy is called **preeclampsia**.
- **Biochemical marker of preeclampsia** is uric acid (>4.5 mg/dL).
- Preeclampsia, when complicated with generalized tonic-clonic convulsion and coma is called **eclampsia**.
- In **pre-monitory stage of eclampsia,** eyeballs roll or are turned to one side and become fixed.
- **Magnesium sulfate** is the drug of choice in **eclampsia to control fits**.

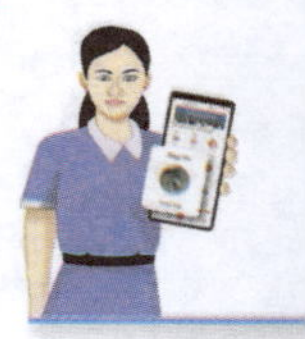

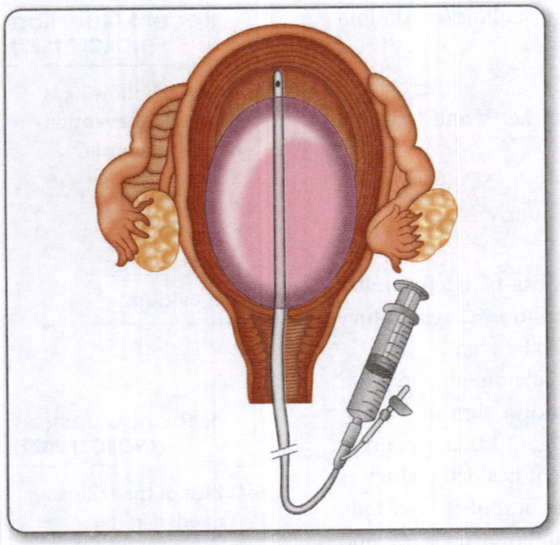

Figure 51: Bakri balloon

- Catheterize the bladder
- Apply fundal pressure and control cord traction to separate the placenta
- Manual removal of placenta is to be done under general anesthesia if placenta does not separate.

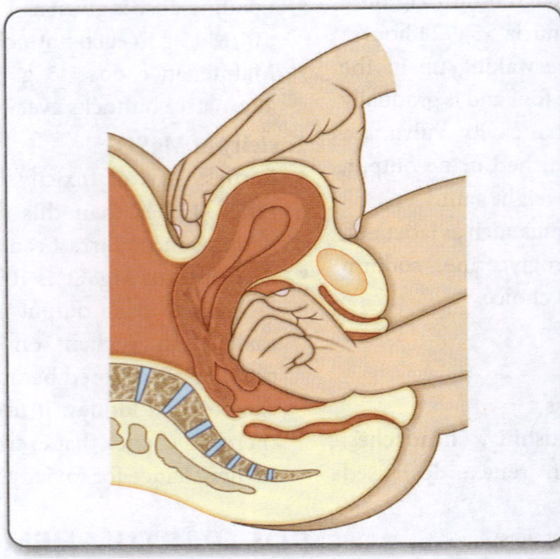

Figure 52: Bimanual massage of the uterus

Clinical Corner

CASE SCENARIO 13:

A nurse is caring for a primigravida receiving magnesium sulfate for pregnancy induced hypertension (PIH). The nurse is conducting assessments every 30 minutes. Which assessment finding would be the most concerning for the nurse?

a. Urine output since the last assessment is 20 mL.
b. Mother's RR is 10 breaths per minute.
c. The FHR measured at 120 beats per minute.
d. The patient's deep tendon reflex is 2+.

Ans. (b) Mother's RR is 10 breaths per minute.

A respiratory rate of 10 bpm is significantly lower than the normal range. This finding suggests respiratory depression, which can be a side effect of magnesium sulfate administration. Respiratory depression can lead to inadequate oxygenation and ventilation, potentially causing respiratory distress or even respiratory arrest. Therefore, it is crucial for the nurse to address this finding promptly and notify the physician to assess and intervene accordingly.

INJURIES TO BIRTH CANAL

Table 16: Types of injuries

Injuries to bony part	Injuries to soft tissue
Injury to symphysis pubis Injury to sacrococcygeal joint Injury to sacroiliac joint	Injury to vulva Perineal tear Laceration of vagina and cervix Rupture of uterus

POINTS TO REMEMBER

- Atonicity of the uterus (80%) is the most common cause of PPH.
- Atonic uterus is flabby and becomes hard on massaging.
- Second most common cause for PPH is trauma.

Recent Question (NORCET 2021)

40. Most common cause of PPH:

a. Placental Abruptio
b. Placenta previa
c. Uterine atony
d. Anemia

Ans. (c) Uterine atony

Uterine atony is responsible for 80% of PPH.

Recent Question (NORCET 2020)

41. Ergometrine is commonly used in the treatment of which of the following condition?

a. PPH
b. APH
c. Cervical incompetence
d. AV Fistula

Ans. (a) PPH

KEY POINTS

- **In PPH**, inj. Oxytocin drip started (10 units in 500 mL of normal saline) at the rate of 40–60 drops/min.
- Oxytocin has a half-life of 3–4 minutes and duration of action is approximately 20 minutes.
- **Synthetic oxytocin** is widely used. It has only got oxytocic effect without any vasopressor (syntocinon, 5 IU/mL) effect.
- **Dangers of oxytocin** are uterine hyperstimulation, uterine rupture, water intoxication, and hypotension.

Vulvar Injuries

Laceration can occur on the vulvar skin posteriorly. Even tear can occur on the inner aspects of labia minora.

Perineal Tear/Perineal Injuries

Gross injury due to mismanaged second stage of labor.

Degree of Perineal Tear

- **First degree:** Limited to vaginal mucosa and skin of the introitus
- **Second degree:** Extends to the fascia and muscles of the perineal body.
- **Third degree:** Trauma involves the anal sphincter.
- **Fourth degree:** Extends into the rectal lumen, through the rectal mucosa.

Central tear: A rare type of tear of the perineum when the head penetrates first through the posterior vaginal wall, then through the perineal body and appears through the skin of the perineum. It usually occurs in patients with contracted outlet.

Causes of Perineal Injury

- Rigid perineum
- Rapid stretching: precipitate delivery, head delivery in breech
- Overstretching of perineum: macrosomia of baby, shoulder delivery, forceps delivery.

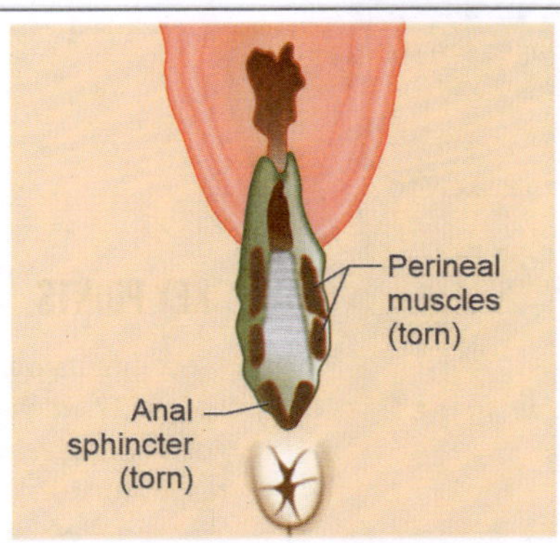

Figure 53: Third-degree perineal tear

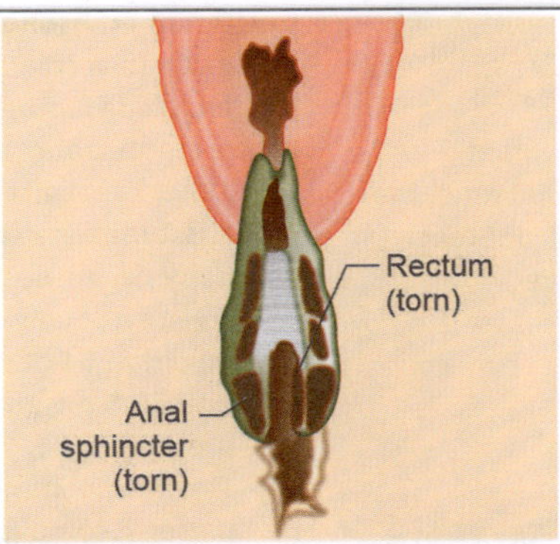

Figure 54: Fourth-degree perineal tear

Prevention of Perineal Tears During Labor

- Perineal massage and warm compresses during labor.
- Perineal support during delivery of presenting part.
- Woman should be discouraged from active pushing at the time of crowning.
- Episiotomy should be performed with all forceps delivery.
- Episiotomy should be performed at an angle of 60° from midline.
- Deliver the head between contraction.

Management of First/Second Degree Tears

- Second degree tear and episiotomy should be sutured.
- Absorbable suture material should be used
- If patient is not on epidural analgesia, inject 1% lignocaine in the perineum for local anesthesia
- **A rectal examination should be done after completion of repair of perineum.**

Management of Third/Fourth Degree Tears

- Repairs must be conducted in operation theatre (OT). It can be done in delivery suite if the patient is on epidural analgesia.
- Rectal examination should be done before commencing repair
- If internal anal sphincter is involved, it should be sutured separately by end-to-end technique with interrupted or mattress sutures
- If external anal sphincter is involved, it can be repaired either by an overlapping or end-to-end method.

Patient education for woman with perineal repair:

- Analgesia
- Perineal hygiene
- Signs and symptoms to be observed for
- Pelvic floor exercise
- Report to midwife/doctor if there develops any complication.

PROLONGED LABOR AND OBSTRUCTED LABOR

Prolonged Labor

- Labor is said to be prolonged when total duration of first and second stage is more than 18 hours
- **Causes:**
  - **First stage:** Failure in cervical dilatation
  - **Second stage:** Non descent of presenting part
- **Prevention:**
  - Early detection of any malpresentation, malposition or congenital abnormality

Recent Question (NORCET 2021)

42. All are the methods used for the removal of placenta, except:
a. Give oxytocin
b. Uterine massage
c. Controlled cord traction
d. Prostaglandin E1

Ans. (d) Prostaglandin E1

Explanation: Prostaglandin E1 is a hormone that can be used to induce labor. It is not used to remove the placenta. The other options, oxytocin, uterine massage, and controlled cord traction, are all used to remove the placenta.

KEY POINTS

- When the combined duration of the first and second stage is less than two hours, it is called **precipitated labor.**
- **Prolonged labor** when the combination of the first and second stage of labor is more than 18 hours.
- Labor is prolonged when the cervical dilatation is less than 1 cm/hr in primi and 1.5 cm/hr in a multi.
- The disparity in the relation between the head and the pelvis is called **cephalopelvic disproportion.**

Recent Question (NORCET 2021)

43. During delivery, there is a laceration in vaginal mucosa involving some perineal muscles, but not involving the anal sphincter. Identify the degree of tear:
a. First
b. Second
c. Third
d. Fourth

Ans. (b) Second

- Use of partograph: Change in position during labor
- Judicious use of augmentation
- **Definitive treatment:** For subnormal uterine activity
  - Amniotomy and/or oxytocin infusion
  - Pain relief by pethidine or epidural analgesia
  - Cesarean section if vaginal delivery is not safe

Obstructed Labor

- Labor is said to be obstructed when the descent of presenting part is arrested because of mechanical obstruction despite having good uterine contraction.
- **Causes:**
  - **Fault in passage:** Cephalopelvic disproportion (CPD), contracted pelvis, soft tissue obstruction like cervical dystocia, tumor, previous operative scar, etc.
  - **Fault in passenger:** Brow presentation, transverse lie, congenital malformations, big baby, locked twins.
- **Bandl's ring**
  - It is also known as pathological ring.
  - It is the constriction between active upper uterine segment and passive lower uterine segment during delivery.
- **Management**:
  - Early detection
  - Cesarean section

PRETERM LABOR AND POST-TERM PREGNANCY

Preterm Labor

- It is defined as uterine contractions occurring after 28 weeks of gestation and before 37 completed weeks of gestation.
- Common signs are palpable uterine contractions, blood discharge, backache, pressure and cramping.
- **Risk factors:**
  - Delivering premature baby in the past
  - Multiple pregnancy (more than one fetus)
  - Cervical incompetence
  - Placental abnormalities (placenta previa)
  - Short interpregnancy interval (less than 6 months)
  - Women younger than 18 years and older than 35 years are at higher risk
  - Pregnancy from invitro fertilization
  - Gestational diabetes
  - Tobacco use and substance use
- **Treatment:**
  - Administer tocolytics to decrease frequency and duration of contraction, postponing delivery.
    - Four example, Oxytocin antagonists (Atosiban).
    - Beta mimetic agents (Ritodrine).
    - Magnesium sulfate.
    - Indomethacin.
  - Glucocorticoid therapy
    - Betamethasone 12 mg I/M 24 hours apart 2 doses
    - Dexamethasone 6mg I/M 12 hours apart 4 doses.

Post-term Pregnancy

- Continuation of pregnancy beyond 2 weeks of expected date of delivery.
- **Maternal risk factors:**
  - Inaccurate estimation of EDD
  - Advanced maternal age
  - Primi para mothers
  - Placental insufficiency
- **Fetal risk factors:**
  - Male fetus
  - Anencephaly
- **Features of postterm newborn:**
  - Absence of vernix caseosa.
  - Placental calcification.
  - Scanty saffron-colored meconium and subsequent oligohydramnios.
  - Overgrown nails.
  - Wrinkled skin appearance in newborn.

Table 17: Facts about preterm and term infants

Preterm infants	Term infants
Poorly developed ear cartilages. Ear may fold easily	Ear Cartilages are well developed
Hair is fine and feathery	Hair is more likely to form firm
Male infant's scrotum in undeveloped, not pendulous Testes may be undescended minimal rugae	Well-developed scrotum Pendulous Testes down in the scrotal sac Rugated
Female infant: Clitoris is prominent; Labia majora poorly developed	Clitoris not prominent Labia majora fully developed
Fine wrinkles in sole	Soles are well and deeply creased
Scarf Sign: The infant's arm is pulled laterally across the chest; in the hypotonic infant (preterm), the elbow will cross the midline This is characteristic feature of infants born before 30 weeks	In a term infant with **normal** tone, the elbow will not reach the midline
Heel to ear maneuver: Heel is brought to ear without resistance	Not possible to bring heel to ear

Clinical Corner

CASE SCENARIO 14:

Nurse Amli was assisting a client with precipitated labor. As an experienced nurse she should anticipate for all the following complications; EXCEPT:

a. PPH
b. Injury to birth canal
c. Intracranial hemorrhage in baby
d. Premature separation of placenta

Ans. (d) Premature separation of placenta

Injury to birth canal, PPH, placenta retention, uterine rupture, infection, fetal hypoxia, intracranial hemorrhage, trauma to fetal skull are the complications of precipitated labor.

KEY POINTS

- Most infants born before 27 weeks of gestation develop respiratory distress syndrome which is associated with surfactant deficiency.
- **Betamethasone** is given to accelerate fetal lung maturity in preterm labor.
- The dose of **vitamin K is 1 mg** for a **term baby**. Single dose given after delivery or within 6 hours of birth. **0.5 mg given for preterm baby**.
- The most common preterm complication is respiratory distress.

PREMATURE RUPTURE OF MEMBRANES

- Spontaneous rupture of membranes beyond 28 weeks of pregnancy but before the onset of labor.
- **Management:**
  - Term PROM
    - Careful observation is made
    - In 90% of cases, spontaneous labor ensues within 24 hours
    - If labor does not start, induction with oxytocin
    - In obstetric indication, Cesarean section is performed
  - **Preterm PROM: Rupture occurs before 37 weeks of pregnancy.**
    - **>34 weeks:** Spontaneous labor ensues within 48 hours otherwise induction with oxytocin
    - Cesarean section for presentation other than cephalic
    - **<34 week:** Conservative attitude
    - **Use of antibiotics:** To minimize risk of infection
    - **Use corticosteroids:** To enhance lung maturity.

PHARMACOLOGY IN OBG

Oxytocic

These are the drugs having power to excite uterine contraction. e.g., oxytocin, ergot derivatives, prostaglandin.

Tocolytic Agent

These are the drugs which inhibit uterine contraction and used to prolong pregnancy in women who experience pre-mature contraction, e.g., magnesium sulfate, calcium channel blockers (Nifedipine), Beta-Adrenergic receptor agonists (terbutaline), Oxytocin inhibitors.

Antihypertensive Drugs

These drugs are used to control high blood pressure when BP is above 160/110. First line drugs of choice in pregnancy are **methyldopa** or **labetalol**. Second line drug is **nifedipine**.

Recent Question (NORCET 2020)

44. Which of the following drug is contraindicated in pregnant women?
a. Heparin
b. Labetalol
c. Dolutegravir
d. Streptomycin

Ans. (d) Streptomycin

Anticonvulsants

- Convulsion in pregnancy is largely due to eclampsia.
- The commonly used anti-convulsants are diazepam, phenytoin and phenobarbitone.
- First choice of anti-convulsant drug is magnesium sulfate.

Table 18: Drugs with power to stimulate urine contraction

Drug	Action	Indication	Contraindication	Side effects	Nursing responsibilities
Oxytocin	Stimulate uterine contraction	Early pregnancy • To accelerate abortion • To stop bleeding after abortion • Later pregnancy • To induce and augment labor • To ripen cervix before induction • Following placenta expulsion as an alternative to ergometrine. • To control PPH	• Heart disease • Contracted pelvis • Malpresentation • Fetal distress • Obstructed labor • Incoordinate uterine contraction	• Uterine hyperstimulation • Uterine rupture • Water intoxication • Hypertension • Fetal distress	• Continuously monitor contraction and discontinue if hyperstimulation occurs • Monitor maternal avital signs and fetal heart rate.
Ergot derivatives (methergine)	Act directly on myometrium producing tetanic contraction of the uterus with complete loss of polarity.	• To stop atonic uterine bleeding • To cut short 3rd stage of labor after expulsion of anterior shoulder.	• High BP • Rh negative factor • Abruptio placenta • Multiple pregnancies before the delivery of last fetus. • Heart disease • Eclampsia or pre-eclampsia	• Nausea • Vomiting • Rise of BP • Interaction with lactation	• Assess maternal vital signs • Asses for lactation process

Contd...

Drug	Action	Indication	Contraindication	Side effects	Nursing responsibilities
Prostaglandin	• PGF2α promotes myometrial contractility • PGE2 helps cervical maturation	• Iinduction of abortion and labor • Cervical ripening • Acceleration of labor • PPH management	• Hypersensitivity • Uterine scar	• Nausea • Vomiting • Diarrhea • Pyrexia • Bronchospasm • When used as abortifacient, extensive lacerations may occur • Tachysystole.	• Same as oxytocin and ergot derivatives

Anticoagulants

Heparin

- It's a weak anticoagulant and it does not cross the placenta. So, it does not lead to any fetal malformation.
- It is the **anticoagulant of choice in the first trimester** (no fetal malformation) and in later weeks of pregnancy. (Since it is a weak anticoagulant patient can deliver at any time).

Warfarin

- It is a strong anticoagulant which can also cause fetal malformation. It may be considered in specific situation **beyond 13 weeks POG.**

OPERATIVE OBG

Dilation and Evacuation

Cervix will be dilated and product of conception will be removed from the uterus.

Indication

- Incomplete abortion
- Inevitable abortion
- Hydatidiform mole
- Medical termination of pregnancy

Complications

Excessive hemorrhage, injury, shock, perforation, sepsis, pelvic inflammation, infertility, cervical incompetency, uterine synechiae.

Suction Evacuation

The product of conception is sucked out from the uterus with the help of a cannula fitted to a suction apparatus.

Indications

- MTP during first trimester
- Inevitable abortion
- Recent incomplete abortion
- Hydatidiform mole

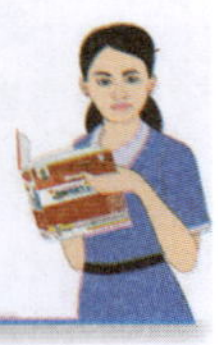

Menstrual Regulation/ Menstrual aspiration

- Aspiration of endometrial cavity within 14 days of missed period in a woman with previous normal cycle.
- Procedure involves the use of suction device or a small tube (canula) to gently remove the lining of uterus (endometrium) and any associated tissue.
- It is typically conducted in cases where a woman desires to regulate her menstrual cycle after a missed period and wishes to prevent or terminate a potential pregnancy.

Hysterotomy

- A form of abortion in which product of conception removed from uterus through the abdominal incision.
- It is like cesarean section but needs a smaller incision.

Indications

- Fibroid in the lower uterine segment
- Mid trimester MTP where other methods are failed
- Cervical cancer with pregnancy
- Uterine anomalies
- Completely low-lying placenta

COMMON GYNECOLOGICAL DISORDERS

Endometriosis

- Common cause of dysmenorrhea, dyspareunia and infertility.
- Endometrium fragments and lodges in other parts of the pelvic cavity.
- Causes inflammation, bleeding, scarring, and adhesions.
- Treated through hormonal therapy, laparoscopic surgery, or major surgical management.

Recent Question (NORCET 2020)

45. As a nurse you are monitoring a patient in immediate postpartum period. You are checking TRP and BP every 15 minutes for first hour. Which value suggest you that there is an excessive blood loss?

a. Increased pulse rate 90–102
b. An increase respiratory rate 18–22
c. Temperature 100.2°F
d. None of the above

Ans. (a) Increased pulse rate 90–102

Polycystic Ovarian Disease (PCOD)

- Characterized by increased testosterone and increased FSH/LH levels.
- In PCOD FSH/LH ratio become 1:2 or 1:3. While in a normal female it is 1:1.
- **Symptoms:**
  - Irregular or no menstrual periods (amenorrhea)
  - Excess body and facial hair (hirsutism), acne, pelvic pain, and infertility.
- **Treatment:**
  - Diet, exercise.
  - Pharmacotherapy includes ethinylestradiol, Cyproterone acetate, metformin.

Menstrual Disorders

- **Amenorrhea** is the absence of menstruation.
- **Primary amenorrhea:** Woman has not begun to menstruate till 16 years of age.
- **Secondary amenorrhea:** Absence of menses for 6 months in a woman who previously had regular menstrual cycle.
- **Dysmenorrhea:** It is painful menstruation.
- **Menorrhagia:** Excessive vaginal bleeding at normal intervals.
- **Metrorrhagia:** Vaginal bleeding between menses. Bleeding may occur as spotting or outright bleeding.
- **Polymenorrhea**: Cyclic bleeding where cycle length is reduced to less than 21 days and remains constant at that frequency.
- **Hypomenorrhea:** C days.
  - **Oligomenorrhea:** Cyclic bleeding where cycle length is increased to more than 35 days.

FIBROID UTERUS

- It is the most common benign and pelvic tumor among females.
- Most common site is uterus
- Most common type of fibroid is intramural.
- Most common sign of this is menorrhagia.

GONORRHEA, SYPHILIS AND PELVIC INFLAMMATORY DISEASE

Gonorrhea

- Infection caused by *Neisseria gonorrheae.* It can be symptomatic with cervicitis and vaginal discharge, or it may be asymptomatic.
- Gonorrhea may lead to pelvic inflammatory disease.

Syphilis

- Syphilis is a systemic disease caused by the bacteria ***Treponema pallidum***.
- If not treated, syphilis may progress from a primary infection characterized by a painless ulcer (chancre), to secondary and tertiary infections.
- Serological tests may be negative in the early stages of infection.

Pelvic Inflammatory Diseases (PID)

- Ascending pelvic infection that involves upper genital tract.
- Commonly caused by bacteria.
- Most common cause of PID is chlamydia followed by Neisseria gonorrhea.
- E-coli cause PID among post-menopausal women.
- PID is a sexually transmitted disease.
- **Signs and symptoms:**
  - Pain ranges from dull aching to severe cramping in lower abdomen.
  - Nausea, elevated temperature, foul smelling, purulent discharge.

Genital TB

- Route of spread: hematogenous
- Most commonly affected site is fallopian tube followed by endometrium
- Most common complication is infertility

CERVICAL CANCER SCREENING

- Cervical intraepithelial neoplasia (CIN) is the precursor lesion to cervical cancer.
- Pap smear test allows early diagnosis of most cases
- Recommendations for cervical cancer screening for women:
  - Annual cervical cytology screening should begin approximately 3 years after initiation of sexual intercourse, but no later than age 21 years.
  - Women younger than 30 years should undergo annual cervical cytology screening.
  - The use of combination cervical cytology and human papillomavirus (HPV) and DNA screening is appropriate for women 30 years and older.
  - Women who underwent **total hysterectomy** for reasons other than cervical cancer no longer need to be screened for cervical cancer.

LACTATION AND FEEDING

Exclusive Breastfeeding

- According to WHO, exclusive breastfeeding means that the infant receives only breast milk. No other liquids or solids are given – not even water – with the exception of oral rehydration solution, or drops/syrups of vitamins, minerals or medicines.
- **WHO and UNICEF** recommend that children initiate breastfeeding within the first hour of birth and be exclusively breastfed for the first 6 months of life.

KEY POINTS

TORCH:

- Acronym of Toxoplasmosis, Rubella, Cytomegalovirus and Herpes Simplex.
- TORCH infections can affect growing embryo and cause congenital anomalies, abnormal fetal development, mental retardation and fetal death.

Recent Question (NORCET 2020)

46. PAP Smear test is used in the diagnosis of:
a. Uterine cancer
b. Cervical cancer
c. Valval cancer
d. Ovarian cancer

Ans. (b) Cervical cancer

Recent Question (NORCET 2021)

47. What is the daily additional calories required for pregnant women?
a. 300 calories
b. 500 calories
c. 100 calories
d. 800 calories

Ans. (a) 300 calories

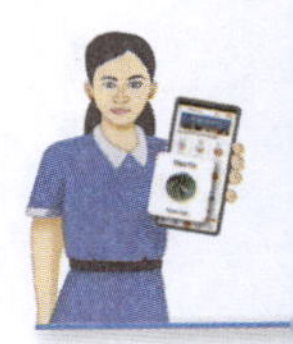

- Extra calories required during lactation is 600 kcal/day.
- Oxytocin is the hormone which helps in milk ejection/galactokinesis/let down reflex.
- Prolactin is the milk producing or galactopoiesis hormone.
- Cabergoline is a drug which decreases the prolactin level.
- Bromocriptine is another drug which reduces the prolactin level. Side effect of this drug is increase in BP.
- Metoclopramide is a drug which increases the prolactin level.

Types of Breast Milk

- **Colostrum**
  - Colostrum is the first stage of breast milk (lasts for several days after delivery)
  - Yellowish in color and rich in nutrients and antibodies
  - High in protein, vitamin A, sodium and chloride; Low in carbohydrate, fat and potassium than the breast milk.
  - **Advantages:** Presence of humoral factors (lactoferrin) and antibodies (IgA, IgG, IgM) provide immunity.
- **Transitional milk**
  - Transitional milk replaces colostrum within four days after delivery
  - It lasts for about two weeks
  - Contains more calories than colostrum
  - Contains lactose, water-soluble vitamins and high levels of fat.
- **Mature milk**
  - Begins to appear at the end of second week after delivery.
  - It is thinner than transitional milk (90% water)
  - **Two types of mature milk:** Foremilk and hindmilk.
  - **Foremilk** occurs at the beginning of feeding (contains vitamin, water and protein)
  - **Hindmilk** forms at the end of the feeding (contains higher level of fat which helps in weight gain of the infant).

Benefits of Breastfeeding

- **For baby**
  - Ideal nutrition for proper growth and development
  - Ideal composition of all required nutrition
  - Less chances of developing diabetes and obesity
  - Presence of antibodies enhances immunity
  - Protection against allergies, respiratory and intestinal infections
- **For mother**
  - Acts as contraceptive (lactation suppresses ovulation)
  - Improves mother-baby bonding
  - Release of oxytocin during breastfeeding helps in uterine involution
  - Weight loss
  - Reduces the risk of cancer of breast, ovary and endometrium.

Correct Positioning

- The baby's head and body should be in straight line
- The baby should be facing the breast
- The baby's nose should be opposite to mother's nipple
- Hold the baby close to the body
- Support the baby's whole body.

Signs of Good Attachment

- Mouth wide open
- Lower lip turned outward
- Baby's chin touching breast
- More of areola visible above the baby's mouth.

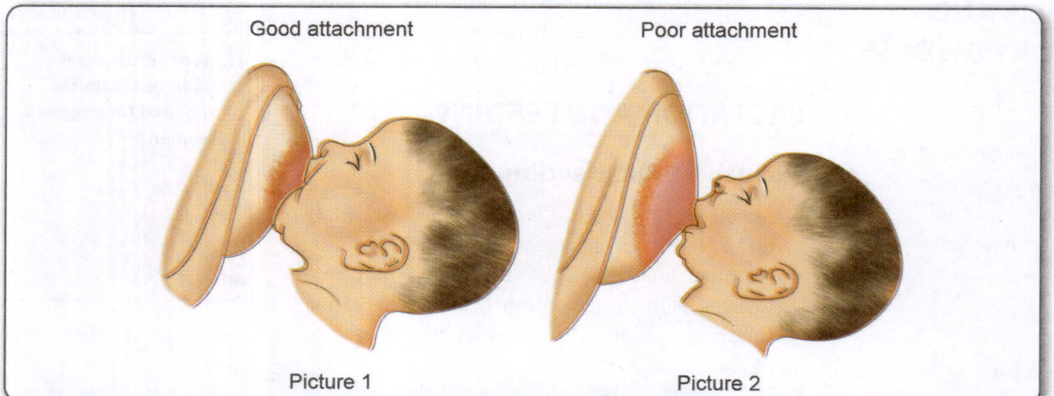

Figure 55: Good and poor attachment

POINTS TO REMEMBER

- **DO NOT** force the baby to take the breast.
- **DO NOT** interrupt feed before baby wants.
- **DO NOT** give any other feeds or water.
- **DO NOT** use artificial teats or pacifiers.

Recent Questions (NORCET 2021)

48. A lactating mother is diagnosed with breast abscess in one of the breasts. Identify the correct measure to be taken by the mother:
a. No breastfeeding by both breasts
b. Continue breastfeeding by opposite breast
c. Give formula feed
d. Give cow milk

Ans. (b) Continue breastfeeding by opposite breast

49. Which of the following is not given to lactating mothers?
a. DMPA
b. POP
c. Mini pills
d. Combined OCPs

Ans. (d) Combined OCPs

Recent Question (NORCET 2022)

50. Which of the following postpartum drugs is safe for breastfeeding mothers?
a. Lithium
b. Captopril
c. Enalpril
d. Hydrochlorothiazide

Ans. (d) Hydrochlorothiazide

KEY POINTS

Management of breastfeeding

- After birth, let the baby rest comfortably on the mother's chest in skin-to-skin contact
- The baby can be put to mother's breast within half hour after birth
- Keep the mother and baby together in bed or within easy reach (rooming-in). **Do not** separate them
- Signs of readiness to breastfeed are baby looking around/moving, mouth open, searching
- Check that position and attachment are correct at the first feed
- Teach the mother correct positioning and attachment for breastfeeding
- Teach the mother how to hold her baby

Contraindications to Breastfeeding

- Mothers on drugs that can be harmful to baby (e.g., Cytotoxics, radioactive isotopes, etc.)
- Babies with birth defects such as cleft lip and cleft palate
- Preterm and very ill babies
- Infant is diagnosed with classic galactosemia
- Mother has suspected or confirmed Ebola virus disease

GTPAL

G – Gravidity

- Number of times woman has been pregnant including current pregnancy irrespective of its outcome.
- Includes miscarriages/abortions
- Twins /triplets count as one

T – Term Births

Child born at 37 weeks or later (twin/triplets count as one)

P – Preterm Births

- Child born between 20 and 37 weeks
- Includes alive or stillborn (twins or triplets count as one)

A – Abortions

Counts as pregnancy

L – Living Children

- Number of living children
- Twin/triplets count individually

Case Examples

A 29-year-old woman is currently 25 weeks pregnant. She had a miscarriage at 12 weeks of gestation three years ago. She has a 4-year-old child who was born at 38 weeks. What is her GTPAL?

Answer: G = 3, T = 1, P = 0, A-1, L = 1

A 30-year-old woman is currently 24 weeks pregnant with twins. She has 8-year-old twins who were born at 36 weeks of gestation, and 10-year-old who was born on 39 weeks of gestation. Five years before, she had a miscarriage at 10 weeks of pregnancy. What is her GTPAL?

Answer: G = 4, T = 1, P = 1, A = 1 L = 3

POINTS TO REMEMBER

- WHO recommends that Mothers known to be HIV-infected (and whose infants are HIV uninfected or of unknown HIV status) should exclusively breastfeed their infants for the first 6 months of life, introducing appropriate complementary foods thereafter, and continue breastfeeding. (Subject to approval by national authorities of countries.)
- In India, National Aids Control Organization (NACO) recommends that HIV-infected women can choose to safely breastfeed their infants with ARV drugs providing protection against transmission of the HIV virus.
- In USA, HIV infected mothers should not breastfeed their infants.

Recent Question

(NORCET 2023)

51. A pregnant client comes to the clinic for her first prenatal examination at 10 weeks. She has been pregnant twice before; the first delivery produced a viable baby girl at 38 weeks 5 years ago; the second pregnancy produced a viable baby boy at 35 weeks 3 years ago. Both children are living and well. What is the GTPAL in this case?

a. 3-2-0-0-2
b. 2-2-0-2-2
c. 3-1-1-0-2
d. 2-1-1-0-2

Ans. (c) 3-1-1-0-2

Golden Points to Remember

- There are the **four openings** in the vestibule:
  1. Urethral
  2. Vaginal orifice and hymen
  3. Opening of Bartholin's duct
  4. Skene's gland
- **Fallopian tube is divided into 4 parts** that is interstitial, isthmus, ampulla, and infundibulum.
- The term **parturition** refers to the process of giving birth to a child including both labor and delivery.
- **A parturient** is a woman in labor.
- Full mature ovum is the largest cell in the body and is about **130 microns in diameter**.
- Release of oocyte (ovum) from the ovary following rupture of mature Graafian follicle and available for conception is known as **ovulation**.
- **Fertilization** is the process of fusion of the spermatozoon with the mature ovum.
- Implantation of fertilized ovum occurs through four stages, i.e., **apposition, adhesion, penetration** and **invasion.**
- The decidua is the endometrial layer of the pregnant uterus.
- Daily urine output of fetus at term is **400–1200 mL**.
- **The green color of amniotic fluid** indicates the presence of **meconium**.
- Amniotic fluid appears **golden color** in case of Rh incompatibility.
- Amniotic fluid appears **dark-brown** color in **intrauterine death.**
- **Embryonic period begins** at 3rd weeks up to 8 weeks' post-conception.
- The fetus is **viable** if born after 28 weeks of gestation.
- At term the weight of fetus varies from **2.5 kg to 3.5 kg** (In India).
- **Hematopoiesis** begins first in the yolk sac by 14th day of conception.
- At term 75–80% of the total hemoglobin is of fetal type HbF.
- At term fetal **IgG level is 10% higher** than the mother.
- The maternal **immunoglobulin G (IgG)** crosses the placenta from 12 weeks of pregnancy onward.
- The umbilical vein carries the oxygenated blood from placenta to fetus.
- Functional closure of **foramen ovale occurs soon after birth** but **anatomical closure** takes place in about one year.
- The weight of the uterus at term is **900–1000 g.**
- The weight of the uterus in non-pregnant state is **60 g**.
- **Dextrorotation** is rotation of uterus on its long axis to the right.
- Irregular, spasmodic and painless contraction without dilatation of cervix is known as **Braxton-Hicks contraction.**
- Braxton-Hicks contraction is **not felt in abdominal pregnancy.**
- Secretion can be squeezed out of breast at **12 weeks.**
- **Chloasma gravidarum or melasma is** pigmentation around the cheek, forehead and around the eyes. Chloasma gravidarum is also known as **pregnancy mask.**
- Pigmented area from xiphisternum to symphysis pubis is called **Linea Nigra**.
- Pigmentary changes take place during the pregnancy due to melanocyte stimulation by anterior pituitary.
- A normal healthy woman should gain about 10–12 kg of weight during pregnancy.
- Water retention at term is **6.5 Liters**.
- Due to elevation of the diaphragm (because of the enlarged uterus), the **heart is pushed upward and outward.**
- **Cardiac output** starts to increase at 5th week of pregnancy.
- Total iron requirement during pregnancy is estimated approximately 1000 mg of elemental iron.
- Hormones essential for **follicular maturation** are FHS and small proportion of LH.
- **Human Chorionic Gonodotrophin (hCG)** is secreted by the syncytiotrophoblast cell.
- During pregnancy preparation of breast is called **mammogenesis.**
- Ejection of breast milk is known as **galactokinesis.**
- **Galactopoiesis** refers to maintenance of lactation.
- Thick yellow secretion from the breast occurs at **16 weeks**.
- On examination the height of uterus remains at:
  - The level of symphysis pubis at **12 weeks of pregnancy**.
  - The level of umbilicus at **24 weeks of pregnancy.**
  - Midway between the symphysis pubis and umbilicus at **16th weeks of pregnancy.**
- Reproductive period of a woman begins at **menarche** and ends in **menopause**.
- The normal period of pregnancy is **280 days (40 weeks).**
- Discoloration and cyanosis of the vulva, vagina, and cervix (Chadwick sign), Goodell's sign, Hegar's sign, uterine enlargement, Braxton Hicks contractions, positive blood pregnancy test are known as **probable signs of pregnancy** (non-specific).
- The positive signs of pregnancy include the detection of a fetal heartbeat, the recognition of fetal movements and visualization of fetus through ultrasound.
- A positive over-the-counter pregnancy test is considered a probable sign of pregnancy.
- Over-the-counter pregnancy tests detect the presence of Human Chorionic Gonadotropin (hCG) hormone.
- Discoloration of the vestibule and anterior wall of vagina is known as **Jacquemier's sign.**
- **Chadwick's sign:** Purplish discoloration of vaginal mucosa visible at 8th week of pregnancy.
- Regular and rhythmic uterine contraction elicited during bimanual examination is known as **palmer's sign.**
- Naegele's formula is used to calculate EDD from LMP. Add 9 calendar months and 7 days to the first day of the last normal period. EDD = LMP + 9 months + 7 days.
- The perception of 1st active fetal movement by women is known as Quickening (feeling of life). It occurs about 18–20 weeks in a **primigravida** and as early as 16 weeks in the **multigravida**.

Contd...

- **Lightening:** Decrease in fundal height a few weeks before onset of labor is known as **lightening (38th week).**
- Lightening is called **Welcome sign** of the baby (38th week).
- Greatest weight gain of the fetus occurs in third trimester of pregnancy.
- Greatest growth in height/length of fetus occurs in second trimester of pregnancy.
- Palpation of the fetal parts is possible at 20th week of pregnancy.
- Active fetal movement can be felt by placing the hand over the uterus by 20th week of pregnancy.
- Fetal heart sound is the most **conclusive clinical sign of pregnancy.**
- Fetal heart starts to beat near to 22 days (3 weeks) after the woman has conceived but the sound is too soft to hear. It can be heard by 6th – 7th week at the earliest through ultrasound.
- **Fetal Heart Tone (FHT) can be observed through Doppler as early as 8–10 weeks and through fetoscope at 18-20 weeks of gestation.**
- Fetal heart tones can usually be detected with a stethoscope between 16 and 20 weeks.
- Uterine shape is changed from cylindrical to spherical after 36th week of pregnancy.
- Crown-rump length of fetus can be detected in ultrasonography at 7th week.
- **Johnson's formula, Hadlock formula and Shephard formula are** used for the estimation of fetal weight.
- Relationship of the long axis of the fetus to the long axis of the centralized uterus or maternal spine is called **fetus lie**.
- **Presentation** is the part of the fetus which occupies the lower pole of the uterus.
- Relation of the denominator to the different quadrant of the pelvis is called **position**.
- Abdominal examinations beyond 28 weeks of pregnancy can reasonably diagnose presentation, position, and attitude of the fetus.
- The formation of swelling due to stagnation of fluid in the layers of the scalp is called **caput succedaneum**.
- Pelvic bone is composed of **four bones:**
  - Two innominate bones,
  - Sacrum, and
  - Coccyx.
- **Female pelvic joints** are two sacroiliac joint, sacrococcygeal joint and symphysis pubic.
- The transverse diameter of the pelvic inlet is 13 cm.
- Systemic supervision of women during pregnancy is called **antenatal care.**
- "Para" is defined as the number of past pregnancies gone beyond period of viability.
- Total number of pregnancies a woman had is called 'Gravida'.
- **Primigravida** is one who is pregnant for the first time.
- The newest guidelines from the WHO recommend that **women** attend 8 Antenatal Clinic (ANC) visits.
- Recommended antenatal visit schedule according to the 2016 WHO ANC model,
  - **Contact 1 – up to 12 weeks**
  - **Contact 2–20 weeks**
  - **Contact 3–24 weeks**
  - **Contact 4–30 weeks**
  - **Contact 5–34 weeks**
  - **Contact 6–36 weeks**
  - **Contact 7–38 weeks**
  - **Contact 8–40 weeks**
- According to WHO FANC Model (old)
  - **Visit 1 - 8–12 weeks of pregnancy**
  - Visit 2 - 24–26 weeks
  - Visit 3 - 32nd week
  - Visit 4 - 36–38 weeks
- Increasing the intake of vegetables, fruits and fluid is the best method to relieve from constipation during pregnancy.
- A sedentary woman needs 1,875 calories per day. **In Addition**, pregnant mother requires 300 calories. Totally pregnant mother requires 2,175 calories per day.
- **Abdominal circumference** is the single measurement which best **reflects fetal nutrition.**
- **Triple test includes** MSAFP, hCG, and uE3. It is used for detection of Down's syndrome. It is performed at **15 to 18 weeks** of pregnancy.
- Expulsion of the viable products of conception out of womb through the vagina into outer world is called **labor.**
- Normal labor also called **Eutocia.**
- Abnormal labor also called **Dystocia.**
- False labor pain is manifested by:
  - Abdominal discomfort
  - Contractions irregular in nature
  - Contraction lessen with activity or rest
  - Cervical dilation is not seen in false pains
  - Pain is relied by enema
- There are the **FOUR** stages of labor: 1. Thinning (effacement) and opening (dilation) of the cervix 2. Baby moving through birth canal 3. Afterbirth 4. Recovery.
- Average duration of **the 1st stage of labor is 12 hours in primigravidae**, and **6 hours in multiparae**.
- Second stage of labor got 2 phases that is **propulsive** and **expulsive**.
- **Pacemaker of the uterine contraction** is situated in the region of the **tubal ostia.**
- Intra-amniotic pressure rises 20 mm Hg during uterine contraction.
- Coordination between fundal contraction and cervical dilatation called **polarity of uterus.**
- Following child birth during which the body tissues, especially the pelvic organs revert back to the pre-pregnant state both anatomically and physiologically. This is called normal **Puerperium.**
- **Puerperium period** starts from after delivery up to the 6 weeks.
- Regeneration of the placental site takes 6 weeks.
- Following delivery, fundus lies about 13.5 cm above the symphysis pubic.
- There are three **types of Lochia.** They are:
  i. Lochia Rubra (1–4 days)

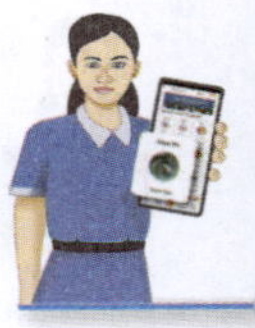

Contd...

ii. Lochia Serosa (5–9 days)
iii. Lochia Alba (10–15 days)

- **Lochia rubra** consists of blood, shreds of fetal membranes and decidua, vernix caseosa, lanugo and meconium.
- The immunoglobulin present in colostrums is **IgA.**
- **Oxytocin** is the major galactokinetic (milk ejection) hormones.
- **Prolactin** appears to be the single most important galactopoietic **(milk production)** hormones.
- Excessive vomiting in 1st trimester is called **Hyperemesis Gravidarum.**
- Abortion is considered before the 20th week of gestation.
- Abortion associated with clinical evidence of infection of the uterus and its contents is called **septic abortion.**
- Missed abortion is also known as **silent abortion**.
- **Incomplete abortion:** In this, fetus is expelled but parts of the placenta and membranes are not expelled.
- Two methods of induction of labor include medical and surgical method.
- An **ectopic pregnancy** is one in which the fertilized ovum is implanted and develops outside the normal endometrial cavity.
- The site of ectopic pregnancy in tube is isthmus, ampullary, and interstitial.
- **Transvaginal sonography (TVS)** gives the most appropriate finding related to ectopic pregnancy.
- Sonography feature of molar pregnancy is **"Snow storm" appearance**.
- Cullen's sign is superficial edema and bruising in the subcutaneous fatty tissue around the umbilicus in ruptured ectopic pregnancy.
- **Hydatidiform mole** is a rare mass or growth that forms inside the uterus at the beginning of a pregnancy. It is a type of **gestational trophoblastic disease (GTD).**
- Hydatidiform mole is also known as **vesicular mole**.
- **Vanishing twin**, also known as fetal resorption, is a fetus in a multigestational pregnancy which dies in utero and is then partially and completely reabsorbed by the twin.
- Miscarriage rate is increased, especially with monozygotic twins.
- In the active management of labor, IM injection of **Ergometrine** (500 mcg in 1 mL) is given **after delivery of the anterior shoulder,** or at the latest, immediately after delivery of the child. In multiple births, it should not be administered until the last child has been delivered.
- **Quadruplets:** Number of the baby is four.
- **Quintuplets:** Number of the baby is five.
- **Polyhydramnios** is a state where liquor amnii exceeds 2000 mL.
- In Polyhydramnios, amniotic fluid index is more than 24 cm (>95th percentile for gestational age).
- **Indomethacin** is given to decrease amniotic fluid.
- Liquor amnii less than 200 mL at term is called **Oligohydramnios.**
- One or more small lobe of placenta placed at varying distance from main placenta is called **placenta succenturiata.**
- Cord attached to the margin of placenta is called **battledore placenta**.
- Cord length less than 20 cm is called short **cord**.
- **HELLP syndrome: H**emolysis, **E**levated **L**iver enzyme, **L**ow **P**latelet count.
- Urinary output less than 400 mL/24 hours in preeclamptic woman is termed oliguria (diminished urinary output).
- The therapeutic level of magnesium sulfate in blood is 4–7 mEq/L.
- Loss of Patellar reflex (deep tendon reflex) is the early warning sign of magnesium toxicity.
- When repeated doses of magnesium sulfate are given parenterally, **knee jerk reflexes** should be tested before each dose. If reflexes are absent, no additional magnesium should be given until reflex return.
- Parenteral administration of magnesium sulfate is contraindicated in patients with heart block or myocardial damage.
- **Calcium gluconate** is the drug of choice to treat magnesium sulfate toxicity.
- Placenta implanted partially or completely over the lower uterine segment is called **placenta previa.**
- **Type II Posterior Placenta Previa** is known as **Dangerous** placenta previa
- Bleeding from or into the genital tract after 28th weeks of pregnancy is called **Antepartum Hemorrhage (APH).**
- In APH **ultrasonography** is the initial procedure either to confirm or to rule out the diagnosis.
- **Betamethasone** is given to accelerate fetal lung maturity in preterm.
- During pregnancy, **anemia** is defined as Hb <10 g/dL.
- **Leishman stain** (study the morphology of the red cells) gives better idea about type of anemia.
- **Mean corpuscular hemoglobin concentration (MCHC)** is the most sensitive index of iron deficiency anemia (<30).
- **Megaloblastic anemia** in pregnancy is always due to folic and B12 deficiency.
- Daily requirement of folic acid in pregnancy is 400 ug/day (4 mg/daily).
- Increase in homocysteine and normal methylmalonate indicates folate deficiency.
- Maternal hyperglycemia during pregnancy can lead to fetal **macrosomia**.
- **Lugol's** solution is used in hyperthyroidism.
- **Streptomycin** crosses placental barrier, so it is contraindicated during pregnancy.
- **Preterm labor** is defined as **regular contractions** of the uterus resulting in changes in the cervix that start before 37 weeks of pregnancy.
- Labor occurs after 20 weeks but before 37 weeks is termed **preterm labor.**
- Pregnancy continuing beyond two weeks of the expected date of delivery (>294 days) is called **post-term or post-maturity**.
- The main clinical significance of post-term maturity is **dysmaturity** or **macrosomia**.

Contd...

- Scar dehiscence means asymptomatic separation of thinning of the scar without involving the peritoneal coat and without any hemorrhage.
- Artificial rupture of membrane is called **Amniotomy**.
- Pelvis is divided into four types—gynecoid, anthropoid, android, and platypelloid.
- The fetus head can be pushed down up to the level of ischial spines and there is no overlapping of the parietal bone over the symphysis pubis. This means **no disproportion.**
- **Constriction ring** is situated at the junction of the upper and lower segment around a constricted part of fetus.
- Both the thighs and legs are partially extended bringing the legs to present at the brim in **footling presentation**.
- When the fetus position is constantly changed after the 36 weeks of pregnancy this stage is called **unstable lie.**
- When the cephalic presentation is complicated by the presence of hand or foot or both alongside the head by the side of breech is called **compound presentation**.
- Cord is lying inside the vagina or outside the vulva following rupture of the membranes is called **cord prolapse**.
- Sims' position should be maintained if cord is prolapsed.
- Abnormally a large-size baby weighing more than 4 kg is considered **macrosomic**.
- **Cleidotomy** is one or both clavicles may be cut with scissors to reduce the shoulder girth.
- **Folic acid supplementation** will reduce the incidence of **Neural Tube Defects (NTD).**
- Blood loss in excess of 500 mL following birth of the baby is called **PostPartum Hemorrhage (PPH)**.
- In atonic hemorrhage the uterus turns flabby and becomes hard on massaging.
- The placenta is said to be retained when it is not expelled out even **30 minutes** after the **birth of the baby.**
- Placenta directly anchored to the myometrium is called **placenta accrete**.
- The uterus is turned inside out partially or completely is called **inversion of uterus**.
- An infection of the genital tract which occurs as a complication of delivery is termed **puerperal sepsis**.
- Rise of temperature **reaching 100.4** or more on two separated occasions at 24 hours apart from first 10 days following delivery is called **puerperal pyrexia**.
- **Dicloxacillin** (500 mg every 6 hourly) is drug of choice in the acute mastitis.
- **Immediate puerperal emergencies** are PPH, shock, postpartum eclampsia, pulmonary embolism.
- After the delivery **molding** subsides within 5 days.
- **Brushfield's spots** (white or greyish brown spots) in the iris is seen in Down's syndrome.
- **Rooming-in** promotes maternal-infant bonding.
- Baby born before completing 37 weeks of gestational age is called **preterm baby.**
- **Asymmetrical Moro reflex** in newborn is associated with brachial plexus, cervical or humerus injuries.
- Progressive thinning and shortening of cervix are defined as effacement.
- The increase in diameter of cervix is called dilation.
- Hundred percent effacement and 10 cm cervical dilation occurs in second stage just before the delivery of fetus.
- **Bishop's score** parameter includes cervical dilatation, effacement, consistency, position and station of head.
- The favorable Bishop's score is 6–13 and unfavorable score is 0–5.
- In **cervicograph** the alter line starts at 3 cm.
- Normal **fetal heart rate** is 110–160 beats/min.
- A significant predictor of fetal well-being is fetal heart rate between 120 and 160 beats/min.
- **Tocolytics** (terbutalin 0.25 mg SC) are used when uterus is hypertonic and there is non-reassuring FHR.
- **Omphalitis** is the inflammation of the umbilical cord; it is also called umbilical sepsis.
- Low level of AFP found in Down's syndrome.
- Down's syndrome is the **trisomy 21**.
- Upward and outward slanting of the eyes with epicanthic folds; short upper lip with small mouth, macroglossia and Mongolian signs are the feature of **Down's syndrome.**
- Uterine tetany could result from the use of oxytocin to induce labor because oxytocin promotes powerful **uterine contractions**.
- Method of **surgical induction of labor** includes ARM and stripping the membranes.
- **Intracervical application of dinoprostone gel** is the gold standard for cervical ripening.
- **Radical mastectomy** refers to removal of breast/s, pectoral muscle, pectoral fascia and nodes.
- **Cessation of menses** in women is due to the inability of the ovary to respond to gonadotropic hormone.
- Main blood supply for uterus is carried out by **Uterine and Ovarian Arteries.**
- **Erb's palsy** is one of the complications of breech delivery. It is characterized by flaccid arms with elbows extended.
- **Intervention** is usually undertaken to help treat or cure a condition. It is a range of motion exercises.
- Morning after pill acts by preventing the implantation of the fertilized ovum if taken within 12 hours' post-intercourse.
- The visual examination of the cervix and vagina by special instruments is called Colposcopy.
- The best time for insertion of IUD is after 2–3 days after the period is over. Intra uterine devices (IUD) insertion is scheduled within 7 days from starting of period. Because internal os is slightly open during the first 7 days of periods and chance of already being pregnant is ruled out in this period.
- The most common problem with IUD is **spontaneous expulsion of device**.
- Mitral stenosis is the valvular lesions that causes a risk of maternal death during labor.
- The main cause of genital warts (Condylomata Acuminata) is Human Papilloma Virus (HPV).
- Genital herpes simplex increases the risk of **cervix cancer**.
- The gold standard for the treatment of hot flushes is **Estrogen administration.** Hot flushes commonly occur due to menopause.

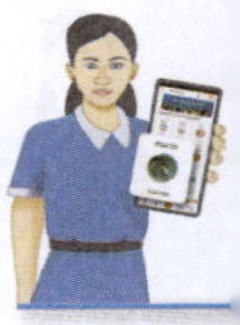

Contd...

- When the posterior bladder wall protrudes downward through the anterior vaginal wall, it is known as cystocele.
- At around 10th day of conception, synthesis of hCG takes place by syncytiotrophoblast cells.
- The fetal blood flow through the placenta is about 500 mL/min.
- Pressure in the umbilical artery is 60 mm/hg.
- Fetus swallows about 400–700 mL of liquor every day.
- The mean cardiac output in fetus is estimated to be 350 mL/kg/min.
- Daily requirement of calcium during pregnancy and lactation averages 1–1.5 g.
- Pregnancy associated plasma protein – A (PAPP – A) is secreted by syncytiotrophoblast and it acts as an immunosuppressant in pregnancy.
- Two site sandwich immunoassay is positive on the first day of the missed period (28th day of cycle).
- **Pseudocyesis** is a psychological disorder where the women have the false belief that she is pregnant although there is no pregnancy exists.
- Johnson's formula, Shepard's formula and Hadlock's formula are used for the **estimation of fetal weight.**
- Expulsion of cervical mucus plug mixed with blood is called **show**.
- Increased thirst in early puerperium is due to the loss of fluid during labor in the lochia, diuresis and perspiration.
- **Endotoxic shock** mostly due to clostridium welchii and Escherichia coli infection.
- **Mifepristone** should not be used in women aged over 35 years, heavy smokers and the clients on long term corticosteroid.
- **The classical triad of symptoms of tubal pregnancy** are abdominal pain, appearance of vaginal bleeding and amenorrhea.
- **Spiegelberg's criteria** is used for the diagnosis of ovarian pregnancy.
- Pregnancy occurring in the rudimentary horn of a bicornuate uterus is called **cornual pregnancy.**
- At 2–3 weeks of gestational age, the neural plate becomes spinal cord and brain in the fetus.
- Differentiation of the external genitalia occurs at the end of the ninth week of gestational age.
- Internal differences in the male and female occur at the end of the seventh week of gestational age.
- When assessing the fundal height, monitor the client for supine hypotension when placed in the supine position.
- In a neonate, the symptoms of methadone withdrawal may begin 7 days to several weeks after birth.
- The mother having a sudden burst of energy is known as **nesting**. It occurs often 24–48 hours before the onset of labor.
- Fetal heart rate fluctuations greater than 25 bpm is called **marked variability.**
- Friedman curve may be used to identify whether a women's cervical dilation during labor is progressing at the expected rate.
- Normal maternal hemoglobin is 11–13 g/dL
- Tidal volume increases throughout pregnancy because of a small degree of hyperventilation that occurs during pregnancy.
- Fibroids, obesity, and polyhydramnios can all increase fundal height and give a false measurement.
- **Nocturnal frequency** a week after delivery may be a sign of a **urinary tract infection (UTI).**
- The quadruple screen is performed between 15 and 18 weeks and assesses for trisomies 13, 18, and 21 and for neural tube defects.
- The one-hour glucose screening is performed between 24 and 28 weeks of pregnancy.
- Amniocentesis is performed between 15 and 20 weeks to confirm diagnosis of Down's syndrome.
- The lack of fetal heart activity in a pregnancy over 6 weeks determines a fetal loss.
- The most significant medical risk that can occur with air travel during pregnancy is deep vein thrombosis, because pregnancy increases the risk of blood coagulation and prolonged sitting produces venous stasis.
- Before providing a specimen for a sperm count, the patient should avoid ejaculation for 48–72 hours.
- Vigorous movement by the fetus followed by no movement may indicate fetal demise and is cause for further assessment.
- Leopold maneuvers are used to assess the fetus's position in utero.
- A high-fiber diet is the first intervention that should be attempted when counseling a woman on the management of hemorrhoids.
- CBC and hemoglobin electrophoresis are both appropriate tests for diagnosing hemoglobinopathies in pregnant women.
- When the fetus is in the breech position, fetal heart tones are best heard at or above the level of the umbilicus.
- The client with placenta previa needs to restrict her activities and may be placed on bed rest. She should avoid sexual intercourse, strenuous activity, and long-distance travel.
- Benign tumors found in the smooth muscle of the uterus are leiomyomas or fibroids.

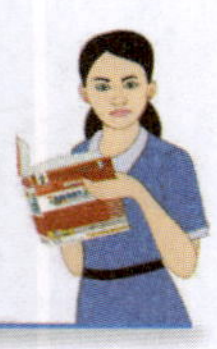

"He who has health has hope; and he who has hope has everything."

—Arabian proverb

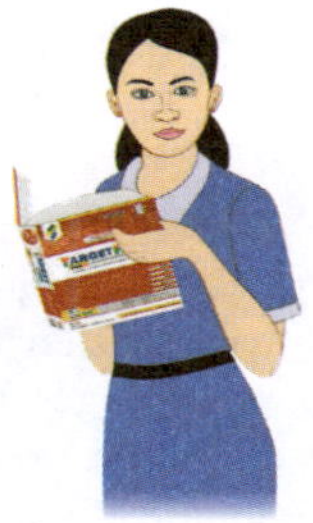

CLINICAL CASE-BASED QUESTIONS

1

The nurse gives Rh_0(D) injection to a 32-year-old primigravida woman presents with 28th week of pregnancy. Which of the following conditions require administering the injection to the woman?

a. Rh positive mother and Rh negative father
b. Rh negative mother and Rh positive father
c. Both parents are Rh negative
d. Both parents are Rh positive

Ans. (b) Rh negative mother and Rh positive father

Explanation: Rh_0(D) injection, also known as Rh immunoglobulin or Rhogam, is administered to prevent the development of Rh isoimmunization in Rh negative mothers during pregnancy. Rh isoimmunization can occur when an Rh negative mother carries an Rh-positive fetus.

In this scenario, the woman is a primigravida (first-time pregnant) and in her 28th week of pregnancy. The injection is necessary when the mother is Rh negative, and the father is Rh positive.

2

The nurse educates a mother-to-be about possible danger signs during the last three months of pregnancy. All of the following findings may be the cause of concern; except:

a. Continuous headache
b. Blurred vision
c. Slight rectal bleeding
d. Marked swelling of hands

Ans. (c) Slight rectal bleeding

Explanation: Slight rectal bleeding is not typically considered a danger sign during the last three months of pregnancy. While any bleeding during pregnancy should be reported to a healthcare professional for evaluation slight rectal bleeding is less likely to be directly related to complications specific to pregnancy.

Other given symptoms such as continuous headache, blurred vision and marked swelling of hands can be indicative of conditions such as pre-eclampsia or gestational hypertension, which can be serious and require immediate medical evaluation.

3

The nurse assesses a pregnant woman who has tested positive for gonorrhea. Which of the following medications should be added by the nurse in the treatment plan?

a. Azithromycin
b. Tetracycline
c. Ceftriaxone
d. Ciprofloxacin

Ans. (c) Ceftriaxone

Explanation: Ceftriaxone and spectinomycin are safe and effective for the treatment of gonorrhea in pregnancy. Tetracycline, and ciprofloxacin are not safe to take during pregnancy. Azithromycin monotherapy for gonorrhea is not recommended.

4

A 32-year-old primigravida woman admitted in Obs-Gyn department due to pre-eclampsia. The woman has a history of diabetes mellitus. Which of the following actions should the nurse take first?

a. Closely monitor the blood pressure of the woman
b. Prepare the woman for child birth
c. Ask the health care provider to prescribe calcium supplements
d. Administer low-dose aspirin as prescribed

Ans. (b) Prepare the woman for child birth

Explanation: Pre-eclampsia is a serious condition characterized by high blood pressure and organ dysfunction during pregnancy. It can be life-threatening to both the mother and the baby. The only definitive treatment for pre-eclampsia is the delivery of the baby and the placenta.

Given the woman's diagnosis of pre-eclampsia, the nurse's priority should be to prepare her for childbirth. This may involve notifying the physician, arranging for necessary interventions such as induction of labor or cesarean section, and ensuring that the delivery environment is ready to provide appropriate care.

5

A 28-year G1 presents to your hospital at 8 weeks of gestation. She has a history of diabetes since age 14. She uses insulin and denies any complications related to her diabetes. Which of the following is the most common birth defect associated to diabetes:

a. Anencephaly
b. Meningomyelocele
c. Sacral agenesis
d. Ventricular septal defect

Ans. (d) Ventricular septal defect

Explanation: Diabetes, particularly poorly controlled diabetes, can increase the risk of various birth defects in infants. Among them, the most commonly associated defect is a ventricular septal defect (VSD). Ventricular septal defect refers to an opening in the septum, the wall that separates the two lower chambers (ventricles) of the heart.

6

A 28 year primigravida presents with pregnancy induced hypertension with blood pressure of 150/100 mm of Hg at 32 weeks of gestation with no other complications. Subsequently, her blood pressure is controlled on treatment. If there are no complications, the pregnancy should be terminated at:

a. 40 completed weeks
b. 37 completed weeks
c. 35 completed weeks
d. 34 completed weeks

Ans. (b) 37 completed weeks

Explanation: In cases of pregnancy induced hypertension without other complications, the general guideline is to consider delivery at around 37 to 38 weeks of gestation. This is because prolonging the pregnancy beyond this point can increase the risk of complications such as pre-eclampsia, fetal growth restriction, and placental abruption.

7

A 32-year-old woman presents with lower abdominal cramping, and pregnancy is confirmed by a positive urine hCG test and a pelvic ultrasound showing a 10-week intrauterine pregnancy. The patient expresses uncertainty about whether to continue the pregnancy. What is the most suitable next course of action?

a. Discuss the situation with the patient's parents.
b. Inform the patient's partner about the situation.
c. Counsel the patient or refer her to an appropriate counselor.
d. Consider terminating the pregnancy.

Ans. (c) Counsel the patient or refer her to an appropriate counselor.

Explanation: It is essential to provide the patient with the necessary support and information to help her make an informed decision regarding her pregnancy. Counseling can help the patient explore her feelings, discuss her concerns, and understand her options. By offering counseling or referring the patient to an appropriate counselor, she can receive professional guidance.

8

A 29-year-old female, 16 weeks pregnant has 2-year-old twins, who were born at 38 weeks gestation and a 6-year-old who was born at 40 weeks, she had no history of abortion what is her GTPAL score?

a. G=3, T=2, P=0, A=0, L=3
b. G=3, T=1, P=0, A=2, L=3
c. G=3, T=2, P=2, A=0, L=3
d. G=3, T=1, P=0, A=0, L=2

Ans. (a) G=3, T=2, P=0, A=0, L=3

Explanation:

G=3 (Gravida: total number of pregnancies)

T=2 (Term births: number of pregnancies delivered at term, which is 37 weeks or more)

P=0 (Preterm births: number of pregnancies delivered before 37 weeks)

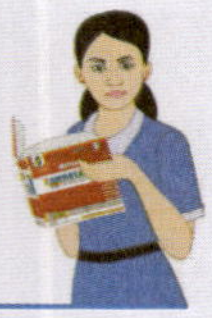

A=0 (Abortions: number of pregnancies that ended before 20 weeks)

L=3 (Living children: number of currently living children)

Therefore, the correct GTPAL score is: G=3, T=1, P=0, A=2, L=3.

9

Nurse Ramya is preparing for a woman health fair. She is aware that the Hormone Replacement Therapy (HRT) is related to:

a. An increased risk for osteoporosis related to bone fracture
b. An increased risk for coronary artery disease (CAD)
c. A decreased risk of deep vein thrombosis (DVT).
d. Decreased risk of breast cancer

Ans. (b) An increased risk for coronary artery disease (CAD)

Explanation: When teaching patients about the risks and benefits of hormone replacement therapy (HRT), it is important to provide accurate information. Research has shown that HRT is associated with an increased risk for coronary artery disease (CAD). HRT is related to decreased risk of osteoporosis, increased risk of DVT, and slightly increased risk of breast cancer.

10

A 32-year-old woman who is 12 weeks pregnant has recently been diagnosed with an autoimmune disease. Which of the following is the only immunoglobulin that will provide protection to the fetus in the womb?

a. IgA
b. IgD
c. IgE
d. IgG

Ans. (d) IgG

Explanation: Gamma globulin replacement therapy and the use of gamma globulin for autoimmune disease have been safe in pregnancy. The essential for maternal IgG to provide an immunoglobulin infusion to the fetus during the third trimester requires that the dose remain sufficient to maintain an adequate plasma IgG level in the mother during the pregnancy.

11

The nurse is conducting an education program for antenatal mothers about the effects of cigarette smoking on fetal development. Which of the following characteristics is associated with babies born to mothers who smoked during pregnancy?

a. Large for gestational age
b. Preterm birth, but appropriate size for gestation
c. Low birth weight
d. Growth retardation in weight and length

Ans. (c) Low birth weight

Explanation: Babies born to mothers who smoke during pregnancy are more likely to have a low birth weight. Cigarette smoking can restrict blood flow through the placenta, reducing the oxygen and nutrient supply to the developing fetus. This can result in impaired growth and development, leading to lower birth weight.

12

On the first postpartum night, a patient requests that her baby be sent back to the nursery so she can get some sleep. The patient is most likely in which of the following phases?

a. Depression phase
b. Letting-go phase
c. Taking-hold phase
d. Taking-in phase

Ans. (d) Taking-in phase

Explanation: The taking-in phase is the first phase of the postpartum period. It typically lasts for 2-3 days. During this phase, the woman is focused on her own needs and recovery. She may be tired, overwhelmed, and need a lot of support. She may also be feeling emotional and may cry easily.

It is common for women in the taking-in phase to ask for help with their baby. They may want their baby to be taken back to the nursery so they can get some sleep. This is a normal request, and it is important to respect the woman's wishes.

13

A 23-year-old patient who is currently in her 27th week of pregnancy has been admitted into the hospital and confined to complete bed rest for six days. Suddenly, she experiences shortness of breath and chest pain. Which of the following conditions is the most likely cause of her symptoms?

a. Myocardial infarction due to a history of atherosclerosis
b. Pulmonary embolism due to deep vein thrombosis (DVT)
c. Anxiety attack due to worries about her baby's health
d. Congestive heart failure due to possible fluid overload

Ans. (b) Pulmonary embolism due to deep vein thrombosis (DVT)

Explanation: During pregnancy, the risk of developing blood clots, particularly in the legs (DVT), is increased. These clots can travel to the lungs, causing a blockage known as a pulmonary embolism. She has been confined to bed rest for six days, which increases her risk of developing DVT. Additionally, she is experiencing shortness of breath and chest pain, which are two of the most common symptoms of pulmonary embolism.

14

A nurse is conducting an assessment on a primipara during her second trimester of pregnancy in a clinic setting. Which of the following physical findings would indicate an abnormality and require further testing?

a. Consistent increase in fundal height
b. Fetal heart rate of 180 bpm
c. Braxton-Hicks contractions
d. Quickening

Ans. (b) Fetal heart rate of 180 bpm

Explanation: The normal fetal heart rate range is between 120 and 160 beats per minute (bpm). A fetal heart rate of 180 bpm is outside of the normal range and would indicate an abnormality. A heart rate of 180 bpm may indicate fetal distress or other underlying conditions, such as fetal arrhythmia or maternal fever.

15

A G2P1 female a known case of polyhydramnios presents to the OG clinic with respiratory distress at 38 weeks of gestation. The obstetrician has planned for the induction of labor. What among the following is a safe method to induce labor in this patient?

a. High rupture of membranes
b. Prostaglandins
c. Abdominal amniocentesis followed by oxytocin drip
d. Low rupture of membrane

Ans. (c) Abdominal amniocentesis followed by Oxytocin drip

Explanation: Polyhydramnios is a condition characterized by an excessive accumulation of amniotic fluid. In cases where polyhydramnios is causing respiratory distress and the patient requires induction of labor, abdominal amniocentesis followed by an oxytocin drip is a safe and effective approach. This procedure helps reduce the pressure on the diaphragm and lungs, alleviating the respiratory distress caused by polyhydramnios. Following amniocentesis, an oxytocin drip can be administered to induce contractions and initiate labor.

16

25-year-old woman suffers from PPH on her second postnatal day. Her APTT and PTT are prolonged while BT, PT and platelet counts are normal. Likely diagnosis is:

a. Acquired hemophilia
b. Lupus anticoagulant
c. Disseminated Intravascular Coagulation
d. Inherited congenital hemophilia

Ans. (a) Acquired hemophilia

Explanation: Acquired hemophilia is a rare condition characterized by the development of autoantibodies called inhibitors against clotting factors, most commonly factor VIII. It can occur in individuals with no previous history of bleeding disorders. Acquired hemophilia is often associated with prolonged activated partial thromboplastin time (APTT) and prolonged partial thromboplastin time (PTT) due to the presence of these inhibitors, while other clotting tests such as bleeding time (BT), prothrombin time (PT), and platelet counts remain normal.

17

A 22-year-old primigravida woman is admitted at 39 weeks' gestation with painless antepartum hemorrhage. On examination uterus is soft nontender and head engaged. The most appropriate management for her would be:

a. Continue to monitor
b. A speculum examination
c. Pelvic examination in OT
d. Tocolysis and sedatives

Ans. (c) Pelvic examination in OT

Explanation: A pelvic examination in the operating theater is typically conducted in cases of painless antepartum hemorrhage (placenta previa) when there is a need for immediate delivery due to significant bleeding or signs of fetal distress. The examination helps assess the severity of the placental abruption and the well-being of the mother and baby.

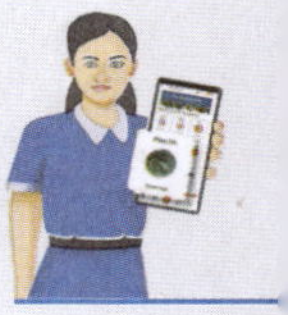

18

A prenatal nurse is giving instructions to a group of pregnant patients on how to prevent toxoplasmosis. Which statement by a patient indicates a need for additional instructions?

a. "I should ensure that meat is well cooked."
b. "I should only drink unpasteurized milk."
c. "I should avoid touching mucous membranes of mouth and nose while handling raw meat."
d. "I should avoid contact with items that may be contaminated with cat feces."

Ans. (b) "I should only drink unpasteurized milk."

Explanation: Drinking unpasteurized milk poses a risk of toxoplasmosis as it can be a potential source of infection. Pregnant women are advised to drink only pasteurized milk to minimize the risk of contracting toxoplasmosis. Therefore, the patient needs further instruction to avoid consuming unpasteurized milk and opt for pasteurized milk instead.

19

A client at 9 weeks' gestation asks the nurse in the prenatal clinic if she can have the chorionic villi sampling (CVS) done at the visit. At what week of gestation should the nurse respond be the best time for the test?

a. Between 8th and 10th weeks
b. Between 10th and 12th weeks
c. Between 12th and 14th weeks
d. Between 14th and 16th weeks

Ans. (b) between 10th and 12th weeks

Explanation: Chorionic villus sampling (CVS) is a prenatal diagnostic test that can be performed between 10th and 13th weeks of gestation. The test involves taking a small sample of cells from the placenta and testing them for genetic abnormalities. The nurse should inform the client that CVS is not recommended before 10 weeks of gestation.

20

Primigravida mother Lucy is on active labor and decided to undergo analgesia. Nurse explained various types of anesthesia available, and client decided to take bilateral pudendal block. After this analgesia, the body part affected is:

a. Abdomen
b. Back
c. Perineum
d. Lower legs

Ans (c) Perineum

Explanation: In pudendal block, local anesthetic is injected into the pudendal canal where the pudendal nerve is located. This allows quick pain relief to the perineum, vulva, and vagina. In spinal anesthesia and epidural anesthesia body below the part of injection is numbed such as abdomen and lower legs.

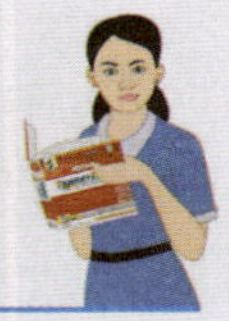

21

During the antenatal visit a primigravida mother complained of backache once she came back to home after work. Which among the following is the correct response from the nurse?

a. It is a normal feeling and nothing to do with it
b. More rest is needed now
c. Practice tailor sitting
d. Practice pelvic floor exercises

Ans. (c) Practice tailor sitting

Explanation: Tailor sit exercise helps you to make your thigh, pelvic, and hip muscles more flexible. This exercise helps to reduce the back pain. All other responses are inappropriate for the situation.

22

Obstetrician ordered triple test for one antenatal mother. Mother asked the nurse regarding the test and nurse educated her about the test. Nurse understood that mother needs more education about the same. Which among the following is not a component of triple test?

a. Maternal serum alpha fetoprotein
b. hCG
c. Unconjugated estriol
d. Inhibin A

Ans. (d) Inhibin A

Explanation: Triple test is a combined biochemical test and it includes Maternal serum alpha fetoprotein, hCG and Unconjugated estriol. This test is done to diagnose down syndrome in which ASAFP and unconjugated estriol are low while hCG is high. Inhibin is another biochemical marker which is not the part of triple test. It is also used to diagnose the fetus with Down syndrome.

23

Nurse educator was taking class of undergraduate nursing students regarding fetal well being. Which among the following parameters is identified by the nursing students as best reflection of fetal nutrition indicating class was effective?

a. Biparietal diameter
b. Abdominal circumference
c. Head circumference
d. Fetal length

Ans. (b) Abdominal circumference

Explanation: Abdominal circumference is the single measurement which reflects fetal nutrition status.

24

An antenatal mother with constipation asked the nurse about the use of castor oil to manage her constipation. Nurse replied that castor oil intake is contraindicated in pregnancy. By keeping this in mind which of the side effects mentioned below made the nurse reply so?

a. It causes sodium and water retention
b. It causes premature contraction
c. It causes potassium retention
d. It leads to fatty liver syndrome

Ans. (b) It causes premature contraction

Explanation: Castor oil is a stimulant laxative which promotes bowel evacuation. But in pregnancy state it may stimulate premature uterine contraction. So it is contraindicated in pregnancy state.

25

Primigravida mother with 15 weeks' period of gestation came to OPD complaining abdominal cramps and passage of several blood clots and diagnosed with inevitable abortion. Which among the following is the priority nursing intervention?

a. Knowledge deficit
b. Severe pain
c. Fluid volume imbalance
d. Ineffective airway

Ans. (c) Fluid volume imbalance

Explanation: Primigravida mother with inevitable abortion and abdominal cramps and bleeding is at risk for fluid volume deficit. Abdominal cramps and pain will be there, but most important nursing diagnosis is fluid volume deficit. Here in the question nothing related to airway is mentioned. So ineffective airway clearance is not an issue here.

26

Doctor ordered internal electronic fetal monitoring to a multiparous woman. Nurse should understand that requirement for electronic fetal monitoring includes all; except:

a. Ruptured membrane
b. Fetal station is at least at -1
c. Cervix has a minimum dilation of 2 cm
d. Woman should provide with pudendal block

Ans. (d) Woman should provide with pudendal block

Explanation: Internal fetal monitoring involves attachment of an electrode to the part of baby's body close to cervix. Except option d all are the prerequisites for internal fetal monitoring.

27

Nurse was going through the file of a client with the diagnosis of pregnancy induced hypertension. What all are the signs and symptoms reported in her file?

a. Proteinuria, weight gain, double vision
b. Proteinuria, vaginal bleeding, and double vision
c. Weight gain, double vision, vaginal bleeding
d. Proteinuria, weight gain, vaginal bleeding

Ans. (a) Proteinuria, weight gain, double vision

Explanation: It is a form of high BP during pregnancy. Signs and symptoms include high blood pressure, proteinuria, swelling in your face and hands, headache that does not go away, vision problems, including blurred vision or seeing spots, pain in your upper right abdomen and trouble in breathing.

28

Doctor ordered oxytocin infusion to a primigravida mother, along with the oxytocin infusion order. What else doctor would order?

a. Intake output monitoring
b. Vaginal bleeding characteristics
c. Nil per orally
d. Fetal monitoring

Ans. (a) Intake output monitoring

Explanation: Oxytocin is a hormone with side effect of water intoxication. Due to this side effect, monitoring of intake and output is needed along with the drug. Fetal monitoring is needed for all women admitted in labor room and not only for women with oxytocin infusion. Oxytocin infusion receiving women would strictly have intake output monitoring.

29

A mother with 39+3 weeks period of gestation is in her second stage of labor. During this stage how frequently the contractions need to be monitored?

a. 5 minutes
b. 10 minutes
c. 15 minutes
d. 30 minutes

Ans. (c) 15 minutes

Explanation: Second stage of labor starts with fully dilated cervix to the delivery of the baby. In this stage nurse needs to monitor strength, frequency, and duration of contraction every 15 minutes. If any maternal or child issue is detected, monitoring needs to be done more frequently.

30

While doing antenatal examination to a client in her first trimester, doctor noticed her fundal height is more than the actual period of gestation. He diagnosed it as gestational trophoblastic disease and ordered ultrasound. What will be the finding in ultrasound?

a. Empty gestational sac
b. Grape like structures
c. Fetus with congenital abnormalities
d. Ectopic pregnancy

Ans. (b) Grape like structures

Explanation: Gestational trophoblastic disease is a condition in which abnormal trophoblast cells grow inside the uterus after conception. It includes hydatidiform mole, invasive mole, choriocarcinoma, etc. Abnormal vaginal bleeding and a uterus that is larger than normal period of gestation are the common findings of this condition. On ultrasound it shows grape like structures.

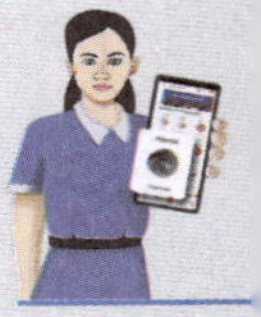

31

Client admitted with labor pain and nurse did vaginal examination for the client. The findings of the PV are cervix 8 cm dilated, 70% effaced and position is +1. Based upon the findings one should understand that presenting part of the fetus is at:

a. 1 cm above the ischial spine
b. At the level of ischial spine
c. 1 cm below the ischial spine
d. At the vagina

Ans. (c) 1 cm below the ischial spine

Explanation: Presenting part location is determined in relation with ischial spine. If the presenting part is at ischial spine then station is zero, if the presenting part is above the ischial spine it is recorded as –1,–2, –3, etc. If the presenting part is below the ischial spine then +1, +2, +3.

32

Client Lucy received her biophysical profile test result for her fetus and the score is 6. Client asked the nurse how to interpret the result. Most appropriate response from the nurse is:

a. Its normal finding and fetus is healthy
b. Need to repeat test after 24 hours
c. High risk for fetal hypoxia
d. Indicates IUD

Ans. (b) Need to repeat test after 24 hours

Explanation: Biophysical profile measures the health status of a fetus. It measures 5 components such as baby's heart rate, muscle tone, movement, breathing, and the amount of amniotic fluid around the baby. Each parameter has a maximum score of 2 and minimum score of zero. So total score for the test is 10 and minimum score for the test is zero. Interpretation of score is as follows, a score of 8 or 10 points means that baby is healthy. A score of 6 or 8 points means that the needs to be retested in 24 hours. A score of 4 or less may mean that the baby is having problems.

33

Obstetrician ordered magnesium sulfate injection to a woman with pre-eclampsia. Nurse should understand that the purpose of this injection for this client is:

a. To reduce blood pressure
b. To reduce proteinuria
c. To prevent seizure
d. To prevent preterm labor

Ans. (c) To prevent seizure

Explanation: Main aim of administering magnesium sulfate injection is to prevent seizure. Magnesium will act like calcium and interrupt signal transmission in hyperstimulated neurological system.

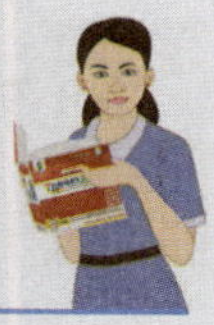

34

Family planning room nurse was educating a woman regarding oral contraceptive. She instructed her to take pills on same time every day. What is the reason behind the statement?

a. To make it as a routine
b. To reduce the side effects of OCPs
c. To maintain hormonal levels in the blood
d. Prevent drug to drug interaction

Ans. (c) To maintain hormonal levels in the blood.

Explanation: Same time intake every day will help to maintain blood level of hormones and thus prevent the hypothalamo-hypophyseal access from secretion of FSH and LH. Thereby prevent the ovulation.

35

Primipara mother came to labor room with the complaint of pain. Nurse assessed the characteristics of pain and reordered it as false pain. Which among the following could have reported by the mother?

a. Pain is in the lower abdomen only
b. Hardening of uterus is there
c. Bag of waters formed
d. Cervix is 4 cm dilated

Ans. (a) Pain is in the lower abdomen only

Explanation: Characteristic of true labor pain includes pain in the lower abdomen, back and radiating to thighs. It is associated with hardening of uterus and cervical dilation. Bag of water also called amniotic sac will be present. Pain is not relieved by enema.

36

Nurse educator was taking class on partograph. At the end of the class, she was evaluating her students. Which statement made by the students indicate that further explanation is needed?

a. In partograph alert line starts at 3 cm of cervical dilation
b. In partograph fetal heart rate is reordered every 30 minutes
c. Each square in cervical dilation part indicates 1 cm dilation
d. Action line is parallel and 4 hours to the right of alert line

Ans. (a) In partograph alert line starts at 3 cm of cervical dilation

Explanation: It is a composite graphical recording of cervical dilatation and descent of head against duration of labor in hours. It also gives information about fetal and maternal condition that are all recorded on single sheet of paper. In partograph alert line starts at 4 cm dilation. All other statements given regarding partograph are correct.

37

Following a class on partograph the nurse educator understands that the class was effective if the student identified which among the following is NOT a component of partograph?

a. Cervical dilation
b. FHR
c. Descent of head
d. Effacement

Ans. (d) Effacement

Explanation: FHR, cervical dilation, descent of the head, contractions per 10 minutes, oxytocin dose, drugs and IV fluids given, pulse and BP of mother, temperature of mother, and urine volume, protein and acetone are the components of partograph.

38

After the delivery of 3000 gm weighing baby by a primipara mother, nurse was waiting for the delivery of the placenta. Nursing student who was witnessing the labor asked the nurse what is the expected weight of placenta? What should be the response from the nurse?

a. 250 g
b. 500 g
c. 600 g
d. 750 g

Ans. (b) 500 gm

Explanation: At the term, expected weight of the placenta is one sixth of the baby's weight. Here the baby's weight is 3000 g and therefore placenta weight will be 500 g.

39

Nurse educator was taking class on ectopic pregnancy. Following class, she asked the students which is the most common site of tubal ectopic pregnancy. Correct response from the group is:

a. Ampulla
b. Isthmus
c. Infundibulum
d. Interstitial

Ans. (a) Ampulla

Explanation: Tubal ectopic pregnancy is the most common type (97%) of ectopic pregnancy. Ampulla (55%) part of the fallopian tube is the most common site for tubal ectopic pregnancy followed by isthmus (25%), infundibulum (18%) and interstitial (2%).

40

While examining a pregnant woman, examiner tapped the cervix with finger and felt there, the fetus floats upward, then sinks back and a gentle tap is felt on the finger. This finding is documented as:

a. Quickening
b. Ballottement
c. Hegar sign
d. Osiander sign

Ans. (b) Ballottement

Explanation: The given examination technique indicates ballottement. Quickening is the fetal movement felt by mother for the first time. Hegar sign is on bimanual examination (two fingers in the anterior fornix and two fingers below the uterus per abdomen), the abdominal and vaginal fingers seem to oppose below the body of uterus. Osiander sign is an **increased pulsation in lateral fornices at 8th week.**

41

After the completion of second stage of labor, the student nurse who was assisting in delivery for the first time, observed lengthening of cord, sudden gush of blood and uterus becoming more globular. Student nurse immediately informed the registered nurse regarding the findings. These signs and symptoms indicate:

a. Primary PPH
b. Baby is about to deliver
c. Placenta separation
d. Atonic uterus

Ans. (c) Placenta separation

Explanation: The given findings like lengthening of cord, sudden gush of blood and uterus becoming more globular are the characteristic signs of placental separation. All the other options are not related to the given observations made by student nurse.

42

Nursing student was going through the labor notes of a mother who delivered 4 hours ago and she noted placenta separated with Duncan mechanism. Based on her knowledge she should understand that this means:

a. Assisted expulsion with fundal pressure
b. Assisted expulsion with controlled cord traction
c. Maternal surface of the placenta presented on expulsion
d. Fetal surface of the placenta presented on expulsion

Ans. (c) Maternal surface of the placenta presented on expulsion

Explanation: Option A and B indicate methods of assisting placental expulsion. Duncan mechanism which is also known as marginal separation presents the maternal surface of the placenta on expulsion. Schultze mechanism which is also known as central separation of placenta presents expulsion of the placenta with the fetal surface foremost.

43

Following preterm delivery nurse was educating mother regarding manual expression of breast milk for her newborn admitted in NICU. Which among the following techniques is the correct option?

a. Ritgen's technique
b. Schulze technique
c. Marmet's technique
d. Duncan technique

Ans. (c) Marmet's technique

Explanation: Marmet's technique is the manual expression and assisting the milk ejection reflex. Ritgen's technique is used to prevent perineal tear. Schulze technique and Duncan technique are used for expulsion of placenta.

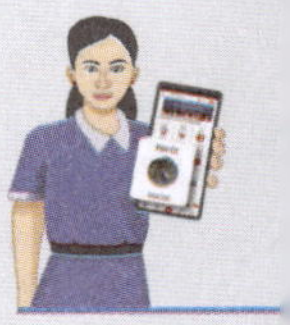

Image-Based Questions

1. Diagnose the underlying disorder shown in the photograph.
(Refer explanation at the end)

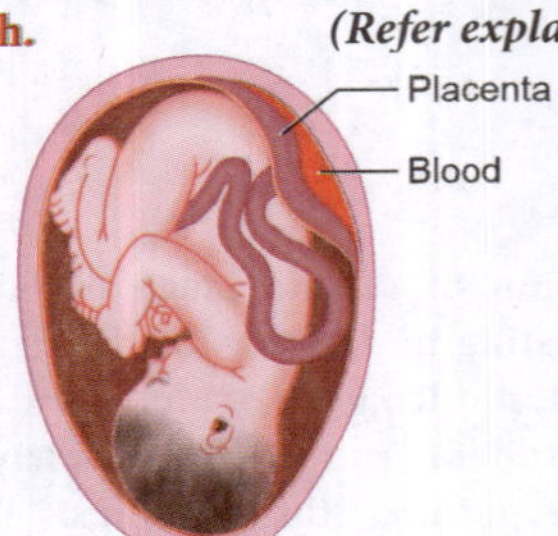

a. Placenta previa
b. Placenta abruptio
c. Atonic uterus
d. Adherent placenta

2. The IUD device used in the image shown below is
(Refer explanation at the end)

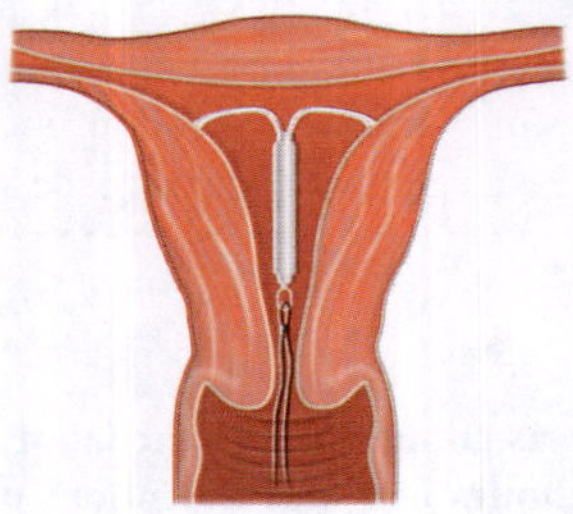

a. Copper-T 375
b. Copper-T 380 A
c. Nova-T
d. Mirena

3. The device/equipment shown in the image is

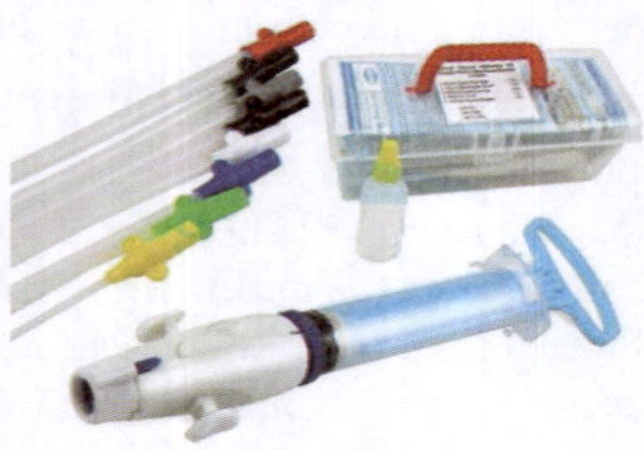

a. Manual vacuum aspiration Kit
b. Malmstorm's vacuum extractor
c. Suction pump
d. Silicon vacuum extractor

4. Use of the instrument shown in the picture is:

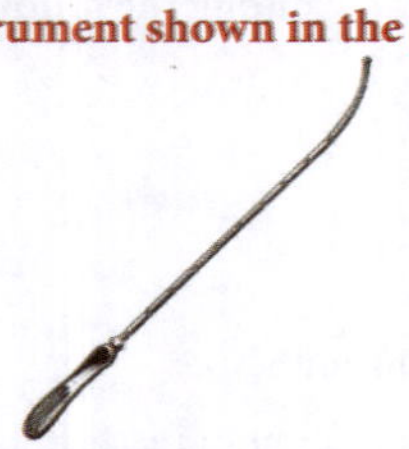

a. To remove tissue from uterine wall
b. To dilate vaginal wall
c. To measure the length and direction of the cervical canal and uterus
d. None of the above

5. Identify the instrument shown in the image.

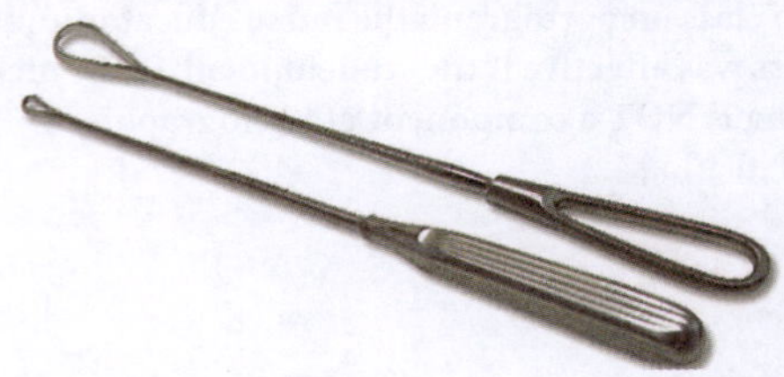

a. Hegar's dilator
b. Vaginal wall retractor
c. Sims uterine sound
d. Sims uterine curette

6. The instrument given in the picture is used for:

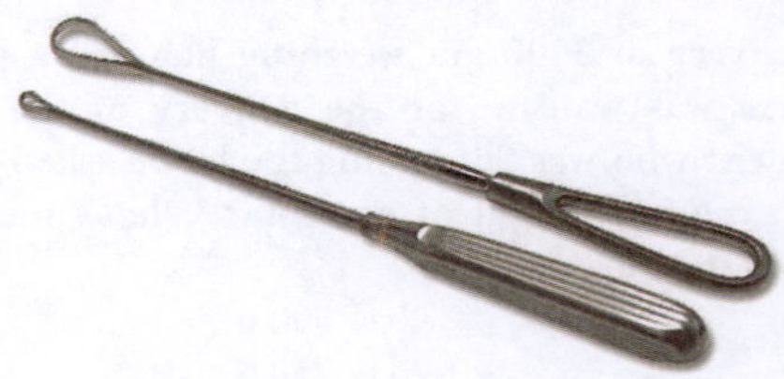

a. Removing tissue from the lining of the uterus
b. D & C procedure
c. Both a & b
d. None of the above

7. Identify the equipment given in the picture.

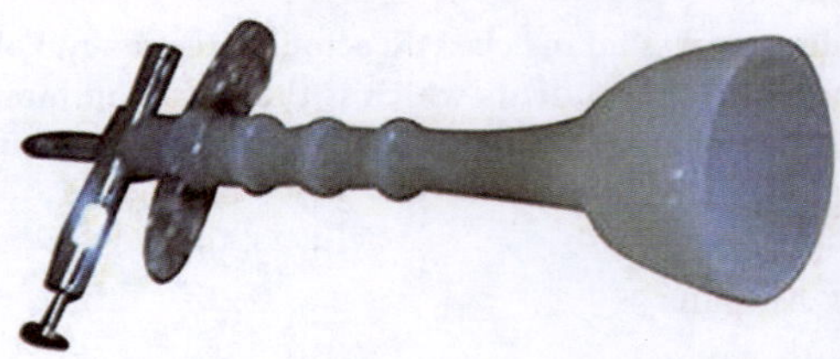

a. Metal cup ventouse
b. Silicon cup ventouse
c. Bird's cup
d. Malmstrom cup

8. Diagnose the condition shown in photograph.
[Recent Question 2012]

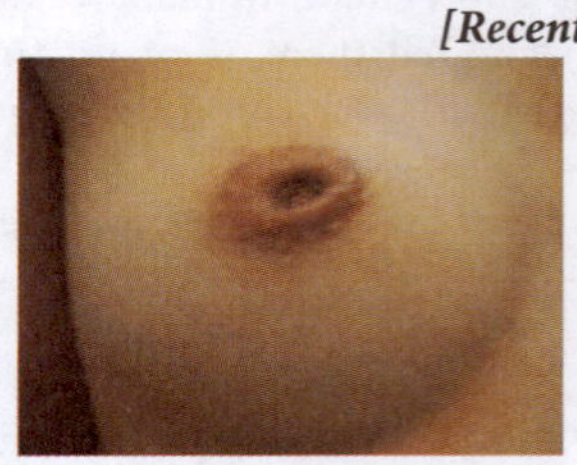

a. Cracked nipple
b. Papilloma of nipple
c. Inverted nipple
d. Retention cyst of a Gland of Montgomery

Ans.

1. b
2. d
3. a
4. c
5. d
6. c
7. b
8. c

[*Courtesy*: PHOTON-20® 3th ed. by Vivek Jain, CBS Publishers and Distributors Pvt Ltd]

9. Identify the procedure shown in the image that is usually done in a labor room.

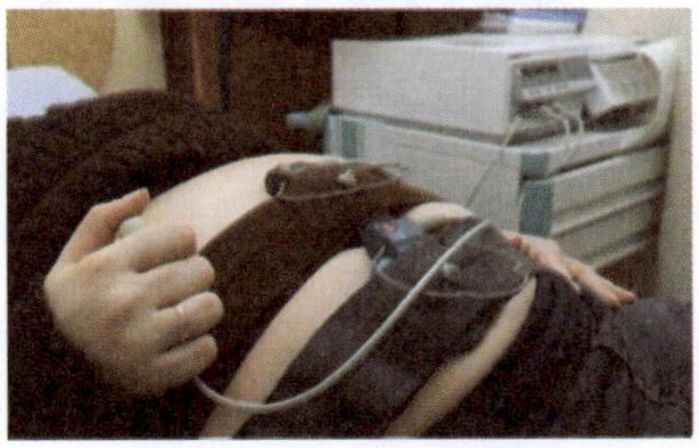

a. Color Doppler b. Amniocentesis
c. NST d. EMG

10. Look at the image below and identify the grip.

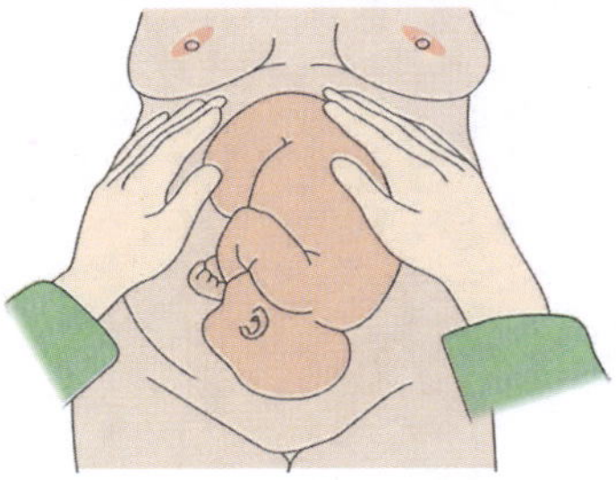

a. Pelvic grip b. Abdominal grip
c. Fundal grip d. Umbilical grip

11. What is the presentation shown in the picture?

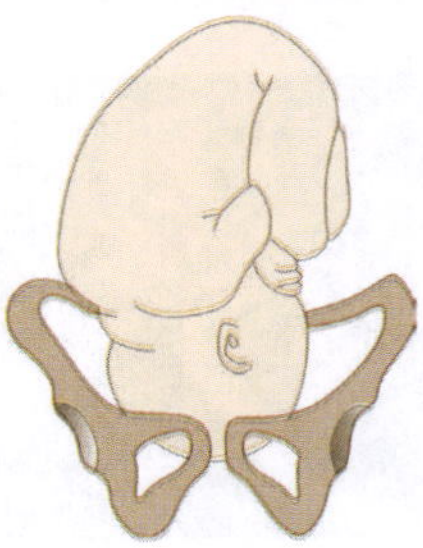

a. LOP b. LOA
c. ROP d. ROA

12. Narrowest part of structure (arrows) shown in the photograph:

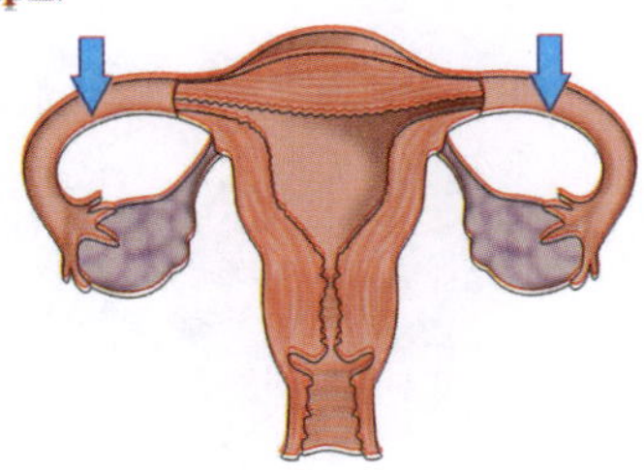

a. Infundibulum b. Interstitium
c. Isthmus d. Ampulla

13. Identify uterine anomaly shown in the photograph.

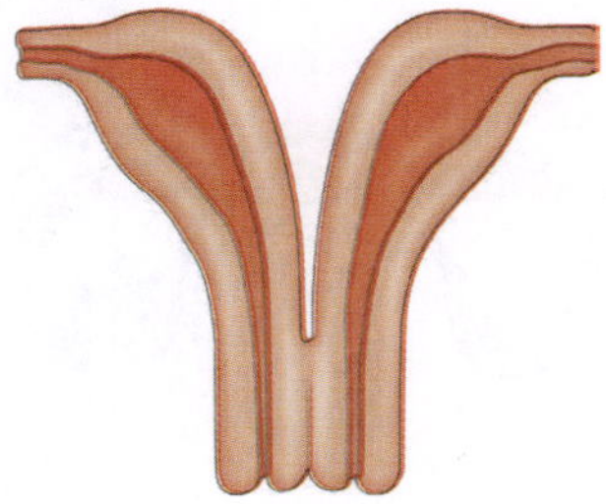

a. Hypoplasia uterus b. Unicornuate uterus
c. Bicornuate uterus d. Uterus didelphus

14. Clinical examination shown in photograph is used to detect:

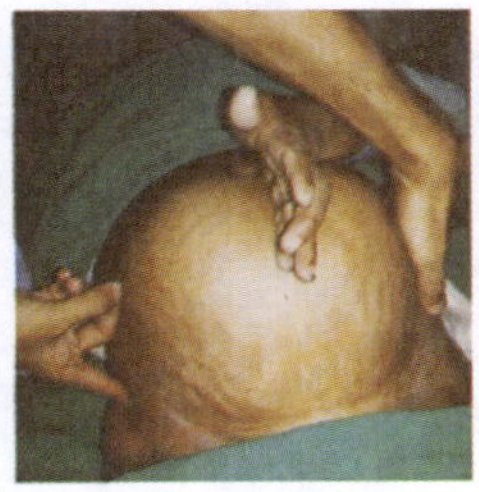

a. Pregnancy b. Hepatomegaly
c. Breech presentation d. Ascites

15. Method shown in photograph is commonly used for screening of:

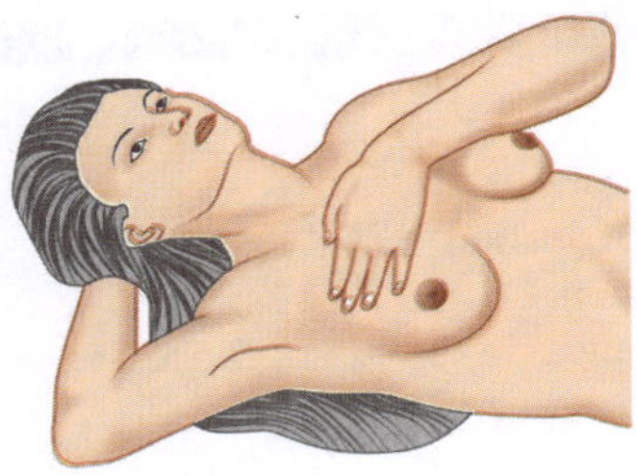

a. Mastitis b. Pleural effusion
c. Breast cancer d. All of these

16. Identify the type of pelvic prolapse (arrow) shown in photograph.

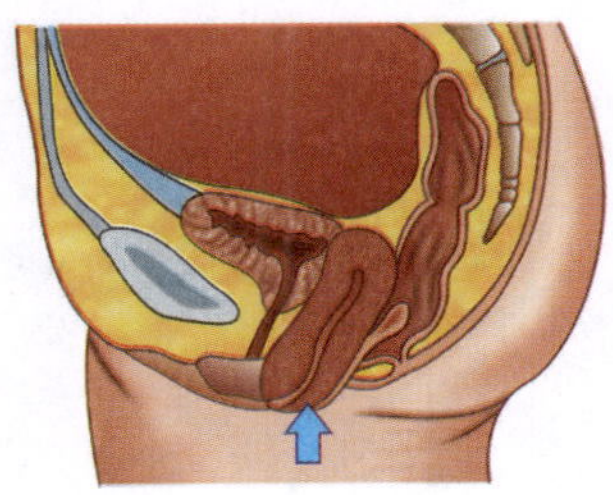

a. Cystocele b. Rectocele
c. Enterocele d. Uterine prolapse

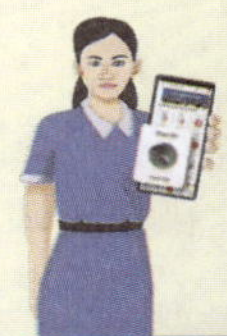

Ans.

9. c
10. c
11. d
12. b
13. d
14. d
15. c
16. d

17. Causes of female fertility are most commonly attributed to:

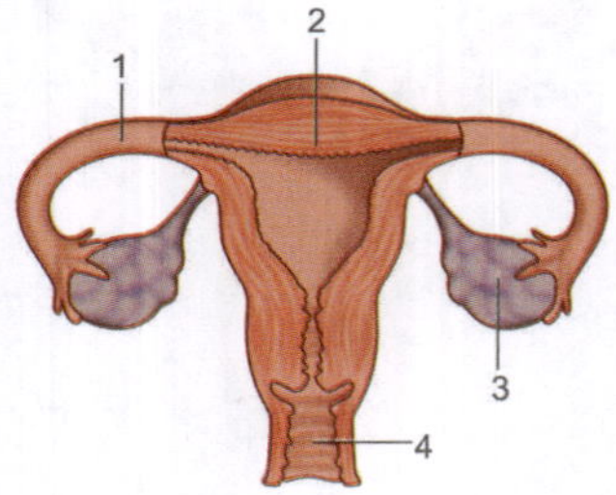

a. 1 b. 2
c. 3 d. 4

18. Gynecological procedure shown in the photograph is:

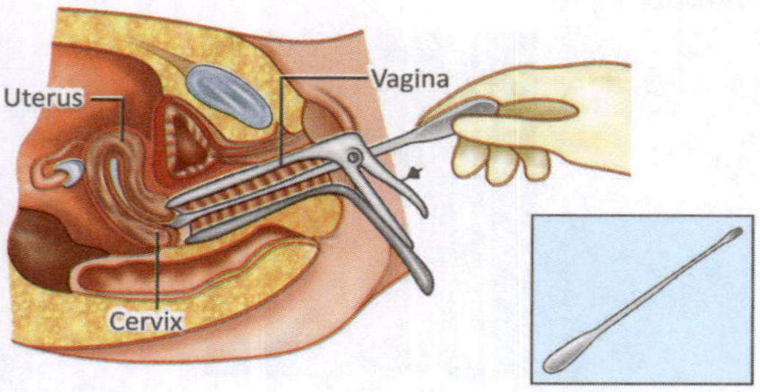

a. Swab of vaginal discharge b. Pap smear
c. VIA test d. Punch biopsy

19. Use of instrument shown in the photograph is:

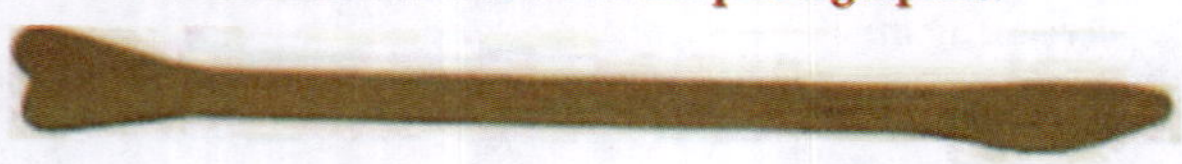

a. Pap smear
b. Cervical dilation
c. Retraction
d. Curetting

20. Largest diameter of fetal skull in photograph is:

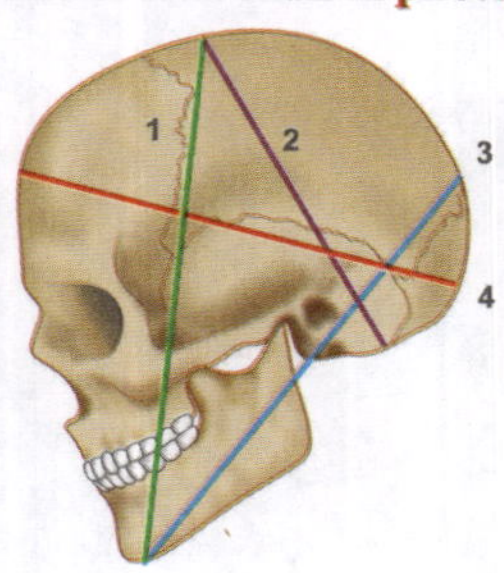

a. 1 b. 2
c. 3 d. 4

21. Pelvis shape type as shown in the photograph is:

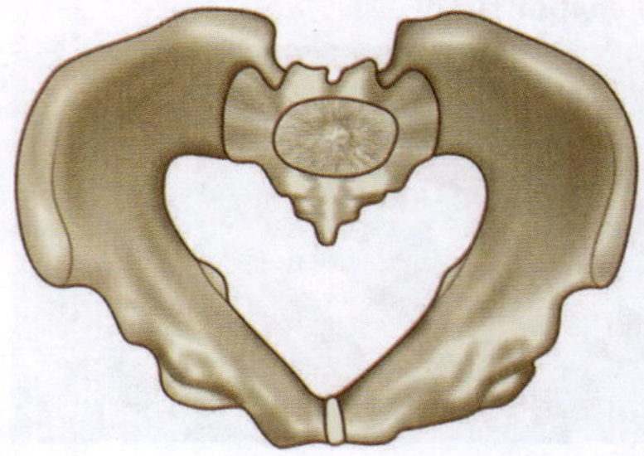

a. Gynecoid b. Android
c. Platypelloid d. Anthropoid

22. Structure 5 in the photograph of breast represents:

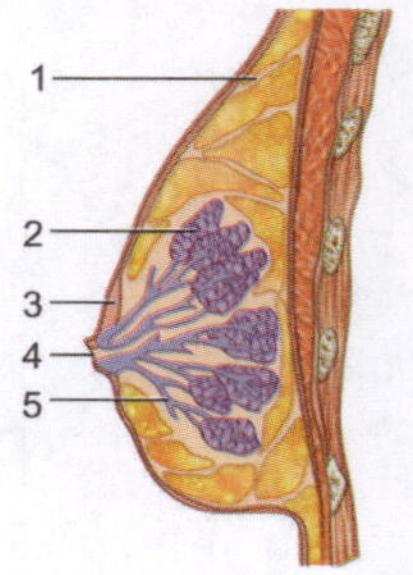

a. Cooper ligament b. Lobule with alveoli
c. Lactiferous duct d. Areolar tissue

23. Identify the type of placenta insertion shown in the photograph.

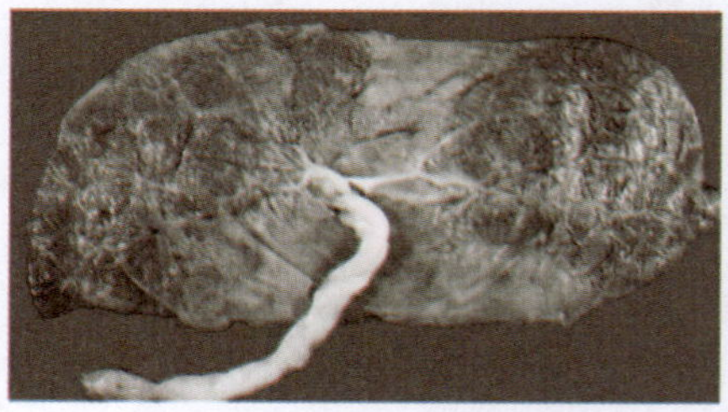

a. Velamentous b. Circummarginate
c. Bilobate d. Circumvallate

24. Clinical sign shown in the photograph is known as:

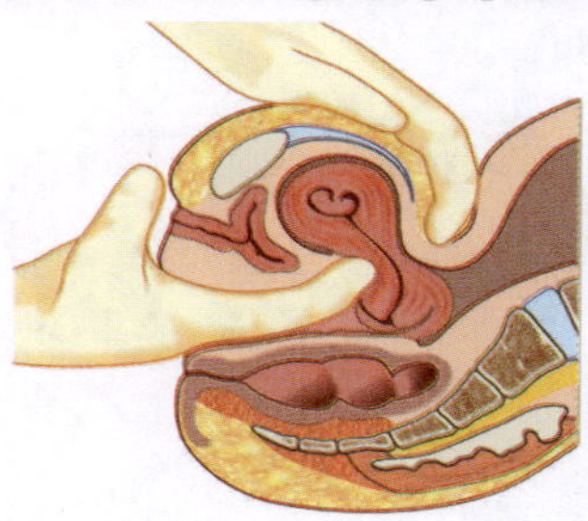

a. Chadwick's sign b. Osiander's sign
c. Palmer's sign d. Hegar's sign

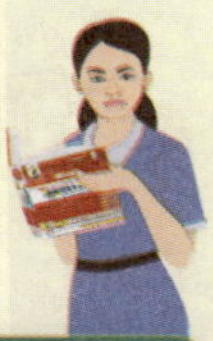

Ans.

17. c
18. b
19. a
20. a
21. b
22. c
23. c
24. d

25. Sign (arrows) shown in the photograph is positive by:

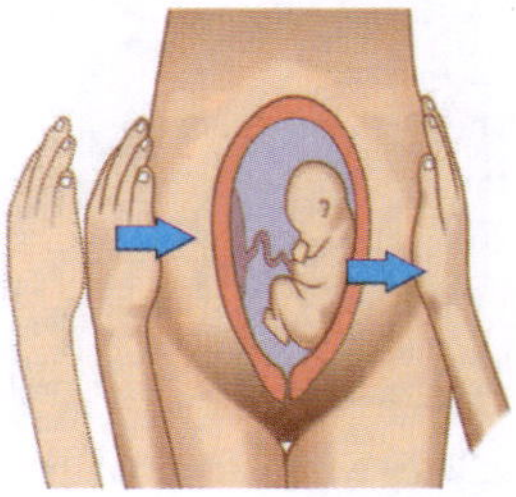

a. 12-14 weeks POG b. 14-16 weeks POG
c. 18-20 weeks POG d. 36-38 weeks POG

26. Identify the diameter '1' shown in the fetal skull photograph.

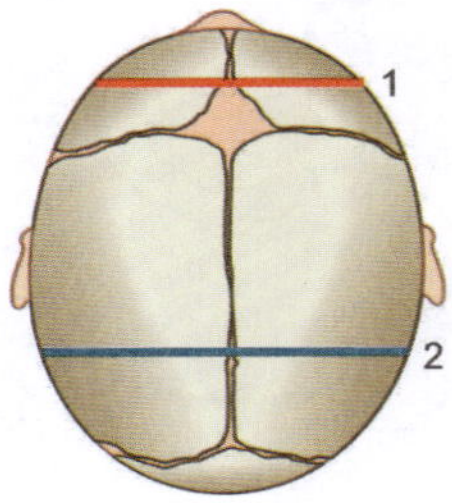

a. Biparietal b. Bitemporal
c. Occipitofrontal d. Mentovertical

27. Maneuver shown in the photograph is known as:

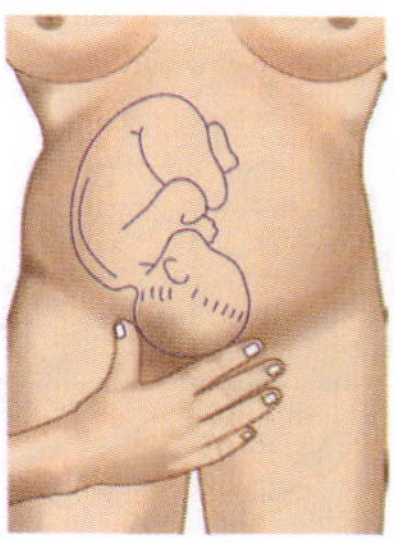

a. Fundal palpation b. Lateral palpation
c. Deep pelvic palpation d. Pawlik's grip

28. Uterine size (arrow) shown in photograph represent gestational age of:

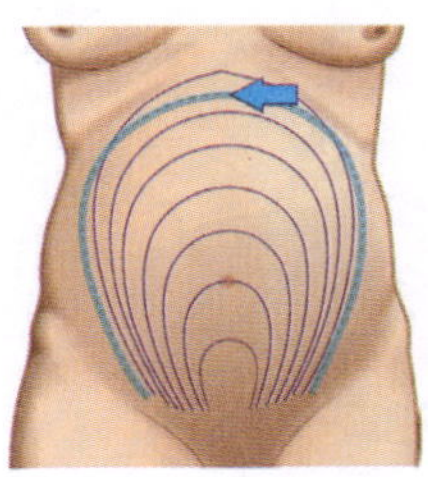

a. 24 weeks POG b. 32 weeks POG
c. 38 weeks POG d. 40 weeks POG

29. Fetal lie type as shown in the photograph is known as:

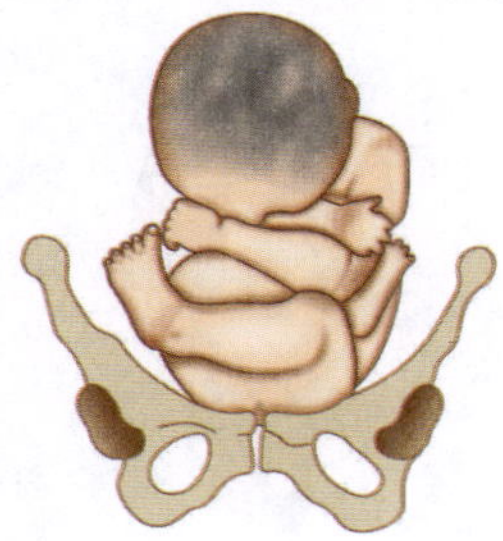

a. Vertex b. Breech
c. Oblique d. Transverse

30. Fetal attitude as shown in the photograph is known as:

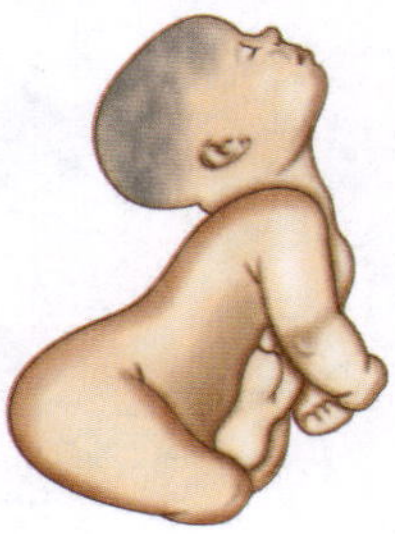

a. Flexed b. Deflexed
c. Partial extended d. Extended

31. Fetal position shown in the photograph is known as:

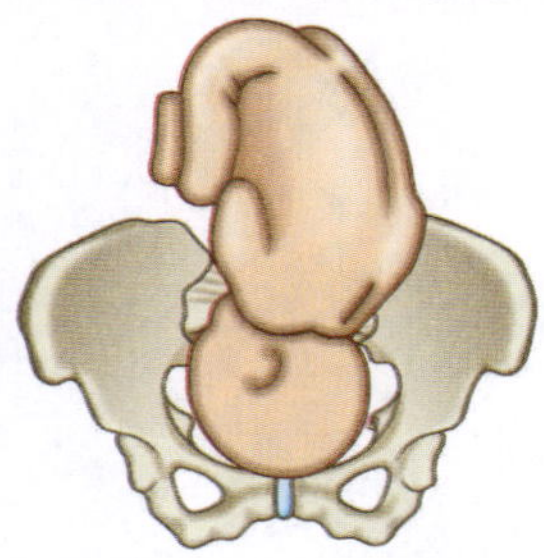

a. Left Occipito-tranverse b. Left Occipito-anterior
c. Occipito-anterior d. Left Occipito-posterior

32. Diagnose the underlying disorder shown in the photograph.

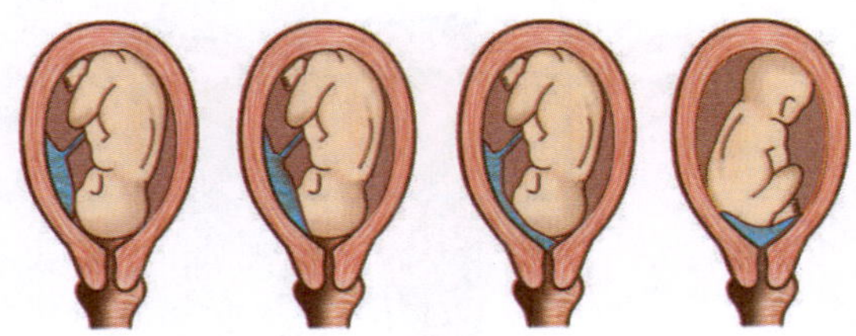

a. Retained placenta b. Adherent placenta
c. Placenta previa d. Abruptio placenta

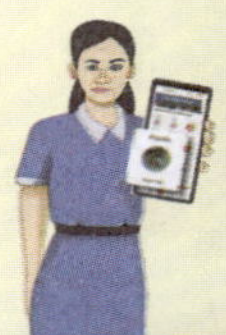

Ans.

25.	c
26.	b
27.	d
28.	d
29.	b
30.	d
31.	b
32.	c

33. Identify the type of placenta praevia as shown in photograph.

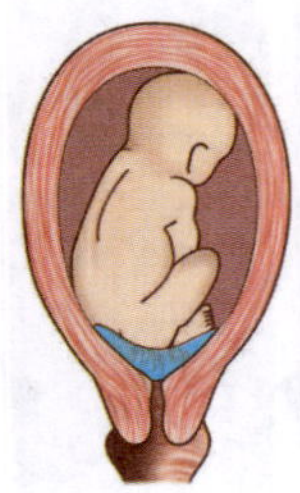

a. I
b. II
c. III
d. IV

34. Stage of labor process shown in the photograph is:

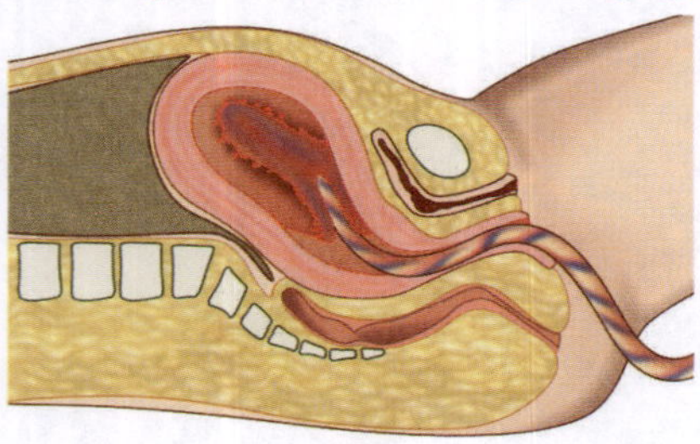

a. First stage Latent phase
b. First stage Active phase
c. Second stage
d. Third stage

35. Presentation of fetus shown in the photograph is:

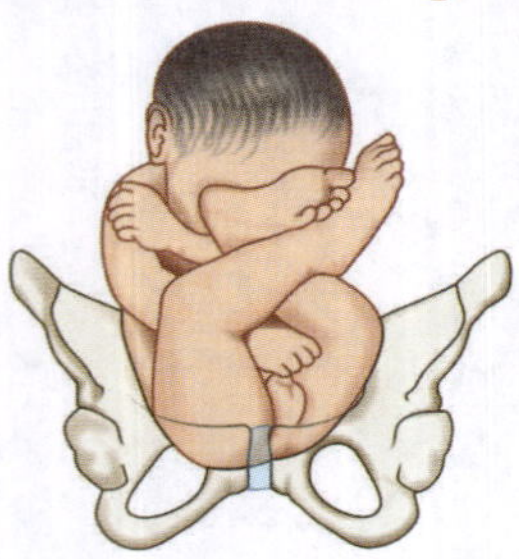

a. Frank breech
b. Complete breech
c. Footling presentation
d. None of these

36. Following are supports of organ (box) in photograph; EXCEPT:

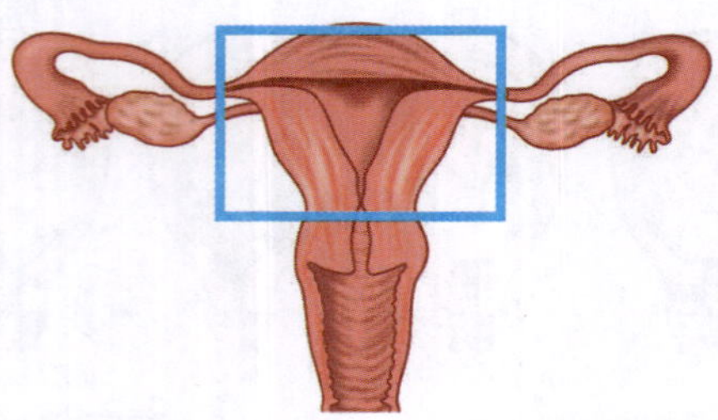

a. Round ligament
b. Tubo-ovarian ligament
c. Utero-sacral ligament
d. Pelvic diaphragm

37. Technique shown in photograph is used for:

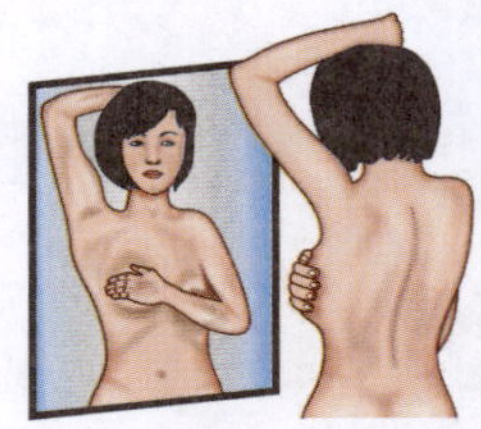

a. Screening axillary lymphadenopathy
b. Screening breast cancer
c. Screening skin carcinoma
d. Screening cervical lymphadenopathy

38. Pelvis shape type as shown in the photograph is:

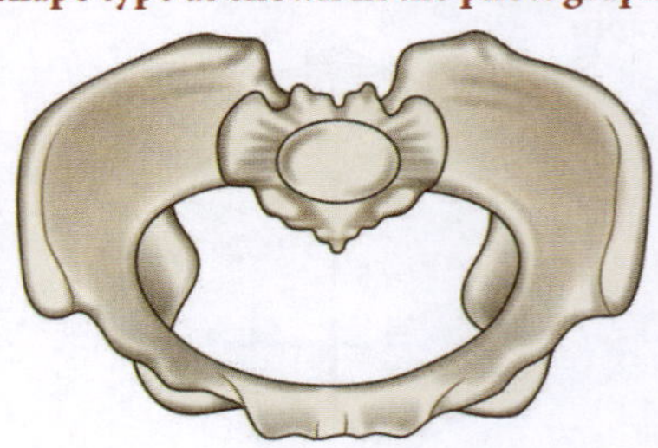

a. Gynecoid
b. Android
c. Platypelloid
d. Anthropoid

39. Measurement of diameter '1' of fetal skull shown in photograph:

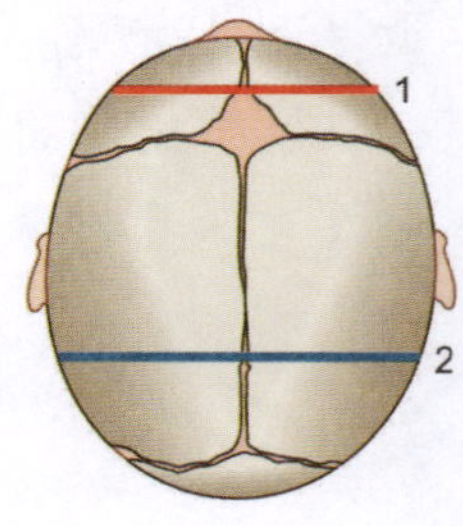

a. 8 cm
b. 9.5 cm
c. 11 cm
d. 13.5 cm

40. Position shown in photograph increases vaginal opening by:

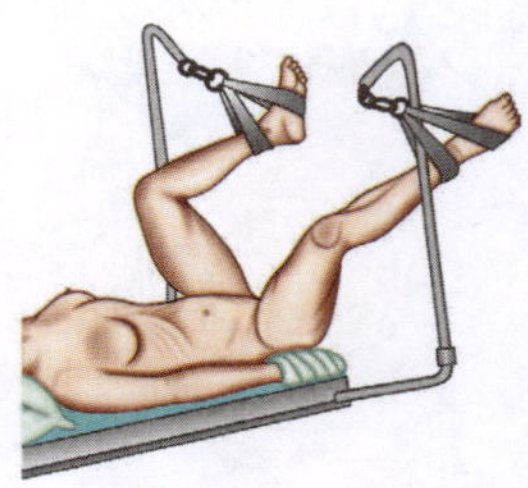

a. 1 cm
b. 2 cm
c. 3 cm
d. 4 cm

Ans.

33. d
34. d
35. a
36. b
37. b
38. c
39. a
40. b

41. Identify the scheme/program/plan launched by Government of India. ***(Refer explanation at the end)***

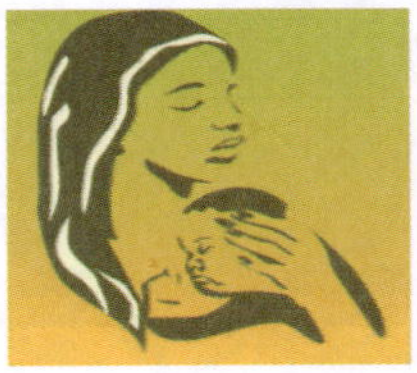

a. Janani Shishu Suraksha Karyakram (JSSK)
b. Kangaroo Mother Care
c. BFHI
d. RCH Program

42. Technique shown in photograph is used for: ***(Refer explanation at the end)***

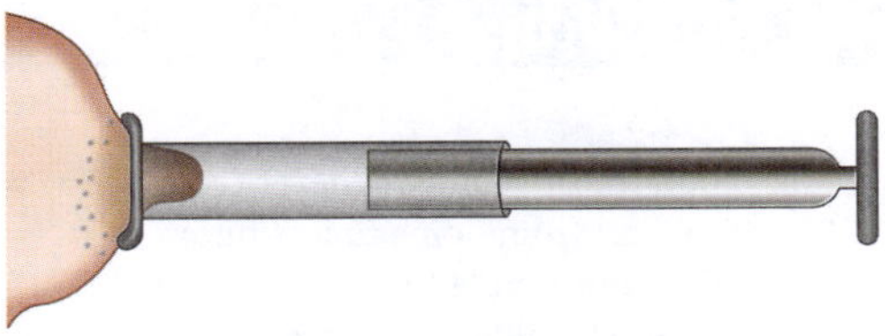

a. Expression of breast milk
b. Retracted nipple
c. Accessory nippple
d. Sore nipples

43. 24-year-old pregnant lady was admitted for Pregnancy-induced-hypertension for monitoring and bed rest. Complication in Supine position (See Photograph) ***[AIIMS May 2017]***

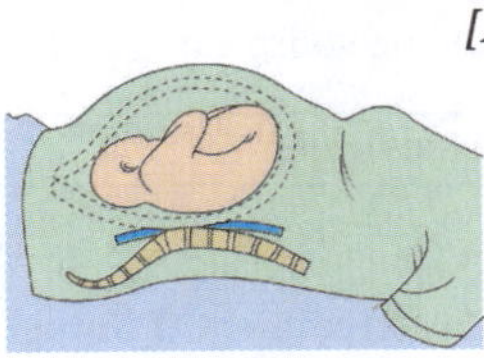

a. Ascending aorta syndrome
b. Supine venacaval syndrome
c. Superior venacaval syndrome
d. Abdominal aorta syndrome

44. Cell cleavage type in Embryo shown in Photograph is: ***[Recent Question 2012]***

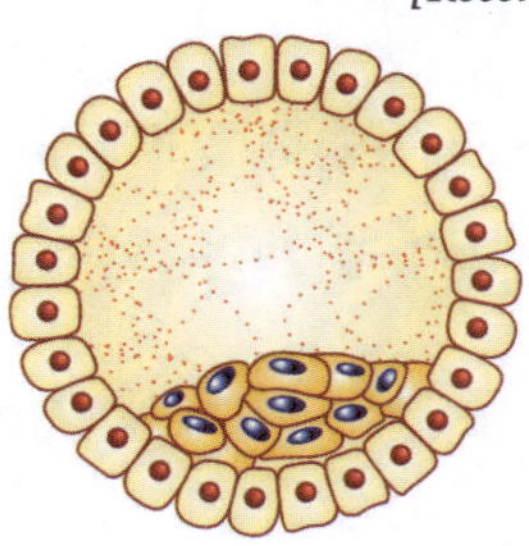

a. Fertilized egg
b. Morula
c. Blastocyst
d. Gastrula

45. Cell cleavage type in Embryo shown in Photograph is:

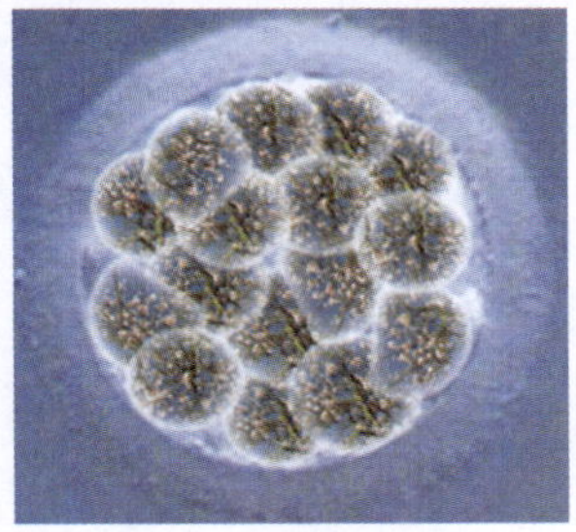

a. Fertilized egg
b. Morula
c. Blastocyst
d. Gastrula

46. Maneuver shown in the Photograph is not done in: ***[Recent Question 2014]***

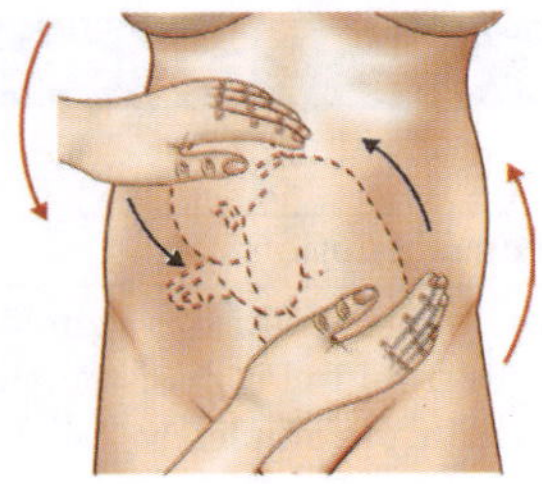

a. Primigravida
b. Flexed breech
c. PIH
d. Anemia

47. Maneuver shown in Photograph is done to evaluate .... in newborn:

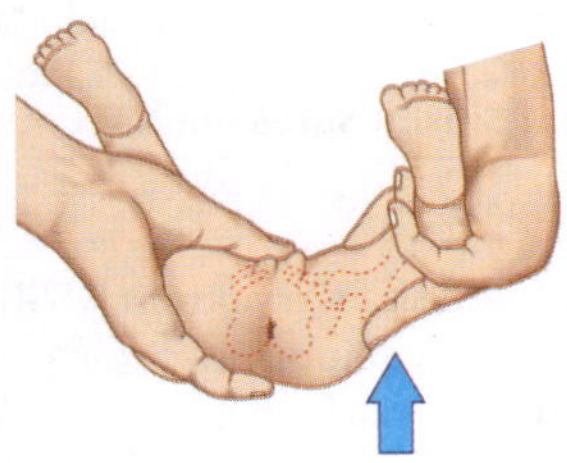

a. Femur fracture
b. Congenital dislocation of hip
c. CTEV
d. Imperforate anus

48. Identify the type of pelvic prolapse (arrow) shown in photograph:

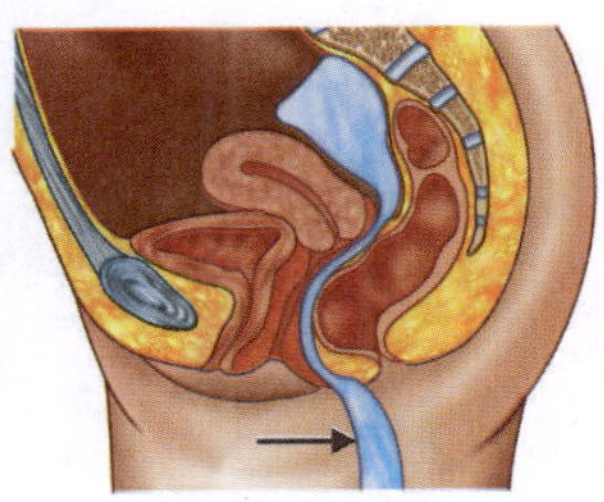

a. Cystocele
b. Rectocele
c. Enterocele
d. Uterine prolapse

Ans.

41. a
42. b
43. b
44. c
45. b
46. c
47. b
48. c

49. Identify the type of Fistula '1' shown in the photograph:

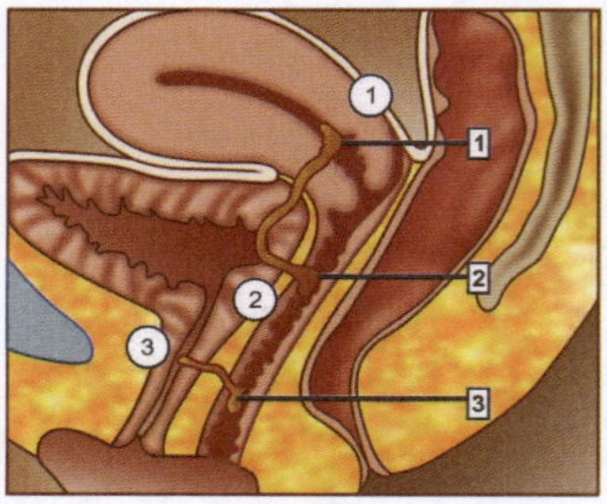

a. Vesicovaginal fistula b. Vesicouterine fistula c. Urethrovaginal fistula d. None of the above

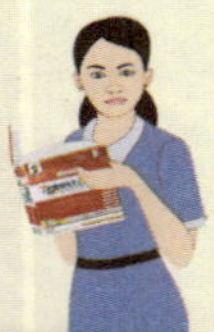

Ans.

49. b

Explanations of Image-Based Questions

1. Ans. (b) Placenta abruptio

Placental abruption is a serious condition in which the placenta separates from the wall of the uterus before birth. It can separate partially or completely.

2. Ans. (d) Mirena

Mirena is a hormonal intrauterine device (IUD) that can provide long-term birth control. The device is a T-shaped plastic frame that's inserted into the uterus, where it releases a type of the hormone progestin. It acts by thickening the mucus in the cervix to stop the sperm from reaching the ovum and thins the lining of the uterus and partially suppress ovulation.

41. Ans. (a) Janani Shishu Suraksha Karyakram (JSSK)

[Ref. Park, 23/e p456]

Janani Shishu Suraksha Karyakram (JSSK) (Photograph)

- **Pregnant women components:**
  - Free deliveries (including cesarean section) in public health institutions
  - Free drugs and consumables
  - Free diet (Normal delivery: 3 days; Cesarean section: 7 days)
  - Free diagnostics
  - Free blood transfusion (whenever required)
  - Free transport from home to institution
- **Child health components:**
  - Nutritional rehabilitation centers (NRCs)
  - Integrated management of neonatal and childhood illnesses (IMNCI):
    - Pre-service IMNCI
    - Facility-based IMNCI (F-IMNCI)
  - Facility based newborn care:
    - Newborn care corner (NBCC)
    - Newborn stabilization unit (NBSU)
    - Special newborn care unit (SNCU)
  - Triage of sick newborns
  - Home-based newborn care (HBNC)

42. Ans. (b) Retracted nipple

[Ref. Ghai, 8/e p154]

Syringe Method of Treatment (Photograph)

- Inverted or retracted nipples makes latching (attachment) difficult to baby
- Treatment is started after birth of the baby
- Nipple is manually everted, stretched & rolled out several times a day
- A plastic syringe is used to draw out to correct the problem

"He who has health has hope; and he who has hope has everything."

—Arabian proverb

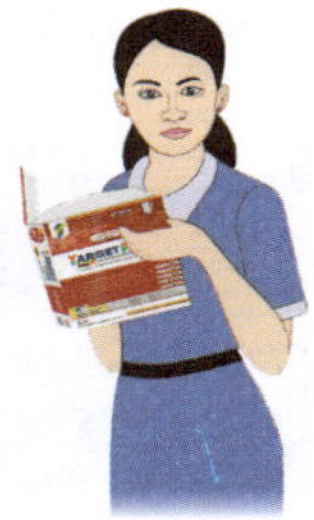

MULTIPLE CHOICE QUESTIONS

(Including Explained and Practice Questions)

ANATOMY OF FEMALE REPRODUCTIVE SYSTEM

1. **Which of the following is not true about female urethra?**
   a. It is about 4 cm long
   b. It is shorter than the male urethra
   c. It is posterior to vaginal orifice
   d. It is straight and offers minor resistance for catheterization

2. **Vulva is composed of which of the following structures?** *New Q*
   a. Vaginal introitus, labia majora, lavia minora and cervix
   b. Clitoris, vestibule and fourchette
   c. Labia majora, labia minora and cervix
   d. Cervix, uterus and ovary

3. **All of the following are the part of vulva, except:**
   a. Bartholin's gland b. Vaginal opening
   c. Mons pubis d. Ampulla

Explanation: The vulva consists of the external female sex organs. The vulva includes the mons pubis, labia majora, labia minora, clitoris, Vestibular bulbs, fourchette, vulval vestibule, urinary meatus, the vaginal opening, and Bartholin's and Skene's vestibular glands. The urinary meatus is also included as it opens into the vulval vestibule.

4. **Nerve supply to vulva is through:**
   a. Ilioinguinal nerve b. Pudendal nerve
   c. Genitofemoral nerve d. All of these

5. **The structure that provides a pad of fatty tissue for the external female genitalia is:**
   a. Perineum b. Labia minora and majora
   c. Mons pubis d. Vulva

6. **Identify the part of uterus among the following?** *(AIIMS Raipur Staff Nurse Grade I-2018)*
   a. Body b. Isthmus
   c. Cervix d. All of these

Explanation: The **uterus** has four major regions: Fundus, Body, Isthmus and cervix. So all three given options are part of uterus.

7. **The most common anatomical position of uterus is:**
   a. Anteverted and antiflexed
   b. Retroverted and retroflexed
   c. Retroverted and antiflexed
   d. Antiverted and retroflexed

Explanation: Normal uterus is anteverted and anteflexed. The normal position is an anteverted uterus, which is tipped forward. The uterine position is also sometimes described in relation to the location of the fundus; that is, an anteflexed uterus, which is normal and where the fundus tilts forward.

8. **The lower uterine segment is formed from the:**
   a. Cervix b. Isthmus and cervix
   c. Body of the uterus d. Isthmus

9. **Structures that support the uterus include:**
   a. Round ligament b. Broad ligament
   c. Cervicovaginal junction d. All of these

10. **The shape of non-pregnant uterus is:**
    a. Globular b. Pear shaped (pyriform)
    c. Oval d. Cylindrical

11. **True support of uterus:**
    a. Broad ligament b. Round ligament
    c. Cardinal ligament d. Uterosacral ligament

12. **Blood supply of the uterus is by:**
    a. Ovarian artery b. Uterine artery
    c. Both a and b d. None of these

13. **The origin of the ovaries is from:**
    a. Genital ridge b. Genital tubercle
    c. Wolffian duct d. Mullerian duct

14. **Ovarian artery is a branch of:**
    a. Renal artery
    b. Internal iliac artery
    c. Abdominal part of the aorta
    d. External iliac artery

15. **Arrange the parts of fallopian tube from medial to lateral order:**
    a. Interstitial b. Isthmus
    c. Ampulla d. Infundibulum
    a. a, b, c, d b. d, c, b, a
    c. a, c, b, d d. b, d, a, c

Explanation: Intramural or interstitial, isthmus, ampulla and infundibulum is the order of arrangement from medial to lateral.

16. **Identify the incorrect statement regarding Fallopian tube:**
    a. Serosa, muscular and mucosa are the layers of fallopian tube
    b. Columnar ciliated epithelium is predominant in fallopian tube
    c. Uterine and ovarian artery supply blood to it
    d. The main function is to produce ova

Explanation: All other statements are correct regarding fallopian tube, but the production of ova is the responsibility of ovary and transportation of it to uterus is the responsibility of fallopian tube.

17. **What happens to the corpus luteum after ovulation if pregnancy does not take place?** *New Q*
    a. Produces a lot of oxytocin.
    b. Degenerates in a short time.
    c. Is maintained intact in the presence of progesterone.
    d. Becomes active and secretes FSH and LH.

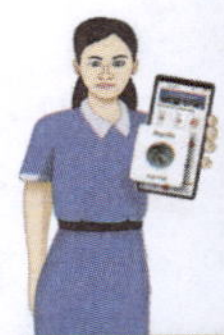

Ans.

1. c
2. b
3. d
4. d
5. c
6. d
7. a
8. b
9. d
10. b
11. c
12. b
13. a
14. c
15. a
16. d
17. b

Explanation: The corpus luteum is a temporary endocrine structure that forms in the ovary after the release of an egg (ovulation). It produces progesterone which is essential for maintaining the lining of the uterus (endometrium) in preparation for pregnancy. If pregnancy does not occur, the corpus luteum will degenerate in a short time, and the levels of progesterone will drop. This will trigger menstruation, which is the shedding of the lining of the uterus.

18. The normal length of the uterine cavity is usually:

a. 5.5-6 cm b. 6.5-7 cm
c. 7.5-8 cm d. 8.5-9 cm

19. Largest cell in the human body is:

a. Myelin cell b. Glial cell
c. Osteocyte d. Ovum

20. The falling down of an organ from its normal anatomical position is termed:

a. Protrusion b. Regurgitation
c. Procidentia d. Hernia

21. A vaginal fistula that opens into the rectum is called: *(LNJP H D 2012)*

a. Rectovaginal fistula b. Enterovaginal fistula
c. Vesicovaginal fistula d. Colovaginal fistula

22. Accumulation of pus in the fallopian tube is known as:

a. Salpingitis b. Pyosalpinx
c. Hydrosalpinx d. Hydro-oopinex

23. The muscle which stretches from the perineum to ischial tuberosity is:

a. Bulbous cavernosum b. Ischiocavernosus
c. Gluteus minimus d. Gluteus maximus

24. Visual examination of the vagina and cervix with an optical magnifying instrument is termed:

a. Proctoscope b. Colposcope
c. Salpingoscope d. Cystoscope

25. A procedure that allows the physician to examine the lining of the bladder is called:

a. Colposcopy b. Urethroscopy
c. Ureteroscopy d. Cystoscopy

26. Inspection of the uterine cavity by endoscopy with access through the cervix is known as:

a. Hysteroscopy b. Salpingoscopy
c. Salpingogram d. Hysterosalpingography

27. Ultrasound is the useful diagnostic method to diagnose the:

a. Endometrial carcinoma b. Cancer cervix
c. Leiomyosarcoma d. Fibroid uterus

28. Inflammation of the fallopian tube is: *(AIIMS Bhopal Nursing Officer, 2018)*

a. Endometritis b. Vaginitis
c. Cervicitis d. Salpingitis

Explanation: Salpingitis is inflammation of fallopian tube. Endometritis is the inflammation of endometrial layer of uterus. Cervicitis is the inflammation of cervix and vaginitis is the inflammation of vagina.

29. At term uterus weight is:

a. 200–300 gm b. 400–500 gm
c. 600–700 kg d. 900–1000 gm

30. Pacemaker of uterine contraction is:

a. Tubal ostia b. SA node
c. AV node d. Purkinje fibers

Explanation: Tubal ostia is the pacemaker of uterine contraction. SA node is the pacemaker of heart.

31. Which among the following is an age-related change that occurs in female reproductive system?

a. Sore nipple
b. Vaginal dryness
c. Decreased risk of vaginal yeast infections
d. Increased level of estrogen

ANATOMY OF BREAST

32. Breast is composed of: *(NCFL 2019) (AP)*

a. Glandular tissues only
b. Connective tissues only
c. Connective and fatty tissues
d. Glandular and fatty tissues

Explanation: Breast is composed of Glandular tissue (special tissue which produces milk) and the collection of fats cells called adipose tissue.

33. Breast is the modification of which gland?

a. Sebaceous gland
b. Endocrine gland
c. Bartholin's gland
d. Sweat gland

34. The skin of the breast is thickest at: *New Q*

a. Superior aspect
b. Lateral aspect
c. Aereola and nipple
d. Base

35. Milk production takes place in which part of the breast?

a. Lobes b. Lobules
c. Mammary duct d. Nipple

36. Approximately how many lobes are present in each breast?

a. 5–10 b. 10–15
c. 15–20 d. 20–25

37. At what week of gestation, breast tissue begins to develop in a fetus?

a. 4 weeks b. 8 weeks
c. 10 weeks d. 12 weeks

MENSTRUAL CYCLE

38. Labor takes place after……day of last menstrual period. *(RRB Feb 2012)*

a. 260 b. 270
c. 250 d. 280

39. Implantation of fertilized egg ideally occurs during the …………..phase of menstrual cycle.

a. Secretory phase
b. Menstrual phase
c. Proliferative phase
d. Ovulation phase

40. The layer of uterus that is sloughed off during menstruation is:

a. Endometrium b. Myometrium
c. Perimetrium d. Serous layer

41. The first episode of menstrual bleeding is called:

a. Thelarche b. Menarche
c. Menopause d. Menorrhea

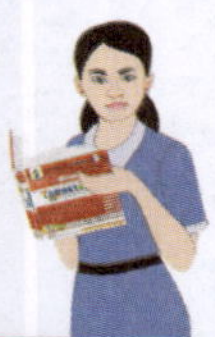

Ans.

18. c
19. d
20. c
21. a
22. b
23. b
24. b
25. d
26. a
27. d
28. d
29. d
30. a
31. b
32. d
33. d
34. d
35. b
36. c
37. a
38. d
39. a
40. a
41. b

42. The phase in which the lining cells of the ovarian follicle are stimulated by luteinizing hormone to develop the corpus luteum, to produce progesterone and estrogen is: *(AIIMS Raipur Grade II 2017)*

a. Menstrual phase b. Proliferative phase
c. Secretory phase d. Follicular phase

FUNDAMENTALS OF REPRODUCTION

43. Vaginal pH is:

a. 3.8-4.5 b. 4.5-6.0
c. 5.0-6.5 d. 6.5-7.5

44. Bartholin gland is found in: *(RRB Feb 2012)*

a. Cervix b. Ovary
c. Vagina d. Uterus

45. Site of fertilization in female reproductive system is: *(RRB Feb 2012)*

a. Ovary b. Cervix
c. Uterus d. Fallopian tube

Explanation: Fertilization occurs at the ampullary part of fallopian tube.

46. Endometrium after conception is known as: *(RRB Feb 2012)*

a. Perimetrium b. Myometrium
c. Decidua d. Prometrium

47. Which chemical present in the acromial tip of sperm facilitates the penetration of zona pellucida of ovum?

a. Hydrochloric acid b. Hyaluronidase
c. Formalin d. Acetyl choline

Explanation: Hyaluronidase is a chemical present in the acromial tip of the sperm which facilitates the penetration of zona pellucida of ovum.

48. After ovulation corpus luteum formed in the ovary releases: *(Staff Nurse G II 2014)*

a. Testosterone b. Aldosterone
c. Progesterone d. Estrogen

49. Fertilized ovum reaches the uterus in:

a. 3-4 days b. 6-8 days
c. 10-12 days d. 12-14 days

50. The first evidence of pubertal development in female is usually manifested as: *(Banaras HU 2015)*

a. Onset of menarche
b. Appearance of breast buds
c. Appearance of axillary and pubic hair
d. Onset of growth spurt

51. Puberty onset in girls starts with:

a. Menarche
b. Growth spurt
c. Menopause
d. Thelarche and growth of pubic hair

52. True regarding primary oocytes is:

a. All primary oocytes are formed in prenatal life
b. All primary oocytes are formed just after the birth
c. All primary oocytes are formed after menarche
d. Primary oocytes are formed just before menstruation

53. The primary oocytes remain suspended in .... Phase of meiosis I.

a. Prophase b. Metaphase
c. Anaphase d. Telophase

54. When the cells in the morula rearrange themselves to form a hollow ball of cells with an inner cell mass, it is known as: *New Q*

a. Zygote b. Blastocyte
c. Ovulation d. Gastrulation

Explanation: When the cells in the morula rearrange themselves to form a hollow ball of cells with an inner cell mass, it is known as a blastocyst.

The blastocyst is an early stage of embryonic development that typically occurs around 4–5 days after fertilization. It is characterized by the formation of a hollow structure with an outer layer called the trophectoderm and an inner cell mass. The fluid-filled cavity within the blastocyst is known as the blastocoel. The blastocyst is important for the implantation process.

55. Seven weeks after the conception, the growing structure inside a uterus is now called: *(RAK MSc 2018)*

a. Zygote b. Embryo
c. Fetus d. Neonate

Explanation:

- Conception to 8th week of gestation – Embryo
- 8th week to delivery – Fetus
- Birth to 4 weeks (28 days) – Neonate
- 4 weeks to 1 year - Infant

56. The phenomenon of mittelschmerz indicates: *(AIIMS BPL NO 2018)*

a. Menstruation b. Ovulation
c. Implantation d. Fertilization

Explanation: Mittelschmerz is one-sided lower abdominal pain and pelvic region associated with ovulation. This occurs roughly midway through a woman's menstrual cycle. The pain can appear suddenly and usually subsides within hours, although it may sometimes last two or three days.

57. Fleeting abdominal pain due to follicular bleeding causing peritoneal irritation is called: *(Safdarjung NO 2018)*

a. Corpus hemorrhagicum
b. Mittelschmerz
c. Corpus luteum
d. Corpus albicans

Explanation: Minor bleeding from the follicle into the abdominal cavity may cause peritoneal irritation and fleeting lower abdominal pain. It is known as **mittelschmerz.**

After ovulation, hemorrhage into the remains of the follicle usually occurs resulting in a structure called a **corpus hemorrhagicum.**

58. When is the best time to achieve pregnancy? *(RAK MSc 2018)*

a. Midway between 7th and 8th day of ovulation
b. Immediately after starting of menses
c. 14 days after the beginning of period
d. 7 days before the next period is expected

Explanation: The best time to achieve pregnancy is 14 days before the next period is expected, if cycle is of 28 days. It is the time of ovulation, i.e., release of ovum and the LH surge precedes before ovulation that provides the best conditions for the fertilization.

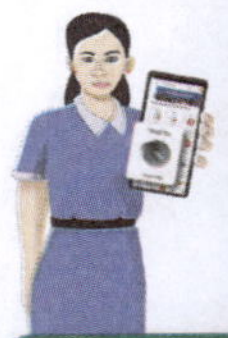

Ans.

42.	c
43.	a
44.	c
45.	d
46.	c
47.	b
48.	c
49.	a
50.	b
51.	d
52.	a
53.	a
54.	b
55.	b
56.	b
57.	b
58.	c

59. The process of maturation of the female egg is termed:
a. Spermatogenesis b. Oogenesis
c. Archiogenesis d. Ovogenesis

60. What is the fertilization life span or viability for oocyte?
a. <12 hours b. 12-24 hours
c. 24-48 hours d. 48-72 hours

61. Spermatozoa is viable for a period of:
a. 12-24 hrs b. 24-48 hrs
c. 48-72 hrs d. Up to 5 days

62. Discharge of ovum from the ovary is referred to as:
a. Maturation b. Ovulation
c. Proliferation d. Nidation

63. By what week of pregnancy do the reproductive organs and genitalia of the baby typically develop? *New Q*
a. 6–8 weeks b. 8–10 weeks
c. 13–16 weeks d. 17–21 weeks

64. Which of the following is the first organ system to develop in the embryo? *New Q*
a. Cardiovascular system b. Nervous system
c. Pulmonary system d. Gastrointestinal system

Explanation: The heart is the first organ to be developed in the fetus. It starts to develop in the third week of pregnancy. The heart of an embryo starts beating at about week 5 of pregnancy. It may be possible to detect the heartbeat at this point using vaginal ultrasound.

65. Risk factors for ectopic pregnancy include all, except: *New Q*
a. Prior history of infertility
b. Prior history of pelvic inflammatory disease
c. Prior history of uterine fibroids
d. Previous tubal surgery

66. Which of the following term refers to infrequent and irregular ovulation:
a. Oligoovulation b. Hypoovulation
c. Polyovulation d. None of these

67. After fertilization of ovum, the initial mitotic division of the zygote results in the formation of:
a. Morula b. Blastomeres
c. Oocytes d. Blastocysts

68. What are the mitotic divisions that a zygote undergoes called? *New Q*
a. Meiosis b. Cleavage
c. Fertilization d. Blastocyte

Explanation: Cleavage is the series of rapid mitotic divisions that a zygote undergoes after fertilization. The zygote divides into two cells, then four cells, then eight cells, and so on. This process of cell division increases the number of cells in the embryo, but it does not increase the size of the embryo.

69. Identify the correct statement regarding implantation:
a. Implantation occurs in anterior or posterior wall of the body near to fundus
b. Implantation occurs on 6th day following fertilization which corresponds to 20th day of regular menstrual cycle.
c. Implantation occurs through four stages apposition, adhesion, penetration and invasion
d. All of the above

Explanation: All the above-mentioned statements are correct regarding implantation. Implantation means fertilized ovum is transferred from site of fertilization to uterus.

70. Implantation of zygote is facilitated by:
a. Trophoblast b. Medulla
c. Cortex d. Blastocysts

71. The outer layer of the blastocyte is called: *New Q*
a. Blastocoel b. Trophoblast
c. Zygote d. Morula

Explanation: The trophoblast is the outer layer of the morula. The trophoblast is responsible for attaching the embryo to the uterine wall. The blastocoel is the fluid-filled cavity inside the morula which provides a space for the embryo to grow and develop.

72. In case of in-vitro fertilization, fertilized ovum transferred into the uterine cavity at:
a. 1–2 cell stage b. 2–4 cell stage
c. 4–8 cell stage d. 16–24 cell stage

73. How many pairs of chromosomes are there in a man? *(RRB Feb 2012)*
a. 24 b. 23
c. 22 d. None of these

74. Corpus luteum is found in: *(RRB Feb 2012)*
a. Fetus b. Placenta
c. Uterus d. Ovary

75. Fusion of sperm and ovum is called: *(RRB Feb 2012)*
a. Fertilization b. Transfusion
c. Combination d. None of these

76. Ischial tuberosity helps for:
a. Bearing of body weight while sitting
b. Normal labor
c. Normal walking
d. Normal standing

77. Basal body temperature will .... following ovulation.
a. Increase b. Decrease
c. No change d. Fluctuation

78. The average age of puberty in girls is:
a. 9–10 years b. 10–12 years
c. 10–14 years d. 14–16 years

79. Time required to reach in two cell stage after fertilization is:
a. 10 hours b. 20 hours
c. 30 hours d. 40 hours

80. Time required to reach in 16 cell stage after fertilization is:
a. 2nd day b. 4th day
c. 6th day d. 8th day

81. Ovulation occurs soon after the formation of:
a. Primary spermatozoa b. Secondary spermatozoa
c. Primary oocyte d. Secondary oocyte

82. Where does oogenesis occurs in human?
a. Inner most layer of ovary b. Outermost layer of ovary
c. Fallopian tube d. Uterus

83. Correct order of oogenesis is:
a. Oogonia → primary oocyte → secondary oocyte → ovulation
b. Primary oocyte → secondary oocyte → oogonia → ovulation
c. Ovulation → primary oocye → secondary oocyte → oogonia
d. Oogonia → ovulation → primary oocyte → secondary oocyte

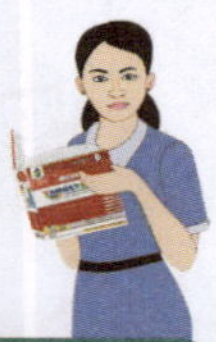

Ans.

59.	b
60.	b
61.	c
62.	b
63.	c
64.	a
65.	c
66.	a
67.	b
68.	b
69.	d
70.	a
71.	b
72.	c
73.	b
74.	d
75.	a
76.	a
77.	a
78.	c
79.	c
80.	b
81.	d
82.	b
83.	a

84. **How many numbers of chromosomes a primary oocyte/primary spermatocyte contains?**
a. 46 b. 44
c. 23 d. 22

85. **Number of chromosomes in secondary oocyte/secondary spermatocyte are:**
a. 46 b. 44
c. 23 d. 22

86. **Sex of the child is determined by the pattern of the sex chromosome supplied by:**
a. Spermatozoon b. Oocyte
c. Morula d. Blastocyst

87. **The correct lineage of a zygote is:** New Q
a. Zygote → Blastomere → Morula → Blastocyst
b. Zygote → Blastula → Morula → Blastocyst
c. Zygote → Morula → Blastomere → Blastocyte
d. Zygote → Blastocyst → Morula → Blastomere

88. **Delayed puberty is:**
a. The absence of testicular development by the age of 14 years in males
b. The absence of breast development by the age of 13 years in females
c. Primary amenorrhea with normal breast development by the age of 15 in females
d. All of the above

89. **Fertilization of two or more ova from the same cycle by sperm from separate acts of sexual intercourse is known as:**
a. Superfetation b. Superfecundation
c. Dizygotic pregnancy d. Monozygotic pregnancy

90. **Total iron requirement for a woman during pregnancy?** New Q
a. 500 mg b. 1000 mg
c. 2000 mg d. 2500 mg

Explanation: The body iron requirement for an average pregnancy is approximately 1,000 mg.

Hallberg (1988) calculated Iron losses during pregnancy:
- 350 mg lost to the fetus and placenta
- 250 mg lost in blood at delivery
- 450 mg required for the large increase in maternal red blood cell mass
- 240 mg basal losses of iron from the body

Hence, Total iron requirements of a pregnancy is about 1,040 mg (excluding blood loss at delivery)

Note: The recommended daily iron intake for pregnant women is around 27–30 mg/day.

PRINCIPAL EVENTS OF EMBRYONIC AND FETAL DEVELOPMENT

91. **A child's heredity is determined at the time of:**
(RRB Feb 2012)
a. Viability b. Delivery
c. Conception d. Infancy

92. **Neural tube/nervous system develops from:**
a. Ectoderm b. Endoderm
c. Mesoderm d. All of these

93. **Closure of neural tube begins at:**
a. Cervical b. Cephalic
c. Podalic d. Lumbar

Explanation: The closure of neural tube begins in the cervical area (in the middle of the embryo) and extends from there in both the cranial and caudal directions.

94. **The heart is developed from:**
a. Paraxial mesoderm
b. Intermediate mesoderm
c. Splanchnopleuric intraembryonic mesoderm
d. Somatoleuric intraembryonic mesoderm

95. **Rectum develops from:**
a. Cloaca b. Hindgut
c. Allantoic remnants d. Urogenital sinus

96. **Small intestine develops from:**
a. Foregut b. Midgut
c. Hindgut d. Endodermal cloaca

97. **Coronary sinus develops from:**
a. Truncus arteriosus b. Conus
c. Sinus venosus d. AV canal

98. **Fetus develops its own blood supply from ....week.**
a. 10th to 12th week b. 12th to 14th week
c. 12th to 16th week d. 12th to 20th week

99. **Daughter cells formed after meiosis I contain .... chromosome.**
a. Polyploid b. Aneuploid
c. Diploid d. Haploid

100. **Which one of the periods of gestation is the most susceptible period for congenital malformations:**
a. 1st week b. 2nd week
c. 3rd week- 8th week d. 9th week-12th week

101. **The physiochemical changes that occur in the sperm to make it capable of fertilizing the ovum is known as:**
a. Spermatogenesis b. Degeneration
c. Capacitation d. Oogenesis

102. **Fetus forms from:**
a. Morula b. Blastocyst
c. Inner cell mass d. Syncytiotrophoblast

103. **At what week embryo can be differentiated as human?**
a. 2nd week b. 4th week
c. 6th week d. 8th week

104. **The mean cardiac output of the fetus at term is:** New Q
a. 100 mL/kg/min b. 200 mL/kg/min
c. 250 mL/kg/min d. 500 mL/kg/min

105. **First of all, fetal heart-sounds can be assessed:**
[AIIMS-2011]
a. Between 2–3 weeks b. Between 8 and 10 weeks
c. Between 10–12 weeks d. Between 16 and 18 weeks

THE PLACENTA AND FETAL MEMBRANES

106. **The thin rim of endometrial stroma overlying the blastocyst is known as:**
a. Decidua capsularis
b. Decidua vera
c. Decidua basalis
d. Decidua parietalis

107. **The cardinal function of decidua is:**
a. Immune response
b. Production of hormones
c. Maintenance of pregnancy
d. None of the above

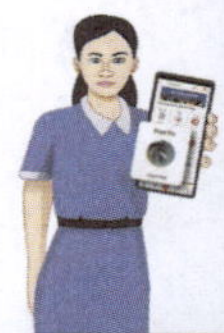

Ans.

84.	a
85.	c
86.	a
87.	a
88.	d
89.	b
90.	b
91.	c
92.	a
93.	a
94.	c
95.	a
96.	b
97.	c
98.	d
99.	d
100.	c
101.	c
102.	c
103.	d
104.	d
105.	b
106.	a
107.	c

108. O_2 and CO_2 are exchanged in the placenta through the process of:
a. Pinocytosis b. Diffusion
c. Facilitated diffusion d. Active transport

109. The following is not a part of conceptus:
a. Amniotic fluid b. Decidua
c. Fetus d. Membrane

110. Characteristic hormone of the placenta is: *(Kerala PSC, Nov 2014)*
a. Estrogen b. Chorionic gonadotropin
c. Corticotrophin d. Oxytocin

111. Normal weight of placenta at term is:*(Staff Nurse G II 2014)*
a. 1/4th of baby weight b. 1/6th of baby weight
c. 500 g d. 900 g

112. The outermost membrane of the placenta is: *(LNJP H D 2012)*
a. Chorion b. Amnion
c. Cotyledons d. Yolk sac

113. Humans placenta fully develop at …… months of pregnancy. *(RRB Feb 2012)*
a. 2 months b. 3 months
c. 1 month d. 4 months

114. Which of the following structures is necessary for maintenance of pregnancy before placental development?
a. Hypothalamus b. Umbilical cord
c. Pituitary d. Corpus luteum

115. The structure that supplies nutrition to the growing ovum before placenta takes the function is:
a. Corpus luteum b. Decidua
c. Myometrium d. Corpus callosum

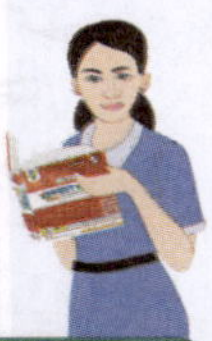

116. About how much blood a mature placenta contains?
a. 250 mL b. 500 mL
c. 700 mL d. 1000 mL

117. Identify the correct statements regarding human placenta:
a. Human placenta is discoid
b. Human placenta is hemochorial
c. Placenta establish connection between mother and baby through umbilical cord
d. All of the above

Explanation: All the above statements are correct regarding human placenta. Placenta develops from two sources, principal component is fetal component named chorion and maternal component named decidua basalis.

118. Placenta shape is:
a. Round b. Global
c. Discoid d. Fusiform

119. Which structure establishes connection between the fetus and mother during intra uterine life?
a. Uterus b. Ampulla
c. Placenta d. Fallopian tube

120. Placenta secretes all the following hormones; EXCEPT:
a. Estrogen *(AIIMS Bhopal Nursing Officer, 2018)*
b. Luteinizing hormone
c. Progesterone
d. Human chorionic gonadotropin

Explanation: Luteinizing hormone is produced by gonadotropic cells in the anterior pituitary gland. All other hormones are secreted by placenta.

121. Umbilical cord is attached to:
a. Fetal surface of placenta
b. Maternal surface of placenta
c. Near to the center of the surface
d. Both a and c

Explanation: Umbilical cord is attached to fetal surface and is attached to center. It is about 40 cm in length usually varies from 30-100 cm.

122. At term approximate placental weight is:
a. 300 gm b. 500 gm
c. 700 gm d. 900 gm

123. Fetal origin of placenta is:
a. 1/5th b. 2/5th
c. 3/5th d. 4/5th

124. Structure that acts as power house of hormone production during pregnancy?
a. Hypothalamus b. Umbilical cord
c. Pituitary d. Placenta

125. The mother's placenta weighs 500 gram. Approximately, how much would be the weight of the full term newborn?
a. 3 kg b. 2 kg
c. 4 kg d. 5 kg

126. The following are the causes of separation of a normally situated placenta; EXCEPT: *(AIIMS Raipur Grade II 2017)*
a. Sudden uterine decompression
b. Defective decidua
c. Supine hypotension syndrome
d. Thrombophilias

ANATOMY OF AMNIOTIC FLUID AND UMBILICAL CORD

127. The average length of umbilical cord is: *(RRB Feb 2012)*
a. 25 cm b. 30 cm
c. 10 cm d. 55 cm

128. Normal volume of amniotic fluid at term is….. mL. *(RRB Feb 2012)*
a. 400–500 mL b. 500–600 mL
c. 600–800 mL d. 1000–1200 mL

129. Functions of the amniotic fluid includes all of the following; EXCEPT:
a. Protection of the fetus from injury
b. Protection of the fetus from infection
c. Temperature maintenance
d. Providing oxygenation to fetus

130. The biochemical and organic compounds present in amniotic fluid are all; EXCEPT:
a. Protein b. Lipid and glucose
c. Urea and creatinine d. Ammonia

131. Amniotic fluid otherwise known as: *(RRB Feb 2012)*
a. Aqueous humor
b. Liquor amnii
c. Liquor chorion
d. None of the above

132. At 12th week of gestation amniotic fluid measures, about:
a. 40 mL b. 50 mL
c. 60 mL d. 70 mL

Ans.
108. b
109. b
110. b
111. b
112. a
113. b
114. d
115. a
116. b
117. d
118. c
119. c
120. b
121. d
122. b
123. d
124. d
125. a
126. b
127. d
128. c
129. d
130. d
131. b
132. b

133. Main carbohydrate in amniotic fluid is: *(CMC Vellore 98)*

a. Glucose b. Fructose
c. Lactose d. Maltose

Explanation: Organic constituents of Amniotic fluid at preterm

- Glucose—20 mg/dL
- Proteins—0.3 mg/dL
- Urea—30 mg/dL
- Non protein nitrogen—30 mg/dL
- Uric acid—9.9 mg/dL
- Creatinine—2 mg/dL
- Lipids—50 mg/dL
- Hormones—Insulin, prolactin, renin

Inorganic constituents of Amniotic fluid at preterm

- Na, K, Cl

134. The functions of amniotic fluid are: *(AIIMS Raipur Grade II 2017)*

a. Protects fetus from jarring and injury
b. Maintains intrauterine temperature
c. Facilitates exchange of nutrients.
d. Protects the placenta and umbilical cord

a. a, b, c b. b, c, d
c. a, c, d d. a, b, c, d

Explanation: The pH of amniotic fluid is 7–7. 5. It serves as a cushion for the growing fetus and also facilitates the exchange of nutrients, water, and biochemical products between mother and fetus. It helps in maintaining intrauterine temperature and protects placenta and umbilical cord. From 10th to the 20th week, amniotic fluid increases from 25 mL to 400 mL.

135. Golden color of amniotic fluid is seen in:

a. Rh- Incompatibility b. Fetal death
c. IUGR d. Fetal distress

136. Identify correct statements regarding amniotic fluid:

a. Maintains optimum temperature of the fetus
b. Contains fetal urine, fetal lanugo and epithelial cells
c. Provides cushion against injury to the fetus
d. All of the above

137. Amniotic fluid volume during pregnancy is:

a. 500–700 mL b. 700–1000 mL
c. 1000–1500 mL d. Above 1500 mL

138. Polyhydroamniosis is a condition when the amniotic fluid volume exceeds more than .... mL.

a. 1000 b. 1500
c. 2000 d. 2500

Explanation: When the volume is more than 2000 mL it is called polyhydroamniosis. If the amniotic fluid volume is less than 200 mL, it is known as oligohydroamniosis.

139. An amniotic fluid index of less than 5 cm indicates: *(Daman & Diu NO 2018)*

a. Anhydramnios b. Hydramnios
c. Polyhydramnios d. Oligohydramnios

Explanation:

- **Oligohydramnios:** Amniotic fluid index of less than 5 cm or 200 mL
- **Polyhydramnios:** An amniotic fluid index more than 25 cm or 2000 mL
- **Anhydramnios:** The absence of the amniotic fluid (liquor amnii)

140. Oligohydramnios is a condition when amniotic fluid is less than: *(RAK MSc 2018)*

a. 75 mL at term b. 100 mL at term
c. 150 mL at term d. 200 mL at term

Explanation: Oligohydramnios is a condition in which amniotic fluid is deficient in amount less than 200 mL at term. Sonographically, oligohydramnios is defined when amniotic Fluid Index (AFI) is less than 5 cm.

141. What is the normal color of amniotic fluid when the bag of water ruptures?

a. As like water b. Bluish
c. Brownish d. Yellowish

(Ref: Hiralal Konar. DC Dutta's Textbook of Obstetrics 9th edition 2018 Jaypee Publications, p. 34.)

Explanation:

- Amniotic fluid is clear liquid as like water
- It never appears bluish
- Dark brown color indicates IUD
- In case of Rh incompatibility, it is Golden yellow color

142. Meconium stained (dark green) amniotic fluid indicates:

a. Respiratory distress
b. Rh incompatibility
c. Post maturity of Fetus
d. Intrauterine Death of Fetus

143. Yellow-colored amniotic fluid indicates:

a. Respiratory distress
b. Rh incompatibility
c. Post maturity of Fetus
d. Hemolytic disease of the newborn

144. Dark red brown amniotic fluid indicates:

a. Respiratory distress b. Rh incompatibility
c. Post maturity of Fetus d. Fetal death

145. Greenish yellow color amniotic fluid indicates:

a. Respiratory distress
b. Rh incompatibility
c. Post maturity of fetus
d. Fetal death

146. Amniotic Fluid Index (AFI) is measured by:

a. Abdominal girth b. Ultrasonography
c. Leopold maneuver d. Ballottement

Explanation: Amniotic Fluid Index is measured with the help of ultrasonography by dividing the abdomen into four quadrants. For dividing the abdomen into four quadrants linea nigra is considered as vertical point and umbilicus is considered as horizontal point.

- In each quadrant, deepest pocket is measured in cm. Sum of all pockets is considered as AFI
- Normal value of AFI varies from 8 cm to 18 cm
- AFI less than 5–6 cm is considered as oligo-hydroamniosis
- AFI more than 20–24 cm is considered as polyhydroamniosis

147. Color of amniotic fluid in post term pregnancy is:

a. Colorless
b. Golden
c. Saffron
d. Brown

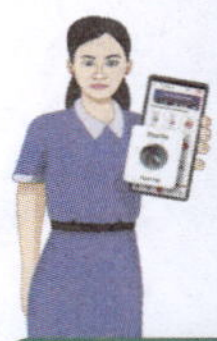

Ans.

133. a
134. d
135. a
136. d
137. b
138. c
139. d
140. d
141. a
142. a
143. d
144. d
145. c
146. b
147. c

Explanation: Color of Amniotic fluid

- **Saffron colored:** Post maturity.
- **Green colored:** Meconium.
- **Golden colored:** Rh isoimmunization.
- **Red colored:** Abruption.
- **Tobacco juice:** Intrauterine death (IUD)
- **White with flakes:** Normal

148. Which one of the following leads to greenish discoloration of the amniotic fluid? *(DSSSB 2013)*

a. Lanugo
b. Hydramnios
c. Vernix
d. Meconium

Explanation: Greenish colored amniotic fluid indicates meconium stained amniotic fluid. It indicates chances of respiratory distress in newborn.

149. All of the following are the effects of polyhydramnios; EXCEPT:

a. Lung hypoplasia
b. Fetal distress
c. Macrosomia
d. Meconium staining and amniotic bands

150. Percentage of water in amniotic fluid is: *(RRB Feb 2012)*

a. 80 b. 90
c. 70 d. 98

151. The function of amniotic fluid is: *(RRB Feb 2012)*

a. Respiration b. Shock protection
c. Endocrine function d. Nutrition

152. Go through the following statements regarding amniotic fluid and find out incorrect statement:

a. Liquor amnii surrounds fetus everywhere except at its attachment with body stalk
b. Amniotic fluid is completely changed and replaced every 3 hours
c. At term the amount of amniotic fluid is 1000-1500 mL
d. Amniotic fluid is colorless and near term it becomes pale straw colored

Explanation: Option c is incorrect. At term the mount of amniotic fluid is about 600-800 mL. All other options are true. Amniotic fluid is colorless and near term it becomes pale straw colored because of the presence of exfoliated lanugo and epidermal cells from skin.

153. Normal umbilical cord contains:

a. One vein and two arteries
b. One artery and two veins
c. One vein and one artery
d. Two arteries and two veins

154. The connection between umbilical vein and inferior vena cava in the fetal life is known as:

a. Umbilical artery b. Ductus venosus
c. Ductus arteriosus d. Pulmonary artery

Explanation: Option b is the correct answer, this vessel has the highest oxygen concentration in the fetal life. Ductus arteriosus is the connection between aorta and pulmonary artery.

155. Polyhydramnios occur in all of the following; EXCEPT:

a. Diabetes mellitus b. Anencephaly
c. Multiple pregnancy d. Renal agenesis of fetus

156. The transmission of infection from the mother to the fetus through placenta is termed: *(DSSSB PHN, 2015)*

a. Iatrogenic b. Teratogenic
c. Nosocomial d. Vertical

FETAL CIRCULATION

157. The umbilical vein carries:

a. Oxygenated blood b. Deoxygenated blood
c. Mixed blood d. All of these

158. After the birth umbilical arteries are called:

a. Ligamentum venosum
b. Umbilical ligament
c. Ligamentum teres
d. Ligamentum arteriosum

Explanation: Medial umbilical ligament is the remnant of distal portion of umbilical artery.

159. In fetal circulation, deoxygenated blood is present in:

a. Umbilical artery b. Umbilical vein
c. Pulmonary artery d. All of these

Explanation: Umbilical artery contains deoxygenated blood. All other blood vessels contain oxygenated blood.

160. Which among the following vessels contains highest oxygen concentration in fetal circulation?

a. Umbilical vein
b. Pulmonary artery
c. Ductus venosus
d. Ductus arteriosus

161. The amount of fetal blood flowing per minute through the placenta at term is:

a. 100–200 mL b. 200–300 mL
c. 300–400 mL d. 500–600 mL

162. Communication between right and left atrium in fetal circulation is known as:

a. Foramen ovale b. Ductus arteriosus
c. Ductus venosus d. Fossa ovalis

163. Communication between aorta and pulmonary artery in fetal circulation is known as:

a. Foramen ovale b. Ductus arteriosus
c. Ductus venosus d. Fossa ovalis

164. Communication between umbilical vein and inferior vena cava in fetal circulation is known as:

a. Foramen ovale b. Ductus arteriosus
c. Ductus venosus d. Fossa ovalis

165. Which of the following is the main cause of Meckel's diverticulum? **New Q** *(AIIMS MG, Faculty 2023)*

a. Vitelline duct of the growing fetus is not fully absorbed during pregnancy.
b. Neural tube of the growing fetus is not fully absorbed during pregnancy.
c. Notochord of the growing fetus is not fully absorbed during pregnancy.
d. Umbilical cord of the growing fetus is not fully absorbed during pregnancy.

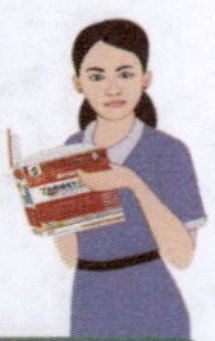

Ans.

148. d
149. c
150. d
151. b
152. c
153. a
154. b
155. d
156. d
157. a
158. b
159. a
160. a
161. d
162. a
163. b
164. c
165. a

166. Main process behind the changes in circulation from fetal period to newborn occurs due to:
a. Clamping of umbilical cord
b. Closure of Ductus Arteriosus
c. Expansion of the lungs
d. Closure of Ductus Venosus

167. Oxygenated blood from placenta goes to fetal heart via:
a. Ductus arteriosus b. Ductus venosus
c. Foramen ovale d. Umbilical artery

168. After birth, in a normal neonate the ductus arteriosus becomes:
a. Venous ligament b. Ligamentum venosum
c. Ligamentum teres d. Ligamentum arteriosum

169. After birth, the umbilical vein collapses and forms:
(Daman & Diu NO 2018)
a. Ligamentum arteriosum b. Ligamentum venosum
c. Ligamentum umbilicus d. Ligamentum teres

Explanation:

Fetal Structure (before birth)	Neonate Structure (after birth)
Foramen ovale	Fossa ovalis
Umbilical vein (intra-abdominal part)	Ligamentum teres
Ductus venosus	Ligamentum venosum
Umbilical arteries and abdominal ligaments	Medial umbilical ligaments, superior vesicular artery (supplies bladder)
Ductus arteriosum	Ligamentum arteriosum

170. After the closure, foramen ovale becomes:
a. Ligamentum venosum
b. Fossa ovalis
c. Ligamentum teres
d. Ligamentum arteriosum

Explanation: The fossa ovalis is a depression in the right atrium of the heart, at the level of the interatrial septum, the wall between right and left atrium. The fossa ovalis is the remnant of a thin fibrous sheet that covers the foramen ovale during fetal development.

171. Uterine artery, is a branch of:
a. Abdominal aorta
b. External iliac artery
c. Femoral artery
d. Internal iliac artery

172. The single umbilical artery is most common in:
a. Oligohydramnios b. Placenta previa
c. Twins d. All of these

Explanation: Monochorionic monozygotic twins is the condition in which there will be single umbilical artery.

ANATOMY AND TYPES OF FEMALE PELVIS

173. The most important muscle of the pelvic floor is:
a. Levator ani muscle b. Ischiocavernosus
c. Bulbocavernosus d. Pubococcygeus

174. The strongest ligament in the female pelvis is:
(RRB Feb 2012)
a. Reverse cervical b. Oblique cervical
c. Transverse cervical d. None of these

175. Number of bones in female pelvis is:
a. 1 b. 2
c. 3 d. 4

Explanation: The pelvis consists of four bones: the right and left hip bones, the sacrum, and the coccyx.

176. Which bone is the part of pelvis?
a. Innominate bone b. Sacrum
c. Coccyx d. All of these

Explanation: All the above-mentioned bones are part of pelvis. Two innominate bones are present. These bones are united by 4 joints such as two sacroiliac joints, sacrococcygeal joint and symphysis pubis.

177. True pelvis is divided as:
a. Inlet, cavity, outlet
b. Brim, cavity, outlet
c. Brim, inlet, outlet
d. Brim, inlet, exit

Explanation: For descriptive purpose, true pelvis can be divided as inlet, cavity and outlet.

178. The innominate bone consists of:
a. Ilium, Ischium, pubis, sacrum and coccyx
b. Ischium, ilium, sacrum and coccyx
c. Ilium, ischium and coccyx
d. Ilium, ischium and pubis

179. The pelvic shape has the poorest prognosis from vaginal delivery is:
a. Platypelloid b. Anthropoid
c. Android d. Gynecoid

180. Which one of the following is the female pelvis?
a. Android b. Gynecoid
c. False pelvis d. Anthropoid

181. Brim of Gynecoid pelvis is.......in shape.
(RRB Feb 2012, RAK MSc 2018)
a. Heart b. Kidney
c. Oval d. Round

Explanation: The shape of brim of gynecoid pelvis is almost round. Gynecoid pelvis is the most suitable pelvis for vaginal delivery.

Table: Comparison of various types of pelvis

	Gynecoid (50% of women)	Android (23% of women)	Anthropoid (24% of women)	Platypel-loid (3% of women)
Brim	Slightly ovoid or transversely rounded	Heart-shaped, angulated	Oval, wider antero-posteriorly	Flattened Antero-posteriorly, wide transversely
	Round	Heart	Oval	Flat

182. The ideal pelvis for child bearing is.....pelvis.
(RRB Feb 2012)
a. Anthropoid b. Platypoid
c. Gynecoid d. Android

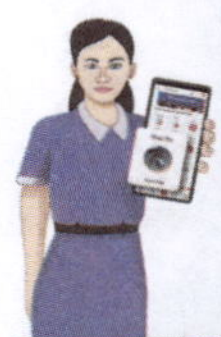

Ans.
166. c
167. b
168. d
169. d
170. b
171. d
172. c
173. a
174. c
175. d
176. d
177. a
178. d
179. c
180. b
181. d
182. c

Explanation: The gynecoid pelvis is more delicate, wider than, and not as high as the male pelvis. The angle of the female pubic arch is wide and round. The female sacrum is wider than the male's and the iliac bone is flatter. The pelvic basin of the female is more spacious and less funnel-shaped.

183. Deep transverse arrest occurs in:
a. Gynecoid pelvis b. Platypelloid pelvis
c. Android pelvis d. Anthropoid pelvis

184. Absence of one sacral ala of pelvis is called:
a. Rickety flat pelvis b. Naegele's pelvis
c. Robert's pelvis d. Kyphotic pelvis

185. The brim of the anthropoid pelvis is…….. shape. *(RRB Feb 2012)*
a. Kidney b. Round
c. Heart d. Oval

186. The type of pelvis in which the features are heart-shaped brim, narrow forepelvis and sciatic notch with prominent ischial spines and suprapubic angle < 90°: *(AIIMS Raipur Grade II 2017)*
a. Gynecoid pelvis b. Android pelvis
c. Anthropoid pelvis d. Platypelloid pelvis

Explanation: Gynecoid pelvis also known as True pelvis is oval at inlet, wide subpubic arch and pelvic brim which is transverse ellipse. Anthropoid pelvis is oval at inlet, pelvic brim is anteroposterior ellipse, suprapubic arch slightly narrowed. Platypoid pelvis is flattened at inlet and has prominent sacrum, pelvic brim is transverse kidney shaped.

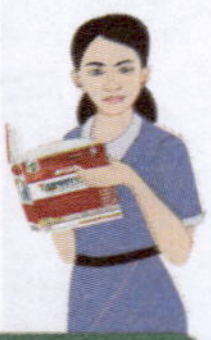

187. The innominate bone of the pelvis is not composed of the:
a. Sacrum b. Ilium
c. Pubis d. Ischium

188. Which one of the following pairs regarding pelvis is not correct? *(Banaras HU 2015)*
a. Gynecoid: Female type
b. Android: Male type
c. Anthropoid: Wedge type
d. Platypelloid: Flat type

189. The suture line between two parietal bones is called: *(Kerala PSC, Nov 2014)*
a. Coronal b. Lambdoidal
c. Frontal d. Sagittal

190. Pelvis is composed of:
a. Innominate bones b. Sacrum
c. Coccyx d. All of these

191. Landmark used while assessing the descend of head during the process of delivery?
a. Ischial spines b. Pubic symphysis
c. Coccyx d. Sacrum

192. Anatomical anterioposterior conjugate is also known as:
a. True conjugate
b. Obstetric conjugate
c. Diagonal conjugate
d. External conjugate

PELVIC DIAMETER

193. The passage of bi-parietal diameter through the pelvic inlet is referred to as:
a. Descent b. Flexion
c. Engagement d. Extension

194. Largest diameter in pelvic inlet is:
a. Anterior Posterior b. Transverse Diameter
c. Oblique Diameter d. None of these

195. Transverse diameter of inlet of pelvis is about:
a. 11 cm b. 12 cm
c. 13 cm d. 14 cm

196. Angle of inclination in human pelvis is:
a. 45° b. Between 55° and 60°
c. 65° d. 75°

197. The pelvic diameter which is measured from the tip of the sacral promontory to the most bulging point on the back of symphysis pubis is known as:
a. Obstetric conjugate b. Diagonal conjugate
c. Anatomical conjugate d. Oblique diameter

198. The pelvic diameter which is measured from middle of sacral promontory to the upper inner surface of the pubic symphysis is known as:
a. Obstetric conjugate b. Diagonal conjugate
c. Anatomical conjugate d. Oblique diameter

199. The distance between middle of sacral promontory to lower inner border of symphysis pubis is known as:
a. Obstetric conjugate
b. Diagonal conjugate
c. Anatomical conjugate
d. Oblique diameter

200. The measurement between one sacroiliac joint and the opposite iliopubic eminence is:
a. Obstetric conjugate
b. Diagonal conjugate
c. Anatomical conjugate
d. Oblique diameter

FETAL SKULL

201. The average Submentovertical diameter is: *(AIIMS Raipur Grade II 2017)*
a. 9.5 cm b. 10 cm
c. 11.5 cm d. 13.5 cm

Explanation:

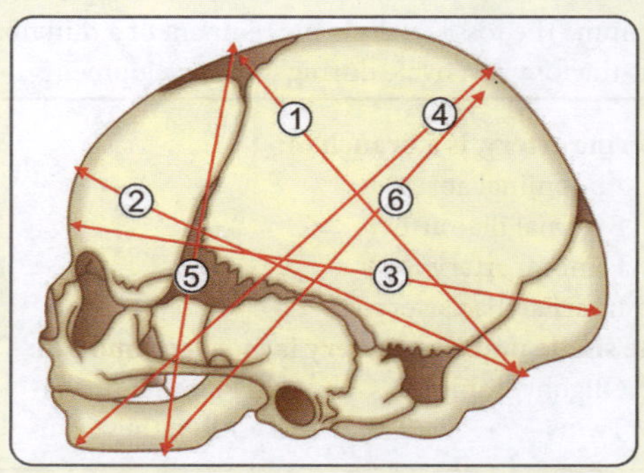

1. Suboccipito-bregmatic—9.5 cm
2. Suboccipito-frontal—10.0 cm
3. Occipito-frontal—11.5 cm
4. Mento-vertical—14 cm
5. Submento-bregmatic—9.5 cm
6. Submento-vertical—11.5 cm

(Ref; D.C. Dutta's Text book of Obstetrics. 7th ed)

Ans.

183. c
184. b
185. d
186. b
187. a
188. c
189. d
190. d
191. a
192. a
193. c
194. b
195. c
196. b
197. a
198. c
199. b
200. d
201. c

202. In the fetal skull, the bregma is found:

(AIIMS Raipur Grade II 2017)

a. At the junction of the sagittal, coronal and frontal sutures
b. At the junction of the lambdoidal and sagittal sutures
c. Between the two halves of the frontal bone
d. Between the frontal bones and parietal bones

Explanation: Posterior fontanelle/Lambda is situated at the junction of Lambdoidal and sagittal sutures. Frontal suture is situated between two halves of frontal bone. Coronal suture is found between frontal and parietal bone.

203. The suture that runs between parietal and frontal bone is:

a. Coronal b. Sagittal
c. Frontal d. Lambdoid

204. The sagittal suture lies between:

a. Occipital bone and two parietal bones
b. Parietal and frontal bone
c. Two frontal bones
d. Two parietal bones

Explanation: Skull contains four sutures. Frontal suture, Coronal suture, Sagittal suture, Lambdoidal suture.

205. The suture that lies between two parietal bone is known as:

a. Sagittal b. Longitudinal
c. Coronal d. Both a and b

Explanation: Suture lies between two parietal bone is known as longitudinal suture which is also known as sagittal suture.

206. Identify correct statements regarding anterior fontanelle:

a. Formed by joining four bones (4 bones or 2 sutures) in the midline
b. Shape is like a diamond
c. Ossified by 18 months of age
d. All of the above

207. Wide gap in the suture is:

a. Diameter
b. Circumference
c. Fontanelles
d. Inlet

208. Soft spot in the skull in between the sutures is known as:

a. Attitude b. Vertex
c. Diameter d. Fontanelle

209. Identify the correct statement(s) regarding posterior fontanelle:

a. It is formed by two sutures or three bones
b. Triangular in shape
c. It generally closes in 6–8 weeks from birth
d. All of the above

210. The diameter extending from the nape of the neck to the center of the bregma is called:

a. Suboccipito bregmatic b. Suboccipito frontal
c. Occipito frontal d. Submentobregmatic

211. Engaging diameter of face presentation is:

a. Mentobregmatic b. Sub-mentobregmatic
c. Mento vertical d. Sub-mentovertical

212. Suboccipitobregmatic diameter measures about:

a. 9.5 cm b. 10 cm
c. 11.5 cm d. 14 cm

213. Suboccipito-frontal diameter measures about:

a. 9.5 cm b. 10 cm
c. 11.5 cm d. 14 cm

214. Occipito frontal diameter measures about:

a. 9.5 cm b. 10 cm
c. 11.5 cm d. 14 cm

215. Mento-vertical diameter measures about:

a. 9.5 cm b. 10 cm
c. 11.5 cm d. 14 cm

216. Submentovertical diameter measures about:

a. 9.5 cm b. 10 cm
c. 11.5 cm d. 14 cm

217. Submentobregmatic diameter measures about:

a. 9.5 cm b. 10 cm
c. 11.5 cm d. 14 cm

218. Biparietal diameter in fetal skull is:

a. 9.5 cm b. 8.5 cm
c. 8 cm d. 7.5 cm

219. Super-subparietal diameter is:

a. 9.5 cm b. 8.5 cm
c. 8 cm d. 7.5 cm

220. Bitemporal diameter is:

a. 9.5 cm b. 8.5 cm
c. 8 cm d. 7.5 cm

221. Bimastoid diameter is:

a. 9.5 cm b. 8.5 cm
c. 8 cm d. 7.5 cm

222. Which of the following is the largest diameter of the fetal skull?

a. Mento vertical
b. Submento vertical
c. Biparietal
d. Suboccipitobregmatic

223. What will be the attitude of head during face and brow presentation?

a. Well flexed
b. Complete extension
c. Adduction
d. Abduction

224. Denominator in vertex presentation?

a. Occiput b. Mentum
c. Frontal eminence d. Sacrum

BREAST EXAMINATION

225. Most common organism responsible for mastitis is:

a. Streptococcus
b. Staphylococcus aureus
c. Meningococcus
d. Pneumococcus

226. Which areolar glands become hypertrophied during pregnancy that remains non- dominating during non-pregnant state?

a. Bulbourethral gland
b. Montgomery's tubercles
c. Lactiferous sinuses
d. Axillary tail

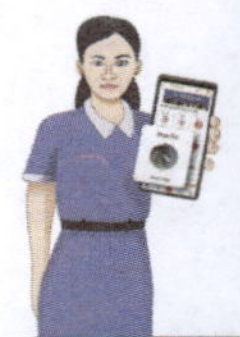

Ans.

202. a
203. a
204. d
205. d
206. d
207. c
208. d
209. d
210. a
211. b
212. a
213. b
214. c
215. d
216. c
217. a
218. a
219. b
220. c
221. d
222. a
223. b
224. a
225. b
226. b

227. Breast self-examination is recommended:
a. Any time during the cycle
b. First day of period
c. 3–5 days after period starts
d. 14 days after period starts

228. Which among the following is the correct statement regarding the breast self-examination in an amenorrhoeic patient?
a. Any time whenever they are free
b. Same day each month
c. Daily examination
d. No examination needed

229. What all are the methods involved in breast self-examination?
a. Inspection and percussion
b. Inspection and auscultation
c. Palpation and inspection
d. Palpation and auscultation

PHYSIOLOGICAL & EMOTIONAL CHANGES DURING PRENATAL PERIOD

230. Constipation may be a problem during pregnancy due to proximity of the rectum and uterus. Rectum is located:
a. In front of the uterus b. At the back of the uterus
c. To the left of the uterus d. Above the uterus

231. Identify the changes occur to the uterus during pregnant state:
a. Hypertrophy and hyperplasia of blood vessels
b. Stretching of muscle fibers
c. Hypertrophy of lymphatic system
d. All of the above

232. Vaginal pH during pregnancy is:
a. Acidic b. Basic
c. Neutral d. Fluctuating

233. The normal vaginal pH during child bearing period is:
a. 4.5 b. 5.7
c. 6.8 d. 7

234. The vaginal pH varies with the range of between:
a. 4–5 b. 5–6
c. 6–7 d. 7–8

235. Changes occur to cervix during pregnancy is:
a. Softening of cervix
b. Hypertrophy and hyperplasia of elastic connective tissues
c. Increased vascularity
d. All of the above

236. Axillary tail, Montogomery's tubercles occur during the time of pregnancy because of the changes in:
a. Skin b. Breast
c. Blood volume d. Uterus

Explanation: Axillary tail occurs because of prolongation of breast tissue under cover of pectoralis major. Montgomery's tubercles are those placed around the nipples, its secretion keeps the areola healthy and moist.

237. Chloasma will appear on .... body part.
a. Breast and nipples b. Cheeks and nose
c. Abdomen d. Limbs

Explanation: The mask of pregnancy technically called melasma or chloasma appears when a steep rise in estrogen levels stimulates excess melanin production (also known as hyperpigmentation).

238. Correct statement regarding changes occurring in the alimentary system during pregnancy is:
a. Increased reflux esophagitis
b. Muscle tone and motility will decrease
c. Risk for peptic ulcer reduces
d. All of the above

239. Correct statement regarding changes occurring in the respiratory system during pregnancy is:
a. Subcostal angle decreases
b. Chest circumference increases
c. Increase in tidal volume d. All of the above

240. Incorrect statement regarding changes which occur during pregnancy is/are: *New Q*
a. Blood volume will increase
b. RBC mass increases to 20–30%
c. Serum albumin level increase
d. Cardiac output increases

Explanation: Physiological changes occurs during pregnancy include:
- Increased blood volume
- Increased RBC mass to 20-30%
- Decreased albumin level (particularly in third trimester). Increased heart rate and stroke volume lead to increased cardiac output.
- Plasma renin levels rise, and atrial natriuretic peptide (ANP) levels tend to fall, leading to systemic vasodilation and increased vascular capacitance.
- Increased glomerular filtration rate (GFR) by about 50%.
- Increased urine frequency.
- Hyperpigmentation of the face, known as melasma.
- Linea nigra, a hyperpigmented line running down the center of the abdomen, may also occur.

241. What is the total weight gain occurring during the course of singleton pregnancy? *(Staff Nurse G II 2014)*
a. 5–7 kg b. 7–9 kg
c. 10–12 kg d. 12–14 kg

Explanation: Expected weight gain during the singleton of pregnancy is 11 kg, in which 1 kg in first trimester and 5 kg each in second and third trimester.

242. Which of the following complaints reported by a 32-week pregnant woman is considered crucial?
a. Heartburn b. Constipation
c. Shortness of breath when climbing up the stairs
d. Frontal and recurring headaches

243. Sodium and water retention occurring during pregnancy because of:
a. Increased ADH b. Increased aldosterone
c. Increased estrogen and progesterone
d. All of the above

ENDOCRINOLOGY ON REPRODUCTION

244. The cause of change in size and appearance of breasts during pregnancy is: *(Safdarjung NO 2018)*
a. Due to the secretion of estrogen and progesterone
b. Because of the weight gain
c. Due to increased metabolic rate that causes the breasts to become larger
d. Cortisol secreted by the adrenal

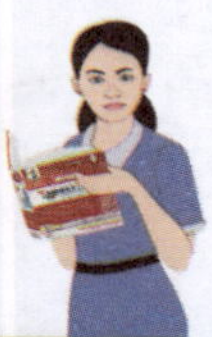

Ans.
227. c
228. b
229. c
230. b
231. d
232. a
233. a
234. a
235. d
236. b
237. b
238. d
239. d
240. c
241. c
242. d
243. d
244. a

Explanation: The secretion of estrogen and progesterone causes the change in size and appearance of breasts during pregnancy. Weight gain causes stretching of breast, not a change in size and appearance.

245. Estrogen and progesterone in birth control pills prevent pregnancy by:

a. Having a positive feedback effect on FSH and LH production
b. Preventing ovulation from occurring
c. Not allowing the endometrium of the uterus to fully develop
d. Preventing the sperms from entering the ovum

246. What all are the changes occur to pituitary gland during pregnancy?

a. Increase in weight and enlarge in size
b. Elevated growth hormone level and serum prolactin level
c. Low level of pituitary gonadotropins
d. All of the above

247. Which of the following hormones inhibits the secretion of follicle stimulating hormone?

a. Progesterone
b. Estrogen
c. Androgen
d. Testosterone

Explanation: **Estrogens** and inhibin B are both inhibitory factors for the secretion of **FSH.** Activin is a promotor of many actions of **FSH** in that it increases **FSH** secretion, promotes ovarian follicular development and inhibits androgen production.

248. A female came to the gynecologist with chief complaints of irregular vaginal bleeding. The nurse knows well that a decrease in ……… hormone is responsible for causing bleeding during the menstrual cycle under physiological condition. New Q (NORCET 2022)

a. Estrogen b. Progesterone
c. FSH d. Thyroxine

249. Gonadotropin releasing hormone (GnRH) stimulates the release of: *(DSSSB 2008)*

a. Follicle stimulating hormone
b. Luteinizing hormone (LH)
c. Growth hormone
d. Both a and b

Explanation: GnRH is a trophic peptide hormone produced by anterior lobe of pituitary and is responsible for the release of follicle-stimulating hormone (FSH) and luteinizing hormone (LH) .

250. Ovulatory function is stimulated by …………gland.

a. Parathyroid
b. Pineal gland
c. Pituitary gland
d. Adrenal gland

251. Location of Graafian follicle is:

a. Uterus b. Fallopian tubes
c. Ovaries d. Cervix

252. Granulosa cells of developing ovarian follicle secretes: *(RRB Feb 2012)*

a. LH b. Progesterone
c. Estrogen d. None of these

253. After ovulation, Graafian follicle become:

a. Corpus luteum b. Placenta
c. Umbilical cord d. Amnion and chorion

Explanation: Graafian follicle is changed to corpus luteum. It will secrete progesterone, 17 alpha progesterone and oestradiol, adrostenedione. At 6th–8th week, there is transfer of function of corpus luteum to the placenta.

254. Hormone responsible for ovulation is: *(Safdarjung NO 2018)*

a. FSH b. LH
c. Estrogen d. Progesterone

Explanation: Luteinizing hormone is a hormone produced by gonadotropic cells in the anterior pituitary gland. In females, an acute rise of LH triggers ovulation and development of the corpus luteum. FSH is responsible for follicle maturation.

255. Time of ovulation corresponds to: *(JIPMER 2012)*

a. Oxytocin level is high
b. Blood level of LH is high
c. Progesterone level is high
d. Endometrial wall is sloughed off

Explanation: Luteinizing Hormone (LH) is a gonadotropin synthesized and secreted by the anterior pituitary gland in response to GnRH. When follicle maturation is complete, an LH surge triggers ovulation.

256. The hormones responsible for the menstrual cycle are: *(Safdarjung NO 2018)*

a. Gonadotropins
b. Estrogen and progesterone
c. Gonadotropins and estrogen
d. Gonadotropins, estrogen and progesterone

Explanation: Gonadotropins (LH and FSH) release from anterior pituitary that stimulates the follicles in the ovary causing the maturation and then final release of the ovum. Growing follicles release the estrogen and progesterone that cause the uterine cells hyperplasia and increase the endometrial thickness of uterus.

257. The large amount of progesterone secreted during the secretory phase of the menstrual cycle is responsible for: *(Safdarjung NO 2018)*

a. The onset of ovulation
b. The regulation of menstruation
c. The incidence of capillary fragility
d. Sustaining the thick endometrium of the uterus

Explanation: Progesterone is important hormone that condition the endometrium by sustaining the thick endometrium in preparation for implantation of a fertilized ovum. Progesterone prepares the uterus for receiving the fertilized ovum.

258. Correct regarding hCG hormone is:

a. Maintenance of corpus luteum till 6 weeks of pregnancy
b. Syncytiotrophoblast of the placenta secrete this hormone
c. 60-70 days of pregnancy hCG reaches maximum level in the blood
d. All of the above

259. Which structure is responsible for secreting progesterone hormone during first six weeks of pregnancy?

a. Corpus luteum
b. Umbilical cord
c. Placenta
d. Decidua basalis

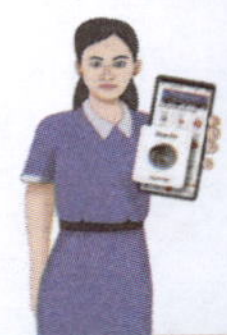

Ans.

245. b
246. d
247. b
248. a
249. d
250. c
251. c
252. c
253. a
254. b
255. b
256. d
257. d
258. d
259. a

260. The hormones responsible for differentiation of male reproductive organs during fetal life; EXCEPT:
a. Dehydroepiandosterone sulfate
b. Dyhydrotestosterone
c. Mullerian duct inhibitor (MDI)
d. Testosterone

261. During the first two months of pregnancy the chief source of estrogen and progesterone is the:
a. Placenta b. Adrenal cortex
c. Corpus luteum d. None of these

262. A hormone that prevents menstruation and maintains pregnancy by sustaining the function of the corpus luteum is: *(AIIMS Raipur Grade II 2017)*
a. Follicle stimulating hormone
b. Luteinizing hormone
c. Gonadotropin releasing hormone
d. Human chorionic gonadotropin hormone

Explanation: Follicle stimulating hormone is essential for pubertal development and plays a key role in function of women's ovaries and men's testes. Luteinizing hormone triggers ovulation in females and development of corpus luteum and in males it stimulates Leydig cell production of testosterone. Gonadotropin releasing hormone is released by the hypothalamus which stimulates the pituitary gland to release the gonadotropin hormones follicle-stimulating hormone (FSH) and luteinizing hormone.

263. Which hormone is essential for the continued activity of follicle stimulating hormone?
a. Progesterone b. Estrogen
c. Androgen d. Testosterone

264. Arachidonic acid in placenta is synthesized under the influence of:
a. Estrogen b. Progesterone
c. Oxytocin d. Phospholipase A2

265. Hormonal influence of menstrual cycle includes:
a. Ovarian hormones
b. Pituitary hormones
c. Hypothalamic releasing hormones
d. All of the above

266. Following are basic elements involved in the uterine contractile systems; EXCEPT:
a. Enzyme adenosine triphosphates
b. Actin
c. Myosin
d. Adenyl-cyclase

267. Hormone responsible for morning sickness is:
a. hCG
b. Oxytocin
c. Prolactin
d. Relaxin

Explanation: High level of serum Human Chorionic Gonadotropin (hCG), estrogen and altered level of immunological states are considered responsible for morning sickness.

268. The hormone responsible for the maintenance of pregnancy is:
a. Estrogen b. Progesterone
c. hCG d. Human placental lactogen

269. Function of progesterone is:
a. Prepare the uterus to receive the fertilized egg
b. Secondary sexual characteristics
c. Milk production
d. Stimulation of ovary

Explanation: Progesterone is hormone secreted by the ovaries, placenta, and adrenal glands that function mainly to regulate the condition of the inner lining (endometrium) of the uterus to receive the fertilized ovum.

270. Chief source of estrogen in the third trimester of pregnancy is:
a. Placenta b. Corpus luteum
c. Ovary d. Pituitary

Explanation: In the early week of gestation, i.e., before the formation of placenta corpus luteum will secrete these hormones but after the formation of placenta, production of estrogen and progesterone is its function.

271. Physiological functions of estrogen include:
a. Responsible for myometrial growth after implantation
b. Stimulates hypertrophy of the endometrium.
c. Decreases the secretion of FSH
d. All of the above

272. Which hormone is responsible for sensitizing the myometrium for oxytocin and prostaglandin?
a. Progesterone b. Estrogen
c. Androgen d. Testosterone

273. Relaxation of smooth muscles and vasodilation occur because of the effect of .... hormone.
a. Endothelin b. Ergometrine
c. Angiotensin II d. Relaxin

Explanation: Relaxin is a hormone that is produced by the ovaries and the placenta during pregnancy. It helps to relax the smooth muscles in the uterus, cervix, and pelvic joints. This allows the uterus to expand during pregnancy and the cervix to dilate during labor. Relaxin also has a vasodilatory effect, which means that it relaxes the blood vessels and increases blood flow.

Endothelin and Angiotensin II are potential vasoconstrictors. Ergometrine is used primarily to induce contractions of the uterus and control postpartum bleeding.

274. Urinary excretion of hCG is maximal between which days of gestation?
a. 50–60 b. 40–50
c. 60–70 d. 30–40

275. The reason for leg cramps in antenatal woman is:
a. Decrease in the serum calcium level
b. Decrease in phosphorus level
c. Retention of salt and fluid
d. Increase in serum progesterone

276. Cervical ripening occurs due to which hormone?
a. Progesterone b. Estrogen
c. Androgen d. Testosterone

277. During pregnancy leucorrhea will increase because of the influence of:
a. Estrogen
b. Progesterone
c. Oxytocin
d. Prolactin

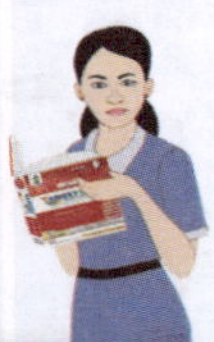

Ans.
260. a
261. c
262. d
263. b
264. d
265. d
266. d
267. a
268. b
269. a
270. a
271. d
272. b
273. d
274. c
275. a
276. b
277. a

Explanation: Increased estrogen during pregnancy leads to hyperplasia of vaginal mucosa which in turn increases the secretions by the endocervical gland.

278. The most common cause of vaginitis in postmenopausal women is:
a. Malignancy
b. Infection
c. Estrogen deficiency
d. Trauma or foreign body

279. Chances of occurrence of osteoporosis will decline in obese patient after puberty, because:
a. Fall in FSH level
b. Fall in LH level
c. Conversion of more androgens into estrogen
d. Due to ore calcium

DIAGNOSIS/SIGNS OF PREGNANCY

280. In urine pregnancy, test hormone played is:
a. Progesterone
b. Estrogen
c. hCG
d. Oxytocin

281. hCG can be detected in blood after conception as early as ….days. *(RRB Feb 2012)*
a. 2 days b. 4 days
c. 9 days d. 15 days

282. Hormone human chorionic gonadotropin can be detected in case of:
a. Pregnancy
b. Hydatiform mole
c. Choriocarcinoma
d. All of the above

Explanation: In all the above mentioned conditions, hCG will be present. In normal pregnancy it will disappear from blood following 2 weeks after delivery.

283. Gestation sac can be seen in ultrasound at ………period of gestation. *(RAK MSc 2018)*
a. 5 weeks b. 6 weeks
c. 8 weeks d. 10 weeks

Explanation: Gestation sac can be seen in ultrasound at 5 weeks of gestation.

Table: Progress of fetal development

Gestational Age (Weeks)	Fetal Structures
4	Chorionic sac
5	Gestation sac
5.5	Yolk sac
6	Fetal pole and cardiac activity
7	Lower limb buds midgut herniation
8	Upper limb buds, stomach
9	Supine, choroid plexus

284. Positive sign of pregnancy is: *(RRB Feb 2012)*
a. Cullen's sign b. Hegar's sign
c. Fetal movement d. Morning sickness

285. Identify correct statements regarding non-stress test (NST):
a. Continuous monitoring of fetal heart rate along with fetal movement (cardiotocography)
b. It will assess the relationship between fetal movement and heart rate
c. FHR acceleration along with fetal movement is expected
d. All of the above

286. Which of the following statements best describes contraction stress test for the pregnant woman: *(Safdarjung NO 2018)*
a. Small amount of oxytocin (Pitocin) is administered during internal fetal monitor to stimulate uterine contraction
b. An external fetal monitor is attached, and the woman ambulates on a treadmill until contractions begin
c. The uterus is stimulated to contract by the use of small amounts of oxytocin (Pitocin) or by the nipple stimulation
d. Uterine contractions are stimulated by Leopold's maneuver's

Explanation: Uterine contractions are stimulated by nipple stimulation or by administering oxytocin in diluted forms. The variation in heart rate is noted through external fetal monitoring system. It is done to assess the uteroplacental insufficiency. Internal fetal monitoring is not done.

287. Contraction stress test (CST) is also known as:
a. Oxytocin challenge test
b. NST
c. Both a and b
d. None of the above

288. CST is used to:
a. Measure the baby's heart rate during uterine contractions
b. Determine the intensity of uterine contraction
c. Determination of maternal wellbeing
d. All of the above

289. Piskacek's sign is:
a. Bluish coloration of the anterior vaginal mucosa
b. Increased pulsation felt through the lateral fornices
c. Cervix become soft as early as 6th week
d. One half of the uterus is more firm than the other half

290. The confirmatory sign early in the pregnancy is:
a. Auscultation of fetal heart rate
b. Ultrasonographic findings
c. Palpation of fetal part
d. All of the above

291. What is the positive sign of pregnancy? *(RAK MSc 2018)*
a. Frequency of micturition
b. Vomiting
c. Braxton Hicks contractions
d. Fetal outline by sonography

Explanation: Positive signs of pregnancy are the signs, which confirm the pregnancy. USG confirms the accurate finding of pregnancy. Frequent micturition and vomiting are presumptive symptoms of pregnancy. Braxton Hicks contraction is probable sign of pregnancy.

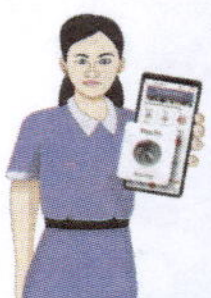

Ans.
278. c
279. c
280. c
281. c
282. d
283. a
284. c
285. d
286. c
287. a
288. a
289. d
290. b
291. d

292. Positive-definite sign of pregnancy is: *(ESIC 2019)*

a. Visualization of fetus by ultrasound
b. Uterine enlargement
c. Amenorrhea
d. Quickening

Explanation: Positive signs of pregnancy are those signs that are definitely confirmed as a pregnancy. They include fetal heart sounds, ultrasound scanning of the fetus, palpation of the entire fetus, palpation of fetal movements, X-ray, and actual delivery of an infant.

293. A positive over-the-counter pregnancy test is considered as: *(NCFL 2019)*

a. Possible sign of pregnancy
b. Presumptive sign of pregnancy
c. Probable sign of pregnancy
d. Positive sign of pregnancy

Explanation: Probable signs of pregnancy include Goodell sign, Chadwick sign, Hegar sign, positive serum and urine samples (Over the counter Urinary Pregnancy Test), Braxton Hicks contractions, and ballottement. Observation of these signs indicates that the woman is most likely pregnant.

294. Which of the following tests can be used to diagnose pregnancy on the first day of the missed period (28th day of cycle)? *(AIIMS Bhopal Nursing Officer, 2018)*

a. Two-site sandwich immunoassay
b. Enzyme-linked immunoassay
c. Agglutination inhibition test
d. Direct latex agglutination test

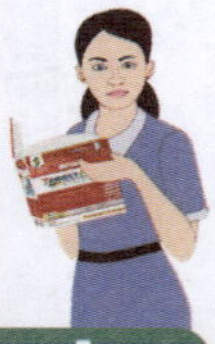

Explanation: Two-site sandwich immunoassay test device designed for the qualitative determination of human chorionic gonadotropin (hCG) concentration in human urine samples, and therefore is an aid in the early detection of pregnancy.

295. At 8 weeks of gestation, the uterus looks like: *(AIIMS Raipur Grade II 2017)*

a. Small unripped pear b. Large orange
c. Size of grape fruit d. Golf ball

Explanation: At 12 weeks uterus looks like grapefruit, at 14–28 weeks uterus looks like size of papaya, at 28–40 weeks uterus looks like watermelon.

296. The uterus has already risen out of the pelvis and is experiencing farther growth into the abdominal area at about: *(RAK MSc 2018)*

a. 8th week of pregnancy
b. 10th week of pregnancy
c. 12th week of pregnancy
d. 18th week of pregnancy

Explanation: Until 12 weeks of pregnancy, the uterus remains as a pelvic organ. At approximately 12 weeks of gestation, the uterus becomes large enough to be palpable just above the pubic symphysis.

297. A nurse is aware that the best place to detect fetal heart sounds in the first trimester of pregnancy?

a. Above the symphysis pubis
b. Above the umbilicus
c. At the umbilicus
d. Below the symphysis pubis

Explanation: Around 10th or 11th week of gestation, it is possible to hear fetal heart rate with an ultrasound fetoscope. To auscultate fetal heart rate, apply conductive gel to the patient's skin, then position the device at midline just above the symphysis pubis and apply firm pressure. A regular stethoscope or fetoscope can detect fetal heart sounds at 18–20 weeks and beyond.

298. With the ordinary stethoscope, the fetal heart sounds can be detected earliest between______ weeks of pregnancy. *(AIIMS Bhopal Nursing Officer, 2018)*

a. 6–8 b. 18–20
c. 24–26 d. 8–10

Explanation: In ordinary stethoscope, the fetal heart sounds can be detected earliest at 18–20 weeks. Through fetal Doppler (Ultrasound), the fetal heartbeat should be audible 95% of the time in 12-week pregnancy, and nearly 100% of the time after 14 weeks.

299. Purple blue tinge of the cervix is: *(DSSSB 2013)*

a. Hegar sign b. Goodell's sign
c. Chadwick's sign d. McDonald's sign

Explanation:

Chadwick's sign: It is a sign of pregnancy consisting of a dark bluish or purplish-red color of the vaginal or cervical mucosa as a result of increased blood supply to the area.

300. Jacquemier's sign is also known as:

a. Osiander's sign
b. Chadwick's sign
c. Goodell's sign
d. Hegar's sign

301. The dusky hue of the vestibule and anterior vaginal wall due to local vascular congestion is called as: *(AIIMS Bhopal Nursing Officer, 2018)*

a. Osiander's sign b. Chadwick's sign
c. Goodell's sign d. Homan's signs

Explanation: Above given definition is Chadwick's sign. It is also known as Jacquemier's sign.

Osiander's sign is vaginal pulsation that mirrors the maternal heart rate as an early sign of pregnancy. Softening of the vaginal portion of the cervix from increased vascularization is known as Goodell's sign. Homan's sign is discomfort behind the knee on forced dorsiflexion of the foot which indicates deep vein thrombosis.

302. The extreme softening of the cervix during the first trimester is known as: *(AIIMS Bhopal Grade-I 2018, RAK MSc 2018)*

a. Chadwick's sign b. Osiander's sign
c. Piskacek's sign d. Goodell's sign

Explanation: It is named after William Goodell. Goodell's sign is a significant softening of the vaginal portion of the cervix due to increased vascularization. This sign occurs at approximately four weeks' gestation.

303. Which of these is a sign of previous childbirth? *(Daman and Diu NO 2018)*

a. Rigid abdominal wall
b. Conical cervix with round external os
c. Ovoid uterus
d. Gaping introitus

Ans.

292. a
293. c
294. a
295. b
296. c
297. a
298. b
299. c
300. b
301. b
302. d
303. d

Explanation: Gaping introitus is a condition in which the vaginal opening is wider which clearly indicates toward previous normal vaginal delivery.

304. Identify the signs which indicate a previous childbirth:
a. Presence of silvery white striae and linea alba
b. Abdominal wall is lax and gaping introitus
c. Perineum is lax and evidence of old scarring indicating previous childbirth
d. All of the above

305. The perception of active fetal movement felt by the mother during pregnancy is known as:
(RRB Feb 2012; JIPMER 2012; Kerala PSC 2014; DSSSB PHN, 2015; AIIMS Bhopal Grade-I 2018)
a. Ballottement b. Engagement
c. Quickening d. Lightening

306. Quickening occurs at: *(LNJP HD 2012)*
a. 8–10 weeks b. 16–20 weeks
c. 12–16 weeks d. 20–24 weeks

Explanation: Quickening is the active fetal movement felt by the mother during pregnancy. A woman who becomes pregnant for the first time typically feels fetal movements at around 18-20 weeks of gestation, whereas multipara women feel fetal movements at around 15-17 weeks of gestation.

307. Regular rhythmic contraction felt during bimanual examination is known as:
a. Quickening b. Hegar's sign
c. Palmer's sign d. Chloasma

Explanation: **Palmer's sign** is a regular rhythmic contraction felt during bimanual examination.

Hegar's sign is a non-sensitive indication of pregnancy in women — its absence does not exclude pregnancy. It pertains to the features of the cervix and the uterine isthmus. It is demonstrated as a softening in the consistency of the uterus, and the uterus and cervix seem to be two separate regions.

- **Chloasma** is a mask of pregnancy when present in pregnant women, it is a tan or dark skin discoloration.
- **Quickening** is the perception of active fetal movement by the mother. It is usually felt about at 18–20 weeks, and about 2 weeks earlier in multipara mother.

308. The first sign seen in pregnancy is: *(RRB Feb 2012)*
a. Quickening b. Amenorrhea
c. Hegar's sign d. None of these

309. Which of the following is an important sign of pregnancy:
a. Increase in the size of breast
b. Alkaline vagina
c. Amenorrhea
d. All of the above

310. Which of the following is not a presumptive sign of pregnancy?
a. Amenorrhea b. Braxton-Hicks contraction
c. Urinary frequency d. Breast changes

311. Which of the following is the early symptom of first trimester of pregnancy?
a. Braxton-Hicks contraction
b. Fetal heart sound can be heard through fetoscope
c. Fetal heart rate through USG
d. Cessation of menstrual cycle

312. Osiander's sign is:
a. Bluish coloration of the anterior vaginal mucosa
b. Increased pulsation felt through the lateral fornices
c. Cervix becomes soft as early as 6th week
d. One half of the uterus is more firm than the other half

313. Pigmented line extending from xiphisternum to the symphysis pubis is termed:
a. Striae gravidarum
b. Linea nigra
c. Striae albicans
d. Linea albicans

Explanation: Linea nigra is a brownish pigmented area in the midline stretching from the xiphisternum to the symphysis pubis and is visible as early as 20th week of gestation.

314. All of the following statements are true regarding Linea nigra; EXCEPT:
a. Brownish black pigmented area in the midline
b. It is probably due to melanocyte stimulating hormone from anterior pituitary
c. Pigmentation disappears after delivery
d. It appears all over the abdomen

Explanation: Linea nigra is a dark vertical line that appears on the abdomen in about 75% of all pregnancies. The brownish streak is usually about a centimeter in width. The line runs vertically along the midline of the abdomen from the pubis to the umbilicus and it may extend till xiphisternum. Linea nigra is due to increased melanocyte-stimulating hormone made by the placenta which also causes melasma and darkened nipples. Linea nigra typically disappears within a few months after delivery.

315. Which sign is considered as welcome sign in pregnancy?
a. Lightening
b. Show
c. Onset of labor pain
d. Quickening

Explanation: Presenting part sink onto the pelvis, this sign is considered as welcome sign of pregnancy as it rule out cephalopelvic disproportion and corresponding conditions that prevent the head from entering in the pelvic inlet.

316. Characteristics of monozygotic pregnancy is:
a. One placenta
b. Sex will be always identical
c. Genetic features will be also same
d. All of the above

317. A patient is transferred to labor room and the nurse identifies that the patient is in first stage of labor. When will the nurse document the progress of labor with respect to the cervical dilation on a partograph? *(NORCET 2022)* **New Q**
a. 4 cm b. 5 cm
c. 7 cm d. 10 cm

318. Identify the correct statements among the following:
a. At birth the uterine body and the cervix ratio is about 1:2
b. At menarche the uterine body and the cervix ratio is about 1:1
c. After menarche the uterine body and the cervix ratio is about 2:1
d. All of the above

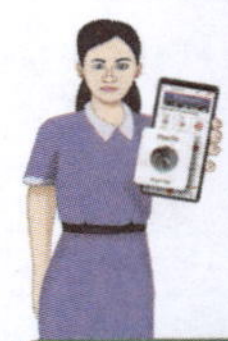

Ans.
304. d
305. c
306. b
307. c
308. b
309. c
310. b
311. d
312. b
313. b
314. d
315. a
316. d
317. b
318. d

ESTIMATION OF EDD & GESTATIONAL AGE

319. LMP of a woman who has 28-day's regular cycle is March 31, 2020. The next ovulation day is most likely to be:
a. April 17, 2020 b. April 15, 2020
c. April 13, 2020 d. April 11, 2020

320. As per embryologist point of view duration of pregnancy is:
a. 10 lunar month b. 9 calendar month +7 days
c. 40 weeks d. 266 days

321. Duration of pregnancy is:
a. 10 lunar months b. 9 calendar months and 7 days
c. 280 days d. All of these

Explanation: Duration of pregnancy can be expressed in all the above given methods and also as 40 weeks, which is calculated from first day of last menstrual cycle. This is called menstrual age or gestational age.

322. The period of gestation, when development of placenta is completed is:
a. 3 weeks b. 12 weeks
c. 16 weeks d. 20 weeks

323. Formula used for calculating expected date of delivery (EDD)
a. Johnson's formula b. Shepard's formula
c. Hadlock's formula d. Naegele's formula

Explanation: EDD is calculated from LMP by adding 7 days to the first day of last menstrual cycle and 9 months to the months.

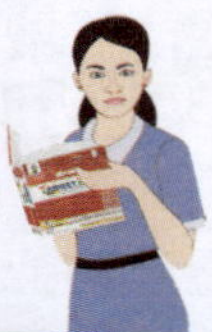

324. How we can estimate EDD?
a. 1st day of last MC + 280 days
b. First day of last MC + 266 days
c. Ovulation day + 280 days
d. Ovulation day + 266 days

325. Calculate EDD if LMP was 7th May 2016:
a. 14th February 2017 b. 14th January 2017
c. 13th February 2017 d. 13th January 2017

Explanation: Adding 7 to the date become 7 + 7 = 14. Adding 9 calendar months become February.

326. First day of last menstrual period is October 19, 2017. What is the expected date of delivery? *(AIIMS Raipur NO 2019)*
a. July 12, 2018 b. July 26, 2018
c. August 12, 2018 d. August 26, 2018

Explanation:
- Naegele's formula - add 9 calendar months and 7 days to the LMP.
- In this example,
  - LMP = 19/10/17 + 9 months = 19/07/18 + 7 days
  - EDD = July 26, 2018

327. Babita's LMP began on June 10. Her EDD should be which of the following?
a. April 17 b. March 17
c. June 22 d. October 12

Explanation: To determine the EDD when the date of the client's LMP is known, use Naegele's formula.

Note: Add 7 days, to the date and 9 months to the month.

328. According to Manisha, her LMP is November 15, 2016, using the Naegele's rule, her EDD is:
a. August 18, 2017
b. August 22, 2017
c. February 22, 2017
d. July 22, 2017

329. A woman is now at 16 weeks of gestation. After how many weeks of gestation the midwife needs to instruct the woman to return for a follow up visit?
a. One b. Two
c. Three d. Four

330. Degree of uterine systole is measured in terms of:
a. Tonus b. Intensity
c. Strength d. Number

331. Height of fundus is midway between umbilicus and xiphisternum at:
a. 24th week b. 26th week
c. 28th week d. 32th week

332. Height of fundus is at the level of umbilicus at:
a. 24th week b. 26th week
c. 28th week d. 30th week

333. The height of a uterus is midway between the symphysis pubis and umbilicus at which week of gestation?
(AIIMS Bhopal Nursing Officer, 2018)
a. 12 weeks b. 8 weeks
c. 16 weeks d. 28 weeks

Explanation:

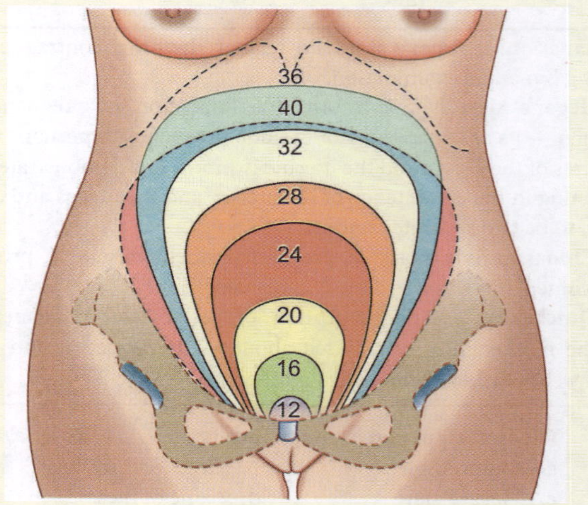

334. First trimester is:
a. First 12 weeks b. 13–28 weeks
c. 29–40 weeks d. None of these

Explanation: First 12 weeks—first trimester
13 to 28 weeks—second trimester
29 to 40 weeks—third trimester

335. Gender determination can be done by …….. POG.
a. 6–12 weeks b. 12–16 weeks
c. 16–18 weeks d. 18–24 weeks

336. Pregnancy is considered full term after how many weeks?
a. 28 weeks b. 32 weeks
c. 36 weeks d. 40 weeks

Ans.
319. c
320. d
321. d
322. b
323. d
324. a
325. a
326. b
327. b
328. b
329. d
330. b
331. d
332. a
333. c
334. a
335. b
336. d

SCREENING TESTS DURING PREGNANCY

337. Indication for hysteroscopy is:
a. Investigation of the cause of irregular bleeding per vaginum
b. Cervical stenosis
c. Fetal monitoring
d. Vaginal fistula

Explanation: Hysteroscopy is a minimally invasive procedure that allows a doctor to see inside the uterus. It is often used to diagnose and treat problems with the uterus, including:
- Abnormal uterine bleeding
- Infertility
- Recurrent pregnancy loss
- To remove Intrauterine devices
- To diagnose and treat endometriosis
- To perform certain uterine surgery.

338. Under USG guidance, fetal blood sampling is performed in the:
a. Umbilical artery
b. Umbilical vein
c. Placenta
d. Iliac vein

339. All of the following can be used to determine a chromosome analysis of the fetus; EXCEPT: *(Banaras HU 2015)*
a. Amniocentesis
b. Chorionic villus sampling
c. Percutaneous umbilical blood sampling (PUBS)
d. Fetal umbilical Doppler velocimetry

340. Diagnostic test used for locating the placenta is:
a. X-ray
b. Ultrasonography
c. Bio-physiological monitoring
d. Coombs test

341. Diagnostic method for determining whether the fallopian tubes in the human female are occluded is:
a. Rubin's test
b. Stress test
c. Ballot test
d. Homan's test

342. A prenatal client with a history of heart disease has been instructed on care at home. Which statement made by the client would indicate that the client understands her needs? *(Safdarjung NO 2018)*
a. There is no restriction on people who visit me
b. I should avoid stressful situations
c. My weight gain is not important
d. I should rest on my right side

Explanation: A prenatal client who has a history of heart disease should be instructed to avoid stressful situations which can aggravate the sympathetic nervous system thereby increasing the risk for acute cardiac emergency. Remaining statements are related to healthy practices but do not directly give idea about patients understanding regarding heart disease.

343. A client is scheduled for amniocentesis. When preparing her for the procedure, nurse should do which of the following?
a. Ask her to void
b. Instruct her to drink 1 L of fluid
c. Place her on her left side
d. Prepare her for IV anesthesia

Explanation: Voiding will decrease the discomfort for doing procedure.

344. Appropriate time for chorionic villus sampling is:
a. 10–12 weeks
b. 14–16 weeks
c. 18–20 weeks
d. 20–22 weeks

Explanation: Option A is the correct answer, amniocentesis timing is 14–16 weeks and that of cordocentesis is 18–20 weeks.

345. Which screening test is not used for cervical cancer? **New Q** *(NORCET 2021)*
a. Colposcopy
b. HPV DNA
c. Pap smear
d. VIA

Explanation: Colposcopy is a procedure used to examine the cervix more closely after an abnormal Pap smear or VIA test. It is not a screening test in itself.

The other three options, HPV DNA, Pap smear, and VIA, are all screening tests for cervical cancer. HPV DNA is a test that looks for the presence of the human papillomavirus (HPV). Visual inspection with acetic acid (VIA) is a simple, inexpensive, and noninvasive screening test for cervical cancer. It is used to detect precancerous lesions and early invasive cancer of the cervix. Pap smear is also a screening test for cervical cancer.

346. The components of triple test include:
a. Maternal serum alpha fetoprotein
b. hCG
c. Unconjugated oestriol
d. All of the above

Explanation: All the above-mentioned are the components of triple screening, which help us to find out down's syndrome, neural tube defect and other chromosomal abnormality present in the fetus. It is performed between 15 and 18 week.

347. Nuchal translucency screening should be done between:
a. 6–10 weeks of pregnancy
b. 11–14 weeks of pregnancy
c. 14–18 weeks of pregnancy
d. 20–22 weeks of pregnancy

348. The purpose of speculum examination is to:
a. Diagnose infections
b. Diagnose premature leaking liquor
c. Study the cervical lesions
d. All of the above

349. While measuring fundal height, client complaining of feeling dizzy and lightheadedness. What is the most appropriate nursing action?
a. Check the vitals of the client
b. Check the fetal heart rate
c. Turn the mother to one side
d. Check the urine protein level

Explanation: While measuring fundal height, woman was on supine position and she was experiencing supine hypotension. By changing her position, i.e., from supine to lateral it will help to remove the compression and restore cardiac output and blood pressure.

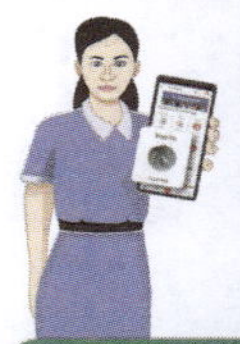

Ans.

337. a
338. b
339. d
340. b
341. a
342. b
343. a
344. a
345. a
346. d
347. b
348. d
349. c

350. During each prenatal checkup, weight, blood pressure and fundal height need to be documented. What is the other parameter that needs to be mentioned?

a. Determining the client's Rh factor
b. Evaluating the client for edema
c. Measuring the client's hemoglobin (Hb) level
d. Obtaining pelvic measurements

Explanation: Edema is an indication for pre-eclampsia during antenatal period.

351. Which of the following prenatal laboratory tests values would the nurse consider as significant?

a. Hemoglobin 12 mg/dL b. Rubella titer 1:5
c. Blood pressure 120/80 d. Protein urea nil

Explanation: Normally rubella titer should be 1:8 or more, a value less than that needs medical care.

352. TORCH indicates:

a. Toxoplasma, rubella, candida and herpes simplex
b. Toxoplasma, rubella, cytomegalovirus and herpes simplex
c. Tetanus, rubella, cytomegalovirus and herpes simplex
d. Tetanus, rabies, CMV, and herpes simplex

ANTENATAL ASSESSMENT OF FETAL WELLBEING

353. Nuchal translucency screening of fetus is done to diagnose:

a. Chromosomal anomalies
b. Congenital heart disease
c. Microcephaly
d. Meningeal abnormalities

354. Instrument used for the collection of pap smear is:

a. Ayre spatula
b. Piper forceps
c. Neville Barnes forceps
d. Simpson's forceps

Explanation: Ayre spatula is a device used to collect Pap smear. It is a wooden spatula with U shaped openings on one side and a flat surface on another.

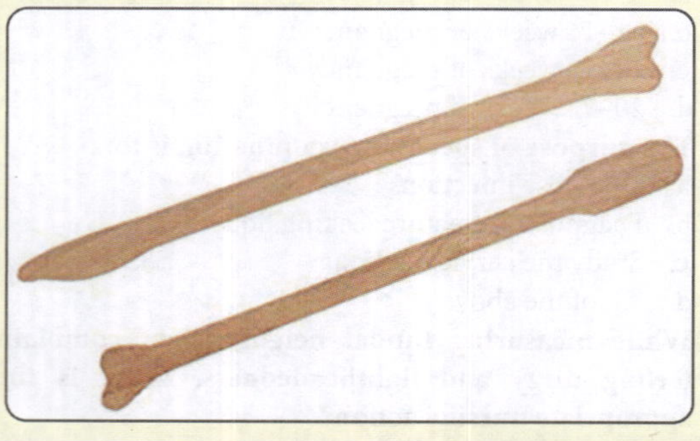

355. A client is scheduled for a Pap smear. The nurse provides instructions to the client regarding preparation for the test. Which of the following is incorrect? *New Q*

a. Suggest applying vaginal creams before procedure to promote comfort
b. Avoid sexual intercourse for 24 hours before the test.
c. Explain that the procedure is painless
d. Avoid vaginal douching for 24 hours before the test

Explanation: Important nursing responsibilities during Pap smear procedure include:

- Explain that the procedure may cause bit discomfort but it is painless.
- **Instruct the client to avoid** having sexual intercourse within 24 hours, douching within 24-48 hours, using a tampon, or applying vaginal creams or lotions. These acts can wash away cellular deposits and change the pH of the vagina.

356. Risk of the damage of fetus by maternal rubella is highest if mother get infected in:

a. 6–12 weeks of pregnancy
b. 16–22 weeks of pregnancy
c. 22–28 weeks of pregnancy
d. 30–36 weeks of pregnancy

357. Which of the following diseases may result in serious teratogenic defect in offspring? *(RAK MSc 2018)*

a. Rubella
b. Rubeola
c. Variola
d. Varicella

Explanation: Rubella or German measles is RNA virus, which is teratogenic and is transmitted by respiratory droplet exposure. The virus affects the fetus to extreme level, if contracted in first trimester. There is increased chances of abortion, congenital malformation, or infant born with rubella. Rubella vaccine cannot be given during pregnancy as it is live attenuated vaccine.

358. Which is the biochemical marker detected in a mother's blood in neural tube defect? *(AIIMS Bhopal Grade-I 2018)*

a. Alpha-fetoprotein b. Ascorbic acid
c. Alkaline phosphatase d. Amino acid

Explanation: Alpha-fetoprotein (AFP) is the first protein marker to be associated with fetal abnormalities that are easily detectable in mother's serum. High level of AFP in the mother's serum is associated with neural tube defect and decreased AFP level in mother's serum is associated with Down's syndrome.

359. Elevated level of maternal serum alpha-fetoprotein (MSAFP) is seen in all the conditions; EXCEPT:

a. Open neural tube defect
b. Rh isoimmunization
c. Anterior abdominal wall defect
d. Down syndrome.

Explanation: Elevated MSAFP is present in all the conditions except Down syndrome. In Down syndrome and gestational trophoblastic disease, MSAFP will decrease.

360. Maternal alpha feto protein level at 20 weeks of pregnancy is 30 ng/mL. Which among the following conditions may present in fetus?

a. Meningocele b. Meningomyelocele
c. Both a and b d. Down syndrome

Explanation: Normal Maternal Serum AFP (MSAFP) at 20 weeks is 74.9 ng/mL (median). Decreased serum AFP is seen in down syndrome, molar pregnancy, spontaneous abortion and Klinefelter syndrome and other chromosomal abnormality. Increased MSAFP indicates risk for neural tube defect.

Ans.

350.	b
351.	b
352.	b
353.	a
354.	a
355.	a
356.	a
357.	a
358.	a
359.	d
360.	d

361. Nuchal fold thickness is present in:
- a. Down's syndrome
- b. Turner syndrome
- c. Klinefelter syndrome
- d. Edward syndrome

362. The best investigation to diagnose anencephaly at 12 weeks of pregnancy is:
- a. X-ray
- b. Amniocentesis
- c. Ultrasonography
- d. Serum AFP

363. WHO recommended minimum/antenatal visits in the developing country is: *New Q*
- a. 3
- b. 4
- c. 6
- d. 8

Explanation: WHO's new antenatal care model increases the number of contacts a pregnant woman has with health providers throughout her pregnancy from four to eight. Antenatal care model with a minimum of eight contacts recommended to reduce perinatal mortality and improve women's experience of care. Source: WHO News release, 7 Nov 2016.

364. What can be the cause of low estradiol level during pregnancy?
- a. Trisomy 18
- b. Down syndrome
- c. Neural tube defect
- d. All of these

365. A significant predictor of fetal well-being is fetal heart rate of: *(ESIC 2019)*
- a. 100–120 beats/min
- b. 180–200 beats/min
- c. 120–160 beats/min
- d. 160–200 beats/min

Explanation: A significant predictor of fetal well-being is fetal heart rate between 120 and 160 beats/min. FHR less than 120 beats/min or more than 160 is a concern.

366. Normal range of fetal heart rate is:
- a. 80–100
- b. 120–160
- c. 120–170
- d. >150

367. The production of the first heart sound is because of which of the following? *(AIIMS Bhopal Nursing Officer, 2018)*
- a. Rushing of blood into ventricle
- b. Closure of semilunar valves
- c. Contraction of atrial musculature
- d. Closure of atrioventricular valves

Explanation: First heart sound s1 is produced due to the closure of atrioventricular valve, i.e., tricuspid valve and bicuspid valve.

368. Cardiac activity of the fetus can be seen through ultrasound by:
- a. 3 weeks
- b. 4 weeks
- c. 5 weeks
- d. 7 weeks

369. Best parameter to assess the gestational age of fetus is:
- a. Biparietal diameter
- b. Length of femur
- c. Crown-rump length
- d. Chest diameter

370. Which of the following fetal defects can be detected by alpha-fetoprotein test?
- a. Fetal distress
- b. Sickle cell anemia
- c. Down syndrome
- d. IUGR

371. Identify the formula which is used for the estimation of fetal weight:
- a. Johnson's formula
- b. Shepard's formula
- c. Hadlock's formula
- d. All of these

Explanation: Johnson's formula, Shepard formula and Hadlock's formula are used to estimate fetal height.

Johnson's formula estimates fetal weight from symphysiofundal height and station of the presenting part.

Shepherd formula uses Abdominal circumference (AC) and Biparietal Diameter (BPD) to estimate fetal weight.

Hadlock's formula estimates fetal weight from AC, BPD and Femur length.

372. Crown rump length of fetus is measured from to:
- a. Coccyx to the heel
- b. Vertex to the heel
- c. Vertex to the coccyx
- d. Head to coccyx

373. The fetus measures 40 cm and weight 1.5 kg expected at .... weeks of pregnancy.
- a. 20
- b. 26
- c. 30
- d. 34

374. Continued bleeding may result to fetal distress. The nurse knows that the fetus is being compromised when she observed or notes which of the following?
- a. Fetal bradycardia
- b. Fetal tachycardia
- c. Fetal thrashing
- d. All of the above

Explanation: These are the signs that a baby is unwell, or is not coping well with the demands of labor. Increase or decrease in the fetal heart rate is considered as distress.

FETUS IN UTERO (LIE, PRESENTATION AND POSITION)

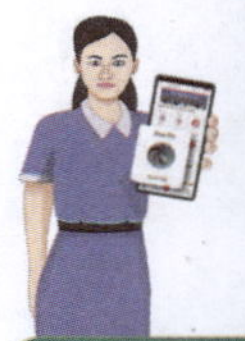

375. Station '0' in descent indicates head is at ....level.
- a. Ischial spine level
- b. Coccyx level
- c. Symphysis pubis level
- d. Ischial tuberosity level

376. Universal attitude is:
- a. Well flexed
- b. Complete extension
- c. Adduction
- d. Abduction

377. Denominator in face presentation:
- a. Occiput
- b. Mentum
- c. Frontal eminence
- d. Sacrum

378. Denominator in brow presentation:
- a. Occiput
- b. Mentum
- c. Frontal eminence
- d. Sacrum

379. Attitude of fetal head in occipito posterior position is: *(Staff Nurse G II 2014)*
- a. Flexion
- b. Adduction
- c. Deflexion
- d. Extension

380. Position of fetus in breech presentation is:
- a. Left sacroanterior
- b. Left mentoanterior
- c. Right occipitoanterior
- d. Left mentoposterior

381. Left occipito posterior position means:
- a. Occiput is placed over the right sacroiliac joint
- b. Occiput is placed over the left sacroiliac joint
- c. Occiput is placed over the right ischial spine
- d. Occiput is placed over the left ischial spine

382. 3rd position of the vertex is also known as:
- a. Right occipito posterior position
- b. Left occipito anterior position
- c. Right occipito anterior position
- d. Left occipito posterior position

Ans.

361. a
362. c
363. d
364. d
365. c
366. b
367. d
368. d
369. c
370. c
371. d
372. c
373. c
374. d
375. a
376. a
377. b
378. c
379. a
380. a
381. b
382. a

383. Internal rotation occurs in normal labor when fetus is at occipito-lateral position:

a. 1/8th of circle b. 2/8th circle
c. 3/8th of circle d. 4/8th circle

384. Station +1 indicates that the presenting part is lying:

a. Slightly below the ischial spine
b. Slightly above the ischial spine
c. High in the false pelvis
d. On the perineum

385. Compound presentation is:

a. Cephalic presentation is complicated by the presence of a hand or a foot or both alongside the head
b. When the presenting part is two buttocks and genitalia
c. In cephalic presentation when the presenting part is face
d. In cephalic presentation presenting part is brow

386. Which one of the following pairs regarding presentation and presenting part in women during labor is not correct? *(Banaras HU 2015)*

a. Cephalic presentation : Chin
b. Face presentation : Face
c. Transverse presentation : Shoulder
d. Breach presentation : Buttock

387. Relationship of the long axis of the fetus to the long axis of the centralized uterus or maternal spine is known as:

a. Lie b. Attitude
c. Denominator d. Position

Explanation: Option A is the correct answer. Attitude is relationship of one part of the body to another. Denominator is bony fixed point on presenting part. Position is the relationship of the denominator to different quadrants of pelvis.

388. Neuromuscular harmony is described in terms of:

a. Attitude b. Contraction
c. Polarity d. Flexion

389. Station of the head is expressed in relation to:

a. Ischial spine b. Pelvic brim
c. Cervix d. Pelvic inlet

Explanation: Station of the head is expressed in terms of ischial spine. At the level of ischial spine, it is termed as 0 station, above which it is indicated in terms of negative numbers such as -1, -2, -3, -4 and -5nd below which are positive numbers such as 1, 2, 3, 4 and 5.

390. What will be the attitude of head during face and brow presentation? *(AIIMS Raipur staff nurse grade I-2018)*

a. Flexion b. Complete extension
c. Adduction d. Abduction

Explanation: Complete extension is the attitude of head in brow presentation. In vertex presentation attitude will be flexion.

391. A woman in labor presents with transverse lie, cervix 4 cm dilated, membrane intact, fetal bradycardia. The treatment of choice is:

a. External cephalic version b. Internal podalic version
c. Cesarean section d. Expectant management

392. In left occiput anterior fetal position, the fetal heart sound is located at: *(AIIMS Bhopal Nursing Officer, 2018)*

a. Around the umbilicus
b. Back towards the mother's flank of the same side
c. Middle of the spino-umbilical line of the same side
d. Below the umbilicus

Explanation:

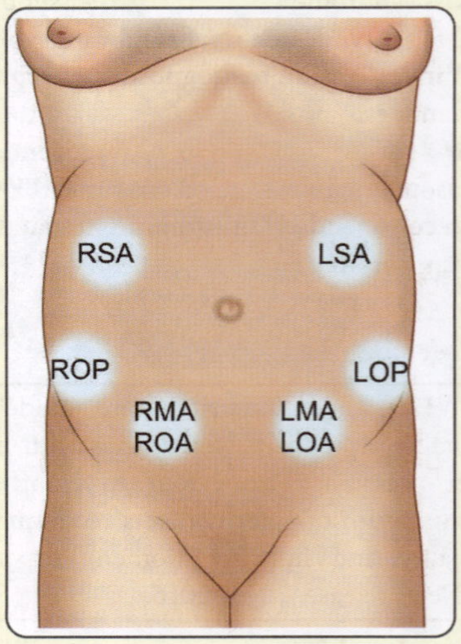

ABDOMINAL EXAMINATION (LEOPOLD MANEUVER)

393. Fundal grip helps to find out:

a. To know the fetal part at the fundus
b. To assess the degree of flexion or attitude
c. To have an idea what the fetal presenting part is
d. To know if engagement occurred or not

Explanation: Fundal grip-to find out the fetal part at fundus

Lateral grip-to find out the location of back, limbs and anterior shoulders.

Pawlik's grip (third leopold)—To have an idea what the fetal presenting part is.

The fourth maneuver is only done if the presentation is in cephalic. The nurse assesses the degree of flexion in this presentation maneuver.

394. Which of the following grips is also known as umbilical grip? *(AIIMS Raipur Staff Nurse Grade I-2018)*

a. Fundal grip b. Lateral grip
c. Pawlik's grip d. Pelvic grip

Explanation: Lateral grip is also known as umbilical grip and the aim of this grip is to identify the fetal back in mother's abdomen.

395. Which of the following is also known as Pawlik's grip?

a. First pelvic grip b. Third leopold
c. Both a and b d. Second leopold

396. Which obstetric grip permits determination of the fetal presentation?

a. Fundal grip b. Lateral grip
c. Pawlik's grip d. Pelvic grip

397. Which obstetrics grip permits determination of the fetal position?

a. Fundal grip b. Lateral grip
c. Pawlik's grip d. Pelvic grip

Ans.

383. b
384. a
385. a
386. a
387. a
388. c
389. a
390. b
391. c
392. c
393. a
394. b
395. c
396. a
397. b

Explanation: The first maneuver (fundal grip) permits determination of the uterine fundus level as well as the fetal presentation. The second maneuver (lateral grip) permits determination of the fetal position.

398. Synonymous of obstetric grip is:
- a. Leopold maneuvers
- b. Fundal grip
- c. Umbilical grip
- d. Pawlik's grip

Explanation: Obstetric grip is also known as Leopold maneuvers which includes fundal grip (first leopold), lateral or umbilical grip (second leopold), Pawlik's grip (third leopold), pelvic grip (fourth leopold)

399. To determine fetal position using Leopold's maneuvers, the first maneuver is to: *(RAK MSc 2018)*
- a. Determine degree of molding
- b. Determine the position of fetus
- c. Determine what part of fetus is in the fundus
- d. Locate the back, arms and legs

Explanation:

Table: Four grips of Leopold's maneuver

Grip	Name	Purpose
First Leopold	Fundal grip	To determine what part of fetus is lying in the fundus
Second Leopold	Lateral or Umbilical grip	To find out the position of back, limbs and the anterior shoulder
Third Leopold	Pawlik's grip or First pelvic grip	To assess the engagement of presenting part
Fourth Leopold	Pelvic grip or Second pelvic grip	To note precise of presenting part, attitude and engagement in vertex presentation.

400. Which of the following obstetric grip is used to assess the descent of head in a pregnant woman?
- a. Fundal grip
- b. Lateral grip
- c. First pelvic grip
- d. Second pelvic grip

401. Painless uterine contractions felt on abdominal palpation occurring every 15 minutes are referred to as:
- a. Braxton Hicks contraction
- b. Quickening
- c. Osiander sign
- d. None of the above

DIFFERENCES BETWEEN TRUE AND FALSE LABOR

402. All of the following are characteristics of false labor pain; EXCEPT:
- a. Contractions are irregular
- b. Contractions felt in abdomen above umbilicus
- c. Bloody show
- d. Fetus is ballotable

403. True labor is characterized by: *(RAK MSc 2018)*
- a. Effacement and dilatation of cervix
- b. Painful uterine contraction
- c. Frequency of contractions increase gradually
- d. All of the above

Explanation: True labor pain is characterized by following symptoms:
- Painful and progressive uterine contraction at regular intervals
- Associated with show
- Progressive effacement and dilatation of cervix
- Frequency of contractions increase gradually
- Formation of bag of membrane
- Decent of the presenting part
- Not relieved by enema, sedatives or by walk
- Pain is felt in the abdomen and radiating to the back.

404. Most reliable indicator of true labor is:
- a. Effacement and dilatation of cervix
- b. Painful uterine contraction
- c. Supra pubic discomfort at regular interval
- d. All of the above

Explanation: Effacement indicates thinning of the cervix which mainly occurs along with dilatation of the cervix.

405. All are the characteristics of true labor pain; EXCEPT:
- a. Intensity and duration of contraction increases progressively
- b. Associated with show
- c. Progressive effacement and dilation of cervix
- d. Pain is confined to lower abdomen and groin

Explanation: Option d is the characteristic of false labor pain and all others are the characteristics of true labor pain.

406. Which of the following is a feature of false labor pain? *(AIIMS Bhopal Grade-I 2018)*
- a. Not associated with the hardening of the uterus
- b. Frequency of contraction increases
- c. Associated with 'show'
- d. Progressive dilation of cervix

Explanation: False labor pain is referred to as Braxton Hicks contractions that occur predominantly in the third trimester but not associated with hardening of uterus. These are typically less painful than those of true labor and also unpredictable, do not occur at regular intervals and do not become more intense over time.

407. False labor manifestation are as follows; EXCEPT: *(ESIC 2019)*
- a. Contraction lessen with activity or rest
- b. Cervix progressively effaced and dilated
- c. Abdominal discomfort
- d. Contractions irregular

Explanation: Progressive effacement and dilated cervix are the features of true labor. All other given manifestations are features of false labor.

408. Which among the following is not a feature of false labor pain? *(AIIMS Bhopal Nursing Officer, 2018)*
- a. Pain is confined to lower abdomen and groin
- b. No effects on dilatation of cervix
- c. Relieved by enema
- d. Formation of bag of waters

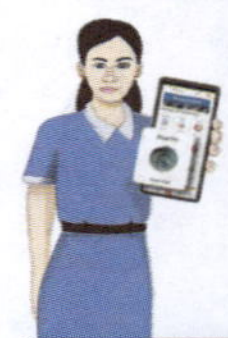

Ans.

398. a
399. c
400. d
401. a
402. c
403. d
404. a
405. d
406. a
407. b
408. d

Explanation: Except option D all other are the characteristics of false labor pain.

False labor pain	True labor pain
Contractions are unpredictable, irregular, vary in length and intensity, unrelated to hardening of the uterus	Contractions are regular and in short intervals, increase in intensity and last longer
Pain is confined to lower abdomen and groin	Pain is felt in the abdomen and radiating to the back
Relieved by enema	Pain will persist irrespective of what we do
There is no formation of bag of water or blood show	Formation of bag of water and bloody show

409. The contraindications of Induction of Labor includes the following; EXCEPT: *(AIIMS Raipur Grade II 2017)*
- a. Placenta Previa
- b. Fetal Macrosomia
- c. Cord presentation
- d. Cephalopelvic disproportion

Explanation: The contraindications include vasa previa, Placenta previa, myomectomy with entry into uterine cavity, previous classical hysterotomy, active genital herpes outbreak, umbilical cord prolapse, or transverse fetal lie.

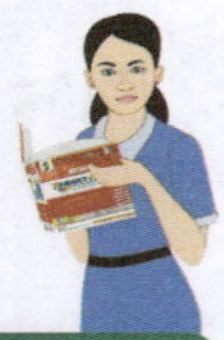

DIFFERENT POSITIONS AND PRESENTATIONS DURING LABOR

410. Denominator in face presentation:
- a. Occiput
- b. Mentum
- c. Frontal eminence
- d. Sacrum

411. General causes of breech presentation is:
- a. Malnutrition
- b. Prematurity
- c. Uterine inertia
- d. Poor bearing down effort

412. The commonest causes of breech presentation is: *(RAK MSc 2018)*
- a. Hydrocephalus
- b. Prematurity
- c. Multipara
- d. Hydramnios

Explanation:
Prematurity is the most common cause of breech presentation as smaller size of fetus and comparatively larger volume of amniotic fluid allow the fetus to undergo spontaneous version (movements) by kicking.

413. Which of the following is a cephalic presentation?
- a. Vertex
- b. Face
- c. Brow
- d. All of these

414. Lateral position is given to pregnant mothers in order to avoid:
- a. Supine hypotension
- b. Orthostatic hypotension
- c. Aspiration
- d. Promotes venous return

Explanation: Lateral position is given to a mother to avoid supine hypotension (postural hypotension). Gravid uterus compresses inferior vena cava when the patient is in supine position and causes hypotension, tachycardia and syncope. This can be avoided by providing lateral position to the client.

415. To promote comfort during labor, Nurse advises a client to assume certain positions and avoid others. Which position may cause maternal hypotension and fetal hypoxia?
- a. Lateral position
- b. Squatting position
- c. Supine position
- d. Standing position

Explanation: In supine position, the weight of the uterine contents presses on the inferior vena cava and slows the venous return of blood to heart, hence leads to maternal hypotension and fetal hypoxia.

416. Which of the following positions should the nurse place the client when the epidural regional block is administered? *(DSSSB 2002)*
- a. Lithotomy
- b. Supine
- c. Prone
- d. Lateral

Explanation: Client should be placed in lateral position or sitting up position.

417. The most unfavorable presentation for vaginal delivery is:
- a. Vertex
- b. Breech
- c. Face
- d. Brow

418. Most common presentation of fetus with anencephaly is:
- a. Breech
- b. Face
- c. Brow
- d. Shoulder

419. The commonest presenting part in cephalic presentation is:
- a. Vertex
- b. Foot
- c. Buttocks
- d. Face

Explanation: The commonest presenting part is vertex in cephalic presentation. It can be face or brow but they are not common.

420. Most common complication associated with breech delivery is:
- a. Abruption placenta
- b. Prolapse cord
- c. Placental retention
- d. Precipitate labor

421. In occipito posterior position, the occiput is towards:
- a. Ischial spine
- b. Sacroiliac joint
- c. Iliopectineal eminence
- d. Pubic symphysis

422. External cephalic version is indicated in:
- a. Breech presentation
- b. Transverse lie
- c. Both a and b
- d. None of these

423. The frequent change of fetal lie and presentation in late pregnancy is known as:
- a. Breech presentation
- b. Footling presentation
- c. Transverse lie
- d. Unstable lie

424. The fetus is in the longitudinal lie with the buttocks or lower extremity entering the pelvis first. This presentation is known as:
- a. Cephalic presentation
- b. Brow presentation
- c. Breech presentation
- d. Sacral presentation

425. Which of the following presentation is a cephalic presentation in which the head is completely extended?
- a. Face presentation
- b. Brow presentation
- c. Breech presentation
- d. Sacral presentation

Ans.

409. b
410. b
411. b
412. b
413. d
414. a
415. c
416. d
417. d
418. b
419. a
420. b
421. b
422. c
423. d
424. c
425. a

426. Which of the following presentation is a cephalic presentation in which the head and neck of the fetus is slightly extended:
a. Face presentation
b. Brow presentation
c. Breech presentation
d. All of the above

427. In frank breech presentation legs will be:
a. One flexed and one extended
b. Both flexed
c. Both extended
d. All of the above

428. Denominator in breech presentation:
a. Occiput b. Mentum
c. Frontal eminence d. Sacrum

NORMAL MECHANISM OF LABOR

429. Progressive thinning and shortening of cervix are defined as: *(AIIMS Nagpur NO 2018)*
a. Expulsion b. Dilation
c. Effacement d. Contraction

Explanation: The processing of thinning of the cervix is known as effacement and the increase in diameter of cervix is called as dilation.

430. It is the visible movement of the head due to untwisting of the neck sustained during internal rotation is:
a. Crowning b. External rotation
c. Restitution d. Torsion of the neck

431. Movement occurred in head to untwist the neck sustained during internal rotation is termed as:
a. Extension b. Restitution
c. Crowning d. External rotation

432. Cardinal movement occur before expulsion is: *(AIIMS 2009)*
a. Engagement b. Crowning
c. Internal rotation d. External rotation

Explanation: External rotation is the cardinal movement which occurs just before the expulsion.

433. What is crowning? New Q *(NORCET 2021)*
a. Rotation at pelvic floor
b. Largest skull diameter fixed that doesn't goes back
c. Largest diameter at ischial spines
d. None of the above

434. Fifth formula is used for assessing:
a. Uterine contraction
b. Progressive descend of the head
c. Fetal well being
d. Labor pain

Explanation: Descent of the head is measured by abdominal palpation and expressed in terms of fifths above the pelvic brim. It is found to be a more reliable way of gauging descent than vaginal examination where large caput formation often leads the inexperienced to confuse scalp descent with skull descent.

435. The realignment of fetal head with the body after the head comes out: *(DSSSB PHN, 2015)*
a. Expulsion b. Descent
c. Engagement d. Restitution

STAGES OF LABOR

436. Which stage of labor is evidenced with effacement of cervix?
a. 1st stage of labor b. 2nd stage of labor
c. 3rd stage of labor d. 4th stage of labor

437. Labor is divided into how many stages?
a. Two b. Three
c. Four d. Five

Explanation: There are total four stages of labor. First stage starts from the onset of true labor pain and ends with the full dilatation of the cervix. Second stage starts from full dilatation of cervix and ends with delivery of the fetus. Third stage starts from delivery of the fetus and ends with expulsion of placenta and membrane. Fourth stage is the observation.

438. A Primigravida patient is admitted to the labor delivery area. Assessment reveals that she is in early part of the first stage of labor. Her pain is likely to be most intense:
a. Around the pelvic girdle
b. Around the pelvic girdle and in the upper arms
c. Around the pelvic girdle and at the perineum
d. At the perineum

Explanation: In pelvic girdle there will be an increase in pressure of presenting part during the labor process.

439. The period between onset of true labor pain up until the cervix is 4 cm dilated is known as:
a. Active phase of labor
b. Latent phase of labor
c. Prolonged phase of labor
d. None of the above

440. Correct sequence in mechanism of labor is:
a. Engagement → descent → flexion → internal rotation
b. Engagement → flexion → crowning → restitution
c. Engagement → decent → internal rotation → flexion
d. Engagement → flexion → extension → crowning

441. Duration of latent phase in primi-gravida is about:
a. 4 hours b. 6 hours
c. 8 hours d. 10 hours

442. What is the reason behind when a patient is advised to walk during her first stage of labor if the membranes are not ruptured?
a. Promote the descent of fetal head
b. Diversion to reduce pain
c. Ensure fetoplacental blood flow
d. Promote placental separation

443. Duration of latent phase in multipara is about:
a. 4 hours
b. 6 hours
c. 8 hours
d. 10 hours

444. Identify correct statement among the following:
a. Cervix will gradually soften, shorten and become thinner, this condition is known as effacement
b. In primigravida effacement precedes dilation of the cervix
c. In multipara both the dilation of cervix and effacement occur simultaneously
d. All of the above

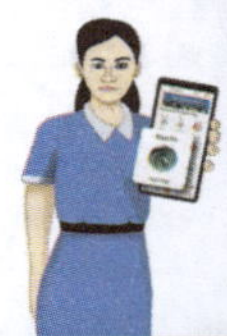

Ans.
426. b
427. c
428. d
429. c
430. c
431. b
432. d
433. b
434. b
435. d
436. a
437. c
438. a
439. b
440. a
441. c
442. a
443. a
444. d

445. In a primi mother average descend in active phase occurs:
a. 1.0 cm/hr b. 1.2 cm/hr
c. 2.0 cm/hr d. 2.2 cm/hr

Explanation: Active phase <1.5 cm/hr

446. First stage of labor is also called
a. Cervical stage b. Expulsive stage
c. Propulsive stage d. Vaginal stage

447. What do you mean by first stage of labor?
a. Onset of true labor pain till full dilation of cervix
b. Full dilation of cervix to expulsion of fetus
c. Expulsion of fetus to expulsion of placenta
d. Observation for at least 1 hour after the expulsion of placenta

448. The expulsion of cervical mucus plug from the vagina, mixed with blood is known as:
a. Amniotic fluid b. Descend
c. Cervical discharge d. Show

449. Other name for normal labor is:
a. Eutocia b. Dystocia
c. Eutonia d. Precipitated labor

450. Primary power of labor is:
a. Abdominal contraction
b. Intrathoracic pressure
c. Pushing effort of the mother
d. Uterine contractions

451. In which stage of labor lower uterine segment will form?
a. 1st stage of labor
b. 2nd stage of labor
c. 3rd stage of labor
d. 4th stage of labor

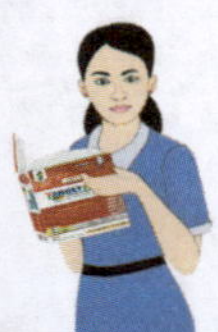

452. All among indicate transition from first stage to second stage; EXCEPT:
a. Increase intensity of uterine contraction
b. Urge to defecate with descent of the presenting part
c. Complete dilation of cervix
d. Relaxation in mother

453. Ripening of the cervix occurs during the:
a. First stage of labor
b. Second stage of labor
c. Third stage of labor
d. Fourth stage of labor

454. Initiation of second stage of labor and cessation of first stage of labor occur when:
a. The baby is delivered
b. The cervix is completely dilated
c. After the delivery of placenta
d. After clamping and cutting the umbilical cord

455. Complete dilation of cervix to birth of a baby is staged as: *(ESIC 2019)*
a. Stage 1 of labor b. Stage 2 of labor
c. Stage 3 of labor d. Stage 4 of labor

Explanation:

- **Stage 1:** Onset of true labor pain to full cervical dilation (9–10 cm)
- **Stage 2:** Complete dilation (9–10 cm) of cervix to birth of a baby
- **Stage 3:** Birth of baby till delivery of placenta
- **Stage 4:** After placental expulsion till 4 hours

456. A 31-year-old multipara is admitted to the birthing room after initial examination reveals her cervix to be at 8 cm, completely effaced (100%), and at 0 station. What phase of labor is she in?
a. Active phase b. Expulsive phase
c. Latent phase d. Transitional phase

Explanation: Transitional phase starts from 8 cm dilatation of the cervix and it is the starting of the second stage of labor.

457. In a primi mother duration of second stage of labor is:
a. 15–30 minutes b. 30–60 minutes
c. 1 hour – 2 hours d. 2–3.5 hours

458. The classical method used in bringing down an arm in breech presentation is called: *(AIIMS Bhopal Grade-I 2018)*
a. Retgen's maneuver
b. Lovset's maneuver
c. Crede's maneuver
d. Pinard's maneuver

Explanation: During breech delivery there may be problem due to the obstructed shoulders. This can occur when arms are raised as the shoulders pass through the mother's pelvis. So, Lovset's maneuver is used for lowering the arm so that the shoulders can descend. Pinard's maneuver is used for breech with extended leg.

459. Criteria for normal labor:
a. Spontaneous in onset
b. Vertex presentation
c. Without undue prolongation
d. All of the above

Explanation: All of the above are criteria for normal labor. Other than these natural termination with minimum aid, without affecting the health of mother and baby is also the criteria for normal labor.

460. Which of the following stages of labor would the nurse assess "crowning"? *(DSSSB)*
a. First stage b. Second stage
c. Third stage d. Fourth stage

Explanation: Birth crowning, which is when baby's head starts to emerge bit by bit during each contraction, occurs during the second stage of labor.

461. 38 weeks' pregnant woman came to clinic and the period of gestation has been confirmed by the ultrasound reports and LMP. She has been started on oxytocin for induction of labor and the nurse notes that the contractions are coming for longer than 70 seconds and she is 3 cm dilated. What should the nurse do next? New Q *(NORCET 2022)*
a. Stop the oxytocin infusion
b. Increase the flow rate
c. Set the drops per minute
d. Document the findings

Explanation: The contractions should last for about 40-60 seconds and should come about every 2–3 minutes. If the contractions are lasting for more than 70 seconds, it is a sign that the woman is receiving too much oxytocin. This can lead to hyperstimulation of the uterus, which can be dangerous for both the mother and the baby.

The nurse should stop the oxytocin infusion and then reassess the woman. If the contractions subside, the nurse can then start the oxytocin infusion again at a lower dose.

Ans.

445. b
446. a
447. a
448. d
449. a
450. d
451. a
452. d
453. a
454. b
455. b
456. d
457. c
458. b
459. d
460. b
461. a

462. Correct statement regarding the onset of labor is:
a. Uterine distention and cervical dilation
b. Accelerated production of estrogen
c. Increased oxytocin and prostaglandin production
d. All of the above

463. The process which reduces surface area at the placental site and is helpful in separation of placenta is known as:
a. Constriction b. Contraction
c. Detachment d. Retraction

464. True labor can be differentiated from false labor in that labor contractions will:
a. Occur immediately after membrane rupture
b. Bring about progressive cervical dilation
c. Be less uncomfortable if client is in side-lying position
d. Stop when the client is encouraged to walk around

465. Uterine contractions are less during the labor, it is termed as:
a. Hypotonia b. Polysystole
c. Hypertonia d. Oligosystole

466. The presence of six or more uterine contractions during a 10-minute period is known as New Q
a. Hypotonia b. Polysystole
c. Hypertonia d. Oligosystole

467. Labor starts with pain and ends with the delivery of: *(RRB Feb 2012)*
a. Umbilical cord b. Fetus
c. Placenta d. None of these

468. A 26-year-old client is admitted to the labor, delivery, recovery, postpartum unit. The nurse completes her assessment and determines the client is in the first stage of labor. The nurse should instruct her: New Q *(NORCET 2022)*
a. To hold her breath during contractions
b. To be flat on her back
c. Not to push with her contractions
d. To push before becoming fully dilated

Explanation: During the first stage of labor, which is characterized by the onset of regular contractions and cervical dilation, it is generally not recommended for the client to actively push until the cervix is fully dilated. This is because premature pushing can increase the risk of cervical trauma and exhaustion. The nurse should instruct the client to relax and breathe through her contractions.

The cervix needs to dilate to its full capacity (typically 10 cm) before the client is encouraged to push during the second stage of labor.

469. In the second stage of labor, the important factor that determines the expulsion of the fetus from birth canal is:
a. Maternal bearing down
b. Cervical dilatation
c. Uterine contractions
d. Adequate pelvic size

470. Characteristic of true labor pain is:
a. Uterine contraction at regular interval
b. Formation of bag of water
c. Pain is not relieved by enema and sedatives
d. All of the above

471. Characteristic of false pain includes:
a. Dull in nature and in lower abdomen and groin
b. No hardening of uterus
c. Relieved by enema and sedatives
d. All of the above

472. A client has been admitted to the labor and delivery unit in active labor. After assessing her, the RN notes that the client's fetus position is left occipital posterior. Which of the following statements best describes what this means to the labor process: New Q *(NORCET 2022)*
a. Decreases the overall time of the labor process
b. Prolongs the client's first stage of labor
c. Decreases the time of the client's first stage of labor
d. Prolongs the client's third stage of labor

473. Expulsion of cervical mucus plug mixed with blood is called:
a. Bleeding per vagina b. Bag of water
c. Show d. Cervical secretion

474. Components of Bishop's cervical scoring system include:
a. Dilatation b. Effacement
c. Consistency d. All of these

475. A primi mother is on first stage of labor and she will be allowed to take only:
a. Liquid diet b. Solid diet
c. Semi solid diet d. NPO

476. In the second stage of labor, which one of the following injections is given to improve uterine contractions? *(DSSB 2013)*
a. Prostaglandin b. Oxytocin
c. Phenergan d. Diazepam

Explanation: Oxytocin is a hormone secreted by posterior lobe of the pituitary and is necessary for uterine contraction. It also helps in milk ejection. So oxytocin reflex is also known as milk ejection reflex.

477. For a patient in active labor, the nurse midwife plans to use an internal electronic fetal monitoring (EFM) device. What must occur before the internal EFM can be applied?
a. The cervix must be dilated fully
b. The fetus must be at 0 station
c. The membranes must rupture
d. The patient must receive anesthesia

Explanation: The membranes must rupture to decrease perinatal mortality and its complication.

478. In normal vaginal delivery, expected blood loss is about:
a. 100–200 mL b. 150–250 mL
c. 200–300 mL d. 300–400 mL

479. A pregnant woman at 38 weeks' gestation is admitted for induction of labor. Her membranes ruptured 12 hours ago. There are no other signs of labor. Which medication should the nurse anticipate for prescription? New Q
a. Oxytocin (Pitocin) b. Estrogen (Premarin)
c. Ergonovine (Ergotrate) d. Progesterone (Prometrium)

Explanation: Oxytocin is a hormone that is used to induce labor. It works by causing the uterus to contract. If the woman's membranes have ruptured, oxytocin is the most likely medication to be prescribed to induce labor.

480. Which of the following stage of labor is called observational stage?
a. Ist stage b. IInd stage
c. IIIrd stage d. IVth stage

481. The primary drug of choice for the active management of third stage of labor is: New Q
a. Ergometrine b. Methergine
c. Oxytocin d. Prostaglandin

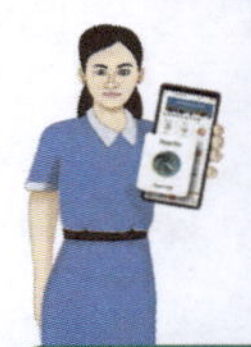

Ans.

462.	d
463.	d
464.	b
465.	a
466.	c
467.	c
468.	c
469.	a
470.	d
471.	d
472.	b
473.	c
474.	d
475.	a
476.	b
477.	c
478.	d
479.	a
480.	d
481.	c

Explanation: WHO Recommendations for active management of the third stage of labor (2012): The use of uterotonics for the prevention of postpartum hemorrhage (PPH) during the third stage of labor is recommended for all births. Oxytocin (10 IU, IV/IM) is the recommended uterotonic drug for the prevention of postpartum hemorrhage.

482. Combined duration of first stage and second stage of labor is more than the arbitrary time limit of 18 hours is known as:
a. Obstructed labor
b. Precipitate labor
c. Prolonged labor
d. Premature labor

483. Progressive descent of the presenting part is arrested due to mechanical obstruction despite of good uterine contraction is known as:
a. Obstructed labor
b. Precipitate labor
c. Prolonged labor
d. Premature labor

484. Causes of prolonged labor include:
a. Uterine inertia
b. Cervical dystonia in fetus
c. Malposition
d. All of the above

485. Criteria of prolonged labor is:
a. Cervical dilatation is less than 1 cm/hr
b. Descent of the presenting part is less than 1 cm/hr
c. Both a and b
d. None of the above

486. Reasons for prolonged labor due to fault in power include:
a. Uterine inertia
b. Incoordinate uterine contraction
c. Both a and b
d. None of the above

487. Reasons for prolonged labor due to fault in passage include:
a. Contracted pelvis
b. Cervical dystonia
c. Pelvic tumor
d. All of the above

488. Reasons for prolonged labor due to fault in passenger include:
a. Malposition
b. Malpresentation
c. Congenital abnormalities
d. All of the above

489. Which stage of labor starts from full dilatation of the cervix, and ends with expulsion of the fetus from birth canal?
a. Fourth stage b. Second stage
c. First stage d. Third stage

490. Major complication in third stage of labor is: *(RAK MSc 2018)*
a. Perineal injuries
b. PPH
c. Subinvolution
d. Uterine rupture

Explanation: Any type of bleeding (more than 500 mL) from birth canal after the birth of baby is called postpartum hemorrhage (PPH). It is the most common complication in third stage of labor.

491. In precipitated labor combined duration of first and second stage will be less than:
a. 1 hour b. 2 hours
c. 3 hours d. 4 hours

492. Expulsion of the fetus within/less than 3 hours of commencement of regular contractions is:
a. Preterm labor b. Precipitate labor
c. Obstruct labor d. Prolonged labor

493. Separation begins at the center of the placenta and slides down the birth canal like a folded umbrella. This method of placental separation referred to as:
a. Duncan mechanism
b. Shultz mechanism
c. Brandt Andrews mechanism
d. Ritgen's maneuver

494. Mismanagement of third stage of labor may lead to:
a. Hyperstimulation of uterus
b. Prolonged labor
c. Inversion of uterus
d. All of the above

495. All are the treatment of choice in precipitate labor; EXCEPT:
a. Administration of ether
b. Administration of magnesium sulfate
c. Oxytocin augmentation
d. Low rupture of membrane

496. Drug of choice to suppress uterine contraction in precipitated labor is:
a. Ether b. Magnesium sulfate
c. Prostaglandin d. Methergine

497. A client is in active labor with twins and the cervix is 5 cm dilated. The nurse observes that contractions are occurring every 7 to 8 minutes in a 30 minute period. The most appropriate action by the nurse would be to:
a. Administer oxygen at 4 liters by mask
b. Note the fetal heart rate patterns
c. Notify the physician immediately
d. Instruct the client to relax during the contractions

Explanation: The client is most likely experiencing hypotonic uterine contractions. The nurse must notify the physician immediately. The usual treatment is oxytocin administration unless cephalopelvic disproportion exists.

PARTOGRAPH

498. Station '0' is indicative of the presenting part being:
a. Slightly above the ischial spine
b. At the level of ischial spine
c. Slightly below the ischial spine
d. On perineum

499. Ms Pavithra, a full term primigravida mother with labor pain got admitted for safe confinement. On PV examination, it was revealed that small part of the head was below the brim of the pelvis and could be lifted out of the pelvis with a deep pelvic grip. What was the descent and engagement of the fetal head? **New Q** *(AIIMS Mangalagiri 2023)*
a. 3/5 b. 4/5
c. 2/5 d. 1/5

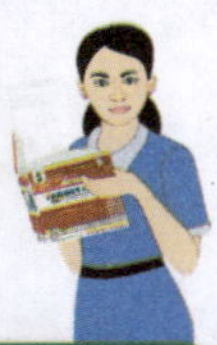

Ans.
482. c
483. a
484. d
485. c
486. c
487. d
488. d
489. b
490. b
491. b
492. b
493. b
494. c
495. c
496. b
497. c
498. b
499. b

Explanation: The amount of descent and engagement of the head is assessed by feeling how much of the head is palpable above the brim of the pelvis.

- **5/5 palpable:** The whole head is above the inlet of the pelvis.
- **4/5 palpable:** A small part of the head is below the brim of the pelvis and can be lifted out of the pelvis with a deep pelvic grip.
- **3/5 palpable:** The head cannot be lifted out of the pelvis.
- **2/5 palpable:** Most of the head is below the pelvic brim.
- **1/5 palpable:** Only the tip of the fetal head can be felt above the pelvic brim. Fully engaged.

500. All among the following are principal movements that occur during labor; EXCEPT:

a. Engagement b. Retraction
c. Crowning d. Restitution

Explanation: Option B retraction is not a principal movement that occurs during labor. Retraction occurs in uterine muscle fibers which means these muscles are shortened permanently. The principal movements occurring during labor are engagement, descent, flexion, internal rotation, crowning, extension, restitution, external rotation and expulsion of trunk.

501. Partograph is also known as:

a. Cervicograph b. Uterograph
c. Ovariograph d. Vaginograph

502. Partograph was first devised by: *(RPSC NG-II, 2007)*

a. Friedman b. AL Mudaliar
c. William Show d. Shirodkar

Explanation: The partograph was designed by **Friedman in 1954** and further **improved by Philpot and Castle** who introduced the alert and action lines to facilitate interventions during labor.

503. Two phases of labor in partograph include:

a. Inertia phase and action phase
b. Active phase and alert phase
c. Active phase and latent phase
d. Inactive phase and active phase

PHARMACOLOGY IN OBG

504. The amount of elemental iron in one iron tablet for mother is: *(AIIMS Bhopal Grade-I 2018)*

a. 60 mg b. 60 g
c. 50 g d. 50 mg

Explanation: The equivalent of 60 mg of elemental iron is 300 mg ferrous sulfate heptahydrate, 180 mg ferrous fumarate or 500 mg of ferrous gluconate.

505. A Nurse is caring for a 16-year-old pregnant client. The client is taking an iron supplement. What should this client drink to increase the absorption of iron?

a. A cup of hot coffee
b. A glass of milk
c. A glass of orange juice
d. Antacid solution

Explanation: Orange is good source of vitamin C and helps in absorption of iron.

506. Which among the following is correct regarding iron supplementation?

a. Take it along with milk
b. Take it along with lemon juice
c. Take it along with water
d. Take it after having food

Explanations: Acidic environment promotes iron absorption. Lemon juice provides acidic medium which promotes absorption of drug. Orange juice can be also taken. Taking iron preparations in empty stomach will also promote its absorption.

507. Most widely used oral iron preparation during pregnancy is.

a. Ferrous gluconate
b. Ferrous sulfate
c. Ferrous fumarate
d. Ferrous succinate

Explanation: Most widely used iron preparation is ferrous sulfate. It contains 200 mg ferrous sulfate which contains 60 mg elementary iron.

508. Injection TT is given to pregnant woman to prevent: *(RRB Feb 2012)*

a. Typhoid b. Maternal tetanus
c. Neonatal tetanus d. Both b and c

Explanation: To prevent them and their neonate from tetanus. (Depends upon previous tetanus vaccination to mother)

509. Drugs and X-rays should be avoided in the ….. trimester of pregnancy. *(RRB Feb 2012)*

a. Second b. First
c. Third d. None

510. Identify the incorrect statement regarding immunization in pregnant woman.

a. Live vaccines are contraindicated in pregnancy
b. Immunization against tetanus can be given
c. Tetanus immunization protects both mother and baby
d. 3 doses of tetanus one in each trimester is recommended

Explanation: Option D is the incorrect statement, live vaccines during pregnancy carry a risk for infection to the unborn baby also. 2 doses of TT immunization is recommended 0.5 mL IM in deltoid region at 6 weeks interval.

511. Which of the following vaccines is contraindicated in pregnancy? *(AIIMS Raipur staff nurse grade I-2018:*

a. Measles
b. Rubella
c. Varicella
d. All of these

Explanation: All the mentioned vaccines are live vaccines and fetus is at risk for developing active infection.

512. As per Govt. of India guidelines, the recommended daily dose of elemental iron for prophylaxis during pregnancy:

a. 50 mg/day for 100 days
b. 50 mg/day for 150 days
c. 100 mg/day for 100 days
d. 100 mg/day for 150 days

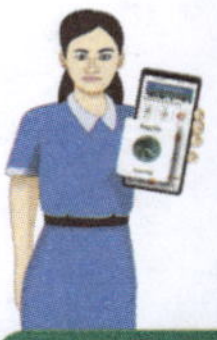

Ans.

500. b
501. a
502. a
503. c
504. a
505. c
506. b
507. b
508. d
509. b
510. d
511. d
512. c

513. A client has come to the clinic for her first prenatal visit. Nurse should include which of the following statements about using drugs safely during pregnancy in her teaching?

a. "All medications are safe after you've reached the 5th month of pregnancy."
b. "Consult with your health care provider before taking any medications."
c. "During the first 3 months, avoid all medications except ones prescribed by your caregiver."
d. "Medications that are available over the counter are safe for you to use, even early on."

Explanation: Most of the drugs can cross the placenta and inhibit normal growth of fetus. So pregnant women must consult with their healthcare provider before taking any medications.

514. Appropriate time for TT immunization in a pregnant woman without previous TT immunization is:

a. At first contact or as early as possible in pregnancy
b. Between 12 and 16 weeks of pregnancy
c. Between 20 and 24 weeks of pregnancy
d. Two weeks before EDD

Explanation:

Table: Tetanus toxoid immunization schedule for women of childbearing age and pregnant women without previous exposure to TT/Td or DTP.

Dose of TT or Td (According to card or history)	When to give	Expected duration of protection
1	At first contact or as early as possible in pregnancy	None
2	At least 4 weeks after TT1	1–3 years
3	At least 6 months after TT2 or during subsequent pregnancy	At least 5 years
4	At least one year after TT3 or during subsequent pregnancy	At least 10 years
5	At least one year after TT4 or during subsequent pregnancy	For all childbearing age year and possibly longer

515. Folic acid deficiency during the pregnancy will lead to:

a. Exstrophy bladder
b. Esophageal atresia
c. Neural tube defect
d. Congenital diaphragmatic hernia

516. How much amount of elemental iron contained by one tablet of ferrous sulfate?

a. 40 mg b. 50 mg
c. 60 mg d. 70 mg

517. Iron and folic acid dose for pregnant women is: *New Q*

a. 60 mg iron, 0.4 mg folic acid
b. 30 mg iron, 0.4 mg folic acid
c. 100 mg iron, 0.3 mg folic acid
d. 60 mg iron, 500 mcg folic acid

518. In which condition oral pills should not be given to a woman?

a. Menstrual problems b. Hypertension
c. Asthma d. Vaginal infection

519. The drug of choice in treatment of typhoid fever during pregnancy is:

a. Quinolones b. Ceftriaxone
c. Levofloxacin d. Norfloxacin

Explanation: Drug of choice for typhoid during pregnancy - 3rd Generation cephalosporins, (e.g., Ceftriaxone) or Ampicillin/ Amoxicillin.

Quinolones are preferred choice in Non-pregnant individuals.

520. Which of the following drugs is safe for the treatment of cholera in pregnant women?

a. Doxycycline b. Chloramphenicol
c. Ofloxacin d. Azithromycin

Ref: CDC. www.cdc.gov/cholera/treatment/antibiotic-treatment.html

Explanation: According to CDC guidelines, Azithromycin is more effective than erythromycin and ciprofloxacin and is an appropriate first line treatment for pregnant women and children.

Tetracycline (Doxycycline) is an effective treatment for cholera and is superior to furazolidone, cholamphenicol and sulfaguanidine but are not recommended during pregnancy.

521. All of the following drugs are unsafe in pregnant women; EXCEPT:

a. Methatexate b. Warfarin
c. Heparin d. ACE inhibitors

522. Which of the following drugs is administered in women with premature spontaneous rupture of membrane before the 37th week of pregnancy?

a. Methergine b. Dexamethasone
c. Captopril d. Magnesium sulfate

523. Management of mastitis includes:

a. Analgesics b. Breast support
c. Antibiotics d. All of these

524. Teratogenic effect of unprescribed drug affects the fetus most commonly in .... trimester.

a. 1st trimester b. 2nd trimester
c. 3rd trimester d. Whole antenatal period

525. The fetus is most likely to be damaged during pregnancy when there is ingestion of drugs during:

a. First trimester b. Second trimester
c. Third trimester d. None of the above

526. The most important observation for a patient in labor in Pitocin augmentation is: *(JIPMER 2012)*

a. Monitoring FHS
b. Monitoring TPR
c. Preparing for emergency CS
d. Monitoring and recording the length of contraction

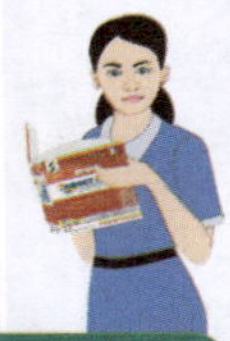

Ans.

513. b
514. a
515. c
516. c
517. d
518. b
519. b
520. d
521. c
522. b
523. d
524. a
525. a
526. d

527. **The primary purpose of administering magnesium sulfate intravenously for a patient who has premature rupture of membrane and has contraction in every 10 minutes is to:** *(AIIMS Bhopal Grade-I 2018)*
   a. Provide sedation
   b. Maintain blood pressure
   c. Inhibit contraction
   d. Improve fetal lung function

Explanation: Magnesium sulfate acts as a tocolytic agent which are used to stop uterine contractions. Tocolytics have no effect on placental perfusion or fetal pulmonary system.

528. **Complication of tocolytic agent is:**
   a. Uterine rupture
   b. Hyperstimulation of uterus
   c. Increased peristaltic movement
   d. Pulmonary edema

Explanation: Pulmonary edema is the most common adverse effect associated with tocolytic agents.

529. **Morphine given to the mother during the process of delivery causes ....in newborn.**
   a. Respiratory depression
   b. Hypoxic ischemia
   c. Intestinal obstruction
   d. Coagulopathy

530. **The hormone that is injected to pregnant women at the time of delivery:** *(RRB Feb 2012)*
   a. Prednisolone b. Progesterone
   c. Oxytocin d. None of these

531. **For what complication should a nurse monitor a patient when an oxytocin infusion is used to induce labor?**
   a. Intense pain b. Uterine tetany
   c. Hypoglycemia d. Umbilical cord prolapse

Explanation: Uterine tetany refers to prolonged uterine contractions during labor due to the infusion of oxytocin. The nurse should monitor a patient for uterine tetany, if occurs, the oxytocin infusion must be stopped to prevent uterine rupture and fetal compromise.

532. **Overstimulated uterus by oxytocin during induction of labor leads to:**
   a. Increased pain with bright red vaginal bleeding
   b. Increased restlessness
   c. Tetanic contractions prolonged for more than 90 sec
   d. Weak contractions prolonged to more than 70 sec

533. **The drug is used to treat premature contractions and delivery is:**
   a. Oxytocin b. Ergot derivative
   c. Prostaglandin d. Tocolytic agents

534. **The best and safest drug for controlling bleeding in dysfunctional uterine bleeding is:**
   a. Estrogen b. Tranexamic acid
   c. Combined pills d. Progesterone

535. **Which of the following drugs is administered when a postpartum client, who is receiving heparin for thrombophlebitis, develops complications related to heparin therapy?**
   a. Vitamin K b. Calcium gluconate
   c. Protamine sulfate d. Aspirin

Explanation: Protamine sulfate is a heparin antagonist. It is administered intravenously to counter the bleeding complications precipitated by heparin overdose.

536. **Which of the following antihypertensives is not safe during pregnancy?**
   a. Labetalol b. ACE inhibitors
   c. Diuretics d. Nifedipine

537. **Prolonged use of methergine induce hypertension and gangrene because of:**
   a. It act directly on myometrium
   b. It has to be used late in the second stage either after the delivery of anterior shoulder or after the delivery of baby
   c. It has a vasoconstrictive action
   d. All of the above

538. **Which of the following is a drug of choice for a pregnant mother with chronic hypertension?** *(AIIMS Bhopal Grade-I 2018)*
   a. Methyldopa b. Atenolol
   c. Diazepam d. Magnesium sulfate

Explanation: Methyldopa is the drug of choice for pregnant mother with chronic hypertension because this drug does not alter the maternal cardiac output or blood flow to the uterus or kidneys, while other drugs like atenolol has been associated with intrauterine growth retardation. Magnesium sulfate is used to treat women with pre-eclampsia. Diazepam is not an antihypertensive drug.

539. **Which of these drugs is contraindicated in a mother in labor with hypertension?** *(Daman & Diu NO 2018)*
   a. Oxytocin b. Prostaglandins
   c. Magnesium sulfate d. Methergine

Explanation: Methergine is a semisynthetic ergot alkaloid used for the prevention and control of postpartum hemorrhage. Methergine is contraindicated in high blood pressure and in pregnancy. So it is contraindicated in a mother in labor with hypertension.

540. **Ergometrine is contraindicated in:**
   a. Diabetes mellitus
   b. Postpartum hemorrhage
   c. Heart diseases
   d. Polyhydramnios

541. **The risk factor for the development of thromboembolic phenomenon in a woman with cardiac disease will be the intake of:**
   a. Antihypertensive drugs
   b. Antiarrhythmic drugs
   c. Intrauterine devices
   d. Steroidal contraceptives

542. **The most common cause of ruptured uterus is:**
   a. Incorrect use of oxytocin
   b. Stimulation of uterus
   c. Twin pregnancy
   d. Precipitate labor

543. **A 47-year-old woman comes to gynecology OPD with complaints of hot flushes after stopping of menstruation. Which of the following drug administration can relieve the 'Hot Flush'?** *New Q*
   a. Fluoxymestrone b. Ethinyl estradiol
   c. Danazol d. Testosterone

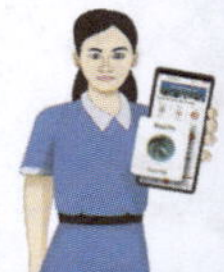

Ans.
527. c
528. d
529. a
530. c
531. b
532. c
533. d
534. b
535. c
536. b
537. c
538. a
539. d
540. c
541. d
542. a
543. b

Explanation: Hot flushes are a common symptom of menopause. They are caused by a decrease in the production of estrogen by the ovaries. When estrogen levels decrease, the body's thermostat becomes more sensitive to changes in temperature, which can lead to hot flushes.

Ethinyl estradiol is a synthetic form of estrogen that can be used to treat hot flushes. It is available in a variety of forms, including oral tablets, transdermal patches, and vaginal rings.

544. Tocolytic agents are used to: *(RAK MSc 2018)*
- a. Enhance the preterm labor
- b. Suppress the preterm labor
- c. Enhance the normal labor
- d. Suppress the normal labor

Explanation: Tocolytic agents are drugs used to delay preterm labor in order to improve perinatal mortality.

545. Oxytocin has a half-life of:
- a. 2–3 minutes
- b. 3–4 minutes
- c. 4–5 minutes
- d. 5–6 minutes

546. Group of drugs that has power to excite uterine contractions are referred to as:
- a. Betamimetics
- b. Steroids
- c. Oxytocics
- d. Tocolytic

547. Contraindication for use of ergometrine/Methergine include:
- a. Suspected pleural pregnancy
- b. Organic cardiac disease
- c. Rh negative mother
- d. All of the above

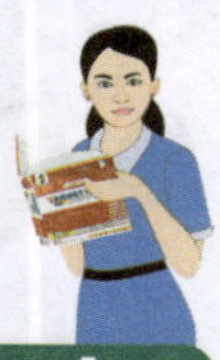

548. Intake of chloramphenicol during pregnancy will lead to:
- a. Gray baby syndrome
- b. Auditory damage
- c. Adrenal suppression
- d. Kernicterus in newborn

549. Which sentence is true regarding ergot derivatives?
- a. They act directly on myometrium
- b. They have has to be used late in the second stage either after the delivery of anterior shoulder or after the delivery of baby
- c. They have has a vasoconstrictive action
- d. All of the above

550. Which of the following is not a side effect of Methergine?
- a. Severe headache
- b. Decreased blood pressure
- c. Difficulty in breathing
- d. Interference with lactation

551. Disadvantages and side effects of prostaglandin include:
- a. Expensive
- b. Tachysystole
- c. Risk for uterine rupture in case of scar
- d. All of the above

552. Which among the following is the major side effect of oxytocin? *(RAK MSc 2018)*
- a. Diuresis
- b. Water retention
- c. Hyperstimulation of uterus
- d. Uterine atony

Explanation: Uterine hyperstimulation is most common side effect. There may be increased duration of uterine contractions or increased frequency (more than 6 contractions per 10 minutes).

553. A nurse should monitor intake and output during oxytocin administration, because the drug: *(Daman & Diu NO 2018)*
- a. Causes toxicity for kidneys
- b. Causes water intoxication
- c. Increases thirst
- d. Induces diuretic effect

Explanation: Oxytocin, due to its ADH like action, causes water intoxication, particularly if given with excessive IV fluid.

554. Complications of oxytocin include:
- a. Uterine hyperstimulation
- b. Uterine rupture
- c. Water intoxication
- d. All of the above

555. Oxytocin is contraindicated in:
- a. Contracted pelvis
- b. Preeclampsia
- c. History of assisted deliveries
- d. PPH

556. Complication of medications used for ovulation induction is:
- a. Increased congenital anomalies
- b. Ovarian hyperstimulation
- c. Endometrial cancer
- d. Ectopic pregnancy

557. Drug of choice to treat infertility due to antisperm antibodies is:
- a. GnRH therapy
- b. Clomiphene citrate
- c. Doxycycline
- d. Dexamethasone

558. Drug of choice to induce ovulation in an infertile female is:
- a. Clomiphene citrate
- b. FSH
- c. GnRH
- d. All of the above

559. Luteal phase defect is treated with:
- a. Progesterone therapy
- b. Estrogen therapy
- c. Testosterone therapy
- d. FSH therapy

560. Ergot derivatives include:
- a. Methergine
- b. Syntometrine
- c. Ergometrin
- d. All of these

561. PGE2 stands for:
- a. Dinoprostone
- b. Oxytocin
- c. Misoprostol
- d. Methergine

562. PGE1 stands for:
- a. Dinoprostone
- b. Oxytocin
- c. Misoprostol
- d. Methergine

563. Major galacokinetic hormone is:
- a. Oxytocin
- b. Prolactin
- c. Estrogen
- d. Progesterone

Explanation: Oxytocin is the hormone which helps in milk ejection, so it is considered as major galactokinetic hormone.

564. Most preferred site for administering inj. Magnesium sulfate is .... muscle.
- a. Deltoid
- b. Ventrogluteal
- c. Vastus lateralis
- d. Dorsogluteal

565. A client is on magnesium sulfate therapy. For the repeated dose administration the nurse need to check:
- a. Urine output >30 mL/hr
- b. Knee jerk reflex are present
- c. Respiration is >12 bpm
- d. All of the above

Ans.

544. b
545. b
546. c
547. d
548. a
549. d
550. b
551. d
552. c
553. b
554. d
555. a
556. b
557. d
558. d
559. a
560. d
561. a
562. c
563. a
564. d
565. d

Explanation: For the subsequent dose administration, the nurse needs to check all the above parameters. If these are not present then toxicity needs to be suspected.

566. The first sign of excessive blood magnesium levels is:
a. Development of cardiac arrhythmias
b. Disappearance of the knee-jerk reflex
c. Increase in respiratory rate
d. Disturbance in sensorium

567. A nurse needs to check the most important parameter if patient is on magnesium sulfate therapy: *(Safdarjung NO 2018)*
a. Urine output >30 mL/hr
b. Presence of knee jerk reflex
c. Respiration is >12 per minute
d. Blood pressure <140 /90 mm Hg

Explanation: Diminished/absence of deep tendon reflex is one of the earliest signs of magnesium toxicity. When a patient receives $MgSO_4$ therapy, the nurse must assess Deep tendon reflexes (knee jerk reflex) frequently. Information from DTRs will help nurses develop judgment about titrating the administration and prevent magnesium toxicity.

568. Antidote of magnesium sulfate is:
a. Calcium gluconate b. Potassium chloride
c. Sodium nitroprusside d. Verapamil

Explanation: Calcium gluconate is the anti-dote of magnesium sulfate. Client on magnesium sulfate therapy should be monitored for deep tendon reflexes hourly. Cardiac and renal function is monitored closely. The urine output should be maintained at 30 mL/ hr because the medication is eliminated through the kidneys.

569. Which drug is used for the management of menorrhagia?
a. Tanexemic acid b. Oral contraceptive pills
c. NSAID d. All of these

570. A primigravida is receiving IV Magnesium sulfate. Which of the following assessment is the priority in this case?
a. Urine for glucose b. Urine for protein
c. Calf tenderness d. Deep tendon reflexes

571. Drug of choice for the management of DUB is:
a. Contraceptive pills
b. Norethisterone acetate
c. 17 alpha ethinyl testosterone
d. All of the above

572. Treatment of choice for endometriosis is:
a. Estrogen and progesterone pill
b. Danazol
c. GnRH analogues
d. All of the above

573. Drug of choice for the management of vaginal trichomoniasis is:
a. Prostaglandin b. Oxytocin
c. Metronidazole d. Gentamycin

574. First antihypertensive drug of choice in obstetric is:
a. Methyldopa b. Atenolol
c. Amlodipine d. ACE inhibitors

575. All are tocolytic agents; EXCEPT:
a. Indomethacin b. Nitric oxide donors
c. Magnesium sulfate d. Diazepam

576. The drug used to prevent circulatory overload during the first stage of labor of a woman with cardiac disease?
a. Betamethasone b. Dexamethasone
c. Furosemide d. Mannitol

577. Vaginal trichomoniasis is best treated with:
a. Systemic antifungal agents
b. Oral metronidazole for the couple
c. Local anesthetics and antifungal agents
d. Local antifungal agents

578. Parameter needs to be monitored in a client receiving Magnesium sulfate is:
a. Half hourly pulse, respiration and BP
b. Deep tendon reflexes every 4 hours
c. Hourly urine output
d. All of the above

579. The nurse administers injection MgSO4 to a woman who is hospitalized with severe pre-eclampsia. What medication would the nurse administer to counter MgSO4 toxicity?
a. Sodium chloride b. Calcium gluconate
c. Epinephrine d. Sodium bicarbonate

580. At what gestational age does the switchover from fetal to adult hemoglobin synthesis begin?
a. 24 weeks b. 30 weeks
c. 36 weeks d. Immediately after birth

581. The drug of choice for Ophthalmia neonatorum is:
a. Ampicillin b. Atropine
c. Gentamycin d. Amoxicillin

582. Oxytocin causes all of the following except:
a. Contraction of uterine muscles
b. Milk ejection
c. Lactogenesis
d. Myoepithelial cell contraction

583. Treatment for gonorrhea includes both ceftriaxone and doxycycline, because:
a. To prevent drug resistance
b. To cure the disease completely
c. Single drug is not successful
d. Chance of coexisting chlamydial infection

584. Which one of the following anti-tuberculosis drugs cannot be given during pregnancy? *(AIIMS Raipur No 2019)*
a. Rifampicin
b. Ethambutol
c. Streptomycin
d. INH

Explanation: Rifampicin, INH and ethambutol are safe during pregnancy. Streptomycin can cause harmful effects in the fetus as it readily crosses the placental barrier.

585. The gold standard for the treatment of hot flushes is: *(AIIMS-BBS SNO 2019)*
a. Oxytocin administration
b. Progesterone administration
c. Estrogen administration
d. Serotonin administration

Explanation: Decrease in level of estrogen is a cause of hot flushes. Hot flushes mean sudden feeling of warmth, usually most intense over the face, neck, chest and profuse sweating. It commonly occurs due to menopause. The gold standard for the treatment of hot flushes is **Estrogen administration.**

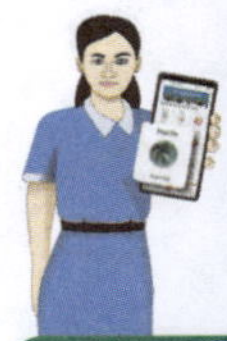

Ans.

566. b
567. b
568. a
569. d
570. d
571. d
572. d
573. c
574. a
575. d
576. c
577. b
578. d
579. b
580. b
581. a
582. c
583. d
584. c
585. c

586. After menopause increased facial hair growth and change in voice occur due to:

a. Fall in FSH level
b. Increase in FSH level
c. Increase in androgen level
d. Decrease in androgen level

587. Which among the following drug will be prescribed by physician for a woman who is experiencing perimenopausal symptoms?

a. Progesterone
b. Estrogen
c. Luteinizing hormone
d. Analgesics

588. Client is not willing to take hormonal replacement therapy after menopause to manage the age related problems, the important management for this client is:

a. Maintaining usual sexual activity
b. Take more dietary fibers and liquids
c. Do regular aerobic, weight-bearing exercise
d. Take multivitamin supplements

589. Which of the following can be used to restore menstrual cycle in a woman with amenorrhea due to polycystic ovarian disease?

a. Danocrine
b. Combined oral pills
c. Progesterone therapy
d. Estrogen therapy

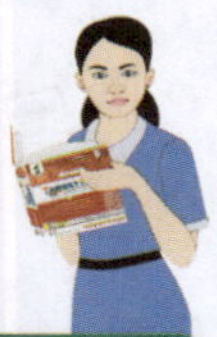

MATERNAL ANALGESIA

590. Which among the following is the potentially harmful side effect of epidural anesthesia?

a. Hypotension b. Headache
c. Decreased urine output d. Increased respiration

Explanation: Hypotension is the potentially harmful side effect of epidural anesthesia as it causes placental insufficiency by decreasing perfusion to the placenta.

591. One of the inhalational anesthetic agents used in labor is Entonox. It is the combination of:

a. 50% oxygen and 50% nitrous oxide
b. 50% oxygen and 50% nitric oxide
c. 50% nitric oxide and 50% nitrous oxide
d. 50% nitrate and 50% oxygen

592. Which among the following statement is INCORRECT regarding paracervical block?

a. It provides pain relief in the first stage of labor.
b. It involves submucosal administration of local anesthetic near the outer rim of cervix.
c. It relieves pain caused by cervical dilation.
d. Perineal infiltration is the other name of paracervical block.

593. Drug of choice for perineal infiltration before episiotomy is:

a. 1% Bupivacaine b. Fentanyl
c. Halothane d. 1% lignocaine

594. Transcutaneous electric nerve stimulation is one of the pain-relieving measures used during delivery. In this method electrodes are placed at:

a. L1-L2 b. L3-L4
c. T10-L1 d. T2-T3

ASSISTED DELIVERIES

595. Failure to deliver the head even after correct and judicious application of forceps raise the suspicion on: *(AIIMS Raipur Grade II 2017)*

a. Cervical dystocia b. Spastic lower segment
c. Constricting ring d. Incoordinate uterine action

Explanation: Cervical dystocia is an abnormal labor as a result of ineffectual dilatation which is caused by inadequate uterine activity, trauma, idiopathic and following surgical procedures. Construction ring is a persistent localized annular spasm of the circular uterine muscles which occurs at any part of the uterus but usually at junction of the upper and lower uterine segments.

596. The indication of forceps delivery is: *(RAK MSc 2018)*

a. Delay in first stage due to hypotonic uterine contraction
b. Delay in first stage due to hypertonic uterine contraction
c. Delay in second stage due to hypotonic uterine contraction
d. Delay in second stage due to hypertonic uterine contraction

Explanation: Objective of forceps application is to cut short second stage of labor; it is also applicable when expulsive efforts are inadequate (hypotonic uterus).

597. Following are the methods of induction of labor; EXCEPT:

a. Artificial rupture of membrane
b. Methergin
c. Oxytocin
d. Prostaglandin

Explanation: Methergin directly acts on the myometrium. It excites uterine contraction which comes so frequent one after the other with increasing intensity that the uterus passes into the state of spasm without relaxation in between. Hence it is not used for induction of labor.

598. Compared to the use of the vacuum extractor, forceps delivery is associated with increased risk of: *(Banaras HU 2015)*

a. Minor facial injuries b. Cephalohematoma
c. Retinal hemorrhage d. Intracranial hemorrhage

599. Instrument of choice for clamping the umbilical cord is:

a. Allis tissue forceps
b. Kocher's hemostatic forceps
c. Long straight hemostatic forceps
d. Multiple toothed vulsellum

600. A primigravida was admitted to the labor room at 40 weeks of gestation for the induction of labor. The obstetrician has planned to induce with misoprostol (PGE_1). What dose to be used? *New Q*

a. 25 mg b. 25 mcg
c. 50 mg d. 50 mcg

601. The therapeutic uses of laparoscopy are:

a. Treatment of endometriosis
b. Tubal ligation
c. Ectopic pregnancy
d. All of the above

602. The management option for primi-mother with Right Occipito Posterior position in second stage of labor is:

a. Immediate cesarean section
b. Forceps application
c. Watchful expectancy
d. Breech extraction

Ans.

586. c
587. b
588. c
589. b
590. a
591. b
592. d
593. d
594. c
595. c
596. c
597. b
598. a
599. b
600. b
601. d
602. c

603. Dangers to the baby from forceps applications are the following; EXCEPT:
a. Intracranial hemorrhage
b. Fracture of the skull bones
c. Brachial palsy d. Facial palsy

604. Mauriceau–Smellie–Veit grip is used to deliver:
a. The extended arms b. The extended legs
c. The extended head d. None of these

605. In which of the following conditions would it be indicated to deliver the baby by forceps:
a. Heart disease
b. Contracted pelvis
c. Cervix fails to dilate completely
d. Presence of meconium-stained fluid in vertex presentation

606. In persistent occipito posterior position the rotation of head is usually done by:
a. Wrigley's forceps b. Kielland's forceps
c. Haig Ferguson's forceps d. Branes nevilli's forceps

607. The fetal head is born by the process of:
a. Crowning b. Restitution
c. Extension d. Internal rotation

608. The indication of forceps delivery is the delay in second stage of labor due to:
a. Hypotonic uterine contraction
b. Hypertonic uterine contraction
c. Poor maternal efforts
d. Placenta previa

609. The suction cup leaves a small swelling on your baby's head during vacuum delivery and is known as:
a. Caput succedaneum b. Cephalohematoma
c. Chignon d. Neonatal tetanus

OPERATIVE OBG

610. An incision made into perineum to enlarge the vagina during delivery is: *(DSSSB PHN, 2015)*
a. Amniotomy b. Episiotomy
c. Cesarean d. Forceps delivery

611. A woman had a midline episiotomy performed at delivery. The primary purpose of the episiotomy is to: *(LNJP H D 2012)*
a. Enlarge the vaginal opening
b. Allow forceps to be applied
c. Eliminate the need for cesarean birth
d. Eliminate the possibility of lacerations

612. Most common incision in episiotomy is: *(AIIMS BBS 2018, NORCET 2021)*
a. Lateral b. Medial
c. J-shaped d. Mediolateral

Explanation: Most common incision in episiotomy is mediolateral. Researches show that mediolateral episiotomy causes less perineal tear as compared to other types of episiotomy hence it is commonly practiced.

613. It is a manipulative procedure designed to change the lie or to bring the comparatively favorable pole to the lower pole of the uterus:
a. Destructive operations b. Evisceration
c. Ventouse d. Version

614. In classical cesarean section more chances of rupture of uterus occur in:
a. Upper uterine segment b. Lower uterine segment
c. Utero cervical junction d. Posterior uterine segment

615. Find out the absolute indication for elective cesarian section:
a. Uncorrectable abnormal lie
b. Placenta previa
c. Previous vertical cesarean section
d. All of the above

Explanation: Absolute indications for cesarian section (it should be done even in the presence of dead fetus) include:
- Previous class C.S. or CS extending to upper segment
- Two or more previous LSCS
- Previous LSCS with malpresentations
- Previous repair of vesicovaginal fistula
- Extreme degree of contracted pelvis
- Placenta previa centralis
- Uncorrectable abnormal lie

616. Previous history of lower segment cesarean section is a significant antenatal history as it can lead to:
a. Abortion b. Antepartum hemorrhage
c. Incompetent cervix d. Uterine rupture

617. During the delivery, the perineal tear extends through the sphincter of the rectum but the rectal mucosa is intact. How would you classify this type of perineal tear? *(Banaras HU 2015)*
a. First-degree b. Second-degree
c. Third-degree d. Fourth-degree

618. The maximum amount of blood lost during delivery is .....mL. *(RRB Feb 2012)*
a. 250 mL b. 100 mL
c. 500 mL d. 300 mL

619. Which instrument is used for dilatation of cervix during D and E procedure?
a. Manual vacuum aspiration syringe
b. Karman's cannula
c. Laminaria tent
d. Uterine curette

620. Two days after having a cesarean birth, a client complains of pain in the right leg. What should be the nurse's initial response? *(AIIMS Raipur NO 2019)*
a. Apply warm soaks
b. Massage the affected area
c. Encourage ambulation and exercise
d. Maintain bed rest and notify the practitioner

Explanation: Temporary nerve irritation or injury can occur with anesthesia, which might cause leg pain after c-section. It is usually resolved within a few days after bed rest. Applying warm soaks and massaging affected area is not recommended. Ambulation and post-natal exercise are encouraged as soon as possible but not an appropriate initial response to the complains of pain.

621. Indications for craniotomy include:
a. Hydrocephalus
b. Interlocking head of twins
c. Cephalic presentation producing obstructed labor with dead fetus
d. All of the above

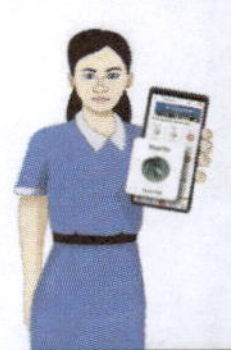

Ans.
603. c
604. c
605. a
606. b
607. c
608. c
609. c
610. b
611. a
612. d
613. d
614. a
615. d
616. d
617. c
618. c
619. c
620. d
621. d

622. A surgical procedure in which the entire breast and axillary lymph nodes are removed is termed as:
a. Radical mastectomy
b. Lobectomy
c. Radical mastectomy with lymphadenectomy
d. Lumpectomy

623. The most common complication after a mastectomy is:
a. Hemorrhage with pain
b. Wound drainage
c. Wound infection
d. Edema and stiffness of the arm

POSTPARTUM NURSING CARE

624. The nurse preparing to administer the Rubella vaccine to a two days postpartum woman. The nurse should caution the client to avoid: *(Safdarjung NO 2018)*
a. Sunlight for 3 days
b. Scratching the injection site
c. Pregnancy for 2–3 months after the vaccination
d. Sexual intercourse for 2–3 months after the vaccination

Explanation: Pregnancy needs to be avoided for 1–3 months as Rubella is live vaccine which can give adverse effect on fetus. This vaccine is usually administered to the client who are IgG negative.

625. Perinatal Period corresponds to:
a. 28 weeks of gestation to 07 days after birth
b. Period of Labor to newborn period
c. Third trimester of pregnancy to newborn
d. 36 weeks of gestation to 3 days after birth

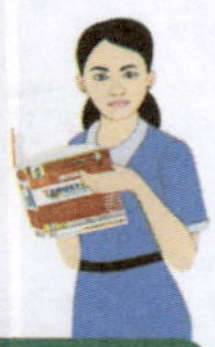

626. Several minutes after a vaginal delivery, nursing assessment reveals gush of blood from the client's vagina, umbilical cord lengthening, and a globular-shaped uterus. Nurse should suspect which condition?
a. Cervical or vaginal laceration
b. Placental separation
c. Postpartum hemorrhage
d. Uterine involution

Explanation: There is mainly 4 signs of placenta separation traditionally. The most reliable sign is the lengthening of the umbilical cord. The uterus takes on a more globular shape and becomes firmer. The uterus rises in the abdomen. The descent of the placenta into the lower segment, and finally into the vagina, displaces the uterus upward and gush of blood occurs.

627. All the following are signs of placental separation and descent; EXCEPT: *(AIIMS BBS NO 2018)*
a. Lengthening of cord
b. Fundus becoming rounder
c. Small fresh blood loss
d. Shortening of cord

Explanation: Lengthening of umbilical cord is a sign of placental separation. Shortening (option d) of cord is just opposite to this statement. So, shortening of cord is the correct answer.

- **Strategy**: Option A and option D are exactly opposite to each other. So any one out of these two is most probably the answer.

628. Mechanism behind placental separation is:
a. Reduction in surface area at the placental site
b. More uterine contraction
c. Increases in the surface area at the placental site
d. All of the above

629. Which among the following parameter needs to be monitored by the nurse following delivery in a woman with stable vital signs?
a. Intake and output
b. Pain level
c. Determine characteristics of lochia
d. Abdominal girth

630. Which of the following lochial findings is expected during the first 24 hours post-delivery?
a. Absence of lochia
b. A greenish discharge with foul odor
c. Bright red color
d. Large clots with lochia

Explanation: Color of the lochia in the first 24 hours is bright red color. Absence of lochia or foul odor indicates infection. Lochia should never contain tissue fragments, membranes or large clots.

631. Duration of puerperium is:
a. 3 weeks
b. 4 weeks
c. 5 weeks
d. 6 weeks

Explanation: Puerperium is the period following childbirth. It begins as soon as the placenta is expelled and lasts for approximately 6 weeks.

632. Lochia secreted following delivery in 1-4 days is known as:
a. Lochia rubra
b. Lochia serosa
c. Lochia alba
d. Leukorrhea

Explanation: Lochia is the vaginal discharge for the first fortnight during puerperium. Lochia rubra red in color (1–4 days), lochia serosa (5–9 days) yellowish, pink or pale brownish. Lochia alba pale white 10–15 days.

633. Reversal of genital organ to its original state is known as:
a. Involution
b. Sub involution
c. Retraction
d. Regression

Explanation: Involution refers to the shrinking or returning of an organ to a former size.

634. The main cause of venous thrombosis in puerperial women is: *(Safdarjung NO 2018)*
a. Increased viscosity of blood due to dehydration
b. Decreased viscosity of blood during labor
c. Stasis of blood in veins due to late ambulation
d. Increase intake of fat in diet

Explanation: Venous stasis in the lower limbs is caused by increased vein distensibility and the gravid uterus acting as a mechanical impediment to venous return. Hypercoagulability, venous stasis and vascular damage are a triad of initiating factors for venous thrombosis. In addition, there are increased levels of most of the circulating clotting factors in preparation for placental separation.

Ans.

622. a
623. d
624. c
625. a
626. b
627. d
628. a
629. c
630. c
631. d
632. a
633. a
634. c

635. Blood and debris discharge from the uterus after delivery is termed: *(DSSSB PHN, 2015)*
a. Septic shock
b. Lochia
c. Pyuria
d. Hematuria

636. The failure of uterus to return to its normal size is: *(DSSSB PHN, 2015)*
a. Involution b. Sub involution
c. Protrusion d. Retraction

637. If the uterus becomes boggy after one hour of delivery, the initial response of the midwife would be to:
a. Notify the physician
b. Check the blood pressure
c. Massage the uterus
d. Observe the amount of bleeding

638. Signs and symptoms of infection in postpartum period would include all the following; EXCEPT:
a. Foul smelling lochia
b. Rapid pulse
c. Generalized rash
d. Discomfort and tenderness of abdomen

639. A 34-year-old female at 38 weeks of gestation delivered a male baby by spontaneous vaginal delivery. What is the interval within which BP should be recorded for the first 2 hours post-delivery? New Q
a. Every 5 min b. Every 15 min
c. Every 30 min d. Every 1 hour

640. Puerperium starts with:
a. Expulsion of fetus
b. Expulsion of placenta
c. Initiation of breastfeeding
d. Onset of labor

641. During involution of uterus, lower uterine segment reverts back to the normal shape and size of the:
a. Cervix b. Isthmus
c. Vagina d. Internal os

642. Commonest cause of puerperal sepsis is:
a. Endometriosis
b. Endometritis
c. Endoparametritis
d. All of these

643. Kegel exercise is done to: *(AIIMS BBS NO 2018)*
a. Strengthening bladder muscle tone
b. Promote fluid intake
c. Prevent urinary infection
d. Assist in toileting

Explanation: Kegel exercise is usually done in the post-natal period for strengthening the pelvic floor and bladder muscle tone. Patient is told to empty the bladder first then to intentionally tighten the pelvic and gluteal muscles 5–10 times in a lying down posture.

644. On the first postpartum (PP) night, a patient requests that her baby be sent back to the nursery so she can get some sleep. The patient is most likely in which of the following phases? New Q
a. Depression phase
b. Letting-go phase
c. Taking-hold phase
d. Taking-in phase

Explanation: The taking-in phase is the first phase of the postpartum period. It typically lasts for 2-3 days. During this phase, the woman is focused on her own needs and recovery. She may be tired, overwhelmed, and need a lot of support. She may also be feeling emotional, and may cry easily.

It is common for women in the taking-in phase to ask for help with their baby. They may want their baby to be taken back to the nursery so they can get some sleep. This is a normal request, and it is important to respect the woman's wishes.

645. Management of atonic uterus include:
a. Massage the uterus b. Methergine
c. Oxytocin infusion d. All of these

646. Lochia is retained, this condition is termed: New Q
a. Lochia rubra b. Lochia Metra
c. Lochia serosa d. Lochia alba

647. Lochia rubra is ....in color.
a. Creamy white b. Pink
c. Red d. Yellowish

648. Following delivery, women are at risk for thrombosis because:
a. Increased blood volume
b. Venous stasis and lack of ambulation
c. Increased cardiac workload
d. Blood loss during delivery

649. Duration of lochia serosa is:
a. 1–4 days b. 2–4 days
c. 5–9 days d. 10–15 days

650. Which of the following interventions is important in postpartum nursing care to promote uterine involution and prevent excessive bleeding? New Q
a. Encouraging early ambulation
b. Administering analgesics for pain relief
c. Applying warm compresses to the perineum
d. Assisting with breastfeeding initiation

Explanation: Encouraging early ambulation is an important intervention in postpartum nursing care to promote uterine involution and prevent excessive bleeding. Early ambulation helps stimulate uterine contractions and aids in the process of the uterus returning to its prepregnancy size and position.

651. Which one of the following findings needs further evaluation and intervention during the first 24 hours of postpartum period?
a. Output exceeds the intake
b. Pulse below the baseline
c. Lochia with foul smell
d. Temperature is 38.6°C

652. Organ subjected to drastic change and stress immediately following delivery is:
a. Hematological b. Pulmonary
c. Musculoskeletal d. Gastrointestinal

653. When performing a postpartum assessment on a patient, a nurse notes the presence of clots in the lochia. The nurse examines the clots and notes that they are larger than 1 cm. Which of the following nursing actions is most appropriate? *(Safdarjung NO 2018)*
a. Document the findings
b. Notify the physician
c. Reassess the client in 2 hours
d. Encourage increased oral intake of fluids

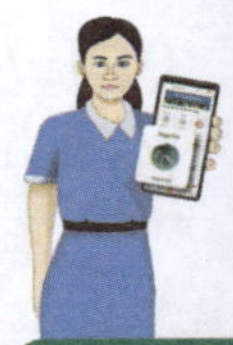

Ans.

635. b
636. b
637. c
638. c
639. b
640. b
641. b
642. b
643. a
644. d
645. d
646. b
647. c
648. b
649. c
650. a
651. c
652. b
653. b

Explanation: The presence of blood clots larger than 1 cm is indicative of hemorrhage, which needs to be notified to the physician/ gynecologist immediately.

654. Which among the following intervention will be helpful in preventing thrombophlebitis following delivery?
a. Elevate the foot end b. Early frequent ambulation
c. Wear elastic stockings d. ROM exercises

655. On 3rd postpartum day Seema noticed some blood stained discharge from the vagina of her newborn female baby. The best response from the nurse is:
a. Call the doctor immediately
b. Reassure the mother that it is a normal finding
c. Send blood sample of the newborn for coagulation studies
d. Assess the newborn for bleeding from other body parts

Explanation: It is a normal finding and is known as pseudo menstruation, it occurs because of the withdrawal of maternal hormones.

656. Which of the following is the most important nursing action when caring for a high risk postpartum client?
a. Psychological support
b. Promoting mother newborn contact
c. Postpartum exercises education
d. Discussing complication and treatment

Explanation: Promoting mother-newborn contact is crucial for all postpartum clients, including high-risk clients. It is essential for establishing bonding, facilitating breastfeeding, and promoting the overall well-being of both the mother and newborn. In addition, it can help to reduce stress and anxiety.

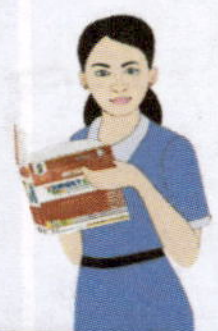

HYPEREMESIS GRAVIDARUM

657. Serial hCG titers is helpful to diagnose:
a. Carcinoma cervix b. Choriocarcinoma
c. Molar pregnancy d. Both b and c

658. Hormone responsible for hyperemesis gravidarum is: *(Staff Nurse G II 2014)*
a. Human chorionic gonadotropin
b. Human placental lactogen
c. Progesterone
d. Relaxin

659. Severe vomiting in pregnancy is known as: *(RRB Feb 2012)*
a. Nausea
b. Hyperemesis gravidarum
c. Morning sickness
d. None of the above

660. Persistent severe vomiting leading to weight loss and dehydration, as a condition occurring during pregnancy is known as:
a. Morning sickness
b. Nausea and vomiting
c. Hyperemesis gravidarum
d. All of the above

661. Most important cause of mortality in obstetrical anesthesia is:
a. Aspiration of vomitus b. Shock
c. Cardiac arrest d. Hypoglycemia

662. Which of the following conditions may lead to hypoglycemia in pregnant women with diabetes?
a. Weight gain b. Hyperemesis
c. Albuminuria d. All of these

HYDATIDIFORM MOLE

663. Hydatidiform mole is an abnormal condition affecting:
a. Amnion b. Chorion
c. Villi d. Blastomere

664. Which among the following can be seen in a partial mole? *(AIIMS Raipur Grade II 2017)*
a. Triploidy b. Haploidy
c. Polyploidy d. Diploidy

Explanation: Partial hydatidiform mole is a type of gestational trophoblastic disease which is characterized by its focal distribution, slower transformation, the presence of an embryo or fetus, and a triploid karyotype. The signs and symptoms of partial hydatidiform mole include abdominal pain, cramps in lower abdomen and vaginal bleeding during pregnancy. The uterus is large for gestational age and fetal heart beat is usually absent.

665. "Snowstorm" pattern on ultrasound with no fetus or gestational sac is the characteristic of:
a. Eclampsia b. Placenta previa
c. Abruption placenta d. Hydatidiform mole

Explanation: Above described ultrasound is the characteristic of hydatidiform mole. In this condition, a rare mass or growth that forms inside the womb (uterus) at the beginning of a pregnancy. It is a type of gestational trophoblastic disease (GTD). The chorionic villi of a molar pregnancy resemble a snowstorm pattern on ultrasound. Bleeding with a hydatidiform mole is often dark brown and may occur erratically for weeks or months.

666. Treatment of hydatidiform mole in a 40-year-old woman is:
a. Hysterotomy b. Hysterectomy
c. Suction evacuation d. Dilatation and Curettage

667. Clinical feature of hydatidiform mole is:
a. Snow storm appearance in USG
b. Elevated levels of hCG
c. Absence of fetal parts and FHS
d. All of the above

668. Gestational trophoblastic disease (GTD) is:
a. Melanoma b. Vesicular mole
c. Fibroid uterus d. Uterine dystocia

669. Molar pregnancy is usually treated by:
a. Antibiotics
b. Surgical suction and evacuation
c. Hysterectomy
d. Oxytocin

670. The most reliable diagnostic procedure for the diagnosis of molar pregnancy is:
a. Biopsy b. Urinary hCG
c. Ultrasound d. Tissue sampling

671. Complications of hydatidiform mole include:
a. Choriocarcinoma
b. Hemorrhage
c. Uterine perforation
d. All of the above

Ans.
654. b
655. b
656. b
657. d
658. a
659. b
660. c
661. a
662. b
663. b
664. a
665. d
666. b
667. d
668. b
669. b
670. c
671. d

672. Complications of hydatidiform mole is; EXCEPT:
a. Development of carcinoma
b. Ascites
c. Acute pulmonary insufficiency
d. Pregnancy Induced Hypertension

673. Trophoblastic tumor marker is:
a. hCG b. Estrogen
c. Progesterone d. FSH

MULTIPLE PREGNANCY

674. Characteristic of dizygotic pregnancy is:
a. Two amnions will be there
b. Sex may be different
c. Genetic features are different
d. All of the above

675. In a multiparous mother duration of third stage of labor is:
a. 10–15 minutes
b. 15–30 minutes
c. 30–45 minutes
d. 45–60 minutes

676. Grand multiparas are at risk for:
a. Malpresentation b. Macrosomia
c. Anemia d. All of these

677. Conjoined twins united in or near the thoracic region is termed as:
a. Thoracopagus b. Pyopagus
c. Craniopagus d. Ischiopagus

678. Conjoined twins united in or near the posterior region are termed:
a. Thoracopagus b. Pyopagus
c. Craniopagus d. Ischiopagus

Explanation:
Pyopagus: Conjoined twins united in or near the posterior region.
Craniopagus: Conjoined twins united in or near the cephalic region.
Ischiopagus: Conjoined twins united in or near the caudal region.

679. Complications of multiple gestation include:
a. Abortion
b. Congenital malformations
c. Low birth weight
d. All of the above

ECTOPIC PREGNANCY

680. Most common site of ectopic pregnancy is:
a. Tubal b. Ovarian
c. Abdominal d. Cervical

Explanation: Ectopic pregnancy is a condition in which fertilized ovum is implanted outside the normal endometrial cavity. Most common site is fallopian tube (97%), in the tubal pregnancy ampulla is the most common part (55%), followed by isthmus (25%), infundibulum (18%), and interstitial (2%). Ovarian ectopic pregnancy is (0. 5%), abdominal is 1%.

681. Which among the following is correct regarding ectopic pregnancy?
a. Risk for subsequent ectopic pregnancies are more
b. Chances of infertility will increase
c. High risk for STD
d. Use of intrauterine devices is contraindicated

682. Which among the following is not a feature of abdominal pregnancy? *New Q*
a. Absence of Braxton Hicks contraction
b. Uterine enlargement and change in consistency
c. Fetal parts and movements are easily palpable.
d. Persistent abnormal position and attitude.

683. In tubal pregnancy, the tube may rupture causing:
a. Sudden knife-like abdominal pain in lower quadrant
b. Painless vaginal bleeding
c. Continuous dull pain in lower abdomen
d. Intermittent abdominal contractions

684. Causes of tubal pregnancy include:
a. Contraceptive failure
b. Tubal surgery and previous tubal pregnancy
c. Pelvic Inflammatory Disease
d. All of the above

685. The most dependable method to diagnose ectopic pregnancy is:
a. Transabdominal ultrasound
b. Transvaginal ultrasound
c. Doppler ultrasound
d. hCG test

686. Which of the following conditions increases the risk of ectopic pregnancy?
a. Salpingitis
b. Uterine infections
c. Pelvic inflammatory disease
d. All of the above

687. Nursing care in a case of a ruptured ectopic pregnancy includes:
a. Monitor for presence and amount of vaginal bleeding
b. Monitor for abdominal distention
c. Monitor for hypovolemia
d. All of the above

688. Ectopic pregnancy is treated with:
a. Normal saline
b. Prostaglandins
c. Methotrexate
d. Oxytocin

689. Low progesterone level can be seen in:
a. Ectopic pregnancy b. Multiple gestation
c. APH d. PPH

ANTEPARTUM HEMORRHAGE

690. Commonest cause of bleeding at term is:
a. Abruptio placenta b. Placenta previa
c. PPH d. Atonic uterus

691. Which of the following is the most common cause of maternal mortality in India?
a. Obstetric hemorrhage b. Malnutrition
c. Anaemia d. Septicemia

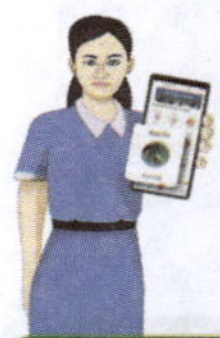

Ans.
672. b
673. a
674. d
675. a
676. d
677. a
678. b
679. d
680. a
681. a
682. b
683. a
684. d
685. b
686. d
687. d
688. c
689. a
690. a
691. a

692. Premature separation of the placenta from the uterine wall before delivery is: *(DSSSB PHN, 2015)*

a. Abruptio placenta b. Placenta previa
c. Fetal distress d. Cord prolapse

693. Identify the danger sign in the antepartum period:

a. Vaginal bleeding b. Blurred vision
c. Leaking amniotic fluid d. All of the above

Explanation: All the above mentioned are danger signs in ante partum period, other than this rapid increase in weight and high BP are also danger signs.

694. Bleeding from or into the genital tract after the 28th week of pregnancy but before the birth of the baby is known as:

a. APH b. IPH
c. IUD d. PPH

Explanation: The 28th week is taken arbitrarily as the lower limit of fetal viability. The main causes are placental bleeding, unexplained and extra placental.

695. In vasa previa, bleeding is likely to occur from:

a. Fetal blood vessels b. Placental site
c. Maternal blood vessels d. Marginal sinus

696. Abruptio placenta occurs in all; EXCEPT:

a. Smokers
b. Pregnancy Induced Hypertension
c. Gestational Diabetes Mellitus
d. Folic acid deficiency

697. Cerclage (encircling cervix with suture) is done for patients with: *(ESIC 2019)*

a. Complete abortion b. Threatened abortion
c. Incomplete abortion d. Incompetent cervix

Explanation: Cerclage (encircling cervix with suture) is done for patients with incompetent cervix. Incompetent cervix refers to impaired retentive power of the cervix (internal OS). Cerclage operation reinforces the weak cervix by a non-absorbable tape, placed around the cervix at the level of internal OS.

698. The purpose of maintaining the Foley catheter in the bladder after a hysterectomy, is to prevent:

a. Infection
b. Bladder distension
c. Stress incontinence
d. Hematuria

699. Which of the following is the disadvantage of using ring pessary for the management of genital prolapsed?

a. It causes dyspareunia
b. It causes vaginitis and ulceration
c. It does not cure stress incontinence
d. All of the above

ABNORMALITIES OF PLACENTA AND CORD

700. The safest position for a lady with cord prolapse in labor is: *(JIPMER 2012; LNJP H D 2012)*

a. Fowler's position b. Prone
c. Supine d. Trendelenburg

701. Placenta attached to lower segment and only the lower margin encroaches into lower uterine segment is known as:

a. Low-lying b. Marginal
c. Incomplete d. Central

702. Placenta previa in which placenta reaches the margin of internal os and not covering it is known as:

a. Low-lying b. Marginal
c. Incomplete d. Central

703. Placenta previa in which placenta partially covers the internal os is known as:

a. Low-lying b. Marginal
c. Incomplete d. Central

704. Placenta previa in which placenta completely covers the internal os is known as:

a. Low-lying b. Marginal
c. Incomplete d. Central

705. Type of placenta previa in which the placenta partially covers the os is:

a. Type I b. Type II
c. Type III d. Type IV

706. Type 1 placenta also known as:

a. Low-lying b. Marginal
c. Incomplete d. Central

707. Type 2 placenta also known as:

a. Low-lying b. Marginal
c. Incomplete d. Central

708. Type 3 placenta also known as:

a. Low-lying b. Marginal
c. Incomplete d. Central

709. Type 4 placenta also known as:

a. Low-lying b. Marginal
c. Incomplete d. Central

710. The term abruptio placenta refers to:

a. Premature delivery of placenta
b. Placenta covers the os partially or marginally
c. Premature separation of placenta after 28 weeks
d. Placenta having additional lobes

711. Cord prolapse seen less commonly in:

a. Complete breech b. Frank breech
c. Kneeling breech d. Footling breech

712. A drop in fetal heart rate that lasts less than 2 minutes and is usually associated with umbilical cord compression is known as:

a. Variable deceleration
b. Prolonged deceleration
c. Early deceleration
d. Late deceleration

713. Uterus with depression at the fundus is called: : *(AIIMS BPL NO 2018)*

a. Uterus didelphys
b. Arcuate uterus
c. Septate uterus
d. Bicornuate

Explanation: An arcuate uterus is characterized by a mild indentation of the endometrium at the uterine fundus. It occurs due to a failure of complete resorption of the uterovaginal septum, and is the most common Mullerian duct anomaly.

714. Cord prolapse is:

a. When umbilical cord comes out of the vagina after delivery
b. Lengthy cord visible first in the USG
c. Cord lying behind the fetus
d. Umbilical cord comes out of the uterus with or before the presenting part of the fetus

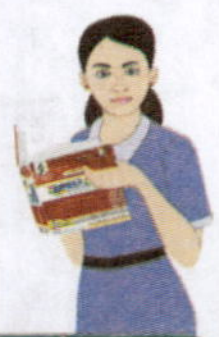

Ans.

692. a
693. d
694. a
695. a
696. c
697. d
698. b
699. d
700. d
701. a
702. b
703. c
704. d
705. c
706. a
707. b
708. c
709. d
710. c
711. b
712. a
713. b
714. d

715. The most appropriate position to place the patient if cord prolapse occurs and the fetus is visible:
a. Left lateral position b. Knee chest position
c. Elevated Sims' position d. Lithotomy position

716. A client with a prolapse uterus is scheduled for a vaginoplasty. Preoperatively the nurse may expect to:
a. Encourage ambulation b. Apply moist compress
c. Elevate the foot of the bed d. Manipulate the procidentia

717. The placenta is said to be retained when it is not expelled out within:
a. 15 minutes b. 30 minutes
c. 45 minutes d. 60 minutes

718. Abdominal hysterectomy is the only intervention to remove retained placenta in:
a. Type III placenta previa b. Type IV placenta previa
c. Placenta accreta d. Uterine inertia

719. The abnormal condition in which the umbilicus is inserted through the membranes of placenta is known as: *(AIIMS Bhopal Grade-I 2018)*
a. Succenturiate b. Battledore
c. Marginal d. Velamentous

Explanation: During pregnancy, normally the umbilical cord inserts into the middle of the placenta as it develops but in velamentous type, the umbilical cord inserts into the fetal membranes (chorioamniotic membranes) then travels within the membrane to the placenta.

720. The placental abnormalities in which, the accessory lobe is developed from the activated villi on the chorionic laeve is: *(AIIMS Raipur Grade II 2017)*
a. Placenta Succenturiata b. Placenta Spuria
c. Placenta extrachorialis d. Placenta marginata

721. The placental abnormalities in which, a thin fibrous ring is present at the margin of the chorionic plate where the fetal vessels appear to terminate is: *(AIIMS Raipur Grade II 2017)*
a. Circumvallate placenta b. Placenta membranacea
c. Placenta marginata d. Placenta spuria

Ref: D.C. Dutta. Textbook of Obstetrics

Explanation: Placenta succenturiata: One or more lobes of the placenta in the size of cotyledon may be placed at varying distance from main placenta margin. These cotyledons are connected to main placenta with small blood vessels. When a small piece of placenta is connected with the main placenta only by membrane without any blood vessel, it is called placenta spuria.

Placenta extrachorialis: Divided into two conditions:
- **Circumvallate placenta:** Fetal surface is divided into central depressed zone surrounded by thickened white ring which is usually complete. Ring is situated at varying distance from margin of placenta. Ring is composed of double folded amnion and chorion.
- **Placenta marginata:** A thin fibrous ring is present at the margin of chorionic plate where the fetal vessels appear to terminate.
- **Placenta membraneous:** Placenta is large and thin and is developed not only from chorionic frondosum but also from chorion laeve. So the wall of ovum is covered by placenta.

722. Premature separation of a normally implanted placenta during the second half of pregnancy, usually with severe hemorrhage is known as: *(DSSSB 2013, Kerala PSC 2014)*
a. Placenta previa b. Ectopic pregnancy
c. Incompetent cervix d. Abruptio placenta

Explanation: Abruptio placenta is defined as the premature separation of the placenta from the uterus. Patients with abruptio placenta, also called placental abruption, typically present with bleeding, uterine contractions, and fetal distress.

723. In which condition, the umbilical cord is attached to the margins of placenta?
a. Battledore placenta b. Circumvallate placenta
c. Placenta membranacea d. Velamentous placenta

Explanation: The given definition refers to battledore placenta. In velamentous placenta, code is inserted into fetal membrane outside the placental margin.

724. One or more lobes of the placenta placed at varying distance from the main placental region is known as:
a. Placenta succenturiata b. Placenta extrachorialis
c. Placenta membranacea d. Battledore placenta

Explanation: Option A is the correct answer. Placenta extrachorialis is of two types (i) circumvallate placenta and (ii) placenta marginata. circumvallate placenta means due to smaller chorionic plate than the basal plate recurrent marginal hemorrhage will occur, and placenta marginata means thin fibrous ring present at the margin of the chorionic plate. Placenta membranacea means placenta is unduly thin and large. Battledore placenta is an abnormality of the cord in which cord is attached to the margin of the placenta.

725. What is velamentous placenta?
a. Fibrous ring present at the margin of placenta
b. Placenta is thin and large
c. Cord is attached to the membranes
d. Cord is attached to the margin of the placenta

Explanation: Option C is the correct answer. Option A is placenta marginata, option B is Placenta membranacea. Option D is battledore placenta.

726. Acordia is:
a. Absence of cord b. Lengthy cord
c. Short cord d. Twisted cord

Explanation: Option A is the correct answer, lengthy cord means abnormal increase in the length of cord and it can be as long as 300 cm. Lengthy cord causes cord prolapse and cord entanglement around the neck. Short cord means cord length less than 20 cm.

727. Morbidly adherent placenta is called as: *(Staff Nurse G II 2014)*
a. Battledore placenta b. Placenta accreta
c. Placenta succenturiata d. Placenta circumvallate

728. Gelatinous substance in the umbilical cord is known as:
a. Wharton's jelly b. True knot
c. False knot d. Vernix caseosa

729. Reason behind false knot in umbilical cord is:
a. Accumulation of Wharton's jelly
b. Accumulation of amniotic fluid
c. Accumulation of blood
d. Dilation of umbilical blood vessels

730. Omphalitis is:
a. Abdominal sepsis b. Placental sepsis
c. Peritoneal sepsis d. Umbilical sepsis

731. Short cord is if the length of the umbilical cord is less than:
a. 10 cm b. 20 cm
c. 30 cm d. 40 cm

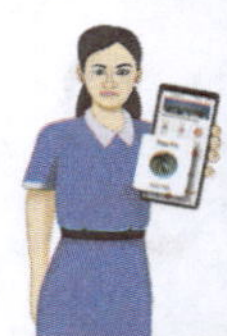

Ans.
715. b
716. b
717. b
718. c
719. d
720. a
721. c
722. d
723. a
724. a
725. c
726. a
727. b
728. a
729. a
730. d
731. b

732. Complications of long umbilical cord include:
a. Cord prolapse b. Cord entanglement
c. Fetal distress d. All of these

733. Most commonly single umbilical artery is seen in:
a. Abruptio placenta b. Placenta previa
c. Multiple births d. Battledore placentae

734. Which of the following clinical presentations would a nurse expect while assessing a patient with abruptio placenta?
a. Rigid, board-like abdomen *(AIIMS Bhopal Grade-I 2018)*
b. Edema in legs
c. Excessive vaginal bleeding
d. Premature rupture of membranes

Explanation: Placental abruption is the premature separation of a normally located placenta from the uterine wall that occurs before delivery of the fetus characterized by excessive vaginal bleeding, uterine tenderness, rapid contractions, abdominal pain and fetal heart rate abnormalities.

735. A client with abruptio placenta is at a risk for developing:
a. Thalassemia
b. Idiopathic thrombocytopenic purpura (ITP)
c. Disseminated intravascular coagulation (DIC)
d. All of the above

736. All the below statements are correct regarding abruptio placenta; EXCEPT:
a. Placenta is in upper segment of the uterus
b. Always revealed bleeding is there
c. Bleeding is dark red in color
d. Painful bleeding is present

Explanation: Option B is related to placenta previa. In abruption placenta, bleeding can be revealed or concealed type.

737. A client arrives at the hospital at 38 weeks of gestation with profuse vaginal bleeding. She states that it occurred suddenly without any contractions. Which condition may the client be experiencing that may require immediate attention? **New Q**
a. Placenta previa b. Abruptio placenta
c. Ruptures uterus d. Concealed abruptio

Explanation: Placenta previa is a condition in which the placenta partially or completely covers the cervix. It can cause painless vaginal bleeding, especially in the third trimester of pregnancy. The bleeding in placenta previa is often bright red and can be sudden and profuse. It is important to note that placenta previa usually does not cause significant pain or contractions.

Abruptio placenta, on the other hand, is the premature separation of the placenta from the uterine wall. It can also result in sudden and severe vaginal bleeding, which is typically dark red and accompanied by abdominal pain or uterine contractions.

The KEYWORD in stem is 'without any contractions', which leads to the answer Placenta Previa.

738. Death of mother in abruptio placenta occurs due to:
a. Infection b. Toxemia
c. Hemorrahage d. Thrombophlebitis

739. The painful vaginal bleeding during the last trimester is caused by:
a. Abruptio placenta b. Frequent intercourse
c. Placenta previa d. Over distension of uterus

740. Obstetrical emergencies include all; EXCEPT:
(LNJP H D 2012)
a. Ectopic pregnancy b. Eclampsia
c. Placenta anterior d. Placenta previa

741. When the placenta lies over the lower uterine segment it is known as:
a. Abruptio placenta
b. Placenta previa
c. Battledore placenta
d. Velamentous placenta

742. Risk factors for placenta previa include:
a. Smoking
b. Placental size
c. Multiparity
d. All of these

743. Clinical feature of placenta previa is/are:
a. Bleeding is always revealed
b. Bright red in color
c. F.H.S. usually present
d. All of the above

744. In placenta previa, vaginal examination should not be done to avoid:
a. Infection
b. Hemorrhage
c. Discomfort
d. Precipitate labor

745. USG of a pregnant women with placenta previa shows that placenta reaches the margin of internal os and is not covering it. The degree of placenta previa is:
a. Low lying
b. Marginal
c. Incomplete
d. Total

Explanation: Option B is the correct answer. In low lying (type 1), major portion of the placenta is in the upper segment and only the lower margin comes into lower segment and is not up to internal os.

Incomplete (type 3 or partial central) Placenta covers the internal os partially.

Total (central or type 4) placenta completely covers the internal os.

746. Which of the following is the usual treatment for partial placenta previa?
a. Heparin therapy
b. Induction of labor with oxytocin
c. Activity limited to bed rest
d. Blood transfusion

Explanation: Activity limited to bed rest, hydration, and careful monitoring of the client's bleeding are the recommended treatment for a client with partial placenta previa.

747. Definitive treatment for grade III placenta previa is:
a. Vacuum delivery b. Blood transfusion
c. Steroid therapy d. Cesarean section

748. Definitive treatment of placenta previa includes:
(RAK MSc 2018)
a. Bed rest b. Supplementary hematinics
c. Use of tocolytics d. Cesarean section

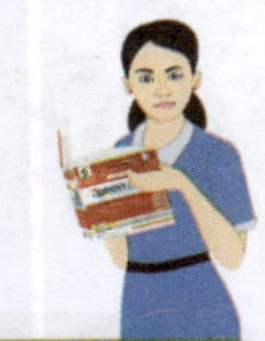

Ans.

732. d
733. c
734. c
735. c
736. b
737. a
738. c
739. a
740. c
741. b
742. d
743. d
744. b
745. b
746. c
747. d
748. d

Explanation:

- Cesarean section is the definitive management for most of the mothers diagnosed with placenta previa.
- Other management strategies in case of placenta previa are as follows:
    - Bed rest to minimize movements of mother
    - Supplementary hematinics are administered to supplement against blood loss.
    - Blood transfusion in case of anemia
    - Use of tocolytics to delay preterm labor
    - Use of cervical cerclage to reduce bleeding
    - Rh immunoglobulin in case of Rh-negative mother.

749. Which of the following is the most important predisposing factor of abruptio placenta?

a. Hypertension in pregnancy
b. Uterine inertia
c. Malnutrition
d. Cephalopelvic disproportion

750. Clinical features of abruptio placenta is:

a. Dark-colored bleeding
b. FHS usually absent
c. Revealed, concealed or mixed type
d. All of the above

751. Cause of fetal death in abruption placenta is:

a. Hypoxia
b. Anoxia
c. Cord tightening
d. Hemorrhage

AMNIOTIC FLUID DISORDERS

752. Which of the following conditions is most likely to cause dyspnea on exertion in a pregnant woman?

a. Abruptio placenta b. Placenta Previa
c. Eclampsia d. Polyhydramnios

753. For ultrasound diagnosis of chronic polyhydramnios, the amniotic fluid index should be:

a. >8 cm b. ≥15 cm
c. ≥18 cm d. >25 cm

754. A woman with 36-week pregnancy is admitted with a diagnosis of polyhydramnios induced respiratory distress. Which of the following is the preferred treatment choice for this client?

a. Use of diuretics
b. Amniocentesis
c. Complete bed rest
d. Artificial rupture of membrane

755. Which of the following is the drug of choice to reduce polyhydramnios?

a. Misoprostol
b. Mifepristone
c. Indomethacin
d. Methergin

756. Polyhydramnios is associated with all of the following conditions; EXCEPT:

a. Esophageal atresia
b. Maternal diabetes
c. Multiple pregnancy
d. Bilateral renal agenesis

ABORTION

757. Modes of induction of mid trimester abortion; EXCEPT:

a. Intra amniotic saline infusion
b. Intra amniotic prostaglandin infusion
c. Menstrual regulation
d. Hysterotomy

758. When are the chances of acute endometritis developing in a woman? *(RRB SSNE 2015)*

a. After menopause
b. After menarche
c. After abortion or childbirth
d. In childhood

759. The safest medical method of termination of pregnancy before 12 weeks is: *(LNJP H D 2012)*

a. Laminaria tent
b. Prostaglandins
c. Suction evacuation
d. Dilation and curettage

760. Abortion is the termination of pregnancy before ...... weeks of pregnancy. *(RRB Feb 2012)*

a. 16th b. 12th
c. 10th d. 24th

761. Abortions during second trimester of pregnancy mainly occur due to:

a. Congenital anomalies of fetus
b. Hormonal deficiency in mother
c. Congenital anomalies of the uterus
d. Malnutrition

762. Which of the following is the method of termination of pregnancy in the second trimester (13 to 20 weeks)? *(AIIMS BPL SNO 2018)*

a. Oxytocin infusion b. Methotrexate
c. Vacuum aspiration d. Mifepristone

Explanation: Oxytocin intravenous infusion is the most successful method to terminate pregnancy in second trimester. The process is achieved as mini labor in second trimester. Oxytocin helps to induce contractions.

Vacuum aspiration, Methotrexate, misoprostol and mifepristone are used for medical abortion up to 12 weeks.

763. A clinical entity where the process of abortion has started but has not progressed to a state from which recovery is impossible is: *(AIIMS Raipur Grade II 2017)*

a. Spontaneous abortion b. Threatened abortion
c. Inevitable abortion d. Missed abortion

Explanation: Spontaneous abortion is non-induced embryonic or fetal death or passage of products of conception before 20 weeks of gestation. Inevitable abortion is characterized by rupture of membranes or cervical dilatation in a previable pregnancy in the presence of vaginal bleeding and contractions. A missed abortion is a miscarriage in which fetus didn't develop or has died but placenta and embryonic tissues are still in uterus.

764. The inevitable abortion distinguished from threatened abortion by:

a. Dilatation of cervical canal
b. Rupture of the membrane
c. Bleeding
d. Uterine contraction

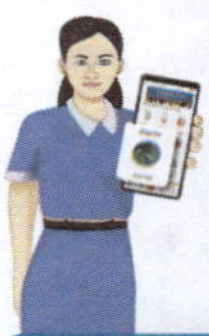

Ans.

749. a
750. d
751. a
752. d
753. d
754. b
755. c
756. d
757. c
758. c
759. b
760. d
761. c
762. a
763. b
764. a

765. A state of miscarriage in which product of conception is retained inside the uterus for a variable period of time is known as: *(AIIMS Raipur Grade II 2017)*

a. Complete abortion b. Incomplete abortion
c. Missed abortion d. Recurrent absorption

Explanation: Complete abortion is one in which all contents are expelled. Incomplete abortion is one in which entire product of conception are not expelled, instead a part of it is left inside the uterine cavity. Recurrent abortion/habitual abortion/recurrent pregnancy loss is three or more consecutive pregnancy losses.

766. Missed abortion is also known as:

a. Complete abortion b. Inevitable abortion
c. Silent miscarriage d. Septic abortion

Explanation: When the fetus is dead and retained inside the uterus for a variable period it is called missed abortion or silent abortion/ early fetal demise.

767. A state of miscarriage in which process has started and progressed to a stage from which continuation of pregnancy is not possible is known as:

a. Missed abortion b. Threatened abortion
c. Inevitable abortion d. Complete abortion

768. Mrs X with 8 weeks of gestation has come to the emergency department with moderate bright red vaginal bleeding. On per-vaginal examination, her cervix is 2 cm dilated. Which of the following terms best describes Mrs X's condition?

a. Incompetent cervix b. Inevitable abortion
c. Threatened abortion d. Missed Abortion

769. A state of miscarriage in which product of conception is completely expelled is known as:

a. Missed abortion b. Threatened abortion
c. Inevitable abortion d. Complete abortion

770. A woman with 20 weeks pregnancy presents with bleeding per vaginum. On speculum examination, the os is open but no products have come out. On P/A examination, uterus size corresponds to 20 weeks. The diagnosis is: *New Q*

a. Missed abortion b. Incomplete abortion
c. Inevitable abortion d. Complete abortion

771. Majority of total abortions occur during:

a. First trimester b. Second trimester
c. Third trimester d. Fourth trimester

772. Signs of inevitable abortion include:

a. Increased vaginal bleeding
b. Aggravation of pain in the lower abdomen
c. Dilated internal os
d. All of the above

773. Signs and symptoms of complete abortion include:

a. Uterus is smaller than the period of amenorrhea
b. Subsidence of abdominal pain and vaginal bleeding
c. Cervical os is closed
d. All of the above

774. A client tells a nurse in prenatal clinic that she has vaginal staining but no pain. Her menstrual history reveals amenorrhea for last two months and pregnancy confirmation after her missed period. On examination, os is closed and uterus corresponds to an 8-week size. Nurse suspects spontaneous abortion. What type of abortion should be suspected in this case? *New Q*

a. Missed b. Threatened
c. Inevitable d. Incomplete

Explanation: A threatened abortion is a pregnancy that is at risk of ending in miscarriage, but the cervix is still closed and the pregnancy tissue has not yet begun to pass. The woman may experience vaginal bleeding, but she may not have any pain.

In the case described, the client has vaginal staining but no pain. Her menstrual history reveals amenorrhea for the last two months and pregnancy confirmation after her missed period. On examination, the os is closed and the uterus corresponds to an 8-week size. These findings are consistent with a threatened abortion.

775. The most common cause of abortion in first trimester:

a. Chromosomal abnormality
b. Trauma
c. Maternal disease
d. RTI

776. ____________ is the most common cause of septic abortion.

a. Pelvic Inflammatory disease
b. Surgical abortion
c. Illegal abortion
d. Sexually Transmitted diseases

777. The most common reason for wilful abortion is:

a. Congenital anomalies in Fetus
b. Birth control
c. Maternal infections
d. Pregnancy as a result of rape

778. Sign of septic abortion includes:

a. Hematuria
b. Polyuria
c. Tenderness of the abdomen
d. All of the above

779. Commonest chromosomal abnormality in early spontaneous abortion is:

a. Monosomy b. Autosomal trisomy
c. Triploidy d. Tetraplody

780. Most appropriate method for abortion in the first trimester of pregnancy is:

a. Mifepristone and Misoprostol
b. Prostaglandin
c. Intrauterine instillation of hypertonic saline
d. Vacuum aspiration

Explanation: In the first trimester, Mifepristone and Misoprostol are the appropriate methods. Prostaglandin, intrauterine instillation of hypertonic saline and vacuum aspirations are preferred in the later trimester.

781. Midterm abortions are commonly due to:

a. Cervical incompetence b. Cervical erosion
c. Cervical laceration d. Cervical infections

782. Complications of abortion include:

a. Infection b. Risk of heavy bleeding
c. Cervical laceration d. All of these

MEDICAL TERMINATION OF PREGNANCY (MTP)

783. In which year, Medical Termination of Pregnancy Act was enacted by the Indian Parliament?

a. 1970 b. 1971
c. 1972 d. 1975

Ans.

765. c
766. c
767. c
768. b
769. d
770. c
771. a
772. d
773. d
774. b
775. a
776. c
777. b
778. c
779. b
780. a
781. a
782. d
783. b

784. The Medical Termination of Pregnancy act came into force in the year: *(Safdarjung NO 2018)*

a. 1964 b. 1962
c. 1972 d. 1966

Explanation: The Medical Termination of Pregnancy Act was enacted by the Indian Parliament in 1971 and came into force from 1 April 1972. The MTP ACT was again revised in 1975. The MTP Act lays down the condition under which a pregnancy can be terminated, the persons and the place to perform it.

785. Indication for termination under MTP ACT is:

a. To save the life of mother
b. Social indication
c. Eugenic
d. All of the above

Explanation: All the above mentioned are the indications for termination of pregnancy under MTP ACT. To save mother means if the continuation of pregnancy causes serious or life threatening complications to mother. Social indication means to prevent grave injury to the physical and mental health of pregnant women. Eugenic means when there is a risk the child will born with serious physical and mental abnormality.

786. MTP methods adopted in first trimester of pregnancy include:

a. Mifepristone and misoprostol
b. Manual vacuum aspiration
c. Dilatation and evacuation
d. All of the above

CONTRACEPTIVE METHODS

787. IUD needs to be removed if .... complication occurs.

a. Excessive bleeding b. Uterine perforation
c. Planning for pregnancy d. All of these

788. Which of the following is a third generation intrauterine device?

a. CuT b. TCu-300
c. TCu-380A d. Progestasert

Explanation: Progestasert is a T-shaped IUD made of ethylene and vinyl acetate copolymer containing titanium dioxide. The vertical stem contains a reservoir of 38 mg progesterone together with barium sulfate dispersed in silicone fluid. The progesterone is released at the rate of 65 µg/day.

789. A couple with one child had been trying, without success for several years to have another child. The following terms would describe the situation:

a. Primary infertility b. Secondary infertility
c. Irreversible infertility d. Sterility

790. Absolute inability to conceive for one or more reason implies: *(AIIMS Bhopal Nursing Officer, 2018)*

a. Sterility b. Fertility
c. Infertility d. Impotence

Explanation: Infertility is the inability to conceive for one or more reason. Sterility means asepsis, free from microorganism. Fertility means potential for reproduction. Impotence means inability to sustain an erection sufficient for sexual intercourse.

791. The index for finding effectiveness of contraception is: *(AIIMS Bhopal Grade-I 2018)*

a. Pearl b. Ponderal
c. Lorentz d. Broca

Explanation: Contraceptive efficacy was measured by the pearl index. Pearl index measures the number of pregnancies that occurs for each contraceptive method if used by 100 women for one year (where a women year is defined as 13 menstrual cycles).

792. Identify the natural method of contraception among the following:

a. Rhythm method b. Coitus interruptus
c. Breastfeeding d. All of these

Explanation: All the above mentioned methods are natural contraceptive methods, temporary methods include condom, intra-uterine devices and steroidal contraception. Permanent methods include vasectomy in male and tubectomy in female.

793. Mini lap is a procedure related to:

a. Family Planning b. Cervical cancer
c. Cesarean section d. Normal labor

Explanation: Mini lap is a procedure related to family planning. In this OPD basis tubectomy will be performed.

794. Identify the emergency contraceptive among the following: *(CGHS 2010)*

a. Prostaglandin b. Progesterone only
c. Mala-D d. Levonorgestrel

Explanation: Levonorgestrel is used as an emergency contraceptive.

795. During suction evacuation in MTP the negative pressure of suction should be:

a. 100–200 mm Hg b. 200–300 mm Hg
c. 400–600 mm Hg d. 700–900 mm Hg

796. All of the following are natural method of birth control; EXCEPT:

a. Coitus interruptus b. Breastfeeding
c. Vasectomy d. Safe period

797. Which of the following is a permanent contraceptive method?

a. Condom b. OCP
c. Tubectomy d. IUD

798. A mother with 9-month baby is planning for tubectomy. What is the ideal time for surgery following menstruation? *(Daman & Diu NO 2018)*

a. Secretory phase
b. Ovulatory phase
c. Menstrual phase
d. Proliferative phase

Explanation: The ideal time for tubectomy is during the Proliferative phase during which the endometrial thickness is about 2–3 mm.

799. Characteristics of a good contraceptive method include all of the following; EXCEPT:

a. It should be effective
b. It should be safe and cost-effective
c. Irreversible
d. No or minimal side effects

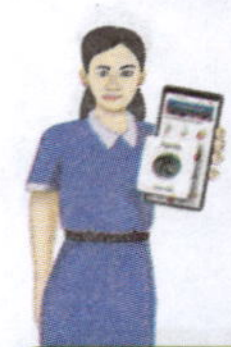

Ans.

784. c
785. d
786. d
787. d
788. d
789. b
790. c
791. a
792. d
793. a
794. d
795. c
796. c
797. c
798. d
799. c

800. Which of the following is a non-surgical method of contraception?
a. Vasectomy b. Tubectomy
c. Copper-T d. Tubal ligation

801. Exclusive breastfeeding can be a contraceptive method for a period of:
a. 1 month b. 3 months
c. 6 months d. 9 months

802. CU-T 380 the number 380 represents:
a. Duration of device
b. Surface area of copper
c. Can be used for 380 intercourse
d. This device was discovered by 380 persons

803. Which IUCD needs to be replaced only after 10 years?:
a. Copper 'T' 200 b. Progestasert *(NCFL 2019)*
c. Cu-'T'380 A d. 'T' Nova 'T'

Explanation:

IUDs	To be replaced in
Cu T 200	4 years
Cu T 380 A	10 years
Multiload Cu 250	3 years
Multiload 375	5 years
Levonorgestrel intrauterine system	7 years

804. Oral contraceptive pills need to be started on:
a. 1st day of menstruation
b. 3rd day of menstruation
c. 5th day of menstruation
d. 7th day of menstruation

805. Absolute contraindication for the use of oral contraceptive pill is:
a. Hypertension
b. Ischemic heart disease
c. Undiagnosed genital tract bleeding
d. All of the above

806. Other than contraception OCP is useful for:
a. Menorrhagia
b. Dysfunctional uterine bleeding
c. Pelvic inflammatory disease
d. All of the above

807. The action of spermicidal agent is to:
a. Prevent the motility of the sperm
b. Kill sperm immediately
c. Render the sperm inactive
d. Prevent sperm from sticking to the uterine wall

808. The contraceptive method advised in clients with molar pregnancy is:
a. Oral contraceptives
b. Barrier method
c. Intrauterine device
d. Norplant

809. All of the following are contraindications for combined oral contraceptive pills; EXCEPT:
a. Diabetes mellitus
b. Previous history of stroke
c. Previous history of thromboembolism
d. Peripheral vascular disease

810. The following contraceptive method would be avoided for a woman who is 38 years old, has 3 children and smokes a pack of cigarette per day is:
a. Cervical cap
b. Diaphragm
c. IUD (Intrauterine device)
d. Oral contraceptives

811. The composition of Mala-N used for spacing pregnancy is:
a. Norgestrel b. Ethinyl estradiol
c. Desogestrel d. Gestodene

812. The dose (in mg) of levonorgestrel and ethinyl estradiol in Mala N is:
a. 0.15 and 0.03 b. 0.8 and 0.03
c. 3.5 and 3.0 d. 3.0 and 3.0

813. Correct regarding the use of vaginal diaphragm is:
a. Introduce it just before ejaculation and remove it after ejaculation
b. Addition of spermicidal jelly has no proved effect on its effectiveness
c. It should be introduced up to 3 hours before intercourse and is to be kept for at least 6 hours after the coital act
d. It should be introduced up to 3 hours before intercourse and should be removed immediately after ejaculation

814. Best method of contraception in a nulliparous woman is:
a. Barrier method b. Rhythm method
c. Intrauterine devices d. Combined oral pills

815. Emergency contraception prevents pregnancy by all of the following mechanisms; EXCEPT:
a. Delaying/inhibiting ovulation
b. Inhibiting fertilization
c. Interrupting an early pregnancy
d. Preventing implantation of the fertilized egg

816. The optimum time to insert intrauterine device is:
a. Prior to menstruation
b. During secretory phase of menstrual cycle
c. Midway to menstruation
d. During menses

817. Hormone replacement therapy after menopause is contra-indicated in:
a. Asthma
b. Diabetes
c. Clients at risk of stroke and thromboembolism
d. Osteoporosis

818. Intrauterine insemination is a treatment of choice for:
a. Cervical stenosis b. Hypospadias
c. Asthenospermia d. All of these

819. The amount of semen usually injected in artificial insemination is:
a. 0.1 mL b. 0.2 mL
c. 0.3 mL d. 0.4 mL

820. Commonly used diagnostic test for infertility among females is:
a. Ultrasonography b. Hysterosalpingogram
c. Pap smear d. Postcoital studies

821. Which among the following contraceptives is associated with lowest risk of transmitting sexually transmitted disease in women?
a. Copper T
b. Condom
c. Injectable hormonal supplements
d. Oral contraceptives

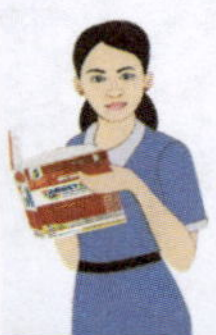

Ans.

800. c
801. c
802. b
803. c
804. a
805. d
806. d
807. b
808. a
809. a
810. d
811. b
812. a
813. c
814. d
815. a
816. d
817. c
818. d
819. c
820. b
821. b

822. The main nursing diagnosis for a 35-year-old female client who has undergone a total vaginectomy is:

a. Social isolation
b. Altered body image
c. Sexual dysfunction
d. Altered coping

Rh INCOMPATIBILITY

823. After determining that a pregnant client is Rh-negative, Gynecologist orders an indirect Coombs' test. What is the purpose of performing this test in a pregnant client? *(RAK MSC 2018)*

a. To determine the fetal blood Rh factor
b. To determine the maternal blood Rh factor
c. To detect maternal antibodies against fetal Rh-negative factor
d. To detect maternal antibodies against fetal Rh-positive factor

Explanation: Pregnant women get a prenatal antibody screening with an indirect Coombs test. It tests the mother's blood to see if there are Anti D antibodies that could pass to and harm her unborn baby. Women who are Rh D negative with a positive anti D antibody screen test are considered Rh alloimmunized.

824. Delayed cord clamping is contraindicated in: New Q

a. Baby born to anemic mother
b. Baby with birthweight >3 kg
c. Rh-incompatibility
d. Preterm baby

Explanation: Rh-incompatibility is the contraindication for delayed cord clamping in order to prevent antibody transfer from mother to fetus.

The other options are not contraindicated for delayed cord clamping.

- **Baby born to anemic mother:** The extra blood from the placenta can help to improve the baby's iron stores.
- **Baby with birthweight >3 kg:** There is no evidence that delayed cord clamping is harmful to babies with birthweights over 3 kg. It may be beneficial for these babies as well.
- **Preterm baby:** Delayed cord clamping is also beneficial for preterm babies. It can help to improve the baby's iron stores and reduce the risk of jaundice.

825. Gravida 2 mother with O negative blood whose husband's blood group is B positive comes to ANC clinic. Which among the following question is most appropriate for the nurse to ask?

a. How many ANC visits you had?
b. What is your LMP?
c. Have you got Anti-D injection during last delivery?
d. What is the age of your first child?

Explanation: This mother is at risk for developing Rh incompatibility, so question related to previous Rh injection during the last delivery is appropriate. Usually RhoGAM injection needs to be given in the ANC period or 72 hours following the delivery.

826. Rh-isoimmunization is given to an Rh-negative pregnant woman if:

a. The first baby born is Rh-negative
b. The husband is Rh-positive
c. The husband is Rh-negative
d. All of the above

827. Rh Negative mother should receive __ globulin. *(ESIC 2019)*

a. RhO (M) globulin
b. RhO (D) immunoglobulin
c. Lecithin/Sphingomyelin
d. Acetylcholinesterase

Explanation: Rh negative mother should receive RhO (D) immunoglobulin. The mother who is Rh negative and baby is Rh positive then the mother should receive Anti D immunoglobin intramuscularly, 300 mcg, within 72 hours of childbirth.

828. Which of the following doses of Rh immunoglobulin RhoGAM is appropriate for a pregnant client at 28 weeks of gestation? *(RAK MSc 2018)*

a. 0.6 mcg in a sensitized client
b. 50 mcg in an unsensitized client
c. 30 mcg in a sensitized client
d. 300 mcg in an unsensitized client

Explanation: A pregnant, Rh unsensitized woman should be administered 300 mcg of RhoGAM at 28 weeks of gestation after indirect Coomb's test. 50 mcg of RhoGAM is usually given after first semester abortion.

829. The following are the complications of Rh isoimmunization; EXCEPT:

a. Hydrops fetalis
b. Kernicterus
c. Anemia
d. Post maturity

830. Blood of choice for exchange transfusion in newborn is:

a. Rh negative blood of same group of baby
b. O negative
c. Both a and b
d. Same blood group of that newborn

Explanation: Rh negative of same blood group is recommended if it is not available then O negative blood should be given.

GESTATIONAL DIABETES MELLITUS (GDM)

831. Hazard associated with gestational diabetes is:

a. Polyhydroamniosis
b. Macrosomia
c. Birth trauma
d. All of these

832. The reason for the development of polyhydroamniosis in a woman with gestational diabetes is:

a. Absence of swallowing reflex in fetus
b. Fetal diuresis
c. Increased transudation
d. Hyperplasia of blood vessels

833. Ketoacidosis occurs due to the deficient intake of:

a. Carbohydrates
b. Protein
c. Fat
d. Minerals

834. After the delivery insulin requirement of a diabetic mother will:

a. Decrease significantly
b. Increase significantly
c. No alteration
d. Insulin can be withdrawn

Explanation: During the delivery process most of the glucose will be consumed as part of metabolism for energy production which significantly reduces the insulin requirement in postpartum period.

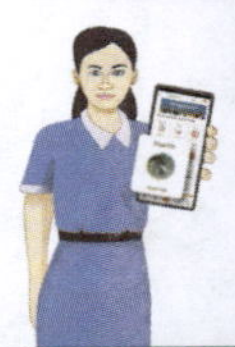

Ans.

822. c
823. d
824. c
825. c
826. b
827. b
828. d
829. d
830. c
831. d
832. b
833. a
834. a

835. Which of the following risk factors is associated with an increased likelihood of developing gestational diabetes mellitus (GDM)? *New Q*

a. Being underweight before pregnancy
b. Having a family history of asthma
c. Being over 35 years of age
d. Having a history of seasonal allergies

Explanation: There are a number of risk factors for GDM, including:
- Being over 35 years of age
- Being overweight or obese
- Having a family history of diabetes
- Having had GDM in a previous pregnancy

836. Maternity Nurse, must be aware that screening for diabetes mellitus in pregnancy is done at: *(NCFL 2019)*

a. 6–17 weeks b. 18–23 weeks
c. 24–28 weeks d. 29–32 weeks

Explanation: Guidelines of American Diabetes Association state that, formal Diabetes testing should be done at 24–28 weeks of gestation. Standard Glucose Tolerance Test (GTT) is done after the overnight fasting (8–14 hours).

837. Which is the most difficult time to control diabetes during maternity cycle?

a. First trimester
b. Second trimester
c. Third trimester
d. Labor & delivery

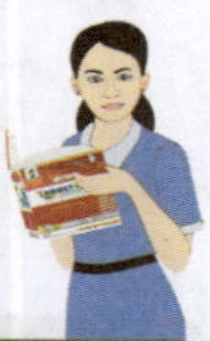

838. At 28 weeks of gestation, a woman is at risk for diabetes as a result of:

a. Increasing human placental lactogen
b. Increasing choriogonadotropin
c. Increasing human somatotropin
d. Decreasing fetal insulin

839. Which of the following is not one of the causes of intrauterine growth retardation?

a. Leucocytosis
b. Pregnancy induced hypertension
c. Gestational diabetes
d. Maternal heart disease

840. Hypoglycemia in a baby of diabetic mother is because of: *(RRB Feb 2012)*

a. Decreased glucagon b. Increased glucagon
c. Increased insulin d. None of these

841. Maternal ketosis is due to deficient intake of:

a. Protein b. Carbohydrate
c. Fat d. Salt

PREELCAMPSIA AND ECLAMPSIA

842. Occurrence of seizures during pregnancy is termed: *(DSSSB PHN, 2015)*

a. Eclampsia b. Preeclampsia
c. Epilepticus d. Myoclonus

843. Hypertensive disorder of pregnancy is: *(RRB Feb 2012)*

a. Stage II HTN
b. Prehypertension
c. Eclampsia
d. None of these

844. A primipara, aged 40 years is hospitalized for severe pregnancy induced hypertension. What can be the first nursing action as the patient got admitted?

a. Start IV for oxytocin administration
b. Record baseline vital signs
c. Administer antihypertensive drugs
d. Collect blood

845. Gestational hypertension is:

a. Hypertension to the extent of 140/90 or more with proteinuria after 20th week of POG
b. Pre-eclampsia complicated with generalized tonic-clonic seizure
c. Sustained raise in BP to 140/90 or more at least two occasions four or more hours apart
d. None of the above

846. The earliest sign of pregnancy-induced hypertension is:

a. Excessive weight gain b. Proteinuria
c. Blurring of vision d. Headache

847. Pre-eclampsia is characterized by all of the following; EXCEPT: *(ESIC 2019)*

a. Seizures
b. Mild facial edema
c. BP greater than 160/110 mm Hg
d. Marked proteinuria.

Ref: The American Congress of Obstetricians and Gynecologists.

Explanation: Pre-eclampsia with the onset of convulsions (**seizure**) is called eclampsia. Pre-eclampsia is characterized by high blood pressure **(SBP ≥140 or DBP ≥90), proteinuria, facial puffiness (mild facial edema)**, rapid weight gain, epigastric and right abdominal pain, visual disturbances, headache, and change in reflexes.

BP greater than 160/110 mm Hg on 2 occasions at least 4 hours apart is a feature of severe pre-eclampsia.

848. The danger of convulsion in a woman with pre-eclampsia ends: *(RAK MSc 2018)*

a. Soon after delivery b. 12 h after delivery
c. 24 h after delivery d. 48 h after delivery

Explanation: The danger of convulsion in a woman with pre-eclampsia starts from the beginning of the labor and ends after 48 hours of the delivery. Patient is closely monitored for next 48 hours for convulsions

849. Which is drug of choice for the management of Eclampsia? *(AIIMS Raipur staff nurse grade I-2018)*

a. Sodium nitroprusside b. Magnesium sulfate
c. Dopamine d. Labetalol

Explanation: Magnesium sulfate ($MgSO_4$) is the agent most commonly used for treatment of eclampsia and prophylaxis of eclampsia in patients with severe pre-eclampsia. It is usually given by either the intramuscular or intravenous routes.

850. Seema at 24 week POG, comes to ANC with complaining of edema in the legs, on examination her BP found to be 145/95 and urine suggestive of proteinuria, what will be the probable diagnosis?

a. Pregnancy–induced hypertension
b. Pre-eclampsia
c. Eclampsia
d. Malignant hypertension

Ans.

835. c
836. c
837. c
838. a
839. c
840. c
841. b
842. a
843. c
844. b
845. c
846. a
847. c
848. d
849. b
850. b

Explanation: Edema, hypertension and proteinuria in the ANC period suggestive of pre-eclampsia. In this condition BP will be of at least 140/90 mm Hg. Pitting edema over the ankles and urine suggestive of proteinuria. If this condition further complicated by seizure attack then it is known as eclampsia.

851. Nurse is caring for a patient who is experiencing eclamptic seizure at present. Which among the following is the priority nursing intervention? *(AIIMS 2016)*
a. Maintain patent airway
b. Administer $MgSO_4$ I/M
c. Start IV fluid
d. Hold the patient tight

Explanation: Priority nursing intervention is to maintain a patent airway. Once seizure is subsided then IV fluids and other medications will come into play.

852. Which out of the following is not a feature of pre-eclampsia? *(Staff Nurse G II 2014)*
a. Seizure b. Edema
c. Hypertension d. Proteinuria

853. Eclampsia is mostly seen at:
a. Antepartum period b. Intrapartum period
c. Postpartum period d. During parturition

854. Bed rest is essential in pre-eclampsia since it:
a. Prevents eclampsia *(RPSC NSg. Tutor 2009)*
b. Mobilizes tissue fluid thereby lowering blood pressure
c. Improves blood circulations and decreases edema
d. Prevents premature labor

855. Premonitory stage of eclamptic seizure is manifested by:
a. Cyanosis
b. Clenched hands
c. Eyeballs roll and are fixed in one direction
d. Looks puffy and comatose

856. In a woman with pre-eclamptic toxemia the danger of convulsion resolved by:
a. Soon after delivery b. 12 hours after delivery
c. 24 hours after delivery d. 48 hours after delivery

857. The Glomerular Filtration Rate (GFR) in pre-eclampsia:
a. Decreases b. Increases
c. Remains the same d. None of these

858. The first assessable objective sign of a convulsion in a client with eclampsia is:
a. Rolling of the eyes to one side with a fixed stare
b. Spots or flashes of light before the eyes
c. Persistent headache and blurred vision
d. Epigastric pain, nausea and vomiting

859. Which of the following finding is expected when assessing a pre-eclamptic woman?
a. Hypotension b. Hematuria
c. Polyuria d. Proteinuria

860. In eclampsia patient becomes unconscious twitching of facial muscles, eye balls roll or are turned to one side and become fixed is known as .... stage.
a. Pre monitory stage b. Tonic stage
c. Clonic stage d. Stage of coma

861. In eclampsia whole body goes into tonic spasm, the trunk opisthotonus, limbs are flexed and hands clenched is known as:
a. Pre monitory stage b. Tonic stage
c. Clonic stage d. Stage of coma

862. In eclampsia voluntary muscles undergo alternative contraction and relaxation, this stage is known as:
a. Pre monitory stage b. Tonic stage
c. Clonic stage d. Stage of coma

863. Clinical manifestation of pre-eclampsia is:
a. Pitting edema b. Proteinuria
c. Both a and b d. None of these

864. Hematological change occurred during pre-eclampsia and eclampsia include:
a. Decreased plasma volume
b. Hemoconcentration
c. Coagulation disorder
d. All of the above

865. Cardiovascular changes occurred during pre-eclampsia and eclampsia include:
a. Generalized vasospasm
b. Increased peripheral vascular resistance
c. Decreased CVP
d. All of the above

866. Renal change occurred during pre-eclampsia and eclampsia includes:
a. Decreased GFR
b. Decreased renal plasma flow
c. Increased serum uric acid
d. All of the above

867. In an eclampsic woman fluid intake should not be more than:
a. Previous 24 hours' urine output
b. Previous 24 hours' urine output + 1000 mL
c. Total blood volume of the patient
d. 10 mL/kg body weight

868. Preeclampsia is:
a. Hypertension to the extent of 140/90 or more with proteinuria after 20th week of POG
b. Preeclampsia complicated with generalized tonic-clonic seizure
c. Sustained raise in BP to 140/90 or more at least two occasions four or more hours apart
d. None of the above

869. Eclampsia is:
a. Hypertension to the extent of 140/90 or more with proteinuria after 20th week of POG
b. Preeclampsia complicated with generalized tonic-clonic seizure
c. Sustained raise in BP to 140/90 or more at least two occasions four or more hours apart
d. None of the above

870. Maternal administration of magnesium sulfate for more than 5-7 days during pregnancy leads to: ***New Q*** *(AIIMS Mangalagiri 2023)*
a. Fetal hypocalcemia b. Fetal hypokalemia
c. Maternal hypertension d. Maternal seizures

Explanation: Continuous administration of magnesium sulfate beyond 5-7 days to pregnant women can lead to hypocalcemia and bone abnormalities in the developing fetus.

871. Which of the following drug is administered to control eclamptic fits?
a. Interferon b. Calcium gluconate
c. Magnesium sulfate d. Magnesium trisilicate

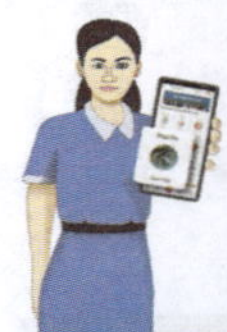

Ans.
851. a
852. a
853. a
854. c
855. c
856. d
857. a
858. a
859. d
860. a
861. b
862. c
863. c
864. d
865. d
866. d
867. b
868. a
869. b
870. a
871. c

POSTPARTUM HEMORRHAGE (PPH)

872. Among the following, the event during pregnancy that requires immediate attention by the physician is: *(AIIMS BPL NO 2018)*

a. Backache b. Frequency of micturition
c. Dependent pedal edema d. Bleeding per vagina

Explanation: Bleeding per vagina in early pregnancy can be sign of abortion, ectopic pregnancy or any other complications. Bleeding is not a usual sign of pregnancy. All other signs are expected during pregnancy.

873. Which of the following is a potential sign or symptom of postpartum hemorrhage (PPH)? *New Q*

a. Abdominal pain
b. Decreased blood pressure
c. Decreased urinary frequency
d. Increased uterine firmness

Explanation: Decreased blood pressure is a common manifestation of postpartum hemorrhage. When there is excessive bleeding, it can lead to a rapid decrease in blood volume, resulting in hypotension (low blood pressure).

Other signs and symptoms of PPH may include excessive or prolonged vaginal bleeding, increased heart rate (tachycardia), pale skin, lightheadedness, and signs of shock.

874. The most frequent causes of maternal death during child birth: *(RRB Feb 2012)*

a. Injection b. Subinvolution
c. Hemorrhage d. None of these

875. The most common cause of Postpartum Hemorrhage (PPH) is:

a. Vaginal lacerations b. Hematological disorders
c. Bleeding disorders d. Uterine atonicity

876. Postpartum hemorrhage is loss of blood which is more than: *(RAK MSc 2018)*

a. 800 mL b. 100 mL
c. 500 mL d. 900 mL

Explanation:

- PPH is defined as amount of blood loss in excess of 500 mL following birth of baby.
- **The average blood loss in:**
  - Normal vaginal delivery: less than 500 mL
  - Cesarean section: 1000 mL
  - Cesarean hysterectomy: 1500 mL

877. Which of the following drug is most commonly used in the management of PPH?

a. Prostaglandins
b. Oxytocin
c. Methergine
d. Estrogen

878. Adverse effect on female sexual functioning in postpartum is:

a. Perinatal lacerations
b. Milk ejection with stimulation
c. Fatigue and exhaustion
d. All of the above

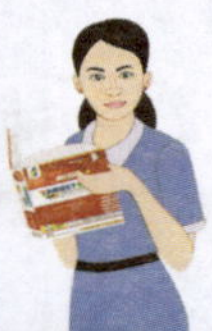

Ans.

872. d
873. b
874. c
875. d
876. c
877. b
878. d
879. d
880. c
881. b
882. a
883. a
884. a
885. a

879. Causes of postpartum hemorrhage include: *(RAK MSc 2018)*

a. Atonic uterus
b. Trauma
c. Blood coagulopathy
d. All of the above

Explanation: Atonicity of uterus is most common cause (80%) of postpartum hemorrhage. At the time of placental separation torn sinuses cannot be effectively compressed by imperfect contraction and retraction of uterine musculature. Other causes are rare (20%), that is traumatic cause, retained tissues and blood coagulopathy.

880. Major complication in third stage of labor is:

a. Atonic uterus b. Retained placenta
c. PPH d. Perineal tear

881. Which of the following is the major cause of pelvic inflammatory disease?

a. Abruptio placenta b. Postpartum hemorrhage
c. Uterine prolapse d. Placenta previa

882. The maternal observation following postpartum hemorrhage are: *(AIIMS Raipur Grade II 2017)*

a. Estimate the total volume of blood lost
b. Record pulse and temperature every 15 minutes
c. Monitor the central venous pressure
d. Administer IV fluids without interruption to combat the fluid loss

a. a, b, d b. b, c, d
c. a, c, d d. a, b, c, d

Explanation: For first hour following birth: Regular assessment of vital signs and uterine tone every 15 minutes. Assessments include estimation of blood loss, fundal height and tone, BP, and pulse.

883. Most common cause of PPH is:

a. Atonic uterus b. Traumatic
c. Retained tissue d. Blood coagulopathy

Explanation: All the above mentioned are the causes of PPH. But the most common cause is atonic uterus. In 80% of the cases the PPH occurs because of the uterine atony.

884. Following delivery nurse suspects atonic PPH in the client, which among the following is the priority nursing intervention?

a. Massage the uterus
b. Administer 10 unit of oxytocin
c. Administer ergometrin
d. Report to the doctor

Explanation: Although, administration of oxytocin helps to arrest PPH through uterine contraction, it is not considered to be a nursing intervention. The priority nursing intervention is to massage the uterus to induce letdown reflex.

885. All of the following drugs can be used in management of postpartum hemorrhage; EXCEPT:

a. Mifepristone b. Misoprostol
c. Syntocinon d. Syntometrine

Explanation: Misoprostol, syntocinon and syntometrine are used for the management of Post Partum Hemorrhage (PPH). Mifepristone in combination with misoprostol is used for Medical Termination of Pregnancy in first trimester of pregnancy. However, Mifepristone is not used for the management of PPH.

886. Primary PPH is:
a. Hemorrhage occurs within 24 hours following the birth of the baby
b. Hemorrhage occurs beyond 24 hours and within puerperium
c. Bleeding occurs after 28 weeks but before the onset of labor pain
d. Bleeding occurs at any time during pregnancy

887. Secondary PPH is:
a. Hemorrhage occurs within 24 hours following the birth of the baby
b. Hemorrhage occurs beyond 24 hours and within puerperium
c. Bleeding occurs after 28 weeks but before the onset of labor pain
d. Bleeding occurs at any time during pregnancy

888. Surgical management for PPH includes:
a. Ligation of uterine artery
b. Ligation of ovarian and uterine artery anastomosis
c. Ligation of anterior division of internal iliac artery
d. All of the above

889. Which of the following condition can place a client at risk for development of postpartum hemorrhage?
a. Twin pregnancy
b. Breech pregnancy
c. Premature rupture of membranes
d. Cesarean delivery

INJURIES TO BIRTH CANAL

890. Bleeding from or into the genital tract after 24 weeks of pregnancy but before the child birth is known as:
a. Antepartum hemorrhage b. Intrapartum hemorrhage
c. Postpartum hemorrhage d. Missed abortion

891. A woman is 37 weeks pregnant and she is bleeding profusely with no pain is suggestive of: *(Safdarjung NO 2018)*
a. Antepartum hemorrhage b. Unavoidable hemorrhage
c. Accidental hemorrhage d. Concealed hemorrhage

Explanation: Woman is 37 weeks pregnant and she is bleeding profusely without pain, it is suggestive of antepartum hemorrhage (APH). Bleeding from or into the genital tract after 24 weeks of pregnancy but before the child birth is known as antepartum hemorrhage.

892. Which of the following you will examine in the placenta to make the diagnosis of antepartum hemorrhage?
a. Infarction b. Calcification
c. Missing abortion d. Blood clots

893. The most common characteristic manifestation of uterine rupture during labor is:
a. Fetal bradycardia
b. Contractions that become stronger and intense
c. Hypertension
d. None of the above

894. Following normal delivery nurses assessing birth canal of a primigravida and found that injuries up to anal sphincter. She recorded this finding as:
a. First degree perineal tear
b. Second degree perineal tear
c. Third degree perineal tear
d. Fourth degree perineal tear

895. All among the following are the causes of perineal injury; EXCEPT:
a. Rigid perineum b. Precipitate delivery
c. Shoulder delivery d. Poor maternal efforts

896. What is the most common cause of traumatic PPH?
a. Pelvic hematoma b. Vulvar injuries
c. Vaginal tear d. Cervical tear

897. Which vaginal portion is more susceptible for tear during labor and delivery?
a. Lower third b. Upper third
c. Middle portion d. Any part

PRETERM LABOR AND POST-TERM PREGNANCY

898. The steroid used in preterm labor helps in:
a. Prevention of jaundice in newborn
b. Prevention of PPH in mother
c. Reducing respiratory distress syndrome
d. Prevention of seizures

899. Baby born before 37 completed week of gestation is known as:
a. Low birth weight baby b. Preterm baby
c. Small for gestational age d. Very low birth weight baby

900. Which among the following is the characteristic of postdate fetuses? *(NIMHANS)*
a. Slethargic and irritable
b. Areola is not pigmented
c. Desquamation of the epidermis
d. Vernixcaseosa covering the body

Explanation: Desquamation of epidermis can be seen in postdate fetuses.

PREMATURE RUPTURE OF MEMBRANES

901. Premature rupture of membrane (PROM) refers to rupture of membrane:
a. Before onset of labor at 37 weeks or beyond
b. Before onset of labor between 28 weeks and 37 weeks of gestation
c. Before 37 completed week of pregnancy
d. More than 24 hours before delivery

902. Term pre-labor rupture of membrane means rupture of membrane:
a. Before onset of labor at 37 weeks or beyond
b. Before onset of labor between 28 weeks and 37 weeks of gestation
c. Before 37 completed week of pregnancy
d. More than 24 hours before delivery

903. Preterm pre-labor rupture of membrane refers to rupture of membrane that occurs:
a. Before onset of labor at 37 weeks or beyond
b. Before 37 weeks of gestation and before onset of labor
c. Before 37 completed week of pregnancy
d. More than 24 hours before delivery

Explanation: Prelabor or Premature Rupture of the Membranes (PROM) refers to rupture of the fetal membranes prior to the onset of regular uterine contractions. It is known as premature rupture of membrane if rupture occurs before the onset of labor at ≥37 weeks of gestation. It is termed as preterm premature rupture of membrane if PROM occurs before 37 weeks of gestation.

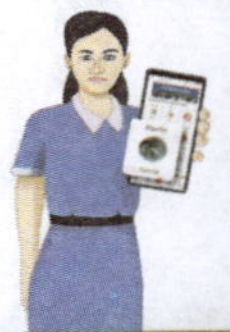

Ans.

886. a
887. b
888. d
889. a
890. a
891. a
892. d
893. a
894. c
895. d
896. d
897. a
898. c
899. b
900. c
901. a
902. a
903. b

904. Prolonged rupture of membrane means rupture of membrane:
- a. Before onset of labor at 37 weeks or beyond
- b. Before 37 weeks of gestation and before onset of labor
- c. Before 37 completed week of pregnancy
- d. More than 24 hours before delivery

905. A vaginal examination reveals that the cervix is 4 cm dilated, with intact membranes and a fetal heart tone rate of 160–170 bpm. The nurse decides to apply an external fetal monitor. The rationale for this implementation is:
- a. The cervix is closed *New Q*
- b. The membranes are still intact
- c. The fetal heart tones are within normal limits
- d. The contractions are intense enough for insertion of an internal monitor

PROLONGED LABOR & OBSTRUCTED LABOR

906. Obstructed labor seen in all; EXCEPT:
- a. Fetal ascites
- b. Congenital equinovarus of fetus
- c. Contracted pelvis
- d. Inter-hydrocephalus of fetus

907. The commonest cause for rupture in uterus is:
- a. Obstructed labor
- b. Postcesarean gestation
- c. Shoulder presentation
- d. Hydramnios

Explanation: The most common cause of uterine rupture is a previous cesarean secuon. This is because the scar tissue from the cesarean section can weaken the uterus and make it more likely to tear.

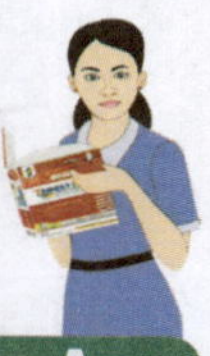

908. The commonest cause of primary dysfunctional labor in primigravida is:
- a. Inadequate uterine contraction
- b. Lack of pain
- c. Cervical dystocia
- d. Macro baby

909. Etiology for contracted pelvis include:
- a. Disease or injuries affecting the pelvis
- b. Short stature of women
- c. Severe infection during childhood
- d. All of the above

COMMON GYNECOLOGICAL DISORDERS

910. All of the following are the common symptoms of perimenopause; EXCEPT:
- a. Irregular periods
- b. Increased libido
- c. Vaginal dryness
- d. Hot flashes

911. Unicornuate uterus refers to:
- a. Menstruation occurs but is not visible due to an obstruction of the outflow tract
- b. Distension of the vagina caused by accumulation of fluid due to congenital vaginal obstruction
- c. Uterus is formed from only one of the paired Müllerian ducts
- d. Complete duplication of uterine horns as well as duplication of the cervix

912. A type of Mullerian duct anomaly in which there is complete duplication of uterine horns as well as duplication of the cervix with no communication between them is known as:
- a. Unicornuate uterus
- b. Bicornuate uterus
- c. Hyperplasia uterus
- d. Uterus didelphys

913. Acquired risk factor for genital prolapse is:
- a. Vaginal delivery with consequent injury to the supporting structures
- b. Congenital weakness of the supporting structures
- c. Malnutrition and aging
- d. Increased weight of the uterus

914. Descent of the uterus toward introitus is known as:
- a. Ist degree uterine prolapse
- b. IInd degree uterine prolapse
- c. IIIrd degree uterine prolapse
- d. IVth degree uterine prolapse

915. The degree of uterine prolapse in which the uterine body descends to lie outside the introitus is:
- a. 1st degree
- b. IInd degree
- c. IIIrd degree
- d. IVth degree

916. Genital prolapse manifestation includes all; EXCEPT:
- a. Difficulty in passing urine
- b. Backache
- c. Difficulty in passing stool
- d. Chancroid

917. What is the cause of primary cervical dystocia?
- a. Rigid cervix
- b. Inefficient uterine contraction
- c. First birth in which external os fail to dilate
- d. All of the above

918. What is the cause of secondary cervical dystocia?
- a. Scarring of the cervix
- b. Post delivery
- c. Postoperative scarring
- d. All of these

919. Cervical incompetence results in:
- a. Second trimester miscarriage
- b. Third trimester miscarriage
- c. Recurrent abortion/preterm labor
- d. All of the above

920. Cephalopelvic disproportion can be assessed with the help of:
- a. Chassar-Moirs method
- b. Munro-Kerr's method
- c. Left-hand grip
- d. All of the above

921. A 40-year-old woman was advised estrogen replacement therapy by the gynecologist. The nurse was directed to educate the woman about the estrogen replacement therapy. Which of the following statement by the nurse indicates that the nurse is aware of the possible complications of estrogen therapy? *New Q*
- a. Estrogen promotes diuresis and weight loss, so increase your fluid intake
- b. You will feel discomfort due to estrogen, so take an analgesic prior to estrogen.
- c. To avoid constipation, you need to increase roughage in your diet
- d. Make sure you keep your clinic appointments, especially your gynecologic checkup.

Ans.

904. d
905. b
906. b
907. b
908. a
909. d
910. b
911. c
912. d
913. a
914. b
915. c
916. d
917. d
918. d
919. d
920. d
921. d

Explanation: Options a, b, and c do not mention any of the possible complications of estrogen therapy.

Option d acknowledges the importance of regular monitoring and follow-up to address any complications or risks associated with estrogen replacement therapy.

922. Semi-Fowler's position is recommended in pelvic inflammatory disease for:

a. Easy observation
b. Promoting drainage to prevent abscesses
c. Easily healing
d. More comfort of the patient

923. Which of the following conditions may be caused by a gonococcal infection?

a. Bartholin's cyst
b. Infertility
c. Pelvic inflammatory disease
d. All of the above

924. Most common hernia in females is:

a. Femoral hernia
b. Inguinal hernia
c. Spigelion hernia
d. Obturator hernia

925. Which of these is not a symptom of vaginal atrophy?

(AIIMS Raipur Grade II 2017)

a. Tightening of vaginal wall
b. Lengthening of vaginal canal
c. Decreased vaginal lubrication
d. Urinary incontinence

Explanation: The symptoms of vaginal atrophy include shortening and tightening of vaginal wall, decreased vaginal lubrication during sexual activity, discomfort with intercourse, light bleeding after intercourse, urinary incontinence, more urinary tract infections, urgency and burning with urination, genital itching, vaginal burning, dryness and discharge.

926. What is the common cause of constipation during pregnancy? *(AIIMS Raipur staff nurse grade I-2018)*

a. Lack of fluid intake
b. Decreased fiber intake
c. Reduced intestinal motility
d. Lack of activity

Explanation: In pregnancy, constipation occurs due to hemorrhages that relax the intestinal muscle and by the pressure of gravid uterus on the intestine.

927. Which of the following instructions should nurse give to a client who is 26 weeks pregnant and complains of constipation?

a. Encourage her to increase her intake of roughage and to drink at least six glasses of water per day
b. Tell her to go to the evaluation unit because constipation may cause contractions.
c. Tell her to ask her caregiver for a mild laxative.
d. Suggest the use of an over-the-counter stool softener

Explanation: Natural remedies will not have any side effect and complication thus, it will help in normal growth and development of fetus.

928. A primigravida client at 25 weeks' gestation visits the clinic and tells the nurse that her lower back aches when she arrives home from work. The nurse should suggest that the client perform:

a. Leg lifting
b. Tailor sitting
c. Side lying
d. Squatting exercises

Explanation: Tailor sitting will help in removing the spasm and congestion which occurs due to pressure of growing fetus to the lower back.

929. Pregnant woman, who is 4 months pregnant asks the nurse how much and what type of exercise she should get during pregnancy. How should nurse counsel her?

a. "Exercise to raise the heart rate above 140 beats/minute for 20 minutes daily
b. "Perform gentle back-lying exercises for 30 minutes daily."
c. "Try high-intensity aerobics, but limit sessions to 15 minutes daily. "
d. "Walk briskly for 10 to 15 minutes daily, and gradually increase this time

Explanation: Walking briskly for 10–15 minutes daily will eliminate pelvic pressure and pain, bloating and discomfort.

930. Which of the following is not advised for a pregnant woman with a complaint of varicose veins?

a. Wear support stockings
b. Stand for long periods
c. Exercise the calf muscles
d. Elevate legs when sitting

931. In pregnancy diagnosis of appendicitis will be late because:

a. Vomiting may misinterpret as hyperemesis
b. ESR and WBC count will be elevated in normal pregnancy as well as appendicitis
c. Location of pain will be shifted to higher level and may misdiagnose as cholelithiasis or renal infection
d. All of the above

932. Supine hypotensive syndrome most commonly seen during ....trimester.

a. 1st Trimester
b. 2nd Trimester
c. 3rd Trimester
d. Whole antenatal period

933. Stillbirth rate includes babies' death after:

(RRB SSNE 2015)

a. 20 weeks
b. 24 weeks
c. 28 weeks
d. 32 weeks

934. A 38-week pregnant mother is complaining of discomfort due to irregularly occurring contraction. The best advice by the nurse is:

a. Lie down in supine position
b. Take some warm drinks
c. Walk around
d. Take some analgesics

Explanation: Patient experiencing Braxton Hicks contractions, it is also known as prodromal labor or practice contractions, or false labor, are sporadic uterine contractions that sometimes start around six weeks into a pregnancy. However, they are not usually felt until the second trimester or third trimester of pregnancy. It can be relieved by walking around until it subsides.

Ans.

922. b
923. d
924. b
925. b
926. c
927. a
928. b
929. d
930. b
931. d
932. c
933. c
934. c

935. Full form of HELLP is:

a. Hemolysis, elevated liver enzymes and low platelet level
b. Hematuria, elevated leucocytes and low pro-thrombin time
c. Hematuria, elevated leucocytes and low partial thromboplastin time
d. Hematuria, elevated leucocytes and low platelet level

936. Pseudocyesis is:

a. False believe of a woman that she is pregnant
b. Abnormal enlargement of uterus
c. False diagnosis that a person is pregnant
d. All of the above

937. All of the following are recognized causes of intrauterine growth retardation (IUGR); EXCEPT: *(RRB Feb 2012)*

a. Hypertension b. Smoking
c. Hypercholesterolemia d. Diabetes

938. During delivery the risk of transmission of maternal infection to the fetus is highest in:

a. Rubella b. Cytomagalo virus
c. Herpes simplex virus d. Human papillomavirus

939. Which one among the following indicates postpartum depression?

a. Suicidal thoughts b. Desire to harm the infant
c. Feeling of worthlessness d. All of these

940. Aerobic organism responsible for puerperal sepsis is:

a. Bacteroides b. Klebsiella
c. Clostridium welchii d. Clostridium

941. The condition where the uterus turns inside out is known as: *(AIIMS Bhopal Grade-I 2018)*

a. Retroversion b. Prolapse
c. Anteversion d. Inversion

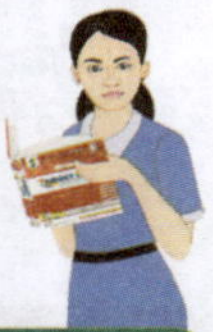

Explanation: Uterine inversion occurs when the placenta fails to detach from the uterus as it exits, pulls on the inside surface, and turns the organ inside out.

Uterine prolapse occurs when pelvic floor muscles and ligaments stretch and weaken, and no longer provide enough support for the uterus. As a result, the uterus slips down into or protrudes out of the vagina.

Anteversion of the uterus refers to the position of the uterus where the long axis of the uterus is bent forward on the long axis of the vagina, against the urinary bladder.

A retroverted uterus means the uterus is tilted backwards toward the rectum.

942. Mrs X, a postnatal mother, admitted with history of fever 102°F, abdominal pain and foul smelling lochia on 8th postnatal day, which of the following complication does this indicate?

a. Puerperal sepsis b. Peritonitis
c. Perineal tear d. Sub involution

943. Infection of genital tract due to complication of delivery is termed as:

a. Puerperal sepsis b. Cervical infection
c. Peritoneal sepsis d. Vaginal infection

944. "Phlegmasia alba dolens" is found in:

a. Breast complication
b. Deep vein thrombosis
c. Placenta previa
d. Pulmonary embolism

Explanation: Phlegmasia alba dolens describes the patient with swollen white leg because of early compromise of arterial blood flow secondary to extensive DVT. This condition is also known as milk leg especially as it affects women in third trimester and postpartum.

945. Chances of acute endometritis is more after:

a. Menopause b. Menarchae
c. Abortion or childbirth d. Infection

946. Pallor, bradycardia, sweating, nausea, hypotension and dizziness occurs when a pregnant woman lies on her back is known as:

a. Malignant hypothermia
b. Orthostatic hypotension
c. Respiratory distress syndrome
d. Supine hypotensive syndrome

947. Nurse caring a high-risk pregnant lady with heart diseases, must know which one of the following valvular lesions cause death during labor? *(NCFL 2019)*

a. Aortic stenosis b. Aortic regurgitation
c. Mitral stenosis d. Mitral regurgitation

Explanation: The typical raise in volume and heart rate in pregnancy is not well tolerated in patients with more than mild mitral stenosis. Hence, Mitral stenosis is the valvular lesions cause death during labor.

Even a severe Aortic Mitral valve regurgitation is usually very well tolerated in pregnancy, unless there is no left ventricular failure. Patients with Aortic stenosis can tolerate pregnancy well with mild or moderate level of obstruction.

948. Vulval cancer can be due to:

a. Fungal infection b. Bacterial infection
c. HPV infection d. All of these

949. Which of the following is the treatment of choice for most benign ovarian tumors?

a. Allowing the tumor for a spontaneous resolution
b. Chemotherapy
c. Radiation therapy
d. Surgical removal

950. The most common type of ovarian cancer is:

a. Adenocarcinomas
b. Endometrial tumors
c. Epithelial ovarian cancer
d. Mucinous adenocarcinomas

951. Commonest benign solid tumor in female is:

a. Fibroid uterus b. Endometriosis
c. Cancer of uterus d. Cervical cancer

952. Fibroid uterus is more common in:

a. Nulliparous women
b. Postmenopausal women
c. Women with multiple sexual partner
d. After 35 years of age

953. Clinical manifestation of fibroid uterus includes:

a. Heavy periods b. Severe abdominal pain
c. Both a and b d. None of the above

954. Complication associated with uterine fibroid is:

a. Persistent menorrhagia leading to anemia
b. Menstrual pain
c. Abdominal cramps
d. All of the above

Ans.

935. a
936. a
937. c
938. c
939. d
940. c
941. d
942. a
943. a
944. b
945. c
946. d
947. c
948. c
949. d
950. c
951. a
952. a
953. c
954. d

955. **Changes occur to the uterus in uterine fibroid is:**
a. Increased surface area of the endometrium
b. Interference with normal uterine contractility
c. Pelvic congestion
d. All of the above

956. **Cause behind infertility in fibroid uterus is:**
a. Ovum production is not there
b. Sperms are malformed
c. Fibroid uterus prevents rhythmic uterine, contraction during intercourse
d. None of the above

957. **Normal lining of the uterus grows outside the uterus is known as:**
a. Cancer of cervix
b. Endometriosis
c. Adenoma of uterus
d. Fibroid uterus

Explanation: A disorder in which tissue that normally lines the uterus grows outside the uterus. With endometriosis, the tissue can be found on the ovaries, fallopian tubes or the intestines. The most common symptoms are pain and menstrual irregularities. Effective treatments, such as hormones and excision surgery, are available.

958. **Common site of endometriosis includes:**
a. Ovary
b. Fallopian tube
c. Intestine
d. All of these

959. **The most common treatment modality for vaginal cancer is:**
a. Chemotherapy
b. Radiotherapy
c. Surgery
d. Complementary therapy

960. **The benign growth in the muscle fibers of the uterus is called as:**
a. Myoma
b. Cyst
c. Congenital anomaly
d. Uterine prolapse

961. **Among the following, which of the following age group women are most vulnerable for vulvar cancer?**
a. 45–60 years
b. 60–70 years
c. 70–80 years
d. Above 80 years

962. **Tingling, numbness and pain in the thumb and fingers of a pregnant women suggestive of which condition?**
a. Osteoporosis
b. Rheumatoid arthritis
c. Carpal tunnel syndrome
d. Calcium deficiency

963. **MMR is:**
a. Maternal death per 1,00,000 live birth
b. Maternal death per 10 thousand live birth
c. Maternal death per 1000 live birth
d. Maternal death per 100 live birth

964. **Which of the following sign in a client indicates thrombophlebitis?**
a. Orthostatic hypotension
b. Shortness of breath when climbing the stairs
c. Diarrhea
d. A painful swelling usually in one leg

965. **Which of the following clinical manifestations suggests the presence of vulvo-vaginal candidiasis?**
a. Mucoid discharge and redness
b. Multiple ulcerative lesions with pruritus
c. Greenish yellow discharge and pruritus
d. Curdy discharge, moist reddened skin and pruritus

966. **Traits are passed on from parents to their offspring by:**
a. Genes
b. Chromosomes
c. Hormones
d. Enzymes

967. **What is the fertility test that requires a couple to have sexual intercourse at the time of ovulation and come for testing 2 to 8 hours after intercourse?** *New Q*
a. Huhner's test
b. Semen analysis
c. Endometrial biopsy
d. Hysterosalpingogram

Explanation: A Huhner's test is a fertility test that evaluates the ability of sperm to move through the cervical mucus and reach the egg. The test is performed by having the couple have sexual intercourse at the time of ovulation. The woman then comes to the clinic 2–8 hours after intercourse for a sample of cervical mucus to be taken. The mucus is then examined under a microscope to see how many sperms are present and how well they are moving.

968. **The incidence of previous cesarean scar rupture is:**
a. 0.5%
b. 0.5–1.0%
c. 1–2%
d. 2-3%

969. **In which of the following condition liquor enters the maternal circulation causing sudden hypotension, hypoxia, dyspnea and often seizures?**
a. Amniotic fluid embolism
b. Pulmonary embolism
c. Obstetrics shock
d. Uterine atony

970. **Commonest cause of vesicovaginal fistula is:**
a. Hysterectomy
b. Vaginal delivery
c. Abdominal surgery
d. Vaginal tuberculosis

971. **Correction of vesicovaginal fistula done at:**
a. During menstruation
b. 5th day of menstruation
c. 3-6 months following delivery
d. After menopause

972. **The commonest cause of uretero vaginal fistula is:**
a. Vaginal tuberculosis
b. Trauma during pelvic surgery
c. Cancer of cervix
d. Hormonal therapy

973. **A postpartum patient was in labor for 32 hours and had ruptured membranes for 24 hours. Which of the following condition is expected in this client?**
a. Endometriosis
b. Endometritis
c. Pelvic thrombophlebitis
d. Salpingitis

Explanation: Endometritis is an infection of the uterine lining and can occur after prolonged rupture of membranes. Caesarean section, prolonged rupture of membranes and long labor with multiple vaginal examinations are important risk factors of endometritis.

974. **State of abnormal uterine bleeding without any clinically detectable organic pelvic pathology and is due to changes in hormone levels is known as:**
a. Menorrhagia
b. Metrorrhagia
c. Dysfunctional uterine bleeding
d. Epimenorrhea

975. **As a management of dysfunctional uterine bleed endometrial resection is done in:**
a. Age over 35
b. Completed her family
c. Not has any significant endometrial pathology such as cancer
d. All of the above

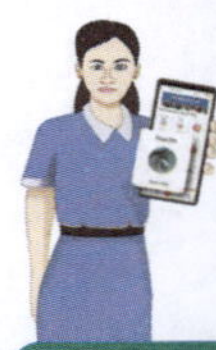

Ans.

955. d
956. c
957. b
958. d
959. c
960. a
961. b
962. c
963. a
964. d
965. d
966. a
967. a
968. a
969. a
970. b
971. c
972. b
973. b
974. c
975. d

976. All are true regarding vernix caseosa; EXCEPT:
a. Secreted by sebaceous gland
b. Mixture of sebum and epidermis
c. Appear like white covering over the skin
d. It is distributed uniformly

977. The primary site of hematopoiesis in the fetus before midpregnancy is:
a. Liver b. Bone
c. Kidney d. Pancreas

978. Lack of ....vitamin is responsible for most of the congenital malformation.
a. Folic acid
b. Riboflavin
c. Niacin
d. Calcium and iron

979. Identify the correct statement regarding kartagener syndrome:
a. It is a rare hereditary disease autosomal recessive caused by a gene defect.
b. There is loss of ciliary function and sperm motility.
c. Primary ciliary dyskinesia and situs inversus are the abnormalities seen along with this condition.
d. All of the above.

980. Which of the following is not a risk factor associated with Macrosomia?
a. Gestational diabetes mellitus
b. Prolonged pregnancy
c. Maternal obesity
d. Short stature

981. It is the alternative of the shape of the forecoming head while passing through the resistant birth passage during labor:
a. Caput succedaneum
b. Molding
c. Cephalhematoma
d. Retinoblastoma

982. Which gland is responsible for initiating the menstrual cycle? *(RAK MSc 2018)*
a. Hypothalamus
b. Anterior pituitary gland (APG)
c. Posterior pituitary gland (PPG)
d. Ovaries

Explanation: Initiation of menstrual cycle is being carried out by hypothalamus. It secretes GnRH which thereby stimulates pituitary gland to secrete FSH and results in follicle development and also secretes LH for releasing ovum from the ovary.

The other options have a role in menstrual cycle but not initiating menstrual cycle.

983. The entire transitional phase between sexual maturity and menopause is called: *(AIIMS BPL NO 2018)*
a. Menarche b. Puberty
c. Thelarche d. Climacteric

Explanation: Climacteric is manifested by a disturbance in the regularity of the menstrual cycle until it ceases completely, which signals the onset of a new period in a woman's life, the menopause. The climacteric generally begins at the ages of 45–54 years, usually at about 47 years of age, and continues for an average of 15–18 months.

984. A 14-year-old girl comes to the gynecologist with her mother as she has not attained menarche. She has a history of an unknown cancer at the age of 10 and had received chemotherapy. What may be the cause for the given scenario? *New Q*
a. Autoimmune ovarian failure
b. Irradiation
c. Etoposide
d. Iatrogenic

Explanation: Etoposide is a medication used in cancer treatment. Girl who is treated with etoposide before puberty is more likely to have delayed menarche and more likely to have irregular menstrual cycles after menarche.

985. Hormone responsible for thelarche is:
a. Estrogen b. Progesterone
c. Oxytocin d. Androgens

986. A permanent cessation of menstruation at the end of reproductive life is called as: *(AIIMS Bhopal Nursing Officer, 2018)*
a. Menarche b. Menopause
c. Precocious puberty d. Thelarche

Explanation: Permanent cessation of menstrual cycle is known as menopause. Initiation of menstruation is known as menarche.

987. Hormonal change occurs in menopause is all; EXCEPT:
a. Fall in serum estradiol level
b. Increase in FSH level
c. Increase in LH level
d. Fall in serum testosterone level

Explanation: In premenopausal women, Estradiol is the main form of estrogen. But serum level significantly falls after menopause. FSH and LH rise after menopause. FSH rise precedes LH rise. FSH is the diagnostic marker for ovarian failure. Androgen level may increase after menopause.

988. Identify the changes occur in female genitalia after menopause:
a. Uterus becomes smaller
b. The vagina become narrower and dry
c. Ovaries become small in size
d. All of the above

989. After menopause in women the chances of her developing osteoporosis increase because of: *(RRB SSNE 2015)*
a. Decrease in estrogen levels
b. Increase in estogen levels
c. Decrease in LH levels
d. Decrease in FSH levels

990. Delayed menopause is:
a. Menopause fails to occur beyond 45 years of age
b. Menopause fails to occur beyond 50 years of age
c. Menopause fails to occur beyond 55 years of age
d. Menopause fails to occur beyond 60 years of age

991. Which of the following is not true about pre-menstrual syndrome? *(AIIMS-BBS SNO 2019)*
a. It occurs during the last half of menstrual cycle
b. It resolves with the onset of menstruations
c. It occurs during the luteal phase
d. It resolves with the onset of ovulation

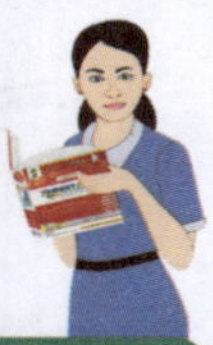

Ans.
976. d
977. a
978. a
979. d
980. d
981. b
982. a
983. d
984. c
985. a
986. b
987. d
988. d
989. a
990. c
991. d

Explanation: Pre-menstrual syndrome (PMS) refers to physical and emotional symptoms that occur in the 1 to 2 weeks before menses. Physical symptoms include breast tenderness, bloating and psychological symptoms include mood swings, anger, etc. It occurs in the last half of menstrual cycle (luteal phase) and typically **ends with the onset of menstrual flow.**

992. Mild premenstrual syndrome can be treated with:
a. Anxiolytics
b. Dietary advice, exercise and evening primrose oil
c. Vitamins and mineral supplements
d. Antidepressants

993. Primary dysmenorrhea cause is:
a. Narrowing of the cervical canal
b. Uterine hypoplasia and contraction
c. Increased vasopressin release
d. All of the above

994. Bleeding between the menstrual period is known as:
a. Menorrhagia b. Metrorrhagia
c. Polymenorrhea d. Dysmenorrhea

995. Absence of a menstrual period in a woman of reproductive age is known as:
a. Hypomenorrhea b. Amenorrhea
c. Dysmenorrhea d. Eumenorrhea

996. Short and scanty periods that lasts for less than 2 days is known as:
a. Amenorrhea b. Hypomenorrhea
c. Menorrhagia d. Metrorrhagia

997. Too frequent menstruation, occurring at any time, but particularly at the beginning and end of menstrual life is known as:
a. Metorrhagia b. Hypomenorrhea
c. Hypermenorrhea d. Epimenorrhea

Explanation: Epimenorrhea is the medical term for too frequent menstruation. It is also known as polymenorrhea.

Epimenorrhea is characterized by menstrual cycles that are shorter than 21 days. This can cause women to have two or more periods in a month.

998. Increased uterine blood flow occurring at regular intervals or loss of more than 80 mL of blood is called as:
(AIIMS BPL NO 2018)
a. Epimenorrhea b. Hypermenorrhea
c. Cryptomenorrhea d. Metrorrhagia

Explanation: Heavy menstrual bleeding or hypermenorrhea is defined as total menstrual flow >80 mL per cycle, or soaking a pad/tampon every 2 hours or less.

999. Epimenorrhea is also known as:
a. Menorrhagia b. Polymenorrhea
c. Metrorrhagia d. Dysmenorrhea

1000. Abnormally heavy bleeding at menstruation is known as:
a. Menorrhagia b. Metrorrhagia
c. Polymenorrhea d. Dysmenorrhea

1001. Menorrhagia is caused by:
a. Fibroid uterus
b. Adenomyosis
c. Dysfunctional uterine bleeding
d. All of the above

1002. A condition in which prolonged or excessive uterine bleeding occurs irregularly and more frequently than normal is known as:
a. Menorrhagia b. Metrorrhagia
c. Menometrorrhagia d. Epimenorrhea

1003. Hypomenorrhea is caused by:
a. Endometrial tuberculosis
b. Malnutrition
c. Uterine synechiae
d. All of the above

1004. Dysmenorrhea is due to:
a. Ovulation
b. Decreased progesterone
c. Increased progesterone
d. Secretory epithelium

1005. Specific manifestation in menopause is:
(Staff Nurse G II 2014)
a. Hot flashes b. Hypotension
c. Hypothermia d. Anorexia

1006. A condition in which the menstruation occurs but is not visible because of an obstruction of the outflow tract is known as:
a. Cryptomenorrhea b. Dysmenorrhea
c. Xerocolpos d. Menorrhagia

1007. Distention of the vagina caused by accumulation of fluid due to congenital vaginal obstruction is known as:
a. Hydro vaginitis b. Hydrocolpos
c. Hydro vaginosis d. Vaginismus

1008. Commonest cause of cryptomenorrhea is:
a. Recto vaginal fistula b. Imperforate hymen
c. Adhesions d. Cervical stenosis

1009. Failure of menses to occur by age 16 years, in the presence of normal growth and secondary sexual characteristics is known as:
a. Primary amenorrhea
b. Secondary amenorrhea
c. Dysmenorrhea
d. Menorrhagia

1010. Secondary amenorrhoea is:
a. Cessation of regular menses for three months
b. Cessation of irregular menses for six months
c. Both a and b
d. Absence of menses for more than one year

1011. Reason behind secondary amenorrhea in polycystic ovarian disease is:
a. More estrogen b. More progesterone
c. More androgens d. More FSH

1012. The most common type of dysmenorrhea is the:
a. Membranous type b. Congestive type
c. Spasmodic type d. Mixed type

1013. The single most important investigation in cases of menorrhagia is:
a. Ultrasound b. Pap smear
c. Pipelle sampling d. Hysteroscopy

1014. Causes of infertility in females includes all of the following; EXCEPT:
a. Hormonal causes
b. Defects of the cervix
c. Ovarian abnormalities
d. Tubal blockage

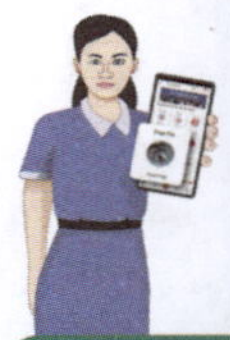

Ans.

992. b
993. d
994. b
995. b
996. b
997. d
998. b
999. b
1000. a
1001. d
1002. c
1003. d
1004. b
1005. a
1006. a
1007. b
1008. b
1009. a
1010. c
1011. c
1012. c
1013. c
1014. b

HIV IN PREGNANCY

1015. Which drug is given to prevent HIV transmission from mother to child/vertical transmission? *(AIIMS Raipur staff nurse grade I-2018)*

a. Nevirapine b. Lamivudine
c. Stavudine d. Abacavir

Explanation: Nevirapine is the drug of choice to prevent transmission of HIV from mother to child. Nevirapine belongs to NNRTI group.

So, all the above-mentioned drugs are contraindicated during pregnancy.

1016. Vertical transmission of HIV is more commonly occurs during:

a. Antenatal period b. Intranatal period
c. Post-natal period d. Equal chance in all stage

Explanation: HIV is more commonly transmitted during intra natal period.

1017. In India, an HIV positive antenatal mother who is on ARV therapy approached the nurse to discuss regarding breastfeeding practices for her newborn after delivery. Which of the following response by the nurse is most appropriate?

a. Encourage exclusive breastfeeding
b. Encourage exclusive replacement feeding
c. Encourage mixed feeding
d. Encourage partial breastfeeding

Explanation: Exclusive breastfeeding is the recommended infant feeding choice for the first 6 months, irrespective of whether mother or infant is provided with ARV drugs for the duration of breastfeeding. Mixed feeding should not be practiced. Only in situations where breastfeeding cannot be done or on individual parents' informed decision, replacement feeding may be considered.

1018. HIV transmission from mother to fetus occurs most commonly during:

a. First trimester
b. Second trimester
c. Third trimester
d. Delivery

1019. ART of choice for the newborn born to HIV positive mother is:

a. Nevirapine b. Lamivudine
c. Indinavir d. Ritonavir

Explanation: The drug of choice is Nevirapine.

1020. Highly contagious perinatal infection among the following is:

a. Pneumococci pneumonia
b. Hepatitis B
c. HIV- AIDS
d. Herpes simplex virus (HSV)

1021. Health education regarding STD include:

a. Avoid multiple sexual partners
b. Always use barrier technique
c. Regularly screen for STD
d. Use different positions during intercourse

GONORRHEA, SYPHILIS & PELVIC INFLAMMATORY DISEASE

1022. Pelvic inflammatory disease can be caused by all of the following; EXCEPT:

a. Illegal abortion
b. Sexually Transmitted Infections
c. Uterine leiomyoma
d. Insertion of an intrauterine contraceptive device.

1023. Which of the following sexually transmitted diseases has a bacterial origin? *(AIIMS Bhopal Nursing Officer, 2018)*

a. Syphilis
b. Hepatitis B
c. Trichomonas Vaginitis
d. Scabies

Explanation:

Disease	Causative organism
Syphilis	Bacteria
Chlamydia	Bacteria
Genital herpes	Virus
Gonorrhea	Bacteria
HIV/AIDS	Virus
HPV	Virus
Trichomoniasis	Parasite

1024. Incubation period for syphilis is:

a. 1 week b. 2 weeks
c. 3 weeks d. 4 weeks

1025. Which among the following perinatal infection does not offer long lasting immunity?

a. Hepatitis B Virus b. Syphilis
c. Toxoplasmosis d. Rubella

1026. VDRL blood test is a screening test for:

a. Anemia b. Syphilis
c. HIV d. Hepatitis B

1027. Before a client with syphilis can be treated the nurse must determine the: *(Safdarjung NO 2018)*

a. Portal of entry
b. Size of the chancre
c. Existence of allergies
d. Name of sexual contacts

Explanation: Penicillin injection is the treatment of syphilis. Allergic reaction to the penicillin can be life threatening. Whenever the patient comes for the penicillin injection, each time antibiotic sensitivity test is to be repeated and if skin reaction is positive for allergic reaction, then the patient can be given alternative therapy as ceftriaxone or erythromycin.

1028. Which among the following condition is seen often in patient with gonorrhea?

a. Trachoma b. Chlamydia
c. Herpes d. Syphilis

Explanation: Most women who are suffering from gonorrhea will be also having chlamydia. So treatment of both condition is required simultaneously.

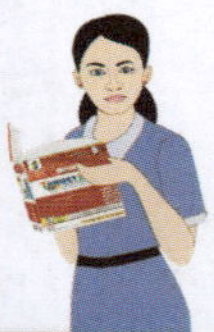

Ans.

1015. a
1016. b
1017. a
1018. d
1019. a
1020. d
1021. a
1022. c
1023. a
1024. c
1025. b
1026. b
1027. c
1028. b

1029. Most commonly transmitted STD among female is:
a. Human Immunodeficiency virus (HIV)
b. Hepatitis B
c. Chlamydia
d. Syphilis

1030. Chlamydia infection leads to:
a. Trachoma
b. Salpingitis
c. Non gonococcal urethritis
d. All of the above

1031. Ophthalmia neonatorum is caused by:
a. Chlamydia trachomatis
b. Neisseria gonorrhea
c. Both a and b
d. None of the above

1032. Lymphogranuloma venereum is caused by …….. organism.
a. Candida Albicans b. Chlamydia Trachomatis
c. Treponema pallidum d. Neisseria gonorrhea

1033. Identify correct statement regarding gonococcal salpingitis:
a. It is a sexually transmitted disease
b. It is usually bilateral infection
c. The symptoms usually appear following menstruation
d. All of the above

1034. Chancroid is caused by:
a. Chlamydia trachomatis
b. Treponema pallidum
c. Neisseria gonorrhea
d. Hemophilus ducreyi

Explanation: Chancroid is a bacterial sexually transmitted disease that causes open sores on or around the genitals of men and women. It is a venereal infection caused by hemophilus ducreyi.

1035. Trial labor is contraindicated in all; EXCEPT:
a. Minor CPD b. Major CPD
c. Elderly primi d. Bad obstetrical history

1036. Which of the following information is appropriate for a pregnant woman who has a positive history of genital herpes but has no lesions during the present pregnancy. *(Safdarjung NO 2018)*
a. You will be isolated from your newborn infant following delivery
b. She will be evaluated at the time of delivery for herpetic genital tract lesions, and if lesions are present a cesarean section will be needed
c. There is little risk to your newborn infant during this pregnancy, birth and following delivery
d. Vaginal deliveries can reduce neonatal infection risks even if you have an active lesion at birth

Explanation: The woman is evaluated for active genital herpes lesions at the time of delivery, and if lesions are present a cesarean delivery will be needed. It is one of the indications of the cesarean section.

1037. Moniliasis is caused by:
a. Candida albicans
b. Chlamydia trachomatis
c. Treponema pallidum
d. Neisseria gonorrhea

1038. Vaginitis is caused by:
a. Trichomoniasis b. Chlamydia trachomatis
c. Treponema pallidum d. Neisseria gonorrhea

1039. Which of the following is not a common cause for vaginitis? *(AIIMS-BBS SNO 2019)*
a. Salmonella b. Trichomonas
c. Candida d. Gardnerella

1040. Inflammation of vagina in postmenopausal women is known as:
a. Toxic shock syndrome
b. Senile vaginitis
c. Chancroid
d. Pelvic inflammatory disease

1041. Postmenopausal yellowish or blood stained vaginal discharge, soreness in the vulva and pruritus vulvae are the manifestations of:
a. Menopause
b. Chancroid
c. Pelvic inflammatory disease
d. Senile vaginitis

1042. Senile vaginitis is caused by:
a. Increased FSH level b. Estrogen deficiency
c. Progesterone deficiency d. LH deficiency

1043. PID is more common among:
a. Menstruating teenagers and multiple sexual partners
b. Using intrauterine devices
c. Absence of contraceptive pill use
d. All of the above

1044. Which of the following is one of the most frequent causes of salpingitis or pelvic inflammatory disease?
a. Chlamydia b. Streptococcus
c. Staphylococcus d. Treponema

1045. What is the site of referred pain when pain is arising from cervix? *(AIIMS Bhopal Nursing Officer, 2018)*
a. Anterior and medial aspect of thigh
b. Upper sacral region
c. Lower sacral region
d. Above the mid-inguinal point

Explanation: Upper sacral region is the site for referred pain which arises from cervix.

1046. Characteristic of vaginal discharge during vaginitis is:
a. Profuse and purulent b. Watery
c. Pus-stained d. Blood-stained

1047. Position given to the patient during vaginal surgery increases the risk for:
a. DVT b. Pulmonary edema
c. Dysrhythmia d. Jaundice

CERVICAL CANCER SCREENING

1048. Cervical cancer staging is primarily based upon:
a. Biopsy b. Age of female
c. Clinical examination d. Marital status

1049. Primary prevention for cervical cancer includes:
a. Raising the age of marriage
b. Use of condom during early intercourse
c. Effective therapy of STDs
d. All of the above

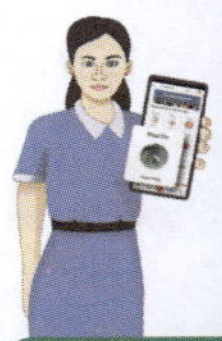

Ans.
1029. c
1030. d
1031. c
1032. b
1033. d
1034. d
1035. a
1036. b
1037. a
1038. a
1039. a
1040. b
1041. d
1042. b
1043. d
1044. a
1045. b
1046. a
1047. a
1048. c
1049. d

1050. Complications of hysteroscopy include:

a. Hemorrhage b. Uterine perforation
c. Infections d. All of these

1051. As per the guidelines of American Cancer Society, for a woman aged 45–54 years, a mammography is recommended:

a. Once a year b. Once in two years
c. Once in five years d. Once in ten years

1052. Early identification of cervical cancer can be done by:

a. HPV vaccine b. Colposcopy
c. Pap smears d. Ultrasonogram

1053. Which of the following surgery is appropriate for stage I and stage II cervical cancer?

a. Bilateral salpingo-oophorectomy
b. Simple total abdominal hysterectomy
c. Radical hysterectomy
d. Bilateral salpingectomy

1054. Predisposing factor for developing cervical cancer is:

a. 45-year-old nullipara
b. 45-year-old multipara
c. 36-year-old who had first child at 22 years
d. 30-year-old who is on oral contraceptives

1055. Cancer of the cervix is caused by ________ infection.

a. Treponema pallidum b. Trichomonas vaginalis
c. Neisseria gonorrheae d. Human papillomavirus

ANEMIA IN PREGNANCY

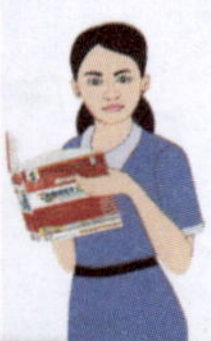

1056. Which of the following conditions is common in pregnant clients in the 2nd trimester of pregnancy? *(RAK MSc 2018)*

a. Breast abscess b. Metabolic acidosis
c. Physiologic anemia d. Respiratory alkalosis

Explanation: Hb level of antenatal mother goes down in second trimester and gradually rise in third trimester. As a result of plasma volume, increase in Hb dilution takes place. The demand of iron is increased specially in 2nd trimester. Thus, mother experiences physiologic anemia.

1057. Most important risk factor for puerperal sepsis include:

a. Lack of breastfeeding
b. Malnutrition and anemia during pregnancy
c. Unclean deliveries
d. Tetanus neonatorum

1058. The causes of physiological anemia in pregnancy is: *(RRB Feb 2012)*

a. Hemodilution b. Hemolysis
c. Hematopoiesis d. None of these

1059. Physiological anemia during pregnancy is a result of: *(LNJP H D 2012, RAK MSc 2018)*

a. Increased blood volume
b. Increased detoxification demands on mother's liver
c. Decreased dietary intake
d. Decreased erythropoiesis after first trimester

1060. Fall in hematocrit value is observed during pregnancy because:

a. Hemodilution
b. Hemoconcentration
c. Blood loss
d. Due to progesterone hormone

Explanation: The disproportionate increase in plasma and RBC volume produce a state of hemodilution which leads to fall in hematocrit during pregnancy.

1061. Adolescent pregnant mother is at risk for ...... complication during pregnancy.

a. Iron deficiency anemia b. Pre eclampsia
c. Eclampsia d. Diabetic mellitus

Explanation: Most commonly observing complication among pregnant adolescent mother is iron deficiency anemia.

1062. As per WHO, anemia in pregnancy is diagnosed if the hemoglobin level is:

a. <10 g/dL b. <11 g/dL
c. <12 g/dL d. <13 g/dL

Ref: https://www.who.int/vmnis/indicators/haemoglobin.pdf

Explanation: As per WHO, Anemia in pregnancy will be diagnosed if the hemoglobin level is <12 g/dL in a non-pregnant woman. But during pregnancy hemodilution occurs, so hemoglobin less than 11 gm/dL is considered as anemia during pregnancy.

1063. Which of the following hemoglobin value denotes anemia in a pregnant woman?

a. Hb 10 g/dL b. Hb 11 g/dL
c. Hb 12 g/dL d. Hb 13 g/dL

Explanation: Indian Council of Medical Research considers hemoglobin (Hb) level below 10.9 g/dL as cutoff point for anemia during pregnancy.

LACTATION AND FEEDING

1064. During which week of Pregnancy for the first time breast milk can be squeezed? *(AIIMS Raipur Staff Nurse Grade I-2018)*

a. 6th week b. 12th week
c. 18th week d. 24th week

1065. Which among the following is the appropriate measure for reducing the breast tenderness in the first trimester of pregnancy?

a. Wash breast with warm water and keep it dry
b. Wear tight clothes to support the breast
c. Expose the breast to air 2 hourly
d. Wash with soap and water 4 hourly

Explanation: Option A is the correct answer, soap use should be minimized and soap should not be applied in the areola because it will cause dryness.

1066. Calcium requirement during pregnancy is:

a. 1.5 gm/day b. 2.0 gm/day
c. 2.5 gm/day d. 3.0 gm/day

Explanation: According to WHO 1.5–2.0 gm oral elemental calcium.

1067. Additional amount of calorie that should be taken by a pregnant woman: *[NCFL 2019; RUHS-Pre MSc. 2007]:*

a. 300 Kcal
b. 500 Kcal
c. 1000 Kcal
d. 100 Kcal

Ans.

1050. d
1051. a
1052. c
1053. c
1054. b
1055. d
1056. c
1057. b
1058. a
1059. a
1060. a
1061. a
1062. b
1063. a
1064. b
1065. a
1066. a
1067. a

1068. Which of the following dietary supplements should be recommended for a pregnant woman who is on heparin therapy?

a. Folic acid b. Zinc
c. Potassium d. Calcium

1069. During a routine prenatal visit, a pregnant client reports heartburn. To minimize her discomfort, nurse should include which suggestion in the plan of care? *(RAK MSc 2018)*

a. Drink more citrus juice b. Eat small, frequent meals
c. Limit fluid intake sharply d. Take sodium bicarbonate

Explanation: To minimize heartburn, patient is advised to avoid overeating and not to go to the bed immediately after having food. Patient can eat small food in frequent intervals.

1070. Which among the following food group is the most preferred food group by pregnant mothers?

a. High fat and low protein.
b. High protein and low carbohydrate.
c. High protein and low fat.
d. High carbohydrate and high fat.

1071. According to WHO, when should the mother starts, breastfeeding to the infant? *(RAK MSc 2018)*

a. Within 30 minutes after birth
b. Within 18 hours after birth
c. After infant's condition stabilizes
d. Within a day after birth

Explanation: As per WHO criteria breastfeeding should be started soon after birth (within 30 minutes to 1 hour). It helps in thermoregulation of baby by skin to skin contact. Release of oxytocin during breastfeeding helps in control of uterine bleeding. Other options are distractors.

1072. The advantages of breastfeeding include the following; EXCEPT: *(AIIMS Raipur Grade II 2017)*

a. Promotion of gastrointestinal function
b. Fostering immune defense
c. Nutritional imbalance d. Economic advantage

Explanation: The advantages of breastfeeding for mother and baby include stronger bones, long term protection, lower SIDS, calorie incinerator, cheap, less risk of cancer, etc.

1073. Benefits of breastfeeding include all; EXCEPT: *(NCFL 2019)*

a. It provides nutrients
b. Colostrum provides a high level of immune protection
c. Less prone for gastrointestinal infection
d. It provides adequate iron to premature newborn

Explanation: Human milk contains little iron, so infants who are exclusively breastfed are at increased risk of iron deficiency after four months of age. The iron storage in preterm infant is less because Iron is mostly accumulated during the third trimester of gestation.

1074. Which of the following measures would the nurse include in the teaching plan about the method to prevent breast engorgement in postpartum period? *(RAK MSc 2018)*

a. Breastfeeding neonate at frequent intervals
b. Decreasing fluid intake for the first 24–48 hours
c. Feeding the neonate, a maximum of 5 minutes per side on the first day
d. Wearing a supportive brassiere with nipple shields

Explanation: Breast engorgement is accumulation of milk in alveoli of breast. It indicates poor breastfeeding so a nurse will teach the client to breastfeed the neonate in frequent intervals in correct position.

1075. Endocrine control of lactation can be seen in:

a. Lactogenesis b. Galactokinesis
c. Galactopoiesis d. All of these

Explanation: Endocrine control of lactation can be seen in Lactogenesis, Galactokinesis, Galactopoiesis and mammogenesis. Mammogenesis means preparation of breast, lactogenesis means synthesis and secretion of milk, galactokinesis means ejection of milk and galactopoiesis means maintenance of lactation. All these are the endocrine control and preparation for lactation.

1076. Let down reflex is also known as:

a. Milk secreting reflex b. Milk ejection reflex
c. Rooting reflex d. Sucking reflex

Explanation: Let down reflex or milk ejecting reflex is produced by oxytocin hormone. It helps in the milk ejection from breast tissue.

1077. Lochia is:

a. Change in vital sign after delivery
b. Vaginal discharge after giving birth
c. Going back of the body to pre-pregnant state
d. Decrease in pigmentation

Explanation: Lochia is the vaginal discharge after giving birth (puerperium) containing blood, mucus, and uterine tissue. Lochia discharge typically continues for 4–6 weeks after childbirth, which is known as the postpartum period.

1078. Drug used to improve the milk production is: *New Q*

a. Metoclopramide b. Sulpiride
c. Dopamine d. All of these

Explanation: Metoclopramide 10 mg TDS will improve the milk production by increasing the prolactin level. Sulpiride, dopamine antagonist has also been found effective.

1079. Immunoglobulin present in breast milk is:

a. IgA b. IgD
c. IgG d. IgM

Explanation: IgA provides immunological defence to the newborn and is present in breast milk.

1080. Only immunoglobulin which can cross the placenta is:

a. IgA b. IgM
c. IgG d. IgE

1081. As per WHO, breastfeeding needs to be initiated within .... after delivery.

a. 20 minutes b. 30 minutes
c. 45 minutes d. 60 minuets

Explanation: Breastfeeding needs to be initiated within 30 minutes following delivery.

1082. The hindmilk is rich in:

a. Fats and vitamins
b. Vitamins and minerals
c. Fats and energy
d. Proteins and energy

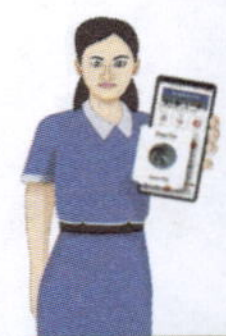

Ans.

1068. d
1069. b
1070. c
1071. a
1072. c
1073. d
1074. a
1075. d
1076. b
1077. b
1078. a
1079. a
1080. c
1081. b
1082. c

1083. The milk secreted, 2 weeks after delivery of the baby is known as:
a. Colostrums b. Mature milk
c. Transitional milk d. Foremilk

1084. Lactose present in a milk is a: *(Banaras HU 2015)*
a. Polysaccharide b. Disaccharide
c. Heteropolysaccharide d. Monosaccharide

1085. Which one of the following is a major protein present in human milk? *(Banaras HU 2015)*
a. Lactalbumin b. Lactoglobulin
c. Casein d. Lactoferrin

1086. The pituitary hormone that stimulates secretion of milk is: *(JIPMER 2012; RRB Feb 2012)*
a. Prolactin b. Oxytocin
c. Estrogen d. Progesterone

1087. Milk ejection occurs due to the hormone:
a. Prolactin b. Estrogen
c. Vasopressin d. Oxytocin

1088. The phase of ejection of milk is called:
a. Mammogenesis b. Lactogenesis
c. Galactopoiesis d. Galactokinesis

1089. Which of the following responses is expected in a mother when the baby is sucking the breast? *(Banaras HU 2015)*
a. Increase of adrenaline
b. Increase of prolactin-inhibiting factor
c. Increase of hypothalamic dopamine
d. Increase of oxytocin

1090. The practice of keeping mother and child together immediately after birth is known as: *(LNJP H D 2012)*
a. Rooming in b. Bonding
c. Puerperium d. Lying in

1091. The process of milk synthesis and secretion from the breast alveoli is called:
a. Mammogenesis b. Lactogenesis
c. Galactokinesis d. Galactopoiesis

1092. During postpartum stage, which of the following medicines can be used to suppress lactation?
a. Oxytocin b. Levonorgestrel
c. Bromocriptine d. Both b and c

1093. Breast engorgement occurs due to:
a. Poor sucking by the baby
b. Over production of breast milk
c. Accumulation in milk ducts
d. All of the above

1094. Which among the following sequences indicates correct mechanism behind lactational amenorrhea?
a. Increased prolactin level → inhibits ovarian response to FSH → less follicular growth → hypoestrogen state → No menstrual cycle
b. Increased prolactin level → suppress the release of LH → No LH surge → Anovulation
c. Both a and b
d. None of the above

1095. When the normal delivery breastfeeding needs to be initiated?
a. Soon after delivery b. 15 minutes after delivery
c. 30 minutes after delivery d. 1 hour after delivery

1096. The most significant constituent of human breast milk by weight is:
a. Carbohydrate b. Water
c. Protein d. Fat

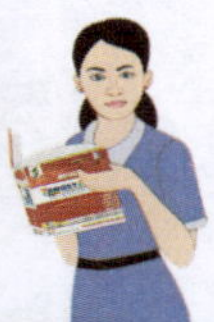

Ans.
1083. b
1084. b
1085. c
1086. a
1087. d
1088. d
1089. d
1090. a
1091. b
1092. c
1093. d
1094. c
1095. a
1096. b
1097. a
1098. d
1099. b
1100. c
1101. a
1102. b
1103. d
1104. a

GTPAL

1097. Gravida indicates:
a. Pregnancy state both present and past
b. State of previous pregnancy beyond the period of viability
c. The number of babies has
d. All of the above

1098. A woman who is pregnant for the first time.
a. Primipara b. Multipara
c. Nuligravida d. Primigravida

1099. A woman who has never completed the pregnancy beyond the stage of viability is known as:
a. Primipara b. Nullipara
c. Nulligravida d. Primigravida

1100. Woman who has never been pregnant is:
a. Primipara b. Nullipara
c. Nulligravida d. Primigravida

1101. A female who has given birth to one viable child is termed: *(RAK MSc 2018)*
a. Primipara b. Multipara
c. Nulligravida d. Primigravida

Explanation:
- The pregnancy beyond the period of viability is called parity. A woman who has given birth to one viable child will be referred to as Primipara.
- **Multipara:** A mother who has completed two or more pregnancies to the stage of viability.
- Primigravida is the woman who has been pregnant for the first time. Gravida (G) denotes a pregnant state (number of times female has been pregnant) both present and past, irrespective of period of gestation.
- **Nulligravida:** A woman who has not now and never been pregnant.

1102. Rama is pregnant for the first time and at 12 weeks POG, her USG is suggestive of twin pregnancy. Her gravida is:
a. Gravida 0 b. Gravida 1
c. Gravida 2 d. Gravida 1+1

Explanation: Rama is pregnant for the first time so gravida 1. Even if the woman is having twin pregnancy it will be considered as gravida 1.

1103. Sheela comes to the ANC clinic for her 2nd antenatal visit. Her history is suggestive of 2 previous abortions and one term delivery. Her gravida and parity is:
a. G1P1 b. G2P1
c. G3P1 d. G4P1

Explanation: Sheela has history of 2 abortions, one term delivery and presently she is pregnant so gravida is 4. Since she has only one term delivery her para is still 1.

1104. G3P 1 +2 means:
a. Three time pregnant with 1 viable birth and 2 abortions
b. Three time pregnant with 1 abortion and 2 viable births
c. Three time pregnant with 1 single baby and 2 twins
d. Three time pregnant with 1 twin delivery and 2 abortions

Explanation: G3 means three time pregnant, P1+2 means 1 viable birth and 2 miscarriages (abortion).

1105. Grand multipara is:
- a. Pregnant woman with previous history of four or more births
- b. Pregnant woman with first pregnancy at the age of 30 or above
- c. Pregnant woman with previous history of 2 abortions
- d. Woman with pregnancy at the age of 18 years

1106. Elderly primigravida is defined as: *(RAK MSc 2018)*
- a. Woman having her first pregnancy above the age of 25
- b. Woman having pregnancy above the age of 30
- c. Woman having her first pregnancy below the age of 18
- d. Woman having her first pregnancy above the age of 35

Explanation: Women having pregnancy above the age of 35 years are considered elderly primigravida (FIGO classification). Women having their first pregnancy below the age of 18 years are called adolescent mothers.

CARE OF NEWBORN

1107. A newborn who is above the 90th percentile on the Intrauterine Growth Curve is termed: *(DSSSB PHN, 2015)*
- a. Post-term baby
- b. Large for gestational age
- c. Small for gestational age
- d. Preterm baby

1108. Mother has given with opioid during labor process, which among the following drugs most commonly ordered by doctor for the newborn baby?
- a. Naloxone
- b. Morphine
- c. Calcium gluconate
- d. Adrenaline

Explanation: Use of opioid causes respiratory depression in newborn baby. The antedote naloxone will be ordered by the doctor for newborn baby.

1109. Among the following, which sign indicates that newborn is adapting well with the external environment?
- a. Nasal flare
- b. Chest in drawing
- c. Retractions
- d. Respiration rate 40-60 breaths/min

Explanation: Respiratory rate of 40-60 breaths/min is normal in newborn and is showing the adaptation with extra uterine environment.

1110. A neonate has been diagnosed with cephalohematoma. Which is the incorrect statement regarding the diagnosis?
- a. Collection of blood between pericranium and flat skull bone
- b. It is never present at the time of birth
- c. Swelling is limited by the suture line
- d. It involves swelling of the tissue over the presenting part of the head

Explanation: Option d is the statement related to caput succedaneum. All other statements are correct in relation to cephalohematoma.

1111. Newborn at risk for developing RDS is:
- a. Newborn with period of gestation < 30 week
- b. Newborn of diabetic mother
- c. Newborn who passed meconium in the uterus
- d. All of the above

Explanation: In all the above conditions newborn is at risk for developing RDS.

1112. Neonates born to woman infected with hepatitis B should undergo which treatment:
- a. Hepatitis B vaccine at birth and 1 month
- b. Hepatitis B immune globulin at birth, no hepatitis B vaccine
- c. Hepatitis B immune globulin within 48 hours of birth and Hepatitis B vaccine at 1 month
- d. Hepatitis B immune globulin within 12 hours of birth and Hepatitis B vaccine at birth, 1 month, 6 months

Explanation: Hepatitis B immune globulin should be given as soon as possible after birth but within 12 hours.

1113. Which of the following findings in a newborn baby girl is normal? *(LNJP H D 2012)*
- a. Bleeding from umbilicus
- b. Respiratory rate of 70/minute at rest
- c. Yellow skin tone at 12 hours of age
- d. Passage of meconium within the first 24 hours

1114. Average birth weight of an Indian baby is: *(RRB Feb 2012)*
- a. 3.5 kg
- b. 2 kg
- c. 4 kg
- d. 3 kg

1115. Human fetus has a coat of hair called: *(RRB Feb 2012)*
- a. Lanugo
- b. Vernix
- c. Striac
- d. None of these

1116. The killing of a newborn child by its parents is called: *(RRB Feb 2012)*
- a. Restitution
- b. Infanticide
- c. Neocide
- d. Infantism

1117. Newborn baby automatically turns the face towards the stimulus and makes sucking. This reflex is known as:
- a. Startle reflex
- b. Rooting reflex
- c. Glabellar reflex
- d. Corneal reflex

1118. Serious danger associated with LBW baby is:
- a. Respiratory distress
- b. Feeding problem
- c. Thermoregulation problem
- d. Hemorrhage

1119. A diabetic female at 40 weeks of gestation delivered a baby by elective cesarean section. Soon after birth the baby developed respiratory distress. The diagnosis is:
- a. Transient tachypnea of the newborn
- b. Congenital diaphragmatic hernia
- c. Tracheoesophageal fistula
- d. Hyaline membrane disease

Explanation: Transient tachypnea of the newborn (TTN) is a common respiratory condition that occurs shortly after birth, usually in term or near-term infants. It is characterized by rapid breathing (tachypnea) and signs of respiratory distress.

In the given scenario, the baby's respiratory distress is likely due to transient tachypnea. This condition can occur in infants delivered by cesarean section, especially if there was limited exposure to the normal squeezing of the birth canal, which helps expel fluid from the lungs. The baby may have retained fluid in the lungs, leading to respiratory symptoms.

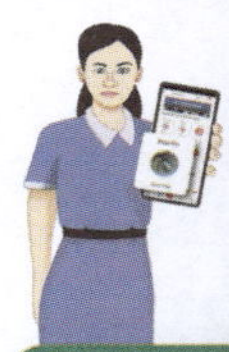

Ans.

1105. a
1106. d
1107. b
1108. a
1109. d
1110. d
1111. d
1112. d
1113. d
1114. d
1115. a
1116. b
1117. b
1118. a
1119. a

"If you would live long, open your heart."
—Bulgarian

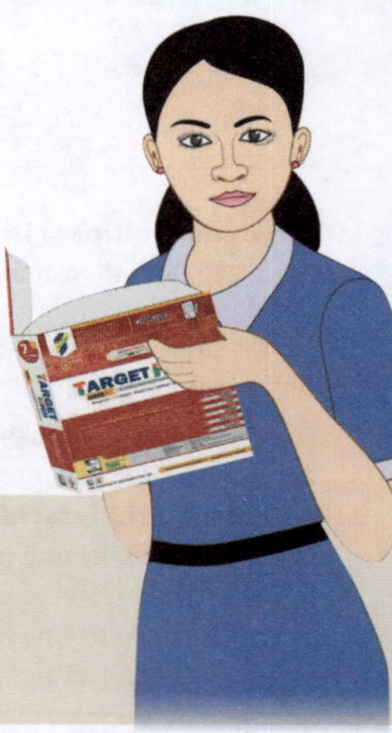

CHAPTER 8

APPLIED MICROBIOLOGY

SYNOPSIS

HISTORICAL PERSPECTIVES OF MICROBIOLOGY

- **Microbiology:** It is the study of microorganism which is only visible through microscope.
- Aristotle (384-322) and others believed that living organisms could develop from non-living materials.
- Rogen bacon in 13th century described that the disease caused by a minute "seed" or "germ".
- **Antony van Leeuwenhoek (1632–1723)**
  - Descriptions of protozoa, basic types of bacteria, yeasts, and algae.
  - The first to see and describe bacteria and their characteristic morphology.
  - Father of bacteriology and protozoology.
  - In 1676, he observed and described microorganisms such as bacteria and protozoa as "animalcules".
- **1798:** Edward Jenner introduces the concepts of vaccination using cowpox material to prevent small pox.
- **Louis Pasteur:**
  - He coined the term "microbiology", aerobic, anaerobic.
  - He disproved the theory of spontaneous germination.
  - He contributed to the development of the first vaccines for the immunization against rabies, anthrax, and chicken cholera.
  - He described the scientific basis for fermentation, winemaking, and the brewing of beer and pasteurization.
  - Pasteur postulated the **germ theory of disease,** which states that microorganisms are the causes of infectious disease.
- **Joseph Lister (1827–1912)**
  - He is the father of antiseptic surgery.
- **Robert Koch**
  - Discovered causative agent for anthrax, tuberculosis, and cholera.
  - His discoveries, in combination with those of Pasteur, established the germ theory of disease
- **Edward Jenner (1749–1823)**
  - First to prevent small pox.
  - He discovered the technique of vaccination.
- **Alexander Fleming**
  - Discovered penicillin in 1929, an antibiotic produced by a fungus that inhibits bacterial growth.
- **Paul Ehrlich:** In 1882 he reported the acid-fastness of tubercle bacillus.

THE NORMAL BACTERIAL FLORA OF HUMAN BODY

Resident Flora

These organisms are relatively fixed and regular type of organism found at a given body site. They perform functions such as synthesis of vitamin K, absorption of nutrient, breakdown of nutrients, etc.

Transient Flora

These are non-pathogenic and potentially pathogenic organisms. These microorganisms do not produce disease under normal circumstances. But if normal flora is destroyed and immune system is weak then they may produce disease.

KEY POINTS

- **Louis Pasteur** (1822-1895) is considered the father of microbiology.
- **Louis Pasteur introduced sterilization** technique and stem sterilizer, autoclave and hot air oven.
- **Louis Pasteur** introduced first live-attenuated vaccine.
- **Robert Koch** is known as the **father of bacteriology.**
- **Robert Koch** introduced **staining technique.**
- **Robert Koch** discovered anthrax bacillus, tubercle bacillus and the cholera vibrios.
- **Joseph Lister** introduced antiseptic surgery.
- **Karl Landsteiner** discovered **ABO blood groups.**
- **Alexander Fleming** discovered the drug **penicillin.**

Normal Flora

Table 1: Normal flora of various body sites

Body site	Name of normal flora
Eye (conjunctiva)	*Corynebacterium xerosis*, coagulase negative staphylococci, nonhemolytic streptococci,
Mouth and upper respiratory tract	*Streptococcus viridans*, diphtheroids, coagulase negative staphylococci, anaerobic cocci, anaerobic spirochaetes, bacteroides, anaerobic cocci, *fusobacterium*.
Gastrointestinal tract	Lactobacilli, anaerobic streptococci, *Clostridium*, *Bacteroides*
Genitourinary	*Mycobacterium smegmatis*, alpha hemolytic streptococci, lactobacilli, *Gardnerella vaginalis*, and *Bacteroides spp*, anamerobic streptococci, clostridia, *Ureaplasma urealyticum*
Skin	*Staphylococcus epidermis* (major), *Staphyloccocus aureus,* Micrococci, Diphtheroids, Propionibacterium, Yeast *(Candida sp.)*

STAINING TECHNIQUES

- **Simple stain**: Methylene blue
- **Negative stain**: Negative stain produces uniform colored background against which uncolored organism strands out, e.g., India ink preparation.
- **Impregnation stains**: Cells and structures that are too thin to be visualized by the light microscope can be rendered visible by impregnation of silver on their surface.

Differential Stain

- Gram's stain
- Acid-fast stain
- Albert's stain

Gram's Stain

- Developed by Christian Gram in 1884.
- It is used to study morphology of bacteria.
- When bacteria are treated with basic dyes such as methyl violet, crystal violet or gentian violet and then with iodine, they retain their color even after decolorization with alcohol/acetone. The microorganisms which retain the color and appear violet in color are called Gram-positive bacteria. On the other hand, the microorganism decolorized will be seen with the help of a counter stain that give them red/pink color and are called Gram-negative.

Acid-Fast Stain

- Normal dyes do not penetrate Mycobacterium. Therefore, the dye containing phenol and application of heat enables it to penetrate the cell wall of mycobacteria. Once the bacteria are stained then they withstand the action of powerful decolorizing agent for a considerable duration of time.
- Acid-fast bacilli (AFB) appear as bright-red structure, whereas tissue, other organisms are seen as blue/green depending upon the counterstain used.

Albert's Stain

- It is used to stain the volutin granules of **diphtheria bacilli**.
- These granules have intense affinity towards basic dyes.

TYPES OF MICROSCOPE

- Light microscopes (Compound microscope)
- Fluorescence microscope
- Dark ground microscope
- Phase contrast microscope
- Interference microscope
- Electron microscope

CULTURE MEDIA

Solid Media, Liquid Media and Semisolid Media

- In culture media, agar is the agent used for solidifying purpose.
- By varying the concentration of sugar, media can be prepared as solid/semisolid.
- Solid media, e.g., blood agar, chocolate agar, MacConkey's agar.
- Liquid media, e.g., nutrient broth, peptone water, sugar media and enrichment media.

Aerobic and Anaerobic Media

Aerobic

- To promote the growth of aerobic organisms, aerobic media is used.
  Example: *E. coli, Salmonella serotypes, Mycobacterium tuberculosis,* etc.

Anaerobic

- Organisms that are unable to use oxygen are known as anaerobic organisms.
- Roberston's cooked meat (Cooked meat broth) media is used to grow anaerobic organism of anaerobic organisms:
  Examples: *Clostridium spp, Bacteroides spp, Peptococcus spp, Pepto-streptococcus spp.*
  Examples of anaerobic media: Leaked blood agar, brain heart infection broth with thioglycollate.

KEY POINTS

Advantages of normal flora:

- Normal flora competes with pathogens for colonization sites.
- It produces substance that inhibit pathogens.
- Normal flora stimulates local immunity.
- Production of vitamins in intestines

Disadvantages of normal flora:

- Source of opportunistic infection in immunosuppressed patients.
- **Oral cavity:** Normal flora of oral cavity causes Plaque formation and dental disease.
- **GI tract:** Causes gastric and duodenal ulcer (e.g., *H. pylori*). Transfer of antibiotic resistance to pathogens
- **Colon:** Production of pathogens. Associated with colon cancer

Enriched Media

- Substances like blood (The most common sheep blood), serum and egg are added to basic media to prepare enriched media.

Example: Blood agar, chocolate agar, Lowenstein-Jensen medium.

Selective Media

- As the name indicates these media selectively inhibit the growth of some microorganisms and permit the isolation of some other microorganisms. These are solid media.

Example: Thiosulphate citrate bile sucrose (TCBS): This medium is used for isolation of *Vibrio cholerae.*

Mannitol salt agar (MSA): This medium is used for isolation of *Staphylococcus aureus*

Enrichment Media

- These media favor the growth of wanted microorganisms and inhibit the growth of unwanted microorganisms. These are liquid media.

Example: Selenite F broth promotes the growth of Salmonella serotype Typhi.

Indicator/Differential Media

- When microorganisms are incorporated to these kind of media different microorganisms show different characteristics.

Example: On MacConkey's medium, lactose fermenters like *E. coli* form pink colonies while non-lactose fermenters like serotype Typhi for pale yellow colonies.

Transport Media

- These media maintain the viability of microorganisms present in the specimen without supporting the growth of any organisms, so that no microorganism overgrows another or dies out.

Example: Thioglycolate broth is for strict anaerobes.

Sugar Media

To a basal medium any fermentable substances such as glucose, lactose or glycerol is added then it is known as sugar media.

Storage Media

Bacteria are best preserved by lyophilization. But for preservation and storage for a few months or so, they can be stab inoculated on semisolid agar or dorset egg medium followed by incubation. When growth appears they can be stored in refrigerator.

KEY POINTS

- **Transport medium** is a special medium which inhibits self-destruction and multiplication of microbes but maintains "status quo" condition.
- Venkataraman Ramakrishna (VR) medium is transport media used for V. cholerae.

Recent Question (NORCET 2022)

1. **Effective disinfectant for COVID in hospital settings is:**
   a. Hydrochloric acid
   b. Sodium hypochlorite
   c. Sulfuric acid
   d. Phenol

Ans. (b) Sodium hypochlorite

BIOCHEMICAL REACTIONS

Table 2: Various tests and their biochemical reactions

Reaction	To know
Carbohydrate fermentation test	Ability of an organism to ferment
Indole test	Ability of an organism to decompose amino acid tryptophan to indole
Citrate test	Ability of an organism to utilize citrate as sole source of carbon for metabolism with resulting growth and alkalinity.
Klinger's agar/triple sugar iron agar test	Ability of an organism to use specific carbohydrate incorporated into the media
Phenylalanine Deaminase test	Ability of an organism to deaminate phenylalanine to phenyl pyruvic acid
Urease test	Ability of an organism to split urea using urease with resulting alkalinity
Nitrate reduction test	To determine the presence of enzyme nitrate reductase in an organism
Oxidase test	Used to determine the presence of enzyme oxidase in an organism
Catalase test	Used to check the presence of enzyme catalase in an organism

GENERAL GUIDELINES FOR COLLECTING CULTURE SPECIMEN

- Try to obtain specimen always from the patient before the initiation of antimicrobial agent.
- Personal protection needs to be ensured by the healthcare professional whoever is collecting the specimen.
- Quantity of the specimen should be adequate to carry out the specific test ordered.
- Blood culture bottle should not be refrigerated once the blood sample is added to it. Keep it in incubator at 37°C or at room temperature.
- CSF sample (except those for viral culture) should not be refrigerated. Keep it in the incubator at 37°C.
- Midstream urine sample needs to be collected as sample and if any delay in sending to the laboratory, keep it in refrigerator.
- Sample collected for viral culture needs to be transported in ice medium.

Guidelines for other samples like throat, stool sample, sputum sample needs to be incorporated.

KEY POINT

Culture media are sterilized by autoclaving method.

Types of Disinfectant/Antiseptic

Table 3: Types of disinfectant/antiseptic

Types	Examples
Alcohol	70% alcohol
Aldehydes	Formaldehyde (3–8%), gluteraldehyde (2%)
Biguanides	Chlorhexidine
Halogen releasing agent	Hypochlorites (1–2%), povidone-iodine
Phenols	Chloroxylenol, hexachlorophene
Heavy metal derivatives	Salt of heavy metal such as silver and mercury
Peroxygen	Hydrogen peroxide

- All the articles are to be cleaned with soap and water before disinfecting it.
- **Sterilization:** It destroys or removes all microorganisms including spores.
- HIV, HBV and HCV are the three important blood-borne pathogens that affect the healthcare workers (HCWs).
- Immunity is a state of resistance to microorganism and their products.
- WBCs are responsible for immune response.
- Immunity against disease condition can be natural (innate) or acquired (adaptive).

KEY POINTS

- A chemical agent that inhibits bacterial growth is called **bacteriostat**.
- A chemical agent that kills bacteria is called **bactericidal**.
- T cells are responsible for cell-mediated immunity.
- B lymphocytes are responsible for humoral immunity or antibody-mediated immunity.
- **Pleomorphic Bacteria** have variable shape (bacteria with changeable shape).
- Spherical bacteria occurring in clusters are called *Staphylococcus*
- **Vibrio cholerae** are **coma-shaped** bacilli.

CLASSIFICATION OF BACTERIA

Shapes and Arrangement of Bacteria

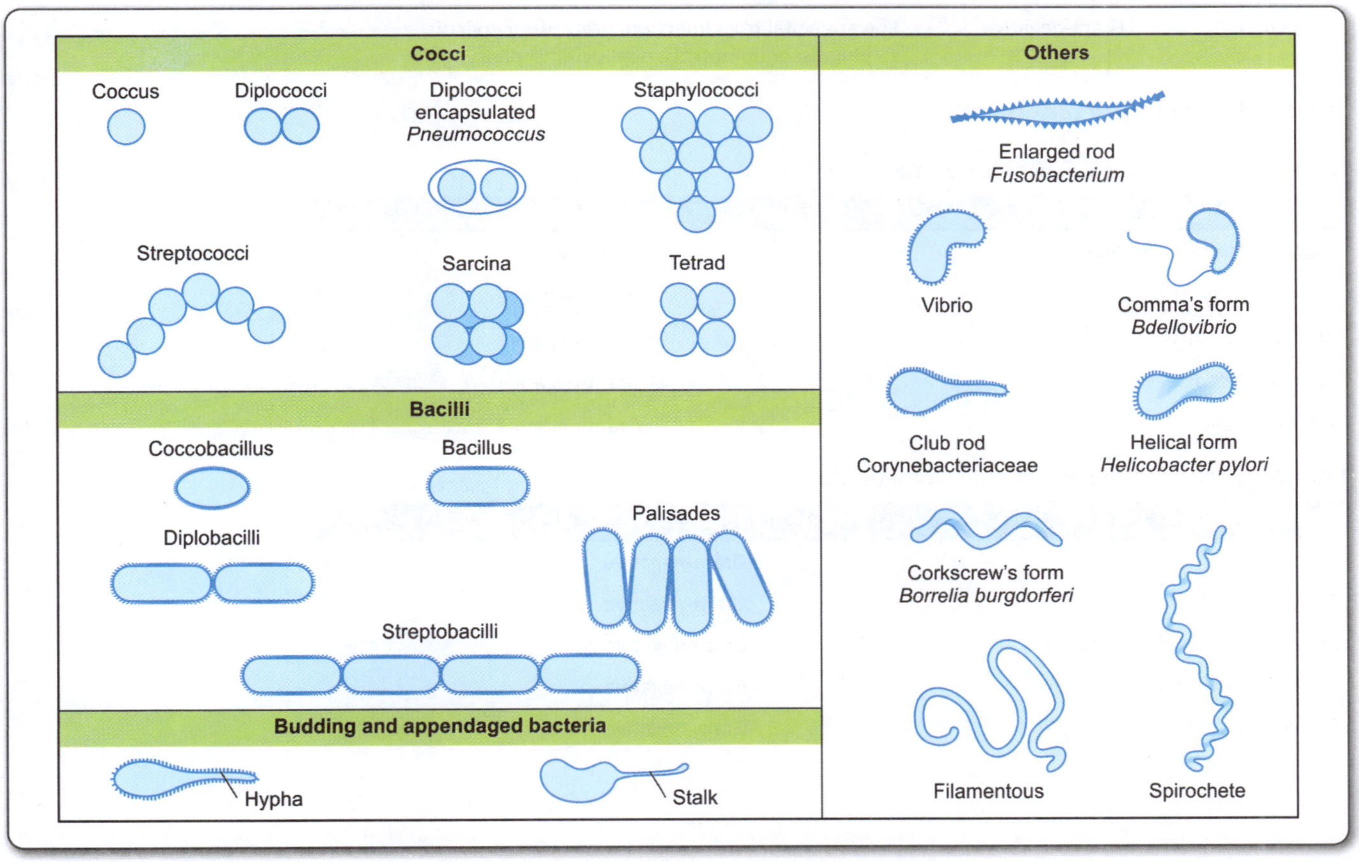

Figure 1: Bacterial morphology

Gram-Positive and Gram-Negative Bacteria

Table 4: Gram-positive and Gram-negative bacteria

Gram-positive bacteria	Gram-negative bacteria
• *Staphylococcus* • *Streptococcus* • *Pneumococcus* • *Mycobacterium* • *Clostridium tetani* • *Bacillus anthracis* • *Lactobacillus*	• *Neisseria gonorrhoeae* • *Neisseria meningitidis* • *Pseudomonas* • *Vibrio cholerae* • *Salmonella* • *Escherichia coli* • *Shigella* • *Brucella*

The Medically Important Cocci

Table 5: Diseases with their causative cocci

Cocci	Types	Diseases
Staphylococcus	Gram-positive	*Staphylococcus aureus:* breast abscess, wound infection, pneumonia, acute osteomyelitis, meningitis, endocarditis, renal abscess, food poisoning,
Streptococcus	Gram-positive	Sore throat, scarlet fever, pyoderma, acute rheumatic fever, glomerulonephritis, pharyngitis,
Enterococcus	Gram-positive	Bacteremia, surgical wound infection, urinary tract infection, endocarditis
Pneumococcus	Gram-positive	Acute bacterial meningitis, otitis media, conjunctivitis, sinusitis, empyema, peritonitis
Meningococcus	Gram-negative	Septicemia, meningitis,
Gonococcus	Gram-negative	Lower genital tract infection, urethritis, cervicitis, salpingitis, endometritis, epididymitis, pharyngitis

The Medically Important Bacilli

Table 6: Bacilli associated with respiratory tract infection

Microorganisms	Types
Corynebacterium diphtheria	Gram-positive
Hemophilus influenzae	Gram-negative
Bordetella pertussis	Gram-negative
Legionnaire's disease	Gram-negative
Klebsiella species	Gram-negative

Table 7: Bacilli associated with infections of intestinal wall

Microorganisms	Types
E. coli	Gram-negative
Typhoid, paratyphoid	Gram-negative
Dysentery bacilli (*Shigella spp*)	Gram-negative
Proteus spp normal	Gram-negative
Pseudomonas normal	Gram-negative

KEY POINTS

- **Acetone** is the decolorizing agent used in Gram staining.
- ***E. coli*** is a Gram negative motile bacillus.
- *E. coli* is the most common cause of Urinary Tract Infection (UTI).
- *Staphylococcus aureus* is a Gram-positive cocci associated with infective endocarditis in IV drug users.
- ***Clostridium perfringens*** causes gas **gangrene.**
- ***Clostridium botulinum*** is spore forming, non-motile, encapsulated bacterium. It causes **food poisoning.**

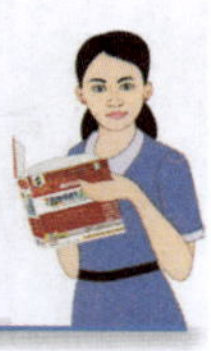

Spore-bearing Medically Important Bacilli

Table 8: Diseases and their causative spore-bearing bacilli

Microorganisms	Types	Diseases
Clostridium tetani	Gram-positive	Tetanus
Clostridium perfringens	Gram-positive	Gas gangrene
Clostridium botulinum	Gram-positive	Botulism (food poisoning)
Clostridium difficile	Gram-positive	Pseudomembranous colitis
Bacillus anthracis	Gram-positive	Anthrax

Bacilli Derived from Infected Animal

Table 9: Diseases and their causative bacilli

Microorganisms	Types	Diseases
Plague bacillus	Gram-negative	Plague
Brucella spp	Gram-negative	Brucellosis

The Causative Organisms

Table 10: Diseases and their causative organisms

Microorganism	Types	Disease
Vibrio cholerae	Gram-negative	Cholera
Campylobacters	Gram-negative rods	Diarrhea
Helicobacter pylori	Gram-negative	Gastric/Duodenal ulcer
Bacteroides	Gram-negative	Abdominal, brain and lung abscess

Diagnostic Tests Done

Table 11: Various diseases and their diagnostic tests

Diagnostic tests	Diseases
Paul-Bunnelf test	Infectious Mononucleosis
Mantoux test	Tuberculosis (TB)
Schick test	Diphtheria
Widal test	Typhoid
VDRL test	Syphilis
Dick Test	Scarlet fever
Weil-felix reaction	Typhus fever

VIRUS

- It is the smallest known infective agents.
- Virus carry its own genetic information in the form of DNA or RNA.
- Genome is protected by an outer protein coat (capsid) composed of capsomers.
- The stages of viral replication are adsorption, entry into cells, uncoating, biosynthesis, virion assembly and release
- It has no metabolic activity outsides the host cell.
- Viruses vary in shape from the simple helical and icosahedral to more complex structures.
- Antibiotics have no effect on viruses, but antiviral drugs have been developed to treat life-threatening infections.
- Vaccines that produce lifelong immunity can prevent some viral infections.

KEY POINTS

- ***T. pallidum*** is the causative agent of **syphilis.**
- **VDRL** (Venereal Disease Research Laboratory) test is done for the **diagnosis of syphilis.**
- **Poxviruses are the largest** and most complex of all viruses.
- **Hepatitis B** is caused by **DNA virus** and all other types of hepatitis are caused by RNA viruses.
- **Most common cause of diarrhea in children in the age group of 6–24 months: Rotavirus**
- Most common cause of Acute Hemorrhagic Conjunctivitis: Enterovirus (70%).
- The main cause of **genital warts** (Condylomata Acuminata) is human papilloma virus (HPV).
- HIV is called retrovirus.

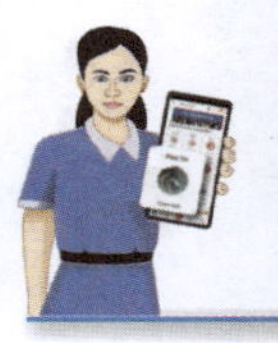

FUNGUS

- Fungi constitute a large, diverse group of heterotrophic organisms, most of which found as saprophytes in the soil and on decaying plant material.
- Fungi classified into yeasts, yeast-like, molds and dimorphic fungi.
- Mycoses can be classified into superficial, subcutaneous, systemic, and opportunistic.
- Candidiasis is the most common mycosis involving skin and its appendages, mucosa and internal organs.

PARASITES

- These are an animal or plant which lives in or upon another organism and derives its nutrient directly from it.
- Parasites are classified as protozoa (unicellular organisms) and helminths (multicellular organisms).
- Parasites exist in three morphological forms trophozoite, precyst and cyst.

KEY POINTS

- **Definitive host - sexual** replication of parasite occurs.
- **Intermediate host - asexual** replication of parasite occurs

Golden Points to Remember

- Bacterial cell division occurs by **binary fission.**
- **Hot air oven is a dry heat** sterilization method while **autoclave is moist heat** sterilization method.
- Temperature and time required in **hot air oven is 160°C for one hour or 180°C for 2 minutes** for sterilization.
- Temperature and time required in **autoclave** is **121°C for 30 minutes at a pressure of 15 pounds** per square inch.
- **Filtration** is a method adopted to sterilize sera, sugar and antibiotic solutions.
- A **parasite** is a microorganism which lives on a living host and derives nutrition from the host without any benefits to the host. It causes disease in the host.
- **Antigen** is a substance introduction of this into the body evoke immune reaction.
- **Clostridial pathogenicity** is mainly because of the production of **exotoxin.**
- Mycoplasma differ from other bacteria because they lack a rigid cell wall.
- **Mycoplasma** are the **smallest free living** microorganism.
- **HBsAg** is also called Australia antigen.
- **Definitive host** in which **sexual** replication of parasite occurs.
- **Intermediate host** in which **asexual** replication of parasite occurs.
- **Louis Pasteur** proposed the **germ theory** of disease.
- **Robert Koch** proved/confirmed the germ theory of disease.
- **Mycobacterium leprae** was the first bacterium identified causing disease in humans.
- Mycobacterium tuberculosis is also known as **Koch's bacillus.**
- **Antony Van Leeuwenhoek** developed **microscope** first time.
- **Knoll and Ruska** developed **electron microscope.**
- In bacteria, **mesosome** is responsible for **respiration**, cell division and sporulation.
- Capsule of the bacteria helps it to enable adherence to surface, protection against phagocytosis, and prevents desiccation and provides nutrients.
- Bacteria that are unable to synthesize their own food materials are called **Heterotrophs.**
- Mesophilic bacteria grow best between 25°C and 40°C temperature.
- **Differential staining** gives different colors to different bacteria.
- **Hanging Drop Method** is used to observe the **motility of a microbe.**
- **Blood and Bone Marrow Sample** should be incubated at **37°C** during storage prior to processing.
- Bacteria that thrive in high temperature (40°C–70°C) are called **thermophilic.**
- **Non-motile small appendages** on the surface of bacteria which help in transfer of DNA from one cell to another during conjugation are called **sex pili.**
- **Nosocomial infection** is those infections acquired by a person after 48 hours of hospital stay. The infection should neither be present nor in its incubation period when the patient at the time of admission.
- The interval between exposure to infection and the appearance of the first symptoms is called **incubation period.**
- When a patient is already suffering from an infection acquires another infection from another patient or source is called **cross infection.**
- Organisms that live in an intimate non-parasitic relationship with the host are called **commensal.**
- **Bacteremia** is the presence of pathogenic bacteria in the blood.
- A disease transmitted by direct contact is called **contagious infection.**
- **Physician-induced infections** resulting from investigative, therapeutic and other procedure, like surgery is called **iatrogenic infection.**
- **Autoclaving** is the **most reliable** method of sterilization.

Contd...

- **Bacillary dysentery** is commonly caused by ***Shigella spp.***
- ***Salmonella serotype Typhi*** causes **typhoid fever**.
- **Widal test** is the specific diagnostic test for **typhoid fever.**
- ***Staphylococcus epidermidis*** is normal skin commensal but may act as an opportunistic pathogen in prosthetic heart valves, intraperitoneal catheters leading to septicemia and sub-acute endocarditis.
- **Leprosy** also known as **Hansen's disease.**
- ***Coxiella burnetii*** is the causative agent of **Q fever.**
- **Rubella infection to mother in the first trimester** of pregnancy may cause **fetal death or congenital defect** in the child.
- **Tsetse fly (sandfly)** transmit the condition known as **Sleeping sickness** which is caused by ***Trypanosoma brucei gambiense.***
- **Vector** is responsible for spreading disease from one individual to another.
- **Filariasis** is caused by ***Wuchereria bancrofti.***
- ***Plasmodium*** is an organism of **phylum Sporozoa.**
- **Intact skin, mucous membrane and their secretions, and normal microbial flora** are body's nonspecific **first line resistance** against an infection.
- **Inflammation, Fever and phagocytic WBC** are body's non-specific **second line defense** mechanism.
- **Antibodies** are the part of specific **third line defense.**
- Neutrophils and monocyte have **phagocytic action.**
- **Basophils release histamine** to play role in inflammatory reaction.
- When the cells are invaded by a virus, they produce **Interferon.**
- A person acquire immunity after suffering from an infectious disease, this type of immunity is known as **natural active immunity.**
- **Natural passive immunity** occurs when infant gets antibodies from his mother through placenta and colostrum.
- Diphtheria is caused by *Corynebacterium diphtheriae.*
- **Intradermal route** is used for **diphtheria toxin injection** in Schick test. It is injected in left forearm.
- Tuberculin test is based on type 4 hypersensitivity.
- **Ziehl-Neelsen** stain is also known as **acid-fast stain.**
- In **Mantoux test,** purified protein derivative (PPD) is injected intradermaly. Erythema, edema and Induration more than 10 mm in diameter is suggestive of positive mantoux test.
- Organisms that originate from outside the body of the patient are known as **exogenous.**
- **Fomites:** The objects contaminated with pathogenic microorganisms.
- **Mutation** is the alteration in genetic material.
- **Pasteurization of milk:**
  - **HTST (High Temperature Short Time) of flash method:** The milk is heated to 72°C (161°F) for 15 seconds.
  - **Holder method: The milk is heated to** 63°C and holding this for 30 minutes.
- **Black, yellow, red and blue** are the color codes used in biomedical waste management.
- ***Staphylococcus aureus*** is a non-motile organism.
- Hepatitis A, polio, typhoid is mainly transmitted by **fecal-oral route.**
- ***Ascaris lumbricoides*** is also known as round worm.
- ***P. ovale*** is a species which is rarely reported in India.

Image-Based Questions

1. Microbiologist shown in photograph is credited with discovery of: *[Recent Question 2013]*

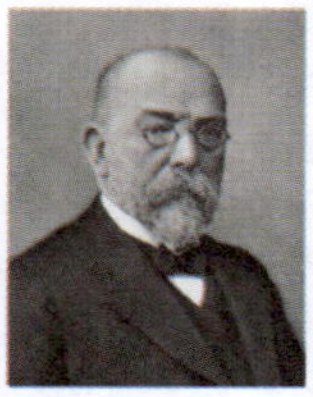

a. Sarcoma virus
b. Mycobacterium tuberculosis
c. HIV virus
d. Mycobacterium leprae

2. Identify the instrument shown in the photograph.

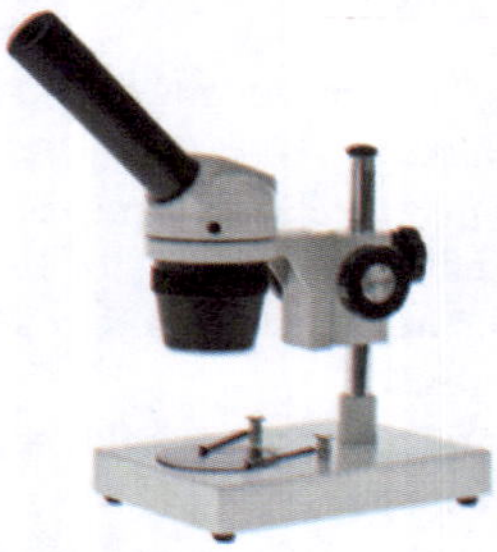

a. Electron microscope
b. Compound microscope
c. Dissecting microscope
d. Confocal microscope

3. Identify the scientist shown in photograph. *[Recent Question 2013]*

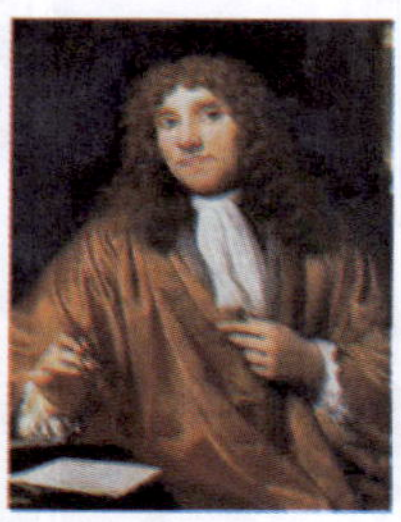

a. Edward Jenner
b. Louis Pasteur
c. James Lind
d. Antonie van Leeuwenhoek

4. Identify the bacterial shape as shown in the photograph.

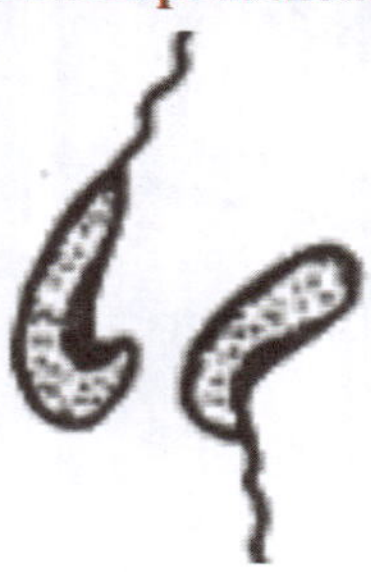

a. Bacillus
b. Vibrio
c. Spirillum
d. Spirochaete

5. Identify the type of Flagellar arrangement in Bacterium depicted in photograph.

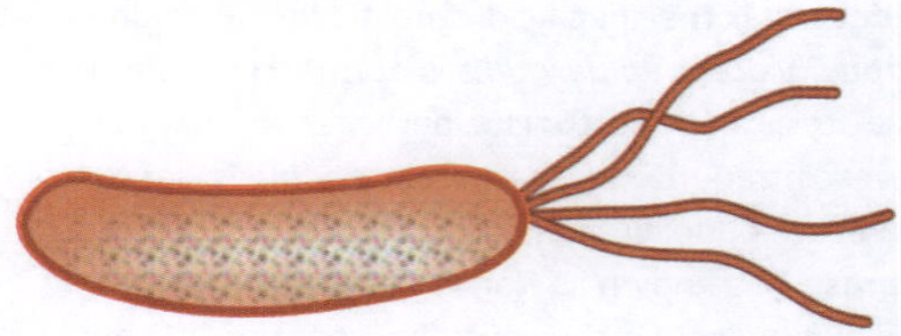

a. Monotrichous
b. Peritrichous
c. Lophotrichous
d. Amphilophotrichous

6. Identify the following culture media.

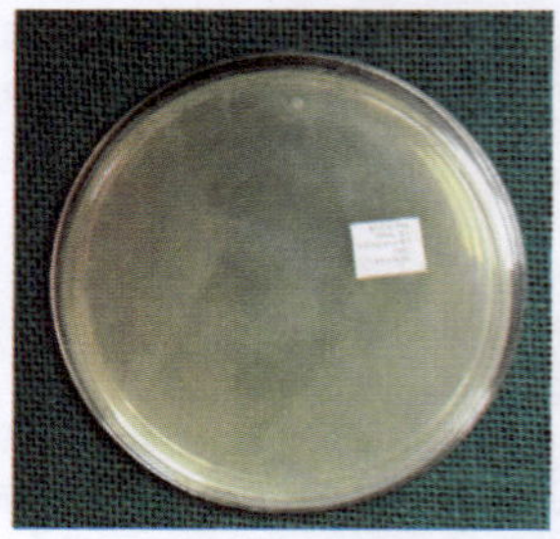

a. Nutrient agar
b. Blood agar
c. Chocolate agar
d. MacConkey agar

7. Identify the following culture media.

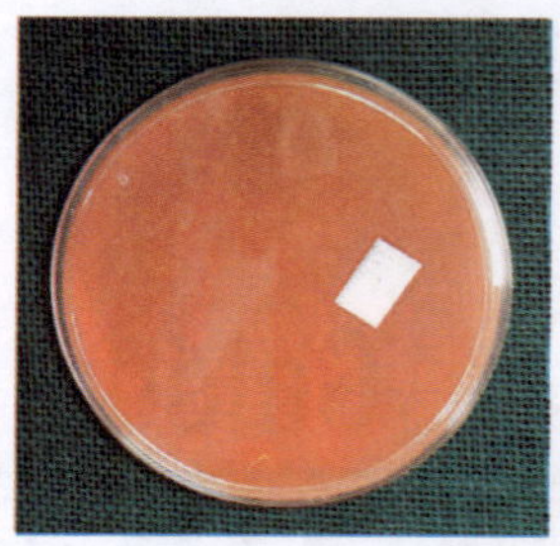

a. Nutrient agar
b. Blood agar
c. Chocolate agar
d. MacConkey agar

8. Identify the following culture media.

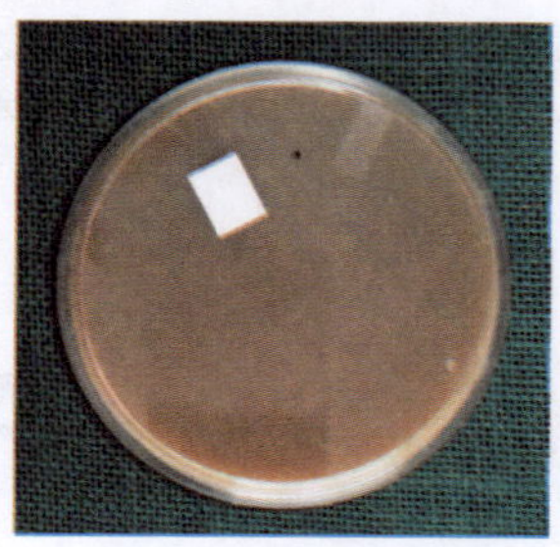

a. Nutrient agar
b. Blood agar
c. Chocolate agar
d. MacConkey agar

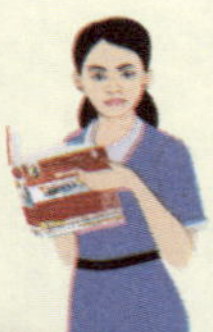

Ans.

1. b
2. c
3. d
4. b
5. c
6. a
7. b
8. c

[*Courtesy*: PHOTON-20® 3th ed. by Vivek Jain, CBS Publishers and Distributors Pvt Ltd]

9. Identify the instrument shown in the photograph.

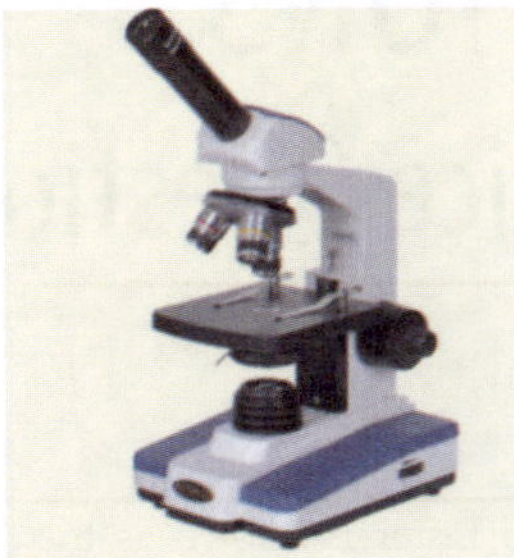

a. Electron microscope
b. Compound microscope
c. Dissecting microscope
d. Confocal microscope

10. Instrument shown in photograph is sterilized by: *[Recent Question 2013]*

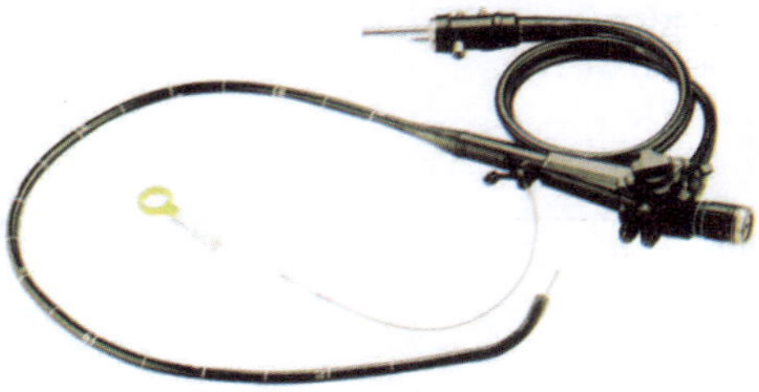

a. Formalin
b. Autoclaving
c. Boiling
d. Glutaraldehyde

11. Temperature used by the instrument shown in photograph is usually: *[Recent Question 2014]*

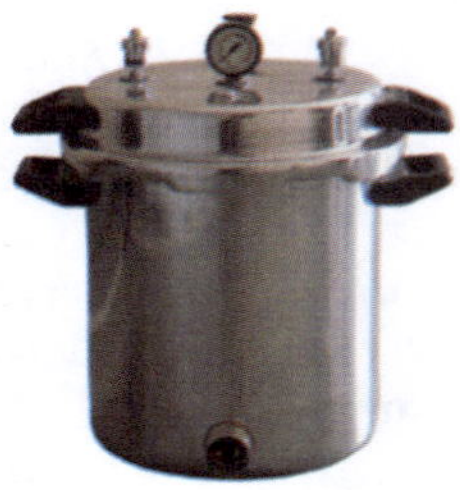

a. 121°C
b. 160°C
c. 1050°C
d. 2000°C

12. False about structure (Arrow) shown in photograph is:

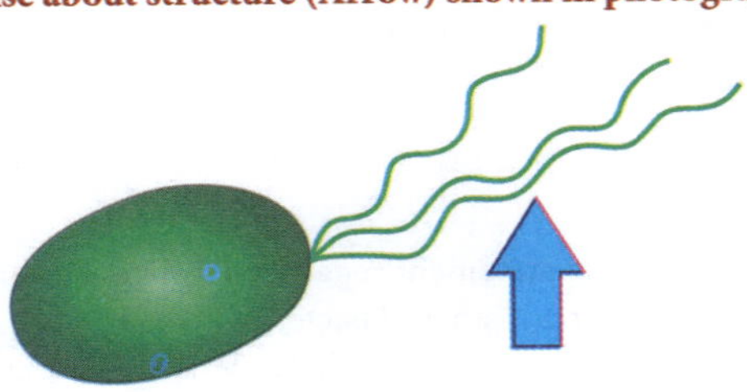

a. Locomotion
b. Attachment
c. Proteinaceous
d. Antigenic

13. Condition shown in photograph is caused by: *[Recent Question 2013]*

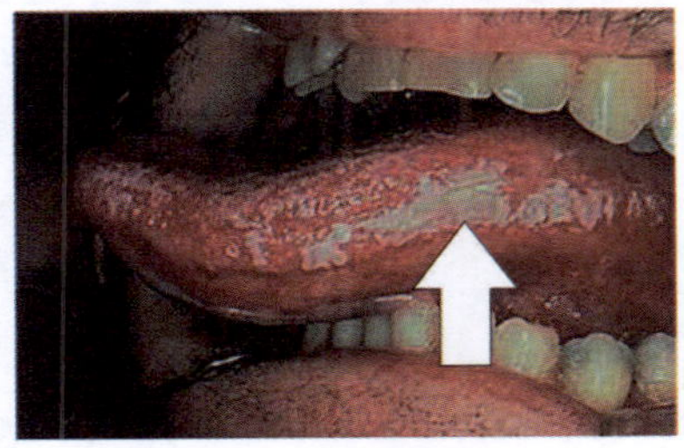

a. HSV
b. EBV
c. CMV
d. HPV

14. Most common virus affecting the Gland (Encircled) as shown in photograph is: *[Recent Question 2012]*

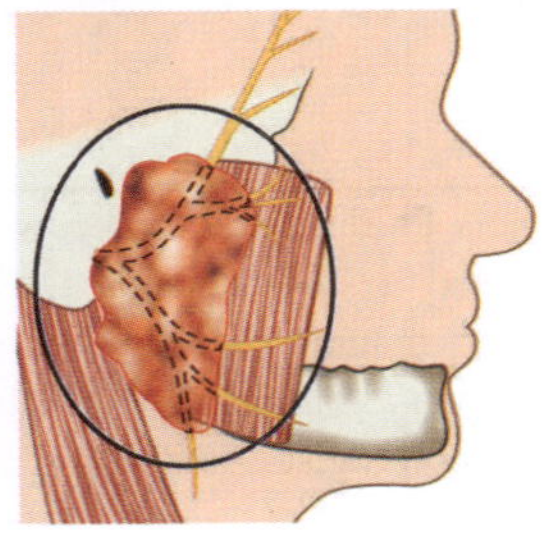

a. Varicella virus
b. Measles virus
c. Mumps virus
d. Rubella virus

15. Machine shown in photograph is used for:

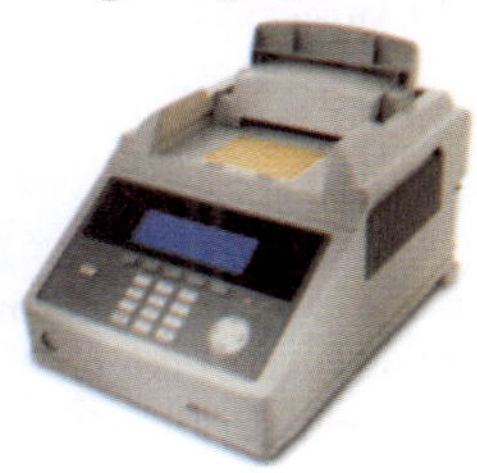

a. Hb, TLC, DLC
b. Culture, Sensitivity testing
c. Polymerase chain reaction PCR)
d. Electron microscopy

16. The bacteria shown in the microscopic image below is most likely:

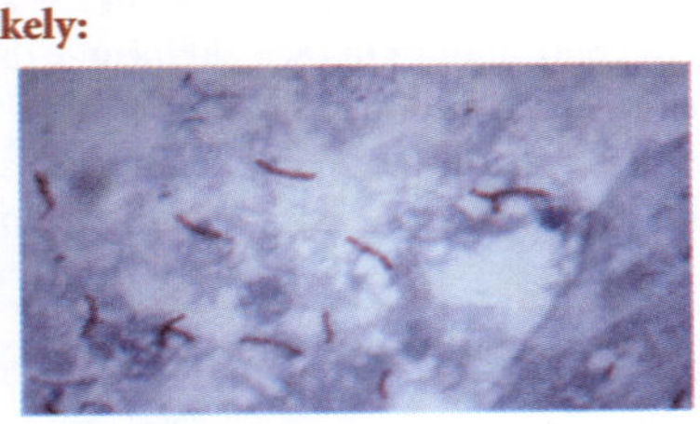

a. Streptococcus aureus
b. Staphylococcus perfringens
c. Clostridium tetanus
d. Mycobacterium tuberculosis

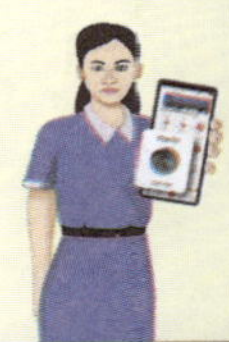

Ans.

9.	b
10.	d
11.	a
12.	b
13.	b
14.	c
15.	c
16.	d

"A man's health can be judged by which he takes two at a time - pills or stairs."

—Joan Welsh

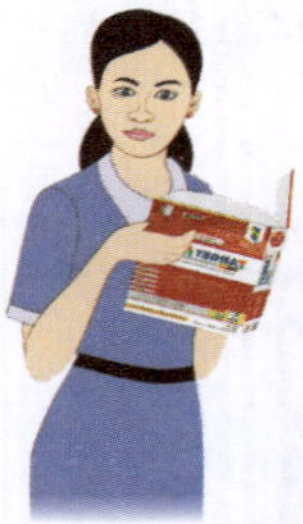

MULTIPLE CHOICE QUESTIONS

(Including Explained and Practice Questions)

INTRODUCTION & HISTORICAL PERSPECTIVES

1. Which of the following pioneers of Microbiology is credited with the discovery of microorganisms using high quality magnifying lenses (early microscopes)?

(Safdarjung NO 2018)

a. Antonie van Leeuwenhoek
b. Louis Pasteur
c. Robert Hooke
d. Robert Koch

Explanation: Antonie Philips van Leeuwenhoek discovered microorganism. He used a simple single lens device with good magnification. By using magnifying lenses, he discovered micro-organisms and also known as Father of Microbiology and therefore, known as the first microbiologist. He discovered protozoa and also improved the microscope.

2. The vaccination was first performed by:

(Banaras HU 2015)

a. Jonas Salk   b. Edward Jenner
c. Louis Pasteur   d. Alexander Fleming

3. Father of antiseptic surgery is:

a. Louis Pasteur
b. Robert Koch
c. Antonie van Leeuwenhoek
d. Lister

4. Which among the following is a contribution by Louis Pasteur in the field of microbiology?

a. Techniques of Pasteurization
b. Process of Fermentation
c. Rabies, cholera and anthrax vaccine
d. All of the above

5. Father of modern microbiology is:

a. Robert Koch   b. Edward Jenner
c. Louis Pasteur   d. Joseph Lister

Explanation: Louis Pasteur is widely regarded as the father of modern microbiology. His contributions to the field include the development of the germ theory of disease, the process of pasteurization, and the discovery of the principles of vaccination. Pasteur's experiments and discoveries paved the way for advancements in the understanding of microorganisms and their role in causing diseases.

6. Who is known as "Father of Antiseptic Surgery"?

a. Robert Koch
b. Joseph Lister
c. Paul Ehrlich
d. Antony Van Leeuwenhoek

Explanation: Joseph Lister is known as the "Father of Antiseptic Surgery." He revolutionized surgical practices by introducing antiseptic techniques to prevent infection during surgeries. Lister promoted the use of carbolic acid (phenol) as an antiseptic to sterilize surgical instruments and clean wounds, significantly reducing the risk of infections and improving patient outcomes.

7. Who is known as "Father of Bacteriology"?

a. Robert Koch
b. Joseph Lister
c. Paul Ehrlich
d. Antony Van Leeuwenhoek

Explanation: Robert Koch is known as the "Father of Bacteriology." He made significant contributions to the field by discovering the causative agents of several diseases, including anthrax, tuberculosis, and cholera.

8. The main difference between Prokaryotic and Eukaryotic cell is absence of:

a. True nucleus   b. Genetic material
c. Plasma membrane   d. Flagella

9. The discovery that led to the development of first antibiotic was made by:

a. Robert Koch   b. Alexander Fleming
c. Joseph Lister   d. Antonie van Leeuvenhoek

10. Who accidently discovered fungus Penicillium that produces a substance which destroys staphylococci?

(AIIMS BPL NO 2018)

a. Alexander Domagk   b. Eduard Buchner
c. Karl Popper   d. Alexander Fleming

11. Penicillin was discovered by:

a. Robert Koch   b. Alexander Fleming
c. Joseph Lister   d. Antonie van Leeuwenhoek

12. Life cycle of malarial parasite was first described by:

(RPSC NG-II Exam. 2007)

a. Joseph Lister   b. Alexander Fleming
c. Robert Koch   d. Ronald Ross

13. Germ theory was proposed by:

a. Pasteur
b. Koch
c. Landsteiner
d. Lister

14. Identify correct statement regarding Robert Koch:

a. He is known as father of bacteriology
b. The causative organism of cholera, Vibrio cholera was identified by him
c. He discovered hypersensitivity phenomenon
d. All of the above

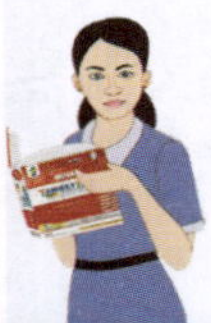

Ans.

1. a
2. b
3. d
4. d
5. c
6. b
7. a
8. a
9. b
10. d
11. b
12. d
13. a
14. d

CLASSIFICATION OF BACTERIA

15. A cluster of polar flagella is called: *(Safdarjung NO 2018)*

a. Lophotrichous
b. Amphitrichous
c. Monotrichous
d. Peritrichous

Explanation:

- **Lophotrichous:** The flagella are present in the form of cluster at one pole.
- **Amphitrichous:** When a single or clusters of flagella are present at both ends.
- **Monotrichous:** When a single polar flagellum is present on a bacteria.
- **Peritrichous:** When flagella are lateral and surround whole surface of bacteria.
- **Atrichous:** No flagella

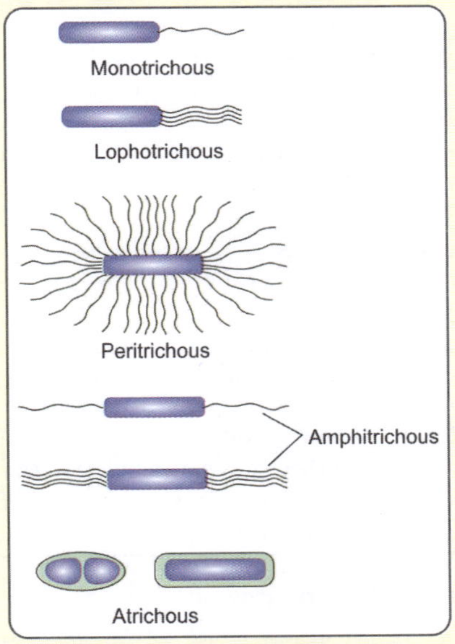

Figure: Types of flagellar arrangement in bacteria

16. Depending upon their oxygen requirement and metabolism Vibrio Cholerae species are: *(Safdarjung NO 2018)*

a. Obligate aerobes
b. Facultative anaerobes
c. Obligate anaerobes
d. Microaerophilic

Explanation: *Vibrio cholerae* are aerobes and facultative anaerobes. Facultative anaerobe is organism which forms ATP by aerobic respiration in presence of oxygen, but is capable of switching to fermentation or anaerobic respiration in absence of oxygen.

17. All of the following occur in the stationary phase of bacterial growth curve; EXCEPT: *(Safdarjung NO 2018)*

a. Cells show uniform and regular staining
b. Cells show presence of intracellular storage granules
c. Spores are seen
d. Exotoxins are formed

Explanation: In the stationary phase, the bacteria may turn Gram negative from Gram positive. All other statements regarding stationary phase of bacterial growth are true.

18. Which of the following is the unit of measurement in bacteriology? *(AIIMS BPL NO 2018)*

a. Joule
b. Newton
c. Micron
d. Pascal

Explanation: 1 micron = one thousandth of a millimeter. It is the unit used in bacteriology.

19. Nutritional dependent bacteria are called: *(AIIMS BPL NO 2018)*

a. Heterotrophs
b. Autotrophs
c. Chemotrophs
d. Phototrophs

Explanation: Heterotrophs do not make their own food so depend on other sources of energy.

Autotrophs make their own food. Chemotrophs use chemicals to prepare their food. Phototrophs use photosynthetic pigments to prepare food.

20. A food item commonly associated with Bacillus cereus food poisoning is: *(AIIMS-BBS SNO 2019, ESIC 2019)*

a. Honey
b. Green beans
c. Baked potato
d. Fried rice

Explanation: *Bacillus cereus* is a toxin-producing bacteria that is one of the most common causes of food poisoning, also called "fried rice syndrome". The bacteria are contacted from fried rice dishes that have been kept at room temperature for hours.

21. The division of bacterial cells and the exponential increase in their number are indicative of which phase? *(AIIMS BPL NO 2018)*

a. Lag phase
b. Stationary phase
c. Phase of decline
d. Logarithmic phase

Explanation: Logarithmic phase, also known as exponential phase is a period described by cell doubling. The number of new bacteria appearing per unit time is proportional to the present population.

22. Example of acid fast bacilli? *(RRB Feb 2012)*

a. E. coli
b. Mycobacterium
c. Clostridium
d. None of these

23. Mycobacterium leprae is also known as:

a. Golden bacilli
b. Koch's bacillus
c. Magical bacilli
d. Hansen's bacilli

24. Drug of choice to treat leprosy is:

a. Rifampicin
b. Acyclovir
c. Zidovudine
d. Dapsone

25. Mycobacterium tuberculosis is also known as:

a. Golden bacilli
b. Koch's bacillus
c. Magical bacilli
d. Hansen's bacilli

26. All of the following are acid-fast organisms; EXCEPT:

a. Mycobacterium tuberculosis
b. Nocardia
c. Isospora belli
d. Staphylococcus

27. Bacterial structure involved in respiration is:

a. Ribosome
b. Pili
c. Mesosome
d. Flagella

Ans.

15.	a
16.	b
17.	a
18.	c
19.	a
20.	d
21.	d
22.	b
23.	d
24.	d
25.	b
26.	d
27.	c

28. Identify correct statement regarding bacteria:

a. Respiration, cell division and sporulation are the functions of mesosome in bacteria
b. Capsule in bacteria enables adherence to surface and protection against phagocytosis
c. Heterotrophs are the bacteria that are unable to synthesize their own food materials
d. All of the above

29. Correct regarding cocci are:

a. Cocci are spherical shaped bacteria
b. Cocci present in chain is known as streptococci
c. Cocci present in the shape of grapes is known as staphylococci
d. All of the above

30. Coma shaped bacteria are known as:

a. Staphylococci b. Streptococci
c. Vibrio d. Bacillus

31. MRSA is mediated due to:

a. Plasmid b. Chromosome
c. Transposons d. None of these

32. Which one of the following is post streptococcal sequelae:

a. Acute rheumatic fever
b. Cellulitis
c. Pharyngitis
d. Impetigo

33. Acid fast staining is used to detect:

a. Mycobacterium TB b. C. tetani
c. HIV/AIDS d. Meningococci

34. Gas gangrene is caused by:

a. Clostridium tetani
b. Clostridium botulism
c. Corynebacterium diphtheriae
d. Clostridium perfringens

35. Food poison is caused by:

a. Clostridium perfringens
b. Clostridium botulism
c. Corynebacterium diphtheriae
d. Clostridium tetani

36. Incubation period for primary syphilis:

a. 1–2 days b. 1–2 weeks
c. 1 month d. 3 months

37. The causative agent of Tuberculosis (TB) is: *(RPSC Nsg. Tutor 2009)*

a. Mycobacterium tuberculosis
b. Mycobacterium leprae
c. Treponema pallidum
d. Borrelia species

38. The causative agent of Syphilis is:

a. Mycobacterium tuberculosis
b. Mycobacterium leprae
c. Treponema pallidum
d. Borrelia species.

39. Lyme disease is caused by:

a. Borrelia vincenti
b. Borrelia burgdorferi
c. Borrelia recurrentis
d. Leptospira interrogans

40. Pathogenic organism in the blood is known as:

a. Toxemia b. Septicemia
c. Bacteremia d. Hemangioma

41. The typical bacterial growth curve shows:

a. 5 phases b. 4 phases
c. 3 phases d. 2 phases

42. Study of bacteria requires the use of:

a. Microscopes b. Telescopes
c. Cystoscopes d. Endoscopes

43. The causative agent of plague is:

a. Mosquito
b. Yersinia pestis
c. Mycobacterium tuberculi
d. Mycobacterium lepare

44. The microorganism that can be acid-fast stained is:

a. Tubercle bacilli b. Lepra bacilli
c. Nocardia d. All of these

45. Characteristic feature of staphylococcus aureus is:

a. It is aerobic
b. It produces golden yellow colonies.
c. Non-sporing
d. All of the above

46. Dental caries are caused by:

a. E. Coli b. Lactobacilli
c. Shigella d. Staphylococci

47. The microorganism closely associated with dental caries is: *(AIIMS-BBS SNO 2019)*

a. *Corynebacterium species*
b. Urea plasma species
c. *Candida albicans*
d. *Streptococcus sanguis*

Explanation: *Streptococcus sanguis* is a type of bacteria commonly found in the oral cavity and is closely associated with the development of dental caries, also known as tooth decay. This bacterium, along with other Streptococcus species, can metabolize sugars from the diet and produce acids as byproducts. These acids can demineralize the tooth enamel, leading to the formation of cavities and dental caries.

48. Thermophilic bacteria grow at: *(ESI Jaipur Exam. 2009)*

a. 25°C b. 30°C
c. 35°C d. 50°C

49. "Klebs Loeffler bacillus" is the name of: *(RPSC NG-II Exam. 2007)*

a. Streptococci
b. Salmonella typhi
c. Corynebacterium diphtheria
d. Meningococci

50. Bacteria belongs to:

a. Prokaryotes b. Eukaryotes
c. Both a and b d. None of these

51. Site of respiration in bacteria is: *(Q wave Vol 2)*

a. Mitochondria
b. Golgi apparatus
c. Cell membrane
d. Cell wall

52. Bacteria that grow between 25°C and 40°C are:

a. Capnophilic
b. Psychrophilic
c. Thermophilic
d. Mesophilic

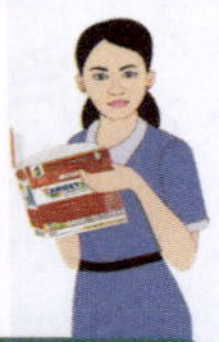

Ans.

28. d
29. d
30. c
31. b
32. a
33. a
34. d
35. b
36. c
37. a
38. c
39. b
40. b
41. b
42. a
43. b
44. d
45. d
46. b
47. d
48. d
49. c
50. a
51. c
52. d

53. Shape of cocci:
a. Rod b. Spherical
c. Comma d. Spiral

54. Which of the following is a Gram-positive cocci? *(AIIMS 2015)*
a. Streptococcus b. Neisseria
c. Escherichia d. Corynebacterium

55. Population doubling time in coliform bacilli is: *(PGI May 2015)*
a. 20 seconds b. 20 minutes
c. 20 hours d. 20 days

56. The following organism is arranged in cubical pockets of eight cocci:
a. Micrococcus b. Sarcina
c. Aerococcus d. Peptostreptococcus

57. Gram-positive bacteria is which is usually sensitive to penicillin is:
a. *Staphylococcus aureus*
b. *Enterococcus faecalis*
c. *Streptococcus pyogenes*
d. *Staphylococcus epidermidis*

58. Streptococci causing neonatal meningitis:
a. Group-A b. Group-B
c. Group-C d. Group-D

59. Which of the following gram positive bacteria is responsible for food poisoning?
a. Mycoplasmas b. Pseudomonas
c. Clostridia d. All of these

60. Methicillin resistance bacteria are:
a. Streptococci b. Pseudomonas
c. Hemophilus d. Staphylococci

61. The organism causing UTI in sexually active women:
a. *Staphylococcus aureus*
b. *Staphylococcus epidermidis*
c. *Staphylococcus saprophyticus*
d. *Streptococcus viridans*

62. Organism that has considerable resistance to antiseptics, disinfectants and antibiotics:
a. *E. coli*
b. Pseudomonas
c. Staphylococci
d. Streptococci

63. Endocarditis in a patient with colon cancer is caused by:
a. *Staphylococcus epidermidis*
b. *Streptococcus bovis*
c. *Streptococcus sanguis*
d. *Streptococcus mutans*

64. Which is a lactose fermenter?
a. *Pseudomonas* b. *Salmonella*
c. *Klebsiella* d. *Shigella*

65. Bacteria associated with dental caries:
a. *Streptococcus mutans*
b. *Streptococcus pyogenes*
c. *Streptococcus faecalis*
d. *Streptococcus agalactiae*

66. Most important cause of traveler's diarrhea is: *(MAH 14)*
a. Enterotoxigenic *Escherichia coli*
b. Enteroinvasive *E. coli*
c. Enterohemorrhagic *E. coli*
d. Enteropathogenic *E. coli*

67. A food commonly associated with bacillus cereus food poisoning is:
a. Fried rice b. Baked potato
c. Green beans d. Honey

68. Gastroenteritis with high fatality is caused by:
a. Campylobacter jejuni
b. Anthrax
c. Salmonella
d. Giardia

69. Organism causing peptic ulcer:
a. *H. pylori*
b. *C. jejuni*
c. *Cl. tetani*
d. *E. coli*

70. Vibrio cholerae was first isolated by:
a. Hoffman b. John Snow
c. Koch d. Ogston

71. Clostridium tetani is:
a. Gram-positive, non-sporing
b. Gram-negative, non-sporing
c. Gram-positive, spore forming
d. Gram-negative, spore forming

72. Increased risk of food borne botulism is associated with:
a. Commercially canned foods
b. Restaurant prepared foods
c. Home canned foods
d. Fried foods

73. The first symptom of tetanus:
a. Trismus
b. Risus sardonicus
c. Opisthotonos
d. Convulsions

74. Waterhouse–Friederichsen syndrome is caused by:
a. Neisseria meningitidis
b. Staphylococcus aureus
c. Pseudomonas aeruginosa
d. Hemophilus influenza

75. The botulism intoxication occurs due to:
a. An endotoxin
b. An exotoxin
c. Neurotoxin
d. Mycotoxin

76. Which of the following is NOT a characteristic of cell wall of a gram positive bacteria? *(AIIMS Bhopal Nursing officer, 2018)*
a. Absent sulfur-containing amino acids
b. Thick cell wall
c. Absent lipids
d. Absent teichoic acid

Explanation: Except option d all the other given options are the characteristic of cell wall of gram positive bacteria.

NORMAL BACTERIAL FLORA OF HUMAN BODY

77. Mechanism of direct transfer of free DNA:
a. Transformation
b. Conjugation
c. Transduction
d. Transposition

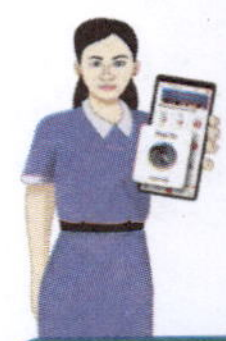

Ans.

53.	b
54.	a
55.	b
56.	b
57.	c
58.	b
59.	c
60.	d
61.	c
62.	a
63.	b
64.	c
65.	a
66.	a
67.	a
68.	b
69.	a
70.	c
71.	c
72.	c
73.	a
74.	a
75.	c
76.	d
77.	a

78. Phage-mediated transfer of DNA from one bacterium to another bacterium is known as:
a. Transformation b. Transduction
c. Transmission d. Conjugation

STAINING TECHNIQUE

79. The most common staining technique used to distinguish between Gram+ve and Gram-ve bacteria is:
a. Gram staining b. Ziehl–Neelsen staining
c. Acid Fast staining d. Albert's staining

80. The most common staining technique used to stain Mycobacteria species is:
a. Gram staining b. Ziehl-Neelsen staining
c. Albert's staining d. Eosin staining

81. Substance used for decolorizing gram stain is:
a. Acetone b. Formaldehyde
c. Glutaraldehyde d. Cidex

82. Stain used in acid fast staining is: *(Q wave Vol 2)*
a. Dilute carbol fuchsin
b. Concentrated carbol fuchsin
c. Methyl violet
d. Iodine

83. Stain used in electron microscopy:
a. Carbol fuchsin b. Phosphotungstic acid
c. Luxol fast blue d. Thioflavin T

84. India ink is used to demonstrate the following part of bacteria:
a. Cell wall b. Nucleus
c. Capsule d. Flagella

85. Which of the following organism can survive pasteurization by Holder method?
a. Mycobacterium b. Brucella
c. Salmonella d. Coxiella burnetii

86. An example for negative staining:
a. Gram staining b. Fontana's staining
c. India ink preparation d. Ziehl-Neelsen technique

TYPES OF MICROSCOPE

87. All are parts of the light microscope; EXCEPT: *(Banaras HU 2015)*
a. Condenser b. Eye-piece
c. Slide with cover slip d. Objective lens

88. Electron microscope use electron for their which property: *(Kerala PSC, Nov 2014)*
a. Wave nature
b. Spin
c. Negative charge of electron
d. None of the above

89. Tissue fixation for electron microscopy is done with:
a. Formaldehyde b. Glutaraldehyde
c. Ziehl–Neelsen stain d. Magnesium sulfate

90. Correct statement regarding microscope is:
a. Electrons are used as a source of illumination in Electron microscope
b. Antonie Van Leeuwenhoek developed microscope first time
c. Knoll & Ruska developed electron microscope
d. All of the above

91. Reflected light is used in:
a. Light microscope b. Phase contrast microscope
c. Dark field microscope d. Electron microscope

92. Resolving power of electron microscope:
a. 1 nm b. 0.1 nm
c. 0.01 nm d. 0.001 nm

93. Which of the following is the unit of measurement in bacteriology? *(AIIMS Bhopal Nursing officer, 2018)*
a. Joule b. Newton
c. Micron d. Pascal

Explanation: Micron is the unit of measurement in bacteriology. Joule is the unit of energy. Newton is the unit of force and Pascal is the unit of pressure.

CULTURE MEDIA

94. In a laboratory cultures, most human pathogens grow best at: *(AIIMS-BBS SNO 2019)*
a. 30°–37°C b. 15°–20°C
c. 38°–50°C d. 20°–30°C

Explanation: Since normal human body temperature is 37°C, the majority of human pathogens grow at this temperature. If the temperature gets hot enough the organisms are denatured and stop functioning.

95. The following method is used to observe the motility of a microbe:
a. Wet mount technique
b. Hanging drop method
c. Dry mount lamination method
d. All of the above

Explanation: Hanging drop method is a special type of wet mount in which a drop of medium containing organism is placed on a microscope cavity slide, often is used to observe motility of bacteria.

96. Antibiotic sensitivity is usually done on: *(Safdarjung NO 2018)*
a. Blood agar b. MacConkey Agar
c. Mueller-Hinton Agar d. Chocolate agar

Explanation: Media for antibiotic sensitivity testing is cation-adjusted Mueller-Hinton Agar and is used to test antibiotics like trimethoprim and sulfonamides. It usually contains: 2.0 g beef extract.

97. The optimum temperature for the growth of most pathogenic bacteria is: *(Banaras HU 2015)*
a. 25°C b. 30°C
c. 37°C d. 42°C

98. Recommended transport medium for stool specimen suspected a contain Vibrio cholerae is:
a. Buffered glycerol saline medium
b. Venkatraman-Ramakrishanan medium
c. Nutrient broth
d. Blood agar

99. Which is an enriched media?
a. Selenite F broth b. Peptone water
c. MacConkey agar d. Chocolate agar

100. Agar concentration required to prepare nutrient agar is:
a. 1–2% b. 4–6%
c. 0.25–0.5% d. 0.5–1%

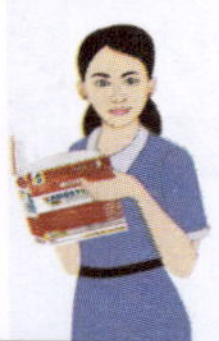

Ans.

78. b
79. a
80. b
81. a
82. b
83. b
84. c
85. d
86. c
87. c
88. a
89. b
90. d
91. c
92. b
93. c
94. a
95. b
96. c
97. c
98. b
99. d
100. a

101. **The media used to grow the microorganisms is known as:**
   a. Culture media b. Culture plate
   c. Culture Tube d. All of these

BIOCHEMICAL REACTIONS OF MICROORGANISMS

102. **Lethal effect of moist heat is due to:** *(AIIMS BPL NO 2018)*
   a. Cutting off of nutrient supply
   b. Damage to DNA
   c. Denaturation of proteins
   d. Toxic to mitochondria

Explanation: Moist heat kills microorganisms by denaturing their proteins as it causes proteins and enzymes to lose their three-dimensional functional shape.

103. **The endotoxic activity of the gram-negative bacteria is due to:** *(AIIMS BPL, AIIMS BBS NO 2018)*
   a. Cell wall b. Glycolipids
   c. Aminoglycosides d. Lipopolysaccharides

Explanation: Lipoprotein are the toxin released on cell wall destruction by the Gram-negative bacteria within its own cell.

104. **Which of the following is the most important biochemical reaction for the production of ATP in microorganisms?** New Q
   a. Fermentation b. Respiration
   c. Photosynthesis d. Hydrolysis

Explanation: Respiration is the most important biochemical reaction for the production of ATP in microorganisms. In respiration, the energy released from the oxidation of organic molecules is used to synthesize ATP.

105. **Jarisch-Harxheimer reaction is common in:**
   a. Tuberculosis b. Gonorrhea
   c. Chlamydia d. Syphilis

106. **Name the first organic acid produced by microbial fermentation:**
   a. Acetic acid b. Lactic acid
   c. Butyric acid d. None of these

107. **Antiviral protein is known as:**
   a. Antibody b. Interferon
   c. Antigen d. Antibody

GUIDELINES FOR COLLECTING CULTURE SPECIMEN

108. **Common specimens collected for the laboratory diagnosis of dermatophytes are all; EXCEPT:**
   a. Nail clippings b. Skin scrapings
   c. Hair d. Urine

109. **Which of the following statement regarding collection of specimen for microbial culture is NOT true?**
   a. Use universal precautions for collecting and handling all specimens
   b. Avoid contamination with indigenous flora
   c. Swabs are convenient but inferior to tissue and fluid
   d. Swabs are sufficient for fungal and mycobacterial culture

Explanation: Swabs are convenient but inferior to tissue and fluid. Tissue and fluid are essential for fungal and mycobacterial culture.

TYPES OF DISINFECTANTS/ANTISEPTIC

110. **The most unreliable method of sterilization is:** *(AIIMS Raipur NO 2019)*
   a. Sunlight b. Drying
   c. Heating d. Filtration

Explanation: Sunlight is a natural method of sterilization. Microbicidal activity is due to presence of UV rays. It is not sporicidal, hence, does not sterilize. So, it is most unreliable sterilization method.

111. **The pressure set in autoclave for sterilization is:** *(DSSSB PHN, 2015)*
   a. 15 lb b. 5 lb
   c. 10 lb d. 20 lb

112. **Biological pesticides are produced by:** *(Staff Nurse G II 2014)*
   a. Bacillus thuringiensis
   b. Agrobacterium tumefaciens
   c. Pseudomonas
   d. Bacillus anthracis

113. **The method of reducing the number of pathogens from any article, surface or medium is known as:** *(ISRO)*
   a. Sterilization b. Incineration
   c. Disinfection d. Lysis

114. **Which of the following is most resistant to sterilization?**
   a. Tubercle bacilli b. Viruses
   c. Spores d. Prions

115. **Endoscope is sterilized by:**
   a. Glutaraldehyde b. Formaldehyde
   c. Atuoclaving d. Hot air oven

116. **Which of the following item is NOT sterilized by antiseptic solution?** *(ESI 2009)*
   a. Suction catheter b. Enema tube
   c. Surgical scissor d. Nasogastric tube

117. **Chemical used for sterilization of heart lung machine is:**
   a. Hypochlorite b. Ethylene oxide
   c. Cidex d. Korsolex

118. **Which parameter is not included in HAI surveillance?**
   a. CA-UTI (catheter associated urinary tract infection)
   b. CLABSI (central line associated bloodstream infection)
   c. VAP (ventilator associated pneumonia)
   d. Open wound infections

119. **Hand rub should not be used in which condition?**
   a. Before touching patient
   b. After touching patient
   c. After touching patient's surrounding
   d. Hands are visibly soiled

120. **How many moments of hand hygiene have been laid down by WHO?**
   a. 5 b. 6
   c. 7 d. 8

121. **Chemical method of sterilization include:**
   a. Ethylene oxide b. Formaldehyde
   c. Hypochlorite d. All of these

122. **Which of the following is most reliable and commonly employed method of sterilization?**
   a. UV rays b. Heat
   c. X-rays d. All of these

123. **Which of the following is moist heat method of sterilization?**
   a. Autoclave b. Hot air oven
   c. Ultraviolet radiation d. Incineration

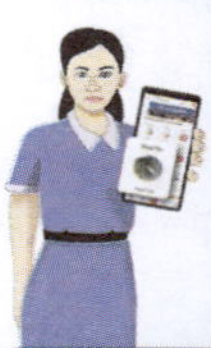

Ans.

101.	a
102.	c
103.	d
104.	b
105.	d
106.	b
107.	b
108.	d
109.	d
110.	a
111.	a
112.	a
113.	c
114.	d
115.	a
116.	c
117.	b
118.	d
119.	d
120.	a
121.	d
122.	b
123.	a

124. Which of the following is used for sterilization of cystoscopes, endoscopes and bronchoscopes?
a. Glutaraldehyde
b. Ethanol
c. Methanol
d. Ethylene oxide

125. Method of sterilization used for culture media is:
a. Autoclave b. Hot air oven
c. Pasteurization d. None of these

126. The method of killing all microorganisms including their spores is known as:
a. Sterilization b. Disinfection
c. Incineration d. Lysis

127. The method of reducing the number of pathogens from any article, surface or medium is called:
a. Sterilization b. Disinfection
c. Incineration d. Lysis

128. Lysol and Dettol are:
a. Buffers b. Disinfectants
c. Salt solution d. None of these

129. Chemical agent that inhibit the growth of microorganism is:
a. Disinfection b. Sterilization
c. Asepsis d. Hygiene

130. Which of the following is moist heat method of sterilization?
a. Boiling b. Autoclaving
c. Hot air oven d. Both a & b

131. Temperature range used for autoclaving is ....
a. 100°C for 10 m b. 100°C for 30 m
c. 121°C for 15 m d. 121°C for 30 m

132. Alcohols, Aldehydes, phenols, etc. are:
a. Chemical methods of sterilization
b. Physical methods of sterilization
c. Dry heat method of sterilization
d. Moist heat method of sterilization

133. Which of the following burns the waste at very high temperatures and thus, reduces its volume?
a. Incinerator
b. Autoclave
c. Hot air oven
d. All of these

134. The disadvantage of incinerator is that it generates:
a. Highly toxic gases
b. UV rays
c. Radioactive rays
d. X-rays

135. Infectious waste after treatment can be disposed of by:
a. Land – filling or deep burial
b. UV rays
c. Radioactive rays
d. X-rays

136. Which of the following substances are formed in the serum and tissue fluids in response to an antigen?
a. Antibodies b. Hormones
c. Enzymes d. All of these

137. Temperature range in pasteurization of milk by holder method is:
a. 75°C for 15 m b. 75°C for 30 m
c. 63°C for 30 m d. 63°C for 15 m

138. Sterilization of endoscope is done: *(ESI Jaipur Exam. 2009)*
a. Carbolic acid
b. Savlon
c. Hypochlorite
d. By 2% glutaraldehyde

139. Asepsis means: *(RPSE NG-II Exam.2010)*
a. Freedom from infection
b. Freedom from sterility
c. Freedom from isolation
d. Freedom from pain

140. The process of prevention of infection, by inhibiting the growth of bacteria in wounds or tissues is called:
a. Antisepsis
b. Sterilization
c. Disinfection
d. Decontamination

141. The following is not sterilized by gamma radiation:
a. Gloves
b. Cadgut
c. Catheter
d. Autoclave

142. Holder's method of sterilization is:
a. Moist heat at 63°C for 30 m
b. Moist heat at 72°C for 15 s
c. Dry heat at 63°C for 30 m
d. Dry heat at 72°C for 15 s

143. Best way of sterilizing disposable plastic syringes is: *(Q wave 2 &3)*
a. UV rays b. Autoclave
c. Gamma rays d. Hot air oven

144. The most suitable disinfectant for decontamination of HIV contaminated endoscope is: *(MH 2014)*
a. 1% sodium hypochlorite
b. 2% glutaraldehyde
c. 5% phenol
d. 70% ethanol

145. Flexible fiber optic endoscopes are sterilized by:
a. Auto clave
b. Cetrimide
c. 2% glutaraldehyde
d. Gamma-radiation

146. Temperature and duration for Flash process of Pasteurization:
a. 77°C for 20 s
b. 100°C for 20 s
c. 63°C for 20 s
d. 63°C for 30 m

147. Sterilization of heat labile media is done by:
a. Filtration
b. Pasteurization
c. Autoclaving
d. Tyndallization

148. The temperature and duration required to kill spores in autoclave:
a. 63°C for 12 m
b. 72°C for 12 m
c. 121°C for 12 m
d. 160°C for 12 m

Ans.
124. a
125. a
126. a
127. b
128. b
129. a
130. d
131. d
132. a
133. a
134. a
135. a
136. a
137. c
138. d
139. a
140. a
141. d
142. a
143. c
144. b
145. c
146. a
147. d
148. c

149. The chemical disinfectant which acts by plasma membrane damage:

a. Chlorine b. Formaldehyde
c. Alcohol d. Phenol

150. The following are disinfectants; EXCEPT:

a. 100% alcohol b. Acridine dyes
c. Isopropyl alcohol d. Halogens

151. Glass wares and syringes are sterilized by:

a. Autoclave b. Steamer
c. Flaming d. Hot air oven

152. Operation theatres are sterilized by:

a. Formaldehyde gas b. Ethylene oxide
c. Carbolic acid d. Chlorine gas

153. Non-disposable syringes are sterilized by:

a. Hot air oven b. Autoclave
c. Incineration d. Steamer

154. Heart lung machines are best sterilized by:

a. Acridine dyes
b. Ethylene oxide gas
c. Isopropyl alcohol
d. 100% alcohol

155. The principle of autoclave is:

a. Oxidative damage
b. Increased level of electrolytes
c. Denaturation and protein coagulation
d. Denaturation and oxidation

156. Plastic syringes are sterilized by:

a. Glutaraldehyde b. Autoclave
c. Hot air oven d. Ionizing radiation

157. Percentage of sodium hypochlorite used for disinfecting HIV infected liquid waste:

a. 1% b. 2%
c. 5% d. 10%

VIRUS

158. Warts are caused by: *(AIIMS Nagpur NO 2018)*

a. Protozoa b. Fungus
c. Viruses d. Bacteria

Explanation: Warts are common benign skin tumors caused by infection with Human Papilloma Virus (HPV), which belongs to the DNA virus group. Warts occur most frequently between the ages of 12 years and 16 years.

159. In majority of the cases the causative organism for sore throat is: *(Banaras HU 2015)*

a. Gonococci b. Staphylococci
c. Meningococci d. Streptococci

160. Which one of the disease is not caused by an acid fast bacilli (AFB)? *(Banaras HU 2015)*

a. Leprosy b. Tuberculosis
c. Nocardiosis d. Typhoid

161. Infection with group A beta hemolytic streptococci can lead to: *(JIPMER 2012)*

a. Hepatitis
b. Meningitis
c. Rheumatoid arthritis
d. Rheumatic fever

162. Viruses are: *(ESIC Chennai May 2012)*

a. One-cell microorganisms with a simple cellular organization whose nucleus lacks a membrane.
b. Pieces of nucleic acid (DNA or RNA) wrapped in a thin coat of protein that replicate only within the cells of living hosts
c. Multicellular organisms that live in or on a host to obtain nourishment without providing any benefit to the host
d. None of the above

163. Common cold is caused by: *(ESIC Chennai May 2012)*

a. Rhinovirus
b. Staphylococcus aureus
c. Shigella
d. Escherichia coil

164. The most common early symptom of hepatitis 'A' is: *(LNJP H D 2012)*

a. Loss of appetite b. Abdominal distention
c. Shortness of breath d. Ecchymosis

165. HIV is a:

a. Retrovirus b. DNA virus
c. Fungus d. Bacteria

166. All of the following are live-attenuated vaccines; EXCEPT:

a. MMR
b. Yellow fever 17D vaccine
c. Salk polio vaccine
d. Sabin polio vaccine

167. Which of the following infectious agents can be transmitted through blood transfusion?

a. HIV
b. Treponema pallidum
c. Toxoplasma gondii
d. All of the above

168. All of the following viruses are transmitted by respiratory route except:

a. Influenza virus
b. Rota virus
c. Respiratory syncytial virus
d. Rhinovirus

169. Zero dose of OPV is given:

a. At one month
b. At birth
c. When child is having diarrhea
d. When child is having polio

170. Most effective mode of transmission of HIV:

a. Sexual b. Blood product
c. Needle/syringe d. Mother of fetus

171. Most common malignancy in AIDS is:

a. Kaposi sarcoma
b. B-cell lymphoma
c. Leukemia
d. Burkitt's lymphoma

172. The most common viral cause of gastroenteritis:

a. Rotavirus b. Norwalk virus
c. Adenovirus d. Hepadnavirus

173. All are true about SARS; EXCEPT:

a. Epidemic is seen in India
b. Spreads by droplet
c. Diagnosed by PCR
d. Caused by a type of coronavirus

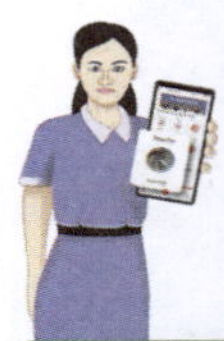

Ans.

149. d
150. a
151. d
152. a
153. a
154. b
155. c
156. d
157. a
158. c
159. d
160. d
161. d
162. b
163. a
164. a
165. a
166. c
167. d
168. b
169. b
170. b
171. a
172. a
173. a

174. Perinatal Hepatitis B transmission is maximum in:
a. 1st trimester b. 2nd trimester
c. 3rd trimester d. During delivery

175. Which Hepatitis virus is associated with highest mortality in pregnancy?
a. Hepatitis A b. Hepatitis B
c. Hepatitis C d. Hepatitis E

176. Hepatitis virus that spreads by fecal-oral route:
a. Hepatitis A b. Hepatitis B
c. Hepatitis C d. Hepatitis D

177. Acute hepatitis B infection is best diagnosed by:
a. HBsAg
b. HBeAg
c. IgM Anti HBc antibody
d. HBcAg

178. The causative agent of AIDS is:
a. Human immunodeficiency virus (HIV)
b. Mycobacterium tuberculi
c. Mycobacterium leprae
d. Treponema pallidum

179. HIV virus belongs to: *(RPSC NG-II Exam. 2007)*
a. Adenovirus b. Retrovirus
c. Flavivirus d. Cyclovirus

180. Most often cells from blood infected by HIV is: *(RPSC Nursing Tutor- 2009)*
a. CD4 T. Lymphocytes
b. Red Blood Cells
c. Monocytes
d. b. Lymphocytes

181. SARS virus is a:
a. Coronavirus b. Lentivirus
c. Calicivirus d. Arenavirus

182. The main cell affected in HIV infection is:
a. CD4 T cell b. CD8 T cell
c. B cell d. Macrophages

183. Range of incubation period in typhoid:
a. 3–21 days
b. 10–30 days
c. 1–3 months
d. 3–6 months

184. Route of administration of influenza vaccine:
a. Intradermal
b. Subcutaneous
c. Per oral
d. Intranasal

185. Incubation period for influenza pandemic H1N1:
a. 12–24 h b. 1–3 days
c. 1–7 days d. 5–10 days

186. Incubation period of mumps:
a. 1–7 days b. 7–14 days
c. 12–24 days d. 21–28 days

187. Who discovered Oral polio vaccine which is used nowadays?
a. Koprowski b. Cox
c. Salk d. Sabin

188. Corneal beading is a complication of:
a. Leprosy
b. AIDS
c. Herpes simplex keratitis
d. Acanthamoeba keratitis

189. Most common site of extra thoracic TB in children:
a. Lymph node b. Skeleton
c. Central nervous system d. Heart

190. Smallest virus is: *(Q wave)*
a. Pox virus b. Herpes virus
c. Parvo virus d. Adeno virus

191. Incubation period of measles:
a. 1–2 days b. 3–6 days
c. 1–7 days d. 9–11 days

192. Yellow fever is caused by:
a. Flavivirus
b. Alphavirus
c. Calcivirus
d. Bunyavirus

193. Chances of perinatal HIV infection to the baby:
a. 0.5–1% b. 30%
c. 50% d. 90%

FUNGUS

194. Tinea pedis is caused by:
a. E. floccosum b. T. rubrum
c. Microsporum d. T. schoenleinii

195. Tenia pedis is more common among:
a. People of cold countries
b. Those wearing occlusive shoes and socks
c. Hospitalized people
d. People who eats fermented food

196. Fungi can be stained by:
a. Glycerine b. Cotton blue
c. Lactophenol d. Phenol

197. Common symptoms of pulmonary (lung) mucormycosis include all; EXCEPT:
a. Cough b. Fever
c. Shortness of breath d. Nasal congestion

Explanation: Symptoms of pulmonary (lung) mucormycosis include:
- Fever
- Cough
- Chest pain
- Shortness of breath

198. Common symptoms of rhinocerebral mucormycosis include all; EXCEPT:
a. Headache
b. Nasal of sinus congestion
c. Black lesions on nasal bridge
d. Cough

Explanation: Symptoms of rhinocerebral (sinus and brain); mucormycosis include:
- One-sided facial swelling
- Headache
- Nasal or sinus congestion
- Black lesions on nasal bridge or upper inside of mouth that quickly become more severe
- Fever

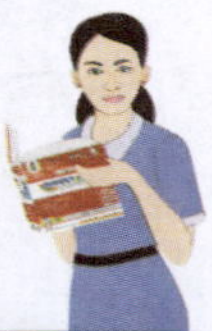

Ans.
174. d
175. d
176. a
177. c
178. a
179. b
180. a
181. a
182. a
183. a
184. d
185. c
186. c
187. d
188. a
189. a
190. c
191. d
192. a
193. b
194. b
195. b
196. b
197. d
198. d

199. Symptoms of gastrointestinal mucormycosis include all; EXCEPT:
- a. Abdominal pain b. GI bleeding
- c. Nausea and Vomiting d. Constipation

200. Which of the following drug is used in the treatment of mucormycosis?
- a. Amphotericin B b. Fluconazole
- c. Voriconazole d. Echinocandins

Explanation: Mucormycosis is a serious infection and needs to be treated with prescription antifungal medicine, usually amphotericin B, posaconazole, or isavuconazole. Other medicines, including fluconazole, voriconazole, and echinocandins, do not work against fungi that cause mucormycosis. Often, mucormycosis requires surgery to remove the infected tissue. (Source: CDC)

PARASITES

201. Microorganisms are living structures of microscopic size, belongs to:
- a. Prokaryotes b. Eukaryotes
- c. Both a & b d. None of these

202. Amoebic dysentery is caused by:
- a. Vibrio cholera b. Shigella
- c. Entamoeba histolytica d. Plasmodium

203. Amoebiasis is caused by: *(AIIMS-BBS SNO 2019)*
- a. Entamoeba histolytica
- b. Toxoplasma gondii
- c. Leishmania donovani
- d. Trypanosoma cruzi

204. Pathogen means *(RPSC Nurse Grade II Exam.2010)*
- a. Microorganism which causes disease
- b. Microorganism which are found in animals
- c. Microorganism which helps in digestion
- d. Microorganism which are found in plants

205. Amphitrichous flagella means:
- a. Flagella all-round the cell
- b. Flagella at both ends
- c. Flagella at one end
- d. Flagella in tufts

206. When Flagella is present all around the cell it is called:
- a. Amphitrichous b. Monotrichous
- c. Peritrichous d. Lophotrichous

207. Rice water stool is associated with DNB 2015:
- a. Cholera b. Bacillary dysentery
- c. Salmonella infection d. Pseudomembranous colitis

RODENTS & VECTORS

208. All of the following are vector bone diseases; EXCEPT:
- a. Malaria b. Filariasis
- c. Rubella d. Chagas disease

209. Which one of the following agents can be used to prevent malaria?
- a. Chloroquine b. Albendazole
- c. Attenuated vaccine d. Chloramphenicol

210. Dengue is caused by:
- a. Alphavirus b. Bunyavirus
- c. Flavivirus d. Hantavirus

211. Infective period of Aedes mosquitoes in dengue:
- a. 1- 2 days b. 8- 10 days
- c. Till next bite d. Till death

212. Scrub typhus is transmitted by:
- a. Louse b. Trombiculid mite
- c. Rat flea d. Soft tick

DIAGNOSTIC TESTS

213. Schick test is used in confirming the diagnosis of: *(Safdarjung NO 2018; DSSSB PHN, 2015)*
- a. Tuberculosis b. Diphtheria
- c. Syphilis d. Scarlet fever

Explanation: Schick test is intradermal test used to assess the immune status of a person susceptible to diphtheria. It is based on the neutralization reaction between specific antigen and antibody against diphtheria toxin.

214. Widal test is performed for identifying: *(DSSSB PHN, 2015)*
- a. Clostridium b. Salmonella
- c. Staphylococcus d. Meningococcal

215. ELISA test is used to detect: *(ESIC Chennai May 2012)*
- a. HIV infection b. Malaria infection
- c. Lung infection d. Cholera infection

216. The Widal test is positive if two antigen titer is more than: *(ESIC Chennai May 2012)*
- a. 1: 70 in an active infection
- b. 1: 160 in an infection
- c. 1: 80 in an active infection
- d. 1: 90 in an active infection

217. VDRL test is performed to diagnose: *(ESIC Chennai May 2012)*
- a. Syphilis b. Pregnancy
- c. Both a and b d. Myasthenia gravis

218. Northern blotting is used for separation of:
- a. DNA b. RNA
- c. Proteins d. None of these

219. A positive tuberculin test is an example of:
- a. Type I hypersensitivity b. Type II hypersensitivity
- c. Type III hypersensitivity d. Type IV hypersensitivity

220. A positive tuberculin test is indicated by and area of induration of:
- a. <5 mm in diameter b. 6–9 mm in diameter
- c. >10 mm in diameter d. No induration

221. Widal test belongs to which of the following types? *(AIIMS BBS NO 2018)*
- a. Precipitation test b. Bacteriolysin
- c. Neutralization d. Agglutination test

Explanation: Agglutination reaction is when a particulate antigen combines with its antibody, the particles are clumped or agglutinated. Widal test is an agglutination test that helps in differentiating the serotypes of non-enteric Salmonella from enteric ones.

222. Diagnostic test used for typhoid fever is:
- a. Blood culture b. Dick test
- c. Schick test d. Widal test

223. Diagnostic test used for TB is:
- a. Mantoux test b. Dick test
- c. Schick test d. Widal test

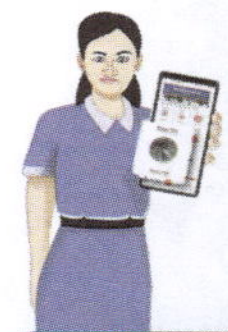

Ans.

199. d
200. a
201. a
202. c
203. a
204. a
205. b
206. c
207. a
208. c
209. a
210. c
211. d
212. b
213. b
214. b
215. a
216. b
217. a
218. b
219. d
220. c
221. d
222. d
223. a

224. Diagnostic test used for scarlet fever is:
a. Mantoux test b. Dick test
c. Schick test d. Widal test

225. Diagnostic test used for typhus fever is:
a. Mantoux test b. Dick test
c. Schick test d. Weil Felix

226. Route of injecting chick test toxin/ purified protein derivative (Mantoux test) is:
a. Intra vascular b. Intradermal
c. Intra muscular d. Subcutaneous

227. Site for injecting test toxin/purified protein derivative (Mantoux test) is:
a. Right upper arm b. Left upper arm
c. Right forearm d. Left forearm

228. Most accurate method of diagnosis of Helicobacter pylori is:
a. Culture
b. Biopsy urease test
c. Histopathology
d. Urea breath test

229. During the window period of patient with AIDS, best diagnostic test is:
a. ELISA b. Western Blot
c. Rapid test d. RT-PCR

230. Best indicator of HIV prognosis:
a. CD4T cell count b. CD8 T cell count
c. HIV RNA d. ELIS

231. ELISA stands for:
a. Enzyme Linked Immunosorbent Assay
b. Enzyme Lipase Immunosorbent Assay
c. Enzyme Linked Immunity Assay
d. Enzyme Lipase Immunity Assay

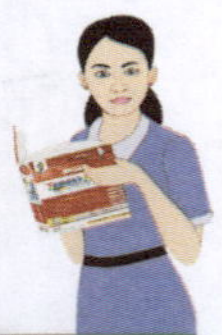

232. Urine sample for culture is collected from: *(RPSC Nursing Tutor- 2009)*
a. First-void urine
b. Last-void urine
c. Either First or Last void urine
d. Midstream urine

233. Usual dose of purified protein derivative in Mantoux test is:
a. 5 IU b. 50 IU
c. 100 IU d. 500 IU

234. Mantoux +ve is induration measuring:
a. >10 mm b. 6–9 mm
c. <5 mm d. >20 mm

235. VDRL is used in the diagnosis of:
a. Syphilis b. HIV
c. Typhoid d. Tuberculosis

HYPERSENSITIVITY AND IMMUNE SYSTEM

236. An example of type IV hypersensitivity is: *(AIIMS-BBS SNO 2019)*
a. Arthus reaction
b. Tuberculin-type reaction
c. Atopy
d. Anaphylactic reaction.

Explanation: Type IV hypersensitivity are cell mediated reactions, initiated by T-lymphocytes and mediated by effector T-cells and macrophages. It takes 48–72 h or longer, after contact with antigen.
- Tuberculin skin test, granulomatous inflammation, etc.

237. Which of the following about active immunity is correct?
a. No lag phase
b. Booster doses are useful
c. Useful in immunodeficient people
d. No memory cells

238. Primary immune response – the correct statement is:
a. Involves IgG
b. Antibody producing cells- Memory B cell
c. No lag period
d. Slow and sluggish

239. Which antibody crosses placenta?
a. IgA b. IgG
c. IgE d. IgM

240. Which is an example of surface Ig?
a. IgA b. IgG
c. IgE d. IgM

241. Type I hypersensitivity is mediated by which of the following immunoglobulins?
a. IgA b. IgG
c. IgM d. IgE

242. Wheal and flare is which type of hypersensitivity reaction?
a. Type I b. Type II
c. Type IV d. Type V

243. Type I hypersensitivity includes all of the following; EXCEPT:
a. Autoimmune hemolytic anemia
b. Anaphylaxis
c. Extrinsic asthma
d. Hay fever

244. Which of the following statement regarding graft rejection is incorrect?
a. First-set rejection usually occurs within 2 weeks after transplantation
b. Second-set rejection occurs months to year
c. Second-set rejection occurs due to immunological memory
d. Hyperacute rejection occurs within minutes to hours

245. Transplantation between members with same genetic constitution is known as:
a. Autograft
b. Isograft
c. Allograft
d. Xenograft

246. Which of the following is live attenuated vaccine?
a. BCG vaccine
b. Rabies vaccine
c. Diphtheria toxoid
d. Tetanus toxoid

247. Which of the following single dose is sufficient for immunization?
a. Live attenuated vaccine
b. Killed vaccine
c. Toxoid s
d. None of the above

248. The infection acquired after 48 h of admission to the hospital is:
a. Hospital Acquired Infection
b. Hospital Associated Infection
c. Nosocomial Infection
d. All of the above

Ans.
224. b
225. d
226. b
227. d
228. d
229. d
230. a
231. a
232. d
233. a
234. a
235. a
236. b
237. b
238. d
239. b
240. a
241. d
242. a
243. a
244. b
245. b
246. a
247. a
248. d

249. Interval between exposure to infection and occurrence of sign and symptoms is known as:
a. Incubation period
b. Prodromal stage
c. Incidence
d. Surveillance

250. Which of the following is used for passive immunization?
a. Human sera and Animal sera
b. Killed vaccine
c. Toxoid
d. Live attenuated vaccine

251. The resistance exhibited by the host against any foreign antigen including microorganisms is:
a. Immunity b. Antigenicity
c. Antibodies d. None of these

252. Which is the only antibody that can cross placenta?
a. IgG b. IgA
c. IgD d. All of these

253. Which antibody is responsible for allergic responses?
a. IgG b. IgA
c. IgD d. IgE

254. When the patient is acquiring infection from another patient it is known as:
a. Cross infection
b. Iatrogenic infection
c. Opportunistic infection
d. Nosocomial infection

255. Infection occurred as a result of investigation or therapeutic procedure is known as:
a. Cross infection b. Iatrogenic infection
c. Opportunistic infection d. Nosocomial infection

256. When the patient is acquiring infection during low immunity state is known as:
a. Cross infection
b. Iatrogenic infection
c. Opportunistic infection
d. Nosocomial infection

257. Disease transmitted by direct contact is known as:
a. Cross infection
b. Contagious infection
c. Opportunistic infection
d. Nosocomial infection

258. Artificial active immunity is produced by:
a. Vaccination
b. Immunoglobulins
c. Human and animal sera
d. None of these

259. The overall resistance in a community is referred as:
a. Herd immunity b. Active immunity
c. Passive immunity d. Innate immunity

260. Antibodies are produced by: *(AIIMS-BBS SNO 2019)*
a. NK cells
b. Neutrophils
c. T lymphocytes
d. B lymphocytes

261. An example for artificial passive immunity:
a. Interferon b. Tetanus immune globin
c. Hepatitis B vaccine d. BCG vaccine

262. True about live vaccination are all; EXCEPT:
a. Latent phase
b. No negative phase
c. Both humoral and cellular response
d. Immunological memory

263. Immunoglobulin that is inactivated at high temperature:
a. IgG b. IgA
c. IgM d. IgE

264. Immunoglobulins are:
a. Glycolipids
b. Glycoproteins
c. Polypeptides
d. Proteoglycans

265. Exotoxins are usually:
a. Protein b. Heat labile
c. More antigenic d. Nonenzymatic

266. True about exotoxins:
a. Produced only by gram positive bacteria
b. Neutralized by antitoxin
c. Less potent than endotoxin
d. Pyrogenic

267. The function of an adjuvant in a vaccine is to enhance its:
a. Distribution
b. Immunogenicity
c. Absorption
d. Shelf life

268. The immunity resulting in the infant, as a result of immunization of a pregnant woman with tetanus toxoid is called:
a. Innate immunity
b. Natural active immunity
c. Artificial active immunity
d. Natural passive immunity

269. Anti-D given to a Rh negative pregnant woman with Rh-positive fetus, before delivery is an example of:
a. Artificial active immunity
b. Artificial passive immunity
c. Natural passive immunity
d. Adoptive immunity

270. Injection of lymphocytes in the treatment of lepromatous leprosy is an example of:
a. Innate immunity
b. Adoptive immunity
c. Natural passive immunity
d. Artificial passive immunity

271. ABO antibodies are:
a. IgG b. IgA
c. IgM d. IgE

272. Anaphylaxis is:
a. Type I Hypersensitivity
b. Type II Hypersensitivity
c. Type III Hypersensitivity
d. Type IV Hypersensitivity

273. Contact dermatitis is:
a. Type I Hypersensitivity
b. Type II Hypersensitivity
c. Type III Hypersensitivity
d. Type IV Hypersensitivity

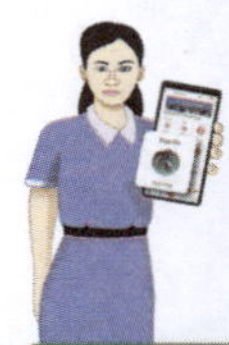

Ans.

249. a
250. a
251. a
252. a
253. d
254. a
255. b
256. c
257. b
258. a
259. a
260. d
261. b
262. b
263. d
264. b
265. a
266. b
267. b
268. d
269. b
270. b
271. c
272. a
273. d

274. Kupffer cells are seen in:
a. Thymus
b. Spleen
c. Liver
d. Lymph node

275. Antibiotic used in Toxic shock syndrome:
a. Vancomycin
b. Cephalosporins
c. Streptomycin
d. Clindamycin

276. Grave's disease belongs to:
a. Type I hypersensitivity
b. Type II hypersensitivity
c. Type III hypersensitivity
d. Type IV hypersensitivity

277. Type of hypersensitivity involved in Rh incompatibility:
a. Type I hypersensitivity
b. Type II hypersensitivity
c. Type III hypersensitivity
d. Type IV hypersensitivity

278. Chemically an antigen may be:
a. Lipid
b. Polysaccharide
c. Protein
d. Any of these

279. Example of cell mediated hypersensitivity:
a. Transfusion reactions
b. Arthus reactions
c. Type II lepra reaction
d. Tuberculin test

280. Tuberculin test is an example of:
a. Type I hypersensitivity
b. Type II hypersensitivity
c. Type III hypersensitivity
d. Type IV hypersensitivity

281. Dose of human tetanus Ig for post exposure prophylaxis:
a. 250–500 units
b. 500–750 units
c. 750–1000 units
d. 1000–1200 units

Ans.
274. c
275. d
276. b
277. b
278. d
279. d
280. d
281. a

"It is health that is real wealth and not pieces of gold and silver."
—Mahatma Gandhi

CHAPTER 9

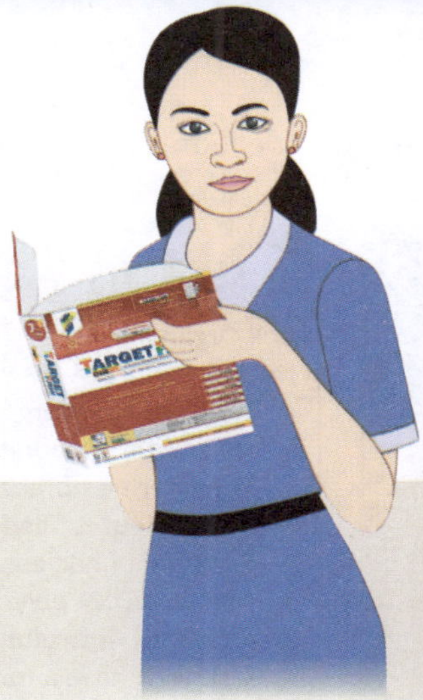

APPLIED BIOCHEMISTRY AND NUTRITION

SYNOPSIS

APPLIED BIOCHEMISTRY

INTRODUCTION

- Biochemistry is the study of chemical processes within a body and related to the living organisms.
- The first enzyme discovered was 'diastase' (now called 'amylase') in the year 1833.
- James Watson, Francis Crick, Maurice Wilkins, and Rosalind Franklin (1950s) co-discovered the **helix structure of DNA.**

THE CELL

- The cell is the structural and functional unit of life.
- Living cells are divided into two groups:
  - Prokaryotes, e.g., Bacteria (unicellular)
  - Eukaryotic cells, e.g., Animal cells, plant cells, fungi and protozoa (unicellular or multicellular)

KEY POINT

- The name Biochemistry was coined in 1903 by a German chemist named Carl Alexander Neuber (1877-1956). He is regarded as "father of modern biochemistry".

Table 1: Differences between prokaryotic cells and eukaryotic cells

Parameters	Prokaryotic cells	Eukaryotic cells
Cell size	Small (1–10 nm)	Large (1 to 10000 times larger in size than prokaryotic cells)
Overall organization	Simple	Complex
Cell wall	Present	Absent
Cell membrane	Present sometimes surrounded by capsule	Present
Nucleus	Single nucleus which contains double helix DNA that is present in a poorly defined region called nucleoid	Well defined nucleus with a membrane and multiple DNA double helices organized into chromatin
Reproduction	Asexual	Sexual
Examples	Bacteria, blue green algae	Animal and plant cells

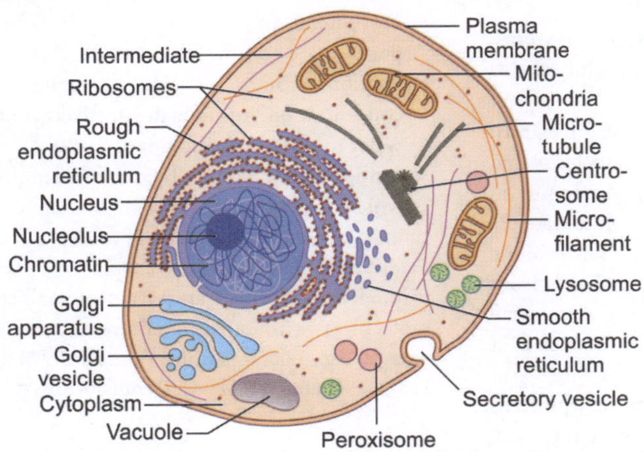

Figure 1: Animal cell structure

KEY POINTS

Cell Organelles

Nucleus

- **Nucleus** is the largest component of the cell, containing DNA organized into separate chromosomes.
- Nucleus is surrounded by nuclear membrane. Nuclear membrane consists of two layers.
- The intermembrane space between inner and outer membrane is known as **perinuclear space (cisterns).**
- The nucleus is filled with nucleoplasm which contains **nucleolus** and **chromatin.**
- Function of nucleus includes control of cell division (DNA replication), protein synthesis.
- DNA and DNA polymerase are the markers of the nucleus.

Endoplasmic Reticulum

- Cisternae have a role in the exchange of materials between the cell and the extracellular fluid.
- **Rough Endoplasmic reticulum (RER):** Also called granular type of endoplasmic reticulum. It contains ribosomes.
- **Smooth Endoplasmic reticulum (SER):** Also called agranular type of endoplasmic reticulum. It does not contain ribosomes. SER has enzymes for biosynthesis of lipids and glycoproteins.
- SER is important in hepatocytes for oxidative metabolism and detoxification of many drugs.
- Glucose-6-phosphatase is a marker enzyme for Endoplasmic reticulum.

Ribosomes

- Ribosomes on the RER are involved in synthesis of proteins for export from the cell.
- Free ribosomes present in the cytoplasm synthesize proteins for use within the cell.

Golgi Apparatus (Golgi complex, Golgi body)

- Golgi apparatus moves molecules from endoplasmic reticulum to their destination.
- It is the site where secretions from other organelles are brought and assembled.
- Newly synthesized proteins are transferred from RER and stored in Golgi apparatus temporarily.

Mitochondria

- Mitochondria are the major organelle of a eukaryotic cell.
- Mitochondria contains its own DNA.
- Mitochondrion produces energy in the form of ATP (Adenosine Triphosphate). So it is called as a **"powerhouse of the cell".**

Lysosomes

- It is a membrane-bound cell organelle and are structurally and chemically spherical vesicles.
- Lysosomes are absent in RBC.
- Lysosomes act as **waste disposal system of the cell.**
- They are responsible for cellular homeostasis.
- They are responsible for autolysis, so it is called as Suicide-bags.

Peroxisomes

- Major function of peroxisomes is in hepatocytes, involved in oxidation of fatty acids.

Cytosol

- It is a colloidal solution of proteins containing nearly 70% water.

Plasma Membrane (cell membrane)

- It is the outer membrane of the cell.
- It is composed of lipids, proteins and carbohydrates.
- Functions include compartmentalization, providing cell shape, cell movement, transport of substances and signal transduction.

TRANSPORT MECHANISMS

There are three types of transport systems, i.e., Diffusion, Facilitated diffusion and Active transport.

- **Diffusion (simple diffusion or passive diffusion):** It is a process in which molecules of a material that move from an area of higher concentration to an area of lower concentration. Some solutes like O_2, N_2, CO_2 and NO, urea move across cell membrane by diffusion. The net movement of molecule from one side to the other side of the cell membrane continues until concentration on both sides is at equilibrium.
  - **Channels** are pore-forming membrane proteins which facilitate flow of ions across secretory and epithelial cells.
  - **Osmosis:** It refers to the spontaneous net movement of solvent molecules through partially permeable (semipermeable) membrane into a region of higher solute concentration. **Aquaporin** selectively conducts water molecules in and out of the cell.
  - **Ionophores:** These are lipid-soluble molecules which facilitate transport of ions across the lipid bilayer of the cell membrane.
- **Facilitated Diffusion:** Transport of solutes through membrane transport proteins (carrier molecules) without expenditure of metabolic energy, e.g., Glucose transporters (GLUT), Cl^-/ HCO_3 exchanger, ATP-ADP translocase.

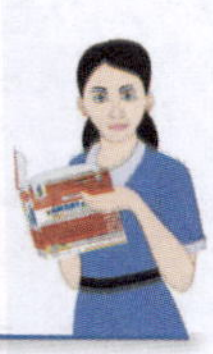

KEY POINTS

- A hypotonic solution is any solution that has a lower osmotic pressure than another solution.
- When the cell is placed into a hypotonic solution it rapidly gains water by osmosis and swells.
- When the cell is placed in the hypertonic solution, it loses water by osmosis and shrinks.

- **Active Transport:** Transport protein moves a specific molecule against the concentration gradient (lower concentration to higher concentration). This process requires energy provided by ATP. It is classified into primary and secondary active transport.

Transport of Large Molecules

- **Endocytosis:** It is a mechanism for the uptake of large molecules such as proteins, polysaccharides, or polynucleotides.
  - **Phagocytosis (cell eating):** Ingestion of bacteria, viruses, etc. It occurs only in specialized cells like macrophages and granulocytes.
  - **Pinocytosis**: Ingestion of liquid into a cell by the budding of small vesicles from the cell membrane.
- **Exocytosis:** It is reverse of endocytosis. It involves release of macromolecules to the exterior of cell.

pH, BUFFERS AND ACID-BASE BALANCE

pH

pH is defined as the negative logarithm ($-\log_{10}$) of the hydrogen ion (H^+) concentration. Low pH indicates higher concentration of H^+ ions; high pH indicates lower H^+ concentration. The scale of pH measurement varies from 0 to 14.

- pH below 7 is considered acidic
- pH equal to 7 is considered neutral
- pH above 7 is considered alkaline.

Acid: It is a substance which releases hydrogen (H^+) ions on dissociation in water.

Base: It is a substance which releases hydroxyl (OH^-) ions in an aqueous solution. The OH^- ions reduce H^+ (acidity) by binding with free H^+ ions.

Amphoteric substances: The substances (E.g., some amino acids and proteins) that can act as acid as well as base are called as Amphoteric substances, e.g. Glycine.

Buffers

Buffer is a solution, which resists change in pH.

- **Plasma Buffers:** Blood plasma has three major buffers:
  - **Phosphate buffer:** Important buffer in the urine
  - **Protein buffer:** It is the largest buffer in the body, e.g., Albumin (blood plasma) and Hemoglobin (intracellular)
  - **Bicarbonate buffer:** Significant buffer in buffering pH in extracellular fluid.

Maintenance of Acid-Base Balance

- Lungs and kidneys stabilize extracellular fluid pH
- **Lungs**: Respiratory system **controls pCO_2** that minimize pH changes in arterial blood
- **Kidney**: Regulates acid-base balance by controlling **bicarbonate reabsorption** and **secreting acid.**

Acid-Base Imbalance

- Normal pH of blood: 7.35–7.45
- Blood pH < 7.35: Acidemia or acidosis
- Blood pH > 7.35: Alkalemia or alkalosis.

KEY POINT

Dialysis is the process of separating molecules in solution by the differences in their rates of diffusion through a semipermeable membrane.

KEY POINTS

- A pH lesşer than 7.35 indicates acidosis.
- A pH greater than 7.45 indicates alkalosis.
- Normal pH of blood: 7.35–7.45
- Normal range of $PaCO_2$: 35–45 mm Hg
- Normal range of P_aO_2: 75–100 mm Hg
- Normal range of HCO_3: 22–26 mEq/L
- Normal range of Oxygen saturation (SPO_2): 95–100%

Table 2: Compensatory responses in different types of acid-base imbalances

Acid-base imbalance	Arterial blood			Compensatory response
	pH	pCO_2	HCO_3	
Respiratory Acidosis	↓	↑	↑	Kidney increases H^+ excretion which in turn increases plasma HCO_3^-
Respiratory Alkalosis	↑	↓	↓	Kidney increases HCO_3^- excretion which in turn decreases plasma HCO_3^-
Metabolic Acidosis	↓	↓	↓	Alveolar hyperventilation
Metabolic Alkalosis	↑	↑	↑	Alveolar hypoventilation

Anion Gap = ($Na^+ + K^+$) – ($Cl^- + HCO_3^-$)

- **Anion gap is a difference between the sum cations ($Na^+ + K^+$) and anions ($Cl^- + HCO_3^-$)**
- **Normal value** anion gap is 12 – 16 mEq/L
- It is most commonly used parameter to establish differential diagnosis for metabolic acidosis.

ENZYMES AND COENZYMES

- All enzymes are protein in nature and have large molecular weights.
- Enzymes are organic molecules that are produced in the living organisms and increase the rate of biochemical reaction.
- Enzymes are not dialyzable, colloidal and thermolabile proteins with highly specific catalytic activity.
- Intracellular enzymes: produced and function within the cell of particular tissue, e.g., Enzymes of citric acid cycle, glycolysis, fatty acid synthesis.

Practice Questions

1. Interpret the following ABG values: pH 7.42, P_aCO_2 40 mm Hg, HCO_3 25 mEq/L.

a. Respiratory alkalosis, compensated
b. Metabolic alkalosis, compensated
c. Metabolic acidosis, uncompensated
d. Normal

Ans. (d) Normal

2. All of the following conditions will cause respiratory alkalosis; EXCEPT:

a. Fever
b. Anxiety
c. Laryngeal obstruction
d. Salicylate toxicity

Ans. (c) Laryngeal obstruction

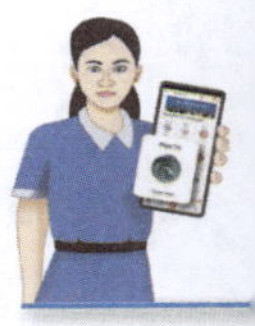

- Extracellular enzymes: Produced by the cells of particular tissue but are liberated and function in other tissues, e.g., Trypsin, Chymotrypsin.

Proenzymes

- Enzymes secreted in their active form are called **zymase**.
- Enzymes secreted in their inactive form is known as **proenzyme** or **zymogen.**
- Proenzyme is converted to active enzyme when it comes in contact with certain activating agents, e.g., Pepsinogen (inactive) is activated into pepsin (active form) by H^+ of gastric juice.

Coenzymes

- A coenzyme is a dialyzable, thermostable, low-molecular weight and organic substance.
- Generally, coenzymes are derivatives of the B complex group of vitamins, e.g., FMN and FAD (derivates of B_2), CoA (derivatives of pyridoxine), Tetrahydrofolate (Folate), etc.

Isoenzymes

- Isoenzymes are generally multiple forms of enzymes. Each of two or more enzymes have identical functions but different structures, e.g., Lactate Dehydrogenase, Creatine Phosphokinase.

Cofactors

- Some enzymes require certain metal ions for their activity. These metal ions are called **cofactors,** e.g., Mg^{2+}, Zn^{2+} or Cl^-.

Classification of Enzymes

- **Oxidoreductase**: Involved in oxidation (addition of oxygen) and/or reduction (removal of hydrogen or electrons) of the substrate, e.g., Alcohol dehydrogenase, Glutathione reductase
- **Transferase:** Catalyze transfer of a particular group from one substrate to another, e.g., Hexokinase, Oxaloacetate transaminase
- **Hydrolase:** It brings about hydrolysis of a substrate with the addition of a water molecule, e.g., Glucose-6-phosphatase, amylase, pepsin
- **Lyase**: It catalzes splitting of a substrate into two products without the addition of water molecule, e.g., Pyruvate decarboxylase, fumarase
- **Isomerase**: Catalyzes the conversion of one isomeric form of the substrate into another, e.g., Alanine racemase
- **Ligase**: Involved in the synthesis of a product by linking two substances together, e.g., Glutamine synthetase.

KEY POINTS

Enzymes

- **Increase in temperature** increases the rate of enzyme catalyzed reaction.
- **Optimum pH** for most of the enzymes is in the neutral range, i.e., around 7.0
- Optimum pH for pepsin is about 2.0 and pancreatic juice is near 8.0.
- Reaction velocity is proportional to the concentration of the enzyme present in the reaction mixture.

Table 3: Major enzymes, their principal sources and diagnostic significance

Enzymes	Principal sources	Increased conditions	Decreased conditions
Acid phosphatase	Prostate and RBC	Carcinoma of prostate	–
Alkaline phosphatase	Liver, bone, placenta and kidney	Obstructive jaundice, rickets, Paget's disease, hyperparathyroidism	–
Aldolase	Skeletal muscle and heart	Muscular dystrophies, acute liver disease	–
Amylase	Salivary glands, pancreas and ovaries	Acute pancreatitis, intestinal obstruction and acute parotitis	Acute liver failure
Ceruloplasmin	Liver	Cirrhosis of liver	Wilson's disease
Choline esterase	Liver	Nephrotic syndrome, organanophosphorous poisoning	Acute liver diseases
Creatine Phosphokinase (CPK)	Skeletal muscles, brain and heart	Myocardial Infarction and muscular dystrophies	–
Glutamate oxaloacetate Transaminase (GPT)	Liver, skeletal muscle, heart, kidney and RBCs	Mycocardial infarction, toxic liver cell necrosis, acute liver diseases, and muscle diseases	–
Gamma-Glutamyl transferase	Liver and kidney	Alcoholism and hepatobiliary diseases	–
Lactate dehydrogenase (isoenzyme)	Heart, liver, skeletal muscle, RBCs and platelets	Acute myocardial infarction, acute hepatitis and muscle disorders	–
Lipase	Pancreas	Acute pancreatitis and pancreatic carcinoma	Liver diseases and diabetes mellitus
5'-Nucleotidase	Hepatobiliary tract	Liver diseases, obstructive jaundice and hepatic carcinoma	–
Trypsin	Pancreas	Acute pancreatic disease	–

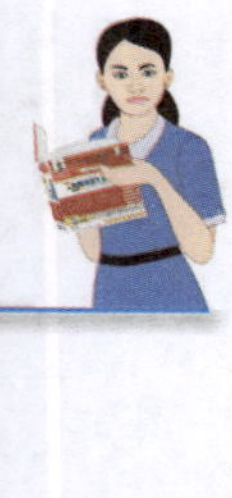

CARBOHYDRATES

- Carbohydrates are the most abundant biological molecules containing Carbon (C), Hydrogen (H) and Oxygen (O) molecules
- Energy production from carbohydrates is 4 kcal/g.

Classification

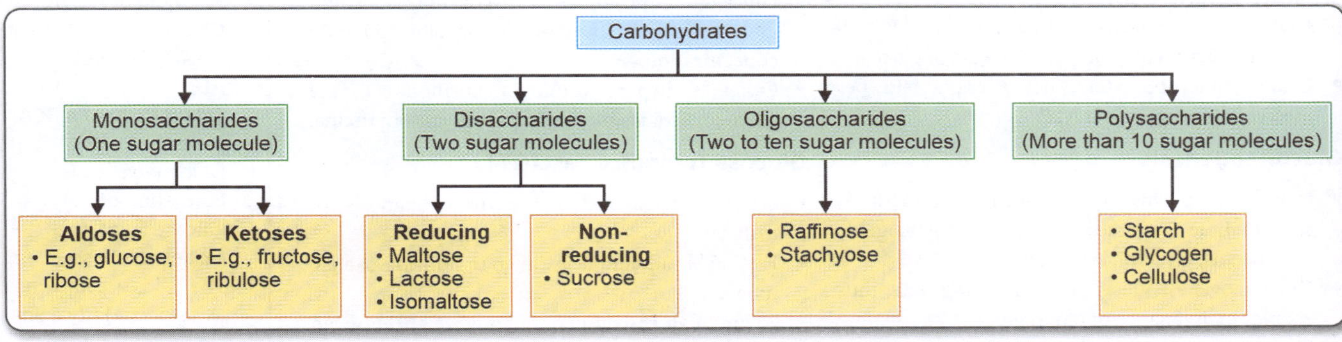

Figure 2: Classification of carbohydrates

- Aldoses: Has aldehyde (–CHO) group on carbon-1, e.g., Glucose
- **Ketoses**: Has ketone (–CO) group at carbon-2, e.g., Fructose
- Trioses are the smallest monosaccharide with 3 carbon atoms, e.g., Glyceraldehyde
- Glucose (dextrose), galactose (constituent of lactose) and fructose are known as **hexoses**
- **Disaccharides (consist of two monosaccharides)**
  - **Sucrose (Cane sugar):** D-Glucose + D-Fructose
  - **Maltose** = D-Glucose + D-Glucose
  - **Lactose (Milk sugar)** = D-Galactose + D-Glucose
- **Polysaccharides**
  - Starch is stored as reservoir of food in cereals and tubers in **plant**
  - Starch consists of two polysaccharide units, i.e., amylase and amylopectin
  - **Glycogen (animal starch)** is found in animals
  - **Cellulose** is a component of cell wall of plants.

Uses of Carbohydrates

- Carbohydrates are the main sources of energy in the body. Brain cells and RBCs are entirely dependent on glucose, an energy source
- Storage form of energy in the body. Stored as glycogen in animals and as Starch in plants
- Glycoproteins and glycolipids are components of cell membranes and receptors.

KEY POINTS

- Carbohydrates are the main energy source of human diet.
- Carbohydrates provide 4 Kcal (calories) per gram.
- Monosaccharides are aldehydes or ketones. They are the simplest forms of carbohydrates in that they cannot be hydrolyzed to smaller carbohydrates.
- Lactose (milk sugar) is a disaccharide (D-galactose + D-glucose).
- Sucrose (cane sugar) is a combination of D-glucose and D-fructose).
- Fructose (monosaccharide) is a fruit sugar.

Digestion of Carbohydrates

Table 4: Digestive enzymes and their action on carbohydrates

Enzymes	Site of action	Action
Salivary amylase	Mouth	Breaks starch/Glycogen into partially hydrolyzed dextrins, oligo-saccharides, isomaltose and maltose
Pancreatic amylase	Small intestine	Breaks partially hydrolyzed dextrins/oligosaccharides into dextrins, maltose, isomaltose, maltotriose
α – Dextrinase	Small intestine	Breaks α – limit dextrins into Maltotriose, glucose
Disaccharidases	Small intestine	
Sucrase	Small intestine	Breaks sucrose into glucose and fructose
Lactase	Small intestine	Breaks lactase into glucose and galactose
Maltase	Small intestine	Maltose into glucose
Isomaltase	Small intestine	Isomaltose into glucose

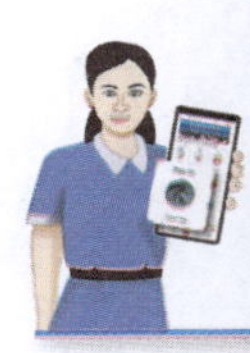

Carbohydrate Metabolism

Glycolysis (Embden-Meyerhof Parnas Pathway)

- Glycolysis is the process of breakdown of glucoses into pyruvic acid (aerobic glycolysis) or lactate (anaerobic glycolysis)
- Under **aerobic conditions**, total yield of **ATP is 10** while the **net yield is 36 per** molecule of glucose
- **Under anaerobic state,** net energy yield per molecule of glucose is 2 ATP.

Gluconeogenesis

- Process of formation of glucose from non-carbohydrate sources such as glucogenic aminoacids, glycerol, lactate, etc.
- Gluconeogenesis takes place in fasting state, thus enables maintenance of blood glucose
- Does not take place in muscle.

TCA Cycle (Tricarboxylic Acid Cycle)

- Also called Citric acid cycle or Krebs cycle
- It is a process of oxidation of Acetyl CoA to CO_2 and H_2O
- **Total ATP yield is 12 ATP** per molecule of acetyl CoA.

Glycogenesis

- Process of conversion of glucose to glycogen
- Glycogenesis is stimulated by insulin.

Glycogenolysis

- Process of conversion of glycogen to either glucose-6-phosphate (in muscle) or free glucose (in liver and kidney).

Regulation of Blood Glucose

- Insulin is the only hormone which has hypoglycemic action
- Insulin lowers blood glucose by facilitating uptake of glucose by extrahepatic tissues and also suppressing glycogenolysis.
- Glucagon promotes glycogenolysis and gluconeogenesis, thus increasing blood glucose concentration.
- Other hyperglycemic hormones are glucocorticoids, growth hormone, and thyroxine.

Glucose Tolerance Test (GTT)

- GTT is performed to confirm diagnosis of diabetes
- Fasting blood sample is drawn in fluoride-oxalate tube
- 75 gm of glucose (1 g/kg of body weight) is given in 200–300 mL of water
- Blood sample is again drawn after 1 hour and 2 hours. Urine sample may also be collected
- Each sample is analyzed and glucose level is plotted against time (glucose tolerance curve)
- In normal individual, the fasting blood sugar should be normal; it increases about 50% within an hour and thereafter returns towards fasting after two hours
- If glucose tolerance curve is normal but there is glycosuria (glucose in urine), it is referred to as **renal glycosuria.**

KEY POINTS

- Carbohydrates form 50–70% of total energy intake in a balanced diet.
- Net yield of ATP in Glycolysis: Aerobic - 36 ATP, Anaerobic - 2 ATP.
- Total ATP yield in TCA cycle is 12 ATP.
- Gluconeogenesis: Formation of glucose from non-carbohydrate sources.
- The lipids are known as esters of fatty acids
- Lipids are insoluble in water.
- One gram of fat provides 9 Kcal of energy.
- Saturated fats tend to be solid at room temperature and mostly from animal sources, while unsaturated fats are usually liquid and mostly from plant sources.
- The three main omega-3 fatty acids are alpha-linolenic acid (ALA), eicosapentaenoic acid (EPA), and docosahexaenoic acid (DHA)
- Omega-3 fatty acids are polyunsaturated fatty acids (PUFA)
- Omega-3 fatty acids significantly reduce blood triglyceride levels

LIPIDS

- Lipid is a heterogeneous group of hydrophobic organic molecules.
- Lipids are insoluble in water and soluble in organic solvent (acetone, alcohol, ether, etc.).

Classification

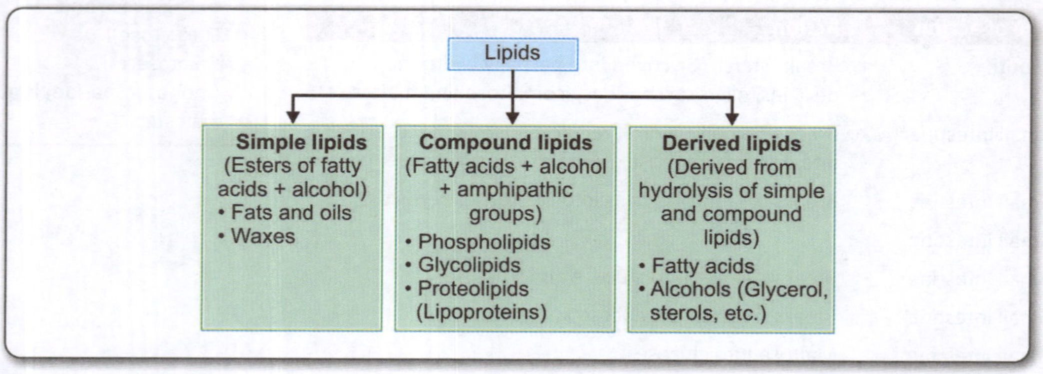

Figure 3: Classification of lipids

KEY POINTS

Lipids

- At room temperature, short chain fatty acids are liquid and long chain fatty acids are solid.
- **Salts of various fatty acids** are used as **soaps** and **emulsifying agents.**
- Hydrogenation of vegetable oil results in the formation of vegetable ghee**.**
- **Saturated fatty acids** end in word "**-anoic**". e.g., Octadecanoic acid.
- **Unsaturated fatty acids** end with **"-enoic".** e.g., Octadecenoic acid.
- **Polyunsaturated fatty acids (PUFA),** i.e., Linolenic acid, linoleic acid and arachidonic acid, form essential components of the diet. They are called **essential fatty acids.** The major sources of PUFA are soybean oil, sunflower oil, groundnut (peanut) oil, etc.
- **Phospholipids** are predominant lipids of a cell membrane. Phospholipids (lecithin) are components of lung surfactants.
- **Phospholipids** are essential component of the bile. It helps in regulation of serum cholesterol.
- **Triacylglycerol** stored in adipose tissue releases free fatty acids during fasting and starvation.
- **Lipids** act as electric insulators in myelin sheath of nervous system**.**

Enzymes Catalyzing the Digestion of Lipids

- **Lingual lipase** is secreted in mouth which converts triglycerides into fatty acids, monoglycerides and glycerol
- Lipase/Colipase, phospholipase, Cholesterol esterase and Retinyl ester hydrolase are secreted in pancreas
- Monoglyceride lipase and licithinase are secreted in small intestine.

Metabolism of Lipids

- The major pathway for catabolism (β-oxidation) of fatty acids occur in the **mitochondria**.
- In β-oxidation, a total of **131 ATP** molecules are produced from one molecule of palmitic acid, however, the **net yield is 129 ATP** because 2 ATPs are used during activation of the fatty acid.
- The process of formation of ketone bodies is called ketogenesis. **Acetoacetate, β-hydroxybutyrate and acetone** are collectively known as ketone bodies.
- **Acetoacetate and β-hydroxybutyrate** are strong acids. Accumulation of these two will lead to metabolic acidosis (ketoacidosis). This occurs in severe diabetes, starvation or on high fat, low carbohydrate diet.
- **Cholesterol** is a metabolic precursor of various substances such as steroid hormones, vitamin D and bile acids and salts.

PROTEINS

- Proteins are nitrogenous organic compounds that are composed of one or more than one long chains of amino acids
- Amino acids are also called building blocks of proteins.

AMINO ACIDS

Amino acids are important dietary sources of nitrogen.

Classification

Based on Structure of their Side Chain

- Neutral amino acids
  - Aliphatic amino acids, e.g., Glycine, Alanine
  - Aromatic amino acids, e.g., Phenylalanine, tyrosine, trypto-phan.
- Acidic amino acids, e.g., Asparagine, Glutamine
- Basic amino acids, e.g., Lysine, arginine, histidine
- Imino acids, e.g., Proline.

Based on Polarity

- Amino acids with polar side chain, e.g., Serine, threonine, tyrosine
- Amino acids with nonpolar side chain, e.g., Glycine, alanine, valine, leucine, etc.

Based on Dietary Requirement

- Essential amino acids
- Semi-essential amino acids
- Non-essential amino acids.

KEY POINTS

- Low Density Lipoprotein (LDL) increases the risk of coronary artery diseases. It is called bad cholesterol.
- High Density Lipoprotein (HDL) decreases, the risk of Coronary Artery Disease (CAD). **Good Cholesterol.**
- Consumption of saturated fats increases the LDL
- Canola oil is high in healthier unsaturated fatty acids.

(NORCET 2023)

Coconut oil is high in saturated fatty acids.

Recent Question
(NORCET 2023)

1. **Which oil is harmful for coronary artery disease**
   a. Coconut oil
   b. sunflower oil
   c. Canola oil
   d. Olive oil

Ans. (a) Coconut oil

Coconut oil is considered harmful for coronary artery disease (CAD) as it is high in saturated fat, which can raise LDL cholesterol levels and contribute to the development and progression of CAD.

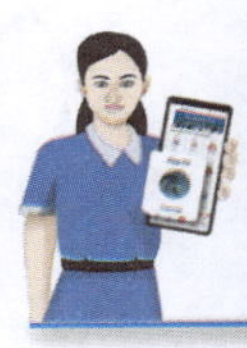

Based on Nutritional Requirement

Table 5: Essential and semi-essential amino acids

Essential amino acids (Cannot be synthesized in the body; to be essentially included in the diet)	
• Isoleucine • Leucine • Lysine • Methionine (Sulfur-containing)	• Phenylalanine • Threonine • Tryptophan • Valine
Semi-essential amino acids (To be essentially included in the diet in certain conditions, e.g., Pregnancy, lactation, high grade fever etc.)	
• Arginine • Histidine	
Non-essential amino acids (Synthesized in the body; not dietary essential)	
• Alanine • Asparagine • Aspartate • Cysteine (sulfur-containing) • Glutamate	• Glutamine • Glycine • Proline • Serine • Tyrosine

Classification

Table 6: Classification of proteins

Simple proteins	Conjugated proteins (Conjugated with non- protein substances)	Derived proteins (Derivates of simple proteins)
• Albumins • Globulins • Glutelins • Prolamines • Sclero-proteins	• Glycoproteins • Lipoproteins • Nucleoproteins • Phosphoproteins • Metalloproteins	• Primary derived proteins (denatured or coagulated proteins • Secondary derived proteins (by cleavage of the peptide bonds)

Transport Proteins and its Functions

Table 7: Molecules transported by transport proteins

Transport proteins	Molecules transported
Albumin	• Copper, Iron, bilirubin, free fatty acids, steroids, heme
Transferrin, ferritin, hemosiderin	• Iron
Ceruloplasmin	• Transport of Copper
Haptoglobin, Hemopexin	• Free hemoglobin
Thyroid binding globulin	• T thyroid hormone
Cortisol binding globulin	• Cortisol
Sex hormone binding globulin	• Androgens, Estrogens

Digestion, Absorption and Metabolism of Proteins

- Digestion of proteins begins in the **stomach** by the action of enzyme pepsin at acidic pH (1.5–2.5) of gastric juice
- Proteolytic enzyme **Pepsin** is secreted in the form of **pepsinogen** (zymogen) by the cells of gastric mucosa. Pepsinogen is activated into pepsin by hydrogen ions of the gastric juice (HCl)
- Trypsin (as trypsinogen), chymotrypsin (as chymotrypsinogen) and carboxypeptidases are secreted by pancreas. These enzymes act on proteolytic products of pepsin in the small intestines.

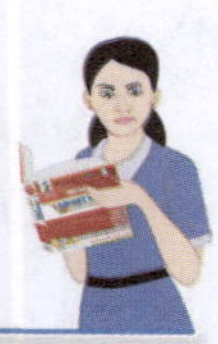

KEY POINTS

- Amino acids are the building blocks of protein.
- Essential amino acids cannot be synthesized in the body. To be essentially included in the diet.
- Type I collagen is the most abundant protein in human body.
- Albumin is the most abundant plasma proteins.
- Albumin comprises 60% of the total serum protein.
- Albumin maintains the oncotic of colloidal osmotic pressure of the blood compartment.

- The end production of digestion of proteins, i.e., amino acids are absorbed from the small intestines
- α-amino group of amino acids can be removed either by **transamination** or **deamination**
- Transamination refers to transfer of α-amino group from an amino acid to keto acid
- Deamination refers to removal of the α-amino group from amino acids
- Ammonia is removed as glutamine from the brain
- Ammonia is removed as urea from the liver (urea cycle)
- **Urea cycle** is the process of converting high toxic ammonia into urea in the liver. Urea is less toxic, water soluble and excretory waste product
- **Phenylketonuria** is a condition due to deficiency of hepatic phenylalanine hydroxylase (autosomal recessive disorder)
- Deficiency of ***tyrosinase*** in the melanocytes causes albinism

VITAMINS, MINERALS AND ELECTROLYTES

Vitamins

- Vitamins are called protective accessory food factors since they are essential for life and well-being.
- Vitamins are classified into water soluble and fat soluble.

KEY POINTS

- The urea cycle or ornithine cycle converts excess ammonia into urea in the mitochondria of liver cells.
- Urea is the chief nitrogenous end product resulting from the metabolic breakdown of proteins.

Recent Question (NORCET 2023)

2. Complications of Thiamine deficiency is:
a. Memory loss
b. Tachycardia
c. Bradycardia
d. Sore throat

Ans. **(a) Memory loss**

POINT TO REMEMBER

Sources, Functions and Deficiency diseases are given in a table form in Appendices.

Table 8: Classification of vitamins

Water soluble vitamins	Fat soluble vitamins
Vitamin C (Ascorbic acid) Vitamin B1 (Thiamin) Vitamin B2 (Riboflavin) Vitamin B3 (Niacin) Vitamin B5 (Pantothenic acid) Vitamin B6 (Pyridoxine) Vitamin B7 (Biotin) Vitamin B9 (Folic acid) Vitamin B12 (Cyanocobalamin) Cholin	Vitamin A (Retinol) Vitamin D • D2 – Ergocalciferol • D3 – Cholecalciferol Vitamin E (Tocoferol) Vitamin K (Menadione)

KEY POINTS

Proteins

- Plasma contains over 300 proteins
- Albumin, globulin and fibrinogen are the major plasma proteins
- Total plasma protein concentration range is 6.3–8.0 g/dL; Albumin – 3.7–5.3 g/dL; globulin – 1.8–3.7 g/dL
- Albumin/Globulin ratio (A/G ratio) is 1.2–2.0:1
- **Albumin** maintains plasma colloidal **osmotic pressure**
- **Hypoalbuminemia** (low plasma albumin) may arise due to protein malnutrition (kwashiorkor/marasmus), malabsorption, chronic liver disease, proteinuria (nephrotic syndrome) or increased catabolism
- **Hyperglobulinemia** (increase in globulin) occurs commonly in advanced liver disease, chronic infectious diseases or multiple myeloma
- Some proteins (e.g., Pepsin and amylase) act as enzymes
- Proteins act as transporters (e.g., Hemoglobin), receptors (e.g., Hormone receptors), storage molecules (e.g., Ferritin).
- On heating or adding strong acids, protein loses its natural structure and gets precipitated. This is known as **denaturation** of proteins
- **Chromatography** is a separation technique used for separating a mixture of chemical substances into its individual components
- **Electrophoresis** is movement of charged particles in solution under the influence of an electric field. This technique is used for separation and quantitative analysis of specific serum proteins, lipoproteins, etc.

Minerals

Sodium

- Sodium (Na^+) is the major extracellular cation
- Normal serum sodium level is 135 – 145 mEq/L
- Na^+ is freely filtered in glomeruli. The filtered sodium is reabsorbed by:
  - Proximal tubules – 70%
  - Loop of Henle – 15%
  - Distal convoluted tubule – 5%
  - Collecting duct – 10%.
- **Functions of sodium:**
  - Fluid and electrolyte balance.
  - Plays a major role in the maintenance of osmotic pressure of body fluids
  - Regulation of acid base balance
  - Maintenance of neuromuscular irritability and excitability (nerve transmission).
  - Maintenance of blood viscosity
  - Helps in absorption of monosaccharide and amino acids.
- **Daily requirement (as sodium chloride) is 5–15 g**
- **Sources:** Main source is common salt. Meat, seafoods, milk and cheese are also good sources of sodium.

Potassium

- Potassium (K^+) is the chief intracellular cation
- Maintenance of normal level of K^+ is essential for life.
- Normal serum potassium level is 3.5 – 5.2 mEq/L
- **Functions**
  - Water and electrolyte balance
  - Regulation of pH of body fluids
  - Maintenance of neuromuscular irritability and excitability
  - Storage of glycogen and cell protein requires K^+
- **Recommended Daily Requirement of potassium for an adult is 4 g.**
- **Sources:** Most of the vegetables (e.g., potato, tomato), dairy products, coffee, cocoa, dried beans, wheat bran, eggs, meat, and fruits (banana, peach, orange).

Calcium

- **Calcium (Ca)** is found in highest concentration in the body
- An adult man contains nearly 1.0–1.2 kg of calcium (99% of it is present in skeletal tissue)
- Normal serum calcium level is 9–11 mg/dL.
- **Calcium absorption**
  - Calcium is absorbed by all parts of small intestine. Most rapid absorptions occur in the acidic medium (duodenum) compared to alkaline medium (remaining part of small intestines).
  - Calcium absorption is impaired in vitamin D deficiency
  - Excess of phosphate reduces calcium absorption.
- **Regulation of serum calcium**
  - Vitamin D increases serum Calcium by promoting intestinal absorption
  - Parathyroid (PTH) hormone plays a vital role in regulation of Ca^{2+}. Low serum calcium leads to increase in the PTH secretion. PTH acts on osteoclasts and promotes transfer of calcium from **bone** tissues to the blood (known as bone resorption)
  - PTH increases reabsorption of calcium by the kidneys
  - Calcitonin lowers serum calcium by promoting deposition of calcium by osteoblasts (opposite to PTH action).
- **Functions**
  - Calcification of growing bones and teeth
  - Maintenance of mature bone
  - Calcium is essential for **blood clotting**
  - Activator for several enzymes
  - Required for contraction of muscles
  - Role in citric acid cycle and glycogen break down.
- Decrease in blood calcium level may result in tetany (abnormal muscle spasm)
- Deficiency of calcium results in rickets in children and osteomalacia in adults
- **Recommended daily requirement is 800 mg for an adult; 1.2 g/day during pregnancy.**

KEY POINTS

- Dietary products are the main sources of calcium.
- Vitamin D promotes intestinal absorption of calcium.
- Parathyroid hormone increases serum calcium by promoting bone resorption and renal reabsorption.
- Calcitonin lowers serum calcium.

Table 9: Minerals, their major functions, sources, RDA, deficiency disorders and toxicity symptoms

Minerals	Biological functions	Sources	Daily requirement	Deficiency disorders	Toxicity symptoms
Calcium (Ca)	Calcification of teeth and bone, blood clotting and cofactor for enzymes, such as adenylate cyclase, glycogen synthase, etc.	Milk and milk products, legumes and dry fruits	800–1200 mg	Tetany, osteoporosis	Renal stones
Phosphorus (P)	Calcification of teeth and bone, component of nucleic acids, regulation of blood pH and activator for enzymes involved in phosphorylation/dephosphorylation	Milk and milk products, eggs, meat, legumes and cereals	1.0–1.5 g	Neuromuscular, skeletal and renal manifestations	—
Iron (Fe)	Component of heme and non-heme proteins, e.g., hemoglobin, catalase, cytochromes, etc.	Meat, green leafy vegetables	10–20 mg	Anemia	Hemosiderosis
Copper (Cu)	Component of many enzymes, such as cytochrome oxidase, ceruloplasmin, tyrosinase, etc., also helps in iron metabolism	Meat, egg and legumes	2–3 mg	Menke's disease, anemia, neutropenia	Wilson disease
Zinc (Zn)	Cofactor for various enzymes, such as carbonic anhydrase, DNA and RNA polymerases, alkaline phosphatase; also has role in insulin secretion and taste development	Meat, seafoods and legumes	10–15 mg	Poor wound healing, growth retardation	Gastrointestinal irritation
Iodine (I_2)	Synthesis of thyroid hormones	Iodized salt, seafoods	50–100 µg	Endemic goiter, myxedema, cretinism	Thyrotoxicosis
Fluoride (F)	Promotes normal bone and teeth development	Drinking water and tea	2–3 mg	Dental caries	Fluorosis
Magnesium (Mg)	Component of the bone structure, in nerve impulse transmission, also acts as cofactor for various ATP-dependent enzymes	Cereals, seafoods, coffee and tea	250–300 mg	Depression, muscle weakness and tetany	Drowsiness and lethargy
Manganese (Mn)	Cofactor for various enzymes, such as hydrolases, decarboxylases, transferases, etc.	Nuts, whole grains and tea	2–5 mg	Bone deformities	Psychotic symptoms
Chromium (Cr)	Regulation of blood glucose	Mushrooms, nuts and black pepper	50–100 µg	Glucose intolerance	Lung cancer
Selenium (Se)	Component of selenoproteins such as glutathione peroxidase	Cereals, fish and meat	50–100 µg	Liver necrosis	Hair loss
Cobalt (Co)	Component of vitamin B_{12}	Liver meat	1–2 µg	Pernicious anemia	Polycythemia, hypothyroidism
Molybdenum (Mo)	Component of flavoprotein containing oxidases such as xanthine oxidase	Pulses and cereals	100–200 µg	Affects growth, causes mental retardation	Anorexia and diarrhea

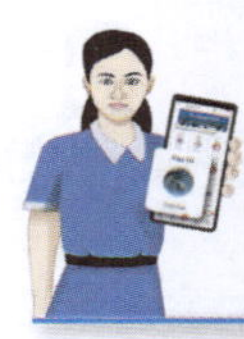

APPLIED NUTRITION

- **Food:** Any substances that are consumed by human or animal for maintaining the health and well-being.
- **Nutrition:** Nutrition is the intake of food, considered in relation to the body's dietary needs.
- **Dietetics**: It is the science that deals with the study of nutrition in health and disease.
- **Nutrients:** Nutrients are the components of food that are essential for normal growth and maintenance of health.
- **Malnutrition:** It is insufficient, excessive, or imbalanced consumption of nutrients.
- **Undernutrition**: Deficient bodily nutrition due to inadequate food intake (hyponutrition)
- **Overnutrition**: Excessive intake of nutrients (hyperalimentation).

CALORIE

- The energy (heat) required to raise the temperature of 1 gram of water through 1°C. It is equal to 4.1868 joules
- 1 Kilocalorie (Kcal) = 1000 Calories, i.e., the energy (heat) required to raise the temperature of 1000 gram (1 kg) of water through 1°C (4.1868 Kilojoules)

Table 10: Caloric values of macronutrients per gram

Macronutrients	Kilocalorie (kcal)/gram
Carbohydrates	4
Proteins	4
Fat	9

METABOLISM

- **Catabolism:** Biochemical processes that break down molecules in an organism are known as catabolism.
- **Anabolism:** Processes that build up complex materials from simpler substances are known as anabolism.
- **Basal Metabolic Rate (BMR):** It is the amount of energy (in calories) that is required to maintain vital body functions while at rest, for example, breathing, blood circulation, cell growth, nerve functions, etc.
- **Facts about BMR**
  - BMR is greatest during first few years of life.
  - Females have 2 to 12% less BMR as compared to males. BMR is increased in pregnancy and lactation.
  - BMR increases in cold climate. BMR increases by 7% with a rise in body temperature by each degree Fahrenheit.
  - Nonvegetarians have 11% more BMR than vegetarians.
  - BMR increases when adrenaline and nonadrenaline is released.
  - Certain drugs (e.g., Caffeine, nicotine) increases BMR.
  - Increased BMR: Hyperthyroidism, Cushing's syndrome, diabetes insipidus, leukemias, polycythemia.
  - Decreased BMR: Hypothyroidism, Addison's disease, hypopituitarism and shock.

Formula to Calculate BMR

Men:

BMR = $66 + (13.7 \times \text{weight kg}) + (5 \times \text{height in cm}) - (6.8 \times \text{age in years})$

Women:

BMR = $65 + (9.6 \times \text{weight kg}) + (1.8 \times \text{height in cm}) - (4.7 \times \text{age in years})$

CLASSIFICATION OF FOODS

Based on chemical composition

- Macronutrients
  - Proteins
  - Fats
  - Carbohydrates
- Micronutrients
  - Vitamins
  - Minerals

Based on Origin of food

- Animal origin (E.g., meat, seafood, etc.)
- Plant origin (E.g., vegetables).

Based on Predominant function

- Body building food, e.g., milk, meat, egg, pulse, etc. (Protein)
- Energy giving food, e.g., sugar, root, tubers, fats and oils (Carbohydrates and fat)
- Protective food, e.g., vegetables, fruits, milk (Rich in Vitamin and minerals).

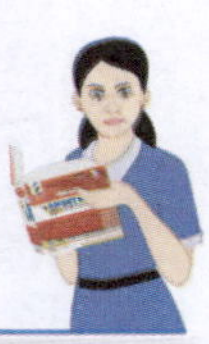

Recent Question (NORCET 2023)

3. What is the range of MUAC for malnutrition?

a. <12.5 cm
b. <11.5 cm
c. <13.5 cm
d. <14.5 cm

Ans. (a) <12.5 cm

Recent Question (NORCET 2021)

4. Which of the following is given to pregnant women to prevent Neural Tube Defect in fetus?

a. Folic acid
b. Calcium tablets
c. Vitamin K
d. Thyroxin

Ans. (a) Folic acid

Recent Question (NORCET 2022)

5. After receiving her dinner tray, a 10-year-old child with insulin-dependent diabetes mellitus expresses a dislike for broccoli and requests corn on the plate instead. The nurse's appropriate response is:

a. "No vegetable exchanges are allowed."
b. "Yes, you may exchange any vegetable for any other vegetable."
c. "Corn and other starchy vegetables are considered to be bread exchanges."
d. "Yes, but only one-half ear is allowed."

Ans. (c) Corn and other starchy vegetables are considered to be bread exchanges.

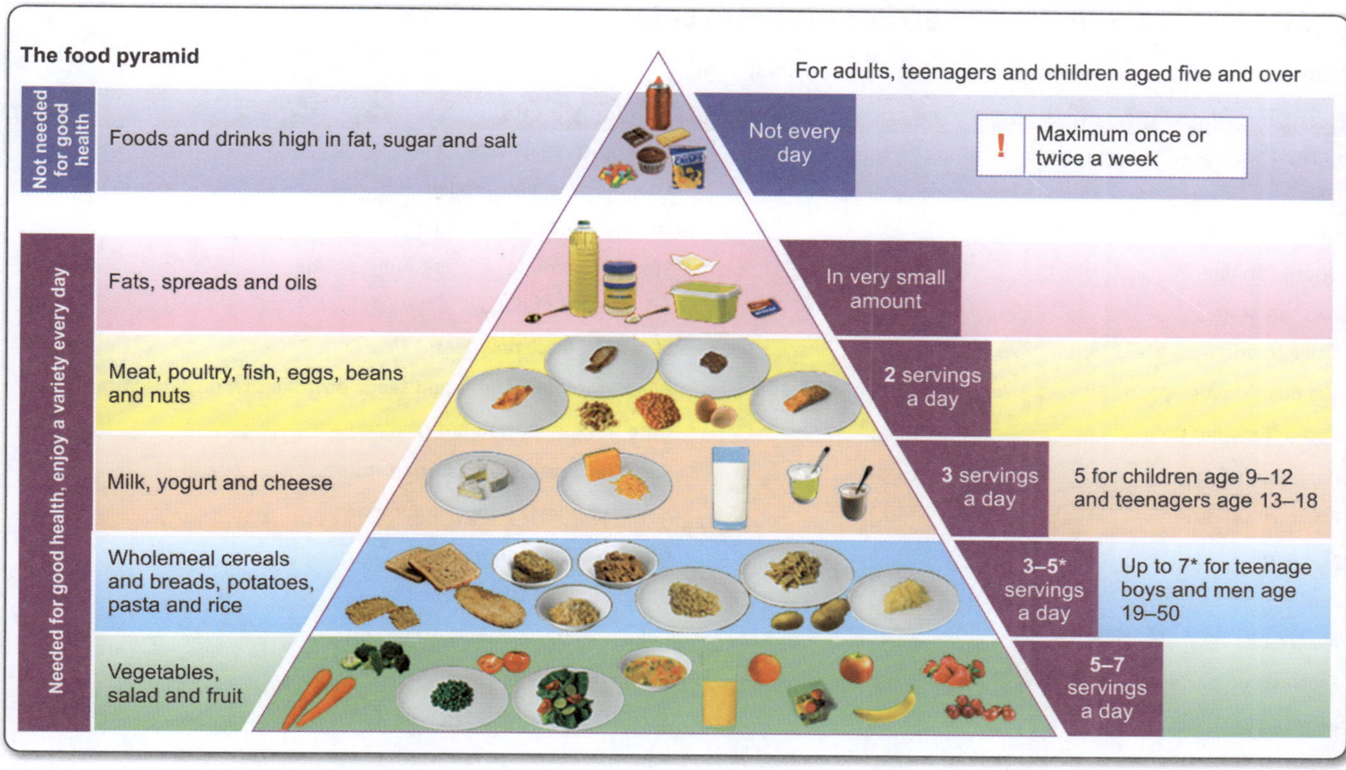

*Daily servings guide—wholemeal cereals and breads, potatoes, pasta and rice

Active	Child (5–12)	Teenager (13–18)	Adult (19–50)	Adult (51+)
Female	3–4	4	4–5	3–4
Male	3–5	5–7	5–7	4–5

Inactive	Teenager (13–18)	Adult (19–50)	Adult (51+)
Female	3	3–4	3
Male	4–5	4–6	4

Drink at least 8 glasses of fluid in a day—water is best

There is no guideline for inactive children as it is essential that all children are active

Figure 4: The food pyramid showing the amount of food products that should be consumed as a balanced diet

FOOD PRESERVATION METHODS

Table 11: Household and commercial methods of preservation

Household methods	Commercial methods
• Refrigeration • Heating • Pickles and Jams • Drying • Smoking • Chemical • Sealing	• Canning and bottling • Machine drying • Preservatives • Freeze drying • Cold storage • Irradiation • Use of antibiotics • Pasteurization

COMMON ADULTERANTS USED IN FOOD MATERIALS

Table 12: Food materials and their respective common adulterants

Food materials	Common adulterants
Cereals such as wheat and rice	Mud, grits, soapstone bits
Dals	Coal tar dyes, khesari dals
Haldi (Turmeric powder)	Lead chromate powder
Dhania powder	Starch, cow dung or horse dung powder
Black pepper	Dried seeds of papaya
Chilli powder	Saw dust, brick powder
Tea dust/leaves	Black gram husk, tamarind seeds powder, saw dust, used tea dust
Coffee powder	Date husk, tamarind husk, chicory
Asafetida (Hing)	Sand, grit, resins, gums, soap stones
Mustard seeds	Seeds of prickly poppy, argemone
Edible oils	Mineral oil, argemone oil
Butter	Starch, animal fat
Ice creams	Cellulose, starch, non-permitted colors
Fresh green packed peas	Green dye
Milk	Extraction of fat, addition of starch and water
Ghee	Vanaspati, mashed potatoes, sweet potatoes
Sweet wines	Diethylene glycol
Honey	High fructose syrup, cane sugar, jaggery
Alcoholic liquors	Methanol
Wheat flour	Excessive sand, dirt, bran and chalk powder
Cumin seeds	Grass seeds colored with charcoal dust

TESTS TO DETECT COMMON ADULTERATION

Table 13: Tests to detect common adulteration in food items

Food items	Test to detect adulteration
Honey	• **Aniline Chloride test** (starch mixed honey turns orange red in color if mixed aniline chloride)
Ghee	• **Iodine solution test** (boil sample and add a drop of iodine solution; sample turns blue if starch was mixed; color disappears if cooled and reappears on heating again)
Black pepper	• Papaya seeds float on **carbon tetrachloride** solution while pure black pepper seeds settles down.
Coriander powder	• Soak in water. Dung will float and can be detected by its foul smell
Pulses	• Heat with **diluted HCL** on simmer for 15 mins. Pink color indicates presence of kesari dal
Chilli powder	• Add sample in a beaker of **Chloroform+carbon tetrachloride**. Brick powder will settle at the bottom
Wheat flour	• Shake sample with dilute Hydrochloride; effervescence indicates chalk
Turmeric powder	• Dissolve sample in 1:7 **sulphuric acid** and filter it. Add 1 to 2 drops of 0.1% **diphenylcarbazide**; A pink color indicates presence of lead chromate
Asafetida (Hing)	• Shake a small quantity with water. **Soap stone** or **other earthly matter** will settle at bottom
Cumin seeds (Jeera)	• Rub the cumin seeds on palms. If palm turns black, adulteration is indicated.

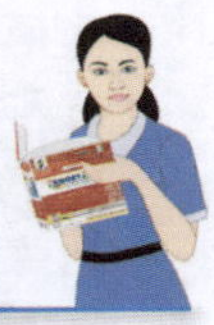

Golden Points to Remember

- The name Biochemistry was coined in 1903 by a German chemist named Carl Alexander Neuber (1877-1956). He is regarded as "father of modern biochemistry"
- The first enzyme discovered was 'diastase' (now called 'amylase') in the year 1833
- James Watson, Francis Crick, Maurice Wilkins, and Rosalind franklin (1950s) co-discovered the **helix structure of DNA**
- The cell is the structural and functional unit of life
- **Nucleus** is the largest component of the cell, containing DNA organized into separate chromosome
- Nucleus is surrounded by nuclear membrane. Nuclear membrane consists of two layers
- Function of nucleus includes control of cell division (DNA replication), protein synthesis
- Glucose-6-phosphatase is a marker enzyme for Endoplasmic reticulum
- Mitochondria produces energy in the form of ATP. So it is called as "power house of the cell"
- Ribosomes on the RER are involved in synthesis of proteins for export from the cell
- Lysosomes act as **waste disposal system of the cell**
- Diffussion is a process in which molecules of a material that move from an area of higher concentration to an area of lower concentration
- Osmosis refers to the spontaneous net movement of solvent molecules through partially permeable (semipermeable) membrane into a region of higher solute concentration
- **Aquaporin** selectively conduct water molecules in and out of the cell
- **Ionophores** are a lipid-soluble molecules which facilitate transport of ions across the lipid bilayer of the cell membrane
- Transport of solutes through membrane transport proteins (carrier molecules) without expenditure of metabolic energy is known as facilitated diffusion
- In Active transport, Transport protein moves a specific molecule against the concentration gradient
- A hypotonic solution is any solution that has a lower osmotic pressure than another solution
- When the cell is placed into a hypotonic solution it rapidly gains water by osmosis and swells
- When the cell is placed in the hypertonic solution, it losses water by osmosis and shrinks.
- Dialysis is the process of separating molecules in solution by the differences in their rates of diffusion through a semipermeable membrane
- A pH lesser than 7.35 indicates acidosis
- A pH greater than 7.45 indicates alkalosis.
- Normal pH of blood: 7.35 - 7.45
- Normal range of PaCO2: 35 to 45 mmHg
- Normal range of PaO2: 75 to 100 mmHg
- Normal range of HCO3: 22 to 26 mEq/L
- Normal range of Oxygen saturation (SPO2): 95-100%
- Lungs and kidneys stabilize extracellular fluid pH
- Respiratory system **controls pCO_2** that minimize pH changes in arterial blood
- **Kidney** regulates acid-base balance by controlling **bicarbonate reabsorption** and **secreting acid.**
- **Anion gap is a difference between the sum cations and anions**
- All enzymes are protein in nature and have large molecular weights
- Enzymes secreted in their active form are called **zymase**
- Enzymes secreted in their inactive form is known as **proenzyme** or **zymogen**
- **Increase in temperature** increases the rate of enzyme catalyzed reaction
- **Optimum pH** for most of the enzymes is in the neutral range, i.e. around 7.0
- Optimum pH for pepsin is about 2.0 and pancreatic juice is near 8.0
- Carbohydrates are the most abundant biological molecules containing Carbon (C), Hydrogen (H) and Oxygen (O) molecules
- Energy production from carbohydrates is 4 kcal/g.
- Aldoses has aldehyde (–CHO) group on carbon-1, e.g. Glucose
- **Ketoses has** ketone (–CO) group at carbon-2, e.g. Fructose
- Trioses are the smallest monosaccharide with 3 carbon atoms, e.g. Glyceraldehyde
- **Disaccharides consist of two monosaccharides**
- **Sucrose is a cane sugar made up of Glucose and Fructose**
- Lactose (milk sugar) is a disaccharide made up of D-Glucose and D-Galactose
- Fructose (monosaccharide) is a fruit sugar
- Starch is stored as reservoir of food in cereals and tubers in **plant**
- Carbohydrate forms 50-70% of total energy intake in a balaneced diet.
- Net yield of ATP in Glycolysis: Aerobic - 36 ATP, Anaerobic - 2 ATP.
- Total ATP yield in TCA cycle is 12 ATP.
- Gluconeogenesis refers to formation of glucose from non-carbohydrate sources.
- TCA cycle is alco called Citric acid cycle or Krebs cycle.
- **Total ATP yield in TCA cycle is 12 ATP** per molecule of acetyl CoA
- Gluconeogenesis is a process of formation of glucose from non-carbohydrate sources such as glucogenic aminoacids, glycerol, lactate etc.
- Gluconeogenesis takes place in fasting state, thus enables maintenance of blood glucose
- Insulin is the only hormone which has hypoglycemic action
- Glucagon promotes glycogenolysis and gluconeogenesis, thus increasing blood glucose concentration
- Glucose Tolerance Test (GTT) is performed to confirm diagnosis of diabetes. In this test, 75 gm of glucose (1g/kg of body weight) is given in 200-300 ml of water
- The lipids are known as esters of fatty acids
- Lipids are insoluble in water.

Contd...

- One gram of fat provides 9 Kcal of energy.
- Saturated fats tend to be solid at room temperature and mostly from animal sources, while unsaturated fats are usually liquid and mostly from plant sources.
- The three main omega-3 fatty acids are alpha-linolenic acid (ALA), eicosapentaenoic acid (EPA), and docosahexaenoic acid (DHA)
- Omega-3 fatty acids are polyunsaturated fatty acids (PUFA)
- Omega-3 fatty acids significantly reduce blood triglyceride levels
- Low Density Lipoprotein (LDL) increases the risk of coronary artery diseases. It is called bad cholesterol.
- High Density Lipoprotein (HDL) decrease the risk of Coronary Artery Disease (CAD). **Good Cholesterol.**
- Consumption of saturated fats increases the LDL
- Coconut oil is high in saturated fatty acids.
- Canola oil is high in healthier unsaturated fatty acids.
- **Salts of various fatty acids** are used as **soaps** and **emulsifying agents**
- Hydrogenation of vegetable oil results in the formation of vegetable ghee
- **Saturated fatty acids** end in word "-**anoic**". e.g. Octadecanoic acid.
- **Unsaturated fatty acids** end with **"-enoic".** e.g. Octadecenoic acid.
- **Polyunsaturated fatty acids (PUFA),** i.e. Linolenic acid, linoleic acid and arachidonic acid, form essential component of the diet. They care called **essential fatty acids.** The major sources of PUFA are soybean oil, sunflower oil, groundnut (peanut) oil etc.
- **Lipids** act as electric insulators in myelin sheath of nervous system
- Proteins are nitrogenous organic compounds that are composed of one or more than one long chains of amino acids
- Amino acids are also called building blocks of proteins.
- Essential amino acids cannot be synthesized in the body. It has to be essentially included in the diet
- Essential amino acids include Isoleucine, Leucine, Lysine, Methionine (sulfur-containing), Phenylalanine, threonine, Tryptophan, and Valine.
- Type I collagen is the most abundant protein in human body.
- Albumin is the most abundant plasma proteins.
- Albumin comprises 60% of the total serum protein
- Albumin maintains the osmotic pressure of the blood compartment
- Digestion of proteins begins in the **stomach** by the action of enzyme pepsin at acidic pH (1.5 – 2.5) of gastric juice
- **Urea cycle** is the process of converting high toxic ammonia into urea in the liver. Urea is less toxic, water soluble and excretory waste product
- The urea cycle or ornithine cycle converts excess ammonia into urea in the mitochondria of liver cells.
- Urea is the chief nitrogenous end product resulting from the metabolic breakdown of proteins
- **Phenylketonuria** is a condition due to deficiency of hepatic phenylalanine hydroxylase (autosomal recessive disorder)
- Albumin, globulin and fibrinogen are the major plasma proteins
- **Albumin** maintains plasma colloidal **osmotic pressure**
- Sodium (Na+) is the major extracellular cation
- Normal serum sodium level is 135 – 145 mEq/L
- **Daily requirement of Sodium is (as sodium chloride) is 5 – 15g**
- Potassium (K+) is the chief intracellular cation
- Normal serum potassium level is 3.5 – 5.2 mEq/L
- **Recommended Daily Requirement of potassium for an adult is 4g.**
- **Calcium** is found in highest concentration in the body
- An adult man contains nearly 1.0 – 1.2 kg of calcium (99% of it present in skeletal tissue)
- Normal serum calcium level is 9 – 11 mg/dl.
- **Recommended daily requirement is 800 mg for an adult; 1.2 g/day during pregnancy**
- Calcium is essential for **blood clotting**
- Dietary products are the main dietary source of calcium.
- Vitamin D increases promotes intestinal absorption of calcium.
- Parathyroid hormone increases serum calcium by promoting bone resorption and renal reabsorption.
- Calcitonin lowers serum calcium.
- Biochemical processes that break down molecules in an organism are known as catabolism
- Processes that build up complex materials from simpler substances are known as anabolism
- **Basal Metabolic Rate** (BMR) is the amount of energy (in calories) that is required to maintain vital body functions while at rest, for example, breathing, blood circulation, cell growth, nerve functions etc.
- BMR is greatest during first few years of life
- BMR is increased in Hyperthyroidism, Cushing's syndrome, diabetes insipidus, leukemias, polycythemia
- BMR is decreased in Hypothyroidism, Addison's disease, hypopituitarism and shock.
- Aniline Chloride test is used to detect adulteration in Honey.
- Iodine solution test is used to detect adulteration in Ghee

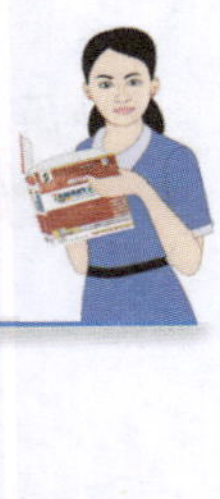

"Ill-health of body or of mind, is defeat. Health alone is victory."

—Thomas Carlyle

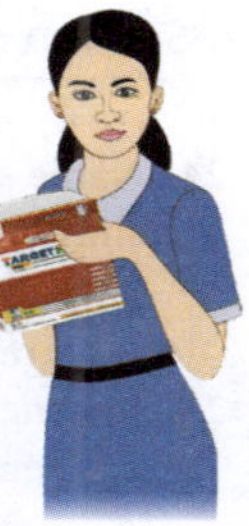

MULTIPLE CHOICE QUESTIONS (Including Explained and Practice Questions)

INTRODUCTION AND ANATOMY OF CELL

1. **Pyknosis is characterized by:** *(Safdarjung NO 2018)*
   a. Nuclear basophilia b. Nuclear shrinkage
   c. Nucleus disintegration d. Nucleolus disintegration

Explanation: Pyknosis is irreversible cell death characterized by nuclear condensation/shrinkage and clumping of chromatin.

2. **The activation of caspases is likely to lead to:** *(Safdarjung NO 2018)*
   a. Apoptotic cell death
   b. Blood coagulation
   c. Mitotic cell division
   d. G1 and S phase of cell cycle

Explanation: Activation of enzymes called Caspases leads to apoptosis which is a pathway of cell death. Caspases are cysteine proteases that help in cleavage of proteins.

3. **Mitosis is a condition of:** *(Banaras HU 2015)*
   a. Cell breakdown
   b. Cell division without reduction
   c. Cell death
   d. Cell division with half chromosomes
4. **Powerhouse of the cell is:** *(ESIC Chennai May 2012)*
   a. Mitochondria b. Nucleus
   c. Golgi bodies d. Cell wall
5. **Chief components of a cell are:**
   a. Carbon, hydrogen, nitrogen and oxygen
   b. Hydrogen, nitrogen, sodium and potassium
   c. Magnesium, potassium, carbon and hydrogen
   d. Helium, nitrogen, calcium and carbon
6. **The aqueous component of the cell, within which various organelles and particles are suspended, is:**
   a. Cytosol b. Cytoplasm
   c. Nucleus d. Cytoblast
7. **Number of mitochondria is less in:**
   a. Red fibers b. Myosin
   c. White fibers d. Actin
8. **Storage house of iron in a cell is:**
   a. WBC
   b. Reticuloendothelial system
   c. Platelet
   d. Ribosome
9. **Cytokines are responsible for:**
   a. Pain b. Touch
   c. Sensation d. Inflammation
10. **Largest organelle of a cell is:**
   a. Golgi apparatus b. Nucleus
   c. Ribosome d. Endoplasmic reticulum
11. **Suicidal bag of cell is:**
   a. Ribosome b. Lysosomes
   c. Vacuole d. Nucleus
12. **Plasma membrane of eukaryotic organisms is made up of:**
   a. Phospholipid bilayer
   b. Phospholipid monolayer
   c. Carbohydrate, protein and fat
   d. Carbon, nitrogen and oxygen
13. **Structure and motility of the cell is maintained by:**
   a. Cartilage b. Microtubules
   c. Nucleus d. Golgi apparatus
14. **Powerhouse of the all human body is:**
   a. Nucleus b. Ribosome
   c. Mitochondria d. Lysosome
15. **Produced form of energy is:**
   a. ATP b. ADP
   c. GTP d. Actin
16. **Cytoplasm refers to:**
   a. Contents of the cell including nucleus
   b. Contents of the cell excluding nucleus
   c. Nucleus of the cell
   d. Nucleus and cytosol of the cell
17. **Protein factory in human cell is:**
   a. Ribosome
   b. Nucleus
   c. Cytoplasm
   d. Golgi apparatus
18. **__________ has no nucleus:**
   a. RBCs b. WBCs
   c. Lymphocytes d. Monocytes
19. **Pinocytosis are:**
   a. Drinking b. Phagocyting
   c. Moving d. RNA production
20. **Phagocytosis is the responsibility of:**
   a. Eosinophil b. Neutrophils
   c. Monocyte d. Lymphocyte
21. **Which of the following order is correct about phases of mitosis cell division?**
   a. Prophase - Anaphase - Telophase - Metaphase
   b. Prophase - Anaphase - Metaphase - Telophase
   c. Prophase - Metaphase - Telophase - Anaphase
   d. Prophase - Metaphase - Anaphase - Telophase
22. **Name the tissue which is widely and abundantly distributed in human body:**
   a. Connective tissue b. Cartilaginous tissue
   c. Lymphoid tissue d. Epithelial tissue
23. **All are loose connective tissues; EXCEPT:**
   a. Areolar b. Reticular
   c. Adipose d. Epithelial

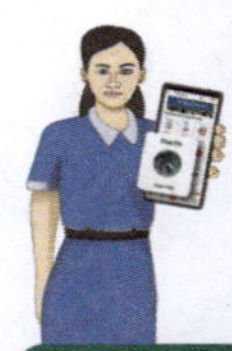

Ans.

1.	b
2.	a
3.	b
4.	a
5.	a
6.	b
7.	c
8.	b
9.	d
10.	b
11.	b
12.	a
13.	b
14.	c
15.	a
16.	b
17.	a
18.	a
19.	a
20.	b
21.	d
22.	a
23.	d

24. Name the epithelium which is most efficient in allowing simple substances across cell:
a. Squamous epithelium b. Simple stratified epithelium
c. Transitional epithelium d. Stratified epithelium

25. Regenerating capacity is more in .... tissue.
a. Muscle b. Epithelial
c. Cartilaginous d. Bone

26. Identify the function of epithelium:
a. Absorption b. Protection
c. Secretion d. All of these

27. Among the following, cuboidal epithelium is seen in:
a. Skin b. Trachea
c. Esophagus d. Thyroid gland

28. Lining of the uterus is made up of:
a. Simple columnar epithelium
b. Ciliated columnar epithelium
c. Simple squamous epithelium
d. Simple cuboidal epithelium

29. Lining of the trachea is made up of:
a. Simple stratified epithelium
b. Stratified columnar epithelium
c. Columnar epithelium
d. Pseudostratified columnar epithelium

30. Epithelium which allows the stretching and distention of hollow organ and helps to accommodate the content:
a. Simple epithelium b. Squamous epithelium
c. Transitional epithelium d. Cuboidal epithelium

31. Among the following, transitional epithelium is present in:
a. Esophagus b. Trachea
c. Urinary bladder d. All of these

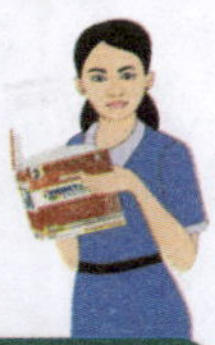

32. Formation of scar tissue is:
a. Fibrosis b. Granulation
c. Adhesion d. Keloid

33. The major function of ciliated epithelium present in the uterine tubes is to facilitate:
a. Implantation of fertilized ova
b. Movement of ova in uterine tube
c. Release of ova from fallopian tube
d. Secretion in endometrium

34. The mucous, serous and synovial membranes are formed by sheets of:
a. Epithelial tissue b. Connective tissue
c. Fibrous tissue d. Nervous tissue

35. Efficient regenerating capacity is more after mechanical friction in:
a. Simple epithelium b. Squamous epithelium
c. Transitional epithelium d. Stratified epithelium

36. Maturation of B-cell lymphocytes takes place at:
a. Blood b. Bone marrow
c. Brain d. Base of the skull

37. Maturation of T-cell lymphocytes takes place at:
a. Thyroid b. Thymus
c. Trachea d. Liver

38. Memory cells are formed from:
a. Neutrophil b. Eosinophil
c. Lymphocytes d. Monocyte

39. Cisternae are the part of .... cellular organ.
a. Endoplasmic reticulum b. Golgi apparatus
c. Lysosome d. Both a and b

40. Cellular organ responsible for destroying foreign material and microorganism is:
a. Nucleus b. Lysosomes
c. Mitochondria d. Vacuole

41. Which of the following organelles is responsible for the production of energy in the form of ATP in human cells? *New Q*
a. Nucleus b. Mitochondria
c. Golgi apparatus d. Endoplasmic reticulum

Explanation: Mitochondria are the organelles responsible for producing energy in the form of ATP in human cells. They are found in all eukaryotic cells, and they are often called the "powerhouses" of the cell.

42. Which of the following is the most abundant type of molecule in the cell membrane? *New Q*
a. Phospholipids b. Proteins
c. Carbohydrates d. DNA

Explanation: Phospholipids are the most abundant type of molecule in the cell membrane. They make up about 50% of the cell membrane.

43. Which organelle is responsible for the detoxification of harmful substances in human cells? *New Q*
a. Nucleus
b. Golgi apparatus
c. Smooth endoplasmic reticulum
d. Lysosomes

Explanation: Lysosomes play a number of important roles in the cell, including: detoxification, Phagocytosis, and autophagy.

44. Epithelial tissues are characterized by: *New Q*
a. High vascularity b. Extracellular matrix
c. Cellularity and polarity d. Cells are loosely packed

Explanation: Epithelial tissues are characterized by being cellular, means they are made up of cells. They are also polarized, means they have a distinct apical (top) and basal (bottom) surface. The apical surface is typically facing the outside of the body or an internal cavity, while the basal surface is attached to a basement membrane.

45. The structure that provides attachment between epithelial cells is called: *New Q*
a. Basement membrane b. Extracellular matrix
c. Desmosomes d. Gap junctions

Explanation: Desmosomes are specialized structures that hold epithelial cells together. They are composed of transmembrane proteins that anchor the cells to each other. Desmosomes are important for maintaining the integrity of epithelial tissues.

46. Mucous membrane of vagina is lined by:
a. Nonkeratinized stratified squamous epithelium
b. Keratinized Stratified Squamous epithelium
c. Columnar cells
d. Cuboidal epithelium

47. Which of the following is both endocrine and exocrine gland?
a. Thyroid b. Pituitary
c. Pancreas d. Adrenal

48. Shrinkage of cell size is known as:
a. Atrophy b. Metastasis
c. Necrosis d. Hypertrophy

Ans.

24.	a
25.	b
26.	d
27.	d
28.	a
29.	d
30.	c
31.	c
32.	a
33.	b
34.	a
35.	d
36.	b
37.	b
38.	c
39.	d
40.	b
41.	b
42.	a
43.	d
44.	c
45.	c
46.	a
47.	c
48.	a

49. Identify cellular adaptation among the following:
a. Hypertrophy b. Atrophy
c. Hyperplasia d. All of these

50. Correct regarding metaplasia is:
a. It is a reversible change
b. It results from the reprogramming of stem cells
c. It makes the cells more resistant to the stem cells
d. All of the above

51. The Golgi apparatus:
a. Is composed of a stack of disc-shaped cisternae.
b. Is involved in the biosynthesis of phospholipid.
c. Contains the enzymes of the glyoxylate cycle.
d. Is involved in the glycosylation of the proteins.

52. The following points about endoplasmic reticulum are true except that:
a. It contains spaces, which serve as channels for transport.
b. It may be either 'rough' or smooth.
c. It plays a role in lipid biosynthesis.
d. It plays a role in the synthesis of carbohydrates.

53. Codons are present on:
a. DNA b. mRNA
c. tRNA d. rRNA

54. The Watson-Crick model of DNA is:
a. Right-handed antiparallel double helix.
b. Left-handed antiparallel double helix.
c. Right-handed parallel double helix.
d. Left-handed parallel double helix.

55. Which of the following cellular organelle serves as the site of protein synthesis?
a. Golgi bodies
b. Endoplasmic reticulum
c. Mitochondria
d. Peroxisomes

56. Which of the following cellular organelle causes autodigestion?
a. Golgi bodies
b. Lysosomes
c. Microsomes
d. Peroxisomes

57. The nitrogenous base absent in DNA is:
a. Uracil b. Cytosine
c. Thymine d. Guanine

58. All these reactions take place inside the mitochondria; EXCEPT:
a. EM pathway
b. Urea cycle
c. Electron transport chain
d. Beta oxidation of fatty acids

59. Eukaryotic plasma membrane is made up of all; EXCEPT:
a. Carbohydrates
b. Triglycerides
c. Lecithin
d. Cholesterol

60. Which of the following occurs in mitochondria and cytosol?
a. Urea cycle
b. Glycolysis
c. Gluconeogenesis
d. HMP shunt pathway

61. Protein synthesis occurs in:
a. Ribosomes b. Golgi apparatus
c. Lysosomes d. Endosomes

62. Protein glycosylation occurs in:
a. ER b. Golgi bodies
c. Mitochondria d. Peroxisomes

63. Mitochondria have:
a. Plasmid DNA b. Circular DNA
c. Single stranded DNA d. Double stranded DNA

64. Synthesis of rRNA takes place in:
a. Cytosol
b. Nucleus
c. Nucleolus
d. Mitochondria

65. Membrane proteins are synthesized in:
a. Free ribosome
b. Bound ribosome
c. Nucleolus
d. Mitochondria

66. RNA is present in:
a. Cytoplasm b. Nucleus
c. Ribosome d. All of these

67. Main function of mitochondria is:
a. Protein synthesis
b. Glycolysis
c. Electron transfer
d. Fat synthesis

68. Estrogen receptors are seen in:
a. Microsomes
b. Membrane bound
c. Nucleus
d. Mitochondria

69. Protein synthesis is sorted out at/by:
a. Ribosomes
b. Mitochondria
c. Golgi apparatus
d. Endoplasmic reticulum

70. In mammalian cells, protein synthesis takes place chiefly at:
a. Smooth endoplasmic reticulum
b. Rough endoplasmic reticulum
c. Nucleus
d. Nucleolus

71. Cellular organelle that stores peroxidases is:
a. Lysosomes
b. Peroxisome
c. Microsomes
d. None of these

72. Secretory proteins are synthesized in:
a. Cytoplasm
b. Endoplasmic Reticulum
c. First in cytoplasm and then in Endoplasmic Reticulum
d. First in Endoplasmic Reticulum and then in cytoplasm

73. Chromosomal studies are done in which stage:
a. Prophase
b. Metaphase
c. Telophase
d. Anaphase

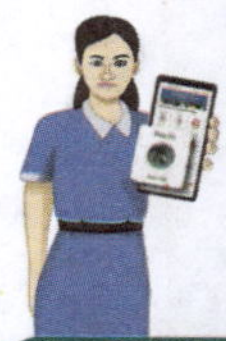

Ans.

49.	d
50.	d
51.	a
52.	d
53.	b
54.	a
55.	b
56.	b
57.	a
58.	a
59.	b
60.	a
61.	a
62.	b
63.	b
64.	c
65.	b
66.	d
67.	c
68.	c
69.	c
70.	b
71.	d
72.	b
73.	b

TRANSPORT MECHANISMS

74. Which of the following mechanisms facilitates transfer of large particles across cell membrane?
a. Active transport
b. Facilitated transport
c. Passive diffusion
d. Phagocytosis

75. Physiological mechanism behind the elimination of carbon dioxide from the body is:
a. Osmosis
b. Facilitated diffusion
c. Simple diffusion
d. Active transport

76. 'Transportation of triglycerides from liver to adipose tissues' is the function of which of the following lipoproteins? *(AIIMS BPL NO 2018)*
a. Low density lipoprotein
b. Intermediate density lipoprotein
c. Very low density lipoprotein
d. High density lipoprotein

Explanation: Liver is mainly responsible for the synthesis of triglycerides. Apo B100 is synthesized by liver around peripheral triglycerides resulting in formation of VLDL secreted from liver into the blood. Thus, VLDL transports triglycerides from liver to peripheral tissues.

77. The pathway through which a cell produces the maximum number ATP molecules is: *(AIIMS-BBS SNO 2019)*
a. Pentose phosphate pathway
b. Glycolysis
c. Lactic acid fermentation
d. TCA cycle

Explanation: TCA cycle produces 38 ATPs (34 ATP from oxidative phosphorylation + 4 ATP from substrate level phosphorylation).

78. Diffusion through a cell membrane does NOT depend on: *(AIIMS BPL NO 2018)*
a. Kinetic energy of the particle
b. Charge of the particle
c. Concentration gradient
d. Size of the particle

Explanation: Diffusion is a passive process that does not depend on the kinetic energy of the particles. Diffusion mostly depends on the carrier proteins embedded in the cell membrane which help in diffusion. Diffusion depends on the charge and size particle and concentration gradient.

79. Water present outside the cells, blood plasma and interstitial space is:
a. ECF
b. ICF
c. Metabolic water
d. All of these

80. The pathway which is considered to be amphibolic is:
a. Glyconeogenesis
b. β-Oxidation
c. Hexose monophosphate shunt
d. Citric acid cycle

81. A major function of the TCA is:
a. Oxidation of acetate to oxaloacetate
b. Oxidation of acetate and reduction of nucleotide coenzymes
c. Generation of heat to maintain body temperature
d. Generation of CO_2 from substrates

82. Net ATP molecules generated in the conversion of glucose to lactate are:
a. 0 b. 2
c. 3 d. 4

83. All the following are substrates for gluconeogenesis; EXCEPT:
a. Palmitic b. Lactic acid
c. Glycerol d. Alanine

84. The urea cycle:
a. Converts urea to uric acid.
b. Converts ammonia to urea.
c. Is an energy-producing pathway.
d. Converts urea to ammonia and carbon dioxide.

85. Glycine is the precursor of all the following; EXCEPT:
a. Epinephrine b. Creatine
c. Haem d. Glutathione

86. The Michaelis-Menten constant 'Km' is:
a. Equal to (1/2)Vmax.
b. Dependent on pH.
c. Dependent on enzyme concentration.
d. Equal to the substrate concentration at half-maximal activity.

87. The rate-limiting step in heme synthesis is catalyzed by:
a. Heme synthase b. δ-ALA synthase
c. δ-ALA dehydratase d. Porphobilinogen deaminase

88. Which of the statements regarding active transport is incorrect?
a. Requires carrier protein
b. Energy dependent
c. Against concentration gradient
d. Transport of water is an example

89. Complete oxidation of one molecule of glucose yields how many ATPs? *(AIIMS Bhopal Nursing Tutor 2014)*
a. 12 b. 24
c. 36 d. 129

90. Gluconeogenesis is inhibited by:
a. Glucagon b. Growth hormone
c. Insulin d. Glucocorticoids

91. Function of HDL is the transport of:
a. Triglycerides from intestine to adipose tissues
b. Cholesterol from liver to peripheral tissues
c. Cholesterol from peripheral tissues to liver
d. Free fatty acids (NEFA) from adipose tissues

92. Function of LDL is the transport of:
a. Triglycerides from intestine to adipose tissues
b. Cholesterol from liver to peripheral tissues
c. Cholesterol from peripheral tissues to liver
d. Free fatty acids (NEFA) from adipose tissues

93. Gamma aminobutyric acid (GABA) is derived from which amino acid?
a. Tyrosine b. Tryptophan
c. Glutamic acid d. Serine

94. Lysine is:
a. Deficient in cereals (rice, wheat)
b. Deficient in pulses (dal, Bengal gram)
c. Mainly glucogenic
d. A non-essential amino acid

Ans.
74. d
75. c
76. c
77. d
78. a
79. a
80. b
81. b
82. b
83. a
84. b
85. a
86. d
87. b
88. d
89. c
90. c
91. c
92. b
93. c
94. a

95. How many ATPs are generated per one rotation of the citric acid cycle? (How many ATPs are produced when one molecule of acetyl CoA is oxidized in TCA cycle?)

a. 2 b. 8
c. 10 d. 15

96. During starvation, all the following substances are increased in blood or tissues; EXCEPT:

a. Ketone bodies b. Epinephrine
c. Glycogen d. Glucagon

97. Death due to cyanide poisoning is a result of:

a. Cyanide hemoglobin complex formation
b. Cyanide inhibiting complex I of respiratory chain
c. Cyanide inhibiting cytochrome oxidase
d. Cyanide blocking oxygen transport in blood

98. Which reaction takes place exclusively in liver?

a. Gluconeogenesis b. Glycolysis
c. Glycogen synthesis d. Albumin synthesis

99. Pentose phosphate pathway produces:

a. ATP b. NADPH
c. Acetyl CoA d. ADP

100. Glycolysis occurs in:

a. Cytosol b. Mitochondria
c. Nucleus d. Lysosome

101. G6PD stands for:

a. Glucose 6 phosphatase dehydratase
b. Glucose 6 phosphate dehydrogenase
c. Glucose 6 phosphodiesterase
d. Glucose 6 phosphate decarboxylase

102. Alcohol is converted into methanol by:

a. Oxidation b. Reduction
c. Transamination d. Decarboxylation

pH, BUFFERS & ACID-BASE BALANCE

103. Which of the following plays a role in maintaining acid-base balance?

a. Sodium b. Potassium
c. Iron d. Both a and b

104. The principal plasma protein responsible for exerting colloidal osmotic pressure is:

a. Hemoglobin b. CRP
c. Albumin d. Haptoglobin

105. In phenylketonuria (PKU), the compound accumulated in the urine is:

a. Homocysteine
b. Tryptophan
c. α-Keto acid
d. Phenylpyruvate

106. The factors that affect electrophoresis of particles are affected by:

a. Change
b. Mass
c. Viscosity
d. Charge and mass

107. Pellagra is due to the deficiency of:

a. Nicotinic acid
b. Pantothenic acid
c. Pyridoxine
d. Biotin

108. Respiratory alkalosis may occur when:

a. A patient hyperventilates
b. There is anemia
c. Chest wall expansion is impaired
d. There is diarrhea

109. The normal pH of human blood is:

a. 7.0–7.1 b. 7.25–7.3
c. 7.35–7.45 d. 7.5–7.55

110. The most important buffer present in the RBCs is:

a. Bicarbonate
b. Protein
c. Phosphate
d. Hemoglobin

Explanation: Hemoglobin is an important intracellular protein buffer present inside the red blood cells (RBC).

111. Compensatory response for respiratory alkalosis involves:

a. Decrease in bicarbonate levels
b. Increase in bicarbonate levels
c. Decrease in pCO_2
d. Increase in pCO_2

112. The primary defect in metabolic acidosis is a reduction in the plasma concentration of:

a. Bicarbonate ions
b. CO_2 levels
c. Phosphate ions
d. Hydrogen ions

113. Retention of sodium in the body leads to:

a. Water retention b. Potassium retention
c. Water loss d. Potassium loss

114. Water depletion occurs in:

a. Adrenal failure b. Burns
c. Hyperventilation d. Small intestinal fistula

115. Which of the following lipids is not present in vegetable oils?

a. Cholesterol
b. Linoleic acid
c. Oleic acid
d. Stearic acid

116. Which one of the following is a dietary essential?

a. Oleic acid b. Palmitic acid
c. Stearic acid d. Linolenic acid

117. Normal serum creatinine level is:

a. 0.2–0.4 mg/dL
b. 0.3–0.6 mg/dL
c. 0.7–1.4 mg/dL
d. 1.4–2.8 mg/dL

118. One deciliter (100 mL) of blood with 15 grams of hemoglobin can carry how much oxygen?

a. 7.5 mL of oxygen
b. 15 mL of oxygen
c. 20 mL of oxygen
d. 30 mL of oxygen

119. Normal specific gravity of urine is:

a. 1.003–1.010
b. 1.010–1.015
c. 1.015–1.025
d. 1.025–1.035

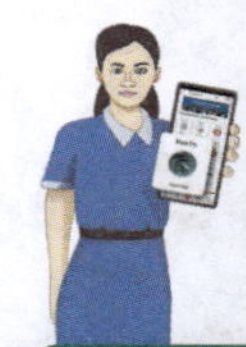

Ans.

95. c
96. c
97. c
98. d
99. b
100. a
101. b
102. b
103. d
104. c
105. d
106. d
107. a
108. a
109. c
110. d
111. a
112. a
113. a
114. c
115. a
116. d
117. c
118. c
119. c

120. Polyuria is a characteristic feature of all the following; EXCEPT:
a. Diabetes mellitus
b. Glomerulonephritis
c. Diabetes insipidus
d. Chronic renal failure

121. Specific gravity of urine increases in:
a. Chronic glomerulonephritis
b. Diabetes mellitus
c. Liver diseases
d. Intake of vegetables

122. Failure of concentrating capacity of urine is assessed by:
a. Urea clearance
b. Water deprivation test
c. Specific gravity of urine after giving water
d. Creatinine level in urine

123. Causes of metabolic alkalosis include the following; EXCEPT:
a. Prolonged vomiting
b. Continuous gastric aspiration
c. Hyperventilation
d. Ingestion of antacids

124. In respiratory acidosis, patient will show which of the following features?
a. A low pCO_2
b. Lowered plasma bicarbonate
c. Reduced rate and depth of respiration
d. Decreased hydrogen ion concentration in plasma

125. Administration of diuretics cause loss of potassium, which may lead to:
a. Metabolic acidosis
b. Respiratory acidosis
c. Respiratory alkalosis
d. Metabolic alkalosis

126. Respiratory acidosis can result from all the following; EXCEPT:
a. Bronchial asthma
b. Narcotic poisoning
c. Poliomyelitis
d. Artificial ventilation

127. In compensated metabolic alkalosis:
a. Respiratory center is stimulated
b. pCO_2 increases
c. pO_2 elevated
d. Urine becomes acidic

128. Secretion of ADH is stimulated by all; EXCEPT:
a. Increased sodium in serum
b. High osmolality of plasma
c. Inability to retain sodium
d. Contraction of ECF volume

129. Buffer system that mainly maintain the pH of body is:
a. Acetate buffer
b. Bicarbonate buffer
c. Phosphate buffer
d. Glycine buffer

130. The normal pH of blood is:
a. 6.8
b. 7.1
c. 7.4
d. 7.9

131. The most important buffer in RBC:
a. O_2 Hb + K Hemoglobinate
b. H_2CO_3 + K HCO_3
c. H_2CO_3 + Na HCO_3
d. H_2 Hb + Nb Hemoglobinate

132. At physiological pH, the most stable amino acid is:
a. Histidine
b. Lysine
c. Arginine
d. Leucine

133. The most important buffer in extracellular fluid is:
a. Hemoglobin
b. Bicarbonate
c. DPG
d. Chloride

134. Anion gap means:
a. Gap in anion molecule
b. Unmeasured anion present in plasma
c. Unmeasured ions
d. Primary deficit of anions

ENZYMES & CO-ENZYMES

135. Regulation of water and sodium in the body is by the action of:
a. Antidiuretic hormone
b. Aldosterone
c. Thirst mechanism
d. All of these

136. All of the following enzymes are found in lysosomes; EXCEPT:
a. Acid phosphatase
b. Cathepsin
c. β-galactosidase
d. Lipoprotein lipase

137. Which of the following is a characteristic of prostaglandins?
a. They do not contain keto or hydroxyl group.
b. They are synthesized from polyunsaturated fatty acids.
c. They contain ring structures with 8 carbons.
d. They are derived from fatty acid with 22 carbons.

138. In DNA, adenine always base pairs with:
a. Guanine
b. Thymine
c. Cytosine
d. Uracil

139. Isoenzymes for a given reaction:
a. Have different substrate specificities.
b. Bind to at least two different substrates.
c. Have identical affinities for the same substrates.
d. Exhibit different electrophoretic mobility.

140. LDH from skeletal muscle is:
a. A catalyst in the rate-limiting step in glycolysis.
b. An allosteric enzyme.
c. Composed of four elements.
d. Identical in composition with cardiac muscle.

141. Which of these serum enzyme activities rises 4–8 hours after AMI?
a. AST
b. ALT
c. CKMB
d. LDH

142. The isoenzyme CK (MB) is specifically increased in blood of patients who have:
a. Skeletal muscle disease.
b. Infective hepatitis.
c. Recent myocardial infarction.
d. Acute pancreatitis.

143. The color of feces is due to the presence of:
a. Biliverdin
b. Stercobilin
c. Bilirubin
d. Porphobilinogen

144. A patient with β-thalassemia trait will have:
a. Elevated HbA2 levels.
b. Elevated level of HbF.
c. Mild hypochromic microcytic anemia.
d. Hemolytic anemia.

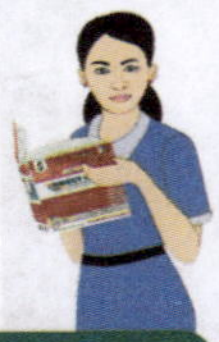

Ans.

120.	b
121.	b
122.	b
123.	c
124.	c
125.	d
126.	d
127.	b
128.	c
129.	b
130.	c
131.	c
132.	a
133.	b
134.	b
135.	d
136.	d
137.	b
138.	b
139.	d
140.	c
141.	c
142.	c
143.	b
144.	c

145. The substance deposited in skin and sclera in jaundice is:
a. Indirect or unconjugated bilirubin
b. Direct or conjugated bilirubin
c. Biliverdin
d. Stercobilin

146. Hepatic disease leads to major elevation of:
a. Biliverdin
b. Total bilirubin
c. Albumin
d. Heme

147. Which substance would increase in plasma if jaundice is diagnosed?
a. Bile acids
b. Bilirubin
c. Stercobilin
d. Urobilin

148. The enzyme used to diagnose acute pancreatitis is:
a. Acid phosphatase
b. Creatinine kinase
c. Alkaline phosphatase
d. Amylase

149. Inulin is used to assess the function of:
a. Liver
b. Thyroid
c. Kidney
d. Gastric

150. The following are indicators of liver function; EXCEPT:
a. Creatinine
b. Bilirubin
c. Albumin
d. Cholestero

151. A person with obstructive jaundice will have all the following conditions; EXCEPT:
a. Hypercholesterolemia
b. Bile salts and pigments in urine
c. Elevated conjugated bilirubin levels
d. Decreased alkaline phosphatase levels

152. IgG:
a. Is found primarily in mucosal secretion
b. Is seen in the primary immune response
c. Promotes phagocytosis and activate complement
d. Has the highest molecular weight

153. The immunoglobulin molecule binds to the antigen via the:
a. Variable region b. Constant region
c. J region d. Fc region

154. Antigens:
a. Are only of polysaccharide in nature
b. Have very low molecular weights
c. Always elicit immune response
d. In the native state are recognized by B cells

155. Glutathione does all the following; EXCEPT:
a. Scavenging peroxides and free radicals
b. Acting as a cofactor for enzymes
c. Participating in the transport of amino acids
d. Forming sulfur conjugates for detoxication of compounds

156. Ketone bodies in urine are identified by:
a. Heat and acetic acid test
b. Rothera's test
c. Benzidine test
d. Benedict's test

157. Ketosis is often seen in:
a. Nephritis
b. Coronary artery disease
c. Muscle degeneration
d. Uncontrolled diabetes mellitus

158. Blood urea level is markedly increased in:
a. Liver diseases b. Renal diseases
c. Cardiac diseases d. Protein intake

159. Heme is converted to bilirubin in:
a. Mitochondria
b. Microsomes
c. Golgi bodies
d. Plasma membrane

160. Bilirubin in serum can be measured by:
a. Van den Bergh reaction
b. Ehrlich's reaction
c. Schlesinger's reaction
d. Fouchet's reaction

161. Congenital hyperbilirubinemia with a bilirubin level of 2.5 mg/dL is suggestive of:
a. Crigler-Najjar syndrome
b. Gilbert's syndrome
c. Dubin-Johnson syndrome
d. Rotor syndrome

162. A person with HbS trait is likely to have:
a. About 90% of hemoglobin as HbS
b. A single band on electrophoresis
c. Sickling at high altitudes
d. Irreversibly sickled cells in peripheral smear

163. Insulin activates:
a. Lipolysis
b. Ketogenesis
c. Gluconeogenesis
d. Glycogenesis

164. Which tissue is most insulin sensitive?
a. Brain b. Liver
c. Adipose tissue d. Cardiac muscle

165. A patient with infective hepatitis is likely to have all the following findings; EXCEPT:
a. Hyperbilirubinemia
b. Bilirubinuria
c. Absence of bile salts in urine
d. Elevated AST

166. An increase in serum unconjugated bilirubin occurs in:
a. Hemolytic jaundice
b. Obstructive jaundice
c. Defect in intestinal absorption
d. Glomerulonephritis

167. Gastric acid secretion is stimulated by all the following; EXCEPT:
a. Hyperglycemia b. Gastrin
c. Vagal stimulation d. Histamine

168. Normal level of albumin in blood is:
a. 1.5–2.5 mg/dL b. 2.5–3.5 mg/dL
c. 2.5–3.5 g/dL d. 3.5–5.0 g/dL

169. Creatinine is synthesized from:
a. Glycine, arginine and methionine
b. Glycine and methionine
c. Ornithine and glycine
d. Thymine and ornithine

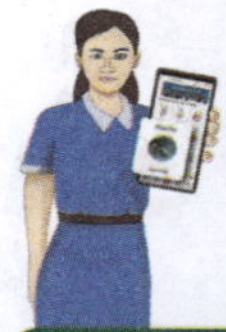

Ans.

145. b
146. b
147. b
148. d
149. c
150. a
151. d
152. c
153. a
154. d
155. b
156. b
157. d
158. b
159. b
160. a
161. b
162. c
163. d
164. c
165. c
166. a
167. a
168. d
169. a

170. The earliest immunoglobulin to be synthesized by the fetus is:

a. IgD b. IgM
c. IgA d. IgE

171. Immunoglobulin which crosses placenta and gives immunity to newborn is:

a. IgG b. IgA
c. IgM d. IgE

172. Thirst is stimulated by:

a. ADH b. Noradrenaline
c. Epinephrine d. Dopamine

173. Atherosclerosis is due to:

a. HDL receptor defect
b. Apoprotein E deficiency
c. Decreased LDL activity
d. Decreased lipoprotein lipase

174. Richest source of triglycerides in blood:

a. HDL b. LDL
c. VLDL d. Chylomicrons

175. In maple syrup urine disease, the amino acid excreted in urine is:

a. Tryptophan b. Arginine
c. Phenylalanine d. Leucine

176. Phenylketonuria is detected by which urine test:

a. Guthrie test
b. Sodium nitroprusside test
c. Blot test
d. Ferric chloride

177. Defect in Phenylketonuria:

a. Phenyl alanine hydroxylase
b. Homogentisate oxidase
c. Pyruvate hydroxylase
d. Fumarylacetoacetate hydroxylase

178. Sickle cell anemia is:

a. Autosomal dominant b. Autosomal recessive
c. X-linked dominant d. X-linked recessive

179. Genetic inheritance of Hemophilia is:

a. Linked dominant b. Linked recessive
c. Autosomal dominant d. Autosomal recessive

180. In fatty liver, lipid which accumulates is:

a. HDL b. Triglycerides
c. Cholesterol d. FFA

CARBOHYDRATES

181. Due to glycolysis in post-mortem muscles, there is accumulation of: *(Safdarjung NO 2018)*

a. Carbon b. Lactic acid
b. Oxygen c. Blood

Explanation:

- In post-mortem muscles, homeostasis is maintained by preservation of ATP concentration.
- Absence of oxygen in the muscles results in anerobic glycolysis of muscle glycogen resulting in post-mortem glycolysis, decreased level of ATP, glycogen lactic acid accumulation and decreased muscle pH.

182. Ketone bodies are synthesized from: *(AIIMS Nagpur NO 2018)*

a. Acetyl CoA b. Cholesterol
c. Phospholipids d. Triglycerides

Explanation: Ketogenesis is the biochemical process through which organisms produce ketone bodies through breakdown of fatty acids and ketogenic amino acids. The 3 ketone bodies, each synthesized from acetyl-CoA molecules, are acetoacetate, acetone, and β-hydroxybutyrate.

183. Tissue forms lactic acid from glucose. This phenomenon is termed: *(Safdarjung NO 2018)*

a. Aerobic glycolysis
b. Oxidation
c. Oxidative phosphorylation
d. Anerobic glycolysis

Explanation: Tissues from lactic acid form glucose. This phenomenon is termed as Anerobic Glycolysis. Under anerobic conditions, lactate or lactic acid is produced as end product from pyruvate.

184. Lecithin on hydrolysis yields all the following; EXCEPT: *(Safdarjung NO 2018)*

a. Glycerol b. Fatty acid
c. Choline d. Glucose

Explanation: Lecithin is present in brain, lungs, nerve cells, sperm and egg yolk. Lecithin is surface active agent and helps in emulsification of fat. Lecithin on hydrolysis produces two molecules of fatty acids, one molecule of glycerol, one molecule of choline and one molecule of phosphoric acid. Glucose is not produced in lecithin hydrolysis.

185. NADPH required for fatty acid synthesis can come from: *(Safdarjung NO 2018)*

a. Hexose monophosphate shunt
b. Oxidative decarboxylation of malate
c. Extra mitochondrial oxidation of isocitrate
d. All of the above

Explanation: The fatty acids are synthesized with starting material as Acetyl CoA and NADPH in the presence of enzyme fatty acid synthases. The NADPH required for this process of fatty acid biosynthesis comes from oxidative decarboxylation of malate. Malate gets oxidized to pyruvate and CO_2, and $NADP^+$ gets reduced to NADPH.

186. Which one of the following is an essential amino acid? *(Banaras HU 2015)*

a. Alanine b. Serine
c. Tryptophan d. Glutamic acid

187. Synthesis of glucose from non-carbohydrate source is referred as: *(DSSSB PHN, 2015)*

a. Glycolysis b. Gluconeogenesis
c. Glycogenolysis d. Glycogenesis

188. Which one of the following sugar concentrations is highest in honey? *(Banaras HU 2015)*

a. Lactose b. Maltose
c. Glucose d. Fructose

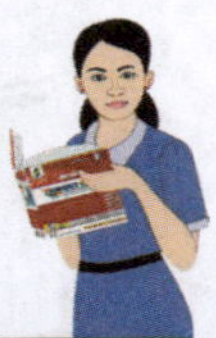

Ans.

170.	b
171.	a
172.	a
173.	b
174.	c
175.	d
176.	a
177.	a
178.	b
179.	b
180.	b
181.	b
182.	a
183.	d
184.	d
185.	b
186.	c
187.	b
188.	d

189. Lactose is made up of:
a. Fructose
b. Glucose
c. Galactose
d. Glucose and galactose

190. Calorific value of carbohydrates is:
a. 4 kcal/gram
b. 9 kcal/gram
c. 5 kcal/gram
d. None of these

191. Which of the following does not contain carbohydrates?
a. Potatoes
b. Rice
c. Daal
d. Vegetable oil

192. Which of the following is not a disaccharide?
a. Sucrose
b. Maltose
c. Lactose
d. Fructose

193. Reducing sugars are differentiated from non-reducing sugars by:
a. Iodine test
b. Molisch's test
c. Seliwanoff's test
d. Benedict's test

194. Sucrose consists of:
a. Glucose + glucose
b. Glucose + fructose
c. Glucose + galactose
d. Glucose + mannose

195. Hydrolysis of maltose will give rise to:
a. Glucose only
b. Glucose and fructose
c. Glucose and galactose
d. Glucose and mannose

196. The normal fasting plasma glucose level is:
a. 40-60 mg/100 mL
b. 70-110 mg/100 mL
c. 120-150 mg/100 mL
d. 160-180 mg/100 mL

197. Benedict's reagent will be reduced by all the following substances seen in urine; EXCEPT:
a. Fructose
b. Galactose
c. Pentose
d. Sucrose

198. Sucrose has glucose &:
a. Maltose
b. Fructose
c. Glycogen
d. Galactose

199. Another name for glucose:
a. Dextrin
b. Dextrose
c. Sucrose
d. Saccharin

200. End product of the action of salivary amylase is:
a. Mannose
b. Maltose
c. Sucrose
d. Fructose

LIPIDS

201. Deficiency of Essential Fatty Acids causes:
a. Dermatitis
b. Growth retardation
c. Reproductive failure
d. All of these

202. Rancidity of fat is due to:
a. Auto oxidation of hydrogenated unsaturated fatty acids
b. Hydrogenation of unsaturated bond
c. Growth of microorganisms
d. None of the above

203. PUFAs are mostly found in:
a. Vegetable oils
b. Animal foods
c. Butter
d. Ghee

204. Linoleic acid is found mostly in:
a. Sunflower oil
b. Corn oil
c. Hemp oil
d. All of these

205. Cholesterol is required for:
a. Formation of bile
b. Precursor for all steroid hormones
c. Formation of vitamin D
d. All of the above

206. The amount of fat in daily energy intake should be:
a. 10–20%
b. 20–30%
c. 30–40%
d. 40–50%

207. A lipid bilayer is permeable to:
a. Urea
b. Potassium
c. Sodium
d. Glucose

208. Biological lipid bilayers contain the following lipids:
a. Cholesterol
b. Linoleic acid
c. Palmitic acid
d. Stearic acid

209. Calories generated per gram of fat is:
a. 4 kcal
b. 5 kcal
c. 8 kcal
d. 9 kcal

210. Cholesterol is synthesized from:
a. Acetyl CoA
b. Maltate
c. Alpha Ketoglutaric acid
d. Oxalate

211. Which cholesterol is designated as "Good Cholesterol"?
a. VIDL
b. LDL
c. HDL
d. IDL

212. Emulsification of lipids in the small intestine requires:
a. Pancreatic lipase
b. Gastric lipase
c. Bile salts
d. Bile pigments

PROTEINS & AMINO ACIDS

213. The most abundant plasma protein is:
a. Albumin
b. Fibrinogen
c. Gelatin
d. Globulin

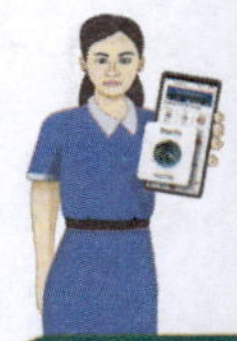

Ans.
189. d
190. a
191. d
192. d
193. d
194. b
195. a
196. b
197. d
198. b
199. b
200. b
201. d
202. a
203. a
204. d
205. d
206. b
207. a
208. a
209. d
210. a
211. c
212. c
213. a

214. Building block of protein is:
a. Glucose b. Lipids
c. Fatty acids d. Amino acids

215. Primary structure of proteins represents: *(Safdarjung NO 2018)*
a. Linear structure of proteins joined by peptide bonds
b. 3-dimensional structure of proteins
c. Helical structure of proteins
d. Sub unit structure of proteins

Explanation:

- Primary structure of proteins represents linear sequence of proteins (known as primary structure) joined by peptide bonds. The structure of proteins is complex and has been divided into four levels, according to organization: Primary, secondary, tertiary and quaternary.
- Tertiary structure of proteins is three dimensional.
- Secondary structure of proteins is helical.
- Subunit structures of proteins is polypeptide chains.

216. Differentiate the essential amino acid in the following: *(DSSSB PHN, 2015)*
a. Proline b. Tyrosine
c. Glycine d. Valine

217. Which nutrient is not found in eggs? *(RRB SSNE 2015)*
a. Carbohydrate and Vitamin-C
b. Protein and calcium
c. Fat and Vitamin-D
d. Protein and Iron

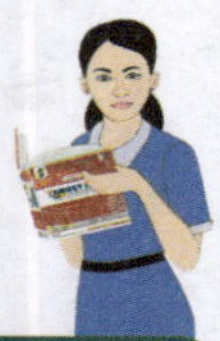

218. Protein deficiency disease is known as: *(ESIC Chennai May 2012; ESIC Chennai May 2012)*
a. Gaucher's disease b. Kwashiorkor
c. Cushing's disease d. None of these

219. Disease kwashiorkor is caused due to deficiency of: *(LNJP H D 2012)*
a. Fats b. Vitamin A
c. Carbohydrates d. Proteins

220. Protein requirement for a pregnant woman per day is …….. grams. *(RRB Feb 2012)*
a. 20 g b. 60 g
c. 30 g d. 100 g

221. Aspartate aminotransferase enzyme*(ESIC Chennai May 2012)*
a. Plays a role in processing proteins
b. Plays a role in metabolism, the process that converts food into energy
c. Both a and b
d. None of the above

222. The technique used for most routine protein and nucleic acid separation is: *(ESIC Chennai May 2012)*
a. Evaporation b. Chromatography
c. Electrophoresis d. Filtration

223. The following essential amino acid(s) is/are deficient in pulses:
a. Leucine b. Methionine
c. Tryptophan d. Methionine and tryptophan

224. Protein of cereals and pulses are:
a. Complete
b. Incomplete
c. Partially complete
d. None of the above

225. The following is included in daily meals to supplement the protein of rice:
a. Vegetables
b. Dal
c. Potatoes
d. Ghee

226. Amino acids of cereals are deficient in:
a. Lysine b. Methionine
c. Cytosine d. Both a and c

227. The amount of protein in daily energy intake should be:
a. 10–15% b. 15–20%
c. 20–25% d. 25–30%

228. Which one of these amino acids cannot have optical isomers?
a. Alanine b. Histidine
c. Threonine d. Glycine

229. Edema due to hypoproteinemia is seen in the following conditions; EXCEPT:
a. Nephrotic syndrome b. Malabsorption syndrome
c. Malnutrition d. Rheumatoid arthritis

230. Which of the following techniques for purification of proteins can be made specific for a given protein?
a. Gel-filtration chromatography
b. Ion-exchange chromatography
c. Electrophoresis
d. Affinity chromatography

231. All the following are sulfur containing amino acids; EXCEPT:
a. Cysteine b. Methionine
c. Homocysteine d. Threonine

232. Non-essential amino acids:
a. Are not seen in tissue proteins
b. Could be synthesized in the body
c. Have no role in body metabolism
d. Have aromatic ring structure

233. Proteins may be denatured irreversibly by:
a. Adding urea
b. Bringing to isoelectric pH
c. Heat coagulation
d. Reduction with mercaptoethanol

234. Proteinuria is seen in all the following conditions; EXCEPT:
a. Acute glomerulonephritis b. Diabetes insipidus
c. Pyelonephritis d. Multiple myeloma

235. Edema due to hypoproteinemia may be seen in all the following clinical conditions; EXCEPT:
a. Protein losing enteropathy
b. Cirrhosis liver
c. Malnutrition
d. Nephrotic syndrome

236. The simplest amino acid is:
a. Tryptophan
b. Valine
c. Glycine
d. Arginine

237. In sickle cell anemia, glutamine in beta chain is replaced by:
a. Arginine b. Alanine
c. Valine d. Methionine

238. In Phenylketonuria the main aim of first line therapy is:
a. Replacement of the defective enzyme
b. Replacement of the deficient product
c. Limiting the substrate for deficient enzyme
d. Giving the missing amino acid by diet

Ans.

214. d
215. a
216. d
217. a
218. b
219. d
220. b
221. c
222. c
223. b
224. b
225. b
226. a
227. b
228. d
229. d
230. d
231. d
232. b
233. c
234. b
235. a
236. b
237. c
238. c

VITAMINS, MINERALS & ELECTROLYTES

239. All of the following are good sources of vitamin A; EXCEPT: *(AIIMS Raipur NO 2019)*

a. White potatoes b. Carrots
c. Apricots d. Egg yolk

Explanation:

- White potatoes do not contain vitamin A. They are rich in carbohydrates.
- Carrots, eggs, apricots are rich sources of vitamin A.

240. Absorption of dietary Iron is enhanced by: *(AIIMS Raipur NO 2019)*

a. Dietary fibers b. Tea
c. Vitamin C d. Calcium

Explanation: Absorption of dietary Iron is enhanced by **Vitamin C.** Iron absorption is inhibited by intake of tea and calcium. Iron absorption is unaffected by dietary fibers.

241. The optimum fluoride concentration in drinking water in India is recommended to be: *(AIIMS-BBS SNO 2019)*

a. 1-2 ppm
b. 3-5 ppm
c. 0.3-0.5 ppm
d. 0.1-0.2 ppm

242. Which of the following vitamins is soluble in water? *(RRB SSNE 2015)*

a. Vitamin A b. Vitamin C
c. Vitamin K d. Vitamin D

243. Identify which is NOT an antioxidant:

a. Vitamin K b. Vitamin E
c. Vitamin A d. Beta carotenes

244. Vitamin B1 is also known as: *(RRB SSNE 2015)*

a. Niacin b. Thiamine
c. Riboflavin d. Pyridoxine

245. Which one of the following vitamins help in wound healing? *(Banaras HU 2015)*

a. Vitamin A b. Vitamin B
c. Vitamin C d. Vitamin D

246. Which of the following symptoms is most commonly associated with Vitamin C deficiency? *(Kerala PSC, Nov 2014)*

a. Photophobia
b. Bleeding gums
c. Muscular hypoxia
d. Conjunctival xerosis

247. Deficiency of vitamin B1 causes: *(Kerala PSC, Nov 2014)*

a. Beriberi
b. Rickets
c. Pellagra
d. Xerophthalmia

248. Deficiency of which vitamin causes scurvy? *(Staff Nurse G II 2014)*

a. Vitamin A b. Vitamin B
c. Vitamin D d. Vitamin C

249. The mineral element which is essential for synthesis of thyroxin is: *(JIPMER 2012)*

a. Sodium b. Iron
c. Iodine d. Chloride

250. Deficiency of which of the following vitamins causes pellagra: *(JIPMER 2012)*

a. Folic acid
b. Vit. D
c. Vitamin B12
d. Niacin

251. Vitamin E is otherwise known as: *(JIPMER 2012)*

a. Retinoic acid b. Tocopherol
c. Calciferol d. Pantothenic acid

252. Bone deformation can occur due to lack of: *(ESIC Chennai May 2012)*

a. Calcium b. Vitamin D
c. Phosphorus d. All of these

253. Vitamin 'D' deficiency may result in: *(ESIC Chennai May 2012)*

a. Rickets b. Night blindness
c. Beriberi d. Scurvy

254. Which of the following vitamins is considered as good for eyes? *(ESIC Chennai May 2012)*

a. B b. C
c. K d. A

255. Vitamin essential for coagulation of blood is: *(ESIC Chennai May 2012)*

a. A b. B
c. K d. D

256. Which one of the following is not a micronutrient?

a. Iodine b. Iron
c. Vitamins d. Protein

257. A person suffering from swollen spongy and bleeding gums is mostly deficient in:

a. Vitamin A b. Vitamin B_1
c. Vitamin C d. Vitamin D

258. The following vitamin functions like a steroid hormone:

a. Vitamin A
b. Vitamin B1
c. Vitamin C
d. Vitamin D

259. The following is called provitamin A:

a. β-Carotene
b. Retinol
c. Vitamin C
d. Pyridoxine

260. A woman who intends to get pregnant is generally given supplements of:

a. Vitamin C b. Folic acid
c. Thiamine d. Niacin

261. Deficiency of the following vitamin causes megaloblastic anemia:

a. Folic acid b. Niacin
c. Iron d. Vitamin E

262. The richest source of calcium is:

a. Sesame seeds
b. Dried small fish
c. Skimmed milk powder
d. None of the above

263. Which of the following is the richest source of potassium?

a. Cabbage
b. Coffee
c. Dal
d. Potatoes

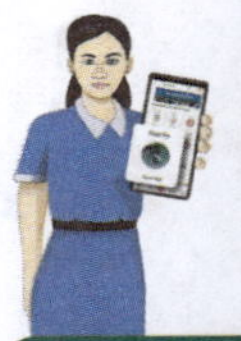

Ans.

239. a
240. c
241. a
242. b
243. a
244. b
245. c
246. b
247. a
248. d
249. c
250. d
251. b
252. d
253. a
254. d
255. c
256. d
257. c
258. d
259. a
260. b
261. a
262. b
263. d

264. Which of the following trace element is essential for the synthesis of insulin?
a. Zinc
b. Cobalt
c. Chromium
d. Copper

265. Germination of seeds increases:
a. Digestive enzymes
b. Vitamin C
c. Vitamin B_1
d. Both a and b

266. The following are called reducing sugars; EXCEPT:
a. Glucose
b. Sucrose
c. Lactose
d. Maltose

267. Which of the following reagent is used for distinguishing a reducing monosaccharide from a reducing disaccharide?
a. Benedict's reagent
b. Fehling's solution
c. Seliwanoff's reagent
d. Barfoed's reagent

268. The following polysaccharides are polymers of glucose; EXCEPT:
a. Amylose
b. Inulin
c. Glycogen
d. Cellulose

269. Milk sugar is called:
a. Lactose
b. Glucose
c. Sucrose
d. Galactose

270. Which one of the following is not a body-building food?
a. Meat
b. Pulses and legumes
c. Fruits
d. Egg

271. Gout is generally associated with:
a. Smoking
b. Low-protein diet
c. Increased xanthine oxidase activity
d. Increased urate deposition in joints

272. In humans, the main end product of purines catabolism is:
a. Ammonia
b. Uric acid
c. Urea
d. β-Alanine

273. A diet of only plant products can lead to:
a. Pellagra
b. Megaloblastic anemia
c. Scurvy
d. Marasmus

274. In adults, a severe deficiency of vitamin D causes:
a. Night blindness
b. Osteomalacia
c. Skin cancer
d. Pellagra

275. Both Wernicke's disease and beriberi can be reversed by administration of:
a. Vitamin C
b. Vitamin A
c. Vitamin B_6
d. Thiamine

276. Which vitamin acts as an antioxidant?
a. Vitamin K
b. Vitamin E
c. Niacin
d. Pyridoxine

277. Cobalt is found in:
a. Vitamin C
b. Vitamin B_{12}
c. Thiamine
d. Folic acid

278. Ceruloplasmin contains:
a. Zinc b. Selenium
c. Copper d. Manganese

279. Deficiency of the following substance causes hypochromic microcytic anemia:
a. Niacin b. Vitamin B_{12}
c. Folate d. Iron

280. In hemochromatosis, the liver gets infiltrated with:
a. Iron b. Copper
c. Manganese d. Zinc

281. Goiter can be prevented by regular intake of:
a. Protein b. Calcium
c. Iodized salt d. Lipids

282. Osmolality of plasma is contributed largely by:
a. Bicarbonate b. Potassium
c. Protein d. Sodium

283. The dominant cation in the intracellular fluid is:
a. Sodium b. Potassium
c. Calcium d. Magnesium

284. Excess of aldosterone causes:
a. Sodium and water retention
b. Increased urinary sodium excretion
c. Hyperkalemia
d. Decreased renal blood flow

285. The following vitamins act as antioxidants; EXCEPT:
a. Vitamin E b. Vitamin D
c. Vitamin A d. Vitamin C

286. Which indicates an abnormal renal function?
a. Blood urea 30 mg/dL
b. GFR = 125 mL/min
c. Serum creatinine 8 mg/dL
d. Urine pH = 6.8

287. Deficiency of vitamin A leads to:
a. Night blindness
b. Rickets
c. Macrocytic anemia
d. Microcytic anemia

288. Deficiency of vitamin D leads to:
a. Night blindness
b. Macrocytic anemia
c. Rickets
d. Microcytic anemia

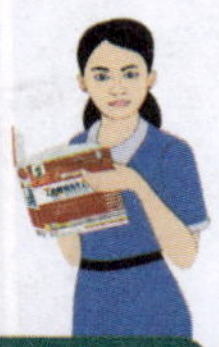

Ans.

264. a
265. d
266. b
267. a
268. b
269. a
270. c
271. d
272. b
273. b
274. b
275. d
276. b
277. b
278. c
279. d
280. a
281. c
282. d
283. b
284. a
285. b
286. c
287. a
288. c

289. The most important biological role for vitamin E is:
a. To produce clotting factors
b. Antidote of selenium poisoning
c. Anticoagulant
d. Antioxidant

290. Large doses of vitamin K in neonates may cause:
a. Rebound bleeding
b. Porphyria
c. Jaundice
d. Cyanosis

291. Deficiency of vitamin K can occur in the following conditions; EXCEPT:
a. Following gastrectomy
b. Prolonged antibiotic therapy
c. Obstructive jaundice
d. Administration of dicoumarol

292. All are good sources of vitamin A; EXCEPT:
a. Pumpkin b. Carrot
c. Mangoes d. Oranges

293. Richest source of vitamin D is:
a. Fresh leafy vegetables
b. Fish liver oil
c. Egg yolk
d. Vegetable oils

294. In thiamine deficiency, serum levels of the following compound are increased:
a. Glycine
b. Pyruvic acid
c. Glutamic acid
d. Transketolase

295. Beriberi is due to the deficiency of:
a. Niacin
b. Thiamine
c. Riboflavin
d. Vitamin B_{12}

296. Glossitis is due to the deficiency of:
a. Niacin
b. Thiamine
c. Riboflavin
d. Vitamin B_{12}

297. The water soluble vitamin synthesized in human body is:
a. Ascorbic acid
b. Pyridoxine
c. Niacin
d. Pantothenic acid

298. Pellagra is due to the deficiency of:
a. Niacin
b. Thiamine
c. Riboflavin
d. Vitamin B_{12}

299. Daily requirement of pyridoxine for an adult is:
a. 2 mg b. 10 mg
c. 20 mg d. 70 mg

300. Vitamin B6 is required for:
a. Conversion of glycine to serine
b. Production of gamma amino butyric acid (GABA)
c. Production of xanthurenic acid
d. Esterification of palmitic acid

301. Daily requirement of vitamin B12 for a normal healthy adult is:
a. 1 mg b. 5 mg
c. 100 mg d. 750 mg

302. Scurvy is due to the deficiency of:
a. Niacin b. Thiamine
c. Riboflavin d. Vitamin C

303. Pernicious anemia is caused by:
a. Inadequate intake of vitamin B_1
b. Absence of hydrochloric acid in gastric juice
c. Absence of intrinsic factor of the gastric juice
d. Overproduction of extrinsic factor

304. A patient who has undergone gastrectomy is likely to develop deficiency of:
a. Vitamin A
b. Vitamin B_{12}
c. Vitamin B_1
d. Vitamin K

305. Absorption of vitamin B12 takes place from:
a. Stomach b. Duodenum
c. Jejunum d. Ileum

306. Normal level of sodium in plasma is:
a. 3.5–5.2 mg/dL
b. 9–11 mg/dL
c. 125–135 mEq/L
d. 135–145 mEq/L

307. Normal level of potassium in plasma is:
a. 3–4 mg/dL
b. 9–11 mg/dL
c. 3.5–5.0 mEq/L
d. 96–106 mEq/L

308. Normal level of chloride in plasma is:
a. 3–4 mg/dL b. 9–11 mg/dL
c. 4–5 mEq/L d. 96–106 mEq/L

309. Iron is deficient in:
a. Cereals (rice, wheat)
b. Maize and corn
c. Pulses (Bengal gram, etc.)
d. Milk

310. The micromineral present in teeth is:
a. Calcium b. Iodine
c. Fluorine d. Manganese

311. Which of the following trace elements has an antioxidant role?
a. Chromium
b. Zinc
c. Selenium
d. Nickel

312. The drug of choice for primary gout is:
a. Allopurinol
b. Aspirin
c. Colchicine
d. Probenecid

313. All are steroids; EXCEPT:
a. Testosterone
b. Vitamin D
c. Cholesterol
d. Thyroxine

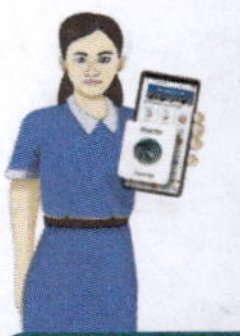

Ans.

289. d
290. c
291. a
292. d
293. b
294. b
295. b
296. c
297. c
298. a
299. a
300. b
301. a
302. d
303. c
304. b
305. d
306. d
307. c
308. d
309. d
310. c
311. c
312. a
313. d

314. In carboxylation of clotting factors by Vitamin K, which amino acid is carboxylated?
a. Glutamate
b. Aspartate
c. Histamine
d. Histidine

315. The vitamin synthesized by bacteria in the intestine is:
a. Vitamin K
b. Vitamin B_1
c. Vitamin D
d. Biotin

316. Among the following, which is the most effective antioxidant?
a. Vitamin B_{12}
b. Vitamin D
c. Vitamin E
d. Vitamin K

317. The major vitamin deficiency in Wernicke's encephalopathy:
a. B_1 b. B_2
c. B6 d. B_{12}

318. Which of the following vitamins prevents autoxidation?
a. Tocopherol
b. Biotin
c. Pyridoxine
d. Vitamin-A

319. Which of the following vitamin deficiency is seen with biliary obstruction?
a. Vitamin K
b. Vitamin B_{12}
c. Vitamin C
d. Vitamin B_2

320. Dermatitis, diarrhea and dementia are seen in deficiency of:
a. Thiamine
b. Riboflavin
c. Niacin
d. Folate

321. Isoniazid induced peripheral neuropathy responds to administration of:
a. B_{12}
b. Riboflavin
c. Pyridoxine
d. Ascorbic acid

322. Which vitamin is most likely to be deficient in patients on treatment with Isoniazid?
a. Vitamin B_1
b. Vitamin B_2
c. Vitamin B_6
d. Vitamin B_{12}

323. Vitamin K is required for:
a. Hydroxylation
b. Chelation
c. Transamination
d. Carboxylation

324. Which of the following is not a feature of niacin deficiency?
a. Diarrhea
b. Red tongue
c. Psychosis
d. Conjunctival congestion

325. Wernicke Korsakoff syndrome is associated with deficiency of enzyme:
a. Transketolase
b. Glucose-6-phosphate dehydrogenase
c. Transaldolase
d. Glucokinase

326. Hemorrhagic disease of the newborn is attributed to the deficiency of:
a. Vitamin A b. Vitamin E
c. Vitamin K d. Vitamin C

327. Hypervitaminosis-A induces damage to:
a. Rough endoplasmic reticulum
b. Mitochondria
c. Microtubule
d. Lysosome

328. Active form of vitamin D is:
a. Calcitriol
b. Secosterol
c. Cholecalciferol
d. 25-Hydroxy cholecalciferol

329. Vitamin required for collagen synthesis:
a. Vitamin A b. Vitamin C
c. Thiamine d. Folic acid

330. Vitamin B_{12} deficiency is not associated with:
a. Megaloblastic anemia
b. Subacute combined degeneration of spinal cord
c. Achlorhydria
d. Microcytic anemia

331. Pyridoxine is given in treatment of:
a. TB b. Malaria
c. Leprosy d. HIV

332. Pyridoxine is:
a. Vitamin B_2 b. Vitamin B_3
c. Vitamin B_6 d. Vitamin B_9

333. Vitamins synthesized by Intestinal bacteria are:
a. A and K b. C and K
c. A and E d. K and B

334. Riboflavin deficiency is assessed by:
a. Transketolase
b. Glutathione reductase
c. PDH
d. None

335. Main function of Vitamin C in the body is:
a. Coenzyme for energy metabolism
b. Regulation of lipid synthesis
c. Involvement as antioxidant
d. Inhibition of cell growth

336. Neurotoxicity is seen with excess of:
a. Vitamin B6 b. Vitamin B12
c. Vitamin B2 d. Vitamin C

337. Glutathione requires which vitamin to act as antioxidant:
a. Vitamin E b. Niacin
c. Vitamin C d. Vitamin A

338. All are true about vitamin E; EXCEPT:
a. Acts as antioxidant
b. Prevents lipid peroxidation of cell membrane
c. Water soluble vitamin
d. Chemically tocopherol

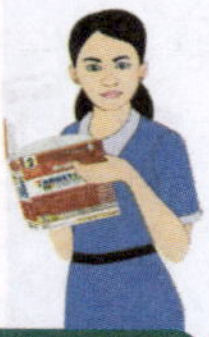

Ans.

314. a
315. a
316. c
317. a
318. b
319. a
320. c
321. c
322. c
323. d
324. d
325. a
326. c
327. d
328. a
329. b
330. d
331. a
332. c
333. d
334. b
335. c
336. a
337. b
338. c

339. Whole wheat is an excellent source of:

a. Vitamin D b. Vitamin C
c. Vitamin A d. Thiamine

340. Vitamin K dependent clotting factors are:

a. II b. VII
c. IX d. X
e. All of the above

341. Vitamin A is stored mainly as retinol esters in:

a. Kidney b. Muscle
c. Liver d. Retina

342. Which of the following pair is NOT correctly matched?

a. Vitamin B_6 — Beriberi
b. Vitamin B_{12} — Pernicious anemia
c. Vitamin C — Scurvy
d. Vitamin D — Osteoporosis

343. In Beriberi, which enzyme activity is measured?

a. Transketolase b. Transaminase
c. Decarboxylase d. Deaminase

344. Not seen in thiamine deficiency:

a. Cerebellar dysfunction b. Amnesia
c. Confabulation d. Nystagmus

345. Both Vitamin K and C are involved in:

a. Synthesis of clothing factors
b. Post-translational modifications
c. Antioxidant mechanisms
d. Microsomal hydroxylation reaction

346. In diarrhea, which of the following supplementation should be done?

a. Iron b. Iodine
c. Zinc d. Calcium

347. In Wilson's disease, copper accumulates in all; EXCEPT:

a. Liver b. Eye
c. Brain d. Spleen

348. Ferritin, the storage form of iron, is stored in all of the following part of body; EXCEPT:

a. Liver b. Spleen
c. Bone marrow d. Hemoglobin

NUTRITION: TERMINOLOGIES

349. IARI stands for: *(Safdarjung NO 2018)*

a. Institute of Agro and Revenue Investigation
b. Indian Agriculture Research Institution
c. India Agriculture Research Institute
d. Indian Agricultural Research Institute

Explanation: IARI stands for Indian Agricultural Research Institute or Pusa Institute. It is meant for research and education in the field of agriculture. Its headquarters is in New Delhi.

350. Which of the following service(s) is/are provided under ICDS programme?

a. Supplementary nutrition
b. Health referrals
c. Nonformal education
d. All of the above

351. IDD programme has been initiated in:

a. Himalayan region
b. Tribal areas
c. South India
d. All over India

352. Mid-day Meal Programme provides meals to children for the following minimum number of days:

a. 275 b. 250
c. 345 d. 200

CALORIE & METABOLISM

353. Adult basal metabolic rate decreases with an increase in: *(AIIMS-BBS SNO 2019)*

a. Muscle mass b. Fever
c. Body fat d. Body surface area

Explanation: BMR rate is the number of calories required to keep your body functioning at rest. BMR decreases with an increase in body fat. Normal BMR in women is 1493 calories, normal BMR in men is 1662 calories.

354. The extra amount of calories required during pregnancy is: *(NCFL 2019)*

a. 300 kcal b. 440 kcal
c. 550 kcal d. 600 kcal

Explanation:

Calories required for a sedentary women	Additional calories in pregnancy	Total
1875 (depends on her physical activity)	300	2175
	Additional calories in breastfeeding	
1875 (depends on her physical activity)	500	2375

355. A nurse must be aware that eating Maize alone may lead to: *(NCFL 2019)*

a. Beriberi b. Pellagra
c. Scurvy d. Phrynoderma

Explanation:

- Pellagra occurs due to the deficiency of the vitamin niacin.
- Maize is rich in vitamins A, B (except niacin), C & folic acid and is a poor source of niacin and tryptophan. Hence, people only on maize diet will suffer from pellagra.

356. The nurse is providing a teaching session to a client who has ulcerative colitis. The nurse will instruct the client for which diet? *(NCFL 2019)*

a. Carbohydrate-consistent diet
b. High-calorie, high-protein diet
c. High-calcium and high potassium diet
d. Low-residue, low-fiber diet

Explanation:

- Ulcerative colitis is the inflammatory bowel disease that mainly affects the large intestine or colon. Symptoms will mimic like irritable bowel syndrome and Crohn's disease. Low residue diet is a low-fiber foods such as egg, fish, white rice, bread, well cooked vegetables without skin/seeds, daily products, poultry, etc. Avoid foods that are high in fiber, whole grains and foods that contain nuts or seeds.
- Low residue diet helps in easy digestion and decreases the bowel movements and thereby it decreases diarrhea.

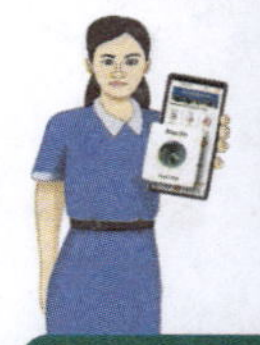

Ans.

339. d
340. e
341. c
342. a
343. a
344. a
345. b
346. c
347. d
348. d
349. d
350. d
351. d
352. b
353. c
354. a
355. b
356. d

357. All the following are foods rich in iron; EXCEPT: *(AIIMS BBS NO 2018)*

a. Spinach b. Fish
c. Milk d. Liver

Explanation:

- 100 gm of raw spinach contains 2.71 mg of iron
- 100 gm of fish contains 28 mg of iron
- 100 gm of liver contains 17 mg of iron
- 100 gm of milk contains 0.04 mg of iron

358. How many calories are there in one gram of fat? *(Safdarjung NO 2018)*

a. 4 b. 12
c. 8 d. 9

359. BMI greater than 30 is considered as: *(DSSSB PHN, 2015)*

a. Overweight
b. Bulimia
c. Obese
d. Stout

360. In which organ does the maximum absorption of Iron take place? *(RRB SSNE 2015)*

a. Stomach b. Small Intestine
c. Colon d. Liver

361. How many calories does 1 gm of fat give? *(JIPMER 2012)*

a. 4 b. 8
c. 10 d. 9

362. Prolonged use of Kesari dal can lead to: *(JIPMER 2012)*

a. Lathyrism b. Gastric upset
c. Gout d. Esophagitis

363. Which of the following nutrients does not provide energy to body?

a. Minerals b. Protein
c. Carbohydrate d. Fat

364. The following digestive enzyme is present in gastric juice:

a. Pepsin
b. Trypsin
c. Chymotrypsin
d. Peptidases

365. Energy required in addition to total calories for a lactating mother from 0-6 months is:

a. + 350 kcal b. + 450 kcal
c. + 550 kcal d. + 600 kcal

366. Basal metabolic rate is measured in:

a. Post-absorptive state
b. Lying down
c. Awake
d. All of the above

367. Obesity is usually assessed by:

a. BMI b. BMR
c. Growth chart d. None of these

368. BMR is affected by:

a. Body temperature b. Body size
c. Gender d. All of these

369. Food energy is measured in:

a. Kilocalories b. Proteins
c. Grams d. None of these

370. The storage form of iron is:

a. Hemeprotein b. Cytochromes
c. Ferritin d. All of these

371. The average water loss in urine is:

a. 500 mL b. 1200 mL
c. 1500 mL d. 1000 mL

372. For planning a balanced diet, it is essential to have:

a. Knowledge of the RDAs b. Physiological status
c. Food groups d. All of these

373. Urine will have abnormal color in all the following conditions; EXCEPT:

a. Melanuria b. Porphyria
c. Creatinuria d. Alkaptonuria

374. Normal urine contains all following; EXCEPT:

a. Glucose b. Ethereal sulfate
c. Bicarbonate d. Creatinine

CLASSIFICATION OF FOOD

375. Highest energy yielding food group is: *(Safdarjung NO 2018)*

a. Carbohydrates b. Fats
c. Sugars d. Protein

Explanation:

Food group	Calories/gram
Fats	9
Carbohydrates (sugars)	4
Protein	4

376. Select the pair which has the same relationship as the pair Iodine: Goiter. *(RRB SSNE 2015)*

a. Mango: Anemia b. Insulin: Diabetes
c. Hormones: Cancer d. Fat: Obesity

377. Which of the following is significantly different between human and cow's milk? *(RRB SSNE 2015)*

a. Proteins and Fat b. Proteins and sugar
c. Proteins and Lactose d. Minerals

378. The best way to retain nutrients while cooking vegetables is:

a. Wash and peel vegetables
b. Avoid soaking in water
c. Drain water after cooking
d. Use shortest cooking time

379. Dietary fiber is rich in:

a. Collagen b. Pectin
c. Starch d. Proteoglycan

FOOD PRESERVATION METHODS

380. The best way of increasing the nutritive value of pulses is: *(AIIMS BBS NO 2018)*

a. Mixing pulses
b. Fortification
c. Parboiling
d. Germination

Explanation: The sprouting breaks down the macromolecules into low molecular weight molecules, which can be easily digested and absorbed in body. Sprouting increases the bioavailability of iron, zinc and calcium. Sprouting reduces the phenol and tannin content in foods.

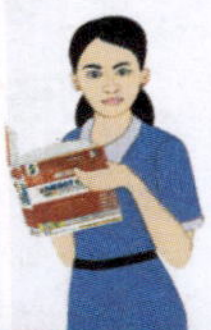

Ans.

357. c
358. d
359. c
360. b
361. d
362. a
363. a
364. a
365. d
366. d
367. a
368. d
369. a
370. c
371. c
372. d
373. c
374. a
375. b
376. b
377. c
378. a
379. b
380. d

"One day in perfect health is much."
—Arabic

CHAPTER 10

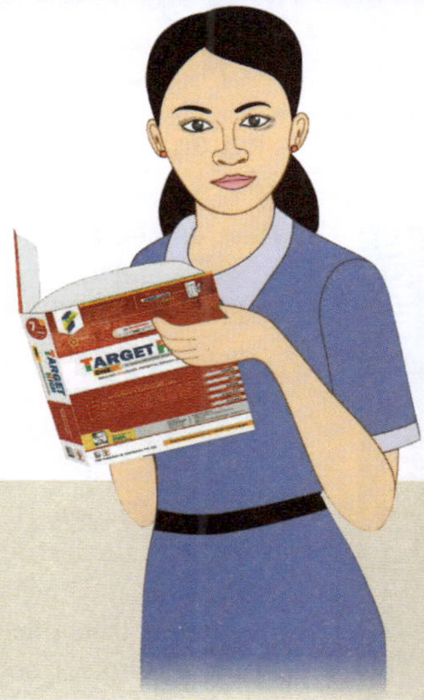

APPLIED SOCIOLOGY AND PSYCHOLOGY

SYNOPSIS

APPLIED SOCIOLOGY

INTRODUCTION

- **Sociology:** The study of social life, social change, and the social causes and consequences of human behavior.
- **Anthropology:** The study of what makes us human.
- **Individual:** An individual is a person with unique identity, may be similar to siblings but not exactly same except in case of twins.
- The word "sociology" was coined by **Auguste Comte**, a French Philosopher in 1839.
- **Auguste Comte** is considered the "Father of Sociology".

SOCIALIZATION

- Socialization is a lifelong process which starts at birth and continues till death. At each distinct phase in life, there are transitions to be made or crises to be overcome.

Importance of Socialization

- Helps an individual to make transitions and adapt to the changing environment.
- Process of socialization includes the elements and agencies of socialization such as family, formal educational system (school, college), peer group, media and technology, religion, government, legal system, and workplace.
- Socialization starts at birth.
- Socialization is innate and unavoidable.

Elements of Socialization

- The **physical** and **psychological heritage** of the individual.
- The **environment** in which he/she is born.
- The **culture** in which an individual's rearing is done.

Features of Socialization

- **Imitation**: It is copying the acts of others.
- **Suggestion:** It is a process of communication in which the suggested idea is accepted without logical grounds.
- **Identification:** In the very early stages, a child cannot make any distinction between himself and his environment. Most of his initial reactions are just natural and spontaneous. As he grows older, he learns to identify through which he satisfies his needs.
- **Language:** Language is the medium of expression.

Phases of Socialization

- **Primary socialization:**
    - It takes place in infancy and childhood.
    - This is the most crucial stage of socialization, as the basic behavior pattern is learnt by the child at this stage.
    - The child internalizes many of the socially approved values, attitudes, beliefs, and behavior patterns of his culture.
    - It is further divided as oral stage, anal stage and oedipal stage.
- **Secondary socialization:**
    - It starts from the later stage of childhood and goes up to maturity.
- **Anticipatory socialization:**
    - It is the kind of learning which describes a person's future roles.
    - Anticipatory socialization makes the individual expect his or her own participation in a social situation by watching how others would behave in that situation.

KEY POINTS

- Sociology emerged as an independent and separate discipline around the middle of the 19th century.
- Merton coined the term anticipatory socialization.

Practice Questions

1. Society is a web of social relationships" is said by ....

a. Maciver
b. Comte
c. Spencer
d. Darwin

Ans. (a) Maciver

2. "Man is a social animal" is said by ....

a. Aristotle
b. Max Weber
c. Mead
d. Karl Max

Ans. (a) Aristotle

3. Who among the following defined socialization as "the process of working together, of developing group responsibility, or being guided by the welfare needs of others"?

a. Ogburn
b. Lundberg
c. Johnson
d. Bogardus

Ans. (d) Bogardus

- **Developmental socialization:**
  - As an individual grows, he changes and molds himself according to the standards and the needs of the society.
- **Resocialization:**
  - It is a process by which one's sense of social values, beliefs, and norms are re-engineered.
  - Resocialization is a kind of learning, which involves the learning of new ways of thinking. Feeling and behaving that are completely different from one's previous way of life.
  - **For example**, resocialization occurs when one converts into a different religion or joins army or is put in a prison.

Individualization Versus Socialization

- ***Individualization*** is the development of oneself through taking decisions by himself and learning to act independently. It is influenced by other external factors like the family, community, and the environment.
- ***Socialization*** is the process by which the individual learns to conform to the norms of the group.

FAMILY

Family is a group of people affiliated either by consanguinity (by birth), affinity (by marriage or other relationships), or by coresidence or combination of these.

Characteristics of Family

- Mating relationship
- Marriage
- Nomenclature system
- Economic provision
- Common habitation

KEY POINT

Internalization of norms is the most important aspect of primary socialisation

Practice Questions

4. Which type of socialization is considered the most essential and basic?

a. Primary socialization
b. Secondary socialization
c. Adult socialization
d. Re-socialization

Ans. (a) Primary socialization

5. During which stage of life does primary socialization take place?

a. Adult stage
b. Pre-natal stage
c. Childhood stage
d. Adolescent stage

Ans. (c) Childhood stage

6. Which of the following aspects is related to a Joint Family?

a. Common property
b. High interaction
c. Big Mess
d. All the above

Ans. (d) All the above

7. What is the term for the marriage of a man with the childless widow of his deceased brother?

a. Levirate
b. Sororate
c. Sororal polygyny
d. Polygyny

Ans. (a) Levirate

Types of Family

Types of family	Advantage	Disadvantage
Nuclear family: This type of family consists of two parents and their children.	• Good personality development among children • Good status of female • Effective family planning • Peace and harmony in family environment • More responsibilities on each family members • Less chance for family conflict	• Economic drawback • Children security issues if both are working parents. • Socialization decreases • Loneliness • Security problem
Joint family/Extended family: It is a type of family structure where several generations of a family, including grandparents, parents, children, and sometimes even aunts, uncles, and cousins, live together under one roof or in close proximity. Multiple nuclear families come together to form a larger household.	• Strong support system for all members • Shared responsibilities • Cultural preservation	• Lack of privacy • Differences and conflicts • Generational gaps • Economic instability • Exploitation

Childless Family

There are couples who either cannot or choose not to have children. Childless families consist of a husband and wife living with each other.

Stepfamily

Because of divorce two separate families can merge into one new unit. It consists of a new husband and wife and their children from previous marriages.

Functions and Role of Family

- Protection, love, and affection
- Reproduction
- Socialization
- Satisfaction of sexual needs
- Economic function

Characteristics of Healthy Family

- Love
- Trust
- Peace
- Patience
- Kindness
- Gentleness
- Self-control
- Discipline

Family Cycle

Stage of family cycle	Description
Single young adult	It is often considered the basic unit of family.
New couple	When the young adults are united by marriage.
Couple with children	When the couple became mother or father through the birth of a child.
Couple with teenagers	As the child grow and become teenager followed by adulthood.
Launching children	The parents help the children to work for the social identity and roles.
Late adulthood	It begins after 65 years of age and beyond.

Basic Needs of Family

- Need for reproduction
- Sexual satisfaction
- Upbringing of children
- Economic needs
- Psychological and emotional needs
- Social needs
- Religion

MARRIAGE

Marriage is the approval of social pattern where by two or more persons establish a family.

Forms of Marriage

- **Monogamy:** A man or woman can have only one mate at a time. It is the most common type of marriage universally recognized.
- **Polygamy**: Practice of having multiple spouses or marital partners simultaneously. It is a form of marriage in which an individual is married to more than one person at the same time. There are two main types of polygamy: (1) polygyny and (2) polyandry.
  - **Polygyny:** It is a form of marriage in which one man marries more than one woman at a given time. Polygyny is more common than polyandry.
  - **Polyandry**: This system permits a woman to have more than one husband. It is of two types: (1) fraternal and (2) nonfraternal. In fraternal, a woman marries to two or more brothers. In nonfraternal, husbands of a woman are not related to each other.

Legislations on Indian Marriage and Family

Legislation	Description
	Before independence
Hindu Widow Remarriage Act of 1856	Permits the wife to marry a second husband after the death of her husband.
Special Marriage Act of 1872	Permitted a couple to get married even if they do not belong to the same endogamous group (i.e. different religion, caste, or communities).
Child Marriage Restraint Act of 1929	Permitted only males above 18 years and females above 15 years to get married.
Hindu Women's Right to Property Act 1937	Permitted the widow to have the same right as her deceased husband in matters of joint family property.
	After independence
Special Marriage Act of 1954	It is an amended form of the Special Marriage Act of 1872. It permits the minimum age of marriage at 21 years for boys and 18 years for girls.
Hindu Marriage Act of 1955	Applies to all members of Hindu society. According to this Act, the word Hindu includes any person who is not a Christian, Muslim, Parsi, or Jew. The Act applies to Hindus, including Hindus, Jains, Buddhists, and Sikhs. Allows divorce with equal rights for women and men.
Hindu Succession Act of 1956	After the death of a man, there is equal division of his property among his widow and children (sons and unmarried daughters).
Dowry Prohibition Act of 1961	Persons involved in giving and accepting dowry are punished. The act includes a fine of 5,000 rupees or imprisonment for six months for dowry demand.

KEY POINTS

- **In Patrilocal family,** the husband lives in the residence of his wife after marriage
- **In Polyandrous system**, a woman can marry more than one husband and keep all of them with herself
- **Endogamy:** A sort of marriage in which both partners are from the same caste, tribe, or race.
- **Exogamy:** A sort of marriage in which the mate comes from a different caste, tribe, or race.
- **Isogamy:** Isogamy refers to marriage between persons from two equal social level families
- **Cohabitation:** When a couple shares a residence but not a marriage, this is referred to as cohabitation.
- **Levirate marriage:** A Levirate marriage occurs when a woman marries her husband's brother after his death.

Practice Question

8. The Special Marriage Act of India allows marriages between individuals of different religions or castes. What is the minimum age for marriage under this Act?

a. 18 years for males and 16 years for females
b. 21 years for males and 18 years for females
c. 21 years for both males and females
d. 18 years for both males and females

Ans. (b) 21 years for males and 18 years for females

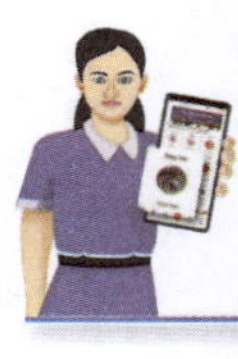

SOCIETY

- Society refers to a group of individuals who share common goals, interests, and values and interact with one another within a specific geographic or social community.
- It is a complex web of social relationships and interactions that shape the norms, beliefs, customs, and institutions within a particular group or community.

Social structure: Social structure is patterned, orderly and enduring form of social relationships that people establish with one another.

Types of Societies

- **Pastoral society:** It consists of religious leaders who help people to solve their problems.
- **Horticultural society:** It consists of individuals who grow farm with fruits, tress, and vegetables in their land.
- **Feudal society:** It consists of landlords who owned the land and allowed farmers, peasants and craftsman to work on their land.
- **Agrarian society:** Individuals with significant agricultural knowledge and cultivated crops in their own land.
- **Industrial society:** It consists of individuals who owned their own business and private industry.
- **Post-industrial society:** It consists of individuals dependent on the communication technology and information.
- **Western society:** It consists of individuals with the democratic belief.
- **Knowledge society:** It consists of individuals dependent on electronic goods capable of storing large capacities of information.
- **Information society:** The society that has allowed the use of computers, telecommunication in their institutions like homes, schools, offices.

Basic Components of Social Structure

There are four basic components of social structure. They are status, roles, group and social institution.

- **Status:** Status refers to the place or position that a person occupies in a system of social relationship.
  There are three types of status:
  1. **Ascribe status:** A social position that is placed on the individual by society, usually on the basis of some inherited characteristics.
  2. **Achieved status**: Attained by a person largely through his or her own effort. One must do something to acquire an achieved status.
  3. **Master status** is a status that dominates others and thereby determines a person's general position within society.
- **Role:** A role is a set of behaviors typically performed by an individual in a particular social situation. **Role conflict** occurs when incompatible expectations arise from two or more social positions that are held by the same person.
- **Group:** It is any number of people with similar norms, values and expectations who regularly and consciously interact. It is important to emphasize that members of a group share same sense of belonging.

Table 1: Classification of social groups

Name	Base of classification	Types of groups
WG Sumner	Socal relationships	• Ingroups • Outgroups
CH Cooley	Social interaction	• Primary group • Secondary group
PA Sorokin	Size	• Horizontal group • Vertical group
CA Ellwood	Membership and durability	• Voluntary • Involuntary • Institutional group • Noninstitutional group • Permanent group • Temporary group
Park and Burgess	Territory	• Territorial • Nonterritiorial

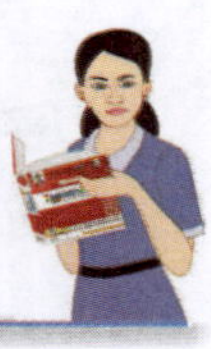

KEY POINTS

- **Agrarian society** primarily based on agriculture, with most people engaged in farming and producing food
- **Traditional society** relies on ancient customs, traditions, and cultural practices
- **Post-industrial society** relies heavily on advanced technology, information, and services
- **Tribal society** is characterized by small, self-sufficient groups of people who rely on hunting and fishing

KEY POINTS

Examples of social status:

- Race or ethnicity is an ascribed status.
- A college degree is an achieved status
- For a well-known celebrity, their celebrity status can be considered a master status.

There are different types of groups:

- **Primary group:** It refers to a small group characterized by intimate, face-to-face association and cooperation.
- **Secondary group**: It refers to a formal, impersonal group in which there is a little social intimacy or mutual understanding.

Table 2: Comparison between primary and secondary groups

Primary group	Secondary group
Generally small	Usually large
Relatively long period of interaction	Shourt duration
Intimate, face-to-face association	Little social intimacy or mutual understanding
Emotional depth in relationships	Relationship gererally superficial
Cooperative, friendly	More formal and impersonal

- **Ingroup:** It can be defined as any group or category to which people feel they belong. Simply put, it comprises everyone who is regarded as "we" or "us". The ingroup may be as narrow as one's family or as broad as an entire society.
- **Outgroup**: It is a group or category to which people feel they do not belong.
- **Reference group**: A group that provides an individual with models of how he or she should behave, dress, live.

- **Social institutions:** They are organized patterns of beliefs and behavior centered on basic social needs. The mass media, the government, the economy, the family and the health care system are all examples of social institutions.

CROWD

When a large number of people gather at one place, it is called crowd.

Characteristics of Crowd

- Crowd is anonymous.
- It is gathering.
- Narrow attention
- Temporary in nature
- Highly influential
- Unity depends up on the interaction among members.

Types of Crowd

Types of crowd	Description
Mob	A group of persons stimulating one another to excitement and losing ordinary rational control over their activity is like that of riots.
Audience	A group of persons who are gathered to witness or receive a particular message.

COMMUNITY

- Community is a group of individuals living together in specific geographical area (e.g. country, village or town) having common religion, norms, beliefs, values and cultural heritage.
- Community has no legal status.
- Every community is socially identified by a name.

Society	Community
It is a network of social relationships including every relationship established among people. Abstract in nature.	It is a group of individuals. Concrete in nature.
A definite geographical area not necessary. It is universal.	A definite geographical area is necessary.
Consists of people with different cultural practices.	Consists of people with same cultural practices.
Common objectives and interests may or may not be present.	Common objectives or interests present among members.
A sense of "we feeling" or community sentiment is not essential.	Community sentiment is vital for the existence of a community.
A society can have one or more than one community.	A community can have only one society.

KEY POINTS

- **A primary group** is characterized by Intimate and enduring relationships with strong emotional ties.
- **A family** consisting of parents and their children is an **example of a primary group.**
- **Secondary group** is formal and goal-oriented relationships for a specific purpose.

Practice Questions

9. The primary group is essential for:

a. Accomplishing specific tasks and achieving goals.
b. Providing emotional support and a sense of belonging.
c. Engaging in formal and impersonal interactions.
d. Establishing professional connections and networking.

Ans. (b) Providing emotional support and a sense of belonging.

10. An example of a secondary group is:

a. A close-knit group of childhood friends.
b. A neighborhood community organization.
c. A team of employees working on a long-term project.
d. A family with parents and their children.

Ans. (c) A team of employees working on a long-term project.

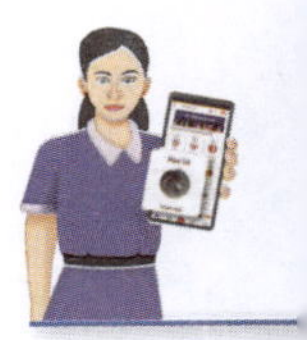

Types of Communities

- **Rural:** Comprising of village area population.
- **Urban:** Comprising of town and city area population.
- **Regional:** Comprises a large area of population which may include both urban and rural population. There is more similarity in the population of a region. India has four regions namely North, South, East and West.

CULTURE

- **Culture:** Culture is the customs, ideas, beliefs, etc. of a particular society, country, etc.
- **Acculturation:** It is a process of cultural contact and exchange through which a person or group comes to adopt certain values and practices of a culture that is not originally their own, to a greater or lesser extent.
- **Assimilation:** When the original culture is wholly abandoned, and the new culture adopted in its place, it is called assimilation.

Characteristics of Culture

- Culture is acquired.
- Culture is a social phenomenon.
- Culture is shared and transmitted.
- Culture is a continuous process.
- Culture is accumulative.
- Culture is indivisible.
- Culture is diverse and dynamic.
- Culture is sensitive and delightful.
- Culture is related to society.

Nature of Culture

- Culture is dynamic based on human experiences from time-to-time.
- A culture is acquired behavior not innate.
- Culture defines attitudes, values and goals of an individual.
- Culture defines myths, legends, and the supernatural powers beyond the explanation of science.
- Culture provides behavior patterns.
- Culture is a continuous process.
- A culture is passed from one generation to other.
- Culture is a qualitative phenomenon.

Strategies and Outcomes of Acculturation

- **Assimilation:** It believes that original culture is less important.
- **Separation:** It is used when little to no importance is placed on grasping the new culture and high importance is placed on maintaining the original culture.

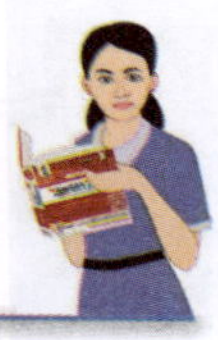

- **Integration:** This strategy is used when both maintaining the original culture and adapting to the new one are considered important.
- **Marginalization:** This strategy is used by those who place no importance on either maintaining their original culture or adopting the new one.
- **Transmutation:** This strategy involves creating a third culture that blends elements of both the original culture and the new culture, emphasizing the importance of both.

SOCIAL CHANGE

Social change is any alterations that occur in social organization that is the structure and functions of the society. —**Kingsley Davis**

Characteristics of Social Change

- Universal phenomenon
- Consists of the modifications or replacements
- Community change
- Not uniform in speed
- Directly related to time
- As essential as a law of nature
- Not predictable
- Not uniform throughout
- Measured in terms of speed of change.

Factors Affecting Social Change

Demogrpahic factors	Size of family, population, migration patterns
Geographical factors	Climate change, floods, earthquake, etc.
Biological factors	Sex, relations, marriage
Cultural factors	Religion, values, beliefs, practices
Technological factors	Inventions, innovations, communication technologies, etc.
Political factors	Political ideologies, government policies, revolutions

Cultural lag: It is the adjustment gap between material and nonmaterial culture.

SOCIAL CONTROL

Social control is the pattern of pressure, which is a society exerts to maintain order and establish rules.

—**Ogburn and Nimkoff**

Classification of Social Control

- **Positive control:** It includes the efforts to encourage ideal or accepted behavior such as rewards, encouragement, praise, etc.

Practice Questions

11. The transmission of cultural elements from one society to another is known as:

a. Cultural assimilation
b. Cultural diffusion
c. Cultural relativism
d. Cultural adaptation

Ans. (b) Cultural diffusion

12. Cultural relativism is the idea that:

a. Cultures can be ranked in terms of superiority.
b. One's own culture is superior to all others.
c. Cultures should be understood and evaluated within their own context.
d. Cultural practices and beliefs should be standardized worldwide.

Ans. (c) Cultures should be understood and evaluated within their own context.

KEY POINTS

- The term "**subculture**" refers to a smaller culture within a larger culture, sharing some distinct traits.
- Ethnocentrism is the belief that **one's own culture is the standard by which all others should be judged.**
- Technological advancements and scientific discoveries can contribute to social change
- Social control refers to **the means and mechanisms used to ensure conformity to social norms.**

- **Negative control:** It includes the efforts to discourage the unwanted behavior like punishment, disapproval, penalty, etc.
- **Direct control:** The control exerted by the family, neighborhood, village elders, religious leaders, etc. are the examples of direct control.
- **Indirect control:** The control exerted by the secondary groups or social systems like folkways, mores, institutions, public opinions, etc. are the common examples of indirect control.

NORMS

Norms are the standardized generalizations concerning expected modes of the behavior.

Types of Norms

- **A prescriptive norm** is positive in form and spells out forms of behavior which role-players are expected to follow means moral values and societal standard norms to be followed.
- **A proscriptive norm** is one which directs a role-player to avoid or abstain from certain type of activity.
- **Formal norms** have generally been written down and involve strict rules for punishment of violators. For example, laws and legal boundaries.
- **Informal norms** are generally understood but are not precisely recorded. For example, folkways, mores, fashion, customs, religion.

- **Folkways:** They are behavior patterns of everyday life which generally arise unconsciously in a large group.
- **Mores:** These are the strong ideas of right and wrong which require certain acts and forbid others.
- **Fashion:** It is an important means of social control as it affects the opinion, believes, speech, dress, music, art and craft and literature.
- **Customs:** These are the ways or methods of acting sanctioned and recognized by society. **—MacIver and Page**
- **Religion:** It is the attitude toward superhuman powers. **—Ogburn and Nimkoff**

SOCIAL STRATIFICATION

A society's categorization of its people into groups based on socioeconomic factors like wealth, income, race, education, ethnicity, gender, occupation, social status, or derived power.

Characteristics of Social Stratification

- Social phenomenon
- Universal
- Ancient
- Diversity

Forms of Social Stratification

Forms of social stratification are caste system and class system.

Table 3: Differences between caste and class

Caste	Class
Specific: The caste system is unique to India, hence it is not universal	**Universal:** The class system is universal in nature
Criteria for classification: Birth is the criteria of the status and not the achievement	**Acquired status:** Status is achieved by the individual
Closed system: Caste system is a closed system. It restricts social mobility	**Open system:** It facilitates social mobility. Individuals can move from the lower class to the upper class
Endogamous group: A caste member has to marry within the group, select the life partner from his own caste system. Intercaste marriages are not permitted	**Exogamous group:** The members are free to select their life partner from any one of the classes
Origin: The caste system is believed to have a divine origin. It is based on Hindu traditions	**Secular:** The class system is secular. It has nothing to do with religion

SOCIAL MOBILITY

The movement of people or group of people from one social status or position to another status or position within a society is known as social mobility. For example, the poor people may become rich.

Types of Social Mobility

- **Vertical social mobility:** The movement of group of people from one social status to another is known as vertical mobility. It involves change in class, occupation and power. Vertical mobility may be upward or downward both.

KEY POINTS

- **Internal social control refers to** individual's fear of negative consequences and punishments that result from violating social norms
- Social norms and values are important in social control because they **Provide guidelines for acceptable behavior.**
- Social mobility refers to the change in a person's social position within a society.
- Caste is a closed system and restricts mobility.
- Class is a open system and facilitates social mobility.

Practice Question

13. Which of the following is an example of informal social control?

a. Police enforcing traffic laws.
b. A teacher reprimanding a student for misbehavior.
c. The court system handing out fines for illegal activities.
d. The government implementing new tax policies.

Ans. (b) A teacher reprimanding a student for misbehavior.

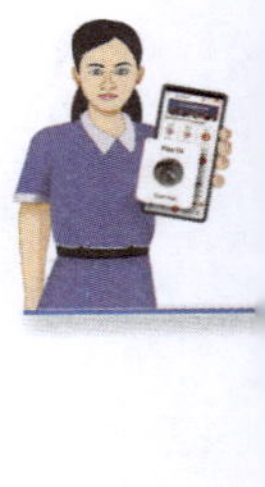

- **Downward social mobility:** The movement of a person or a group from upper to lower social class is called as downward mobility. For example, a businessman may become a bankrupt.
- **Upward social mobility:** The movement of a person or a group from the lower class to upper class. For example, a clerk becomes a bank manager; a farmer becomes a minister, etc.

- **Horizontal social mobility:** It indicates a change in position, without the change of status. For example, a nursing officer working in a hospital may resign from the job and join another hospital as a nursing officer and work in the same capacity.

Factors Influencing Social Mobility

- Motivation
- Education
- Skill training
- Migration
- Industrialization
- Urbanization
- Legislation
- Modernization

SOCIAL PROBLEMS

- Social problems are the behavior pattern or situations that are considered objectionable or undesirable in society.
- It is a condition where there is deviation from social norms.
- Social problems include prostitution, crime, divorce, dowry, juvenile delinquency, drug abuse and addiction, alcoholism, handicapped or disability, population, slums, poverty, etc.

Poverty

Types of Poverty

There are two main classifications of poverty:

1. **Absolute poverty:** Where household income is not sufficient to maintain basic living standards (food, shelter, housing).
2. **Relative poverty:** The economic standard of a household in comparison to the standards of the surrounding population. It is a measure of income inequality.

In India, the poverty line estimation based on the consumption expenditure and not on the income levels.

The National Sample Survey Organisation (NSSO) conducts the survey of household consumer expenditure once every 5 years where the households are asked about their consumption of last 30 days which is then taken as a representative of the general consumption.

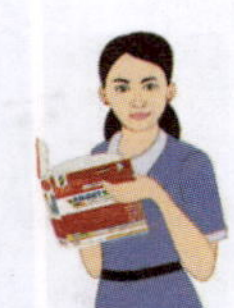

The Planning Commission estimates the incidence of poverty on the basis of the survey findings. On the basis of the 2009 consumption based criteria, the NC Saxena Committee said that 50% of Indians lived below the poverty line.

The household income limit to become a beneficiary under the **BPL (Below Poverty Line)** list is **Rs. 27,000 per year** as per the method authorized by the Union Cabinet.

Per capita daily income of less than Rs. 150 is considered Extreme poverty. According to this figure, 12.4% of Indians are living in extreme poverty.

Rangarajan Committee (2014)

- The committee recommended the poverty line for all India as monthly per capita consumption expenditure **of ₹972 in rural areas and Rs. 1,407 in urban areas**. It also recommended the daily per capita expenditure to **₹47 in urban and ₹32 in rural.**
- Household spending more than the recommended amount is not deemed to be poor while household earning less is termed Below Poverty Line.

Socio-Economic and Caste Census (SECC)—7 criteria to measure deprivation:

1. Households with only one room with no solid walls and roof
2. Households with no adult male aged 15–59
3. Female-headed households
4. Households with differently-abled members
5. Households with no able-bodied members
6. SC/ST households with no literate member above the age of 25
7. Landless households deriving major portion of their income from manual labor.Ref: *Poverty Measurement in India: A Status Update, Ministry of Rural Development Working Paper No. 1/2020*

Poverty Alleviation Programs in India

- **Integrated Rural Development Programme (IRDP):** Provides subsidy and bank credit for productive employment opportunities.
- **Jawahar Rozgar Yojana/Jawahar Gram Samridhi Yojana:** Provides opportunities for the unemployed and underemployed in rural areas through the creation of economic infrastructure and community and social assets.
- **Rural housing—Indira Awaas Yojana:** Provides free housing to Below Poverty Line families in rural areas especially for the households of SC/STs.
- **Food for Work Programme:** Provides food security through wage employment.
- **National Old Age Pension Scheme (NOAPS):** Provides ₹200 per month for 60- to 79-year-old applicants. For applicants aged above 80 years, the amount is ₹500 per month.

Practice Question

14. Formal social control is characterized by:

a. Unwritten rules and customs passed down through generations.
b. Sanctions and punishments enforced by official institutions.
c. The collective beliefs and values of a society.
d. The influence of friends and family on individual behavior.

Ans. (c) Cultures should be understood and evaluated within their own context.

KEY POINTS

Poverty alleviations programs by Govt (UPDATE):

- Prime Minister Street Vendors Atmanirbhar Nidhi PM SVanidhi (2020) - Microcredit facilities for street sellers.
- Pradhan Mantri Shram Yogi Maan Dhan (2019) - for unorganized workers.
- National Nutrition Mission (Poshan Abhiyan) (2018)
- Solar Charkha Mission(2018) - to set up the Solar charkha clusters by providing job to 1 lakh people.
- Pradhanmantri Garib Kalyan Yojana (2016)
- Pradhanmantri Ujjwala Yojana (2016) -supply of LPG connections to the 50 million families from marginalized sections.

KEY POINT

When a person changes his/her occupation or job within the same social class, it is known as **Horizontal mobility**

- **Annapurna Scheme:** Provides 10 kg of free food grains a month for the eligible senior citizens.
- **Sampoorna Grameen Rozgar Yojana (SGRY):** The generation of wage employment, creation of durable economic infrastructure in rural areas and provision of food and nutrition security for the poor.
- **Mahatma Gandhi National Rural Employment Guarantee Act (MGNREGA) 2005:** The Act provides 100 days assured employment every year to every rural household. One-third of the proposed jobs would be reserved for women.
- **National Rural Livelihood Mission: Aajeevika (2011):** Provides jobs with regular income on a monthly basis to the rural poor. Self-help groups are formed at the village level to help the needy.
- **National Urban Livelihoods Mission (NULM):** The NULM works for the urban poor population by organizing them in creating employment through self-help groups, leading to market-based employment.
- **Pradhan Mantri Kaushal Vikas Yojana:** It will focus especially on class X and XII dropouts toward employment.
- **Pradhan Mantri Jan Dhan Yojana:** It is specifically targeted at the poor with no bank account. It aims at direct benefit transfer of subsidy, pension, insurance, etc. This scheme has attained the target of opening 1.5 crore bank accounts among the targeted population.

Housing

- The National Housing Policy 1988
- Pradhan Mantri Awas Yojana (Urban) Mission launched on 25th June, 2015 which intends to provide housing for all in urban areas by year 2022.

Illiteracy

- The right to education is one of the fundamental rights in India.
- International Literacy Day—8th September.
- The Total Literacy Campaign or the **Sarva Shiksha Abhiyan**—launched in 2001 to ensure education for all children in the age group 6–14 years.
- **Kanya Saksharta Protsahan Yojana**—promotes education for tribal girl students.
- **Saakshar Bharat**—provides education for adults in gram panchayats.
- **Shiksha Sahayog Yojana**—provides scholarship to BPL student.
- **Kasturba Gandhi Balika Vidyalaya Yojana**—along with education, this scheme also provides hostel facility for girls.
- The literacy rate of India is 74.04%. For males—82.14% and for females—65.46%.
- Kerala has the highest literacy rate—93.91% , Lakshadweep—92.28% and Mizoram—91.58%
- The lowest literacy rate is in Bihar (63.82%), Arunachal Pradesh (66.95%), and Rajasthan (67.06%).

Prostitution

Prostitution is the practice of habitual and intermittent sexual union, more or less promiscuous, for mercenary inducement. **—Geoffrey May**

Types of Prostitutes

- **Street prostitutes:** They get the customers from the streets.
- **Brothel prostitutes:** They do sexual service for commission in the brothel.
- **Call girl prostitutes:** They work through agent or independently.
- **Miscellaneous:** They work in massage parlors, bars, dance clubs, etc.

Laws and Legislation

- Bombay Prostitution Act, 1923: It states offense if prostitution is practiced in prohibited places.
- Suppression of Immoral Traffic Act (SITA), 1956: It declares punishment for people involved in brothel.

Dowry

- Dowry Prohibition Act, 1961
  - For taking dowry, 5 years imprisonment and Rs. 15,000 fine or equal value of dowry taken.
  - Nonbailable offense for investigation
- Protection of Women from Domestic Violence (2005)—provides protection to women who are victims of domestic violence.

Child Labor

Any child below 14 years of age if made to work as per the adult working hours with minimum wage and posing a risk to their physical and mental health is called child labor.

Child Abuse

- It includes physical, mental, psychological and sexual harm. It also includes neglect of the needs of the child by the primary caregiver.
- ISPCAN— The International Society for Prevention of Child Abuse and Neglect.
- POSCO Act, 2012—The Protection of Children from Sexual Offences.

Juvenile Delinquency

Crime done by the children. Forms/Patterns include gambling, vandalizing, murder, sexual offense, rape, suicide, bullying.

Practice Question

15. Which poverty alleviation scheme in India aims to provide 100 days of wage employment to rural households?

a. NRLM
b. PMAY
c. MGNREGA
d. PMJDY

Ans. (c) MGNREGA

KEY POINTS

- The Pradhan Mantri Awaas Yojana (PMAY) aims to provide **Access to safe and affordable housing for all urban and rural poor.**
- The Pradhan Mantri Jan Dhan Yojana (PM-JDY) primarily focuses on **financial inclusion by offering bank accounts, insurance, and pensions to the unbanked population.**
- Deen Dayal Upadhyaya Grameen Kaushalya Yojana (DDU-GKY) scheme provides skill development training to unemployed youth for enhancing their employability?

KEY POINTS

- **Child laborer:** According to the Indian Constitution, a child laborer is someone who is under the age of 14 and works for a living.
- **Mores:** Mores, such as folkways, are moral judgments that are strongly ingrained in community life.

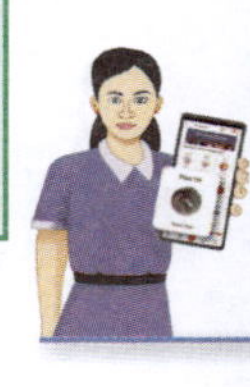

Types of Juvenile Delinquency

- Truancy—escape from school during school hours.
- Vagrancy—wandering

Substance Abuse

- **Tolerance:** In order to get the same desired effect, the amount of substance required increases with time as the body starts tolerating the effect.
- **Dependence** – The stage where the body manifests withdrawal symptoms if a particular substance use is decreased or stopped.
- **Abuse:** Wrong way or method of using a substance leading to significant loss in physical, mental and psychological health of an individual, also leading to neglect of duties and interpersonal problems.

HIV/AIDS

Human immunodeficiency virus/acquired immunodeficiency syndrome (HIV/AIDS) is a significant social problem in India.

POPULATION EXPLOSION

- The total number of individuals occupying an area or making up a whole, is called population.
- India is the second most populated country. As per the United Nations projections, India has overtaken China as most populated country by the end of April, 2023.
- Uttar Pradesh is the most populated state in India.

Demography is the study of population. Some of the methods used to study the population are through:

- Birth rate
- Death rate
- Marriage rate
- Fertility rate
- Sex ratio

Malthusian Theory of Population

- Thomas Malthus stated Principles of Population.
- He observed that as food production and availability increased, so did the population. However, he argued that when population growth outpaced food production, it led to issues like poverty, malnutrition, and diseases, which he referred to as Malthusian catastrophes.

Population Explosion in India

- The year 1921 is referred to as "The Great Divide" in India because it marked a significant shift with low mortality rates and high birth rates.
- At the time of India's Independence in 1947, the population stood at around 34 crores (340 million).
- Population explosion in India started from 1951 onward. According to the 2011 census, India's population reached approximately 121 crores (1.21 billion).
- It is estimated that around 33 births occur every minute in India, indicating a high population growth rate.
- India was the first country to launch a family planning program with the goal of reducing the fertility rate to 2.1 by 2025. Family planning initiatives aim to promote reproductive health and provide access to contraception and reproductive health care services.

URBANIZATION

Urbanization is the term used for the process of shift in population from rural areas to urban areas for employment opportunities, better wages, better education and health facilities. It mostly includes the dominance of nonagricultural occupation.

Classification of Cities on the Basis of Size (as per Census of India 2011)

- **Town:** Comprises 5,000–50,000 people
- **City:** Comprises 50,000 people and above
- **Metropolitan cities:** Comprises population of 4 million or above

Urban agglomeration: It is a continuous urban spread constituting a town and its adjoining outgrowths (OGs) or two or more contiguous towns together with or without outgrowths of such towns.

KEY POINTS

- World population Day is observed on 11 July every year.
- Population explosion refers to a **rapid increase in the population of a region over a short period.**
- Population explosion in India started from 1951 onward.
- High birth rates and fertility rates contribute to population explosion.
- Uttar Pradesh is the most populated state in India.
- The term "gateway drug" refers to a substance that may **lead to the use of more dangerous and addictive substances.**

APPLIED PSYCHOLOGY

INTRODUCTION

Psychology is the scientific study of the human mind and behavior. It explores various aspects of human cognition, emotion, perception, motivation, personality, and social interactions.
Father of Psychology: Wilhelm Wundt (German Psychologist)

PURE PSYCHOLOGY VERSUS APPLIED PSYCHOLOGY

Pure psychology: It is also known as theoretical or academic psychology. It provides framework and theories for the sake of advancing knowledge and understanding in the field.
Applied psychology: It refers to the practical application of psychological principles and theories to address real-world problems and improve people's lives. Applied psychologists utilize the knowledge gained from pure psychology and apply it to specific areas.

BRANCHES OF PURE PSYCHOLOGY

Table 4: Branches of pure psychology and their descriptions

Branch	Description
General psychology	Study of wide range of topics related to human behavior and mental processes.
Abnormal psychology	Study of atypical behavior, thoughts, and emotions. It involves the investigation, understanding, and treatment of psychological disorders and abnormal behavior patterns.
Social psychology	It examines how people's thoughts, attitudes, and behaviors are shaped by social interactions, social norms, group dynamics, and social influence.
Physiological psychology (Biopsychology or Psychobiology)	Understanding how biological processes and structures influence behavior, thoughts, and emotions. It seeks to explore the relationship between the brain, the nervous system, and behavior.
Parapsychology	Parapsychology is a field of study that explores phenomena and experiences that are beyond the scope of conventional scientific understanding. Parapsychologists examine a range of phenomena, including **telepathy** (mind-to-mind communication), **clairvoyance** (perceiving distant or hidden objects or events), **precognition** (knowing future events), **psychokinesis** (influencing objects or events with the mind), near-death experiences, out-of-body experiences, and experiences associated with hauntings and apparitions.
Developmental psychology	It focuses on the study of human development across the life span.
Experimental psychology	It focuses on conducting scientific experiments to study and understand human behavior and mental processes.

BRANCHES OF APPLIED PSYCHOLOGY

Table 5: Branches of applied psychology and their descriptions

Branch	Description
Educational psychology	It applies psychological theories and research to inform educational practices and enhance learning and development.
Clinical psychology	It focuses on the assessment, diagnosis, treatment, and prevention of mental disorders and psychological distress.
Industrial psychology	It applies psychological principles and theories to the workplace and organizations.
Legal psychology	It tries to analyze the behavior of clients, criminals and witnesses.

KEY POINTS

- Psychology is the positive science of behavior. Wilhelm Wundt.
- Applied psychology is concerned with **Applying psychological principles to practical problems**.
- Gestalt psychology was founded in Germany around 1912 by Max Wertheimer and his colleagues.
- Gestalt psychologists believed that the mind should be understood as perceiving whole patterns of sensory activity and the organization of relationships within those patterns.

KEY POINT

Parapsychology describes and explains about the alleged psychic phenomena such as extra sensory perceptions which are present in telepathy, precognition, etc

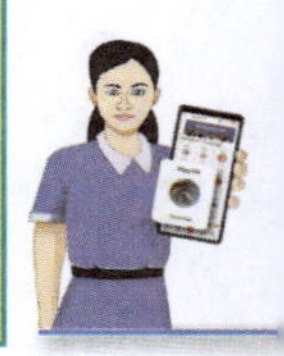

IMPORTANCE OF PSYCHOLOGY FOR NURSES

- To understand patients
- To understand self
- To identify abnormal behavior
- To help patients to adjust and adapt with different hospital environment
- Effective studying.

MIND

Austrian neurologist **Sigmund Freud** introduced the model of human mind.

Three Levels of Mind

1. **Consciousness:** Mental processes and experiences that are currently in our awareness. It includes our thoughts, perceptions, sensations, and feelings that we are actively aware of at any given moment. For example, when we are reading, solving a problem, or having a conversation, we are utilizing our conscious mind.
2. **Preconsciousness (subconsciousness):** Mental processes and information that are not in our immediate awareness but can be accessed relatively easily. It includes memories, stored knowledge, and information that we can bring into consciousness when needed. For example, recalling a phone number.
3. **Unconsciousness:** It contains thoughts, desires, memories, and emotions that are repressed or outside of conscious awareness but still influence our thoughts, feelings, and behaviors. Freud believed that the unconscious mind holds unresolved conflicts, hidden motivations, and unconscious drives that can shape our behaviors and experiences without our conscious knowledge.

Three Components of Mind

1. **Id:**
   - Primitive part of the mind that operates on the **pleasure principle**.
   - It seeks immediate gratification of basic needs, driven by unconscious desires.
   - It disregards social norms and consequences, acting impulsively and irrationally.
   - The id is **focused on satisfying primal urges** like hunger, thirst, and sexuality.
   - It exists from birth and seeks instant gratification without considering morality or societal rules.
2. **Ego:**
   - The ego develops in response to the demands of reality and acts as a mediator between the id and the external world.
   - It operates on the **reality principle** and seeks to find realistic and socially acceptable ways to fulfill the desires of the id.
   - The ego helps to balance the conflicting demands of the id and the superego.
   - It considers the consequences of actions, makes decisions, and attempts to find a compromise between the desires of the id and the restrictions of the superego.
   - The ego also employs defense mechanisms to manage conflicts and protect the individual from anxiety or distress.
3. **Superego:**
   - The superego represents the internalized moral standards and values of society, as well as the individual's conscience.
   - It develops through socialization and the internalization of societal and parental expectations.
   - The superego acts as a moral guide and enforcer, striving for perfection and adherence to **moral and ethical principles**.
   - It includes the individual's sense of right and wrong, societal norms, and idealized standards.
   - The superego can sometimes conflict with the id's desires, leading to feelings of guilt or shame.

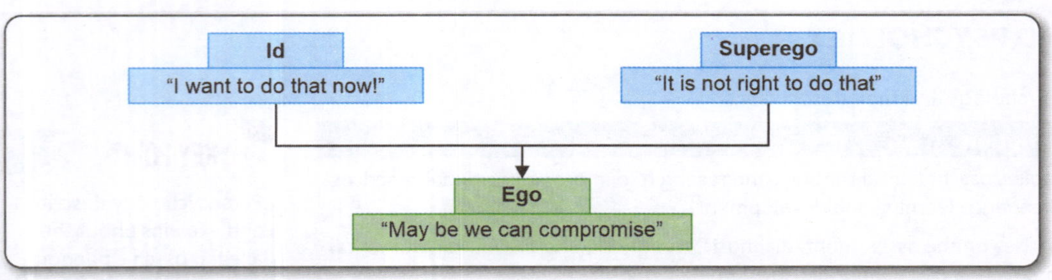

Figure 1: Components of mind

KEY POINT

Sigmund Freud (1856-1939) was an Austrian neurologist and the founder of psychoanalysis, a field of psychology that had a profound impact on the understanding of human behavior and the development of modern psychology.

Practice Questions

16. According to Freud's psychoanalytic theory, the three levels of the mind are:
a. Id, Ego, Superego
b. Unconscious, Subconscious, Conscious
c. Animalistic, Rational, Moral
d. Physical, Emotional, Intellectual

Ans. (b) Unconscious, Subconscious, Conscious

17. The part of the mind that thoughts, memories, and information that are not currently in our awareness but can be readily accessed and brought into consciousness with relative ease is known as:
a. Unconscious mind
b. Subconscious mind
c. Preconscious mind
d. Superego

Ans. (c) Preconscious mind

18. The part of the mind that represents our internalized moral values, societal norms, and conscience is known as the:
a. Unconscious mind
b. Ego
c. Superego
d. Preconscious mind

Ans. (c) Superego

BEHAVIOR

Behavior refers to the observable actions, reactions, or conduct of an individual or organism in response to internal or external stimuli.

Factors Affecting Behavior

- Hereditary/genetics
- Environment
- Early childhood experiences
- Social norms
- Culture
- Religion and faith
- Attitude

ATTENTION

Attention refers to the cognitive process of selectively focusing on specific information or stimuli while disregarding or filtering out others.

Types of Attention

- **Selective attention**: It involves focusing on a particular stimulus or task while ignoring competing or irrelevant stimuli. It **allows us to concentrate** on what is important and filter out distractions.
- **Divided attention**: It refers to the ability to allocate attention to multiple tasks or stimuli simultaneously. It involves **multitasking** and requires the distribution of attentional resources among different demands.
- **Sustained attention:** Sustained attention, also known as **vigilance**, involves maintaining focus and **concentration over an extended period.** It is essential for tasks that require prolonged attention, such as studying or monitoring for potential threats.
- **Executive attention**: It involves the ability to control and manage attentional resources, switch between tasks, and inhibit distractions. It is important for **goal-directed behavior**, decision-making, and cognitive flexibility.

Factors Affecting Attention

- Nature, intensity, and size of stimuli
- Individual differences
- Cognitive abilities
- Motivation
- Arousal levels
- Past experience
- Emotions

PERCEPTION

- Perception refers to the process by which we interpret and make sense of sensory information from our environment.
- It involves organizing and interpreting incoming sensory stimuli to create meaningful experiences and understand the world around us.

Principles of Perception

Gestalt principles: The Gestalt principles describe how our brains naturally organize visual elements into meaningful wholes. These principles include:

- Figure-ground: We perceive objects or figures as distinct from their surrounding background.
- Proximity: Objects that are close together are perceived as belonging to a group.
- Similarity: Objects that are similar in shape, color, or size are perceived as belonging to a group.
- Continuity: We perceive smooth, continuous lines or patterns rather than fragmented or abrupt ones.
- Closure: We tend to fill in missing information to perceive complete objects or figures.

Depth perception: It allows us to perceive the relative distance of objects in three-dimensional space. Key depth cues include:

- Binocular cues: Depth cues that rely on the input from both eyes, such as retinal disparity (slight differences in the images seen by each eye) and convergence (the inward turning of the eyes when focusing on nearby objects).
- Monocular cues: Depth cues that can be perceived with just one eye, such as relative size, overlap (occlusion), texture gradient, linear perspective, and motion parallax.

Size constancy: Size constancy refers to our ability to perceive the true size of an object despite variations in its distance from us.

Perceptual constancy: It is the ability to perceive objects as stable and unchanging despite variations in sensory input.

- Color constancy: We perceive objects as having consistent colors even when the lighting conditions change.
- Shape constancy: We perceive objects as having a consistent shape, even when viewed from different angles.
- Size constancy (mentioned above): We perceive objects as maintaining the same size, even when the distance changes.

Errors in Perception

- **Illusion**: It is the misinterpretation of the perception or an existing stimuli.
- **Hallucination**: Sensory perception occurs in the absence of an existing stimuli.

LEARNING

- Learning refers to the process of acquiring knowledge, skills, behaviors, or attitudes through experience, study, or teaching.

KEY POINTS

- **Executive attention** involves the ability to control and manage attentional resources. It is essential for Goal-directed beahvior.
- **Sustained attention** refers to concentration over an extended period of time.
- **Divided attention** involved multitasking.
- **Selective attention** facilitates concentrating on important thing and filter out distractions.
- **Gestalt principles** describe how our brains naturally organize visual elements into meaningful wholes, such as figure-ground, proximity, similarity, continuity, and closure.
- **Depth perception** allows us to perceive the relative distance of objects in three-dimensional space using binocular and monocular cues.

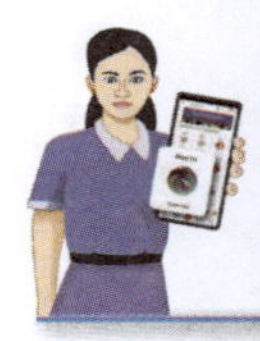

- Learning involves a change in behavior, cognition, or understanding because of experiences and interactions with the environment.

Nature of Learning

- Permanent change in the behavior
- Modification of behavior
- Purposeful and goal directed
- Active process
- Multifaceted

Types of Learning

Stimulus-response learning: It is a type of learning that involves forming associations between specific stimuli and corresponding behavioral responses. It is based on the idea that certain stimuli in the environment can trigger specific responses through repeated pairings or associations.

- **Classical conditioning:**
  - It was first studied by Ivan Pavlov.
  - Classical conditioning typically involves unconditioned stimulus (US), unconditioned response (UR), conditioned stimulus (CS), and conditioned response (CR).
  - An example of classical conditioning is Pavlov's experiment with dogs, where he paired the sound of a bell (conditioned stimulus) with the presentation of food (unconditioned stimulus). Initially, the bell did not elicit salivation (unconditioned response) from the dogs. However, after repeated pairings, the dogs started to salivate (conditioned response) upon hearing the bell alone, even in the absence of the food.
- **Instrumental conditioning:**
  - Also known as operant conditioning.
  - It focuses on the relationship between voluntary behaviors and their outcomes, and how these outcomes influence the likelihood of the behaviors being repeated or modified in the future.
  - Components of instrumental leaning are behavior, consequences (punishment or reinforcement).

Observational learning: It is also known as social learning or modeling, occurs when individuals learn by observing and imitating the behaviors of others.

Cognitive learning: It involves the acquisition of knowledge, skills, or understanding through mental processes such as perception, attention, memory, problem-solving, and reasoning. It encompasses various forms of learning, including concept formation, insight learning, and information processing.

Implicit learning: It refers to the acquisition of knowledge or skills that occur without conscious awareness or deliberate instruction. It often involves learning through exposure to patterns or regularities in the environment.

Laws of Learning

- **Law of readiness**: Learning is most effective when the learner is ready and motivated to learn.
- **Law of exercise**: Repetition or practice is necessary for learning to occur.
- **Law of effect:** Learning is influenced by the consequences or outcomes of one's actions. Positive reinforcement, such as rewards or praise, tends to strengthen learning, while negative consequences can inhibit or discourage learning.
- **Law of primacy:** Initial learning of a concept or skill is particularly important. The first impression or initial learning experience tends to have a strong influence on subsequent learning and retention.
- **Law of intensity:** Emotional or motivational intensity of a learning experience can enhance the learning process. Strong emotions, such as excitement or interest, can increase the attention and engagement of learners, leading to better learning outcomes.
- **Law of recency:** Most recently learned information is most likely to be remembered and recalled. This law highlights the importance of reviewing and revisiting newly learned material to reinforce retention.
- **Law of association:** The law of association emphasizes the role of linking new information or skills with existing knowledge or experiences.
- **Law of transfer:** Learning in one context can be applied or transferred to other situations. Knowledge and skills acquired in one domain can be utilized in a different but related context.
- **Law of use and disuse:** Learned behavior or skill is not used or practiced over time, it becomes weakened or forgotten.

Theories of Learning

- **Trial and error theory of learning:**
  - Developed by E.L. Thorndike (1874–1949).
  - Learning takes place when individuals engage in a series of actions or behaviors and learn from the consequences that follow.
  - The process involves making various attempts or "trials" to achieve a desired outcome and adjusting behavior based on the feedback received.
  - For example, Edward Thorndike's puzzle box experiments.
- **Theory of classical conditioning:**
  - The process of classical conditioning involves the repeated pairing of the conditioned

KEY POINTS

- Operant conditioning, as proposed by BF Skinner. It involves reinforcing desired behaviors with rewards to increase their occurrence.
- Trial and error theory of learning was developed by **EL Thorndike (1874–1949).**
- An example of classical conditioning is Pavlov's experiment with dogs
- Implicit learning involves learning through exposure (experience).

Practice Questions

19. Which law of learning emphasizes that repetition or practice is necessary for learning to occur?

a. Law of readiness
b. Law of exercise
c. Law of effect
d. Law of primacy

Ans. (b) Law of exercise

20. Which law of learning highlights the role of linking new information or skills with existing knowledge or experiences?

a. Law of readiness
b. Law of association
c. Law of intensity
d. Law of transfer

Ans. (b) Law of association

stimulus with the unconditioned stimulus, resulting in the acquisition of the conditioned response.

- This pairing creates an association or link between the stimuli, and eventually, the conditioned stimulus alone is sufficient to produce the conditioned response.
- For example, Ivan Pavlov's dog experiment. (explained above)

- **Theory of operant conditioning:**
  - Also known as instrumental conditioning, is a theory of learning that was developed by BF Skinner, an American psychologist.
  - In operant conditioning, behavior is shaped through the use of rewards and punishments.
  - For example, Skinner box experiment with rats—a hungry rat learned to press a lever in a Skinner box to receive food as a positive reinforcement.
- **Theory of insightful learning:**
  - It emphasizes the role of cognitive processes, problem representation, restructuring, and the emergence of sudden insights or "aha" moments in the learning process.
  - It emphasizes that **learning is a creative and active process**, where learners actively explore, problem-solve, and restructure their understanding through insights.
- **Observational learning:**
  - Observational learning has been studied extensively by psychologist Albert Bandura, who proposed the Social Learning Theory.
  - Bandura demonstrated that individuals can learn new behaviors, attitudes, and emotional responses through observation and imitation of others.
  - He emphasized the importance of modeling, self-efficacy beliefs, and vicarious reinforcement in the process of observational learning.

MEMORY

Memory is the power that we possess to "store" our experiences and to bring them into the field of consciousness sometime after the experiences have occurred. **—William Ryburn, 1956**

Types of Memory

- **Sensory or immediate memory**: Information is stored only for a fraction of seconds. It is of two types.
  - **Iconic memory:** Storage of visual information for a fraction of second comes under this category. For example, when you look at a sparkler and then quickly move it in a circular motion. Even after you stop moving the sparkler, you can still see a trail of light for a brief moment.
  - **Echoic memory:** For example, storage of auditory stimuli for a fraction of second.
- **Short-term or working memory**:
  - Storage of information for 15–30 seconds comes under this category.
  - With the help of repetition of same information again and again, this type of memory may be transferred to long-term memory.
- **Long-term memory:**
  - In this type of memory, storage of information remains for days, months, years and even for a lifetime.
  - This type of memory is again of further two types.
    - **Episodic memory**: Memory is related with the personal information of an individual such as his name, qualifications, date of birth, etc.
    - **Semantic memory**: It includes things that are a common knowledge. Information related to the ideas and concepts that are not drawn from personal experience comes under this category such as 4 multiply by 4 is equal to 16.

Process of Memory

- Learning
- Retention
- Recall
- Recognition

FORGETTING

It is failure at any time to recall an experience; when attempted to do so, or to perform an action previously learned. **—Drever**

Types of Forgetting

- **Normal or natural forgetting**: It is the human nature to forget something in a day to day life because it is not possible to retain each and every thing.
- **Morbid/abnormal forgetting**: Forgetting the unpleasant and painful memory, comes under this category.
- **General forgetting:** When the individual is not able to recall anything that was previously learned, then this type of learning is called general forgetting.
- **Specific forgetting:** Individual forgets only a specific part of his earlier learning in this case.
- **Physical forgetting:** Forgetfulness that occurs due to some physical factors such as age, disease, accident, etc.
- **Psychological forgetting:** Loss of memory due to psychological factors such as stress, fear, etc.

Practice Questions

21. The theory of operant conditioning, developed by BF Skinner, involves shaping behavior through the use of:
a. Direct instruction and memorization
b. Repeated pairing of conditioned and unconditioned stimuli
c. Rewards and punishments
d. Observing and imitating others

Ans. (c) Rewards and punishments

22. Social learning theory was proposed by?
a. BF Skinner
b. Ivan Pavlov
c. Albert Bandura
d. Erik Erikson

Ans. (c) Albert Bandura

KEY POINTS

- Retroactive interference occurs in memory when new information hinders the recall of previously learned information.
- **Semantic memory** includes things that are a common knowledge. For example, Knowing that 5 x 5 = 25.
- **Morbid/abnormal forgetting** refers to forgetting the unpleasant and painful memory

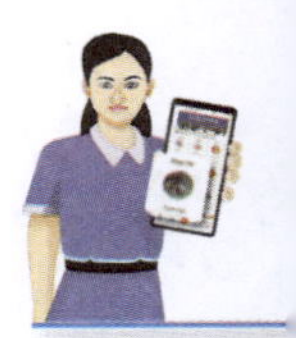

THINKING

Thinking is the cognitive process of mentally processing information, forming ideas, and making sense of the world around us.

Types of Thinking

- **Perceptual or concrete thinking**: This is the simplest form of thinking that is based on the perception of actual or concrete objects and events.
- **Conceptual or abstract thinking:** It is an abstract thinking that requires abstract ideas.
- **Reflective thinking:** Thinking, which aims at solving complex problems comes under this category. It is a higher form of thinking as compared to concrete and abstract thinking. This type of thinking requires logical arrangements of relevant experiences in response to the solution of a problem. As level of thinking does not require any trial and error efforts, hence it is an insightful cognitive approach of learning.
- **Creative thinking:** Thinking is concerned with the construction of new ideas. For example, thinking of scientists and inventors.
- **Critical thinking**: It is the most responsible and skillful thinking that leads to a good judgment. It is a higher order well-disciplined thought process. Here the person discovers the truth by stepping aside from his own personal belief system.
- **Non-directed or associative thinking:** In this type of thinking, the individual thinks without any goal, i.e. he is not having a direction, e.g. day dreaming, fantasy, etc.

REASONING

Reasoning is a stepwise thinking with a purpose or goal in mind. —Garrett

Types of Reasoning

- **Inductive reasoning**: Generalizing based on specific observations or evidence. Example: You wear blue shirt, people give you compliments. Based on this specific observation, you generalize that wearing blue shirt makes more people to give compliments.
- **Deductive reasoning**: Drawing specific conclusions from general principles or premises. Example: Suppose you know all the mammals are "warm-blooded" and that a dog is a mammal. Using deductive reasoning, you conclude that the dog is "warm-blooded".

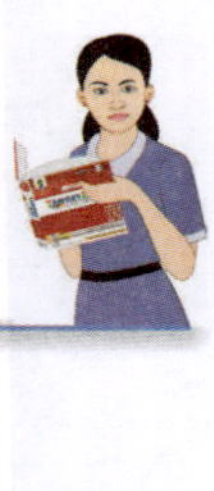

PROBLEM-SOLVING

It is a cognitive process that involves finding solutions to difficult or challenging problems.

Steps in Problem-Solving

- Define the problem
- Gather information
- Analyze the problem
- Generate alternative solutions
- Evaluate and select the best solution
- Implement the solution
- Reflect and learn.

INTELLIGENCE

Intelligence is, "the aggregate or global capacity of individuals to act purposefully, to think rationally, and to deal effectively with his environment".

—**David Wechsler, 1944**

Classification of Intelligence

- **General intelligence:** Overall cognitive ability that underlies all intellectual tasks. It is often measured by tests like intelligence quotient (IQ) tests, which assess various cognitive abilities such as logical reasoning, problem-solving, and verbal comprehension.
- **Emotional intelligence:** Ability to perceive, understand, and manage one's own emotions and the emotions of others. It includes skills like empathy, self-awareness, self-regulation, social awareness, and relationship management.
- **Practical intelligence:** It refers to the ability to apply knowledge and skills effectively in real-world situations.
- **Social intelligence:** It involves understanding and effectively navigating social interactions and relationships.

Intelligence Quotient

IQ = (Mental Age/Chronological Age) × 100

Intelligence Test

- Stanford-Binet Intelligence Scales—applicable to various age groups.
- Wechsler Adult Intelligence Scale (WAIS) — designed to assess intelligence in **adults**.
- Wechsler Intelligence Scale for Children (WISC)—specifically designed for **children aged 6–16 years.**
- Raven's Progressive Matrices—nonverbal test.

STRESS

Stress is a natural physiological and psychological response to perceived threats, challenges, or demands. It is the body's way of preparing itself to cope with a perceived threat or pressure.

The term "stress" in the context of psychology and biology was coined by **Hans Selye**.

Practice Question

23. Which type of thinking involves drawing specific conclusions from general principles?

a. Inductive reasoning
b. Critical thinking
c. Deductive reasoning
d. Creative thinking

Ans. (c) Deductive reasoning

KEY POINTS

- **Hans Selye** is often referred to as the "Father of Stress Research" for his groundbreaking work on the physiological and psychological effects of stress on the human body.
- **General Adaptation Syndrome (GAS):** Selye's most significant contribution to stress research is the concept of the General Adaptation Syndrome (GAS).
- The **Yerkes-Dodson curve,** also known as the Inverted-U model, is a psychological concept that describes the relationship between arousal/stress and performance.

Types of Stress

- **Acute stress:** Stressful events that last only for a short duration.
- **Chronic stress:** Stressful events that extend over time.

Types of Stressors

- **Catastrophic event:** It occurs at times of major disasters or traumatic events, individuals may experience a heightened level of stress known as acute stress reaction.
- **Important life events:** Major life events such as death of loved one cause stress.
- **Daily hassles**: Minor, everyday stressors and inconveniences that individuals encounter in their daily lives.

General Adaptation Syndrome

- It is developed by **Hans Selye**. It has three stages.
  - **Alarm reaction/Flight and fight response**: When a stressor is perceived, the body activates the "fight-or-flight" response, which prepares the individual to confront or flee from the stressor.
  - **Resistance:** In this stage, the body attempts to adapt and cope with the ongoing stressor.
  - **Exhaustion:** In this stage, the body's resources become depleted, and the individual may experience physical, emotional, and psychological exhaustion.

Coping with Stress

- **Emotion-focused coping:** Individuals use to manage and regulate their emotions in response to stressful or challenging situations.
- **Problem-focused coping**: Individuals use to directly address and manage the underlying problem or stressor causing distress. It involves taking practical actions and problem-solving steps to alleviate or resolve the source of stress.
- **Avoidance coping:** Avoiding or minimizing contact with the stressor or the emotions associated with it. Rather than directly confronting the stressor or addressing the underlying problem, individuals may choose to ignore, avoid, or distract themselves from the source of stress.

CONFLICT

Struggle between people with opposing needs, wishes, or demands.

Types of Conflict

- **Interpersonal conflict**: This type of conflict occurs between two or more individuals. It can arise due to differences in opinions, values, or personal interests.
- **Intrapersonal conflict**: It refers to a conflict that takes place within an individual. It involves an internal struggle or dilemma, such as making a difficult decision or dealing with conflicting emotions.
- **Intergroup conflict**: It occurs between different groups or teams. It can arise due to competition for resources, power struggles, or differences in goals and perspectives.
- **Organizational conflict:** This type of conflict occurs within an organization. It may involve conflicts between employees, departments, or management levels. Organizational conflicts can arise due to issues such as leadership styles, organizational changes, or conflicting objectives.
- **Ideological conflict:** It arises from differences in beliefs, values, or ideologies. It can occur between individuals, groups, or even nations, and often involve deeply rooted disagreements about political, religious, or social ideologies.
- **Cultural conflict:** It arises when individuals or groups with different cultural backgrounds clash due to differences in norms, customs, traditions, or worldviews. It can occur on both interpersonal and societal levels.
- **Environmental conflict:** It arises from disputes over the use, management, or protection of natural resources or the environment. This type of conflict can involve various stakeholders, such as communities, governments, and businesses.
- **Role conflict:** It occurs when individuals or groups experience conflicting expectations or demands from different roles they occupy. For example, a person may face conflict between their roles as a parent and an employee.
- **Approach-approach conflict:** When an individual is faced with two desirable options (both positive) or goals but can only choose one. In this conflict, both choices have positive attributes, and the individual is torn between them.
- **Approach-avoidance conflict:** When an individual is faced with a situation or goal that has both positive and negative aspects or outcomes. In this conflict, the individual is attracted to the potential benefits or rewards of the situation but is also repelled by the potential drawbacks or risks.
- **Avoidance-avoidance conflict:** It arises when an individual is faced with two undesirable options or outcomes, and he must choose between them.

For example, student hates to work out his school assignment, but also dislikes the punishment he would receive if he failed to do it. He wants to avoid both the things, if possible.

Conflict Resolution

- **Win-lose approach**: Deciding one solution and leaving behind the other is a win-lose approach.

KEY POINTS

- **Eustress** is a positive stress that can be motivating and beneficial.
- **The fight-or-flight response** is a physiological response to danger or stress.
- The **sympathetic nervous system** is responsible for the **fight-or-flight response**. It releases hormones, such as adrenaline and noradrenaline, that prepare the body to either fight or flee from danger.
- The **parasympathetic nervous system** is responsible for the body's **rest-and-digest** response. It releases hormones, such as acetylcholine, that help the body to relax and recover from stress.
- Type of conflict occurs within an individual and involves an internal struggle or dilemma is known as Interpersonal conflict

- **Lose-lose approach**: When neither person is happy with the outcome, then the lose-lose approach occurs. Issues are never resolved under this approach.
- **Win-win approach**: Mutually acceptable outcome occurs in this approach. This is the most effective method of resolving the conflict.

ATTITUDE

Attitude refers to an individual's mindset, perspective, or outlook toward something or someone.

Factors Influencing Attitude

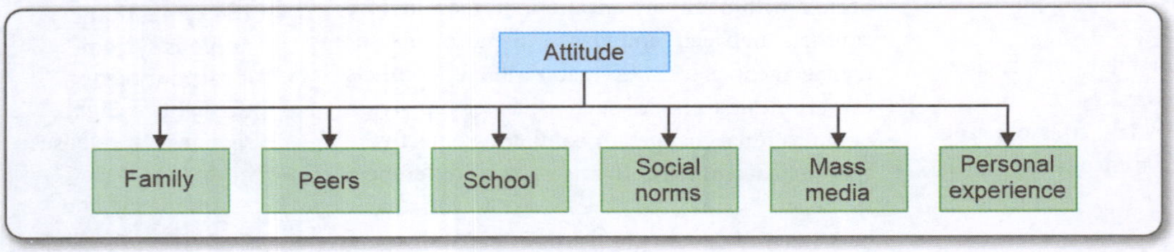

Figure 2: Factors influencing attitude

PERSONALITY

Personality is the total quality of the individual's behavior. —**RS Woodworth**

Approaches to Personality

- **Trait approach:** Individuals differ from one another based on the presence and combination of different traits.
- **Psychobiological approach:** Focuses on the role of biology in determining personality.
- **Social learning approach:** States that our personality is shaped by what we learn from our experiences.
- **Psychodynamic approach:** Freud's theory proposed that childhood sexuality and unconscious motivations influence personality.
- **Humanistic approach:** The ultimate psychological need that arises after basic physical and psychological needs are met and self-esteem is achieved for the motivation to fulfill one's potential.
- Methods of personality assessment have been depicted in Figure 3.

Methods of Personality Assessment

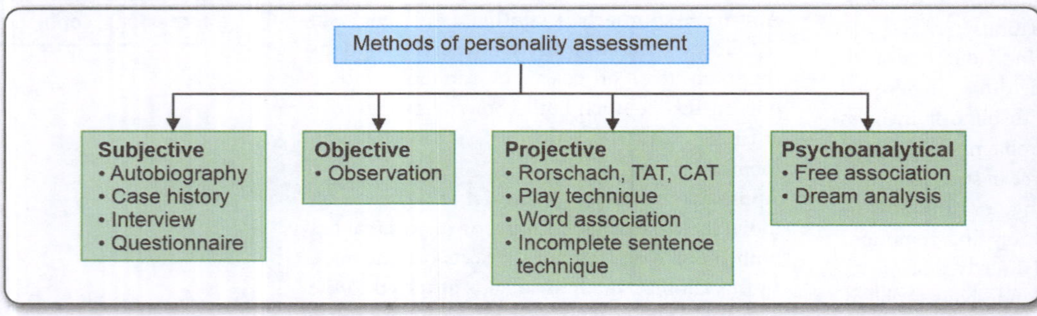

Figure 3: Methods of personality assessment

Sheldon's Personality Types

Sheldon's personality types are based on his somatotype theory, which categorizes individuals into three primary body types: (1) ectomorphs, (2) mesomorphs, and (3) endomorphs (Fig. 4).

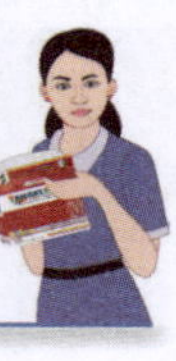

- **Ectomorphs**: Ectomorphs have a leaner and more slender body type. They typically have a fast metabolism, lower body fat, and find it challenging to gain weight or muscle mass. Ectomorphs are often associated with traits such as **being more introverted**, intellectual, and having a preference for solitary activities.
- **Mesomorphs**: Mesomorphs are characterized by a muscular and athletic build. Mesomorphs are often associated with traits such as strength, power, and agility. They are considered to be naturally suited for activities that require **physical performance, such as sports.**

Practice Questions

24. Which of the following approaches to personality focuses on unconscious processes and early childhood experiences?
a. Trait approach
b. Humanistic approach
c. Psychodynamic approach
d. Behavioral approach

Ans. (c) Psychodynamic approach

25. Which of the following approaches to personality emphasizes the influence of genetics and biology on individual differences?
a. Trait approach
b. Humanistic approach
c. Psychodynamic approach
d. Social-cognitive approach

Ans. (a) Trait approach

KEY POINTS

- **Ectomorphs** are often associated with traits such as being more **introverted** and intellectual.
- **Mesomorphs** are considered to be naturally suited for activities that require **physical performance, such as sports.**
- **Endomorphs** are more **relaxed, sociable,** and having a greater affinity for comfort and relaxation

- **Endomorphs**: Endomorphs have a higher proportion of body fat and a rounder physique. They tend to have a softer, curvier appearance and may struggle with weight management. Endomorphs are often associated with traits such as being more **relaxed, sociable**, and having a **greater affinity for comfort and relaxation**.

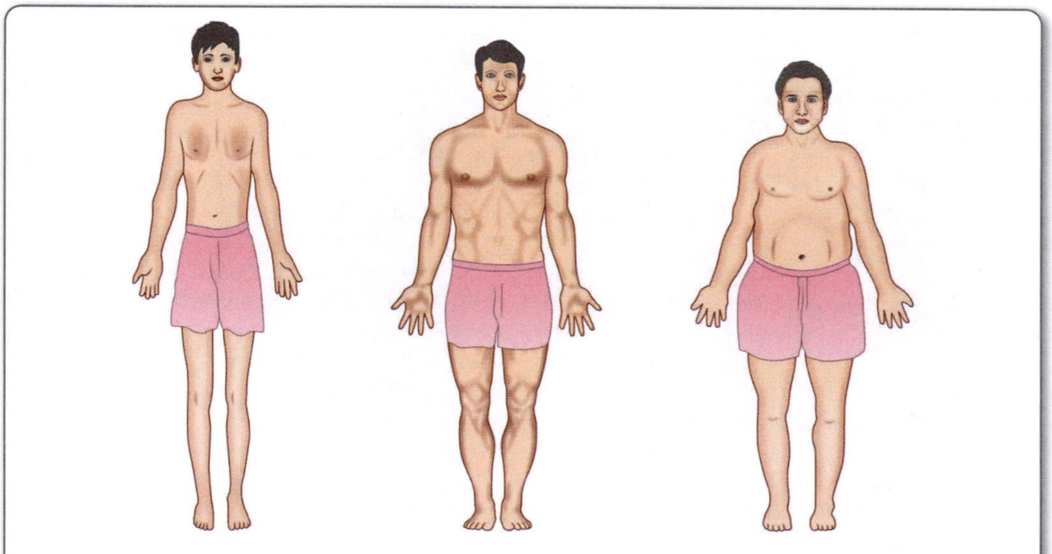

Figure 4: Sheldon's somatotypes, or three body types

Golden Points to Remember

APPLIED PSYCHOLOGY

- The term psychology is derived from the Greek words. Psyche meaning social and meaning logos study.
- Psychoanalytic therapy was developed by **Sigmund Freud**
- Psychology is said to be the scientific study of **Behavior** and **Mental Processes.**
- Wilhelm Wundt is the father of experimental psychology.
- Individual psychology was proposed by Alfred Adler.
- **Geopsychology** deals with the physical environment.
- **First psychology lab** was established by Wilhelm Wundt.
- **Legal Psychology** is the branch of experimental psychology.
- Sensory processing disorders (SPD) are neurological disorders causing difficulties to process information from the five primary sense organs.
- Repression is a psychological defense mechanism that operates in the preconscious part of our mind.
- Besides hearing, the auditory system is involved with gait and balance.
- In resting state, the inside of a neuron has a negative electrical charge.
- The hindbrain comprises the vital medulla oblongata.
- Malfunction of the reticular activating system relates to sleeping sickness.
- Reflex actions are initiated by selective impulses in the spinal cord.
- Trisomy 21 leads to Down syndrome.
- Main function of the myelin is to increase the speed of electrical signal transmission along the axon.
- Conflict is defined as opposition or dispute between persons, groups or ideas.
- Creative thinking comprises four stages in the following sequence: Preparation – Incubation – Illumination – Verification.
- **Id** is pleasure principle, in the unconscious domain. Id seeks immediate gratification of its needs and desires, regardless of the consequences
- Ego is reality principle. Ego seeks to satisfy the id's needs in a way that is realistic and does not conflict with the demands of the external world. The ego is conscious and unconscious.
- **Superego** is principle of idealism. It strives for perfection. The superego is unconscious.
- **Morbid jealousy** is a type of pathological jealousy that is characterized by irrational and excessive fear of being betrayed by a partner.
- An adjustment of human beings to the world and to each other is called **mental health.**
- In adolescence, psychological needs for maintaining health and well-being encompass developing a sense of identity, self-acceptance, autonomy, competence, and relatedness.
- Late adulthood involves psychological needs for ego integrity, social support, and spiritual growth
- **Oedipus complex** (given by Sigmund Freud) is seen in boys of 3–5 years of age
- The **Electra complex** is a psychological term introduced by Carl Jung. It is the counterpart to Freud's Oedipus complex and refers to a girl's feelings of attraction toward her father and rivalry with her mother during her psychosexual development.

Contd...

- Gaining pleasure through activities of discovering the different properties of tools and materials is defined as **explorative play.**
- The **MMPI (Minnesota Multiphasic Personality Inventory)** is used to assess aspects of personality and the existence of components of psychopathology.
- A **cardinal trait** is a dominant and pervasive trait in a person's personality that strongly influences behavior and shapes many aspects of his/her life.
- Most subjective method for measuring personality of a child is Questionnaire method.
- **Thematic Apperception Test (TAT)** of measuring personality is a **Projective technique**
- **Aptitude** is the combination of traits indicating an individual's potential to acquire particular knowledge, skills, or organized responses.
- **Attention** is the ability to produce, select, manage, and maintain sufficient stimulation at a specific amount of time to process any kind of information.
- **Cognition** is a basic mental process like sensation, attention, perception and complex mental operations such as intelligence, reasoning, decision-making, memory and problem-solving.
- A relatively enduring behavioral change brought about by an experience is called **Learning.**
- Thinking which aims at solving complex problems is **Reflective thinking.**
- **Memory images** or traces are present in the mind in the form of **Engrams.**
- **Emotion** is the affective experience tied to inner adjustments, mental-physiological arousal, and outwardly observable behavior in an individual.
- Motivation refers to the states within a person or animal that drives behavior toward some goals
- Primary drive is also known as **biological drive** and is necessary for the survival of the organism.
- Need for achievement and power is an example of secondary motives.
- An individual who is striving to achieve success in professional life is trying to satisfy his personal motives.
- Maslow – hierarchy of needs theory is based on Satisfaction-progression.
- Characteristics of Good Psychological Test are Validity, Reliability, Uniformity, Standardized norms, and Objectivity.
- **Rorschach's Projective Test** is designed to measure unconscious intention.

APPLIED SOCIOLOGY

- The term **Sociology** was coined by a French philosopher, Auguste Comte, in 1839.
- In sociology, **Society** refers to patterns of the norms of interaction
- **Cultural view of Society:** Society is the total social heritage of folkways, mores and institutions, of habits, sentiments and ideals.
- **Talcott Parsons** is one of the most prominent sociologists who proposed the functional view of society.
- A group of people with the same or related occupations is usually termed Professional community.

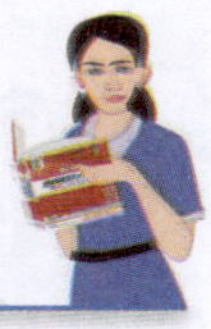

- A community is a social group with some degree of we feeling living in a given area.
- An Association usually is working together of people to achieve a purpose
- Isolation is defined as the absence of communicative interactions or social contact.
- Socialization proceeds throughout the course of life.
- Lenski classified the society into FIVE groups.
- **Norms** are the established standards of behavior that a society upholds. Norms inform individuals how to behave in given situations according to the society.
- **Toleration** favors the assimilation process.
- A phase of maladjustment in which the nonmaterial culture is still fighting to adapt to changing material conditions is referred to as **cultural lag.**
- **Mores** are rules that are judged extremely important for the well-being of a society, generally because they embody people's most valued ideals.
- Resisting social change because it comes from outside of one's group is called **Ethnocentrism.**
- **Cohabitation:** When a couple shares a residence but not a marriage, this is referred to as cohabitation.
- **Conjugal family:** A conjugal family is a family system consisting of spouses and their dependent children.
- **Consanguine family:** A consanguine family is made up of members who are related by blood.
- **Endogamy:** A sort of marriage in which both partners are from the same caste, tribe, or race.
- **Exogamy:** A sort of marriage in which the mates come from different castes, tribes, or races.
- **Isogamy:** Isogamy refers to marriage between persons from two equal social level families.
- **Levirate marriage:** A Levirate marriage occurs when a woman marries her husband's brother after his death.
- **Polygamy:** Polygamy is a form of marriage in which men have more than one wife.
- **Polyandry:** It is a form of marriage in which women have more than one husband.
- **Caste** is a hereditary endogamous social group in which a person's rank and associated rights and obligations are determined by his birth into a certain social group
- **Class:** Max Weber defined a class as a group of people who have similar levels of wealth and income.
- **Social stratification** is a horizontal division of society into higher and lower social units.
- **Acculturation** is the absorption of one cultural group into another, which affects the existing culture and hence changes group identity.
- **Child laborer:** According to the Indian Constitution, a child laborer is someone who is under the age of 14 and works for a living.
- **Folkway:** It is a uniform and common way of living and helping in social control. A folkway describes or draws a line between right and wrong.
- **Social control** is a complete process where a society provides security to its members and conformity to their prospects.

"To keep the body in good health is a duty... otherwise we shall not be able to keep our mind strong and clear."
—Buddha

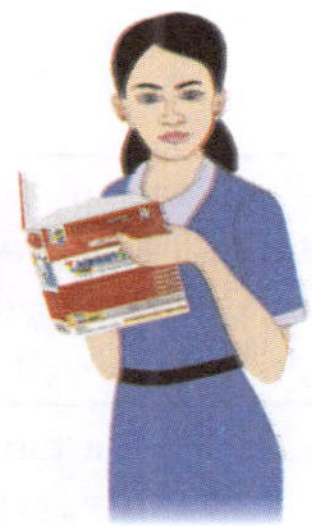

MULTIPLE CHOICE QUESTIONS
(Including Explained and Practice Questions)

APPLIED SOCIOLOGY

INTRODUCTION TO SOCIOLOGY

1. Who coined the term "sociology" and is considered the Father of Sociology?
a. Karl Marx b. Auguste Comte
c. Max Weber d. Emile Durkheim

2. Who stated that "Man is a Social Animal"?
a. Aristotle b. Confucius
c. Plato d. Socrates

3. Which sociologist is known for authoring the book 'Social Organization: A Study of the Larger Mind'?
a. Charles Cooley b. EB Tylor
c. Ferdinand Tönnies d. Émile Durkheim

4. Which of the following school of thought believes that the scope of sociology should be limited to the study of social institutions?
a. Formalistic school
b. Synthetic school
c. Symbolic interactionism
d. Structural functionalism

Explanation: The formalistic school of thought believes that the scope of sociology should be limited to the study of social institutions, while the synthetic school of thought believes that the scope of sociology should be broader and should include the study of social processes and social interactions.

Symbolic interactionism focuses on the meanings that people give to their social interactions. Structural functionalism is a macro-level theory that focuses on the ways in which society is organized and how different parts of society work together to maintain order and stability.

5. Which School of Thought opined that sociology is a general science?
a. Synthetic School c. Vienna School
b. Formalistic School d. Scientific School

Explanation: The synthetic school of thought in sociology believes that sociology is a general science that studies all aspects of social life. This school of thought was founded by **Émile Durkheim**, who argued that sociology should be a science that studies the social facts, or the things that happen in society, that are beyond the control of any individual.

6. Who is associated with the development of positivism, a school of thought in sociology?
a. Bourdieu c. Auguste Comte
b. Emile Durkhein d. Montesquieu

7. CH Cooley is a prominent sociologist in .... School of Thought.
a. Formalistic c. Vienna
b. Mercantilism d. Chicago

8. .... is an impersonal way of control.
a. Informal c. Kinship
b. Formal d. Family

INDIVIDUAL

9. The process of social interaction by which people acquire the knowledge, attitudes, values, and behaviors essential for significant participation in society is called:
a. Culture b. Defining the situation
c. Social communication d. Socialization

10. The process of by which an individual is made independent of the group is called:
a. Individualization b. Growth
c. Development d. Communication

11. Which of the following is not a characteristic of social group?
a. Its members are conscious of shared membership
b. Its members accept certain rights and obligations
c. Its members are a casual collection of people
d. Its members have a distinctive set of interpersonal relations.

12. The response of individuals to one another is:
a. Culture b. Ethos
c. Social interaction d. None of these

FAMILY

13. A group of people whose members are related by marriage, or adoption is a (an):
a. Family b. Institution
c. Friend d. None of these

14. Basic needs of the family include:
a. Need for reproduction
b. Economic needs
c. Psychological and emotional needs
d. All of the above

15. The system under which boys and girls are allowed to mix with each other and are given maximum permissible mixing facility by society before marriage is known as:
a. Probationary marriage
b. Experimental marriage
c. Compassionate marriage
d. None of the above

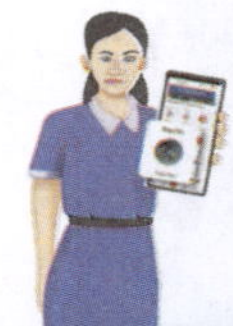

Ans.

1.	b
2.	a
3.	a
4.	a
5.	a
6.	c
7.	d
8.	b
9.	d
10.	a
11.	c
12.	c
13.	a
14.	d
15.	a

Explanation: Probationary marriage is a type of marital arrangement that allows a couple to live together and test their compatibility before legally formalizing the union. The concept is similar to cohabitation or "living together," which is common in many Western societies.

16. If in a family, the offspring inherit the mother's name, the family is called:

a. Matronymic b. Patronymic
c. Matripotestal d. Matrilineal

Explanation: In a matronymic naming system, an individual's last name is derived from the mother's first name. This is the counterpart of a patronymic system where the father's name is inherited.

17. When the offspring inherit the father's name, the family is called:

a. Patronymic b. Patrilineal
c. Patriarchal d. Conjugal

18. In .... family, the husband goes to live in the house of his wife.

a. Matrilineal b. Matriarchal
c. Matrilocal d. Matripotestal

Explanation:

- Matrilocal refers to a family system in which the husband goes to live in the house or community of his wife after marriage. It relates to the residence pattern or living arrangement of the married couple.
- Matriarchal refers to a social system or family structure in which women hold the primary power, authority, and decision-making roles. It is a system where women are the central figures in family and societal leadership.
- A society can be matrilocal, where the husband lives with the wife's family, but not necessarily matriarchal, where women hold dominant positions of power.
- Matrilineal refers to a social or family system in which lineage, inheritance, and descent are traced through the maternal line.

19. Who among the following follows the matrilineal family system?

a. Nairs of Kerala b. Bhils
c. Kadars d. Muslims

20. .... is the family that extends beyond the nuclear family.

a. Extended family c. Nuclear family
b. Joint family d. Neo local family

Explanation: An extended family refers to a family which extends beyond the nuclear family to include grandparents and sometimes other relatives also. It includes relatives such as cousins, aunts, uncles, etc.

MARRIAGE

21. Marriage is:

a. A mating relation between male and female
b. A friendly relation
c. Temporary relation
d. Informal relationship

22. Hindu Marriage Act came into existence from:

a. 1920 b. 1960
c. 1955 d. None of these

23. Marriage by capture is prevalent among the .... tribes of India.

a. Gond b. Santhal
c. Khasi d. Jhang

Explanation: Marriage by capture is a traditional form of marriage among the Gond tribals of India. In this type of marriage, the groom would forcefully take the bride away from her home and family. This would often be done with the help of the groom's friends and family.

Marriage by capture was once a common practice among the Gonds, but it is now becoming less common.

24. According to traditional Hindu law, marriage is a ....

a. Sacrament b. Contract
c. Regulation of prostitution d. None of these

25. .... is the marriage of a man with the childless widow of his deceased brother.

a. Levirate b. Sororate
c. Sororal polygyny d. Polygyny

26. .... may by described as a combination of polygamy and polyandry.

a. Monogamy b. Levirate
c. Sororate d. Group marriage

27. Marriage within the class is known as:

a. Endogamy b. Exogamy
c. Incest taboo d. Sororate

SOCIETY AND SOCIAL GROUPS

28. Acceptance in a group is shown by ....

a. Listening to the group members
b. Probing and questioning the group members
c. Solving the problems of the group
d. Doing things for the group members

29. Which one of the following is a reference group?

a. Occupational group
b. Group taken to evaluate one's own aspect of life
c. A relative longer group
d. A group which allows for social mobility

30. Social group as a method of social work primarily aims at .... .

a. Development of leadership qualities
b. Development of democratic lifestyle
c. Development of capability for adjustment
d. All of the above

31. The main feature of the primary group is ....

a. Face to face relationship
b. Relations are causal
c. It has large membership
d. It governs rules and regulations

32. Which of the following is NOT a primary group?

a. Mob b. Family
c. Gang d. Pear group

33. Responsibility for the choice of program in group work rests with ....

a. Members of the group
b. Group worker
c. The Agency
d. Members of the group with the help of group worker

34. Which one of the following is a 'secondary group'?

a. Nuclear family b. Peer group
c. Association d. Joint family

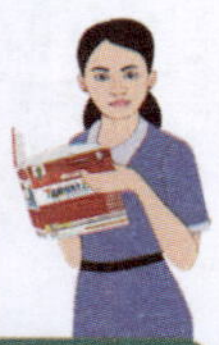

Ans.

16. a
17. a
18. c
19. a
20. a
21. a
22. c
23. a
24. a
25. a
26. d
27. d
28. a
29. b
30. d
31. a
32. a
33. d
34. c

CULTURE

35. Which term refers to the tendency of an individual to view their own culture as superior and to act in a superior manner toward another culture?

a. Ethnocentrism b. Cultural relativism
c. Cultural supremacy d. Acculturation

Explanation: Ethnocentrism is a tendency to judge other cultures based on one's own cultural norms and standards. An individual who is ethnocentric views their own culture as superior and tends to act in a superior manner toward other cultures.

Cultural relativism is the opposite of ethnocentrism and refers to the view that each culture should be judged on its own terms, without imposing one's own cultural standards. Cultural supremacy is not a commonly used term and is not related to the concept of ethnocentrism. Acculturation refers to the process of adapting to a new culture, often as a result of immigration or prolonged contact with a different culture.

36. What is the process of cultural contact and exchange through which a person or group adopts values and practices of a different culture called?

a. Assimilation b. Acculturation
c. Separation d. Marginalization

37. Which characteristic of culture refers to the fact that it is continuously evolving and changing?

a. Culture is acquired.
b. Culture is diverse and dynamic.
c. Culture is indivisible.
d. Culture is accumulative.

38. Which strategy of acculturation involves abandoning the original culture and fully adopting the new culture?

a. Assimilation b. Separation
c. Integration d. Marginalization

39. Which outcome of acculturation involves placing equal importance on maintaining the original culture and adapting to the new one?

a. Assimilation b. Separation
c. Integration d. Marginalization

SOCIAL CHANGE

40. Cultural lag:

a. Refers to new forms of social disintegration.
b. Is the adjustment gap between material and nonmaterial culture.
c. Occurs when the dominant group forces changes upon the subordinate group.
d. Is society's way of avoiding the social problems that ensue from social change.

41. Which among the following is not a component of culture?

a. Beliefs b. Values
c. Signs d. Development

42. Which of the following is deliberately formed?

a. Community b. Society
c. Association d. None of these

43. According to Ogburn, the rate of change in material culture is:

a. The same as that of nonmaterial culture
b. Faster than that of nonmaterial culture
c. Slower than that of nonmaterial culture
d. None of the above

SOCIAL CONTROL

44. The term "control" involves:

a. The idea of restraint or direction
b. Overtone to a culture
c. System of land reforms
d. Manipulation of emotions

45. Which of the following is not true about the term "control"?

a. The idea of restraint or direction
b. Process or technique of control
c. It stands on the way of democracy
d. It involves exertion of power and authority

46. All of the following are true about social control; except:

a. The idea of restraint and direction
b. Includes formal and informal modes which have an impact on others
c. It is grounded in the norms and values
d. Social control is always oppressive

47. Ultimate basis of social control is:

a. Social organization b. Social mobility
c. Social class d. Social change

48. In our modern times:

a. Every society is exclusively competitive
b. No society is either exclusively competitive or exclusively cooperative
c. Every society is exclusively cooperative
d. Societies alternate between being exclusively competitive or cooperative.

49. A norm is a:

a. Specific guide to action
b. Culture of society
c. Guideline for socialization
d. Guideline for social interaction

50. Norms are enforced by:

a. Positive sanction
b. Negative sanction
c. Order
d. Positive and negative sanction

51. Norms are imposed through .... means of social control.

a. Formal and legal b. Formal and informal
c. Cultural d. Informal and legal

52. A value is a belief that something is:

a. Moral b. Very productive in society
c. Good and desirable d. Cultural

53. Which type of control is typically associated with bureaucratic organizations?

a. Control by officials b. Informal control
c. Formal control d. Judicial control

SOCIAL STRATIFICATION

54. Social stratification is:

a. A system in which people can change their status with relative ease.
b. Based entirely on self-classification.
c. The ranking or grading of individuals and groups into hierarchical layers.
d. A consequence of human nature.

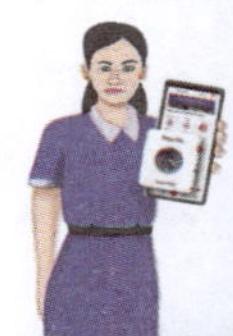

Ans.

35. a
36. b
37. b
38. a
39. c
40. b
41. d
42. c
43. b
44. a
45. c
46. d
47. a
48. b
49. a
50. d
51. b
52. c
53. c
54. c

55. The process of movement of people of a group from one social status to another is called:
a. Movement b. Social differentiation
c. Social stratification d. Social mobility

56. Which of the following is not a major cause of social stratification?
a. Social tensions b. Access to resources
c. Natural calamities d. Economic disparities

Explanation: "Social tensions" can refer to conflicts, disputes, or disagreements between individuals or groups within a society. While social tensions can be a result of social stratification, they are not considered a direct cause of social stratification itself.

57. Division of society on the basis of class is:
a. Peculiar to few affluent societies
b. Of comparatively recent origin
c. Found in all societies since ancient time
d. Exclusive to business community

58. Who defined social class as a portion of community marked off from the rest by social status?
a. MacIver and Page b. Ogburn
c. Nimkoff d. Comte

59. Which one of the following is not true about social class?
a. Social class is often determined by an individual's economic position
b. Social class is closely tied to power and influence within a society
c. Social class influences an individual's lifestyle and consumption patterns
d. Social class is fixed and unchanging

60. Which one of the following does not fit in the characteristic of social class?
a. Each class has certain privileges
b. It represents vertical division of society
c. Social class comes into being due to social stratification
d. Members within a social class share identical experiences, values, and lifestyles

SOCIAL PROBLEMS

61. Which of the following is not characteristic of social problem?
a. Generally regarded harmful for the society
b. It has effect on a large section of a society
c. Develops gradually and slowly
d. Easily resolved through individual effort

62. Which of the following is not source of social problem?
a. Social change b. Poverty
c. Personal development d. Personal disorganization

63. Density of population is very much related to:
a. Climate b. Political system
c. Environmental study d. Economic condition

64. Which is an institution to rehabilitate juvenile delinquents?
a. Juvenile Courts b. Remand Homes
c. Foster Homes d. All of these

65. All of the following are the causes of rapid growth of population in India; except:
a. Peaceful conditions
b. Excess birth over death
c. Progress in medical facilities
d. Declining fertility rate

66. What is the effect of overpopulation?
a. Population and poverty b. Low per capita income
c. Shortage of food d. All of these

67. Poverty is a:
a. Social problem b. Economic problem
c. Political problem d. Religious problem

Explanation: Poverty is generally regarded as a social problem. It is a condition in which individuals or communities lack the resources, capabilities, and opportunities necessary for a minimum standard of living. While poverty has economic dimensions and is often linked to economic challenges, it is not solely an economic problem.

COMMUNITY

68. The three-tier system of Panchayati Raj was recommended by:
a. Kaka Kalekar Committee
b. Simon Commission
c. Balwant Rai Mehta Committee
d. Jai Prakash Narain Committee

Explanation: The three-tier system of Panchayati Raj in India was recommended by the Balwant Rai Mehta Committee. The committee was formed in 1957 with the objective of studying and making recommendations on the functioning of local self-governments, particularly at the rural level. The committee, headed by Balwant Rai Mehta, submitted its report in 1957, which laid the foundation for the establishment of a three-tier system of Panchayati Raj institutions in India.

69. Unlike village community, urban society lacks in:
a. Secondary social control b. Social tolerance
c. Self sufficiency d. All of these

70. Social distance in a city is due to:
a. The size of city
b. The distance between residences
c. The social heterogeneity
d. The traffic problem in city

71. The spatial feature of urbanization in India has been:
a. Localized in nature b. Balanced
c. Both a and b d. None of these

72. Which is not a feature of urban life?
a. Loss of humanistic value b. Impersonal relationship
c. Informal ties d. Competition

73. Who developed the concept of urbanism as a way of life?
a. Louis Wirth b. Fisher
c. Louis Coser d. Comte

74. The world's first cities appeared around ....
a. 3500 BC b. 300 BC
c. 2000 BC d. 100 AD

75. Which among the following was an exclusive university town?
a. Taxila b. Pataliputra
c. Nalanda d. Kashi

76. Which of the following is not one of the features of urban community?
a. Face to face relationships
b. Complex life
c. Materialistic
d. Glamour in life

Ans.

55.	d
56.	a
57.	c
58.	a
59.	d
60.	d
61.	c
62.	c
63.	a
64.	d
65.	d
66.	d
67.	a
68.	c
69.	c
70.	c
71.	a
72.	c
73.	a
74.	a
75.	c
76.	a

APPLIED PSYCHOLOGY

INTRODUCTION TO PSYCHOLOGY

77. The branch of psychology that deals with the analysis of behavior of clients, criminals and witnesses is known as:
a. Military psychology
b. Counseling psychology
c. Legal psychology
d. Judicial psychology

78. The branch of psychology that deals with the individuals' behavior at work is known as:
a. Occupational psychology
b. Organizational psychology
c. Job psychology
d. Institutional psychology

79. All of the following are types of applied psychology; except:
a. Occupational psychology
b. Educational psychology
c. Forensic psychology
d. Developmental psychology

80. Who defined Psychology as "a scientific study of conscious experience"?
a. William James
b. Wilhelm Wundt
c. Pastorino and Portillo
d. William McDougall

81. Psychology is defined as the scientific study of:
a. People and things
b. Emotions and beliefs
c. Perception and religion
d. Mind and behavior

82. Most human behavior:
a. Can be easily explained
b. Has multiple causes
c. Stems from unconscious desires
d. Depends on social influence

83. Psychology is a:
a. Natural science
b. Physical science
c. Biological science
d. Social science

84. Psychology as a 'Science of Mind' is defined by:
a. Psychoanalysts
b. Behaviorists
c. Functionalists
d. Ancient Greek Philosophers

85. 'Psychology' as the scientific study of activities of organism in relation to its environment is defined by:
a. J.B Watson
b. Sigmund Freud
c. Woodworth
d. William James

86. Abnormal psychology is mainly the study of:
a. Normality of mind
b. Unconscious level of mind
c. Subconscious level of mind
d. Abnormality of mind

STRUCTURE OF THE MIND

87. In Freud's psychoanalytic theory of personality, the pleasure principle is the driving force of the ....
a. Id b. Ego
c. Superego d. All of these

88. .... is the component of personality that deals with the demands of reality.
a. Id b. Ego
c. Superego d. All of these

89. In Freud's topographic model, the 'çensor' guards the border between . . .
a. The conscious and the preconscious
b. The conscious and the unconscious
c. The preconscious and the unconscious
d. The ego and the Id

90. According to Freud, the odd, magical quality of dreams reflects the influence of . . .
a. Primary process thinking
b. Secondary process thinking
c. The 'dream work'
d. Defense mechanisms

91. Which of the following statements is true about the ego, according to Freud?
a. It exists prior to the Id
b. It follows the 'pleasure principle'
c. It lends its libidinal energy to the superego
d. It follows the 'reality principle'

92. Which Freudian defense mechanism does this statement illustrate: 'I'm not jealous, you are'?
a. Projection b. Repression
c. Sublimation d. Denial

93. One of these four lists contains concepts from Freud's topographic, structural and genetic models, in that order. Which is it?
a. Unconscious, ego, and repression
b. Unconscious, id, and reaction formation
c. Preconscious, superego, and regression
d. Preconscious, superfly, and fixation

94. Which of the following is not a weakness of psychoanalytic evidence?
a. It is subjectivity
b. It is limited quantity
c. It is vulnerability to suggestion
d. It is lack of public availability

95. A trance-like state in which a person is highly responsive to suggestions and can experience an altered state of consciousness:
a. Hypernosis b. Hypnosis
c. Stress d. Depression

96. Freud emphasized the role of ________ in shaping people's personality.
a. Free will
b. Unconscious desires
c. Hormones
d. Group influence

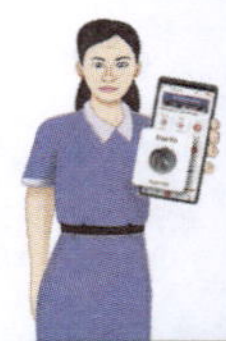

Ans.

77.	c
78.	a
79.	d
80.	b
81.	b
82.	b
83.	a
84.	a
85.	c
86.	d
87.	a
88.	b
89.	c
90.	a
91.	d
92.	a
93.	c
94.	b
95.	b
96.	b

Explanation: Freud emphasized the role of unconscious desires in shaping people's personality. According to Freud's psychoanalytic theory, a significant part of an individual's thoughts, feelings, and motivations are driven by unconscious processes and desires. These desires can be sexual, aggressive, or even simply the desire to avoid pain.

97. What is the name of Freud model of the mind which comprises the Id, Ego and Superego?
a. Structural model b. Unconscious model
c. Topographical model d. Genetic model

98. According to Freud model, what is the consequence of the physical inability of women to overcome penis envy and the reason their personality would never fully develop?
a. Their id could never fully develop
b. Their superego could never fully develop
c. Their ego could never fully develop
d. All of the above

Explanation: According to Freud's psychoanalytic theory, penis envy refers to the supposed desire that women have for possessing a penis, which they believe men have and they lack. Freud theorized that women experience a sense of inferiority and develop an unresolved conflict because of this perceived physical inadequacy. He suggested that this unresolved conflict could lead to women having an underdeveloped ego, which is responsible for mediating between the demands of the id (primitive desires) and the superego (internalized moral standards).

99. Which layer of human mind stores the information gained by experience or learning?
a. Unconsciousness b. Preconsciousness
c. Id d. Ego

Explanation: The preconscious is a level of awareness that lies between the conscious and unconscious. It contains information that is not currently in our awareness, but that can be easily brought to mind. The preconscious is also where information is stored that we have learned through experience or education. This information can be accessed and used by the conscious mind when we need it.

PSYCHOLOGY OF HUMAN BEHAVIOR

100. All of the following are types of conflict; except:
a. Intrapersonal b. Manifest
c. Interpersonal d. Intragroup

101. Adaptive mechanism of giving excuses when a person cannot solve a problem:
a. Projection b. Substitution
c. Rationalization d. Compensation

102. In which defense mechanism anxiety is expressed through physical symptoms?
a. Projection b. Regression
c. Conversion d. Hypochondriasis

103. The involuntary blocking of unpleasant feeling and experiences from one's awareness is known as ....
a. Displacement b. Repression
c. Regression d. Suppression

104. Most commonly used defense mechanism by a physically abusive individual is:
a. Transference b. Manipulation
c. Displacement d. Reaction formation

105. Imposing one's own weaknesses on others is a defense mechanism, which is known as:
a. Projection b. Intellectualization
c. Suppression d. Displacement

106. Finding a logical reason for the things that one wants to do 'sour grapes' mechanism is: New Q
a. Projection b. Rationalization
c. Identification d. Sublimation

ATTENTION AND PERCEPTION

107. Which type of attention is primarily involved in multitasking?
a. Selective Attention
b. Sustained Attention
c. Executive Attention
d. Divided Attention

108. Sustained attention is crucial for which of the following activities?
a. Switching between tasks quickly
b. Concentrating on a lecture for a long period
c. Ignoring irrelevant stimuli to focus on a specific task
d. Distributing attentional resources among different tasks

109. Which type of attention involves controlling and managing attentional resources and inhibiting distractions, and is important for goal-directed behavior, decision-making, and cognitive flexibility?
a. Selective Attention b. Sustained Attention
c. Executive Attention d. Divided Attention

110. What does the Gestalt principle of proximity state?
a. Objects that are similar in shape are perceived as belonging to a group
b. Objects that are close together are perceived as belonging to a group
c. We perceive smooth, continuous lines rather than fragmented ones
d. We fill in missing information to perceive complete objects

111. Which of the following is a binocular cue for depth perception?
a. Texture gradient b. Retinal disparity
c. Relative size d. Motion parallax

112. What is the phenomenon where we perceive an object as having a consistent color even when the lighting conditions change?
a. Shape constancy b. Size constancy
c. Color constancy d. Continuity

113. Which of these describes an illusion?
a. A sensory perception occurring in the absence of an existing stimuli
b. The misinterpretation of the perception of an existing stimuli
c. The ability to perceive objects as stable and unchanging despite variations in sensory input
d. The ability to perceive the true size of an object despite variations in its distance from us

LEARNING

114. Maturation merely provides a biological pace for:
a. Memory to occur b. Growth to occur
c. Learning to occur d. Thinking to occur

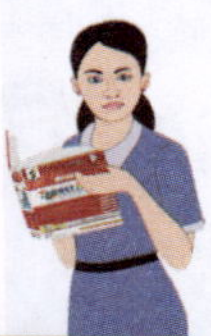

Ans.

97.	a
98.	c
99.	b
100.	b
101.	c
102.	c
103.	b
104.	c
105.	a
106.	b
107.	d
108.	b
109.	c
110.	b
111.	b
112.	c
113.	b
114.	b

Explanation: Maturation refers to the biological process of development and growth that occurs naturally and unfolds according to a predetermined sequence. It involves changes in physical, cognitive, and emotional domains.

115. Symbolic concepts become more readily available for use in:
a. Dreams b. Imagination
c. Learning d. Thought

116. Which term refers to the mental activities involved in the acquisition, processing, organization and use of knowledge?
a. Emotion b. Cognition
c. Feeling d. Imagination

117. In which type of memory, the materials are stored for later retrieval?
a. Rote memory
b. Sensory memory
c. Short-term memory (STM)
d. Long-term memory (LTM)

118. With development, children's memory relies more heavily on:
a. Imagination b. Symbolic concepts
c. Gestures d. Experiences

119. Perception is:
a. An analytic representation of the world
b. An appropriate representation of the world
c. An adequate representation of the world
d. A native representation of the world

Explanation: Perception is defined as an appropriate representation of the world. This means that our perceptions are what we use to make sense of the world around us. Our perceptions are shaped by our experiences, our beliefs, and our expectations. This means that two people can have very different perceptions of the same event.

120. The capacity to learn and adapt to the requirements for survival in one's culture is called:
a. Intelligence b. Memory
c. Emotion d. Learning

121. The last stage of creative thinking is:
a. Verification b. Evaluation
c. Incubation d. Preparation

122. Which law of learning states that learning is most effective when the learner is ready and motivated?
a. Law of Readiness b. Law of Exercise
c. Law of Effect d. Law of Primacy

123. According to the law of effect, learning is influenced by:
a. Repetition or practice
b. Consequences or outcomes
c. Emotional intensity
d. Association with existing knowledge

124. Which of the following laws of learning suggests that knowledge and skills acquired in one context can be applied to other situations?
a. Law of Primacy b. Law of Transfer
c. Law of Association d. Law of Effect

125. Which law of learning emphasizes the importance of repetition or practice for effective learning?
a. Law of Readiness
b. Law of Exercise
c. Law of Effect
d. Law of Recency

126. Who developed the trial and error theory of learning?
a. Ivan Pavlov b. BF Skinner
c. Albert Bandura d. Edward Thorndike

Explanation:
- **Edward Thorndike** – Trial and Error theory of learning
- Ivan Pavlov – Classical conditioning
- BF Skinner – Operant conditioning
- Albert Bandura – Observational learning

127. The process of classical conditioning involves:
a. Shaping behavior through rewards and punishments
b. Making various attempts or "trials" to achieve a desired outcome
c. Pairing a conditioned stimulus with an unconditioned stimulus
d. Active exploration and problem-solving through insights

128. The theory of operant conditioning, developed by BF Skinner, involves shaping behavior through:
a. Making various attempts or "trials" to achieve a desired outcome
b. Pairing a conditioned stimulus with an unconditioned stimulus
c. Rewards and punishments
d. Cognitive processes and insights

MEMORY

129. Which type of memory stores visual information for a fraction of a second?
a. Sensory memory b. Short-term memory
c. Iconic memory d. Echoic memory

130. Which type of memory stores auditory stimuli for a fraction of a second?
a. Episodic memory b. Short-term memory
c. Iconic memory d. Echoic memory

131. Which type of memory involves the storage of information for 15-30 seconds?
a. Sensory memory b. Short-term memory
c. Iconic memory d. Echoic memory

132. What type of memory retains personal information such as one's name, qualifications, and date of birth?
a. Episodic memory b. Semantic memory
c. Sensory memory d. Short-term memory

133. Which process of memory involves the ability to retrieve previously learned information?
a. Learning b. Retention
c. Recall d. Recognition

FORGETTING

134. When an individual is unable to recall anything that was previously learned, it is referred to as:
a. Normal forgetting b. Morbid forgetting
c. General forgetting d. Specific forgetting

135. Loss of memory due to factors such as stress or fear is referred to as:
a. Normal forgetting b. Morbid forgetting
c. General forgetting d. Psychological forgetting

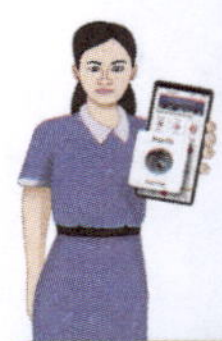

Ans.

115.	d
116.	b
117.	d
118.	b
119.	b
120.	a
121.	a
122.	a
123.	b
124.	b
125.	b
126.	d
127.	c
128.	c
129.	c
130.	d
131.	b
132.	a
133.	c
134.	c
135.	d

136. Which type of forgetting involves the loss of memory for only a particular part of earlier learning?
a. Normal forgetting
b. Morbid/abnormal forgetting
c. General forgetting
d. Specific forgetting

THINKING AND REASONING

137. Which type of thinking aims at solving complex problems and requires logical arrangement of relevant experiences?
a. Perceptual or concrete thinking
b. Conceptual or abstract thinking
c. Reflective thinking
d. Creative thinking

138. 'Daydreaming and fantasy' are types of:
a. Perceptual thinking b. Reflective thinking
c. Non-directive thinking c. Creative thinking

Explanation: In non-directive or associative thinking, the individual's thoughts wander without specific goal or direction. Day-dreaming and fantasy are examples of non-directive thinking.

139. Which type of thinking involves responsible and skillful thought process leading to good judgment?
a. Reflective thinking b. Creative thinking
c. Critical thinking d. Nondirected thinking

140. If it is known that all flowers need sunlight to grow, and roses are a type of flower, what can you deduce using deductive reasoning?
a. Roses need sunlight to grow.
b. Roses do not need sunlight to grow.
c. Roses are not flowers.
d. Not all flowers need sunlight to grow.

141. If you conclude that a dog is warm-blooded because all mammals are warm-blooded and a dog is a mammal, what type of reasoning are you using?
a. Inductive reasoning b. Deductive reasoning
c. Creative reasoning d. Critical reasoning

142. Which type of reasoning involves generalizing based on specific observations or evidence?
a. Inductive reasoning b. Deductive reasoning
c. Creative reasoning d. Critical reasoning

CONFLICTS

143. Which type of conflict arises from differences in beliefs, values, or ideologies?
a. Organizational conflict b. Role conflict
c. Ideological conflict d. Interpersonal conflict

144. What does Approach-approach conflict refer to?
a. Facing a situation with both positive and negative aspects
b. Having to choose between two undesirable options
c. Being faced with two desirable options but can only choose one
d. Experiencing conflicting expectations from different roles

145. When both parties involved in a conflict are unhappy with the outcome, which approach has likely been used?
a. Win-lose approach b. Lose-lose approach
c. Win-win approach d. None of these

Explanation: Lose-lose approach is described as an outcome where neither party is happy with the resolution of the conflict.

146. A conflict that arises due to differences in norms, customs, traditions, or worldviews is known as:
a. Intrapersonal conflict b. Environmental conflict
c. Cultural conflict d. Role conflict

Explanation: Cultural conflict is type of conflict that emerges when individuals or groups with different cultural backgrounds clash due to differences in norms, customs, traditions, or worldviews.

147. If a student dislikes working on a school assignment but also doesn't want to face punishment for not doing it, which type of conflict is he experiencing?
a. Approach-approach conflict
b. Approach-avoidance conflict
c. Avoidance-avoidance conflict
d. Role conflict

Explanation: Avoidance-avoidance conflict arises when an individual is faced with two undesirable options or outcomes and must choose between them.

PERSONALITY

148. One trait that dominates a personality so much that it influences nearly everything a person does is a:
a. Global Trait b. Cardinal Trait
c. Specific trait d. Central Trait

Explanation: A cardinal trait is a dominant and pervasive characteristic that shapes and defines a person's behavior across various situations and contexts. It is the central organizing principle of a person's personality and influences a wide range of behaviors and actions.

149. Who is the pioneer that proposed the 16 basic dimensions of normal personality and devised a questionnaire (16PF) to measure them?
a. Carl Jung b. Raymond Cattell
c. Julian Rotter d. Gordon Allport

150. Sheldon proposed three different types of traits. The trait that would best describe a football player would be:
a. Mesomorph b. Endomorph
c. Ectomorph d. Activomorph

Explanation:
- Sheldon proposed a somatotype theory, which categorized individuals into three basic body types: mesomorphs, endomorphs, and ectomorphs.
- **Mesomorphs** are characterized as having a muscular and athletic build, which is often associated with traits such as strength, power, and agility. Football players typically require physical attributes that align with the mesomorphic body type.
- **Endomorphs** tend to have a higher proportion of body fat and a rounder physique.
- Ectomorphs have a leaner and more slender body type.
- **Activomorph** is not a recognized term in Sheldon's somatotype theory.

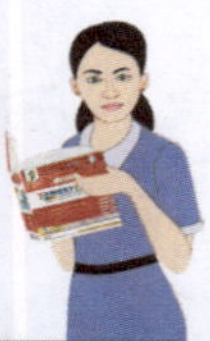

Ans.

136. d
137. c
138. c
139. c
140. a
141. b
142. a
143. c
144. c
145. b
146. c
147. c
148. b
149. b
150. a

151. The idea that you can assess someone's personality by studying their face is called:

a. Phrenology b. Physiology
c. Somatology d. Physiognomy

Explanation: Physiognomy is the practice of trying to determine an individual's character, personality traits, or temperament by analyzing facial features, such as the shape of the face, the placement of facial features, or the expressions displayed.

152. The ________ complex is to girls as the ________ complex is to boys.

a. Electra, Oedipus b. Oedipus, Electra
c. Oral, phallic d. Phallic, oral

153. Which of the following is NOT one of the Big Five traits?

a. Sense of humor b. Openness to experience
c. Conscientiousness d. Extraversion

Explanation: The Big Five traits, also known as the Five-Factor Model, are a widely accepted framework for describing and measuring personality traits. The Big Five traits include (i) openness to experience, (ii) conscientiousness, (iii) extraversion, (iv) agreeableness, and (v) neuroticism (also known as emotional stability)

INTELLIGENCE

154. David Wechsler defines intelligence as:

a. The psychological potential to solve problems
b. What intelligence tests measure
c. Being able to behave in a consistent way
d. The global capacity to act purposefully, think rationally and deal effectively with the environment

155. The belief that 'intelligence is a general ability' is a result of the work of:

a. Binet b. Gardner
c. Sternberg d. Spearman

156. If it is demonstrated that an intelligence test discriminates against certain ethnic groups, then it can be said that the test:

a. Is reliable
b. Has used a standardization sample
c. Is valid
d. Has culture bias

157. According to Sternberg, intelligence is:

a. Made up of three different independent intelligences
b. A single, general underlying ability.
c. Made up of eight or more independent mental abilities
d. A single, specific ability which cannot be measured by traditional intelligence tests

Explanation: According to Robert Sternberg, intelligence is made up of three independent intelligences: Analytical intelligence, Creative intelligence, and Practical intelligence.

158. If an intelligence test measures consistently what it is supposed to be measuring each time it is used, then it is said that the test is:

a. Based on a normal distribution
b. Standardized
c. Valid
d. Reliable

Explanation: Reliability is the consistency of a measure. A reliable test will produce similar results when it is administered to the same person on different occasions. In other words, a reliable test will measure what it is supposed to measure consistently.

159. In terms of intelligence:

a. Identical twins are more similar to one another than are fraternal twins
b. Fraternal twins are more similar to one another than are non-twin siblings
c. Adopted children are more similar to their biological parents than their adoptive parents
d. All of the above statements are true

160. What does IQ stand for?

a. Investment in education quotient
b. Intellect quotient
c. Intelligence quotient
d. Intelligence question

161. The current Stanford-Binet Intelligence Test is descended from the test developed by Binet and Simon:

a. In early 1900s b. In early 1800s
c. In early 1600s d. In early 1700s

Explanation: The test developed by Alfred Binet and Theodore Simon was called the Binet-Simon Scale. It was the first intelligence test ever developed, and it is considered to be the grandfather of all modern intelligence tests. The Binet-Simon Scale was developed in France in **1905**. The first version of the Stanford-Binet Intelligence Scale developed by Lewis Terman was published in **1916**. It was a revision of the Binet-Simon Scale.

162. The process of encoding, storing, and retrieving information in memory is known as: *New Q*

a. Perception b. Learning
c. Cognition d. Recall

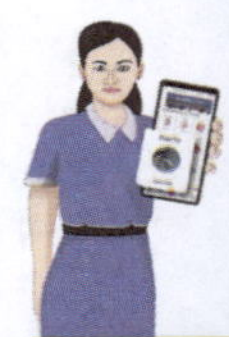

Explanation: Overall, memory processing is a complex cognitive function that allows us to encode, store, and retrieve information, forming the basis for learning, knowledge acquisition, and everyday cognitive activities.

163. Magical thinking is chiefly seen in: *(AIIMS BBS 2016)*

a. Adolescents b. Toddlers
c. Preschoolers d. Infants

Explanation: Magical thinking is a stage that occurs between the 2 and 7 years of age. Age group from 1-3 years is known as toddlers and age group from 3–5 years is known as preschoolers. The prime time for fantasy (magical thinking) is during preschool age (around 5 years) than toddler age. At this developmental stage, children believe in fantastic characters so much that they truly believe they accompany them every day. For example, they believe that the mountains can move and due to this, they can enjoy authentic adventure when they are in a moving car.

164. The first task in psychology is to carefully observe and objectively describe: *(IGNOU PB BSc 2016)*

a. Behavior b. Personality
c. Social institution d. Motivation

Explanation: The first task in psychology is to make accurate observations about behavior. This means that psychologists must first describe behavior. Rest of the options are irrelevant to the statement given above.

Ans.

151. d
152. a
153. a
154. d
155. d
156. d
157. a
158. d
159. d
160. c
161. a
162. c
163. c
164. a

165. Aptitudes are defined as: *(IGNOU PB BSc 2016)*

a. Preferences to perform certain activities
b. High level of achievement in an area
c. Skills one brings to a given task
d. Abilities of individual to learn in specific endeavor

Explanation: Aptitude is a component of a competence to do a certain kind of work at a certain level. Outstanding aptitude can be considered "talent". An aptitude may be physical or mental. Aptitude is outcome of both inborn and hereditary potential to do certain kinds of work whether developed or undeveloped.

166. Gradual disappearance of conditioned response to stimuli is referred to as: *(JIPMER 2015)*

a. Negative conditioning b. Extinction
c. Delayed conditioning d. Elimination

Explanation:

Extinction	Extinction is the gradual weakening and disappearance of a conditioned response
Negative conditioning	Negative conditioning is the removal of a stimulus after a response.
Delayed conditioning	A form of classical conditioning in which the conditioned stimulus precedes the unconditioned stimulus by a significant time period and the organism learns to withhold its conditioned response
Elimination	Elimination is an aversive stimulus or punishment during which the client is removed from the environment when the desired behavior is being exhibited.

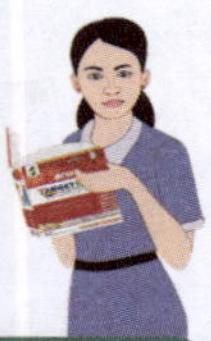

Ans.

165. d
166. b
167. a
168. a
169. a
170. a
171. c

167. Ego works based on the: *(DSSSB PHN, 2015)*

a. Reality b. Pleasure
c. Perfection d. Conscience

Explanation: The id, ego, superego are the names for the three parts of the structure of human personality given by psychoanalytical theory. Ego is the realistic part that mediates between the desires of the id and the superego. The id is the primitive instinctual part of mind which operates on pleasure principle. The superego (perfection) is the aspect of personality that holds all of our internalized moral standards and ideals that we acquire from both parents and society.

Structure of personality	Principle
Id	Pleasure
Ego	Reality
Superego	Perfection

168. Psychology is a: *(Safdarjung NO 2018)*

a. Natural science b. Physical science
c. Biological science d. Social science

Explanation: Psychology is a natural science. "Natural science" means a branch of science that is concerned with the description, prediction and understanding of natural phenomena (based on observation and empirical evidence) -- and it can be seen in psychology.

169. Psychology as a 'Science of Mind', is defined by: *(Safdarjung NO 2018)*

a. Psychoanalysts b. Behaviorists
c. Functionalists d. Ancient Greek Philosophers

Explanation:

School/System of Psychology	Definition
Psychoanalysts	Psychoanalysis is the school of psychology that focuses on treating mental disorders by recognizing the relationships between the conscious mind and the unconscious mind. Proponent of this school of psychology is William James.
Functionalists	Functionalists focused on the purpose of consciousness and behavior.
Behaviorists	A school of psychology that confines itself to the study of observable and quantifiable aspects of behavior and excludes subjective phenomena, such as emotions or motives.
Ancient Greek philosophers	Study of mind as a function of bodily processes. They are due to brain pathology.

170. EB Titchener (1867-1927) defined 'Psychology' as the science of: *(Safdarjung NO 2018)*

a. Conscious Experience b. Science of Mind
c. Science of Experience d. Science of Soul

Explanation: EB Titchener coined the terms: structural psychology and functional psychology. **Titchener** concluded that there are three essential elements that make up all **conscious experiences**: feelings, sensations, and images.

Table: Other definitions along with their authors

Definition of Psychology	Given by
Science of Mind	William James
Science of Soul	Rudolf Geöckle
Science of Experience	Carl Rogers Abraham Maslow

171. 'Psychology' as the scientific study of activities of organism in relation to its environment is defined by: *(Safdarjung NO 2018)*

a. JB Watson b. Sigmund Freud
c. Woodworth d. William James

Explanation:

Table: Definition of psychology given by various theorists

Theorists	Definition of Psychology
Woodworth	Psychology' as the scientific study of activities of organism in relation to its environment.
William James	Psychology as Study of Mind
Sigmund Freud	This school of thought emphasized the influence of the unconscious mind on behavior.
JB Watson	Scientific study of behavior and mental processes.

"Ill-health of body or of mind, is defeat. Health alone is victory."

—Thomas Carlyle

CHAPTER 11

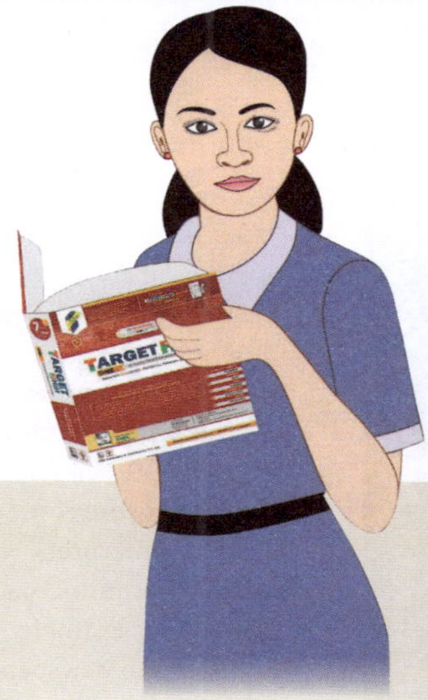

NURSING RESEARCH AND STATISTICS

SYNOPSIS

INTRODUCTION

Nursing research provides evidence used to support nursing practices, education, administration and management.

DEFINITION

Nursing research is a planned attempt to increase nursing knowledge by the discovery of new facts through systematic enquiry.

STEPS IN THE QUANTITATIVE RESEARCH PROCESS

Conceptual Phase

- Formulating and delimiting the problem.
- Reviewing the literature.
- Developing a theoretical framework.
- Identifying the research variables.
- Formulating hypotheses.

Design and Planning Phase

- Selecting a research design.
- Specifying the population.
- Operationalizing the variables.
- Conducting the pilot study/making revisions.

Empirical Phase

- Selecting the sample
- Collecting the data
- Organizing data for analysis

Analytic Phase

- Analyzing the data
- Interpreting the results

Dissemination Phase

- Communicating results

STEPS IN THE QUALITATIVE RESEARCH PROCESS

- Define/clarify broad topic
- Review of the literature
- Identify site/setting
- Obtain access
- Obtain and test equipment
- Begin data collection/analysis
- Identify themes/categories
- Triangulation/saturation
- Formulate hypotheses/theories
- Communicate findings

RESEARCH PROCESS

Research Problem

- It is the first step in research process.
- A research problem is a question that researcher wants to answer or a problem that a researcher wants to solve.
- Research problem to be developed, components etc

Review of Literature

Review of Literature (ROL) is a systematic way of presentation of relevant references along with brief findings in the specific juncture for the proposed study or research proposal.

Sources of Review of Literature

- **Primary sources:** A primary source provides direct or first-hand evidence about an event, object, person, or work of art. Examples include:
  - Historical and legal documents
  - Original research articles found in Scholarly journals
  - Published thesis
  - Eyewitness accounts
  - Results of experiments

Recent Questions (INC PhD 2020)

1. Which among the following is not an appropriate research area?

a. Abortion mortality as a method of contraceptive
b. Postpartum contraceptive methods
c. Initiation of breastfeeding immediately after delivery
d. Low birth weight babies and their outcomes

Ans. (a) Abortion mortality as a method of contraceptive.

2. In Vancouver style et al is used after how many authors?

a. 3
b. 6
c. 8
d. 10

Ans. (b) 6

KEY POINT

A research proposal is a document proposing a research project.

- Statistical data
- Pieces of creative writing
- Audio and video recordings, speeches, and art objects
- Interviews, surveys, and fieldwork
- Internet communications via E-mail, blogs, LISTSERV, and newsgroups

- **Secondary sources:** Secondary sources describe, discuss, interpret, comment upon, analyze, evaluate, summarize, and process primary sources. For example:
  - Articles in newspapers or popular magazines.
  - Book or movie reviews.
  - Articles found in scholarly journals that discuss or evaluate someone else's original research.
- **Types of sources**
  - **Print sources:** Information gathered from printed materials including journals, magazines, textbooks, etc.
  - **Electronic sources:** Information gathered from electronic media such as internet, CD, online journals, blogs, etc. Some of the electronic databases for nursing research are given below.
  - **Ovid MEDLINE:** Literature in the fields of medicine, nursing, dentistry, and preclinical sciences.
  - **Ovid CINAHL (Cumulative index to Nursing allied Health Literature):** Literature related to nursing and allied health disciplines including medical records, physical and occupational therapy.
  - **PubMed:** The US National library of medicine database of biomedical citation and abstracts that is searchable on the website at no cost.
  - **MEDLINE** is the largest component of Pubmed.
  - Cochrane Library.

Research Variables

A **variable** is a measurable characteristic that varies. It may change from group to group, person to person, or even within one person over time.

- **Dependent variables:** These are the variables which changed according to the independent variable, e.g., A study to assess the effect of hand grip exercises on BP of prehypertensive client. Here dependent variable is BP of prehypertensive client.
- **Independent variables:** These are the variables manipulated by the researcher. Researcher has good control over these variables, e.g., A study to assess the effect of hand grip exercises on BP of pre-hypertensive client. Here independent variable is hand grip exercises

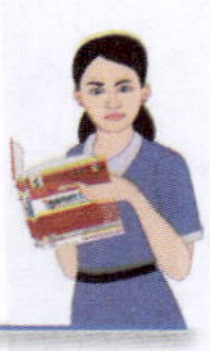

- **Extraneous variables:** These are factors in the research environment which may have an effect on the dependent variable(s) but which are not controlled. Extraneous variables may damage a study's validity, making it impossible to know whether the effects were caused by the independent or some extraneous (not measured) factor. If they cannot be controlled, extraneous variables must at least be taken into consideration when interpreting results.
- **Confounding variables:** Extraneous variables become confounding variable if there is an academic evidence that the extraneous variable (which was not measured in the study) has influence (or relationship) on dependent variable.
- **Continuous variables:** These variables can take an infinite range of values along a continuum, e.g., weight in kg.
- **Discrete variables:** They are having a finite number of values between two points, e.g., number of children
- **Categorical variables:** They do not represent quantity or numerical value, e.g., Nominal variable: Gender (male, female), Religion (Hindu, Muslim, Christian), etc.
- **Ordinal variables:** Severity of disease (mild, moderate, severe), Socio-Economic status, e.g., poor, middle class, upper middle class, affluent.

Examples to Explain all These Four Variables

- **Study title:** The impact of teaching style (lectures/seminars) on exam performance of students.
- **Independent variable (IV):** Teaching style (either lectures or seminars).
- **Dependent variable (DV):** Exam performance of students (statistics exam ranging from 0 :o 100 marks).
- **Extraneous variables:** Quality of lecturer and tiredness of students; the researcher was not indented to measure these variable in his/her research.
- **Confounding variables:** If researcher found academic evidence (from research articles from scholarly journals) that quality of the teacher or tiredness of student will affect the exam performance, then **these two variables may be called confounding variables**. Because the researcher cannot be sure that only the independent variable (teaching style) has caused changes in students' performance.

Objectives

- A research objective is a clear, concise, declarative statement which provides direction to investigate the variables.
- The objectives of a research project summarize what is to be achieved by the research.

Characteristics of research objectives:

- A well-framed objective will be SMART
  - S - Specific
  - M - Measurable
  - A - Attainable
  - R - Realistic
  - T - Time-bound

KEY POINTS

- **A literature review is** everything that is known about subject.
- In quantitative research studies**,** the literature review should occur early in the research process.

Recent Question (INC PhD 2020)

3. Characteristics of research objective are all; EXCEPT:
a. Measurable
b. Testability
c. Time bound
d. Equivocal

Ans. (d) Equivocal

KEY POINT

A research objective must be SMART (Specific, Measurable, Attainable, Realistic and Time-bound).

Types of research objectives:

- **General objectives:** Broad statement of what is to be achieved.
- **Specific objective:** General objectives are broken into number of small and short-term objectives.
- **Primary objectives:** The primary research objective should focus on the core variable stated in the problem statement.
- **Secondary objectives:** Secondary objectives are other constructs being tested by the study that could clarify findings from the primary objective.

Hypothesis

It is statement which reveals the expected relationship among two or more variables under study. A clearly stated hypothesis explains:

- The variables under study
- Population
- Proposed outcome of the study
- Level of significance.

Types of Hypothesis

Simple Vs Complex

- Simple hypothesis is one which explains the relationship between two variables, e.g., handgrip exercise among pre-hypertensive client help to decrease the BP reading.
- Complex hypothesis is one which explains the relationship between more than two variables, e.g., knowledge regarding newborn care is higher among the nurses who all are working in labor room and having more experience than the nurses who all are working in other area and less experience.

Directional and Non-directional Hypothesis

Directional Hypothesis

- It not only specifies the existence of relationship between variables but also specifies the direction of relationship between the variables.
- The direction of relationship can be positive and negative.
- The following example explains the positive relationship, e.g., nurses with good knowledge regarding organ donation have positive attitude towards organ donation.

Non-directional Hypothesis

It only specifies the existence of relationship between variables and does not specify the direction of relationship. There is a relationship between knowledge and attitude regarding organ donation among nurses.

Associative and Causal Hypothesis

Associative hypothesis explains the relationship between two variables in the natural setting without any manipulation. Lower the level of hemoglobin level, higher the incidence of infection among cancer patients.

Causal Hypothesis: It explains the cause and effect relationship between two or more independent and dependent variables, e.g., prevalence of ventilator associated pneumonia is less among the patient who all are receiving oral care using betadine as compared to the patient who all are receiving oral care using hydrogen peroxide.

Null Hypothesis and Research Hypothesis

Null hypothesis states that there is existence of no relationship between variables. It is used for statistical testing and interpretations. Research hypothesis states that there is existence of relationship between the variables.

- **Research hypothesis:** There will be positive correlation between LDL value and systolic blood pressure of adult patients.
- **Null hypothesis:** There will be no correlation between blood cholesterol levels and blood pressure of patients.

RESEARCH DESIGNS

- **Quantitative**
  - Experimental
    - True experimental
    - Quasi-experimental
    - Pre-experimental
  - Non-experimental
    - Descriptive
    - Survey
    - Correlational
    - Methodological
    - Comparative
    - Explorative
    - Case-control studies
    - Cohort studies
- Qualitative
    - Grounded theory approach
    - Phenomenological study
    - Ethnography
    - Case study method

Quantitative v/s Qualitative Research

In quantitative research, the variables are measured and quantified whereas in qualitative research, the variables are not quantified.

Nutshell of Experimental Designs

- **Experimental:** Manipulation + Control + Randomization
- **Quasi-experimental:** Manipulation + Control/ Randomization
- **Pre-experimental:** Manipulation only

KEY POINTS

- Realistic expectation which is something that we believe to be true is known as Assumption.
- **Hypothesis** is a statement of tentative prediction of relationship between two variables.
- **Simple hypothesis** – predicts relationship between two variables.
- **Complex hypothesis** – predicts relationship between more than two variables.
- **Null hypothesis** – states that there is no relationship between variables.
- **Directional hypothesis** – Statement specifies the direction of change, e.g., exercise therapy will **reduce** weight in obese individuals.
- **Non-directional hypothesis** – statement does not specify the direction of change. For example, Vitamin C administration **affects** iron absorption in the guts.
- A "Research Design" is a framework or blueprint for conducting the research.
- Experimental research methods are useful in establishing cause and effect relationship.
- True experimental research is the most accurate form of experimental research design.

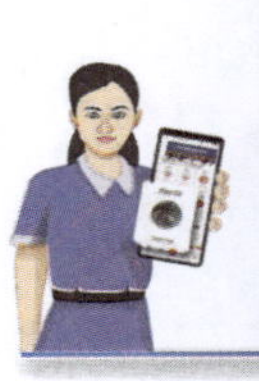

Quantitative Research Approach

- The researcher plays an active role by introducing the intervention.
- Characteristics of true experiments are:
  - **Manipulation:** Experimenter does something to at least some subjects (experimental manipulation/intervention).
  - **Control:** Experimenter introduces controls over the experimental situation. Control can be achieved.
  - Manipulating:
    - Randomizing.
    - Carefully preparing experimental protocols.
    - And/or using a control group.
  - **Characteristics-Manipulation, Control, Randomization:** Experimenter assigns subjects to a control or experimental group on a random basis. Methods of randomization includes flipping a coin, matching, draw of lots (pulling names from a hat), table of random numbers, cluster randomization **(reduces possibility of contamination)**, and Computer-generated random numbers.

Basic Experimental Designs (True Experimental)

- Pretest post-test design (before-after design; **classic experimental design**).
- Post-test only design (after-only design).
- Solomon four- group design.
- Factorial design.
- Randomized block design.
- Crossover design (repeated measure design).

Pretest Post-Test Design

Table 1: Schematic presentation of pretest–post-test design

Group	Pretest	Intervention	Post-test
R C	O_1		O_2
R E	O_1	x	O_2

R-Randomization; C-Control; E-Experimental; O1-Pretest Observation; X-Intervention, O_{2-} Post-test observation

- Classic experimental design and it is most commonly used in nursing research.
- Two randomized groups; One group receives the experimental treatment and the other group receives no treatment, a placebo treatment, or the usual treatment.
- Treatment is under the control of the researcher.
- The dependent variable is measured twice, before and after the manipulation of the independent variable.
- Comparison of the post-test scores allows determining the effect of the independent variable.

Post-Test Only Design

Table 2: Post-test only design (after-only design)

Group	Pretest	Intervention	Post-test
R C			O
R E		x	O

R-Randomization; C-Control; E-Experimental; O-Post-test Observation; X-Intervention

- For both the groups, observation was done only after intervention was administered to experimental group.

Solomon Four Group Design

Table 3: Solomon four group design

Group	Pretest	Intervention	Post-test
RC	O_1		O_2
RC			O_2
RE	O_1	x	O_2
RE		x	O_2

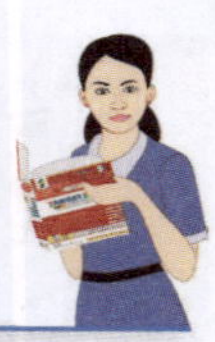

KEY POINTS

- Correlational research is a type of descriptive research.
- Qualitative research designs include phenomenology, ethnography, grounded theory, historical research, and case study.
- **Triangulation** refers to the use of multiple **methods** or data sources in qualitative **research** to develop a comprehensive understanding of phenomena.

Recent Question
(INC PhD 2020)

4. Which among the following objectives reflects experimental design?

a. Knowledge level of primi mother about newborn care
b. Effect of CBT among HD patients to decrease anxiety
c. Comparison of antenatal care knowledge among primi mothers and multi gravida mothers
d. Assess the medication error committed by a newly joined staff at 0 months and 6 months

Ans. (b) Effect of CBT among HD patients to decrease...

KEY POINT

Internal & external validity of research study:
Internal validity: The extent to which it can be inferred that the independent variable caused or influenced the dependent variable.
External validity: The generalizability of the observed relationships across samples, settings, or time.

R-R Randomization; RC-Control; RE-Experimental; O_1-Pretest Observation; X-Intervention, O_2- Post-test observation

- Involves two experimental groups and two control groups.
- One experimental and one control group are administered pretest and other groups are not.
- Allows the effects of pretest measure and intervention to be segregated.

Factorial Design

Table 4: Factorial design

Intervention	A1	A2
B1	A1B1	A2B1
B2	A1B2	A2B2
B3	A1B3	A2B3

A1- Treatment 1; A2-Treatment 2; B1, B2, B3-Different levels of treatment

- Used to manipulate two or more independent variables simultaneously.
- Independent Variables - Factors.
- Each factor – levels (two or more).
- Treatment condition – cell (Box); for e.g., A1B1 refers to subject receiving treatment 1 (A1) at the level of B1 (once a day).
- Designs can be 2 × 2, 2 × 3, 3 × 3, 3 × 4 example of factorial design.

Randomized Block Design

Table 5: Randomized block design

	Male (B1)	Female (B2)
Intervention -A1	A1B1	A1B2
Intervention - A2	A2B1	A2B2

- It is also similar to factorial design.
- There are two treatments and two factors but one factor is not experimentally manipulated -Blocking variable: **Gender is the blocking variable in the above example**
- Designs can be 2 × 2, 2 × 3, 2 × 2 × 2.

Crossover Design (Repeated Measure or Counterbalanced Design)

- Involves exposure of same subjects to more than one experimental treatment
- Subjects are randomly assigned to different orderings of treatment.
- Subjects serve as their own control.
- **Extremely powerful design** but inappropriate for certain types of research due to problem of carry-over effects.

E.g., patient A is randomized to receive Treatment #1 for a period of time. After completing Treatment #1, the patient then "crosses over" and receives Treatment #2.

Quasi-Experiments

- Like true experiments, involve the manipulation of an IV, i.e., an intervention.
- However, these designs lack either randomization or control.
- Facilitate search for knowledge and examination of causality in situations in which complete control is not possible.
- Developed to control as many threats to validity as possible.

Important Note

Design	Characteristics
Non-experimental	No manipulation
True experimental	Manipulation + Control + Randomization
Quasi-experimental	Manipulation + Some control (No randomization)
Pre-experimental	Manipulation only (no control/randomization)

Recent Questions
(INC PhD 2020)

5. Researcher planned to assess medication error committed by newly recruited nurses. For this, researcher recruited a group of nurses and assessed them at 0 month, 6 months and 8 months. Which among the following is the most appropriate study design for this study?
 a. Cross over
 b. Retrospective comparative
 c. Repeated measure design
 d. Cross sectional design

Ans. (c) Repeated measure design

6. RCT results informed in which of the following formats?
 a. PERT
 b. MOOSE
 c. CONSORT
 d. CINHAL

Ans. (c) CONSORT

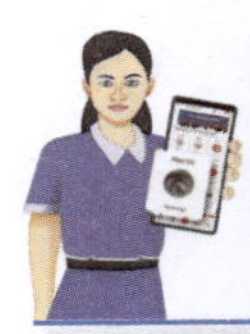

Quasi-Experimental Designs (Controlled Trials without Randomization)

- Non-equivalent control group pretest-post-test design
- Non-equivalent control group post-test only design (pre experimental).
- **Design-interrupted time series design (one group):** Information is collected over an extended period and an intervention is introduced during that period. Seasonal variations or other cyclical influences can be interpreted as treatment effects.

O1	O2	O3	O4	X	O5	O6	O7	O8

- Time series non-equivalent control group design (two group but not randomized).

O1	O2	O3	O4	X	O5	O6	O7	O8
O1	O2	O3	O4		O5	O6	O7	O8

- Time series with multiple institutions of treatment: Multiple treatments will be implemented over an extended period of data collection.

O1	O2	X	O3	O4	X	O5	O6	X	O7	O8

- Time series with intensified treatment: In this design treatment is intensified over a period of time.

O1	O2	X	O3	O4	X	O5	O6	X	O7	O8
O1	O2	X	O3	O4	X +1	O5	O6	X+2	O7	O8

- Time series with withdrawn and reinstituted treatment: Treatment is instituted and withdrawn alternatively between observations over a period of time.

O1	O2	X	O3	O4	(-X)	O5	O6	X	O7	O8

Limitations of Quasi-experiments

- Several rival hypotheses competing with intervention as explanation for the results.
- Take the weaknesses into account in interpreting results.
- Conclusion depends on part of human judgment rather than more objective criteria, cause and effect inferences may be less convincing.

Qualitative Research Designs

- Qualitative research is defined as "the study of the nature of phenomena".
- Qualitative research designs are "rooted in the naturalistic paradigm".
- In qualitative research, the research process is inductive, rather than deductive, and begins with broad exploratory aims.
- Types of qualitative research designs most often used to conduct nursing research include:
  - Phenomenology
  - Grounded theory
  - Ethnography
  - Narrative inquiry
  - Case study.
- **Phenomenology:** Phenomenological study attempts to capture lived experiences of the people about a phenomenon. The purpose of phenomenological research is to describe specific phenomena of interest as they are lived and experienced by individuals. For e.g., "what are the experiences of siblings living with an intellectually challenged child?".

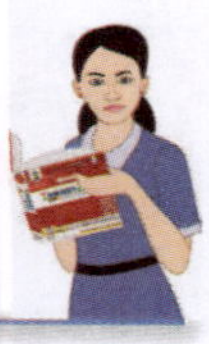

- **Grounded theory:** It is an inductive technique developed for health-related topics by Glaser and Strauss (1967). The theory is "grounded" in actual data, which means the analysis and development of theories happen after the data are collected.
- **Ethnography:** Often used in the social sciences. Data collection is often done through participant observation, interview, question, etc. Ethnography focuses on culture of group of the people.
  - Macro-ethnography - researches on broadly defined culture, e.g., The Dravidian culture.
  - Micro-ethnography - focuses on more narrowly defined ones, e.g., The culture of slum dwellers.
- **Narrative enquiry:** It involves individual narrative accounts and the interpretation of their meaning. Narrative accounts can be collected from different groups of people or individuals.
- **Case study:** Case study is useful for trying to test theoretical models by using them in real world situation.
- **Historical research:** Systemic collection and objective evaluation of data related to past occurrences. It usually includes identification of origin, date, evidence of location, recognition of authorship, attribution to credibility, etc.
- Data collection methods in qualitative research:
  - Observations
  - Interviews (individual or group)
  - Focused group discussion
  - Textual or visual analysis (e.g, from books or videos).

Descriptive Research Designs

Refer to "Community Health Nursing" synopsis for details on descriptive research designs.

Recent Questions (INC PhD 2021)

7. Which among the following research design is appropriate to study lived experience?

a. Phenomenology
b. Ethnography
c. Grounded theory
d. Case study

Ans. (a) Phenomenology

8. Data collection occurs in qualitative study at______

a. Lab setting
b. Natural setting
c. Classroom
d. Clinical area

Ans. (b) Natural setting

MIXED METHOD RESEARCH

Mixed methods research is an approach that involves collecting and analysing both quantitative and qualitative data.

This approach allows researchers to gain a more comprehensive understanding of the research question by combining the strengths of both methods.

Mixed Method Designs

There are Four major types of mixed method research designs:

Here below mentioned, all capital letters for dominant strand and all lower case letters for non-dominant strand sequence. An arrow is used for sequential designs and + is used for concurrent designs.

1. The convergent parallel design (QUAL + QUAN)
2. The explanatory sequential design [QUAN >> qual) OR quan >>QUAL]
3. The exploratory sequential design [QUAL >>quan OR qual >> QUAN]
4. The embedded design: [QUAL (quan) or QUAN (qual)]

Meta-Analysis

- In 1976, **Gene Glass** coined the term 'meta-analysis' to refer to 'the statistical analysis of a large collection of analysis results from individual studies for the purpose of integrating the findings.
- Meta-analysis is a consolidated and quantitative review of a large, and often complex, sometimes apparently conflicting, body of literature.
- Rigorously conducted meta-analyses are useful tools in evidence-based nursing/medicine
- Each study is a "case" in the meta-analysis, whereas each subject is a "case" in other research designs.
- Effect Size (ES) is the "dependent variable" in the meta-analysis.
- Funnel-Plot, Fail-safe N and Egger test are the approaches to avoid publication bias in meta-analysis.

Forest Plot

- The graphical display of results from individual studies on a common scale is a "Forest plot".
- Each row represents an individual study.

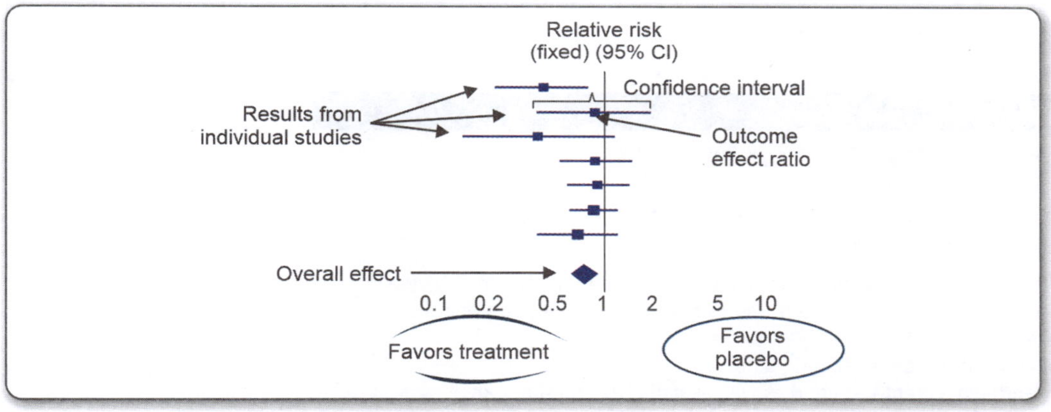

Figure 1: Forest plot diagram

Levels of Scientific Evidence

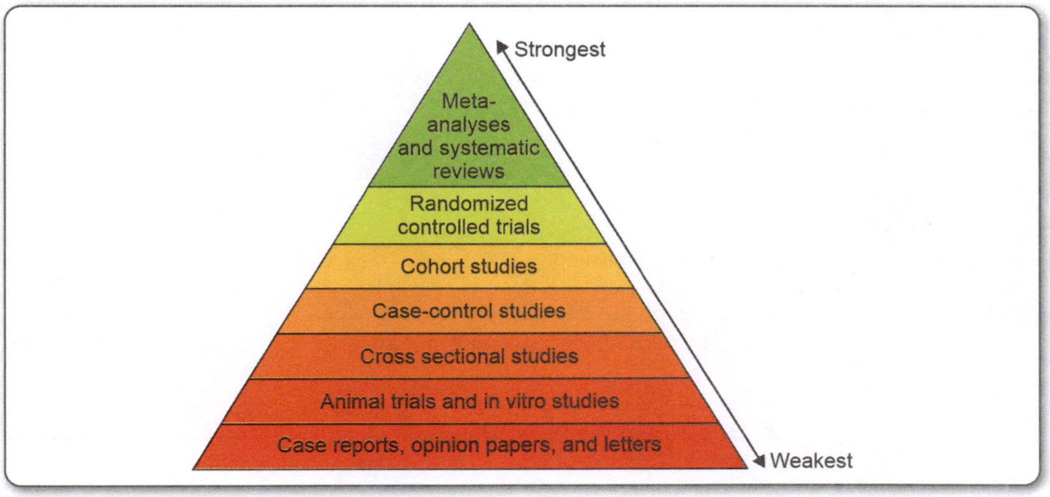

Figure 2: Hierarchy of scientific evidence

Mixed methods:

- **The convergent parallel design:** simultaneous collection and analysis of both quantitative and qualitative data
- **The explanatory sequential design:** Collection and analysis of Quantitative data first, then qualitative data
- **The exploratory sequential design:** collects and analyses qualitative data followed by quantitative data
- **The embedded design:** The qualitative method may be embedded within the quantitative method, or the quantitative method may be embedded within qualitative method.

KEY POINTS

- Forest plot diagrams are used in meta-analyses and systematic reviews to visually present the results of multiple studies on a specific topic.
- In a forest plot, the "I-square" (I2) is a statistical measure used to assess the heterogeneity or variability of effect sizes among the studies included in a meta-analysis

MAJOR TYPES OF DATA COLLECTION METHODS

- **Self-reports:** By questioning people. For e.g., attitude, knowledge, economic status, etc.
- **Observation:** By observing people. For e.g., non verbal communication, sleep wake cycle, facial expressions, injection technique, etc.
- **Biophysiologic measures:** Requires technical instruments; most accurate method of data collection, e.g., Height, weight, Blood pressure, etc.
  - **In vivo:** Performed on or with people or living organisms.
  - **In vitro:** Data gathered and then subjected to laboratory analysis.

Types of Qualitative Self-Reports

- **Unstructured interviews:** Interview conducted without any planned/prepared questions.
- **Semi-structured interviews:** Interview conducted with open ended questions.
- **Focus group interview:** In a focus group interview, a group of four or more people is assembled for a discussion.
- **Joint interview:** In phenomena that involve a relationship between two or three people, or that requires understanding the perspective of more than one person.
- **The Think-Aloud method:** This is a qualitative method that has been used to collect data about cognitive processes, such as thinking, problem solving, and decision making.
- **Photo elicitation interview:** It involves an interview stimulated and guided by photographic images.
- **Self-report narrative on the internet:** A potentially rich data source for qualitative researcher involves narrative self-reports available on or through internet.
- **Life histories, oral history, and critical incidents.**
- **Diaries and Journals.**

Quantitative Self-Reports

- A researcher collecting structured self-report data for a quantitative study almost always uses a **form**, written instrument.

POINT TO REMEMBER

- Single blind studies involve masking one group (either participants or investigator) and double blind studies involve masking of two groups (both participants and investigator)
- Partially randomized patient preference design involves randomizing patient without treatment preference and Randomized consent (Zelen design) randomizes prior to informed consent.

Table 6: Types of close-ended questions

Type	Examples
Dichotomous question	Question with two options Had your breakfast today? Yes/No
Multiple choice question	More than two option will be there. Capital of India is .... New Delhi, Mumbai, Kolkata, Bengaluru
Cafeteria question	People with different opinions can select any answer which is matching with their idea. Select your view regarding estrogen replacement among the following: Estrogen replacement should be banned. Estrogen replacement has good as well as bad effect on the body. Estrogen replacement has a lot of beneficial effect. In long-term point of view estrogen has only bad effect on the body.
Rank order question	In this type of question, clients will be asked to rank their interest/ opinion. Arrange the following needs of human being as per your priority? Oxygen, shelter, water, job, family
Forced choice question	It makes the respondents choose a response option that indicates a definitive opinion. Blood donation will be helpful to have a healthy lifestyle: Strongly agree/Agree/Disagree/Strongly disagree
Rating question	On a scale, respondent asked to rate their response, Indicate your hospital satisfaction in a 1-10 scale 0 means least satisfaction and 10 means highly satisfied

Q-Sort Technique/Q-Methodology

- Q methodology **(Stephenson, 1975)** uses a **Q-sort** procedure, which involves sorting a deck of cards according to specified criteria.
  - In Q-sort participants are presented with a set of statement card
  - Participants are asked to sort the cards along a particular dimension, such as approve/ disapprove.
  - The numbers of cards are typically 60 to 100.
  - Cards are sorted into 9 or 11 piles.

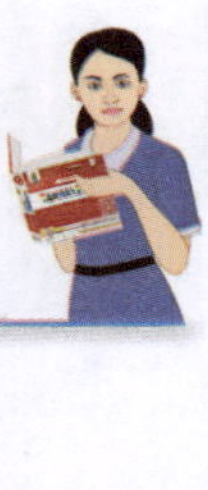

Recent Questions
(INC PhD 2020)

9. Mixed method research includes all; EXCEPT:
a. Embedded design
b. Emergent design
c. Triangulation design
d. Cross over design

Ans. (d) Cross over design.

10. Length of Visual analogue scale is, usually
a. 5 cm
b. 10 cm
c. 15 cm
d. 20 cm

Ans. (b) 10 cm

Delphi Technique

- The Delphi technique is used to measure the judgments of a group of experts for the purpose of making forecast.
- **Three types:**
  - **Classic Delphi**: Focus is on reaching on consensus.
  - **Policy Delphi**: The aim is not consensus but rather to identify and understand a variety of view point.
  - **Decision Delphi**: The panel consists of individuals in decision making.

Likert Scale

- A Likert Scale is an ordinal scale format that asks respondents to indicate the extent to which they **agree or disagree** with the opinion expressed by the statement.
- Likert scale is also called **rating scale.**
- An ideal Likert Scale will have seven point responses.
- Likert Scale with odd number of (3, 5, 7.9 and so on) points responses will have more reliability than the scale with even number of responses.

Semantic Differential Scale

- The Semantic Differential (SD) scale measures attitude and beliefs.
- A SD scale consists of two opposite adjectives such as effective/ineffective, good/bad, important/ unimportant or strong/weak that captures a person's attitudes and/or feelings about a given object.

Visual Analogue Scale (VAS)

- The VAS is a straight line, the end anchors of which are labeled as the extreme limits of the sensation or feeling being measured.
- They are used to measure subjective experiences, such as pain, fatigue, nausea and dyspnea. E.g., pain scale (Graphical rating scale).

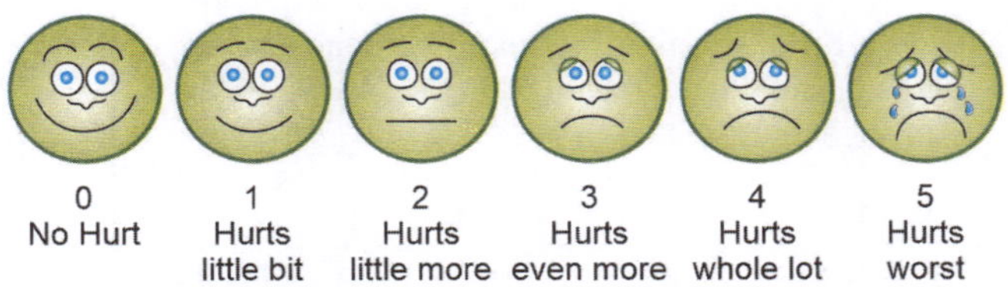

Figure 3: Example of graphic rating scale

Validity and Reliability of Scales

- **Validity:** Validity of the scale refers to the extent to which the scale measures what is intended to be measured.
  - **Face validity:** Face validity considers how suitable the content of a test seems to be on the surface. It's similar to content validity, but face validity is a more informal and subjective assessment.
  - **Construct validity:** The degree to which key constructs are adequately captured in the tool for measuring study variable.
  - **Content validity:** Content validity assesses whether a test is representative of all aspects of the construct. To produce valid results, the content of a test, survey or measurement method must cover all relevant parts of the subject it aims to measure.
  - **Criterion validity:** Criterion validity evaluates how closely the results of the test correspond to the results of a different test (another tool).
- **Reliability:** Reliability of the scale refers to consistency of the tool to measure the variable on repeated administration.
  - **Test-retest reliability:** It refers to the degree to which **test** results are consistent over time. In order to measure **test-retest reliability**, we must give the same **test** to the same individuals on two occasions and correlate the scores.
  - **Inter-rater reliability: Inter-rater reliability**, **inter-rater** agreement, or concordance is the degree of agreement among raters. It gives a score of how much homogeneity, or consensus, there is in the ratings given by judges.
  - **Split-half reliability:**. If the two halves of the test provide similar results, then this would suggest that the test has internal **reliability.** A test can be **split** in **half** in several ways, e.g., first **half** and second **half**, or by odd and even numbers.
  - **Internal consistency: Internal consistency** is typically a measure based on the correlations between different items on the same test.
  - **Parallel forms reliability:** It is a measure of reliability obtained by administering different versions of an assessment tool.

Recent Question (INC PhD 2020)

11. Which among the following tools is appropriate to collect data related to social status?
a. Rating scale
b. Observation
c. Interview
d. Check list

Ans. (c) Interview

KEY POINT

Bio-physiological method of data collection is the most reliable and accurate method.

Recent Question (INC PhD 2021)

12. Bipolar scale is an example of:
a. Semantic differential scale
b. Visual analogue scale
c. Likert scale
d. Delphi technique

Ans. (a) Semantic differential scale

Recent Questions (INC PhD 2020)

13. Researcher conducted a study, and he wants to generalize his findings to the population. Which type of population is this?
a. Target population
b. Accessible population
c. Available population
d. Research subject only

Ans. (a) Target population

14. Which of the following strategies will decrease sampling error?
a. Non-probability sampling method
b. Decrease sample size
c. Increase sample size
d. Use convenient sampling technique.

Ans. (c) Increase sample size.

SAMPLE AND SAMPLING TECHNIQUE

- **Sampling:** Sampling is the process of selecting a small number of elements from a larger defined target group of elements.
- **Population:** A complete set of persons or objects that possess some common characteristics of interest to the researcher.
- **Target population** is made up of the group of people or objects to which the researcher wishes to generalize the findings of the study.
- **Actual population** is that group that is actually available for study by the researcher.
- **Sample:** A subset of population that is selected to represent the population.
- **Sampling frame:** A sample frame is a list that includes every member of the population from which a sample is to be taken.
- **Sampling error:** It is any type of bias that is attributable to mistakes in either drawing a sample or determining the sample size.
- **Representative sample:** A representative sample has all the important characteristics of the study population from which it is drawn.

Steps of Sampling Process

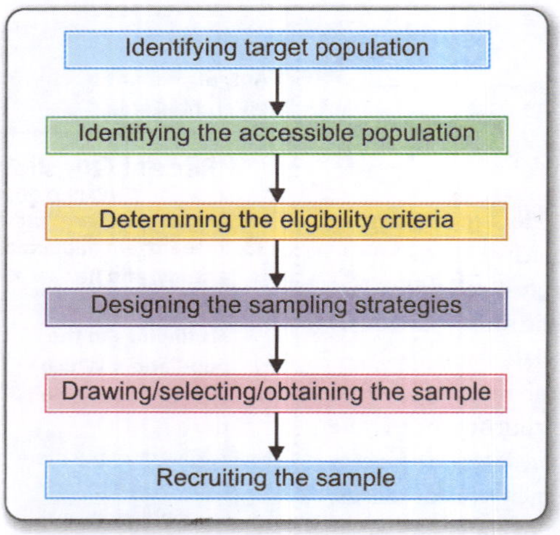

Figure 4: Steps of sampling process

Types of Sampling Methods

- Probability sampling
  - Simple random sampling
  - Systematic random sampling
  - Stratified random sampling
  - Cluster sampling
- Nonprobability sampling
  - Convenience sampling
  - Judgment sampling (purposive sampling)
  - Quota sampling
  - Snowball sampling

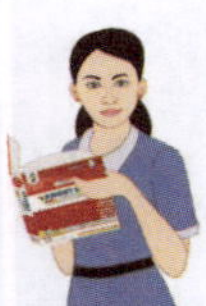

Probability Sampling

This involves random selection of elements from a population. Each subject has equal chance of being selected for the research study.

Simple Random Sampling

Researchers establish a sampling frame, from which the sample will be chosen. It is used in situations where the **number of sampling units is relatively small.** Lottery method may be used to select subjects from sampling frame.

Systematic Random Sampling

The defined target population is ordered and the sample is selected according to position using a skip interval. Skip interval (k) is the standard distance between elements chosen for the sample. For example, you want sample of 8 houses (n) from a street of 120 houses (N).

Sampling interval (k) = N/n
K = 120/8
= 15

Every 15th house is chosen after a random starting point between 1 and 15. If the random starting point is 11, then the houses selected are 11, 26, 41, 56, 71, 86, 101, and 116.

Stratified Random Sampling

- The population is divided into different subgroups and samples are selected from each subgroups.
- The population is divided into groups, based on some characteristics. The groups are called **strata.**
- Divide the target population into homogeneous strata.
- Draw random samples from each stratum.
- Combine the samples from each stratum into a single sample of the target population.

Example: Suppose we conduct a national survey. We might divide the population into groups or strata, based on geography —North, East, South, and West. Then, within each stratum, we might randomly select survey respondents.

Cluster Sampling

- The entire population of interest is divided into groups, or clusters.
- With cluster sampling, every member of the population is assigned to one and only one group.
- Each group is called a cluster. Each cluster must be mutually exclusive.
- A sample of clusters is chosen, using a probability method.
- Only individuals within sampled clusters are surveyed.
- After clusters are selected, then all units within the clusters are selected.

KEY POINTS

- **Reliability** refers to degree of consistency or accuracy with which an instrument measures for which it is designed to measure.
- **Validity:** Degree to which an instrument measures what it is intended to measure
- The aggregate of individuals who are accessible to the researcher from which the samples are selected for the research study is known as **accessible population.**
- The aggregate of individuals for which the researcher wants to generalize the findings of research study is known as **target population.**

POINT TO REMEMBER

Difference between Stratified sampling and Cluster sampling: With stratified sampling, the sample includes elements from each stratum. With cluster sampling, in contrast, the sample includes elements only from sampled clusters.

Non-probability Sampling

Non-probability sampling technique is a method, where sample is selected by nonrandom method.

- **Convenient sampling:** Researcher selects a sample which is most readily or more conveniently available to the researcher. This kind of sampling technique is also called **accidental sampling** technique. This is considered to be the weakest method of sampling technique.
- **Snowball sampling:** participants or the members of sample are requested to refer other people who may meet the eligibility criteria set by the researcher to participate in the research study but are inaccessible to the researcher. This method is also referred as **chain sampling** or **network sampling,** e.g., The researcher may identify, one or two **drug addicts** and then ask them to get more **drug addicts** through their contacts.
- **Quota sampling:** The researcher divides the population into various homogenous segments or quotas or subgroups. The researcher selects sample from each segment or each quota by convenient sampling technique.
- **Purposive sampling (Judgmental sampling):** The researcher draws a sample with a specific purpose that is associated with the research study.

Sampling in Mixed Method Research

- Identical sampling
- Parallel sampling
- Nested sampling

Determinants of Sample Size

- Type of analysis to be employed
- The level of precision needed
- Level of significance for testing hypothesis
- Population homogeneity/heterogeneity
- Available resources
- Sampling technique used.
- Effect size of previous similar studies.

Reference and Citations

Citation

- A citation is a **reference to the source of information (published or unpublished) used in the research article/dissertation**
- A citation is an abbreviated alphanumeric expression embedded in the body of a research work/article that refers to bibliographic references section.

Some reference style in practice

Field	Recommended reference style
Medical, nursing and health sciences	Vancouver, APA
Education	APA
Arts	Harvard, Chicago, MLA, APA

Recent Questions (INC PhD 2020)

15. Sampling method used in a population showing linear trend is:

a. Simple random method
b. Stratified random method
c. Cluster sampling method
d. Systematic random sampling

Ans. (b) Stratified random method.

Explanation: Stratified sampling is best for linearly trended population. Next best is systematic sampling.

16. Out of 3000 accessible population researcher needs 150 sample. What is the k value?

a. 15
b. 20
c. 30
d. 50

Ans. (b) 20

Explanation:
k = Population size/sample size
= 3000/150 = 20

Recent Question (INC PhD 2021)

17. Participant refer to a new participant for the study. This type of sampling technique is known as:

a. Convenient sampling
b. Snow ball sampling
c. Quota sampling
d. Purposive sampling

Ans. (b) Snow ball sampling

Vancouver reference style:

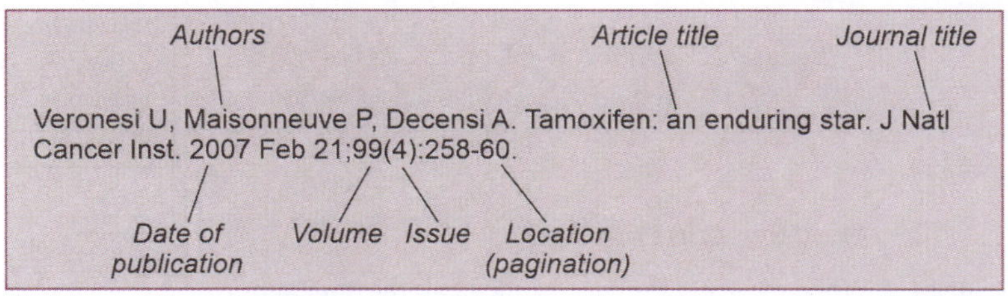

Figure 5: Parts of Vancouver reference style (journal article)

Table 7: Types of articles and referencing styles

Type of article	Example reference
Journal article- one author	Rourke E. Severe depression in old age. Med Today. 2012 Dec;3(12):40-47.
Journal article – two authors	Rourke E, Hussain R. Learning on the job: metaphors of choreography and the practice of sex in sex-on-premises venues. Venereology. 2010;13(1):27-36.
Journal article – two to six authors	Rourke E, Hussain R, Bishara J, Pitlik S, Leibovici L, Paul M. Treatment of human brucellosis: systematic review and meta-analysis of randomised controlled trials. Br Med J (Clin Res Ed). 2018 Apr 29;336(7646):701-4
Journal article-more than six authors	Rourke E, Hussain R, Bishara J, Shield J, Taylor CT, Smith IL, et al. Hendra virus infection in veterinarian. Med J Aust. 2010 Oct 20;185(10):562-64.

Note: The article mentioned is an example and not original references.

*If the work you need to reference has more than six authors, **you should list the first six authors, followed by et al.**

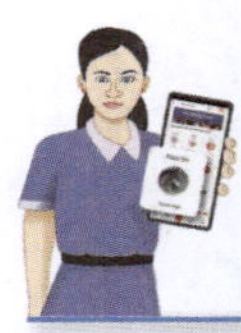

APA reference style

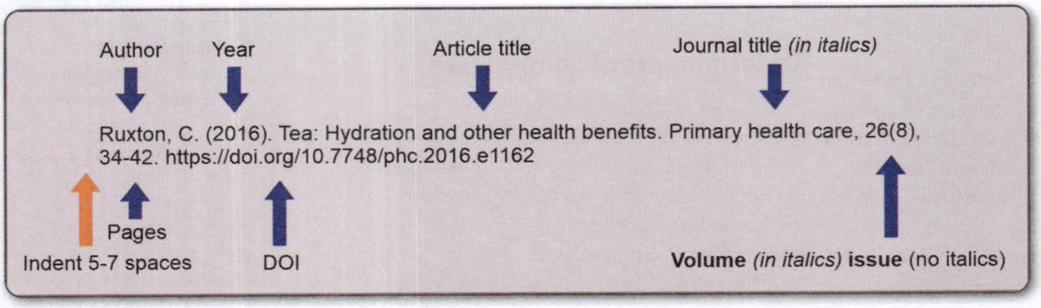

Figure 6: Parts of APA reference style (Journal article)

ETHICS IN RESEARCH

Ethics: What is right and what is wrong?

- **Principles of beneficence**
  - Establishing the positive risk benefit ratio.
  - A potential risk of the research study must be carefully assessed.
  - Participants are protected from any harmful effect of research activity.
- **Principles of respect of human dignity**
  - This principle emphasizes on the freedom of choice, where participants have right to accept or reject to be a part of the research study.
  - Participants have full right to question the researcher for any additional information.
  - Participants have right to quit from the study at any stage of the research study.
  - A fully informed consent must be obtained from the participant. In case of the fetus, child, psychological, neurological or physical inability the informed consent can be obtained from parents or legal guardians.
- **Principle of justice**
  - This ethical principle directs the researchers to abide by the participant's right of fair treatment and maintenance of privacy.
- **Principle of non-maleficence:** Do no harm.
- **Principle of autonomy:** Participants can make his own decisions about whether to participate in research.

DATA ANALYSIS AND INTERPRETATION

Types of Data

- **Ungrouped and grouped**
  - **Ungrouped data** is presented individually, e.g., Weight of 11 patients visited OPD. Mr. Ram, 60 kg; Kapoor, 55 kg; Amit-72 kg, etc.
  - **Grouped data** is presented as groups consisting of identical data by frequency, e.g.,

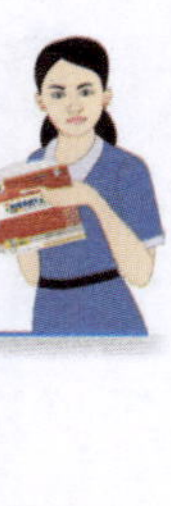

Systolic blood pressure	Frequency
90–100	5
101–110	9
111–120	12
121–130	10

Class Interval

While grouping the data, there are two types of class intervals used, i.e.,

- Inclusive class interval
- Exclusive class interval

Inclusive Class Interval

When the lower and the upper class limit are included in the class interval:

e.g., class A 0–15 B 16–30 C 31–45

For Class B,

Lower class boundary = 15.5 Upper class boundary = 30.5

Inclusive class interval = Upper class boundary – lower class boundary
= 30.5 – 15.5
= 15

Exclusive Class Interval

When the lower limit is included, but the upper limit is excluded:

e.g., class A 0–15 B 15–30 C 30–45

For Class B

Lower class limit (LCL) = 15
Upper class limit (UCL) = 30 (not included)
Exclusive class interval = UCL – LCL
= 30 – 15
= 15

Difference: In exclusive class intervals, the upper class limit is excluded from the class (It is added to the next class).

In inclusive class intervals, both lower and upper class limits are included in the same class, i.e., it will fall between upper and lower class boundaries.

Recent Questions (INC PhD 2020)

18. While conducting research activity, ethics are needed to be kept in mind always because
a. They protect the human subjects
b. They protect the researcher
c. They protect the ethics committee
d. They protect the institution

Ans. (a) They protect the human subjects

19. Someone who is copying the original research work done by others is known as
a. Cheating
b. Plagiarism
c. Copying
d. Fidelity

Ans. (b) Plagiarism

KEY POINT

A dichotomous variable is a nominal variable that has only two categories or values. Example: Gender (male and female).

Qualitative and Quantitative Data

- **Qualitative:** Non-numerical, based on nominal or ordinal scale, e.g., Gender (male/female), religion (Hindu/Muslim/Christian).
- **Quantitative:** Numerical or based on numbers, e.g., Height in cm, weight in kg.

Continuous and Discrete

- **Continuous:** Data for which unlimited number of possible values exist, e.g., Height, weight. (includes decimals).
- **Discrete:** Data for which distinct categories and a limited number of possible values exist, e.g., Number of children in a family.

Variables

- A **variable** is **defined** as anything that has a quantity or quality that varies from person to person. For example. Age of the patients.
- **Qualitative variables:** Variables that can take a few values, that are not measurable, but are only attributes or qualities and are called 'Qualitative Variables', e.g., Gender (male, female), Religion (Hindu, Muslim, Christian, etc.)
- Since Qualitative variables can take a few values or categories, they are also called **categorical variables.**
- **Quantitative variables:** Quantitative variables are measurable and can take any value on a continuous spectrum. They are also called **Continuous variables. Examples:** Blood sugar, serum creatinine, age, income, height, weight, etc.

Types of Variables

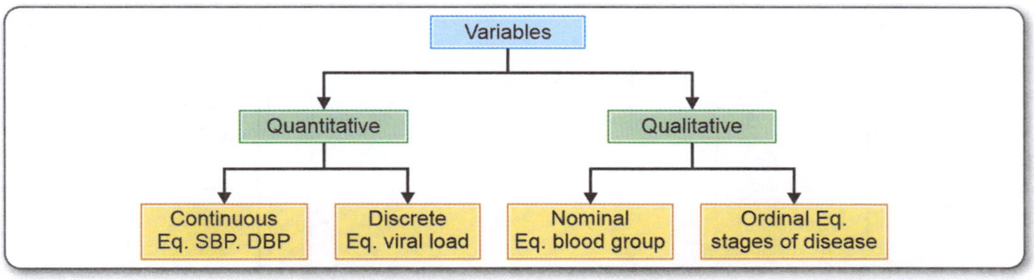

Figure 7: Types of variables

Scales of Measurements

- Categorizing subjects into different groups (*grouping by gender, religion*), then ***Nominal* scale** is the way to go.
- **Dichotomous scale:** Where data is divided into only two categories or group, e.g., Male or female.
- If you can rank ordering people along some dimension, then **Ordinal scale** is best (*ranking basketball teams, SES*).
- To quantify a trait on a scale where the distance between ranks is same, then the **Interval scale** is the way (*temperature*).
- To measure something on a scale where there is a true zero point, then a **Ratio scale** should be used (*weight, pulse, Hb*).

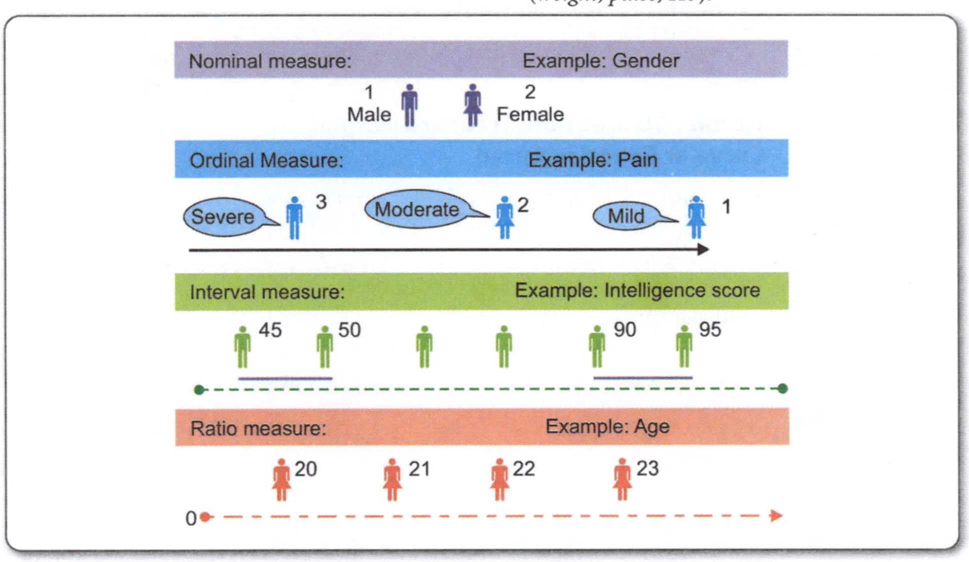

Figure 8: Scales of measurements

Recent Question
(INC PhD 2020)

20. Which of the following is a nominal variable?
a. Weight
b. Anxiety level
c. Number of children
d. Gender

Ans. (d) Gender

KEY POINTS

- **Ratio** represents continuous values. The degree of difference and ratio between each item can be measured. **Examples:** height, weight, distance.
- Ratio scale has a constant interval and a true zero point.

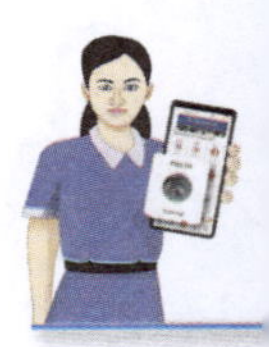

Strength of Measurement Scales

Weaker ⟵ Nominal – Ordinal – Interval – Ratio ⟶ Stronger

Table 8: Measurement scales and their strength

OK to compute....	Nominal	Ordina l	Interval	Ratio
Frequency distribution	Yes	Yes	Yes	Yes
Median and percentiles	No	Yes	Yes	Yes
Add or subtract	No	No	Yes	Yes
Mean, SD, standard error of the mean	No	No	Yes	Yes
Ratio, or coefficient of variation	No	No	No	Yes

NUMERICAL DATA PROPERTIES AND MEASURES

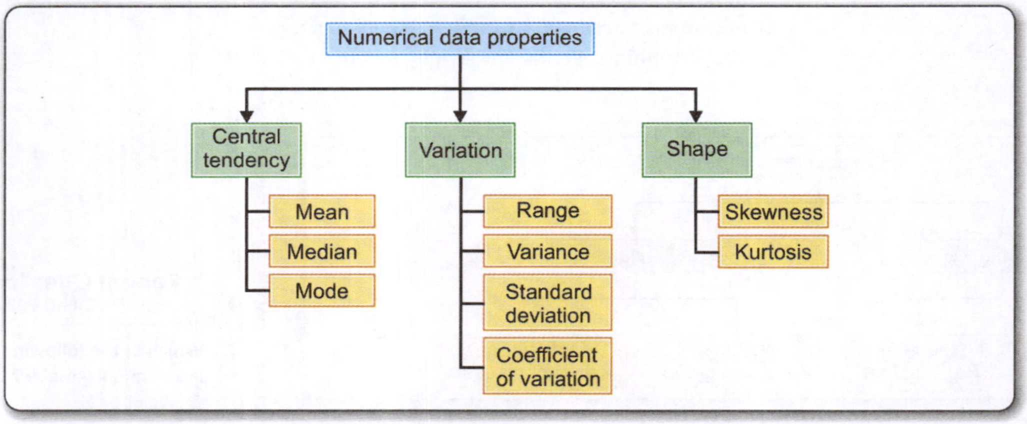

Figure 9: Numerical data properties

Central Tendencies

Mean

Stable average, which is based on all observations. Calculated for quantitative data, measured in interval/ratio level.

Median

Score that divides a distribution exactly in half. Exactly 50% of the data fall above the median and 50% below. To determine the median, sort the data and find the midpoint.

Mode

Mode is the **most frequently** occurring observation. Mode is not affected by extreme values.

Variation

Measures of Dispersion

- **Range:** Difference between the highest and lowest data points.
- **Variance, SD:** Standard Deviation is the square root of variance. SD gives us an idea of 'spread' of dispersion. Larger the SD, greater the dispersion of values about mean.
  It is the best and **most frequently used measure of dispersion.**

Probability Curve; Normal Curve

In a normally distributed data, **Mean = Median = Mode**

Normal Distribution: Standard Normal Curve or Gaussian Curve

- *Smooth, bell-shaped, perfectly symmetrical curve, based on an infinitely a large number of observations.*
- Total area of the curve is 1; its mean is zero; and its standard deviation is 1.
- *Mean, median and mode all coincide.* Mean divides the area under the curve into 2 equal halves.

KEY POINT

Standard Deviation (SD) is primarily used with mean values to provide descriptive statistics for parametric tests. Interquartile range (IQR) is primarily used with median values to provide descriptive statistics for non-parametric tests.

Recent Question
(NORCET 2020)

21. Difference between smallest and largest value is known as:

a. Mean
b. Average
c. Range
d. Standard deviation

Ans. (c) Range

- A random variable (x) is standardized when it has been adjusted so that its mean = 0 and SD = 1.
- ***Standardization*** = (x-)/σ.

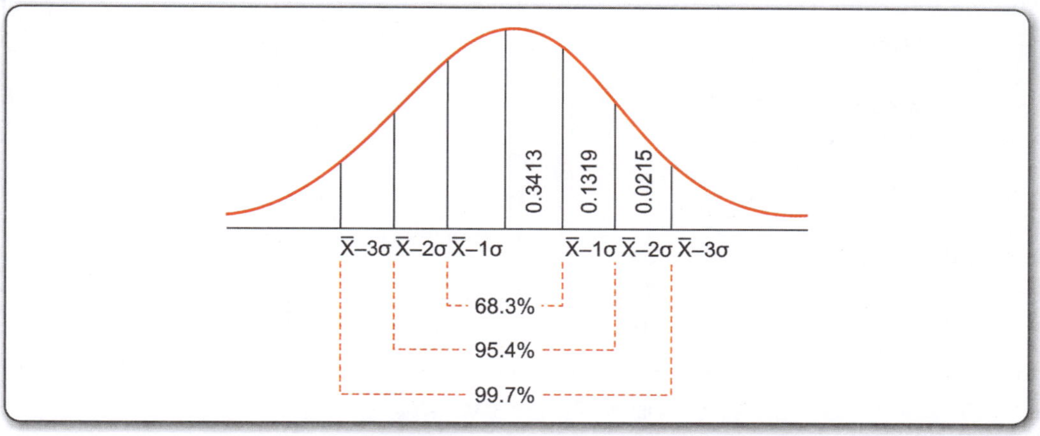

Figure 10: Standard normal curve

Shape

Kurtosis and Skewness

Table 9: Skewness and its interpretations

Skewness	Interpretation
Positive (Mean>Median)	Tail is toward right. Large number of low scores and small number of high scores.
Negative (Mean<Median)	Tail is toward left. Large number of high scores, small number of low scores.

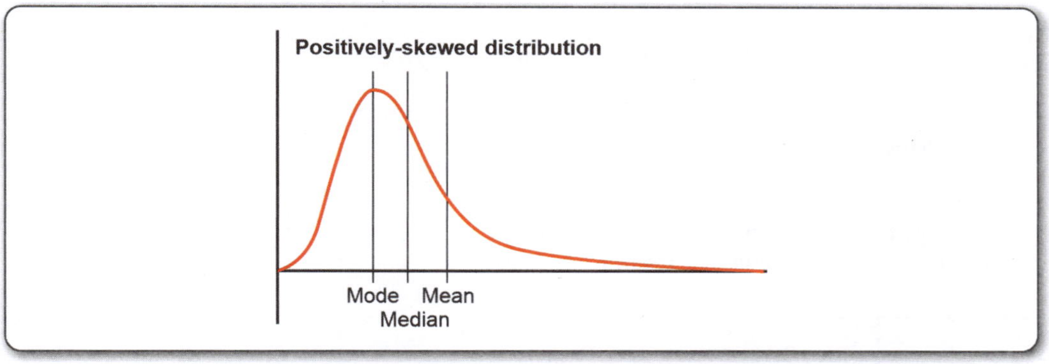

Figure 11: Positively-skewed distribution curve

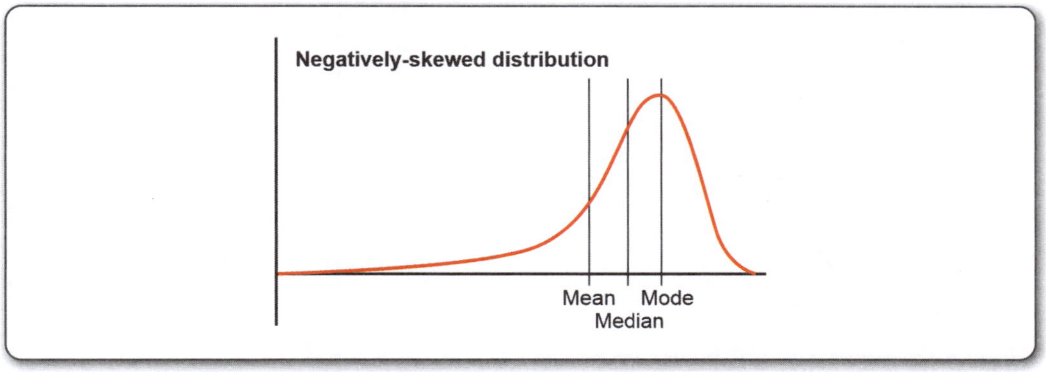

Figure 12: Negatively-skewed distribution curve

KEY POINTS

- Data points in a normal distribution are more likely to fall closer to the mean.
- 68.3% of all data points will be within ±1SD from the mean
- 95.4% of all data points will be within + 2SD from the mean
- 99.7% of all data points will be within ±3SD
- If mean is more than the median, then the data is said to be positively skewed.
- In a positively skewed data distribution Mode < Median < Mean.
- If mean is less than the median, then the data is said to be negatively skewed.
- In a negatively skewed data distribution Mean < Median < Mode.

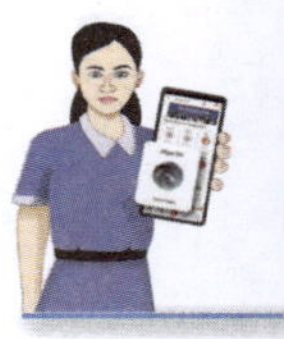

Histogram

Presentation of Statistical Data

- It is a pictorial diagram of frequency distribution used for continuous and ordered data.
- It has a series of blocks adjacent to each other *with no intervening space and area of each block is proportional to the frequency.*
- Class intervals are given along the horizontal axis and frequencies along the vertical axis.
- **Frequency polygon** (an area diagram) *is formed by joining the mid-points of the histogram blocks.*
- Frequency curve
  - If number of observations is very large and group interval is reduced and frequency polygon loses its angulations resulting in a smooth curve known as frequency curve.

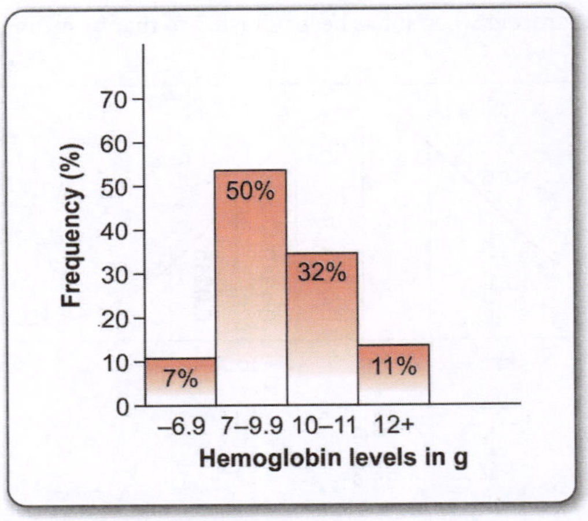

Figure 13: Histogram

> **KEY POINT**
> Scatter plot diagram is used to illustrate correlation.

Line Diagram

- Line diagrams are used to show the trend of events with the passage of time.

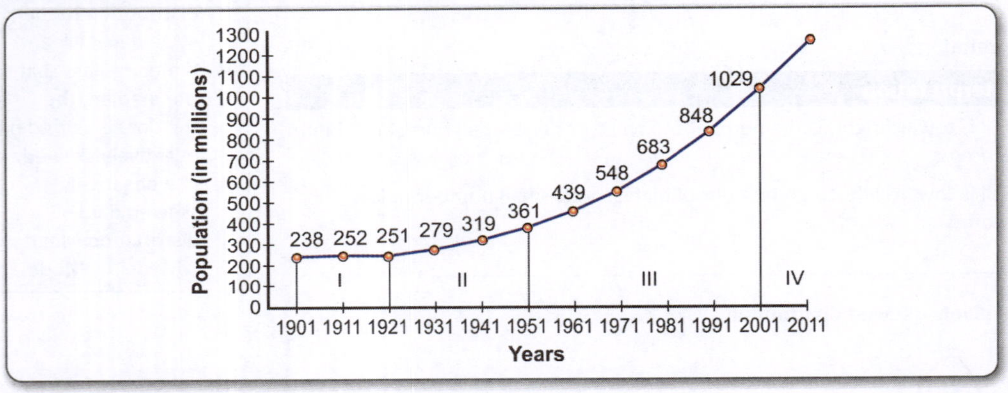

Figure 14: Line diagram

- **Cumulative frequency curve or *Ogive***
  - *It is a line diagram, showing cumulative frequency distribution of quantitative data.*
  - Curve is plotted by taking the variable on X axis and cumulative frequency on Y axis.
  - Median can be calculated from Ogive.

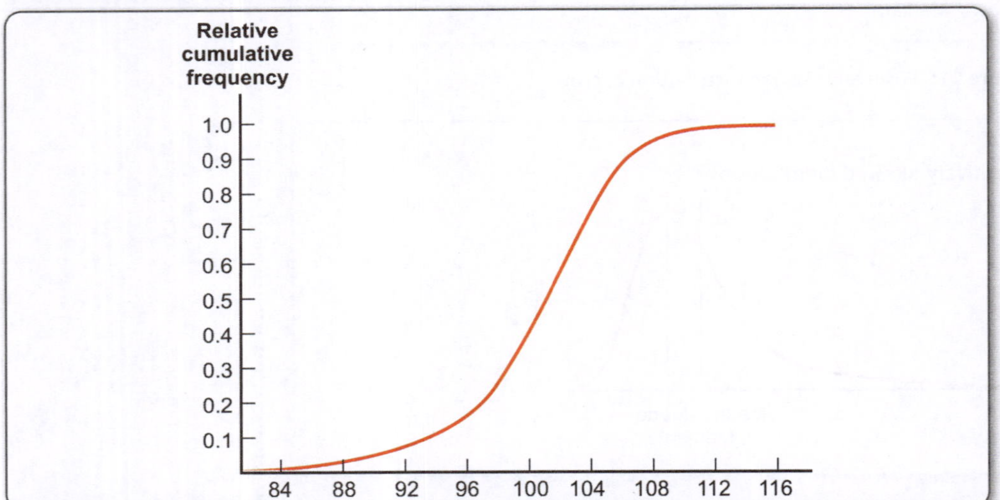

Figure 15: Cumulative frequency curve

Pie Charts

Serum Sodium concentration 1000 people

- Areas of segments of a circle (*depends upon the angle at center)* are compared.
- Considered inferior to bar charts. It is often necessary to indicate percentages in segments.

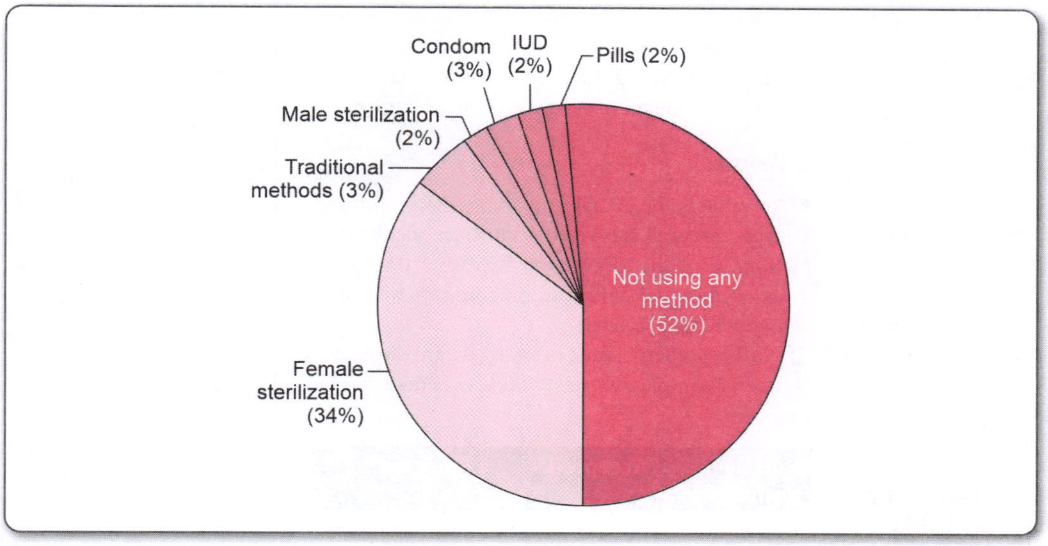

Figure 16: Pie chart

- Pictogram (a form of bar chart):
  - Used to present data to "man on street" or layman who cannot understand orthodox charts.
  - Small pictures or symbols are used to present data.
  - Fractions of picture can be used to represent numbers smaller than the value of a whole symbol.

Recent Question (NORCET 2023)

22. If relative risk is 1 what it indicates?

a. No association
b. Negative association
c. Positive association
d. Positive Correlation

Ans. (a) No association

A relative risk of 1 means that there is no significant difference in the risk of an outcome between the exposed and unexposed groups. It suggests that the exposure (e.g., a risk factor) is not associated with an increased or decreased risk of the outcome (e.g., a disease or health condition)

APPLICATION OF INFERENTIAL STATISTICS

Test of Significance

Table 10: Test of significance

Attribute	Types of data	Distribution	Number of groups	Statistical test
Unpaired groups or ≥2 independent sample/ group	Quantitative	Parametric	2 groups	Unpaired 't' test
			>2 groups	One way ANOVA
		Non-parametric	2 groups	Mann Whitney
			>2 groups	Kruskal wallis
	Qualitative (Categorical) >2 groups		2 groups	Chi Square, Fisher exact
			Chi Square	
Paired Groups (e.g., Before and After)	Quantitative	Parametric	2 groups	Paired 't' test
			>2 groups	Repeated measures ANOVA
		Non-parametric	2 groups	Mann Wilcoxon
			>2 groups	Friedman's test
	Qualitative (Categorical) >2 groups		2 groups	Mc Nemar test
			Cochran's Q test	
Looking for an association between two variables	Quantitative	Both variables are parametric	Pearson's Correlation Coefficient 0 = No correlation, +ve=Direct Correlation, -ve = Inverse correlation	
		Both variables are non-parametric	Spearman's rank correlation coefficient, **Kendall's** test	
	Qualitative (Categorical)	2 × 2 data	Risk Ratio	
		Otherwise	Chi square for trend, Logistic regression	

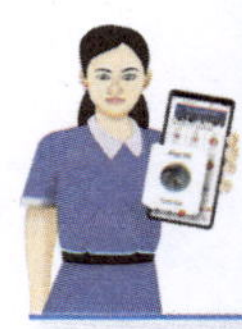

Student 't' Test (Devised by WS Cassette)

- Based on *"t" distribution* (a continuous, symmetrical, bell shaped, unimodal distribution of infinite range similar in shape to normal distribution, but more spread out).
- Used to find the significance of difference between two means, when sample size is less than 30.
    - **Student t test for single small sample →** compares a single sample mean with population mean.
    - **Student t test for independent samples (Unpaired t test)** compares mean of 2 small samples
    - **Student t test for paired samples** (**Paired t test**) compares mean of 2 small paired samples (before and after)
- Used to evaluate the null hypothesis for continuous (quantitative) variables (e.g., height, weight, BP).

Chi-Square Test (χ^2) -Developed by Karl Pearson

- It is a nonparametric test *used for qualitative data* in form of proportions.
- It is an alternate method of testing the significance of difference between two proportions.
- Used as a test of goodness of fit (whether observed frequency distribution differs from theoretical distribution (i.e., normal, binomial or Poisson) by chance or sample is from a different population)
- *Advantage*: This can also be used when more than two groups are to be compared.

Yates correction: Applied when the expected frequency in any cell of the 2 × 2 contingency table is less than 5. It decreases the likelihood of type I error.

Spearman's Rank Correlation Coefficient (RHO)

- Used when measurements are in terms of ranks
- *It is used* to determine whether there is a *monotonic relation between 2 variables* (i.e., Increase in one is associated with increase or decrease in other)
- Value of Rho ranges between – 1 [Inverse or negative relationship] and + 1 [Positive relationship]Q
    - Values between – 0.1 to – 0.3 and 0.1 to 0.3 → indicate *weak relationship*
    - Values between – 0.3 to – 0.5 and 0.3 to 0.5 → indicate *moderate relationship*
    - Values < – 0.5 and > 0.5 → indicate *strong relationship*

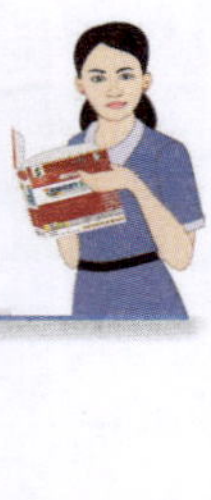

Degree of Freedom [DF]

- In chi square test, ***DF = (c - 1) (r - 1)***; c = Number of columns; n = Number of rows
- In unpaired ' t' test, DF = n1+ n2 – 2, where n1 and n2 are number of observation in each series.
- In paired 't' test, DF = n-1
- In testing the significance of correlation, DF = n – 2, n is the number of paired measurements.

p Value

- 'p' value is the actual probability of committing type 1 error. It is based on statistical calculation.
- If, p < α (usually taken as 5% or 0.05), the association is statistically significant and null hypothesis is rejected.

Null hypothesis assumes no significant difference between 2 samples, whatever difference occurs is by chance.

Null Hypothesis	Accepted	Rejected
True	Correct conclusion	Type I (α) error
False	Type II (β) error	Correct conclusion

Type I Error or α Error

- *Rejecting a null hypothesis when actually it is true* (a statistically significant difference is found between two groups when actually there is no difference).
- If null hypothesis is false, there can be no type I error.
- Probability of a type I error is equal to alpha.
- Multiple comparisons and repeated testing for significance increase likelihood of type I error. Type I error is important in *sample size determination and* statistical testing for significance.

Type II Error or β Error

- *Acceptance of a null hypothesis as true when actually it is false.*
- The study fails to find a statistically significant difference when actually there is a difference.
- If null hypothesis is true, there can be no type II error.
- Probability of a type II error is equal to beta.
- *It is inversely related to type I error.*

Type II error or β error is used to determine the power of study = 1 – β

KEY POINTS

- Chi-square test is a non-parametric test used to find out association between two unrelated categorical variables.
- McNemer test is used to find out relationship between two related categorical variables.
- Independent sample 't' test or student's t test or unpaired 't' test is used to compare means of two independent groups. For example, to compare the mean hemoglobin level of males and females.
- One-way ANOVA is used for comparison of means between three or more independent groups.
- Sphericity assumption in repeated measures one-way ANOVA is tested using the **Mauchly's test.**
- **The *F-statistic* is calculated in ANOVA.**
- Paired 't' test is used for comparison of means of two related (paired) observation from the same group. For example, to compare pre-test and post-test hemoglobin level of same group.
- Repeated measures ANOVA is used for comparison of means of three or more observation of same group.

Power of a trial *is the probability that the study would reject a null hypothesis as false when it is actually false.*

- It is the ability to detect a true difference in outcome between control arm and intervention arm.
- *Conventionally power of a study is taken as 0.8* Q, i.e., a study that has less than 80% chance of detecting a false null hypothesis is unacceptable.

As sample size increases power of study increases. Power is a determinant of sample size in clinical trials.

Cronbach's α (alpha) is a measure of *internal consistency or reliability.* Alpha varies from 0 to 1.

Cronbach's	≥ 0.9	0.9 > α ≥ 0.8	0.8 > α ≥ 0.7	0.7 > α ≥ 0.6	0.6 > α ≥ 0.5	α < 0.5
Internal consistency	Excellent	Good	Acceptable	Question-able	Poor	Unacceptable

Parametric and Non-parametric Test

Parametric test is the test which makes assumptions about parameters of population distribution from which data are drawn, while non-parametric test is that which makes no such assumptions.

Table 11: Difference between parametric and non-parametric test

Parametric tests	Non-parametric test
Z test, 1-sample t test	Wilcoxon Signed Rank
Paired (Dependent)sample t test	Mann-Whitney
2(independent) sample t test	Kruskal-Wallis
1-way Anova	Friedman
2-way Anova	Chi-square test of independence

Pearson Correlation Coefficient

- Pearson correlation coefficient shows linear correlation between two continuous variables.
- The Pearson correlation is also known as the "product moment correlation coefficient".
- The correlation coefficient value (r) ranges between −1 to +1.
- The r value close to +1 shows strong positive correlation.
- The r value close to −1 shows strong negative correlation.
- Value close to zero shows very weak or no correlation.
- 0 indicates no correlation.
- +1 indicates perfect positive correlation.
- −1 indicates perfect negative correlation.

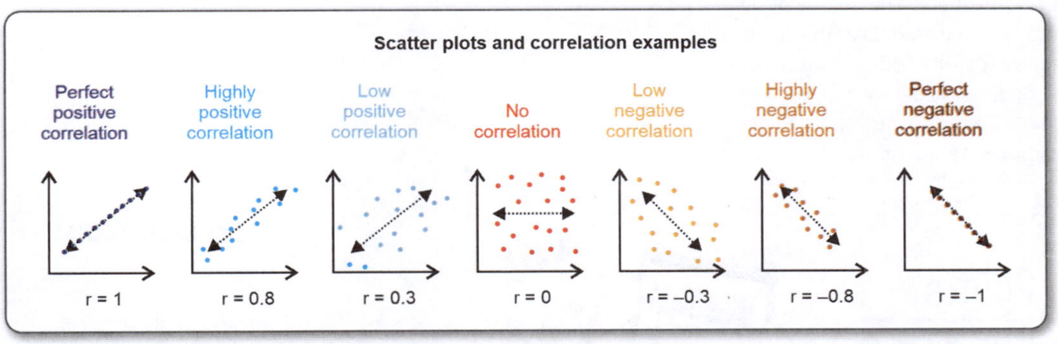

Figure 17: Scatter plots and correlation examples

KEY POINTS

- Pearson correlation is used to find linear relationship between two normally distributed continuous variables.
- Spearman correlation is used when the data is not normally distributed.
- Correlation values (r) fall on scale between −1 and +1. Value close to ±1 indicates strongest correlation. The value that is farthest from ±1 indicates weakest or no correlation.

Recent Question
(NORCET 2020)

23. For formula for calculating degree of freedom in Chi-square test is:

a. (r − 1) (c − 1)
b. r × c
c. (r + 1) (c + 1)
d. (r − 1) (c + 1)

Ans. (a) (r − 1) (c − 1)

KEY POINTS

- t-test and ANOVA (F test) are parametric tests.
- Chi-square test, Mann-Whitney U test, Wilcoxon rank sum test, Kruskal-Wallis H test are non-parametric tests.

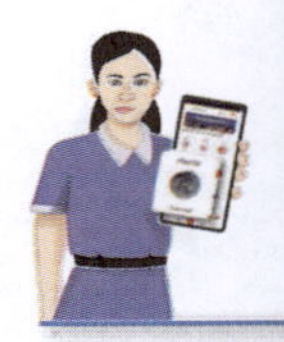

Golden Points to Remember

- **Attrition** means progressive loss of data in research. It occurs when cases are lost from a sample over time or over a series of sequential processes.
- **Hawthorne effect:** The subject in a research study behaves in a particular manner because they are aware that they are being observed.
- **External validity** denotes the results of a study which can **be generalized across the situations, stimuli and people.**
- **Internal validity** refers to the extent in which the evidence supports the claim in regard to cause and effect, **within the context of that study.**
- A pilot study is a research study conducted on a small scale before the intended study.
- A careful appraisal of the strengths and weaknesses of the study is known as **Research critique.**
- Conceptual definition provides the theoretical meaning of a variable and is often derived from a theorist's definition of a related concept.
- **Hawthorne effect:** Tendency of subjects to perform better when they are aware that they are being observed.
- **Experimental effect:** Researcher's characteristics, mannerisms or behavior may influence subject behavior.
- **Reactive effect:** Reactive effect of pretest occurs when subjects have been sensitized to the treatment because of taking a pretest.
- **Novelty effect:** When a treatment is new, subjects and researcher might behave in different ways.
- The word statistics was first used by a German scholar **Gottfried Achenwal**.
- **Nominal** measurement consists of categories that are not more or less than each other but are different from one another. Example: **gender:** male, female. **Religion:** Hindu, Muslim, Christian.
- **Ordinal** level of measurement ranks items based on their relative standing on a specific attribute. The degree of difference between items cannot be measured. **Examples:** Income: low, middle, upper. Disease status: Mild, Moderate, Severe.
- **Interval scale:** The degree of difference between items can be measured but the ratio between them cannot be measured. Zero is arbitrary. **Examples**: temperature, pH.
- Mean, median and mode are **measures of central tendency.**
- **Median** is the point on a numerical scale above which and below which 50% of cases falls.
- 50th percentile is equivalent to Median.
- Median is the middle value of a data set. Commonly used for description of data with non-normal distribution.
- IQR refers to Inter-Quartile Range. It is the deference between 25th percentile and 75th percentile of a data set.
- Mode is the value which has highest frequency.
- Mean is the average of all the values. Most commonly used parameter in a normally distributed data.
- Range, standard deviation and variance are **measures of dispersion.**
- The **range** of a set of data is the difference between the highest and lowest values in the set.
- The **standard deviation** is a statistic that measures the dispersion of a dataset relative to its mean.
- Standard deviation is square root of variance; or variance is square of standard deviation.
- The formula to calculate degree of freedom (df) in Chi-square test is **(c – 1) (r – 1).**
- The formula to calculate degree of freedom (df) in t-test is n-1.
- Probability values fall on scale between **0 and 1.**
- **Type I error (α) occurs** when a true null hypothesis is rejected.
- A Type-I error refers to **False positive (similar to wrong diagnosis).**
- Type II error (β) occurs when one fails to reject a null hypothesis that is actually false.
- A type-II error refers to **False negative (Similar to missed diagnosis).**
- p value refers to probability of type-1 error (α).
- The sensitivity of a statistical test is measured by its power. Power refers to $1 - \beta$.

Image-Based Questions

1. **SpO$_2$ measurement taken with and without micropore in a pediatric population is depicted in the following scattered plot diagram. Which of the following is true?** ***[AIIMS November 2016]***

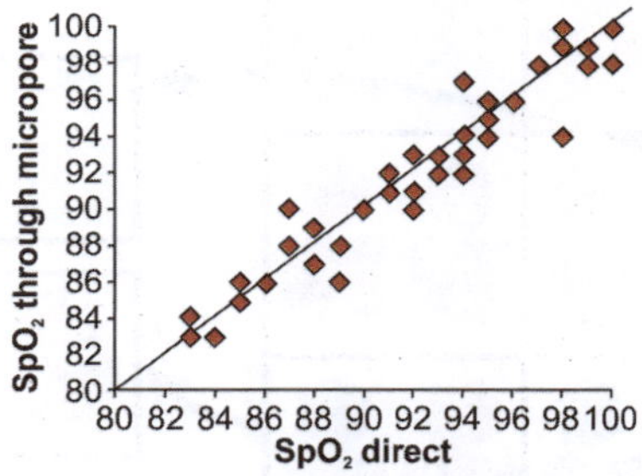

a. There is no agreement between two measurements
b. There is a negative correlation between two measurements
c. There is no association between the two measurements
d. There is a positive correlation between two measurements

2. **Identify the statistical diagram shown in photograph.** ***[Recent Question 2017]***

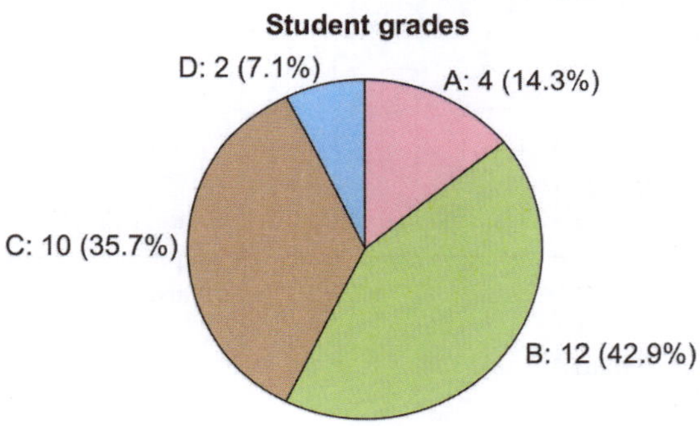

a. Pie chart
b. Pictogram
c. Scatter diagram
d. Ogive

3. **In the diagram depicted here, how much is the area between points A & B, on either side of the mean?** ***[Recent Question 2016]***

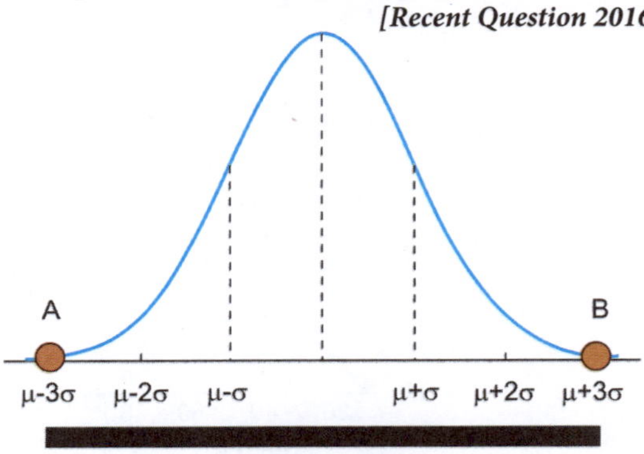

a. 68.3%
b. 95.4%
c. 99.7%
d. 102.5%

4. **In the following type of distribution.** ***[Recent Question 2016]***

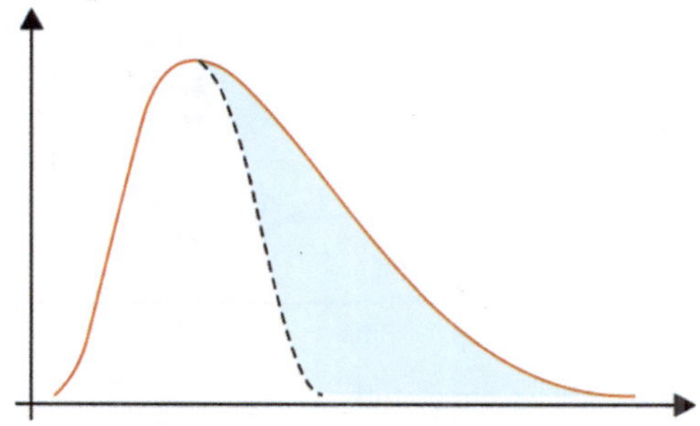

a. Mean = Median = Mode
b. Mean > Median > Mode
c. Mode > Median > Mean
d. Median > Mode > Mean

5. **Identify the epidemiological study design.** ***[Recent Question 2014]***

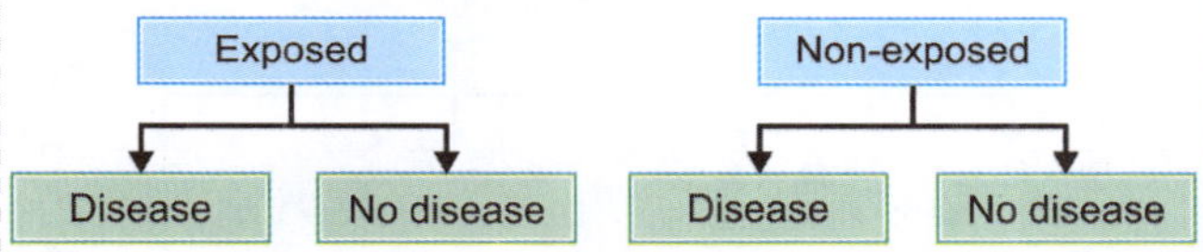

a. Cohort study
b. Case Control study
c. Cross Sectional study
d. Nested Case Control study

6. **Identify the epidemiological study design.** ***[Recent Question 2013]***

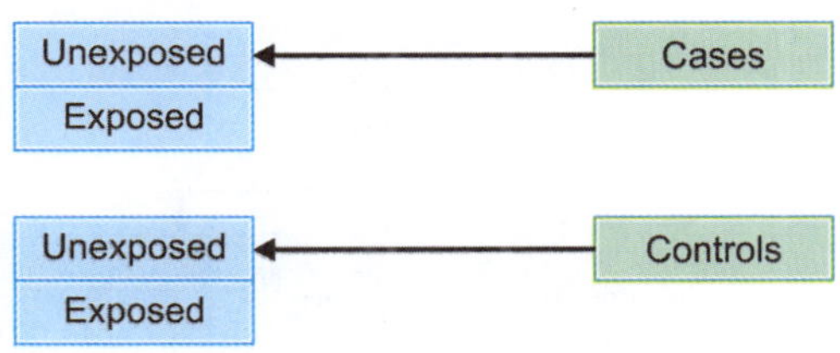

a. Cohort study
b. Case Control study
c. Cross Sectional study
d. Nested Case Control study

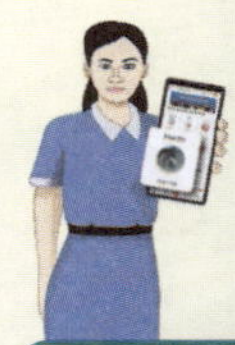

Ans.

1. d
2. a
3. c
4. b
5. a
6. b

[*Courtesy*: PHOTON-20® 4th ed. by Vivek Jain, CBS Publishers and Distributors Pvt Ltd]

7. Identify the epidemiological study design.

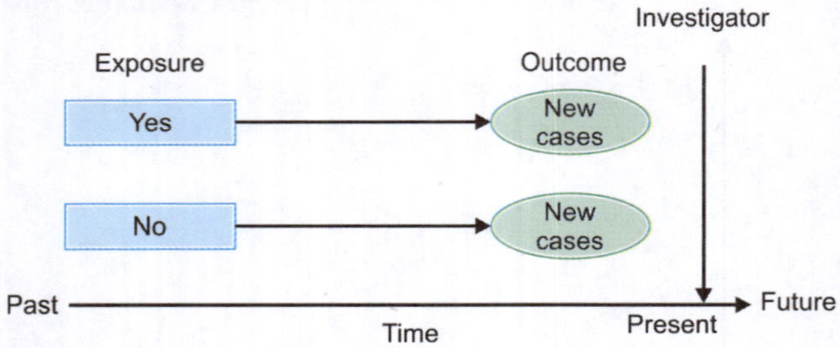

a. Prospective Cohort study
b. Case Control study
c. Retrospective Cohort study
d. Nested Case Control study

8. Identify the epidemiological study design.

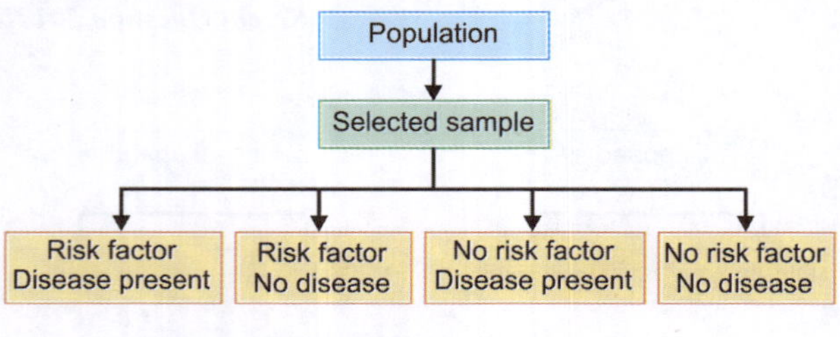

a. Prospective Cohort study
b. Cross Sectional study
c. Retrospective Cohort study
d. Nested Case Control study

9. Identify the epidemiological study design.

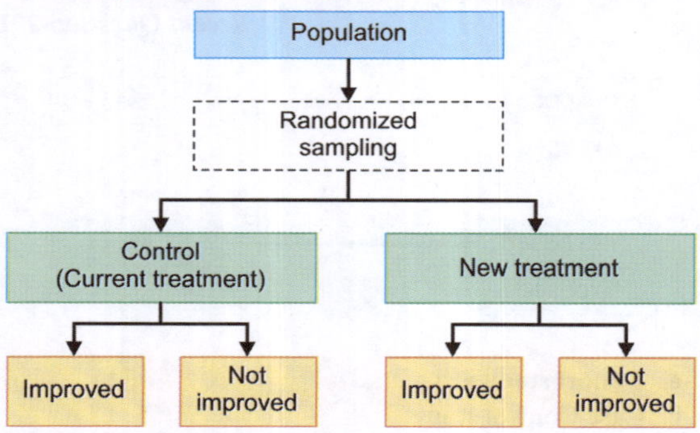

a. Prospective Cohort study
b. Meta-analysis
c. Retrospective Cohort study
d. Randomized Control Trial

10. Type of sampling shown in figure is:
[Recent Question 2015]

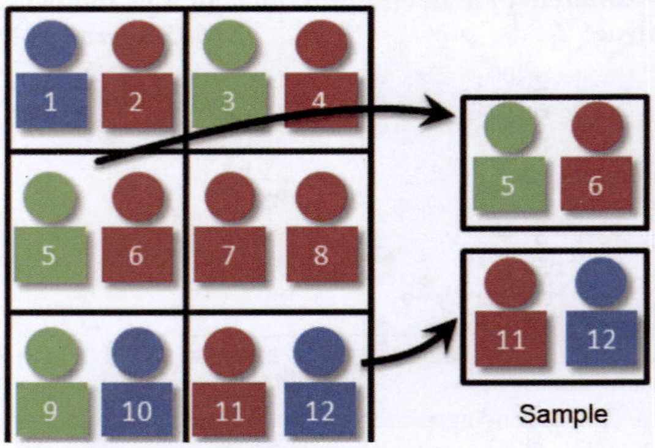

a. Simple random sampling
b. Systematic random sampling
c. Stratified random sampling
d. Cluster random sampling

11. Identify parameter represented by 'Black arrow'.

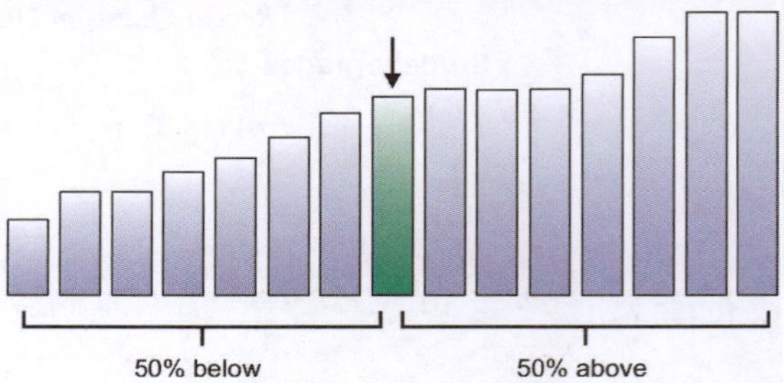

a. Mean
b. Median
c. Mode
d. Range

12. Identify the statistical diagram shown.

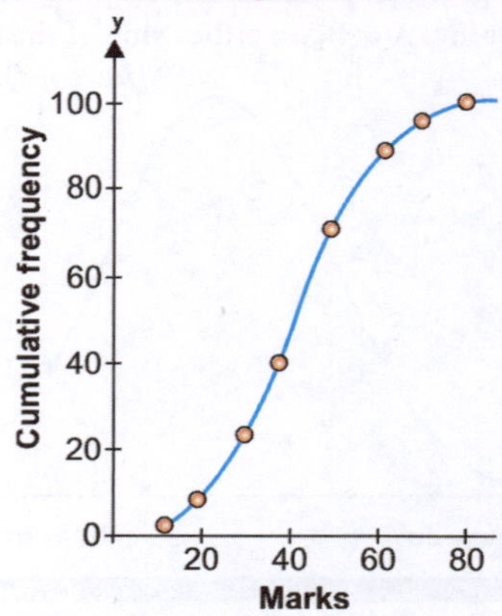

a. Frequency polygon
b. Histogram
c. Line diagram
d. Ogive

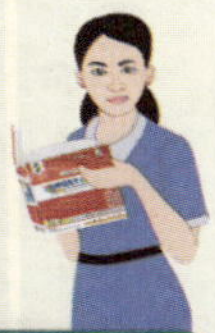

Ans.

7. c
8. b
9. d
10. d
11. b
12. d

13. Identify the statistical diagram shown.
[Recent Question 2014, 2016]

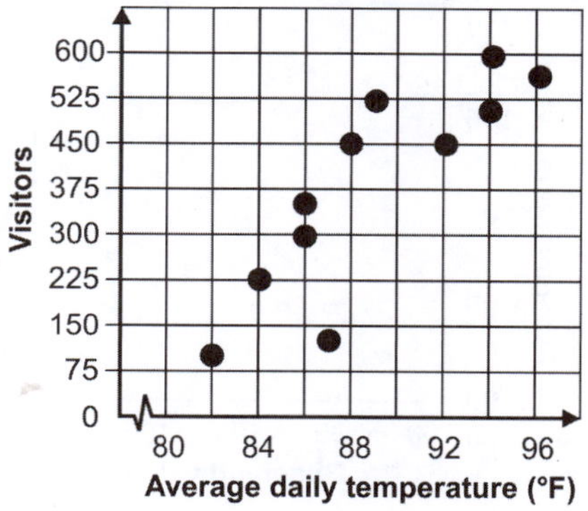

a. Scatter diagram
b. Cumulative frequency diagram
c. Line diagram
d. Pictogram

14. In the given scatter diagram, correlation coefficient 'r' will lie between
[Recent Question 2014]

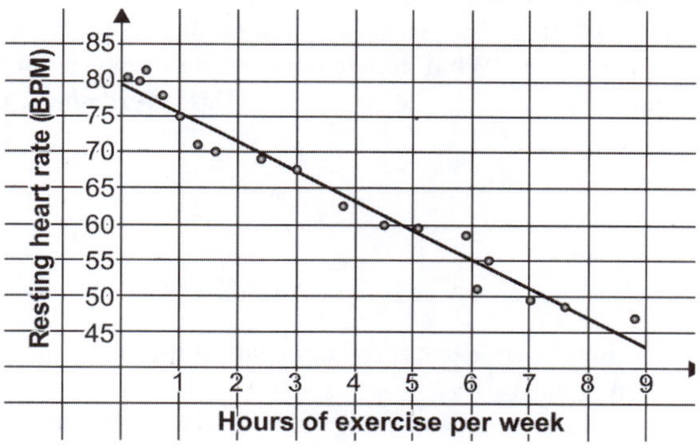

a. 0 and 1
b. 0 and –1
c. 1 and –1
d. 0 and 100

15. Identify the statistical diagram shown.
[Recent Question 2013]

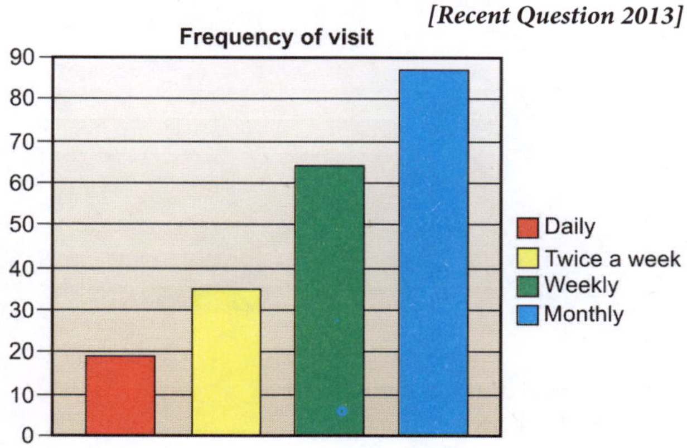

a. Histogram
b. Pie chart
c. Bar diagram
d. Ogive

16. Identify the statistical diagram shown.

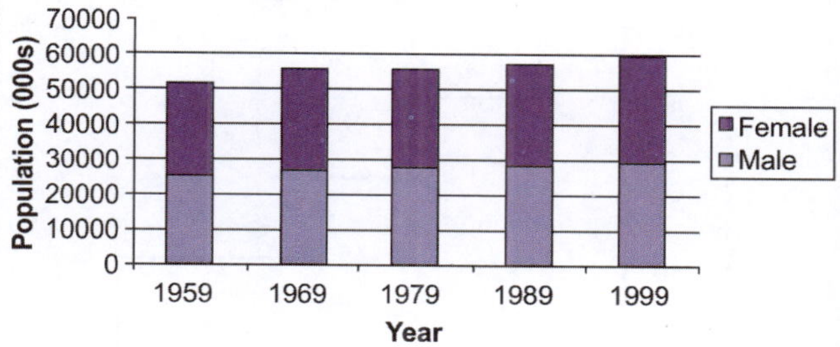

a. Simple bar chart
b. Multiple bar chart
c. Cluster bar chart
d. Component bar chart

17. Identify the diagram shown. *[Recent Question 2012]*

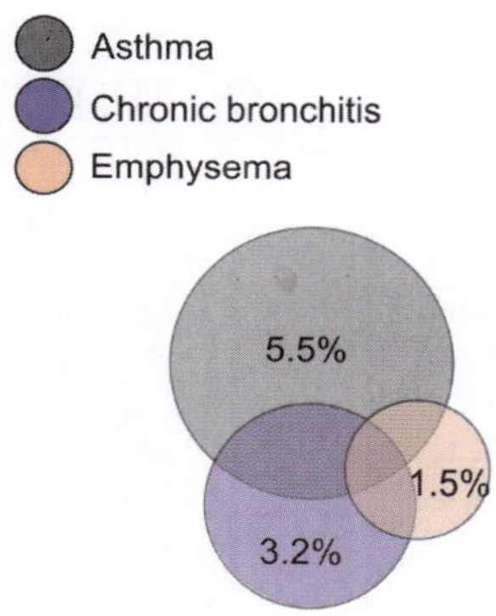

a. Stem and leaf plot
b. Pie chart
c. Venn diagram
d. Flow chart

18. Identify the diagram shown.

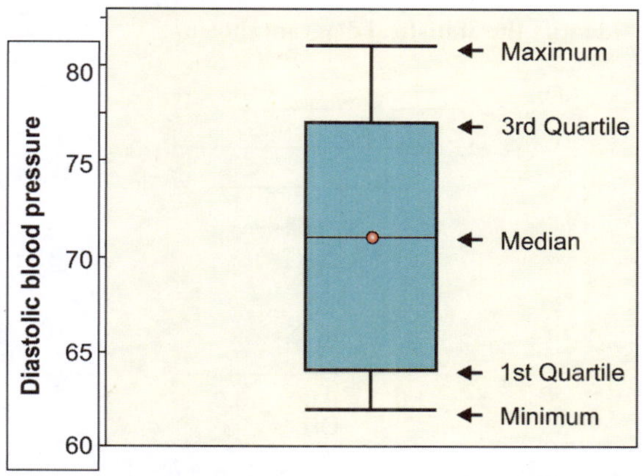

a. Stem and leaf plot
b. Box and Whisker plot
c. Venn diagram
d. Pictogram

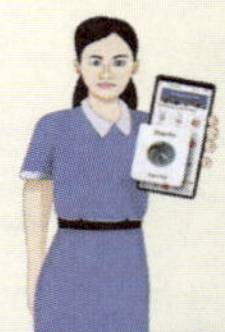

Ans.

13. a
14. b
15. c
16. d
17. c
18. b

19. Identify the diagram shown.

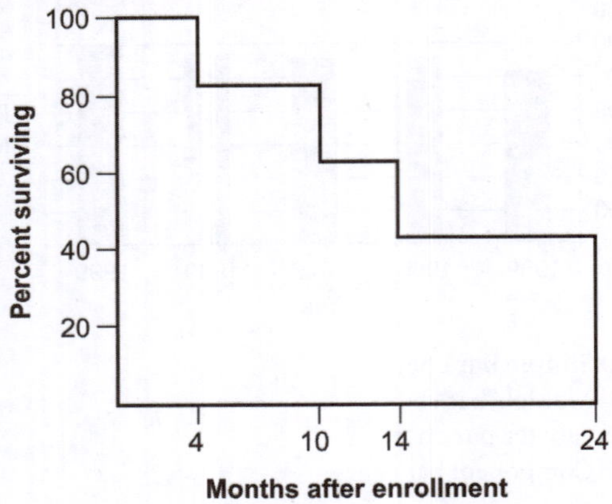

a. Histogram
b. Line diagram
c. Box and Whisker plot
d. Kaplan Meier plot

20. Identify formula shown in picture.

$$\chi_c^2 = \Sigma \frac{(O_i - E_i)^2}{E_i}$$

a. Paired Students' t test
b. ANOVA test
c. Mean test
d. Chi square test

21. Identify the Statistical diagram shown.

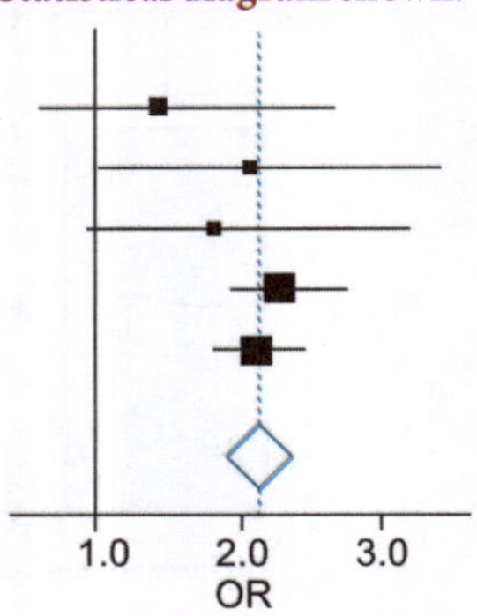

a. Funnel plot
b. Forest plot
c. Spaghetti plot
d. Mosaic plot

22. Identify the Statistical diagram shown.

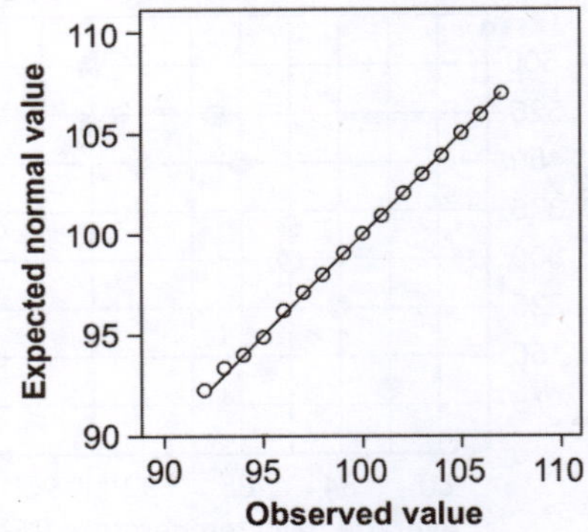

a. Funnel plot
b. Dot plot
c. Spaghetti plot
d. Q-Q plot

23. A study was conducted to see the effect of pulse oximeter readings in neonates with and without microspore. A plot between the two values was made as shown in the figure below. What conclusion can be drawn from the plot? *[AIIMS November 2016]*

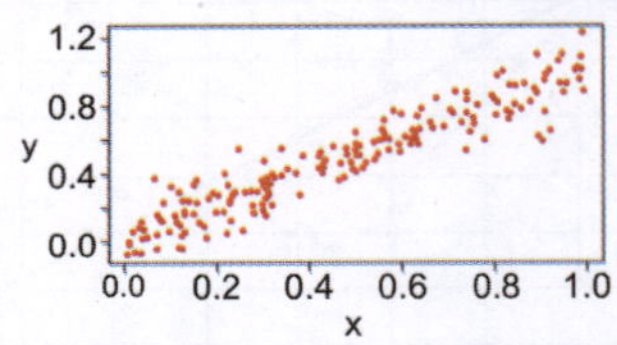

a. There is a positive correlation with constant 3% increase in Y-axis value.
b. There is a constant negative correlation between two variables.
c. There is a constant positive correlation between two variables.
d. There is no correlation.

24. Identify the distribution shown. *[Recent Question 2015]*

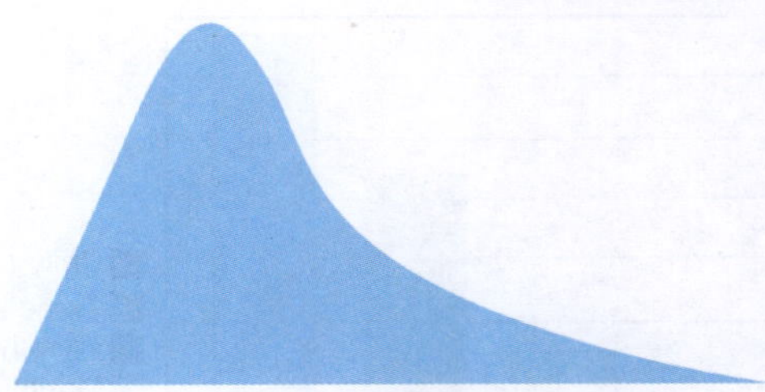

a. Normal distribution
b. Right-skewed distribution
c. Left-skewed distribution
d. Poisson's distribution

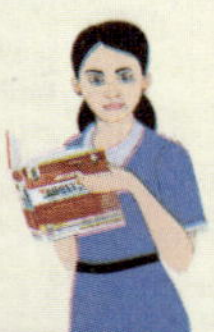

Ans.

19. d
20. d
21. b
22. d
23. c
24. b

25. Identify the statistical diagram shown.

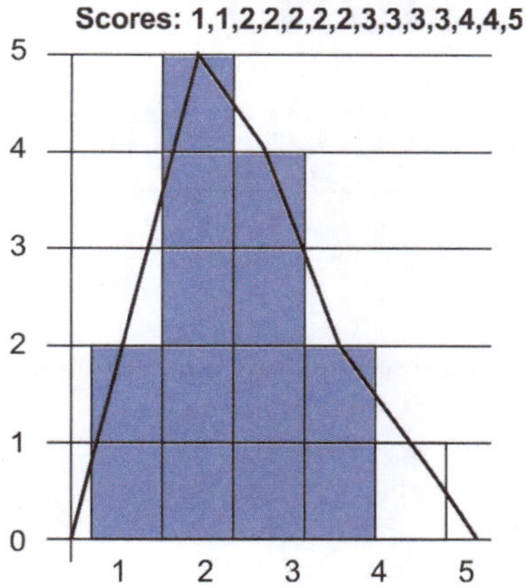

a. Histogram b. Frequency polygon
c. Line chart d. Ogive

26. Identify the statistical diagram shown.

[Recent Question 2014]

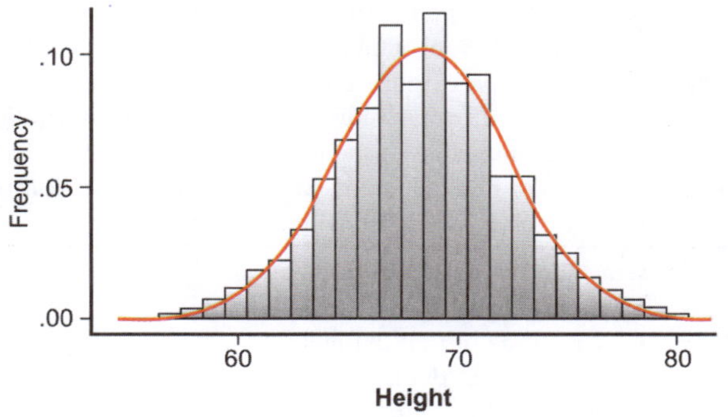

a. Frequency polygon b. Histogram
c. Frequency curve d. Ogive

27. Identify the statistical diagram shown.

[Recent Question 2014]

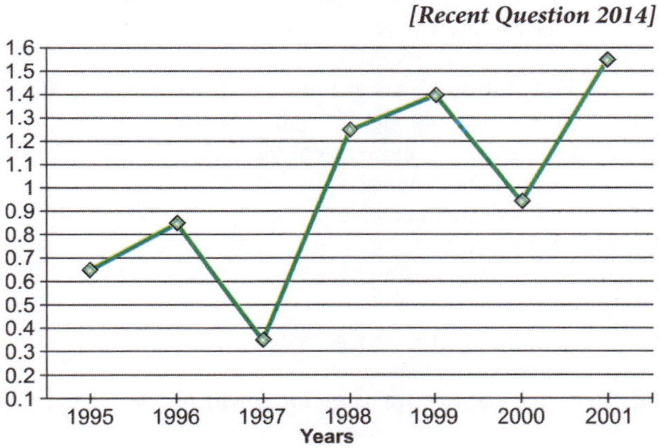

a. Frequency polygon b. Histogram
c. Line diagram d. Ogive

28. Type of sampling shown in figure is:

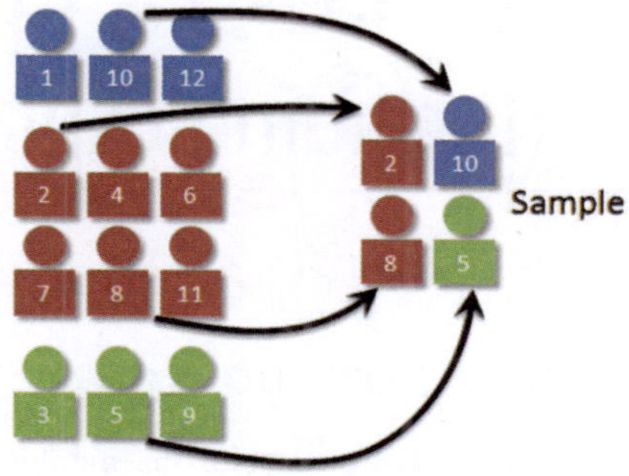

a. Simple random sampling
b. Systematic random sampling
c. Stratified random sampling
d. Cluster random sampling

29. Identify the diagram shown in figure.

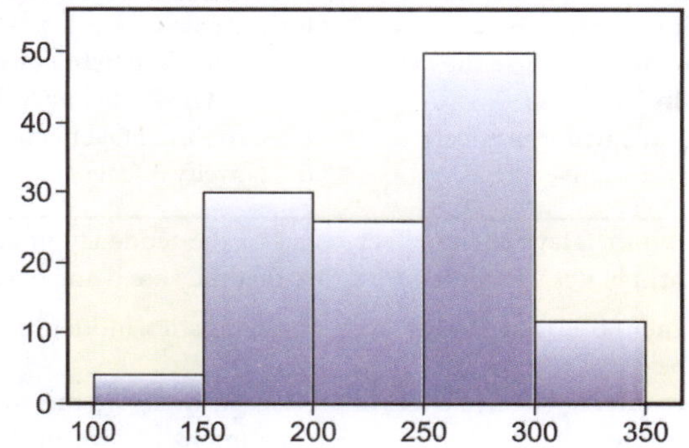

a. Simple bar chart b. Frequency diagram
c. Component bar chart d. Histogram

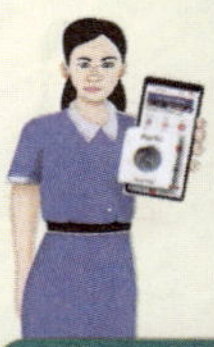

Ans.

25. b
26. c
27. c
28. c
29. d

"Health is the greatest of all possessions; a pale cobbler is better than a sick king."
—Isaac Bickerstaff

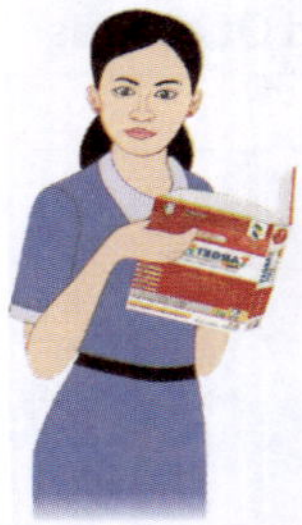

MULTIPLE CHOICE QUESTIONS
(Including Explained and Practice Questions)

INTRODUCTION & DEFINITIONS

1. The terminology used to explain the number of subjects recruited to participate in a study decline during a course of the project: *(AIIMS Raipur NO 2019)*
a. Variability　　b. Heterogenetic
c. Homogeneity　　d. Attrition

Explanation: Attrition means "wearing away" or progressive loss of data in research. It occurs when cases are lost from a sample over time or over a series of sequential processes. Sample attrition is commonly expected in a longitudinal studies or experimental studies.

2. The subject in a research study behaves in a particular manner because they are aware that they are being observed. This is called: *(AIIMS Raipur NO 2019)*
a. Hawthorne effect　　b. Experimental effect
c. Reactive effect　　d. Novelty effect

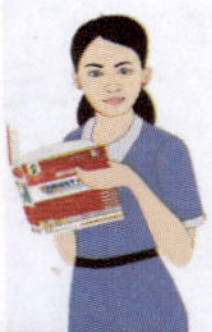

Explanation: **Hawthorne effect** refers to the tendency of subjects to perform better when they are aware that they are being observed.

Experimental effect: Researcher's characteristics influence subject behavior.
Reactive effect: Reactive effect of pretest sensitivity on the posttest.
Novelty effect: Subjects and researcher might behave in different ways when exposed to new treatment.

3. A nurse who reads research articles and incorporates research findings into clinical practice is a:
a. Consumer
b. Primary investigator
c. Co-investigator
d. Collaborator

4. Contributions of Florence Nightingale to nursing research is:
a. Case study approach
b. Conceptual Framework for research
c. Data collection and analysis
d. Qualitative research method

5. The researcher uses which portion of the research report to capture the reader's attention?
a. Abstract　　b. Methodology
c. Results　　d. Review of Literature

6. The sentence "The purpose of this study was to examine the relationship between knowledge and pre-operative anxiety among patients undergoing abdominal surgery" would most likely be found in which chapter of a research dissertation?
a. Introduction
b. Review of Literature
c. Methodology
d. Data Analysis and Interpretation

7. Feasibility of a research study is determined by examining:
a. Investigator's credibility
b. Availability of subjects
c. Importance of research problem
d. Previous research evidences

8. The researcher has written in his research proposal that written permission has been obtained from two local hospitals to access their staff nurses for data collection. This is an example of what aspect of a research:
a. Reliability　　b. Validity
c. Ethics　　d. Feasibility

Explanation: Validity and reliability are related to assessment of measurement tools for its appropriateness and consistency respectively. Obtaining permission from a hospital to access their employees for data collection is part of feasibility in conducting the research. Obtaining permission from study participants and institutional ethical committee (including hospital ethics committee) are related to ethical aspect of a research study. So, obtaining permission from hospitals is more closely associated with feasibility than ethics.

9. "Abstract" in research is defined as:
a. Specific and particular
b. General and not well-defined
c. Precise and well-defined
d. Concrete and specific

10. Who is the first nurse researcher?
a. Martha Rogers　　b. Dorothea Orem
c. Florence Nightingale　　d. Sr. Callista Roy

11. Condition or characteristic that can take on different values or categories is called a:
a. Constant
b. Variable
c. Cause-and-effect relationship
d. Descriptive relationship

12. All of the following are examples of grand theory; EXCEPT:
a. Interpersonal Model
b. Community Empowerment Model
c. Health Belief Theory
d. Maslow's Hierarchy Needs Theory

13. The theories are:
a. Based on preexisting facts
b. Testable
c. Formulated prior to research
d. Derived from issues

14. Inductive theories are based on conclusion drawn by:
a. Testing theories
b. Moving from general to specific
c. Moving from specific to general
d. General observations

Ans.

1.	d
2.	a
3.	a
4.	c
5.	a
6.	a
7.	b
8.	d
9.	b
10.	c
11.	b
12.	b
13.	b
14.	c

15. Theories are
a. Already existing
b. Formulated and keep on changing
c. Stagnant and never change
d. None of the above

16. Research paradigm is:
a. Conceptual framework
b. Theoretical framework
c. Study framework
d. None of the above

17. Nursing research can be based on:
a. Only nursing theories
b. Theories from other disciplines
c. Both a and b
d. None of the above

18. A study of experiences is called:
a. Phenomenology b. Ethnography
c. Action research d. Grounded theory

19. The group of study participants that does not receive the intervention is known as:
a. Control group b. Experimental group
c. Randomized group d. Subjects

20. Subset of a population is called as:
a. Study population b. Target population
c. Sample d. Unit

21. The first annotated index of nursing research was the work of:
a. Dorothea Orem b. Florence Nightingale
c. Denise Polit d. Virginia Henderson

22. Who was the first to use the word "Statistics"?
(Safdarjung NO 2018)
a. Gottfried Achenwall b. Prof. Horace Secrist
c. Croxton and Cowden d. Gelan

Explanation: The word statistics was first used by a German scholar Gottfried Achenwall in the middle of the 18th century as the science of statecraft concerning the collection and use of data by the state.

23. The indices calculated from a sample is called as:
a. Parameter b. Statistics
c. Conclusion d. Inference

24. The method of statistics that is used to draw conclusion from a data collected from a sample of population instead of entire population is referred as:
a. Descriptive statistics b. Inferential statistics
c. Census statistics d. Population survey

25. The statistical approach used to test whether the outcome of the study is a result of factors planned within design of the study is called:
a. Analytical statistics b. Descriptive statistics
c. Inferential statistics d. All of these

26. The statistical method that is used to explain and summarize a specific set of data is known as:
a. Inferential statistics b. Descriptive statistics
c. Theme identification d. None of these

27. Health Adjusted Life Expectancy is a measure of:
a. Mortality b. Disability
c. Fertility d. Reproduction Rate

28. Number of existing cases of a disease during a given time interval gives:
a. Point prevalence b. Incidence
c. Period prevalence d. None of these

29. The number of new cases that occur within a specific population within a defined time interval is:
a. Incidence b. Point Prevalence
c. Period prevalence d. Lifetime Prevalence

30. Full form of SPSS is:
a. Statistical Package for Social System
b. Statistical Programme for Social Sciences
c. Statistical Package for Social Sciences
d. Statistical Programme for Scientific Studies

STEPS & PHASES IN RESEARCH PROCESS

31. Which of the following is NOT a common feature of both research process and nursing process?
a. Identifies new information
b. Involves critical thinking
c. Has a broader focus
d. Utilizes complex thinking

Explanation: Research has a broader focus and involves generalizability of findings, whereas nursing process is client-focused and not generalized to all patients/population. Other three features are common to research and nursing process.

32. The specific aim or goal of the research study based on the identified problem is termed as:
a. Purpose b. Assumptions
c. Operational definition d. Methodology

33. The first step of the Research Process is to:
a. Prepare the Research Design
b. Complete Data Collection and Analysis
c. Formulate the Research Questions
d. Prepare the Report

34. Which of the following is not the purpose of pilot study?
a. Tool refinement
b. Fine tune the data collection process
c. Help in sample size calculation
d. Drawing final inferences

35. PICO means:
a. Population, intervention, comparison, outcome
b. Prevalence, incidence, cohort, observation
c. Polio, influenza, chickenpox, ovulation
d. Patient, injection, catheterization, operation

36. The initial and one of the most significant steps in conducting the research process is:
a. Defining the research variables
b. Identifying the research problem
c. Stating the research purposes.
d. Determining the feasibility of the study

37. Problem identification in the research process would be equivalent to which step in the nursing process?
a. Nursing assessment b. Planning
c. Implementation d. Evaluation

38. The major objective of conducting a basic research is to:
a. Develop knowledge for immediate use
b. Develop theories and principles
c. Make a decision
d. Provide a solution for existing problems

39. The development of a solid foundation of reliable knowledge is typically built from:
a. Action research b. Basic research
c. Developmental research d. Methodological research

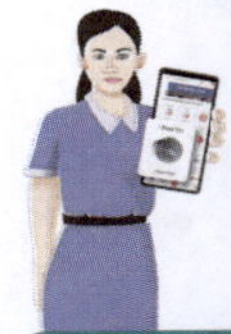

Ans.

15.	b
16.	a
17.	c
18.	a
19.	a
20.	c
21.	d
22.	a
23.	b
24.	b
25.	c
26.	b
27.	b
28.	c
29.	a
30.	c
31.	c
32.	a
33.	c
34.	d
35.	a
36.	b
37.	a
38.	b
39.	b

40. The deductive approach in writing protocol involves:
a. Moving from general concept to a specific one
b. Moving from specific and then expands to overall plan
c. Moving from precise to wide-ranging
d. Moving from meticulous to specific

41. Problem identification in the research process is similar to which step of the nursing process?
a. Data interpretation b. Goal identification
c. Nursing diagnosis d. Identifying solutions

Explanation: Identification of a research problem is the first and most important step in research process. It can be compared to assessment and nursing diagnosis step of the nursing process.

42. The planning step in the nursing process is similar to which step in the research process?
a. Data collection
b. Design
c. Implementation
d. Goal identification

43. Which of the following research steps is completed first?
a. Determining the population
b. Identification of a problem
c. Formulation of research question or hypothesis
d. Literature review

44. The only step involved in qualitative research process is:
a. Getting entry into research setting
b. Random selection of sample
c. Using a structured questionnaire for data collection
d. Using inferential statistics for analysis of data

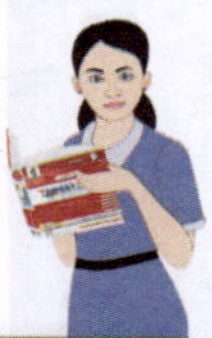

45. Which of the following statement is TRUE?
a. An aim can have only one objective
b. Objectives have no link with methodology
c. Objectives have no link with study title
d. Objectives are subsidiary to aims

46. Who proposed the theory of interpersonal relationship?
a. Orem b. Abdullah
c. Peplau d. Jean Watson

47. Theory of theory is termed:
a. Grand theory b. Meta theory
c. Systematic theory d. Middle range theory

48. After the research is completed, a meeting of a researcher with study participants that ensures their understanding of the reasons for the procedures used in the study is known as:
a. Explanation b. Debriefing
c. Informing d. Research meeting

49. A small-scale trial run of a research study is referred to as:
a. Minor project b. Pilot study
c. Miniature study d. Sample study

50. Assumption and delimitation are identified in which stage of research process?
a. Planning b. Implementing
c. Writing report d. Critiquing

RESEARCH PROBLEM

51. The most important source for identification of a research problem is:
a. Nursing practice
b. Nursing practice guidelines and protocols
c. Nursing textbooks
d. Nursing code of ethics

52. Which of the following describes what a problem is?
a. Usually a question that needs to be answered
b. The aim of the study
c. Direction and form of the study
d. Predictor of relationship between two or more variable

53. Discrepancy between what is known and what ought to be known is described as:
a. Research results b. Research phenomenon
c. Research objective d. Research problem

54. Which of the following is NOT considered as component of the research problem?
a. Research instruments b. Variables of the study
c. Study population d. Research setting

REVIEW OF LITERATURE

55. A literature review is: *(RAK MSc 2018)*
a. Everything that is known about subject
b. An analytical summary of research findings
c. All approved data on a research topic
d. A compilation of all positive results of research

Explanation: A literature review is everything that is known about subject.

The purpose of a good literature review is to get thorough familiarity with available evidence about the subject of study.

Review of literature is not an analytical summary of research findings or the positive results

56. In quantitative research process, the literature review should occur: *(RAK MSc 2018)*
a. Near the end of research process
b. Shortly before the analysis of the problem
c. Early in the research process
d. None of the above

Explanation: Investigators usually undertake a thorough literature review as an early step in a research study. Once the researcher has identified a potential research problem, the next step is to review the related literature. The main purpose of literature review is to keep the reader up-to-date with the research done on the selected topic.

57. The purpose of a literature of review is to:
a. Define the problem
b. Identify strengths and weaknesses of previous studies
c. Help in operational definition
d. All of the above

58. Which of the following is considered to be the highest quality type of literature?
a. Research articles in a peer-reviewed journal
b. Secondary sources
c. Books
d. Research reports in a conference proceeding

59. The most useful abstracting index for nursing literature is:
a. ERIc b. CINAHL
c. Pubmed d. Psych INFO

60. Index that provide the largest number of relevant nursing sources is:
a. International Nursing Index
b. Cumulative Index to Nursing & Allied Health Literature
c. Nursing Studies Index
d. Cochrane Database

Ans.

40.	a
41.	c
42.	b
43.	b
44.	a
45.	d
46.	c
47.	b
48.	b
49.	b
50.	a
51.	a
52.	a
53.	d
54.	a
55.	a
56.	c
57.	d
58.	a
59.	b
60.	b

61. In the following APA formatted reference, what does the 23 refer to? "Derwing, T. M., Rossiter, M. J., & Munro, M. J. (2002). Teaching native speakers to listen to foreign-accented speech. Journal of Multilingual and Multicultural Development, 23(4), 245-259.":

a. Volume number b. Issue number c. Page number d. Chapter number

Explanation: The components of APA reference style is depicted in the image below.

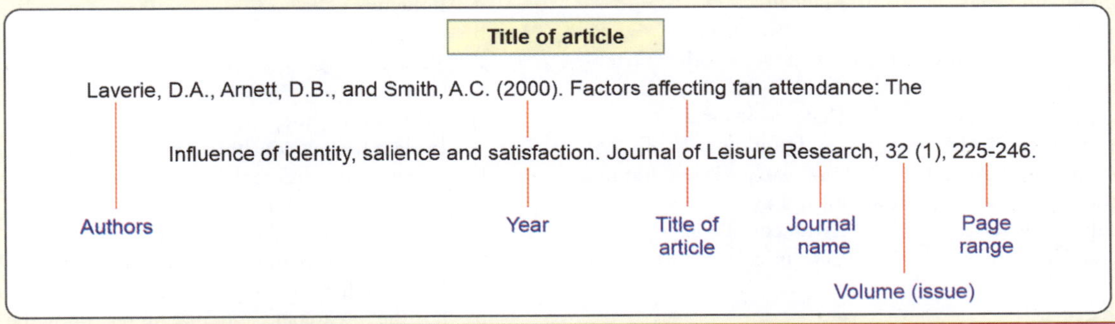

62. Which of the following is TRUE regarding writing review of literature?

a. Avoid long paragraphs
b. Avoid short paragraphs
c. Avoid link between connected paragraphs
d. Avoid pointing out gaps between literature

63. Which of the following is NOT TRUE of computer based pubmed search?

a. Keywords are unrelated to MeSH
b. Boolean operators 'AND' or 'NOT' can be used
c. Google search for Pubmed then proceed further
d. Search can be limited by years

64. All of the following techniques deals with extraneous variables in quantitative research; EXCEPT:

a. Randomization
b. Repeated measures
c. Homogeneity
d. Bracketing

65. Which of the following is considered as a bibliography data-base for biomedical literature?

a. Google
b. Medline
c. MSN search
d. SAFARI

66. Which of the following is considered as a nursing and allied health sciences database?

a. Medline b. Pubmed
c. CINAHL d. Ovid plus

67. The word theory is derived from:

a. Theoria b. Theoryia
c. Theoretical d. Theorium

68. All of the following are the building blocks of theory; EXCEPT:

a. Conceptual definition
b. Theoretical propositions
c. Construct
d. Concept

69. Development of conceptual framework in quantitative research is mainly:

a. Before literature review b. During literature review
c. Before data analysis d. After data analysis

RESEARCH VARIABLES & EXAMPLES

70. The process of drawing a specific conclusion from a set of ideas is known as:

a. Inductive reasoning b. Deductive reasoning
c. Idealism d. Logical reasoning

71. A variable that is presumed to cause a change in another variable is called:

a. Dependent variable b. Independent variable
c. Intervening variable d. Active variable

72. The variable in an experiment that is known from the start and does not change is called:

a. Dependent variable b. Extraneous variable
c. Independent variable d. Confounding variable

73. The variable which is influenced by the intervention of the researcher is called:

a. Independent b. Dependent
c. Discrete d. Extraneous

74. The variable that is manipulated in an experiment is called:

a. Independent variable b. Dependent variable
c. Criteria variable d. Controller variable

75. A researcher studied the effect of a scheduling assignment on nurses' morale, the scheduling assignment would be referred to as:

a. Active variable b. Independent variable
c. Dependent variable d. Interfering variable

76. Identify the dependent variable in the following statement: "Hypertensive patients who receive exercise therapy report better blood pressure control and require less drug dose than hypertensive patients not receiving exercise therapy.":

a. Blood pressure b. Exercise therapy
c. Hypertensive patients d. All of these

77. Identify the independent variable in the following research statement: "A study on effectiveness of exercise therapy on sleep hygiene among undergraduate nursing students"

a. Exercise therapy b. Sleep hygiene
c. Undergraduate students d. Students

78. Variable that is irrelevant in an investigation and needs to be controlled is called:

a. Indirect variable
b. Active variable
c. Dependent variable
d. Extraneous variable

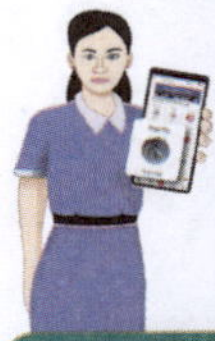

Ans.

61.	a
62.	a
63.	a
64.	d
65.	b
66.	c
67.	a
68.	a
69.	b
70.	b
71.	b
72.	c
73.	b
74.	a
75.	b
76.	a
77.	a
78.	d

79. Biasness of a study can be reduced by controlling which of the following variables?
a. Extraneous b. Independent
c. Dependent d. Demographic

80. __________ refers to the influence of a single independent variable.
a. Confounding effect b. Main effect
c. Extraneous effect d. Proactive effect

81. Variable that changes due to the influence of another variable is known as the:
a. Independent variable b. Dependent variable
c. Extraneous variable d. Confounding variable

82. The variables that are not studied in the experiment but may affect the dependent variable are known as:
a. Independent variable b. Extraneous variable
c. Dependent variable d. Categorical variable

HYPOTHESIS

83. Which scientific method focuses on testing hypotheses developed from theories?
a. Deductive method b. Inductive method
c. Hypothesis method d. Pattern method

84. Which scientific method often focuses on generating new hypotheses and theories?
a. Deductive method b. Inductive method
c. Hypothesis method c. Pattern method

85. Identify the type of hypothesis from the following statement: "Two hourly position change is more effective than four hourly position change in prevention of pressure ulcer in bed-ridden patients."
a. Simple, research b. Simple, directional
c. Complex, casual d. Complex, associative

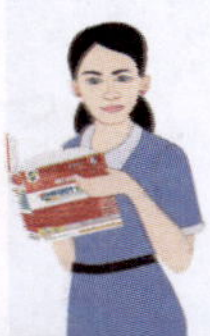

86. Identify the type of hypothesis from the following statement: "Emotional well-being is influenced by the self-esteem, degree of social support and financial status in women breast cancer survivors."
a. Simple, research b. Simple, directional
c. Complex, non-directional d. Complex, directional

87. Identify the type of hypothesis from the following statement: "The lower the blood sugar level, the lesser is the risk of infection among diabetic patients"
a. Simple, associative
b. Simple, causal
c. Causal, null
d. Causal, directional

88. Identify the type of the following hypothesis. "Hypertensive patients who receive exercise therapy report better blood pressure control and require less drug dose than hypertensive patients not receiving exercise therapy.":
a. Simple, directional hypothesis
b. Simple, non-directional hypothesis
c. Complex, non-directional hypothesis
d. Complex, directional hypothesis

89. What type of hypothesis is the following? "High-fiber diet is related to increased bowel movement and lower cholesterol levels.":
a. Complex, directional, causal
b. Complex, directional, associative
c. Simple, non-directional, research
d. Simple, directional, causal

90. Statement of the expected relationship between two or more variables is known as the:
a. Assumption b. Hypothesis
c. Problem statement d. Research question

91. The hypothesis that begins with specific observations and move towards generalizations, is called as:
a. Inductive
b. Deductive
c. Simple
d. Complex

92. Hypothesis does not:
a. Explain the relationship between variables
b. Measures the differences between variables
c. Give direction to data collection
d. Give direction to data analysis

93. Which of the following is not true for hypothesis?
a. It is a prediction of relationship between variables
b. It is the researcher's anticipation regarding the study
c. A hypothesis is a tentative generalization
d. It cannot be tested

94. Which of the following statements meets the criteria for the complex hypothesis?
a. There is significant negative correlation between years of experience and level of burnout symptoms of nurses
b. Music therapy reduces the anxiety among post-operative CABG patients
c. Balanced diet and regular exercise decrease the incidence of postpartum depression
d. Female nurses have higher job satisfaction compare to male nurses

95. Pair of hypotheses that are similar to each other is:
a. Simple and complex
b. Associative and causal
c. Directional and non-directional
d. Research and null

96. 'Demonstration method of teaching is more effective than video assisted teaching to teach nursing procedures' is an example of:
a. Directional hypothesis
b. Complex hypothesis
c. Non-directional hypothesis
d. Null hypothesis

97. 'There is no difference in the anxiety level of children of high IQ and those of low IQ' is an example of a:
a. Directional hypothesis
b. Non-directional hypothesis
c. Null hypothesis
d. Simple hypothesis

98. Which of the followings statement best describes the term 'research hypotheses'?
a. It is formulated prior to a review of the literature
b. It is a statement of predicted relationships between two or more variables
c. It is a statement of known fact
d. All of the above

99. Hypotheses are often generated as the data are collected, interpreted, and analyzed in which type of research studies?
a. Quantitative research studies
b. Qualitative research studies
c. Prospective cohort studies
d. Comparative studies

Ans.

79.	a
80.	b
81.	b
82.	b
83.	a
84.	b
85.	b
86.	c
87.	a
88.	d
89.	b
90.	b
91.	a
92.	b
93.	d
94.	c
95.	b
96.	a
97.	c
98.	b
99.	b

100. The statement of beliefs and ideas which are considered to be true are known as: *(RAK MSc 2018)*

a. Hypothesis b. Assumption
c. Conceptual definition d. Operational definition

101. Realistic expectation which is something that we believe to be true is: *(AIIMS Raipur NO 2019)*

a. Hypothesis
b. Conceptual framework
c. Assumption
d. Concepts

Explanation: Assumption is a statement on principles that are taken as truth based on a person's values and beliefs. In simple terms, it is a statement that is taken for granted or are considered to be true, even though they have not been actually scientifically tested or validated.

Hypothesis: It is a formal tentative statement of the expected relationship between two or more variables.

102. Basic principles that are accepted as being true on the basis of logic or reason, without proof or verification is referred as:

a. Hypothesis b. Assumptions
c. Constructs d. Propositions

103. Which of the following term describes the boundaries that the researcher has set for the study?

a. Assumption
b. Hypothesis
c. Conceptual framework
d. Delimitation

104. Those restrictions that the researcher places on the study before gathering data are called:

a. Assumptions
b. Limitations
c. Delimitations
d. Hypothesis

105. Which of the following is true about delimitations?

a. These are the shortcomings of a study.
b. These are the boundaries we set to our study before its start
c. These are the potential weaknesses in the study.
d. These include the drop out of the subjects.

RESEARCH APPROACH & DESIGNS

106. All the following are qualitative research methods; EXCEPT: *(AIIMS BBS NO 2018)*

a. Phenomenology b. Ethnography
c. Grounded theory d. Correlation

Explanation: Qualitative research designs include historical research, phenomenology, ethnography, grounded theory, case study, and triangulation method.

Correlation research is a quantitative, non-experimental research, which involves the study of two variables and their correlation with each other in natural settings.

107. Examining cause and effect relationship between variables under highly controlled conditions is: *(AIIMS BBS NO 2018)*

a. Correlational research
b. Experimental research
c. Descriptive research
d. Quasi-experimental research

Explanation: Cause and effect refer to a relationship between two variables in which one variable causes change in the other variable. Example. Regular exercise (cause) leads to weight loss (effect).

Experimental research methods are useful in establishing cause and effect relationship. True experimental research is the most accurate form of experimental research design to establish cause and effect.

Quasi-experimental does not have controlled conditions. Correlational and descriptive researches are nonexperimental researches.

108. A blueprint for the conduction of study is: *(Daman & Diu NO 2018)*

a. Pilot study b. Research hypothesis
c. Research design d. Data collection tool

Explanation: A research design is a framework or blueprint for conducting the research. It specifies the details of the procedures necessary for obtaining the information.

109. Which of these designs is used to estimate the prevalence of osteoporosis? *(Daman & Diu NO 2018)*

a. Cross-sectional
b. Quasi experimental
c. Cross-over
d. Factorial

Explanation: Quasi experimental, cross-over and factorial designs are methods of experimental research in which the researcher is interested to test the effectiveness of an intervention. Whereas cross-sectional studies collect data from subjects at only one point in time. It is usually carried out to assess the prevalence of specific disease or awareness on specific variable under study.

110. A careful appraisal of the strengths and weaknesses of the study is: *(RAK MSc 2018)*

a. Research proposal
b. Action research
c. Research critique
d. Evidence-based practice

Explanation: **Research critique** is a systematic way of objectively reviewing a research study to highlight both its strengths and weaknesses.

A research proposal is a document proposing a research project. **Action research** is a type of research method and **evidence-based practice** refers to the use of current research evidences in nursing/medical practice.

111. The final step of the research process for a researcher is to: *(Safdarjung NO 2018):*

a. Utilize the findings
b. Analyze the data
c. Interpret the findings
d. Communicate the findings

Explanation: As per the phases and steps of research process, the options given above can be sequentially organized as – *analyze the data, interpret the findings, communicate the findings and then utilize the findings.*

Utilization of the research findings is the final step a researcher can do.

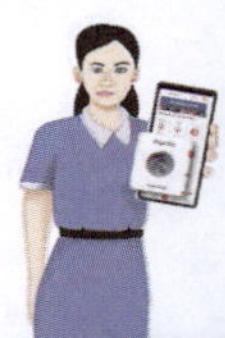

Ans.

100. b
101. c
102. b
103. d
104. c
105. b
106. d
107. b
108. c
109. a
110. c
111. a

112. Which of the following is NOT TRUE about the characteristics of a good research? *(Safdarjung NO 2018)*

a. Conducted using large amount of funds
b. Orderly and systematic process
c. Finding solution of problem
d. Begin with clearly defined purposes

Explanation: Parsimony is one of the characteristics of scientific research. Research must be conducted in simple and economic manner. Using large amount of funds to conduct research is not cost effective and feasible.

113. Quantitative and qualitative research approaches are particularly useful in nursing because they:

a. Require less resources
b. Are easy to implement
c. Generates different types of nursing knowledge
d. Are both process oriented

114. A researcher conducts a smaller study of the planned study to identify any problematic areas before implementing a planned large scale research investigation. This smaller study is known as: *New Q*

a. Abstract study
b. Exploratory study
c. Pilot study
d. Pretest

115. A research study framework reflects the:

a. Researcher's "theory" or idea about the study
b. Study design
c. Methodology
d. Data collection plan

116. As a professional, a nurse can do research for varied reason; except:

a. Professional advancement
b. To validate the results of new nursing modalities.
c. For financial gains
d. To improve nursing care

117. Which of the following is not the element of a research statement?

a. Research design
b. Research instrument
c. Population
d. Setting

118. The central concepts of conceptual models in nursing includes:

a. Head, heart and hand
b. Human, health, disease and environment
c. Man, health, environment and nursing
d. Agent, host, reservoir and environment

119. Which of the following is characteristic of qualitative research?

a. Generalization to the population
b. Random sampling
c. Unique case orientation
d. Application of statistics for analysis

120. Research in which the investigator plays an active, interactive role is called:

a. Action research
b. Interventional research
c. Inferential research
d. Interactive research

121. Which of the following would be in the introduction section of a research proposal?

a. Data analysis procedure
b. Description of an instrument
c. A time frame
d. Statement of purpose

122. Which of the following would not be in a research proposal?

a. Budget
b. Time frame
c. Methods
d. Results

123. A research proposal is best described as a:

a. Framework for data analysis
b. Written account of the plan for the intended study
c. Description of ethical perspective of the study
d. Argument for the merit of the study

124. Which of the following is the purpose of a research proposal?

a. Guide for conducting study
b. Saves money of the funding agency
c. Prevents evaluation by others in doing study
d. Helps in solving problems after conclusion of data analysis

125. A good research proposal will always:

a. Focus on addressing the research objectives
b. Focus on specific style of writing references
c. Consider all possible research that had previously been done on the topic
d. Provide researchers names and address

126. Which of the following type of studies is an example of qualitative research method?

a. Cross sectional design
b. Correlational studies
c. Ethnography
d. Survey design

127. Which of the following types of research study involve at least some control by the researcher to evaluate the intervention?

a. Correlational
b. Descriptive
c. Cohort study
d. Quasi-experimental

128. Which of the following type of research involves high researcher control, random sampling, and laboratory setting?

a. Cohort study
b. Case control study
c. True Experimental
d. Quasi experimental

129. Research questions: "Does motivational counseling before discharge by nurses improve patients' compliance with their drug regimens?"
Which of the following research is appropriate to answer this research question?

a. Applied research
b. Basic research
c. Descriptive research
d. Phenomenological research

130. A researcher investigates the effect of foot massage on sleep quality of patients. This study would be described as:

a. Applied research
b. Basic research
c. Grounded theory approach
d. Phenomenological research

131. Applied research seeks to solve a clinical problem in:

a. Natural setting
b. Laboratory setting
c. Controlled setting
d. Simulated setting

132. Which of the following is the best way to achieve scientific rigor in quantitative research?

a. Following a strict time frame
b. Extent of precision and control exerted by the methodology
c. Degree of determination in data collection
d. Analytical methods used to interpret and conclude the study

Ans.

112. a
113. c
114. c
115. a
116. c
117. b
118. c
119. c
120. b
121. d
122. d
123. b
124. a
125. a
126. c
127. d
128. c
129. a
130. a
131. a
132. b

133. Quantitative research is a process to:
a. Describe lived experiences of people
b. Develop theories and hypothesis
c. Evaluate theories and hypothesis
d. Obtain feelings and beliefs of the people

134. All of the following are the purpose of evidence-based practice; EXCEPT:
a. To abolish wrong practices
b. To improve quality of patient care
c. To obtain more research funds from agencies
d. To improve the patient-care outcome

135. Barriers of evidence-based practice includes all of the following; EXCEPT:
a. Lack of knowledge
b. Lack of scientific literature
c. Lack of skills in conducting computer based literature search
d. Lack of time to read literature

Explanation: The most important individual barriers to implementation of EBP are lack of time to read literature (due to higher work load), lack of ability to work with computer, lack of knowledge or language proficiency are the common barriers of evidence based practice.

There is no dearth of scientific literature in nursing science with online and printed sources. So, it is not a barrier in EBP.

136. All of the following are steps of quantitative research; EXCEPT:
a. Formulation of research problem
b. Formulation of research questions
c. Data analysis
d. Systemic review of research study

137. Find the odd one out regarding the typical characteristics of a research objective:
a. Observable b. Measurable
c. Achievable d. Verifiable

138. What the acronym SMART specifies, that the objectives should be?
a. Specific, measurable, achievable, realistic, and timely
b. Simple, modifiable, applicable, realistic, technical
c. Small, measurable, applicable, reliable, timely
d. Sensitive, matching, affordable, robust, testable

139. All the following statements are correct regarding objectives; EXCEPT:
a. An objective is a statement in specific and measurable terms
b. Objectives have a broader perspective than aims.
c. Objectives lay out how the researcher plans to accomplish the aims
d. A research study may include a number of objectives

140. The statement "to compare the knowledge of primigravida and multigravida women regarding breast feeding practices" is described as research:
a. Assumption b. Hypothesis
c. Objective d. Problem

141. Which of the following section of research report describes the study subjects in detail?
a. Introduction
b. Background
c. Methodology
d. Data analysis and Discussion

142. In a peer-reviewed journal, the articles are published on the basis of:
a. Subjective discretion of the editors
b. Number of authors listed
c. Sincerity of the authors listed
d. Comments of the reviewers

143. The sources to develop a conceptual framework includes all of the following; EXCEPT:
a. Researcher's own experiences
b. Historical evidences
c. Previous research evidences
d. Theoretical concepts

144. Phenomenological study involves all the following features; EXCEPT:
a. Bracket out b. Manipulation
c. Description d. Analysis

145. The method that focuses on description and interpretation of cultural behavior is referred as:
a. Phenomenology
b. Ethnography
c. Grounded theory
d. Symbolic interactionism

146. The research design in which the area of inquiry is the manner by which people make sense of social interactions:
a. Symbolic interactionism
b. Phenomenology
c. Grounded theory
d. Case study

147. The area of inquiry in grounded theory approach is:
a. Lived experiences
b. Social structural processes within social setting
c. Holistic view of culture
d. All of the above

148. Use of multiple referents to draw conclusions about what constitutes the truth is termed as:
(INC consortium PhD Entrance 2011)
a. Data verification b. Cross reference
c. Error measurement d. Triangulation

149. Who coined the term 'triangulation' in research?
a. Hungler b. Stuart
c. Denzin d. Polit

150. The primary objective of an experimental research is to detect the effect produced by:
a. Extraneous variable b. Confounding variable
c. Independent variable d. Dependent variable

151. Which of the following research design mandatorily requires randomization, control and manipulation?
a. Explorative study
b. Quasi-experimental design
c. True experimental design
d. Pre-experimental design

152. Properties of true experimental research study are the following; EXCEPT:
a. Manipulation b. Control
c. Matching d. Randomization

153. The type of research that has a control over variables, manipulates variables and uses purposive sampling, is known as:
a. Nonexperimental b. Pre-experimental
c. Quasi experimental d. True experimental

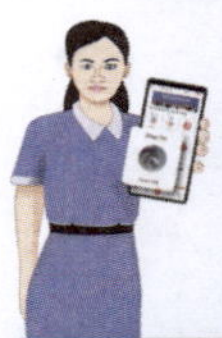

Ans.
133. c
134. c
135. b
136. d
137. d
138. a
139. b
140. c
141. c
142. d
143. b
144. b
145. b
146. a
147. b
148. d
149. c
150. c
151. c
152. c
153. c

154. Study participants (subjects) are randomly assigned into two groups. One group of subjects is administered a treatment and is then compared, on the dependent variable, with another group of subjects who did not receive the treatment. This research design is known as:

a. Pretest-posttest design b. Posttest-only design
c. Pre-experimental design d. Time series design

155. A type of observational study that involves data collection from a population, or a representative subset, at one specific point in time is known as:

a. Cross-sectional study
b. Longitudinal study
c. Retrospective study
d. Prospective cohort study

156. Rate of incidence is best studied by:

a. Retrospective studies b. Prospective studies
c. Cross sectional d. Case control

157. The type of research focused on finding a solution to an immediate practical problem is termed as:

a. Basic research b. Applied research
c. Explanatory research d. Descriptive research

158. Case studies may concern an in depth examination of:

a. Individuals b. Groups of people
c. Institutions d. All of these

159. Repeated-measures design is also known as:

a. Crossover design b. Solomon four-group design
c. Time series design d. With-in subjects design

160. Sensitization of research participants to a pretest can be controlled by ________ research design.

a. Cross over design b. Solomon four-group
c. Case control study d. Pre-experimental

161. Ex-post facto studies are known as:

a. Experimental study b. Causal comparative
c. Cross-sectional study d. Retrospective

162. 'Lived experience of surviving an earth quake'. This title would indicate which of the following types of qualitative research?

a. Historical
b. Ethnographic
c. Grounded theory approach
d. Phenomenological

163. When a researcher starts with the dependent variable and moves backward in time, it is called as:

a. Prospective research
b. Retrospective research
c. Cross sectional research
d. Ex-post facto research

164. Large sample size is required for:

a. Ethnography research
b. Correlational research
c. Grounded theory approach
d. Phenomenological research

165. Section of research report that includes interpretation and evaluation of the results of the research is:

a. Abstract b. Methods ad material
c. Results d. Discussion

166. Which of the following is NOT one of the seven major parts to the research report?

a. Results b. Footnotes
c. References d. Discussion

167. Which of the following is true about writing a conclusion of a research report?

a. Can introduce new information
b. Must be based only on material presented in the report
c. It is the same as the abstract
d. Should focus only on the objectives of the research

168. Which is TRUE of the abstract?

a. Is usually placed after the methods
b. It summarizes the study
c. Is generally of >500 words
d. Does not mention methods and objectives

169. Best strategy to promote research utilization among nurses is:

a. Train and equip nurses with the knowledge of evidence based practice
b. Research collaboration among nurse researcher and nurses clinicians
c. Motivating nurses to read, review, participate in research
d. All of the above

170. Studies that produce basic estimates of the rates of disorder in a general population and its subgroups is referred as:

a. Qualitative epidemiology
b. Analytic epidemiology
c. Experimental epidemiology
d. Descriptive epidemiology

171. Which of the following type of research focused on finding a solution to an immediate practical problem?

a. Basic research b. Applied research
c. Explanatory research d. Descriptive research

172. Cohort study is also known as:

a. Prospective study b. Forward looking study
c. Incidence study d. All of these

173. The most objective approach to obtain nursing knowledge is through:

a. Experience b. Text books
c. Trial and error d. Scientific research

174. Relative risk is calculated in: *(ESIC 2019)*

a. Cross sectional study b. Cohort study
c. Case control study d. None of these

175. Which of the following is a type of prevalence rate?

a. Period prevalence b. Time prevalence
c. Duration prevalence d. Interval prevalence

176. The evidence to assert, whether or not, experimental treatment/condition has made the difference refers to: *(NCFL 2019)*

a. External validity b. Internal validity
c. Criterion validity d. Construct validity

Explanation: Internal validity is the validity refers to the extent in which the evidence supports the claim in regard to cause and effect, within the context of that study.
External validity refers to generalizability of the study findings across the situations, stimuli and people.

DATA COLLECTION METHODS

177. Which of the following is NOT a method of data collection? *(RAK MSc 2018)*

a. Interviews b. Experiments
c. Questionnaires d. Observations

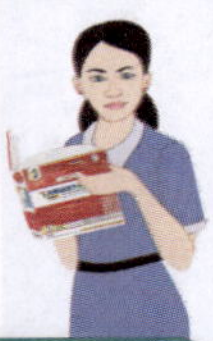

Ans.

154. b
155. a
156. b
157. b
158. d
159. a
160. b
161. b
162. d
163. b
164. b
165. d
166. b
167. b
168. b
169. d
170. d
171. b
172. d
173. d
174. b
175. a
176. b
177. b

Explanation: Observation, interview, questionnaires and bio-physiological measures are the common methods of data collection in research, whereas the term experiment refers to a type of research study.

178. Which of the following is NOT the element of an informed consent? *(Safdarjung NO 2018)*

a. Purpose of study
b. Offer answer only for selected questions
c. Subject selection process
d. Alternative procedures if any, are disclosed

Explanation: Informed consent is a voluntary agreement to participate in research. It is not merely a form that is signed but is an educational process, in which the subject has an understanding of the research and its risks. Offering answers only for selected questions will not complete the educational process of understanding of the research process.

Informed consent is essential before enrolling a participant and ongoing once enrolled.

The basic elements of the consent process include:

- Full disclosure of the nature of the research, **purpose of study** and the participant's involvement.
- **Subject selection process** and adequate comprehension on the part of the potential participant, and
- The participant's voluntary choice to participate.

179. Which of the following is an example of inductive reasoning?

a. Reasoning from all hypertensive patients to a single hypertensive patient
b. Reasoning from a single depressive patient to all depressive patients
c. Using a standard nursing care plan for a specific patient
d. All of the above

180. Study participants in a research study of quality of life (QOL) in Older Adults living in Nursing homes were asked to fill a questionnaire. Which of the following would be a likely assumption the researcher made in relation to this study?

a. Subjects will complete every item on the questionnaire
b. All older adults who are asked to fill the questionnaire will complete the questionnaire
c. Participants are able to identify a personal awareness of QOL
d. QOL is an important issue among older adults in living in nursing homes

181. In the review of literature report of a study on elder abuse, the researcher stated two previous studies suggesting that older persons aged above 80 years are more likely to be abused than older persons aged less than 80 years. This information suggests the current study is significant because it:

a. Influences policy making on older persons
b. Challenges existing evidence on elder abuse
c. Builds on previous research
d. Addresses multidisciplinary concerns on elder abuse

182. Which of the following is TRUE?

a. Problem statement is why study is being done
b. Research purpose is what will be examined in the study
c. Research questions provide greater focus to research
d. Research feasibility ignores the money aspect

183. A researcher is planned to study mistreatment of older persons. The research designs the study where data collection is to be conducted at older person's home. Which type of setting is this?

a. Partially controlled, clinical
b. Highly controlled, clinical
c. Natural, field
d. Highly controlled, field

184. Which of the following is the criteria of primary source of literature?

a. Interview based primary data only
b. Record based data
c. Original articles published in a journal
d. Meta-analysis data published in a journal

185. A critical aspect of beginning a database search for relevant literature on a topic of interest involves identifying:

a. Reference management software
b. Electronic journals
c. Keywords
d. Existing knowledge

186. A method of data collection in which several rounds of questionnaires are mailed to a panel of experts, focusing on their opinions or judgment concerning a specific topic of interest is:

a. Focus group interview
b. Meta-analysis
c. Delphi technique
d. Systematic analysis

187. A survey measuring individuals across a period of time is called:

a. Longitudinal Survey
b. Cross-sectional Survey
c. Intervention Survey
d. Experimental Survey

188. Which of the following statement is true about cross-sectional survey study?

a. High in internal validity and low in reliability
b. High in reliability but low in internal validity
c. High in reliability and internal validity
d. Low in reliability and internal validity

189. Which type of validity of any test/tool is determined by comparing it with a Gold Standard?

a. Content validity
b. Criterion validity
c. Concurrent Validity
d. Construct validity

190. The terms repeatability, precision, reproducibility, and consistency are used to indicate:

a. Validity
b. Sensitivity
c. Specificity
d. Reliability

191. A Likert scale is best described as a list of:

a. Open-ended items (questions) with unlimited responses
b. Closed-ended items with a fixed number of alternative responses
c. Open-and closed-ended items with variable responses
d. Closed-ended items with a dichotomous response

192. The degree with which all items on a scale measure the same variable is:

a. Validity
b. Equivalence
c. Homogeneity
d. Stability

193. Reliability is mostly a matter of ____________, while validity is mostly about.

a. Consistency, accuracy
b. Accuracy, consistency
c. Similarity, dissimilarity
d. Similarity, consistency

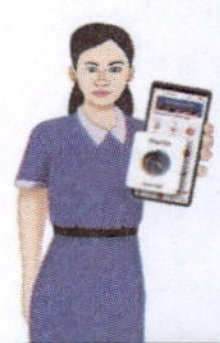

Ans.

178.	b
179.	b
180.	c
181.	c
182.	c
183.	c
184.	c
185.	c
186.	c
187.	a
188.	b
189.	b
190.	d
191.	b
192.	c
193.	a

194. The degree to which the researcher feels that this was a worthwhile project is known as:
a. Reliability
b. Internal validity
c. External validity
d. Concurrent validity

195. Cronbach's α measure of reliability indicates which of the following characteristics of a research tool:
a. Equivalency reliability
b. Stability reliability
c. Internal consistency
d. Inter-rater reliability

196. Which of the following procedures used to derive the stability index of a research tool?
a. Inter-rater reliability
b. Internal consistency
c. Cronbach's alpha
d. Test-retest reliability

197. The adequacy of an instrument in differentiating between the performance or behavior on some future criterion is termed as:
a. Predictive validity
b. Concurrent validity
c. Content validity
d. Construct validity

198. Which of the following is considered as a threat to internal validity of a research?
a. The Hawthorne effect
b. Maturation effect
c. Experimenter effects
d. All of these

199. Which of the following data collection method is most reliable?
a. Self-reports
b. Observation
c. Biophysiologic measures
d. Questionnaires

200. Identify the correct sequence of data collection:
a. Contact, inform, consent, collect
b. Contact, consent, inform, collect
c. Inform, contact, consent, collect
d. Contact, inform, collect, consent

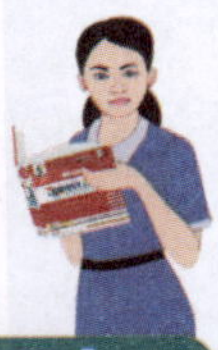

201. In research, Maturation threat is a threat to:
a. External validity
b. Internal validity
c. Factor validity
d. Content validity

202. The term which refers to the extent to which the results of the study can be generalized to the larger population:
a. Internal validity
b. Predictive validity
c. External validity
d. Content validity

203. An approach to construct validity that involves assessing the degree to which two methods of measuring a construct are similar is referred as:
a. Discriminant validity
b. Concurrent validity
c. Convergent validity
d. Divergent validity

204. The degree to which scores of an instrument are correlated with some external criterion measured at the same time:
a. Factor validity
b. Construct validity
c. Content validity
d. Concurrent validity

205. The criteria for validity of a screening test is:
a. Accuracy
b. Predictability
c. Sensitivity and specificity
d. Cost effectiveness

206. Internal consistency measures include:
a. Split-half reliability
b. Kuder-Richardson coefficient
c. Cronbach's alpha
d. All of the above

207. A statistical measure of inter-rater reliability is:
a. Cohen's Kappa
b. Cronbach's α
c. Kuder-Richardson coefficient
d. Odds-ratio

208. Which of the following differentiate true experimental research from quasi-experimental research?
a. Manipulation of independent variable
b. Use of non-probability sampling technique
c. Random allocation of subjects to groups
d. Large sample size

209. The power analysis is used to determine _______ in quantitative research studies.
a. The level of significance
b. The sample size
c. The Internal validity
d. The reliability

210. In qualitative research, the sample size is determined by:
a. Power analysis
b. The 'rule of 30'
c. The 'rule of 60'
d. Data saturation

211. The reliability that indicates the consistency of test scores over time is referred to:
a. Parallel form reliability
b. Inter-rater reliability
c. Test-retest reliability
d. Internal consistency

212. All of the following are type of reliability; EXCEPT:
a. Inter-rater
b. Internal consistency
c. Concurrency
d. Test-retest

213. The validity that refers to the extent to which a measure is related to an outcome is:
a. Convergent validity
b. Expert validity
c. Criterion-related validity
d. Content reliability

214. The consistency of measurement based on the correlation between scores on two similar forms of the same test taken by the same subject is known as:
a. Test-retest reliability
b. Equivalent forms reliability
c. Inter-rater reliability
d. Internal consistency

215. Which of the following is NOT an advantage of the observation method?
a. There is no recall bias provided it is planned
b. It provides direct information about behavior of the individuals and groups
c. It permits evaluators to enter into and understand circumstances/context
d. It introduces the subjective bias

216. A method in which several rounds of questions are given to a panel of experts is called:
a. Q-methodology
b. Meta-analysis
c. Delphi technique
d. Content analysis

217. When constructing a questionnaire which of the following is NOT one of the principle?
a. Do not use "leading" or "loaded" questions
b. Avoid double barreled questions
c. Avoid double negative questions
d. Avoid using multiple items to measure single construct

218. The interview technique that allows the questions to emerge from the immediate context or course of things is known as:
a. Structured quantitative interview
b. Formal interview guide approach
c. Informal conversational interview
d. Standardized open-ended interview

Ans.

194. b
195. c
196. d
197. a
198. d
199. c
200. a
201. b
202. c
203. c
204. d
205. c
206. d
207. a
208. c
209. b
210. d
211. c
212. c
213. c
214. b
215. d
216. c
217. d
218. c

219. A nurse researcher get herself transferred to pediatric ICU (PICU) to be able to observe and collect data from nurses of PICU on needle stick injury. The researcher is using the role of:
a. Participant-as-observer b. Complete participant
c. Complete observer d. Formal observer

220. Qualitative data analysis requires the categorization and indexing of texts or videos. The labels that are given to sections of the text and video material are known as:
a. Data points b. Memos
c. Data codes d. Units of analysis

221. The discussion section is characterized by which one of the followings?
a. The researcher's reporting of the statistical results.
b. A brief conclusion and description of statistical tests
c. Repeating all of the literature listed in the literature review
d. The researcher's interpretation of the results.

222. In which section the reporting accuracy of numerical information is most critical?
a. Discussion b. Review of literature
c. Limitations d. Results

223. Identify the correct order of a quantitative research report?
a. Literature review, results, methods, discussion
b. Literature review, methods, results, discussion
c. Discussion, Literature review, methods, results
d. Methods, results, literature review, discussion

224. Which of the followings is in a research report but not in a proposal?
a. Title page b. Abstract
c. Findings d. Supporting material

225. Which of the following parts of a journal article is read the most?
a. Results b. Discussion
c. Introduction d. Abstract

226. Ideally the abstract of the research article should be limited to:
a. 100 words b. 100–150 words
c. 150–250 words d. 250–500 words

227. Which of the following communication channel is appropriate for dissemination of research finding to largest target group?
a. Thesis/dissertation
b. Oral or poster presentation in conference
c. Newsletter
d. Scientific Journal articles

228. Which of the following statement is true about 95% Confidence Interval (CI)?
a. 95% probability the population parameter lies within the interval
b. 95% probability the population parameter lies outside the interval
c. 5% probability the population parameter lies within the interval
d. All of the above statements are true

229. In exclusive type of class interval the value 30 will be put under:
a. 20-30 b. 30-40
c. Either A or B d. Both A and B

230. The Census is conducted once in every:
a. 5 years b. 8 years
c. 10 years d. 15 years

231. Coding, data reduction, theme, and data saturation are the terms associated with:
a. Quantitative study b. Qualitative study
c. Cross-over study d. Randomized control trial

Explanation: Coding refers to break down and labeling of large amounts of data. Data reduction means using coding to reduce data. Theme is abstract idea or concept. Data saturation means information gets redundant. The above said terms are associated with qualitative research studies.

SAMPLE & SAMPLING TECHNIQUES

232. Probability sampling includes all the following techniques; EXCEPT: *(AIIMS Raipur NO 2019)*
a. Systematic sampling b. Simple random sampling
c. Purposive sampling d. Cluster sampling

Explanation: Purposive sampling or judgmental sampling is a non-probability sampling technique. Subjects are chosen with a specific purpose in mind. **Example:** A study is focused on the victims of a sexual assault. Purposive sampling technique is used to find and collect the subjects who were victims of sexual assault.

Other options are type of probability sampling technique where each of the subject in the population gets equal chance to be selected as a sample.

233. From which of these populations does a researcher select the actual study samples? *(Daman & Diu NO 2018)*
a. Accessible b. Target
c. Universal d. Scientific

Explanation: **Accessible population:** The aggregate of individuals who are accessible to the researcher from which the samples are selected for the research study. In simple words, it is a population the researchers get access for study. Target population refers to aggregate of individuals to which the researcher wants to generalize the findings of research study.

234. A researcher is using random sampling method to decrease the sampling bias in a research study. This is done to achieve:
a. Manipulation
b. Data collection
c. Control
d. Encourage participation of subjects

235. Which of the following level of evidence is placed at the top of the hierarchy of evidence? New Q
a. A consensus of opinion from experts of the subject
b. Meta-analysis of multiple randomized clinical trials
c. Results from a single well-controlled experimental study with a large sample size
d. Results from a well-designed cohort studies

236. Theoretical sampling is considered as a critical feature of:
a. Grounded theory b. RCT
c. Methodological design d. Developmental research

237. The process of selecting a small group from a larger group is known as:
a. Triangulation
b. Cross matching
c. Sampling
d. Trimming

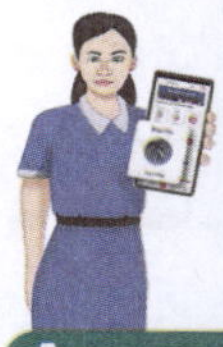

Ans.

219.	a
220.	b
221.	d
222.	d
223.	b
224.	c
225.	d
226.	c
227.	d
228.	a
229.	b
230.	c
231.	b
232.	c
233.	a
234.	c
235.	b
236.	a
237.	c

238. Whole group of people or objects to which the researcher wishes to generalize the study findings and which meet a set of criteria of interest to researcher is known as:

a. Study population b. Sample population
c. Target population d. Sampling frame

239. Which of the following is NOT TRUE of probability sampling technique?

a. Each unit has an equal chance of selection
b. Generate unbiased estimation of population
c. Produce a sample that resembles population as closely as possible
d. Avoids use of sampling frame

240. All of the following are random sampling methods; EXCEPT:

a. Snow ball sampling b. Simple random sampling
c. Stratified sampling d. Cluster sampling

241. Which is TRUE of the stratified random sampling technique as compared to Simple Random Sampling (SRS)?

a. It is used for homogenous population
b. It is less accurate than simple random sampling.
c. It is time consuming
d. Its analysis is easier than simple random sampling.

242. A sample in which each element has an equal likelihood of inclusion is a:

a. Biased sample b. Snowball sample
c. Probability sample d. Quota sample

243. A sample which involves a random start and then proceeds with every kth element from then onwards is:

a. Simple random sampling
b. Stratified random sampling
c. Systematic sampling
d. Snowball sampling

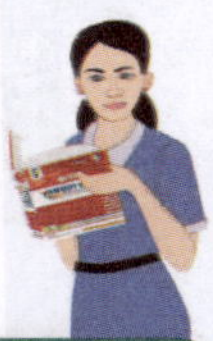

244. Which of the following sampling methods is the best way to select a group of people for a study if one is interested in generalizing it to the larger population?

a. Convenience sampling
b. Quota sampling
c. Purposive sampling
d. Random sampling

245. Which of the following is NOT a form of non-probability sampling?

a. Snowball sampling b. Convenience sampling
c. Quota sampling d. Systematic sampling

246. A type of non-probability sampling is:

a. Simple random b. Systematic
c. Purposive d. Cluster

247. Cluster sampling technique is also known as:

a. Simple random sampling b. Multistage sampling
c. Quota sampling d. Snow ball sampling

248. Snowball sampling is also known as:

a. Chain sampling b. Cluster sampling
c. Quota sampling d. Stratified sampling

249. A non-probability sampling technique where research participants recruit other participants?

a. Stratified b. Convenience
c. Cluster d. Snowball

250. In a study to establish "Relationship between hypertension and cardiac disease", the participants are the inpatients of a Cardiac Clinic, who are willing to participate in the study. The 'Sampling Technique' should be:

a. Convenience sampling b. Simple random sampling
c. Stratified sampling d. Cluster sampling

251. When each member of a population has an equal probability of being selected for a sample, it is called:

a. Convenient sampling
b. Purposive sampling
c. Simple random sampling
d. Cluster sampling

252. For a research study, a total of 30 nursing faculties are randomly selected from a random sample of three nursing colleges in a region. This is an example of:

a. Simple random sampling
b. Cluster sampling
c. Purposive sampling
d. Snow ball sampling

253. A researcher has decided to assess blood pressure from all of the patients who attended the Medicine OPD over a month period of time. This is an example of:

a. Stratified random sampling
b. Snow ball sampling
c. Convenience sampling
d. Quota sampling

254. Which of the following is a non-probability sampling?

a. Cluster sampling b. Systematic sampling
c. Quota sampling d. All of these

255. Which of the following sampling technique is least likely to draw a representative sample from the population?

a. Cluster sampling
b. Convenience sampling
c. Systematic sampling
d. Stratified random sampling

256. On a given day a hospital had 50 admissions with about 20 girls and 30 boys, out of which 10 girls and 20 boys needed surgery. What is the probability of picking up a person requiring surgery?

a. 2/6 b. 3/5
c. 1/2 d. 6/25

Explanation: Out of 50 patients, 30 requires surgery. So, the probability of picking up a person requiring surgery from 50 is 30/50. It is equal to 3/5.

ETHICS IN RESEARCH

257. The principles of ethics in nursing research include:

a. Beneficence
b. Respect for human dignity
c. Justice
d. All of the above

258. Code of Ethics for Nurses in India is given by:

a. Indian Nursing Council
b. Nursing Research Society of India
c. Indian Professional Nurses Association
d. Trained Nurses Association of India

259. An explicit guarantee by a researcher to a subject whereby the subject is assured that any information provided to the researcher cannot be attributed back to that subject:

a. Anonymity b. Blinding
c. Confidentiality d. Confrontation

260. Which of the following term refers to the process of obtaining a 12-year-old child's agreement for participation in the study?

a. Informed assent b. Consent of a minor
c. Collateral consent d. Minor agreement

Ans.

238. c
239. d
240. a
241. c
242. c
243. c
244. d
245. d
246. c
247. b
248. a
249. d
250. a
251. c
252. b
253. c
254. c
255. b
256. b
257. d
258. a
259. c
260. a

261. Which one is not the Fundamental guiding principles of ethics?
a. Respect for patient and their autonomy
b. Maleficence
c. Beneficence
d. Justice

262. Which of the following is not required in consent form?
a. Address of researcher b. Name of researcher
c. Phone no. of the researcher d. Income of the researcher

TYPES OF DATA

263. A method of integrating the findings of prior research studies using statistical procedures is:
a. Meta-analysis b. Content analysis
c. Secondary analysis d. Systematic analysis

264. Which of the following is a characteristic of a qualitative research?
a. Deductive process b. Inductive process
c. Fixed research design d. Manipulation

265. Which of the following design is involved in Qualitative research?
a. Emergent design b. Comparative design
c. Prospective cohort d. Quasi design

266. The guiding principle to decide sample size in qualitative research is:
a. Data saturation b. Number of variables
c. Power of the study d. Theme identification

267. The method of deriving a complex array of data from a variety of sources, using variety of methods in qualitative research is referred as:
a. Triangulation b. Bricolage
c. Verification d. Cross-analysis

Explanation: In qualitative research, triangulation refers to the process of collecting and analyzing data from multiple sources and using various methods to gain a more comprehensive and accurate understanding of the research topic. It involves combining different data collection techniques, such as interviews, observations, and document analysis, and comparing findings from different sources to validate and corroborate the results.

268. Which of the following is involved in quantitative research?
a. Phenomenology b. Ethnography
c. Clinical trial d. Grounded theory

269. A process that renders data into numbers that can be entered into a database is:
a. Matrixing b. Coding
c. Transcribing d. Editing

270. Which of the following terms best describes data which was originally collected at an earlier time by a different person for a different purpose?
a. Primary data b. Secondary data
c. Experimental data d. Basic data

271. Secondary data may include which of the following?
a. Official documents b. Personal documents
c. Archived research data d. All of these

272. Open-ended questions provide primarily which of the following type of data?
a. Confirmatory data b. Qualitative data
c. Predictive data d. None of these

273. The process of transforming qualitative research data from written or tape recorded interviews into typed text is called:
a. Segmenting b. Coding
c. Transcription d. Memoing

VARIABLES & SCALES OF MEASUREMENTS

274. The extent (or degree) to which a tool measures what it is supposed to measure is known as? *(Daman & Diu NO 2018)*
a. Reliability b. Validity
c. Specificity d. Stability

Explanation: Validity is the extent to which an instrument or test or tool measures what it is supposed to measure. An instrument is said to be valid if it measures what the researcher intends to measure.
Reliability refers to the consistency of measurement.

275. The accuracy and consistency in measurement of an instrument refers to: *(AIIMS Raipur NO 2019)*
a. Validity b. Analysis
c. Appropriability d. Reliability

276. The degree of consistency with which an instrument measures the attribute it is supposed to be measuring is called:
a. Validity b. Reliability
c. Sensitivity d. Objectivity

Explanation: **Reliability** refers to degree of consistency or accuracy with which an instrument measures for which it is designed to measure.
Validity: Degree to which an instrument measures what it is intended to measure.
Analysis: Method of organizing, sorting, scrutinizing data to answer research question.
Appropriability is a distractor.

277. The purpose statement of a research study should identify the study variable(s) and:
a. Design of the study b. Data collection tools
c. Statistical methods d. Population

278. Likert scale is:
a. Ordinal scale b. Normal scale
c. Variance scale d. Categorical scale

279. In research, how a variable or concept will be defined and measured in the study is termed as:
a. Assumption b. Hypothesis
c. Operational definition d. None of these

280. The statement below is an example of which of the following? "In this study, patient satisfaction is reflected as a score between 0 and 100 on nursing care satisfaction scale":
a. Problem statement b. Assumption
c. Associative hypothesis d. Operational definition

281. All of the following are component of a research hypothesis; EXCEPT:
a. Independent variables b. Dependent variables
c. Study population d. Extraneous variables

282. Which of the following variable can be measured on a nominal scale?
a. Height of the patient in cm
b. IQ score of the patient
c. Gender of the patient
d. Hemoglobin level of the patient

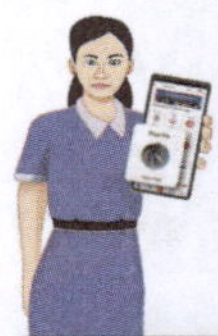

Ans.
261. b
262. d
263. a
264. b
265. a
266. a
267. a
268. c
269. b
270. b
271. d
272. b
273. c
274. b
275. d
276. b
277. d
278. a
279. c
280. d
281. d
282. c

283. Marital Status and religion are measured on:
a. Nominal scale of measurement
b. Ordinal scale of measurement
c. Interval scale of measurement
d. Ratio scale of measurement

284. Which of the following scale of measurement has an absolute zero?
a. Nominal b. Ordinal
c. Interval d. Ratio

285. Which of the following scale of measurement is appropriate to measure the weight (in kg) of the patient?
a. Ordinal scale b. Nominal scale
c. Ratio scale d. Interval scale

286. Measurement of body temperature is an example of:
a. Physiological measurement
b. Biological measurement
c. Biophysical measurement
d. All of the above

287. Age is an example of:
a. Continuous variable b. Discrete variable
c. Categorical variable d. Nominal variable

288. Gender is an example of:
a. Dichotomous variable
b. Discrete variable
c. Ordinal variable
d. Quantitative variable

289. Which of the following variables is measured on the ordinal scale?
a. Type of anemia b. Severity of anemia
c. Hemoglobin in gm% d. Serum ferritin level

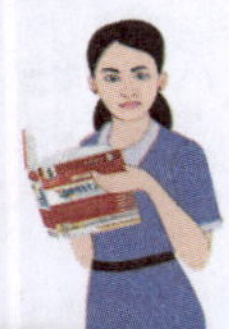

290. Which of the following is an example of dichotomous variable? *(AIIMS M.Sc Nursing Entrance 2008)*
a. Age b. Gender
c. Educational status d. Occupation

291. The term which refers to the validity of a research in which the difference in the dependent variable is actually a result of the independent variable:
a. Construct validity b. Conclusion validity
c. Internal validity d. External validity

292. Which of the following could not be measured directly?
a. Blood pressure b. Hope
c. Temperature d. Weight

293. In Vancouver's style of reference writing, et al. is used if the author number exceeds:
a. 1 b. 2
c. 6 d. 7

294. A coefficient of correlation value of "r = +0.8" indicates:
a. Strong direct relationship between two variables
b. Strong inverse relationship between two variables
c. Insignificant association between two variables
d. One variable is the cause of the other variable

295. Type of graphical presentation data used to explain correlation between dependent and independent variable is:
a. Bar diagram
b. Histogram
c. Scatter plot
d. Frequency polygon

296. Which of the following scale of measurement has an absolute zero? *(RAK MSc 2018)*
a. Nominal b. Ordinal
c. Interval d. Ratio

Ans.

283. a
284. d
285. c
286. d
287. a
288. a
289. b
290. b
291. c
292. b
293. c
294. a
295. c
296. d
297. a
298. b
299. c
300. c

Explanation:

- **Ratio scale:** This scale has a constant interval and a true zero point. Example: height, weight, hemoglobin level.
- **Interval scale:** It has equal unit with an arbitrary zero point. There is a natural order that exists, no absolute zero and has negative value. Example: Fahrenheit scale of temperature, pH and intelligence score.
- **Nominal scale:** Categorical scale with non-numerical characteristics, e.g., gender, blood group, religion, etc.
- **Ordinal scale:** These variables are dealt with their relative differences rather than with quantitative differences. The data can be ordered, e.g., mild, moderate, severe.

297. Which measurement denotes subjects from the heaviest to the lightest? *(AIIMS Raipur NO 2019)*
a. Ordinal b. Ratio
c. Nominal d. Interval

Explanation:

- Ordinal level ranks objects based on their relative standing on a specific attribute. Ordinal scale is that reports the ranking and ordering of the data without actually establishing the degree of variation between them.
  Example: Income: low, middle, upper

298. Which of the following is an example of dichotomous variable? *(RAK MSc 2018)*
a. Age b. Gender
c. Educational status d. Occupation

Explanation:

- A dichotomous variable is a nominal variable that have only two categories or values. Among the given options, gender has only two categories, i.e., male and female.
- Age is a continuous (quantitative) variable which can take any number of values.
- Educational status and occupation are considered as categorical variables but can take more than two values.
  Clue: 'Di' means two. Dichotomous variables have only two levels in the category.

299. Which is the point on a numerical scale above which and below which 50% of cases falls? *(AIIMS Raipur NO 2019)*
a. Central Tendency b. Mode
c. Median d. Mean

Explanation:

- **Median** is the middle most value when data is arranged in ascending order of magnitude. The middle value divides the number of observation in the data into two equal parts. M = n + 1/2
- **Mean:** Most commonly used, it is sum of all the values, divided by number of values.
- **Mode**: Value which has the highest frequency.
- Mean, median and mode are the parameters of central tendency.

300. Correlation is a method used to determine if:
a. Variable X Causes variable Y
b. Variable Y causes variable X
c. Variable X and Y vary together
d. Variable X and Y are parallel

301. A researcher reported the correlation between variables X and Y is r = 0.6. Which of the following interpretation is correct?
- a. The X-variable explains 60% of the variability in the Y-variable.
- b. The X-variable explains 40% of the variability in the Y-variable.
- c. The X-variable causes negative changes in 60% of the Y-variable.
- d. The X-variable is equal to 60% of the Y-variable.

302. Statistical procedure that is used to predict the value of a dependent variable based on the value of one or more independent variable is known as:
- a. Repeated measures ANOVA
- b. Regression analysis
- c. General linear model
- d. Q-Sort Analysis

303. A systematic method for continuous monitoring of diseases in a population, in order to be able to detect changes in disease patterns and then to control them is:
- a. Surveillance
- b. Conditional probability
- c. Screening
- d. Prevalence

304. Incidence Rate as a measure of morbidity includes the occurrence of:
- a. All old cases of disease
- b. All new cases of disease
- c. All old and new cases of disease
- d. All of the above

305. Comparative values between two amounts is called as:
- a. Ratio
- b. Coefficient
- c. Variance
- d. None of these

306. All of the following are quantitative variables; EXCEPT:
- a. Serum cholesterol
- b. Weight
- c. Gender
- d. Celsius temperature scale

307. Study title: "The effects of gender and smoking habits compared to amount of dental caries are the:
- a. Constant variable
- b. Independent variable
- c. Dependent variable
- d. Extraneous variable

CENTRAL TENDENCIES

308. The value of highest frequency in the data is: *(AIIMS Nagpur NO 2018)*
- a. Mode
- b. Mean
- c. Standard deviation
- d. Median

Explanation: **Mode** is the number which appears most often (Highest frequency) in a set of numbers.

Example: in {6, 3, 9, 6, 6, 5, 9, 3} the Mode is 6 (it occurs most often).

309. Identify the mode of the following values: *(RAK MSc 2018)*
6, 3, 5, 6, 8, 9, 4, 6, 7, 6, 8, 6
- a. 3
- b. 8
- c. 6
- d. 7

Explanation: Dataset: 6, 3, 5, 6, 8, 9, 4, 6, 7, 6, 8, 6

Step 1: Arrange it in an ascending order
3, 4, 5, 6, 6, 6, 6, 6, 7, 8, 8, 9

Step 2: Identify the most frequently occurred value in the dataset
Value '6' repeated 5 times in the given dataset.

So, the mode is '6'.

310. The measure of central tendency that represents the score most occurring in a distribution of scores is called: *(RAK MSc 2018)*
- a. Mean
- b. Mode
- c. Variable
- d. Median

Explanation: The mode is the most frequently occurring score value in a given dataset.
- For example, in the following dataset
- 5, 8, 12, 13, 15, 15, 15, 16, 16, 18 19
- 15 is the most frequently occurring value (3 times). So, number 15 is considered as mode in this dataset.
- Mean is the average of a given dataset.
- Median is a middle value of a given dataset.
- Variable is defined as any value which varies and is not related to central tendency.

311. Which of the following is the formula for range? *(RAK MSc 2018)*
- a. H + L
- b. L × H
- c. L − H
- d. H − L

Explanation: Range is a measure dispersion of a dataset. The **range** of a set of data is the difference between the highest and lowest values in the set. To find the **range**, first order the data from least to greatest. Then subtract the smallest (L) value from the largest value (H) in the set. It is given in formula as H-L.

Example:
Question: Calculate range for a given data set: 9, 8, 5, 3, 6, 11, 13, 18.
Answer:
Step 1: arrange it in ascending order
i.e. 3, 5, 6, 8, 9, 11, 13, 18
Highest value (H) = 18
Lowest value (L) = 3
Range = H - L
Range = 18- 3 = 15

312. Identify the mode of the following series: 6, 3, 5, 6, 7, 8, 9, 4, 3, 6, 6, 8, 9, 6.
- a. 3
- b. 6
- c. 8
- d. 9

313. Calculate the mean of 2, 4, 5, 6, 7.
- a. 4.2
- b. 4.4
- c. 4.6
- d. 4.8

314. What is the median of the following ungrouped data: 18, 6, 12, 10, 14, 5, 9?
- a. 10
- b. 9
- c. 12
- d. 18

315. The measure of central tendency measures the following characteristic:
- a. Dispersion
- b. Asymmetry
- c. Average
- d. Spread

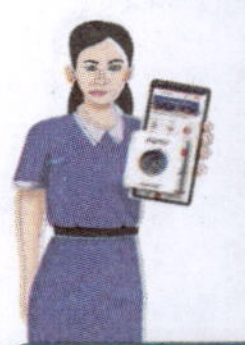

Ans.

301.	a
302.	b
303.	a
304.	b
305.	a
306.	c
307.	c
308.	a
309.	c
310.	b
311.	d
312.	b
313.	d
314.	a
315.	c

316. If mean is less than the median, then the data is said to be:
a. Positively skewed
b. Negatively skewed
c. Equitable distribution
d. Normal distribution

317. Which of the following is true about a negatively skewed data distribution?
a. Mean < median < Mode
b. Mode > median > Mean
c. Median > Mean > Mode
d. Mean = Median = Mode

318. 50th percentile is equivalent to:
a. Mean b. Median
c. Mode d. Range

319. The proportion of observations fall above the median is:
a. 60% b. 50%
c. 75% d. 95%

320. A measure of central tendency which is calculated by numbers arranged in ascending or descending order is:
a. Standard deviation b. Range
c. Median d. Mode

321. Which measure of central tendency is Influenced by extreme scores and skewed distributions?
a. Mean b. Median
c. Mode d. Range

322. Which of the following measures of central tendency is most appropriate to be considered when the data has significant variability?
a. The Mean b. The Median
c. The Mode d. Variance

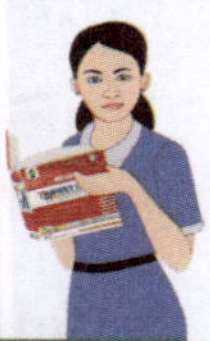

323. The measure of central tendency that represents the score most occurring in a distribution of scores is called:
a. Mean b. Mode
c. Variable d. Medium

324. The measure of Central Tendency that represents the exact middle of a set of scores is:
a. Mode
b. Mean
c. Normal Distribution
d. Median

325. The Measure of Central Tendency that is computed by summing all the scores of a study and dividing by the number of subjects is called the:
a. Medium b. Mode
c. Normal Distribution d. Mean

326. The most frequently occurring number in a set of values is called the:
a. Variance b. Mean
c. Mode d. Median

327. The measure of central tendency that is preferred when the data is severely skewed is:
a. Mean b. Mode
c. Median d. Variance

328. The mean and standard deviation (SD) for following data: 12, 16, 18, 14, 10, 20 *New Q*
a. 15 and 3.7, respectively
b. 14 and 3.4, respectively
c. 15 and 2.7, respectively
d. 14 and 2.7, respectively

Explanation:

Data Set: 12, 16, 18, 14, 10, 20

- **Step 1:** Calculate the mean
  Mean (Average) = Sum of all values/Total number of values
  Mean = (12 + 16 + 18 + 14 + 10 + 20)/6 = 90/6 = 15
- **Step 2:** Calculate the differences between each value and the mean, and square the differences.
  2–15 = –3
  16–15 = 1
  18–15 = 3
  14–15 = –1
  10–15 = –5
  20–15 = 5
  Square each difference:
  (–3)*2 = 9
  1*2 = 1
  3*2 = 9
  (–1)*2 = 1
  (–5)*2 = 25
  5*2 = 25
  Sum of ((X - Mean)*2) = 9 + 1 + 9 + 1 + 25 + 25 = 70
- **Step 3:** Calculate the variance using the n-1 formula
  Variance = Sum of ((X – Mean)^2) / (N – 1)
  Variance = 70 / (6 – 1) = 70 / 5 = 14
- **Step 4:** Calculate the standard deviation using the square root of the variance
  SD = Square root of the Variance
  SD = Square root of 14 ≈ 3.74

Therefore, the standard deviation (SD) for the given data set is approximately 3.7.

329. The best measure of central tendency in a normally distributed continuous data is:
a. Mean
b. Median
c. Mode
d. Range

330. Median of the following data will be: 10, 9, 8, 12, 8, 7, 5:
a. 8.75 b. 8
c. 9 d. 10

331. Mean, Medium and Mode are:
a. Measure of dispersion
b. Measure association between two variables
c. Test of significance
d. Measure of central tendency

VARIATION & SHAPE IN DATA DISTRIBUTION

332. Linear relationship between two quantitative (continuous) variables can be best presented by:
a. Frequency polygon
b. Scatter plot diagram
c. Histogram
d. Pie diagram

333. The characteristics of an ideal curve is/are:
a. It is bell shaped
b. Mean, median and mode do not coincide
c. It is asymmetrical around the mean
d. All of the above

Ans.

316.	b
317.	a
318.	b
319.	b
320.	c
321.	a
322.	b
323.	b
324.	d
325.	d
326.	c
327.	c
328.	a
329.	a
330.	b
331.	d
332.	b
333.	a

334. Which of the following is a measure of dispersion? *(Daman & Diu NO 2018)*

a. Mean b. Mode
c. Standard deviation d. Median

Explanation: The measures of dispersion refers to variation among the values in the given set of data. The most commonly used measures of dispersion are range, mean deviation and standard deviation. Other options given are parameters of central tendencies.

335. Spread of dispersion is expressed by: *(AIIMS Jodhpur SNO 2018)*

a. Mean b. SD
c. Mode d. Median

336. Relationship between weight in kg and height in cm can be showed in: *(AIIMS Jodhpur SNO 2018)*

a. Bar diagram b. Scattered plot
c. Histogram d. Pie chart

337. Correlation is strongest: *(AIIMS Jodhpur SNO 2018)*

a. – 1.00 b. – 0.95
c. + 0.90 d. + 0.10

338. The square root of the variance is:

a. Standard deviation b. Standard error
c. Z Score d. Variance

339. Which of the following is NOT a measure of variability?

a. Median b. Variance
c. Standard deviation d. Range

340. Which of the following is NOT a measure of dispersion?

a. Variance b. Mode
c. Standard deviation d. Range

341. The degree of flatness or peakedness of a graph of a frequency distribution is termed as:

a. Kurtosis b. Skewness
c. Standard deviation d. Variance

342. Standard deviation is a measure of:

a. Chance
b. Central tendency
c. Deviation from mean value
d. None of these

343. Probability values fall on scale between:

a. 0 and 1
b. –1 to +1
c. 0.001 to 1
d. 0.05 to 0.001

344. Which of the following is a measure of dispersion?

a. Mean
b. Median
c. Mode
d. Variance

345. A large standard deviations in a data set suggest that:

a. Scores are probably widely scattered.
b. There is very little difference among scores.
c. Mean, median and mode are the same
d. The scores are normally distributed.

346. Which measure of dispersion is best suited for comparing the variability between two normally distributed data sets? *New Q*

a. Range
b. Interquartile range
c. Standard deviation
d. Weighted mean

Explanation: The measure of dispersion that is best suited for comparing the variability between two normally distributed data sets is the standard deviation. The standard deviation provides a measure of the average deviation of data points from the mean and takes into account the entire distribution of values. The range and interquartile range only consider the extremes or the central portion of the data, respectively, hence suitable for non-parametric distribution. The weighted mean is a measure of central tendency and does not directly assess variability.

347. Which of the following is not a characteristic of normal distribution?

a. Symmetric b. Bell-shaped
c. Mean = median = mode d. Negative skewness

348. A statistic which describes the interval of scores bounded by the 25th and 75th percentile ranks is:

a. Inter quartile range b. Confidence Interval
c. Range d. Variance

349. X is the symbol of:

a. Median b. Mode
c. Mean d. Range

350. In a normal distribution curve, how many percentage of the data (area) fall within two standard deviation of the mean:

a. 68.2% b. 90.6%
c. 95.4% d. 99.6%

351. In a normally distributed data, approximately what percentage of score fall within one standard deviation of the mean?

a. 34% b. 68%
c. 95.4% d. 99.6%

352. All of the following are the measures of dispersion; EXCEPT:

a. Variance b. Median
c. Standard deviation d. Range

353. Which among the following is not a characteristics of a Normal probability curve? *New Q*
(AIIMS MG, Faculty Entrance 2022)

a. It is a bell shaped curve
b. Mean = Median = Mode
c. The curve is asymptotic
d. Normal curve is platykurtic

Explanation:

- A platykurtic distribution has a lower peak and wider bell shape. It will also have longer and shorter tails than a normal distribution.
- **Characteristics of Normal probability curve include:**
  - It is a bell shaped curve.
  - The curve is symmetric at the center (i.e., around the mean).
  - The curve is asymptotic. "**Asymptotic** to the x axis" means that a function or curve is approaching the x axis

354. The two most important parameters used for describing a normally distributed continuous variable are:

a. Mean and standard deviation
b. Median and Range
c. Mean and Variance
d. Median and standard deviation

355. Regression line is used to:

a. Determine if any x-values are outliers
b. Determine if any y-values are outliers
c. Estimate the change in y for every ten unit change in x
d. Estimate the change in y for a one-unit change in x

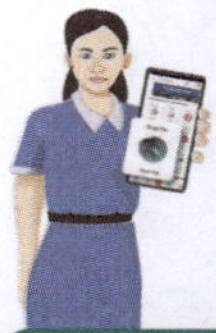

Ans.

334. c
335. b
336. b
337. a
338. a
339. a
340. b
341. a
342. c
343. a
344. d
345. a
346. c
347. d
348. a
349. c
350. c
351. b
352. b
353. d
354. a
355. d

356. Correlation is measured between:

a. –1 to +1 b. 0 to 1
c. 0 to –1 d. 0.001 to 0.05

357. Which of the following correlation coefficients would indicate the strongest relationship between anxiety and exam performance?

a. r = 0.50 b. r = –0.50
c. r = –0.55 d. r = –1.20

358. Which of the following statement is NOT TRUE about confidence intervals (CI)?

a. The intervals give a range of values within which the true value will lie
b. A 95% confidence interval has a 0.95 probability of containing the population mean
c. A 95% confidence interval does not mean that 95% of the sample data lie within the interval
d. The intervals give estimation about relationship between two variables with 95% confidence

359. Confidence Interval (CI) will be the widest for a particular data set if it is calculated for:

a. 50% CI b. 90% CI
c. 95% CI d. 99% CI

360. 95% confidence interval refers to:

a. Considering 1 out of 20 chances are taken to be wrong.
c. Considering 95 out of 100 chances are taken as wrong
b. Considering 1 out of 100 chances are taken as wrong.
d. Considering 5 out of 20 chances are taken as wrong.

361. Which of the following value of Relative Risk indicates the strong association between cause and effect?

a. 1 b. –1
c. 0 d. None of these

362. In a normally distributed area, how much of the sample is included in 1.95 SD?

a. 99% b. 95%
c. 68% d. 65%

363. A normal distribution curve depends on:

a. Mean and sample size
b. Range and sample size
c. Mean and standard deviation
d. Median and Range

364. If r = 1.20 it means:

a. Strong positive correlation
b. Negative correlation
c. No correlation
d. It is a wrong statement

Explanation: Correlation (r) ranges from –1 to +1 where –1 corresponds to perfect negative correlation and +1 corresponds to perfect positive correlation. So, there is no possibility of r = 1.2, hence, it is a wrong statement.

365. Attributable risk means:

a. Fatality of a disease
b. Disease risk ratio between exposed and non-exposed
c. Risk difference between exposed and non-exposed
d. Communicability of a disease

366. Effect size is used to calculate:

a. Reliability b. Sample size
c. Internal consistency d. Predictive validity

367. Strong correlation is signified by a correlation coefficient of:

a. Zero b. 1
c. <1 d. >1

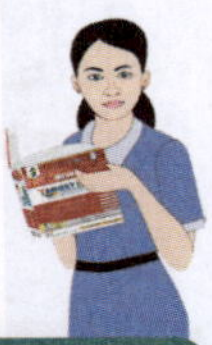

Ans.

356. a
357. c
358. d
359. d
360. a
361. a
362. b
363. c
364. d
365. c
366. b
367. b
368. b
369. b
370. b
371. b
372. b
373. a
374. a
375. d
376. b

368. Mosquito density decreases as height increases in:

a. Positive correlation b. Negative correlation
c. Bidirectional d. Zero correlation

369. In a study, variation in cholesterol was seen before and after giving a drug. The test which would give its significance is:

a. Unpaired t – test b. Paired t - test
c. Chi-square test d. Fisher test

370. Mean hemoglobin of a sample of 100 pregnant women was found to be 10 mg% with a SD of 1 mg%. The SE of the estimate would be:

a. 0.01 b. 0.1
c. 1 d. 10

Explanation: For a given sample size, the standard error equals the standard deviation divided by the square root of the sample size.

In this example,

SE = $\sqrt{SD/n}$
= $\sqrt{1/100}$
= $\sqrt{0.01}$
SE = 0.1

371. After applying a statistical test, an investigator gets the 'p value' as 0.01. It means that:

a. The probability of finding a significant difference is 1%
b. The probability of declaring a significant difference, when there is truly no difference, is 1%
c. The difference is not significant 1% times and significant 99% times
d. The power of the test used is 99%

372. Mean bone density amongst two groups of 50 people each is compared with each other. The test of significance used would be:

a. Paired 't' test b. Student 't' test
c. Analysis of variance d. Chi-Square test

373. When do the variables follow standard normal distribution?

a. Mean = Median
b. Median = Variance
c. Mean = 2 × Median
d. Standard deviation = 2 × variance normal curve

374. How much population falls between median and median plus one standard deviation in a normal distribution?

a. 0.34 b. 0.68
c. 0.17 d. 0.47

375. Measures of dispersion all; EXCEPT:

a. Range b. Mean or average deviation
c. Standard deviation d. Correlation and regression

376. A chest physician observed that the distribution of forced expiratory volume (FEV) in 300 smokers had a median value of 2.5 L with the 1st and 3rd quartiles being 1.5 & 4.5 L respectively. Based on this data now many persons in the sample are expected to have a FEV between 1.5 and 4.5 L:

a. 75 b. 150
c. 225 d. 300

Explanation: Median is 50th percentile. 1st and 3rd quartiles are 25th and 75th percentile respectively.

In the given question, sample size = 300.

So, participants between each quartile = 300/4
= 75

Participants between 1st and 3rd quartile = participants between 1st and 2nd quartile +
Participants between 2nd and 3rd quartile = 75 + 75
= 150

377. Mean and standard deviation can be worked out only if the data is on:
a. Interval/Ratio scale b. Dichotomous scale
c. Nominal scale d. Ordinal scale

378. Frequency distribution in quantitative data is studied by?
a. Histogram b. Line diagram
c. Pie diagram d. Ski diagram

379. Graph to correlate two quantitative data is:
a. Histogram b. Scatter diagram
c. Line diagram d. Frequency curve

380. Distribution of continuous data can be best represented by:
a. Pie chart b. Pictogram
c. Histogram d. Line diagram

381. Descriptive and inferential studies fall into which of the following type of result?
a. Qualitative
b. Quantitative
c. Correlation
d. Central tendency

382. Content Analysis refers to:
a. Reading books time and again for in-depth content
b. Interpretation of qualitative data
c. Interpretation of quantitative data
d. Presentation of quantitative data

383. Categorization scheme refers to:
a. Overlapping of groups to find a result
b. Set groups in order that do not overlap
c. Cross checking of groups
d. All of the above

DIAGRAMMATIC PRESENTATION OF DATA

384. Best method to show trend of events with passage of time is:
a. Line diagram
b. Bar diagram
c. Histogram
d. Pie chart

385. Best way to plot the change of incidence of disease over time is:
a. Histogram b. Line chart
c. Scatter diagram d. Ogive

386. The diagram that is used to visually examine the linear relationship between two continuous variables is known as:
a. Pie chart b. Frequency polygon
c. Scatterplots d. Histogram

387. Which of the following is a type of bar graph?
a. Polygon b. Pie chart
c. Histogram d. Line graph

388. Which of the following data presentation method uses angle for construction?
a. Table b. Pie graph
c. Bar chart d. Frequency

TEST OF SIGNIFICANCE

389. The sensitivity of a statistical test is measured by its:
a. Sample size
b. Power
c. Type of hypothesis
d. Sampling technique

390. Which of the following component is NOT required for estimating power (1-beta) of a study?
a. The effect size b. Sample size
c. Standard deviation d. Level of significance (alpha)

391. The values that mark the boundaries of the confidence interval is:
a. Margin of error b. Standard error
c. Confidence limits d. Confidence intervals

392. Which of the following is a NOT a parametric statistical test?
a. t-test b. ANOVA
c. Pearson Correlation d. Mann-Whitney U-test

393. The correct formula to calculate degree of freedom (df) in Chi-square test is:
a. n – 1 b. n – 2
c. (c – 1) (r – 1) d. n (n – 1)

394. The degree of freedom (DF) while computing Chi-square test for a 3 × 3 contingency table is:
a. Two b. Four
c. Six d. Nine

395. How many degrees of freedom would a table with 2 rows and 3 columns have?
a. 1 b. 2
c. 3 d. 4

396. Chi-square test, how many degrees of freedom would a table with 2 rows and 2 columns have?
a. 1 b. 2
c. 3 d. 4

397. All of the following are the method of obtaining vital statistics; EXCEPT:
a. Registration method
b. Census enumeration
c. Operational research method
d. Analytical method

398. In biomedical research survival analysis is typically used to evaluate:
a. Incidence of a disease b. Point Prevalence
c. Lifetime Prevalence d. Life expectancy

399. Which of the following is a measurement of fertility?
a. Maternal Mortality rate b. Reproductive rate
c. Under fiver mortality rate d. Maternity morbidity rate

400. Kruskal-Wallis test is used to:
a. Test the difference between two independent group means
b. Test the difference among the means of 3 or more related groups
c. Test the difference among the means of 3 or more independent groups
d. Test the difference in ranks of scores of 3 or more independent groups

401. Z score criteria is applicable to:
a. Normal distribution b. Skewed deviation
c. Chi-square test d. Paired 't' test

402. Odds ratio is related to:
a. Relative risk b. Incidence
c. Prevalence d. Attributable risk

403. Height of group of 20 Boys aged 10 years was 140 ±13 cm & 20 girl of same age was 135 cm ±7cm to test the statistical significance of difference in height, test applicable is:
a. *Chi square* b. Z - test
c. T - test d. F - test

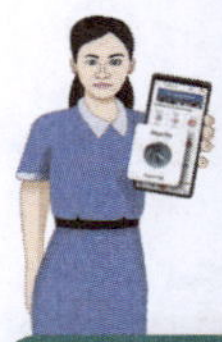

Ans.

377. a
378. a
379. b
380. c
381. b
382. b
383. b
384. a
385. b
386. c
387. c
388. b
389. b
390. c
391. c
392. d
393. c
394. b
395. b
396. a
397. c
398. d
399. b
400. d
401. a
402. a
403. c

404. Which is the best method to compare the results obtained by a new test and a gold standard test?

a. Correlation study
b. Regression study
c. Bland and Altman analysis
d. Kolmogorov-Smirnov test

405. Appropriate statistical method to compare two means is:

a. Chi square test
b. Students T test
c. Odd ratio
d. Correlation coefficient

TYPE I AND TYPE II ERRORS

406. A type-II error refers to:

a. False positive
b. False negative
c. True positive
d. True negative

407. While testing the hypothesis, fail to reject the null hypothesis when the null hypothesis is actually false is known as:

a. Type-I error
b. Type-11 error
c. Sampling error
d. Standard error

408. Type I errors in research occur when:

a. The null hypothesis is rejected but it should have been retained.
b. The null hypothesis is accepted but it should have been rejected
c. The null hypothesis is not rejected due to sampling error
d. The obtained p-value is higher than 0.05.

409. While testing the hypothesis, rejecting the null hypothesis when the null hypothesis is actually true is known as:

a. Type-I error
b. Type-11 error
c. Sampling error
d. Standard error

PARAMETRIC & NONPARAMETRIC TESTS

410. A nurse researcher wanted to compare the male and female patients on their level of satisfaction of nursing care provided to them. The level of satisfaction was measured as 'satisfied' or 'not-satisfied'. Which of the following statistical method is appropriate to associate the gender and satisfaction level of patients?

a. T-test
b. Chi-square test
c. Correlation coefficient
d. ANOVA

411. Linear relationship between height (in cm) and weight (in kg) of the patients can be analyzed:

a. t-test
b. Range of variation
c. Correlation coefficient
d. ANOVA

412. Association between height (short, average or tall) and weight (underweight, normal or overweight) can be calculated using:

a. t-test
b. ANOVA
c. Chi Square test
d. Correlation coefficient

413. To analyze the relationship between Systolic blood pressure (in mm of hg) and weight (in kg) in a sample of 100 patients, we could use:

a. Paired t-test
b. Correlation coefficient
c. Chi-squared test
d. One-way ANOVA

414. Which of the following is a non-parametric test?

a. ANOVA
b. Chi-squared test
c. Independent t-test
d. Paired t-test

415. Which of the following is a parametric test?

a. Paired t-test
b. Chi-squared test
c. Mann-Whitney U test
d. Wilcoxon signed rank sum test

416. Which of the following is NOT an assumption made by parametric tests?

a. Sample scores a have been drawn from a normally distributed population
b. The samples are assumed to have the same variance
c. Outcome variable is measured on an interval or ratio scale
d. Outcome variable is measured on a nominal or rational scale

417. Which of the following is a true statement about non-parametric tests?

a. They are used to analyze data that are normally distributed.
b. Paired t-test is a nonparametric test.
c. They are used to analyze data that are not normally distributed.
d. They can be used only when the data is collected from a random sample of subjects

418. What is NOT TRUE about Yate's Correction in Chi-square test?

a. Applied when there is two categorical variables are compared.
b. Applied when there is 2×2 contingency table is used
c. Recommended when there is less than 5 numbers are there is contingency cells
d. It is used when normality assumption is not satisfied.

419. One-way ANOVA (Analysis of Variance) test is used to:

a. Test the difference between two independent group means
b. Test the difference among the means of 3 or more related groups
c. Test the difference among the means of 3 or more independent groups
d. Test the difference in ranks of scores of 3 or more independent groups

420. Unpaired t test is used to:

a. Test the difference between two independent group means
b. Test the difference among the means of two related groups
c. Test the difference among the means of 3 or more independent groups
d. Test the difference in ranks of scores of 3 or more independent groups

421. Paired t test is used to:

a. Test the difference between two independent group means
b. Test the difference among the means of two related groups
c. Test the difference among the means of 3 or more independent groups
d. Test the difference in ranks of scores of 3 or more independent groups

422. Which of the following statistical test is appropriate to find difference in the IQ score of men and women who fall into one of three different age group?

a. One-way ANOVA
b. 2 by 3 Factorial ANOVA
c. Repeated measures ANOVA
d. Multiple regression

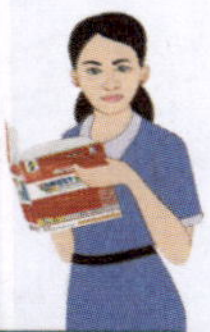

Ans.

404. c
405. b
406. b
407. b
408. a
409. a
410. b
411. c
412. c
413. b
414. b
415. a
416. d
417. c
418. d
419. c
420. a
421. b
422. b

"**Health is the greatest of all possessions; a pale cobbler is better than a sick king.**"

—Isaac Bickerstaff

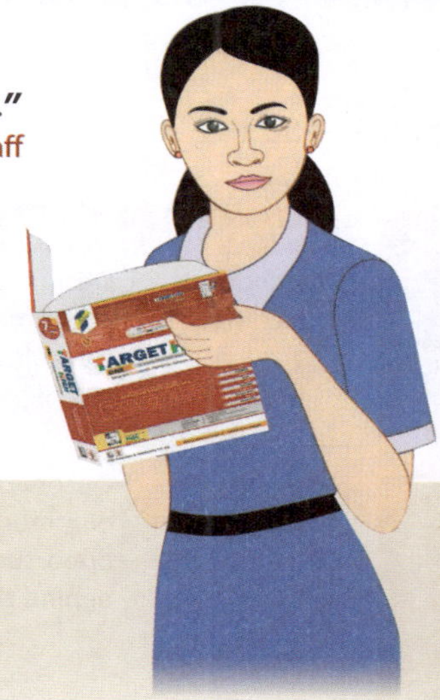

CHAPTER 12

NURSING EDUCATION

SYNOPSIS

EDUCATION

It brings change in behavior of an individual in a desirable manner. It aims at all-round development of an individual.

Philosophies of Education

The term 'Philosophy' has been derived from two words, i.e., "philos" means 'love' and "sophia" means 'wisdom'. Philosophy means love for wisdom.

Traditional Philosophies

Table 1: Traditional Philosophies: Some facts

Character	Naturalism	Idealism	Pragmatism (Experimentalism)	Realism
Exponents	• **Aristotle** • JJ Rousseau	• **Plato** is father of Idealism • Socrates, Kant, Hegel, Guru Nanak, Tagore, Mahatma Gandhi, Dayananda and others.	• **William James** is the father of Pragmatism • **John Dewey**, S. Kil Patrick • Margaret H and Mead	• J Friedrich Herbert • Herbert Spencer • Franklin Bobbitt
Fundamental principles	• Separate nature from God • Human life is part of nature • Emphasize 'matter and the physical world' • Ignore spirituality and supernaturalism	• Ideas or thoughts make up fundamental reality • Ultimate reality is spiritual rather than physical, mental or material • The only real things are mental entities, not physical things	• It is the product of practical experiences of life • Based on practical utility. • Emphasize is on action rather than on thought • Experimental method of science	• Correspondence and sensation (as we see it). • What is true and real in daily life is admissible • Opposes to idealism • Against spiritualism
Aims of Education	Self-realization, Self-expression, Self-preservation, Struggle for existence	Idealism emphasizes the glory and grandeur of human life.	Creation of new values, activity and experience, personal and social adjustment, reconstruction of experience, all-round personality development	Man leads a happy and comfortable life through education. To develop memory of the child.
Curriculum	No fixed curriculum. Every child has the right to determine his/her curriculum. Learn directly from nature through experience	Based upon ideas and ideals. Language, literature, social studies, science and mathematics are included	Curriculum is fixed in advance at the beginning itself. Utilitarian curriculum includes subjects that impart knowledge and various types of skills. Practical subjects like social studies, physics, maths and hygiene are included at later stage.	Subjects of physical world: mathematics, science and social science

Contd...

Character	Naturalism	Idealism	Pragmatism (Experimentalism)	Realism
Methods of teaching	Observation and experimental methods (Learning by doing)	Self-activity, play way method, project method. **Kindergarten** method. Discussion, lecture, questioning and imitation.	Project method Practical/experiments Handling of objects, tools and making things	Demonstrate, Recite
Role of teacher	Observer, supplier of materials and opportunities (role is behind the scene)	Teacher has to be specialist in knowledge. Teacher's personality is a source of inspiration for students.	Teacher will not impose anything on child. Teacher will facilitate students to be experimenter and discoverer	Displays, imparts knowledge.

Modern Contemporary Philosophies

- **Existentialism**: This philosophy emphasizes the existence of the humans as a free and responsible agent determining their own development through acts of the will. It is the youngest of all philosophy, primarily built upon the work of contemporary scholars of the 20th century. Chief exponents are **Søren Kierkegaard**, **Karl Jaspers** and **Jean–Paul Sartre**
- **Progressivism**: It is the advocacy of improvement of society by reform. Progressivism revolves around the students' needs, including teaching students to be good citizens as well as good learners. Exponents are John Dewey, William James, G Thomas Lawrence.
- **Behaviorism:** It believes that the learning is a result of environmental conditioning. Exponents are Ivan Pavlov (classical conditioning), Skinner (Operant conditioning), John Watson, and Edward Lee Thorndike (connectionism)
- **Humanism**: It emphasizes the value of human beings and generally prefers critical thinking and evidence (rationalism and empiricism) over superstition. The humanist emphasizes on literature. Key proponents of humanism include **Carl Rogers** and **Abraham Maslow**.
- **Experimentalism:** Experimentalism believes that things are constantly changing. Chief proponent is John Dewey.
- **Eclecticism:** It is the process of pulling out and putting together of the good ideas and concepts of various philosophies of education.
- **Reconstructionism:** It emphasizes the addressing of social questions and a quest to create a better society and worldwide democracy. Theodore Brameld was the founder of reconstructionism.
- **Essentialism**: Essentialism refers to the "traditional" or "Back to the Basics" approach to education.

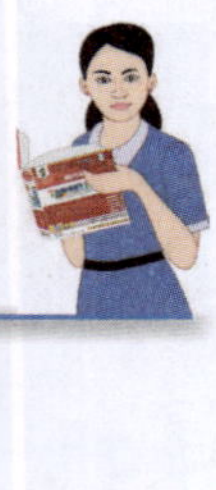

INDIAN NURSING COUNCIL (INC)

- Indian Nursing Council is a national regulatory body for nurses and nursing education in India. Indian Nursing Council is an autonomous body under the Government of India.
- Indian Nursing Council was established by Government of India under section 3(1) of the INC Act 1947.
- Important functions of INC:
  - To maintain uniform standard of nursing education in India
  - To prescribe the syllabus and regulations for nursing programs
  - To recognize the qualifications for the purpose of registration and employment
  - To advise State Nursing Councils, Central Government, State Governments, and Examining boards regarding Nursing education in India
- Minimum required physical facilities for a nursing college with an intake of 60 students (Key points)
  - Teaching block
    - Lecture hall: 4 × 1080 = 4320 sq. ft
    - Nursing foundation lab: 1500 sq. ft
    - Other labs (nutrition, CHN, OBG/ Pediatric, pre-clinical science): 900 sq. ft each
    - Library: 2400 sq. ft
    - Staff Room: 1000 sq. ft
    - Faculty Room: 2400 sq. ft
    - A.V Aids room: 600 sq. ft
    - Total area (Teaching block): 23720 sq. ft
  - Hostel Block
    - Rooms (single/double): 24000 sq. ft
    - One toilet and one bathroom for every 5 students
    - Recreation room: 500 sq. ft
    - Dining Hall : 3000 sq. ft

KEY POINTS

- **Plato** is the Father of Idealism. Other proponents of Idealism include Socrates, Kant, Hegel, Guru Nanak, Tagore, Mahatma Gandhi, Dayananda and others.
- **Aristotle and JJ Rousseau** are the proponents of Naturalism.
- **Naturalism** emphasizes 'matter and the physical world'. It ignores spirituality and supernaturalism.
- **William James** is the Father of Pragmatism. Other proponents of pragmatism include **John Dewey** and S. Kil Patrick.
- Pragmatism emphasizes action rather than thought.
- J Friedrich Herbert, Herbert Spencer and Franklin Bobbitt are proponents of Realism.
- Idealism believes that ultimate goal of human activities is the realization of human mind in his or herself.

- Kitchen and store: 1500 sq. ft
- Reading room: 250 sq. ft
- Total area (hostel block): 30750 sq. ft
- Total area required: 23720 + 30750 = 54470 sq.ft

- Teaching faculty requirement for nursing colleges/schools
  - Teacher: Student ratio is 1:10

NURSING PROGRAMS IN INDIA

Table 2: Important points of nursing programs

Nursing programs	Training duration	Examinations	Registration
Auxiliary Nurse and Midwife (ANM)	2 years	Nursing Examination Board	R. ANM
General Nursing & Midwifery	3 and 1/2 years 3 years from 2015-2016	Nursing Examination Board	R.N and R.M
BSc (Basic)	4 years	University	R.N & R.M
BSc (Post Basic)	Regular: 2 years Distance: 3 years	University	Additional Qualification
MSc	2 years	University	Additional Qualification
MPhil	1 year (Full time) 2 years (part time)	University	Additional Qualification
PhD	3-5 years	University	Additional Qualification

Source: Indian Nursing Council

NURSING EDUCATION IN INDIA

- BSc Nursing program was first started in India in the year 1946 in Christian Medical College (CMC), Vellore and Rajkumari Amrit Kaur (RAK) College of Nursing at Delhi University.
- Masters of Nursing (MSc) was started at RAK College of Nursing in 1959 and in 1969 in CMC Vellore.
- M.Phil in Nursing program was started at RAK College of Nursing in the year 1986 as a regular and part time course.
- PhD program in Nursing was first started in India in 1992

INTERNATIONAL COUNCIL OF NURSES (ICN)

- **ICN** was founded in 1899.
- ICN is a federation of more than 130 National Nurses Associations (NNAs). There is one voting member from each member association.

STATE NURSING COUNCILS IN INDIA

- Functions include:
  - Granting recognition to nursing colleges/schools and conduct regular inspections
  - Registration of qualified nurses with valid degree/diploma/certificates
- There are 23 state nursing councils in India.
- Tamil Nadu Nursing and Midwives Council (TNMC) is the earliest Nursing Council in South-East Asia (1926).

TRAINED NURSES ASSOCIATION OF INDIA (TNAI)

- TNAI was established in the year 1908.
- TNAI got affiliated with International Council of Nurses (ICN) in the year 1912.
- The Government of India has recognized TNAI as a service organization in 1950.
- Key office bearers as on June, 2018.
  - President: Dr Roy K George
  - Secretary General: Mrs Evelyn P Kannan
- The Postal Department of the Government of India honored TNAI by releasing a stamp in the name of TNAI in **2011**.

CURRICULUM

- **Curriculum:** "A systematic arrangement of the sum total of selected experiences planned by a school or a defined group of students to attain the aims of a particular educational program"

  – Florence Nightingale
- **The four Cs of Curriculum are:**
  - Cooperative
  - Continuous
  - Comprehensive
  - Concrete

Practice Question

1. The philosophy of education in which treatment of things is based solely on their practical utility is called_____.

a. Realism
b. Idealism
c. Naturalism
d. Pragmatism

Ans. (d) Pragmatism

TNAI

KEY POINTS

- As on Aug 2021, The president of TNAI is Dr. Roy K George.
- General Secretary - Mrs. Evelyn P. Kannan.
- The TNAI's International Training Center (for skill training) was inaugurated on 14th April, 2018.
- The Nurse Practitioner in Critical Care Nursing was started in India in the academic year of 2017-18.

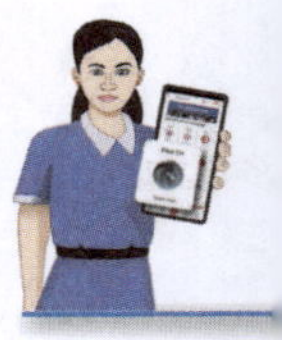

- **Levels of curriculum planning**
  - **Societal curriculum:** Planned for large group of students in a specific program, e.g., GNM or BSc Nursing.
  - **Institutional curriculum:** Planned for a group of students who will study in a particular institution for specific period of time.
  - **Instructional curriculum:** Consists of content and activities planned for a specific period of time (day by day and week by week).
- **Phases of curriculum development**
  - Development phase: Planning and developing
  - Implementation phase: Management and implementation
  - Evaluation phase: Assessment of teaching and learning process

EDUCATIONAL OBJECTIVES

Educational or learning objectives is defined as "Desired end results or anticipated end results"

Taxonomy of Educational Objectives

It is a systematic organization of objectives into three domains, i.e.,

- **Cognitive domain (Knowledge)**
- **Conative or psychomotor domain (Skill)**
- **Affective domain (Attitude)**

Bloom's Taxonomy of Educational Objectives (1956)

- It is one of the most widely used ways of organizing levels of expertise.
- **Cognitive Domain**
  - The cognitive domain involves knowledge and the development of intellectual skills
  - This includes knowledge, comprehension, application, analysis, synthesis and evaluation
- **Conative (psychomotor) domain**
  - Psychomotor domain includes physical movement, coordination, and use of motor-skill areas.
- **Affective Domain**
  - Affective domain includes the manner in which we deal with things emotionally, such as feelings, values, appreciation, and attitudes.

Recent Questions (INC PhD 2020)

1. Basic cognitive domain verb among the following is:
   a. Receiving
   b. Responding
   c. Applying
   d. Organizing

Ans. (c) Applying

2. Which among the following shows higher level of domain verb?
   a. Remembering
   b. Receiving
   c. Imitation
   d. Creating

Ans. (d) Creating

3. Nursing student working is a palliative care setting spent her time with the patient who all are in the end stage of the life. She always spent time with dying patient's last 5-10 min. What kind of educational domain verb she achieved?
   a. Characterization
   b. Receiving
   c. Responding
   b. Valuing

Ans. (a) Characterization

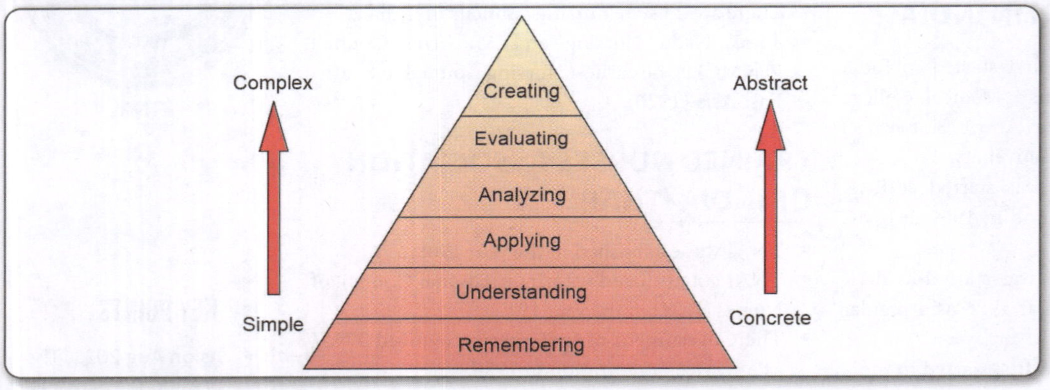

Figure 1: Cognitive domain

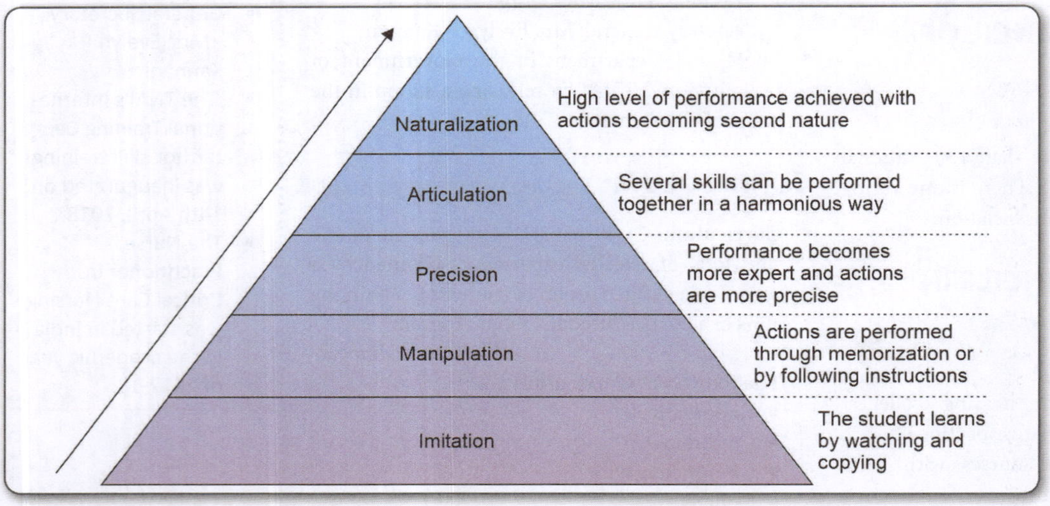

Figure 2: Psychomotor domain (Based on Dave, 1975)

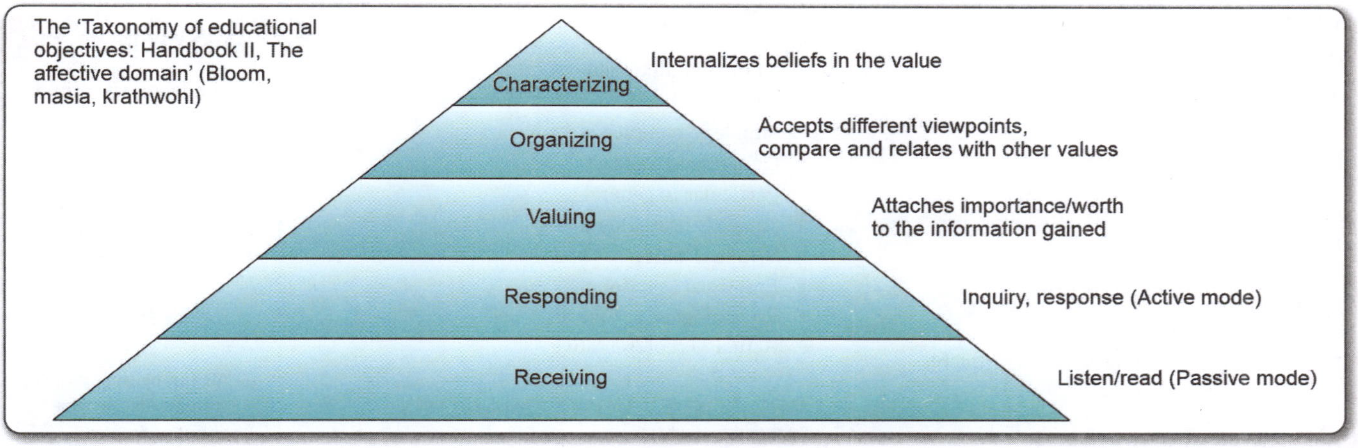

Figure 3: Affective domain

AUDIO-VISUAL AID

Audio-visual-aid: It is an instructional device in which message can be heard as well as seen.

Classification of A-V Aids

Auditory Aids

Radio, recordings, mike, programs, megaphone, and gramophone

Visual Aids

- **Non-projected/unprojected:** Model, 3-D materials, pictures, charts, flannel graph, boards, cartoons, maps, photographs, flashcards, illustrations, posters and printed materials.
- **Projected aids:** Epidiascope, slide projector, overhead projector, film projector, opaque projector.
- **Audio-visual aids:** Television, video, sound motion picture.
- **Aid through activity:** Field trip, models, collection of material and exhibition.
- **Traditional media**: Puppets, dramas, folk songs and folk dance.

Table 3: Two- and three-dimensional AV aids

Two-dimensional AV aids	Three-dimensional AV aids

• Printed materials
• Chart
• Posters
• Graph
• Photos and map
	• Model
	  ▪ Solid model (Globe, clay model)
	  ▪ Cutway and X-ray models, e.g., Cross sectional model of human body
	  ▪ Working models (Circulatory system model with working motor)
	  ▪ Sand models (community area, forest area)
	  ▪ Scale models (models of organs of body)
	• Exhibit
	• Specimen
	• Mock-up
	• Moulage
	• Objects
	• Realia (Natural and preserved)
	• Diorama
	• Puppets

KEY POINTS

- The most commonly available aid in the classroom situation is blackboard
- **Black, Blue** and **Green** are best colors to write on the transparencies
- Flannel boards are covered with rough khadi. The cut outs, drawings and other illustrations are placed on the board.
- Epidiascope is the projected aid for projecting opaque objects
- Flash card is a method which consists of series of cards that are flashed one after another. Sizes of the cards are
  10" x 12" or 22" x 28"
- Flashcards are ideal for a group of 20–30 people

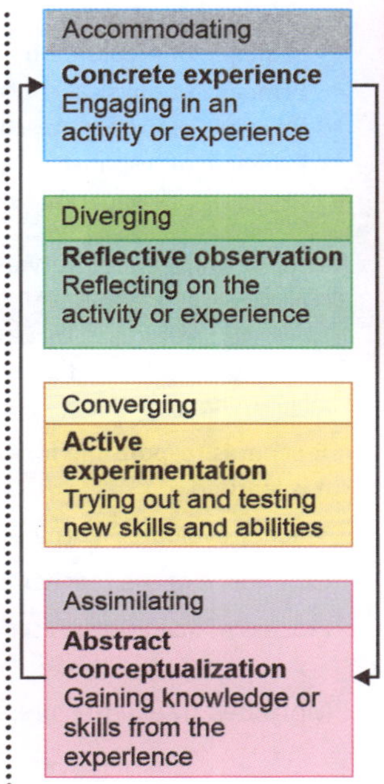

Cycle of Kolb's learning styles

Recent Question
(AIIMS Bibinagar, Faculty 2023)

4. In which phase of microteaching does the teacher get trained on the skills and components of teaching through lectures, discussion, illustration, and demonstration of the skill by experts?

a. Transfer phase
b. Evaluation phase
c. Skill acquisition phase
d. Knowledge acquisition phase

Ans. (d) Knowledge acquisition phase

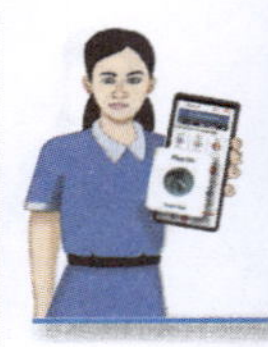

Characteristics of Good Teaching A-V Aids

- Meaningful
- Purposeful
- Accuracy in every aspect
- Simple
- Cheap
- Improvised
- Large size
- Up-to-date
- Easily portable
- According to mental level of the students
- Motivates the learners

Principles of A-V Aids

- Principle of selection
- Principle of preparation
- Principle of physical control
- Principle of proper presentation
- Principle of response
- Principle of evaluation

MAXIMS OF TEACHING

- Known to unknown
- Easy to difficult
- Simple to complex
- Concrete to abstract
- Particular to general
- Analysis to synthesis
- Whole to parts
- Empirical to rational
- Psychological to logical
- Actual to representative

PEDAGOGY VS ANDRAGOGY

- **Pedagogy:** Pedagogy is the study and theory of the methods and principles of teaching. It is a child-focused teaching approach.
- **Andragogy:** It refers to method and principles used in adult education.

KEY POINTS

- Pedagogy is a child-focused teaching approach.
- Andragogy is adult-focused teaching approach.

Recent Questions (INC PhD 2021)

5. All among the following statements are true about andragogy; EXCEPT:

a. They are participating in learning process for specific needs and reason
b. They possess their own preferred learning style.
C. Continuous motivation and reinforcement are needed
d. They have broad and diverse range of experience

Ans. (c) Continuous motivation and reinforcement are needed.

6. Group discussion is suitable for a group of .... people.

a. 3–6
b. 4–8
c. 6–12
d. 10–16

Ans. (c) 6–12

Table 4: Differences between pedagogy and andragogy

Pedagogy	Andragogy
The learner is dependent upon the instructor for all learning	Self-directed learning
Teacher is responsible for what is taught and how it is learned	Learner is responsible for his own learning
Teacher evaluates learning	Self- evaluation
Experience of the teacher is most influential	Adults are rich resource for one another
Process of acquiring prescribed subject matter	Learners perform a task, solve problem relevant to real-life tasks
Motivated by external pressures	Self-motivating factors: recognition, better quality of life, etc.

PRINCIPLES OF TEACHING

- Principle of **C**reativity
- Principle of **L**ooking ahead
- Principle of **F**lexibility and cooperation
- Principle of **D**iagnostic and remedial teaching
- Principle of **L**inking teaching with actual life
- Principle of **P**lanning
- Principle of **A**im
- Principle of **I**nterest or motivation
- Principle of **S**ympathy and kind atmosphere
- Principle of **A**ctivity or learning by doing

Teaching Methods

Table 5: Teaching methods and its significance

Teaching methods	Significance
Lecture method	• Controlled and information centered approach • Teacher talks and Students are passive listeners • The teacher transmits information to a large group (Ideal for a large group of students) • Also known as **"autocratic teaching strategy"** • **Most commonly** used method of teaching

Contd...

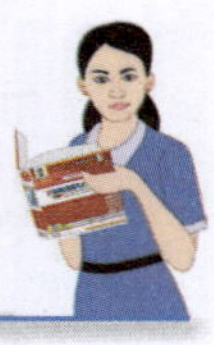

Recent Question (INC PhD 2020)

7. Didactic method of teaching is:

a. Lecture
b. Group discussion
c. Demonstration
d. Role play

Ans. (a) Lecture

Teaching methods	Significance
Seminar	• Group of people coming together for the discussion and learning of specific technique and topics. • It involves paper reading of a theme and followed by the discussion to clarify the complex aspect of the theme.
Symposium	• Group of individuals comes together to solve problems of a given subject in a specified time
Panel discussion	• Group of 6-8 qualified experts discuss a topic in front of an audience
Demonstration	• Taught by "exhibition and explanation" • Most commonly used Student-centered teaching method in Nursing • **Best method** to teach nursing skills
Laboratory method	• First- hand experience of learning situation • Helps to understand and test concept • Promote insight through practical exercise
Role-play	• Spontaneous acting out of roles in the context of human relations situations, e.g., Sociodrama, psychodrama • Best method for health education (attitude related awareness programs) of community people
Programmed instruction	• Planned sequence of experiences, leading to proficiency in terms of stimulus response relationship (Espich JE and Williams B.)
Individualized instruction	• Learners are allowed to work/learn at their own pace. • The instructions are tailored as per the needs and abilities of the learner.
Discussion method	• A cooperative problem-solving activity seeking consensus for solution of a problem • Maximum participation of students is possible
Team teaching	• A team of teachers working together with a single group of students • Multiple talents and resources are pooled for the benefit of learners.
Simulated teaching	• A form of experiential learning • Teaching process is displayed artificially by simulating actual life situation
Microteaching	• A technique aimed to prepare student-teachers to the real classroom setting • Student-teacher teaches a small group of **4-6 learners** for a length of **5-10 minutes**
Assignment method	• This method comprises of guided information, self-learning, writing skills, and organization of knowledge
Problem-solving method	• Learners are confronted with real problems and provided with opportunity and freedom to solve the problems
Project method	• Problem-oriented method which is directed and planned by the learner himself
Case study	• The most effective clinical teaching method • Comprehensive study of a patient with a disease condition
Workshop	• Experienced people and experts come together to find solutions to problems encountered in their work situations • Participants have an active role
Puppet show	• Puppet show can help boost creativity and imaginations of the learners
Educational field trips	• Taking students on field trips (learning excursion outside the classroom) and providing them opportunity to experience in real-life settings and making learning more effective
Clinical teaching	It includes: • Client family-centered approach • Conference ▪ Clinical conference ▪ Group conference ▪ Staff conference ▪ Nursing care conference ▪ Individual conference ▪ Team conference

Contd...

Recent Questions
(INC PhD 2020)

8. Which of the following strategies can bridge gap between education and practice in nursing?
a. Dual role
b. Guidance
c. Preceptorship
d. Supervision

Ans. (a) Dual role

9. Clinical Preceptors need
a. Good clinical skill
b. Good research knowledge
c. Punishment capacity
d. Poor communication

Ans. (a) Good clinical skill

Recent Questions
(INC PhD 2021)

10. Which among the following is the most appropriate method for teaching NG intubation?
a. Lecture
b. Role play
c. Demonstration
d. Clinical rounds

Ans. (c) Demonstration

11. To teach the general public and students regarding social issues which among the following is the appropriate method of teaching?
a. Symposium
b. Role play
c. Demonstration
d. Seminar

Ans. (b) Role play

POINT TO REMEMBER

Selection of clinical teaching method must be in accordance with the teacher's ability to use it effectively and creatively.

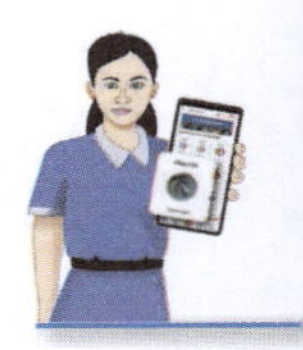

Teaching methods	Significance
	• Bedside clinic • Nursing rounds • Ward-teaching program • Ward class • Ward clinics • Case method • Assignments • Brain storming method • Group discussion • Demonstration method • Laboratory method • Process recording • Health talks • Problem-solving • Observation

POINT TO REMEMBER

Nursing round method is applicable for only small group of students.

EVALUATION

- **Evaluation:** Pupil's qualitative progress and behavioral changes (value judgement) are tested, e.g., Very good, good, bad, etc.
- **Measurement:** Refers to quantitative description of pupil's attainment in a subject, e.g., Exam score in a specific subject.
- **Assessment:** "Assessment in education is the process of *gathering, interpreting, recording,* and *using* information about pupils' responses to an educational task." **– Harlen et al (1992).**
- **Criterion referenced assessment:** It determines whether each student has achieved specific skills or concepts. Each individual is compared with a pretest standard for acceptable achievement. Focus is on whether the student could perform that task with the preset criteria, e.g., Driving test
- **Norm referenced assessment:** Compare students to what is normal for that age, class and course. Percentile rank is preferred.
- **Formative Assessment:** With formative assessments, students are evaluated during the work process and the focus is on improving the process. Majority of formative assessment are informal, e.g., Teacher's assessment of seminar presentation.
- **Summative Assessment:** With summative assessments, students are evaluated upon completion of the work and the focus is on the final product, **e.g., Final University exam**

The methods used for the assessment of knowledge are:

- **Subjective type:** Essay type, narrative type, comparison, amplification, precise writing, short notes.
- **Objective type:** MCQ, matching type, fill in the blanks, sentence completion type, Problem-solving type and situational.

Recent Question (INC PhD 2020 & 2021)

12. Anecdotal record means:

a. Whatever teacher heard about the student
b. Teachers' observation about student
c. Students' own description about certain activities
d. Seniors, juniors, and peer group observation about student

Ans. (b) Teachers' observation about student.

Table 6: Methods of evaluation and instruments used for evaluation for domains of learning

Domain	Methods	Instruments/Tools
Cognitive/ Knowledge	Written	Essay type questions Short answer questions Multiple choice questions
	Oral	Viva Voice
Psychomotor/ Skill	Observation	Traditional practical examinations
		OSCE
		OSPE
		Checklist, nursing process
Affective/ Attitude	Observation Self-reported	Behavioral scales: anecdotal records, personal records, cumulative records, communication, group discussion, process recording, etc.
		Psychological scales: Likert Scale (summative scales), semantic differential scale, sociometry, Scalogram

Abbreviations: OSCE, objective structured clinical Examination; OSPE, objective structured practical examination

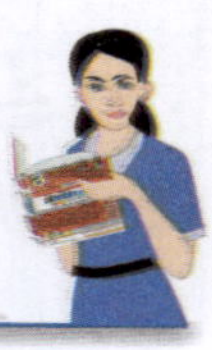

KEY POINTS

Objective structured clinical examination (OSCE)

It is a multidimensional practical examination of clinical skills, as a tool for assessing clinical competence.

The steps in designing and implementing an OSCE:

- Have Set of CLEAR OBJECTIVES
- Identify the PRACTICAL aspects
- Select the TASK
- Break into SUB-TASKS
- Assign SCORES (WEIGHTS) for each sub task
- Set up STATIONS
- CONDUCT after orienting students and examiners
- Make NOTES of the process and review
- ANALYZE the results and use the same for student assessment

Item Analysis

It is a statistical technique which is used for selecting and rejecting the items of the objective test (MCQs) on the basis of their difficult value and discriminated power.

Statistical Method Used

1. **Difficulty Index or Facility value – (item difficulty):**
   - The facility value of an item is defined as the proportion or percentage of the examinees who have answered the item correctly
   - Difficulty Index ranges from 0 – 100%;
     - Easy – ≥ 85%
     - Medium – 51%-84%
     - Hard - ≤ 50
2. **Discriminative index (DI)–(item discrimination):** It is the ability of an item to discriminate between skilled and unskilled examinees
   - DI ranges from -> -1 to +1
   - ≥ 0.35 – GOOD
   - <0.2 – 0.35> – INTERMEDIATE
   - ≤ 0.2 - UNACCEPTABLE

- **Distracter efficiency:** Distracter should be PLAUSIBLE. Any distracter that is not picked by at least 5% of student–is not a good distracter.

CONTINUING NURSING EDUCATION(CNE)

It provides the opportunity for working professionals to continue their learning and remain abreast of the developments in their field.

Roles of the Nurse as CNE Educator

- Frequently assesses learning needs of the nurses
- Applies adult learning principles
- Uses teaching techniques that empower nursing staff
- Sensitive to the learning deficits of the nursing staff and creatively minimize these difficulties
- Prepares the nurses readily regarding knowledge and skill deficits
- Actively seeks out teaching opportunities for nurses

IN-SERVICE EDUCATION

A program of instructions or training provided by an agency or institution for its employees. The program is held in the institution or agency and is intended to increase the skills and competencies of the employees in a specific area.

Table 7: Differences between continuing nursing education and in-service education

Continuing nursing education	In-service education
To enhance overall knowledge and practice skills (update)	Meets requirement needed to function in a specific work setting.
Example: Conferences, Workshops, Symposiums, etc.	**Example:** Demonstration of new equipment, review of newly implemented protocol, etc.
Broad scope	Narrow scope
Usually a planned program	Often spontaneous
Conducted in different settings	Conducted in work setting
Responsibility of individual	Responsibility of an organization

JOHARI WINDOW

- Johari Window was developed by Joseph Luft (1916–2014) and Harrington Ingham (1916–1995) in 1955.
- The Johari Window is a **technique that aims to help people understand their emotional and physical relationship with themselves and other people**.
- The window consists of four segments (or panes) of human interaction: **open, hidden, blind and unknown**.

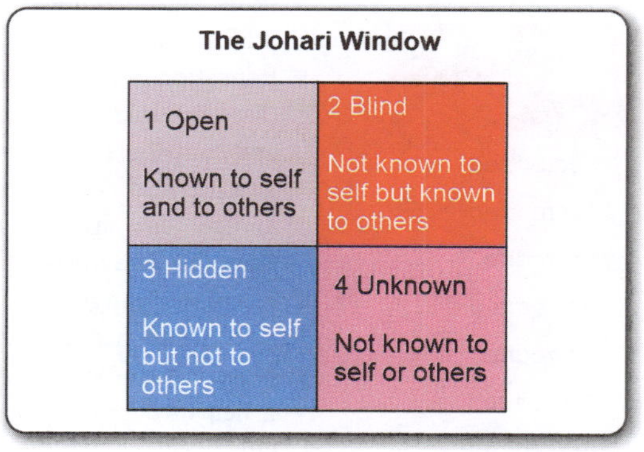

Recent Question
(INC PhD 2020

13. Which among the following is not a principle of question making?
a. Question should be clear
b. Question should be unambiguous
c. Avoid sensitive questions
d. Use double negative question

Ans. (d) Use double negative question.

KEY POINT

Approaches to in-service education:
- In-service education is a planned educational activities provided in a job setting.

KEY POINT

OSLER– Objective Structured Long Examination Record: It is a modification of the long-case clinical examination mainly used in medical education. It is a 10-item analytical record.

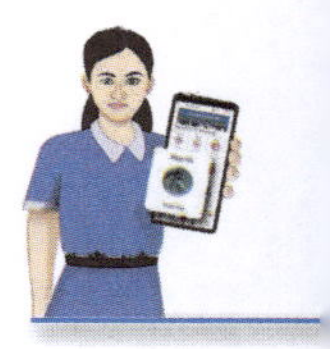

- Application in Nursing
  - Self-awareness gives the nurse a skill to establish relationship with patients and co-workers with different values, beliefs and principles
  - It helps in building team work

ACCREDITATION IN HIGHER EDCUATION

- Accreditation refers to **a voluntary review process of educational programs** by a professional organization
- "Accreditation is the process whereby an organization/agency recognizes a college or university or a program of study having met certain predetermined qualifications and standard." – Selden
- **Purpose:** Administration requirements, recognition, to bring uniform standards in nursing education, institutional self-improvement.
- **Advantage:** Standards in education and statutory power to punish wrong doers
- **Disadvantage:** Time consuming and expensive
- Some important accrediting agencies in higher education
  - INC (Indian Nursing Council)
  - MCI (Medical Council of India)
  - DCI (Dental Council of India)
  - PCI (Pharmacy Council of India)
  - UGC (University Grants Commission)
  - NAAC (National Assessment and Accreditation Council)
  - AICTE (All India Council for Technical Education)
- The NAAC was established in 1994 as an autonomous institute of the UGC. The prime agenda of NAAC is to assess and accredit institutions of higher learning with all objective of helping them to work continuously to improve the quality of education.
- NAAC grades range from A++ (highest) to D.

Table 8: NAAC grading scale

Range of institutional CGPA	Letter Grade	Performance descriptor
3.51–4.00	A++	Accredited
3.26–3.50	A+	Accredited
3.01–3.25	A	Accredited
2.76–3.00	B++	Accredited
2.51–2.75	B+	Accredited
2.01–2.50	B	Accredited
1.51–200	C	Accredited
1.50	D	Not accredited

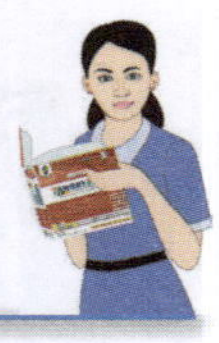

EDUCATIONAL LEARNING THEORIES

Four theories of learning are:

1. **Classical conditioning:** Classical conditioning **(learning through association)** is discovered by Pavlov. Two stimuli are linked together to produce a new learned response in a person or animal. An automatic conditioned response is paired with a specific stimulus, e.g., Pairing an anxiety-provoking situation, such as performing in front of a group, with pleasant surroundings helps the student learn new associations.
2. **Operant conditioning:** In operant conditioning, new or continued behaviors are impacted by new or continued consequences, e.g., A student tends to complete his/her homework daily; because he/she knows that he/she will be rewarded with a candy.
3. **Cognitive theory:** Cognitive Learning Theory explains how we process information when we learn. Learner is an active participant in this process.
4. **Social learning theory:** Social learning theory suggests that social behavior is learned by observing and imitating the behavior of others, e.g., Children learn by imitating family members and television characters.

INNOVATIVE METHODS OF TEACHING

- **Flipped classroom:** A flipped classroom is an **instructional strategy** and a type of blended learning. It aims to increase student engagement and learning by having students complete readings at their home and work on live problem-solving during class time.
- **Brainstorming:**
  - It is a problem-solving activity where students build on or develop higher order thinking skills. It encourages creative thought and critical thinking.
  - Education brainstorming is a group of activity that encourage the student to focus on a topic and contribute to the free flow of ideas
  - Teacher begins a session by posing a question and students are encouraged to **express their thoughts and ideas.**
- **Concept mapping:**
  - A concept map is a visual organization and representation of knowledge.
  - It helps students to organize new information effectively.
  - It helps students to make meaningful connections between main idea.

KEY POINTS

Flipped class room

- This method of teaching is just opposite to the traditional teaching method.
- Students introduced to a new topic during out of the class time usually at home setting
- Classroom is for interactive sessions and discussion regarding the new topic.
- Flipped classroom typically involves a blend of online and face-to-face learning

Golden Points to Remember

- BSc Nursing program was first started in India in the year 1946 in Christian Medical College. (CMC), Vellore and Rajkumari Amrit Kaur (RAK) College of Nursing at Delhi University.
- MSc nursing program was first started at RAK College of Nursing in the year 1959.
- MPhil in Nursing program was started at RAK College of Nursing in the year 1980.
- Doctorate or PhD program in Nursing was first started in India in 1992.
- Idealism believes "Ultimate reality is spiritual rather than physical, mental rather than material".
- Translating the message into verbal and non-verbal symbols to communicate with the receiver is called Encoding.
- The reproduction of the essential features of a real-life situation is called **Simulation.**
- **Cognitive domain** has different levels, like knowledge, comprehension, application, analysis, synthesis and evaluation.
- **Psychomotor skills** refer to performance of a particular act automatically and with a high degree of efficacy. Three levels are imitation, control and automatism.
- **Affective domain** deals with emotions or feelings indicated by words. Three levels are attention, response, internalization.
- The best method to teach a patient any skills, such as using inhaler, is done by Demonstration.
- In panel discussion, group of 6-8 qualified experts discuss a topic in front of an audience.
- In microteaching, student-teacher teaches a small group of **4–6 learners** for a length of **5–10 minutes.**
- Learning that is carried out in the affective domain is Passive Learning.
- Unit planning provides sound basis of Evaluation.
- **Questions that require the respondents to make a choice between more than two responses called Multiple Choice Questions.**
- The best method to teach a patient any skills, such as using spirometry, is done by Demonstration.
- Health education by a nurse to a group of people can be termed as Small Group Communication.
- Learning that is carried out in the affective domain is called Passive Learning.
- **Summative evaluation**: The type of assessment where the outcome is evaluated at the end of academic years.
- **Formative evaluation:** The type of assessment where the outcome is evaluated frequently throughout the year.
- **Criterion referenced assessment evaluates students against** pretest standard for acceptable achievement. Example: Driving test.
- **Program evaluation:** The systematic assessment of the operation and or outcomes of a program or policy, compared to set.
- Behavioral objectives model is also referred to as product model.
- **Teacher: Student** ratio recommended by Indian Nursing Council is **1:10.**
- **The four Cs of Curriculum are:** Cooperative, Continuous, Comprehensive and Concrete.

"The groundwork for all happiness is good health."
—Leigh Hunt

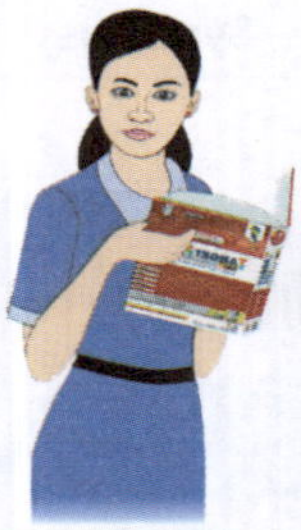

MULTIPLE CHOICE QUESTIONS
(Including Explained and Practice Questions)

HISTORY OF NURSING EDUCATION IN INDIA

1. MPhil in Nursing program was started at RAK College of Nursing in the year: *New Q*

a. 1972 b. 1980
c. 1986 d. 1992

2. PhD program in Nursing was first started in India in: *New Q*

a. 1980 b. 1985
c. 1992 d. 1996

3. National Consortium for PhD in Nursing in India was initiated by: *New Q*

a. AIIMS, New Delhi
b. RAK College of Nursing, New Delhi
c. Indian Nursing Council
d. IGNOU

4. In India, the first four-year basic Bachelor Degree nursing program was established in:

a. 1920 b. 1940
c. 1946 d. 1955

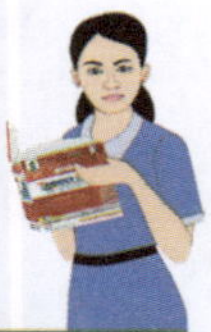

Explanation: The first four-year Basic BSc program was established in 1946 at RAK College of Nursing in Delhi and CMC College of Nursing in Vellore.

Ans.

1.	c
2.	c
3.	c
4.	c
5.	c
6.	c
7.	b
8.	a
9.	a
10.	c
11.	b
12.	c
13.	a
14.	b
15.	a
16.	a

REGULATORY AND PROFESSIONAL BODIES

5. The function of Indian Nursing Council is to:

a. Arrange for university inspections of colleges in respective states
b. Financial assistance to conferences and seminars conducted by nursing colleges
c. Make policies for Nursing Education and Practice
d. Recruit nursing personnel in hospitals

6. Trained Nurses Association of India (TNAI) was formed in the year:

a. 1928 b. 1947
c. 1908 d. 1890

7. The International Council of Nurses (ICN) was established in the year: *(Tutor Exam 2015, AIIMS, Rishikesh)*

a. 1869 b. 1899
c. 1928 d. 1905

8. The International Council of Nurses (ICN) is headquartered in:

a. Geneva, Switzerland
b. Washington, US
c. New York, US
d. London, UK

NURSING PROGRAMS IN INDIA

9. In India, first MSc Nursing programme was started in RAK college in the year: *(Tutor Exam 2015, AIIMS, Rishikesh)*

a. 1959 b. 1948
c. 1946 d. 1970

EDUCATIONAL OBJECTIVES

10. Who stated "education is not a preparation for life; education is life itself"?

a. Jean Piaget
b. Socrates
c. John Dewey
d. Mahatma Gandhi

11. "Democracy and Education" (1916) was authored by:

a. Sigmund Freud b. John Dewey
c. Jean Piaget d. Jawaharlal Nehru

12. The interaction analysis category system in education for increasing the teacher effectiveness was developed by:

a. Amidon b. Simon
c. Flander d. Richard Over

13. Who stated that "Man is born free but every-where he is in chains"?

a. Jean Jacques Rousseau b. Sigmund Freud
c. John Dewey d. Jean Piaget

14. "By 'Education' I mean an all-round drawing out of the best in child and man body, mind and spirit". This quotation is given by:

a. Rabindranath Tagore b. Mahatma Gandhi
c. Sarvepalli Radhakrishnan d. Jawaharlal Nehru

15. The cognitive domain in educational objectives refers to: *(AIIMS Raipur NO 2019):*

a. Knowledge b. Attitude
c. Skills d. Behavior

Explanation: There are three domains of educational objectives that are cognitive, conative and affective.

- **Cognitive domain:** It has different levels like knowledge, comprehension, application, analysis, synthesis and evaluation.
- **Psychomotor domain:** Related to skills. Three levels are imitation, control, and automatism.
- **Affective domain:** Dealing with emotions or feelings (behavior). Three levels are attention, response, internalization.

16. A principle of adult learning is:

a. Learning is self-directed b. Learning by doing
c. Learning by imposition c. Learning by imitation

17. Affective domain of Bloom's taxonomy includes all; EXCEPT:

a. Valuing b. Responding
c. Organization d. Synthesis

Explanation: Affective domain is categorized into five subdomains, which include: Receiving, Responding, Valuing, Organization, Characterization.

Synthesis is a subdomain of Knowledge domain.

18. One of the areas of 'Learning Objective' in Bloom's Taxonomy is:

a. Application b. Cognitive
c. Communication d. Intellectual

Explanation: Bloom's Taxonomy is a framework used to classify learning objectives based on the cognitive processes involved. It categorizes learning objectives into different levels, including remembering, understanding, applying, analyzing, evaluating, and creating.

19. Cognitive domain of Bloom's Taxonomy includes all; EXCEPT:

a. Analysis b. Criticism
c. Evaluation d. Synthesis

20. Conative domain of Bloom's Taxonomy includes ....

a. Application of knowledge b. Skilled movements
c. Reflex movements d. Perceptual activities

21. Affective domain of Bloom's Taxonomy includes:

a. Receive b. Respond
c. Value d. All of these

22. Psychomotor domain of Bloom's Taxonomy includes all; EXCEPT:

a. Imitation b. Application
c. Develop precision d. Manipulation

23. Factors that affect the human behavior are:

a. Experience, dignity, values, attitude
b. Knowledge, motivation, attitudes, values
c. Knowledge, belief, dignity, values
d. Knowledge, belief, attitudes, values

24. Nursing Educational Research is required to:

a. Improve self-image of nursing professionals
b. Ensure evidence-based nursing practice
c. Persuade young people to come into nursing profession
d. Uphold professional dignity

EDUCATIONAL MEDIA (AV AIDS)

25. The reproduction of the essential features of a real-life situation is called: *(AIIMS Raipur NO 2019)*

a. Exhibition b. Module
c. Simulation d. Demonstration

Explanation: A simulation is an approximate imitation of the operation of a process or system. The model is a well-defined description of the simulated subject, and represents its key characteristics. Simulation is one of the best methods to teach clinical skills for nursing students.

26. Video conferencing can be classified as one of the following types of communication: *(AIIMS Raipur NO 2019)*

a. Visual one-way b. Audio-Visual one-way
c. Audio-Visual two-way d. Visual two-way

Explanation: Video conferencing means to conduct a conference between two or more participants at different sites by using networks to transmit audio-video data. So, video conferencing is an audio-visual two-way type of communication.

27. One form of graphic presentation for health education is: *(AIIMS Nagpur NO 2018)*

a. Notice board b. Charts
c. Poster d. Blackboard

Explanation: A **chart** is a graphical representation of data, in which "the data are represented by symbols, such as bars in a bar chart, lines in a line chart, or slices in a pie chart." **Poster** consists textual and graphic elements, images which designed to be eye catching and informative.

28. Which of the following is NOT a visual aid used in health education? *(AIIMS-BBS SNO 2019)*

a. Textbooks b. Posters
c. Film strips d. Audio cassettes

29. Facts and ideas arranged for expressing the process or development of an issue to the point of its resolution over a period of time is:

a. Narration chart b. Strip chart
c. Cycle chart d. Evolution chart

30. A map that describes the political divisions of the world, continents and nations is known as:

a. Physical map b. Relief map
c. Political map d. Weather map

31. Which of the followings is NOT an activity aid?

a. Field trip b. School museum
c. Role play d. Graphs

32. An equipment that projects the real magnified image on a screen directly from pictures and drawings on paper is:

a. Slide projector b. LCD projector
c. Episcope d. Microscope

33. Most common AV aid used for educating general public is:

a. Audio tape b. Radio
c. CD system d. Tape recorder

34. The most essential body language in classroom teaching is:

a. Eye contact b. Controlled movement
c. Humorous d. Straight posture

35. Which of the following is the most popular method of delivering distance learning courses at present?

a. Video conferencing b. Web-based learning
c. Teleconferencing d. Internet

36. An overhead projector works by:

a. Refraction of light b. Reflection of light
c. RGB color method d. CMYK color method

37. The blind spots of the blackboard are in the:

a. Lower third part of the board
b. Corners of the board
c. Lower one fourth of the board
d. Upper left side of the board

38. Which one of the following is NOT a part of electronic media?

a. Radio b. Brochure
c. Film d. Television

39. The oldest and cheapest audio-visual aid that is widely accepted in teaching is:

a. Charts b. Chalkboard
c. Flip cards d. PPT

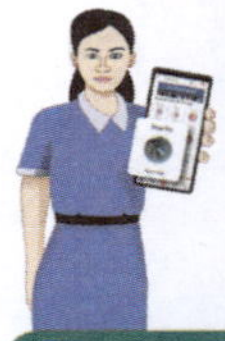

Ans.

17. d
18. b
19. b
20. a
21. d
22. b
23. d
24. b
25. c
26. c
27. b
28. d
29. a
30. c
31. d
32. c
33. b
34. a
35. c
36. b
37. b
38. b
39. b

40. Mock up is one of the examples of:
a. 3 - Dimensional aid b. Project aid
c. Field trip d. None of these

41. The ideal size of a flashcard should be:
a. 10” × 12” or 22” × 28” in size
b. 12” × 12” or 20” × 20” in size
c. 8” × 12” or 18” × 24” in size
d. 11” × 16” or 21” × 26” in size

42. A board which is used both for informational and educational purposes is called:
a. Whiteboard b. Blackboard
c. Flannel board d. Bulletin board

PRINCIPLES & MAXIMS OF TEACHING

43. Which of the following is NOT the maxim of teaching?
a. Known to unknown b. Complex to simple
c. Concrete to abstract d. Analysis to synthesis

PEDAGOGY VS ANDROGOGY

44. Andragogy refers to:
a. Child learning b. Adult learning
c. Learning by doing d. Practical learning

PRINCIPLES OF TEACHING

45. Which of these is NOT a conventional philosophy?
a. Idealism b. Naturalism
c. Pragmatism d. Existentialism

46. Which philosophy believes that ultimate goal of human activities is the realization of human mind in his or herself?
a. Idealism b. Pragmatism
c. Realism d. Existentialism

47. Which of the following is not the principle of Lesson Planning?
a. Flexible
b. Mastery and adequate training on the topic
c. Active student participation
d. Single teaching method

48. In which type of objective, breaking down of professional functions into components (activities) is done that together indicate the nature of the functions?
a. Central b. Specific
c. Intermediate d. Tertiary

49. Which philosophical thought states that ‘ultimate reality is spiritual rather than physical, mental rather than material’? ***(Tutor Exam 2015, AIIMS, Rishikesh)***
a. Idealism b. Realism
c. Pragmatism d. Spiritualism

50. John Dewey was a proponent of:
a. Spiritualism b. Idealism
c. Realism d. Pragmatism

51. Who among the following proposed that education be designed on the basis of a theory of experience?
a. Socrates b. John Dewey
c. Aristotle d. Jean Piaget

52. All of the following are traditional philosophies of education; EXCEPT:
a. Idealism b. Pragmatism
c. Naturalism d. Essentialism

METHODS OF TEACHING

53. The best method to teach a patient any skills, such as using inhaler, is by: ***(AIIMS BBS NO 2018):***
a. Lecture b. Demonstration
c. Discussion d. Panel session

Explanation: The best method to teach a patient any skills, is by doing and showing the things. Demonstration is the process of performing the procedure the way teacher expects the learner to practice.

54. Which of the following is NOT an autocratic method of teaching?
a. Lecture b. Demonstration
c. Discussion d. Tutorial

55. Teaching method in which students learn to do critical thinking through discussion and interaction and develop higher analytical cognitive skills is:
a. Seminar b. Symposium
c. Panel discussion d. Lecture

Explanation: A seminar is a teaching method in which a small group of students meets with a teacher or other expert to discuss a particular topic. The seminar is typically led by the teacher/mentor or expert, but the students are encouraged to participate in the discussion and ask questions.

56. Which of the following is not a clinical method of teaching?
a. Case methods/case study b. Nursing rounds and reports
c. Process recording d. Seminar

57. Method of teaching in which an excursion to the patient’s area is arranged to provide learning experience to the students is:
a. Case presentation b. Nursing rounds
c. Morning report d. Process recording

58. A written verbatim account of a visit for the purpose of bringing out the interplay between the patient and the nurse:
a. Morning report b. Evening report
c. Case study d. Process recording

59. The most essential quality of an effective teacher is:
a. A strict personality
b. Communication skill
c. Friendly attitude
d. Superior knowledge of the subject

60. Which method of teaching would be most suitable to teach nursing care of children with “Mental Retardation” for a class of 100 nursing students?
a. Group discussion b. Lecture cum discussion
c. Problem-solving d. Web-based learning

61. A group of 10 people are speaking on a topic of common interest in an educational programme. This method is best known as:
a. Workshop b. Panel discussion
c. Group discussion d. Lecture

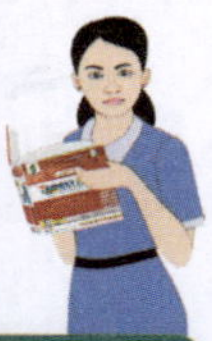

Ans.

40.	a
41.	a
42.	d
43.	b
44.	b
45.	d
46.	a
47.	d
48.	d
49.	a
50.	d
51.	b
52.	d
53.	b
54.	c
55.	a
56.	d
57.	b
58.	d
59.	b
60.	c
61.	c

62. **All that is learnt during educational activities that is not a designated part of official curriculum is known as the:**
 a. Extra curriculum b. Observed curriculum
 c. Hidden curriculum d. Experienced curriculum
63. **The demonstration on "Neurological examination" would be most useful, if done in a group of:**
 a. 10 b. 20
 c. 25 d. 30
64. **Which one of the following is NOT among the maxims of Teaching?**
 a. Analysis to synthesis b. General to particular
 c. Easy to difficult d. Concrete to abstract
65. **Lesson plan is prepared by the:**
 a. Teacher b. Administrator
 c. Student d. Principal
66. **Which one of the following is not a quality of a good teacher?**
 a. Good Motivator b. Intolerance
 c. Leadership d. Mastery of the content
67. **Which of the following learning domain is a skill domain?**
 a. Cognitive b. Affective
 c. Conative d. None of these
68. **Which of the following learning domains influence nursing practice?**
 a. Cognitive and conative
 b. Conative and affective
 c. Affective and cognitive
 d. Cognitive, conative and affective
69. **Panel discussion method was introduced by:**
 a. William James b. Harry A. Overstreet
 c. W.F. Skinner d. Jean Piaget
70. **Preferably, panel discussion consists of:**
 a. 3–5 members b. 4–8 members
 c. 6–9 members d. 6–10 members
71. **Role of the participants in seminars include:**
 a. Observe the speaker
 b. Observe and note the information
 c. Analyze, discuss and critique the content
 d. Listen to the speeches and prepare an article for publication
72. **Who decides the topic of any seminar?**
 a. Secretary
 b. Participants
 c. Chairperson
 d. Organizer
73. **Ideally, the duration of a seminar presentation is:**
 a. 20-30 minutes
 b. 30-45 minutes
 c. 45-60 minutes
 d. 60-120 minutes
74. **The duration of micro-teaching is:**
 a. 2-5 minutes
 b. 5-10 minutes
 c. 10-15 minutes
 d. 15-20 minutes.
75. **Conference is a type of:**
 a. Discussion
 b. Group discussion
 c. Lecture
 d. Work shop
76. **The type of teaching method that allows learning the first hand information to the student is:**
 a. Group discussion
 b. Program instruction
 c. Field trip
 d. Nursing care studies
77. **Case method is a:**
 a. Lecture method
 b. Clinical method
 c. Individual discussion
 d. Demonstration method
78. **All of the following are a method of clinical teaching; EXCEPT:**
 a. Simulation
 b. Nursing round
 c. Case discussion
 d. Case method
79. **Common topics preferred for symposiums are related to:**
 a. Recent trends in nursing
 b. Controversies in nursing
 c. Innovations in nursing
 d. Emergency conditions
80. **Which of the following is a discussion method in which the participants have the opportunity for direct conversation with the speaker?**
 a. Seminar
 b. Conference
 c. Lecture
 d. Symposium
81. **Syllabus is a part of:**
 a. Student
 b. College
 c. Institution
 d. Curriculum
82. **Which of the following learning domain is skill domain?**
 a. Psychomotor
 b. Cognitive
 c. Attitude
 d. Affective
83. **One of the objectives of microteaching is:**
 a. To learn the knowledge through peer group
 b. To learn the skills through feedback
 c. To enable the teacher trainee to learn and incorporate the new teaching skills under controlled condition
 d. To learn to complete the task within time
84. **A group of 6-8 qualified experts discusses a topic in front of an audience. This is known as:**
 a. Group discussion b. Panel discussion
 c. Symposium d. Webinar
85. **The most important step to consider while giving health education to a community is:**
 a. Participation of doctors
 b. Knowing of local needs
 c. Health education
 d. Community discussion
86. **Which domain of objectives is not being evaluated through our present system of examination?**
 a. Cognitive b. Conative
 c. Affective d. All of these

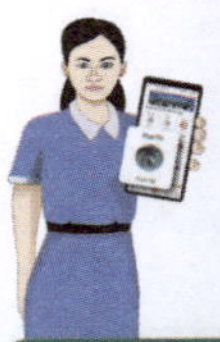

Ans.

62.	c
63.	a
64.	b
65.	a
66.	b
67.	c
68.	d
69.	b
70.	b
71.	c
72.	d
73.	d
74.	b
75.	a
76.	c
77.	b
78.	a
79.	b
80.	d
81.	d
82.	a
83.	c
84.	b
85.	b
86.	c

87. Which of the following would be the best teaching method to increase awareness of rural population towards small family?
a. Charts
b. Role playing
c. Film show
d. Television

88. Students who ask questions in the classroom should be:
a. Advised to meet the teacher personally after the class
b. Encouraged to find answers independently
c. Encouraged to continue asking questions
d. Reprimanded for misbehavior

89. Participation of men and women factory workers together in an educational program on "Safe Sex" would first depend on the:
a. Consideration of the factory owner
b. Culture of that particular social group
c. Comfort of the Health Educator
d. Convenience of the factory manager

90. The purpose of Lesson Planning is to:
a. Complete the prescribed syllabus
b. Ensure complete learning of the topic
c. Promote attention of student
d. Provide written notes to students

91. Which of the following factor should the teacher always consider while writing outcomes and objectives for technology-enhanced lessons?
a. Teaching methods to be used
b. Technology skills to be learned
c. Skills and attitude to be learned
d. All of the above

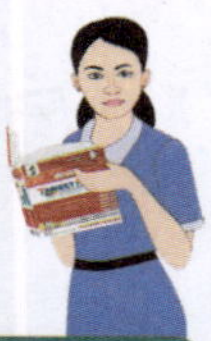

EVALUATION/ASSESSMENT METHODS

92. Unit planning provides sound basis of: *(AIIMS Nagpur NO 2018)*
a. Implementation
b. Planning
c. Re-planning
d. Evaluation

Explanation: Unit planning may be defined as comprehensive series of the related content and meaningful educational activities, so developed as to achieve pupil's purposes, provide significant educational experiences which result in appropriate behavioral changes. It provides basis of evaluation.

93. The educational assessment that is generally carried out throughout a course or project is known as:
a. Criterion-referenced assessment
b. Continuous assessment
c. Formative assessment
d. Summative assessment

94. The educational assessment that is generally carried out at the end of the course is known as:
(OR)
The type of assessment where the outcome is evaluated at the end of academic year is: *(AIIMS Raipur NO 2019)*
a. Summative evaluation
b. Formative evaluation
c. Periodical evaluation
d. Program evaluation

Explanation: Summative evaluation: The outcome is evaluated at the end of academic year. It is a certifying evaluation designed to develop competent personnel from practicing.
Formative evaluation: It is an in-process evaluation of student through the course., e.g., Class tests.
Periodical evaluation: Weekly and monthly evaluation. It is schedule to re-occur.
Program evaluation: The systematic assessment of outcomes of a program or policy

95. Which of the following is not the purpose of assessment?
a. Certification
b. Safeguarding public
c. Monitoring the program
d. Safeguarding educational institution

96. The important characteristic of assessment tool that helps us know about whether the tool measures what it is intended to measure is:
a. Validity
b. Objectivity
c. Reliability
d. Practicability

97. A type of validity in which the test scores correlates with another construct related to what is being tested is called:
a. Content validity
b. Construct validity
c. Face validity
d. Criterion validity

98. The method used to establish reliability of a tool is:
a. Chi-square test
b. Fisher's exact test
c. Split half test
d. Paired t test

99. Which of the following tool can be used for assessing student's ability to perform suctioning?
a. Likert scale
b. Checklist
c. Semantic differential scale
d. Critical incident technique

100. The purpose of taking return demonstration from students after a teaching session of demonstration of nursing procedure is to:
a. Fulfill syllabus norm
b. Ensure safe Nursing practice
c. Follow institutional policy
d. Identify mistakes

101. Before the nursing students start their clinical postings, the supervising teacher needs to:
a. Help students to identify their own 'Learning Objectives'
b. Inform students about make-up duty for their absence during clinical postings
c. Instruct students to help doctors in treating patients
d. Instruct to bring text books along with them

102. The uniform method of assessing students' overall learning would be:
a. Objective structured clinical evaluation
b. Case method
c. Group Project
d. Viva Voce

103. ________ is an example of Criterion-referenced assessment.
a. IQ test
b. Wechsler Intelligence Scale for Children (WISC)
c. Driving test
d. Graduate Record Examination (GRE)

Ans.
87. b
88. c
89. b
90. b
91. c
92. d
93. c
94. a
95. d
96. a
97. b
98. c
99. b
100. b
101. a
102. a
103. c

104. Which of the following is NOT a problem-solving approach?
a. Inductive approach b. Logical approach
c. Reasoning approach d. Deductive approach

105. List of items with appropriate columns meant to be observed by the observer is known as:
a. Questionnaire b. Checklist
c. Ranking item d. Anecdotal record

106. Problem solving evaluation enables the teacher to assess the students':
a. Critical thinking b. Emotional status
c. Adaptability d. Adjustability

107. Multiple choice questions consist of:
a. A statement with a blank space
b. A problem and a list of solutions
c. Assertion and reason
d. An open ended question without distractors

108. When assessing the academic achievement of the students, which of the following factors is most important to consider:
a. The students' current performance level
b. The students' interest in education
c. The students' prior opportunities to learn
d. The students' ability to learn

GUIDANCE AND COUNSELING

109. Who plays a proactive role in counseling?
a. Counselee b. Counselor
c. Administrator d. Referee

110. Listening in counseling is what process?
a. Passive process b. Dual process
c. Active process d. Lengthy process

111. The final step of directive counseling is:
a. Prognosis b. Synthesis
c. Follow-up d. Diagnosis

112. The test that is intended to measure the learnt knowledge and skill is:
a. Aptitude test b. Achievement test
c. Ability test d. Observation

113. Trustworthiness of the counselor is termed as:
a. Fidelity b. Justice
c. Autonomy d. Intelligence

114. Number of phases in counseling process is:
a. 2 - 3 b. 5
c. 7 d. 8

115. Counseling should be done by a:
a. Teacher b. Parent
c. A trained counselor d. Any of these

116. Guidance is provided by:
a. Teachers b. Parents
c. A trained guide d. Any experienced person

COMMUNICATION PROCESS

117. The nurse lean towards the patient in the communication to:
a. Maintain eye contact b. To comfort the patient
c. Show genuine interest d. Show courtesy

118. Non-verbal communication includes:
a. Phrases b. Gestures
c. Information d. Words

119. The communication phase that is facilitated by knowledge of the patients is known as:
a. Message heard b. Thinking of a message
c. Decoding the message d. All of these

120. All are important elements of communication process; EXCEPT: *(SAFDARJUNG NO 2018)*
a. Sender and receiver b. Referent and message
c. Channel and feedback d. Time and environment

Explanation: Communication is an ongoing process where time is not considered during communication.

Elements of communication are sender, referent (motivates the sender or receiver to share information) receiver, message, channel of communication and feedback from receiver.

121. Health education by a nurse to a group of people can be termed as: *(Safdarjung NO 2018)*
a. Small group communication
b. Interpersonal communication
c. Intrapersonal communication
d. Public communication

Explanation: Health education is an example of small group communication. Where communication is between nurse and group of people.

122. Translating the message into verbal and non-verbal symbols to communicate the receiver means: *(Safdarjung NO 2018)*
a. Encoding b. Decoding
c. Channel d. Feedback

Explanation: Encoding: The message is theoretical and intangible, its further passing requires use of certain symbols such as words, actions or pictures, etc. This process of conversion of message into the symbols is the process of encoding.

Decoding means interpretation. The receiver decodes the encoded message to understand the meaning of it.

123. Aspect of verbal communication includes:
a. Vocabulary b. Postures
c. Art and music d. Messages within message

124. Barrier of communication includes:
a. Information overload b. Exploring
c. Focusing d. Summarizing

125. Communication is described as the "matrix for all thought and relationships between persons" said by:
a. William Scott b. Murray and Zentner
c. GG Brown d. WH Newman

126. Mental processing of the message and understanding the senders' message is:
a. Decode b. Encode
c. Feedback d. Imagination

127. A technique whereby to repeats the main message the client has expressed is:
a. Listening b. Restating
c. Clarification d. Reflection

128. If a person is communicating with his friend on telephone, it is referred to as:
a. Intrapersonal communication
b. Interpersonal communication
c. Media communication
d. Mass communication

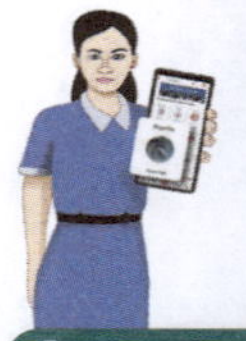

Ans.

Q	Ans
104.	b
105.	b
106.	a
107.	b
108.	c
109.	a
110.	c
111.	c
112.	b
113.	a
114.	b
115.	c
116.	d
117.	c
118.	b
119.	c
120.	d
121.	a
122.	a
123.	a
124.	a
125.	b
126.	a
127.	b
128.	b

129. Special words or expressions used by a profession or group that are difficult for others to understand are known as:

a. Equivocal terms b. Jargon
c. Technical terms d. Code language

130. An automatic psychological process of receiving aural stimuli is known as:

a. Listening b. Hearing
c. Understanding d. Speaking

131. In the communication process to encode means to:

a. Convert coded language into meaning
b. Translate ideas into a code
c. Infer the jargons
d. Analyze the code

132. Which of the following is an example of a non-verbal communication?

a. Vernacular language b. Smile
c. Jargon d. Slang

133. The one who receives the message is known as:

a. Encoder b. Decoder
c. Communicator d. Mediator

134. The health communication is:

a. Teacher centric
b. One of the costly methods of imparting information
c. Process oriented
d. Not includes relationship building

135. An effective communication should be:

a. One-way process b. Two-way process
c. Directive d. Three-way process

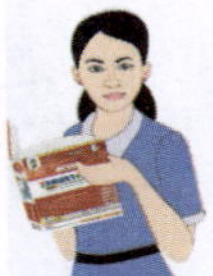

INTERPERSONAL COMMUNICATION AND RELATIONSHIP

136. Another name for interpersonal communication is:

a. Mass communication
b. Face to face public communication
c. Dyadic communication
d. Virtual reality

137. Which of the following is an example of mediated communication?

a. A newscaster delivers the weather report on the 6 o'clock news
b. Two friends gossip with one another
c. Students work on the class project together
d. A politician addresses a nominating convention

138. Comparing with small group communication, in organizational communication:

a. Feedback is easier and more immediate
b. Communication roles are more formal
c. Message can be better adapted to the specific needs of the receiver
d. People are closer to one another in space

139. As per the principles of communication "interpersonal communication is irreversible" means:

a. Once a word goes out of your mouth you can never swallow it again
b. Once created, communication has the physical property of matter, it can't be uncreated
c. Once communication begins, it never loops back on itself
d. All of the above

140. According to the statement "communication is interaction perspective", feedback is:

a. Never intentional b. Sometimes unintentional
c. Always intentional d. Seldom useful

141. A set of social rules that specify appropriate and inappropriate behavior in the given specific situations is known as:

a. Beliefs b. Rules
c. Norms d. Moral values

142. One of the most important reinforcing factors for a behavior to happen or to avoid:

a. Distant relatives influence
b. Change in the political parties of that particular area
c. Peer group
d. Imprisonment

143. Which of the following theories directly relates to behavior change?

a. PEN - 3 model b. Health Illness continuum
c. Rogers' theory d. McNileimers rule

144. An observational method used frequently in classroom or learning settings in which the observer summarizes a single developmental incident after the event has occurred is known as:

a. Anecdotal report b. Observational report
c. Contingency record d. Incident report

HUMAN RELATIONS

145. Maslow's Hierarchy of needs include:

a. Self-actualization b. Self-esteem
c. Physiological d. All of these

146. According to Maslow's hierarchy of needs, the highest level is:

a. Physiological needs b. Safety and Security
c. Love and affection d. Self-actualization

147. Which of the following is a characteristic of private relationships?

a. Extrinsic rewards
b. Normative rules
c. Use of particularistic knowledge
d. Substitutability

148. Basic components of attitude include all; EXCEPT:

a. Emotional component b. Informational component
c. Behavioral component d. Spiritual component

Ans.

129. b
130. a
131. b
132. b
133. b
134. c
135. b
136. c
137. a
138. b
139. d
140. b
141. c
142. c
143. a
144. a
145. d
146. d
147. c
148. d

"Better ten times ill than one time dead."
—Yiddish

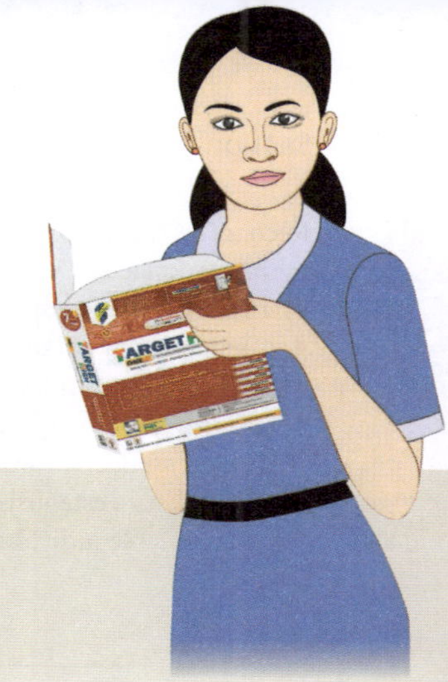

CHAPTER 13

NURSING ADMINISTRATION AND MANAGEMENT

SYNOPSIS

ORGANIZATION

A systematic arrangement of people brought together to accomplish some specific purpose/goal.

ADMINISTRATION

It is the organization and direction of human and material resources to achieve desired goals. (Pfiffner & Presthus)

MANAGEMENT

Process of getting things done efficiently and effectively through and with other people.

Levels of Management

- Top Managers
- Middle Managers
- First-Line Managers

Theories of Management

1. Classical Management Perspective
2. Behavioral Management Perspective
3. Quantitative Management Perspective

1. Classical Management Perspective

It includes both scientific management and administrative management.

- Concerned with improving the performance of individual workers (i.e., efficiency).
- A theory that focuses on managing the organization as a whole.

Scientific Management

Frederick Taylor

- Father of scientific management
- Replaced the old rule-of-thumb method.
- Believed in selecting, training, teaching and developing workers.
- Used time study, standards planning, exception rule of management, slide-rules, instruction cards, incentives, etc.

Frank and Lillian Gilbreth

- Reduced number of movements in bricklaying, resulting in increased output of 200%.

Henry Gantt

- Developed other techniques, including the Gantt chart, to improve working efficiency through planning/scheduling.

Administrative Management Theory

- Focuses on managing the organization.

Henri Fayol

- Wrote General and Industrial Management
- Helped to systematize the practice of management
- First to describe management as planning, organizing, leading and controlling.

Fayol's 14 Principles of Management

- Division of labor
- Authority
- Discipline
- Unity of command
- Unity of direction
- Subordination of individuals to the common good
- Remuneration
- Centralization
- Scalar chain
- Order
- Equity
- Stability
- Initiative
- *Esprit de corps*

2. Behavioral Management Perspective

- Emphasizes individual attitudes and behaviors and group processes.

KEY POINTS

- The administration is defined as an act of administering the whole organization by a group of people. (Top Level)
- Management is a systematic way of managing people and things **within the organization**. (Middle and lower level)

Practice Question

1. Which of the following is NOT one of the Fayol's principles of Management?

a. Centralization
b. Formal rules
c. Division of labor
d. Discipline

Ans. (b) Formal rules

- Recognizes the importance of behavioral processes in the workplace.
- **The Hawthorne Studies**
  - *Conducted by Elton Mayo and associates at Western Electric (1927–1935)*
  - *Group study: The effects of a piecework incentive plan on production workers*
    - Workers established informal levels of acceptable individual output.
    - Over-producing workers were labeled "rate busters" and under-producing workers were considered "chiselers."
  - *Interview program*
    - Confirmed the importance of human behavior in the workplace.
- ***Human Relations Movement***
  - Perspective that workers respond primarily to the social context of work
  - Abraham Maslow
    - Posited a hierarchy of needs

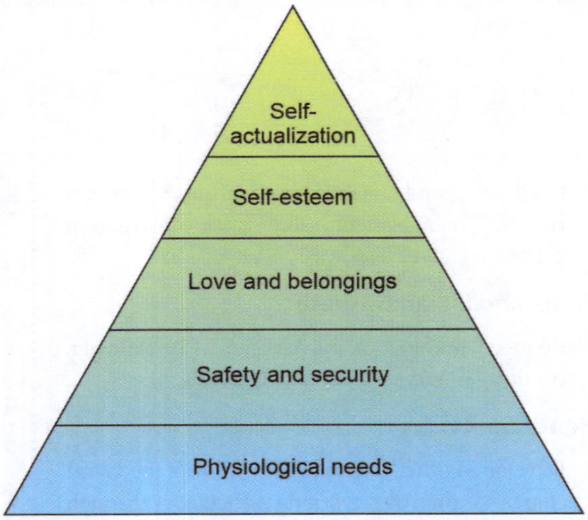

Figure 1: Hierarchy of needs

Douglas McGregor

- Proposed Theory X and Theory Y concepts of managerial beliefs.

Theory X

- People do not like work and try to avoid it.
- People do not like work, so managers have to control, direct, coerce, and threaten employees to get them to meet organizational goals.
- People prefer to be directed, to avoid responsibility and to want security; they have little ambition.

Theory Y

- Work is a natural part of people's lives.
- People are internally motivated by commitment.
- People are committed to goals to the degree they receive rewards.
- People will seek and accept responsibility.
- People have the capacity to be innovative.
- People are bright, but mostly under-utilized.

Max Weber Theory of Bureaucracy

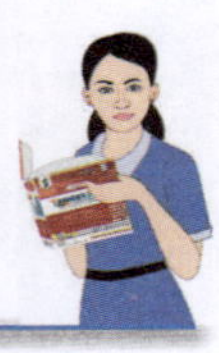

Used to describe a structure based on sociological concept of rationalization of collective activities.

Features of Bureaucracy

- Clear division of labor
- Hierarchical management of position
- Formal rules and regulation
- Impersonal relationship
- Employment based entirely on technical competence.

Organizational Behavior

- A contemporary field focusing on behavioral perspectives of management.
- Organizational behavior research
  - Job satisfaction
  - Job stress
  - Motivation and leadership
  - Group dynamics and organizational politics
  - Interpersonal conflict
  - Design of organizations
- **Five Functions of Management**
  i. Planning
  ii. Organizing
  iii. Coordinating
  iv. Directing
  v. Controlling

Practice Question

2. All of the following are the elements of management; EXCEPT:
a. Controlling
b. Organizing
c. Staffing
d. Commanding

Ans. (d) Commanding

KEY POINTS

- The Famous 14 Principles of management was proposed by Henry Fayol
- "Esprit de corps" refers to **Sense of belonging.** It is one of the Fayol's 14 principles of management.
- Theory X and Theory Y of management were proposed by Douglas McGregor
- Father of Scientific Management is **Frederic Winslow Taylor.**
- **Max Weber:** Theory of Bureaucracy.

Recent Question (INC PhD 2020)

1. Successive levels of authority in an organization represents
a. Hierarchy
b. Span of control
c. Unity of command
d. Division of labor

Ans. (a) Hierarchy

- **Organizing**
  - Management function of setting up the group, allocating resources, and assigning work to achieve goals.
- **Organization chart**
  - Uses boxes to represent the various positions or departments in an organization.
  - Lines connecting the boxes indicate who reports to whom.
- **Authority**
  - The right to perform a task or give orders to someone else.
- **Line Authority**
  - The right to carry out tasks and give orders related to the organization's primary purpose.
- **Staff Authority**
  - The right to advise or assist those with line authority.
- **Functional Authority**
  - The right given by higher management to specific staff personnel to give orders concerning an area in which the staff personnel have expertise.
- **Delegating:** Giving another person the authority and responsibility to carry out a task.

Elements of Administration

As per Luther Gulick elements of administration are POSDCORB

P	planning
O	organization
S	staffing
D	directing
CO	coordinating
R	reporting
B	budgeting

Comparing Formal and Informal Organization

Table 1: Comparison between formal and informal organization

Characteristics	Formal organization	Informal organization
Structure		
• Origin	Planned	Spontaneous
• Rationale	Rational	Emotional
• Characteristics	Stable	Dynamic
Position terminology	Job	Role
Goals	Profitability of service to society	Member satisfaction
Influence		
• Base	Position	Personality
• Type	Authority	Power
• Flow	Top-down	Bottom-up
Control mechanisms	Threat of firing, demotion	Physical or social sanctions (norms)
Communication		
• Channels	Formal channels	Grapevine
• Networks	Well defined, follow formal lines	Poorly defined, cut across regular channels
• Speed	Slow	Fast
• Accuracy	High	Low
Charting the organization	Organization chart	Sociogram
Miscellaneous		
• Individuals included	All individuals in work group	Only those "acceptable"
• Interpersonal relations	Prescribed by job description	Arise spontaneously
• Leadership role	Assigned by organization	Result of membership assignment
• Basis for interaction	Functional duties or position	Personal characteristics, ethnic background, status
• Basis for attachment	Loyalty	Cohesiveness

Recent Question (NORCET 2021)

2. PDSA stands for:

a. Plan, do, study, act
b. Plan, define, simplify, act
c. Plan, define, simplify, assume
d. Perform, due, simplify, act

Ans. (a) Plan, do, study, act

KEY POINTS

- The communication in which managers interact with people in other departments in the organization who are NOT at the same level in the hierarchy as them is called **diagonal communication.**
- **Vertical communication:** Information flows between or among subordinates and superiors of the organization.
- **Horizontal communication:** Exchange of information across departments at same level in an organization (similar hierarchical departments).
- Horizontal communication is also known as **lateral communication.**
- **Upward communication:** Communication proceeds from lower level to upper level.
- Assertiveness allows for objective responses.

3. Quantitative Management Perspective

- This theory is concerned with applying quantitative management tools focusing on decision making, economic effectiveness, mathematical models and the use of computer.
- Management science, operations management, and management informational system are its branches.

LEADERSHIP

Theories on Leadership

- **Trait theories:** Individual with certain trait or characteristic become leader.
- **Leadership style theories:** Leadership style form most significant basis for effective leadership.
- **Trait and situational match theory:** When certain trait match with particular situation leadership become most effective.
- **Leadership style and situational theory:** When certain leadership style match with particular situation leadership become effective.
- **Greatman theory:** According to this certain people are born with certain characteristics to become a leader.
- **Charismatic theory:** People become leaders because they have charisma, because of this other people feels better in their presence and they will get emotional support and inspiration from leaders.
- **Situational theory:** Different situation require different trait to become leaders. So, a person who is leader at one situation may become follower at another situation.
- **Contingency theory:** According to this leader's role depends upon three situation and are—(1) leader-member relation, (2) task structure and (3) position power.
  - Leader-member relation means the faith and loyalty group members possessed towards the leader.
  - Task structure is said to be high if it is easy to define and measure a task in terms of goal clarity, extent to which the decision can be verified, multiplicity of goal path and specificity of solution. If not, then task structure is low.
  - Position power: It means the power which they are obtaining by sitting in a specified position or a chair.
- **Path goal theory:** As per this, leader facilitates the followers to accomplish goal by minimizing the obstruction and rewarding them for the accomplishment of the task.

Leadership Styles

- **Autocratic leadership:** Leader has strong control over the group and takes decision.
- **Democratic leadership:** Leader acts as a facilitator and encourages the group to take decision
- **Laissez fare leadership:** Leader participates minimally and acts as a resource person or consultant.
- **Participative leadership:** In this style functions are distributed among all the group members.

Leadership Style in Nursing

- Charismatic leadership
- Authoritarian leadership
- Democratic or participative leadership
- Laissez fare leadership
- Situational leadership
- Transactional leadership

BUDGETING

- Budget is the forecast of the resources required to deliver the services offered by the organization.
- A budget is a financial plan that includes estimated expenses as well as income for a period of time.
- Principles of budgeting:
  - Sound financial management
  - Based on objectives and polices
  - Financial and non-financial resources
  - Planned in advance
  - Consistent delegation
  - Coordination efforts
  - Adequate checks and balances
  - Appropriate to the nature of business
  - Under directions and supervision
  - Quality and quantity evaluation.
- Types of budget:
  - **Incremental budget:** A budget which is prepared using a previous period's budget or actual performance as a basis with incremental amounts added for the new budget period.
  - **Programme budget:** This type of budget includes expenses and revenues related to one specific project.
  - **Open-ended budget:** This is when a firm has pending transactions that will occur near the end of the accounting period, and the budget will not change until these are accounted for.
  - **Production budget:** The production budget calculates the number of units of products that must be manufactured.
  - **Cash budget:** A cash budget is an estimation of the cash flows of a business over a specific period of time.
  - **Flexible budget:** A flexible budget is a budget that adjusts or flexes with changes in volume or activity.
  - **Zero-based budget:** Zero-based budgeting (ZBB) is a method of budgeting in which all

Recent Question
(INC PhD 2020)

3. Power due to position is
a. Expert
b. Legitimate
c. Coercive
d. Reward

Ans. (b) Legitimate

KEY POINTS

- The leadership style in which the leader alone determines policies and makes plans is **Autocratic.**
- Whole team is involved in formulating decision in **democratic leadership.**
- **Laissez-faire leadership** (delegative leadership): Leader is hands-off and allows group members to make the decisions. The leader has absolutely no control.

expenses must be justified for each new period. This approach requires organizations to build their annual budget from zero each year to help verify that all components of the annual budget are cost-effective, relevant, and drive improved savings.

- **Rollover budget:** A *rollover budget* is when the budget category totals rollover into the following budget cycle.
- **Fixed ceiling budget:** A fixed budget is a financial plan that is not modified for variations in actual activity.
- **Capital expenditure budget:** A capital expenditure budget is a formal plan that states the amounts and timing of fixed asset purchases by an organization.

MATERIAL MANAGEMENT

It is a scientific technique, concerned with Planning, Organizing and Control of flow of materials, from their initial purchase to destination.

Aims of Material Management

To Get

- The right quality
- Right quantity of supplies
- At the Right time
- At the Right place
- For the Right cost

Purpose of Material Management

- To gain economy in purchasing
- To satisfy the demand during period of replenishment
- To carry reserve stock to avoid stock out
- To stabilize fluctuations in consumption
- To provide reasonable level of client services.

Objectives of Material Management

Primary

- Right price
- High turnover
- Low procurement
- Storage cost
- Continuity of supply
- Consistency in quality
- Good supplier relations
- Development of personnel
- Good information system

Secondary

- Interdepartmental
- Forecasting
- Product improvement
- Standardization
- Make or buy decision
- New materials and product
- Favorable reciprocal relationship

Basic Needs of Material Management

- To have adequate stock of material when required.
- To spend minimum money for high quality material.
- To reduce the inventory investment and to operate it efficiently.

Functional Areas of Material Management

- Purchasing
- Central service supply
- Central stores
- The print shops
- The pharmacy
- Dietary and linen services

INVENTORY CONTROL

It means stocking adequate number and kind of stores so that the materials can be available whenever and wherever required. Scientific inventory control results in optimal balance.

Functions of Inventory Control

- To provide maximum supply service, consistent with maximum efficiency and optimum investment.
- To provide cushion between forecasted and actual demand for a material

Always Better Control (ABC) Analysis

Items are divided into three categories named A, B and C.

A items are high value items, B items are intermediate value and C items are low value items.

- **Item A:** These are important items and it is about 10–20% of inventory items and consume 50–60% of the inventory cost. These items are having tight control and is managed by top level manager.
- **Item B:** These are 30–40% of all inventory items and consume 30–40% of the total inventory cost. These are important items but not critical. **These items are having moderate control and is managed by middle level manager.**
- **Item C:** Item C account for 40–50% of all inventory items and needs 5–10% of the total inventory cost. These items are having low level control and is managed by low level manager.

Recent Question
(INC PhD 2020)

4. Budget which shows income and expenditure is known as
a. Capital budget
b. Revenue budget
c. Operational budget
d. Fixed budget

Ans. (b) Revenue budget

VED Analysis

V = Vital
E = Essential
D = Desirable

- Vitals means shortage of the item cannot be tolerated.
- Essential items are those items, shortage of which can be tolerated for a short period.
- Desirable items are those items, shortage of which will not adversely leave any impact.

FSN Analysis

Based on Utilization

- Fast moving
- Slow moving
- Nonmoving

Nonmoving items must be periodically reviewed to prevent expiry and obsolescence.

HML Analysis

Based on Cost per Unit

- Highest
- Medium
- Low

This is used to keep control over consumption at departmental level for deciding the frequency of physical verification.

STAFF DEVELOPMENT

Activities involved in staff development are as follows:

- Induction training
- Job orientation
- In-service education
- Continuing education

Induction Training

During the first 2–3 days of duty the employee is given with brief explanation of policies, regulations, philosophy and standard.

Job Orientation

New employee is given with orientation regarding job responsibilities. work place, client and coworker.

In-service Education

Ongoing job instructions are given to employees to enhance their work performance.

Continuing Education

It's a planned activity directed towards meeting learning needs of a the nurse following basic nursing education exclusive of full time formal post-basic education.

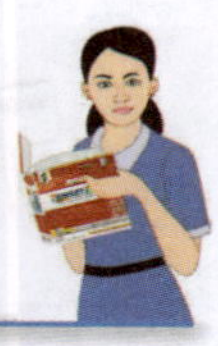

QUALITY MANAGEMENT

Quality is defined as proper performance (according to standards) of interventions that are known to be safe, that are affordable to the society in question, and that have the ability to produce an impact on mortality, morbidity, disability and malnutrition.

- **Quality management** can be considered to have four main components: quality planning, quality control quality assurance and quality improvement.
- **Quality management** uses quality assurance and control of processes as well as products to achieve more consistent quality.

Principles of Quality Management

- Customer focus
- Leadership
- Involvement of people
- Process approach
- System approach to management
- Continual improvement
- Factual approach to decision making
- Mutually beneficial supplier relationships

Approaches for a Quality Assurance Programme

- Credentialing
- Licensure
- Accreditation
- Certification

Credentialing

Credentialing refers to a type of designation, award, status, recognition, or ***seal of approval*** to the individuals or organizations.

It is the formal reorganization and establishing qualification of licensed individual.

Licensure

It is granting permission to the individual for the entry and exit from a particular profession. Licensure helps to ensure the quality professional practice.

Accreditation

Accreditation is a process in which certification of competency, authority, or credibility is awarded to an agency or organization.

Assessment is done by an independent agency.

Agency's physical structure, organizational structure and personnel qualifications are assessed.

The aim of accreditation is to encourage organizational development.

Example: NABH and NAAC accreditation for Hospitals and Universities/Educational institutes respectively.

KEY POINTS

- **Cost-benefit analysis** is the most popular economic evaluation tool used for program priority setting.
- The cost covering the salaries of the staff and machinery/equipment is termed Fixed cost.
- Inventory control is the process of maintaining the optimum needed quantity that is sufficient for the smooth operation of the organization.
- **Procurement:** Process of selecting vendors, establishing payment terms, selection, negotiation, and purchasing of goods.
- The time that elapses between placement of an order and delivery of the material is termed **Lead Time**.
- VED stands for Vital, Essential and Desirable.
- **FSN** stands for fast-moving, slow-moving and non-moving items.
- In FSN analysis, items are classified on the basis of rate of consumption.
- Delegation refers to assignment of any responsibility or authority to another person to carry out specific activities.
- The purpose to conduct staff training is to improve communications, staff morale, and quality of work.

Certification

It is a process of providing with an official document attesting to a status or level of achievement.

- **Example:** Professional certification, trade certification, etc.

Quality Assurance Methods

Peer Review

It means quality of work or a product is cross-checked by the members of same professional group. Peers can identify errors or problem fastly and easily than any other one and can be corrected.

Standards can be classified and formulated according to frames of references used for setting and evaluating nursing care services.

Structure Standard

A structural standard involves the 'set-up' of the institution. They refer to the organizational structure in which nursing is implemented. In this it will measure whether the structure is adequate, reliable and desirable.

Process Standards

Process standards describe the behaviors of the nurse at the desired level of performance.

A process standard involves the activities concerned with delivering patient care.

Outcome Standards

- Outcome standards refer to the description of the results of nursing activity in terms of the change that occurs in the patient.
- This change may be due to nursing care, medical care or as a result of variety of services offered to the patient.
- Outcome standards reflect the effectiveness and results rather than the process of giving care.

NURSING AUDIT

- Nursing audit is a method which systematically examines the quality of nursing care **(Elison).**
- Nursing audit evaluates the nursing functions to help to appraise and improve the quality of patient care as per the standards and criteria laid down by the experts.
- Nursing audit committee.
- Audit committee is needed to establish criteria and process for quality assurance and to evaluate care, make recommendations and do follow ups.

NORMS OF STAFFING (SIU—STAFF INSPECTION UNIT)

- Nurse patient ratio as per SIU norms.

Table 2: Wards and their nurse patient ratio

Ward	Nurse patient ratio
General Ward	1 : 6
Special Wards (pediatrics, burns, neurosurgery, cardiothoracic, neuromedicine, nursing home, spinal injury, emergency wards attached to casualty)	1 : 4
ICU	1:1 (Nothing mentioned about the shifts)
OT	Major: 2 nurses per table Minor: 1 nurse per table
Labor Room	1 nurse per table

- One Nursing sister (in-charge) for every 3.6 staff nurses.
- One ANS for every 4.5 nursing sisters.
- One DNS for every 7.5 ANS.
- Nursing superintendent for every 250–500 beds.
- CNO for 500 or more bedded hospitals.

NORMS OF (AS PER INC AND TNAI)

Chief nursing officer	1:500
Nursing superintendent	1:400 or above
DNS	1:300 and additionally one for every 200 beds
ANS	1 for 100–150 beds or 3–4 wards
Ward sister	1 for 25–30 bed or one ward. 30% leave reserve

Contd...

Recent Question (INC PhD 2020)

5. Steps involved in job description include all; EXCEPT:
a. Job summary
b. Job appraisal
c. Working conditions
d. Skills and specification

Ans. (b) Job appraisal

Practice Question

3. The process of assessing staff members for their contribution to the organization is
a. Peer-review
b. Job review
c. Performance appraisal
d. Job assessment

Ans. (c) Performance appraisal

Recent Question (AIIMS Bibinagar, Faculty 2023)

6. What is a systematic process of collecting information related to a specific job called?
a. Rating scale
b. Q-sort technique
c. Job description
d. Job analysis

Ans. (d) Job analysis

KEY POINTS

- Quality assurance is concerned with standard of practice.
- Quality indicator is the best to determine whether high quality care is being delivered.
- An organization's ability to meet analytical specifications for precision and accuracy is referred to as quality control.
- The audit which is conducted between two regular audits is known as "Interim Audit".

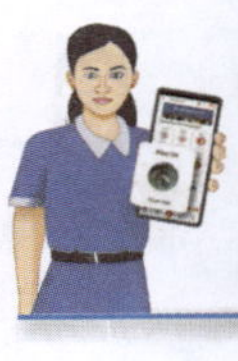

Staff nurse	
General ward (teaching hospital)	1:3
General ward (non-teaching hospital)	1:5–30% leave reserve
OPD and emergency	1:100
ICU	1:1

- It is suggested that for 250 bed hospital there should be One Infection Control Nurse (ICN).

TEACHER-STUDENT RATIO FOR NURSING PROGRAMS AS PER INDIAN NURSING COUNCIL (INC)

- 1 teacher: 10 students for BSc Nursing and GNM courses.
- 1 teacher: 5 students for MSc Nursing courses.

Recent Questions
(AIIMS Bibinagar, Faculty 2023)

7. A planned learning experience provided by employing an agency for the improvement of employees is known as:
a. Career planning
b. Democratic management
c. In-service education
d. Job description

Ans. (c) In-service...

8. Evaluations conducted on behalf of patients who are still undergoing care is called:
a. Retrospective nursing audit
b. Concurrent nursing audit
c. Closed chart audit
d. Prospective nursing audit

Ans. (b) Concurrent...

Golden Points to Remember

- Mission statement is a broad statement of an organization that specifies how it will achieve its goals.
- **Henri Fayol:** 14 principles of management.
- Performance appraisal is the way of acknowledging the performance of an employee.
- Source of income in budgeting terms is called **Revenue.**
- Headquarters of International Nursing Council is in **Geneva.**
- Patient care method in which patient care areas provide various levels of care Progressive patient care. E.g. Step down units.
- Purpose of recruitment is to provide a pool of potentially qualified candidates for job.
- Individuals who do NOT make decision unit they are aware of all the facts pertaining to a certain situation are called **open minded.**
- SWOT stands for strengths, weaknesses, opportunities and threats.
- The most crucial phase of group dynamics is storming phase.
- Ward in-charge Nurse (head nurse) is responsible for inventory control at lower managerial level.
- **Replacement:** There must be a regular system of replacing certain items when they are broken or of no use before new ones are supplied.
- **Procurement:** Process of selecting vendors, establishing payment terms, strategic vetting, selection, negotiation and purchasing of goods.
- **Storage:** Materials stored in an appropriate place in a correct way.
- **Democratic leadership**: Whole team is involved in formulating decision.
- **Autocratic leadership:** Leader alone establishing policies and making plans. The criteria used by him is "Do what I say or else..."
- **Laissez-faire leadership:** This is also known as delegative leadership in which leaders are hands-off and allow group members to make the decisions. The leader has absolutely no control.
- Leaders have followers whereas managers do not have followers.
- World Health Organization (WHO) was constituted in the year 1947.
- WHO is headquartered in Geneva, Switzerland.
- The International Council of Nurses (ICN) was established in the year 1899.
- The International Council of Nurses (ICN) is headquartered in Geneva, Switzerland.
- Quality indicators is the best to determine whether high quality care is being delivered.
- An organization's ability to meet analytical specifications for precision and accuracy is referred to as **quality control.**
- Procedure manual is a written document which guides rationalized nursing measures.
- A planned schedule of duty hours of nurses is referred to as Duty Roaster.
- **The INC standard for Teacher:** UG Students ratio for nursing colleges is 1:10.
- National Health Policy is announced by Government of India in the year 1982.

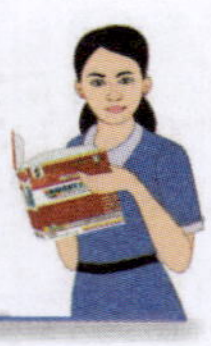

"As I see it, every day you do one of two things: build health or produce disease in yourself."
—Adelle Davis

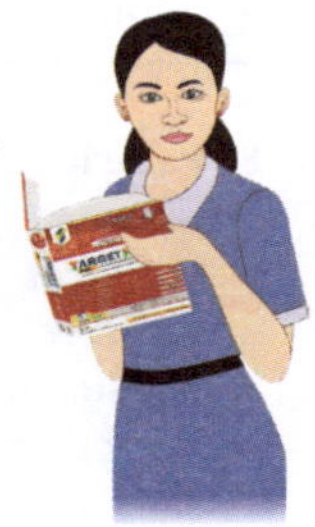

MULTIPLE CHOICE QUESTIONS

(Including Explained and Practice Questions)

INTRODUCTION TO NURSING ADMINISTRATION & MANAGEMENT

1. Which of the following is NOT the principle of organization? *(RAK MSC 2018)*

a. Hierarchy
b. Delegation
c. Span of control
d. Pervasiveness

Explanation: Pervasiveness is not the principle of the organization. There are six principles of organization given by Henri Fayol (1947)

- Hierarchy
- Span of control
- Integration Vs Disintegration
- Centralization Vs Decentralization
- Unity of Command
- Delegation

2. The level of conversation in which no sharing of oneself occurs is: *(AIIMS-BBS SNO 2019)*

a. Level 1: Open conversation
b. Level 5: Cliché conversation
c. Level 4: Reporting of facts
d. Level 2: Spontaneous conversation

Explanation:

- **Level 5 (cliché' conversation)** It is very superficial communication, where there is no communication about their self and everyone remains safe in conversation.
- **Level 1 (Open conversation)** This happens in emotionally open and honest communication.
- **Level 2 (Spontaneous conversation)** Spontaneous thought like what is felt about situation is shared.
- **Level 3 (My ideas or judgment)** Own ideas and opinion are shared.
- **Level 4 (Reporting of facts)** Share facts and expose almost nothing about personal.

3. Which of the following function the LEAST important to a nurse manager? *(RAK MSc 2018)*

a. Decision-making
b. Manipulating people
c. Monitoring subordinates
d. Effective leading

Explanation: Role of Nurse as a Manager include all except manipulating the people, as manipulation involves managing or influence skillfully, especially in an unfair manner.

4. Professional negligence is legally termed as: *(AIIMS Raipur NO 2019)*

a. Crime
b. Assault
c. Malpractice
d. Slander

Explanation:

- Malpractice is a professional liability based on negligence and includes professional misconduct, breach of duty or standard of care, illegal or immoral conduct or failure to exercise reasonable skill, all of which lead to harm.
- **Crime** is an offence and is punishable by law.
- An assault is the act of inflicting physical harm or unwanted physical contact upon a person.
- **Slander** refers to crime of making false spoken statement damaging to a person's reputation.

5. The process that enables one to access a nurse or a physician via telephone or computer is called: *(AIIMS BPL NO 2018)*

a. Telehealth
b. E-Medicine
c. Quality assurance
d. Distant consultation

Explanation: Telehealth involves the distribution of health-related services and information via electronic information and telecommunication technologies. Distance consultation comes under the ambit of telehealth. **E-medicine** refers to electronic collection of medical information and record about the person that can be stored in the computer.

6. The commission or omission of an act that a reasonably prudent person would have performed in a similar situation thus causing harm to another person is called: *(AIIMS BPL NO 2018)*

a. Negligence
b. Libel
c. Slander
d. Assault

Explanation: An unintentional tort is one that is negligent, as opposed to intentional torts, which are torts done deliberately. Intentional torts include assault, battery, false imprisonment, intentional infliction of emotional distress, libel, slander and trespassing.

7. Which of the following situation is considered as an intentional tort? *(Safdarjung NO 2018)*

a. Nurse miscounts the gauze pads during a surgery.
b. Nurse divulges private information about the patient to media.
c. Nurse causes a burn when applying a warm soak to legs.
d. Nurse fails to monitor blood pressure when administering an anti-hypertensive to drugs.

Explanation: Nurse divulges private information about the patient to media is to be considered as intentional tort. Intentional tort is a civil wrong performed by a person knowingly and the person was also aware of the possible consequences of his/her act.

Miscounting the gauze pads, failure to monitor the vital signs and causing burns while applying warm soakage are examples of negligence or malpractice.

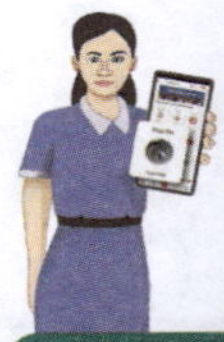

Ans.

1.	d
2.	b
3.	b
4.	c
5.	a
6.	a
7.	b

8. False harmful written report is called: *(Kerala PSC, Nov 2014)*

a. Libel b. Slander
c. Tort d. Felony

9. Nursing management research should focus on:

a. Patient treatments b. Patient care
c. Patient complaints d. Quality assurance

10. The study of how people interact within groups and its principles are used to make businesses operate more effectively is known as:

a. Classic Theory
b. Humanistic Behavior
c. Organizational Behavior
d. Holistic Behavior Concept

11. It is the way in which people work one another in a coordinal manner recognizing other's needs, views, values and temperaments.

a. Personal Relation b. Human Relation
c. Family Relation d. Formal Relation

12. Skilled communication of ideas to the various members of the public with objectives of producing a desired result is referred to as:

a. Human Relation
b. Public Relation
c. Behavior
d. Therapeutic Communication

THEORIES OF MANAGEMENT

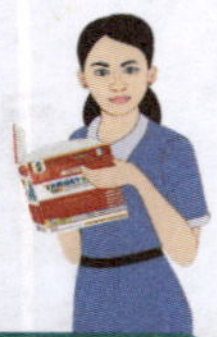

13. Who has given 14 principles of management? *(RAK MSC 2018)*

a. Daniel Fraud b. Mary Follett
c. Henri Fayol d. Florence Nightingale

Explanation: Henri Fayol described the 14 principles of management.

1. Division of work	8. Equity
2. Centralization	9. Unity of direction
3. Authority and Responsibility	10. Stability of Tenure
4. Scalar Chain	11. Interest
5. Discipline	12. Initiative
6. Order	13. Remuneration
7. Unity of Command	14. Esprit De Corp

14. Two-factor theory (Motivation-Hygiene theory) of management was proposed by: *(AIIMS-BBS SNO 2019)*

a. Frederick Herzberg b. W. Edwards Deming
c. Frederick Taylor d. Elton Mayo

Explanation:

Name	Contribution
Max Weber	Theory of Bureaucracy
Henri Fayol	14 principles of management
Frederic Winslow Taylor	Father of scientific management
Elton Mayo	Human relation motivation theory-including **Hawthorne effect.**

15. Which of the following theories stresses the importance of change within organizations? *(AIIMS-BBS SNO 2019)*

a. Neoclassical Theory b. Classical Theory
c. System Theory d. Chaos Theory

Explanation: Chaos theory incorporates principles of quantum mechanics. It stresses the importance of change within organizations.

16. Which of the following action guiding theory explains that the rightness or wrongness of an action depends on the consequences of the action? *(AIIMS BBS NO 2018)*

a. Utilitarian b. Deontological
c. Nonmaleficence d. Beneficence

Explanation: Utilitarian (ethical) theory is proposed by Jeremy Bentham and John Stuart Mill. This theory guides an individual to what to do in specific situation. An action is right if promotes happiness and will be considered wrong if it is against happiness. So, this theory explains about rightness and wrongness of any action depends on its consequences.

17. The ethical principle, which shows obligation to tell the truth is: *(AIIMS Raipur NO 2019)*

a. Autonomy b. Veracity
c. Fidelity d. Beneficence

Explanation:

- The ethical principle which shows obligation to tell the truth is **veracity.**
- **Autonomy:** Refers to the right to make one's own decisions.
- **Fidelity:** It means to keep a promise.
- **Beneficence**: Refers to taking positive actions to help others.

18. "Esprit de corps" refers to: *(AIIMS Raipur NO 2019)*

a. Sense of achievement b. Sense of humor
c. Sense of belonging d. Sense of morality

Explanation:

- "Esprit de corps" refers to **Sense of belonging.** It means promotion of team spirit brings the organization a feel of unity. It is one of the Fayol's 14 principles of management.

19. Source of income in budgeting terms is called: *(AIIMS Raipur NO 2019)*

a. Capitation b. Cash flow
c. Profit d. Revenue

Explanation: Source of income in budgeting terms is called as **Revenue.**

Cash flow refers to projecting how and when cash comes in and flows out of a business within a specified time period. **Capitation** means fixed, prearranged monthly payments. **Profit** refers to projected net revenue that will permit the company in attaining its goals.

20. The number of people directly reporting to any one manager or officer is known as: *(RAK MSc 2018)*

a. Line organization b. Scalar chain
c. Span of control d. Staffing

Explanation: Span of control is one of the principles in organization, where span of control depicts the number of employees that can be handled by a single manager; the number of people who report to one manager in the hierarchy.

Ans.

8.	a
9.	b
10.	c
11.	b
12.	b
13.	c
14.	a
15.	d
16.	a
17.	b
18.	c
19.	d
20.	c

21. An answerability of a subordinate to his/her superior for performance of the assigned tasks is known as: *(RAK MSc 2018)*
- a. Responsibility
- b. Accountability
- c. Authority
- d. Delegation

Explanation: An answerability of a subordinate to his/her superior for performance of the assigned tasks is known as Accountability. Accountability, means that the employee or subordinate is held responsible for successfully completing the task and will have to at least explain why they failed to do so.

22. Who is known as the Father of Scientific Management? *(AIIMS-BBS SNO 2019)*
- a. Max Weber
- b. Henri Fayol
- c. Frederic Winslow Taylor
- d. Elton Mayo

23. Theory X and theory Y of management was proposed by:
- a. William Ouchi
- b. Douglas McGregor
- c. Mary Follett
- d. Frederick Taylor

24. Hawthorne experiments were conducted by:
- a. Edwards Deming
- b. Elton Mayo
- c. Henry Ford
- d. F.W Taylor

25. "When managers make a decision, they must take into account all aspects of the current situation and act on those aspects that are key to the situation at hand". This is stated by which of the following management theory?
- a. Theory X
- b. Contingency Theory
- c. Chaos Theory
- d. Frederick Taylor

26. Mr. Anoop is a person who has natural dislike for work. He avoids responsibility and has to be forced to do his work. He also has ambition. Which of the following theory best explains this scenario his character?
- a. Theory X
- b. Theory Y
- c. Contingency theory
- d. Two factor theory

27. Mrs. Renuka, a CHC head nurse, is highly motivated to work. She will take responsibility is also very open and will make changes if necessary. She needs very little or no direction and will work on her own. Which of the following theories best describes her character?
- a. Theory X
- b. Theory Y
- c. Contingency theory
- d. System theory

28. Characteristics of good reporting includes:
- a. Fact
- b. Accuracy
- c. Legibility
- d. All of these

29. With reference to elements of administration, POSDCORB stands for:
- a. Planning, Observing, Staffing, Directing, Controlling, Reporting, and Budgeting
- b. Preparation, Organizing, Staffing, Directing, Controlling, Reporting and Budgeting
- c. Planning, Organizing, Staffing, Directing, Coordinating, Reporting, and Budgeting
- d. Preparation, Observation, Staffing, Directing, Coordinating, Reporting and Budgeting

30. Which of the following is a characteristic of Theory X?
- a. Highly-motivated employees
- b. Employees will take their own responsibility and do not need to be coerced to work
- c. Employees inherently dislikes work
- d. Employees will do his work no matter what

31. The authority flows from top to bottom is referred to as:
- a. Span of control
- b. Scalar chain
- c. Line organization
- d. Lateral organization

32. Functions of management includes:
- a. Planning
- b. Organizing
- c. Controlling
- d. All of these

33. Principles of organization includes:
- a. Hierarchy
- b. Delegation
- c. Span of control
- d. All of these

34. A nurse who integrates body—mind-spirit principles in clinical practice is known as:
- a. Nurse specialist
- b. Nurse Administrator
- c. Holistic nurse
- d. Nurse Practitioner

35. Behavioral objectives model is also referred as:
- a. Process model
- b. Product model
- c. Interpersonal model
- d. Biological model

36. Those institutions that are systematically organized and purposely set up is known as:
- a. Formal agency
- b. Governmental agency
- c. Service agency
- d. Technical agency

37. If a Head nurse asks her staff nurse to compile a report on incidence of needle stick injury in the ward, which form of communication it will be?
- a. Upward communication
- b. Intrapersonal communication
- c. Downward communication
- d. Lateral communication

38. The process to decide whether the functioning of an organization is 'Good' or 'Bad' is known as:
- a. Inspection
- b. Audit
- c. Quality Assurance
- d. Inventory

39. An organization's ability to meet analytical specifications for precision and accuracy is referred to as:
- a. Quality improvement
- b. Quality assurance
- c. Quality control
- d. Benchmarking

40. Which of the following is incorrect regarding system approach in management?
- a. The organization is viewed as a whole or as a system
- b. The organization is viewed as a unified and purposeful system
- c. System approach is proposed by quantitative school of management
- d. The whole is greater than the sum of its parts

41. Which of the following term refers to communication between similar hierarchical departments?
- a. Downward
- b. Lateral
- c. Diagonal
- d. Vertical

42. The theory in which, the traditional view of the work force holds that workers are inherently lazy, self-centred, and lacking ambition.
- a. Chaos theory
- b. Theory X
- c. Theory Y
- d. Contingency theory

43. A goal-directed and innate patterns of behavior that are not the result of learning or experience is known as:
- a. Inspirational Theory
- b. Guided Theory
- c. Instinct Theory
- d. Drive Theory

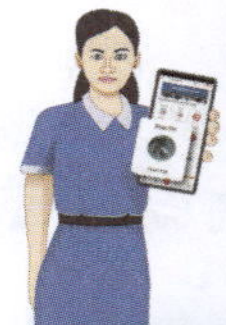

Ans.

21.	b
22.	c
23.	b
24.	b
25.	b
26.	a
27.	b
28.	d
29.	c
30.	c
31.	c
32.	d
33.	d
34.	c
35.	b
36.	a
37.	c
38.	c
39.	c
40.	c
41.	b
42.	b
43.	c

44. Which of the following model is based around the concept of providing economic security for employees through wages and other benefits that will create employee loyalty and motivation?

a. Autocratic Model
b. Custodial Model
c. Supportive Mode
d. Collegial Model

45. In which model, employees depend on each other cooperatively and work as a team with enthusiasm and self-discipline to do the task?

a. Humanistic Model
b. Modern Organizational Model
c. Collegial Model
d. Behavioral or Neoclassical Model

46. Below are the Fayol's 14 Principles of Management; EXCEPT:

a. Authority
b. Discipline
c. Unity of work
d. Unity of direction

47. Hertzberg classified the needs into two broad categories namely:

a. Hygiene factors and improving factors
b. Hygiene factors and motivating factors
c. Hygiene factors and successful factors
d. Hygiene factors and leadership factors.

48. Which of the following theorist said "workers are inherently motivated and eager to accept responsibility. An appropriate management style is to focus on creating a productive work environment coupled with positive rewards and reinforcement".

a. Hertz Berg
b. McGregor's
c. Path Goal
d. Behavior

49. Which of the following theory suggests that behavior is guided by biological needs and learned ways of reducing drives arising from those needs?

a. Drive Reduction Theory
b. Incentive Theory
c. Theory X
d. Theory Y

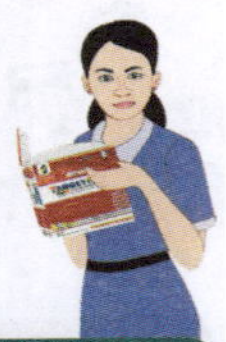

THEORIES AND STYLES OF LEADERSHIP

50. A public health nurse in the health center behaves like a dictator and uses position power to get her work done. She makes all the decisions and does not involve her subordinates in decision making. Which style of leadership BEST describes her? *(RAK MSC 2018)*

a. Autocratic
b. Democratic
c. Bureaucratic
d. Laissez faire

Explanation: In autocratic leadership style, the leader assumes complete control over the decisions and activities of the group.

51. The leadership style in which the leader alone determines policies and make plans is: *(AIIMS Raipur NO 2019)*

a. Democratic
b. Autocratic
c. Rewarded
d. Laissez-faire

Explanation: Leadership styles:

- **Autocratic:** Leader alone establishes policies and makes plans. The criteria used by him is "Do what I say or else..."
- **Democratic:** Whole team is involved in formulating decision.
- **Laissez-faire** (Delegative leadership) Leaders allow group members to make the decisions. The leader has absolutely no control.
- **Rewarded** is not a type of leadership style.

52. Leadership is important for the success of any organization. The following are important elements in leadership; EXCEPT: *(RAK MSC 2018)*

a. There must be a leader and followers in the organization
b. The leader is usually autocratic
c. There is unequal distribution of power between the leader and the followers
d. Leaders can influence the followers by their behavior.

Explanation: Leadership is an ability to influence an individual or group in order to maintain the morale of the group. Leader has followers. Leaders counsel the employees and develop team spirit. Here they have considerable freedom of action, which is usually not there in autocratic type of leadership.

53. Acknowledging the performance of an employee is through the way of: *(AIIMS Raipur NO 2019)*

a. Self-assessment
b. Performance appraisal
c. Rewards
d. Appreciation

Explanation: Acknowledging the performance of an employee is through the way of **Performance appraisal. Performance appraisal** is a periodic formal evaluation of how well personnel have performed their duties during a specific period. The outcome of performance appraisal is used to determine the reward, promotion, etc.

54. The style of leadership that dominates and commands the group is: *(DSSSB PHN, 2015)*

a. Autocratic
b. Democratic
c. Situational
d. Laissez-faire

55. Which type of leadership theories considers that the people inherit certain qualities that make them better suited to leadership?

a. Learning theories
b. Trait theories
c. Behavioral theories
d. "Great Man" theory

56. The tendency to over-rate an employee's performance is known as:

a. Positive effect
b. Halo Effect
c. Hawthorn Effect
d. Biasness

57. Which of the following is the best leadership style in a crisis situation where a quick decision making and implementation is required?

a. Democratic
b. Authoritarian
c. Bureaucratic
d. Laissez-faire

58. Which of the following characteristics is NOT a characteristic feature of Laissez-faire leadership?

a. Very little guidance from leaders
b. There is little time for group decision-making
c. Complete freedom for followers
d. Leaders provide the resources needed

59. Moderate control, motivation, awards, interactive communication, and group decision making are the characteristic features of:

a. Authoritarian leader
b. Democratic leader
c. Laissez – faire leader
d. Autocratic leader

60. A method of negotiation in which employees use authorized union representatives to engage in talks with authority is known as:

a. Collective bargaining
b. Leadership
c. Group dynamics
d. Advocacy

Ans.

Q	Ans
44.	b
45.	c
46.	c
47.	b
48.	b
49.	a
50.	a
51.	b
52.	b
53.	b
54.	a
55.	b
56.	b
57.	b
58.	b
59.	b
60.	a

61. Authority means:
- a. Right to command
- b. Right to reprimand
- c. Right to use and abuse power
- d. Right to perform duty

62. Which of the following power refers to the ability of a leader to influence a follower because of the follower's loyalty and admiration?
- a. Coercive power
- b. Referent power
- c. Legitimate power
- d. Authoritative power

63. The nurse in-charge of the ward says my staff has done the right thing in the right time. What type of statement is this?
- a. Aggressive
- b. Harsh
- c. Assertive
- d. Passive

64. Which of the following is the ideal way for a standard organization to retain the motivation of its competent employees?
- a. Competent pay scale
- b. Transparent policies
- c. Free education for children
- d. Free health care facilities

65. Assignment of any responsibility or authority to another person to carry out specific activities is known as:
- a. Promotion
- b. Delegation
- c. Deputation
- d. All of these

66. Leadership style in which all the rights to make decisions is fully given to the worker is known as:
- a. Laissez – fair
- b. Autocratic
- c. Democratic
- d. Authoritarian

67. Which of the following is NOT a characteristics of a leader:
- a. Has position authority not formal authority
- b. Administers rather than innovates
- c. Influences followers instead of giving instructions
- d. Has followers but no subordinates

68. Which of the following is NOT a characteristic of an authoritarian leader?
- a. Do not consult subordinates to make decision
- b. Listen to the employees of the organization
- c. One-way communication is preferred
- d. Instruct his employees exactly what he wants

69. Which of the following is not a role of supervisors?
- a. Informing employees regarding organizational policies
- b. Train the employees
- c. Authoritative
- d. Mentor to juniors

70. Which of the following attributes is least likely to be cause of conflict in administration?
- a. Authority
- b. Needs
- c. Perception
- d. Power

71. The team member who gets the team members moving in the right direction is known as:
- a. Coordinator
- b. Controller
- c. Recorder
- d. Mobiliser

72. A team member who always prefers everyone in the group to follow what he propose is a:
- a. Active member
- b. Criticizer
- c. Pleaser
- d. Controller

73. Once a problem is formulated, the next step is to:
- a. List all possible solutions
- b. Decide what is critical in the decision
- c. Select an alternative choice
- d. Compare all possible solutions

74. Managers have the ability, authority and power to control their employees. However, the employee's performance in this model will be much lower than expected. This is the feature of which of the following model?
- a. Autocratic Model
- b. Custodial Model
- c. Collegial Model
- d. Supportive Model

75. All the following are said to be the quality of a leader; EXCEPT:
- a. Inspire
- b. Develop
- c. Administer
- d. Innovates

76. Theory focuses on individual characteristics of successful leader:
- a. Trait Theory
- b. Managerial Grid
- c. Contingency Theory
- d. Behavior Theory

MATERIAL MANAGEMENT & INVENTORY CONTROL

77. Stocking adequate numbers and kinds of stores, so that the required material is available whenever necessary is: *(AIIMS Raipur NO 2019)*
- a. Replacement
- b. Procurement
- c. Storage
- d. Inventory control

Explanation:
- **Inventory control** is the process of maintaining the optimum needed quantity (stocks) that is sufficient for the smooth operation of the organization.
- **Replacement:** System of replacing certain items.
- **Procurement:** Process of purchasing of goods.
- **Storage:** Storage of materials at an appropriate place.

78. VED stands for: *(AIIMS Nagpur NO 2018)*
- a. Valuable, Essential, Desirable
- b. Valuable, Estimated, Desirable
- c. Vital, Essential, Desirable
- d. Vital, Estimated, Desirable

Explanation: VED analysis is a technique in inventory control. It divides inventory into three groups: **vital items, essential items and desirable items.**

79. Checking the equipment and supplies periodically is known as:
- a. Item analysis
- b. Investigation
- c. Inventory
- d. Indent

80. The process of linking each item of expenditure to its justified purpose is known as:
- a. Cost analysis
- b. Cost Saving
- c. Cost Accounting
- d. Value Analysis

81. In budgeting terms, the source of income is known as:
- a. Capitation
- b. Revenue
- c. Budget
- d. Profit source

82. Inventory refers to:
- a. Detailed list of all articles in the ward, their specifications and standard quantity
- b. List of articles borrowed from a central supply
- c. List of articles for repair or replacement
- d. List of obsolete materials

83. The institutional budget that forecasts revenues and expenses for a period beyond the current year is referred as:
- a. Forecast budget
- b. Rollover budget
- c. Flexible budget
- d. Predictive budget

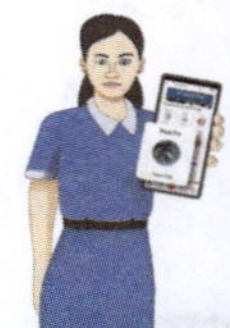

Ans.

Q	Ans
61.	a
62.	b
63.	c
64.	b
65.	b
66.	a
67.	b
68.	b
69.	c
70.	a
71.	a
72.	d
73.	b
74.	a
75.	c
76.	a
77.	d
78.	c
79.	c
80.	c
81.	b
82.	a
83.	b

84. All of the following are included in the calculation of the operating budget; EXCEPT:
a. Staff salary
b. New building construction costs
c. Bonus for staff
d. Travel allowances

85. Which of the following is a pre-requisite for budget preparation is?
a. Availability of resource
b. Check the insufficient budget
c. Estimation of income and expenditure
d. Review of requirements

86. Which of the following services is responsible for central supply in the hospital?
a. Pharmacy services b. Supported services
c. Diagnostic services d. Therapeutic services

87. Radiology department is a part of:
a. Informational services b. Therapeutic services
c. Diagnostic services d. Medical services

88. In which of the following method of inventory control, the items are classified on the basis of rate of consumption?
a. ABC analysis b. HML analysis
c. FSN analysis d. VED analysis

89. In material management, the time that elapses between placement of an order and delivery of the material is termed as:
a. Waiting time b. Lead time
c. Execution time d. Reorder time

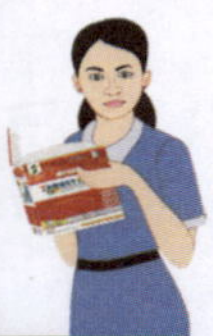

90. The cost covering the salaries of the staff, and machinery/equipment is termed as:
a. Total cost b. Flexible cost
c. Operative cost d. Fixed cost

91. What is the most popular economic evaluation tool used for program priority setting?
a. Risk-benefit analysis b. Cost-efficiency analysis
c. Cost-benefit analysis d. Cost analysis

92. The type of budget that compares the performance of the activities with the budget utilization is known as:
a. Operating budget
b. Utilization budget
c. Program performance budget
d. Incentive budget

93. The type of budgeting technique that requires items to be justified from the beginning without regarding the expenditure in the past is called:
a. Incremental budgeting b. Operating budgeting
c. Rolling budget d. Zero-based budgeting

HEALTH ECONOMICS

94. Which of the following occupation accounts for the highest percentage of workers in the national health services?
a. Doctors
b. Nurses
c. Technical staff
d. Ambulance staff

95. Increased life expectancy is closely associated with:
a. Reduction in exercise
b. Reduced spending on pharma research
c. Increased per capita health spending
d. Reduced Gross enrollment ratio

96. National Health Policy, 2017 aims to increase public health expenditure to:
a. 2.5% of the GDP by 2025 b. 5% of the GDP by 2025
c. 2.5% of the GDP by 2030 d. 2.5% of the GDP by 2020

97. In Budget 2021, India's public expenditure on healthcare stood at:
a. 1.2% of GDP b. 2.4% of GDP
c. 3.2% of GDP d. 4.1% of GDP

98. Out of Pocket Expenditures (OOPE) are expenditures directly made by households at the point of receiving health care. The OOPE on health is highest in:
a. Tamil Nadu b. Kerala
c. Gujarat d. Uttar Pradesh

99. Per capita total health expenditure is maximum in:
a. Tamil Nadu b. Kerala
c. Maharashtra d. Gujarat

Source: NHA, 2016-17

STAFF DEVELOPMENT

100. Purpose of recruitment is to: *(AIIMS Raipur NO 2019)*
a. Provide a pool of potentially qualified candidates for job
b. Interview and promote the candidate
c. Do staff promotion and training
d. Minimize labor turns over in the organization

Explanation: Recruitment means providing a pool of potentially qualified candidates for job situation. It is the process of actively seeking out or attracting applicants for existing positions.

101. During a performance appraisal, if the head nurse commits an error, it is called: *(AIIMS BPL NO 2018)*
a. Horns effect b. Halo effect
c. Paired comparison d. Central tendency error

Explanation: During performance appraisal there are several errors that take place by supervisor, one of them is Halo effect. When a single positive or negative dimension of a subordinate's performance is allowed to influence the supervisor's rating of that subordinate on other dimensions, a halo effect is operating. For example: the supervisor likes Tom because he is very cooperative.

102. Experienced nurse introducing an employee to new responsibilities through teaching and guidance is called: *(AIIMS BBS NO 2018)*
a. Mentorship b. Preceptorship
c. Professionalism d. Leadership

Explanation: Preceptorship is termed when an experienced person instructs and guides a person about his duties and skills in a particular field.

Mentorship is defined as guiding someone to improve skills.

103. The manager gives incentive for one employee on their extra effort on new project, the power which is used in this situation is: *(Safdarjung NO 2018)*
a. Coercive b. Reward
c. Legitimate d. Expert

Explanation: Reward is when employee is provided with monitory or non-monitory incentives for good performance as a positive reinforcement.

Ans.

84.	b
85.	c
86.	b
87.	c
88.	c
89.	b
90.	d
91.	c
92.	c
93.	d
94.	b
95.	c
96.	a
97.	a
98.	d
99.	b
100.	a
101.	b
102.	b
103.	b

104. The responsibilities of employees that is standardized by an organization is referred as:
a. Job specification
b. Job analysis
c. Job description
d. Job standardization

105. The purpose to conduct staff training is to:
a. Improve quality of work
b. Improve staff morale of staffs
c. Help improve communication
d. All of the above

106. The planned educational experiences provided within job setting is known as:
a. In service education
b. Developmental education
c. Additional education
d. Specialized education

107. The evaluation of the training program should include all of the following; EXCEPT:
a. Feedback from learners
b. Attention of learners
c. Performance tests
d. Learner's behavior change

108. In nursing services administration, who is responsible for inventory control at lower managerial level?
a. Staff nurse
b. Head nurse
c. Assistant Nursing Superintendent
d. Nursing Superintendent

109. The continuing process of measuring services, products, and practices of an organization against the strongest competitors in quality control and quality assurance is known as:
a. Auditing
b. Benchmarking
c. Quality assurance
d. Quality improvement

110. Which of the following is the first step in job evaluation?
a. Job specification
b. Job assessment
c. Job description
d. Job analysis

111. On the job instruction that is given to staff nurses to improve their performance is known as:
a. Induction training
b. In-service education
c. Job stimulation
d. Bridging course

PLANNING

112. Which of the following is NOT a step of planning? *(AIIMS BPL NO 2018)*
a. Briefing
b. Execution
c. Strategic healthcare planning
d. Needs identification

Explanation: Briefing, strategic health care planning and need identification are all the part of planning process. Execution refers to implementation of plan.

113. The method of setting formal guidelines before starting a work is known as:
a. Planning
b. Coordinating
c. Execution
d. Assessment

114. While planning for a new Hospital, the most important factor to keep in mind is the:
a. Organizational profits
b. Health Care System
c. Patients' Comfort
d. Unit Facilities and organizational convenience

115. The first step in planning is:
a. Measurement of social marketing plans.
b. Assessment of learning objectives
c. Assessment of existing health needs and problems.
d. Determination of practice settings.

116. The planning cycle includes all of the following; EXCEPT:
a. Developing a plan
b. Designing the job
c. Evaluating the plan
d. Determining the indicators of monitoring and evaluation

DIRECTING AND LEADING

117. Individuals who do not make decision until they are aware of all the facts pertaining to a certain situation are called: *(AIIMS-BBS SNO 2019)*
a. Introvert
b. Open minded
c. Extrovert
d. Judgmental

Explanation: Open-minded individuals have willingness to try new things, or to hear or consider new ideas. They do not make decision unit they are aware of all the facts pertaining to a certain situation.

118. A surgical patient in his unit has a fall from his bed on the 2nd post-operative day and accidentally the feeding tube dislodged from the nose; on assessment the patient was looking irritable and reported pain in the area of surgical incision. The above-mentioned issue was to be documented as an unusual event as it occurred at the health care facility. Being a nurse, which of the following report do you consider in reporting? *(AIIMS BPL NO 2018)*
a. Employee incident report
b. Offense incident report
c. Patient incident report
d. Shift incident report

Explanation: **Patient incident report** is also known as accidental report which is the documentation of the incidence or any accident in detail that has to be filled in the nursing superintendent cabin and should contain complete information of the patient (name and age) along with the place and time of accident and whether any preventive actions were taken or not by the nurse. This can be used for preventing reoccurrence of such accidents in future.

119. Leader assuming complete control over the decisions and activities of the group is called: *(AIIMS BBS NO 2018)*
a. Transformational leadership
b. Laisser-faire leadership
c. Autocratic leadership
d. Democratic leadership

Explanation: **Autocratic leadership** is one kind of leadership in which leader controls the group and all decisions are taken by leader without getting inputs from group members.

120. All the following are conflict resolution strategies except: *(AIIMS BBS NO 2018)*
a. Collaborating
b. Resistance
c. Smoothing
d. Avoiding

Explanation: Resistance is the refusal to accept or comply with something. Resistance increases conflict by increasing dissatisfaction in group. Conflict resolution strategies are avoiding, collaborating, smoothing, repression, and sharpening.

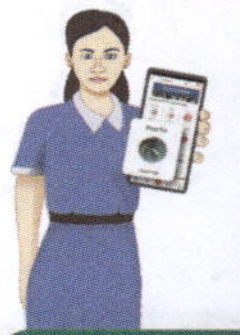

Ans.

104.	c
105.	d
106.	a
107.	b
108.	b
109.	b
110.	d
111.	b
112.	b
113.	a
114.	c
115.	c
116.	b
117.	b
118.	c
119.	c
120.	b

121. Which of the following teaching methods is useful for learning a skill? *(Kerala PSC, Nov 2014)*

a. Lecture b. Demonstration
c. Seminar d. Symposium

122. A broad statement of an organization that specifies how it will achieve its goals is:

a. Aims and goals b. Policy statement
c. Vision statement d. Mission statement

123. The group effort required to achieve a common organizational goal is:

a. Supervision b. Direction
c. Coordination d. Organization

124. A type of patient care assignment, which requires giving complete nursing care to a specific number and category of patients, during the scheduled duty hours is known as:

a. Team nursing
b. Task nursing
c. Individual Care Assignment
d. Organizational Nursing

125. The type of nursing care assignment that is best suited in an Intensive Care Unit is:

a. Functional method b. Case method
c. Task method d. Team method

126. The primary purpose of legislation is to protect the:

a. Hospital authority b. Nursing staff
c. Patient d. Patient and staff nurse

127. An answerability of a subordinate to his/her superior for performance of the assigned tasks is known as:

a. Answerability b. Responsibility
c. Accountability d. Appraisal

128. In which of the following situation, implied consent is required?

a. Routine lab test b. Emergency situation
c. Routine treatment d. Minor client

129. Coordination of the end of life care is known as:

a. Palliative care b. Critical care
c. Hospice management d. Rehabilitative care

130. Which of the following committee recommended the implementation of PHCs under public health care system in India?

a. Kartar Singh Committee
b. Bhore Committee
c. Mudaliar Committee
d. High Power Committee

131. Delegation of authority by an in-charge nurse to her staff nurse is an example of:

a. Upward delegation b. Downward delegation
c. Sideward delegation d. Lateral delegation

132. The administrative head of the College of Nursing is:

a. Chairman of the college b. Principal
c. CNO d. Nursing Superintendent

133. A written document which guides rationalized nursing measures is referred as:

a. Policy manual b. Procedure manual
c. Protocol d. Service manual

134. The professional body responsible for recognition and monitoring of Nursing colleges in India is:

a. Trained Nurses Association of India
b. Indian Nursing Council
c. National Institute of Health and Family Welfare
d. World Health Organization

135. A team member who does not want to contribute out of a fear of making a mistake is referred as:

a. Pleaser b. Passive member
c. Criticizer d. Active member

136. Assertiveness allows for:

a. Apologetic responses
b. Passive responses
c. Objective responses
d. Aggressive responses

137. Assertive communication is a way of communicating that allows a person to:

a. Avoid problems by being submissive
b. Underestimate the rights of the other person
c. Express themselves in direct and honest ways, without violating the rights of others
d. Avoid conflict by remain silent

138. All of the following are characteristics of assertive techniques; EXCEPT:

a. Ability to express honestly
b. Winning the situation
c. Mutual respect and their rights
d. Objectiveness in interaction

139. Advantages of being assertive includes all; EXCEPT:

a. It helps an individual to achieve goals
b. It helps an individual to win
c. It helps an individual to communicate without hurting others
d. It helps to recognize their one's rights

140. All of the following are styles of behavior; EXCEPT:

a. Aggression b. Assertion
c. Passive d. Conflict

141. Characteristics feature of passive person is that they are:

a. Defensive b. Emotionally expressive
c. At a loss for words d. Too demanding

142. Which of the following term refers to the degree to which decision making is concentrated at a single point in the organization?

a. Centralization
b. Subordination
c. Line of control
d. Delegation

143. In paper presentation, a presenter presents a topic to the audience. After presentation, the audience can ask questions about the topic. Which of the following type of communication pattern is used here?

a. Vertical Communication
b. Formal Communication
c. Socratic Communication
d. One-way Communication

144. Focus group discussion (FGD), panel discussion, symposium are examples of:

a. One-way communication
b. Socratic communication
c. Informal communication
d. Vertical communication

145. In which stage of group development individuals often challenge goals and struggle for power occurs:

a. Norming b. Performing
c. Storming d. Forming

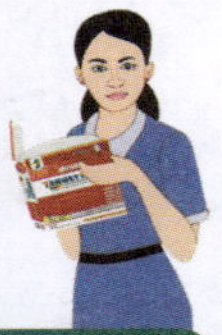

Ans.

121. b
122. d
123. c
124. c
125. b
126. d
127. c
128. b
129. c
130. b
131. b
132. b
133. b
134. b
135. b
136. c
137. c
138. b
139. b
140. d
141. c
142. a
143. c
144. b
145. c

146. In which stage of group development individuals often confused because roles are not clear and there is no leader present in group.

a. Norming b. Performing
c. Storming d. Forming

147. A competitive bargaining strategy in which one party gains only if the other party loses something is known as:

a. Cooperative bargaining b. Productive bargaining
c. Distributive bargaining d. Collective bargaining

148. Most common type of bargaining process similar to the problem solving process, in which both parties are trying to reach to beneficial alternatives where it will lead to win-win situation.

a. Distributive b. Integrative
c. Productive d. Collective

149. All of the following are the purposes of public relation officer; EXCEPT:

a. Keeping the public informed about the availability of health care services.
b. Giving the clientele information on the procedural aspects of health care.
c. Disclosing the treatment details of individual patients
d. Communicating the benefits of healthcare services

150. Qualities of Public Relation Officer (PRO) include all of the following; EXCEPT:

a. Infinite capacity to persist.
b. Ability to communicate effectively in written and verbal form
c. Should be an introvert personality in order to maintain confidentiality of vital information.
d. Pleasant voice and ability to speak in public.

HUMAN RESOURCE MANAGEMENT

151. Human Resource Development is closely associated with:

a. Budgeting b. Staffing
c. Directing d. Planning

152. In recruitment process, a higher job position is open to all the qualified candidates who may wish to apply is known as:

a. Recruitment by promotion
b. Direct recruitment
c. Indirect recruitment
d. Recruitment by deputation

153. Which of the following department is responsible for recruitment, hiring employees and employee benefits?

a. Human Resource Department
b. Accounts Department
c. Financial Department
d. Information system Department

154. All of the following activities are a part of Staff Recruitment Process; EXCEPT:

a. Advertisement and Interview
b. Guidance and Counseling
c. Selection and Training
d. Interview and Selection

155. Human resource planning does not include:

a. Staff appraisal
b. Demand forecasting
c. Supply forecasting
d. Preparing a plan of action

156. "Workers must be paid a fair wage for their services", which of the following example correctly suit for this principle?

a. Subordination b. Remuneration
c. Fairness d. Delegation

QUALITY MANAGEMENT (CONTROLLING)

157. Hospital has to keep MLC record up to:

(AIIMS Raipur NO 2019)

a. 1 year b. 5 years
c. 10 years d. 15 years

158. Which of following rate is applied to calculate "The total number of deaths occurring in a hospital after 48 hours of admission for a period (divided by) total number of discharges including death (minus) death under 48 hours for the same period in a hospital multiplied by 100"?

(Safdarjung NO 2018)

a. GDR b. NDR
c. TBOR d. OR

Explanation: NDR: Net Death Rate (institutional death rate) The ratio of the total number of deaths occurring in the hospital, 48 hours or more after admission, for a period to the total number of discharges and deaths, 48 hours and over, for that period.

The formula for figuring the percentage is:

$$\frac{\text{Deaths (including newborn) minus those under 48 hours for a period}}{\text{Total number of discharges (including deaths and newborn) minus deaths less than 48 hours for the period}} \times 100$$

GDR (Gross death rate or hospital death rate) The proportion of inpatient hospitalizations that end in death, usually expressed as percentage.

159. A written record related to total number of patients' in hospital on daily basis is called:

a. Census b. Anecdotes
c. Patient attendance record d. OPD record

160. Minimum age required for a candidate to join BSc Nursing (Degree) course is:

a. 16 years b. 17 years
c. 18 years d. 19 years

161. Which of the following is the best indicator to determine whether high quality care is being delivered?

a. Audit report
b. Quality indicators
c. Report of quality assurance agencies
d. Vital indicators

162. In India, legal responsibility related to patient care in hospital falls on:

a. Nurses b. Doctors
c. Hospital d. Health Insurance Company

163. The department that is responsible for maintaining copies of all records related to patient is:

a. Information System Department
b. Medical Record Department
c. Nursing Information system department
d. Department of Hospital Information System

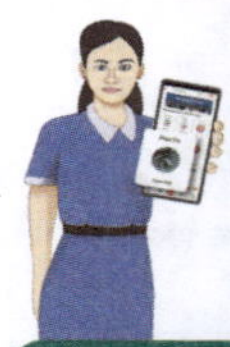

Ans.

146. d
147. c
148. b
149. c
150. c
151. b
152. b
153. a
154. b
155. a
156. b
157. c
158. b
159. a
160. b
161. b
162. b
163. b

164. First contact of patients with a hospital is usually with:

a. Nursing information department
b. Accounts department
c. Admissions department
d. Medical record department

165. Which of the following hospital services is concerned with policies and procedural activities?

a. Nursing services
b. Medical services
c. Administrative services
d. Informational services

166. Quality assurance is concerned with:

a. Adequacy of care
b. Standard of practice
c. Practice ratings
d. Organizational practice

167. All India Institute of Medical Sciences (AIIMS), New Delhi is an example of:

a. Tertiary care teaching cum research hospital
b. General Hospital
c. Specialized Hospital
d. Corporate Hospital

168. Which of the following is NOT a component of a nursing diagnosis?

a. Effect and Relationship
b. Outcome and Evidence
c. Cause and Effect
d. Effect and Evidence

169. The major purpose of Hospital Information System (HIS) is to achieve the best possible support of patient care and administration by:

a. Use of information technology
b. Personal health record
c. Nursing process
d. Electronic data processing

PROGRAM EVALUATION REVIEW TECHNIQUE (PERT) & ACTIVITY

170. The assessment method that occur after the patient has been discharged is: *(Safdarjung NO 2018)*

a. Concurrent Evaluation
b. Auditing
c. Retrospective evaluation
d. Quality assurance

Explanation: Retrospective evaluation is a type of assessment that is done to find out whether goals are met in hospital after the discharge of the patient.

Concurrent evaluation: Continuous assessment process when patient is in the hospital.

Auditing: Systematic assessment of records, documents of a unit or organization.

Quality assurance: Evaluation of patient care by developing standards of care and implementing mechanisms to see whether they met.

NURSING AUDIT

171. The collection of information from nursing records and through other evidences about patient care is called: *(AIIMS BPL NO 2018)*

a. Nursing audit
b. Medical audit
c. Inspection
d. Accreditation

Explanation: Nursing audit is a systematic evaluation of nursing records and evidences about patient care. Medical audit refers to audit of medical care from medical care. Systematic review of medical care in order for improvement and analysis.

172. The professional body that is responsible for control and maintenance of standards of nursing in India is:

a. Trained Nurses association of India (TNAI)
b. Medical Council of India (MCI)
c. India Nursing Council (INC)
d. All India Federation of Nurses (AIFN)

173. Certification refers to providing official document to:

a. Attesting level of achievement
b. Rating standards
c. Auditing outcome
d. Both a & b

174. National Health Policy is announced by Government of India in the year:

a. 1950
b. 1978
c. 1982
d. 1990

175. Which of the following is an Indian health care accrediting agency?

a. Joint Commission International (JCI)
b. National Accreditation Board for Hospitals & Healthcare Providers (NABH)
c. Joint Commission on Accreditation of Healthcare (JCAH)
d. International Society for Quality in Health Care (ISQHC)

176. Accreditation refers to:

a. Making assessment
b. Ensuring Quality
c. Meeting standards
d. Cost effective care

177. Evaluation is done:

a. At the end of the program
b. At regular intervals
c. By drawing comparison between planning and achievement
d. To determine whether the policy is being correctly implemented.

STAFFING NORMS (SIU & INC)

178. According to Indian Nursing Council (INC), the nurse-patient ratio in Intensive Care Unit should be maintained at:

a. 1:1
b. 1:2
c. 1:3
d. 1.4

179. The INC standard for Teacher: UG Students ratio for nursing colleges is:

a. 1: 5
b. 1:10
c. 1:12
d. 1:15

180. As per INC recommendation, the ideal Nurse: Patient ratio in a Hospital General Ward should be:

a. 1:1
b. 1:5
c. 1:10
d. 1:15

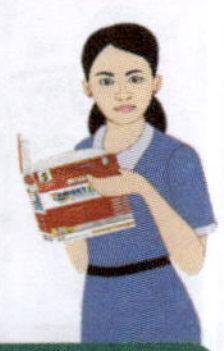

Ans.

164. c
165. c
166. b
167. a
168. b
169. a
170. c
171. a
172. c
173. a
174. c
175. b
176. b
177. b
178. a
179. b
180. b

181. As per the Staff Inspection Unit (SIU), the recommended Nurse: Patient ratio in a Hospital General Ward should be:

a. 1:2 b. 1:5
c. 1:6 d. 1:10

182. The most crucial phase of group dynamics is:

a. Forming b. Norming
c. Storming d. Performing

ROLE OF NURSE AS A MANAGER

183. Patient care method in which patient care areas provide various levels of care: *(AIIMS Raipur NO 2019)*

a. Team nursing b. Progressive patient care
c. Case method d. Primary nursing care

Explanation: Progressive patient care units also called as intermediate care or step-down units, provide a transition between the ICU and the general unit or discharge.

184. Which of the following is INCORRECT about SWOT analysis for decision making? *(AIIMS-BBS SNO 2019)*

a. S is for strengths
b. W is for weaknesses
c. O is for opportunities
d. T is for time

Explanation:

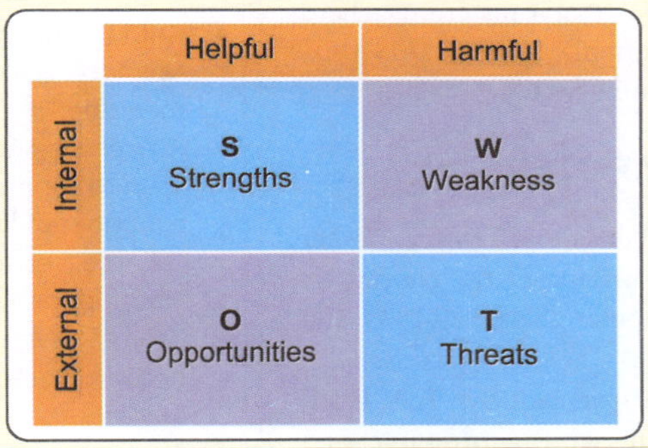

185. The communication in which managers interact with managers, physicians and groups of people in other departments in the organization who are NOT at the same level in the hierarchy as them is called: *(AIIMS-BBS SNO 2019)*

a. Vertical communication b. Horizontal communication
c. Diagonal communication d. Upward communication

Explanation: Diagonal communication is held between different structures of a business firm. It is between higher and lower sectors of a business firm. It is also known as cross-functional communication.

186. Group strength and group bonding that hold the group members together, thereby sustaining them, are together known as: *(AIIMS BPL NO 2018)*

a. Group structure b. Group goals
c. Cohesiveness d. Temporal change

Explanation: Group cohesiveness (also called group cohesion and social cohesion) arises when bonds link members of a social group to one another and to the group as a whole.

187. The phenomenon of a nurse respecting a patient's rights to make decisions about his health and health care is called: *(AIIMS BBS NO 2018)*

a. Human dignity b. Integrity
c. Autonomy d. Altruism

Explanation: Autonomy is the right to self-determination, and it is one of the ethical principle of nursing. Autonomy refers to the right of patients to make decisions about their medical care without their health care provider trying to influence the decision.

188. There are several differences between a leader and a manager. Which of the following manager does not have? *(RAK MSc 2018)*

a. Formal authority b. Subordinates
c. Followers d. Responsibility

Explanation: The manager never has any followers, whereas the leader has followers.

Table: Differences between leader and manager

Characteristics	Leader	Manager
Formal rights	A leader has no formal rights	A manager has certain formal rights
Followers/ subordinates	**A leader has followers**	A manager has subordinates
Functions	A leader is to guide and motivate his followers	A manager is to plan, organize, staff direct, motivate and control
Necessity	Leadership is not a necessity for an organization	Managership is a necessity for an organization
Scope	Leadership is a part of managerial functions. Thus, its scope is limited	Managership is a wider terms and includes leadership
Mutual relationship	All leaders are not managers	All managers are leaders

189. The nurse manager requires several skills to be effective in her work. Which of the following skills is the most important skill to be an effective nurse manager at all levels of management? *(RAK MSc 2018)*

a. Technical skills b. Conceptual skills
c. Human skills d. Supervisory skills

Explanation: Human skills: Interpersonal skills or human skills are required to speak with patients, relatives and health team members. It is important for nurse managers to be the leading example in the health team.

190. Supervision is an important function of management. Which of the following is not a characteristic/function of a supervisor? *(RAK MSc 2018)*

a. It can be seen as overseeing someone's work
b. Ensures that subordinates carry out their activities effectively
c. Acting as a mentor to the subordinates
d. Is always related to checking of subordinate's work

Explanation: Checking of subordinate's work is not a function of supervisor. Subordinates check the work, but supervisors give guidance on how to work, hence this is not the characteristic of supervision. All other statements are related to functions of a supervisor.

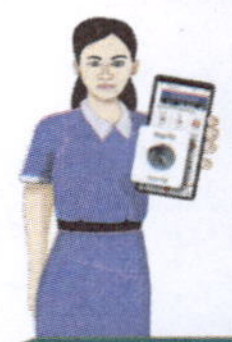

Ans.

181. c
182. c
183. b
184. d
185. c
186. c
187. c
188. c
189. c
190. d

"An ounce of prevention is worth a pound of cure."

—Unknown

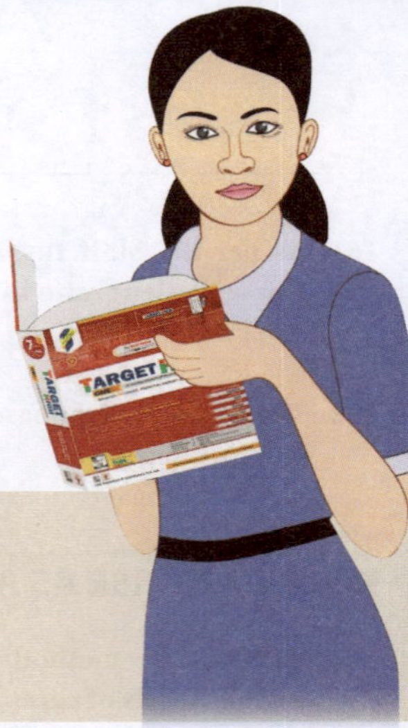

CHAPTER 14

COMPUTER/HEALTH AND NURSING INFORMATICS

SYNOPSIS

BASIC KEY TERMS

- **Access:** To gain entry to data or reading the data.
- **Analog:** Using signals or information represented by a continuously variable physical quantity such as spatial position, voltage, etc.
- **ASCII:** American Standard Code for Information Interchange.
- **Backup:** Saving any data or information for future.
- **Bios:** Controls input and output operations.
- **Binary:** A **binary** digit, or bit, is the smallest unit of data in computing. It is represented by a 0 or a 1.
- **Bit:** The smallest unit of data in binary.
  - 8 bits = 1 byte
  - 4 bits = 1 nibble
- **Byte**: Byte is a group of binary digits or bits (usually eight) operated on a single unit. A byte is considered as a unit of a memory size.

  8 bits = 1 byte
  1024 Bytes = 1 kilobyte (KB)
  1024 KB = 1 Megabyte (MB)
  1024 MB = 1 Gigabyte (GB)
  1024 GB = 1 Terabyte (TB)
  1000 TB = 1 Petabyte
- **Cache:** It is a hardware or software component that temporarily stores data so future requests for that data can be served faster.
- **CD ROM** (Compact Disk Read Only Memory): From CD ROM, the data can only be read but not edited, manipulated, or deleted.
- **Chip:** Chip is a short form for 'microchip'. It is a small piece of semiconducting material implanted with an integrated circuit.
- **Code:** Language expressed or understood by the computer.
- **DOS (Disk Operating System):** It is a command based operating system that runs from a hard disk drive. Most commonly refers to MS-DOS (Microsoft Disk Operating System).

HISTORY OF COMPUTERS

- **Charles Babbage** is considered as the "father of the computer". He originated the concept of a programmable computer (between 1833 and 1871).
- **Microprocessor** was invented by **Ted Hoff, Stanley Mazor and Federico Faggin** (at Intel Inc) in **1970**.
- **Microcomputer** was invented by **H. Edward Roberts in 1975**.

KEY POINTS

- A hard disk is divided into tracks which are further subdivided into sectors.
- The central processing unit consists of Control unit, ALU and CPU.
- RAM (Random Access Memory) is a volatile memory.
- Router is a device used to connect a number of LANs (Local Area Networks).
- Fiber optic cable is used as a high speed network backbone media.
- A bit is the smallest unit of the information.
- Buffer is the temporary storage that can be used to compensate for a difference in data rate and data flow between devices.

GENERATIONS OF COMPUTERS

Table 1: Computer generation, period, features and examples

Generation	Period	Features	Examples
First generation	1940–1955	**Vacuum tubes** and **magnetic tapes** Slow in speed Very huge in size Limited storage size Punched cards were used to input the data. Processing time for calculation was **milliseconds**	ENIAC, EDVAC, UNIVAC 1
Second generation	1955–1964	Used **Transistor** for electronic circuitry. Large in size, relatively slow and expensive Needed air conditioned room as they got heated up very quickly Processing time was **microseconds**	IBM, 1401, RCA501, Honeywell 200, etc.

Contd...

Generation	Period	Features	Examples
Third Generation	1964–1975	Used **integrated circuits (ICs)** Keyboards and monitors were invented for input and output Operating system (OS) was designed. PASCAL (high level language) was developed. Processing time was **nanoseconds**	IBM 360 series and 370 series
Fourth Generation	1975–1980	Used **Microprocessor** Several input devices were introduced. For example, Mouse, scanners, microphones, etc. Magnetic disk was used as primary external storage device Graphical user Interface (GUI) was developed	IBM personal computers, Apple Macintosh, HP 3000
Fifth Generation	1980–till date	Many new inventions such as laptops, tablets, smartphone, etc. New features include artificial intelligence, natural language processing, user friendly interface, voice command input	Desktop, Laptops, Notebook, Tablets, Supercomputers, etc.

CLASSIFICATION OF COMPUTERS

Based on Function

- **Digital computers:** They operate on inputs that are converted into binary digits (0 or 1). Most of the computers available today are digital computers.
- **Analog computers:** Process analog data, which is of continuous nature as input. Such data includes pressure, voltage, temperature, speed, etc. It measures continuous changes in specific physical quantity, e.g., Speed is measured by the speedometer of a car.
- **Hybrid computers:** Hybrid computers exhibit features of both digital and analog computers. They are highly accurate and very fast in speed. They take analog signals and convert them into digital.

Based on Size and Capacity

- **Mainframe computers** (introduced in 1950s): They are used primarily by large organizations for critical applications (bulk data processing). They are known for their large size, amount of storage, processing power and high level of reliability.
- **Minicomputers** (introduced in 1960s): Much smaller than mainframe computers.

Used in computer-aided designing and small organizations.

- **Micro computers/personal computers** (introduced in the 1980s): Smaller in size and portable. They were single user systems for everyday activities like calculations, documentations, designing and presentations.
- **Supercomputers:** Most powerful and the largest computers. They are made for specific tasks such as defense system, weather forecasting, and complex scientific research.

HARDWARE AND SOFTWARE

Hardware

Hardware refers to the physical parts of the computer system. For example, CPU (central processing unit), Monitor, Keyboard, mouse, etc.

Structure and Parts of Computer

The basic structure of computer comprises of input devices/units, central processing and output devices/units.

KEY POINTS

- The physical component of the computer that anyone can touch is known as "hardware".
- Silicon is the primary element in computer chips.
- A pixel is the smallest portion of the screen. Entire screen is made by putting millions of pixels together in a matrix form.
- Three color dots form a color pixel on a screen, and these are the following color dots: red, blue, and green.
- In fourth generation computer, data is stored on the floppy diskette in magnetism form.

Table 2: Parts of hardware devices

Parts	Devices
Input devices/unit	• Mouse • Keyboard • Scanner • Microphone • Web/video camera • Joystick • Light pen • Trackball • Bar code reader • Touch screen • Graphic tablet • Magnetic ink character reader (MICR) • Optical Mark recognition (OMR)

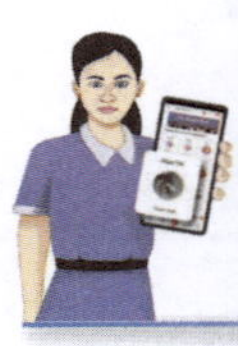

Contd...

Parts	Devices
Central processing unit	Memory unit • Internal: RAM (Random Access Memory): temporary storage • External: ROM (Read Only Memory): permanent storage • Control Unit: It draws information from memory and decodes it for further execution Arithmetic Logic Unit (ALU): It is the decision maker of CPU
Output devices/unit	• Monitors • Printers • Plotters • Speaker/Head phone

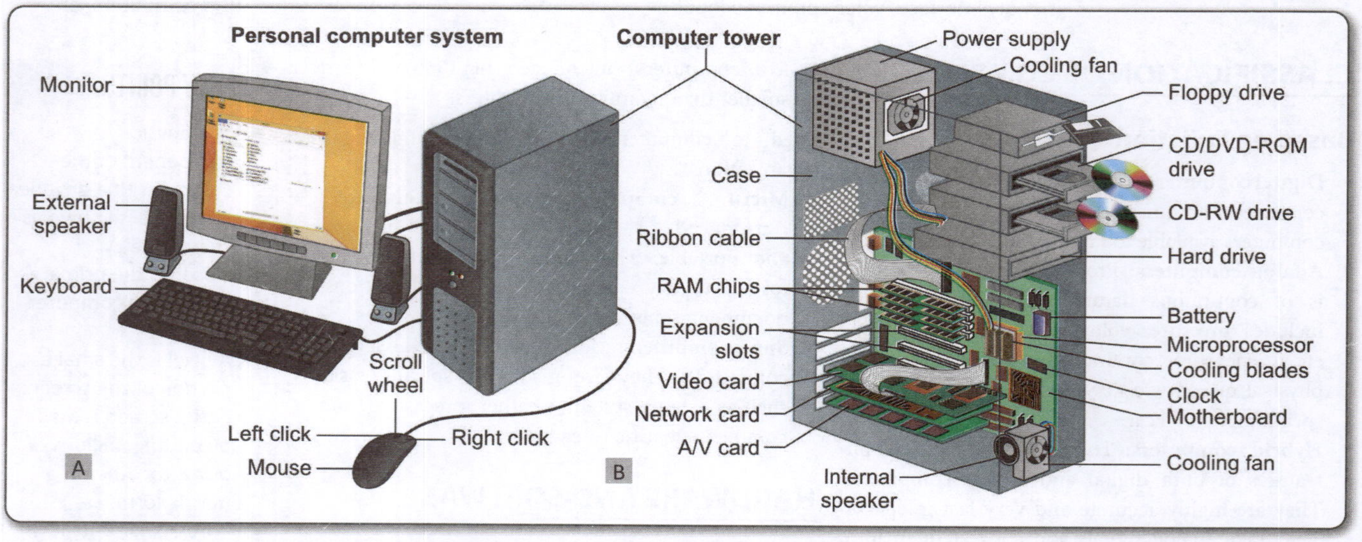

Figures 1A and B: (A) Structure and parts of computer; (B) Components of CPU

Uses of Computers in Healthcare System

- Computer-aided teaching and testing
- Patient management system/Hospital Information System
- Telemedicine
- Telenursing
- Nursing informatics

Nursing Informatics

Nursing informatics is the specialty that integrates **nursing** science with information and communication technologies to define, identify, and communicate data, information, knowledge, and wisdom in nursing practice. (Adapted from *IMIA Special Interest Group on Nursing Informatics 2009)*

Software Programs

There are three types of programs:

- **Application programs** (programs used by users to perform task)
  E.g., MS-Word, MS-Excel, Adobe Photoshop, SPSS, etc.
- **System software** (an interface between user and computer)
  - Operating system. For example, Microsoft windows, MS-DOS, Ubuntu, LINUX,
  - Utility program
- **Driver programs:** This program communicates between input/output devices and computer. E.g., Installation software for hardwares or such as printer, scanner, etc.

KEY POINTS

- Spreadsheet programs (e.g., MS-excel) help to calculate numbers related to rows and columns.
- MS PowerPoint is used to prepare presentations.
- MS word is a word processing application software.

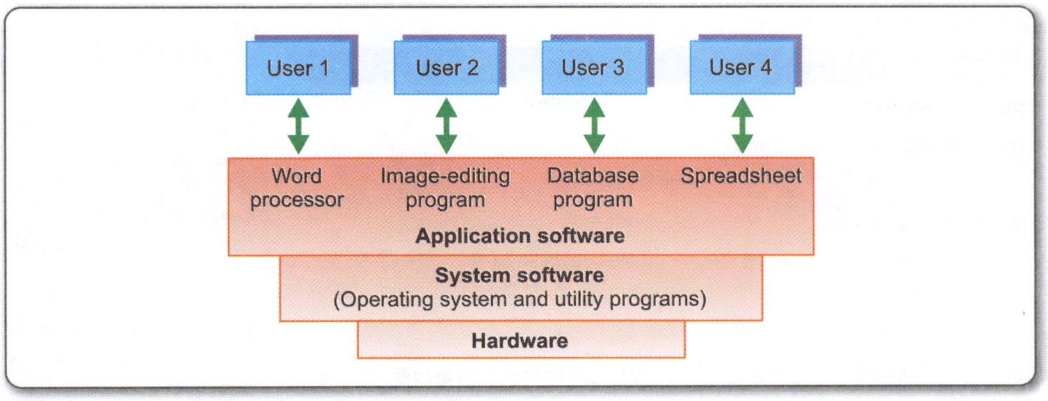

Figure 2: Hierarchy of computer software

Types of Operating Systems (OS)

Table 3: Types of operating systems

Operating system	User	Type
UNIX	Multi-user; multi-tasking	Network OS
Linux	Multi-user; multi-tasking	Network OS
DOS	Single-user; single tasking	Desktop OS
Mac OS	Single-user; multi-tasking	Desktop OS
MS Windows	Single-user; multi-tasking	Desktop OS
Palm OS/Pocket OS/Android/IOS	Single-user; multi-tasking	Mobile OS

Application Software (Application Programs)

An **application** is any program, or group of programs, that is designed for the user.

Common Application Software and its Uses

Table 4: Application software with example

Application software/package	Example
Word processors	MS-Word (MS-Office) Word pad Notepad Open Office
Spreadsheets	MS-Excel (MS-Office) Open Office Apple Numbers
Presentation software	MS-PowerPoint Keynotes
Databases	Oracle, MS Access, FoxPro
Image editors	Adobe Photoshop MS Paint Google Picasa
Web Browsers	Internet Explorer (by Microsoft) Mozilla Firefox Safari (by Apple) Chrome (by Google)
Statistical Packages	SPSS (Statistical Package for Social Science) Epi info (by CDC) SAS (Statistical Analysis System) STATA
PDF Reader/Editor	Adobe Acrobat Reader
File storage services	Google Drive Drop box

KEY POINTS

Artificial intelligence (AI) in nursing:

- AI is rapidly transforming the healthcare industry, including Nursing.
- AI in Nursing can be useful for
  - Clinical decision support
  - Patient monitoring
  - Remote patient monitoring
  - Education and Training
  - Research

Potential challenges with (AI) in nursing:

- Data privacy and security
- Bias - Algorithms can be biased and insensitive to human feelings.
- Interpretability: AI algorithms can be complex and difficult to interpret

KEY POINTS

File extensions for files:

- Notepad files - .txt
- Word pad files - .rtf
- MS word files - .doc & .docx
- MS excel - .xls & xlsx
- MS PowerPoint - .ppt & .pptx
- Portable Document Format (PDF) file - .pdf
- MS Paint file - .bmp
- Image files - .jpeg, .tiff
- Video files - .mp4, .mpeg, .mkv, .avi
- SPSS data file - .sav
- SPSS output file - .spv

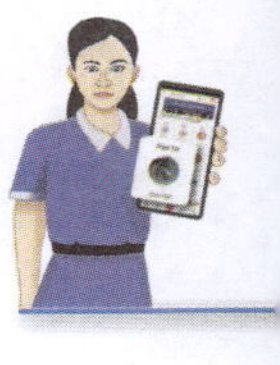

Table 5: Commonly used windows shortcut keys

Shortcut key	Action
To open windows help and support	Windows + F1
To open help menu of current application (currently running)	F1
To open start menu	Ctrl + Esc
To quit active application or close current window	Alt + F4
To open the run menu	Windows key + R
To open explorer	Windows key + E
To switch between open programs	Alt + Tab
To maximize the current window	Windows key + up arrow
To open task manager	Ctrl + Shift + Esc
To open search for files and folders	Windows key + F
To minimize all windows	Windows key + M

Table 6: Commonly used MS-Word shortcut keys

Shortcut key	Action
F1	To get help or use office assistant
Ctrl + A (Control and A)	To select all in the current document
Ctrl + C	To copy all the selected item or text
Ctrl + X	To cut all the selected item or text
Ctrl + V	To paste the copied item or text
Ctrl + B	Bold the selected text
Ctrl + F	Displays the Find dialog box to search the current document
Ctrl + G	Displays the Go To dialog box to search for a specific location in the current document
Ctrl + H	Displays the Replace dialogue box
Ctrl + I	Italicize the text
Ctrl + J	Switch a paragraph between Justify and left alignment
Ctrl + L	Left align a paragraph
Ctrl + N	Opens a new blank document
Ctrl + O	Opens 'open' dialogue box for opening an existing file
Ctrl + P	Prints a document
Ctrl + R	Switch the alignment of the paragraph between right and left
Ctrl + S or Shift + F12 Key	Saves the document
Ctrl + U	Underlines the selected text
Ctrl + Y	Redo the last action
Ctrl + Z	Undo the last action
Ctrl + Enter	Insert a page break
F9 Key	Refresh (**NOTE:** F5 is the shortcut key for refresh in windows and internet explorer)

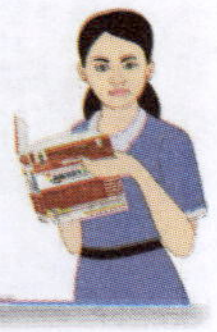

KEY POINTS

AI ChatBots

Conversational AI or chatbots, are computer programs that are designed to simulate conversation with human users.

Some ChatBot that are currently being used include:

ChatGPT:

- It is a chatbot developed by OpenAI.
- It is a large language model (LLM) that is trained on a massive dataset of text and code.
- ChatGPT can generate text, translate languages, write different kinds of creative content, and answer your questions in an informative way.

Bard

- Bard is a chatbot developed by Google AI.
- It is also a large language model that is trained on a massive dataset of text and code.
- Bard can generate text, translate languages, write different kinds of creative content, and answer your questions in an informative way.

Table 7: Commonly used MS-excel shortcut keys

Shortcut key	Action
F1	To get help or use office assistant
F2	Edit the active cell
Ctrl + A (Control and A)	Select all content in the worksheet
Ctrl + Space	Select an entire column in a worksheet
Shift + Space	Select an entire row in a worksheet
Ctrl + C	Copy the highlighted selection
Ctrl + X	Cut the highlighted selection
Ctrl + V	Paste the copied selection
Ctrl + B	Bold the highlighted selection
Ctrl + F	Displays find dialogue box to search the active document
Ctrl + Space	Select an entire column in a worksheet
Shift + Space	Select an entire row in a worksheet
Ctrl + I	Italicize the highlighted selection
Ctrl + Shift + %	Apply the Percentage format
Ctrl + Page up	Move to a previous sheet in a workbook
Ctrl + P	Move to a next sheet in a workbook
Ctrl + S or Shift + F12 Key	To save the document
Ctrl + U	To underline the highlighted selection
Ctrl + Y	Redo last action
Ctrl + Z	Undo last action

Table 8: Common file extensions

File type	File extensions	File type (category)
Text file/spread sheet extensions	.doc	Word document (MS word 97-2003 version)
	.docx	Word document (MS word 2007 or latest version)
	.xls	Excel Spreadsheet (MS Excel 97-2003)
	.xlsx	Excel spreadsheet (MS Excel 2007 or latest)
	.pdf	Document file (Portable document format used by Acrobat reader);
	.rtf	Rich Text Format (word file); opens in WordPad or MS word
Image file extensions	.bmp	Bit mapped picture (standard windows format for picture; used by MS Paint)
	.jpg/jpeg	Joint photographic expert group; picture format; used for web graphics
	.gif	Graphics Interchange Format; Used for web graphics; compressed format for web use
	.psd	Photoshop document: Image file format for Adobe Photoshop
	.tiff	Tagged Image File Format; High quality image format (uncompressed)

Contd...

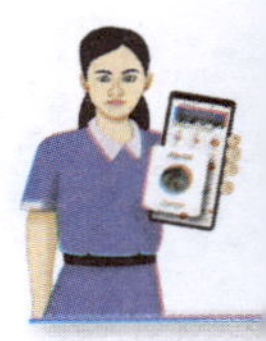

File type	File extensions	File type (category)
Video file extensions	.avi	Audio-Video Interleave; windows standard for video files
	.mpg	Motion pictures experts group; high quality video file format
	.mp4	Video file format
Audio file extensions	.wav	"Wave Sound" the Windows standard for audio files
	.mp3	Compressed audio file
Other formats	.ppt	PowerPoint presentation (MS PowerPoint 97-2003)
	.pptx	PowerPoint presentation (MS PowerPoint 2007 or latest version)
	.exe	Executable program file
	.fla	Editable flash file
	.htm or .html	Hyper Text Markup Language; for internet documents; opens in web browser

COMPUTER NETWORKING

Key Terms

- **ISP:** Stands for Internet Service Provider. An ISP provides access to the Internet.
- **WSP:** Stands for Wireless Service Provider. WSP provides users a wireless access to internet.
- **LAN:** Stands for Local Area Network. It refers to a network or a portion of a network that is not publicly accessible to the greater internet. For example, Home or Office network.
- **WAN**: Stands for Wide Area Network. It means a network that is much more extensive than a LAN. WAN is usually reachable through internet.
- **Servers**: Servers are a storage point required to transfer the data through internet.
- **Clients**: A computer or workstation that is capable of obtaining information and application is known as client.
- **Modem**: A modem (Modulator – Demodulator) is a hardware device that modulates one or more carrier signals to encode and decode digital information.
- **DNS**: Stands for Domain Name System. It is used to convert the domain name into related IP address.
- **Wi-Fi:** Wi-Fi is a popular wireless networking technology that provides users with wireless Internet and network connections (through devices using IEEE 802.11 standards).
- **Bluetooth**: Bluetooth is a short-range wireless communication technology that allows devices such as mobile phones, computers, and peripherals to transmit data or voice wirelessly over a short distance.

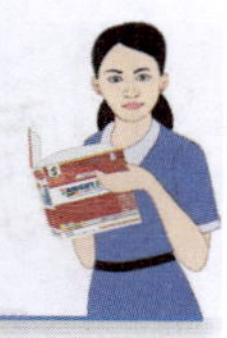

Methods of Internet Access

- **Wired access**
  - Dial-up connection
  - Digital Subscriber Line (DSL)
  - Cable Modem (Cable Internet Access)
  - Integrated Services Digital Network (ISDN)
  - Fiber to Home
- **Wireless access**
  - WiMax
  - Wireless ISP
  - Mobile Broadband
  - GPRS (General Packet Radio Service)
  - Satellite Broadband

Network Topology

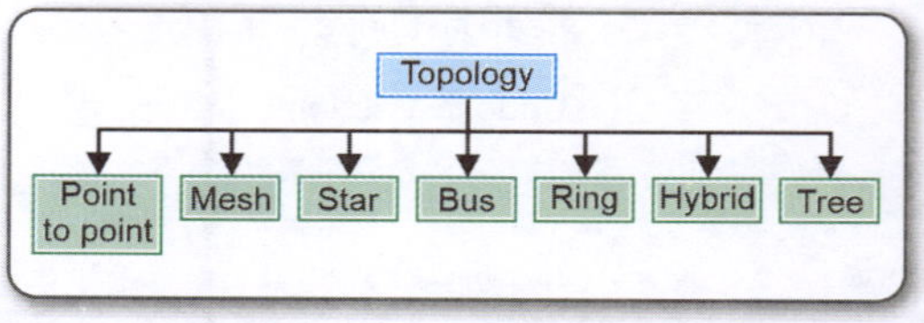

Figure 3: Types of network topology (Flowchart)

Web/Internet Key Terminologies

- **HTML:** Stands for Hyper Text Markup Language. Standard language (basic) which is used to create web pages.
- **HTTP:** Stands for Hyper Text Transfer Protocol. It is a protocol used to transfer files in web (World Wide Web).
- **HTTPS:** Stands for Hyper Text Transfer Protocol Secure. This is secured protocol which keeps the information safe from hackers.
- **Internet:** Internet refers to network of networks which connects millions of computers around the globe.
- **WWW:** Stands for World Wide Web. WWW is a global collection of documents and other resources, linked by hyperlinks and URLs.
- **URL:** Stands for Uniform Resource Locator. It is otherwise known as web address. It is used to specify addresses on the World Wide Web.

KEY POINTS

- The star topology is the best network topology for large businesses because it is simple to control and coordinate from the central computer.
- In Optic fiber cable, the transmission of data occurs in the form of light, so optic fiber provides higher data transfer speed than other cables.
- 1000 Mbps is the max data transfer rate for optical fiber cables.
- The term FTP stands for File transfer protocol.
- A file server allows LAN users to share the data. It acts as a medium for data transfer.
- World Wide Web (WWW) creates a collection of hyper-linked documents on the Internet.
- A URL (Uniform Resource Locator) is a database connection that describes the database's location on a computer network and the retrieval process.

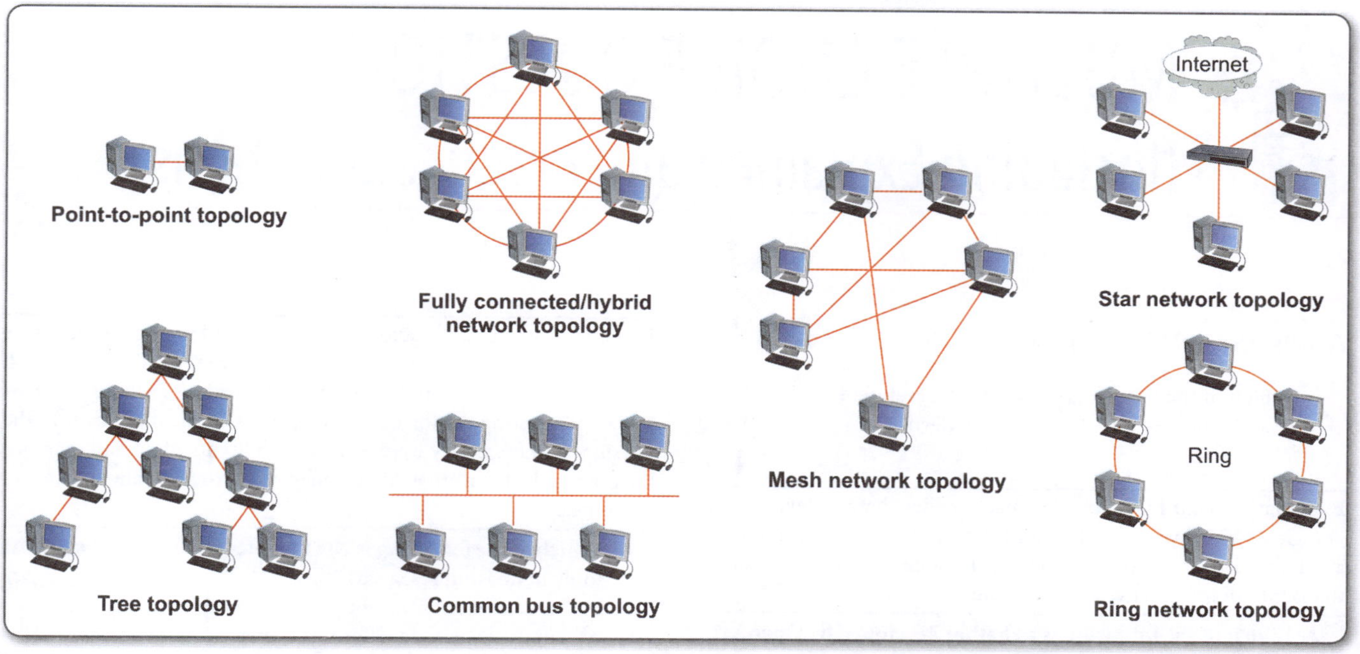

Figure 4: Types of network topology

- **IP Address**: Stands for Internet Protocol Address. An IP address is a logical address that is assigned by software residing in a server or router. For example, 1.120.12.85 could be an IP address. Each number can be zero to 255.
- **Firewall**: Firewall is a network security system.
- **Computer virus**: A computer virus is a type of malicious software program (malware) that, when executed, replicates itself by modifying other computer programs and inserting its own code. When this replication succeeds, the affected areas are then said to be "infected" with a computer virus.
- **Antivirus software**: Antivirus software or anti-malware is a computer program used to prevent, detect, and remove malware or computer virus.
- **Phishing**: Phishing is the attempt to obtain sensitive information such as usernames, passwords, and credit card details (and money), often for malicious reasons, by disguising as a trustworthy entity in an electronic communication like E-mail.
- **Whaling**: Whaling is a specific kind of malicious hacking within the more general category of phishing, which involves hunting for data that can be used by the hacker.
- **Spamming**: Use of electronic messaging systems like e-mails to send unwanted bulk messages (Junk mails).

Golden Points to Remember

- **Charles Babbage** is considered as the "father of the computer". He originated the concept of a programmable computer between 1833 and 1871.
- **Microprocessor** was invented by **Ted Hoff, Stanley Mazor and Federico Faggin** (at Intel Inc) in **1970**
- **Microcomputer** was invented by **H Edward Roberts in 1975**
- **Digital computers** operate on inputs that are converted into binary digits (0 or 1).
- Analogue computers process analogue data, which is of continuous nature as input
- Hybrid computers exhibit features of both digital and analog computers
- ALU stands for Arithmetic Logic Unit
- ALU is responsible for performing mathematical operations
- Brain of the computer system is CPU
- Bit is The smallest unit of data in binary.
- Eight bits are equal to one byte. Four bits are equal to one nibble
- A **binary** digit, or bit, is the smallest unit of data in computing. It is represented by a 0 or a 1.
- The list of coded instruction is called Computer Program
- Cache is a hardware or software component that temporarily stores data so future requests for that data can be served faster
- A hard disk is divided into track which are further subdivided into sectors.

and many more

"Sometimes the remedy is worse than the disease."

—Francis Bacon

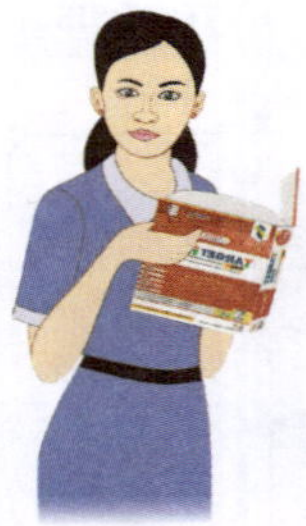

MULTIPLE CHOICE QUESTIONS

(Including Explained and Practice Questions)

ARTIFICIAL INTELLIGENCE

1. Which of the following is a chatbot developed by Google AI? *New Q*

a. Chatbot b. Meena
c. Xiaoice d. Bard

Explanation: Bard is a large language model chatbot developed by Google AI. Bard was launched on February 6, 2023. It is trained on a massive dataset of text and code, and is able to hold conversations that are both informative and engaging.

2. Which of the following is a chatbot developed by OpenAI? *New Q*

a. Xiaoice b. Bard
c. ChatGPT d. LaMDA

Explanation: ChatGPT is a chatbot developed by OpenAI. It is trained on a massive dataset of text and code, and is able to hold conversations that are both informative and engaging.

Xiaoice is a chatbot developed by Microsoft Research China, Bard is a chatbot developed by Google AI, and LaMDA is a chatbot developed by Google AI.

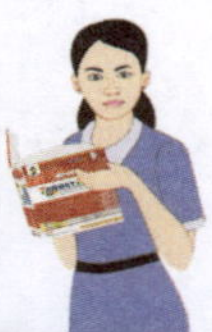

Ans.

1. d
2. c
3. d
4. c
5. b
6. b
7. a
8. c
9. c

3. Which of the following is NOT a potential benefit of Artificial Intelligence in nursing? *New Q*

a. Improved accuracy of diagnoses
b. Increased efficiency of care delivery
c. Personalized care
d. Increased workload for nurses

4. All of the following are potential risks of AI in nursing; EXCEPT: *New Q*

a. AI could be used to make biased decisions about patients.
b. AI could be used to replace nurses in the workforce.
c. AI may increase the cost of care delivery
d. AI could be hacked and used to harm patients.

Explanation: The potential risks of AI in nursing include the possibility of biased decision-making, the potential replacement of nurses in the workforce, and the risk of AI being hacked and used to harm patients. However, it is not directly associated with increasing the cost of care delivery. In fact, AI has the potential to streamline processes and improve efficiency, which could potentially reduce costs.

5. The following are the most important things for nurses; to prepare for the future of AI in nursing; except: *New Q*

a. Learn about the different applications of AI in nursing.
b. Resist the introduction of AI as it is a potential threat to nursing workforce
c. Be critical to the use of AI in nursing.
d. Be open to the idea of using AI in their practice.

Explanation: Nurses should be proactive in preparing for the future of AI in nursing by learning about the different applications of AI, being critical of its use, and being open to the idea of using AI in their practice. Resisting the introduction of AI as a potential threat to the nursing workforce may hinder nurses' ability to adapt and embrace the potential benefits that AI can offer in improving patient care and outcomes.

6. Which of the following is NOT a potential benefit of using AI tools in nursing research? *New Q*

a. Increased efficiency of data collection and analysis
b. Increased workload for researchers
c. Improved accuracy of research findings
d. Personalized research

Explanation: Increased workload for researchers is not a potential benefit of using AI tools in nursing research. AI can actually help to reduce the workload for researchers by automating tasks and providing support for data analysis.

7. Which of the following is a potential benefit of using AI in nursing research? *New Q*

a. Increased accuracy in data analysis
b. Decreased need for human involvement
c. Reduction in ethical considerations
d. Limited applicability in complex research studies

Explanation: The use of AI in nursing research can provide increased accuracy in data analysis. AI algorithms can process large amounts of data quickly and efficiently, allowing for more precise analysis and identification of patterns or trends that may not be easily recognizable by human researchers.

8. How can AI be utilized in data analysis for nursing research? *New Q*

a. Identifying research participants
b. Generating research hypotheses
c. Analyzing large datasets for patterns and trends
d. Conducting literature reviews

Explanation: AI can be utilized in data analysis for nursing research by analyzing large datasets for patterns and trends. This can help researchers uncover new insights, identify associations, and make predictions based on the data.

9. How can researchers best use AI tools to improve nursing research? *New Q*

a. By using AI to automate tasks and free up time for researchers to conduct more research.
b. By using AI to help researchers to make better decisions about research design and analysis.
c. By using AI to collect and analyze data to improve the quality of research findings.
d. By using AI to make research findings more accessible to the public.

10. Which of the following is NOT a potential benefit of using AI in high fidelity simulation learning in nursing? *New Q*

a. AI can be used to create more realistic and immersive simulations.
b. AI can be used to replace human instructors.
c. AI can be used to track learner progress and identify areas for improvement.
d. AI can be used to provide feedback to learners in real time.

Explanation: AI can be used to supplement human instructors, but it is not yet possible for AI to fully replace human instructors. Human instructors are still needed

BASIC KEY TERMS

11. Which one of the following competencies is not included as expected outcome after teaching the subject nursing informatics? *(AIIMS Raipur NO 2019)*

a. Basic computer skills
b. Information literacy
c. Basic informatics competencies
d. Advance informatics competencies

Explanation: **Advance nursing informatics** competencies are not included as expected outcome or the objective of the subject nursing informatics as only a basic knowledge in computer skills, information literacy and informatics is required to provide technology-based services to the patient.

12. If a computer provides database services to others, then it will be known as: *(AIIMS Raipur NO 2019)*

a. Web server
b. Application server
c. Database server
d. FTP server

Explanation: A database server has an application that helps to provide database services to other computers. **Web server** provides web pages. **Application server** serves dual purpose, it can create web applications as well as provide them the servers to run. **FTP server** helps in transferring of data among different computers present in a network.

13. A computer must have: *(AIIMS Raipur NO 2019)*

a. Microsoft office
b. Operating System
c. Internet connectivity
d. An antivirus

Explanation: A computer must have an operative system to run. Operating system is called the manager of the computer system resources. Operating system acts as a liaison between the computer and the humans. Some of the common disk operating systems are: Windows, Disk operating system (DOS), Unix or Xenix and Linux.

Microsoft office and antivirus are applications that are not mandatory to run a computer. Internet connectivity is not mandatory to operate a computer.

14. The _____ manages and coordinates the functions of the entire computer system. *(AIIMS BPL NO 2018)*

a. Control unit (CU)
b. Arithmetic logic unit (ALU)
c. Hard disk drive
d. Registers

Explanation: Control unit (CU) coordinates the functions of computer system. The information stored in the memory unit (e.g., hard disk drive) is extracted, decoded and executed by the **control unit**. Control unit demands help from ALU whenever required. CPU contains **registers** where processing of arithmetic operations of data occurs.

15. What is computer booting? *(AIIMS BPL NO 2018)*

a. Loading operating system into memory to make the computer system ready to use
b. Defragmenting the hard disk drive
c. Deleting the operating system
d. Formatting the hard disk drive

Explanation: The startup process of computer system is termed "Booting". In this, the computer system checks whether all the devices are connected properly or not. This is done by a small program in ROM.

16. _______________ use diagnostic routines to test system for equipment failure. *(AIIMS Nagpur NO 2018)*

a. Managing task
b. Managing files
c. Booting
d. Formatting

Explanation: **Booting** uses diagnostic routines to test system for equipment failure. The startup process of computer system is termed "Booting". This happens before an operating system comes into action.

17. Using ____________ button, you can move around the worksheet. *(AIIMS Nagpur NO 2018)*

a. Start
b. Scroll
c. Formatting
d. All of these

18. Clinical and technological advancements in nursing by application of computer and information science is called: *(AIIMS Nagpur NO 2018)*

a. Nursing informatics
b. Nursing diagnosis
c. Nursing procedure
d. Nursing reference

Explanation: **Nursing informatics** is called the clinical and technological advancements in nursing by application of computer and information science. Nursing informatics is amalgamation of nursing science, computer science and information science.

Nursing diagnosis, procedures and references are not technology based concepts hence they are incorrect.

19. The tracks on the disk surface are divided into invisible segments called: *(AIIMS Nagpur NO 2018)*

a. Surface
b. Sector
c. Segments
d. None of these

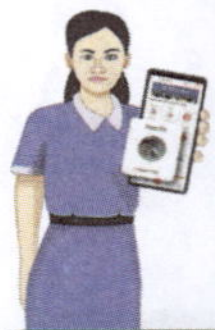

Ans.

10.	b
11.	d
12.	c
13.	b
14.	a
15.	a
16.	c
17.	b
18.	a
19.	b

Explanation: Sectors are the tracks on the disk surface that are divided into invisible segments.

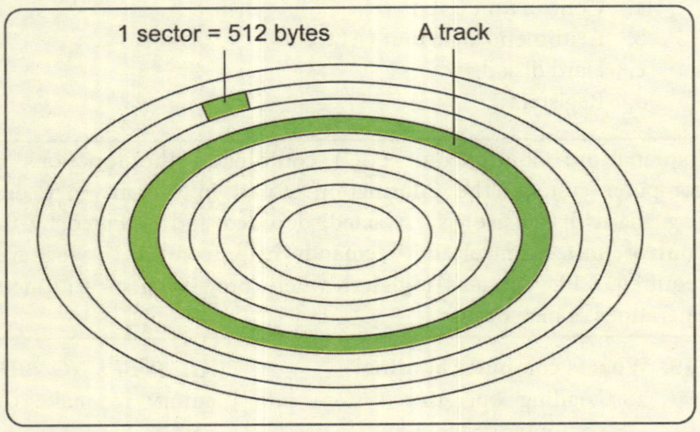

20. The data that is produced as a result of processing by the CPU is known as: *(AIIMS Nagpur NO 2018)*

a. Scanning
b. Output
c. Input
d. None of these

Explanation:

- **Output** is produced as a result of processing by the CPU. Output devices enable the user to obtain the data which was entered through an input device and processed by CPU by converting the binary codes back into the language the user can read and understand.
- **Scanning** is done by the scanner and is a type of **input**. Hence, **all other options** are incorrect.

21. The full form of CLI: *(AIIMS Nagpur NO 2018)*

a. Command Line Interspace
b. Command Line Interface
c. Common Line Interface
d. Common Line Interspace

Explanation: CLI stands for **Command Line Interface**. It is an interface between user and computer that is based on text.

22. One or more users simultaneously on two or more processors are known as: *(AIIMS Nagpur NO 2018)*

a. Time sharing
b. Multiprogramming
c. Multitasking
d. Multiprocessing

Explanation: Multiprocessing is the term used when one or more users simultaneously work on two or more processors. It uses two or more CPU within a single computer system.

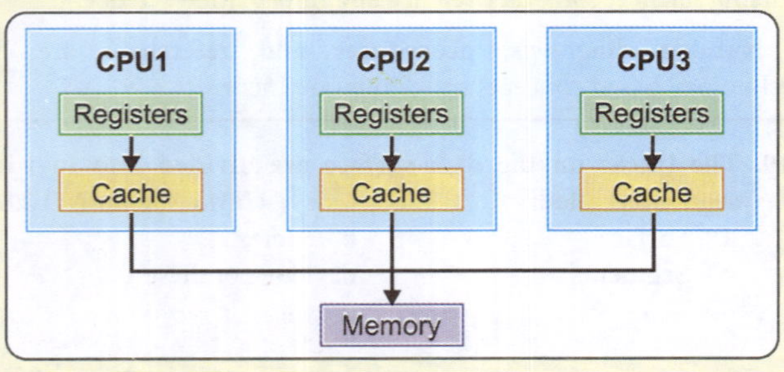

Figure: Multiprocessing

23. Hypertext is a text that: *(Safdarjung NO 2018):*

a. Appears as superscript
b. Contains links to another document
c. Appears above normal text
d. Has images embodied in the text

Explanation: Hypertext is a text displayed on a computer display or other electronic devices with reference to other text (document) that the reader can immediately access. Hypertext documents are interconnected by hyperlinks, which are typically activated by a mouse click, key press or by touching the screen.

24. What is the process of starting the computer called?

a. Booting
b. Shut down
c. Restart
d. Memory

25. CPU stands for:

a. Control of Power Unit
b. Central Program Unit
c. Central Processing Unit
d. Central Power Unit

26. It is an excellent program for calculation:

a. M.S. Word
b. M.S. Power Point
c. M.S. Excel
d. M.S. DOS

27. The small graphical buttons in Windows, which represent folders, data files, program files, etc.

a. Programs
b. Orientation
c. Presentation
d. Icons

28. What is the function of Slide Show Button?

a. Edit a slide
b. Insert a picture in the slide
c. View the slide show
d. Give animation effect to the slide

29. To create a folder on the desktop:

a. Left click on your desktop, click folder, new
b. Open a Word processor, click file, new
c. Right click on your desktop, click new, folder
d. Open my computer, control panel, click new folder

30. Slides can have:

a. Title, text, graphs
b. Drawn objects, shapes
c. Clipart, drawn art, visual
d. All of the above

31. Right-justified text is aligned on:

a. Left margin
b. Between the Left and right margin
c. Right margin
d. Center

32. The function of inserting the content of the clipboard at the insertion point is called:

a. Cut
b. Copy
c. Paste
d. Delete

33. A document for storing and calculating numerical data mainly used for financial planning and accounting:

a. Accounts
b. Spreadsheet
c. Business
d. Template

34. The function of checking the spelling is called:

a. Grammar check
b. Accessing
c. Formatting
d. Spell-check

35. To Boot/Boot up a computer means:

a. Start the computer
b. Install a program
c. Shut Down the computer
d. Restart the computer

Ans.

20. b
21. b
22. d
23. b
24. a
25. c
26. c
27. d
28. c
29. c
30. d
31. c
32. c
33. b
34. d
35. a

36. **What is it called when you remove some information from a file or remove a file from the disk?**
    a. Save b. Edit
    c. Delete d. Highlight
37. **What do you do to enlarge an area of a document for easy viewing?**
    a. Flip b. Trash
    c. Zoom d. View
38. **A ____________ can have multiple slides.**
    a. Windows b. Presentation
    c. Computer d. File
39. **An __________ has a four sided boundary around it.**
    a. Cursor b. Work sheet
    c. Excel d. Active cell
40. **M.S. DOS works on:**
    a. Command prompt b. Codes
    c. Mouse d. Copy
41. **The ______________ option is used to reverse the last action performed on the document.**
    a. Cut b. Close
    c. Save d. Undo
42. **Print option is under the ______________ menu.**
    a. Edit b. View
    c. File d. Format
43. **Users manipulators that make the computer work:**
    a. Hardware b. Software
    c. Peopleware d. Electronic
44. **A unit of data in the binary numbering system:**
    a. Hexadecimal b. Numeral
    c. Bits and bytes d. None of these
45. **A class of computer that operates on continuous physical or electrical magnitudes, measuring ongoing continuous analog quantities such as voltage, current, temperature and pressure:**
    a. Analog b. Digital
    c. Hybrid d. None of these
46. **A class of computer that operates on discrete discontinuous numerical digits using the binary numbering system:**
    a. Analog b. Digital
    c. Hybrid d. None of these
47. **A class of computers that contains features of both analog and digital computer:**
    a. Digital b. Analog
    c. Hybrid d. Electronic
48. **Modem is short form of:**
    a. Modulating and demodulating device
    b. Model and demodeling device
    c. Modulating and decoding device
    d. None of the above
49. **Topology comes from the Greek Word *topos*, which means:**
    a. Land b. Connection
    c. Geography d. Communication

HISTORY & GENERATIONS OF COMPUTERS

50. **__________ designed the first modern computer.**
    a. Abacus
    b. Bill Gates
    c. Charles Babbage
    d. APJ Abdul Kalam
51. **A type of computer that is small, special function computer that was introduced in the 1990's:**
    a. Supercomputers b. Mainframes
    c. Microcomputer d. Hand-held computer
52. **Who is known as 'Father of Computer'?**
    a. Vint Cerf b. Bill Gates
    c. Charles Babbage d. Mark Zuckerberg
53. **Which of the following is the chief component of first generation computer?**
    a. Transistors
    b. Vacuum Tubes and Valves
    c. Integrated Circuits
    d. Diodes

CLASSIFICATION OF COMPUTERS

54. **____________ is the onscreen area where all the icons, windows and dialog boxes are displayed.** *(AIIMS Nagpur NO 2018)*
    a. Drives b. Desktop
    c. Screen d. My computer
55. **Different network can be linked using:** *(Safdarjung NO 2018)*
    a. A remote PC b. A router PC
    c. A disk server d. Modem

Explanation: A router PC makes the packets travel through it. Packets transmit from one router to another over the internet till it reaches its destination as per the IP protocol. Each packet can take different router to travel. This helps to link different networks.

56. **The physical components of a computer are referred to as:**
    a. Hardware b. Software
    c. Peopleware d. Electronic
57. **A ___________ is a set of cooperative interconnected computers for the purpose of information exchange.**
    a. Networking b. Network
    c. Topology d. Server

COMPUTER HARDWARE

58. **A storage device, which loses data when power supply is stopped, is called____ memory.** *(AIIMS BPL NO 2018)*
    a. Volatile b. Static
    c. Dynamic d. Secondary

Explanation: RAM is known as "random access memory", which is a **"volatile"** memory as it is a type of temporary memory on which one can read and write, once reading and writing is done. **Static** RAM (SRAM) and **Dynamic** RAM (DRAM) are two types of RAM. **Secondary** memories (e.g., hard disk) are permanent memories; hence they do not lose data when power supply is stopped.

59. **An extremely fast memory that works as an intermediary between CPU and main memory is called:** *(AIIMS BBS NO 2018)*
    a. DRAM b. Cache
    c. EPROM d. Blu-ray disk

Explanation: **Cache** is an extremely fast and short term memory that works as an intermediary between CPU and main memory. This stores the previously visited Web pages on the hard drive and RAM.

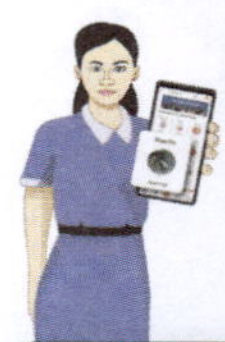

Ans.

36.	c
37.	c
38.	b
39.	d
40.	a
41.	d
42.	c
43.	c
44.	c
45.	a
46.	b
47.	c
48.	a
49.	c
50.	c
51.	d
52.	c
53.	b
54.	b
55.	b
56.	a
57.	b
58.	a
59.	b

60. The time it takes to spin the specified sector of hard disk under the read/write head is called: *(AIIMS BBS NO 2018)*

a. Latency b. Response time
c. Seek time d. Data transfer rate

Explanation: **Seek time** is the time that the hard disk controller takes to find a part of stored data.

61. ______________ is the device that sends the information about the direction or angle of the stick to the device or application it is controlling. *(AIIMS Nagpur NO 2018)*

a. Scanner b. Joystick
c. VDU d. Mouse

Explanation: **Joystick** is the input device that sends the information about the direction or angle of the stick to the device or application it is controlling. It is also a pointing device like mouse that controls the movement of the cursor. It has two buttons called "triggers". It is used to play video games. They may have one or more push buttons.

62. Devices such as the monitor, speaker and printer are known as:

a. Input b. Output
c. Processing d. Storage

63. What do the letters ROM stand for?

a. Random Organized Memory
b. Read Only Memory
c. Right Only Memory
d. Ready Optional Memory

64. What is the function of the backspace key?

a. Deletes the previous Word
b. Deletes one character to the right of the cursor
c. Deletes the next character
d. Deletes one character to the left of the cursor

65. Which of the following is an input device?

a. Speaker b. Printer
c. Mouse d. Monitor

66. Which one is a storage device?

a. Speaker b. Headphones
c. Compact Disk d. Modem

67. Computer is an ______________ machine that works under the control of stored programs.

a. Electrical b. Electronic
c. Clinical d. Hydraulic

68. You can delete a file by clicking it and pressing the ______________ key.

a. Shift b. Control
c. Caps lock d. Delete

69. It is referred to as the brain of the computer:

a. Output device b. Memory
c. Input device d. CPU

70. The type of memory that storage is not erased even if computer is turned off is called:

a. RAM b. ROM
c. CPU d. ALU

71. The working memory that is used for primary storage is referred to as:

a. RAM B. ROM
c. CPU d. ALU

72. For a computer to work, it must have a way of receiving commands. This is done through the use of:

a. Diskettes b. Printer
c. CPU d. Input devices

73. What is the most commonly used input device?

a. Keyboard and mouse
b. Keyboard and scanner
c. Scanner and mouse
d. Scanner and keyboard

74. A type of hardware that is used to output the results processed by the computer is called:

a. Input device b. Output device
c. Storage d. Process

75. Computer process is done using what device in the computer:

a. Input device b. Output device
c. CPU d. Storage media

76. CD-ROM, Hard drive, USB disk and diskettes are types of:

a. Input device
b. Output device
c. Process
d. Storage media

77. A type of storage media that has very high speed and high density that can store large capacity of files:

a. USB disk b. Diskette
c. CD ROM d. Hard drive

78. ______________ is an electronic device capable of handling large arithmetic and logical operations:

a. Calculator
b. Arm machine
c. Cash register machine
d. Computer

79. Which of the following are components of CPU?

a. Control unit, keyboard
b. Control unit, monitor
c. Arithmetic logic unit, mouse
d. Arithmetic logic unit, control unit

80. RAM stands for:

a. Read Access Memory
b. Random Access Memory
c. Remote Access Memory
d. Ready Access Memory

81. In computer, where is RAM located?

a. Hard Disk b. Mother board
c. SMPS d. Processor

82. ALU stands for:

a. Arithmetic Logic Unit
b. Arithmetic Logarithmic Unit
c. Arithmetic Local Unit
d. Analog Logic Unit

83. In computer, saved files are stored at:

a. Cache b. RAM
c. Hard disk d. SMPS

84. Which of the following is used to make computer chips?

a. Copper
b. Iron
c. Silicon
d. Aluminum

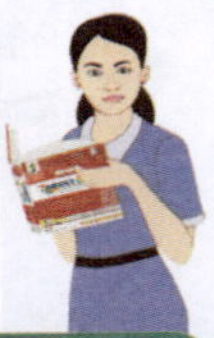

Ans.

60. c
61. b
62. b
63. b
64. d
65. c
66. c
67. b
68. d
69. d
70. b
71. a
72. d
73. a
74. b
75. c
76. d
77. d
78. d
79. d
80. b
81. b
82. a
83. c
84. c

85. **Find out the odd one:**
   a. Mouse b. Scanner
   c. Keyboard d. Printer

86. **Which of the following storage devices can store maximum amount of data?**
   a. Floppy Disk b. Hard Disk
   c. DVD d. Blue-ray Disk

SOFTWARE PROGRAMS

87. **Software designed for a specific purpose is called:** *(Safdarjung NO 2018)*
   a. System software b. Compiler
   c. Specific software d. Application software

Explanation: **Application software** is goal directed software. They are developed specifically to solve a purpose. Application software helps in performing a number of tasks in a coordinated manner in which data-base program performs the function of collecting, organizing and analyzing the data. **Examples:** MS Word, MS Excel, MS-PowerPoint, etc.

88. **Which of the following best describes virtual reality (VR)?** *(AIIMS Raipur NO 2019)*
   a. It brings the learner to another reality even if it is not existing
   b. It provides a case study
   c. It creates competition to all participants
   d. It simulates different cases and situations

Explanation: **Virtual reality** brings the learner to another reality through simulation in which the computer generates a situation which is not real, and it enables the user to interact with the unreal environment.

89. **Which of the following is the valid cell address corresponding to the seventh row and eighth column of a worksheet?** *(AIIMS BPL NO 2018)*
   a. H8 b. H7
   c. 7H d. 78

Explanation: In a worksheet, row is denoted by number (1, 2, 3 and so on) and column is denoted by alphabets (A, B, C.. and so on). Cell address changes based on relative position of rows and columns. The cell address is denoted as column name followed by the row name. So the answer is H7.

90. **____ is used to copy formatting styles of a selected text and apply to other texts in a word document.** *(AIIMS BPL NO 2018)*
   a. Autocorrect b. Format painter
   c. Mail merge d. Marco

Explanation: Format painter is a feature that enables the user to "copy formatting" from one place and applying it to another.

91. **Using a computer to determine solution aids in decision making is called:** *(AIIMS BPL NO 2018)*:
   a. Models b. Decision tree
   c. Simulations d. Linear programming

Explanation: Linear programming is a technique to get the desired solution, taking in consideration the actively working constraints by formulating the problem into a mathematical model. This helps in the decision-making process.

92. **The size of a 12-point text in MS-word is equivalent to:** *(AIIMS BBS NO 2018)*
   a. 1/6 inch b. 1/4 inch
   c. 1/2 inch d. 1/3 inch

Explanation:
- 72 points = 1 inch, hence,
- 1/6 inch = 12 points
- 1/4 inch = 18 points
- 1/2 inch = 36 points
- 1/3 inch = 24 points

93. **Computer programs that make the computer work:**
   a. Hardware b. Software
   c. Peopleware d. Electronic

94. **What type of software that supervises the computer's system resources?**
   a. Network Software b. Application Software
   c. Operating System d. Internet Software

95. **A type of software that is designed to help perform singular or multiple related specific tasks:**
   a. Network Software b. Application Software
   c. Operating System d. Internet Software

96. **Windows, Linux and Ubuntu is an example of:**
   a. Application Software b. Network Software
   c. Operating system d. None of these

97. **A program that allows users to access resources from the web is referred to as:**
   a. MS Word b. Photoshop
   c. MS Access d. Web browser

98. **__________ is a matter of the user's freedom to copy, run, distribute, study, change and improve the software.**
   a. Free software b. Licensed software
   c. System software d. None of these

99. **__________ are raw facts that are without meaning:**
   a. Data b. Database
   c. Tables d. Information

100. **Processed data is known as:**
   a. Data b. Database
   c. Tables d. Information

101. **In MS-Access, what data type that is equivalent to alpha numeric?**
   a. Currency b. Character
   c. Text d. Logical

102. **What data type is appropriate for entries in a form of amount or money?**
   a. Currency b. Character
   c. Text d. Logical

103. **What data type that outputs for only two results?**
   a. Currency b. Character
   c. Text d. Logical

104. **Computer program used to input store, modify, process and access data in a database is referred to as:**
   a. Office Applications b. DBMS
   c. RDBMS d. Antivirus

105. **A computer program or a set of instructions that, when executed cause the computer to open or start a specific computer program or function:**
   a. Data file b. Processing file
   c. Text file d. Office file

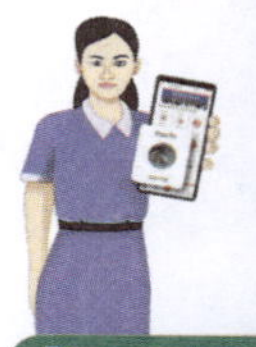

Ans.

85.	d
86.	b
87.	d
88.	a
89.	b
90.	b
91.	d
92.	a
93.	b
94.	c
95.	b
96.	c
97.	d
98.	a
99.	a
100.	d
101.	c
102.	a
103.	d
104.	b
105.	b

106. A program that is used to upload files to and download from distant computer:

a. Http b. URT
c. Ftp d. Utp

107. FTP means:

a. Free transfer pass
b. File transfer protocol
c. File transmission protocol
d. File transmission pass

108. A set of data elements (values) that is organized using a model of vertical columns (which are identified by their name) and horizontal rows:

a. Database b. Records
c. Table d. Fields

109. Data in computer is stored and transferred in:

a. Binary form
b. Decimal form
c. Alphabetical form
d. Alphanumerical form

110. LINUX is a/an:

a. Application software
b. Operating system
c. Antivirus program
d. Malware

111. MS-Word is a/an:

a. Application software
b. Operating system
c. Hardware
d. Malware

112. One byte is equal to:

a. 2 bits b. 8 bits
c. 16 bits d. 32 bits

113. 1 Mega Byte (MB) is equal to:

a. 1024 Bits b. 1024 Bytes
c. 1024 Kilo bytes d. 1024 Giga bytes

114. If the displayed system date and time is wrong, you can reset it using:

a. Write file b. Task Manager
c. Debugging d. Control panel

115. Microsoft windows is a/an:

a. Word processing software
b. Operating system
c. Database program
d. Statistical package

116. SPSS is a/an:

a. Operating system
b. Statistical package
c. Data base
d. Word processor

117. Which of the following is not an application software?

a. MS-Word
b. Adobe Photoshop
c. SPSS
d. Linux

118. Which of the following windows do not have start button?

a. Windows 97
b. Windows XP
c. Windows Vista
d. Windows 8

119. Which of the following is the latest version of Microsoft windows?

a. Windows Vista
b. Windows 8.0
c. Windows 8.1
d. Windows 10

120. Which of the following functions in MS-Word enables the user to send same letter to different persons?

a. Macros
b. Mail merge
c. Template
d. Address block

121. Intersection of rows and columns is known as:

a. Data b. Schema
c. Table d. Cell

122. Which of the following functional keys is used to check spellings in MS-Word?

a. F1 b. F3
c. F5 d. F7

123. Which of the following term refers to the Word processing task associated with changing the appearance of a document?

a. Editing
b. Writing
c. Formatting
d. Printing

124. The term gigabyte refers to:

a. 1024 bytes
b. 1024 kilobytes
c. 1024 megabytes
d. 1024 Terabytes

125. The smallest font size available in Font Size tool on formatting tool bar of MS-Word is:

a. 4 b. 8
c. 10 d. 12

126. The largest font size available in Font Size tool on formatting tool bar of MS-Word is:

a. 32 b. 48
c. 72 d. 96

127. PDF stands for:

a. Portable Document Format
b. Portable Document File
c. Public Document Format
d. Private Document Format

128. PowerPoint presentations are widely used as:

a. Note outlines for teachers
b. Project presentations by students
c. Communication planning
d. All of the above

129. In slide layout panel of MS-PowerPoint, how many layouts are available for text layout by default?

a. 4 b. 7
c. 10 d. 12

130. In PowerPoint, which of the following helps to create presentation by selecting readymade font color and graphics effects?

a. Presentation template
b. Design template
c. Slide master
d. Automatic animation scheme

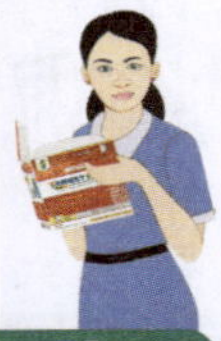

Ans.

106.	c
107.	b
108.	c
109.	a
110.	b
111.	a
112.	b
113.	c
114.	d
115.	b
116.	b
117.	d
118.	d
119.	d
120.	b
121.	d
122.	d
123.	c
124.	c
125.	b
126.	c
127.	a
128.	d
129.	a
130.	b

131. In a PowerPoint presentation:
a. Image can be inserted but not movie clips
b. Movie clips can be inserted but not Image
c. Both cannot be inserted
d. Both can be inserted

132. In MS-Word, autocorrect option was designed to replace:
a. Misspelled Words
b. Grammatically incorrect Words
c. Repetitive Words
d. Abbreviations

133. In MS-Word, END key is used to move the cursor to:
a. End of the line
b. End of the page
c. End of the document
d. None of these

USES OF COMPUTERS IN HEALTHCARE SYSTEM

134. In telemedicine terms, the hub is: *(AIIMS Raipur NO 2019)*
a. A physical line of communication
b. The patient on the receiving end who is in his/her home
c. The provider reaching out from a primary clinical site
d. The provider on the receiving end at a remote site

Explanation: **Telemedicine** hub refers to the primary clinical site from where the health provider renders health services to the remote places.

135. Which of the following is NOT true about nursing informatics? *(AIIMS-BBS SNO 2019)*
a. It is not a multidisciplinary science practice
b. It is specific to nursing and nursing practice
c. Graves and Corcoran provided the first definition
d. It is not to be equated with the generic term informatics

Explanation: Nursing informatics is a field of nursing that incorporates nursing, computer and information sciences to maintain and develop medical data and systems to support the practice of nursing, and to improve patient care outcomes. It is a multidisciplinary science practice.

136. Hospital information system helps nurses to prevent prescription errors by: *(AIIMS Nagpur NO 2018)*
a. Preventing side effects
b. Avoiding transcribing orders
c. Providing right dosage
d. Providing right dilution

Explanation: Hospital information system helps nurses to prevent prescription errors by **avoiding transcribing orders** as with this system, the nurse does not have to transfer the physician's orders to other health departments, specifically medication administration record. This enhances compliance and minimizes errors.

137. The collection and integration of various pieces of hardware and software and the human resources that meet the data collection, storage, processing and report generation needs of an organization is known as:
a. Computer systems
b. Information systems
c. Network systems
d. Management information systems

138. A type of information systems that provides managers information about their business operations is known as:
a. Transaction systems
b. Excision systems
c. Physiologic systems
d. Management information systems

139. A system that is used to process predefined transactions and produce predefined reports is referred to as:
a. Transaction systems
b. Decision support systems
c. Physiologic monitoring systems
d. Management information systems

COMMONLY USED SHORTCUT KEYS

140. Keyboard shortcut to make a paragraph center aligned in MS-Word document is: *(AIIMS BPL NO 2018)*
a. Ctrl + E b. AlT + E
c. Ctrl + X d. Ctrl + A

Explanation: Shortcut keys for alignment includes:
- **Ctrl + E:** Center aligned
- **Ctrl + J:** Justified
- **Ctrl + L:** Left aligned
- **Ctrl + R:** Right aligned

Other options are not related to alignment
- **Alt + E:** Shortcut helps to open the edit options in the present program
- **Ctrl + X:** Shortcut used to cut the selected text/image/file
- **Ctrl + A:** Shortcut used to select all the content in the document

141. The ____________ key is used to erase the character to the right of the cursor.
a. Delete b. Erase
c. Backspace d. ESC

142. In MS-Word, by pressing which of the following keys we can move to the beginning of the first page of the document?
a. Shift + home b. Control + home
c. Alt + home d. Shift + control + home

143. Which of the following commands used to select all the text in a document?
a. Control + A b. Control + C
c. Control + V d. Control + X

144. Which of the following commands is used to copy the selected text?
a. Control + A b. Control + C
c. Control + X d. Control + Z

145. Which of the following commands is used to open a new blank Word document?
a. Control + M b. Control + N
c. Control + O d. Control + X

146. Which of the following functional keys is used to start a slide show in a PowerPoint presentation?
a. F1 b. F2
c. F3 d. F5

147. In MS-Word, F12 is a short cut key for:
a. Save b. Save as
c. Open d. Close

148. Which of the following short cut keys is used to convert the selected text into capital letters in MS-Word?
a. Control + F3 b. Shift + F3
c. Control + F3 d. Shift + F5

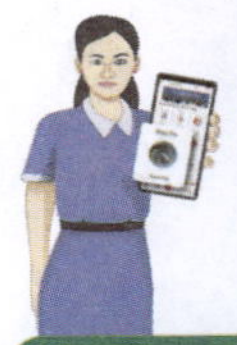

Ans.

131. d
132. a
133. a
134. c
135. a
136. b
137. b
138. d
139. a
140. a
141. a
142. b
143. a
144. b
145. b
146. d
147. b
148. b

COMMON FILE EXTENSIONS

149. A document, written in HTML which contains automated links to other documents is referred to as:
a. HTML b. URL
c. Hypertext d. Highlights

150. Files that contain data that have been captured and stored on a computer using a software program:
a. Data file b. Executable file
c. Text file d. Processing file

151. Which of the following type of files uses JPG as an extension?
a. Video b. Image
c. Word d. PowerPoint

152. Which of the following is the extension used in Word file created by MS-Word 97-2003?
a. .doc b. .docx
c. .txt d. .txts

153. Which of the following is the extension used in Word file created by MS-Word 2007 or latest?
a. .doc b. .docx
c. .txt d. .txts

154. Which of the following file formats can be added to a PowerPoint show?
a. .jpg b. .mpeg
c. .gif d. All of these

COMPUTER NETWORKING

155. The art and science of creating networks is referred to as:
a. Networking b. Network
c. Topology d. Server

156. The computer that provides resources to a network is called:
a. Networking b. Network
c. Topology d. Server

157. The computer that access shared resources on the network is referred to as:
a. Peer b. Server
c. Client d. Mainframe

158. The basic building block of any computer networks that can range from simple to complex connection is referred to as:
a. Local Area Network b. Metropolitan area network
c. World wide web d. Communication

159. __________ is a network topology or circuit arrangement in which all the nodes of the computers are directly attached to a line.
a. Star b. Ring
c. Bus d. Mesh

160. This topology is centralized structure where all computers are connected through a central computer:
a. Star b. Ring
c. Bus d. Mesh

161. What cable is used to connect star topology?
a. Twisted pair cable b. Coaxial cable
c. Fiber Optics d. All of these

162. In star topology, the computers are using UTP cables connected in a ____________ to share resources.
a. Cables b. Network interface card
c. Hub d. Outer

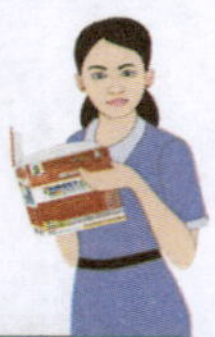

Ans.
149. c
150. a
151. b
152. a
153. b
154. d
155. a
156. d
157. c
158. a
159. c
160. a
161. d
162. c
163. d
164. c
165. d
166. b
167. b
168. a
169. c
170. a
171. c

WEB/INTERNET KEY TERMINOLOGIES

163. Identify the odd term out: *(Safdarjung NO 2018)*
a. Front page express b. Composer
c. Web Page Editor d. World Wide Web

Explanation: Front page express, composer and web page editor are having one similarity that they are all web editing software, whereas World Wide Web (WWW) is a chain of interconnected servers that stores a large number of information and send files across the internet.

164. The domain name in a URL refers to the: *(Safdarjung NO 2018):*
a. Protocol b. File name
c. Server d. Directory

Explanation: URL stands for "Uniform Resource Locator." URL helps the user to locate the Web page. URL consists of:

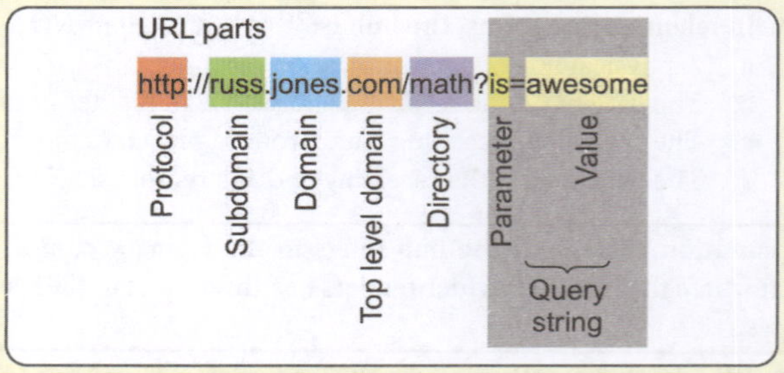

File name follows directory. Domain name refers to main web page or particular server.

165. The language that is used to create hypertext documents is known as:
a. WWW b. url
c. http d. html

166. The text in a web document that if clicked would open another document in the internet is called:
a. HTML b. Hyperlink
c. Hypertext d. URL

167. There are 3 parts of an email address. What are these parts?
a. Caller id, name of network, domain name
b. User id, name of network, domain name
c. Caller id, name of computer, domain name
d. User id, name of computer, domain name

168. What can HTML do?
a. Create web pages b. Send email
c. Transfer files d. Download files

169. ________________ is one of the protocols used in the internet for terminal emulation program that is part of the TCP/IP protocols.
a. HTTP b. HTML
c. Telnet d. FTP

170. WWW stands for:
a. World Wide Web b. Wide World Web
c. Web World Wide d. Wide Web World

171. URL stands for:
a. Universal Resource Locator b. Universal Resource Link
c. Uniform Resource Locator d. Uniform Resource Link

"**One day in perfect health is much.**"
—Arabic

CHAPTER 15

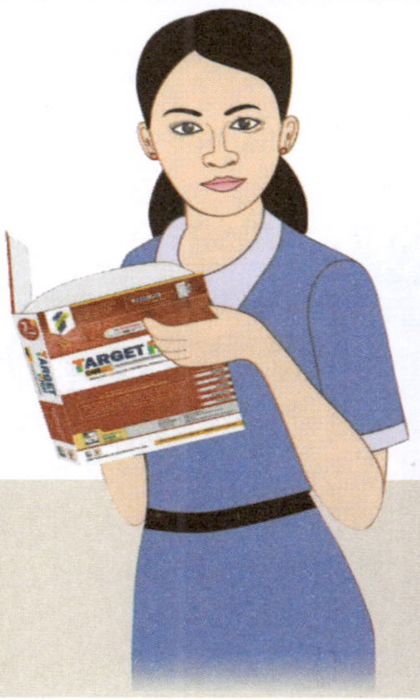

FORENSIC NURSING AND INDIAN LAWS

SYNOPSIS

INTRODUCTION

- Forensic nurses provide comprehensive care to individuals who have experienced violence, trauma, or are involved in legal proceedings.
- Forensic nurses work in various settings such as hospitals, clinics, correctional facilities, and forensic laboratories.
- Forensic nursing requires a unique set of skills, combining medical knowledge, evidence collection, and legal understanding.

IMPORTANCE

- Collection and preservation of evidence related to crimes, accidents, or abuse cases.
- To gather physical evidence, document injuries, and provide detailed reports for legal purposes. This can involve photographing injuries, collecting DNA samples, and maintaining chain of custody for evidence.
- To provide compassionate care to victims of violence or trauma, including sexual assault, domestic violence, child abuse, and elder abuse.
- To prepare thorough assessments, provide medical treatment, offer emotional support, and connect patients with appropriate resources for counseling and follow-up care.
- To collaborate with multidisciplinary teams, including law enforcement personnel, social workers, psychologists, and legal professionals.

AREAS OF FORENSIC NURSING PRACTICE

- Intimate partner violence
- Child abuse/maltreatment
- Elder abuse
- Sexual assault
- Death investigation
- Correctional nursing

SCOPE AND PRACTICE OF FORENSIC NURSING

- Forensic evidence collection
- Sexual assault nurse examiner
- Documentation and reporting of findings and observation
- Injury assessment and documentation
- Expert witness testimony
- Collaborative role
- Community education and advocacy

MILESTONES IN FORENSIC NURSING

- **1982:** The International Association of Forensic Nurses (IAFN) was established.
- **1995:** The American Nurses Association recognized forensic nursing as a nursing specialty.
- **2021:** Indian Nursing Council introduced forensic nursing as a subject in the graduate nursing program.

KEY POINTS

- Forensic nursing is a specialty within the nursing profession that focuses on the application of nursing knowledge to the legal system.
- Forensic nurses work in collaboration with law enforcement, legal professionals, and other healthcare providers.
- The history of forensic nursing can be traced back to the early 1900s, when nurses began to work in prisons and jails.
- In the 1960s, nurses began to work in the field of child abuse, and in the 1970s, nurses began to work in the field of sexual assault.
- The International Association of Forensic Nurses (IAFN) was established in 1982.
- In 2021, Indian Nursing Council introduced Forensic Nursing as a subject in their Under Graduate curriculum.

SUBSPECIALTIES IN FORENSIC NURSING

Table 1: Subspecialties and their descriptions

Subspecialty	Description
Sexual assault nurse examiners (SANEs)	Providing comprehensive care to individuals who have experienced sexual assault or rape. They are trained in forensic evidence collection, conducting sensitive interviews, and providing medical and psychological support to survivors.
Forensic psychiatric nurses	Work with individuals involved in the legal system who have mental health issues. They assess and treat mental health conditions, provide counseling, and therapy, and assist in determining the mental competency of individuals involved in legal proceedings.
Forensic nurse death investigators	Nurses work closely with medical examiners or coroners to investigate deaths that are suspicious, violent, or unexpected. They assist in the collection of evidence, document injuries, and provide expert input on the medical aspects of death investigations.
Forensic nurse consultants	Provide expert advice and consultation on forensic nursing matters. They may assist with legal cases, review medical records, provide expert testimony, and offer guidance on policies and protocols related to forensic nursing practice.
Forensic nurse educators	They are responsible for teaching and training aspiring forensic nurses. They develop and deliver educational programs, design curriculum, and provide guidance on forensic nursing practice.
Forensic nurses in correctional settings	Nurses work within prisons, providing health care services to individuals who are incarcerated. They assess and treat injuries, conduct health screenings, address mental health concerns, and provide support for inmates within the criminal justice system.
Legal nurse consultants	They bridge the gap between health care and the legal system. They provide expertise and analysis on medical-legal cases, review medical records, assist with case preparation, and offer guidance on health care standards and regulations within legal contexts.

ETHICAL ISSUES IN FORENSIC NURSING

Table 2: Ethical issues and their descriptions

Ethical issues	Description
Confidentiality and privacy	Forensic nurses often work with sensitive and confidential information related to victims, perpetrators, and legal cases. They must maintain strict confidentiality and privacy while balancing the need to share pertinent information with law enforcement and legal authorities to ensure public safety and facilitate justice.
Informed consent	Obtaining informed consent can be challenging in forensic nursing, especially in cases involving victims of violence or trauma. Forensic nurses must ensure individuals fully understand the purpose, risks, and benefits of any procedures or interventions, while taking into account their emotional and psychological state.
Autonomy and decision-making	Forensic nurses may encounter situations where individuals' autonomy and decision-making capacity are compromised due to trauma, mental health issues, or other factors. Balancing respect for autonomy with the duty to protect vulnerable individuals can be ethically complex.
Dual roles and conflicts of interest	Forensic nurses may face situations where they have dual roles or conflicting responsibilities. For example, they may be both a health care provider and a forensic expert witness. Managing potential conflicts of interest and ensuring objectivity and integrity is essential in such cases.

Contd...

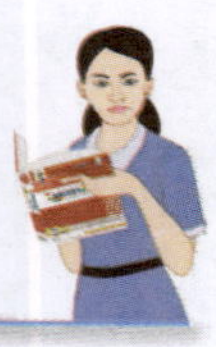

KEY POINTS

The roles of the forensic nurse include:
- Collecting and analyzing evidence
- Providing care to victims of crime:
- Testifying in court

KEY POINTS

- Forensic nurse death investigators are nurses who work closely with medical examiners or coroners to investigate deaths that are suspicious, violent, or unexpected.
- Forensic psychiatric nurses work with individuals involved in the legal system who have mental health issues.
- Sexual Assault Nurse Examiners (SANEs) provide comprehensive care to individuals who have experienced sexual assault or rape.
- Forensic nurses in correctional settings work within prisons and provide healthcare services to individuals who are incarcerated.

KEY POINT

Obtaining informed consent can be challenging in forensic nursing, especially in cases involving victims of violence or trauma.

Ethical issues	Description
Cultural sensitivity and diversity	Forensic nurses work with diverse populations, and cultural sensitivity is crucial in providing equitable care. Respecting cultural beliefs, practices, and norms while ensuring the safety and well-being of individuals can present ethical challenges.
Professional boundaries	The nature of the work may involve intimate examinations, sensitive conversations, and emotional support. Forensic nurses must establish and maintain professional boundaries to ensure ethical practice and prevent any exploitation or misconduct.
Justice and fairness	Forensic nursing is inherently connected to the pursuit of justice. Ensuring fairness, impartiality, and upholding the principles of justice is paramount.
Duty to report	Forensic nurses have a legal and ethical duty to report certain incidents, such as child abuse or certain types of violence. However, dilemmas can arise when considering the potential consequences and impact of reporting, particularly in cases where the victim may be at risk or reluctant to involve the legal system.

FORENSIC TEAM

Forensic team is a multidisciplinary group of professionals who work together to provide comprehensive care, support, and expertise in forensic cases.

Table 3: Forensic team members and their functions

Team member	Function
Medical examiners/Forensic pathologists	These professionals are responsible for conducting autopsies and determining the cause and manner of death in cases of suspicious or violent deaths.
Forensic nurses	They provide direct care to individuals affected by violence or trauma, conduct forensic assessments, collect evidence, and provide support throughout legal proceedings.
Law enforcement officers	Police officers and detectives work closely with forensic nurses to investigate crimes, gather evidence, and ensure the safety and well-being of individuals involved.
Legal professionals	Attorneys, prosecutors, and defense lawyers are involved in forensic cases.
Psychologists/Psychiatrists	They assess and treat individuals affected by trauma, provide counseling, and offer expert opinions on the psychological impact of the events.
Social workers/counselors	They assist with crisis intervention, safety planning, and connecting individuals with appropriate community services.
Forensic scientists	Forensic scientists analyze and interpret physical evidence collected by forensic nurses, such as DNA samples, fingerprints, or ballistics.
Victim advocates	They are professionals who work to ensure the rights, needs, and well-being of victims are addressed throughout the forensic process.

KEY POINTS

- Types of Legal inquest procedure include Police inquest and Magistrate inquest.
- Police inquest is conducted by a police officer, usually a senior investigating officer.
- Magistrate inquest is conducted by a coroner, who is a judicial officer.

KEY POINT

When photographing forensic evidence, it is important to capture two images of each finding.

EVIDENCE AND SAMPLE COLLECTION IN FORENSIC NURSING

Locard's Principle

- Formulated by forensic scientist **Dr Edmond Locard.**
- When a person or object comes into contact with another person or object, there will be an exchange of materials between them. This principle forms the basis of forensic science and is often summarized as "Every contact leaves a trace".

Chain of Custody

It refers to the chronological documentation and control of the handling, transfer, and storage of physical or digital evidence.

KEY POINT

In cases of hanging (in suicide), ligature marks are typically oblique, continuous around the neck, and located below the thyroid cartilage in suicides.

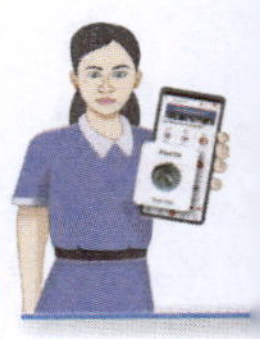

Types of Samples in Forensic Nursing

- **Biological samples**: Any organic material or substance that contains biological matter and can be collected from a person, crime scene, or other relevant sources for forensic analysis. These samples often contain genetic material, such as DNA, which can provide valuable information for identification. For example, blood, saliva, semen, urine, hair, fingernail clippings, tissue samples, and biological swabs from various body surfaces.
- **Trace evidence**: Small amount of material or evidence left behind at a crime scene or found on a person that is often not readily visible or easily detectable. For example, fiber from clothes, soil, glass fragment, hair, paint chips, soil or dirt, gunshot residue.
- **Digital evidence:** It refers to any form of electronic data or information that can be collected and analyzed in the context of a forensic investigation. For example, e-mails, text messages, photographs, videos, social media posts, internet browsing history, etc.

COMPREHENSIVE FORENSIC NURSING CARE

The aim of this is to promote healing, facilitate recovery, and assist in the process of justice while considering the unique needs and circumstances of each individual and their cultural background.

Physical Aspects

- Assess and treat physical injuries resulting from violence or trauma.
- Provide medical interventions, administer medications, and perform forensic examinations to document injuries and collect evidence.
- Ensure the physical safety and well-being of the victims, addressing immediate medical needs and promoting healing.

Psychosocial Aspects

- Recognize and address the emotional and psychological impact of the traumatic event on the victims and their families.
- Provide trauma-informed care, offer emotional support, and facilitate access to counseling or therapy services.
- Assess for symptoms of post-traumatic stress disorder (PTSD), anxiety, depression, and other psychological effects, and collaborate with mental health professionals for comprehensive care.

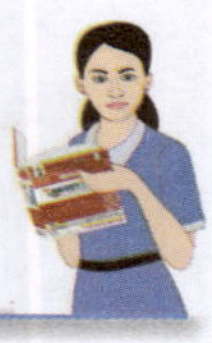

Cultural and Spiritual Aspects

- Respect and consider the cultural and spiritual beliefs and practices of the victims and their families.
- Provide care that is culturally sensitive and appropriate.
- Collaborate with cultural liaisons, interpreters, or spiritual advisors to ensure the provision of culturally competent care.

Legal Aspects

- Document injuries and collect evidence in a manner that adheres to legal requirements, ensuring chain of custody.
- Collaborate with law enforcement, provide expert testimony in court, and assist with the understanding and navigation of the legal process for the victims and their families.
- Advocate for the rights of the victims and work toward ensuring justice.

VIOLENCE

Violence refers to intentional acts of harm or aggression inflicted upon individuals, often resulting in physical, psychological, or emotional trauma.

Types of Violence

- **Interpersonal violence**: It refers to acts of physical, sexual, psychological, or emotional harm inflicted upon individuals by others. For example, physical assault, domestic violence, sexual assault, child abuse, elder abuse, bullying, and human trafficking.
- **Intimate partner violence:** Violence that occurs within intimate relationships, including physical, sexual, or emotional abuse. It is also a type of interpersonal violence.
- **Community violence**: It involves violence occurring within communities, such as gang-related violence, riots, or acts of terrorism.
- **Self-directed violence**: This refers to intentional self-harm or suicidal behaviors exhibited by individuals.
- **Workplace violence**: Violence that occurs in health care settings, including assaults on health care professionals by patients or their family members.
- **Collective violence:** It refers to acts of violence committed by large groups or organized entities against other groups, communities, or societies. For example, riots, mob violence, acts of terrorism, ethnic or religious conflicts, and warfare.

Major Causes of Violence

- Patriarchy
- Gender inequality
- Poverty
- Drug abuse (including alcohol)

KEY POINTS

- Locard's principle is a fundamental concept in forensic science.
- Locard's principle states that "Every contact leaves a trace," meaning that whenever two objects come into contact, there is a transfer of materials between them.

Practice Questions

1. When providing forensic nursing care to a victim of violence, the immediate priority is to:

a. Document all injuries and evidence for legal proceedings
b. Notify law enforcement and initiate criminal investigations
c. Ensure the safety and well-being of the victim
d. Conduct psychological assessments to assess trauma

Ans. (c) Ensure the safety and well-being of the victim

2. As a forensic nurse caring for a victim of violence, the appropriate action to preserve forensic evidence is to:

a. Clean and sanitize all wounds and injuries thoroughly
b. Discard any clothing or items with potential evidence
c. Take photographs and collect swabs of any bodily fluids or evidence
d. Administer pain medications to minimize discomfort

Ans. (c) Take photographs and collect swabs of any bodily fluids or evidence

Sources of Data on Violence in India

- **The National Crime Records Bureau (NCRB):** The NCRB is a government agency that collects data on crime in India.
- **The National Family Health Survey (NFHS):** Collecting data on various topics including domestic violence.
- Nongovernmental organizations (NGOs)
- Media reports (less reliable).

Summary of Data on Crimes in India (2021) as per NCRB

- No. of murder cases: 29,272
- Attempt to commit murder: 55,672
- No. of culpable homicide not amounting to murder: 3,807
- Causing death by negligence: 146,195
- Deaths due to medical negligence: 142
- Dowry deaths: 6,753
- Abetment of suicide: 9,361
- Attempt to commit suicide: 1,863
- Sexual harassment: 17,539
- Crime against women-related acts: 15,781
- No. of POCSO cases: 53,874

SEXUAL ABUSE

- It refers to any nonconsensual or unwanted sexual act or behavior inflicted upon an individual.
- It involves engaging in sexual activities without the informed and voluntary consent of one or more parties involved.

Types of Sexual Abuse

- **Sexual assault:** Any nonconsensual sexual act, including penetration or attempted penetration, unwanted touching, or coerced sexual activity.
- **Rape:** Nonconsensual sexual intercourse involving penetration, often accompanied by force, threats, or coercion.
- **Child sexual abuse:** Sexual exploitation or molestation of a child, including any sexual activity with a minor who cannot legally provide informed consent.
- **Sexual harassment:** Unwanted sexual advances, comments, or behaviors that create a hostile or intimidating environment.
- **Intimate partner sexual violence:** Nonconsensual sexual acts committed by an intimate partner, including within the context of domestic violence or abusive relationships.

Importance of Forensic Nursing in Sexual Abuse

Aims to provide compassionate and evidence-based care, contribute to justice and legal proceedings, and promote healing and recovery for survivors.

- Forensic assessment
- Evidence collection
- Trauma-informed care
- Treatment and referral
- Legal collaboration
- Advocacy and prevention

Posterior fourchette sustains the most injury during a sexual assault involving penile penetration only.

DEATH

Types of Death

- **Natural death:** It refers to death resulting from disease, illness, or medical conditions not caused by external factors.
- **Accidental death:** It occurs because of an unintentional event or mishap, such as car accidents, falls, drownings, or drug overdoses.
- **Suicidal death:** It occurs when an individual intentionally takes their own life.
- **Homicidal death**: It refers to death caused by the intentional actions of another person.
- **Undetermined death:** In some cases, the cause and manner of death may remain undetermined despite thorough investigations.

FUNDAMENTAL RIGHTS

Fundamental rights, also known as human rights or constitutional rights, are the basic rights and freedoms that are inherent to all individuals by virtue of their humanity.

- **Articles 12–35** contained in **Part III of the Constitution** deal with Fundamental Rights.
- The Indian Constitution guarantees six fundamental rights to its citizens. These rights are:
  1. Right to Equality (Articles 14–18)
  2. Right to Freedom (Articles 19–22)
  3. Right against Exploitation (Articles 23–24)
  4. Right to Freedom of Religion (Articles 25–28)
  5. Cultural and Educational Rights (Articles 29–30)
  6. Right to Constitutional Remedies (Articles 32–35)

RIGHTS OF VICTIM

- The rights of a victim refer to the entitlements and protections afforded to individuals who have experienced harm, whether it be physical, psychological, or emotional, as a result of a crime or violation.
- These rights aim to ensure that victims are treated with dignity, respect, and fairness throughout the criminal justice process and beyond.

Rights

- Right to Information
- Right to Protection and Safety

KEY POINTS

Overview of POCSO Act

- The Protection of Children from Sexual Offences (POCSO) Act, 2012 is a comprehensive law enacted by the Government of India to protect children from offenses of sexual assault, sexual harassment and pornography.
- The primary objective of the POCSO Act is to provide a child-friendly legal framework for the protection, care, and support of children who are victims of sexual abuse and exploitation.
- **Definitions and scope**: The act defines various forms of sexual offenses against children, including child sexual abuse, child pornography, and the use of a child in explicit conduct. It covers all persons, including family members, neighbors, and acquaintances who commit such offenses.
- The Act defines a child as a person below the age of 18 years. The POCSO Act provides for a number of safeguards for children, including:
  - A child-friendly reporting mechanism
  - Special Courts to try cases under the Act
  - Protection of the identity of the child
  - Speedy trial of cases
  - Stringent punishment for offenders

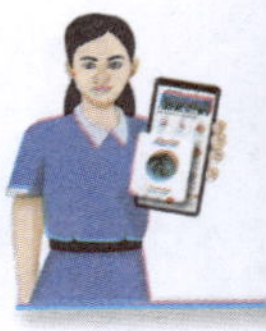

- Right to Participation
- Right to Privacy
- Right to Support and Assistance
- Right to Restitution
- Right to Speedy Justice
- Right to Fair Treatment
- Right to Consultation
- Right to Appropriate Accommodation

RIGHTS OF ACCUSED

The rights of the accused, also known as the rights of the defendant, are a set of legal protections granted to individuals who are facing criminal charges.

Rights

- Presumption of Innocence
- Right to Legal Representation
- Right to a Fair Trial
- Right to Confront Witnesses
- Right to Remain Silent
- Right to Due Process
- Protection against Double Jeopardy
- Protection against Cruel and Unusual Punishment
- Right to Bail
- Right to Appeal

HUMAN RIGHTS COMMISSION

- The Human Rights Commission, also known as the Human Rights Institution, is an independent organization or government agency tasked with promoting and protecting human rights within a specific country or jurisdiction.
- These commissions play a crucial role in upholding human rights standards, advocating for the rights of individuals and groups, and addressing human rights violations.
- In India, the National Human Rights Commission (NHRC) was established on October 12, 1993, under the Protection of Human Rights Act, 1993.
- **Shri Justice Arun Kumar Mishra** is the Chairman of National Human Rights Commission of India, **w.e.f 02.06.2021.**

Functions of Human Rights Commission

- Monitoring and Investigation
- Promotion and Education
- Policy Development and Advocacy
- Complaint Handling and Redress
- Research and Reporting
- Collaboration and Cooperation
- Capacity Building
- Public Engagement and Consultation

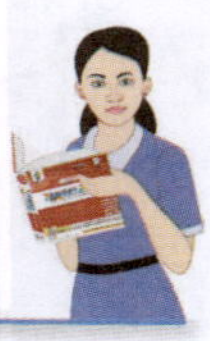

INDIAN NURSING COUNCIL ACT

The Indian Nursing Council Act, 1947 is an Act of Parliament of India that established the Indian Nursing Council (INC) and empowered it to regulate the nursing profession in India.

The INC is a statutory body that is responsible for maintaining standards of nursing education and practice, and for registering nurses and midwives in India.

The act gives statutory powers to the council to maintain uniform standards and regulation of nursing education all over the country.

Functions of the INC

- To establish and monitor uniform standards of nursing for nurse midwifes, ANM, and health visitors' education by doing inspection of the institutions.
- To recognize the qualification(s) under section 10(2)(4) of the Indian Nursing Council Act, 1947 for the purpose of registration and employment in India and abroad.
- To prescribe minimum standards of education and training in various nursing programs.
- To prescribe the syllabus and regulations for nursing programs under section 16 of the Indian Nursing Council Act, 1947.
- Power to withdraw the recognition of qualification under Section 14 of the Indian Nursing Council Act, 1947 in case the institution fails to maintain its standards under Section 14(1)(b) of the Act.
- To recognize Degree/Diploma/Certificate awarded by Foreign Universities.
- To give approval for registration of Indian and Foreign Nurses possessing foreign qualification.
- To maintain Indian Nurses Register for registration of nursing personnel.
- To advise the State Nursing Councils, Examining Boards, State Governments and Central Government in various important items regarding nursing education in the country.
- To prescribe code of ethics and professional conduct.
- To regulate the policies of training of nursing programs in the field of nursing to improve the quality of nursing education.
- To promote research in nursing.

Council of Members

- INC has a council of members as prescribed in the act.
- The President of the Council shall be elected by the members of the Council from among themselves.

- **Child-friendly procedures**: The act incorporates child-friendly procedures for recording the statement of the child, including the provision for video recording of the child's statement to minimize trauma and ensure a safe and comfortable environment for the child during the legal process.
- **Special courts**: The POCSO Act mandates the establishment of special courts exclusively for the trial of offenses under the act.
- **Protection of identity and privacy**: The POCSO Act emphasizes the protection of the identity and privacy of the child victim throughout the legal proceedings. It prohibits the publication of the child's identity and ensures that the child's privacy is maintained during investigation, trial, and reporting.
- **Presumption of guilt**: The POCSO Act introduces a legal presumption that the accused is presumed to be guilty unless proven innocent, shifting the burden of proof onto the accused.
- **Penalties and punishments**: The act prescribes stringent punishments for offenders. It categorizes offenses based on their severity, and the penalties can include imprisonment ranging from a minimum of 3 years to life imprisonment, along with fines.

- An elected or nominated member, other than a nominated President, shall hold office for a term of five years from the date of his election or nomination or until his successor has been duly elected or nominated, whichever is longer.

Executive Committee

- The Executive Committee shall consist of nine members, of whom seven shall be elected by the Council from among its members.
- The President and Vice President of the Council shall be members ex officio of the Executive Committee, and shall be President and Vice President, respectively, of that Committee.

Indian Nurses Register

- The Indian Nurses Register is a register maintained by the Council, containing the names of nurses, midwives, auxiliary nurse-midwives, and health visitors enrolled on any State register.
- The Secretary of the Council is responsible to keep the Indian Nurses Register in accordance with the provisions of this Act, and from time to time, to revise the register and publish it in the Gazette of India.
- The register shall deemed to be a public document within the meaning of Indian Evidence Act, 1872.
- **Supply of copies of State registers**: Each State Council shall supply 20 printed copies of the State register to the INC as soon as may be after the **1st day of April of each year** and inform the Council without delay of all additions to, and other amendments in, the State register made from time to time.

STATE NURSING REGISTRATION COUNCIL

- State council means a Council (by whatever name called) constituted under the law of a State to regulate the registration of nurses, midwives or health visitors in the State.
- There are 28 State Nursing Registration Councils (SNRCs) in India, each responsible for registering nurses and midwives within its state.
- The SNRCs are responsible for:
    - Registering nurses and midwives
    - Maintaining a register of nurses and midwives
    - Enforcing the Nursing Act and Rules
    - Promoting the standards of nursing education and practice
- The first state nursing council in India was the Madras Nursing Council, which was constituted in 1926. The Bombay Nursing Council was constituted in 1935.

OVERVIEW OF THE INDIAN JUDICIAL SYSTEM AND LAWS

Hierarchy of Courts

Supreme Court of India

- The highest judicial authority in the country, responsible for interpreting the constitution and acting as the final appellate court for both civil and criminal cases.
- It is located in New Delhi and acts as the final appellate court.
- It hears appeals from High Courts and has the power to review and revise their decisions.

High Courts

- Each state in India has a High Court, which has jurisdiction over the state and serves as the highest appellate court within that jurisdiction.
- High Court judges hear appeals from District Courts and have the power to revise and review their judgments.

District Courts

- These courts are in every district of the country and handle both civil and criminal cases.
- They are presided over by Judicial Magistrates, including Judicial Magistrate First Class (JMFC), and handle both civil and criminal cases.

Laws and Legal Framework

- **Constitution of India:** The Constitution is the supreme law of the land and provides the framework for governance and protection of fundamental rights. It sets out the structure of the government, division of powers, and fundamental rights and duties of citizens.
- **Civil law:** Indian civil law includes various acts and statutes governing contracts, property, family matters, succession, and other civil disputes.
- **Criminal law:** Criminal law in India is primarily governed by the Indian Penal Code (IPC), which defines and punishes criminal offenses. Additionally, the Criminal Procedure Code (CrPC) provides the procedural framework for criminal proceedings.
- **Personal laws:** India recognizes personal laws for different religious communities in matters of marriage, divorce, inheritance, and other personal affairs. These personal laws are based on religious scriptures, customs, and community practices.

Legal Procedures

- **Adversarial system**: India follows an adversarial system of justice, where two opposing parties present their arguments before a judge who acts as an impartial adjudicator.

- The POCSO Act has been amended twice, in 2018 and 2019. The amendments have increased the punishment for offenses under the Act and have also provided for more stringent safeguards for children.
- **Rehabilitation and support**: The act recognizes the need for the physical, emotional, and psychological rehabilitation and support of child victims. It provides for the establishment of special cells or agencies to coordinate and provide support services, such as medical care, counseling, and legal aid, to the child victims and their families.
- Number of POCSO cases registered in India in the year 2021: **53,874** (Source: NCRB)

KEY POINT

The subjective response experienced by the surviving loved ones is called Bereavement

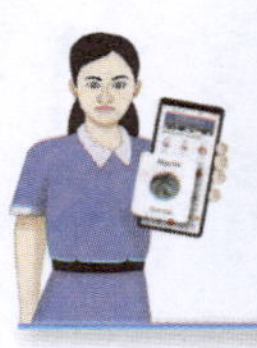

- **Trial process**: Trials can be conducted in both civil and criminal cases. Parties present evidence, call witnesses, and make arguments. In criminal cases, guilt must be proven beyond a reasonable doubt, while civil cases require a preponderance of evidence.
- **Appellate process**: Parties dissatisfied with the decision of a lower court can appeal to a higher court within the hierarchy, seeking a review of the decision based on legal errors or new evidence.

Judicial Independence

- **Independence of the judiciary**: The judiciary in India is independent of the executive and legislative branches of government. Judges are appointed through a rigorous process and are meant to be impartial and free from external influence.

  As on June, 2023, the method of appointment of judges in high courts and supreme courts in India is through the **collegium system.**
- **Judicial activism**: The Indian judiciary has played an active role in interpreting laws and protecting fundamental rights. It has issued landmark judgments on various socio-political issues and has been instrumental in shaping public policy.

CIVIL CASE PROCEDURE

1. **Filing the complaint**: The plaintiff (the person bringing the case) files a written complaint, known as a plaint, before the appropriate civil court. The **plaint** outlines the facts of the case, the relief sought, and the legal grounds for the claim.
2. **Issuance of summons**: The court reviews the plaint and, if satisfied, issues a summons to the **defendant** (the person against whom the case is filed). The summons informs the defendant about the case and directs them to appear in court on a specified date.
3. **Pleadings**: The defendant submits a written statement, known as a written statement of defense, in response to the plaint.
4. **Evidence**: Both parties present their evidence, including documents, witnesses, and other forms of evidence, to support their claims or defenses. The court examines and considers the evidence presented by both sides.
5. **Arguments:** After the evidence is presented, the parties make their arguments before the court, presenting their interpretation of the law and their case.
6. **Judgment**: The court examines the evidence, arguments, and applicable laws before delivering its judgment. The judgment may involve granting or denying the relief sought by the plaintiff and may include awards of damages or specific performance, among other remedies.

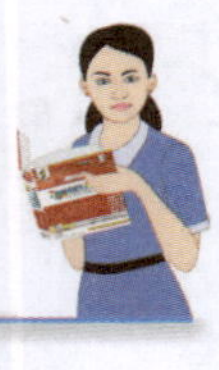

CRIMINAL CASE PROCEDURE

- **Filing the FIR:** In a criminal case, the first step is the filing of the First Information Report (FIR) with the police, which contains details of the alleged criminal offense.
- **Investigation:** Upon receiving the FIR, the police investigate, gather evidence, and identify potential witnesses. If sufficient evidence is found, the police may file a charge sheet, also known as a police report, before the appropriate criminal court.
- **Charges framing:** The court examines the charge sheet and frames charges against the accused. The charges specify the offenses allegedly committed by the accused.
- **Trial:** The trial commences, and both the prosecution and the defense present their respective cases. Witnesses are examined, and evidence is presented before the court.
- **Arguments**: After the presentation of evidence, the prosecution and the defense make their arguments, summarizing their case and interpreting the law.
- **Judgment:** The court evaluates the evidence, arguments, and applicable laws before delivering its judgment. If the accused is found guilty, the court determines the appropriate punishment.

INDIAN PENAL CODE (IPC)

- The IPC is a comprehensive code that defines various criminal offenses and prescribes punishments for those offenses.
- It covers a wide range of crimes, including offenses against the person, property, public order, morality, and more.
- The IPC serves as a primary source of criminal law in India.

CRIMINAL PROCEDURE CODE (CrPC)

- Criminal Procedure Code is a procedural law that governs the investigation and trial of criminal cases in India.
- It provides the framework for the conduct of investigations, arrest, bail, trial proceedings, and appeals.
- This ensures fairness and adherence to legal procedures in criminal cases.

INDIAN EVIDENCE ACT

- It governs the rules and principles relating to the admissibility and assessment of evidence in Indian courts.
- It lays down guidelines for the examination and cross-examination of witnesses, the production and proof of documents, and the relevancy and weight given to different types of evidence during trial proceedings.

KEY POINTS

- The judiciary in India is independent of the executive and legislative branches of government
- Supreme court of India is the highest judicial authority in the country.
- Each state in India has a High Court, which has jurisdiction over the state
- High Court judges hear appeals from District Courts
- Criminal law in India is primarily governed by the Indian Penal Code (IPC)
- The Criminal Procedure Code (CrPC) provides the procedural framework for criminal proceedings
- As on July, 2023, the method of appointment of judges in high courts and supreme courts in India is through the **collegium system.**

Practice Questions

3. Which step marks the initiation of a criminal case in India?

a. Charges framing
b. Trial
c. Filing the FIR
d. Investigation

Ans. (c) Filing the FIR

4. The Indian Penal Code (IPC) primarily deals with:

a. The conduct of investigations and trial proceedings
b. The rules and principles of evidence admissibility
c. Prescribing punishments for criminal offenses
d. The framework for criminal procedure

Ans. (c) Prescribing punishments for criminal offenses

Golden Points to Remember

- Forensic nursing is a specialized area of nursing that involves the application of nursing knowledge and skills in legal and investigative contexts.
- Forensic nurses provide comprehensive care to individuals who have experienced violence, trauma, or are involved in legal proceedings.
- A forensic nurse has advanced knowledge of forensic evidence collection and preservation.
- The International Association of Forensic Nurses (IAFN) was established in 1982.
- Indian Nursing Council introduced forensic nursing as a subject in the graduate nursing program in 2021.
- Forensic psychiatric nurses work with individuals involved in the legal system who have mental health issues.
- Forensic nursing is inherently connected to the pursuit of justice. Ensuring fairness, impartiality, and upholding the principles of justice are paramount.
- When photographing forensic evidence, it is important to capture two images of each finding.
- **Locard's principle:** When a person or object comes into contact with another person or object, there will be an exchange of materials between them. Summarized **as "Every contact leaves a trace".**
- Chain of custody refers to the chronological documentation and control of the handling, transfer, and storage of physical or digital evidence.
- **Biological samples:** Any organic material or substance that contains biological matter and can be collected from a person, crime scene, or other relevant sources for forensic analysis.
- **Trace evidence:** Small amount of material or evidence left behind at a crime scene or found on a person that is often not readily visible or easily detectable. E.g., hair, cloth fibers, etc.
- **Digital evidence** refers to any form of electronic data or information that can be collected and analyzed in the context of a forensic investigation.
- When providing forensic nursing care to a victim of violence, the immediate priority is to ensure the safety and well-being of the victim.
- Sexual abuse refers to any nonconsensual or unwanted sexual act or behavior inflicted upon an individual.
- Child sexual abuse refers to sexual exploitation or molestation of a child, including any sexual activity with a minor who cannot legally provide informed consent.
- **Posterior fourchette** sustains the most injury during a sexual assault involving penile penetration only.
- **Articles 12–35** contained in **Part III of the Constitution** deal with Fundamental Rights.
- The Indian Constitution guarantees six fundamental rights to its citizens: 1. Right to Equality, 2. Right to Freedom, 3. Right against Exploitation, 4. Right to Freedom of Religion, 5. Cultural and Educational Rights, 6. Right to Constitutional Remedies.
- The rights of a victim refer to the entitlements and protections afforded to individuals who have experienced harm.
- In India, the National Human Rights Commission (NHRC) was established on October 12, 1993, under the Protection of Human Rights Act, 1993.
- **Shri Justice Arun Kumar Mishra** is the Chairman of National Human Rights Commission of India, **w.e.f 02.06.2021. (As on July 2023)**.
- The Protection of Children from Sexual Offences (POCSO) Act, 2012 is a comprehensive law enacted by the Government of India to protect children from offences of sexual assault, sexual harassment and pornography.
- The POCSO Act has been amended twice, in 2018 and 2019.
- The Indian Nursing Council Act, 1947 is an Act of Parliament of India that established the Indian Nursing Council (INC) and empowered it to regulate the nursing profession in India.
- The President of the INC shall be elected by the members of the Council from among themselves.
- The Secretary of the Council is responsible to keep the Indian Nurses Register in accordance with the provisions of this Act.
- There are 28 State Nursing Registration Councils (SNRCs) in India, each responsible for registering nurses and midwives within its state.
- The first state nursing council in India was the Madras Nursing Council, which was constituted in 1926. The Bombay Nursing Council was constituted in 1935.
- The National Nursing and Midwifery Commission Bill 2023 (NNMC 2023) was passed in Lok Sabha on July 28. NNMC was passed in Rajya Sabha on 08 August 2023.
- The highest judicial authority in the country is the Supreme Court.
- Each state in India has a High Court, which has jurisdiction over the state and serves as the highest appellate court within that jurisdiction.
- The Constitution is the supreme law of the land and provides the framework for governance and protection of fundamental rights.
- Criminal law in India is primarily governed by the **Indian Penal Code (IPC),** which defines and punishes criminal offenses.
- The Criminal Procedure Code (CrPC) is a procedural law that governs the investigation and trial of criminal cases in India.
- Indian Evidence Act governs the rules and principles relating to the admissibility and assessment of evidence in Indian courts.

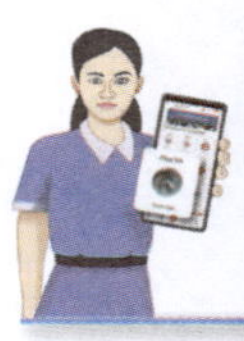

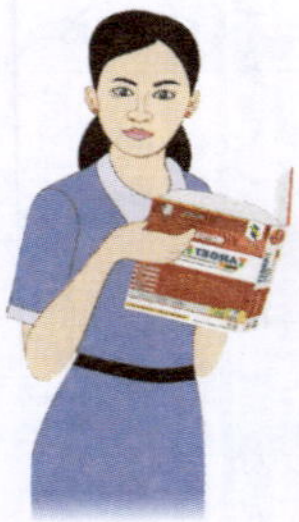

"To keep the body in good health is a duty... otherwise we shall not be able to keep our mind strong and clear."
—Buddha

MULTIPLE CHOICE QUESTIONS

(Including Explained and Practice Questions)

INTRODUCTION TO FORENSIC NURSING

1. Indian Nursing Council introduced forensic nursing as a subject in the graduate nursing program in the year:
   a. 2016
   b. 2018
   c. 2021
   d. 2023

2. The International Association of Forensic Nurses (IAFN) was established in the year:
   a. 1965 b. 1982
   c. 1995 d. 2001

3. Which of the following statement regarding the responsibilities of a forensic nurse is incorrect?
   a. "The forensic nurse only cares for dead patients."
   b. "The forensic nurse provides expert testimony at court trial."
   c. "Forensic nurse provides compassionate care to victims of violence or trauma"
   d. "Forensic nurse gathers physical evidence, documents injuries, and provides detailed reports for legal purposes."

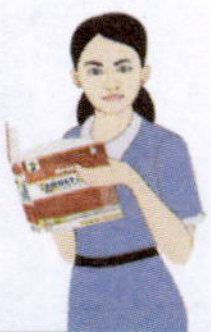

ETHICAL ISSUES IN FORENSIC NURSING

4. In forensic nursing, what ethical issue arises when balancing the need to maintain confidentiality and privacy with the obligation to share relevant information with law enforcement and legal authorities?
   a. Informed Consent
   b. Dual Roles and Conflicts of Interest
   c. Confidentiality and Privacy
   d. Cultural Sensitivity and Diversity

5. When providing care, what ethical challenge may arise in respecting beliefs and practices while ensuring the safety and well-being of individuals?
   a. Safety and privacy
   b. Duty to report
   c. Cultural sensitivity and diversity
   d. Autonomy and decision-making

FORENSIC TEAM

6. Which member of the forensic team is responsible for conducting autopsies and determining the cause and manner of death in cases of suspicious or violent deaths?
   a. Medical Examiners/Forensic Pathologists
   b. Forensic Nurses
   c. Forensic scientists
   d. Psychologists/Psychiatrists

7. Which of the following forensic team members are primarily responsible for crisis intervention, safety planning, and connecting individuals with appropriate community services?
   a. Medical examiners
   b. Victim advocates
   c. Forensic nurses
   d. Social workers/Counselors

8. Which sub-specialty of forensic nursing involves working closely with medical examiners or coroners to investigate suspicious, violent, or unexpected deaths?
   a. Legal Nurse Consultant
   b. Forensic Psychiatric Nurse
   c. Forensic Nurse Death Investigator
   d. Forensic Nurse Consultant

9. Which forensic nurse is responsible for conducting screenings of sexual predators?
   a. Legal nurse consultant
   b. Forensic psychiatric nurse
   c. Sexual assault nurse examiner
   d. Forensic Nurse Death Investigator

Explanation: The role of the forensic psychiatric nurse involves conducting sexual predator screening. Sexual assault nurse examiners are responsible for gathering evidence from victim of sexual abuse. Legal nurse consultants are involved in investigating care delivery outcomes. Forensic nurse death investigator works closely with medical examiners or coroners to investigate suspicious, violent, or unexpected deaths.

10. The responsibilities of the legal nurse consultant (LNC) include all; except:
   a. Representing patients in a court of law
   b. Creating timelines of health care events
   c. Organizing and analyzing medical records
   d. Identifying when standards of care are met or breached

11. While testifying in court proceedings, the legal nurse consultant (LNC) should do all; except:
   a. Respond confidently
   b. Avoid becoming angry
   c. Answer questions quickly
   d. Refrain from saying "I believe"

Explanation: While testifying in court proceedings, It is important to take a brief moment to carefully formulate and provide an answer to a question, as responding too quickly increases the chances of misspeaking or providing inaccurate information. The LNC should respond confidently, avoid becoming angry, refrain from saying "I believe", and sit with hands resting on the lap.

Ans.

1. c
2. b
3. a
4. c
5. c
6. a
7. d
8. c
9. b
10. a
11. c

12. All of the following activities are included in the forensic nurse's role; except:
 a. Collecting evidence
 b. Conducting autopsy
 c. Providing expert testimony
 d. Documentation of injuries

Explanation: The responsibilities of a forensic nurse in the field include evidence collection, enhancing assessment skills in relation to injuries and abuse, offering expert testimony, and acquiring proficiency in documenting injuries. The responsibility of conducting an autopsy typically falls under the jurisdiction of a forensic pathologist, rather than a forensic nurse.

13. All of the following cases require the involvement of forensic nurse in the emergency room; except:
 a. Victim of suspected homicide
 b. College student reporting rape
 c. Student who has sued for malpractice
 d. Older adult with signs of abuse

Explanation: Forensic nurses in the emergency department play a crucial role in providing care to individuals involved in various crimes, such as homicide, rape, elder abuse, and assault during violent incidents like robbery. However, it is important to note that addressing a person who has filed a malpractice lawsuit is not within the immediate scope of the forensic nurse's role in the emergency room.

EVIDENCE COLLECTION AND DOCUMENTATION

14. What is the first step in preserving evidence at a crime scene?
 a. Contacting law enforcement.
 b. Thoroughly cleaning the victim's skin.
 c. Identifying the nature and origin of the injuries.
 d. Drying the victim's clothing and placing in an individual evidence bag.

Explanation: The first crucial step in effective evidence preservation is to determine the nature (e.g., physical, sexual, emotional) and origin (e.g., accident, neglect, violence, torture, drug-related) of the injuries. This identification helps guide the collection process and enables the retrieval of specific forensic evidence.

15. Locard's principle in forensic science is based on the idea that:
 a. Every contact leaves a trace
 b. DNA is the most valuable evidence
 c. Chain of custody is essential in evidence handling
 d. Biological samples are the most reliable evidence

Explanation: Locard's principle states that when a person or object comes into contact with another person or object, there will be an exchange of materials between them. This principle forms the basis of forensic science and is often summarized as "Every contact leaves a trace".

16. Which of the following is not an example of transient evidence?
 a. Blood samples
 b. The smell of alcohol
 c. Swelling of the wrists
 d. Upper arm tenderness

Explanation: Transient evidence refers to temporary elements that are subject to change or disappearance. Examples include body odors, smell of alcohol, as well as physical states like swelling, edema, tenderness, or pain. On the other hand, tangible evidence consists of physical items such as blood samples and photographs.

17. Which of the following fluids are commonly collected for DNA analysis in forensic nursing?
 a. Blood
 b. Saliva
 c. Semen
 d. All of the above

18. What does chain of custody refer to in forensic investigations?
 a. Chronological documentation and control of evidence handling, transfer, and storage
 b. Chronological analysis of biological samples for DNA identification
 c. Orderly collection of trace evidence from crime scenes
 d. Integration of digital and manual analysis of sample

19. In forensic nursing, the collection of evidence from bite marks serves which purpose?
 a. Identifying the motive behind the crime.
 b. Establishing a strong legal case.
 c. Determining the timeline of the assault.
 d. Facilitating perpetrator identification through DNA-tested saliva.

20. Which of the following is NOT a benefit of digital photographic documentation in forensic nursing?
 a. Inability to alter the original image
 b. Ability to review images and reshoot
 c. Ease of distribution during legal proceedings
 d. Enhanced control of the evidence chain of custody

Explanation: Digital images can be altered. This is because they are stored in a digital format, which means that they can be edited or manipulated using software. This is why it is important to use a secure method of storing and managing digital images.

21. Which type of wounds are indicated by multiple parallel superficial criss-crossing patterns?
 a. Accidental wounds
 b. Fabricated wounds
 c. Suicidal wounds
 d. Homicidal wounds

Explanation: Suicidal wounds often exhibit a characteristic feature known as hesitation marks. These are typically superficial and irregular wounds caused by hesitation or uncertainty during a suicide attempt. The individual may repeatedly inflict shallow cuts or scratches in a criss-crossing pattern, indicating a struggle or reluctance to cause deep or fatal injuries.

22. Which of the following is an example of trace evidence in forensic nursing?
 a. Blood samples
 b. DNA swabs
 c. Soil or dirt
 d. Digital photographs

Explanation: Soil or dirt collected from crime scene is considered to be trace evidence. Blood samples and DNA swabs are considered to be biological samples. Digital photographs are digital evidence.

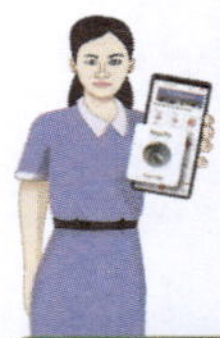

Ans.

12.	b
13.	c
14.	c
15.	a
16.	a
17.	d
18.	a
19.	d
20.	a
21.	c
22.	c

23. Which of the following is not one of the key components of forensic documentation?

a. Photography
b. Written documentation
c. Diagrammatic documentation
d. Diascopy

Explanation: Forensic documentation typically involves photography, written documentation, and diagrammatic documentation. Diascopy is not a component of a forensic documentation. Diascopy is a diagnostic technique used in dermatology to assess the blanching or persistence of skin lesions under pressure. It involves applying pressure to a skin lesion with a glass slide or a finger and observing the resulting changes in color.

24. What information does a medicolegal report typically contain?

a. Details of identification signs
b. Report on filed cases
c. Documentation of injuries
d. Information regarding fingerprints

Explanation: A medicolegal report primarily focuses on documenting injuries observed during the medical examination. This includes a detailed description of the nature, extent, and location of the injuries sustained by the individual.

25. An autopsy report is typically written in:

a. Single copy on the same day
b. Single copy on the next day
c. Duplicate
d. Triplicate

Explanation: An autopsy report is commonly prepared in triplicate using carbon papers, meaning that three identical copies of the report are generated. One copy is retained in the records of the medical examiner's office or the institution conducting the autopsy. The other two copies are distributed to relevant parties involved in the case, such as law enforcement agencies, legal professionals, or other authorized individuals.

26. When documenting gunshot wounds, what action should nurses take?

a. Identify the type of firearm used.
b. Identify the entry and exit wounds
c. Remove bullets or fragments with plastic-shielded forceps with caution
d. Remove gunshot powder residue with damp cotton swab

Explanation: When documenting gunshot wounds, nurses should handle and preserve any bullets or fragments with caution, using plastic-shielded forceps. It is important not to attempt to identify entrance or exit wounds unless stated by the patient, and guessing the caliber of the bullet should be avoided to ensure accurate reporting.

FORENSIC NURSING CARE

27. When assessing the level and nature of collaboration during an interview with a forensic patient, what should be taken into consideration?

a. Availability of law enforcement officers
b. Waiting time for triage of other patients
c. Applicable hearsay exceptions in the law
d. Nature of the crime and the need for evidence preservation

28. Which of the following is NOT a goal of forensic interviewing?

a. To obtain accurate and reliable information.
b. To build rapport with the patient.
c. To protect the patient's rights.
d. To help the patient heal.

29. Which of the following is NOT a good practice when interviewing a forensic patient?

a. Asking open-ended questions
b. Using leading questions
c. Offering support and comfort
d. Avoiding distractions

Explanation: Leading questions are questions that suggest the answer to the question. These types of questions should be avoided when interviewing a forensic patient because they can lead the patient to provide inaccurate or unreliable information.

30. Which of the following is a common misconception about forensic interviewing?

a. That it is easy
b. That it is always successful
c. That it is always necessary
d. That it is always done by law enforcement

Explanation: Forensic interviewing can be done by a variety of professionals, including law enforcement officers, social workers, and mental health professionals. It is important to choose an interviewer who has experience and training in forensic interviewing.

31. During the orientation of a new nurse at a prison/correctional facility, which information will be included?

a. Inmates can be issued medical supplies safely
b. Nurses are subject to manipulation by inmates
c. Delivery of nursing care is a priority over personal safety
d. Nurses may be required to provide care to inmates in a locked and enclosed environment

Explanation: During the orientation of new nurses at a correctional facility, they will be informed about the potential for inmates to manipulate them. Nurses should prioritize their personal safety and be aware of the possibility that medical supplies can be used as weapons by inmates. Additionally, nurses should understand that they should never be confined or locked in an environment alone with an inmate.

32. Forensic nurse is conducting an education session on the treatment of communicable diseases among inmates of a correctional facility. The nurse will include all of the following diseases; except:

a. HIV
b. Hepatitis
c. Meningitis
d. Tuberculosis

Explanation: In the imprisoned population, HIV, hepatitis, and tuberculosis pose significant concerns due to factors like drug misuse, sexual activity, and tattooing. However, meningitis is not considered a major concern in this population.

VIOLENCE

33. The most common type of elder mistreatment is:

a. Financial abuse
b. Sexual abuse
c. Neglect
d. Physical abuse

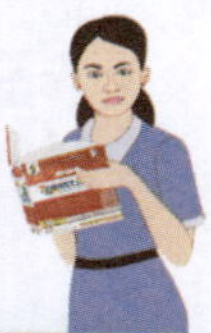

Ans.

23. d
24. c
25. d
26. c
27. d
28. d
29. b
30. d
31. b
32. c
33. c

34. Which type of violence involves violence occurring within communities, such as gang-related violence or acts of terrorism?

a. Interpersonal violence
b. Intimate partner violence
c. Community violence
d. Self-directed violence

35. Domestic violence is an example of:

a. Community violence
b. Self-directed violence
c. Interpersonal violence
d. Collective violence

Explanation: Interpersonal violence refers to acts of physical, sexual, psychological, or emotional harm inflicted upon individuals by others. Examples are physical assault, domestic violence, sexual assault, child abuse, elder abuse, bullying, and human trafficking.

36. Which type of violence refers to violence occurring within the health care setting, including assaults on health care professionals by patients or their family members?

a. Interpersonal violence
b. Workplace violence
c. Community violence
d. Self-directed violence

37. Which of the following source provides reliable data on violence in India?

a. Media reports
b. National Crime Records Bureau (NCRB)
c. Nongovernmental organizations (NGOs)
d. Personal opinions

SEXUAL ABUSE

38. All of the following activities are performed by the sexual assault nurse examiner (SANE); except:

a. Collect forensic evidence
b. Conduct detailed physical examination
c. Objectively care for sexual assault victims
d. Identify a victim's future medical needs and associated costs

Explanation: SANE is trained in forensic evidence collection, conducting detailed physical examination, conducting sensitive interviews, and providing medical and psychological support to survivors.

39. What is the primary goal of forensic nursing in sexual abuse cases?

a. Providing trauma-informed care
b. Collecting evidence for legal proceedings
c. Treating and referring survivors for appropriate care
d. Collaborating with legal professionals

Explanation: The primary goal of forensic nursing in sexual abuse cases is collecting evidence for legal proceedings. Forensic nurses are specially trained to collect evidence from sexual assault survivors in a way that is both sensitive and legally sound. They also provide emotional support and referrals to other resources as needed but the primary goal is to collect evidence.

40. What is the term for nonconsensual sexual acts committed by an intimate partner?

a. Forced sex
b. Sexual harassment
c. Intimate partner sexual violence
d. Rape

41. Which of the following best describes sexual harassment?

a. Nonconsensual sexual intercourse involving penetration
b. Unwanted sexual advances, comments, or behaviors
c. Sexual exploitation or molestation of a child
d. Any nonconsensual sexual act or unwanted sexual behavior

42. POCSO Act stands for:

a. Prevention of Children from Sexual Offences
b. Prevention of Children from Sexual Outrages
c. Protection of Children from Sexual Offences
d. Protection of Children Safety and Offences

43. The POCSO Act was enacted by the Government of India to protect children from offences of sexual assault, sexual harassment and pornography in the year:

a. 2005
b. 2012
c. 2014
d. 2016

Explanation: The Protection of Children from Sexual Offences (POCSO) Act, 2012 is a comprehensive law enacted by the Government of India to protect children from offences of sexual assault, sexual harassment and pornography. The POCSO Act has been amended twice, in 2018 and 2019. The amendments have increased the punishment for offences under the Act and have also provided for more stringent safeguards for children.

44. What is the age criteria for defining a child under the POCSO Act?

a. Below 12 years
b. Below 16 years
c. Below 18 years
d. Below 21 years

45. What does the POCSO Act emphasize regarding the identity of child victims?

a. Publication of the child's identity is allowed for investigation purposes.
b. The media may be allowed to publish child's identity after the trial
c. The child's identity is disclosed to the accused during trial.
d. The child's privacy is maintained during investigation, trial, and reporting

DEATH

46. For which type of deaths are medicolegal investigations conducted?

a. Natural and anticipated deaths
b. Sudden, unexpected, non-natural deaths
c. Deaths related to public health emergencies
d. Deaths occurring within institutional settings

47. All of the following are the manners of death that can be listed on a death certificate; except:

a. Suicide
b. Natural
c. Homicide
d. Chronic disease

Explanation: Chronic disease is not classified as a specific manner of death. The five recognized manners of death that can be listed on a death certificate are suicide, natural, accident, homicide, and undetermined.

48. What is the most commonly used type of chemical for suicide in India?

a. Psychotropic drugs
b. Petrochemicals
c. Pesticides
d. Muscarines

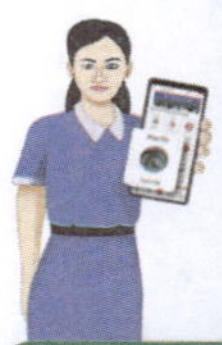

Ans.

34. c
35. c
36. b
37. b
38. d
39. b
40. c
41. b
42. c
43. b
44. c
45. d
46. b
47. d
48. c

Explanation: As per NCRB report, 2021, 25.1% of suicide in India is by consuming poison. Among these, nearly three fourth of the death by self-ingestion of poisoning is due to consumption of pesticides.

49. Most common method of suicide in India as per National Crime Records Bureau Report, 2021 is:

a. Pesticides b. Hanging
c. Drowning d. Self-immolation

Explanation: Suicide by 'Hanging' (57.0%), Consuming 'Poison' (25.1%), 'Drowning' (5.1%) and 'Self Immolation' (2.6%) were the prominent means of committing suicides (NCRB report, 2021).

50. Death caused by the intentional actions of another person is referred to as:

a. Homicidal death b. Undetermined death
c. Suicidal death d. Accidental death

FUNDAMENTAL RIGHTS AND RIGHTS OF VICTIMS

51. Which part of the Indian Constitution contains the Fundamental Rights?

a. Part I b. Part II
c. Part III d. Part IV

52. Which article of the part III of the Indian Constitution deals with fundamental rights of an individual?

a. Article 1 to 3
b. Article 3 to 12
c. Article 12 to 35
d. Article 15 to 40

53. Which right ensures that victims are provided with relevant and timely information about their case and the criminal justice process?

a. Right to Protection and Safety
b. Right to Participation
c. Right to Information
d. Right to Privacy

54. Which right ensures that victims are treated respectfully throughout the criminal justice process?

a. Right to Support and Assistance
b. Right to Fair Treatment
c. Right to Restitution
d. Right to Speedy Justice

55. Which right ensures that victims have the opportunity to express their views and concerns during legal proceedings?

a. Right to Privacy
b. Right to Participation
c. Right to Consultation
d. Right to Appropriate Accommodation

56. Which act established the National Human Rights Commission (NHRC) in India?

a. Protection of Human Rights Act, 1993
b. Human Rights Commission Act, 1950
c. Human Rights Commission Act, 1993
d. National Human Rights Act, 1993

Explanation: In India, the National Human Rights Commission (NHRC) was established on October 12, 1993, under the Protection of Human Rights Act, 1993. **Shri Justice Arun Kumar Mishra** is the Chairman of National Human Rights Commission (NHRC), **w.e.f 02.06.2021.**

NURSING COUNCIL ACT

57. The Indian Nursing Council Act, 1947 empowers the Indian Nursing Council (INC) to:

a. Regulate the hospital services in India
b. Establish uniform standards for nursing education and practice
c. Monitor the hospitals for quality of health care in India
d. Accredit hospitals and clinics in India

58. Indian Nursing Council prescribes the syllabus and regulations for nursing programs under which section of the Indian Nursing Council Act, 1947?

a. Section 3 b. Section 8
c. Section 16 d. Section 20

59. The president of the Indian Nursing Council shall be:

a. Appointed by the Ministry of Health and Family Welfare, Govt of India
b. Appointed through a direct recruitment by UPSC
c. Elected by the Registered Nurses across the country
d. Elected by the members of the council among themselves

60. The executive council of Indian Nursing Council consists of:

a. 7 members b. 9 members
c. 12 members d. 29 members

61. Who is responsible to keep the Indian Nurses Register in accordance with the provisions of the council?

a. The president, INC b. The vice president, INC
c. The secretary, INC d. The joint secretary, INC

62. Which of the following statement is incorrect regarding Indian Nurses Register?

a. The register shall be deemed to be a public document within the meaning of Indian Evidence Act, 1872.
b. Each State Council shall supply 20 printed copies of the State register to the INC
c. The Secretary of the Indian Nursing Council is responsible to keep the Indian Nurses Register
d. The President of the council is responsible for publishing the Register in the Gazette of India.

63. In which year was the Madras Nursing Council, the first state nursing council in India, constituted?

a. 1908 b. 1926
c. 1945 d. 1947

OVERVIEW OF THE INDIAN JUDICIAL SYSTEM AND LAWS

64. What is the supreme law of the land in India?

a. Indian Penal Code
b. Code of Criminal Procedure
c. Constitution of India
d. Personal Laws

65. Which legal system does India follow, where two opposing parties present their arguments before a judge?

a. Inquisitorial system
b. Adversarial system
c. Mediation system
d. Arbitration system

Explanation: India follows an adversarial system of justice, where two opposing parties present their arguments before a judge who acts as an impartial adjudicator.

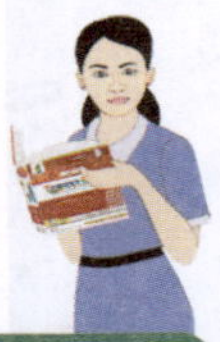

Ans.

49.	b
50.	a
51.	c
52.	c
53.	c
54.	b
55.	b
56.	a
57.	b
58.	c
59.	d
60.	b
61.	c
62.	d
63.	b
64.	c
65.	b

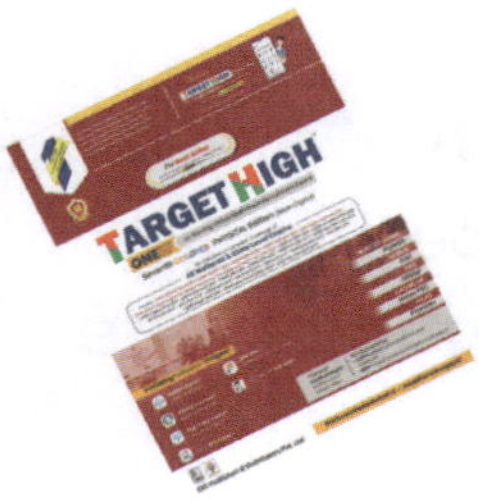

Read from **TARGET HIGH** *Book*

Section B

Previous Year Papers

(18 Papers in Book + 119 Paper in **Target High** Digital Lite)

PAPERS COVERED *(IN BOOK)*

1. NORCET (June) 2023 (Memory Based) (NEW)
2. AIIMS Jodhpur (SNO) 2023 (NEW)
3. AIIMS Bibinagar (Tutor) 2023 (NEW)
4. AIIMS Bibinagar Associate Professor 2023 (NEW)
5. Sree Chitra Tirunal Institute for Medical Science and Technology (NO) 2023 (NEW)
6. Uttar Pradesh University of Medical Sciences (NO) 2023 (NEW)
7. NORCET (NO) 2022 (Memory Based) (NEW)
8. Staff Nurse Examination Himachal Pradesh 2022 (NEW)
9. Western Coalfields Limited 2022 (NEW)
10. Odisha Subordinate Staff Selection Commission (NO) 2022 (NEW)
11. Gujarat Nursing Service (Nursing Officer/Principal) 2022 (NEW)
12. NORCET (NO) 2021 (Memory Based) (NEW)
13. CNCI (NO) 2021
14. NORCET (NO) 2020
15. Combined AIIMS (NO) (Bhopal, Jodhpur, Patna & Raipur) 2020
16. AIIMS Nagpur (NO) 2020
17. AIIMS Patna (NO) 2020
18. Nursing Officer Exam, JIPMER 2020

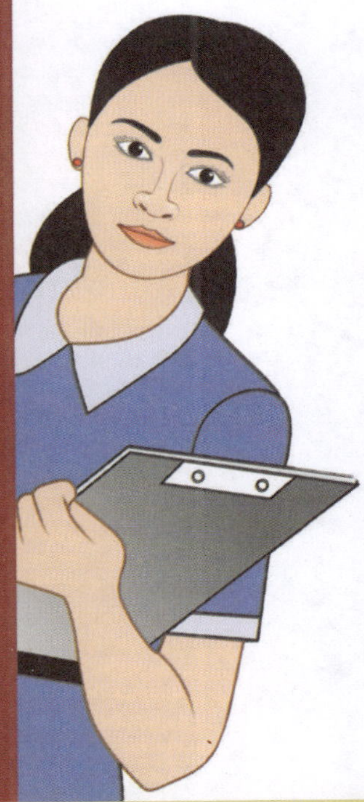

Papers Covered in
Nursing Next Live>
TARGET HIGH Digital Lite

Turn overleaf

Practice from

TARGET HIGH

Digital

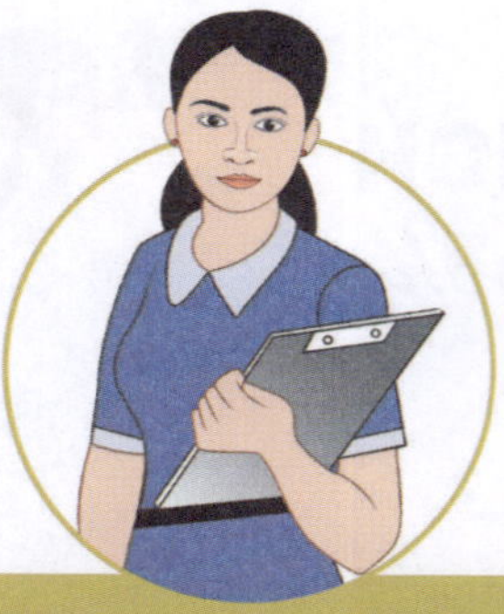

Practice, Practice & Practice

Now Attempt Papers in

Review & Practice Mode

PAPERS COVERED *(in Target High Digital Lite)*

1. NORCET (June) 2023 (Memory Based) (NEW)
2. AIIMS Jodhpur (SNO) 2023 (NEW)
3. AIIMS Bibinagar (Tutor) 2023 (NEW)
4. AIIMS Bibinagar Associate Professor 2023 (NEW)
5. Sree Chitra Tirunal Institute for Medical Science and Technology (NO) 2023 (NEW)
6. Uttar Pradesh University of Medical Sciences (NO) 2023 (NEW)
7. NORCET (NO) 2022 (Memory Based) (NEW)
8. Staff Nurse Examination Himachal Pradesh 2022 (NEW)
9. Western Coalfields Limited 2022 (NEW)
10. Odisha Subordinate Staff Selection Commission(NO) 2022 (NEW)
11. Gujarat Nursing Service 2022 (Nursing Officer/Principal) (NEW)
12. NORCET (NO) 2021 (Memory Based) (NEW)
13. Combined AIIMS (NO) (Bhopal, Jodhpur, Patna & Raipur) 2020
14. AIIMS Raipur (Lecturer) 2021
15. AIIMS NORCET 2020
16. AIIMS Nagpur (Nursing Officer) 2020
17. AIIMS Patna (Nursing Officer) 2020
18. AIIMS Raipur (Nursing Officer) 2019
19. AIIMS Bhatinda (Nursing Officer) 2019
20. AIIMS Raipur (Nursing Officer) 2019; Shift 1
21. AIIMS Raipur (Nursing Officer) 2019; Shift 2
22. AIIMS Raipur (Nursing Officer) 2019; Shift 3
23. AIIMS Bhubaneshwar (Senior Nursing Officer) 2019
24. AIIMS New Delhi (Nursing Officer) 2019
25. AIIMS New Delhi (Nursing Officer) 2018
26. AIIMS Nagpur (Nursing Officer) 2018
27. AIIMS Jodhpur (Senior Nursing Officer) Grade I: 2018
28. AIIMS Bhopal (Senior Nursing Officer) 2018
29. AIIMS Bhopal (Nursing Officer) 2018; Shift 1
30. AIIMS Bhopal (Nursing Officer) 2018; Shift 2
31. AIIMS Mangalagiri (Nursing Officer) Grade-II; 2018; Shift 2
32. AIIMS Bhubaneswar (Nursing Officer) 2018
33. AIIMS Raipur (Nursing Officer) 2017; Shift 1
34. AIIMS Raipur (Nursing Officer) 2017; Shift 2
35. AIIMS Raipur (Nursing Officer) 2017; Shift 3
36. AIIMS Raipur (Nursing Tutor) 2017
37. AIIMS Jodhpur & Rishikesh (Nursing Officer) 2017
38. AIIMS Raipur (Senior Nursing Officer) 2017
39. AIIMS Bhopal (Nursing Officer) 2016
40. AIIMS New Delhi (Nursing Officer) 2016
41. AIIMS Bhopal (Senior Nursing Officer) 2016
42. CNCI (Nursing Officer) 2021
43. BFUHS 2021
44. ESIC Paramedical 2019; Shift 1
45. ESIC Paramedical 2019; Shift 2
46. ESIC (Nursing Officer) 2016; Shift 1
47. ESIC (Nursing Officer) 2016; Shift 2
48. ESIC (Nursing Officer) Banglore Shift 1: 2016
49. ESIC (Nursing Officer) Banglore Shift 2: 2016
50. ESIC (Nursing Officer) Delhi 2016
51. ESIC (Nursing Officer) Banglore 2013
52. ESIC (Nursing Officer) Chennai 2012
53. ESIC (Nursing Officer) Grade II: 2011
54. ESIC (Nursing Officer) Ahmedabad 2011
55. Kerala PSC 2021
56. Kerala PSC (Nursing Officer) 2017
57. Kerala PSC (Nursing Officer) 2016
58. Kerala PSC (Nursing Officer) 2014
59. Kerala PSC (Nursing Officer) Grade II: 2011
60. Kerala PSC (Nursing Officer) Set C: 2011
61. Kerala PSC (Nursing Officer) 2010
62. BHU (Nursing Officer) 2019
63. BHU (Nursing Officer) 2018
64. BHU (Nursing Officer) 2016
65. BHU (Nursing Officer) 2015
66. Safdarjung (Nursing Officer) 2019
67. Safdarjung (Nursing Officer) 2018
68. JIPMER (Nursing Officer) 2020
69. JIPMER (Nursing Officer) 2013
70. JIPMER (Nursing Officer) 2012
71. UK State MSc (Nursing Officer) 2016
72. UK Nursing Tutor (Paper 1- Set B)
73. RRB (Nursing Officer) 2019; Shift 1
74. RRB (Nursing Officer) 2019; Shift 2
75. RRB (Nursing Officer) 2019; Shift 3
76. RRB (Nursing Officer) 2019; Shift 4
77. RRB (Nursing Officer) 2019; Shift 5
78. RRB Paramedical PHN 2015
79. RRB (Nursing Officer) 2015; Set A
80. RRB (Nursing Officer) 2015; Set B
81. RRB (Nursing Officer) 2015; Set C
82. RRB Secunderabad (Senior Nursing Officer) 2015
83. RRB (Nursing Officer) 2012
84. HPSSC (Nursing Officer) 2016
85. HP (Nursing Officer) 2016
86. RAK MSc Entrance Exam 2018
87. RAK New Delhi Entrance Exam 2017
88. GMCH (Nursing Officer) 2019
89. GMCH (Nursing Officer) 2016
91. Northern Coal Field Limited, Singrauli (Nursing Officer) 2019
92. PGIMER Chandigarh (Nursing Officer) 2016
93. CHO Haryana 2021
94. CHO Rajasthan 2020
95. CHO Madhya Pradesh 2020
96. CHO Madhya Pradesh 2019 Shift-1
97. CHO Uttar Pradesh 2018
98. RUHS MSc Nursing Entrance Exam 2018
99. RUHS MSc Nursing Entrance Exam 2016
100. RUHS Post Basic Basic Nursing Entrance Exam 2016
101. LNJP Hospital Delhi (Nursing Officer) 2012
102. DSSSB Shift I (NO) 2019
103. DSSSB Shift II (NO) 2019
104. DSSSB PHN 2015
105. DSSSB ANM 2015
106. Jhalawar Hospital and Medical College Society 2012
107. TNPSC Maternal and Child Health Officer 2015
108. RML Hospital (Nursing Officer) 2011
109. Insurance Medical Services (Nursing Officer) 2004
110. RRC (Nursing Officer) 2012
111. SCTIMST (Nursing Officer) 2015
112. Rohtak (Nursing Officer) 2020
113. NIMHANS (Nursing Officer) 2019 (Memory Based)
114. SKIM (Nursing Officer) 2020 Paper
115. Gujarat Staff (Nursing Officer) 2021
116. Jr. Grade Nurse/Jr. Staff Nurse/Jr. Nurse 2020
117. UPPSC Staff Nurse 2021
118. Uttarakhand Assistant Professor 2021
119. Daman & Diu (NO) 2018

"Sometimes the remedy is worse than the disease."
—Francis Bacon

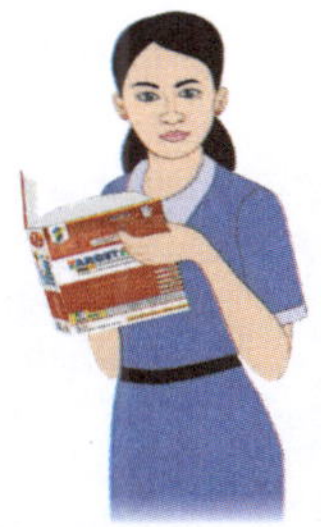

NORCET (June) 2023 (Memory Based)

1. Which oil is harmful for coronary artery disease?
a. Coconut oil b. Sunflower oil
c. Safflower oil d. Olive oil

2. When performing a cardiovascular assessment, the nurse notes that patient needs to sit upright to breathe. This behavior is most indicative of:
a. Pericarditis b. Anxiety
c. Congestive heart failure d. Angina

3. The child with iron poisoning is given IV deferoxamine mesylate (Desferal). Following administration, the child suffers hypotension, facial flushing, and urticaria. The initial nursing intervention would be to:
a. Discontinue the IV
b. Stop the medication, and begin a normal saline infusion
c. Take all vital signs, and report to the physician
d. Assess urinary output, and if it is 30 mL an hour, maintain current treatment

4. Which of the following is the classical CSF finding seen in Tuberculous meningitis?
a. Increased protein, decreased sugar, increased lymphocytes
b. Increased protein, sugar and lymphocytes
c. Decreased protein, increased sugar and lymphocytes
d. Increased sugar, protein and neutrophils

5. A patient is admitted in emergency with a suspected fracture of neck of femur. While assisting, the nurse will place the patient in which of the following position?
a. External rotation less than 45°.
b. External rotation more than 45°.
c. Internal rotation less than 45°.
d. Internal rotation more than 45°.

6. Patient develops type 2 respiratory failure. What could be the possible cause associated with it?
a. Interstitial lung disease b. Flail chest
c. Pulmonary edema d. ARDS

7. A client develops severe dyspnea after 100 meter of running. Using the mMRC Dyspnea scale, the client will be categorized into which grade to assess degree of baseline functional disability due to dyspnea?
a. Grade 0 b. Grade 1
c. Grade 2 d. Grade 3

8. You have to assess the blood sugar level of your patient by using glucometer. The appropriate nursing action from the following is:
a. Do not clean the site with alcohol swab
b. Check blood glucose level twice to obtain accurate reading
c. Wipe the first drop of blood and use second to measure the reading
d. First prick the finger and then connect the glucometer strip into the device.

9. Polyuria is the characteristic feature of all of the following; except:
a. Diabetes mellitus b. Diabetes insipidus
c. Glomerulonephritis d. Chronic renal failure

10. How much Energy (Kcal) is provided by 500 mL of 5% Dextrose?
a. 50 Kcal b. 100 Kcal
c. 150 Kcal d. 200 Kcal

11. Osmolarity of plasma in normal adult is:
a. 260-270 mOsm/L b. 320-330 mOsm/L
c. 280-290 mOsm/L d. 300-310 mOsm/L

12. What is the diagnostic test for enteric fever in 2nd week?
a. Widal test b. Blood culture
c. Stool test d. Sputum test

13. All of the following can be seen in dengue hemorrhagic fever; except:
a. Fever b. Thrombocytopenia
c. Leukocytosis d. Increased hematocrit count

14. While providing care to a 5-year-old child, the nurse noticed that the patient is experiencing seizures. Select the priority nursing intervention during seizure.
a. Maintain the patient in lying position, flat surface: turn head to side during seizure activity, give IV midazolam in appropriate dose and begin infusion of IV anticonvulsant
b. Maintain the patient in supine position, give supplemental oxygen, and start IV midazolam in an appropriate dose
c. Maintain the patient in lying position, flat surface; turn head to side during seizure activity; loosen clothing from neck or chest and abdominal areas; suction as needed; supervise supplemental oxygen or bag ventilation
d. Maintain the patient in supine position, flat surface; turn head to side during seizure activity, provide supplemental oxygen and inform the doctor on duty

15. The nurse finds out the Serum potassium level of his patient is 6.5 mEq/L. Which changes on a patient's electrocardiogram (ECG) reflect hyperkalemia?
a. Tall peaked T waves b. Narrow QRS complex
c. Tall P waves d. Normal P-R interval"

16. Which of the following is used in the management of hyperkalemia?
a. Insulin with glucose
b. Sodium bicarbonate
c. Potassium chloride
d. Magnesium sulfate

17. Osler's nodes are the features of which of the following?
a. Rheumatic endocarditis
b. Endocarditis
c. Osteoarthritis
d. Rheumatic heart disease

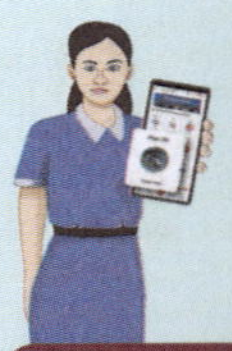

Ans.

1. a
2. c
3. b
4. a
5. a
6. b
7. a
8. c
9. c
10. b
11. c
12. a
13. c
14. c
15. a
16. a
17. b

18. Duke criteria are followed in:
a. Infective endocarditis
b. Complete heart block
c. Rheumatoid heart diseases
d. Rheumatoid arthritis

19. Which one of the following should be used following administration of barium enema?
a. Antacid b. Laxative
c. Analgesics d. Fruit Juice

20. If the trait in the pedigree is autosomal recessive and subject to complete penetrance, which of the following is true?

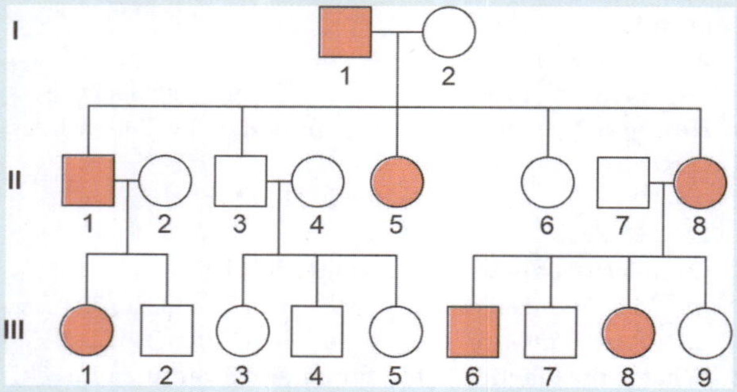

a. Individual I-2 must be heterozygous
b. Individual II-1 might be heterozygous
c. Individual II-3 must be heterozygous
d. Individual III-2 might be heterozygous

21. A client presents to the dermatology OPD with the complaint in the groin area. The examination findings include a small red scaly rash in the groin area extended to the inner thigh and buttocks area. The client is infected with jock itch. Identify the exact diagnosis based on his clinical image given below.

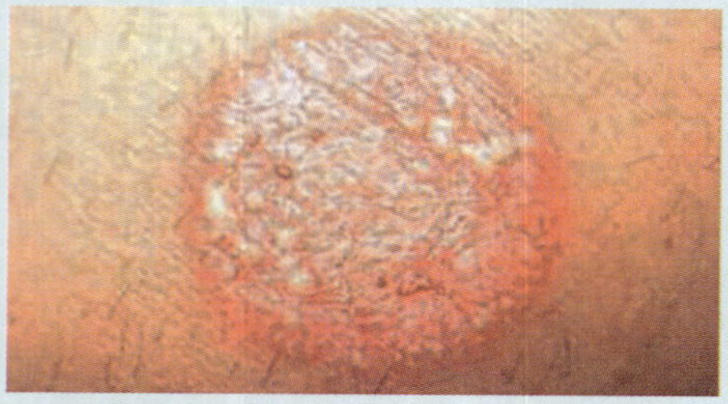

a. Tinea pedis b. Tinea cruris
c. Tinea capitis d. Tinea corporis

22. Identify the condition shown in the given image of X-ray.

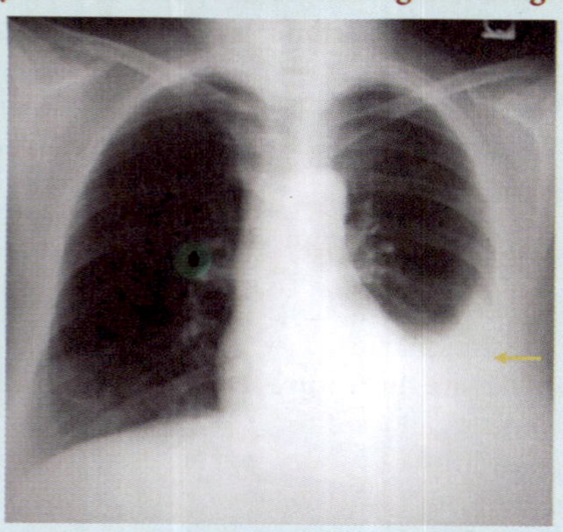

a. Pneumothorax b. Pleural effusion
c. Pleurisy d. Pulmonary infarction

23. Which symptom is NOT commonly seen in right sided heart failure?
a. Crackles b. Nocturia
c. Jugular vein distension d. Weight gain

24. Honey bee lesion seen in the given below image is a characteristic feature of which disease condition?

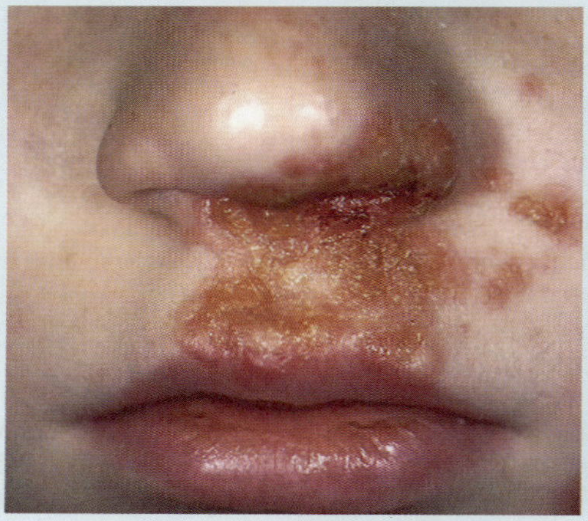

a. Impetigo b. Dermatitis
c. Urticaria d. None of these

25. Which perfusion pressure is ideally maintained in patient with traumatic brain injury?
a. 60–70% b. 70–80%
c. 80–90% d. 90–95%

26. The cause of endocarditis is:
a. Proteus
b. Beta hemolytic Streptococcus
c. Pseudomonas
d. E. coli

27. Trendelenburg gait is seen in which of the following condition?
a. Hip abductor weakness.
b. Gluteus medius muscle weakness
c. Coxa vera
d. All of the above

28. The most common cause of pyogenic meningitis in adults is:
a. N. meningitidis
b. E. coli
c. Beta hemolytic streptococcus
d. Haemophilus influenzae type B

29. A pregnant client comes to the office for her first prenatal examination at 10 weeks. She has been pregnant twice before; the first delivery produced a viable baby girl at 39 weeks 3 years ago; the second pregnancy produced a viable baby boy at 36 weeks 2 years ago. Both children are living and well. Using the GTPAL system to record her obstetrical history, the nurse should record:
a. 3-2-0-0-2 b. 2-2-0-2-2
c. 3-1-1-0-2 d. 2-1-1-0-2

30. A 35-weeks-pregnant client is undergoing a nonstress test (NST). During the 20-minute examination, the nurse notes three fetal movements accompanied by accelerations of the fetal heart rate, each 15 bpm, lasting for 15 seconds. The nurse interprets this test to be:
a. Nonreactive
b. Reactive
c. Positive
d. Negative

Ans.
18. a
19. b
20. c
21. b
22. b
23. a
24. a
25. a
26. b
27. d
28. a
29. c
30. b

31. A pregnant client continues to visit the clinic regularly during her pregnancy. During one of her visits while lying supine on the examining table, she tells the RN that she is becoming light-headed. The RN notices that the client has pallor in her face and is perspiring profusely. The first intervention the RN should initiate is to:

a. Place the examining table in the Trendelenburg position
b. Assess the client to see if she is having vaginal bleeding
c. Obtain the client's vital signs immediately
d. Help the client to a sitting position

32. A patient in 28-week gestation is receiving labetalol and magnesium sulfate for her pre-eclampsia treatment. On checking her BP, you find that it is 86/56. The most likely cause of this finding is:

a. False BP reading
b. Accidental overdose of labetalol
c. Patient is anxious
d. Magnesium toxicity

33. A pregnant woman at 28 weeks of gestation visited antenatal clinic at a primary health center for the first time. Her hemoglobin level was found to be 9 g. The management will include:

a. Tablet iron folic acid—one tablet (containing 60 mg elemental iron and 500 microgram of Folic acid) daily
b. Tablet iron folic acid—one tablet (containing 50 mg elemental iron and 500 microgram of Folic acid) weekly
c. Blood Transfusion
d. Tablet iron folic acid—two tablet (containing 60 mg elemental iron and 500 microgram of Folic acid) daily

34. The given below statements are true about DMPA (Antara); except:

a. It is injectable
b. It is irreversible
c. Can be used in 15–45 years of age group
d. Provided by Government of India for free

35. A client is admitted in hospital for induction of labor owing to gestational age of 42 weeks confirmed by dates and ultrasound. When she has dilated 3 cm she has contractions of 70 sec. She is receiving IV oxytocin. Nurse priority intervention should be?

a. Stop IV oxytocin Infusion
b. Notify physician
c. Prepare for delivery
d. Check FHR

36. A pregnant woman in active labor experienced spontaneous rupture of membrane. What will be the priority nursing intervention?

a. FHR assessment
b. Amniotic fluid color
c. Vital Signs of mother
d. Call the doctor

37. The nurse is performing a postdelivery assessment of a patient 2 hours after postpartum. The nurse documented that the uterus is soft and feels deviated toward right side, fundus two fingers above umbilicus. What will be the possible cause of this condition?

a. Hemorrhage
b. Involution
c. Infection
d. Bladder distention

38. After normal vaginal delivery, a woman is shifted to post-operative ward. What is the first priority?

a. Observe bleeding and color of lochia
b. Start IV fluid
c. Check vital signs
d. Check pain level.

39. A client is being discharged with albuterol (Proventil) and beclomethasone dipropionate (Vanceril) to be administered *via* inhalation three times a day and at bedtime. Client teaching regarding the sequential order in which the drugs should be administered includes:

a. Glucocorticoid followed by the bronchodilator
b. Bronchodilator followed by the glucocorticoid
c. Alternate successive administrations
d. According to the client's preference

40. Atropine can be used topically; except in:

a. Cataract
b. Corneal ulcer
c. Uveitis
d. Acute congestive glaucoma

41. A patient has type 1 diabetes mellitus. He came in emergency in condition of DKA. His blood glucose level is 550 mg/dL. What is the priority nursing action?

a. Start regular insulin infusion with normal saline
b. Start NPH insulin
c. Give sweet juice
d. Start Dextrose 50%

42. Which of the following is a longest acting basal insulin?

a. Lispro
b. Aspart
c. Glargin
d. Degludec

43. Administration of which antibiotic does not require a sensitivity test?

a. Metronizadole
b. Amoxicillin
c. Cefoparazone
d. Merepenem

44. Patient is posted for mastectomy and the surgical ward nursing officer has given test dose of antibiotic to check any reaction. After 10 minutes, the patient complains of redness and itching at the test dose administration site. Nurse documents that patient developed drug-induced urticaria. Which of the following drug is not recommended in case of drug-induced urticaria?

a. Corticosteroid
b. Epinephrine
c. Chlorpromazine
d. Hydrocortisone

45. Xpert MTB/RIF assay gives information about:

a. Detection of rifampicin resistance alone
b. Detection of mtb and patient MDR TB
c. Detection of mtb alone
d. Detection of mtb and resistance to 2nd line anti TB drugs

46. Opioid tolerance develops rapidly to all of the following, except:

a. Euphoria
b. Respiratory depression
c. Sedation
d. Constricted Pupils

47. Which of the following drug is not used in CKD?

a. Furosemide
b. Hydrochlorothiazide
c. Spironolactone
d. Chlorthalidone

48. Which of the following is associated with ranitidine; except:

a. Should be taken with antacid
b. Smoking affects the action
c. Side effect of Rantac is diarrhea
d. Confusion develops with Rantac

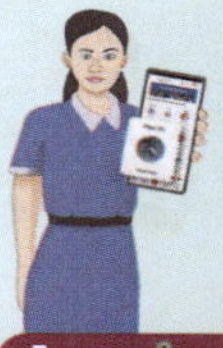

Ans.

31. d
32. d
33. d
34. b
35. a
36. a
37. d
38. c
39. b
40. d
41. a
42. d
43. a
44. c
45. a
46. d
47. c
48. a

49. What you will do to increase absorption of percutaneous nitroglycerin?
a. Apply near heart
b. Apply in non-hairy area
c. Apply over bony prominence
d. Apply on abdomen

50. Patient has BP of 155/88, pulse 86 and respiration 20. You administered nitroglycerin by IV route. Which of the following is expected response of the drug?
a. BP 160/70, pulse 98, RR - 20
b. BP 90/60, pulse 48, respiration 24
c. BP 88/56, pulse 92, respiration 20
d. BP 170/82, pulse 60, respiration 24

51. If there is a control over drugs and cigarette shops around school, it is aimed at
a. Supply reduction
b. Demand reduction
c. Harm reduction
d. Risk reduction

52. Patient with digoxin should be checked for which electrolyte?
a. Potassium
b. Calcium
c. Magnesium
d. Sodium

53. A long acting NTG drug must be administered at what time for patient with nocturnal angina?
a. Noon
b. Evening
c. Early morning
d. Bedtime

54. Aspirin is prescribed for all; except:
a. Liver cancer
b. Brain tumor
c. MI
d. Stroke

55. A 35-year-old farmer brought to emergency with history of multiple time vomiting, loose stool and breathlessness for two hours while he was fumigating his crops. On examination, he was drowsy and had excessive salivation, involuntary defecation, pulse rate 46/min, BP-90/60 mm Hg, respiratory rate-14/minute, pupils-bilaterally constricted, twitching in bilateral calf muscles. Chest auscultation revealed bilateral crackles. What is likely poisoning?
a. Opioids
b. Aluminum Phosphide
c. Arsenic
d. Organophosphorus

56. In case of pediatrics immunization, which muscle is preferable for IM injection?
a. Vastus lateralis
b. Deltoid
c. Dorsogluteal
d. Ventro Gluteal

57. Which of the following has low risk of sudden infant death syndrome?
a. Baby who sleeps on his back
b. History of previous baby who had sudden infant death syndrome.
c. Baby with prenatal drug exposure
d. Baby who is premature

58. Phototherapy for an infant of age 90 hours should be instituted when the total serum bilirubin level is?
a. 12.5 g b. 20 g
c. 15 g d. 10 g

59. A newborn nursery notes that a 36-hour-old baby is jaundiced. Phototherapy has been initiated. Which of the following nursing interventions will be most therapeutic?
a. Maintain a warm ambient environment
b. Have the mother feed the baby frequently
c. Have the mother hold the baby skin to skin
d. Place the baby naked by a closed sunlight window

60. What is the management of a baby born to a a mother who was on ART during the antenatal period?
a. Exclusive breastfeeding, nevirapine for 6 weeks
b. Exclusive replacement feeding, nevirapine for 6 weeks
c. Exclusive breastfeeding, nevirapine for 12 weeks
d. Exclusive replacement feeding, nevirapine for 12 weeks

61. In tracheoesophageal fistula, which position is preferred?
a. Prone
b. Head end elevation at 30 degree
c. Supine
d. Lateral

62. All of the following are the early signs and symptoms of meningitis, except in infant?
a. Poor feeding b. Tensed fontanel
c. Vomiting and irritability d. High pitched cry

63. What is the targeted oxygen saturation in both preterm and term neonates receiving oxygen therapy?
a. 81-92% b. 91-95%
c. 95-100% d. None of these

64. What is the weight-for-height z-score or SD of MUAC for acute malnutrition according to the growth chart?
a. <-2 SD
b. <-3 SD
c. >2 SD
d. Equal to 2 SD

65. If a child has done routine immunization of DPT and after giving injection, the child develops fever, swelling over the vaccine site, then nurse gives what advice to parents?
a. It is normal reaction, nothing to do
b. It is mild reaction, advise to call the Doctor
c. Tell to withhold next dose of DPT
d. Refer child to emergency department

66. What the SpO_2 level in newborn in first 5 minutes?
a. 60-65
b. 70-75
c. 80-85
d. 90-95

67. Which of the following is the correct height velocity in children aged 2—10 years?
a. 8–18 cm/year
b. 4–6 cm/year
c. 2–4 cm/year
d. 6–8 cm/year

68. Which of the following is not a sign of dehydration in an infant?
a. Perianal excoriation
b. Delayed skin pinch
c. Dry mouth
d. Drying of tears

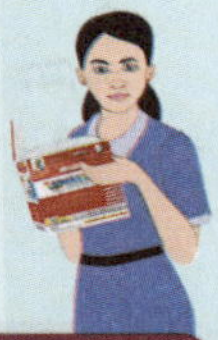

Ans.

49. b
50. c
51. a
52. a
53. b
54. a
55. d
56. a
57. a
58. c
59. b
60. a
61. b
62. b
63. b
64. a
65. a
66. c
67. b
68. a

69. A baby at 3 years will be considered for having developmental delay if he or she:
a. Cannot hop on one foot
b. Cannot catch ball reliably
c. Cannot hold spoon effectively
d. Cannot copy a square

70. Up to which age, height of the child is measured in lying down posture?
a. 12 months b. 18 months
c. 24 months d. 36 months

71. An image of the baby is shown with different zones of bilirubin level. How much bilirubin level in baby is likely to have up to 3rd zone?

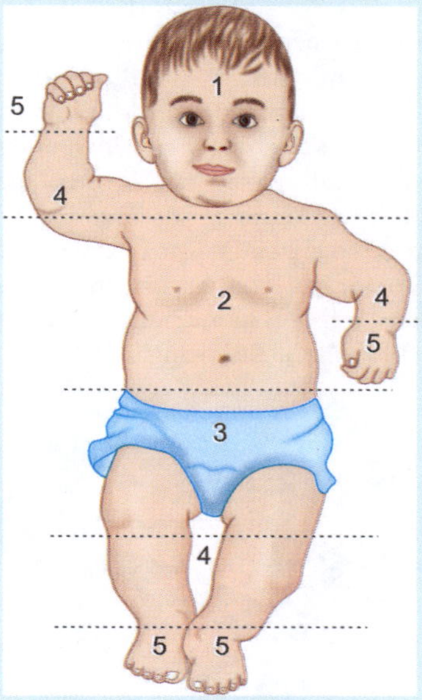

a. 4-6 mg/dL
b. 9-12 mg/dL
c. 13-16 mg/dL
d. 15-20 mg/dL

72. An 8-year-old child comes to the physician's office complaining of swelling and pain in the knees. His mother says, "the swelling occurred for no reason, and it keeps on getting worse." The initial diagnosis is Lyme disease. When talking to the mother and child, questions related to which of the following would be specific to include in the initial history?
a. A decreased urinary output and flank pain
b. A fever of over 100°F occurring over the last 2-3 weeks
c. Circular or oval-shaped rash that looks like a Bull's eye
d. Headaches, malaise, or sore throat

73. A newborn baby had lumbosacral meningocele. Till the period of surgery, the sac should be well protected by covering it with a sterile gauze piece soaked in:
a. Spirit b. Normal Saline
c. Methylene Blue d. Betadine

74. What is the dose of adrenaline in neonates in CPR?
a. 0.5 mg/kg (1: 10,000 dilution)
b. 0.05 mg/kg (1 mL of 1:10,000 dilution
c. 0.1 mg/kg (1:1000)
d. 0.1 mg/kg (1: 10,000)

75. When teaching a mother of a 4-month-old with diarrhea about the importance of preventing dehydration, the nurse would inform the mother about the importance of feeding her child:
a. Fruit juices
b. Diluted carbonated drinks
c. Soy-based, lactose-free formula
d. Regular formulas mixed with electrolyte solutions

76. Which of the following is true about Kangaroo Mother care?
a. Exclusive breastfeeding, Early discharge, Belongingness
b. Exclusive breastfeeding, Early discharge, Prevention of Infection
c. Exclusive breastfeeding, Early discharge, Prevention of hypothermia
d. Exclusive breastfeeding, Early discharge, Supplementary nutrition

77. Which of the following findings in newborn requires immediate nursing intervention?
a. Hemoglobin 17 g/dL b. Blood glucose 30 mg/dL
c. Platelets 2.5 lakh/mm^3 d. WBC 18000/mm^3

78. Which of the following statement is true about precocious puberty?
a. Precocious puberty is early puberty
b. It happens when GNRH releases early.
c. In girls, breasts develop at an atypically early age along with growth spurts.
d. All of the above

79. A client with a C-3–4 fracture has just arrived in the emergency room. The primary nursing intervention is:
a. Stabilization of the cervical spine
b. Airway assessment and stabilization
c. Confirmation of spinal cord injury
d. Normalization of intravascular volume

80. When evaluating a client with symptoms of shock, it is important for the nurse to differentiate between neurogenic and hypovolemic shock. The symptoms of neurogenic shock differ from hypovolemic shock in that:
a. In neurogenic shock, the skin is warm and dry
b. In hypovolemic shock, there is bradycardia
c. In hypovolemic shock, capillary refill is less than 2 seconds
d. In neurogenic shock, there is delayed capillary refill

81. A client with a diagnosis of C-4 injury has been stabilized and is ready for discharge. Since this client is at risk of autonomic dysreflexia, he and his family should be instructed to assess for and report:
a. Dizziness and tachypnea
b. Circumoral pallor and lightheadedness
c. Headache and facial flushing
d. Pallor and itching of the face and neck

82. A 30-year-old male patient presented to Surgery OPD with complaint of bleeding per rectum. History is suggestive of hemorrhoids. What will be the confirmatory test in OPD?
a. Proctoscopy
b. Sigmoidoscopy
c. Digital rectal examination
d. USG whole abdomen

83. Surgical checklist includes all; except:
a. Time in b. Time out
c. Sign in d. Sign out

Ans.

69.	c
70.	c
71.	b
72.	c
73.	b
74.	b
75.	c
76.	c
77.	b
78.	d
79.	b
80.	a
81.	c
82.	c
83.	a

84. The procedure in which the following instrument is used?

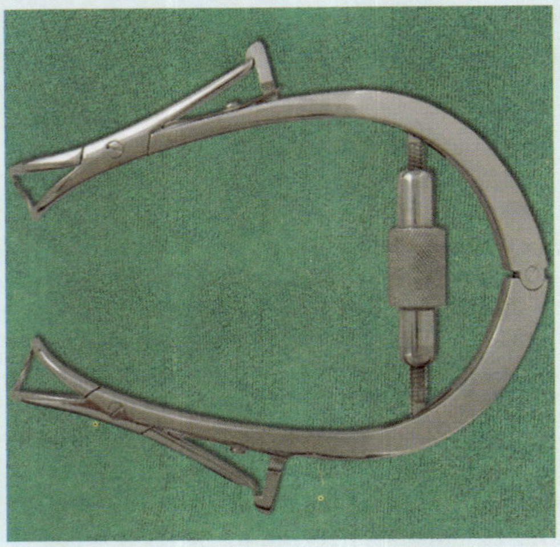

a. Abdominal surgery b. Thyroidectomy
c. Whipple surgery d. Orthopedic surgery

85. A 30-year-old woman presents in emergency with ruptured gallbladder. Emergency open cholecystectomy surgery performed in the hospital. On the second postoperative day, she begins to complain of cramping abdominal pain without vomiting. She has a temperature of 99.5°F, blood pressure is 128/84 mm Hg, and pulse is 82/min. Her physical exam is significant for absent bowel sounds, a mildly distended abdomen with mild diffuse tenderness without rebound or guarding. Which of the following would most likely be the suspected complication associated with this clinical finding?

a. Peritonitis b. Gastritis
c. Evisceration d. Dehiscence

86. A patient presented with swelling in front of neck in midline which moves on deglutition. Which among the following will be the LESS likely diagnosis?

a. Thyroglossal Cyst
b. Solitary thyroid nodule in isthmus
c. Subhyoid bursitis
d. Lipoma

87. Which type of lung cancer is more commonly seen in non-smokers?

a. Adenocarcinoma b. Squamous cell carcinoma
c. Small cell carcinoma d. Large cell carcinoma

88. Which of the following laboratory findings is less likely to be seen when a patient presents with trauma?

a. Urinary retention b. Increased sodium
c. Increased creatinine d. Elevated creatine kinase

89. Cause of decreased peripheral vascular resistance is:

a. Cardiogenic shock b. Hypovolemic shock
c. Neurogenic shock d. Pulmonary embolism

90. If child has to be posted for surgery, then for overnight fasting which solution is given?

a. DNS b. 5% Dextrose
c. ½ dextrose d. RL

91. In split thickness skin grafting, what all layers of skin are present?

a. Epidermis only
b. Epidermis and entire dermis
c. Epidermis and superficial dermis
d. Tissue and cartilage

92. Which of the following sutures needle is preferred for fixing a drain?

a. Reverse cutting needle b. Cutting needle
c. Round body needle d. Taper body needle

93. Which blade is used for incision and drainage?

a. 10 b. 11
c. 12 d. 15

94. Consider the following fertility related statistics. The mortality rate of women in reproductive age is not taken into consideration while calculating which of these statistics?

1. Total fertility rate 2. Gross reproductive rate
3. Net reproduction rate 4. General fertility rate

a. 1, 2, 3 b. 1, 3, 4
c. 2, 3, 4 d. 1, 2, 4

95. Which committee depict rural three trier system?

a. Shrivastav committee b. Bhore committee
c. Kartar Singh committee d. Mudaliar committee

96. Epigastric artery is the branch of which of the following?

a. Internal iliac artery b. External iliac artery
c. Internal gastric Artery d. External gastric Artery

97. The patient is having an IV line in external jugular vein and as per the doctor orders, the nurse has to administer a drug through that IV line. The nurse is well aware that the drug will travel through the following structure to reach up to the heart?

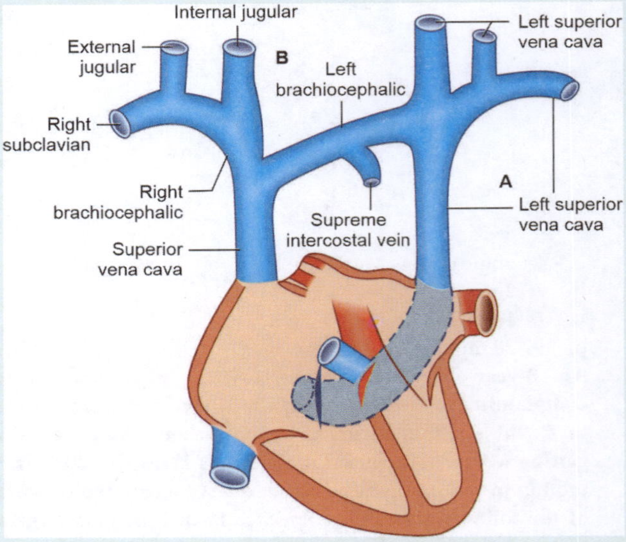

a. EJV - subclavian vein - IJV - heart
b. EJV - IJV - brachiocephalic vein - heart.
c. EJV - Brachiocephalic vein - SVC - heart.
d. EJV - IJV - subclavian vein - brachiocephalic vein - heart.

98. Complication of thiamine deficiency is:

a. Memory loss b. Tachycardia
c. Bradycardia d. Sore throat

99. If relative risk is 1. what does it indicates?

a. No association b. Negative association
c. Positive association d. Positive Correlation

Explanation: *For detail explanation refer Nursing Research Synopsis*

100. A patient can move her extremities in normal manner but she can't move against resistance. What is her muscle strength testing score?

a. 1 b. 2
c. 3 d. 4

Ans.

84. b
85. a
86. d
87. a
88. b
89. c
90. a
91. c
92. a
93. b
94. d
95. a
96. b
97. c
98. a
99. a
100. c

101. Incorrect statement from the following is:
a. Bed sore can be prevented by 2 hourly positioning
b. Most commonly affected part is sacrum
c. Air mattress can prevent bed sore
d. Early stage bed sore can be managed by minimal wound dressing and reducing pressure to affected side

102. Ratio of chest compression to ventilation/minute in neonates?
a. 90:30 b. 3:1
c. 15:2 d. 30:2

103. 500 mL of 5% Dextrose is to be administered in 5 hours with burette set. Calculate the flow rate (mL/h)
a. 50 b. 100
c. 80 d. 200

104. After starting blood transfusion, patient develops chills after 30 minutes. What is the first nursing action?
a. Stop the transfusion
b. Slow the transfusion
c. Administer antihistaminic
d. Inform the doctor

105. A first aid provider found an adult victim who is unresponsive with no pulse and gasping. The single rescuer has activated the emergency medical service. After starting the chest compression, how frequently the rescuer needs to assess the patient for the sign of pulse?
a. After 5 cycles of CPR b. After 10 cycles of CPR
c. After 2 minutes d. Both a and c

106. The nurse provides care to a patient with an endotracheal tube and positive pressure mechanical ventilation. Which of the following observation requires intervention by the nurse?
a. The intern nurse drains ventilator tubing condensation toward the endotracheal tube connection
b. The patient gags and bites the endotracheal tube
c. The intern nurse reports that the patient's weight has increased 1.3 kg over past 72 hours
d. The endotracheal tube cuff pressure is 22 cm H2O

107. A nurse taking care of a patient with chest tube drainage suddenly notices that there is no fluctuation in the water seal tube. Which of the following action should the nurse take first?
a. Turn the patient to the unaffected side
b. Inform the physician
c. Check the tubing to ensure there is no kinking
d. Start milking the chest tube

108. After a liver biopsy, the best position for the client is:
a. High Fowler b. Prone
c. Supine d. Right lateral

109. Normal blood pressure of adult person:
a. 150/90 b. 60/40
c. 110/50 d. 120/80

110. The steps of urinary catheterization to a female client are:
a. Clean the site with betadine - apply lubricant on tip of catheter - Insert catheter - check for urine - inflate the balloon
b. Apply lubricant on tip of catheter - clean the site with betadine - insert catheter - inflate the balloon - check for urine
c. Clean the site with betadine - apply lubricant on tip of catheter - insert catheter - inflate balloon - check for urine
d. Insert Catheter---Clean the site with betadine----Apply lubricant on the tip of catheter----Check urine---- Inflate balloon.

111. What is the frequency of tuning fork used in the clinical setting?
a. 256 b. 512
c. 1024 d. 3048

112. Gastric lavage procedure should be avoided in which of the following situation?
a. Kerosene Poisoning
b. Arsenic Poisoning
c. Organophosphate Poisoning
d. Ethanol Poisoning

113. The type of fluid which cause water to shift from cells into blood stream?
a. Hypotonic b. Hypertonic
c. Isotonic d. Albumin

114. What is the best position to keep a 12-year-old child after a lumbar puncture to assess CSF?
a. Semi-Fowler's so that the child can watch TV and be entertained
b. Supine position for several hours so as to prevent a headache
c. On her right side to prevent leak of CSF
d. Prone for two hours to prevent vomiting and aspiration

115. Feeling of loss and sadness, loneliness is seen in which stage of Kubler-Ross model?
a. Bargaining b. Acceptance
c. Depression d. Denial

116. All are criteria for high quality CPR; except:
a. Rate of compression 100–120/min
b. High ventilation
c. Minimal interruption
d. Allow complete chest recoil

117. A spill incident occurred in surgical unit. Which of the following statement is true while disinfecting the spill?
a. Once prepared can be used for a maximum duration of 7 days
b. 1% glutaraldehyde is used commonly
c. Dilute with water in 1:5 ratio before every use
d. Minimum contact period for disinfection is 20 minutes

118. As per the schedule, OT list nurse Reena has to scrub for the next laparoscopic cholecystectomy surgery. Arrange the given below activity in ascending order which the nurse reena will perform to get ready for the surgery?
1. Wear gloves
2. Scrubbing
3. Wear gown
4. Arrange and count instrument

a. 4, 2, 1, 3 b. 2, 1, 3, 4
c. 2, 3, 1, 4 d. 4, 1, 2, 3

119. You are instructing a female client about clean catch urine sample and ask her to clean the perineum before collecting the sample. Which statement by the nurse indicates her complete knowledge regarding clean catch urine specimen?
a. Clean the whole perineal area.
b. Clean the labia majora from back to front.
c. Clean the labia minora from front to back.
d. Clean the labia minora from back to front

120. All are true about hand hygiene; Except:
a. Cut short nails
b. Handwash for 40 sec
c. Don't use artificial nails
d. Use alcohol-based hand rub when hands are visibly soiled

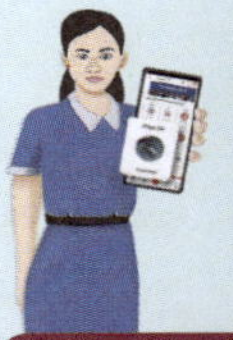

Ans.

101. d
102. a
103. b
104. a
105. d
106. b
107. c
108. d
109. d
110. a
111. b
112. a
113. b
114. b
115. c
116. b
117. d
118. c
119. c
120. d

121. For which exposure, postexposure prophylaxis is not given?
a. HIV b. Hep-b
c. Hep-c d. Tetanus

122. During cardiopulmonary resuscitation, external cardiac compression is given over:
a. Upper third of sternum
b. Mid third of sternum
c. Lower one third of sternum
d. Precordium overall

123. Which of the following findings is documented by the assigned nurse while auscultating the breath sound of a client with hemothorax?
a. Absent breath sound in affected lung
b. Dull sound with tympanic
c. Dull sound with resonance
d. Hyperresonance

124. Which of the following is the priority intervention to be performed in a client experiencing sudden cardiac arrest?
a. Chest compression b. Check for consciousness
c. Check for pulse d. Check for breath

125. All of the following are moments of hand hygiene; except:
a. Before touching the patient
b. After touching the patient
c. Before touching the patient surrounding
d. Before any aseptic procedure

126. Identify the image of the oxygen device given below?

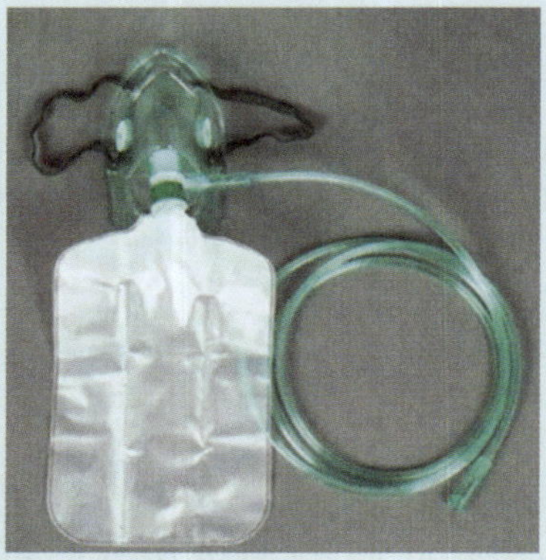

a. Non-re-breather mask
b. Venturi mask
c. Partial rebreathing mask
d. Face mask

127. Select suitable figure from the four alternatives that would complete the figure matrix.

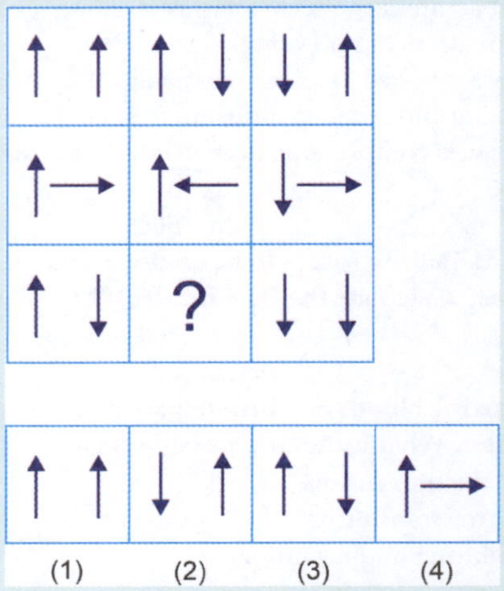

a. 1 b. 2
c. 3 d. 4

128. Which of the following city name is changed to Sambhajinagar?
a. Ahmad Nagar
b. Aurangabad
c. Pune
d. Nashik

129. Snow festival is arranged in which place?
a. Himachal
b. J & K
c. Laddak
d. Sikkim

130. Which country is not a part of G20?
a. Brazil
b. Pakistan
c. Russia
d. China

131. CDFI, EFHK, GH_M?
a. J b. K
c. L d. I

132. 8' 9 145......which one is following is related this???
a. 6 '8' 104 b. 9' 10' 210
c. 6' 7' 85 d. 7' 8' 57

133. SWOT analysis stands for the following; except:
a. S - strength b. W - weakness
c. O - opportunities d. T - Time

Ans.

121. d
122. c
123. a
124. a
125. c
126. a
127. a
128. b
129. b
130. b
131. a
132. c
133. d

"**One day in perfect health is much.**"
—Arabic

AIIMS Jodhpur (SNO) 2023

1. Following a road accident, a patient was admitted to the neurosurgery ICU due to a head injury. During the assessment, the patient opens his eyes to painful stimuli but not to verbal stimuli. He answers questions by making incomprehensible sounds and localzses the site of the painful stimulus. His GCS score will be:

a. 9 b. 8
c. 6 d. 7

2. A short-term goal for a patient with Alzheimer's disease is:

a. Regained sensory perception and cognitive function
b. Increased self-esteem and improved self-concept
c. Improved problem solving in activities of daily living
d. Improved functioning in the least restrictive environment

3. The primary fever in malaria corresponding to the development of the parasites in the red blood cells comprise all of the following; except:

a. Hot stage b. Relapse stage
c. Sweating stage d. Cold stage

4. What is the function of mRNA?

a. Escorts amino acid to ribosome
b. Carries message for protein synthesis
c. Helps form the ribosomes
d. Bonds with new strand

5. Second component (other than NST) in Modified Biophysical Profile is:

a. Fetal breathing movements
b. Amniotic fluid index
c. Fetal movements
d. Fetal tone

6. What is the best position for a patient in anaphylactic shock?

a. Supine with legs elevated
b. High fowler's
c. Semi fowler's
d. Lateral recumbent

7. The year 2023 has been declared as The International Year of:

a. Fruits b. Cereals
c. Nuts d. Millets

8. Regarding the placement of leads when recording ECG all of the following are correct; except:

a. V4-7th intercostal space at the midclavicular line
b. V3-linear midpoint between V2 and V4
c. V2 4th intercostal space left margin of sternum
d. V1-4th intercostal space- right margin of sternum

9. Low molecular weight heparin should be administered:

a. Intradermally
b. Intravenously
c. Subcutaneously
d. Intramuscularly

10. Beta-thalassemia is an autosomal recessive disorder. It is characterized by reduced hemoglobin levels in the body and is also known as:

a. Aplastic anaemia b. Sickle cell anemia
c. Cooley's anemia d. Hemolytic anemia

11. Epigenic factors play an important role in schizophrenia. In genetically vulnerable people, environmental factors may increase the risk and trigger schizophrenia. Which of the following statements is true?

a. Social companionship increases the risk of schizophrenia
b. Living in poverty does not increase the risk of schizophrenia.
c. Childhood trauma such as poverty or abuse can trigger schizophrenia
d. People living in rural areas are more vulnerable

12. Identify the contraceptive device shown in the given picture.

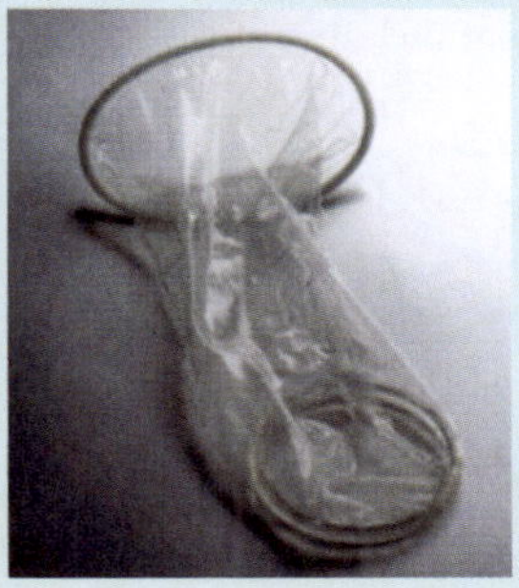

a. Female condom b. Diaphragm
c. Vaginal sponge d. Male condom

13. A nurse posted in a paediatric cardiology unit noted that the assessment findings of an infant reveal a continuous machinery murmur on the auscultation of the heart and signs of heart failure. She identifies that the infant has which of the following congenital cardiac defects?

a. Atrial septal defect b. Aortic stenosis
c. Ventricular septal defect d. Patent ductus arteriosus

14. At the central level, the Union Ministry of Health and Welfare is headed by a cabinet minister, a minister of state and a deputy health minister. These are political appointments and have a dual role to serve political as well as administrative responsibilities for health. One of the functions in the union list is:

a. To organize family welfare program through family welfare centers
b. International health relations and quarantine
c. Prevention of extension of communicable diseases from one unit to another
d. Regulation and development of medical, nursing and other allied health professions

Ans.

1. a
2. d
3. b
4. b
5. b
6. a
7. d
8. a
9. c
10. c
11. c
12. a
13. d
14. d

15. You have collected pus sample from a purulent lesion on the skin of a patient. You have sent the sample for gram staining. The microbiologist reports Staphylococci seen. Which of the below shapes of bacteria must the microbiologist have seen?

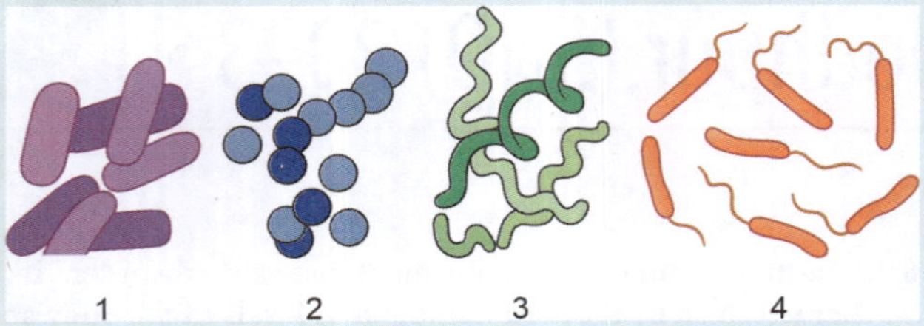

a. 4 b. 2
c. 1 d. 3

16. _____________ is an example of secondary prevention.

a. Treatment of the disease and rehabilitation
b. Proper disposal of garbage
c. Screening and case finding
d. Encouraging physical exercise

17. On physical examination of a patient's chest, a nurse observed a 'barrel chest'. A barrel chest is usually associated with:

a. Emphysema b. Kyphoscoliosis
c. Marfan syndrome d. Nickets

18. The 'Food Guide Pyramid' is a nutritional educational guide that emphasizes the importance of foods from different food groups. Which of the given statements is/are correct?

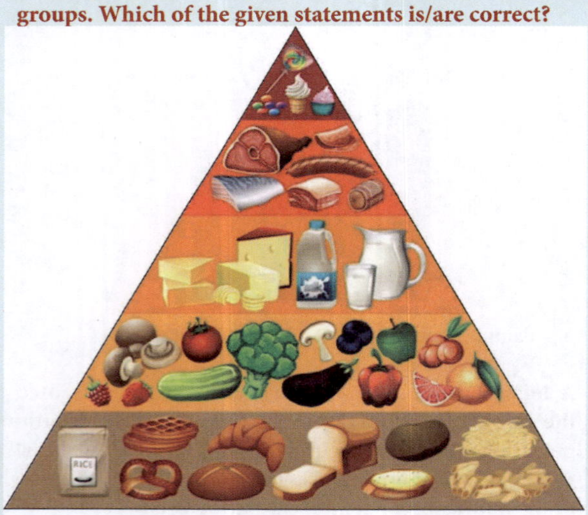

The food guide pyramid

1. Each of the food groups (shown in the picture) provides some of the nutrients required.
2. Each of the food groups provides all the nutrients required.
3. Foods in one group cannot replace those in another.
4. Food groups toward the top of the pyramid are increasingly more important.

a. Only 1 and 4
b. Only 2
c. Only 2 and 4
d. Only 1 and 3

19. The optimal target for patients with diabetes mellitus is maintaining a glycated hemoglobin (HbA1c) at:

a. Above 6.5%
b. Below 6.5%
c. Above 9%
d. Below 9%

20. Which of the following types of research involves at least some control by the researcher to implement the study treatment?

a. Correlational b. Experimental
c. Descriptive d. Quasi-experimental

21. Identify the fontanel indicated by the arrow.

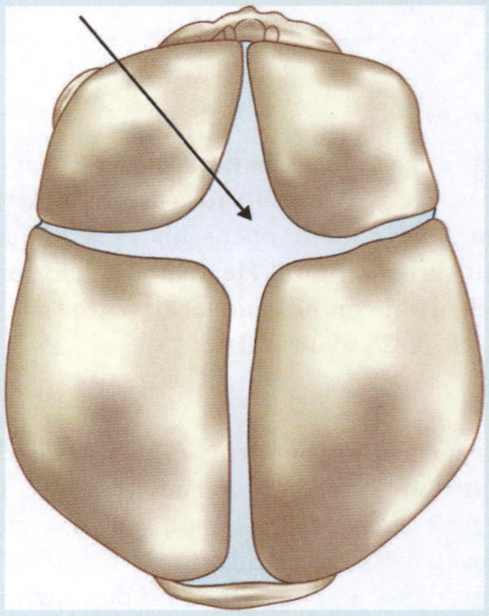

a. Anterior fontanel b. Posterior fontanel
c. Temporal fontanel d. Occipital fontanel

22. Children with Down's syndrome have what is known as brachycephaly. This means that the shape of the back of the head is:

a. Pointed b. Rounded
c. Flattened d. Pyramidal

23. The nurse manager needs to buy six new hospital beds for the unit. What type of budget will be used for this expenditure?

a. Capital budget b. Revenue budget
c. Operating budget d. Salary budget

24. If the calculated Chi square value in hypothesis testing is greater than the critical Chi value, then:

a. Reject null hypothesis
b. Do nothing
c. Do not reject null hypothesis
d. Estimate again

25. A probability distribution that is symmetric about the mean, showing that the data near the mean are more frequent in occurrence then the data far from the mean, is known as:

a. Normal distribution b. Poisson distribution
c. Skewed distribution d. Binomial distribution

26. A suprapubic cystostomy with a malecot catheter has been ordered for a patient. Which of the given catheters, in the images would you keep in your tray?

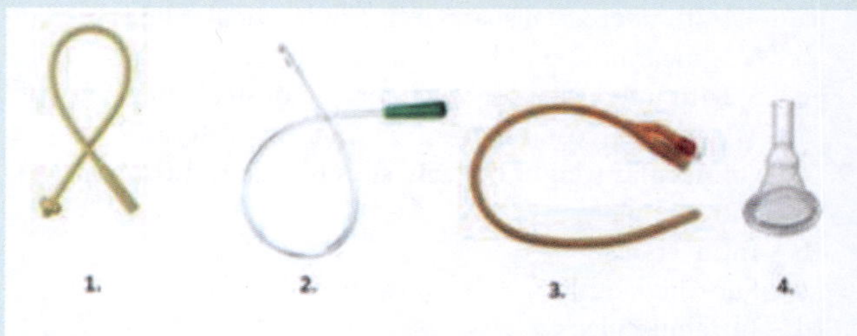

a. 1 b. 2
c. 3 d. 4

Ans.

15.	b
16.	c
17.	a
18.	d
19.	b
20.	d
21.	a
22.	c
23.	a
24.	a
25.	a
26.	a

27. Hospital information systems (HIS) is introduced in a hospital to support tasks like patient care and administration of a hospital. The nurses are expected to have a cultural lag which can overcome by which of the following?
  a. The organization should recruit new nurses who are trained in HIS.
  b. The organization should leave the nurses to learn or not learn HIS.
  c. The organization should invest in equipment and training the nurses.
  d. The organization should refine policies to force the nurses to adapt to the change.

28. When an antigen is mixed with its corresponding antibody at a suitable pH and temperature, antigen-antibody reaction causes clumping of particles together. This reaction is known as:
  a. Agglutination reaction b. Precipitation reaction
  c. Complement fixation d. Immunofluorescence

29. The misunderstanding or misinterpretation of the meaning which restricts effective communication is known as:
  a. Emotional barrier b. Physical barrier
  c. Semantic barrier d. Cultural barrier

30. A nurse posted in the postnatal ward is going around assessing patients. Which among the following postpartum women will need Rh (D) immune globulin (RhoGAM) before discharge?
  a. An Rh-negative primigravida with an Rh-positive infant
  b. An Rh positive primigravida with an Rh-positive infant
  c. An Rh-negative primigravida with an Rh-negative infant
  d. An Rh-positive primigravida with an Rh-negative infant

31. Suppose you were a nurse who was posted in the COVID-19 screening area where RT-PCR testing was conducted. Which transport media was used in the transport tube of COVID-19 swabs?
  a. PCR b. VVM
  c. RAT d. VTM

32. An example of inductive reasoning is:
  a. Reasoning from all chronically ill patients to a single chronically ill patient
  b. Reasoning from a single diabetic patient to all diabetic patients
  c. Using a computerized nursing care plan to care for insulin-dependent diabetic patients
  d. Using a standard nursing care plan to care for a specific patient

33. A nurse posted in the paediatric ward was doing a dehydration assessment for a child admitted with complaints of diarrhea. The nurse noted that the child was unconscious, and he had sunken eyes, skin pinch going back very slowly. Also, the child was not able to drink fluids. Based on these observations, what should the nurse categorize this dehydration as?
  a. No dehydration b. Mild dehydration
  c. Moderate dehydration d. Severe dehydration

34. The main features of the rural community are that the rural community is closely associated with:
  a. Direct effect of natural elements like rains, drought, heat, on their lives
  b. Remote from nature
  c. Work in closed environment
  d. Work in different occupations and contact is less between members

35. A client is admitted to the ward at 4 pm. She is posted for hemorrhoidectomy the next day morning. The nurse is expected to record the assessment of her vital signs. Before checking the blood pressure, the most important principle the nurse has to follow is:
  a. Prepare the equipment and supplies
  b. Explain the procedure to the client
  c. Wash hands
  d. Position the client

36. The kidneys are located __________ on the posterior abdominal region.
  a. Supraperitoneally
  b. Infraperitoneally
  c. In peritoneal cavity
  d. Retroperitoneally

37. While conducting delivery of a woman, a midwife suddenly finds that the internal rotation of shoulders is not occurring even after good uterine contractions. To release the anterior shoulder, she is performing which of the following manoeuvers in the given picture?

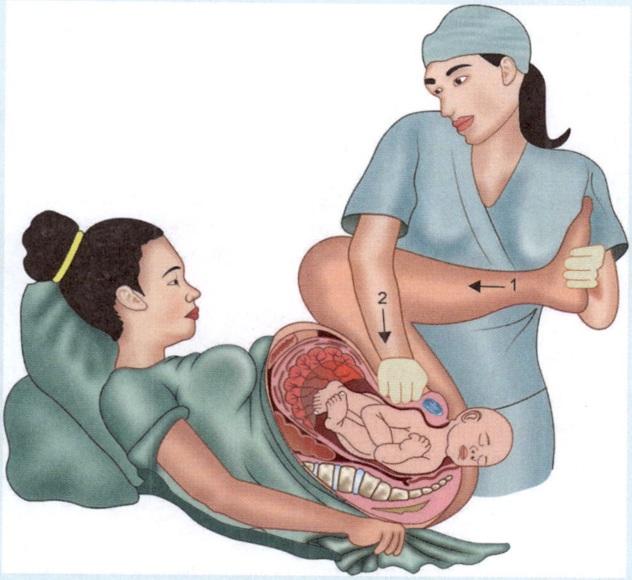

  a. Corkscrew manoeuvre
  b. Lovset's manoeuvre
  c. McRoberts manoeuvre
  d. Rubin manoeuvre

38. A nurse working in a ward notices that blood has spilled on the floor during blood collection. The spill covers an area of more than 20 cm. The nurse asked the housekeeping staff to clean the spill on the floor. What would the recommended disinfectant used for handling this spill be?
  a. 1:100 dilution of 5% sodium hypochlorite
  b. 1:2 dilution of 2% bleach solution
  c. 1:5 dilution of 5% bleach solution
  d. 1:10 dilution of 5% of sodium hypochlorite

39. Which type of coping strategy is most effective during a stressful circumstance that cannot be changed?
  a. Emotion focused coping
  b. Avoidance
  c. Problem focused coping
  d. Coping flexibility

Ans.

27. c
28. a
29. c
30. a
31. d
32. b
33. d
34. a
35. b
36. d
37. c
38. d
39. a

40. Identify the instrument shown in the picture below.

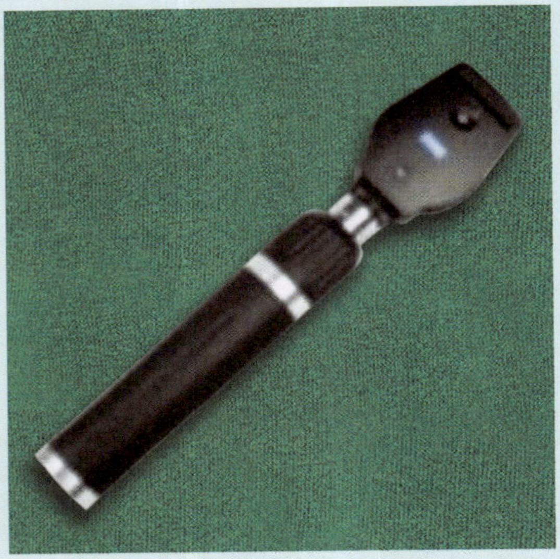

a. Otoscope
b. Arthroscope
c. Sigmoidoscope
d. Ophthalmoscope

41. During discharge teaching a patient with depression, the psychiatric nurse informed him to avoid foods containing tyramine—such as cheese, milk, wine, preserved meats and avocados—to prevent a hypertensive crisis. Which class of antidepressant drugs are prescribed to the patient?

a. Selective serotonin reuptake inhibitors
b. Tricyclic antidepressants
c. Selective norepinephrine reuptake inhibitors
d. Monoamine oxidase inhibitors

42. A nurse is going to administer ear drops to a 30-year-old patient suffering from otitis media. The most appropriate method to administer the ear drops to this patient is by:

a. Separating the palpebral fissures with a clean gauze pad
b. Pulling the pinna up and back
c. Pulling the tragus up and back
d. Pulling the pinna down and back

43. Given below is an ECG of a patient with chest pain due to ischemic heart disease. The ECG shows:

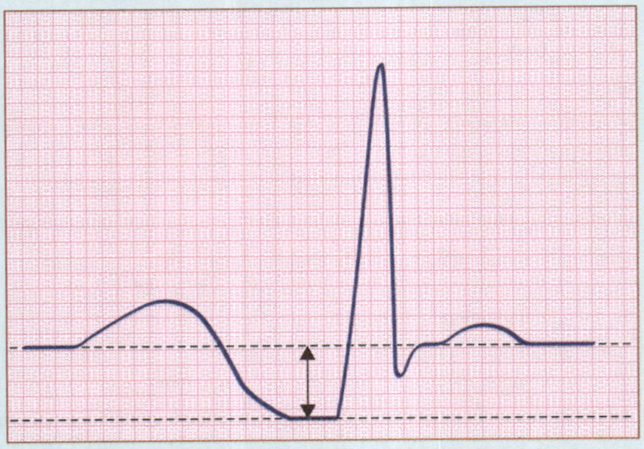

a. T-wave inversion
b. Increased PR Interval
c. ST depression
d. Increased QRS interval

44. Acid fast staining used in the below slide showing mycobacterium tuberculi is named:

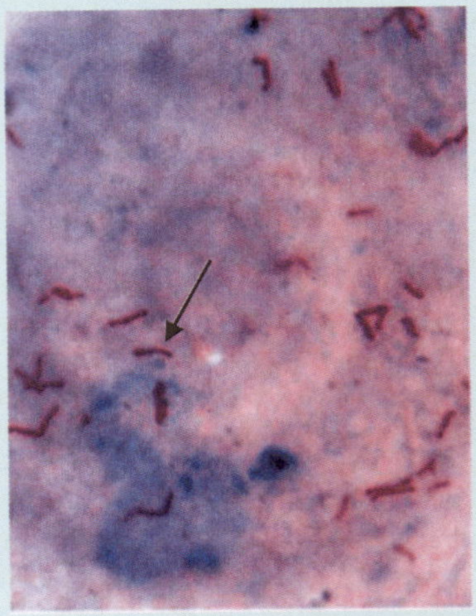

a. Gram staining
b. Albert's staining
c. Giemsa staining
d. Ziehl-Neelsen staining

45. A normal man marries a woman with color blindness. Their children would be:

a. Color blind sons and carrier daughters
b. Normal daughters and normal sons
c. Normal sons and carrier daughters
d. Color blind daughters and carrier sons

46. During a home visit by a community health nurse, a middle-aged woman reported to the nurse that she has had weakness, fatigue, dyspnea and headache for the past three months. On physical examination, the nurse noted spoon-shaped fingernails and a heart rate of 120/minute. Based on these findings, the nurse documented that the woman may have.

a. Folic acid deficiency anaemia
b. Aplastic anaemia
c. Iron deficiency anaemia
d. Hemolytic anaemia

47. Identify the larva of the mosquito shown in the given picture.

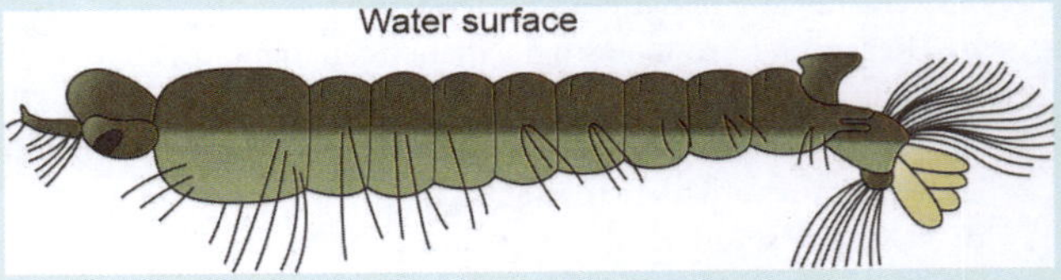

a. Mansonia
b. Aedes
c. Anopheles
d. Culex

48. Patient X came to the emergency department with a history of road traffic accidents. The triage nurse assessed the patient and shifted him to the red area. During the assessment, she found that the patient had fractured a segment sinking into the chest with inspiration and expanding of the chest wall with expiration, opposite the normal chest wall mechanics. Which of the following abnormalities would have been noted by the nurse and what would this abnormality indicate?

a. Pectus carinatum; chest trauma
b. Barrel chest; rib fracture
c. Pectus excavatum; chest trauma
d. Flail chest; rib fracture

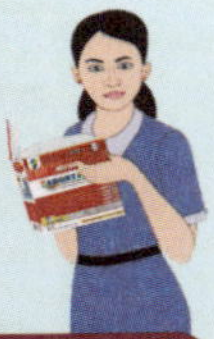

Ans.

40.	d
41.	d
42.	b
43.	b
44.	d
45.	a
46.	c
47.	c
48.	d

49. The first drug of choice to treat an anaphylactic reaction is:

a. Corticosteroids
b. Epinephrine
c. Antihistamines
d. Bronchodilator

50. To use a t-test, the dependent variable must have:

a. Nominal or interval data
b. Interval or ratio data
c. Ordinal or interval data
d. Ordinal or ratio data

51. According to the biomedical waste management of India, category 1 of waste, including human anatomical waste, should be disposed by:

a. Disposal in municipal landfill
b. Disinfection by chemical treatment
c. Incineration
d. Local autoclaving

52. When ventilation exceeds perfusion, it leads to which of the following?

a. Dead space
b. Silent unit
c. Pneumothorax
d. Shunt

53. Glomerulonephritis is a kidney disorder that affects the glomeruli. It is usually characterized by edema, hypertension and:

a. WBC in urine
b. Dysuria
c. Polydipsia
d. Hematuria

54. A problem-based learning is student centred learning strategy in which students collaboratively solve the problems and this reflects on their experience. One important component is:

a. Presentation of real-world situation or problem from ordinary life
b. Focus the educational program
c. Careful inspection of methods
d. Flexible approaches to learning

55. The blood groups in individuals are different due to the specific:

a. Antigens on the surface of WBCs
b. Antibodies on the surface of WBCs
c. Antigens on the surface of RBCs
d. Antibodies on the surface of RBCs

56. Benzimidazole used in treatment of parasitic infections is :

a. An antifungal drug
b. None of the given option
c. A broad-spectrum antibiotic
d. A broad-spectrum anthelmintics

57. Which of the following is an important principle of delegation?

a. Delegation is the same as work allocation
b. No transfer of authority exists when delegating
c. When delegating, you must transfer authority
d. Responsibility is not transferred with delegation

58. Which of the following statements is incorrect with respect to portal vein?

a. Portal blood is rich in nutrients.
b. Portal blood is rich in oxygen.
c. Portal blood comes from the gastrointestinal system.
d. Portal circulation constitutes 80% of the circulation to the liver.

59. A patient with COAD has to be put on oxygen using a face mask. Identify the type of mask shown in the picture below.

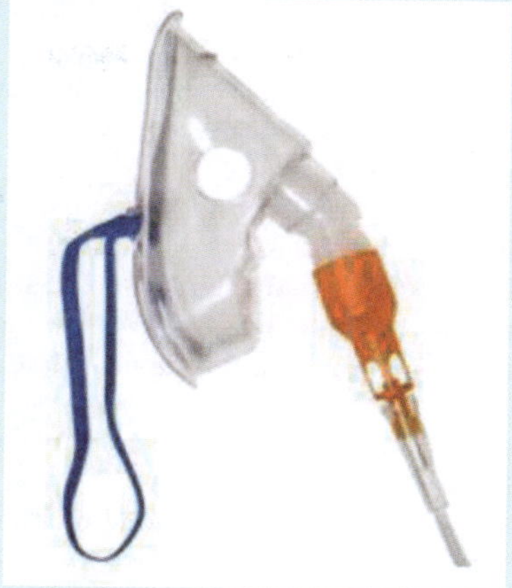

a. CPAP mask
b. Simple face mask
c. Face mask with reservoir bag
d. Venturi mask

60. Water hammer pulse is seen in:

a. Mitral stenosis
b. Left ventricular failure
c. Aortic stenosis
d. Aortic regurgitation

61. Doctors and nurses, who are in direct contact with patients and their relatives, have opportunities for much individual health education. What is the biggest advantage of individual health education?

a. It depends upon the personality and reputation of the speaker.
b. It can be costly and time consuming.
c. We can discuss, argue and persuade the individual to change his behavior.
d. It is very useful in reaching large number of people

62. The lab report of a patient is detailed below:

pH	7.12
HCO3-	1mmol/L
PCO_2	18mm Hg

Which of the following is the primary acid base disorder?

a. Metabolic alkalosis
b. Metabolic acidosis
c. Respiratory alkalosis
d. Respiratory acidosis

63. Which of the following is a stage in the stages of change model?

a. Deliberation
b. Meditation
c. Study
d. Contemplation

64. A 54-year-old man presented in the emergency department with polyphagia and polydipsia. He also complained of headaches, malaise and some visual changes. The assessment showed signs of dehydration and some additional symptoms. The nurse reported to the physician that the patient may have diabetic ketoacidosis. Which of the following additional symptoms might the nurse have noted?

a. Decreased respirations and increased urine output
b. Kussmaul respirations and fruity odor on the breath
c. Cheyne-stokes respirations and foul-smelling urine
d. Biot respirations and severe abdominal pain

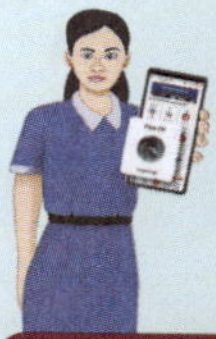

Ans.

49.	b
50.	b
51.	c
52.	a
53.	d
54.	a
55.	c
56.	d
57.	c
58.	b
59.	d
60.	d
61.	c
62.	b
63.	d
64.	b

65. According to WHO, the most cost-effective way to stop the spread of TB in communities with a high incidence is by curing it. The best curative method for TB is known as DOTS. One of its components is:

a. Standardzsed treatment regimen directly of eighteen months observed by a healthcare worker
b. Patients will buy the drugs
c. Case detection by sputum smear microscopy
d. Health for all by 2000 AD

66. A physician has prescribed Tab Atenolol 25 mg for a patient. On assessment the nurse finds that the patient's systolic blood pressure is 90 mmHg. The appropriate nursing action would be:

a. Advise the patient to increase sodium intake
b. Monitor serum potassium levels
c. Administer the drug and continue monitoring the blood pressure
d. Withhold the drug and notify the prescriber

67. The T-wave in ECG represents:

a. Ventricular repolarization
b. Time needed for sinus node stimulation
c. Total time for ventricular depolarization
d. Repolarization of Purkinje fibers

68. A client is admitted with acid attack burns on his face and eyes. The nurse understands that the client has great risk for which of the following complications?

a. Development of glaucoma
b. Bacterial infections
c. Long-term morbidity
d. Contracture

69. While doing bedside rounds, a nurse posted in the pediatric urology ward saw a 5-year-old child. On being asked about the child's medical history, the child's mother said that the child had recently had a streptococcal throat infection. She also reported periorbital and facial edema, decreased urine output and hematuria. The child's blood pressure was 156/98 mm of Hg and lab investigations showed increased blood urea nitrogen level and creatinine level and increased anti-streptolysin O titer. Based on these inputs, what may be the probable diagnosis of the child?

a. Polycystic kidney disease
b. Nephrotic syndrome
c. Glomerulonephritis
d. Hemolytic uremic syndrome

70. The main objective of National Iodine Deficiency Disorders Control Program in India is:

a. Development of guidelines on control
b. Supply of iodized salt in place of common salt
c. Early detection of iodine deficiency
d. Behavior change communication

71. A 30-year-old patient was brought to the emergency department. On examination, the triage nurse noticed that his respiratory rate was 36/ minute, and he had a nonproductive cough. History also revealed that he recently had a cold. After lung auscultation and analysis of examination findings, she suspected the probability of asthma. Which of the following lung auscultation findings suggested that he may have bronchial asthma?

a. Pericardial friction rub
b. Low pitched murmurs
c. Inspiratory and expiratory wheezes
d. Pleural friction rub

72. A patient was brought to the emergency ward with numbness and weakness on one side of his body, slurred speech, difficulty in walking and dizziness. After taking a CT scan, the doctor diagnosed it as an embolic stroke. Which of the following conditions places the client at the risk of a thromboembolic stroke?

a. Atrial fibrillation
b. Guillain-Barré syndrome
c. Multiple sclerosis
d. Bradycardia

73. Which of the following tarsal bones is most commonly fractured?

a. Cuboid bone
b. Navicular bone
c. Talus
d. Calcaneus

74. In India, unsafe drinking water and lack of basic sanitation are the leading causes for:

a. Asthma
b. Respiratory problems
c. Heart disease and diabetes
d. Diarheal diseases and cholera

75. While recording the weight of a 2-year-old boy on the WHO growth chart, a nurse notes that the weight curve is below -2 SD. The nurse interprets this as:

a. Overweight for his age
b. Under nutrition
c. Severely underweight
d. Normal weight for his age

76. A2-year-old child is brought to the pediatric OPD with the complain of failure to thrive. On assessment, the nurse observes that the child weighs less than 35D, as per WHO growth chart, and MUAC (Mid-Upper Arm Circumference) is less than 11 cm. What would the nurse expect for this childs?

a. Moderate acute malnutrition
b. Acute malnutrition
c. Chronic malnutrition
d. Severe acute malnutrition

77. CDC recommends children get two doses of MMR vaccine, starting with the first dose at 12 through 15 months of age, and the second dose at:

a. 4–6 years of age
b. 10–12 years of age
c. 2–3 years of age
d. 6–8 years of age

78. A patient has been received in the emergency department of a hospital with history of head injury. The nurse in the ER makes a quick neurological assessment of the patient using Glasgow Coma Scale. Her assessment findings are shown in the given table. What will you interpret based on the given table?

Name: ABCD **Age:** 28 years **CR no.:** 123456		
Behavior	**Response**	**Score**
Eye opening response	Opens eyes to pain	2
Verbal response	Speaks inappropriate words	3
Motor response	Abnormal flexion is observed	3
Total GCS score		**8**

a. Moderate brain injury
b. No neurological deficit
c. Severe brain injury
d. Mild brain injury

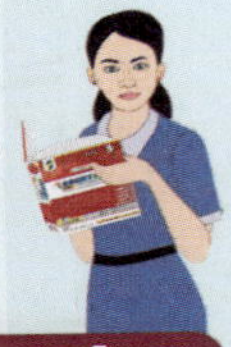

Ans.

65. c
66. d
67. a
68. a
69. c
70. b
71. c
72. a
73. d
74. d
75. b
76. d
77. a
78. c

79. A patient was presented to the pediatric OPD with fever, malaise, coryza, cough and conjunctivitis. There were small red spots with a bluish-white center and a red base located on the buccal mucosa and nurse documented this finding. What are these spots called and what are the spots indicative of?

a. Koplik's spots; diphtheria
b. Brush field spots; measles
c. Bull neck spots; diphtheria
d. Koplik's spots; measles

80. A shortened PR interval, slurring (called a delta wave) of the initial QRS deflection, and prolonged QRS duration are characteristics of:

a. Atrial tachycardia
b. Wolff-Parkinson-White (WPW) syndrome
c. Myocardial ischemia
d. Left bundle branch block

81. The ideal time when the nurse asks the patient to bear down during second stage of labor is:

a. When the fetal head starts to distend the perineum
b. In between the contractions
c. When the patient feels strong
d. When the cervix is fully dilated

82. The leadership style adopted to make crucial decisions that need to be made on the spot, when dealing with inexperienced and new team members and there's no time to wait for team members to gain familiarity with their role, is known as:

a. Democratic b. Participatory
c. Authoritative d. Coaching

83. The part of the colon that absorbs the remaining water and other key nutrients from the indigestible material, solidifying it to form stool is:

a. Ascending colon b. Descending colon
c. Rectum d. Transverse colon

84. Identify the study design given in the picture.

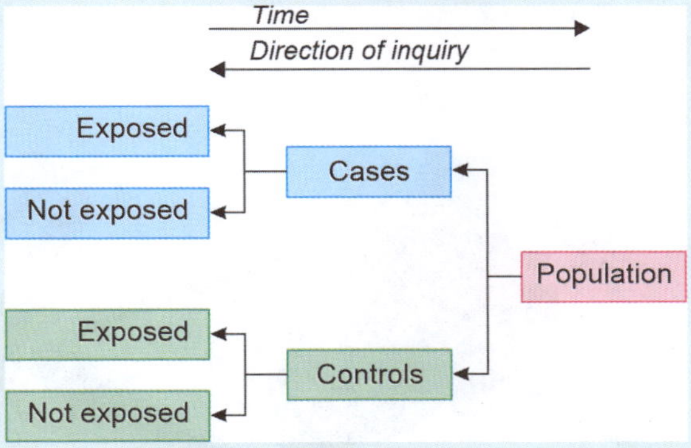

a. Nested case control study
b. Retrospective cohort study
c. Case-control study
d. Prospective cohort study

85. A nurse is headed to work with her friend on a bus. Suddenly, she notices blood coming from her friend's nose. What is the first line of management that the nurse can use in this situation?

a. Do not touch the nose and immediately go to the hospital
b. Pinch the nose with sterile gauze
c. Pinch the nose and move forward
d. Pinch the nose and move backward

86. A woman visits the pediatrics OPD with her 2-year-old toddler with complaints of sudden stoppage of breath in the child initiated by a provocative event. All the following are true about breath holding spells; except:

a. They occur during inspiration
b. Cyanosis may/may not occur
c. They are involuntary
d. Bradycardia may occur

87. A nurse plans to teach a postpartum mother the prevention of breast engorgement. Which of the following measures would the nurse include in her teaching plan?

a. Breastfeed the neonate at regular intervals
b. Decrease the intake of fluid during the first 24 to 48 hours
c. Massage the breast vigorously before feeding
d. Use nipple shields while feeding the neonate

88. A nurse is posted in the pediatric immunization clinic. She notices a child who is very active. He is climbing stairs in the playroom, walking forward and turning pages in a book. Based on these observations, what may be the approximate age of the child?

a. 18–24 months b. 8–10 months
c. 10–12 months d. 6–9 months

89. The leakage of blood backward through the mitral valve each time the left ventricle of the heart contracts, is known as:

a. Mitral regurgitation b. Mitral prolapse
c. Mitral stenosis d. Mitral systole

90. A client has an infection spreading through droplets. The nurse is ready to check the client's temperature. Which of the following should the nurse use to control the spread of infection?

a. Mask b. Goggles
c. Gloves d. Gown

91. The nurse is preparing for the physical examination of a newly admitted client. The assessment tray should contain all the following; except:

a. Sphygmomanometer b. Thermometer
c. Fundoscope d. Stethoscope

92. The Down's syndrome is a congenital chromosome abnormality and is also known as:

a. Trisomy 20 b. Trisomy 18
c. Trisomy 31 d. Trisomy 21

93. There are various techniques that are used to preserve foods and prevent foods from spoiling. Which of the following is the most common and best method?

a. Freeze drying b. Fermentation
c. Freezing d. Heating

94. Infant Mortality Rate (IMR) is the ratio of deaths under 1 year of age to:

a. A rate per 100 live births b. A rate per 1000 live births
c. A rate per 10 live births d. A rate per 10,000 live births

95. A tumour of the adrenal medulla (Pheochromocytoma) is associated with an increased production of which hormone?

a. Glucocorticoids b. Mineralocorticoids
c. Androgen d. Epinephrine

96. The nurse manager compares the actual results of the budget with the projected results of the budget. What budgeting process is this?

a. Controlling b. Incremental budgeting
c. Revenue sharing d. Variable budgeting

Ans.

79. d
80. b
81. a
82. c
83. a
84. c
85. c
86. a
87. a
88. a
89. a
90. a
91. c
92. d
93. d
94. b
95. d
96. a

97. A group of subcortical nuclei within the brain called basal ganglia helps a person perform which of the following important functions?
 a. Unconditional learning b. Emotional behaviors
 c. Involuntary motor activity d. Learning impairment

98. A terminally ill 70-year-old lady has fears of being alone and constantly wants someone near her. Which of the following actions by the nurse would be most appropriate to deal with her loneliness?
 a. Place her near the window so that she can see nature.
 b. Plan to spend more time with her holding her hands and listening to her.
 c. Put on the television in her room and ask her to watch some programs.
 d. Explain her that she has to keep her mind active and focused.

99. A leader can be effective in one circumstance and can be ineffective in another circumstance. This is a leader's ability to adapt, which can be their most important tool in the workplace. This theory of leadership is known as:
 a. Strategic
 b. Democratic
 c. Contingency
 d. Autocratic

100. All of the following are local manifestations of inflammation; except:
 a. Redness
 b. Increased WBC count
 c. Warmth
 d. Pain

Ans.
97. b
98. b
99. c
100. b

"After dinner rest a while; after supper walk a mile."
—T. Cogan

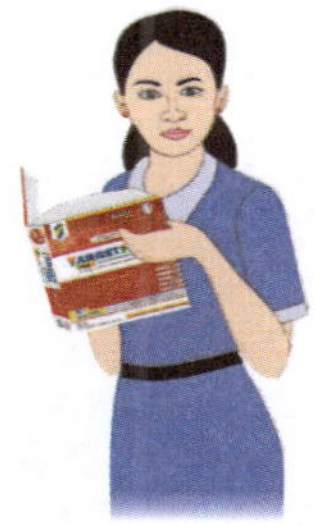

AIIMS, Bibinagar (Tutor) 2023

1. The anatomical structure in foetal circulation that allows the entry of blood from the right atrium to the left atrium is:
a. Umbilical artery b. Foramen ovale
c. Ductus arteriosus d. Ductus venosus

2. The size of bacteria is usually expressed in terms of:
a. Nanometers b. Millimicrons
c. Angstroms d. Micrometers

3. The color code used in the IMNCI case management process for urgent referral is:
a. Red b. Pink
c. Green d. Yellow

4. The structure that prevents atrioventricular valves opening upward into the atria during the ventricular systole is ___________.
a. Papillary muscles b. Chordae tendineae
c. Purkinje fibre d. Intercalated discs

5. Which of the following is NOT an essential function of a family?
a. Transmission of caste system to next generation
b. Regulation of sexual reproduction
c. Teach children to socialize
d. Ensure economic stability

6. A systematic inquiry into principles of right and wrong conduct is known as:
a. Ethics b. Values
c. Law d. Justice

7. ___________ is the type of attention that facilitates an individual to change his focus and attention between two or more stimuli.
a. Divided attention b. Focused attention
c. Selective attention d. Altering attention

8. The type of placenta previa which is known as dangerous placenta previa is:
a. Central placenta previa
b. Type II posterior placenta previa
c. Marginal placenta previa
d. Type II anterior placenta previa

9. The type of joint found between the skull bones is:
a. Cartilaginous joint b. Synovial joint
c. Fibrous joint d. Hinge joint

10. What is the Intelligence Quotient (IQ) of an individual with the mental age of 30 and chronological age of 25?
a. 100 b. 123
c. 83 d. 120

11. The type of programmed instruction in which the learner moves from one frame to another until he completes the program and the responses are controlled by the programmer from a far place is:
a. Intrinsic programming b. Branching programming
c. Linear programming d. Remediation

12. The type of microscope that enables observation of living cells at extremely high magnification and resolution under physiological condition is:
a. Scanning electron microscope
b. Atomic force microscope
c. Compound microscope
d. Transmission electron microscope

13. The hammershaped bone of the middle ear which contacts with the tympanic membrane is:
a. Malleus b. Incus
c. Cochlea d. Stapes

14. Which of the following is NOT a principal component of the integrated practice model of forensic nursing science?
a. Clarification of roles b. Role identification
c. Role expectations d. Role behavior

15. General intelligence theory was described by:
a. Louis Thurstone b. Charles Spearman
c. Jerome Bruner d. Howard Gardner

16. Which of the following is a rich dietary source of Vitamin D?
a. Broccoli b. Oily fish
c. Squid d. Octopus

17. The route of administration in which the drug is rubbed into the skin to get absorbed to produce a systemic effect is:
a. Inunction b. Dermojet
c. Iontophoresis d. Topical application

18. Which of the following etiological factors is associated with post-mature babies?
a. Maternal uterine anomalies
b. Foetal adrenal hyperplasia
c. Anencephaly
d. Maternal low socio-economic status

19. The side effect caused by all statins is:
a. Stroke b. Hypersomnia
c. Myocardial infarction d. Muscle tenderness

20. Which of the following is a plasma-derived chemical mediator of acute inflammation?
a. Histamine b. Prostaglandins
c. Cytokines d. Kinins

21. The factor that delays wound healing is:
a. Young age b. Neutrophilia
c. Increased zinc intake d. Movement of affected area

22. Which of the following is a cause for orthostatic hypotension?
a. Lack of fluid intake b. Peripheral vasoconstriction
c. Fluid loss d. Peripheral vasodilatation

23. Immunization against which of the following maternal infections is a primary prevention measure for mental retardation?
a. Mums b. Rubella
c. Tetanus d. Measles

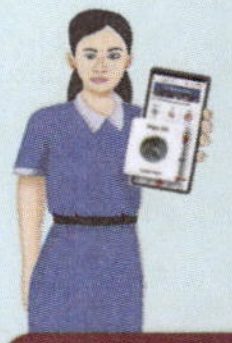

Ans.

1.	b
2.	d
3.	b
4.	b
5.	a
6.	a
7.	d
8.	b
9.	c
10.	d
11.	c
12.	b
13.	a
14.	b
15.	b
16.	b
17.	a
18.	c
19.	d
20.	d
21.	d
22.	d
23.	b

24. The least nephrotoxic drug among aminoglycosides is:
a. Gentamicin b. Kanamycin
c. Neomycin d. Streptomycin

25. Erb's paralysis of a newborn is a result of injury to the:
a. 2nd and 3rd cervical spinal nerves
b. 7th cervical and 1st thoracic spinal nerves
c. 5th and 6th cervical spinal nerves
d. 3rd and 4th cervical spinal nerves

26. The bacteria that can causes acute diarrhoeal disease is:
a. E. hystolytica b. Trichomoniasis
c. Salmonella d. Trichuriasis

27. The stage of General Adaptation Syndrome of stress in which the body begins to repair itself and tries to maintain its equilibrium is:
a. Activation stage b. Resistance stage
c. Alarm stage d. Exhaustion stage

28. The body of legal principles that has evolved from court decisions is known as:
a. Constitutional law b. Statutory law
c. Administrative law d. Common law

29. The investment is considered good if the cost-to-benefit ratio is:
a. >1 b. <1
c. >2 d. 0

30. A formal tentative statement about the expected relationship between two or more variables under the study is:
a. Hypothesis b. Variable
c. Delimitation d. Assumption

31. The structural protein in which the double helix structure of DNA is twisted and wrapped to maintain its heavily coiled three-dimensional shape is:
a. Histones b. Adenine
c. Chromatin d. Nucleotide

32. The initial role of the field forensic epidemiology was investigation related to:
a. Medical misadventures b. Bioterrorism
c. Industrial accidents d. Drug prevention

33. Imipramine, an antidepressant drug, belongs to the classification of:
a. Selective Serotonin Reuptake Inhibitors
b. Atypical antidepressants
c. Dopaminergic antidepressants
d. Tricyclic antidepressants

34. The indication for precordial thump is:
a. Choking b. Hypovolemic shock
c. Pericardial effusion d. Ventricular tachycardia

35. Which of the following is NOT a quality of a professional nurse?
a. Good physical health b. Technical competence
c. Self-belief d. Pessimism

36. The minor disorder that is commonly seen among artificially fed newborn babies is:
a. Erythema toxicum b. Ammonia dermatitis
c. Pathological jaundice d. Atopic dermatitis

37. The most common cause of traveller's diarrhea worldwide and diarrheal disease in children in developing countries is:
a. Rota virus b. Salmonella
c. Shigella dysenteriae d. Escherichia coli

38. The level of measurement that has magnitude, equal interval and an absolute zero point is:
a. Ordinal measurement b. Interval measurement
c. Nominal measurement d. Ratio measurement

39. The form of prostaglandin mainly produced from foetal membrane is:
a. PGD2 b. PGE1
c. PGI2 d. PGF2 α

40. Vertebrae are what kind of bones?
a. Flat bones b. Short bones
c. Sesamoid bones d. Irregular bones

41. An individual believing that he is being malevolently treated is known as:
a. Delusion of jealousy
b. Delusion of persecution
c. Hebephrenic schizophrenia
d. Delusion of grandiosity

42. Which of the following is a clinical feature of complete abortion?
a. Fresh vaginal bleeding b. Bulky uterus
c. Closed cervical OS d. Severe abdominal pain

43. The digestion of carbohydrates takes place mainly in the:
a. Stomach b. Small intestine
c. Large intestine d. Mouth

44. The benefit of job analysis includes the following; except:
a. Determining educational qualification
b. Determining the experience required
c. Determining the skills needed
d. Determining the duties and responsibilities

45. Which of the following is an indication for intra-arterial administration of drugs?
a. Skin and soft tissue infections
b. Local malignancies
c. Rheumatoid arthritis
d. COPD

46. The area between the lungs, occupied by the heart, great vessels, trachea and esophagus is known as:
a. Hilum b. Diaphragm
c. Mediastinum d. Pleural cavity

47. Resistance to which of the following antitubercular drugs is considered multidrug resistant TB?
a. Isoniazid and Rifampicin
b. Pyrazinamide and Ethambutol
c. Isoniazid and Pyrazinamide
d. Rifampicin and Streptomycin

48. Which of the following sets of responses promotes effective problem solving?
a. Low incubation and low cognitive workload
b. Long incubation and low cognitive workload
c. Low incubation and high cognitive workload
d. Long incubation and high cognitive workload

49. Which of the following is a rich dietary source of Vitamin K?
a. Green leafy vegetables b. Fish
c. Egg d. Carrot

50. The stage of group development in which the group members actively discuss and formulate an action plan is:
a. Forming b. Norming
c. Storming d. Performing

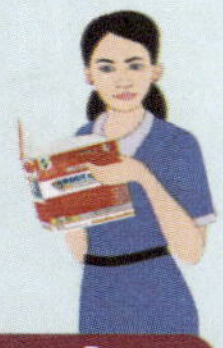

Ans.
24. d
25. c
26. c
27. b
28. d
29. a
30. a
31. a
32. b
33. d
34. d
35. d
36. b
37. d
38. d
39. d
40. d
41. b
42. c
43. b
44. d
45. b
46. c
47. a
48. b
49. a
50. b

51. A planned automation system influences the following in an organization; except:
a. Work efficiency b. Monitoring
c. Cost-effectiveness d. Conflicts

52. Which of the following is NOT a function of state nurses registration council?
a. Accredit nursing institutions
b. Maintenance of the Indian nurses register
c. Prescribe the rules of conduct and take disciplinary action
d. Provide legal protection to the members

53. The goal of palliative care is to:
a. Fasten the cure of the patient
b. Hasten the death of the suffering patient
c. Improve the quality of life of the patient by symptomatic management
d. Increase the longevity of the patient

54. Which of the following is NOT a cause for hypersomnia?
a. Narcolepsy b. Kleine–levin syndrome
c. Sleep apnoea d. Dysthymia

55. Which semi-essential amino acid synthesis is decreased during pregnancy and lactation?
a. Tyrosine b. Tryptophan
c. Arginine d. Methionine

56. The key regulatory enzyme of cholesterol synthesis is:
a. HMG – CoA reductase b. Lanosterol
c. Cyclase d. NADPH

57. Which of the following is associated with decrease in pulse rate?
a. Short and stout physique
b. Tall and slender physique
c. Fever
d. Pain

58. Which of the following is NOT an agency of socialization?
a. Meditation b. Family
c. Mass media d. Peers

59. Which of the following measure is NOT a usual means to prevent hospital-acquired infections?
a. Use of air filtration b. Use of ultraviolet lights
c. Use of PPE d. Use of antibiotics

60. Short scenarios in a written or pictorial form that are intended to elicit responses about people's beliefs and perception are known as:
a. Anecdotes b. Projective technique
c. Vignettes d. Q sorts

61. ________ is the hormone that helps in reabsorption of sodium, chloride and water in the renal tubules to maintain the water balance.
a. Thyroxin b. Aldosterone
c. Growth hormone d. Calcitonin

62. Which of the following is the constituent of Mala N?
a. D–Norgestrel
b. Norethisterone Acetate
c. Gossypol
d. Medroxy Progesterone Acetate

63. Gomez classification system is used in children for the assessment of:
a. Anaemia
b. Protein energy malnutrition
c. Vitamin deficiency
d. Calcium deficiency

64. ________ is the loss of sense of smell.
a. Ageusia b. Achalasia
c. Allele d. Anosmia

65. The pacemaker cells that originate peristaltic contractions of ureters to propel urine from the kidneys to the bladder are located in_________.
a. Detrusor muscles b. Nephrons
c. Major calyces d. Minor calyces

66. Nursing informatics and technological advances result in the following; except:
a. Improved health outcome
b. Improved direct care process
c. Multi-mode communication
d. Complex working pattern

67. Which phase of disaster management involves the development of crisis and emergency response protocol?
a. Prevention phase b. Response phase
c. Preparedness phase d. Recovery phase

68. The process by which individuals and groups are ranked in a more or less enduring hierarchy of status is known as:
a. Social agency b. Social classification
c. Social stratification d. Social mobility

69. The extensor muscle of the elbow joint is/are called:
a. Biceps b. Triceps
c. Brachialis d. Teres minor

70. Which of the following can cause secondary osteoporosis?
a. Oral corticosteroids b. Menopause
c. Increasing age d. Estrogen supplementation

71. Which of the following is NOT an integral component of nursing informatics?
a. Information science b. Forensic science
c. Nursing science d. Computer science

72. The most common symptom of peptic ulcer is:
a. Increased appetite
b. Abdominal pain with burning sensation
c. Weight gain
d. Dysphagia

73. Which of the following acts as a competitive inhibitor of Xanthine oxidase and used in the treatment of gout?
a. Malonate b. Iodoacetamide
c. Succinate d. Allopurinol

74. ________ is a type of turn used in the application of bandage to the body parts that are not uniform in circumference.
a. Figure of eight b. Reverse spiral turn
c. Spiral turn d. Circular turn

75. The ethical theory that defines ethical behavior as acts that assure the greatest possible good for the greatest number of individuals is:
a. Ethical relativism b. Utilitarianism
c. Egoism d. Ethical formalism

76. _________ is the value that is acceptable by people in a civilized society and helps to choose the right way for a healthy society.
a. Spiritual value b. Ethical value
c. Social value d. Moral value

77. The joints seen in cardiac muscles that help in spreading impulses from one cell to another are known as:
a. Intercalated discs b. Purkinje fibres
c. Chordae tendineae d. Fibrous skeleton

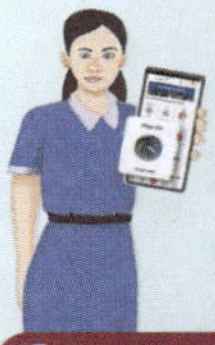

Ans.

Q.	Ans
51.	d
52.	b
53.	c
54.	d
55.	c
56.	a
57.	b
58.	a
59.	d
60.	c
61.	b
62.	b
63.	b
64.	d
65.	d
66.	d
67.	c
68.	c
69.	b
70.	a
71.	b
72.	b
73.	d
74.	b
75.	b
76.	d
77.	a

78. The lipoprotein formed from the monoglycerides and fatty acids that are absorbed into the blood stream is:
a. Micelles b. Diglycerides
c. Chylomicron d. Glycolipids

79. Which of the following is NOT a component of Hayem's fluid used in RBC estimation?
a. Mercuric chloride b. Sodium sulfate
c. NaCl d. Acetic acid

80. The intake of which of the following foods should be limited for a person on a low potassium diet?
a. Strawberry b. Apple
c. Cucumber d. Potato

81. The type of breech presentation that is common among primigravida mothers is:
a. Knee presentation b. Footling presentation
c. Flexed breech d. Frank breech

82. The school of philosophy where there is a blend or synthesis of diverse philosophy is:
a. Eclecticism b. Essentialism
c. Progressivism d. Pragmatism

83. The part of the ear that helps in maintaining balance is:
a. Vestibule b. Middle ear
c. Cochlea d. Tympanic cavity

84. A brief description about the content of the literature and evaluative comments about its usefulness is known as:
a. Abstract b. Bibliography
c. Citation d. Annotation

85. ___________ is an approach that facilitates a solution for a disagreement.
a. Accommodation b. Conflict resolution
c. Collaboration d. Compromising

86. There are _____ parathyroid glands present in a human being.
a. 4 b. 3
c. 6 d. 2

87. The concept of cultural lag was introduced by:
a. Auguste Comte b. Carl Rogers
c. Max Weber d. William F Ogburn

88. The type of nursing audit which monitors finance, nursing service, medical records and environment is:
a. Outcome audit b. Process audit
c. Financial audit d. Structure audit

89. A formal system designed to provide timely and necessary information to planners for making decisions is:
a. Records and Reports
b. Management information System
c. Health Information System
d. Surveillance

90. The metabolism of a drug during its passage from the site of absorption to systemic circulation is known as:
a. Bio availability b. First pass effect
c. Bio equivalence d. Auto induction

91. Select the most appropriate meaning of the given proverb: 'Too many cooks spoil the broth.'
a. When many cooks work together, the food is delicious
b. A job gets done quickly when there are more people to help
c. A job is not done well when too many people are involved
d. Some dishes can be cooked well only by expert cooks

92. Select the most appropriate option to fill in the blank.
She went ____bed late yesterday night.
a. On b. In
c. For d. To

93. Select the most appropriate option to fill in the blanks.
Northern Florida is cold in January, and I walk fast for _______ but also because, although the neighbourhood is antique, it is not ________ safe.
a. Exercise; luckily b. Warmth; perfectly
c. Habit; unusually d. Comfort; deliberately

94. Select the most appropriate option to fill in the blanks.
Hugo told me once that fall was his _______ time of the year. He told me to hold leaves as ______ as you would a pretty girl's hand.
a. Precious; quietly b. Delighted; softly
c. Favorite; delicately d. Enjoyable; sternly

95. Select the most appropriate synonym of the given word: Demure.
a. Perfect b. Timid
c. Buoyant d. Attractive

96. Select the most appropriate meaning of the given idiom: In one's true colors.
a. As a person really is b. In a disguise
c. As one pretends to be d. In a happy mood

97. Sentences of a paragraph are given below in jumbled order. Arrange the sentences in the correct order to form a meaningful and coherent paragraph.
A. An artist once discovered a valuable possibility in this street.
B. In a little district west of Washington Square, the streets have run crazy and broken themselves into small strips called 'places'.
C. One street crosses itself a time or two.
D. These 'places' make strange angles and curves.
a. BADC b. BCDA
c. BACD d. BDCA

98. Select the most appropriate option to fill in the blank.
His gym equipment _____ a lot of room.
a. Takes up b. Takes away
c. Takes off d. Takes in

99. Select the most appropriate ANTONYM of the given word: Agile.
a. Energetic b. Humble
c. Brisk d. Sluggish

100. Sentences of a paragraph are given below in jumbled order. Arrange the sentences in the correct order to form a meaningful and coherent paragraph.
A. Vidyavan reached home and asked his father if he liked the precious jewel he sent through Lakshapathi.
B. Much to his surprise, his father said that he did not receive any gift.
C. But he hadn't mentioned anything about the jewel.
D. The old man (Vidyavan's father) then said that Lakshapathi had come to see him and also informed him that his son (Vidyavan) was happy in Magadha.
a. ABDC b. ACBD
c. ADCB d. ABCD

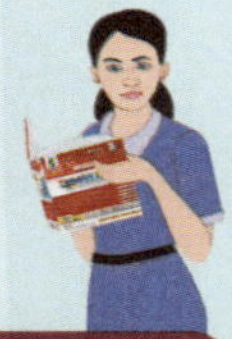

Ans.
78. c
79. d
80. d
81. d
82. a
83. a
84. d
85. b
86. a
87. d
88. d
89. b
90. b
91. c
92. d
93. b
94. c
95. b
96. a
97. d
98. a
99. d
100. a

"Sometimes the remedy is worse than the disease."
—Francis Bacon

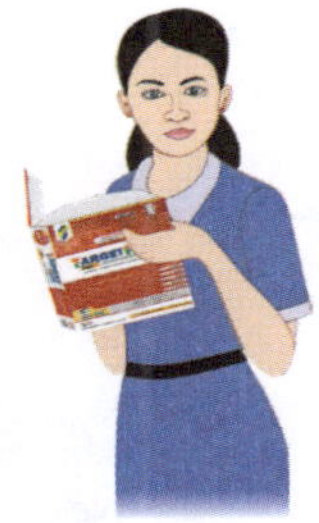

AIIMS, Bibinagar Associate Professor 2023

1. Which of the following is a common disorder for a child with Cushing syndrome?
a. Respiratory acidosis
b. Metabolic alkalosis
c. Metabolic acidosis
d. Respiratory alkalosis

2. All of the following statements are true about SIADH lab values; except:
a. SIADH cause increased urine osmolarity
b. SIADH cause elevated urine sodium concentration
c. SIADH cause decreased plasma osmolarity
d. SIADH cause increased plasma osmolarity

3. What is the diagnosis code of dual-role transvestism in ICD-10?
a. F 64.3
b. F 64.2
c. F 64.0
d. F 64.1

4. Self-care deficit theory was developed by:
a. Betty Neuman
b. Florence Nightingale
c. Virginia Henderson
d. Dorothea Elizabeth Orem

5. Maternal administration of magnesium sulfate for longer than 5-7 days during pregnancy leads to:
a. Fetal hypocalcemia
b. Fetal hypokalemia
c. Maternal hypertension
d. Maternal seizures

6. Which of the following is an important role of a nurse in milieu therapy?
a. Helps in attitude therapy
b. Helps in assisting ECT or other brain stimulation therapy
c. Helps to manage the environment
d. Helps in assisting Eye Movement Desensitization and Reprocessing (EMDR) therapy

7. Intracranial herniation that occurs when brain tissue is displaced under the falx cerebri is called:
a. Uncal herniation
b. Subfalcine herniation
c. Disk herniation
d. Inguinal herniation

8. Which of the following is a FALSE statement regarding Ayushman Bharat?
a. Only two members in a family are eligible for this scheme
b. It is the world's largest health insurance/assurance scheme fully financed by the government
c. It provides a cover of ₹5 lakh per family per year for secondary and tertiary care hospitalization across public and private empanelled hospitals in India
d. It covers up to 3 days of prehospitalization and 15 days posthospitalisation expenses such as diagnostics and medicines

9. Which of the following tests is used to detect deep vein thrombosis?
a. D-dimer tests
b. Immunosorbent assay
c. ELISA test
d. WIDAL test

10. Arteriovenous malformation causes pain, bleeding or ulcers in which stage of Schöbinger staging system?
a. Stage I (quiescence)
b. Stage III (destruction)
c. Stage II (expansion)
d. Stage IV (decompensation)

11. Which of the following is the main cause of hypercalcemia?
a. Decreased parathyroid hormone (PTH)
b. Decreased antidiuretic hormone (ADH)
c. Increased antidiuretic hormone (ADH)
d. Increased parathyroid hormone (PTH)

12. A planned learning experience provided by employing an agency for the improvement of employees is known as:
a. Career planning
b. Democratic management
c. In-service education
d. Job description

13. Which type of leadership style is the least intrusive and ensures that the decision-making authority lies with the team members?
a. Democratic leadership
b. Strategic leadership
c. Autocratic leadership
d. Laissez-faire leadership

14. Ankylosing spondylitis leads to:
a. Inflammation of the spine
b. Inflammation of the sacrum
c. Inflammation of the coccyx
d. Inflammation of the xiphisternum

15. Ms. Pavithra, a full term primigravida mother with labor pain got admitted for safe confinement. On PV examination it was revealed that small part of the head was below the brim of the pelvis and could be lifted out of the pelvis with a deep pelvic grip. What was the descent and engagement of the foetal head?
a. 3/5
b. 4/5
c. 2/5
d. 1/5

16. Which of the following is NOT a cause of Systemic Lupus Erythematosus (SLE)?
a. Vitamin deficiency
b. Immunological factor
c. Environmental factor
d. Genetic factor

17. Which of the following is a multi-dimensional pain assessment tool with three main components as sensory intensity, the cognitive evaluation of pain and the emotional impact of pain?
a. Visual Analogue Scale (VAS)
b. McGill Pain Questionnaire (MPQ)
c. FLACC scale
d. Numeric Rating Scale (NRS)

18. All of the following are the advantages of a Gantt chart; except:
a. Helps to unsplit the activities by status of the task
b. Helps to schedule the tasks with start date and end date
c. Helps to understand the percentage of work or tasks remaining
d. Helps to understand the percentage of task completion

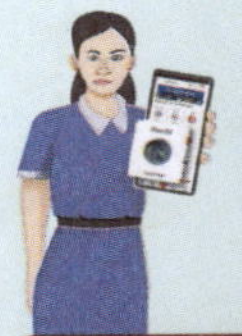

Ans.

1. b
2. d
3. d
4. d
5. a
6. c
7. b
8. a
9. a
10. b
11. d
12. c
13. d
14. a
15. b
16. a
17. b
18. a

19. Which one of the following is the preferred site for thoracentesis procedure performed in the upright or seated position?
- a. Posterior mid-scapular line
- b. Posterior mid-clavicular line
- c. Midaxillary line
- d. Near the 6th rib

20. Failure to develop the caudal end of the neural tube resulting in a protrusion with cerebrospinal fluid, meninges, overlying skin, and not having the spinal cord as its content is called:
- a. Meningocele
- b. Macrocephaly
- c. Hydrocephalus
- d. Cephalohematoma

21. What is osteoclast?
- a. Cells that absorb new bone
- b. Cells that make new bone
- c. Cells that make old bone
- d. Cells that absorb old bone

22. Which of the following kidney stones are very rare and occur due to an inborn congenital disorder?
- a. Calcium oxalate stones
- b. Struvite stones
- c. Cystine stones
- d. Uric acid stones

23. What is the recommended energy levels used to perform synchronized cardioversion?
- a. 50–200 joules
- b. 100–400 joules
- c. 10–30 joules
- d. 30–60 joules

24. All of the following are the symptoms of bulbar palsy, except:
- a. Dysphonia
- b. Drooling
- c. Dysphagia
- d. Dyspnea

25. Which of the following is a true statement regarding Mann Whitney U test?
- a. It is a nonparametric test to compare outcomes between two dependent groups.
- b. It is a parametric test to compare outcomes between two independent groups.
- c. It is a parametric test to compare outcomes between two dependent groups.
- d. It is a nonparametric test to compare outcomes between two independent groups.

26. Chorionic villus sampling (CVS) is a diagnostic test used to detect:
- a. Edward's syndrome
- b. Cystic fibrosis
- c. Neural tube defect
- d. Cardiac abnormality

27. Which of the following clinical teaching methods is defined as a written record of an interaction between a nurse and a client?
- a. Nursing rounds
- b. Nursing care conference
- c. Case presentation
- d. Process recording

28. HLA typing is also known as:
- a. Blood bonding
- b. Tissue typing
- c. Organ matching
- d. Cross matching

29. What is the main purpose of Spearman's Rank correlation coefficient technique?
- a. Used for quantitative data
- b. To determine the setting of study
- c. To determine study population and sample size
- d. To summarize the strength and direction of a relationship between two variables.

30. Cancer that form in bones and soft tissues, including muscle, fat, blood vessels, lymph vessels, and fibrous tissue is called:
- a. Leukemia
- b. Sarcoma
- c. Melanoma
- d. Carcinoma

31. Which chemotherapeutic drug is essential to maintain the topology of the DNA?
- a. Topoisomerase inhibitor
- b. Monoclonal antibodies
- c. Antitumor antibiotics
- d. Alkylating agents (or) DNA-damaging agents

32. Which of the following is the main goal of pilot study?
- a. To assess feasibility
- b. To check the study population
- c. To assess the variables
- d. To test hypotheses about the effects of an intervention

33. What is POSDCORB in nursing management?
- a. Planning, Organizing, Staffing, Developing, Coordinating, Recording and Bargaining
- b. Planning, Organizing, Staffing, Directing, Coordinating, Reporting and Budgeting
- c. Preparing, Orientation, Staff, Delegation, Communication, Recording and Budgeting
- d. Planning, Orientation, Staff, Delegation, Communication, Recording and Balancing

34. According to Marie Jahoda, all of the following statements are correct regarding ideal mental health; except:
- a. Capability for growth and development
- b. Accurate perception of reality
- c. Dependence on each other
- d. Positive view of self

35. How many muscle tendons connect to the shoulder to make up the rotator cuff muscle?
- a. Five
- b. Two
- c. Four
- d. Three

36. A type of brain injury that is common among people who drink a lot of alcohol is:
- a. Brain aneurysm
- b. Wernicke encephalopathy
- c. Carbon monoxide poisoning
- d. Anoxic brain injury

37. Which of the following parasitic organism causes hydatid cyst of the liver?
- a. Trichomonas
- b. *Echinococcus granulosus*
- c. Toxocara canis
- d. Trichinella spiralis

38. A field of nursing that extends and expands the boundaries of nursing's scope of practice, contributes to nursing knowledge, and promotes the advancement of the profession is known as:
- a. Distance learning
- b. Continuing nursing education
- c. In-service education
- d. Advanced nursing practice

39. What is the normal central venous pressure?
- a. 8–12 mm Hg
- b. 2–6 mm Hg
- c. 10–16 mm Hg
- d. 4–8 mm Hg

40. The integration of best research evidence with the best available scientific research, clinical expertise and patient values is known as:
- a. Advanced nursing practice
- b. Effective management
- c. Nursing administration
- d. Evidence-based practice

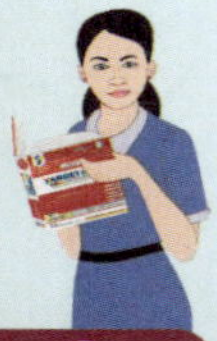

Ans.

19.	a
20.	a
21.	d
22.	c
23.	a
24.	d
25.	d
26.	a
27.	d
28.	b
29.	d
30.	b
31.	a
32.	a
33.	b
34.	c
35.	c
36.	b
37.	b
38.	d
39.	a
40.	d

41. Percutaneous coronary intervention (PCI) is also known as:
a. Angiogram
b. Maze surgery
c. Angioplasty with stent
d. Coronary artery bypass graft (CABG)

42. Miss Geetha, a 26-year-old woman got admitted in emergency ward and diagnosed as third-degree burns with interrupted skin barrier, lead to which of the following complication?
a. Obstructive shock b. Distributive shock
c. Hypovolemic shock d. Cardiogenic shock

43. Abnormal insertion of umbilical cord on the edge of the placenta along with the chorioamniotic membrane is known as:
a. Vasa previa b. Velamentous placenta
c. Placenta fenestrata d. Battledore placenta

44. What is PDCA model in quality assurance?
a. Planning, Doing, Checking and Acting
b. Preparation, Documentation, Case Analysis and Applying
c. Planning, Doing, Clarifying, and Assuring
d. Preparation, Documentation, Checking, and Applying

45. Which of the following diets is recommended for patients who have undergone peritoneal dialysis?
a. High sodium diet b. High calcium diet
c. High calorie diet d. High potassium diet

46. When the body's immune system mistakenly attacks the peripheral nerves in the body, it is known as:
a. Carpal tunnel syndrome
b. Meralgiaparesthetica
c. Galloway mowat syndrome
d. Guillain-Barré syndrome

47. What does the word 'N' denote in TNM classification of cancer?
a. Number of nearby organs that have cancer
b. Number of nearby tumours
c. Not knowing the exact location of cancer
d. Number of nearby lymph nodes that have cancer

48. Removal of excess skin and fat from the eyelids is called:
a. Phacoemulsification
b. Lasik eye surgery
c. Argon laser trabeculoplasty (ALT)
d. Blepharoplasty

49. In which year was IMNCI implemented in India?
a. 2018 b. 2003
c. 2013 d. 1993

50. Which of the following is a Quasi-experimental design with control groups?
a. One Group Post-test-Only Design
b. Post-test-Only Design with Nonequivalent Groups
c. The One-Group Pre-test-Post-test Design using a Non-equivalent Dependent Variable
d. One-Group Pre-test-Post-test Design

51. According to Tamil Nadu Nurses and Midwives Council, how many credit hours is mandatory for license renewal?
a. 50 hours b. 150 hours
c. 100 hours d. 200 hours

52. In cyanotic congenital cardiac defects, which of the following is called left heart obstructive lesions?
a. Tricuspid atresia b. Critical aortic stenosis
c. Tetralogy of Fallot d. Critical pulmonary stenosis

53. Which of the following statements is FALSE regarding electrolytes?
a. Balances your body's acid/base (pH) level
b. Moves nutrients into your cells
c. Helps in blood production
d. Balances the amount of water in your body

54. When was the National AIDS Control Programme Phase IV (NACP-IV) launched?
a. 2002–2007 b. 2012–2017
c. 2017–2022 d. 2007–2012

55. Which of the following disorders is NOT a category of psychosis?
a. Hallucination
b. Disorganized behavior
c. Phobia
d. Delusion

56. All of the following are the causes of lower GI bleeding; except:
a. Inflammatory bowel disease
b. Diverticular disease
c. Proctitis
d. Peptic ulcer

57. What is PET process in evidence-based practice?
a. Practicability, empirical, and technical
b. Practice question, explanation, and translation
c. Practice question, evaluation, and termination
d. Practice question, evidence, and translation

58. Which of the following is NOT a type of attitude scale?
a. Guttman scale b. Q-sort scale
c. Thurstone scale d. Likert scale

59. An incision made on each side of the scrotum to reach the vas deferens in vasectomy procedure is called:
a. No-scalpel vasectomy
b. Conventional vasectomy
c. Scalpel vasectomy
d. Non-conventional vasectomy

60. Esophageal varices is most common in patients with:
a. Gastroesophageal reflux disease (GERD)
b. Liver disease
c. Tracheaoesophageal fistula
d. Kidney disease

61. Which of the following is NOT a possible cause of malabsorption syndrome?
a. Celiac disease b. Crohn's disease
c. Hydrocele d. Cystic fibrosis

62. Geetha, a 6-year-old girl had severe diarrhea and her body lost too much of sodium bicarbonate. This led to:
a. Hyperchloremic acidosis
b. Calcemic acidosis
c. Diabetic ketoacidosis
d. Lactic acidosis

63. When does acute rejection occur?
a. Any time from the first week after the transplant to 3 months afterward
b. Any time from the sixth month after the transplant to 9 months afterward
c. Any time from 3 months after the transplant to 6 months afterward
d. Can take place over many years

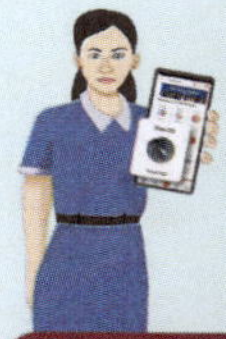

Ans.

41. c
42. c
43. b
44. a
45. c
46. d
47. d
48. d
49. b
50. b
51. b
52. b
53. c
54. b
55. c
56. d
57. d
58. b
59. b
60. b
61. c
62. a
63. a

64. The acronym FAST is used to assess stroke. What is FAST?
a. Face, Arm, Speech, Time
b. Fast, Arrival, Steady, Time
c. Face, Assess Reflex, Smart, Treatment
d. Fast, Act, Sit, Treatment

65. Which type of analgesics are commonly used in ICU?
a. NSAID
b. Antiepileptic drugs
c. Non-opioid analgesics
d. Opioid analgesics

66. A type of blood cancer that affects the plasma cells in bone marrow is called:
a. Lymph adenoma
b. Multiple myeloma
c. Lymphoma
d. Leukemia

67. What is hypophosphatemia?
a. Serum phosphate is 10 mg/dL
b. Serum phosphate less than 2.5 mg/dL
c. Serum phosphate is 7 mg/dL
d. Serum phosphate is 12 mg/dL

68. The classic sign of duodenal atresia in USG finding is:
a. Seashore sign
b. Cracked pot sign
c. Double bubble sign
d. Curtain sign

69. Which of the following is the main cause of Meckel's diverticulum?
a. Vitelline duct of the growing fetus is not fully absorbed during pregnancy.
b. Neural tube of the growing fetus is not fully absorbed during pregnancy.
c. Notochord of the growing fetus is not fully absorbed during pregnancy.
d. Umbilical cord of the growing fetus is not fully absorbed during pregnancy.

70. All of the following are the causative organisms of urethritis, except:
a. *Taenia solium*
b. *Mycoplasma genitalium*
c. *Neisseria gonorrhoea*
d. *Chlamydia trachomatis*

71. What is a systematic process of collecting information related to a specific job called?
a. Rating scale
b. Q-sort technique
c. Job description
d. Job analysis

72. Karthik, a 2-year old boy got admitted. After physical examination the nurse finds that the child has protruded abdomen, visible ribs, head seems larger than body, very little hair, very weak, wrinkled skin and looks like an old man in appearance. What is the probable diagnosis?
a. Congenital abnormality
b. Severe dehydration
c. Crohn's disease
d. Marasmus

73. In which phase of microteaching does the teacher get trained on the skills and components of teaching through lectures, discussion, illustration, and demonstration of the skill by experts?
a. Transfer phase
b. Evaluation phase
c. Skill acquisition phase
d. Knowledge acquisition phase

74. Which of the following is not a type of gastric analysis?
a. Antibody Antigen Test
b. Augment Histamine Test Meal
c. Penta-gastrin Stimulation Test
d. Fractional Test Meal

75. Which of the following is called galactokinetic hormone?
a. Progesterone
b. Human chorionic gonadotropin (hCG)
c. Prolactin
d. Estrogen

76. Which type of patient classification system describes different patient care levels in general terms, such as 'Minimum, Moderate, or Maximum care'?
a. Prototype
b. Care interaction
c. Case study
d. Summative task

77. All of the following are the complications of leptospirosis; except:
a Meningitis
b. Renal failure
c. Spina bifida
d. Liver failure

78. In Vincent's infection, ulceration is commonly present in the:
a. Stomach
b. Bronchus
c. Palate
d. Esophagus

79. In which year RNTCP was renamed as the National TB Elimination Program (NTEP)?
a. 2015
b. 2020
c. 2010
d. 2025

80. Mr Bala was admitted in hospital with complaints of sudden chest pain and shortness of breath. After physical examination the nurse reveals the clinical findings as hyperresonance of chest during percussion. What is the diagnosis of the patient?
a. Lung cancer
b. Pneumothorax
c. Atelectasis
d. Hemothorax

81. A type of paroxysmal supraventricular tachycardia that results due to the presence of a re-entry circuit within or adjacent to the AV node is:
a. Atrioventricular Nodal Re-entrant Tachycardia (AVNRT)
b. Wolff–Parkinson–White (WPW) Syndrome
c. Junctional Ectopic Tachycardia (JET)
d. Accelerated Junctional Rhythm and Junctional Tachycardia

82. Which type of MRI visualizes how water molecules pass through parts of the brain during metastasis?
a. Magnetic resonance angiography (MRA)
b. Diffusion tensor imaging
c. Infusion tensor imaging
d. Magnetic resonance venography (MRV)

83. Which one of the following option is false regarding objective structured clinical examination?
a. Inexpensive
b. Safety and availability
c. Uniformity
d. Allows teaching audit

84. Evaluations conducted on behalf of patients who are still undergoing care is called:
a. Retrospective nursing audit
b. Concurrent nursing audit
c. Closed chart audit
d. Prospective nursing audit

85. Medullary Cystic Kidney Disease (MCKD) is an:
a. Autosomal recessive disorder
b. Allosomal dominant disorder
c. Autosomal dominant disorder
d. Allosomal recessive disorder

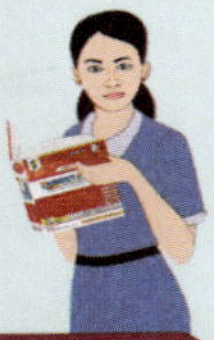

Ans.

64. a
65. d
66. b
67. b
68. c
69. a
70. a
71. d
72. d
73. d
74. a
75. c
76. a
77. c
78. c
79. b
80. b
81. a
82. b
83. a
84. b
85. c

86. A technique used to arrange raw material orders from suppliers based on the production schedules to reduce inventory costs is called:
a. Ved analysis
b. Safety stock inventory management
c. Abc analysis
d. Just in time inventory management

87. All of the following are types of non-probability sampling; except:
a. Cluster
b. Convenience
c. Purposive
d. Snowball

88. All of the following statements are benefits of advanced health; except:
a. Demonstrate incompetence in the written documentation, computer charting and oral presentation of health assessments
b. Appropriately utilize and interpret assessment strategies including: clinical interviewing, physical examination techniques, diagnostic procedures and common laboratory testing in health assessment of individuals
c. Demonstrate sound critical thinking, diagnostic reasoning, and clinical decision-making skills in obtaining, interpreting and integrating health assessments
d. Integrate developmental, socio-cultural, pathophysiological and psychosocial theoretical perspectives with empirical and experiential, practical knowledge for comprehensive health assessment

89. In aortic valve regurgitation, some blood leaks back to which part of the heart?
a. Right ventricle
b. Left atrium
c. Left ventricle
d. Right atrium

90. Chromosomal microarray is also called:
a. Fluorescence in situ hybridization (fish)
b. Amniocentesis
c. Molecular karyotyping
d. Chorionic villus sampling (CVS)

91. How long does the first period of Rapid Eye Movement (REM) sleep last?
a. 10 minutes
b. 15 minutes
c. 20 minutes
d. 5 minutes

92. Necrosis occur on the cells of anterior pituitary gland following significant post-partum bleeding, hypovolemia, and shock is called:
a. Sheehan syndrome
b. Cumming syndrome
c. Zika syndrome
d. Angelman syndrome

93. The three parameters used in MELD score (Model for End-stage Liver Disease) are:
a. Clotting time, glomerular filtration rate, intake and output factor
b. Ldl, hdl and triglycerides
c. Sodium bicarbonate, oxygen saturation, PCO_2
d. Total bilirubin, prothrombin time and creatinine

94. The two principal measures used in item analysis are:
a. Item analysis and item management
b. Item difficulty and item management
c. Item difficulty and item discrimination
d. Item arrangement and item division

95. Which analgesic is commonly used for cancer patients with severe pain?
a. Non-steroidal Anti-inflammatory Drugs (NSAID)
b. Opioid medicine
c. Acetylated salicylates
d. Non-acetylated salicylates

96. Which part of the brain is affected in dyskinetic cerebral palsy?
a. Medulla oblongata
b. Motor cortex
c. Cerebellum
d. Basal ganglia

97. In muscular dystrophy, which of the following proteins gets damaged?
a. Tubulin
b. Pikachurin
c. Myosin
d. Dystrophin

98. Radiation used before surgery to shrink the tumour is called:
a. Radiosensitizer
b. Adjuvant therapy
c. Neoadjuvant therapy
d. Palliative radiation

99. Which of the following is NOT a component of biomechanics?
a. Balance
b. Motion
c. Force
d. Rest

100. Which of the following is an adequate level of vitamin D?
a. 30 nmol/l
b. 50 nmol/l
c. 125 nmol/l
d. 20 nmol/l

Ans.

86. d
87. a
88. a
89. c
90. c
91. a
92. a
93. d
94. c
95. b
96. d
97. d
98. c
99. d
100. b

"He who has health has hope; and he who has hope has everything."
—Arabian proverb

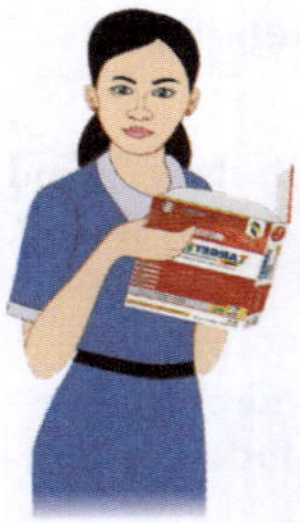

Sree Chitra Tirunal Institute for Medical Science and Technology (NO) 2023

1. The nurses are participating in a health fair at the local mall and are giving influenza vaccine to senior citizens. What level of prevention are the nurses practicing?
a. Primary prevention
b. Secondary prevention
c. Tertiary prevention
d. Quaternary prevention

2. Nursing care provided that is supported by reliable research is known as:
a. Evidence-based practice
b. Theory-based practice
c. Knowledge-based practice
d. Historical practice

3. Who decreased mortality by improving sanitation in the battlefields, resulting in a decrease of illness and infection?
a. Florence Nightingale
b. Clara Barton
c. Dorothea Dix
d. Lillian Wald

4. Which of the following are the four basic techniques of physical examination?
a. Interview, inspection, percussion, resonance
b. Inspection, palpation, percussion, auscultation
c. Interview, subjective data, objective data, closure
d. Inspection, palpation, percussion, tapping

5. Which of the following terms denotes patient's inability to void even though the kidneys are producing urine that enters the bladder?
a. Urgency
b. Retention
c. Oliguria
d. Dysuria

6. Cheyne-Stokes respiration describes:
a. Rapid breathing
b. Difficult breathing
c. Moist or stertorous breathing
d. Periods of apnea and hyperventilation

7. The angle of insertion for an intramuscular injection is:
a. 90°
b. 30°
c. 160°
d. 180°

8. The purpose of making mitten corners while doing bed making is:
a. To keep bed linen secure
b. To provide warmth
c. To prevent cross infection
d. To prevent foot drop

9. One example of isotonic solution is:
a. 0.9% NaCl
b. 0.45 % NaCl
c. 3% NaCl
d. 5 % NaCl

10. The nurse is preparing to take a pulse on a patient who is receiving digoxin (Lanoxin), which affects the heart rate. This assessment needs to be completed prior to the medication administration. Which skill is correct when assessing the pulse of this patient?
a. A radial pulse taken for 15 seconds.
b. A femoral pulse taken for 15 seconds.
c. A carotid pulse taken for a full minute.
d. An apical pulse taken for a full minute.

11. Supination is:
a. Turn lower arm and hand so palm is down
b. Turn lower arm and hand so palm is up
c. Turn palm toward the inner aspect of forearm
d. Tum fingers position to midline

12. Which of the following is an indication for a binder to be placed around a surgical patient with new abdominal wound?
a. Collection of wound drainage
b. Providing support to abdominal tissues when coughing and walking
c. Reduction of abdominal swelling
d. Stimulation of peristalsis

13. Which of the following is the most effective way to break the chain of infection?
a. Hand hygiene
b. Wearing gloves
c. Placing patients in isolation
d. Providing private rooms for patients

14. When the patient develops dyspnea, what is the first intervention that is to be carried out?
a. Take blood pressure
b. Elevate the foot of the bed
c. Remove pillows from the head
d. Elevate the head of the bed

15. While giving oral medication_____ position is essential to prevent aspiration.
a. High Fowler's
b. Left lateral
c. Sim's
d. Supine

16. The test considered the gold standard to detect COVID-19 is:
a. The reverse transcription-polymerase chain reaction (RTPCR) test
b. Rapid antigen test
c. Cartridge based nucleic acid amplification test
d. Rapid diagnostic test

17. The nurse is giving discharge instructions to a newly diagnosed diabetic. The nurse discusses with the patient what the dietary intake should be. This is an example of which health care service?
a. Illness prevention
b. Restorative care
c. Health promotion
d. Tertiary care

18. The multidisciplinary care model used to move patients efficiently from admission to discharge is callled:
a. Team nursing
b. Nursing process
c. Interdisciplinary care
d. Case management

19. The leading cause of cognitive impairment in old age is:
a. Stroke
b. Malnutrition
c. Alzheimer's disease
d. Loss of cardiac reserve

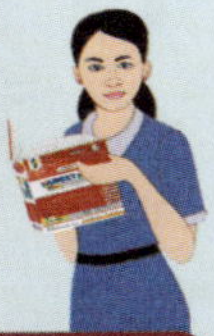

Ans.

1. a
2. a
3. a
4. b
5. b
6. d
7. a
8. a
9. a
10. d
11. b
12. b
13. a
14. d
15. a
16. a
17. c
18. d
19. c

20. A patient needs to learn to use a walker. Which domain is required for learning the skill?
a. Affective domain b. Cognitive domain
c. Attentional domain d. Psychomotor domain

21. The nurse is caring for a patient with pneumonia who has severe malnutrition. The nurse recognizes that, because of the nutrition status, the patient is at increased risk of:
a. Cardiac disease b. Sepsis
c. Diarrhea d. Insomnia

22. An elderly patient comes to the hospital with complaints of severe weakness and diarrhea for several days. It is important to assess which one of the following problems initially?
a. Malnutrition b. Dehydration
c. Skin breakdown d. Incontinence

23. When assessing the lower extremities for arterial function, which intervention should the nurse perform?
a. Assessing the medial malleoli for pitting edema
b. Performing allen's test
c. Assessing the Homans test
d. Palpating the pedal pulses

24. While auscultating the adult patient's lungs, the nurse hears loud, bubble sounds during inspiration that do not disappear after the patient coughs. Which finding should the nurse document from the lung assessment?
a. Rhonchi b. Coarse crackles
c. Sibilant wheeze d. Pleural friction rub

25. A patient's effort to manage psychological s!ress is known as:
a. Secondary appraisal b. Coping
c. Primary appraisal d. Distress

26. The nurse assists a patient in connecting a stressful event with the patient's reaction to the event. This approach is known as:
a. Evaluative care b. Problem solving
c. Situational intervention d. Crisis intervention

27. The normal Potassium level in the blood for adults is:
a. 2–3 mEq/L
b. 2.9–6.2 mEq/L
c. 3.5–5.2 mEq/L
d. 3.4–6.8 mEq/L

28. Before the nurse washes hands when leaving an isolation room, what is the last thing that is removed?
a. Head cover b. Mask
c. Gown d. Goggles

29. To remove a glove that is contaminated, what should the nurse do first?
a. Grasp the outside of the cuff or palm of the glove and pull it away from the hand without touching the wrist or fingers
b. Put the thumb inside the wrist to slide the glove over the hand with minimal touching of the hand by the other gloved hand
c. Pull the glove off the back of the hand until it slides off the entire hand and discard it
d. Rinse the gloves before removing them to minimize the contamination factor.

30. Which one of the following is a common condition that causes numbness, tingling, and pain in the hand and forearm?
a. Carpal tunnel syndrome
b. Tarsal tunnel syndrome
c. Bell's palsy
d. Dystonia

31. Night blindness is caused due to the deficiency of vitamin:
a. A b. D
c. E d. K

32. Which one of the following vitamins is not fat-soluble?
a. A b. D
c. B d. K

33. Which of the following is the most sensitive indicator of changes in neurologic status?
a. Loss of consciousness b. Memory
c. Pain d. Vascular flow

34. Patients with bacterial meningitis demonstrate, which one of the following?
a. Decreased CSF glucose level
b. Increased CSF glucose level
c. Decreased CSF protein level
d. Increased CSF magnesium level

35. Transsphenoidal approach is used in the excision of which type of tumors?
a. Glial tumors b. Pituitary tumors
c. Oligodendrogliomas d. Acoustic neuromas

36. Which of the following is an incorrect match?
a. Dysphagia: inability to speak
b. Hemiparesis: weakness
c. Hemiplegia: paralysis
d. Aphasia: inability to communicate

37. Phenytoin, carbamazepine, and valproate are drugs classified under the category:
a. Neuromuscular blocking agent
b. Antiepileptic drugs
c. Antidepressants
d. Antipsychotic drugs

38. Cholinergic crisis occurs because of over medication in which of the following conditions?
a. Myasthenia gravis
b. Guillain-Barre syndrome
c. Creutzfeldt-Jakob disease
d. Amyotrophic lateral sclerosis

39. One of the primary nursing objectives in a client with a Cerebrovascular accident is maintenance of the airway. To achieve this objective, the nurse should initially place the client in the:
a. Prone position b. Lateral position
c. Supine position d. Trendelenburg position

40. The client diagnosed with atrial fibrillation hasexperienced a transient ischemic attack. Which of the following medication would the nurse anticipate being ordered for client at discharge?
a. An oral anticoagulant medication
b. A beta-blocker medication
c. An antihyperuricemia medication
d. A thrombolytic medication

41. Which one of the following is a primary brain tumor?
a. Cerebral angioma b. Glioma
c. Fibroadenoma d. Wilm's tumor

42. A CT scan of the head shows a collection of blood between the skull and dura mater. Which type of head injury does this finding suggest?
a. Subdural hematoma b. Subarachnoid hemorrhage
c. Epidural hematoma d. Contusion

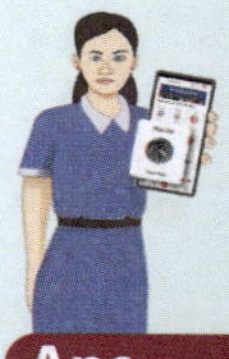

Ans.

20.	d
21.	b
22.	b
23.	d
24.	b
25.	b
26.	d
27.	c
28.	b
29.	a
30.	a
31.	a
32.	c
33.	a
34.	a
35.	b
36.	a
37.	b
38.	a
39.	b
40.	a
41.	b
42.	c

43. Signs of increased intracranial pressure are:
a. Weak rapid pulse, normal blood pressure, fever, lethargy
b. Rapid weak pulse, fall in blood pressure, low temperature
c. Slow bounding pulse, raising blood pressure, high temperature
d. Slow bounding pulse, fall in blood pressure, low temperature

44. The nurse is assessing a client with tentative diagnosis of brain tumor. What would the nurse anticipate the client's primary complaint to be?
a. Decreased appetite b. Frequent insomnia
c. Recurrent headache d. Peripheral edema

45. Temporary paralysis of seventh cranial nerve that causes paralysis only of the affected side of face occurs in:
a. Bell's palsy b. Trigeminal neuralgia
c. Myelitis d. Multiple sclerosis

46. The correct angle for 'Head of the bed' elevation in ventilated patients to decrease respiratory complications:
a. Between 20 and 30°
b. Between 30 and 45°
c. Between 45 and 60°
d. 90°

47. Which layer encloses the valves of the heart?
a. Pericardium b. Myocardium
c. Epicardium d. Endocardium

48. Which two valves of the heart open during ventricular contraction of the heart?
a. Aortic and tricuspid valves
b. Pulmonic and aortic valves
c. Pulmonic and tricuspid valves
d. Aortic and mitral valves

49. The amount of resistance to ejection of blood from ventricle is called:
a. Preload b. Ejection fraction
c. Afterload d. End diastolic pressure

50. Which of the following blood vessels has two major branches: Circumflex artery and anterior descending artery?
a. Posterior interventricular artery
b. Right pulmonary artery
c. Right coronary artery
d. Left coronary artery

51. T wave in the ECG graph represents:
a. Ventricular depolarization
b. Atrial depolarization
c. Ventricular repolarization
d. Atrial repolarization

52. Which diagnostic test can measure the size and ejection fraction of heart?
a. Electrocardiography
b. Echocardiography
c. Treadmill test
d. Barium swallow

53. After cardiac catheterization, immediate priority nursing intervention is:
a. Check for distal pulses and bleeding from site
b. Provide bed rest for 4-6 hours and move the extremities every hourly
c. Ensure patient safety by helping him get out of the bed
d. Instruct to drink adequate fluid to flush out the contrast agent if used

54. Osler nodes and Janeway lesions are manifestations of:
a. Myocarditis b. Endocarditis
c. Pericarditis d. Aortic regurgitation

55. With aging, the blood pressure is often higher due to:
a. Loss of muscle mass
b. Change in exercise and diet
c. Decreased peripheral resistance
d. Decreased elasticity in arterial walls

56. People with mechanical valves require to take these medications lifelong:
a. Antipyretics b. Analgesics
c. Anticoagulants d. Antibiotics

57. Which of the following sign is positive in deep vein thrombosis?
a. Roman's sign b. Jacquemier's sign
c. Kernig's sign d. Hegar's sign

58. Which one of the following cardiac rhythm is nonshockable?
a. Ventricular tachycardia
b. Ventricular fibrillation
c. Pulseless electrical activity
d. Pulseless ventricular tachycardia

59. Which one of the following represents the full form of AED?
a. Autonomous External Defibrillator
b. Automated Extracorporeal Defibrillator
c. Automated External Desynchronizer
d. Automated External Defibrillator

60. The inotropic medication primarily:
a. Decreases afterload
b. Increases the force of contraction
c. Decreases preload
d. Decreases heart rate

61. Which of the following ECG findings alerts the nurse that the client needs an antiarrhythmic?
a. Normal sinus rhythm
b. Sinus bradycardia
c. Sinus arrhythmia
d. Frequent ventricular ectopy

62. A nurse performed an ECG. At the time of interpretation, she found that it is a normal sinus rhythm. The normal duration of the QRS complex is:
a. 0.08–0.10 Second b. 0.2–0.8 Second
c. 0.8–1.2 Second d. 1.2–2.0 Second

63. The nurse needs to inform the cardiac surgeon immediately when she observes which one of the following parameters during the first postoperative day of a patient who has undergone Coronary Artery Bypass Grafting?
a. Urine output <0.5 mL/kg/h
b. Temperature of 99°F
c. Chest drainage of 100 mL over 4–6 hours
d. Discomfort at the incision site

64. A patient reports that he experiences chest pain whenever he performs activities, but it is relieved by taking rest. This is an example of:
a. Unstable Angina b. Stable Angina
c. Variant Angina d. Prinzmetal Angina

65. Rheumatic heart disease results from rheumatic fever which is caused by:
a. Bacterial infection b. Protozoal infection
c. Viral infection d. Fungal infection

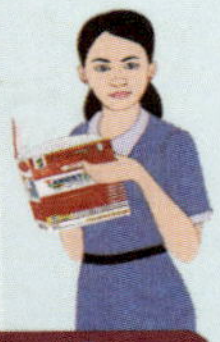

Ans.

43. c
44. c
45. a
46. b
47. d
48. b
49. c
50. d
51. c
52. b
53. a
54. b
55. d
56. c
57. a
58. c
59. d
60. b
61. d
62. a
63. a
64. b
65. a

66. Heart valve affected most by rheumatic fever is:
a. Tricuspid valve b. Mitral valve
c. Aortic valve d. Pulmonary valve

67. Diagnostic criteria used for infective endocarditis is:
a. Jones criteria b. NYHA classification
c. Dukes criteria d. Rockall criteria

68. Reticular activating system controls which one of the following?
a. Consciousness b. Reflex action
c. Memory d. Speech and vocabulary

69. Most used site for test dose of medications is:
a. Forearm b. Gluteal region
c. Deltoid muscle d. Fingertips

70. The pneumatic bed is used to prevent:
a. Joint pain b. Pressure ulcer
c. Back pain d. Hip pain

71. A client with Parkinson's disease is experiencing anorexia and vomiting since the beginning of treatment with levodopa. What should be the initial action?
a. Assess his food preference
b. Monitor blood pressure
c. Hold medication
d. Administer medication with food

72. Core body temperature is highest in the:
a. Early morning b. Noon
c. Late afternoon d. Night

73. Which one of these is not a cardiac biomarker?
a. Alkaline phosphatase b. Creatinine kinase
c. Troponin d. Myoglobin

74. A patient presents to the emergency department with blood pressure 180/130 mmHg, headache, and confusion. Which additional finding is consistent with diagnosis of hypertensive emergency?
a. Retinopathy b. Bradycardia
c. Jaundice d. Urinary retention

75. The nurse plans for rest period during the complete bed bath procedure to a patient to avoid which one of the following cardiovascular effects?
a. Increase in oxygen consumption
b. Decrease in blood supply to the skin
c. Decrease in preload
d. Increase in afterload

76. Cushing's triad refers to a set of signs that are indicative of:
a. increased intra-abdominal pressure
b. increased intra-thoracic pressure
c. increased intra-ocular pressure
d. increased intracranial pressure

77. Which one of the following is a type of generalized seizure?
a. Absence seizure b. Pseudo seizure
c. Partial seizure d. Complex partial

78. Which of the following is a non-drug therapy for children with epileptic seizure?
a. Ketogenic diet b. High protein diet
c. Low fat diet d. High fiber diet

79. Sound created by turbulent abnormal blood flow of heart, heard during auscultation:
a. Friction rub
b. Gallop
c. Murmurs
d. Rasping

80. Which one of the following is the sound that provides the systolic pressure reading and is the first Korotkoff sound (Phase 1) heard as the pressure in the blood pressure cuff is released?
a. A sharp tapping sound
b. A swishing/whooshing sound
c. A thump
d. A soft, blowing, muffled sound

81. Which of the following treatment strategies have been shown to improve the outcome in patients diagnosed to have Guillain-Barre syndrome?
a. Heat therapy b. Immobilization
c. Anticholinesterases d. Plasmapheresis

82. Parkinson's disease includes all these symptoms; except:
a. Bradykinesia and loss of postural reflexes
b. Stiff limbs
c. Thunderclap headache
d. Tremors of hand, arms, legs, jaw, and face

83. Which term would the nurse use to document pain at one site that is perceived in another site?
a. Referred pain b. Phantom pain
c. Intractable pain d. Aftermath of pain

84. The two main factors for determining blood pressure are peripheral resistance, and which one of the following?
a. Cardiac output b. Age
c. Pulse pressure d. Pulse deficit

85. In infectious diseases such as hepatitis B and C, a reservoir for pathogens is:
a. The blood b. The urinary tract
c. The respiratory tract d. The reproductive tract

86. Involvement of which of the following structures will lead to right-sided hemiplegia and aphasia?
a. Left middle cerebral artery
b. Vertebral artery
c. Brain stem
d. Right middle cerebral artery

87. For doing nasotracheal suctioning, the catheter should be inserted during which of the following patient activities?
a. Swallowing b. Inhaling
c. Exhaling d. Retching

88. Which of the following is the organism that causes peptic ulcer disease?
a. Staphylococcus b. Corynebacterium
c. Helicobacter pylori d. Streptococcus

89. Which of the following is the drug of choice to treat anaphylaxis?
a. Atropine b. Sodium bicarbonate
c. Digoxin d. Epinephrine

90. Which of the following is the earliest manifestation of inadequate oxygenation?
a. Vomiting
b. Bradycardia
c. Restlessness
d. Hypotension

91. The principle of fairness is known as:
a. Advocacy
b. Autonomy
c. Justice
d. Accountability

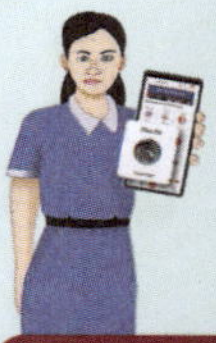

Ans.

66.	b
67.	c
68.	a
69.	a
70.	b
71.	d
72.	c
73.	a
74.	a
75.	a
76.	d
77.	a
78.	a
79.	c
80.	a
81.	d
82.	c
83.	a
84.	a
85.	a
86.	a
87.	b
88.	c
89.	d
90.	c
91.	c

92. The appendix is in:
a. The left antecubital fossa
b. The left iliac fossa
c. The right antecubital fossa
d. The right iliac fossa

93. The oxygen cylinder color code in India is:
a. Black body and white shoulder
b. Black
c. Green body and white shoulder
d. Light blue

94. fMRI stands for:
a. Fast Magnetic Resonance Imaging
b. Fundamental Magnetic Resonance Imaging
c. Fractional Magnetic Resonance Imaging
d. Functional Magnetic Resonance Imaging

95. Kussmaul breathing is a deep and labored breathing pattern often associated with:
a. Diabetic ketoacidosis
b. Hepatitis
c. Hepatomegaly
d. Acute Renal Failure

96. RBSK full form:
a. Rashtriya Bal Shramik Karyakram
b. Rashtriya Bal Suraksha Karyakram
c. Rashtriya Bal Swasthya Karyakram
d. Rashtriya Bal Shramik Kalyan

97. The natural pacemaker of the heart is:
a. AV node
b. SA node
c. Purkinje fiber
d. Bundle of His

98. Short shuffling gait is characteristically seen in:
a. Alzheimer's disease
b. Parkinson's disease
c. Multiple sclerosis
d. Myasthenia gravis

99. What is a 1% solution?
a. 10 mg in 1 mL
b. 1 mg in 1 mL
c. 100 mg in 1 mL
d. 0.10 mg in 1 mL

100. Spinal cord is continuous with which part of the brain?
a. Medulla oblongata
b. Cerebrum
c. Midbrain
d. Pons

Ans.

92. d
93. a
94. d
95. a
96. c
97. b
98. b
99. a
100. a

"It is health that is real wealth and not pieces of gold and silver."
—Mahatma Gandhi

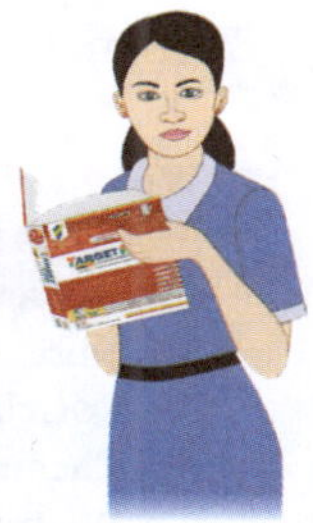

Uttar Pradesh University of Medical Sciences (NO) 2023

1. The normal range of clotting time by capillary tube method is:

a. 2 to 8 minutes
b. 24 to 48 hours
c. 2 to 8 seconds
d. 12 to 18 hours

2. To deliver high-quality care in a tertiary hospital, the manpower required is:

a. A team of doctors and staff nurses
b. Staff nurse and pharmacist
c. An interprofessional team of doctors, nurses, pharmacists, occupation therapists and social workers
d. Nursing administrator and staff nurse

3. The reason for pulling the auricle down and back while instilling ear drops to a child less than 3 years of age is:

a. To avoid adverse effects
b. To treat infection and inflammation
c. That the ear canal is straighter for children at this age
d. To avoid perforation of ear drum

4. Mr. Nanda Kishore Yadav, a 52-year-old, was admitted with a stab injury due to communal riots and undergoes a cholecystectomy and is being discharged after recovery. Since he is an employee of a private company and the bill will be cleared from the company, the company is demanding access to his case file. The most appropriate action of the nurse will be to:

a. Inform the company that the access of the health records can be provided only to his relatives
b. Refuse access to his health records
c. Inform the company to obtain permission from the hospital authorities to provide access to the health records
d. Provide access to his health records

5. All of the following are the primary prevention methods of hypertension; except:

a. Early case detection
b. Dietary sodium restriction
c. Weight reduction
d. Increased physical activity

6. In which position should a nurse place a patient while preparing the patient for thoracentesis?

a. Supine position
b. Prone position
c. Sitting position
d. Lateral position

7. Which of the following Five-Year plans introduced 'Target-Free Approach' in National family welfare program?

a. Fifth Five-Year Plan
b. Sixth Five-Year Plan
c. Seventh Five-Year Plan
d. Eighth Five-Year Plan

8. During the health educating on anticoagulation therapy for the patient with valve replacement surgery with a mechanical valve, which of the following statements by the nurse about the therapeutic level of the drug is correct?

a. Maintain international normalized ratio of 3.5-4.5
b. Maintain international normalized ratio of 1
c. Maintain international normalized ratio of 2.5-3
d. Maintain international normalized ratio of 1.5-2.5

9. Which of the following is the function of the State Nursing Councils in India?

a. To promote the development of strong national associations
b. To provide registration for foreign nurses
c. To prescribe rules of conduct, take disciplinary actions
d. To prescribe curricula for nursing education

10. The nurse is taking care of an aggressive patient. Which of the following nursing actions is a part of nursing assessment in the nursing process?

a. Asking about the previous history of the aggressive behavior
b. Removing all the sharp instruments from the environment
c. Writing nursing diagnosis as 'Risk for violence'
d. Maintaining the calm and cool environment

11. In rural area plains, one subcenter is established for:

a. 5000 people
b. 3000 people
c. 10,000 people
d. 2000 people

12. Client X, on admission to hospital with severe pain, has a decreased blood pressure. What is the rationale for the decreased blood pressure?

a. Increased cardiac output
b. Vasoconstriction of the arterioles
c. High metabolic rate
d. Vasodilation of the arterioles

13. After heart surgery, which type of pacing is used to manage bradydysrhythmias or tachydysrhythmias in the early postoperative period?

a. Permanent pacing
b. Transcutaneous pacing
c. Transvenous pacing
d. Epicardial pacing

14. Which of the following is NOT a type of blood cell?

a. Leukocytes
b. Platelets
c. Plasma
d. Erythrocytes

15. The drug of choice for chemoprophylaxis of cholera is:

a. Streptomycin
b. Amoxycillin
c. Paracetamol
d. Tetracycline

16. ALL of the following are barrier methods of contraception except:

a. Diaphragm
b. Condom
c. Vaginal sponge
d. Intrauterine device

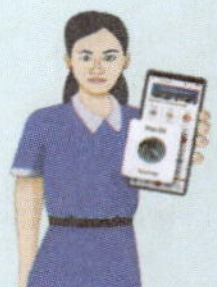

Ans.

1.	a
2.	c
3.	c
4.	c
5.	a
6.	c
7.	d
8.	c
9.	c
10.	a
11.	a
12.	d
13.	d
14.	c
15.	d
16.	d

17. Which of the following tests assess high-level cognitive processes such as attention, perseverance, abstract thinking, CF and set shifting?
a. Observation method
b. Rorschach inkblot test
c. Thematic apperception test
d. Wisconsin card sorting test

18. Which movement aids in the birth of after-coming head of breech?
a. Extension b. Rotation
c. Deflexion d. Flexion

19. The nurse reviews the lab report of a patient with schizophrenia, who is taking Clozapine 25mg QD. His report shows a WBC count of 1500 per mcL. Based on the findings, which of the following orders should the nurse expect from the psychiatrist?
a. Discontinue Clozapine
b. Continue with the same dose of Clozapine
c. Increase the dose of Clozapine
d. Decrease the dose of Clozapine

20. All of the following are legal guidelines for documentation; except:
a. Begin each entry with date and time and end with your signature
b. Do not leave blank space or lines in a written nurses' progress note
c. Record all written entries legibly and in black ink
d. Always record critical comments about a patient

21. In which type of measurement can the attributes be rank ordered?
a. Ratio b. Ordinal
c. Nominal d. Interval

22. A hospital utilizes many rubber goods such as hot water bags, gloves etc. Care of rubber goods increases durability. Rubber goods are stored without folding repeatedly to:
a. Prevent cracks in the rubber goods
b. Prevent from melting due to heat
c. Reduce the occupying space
d. Prevent from infestations

23. If $x = \frac{1}{4}y$ and $y = \frac{1}{4}z$, than x : y : z is equal to:
a. 1 : 4 : 16 b. 2 : 4 : 16
c. 3 : 2 : 16 d. 4 : 2 : 16

24. Increased serum chloride levels are seen in all of the following; except:
a. Renal tubular acidosis b. Severe diarrhea
c. Water intoxication d. Cushing syndrome

25. Identify the noninvasive treatment modality which uses MRI strength magnetic pulses to stimulate focal areas of the cerebral cortex to treat depression.
a. Transcranial magnetic stimulation (TMS)
b. Deep brain stimulation
c. Vagus nerve stimulation
d. Light therapy

26. Select the most appropriate meaning of the given idiom. Our English teacher always forbids us from being idle at home and advises us to be up and doing.
a. Indolent b. Lacklustre
c. Languid d. Lively

27. Good housekeeping is basic essential of nursing care. A well managed housekeeping aims to:
a. Increase the patient turnover
b. Increase the hospital acquired infections
c. Increase the days of hospitalization of patients
d. Increase the hospital management cost

28. Select the most appropriate option to fill in the blank. Neither Ramesh nor Sheetal ______________ present at the meeting.
a. Are b. Was
c. Is being d. Were

29. The process of managing several projects, often with the intention of improving an organization's performance, is known as:
a. Project management b. Transformational leadership
c. Nursing management d. Program management

30. The nurse is taking care of a suicidal client. Which of the following nursing actions indicates a part of the evaluation in the nursing process?
a. Obtaining a short-term contract from the client that he/she discusses suicidal feelings with nurses
b. Determining that nursing interventions are appropriate to achieve the goal
c. Finding the mental status of the client
d. Keeping the environment safe

31. Where is Central Food Technological Research Institute (CFTRI) located?
a. Lucknow b. Hyderabad
c. Coonoor d. Mysore

32. What is the appropriate solution for cleaning the wound initially?
a. Soap and water b. Alcohol
c. Hydrogen peroxide d. Plain water

33. For a successful demonstration method, the teacher:
a. Need not involve students in demonstration
b. Needs to plan all the activities in great detail and rehearse them
c. Should proceed with the demonstration as quickly as possible after the lecture
d. Should never break down the demonstration into a simple step-by-step pattern

34. During the learning process, if repeated application of stimulus evokes greater and greater response, then it is called:
a. Priming b. Conditioned response
c. Habituation d. Sensitization

35. Pipes P and Q can fill a completely empty tank in 54 minutes and 72 minutes respectively, when opened independently. Pipe R can empty the completely filled tank in 48 minutes. Initially all the three pipes P, Q and R, are opened simultaneously. After how much time (in minutes) pipe R be closed so that the tank will be completely filled in a total time of 45 minutes?
a. 36 b. 22
c. 45 d. 29

36. The basic characteristic of an exhibition is:
a. A play activity
b. That it should have a central theme that focuses on a particular concept
c. Used in higher classes
d. That the teacher is the leader

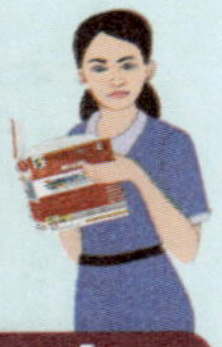

Ans.

17. d
18. d
19. a
20. d
21. a
22. a
23. a
24. c
25. a
26. d
27. a
28. b
29. d
30. b
31. d
32. a
33. b
34. d
35. b
36. b

37. A thyroid function test is commonly ordered as a baseline with lithium treatment:
a. Because thyroid-stimulating hormone interferes with the metabolism of lithium
b. Because lithium decreases the level of thyroid-stimulating hormone
c. Because lithium increases the level of thyroid-stimulating hormone
d. To confirm that the patient's mood has improved

38. Any newly hospitalized patient exhibits increased anxiety because of which of the following reasons?
a. Loss of personal freedom and identity
b. Unfamiliar health personnel
c. Hospital routines and investigations
d. Increased risk of infection and unsafe environment

39. Ram travelled by car and covered the first 175 km in 4 hours and the next 275 km in 5 hours. What is his average speed (in km/h) for the entire trip?
a. 45 b. 55
c. 60 d. 50

40. All of the following drugs improve milk production in a mother; except:
a. Metoclopramide
b. Sulpiride
c. Bromocriptine
d. Domperidone

41. The apparatus used to record blood pressure is:
a. Ergometer
b. Sphygmomanometer
c. Ergograph
d. Thermometer

42. In the context of music, a 'Saptak' contains __________ pure/ unadulterated notes.
a. 15 b. 11
c. 7 d. 18

43. What is the gold standard for the diagnosis of neonatal sepsis?
a. Complete blood count
b. Immature to Total neutrophil count (I/T ratio)
c. Absolute neutrophil count
d. Blood culture

44. The measures of social differentiation include all of the following; except:
a. Income
b. Religion
c. Marital state
d. Education

45. One housekeeping lady suddenly got burned while cleaning the toilet with chemical agents. What should be the first aid management for her?
a. Wash the area with plenty of water.
b. Immediately cover the area with a piece of clean cloth.
c. Apply antiseptic cream.
d. Immediately go to the physician for checkup.

46. HIV post-exposure prophylaxis (PEP) should be started within how many hours after the person's exposure?
a. 48 hours
b. 12 hours
c. 72 hours
d. 24 hours

47. When used in the context of nursing, which quadrant of the Johari window has nonproductive space for individuals which hinders communication with each other?
a. Quadrant 3 - Hidden area
b. Quadrant 1 - Open area
c. Quadrant 2 - Blind area
d. Quadrant 4 - Unknown area

48. The Continuous Performance Test is the most common research paradigm used to examine __________.
a. Modes of processing
b. Sustained attention
c. Language dysfunction
d. Selective attention

49. Thinking in which the thoughts are largely narcissistic and egocentric, with emphasis on subjectivity rather than objectivity, is called:
a. Automatism
b. Autistic thinking
c. Ataxia
d. Agnosia

50. A client addicted to alcohol makes a statement to the nurse, "I do not have a problem with alcohol. I can quit whenever I want." Which of the following nursing diagnoses is appropriate for this patient?
a. Disturbed thought processes
b. Disturbed sensory perception
c. Ineffective denial
d. Impaired verbal communication

51. The normal puerperium usually lasts for up to:
a. 8 weeks
b. 6 weeks
c. 2 weeks
d. 4 weeks

52. The indicators that suggest that development is seriously disordered in a child includes all of the following; except:
a. Persistently low muscle tone or floppiness
b. Persistent toe walking
c. No speech by 18 months
d. Climbing stairs with two feet per step by 2 years

53. The importance of accreditation for higher education institution is to ensure:
a. Licensure
b. Quality standards
c. Political advancement
d. Registration

54. Antigens are usually _____ in nature.
a. Fats b. Proteins
c. Disaccharides d. Monosaccharides

55. Select the most appropriate option to fill in the blank. Rama got annoyed ____________ his brother for being late.
a. on b. with
c. at d. by

56. A & B means 'A is the mother of B'
A% B means 'A is the son of B'
A @ B means 'A is the sister of B'
A = B means 'A is the brother of B'
If H and Y @ Z % D = K & M, then how is K related to Y?
a. Father's sister
b. Mother's sister
c. Sister's father
d. Father's mother

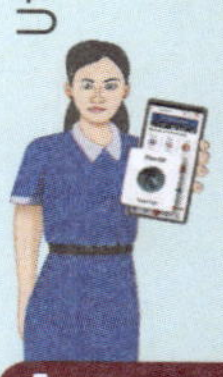

Ans.

37. c
38. a
39. d
40. c
41. b
42. c
43. d
44. c
45. a
46. c
47. c
48. b
49. b
50. c
51. b
52. d
53. b
54. b
55. b
56. a

57. The best method to assess temperature of a neonate is:

a. By keeping a thermometer in the mouth in a horizontal line with the body so that the tip of the thermometer faces the tongue
b. By keeping a thermometer in the axilla in a horizontal line with the body so that the tip of the thermometer faces the axilla
c. By keeping a thermometer in the rectum in a horizontal line with the body
d. By keeping a thermometer in the eardrum in a horizontal line with the body so that the tip of the thermometer faces the axilla

58. The person who manages both patient care and nursing care in health care services is called:

a. The Nursing Administrator
b. The Nurse Practitioner
c. The Nursing Supervisor
d. The Nurse Educator

59. What is the early sign of subgaleal hemorrhage?

a. Hyperbilirubinaemia
b. Anaemia and Hypovolemic shock
c. Decreasing head circumference
d. Forward and lateral positioning of a newborn's ears

60. Which of the following is the appropriate nursing intervention for the client with suicidal ideation?

a. Keeping sharp instruments out of reach of the patient
b. Determining the goal that the client will discuss the suicidal idea with the nurse by discharge
c. Determining whether the interventions provided are adequate to minimize the patient's suicidal ideas
d. Forming the nursing diagnosis as 'Risk for self-directed violence'

61. The original and firsthand data collected by the researcher is known as:

a. Interview data b. Secondary data
c. Primary data d Tertiary data

62. The Benton Visual Retention Test is used to assess____.

a. Executive functioning
b. Nonverbal memory
c. Language
d. Verbal memory

63. The process of starting other foods and fluids when breast milk alone is no longer sufficient to meet the nutritional requirements of infant is known as:

a. Complementary feeding
b. Exclusive breastfeeding
c. Demand feeding
d. Substitute feeding

64. The energy value of foods has long been expressed in terms of:

a. Kilocalorie b. Joules
c. Ampere d. Newton

65. Rehan, a 4-year-old male was brought to the pediatric OPD and presented with limited self-expression, crying and facial expression. Rehan's mother Mrs. Fathima enquired with the nursing officer the factor affecting her son's communication. The response of the nursing officer will be:

a. Emotional b. Developmental
c. Socio-cultural d. Physical

66. What is the importance of citrate in the WHO oral rehydration solution?

a. Increased shelf life b. Cheaper
c. Tastier d. Nutritious

67. A public health nurse was diagnosed to have HBeAg and HBsAg in the serum. Most likely, which of the following does she have?

a. Recovery from hepatitis B
b. Acute infectious hepatitis B
c. HBV+HBE coinfection
d. Chronic hepatitis

68. ______________ is a macrovascular complication of Diabetes Mellitus.

a. Diabetic retinopathy b. Diabetic neuropathy
c. Diabetic nephropathy d. Coronary heart disease

69. The final stage of development in the expanding social radius of maturing individuals during adulthood is:

a. Intimacy b. Generativity
c. Identity d. Integrity

70. The condition in which a stone is formed in the ducts of salivary glands is known as:

a. Sialorrhoea b. Xerostomia
c. Mumps d. Sialolithiasis

71. A procedure to measure the amount of energy an individual expends by calculating the respiratory gas exchange is known as:

a. Calorific value
b. Dietary thermogenesis
c. Indirect calorimetry
d. Direct calorimetry

72. The type of staining technique that gives different colors to different bacteria is known as:

a. Complex stain b. Impregnation stain
c. Differential stain d. Simple stain

73. The hormone that is mainly responsible for coping and adaptation during acute stress is:

a. Cortisol b. Insulin
c. Growth hormone d. Thyroxine

74. The most common malpresentation is:

a. Breech presentation
b. Transverse lie
c. Face presentation
d. Shoulder presentation

75. The normal prothrombin time is:

a. 2 – 4 minutes b. 4 – 8 minutes
c. 12 – 16 seconds d. 12 – 16 minutes

76. All of the following are functions of fat; except:

a. They are necessary for conversion of carotene to vitamin A.
b. They are concentrated sources of energy.
c. They are a major source of energy for the body.
d. They help in absorption of vitamin D.

77. Which of the following muscles allow fast movements and movements against resistance in the radioulnar joint?

a. Biceps brachii b. Pronator teres
c. Latissimus dorsi d. Quadriceps femoris

78. Which of the following is an amplifier host in Japanese encephalitis?

a. Monkey b. Horse
c. Pigs d. Dogs

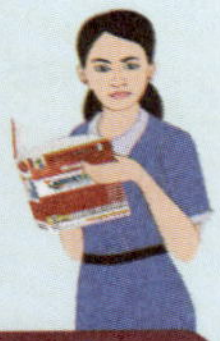

Ans.

57. b
58. a
59. d
60. a
61. c
62. b
63. a
64. a
65. b
66. a
67. b
68. d
69. d
70. d
71. c
72. c
73. a
74. a
75. c
76. a
77. b
78. c

79. What is the probable rate of anterior rotation of occiput if labor progresses uneventfully in occipito-posterior position?

a. 90% b. 30%
c. 70% d. 50%

80. The Deccan Plateau lies entirely to the south of the river ______.

a. Narmada b. Pamba
c. Periyar d. Kaveri (Cauvery)

81. Intrauterine pressure below 25 mm Hg during contraction is a characteristic feature of:

a. Uterine inertia
b. Constriction ring
c. Spastic lower segment
d. Incoordinate uterine action

82. A patient with a diabetic foot is about to get discharged from the hospital. Which of the following comprises effective interdisciplinary discharge planning?

a. Ensure that the hospital bills are paid by the patient/family members.
b. Ensure that all the medication instructions are given to the patient and his family members.
c. Ensure that there is a written order for discharge from the physician/treating team.
d. Ensure that the nurse educator, dietician and physician provide the right information to manage his condition.

83. The three main components of cardiopulmonary resuscitation (CPR) include all of the following;except:

a. Circulation b. Digestion
c. Breathing d. Airway

84. Which of the following is NOT a sign of severe illness in infants?

a. Difficult breathing
b. Mild chest indrawing
c. Fast breathing
d. Inability to breastfeed

85. How long should the nurse wait before making further measurements after releasing the pressure completely in the cuff and estimating the systolic pressure?

a. 60–120 seconds b. 40 seconds
c. 10–20 seconds d. 25–30 seconds

86. All of the following statements related to gastrostomy are correct; except:

a. Parenteral nutrition can be given through gastrostomy
b. Nutrients are sent into the gastrointestinal tract through a feeding tube
c. It is the creation of an artificial external opening into the stomach
d. Enteral nutrition can be given through gastrostomy

87. The most important function of red blood cells is:

a. To act as antiparasitic and antiallergic
b. To transport oxygen from lungs to the tissues
c. To prevent bleeding by Hemostasis
d. To provide first line of defense

88. Select the term from among the given options that can replace the question mark (?) in the following series. PPR-4, NRP-12, LTN-39, JVL-103, ?

a. HXH-226 b. IXK-224
c. HXJ-228 d. HXL-220

89. What do you mean by abdominal thrusts?

a. It is a technique to apply abdomen binder for a postoperative patient.
b. A first-aider stands behind the victim, with arms wrapped around the victim's waist and make a fist using two hands and press in with quick inward and outward thrusts.
c. Instruct the victim to give abdominal pressure.
d. A technique used by the doctor to press the abdomen.

90. Which of the following approaches emphasires the importance of human relations in nursing?

a. Therapeutic communication
b. Cost effective approach
c. High-tech, high-touch approach
d. Comprehensive care approach

91. The major mineral element of the body is:

a. Iron b. Sodium
c. Potassium d. Calcium

92. The example for distributive shock among the following shock types is:

a. Anaphylactic shock b. Burn shock
c. Surgical shock d. Hemorrhagic shock

93. Which of the following option is equal to $(5^3 \times 5^{-10} \times 5^{-20} \times 5^{11} \times 5^{16})^{200}$?

a. 25 b. 0
c. 1 d. 5

94. The nurse teaches a student nurse to keep in mind the following points while monitoring blood pressure. Which of the following is miscommunicated to the student?

a. The patient is asked not to talk during measurements.
b. The cuff bladder should be centred over the brachial artery.
c. Initial recordings are made on both arms, and subsequent measurements are taken on the arm with the lower pressure.
d. The cuff bladder width should be at least 40% and length at least 80% of limb circumference.

95. The most important factor for successful induction of labor include:

a. Elderly primigravidae b. Bishop score >6
c. Small foetus d. Maternal BMI>25

96. Which of the following is NOT a basic strategy for health promotion?

a. Mediating b. Advocacy
c. Enabling d. Forcing

97. Which of the following organisms is an obvious source of hospital infection that grows in hand lotions?

a. Pseudomonas b. Staphylococci
c. E. coli d. Streptococci

98. The type of statistics that deals with enumeration, organization and graphical representation of data is called ______.

a. Applied statistics b. Descriptive statistics
c. Deferential statistics d. Inferential statistics

99. A family planning procedure where aspiration of uterine contents is done within 6-14 days of missed period is called______.

a. Menstrual induction
b. Induced abortion
c. Menstrual extraction
d. Menstrual regulation

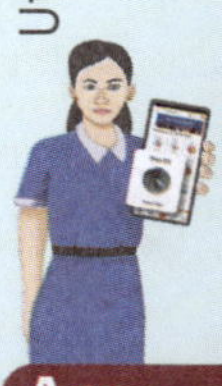

Ans.

79.	a
80.	a
81.	a
82.	d
83.	b
84.	b
85.	a
86.	a
87.	b
88.	c
89.	b
90.	a
91.	d
92.	a
93.	c
94.	c
95.	b
96.	d
97.	a
98.	b
99.	d

100. What is the first nursing action to be taken when infiltration or extravasation is observed (signs include erythema, pain, oedema, blanching, streaking on the skin along the vein, and darkened area at the insertion site)?

a. Infusing an antidote b. Stop the infusion
c. Remove the IV line d. Elevate the extremity

101. Which of the following is a part of planning in the nursing process?

a. Evaluation b. Short-term goals
c. Subjective data d. Objective data

102. All of the following are fat soluble vitamins; except:

a. Vitamin B12 b. Vitamin D
c. Vitamin A d. Vitamin K

103. Which of the following is an example of a clinical assessment of nutritional status?

a. Food frequency questionnaire
b. Checking level of nutrients in a person's blood
c. Asking a client about symptoms of deficiency
d. MUAC

104. The most frequently used communication channel is ________.

a. Written channel b. Visual channel
c. Auditory channel d. Tactile channel

105. The nurse is caring for a patient with a suicidal attempt. Which of the following nursing actions is a part of outcome identification in the nursing process?

a. Getting a short-term contract from the patient that he/she will seek help from the nurse whenever he/she has suicidal thoughts
b. Preparing a safe environment for the patient
c. Forming a goal the patient will not harm him self during hospitalization
d. Collecting the family history of the patient

106. A swelling over the scalp which is present at birth or just after birth in case of vaginal delivery is known as:

a. Encephalocele b. Meningocele
c. Caput succedaneum d. Hydrocephalus

107. Nurses must keep the medico-legal issues under consideration for admission and discharge, to safeguard themselves and the healthcare agency. Which of the following is a medico-legal issue involving discharge?

a. Handing over the patient records to the legal authority without written permission from the treating physician
b. Keeping the discharge note under lock and key until handed over to the concerned patient
c. Duly assessing the patient for the readiness of discharge
d. Ensuring that the written order of the discharge or referral from the hospital is duly signed by the treating physician

108. For a woman presenting with occipitoposterior position, vaginal examination is performed on rupture of the membrane with an unengaged foetal head to rule out:

a. Placenta previa
b. Cord prolapse
c. Cervical effacement
d. Adequacy of pelvis for childbirth

109. The stage that begins with full dilation of cervix and ends with expulsion of the foetus is:

a. Third stage b. First stage
c. Fourth stage d. Second stage

110. The two important diagnostic criteria of pre-eclampsia is:

a. Hypertension and proteinuria
b. Hypertension and increased cholesterol level
c. Oedema and increased blood urea level
d. Hypertension and increased blood glucose level

111. Which of the following is the traditional site for IM injection?

a. Dorsogluteal b. Deltoid
c. Vastus lateralis d. Ventrogluteal

112. In cardioversion, the electrical impulse discharges at _____ by the defibrillator which is synchronized with the ECG on a cardiac monitor.

a. QRS complex b. T wave
c. PR interval d. P wave

113. The capillary tube method is used routinely in clinical laboratories to estimate:

a. Activated partial thromboplastin time
b. Prothrombin time
c. Clotting time
d. Bleeding time

114. As per Article 151 (2) of the constitution of India, 'reports of the comptroller and auditor-general of India relating to the accounts of a state shall be submitted to the ______, who shall cause them to be laid before the legislature of the state'.

a. President of the union
b. Chairman of the state legislative council
c. Governor of the state
d. Chief Minister of the state

115. In an emergency situation of injury, which of the following types of care is applicable?

a. Tertiary care b. Primary care
c. Immediate care d. Secondary care

116. In the human cardiac conductive system, which of the following is considered as the natural pacemaker of the heart?

a. Atrioventricular node b. Bundle of His
c. Purkinje fibers d. Sinoatrial node

117. A registered midwife certified by INC usually provides ________.

a. Direct patient care, and educates, consults and conducts research
b. Health care to a group of patients in an outpatient or community based setting
c. Care to the mother during prepartum, intrapartum and postpartum periods
d. Specialized care to the victims of trauma

118. A nurse checks the blood pressure of an adult client admitted into the emergency room.
Which of the findings would be a cause for concern and has to be reported immediately?

a. A systolic pressure of 130 mm Hg
b. A diastolic pressure of 90 mm Hg
c. A diastolic pressure of 78 mm Hg
d. A systolic pressure of 90 mm Hg

119. Suppositories can be inserted in all of the following; except:

a. The vagina b. The urethra
c. The axilla d. The rectum

120. Which of the following is the most reliable pulse in infants?

a. Carotid pulse b. Dorsalis pedis pulse
c. Apical pulse d. Radial pulse

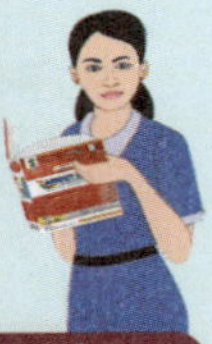

Ans.

100. d
101. b
102. a
103. c
104. c
105. c
106. c
107. a
108. b
109. d
110. a
111. a
112. a
113. c
114. c
115. c
116. c
117. c
118. d
119. c
120. c

121. The theory that views intelligence as mostly a culturally specific cognitive process is:
a. Script theory b. Piaget's theory
c. Kohlberg's theory d. Vygotsky's theory

122. Which of the following is an example of a long-term goal?
a. The client will verbalize the understanding that the sensory disturbance results from his/her illness and demonstrate ways to interrupt hallucinations.
b. The client will willingly attend therapy activities accompanied by a trusted staff member within one week.
c. Within a week, the client will recognise signs of increasing anxiety and agitation and report to staff for assistance.
d. The client will discuss the content of hallucinations with the nurse or therapist within one week.

123. While choosing interventions in a nursing care plan, the most important factor to be considered is:
a. The capability of the nurse
b. The feasibility of doing the interventions
c. The desired patient outcome
d. Acceptability to the patient

124. Which of the following is the leading cause of blindness in the Indian population?
a. Glaucoma b. Refractive error
c. Cataract d. Corneal pathologies

125. Ms. Sunitha hands over her patient to Ms. Manjula after her duty. Ms. Manjula also asks a few questions regarding patient conditions, medications, care and feeding, etc. The type of communication between these nurses will be:
a. Intrapersonal b. Public communication
c. Transpersonal d. Interpersonal

126. Nonfatal complications of measles include:
a. Encephalitis
b. Conjunctivitis, otitis media and mouth ulcers
c. Pneumonia
d. Laryngotracheitis

127. A nurse injects a small amount of an antibiotic intra-dermally/subcutaneously and observes for hypersensitivity reaction. Which of the following ethical terms best describes this act?
a. Beneficence b. Nonmaleficence
c. Justice d. Autonomy

128. The dye commonly mixed with bacteria in negative staining is:
a. Methylene blue b. Indian ink
c. Crystal violet d. Neutral red

129. Which of the following is the most effective way to control the transmission of an infectious agent?
a. Taking vaccination for all pathogens
b. Practising isolation precautions
c. Practising meticulous hand hygiene
d. Identifying the infectious agent

130. The components of attention traditionally used to describe cognitive deficits include all of the following; except:
a. Selectivity b. Memory
c. Capacity d. Sustained concentration

131. What is the range of normal serum cholesterol?
a. More than 400 mg/dL
b. 350 – 400 mg/dL
c. 150 – 200 mg/dL
d. 250 – 300 mg/dL

132. In which of the following teaching methods, one teacher presents the new material to the students while the other teacher constructs a concept map on the overhead projector as the students listen to the presenting teacher?
a. Team teaching b. Concept map
c. Demonstration d. Symposium

133. A nurse collects blood samples at the time of admission and sends to the laboratory for testing as per the prescription of the physician. The patient is interested to know the tests that will be done with the blood collected. The nurse's appropriate action will be:
a. To inform about all the blood investigations
b. To tell only about the special investigations and hide the routine investigations
c. To not inform about any of the blood investigations
d. To tell only about the routine investigations and hide the special investigations

134. Triad symptoms of depression include:
a. Suicidal ideas, hopelessness and decreased appetite
b. Worthlessness, disturbed sleep and delusions
c. Pervasive sadness, anhedonia and decreased psychomotor activity
d. Monotonous voice, preoccupations and poor memory

135. The desirable level of total cholesterol, LDL and triglyceride levels is less than ______, ______ and ______, respectively.
a. 200, 130, 150 b. 270, 200, 220
c. 250, 180, 200 d. 300, 230, 250

136. The process by which a nongovernmental or private body evaluates the quality of a higher, education institution as a whole or of a specific educational programme, in order to formally recognize it as having met certain predetermined minimal criteria or standards is known as ____________.
a. Standardization b. Licensure
c. Registration d. Accreditation

137. As per the Wechsler Intelligence Scale, if an individual scores an IQ of 90–109, then that individual is categorized as:
a. Average b. Superior
c. High average d. Low average

138. Learning through conditioned stimulus is called:
a. Pavlovian learning b. Operant learning
c. Motivational learning d. Punishment learning

139. While assessing a puerperal woman, a midwife observes pain in the calf muscles on dorsiflexion of the foot. Which of the following signs is the midwife eliciting?
a. Linton's sign b. Neuhof's sign
c. Homan's sign d. Moses sign

140. A nurse attends a ward-based education program on how to insert an intubation tube for an unconscious patient. This can be categorized as which type of education?
a. In-service education
b. Induction program
c. Continuing education
d. Graduate education

141. In case of emergency wound bandaging, the knot should be _______.
a. Over the wound
b. On the right side of the wound
c. Below the wound
d. Away from the wound

Ans.

121. d
122. a
123. c
124. c
125. d
126. b
127. b
128. b
129. c
130. b
131. c
132. a
133. a
134. c
135. a
136. d
137. a
138. a
139. c
140. a
141. a

142. Which of the following clinical assessment findings gives the nurse a clue about the risk of cephalopelvic disproportion in a woman?

a. Primigravidae
b. Twin gestation
c. Obesity
d. Short stature

143. Select the combination of letters that when sequentially placed in the blanks of the given series will complete the series.

F H _ B E _ T _ H N _ E W _ F H _ B _ W T

a. N E T F B N E
b. N W F B T N E
c. W N F E T N B
d. N W F B T N H

144. In the ________________ mode of mechanical ventilation, mechanical breaths are delivered at a preset frequency, but the machine tries to deliver these breaths in response to the patient's spontaneous inspiratory efforts.

a. Assist control ventilation
b. Controlled mandatory ventilation
c. Supported ventilation
d. Synchronized intermittent mandatory ventilation

145. The acid-base disorder that occurs due to hyperventilation at high altitude is:

a. Respiratory alkalosis
b. Respiratory acidosis
c. Metabolic acidosis
d. Metabolic alkalosis

146. The primary action of parathyroid hormone is:

a. To increase the level of calcium
b. To decrease the level of glucose
c. To increase the level of phosphate
d. To decrease the level of calcium

147. Select the most appropriate meaning of the underlined proverb in the following sentence.

The local tourist guide kept arguing with the historian throughout the journey. It is ultimately the empty vessels that make much noise.

a. People who enquire into other's work fail miserably in life.
b. People must always be careful instead of showing bravery to others.
c. A person's character can be judged by his/her outer appearance.
d. People with least knowledge often speak the loudest.

148. If 2 is added to each even digit and 1 is subtracted from each odd digit in the number given below, what will be the product of digits which are second from the left and third from the right in the new number thus formed?

(Left) 49726536 (Right)

a. 6
b. 32
c. 48
d. 64

149. Select the most appropriate option to fill in the blank.

______ she reached the port, when her ferry arrived.

a. Hardly how
b. -Hardly had
c. How hardly
d. Had hardly

150. All of the following are examples for parenteral route of drug administration; except:

a. Sublingual
b. Intramuscular
c. Intravenous
d. Subcutaneous

151. The disorder in which the symptoms of schizophrenia and mood disorders are prominently present within the same episode is known as:

a. Induced delusional disorders
b. Persistent delusional disorders
c. Acute and transient psychotic disorders
d. Schizoaffective disorder

152. Which of the following is a precise X-ray beam that takes cross-sectional images layer by layer?

a. Single-Photon Emission Computed Tomography (SPECT)
b. Computed Tomography (CT) scan
c. Positron Emission Tomography (PET)
d. Magnetic Resonance Imaging (MRI)

153. An in-depth study of a particular research problem rather than a sweeping statistical survey, which is useful when not much is known about a phenomenon is called:

a. Experimental design
b. Time series design
c. Quasi-experimental design
d. Case study design

154. In 1919, Gandhiji gave a call for satyagraha against the ______ that the British had just passed.

a. Indian Press Act
b. Rowlatt Act
c. Indian Councils Act
d. Government of India Act

155. While performing physical examination of a child, the nurse finds difficulty in palpating femoral pulses. Which of the below-mentioned conditions should the nurse suspect for the child?

a. Tricuspid atresia
b. Coarctation of aorta
c. Atrial septal defect
d. Ventricular septal defect

156. As per the Census of India 2011, sex ratio in the country has ______ per thousand males in 2001 to 943 females per thousand males in 2011.

a. Increased from 856 females
b. Decreased from 973 females
c. Increased from 933 females
d. Decreased from 1084 females

157. Prophylactic administration of vitamin A in a child is an example of:

a. Rehabilitation
b. Specific protection
c. Treatment
d. Health promotion

158. The graph that represents the data of a cumulative frequency distribution is a/an __________.

a. Spot map
b. Pie diagram
c. Line graph
d. Ogive

159. In a diabetic woman, the presence of ketone bodies in urine with kussmaul breathing is suggestive of:

a. Diabetic ketoacidosis
b. Respiratory acidosis
c. Metabolic alkalosis
d. Hyperosmolar coma

160. Quality documentation has all of the following characteristics; except:

a. Sticking to the facts
b. Complete information within a recorded entry
c. Timely entries on the patient's ongoing care
d. Recording not only objective information, but also subjective information by the nurse

161. The Western Dedicated Freight Corridor of India, when complete, will connect Jawaharlal Nehru Port Trust (JNPT) in Maharashtra to ______ in Uttar Pradesh (as per information available from the Ministry of Railways on 08 Feb 2023).

a. Khurja
b. Tundla
c. Dadri
d. Saharanpur

162. Which type of bilirubin is increased in obstructive jaundice?

a. Bilirubin diglucuronide
b. Unconjugated bilirubin
c. Indirect bilirubin
d. Direct bilirubin

Ans.

142. d
143. b
144. d
145. a
146. a
147. d
148. b
149. b
150. a
151. d
152. b
153. d
154. b
155. b
156. c
157. b
158. d
159. a
160. d
161. c
162. d

163. As per Haj Policy 2023, out of the total number of 'Haj' seats allocated to the Government of India, ______ will be allocated to the Haj Committee of India.

a. 50% b. 60%
c. 20% d. 80%

164. A PAP smear and colposcopic examination for the early detection of cervical cancer and papilloma virus infection is an example of:

a. Primary prevention
b. Secondary prevention
c. Tertiary prevention
d. Primordial prevention

165. Mrs. Mamata Das, a 38-year-old female, is admitted to the hospital with a history of RTA and multiple fractures. This type of admission is referred to as:

a. Emergency admission b. Long term admission
c. Therapeutic admission d. Diagnostic admission

166. The theory that focusses primarily on logical deductive reasoning with little attention to social intelligence and emotional intelligence is:

a. Script theory b. Kohlberg's theory
c. Vygotsky's theory d. Piaget's theory

167. While performing the Weber test, a vibrating tuning fork is placed in the middle of the top of the child's head. What response from the child is considered as normal?

a. Hearing sound in the right ear
b. Hearing no sound in both the ears
c. Hearing sound equally in both the ears
d. Hearing sound in the left ear

168. As per the ESI scheme, the contributions of the employer and employee for financial support are ______ and ______ of the wages, respectively.

a. 2% and 3% b. 3% and 2%
c. 4.75% and 1.75% d. 1.75% and 4.75 %

169. The premonitory stage of postpartum eclampsia can be recognized by all of the following features; except:

a. Eye balls roll and become fixed
b. Twitching of muscles of face, tongue and limbs
c. The tongue protrudes between the teeth
d. The patient becomes unconscious

170. The Apgar score is an objective method of evaluating the condition of:

a. A foetus b. A toddler
c. An adult d. A newborn

171. Where does the absorption of calcium take place?

a. Ileum
b. Jejunum
c. Antrum of stomach
d. Duodenum

172. Which two numbers should be interchanged to make the following equation correct?

$14 \times 12 - 8 + 28 \div 4 = 107$

a. 8 and 4 b. 14 and 8
c. 12 and 28 d. 12 and 8

173. The capacitance vessels are:

a. Arteries b. Arterioles
c. Veins d. Capillaries

174. The basic unit in all societies is:

a. Family b. Caste
c. Religion d. Income

175. In which stage of erythropoiesis does a cytoplasm become polychromatic?

a. Reticulocyte stage
b. Intermediate normoblast stage
c. Early normoblast stage
d. Pronormoblast stage

176. The therapy used for relieving seasonal depression is called:

a. Relaxation therapy b. Light therapy
c. Occupational therapy d. Milieu therapy

177. Mr. Basavaraj Gowda, a patient, is planned for discharge tomorrow. Mr. Velayudhan informed this to Mrs. Sangeeta, a nursing officer. In the process of communication, the role of Mr. Velayudhan is that of a:

a. Receiver b. Message
c. Referent d. Sender

178. Superantigens are the antigens that activate a large fraction of:

a. T cells b. B cells
c. IgA d. IgG

179. Which of the following is NOT a function of the Indian Nursing Council to maintain standards in nursing education?

a. Initiating, prescribing, guiding and supervising the different levels of nursing education
b. Recognizing and approving various institutions for conducting different nursing educational programs
c. Prescribing of syllabi
d. Recognizing any qualifications related to nursing, irrespective of adequacy of training

180. In February 2023, an Indian shooter ______ won the gold medal in the 10 m air rifle individual event at the ISSF Shooting World Cup at Cairo.

a. Udhayveer Sidhu b. Rudrankksh Patil
c. Bhowneesh Mendiratta d. Swapnil Kusale

181. The role of the Trained Nurses Association of India is to:

a. Provide registration for foreign nurses
b. Improve the living and working conditions of nurses
c. Prescribe curricula for nursing education
d. Promote the development of strong national associations

182. A teacher must consider the principle of individual difference in order to:

a. Adopt a suitable teaching technique and standard
b. Complete the course on time
c. Distribute study materials
d. Assess student performance

183. A known diabetic patient who has stopped taking insulin for the past three days has been admitted in the casualty ward with altered sensorium, dehydration and kussmaul breathing.

The first investigation to be done for this patient is:

a. Complete hemogram and blood urea
b. Liver function test and clotting time
c. ECG and lipid profile
d. Blood sugar and urine for acetone

184. ______ was conferred with the Padma Vibhushan Award 2023 by the Government of India for his contribution in the field of Science and Engineering.

a. Ganesh Nagappa Krishnarajanagara
b. Mahendra Pal
c. Khadar Valli Dudekula
d. Srinivasa Varadhan

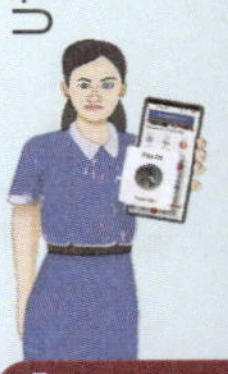

Ans.

163. d
164. b
165. a
166. d
167. c
168. c
169. c
170. d
171. d
172. d
173. c
174. a
175. b
176. b
177. d
178. a
179. d
180. b
181. b
182. a
183. d
184. d

185. Mrs. Salaluddhin, a nursing supervisor, visits the ward where Ms. Kavitha is performing a Ryle's tube feeding to a bedridden patient. In response to the nursing supervisor's presence, the feeding syringe slips from the hands of Ms. Kavita. Mrs. Salaluddhin stares at her and walks out of the ward. The type of communication in this situation is referred to as:

a. Empathetic communication
b. Meta communication
c. Verbal communication
d. Nonverbal communication

186. Which of the following statements is incorrect with respect to physiological responses to stress?

a. Acute stressors elicit a decrease in the markers of inflammation like IL-6.
b. Acute stressors elicit a decrease in cellular immune response.
c. The Hypothalamic-Pituitary Axis (HPA) response to stress varies according to the nature of stress.
d. Stressors of many kinds activate the noradrenergic system in the brain, most notably in the locus coeruleus, and cause the release of catecholamines.

187. A primigravida woman has delivered a male baby and is bleeding profusely after expulsion of the placenta. The midwife's diagnosis is PPH. What should be the midwife's immediate next step?

a. Call for help
b. Catheterization of the bladder
c. Examining the expelled placenta
d. Massaging the uterus

188. According to IMNCI, the danger signs for a sick child from two months to five years include:

a. Lethargy/unconsciousness, inability to drink/breastfeed, ear problems and malnutrition
b. Convulsions, lethargy/unconsciousness, inability to drink/breastfeed and ear problems
c. Convulsions, lethargy/unconsciousness, inability to drink/breastfeed and vomiting
d. Convulsions, lethargy, fever and diarrhea

189. Who among the following is popularly known as the Father of Yoga?

a. Charaka b. Atreya
c. Maharishi Patanjali d. Sushruta

190. Which of the following is the most commonly used irrigation solution and its temperature?

a. Sterile water, 100°F b. Normal saline, 100°F
c. Sterile water, 98.6°F d. Normal saline, 98.6°F

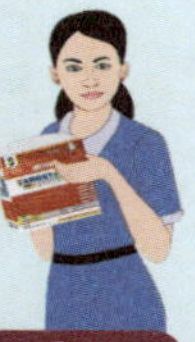

Ans.

185. d
186. a
187. a
188. c
189. c
190. d
191. d
192. c
193. a
194. b
195. c
196. c
197. d
198. a
199. a

191. Each of the letters given below has been assigned a number. Select the combination of numbers such that the corresponding letters when arranged accordingly will form a meaningful word.

1	2	3	4	5	6	7
T	S	E	C	Y	A	S

a. 6, 4, 2, 1, 3, 7, 5 b. 3, 2, 4, 1, 6, 7, 5
c. 3, 4, 2, 6, 1, 7, 5 d. 3, 4, 2, 1, 6, 7, 5

192. Which of the following is the drug of choice for treatment of OCD?

a. Lithium b. Diazepam
c. Fluoxetine d. Carbamazepine

193. The benefits of maternal administration of glucocorticoids in preterm labor is to:

a. Help in fetal lung maturation
b. Maintain integrity of foetal membranes
c. Arrest the uterine contractions
d. Prevent foetal infections

194. Deficiency of alpha antitrypsin may predispose a patient to:

a. Emphysema
b. Chronic obstructive pulmonary disease
c. Bronchitis
d. Pneumothorax

195. Where could they keep their caterpillars?

a. In the carpenter's shop b. In the gymnasium
c. In a shed d. In a house

196. What care had to be taken in feeding caterpillars?

a. Leaves must be green b. Leaves must be wet
c. Leaves must be dry d. Leaves must be soft

197. What kinds of boxes were made for the caterpillars?

a. With sawdust
b. With wood
c. With cardboard
d. With glass fronts and air holes

198. Do all the caterpillars need sawdust?

a. No; only those kinds which spin their spittle into sawdust tombs
b. No; only those kinds which spin their own cocoons
c. No; only those kinds which spin others cocoons
d. No; only those kinds which make their own cocoons

199. How did they gas the butterflies they caught?

a. By mixing cut laurel with water in jam jars
b. By mixing water with sawdust
c. By mixing sawdust with mud
d. By mixing chrysalis with water

"Sometimes the remedy is worse than the disease."

—Francis Bacon

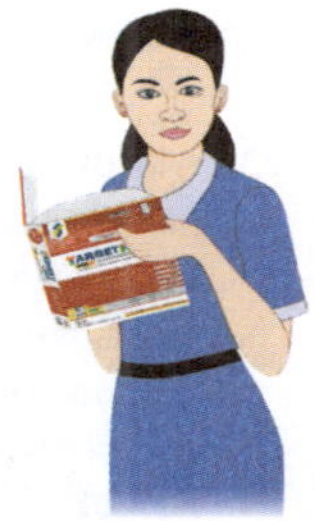

NORCET (NO) 2022 (Memory Based)

1. Which of the following is not included in the National Vector Borne Disease Control Program?

a. Malaria b. Dengue
c. Plague d. Filariasis

2. All of the following vaccines are given IM; except:

a. Hep B b. DPT
c. PCV d. MMR

3. Which of the following vaccines is most freeze sensitive vaccine?

a. MMR b. DPT
c. Hep B d. TT

4. Which of the following muscles is the site for DPT vaccination?

a. Ventrogluteal b. Vastus lateralis
c. Deltoid d. Dorsogluteal

5. Iron and folic acid dose for pregnant women:

a. 60 mg iron, 0.4 mg folic acid
b. 30 mg iron, 0.4 mg folic acid
c. 100 mg iron, 0.3 mg folic acid
d. 60 mg iron, 500 mcg folic acid

6. Night blindness is due to the deficiency of:

a. Vitamin A b. Vitamin C
c. Vitamin D d. Vitamin B_{12}

7. Which of the following vaccines is kept in freezer compartment of the refrigerator?

a. Measles b. DPT
c. Hep B d. OPV

8. Screening of depression at community level is an example of:

a. Secondary prevention
b. Primary prevention
c. Rehabilitation
d. Tertiary prevention

9. A study was done to identify the number of typhoid cases due to exposure from a common well in the village groups formed of carriers and diseased people. What type of study design is represented here?

a. Cohort study b. Cross-sectional study
c. Case-control study d. Field trial

10. Wernicke's and Korsakoff in alcoholic patient occur due to the deficiency of:

a. Thiamine deficiency b. Vitamin C
c. Vitamin D d. Vitamin A

11. Sciatic nerve damage occurs due to IM injection given at which of the following muscles?

a. Dorsogluteal b. Vastus lateralis
c. Ventrogluteal d. Deltoid

12. According to WHO, hypothermia in newborn is defined below:

a. 36.5°C b. 37°C
c. 36.9°C d. 37.2°C

13. Primary prevention strategy for cervical cancer is:

a. HPV vaccine
b. Medications
c. Health education
d. Screening for cervical cancer

14. Rickets in children is caused by:

a. Vitamin D deficiency b. Vitamin C
c. Vitamin A d. Vitamin B_{12}

15. The disease caused by the rat flea is:

a. Murine typhus b. Epidemic typhus
c. Japanese encephalitis d. Chagas disease

16. During child CPR, chest compressions should be given at:

a. Upper half of sternum b. Xiphisternum
c. Lower half of sternum d. Below sternum

17. A client undergoes mastoidectomy. When the client returns to the unit postoperatively, the client has difficulty drinking without drooling. It is most important for the nurse to take which action?

a. Re-assure patent as this is a normal finding
b. Assess patient's ability to whistle
c. Notify the physician.
d. Suction the secretions

18. Which of the following is helpful in prevention of pre-eclampsia?

a. Ascorbic acid
b. Vitamin E
c. Calcium
d. Vitamin A

19. All among the following are the emergency contraceptives; except:

a. Danazol b. Levonorgestrel
c. Cu T d. Mifepristone

20. Skin of a patient with Addison's disease appears:

a. Yellow b. Bronze
c. Black d. Gray

21. A pregnant woman at 38 weeks came to clinic and the period of gestation has been confirmed by the ultrasound reports and LMP. She has been started on oxytocin for induction of labor and the nurse notes that the contractions are coming for longer than 70 seconds and she is 3 cm dilated. What should the nurse do next?

a. Stop the oxytocin infusion
b. Increase the flow rate
c. Set the drops per minute
d. Document the findings

22. Severely dehydrated child exhibits:

a. Sunken eyes
b. Skin goes back very slowly (in more than 2 seconds)
c. Eagerly drinks water
d. Irritable

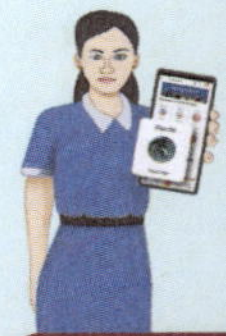

Ans.

1.	c
2.	d
3.	b
4.	b
5.	d
6.	a
7.	d
8.	a
9.	b
10.	a
11.	a
12.	a
13.	a
14.	a
15.	a
16.	c
17.	b
18.	c
19.	a
20.	b
21.	a
22.	b

23. All of the following statements are indicative of perfect latching; except:
- a. Baby's mouth wide open
- b. Lower areola is more visible than upper areola
- c. Baby's chin with mother breast
- d. Lower lip turn outwards

24. All of the following are included in the surgical safety checklist; except:
- a. Name of the surgeon and anesthetic
- b. Confirm the site
- c. Confirm the specimen labeling for transport biopsy
- d. Confirm the patient blood group

25. Patients taking MAO are not allowed to consume tyramine rich food as it causes:
- a. Diarrhea
- b. Hypertensive crisis
- c. Delayed drug effect
- d. Apnea

26. All of the following are included in the ventilator-associated pneumonia bundle care; except:
- a. Head elevated at 30°
- b. Sedation vacation
- c. Antibiotic prophylaxis
- d. Supraglottic suctioning

27. The priority nursing action in case of needle stick injury includes:
- a. Inform the physician
- b. Press the injured site to squeeze blood
- c. Wash the area with copious amount of water
- d. Press the area to stop bleeding

28. A 40-week pregnant woman came to the clinic. NST is performed for 20 minutes and shows two fetal movements which is followed by acceleration lasting for 15 seconds. Interpret the findings:
- a. Positive
- b. Negative
- c. Reactive
- d. Nonreactive

29. A person has a central venous catheter in place. Which of the following data can be assessed with this?
- a. Central venous pressure
- b. Blood pressure
- c. Urine output
- d. Pulse pressure

30. A patient who was on intravenous fluid therapy develops pain, redness and warmth at the site of peripheral cannula. This indicates:
- a. Venous spasm
- b. Phlebitis
- c. Infiltration
- d. Extravasation

31. In assessing the nature of the stool of a client who has cystic fibrosis, what would the nurse expect to see?
- a. Clay-colored stools
- b. Steatorrhea stools
- c. Dark brown stools
- d. Blood-tinged stools

32. A female came to the gynecologist with chief complaints of irregular vaginal bleeding. The nurse knows well that a decrease in this hormone is responsible for causing bleeding during the menstrual cycle under normal physiological condition:
- a. Estrogen
- b. Progesterone
- c. FSH
- d. Thyroxine

33. What is the complication of liver biopsy in children?
- a. Bleeding
- b. Bile leak
- c. Pneumothorax
- d. Prolonged drainage of ascitic fluid

34. When does the child identify gender?
- a. 7 – 8 years
- b. 3 years
- c. At puberty
- d. 6 years

35. A patient presents with tension pneumothorax. What will be the priority nursing intervention?
- a. Wide bore needle in 2nd mid clavicular space followed by chest tube drainage
- b. Providing prone position
- c. Giving chest physiotherapy
- d. Providing pain medication

36. Which of the following is a nonabsorbable suture?
- a. Chromic catgut
- b. Polyglactin
- c. Polypropylene
- d. Monocryl

37. The normal urine output in adult in 24 hours is:
- a. 2000 mL
- b. 1500 mL
- c. 500 mL
- d. 2500 mL

38. The concentration of sodium chloride in isotonic solution is -----.
- a. 9%
- b. 0.09%
- c. 0.9%
- d. 19%

39. A patient admitted in emergency department with burn on one upper limb and full back. According to rule 9, calculate the burn area:
- a. 18%
- b. 27%
- c. 9%
- d. 36%

40. This is the classic ECG change in MI (myocardial infarction):
- a. ST-segment elevation
- b. Negative T-waves
- c. Development of an abnormal Q wave
- d. All of the above

41. In clinical setup, KCL bolus is contraindicated because:
- a. It may lead to cardiac arrest and sudden death.
- b. It leads to hypotension only.
- c. It may damage the veins of the patient.

42. Which of the following is needed in the management of the PIH?
- a. Vitamin C
- b. Vitamin E
- c. Folic acid
- d. Calcium

43. Most common congenital malformation in overt diabetes in pregnancy:
- a. Ventricular septal defect
- b. Sacral agenesis
- c. Tetralogy of Fallot
- d. Atrial septal defect

44. A female patient underwent modified radical mastectomy. She develops winging of the scapula. It is due to the damage to:
- a. Long intrathoracic nerve
- b. Intercostal brachial nerve
- c. Phrenic nerve
- d. Axillary nerve

45. To ensure proper client education, the nurse should teach the client taking sublingual nitroglycerine to expect which of the following responses with administration?
- a. Stinging, burning when placed under the tongue
- b. Temporary blurring of vision
- c. Generalized urticaria with prolonged use
- d. Urinary frequency

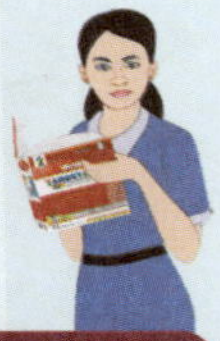

Ans.

23. b
24. d
25. b
26. c
27. c
28. c
29. a
30. b
31. b
32. b
33. a
34. a
35. a
36. c
37. b
38. c
39. b
40. d
41. a
42. d
43. a
44. a
45. a

46. At what point blood pressure is considered "high"?

a. 120/80 mm Hg b. 130/80 mm Hg
c. 140/90 mm Hg d. 210/120 mm Hg

47. Solution used for disinfection in a COVID patient is:

a. Hydrochloric acid
b. Sodium hypochlorite
c. Sulfuric acid
d. Phenol

48. Most infectious disease leading to mortality in children worldwide:

a. Diarrhea
b. Pneumonia
c. Acute epiglottitis
d. CROUP

49. Lactulose is prescribed for the patient suffering from liver cirrhosis so as to:

a. Prevent hepatic encephalopathy
b. Decrease production of bilirubin
c. Increase lactulose level in blood
d. Increase breakdown of bilirubin

50. Example of post-traumatic stress syndrome (PTSD) includes:

a. Divorce b. Gunshot
c. Financial loss d. All of these

51. Which measure is used for growth monitoring at Anganwadi center?

a. Weight for height
b. MUAC
c. Skin fold thicknesses
d. Weight for age

52. National Institute of Nutrition is situated in:

a. Hyderabad b. Bangalore
c. New Delhi d. Chandigarh

53. Vitamin D deficiency in children results in:

a. Scurvy b. Night blindness
c. Rickets d. Beriberi

54. Which of the following disease is caused by the rat flea?

a. Endemic typhus b. Tick typhus
c. Sleeping sickness d. Typhoid

55. Which of the following postpartum drugs is safe for breastfeeding mothers?

a. Lithium b. Captopril
c. Enalpril d. Hydrochlorothiazide

56. Primary prevention for CA Cervix can be done by:

a. HPV vaccine b. Pap smear
c. Drug therapy d. Preventing complications

57. Which bank plays a primary role in managing and governing the financial system of the country?

a. HDFC b. RBI
c. SBI d. PNB

58. Complete the sequence

1 2 3 5 8 13……

a. 20 b. 21
c. 15 d. 23

59. The following are the rivers in Punjab; except:

a. Beas b. Yamuna
c. Jhelum d. Ganga

60. Which of the following image is present behind the 2000 rupees note?

a. Red fort b. Hampi
c. Ellora Caves d. Mangalyaan

61. Identify the name of the following image:

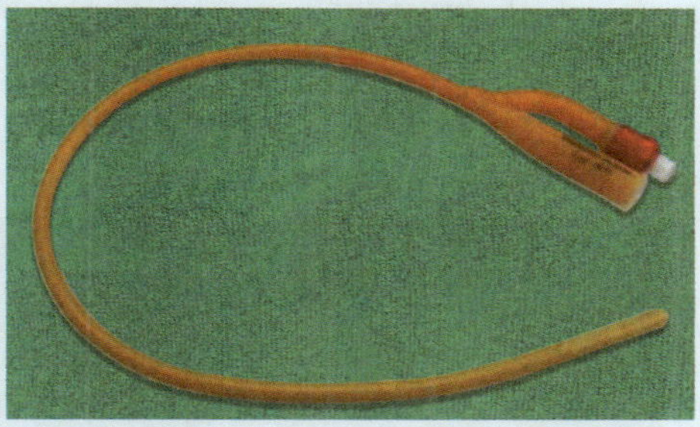

a. Suction catheter b. Suprapubic catheter
c. Foleys catheter d. Robinson catheter

62. Which is the correct placement of simple oxygen mask in pediatric patients?

a. 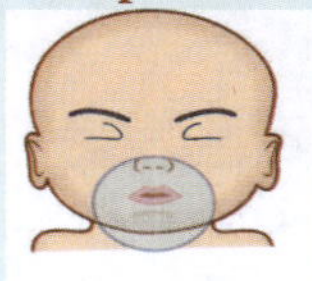 b. 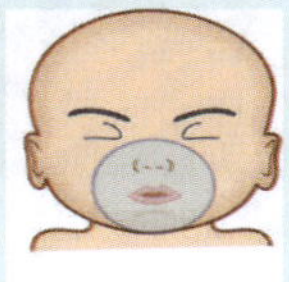

c. 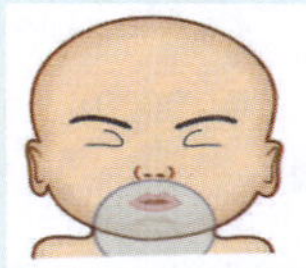 d. 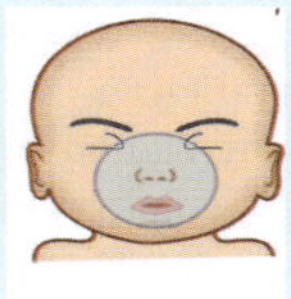

63. Identify the following inheritance pattern:

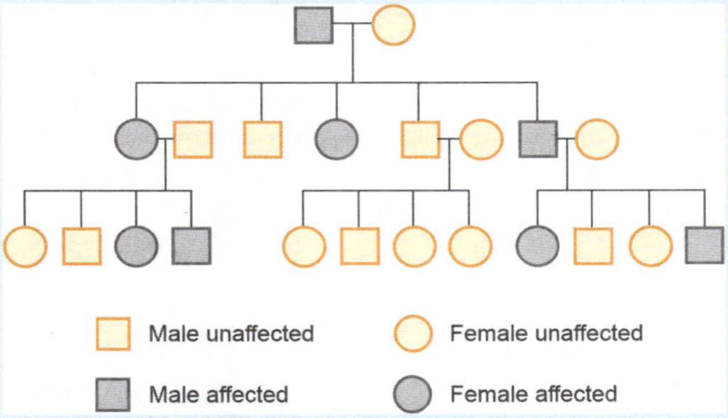

a. Autosomal dominant b. Autosomal recessive
c. X-linked recessive d. X-linked dominant

64. Which gas is used in laparoscopy procedure?

a. CO_2 b. CO
c. Oxygen d. Nitrogen

65. Most indicative of correct NG tube placement is:

a. Acid pH 3.8
b. Absence of respiratory distress
c. Marking visible just above nasal area
d. Tape secured tightly

66. The following techniques should never be used to confirm the location of an NG tube:

a. 'Whoosh' test: auscultation of air insufflated through the feeding line
b. Using the absence of respiratory discomfort as a sign that position is appropriate
c. Keeping an eye on the bubbling at the tube's end
d. Observing the appearance of NG tube aspirate

Ans.

46. b
47. b
48. b
49. a
50. b
51. b
52. a
53. c
54. a
55. d
56. a
57. b
58. b
59. d
60. d
61. c
62. b
63. a
64. a
65. a
66. a

67. Doctor orders the removal of the NG tube for a patient. The nurse follows the order and removes it. She knows that after the removal of NG tube, it has to be discarded in:

a. Yellow bin b. Red bin
c. Blue bin d. Black bin

68. Identify the following logo:

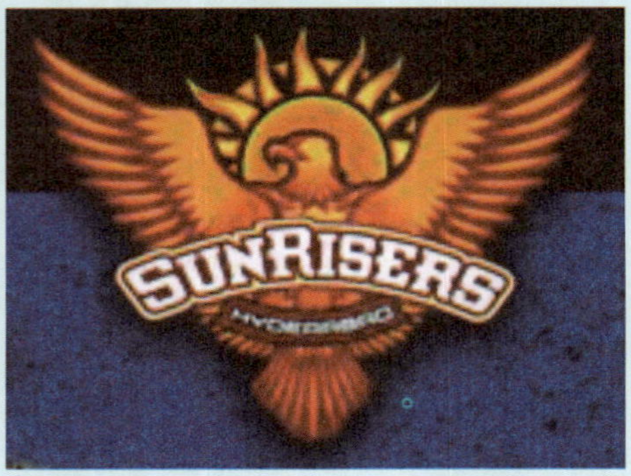

a. Mumbai b. Chennai
c. Rajasthan d. Hyderabad

69. Recommended dose of Adrenaline used for neonatal resuscitation is:

a. 0.01 mg/kg/body weight (0.1 mL/kg, 1:10000)
b. 1 mg/kg body weight (1 mL, 1:1000)
c. 0.1 mg/kg body weight (0.1 mL, 1:10000)
d. 0.5 mg/kg body weight (0.1 mL/kg, 1:1000)

70. A patient who has undergone thyroidectomy shows the symptoms of carpopedal spasm. Which medication is to be administered to this patient?

a. Calcium carbonate b. Calcium gluconate
c. Calcium lactate d. Calcium citrate

71. All of the following help in the absorption of iron; except:

a. Curd b. Sprouts
c. Amla d. Orange

72. Anthracosis is due to:

a. Coal dust b. Silicon
c. Cotton d. Sugarcane

73. Current Vice President of India is:

a. Droupadi Murmu b. Jagdeep Dhankar
c. Uday Umesh Lalit d. Narendra Modi

74. Current Chief Justice of Supreme Court is:

a. N.V. Ramana b. Jagdeep Dhankar
c. Uday Umesh Lalit d. Lalit Modi

75. Aurangabad is also known as:

a. Sambhajinagar b. Dharashiv
c. Motinagar d. Mojhpur

76. Identify the disease in the following image:

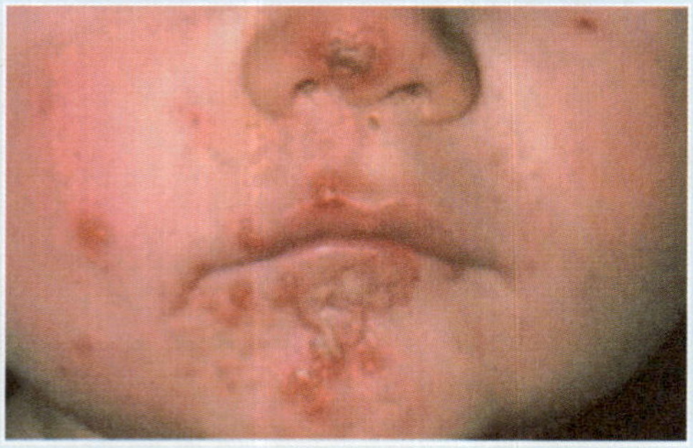

a. Impetigo b. Lupus erythematosus
c. Roseola infantum d. Varicella

77. Identify the disease in the following image:

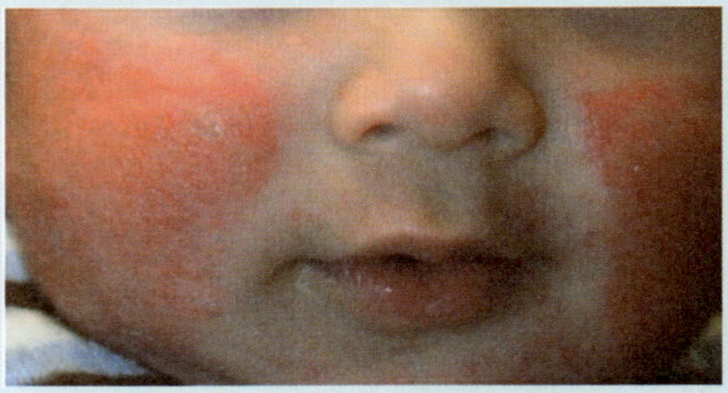

a. Atophic dermatitis b. Impetigo
c. Acne vulgaris d. Juvenile psoriasis

78. The endemic disease that occurs every 4 years of interval is called:

a. Secular trend b. Time trend
c. Periodic trend d. Cyclic trend

79. Which of the following muscles is the site for DPT in infants?

a. Ventrogluteal b. Vastus lateralis
c. Deltoid d. Dorsogluteal

80. Most common size of indwelling urinary catheter in adult females:

a. 5 to 8 fr b. 10 to 12 fr
c. 14 to 16 fr d. 16 to 18 fr

81. Night blindness is due to the deficiency of:

a. Vitamin A b. Vitamin B_1
c. Vitamin C d. Vitamin B_{12}

82. JSSK was introduced in the year:

a. 1995 b. 2000
c. 2011 d. 1980

83. The difference between systolic and diastolic blood pressure is known as:

a. Pulse difference b. Cardiac pressure
c. Systolic pressure d. Pulse pressure

84. Identify an example of age-independent anthropometry.

a. MUAC b. Weight
c. Head circumference d. Chest circumference

85. Most common area affected in trichotillomania is:

a. Scalp b. Face
c. Arms d. Eyelashes

86. Cleft lip baby diet postsurgery must include:

a. Fruit pulp b. Crackers
c. Purees d. Cold cereals

87. Nurses Day theme 2021 was:

a. Nurses: a voice to lead - a vision for future healthcare.
b. Nurses: a voice to lead - nursing the world to Health.
c. Nurses: a voice to lead - health for all.
d. Nurses: a voice to lead - health is a human right.

88. Total parenteral nutrition (TPN) fluid is of which type:

a. Isotonic b. Hypotonic
c. Hypertonic d. None of these

89. Male infertility is common complication of:

a. Measles b. Chicken pox
c. Mumps d. Rubella

90. A patient transferred to labor room and the nurse identifies that the patient is in first stage of labor. When will the nurse document the progress of labor with respect to the cervical dilation on a partograph?

a. 4 cm b. 5 cm
c. 7 cm d. 10 cm

Ans.

67.	b
68.	d
69.	a
70.	b
71.	a
72.	a
73.	b
74.	c
75.	a
76.	a
77.	a
78.	d
79.	b
80.	c
81.	a
82.	c
83.	d
84.	a
85.	a
86.	c
87.	a
88.	c
89.	c
90.	b

91. A patient is prescribed 2000 mL of D5½ NS that should be administered within 24 hours with a microdrip set. Calculate the drop rate.

a. 33 b. 42
c. 66 d. 83

92. You have received a victim with a history of fall from 3rd floor and on examination, the victim is unresponsive. Which method the nurse will use to assess the airway in this victim?

a. Jaw thrust maneuver
b. Head-tilt-chin lift maneuver
c. Heimlich maneuver
d. None of the above

93. A person believes that he is God and he has all the powers. He is exhibiting:

a. Delusion of reference b. Delusion of grandeur
c. Delusion of persecution d. Nihilistic delusion

94. Mantoux test is done on a patient who has been suffering from HIV. What value of induration indicates the TB infection in the patient?

a. 5 b. 7
c. 11 d. 15

95. Tell the odd one out:

Kind: Thoughtful: Ambient: Gracious

a. Thoughtful b. Ambient
c. Gracious d. Kind

96. Patient in ED is admitted with a history of chemical burns. What is the priority nursing intervention?

a. Wash with running water
b. Call doctor
c. Apply povidone cream
d. Apply antibiotic cream

97. A patient with circumferential burn comes to the emergency. The patient should be assessed for which complication?

a. Absent peripheral pulse b. Fluid status
c. Urine output d. Engorged neck veins

98. Schizophrenia life expectancy is.....years less than the general population.

a. 2 – 5 years b. 8 – 10 years
c. 11 – 20 years d. 1 – 2 years

99. A young male with a movable and painless lump came to the OPD. Identify the condition:

a. Lipoma b. Myoma
c. Subcutaneous lesion d. Hive

100. All of the following are included in surgical safety checklist, except:

a. Sign-in b. Sign-out
c. Time-in d. Time-out

101. All among the following are seen in anorexia nervosa; except:

a. Myocardial hypertrophy b. Osteoporosis
c. Electrolyte imbalance d. Menorrhagia

102. A patient has asthma and is prescribed albuterol and beclomethasone. Which of the following statements indicates that the patient needs no further teaching regarding the use of inhalational agents?

a. First administer the Albuterol, and then 5 minutes later, administer the beclomethasone.
b. First administer the beclomethasone, and then immediately administer the Albuterol.
c. First administer the beclomethasone, and then 5 minutes later administer the Albuterol.
d. First administer the Albuterol and, then 1 minute later administer the beclomethasone.

103. A 16-year-old student has a long history of bronchial asthma and has experienced several severe asthmatic attacks during the school year. The school nurse is required to administer 0.2 mL of 1/1000 solution of epinephrine SC during an asthma attack. How does the school nurse evaluate the effectiveness of this intervention?

a. Increased pulse rate
b. Increased expectorate of secretions
c. Decreased inspiratory difficulty
d. Increased respiratory rate

104. A person has a poultry farm and sells eggs and buys food. One kg is equal to Rs 20. He sells one egg for Rs 4.5. How much eggs should be sold for buying 5 kg food? (Arithematics)

a. 22.22 b. 23.22
c. 24.22 d. 25.22

105. What is the compression to ventilation ratio in infant during neonatal resuscitation?

a. 3:1 b. 15:2
c. 1:3 d. 1:5

106. Identify the following image:

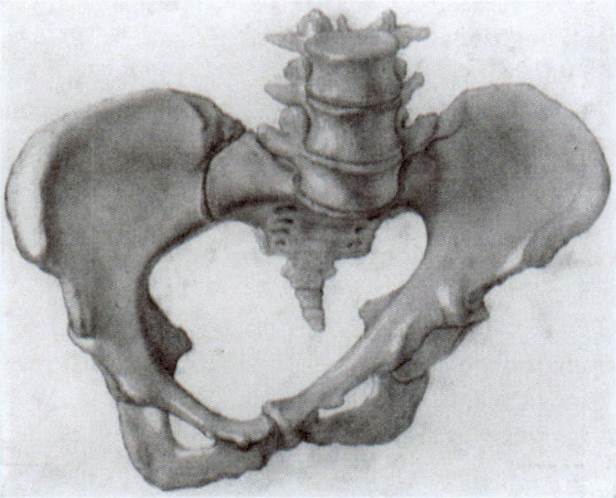

a. Naegele's Pelvis b. Robert's Pelvis
c. Scoliotic Pelvis d. Android Pelvis

107. Identify the following image:

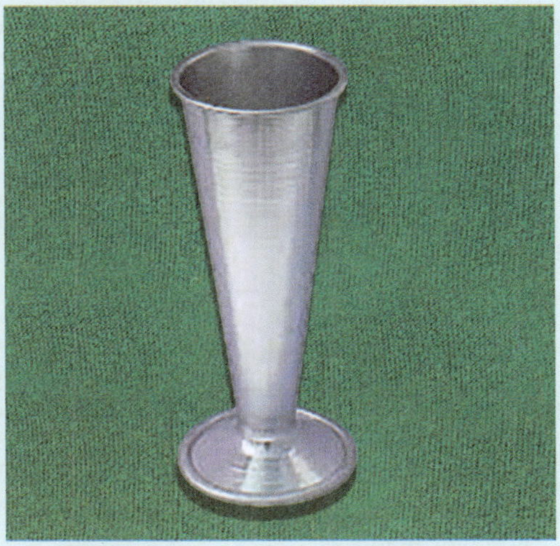

a. Stethoscope b. Pinard fetoscope
c. Doppler d. Endoscope

108. A patient with diabetes mellitus is on regular insulin and insulin was administered at 9:00 am. By what time will it take to reach its peak level?

a. 10:30 am b. 12:00 noon
c. 04:00 pm d. 10:30 am

Ans.

91. d
92. a
93. b
94. a
95. b
96. a
97. a
98. c
99. a
100. c
101. d
102. a
103. c
104. a
105. a
106. a
107. b
108. b

109. Identify the given instrument:

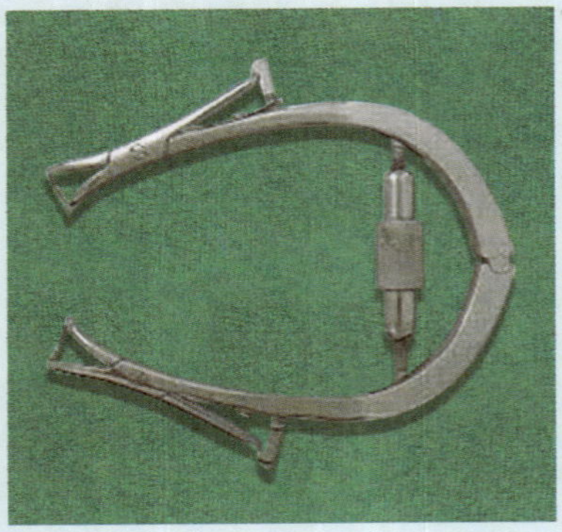

a. Jolls retractor
b. Omni-tract wishbone retractor
c. Balfour abdominal retractor
d. Richardson retractor

110. A low birth weight baby is:

a. <1500 g b. <500 g
c. <2500 g d. <1000 g

111. Normal healthy adult person pulse range is:

a. 60–80 beats/minute b. 60–100 beats/minute
c. 70–110 beats/minute d. 40–90 beats/minute

112. Life span of contraceptive device Cu-T 380 A is:

a. 10 years b. 5 years
c. 7 years d. 15 years

113. When is World Patient Safety Day Celebrated?

a. 17th September b. 27th September
c. 24th September d. 20th September

114. Formula for measuring the ET tube size in children?

a. (Age in years/ 4) + 4
b. (Age in years/36 month) + 4
c. (Age in years/18 month) + 4
d. (Age in years/6) + 3.5

115. Which among the following is seen in multiple sclerosis?

a. Bradykinesia b. Loss of consciousness
c. Rhythmic shaking d. Speech changes

116. Which among the following is a priority management technique used in myasthenia gravis?

a. Maintain balance between sleep and rest
b. Maintain hygiene
c. Maintain hydration
d. Maintain respiratory function

117. After school bus accident, a nurse should give the first priority to which patient?

a. A patient with leakage of clear fluid from the ear
b. A patient with hematoma on head
c. A patient with 2-inch scalp laceration
d. A patient showing clear pupillary reaction with light

118. Which sign is the most indicative of myasthenia gravis?

a. Propulsive gait
b. Drooping of one or both eyelids
c. Waddling gait
d. Pill-rolling tremor

119. To measure the required length of nasogastric tube, measurements should be taken from the patient's:

a. Ear to xiphisternum
b. Nose to ear to xiphisternum
c. Nose to xiphisternum
d. Angle of the jaw to xiphisternum

120. Identify the use of the instrument that is shown in the following image:

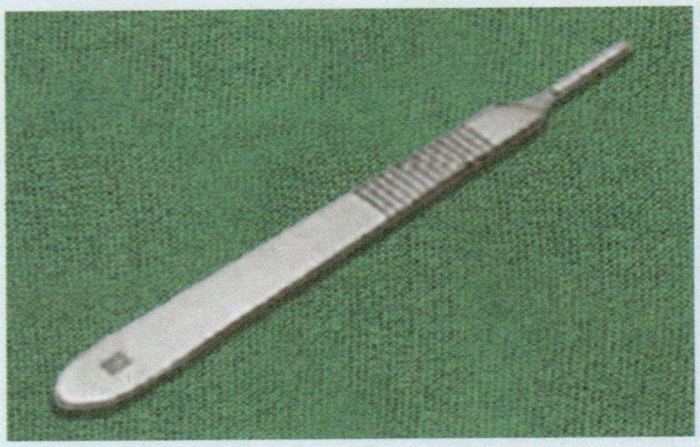

a. Used for fixing surgical blade
b. Dissection of the tissues
c. Used for cutting the skin
d. Used for ear examination

121. A client receiving parenteral nutrition (PN) complains of a headache. The nurse notes that the client has an increased blood pressure, bounding pulse, jugular vein distention and crackles bilaterally. The nurse determines that the client is experiencing which complication of PN therapy?

a. Sepsis
b. Air embolism
c. Hypervolemia
d. Hyperglycemia

122. A hospital caught fire. What will be the priority nursing intervention in this case?

a. Evacuate the patient
b. Use the fire extinguisher
c. Shut off the oxygen supply
d. Call fire department

123. According to Schneider, all of the following symptoms in schizophrenia patients are known as first rank symptoms; except:

a. Auditory hallucination
b. Visual hallucination
c. Thought echo
d. Thought broadcast

124. Identify the image given below:

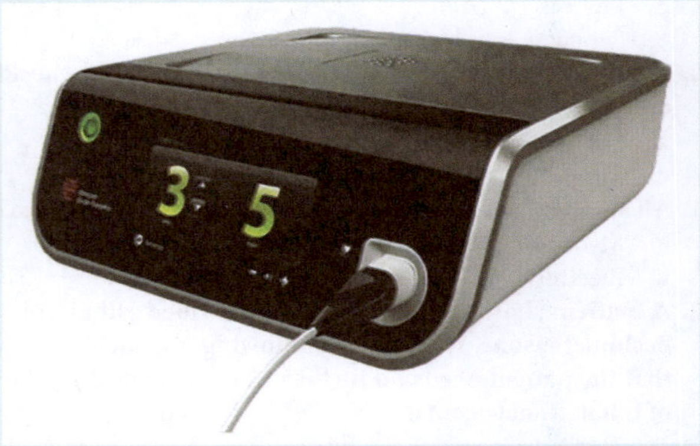

a. Harmonic scalpel b. Monopolar cautery
c. Bipolar cautery d. Defibrillator

125. The newborn passes the meconium within:

a. 6 hours b. 12 hours
c. 24 – 48 hours d. 96 hours

Ans.

109.	a
110.	c
111.	b
112.	a
113.	a
114.	a
115.	d
116.	d
117.	a
118.	b
119.	b
120.	a
121.	c
122.	c
123.	b
124.	a
125.	c

126. Identify the surgical blade:

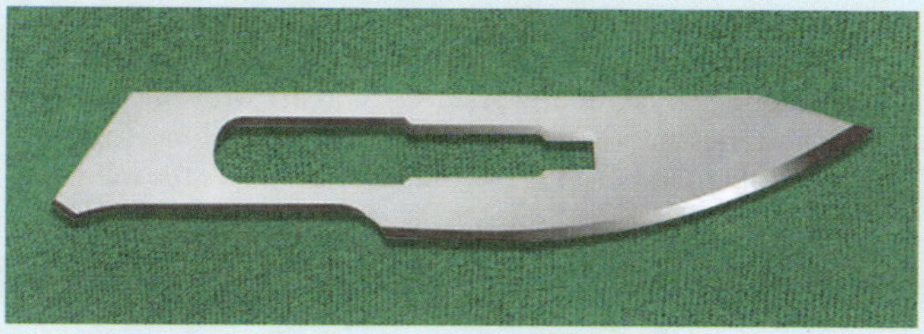

a. 23 number b. 11 number
c. 12 number d. 15 number

127. Which of the following is given to prevent NTD in pregnant females?
a. Folic acid
b. Calcium tablets
c. Vitamin K
d. Thyroxin

128. The antilarval method includes:
a. Rosemary
b. Citronella Geranium
c. Gambusia affinis
d. Malathion

129. Earthquake is measured by which scale?
a. Richter scale
b. Moment magnitude scale
c. Modified Mercalli scale
d. None of the above

130. All of the following result in delirium; except:
a. Benzodiazepines withdrawal
b. Opioid withdrawal
c. Hyponatremia
d. Depression

131. PQLI (The Physical Quality of Life Index) is all; except:
a. Life expectancy at one year of age
b. Literary rate
c. IMR
d. Income

132. Which test is used to check whether freeze-sensitive vaccines have been damaged by exposure to temperatures below 0 °C?
a. Stick test b. Shake test
c. Shick test d. Shock test

133. Egg contains all; except:
a. Vitamin C
b. Vitamin A
c. Whole protein
d. Carbohydrate

134. Vaccine given at birth; except:
a. BCG b. OPV
c. Hepatitis B d. IPV

135. After a 10-year-old child with insulin-dependent diabetes mellitus receives her dinner tray, she tells the nurse that she hates broccoli and wants some corn on the cob. The nurse's appropriate response is:
a. "No vegetable exchanges are allowed."
b. "Corn and other starchy vegetables are considered to be bread exchanges."
c. "Yes, you may exchange any vegetable for any other vegetable."
d. "Yes, but only one-half ear is allowed."

136. A 26-year-old client is admitted to the labor, delivery, recovery, postpartum unit. The nurse completes her assessment and determines the client is in the first stage of labor. The nurse should instruct her:
a. To hold her breath during contractions
b. To be flat on her back
c. Not to push with her contractions
d. To push before becoming fully dilated

137. A 6-month-old infant has developmental delays. His weight falls below the 5th percentile when plotted on a growth chart. A diagnosis of failure to thrive is made. What behaviors might indicate the possibility of maternal deprivation?
a. Responsive to touch, wants to be held
b. Uncomforted by touch, refuses bottle
c. Maintains eye-to-eye contact
d. Finicky eater, easily pacified, cuddly

138. A 7-year-old child is brought to the ER at midnight by his mother after symptoms appeared abruptly. The nurse's initial assessment reveals a temperature of 104.5°F (40.3°C), difficulty swallowing, drooling, absence of a spontaneous cough, and agitation. These symptoms are indicative of which one of the following?
a. Acute tracheitis
b. Acute spasmodic croup
c. Acute epiglottitis
d. Acute laryngotracheobronchitis

139. Which one of the following is considered a reliable indicator for assessing the adequacy of fluid resuscitation in a 3-year-old child who suffered partial- and full thickness burns to 25% of her body?
a. Urine output b. Edema
c. Hypertension d. Bulging fontanelle

140. The nurse is assessing and getting a history from a client treated for depression with a monoamine oxidase (MAO) antidepressant. The most serious side effect associated with this antidepressant and the ingestion of tyramine in aged foods may be:
a. Hypertensive crisis b. Severe rash
c. Severe hypotension d. Severe diarrhea

141. After the fetal activity test (nonstress test) is completed, the RN is looking at the test results on the monitor strip. The RN observes that the fetal heart accelerated 5 beats/min with each fetal movement. The accelerations lasted for 15 seconds and occurred 3 times during the 20-minutes test. The RN knows that these test results will be interpreted as:
a. A reactive test b. A nonreactive test
c. An unsatisfactory test d. A negative test

142. The most important reason to closely assess circumferential burns at least every hour is that they may result in:
a. Hypovolemia
b. Renal damage
c. Ventricular arrhythmias
d. Loss of peripheral pulses

143. A schizophrenic client who is experiencing thoughts of having special powers states that "I am a messenger from another planet and can rule the earth." The nurse assesses this behavior as:
a. Ideas of reference b. Delusions of persecution
c. Thought broadcasting d. Delusions of grandeur

Ans.
126. a
127. a
128. c
129. a
130. d
131. d
132. b
133. d
134. d
135. b
136. c
137. b
138. c
139. a
140. a
141. a
142. d
143. d

144. A 56-year-old client is admitted to the psychiatric unit in a state of total despair. She feels hopeless and worthless, has a flat affect and very sad appearance, and is unable to feel pleasure from anything. Her husband has been assisting her at home with the housework and cooking: however, she has not been eating much, lies around or sits in a chair most of the day, and is becoming confused and thinks her family does not want her around anymore. In assessing the client, the nurse determines that her behavior is consistent with:

a. Transient depression
b. Mild depression
c. Moderate depression
d. Severe depression

145. A newborn infant is exhibiting signs of respiratory distress. Which of the following would the nurse recognize as the earliest clinical sign of respiratory distress?

a. Cyanosis
b. Increased respirations
c. Sternal and subcostal retractions
d. Decreased respirations

146. A 16-year-old client with anorexia nervosa is on an inpatient psychiatric unit. She has a fear of gaining weight and is refusing to eat sufficient amounts to maintain body weight for her age, height, and stature. To assist with the problem of powerlessness and plan for the client to no longer need to withhold food to feel in control, the nurse uses the following strategy:

a. Establish a structured environment with routine tasks and activities. Also, serve meals at the same time each day.
b. Distract the client during meals to get her to eat because she must take in sufficient amounts to keep from starving.
c. Do frequent room checks to be sure that the client is not hiding food or throwing it away.
d. Listen attentively and participate in in-depth discussions about food, because these actions may encourage her to eat.

147. A client has been admitted to the labor and delivery unit in active labor. After assessing her, the RN notes that the client's fetus position is left occipital posterior. Which of the following statements best describes what this means to the labor process?

a. Decreases the overall time of the labor process
b. Prolongs the client's first stage of labor
c. Decreases the time of the client's first stage of labor
d. Prolongs the client's third stage of labor

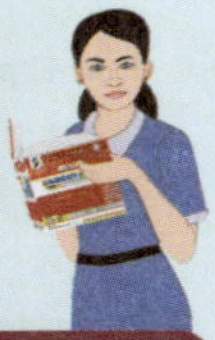

Ans.

144. d
145. c
146. a
147. b

"One day in perfect health is much."
—Arabic

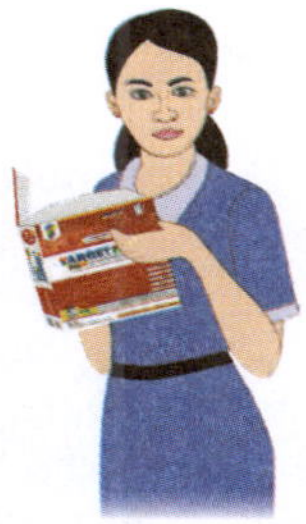

Staff Nurse Examination Himachal Pradesh 2022

1. **The most preferred intramuscular injection site for children and infants is:**
   a. Deltoid site b. Dorso-gluteal site
   c. Ventrogluteal site d. Vastus lateralis site
2. **Which of the following nursing interventions would be most important for determining fluid balance in a client with end stage renal failure?**
   a. Monitor urine specific gravity
   b. Measure fluid intake
   c. Weigh daily
   d. Record frequency of bowel movements
3. **Which of the following ethical principles refers to the duty not to harm?**
   a. Beneficence b. Nonmaleficence
   c. Fidelity d. Veracity
4. **Skin breaks, abrasion, blister or shallow crater, edema, and infection are:**
   a. Stage-I pressure ulcer
   b. Stage-II pressure ulcer
   c. Stage-III pressure ulcer
   d. Stage-IV pressure ulcer
5. **Which of the following is considered the most important aspect of hand washing?**
   a. Soap b. Water
   c. Friction d. Time
6. **Color coding for nitrous oxide cylinder is:**
   a. Black
   b. Black with white shoulders
   c. French blue
   d. Gray
7. **A child who is being treated for leukemia develops stomatitis. Which of the following nursing care measures is essential?**
   a. Using dental floss to clean the teeth
   b. Frequent cleaning of the mouth with an astringent mouthwash
   c. Use of an overbed cradle
   d. Swabbing the mouth with moistened cotton swabs
8. **Partial or complete separation of wound edges is called:**
   a. Abscess formation
   b. Wound dehiscence
   c. Wound evisceration
   d. Fistula
9. **During administration of the enema, if the patient complains of abdominal cramps, what should the nurse do?**
   a. Stop giving enema
   b. Continue giving enema
   c. Slow the rate of giving enema
   d. Administer analgesic
10. **What is the main purpose of the cardiac bed?**
    a. To increase the appetite
    b. To relieve dyspnea
    c. To keep the patient warm
    d. To increase circulation
11. **The technique used to prevent cross infection is known as:**
    a. Nursing care b. Barrier nursing
    c. Actual nursing d. Preventive nursing
12. **A system of family-centered care to dying patients is known as:**
    a. Hospital
    b. Hospice
    c. Nursing home
    d. Day care center
13. **Which of the following assessment findings should alert the nurse that the elderly client should be evaluated for pernicious anemia?**
    a. Clubbing of the nails
    b. Bloody stools
    c. Beefy-red tongue
    d. Enlarged lymph nodes
14. **What is the primary reason for administering the iron using the Z track technique?**
    a. It prevents pain at injection site
    b. It prevents staining of the skin
    c. It improves the amount of absorption
    d. It increases the speed of onset of action
15. **Which nursing intervention is appropriate to prevent pulmonary embolus in a patient who is prescribed bed rest?**
    a. Limit the client's fluid intake
    b. Encourage deep breathing and coughing
    c. Use the knee gatch when the client is in bed
    d. Teach the patient to move legs in bed
16. **Which of the following nursing intervention is appropriate when an IV infusion infiltrates?**
    a. Elevate the site
    b. Discontinue the infusion
    c. Attempt to flush the tube
    d. Apply warm, moist compress
17. **Which of the following conditions has an increased risk for developing hyperkalemia?**
    a. Crohn's disease
    b. Cushing's disease
    c. Chronic heart failure
    d. End-stage renal disease
18. **A circumscribed raised lesion that contains pus which may be formed as a result of purulent changes in a vesicle is:**
    a. Macule b. Papule
    c. Nodule d. Pustule

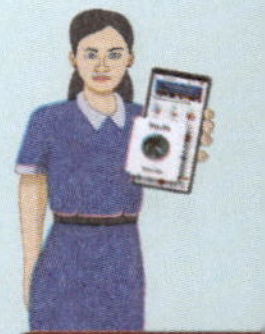

Ans.

1.	d
2.	c
3.	b
4.	b
5.	c
6.	c
7.	d
8.	b
9.	a
10.	b
11.	b
12.	b
13.	c
14.	b
15.	d
16.	b
17.	d
18.	d

19. According to Maslow's hierarchy of human needs, the highest level is:
a. Safety and security
b. Belongingness and affection
c. Esteem and self-respect
d. Self-actualization

20. Which of the following is the appropriate nursing intervention for a patient with a terminal illness who is passing through the 'acceptance stage'?
a. Encouraging the patient to cry
b. Encouraging unrestricted visitors
c. Explaining the patient what is being done
d. Being around though not speaking

21. Myocardial infarction (MI) is also known as:
a. Angina pectoris b. Heart attack
c. Dysrhythmia d. Heart Failure

22. Nitroglycerine is a:
a. Vasodilator
b. Diuretic
c. Cardiac Glycoside
d. Angiotensin converting enzyme

23. Sinoatrial node is located at:
a. Upper posterior wall of the right atrium
b. Lower posterior wall of the right atrium
c. Upper anterior wall of the right atrium
d. Lower anterior wall of the right atrium

24. The normal QRS interval is:
a. 0.06 to 0.10 seconds
b. 0.1 to 0.15 seconds
c. 0.12 to 0.16 seconds
d. 0.14 to 0.18 seconds

25. Holter monitoring, a noninvasive recording of ECG to match the abnormalities with symptoms is done up to:
a. 12 hours b. 48 hours
c. Four days d. One week

26. Treadmill protocol I is related to:
a. Coronary artery bypass graft
b. Echocardiogram
c. Angiogram
d. Exercise ECG test

27. Sinus tachycardia is treated by:
a. Dilantin b. Derriphyllin
c. Furosemide d. Atenolol

28. Which of the following is the quickest source of energy?
a. Dal rice
b. Slice of bread
c. Glass of orange juice
d. Glass of milk

29. The reason for polyurea is best defined as:
a. Lack of urine formation
b. Diminished ability of the kidneys to concentrate the urine
c. Passing too much urine at night
d. Dark colored urine

30. Glasgow Coma Scale is scored between:
a. 5–12 b. 7–18
c. 11–25 d. 3–15

31. Color of stool of patients having gastrointestinal bleeding will be:
a. Black b. Dark green
c. Clay d. Light brown

32. Paraplegia means:
a. Paralysis of one side of the body
b. Paralysis of the lower limbs
c. Paralysis of all four limbs
d. Impaired strength in the whole body

33. Tuberculin test is considered positive if induration is more than:
a. 2 mm b. 4 mm
c. 6 mm d. 10 mm

34. When recording blood pressure, the sounds which are heard with a stethoscope placed over the artery are termed:
a. Wheeze b. Murmurs
c. Crackle sounds d. Korotkoff sounds

35. Passive acquired immunity is obtained by:
a. Exposure to a disease
b. Immunization with antigen
c. Recovering from a disease
d. Giving an antitoxin or antiserum

COMMUNITY HEALTH NURSING

36. Incidence of a disease is defined as:
a. Number of old cases of the disease present during a specific period in a given population.
b. Number of total cases of disease existing in a given population at a given point of time.
c. Number of old plus new cases of disease existing in given population during given time period.
d. Number of new cases of disease occurring in a given population.

37. Oral rehydration solution contains all, except:
a. Calcium lactate b. Sodium chloride
c. Potassium chloride d. Glucose

38. Which of the following is secondary level of prevention?
a. Health promotion
b. Early diagnosis and treatment
c. Disability limitation
d. Rehabilitation

39. A woman in reproductive years is recommended to conduct 'Self-Breast Examination' to screen breast cancer as per the following schedule:
a. Whenever she gets time
b. Once in a month just before menstruation
c. Once a month on 6 to 8 days of menstruation
d. Any day in a month

40. Which of the following is not the route of transmission of hepatitis B?
a. Feco-oral route
b. Parenteral route
c. Sexual transmission
d. Perinatal transmission

41. The following are the beneficiaries of Integrated Child Development Scheme; except:
a. Children up to six years of age
b. Adolescent boys
c. Adolescent girls
d. Pregnant and lactating mothers

42. Definite host of Malarial Parasite is:
a. Man b. Mosquito
c. Pig d. Sand fly

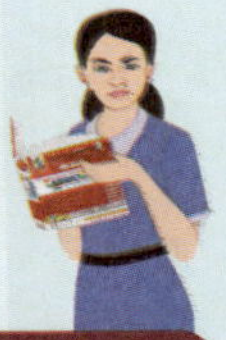

Ans.

19. d
20. d
21. b
22. a
23. a
24. a
25. b
26. d
27. d
28. c
29. b
30. d
31. a
32. b
33. d
34. d
35. d
36. d
37. a
38. b
39. c
40. a
41. b
42. b

43. A substance which is added to lower the quality of food is known as:
a. Preservative b. Fertilizer
c. Adulterant d. Supplement

44. An organism that is capable of invading and multiplying in the body of the host is the:
a. Causative agent b. Reservoir
c. Support d. Carrier

45. Anyone who is experiencing cough for 2 weeks, fever and weight loss should:
a. Get screened for tuberculosis
b. Get treatment for viral fever
c. Get treatment for pneumonia
d. Get screened for cancer

46. Which hormone is primarily responsible for milk ejection?
a. Estrogen b. Progesterone
c. Oxytocin d. Prolactin

47. Which of the following are the components of the cervical examination during labor?
a. Dilation, Effacement and Station
b. Presentation, Station and Dilation
c. Dilation, Presentation and Effacement
d. Station, Dilation and Descent

48. The narrowest part of fallopian tube is:
a. Infundibulum
b. Conceal
c. Ampulla
d. Interstitial portion

49. The white line formed in the lower part of abdomen during pregnancy is known as:
a. Linea nigra
b. Striae gravidarum
c. Pregnancy mask
d. None of the above

50. Before birth, which of the following structures connect the right and left auricles of the heart?
a. Umbilical vein b. Foramen ovale
c. Ductus arteriosus d. Ductus venous

51. A client in her third trimester tells the nurse, "I'm constipated all the time". Recommended intervention is:
a. Daily enemas
b. Laxatives
c. Increased fiber intake
d. Decreased fluid intake

52. In which of the following conditions can the causative agent pass through the placenta and affect the fetus in utero?
a. Gonorrhea b. Rubella
c. Candidiasis d. Moniliasis

53. Expulsion of cervical mucus mixed with blood is called:
a. Serous b. Hemorrhage
c. Shaw d. Vaginal discharge

54. The common normal site of implantation of blastocyst in the uterus is:
a. Upper uterine portion
b. Mid-uterine area
c. Lower uterine area
d. Lower cervical segment

55. When breastfeeding should be started after normal delivery?
a. Soon after delivery b. After 2 hours
c. After 6 hours d. After 4 hours

56. Which of the problems is least likely to occur in small for gestation (SGA) newborn whose weight is 2.3 kg?
a. Hypoglycemia
b. Polycythemia
c. Brachial plexus palsy
d. Asphyxia

57. Treatment modalities during precipitous labor include all, except:
a. Suppression of uterine contraction
b. Episiotomy
c. Oxytocin augmentation
d. Careful conduction of controlled delivery

58. Pre-eclampsia can be cured by:
a. Antihypertensives
b. Diet alone
c. Decrease fluid intake
d. Delivery of baby

59. Fetal blood sampling is performed under ultrasound guidance by inserting a needle in the:
a. Cephalic vein b. Umbilical artery
c. Iliac vein d. Umbilical vein

60. The third stage of labor usually lasts about:
a. 5 minutes b. 15 minutes
c. 2 minutes d. 60 minutes

CHILD HEALTH NURSING

61. On second postoperative day after repair of cleft palate, which is the suitable method of feeding?
a. Cup
b. Straw
c. Rubber tipped syringe
d. Large holed nipple

62. A child up to five years of age should get how many doses of Vitamin A?
a. 3 b. 5
c. 7 d. 9

63. Taste perception of baby develops at what age?
a. Birth
b. 4 months
c. 6 months
d. 8 months

64. Head control is possible in an infant by which month?
a. 1 b. 2
c. 3 d. 6

65. What is the normal heart rate at birth?
a. 120–160/minutes b. 100–120/minutes
c. 160–180/minutes d. Less than 100/minutes

66. What is the earliest sign of rickets?
a. Rickety rosary b. Craniotabes
c. Bowlegs d. Harrison's groove

67. Exclusive breastfeeding is recommended at least for how many months?
a. 4 months b. 6 months
c. 9 months d. 1 Year

68. A six-month-old child is suspected of having intussusception, a nurse should expect the child to undergo which of the following procedures?
a. Colonoscopy b. Rectal Biopsy
c. Barium enema d. X-ray abdomen

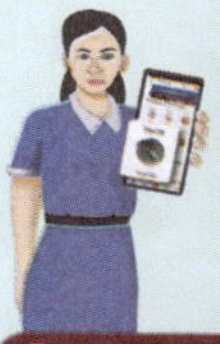

Ans.

43. c
44. a
45. a
46. c
47. a
48. d
49. b
50. b
51. c
52. b
53. c
54. a
55. a
56. c
57. c
58. d
59. d
60. b
61. a
62. d
63. a
64. c
65. a
66. b
67. b
68. d

69. What is the treatment of choice in IMNCI (Integrated Management of Neonatal and Childhood Illness) for a child with severe dehydration?
a. Penicillin
b. Gentamicin
c. Ampicillin and gentamicin
d. Fluid replacement therapy

70. Which deficiency leads to neural tube defects in newborn?
a. Iron deficiency
b. Folic acid deficiency
c. Vitamin B12 deficiency
d. Calcium deficiency

71. It is generally considered that 'cognitive behavioral therapy' changes:
a. Thought process
b. Behavior
c. Thoughts and behavior
d. Intelligence

72. Empathy involves:
a. Feeling sorry for someone
b. Putting others before you
c. Putting you in someone else's shoes
d. Putting you before others

73. The following are the complications of ECT, except:
a. Post ECT confusion
b. Headache
c. Diarrhea
d. Memory loss

74. Sleep disorder in children is due to which of the following reasons:
a. Loss of appetite
b. Bright light
c. Insecurity
d. Constipation

75. Disaster is which type of crisis?
a. Adventitious
b. Maturational
c. Situational
d. All of the above

76. Atheromatous changes of blood vessels affect early in:
a. Kidney
b. Heart
c. Liver
d. Spleen

77. Hypertrophy is:
a. Increase in cell number
b. Increase in cell size
c. Decrease in cell number
d. Decrease in cell size

78. Pharmacokinetics is the branch that is related to:
a. Drug manufacturing
b. Drug designing
c. Passage of drugs through the body
d. Effect of drugs on the body

79. A partial agonist has:
a. Full affinity and intrinsic activity
b. Full affinity but less intrinsic activity
c. Full intrinsic activity but less affinity
d. Activity opposite to agonist

80. Alpha 1 adrenergic receptors are:
a. Ligand gated ion channels
b. Enzyme linked receptors
c. G-protein coupled receptors
d. Gene based receptors

81. Hypoglycemia is caused when glucose level falls below:
a. 80 mg %
b. 70 mg%
c. 60 mg%
d. 40 mg%

82. Lipids are:
a. Heterogeneous group of compounds, actually or potentially related to fatty acids
b. Soluble in nonpolar organic solvents
c. Insoluble in water
d. All of the above

83. Which of the following vegetarian food supplements the protein with rice?
a. Vegetables
b. Pulses
c. Fruits
d. Nuts

84. The richest natural source of vitamin A is:
a. Carrot
b. Butter
c. Peas
d. Cod liver oil

85. Daily requirement of Vitamin C for adults is:
a. 10 mg
b. 40 mg
c. 50–100 mg
d. 100–300 mg

MICROBIOLOGY

86. Nonessential amino acid is:
a. Tyrosine
b. Phenylalanine
c. Lysine
d. Threonine

87. Glycemic index is defined as:
a. Glucose control in last 3 months
b. Measure of the change in the blood glucose following ingestion of proteins
c. Measure of the change in the blood glucose following ingestion of carbohydrate
d. Measure of the change in the blood glucose following ingestion of fats

88. Spherical bacteria occurring in cluster are called:
a. Staphylococci
b. Streptococci
c. Pneumococci
d. Cocobacilli

89. The media to grow bacteria is known as:
a. Nutrition media
b. Culture media
c. Culture forum
d. Culture biosphere

90. Amphitrichous flagella means:
a. Flagella all-round the cell
b. Flagella at both ends
c. Flagella at one end
d. Flagella in tufts

91. How is random sampling effective?
a. Reasonably accurate
b. An economical method of data collection
c. Free from personal biases
d. All of the above

92. In order to pursue the research, which of the following is priorly required?
a. Developing a research design
b. Formulating a research question
c. Deciding about the data analysis procedure
d. Formulating a research hypothesis

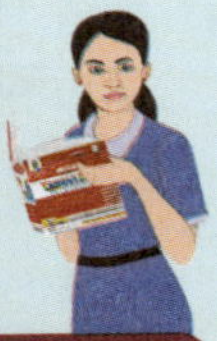

Ans.

69. d
70. b
71. c
72. c
73. c
74. c
75. a
76. b
77. b
78. c
79. b
80. c
81. b
82. d
83. b
84. d
85. c
86. a
87. c
88. a
89. b
90. b
91. d
92. b

93. Which one among the following statement is true in the context of the testing of hypotheses?

a. It is only the alternative hypotheses that can be tested.
b. It is only the null hypotheses that can be tested.
c. Both the alternative and the null hypotheses can be tested.
d. Both the alternative and the null hypotheses cannot be tested.

94. What are the conditions in which Type-I error occurs?

a. The null hypotheses get accepted even if they are false.
b. The null hypotheses get rejected even if they are true.
c. Both the null hypotheses as well as alternative hypotheses are rejected.
d. None of the above.

95. What is 'Mode' in statistics?

a. Average of all numbers
b. Middle point of all numbers
c. Largest number
d. The number repeated most frequently

GENERAL KNOWLEDGE

96. In which district is Shirgul Devta worship famous?

a. Sirmour
b. Kangra
c. Chamba
d. Kullu

97. Kalatop Wildlife Sanctuary is located in which place?

a. Una
b. Lahaul
c. Kinnaur
d. Chamba

98. Chandra and Bhagha rivers meet at which place to form the Chenab River?

a. Tandi
b. Kaza
c. Keylong
d. Manali

99. What is the literacy rate of Himachal Pradesh as per Census 2011?

a. 82.80%
b. 84.80%
c. 68.80%
d. 73.20%

100. Which hill pass connects internal and external Seraj?

a. Kugti
b. Jalori
c. Kalicho
d. Chobu

Ans.

93. b
94. b
95. d
96. a
97. d
98. a
99. a
100. b

"After dinner rest a while; after supper walk a mile."

—T. Cogan

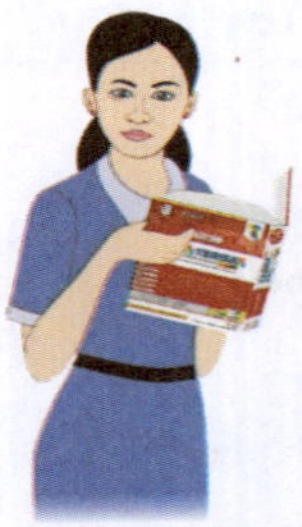

Western Coalfields Limited 2022

1. What is the biological function of copper?
a. Helps in muscle contraction.
b. Cofactor for several enzymes
c. Helps in the transmission of nerve impulses.
d. Involved in the synthesis of thyroid hormones.

2. Which are the risk factors for hearing loss ?
a. Congenital malformation
b. Recurrent ear infection
c. Bacterial meningitis
d. All of the above

3. What provides the framework of synthesis of the cancellous bone tissue within metaphysis?
a. Diaphyis plate b. Epiphysis plate
c. Epiphyseal plate d. Metaphysical

4. Which muscle turns the palm upward or anterior?
a. Pronator teres b. External anal sphincter
c. Obturator externus d. Supinator

5. Why hand wash is a very important step in the procedure for care of wound?
a. To avoid any further injury
b. To cover the wound and quicken healing
c. To prevent cross contamination
d. T0 help remove extra moisture from the wound

6. Which among the following drug is obtained from leaves?
a. Digitoxin b. Tubocurarine
c. Emetine d. Vincristine

7. Which of the following is not one of the national health program in India?
a. Chinese Encephalitis Control Program
b. Kala-Azar Control Program
c. National Diabetes Control Program
d. Universal Immunization Program

8. Identify the Incorrect activity during first aid for serious burns.
a. Do not open blisters, treat for shock.
b. Do not apply ointment or any other home remedy.
c. If the hands are involved, keep them above the level of victim's heart.
d. Give a strong solution of salt and soda.

9. What is an example of monera microorganisms?
a. Eubacteria b. Protozoans
c. Invertebrates d. Mosses and ferns

10. What is the most common cause of malaria in India?
a. Plasmodium vivax
b. Plasmodium ovale
c. Plasmodium primaquine
d. Plasmodium merel

11. Which among the following is not one of the characteristic of society?
a. Likeless b. Difference
c. Interpendence d. Conflict

12. How should heartburn in the mid chest region during pregnancy be managed?
a. Sit or lie down when she feels slight dizziness
b. Exercising the calf muscles by rising on the toes
c. Sleeping with more pillows than usual
d. Never prescribe antacid for severe cases.

13. What should be the correct approach of nurse staff to violence, one of the psychiatric emergencies?
a. Approach the patient from front if she is to be restrained.
b. Provide low calorie diet.
c. Have a nonthreatening approach and do not challenge the patient.
d. Reduce environmental structures.

14. Which of the following genetic condition has the characteristic features of extra fingers and/or toes?
a. Huntington disease b. Hypercholesterolemia
c. Polydactyly d. Achondroplasia

15. Which is the anti-larval measure for mosquito control?
a. Screening
b. Genetic control
c. Environmental control
d. Residual sprays

16. Which of the following field of applied microbiology deals with exploration for microbial life in outer space?
a. Public health microbiology
b. Air microbiology
c. Industrial microbiology
d. Exomicrobiology

17. Which of the following tool in MS Excel predicts a value based on the forecast for the prior period, adjusted for the error in that prior forecast?
a. Exponential smoothing b. Moving average
c. Descriptive statistics d. Correlation covariance

18. Who is the father of sociology?
a. Max Weber b. Auguste Comte
c. Karl Max d. Herbert Spencer

19. How many vertebrae are in thoracic ?
a. 5 b. 12
c. 7 d. 8

20. What is the shape of Bacillus tuberculosis bacteria?
a. Ellipsoidal/Spherical b. Filamentous
c. Rod-shaped d. Vibrio or Coma

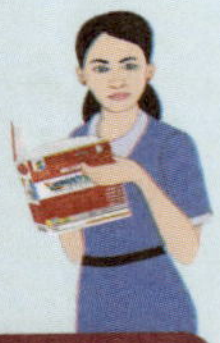

Ans.

1. b
2. d
3. c
4. d
5. c
6. a
7. a
8. d
9. a
10. a
11. a
12. c
13. c
14. c
15. c
16. d
17. a
18. b
19. b
20. c

21. Aedes (Vector), Virus (Cause) are associated to which disease?
a. Japanese Encephalitis b. Filaria
c. Dengue d. Kala azar

22. Which of the following are established covering a population of 1,00,000?
a. Primary health centers b. Sub-center level
c. Anganwadi center d. Community health center

23. Which of the following eye injury may be due to heat or chemicals?
a. Abrasion b. Foreign body
c. Burns d. Contusion

24. ______ is a fracture in the newborn child due to injury during delivery.
a. Birth fracture b. Labor fracture
c. Pathological fracture d. Green stick fracture

25. ________ is the part of the fetus in the lower pole of the uterus.
a. Presentation b. Position
c. Denominator d. Attitude

26. Which of the following is one of the commonly used bibliography database?
a. ESIC b. CINAHL
c. AIDSINE d. CANCLIT

27. Which malignant type neoplasm is used for cancer of the epithelial tissues such as skin or stomach lining?
a. Carcinoma b. Sarcoma
c. Leukemias d. Lymphomas

28. What is called to the relationship between drug concentration and time?
a. Pharmacokinetics b. Pharmacodynamics
c. Pharmacogenomics d. Pharmacovigilance

29. In which technique of cancer detection, low energy beam are used and films of the soft breast tissue are taken without the use of a radio-opaque medium?
a. Mammography b. Xerography
c. Thermography d. Computed Tomography

30. Which of the following statement is correct for the Nurse clinician?
a. Broad practice base
b. May function in a clinical or community setting
c. Strict regulations for practice as a Nurse Specialist
d. Must have formal academic preparation at postgraduate level in a University

31. Which among the following tissue is found in brain and spinal cord?
a. Nervous tissue b. Epithelial tissue
c. Muscle tissue d. Connective tissue

32. Which among the following belongs to dsRNA virus?
a. Rice dwarf b. Rhabdovirus
c. Mosaic virus d. Parvovirus

33. Which among the following is one of the laboratory finding of dengue shock syndrome(DSS)?
a. Thrombocytopenia < 100000 cells/ mm^3
b. No evidence of plasma leakage
c. Leucocytosis
d. Hemoatocrit elevation more than 10%.

34. What can be defined as the field that deals with any genetic condition that occurs due to changes in the nucleotide sequence of DNA representing a gene?
a. Pharmacogenetics b. Somatic cell genetics
c. Population genetics d. Molecular genetics

35. What indicates the number of deaths between 1 and 4 years in a year per 1000 children?
a. Postnatal mortality rate b. Neonatal mortality rate
c. Infant mortality rate d. Child mortality rate

36. What is true about law of segregation?
a. Members of the gene pair segregation and pass to different gametes
b. This law applies to genes on homologous chromosomes
c. The exception to the law is an event of nondisjunction
d. All of the above

37. One or more users simultaneously on two or more processors are known as______.
a. Multiprogramming b. Multiprocessing
c. Time sharing d. Multitasking

38. Mental experiences operate on different levels of awareness. The level that best portrays one's attitude, feelings and desires is the __________.
a. Conscious b. Unconscious
c. Preconscious d. Foreconscious

39. Which of the following nasal dysfunction is commonly due to degenerative changes in skeletal framework of nose?
a. Polydipsia b. Nasal Obstruction
c. Rhinorrhea d. Epistaxis

40. Which of the following strategy has been formulated as per HFA/2000, defined by World Health Assembly?
a. To achieve a net reproduction rate of two.
b. To reduce the crude birth rate from the level of 33 per 1000 population to 25.
c. Reduction of infant mortality from the level of 125 to below 60.
d. To raise the expectation of life at birth from the level of 52 years to 80.

41. What is the function of Nucleic acids?
a. Primary source of energy.
b. Constituents of the plasma membrane.
c. Hereditary factor
d. Form structural components like myosin of muscles

42. ________is relatively a large area of psychology which deals with the fundamental rules, principles and theories of psychology in relation to the study of behavior of normal adult human beings.
a. Social psychology
b. Physiological psychology
c. General psychology
d. Development psychology

43. Which is the most common type of hepatic cirrhosis?
a. Postnecrotic cirrhosis b. Biliary cirrhosis
c. Alcoholic cirrhosis d. Medicine cirrhosis

44. Figure out the micronutrient from the following:
a. Protein
b. Fat
c. Mineral
d. Carbohydrate

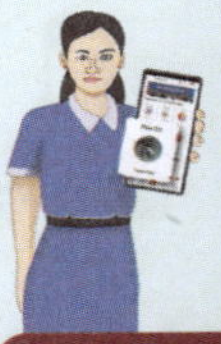

Ans.

21. c
22. d
23. c
24. a
25. a
26. b
27. a
28. a
29. a
30. a
31. a
32. a
33. a
34. d
35. d
36. d
37. b
38. b
39. b
40. c
41. c
42. c
43. c
44. c

45. What are the plasma antibodies of blood type -B?
a. Anti-B
b. Anti-A
c. Anti-O
d. Anti-A, Anti-B

46. Which among the following is said to be twin sister of sociology?
a. Psychology
b. Anthropology
c. Political science
d. Economics

47. Which among the following defences mechanism is related to the given example?
"During lunch at a restaurant, Mark is angry at his older brother, but does not express it and instead is verbally abusive to the server."
a. Displacement
b. Reaction formation
c. Regression
d. Sublimation

48. What is the use of ears for the evaluation of various body systems in children?
a. Palpation
b. Inspection
c. Auscultation
d. Intugementory

49. In operant conditioning, something is added to decrease the likelihood of a behavior, this is said as ______.
a. Positive reinforcement
b. Positive punishment
c. Negative reinforcement
d. Negative punishment

50. Which among the following mental and behavioral disorder group includes mental and behavioral disorders that are the persistent expression of an individual's characteristic lifestyle and mode of relating to self and others?
a. Disorder of Adult Personality and Behaviour
b. Neurotic, Stress Related and Somatoform Disorders
c. Organic (Symptomatic) Disorders
d. Behavioural and Emotional Disorders with Onset usually Occurring in Childhood and Adolescence.

51. ________ helps you overcome concrete, straightforward problems.
a. Crystallized intelligence
b. Fluid intelligence
c. Competence intelligence
d. Levelled intelligence

52. What is the nutritional class of fungi, according to the Whittaker five-kingdom concept?
a. Phototrophic
b. Chemoautotrophic
c. Heterotrophic
d. Homerotrophic

53. All of the following are the nursing intervention for alcohol withdrawal delirium, except:
a. Speak in a calm and quiet voice
b. Change the nursing staff as frequently as possible
c. Provide a calm environment, minimizing noise
d. Provide seclusion, and restraints as necessary

54. Which are the parts of stethoscope?
a. Bell
b. Ear piece
c. Tubing
d. All of the above

55. Which of the following statement is correct for false labor contractions?
a. Increase in duration, frequency, and intensity.
b. Continue no matter what the women's level of activity.
c. Begin irregularly but become regular and predictable.
d. Felt first abdominally and remain confined to the abdomen.

56. What should be the usual amount of enema solution for infant?
a. 500 mL
b. 300–500 mL
c. 250–350 mL
d. Less than 250 mL

57. What is the function of phosphorus?
a. Development of bones and teeth
b. Regulations of pH of body fluids.
c. Regulation of muscle contraction.
d. Role in transmission of nerve impulses.

58. _______ is the name given to the endometrium during pregnancy.
a. Amniotic cavity
b. Inner cell mass
c. Trophoblast
d. Decidua

59. Which of the following is a fat soluble vitamin?
a. Pyridoxine (vitamin B6)
b. Ascorbic acid (vitamin C)
c. Tocopherol (Vitamin E)
d. Thiamine (vitamin B1)

60. Which of the following hearing aids are fully programmable with most of the functions automatically controlled?
a. Analogue technology based
b. Semi-digital based
c. Part programmable hearing aids
d. Digital hearing aids

61. Identify an incorrect measure for essential newborn care to child health.
a. Place the newborn next to the mother to get the breast and warmth
b. Dry the newborn as soon as possible
c. Cut the cord when it becomes thin and dark
d. Wrap the newborn in a dry towel to prevent heat loss from the body

62. Which among the following is one of the late side effect of external radiation therapy?
a. Cystitis
b. Radiation-induced heart disease
c. Radiation pneumonitis
d. Fibrosis

63. What type of nomenclature of drugs are catchy and easy to remember?
a. Chemical name
b. Generic name
c. Proprietary name
d. Non-proprietary name

64. Which is the correct general toxicity for antimetabolites chemotherapy?
a. Bone marrow suppression
b. Stomatitis
c. Pulmonary abnormalities
d. Neurotoxicity

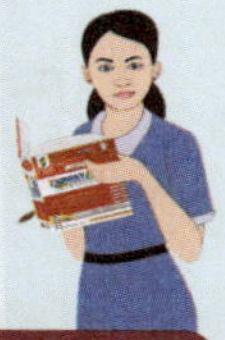

Ans.

45. b
46. b
47. a
48. c
49. b
50. a
51. a
52. c
53. b
54. d
55. d
56. d
57. a
58. d
59. c
60. d
61. c
62. d
63. c
64. a

65. Which of the following health care system is one of the indigenous systems of medicine?

a. Hospitals b. Polyclinics
c. General practitioners d. Siddha

66. Which among the following is a nutritional problem in India?

a. Xerophthalmia
b. Leprosy
c. Acute respiratory disease
d. AIDS

67. Identify the function of DGHS (Directorate General of Health services).

a. To consider and recommend broad guidelines for health policies
b. To make proposal for medical and health legislation for the country as a whole.
c. To make recommendation to the central government regarding distribution of available grants-in-aid for health purposes to the States.
d. International health relations and quarantine

68. What is the causative organism for whooping cough?

a. *Salmonella typhi* b. *Vibrio cholerae*
c. *Sarcoptes scabiei* d. ***Bordetella pertussis***

69. Which of the following bacterial structures is involved in attachment to cell surface?

a. Flagella b. Fimbriae
c. Capsule d. Mesosomes

70. Inflammation of the inner ear is known, as________.

a. Labyrinthitis b. Menieres disease
c. Tinnitus d. Positional vertigo

71. Elon Musk recently acquired Twitter at what price?

a. USD 44 billions b. USD 41 billions
c. USD 40 billions d. USD 35 billions

72. In the question below is given a statement followed by two conclusions numbered I and II. You have to assume everything in the statement to be true, then consider the two conclusions together and decide which of them logically follows beyond a reasonable doubt from the information given in the statement.

Statement:

In a test match, the total runs made by a team were 300. Out of these, 240 runs were made by bowlers.

Conclusions:

I. 80% of the team consists of bowlers.

II. The opening batsmen were bowlers.

a. Only conclusion I follows
b. Only conclusion II follows
c. Either I or II follows
d. Neither I nor II follows

73. Find the odd one out.

a. America b. Asia
c. Africa d. Antartica

74. What will come in the place of "?" in the following question? BCD: DEF :: LMN: ?

a. PQO b. NOP
c. QPO d. PON

75. Which of the following option explains the idiom, 'Blowing his own trumpet' best'?

a. Flatters b. Praises others
c. Praises himself d. Admonishes others

76. Name the country that launched the world's first fully-fledged 5G mobile network nationwide.

a. Japan b. Turkey
c. India d. South Korea

77. A person who composes a sequence of steps and movements of dances is _______.

a. Dancer b. Cinematographer
c. Animator d. Choreographer

78. A polyclinic always has ______.

a. Nurse b. Chemist shop
c. Bed d. Doctor

79. A, B, C, D and E are sitting horizontally on the top of the bench. A is sitting with E, who is on the left end of the bench, C is on the second position from the right, A is to the right of B and E, A and C are sitting together. Figure out the sitting position of A.

a. Between B and D
b. Between E and D
c. Between B and C
d. Between C and E

80. Which doctor discovered function of heart?

a. William Harvey b. Robert Koch
c. Felix Hoffman d. Aaron Glassman

81. Which one of the following appointments is not under the authority of the President of India?

a. Chief of the Army Staff
b. Speaker of Lok Sabha
c. Chief Justice of India
d. Chairman of Finance Commission

82. Which country will host the 2023 Men's Hockey World Cup?

a. The Netherlands b. Spain
c. India d. Brazil

83. Which number should come next?
46, 44, 40, 38, 34, ______

a. 30 b. 32
c. 33 d. 36

84. If P is the brother of Q, Q is the sister of R, and R is the father of S. How S is related to P?

a. Brother
b. Sister
c. Nephew
d. Cannot be determined

85. Where was the QUAD summit 2022 held?

a. New Delhi, India
b. Tokyo, Japan
c. Moscow, Russia
d. Canberra, Australia

86. Arrange the words given below in a meaningful sequences (1) Cut, (2) Wear, (3) Mark, (4) Stitch, (5) Iron

a. 4, 1, 5, 2, 3
b. 3, 1, 4, 5, 2
c. 1, 3, 2, 4, 5
d. 2, 4, 3, 1, 5

87. Who has become the first Indian-origin Prime Minister of the UK?

a. Krupesh Hirani
b. Rishi Sunak
c. Seema Malhotra
d. Shami Chakrabarti

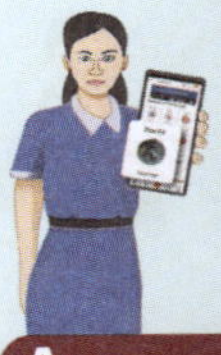

Ans.

Q.	Ans.
65.	d
66.	a
67.	d
68.	d
69.	b
70.	a
71.	a
72.	d
73.	a
74.	b
75.	c
76.	d
77.	d
78.	d
79.	c
80.	a
81.	b
82.	c
83.	b
84.	d
85.	b
86.	b
87.	b

88. In this question below, are given two statements followed by two conclusions numbered I and II. You have to take the given two statements to be true even if they seem to be vary from commonly known facts. Read these two conclusions and then decide which of the given conclusions logically and analytically follows from the given two statements?

Statements:

All goats are flowers.

No flower is book.

Some books are pens.

Conclusions:

I. Some pens are goats

II. No pen is goat

a. If only conclusion I follows.
b. If only conclusion II follows.
c. If either conclusion I or II follows.
d. If both conclusions I and II follow.

89. From which among the following Veda the Gayatri Mantra was first recorded?

a. Samaveda
b. Upanishad
c. Rigveda
d. Yajurveda

90. Complete the second pair in which both the elements bear the same relationship as in the first pair. FILM: 10 : : HOTEL:?

a. 14
b. 16
c. 12
d. 20

91. Identify an element with lowest melting point.

a. Argon
b. Sulfur
c. Titanium
d. Zinc

92. Mannu travelled ____ her mother all ___ the world when she was 8 years old.

a. For, around
b. With, around
c. With, over
d. By, above

93. "She has finished her assignment." (change voice)

a. Her assignment has been finished by her
b. Her assignment was finished by her
c. She has been finishing her assignment
d. Her assignment was finished

94. What is the maximum number of Lok Sabha parliamentary contituencies in the country?

a. 539 b. 543
c. 238 d. 552

95. Change of speech:

Martha said, "I am going to Mexico next year."

a. Martha said that she had been going to Mexico next year.
b. Martha said that she was going to Mexico next year.
c. Martha said that she had gone to Mexico next year
d. Martha said that she will be going to Mexico next year.

96. Antonym of the word "Abolish" is ______.

a. Institute
b. Stamp out
c. Rescind
d. Suppress

97. Find the correctly spelt word from the following.

a. Crystallization
b. Controvertial
c. Interogation
d. Rehabilitation

98. Arrange the given words in a logical sequence: (1) Plan (2) Shop (3) Mall (4) Drive (5) Return

a. 52134
b. 14325
c. 52314
d. 51234

99. Synonym of the word "Awkward" is _____.

a. Dexterous b. Urbane
c. Blundering d. Convenient

100. Ram searched a hotel in booking site which has: (A) posh, air-conditioned, (B) the guest, (C) are available for, (D) fully furnished rooms.

a. ABCD
b. ADCB
c. ACBD
d. ABDC

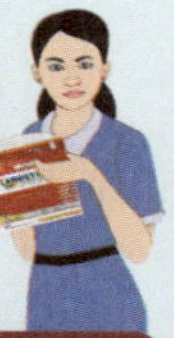

Ans.

88. c
89. c
90. c
91. a
92. b
93. a
94. b
95. b
96. a
97. d
98. b
99. c
100. b

"**Sometimes the remedy is worse than the disease.**"

—Francis Bacon

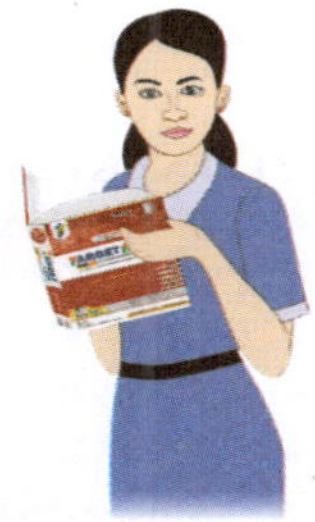

Odisha Subordinate Staff Selection Commission (NO) 2022

1. $\frac{\sqrt{18}+\sqrt{162}}{\sqrt{72}} = ?$
   - a. 2
   - b. $2\sqrt{3}$
   - c. $3\sqrt{2}$
   - d. $\frac{2}{\sqrt{3}}$

2. **A car covers the first 50 km of its journey in 75 minutes and the remaining 30 km in 25 minutes. What is the average speed of the car?**
   - a. 40 km/h
   - b. 48 km/h
   - c. 54 km/h
   - d. 60 km/h

3. **The greatest 4-digit number exactly divisible by 15, 20 and 25 is:**
   - a. 9990
   - b. 9900
   - c. 9995
   - d. 9000

4. **If a number is 50% more than the other, how much per cent is the second number less than the first?**
   - a. 16½%
   - b. 20%
   - c. 33⅓%
   - d. 50%

5. **'A' can do ¼ of a work in 6 days and 'B' can do ⅔ of the work in 12 days. In how many days both 'A' and 'B' together can do the work?**
   - a. 4 days
   - b. $7\frac{1}{5}\%$
   - c. $10\frac{2}{7}$ days
   - d. 12 days

6. **On selling an article for ₹900, the loss is 25%. To make a profit of 25%, the article must be sold at:**
   - a. ₹1125
   - b. ₹1200
   - c. ₹1375
   - d. ₹1500

7. **The average of 20 numbers is 48. If two numbers, namely, 53 and 70 are discarded, what is the average of the remaining numbers?**
   - a. 47.5
   - b. 46.5
   - c. 45.5
   - d. 45

8. **If a man spends 5/8 part of money and again earns 1/3 part of the remaining money, what part of his money is with him now?**
   - a. 3/8
   - b. 3/4
   - c. 1/4
   - d. 1/2

9. **A number exceeds 30% of itself by 49. The number is:**
   - a. 56
   - b. 63
   - c. 70
   - d. 210

10. **Two numbers are in the ratio 3:8. If larger number is 40 more than the smaller number, then the product of the number is:**
    - a. 1536
    - b. 1636
    - c. 1736
    - d. 1836

11. **Select the correct passive form of the following sentence. They say that elephants have good memories.**
    - a. They are said to have good memories.
    - b. They have said that elephants have good memories.
    - c. Elephants are said to have good memories.
    - d. None of these.

12. **Select the appropriate preposition to fill in the blank. Chairs are made ________ wood.**
    - a. from
    - b. on
    - c. in
    - d. of

13. **Choose the correct meaning of the underlined word: He is a novice in the trade.**
    - a. Expert
    - b. New
    - c. Experienced
    - d. Old

14. **Fill in the blank with appropriate word. He is slow _______ he is steady.**
    - a. And
    - b. Or
    - c. Because
    - d. None of these

15. **Select the correct articles and fill in the blanks. I found _______ book last night, _______ book is very useful.**
    - a. the, a
    - b. the, the
    - c. a, the
    - d. a, a

16. **A nurse is performing CPR on an adult patient. When performing chest compressions, the nurse understands the correct hand placement is located over the:**
    - a. Upper half of the sternum
    - b. Upper third of the sternum
    - c. Lower half of the sternum
    - d. Lower third of the sternum

17. **The client presents with severe rectal bleeding, 16 diarrheal stools a day, severe abdominal pain, tenesmus and dehydration. Because of these symptoms, the nurse should be alert for which other problem associated with disease?**
    - a. Crohn's disease
    - b. Ulcerative colitis
    - c. Diverticulitis
    - d. Peritonitis

18. **Side effect of oral contraceptives are all; except:**
    - a. Irregular bleeding
    - b. Headache
    - c. Venous thrombosis
    - d. Increased risk of ovarian cancer

19. **A freshly prepared ORS solution should not be used after:**
    - a. 4 hours
    - b. 6 hours
    - c. 12 hours
    - d. 24 hours

20. **To do percussion and postural drainage of lungs in bronchiectasis, what body position of the patient, a nurse should use?**
    - a. Supine position
    - b. Prone position
    - c. Decubitus position
    - d. Semi fowler's position

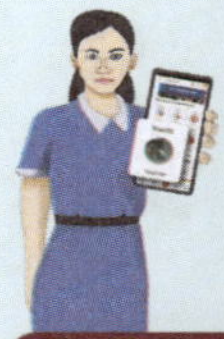

Ans.

1.	a
2.	b
3.	b
4.	c
5.	c
6.	d
7.	b
8.	d
9.	c
10.	a
11.	c
12.	d
13.	b
14.	d
15.	c
16.	c
17.	b
18.	d
19.	d
20.	b

21. ESR is considered to be the measure of which of the following blood physical-chemical property?
a. Stability of colloid solution
b. Blood suspension properties
c. Volume of blood cellular part
d. Blood product

22. Most effective mode of transmission of HIV:
a. Sexual b. Blood product
c. Needle/syringe d. Mother of fetus

23. A nurse observes that the fingers of the casted forearm of patient with fracture ulna are pale, cool and capillary refill is delayed. She has to interpret it as:
a. Nerve impairment is developing in the fingers
b. Arterial blood supply to the fingers is reduced
c. A normal finding
d. Venous stasis occurring in the fingers

24. The drug that increases both systolic and diastolic blood pressure for prolonged period is:
a. Dopamine b. Ephedrine
c. Epinephrine d. Dobutamine

25. A major goal for the client during first 48 hours after a severe burn is to prevent hypovolemic shock. The best indicator of adequate fluid balance during this period is:
a. Elevated hematocrit levels
b. Urine output of 30 to 50 mL/hour
c. Change in level of consciousness
d. Estimate of fluid loss through burn eschar

26. When the patient is acquiring infection from another patient, it is known as ______________.
a. Cross infection b. Iatrogenic infection
c. Opportunistic infection d. Nosocomial infection

27. Drug of choice to treat leprosy is______________.
a. Rifampicin b. Acyclovir
c. Zidovudine d. Dapsone

28. Following vasectomy for family planning, a patient should be advised to use some other method of contraception, till:
a. Removal of all sutures
b. Pain completely subsides
c. Two weeks
d. Eight weeks

29. Paracetamol is an:
a. Antipyretic b. Antitussive
c. Antibiotic d. Antiemetic

30. During ABG analysis, blood is collected from:
a. Artery b. Vein
c. Capillary d. It can be taken from any site

31. A one-year-old child presented to OPD with the history of short stature, tiredness and constipation. Examination revealed a palpable goiter. Serum T4 was decreased and TSH levels were increased. Which is the most probable diagnosis?
a. Thyroid dysgenesis
b. Thyroid dyshormonogenesis
c. TSH receptor blocking antibody
d. Central hypothyroidism

32. A client is admitted to the psychiatric unit of a local hospital with chronic undifferentiated schizophrenia. During the next several days, the client is seen laughing, yelling and talking to herself. This behavior is characteristic of:
a. Delusion b. Looseness of association
c. Illusion d. Hallucination

33. Which is the most common side effect of copper-T among the following?
a. Pain b. Bleeding
c. Perforation d. Ectopic pregnancy

34. Which among the following condition is required for repeated blood transfusion?
a. Iron deficiency anemia
b. Pernicious anemia
c. Thalassemia
d. Vitamin B12 deficiency anemia

35. To avoid pulling the urinary catheter, nurse should tape the catheter on patient's:
a. Upper thigh b. Lower thigh
c. Hind leg d. Foot

36. Which among the following is correct regarding iron supplementation?
a. Take it along with milk
b. Take it along with lemon juice
c. Take it along with water
d. Take it after having food

37. A baby is admitted into the hospital with a history of projectile vomiting after each feeding. On examination, it is found that the pyloric sphincter is thickened and does not open readily. Because of the baby's loss of gastric juice, his blood probably indicates:
a. Acidosis b. Leukocytosis
c. Alkalosis d. An excessively low pH

38. Best test to detect iron deficiency in community is:
a. Transferrin
b. Serum ferritin
c. Serum iron
d. Hemoglobin

39. A client with chronic schizophrenia who takes neuroleptic medication is admitted to the psychiatric unit. Nursing assessment reveals rigidity, fever, hypertension and diaphoresis. These findings suggest which life-threatening reaction?
a. Tardive dyskinesia b. Dystonia
c. Neuroleptic d. Akathisia

40. What do you mean by first stage of labor?
a. Onset of true labor pain till full dilation of cervix
b. Full dilation of cervix to expulsion of fetus
c. Expulsion of fetus to expulsion of placenta
d. Observation for at least 1 hour after the expulsion of placenta

41. Gallow's traction is used for:
a. Fracture shaft of femur b. Fracture neck of femur
c. Fracture humerus d. Fracture tibia

42. While giving NG tube feeding, which of the following nursing actions prevents complications?
a. Advance tube 2 cm
b. Flush with 20 mL of air
c. Provide high fowler's position
d. Plug the air vent during feeding

43. When teaching a patient, who has a diagnosis of schizophrenia about success - independent living in the community, a nurse should encourage the patient to:
a. Establish a structured daily routine
b. Spend time alone
c. Plan a program of self-fulfillment
d. Discontinue dedication when symptoms disappear

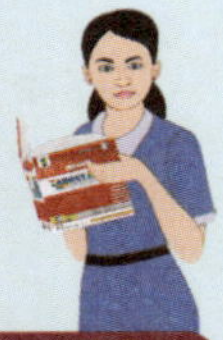

Ans.

21. b
22. b
23. b
24. b
25. b
26. a
27. d
28. d
29. a
30. a
31. b
32. d
33. b
34. c
35. a
36. b
37. c
38. b
39. c
40. a
41. a
42. c
43. a

44. In an infant, the important clinical finding which makes one to suspect increased intracranial tension is:
a. Fever
b. Sunken eyes
c. Tachypnea
d. Bulged anterior fontanel

45. A client is to receive 2000 mL of IV fluid in 12 hours. The drop factor is 10 gtt/mL. At how many drops per minute should the flow rate be set?
a. 22 drops/minute b. 24 drops/minute
c. 26 drops/minute d. 28 drops/minute

46. When taking apical pulse, where should the nurse place the stethoscope?
a. Just to the left of the median point of the sternum.
b. In the 5th intercostal space at the left midclavicular line.
c. Between 6th and 7th ribs at the left mid axillary line.
d. Between 3rd and 4th ribs and to the left the sternum.

47. A 55-years-old male patient who is diagnosed with evolving myocardial infarction (MI) insists on going home. The nurse encourages the patient to be admitted because the greatest risk within the first 24 hours of sustaining an MI is:
a. Heart failure
b. Sudden death
c. Pulses embolism
d. Ventricular aneurysm

48. Iron is deficient in:
a. Cereals (rice, wheat) b. Maize and corn
c. Pulses (Bengal gram, etc.) d. Milk

49. The nurse must know that the most accurate oxygen delivery system available is:
a. The venturi mask
b. Nasal cannula
c. Partial nonrebreather mask
d. Simple face mask

50. During home visit, Nurse Mala found no signs of dehydration in a 7-week-old child who had diarrhea for last 2 weeks. The child is having:
a. Persistent diarrhea b. Acute diarrhea
c. Dysentery d. Severe dysentery

51. Glucose is added in ORS to:
a. Improve taste
b. Decrease bacterial colonization of GIT
c. Increase the stability
d. Increase the absorption of sodium

52. For IM injection, the nurse should insert the needle into the muscle at angle of:
a. 15° b. 30°
c. 45° d. 90°

53. Nurse is about to catheterize bladder of a pregnant lady. She should be aware that all the following facts about female urethra are true; except:
a. It is about 1.5 inches in length.
b. It is posterior to vaginal orifice.
c. It is pierces through urogenital diaphragm.
d. It is straight and offers minor resistance for catheterization.

54. An ABG analysis report shows: pH-7.20; PCO$_2$-35mm Hg$_3^-$-20mEq/L. These findings are suggestive of:
a. Metabolic acidosis
b. Metabolic alkalosis
c. Respiratory alkalosis
d. Respiratory acidosis

55. Phenylketonuria is detected by which urine test?
a. Guthrie test
b. Sodium nitroprusside test
c. Blot test
d. Ferric chloride

56. A client is scheduled for a bronchoscopy. When teaching the client what to expect afterward, the nurse's highest priority of information would be:
a. Food and fluids will be withheld for at least 2 hours.
b. Warm saline gargles will be done q2h.
c. Coughing and deep-breathing exercises will done q2h.
d. Only ice chips and cold liquids will be allowed initially.

57. The elbow is ________ to the wrist.
a. Distal b. Lateral
c. Ventral d. Proximal

58. Which of these diseases cause predominately sensory loss?
a. Guillain-Barre syndrome
b. Diphtheria
c. Lead poisoning
d. Diabetes

59. A client is experiencing anxiety attack. The most appropriate nursing intervention should include:
a. Turning on the television
b. Leaving the client alone
c. Staying with the client and speaking in short sentences
d. Ask the client to play with other clients

60. Which of the action could aggravate the cause of flare ups in a patient with pruritus?
a. Sleeping in cool and humidified environment
b. Daily bathes with fragrant soap
c. Using clothes made fragrant soap
d. Increasing fluid intake

61. All of the following nursing interventions are correct when using the Z-track method of drug injection; except:
a. Prepare the injection site with alcohol
b. Use a needle that is at least 1 inch long
c. Aspirate for blood before injection
d. Rub the site vigorously after the injection to promote absorption

62. A parent brings a toddler, aged 18 months, to the clinic for a regular check-up. When palpating the toddler's fontanels, what should the nurse expect to find?
a. Closed anterior fontanel and open posterior fontanel
b. Open anterior fontanel and closed posterior fontanel
c. Closed anterior posterior fontanels
d. Open anterior and posterior fontanels

63. Which of the following item is not sterilized by antiseptic solution?
a. Suction catheter b. Enema tube
c. Surgical scissor d. Nasogastric tube

64. Main function of vitamin C in the body is:
a. Coenzyme for energy metabolism
b. Regulation of lipid synthesis
c. Involvement as antioxidant
d. Inhibition of cell growth

65. An infant is to receive thyroxin, 0.35 mg once a day orally. The medication is available in elixir form 0.25 mg/mL. How much elixir should the nurse administer?
a. 1.4 mL b. 1.3 mL
c. 2.4 mL d. 1.0 mL

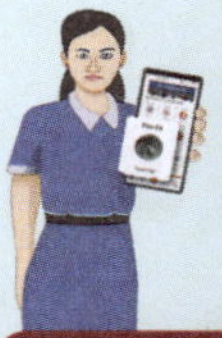

Ans.

44.	d
45.	d
46.	b
47.	b
48.	d
49.	c
50.	a
51.	d
52.	d
53.	b
54.	a
55.	a
56.	a
57.	d
58.	d
59.	c
60.	b
61.	d
62.	c
63.	c
64.	c
65.	a

66. Light rays entering the eye is controlled by:
a. Pupil b. Iris
c. Cornea d. Lens

67. In HIV, maximum risk of transmission is by:
a. Homosexual b. Blood
c. Heterosexual d. Needle prick

68. Inadequate intake by the pregnant woman of which vitamin can cause neural tube detect?
a. Folic acid b. Thiamine
c. Niacin d. Riboflavin

69. Which of the following factor may affect the drug absorption rate from IM injection site?
a. Muscle tone
b. Muscle strength
c. Amount of body fat at injection site
d. Blood flow to the injection site

70. 60-year-old man had undergone cardiac bypass surgery 2 days back. Now, he started forgetting things and was not able to recall names and phone numbers of his relatives. What is the probable diagnosis?
a. Depression
b. Post-traumatic psychosis
c. Cognitive dysfunction
d. Alzheimer's disease

71. Which of the following is significantly different between human and cow's milk?
a. Proteins and fat
b. Proteins and sugar
c. Proteins and lactose
d. Minerals

72. The most common type of ovarian cancer is:
a. Adenocarcinomas
b. Endometrial tumors
c. Epithelial ovarian cancer
d. Mucinous adenocarcinomas

73. Which should be the temperature of delivery room to maintain warmth for a neonate?
a. 21–24°C b. 25–28°C
c. 28–30°C d. Above 30°C

74. Geeta returns from the Postanethesia Care Unit (Recovery Room) with a nasogastric tube in place following a gallbladder surgery. She continues to complain of nausea. Which action would the nurse take?
a. Call the physician immediately
b. Administer the prescribed antiemetic
c. Check the patency of nasogastric tube for any obstruction
d. Change the patient's position

75. The substance deposited in skin and sclera in jaundice is:
a. Indirect or unconjugated bilirubin
b. Direct or conjugated bilirubin
c. Biliverdin
d. Stercobilin

76. MTP can be done up to:
a. 12 weeks b. 16 weeks
c. 20 weeks d. 10 weeks

77. Which hormone is responsible for the secretion of milk after parturition?
a. ICSH b. Prolactin
c. ACTH d. Oxytocin

78. A thirty-year-old patient has an ulcer over lateral malleolus. Nurse caring for this patient understands, the pain of the patient is due to:
a. Edema b. Exudate
c. Infection d. Ischemia

79. When is the best time to achieve pregnancy?
a. Midway between 7 and 8 day of ovulation
b. Immediately after starting of menses
c. 14 days after the beginning of period
d. 7 days before the next period is expected

80. A patient gives a history that she has missed a single dose of her combined oral contraceptive pill. Which of the following will you advise her?
a. Continue with the course without regard to the missed dose.
b. Take 2 pills the next day and continue with the course. c. Take 2 pills every day for the remaining part of the course.
d. Discontinue the course and use an alternative method of contraception.

81. After receiving report, which of the following patients should the nurse see first?
a. A patient in sickle-cell crisis with an infiltrated IV.
b. A patient with leukemia who has received one-half unit of packed cells.
c. A patient scheduled for a bronchoscopy.
d. A patient complaining of a leaky colostomy bag.

82. As a safety alert, the nurse is aware that the following medication is never given directly intravenously.
a. Potassium chloride
c. Dextrose
b. Lasix
d. Calcium gluconate

83. Depression:
a. Is a normal part of aging.
b. Is not a normal process of aging.
c. Includes symptoms, such as loss of interest, sadness, weight loss and worthless feelings.
d. b and c are the correct answers.

84. Which of the following signs will indicate that a young child is suffering from severe pneumonia?
a. Dyspnea b. Wheezing
c. Fast breathing d. Chest indrawing

85. Human milk is rich in all; except:
a. Vitamin A b. Vitamin C
c. Iron d. Vitamin E

86. The nutrient that provides the body's preferred energy source:
a. Fat b. Protein
c. Vitamin d. Carbohydrate

87. DOTS is used in the treatment of:
a. Tuberculosis b. Leprosy
c. Malaria d. Filaria

88. Which of the following condition is manifested by increased intraocular pressure?
a. Cataract b. Conjunctivitis
c. Dacryocystitis d. Glaucoma

89. Inspection of the uterine cavity by endoscopy with access through the cervix is known as:
a. Hysteroscopy b. Salpingoscopy
c. Salpingogram d. Hysterosalpingography

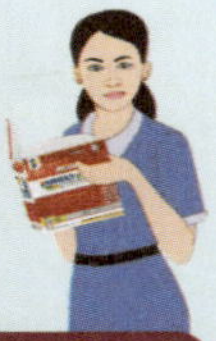

Ans.

66.	a
67.	b
68.	a
69.	d
70.	c
71.	c
72.	c
73.	b
74.	c
75.	b
76.	c
77.	b
78.	d
79.	c
80.	b
81.	a
82.	a
83.	c
84.	d
85.	c
86.	d
87.	a
88.	d
89.	a

90. Identify the high-risk infant among the following:
a. Infant with birth weight 2.5 kg
b. Infant on artificial feeding
c. Infant with birth weight 2 kg
d. Infant with Apgar score 8

91. Most common site of extrathoracic TB in children:
a. Lymph node
b. Skeleton
c. Central nervous system
d. Heart

92. A nurse is caring an anemic patient. What finding should suggest her that it is acute blood loss anemia?
a. Exertional dyspnea
b. Easy fatigue on exertion
c. Bradycardia at rest
d. Postural hypotension

93. Which is the common nutritional problem associated with down syndrome?
a. Obesity
b. Kwashiorkor
c. Marasmus
d. Vitamin A deficiency

94. Nurse has to apply erythromycin ointment to a newborn child. Which area of eye she is supposed to place it?
a. On the cornea
b. Under the eyelid
c. Lower conjunctiva
d. Upper conjunctiva

95. Which of the following is a specific investigation to detect seizures?
a. CT scan
b. MRI scan
c. EEG
d. X-ray

96. An adult has just been brought in by ambulance after a motor vehicle accident. When assessing the client, the nurse would expect which of the following manifestations could have resulted from sympathetic nervous system stimulation?
a. A rapid pulse and increased respiratory rate
b. Decreased physiologic functioning
c. Rigid posture and altered perceptual focus
d. increased awareness and attention

97. The client has clear drainage from the nose and ears after a head injury. How can the nurse determine if the drainage is CSF?
a. Measure the pH of the fluid
b. Measure the specific gravity of the fluid
c. Test for glucose
d. Test for chlorides

98. Which of the following tools does a nurse use to assess the cognitive function of a client?
a. Ishihara polychromatic plates
b. Rorschach Ink blot test
c. Mini-mental status examination
d. Goldberg Depression Scale

99. The drug which is used to create aversion in alcohol dependence is:
a. Apomorphine
b. Propanolol
c. Diazepam
d. Disulfiram

100. A nurse is performing CPR on an adult patient. When performing chest compressions, the nurse understands the correct hand placement is located over the:
a. Upper half of the sternum
b. Upper third of the sternum
c. Lower half of the sternum
d. Lower third of the sternum

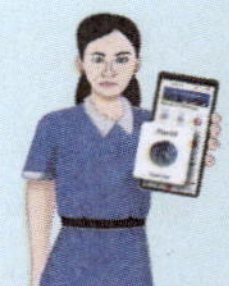

Ans.

90. c
91. a
92. d
93. a
94. c
95. c
96. a
97. c
98. c
99. d
100. c

"One day in perfect health is much."
—Arabic

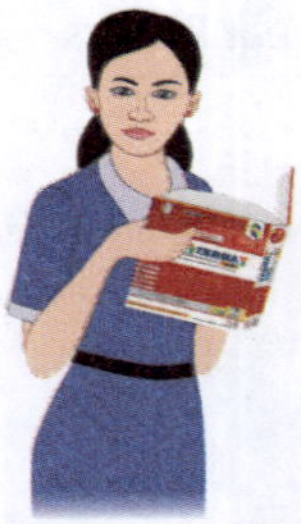

Gujarat Nursing Service (Nursing Officer/Principal) 2022

1. Above the sternum, the right and left jugular vein are united by the transverse vein called:
- a. Jugular arch
- b. Deep Cervical arch
- c. Transverse jugular plexus
- d. Suboccipital plexus

2. Pentavalent vaccine contains:
- a. DPT, hepatitis B and Haemophilus influenzae B
- b. DPT, OPV and Haemophilus influenzae B
- c. IPV, OPV, DPT
- d. IPV, hepatitis B and Haemophilus influenzae B

3. Flash cards contain a picture or diagram and card size is:
- a. 10 inch × 12 inch
- b. 10 inch × 15 inch
- c. 12 inch × 20 inch
- d. 12 inch × 15 inch

4. The variable other than independent variable that could cause a change in the dependent variable is known as:
- a. Extraneous variable
- b. Intervening variable
- c. Predictor variable
- d. Target variable

5. The cup shaped depression in the lateral surface of the Hip bone is:
- a. Ileum
- b. Iliac crest
- c. Greater trochanter
- d. Acetabulum

6. Leishmaniasis are group of:
- a. Air borne diseases
- b. Bacterial diseases
- c. Cestode infections
- d. Protozoal diseases

7. Trisomy-21 is seen in:
- a. Turner's syndrome
- b. Down syndrome
- c. Klinefelter syndrome
- d. Triple-X syndrome

8. A testable or expected relationship between two or more than two variables which are measurable or potentially measurable, is called:
- a. Hypothesis
- b. Reliability
- c. Assumption
- d. Variable

9. Diencephalon consists of:
- a. Basal ganglia and thalamus
- b. Thalamus and medulla
- c. Thalamus and hypothalamus
- d. White matter and cerebrum

10. A particular ECG change observed in hypokalemia is:
- a. ST-segment elevation
- b. U wave, which is a position deflection after the T wave
- c. Tall peaked T wave
- d. Widening of the QRS complex and increased amplitude

11. Normally how much percentage a child during his first year of life gains weight from its birth weight?
- a. 100%
- b. 150%
- c. 200%
- d. 250%

12. During anemia in pregnancy, the total iron binding capacity is elevated to:
- a. 100-200 ug/L
- b. 300-400 ug/L
- c. 700-900 ug/L
- d. 1000-1500 ug/L

13. The right coronary artery ends by:
- a. Circumflex branch of LCA
- b. Infundibulum of right ventricle
- c. Ascending aorta
- d. Intraventricular septum

14. The solvent used for dilution of BCG vaccine is:
- a. Normal saline
- b. Distilled water
- c. Dextrose 5%
- d. Tap water

15. The sudden jerk of limb or muscle group is:
- a. Dystonia
- b. Myoclonus
- c. Athetosis
- d. Ballismus

16. An antenatal mother with 34 weeks of gestation admitted with sudden vaginal bleeding, mild abdomen and back pain, tender uterus and dark red clotted blood. The clinical symptoms suggest:
- a. H-Mole
- b. Placenta Previa
- c. Abruptio Placenta
- d. Ectopic Pregnancy

17. The narrow part of larynx at the level of vocal cords is:
- a. Vestibule
- b. Rima glottidis
- c. Infraglottic part
- d. Cricoarytenoids

18. The method used to remove temporary hardness of water is:
- a. Base exchange process
- b. Permutit method
- c. Clark's method
- d. Chlorination

19. Kernig's sign is observed in:
- a. Meningeal irritation
- b. Fracture
- c. Neural tube defects
- d. Respiratory disorder

20. The beginning gestational trophoblastic changes of the chorionic villi is called:
- a. Choriocarcinoma
- b. Trophoblastic carcinoma
- c. Hydatidiform mole
- d. Invasive mole

21. The muscle which flexes both the hip and knee joints is:
- a. Sartorius
- b. Quadriceps femoris
- c. Gluteus maximus
- d. Vastus medialis

22. A patient is on DOTS therapy and his urine color turns to red, this happens due to intake of:
- a. Rifampicin
- b. Streptomycin
- c. Ethambutol
- d. Pyrazinamide

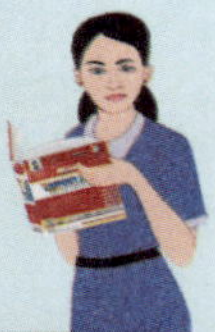

Ans.

Q	Ans
1.	a
2.	a
3.	a
4.	a
5.	d
6.	d
7.	b
8.	a
9.	c
10.	b
11.	c
12.	b
13.	a
14.	a
15.	b
16.	c
17.	b
18.	c
19.	a
20.	c
21.	a
22.	a

23. Dipping palpitation is used commonly in the case of:
a. Ascites
b. Jaundice
c. Intestinal obstruction
d. Renal failure

24. The major complications that can occur due to the presence of carcinoma cervix in pregnant women are:
a. Irregular vaginal bleeding, PROM, preterm labor
b. Vaginal discharge, hypertension, postmaturity
c. Continuous vaginal bleeding, uterine fistula, postcoital bleeding
d. PROM, hypotension, IUGR

25. The natural pacemaker of the heart is:
a. Atrioventricular node
b. Bundle of His
c. Sinoatrial node
d. Purkinje fibers

26. Patient with prolonged rest and restricted movement developed a deformity called:
a. Foot drop
b. Foot elevation
c. Foot debridement
d. Paralysis

27. Failure of fusion of two halves of the neural arch is called:
a. Anencephaly
b. Spina bifida
c. Encephalocele
d. Spinal dysraphisms

28. Isthmorrhaphy is a treatment choice for:
a. Premature rupture of membrane
b. Hydramnios
c. Incompetent Cervix
d. Chorioamnionitis

29. The hormone produced from the adrenal cortex is:
a. Adrenaline
b. Calcitonin
c. Aldosterone
d. Epinephrine

30. Which one of the following is not a secondary skin lesion?
a. Scales
b. Keloid
c. Wheal
d. Lichenification

31. The 'key to auscultation of the heart' is called:
a. First heart sound S1
b. Second heart sound S2
c. Third heart sound S3
d. Fourth heart sound S4

32. Implantation of the fetus in any site other than a normal uterine location is called:
a. Ectopic pregnancy
b. Multiple pregnancy
c. H-Mole
d. Molar pregnancy

33. The communication between the nasopharynx and the oropharynx is called:
a. Nasal cavity
b. Nasopharynx isthmus
c. Choanae
d. Pharyngeal isthmus

34. Calorie provided to all students through mid-day meal program:
a. 100 calories, 2–10 g of fats
b. 700 calories, 20 g of proteins
c. 200 calories, 4–12 g of proteins
d. 500 calories, 6–10 g of fats

35. The recommended temperature for storage of polio vaccine is:
a. 40°C
b. -20°C
c. -15°C
d. 4°C

36. Abruptio placenta is:
a. Deeply penetrated placenta
b. Placenta lying in the lower uterine wall
c. Separation of placenta following delivery
d. Premature separation of normally implanted placenta

37. A state of disequilibrium and a lack of social solidarity is:
a. Social conflict
b. Communalism
c. Poverty
d. Social disorganization

38. Dukoral vaccine is used for:
a. Diarrheal disease
b. Hepatitis D
c. Cholera
d. Pneumococcal meningitis

39. Amount of oxygen administered to infants by nasal catheter per minute:
a. 4 liters
b. 5 liters
c. 2.5 liters
d. 1 liter

40. A patient with a missed menstrual period and nausea has which sign of pregnancy?
a. Probable sign
b. Positive sign
c. Presumptive sign
d. Questionable

41. Recognized or accepted ways of behaving in the society is:
a. Tradition
b. Custom
c. Social control
d. Folkways

42. Artemisinin-based Combination Therapy (ACT) is recommended for all patients who are suspected of:
a. Malaria
b. Cholera
c. Filariasis
d. Zoonosis

43. The condition usually diagnosed with Wangensteen-Rice X-ray is:
a. Esophageal Atresia
b. Pyloric stenosis
c. Anorectal malformation
d. Cleft lip

44. The relationship of the long axis of the fetus to the long axis of the uterus is:
a. Lie
b. Presentation
c. Position
d. Attitude

45. Liberty, equality and fraternity are the basic principles of:
a. Democracy
b. Marriage
c. Family
d. Socialization

46. The disease imported in a country, which was not otherwise present:
a. Epornithic disease
b. Zoonotic disease
c. Exotic disease
d. Epizootic disease

47. The following one is not a sign of severe dehydration in children:
a. Lethargic or unconscious
b. Skin pinch goes back readily
c. Unable to drink poorly
d. Sunken eyes

48. The purpose of root cause analysis (RCA) is to:
a. Identify appropriate solution
b. Discovering the problem area
c. Looking for effect relationship
d. Give short-term relief from the problem

49. Low specific gravity of the urine is observed in:
a. Diabetes mellitus and nephrosis
b. Dehydration and fever
c. Renal failure and diabetes insipidus
d. Diarrhea and glycosuria

Ans.

23.	a
24.	a
25.	c
26.	a
27.	b
28.	c
29.	c
30.	c
31.	b
32.	a
33.	d
34.	b
35.	b
36.	d
37.	d
38.	c
39.	d
40.	c
41.	d
42.	a
43.	c
44.	a
45.	a
46.	c
47.	b
48.	a
49.	c

50. The device used to maintain sterile environment while working with microorganism is:
a. Laminar air flow b. Microwave
c. Incubator d. Humidifier

51. Phocomelia is a condition of:
a. Congenital absence of limb
b. Congenital absence of nail
c. Congenital dislocation of limb
d. Congenital disease of heart

52. The primary goal in International Patient Safety Goal (IPSG) is:
a. Improve safety of high- alert medication
b. Identify patients correctly
c. Improve communication
d. Reduce the risk of health care associated infection

53. A patient is brought to the emergency department with severe respiratory distress. Which method of temperature measurement would be the most appropriate?
a. Oral temperature with an electric thermometer
b. Axillary with an electronic thermometer
c. Temporal artery
d. Rectal temperature

54. The term full-blown AIDS refers to:
a. Survival period
b. Total destruction of immune system
c. Positive response to retroviral therapy
d. Primary stage of AIDS

55. Misperception of external stimuli is:
a. Illusion b. Hallucination
c. Agitation d. Delusion

56. The process of comparing a patients' new medication order with all the medications the patient had been taking prior to changing level of care is:
a. Medication error
b. Medication reconciliation
c. Errors of proficiency
d. Execution measures

57. Dyspnea that occurs within minutes after lying down is termed:
a. Platypnea b. Orthopnea
c. Dyspnea d. Palpitation

58. Travelers diarrhea is caused by:
a. Enteropathogenic *E. coli*
b. Enterotoxigenic ***E. coli***
c. Enteroinvasive *E. coli*
d. Verotoxigenic *E. coli*

59. Korsakoff syndrome is associated with:
a. Poisoning b. Drug abuse
c. Morphine overdose d. Chronic alcoholism

60. LAMA stands for:
a. Discharge against medical advice
b. Leaving against medical advice
c. Leaving along with medical advice
d. Leaving along with medical assistance

61. Water hammer pulse is also called:
a. High volume pulse
b. Collapsing pulse
c. Low volume pulse
d. Regular irregular pulse

62. The most infectious form of leprosy is:
a. Tuberculoid leprosy
b. Borderline tuberculoid leprosy
c. Mid-borderline leprosy
d. Lepromatous leprosy

63. Tactile hallucination is:
a. Sensation of being touched, pricked or tangled
b. Experiencing unpleasant taste
c. Visual sensation where the person feels that the objects or a person seen is reduced in size
d. Destination of body image

64. Medicolegal cases (MLC) should be recorded on the patient case sheet:
a. With red ink on the right-hand top corner
b. With red ink on the left-hand corner
c. No need to highlight
d. With any ink

65. Using strader's seven step decision making process, the nurse needs to first identify the purpose. What must the nurse do next?
a. Decide who will be involved in the decision
b. Enlist the cooperation of the client
c. Set the criteria
d. Identify solutions

66. The most important specimen for isolation of Salmonella typhi culture in first week of enteric fever is:
a. Blood b. Urine
c. Stool d. CSF

67. ECT is currently indicated as a line of treatment in the following conditions; except:
a. Catatonic schizophrenia
b. Severe depression with psychosis
c. Manic depressive psychosis
d. Obsessive compulsive disorder

68. The specialty that integrates nursing science with multiple information and analytical sciences to identify, define, manage and communicate data, information, knowledge and wisdom in nursing practice is:
a. Telenursing b. Telehealth
c. Nursing informatics d. Health technology

69. In the daily practice of nursing, nurses use critical thinking in:
a. Setting priorities for the day
b. Every decision that is made
c. Calling the pharmacy to obtain a medication
d. Checking supplies in the client's room

70. The common name for Taenia Saginata is:
a. Armed tapeworm b. Beef tapeworm
c. Pork tapeworm d. Trematodes

71. All are true about conversion disorder; except:
a. Presence of secondary gain
b. Onset in late age
c. Patient does not consciously produce symptom
d. Relation with stress

72. The competency of nursing informatics specialists is determined through studying the following categories, except:
a. Computer skills
b. Informatics knowledge
c. Informatics skills
d. Health technology

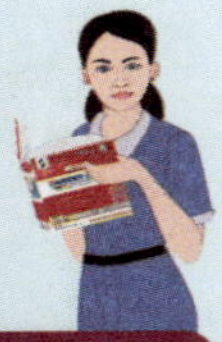

Ans.

50.	a
51.	a
52.	b
53.	c
54.	b
55.	a
56.	b
57.	b
58.	b
59.	d
60.	b
61.	b
62.	d
63.	a
64.	a
65.	c
66.	a
67.	d
68.	c
69.	a
70.	b
71.	b
72.	d

73. When nurses assist clients in exploring their lifestyle habits and health behaviors to identify health risks, nurse are most likely to use which of the following model?
a. Medical model b. Wellness model
c. Psychosocial model d. Physiological model

74. Protamine sulphate is antidote of:
a. Warfarin b. Vitamin K
c. Heparin d. Paracetamol

75. The formula for calculation of IQ is expressed as:
a. IQ=CA/MA × 100 b. IQ=MA/CA × 100
c. IQ=age × 100/CA d. IQ=age × 100/MA

76. Healthcare informatics and technology can help nurses in:
a. Quality control
b. Reduce medication side effects
c. Increase communication and efficiency
d. Manpower planning

77. In Hildegard Peplau's interpersonal relations model, the focus is on which of the following?
a. Individual b. Community
c. Large society d. Family

78. The earliest immunoglobulin to be synthesized by the fetus is:
a. Ig M b. Ig A
c. Ig G d. Ig E

79. Ms Pooja, a school girl, has started experiencing fear about studying in school. She has been reporting headaches and stomachaches and has missed several classes in the few weeks. Her illness is:
a. Dissociative disorders b. Phobic disorders
c. Somatization disorder d. Generalized anxiety disorder

80. As per Indian Nursing Council norms for B.Sc. nursing program, the size of the Hospital/Nursing Home for affiliation should not be less than:
a. 100 beds b. 30 beds
c. 150 beds d. 250 beds

81. The central focus in decision making of care in nursing process is:
a. Nurse b. Doctor
c. Patient d. Family member

82. Generation time of Mycobacterium tuberculosis is:
a. 10 hours b. 20 hours
c. 20 days d. 10 days

83. Light Therapy is mainly indicated for:
a. Seasonal Affective Disorder (SAD)
b. Glaucoma
c. Anxiety disorder
d. Phobia

84. A synergetic relationship between a beginning nurse and a nurse with multiple years of experience is:
a. Induction program
b. Nurse mentorship
c. Interpersonal relationship
d. Faculty orientation program

85. Nursing interventions for chronic glomerulonephritis patient when hospitalized include the following; except:
a. Observe for changes in fluid and electrolyte states
b. Monitor signs of deterioration of renal function
c. Reporting of cardiac and neurologic status changes
d. Don't allow patient to verbalize as it increases anxiety level

86. Wrong statement about Albendazole is:
a. Poor CSF penetration
b. Contraindicated in pregnancy
c. Use in neurocysticercosis
d. Can cause hepatotoxicity

87. Relaxation therapies include all; except:
a. Meditation b. Deep breathing exercise
c. Yoga d. Catharsis

88. The application for patent can be filed by any of the following persons, either alone or jointly with any other person; except:
a. True and first inventor
b. True and first inventor's assignee
c. Legal representative of deceased true and first inventor or his/her assignee
d. Organization only

89. Terminal insomnia is:
a. Difficulty in falling sleep b. Difficulty in staying asleep
c. Premature awakening d. Dreaming during sleeping

90. IV diazepam has which of the following effects that is not seen by other routes?
a. Analgesia b. Coronary dilation
c. Hypotension d. Diazepam

91. The optimal size for group therapy is:
a. 15–20 members b. 8–10 members
c. 20–25 members d. 15–25 members

92. Rights are afforded to inventors and creators under the umbrella of:
a. Intellectual property rights
b. Patent
c. Inventors property rights
d. Patent property rights

93. Nursing theory focuses on clinical nursing practice, which is:
a. Prescriptive theory b. Descriptive theory
c. Developmental theory d. Systems theory

94. Dextromethorphan could not be given with:
a. Paracetamol b. Atropine
c. MAO inhibitor d. SSRIs

95. The drug of choice for mood disorder is:
a. Chloropromazine b. Imipramine
c. Lithium d. Donepezil

96. Nurses who provide knowledgeable, competent, and safe care to people of diverse cultures to themselves and others are:
a. Cultural competent nurses
b. Transcultural nurses
c. Transculture competent nurse
d. Holistic nurses

97. Altered health maintenance is an example of:
a. Collaborative problem b. Interdisciplinary problem
c. Medical problem d. Nursing problem

98. Heparin is:
a. Only in-vivo anticoagulant
b. Only in-vitro anticoagulant
c. Oral anticoagulant
d. Parenteral anticoagulant

99. Alexithymia is:
a. Feeling of intense rapture
b. Pathological sadness
c. Inability to recognize and describe feelings
d. Inappropriate mood

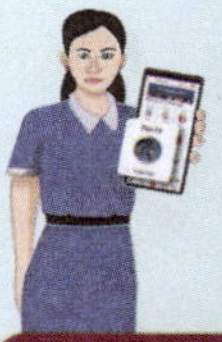

Ans.

73.	b
74.	c
75.	b
76.	c
77.	a
78.	a
79.	c
80.	a
81.	c
82.	b
83.	a
84.	b
85.	d
86.	a
87.	d
88.	d
89.	c
90.	b
91.	b
92.	a
93.	a
94.	c
95.	c
96.	b
97.	d
98.	d
99.	c

100. Translational research is also known as:
- a. Bench to bedside
- b. Classroom to bedside
- c. Evidence-based practice
- d. Basic research

101. The leading cause of cognitive impairment in old age is:
- a. Stroke
- b. Malnutrition
- c. Alzheimer's disease
- d. Loss of cardiac reserve

102. Drug of choice to intact early ectopic pregnancy is:
- a. Methotrexate
- b. Mifeprin
- c. Alfa interferon
- d. Efudix

103. Truth-telling about the disease and its prognosis to terminally ill patients, in such situation which ethical principal is followed by a nurse?
- a. Confidentiality
- b. Fidelity
- c. Justice
- d. Veracity

104. A reliable and generalizable predictive scale to identify patients at risk of difficult intravenous access is:
- a. A-DIVA scale
- b. DIA scale
- c. RDIA scale
- d. RDIVA scale

105. A painful emotional state which results from a tension between opposed and contradictory wishes is called:
- a. Regression
- b. Resolution
- c. Conflicts
- d. Climate

106. When the drug is introduced in the bone marrow, the route is called:
- a. Intraperitoneal
- b. Intrathecal
- c. Intramedullary
- d. Intra-arterial

107. The patient was admitted to the hospital for an outpatient surgical procedure. Discharge was on the same day, and recovery continued at home. This is an example of what type of health care?
- a. Primary
- b. Secondary
- c. Tertiary
- d. Quarterly

108. The Braden scale uses score from less than or equal to 9 to and as high as 23. The lower the number:
- a. The higher the risk is for developing an acquired ulcer or injury.
- b. The lower the risk is for developing an acquired ulcer or injury.
- c. The medium the risk is for developing an acquired ulcer or injury.
- d. No risk is for developing an acquired ulcer or injury.

109. The degree to which individuals like or are attracted to other members of the group or to people who attempt to influence them is:
- a. Group dynamics
- b. Group cohesiveness
- c. Group behavior
- d. Group culture

110. Quantity of adrenaline in 100 mL of 1 in 1000 solution is:
- a. 1 g
- b. 10 g
- c. 0.1 g
- d. 100 g

111. The theory that emphasizes the importance of cooperation and participation in the workplace is:
- a. Chaos theory
- b. Systems theory
- c. Classical theory
- d. Neoclassical theory

112. The effect that refers to a phenomenon in which participants alter their behaviour as a result of being part of an experiment or study is:
- a. Hawthorne effect
- b. Normality effect
- c. Observational effect
- d. Qualitative effect

113. Reward that satisfies a biological need is called:
- a. Negative reinforcers
- b. Positive reinforcers
- c. Secondary reinforcers
- d. Primary reinforcers

114. Lysergic acid Diethylamide (LSD) is a product of:
- a. Cocoa
- b. Opium
- c. Cannabis sativa
- d. Claviceps purpurea

115. The least likely to be used by a cognitive therapist in treating a client is:
- a. Giving the client homework
- b. Arguing with client's statement
- c. Repeating what the client has said without its interpretation
- d. Pointing out irrational beliefs to the client

116. The means of protecting health information authorized by the individual is:
- a. Voting
- b. Privacy
- c. Admitting
- d. Sorting

117. When an apple is offered to a child, he thinks for a moment and at once refuses to take it, his thinking refers to:
- a. Perceptual
- b. Divergent
- c. Convergent
- d. Reflective

118. 5% glucose saline mean:
- a. 0.5 glucose and 0.45 g sodium chloride in each 100 mL
- b. 5 g of glucose and 0.9 g of sodium chloride in each 100 mL
- c. 5 g of glucose and 0.45 g of sodium chloride in each 100 mL
- d. 0.5 g glucose and 0.9 g sodium chloride in each 100 mL

119. The administrative effort to enhance the quality services and practices in an organization is:
- a. Quality improvement
- b. Quality indicator
- c. Quality assurance
- d. Quality control

120. Computerized provider order entry (CPOE) system are now designed with which of following?
- a. Patient information
- b. Health information
- c. Drug safety software that has safeguards for dosing, duplication of therapies, and drug-drug interaction (DDI) checking
- d. All of the above

121. A secondary reinforce is defined as:
- a. A consequence that goes unnoticed by the learner
- b. Another term to refer to punishment
- c. Something that has been paired with a primary reinforce
- d. A stimulus that satisfies biological needs

122. 5% dextrose in normal saline is:
- a. Isotonic
- b. Hypotonic
- c. Hypertonic
- d. Neutral

123. The values and attitudes of the employees of an organization that has an impact on the development of an unique social and psychological work setting of an organization is:
- a. Organizational climate
- b. Organizational culture
- c. Organizational effectiveness
- d. Organizational change

124. Information Technology which has been used to generate pertinent medical evidence.
- a. Mine the literature
- b. Personal health records
- c. Claims, and organizational records
- d. All of the above

Ans.

100. a
101. c
102. a
103. d
104. a
105. c
106. c
107. b
108. a
109. b
110. c
111. d
112. a
113. d
114. d
115. c
116. b
117. a
118. b
119. c
120. c
121. c
122. c
123. b
124. d

125. One of the following is not a simple protein:
a. Albumins
b. Glutelins
c. Prolamins
d. Glycoprotein

126. Vitamin which is also known as antisterility vitamin:
a. Vitamin C
b. Vitamin E
c. Vitamin A
d. Vitamin K

127. The systematic analysis of the data related to the task and the time required to complete each task in a given project is:
a. Critical path method
b. Program evaluation and review technique
c. Management by objective
d. Gantt chart

128. The goal of Electronic Health Record standard is, which of the following?
a. Promote technical innovation using adopted standards
b. Keep implementation costs as high as reasonably possible
c. Promote noninteroperability
d. Discourage participation

129. The functional unit of muscle is:
a. Fiber cell
b. Sarcomere
c. Myofibril
d. H band

130. Quantitative reduction of bone mass is seen in:
a. Giant cell tumor
b. Bone tumor
c. Osteoporosis
d. Osteomyelitis

131. Lacking of clear information about the role expected is:
a. Role
b. Role expectation
c. Role conflict
d. Role ambiguity

132. One of the following is a nonparametric test:
a. ANOVA
b. Student's t-test
c. Chi-squared test
d. Z-test

133. The movement of solvent from a region of lower solute concentration to a region of higher solute concentration through a semipermeable membrane is:
a. Osmosis
b. Diffusion
c. Permeability
d. Active transport

134. Impairment in motor or sensory functions of the lower extremities is called:
a. Quadriplegia
b. Strokes
c. Paraplegia
d. Hemiplegia

135. Influencing people to follow you and to work willingly for the achievement of a common goal is called:
a. Management
b. Delegation
c. Counseling
d. Leadership

136. Which of the following sentence is true about confidence intervals?
a. The intervals give a range of values within which the true value will lie.
b. 95% confidence interval means that 95% of all observed values fall within that interval.
c. They indicate the presence or otherwise of a statistical difference between two groups.
d. The intervals are larger with smaller sample size.

137. According to the chemical nature of the carbonyl group monosaccharides are divided into:
a. Pentose and Hexoses
b. Aldoses and Ketoses
c. Trioses and Tetroses
d. Pentoses and Tetroses

138. Cola- or tea-colored urine indicates:
a. Alka proteinuria
b. Extravascular hemolysis
c. Inflammation of the kidneys
d. Acute pyelonephritis

139. The document that identifies the qualification and attributes required to perform a job is:
a. Job withdrawal
b. Job specification
c. Job satisfaction
d. Job content

140. You calculate a 95% confidence interval, what does it mean:
a. You can be "95% confidence" that your interval will include the population parameter.
b. You can be "5% confidence" that your interval will not include the population parameter.
c. The process you used will capture the true parameter 95% of the time in the long run.
d. All of the above statements are true.

141. The end product of glycolysis under anaerobic conditions is:
a. Lactic acid
b. Pyruvic acid
c. Acetoacetic acid
d. Oxaloacetic acid

142. Staghorn stone is mainly composed of:
a. Calcium phosphate
b. Magnesium, ammonium and phosphate
c. Uric acid
d. Calcium, phosphate and Calcium oxalate

143. Assignment of any responsibility and authority to another person is called:
a. Delegation
b. Declaration
c. Management
d. Planning

144. A type-II error is also known as:
a. False positive
b. False negative
c. Double negative
d. Positive negative

145. Glycerol is the backbone of:
a. Glycerophospholipid
b. Sphingophospholipid
c. Glycolipids
d. Cholesterol esters

146. Seminoma testis is a:
a. Germ cell tumor
b. Vascular tumor
c. Epithelial tumor
d. Mesothelial tumor

147. Following death, the response experienced by the loved ones is called:
a. Grief
b. Mourning
c. Compliance
d. Bereavement

148. Among the following which is not a type of reliability:
a. Split-half
b. Content
c. Internal consistency
d. Test-retest

149. Mineral lacking in milk is:
a. Calcium
b. Iron
c. Sodium
d. Potassium

150. 'Hobnail' appearance on the surface of the liver is seen in:
a. Liver cancer
b. Liver cirrhosis
c. Liver abscess
d. Liver fibrosis

151. The mineral which acts as a cofactor for other enzyme is:
a. Iron
b. Copper
c. Potassium
d. Sodium

152. The following principle is followed to determine the sample size for qualitative research.
a. The 'thumb rule'
b. The 'rule of 30'
c. Data saturation
d. Power analysis

153. MacCallum plaque is seen in:
a. Atherosclerosis
b. Rheumatoid heart disease
c. Rheumatic heart disease
d. Coal worker's pneumoconiosis

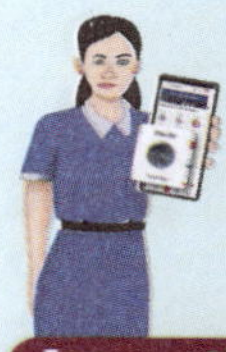

Ans.

Q.	Ans.
125.	d
126.	b
127.	b
128.	a
129.	b
130.	c
131.	d
132.	c
133.	a
134.	c
135.	d
136.	a
137.	b
138.	c
139.	b
140.	d
141.	a
142.	b
143.	a
144.	b
145.	a
146.	a
147.	a
148.	b
149.	b
150.	b
151.	c
152.	c
153.	c

154. The enzyme which helps for the digestion of fat after emulsification is:
a. Renin b. Amylase
c. Lipase d. Trypsin

155. The type of shock uncounted in case of road traffic accidents with the significant hemorrhage is:
a. Septic shock b. Neurogenic shock
c. Hypovolemic shock d. Cardiogenic shock

156. The death caused by obstruction of the cavities of nose and mouth by a bed clothing, a pillow or a cushion is called:
a. Strangulation b. Smothering
c. Asphyxia d. Gagging

157. During lactation, the additional caloric requirement of mother is:
a. +100 cal/day b. +330-400 cal/day
c. 2300 cal/day d. 2700 cal/day

158. Atrophy is:
a. Increased size of a tissue
b. Normal multiplication of tissue
c. Reduced size of an organ or tissue
d. Increased number of cells in an organ

159. Artificial method of preserving the dead body is called:
a. Embalming b. Ossification
c. Autopsy d. Dispatching

160. The probability or ratio of dying between birth and first birthday expressed per 1000 live births is:
a. Child mortality rate b. Under -five mortality rate
c. Postnatal mortality rate d. Infant mortality rate

161. One of the following studies would require the largest sample size:
a. Correlational b. Ethnography
c. Ground theory d. Phenomenological

162. Sentinel surveillance indicates:
a. Identifying high risk group
b. Surveillance of water population
c. Surveillance of environmental control
d. Monitoring of rate of occurrence of specific diseases

163. "TIGH" means:
a. Time, incidence, goal and hormones
b. Tetanus immune globulin, human
c. Total intake of growth hormone
d. Time, immune globulin G, health

164. The basics for primary healthcare was laid down by:
a. Mudaliar Committee b. Bhore Committee
c. Kartar Committee d. Srivastava Committee

165. The study of how to use computer to capture the data and provide to the better for clinical and research purpose is:
a. Case management b. HMS
c. Informatics d. Computer and Technology

166. A trained community based link worker at village level who acts as a bridge between the Government functionaries and tribal -nontribal population is:
a. ANM b. ASHA
c. MPHW(M) d. MPHW (F)

167. The blueprint of an educational program is:
a. Curriculum
b. Lesson plan
c. Master rotation plan
d. Time table

168. One of the specific objectives of mother and child health(MCH) is:
a. Promotion of the physical and psychological development of the child
b. Care of the child
c. Health care and education of the child
d. Child care and mother safety

169. Vibrations of speech felt as tremors of the chest wall felt during palpation is:
a. Fremitus b. Egophony
c. Crackles d. Compliance

170. The vitamin which is produced by the bacteria living in the colon is:
a. Vitamin K b. Vitamin A
c. Vitamin B d. Vitamin D

171. Transplant rejection is an example of:
a. Type 4 hypersensitivity
b. Type 2 hypersensitivity
c. Type 3 hypersensitivity
d. Type 1 hypersensitivity

172. Management of conjunctivitis includes the following; except:
a. Eye irrigation
b. Warm Compresses
c. Rubbing affected eye with moist wash cloth
d. Eye lid cleaning

173. Most important aspect of management of burn injury in first 24 hours is:
a. Dressing b. Antibiotic therapy
c. Fluid resuscitation d. Plastic surgery

174. In quantitative research studies, the power analysis is used to:
a. Set the level of significance
b. Test the internal validity
c. Estimate the sample size
d. Determine the reliability

175. The principle of adult learning is:
a. Needs assessment and safety in the training environment
b. Vocation or professional training
c. Remedial classes
d. Personal enrichment program

176. Cognitive domain in Bloom's taxonomy includes all the following; except:
a. Synthesis b. Criticism
c. Knowledge d. Comprehension

177. The essential components of experimental or interventional research designs are:
a. Hypothesis, assumption and intervention
b. Pre-test post-test, control and variable
c. Experiment control and hypothesis
d. Randomization, control and manipulation

178. "Education is not a preparation for life; education is life itself" stated by:
a. Mahatma Gandhi b. Bertrand Russell
c. Helen Keller d. John Dewey

179. The failure to meet an ordinary standard of care resulting in injury to the patient or plaintiff is called:
a. Negligence
b. Malpractice
c. Defamation
d. False imprisonment

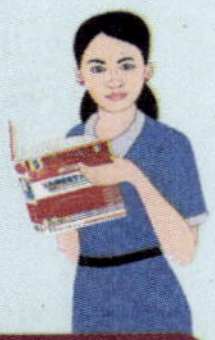

Ans.

154. c
155. c
156. b
157. b
158. c
159. a
160. d
161. a
162. d
163. b
164. b
165. c
166. b
167. a
168. a
169. a
170. a
171. a
172. c
173. c
174. c
175. a
176. b
177. d
178. d
179. a

180. One of the following is known as the protein factory of cells:
a. Ribosomes b. Cytoplasm
c. Golgi bodies d. DNA

181. Framework that explains relationship between concepts and links, concepts from various theories, research findings and experience of researcher is:
a. Conceptual framework
b. Study framework
c. Both conceptual and study framework
d. Theoretical framework

182. A deep partial thickness injury involves the distraction of the epidermis and upper layers of the dermis and injury to deeper portions of the dermis, thus injury in burn is classified as:
a. Second degree b. First degree
c. Third degree d. Fourth degree

183. A type of educational assessment which is generally carried out throughout a course or project is:
a. Summative assessment
b. Formative assessment
c. Criterion-referenced assessment
d. Impassive assessment

184. The basic element of a theory or research that is used to explain and interpret facts is:
a. Empirical indication b. Concept
c. Relational statement d. Hypothesis

185. All are the interventions to control the ICP in a patient with head injury, except:
a. Elevate the head of the bed to 30°
b. Frequent repositioning of the patient
c. Maintain normal body temperature
d. Maintain fluid restriction

186. A type of sampling in which the population is first divided into two or more subsets based on some characteristics is called:
a. Simple random sampling
b. Systematic random sampling
c. Stratified random sampling
d. Nonprobability sampling

187. A disorder of localized increased bone remodeling, most commonly affecting the skill, fever, tibia, pelvic bones and vertebrae is:
a. Paget's disease b. Osteomyelitis
c. Kyphosis d. Osteomalacia

188. Experimental studies differ from other research approaches because of the:
a. Exposure of all the subjects to the treatment
b. Conduct of the study in a laboratory
c. Controlled manipulation of at least one treatment variable
d. Easy availability of human subjects

189. A well-known reflex, indicative of CNS disease affecting the corticospinal tract is:
a. Patellar reflex b. Deep tendon reflex
c. Babinski response d. Brachioradialis reflex

190. The research critique in nursing study is a careful appraisal of the:
a. Quality of a research study
b. Strength and weakness of research study
c. Research exposure of the researcher
d. Strength and weakness of assumption and hypothesis

191. A malignant proliferation arising from the epidermis is:
a. Basal cell carcinoma
b. Squamous cell carcinoma
c. Keloids
d. Malignant Melanoma

192. One of the earliest symptoms of Vit. A deficiency is:
a. Nyctalopia b. Xerophthalmia
c. Bitot's spot d. Keratomalacia

193. A clinical syndrome of unknown cause involving the peripheral and cranial nerves is:
a. Bell's palsy
b. Polyneuropathies
c. Guillain – Barre Syndrome
d. Peripheral neuropathies

194. The most important health functionary link between rural poor and good health care under "Integrated Child Health Development Scheme" (ICDS) is:
a. Village health guide
b. Multipurpose health worker
c. Auxiliary nurse midwife
d. Anganwadi health worker

195. A defect in the transmission of impulses from nerve to muscle cells due to loss of available or normal receptors on the postsynaptic membrane of the neuromuscular junction is called:
a. Alzheimer's disease b. Huntington's disease
c. Myasthenia Gravis d. Parkinson's disease

196. A legal wrong committed against a person his or her rights, or property, intentional, wilfully committed without just cause is:
a. Tort law b. Constitution law
c. Criminal law d. Contract law

197. One of the cranial nerves whose function is the movement of sternocleidomastoid and trapezius muscle is:
a. Cranial nerve XI b. Cranial nerve VI
c. Cranial nerve V d. Cranial nerve VII

198. A sampling method in which the researcher handpicks the sample is called:
a. Convenient sampling b. Purposive sampling
c. Quota sampling d. Cluster sampling

199. Ringworm of the scalp, a contagious fungal infection is:
a. Tinea Capitis b. Tinea Unguium
c. Tinea Corporis d. Tinea Pedis

200. Wrongful killing of a human being without justification or excuse is:
a. Noncriminal homicide b. First degree murder
c. Excusable homicide d. Felonious homicide

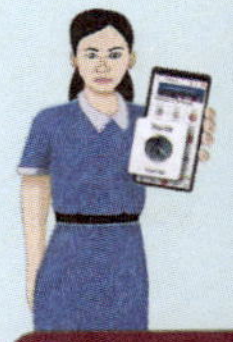

Ans.
180. a
181. a
182. a
183. b
184. b
185. b
186. c
187. a
188. c
189. c
190. b
191. b
192. a
193. c
194. d
195. c
196. a
197. a
198. a
199. a
200. d

"After dinner rest a while; after supper walk a mile."

—T. Cogan

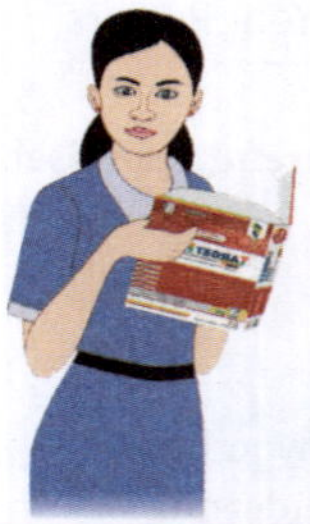

NORCET (NO) 2021 (Memory Based)

1. Which of the following color code is not included in triage?
a. Black b. Blue
c. Green d. Red

2. The side effect of chloramphenicol drug is:
a. Bone marrow suppression
b. Epilepsy
c. Osteoporosis
d. Weight gain

3. Normal respiration in adults is:
a. 10 beats/min b. 14 beats/min
c. 30 beats/min d. 8 beats/min

4. The full form of DPT is:
a. Dengue, pertussis, tetanus
b. Diphtheria, pneumonia, tetanus
c. Diphtheria, pertussis, tetanus
d. Diphtheria, pertussis, typhoid

5. What is the dose of iron and folic acid in the Anemia Mukt Bharat Scheme?
a. 50 mg and 500 mcg b. 60 mg and 500 mcg
c. 50 mg and 400 mcg d. 40 mg and 500 mcg

6. What is baking powder?
a. Sodium chloride b. Sodium bicarbonate
c. Potassium bicarbonate d. Potassium chloride

7. The most common type of episiotomy is:
a. Right mediolateral b. J shaped
c. Lateral d. Median

8. Which of the following blood group is a universal donor?
a. O positive b. O negative
c. AB positive d. AB negative

9. A harsh, vibratory sound that occurs due to the narrowing of the upper airway, heard most prominently when inhaling is known as:
a. Stridor b. Wheezing
c. Rhonchi d. Snoring

10. Rapid and weak pulse is known as:
a. Bounding pulse b. Thready pulse
c. Strong pulse d. None of these

11. Chances of PTSD are most common in:
a. Divorce
b. Diagnosis of cancer
c. Facing gunshot (means someone puts the gun on skull)
d. Bank robbery

12. Projective technique is used for the assessment of:
a. Memory b. Intelligence
c. Knowledge d. Personality

13. What differentiates mania from hypomania?
a. Psychotic symptoms
b. Reduced sleeping time
c. Effect on work
d. Need for hospital admission

14. Which screening test is not used for cervical cancer?
a. Colposcopy b. HPV DNA
c. Pap smear d. VIA

15. Mr X does not use a car while going out, scared of using lifts. He avoids going in public places and keeps the doors open while in a closed room. He finds it uncomfortable to leave the house alone, so he always takes a family member along whenever he goes out. What will be the probable diagnosis?
a. Claustrophobia b. Agoraphobia
c. Public phobia d. Aerophobia

16. Which vaccine is not included in Indradhanush Program?
a. DPT b. Hepatitis B
c. Pneumococcal vaccine d. Measles

17. Which of the following is the longest bone of the body?
a. Femur b. Tibia
c. Fibula d. Radius

18. Which of the following is the "Breast bone" in the following bones?
a. Sternum b. Ribs
c. Clavicle d. Vertebrae

19. Which among the following is most common in patient with schizophrenia.
a. Thought broadcasting b. Visual hallucinations
c. Thought block d. Delusion of persecution

20. A person is saying his family members are dying. He is also decaying, nothing exists in the world. What could be the probable diagnosis?
a. Delusion of persecution b. Paranoid delusion
c. Nihilistic delusion d. Delusion of reference

21. In which color bag placenta is discarded?
a. Red b. Yellow
c. Blue d. Black

22. Which measure is used for growth monitoring at Anganwadi center?
a. Weight for height b. MUAC
c. Skin fold thicknesses d. Weight for age

23. Which of the following is not a sign of good attachment?
a. Upper side areola more exposed than lower
b. Widely open mouth
c. Chin touches the breast
d. Lower lip move inward

24. What is the range of MUAC for malnutrition?
a. <12.5 cm b. <11.5 cm
c. <13.5 cm d. <14.5 cm

25. A cotton ball infected with pus is discarded in which colored bin?
a. Yellow
b. Black
c. Red
d. Blue

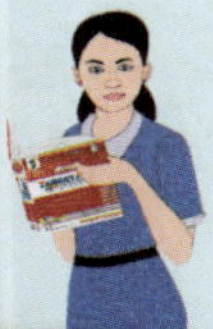

Ans.

1. b
2. a
3. b
4. c
5. b
6. b
7. a
8. b
9. a
10. b
11. c
12. d
13. d
14. d
15. a
16. c
17. a
18. a
19. d
20. c
21. b
22. d
23. d
24. a
25. a

26. A fluid that causes shifting of fluid from cells to blood:
a. Hypertonic b. Hypotonic
c. Isotonic d. Isotope

27. Signs of fluid overload:
a. Elevated JVP b. Collapsed Jugular vein
c. Thready pulse d. Irregular pulse

28. An alcoholic patient is administered disulfiram. How long can the disulfiram-ethanol reaction (DER) last?
a. 24 hours b. 36 hours
c. 96 hours d. 1 week

29. Covishield vaccine is contraindicated in:
a. Previous allergy to first dose of covishield
b. History of carcinoma
c. History of pollen allergy
d. History of radiation therapy

30. Bluish discoloration of vagina and cervix in the first trimester is known as:
a. Chadwick b. Osiander's
c. Hegar d. Goodell

31. Which preservative is used during packing of catgut?
a. Formaldehyde b. Glutaraldehyde
c. Isopropyl alcohol d. Sodium hypochlorite

32. A patient comes with the diagnosis of COPD. True about oxygen administration in this patient is/are:
1. Use Venturi mask at 28% (not >6 lit/min)
2. Use the nasal cannula with flow rate of not >4 lit/min
3. Maintain the SPO2 in between 88 and 92%
4. Maintain oxygen flow rate at 8 to 12 L/min

a. All are true b. 2, 3 and 4 are true
c. Only 1 and 2 are true d. 1, 2, 3 are true

33. Positive Stallworthy sign is seen in which of the following conditions?
a. Abruptio Placenta b. Placenta Previa
c. Placenta Succenturiata d. Placenta Bilobata

34. Intramuscular injection is given at which angle?
a. 30° b. 60°
c. 90° d. 15°

35. Which of the following muscles is the site for 2nd dose of DPT?
a. Ventrogluteal b. Vastus lateralis
c. Deltoid d. Dorsogluteal

36. SSPE is the complication of which of the following disease?
a. EBV b. Measles
c. Varicella d. Mumps

37. Which of the following is the most common cause of UTI in children?
a. ***E. coli*** b. Proteus
c. *S. aureus* d. Pneumococcus

38. What is crowning?
a. Rotation at pelvic floor
b. Largest skull diameter fixed that doesn't go back
c. Largest diameter at ischial spines
d. None of the above

39. All indicators are age independent; except:
a. Chest circumference b. BMI
c. Weight for height d. MUAC

40. Diseases that occur in 5 to 7 years of interval are called:
a. Secular trend
b. Time trend
c. Periodic trend
d. Cyclic trend

41. Which of the following best describes COVID-19?
a. Pandemic b. Endemic
c. Epidemic d. Sporadic

42. Which of the following is not a symptom of multisystem involvement in COVID-19?
a. Fever b. Rash
c. Pruritic conjunctivitis d. Shock

43. Which of the following is NOT included in surgical safety checklist?
a. Before induction of anesthesia
b. Before skin incision
c. After skin incision
d. Before leaving the operative room

44. Which of the following foods contain high dietary fiber?
a. Orange b. Wheat
c. Spinach d. Green gram

45. Caudal regression syndrome is seen in:
a. Gestational HTN b. Gestational diabetes
c. Eclampsia d. None of these

46. A female reported with excessive vomiting and diagnosis of complete mole. Which of the following is true about complete mole?
a. Decrease HCG level
b. It will be triploid
c. The genotype will be 46(xx)
d. Height of uterus less than gestational age

47. Which of the following is NOT a feature of pre- eclampsia?
a. Hypertension b. Proteinuria
c. Polyuria d. Hypotension

48. A patient has a respiratory rate of 36/min, this condition is known as:
a. Eupnea b. Dyspnea
c. Bradypnea d. Tachypnea

49. What will be prescribed to the mother to prevent neural tube defect (NTD) in fetus?
a. B_6 b. B_{12}
c. B_2 d. Folic acid

50. A patient of RTA with head injury comes to the hospital. You assess the patient by using GCS and the patient score is 9. What is the range of GCS?
a. 15 and 5 b. 10 and 0
c. 15 and 3 d. 15 and 0

51. Partial obstruction of trachea by epiglottis results in:
a. Snoring b. Stridor
c. Rhonchi d. Wheezing

52. Which of the following is a potential issue associated with the incorrect use of a spacer in a Metered Dose Inhaler (MDI)?
a. Impaired drug delivery to the lungs
b. Difficulty in coordinating inhalation
c. Reduced deposition of drug in the mouth
d. Increased risk of mouth infection

53. Exclusive breastfeeding should be continued up to which age?
a. 4 months b. 6 months
c. 8 months d. 12 months

54. Which of the following is NOT included in active management of the 3rd stage of labor?
a. Uterine fundal massage after expulsion of placenta
b. Controlled cord traction
c. Administration of Uterotonic
d. Delayed cord clamping

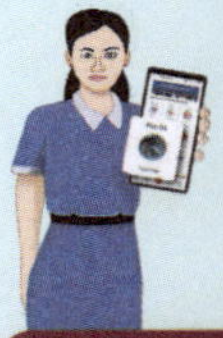

Ans.

26. a
27. a
28. d
29. a
30. a
31. c
32. d
33. b
34. c
35. c
36. b
37. a
38. b
39. a
40. d
41. a
42. c
43. c
44. c
45. b
46. c
47. d
48. d
49. d
50. c
51. d
52. a
53. b
54. d

55. Which of the following gas is used to create pneumoperitoneum during surgery?
a. Oxygen
b. Carbon dioxide
c. Nitrogen
d. Nitrous oxide

56. During the surgery of breast cancer, the breast surgeon needs to take a sentinel lymph node biopsy. Which of the following procedures will be used by the surgeon to take a biopsy?
a. Gamma probe
b. Laparoscope
c. Endoscope
d. Colposcope

57. Choice of fluid in children with moderate dehydration is:
a. D 5% b. D 10%
c. Normal saline d. NS 5%

58. Which among the following causes the occurrence of symptoms of bipolar disorder?
a. Physical activity
b. Return on previous performance level of work
c. Reduced sleep
d. None of the above

59. PDSA stands for:
a. Plan, do, study, act
b. Plan, define, simplify, act
c. Plan, define, simplify, assume
d. Perform, due, simplify, act

60. What is the typical urine output of a healthy adult?
a. 100 mL b. 500 mL
c. 1500 mL d. 2500 mL

61. Premature babies have more chances of hypothermia because of all of the following, except:
a. Cold environment
b. Less developed epidermis
c. Less brown fat
d. Small body surface area in comparison to weight

62. Which of the following is not included in Mission Indradhanush?
a. Measles b. DPT
c. PCV d. Hepatitis B

63. Which type of bandage is used for the ankle joint?
a. Spiral b. Reverse spiral
c. Figure of 8 d. Circular

64. What a nurse will not do while administering KCl?
a. Mix in the NS saline and slow infusion
b. Give some fruits juice
c. Monitoring of intake and output
d. Administer the KCl bolus

65. India crossed 100 crore Covid vaccination on:
a. 19th October, 2021
b. 20th October, 2021
c. 21st October, 2021
d. 22nd October, 2021

66. Cannula used for blood transfusion is:
a. 18G b. 21G
c. 22G d. 23G

67. Length of child doubles by:
a. 2 years b. 3 years
c. 4 years d. 5 years

68. According to Govt. of India, the emergency contraceptive is:
a. Levonorgestrel 1.5 mcg
b. Levonorgestrel 1.5 mg
c. Levonorgestrel 150 mg
d. Progestogen-only pill (POPs)

69. Which of the following is not given to lactating mothers?
a. DMPA
b. POP
c. Mini pills
d. Combined OCPs

70. Cu-T is NOT inserted in:
a. Unexplained vaginal bleeding
b. Multiparous female
c. After delivery
d. Anemia

71. Which muscle has no role in episiotomy?
a. Ischiocavernosus
b. Superior transverse perineal muscles
c. Deep transverse perineal muscles
d. Bulbospongiosus

72. Which of the following is not a symptom of acute renal failure?
a. Hyponatremia
b. Hypokalemia
c. Metabolic alkalosis
d. Metabolic acidosis

73. If a nurse is using 4 size of ET tube, which size of suction catheter will be used by her?
a. 6 fr b. 8 fr
c. 10 fr d. 12 fr

74. A nurse measures the temperature of the child as 38.2°C. What will be his temperature in Fahrenheit?
a. 101.4°F b. 102.6°F
c. 100.7°F d. 99.8°F

75. What does fr indicate in 20 fr of urinary catheter?
a. Inner circumference of catheter
b. Outer circumference of catheter
c. Radius of catheter
d. Length of catheter

76. Bandl's ring is known as a pathological ring, if there is:
a. Precipitatous labor b. Obstructed labor
c. Deep transverse arrest d. None of these

77. What is correct about the use of AED?
a. Used for cardiac arrest patient by medical professionals
b. Used for elderly patients in cardiac arrest by a person with medical training
c. Not used for child below 8 years age and by a medical personnel
d. It can be used for any age group by any person.

78. In an emergency, patient is admitted with cardiac arrest. Which pulse is used to assess PR in the patient?
a. Carotid b. Brachial
c. Apical d. Femoral

79. Which of the following site is NOT used in emergency for infusion?
a. Medial end of clavicle b. Distal end of tibia
c. Distal end of femur d. Proximal end of tibia

80. Recommended duration of hand-rub by WHO is:
a. 20 sec to 30 sec b. 40 sec to 60 sec
c. 1 min to 3 min d. 3 min to 5 min

Ans.

55. b
56. a
57. c
58. b
59. a
60. c
61. d
62. c
63. c
64. d
65. c
66. a
67. c
68. b
69. d
70. a
71. a
72. c
73. b
74. c
75. b
76. b
77. d
78. a
79. a
80. a

81. Disinfection of elastic endoscope is done by using:
a. Ethylene oxide
b. Glutaraldehyde
c. Formaldehyde
d. Hydrogen peroxide

82. Transmission based precautions are:
a. Airborne, contact and universal precautions
b. Airborne, droplets and contact precautions
c. Universal precaution, vaccination, prevention of needlestick injury
d. PPE, airborne and contact precautions

83. During doffing, PPE is removed in which order?
a. Goggles, mask, gloves, gown
b. Gown, mask, goggles, gloves
c. Mask, goggles, gloves, gown
d. Gloves, gown, goggles, mask

84. During delivery, there is a laceration in vaginal mucosa involving some perineal muscles, but not involving the anal sphincter. Identify the degree of tear:
a. First b. Second
c. Third d. Fourth

85. A placenta that is partially or completely attached to myometrium without disturbing the decidua is called:
a. Placenta accreta b. Increta
c. Percreta d. Placenta succunturiata

86. The life expectancy of patients with schizophrenia is reduced by:
a. 10 to 20 years of age b. 20 to 30 years of age
c. 30 to 40 years of age d. 15 to 25 years of age

87. Complete bowel obstruction results in all; except:
a. Bilious vomiting b. Infection
c. Diarrhea d. Abdominal pain

88. Which antiepileptic is given by intranasal route in an emergency?
a. Valproate b. Midazolam
c. Phenytoin d. Gabapentin

89. A lactating mother is suffering from mastitis and she went to the clinic for the check-up. After the assessment, breast abscess is diagnosed in one of the breast. Identify the measure taken by the mother:
a. No breastfeeding by both breasts
b. Continue breastfeeding by opposite breast
c. Give formula food
d. Give cow milk

90. How a nurse will administer an injection of dextran iron to a patient?
a. At an angle of 45° intramuscularly
b. Pull the skin lateral toward site of injection
c. Use Z track technique
d. Remove the needle at 45°

91. In the context of vital signs assessment, which of the following is considered the fifth vital sign:
a. RR b. HR
c. BP d. Pain

92. Which congenital heart disease is associated with minimum chances of heart failure?
a. Transposition of great arteries
b. ASD
c. VSD
d. Patent ductus arteriosus

93. Hormone responsible for lactation:
a. Prolactin b. GH
c. FSH d. HCG

94. The difference between systolic and diastolic blood pressure is called:
a. Pulse pressure b. Pulse deficit
c. Auscultatory gap d. Korotkoff sounds

95. What is the daily additional calories required for pregnant women?
a. 300 calories b. 500 calories
c. 100 calories d. 800 calories

96. Iron and folic acid dose in pregnant woman is:
a. 60 mg iron, 0.4 mg folic acid
b. 30 mg iron, 0.4 mg folic acid
c. 100 mg iron, 0.3 mg folic acid
d. 60 mg iron, 0.2 mg folic acid

97. Stallworthy sign is seen in:
a. Posterior placenta previa b. Hydatidiform mole
c. APH d. PPH

98. Which is a high pitched lung sound?
a. Wheezes b. Rhonchi
c. Rales d. Coarse crackles

99. In typhoid what type of fever is common?
a. Step ladder fever b. Intermittent fever
c. Continuous fever d. Relapsing fever

100. Most common cause of PPH:
a. Placental Abruptio b. Placenta previa
c. Uterine atony d. Anemia

101. HPV vaccine is used to prevent which of the following cancer?
a. Cervical cancer b. Breast cancer
c. Stomach cancer d. Lung cancer

102. All are the methods used for the removal of placenta; except:
a. Give oxytocin b. Uterine massage
c. Controlled cord traction d. Prostaglandin E1

103. Complementary feeding starts at:
a. 3 months b. 6 months
c. 9 months d. 12 months

104. India started COVID-19 vaccination with COVAXIN on:
a. 16 January, 2021 b. 10 January, 2021
c. 16 March, 2021 d. 18 May, 2021

105. Identify the following image:

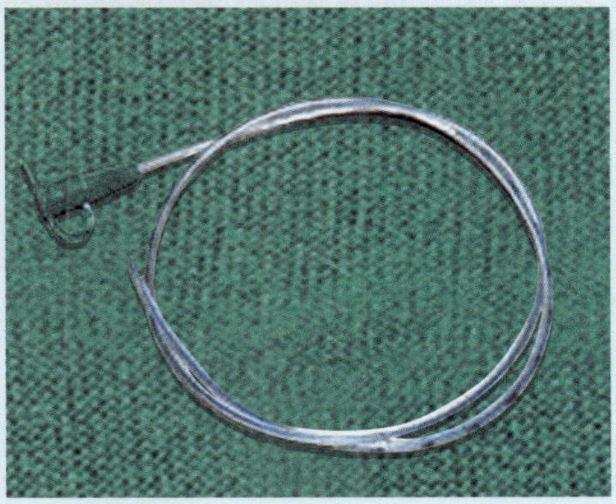

a. NG tube
b. Child feeding tube
c. ET tube
d. Suction tube

Ans.

81. a
82. b
83. d
84. b
85. a
86. d
87. c
88. b
89. b
90. c
91. d
92. a
93. a
94. a
95. a
96. a
97. a
98. a
99. a
100. c
101. a
102. d
103. b
104. a
105. a

106. Identify the following image:

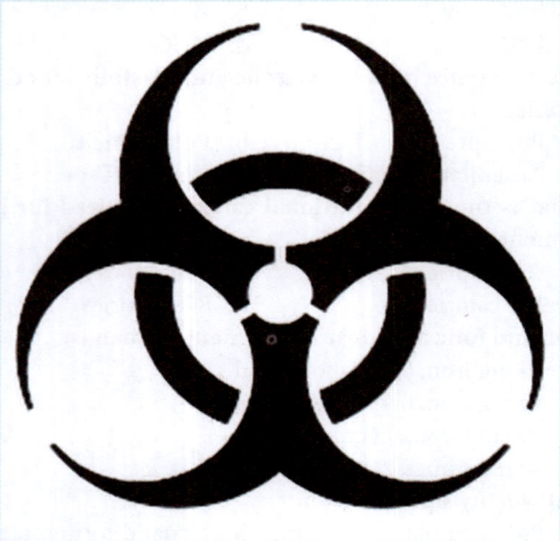

a. Biohazard
b. Radiation
c. Cytotoxic
d. BMW

107. Identify the following image:

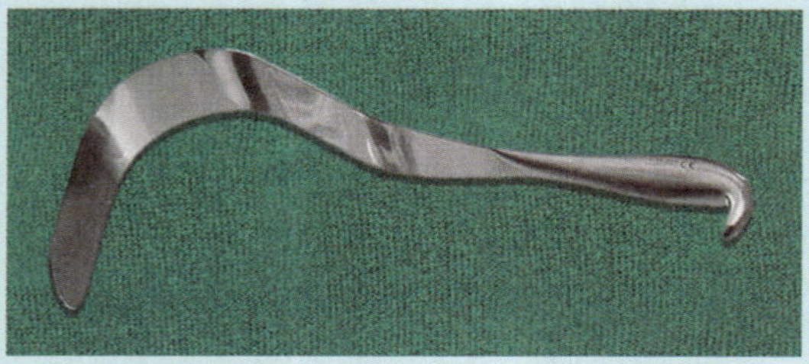

a. Deaver retractor
b. Hohmann retractor
c. Senn retractor
d. Ribbon retractor

108. Self-retainable catheter is:

a. Malecot catheter
b. Rubber catheter
c. Ryle's tube
d. Robinson catheter

109. A patient with blood transfusion has a light headache, chills and rashes. What nurse will expect to be ordered to the patient?

a. Adrenaline and noradrenaline
b. Atropine and adrenaline
c. Atropine and dexamethasone
d. Adrenaline and hydrocortisone

110. A child reported in emergency with acute bronchospasm and has a history of bee sting. What is the most preferred route of adrenaline administration?

a. Intraosseous
b. Intramuscular
c. Subcutaneous
d. Intratracheal

111. The difference between apical pulse and radial pulse is called:

a. Atrial flutter
b. Atrial fibrillation
c. Pulse deficit
d. Sinus bradycardia

112. What is chest compression and ventilation ratio in neonatal resuscitation?

a. 3:1 b. 4:1
c. 1:1 d. 1:2

113. All of the following are used in raised ICP; except:

a. Mannitol b. Sedation
c. Hyperventilation d. IV Dextrose 5%

114. A 20-year-old man admitted in the hospital with massive hemorrhage due to RTA. Which cannula the nurse will use?

a. 20G b. 18G
c. 26G d. 23G

115. A female with scalded burn comes to the hospital. What is the fluid of choice for initial stage fluid replacement?

a. NS b. RL
c. D5% d. D10%

116. Which is not used for induction of labor with a history of previous LSCS?

a. Prostaglandin b. Amniotomy
c. Oxytocin d. Stripping of membranes

117. In which condition gastric lavage is contraindicated?

a. Corrosive poisoning
b. Salicylate poisoning
c. Medication poisoning
d. None of the above

118. A baby admitted in hospital with the complaint of foreign body aspiration. The nurse will do:

a. 5 back slap 5 chest thrust
b. 2 back slap 2 chest thrust
c. Heimlich maneuver
d. CPR

119. Identify the correct method of inserting urinary catheter in a neonate:

a. 12 fr is appropriate size for catheterization in neonate
b. No requirement of jelly
c. Inflate the balloon after insertion of entire catheter
d. Inflate the balloon when urine seen, no matter location of catheter

120. Weight of infant quadruples by:

a. 1 year b. 2 years
c. 3 years d. 4 years

121. A 50-year-old patient with 54% burn is admitted in the hospital. According to Wallace rule of 9, how many % is given to perineum?

a. 1% b. 2%
c. 4.5% d. 9%

122. Identify the following image:

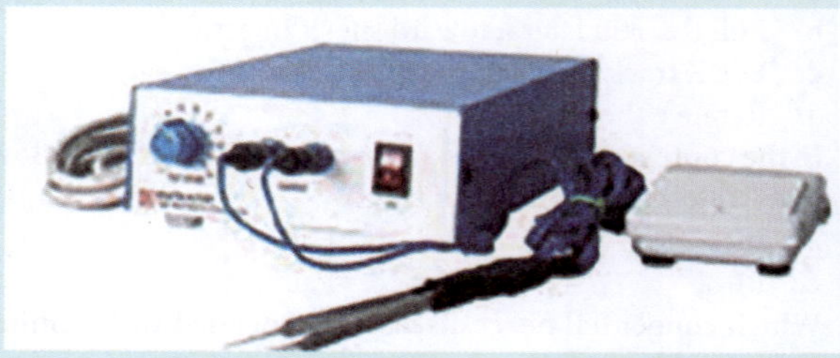

a. Bipolar cautery
b. Monopolar cautery
c. Electric pencil
d. None of the above

Ans.

106. a
107. a
108. a
109. d
110. b
111. c
112. a
113. d
114. b
115. b
116. a
117. a
118. a
119. d
120. b
121. a
122. a

123. Identify the image:

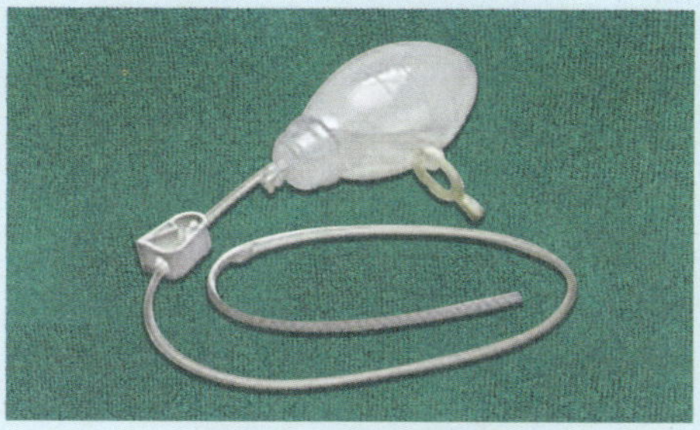

a. Penrose drain
b. Hemovac drain
c. Jackson Pratt drain
d. None of these

124. India's 1st indigenous COVID vaccine is:

a. Covaxin
b. Covishield
c. Moderna
d. Sputnik

125. Identify the number of surgical blade:

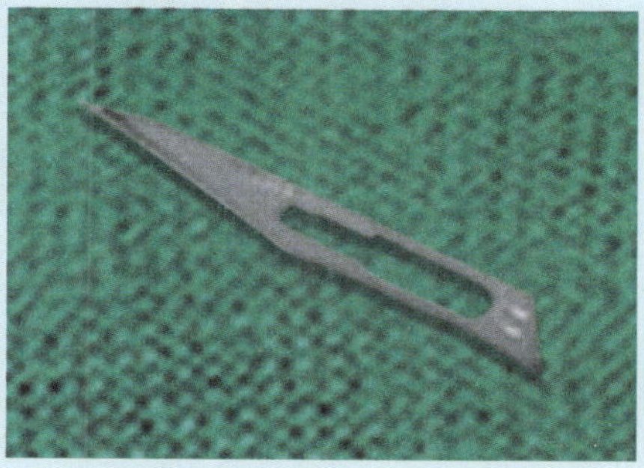

a. 10
b. 11
c. 15
d. 20

126. The protection period provided by Cu-T 380 A is:

a. 10 years
b. 20 years
c. 15 years
d. 5 years

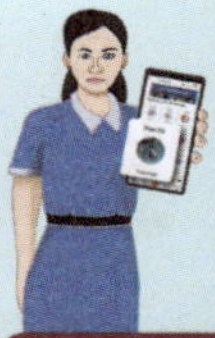

Ans.

123. c
124. a
125. b
126. a

"Sometimes the remedy is worse than the disease."
—Francis Bacon

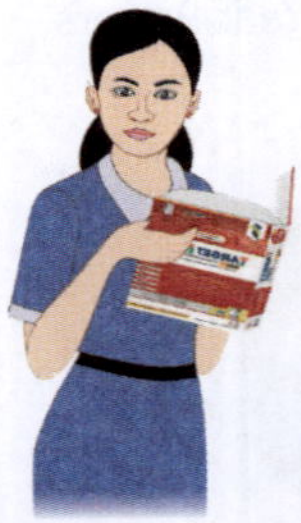

CNCI (NO) 2021

1. Name the non-stimulant drug with Norepinephrine reuptake inhibiting action used in the treatment of ADHD.
a. Atomoxetine b. Dexamphetamine
c. Methyl Phenidate d. Pimozide

2. How should a nurse administer an iron injection to an adult?
a. Intradermal in the forearm
b. Subcutaneous in the arm
c. Z track intramuscular in the gluteal
d. Intramuscular in the deltoid

3. The expected height of a normal child at 12 months is:
a. 45 cm b. 50 cm
c. 75 cm d. 100 cm

4. Increased depth of breathing with normal respiratory rate is called:
a. Kussmaul's breathing b. Bradypnea
c. Orthopnea d. Hyperpnea

5. A nurse enters a room and finds a patient lying on the floor. Which action should the nurse perform first?
a. Assist the patient back to bed
b. Establish whether the patient is responsive
c. Ask the patient what happened
d. Call for help to get the patient back in bed

6. The neural tube defect among newborns can be prevented by providing:
a. Iron to the mother in third trimester
b. Folic acid to mother in first trimester
c. Iron and folic acid throughout pregnancy
d. Vitamin K to the mother in first trimester

7. What is hyperemesis gravidarum?
a. Morning sickness b. Lethargy
c. Excessive vomiting d. Excessive loose motion

8. Which position is suitable for an unconscious patient while performing mouth care?
a. Fowler's position b. Knee chest
c. Supine d. Side lying

9. Mr. Sharma developed features of depression after his divorce. Here divorce is considered as:
a. Precipitating factor
b. Perpetuating factor
c. Predisposing factor
d. Personality factor

10. A baby whose birth weight is 3 kg, what will be his required weight at the age of 4 years?
a. 6 kg b. 12 kg
c. 14 kg d. 16 kg

11. Which anti-tuberculosis drug causes poor vision and difficulty in color perception?
a. Streptomycin b. Ethambutol
c. Rifampicin d. Pyrazinamide

12. The act of rubbing an oil onto the skin to produce a local effect is known as:
a. Injection b. Inhalation
c. Inunction d. Infusion

13. A 50-year-old man presents with sudden onset of dyspnea, breathlessness and chest pain. Examination shows tachypnea, hypotension, cyanosis, jugular vein distension, tachycardia and low-grade fever. The most likely diagnosis is:
a. Acute MI
b. Acute attack of bronchial asthma
c. Stroke
d. Pulmonary embolism

14. While providing care to a patient with Hepatitis, the nursing officer should take special precautions to:
a. Prevent droplet spread of infection
b. Use caution when bringing food for patient
c. Wear mask and gown before entering the room
d. Use gloves when removing the patient's bed pan

15. The term Aphakia means:
a. Inflammation of lens b. Absence of lens
c. Enhancement of lens d. Lens disease

16. The uterine fundus height of a pregnant patient is at the level of the umbilicus, her pregnancy is about:
a. 10 to 12 weeks b. 14 to 16 weeks
c. 20 to 24 weeks d. 30 to 32 weeks

17. As a nurse you are monitoring a patient in immediate postpartum period. You are checking TRP and BP every 15 minutes for first hour. Which value suggests you that there is an excessive blood loss?
a. Increased pulse rate 90 – 102
b. An increased respiratory rate 18 – 22
c. Temperature 100.2° Fahrenheit
d. None of the above

18. While assessing Mr. Gupta with Braden Scale, the score attained was 8 which indicates that the risk of developing pressure sore for Mr. Gupta is:
a. Mild b. Moderate
c. High d. Very High

19. What is the name of the opening that connects two atria of fetal heart?
a. Ductus arteriosus
b. Ductus venosus
c. Foramen ovale
d. Ligamentum teres

20. In which of the following genetic condition, Karyotype 47, XXY is seen?
a. Down's syndrome
b. Klinefelter's syndrome
c. Edward's syndrome
d. Patau's syndrome

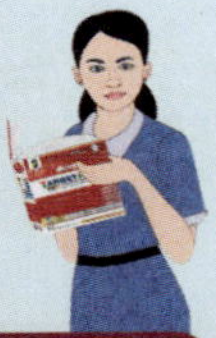

Ans.

1.	a
2.	c
3.	c
4.	d
5.	b
6.	b
7.	c
8.	d
9.	a
10.	d
11.	b
12.	c
13.	d
14.	d
15.	b
16.	c
17.	a
18.	d
19.	c
20.	b

***Disclaimer:** The questions are prepared by memory-based recall from candidates who attended the examination.*

21. Which statement among the following is true as far as maturation of Graafian follicle is concerned?
a. Maturation is influenced by both FSH and LH
b. Maturation is only influenced by FSH
c. Maturation is only influenced by LH
d. Maturation is only influenced by progesterone

22. What immediate nursing intervention will you take in case of blood transfusion reaction?
a. Inform the physician
b. Inform the blood bank
c. Monitor vital signs
d. Stop the transfusion and monitor the vital signs

23. As a staff nurse you are caring a patient with Psoriasis. Salicylic acid is prescribed to the patient. Which finding indicates the presence of systemic toxicity from this medication?
a. Respiration decreased b. Tinnitus
c. Constipation d. Diarrhea

24. Phlebostatic axis is the point at intersection of:
a. Mid-axillary line and line drawn through forth intercostal space
b. Anterior axillary line and sixth intercostal space
c. Posterior axillary line and fifth intercostal space
d. Anterior axillary line and fourth intercostal space

25. Name of the receptor on epidermis that transmits stimuli to the axon through a chemical synapse.
a. Langerhans cells
b. Merkel cells
c. Woodzer cells
d. Berger cells

26. Administration of Mesna with a chemotherapy agent helps in:
a. Favoring the destruction of cancer cells
b. Protecting the cells
c. Preventing formation of uric cells
d. Increasing production of WBC

27. Your patient complains of dry mouth with swallowing difficulty. Which among the following drugs can produce these side effects when administered in the above condition?
a. Dicyclomine b. Pyrantel Pamoate
c. Griseofulvin d. Naloxone

28. Uterine polarity is:
a. The neuromuscular disharmony between the two uterine segments throughout labor
b. The neurochemical disharmony between the two segments of the uterus throughout labor
c. The neuromuscular harmony between the two uterine segments throughout labor
d. The muscular disharmony between the two uterine segments during labor

29. Medical treatment of coronary artery disease includes which of the following procedure?
a. Cardiac catheterization
b. Oral medication administration
c. Coronary artery bypass grafting
d. Percutaneous transluminal coronary angioplasty

30. Which of the following causative organism is responsible for Moniliasis?
a. Candida albicans b. Tinea cruris
c. Staphylococcus aureus d. Gonococci

31. A 30-year-old pregnant woman is diagnosed with pulmonary tuberculosis. Which of the following anti tuberculosis drug should not be given?
a. INH b. Rifampicin
c. Streptomycin d. Ethambutol

32. A disorder of thought in which patient has a false and fixed belief that members of his family are trying to kill him is:
a. Delusion of persecution b. Delusion of grandeur
c. Nihilistic disorder d. Delusion of guilt

33. Kernicterus, which may occur as a complication of jaundice is a pathological condition of:
a. Liver b. Brain
c. Kidney d. Heart

34. Munson's sign is a characteristic of advanced case of:
a. Keratoconus b. Cataract
c. Strabismus d. Diabetic Retinopathy

35. Rose Bengal test is used in the diagnosis of:
a. Brucellosis b. Byssinosis
c. Whooping cough d. Bronchiectasis

36. Which of the following neurotransmitters is deficient in depression?
a. Serotonin b. 5 HT
c. GABA d. Both a and b

37. A patient receiving IV fluids develops warm tenderness, erythema and pain at the site. The nurse suspects which of the following?
a. Fluid overload b. Sepsis
c. Phlebitis d. Infiltration

38. Station in obstetric pelvis is related to:
a. Iliac spine b. Ischial spine
c. Coccyx d. Ileum spine

39. Inflammation of tissues surrounding the nail is known as:
a. Clubbing b. Koilonychia
c. Paronychia d. Onycholysis

40. Name the neurological disorder characterized by the loss of the ability to execute or carry out skilled movements and gestures, despite having the desire and the physical ability to perform them.
a. Anhedonia b. Apraxia
c. Apathy d. Amnesia

41. The heat regulatory center of the body is located at:
a. Medulla oblongata b. Thalamus
c. Limbic system d. Hypothalamus

42. The nurse administers ear drop to a 7-year-old child. How does the nurse pull the patient's ear?
a. Outward b. Backward
c. Upward and Backward d. Backward and Downward

43. Which of the following is not an isotonic fluid?
a. 0.9%
b. RL
c. Dextrose 5% in water
d. Dextrose 5% in normal saline

44. Meniere's disease is related to:
a. Eye
b. Ear
c. Respiratory system
d. Digestive system

45. The space between arachnoid and pia mater is called:
a. Epidural b. Subdural
c. Subarachnoid d. Extradural

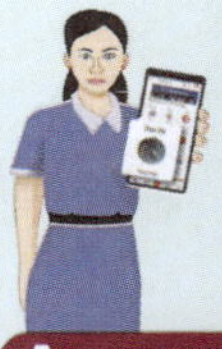

Ans.

21. a
22. d
23. b
24. a
25. b
26. b
27. a
28. c
29. b
30. a
31. c
32. a
33. b
34. a
35. a
36. a
37. c
38. b
39. c
40. b
41. d
42. c
43. d
44. b
45. c

46. Which assessment indicates the nurse about development of cardiogenic shock in MI patient in ICU?
a. Bradycardia
b. Increased blood pressure
c. Oliguria
d. Warm and flushed skin

47. According to Freud, which component of personality operates according to the reality principle?
a. ID
b. Ego
c. Super ego
d. Trust

48. Which is not a cause of APH?
a. Placenta previa
b. Cord presentation
c. Abruptio placentae
d. Rupture of uterus

49. Cord clamping is delayed by 1-3 minutes in neonates because:
a. Prevents anemia in women
b. Placenta separates easily
c. Prevents jaundice in neonate
d. Neonate gets cord blood

50. Which of the following causative organism is responsible for syphilis?
a. Human immune deficiency virus
b. Sarcoptes scabi
c. Neisseria gonorrhea
d. Treponema pallidum

51. Warning signs of lung cancer include persistent cough, bloody sputum, dyspnea and which of the other following symptoms?
a. Dizziness
b. Generalized weakness
c. Hypotension
d. Recurrent pleural effusion

52. At the time of diagnosis of Hodgkin's lymphoma, which of the following areas is often involved?
a. Back
b. Neck
c. Chest
d. Groin

53. Which of the following is a malignant tumor of the connective tissue?
a. Sarcoma
b. Carcinoma
c. Osteoma
d. Glaucoma

54. Which of the following is suggested as surgical intervention for Ca Prostate?
a. Radical prostatectomy
b. Bilateral orchiectomy
c. Transurethral resection of prostate (T.U.R.P)
d. Transurethral resection of bladder tumor (T.U.R.B.T)

55. Which type of cancer has poorest prognosis given below?
a. Leukemia
b. Breast cancer
c. Pancreatic cancer
d. Lymphoma

56. Which of the following is the feature of benign tumor?
a. Infiltrative type of growth
b. Metastasis is present
c. Contained within a capsule
d. Grows rapidly

57. The patient with cancer is receiving chemotherapy and develops thrombocytopenia. The nurse identifies which intervention as the highest priority in the nursing plan of care?
a. Ambulation three times a day
b. Monitoring a platelet count
c. Monitoring temperature
d. Monitoring for pathological factors

58. In the patient with terminal lung cancer, the focus of nursing care is on which of the following nursing interventions?
a. Prepare the patient's will
b. Provide nutritional support
c. Provide emotional support
d. Provide pain control

59. Mrs. Sharma with advanced breast cancer is prescribed tamoxifen (Nolvadex). When teaching the patient about this drug, the nurse should emphasize the importance of reporting which adverse reaction immediately?
a. Hearing loss
b. Headache
c. Vision changes
d. Anorexia

60. Kaposi's sarcoma is the type of cancer which is common in people with:
a. Kidney failure
b. Liver cirrhosis
c. Kangri cancer
d. HIV

61. Which of the following is a malignant tumor of the bone?
a. Fibrosarcoma
b. Lipoma
c. Osteogenic sarcoma
d. Osteoma

62. A male patient is receiving external radiation to the neck for cancer of the larynx. The most likely side effect to be expected is:
a. Dyspnea
b. Diarrhea
c. Sore Throat
d. Constipation

63. Which of the following is a diagnostic test for the diagnosis of prostate cancer?
a. Digital rectal examination
b. Prostate specific antigen (PSA)
c. Prostate biopsy
d. All of the above

64. The presence of which protein in urine is suggestive of the diagnosis multiple myeloma?
a. Fibronectin
b. Elastin
c. Bence-Jones proteins
d. Collagen

65. The patient with leukemia is receiving busulfan (Myleran) and allopurinol (Zyloprim). The nurse tells the patient that the purpose of the allopurinol is to prevent:
a. Alopecia
b. Hyperuricemia
c. Vomiting
d. Nausea

66. A nurse is teaching a patient who suspects that she has a lump in her breast. The nurse instructs the patient that a diagnosis of breast cancer is confirmed by:
a. Breast self-examination
b. Mammography
c. Chest X-ray
d. Fine needle aspiration

67. Common cancer of oral cavity is:
a. Adenocarcinoma
b. Squamous cell carcinoma
c. Sarcoma
d. Melanoma

68. A 36-year-old man with lymphoma presents with signs of impending septic shock 9 days after chemotherapy. The nurse could expect which of the following to be present?
a. Flushing, decreased oxygen saturation, mild hypotension
b. Low grade fever, chills, tachycardia
c. Elevated temperature, oliguria, hypotension
d. High grade fever, normal blood pressure, increased respirations

69. In staging and grading neoplasm TNN system is used. TNM stands for?
a. Time, neoplasm, mode of growth
b. Tumor, node, metastasis
c. Tumor, neoplasm, mode of growth
d. Time, node, metastasis

70. A patient has undergone external radiation therapy. The expected side effects include the following apart from:
a. Hair loss
b. Ulceration of oral mucous membranes
c. Constipation
d. Headache

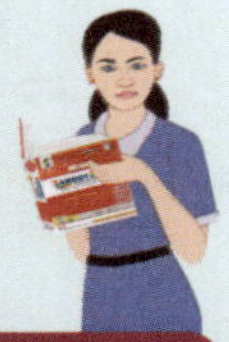

Ans.

46.	c
47.	b
48.	b
49.	d
50.	d
51.	d
52.	b
53.	a
54.	a
55.	c
56.	c
57.	b
58.	d
59.	c
60.	d
61.	c
62.	c
63.	d
64.	c
65.	b
66.	d
67.	b
68.	b
69.	b
70.	c

CNCI (NO) 2021

71. Skin reactions are common in radiation therapy. Nursing responsibilities on promoting skin integrity should be promoted apart from:
   a. Avoiding the use of ointments, powders and lotion to the area
   b. Using soft cotton fabrics for clothing
   c. Washing the area with a mild soap and water and patting it fry, not rubbing it
   d. Avoiding direct sunlight or cold

72. Radiation protection is very important to implement when performing nursing procedures. When the nurse is not performing any nursing procedures, what distance should be maintained from the patient?
   a. 1 feet
   b. 2 feet
   c. 2.5 feet
   d. 3 feet

73. A patient is taking cyclophosphamide for the treatment of the lymphoma. The nurse is very cautious while administering the medication because this drug poses the fatal side effect of:
   a. Alopecia
   b. Myeloma
   c. CNS toxicity
   d. Hemorrhagic cystitis

74. Specific classification of the chemotherapeutic agent, Vincristine is:
   a. Hormone modulator
   b. Mitotic inhibitor
   c. Antineoplastic antibiotic
   d. Antimetabolite

75. A 25-year-old patient is inquiring about the method or ways to detect cancer earlier. The nurse least likely identifies this method by stating:
   a. Annual chest X-ray
   b. Annual pap smear for sexually active women only
   c. Annual digital rectal examination for persons over age of 40
   d. Yearly physical and blood examination

76. All are recognized tumor markers; EXCEPT:
   a. Beta hCG
   b. Beta-2-microglobulin
   c. Alpha fetoprotein
   d. Acid phosphatase

77. Least amenable to screening is:
   a. Breast
   b. Cervix
   c. Oral cavity
   d. Lung

78. In which of the following head/neck cancers, is lymph node metastasis least common?
   a. Tongue
   b. Bucal Mucosa
   c. Hard Palate
   d. Lower alveolus

79. Secondaries of all the following cause osteolytic lesions; EXCEPT:
   a. Prostate
   b. Kidney
   c. Bronchus
   d. Thyroid

80. Treatment of bone metastasis is by:
   a. Samarium 153
   b. I-131 with tositumomab
   c. P-32
   d. Yttrium

81. Hypercalcemia associated with malignancy is most often mediated by:
   a. PTH b. PTH-rp
   c. IL-6 d. Calcitonin

82. A patient with leukemia on chemotherapy develops acute lower abdominal pain associated with anemia, thrombocytopenia and leucopenia. Which of the following is the clinical diagnosis?
   a. Appendicitis
   b. Leukemic colitis
   c. Perforation peritonitis
   d. Neutropenic Colitis

83. Drug used for estrogen dependent breast cancer is:
   a. Tamoxifen
   b. Clomiphene citrate
   c. Estrogen
   d. Adriamycin

84. All are removed in Radical mastectomy; EXCEPT:
   a. Pectoralis major
   b. Pectoralis minor
   c. Axillary lymph node
   d. Supraclavicular node

85. Estrogen receptor studies in carcinoma Breast is done on:
   a. Blood b. Urine
   c. Tumor tissue d. Ovary

86. Complications of total thyroidectomy include all; EXCEPT:
   a. Hoarseness
   b. Airway obstruction
   c. Hemorrhage
   d. Hypercalcemia

87. In the post-operative room after the thyroid surgery, patient developed breathlessness and the wound was seen bulging with blood stained. What would be the first thing to do?
   a. Tracheostomy
   b. Cricothyroidotomy
   c. Laryngoscopy and intubation
   d. Remove the stitch and take the patient to OT

88. After Cholecystectomy, there was 50 ml bile output from the drain on the first post-operative day management is:
   a. Intrabiliary stent
   b. Immediate exploration
   c. T-tube drainage
   d. Observation

89. Which maneuver is done to temporarily stop inadvertent bleeding during cholecystectomy?
   a. Patey
   b. Pringle
   c. Kocher
   d. Billroth

90. The following anastomosis are done in whipple procedure; EXCEPT:
   a. Hepatico-jejunostomy
   b. Pancreato gastrectomy
   c. Gastro jejunostomy
   d. Jejuno-jejunostomy

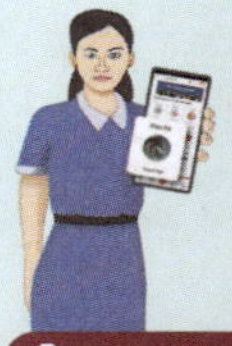

Ans.

71. c
72. d
73. d
74. b
75. b
76. d
77. d
78. c
79. a
80. a
81. b
82. d
83. a
84. d
85. c
86. d
87. d
88. d
89. b
90. d

91. The most likely cause of fluctuating jaundice in a middle aged/elderly man is:

a. Periampullary cancer b. Liver fluke infestation
c. Choledochal cyst d. Carcinoma head of pancreas

92. Most common cause of upper GI bleeding:

a. Gastric ulcer b. Esophageal varices
c. Gastritis d. Carcinoma stomach

93. A 60-year-old man suffering from left colon cancer presented with acute left colonic obstruction and the treatment is:

a. Primary resection and Hartman procedure
b. Defunctioning colostomy
c. Right hemicolectomy
d. Resection and end to end anastomosis

94. BCG is used in the treatment of:

a. Carcinoma cervix
b. Carcinoma colon
c. Carcinoma of urinary bladder
d. All of the above

95. Most radiation-sensitive testicular tumor is:

a. Seminoma b. Teratoma
c. Interstitial cell tumor d. None of the above

96. Most common site to put a chest drain in case of pleural effusion?

a. 2nd intercostal space mid-clavicular line
b. 7th intercostal space mid-clavicular line
c. 5th intercostal space in mid-axillary line
d. 5th intercostal space just lateral to vertebral column

97. Virus causing head and neck cancer:

a. EBV b. HSV
c. HPV d. HBV

98. All these are feeding tubes; EXCEPT:

a. Freca tube b. Ryles tube
c. PEG tube d. T Tube

99. All these are types of esophageal surgeries; EXCEPT:

a. Ivor Lewis b. McKeown
c. Transhiatal d. Cytoreductive

100. AFP is raised in ___________:

a. Ca prostate b. HCC
c. Ca lung d. Ca colon

Ans.

91. a
92. a
93. a
94. c
95. a
96. c
97. a
98. d
99. d
100. b

"After dinner rest a while; after supper walk a mile."

—T. Cogan

NORCET (NO) 2020

1. **A nurse was giving instruction to a postpartum mother of a newborn with hyperbilirubinemia. Which of the following is an appropriate instruction?**
   a. Withhold breastfeeding if phototherapy is continued
   b. Substitute breastfeeding with formula feeding
   c. Continuous breastfeeding every second hourly
   d. Routine supplementary feeds are recommended
2. **While performing an endotracheal tube (ET) suction, the nurse observed that the client is having sudden severe tachycardia. Which of the following should be the immediate response of the nurse?**
   a. Continue the suction
   b. Stop suction and perform re-oxygenation
   c. Hyperoxygenate before suctioning
   d. Call the physician
3. **A pregnant woman visiting antenatal clinic complains that she gets frequent leg cramps and pain during night. Which of the following is an appropriate intervention to be suggested for the client?**
   a. Dorsiflexion with knee extension exercise
   b. Complete bed rest is advised
   c. Use of compression stockings
   d. All of the above
4. **A 32-year-old male patient is admitted to an acute care psychiatric ward. The patient started showing aggressive tantrum. Which of the following actions by the nurse is a priority?**
   a. Wait until the patient calms down on his own
   b. Administer sedatives SOS
   c. Warn the patient not to do such aggressive act
   d. Call for help to settle down situation
5. **Which of the following drug causes red color urine?**
   a. Streptomycin b. Rifampicin
   c. Ethambutol d. Isoniazid
6. **A 65-year-old patient admitted in a long-term care facility has developed pressure ulcer. On assessment, the nurse found that the bone is visible and palpable on the wound site. The nurse knows that the stage of the pressure ulcer is:**
   a. Stage-I b. Stage-II
   c. Stage-III d. Stage-IV
7. **The bullet train project in India is launched with the support of which of the following country?**
   a. Russia b. Germany
   c. Japan d. Korea
8. **During post-operative care of an infant with a cleft palate repair, the nurse should position the baby in which of the following positions?**
   a. On side lying position b. In an infant seat
   c. Prone d. Supine
9. **What is the color coding of the bag used in hospitals to dispose of human anatomical wastes such as body parts?**
   a. Red b. Black
   c. Yellow d. Blue
10. **The vaccine that forms blister and leaves permanent scar in babies is:**
    a. DPT b. BCG
    c. Measles d. Pentavalent
11. **Identify the device/instrument shown in the photograph:**

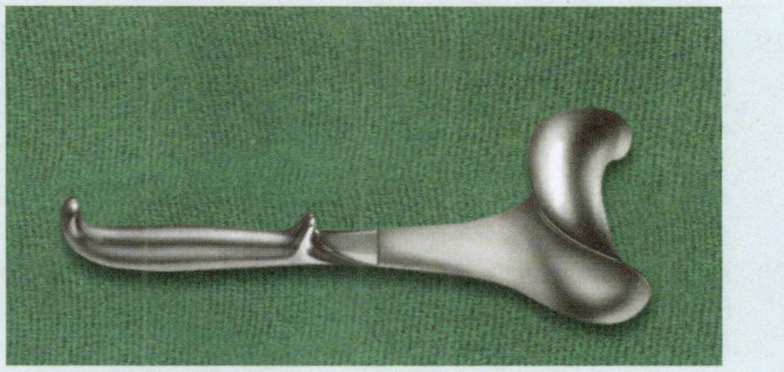

    a. Doyen's retractor
    b. Deaver retractor
    c. Anterior vaginal wall retractor
    d. HSG canula
12. **The pelvic shape that has the poorest prognosis from vaginal delivery is:**
    a. Platypelloid b. Anthropoid
    c. Android d. Gynecoid
13. **Which of the following colored IV cannula is used for Infant?**
    a. Grey b. Pink
    c. Yellow d. Green
14. **Amputation that includes all levels of thigh amputations from the hip to the knee joint is known as:**
    a. Transfemoral amputations
    b. Transtibial amputations
    c. Lower limb amputation
    d. Hip disarticulation amputation
15. **Therapeutic use of paracetamol is:**
    a. Prevent nausea and vomiting
    b. Pain relief
    c. Motion sickness
    d. All of the above
16. **Surgical complications that result from foreign materials such as surgical sponge or gauze piece accidentally left inside patient's body is known as:**
    a. Surgical hemostatic syndrome
    b. Gossypiboma
    c. Idiopathic necrosis
    d. Gossypium hirsutum

Ans.

1. c
2. b
3. a
4. d
5. b
6. d
7. c
8. c
9. c
10. b
11. a
12. c
13. c
14. a
15. b
16. b

Disclaimer: *The questions are prepared by memory-based recall from candidates who attended the examination.*

17. Which of the following position is advised to relieve cord compression during labor?
a. Supine b. Right lateral
c. Trendelenburg d. Lithotomy

18. What is the cerebral tissue perfusion pressure if Blood Pressure is 90/60 and ICP is 18?
a. 42 mm Hg b. 52 mm Hg
c. 60 mm Hg d. 72 mm Hg

Explanation:
CPP = MAP – ICP
MAP = [SBP + 2(DBP)]/3
MAP = [90 + 2(60)/3
= 210/3
MAP = 70 mm Hg

CPP = MAP – ICP
= 70 – 18
= 52 mm Hg

19. All of the following signs and symptoms are indicative of increased intracranial pressure in children; EXCEPT:
a. Nausea
b. Vomiting
c. Extreme irritability
d. Decreased Pulse pressure

20. In solar system, which of the following is the third planet from the sun?
a. Venus b. Earth
c. Saturn d. Mercury

21. What is the suction pressure applied while performing endotracheal tube suction in an adult patient?
a. 40-60 mm Hg
b. 50-75 mm Hg
c. 60-100 mm Hg
d. 100-120 mm Hg

22. What is the national currency of the United Kingdom?
a. Yen b. Euro
c. Pound d. Dollar

23. Which country supplied Rafale jets to India?
a. Germany b. USA
c. France d. Italy

24. Used nasogastric tube has to be discarded in:
a. Yellow bag b. Red bag
c. Blue bag d. Black bag

25. Drug allergy is usually tested with an intradermal injection of small dose of a drug. Which of the following is the reason for using intradermal route for testing drug allergy?
a. Slow absorption of drug
b. Easy to administer the drug
c. Less painful
d. All of the above

26. Which of the following vaccine should not be frozen and should be discarded if frozen?
a. OPV b. Measles
c. DPT d. MMR

27. Which of the following antibiotic does not require test dose before administration?
a. Augmentin b. Penicillin
c. Ciprofloxacin d. Sulbactum

28. Identify the instrument given in the image:

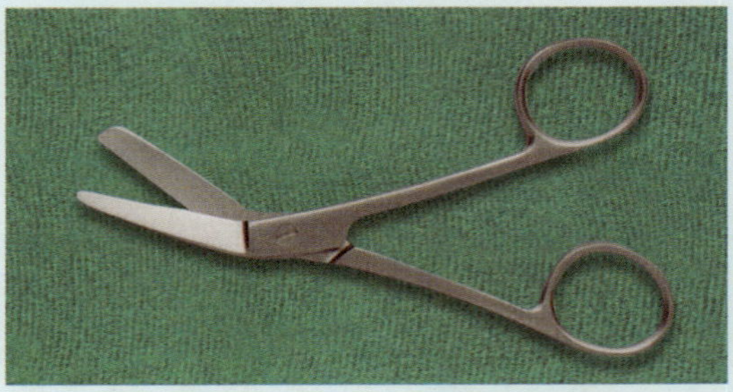

a. Surgical scissor b. Episiotomy scissor
c. Cord cutting scissor d. Mayo scissor

29. Murphy's sign is seen in which of the following disease condition?
a. Liver abscess b. Splenomegaly
c. Peritonitis d. Acute cholecystitis

30. Patients scheduled for surgery are instructed to remove nail polish. What is the reason for removing nail polish before surgery?
a. To observe clubbing of fingers
b. To detect cyanosis caused by low oxygen level
c. Both a and b
d. None of the above

31. Which of the following gas is most pungent smelling?
a. Sevoflurane b. Isoflurane
c. Both are equally pungent d. Benzene

32. A 7-year-old child is intermittently bedwetting at least 2 times a week. The nurse anticipates which of the following drug to be prescribed by the physician?
a. Desmopressin b. Diazepam
c. Methylphenidate d. Fluoxetine

33. Identify the equipment given in the image:

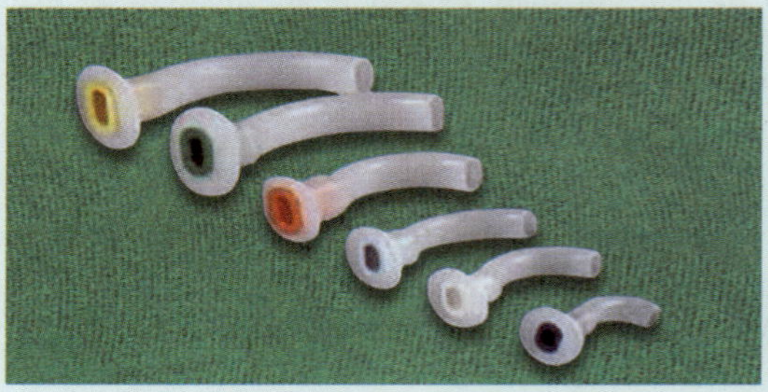

a. Nasopharyngeal airway b. Guedel airway
c. Tracheostomy tube d. Tongue depressor

34. Identify the image given below:

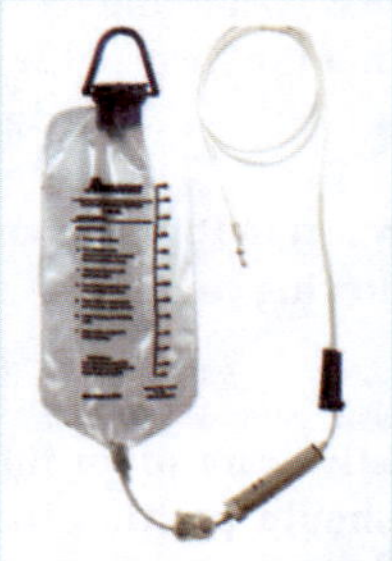

a. IV fluid bag
b. Enteral feeding bag
c. Peritoneal dialysis bag
d. Enema bag

Ans.

17.	c
18.	b
19.	d
20.	b
21.	d
22.	c
23.	c
24.	b
25.	a
26.	c
27.	c
28.	b
29.	d
30.	b
31.	b
32.	a
33.	b
34.	b

35. Catgut is banned in Europe and Japan. The reason for the ban is due to concern over the risk of developing:
a. Cancer due to carcinogenic ingredients
b. Bovine Spongiform Encephalopathy (BSE)
c. Necrotic lesions
d. None of the above

36. As per The Mental Healthcare Act 2017, which of the following statement is NOT TRUE regarding ECT therapy?
a. ECT should not be used without muscle relaxant
b. ECT should not be used without anesthesia
c. ECT therapy will not be performed for minors
d. Direct ECT can be given with the consent of the patient

37. The leading anatomical part of the fetus closest to the pelvic inlet of the birth canal refers to:
a. Presentation b. Lie
c. Denominator d. Position

38. The diameter that is being assessed in the given image is:

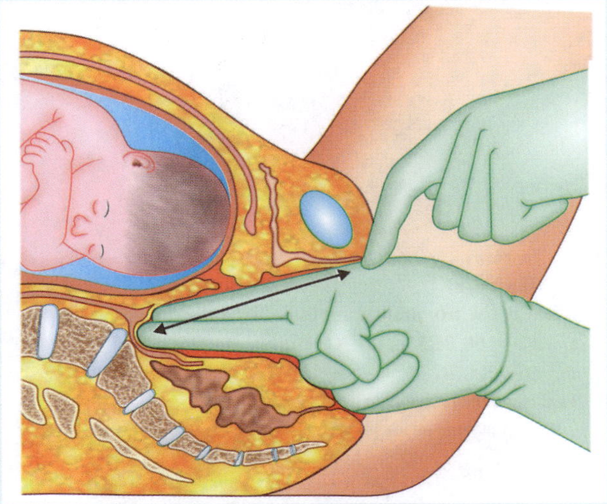

a. Obstetrical conjugate
b. Anatomical conjugate
c. True conjugate
d. Diagonal conjugate

39. The southernmost state of India is:
a. Kerala b. Tamil Nadu
c. Andhra Pradesh d. Karnataka

40. A nurse caring for a HIV positive patient got an accidental needle stick injury. Which of the following is an appropriate immediate action following needle stick injury?
a. Squeeze the wound to bleed it
b. Wash the wound and surrounding skin with soap and rinse
c. Use bleach or alcohol to clean the wound
d. Put the pricked finger in mouth

41. Which of the following color bag is used to discard resection of gangrene part of the patient?
a. Red b. Blue
c. Yellow d. Black

42. Ergometrine is commonly used in the treatment of which of the following condition:
a. PPH
b. APH
c. Cervical incompetence
d. AV Fistula

43. Jackson Pratt drain was used in all of the following surgeries, EXCEPT:
a. Thoracic surgery
b. Head and neck surgery
c. Abdominal surgery
d. Breast reduction and breast reconstruction surgery

44. Oral white patches which are commonly seen in infants and bleed on touching are:
a. Pancytopenia b. Leukoplakia
c. Leucopenia d. Myeloma

45. Which of the following is a function of fallopian tube?
a. Implantation b. Fertilization
c. Sperm production d. Ovum production

46. How to measure the uterine contraction of the pregnant lady who is on labor pain?
a. Asking question to the lady
b. By using pantograph
c. Assess by placing the hand on abdomen
d. Assess by performing Leopold's maneuver

47. What is the normal CVP pressure?
a. 1-2 mm hg b. 2-6 mm hg
c. 3-8 mm hg d. 5-8 mm hg

48. Premature destruction of RBC's were seen in which of the following conditions?
a. Sickle cell anemia
b. G6PD Deficiency
c. Systemic lupus erythematosus
d. Guillain-Barre Syndrome

49. Identify the size of scalpel blade in the following image:

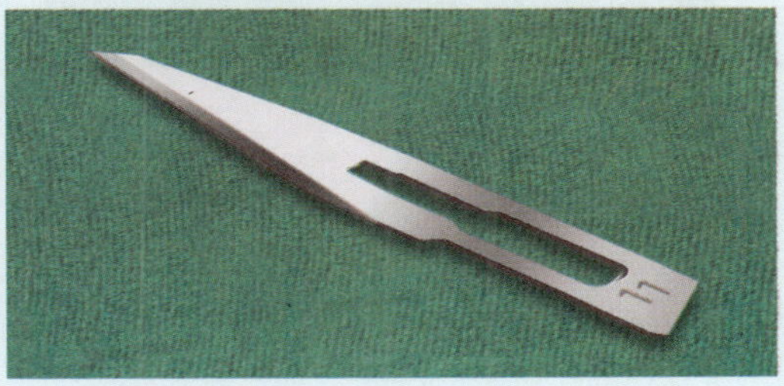

a. 10 b. 11
c. 12 d. 13

50. Identify the X-ray image:

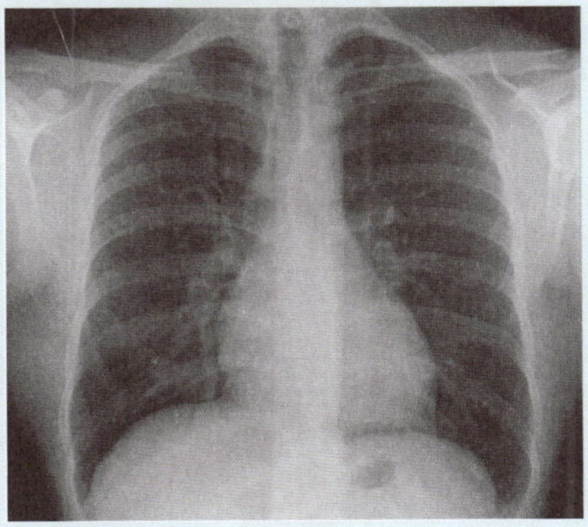

a. Pneumothorax
b. Tetrology of fallot
c. Flail chest
d. Hiatal hernia

Ans.

35.	b
36.	d
37.	a
38.	d
39.	b
40.	b
41.	c
42.	a
43.	b
44.	b
45.	b
46.	c
47.	b
48.	b
49.	b
50.	a

51. Identify the given condition in the image:

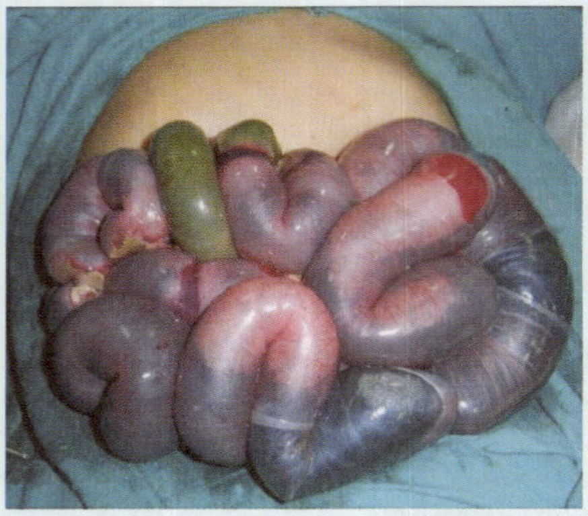

a. Omphalocele
b. Gangrenous colon
c. Crohn's disease
d. Abdominal hernia

52. Identify the instrument:

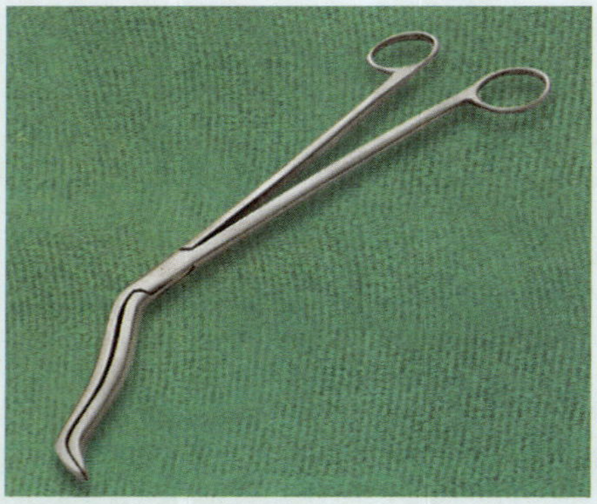

a. Kelly Hemostatic Forceps
b. Cheatle forceps
c. Sponge holder forceps
d. Magill forceps

53. A female in labor room with cord prolapse should be given which of the following position?

a. Semi-Fowler's
b. Prone position
c. Lithotomy position
d. Knee chest position

54. Identify the position of fetus shown in the given image:

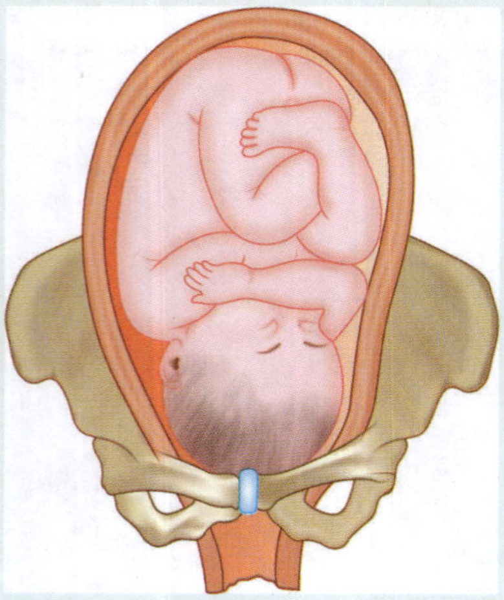

a. Left occiput anterior
b. Left occiput posterior
c. Right occiput anterior
d. Right occiput posterior

55. What is the size of IV cannula shown in the image?

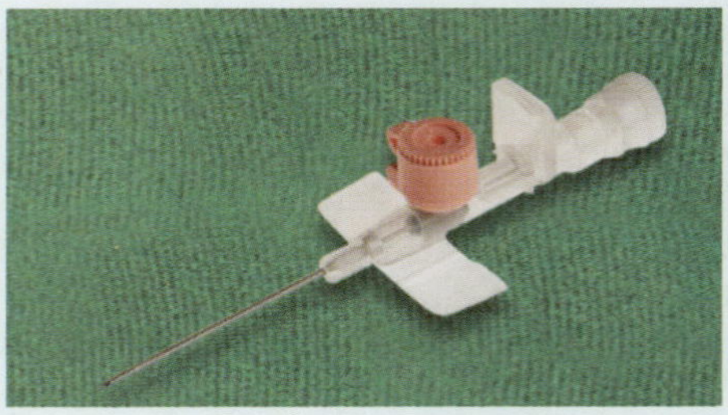

a. 18G
b. 20G
c. 22G
d. 24G

56. Identify the pulse site in the image:

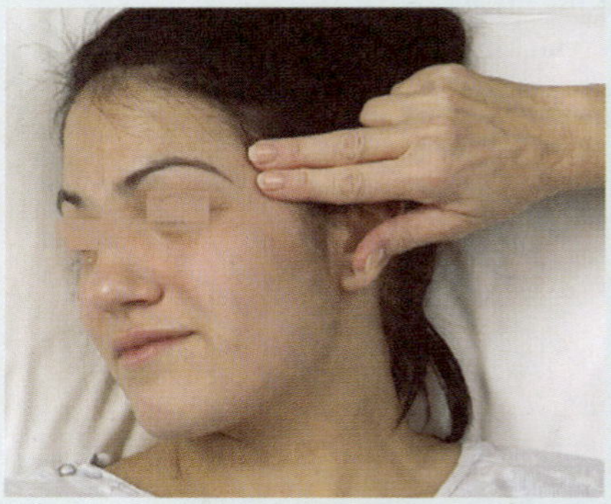

a. Carotid
b. Occipital
c. Temporal
d. Popliteal

57. What is the normal neonatal heart rate?

a. 120-160 BPM
b. 100-120 BPM
c. 160-200 BPM
d. 80-100 BPM

58. The needle in the image is used for:

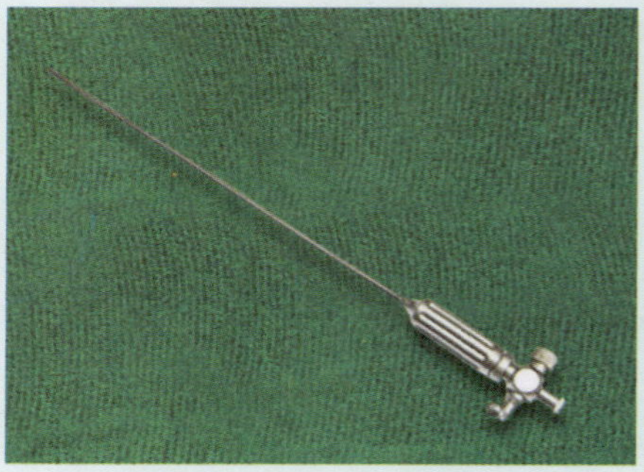

a. Bone marrow biopsy
b. Laparoscopic procedure
c. Lumbar puncture
d. Blood sampling

59. Dichotic notch of the arterial wave form indicates:

a. Increased resistance to blood flow
b. Sudden fall in blood pressure
c. Opening of aortic valve
d. Closure of aortic valve

60. While giving CPR what is the correct position of hand?

a. Above the chest
b. Above the nipples
c. Just below the nipple
d. Lower half of the sternum

61. Which of the following is the first discovered vaccine?

a. Chicken Pox
b. Rabies
c. Small pox
d. H1NI Flue

Ans.

51. b
52. b
53. d
54. d
55. b
56. c
57. a
58. b
59. d
60. d
61. c

62. Which of the following vitamin deficiency will cause pernicious anemia?

a. Vitamin B12 b. Folic acid deficiency
c. Serum Iron deficiency d. Calcium deficiency

63. Who is the director of AIIMS, New Delhi ? ***(As on September 2020)***

a. Dr. Gitanjali Batmanaben
b. Dr. Vikas Bhatia
c. Dr. Ravi Kant
d. Dr. Randeep Guleria

64. Who is at present the CEO of Google? *(As on September 2020)*

a. Mark Zuckerberg b. Sunder pichai
c. Satya Nadella d. Timothy Donald Cook

65. What is the name of space agency of India?

a. NASA b. ISRO
c. WIPRO d. CBI

66. Who is the president of Turkey at present?

a. Recep Tayyip Erdogan
b. Vladimir Putin
c. Yoshihide Suga
d. Justin Trudeau

67. The machine shown in the image is used for:

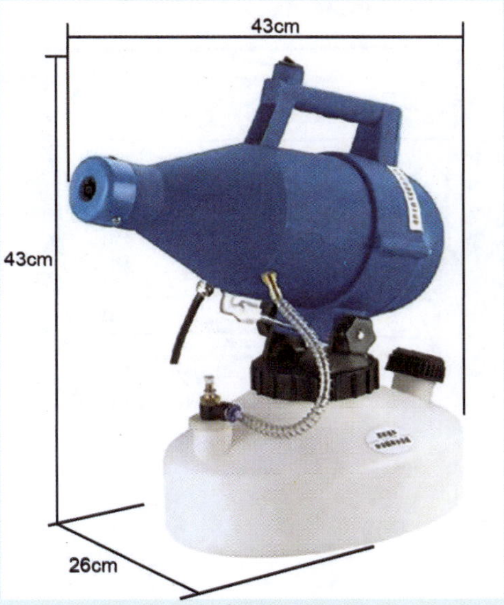

a. Hot wave autoclave b. Sonicator
c. Fumigation d. HEPA filter

68. Corona virus has spread worldwide. This is known as:

a. Epidemic b. Pandemic
c. Zoonotic d. Endemic

69. Corona virus outbreak was first seen in:

a. Wuhan city in china b. India
c. UK d. Turkey

70. A patient is taking furosemide as a diuretic. Which of the following is to be included in the diet of the patient?

a. Nuts b. Vegetable soups
c. Raw vegetables d. Banana

71. Silent MI is commonly seen in:

a. CKD b. HTN
c. Diabetes mellitus d. COPD

72. Who was the founder of Red Cross Society?

a. Louis Appia b. Gustave Moynier
c. Théodore Maunoir d. Henry Dunant

73. Which of the following is incorrect about bedsore?

a. Mobilization will affect bedsore
b. Moisture will affect bedsore
c. Friction force will affect bedsore
d. Nutritional status does not affect bedsore

74. Which of the following drug is contraindicated in pregnant lady?

a. Heparin
b. Labetalol
c. Dolutegravir
d. Streptomycin

75. Lorazepam challenging test is done to validate the diagnosis of:

a. Catatonia b. Stupor
c. Dementia d. Depression

76. Identify the image:

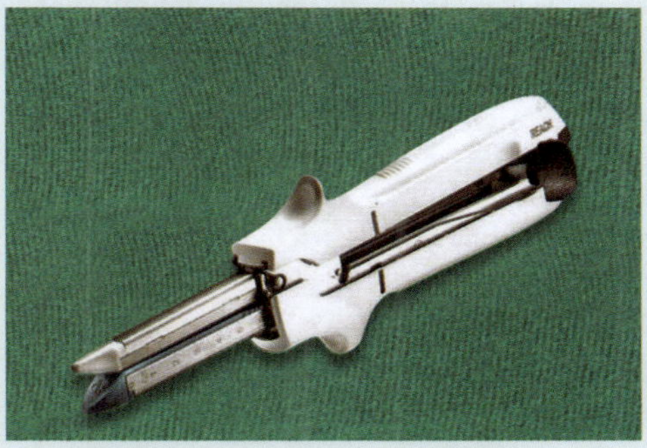

a. Linear stapler b. Punch biopsy
c. Bone marrow needle d. Trochar

77. Identify the image:

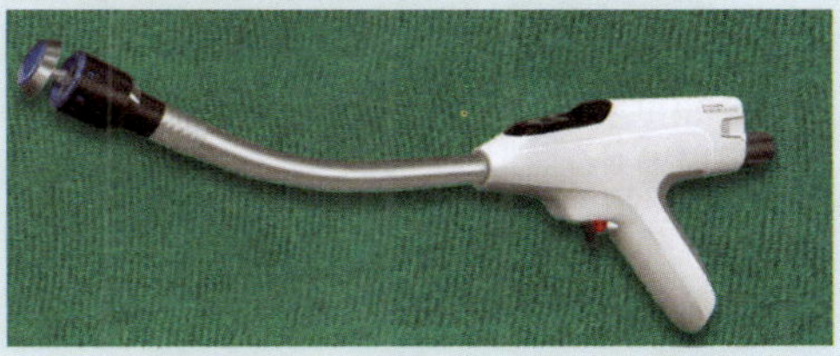

a. Circular stapler b. Vein viewer
c. Biopsy gun d. Trochar

78. Diagnostic test used for DIC:

a. PT b. INR
c. PT, aPTT d. DCT, ICT

79. Antimicrobial dressing is composed of which of the following metal?

a. Copper b. Zinc
c. Sodium d. Silver

80. Which among the following is added with ORS to control diarrhea?

a. Copper
b. Calcium
c. Zinc
d. Potassium

81. After 2 hours of birth, baby has acrocyanosis. What should the nurse do?

a. Inform the physician
b. Intubate the infant
c. Document the finding
d. Give oxygen

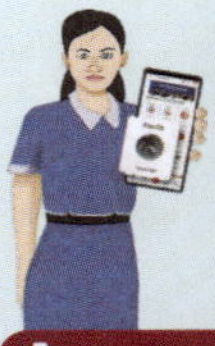

Ans.

62.	a
63.	d
64.	b
65.	b
66.	a
67.	c
68.	b
69.	a
70.	d
71.	c
72.	d
73.	d
74.	d
75.	a
76.	a
77.	a
78.	c
79.	d
80.	c
81.	c

82. Identify the image given below:

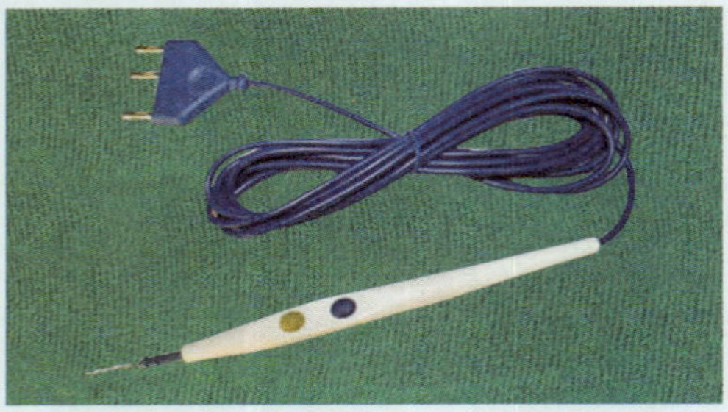

a. Monopolar cautery b. Bipolar cautery
c. Harmonic scalpel d. Surgical scalpel

83. Which hormone regulates calcium and phosphate?

a. Parathyroid Hormone b. TSH
c. FSH d. LH

84. At which week mother feels movement of the baby:

a. 10-12 Weeks b. 12-14 Weeks
c. 14-16 Weeks d. 18-20 Weeks

85. Which electrolyte causes atrial depolarization?

a. Sodium b. Potassium
c. Calcium d. Phosphate

86. Identify the pelvic grip shown in the image:

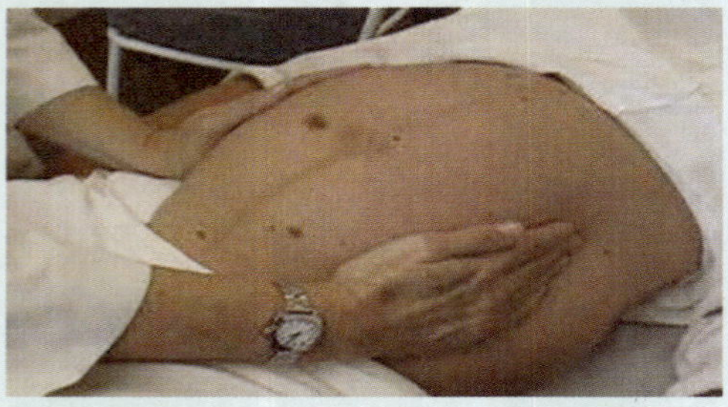

a. Fundal grip b. Lateral grip
c. Pawlik grip d. Deep pelvic grip

87. Blue color pipelines in OT is used to deliver:

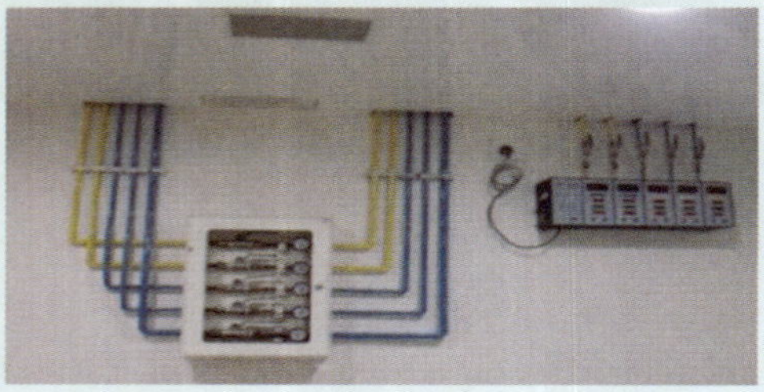

a. Oxygen b. Medical air
c. Vacuum d. Nitrous oxide

88. Lignocaine is used to treat:

a. MI b. Angina
c. CAD d. Arrhythmia

89. Bandaging of lower legs should be started from:

a. Ankle b. Foot
c. Knees d. Fingers

90. Pain in the Mc Burneys point is a characteristic of:

a. Cholelithiasis b. Appendicitis
c. Urolithiasis d. Nephrolithiasis

91. Surgical glove will be discarded in which color biomedical bag:

a. Yellow b. Block
c. Green d. Red

92. Distended jugular vein is seen in:

a. Decreased CVP
b. Increased CVP
c. Increased BP
d. Decreased BP

93. The assessment of acute malnutrition in children is done by:

a. Height
b. Weight
c. BMI
d. Weight for Height

94. Diminished lung sounds and pain during inspiration is a classical sign of:

a. Hemothorax
b. Pneumothorax
c. Pyothorax
d. Chylothorax

95. Find the next number in the series 10, 9, 7, 4:

a. 3 b. 2
c. 1 d. 0

96. Which IV fluid you will give with packed RBC?

a. 3% NaCl b. 5% Dextrose
c. RL d. Normal Saline

97. Identify the following image:

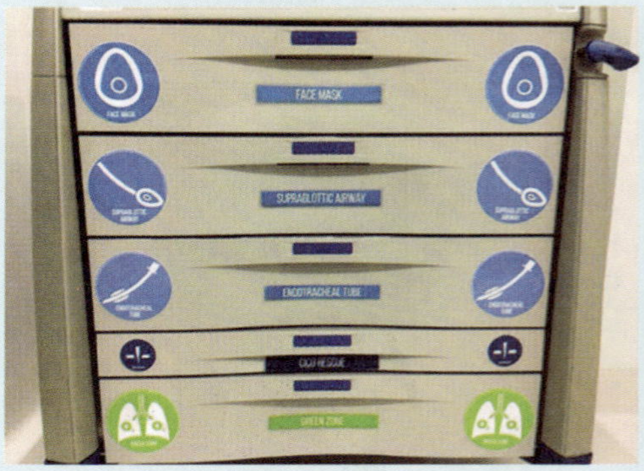

a. Anesthesia trolley
b. Airway cart
c. Defibrillator
d. Bronchoscopy trolley

98. Clonidine is used to:

a. Increase Low BP
b. Decrease High BP
c. Increase Pulse rate
d. Decrease Pulse rate

99. The ET Tube size 5.5 is used for:

a. Infants b. Adults
c. Children d. Geriatric

100. Which of the following vitamin deficiency leads to bleeding gums?

a. Vitamin C b. Vitamin A
c. Vitamin B d. Vitamin K

101. Which among the following is an output device?

a. Printer b. Joystick
c. Camera d. Keyboard

102. PDS suture is an example of:

a. Natural absorbable suture
b. Synthetic absorbable suture
c. Synthetic Non absorbable suture
d. Natural Non absorbable suture

Ans.

82. a
83. a
84. c
85. a
86. b
87. d
88. d
89. b
90. b
91. d
92. b
93. d
94. b
95. d
96. d
97. b
98. b
99. c
100. a
101. a
102. b

103. After death of a person, how long cornea can be preserved?
a. 2 Hours b. 6 Hours
c. 8 Hours d. 12 Hours

104. Which snake venom causes rapid DIC?
a. Cobra b. Krait
c. Viper d. Bandy-Bandy

105. The primary action of injection paracetamol is:
a. Antiemetic
b. Anti-motility
c. Anti-inflammatory
d. Antipyretic

106. Identify the position shown in the image:

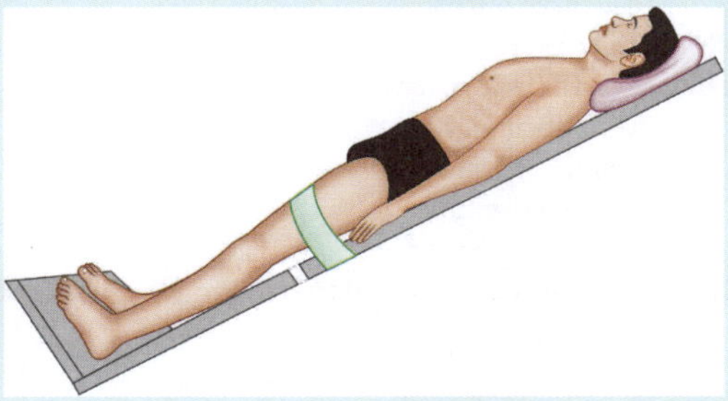

a. Trendelenburg b. Reverse Trendelenburg
c. Lithotomy d. Sims position

107. Nicotine replacement therapy is used for:
a. Smoking cessation
b. Alcohol withdrawal
c. Opioid withdrawal
d. Pontine hemorrhage

108. Difference between smallest and largest value is known as:
a. Mean b. Average
c. Range d. Standard deviation

109. Which electrolyte is closely monitored in digoxin administration?
a. Sodium b. Calcium
c. Potassium d. Phosphate

110. Identify the placental removal technique shown in the image:

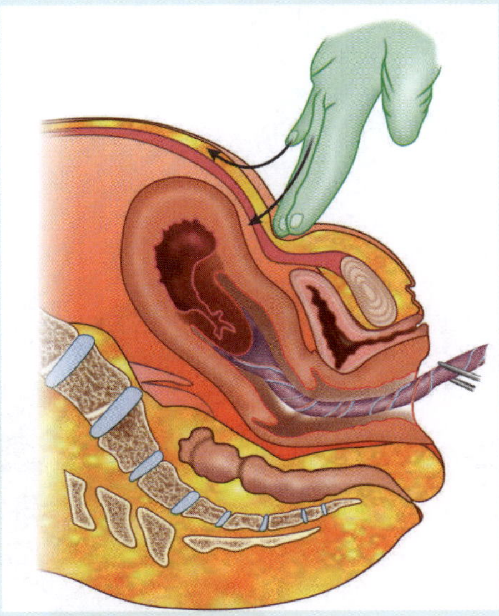

a. Manual removal
b. Cord traction by doctor
c. Expulsion of placenta by fundal pressure
d. Cesarean session

111. Which of the following is not used before ECT Procedure?
a. Have light meal before the procedure
b. Premedication with anticholinergics
c. NPO
d. Wash the oils from hair

112. Identify the investigation image shown below:

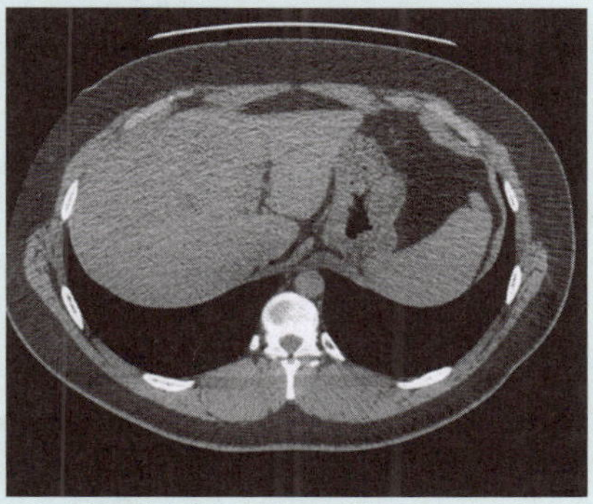

a. CT brain
b. MRI brain
c. CT KUB
d. MRI KUB

113. What is meant by posthumous child?
a. Abused child
b. Child who lost the parents after birth
c. Childbirth after death of the biological parent
d. Child who doesn't have mother

114. Use of vaporizers in OT is to:
a. Maintain required humidity in OT
b. Make sure required number of air exchange occurred in OT
c. Deliver given concentration of volatile anesthetic agent
d. Disinfect environmental air in OT

115. Which of the following antipsychotic drug causes hyperprolactinemia?
a. Clozapine b. Risperidone
c. Quetiapine d. Olanzapine

116. Clinically used form of lithium is
a. Lithium Oxalate b. Lithium Disodium
c. Lithium Carbonate d. Lithium Permanganate

117. Which blood group is known as universal recipient?
a. O Negative b. O Positive
c. AB Positive d. AB Negative

118. Identify the following image:

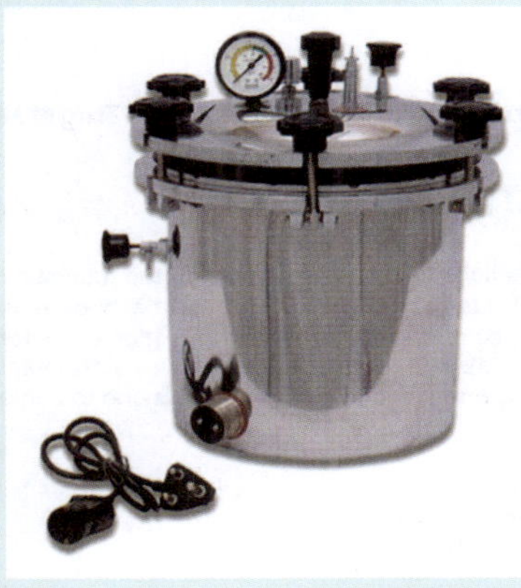

a. Boiler b. Autoclave
c. Fumigator d. Vaccine container

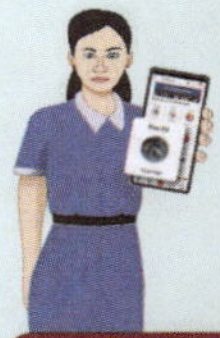

Ans.

103.	b
104.	c
105.	d
106.	b
107.	a
108.	c
109.	c
110.	c
111.	a
112.	c
113.	c
114.	c
115.	b
116.	c
117.	c
118.	b

119. Heimlich maneuver is used to treat:
- a. Lower airway obstruction
- b. Nasal obstruction
- c. Tracheal obstruction
- d. Upper airway obstruction

120. Extra calories needed during second trimester of pregnancy is:
- a. 300 Kcal/day
- b. 500 Kcal/day
- c. 600 Kcal/day
- d. 700 Kcal/day

121. Which is not an adverse effect of clozapine?
- a. Weight gain
- b. Hypersalivation
- c. Hepatotoxicity
- d. Tachycardia

122. Use of epinephrine will cause which of the following symptoms?
- a. Bradycardia
- b. Tachycardia
- c. Increased BP
- d. Tachypnea

123. In which of the following vaccine, cold chain must be maintained?
- a. Killed vaccine
- b. Live vaccine
- c. Toxoids
- d. Serums

124. Which of the following is not transmitted by needle stick injury?
- a. HIV
- b. Hepatitis B
- c. Scrub Typhus
- d. Hepatitis C

125. Cyanotic spell is seen in:
- a. Atrial septal defect
- b. Ventricular septal defect
- c. Tetralogy of Fallot
- d. Trans position of arteries

126. Side effect of clozapine includes:
- a. Agranulocytosis
- b. Nausea
- c. Vomiting
- d. Diarrhea

127. Which of the following is primary prevention in skin cancer?
- a. Applying sunscreen creams and lotions while going out
- b. Professional skin examination and self-skin examination
- c. Early diagnosis and initiation of treatment for skin cancer
- d. Health education regarding treatment compliance of chemotherapy

128. Most painful type of burns is:
- a. First-degree burns
- b. Second-degree burns
- c. Third-degree burns
- d. Fourth-degree burns

129. Scrubbing will be considered as:
- a. Chemical disinfection
- b. Physical disinfection
- c. Physical sterilization
- d. Chemical sterilization

130. Which states border is not connected to Madhya Pradesh?
- a. Maharashtra
- b. Gujarat
- c. Rajasthan
- d. Odisha

131. Which of the following is not a social media platform?
- a. Twitter
- b. Instagram
- c. Facebook
- d. Windows

132. Atrio-Venous fistula is assessed for:
- a. Giving IV medication
- b. Blood sampling
- c. Arterial BP
- d. Patency

133. PAP Smear test is used in the diagnosis of:
- a. Uterine Cancer
- b. Cervical Cancer
- c. Valval Cancer
- d. Ovarian Cancer

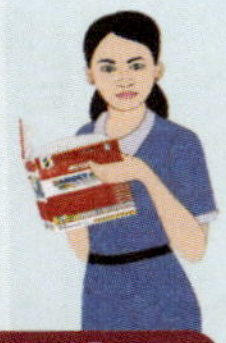

Ans.

119. d
120. a
121. c
122. b
123. b
124. c
125. c
126. a
127. a
128. b
129. b
130. d
131. d
132. d
133. b

"It is health that is real wealth and not pieces of gold and silver."

—Mahatma Gandhi

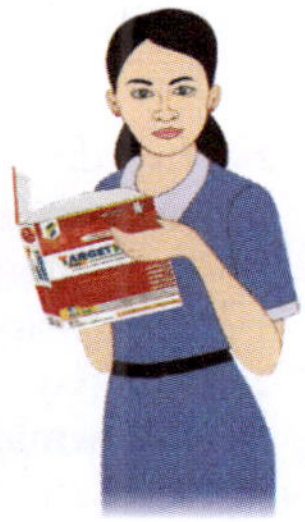

Combined AIIMS (NO) (Bhopal, Jodhpur, Patna & Raipur) 2020

1. The position used for most of the gynecological procedures, is:

a. Lithotomy position b. Supine position
c. Prone position d. Sims' position

2. Thyroid eye disease (TED) is also known as:

a. Graves Orbitopathy
b. Hashimoto's Disease
c. Goiter
d. Thyroid nodules

3. How many items are included in the WHO surgical safety checklist: SITOSO?

a. 18 items b. 19 items
c. 20 items d. 30 items

4. Which of the following code is associated with cardiac arrest during medical emergency?

a. Code Blue b. Code Black
c. Code Green d. Code Red

5. In iron deficiency anemia, the fingernails become spoon shaped, this condition is referred to as:

a. Koilonychia b. Paronychia
c. Bleb d. Felon

6. How is blood loss measured in Post-partum hemorrhage?

a. By estimating blood loss in number of pads and by weighing the sponges absorbed with blood.
b. By monitoring pulse rate and blood pressure.
c. By monitoring hematocrit count.
d. All of the above

7. SCD (Sequential Compressive Device) used for treatment of DVT patients, ensures:

a. Formation of thrombus within the deep veins
b. Walking and preventing blood clots
c. Prevents patients from hypothermia
d. None of the above

8. The traction used for cervical spine injury:

a. Halo traction b. Skin traction
c. Skeletal traction d. All of these

9. In operation theater during cauterization, the electric current passing from a single electrode is called:

a. Bovie cautery b. Mono polar cautery
c. Bipolar cautery d. Both (a) and (b)

10. Tracheostomy is done in which tracheal ring?

a. Between 1st and 2nd tracheal ring
b. Between 2nd and 3rd tracheal ring
c. Between 3rd and 4th tracheal ring
d. None of the above

11. The instrument used for measuring fetal heart rate (FHR):

a. Pinard Stethoscope
b. Proctoscope
c. Endoscope
d. Both (a) and (b)

12. The type of cyanosis seen in PDA is:

a. Differential cyanosis b. Central cyanosis
c. Peripheral cyanosis d. All of these

13. Fetal monitoring machine is used to:

a. Record heartbeat of fetus
b. Record respiratory rate of fetus
c. Record contractions of mother's uterus.
d. Both (a) and (c)

14. The device used to maintain the patency of the oral airways:

a. Guedel Airway b. Nasopharyngeal Airway
c. Endotracheal Intubation d. All of these

15. Measurement of arterial blood gas shows pH: 7.2, $PaCO_2$: 70 mm Hg, HCO_3 : 27 mmol/L and PaO_2 : 59 mm Hg. Interpret this:

a. Respiratory acidosis b. Respiratory alkalosis
c. Metabolic acidosis d. Metabolic alkalosis

16. What is the antidote of narcotics?

a. Naloxone b. Flumazenil
c. Digibind d. Atropine sulfate

17. With which of the following, the "Indradhanush scheme" is associated with:

a. Immunization
b. Sanitation
c. Mid-day meal programme
d. All of the above

18. Antidote for heparin is:

a. Naloxone b. Flumazenil
c. Digibind d. Protamine sulfate

19. The infant's weight becomes triple from birth weight in:

a. 1 year b. 2 years
c. 3 years d. None of these

20. Lumbar puncture is done at:

a. Between the lumbar vertebrae L-3/ L-4
b. Between the lumbar vertebrae L-4/ L-5
c. Between the lumbar vertebrae L-5/ S-1
d. All the above

21. Ishihara chart is used for the assessment of:

a. Night blindness b. Color vision
c. Both (a) and (b) d. None of these

22. In second degree bedsore, there is an involvement of:

a. Epidermis and dermis
b. Dermis and subcutaneous tissues
c. Subcutaneous tissues and muscles
d. All of the above

23. Which of the following is the cardinal sign of pyloric stenosis?

a. Projectile Vomiting
b. Fever
c. Diarrhea
d. Constipation

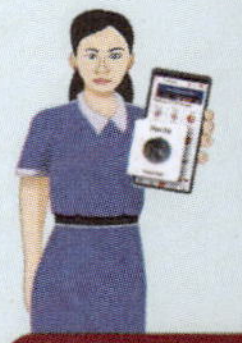

Ans.

1. a
2. a
3. b
4. a
5. a
6. d
7. b
8. a
9. b
10. b
11. a
12. a
13. d
14. a
15. a
16. a
17. a
18. d
19. a
20. d
21. b
22. a
23. a

Abbreviation: NO, Nursing Officer

***Disclaimer:** The questions are prepared by memory-based recall from candidates who attended the examination.*

24. In the following, all are the contraindications for measurement of rectal temperature; EXCEPT:
a. Colon surgery b. Hemorrhoid and piles
c. Diarrhea d. Constipation

25. The core temperature is measured from which of the following sites?
a. Rectum b. Tympanic membrane
c. Axilla d. Both (a) and (b)

26. The antidote used for heroin poisoning is:
a. Naloxone b. Flumazenil
c. Digibind d. Protamine sulfate

27. For which of the following there is no vaccine available?
a. Hib b. HIV
c. Polio d. None of these

28. According to hospital's protocol during emergency situation "code pink" is used for which condition?
a. Infant and child abduction
b. Disastrous situation
c. Bomb threat nearby
d. Fire in hospital

29. What is the early sign of increased ICP (Intracranial pressure)?
a. Altered level of consciousness
b. Decreased level of consciousness
c. Bradycardia
d. All of the above

30. What is the purpose of using succinylcholine during the Electroconvulsive therapy?
a. Reduction in oral secretions
b. Muscle relaxant
c. Muscle contraction
d. Both (b) and (c)

31. Which gauze cannula is commonly used for blood transfusion?
a. 16 G - Gray color b. 18 G - Green color
c. 22 G - Blue color d. 23 G - Orange color

32. Which drug should be used for rinsing the syringe before taking blood sample for ABG analysis?
a. Heparin b. Dobutamine
c. Dopamine d. Adrenaline

33. Which is the appropriate nursing action by nursing officer after taking ABG sample from radial artery?
a. Put pressure on the site for 5 minutes with sterile pad
b. Clean with alcohol swabs
c. Cover site with cloth-piece
d. None of the above

34. Chhaya oral contraceptive pills (OCP) is:
a. Non-hormonal and non-steroidal
b. Hormonal and steroidal
c. Non-hormonal and steroidal
d. None of the above

35. A 27-year-old female, 16-week pregnant, has 2-year-old twins, who were born at 39 weeks gestation and a 5-year-old who was born at 40 weeks, she had no history of abortion what is her GTPAL score?
a. G=3, T=2, P=0, A=0, L=3
b. G=3, T=1, P=0, A=2, L=3
c. G=3, T=2, P=2, A=0, L=3
d. G=3, T=1, P=0, A=0, L=2

36. How many faces are there in Wong-Baker facial pain rating scale?
a. 8 faces b. 6 faces
c. 10 faces d. 5 faces

37. Which of the following is the warning sign post renal transplantation?
a. Decreased urine output b. Increased urine output
c. Pale color urine d. Both (a) and (b)

38. All of the following are antiplatelet medications; EXCEPT:
a. Aspirin b. Clopidogrel
c. Cangrelor d. Canglob

39. Another name for Cidex solution is:
a. Glutaraldehyde b. Formaldehyde
c. Carbaldehyde d. Carboxaldehyde

40. At how much interval BP measurement for a mother should be done during second stage of labor?
a. 15–20 minutes b. 30 –40 minutes
c. 50–60 minutes d. 60–90 minutes

41. Which solution is used for management of blood spillage?
a. Sodium hypochlorite 0.5%
b. Sodium bicarbonate 0.5%
c. Potassium hypochlorite 0.5%
d. Potassium chloride 0.5%

42. As per BMW management and according to WHO, infected cotton sponge is discarded into which color-coded bag?
a. Yellow Bag b. Red Bag
c. Black Bag d. Blue Bag

43. As per BMW management and according to WHO, infected syringe without needle is discarded into which color-coded bag?
a. Yellow bag b. Red bag
c. Black bag d. Blue bag

44. A patient's blood pressure suddenly drops, what is expected from on-duty nursing officer, that which drug will doctor order that is to be administered immediately?
a. Dopamine b. NORAD
c. Both (a) and (b) d. None of these

45. Number of teeth in a 3-year old child is:
a. 20 temporary teeth b. 25 temporary teeth
c. 12 temporary teeth d. 16 temporary teeth

46. According to psychosocial theory of Erikson, which behavior is seen in toddler age group?
a. Autonomy vs. shame b. Generativity vs. stagnation
c. Ego integrity vs. despair d. Trust vs. mistrust

47. When does the posterior fontanel close in the baby?
a. 2 to 3 months b. 2 to 3 years
c. 2 to 3 weeks d. 2 to 3 days

48. In which type of solution does the fluid shift from tissues to blood?
a. Hypertonic solution b. Hypotonic solution
c. Isotonic solution d. None of these

49. Fluid volume deficit or hypovolemia describes the loss of:
a. Intracellular fluid b. Extracellular fluid
c. Capsular fluid d. Both (a) and (b)

50. What is the action of vagus nerve stimulation on heart rate?
a. Decreases heart rate b. Increases heart rate
c. Normal heart rate d. None of these

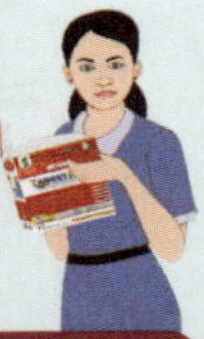

Ans.
24. d
25. d
26. a
27. b
28. a
29. a
30. b
31. b
32. a
33. a
34. a
35. a
36. b
37. a
38. d
39. a
40. c
41. a
42. a
43. b
44. c
45. a
46. a
47. a
48. a
49. b
50. a

51. A patient suddenly develops respiratory difficulties such as dyspnea, what is the first priority of the nursing officer?
a. Raise the head of bed for Fowler's position and administer oxygen
b. Only administer oxygen
c. Check oxygen saturation of client
d. Give Semi-Fowler's position

52. A Nursing officer is working in eye ward. A doctor ordered for a specific eye disease an ointment and an eye drops, a prudent nursing officer should administer which type of medicine first?
a. Eye drops b. Eye ointment
c. Both simultaneously d. None of these

53. The bluish discoloration of the cervix, vagina that is observed as early as 6–8 weeks after conception is called:
a. Chadwick sign b. Osiander sign
c. Homans sign's d. None of these

54. What is the colostomy size for a client whose stoma diameter is of 27 mm size?
a. 29 mm b. 28 mm
c. 27 mm d. 30 mm

55. The preferred site for intramuscular injection in infants is:
a. Anterolateral portion of vastus lateralis muscle
b. Posterior portion of vastus lateralis muscle
c. Dorsogluteal muscle
d. Ventrogluteal site

56. The route of Mantoux skin test is:
a. Intramuscular b. Intravenous
c. Intradermal d. Subcutaneous

57. In a normal client the maximum time for checking pulse rate is:
a. 1 minute b. 2 minutes
c. 3 minutes d. 4 minutes

58. How many chest compressions should be given in one minute during CPR, when two rescuers are present?
a. 100 compressions per minute
b. 120 compressions per minute
c. 130 compressions per minute
d. 80 compressions per minute

59. Which is the primary assessment done when patients BP fall during labor?
a. Assess vital signs of client
b. Assess the weight of client
c. Assess the blood pressure of client
d. Both a and b

60. All of the following are the benefits of KMC (Kangaroo mother care); EXCEPT:
a. To maintain temperature of the baby
b. To promote bonding between mother and baby
c. To stimulate the hormones like prolactin, oxytocin
d. To increase the hormones like growth hormone

61. Which of the following medication is used in PPH (Post-Partum Hemorrhage)?
a. Oxytocin b. Epinephrine
c. Norepinephrine d. Dobutamine

62. The normal value of serum lithium test is:
a. 0.6 –1.2 mmol/L
b. 0.10 – 3.2 mmol/L
c. 1–1.8 mmol/L
d. 1.2–2.2 mmol/L

63. Which position is given to a client by nursing officer, who has been brought from OT after craniotomy surgery?
a. Low Fowler's position with head elevated at a 30-degree angle
b. Semi-Fowler's position with head elevated at a 45-degree angle
c. High Fowler's position with head elevated at a 90-degree angle
d. All of the above

64. All are the cardinal sign of Pre-eclampsia; EXCEPT:
a. Proteinuria b. Increased blood pressure
c. Edema d. Weight loss

65. Which of the following changes are seen in ECG reading, in patients with hyperkalemia?
a. Tall and peaked T wave b. Shortened QT interval
c. Prolong PR interval d. All of these

66. What is contraindicated in male patient reporting the symptoms of redness and ecchymosis in the scrotum region?
a. Prolonged catheterization
b. Scrotal support
c. Rest and comfort
d. Use of ice packs

67. Which of the following method is used for high flow oxygen administration:
a. High flow nasal cannula (HFNC)
b. Non re-breather face mask
c. Simple face mask
d. Nasal prongs

68. All of the following are goals in the management of massive blood transfusion; EXCEPT:
a. Early recognition of blood loss
b. Maintenance of tissue perfusion
c. Restoration of blood volume and hemoglobin
d. Replacement of >1 blood volume in 8 hours

69. The ratio of mixing bleaching powder and water for acting as a disinfectant is:
a. 1:15 b. 1:20
c. 1:10 d. 1:30

70. In suture holding position, the tip of the needle should penetrate the skin perpendicularly about________ from the wound edge.
a. 2–4 mm b. 5–10 mm
c. 12–15 mm d. 18–20 mm

71. In DPT vaccine 'P' stands for:
a. Pertussis b. Polio
c. Pneumonia d. Pancreatitis

72. Therapeutic use of streptokinase is:
a. Lysis of thrombi in coronary artery
b. Lysis of pulmonary emboli
c. Restoration of cannula patency
d. All of the above

73. What is the drug of choice for alcohol withdrawal symptoms?
a. Chlordiazepoxide b. Labetalol
c. Metoclopramide d. Digoxin

74. Anganwadi worker is supervised by:
a. Mukhya sevika
b. Male health worker
c. Both (a) and (b)
d. None of the above

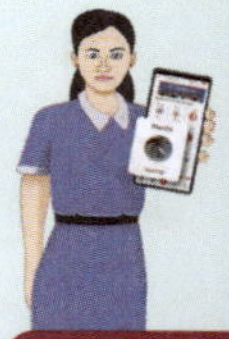

Ans.

51.	a
52.	a
53.	a
54.	a
55.	a
56.	c
57.	a
58.	a
59.	a
60.	d
61.	a
62.	a
63.	a
64.	d
65.	d
66.	a
67.	a
68.	d
69.	c
70.	b
71.	a
72.	d
73.	a
74.	a

75. All of the following are used as treatment modalities of Deep Vein Thrombosis (DVT); EXCEPT:
a. Use of low molecular weight heparin (LMWH)
b. Stockings
c. Intermittent pneumatic compression (IPC)
d. Maximizing invasive procedures

76. Which antipsychotic medications cause amenorrhea?
a. Haloperidol b. Paroxetine
c. Sertraline d. Citalopram

77. Early sign of Vitamin A deficiency is:
a. Myopia
b. Hypermetropia
c. Presbyopia
d. Nyctolopia

78. Parkinson's disease is characterized by deficiency of__________ neurotransmitter.
a. Dopamine b. Acetylcholine
c. Serotonin d. GABA

79. What is an early sign of hypovolemic shock?
a. Loss of blood volume up to 15%
b. Loss of blood volume up to 30%
c. Loss of blood volume up to 60%
d. Loss of blood volume up to 80%

80. Which of the following is the cardinal sign of pulmonary edema?
a. Crackling sound b. Cough
c. Weight loss d. Diaphoresis

81. Which of the following are the correct steps of handwashing?
a. Rub palm to palm — Right palm over left dorsum with fingers interlacing — Palm to palm with interlacing — Back of fingers with interlocking — Rotational rubbing of thumbs and fingertips — Rinse hands
b. Right palm over left dorsum with fingers interlacing — Palm to palm with interlacing back of fingers with interlocking — Rotational rubbing of thumbs and fingertips
c. Rub palm to palm — Palm to palm with interlacing — Back of fingers with interlocking rotational rubbing of thumbs and fingertips — Rinse hands
d. None of the above

82. Which of the following drug causes EPS (Extra Pyramidal Symptoms)?
a. Antipsychotics b. SSRI
c. Mood stabilizers d. Anti-anxiety drugs

83. Which of the following vitamin deficiency causes Bitot's spot and Xerophthalmia?
a. Vitamin D b. Vitamin K
c. Vitamin A d. Vitamin E

84. The first sign of infection is:
a. Fever b. Nausea
c. Diarrhea d. All of these

85. How long do contractions last during second stage of labor at an interval of 3–5 minutes of rest?
a. 20–30 seconds b. 45–90 seconds
c. 100–120 seconds d. None of these

86. The incubation period of *Taenia solium* is:
a. 6 to 8 weeks b. 10 to 12 weeks
c. 14 to 20 weeks d. 20 to 24 weeks

87. High Potassium diet should be avoided in patient's with:
a. CKD b. Diabetes mellitus
c. Renal failure d. Both (a) and (c)

88. Which of the following are the causes of delirium?
a. Brain tumor b. Head trauma
c. Alcohol consumption d. All of these

89. Paranoid thoughts are described as:
a. Hallucinations b. Delusions
c. Illusions d. Anxiety disorders

90. Emergency treatment for cocaine toxicity seeks to stabilize:
a. Kidney functioning b. Body temperature
c. Heart functioning d. All of these

91. Spinal tap is also known as:
a. Pleural tap b. Abdominal tap
c. Lumbar puncture d. All of these

92. If 'P' wave is absent in ECG rhythm, it is an indication of:
a. Sinus arrest b. Atrial fibrillation
c. Both (a) and (b) d. None of these

93. The following conditions can be diagnosed using chest X-ray; EXCEPT:
a. Pneumonia b. Interstitial lung disease
c. Heart failure d. Cell tumor

94. The common side effect of CPAP mask is:
a. Claustrophobia b. Hydrophobia
c. Acrophobia d. Nomophobia

95. The side effects of Tri-cyclic antidepressants (TCA) drugs are:
a. Dry mouth b. Blurred vision
c. Constipation d. All of these

96. The antidote of Paracetamol poisoning is:
a. N-acetylcysteine b. Morphine
c. Warfarin d. Heparin

97. The sports that should be avoided in hemophilia is:
a. Swimming b. Golf
c. Badminton d. Wrestling and boxing

98. Which form of chlorine preparation is used to reduce the bacterial residue in water?
a. Sodium hypochlorite b. Chlorine bleach
c. Calcium hypochlorite d. All of these

99. What is the incubation period of Ascariasis?
a. 2–3 weeks b. 4–8 weeks
c. 9–10 weeks d. None of these

100. All among the following are killed vaccines; EXCEPT:
a. Salk vaccine b. Cholera vaccine
c. Typhoid vaccine d. MMR

101. The X-ray finding in a patient with pleural effusion reveals that fluid starts to build up as a result of gravity in:
a. Costophrenic angle b. Anterior angle
c. Lateral angle d. None of these

102. CAGE questionnaire is used for which of the following behavioral disorders?
a. Alcohol screening
b. Heroine screening
c. Opioid screening
d. Naloxone screening

103. Which of the following are characteristic feature of malnutrition?
a. Stunting, wasting, underweight, and micronutrient deficiency
b. Protein and energy deficiency
c. Kwashiorkor, Marasmus and stunting
d. Low weight for age, weight loss and vomiting

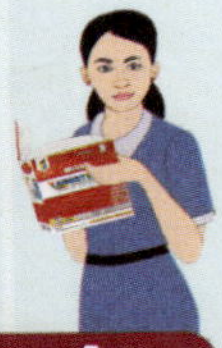

Ans.

75.	d
76.	a
77.	d
78.	a
79.	a
80.	a
81.	a
82.	a
83.	c
84.	a
85.	b
86.	b
87.	d
88.	d
89.	b
90.	d
91.	c
92.	c
93.	d
94.	a
95.	d
96.	a
97.	d
98.	d
99.	b
100.	d
101.	a
102.	a
103.	a

104. In healthy adults, the normal plantar flexion causes a:
a. Downward response of hallux (Flexion)
b. Dorsiflexion of hallux
c. Both (a) and (b)
d. None of the above

105. Surgical procedure used to correct a deviated nasal septum is:
a. Septoplasty b. Annuloplasty
c. Valvuloplasty d. None of these

106. What is the size of needle for Intramuscular (IM) injection in adults?
a. 19–25 gauge
b. 25–27 gauge
c. 22–25 gauge
d. All of the above

107. The breastfeeding should be initiated within ________ after the delivery.
a. 1 hr b. 2 hrs
c. 3 hrs d. 4 hrs

108. A nurse at ICU setting is doing suctioning for a client to remove excessive secretions from the mouth. She should know that the maximum time for suctioning according to the protocol is not to exceed:
a. More than 10 seconds b. More than 5 seconds
c. More than 8 seconds d. More than 20 seconds

109. During CPR after how many cycles does a rescuer change?
a. 5 cycles b. 4 cycles
c. 3 cycles d. 2 cycles

110. Which position a pregnant woman must be given for blood pressure monitoring during last trimester?
a. Trendelenburg position b. Fowler's position
c. Supine position d. Left lateral position

111. Which of the following oral contraceptive pills is an emergency contraceptive method?
a. Chhaya OCP b. Unwanted 72
c. Saheli OCP d. All of these

112. A patient is hungry; he/she suddenly falls down on the floor, what would be the first action of the Nursing officer upon this situation?
a. Check for pulse and breathing
b. Wait for patient to get conscious
c. Do nothing
d. None of the above

113. The vaccine that is contraindicated in pregnancy is (OBG):
a. MMR b. Varicella zoster
c. Both (a) and (b) d. TT

114. What is the best time of insertion of Intrauterine Contraceptive Devices (IUCD)?
a. Starting of menstrual cycle
b. Mid cycle insertion
c. After completion of menstrual cycle
d. None of the above

115. ICDS (Integrated Child Development Services) program was launched in the year:
a. 1975 b. 1980
c. 1992 d. 1995

116. The correct sequence of cardiopulmonary Resuscitation (CPR) is:
a. CAB b. ABC
c. ACB d. None of these

117. The common veins used for placement of central line are all; EXCEPT:
a. Internal jugular vein b. Subclavian vein
c. Femoral vein d. Tibial vein

118. A patient with low urine specific gravity will have all the following characteristics; EXCEPT:
a. Deficit fluid volume b. Excess fluid volume
c. Rebounding pulse d. Weight gain

119. During organ transplantation the living donor must give consent related to all components; EXCEPT:
a. Consent process b. Health Evaluation process
c. Surgical procedure d. No follow up

120. Tongue fall is the main cause of:
a. Central sleep apnea b. Obstructive sleep apnea
c. Both (a) and (b) d. None of these

121. All of the following are the tools of behavioral assessment; EXCEPT:
a. Vineland adaptive behavior scale
b. Vanderbilt assessment scale
c. Vanderbilt digestive center scale
d. Behavior assessment system for children

122. Positive end expiratory pressure (PEEP) is:
a. Alveolar pressure above atmospheric pressure
b. Atmospheric pressure above alveolar pressure
c. Atmospheric pressure above osmotic pressure
d. None of the above

123. Before a surgery to take place, what is the allowable or estimated profuse blood loss in a female patient weighing 60 kg, if her initial hematocrit is 45% and final hematocrit is 30%?
a. 1200 mL b. 1300 mL
c. 1500 mL d. 1600 mL

Explanation:

Formula to calculate allowable blood loss is ABL = [EBV × (Hi – Hf)]/Hi

Where, EBV = Estimated blood volume; Hi = Initial hematocrit; Hf = Final hematocrit.

Estimated blood volume = Weight × 65 mL (for adult woman)

In this case EBV = 65 × 60 = 3900 mL.

Now, apply into the formula:
- ABL = [3900 × (45 – 30)]/45
- ABL = 1300 mL

124. All the principles should be followed while transferring patient to OT table; EXCEPT:
a. Ensure safe transfer from bed to transportation device
b. Ensure safe transfer to pre-operative area
c. Ensure prevention of falls from OT table
d. Ensure safety in recovery room /post-operative ICU

125. All of the following are complications of spinal cord injury (SCI); EXCEPT:
a. Risk of UTI
b. Gonorrhea
c. Flaccidity and spasticity
d. Autonomic hyperreflexia

126. All of the following bones are present in anatomical segment of leg; EXCEPT:
a. Femur b. Fibula
c. Shin bone d. Chin bone

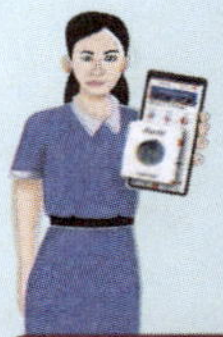

Ans.

104. a
105. a
106. a
107. a
108. a
109. a
110. d
111. b
112. a
113. c
114. b
115. a
116. a
117. d
118. a
119. d
120. a
121. c
122. a
123. b
124. d
125. b
126. d

127. The floor of mouth is formed by _________ muscle.

a. Stylopharyngeus muscle b. Mylohyoid muscle
c. Extensor halluces muscle d. Medial rectus muscle

128. What is the ratio of adrenaline solution in 1 mg/mL of injection?

a. 1:1000 b. 1:2000
c. 1:3000 d. 1:4000

129. Who discovered catgut suture?

a. Galen of Pergamon b. Louis Pasteur
c. Robert Hooke d. Linda Richards

130. 100 mL fluid is given to patient and patient's CVP is 3 mm Hg, then what is the next intervention?

a. Give more fluids b. Restrict fluids
c. Do nothing d. None of these

131. A client name Rohan with weight 65 kg with pulmonary edema is ordered heparin 10 units/kg/hr. How much units of heparin should he receive each hour?

a. 450 Units/hr b. 550 Units/hr
c. 650 Units/hr d. 750 Units/hr

132. The sutures used to close deep, multi-layer lacerations are:

a. Vicryl suture b. Dexon suture
c. Monocryl suture d. All of these

133. When does the infant's weight get double in relation to birth weight?

a. 5 months b. 8 months
c. 10 months d. 12 months

134. Identify the instrument device name that provides positive pressure ventilation:

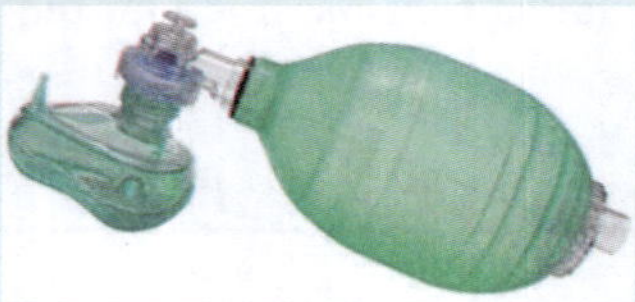

a. Non-rebreather mask b. Hudson mask
c. AMBU bag d. Venturi mask

135. Identify the instrument device name:

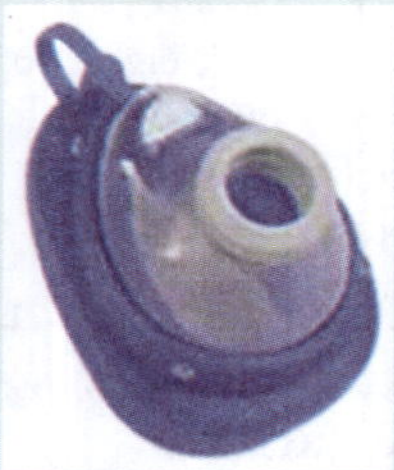

a. Tracheostomy mask b. Face mask
c. Partial rebreather mask d. Venturi mask

136. Identify the disorder presented in the X-ray:

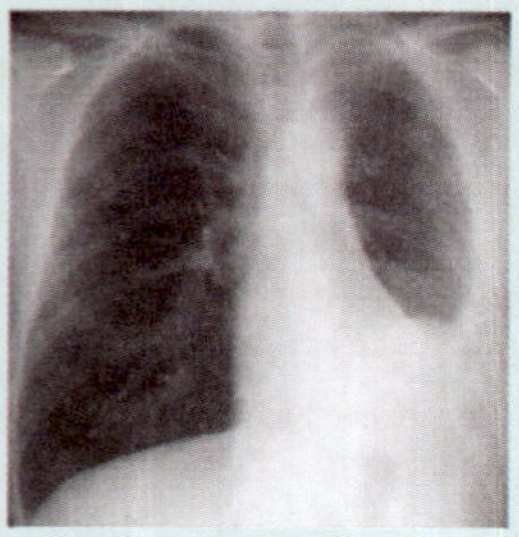

a. Pleural effusion b. Right sided pneumonia
c. Pericarditis d. Bronchiectasis

137. Identify the sign and what deficiency caused it:
(For Video refer NN App Target High Extra Edge Section)

a. Chvostek's sign: Hypocalcemia
b. Trousseau sign: Hypocalcemia
c. Carpopedal spasm: Hypocalcemia
d. None of the above

138. Identify the procedure demonstrated in the video:
(For Video refer NN App Target High Extra Edge Section)

a. Endotracheal intubation
b. Guedel's airway insertion
c. Laryngeal mask airway insertion
d. Oropharyngeal airway

139. Identify the anatomical structure:

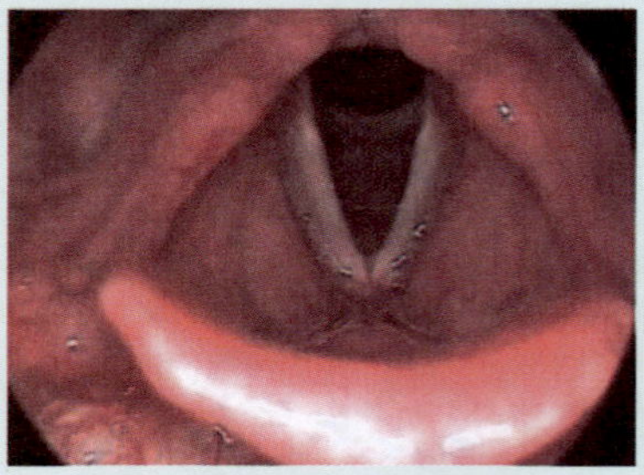

a. Epiglottis with trachea b. Cervix
c. Esophagus opening into stomach
d. Pharynx

140. Identify the condition shown in image:

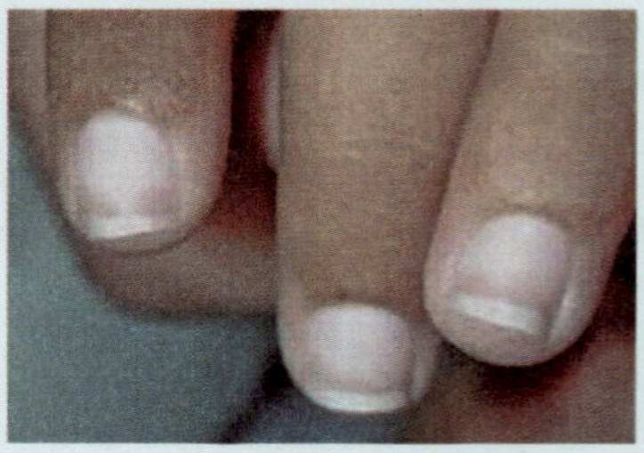

a. Koilonychia b. Spoon-shaped nails
c. Anemic nails d. Paronychia

141. Identify the condition:

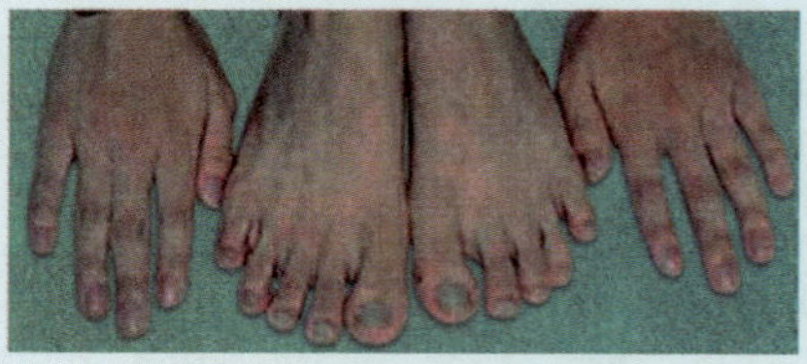

a. Differential cyanosis b. Central cyanosis
c. Peripheral cyanosis d. Extremity cyanosis

142. The condition presented below is caused due to:

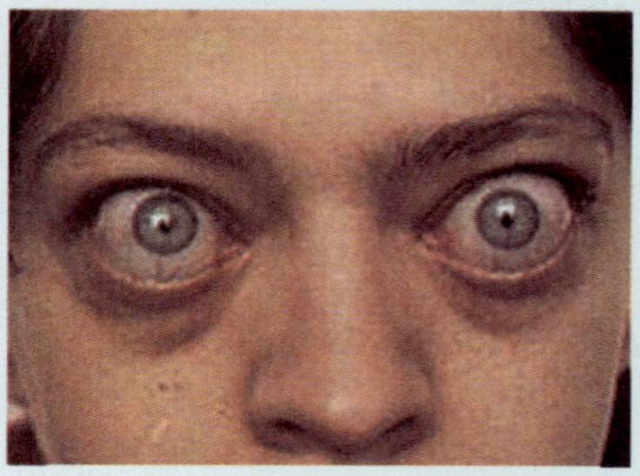

a. Glaucoma b. Hyperthyroidism
c. Hypothyroidism d. Hypopituitarism

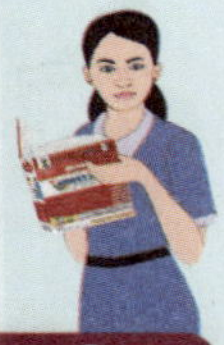

Ans.

127. b
128. a
129. a
130. a
131. c
132. d
133. a
134. c
135. b
136. a
137. b
138. a
139. a
140. c
141. a
142. b

143. Identify the ECG strip:

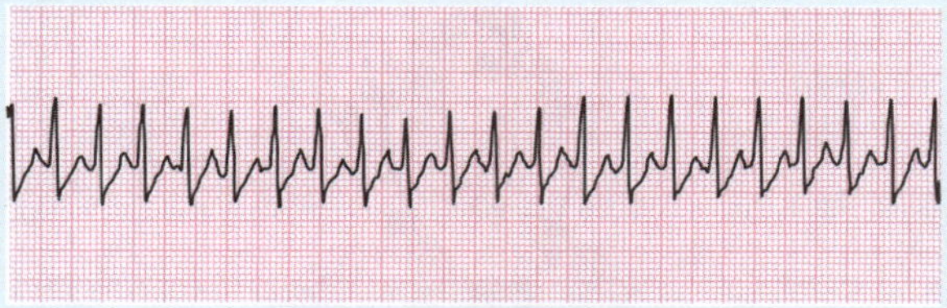

a. Atrial fibrillation
b. Ventricular fibrillation
c. Supraventricular tachycardia
d. First degree AV block

144. The device shown in the image is used in the management of which condition?

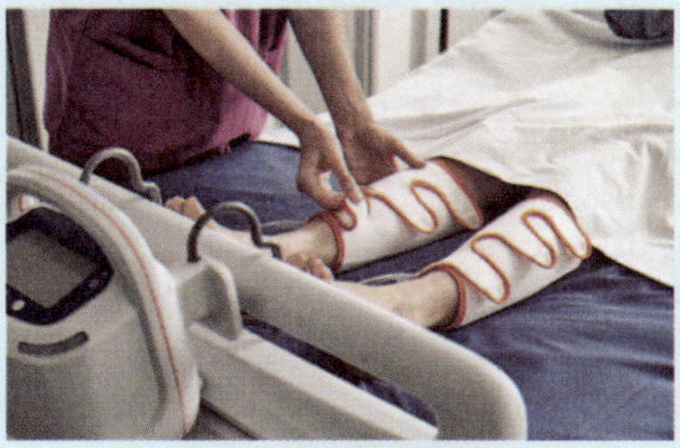

a. Varicose veins b. Hypothermia
c. Cellulitis d. DVT

145. Waxy or cheese-like white substance found coating the skin of newborn human baby is known as:

a. Lanugo b. Vernix caseosa
c. Caput succedaneum d. Amniotic fluid

146. Identify the device shown here:

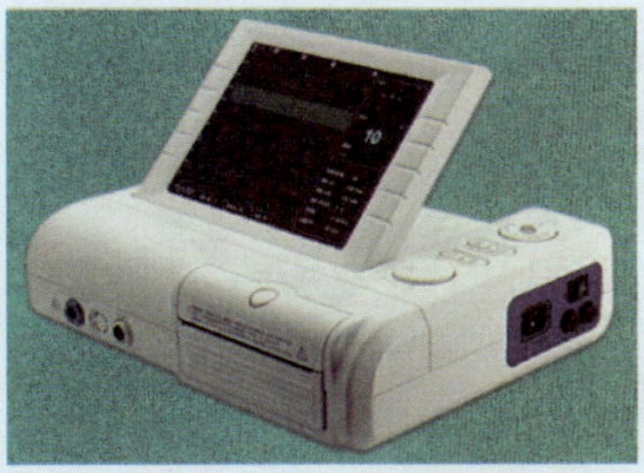

a. CTG machine b. ECG monitor
c. Ultrasound machine d. Ventilator machine

147. Identify the procedure performed on a patient as shown in photograph:

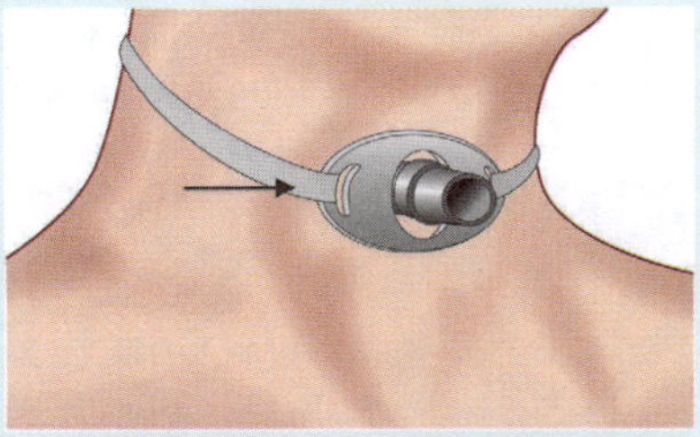

a. Cricothyroidotomy b. Tracheostomy
c. Intubation d. Hoodectomy

148. First sign of immunosuppressed patient is:

a. Vomiting and Nausea b. Headache
c. Fever d. Dizziness

149. Identify the image procedure name:

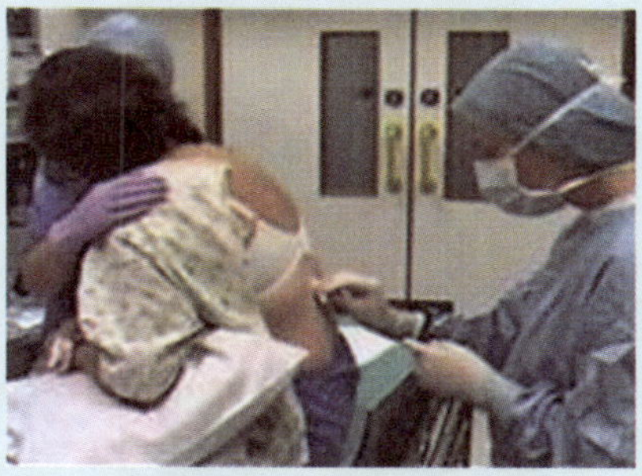

a. Spinal anesthesia b. Thoracotomy
c. Local anesthesia d. Lumbar puncture

150. Sounds in congestive heart failure are:

a. Rhonchi b. Wheezes
c. Pleural rubs d. Crackles

151. What is minimum distance between insulin injection site?

a. 2 cm b. 2.5 cm
c. 1.5 cm d. 3 cm

152. In acetaminophen toxicity nurse observes:

a. Transaminase levels b. Troponin levels
c. Complete blood count d. EEG changes

153. What is the name of this retractor?

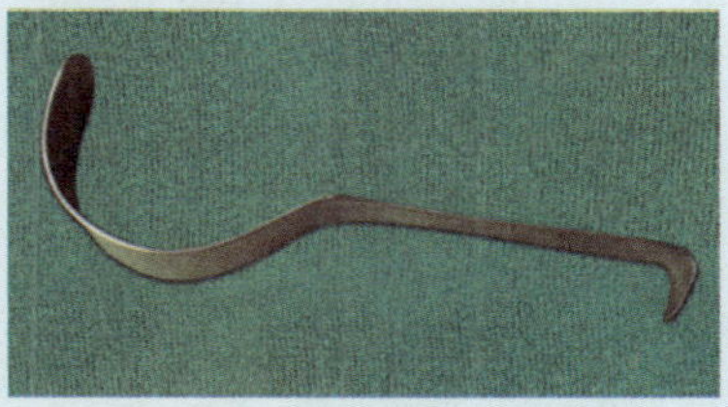

a. Deaver's retractor b. Langenbeck retractor
c. Czerny retractor d. Thomson retractor

154. Identify the procedure shown in the image:

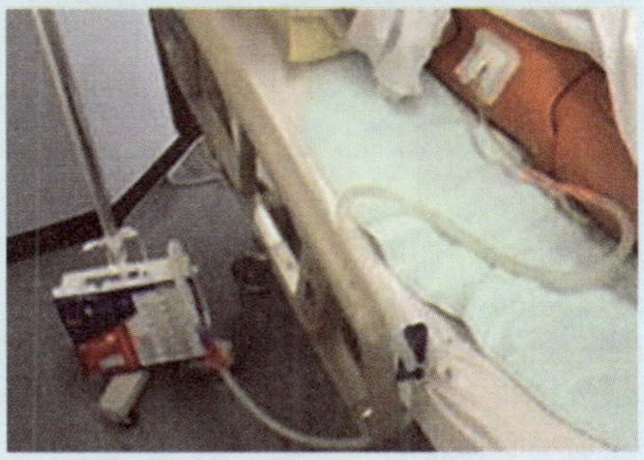

a. Water seal drainage system
b. Thoracentesis
c. Catheterization
d. Bronchoalveolar lavage

155. Identify the encircled part of wave form:

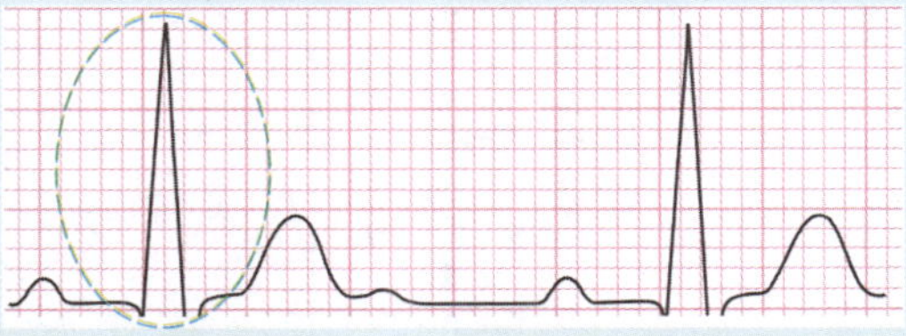

a. PQR complex b. RS wave
c. QRS complex d. T wave

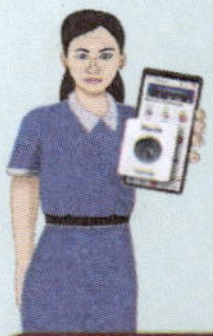

Ans.

143. c
144. d
145. b
146. a
147. b
148. c
149. a
150. d
151. b
152. a
153. a
154. a
155. c

156. Identify the device in the image:

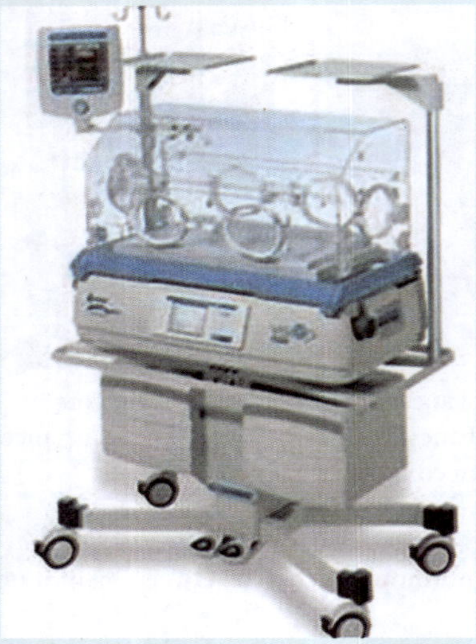

a. Phototherapy machine
b. Incubator
c. Ventilator
d. None of the above

157. All of the following can alter the reading of the below mentioned device; EXCEPT:

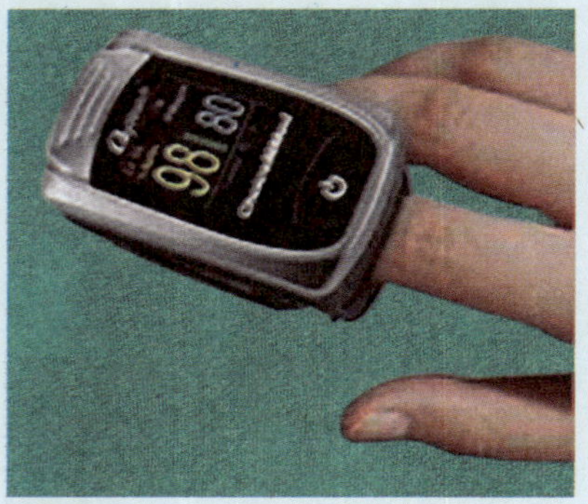

a. Nail polish
b. Intravascular dyes
c. Carboxyhemoglobin
d. Oxyhemoglobin

158. CVP is elevated in all the following conditions; EXCEPT:

a. Hypovolemic shock
b. Overhydration
c. Heart failure
d. Positive pressure breathing

159. Diagnose the underlying medical disorder by ECG change in photograph:

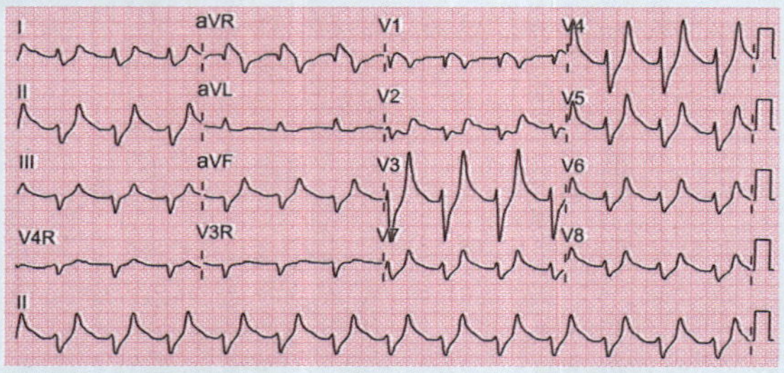

a. Hypokalemia b. Hypercalcemia
c. Hypocalcemia d. Hyperkalemia

160. Identify the image:

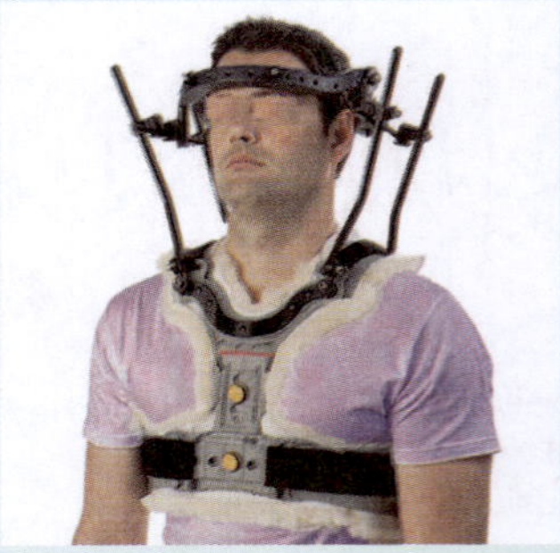

a. Halo traction b. Facet joint traction
c. Thoracic traction d. Lumbar traction

161. Food contraindicated with CRF and spironolactone:

a. Carrots b. Papaya
c. Banana d. Maize

162. Schizotypal disorder is characterized by:

a. Severe social anxiety b. Manic attacks
c. Suicidal tendency d. Hallucinations

163. The image below represents:

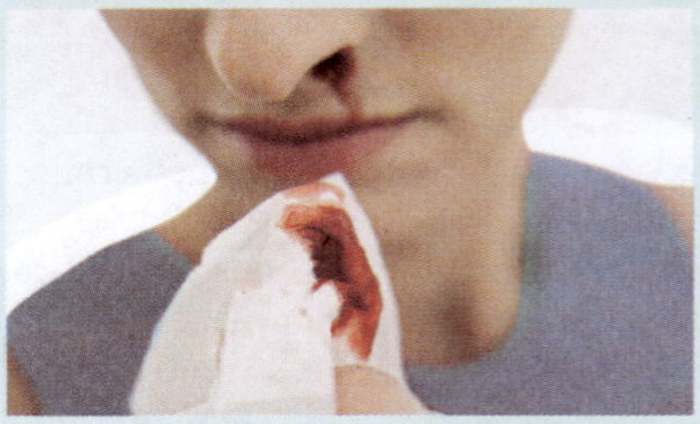

a. Hemoptysis b. Nasal laceration
c. Hematemesis d. Epistaxis

164. The contraindications of the procedure shown in the following image is:

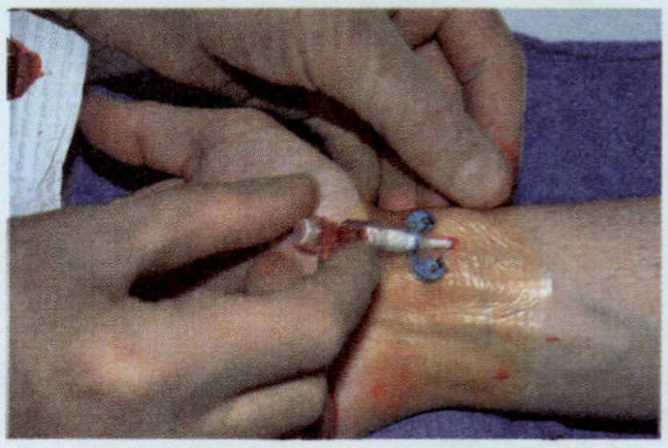

a. Pulse pressure variation b. Hyperkalemia
c. Positive Allen's test d. Ventilated patients

165. The condition shown in the following image is seen in all; EXCEPT:

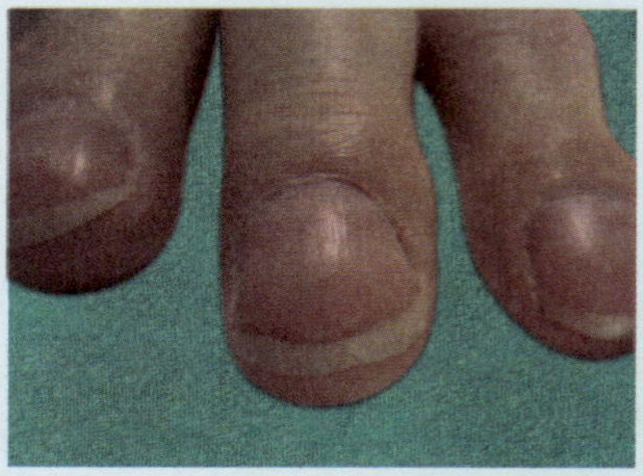

a. Tetralogy of Fallot b. Cystic fibrosis
c. Bronchiectasis d. Raynaud's disease

Ans.

156. b
157. d
158. a
159. d
160. a
161. c
162. a
163. d
164. c
165. d

166. Highest concentration of O_2 is with:

a. Face mask b. Nasal prong
c. Venturi mask d. Rebreathing mask

167. The suture shown in the image is:

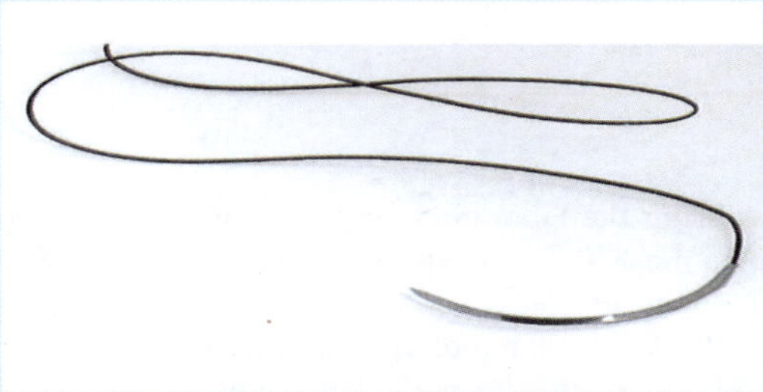

a. Nylon suture b. Plain catgut
c. Prolene d. Cotton

168. In a 50 over match, the chasing team scored 5 runs per over in the first 30 over. Required run rate is 10 runs per over. What is the score of first team?

a. 350 b. 349
c. 250 d. 399

169. The cost of 2 tables is equal to that of 5 chairs and the cost of 10 tables and 10 chairs together is 7000. The total cost of 4 tables and 2 chairs is:

a. 2400 b. 3000
c. 2000 d. 2800

170. A pen is sold at ₹90 with a loss of 10%. At which price it should be sold to make a profit of 10%?

a. 100 b. 110
c. 120 d. 130

171. Which printer is very commonly used for desktop publishing?

a. Laser Printer b. Inkjet Printer
c. Daisy Wheel Printer d. Dot Matrix Printer

172. Personnel who design, program, operate and maintain computer equipment are called:

a. Console operator
b. Programmer
c. Peopleware
d. System analyst

173. The most recent version of Mac OS is based on the ________ operating system.

a. Windows b. Linux
c. Unix d. CMOS

174. What is the shortcut key to display field codes?

a. Alt + F9
b. Ctrl + F9
c. Shift + F9
d. Space + F9

175. Which of the following helps to reduce spelling error in the document?

a. Auto Format b. Auto Correct
c. Smart Tags d. Auto Text

Ans.

166. c
167. a
168. b
169. a
170. b
171. a
172. c
173. c
174. a
175. b

"He who has health has hope; and he who has hope has everything."

—Arabian proverb

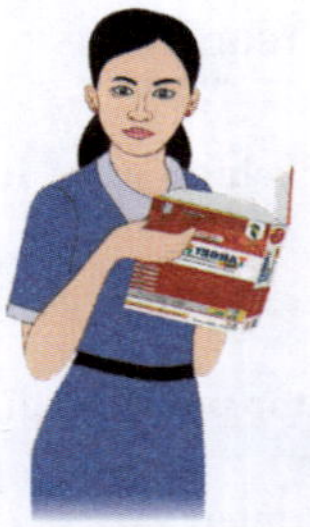

AIIMS Nagpur (NO) 2020

SECTION : SUBJECT KNOWLEDGE OF CONCERNED POST NURSING

1. An order for prednisolone reads 10 mg four times a day. The dose for the child is 2 mg/kg/day. How many pounds does the child weigh?

a. 36 pounds b. 40 pounds
c. 46 pounds d. 44 pounds

2. Which type of leadership theories consider people inherit certain qualities that make them better suited to leadership?

a. Situational theories
b. Contingency theories
c. Trait theories
d. Behavioral theories

3. An acid-fast bacillus which is pathogenic:

a. Bacillus pertussis
b. Corynebacterium diphtheriae
c. Salmonella typhi
d. Mycobacterium leprae

4. Which of the following helps prevent water loss through skin?

a. Keratin b. Melanin
c. Collagen d. Carotene

5. In depression, there is deficiency of:

a. Dopamine b. Acetylcholine
c. GABA d. 5-HT

6. What is the major nursing responsibility when administering sulfonamide preparation?

a. Weigh the child daily
b. Monitor child's temperature
c. Give milk with medication
d. Administer the drug at prescribed times

7. Based on the knowledge of electroconvulsive treatment, the nurse explains to the student nurses that atropine is given before the treatment primarily to:

a. Increase body secretions
b. Minimize intestinal contractions
c. Decrease anxiety
d. Prevent aspiration

8. These agents decreases intestinal muscle tone to slow passage of feces:

a. Cathartics
b. Antidiarrheal opiate agents
c. Hypertonic
d. Laxatives

9. Ketone bodies are found in urine of patients with uncontrolled diabetes due to:

a. Increased metabolism of protein
b. Increased metabolism of fat
c. Impaired kidney function
d. Decomposition of excess sugar in blood

10. Assessing the laboratory findings which results would the nurse most likely to expect to find in a client with chronic renal failure?

a. BUN 10 to 30 mg/dl, creatinine 0.5 to 1.5 mg/dl
b. BUN 35 to 40 mg/dl, Potassium 3.5 mEq/L, Ph 7.35, decreased serum calcium
c. BUN 15 mg/dl, increased serum calcium, creatinine 1.0 mg/dl
d. Decreased serum calcium, blood pH 7.2, Potassium 6.5 mEq/L

11. The ability of a person to readily recover from stressful situations is called:

a. Resilience b. Androgyny
c. Hardiness d. Mental freedom

12. Epidemic dropsy is due to:

a. Ergot b. BOAA
c. Aflatoxin d. Sanguinarine

13. Inadequate intake by the pregnant woman of which vitamin can cause neural tube defect?

a. Niacin b. Folic acid
c. Thiamine d. Riboflavin

14. A method in which several rounds of questions are given to a panel of experts is called:

a. Meta-analysis b. Delphi technique
c. Q-sort methodology d. Content analysis

15. Socialization into one's primary culture as a child is known as:

a. Enculturation b. Acculturation
c. Biculturation d. Assimilation

16. Additional defects associated with exstrophy of bladder is:

a. Congenital heart disease b. Pubic bone malformation
c. Absence of one kidney d. Imperforate rash

17. 7.0 is the normal pH of the:

a. Urine
b. Blood in the renal artery
c. Blood in the testicular vein
d. Fluid within a typical cell

18. Which one of the following statements is not applicable to using an evidence-base in nursing practice?

a. Evidence used in nursing practice must be appraised for its validity and applicability.
b. To ensure the best quality of care given to patients
c. The use of research evidence in nursing practice does not need to be evaluated after it is used or implemented.
d. To ensure that nursing decisions are based on the best quality of evidence.

19. Which of the following means translating the message into verbal and non-verbal symbol to communicate the receiver?

a. Decoding b. Feedback
c. Channel d. Encoding

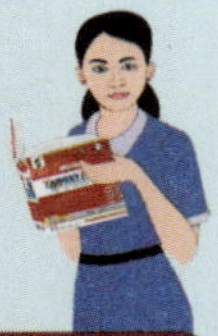

Ans.

1. d
2. c
3. d
4. a
5. d
6. d
7. d
8. b
9. b
10. d
11. a
12. d
13. b
14. b
15. a
16. b
17. d
18. c
19. d

Abbreviation: NO, Nursing Officer

Disclaimer: *The questions are prepared by memory-based recall from candidates who attended the examination.*

20. The junction at which an impulse travels from one neuron to another is called:

a. Axon b. Synapse
c. Nerve message d. Stimulus

21. When using non-verbal communication in a nurse-client relationship, the nurse must be aware of:

a. Contradictions to the clients
b. The client's development level
c. Ethnic background
d. Nervous hand movements

22. Intrinsic factor of castle is secreted by:

a. Mucus cells b. Chief cells
c. Parietal cells d. B cells

23. Hygiene factors and motivational factors are key concepts in:

a. Goal setting theory
b. Maslow's hierarchy of needs
c. Herzberg's two factor theory
d. Expectancy theory

24. A 34-year-old woman complains about pain due to lower abdominal cramping, urine hCG is positive and pelvic ultrasound reveals a 10-week intrauterine pregnancy. The patient states that she is not sure whether to keep the pregnancy. Which of the following is the most appropriate next step in management?

a. Counsel the patient or refer to an appropriate counselor
b. Termination of pregnancy
c. Inform the patient's parents
d. Inform the patient's partner

25. Nursing care that is based on identifying and meeting the needs of a patient is called:

a. Client-oriented b. Goal-oriented
c. Hegar's sign d. Prioritization

26. Which of the following techniques are examples of non-therapeutic communication?

a. Restating b. Giving advice
c. Focusing d. Paraphrasing

27. A 45 days old infant shows development of icterus and two days' later symptoms and signs of acute liver failure appeared. Child was found to be +ve for HbsAg. The mother was also HbsAg carrier. The mother's hepatitis B serological profile is likely to be:

a. HbsAg and Ab +ve
b. HbsAg and anti Hbe Ab +ve
c. HbsAg +ve only
d. Mother infected with mutant HBV

28. The spinal cord is made up of 7 cervical vertebrae, 5 lumbar vertebrae, 4 or 5 fused sacral vertebrae, 4 or 5 coccygeal vertebrae and how many thoracic vertebrae?

a. 8 b. 5
c. 12 d. 10

29. Elements of primary healthcare are the following; EXCEPT:

a. Health education
b. Cost effectiveness
c. Provision of essential drugs
d. Intersectoral coordination

30. One function of parasympathetic nervous system is:

a. Contraction of hair muscles
b. Stimulating of sweat gland
c. Acceleration of heart beat
d. Constriction of pupil

31. Which of the following is most appropriate intervention to reduce stress in a preterm infant at 32 weeks gestation?

a. Tactile stimulation until signs of over stimulation develop
b. Sensory stimulation including several senses at a time
c. Kangaroo care
d. An attitude of extension when prone or side lying

32. Passive immunity against tetanus is obtained by the administration of:

a. TT b. DPT
c. DT d. Tetanus immunoglobulin

33. A nurse demonstrates caring, sincerity, empathy and trustworthiness:

a. Ethical nurse-patient interaction
b. Legal nurse-patient interaction
c. Therapeutic nurse-patient interaction
d. Emotional nurse-patient interaction

34. Lactated Ringer's solution is contraindicated in:

a. Lactic acidosis
b. Fluid lost as bile or diarrhea
c. Burns
d. Hypovolemia

35. Acute illness refers to an illness that:

a. Is synonymous with disease
b. Has a short duration and is severe
c. Causes and irreversible condition
d. Is longer than 6 months, and can also affect functioning in any dimension

36. Major approaches in problem solving are:

a. Inductive, deductive, initiative, synthetic
b. Inductive, deductive, purposive, synthetic
c. Inductive, deductive, analytic, synthetic
d. Inductive, deductive, active, analytic

37. The continuing process of measuring services, products and practices of an organization against the strongest competitors in quality control and quality assurance is known as:

a. Benchmarking b. Auditing
c. Quality Assurance d. Quality Improvement

38. Nurse's main priority assessment while caring for the client having spontaneous abortion:

a. Dehydration b. Hypertension
c. Subinvolution d. Hemorrhage

39. 22-year-old Megha comes to the doctor because of a missed menstrual period. She has hypothyroidism for which she takes thyroxine; she has an artificial heart valve, for which she takes Coumadin, and she recently started tetracycline for acne. Urine human chorionic gonadotropin (hCG) is positive. Which of the following medication should the patient continue to take during pregnancy?

a. Thyroxine
b. Coumadin
c. Tetracycline
d. Oral contraceptive pill (OCP)

40. An infant is to receive thyroxin sodium, 0.35 mg once a day orally. The medications is available in elixir from 0.25 mg/mL. How much elixir should the nurse administer?

a. 1.3 mL b. 1.0 mL
c. 2.4 mL d. 1.4 mL

41. Vaccines and toxoids produce:

a. Acquired immunity b. Active immunity
c. Natural immunity d. Passive immunity

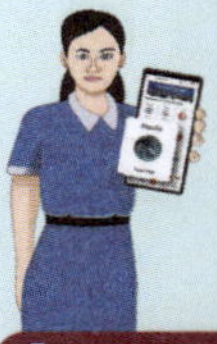

Ans.

20. b
21. d
22. c
23. c
24. a
25. a
26. b
27. a
28. c
29. b
30. d
31. c
32. d
33. c
34. a
35. b
36. c
37. a
38. d
39. a
40. d
41. b

42. The characteristic of an ideal normal distribution curve is/are:

a. Mean, median and mode do not coincide
b. Prescription
c. Bell shaped
d. Its symmetrical around the mean

43. The best and safest method of sterilization is:

a. Boiling for 30 minutes
b. Flaming
c. Autoclaving
d. Immersion in chemical germicide

44. Eugenics means:

a. Genetic preventive measures
b. Improvement of genetic endowment
c. Improvement of environment
d. Genetic counseling

45. Inhibin is secreted by:

a. Corpus luteum b. Stroma
c. Leydig cells d. Surface epithelium

46. Modern concept of chemotherapy was proposed by:

a. Paul Ehrlich b. Frankel
c. Metchnikoff d. Joseph Lister

47. Disposal of expired and cytotoxic drugs is by:

a. Chemical treatment
b. Municipal waste
c. Separate landfill disposal
d. Autoclaving

48. Which is the most relevant knowledge about oxygen administration to a client with COPD?

a. Blood gases are monitored using a pulse oximeter.
b. Oxygen is administered best using a non-rebreather mask
c. Hypoxia stimulates the central chemoreceptors of the medulla that makes the client breath.
d. Oxygen at 1-2 L/min is given to maintain the hypoxic stimulus for breathing.

49. The following develops as a result of a nurse's experience in a specific clinical area, the time the nurse has been in practice, and the quality of relationships the nurse has formed with clients:

a. Personal ethics b. Leadership
c. Ability to delegate care d. Knowing clients

50. OSCE Means:

a. Objective subjective clinical examination
b. Observation subject clinical examination
c. Objective structured clinical examination
d. Observation structured clinical examination

51. Acid medium of vagina maintained by:

a. Trichomonas vaginalis b. E. coli
c. Staphylococci d. Döderlein's bacilli

52. Rorschach Inkblot test, Thematic apperception test are based on the phenomenon of:

a. Transference b. Identification
c. Observation d. Projection

53. The patient has to undergo a loop electrosurgical excision procedure (LEEP), which of the following represents the potential long-term complications from this procedure?

a. Cervical incompetence and cervical stenosis
b. Hernia and intraperitoneal adhesions
c. Abscess
d. Constipation

54. Causative organism of infectious mononucleosis is:

a. Cytomegalovirus b. Toxoplasma
c. Epstein-Barr virus d. Varicella zoster virus

55. The visceral pleura is:

a. The fluid around the lungs
b. The thinnest portion of the peritoneum
c. The membrane lining surface of the lungs
d. The membrane lining the wall of the thoracic cavity

56. Lochia alba follows lochia serosa and usually lasts from the 1st to 3rd week PP. What is lochia?

a. Creamy white-brown, contains decidual cells, may have stale odor
b. Brown to red contains decidual cells and leukocytes
c. Creamy white-brown, stale order
d. Brown to red, tissue fragments, odor

57. Before the placenta functions the corpus luteum is the primary source of synthesis of which of the following hormones:

a. Cortisol and thyroxine
b. Estrogen and progesterone
c. T4 and TSH
d. LH and FSH

58. Maize is deficit in:

a. Tryptophan b. Threonine
c. Methionine d. Leucine

59. The system of evaluation where an employee is measured against his/her co-worker is called:

a. Reports
b. Graphic records
c. Critical incidents
d. Ranking

60. Nursing has a code of ethics that professional registered nurses follow and:

a. Protect the client from harm
b. Ensure identical care to all clients
c. Define the principles by which nurses provide care to their clients
d. Improve self-health care

61. Calorie intake of 1-year-old child:

a. 1000 kcal/day b. 800 kcal/day
c. 1200 kcal/day d. 1500 kcal/day

62. What is the full form of ACTH?

a. Angiotensin converting hormone
b. Adrenocorticotropic hormone
c. Acetylcholine
d. Angiotensin converting enzyme

63. Which mode of clinical application for qualitative research is considered to be the sharing of qualitative findings with the patient?

a. Assessment of progress
b. Coaching
c. Anticipatory guidance
d. Empathy

64. The nurse is informed that a client with a large surgical incision is being transferred from the intensive care unit to the surgical unit. What medication does the nurse anticipate the physician will order for this client?

a. Ascorbic acid b. Mephyton
c. Vitamin B12 complex d. Vitamin A

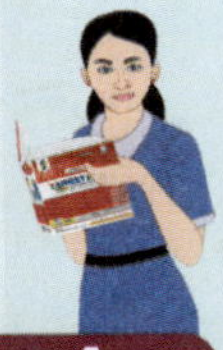

Ans.

42. c
43. c
44. b
45. a
46. a
47. c
48. d
49. d
50. c
51. d
52. d
53. a
54. c
55. c
56. a
57. b
58. a
59. d
60. c
61. a
62. b
63. c
64. a

65. How does audit differ from research?
a. It does not increase our understanding of the topic itself or allows us to transfer the results to other situations
b. It is more likely to be applicable to nursing
c. It can be carried out on inanimate objects
d. It does not need as many people to collect the information

66. The genetic material, deoxyribonucleic acid (DNA) is contained in:
a. Chromatin b. Chromosome
c. Nucleoli d. Nucleus

67. What is the most serious complication of meningitis in young children?
a. Peripheral circulatory collapse
b. Blindness
c. Communicating hydrocephalus
d. Epilepsy

68. Motilin is secreted by cells in:
a. Liver b. Esophagus
c. Pancreas d. Ileum

69. Modified ECT is not given frequently on routine practice because of:
a. Non-availability of anesthetist
b. Respiratory difficulties
c. Osteoporosis
d. Myocardial infarction

70. Thiamine has been prescribed for an alcoholic patient. The rationale for administration of this medication is the prevention of:
a. Wernicke-Korsakoff syndrome
b. Alcohol withdrawal syndrome
c. Alcoholic dementia
d. Huntington's disease

71. When palpating the abdomen of hypertrophic pyloric stenosis infant, the Nurse finds:
a. An olive-sized mass in right upper abdomen
b. Marked tenderness around the abdomen
c. Distended colon
d. Rhythmic peristaltic waves in the lower abdomen

72. Which of the following is a differentiating test between mucus and cerebrospinal fluid (CSF) from a nasal discharge?
a. Glucose b. Specific gravity
c. Microorganism d. Protein

73. All of the following are a good source of Omega 3 PUFA; EXCEPT:
a. Mustard oil b. Fish oil
c. Corn oil d. Ground oil

74. The situation in which individuals have excessive worry or belief that they are suffering from a physical illness despite lack of medical evidence is known as:
a. Somatoform disorder b. Phobic disorder
c. Dissociative disorder d. Pain disorder

75. Which of the following intervention demonstrates the nurse understand about the newborn's thermoregulatory ability?
a. Inspecting the newborn's umbilical cord
b. Obtaining an APGAR score
c. Placing the newborn under a radiant warmer
d. Suctioning with a bulb syringe

76. Oligohydramnios is related with which of the following condition?
a. Esophageal atresia b. Renal Agenesis
c. Anencephaly d. Down's syndrome

77. Using precise methods to investigate problems and arrive at solutions is called:
a. Scientific problem solving
b. Trial and error
c. Critical thinking
d. Planning and execution

78. The famous 14 Principles of Management was first defined by:
a. Adam Smith b. Henri Fayol
c. Elton Mayo d. James Watt

79. The following delusions are common in depression; EXCEPT:
a. Delusion of poverty
b. Delusion of grandeur
c. Delusion of persecution
d. Delusion of nihilism

80. Sunken fontanelle is a sign of:
a. Dehydration b. Hydrocephalus
c. Down's syndrome d. Turner's syndrome

SECTION: GENERAL APTITUDE AND GENERAL AWARENESS

81. Study the below series and identify which number can come in place of "?"
4, 5, 7, 9, 13, 15, 19, 21, 25, ?, 33, 39
a. 31 b. 29
c. 27 d. 33

82. Select the figure that will come next in the following figure series.

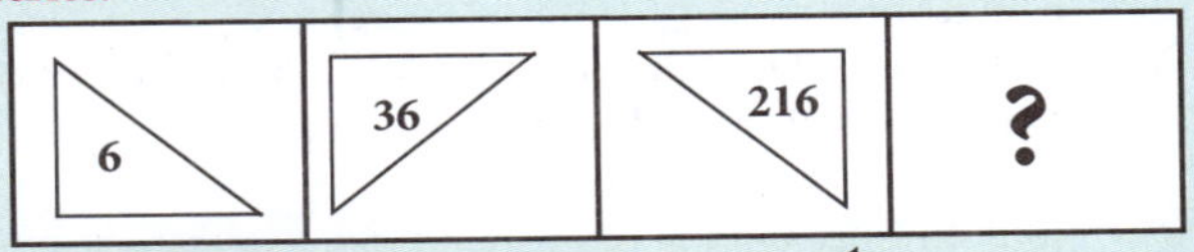

a. 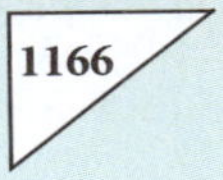

b. 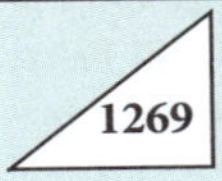

c. 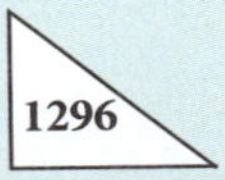

d. 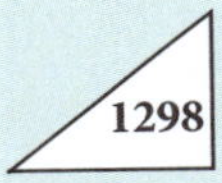

83. The 'Simon Commission' was a group of _______ British Members of Parliament.
a. 7 b. 5
c. 11 d. 3

84. Identify the country which is situated in South America from the following:
a. Nigeria b. Brazil
c. Mexico d. Mongolia

85. The famous monument 'Gol Gumbaz' is located in:
a. Bijapur, Karnataka b. Jaipur, Rajasthan
c. Nashik, Maharashtra d. Hyderabad, Telangana

86. Read the below statements taking them as true even if they seem to be at variance from the commonly known facts. Then choose the option that represents the conclusion that can be definitely drawn from these statements.
Statements:
(i) Some parrots are donkeys.
(ii) All donkeys can sing.
a. No singer is a donkey
b. All donkeys are parrots
c. No parrot can sing
d. Some parrots can sing

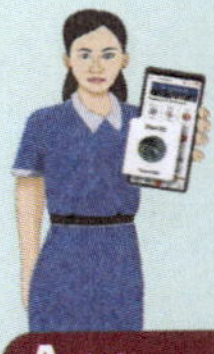

Ans.
65. d
66. d
67. c
68. d
69. a
70. a
71. a
72. a
73. a
74. a
75. c
76. b
77. a
78. b
79. b
80. a
81. a
82. c
83. a
84. b
85. a
86. d

87. Headquarter of UNESCO is situated in:
a. Sydney
b. London
c. Paris
d. New York

88. The given list of words have some aspect in common: Burma, Thailand, Cambodia, Mauritius, Malaysia, Singapore, Philippines, Brunei, Vietnam, Indonesia. Choose the one which is least like other words and is the odd one out.
a. Burma
b. Brunei
c. Cambodia
d. Mauritius

89. The '24th World Energy Congress' was held in September 2019 at:
a. Toronto
b. Shanghai
c. Moscow
d. Abu Dhabi

90. If 4 is related to 64 and 5 is related to 100 in the same way 7 is related to ______.
a. 196
b. 49
c. 98
d. 169

SECTION: BASIC COMPUTER KNOWLEDGE AND NURSING INFORMATICS

91. Clinical information, such as order sets and patient education material, should be reviewed at least:
a. Annually
b. Monthly
c. Biannually
d. Biennially

92. When designing a web page that should appeal to both males and females, a good choice of background color is:
a. Orange
b. Blue
c. Brown
d. Grey

93. Which of the following options best describes the truthfulness of the following statements?
(i) Windows XP is an operating system.
(ii) Both Unix and Linux are multitasking operating system.
a. (i) True, (ii) False
b. (i) True, (ii) True
c. (i) False, (ii) True
d. (i) False, (ii) False

94. In respect to patient data in database, the most important factor is:
a. Transferability
b. Accessibility
c. Security
d. Relevance

95. Which of the following is the primary reason for conducting end-user testing?
a. Identify user competencies
b. Identify errors
c. Determine on going education needs
d. Determine volume capacity

96. In MS-PowerPoint 2016, "Chart" appears under ______ Menu tab.
a. Design
b. Review
c. View
d. Insert

97. How many different unique codes can be generated using 5-bits?
a. 64
b. 32
c. 8
d. 16

98. How many nibbles are in 128 bytes?
a. 64
b. 1024
c. 512
d. 256

99. What is the shortcut key for making the text look darker in MS-Word?
a. CTRL+Z
b. CTRL+B
c. CTRL+I
d. CTRL+Y

100. When doing system analysis and gathering information, the first tool is often an:
a. RFI
b. RFP
c. RFT
d. RFQ

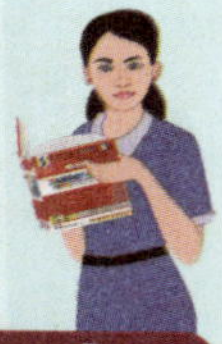

Ans.

87.	c
88.	d
89.	d
90.	a
91.	d
92.	d
93.	b
94.	b
95.	b
96.	d
97.	b
98.	d
99.	b
100.	a

"He who has health has hope; and he who has hope has everything."

—Arabian proverb

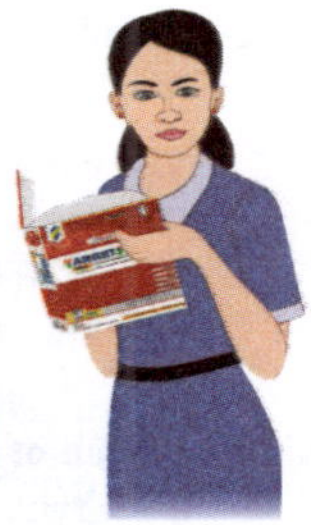

AIIMS Patna (NO) 2020

SECTION: ANATOMY AND PHYSIOLOGY

1. **The apex of the heart is formed mostly by the:**
   a. Left ventricle b. Right atrium
   c. Left atrium d. Central ventricle
2. **Which of the following is the largest cranial nerve?**
   a. Cranial VI b. Cranial nerve X
   c. Cranial nerve VII d. Cranial nerve V
3. **Tarsals of the ankles are examples of which type of bone?**
   a. Short bones b. Sesamoid bones
   c. Long bones d. Pneumatic bones
4. **How many bones are there in the lower extremities in a normal adult?**
   a. 58 b. 62
   c. 64 d. 60
5. **What is the approximate maximum air volume in the lung for normal healthy adult?**
   a. 2400 mL b. 3000 mL
   c. 300 mL d. 6000 mL
6. **Carpometacarpal joint is an example of which of the following types of joints?**
   a. Hinge b. Ball and socket
   c. Pivot d. Saddle
7. **Which of the following layers of the adrenal gland secretes glucocorticoids?**
   a. Adrenal medulla b. Zona glomerulosa
   c. Zona reticularis d. Zona fasciculata
8. **Which of the following is an example of ball-and-socket joints?**
   a. Skull joint b. Thumb joint
   c. Hip joint d. Elbow joint
9. **What is the synonym of Clotting Factor II?**
   a. Christmas factor b. Fibrinogen
   c. Calcium d. Prothrombin
10. **Which of the following quadriceps femoris muscles help in flexion of the thigh?**
    a. Rectus femoris b. Vastus medialis
    c. Vastus intermedius d. Vastus lateralis
11. **Which of the following part of the brain controls body temperature?**
    a. Hypothalamus b. Hippocampus
    c. Pons d. Amygdala
12. **How many pairs of cervical nerves are there in the spinal cord?**
    a. 5 b. 9
    c. 8 d. 12
13. **The elbow is an example of a ______ joint.**
    a. Hinge b. Pivot
    c. Condyloid d. Planar
14. **The expanded ends of a long bone are called:**
    a. Tubercle b. Epicondyle
    c. Diaphysis d. Epiphyses
15. **The posterior pituitary consists mainly of ______.**
    a. Beta cells b. C cells
    c. T cells d. Neuronal projections
16. **Which of the following hormones is NOT secreted from the anterior pituitary?**
    a. Adrenocorticotropic b. Prolactin
    c. Human growth hormone d. Oxytocin
17. **A ______ is a cell that manufactures and stores the protein keratin.**
    a. Keraticellyte b. Keracyte
    c. Keratinocyte d. Keratolytic
18. **Which of the following is an example of synarthrosis joint?**
    a. Fibrous joints of the skull sutures
    b. Wrist joints
    c. Hip joints
    d. Elbow joint
19. **Which one of the following hormones inhibits release of growth hormone?**
    a. Dopamine
    b. Somatotropin
    c. Somatostatin
    d. Thyrotropin inhibiting hormone
20. **Oxytocin is mainly involved in which of the following functions?**
    a. Motor skills
    b. Childbirth and lactation
    c. Growth and mental ability
    d. Regulation of blood pressure

SECTION: MICROBIOLOGY

21. **Which of the following is NOT related to MMR vaccine?**
    a. Rubella b. Measles
    c. Rickets d. Mumps
22. **Who among the following devised the autoclave used for sterilization?**
    a. Charles Chamberland b. Robert Koch
    c. Edward Jenner d. Anton van Leeuwenhoek
23. **Widal, a serological test, is used to detect the presence of which of the following pathogenic microorganisms?**
    a. E. coli
    b. Mycobacterium tuberculosis
    c. Haemophilus influenzae
    d. Salmonella typhi

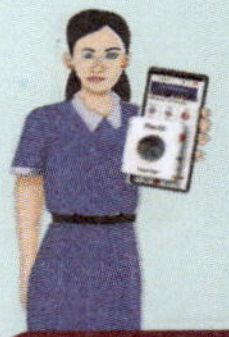

Ans.

1. a
2. d
3. a
4. b
5. d
6. d
7. d
8. c
9. d
10. a
11. a
12. c
13. a
14. d
15. d
16. d
17. c
18. a
19. c
20. b
21. c
22. a
23. d

Abbreviation: NO, Nursing Officer

Disclaimer: *The questions are prepared by memory-based recall from candidates who attended the examination.*

24. The causative agent of Lyme disease is:
a. Rickettsia prowazekii
b. Alphavirus
c. Borrelia burgdorferi
d. Trypanosoma brucei gambiense

25. Which of the following microorganisms causes gonorrhea?
a. Stylus gonorrhea
b. Streptococcus pneumoniae
c. Stereotyoist gonorrhea
d. Neisseria gonorrhea

26. What is the optimum temperature in an autoclave to achieve sterility?
a. 121°C for 30 m
b. 60°C for 30 m
c. 34°C for 30 m
d. 27°C for 20 m

27. Which of the following involves the introduction of antibodies into the body from an animal or person already immune to the disease?
a. Active immunity
b. Artificially acquired passive immunity
c. Naturally acquired passive immunity
d. Innate immunity

28. Type I hypersensitivity is mediated by:
a. IgG
b. IgE
c. IgM
d. IgA

29. Rod-shaped bacteria are called:
a. Cocci
b. Clusters
c. Bacillus
d. Spirochetes

30. Which of the following is true about IgM?
a. It is not produced by vertebrates.
b. It forms the initial immune response.
c. It is not an isotypes of antibody.
d. It is the smallest antibody.

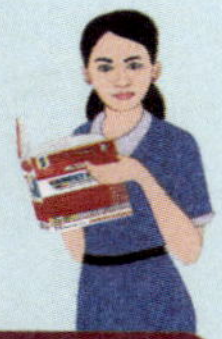

SECTION: SOCIOLOGY

31. As per 2011 census survey, ______ per cent of the population of India suffer from disability (in the identified 8 categories).
a. 2.21
b. 1.2
c. 2.5
d. 3.1

32. Who is considered as the Father of Sociology?
a. Auguste Comte
b. MacIver
c. Emile Durkheim
d. Kingsley Davis

33. Which of the following is not a stage of socialization?
a. Oral stage
b. Despair stage
c. Oedipal stage
d. Latency stage

34. Caste status is an example of which of the following status?
a. Monetary
b. Ascribed
c. Achieved
d. General

35. The general process of acquiring culture is referred to as:
a. Dispersion
b. Diffusion
c. Socialization
d. Acculturation

36. Socialization is a process involving:
a. Declaring everything as belonging to society
b. Setting up the social norms
c. Inducting people to adapt in society
d. Normalization of criminals and anti-social elements

37. Who said that man is a social animal?
a. MacIver
b. Auguste Comte
c. Aristotle
d. Ginsberg

38. Any small group marked by continuous close interaction of a highly personal and emotionally supportive nature is called a/an ______ group.
a. Reference
b. Secondary
c. Primary
d. Interest

39. Polyandry means:
a. A form of marriage that joins one female with more than one male
b. A form of marriage that joins one male with more than one female
c. A form of marriage that joins one female with one male
d. Getting married in the same blood group

40. Providing education to the school, college and street children on prevention of drug addiction is an example of ______ prevention.
a. Primordial
b. Tertiary
c. Primary
d. Secondary

SECTION: NURSING FOUNDATIONS

41. Lack of oxygen in the blood stream is called:
a. Hypoxaemia
b. Cyanosis
c. Hypoxia
d. Anoxaemia

42. Under normal circumstances, concentration of oxygen in inspired air is about ______ per cent.
a. 100
b. 6
c. 29
d. 21

43. As per Kübler-Ross stages of grieving, refusing to believe that loss is happening/has happened is called:
a. Bargaining
b. Denial
c. Acceptance
d. Depression

44. Which of the following organ is one of the primary regulators of body fluid and electrolyte balance?
a. Intestine
b. Kidney
c. Stomach
d. Lungs

45. What is the approximate normal level of haematocrit/packed cell volume in men?
a. 5% to 15%
b. 60% to 70%
c. 40% to 50%
d. 20% to 35%

46. Which of the following tests need to be performed before radial artery cannulation to evaluate radial and ulnar arterial patency?
a. Coop's test
b. Allen's test
c. Capillary refill test
d. Buerger's test

47. A group of symptoms is known as:
a. Signs
b. Syndrome
c. Clinical manifestations
d. Group symptoms

48. Rhythmic waxing and waning of respiration is called:
a. Hypoventilation
b. Orthopnoea
c. Hyperventilation
d. Cheyne-Stokes respiration

49. A bedridden patient is having intact skin at the sacral region, and the symptoms of warmness, pain and firm skin at the site. What is the stage of bedsore?
a. Stage III
b. Stage II
c. Stage I
d. Stage IV

Ans.

24.	c
25.	d
26.	a
27.	b
28.	b
29.	c
30.	b
31.	a
32.	a
33.	b
34.	b
35.	c
36.	c
37.	c
38.	c
39.	a
40.	a
41.	a
42.	d
43.	b
44.	b
45.	c
46.	b
47.	b
48.	d
49.	c

50. Following death, the subjective response experienced by the surviving loved ones is called:
a. Bereavement b. Mourning
c. Compliance d. Grief

51. Which of the following electrolytes does insulin help to move into the cells?
a. Bicarbonates b. Chloride
c. Carbonates d. Potassium

52. Temperature of 98.7 degree Fahrenheit is approximately equal to ______ degree Celsius.
a. 38.16 b. 37.56
c. 37.06 d. 36.52

53. Difference between systolic and diastolic blood pressure is called:
a. Pulse range b. Pulse length
c. Pulse deficit d. Pulse pressure

54. Formula to calculate BMI is:
a. Weight in kg divided by square of height in meters
b. Weight in kg divided by height in feet
c. Weight in kg divided by square of height in feet
d. Weight in kg divided by height in meters

55. Which of the following equipment is used for the examination of the ear?
a. Ophthalmoscope b. Laryngoscope
c. Otoscope d. Proctoscope

56. The specific gravity of the urine normally ranges approximately from:
a. 1.8 to 2.0 b. 1.5 to 1.8
c. 0.75 to 1.00 d. 1.01 to 1.025

57. Insertion of a tube inside the stomach through the nose is called nasogastric:
a. Irrigation b. Intubation
c. Extubation d. Urigation

58. Intravenous solution of 0.45% sodium chloride is a/an ______ solution.
a. Colloid
b. Hypertonic
c. Hypotonic
d. Isotonic

59. ______ is the process of introducing a disinfectant solution to the internal environment of the body when someone passes away.
a. Eubacterium b. Revaccination
c. Embalming d. Rinsing

60. ______ enema is also called antispasmodic enema.
a. Cold b. Carminative
c. Antihelminthic d. Oil

61. HbA1c (glycated hemoglobin) value reflects the blood glucose levels in the past ______ months.
a. 1 b. 7
c. 3 d. 9

62. The sudden fall of temperature from high to normal within a few hours is called:
a. Hypothermia b. Lysis
c. True crisis d. False crisis

63. In a healthy individual, weighing 70 kg at rest, the stroke volume is about:
a. 150 mL
b. 100 mL
c. 50 mL
d. 70 mL

64. The fever in which temperature remains above normal throughout the day and fluctuates more than 2 degree Fahrenheit is known as ______ fever.
a. Lysis b. Remittent
c. Inverted d. Intermittent

65. The site of pulse in the neck is called:
a. Temporal b. Radial
c. Carotid d. Popliteal

66. The gradual decrease in body's temperature after death is called:
a. Stiff mortis b. Algor mortis
c. Rigor mortis d. Livor mortis

67. The discoloration that appears in the dependent areas of the body after death is called:
a. Rigor mortis b. Livor mortis
c. Algor mortis d. Stiff mortis

68. Kussmaul breathing is associated with:
a. Heart failure b. Diabetic ketoacidosis
c. Bronchial asthma d. Atelectasis

69. Absorptive dressings are intended to:
a. Absorb nutrients for the wound
b. Remove drainage from the bed sore
c. Gather moisture from the atmosphere to keep the wound cool
d. Absorb blood from veins

70. Which of the following medication orders are for every other day?
a. qod b. qh
c. qd d. bid

71. A patient is to receive 1000 mL of IV fluid in 6 h. The drop factor is 15 drops per mL. At approximately how many drops per minute should the flow rate be set?
a. 42 drops/m b. 21 drops/m
c. 55 drops/m d. 33 drops/m

72. In which of the following positions is the patient at greatest risk of shearing force?
a. Semi-Fowler's position b. Lying supine in bed
c. Trendelenburg position d. High-Fowler's position

73. Movement of the joints away from the mid-line of the body is called:
a. Addiction b. Adhesion
c. Adduction d. Abduction

74. What does the term Cheilosis mean?
a. Cracking of lips
b. Bad breath
c. Inflammation of the gums
d. Inflammation of the tongue

75. Breathing that is normal in rate and depth is called:
a. Bradypnea b. Tachypnea
c. Apnea d. Eupnea

76. Stiffness in the body that occurs after 2 to 4 h after death is called:
a. Livor mortis b. Algor mortis
c. Stiff mortis d. Rigor mortis

77. Which of the following is NOT an example of dry cold application?
a. Cold compress
b. Ice pack
c. Ice cradle
d. Ice bag

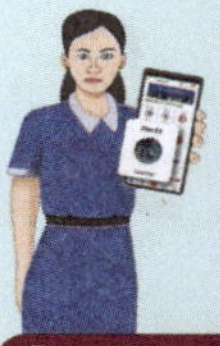

Ans.

50. a
51. d
52. c
53. d
54. a
55. c
56. d
57. b
58. c
59. c
60. b
61. c
62. c
63. d
64. b
65. c
66. b
67. b
68. b
69. b
70. a
71. a
72. d
73. d
74. a
75. d
76. d
77. a

78. The main intracellular cation is:
a. Zinc b. Chloride
c. Potassium d. Halide

79. Inflammation of the oral mucosa is known as:
a. Gingivitis b. Glossitis
c. Parotitis d. Stomatitis

80. Which of the following medication orders is administered immediately and only once?
a. Single order b. PRN order
c. Stat order d. Standing order

SECTION : COMMUNITY HEALTH NURSING-I

81. Koplik's spots are the clinical feature of:
a. Cholera b. Chickenpox
c. Measles d. Pertussis

82. One CHC covers a population of ______ in hilly areas.
a. 80000 b. 10000
c. 30000 d. 50000

83. The number of all current cases of a disease at one point of time is called:
a. Period prevalence b. Point incidence
c. Point prevalence d. Time prevalence

84. In which year was the Rashtriya Swasthya Bima Yojana (RSBY) introduced?
a. 2006 b. 2008
c. 2007 d. 2005

85. Hardness of water is expressed as:
a. PPL b. mg/L
c. mEq/ML d. mg%

86. The route of administration of hepatitis B vaccine is:
a. Intramuscular b. Subcutaneous
c. Intrathecal d. Intradermal

87. The constant presence of a disease or infection within a given geographic area is called:
a. Sporadic b. Endemic
c. Pandemic d. Epidemic

88. The denominator used to calculate crude birth rate is:
a. School-going population
b. Live births in that year
c. Mid-year population in that year
d. Population aged 18 years or above

89. What was the theme of World Health Day 2019?
a. Halt the rise: beat diabetes
b. Healthy heart beat: healthy blood pressure
c. Food safety
d. Universal health coverage: everyone, everywhere

90. What is the minimum contact time required for the chlorination of water to take place?
a. 10 m b. 90 m
c. 60 m d. 30 m

SECTION : NUTRITION

91. Which of the following digestive enzymes present in gastric juice is primarily responsible for breaking down proteins?
a. Trypsin b. Pepsin
c. Peptidases d. Chymotrypsin

92. Emulsification of lipids in the small intestine requires:
a. Gastric lipase b. Pepsin
c. Pancreatic lipase d. Bile salts

93. Which of the following nutrient provides energy to the body?
a. Fat b. Zinc
c. Vitamin A d. Vitamin D

94. Which of the following is precursor to vitamin A?
a. Pyridoxine b. Beta-carotene
c. Thiamine d. Retinol

95. An average healthy person with no diseases should ideally get ______ of his/her daily calorie requirements from healthy fats.
a. 50% to 60% b. 70% to 80%
c. 20% to 30% d. 5% to 10%

96. In which organ does the absorption of iron takes place?
a. Colon
b. Duodenum in small intestine
c. Liver
d. Stomach

97. Vitamin B1 is also known as:
a. Pyridoxine b. Thiamine
c. Riboflavin d. Niacin

98. Which of the following trace elements is essential for the synthesis of insulin?
a. Cobalt b. Iron
c. Zinc d. Sodium

99. Which of the following is an essential amino acid?
a. Niacin b. Thiamine
c. Pyridoxine d. Valine

100. Calories generated per gram of fat is approximately:
a. 4 kcals b. 15 kcals
c. 1 kcals d. 9 kcals

SECTION: MEDICAL SURGICAL NURSING

101. Which of the following drugs is a proton pump inhibitor?
a. Ranitidine b. Famotidine
c. Pantoprazole d. Sucralfate

102. Diabetes insipidus is caused by the deficiency of which of the following hormones?
a. Antidiuretic b. Glucagon
c. Insulin d. Renin

103. The name of the surgery in which there is removal of duodenum, head of pancreas, gallbladder and bile ducts is called:
a. Appendectomy b. Lumpectomy
c. Discectomy d. Pancreatoduodenectomy

104. Bell's Palsy is a disorder of the ______ cranial nerve.
a. 3rd b. 7th
c. 9th d. 5th

105. The most common side effect of thrombolytic therapy is:
a. Metabolic abnormalities
b. Internal bleeding
c. Compartment syndrome
d. Acute renal failure

106. Which type of solution causes water to shift from the cells into the plasma?
a. Alkaline b. Hypotonic
c. Acidic d. Hypertonic

107. An individual with which of the following blood groups is a universal donor?
a. A –ve b. B +ve
c. AB +ve d. O –ve

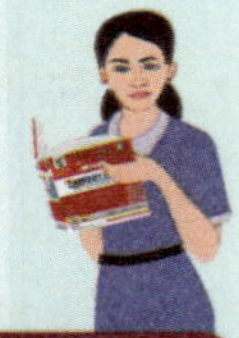

Ans.

78.	c
79.	d
80.	c
81.	c
82.	a
83.	c
84.	b
85.	b
86.	a
87.	b
88.	c
89.	d
90.	d
91.	b
92.	d
93.	a
94.	b
95.	c
96.	b
97.	b
98.	c
99.	d
100.	d
101.	c
102.	a
103.	d
104.	b
105.	b
106.	d
107.	d

108. The loss of urine resulting from cognitive or environmental factors is the manifestation of:
a. Overflow incontinence
b. Functional incontinence
c. Urge incontinence
d. Reflex incontinence

109. While assessing the level of consciousness of a patient using Glasgow Coma Scale, which of the following score represents the best motor response from the patient?
a. 3 b. 4
c. 5 d. 6

110. The loss of ability to recognize objects is called:
a. Dysarthria b. Alexia
c. Ataxia d. Agnosia

111. Which of the following is glandular tissue cancer?
a. Liposarcoma b. Adenocarcinoma
c. Neuroblastoma d. Osteogenic sarcoma

112. The cell-mediated immunity is carried out by:
a. Red blood cells b. T lymphocytes
c. B lymphocytes d. CD4 cells

113. The lateral S-shaped curvature of the spine is called:
a. Scoliosis b. Musculosis
c. Kyphosis d. Lordosis

114. _____ is a radiological examination using a minimal and safe amount of radiation to allow visualization of breast masses.
a. Computed tomography scan
b. Lymphangiogram
c. Angiogram
d. Mammogram

115. Barium enema is used mainly for radiological examination of the:
a. Brain b. Colon
c. Heart d. Oral cavity

116. While doing colostomy irrigation, the height of the irrigation bag should be around:
a. 18 inches b. 24 inches
c. 12 inches d. 36 inches

117. Which one of the following procedures is used to correct otosclerosis?
a. Myringoplasty b. Myringotomy
c. Mastoidectomy d. Stapedectomy

118. The term pyrosis is related to:
a. Heartburn b. Pus formation
c. Dysphagia d. Dyspepsia

119. The drugs used to constrict the pupils are:
a. Mydriatics b. Sulphonamides
c. Antibiotics d. Miotics

120. Which of the following parts of an eye alters the size of the pupil to regulate the amount of light entering the eye?
a. Lens b. Cornea
c. Retina d. Iris

121. The type of incontinence in which there is constant dribbling of urine and is associated with urinating frequently and in small amount is called:
a. Overflow incontinence b. Stress incontinence
c. Functional incontinence d. Urge incontinence

122. Using the 'rule of nine', estimated burn size in an adult having burn injury to chest and stomach is _______ per cent.
a. 18 b. 27
c. 36 d. 9

123. Which among the following is a colloid solution?
a. 0.9% normal saline b. Dextran
c. 0.45% normal saline d. 25% dextrose

124. Which of the following results from severe allergic reaction producing overwhelming systemic vasodilation and relative hypovolemia?
a. Hypovolemia shock b. Anaphylactic shock
c. Neurogenic shock d. Septic shock

125. Which of the following enzymes converts fats into fatty acids and glycerol?
a. Bile b. Trypsinogen
c. Salivary amylase d. Lipase

126. The movement of particles from region of higher concentration to region of lower concentration is called:
a. Diffusion b. Filtration
c. Osmosis d. Hydrolysis

127. In acute pancreatitis, the levels of which of the following enzymes remain elevated for 7-14 days?
a. Urine amylase
b. Serum amylase
c. Serum alkaline phosphatase
d. Serum lipase

128. Which of the following is NOT a manifestation of interstitial cystitis (IC)?
a. Frequency b. Incontinence
c. Urgency d. Pelvis pain

129. The disease that occurs due to the defect in the genes of one or other parent and is transmitted to the offspring is known as _______ disease/disorder.
a. Congenital b. Organic
c. Hereditary d. Allergic

130. Tonometry is the method of measuring the:
a. Pressure inside the lungs
b. Pressure inside the ear
c. Intraocular pressure
d. Blood pressure

131. Hemophilia is associated with:
a. Chromosome 11 b. Y chromosome
c. Chromosome 21 d. X chromosome

132. After a renal transplant, the rejection that occurs within minutes is called:
a. Hyper acute rejection b. Chronic rejection
c. Acute rejection d. Sub-acute rejection

133. Which of the following drugs is used for the dilation of pupil?
a. Tropicamide b. Betamethasone
c. Levofloxacin d. Gentamicin

134. What is the minimum possible score of Glasgow Coma Scale?
a. 3 b. 1
c. 2 d. 0

135. The voice box is known as:
a. Larynx b. Diaphragm
c. Bronchioles d. Pharynx

136. The most serious complication of deep vein thrombosis (DVT) is a blockage known as:
a. Formation of venous ulcers
b. Chronic occlusion of veins
c. Gangrenous development of veins
d. Pulmonary embolism

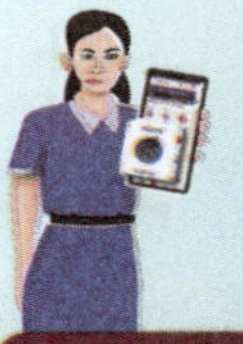

Ans.

108. b
109. d
110. d
111. b
112. b
113. a
114. d
115. b
116. a
117. d
118. a
119. d
120. d
121. a
122. a
123. b
124. b
125. d
126. a
127. d
128. b
129. c
130. c
131. d
132. a
133. a
134. a
135. a
136. d

137. Painful swallowing is known as:
a. Dysphasia b. Odynophagia
c. Ataxia d. Dyspepsia

138. The antidote of warfarin is:
a. Protamine sulfate b. Vitamin K
c. Heparin d. Acetyl cysteine

139. The most common lung cancer seen in non-smokers is:
a. Small cell carcinoma b. Adenocarcinoma
c. Large cell carcinoma d. Squamous cell carcinoma

140. The presence of stones in the urinary tract is called:
a. Kidney lithiasis b. Stone lithiasis
c. Urolithiasis d. Cholelithiasis

SECTION: PSYCHIATRIC NURSING

141. The act of purging or purification of emotions is called:
a. Compulsion b. Catharsis
c. Cataplexy d. Confabulation

142. Which of the following is expected in a patient who is diagnosed with an organic mental disorder?
a. Intact memory
b. Appropriate behavior
c. Disorganization of thoughts
d. Orientation to person, place and time

143. According to Erikson's eight stages of development, initiative vs. guilt take place at:
a. 20–25 years b. 10–15 years
c. 13–19 years d. 3–5 years

144. Which of the following is NOT a sign/symptom of the obsessive-compulsive disorder?
a. No fear of self-harm b. Fear of germs or dirt
c. Obsessive thoughts d. Compulsive acts

145. Which one of the following is derived from the plant 'Cannabis sativa'?
a. Cocaine b. Morphine
c. Ganja d. Opium

146. False sensory perception without real external stimulus is known as:
a. Hallucination b. Illusions
c. Delusions d. Thought insertion

147. A patient admitted in the psychiatric ward refused to eat her lunch stating that the food is poisoned. This kind of response is an example of:
a. Hallucination b. Sympathy
c. Illusions d. Delusions

148. The La Belle indifference is related to:
a. Conversion reaction
b. Obsession compulsions disorder
c. Anxiety disorder
d. Phobic anxiety

149. The disulfiram therapy is indicated in:
a. Acute intoxication
b. Cannabis dependence
c. Anxiety disorder
d. Chronic alcoholism

150. A person suffering from ______, a severe anxiety disorder, is able to speak freely with certain people only and is not able to speak with others, especially with certain social groups such as classmates at school.
a. Mutism b. Aphasia
c. Selective mutism d. Epilepsy

SECTION: MIDWIFERY AND GYNECOLOGICAL NURSING

151. Ovulation in a female with a 36-days cycle occurs between:
a. 30th – 34th day b. 14th – 18th day
c. 8th – 12th day d. 20th – 24th day

152. The condition where the uterus turns inside out is called:
a. Uterine Inversion b. Prolapse
c. Anteversion d. Retroversion

153. The graphical record of maternal and fetal data against time during labor on a single sheet of paper is called:
a. Ultrasonogram b. Tocogram
c. Cardiotocogram d. Partogram

154. The most common genital prolapse is:
a. Rectocele b. Cystocele
c. Procidentia d. Enterocele

155. The first stage of labor is characterized by:
a. Crowning of the head
b. Expulsion of the fetus till the placenta
c. Dilatation of cervix
d. Delivery of the placenta

156. The length of the fallopian tube ranges from:
a. 22-27 cm b. 7-12 cm
c. 28-31 cm d. 2-7 cm

157. The shape of the brim in anthropoid pelvis is:
a. Triangular with base towards sacrum
b. Square
c. Well-rounded
d. Oval

158. The suture that separates the parietal bone from the tabular portion of the occipital bone is called:
a. Lambdoid suture b. Frontal suture
c. Sagittal suture d. Coronal suture

159. Urine formation usually begins towards the end of the ______ and continues throughout fetal life.
a. 3-5 weeks b. 2-3 weeks
c. 21-22 weeks d. 11-12 weeks

160. The settling of fetal head into the brim of the pelvis is called:
a. Crowning of head b. Lightening
c. Engagement d. Descent

161. Which of the following is the common site of fertilization?
a. Interstitial b. Isthmic
c. Ampulla d. Infundibulum

162. At about ______ of gestation, the height of the uterus is at the level of umbilicus.
a. 6-8 weeks b. 3-5 weeks
c. 20-22 weeks d. 10-12 weeks

163. The ovarian cycle is initiated by:
a. Progesterone b. Follicle stimulating hormone
c. Endorphins d. Estrogen

164. The most common cause of non-engagement at term in primigravida is:
a. Cephalopelvic disproportion (CPD)
b. Breech presentation
c. Hydramnios
d. Brow presentation

165. What is the correct sequence of mitosis?
a. Prophase, Metaphase, Anaphase, Telophase
b. Anaphase, Prophase, Metaphase, Telophase
c. Telophase, Anaphase, Prophase, Telophase
d. Metaphase, Anaphase, Prophase, Telophase

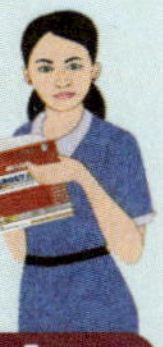

Ans.

137. b
138. b
139. b
140. c
141. b
142. c
143. d
144. a
145. c
146. a
147. d
148. a
149. d
150. c
151. d
152. a
153. d
154. b
155. c
156. b
157. d
158. a
159. d
160. b
161. c
162. c
163. b
164. a
165. a

166. The uterine fibroid is associated with:

a. Endometriosis b. Amenorrhea
c. Ovarian cancer d. PID

167. Inflammation of the fallopian tube is called:

a. Endometritis b. Vaginitis
c. Salpingitis d. Cervicitis

168. The most common site of ectopic pregnancy is:

a. Ampullary region in the fallopian tube
b. Cervix
c. Abdomen
d. Ovary

169. The darkening of the skin over the forehead, bridge of nose or cheekbones during pregnancy is called:

a. Chloasma b. Chadwick's sign
c. Hegar's sign d. Linea nigra

170. The approximate average weight of placenta at birth is:

a. 300 g b. 400 g
c. 508 g d. 600 g

171. Which of the following hormones is increased in Polycystic Ovarian Syndrome?

a. 17-OH progesterone
b. Luteinizing Hormone (LH)
c. Follicle Stimulating Hormone (FSH)
d. Thyroid Stimulating Hormone (TSH)

172. The early puerperium extends:

a. Until twelve weeks of postpartum
b. Up to first year of delivery
c. Until the thirteen weeks of postpartum
d. Until the first week of postpartum

173. Which one of the following is seen in preeclampsia?

a. Facial hair
b. Hypotension
c. Weight loss
d. Proteinuria

174. A normal umbilical cord contains:

a. One artery and five veins
b. Two arteries and one vein
c. Five arteries and two veins
d. Two arteries and ten veins

175. Oxygenated blood from placenta returns to the fetus via the:

a. Superior vena cava
b. Inferior vena cava
c. Umbilical vein
d. Ductus arteriosus

176. Post-term pregnancy is a pregnancy which continues beyond:

a. 294 days
b. 250 days
c. 200 days
d. 170 days

177. What is the ideal average newborn's head circumference at birth?

a. 75 cm b. 35 cm
c. 55 cm d. 15 cm

178. Which of the following indicates relationship of long axis of the fetus to that of mother?

a. Fetal lie
b. Fetal presentation
c. Fetal attitude
d. Fetal position

179. The outer most membrane of placenta is called:

a. Yolk sac b. Chorion
c. Amnion d. Meningitis

180. Peg cells are seen in the:

a. Intestine b. Fallopian tubes
c. Stomach d. Vagina

181. Which of the following is the most important tumor marker to diagnose carcinoma of ovary?

a. Serum human chorionic gonadotropin
b. CA 125
c. Human placental lactogen
d. Serum alpha fetoprotein

182. The onset of menstruation is called:

a. Menopause
b. Menarche
c. Andropause
d. Ovarian cycle

183. Of the 6-7 million oocytes available, how many are released during ovulation?

a. 3000 to 4000
b. 400 to 500
c. 2000 to 3000
d. 100 to 200

184. During the active phase of labor, the cervical dilatation per hour in primigravidas is approximately:

a. 1.2 cm
b. 1.9 cm
c. 2.3 cm
d. 2.5 cm

185. The correct sequence of development of puberty in girls is:

a. Menarche, Pubarche, Thelarche
b. Thelarche, Pubarche, Menarche
c. Thelarche, Menarche, Pubarche
d. Pubarche, Menarche, Thelarche

186. Postpartum hemorrhage is the condition in which there is loss of more than ______ mL vaginal blood.

a. 100 b. 50
c. 10 d. 500

187. The normal APGAR score of a new born is:

a. 7 and above
b. 3 to 4
c. 4 to 6
d. Below 3

188. Which of the following is NOT a feature of HELLP syndrome?

a. Raised liver enzymes
b. Eosinophilia
c. Thrombocytopenia
d. Hemolytic anemia

189. The first perception of active fetal movement felt by the mother during pregnancy is known as:

a. Engagement
b. Hastening
c. Quickening
d. Lightening

190. The maneuver commonly used to manage shoulder dystocia is:

a. Rosette maneuver
b. McRoberts maneuver
c. Jeff Marshal maneuver
d. MacMillan maneuver

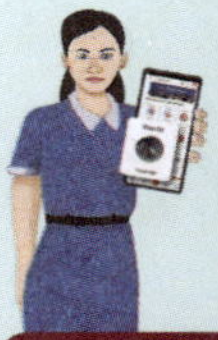

Ans.

166. a
167. c
168. a
169. a
170. c
171. b
172. d
173. d
174. b
175. c
176. a
177. b
178. a
179. b
180. b
181. b
182. b
183. b
184. a
185. b
186. d
187. a
188. b
189. c
190. b

SECTION: PEDIATRIC NURSING

191. Which of the following is the most common cause of ophthalmic neonatorum?
- a. Candida albicans
- b. Staphylococcus aureus
- c. Neisseria gonorrhea
- d. Streptococcus

192. Which of the following is NOT a part of the Tetralogy of Fallot (TOF)?
- a. Patent ductus arteriosus
- b. Right ventricular hypertrophy
- c. Overriding of aorta
- d. Pulmonary stenosis

193. An injury to the upper brachial plexus results in:
- a. Facial palsy
- b. Phrenic nerve palsy
- c. Klumpke's palsy
- d. Erb's palsy

194. Which of the following is the ideal age for closure of the anterior fontanel of a child?
- a. 18 to 24 months
- b. 6 to 8 months
- c. 6 to 8 weeks
- d. 18 to 24 weeks

195. Which of the following is NOT a complication of measles?
- a. Laryngitis
- b. Conjunctivitis
- c. Atrial Septal Defect
- d. Encephalitis

196. The most common type of leukemia seen in children is:
- a. Acute lymphoblastic leukemia (ALL)
- b. Chronic lymphoid leukemia (CLL)
- c. Acute myeloid leukemia (AML)
- d. Chronic myeloid leukemia (CML)

197. Which one of the following is NOT a characteristic of Attention Deficit Hyperactivity Disorder (ADHD)?
- a. Inattention
- b. Impulsivity
- c. Difficulty in eating
- d. Over activity

198. Which of the following is NOT a clinical manifestations of Trisomy 21?
- a. Flat nasal bridge
- b. Protruding tongue
- c. Long hands and fingers
- d. Small nose

199. Which of the following conditions can result in a hairy patch on the back of children?
- a. Epilepsy
- b. Hydrocephalus
- c. Spina bifida occulta
- d. Ricket

200. The Baby-Friendly Hospital Initiative (BFHI) was launched jointly by:
- a. WHO and Red Cross
- b. WHO and FAO
- c. UNICEF and WHO
- d. UNICEF and FAO

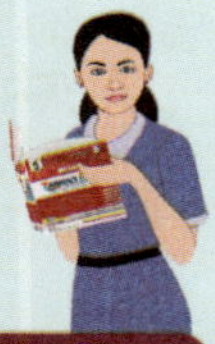

Ans.

191. c
192. a
193. d
194. a
195. c
196. a
197. c
198. c
199. c
200. c

"After dinner rest a while; after supper walk a mile."

—T. Cogan

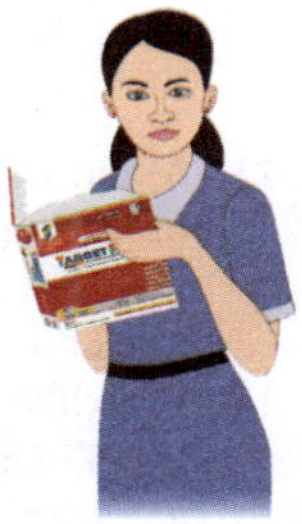

Nursing Officer Exam, JIPMER 2020

1. Nurse Linda was monitoring a 35-year-old male patient who was receiving blood transfusion. On assessment, the nurse found that the respiratory rate is 24 and blood pressure is 90/60. Which of the following is the priority action by the nurse?

a. Slow the infusion rate
b. Immediately flush IV line with normal saline
c. Immediately stop the transfusion
d. Notify the doctor

2. Full form of NITI Aayog is:

a. National Institution for Transforming India
b. National Institution for Transformation of Industries
c. National Income Transformation Initiatives
d. National Institution for Technical Initiatives

3. Which of the following condition is an example of acute organic mental disorder?

a. Schizophrenia
b. Delirium
c. Manic psychosis
d. Obsessive compulsive disorder

4. A nurse is analyzing the serum laboratory report for a client diagnosed with lung cancer that has metastasized to the pelvic bone. Which of the following laboratory findings is expected?

a. Elevated calcium
b. Decreased hemoglobin
c. Elevated creatinine (Scr)
d. Elevated creatine kinase (CK)

Explanation: Hypercalcemia of malignancy is a common finding in patients with cancer, affecting up to 44.1% of patients. It is important to note that hypercalcemia of malignancy is particularly common in cases of advanced stage cancer. The major mechanism, accounting for approximately 80% of malignancy-related hypercalcemia, is mediated by the production of Parathyroid hormone related protein.

5. A patient has underwent a C5–C6 anterior cervical discectomy. Which priority nursing diagnosis should a nurse document in the plan of care of this patient?

a. Potential impaired tissue perfusion
b. Impaired skin integrity related to surgical incision
c. Risk for infection
d. Potential ineffective breathing pattern

6. Nurse Linda is assessing a patient who visited OPD with tentative diagnosis of a hematological disorder. She noted that the patient has smooth and reddened tongue and ulcers at the corners of the mouth. Which of the following Laboratory findings is most likely in this patient?

a. Low hemoglobin
b. Elevated red blood cells (RBCs)
c. Prolonged prothrombin time (PT)
d. Low white blood cells (WBCs)

Explanation: Ulcers at the corners of the mouth (angular cheilosis), a smooth and reddened tongue, and a decreased hemoglobin/RBCs are signs of iron-deficiency anemia. Elevated red blood cells (RBCs) is seen in polycythemia vera. Prolonged Prothrombin time (PT) is associated with clients taking anticoagulants or experiencing a coagulation disorder. Ulcers, if infected, would increase the WBC count.

7. A 60-year-old male patient who had a left total hip replacement was discharged from the hospital one month before. He called the nurse reporting acute constant pain in the left groin and hip area and feeling like the left leg is shorter than the right. The nurse advises the client to come to the hospital immediately suspecting which of the following complication:

a. Aseptic loosening of the prosthesis
b. Deep vein thrombosis (DVT)
c. Dislocation of the prosthesis
d. Wound infection

8. Nurse Linda is caring for a child with hydronephrosis. Which assessment should a nurse perform to obtain the most accurate determination of fluid balance in this child?

a. Measuring the client's intake and output
b. Weighing the client
c. Assessing for edema
d. Evaluated serum electrolyte levels

Explanation: Measuring the child's weight daily on the same scale is most accurate. Intake-Output chart also provides data on fluid balance but there is additional fluid lost through, lungs, skin and Gastrointestinal tract that cannot be accurately measured. So, weight the client is most appropriate answer.

9. AFP is elevated in which of the following conditions?

a. Omphalocele
b. Gastroschisis
c. Down syndrome
d. Spina bifida occulta

10. Abnormal copper accumulation is seen in which of the following disease?

a. Wilson's disease
b. Parkinson's disease
c. Sjögren disease
d. Hemochromatosis

11. Which of the following location is appropriate to screen for jaundice in a child?

a. Skin over sacrum
b. Skin of abdomen
c. Ear pinna
d. Nail bed

12. Which of the following damage is most likely to occur during direct laryngoscopy?

a. Gingival laceration
b. Damage to maxillary incisors
c. Damage to arytenoid cartilage
d. Damage to mandibular molars

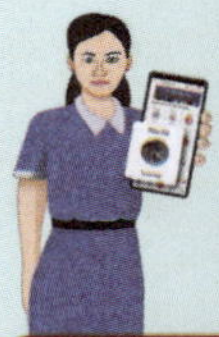

Ans.

1. c
2. a
3. b
4. a
5. d
6. a
7. c
8. b
9. d
10. a
11. b
12. c

Disclaimer: *The questions are prepared by memory-based recall from candidates who attended the examination.*

13. A patient is suffering from hematemesis. Which of the following is the best diet option for this patient?

a. Solid diet b. Liquid diet
c. Low-Fiber diet d. NPO

14. Which of the following antihypertensive drug is contraindicated in gestational hypertension?

a. Nifedipine b. Enalapril
c. Labetalol d. Methyldopa

15. Sign and symptoms of fluoride deficiency include:

a. Weak bone
b. Yellow-brown staining of teeth
c. Dermatitis
d. Joint stiffness

Explanation: Reducing the amount of fluoride in the body leads to the appearance of children dental caries, while in adults most likely to osteoporosis (weak bone). Signs of excess fluoride in the body are dermatitis, spots on teeth as the enamel gets yellow-brown color. Large amounts of fluoride intake over a longer period of time can lead to bone fluorosis. In this case appetite decreases and joints become stiff and painful.

16. World Leprosy Day in 2020 is on:

a. 17 January b. 26 January
c. 3 March d. 17 April

Explanation: World Leprosy Day is observed internationally every year on the last Sunday of January to increase the public awareness of the Leprosy or Hansen's disease. It was observed on Sunday 26th January 2020. The goal for World Leprosy Day is to raise the awareness of a disease that many people believe has been eliminated.

17. 31st National Road Safety Week was observed on:

a. 4th to 10th January 2020
b. 11th to 17th January 2020
c. 3rd to 9th February 2020
d. 10th to 16th February 2020

Explanation: National Road Safety Week in India is organized every January by the National Safety Council of India (NSC). The Ministry of Road Transport & Highways, Government of India has announced the observance of 31st National Road Safety Week from 11th to 17th January 2020.

18. Complication of high flow oxygen in pre-term neonate includes:

a. Acidosis b. Neonatal conjunctivitis
c. Retinal detachment d. Retrolental fibroplasia

Explanation: Retinopathy of prematurity (ROP), also called retrolental fibroplasia (RLF) and Terry syndrome, is a disease of the eye affecting prematurely born babies generally having received neonatal intensive care, in which oxygen therapy is used due to the premature development of their lungs.

19. When the patient is undergoing surgery under general anesthesia, which of the following parameter is the first priority?

a. Reflexes
b. Urine output
c. ABG values
d. Vital signs including SPO_2 with pulse oximeter

20. Who discovered the value of π?

a. Archimedes b. Pythagoras
c. Hipparchus d. Aristotle

21. Which of the following medications is administered to a patient preoperatively to prevent infections?

a. Antihypertensives b. Antibiotic
c. Antitussive d. Antihistamine

22. Which of the following chemotherapeutic agent is known as monoclonal antibody?

a. Rifaximin b. Interferon
c. Rituximab d. Indinavir

Explanation: Rituximab, the first monoclonal antibody approved for the treatment of cancer, is safe and effective in treating patients with relapsed or refractory, CD-20 positive, B-cell, low-grade or follicular non-Hodgkin's lymphoma.

23. Epilepsy awareness day is observed on:

a. March 7 b. March 26
c. April 7 d. April 26

Explanation: Purple Day is an international grassroots effort dedicated to increasing awareness about epilepsy worldwide. On March 26th annually, people in countries around the world are invited to wear purple and host events in support of epilepsy awareness.

24. Pradhan Mantri Jan Dhan Yojana was launched on:

a. 26 January 2014 b. 28 August 2014
c. 26 January 2015 d. 15 August 2015

Explanation: Pradhan Mantri Jan Dhan Yojana (PMJDY), is financial inclusion program of Government of India open to Indian citizens (minor of age more than 10 can also open account with guardian to manage it). Jan Dhan Yojana was announced by the Honorable Prime Minister Narendra Modi on 15 August 2014 and the scheme was launched on 28 August 2014.

25. Nurse Linda had just received a postoperative total hip replacement client from the recovery unit. Which of the following position is appropriate for this client?

a. On the non-operative side or supine position with legs abducted with a help of pillow
b. On the non-operative side or supine position with legs adducted
c. Side lying position with affected leg externally rotated
d. Side lying position with affected leg internally rotated

26. Which of the following radiopaque substance is used in Copper-T devices?

a. Magnesium sulfate b. Barium sulfate
c. Polyethylene glycol d. Iodine

27. 10% of 255 is:

a. 0.255 b. 2.55
c. 25.5 d. 25.0

28. 200% of a number is 140. Then what is 160% of that number?

a. 70 b. 112
c. 224 d. 242

29. A 39-year-old male patient is admitted to the Emergency Department with dyspnea, tachypnea and pink, frothy sputum. The nurse determines that the patient is experiencing:

a. Neck trauma b. Lung abscess
c. Pulmonary embolism d. Cor pulmonale

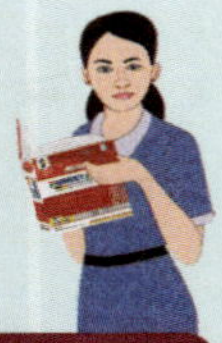

Ans.

13. d
14. b
15. a
16. b
17. b
18. d
19. d
20. a
21. b
22. c
23. b
24. b
25. a
26. b
27. c
28. b
29. c

30. All of the following side effects are expected in a patient with oral cancer who is receiving radiation therapy; EXCEPT:
a. Mucositis b. Xerostomia
c. Trismus d. Oral fluorosis

31. All of the following are features of leukemia; EXCEPT:
a. Anemia b. Polycythemia
c. Neutropenia d. Thrombocytopenia

32. Which of the following assessments has the highest priority in patient who has returned to the nursing unit following right nephrectomy?
a. Tolerance for sipping clear liquids
b. Ability to turn side to side
c. Temperature
d. Hourly urine output

33. Which of the following drug is contraindicated in a patient with thyroid storm?
a. Tapazole b. Propylthiouracil
c. Inderal d. Aspirin

34. Which of the following drug is more likely to cause oral aphthous ulcers?
a. Dexamethasone b. Triamcinolone
c. Benzocaine d. Diclofenac

35. Which of the following neurological side effect is anticipated in an elderly patient who is on NSAID?
a. Cognitive dysfunction b. Tremors
c. Ataxia d. Pseudoparkinsonism

36. All of the following are the features of left-sided heart failure; EXCEPT:
a. Pulmonary congestion b. Tachycardia
c. Orthopnea d. Distended jugular veins

37. Ventilator associated pneumonia is defined as pneumonia that occur ____hours or after ET intubation.
a. 12 h b. 24 h
c. 36 h d. 48 h

38. Position used while inserting NG tube is:
a. Supine b. High Fowler's
c. Low Fowler's d. Side lying

39. All of the following are the features of angina pectoris; EXCEPT:
a. Generalized body pain
b. Jaw aches
c. Pain precipitated by exercise or heavy meals
d. Chest tightness

40. Who is the Father of Green Revolution in India?
a. C Subramaniam
b. M S Swaminathan
c. Varghese Kurien
d. Arun Krishnan

41. The first case of Corona-virus was reported from:
a. Wuhan City, China b. Madrid, Spain
c. Rome, Italy d. New York, USA

42. 2, 1, ½, ¼, ... which number is next in the series?
a. 1/6 b. 1/8
c. 1/12 d. 1/16

43. 4, 7, 12, 19, 28, ... which number is next in the series?
a. 37 b. 39
c. 41 d. 43

44. What will be the net discount percentage of three successive discounts of 30%, 20%, and 10% on a product?
a. 40% b. 50.4%
c. 49.6% d. 60%

45. National aquatic animal of India is:
a. Sardine b. Blue whale
c. River dolphin d. King fish

46. Swachh Bharat Abhiyan was launched in India on:
a. 15 August 2014 b. 2 October 2014
c. 26 January 2015 d. 15 August 2015

47. The theme for International Nurses Day 2019 was:
a. Nurses: A voice to lead – Health is a human right
b. Nurses: A voice to lead – health for all
c. Nurses: A voice to lead – Achieving the sustainable development goals
d. Nursing the world to health

48. All of the following specimens are used for Corona-virus test; EXCEPT:
a. Nasopharyngeal swab specimen
b. Oropharyngeal swab specimen
c. Anterior nares (nasal swab) specimen
d. Urine sample

49. As per standards of American Society of Anesthesiologists, the preoperative fasting criteria for breast milk in infants is:
a. 2 h b. 4 h
c. 6 h d. 8 h

50. A patient is brought to postoperative ward after an emergency gastric surgery. The patient has nasogastric tube inserted for gastric decompression. The drainage from NG tube is normal if it:
a. Returns brown-liquid in color
b. Returns greenish-yellow in color
c. Has an alkaline pH level
d. Measures volume of less than 20 mL

51. A patient is brought to the emergency department after a road traffic accident. The patient's motor score is 2 on GCS. This means the patient response is:
a. Decerebrate response b. Decorticate response
c. Withdraws from touch d. Withdraws to pain

52. All of the following are types of lochia; EXCEPT:
a. Alba b. Serosa
c. Serum d. Rubra

53. A nurse has just performed an NG tube insertion procedure. Most accurate method for confirming the NG tube placement is:
a. X-ray
b. Auscultation
c. Observing patient for coughing aspiration of content and pH monitoring
d. Dip in a bowel of water

54. A patient is brought to the recovery room post thyroidectomy surgery. Which of the following is the most appropriate method to observe for further bleeding?
a. Observe for hemorrhage at operative site and back of neck and shoulder
b. Observe dressing for any leakage of blood
c. Observe the drainage tube for signs of bleeding
d. Observe whether the patient is frequently swallowing

55. A patient's Foley catheter was removed 24 h before. On assessment, the nurse found that the urine output is less than expected volume. Which of the following is the priority nursing action?
a. Administer Inj. Lasix 10 mg IV
b. Ambulate the patient
c. Check bladder for extension
d. Notify the doctor

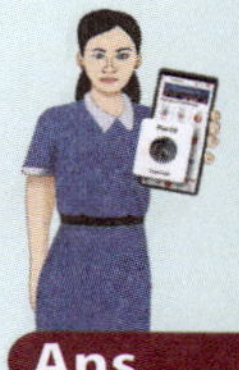

Ans.

30. d
31. b
32. d
33. d
34. d
35. a
36. d
37. d
38. b
39. a
40. b
41. a
42. b
43. b
44. c
45. c
46. b
47. a
48. d
49. b
50. b
51. a
52. c
53. a
54. a
55. c

56. Following delivery nurse suspect atonic PPH in the client, which among the following is the priority nursing intervention?

a. Massage the uterus
b. Administer 10 unit of oxytocin
c. Administer ergometrine
d. Report to the doctor

Explanation: Although, administration of oxytocin helps to arrest PPH through uterine contraction, it is not considered to be a nursing intervention. The priority nursing intervention is to massage the uterus to induce letdown reflex

57. Which of the following drug is contraindicated in a patient with congestive heart failure?

a. Diltiazem
b. Digoxin
c. Furosemide
d. Captopril

58. An unconscious patient is brought to the emergency room after a road traffic accident. Which of the following is the priority intervention in this patient?

a. Assess for level of consciousness
b. Assess vital signs
c. Airway management
d. Management of bleeding

59. Which of the following sign is seen in pancreatitis?

a. Kernig's sign
b. Murphy sign
c. Cullen sign
d. Psoas sign

Explanation: Cullen sign is a hemorrhagic discoloration of the umbilical area due to intraperitoneal hemorrhage from any cause; one of the more frequent causes is acute hemorrhagic pancreatitis. Grey Turner sign is a discoloration of the left flank associated with acute hemorrhagic pancreatitis.

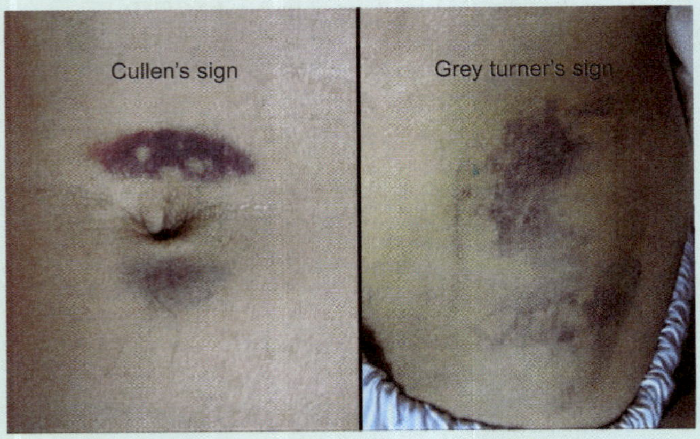

60. Which of the following method is most effective in prevention of teeth discoloration while administering iron syrup?

a. Dilute syrup with a glass of water
b. Mix iron syrup with glass of lemon juice
c. Give syrup through straw
d. Rinse mouth with water after ingestion of syrup

61. All of the following are the signs of respiratory acidosis; EXCEPT:

a. Headache
b. Blurred vision
c. Confusion
d. High alertness

62. A patient's ABG report is as follows: pH- 7.48, PCO_2–32, PO_2 – 88, HCO_3^- 24. Interpret the acid-base imbalance:

a. Respiratory acidosis
b. Respiratory alkalosis
c. Metabolic acidosis
d. Metabolic alkalosis

63. Guerin sign is most commonly seen in:

a. Maxillofacial trauma
b. Basilar skull fracture
c. Clavicle fracture
d. Cervical fracture

Explanation: Guerin sign is bruising in the palate in the region of the greater palatine arteries. Guerin sign is present and characterized by ecchymosis in the region of greater palatine vessels. It is present in mid-facial fracture or maxillofacial fracture.

64. Most common cause of urinary tract infection is:

a. E. coli
b. Staphylococcus
c. Streptococcus
d. Pneumococcus

65. According to WHO, surgical site infections occur at surgical site within:

a. 7 days
b. 15 days
c. 30 days
d. 42 days

Explanation: Surgical site infections are defined as infections that occur 30 days after surgery with no implant, or within 1 year if an implant is placed and infection appears to be related to surgery.

66. Most common complication of respiratory system after abdominal surgery is:

a. Bronchitis
b. Emphysema
c. Atelectasis
d. Pneumonia

67. Antibiotic prophylaxis before dental procedure is mainly given for the prevention of:

a. Surgical site infection
b. Infective endocarditis
c. GI infection
d. Ear infection

Explanation: Antibiotic prophylaxis has been used in dentistry for patients at risk of infective endocarditis or prosthetic joint infection. The scientific rationale for prophylaxis was to eliminate or reduce transient bacteremia caused by invasive dental procedures.

68. A patient is scheduled for an elective surgery. All of the following are important nursing responsibilities one day before surgery; EXCEPT:

a. Patient education
b. Obtaining consent
c. PAC check-up
d. Rehabilitation planning

69. A patient with a diagnosis of End Stage Renal Disease (ESRD) is admitted in ICU. All of the following are appropriate nursing diagnosis for this patient; EXCEPT:

a. Fluid volume excess
b. Decreased RBC
c. Electrolyte imbalance
d. Impaired immune function

70. A patient is brought to ICU from nephrology department. Nurse on duty noticed that there is bleeding from sheath site from right hand. Which of the following is the priority nursing action in this situation?

a. Call to dialysis room and ask dialysis nurse for help
b. Check blood pressure immediately
c. Immediately apply pressure on bleeding site with sterile gauze
d. Inform the doctor

71. Most common cause of upper respiratory infection is:

a. Adenovirus
b. Rhinovirus
c. Influenza virus
d. Enterovirus

Ans.

56. a
57. a
58. c
59. c
60. c
61. d
62. b
63. a
64. a
65. c
66. c
67. b
68. d
69. d
70. c
71. b

72. The patient's blood type is B negative. A nurse informs the family members that packed red blood cells (PRBCs) could likely be used by family members whose blood type:

a. A positive b. B positive
c. B negative d. AB negative

73. Treatment for hemophilia will likely include periodic self-administration of:

a. Fresh frozen plasma b. Factor concentrates
c. Whole blood d. Platelets

74. Which of the following blood pressure reading of a child aged between 3 and 5 years is considered abnormal?

a. 96/42 mm Hg b. 105/60 mm Hg
c. 112/65 mm Hg d. 115/66 mm Hg

75. In a patient with suspected head injury, frequent assessments are performed to determine if a client is developing increased intracranial pressure (ICP). Which of the following option correctly describes the outcome if there is increased ICP?

a. Increased in cerebral perfusion
b. Displacement of brain tissue
c. Improved brain tissue oxygenation
d. Increase in serum pH

76. Which of the following finding is expected in patient with diabetes insipidus (DI)?

a. Hyperglycemia
b. Increased urinary output
c. Increased urine specific gravity
d. Altered level of consciousness

77. A 70-year-old female patient is scheduled for surgery in two hours. Which of the following laboratory finding warrant the most immediate notification of the physician?

a. Prothrombin time 22 seconds
b. Hemoglobin 11 g/dL
c. Creatinine 1.0 mg/dL
d. Potassium 4.6 mEq/dL

78. Which of the following laboratory test result is most important to evaluate when preparing to administer digoxin in a pediatric client who has Congestive Heart Failure (CHF)?

a. Serum magnesium levels
b. Serum potassium levels
c. Serum sodium levels
d. Serum chloride levels

79. Which of the following is an appropriate instruction for a client who is scheduled for an outpatient electroencephalogram (EEG)?

a. NPO for at least 6 hours prior to the procedure
b. Removing all hairpins
c. Instruct to have some of the scalp shaved
d. Draw blood sample for glucose level 2 hours before schedule procedure

80. The earliest sign of increased ICP is:

a. Pupillary reflex changes
b. Changes in LOC
c. Altered sensation
d. Decreased blood pressure

81. Which of the following symptom occurs most frequently in a patient with acute pyelonephritis which should be monitored by the nurse?

a. Rebound tenderness in left lower abdomen
b. Flank pain on the affected side
c. Abnormally low pulse rate
d. Low-grade fever

82. A first year nursing student is asked to demonstrate assessment of blood pressure in an adult client with a manual sphygmomanometer. The student nurse places the bell diaphragm of the stethoscope over the brachial artery and pumps the cuff up to 160 mm Hg. The valve is released to allow a drop of 2 mm Hg per second. At 145 mm Hg the student nurse hears the first tapping sound. The sound becomes muffled at 130 mm Hg. The sound changes to a soft thumping at 120 mm Hg. The sound fades to a muffled blowing sound at 100 mm Hg and is last heard at 88 mm Hg. There is silence at 84 mm Hg. The nurse should document the blood pressure as:

a. 130/84 mm Hg b. 145/84 mm Hg
c. 145/88 mm Hg d. 130/88 mm Hg

83. The purpose of plasmapheresis is in patients with Guillain-Barré syndrome is to:

a. Restore albumin levels in the blood
b. Remove circulating antibodies in the blood
c. Remove excess fluid from the bloodstream
d. All of the above

84. A nurse has received a patient who has underwent a surgical procedure under conscious sedation. Which of the following assessment is most important for a nurse to make postoperatively in this patient?

a. Pain assessment
b. Urine output
c. Ability to swallow liquids
d. Rate and depth of breathing

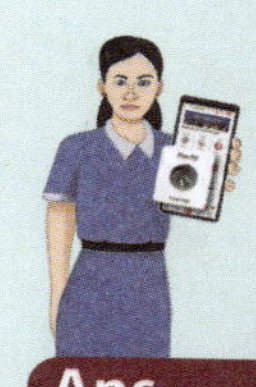

85. A 30-year-old patient in stage-1 labor is breathing rapidly and having difficulty coping with the contractions. Which of the following acid-base imbalance is expected in this patient?

a. Metabolic alkalosis b. Metabolic acidosis
c. Respiratory alkalosis d. Respiratory acidosis

86. Nurse Linda was caring for a patient who has had stroke. The patient gazes at nurse but has difficulty in producing speech in response to the nurse's questions. The patient follows instructions without any problem. The patient is displaying symptoms of:

a. Global aphasia b. Receptive aphasia
c. Expressive aphasia d. Mixed aphasia

87. A 45-year-old patient who underwent exploratory laparotomy five days before has presented with abdominal pain, distended abdomen, absence of flatus, and absent bowel sounds. This is an indication of which of the complication that is likely to occur:

a. Paralytic ileus b. Acute peritonitis
c. Wound dehiscence d. Surgical site infection

88. By what age a child is expected to begin to use simple words to communicate needs?

a. 6 to 9 months b. 10–12 months
c. 1 to 2 years d. 2 to 3 years

89. Normal visual acuity for a four-year-old child is:

a. 20/40 b. 20/60
c. 20/20 d. 20/30

90. A nurse administered phenylephrine eye drops for preparing a patient for ophthalmoscopic examination. Which of the following assessment finding should a nurse expect after administration of eye drops?

a. Constriction of pupil b. Hypotension
c. Pupil mydriasis d. Pupil miosis

Ans.

72.	c
73.	b
74.	a
75.	b
76.	b
77.	a
78.	b
79.	b
80.	b
81.	b
82.	c
83.	b
84.	d
85.	c
86.	c
87.	a
88.	b
89.	c
90.	c

91. **Which of the following manifestation is least expected in a patient presents with meningioma and symptoms of increased intracranial pressure?**
   a. Papilledema
   b. Pyrexia
   c. Headache
   d. Vomiting

92. **The definitive diagnosis of Peptic Ulcer Disease (PUD) is:**
   a. Urea breath test
   b. Upper GI endoscopy with biopsy
   c. Barium contrast X-ray
   d. The string test

93. **Which of the following site is best for the nurse to plan to administer monovalent Hep-B (hepatitis B vaccine) intramuscularly to a newborn?**
   a. Deltoid
   b. Vastus lateralis
   c. Ventrogluteal
   d. Dorsogluteal

94. **While a healthcare team performing the respiratory arrest resuscitation, it is determined that a nurse did not open the valve to the oxygen tank and the client had not been receiving oxygen. Which of the following ethical principle involved in this situation?**
   a. Battery
   b. Nonmaleficence
   c. Fidelity
   d. Beneficence

95. **Which lobe is responsible for touch?**
   a. Frontal
   b. Temporal
   c. Parietal
   d. Occipital

96. **An aged client with diabetes mellitus complaining of a painless peripheral loss of vision is at risk for:**
   a. Cataract
   b. Uveitis
   c. Open-angle glaucoma
   d. Closed-angle glaucoma

Explanation: **Open-angle glaucoma** means that the angle where the iris meets the cornea is as wide and open as it should be. Loss of peripheral or side vision is usually the first sign of glaucoma.
Angle-closure glaucoma presents with eye pain with nausea and sudden visual disturbance.

97. **Initial nursing action after the birth of a preterm baby with Apgar score 8 is:**
   a. Weight the baby
   b. Do suction
   c. Inform the family members about the birth and sex of the baby
   d. Receive the baby in a prewarmed towel and dry the baby

98. **Which of the following is used for visual assessment of neonatal jaundice?**
   a. Wallace rule
   b. Kramer's rule
   c. Lund-Browder chart
   d. Rule of nine

99. **In terms of response to fire accidents in hospital, what is R.A.C.E. stands for:**
   a. Rescue, Alarm, Control, Exit
   b. Rescue, Alarm, Contain, Extinguish
   c. Rescue, Alert, Control, Exit
   d. Rescue, Alert, Control, Extinguish

100. **Which of the following is the most important initial care when chemical burn is suspected?**
   a. Immediately cover the burn area
   b. Remove all the dressings
   c. Provide the calm environment
   d. Excessive flushing with water for 20-30 minutes

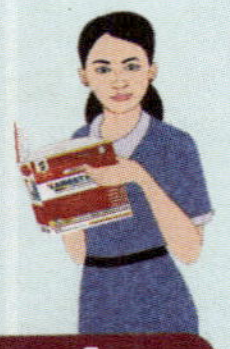

Ans.

91.	b
92.	b
93.	b
94.	b
95.	c
96.	c
97.	d
98.	b
99.	b
100.	d